NUTRITION IN PEDIATRICS 4

BASIC SCIENCE • CLINICAL APPLICATIONS

NUTRITION IN PEDIATRICS 4

BASIC SCIENCE • CLINICAL APPLICATIONS

CHRISTOPHER DUGGAN, MD, MPH
Associate Professor of Pediatrics
Harvard Medical School
Associate Professor in the Department of Nutrition
Harvard School of Public Health
Director, Clinical Nutrition Service
Division of Gastroenterology and Nutrition
Children's Hospital, Boston
Boston, Massachusetts

JOHN B. WATKINS, MD
Associate Professor of Pediatrics
Harvard Medical School
Division of Gastroenterology and Nutrition
Children's Hospital, Boston
Boston, Massachusetts

W. ALLAN WALKER, MD
Conrad Taff Professor of Nutrition
Professor of Pediatrics
Harvard Medical School
Chief, Mucosal Immunology Laboratory
Pediatric Gastroenterology and Nutrition Unit
Massachusetts General Hospital for Children
Boston, Massachusetts

2009

PEOPLE'S MEDICAL PUBLISHING HOUSE—USA
SHELTON, CONNECTICUT

People's Medical Publishing House—USA, Ltd.
2 Enterprise Drive, Suite 509
Shelton, CT 06484
Tel: 203-402-0646
Fax: 203-402-0854
E-mail: info@pmph-usa.com

PMPH-USA

08 09 10 11 12 / IPP / 9 8 7 6 5 4 3 2 1

ISBN 978-1-55009-361-2
Printed in India by International Print-O-Pak
Managing Editor: Patricia Bindner Typesetter (1st Printing): Aptara
Cover Designer: Alex Wheldon Typesetter (2nd Printing): diacriTech

Sales and Distribution

Canada
McGraw-Hill Ryerson Education
Customer Care
300 Water St.
Whitby, Ontario L1N 9B6
Tel: 1-800-565-5758
Fax: 1-800-463-5885

Foreign Rights
John Scott & Company
International Publishers' Agency
P.O. Box 878
Kimberton, PA 19442
Tel: 610-827-1640
Fax: 610-827-1671
E-mail: jsco@voicenet.com

Japan
United Publishers Services Limited
1-32-5 Higashi-Shinagawa
Shinagawa-Ku, Tokyo 140-0002
Tel: 03 5479 7251
Fax: 03 5479 7307

UK, Europe, Middle East
McGraw-Hill Education
Shoppenhangers Road
Maidenhead
Berkshire, England SL6 2QL
Tel: 44-0-1628-502500
Fax: 44-0-1628-635895
www.mcgraw-hill.co.uk

Singapore, Malaysia, Thailand, Philippines, Indonesia, Vietnam, Pacific Rim, Korea
McGraw-Hill Education
60 Tuas Basin Link
Singapore 638775
Tel: 65-6863-1580
Fax: 65-6862-3354

Australia, New Zealand
McGraw-Hill Australia
Pyt LtdLevel 2, 82 Waterloo Road North Ryde, NSW, 2113 Australia
Customer Service Australia
Phone: +61 (2) 9900 1800
Fax: +61 (2) 9900 1980
E-mail: cservice_sydney@mcgraw-hill.com

Customer Service New Zealand
Phone (Free Phone): +64 (0) 800 449 312
Fax: (Free Phone): +64 (0) 800 449 318
Email: cservice@mcgraw-hill.co.nz

Mexico and Central America
ETM SA de CV
Calle de Tula 59
Colonia Condesa
06140 Mexico DF, Mexico
Tel: 52-5-5553-6657
Fax: 52-5-5211-8468
E-mail: editoresdetextosmex@prodigy.net.mx

Brazil
Tecmedd Importadora E Distribuidora De Livros Ltda.
Avenida Maurílio Biagi, 2850
City Ribeirão, Ribeirão Preto – SP – Brasil
CEP: 14021-000
Tel: 0800 992236
Fax: (16) 3993-9000
E-mail: tecmedd@tecmedd.com.br

India, Bangladesh, Pakistan, Sri Lanka
CBS Publishers & Distributors
4596/1A-11, Darya Ganj
New Delhi-2, India
Tel: 23271632
Fax: 23276712
E-mail: cbspubs@vsnl.com

Notice: The authors and publisher have made every effort to ensure that the patient care recommended herein, including choice of drugs and drug dosages, is in accord with the accepted standard and practice at the time of publication. However, since research and regulation constantly change clinical standards, the reader is urged to check the product information sheet included in the package of each drug, which includes recommended doses, warnings, and contraindications. This is particularly important with new or infrequently used drugs. Any treatment regimen, particularly one involving medication, involves inherent risk that must be weighed on a case-by-case basis against the benefits anticipated. The reader is cautioned that the purpose of this book is to inform and enlighten; the information contained herein is not intended as, and should not be employed as, a substitute for individual diagnosis and treatment.

Cover Photo Caption and Acknowledgement
"Severe protein energy malnutrition, before and after nutritional rehabilitation.
Photo courtesy of Dr. Mary Penny of the Instituto de Investigación Nutricional, Lima, Perú."

PREFACE TO THE FOURTH EDITION

The critical role of nutrition in determining health and well-being is increasingly appreciated by scientific and lay audiences alike. Although much interest and excitement has rightly followed the sequencing of the human genome, fundamental aspects of health and disease are strongly related to the "nutritional environment" (i.e., nutritional status and dietary intake of the host) in which these genetic functions are expressed. It seems very likely that the vast range of health outcomes observed among humans is due to a combination of both genetic susceptibility to diseases as well as the very complex external environment, the most important component of which is nutritional status.

This fourth edition of *Nutrition in Pediatrics: Basic Science and Clinical Applications* represents a continuing effort to establish a comprehensive and accessible approach to pediatric nutrition. Perhaps the most important recent development in the field has been the epidemic of obesity, a phenomenon that threatens the health and well-being of current as well as future generations of children and adults. Accordingly, we have created an entirely new section for the fourth edition entitled Obesity and Energy Balance. Chapters reviewing the epidemiology, pathophysiology, treatment, prevention, and complications of obesity are now presented in a logical and coherent manner.

Although the rest of the general outline (General Concepts, Physiology and Pathophysiology, Perinatal Nutrition, Nutritional Aspects of Specific Disease States, and Approach to Nutritional Support) has been maintained from the third edition, we have made several other significant changes to the textbook. Ongoing data concerning the critical role of perinatal nutrition and specifically the fetal origins of adult health are addressed in several updated chapters. Owing to its critical importance in erythrocyte and systemic health, a new chapter on iron has been added. Chapters on diseases of increased incidence have also been added, including new reviews on the topics of Food Allergies, Celiac Disease, Feeding Difficulties, and the Outpatient Care of the Low Birth Weight Infant. Significantly revised and updated chapters populate the rest of the text, especially in the fields of the dietary reference intake, complementary feeding, the metabolic syndrome, and many others. Chapters addressing nutritional considerations in international health, macro- and micronutrients, perinatal nutrition, and multiple pediatric diseases have been updated and revised. As in past editions, comprehensive appendices are included that serve the reader by collating important tools for nutritional assessment, nutritional requirements, and enteral products. Finally, a new font and layout has been selected for this edition, which presents both text and graphs in an efficient and clean manner.

We express sincere thanks and appreciation to Ms. Suzzette McCarron for her unfailing organizational talents and communications skills. Without her extensive efforts, this edition would not have been possible.
The editors are also grateful to Mr. Brian Decker, Ms. Patricia Bindner, and the able staff of BC Decker Publishing Company for their help and "behind-the-scenes" efforts in the publication of this textbook.
Finally, we sincerely thank the dozens of authors who contributed countless hours of writing and research for the completion of this text. Their expertise and labors constitute the heart of this book.

Christopher Duggan
John B. Watkins
W. Allan Walker

DEDICATIONS

To the successful growth and nourishment of Michael, Brendan, and Emily Duggan, as well as that of children in Boston, Bangalore, Cairo, Dar es Salaam, Lima, and other places around the world.

Christopher P. Duggan, MD

To our grandchildren, Mariposa, Lillie, and Gwen, and their nine partners in "Friendship." In memory of Harvey R. Colten MD.

John B. Watkins, MD

To my grandchildren, Douglas and Lena Sandler and Giselle and Kathryn Walker, paradigms of healthy nutrition in children.

W. Allan Walker, MD

CONTENTS

PART III
PERINATAL NUTRITION

PART IV
OBESITY AND ENERGY BALANCE

PART V
NUTRITIONAL ASPECTS OF SPECIFIC DISEASE STATES

CONTRIBUTORS

Stephanie H. Abrams, MD
Assistant Professor of Pediatrics
Baylor College of Medicine
Division of Gastroenterology, Hepatology and Nutrition
Texas Children's Hospital
Houston, Texas
Nutritional Assessment of the Hospitalized Patient

John P. Ackerman, PhD
Post Doctoral Fellow
Department of Pediatrics
University of Maryland School of Medicine
Baltimore, Maryland
Neuropsychological Development

Jane Allen, PhD, DipNutrDiet.
Clinical Senior Lecturer
Department of Pediatrics and Child Health
Children's Hospital, Westmead
The University of Sydney
Sydney, Australia
Exocrine Pancreatic Disease Including Cystic Fibrosis

Diane Anderson, PhD, RD
Associate Professor of Pediatrics
Section of Neonatology
Baylor College of Medicine
Houston, Texas
The Low-Birth-Weight Infant: Inpatient Care

Magdalena Araya, MD, PhD
Professor
Department of Pediatric Clinical Nutrition
University of Chile
Santiago, Chile
Childhood Malnutrition: Prevention and Control at the National Level

Mona Bajaj-Elliott, BSc(Hons), PhD
Senior Lecturer
Institute of Child Health
Division of Infectious Diseases and Microbiology
University College London
London, England
Nutrition and Gene Expression

David J.P. Barker, FRS
Professor
Food Choice Group
DOHaD Division
University of Southampton, Princess Anne Hospital
Southampton, England
Human Growth and Disease in Later Life

Frederick C. Battaglia, MD
Professor Emeritus
Department of Pediatrics and Obstetrics-Gynecology
Perinatal Research Center
University of Colorado at Denver and Health Sciences Center
Aurora, Colorado
Amino Acid Nutrition In Utero: Placental Function and Metabolism

Lori J. Bechard, MEd, RD, LDN
Clincial Nutrition Specialist
Division of Gastroenterology and Nutrition
Clinical Nutrition Service
Children's Hospital, Boston
Boston, Massachusetts
Body Composition and Growth
Cancer Treatment

Gerard T. Berry, MD
Professor of Pediatrics
Harvard Medical School
Division of Genetics
Children's Hospital, Boston
Boston, Massachusetts
Inborn Errors of Metabolism and the Liver

Julie Bines, MD, FRACP
Professor of Pediatrics
University of Melbourne
Melbourne, Australia
Enteral Nutrition

Maureen M. Black, PhD
John A. Scholl Professor of Pediatrics
University of Maryland School of Medicine
Baltimore, Maryland
Neuropsychological Development

Nancy E. Blazar, RD, LD
Private Practice
Cleveland, Ohio
Adolescence: Healthy and Disordered Eating

Jean Louis Bresson, MD
Professor of Nutrition
Descartes Medical School
Paris, France
Energy Metabolism and Requirements in Health and Disease

Kenneth H. Brown, MD
Professor and Director
Program in International Nutrition
Department of Nutrition
University of California Davis
Davis, California
Complementary Feeding

TYLER BURPEE, MD
Research Fellow
Division of Gastroenterology and Nutrition
Children's Hospital, Boston
Boston, Massachusetts
Diarrheal Diseases

ELLEN BUTENSKY, PHD, PNP
Assistant Research Scientist
Department of Gastroenterology and Nutrition
Children's Hospital and Research Center at Oakland
Oakland, California
Nutritional Anemias

BENJAMIN CABALLERO, MD, PHD
Professor
Department of Nutrition
Center for Human Nutrition
Johns Hopkins Bloomberg School of Public Health
Baltimore, Maryland
International Nutrition

ARCHNA G. CALFEE, MD
Attending Pediatrician
Department of Pediatrics
St. Anne's Hospital
Charleton Memorial Hospital
Fall River, Massachusetts
The Adolescent Athlete: Performance-Enhancing Drugs and Dietary Supplements

RYAN P. CALFEE, MD
Clinical Instructor of Orthopedic Surgery
Department of Orthopedic Surgery
Brown University School of Medicine
Providence, Rhode Island
The Adolescent Athlete: Performance-Enhancing Drugs and Dietary Supplements

SUSAN J. CARLSON, MMSC, RD, CSP, LD, CNSD
Neonatal Dietitian
Department of Food and Nutrition Services
University of Iowa Hospitals and Clinics
Iowa City, Iowa
The Term Infant

LETICIA CASTILLO, MD
Associate Professor of Pediatrics
Baylor College of Medicine
Section of Critical Care
Texas Children's Hospital
Houston, Texas
Macronutrient Requirement for Growth: Protein/Amino Acid

LINGTAK-NEANDER CHAN, PHARMD, BCNSP
Associate Professor
Pharmacy and Graduate Program in Nutritional Science
University of Washington
Seattle, Washington
Drug Therapy and Role of Nutrition

TIEN-LAN CHANG, MD, FAAP
Instructor in Pediatrics
Harvard Medical School
Boston, Massachusetts
Standard and Specialized Enteral Formulas

MELANIE V. CONNOLLY, MSC, RD, LDN, CNSD
Clinical Nutrition Specialist
Division of Gastroenterology and Nutrition
Children's Hospital, Boston
Boston, Massachusetts
Special Diets
APPENDIX I: Nutritional Assessment
APPENDIX II: Nutritional Requirements
APPENDIX III: Enteral Products

SUSANNA CUNNINGHAM-RUNDLES, PHD
Professor of Immunology
Department of Pediatrics
Division of Hematology/Oncology
Weill Medical College
Cornell University Medical Center
New York, New York
Malnutrition and Host Defense

DANITA I. CZYZEWSKI, PHD
Assistant Professor of Psychiatry and Behavioral Sciences
Baylor College of Medicine
Houston, Texas
Feeding Difficulties

STEPHEN R. DANIELS, MD, PHD
Professor and Chairman
Department of Pediatrics
University of Colorado School of Medicine
Denver, Colorado
Dietary Reference Intakes

SARAH DE FERRANTI, MD, MPH, FAAP
Instructor in Pediatrics
Harvard Medical School
Department of Cardiology
Children's Hospital, Boston
Boston, Massachusetts
Complications of Obesity: Metabolic Syndrome
Hyperlipidemia and Cardiovascular Disease Risk

HANS DEMMELMAIR, PHD.
Professor
Division of Metabolic Diseases and Nutritional Medicine
Dr. von Hauner Children's Hospital
Ludwig-Maximilians-University of Munich
Munich, Germany
Macronutrient Requirements for Growth: Fats and Fatty Acids

ANNE DONNET-HUGHES, BSC(HONS), PHD
Senior Scientist
Department of Nutrition and Health
Nestlé Research Center
Lausanne, Switzerland
Protective Properties of Human Milk

Sharon M. Donovan, PhD, RD
Professor and Melissa M. Noel Endowed Chair
in Nutrition and Health
Department of Food Science and Human Nutrition
University of Illinois
Urbana, Illinois
Human Milk: Nutritional Properties

Martha V. Douglas-Escobar, MD
Perinatology-Neonatology Fellow
Department of Pediatrics
Division of Neonataology
University of Florida
Gainesville, Florida
Gastrointestinal Development: Implications for Infant Feeding

Christopher Duggan, MD, MPH
Associate Professor of Pediatrics
Harvard Medical School
Associate Professor in the Department of Nutrition
Harvard School of Public Health
Director, Clinical Nutrition Service
Division of Gastroenterology and Nutrition
Children's Hospital, Boston
Boston, Massachusetts
Cancer Treatment
Diarrheal Diseases
Failure to Thrive: Malnutrition in the Pediatric Outpatient Setting

Johanna T. Dwyer, DSc, RD
Professor of Medicine and Community Health
Director Friedman School of Nutrition Science
Tufts New England Medical Center
Boston, Massachusetts
Community Nutrition and Its Impact on Children: Developed Countries

Kenneth Ellis, PhD
Professor of Pediatrics
Baylor College of Medicine
Houston, Texas
Body Composition and Growth

Paul D. Fadale, MD
Associate Professor of Orthopedic Surgery
Department of Orthopedic Surgery
Division of Sports Medicine
Brown University School of Medicine
Providence, Rhode Island
The Adolescent Athlete: Performance-Enhancing Drugs and Dietary Supplements

Wafaie Fawzi, MD, DrPH
Professor of Nutrition and Epidemiology
Harvard School of Public Health
Boston, Massachusetts
Vitamins

Samuel J. Fomon, MD
Professor of Pediatrics
Fomon Infant Nutrition Unit
University of Iowa
Iowa City, Iowa
The Term Infant

Maria-Luisa Forchielli, MD, MPH, FACG
Assistant Professor of Pediatrics/GI Nutrition
University of Bologna Medical School
Bologna, Italy
Enteral Nutrition

Thomas M. Foy, MD
Associate Professor of Pediatrics
Division of Gastroenterology and Hepatology
St. Louis University School of Medicine
St. Louis, Missouri
Feeding Difficulties

A. Lindsay Frazier, MD, ScM
Assistant Professor of Pediatrics
Department of Pediatrics
Harvard Medical School
Dana Farber Cancer Institute
Boston, Massachusetts
Cancer Prevention

Kevin J. Gaskin, MD, FRACP
James Fairfax Professor of Pediatric Nutrition
Department of Paediatrics and Child Health
Faculty of Medicine
University of Sydney
Sydney, Australia
Exocrine Pancreatic Disease Including Cystic Fibrosis

Catherine M. Gordon, MD, MSc
Associate Professor of Pediatrics
Harvard Medical School
Divisions of Endocrinology and Adolescent Medicine
Boston, Massachusetts
Adolescence: Bone Disease

Kathleen S. Gorman, PhD
Professor of Psychology
Feinstein Center for a Hunger Free America
University of Rhode Island
Kingston, Rhode Island
Nutrition and the Behavior of Children

Olivier-Jean Goulet, MD, PhD
Professor
Department de Pediatrie, Gastroenterology et Nutrition
Hôpital Necker-Enfants Malades
Paris, France
Intestinal Failure, Short Bowel Syndrome, and Intestinal Transplantation

Kathleen M. Gura, PharmD, BCNSP, FASHP
Assistant Professor of Pharmacy Practice
Massachusetts College of Pharmacy and Health Sciences
Clinical Pharmacy Specialist
Gastroenterology and Nutrition
Children's Hospital, Boston
Boston, Massachusetts
Drug Therapy and the Role of Nutrition

Colleen Hadigan, MD, MPH
Staff Clinician
National Institute of Allergy and Infectious Diseases
Laboratory of Immunoregulation
National Institute of Health
Bethesda, Maryland
Pediatric HIV Infection

K. Michael Hambidge, MD, ScD
Professor Emeritus
Division of Pediatric Nutrition
University of Colorado School of Medicine
Denver, Colorado
Trace Elements

Paul Harmatz, MD
Associate Gastroenterologist
Department of Gastroenterology and Nutrition
Children's Hospital and Research Center Oakland
Oakland, California
Nutritional Anemias

William Harmon, MD
Professor of Pediatrics
Harvard Medical School
Division of Nephrology
Children's Hospital, Boston
Boston, Massachusetts
Persistent Renal Disease

William W. Hay, Jr., MD
Professor of Pediatrics
Division of Perinatal Medicine and Biology
University of Colorado School of Medicine
Aurora, Colorado
Development of the Fetus: Carbohydrate and Lipid Metabolism

Catherine Hayes, DMD, DMSc
Assistant Professor
Department of Oral Health Policy and Epidemiology
Harvard University School of Dental Medicine
Boston, Massachusetts
Function and Nature of the Components in the Oral Cavity

William C. Heird, MD
Professor of Pediatrics
Children's Nutrition Research Center
Baylor College of Medicine
Houston, Texas
Nutritional Management of Preterm Infants Postdischarge

Kristy M. Hendricks, DSc, RD
Associate Professor
Tufts University School of Medicine
Jaharis School of Nutrition Science and Policy
Tufts University
Boston, Massachusetts
Community Nutrition and Its Impact on Children: Industrialized Countries

Robert Heuschkel, MB, BS, MRCPCH
Clinical Lead and Consultant Pediatric Gastroenterologist
Centre for Pediatric Gastroenterology
Royal Free Hospital
London, England
Inflammatory Bowel Disease

Ann Ashworth Hill, PhD
Emeritus Professor of Community Nutrition
London School of Hygiene and Tropical Medicine
University of London
London, England
Childhood Malnutrition: Prevention and Control at the National Level

Daniel J. Hoffman, PhD
Assistant Professor of Nutritional Sciences
Rutgers University
New Brunswick, New Jersey
Energy and Substrate Regulation in Obesity

Alison G. Hoppin, MD
Instructor in Pediatrics
Department of Pediatrics
Harvard Medical School
Massachusetts General Hospital
Boston, Massachusetts
Evaluation and Management of Obesity

Melissa Hurwitz, MD
Assistant Professor of Pediatrics
Stanford University School of Medicine
Division of Pediatric Gastroenterology, Hepatology and Nutrition
Lucile Salter Packard Children's Hospital
Palo Alto, California
Parenteral Nutrition

Tom Jaksic, MD, PhD
Associate Professor of Surgery
Harvard Medical School
Children's Hospital, Boston
Boston, Massachusetts
The Critically Ill Child

Doron D. Kahana, MD
Fellow
Department of Pediatrics, Division of Gastroenterology and Nutrition
David Geffen School of Medicine at UCLA
Los Angeles, California
Carbohydrate Absorption and Malabsorption

Daniel S. Kamin, MD
Instructor in Pediatrics
Harvard Medical School
Division of Gastroenterology and Nutrition
Children's Hospital, Boston
Boston, Massachusetts
Intestinal Failure, Short Bowel Syndrome, and Intestinal Transplantation

Ciaran P. Kelly, MD
Associate Professor of Medicine
Harvard Medical School
Beth Israel Deaconess Medical Center
Boston, Massachusetts
Celiac Disease

Deirdre Kelly, FRCP, FRCPI, FRCPCH, MD
Professor of Hepatology
Department of Paediatrics
University of Birmingham
Birmingham, England
Acute and Chronic Liver Disease

Lisa C. Kemlage, MS, RD
Registered Dietitian
Glycogen Storage Disease Program
Department of Pediatrics
University of Florida College of Medicine
Gainesville, Florida
Glycogen Storage Disease

John A. Kerner Jr, MD
Professor of Pediatrics
Stanford University School of Medicine
Division of Pediatric Gastroenterology, Hepatology and Nutrition Lucile Salter Packard Children's Hospital
Palo Alto, California
Parenteral Nutrition

Amina Khambalia, MSc
Ph.D. Candidate
Division of Gastroenterology, Hepatology and Nutrition
University of Toronto
Toronto, Ontario, Canada
Iron

Brian D. Kineman, MS
Senior Nutrition Scientist
Mead Johnson Nutritionals
Nutrition Science and Technology Policy
Department of Food Service and Human Health
Evansville, Indiana
Food Safety

Ronald E. Kleinman, MD
Charles Wilder Professor of Pediatrics
Harvard Medical School
Physician-in-Chief and Chair
Department of Pediatrics
Massachusetts General Hospital for Children
Boston, Massachusetts
Standard and Specialized Enteral Formulas

Martin Kohlmeier, MD
Research Professor
Department of Nutrition
University of North Carolina
Chapel Hill, North Carolina
Dietary Supplements and Nutraceuticals

Professor Berthold Koletzko, MD
Professor of Pediatrics
Division of Metabolic Diseases and Nutritional Medicine
Ludwig Maximilians University
Munich, Germany
Macronutrient Requirements for Growth: Fats and Fatty Acids

Nancy F. Krebs, MD, MS
Professor of Pediatrics
Division of Pediatric Nutrition
University of Colorado School of Medicine
Denver, Colorado
Trace Elements

Kathrin Krohn, MD
Division of Metabolic Diseases and Nutrition
Dr. von Hauner Children's Hospital
University of Munich
Munich, Germany
Macronutrient Requirements for Growth: Fats and Fatty Acids

Roland Kupka, ScD
Research Scientist
Department of Nutrition
Harvard School of Public Health
Boston, Massachusetts
Vitamins

Robert M. Lawrence, MD
Clinical Associate Professor
Department of Pediatrics
University of Florida
Gainesville, Florida
Approach to Breast-Feeding

Ruth A. Lawrence, MD, FAAP, FABM, FAACT
Professor of Pediatrics and Obstetrics/Gynecology
Department of Pediatrics
Division of Neonatology
Rochester School of Medicine
Rochester, New York
Approach to Breast-Feeding

Carine M. Lenders, MD, MS
Assistant Professor of Pediatrics
Boston University School of Medicine
Boston Massachusetts
Nutritional Epidemiology

Lynne L. Levitsky, MD
Associate Professor of Pediatrics
Harvard Medical School
Division of Pediatric Endocrinology
Massachusetts General Hospital
Boston, Massachusetts
Macronutrient Requirements for Growth: Carbohydrates

Alice H. Lichtenstein, DSc
Gershoff Professor of Nutrition Science and Policy
Gerald J.and Dorothy R. Friedman School of Nutrition Science and Policy
Director and Senior Scientist, Cardiovascular Nutrition Laboratory
Jean Mayer USDA Human Nutrition Research Center on Aging
Tufts University
Boston, Massachusetts
Dietary Reference Intakes

Clifford W. Lo, MD, MPH, ScD
Assistant Professor of Pediatrics
Harvard Medical School
Division of Gastroenterology and Nutrition
Children's Hospital, Boston
Boston, Massachusetts
Laboratory Assessment of Nutritional Status

Keith J. Loud, MDCM, MSc, FAAP
Assistant Professor of Pediatrics
Northeastern Ohio Universities College of Medicine
Rootstown, Ohio
Adolescence: Bone Disease

Bertram Lubin, MD
Adjunct Professor of Pediatrics
Department of Pediatrics
Division of Hematology
University of California, San Francisco
San Francisco, California
Nutritional Anemias

Alan Lucas, MD, FRCP, FMed, SCI
Professor
MRC Childhood Nutrition Research Center
Institute of Child Health
Great Ormond Street Hospital for Children
London, England
Pediatric Nutrition: A Distinct Subspecialty

William C. MacLean Jr, MD, CH, FAAP
Vice President
Department of Medicine and Regulatory Affairs
Ross Products Division, Abbott Laboratories
Columbus, Ohio
Pediatric Nutrition: A Distinct Subspecialty

Jennifer Maloney, MD
Clinical Instructor
Pediatric Allergy and Clinical Immunology
Mount Sinai Medical Center
New York, New York
Food Allergies

Asim Maqbool, MD
Assistant Professor of Pediatrics
University of Pennsylvania School of Medicine
Division of Gastroenterology, Hepatology and Nutrition
Children's Hospital of Philadelphia
Philadelphia, Pennsylvania
Clinical Assessment of Nutritional Status

Robert Markowitz, MD
Instructor in Pediatrics
Harvard Medical School
Children's Hospital, Boston
Boston, Massachusetts
Failure to Thrive: Malnutrition in the Pediatric Outpatient Setting

Martin G. Martin, MD, MPP
Professor of Pediatrics
David Geffen School of Medicine at UCLA
Division of Gastroenterology
Mattel Children's Hospital
Los Angeles, California
Carbohydrate Absorption and Malabsorption

David F. McNeeley, MD, MPHTM
Fellow, Pediatric Infectious Disease
Division of Pediatric Infectious Disease
Cornell Medical College-New York Hospital
New York, New York
Malnutrition and Host Defense

Nilesh M. Mehta, MD, DCH, MRCPCH
Instructor in Anesthesia
Harvard Medical School
Division of Critical Care Medicine
Children's Hospital, Boston
Boston, Massachusetts
The Critically Ill Child

Elizabeth Metallinos-Katsaras, PhD, RD
Associate Professor of Nutrition
School for Health Studies
Simmons College
Boston, Massachusetts
Nutrition and the Behavior of Children

Aeri Moon, MD
Assistant Professor of Pediatrics
Division of Hematology/Oncology
Weill Cornell Medical College
Division of Pediatric Gastroenterology
New York-Presbyterian Hospital
New York, New York
Malnutrition and Host Defense

Erika K. Nakamoto, MS
Nutritional/Research Biochemist
Department of Defense (DoD), Combat Feeding Directorate
Natick Soldier Research, Development, and Engineering Center
Natick, Massachusetts
Cancer Prevention

Linda P. Nelson, DMD, MScD, FACD
Assistant Professor of Pediatric Dentistry
Department of Developmental Biology
Division of Pediatric Dentistry
Harvard School of Dental Medicine
Boston, Massachusetts
Function and Nature of the Components in the Oral Cavity

Josef Neu, MD
Professor of Pediatrics
Division of Neonatology
University of Florida College of Medicine
Shands Children's Hospital
Gainesville, Florida
Gastrointestinal Development: Implications for Infant Feeding

Ellis J. Neufeld, MD, PhD
Associate Professor of Pediatrics
Harvard Medical School
Division of Hematology/Oncology
Children's Hospital, Boston
Boston, Massachusetts
Hyperlipidemia and Cardiovascular Disease Risk

Irene E. Olsen, PhD, RD
Assistant Professor of Bioscience and Biotechnology
Drexel University
Philadelphia, Pennsylvania
Clinical Assessment of Nutritional Status

Stavroula K. Osganian, MD, ScD
Assistant Professor of Pediatrics
Harvard Medical School
Division of Endocrinology
Children's Hospital, Boston
Boston, Massachusetts
Complications of Obesity: Metabolic Syndrome

Mary E. Penny, MA, MB, ChB, MRCP
Researcher and Director
Instituto de Investigacion Nutricional
Lima, Peru
Protein-Energy Malnutrition: Pathophysiology, Clinical Consequences, and Treatment

Maryanne Quinn, MD
Instructor in Pediatrics
Harvard Medical School
Division of Endocrinology
Children's Hospital, Boston
Boston, Massachusetts
Diabetes Mellitus

Samuli Rautava, MD, PhD
Post Doctoral Research Fellow
Mucosal Immunology Laboratory
Massachusetts General Hospital
Boston, Massachusetts
Immunophysiology and Nutrition of the Gut

Timothy R.H. Regnault, PhD
Assistant Professor of Obstetrics and Gynecology
University of Western Ontario
London, Ontario
Amino Acid Nutrition In Utero: Placental Function and Metabolism

David B. Rhoads, PhD
Assistant Professor of Pediatrics
Harvard Medical School
Pediatric Endocrine Unit
Massachusetts General Hospital
Boston, Massachusetts
Macronutrient Requirements for Growth: Carbohydrates

J. Marc Rhoads, MD
Professor of Pediatrics
Division of Gastroenterology and Nutrition
University of Texas-Houston Medical School
Houston, Texas
Nutrition and Humoral Regulation of Growth

Susan B. Roberts, PhD
Scientist, Energy Metabolism Laboratory
USDA Human Nutrition Research Center
Tufts University
Boston, Massachusetts
Energy and Substrate Regulation in Obesity

Nancy M. Rodig, MD
Instructor in Pediatrics
Harvard Medical School
Division of Nephrology
Children's Hospital, Boston
Boston, Massachusetts
Persistent Renal Disease

Ellen S. Rome, MD, MPH
Assistant Professor of Pediatrics
Section Head in Adolescent Medicine
The Cleveland Clinic
Cleveland, Ohio
Adolescence: Healthy and Disordered Eating

Rachel M. Roth, MD
Cleveland Clinic
Lerner College of Medicine
Case Western Reserve University
Cleveland, Ohio
Macronutrient Requirement for Growth: Protein/Amino Acid

William E. Russell, MD
Associate Professor of Pediatrics and
Cell and Developmental Biology
Department of Pediatrics
Vanderbilt University Medical Center
Division of Endocrinology
Monroe Carell Jr.
Children's Hospital at Vanderbilt
Nashville, Tennessee
Nutrition and Humoral Regulation of Growth

HUGH SAMPSON, MD
Professor of Pediatrics
Division of Allergy and Immunology
Mount Sinai School of Medicine
New York, New York
Food Allergies

IAN R. SANDERSON, MD, MSc, MRCP
Professor of Pediatrics
Adult and Pediatric Gastroenterology
Institute of Cell and Molecular Science
London, England
Nutrition and Gene Expression

RICHARD J. SCHANLER, MD
Associate Chairman
Department of Pediatrics
Chief, Neonatal-Perinatal Medicine
Schneider Children's Hospital at North Shore
Manhasset, New York
The Low-Birth-Weight Infant: Inpatient Care

EDUARDO J. SCHIFFRIN, MD, PHD
Medical Advisor
Department of Research and Development
Nestlé Nutrition
Vevey, Switzerland
Protective Properties of Human Milk

THERESA O. SCHOLL, PHD, MPH
Professor of Obstetrics and Gynecology
University of Medicine and Dentistry of New Jersey
Stratford, New Jersey
Maternal Nutrition and Pregnancy Outcome

JAMES H. SHAW, DMD, PHD
Professor of Nutrition Emeritus
Harvard University School of Dental Medicine
Newton Center, Massachusetts
Function and Nature of the Components in the Oral Cavity

ROBERT J. SHULMAN, MD
Professor of Pediatrics
Baylor College of Medicine
Section of Gastroenterology and Nutrition
Texas Children's Hospital
Houston, Texas
Nutritional Assessment of the Hospitalized Patient

KENDRIN SONNEVILLE, MS, RD, LDN
Doctoral Student
Department of Nutrition
Harvard School of Public Health
Clinical Nutrition Specialist
Children's Hospital, Boston
Boston, Massachusetts
Popular Diets for Obesity

NANCY SPINOZZI, RD, LDN
Clinical Nutrition Service and
Division of Nephrology
Children's Hospital Boston
Boston, Massachusetts
Persistent Renal Disease

VIRGINIA A. STALLINGS, MD
Professor of Pediatrics
Department of Pediatrics
University of Pennsylvania School of Medicine
Philadelphia, Pennsylvania
Clinical Assessment of Nutritional Status
Developmental Disabilities

MELANIE A. STUART, MS, RD
Private Practice
Goose Creek, South Carolina
Community Nutrition and Its Impact on Children: Industrialized Countries

RICARDO UAUY, MD, PHD
Professor
Department of Public Health Nutrition
Instituto de Nutrición y Tecnología de los Alimentos (INTA)
University of Chile
Santiago, Chile
Childhood Malnutrition: Prevention and Control at the National Level

MARTIN H. ULSHEN, MD
Professor of Pediatrics
Division of Pediatric GI and Nutrition
Duke University Medical Center
Durham, North Carolina
Carbohydrate Absorption and Malabsorption

ANGELINA I. VALLADARES, MD
Fellow
Department of Pediatrics
Division of Endocrinology
University of Florida College of Medicine
Gainesville, Florida
Glycogen Storage Disease

CHARLES P. VENDITTI, MD, PHD
Investigator
Genetic Disease Research Branch
National Human Genome Research Institute
Bethesda, Maryland
Inborn Errors of Metabolism and the Liver

EDUARDO VILLAMOR, MD, DRPH
Assistant Professor of International Nutrition
Departments of Nutrition and Epidemiology
Harvard School of Public Health
Boston, Massachusetts
Vitamins

W. ALLAN WALKER, MD
Conrad Taff Professor of Nutrition, Professor of Pediatrics
Harvard Medical School
Chief, Mucosal Immunology Laboratory
Pediatric Gastroenterology and Nutrition Unit
Massachusetts General Hospital for Children
Boston, Massachusetts
Immunophysiology and Nutrition of the Gut
Protective Properties of Human Milk

KAREN WARMAN, MS, RD, LDN
Clinical Nutrition Specialist
Clinical Nutrition Service
Division of Gastroenterology and Nutrition
Children's Hospital Boston
Boston, Massachusetts
Diabetes Mellitus

JOHN B.WATKINS, MD
Associate Professor of Pediatrics
Harvard Medical School
Division of Gastroenterology and Nutrition
Children's Hospital, Boston
Boston, Massachusetts
Failure to Thrive: Malnutrition in the Pediatric Outpatient Setting

DAVID A. WEINSTEIN, MD, MMSc
Associate Professor of Pediatrics and Director
Glycogen Storage Disease Program
Division of Endocrinology
University of Florida College of Medicine
Gainesville, Florida
Glycogen Storage Disease

DASCHA C WEIR, MD
Research Fellow
Division of Gastroenterology and Nutrition
Children's Hospital, Boston
Boston, Massachusetts
Celiac Disease

GERARDO WEISSTAUB, MD, MSc
Instructor
Department of Pediatric Clinical Nutrition
Instituto de Nutrición y Tecnología de los Alimentos (INTA)
University of Chile
Santiago, Chile
Childhood Malnutrition: Prevention and Control at the National Level

WALTER C. WILLETT, MD, DRPH
Frederick John Star Professor of
Epidemiology and Nutrition
Harvard School of Public Health
Boston, Massachusetts
Nutritional Epidemiology

JOSEPH WOLFSDORF, MB, BCH
Professor of Pediatrics
Harvard Medical School
Division of Endocrinology
Children's Hospital, Boston
Boston, Massachusetts
Diabetes Mellitus

CATHERINE E. WOTEKI, PHD, RD
Global Director of Scientific Affairs
Mars, Incorporated
McLean, Virginia
Food Safety

MELISSA WRIGHT, RD, LDN
Clinical Nutrition Specialist
Division of Gastroenterology and Nutrition
Children's Hospital, Boston
Boston, Massachusetts
Laboratory Assessment of Nutritional Status

EMILY WROE, BA
Medical Student
Harvard Medical School
Boston, Massachusetts
Body Composition and Growth

STEVEN H. ZEISEL, MD, PHD
Professor of Nutrition
School of Public Health
University of North Carolina at Chapel Hill
Chapel Hill, North Carolina
Dietary Supplements and Nutraceuticals

BABETTE ZEMEL, PHD
Associate Professor of Pediatrics
Division of GI and Nutrition
Children's Hospital of Philadelphia
Philadelphia, Pennsylvania
Developmental Disabilities

EKHARD ZIEGLER, MD
Professor of Pediatrics
University of Iowa Hospitals and Clinics
Iowa City, Iowa
The Term Infant

STANLEY H. ZLOTKIN MD, PHD, FRCPC
Professor of Pediatrics
University of Toronto
The Hospital for Sick Children
Division of Gastroenterology, Hepatology and Nutrition
Toronto, Ontario, Canada
Iron

I GENERAL CONCEPTS

1

Pediatric Nutrition: A Distinct Subspecialty

William C. MacLean Jr, MD, CH, FAAP
Alan Lucas, MD, FRCP, FMed Sci

Scientific interest in nutrition has a long history.[1–3] Balance studies were conceived by Sanctorius in the 1620s. Lavoisier researched the oxidation of foods and Magendie discovered that protein was necessary for survival two centuries ago. In 1838, Franz Simon produced his classic dissertation, in Latin, on human milk biochemistry, which for the first time underpinned a rational basis for infant nutrition. It was over 100 years ago, in the late nineteenth century, that Rubner defined the energy content of foods and constructed the first calorimeter for measuring energy expenditure. By the early twentieth century, we already had a broad understanding of nutrient needs and an increasing understanding of micronutrients and of the effects of specific deficiencies. (Funk coined the term "vitamines" in 1912.) Sophisticated metabolic research on animals fed by continuous intravenous infusion flourished in the first three decades of the last century, and as early as 1944, we saw the first case of a child, age 5 months, fed successfully via the intravenous route.

In parallel with this long-term development of nutritional science has been an equally long-term appreciation of the clinical and public health importance of infant and child nutrition. In the earliest part of the last century, and well before, nutrition was a prominent and vital part of caring for infants. Unquestionably, in the eyes of early clinicians, how and what the infant was fed during health and illness were primary determinants of survival. The infant mortality rate in the United States in 1900 was 165 per 1,000.[1] The unacceptably high rate and the variability from one area of the country to the other related primarily to mode of feeding in infancy.

At that time, pediatrics, both as an academic specialty and in everyday practice, was in its own infancy. At the turn of the nineteenth century, there were probably fewer than a dozen practitioners in the United States who were exclusively devoted to pediatrics.[2] In the first presidential address to the American Pediatric Society in 1889, Abraham Jacobi discussed the rationale for having the specialty of pediatrics distinct from internal medicine: "Pediatrics deals with the entire organism at the very period during which it presents the most interesting features to the student of biology and medicine ... there is scarcely a tissue or an organ which behaves exactly alike at different periods of life."[2]

A review of the topics covered in the annual presidential addresses to the American Pediatric Society during its first 35 years shows a frequent return to nutrition and nutrition-related subjects. In 1924, David M. Cowie suggested that feeding in infancy was then sufficiently based on sound physiologic principles and that pediatrics needed to focus more on nutrition and metabolism, among other things, of the older child.[2] By 1940, when the eleventh edition of *Holt's Diseases of Infancy and Childhood* was published, the editors unhesitatingly stated, "Nutrition in its broadest sense is the most important branch of pediatrics. A knowledge of its fundamental principles is essential to the physician if he is to apply preventive and corrective measures intelligently."[4]

WHY HAS PEDIATRIC NUTRITION NOT EMERGED AS A DISTINCT SUBSPECIALTY?

Given that nutrition is the oldest branch of pediatrics based on centuries of major research, it seems paradoxical that it has never emerged as a formal, distinct academic discipline. Indeed, considering its roots in and fundamental relationships to that which makes pediatrics unique—growth and maturation—why has nutrition taken a back seat to other subspecialties? The decline in the importance of nutrition in pediatrics can be explained in two ways.

First, the urgency that fostered nutrition research and the illnesses that made nutrition a prominent part of pediatric practice decreased progressively during the last century. The causes of infantile scurvy and rickets and other deficiency diseases were delineated during the early decades of the twentieth century. In fact, with the exception of iron deficiency, primary nutritional deficiencies are now virtually unknown in the United States and other developed countries, and infant mortality rates relate more to the general level of socioeconomic development than to nutritional practices. With the advent of refrigeration and appropriate milk processing technology, survival of artificially fed infants in clean environments is now the norm.

Second, pediatrics has followed the path taken by internal medicine and surgery; the past 40 years have seen the growth of "organ-based" subspecialties: pediatric cardiology, neurology, nephrology, and so on, and, more recently, gastroenterology. The result of this evolutionary course was to imbed clinical nutrition in a variety of "organ-focused" subspecialty areas. This arguably fostered a disease-specific orientation to nutrition and fragmentation of nutrition practice and research. Thus, enteral feeding has come under the wing of gastroenterologists, parenteral nutrition has interested gastroenterologists and pediatric surgeons as well, aspects of growth have fallen into the domain of endocrinology, neonatal nutrition has been taken on by neonatologists, eating disorders by psychologists and psychiatrists, food allergy by allergists and physicians in respiratory medicine, and so forth. This fragmentation and multiple ownership of pediatric nutrition have hindered development of the field as a distinct entity.

WHY IS PEDIATRIC NUTRITION REEMERGING IN IMPORTANCE?

In the past, the major focus in the field of nutrition has been one of meeting nutrient needs and the prevention of nutrient deficiencies. There has now been a fundamental sea change in orientation in this field. The major current interest in nutrition is its impact on health.[5] Our new understanding of the potential biologic impacts of nutrition on health has led us to frame two key new questions: Does nutrition matter in terms of patients' responses to their disease? Does it matter for long-term health and development?

With regard to the first, increasing evidence now indicates that good nutritional care may improve the clinical course of disease, reduce hospital stay, reduce the need for more expensive treatments, and, indeed, result in major reduction in health care costs. Such benefits of nutritional care are emerging over a broad range of pediatric domains such as gastroenterology (eg, Crohn's disease, short-bowel syndrome), surgery, renal medicine, care of disabled children (eg, cerebral palsy), infectious disease (eg, human immunodeficiency virus [HIV]), and oncology. Neonatology provides good examples of the effects of good nutrition on clinical course: Nutritional practices may have a major influence on the incidence of life-threatening diseases (necrotizing enterocolitis and systemic sepsis),[6] may influence the need for expensive and potentially hazardous parenteral nutrition, and may significantly impact length of hospital stay.

However, the factor that has most influenced the reemergence of interest in pediatric nutrition is the increasing evidence for its effects on long-term health and development. The idea that early nutrition could have long-term consequences is part of a broader concept concerning the impact of early life events in general. To focus attention in this area, Lucas proposed using the term "programming,"[7] the idea that a stimulus or insult applied during a critical or sensitive period of development could have a long-lasting or lifetime impact on the structure or function of the organism. The first description of programming during a sensitive or critical period of development was by Spalding, who in 1873 defined the critical period for imprinting in newborn chicks.[8] Since then, developmentalists have described numerous examples of short-lived stimuli—both endogenous and exogenous—that have had lifetime effects.

What is the evidence that nutrition may behave in this programming way? Since the first studies by McCance in the 1960s, the evidence for such programming in animals is overwhelming. Brief periods of experimental nutritional manipulation in early life influence in adult life many outcomes of potential relevance to humans,[9] including blood pressure, insulin resistance, blood lipids, vascular disease, body fatness, bone health, gut function, endocrine status, learning, behavior, and longevity.[9–13] Nutritional programming effects have been seen in all species studied, including nonhuman primates.[10,11]

In the past 25 years, increasing evidence has shown that humans, like other species, may be highly sensitive to early nutrition in terms of later health outcomes. Deficiencies of single nutrients at critical periods can have long-lasting effects. Animal studies have documented the role of zinc deficiency in the development of neural tube defects in the fetus. Choline deficiency in the rat in utero or in the early weeks of life has long-term effects on brain function, specifically memory.[14] Decreased folic acid intake in the periconceptional period also has been linked to neural tube defects in the human.[15]

Iron is another trace element that appears to play a critical role in development. Iron deficiency in rats, for example, produces reversed sleep cycles, altered pain threshold, and difficulty in learning. Dopamine D_2 receptors also are decreased. When the iron-deficient diet is begun at 10 days of age, later iron repletion is unable to reverse these defects completely.[16] In the human, the mechanisms of the detrimental effects of severe iron deficiency in early childhood on subsequent mental development are yet to be elucidated, but several studies suggest that such effects may be permanent and may affect both cognitive ability and behavior.[17–19] On a molecular level, it is possible that iron is required at a critical time for the expression of one or several genes, and if this opportunity is lost, iron sufficiency is unable to reverse the path of development.

Many observational studies have linked growth, size, or nutrition in early life to the types of health outcome influenced by early nutrition in animals. Human studies now point to effects of birth weight, early growth rate, and weight at 1 or 2 years of age on such outcomes as bone mass and coronary events in later life.[20–22] Such observational data might be confounded, but in more recent years, there has been long-term investment in randomized intervention studies. These trials have now shown that early diet during obesity, bone health, and cognitive performance.[9,22–24]

The effects of brief early nutritional interventions are often surprisingly large. Studies in the preterm infant show that feeding a standard versus preterm formula for just 1 month may result in a 12-point deficit in verbal IQ (in males) and a more than doubling of motor or cognitive impairment (both sexes) 7 to 8 years later.[22] In the same population, random assignment to banked donated breast milk rather than infant formula resulted in a reduction in diastolic blood pressure 13 to 16 years later of a magnitude greater than that induced by nonpharmacologic interventions used to manage hypertension in adult life (weight loss, exercise, salt restriction).[23] A small follow-up study of full-term infants who had been randomized to be fed infant formula with or without added arachidonic acid and docosahexaenoic acid for the early months of life found that diastolic blood pressure was significantly lower at 6 years of age in previously supplemented infants.[25] These data require confirmation with larger numbers of subjects. Such data have major biologic and public health implications. They show that nutrition cannot simply be seen in terms of meeting nutritional needs. Rather, nutrition emerges as a major environmental influence on the genome, influencing lifetime health. It is also apparent that there is now a new onus on health professionals to ensure proper nutrition to optimize the short- and long-term health of sick individuals and healthy populations.

RATIONALE FOR A SEPARATE DISCIPLINE

Viewed in the historical context of a changing subspecialty paradigm and a new appreciation of nutrition's role at the molecular level with profound implications for health, the time would seem right for nutrition to be recognized as a distinct area of pediatric practice. But what other criteria should be fulfilled for nutrition to be formally developed as a pediatric subspecialty? Two questions must be addressed: Is there a defined area of pediatric care that requires specific nutritional expertise and are there readily identifiable deficiencies in current pediatric nutritional patient teaching and research that would benefit from such a development?

Defined Area of Expertise

There is a defined area of pediatric care that requires nutritional expertise. Nutritional advice is one of the most common categories of advice sought by parents. Nutritional management problems are possibly the most common problems in pediatric hospital practice; virtually every sick premature infant and a high proportion of sick older children could benefit from specific and expert nutritional attention. Walk on any general ward and the number of patients needing advice from a pediatric cardiologist, nephrologist, or gastroenterologist will be far exceeded by those who would benefit from sound nutritional care.

However, beyond the routine practice of what we know, there are potentially important areas of new expertise that need to be sewn into nutrition practice. Just as a field such as cardiology owes its specialty status in part to the development of specialized techniques—catheterization, diagnostic imaging, etc—so could pediatric nutrition be underpinned by new tools awaiting exploitation in a clinical setting.[7] Isotope probes are available for exploring metabolic process and energy expenditure. Body composition devices (dual X-ray absorptiometry, impedance, isotope dilution, air displacement plethysmography, three-dimensional photonic scanning, ultrasonography, magnetic resonance imaging, etc) are ready to be pioneered in the complex management of sick infants and children. They are also likely to prove useful in the assessment of the impact of public health policy on the nutritional status of the childhood population (for instance, the value of interventions to reduce obesity, which are currently monitored by inappropriately nonspecific and crude methods). New tools are also available to measure and plot growth that will make the diagnosis and management of growth disorders, failure to thrive, and overweight less arbitrary and more precise. Such techniques require trained specialists.

Deficiencies in Patient Care

Subspecialists trained in pediatric nutrition would improve patient care. Specialty advice in nutrition is often sought from physicians whose primary interest is in another area.[26] This results in fragmentation of care and creates a lack of uniformity in how conditions are managed. A "standard of practice" does not exist. Nutrition knowledge has exploded to the point where clinicians in individual subspecialties no longer can be expected to have a comprehensive grasp of all aspects relevant to their own increasingly complex practice. There is an increasing number of children with obesity and latent or overt metabolic syndrome, which will complicate the course of other diseases. In addition, there continues to be a high percentage of inpatients in any general or pediatric hospital who are found to be malnourished by "world-class" criteria as a result of their primary disease. With efforts to contain costs and the move to home care, patients often are leaving hospital with more profound nutritional deficits than before, and the situation can be expected to become worse.

For many years in the United States, parenteral nutrition support in many hospitals was overseen by the surgical service, whereas enteral nutrition was handled by virtually any pediatrician. Even with the advent of nutrition support teams, most of the physicians involved have acquired their nutritional skills in an ad hoc fashion. If consultation about enteral nutrition is needed, the gastroenterologist, by default, has assumed responsibility and is likely to be called. To be sure, gastroenterology and nutrition are closely linked, and most pediatric gastroenterologists have considerable expertise in nutrition, especially as it affects their "organ system." But the pediatric gastroenterologist should not be expected to be well versed in all areas of nutrition, because only a small part of nutrition science and practice is related directly to gastroenterology.

Deficiencies in Teaching

Teaching of nutrition in medical schools also is fragmented at best: "To almost everyone expressing an opinion about the teaching of nutrition in medical schools, it appears to be entirely unsatisfactory. Rare successes prove to be ephemeral and crucially dependent on individual commitment and outside funding."[27] In most medical schools, the basic science pertaining to nutrition is embedded in biochemistry and, perhaps, physiology. A survey of 126 US medical schools in 2004 found that a separate course in nutrition was required in only 32 of the 106 schools responding.[28] Formal teaching of clinical nutrition is nearly nonexistent. The same survey reported that the average contact hours of required nutrition instruction in the third and fourth years of medical school was 5.1 ± 0.7 hours. What teaching there is generally done as a part of primary care rotations or by subspecialists in other areas in pediatrics. Many medical students never observe breast-feeding and are never trained to make up a formula feed. Most house staff leave training with less than adequate understanding of the physiology and management of breast-feeding, the composition and appropriate use of standard or special infant formulas, or the appraisal of simple feeding problems and the rationale for nutrition advice or care during the second 6 months of life and beyond. Public health and preventive nutrition are equally neglected. The provision of 5-year Nutrition Academic Awards to 21 US medical schools since 1998 to foster nutrition education during medical school is a step in the right direction and appears to have produced a number of innovative approaches in nutrition education.[29] The 2004 survey previously referred to, however, concluded the following: "With the move to a more integrated curriculum and problem-based learning at many medical schools, a substantial portion of the total nutrition instruction is occurring outside courses specifically dedicated to nutrition. The amount of nutrition education in medical schools remains inadequate."[28,*]

Nutrition education and practice continue to relate primarily to organ-based specialties. Although this may be acceptable from the point of view of clinical practice, from the point of view of research it will ultimately impede inquiry into the important areas.

Deficiencies in Research

The area that perhaps stands to gain most from the development of nutrition as a distinct discipline is research. Although basic laboratory and animal research in nutrition has been active, the key clinical research questions in pediatric nutrition are unlikely to be addressed as long as nutrition is divided among the traditional specialties. This is so because the orientation toward disease of most subspecialties will favor research to answer questions related to therapeutic dietetics (ie, treatment of disease). With infant survival from a nutritional point of view assured in most Western countries, the issue of how early nutrition should be optimized in terms of its effects on later health becomes of paramount importance.

The objective for clinical research in any field of health policy or clinical practice should be to prove outcome benefits for recommended approaches to management, generally by use of formal clinical trials that test the safety and efficacy of the intervention. This would be standard in established clinical areas. Thus, whether or not a clinician should treat high blood pressure, remove a malignancy rather than give chemotherapy, or repair a heart defect at birth rather than later in childhood and other decisions depend on proven clinical benefit for each management option. For example, physicians routinely treat high blood pressure precisely because lowering blood pressure has been shown to reduce morbidity and mortality from cardiovascular disease.

Research in childhood nutrition has been largely unsatisfactory in this respect. Dietary recommendations fluctuate as new expert groups examine the data. The data that underpin the recommendations for dietary reference nutrient intakes in adults are often inadequate, and recommendations for children frequently are based on even less secure data. In addition, research over the past 50 years has largely failed to address adequately whether adhering to the nutritional recommendations made by ad hoc groups and governmental bodies confers outcome benefits.[7] The critical issue of whether early nutrition, either in health or in disease, influences long-term health or development has, until the last two decades, barely been approached in formal studies. Thus, most recommendations of expert bodies on fundamental areas of practice are based largely on theoretic considerations derived from short-term physiologic experiments and epidemiologic studies rather than on outcome findings from intervention trials. Both physiology and epidemiology can be useful in identifying questions and framing hypotheses for such outcome trials, but neither can replace them.

The paucity of clinical outcome studies in pediatric nutrition contrasts sharply with the major research investment that has been made in pediatric nutritional physiology. Possibly more research effort has been applied here than in any other area of pediatrics. For instance, as far back as 1953, Macy and colleagues summarized the contents of 1,500 publications on the composition of breast milk—just one small area of infant nutrition.[30] The profusion of pediatric nutritional studies in the face of the paucity of outcome data justifying clinical practice suggests that clinical pediatric nutritional research has lacked direction. This lack of research direction, not seen to nearly the same extent in the recognized pediatric specialties, can be traced in part to the absence of guidance on research priorities from specialists trained in nutrition and from centers of excellence in pediatric nutrition.

CONCLUSION

Like the blind men approaching the elephant, each subspecialty comes up with a different view of nutrition. Each subspecialty creates a paradigm that determines how questions are framed and results are interpreted. Depending on one's primary interest, taurine may be thought of as a critical nutrient for neural development and function, a primary determinant of bile acid conjugation, or an osmoregulator of the brain during dehydration. Someone needs to see the elephant for what it is—to collate our knowledge in the field of nutrition, understand its significance for development, and apply it to clinical practice.

Functional specialties in medicine increasingly are interacting in a matrix fashion with organ-based specialties. Clinical nutrition fits comfortably into this new paradigm. The time appears to be right to foster clinical nutrition within pediatrics as a unique discipline. Such a development would address currently identifiable deficiencies in patient care, training, and, especially, research in clinical nutrition.

*For a comprehensive look at the state of nutrition education in medical school curricula, see "An evidenced-based approach to medical nutrition education. Am J Clin Nutr 2006;83:929S–87S."

REFERENCES

1. Cone TE, Jr. History of American Pediatrics. Boston: Little, Brown; 1979.
2. Pearson HA. The Centennial History of the American Pediatric Society 1888–1988. New Haven, CT: Yale University Printing Service; 1989.
3. Kleinman RE, Barness LA, Finberg L. History of pediatric nutrition and fluid therapy. Pediat Res 2003;54:762–72.
4. Holt LE, McIntosh R. Holt's Diseases of Infancy and Childhood, 11th edition. New York: D. Appleton-Century; 1940.
5. Lucas A. Pediatric nutrition as a new subspecialty: Is the time right? Arch Dis Child 1997;76:3–6.
6. Lucas A, Cole TJ. Breast milk and neonatal necrotizing enterocolitis. Lancet 1990;336:1519–23.
7. Lucas A. Programming by early nutrition in man. In: Bock G, Whelan J, editors. The Childhood Environment and Adult Disease. CIBA Foundation Symposium 156. Chichester, UK: Wiley; 1991. p. 38–55.
8. Spalding DA. Instinct with original observations on young animals. Macmillan's Mag 1873;27:282–93; reprinted Br J Anim Behav 1954;2:2–11.
9. Lucas A. Programming by early nutrition: An experimental approach. J Nutr 1998;128:401S–6S.
10. Lewis DS, Mott GE, McMahan CA, et al. Deferred effects of preweaning diet on atherosclerosis in adolescent baboons. Arteriosclerosis 1988;8:274–80.
11. Mott GE, Jackson EM, McMahan CA, McGill HC, Jr. Cholesterol metabolism in adult baboons is influenced by infant diet. J Nutr 1990;120:243–51.
12. Dobbing J. Vulnerable periods in developing brain. In: Dobbing J, editor. Brain, Behavior, and Iron in the Infant Diet. New York: Springer-Verlag; 1990. p. 1–18.
13. Symonds ME, Gardner DS. Experimental evidence for early nutritional programming of later health in animals. Curr Opin Clin Nutr Metab Care 2006;9:278–83.
14. Zeisel SH. Nutritional importance of choline for brain development. J Am Coll of Nutr 2004;23:621S–6S.
15. Centers for Disease Control and Prevention. Recommendations for the use of folic acid to reduce the number of cases of spina bifida and other neural tube defects. Morb Mortal Wkly Rep 1992;41:1–7.
16. Youdim MBH. Neuropharmacological and neurobiochemical aspects of iron deficiency. In: Dobbing J, editor. Brain, Behavior, and Iron in the Infant Diet. New York: Springer-Verlag; 1990. p. 83–99.
17. Lozoff B. Has iron deficiency been shown to cause altered behavior in infants? In: Dobbing J, editor. Brain, Behavior, and Iron in the Infant Diet. New York: Springer-Verlag; 1990. p. 107–25.
18. Walter T. Iron deficiency and behavior in infancy: A critical review. In: Dobbing J, editor. Brain, Behavior, and Iron in the Infant Diet. New York: Springer-Verlag; 1990. p. 135–50.
19. Lozoff B, Beard J, Connor J, et al. Long-lasting neural and behavioral effects of iron deficiency in infancy. Nutr Rev 2006;64:S34–43.
20. Dennison EM, Syddall HE, Sayer AA, et al. Birth weight and weight at 1 year are independent determinants of bone mass in the seventh decade: The Hertfordshire cohort study. Pediatr Res 2005;57:582–6.
21. Barker, DJP, Osmond C, Forsén TJ. Trajectories of growth among children who have coronary events as adults. N Engl J Med 2005;353:1802–9.
22. Lucas A, Morley R, Cole TJ. Randomized trial of early diet in preterm babies and later intelligence quotient. BMJ 1998;317:1481–7.
23. Singhal A, Cole TJ, Lucas A. Early nutrition in preterm infants and later blood pressure: Two cohorts after randomized tri als. Lancet 2001;357:413–9.
24. Fewtrell MS, Prentice A, Jones SC, et al. Bone mineralization and turnover in preterm infants at 8–12 years of age: The effect of early diet. J Bone Miner Res 1999;14:810–20.
25. Forsyth JS, Willatts P, Agostoni C, et al. Long chain polyunsaturated fatty acid supplementation in infant formula and blood pressure in later childhood: Follow up of a randomized controlled trial. BMJ 2003;326:953.
26. Committee on Clinical Practice Issues in Health and Disease. The role and identity of physician nutrition specialists in medical school affiliated hospitals. Am J Clin Nutr 1995;61:264–8.
27. McLaren DS. Nutrition in medical schools: A case of mistaken identity. Am J Clin Nutr 1994;59:960–3.
28. Adams KM, Lindell KC, Kohlmeier M, Zeisel SH. Status of nutrition education in medical schools. Am J Clin Nutr 2006;83:941S–44S.
29. Van Horn L. The Nutrition Academic Award. Am J Clin Nutr 2006;83:936S–40S.
30. Macy IG, Kelly HJ, Sloan RE. The Composition of Milks. Publication No. 254. Washington, DC: National Research Council; 1953.

2

Clinical Assessment of Nutritional Status

Asim Maqbool, MD
Irene E. Olsen, PhD, RD
Virginia A. Stallings, MD

Nutritional assessment is an integral part of patient care since nutritional status affects a patient's response to illness. Attention to nutritional status is especially important in pediatric patients as they are also undergoing the complex processes of growth and development, which are influenced by the genetic makeup of the individual and coexisting medical illness in addition to nutritional status. Thus, the assessment of nutritional and growth status is an essential part of clinical evaluation and care in the pediatric setting.

The assessment should allow for the early detection of both nutrient deficiencies and excesses. There is no single nutrition measurement that is best; therefore, a combination of different measures is required. Growth is an important indicator of health and nutritional status of a child, and a variety of growth charts are currently available to help with the assessment of growth. These include the 2000 Centers for Disease Control and Prevention (CDC) growth charts that represent the US population and the 2006 World Health Organization (WHO) growth charts. Each growth measurement performed needs to be accurate and obtained at regular intervals. These longitudinal data will help identify at-risk patients and will allow the monitoring of a patient's clinical response to nutritional therapy.

During infancy, childhood, and adolescence, many changes in growth and body composition occur. Therefore, clinicians must understand normal growth to recognize abnormal patterns. Clinicians also need to recognize the nutritional changes that occur with acute and chronic disease. With the epidemic of pediatric obesity, the proper identification of the overweight or obese patient is also important. A brief nutritional screening assessment may be used to identify patients in need of an in-depth assessment. A typical nutritional screening includes a brief medical and dietary history (including feeding ability), anthropometric measurements (eg, weight, stature), and possibly laboratory data. A full nutritional assessment includes more detailed medical and dietary histories (including a measure of dietary intake), a complete physical examination, further anthropometric and body composition measurements, sexual and skeletal maturation, laboratory data, and the estimation of nutritional requirements. A clinician's global assessment of the child based on these objective data in addition to his or her clinical judgment is also important to consider in determining nutritional status.[1] Most often, health care professionals work as a team in gathering the information for the assessment of nutritional status of children. (see Chapter 18, "Drug Therapy and Role of Nutrition" for details)

MEDICAL HISTORY

Obtaining the medical history is central to the nutritional assessment. Past and present medical information, including the duration of the current illness, relevant symptoms, diagnostic tests and therapies (eg, chemotherapy, radiation), and medications, is documented. Because nutritional abnormalities are often associated with certain disease states, it is essential to identify underlying medical conditions and the concomitant medication history. Medications can cause nutritional deficiencies (eg, methotrexate as a competitive antagonist of folic acid metabolism) and drug–nutrient interactions (eg, phenytoin and tube feedings; Table 1). Drug–nutrient interactions may occur between drugs (prescription and nonprescription) and foods, beverages, and dietary and vitamin/mineral supplements. Alterations in drug metabolism and absorption by food or pharmacologic interactions may be clinically significant.[2]

Table 1 Examples of Some Common Drug–Nutrient Interactions

Drug	Nutrient
Amphotericin B	Hypokalemia, hypomagnesemia
Antacids	Vitamin D and iron deficiency, hypophosphatemia
Phenobarbital	Vitamin D deficiency
Cholestyramine	Vitamin A, D, E, and K malabsorption
Cyclosporine	Elevated triglycerides, hypokalemia, hypomagnesemia
H2 blockers	Iron deficiency
Methotrexate	Folate deficiency
Phenytoin	Folate deficiency
Corticosteroids	Hyperglycemia, hypophosphatemia
Sucralfate	Hypophosphatemia
Sulfasalazine	Folate deficiency
Trimethoprim	Folate deficiency
6-Mercaptopurine	Purine metabolism (DNA synthesis/repaire)

Past medical history should also include information regarding previous acute and chronic illness, hospitalizations, and operations. The history of past growth patterns (with previous growth charts, as possible), onset of puberty (for the child and other biological family members), and a developmental history (including feeding abilities) may also be included. Family history should include a medical history as well as the family's social and cultural background, especially as related to diet therapy and the use of alternative and complementary medicine. The review of systems includes oral motor function, dental development, and gastrointestinal symptoms such as vomiting, gastroesophageal reflux, diarrhea, and constipation.

PHYSICAL EXAMINATION

Physical examination includes anthropometrics (see below), including weight, stature, head circumference, and arm measures. The frequency of measurements of well children (Table 2) follows the recommendations of the American Academy of Pediatrics.[3] The pattern of measurement for hospitalized patients depends on the age of the patient, illness, and degree of nutritional intervention (see Table 2). Nutritional assessments for patients with complex chronic disease states should be conducted every 1 to 2 months and less often in those with milder disease (every 6 to 12 months). The general physical examination includes an assessment of the patient's general condition and close examination of skin, hair, and teeth (see Table 3). This includes an assessment for pallor, clinical assessment of body fat stores, wasting of muscle mass, edema, skin rash, thinning of hair, and evidence of specific nutritional deficiencies. Examples of specific signs include the flag sign or the loss of hair color associated with a period of malnutrition, followed by recovery with a return of normal hair color and texture to normal. Vitamin A deficiency causes follicular hyperkeratosis and night blindness. It is unusual to see classic signs of marasmus and kwashiorkor in developed countries. Examination of specific organ systems and obtaining medical record information is helpful in assessing the severity of the underlying disease process. It is also important to consider the clinician's clinical judgment in the assessment of nutritional status.[1] Documenting sexual development

Table 2 Suggested Schedule for Growth Assessments in Hospitalized and Healthy Children

Age	Weight	Height	Head Circumference
Hospitalized			
Preterm	Daily	Weekly	Weekly
Full term to 12 months	3×/wk	Monthly	Monthly
1 to 2 yr	3×/wk	Monthly	Monthly
2 to 20 yr	2×/wk	Monthly	As indicated
Outpatient well-child visit			
0 to 2 mo	Monthly	Monthly	Monthly
2 to 6 mo	Every 2 mo	Every 2 mo	Every 2 mo
6 to 24 mo	Every 3 mo	Every 3 mo	Every 3 mo
2 to 6 yr	Annually	Annually	–
6 to 10 yr	Every 2 yr	Every 2 yr	–
11 to 20 yr	Annually	Annually	–

Adapted from the American Academy of Pediatrics.

Table 3 Selected Clinical Findings Associated with Nutritional Inadequacies

Area of Examination	Finding	Considered Nutritional Inadequacy
General	Underweight; short stature	↓Calories
	Edematous; decreased activity level	↓Protein
	Overweight	↓Calories
Hair	Ease of pluckability; sparse, depigmented; lack of curl; dull, altered texture; flag sign	↓Protein
Skin (general)	Xerosis, follicular keratosis	↓Vitamin A
	Symmetric dermatitis of skin exposed to sunlight, pressure, trauma	↓Niacin
	Edema	↓Protein
	Petechiae, purpura	↓Ascorbic acid
	Scrotal, vulval dermatitis	↓Riboflavin
	Generalized dermatitis	↓Zinc, essential fatty acids
	Erythematous rash around mouth and perianal area	↓Zinc
Skin (face)	Seborrheic dermatitis in nasolabial folds	↓Riboflavin
	Moon face; diffuse depigmentation	↓Protein
Subcutaneous tissue	Decreased	↓Calories
	Increased	↓Calories
Nails	Spoon-shaped; koilonychia	↓Iron
Eyes	Dry conjunctiva; keratomalacia; Bitot's spots	↓Vitamin A
	Circumcorneal injection	↓Riboflavin
Lips	Angular stomatitis	↓Riboflavin, Iron
	Cheilosis	↓B-complex vitamins
Gums	Swollen, bleeding	↓Vitamin C
	Reddened gingiva	↓Vitamin A
Teeth	Caries	↓Fluoride
	Stained teeth	↓Iron supplements
	Mottled, pitted enamel	↓Fluoride
	Hypoplastic enamel	↓Vitamins A, D
Tongue	Glossitis	↓Niacin, folate, riboflavin, vitamin B_{12}
Skeletal	Costochondral beading	↓Vitamins C, D
	Craniotabes; frontal bossing; epiphyseal enlargement	↓Vitamin D
	Bone tenderness	↓Vitamin C
Muscles	Decreased muscle mass	↓Protein, calories
	Tender calves	↓Thiamin
Neurologic	Ophthalmoplegia	↓Thiamin, Vitamin E
	Hyporeflexia	↓Vitamin E
	Ataxia, sensory loss	↓Vitamins B_{12}, E
Endocrine and other	Hypothyroidism	↓Iodine
	Glucose intolerance	↓Chromium
	Altered taste	↓Zinc
	Delayed wound healing	↓Vitamin C, zinc

Adapted from reference 4.

by Tanner staging is a routine part of the nutritional assessment of adolescents (see below). For a summary of signs and symptoms of specific nutritional abnormalities, see Table 3.

DIETARY HISTORY

The dietary history is an essential component of the nutritional assessment. The dietary history provides information not only on the amount and quality of food consumed, but also on the eating patterns and behaviors of the family. This part of the nutritional assessment also provides information on the number of meals, snacks, and beverages consumed; special foods eaten by the child and family; vitamin and mineral supplements ingested regularly; food allergies; intolerances; and unusual feeding behaviors. The child and family are asked about psychosocial factors that impact on food selection and intake, including family history, socio-economic status, and use of the Special Supplemental Nutrition Program for Women, Infants, and Children (WIC) and supplemental food programs, parent/caretaker's perception of the child's nutritional status, religious and cultural considerations. Food-related factors may affect dietary intake and include food allergies, intolerances, self-imposed and/or prescribed diets, and feeding skills. These factors are also noted in the assessment.

The assessment of the dietary intake of breast-fed infants is more difficult because the volume of milk consumed cannot be directly measured. An estimate is obtained by weighing the infant before and after feeds and using a conversion factor of 1 mL volume of breast milk consumed for each gram of weight gained. In formula-fed infants, the clinician should inquire about both the amount and type of formula consumed and the details of the method of preparation (concentrates, powders, modular additives).

The quantity and quality of dietary intake are assessed by prospective food records (with weighed or estimated food portions), retrospective 24-hour recalls (previous 24 hours or of a "typical" 24-hour period), or food frequency questionnaires.[5] The prospective food records are usually carried out for 3 to 7 days (including a combination of weekend and weekdays) and provide the most accurate assessment of actual intake. However, food records are used most often in the research setting because they are labor intensive and time consuming. As available, these records are analyzed and compared to the dietary reference intakes (DRIs) (see below) using a computerized nutrient analysis program. A limitation of food records is that parents tend to forget to record all foods eaten or modify feeding practices to be more healthy which may lead to underestimates of intake.[6] The retrospective 24-hour diet recall provides a quicker assessment of dietary intake. For a 24-hour recall, the child/parent is asked to recall what and how much the child ate and drank over the past 24 hours. Recall accuracy depends on the child/parent's memory and ability to estimate portion sizes. Also, because this is only one day of intake, it may not be representative of the usual intake. When the child's intake is affected by acute illness, a 24-hour recall of a "typical day" is more useful to estimate usual intake. The 24-hour recall tends to underestimate usual energy intake yet may over report intake of infants and toddlers.

Another way of assessing dietary intake is the food frequency questionnaire method. These questionnaires collect information on both the frequency and amount consumed of specific foods and are useful in the clinical setting to identify usual eating patterns. A limitation of the food frequency questionnaires is that the amounts of food and thus intake of energy and some nutrients are often overreported.[6] All of these methods of dietary assessment are somewhat limited owing to gaps in the nutrient databases, which lack information about bioavailability, presence of inhibitors and enhancers of absorption, and nutrient availability of specific nutrients of interest.[7]

The most commonly used method of dietary assessment in hospitalized patients is the calorie count. This is a variation of the prospective food records as the amount of food consumed from a known quantity of food (as specified by a menu or list) is recorded. The accuracy of the calorie count assessments is limited by the number of individuals required for the completion of these forms throughout a 24-hour period (eg, the dietitian, the nurse for each shift, the child's family, the child). However, calorie counts are a useful part of nutritional assessment follow-up because these provide a rough assessment of the patient's appetite, intake, and compliance with nutrition recommendations.

ANTHROPOMETRICS AND BODY COMPOSITION

At a minimum, nutritional assessment of a child includes a measured weight, length or height, and head circumference (birth to age 3 years), and these measurements are followed over time to assess short- and long-term growth and nutritional status. For children with chronic disease, a midarm circumference (MAC) and triceps skinfold (TSF) thickness are also part of the assessment to determine body fat and protein stores. In addition, a dual-energy X-ray absorptiometry (DXA) scan may be added to more thoroughly assess body composition (percent fat, lean body, and fat mass) and bone mineral density (BMD) (see Chapter 4, "Body Composition and Growth").

Accurate and reliable anthropometric and body composition measurements require the proper equipment and techniques. Training and practice in anthropometric technique cannot be overemphasized. All growth measures should be taken in triplicate and used as an average. The clinician's assessment for a child depends on the quality of these data. Equipment requirements for each measure are discussed below.

WEIGHT

Weight is a measure of overall nutritional status with age, sex, and height/length required for optimal interpretation. Weight is determined using a digital or beam balance scale. Until the child is approximately 24 months or can cooperate and stand independently, a pan version of the scale is used. Weight should be measured in light or no clothing and without a diaper for infants. It is important that the scale is zeroed prior to each measurement and is calibrated using known weights at least monthly or on movement of the scale.[8] Weights are recorded to the nearest 0.01 kg in infants and 0.1 kg in older children.

STATURE: LENGTH OR HEIGHT

A measure of stature is important for monitoring long-term nutritional status. Recumbent length is measured using a length board for children from birth to 2 or 3 years. The measurement of length requires two individuals. The first person positions the infant straight on the board so that the infant's head is against the headboard and in the Frankfort horizontal plane.[8] The Frankfort plane is the anatomic position when the lower margin of the orbit and the upper margin of the auditory meatus are in line. The second person holds the infant's knees flat to the table and heels flat against the movable footboard.[9] For children able to stand independently and cooperate, height is measured using a stadiometer, with a moveable headboard at a fixed 90° angle to the back of the stadiometer. The child is measured barefoot or in thin socks and in minimal clothing to allow the observer to check for correct positioning. For the measurement, the child stands erect, feet together, heels, buttocks, and back of head touching the stadiometer, and looking ahead in the Frankfort horizontal plane.[8] Because length overestimates height by approximately 0.5 to 1.5 cm,[10] it is essential to record the method of measurement during the transition from recumbent length to standing height. The change to standing height is also accompanied by the transition to pediatric (2 to 18 years) growth charts (see below). Both length and height measurements are recorded to the nearest 0.1 cm.

For children in whom stature measurements are not possible owing to physical constraints (eg, contractures, nonambulatory), alternative measures are available. Upper arm and lower leg lengths provide reliable and valid indexes of stature in children.[11,12] These measurements are conducted using sliding calipers in infants and an anthropometer for children. All measurements are recorded to the nearest 0.1 cm.

The shoulder to elbow length is used for the upper arm measurement.[11,12] In infants (birth to 24 months), the arm is bent to a 90° angle and the measurement is taken from the superior lateral surface of the acronium to the inferior surface of the elbow.[9] For older ages (2 to 18 years), the arm should hang in a relaxed position at the side, and the distance between the superior lateral surface of the acronium to the tip of the radius is measured.[9] Lower leg length is measured as the knee to heel length[9] for infants (0 to 24 months) and as a calf length[9,13] in older children (2 to 18 years). For infants, the superior surface of the knee to the heel is measured while the leg is bent at a right angle at the hip, knee, and ankle.[9] In older children, the medial tip of the tibia to the distal tip of the medial malleolus is measured while that leg is crossed over the opposite knee.[9,13] The right-side extremity should be measured for these alternative stature estimates.[9] If there are asymmetric extremity abnormalities, the measurement should be taken on the least affected side.

HEAD CIRCUMFERENCE

Head growth, primarily owing to brain development, is most rapid within the first 3 years of life. Routine measurement of head circumference (the frontal occipital circumference) is a component of the nutritional assessment in children up to age 3 and longer in children who are at high nutritional risk. Head circumference is a less sensitive indicator of short-term nutritional status than weight and height because brain growth is generally preserved in cases of nutritional stress. Head circumference is not a helpful nutritional status measure in children with hydrocephalus, microcephaly, and macrocephaly.

Head circumference is measured using a flexible, nonstretch tape measure. The circumference should be taken at the maximum distance around the head, which is found by placing the measuring tape above the supraorbital ridge and extending around the occiput.[9,14] Care should be taken to keep the tape measure flat against the head and parallel on both sides. The measurements should be recorded to the nearest 0.1 cm.[14]

GROWTH CHARTS AND TABLES

Serial measurements are essential for optimal assessment of short- and long-term growth and nutritional status. A number of growth charts and tables are available for the comparison of weight, stature, and head circumference with reference populations by age and sex. Weight is also assessed relative to a child's height (weight for height, weight for height[2] or body mass index [BMI]) for an additional assessment. The types of charts and tables available for clinical assessment in infants and children are reviewed.

PREMATURE INFANT GROWTH CHARTS

For infants born prematurely, a variety of charts are available for the assessment of growth. Intrauterine growth-based charts are preferred over postnatal growth-based charts as the pattern and rate of normal intrauterine growth are the standard for growth of premature infants.[15] Growth measurements are plotted based on corrected gestational age for the first 12 months of life. In clinical practice, the use of corrected gestational age may continue to 24 to 36 months, depending on the child's size and growth. The Lubchenco growth charts (see Appendix I, Figure I-24) are widely used owing to ease of clinical use (weekly age intervals, commonly used percentiles) and include charts for weight, length, and head circumference.[16,17] The Babson charts (see Appendix I, Figure I-23) are presented in biweekly age intervals from 26 to 40 weeks gestation and as standard deviations, rather than percentiles, so they are used less in clinical care.[18] More recently, weight charts based on large national datasets of fetal growth have been published.[19,20] In 2003 a set of growth charts that span the intrauterine and postnatal period from 22 to 50 weeks gestational age was published.[21] These charts for weight, length and head circumference provide weekly age intervals and the 3rd to 97th percentiles of growth. These charts are made up of data from several different studies conducted in and outside of the United States. Thus as noted by the author, the generalizability of these growth charts may be limited by the heterogeneity of the data used. There is still a need for more up-to-date reference standards for the assessment of weight, length and head circumference in preterm infants based on a large, contemporary, prospective study of growth using research quality measurement techniques.

Once a preterm infant reaches 40 weeks corrected gestational age, it is appropriate to monitor growth on the new CDC growth charts.[22] Former premature infants are plotted on these charts based on their corrected gestational age (as above). Although all premature infants may not achieve "good" placement on these growth charts, these charts provide the appropriate goal for growth. Also available are the Infant Health and Development Program (IHDP) charts for low birth weight (LBW, 1,501 to 2,500 g) and very low birth weight (VLBW, <1,500 g) premature infants for boys[23,24] and girls[25,26] and the National Institute of Child Health and Human Development (NICHD) Neonatal Research Network Growth Observational Study[27] projected growth charts and tables for VLBW infants (available online: (<http://neonatal.rti.org> as well as in Appendix I, Figures I-25, 26, and 27). These charts provide a comparison of how an LBW or VLBW premature infant grows relative to two reference populations of similar infants. The IHDP and NICHD postnatal charts represent actual, not ideal, patterns of growth for former premature infants. Therefore, these charts may be used in conjunction with but not in place of the CDC growth charts.

GROWTH CHARTS

2000 CDC Growth Charts

In 2000, the CDC and National Center for Health Statistics (NCHS) released an updated set of growth charts called the CDC growth charts (see Appendix I, Figures I-1 to I-10).[22] Changes to the previously used 1977 NCHS growth charts[28] included (1) BMI (kg/m^2) charts for boys and girls (2 to 20 years); (2) 3rd and 97th percentiles for all charts and 85th percentile for the weight-for-stature and BMI-for-age charts; (3) improved transition from recumbent length to standing height measurements in the stature charts; (4) increased age range from 18 to 20 years; and (5) the use of a combination of breast- and formula-fed infants to establish the reference growth patterns.[22] These charts are available for boys and girls ages 0 to 36 months for weight, length, and head circumference by age and weight for length and ages 2 to 20 years for weight, height, and BMI for age and weight for height. Further details on the CDC growth charts, including data exclusions are reviewed in the 2000 CDC. Report.[22] The CDC growth charts are available on the Internet (<www.cdc.gov/growthcharts>).

2006 WHO Growth Charts

Following a comprehensive review of anthropometric references, the WHO undertook the Multicentre Growth Reference Study to generate newer growth reference standards. Data were gathered from healthy infants and children from Brazil, Ghana, India, Norway, Oman, and the United States. The study was designed to gather data reflecting healthy children living under conditions (breast-fed, nonsmoking environments) favorable to fully achieving growth according to their growth potential. The data combined a longitudinal follow-up from birth to 24 months as well as a cross-sectional survey of children between birth and 71 months. The growth standards derived are prescriptive rather than descriptive; that is, for how children should grow as opposed to how they grew at a particular time and place, thereby underscoring that the new growth charts are consistent with growth outcomes occurring under the best health practices. These new, 2006 reference standards include length/height for age, weight for age, weight for length/height, and BMI by age for children from birth to 60 months old.[29]

When comparing the 2000 CDC growth charts to the 2006 WHO growth charts, several differences are notable. The CDC growth charts reflect a heavier and shorter sample than the WHO growth chart, resulting in lower rates of undernutrition (with the exception of the first 6 months of life), and higher rates of overweight and obesity (when based on the WHO standards). The differences in methodology and number of subjects sampled at younger ages in generating the WHO growth charts as compared to the CDC growth charts result in healthy, breast-fed infants tracking along the WHO growth charts with respect to weight for age mean Z-scores, while appearing to falter on the CDC growth charts, from the age of two months onwards. Other important differences are with respect to weight for length curves; the WHO curves start earlier and extend longer than the CDC curves, to facilitate assessment of populations with elevated rates of stunting, and the assessment of tall children unable to stand (for whatever reason), respectively. In summary, the WHO charts appear to capture the rapidly changing growth patterns of infancy. It is noteworthy that the growth trends of US children track along the median of the WHO growth charts, which may render them quite relevant to the US pediatric population.[30] These growth curves are included in Appendix I.

Incremental Growth Velocity

Reference data are also available for incremental growth velocity for boys and girls in weight, stature, and head circumference from 0 to 18 years (see Appendix I, Tables I-5 to I-6).[31–35] These data are presented in time intervals (1, 3, or 6 months) and approximate growth over time by percentile (3rd to 97th or 5th to 95th percentiles). In clinical practice, the incremental tables for weight, length, and head circumference[31,34,35] are helpful in the assessment of former premature infants and other children with growth failure from any cause. The growth increments are easily divided into daily, weekly, or monthly weight gain goals. This method of growth assessment is more sensitive in detecting growth faltering or catchup growth than the growth charts that assess static growth status at one point in time based on cross-sectional data.

Growth charts for the assessment of height and height velocity in relation to the stage of sexual maturity based on US reference data are also available (see Appendix I, Figures I-21 and I-22).[36] These charts provide height growth for early, middle, and late maturers by sex and age at which peak height velocity was reached and explain some of the variation in growth related to different stages of puberty. Height velocity charts are often used in the care of children with poor growth and chronic illnesses.

Special Growth Charts

Although the CDC growth charts are recommended for the growth and nutritional assessment of all children, a number of disease-specific charts have been published (eg, achondroplasia, Brachmann–de Lange syndrome, cerebral palsy, Down syndrome, Marfan syndrome, myelomeningocele, Noonan's syndrome, Prader–Willi syndrome, sickle cell disease, Silver–Russell syndrome, Turner's syndrome, Williams syndrome; see Appendix I, Table I-8). Weight- and height-for-age growth charts are available for boys and girls ages 0 to 36 months and 2 to 18 years based on a large sample of children with Down syndrome.[37,38] However, many other special growth charts are based on small samples of children and include children with suboptimal nutritional status. Disease-specific charts may be helpful to use in conjunction with the CDC growth charts for comparison to peer groups. See Appendix I, Figures I-28 to I-50 for growth curves for a variaty of medical and genetic conditions.

A set of growth charts is also available for the assessment of alternate stature measures,[11,12] including upper arm length (infants 0 to 24 months, girls 3 to 16 years, boys 3 to 18 years) and lower leg length (infants 0 to 24 months, girls 3 to 16 years, boys 3 to 18 years). Similar to other measures of stature, these linear growth measures are used along with weights to help determine a child's nutritional status.[9]

ASSESSMENT OF ANTHROPOMETRICS

Nutritional status indices are essential for the clinical interpretation of the growth measurements. Every nutritional assessment requires one or more of the following indices for interpretation.

Percentiles for Age and Sex

When each of the growth measures is plotted on a growth chart, a percentile or rank of the individual compared to the reference population is determined. For example, the 25th percentile weight for age means that the individual weighs the same or more than 25% of the reference population of the same age and sex, and the 75th percentile weight for age means that the individual weighs the same or more than 75% of the reference population of the same age and sex.[10] Percentiles are easily interpreted and used clinically. Available growth charts provide reference growth of children ranging from the 5th to 95th percentiles and now the 3rd to 97th percentiles. In clinical practice, the 5th to 95th percentile growth charts continue to be used in the screening and follow-up of healthy children, whereas the 3rd to 97th percentile growth charts may be used for children with chronic illness or at nutritional risk. Weight-for-age and height-for-age percentiles are also used to screen for malnutrition using published classifications (see Appendix I, Table I-7). Percent ideal body weight (IBW), based on appropriate height and weight-for-age (see below), is often used as an indicator of wasting or obesity. Height-for-age percentiles are an adequate measure of long-term nutritional status and are used for screening in healthy children with low height-for-age reflecting stunting. Height-for-age is generally interpreted as short (<5th percentile), normal (5 to 95th percentile), and tall (>95th percentile).

Genetic Growth Potential: Midparental Height

In the assessment of a child's stature, it is helpful to estimate the genetic potential for stature as determined by the biologic parents' adult height.[39] This is of particular interest in the child with short stature since it is important to determine if the child is healthy but short owing to family genetic background, disease, and/or poor nutrition. An adjustment for parental height is used for a child's length (0 to 36 months) or height (3 to 18 years) and is based on the mean of the height of both biologic parents. This allows adjustments to the child's stature for tall or short parents. The corrections are based on the Fels Institute and older NCHS data[40] and therefore are used in conjunction with the 1979 NCHS growth charts. Parental height adjustment is appropriate for use with most of the parents and children in the United States; however, it should not be used when the parents do not meet their genetic potential for height (eg, in situations of poor health and/or nutritional status during the parental childhood or adolescence).[39]

Weight for Height

Weight relative to height provides different information on the growth and nutritional status in an individual than either weight-for-age or height-for-age alone. Weight-for-height helps to determine and classify the nutritional status in the individual patient.[41] For children 0 to 6 years of age, weight-for-height is most frequently assessed by determining a percentile on the CDC growth charts.[22] Weight-for-height is generally interpreted as underweight (<5th percentile), within normal variation (5th to 95th percentile), and overweight (>95th percentile) and is used in screening healthy children. Weight-for-height measures are also used for screening classification of protein-calorie malnutrition (see Appendix, Table I-5 to I-6).

BMI is another measure of weight relative to height. The CDC growth charts provide BMI for age and sex from age 2 to 20 years.[22,42] With the availability of these new charts, BMI will be used more frequently as an assessment tool for children. However, because both weight and height in children change over time, unlike in adults, there is no fixed BMI value for the diagnosis of obesity in children (eg, BMI $\geq$ 30). The BMI percentile must be used for interpretation. In the United States, the 85th and 95th BMI percentiles for age and sex are used to define "at risk of overweight" and "overweight" in children.[43] From the International Obesity Task Force, cutoff points for BMI to define overweight and obesity in children based on cross-sectional growth studies from six countries (Brazil, Great Britain, Hong Kong, the Netherlands, Singapore, the United States) are also available.[44] Another study found similar predictions of underweight and overweight in children and adolescents (2 to 19 years) using the BMI-for-age and weight-for-height classifications.[45]

BMI at the lower end of the reference range reflects both low fat and lean mass. At the higher range of BMI, other components that comprise fat-free mass may influence the relationship of BMI to fat mass, and these vary with age in children. BMI is not a perfect measure of adiposity, since height is not fully independent of weight. Stature has been postulated to affect BMI, and in populations with taller stature, BMI may overestimate the prevalence of obesity.[46] A recent study comparing techniques to evaluate adiposity (BMI, isotopic dilution, skin fold equations) in stunted and non-stunted children concluded that BMI predicted percent body fat in both groups of children.[47] An additional study showed that the relationship between BMI and adiposity varied across different populations.[48] BMI should be interpreted with caution in certain clinical conditions including edema, pregnancy, in individuals with a high tumor burden, as well as in individuals with increased lean body mass such as in well-developed athletes. BMI is a screening tool to identify children and adolescents at risk for overweight or obesity and further assessments to determine adiposity should be considered as clinically indicated.

Percent Ideal Body Weight

Percent IBW has been used as an indicator of nutritional status. In clinical practice, percent IBW may be used to classify the degree of over- or undernutrition. An example of a set of clinical classifications is >120% IBW as obese; 110 to 120% IBW as overweight; 90 to 110% IBW as normal range; 80 to 90% IBW as mild wasting; 70 to 80% IBW as moderate wasting; and <70% IBW as severe wasting. IBW is also used as a clinical weight goal in the nutritional rehabilitation of a child.

Percent IBW should be used with caution. A recent study[49] compared the use of BMI percentiles and % IBW to screen for malnutrition in children with cystic fibrosis using data from the cystic fibrosis patient registry. Among children with stature between 25th and 75th percentiles, both percent IBW and BMI yielded similar estimates of ideal weights, for the classification of malnutrition. However, compared with the BMI, percent IBW underestimated the severity of malnutrition in children with short stature (height <25th percentile) whereas the opposite trend was found for the subjects with tall stature (height >75th percentile). These findings support use of BMI in lieu of percent IBW for the classification of pediatric malnutrition.

Percent Weight Loss

Percent of usual body weight loss is an important clinical indicator of nutritional status and nutritional risk. Percent weight loss is calculated as [(previous weight – current weight)/previous weight – 100]. A 5% or greater weight loss in 1 month may be considered an indicator of nutritional risk in children.

Growth Velocity

Growth velocity (change in the growth parameter over time) is useful to detect a change in nutritional status and to monitor the effectiveness of nutritional and medical therapy. As discussed above, age- and sex-specific charts and tables are available for the evaluation of weight, stature, and head circumference growth over time.[31–36]

Body Composition

In children with many acute and chronic diseases, the nutritional assessment requires measurement of body composition (body fat and protein stores) in addition to weight, stature, and head circumference (see Chapter 4, "Body Composition and Growth").

Midarm Circumference

MAC can be used as a measurement of growth, an index of energy and protein stores and can provide information on fat patterning.[14] The measurement is taken at the midpoint of the upper arm, located halfway between the lateral tip of the acromion and the olecranon when the arm is flexed at a 90° angle (measured and marked). For the MAC measurement, the child should be upright with the arm relaxed by the side. A flexible, nonstretch measuring tape is placed perpendicular to the long axis of the arm, tightened around the arm, and recorded to the nearest 0.1 cm.[14] This measurement should be taken in triplicate and used as an average.

Triceps Skinfold Thickness

The TSF thickness is an indicator of subcutaneous fat (energy) stores and total body fat, and provides information on fat patterning.[50] For the measurement, the child should be upright with the arm relaxed at the side. The TSF thickness is measured at the midpoint of the upper arm (defined above) over the center of the triceps muscle on the back of the arm (measured and marked beforehand). The anthropometrist lifts the skinfold with the thumb and index finger, approximately 1 cm above the marked midpoint, and places the calipers at the marked point. Four seconds after the handles of the calipers are released, the measurement is taken and the calipers are removed. This measurement should be taken in triplicate, used as an average, and recorded to the nearest 0.1 cm.[9]

Reference data (age and sex specific) are available for the assessment of MAC and TSF thickness as a percentage[51] (see Appendix I, Tables I-1 to I-4). The MAC and TSF measurements (in mm) are used to calculate upper arm muscle area and fat area (formulas below).[9,51] These are clinical indicators of total body stores of muscle and fat.[9]

Upper arm muscle area (cm^2) = $[MAC\ (cm) - (TSF\ (cm) \times \Pi)]^2/(4 \times 7\Pi)$, where $\Pi = 3.14$.

Upper arm fat area (cm^2) = upper arm area (cm^2) − upper arm muscle area (cm^2), where upper arm area (cm^2) = $MAC^2/(4 \times \Pi)$.

Dual-Energy X-ray Absorptiometry

DXA is a noninvasive measurement of BMD. It is an indirect, low-radiation measurement that has increasing clinical utility. DXA scans are performed on the lumbar spine, hips, and whole body in adults and on the lumbar spine and whole body in infants, children, and adolescents. Although primarily used for the assessment of bones, whole-body scans also provide body composition measures of fat-free mass, fat mass, and percent body fat.[52] In addition, the DXA scans provide information on bone mineral content (BMC) in grams per centimeter or BMD in grams per square centimeter in different regions of the skeleton or the whole body. Values for the lumbar spine are used to assess bone health and are compared with reference data in healthy age- and sex-matched infants, children, and adolescents. Usually, an anteroposterior view of the lumbar vertebrae L1 to L4 or L2 to L4 is used for clinical interpretation. It takes approximately 20 minutes to complete both DXA scans (lumbar spine and whole body), including time for positioning. Younger children are measured while asleep, or sedation may be considered. Results for BMC and BMD are assessed using a z-score (standard deviation score), which compares the individual with the reference database. A z-score of 0 is the mean (similar to the 50th percentile on a growth chart) for the reference data, with +1, +2, −1, and −2 representing plus and minus 1 and 2 standard deviations from the reference mean. These results are expressed as z-scores and percent predicted. The WHO has defined osteoporosis in young, white, adult women as a BMD T-score of −2.5 or less (ie, 2.5 or more standard deviations below the reference mean).[53] A diagnostic criterion for men, children, and other races is not yet available.[53] In clinical practice, children with z-scores of −2 to +2 are considered to have normal BMD, whereas a z-score of −1 to −2 is in the low normal group. A z-score of −2 to −3 is considered in the reduced range, whereas a value of −3 or less is considered to be in the significantly reduced range; z-scores less than −2 are considered in the fracture range (Table 4).

The quality of the DXA–BMD reference datasets available for children is a limitation of this method. The sample sizes are low, and there is minimal detail for children across various pubertal groups. Additionally, these reference data are not heterogeneous nor representative of the ethnic diversity of the US population.[54] Further, the importance of considering other factors, such as a child's stature and pubertal maturity in the interpretation of measures of bone health has been suggested,[55–59] yet currently these also are not considered in the clinical setting. Longitudinal reference data that are representative of healthy, children from the US National Institutes of Health's Bone Mineral Density in Childhood Study[60] are currently pending.

Table 4 Suggested Bone Health Assessment by Dual-Energy X-ray Absorptiometry

z-Score	Interpretation	Repeat Measurements
2 or greater	Increased	Annually
+2 to −2	Normal	If clinical status changes
−1 to −2	Low normal	Every 1 to 2 yr
−2 to −3	Reduced	Annually
−3 or less	Significantly reduced	Every 6 to 12 mo

The advantages of the DXA are the low radiation exposure, fast scan time, and noninvasive nature. The precision of the instrument is excellent. The radiation dose is small (<1 mrem, Hologic Delphi Clinical Bone Densitometer product specifications) or less than that received during a standard airline flight across the United States.[61] The frequency of measurements depends on the clinical needs (see Table 4). Patients with poor BMD measurements may benefit from scans every 6 to 12 months after the baseline assessment. Those individuals with values in the low normal range but with risk factors may need testing every 1 to 2 years. At-risk patients include those with chronic illness (eg, inflammatory bowel disease, cystic fibrosis, celiac disease), poor growth, and reduced physical activity and those receiving chronic medications (eg, corticosteroids, anticonvulsants). A limitation of DXA in the assessment of body composition is that provides a two-dimensional assessment of three-dimensional structures, including the complex structure of bone.

A newer technique providing data on both cortical and trabecular bone is quantitative computed tomography (QCT). This test describes volumetric BMD and also differentiates between cortical and trabecular bone. Special high-resolution scanners have been developed to decrease radiation exposure for the peripheral skeleton, and this is currently a research tool. Bone health in children and adults is altered by intakes of calcium and vitamin D and weight-bearing physical activity. It is important to be aware of the risk factors for bone disease in children, including conditions such as chronic diarrhea, lactose intolerance, poor dietary intake, fat malabsorption, decreased physical activity, and the use of steroid medications.

Air Displacement Plethysmography

Air displacement plethysmography offers a newer alternative for the assessment of body composition that is safe, noninvasive and fast. There are two commercially available plethysmographs from Life Measurement, Inc. (Concord, CA): the BOD POD® for use in children and adults and the more recently available PEA POD® for use in infants up to 6 months of age. This method requires the subject to sit (BOD POD) or lie (PEA POD) within a closed chamber in minimal, close fitting or no clothing, respectively. The subject's volume is estimated indirectly by measuring the volume of air that he or she displaces inside an enclosed chamber.[62] This volume is used to compute body density (body mass or weight/body volume) and in turn fat mass (kg), fat-free mass (kg) and percent body fat.[63] Overall, the BOD POD[62,64] and PEA POD[63] have been reported to provide reliable and valid estimates of body composition; however, neither plethysmograph are widely available in the clinical setting at this time.

SEXUAL AND SKELETAL MATURATION

Because body composition and the rate of growth vary throughout childhood and adolescence, it is important to consider sexual/pubertal and skeletal maturation when assessing an individual patient's anthropometric measurements. For example, a small child who is physically immature (based on sexual and skeletal development) is less of a nutritional concern than a child who is small and appropriately mature for age. The physically immature child with likely growth delay has the potential to catchup to the size of her peers once she advances in maturity.

Sexual maturity is assessed using the Tanner staging system by the clinician physical examination[65] or as a pubertal self-assessment form completed by the child/parent.[66–69] Staging (1 to 5) is based on breast and pubic hair development for girls and genital and pubic hair development for boys (see Appendix I, Figures I-17 to I-20).

Skeletal maturation (or bone age) is the second method for assessment of physical maturity. Bone age is assessed by a left-hand-wrist radiograph and scored using the standards developed by Greulich[70] or the newly revised TW3 method developed by Tanner and colleagues.[71] Bone age provides a measure of "how far a given individual has progressed along his or her road to full maturity"[72] regardless of chronologic age. Sexual and skeletal maturity provide a measure of physical maturity and are valuable in formulating the nutritional assessment of children and adolescents.

LABORATORY TESTS

Laboratory testing is a helpful but less essential part of a nutritional assessment in most children and is presented in detail in Chapter 3, "Laboratory Assessment of Nutritional Status." Nutritional information can be obtained from plasma, serum, urine, stool, hair, and nail samples. The latter two are rarely used clinically. Depending on the underlying medical condition and related nutritional problems from the history and physical examination, a focused laboratory assessment may be obtained. Serum albumin and prealbumin reflect the adequacy of protein and calorie intake. Because the half-life of albumin is 14 to 20 days, it also reflects longer-term protein stores. The shorter half-life of prealbumin (2 to 3 days) is a better short-term indicator of calorie and protein intake. However, the usefulness of prealbumin in the hospitalized patient may be limited by the fact that it is decreased in the setting of stress, sepsis, and acute illness. Checking a C-reactive-protein level may help identify when the low prealbumin level is related to stress. Anemia can be attributable to multiple nutritional deficiencies (eg, iron, vitamin B_{12}, folate, vitamin C, protein, and vitamin E), and a careful analysis of the red blood cell indices and peripheral blood smear will help to determine what further nutritional laboratory tests should be obtained (eg, iron studies, vitamin levels). In premature infants, nutritional anemias can be attributable to iron, vitamin E, and copper deficiencies. Nutritional tests to check for bone health may include serum calcium, phosphorus, alkaline phosphatase, magnesium, and 25-hydroxyvitamin D. Additional information on bone health may be obtained from a parathormone level, radiography, and DXA scan. Specific vitamin and mineral levels can be checked when deficiency or excess states are suspected. A urine analysis, along with serum electrolytes, is useful in assessing the hydration status of the patient. See Table 3 for a list of selected clinical findings related to nutritional inadequacies and Chapter 3, "Laboratory Assessment of Nutritional Status" for a more in-depth look at laboratory assessment of nutritional status.

NUTRITIONAL REQUIREMENTS

The estimation of nutritional requirements is the last step in a nutritional assessment. Recommendations for calorie and protein intake, as well as specific vitamins and minerals, are needed for patient care (see Chapter 8, "Trace Elements," Chapter 9, "Iron," and Chapter 10, "Vitamins"). The history (medical and dietary), physical examination, and anthropometric and laboratory data obtained are used to help estimate these nutritional requirements. These provide a starting point for nutritional therapy and are modified over time based on the patient's ongoing health status and response to nutritional therapy. The adequacy of the nutritional therapy provided should be vigilantly monitored in children with failure to thrive and obesity, and in those patients with conditions requiring enteral or parenteral nutrition.

There are a number of methods to estimate caloric needs of children in the clinical setting, including the DRIs for estimates of total energy needs, the WHO and Schofield prediction equations for estimates of resting energy expenditure (REE), and a direct measurement of REE. In 1989, the National Research Council published the Recommended Dietary Allowances (RDAs) to provide information about the nutrient needs of infants, children, and adolescents, in addition to adults. Longitudinal average dietary intake consistent with good health and appropriate growth in healthy children were used for these estimates.[73] The 1989 RDAs now have been replaced by a more comprehensive set of guidelines called the DRIs. In addition to the RDAs, the DRIs include estimated average requirements, adequate intakes, and tolerable upper intake levels for most nutrients.[74] The DRIs are used in Canada and the United States, and nutrient intakes at the suggested levels promote nutrient function, biological and physical well-being, and disease prevention.[74] DRIs are available for vitamins, minerals (see Chapter 8, "Trace Elements," Chapter 9, "Iron," and Chapter 10, "Vitamins"), energy, and macronutrient recommendations (see Chapter 5, "Macronutrient Requirements For Growth: Carbohydrates," Chapter 6, "Macronutrient Requirements for Growth: Protein and Amino Acids," and Chapter 7, "Macronutrient Requirements for Growth: Fat and Fatty Acids"). Generally, the DRIs provide for the nutritional needs of the healthy individual and population. Therefore, DRIs may require adjustments in the clinical setting because they do not address energy or nutrient requirements for individuals who are malnourished or have acute/chronic disease.

Both the Food and Nutrition Board DRI and the Food and Agricultural Organization of the WHO assessments for energy requirements in children 0 to 2 years are estimated from prediction equations derived from total energy expenditure (TEE, by the double-labeled water methods) and energy needs for tissue deposition for growth "at rates consistent with good health."[75] For children at this young age, estimated energy requirements (EER) vary based on weight. The EER for children 3 to 8 years and 9 to 18 years are also from TEE and energy deposition costs (20 and 25 kcal/d, respectively) and are based on age, weight, height, and level of physical activity (see the Appendix Table II-5). The important role of moderate physical activity in achieving and maintaining the appropriate energy balance for optimal health is emphasized in these new recommendations. Levels of physical activity are categorized into four levels: sedentary, low active, active, and very active.[75,76] EER equations also are available for use in children ages 3 and above who are at "risk of overweight" defined as a BMI > 85th percentile and "overweight" as a BMI > 95th percentile.[43] DRIs provide an estimate of total energy needs in kcal/d and may be adjusted based on nutritional, medical, and growth needs of the individual patient.

The WHO and Schofield REE equations offer another method to estimate energy requirements. The WHO recommendations are based on the evaluation of several thousands of children and are clinically useful. The WHO equations (see Appendix, Table II-14) calculate REE by sex, age, and weight groups and approximate the basal metabolic rate.[77] Total daily energy needs are then estimated by multiplying the REE by a factor to adjust for physical activity, medical status, and/or the need for catchup growth. The Schofield equations (see the Appendix Table II-14) use sex, age, weight, and height of the child and may more accurately predict REE in children with altered growth and body composition (ie, failure to thrive and obesity).[78] Schofield REE estimates are also adjusted for the patient's activity, stress, and growth needs (see Table 5) to approximate total daily energy needs.

The new DRI equations to estimate energy requirement take into account the TEE plus energy deposition for new tissue.[74] For children and adolescents, these also factor in weight, height, and energy needs to sustain growth. Recommendations are made by life stage and gender, and include EER equations for pregnant and lactating women. Equations for EER that account for weight maintenance in overweight individuals from 3 years of age and older are provided.[75]

Table 5 Disease and Physical Activity Factors for Adjustment of Resting Energy Expenditure (REE)

REE factor	Disease and Activity Factors
×1.0–1.1	Well-nourished children, sedated on ventilator, extracorporeal membrane oxygenation; minimal Stress
×1.3	Well-nourished children with decreased activity, minor surgery, mild-to-moderate sedation; minimal stress
×1.5	Ambulatory child with mild-to-moderate stress Inactive child with sepsis, cancer, trauma, extensive surgery Minimally active child with malnutrition and catch-up growth requirements
×1.7	Active child with catch-up growth requirements Active child with severe stress

Adapted from reference 79.

The current DRI for EER provide additional guidance beyond the 1985 FAO/WHO/UNU report for energy requirements with respect to catchup growth in undernourished or stunted children,[75] based on limited data. Similarly, the 2001 FAO/WHO/UNU report on human energy requirements does not specifically address energy requirements for children recovering from moderate or severe malnutrition or chronic illnesses. Direction with respect to caloric replacement to allow for twice normal growth rate for children 6 to 24 months of age is provided.[75] Similar to the new WHO growth charts, the emphasis in the WHO report is prescriptive as opposed to descriptive. Thus, it indicates how individuals should grow in response to appropriate energy intake in optimal conditions rather than reflect how they were observed to grow with inadequate energy intake or excess.

The physical activity level (PAL) variable in these energy equations from both the DRI and WHO do not address energy needs for children with degrees of malnutrition or suffering from chronic illnesses. Currently, the best clinical way to determine an individual's REE and daily energy needs is by indirect calorimetry; however, this method is not readily available in all clinical settings. This technique measures oxygen consumption and carbon dioxide production when the child is resting in the early morning, typically after an age-appropriate fast (usually 12 hours). Sedation may be required for younger children. Results are currently expressed in kcal/d and have been compared to the previous WHO/Schofield equations.[80]

Table 5 provides an example of PAL adapted to estimate energy requirements in children with different types of illnesses and corresponding expected physical activity. Further work is required to examine the newer EER equations with respect to different severity of malnutrition, acute and chronic illnesses in children compared to calorimetric methods. Future recommendations regarding REE adjustment factors for disease states and physical activity are needed.

In summary, for the estimation of energy needs in the clinical setting, an REE based on indirect calorimetry is preferred for children with complex medical and nutritional needs. If an REE measurement cannot be obtained, then the WHO or Schofield equations are recommended. These estimates of REE are then adjusted based on activity, stress, and growth for an estimate of total daily energy needs for the individualized patient. As above, the new DRIs for total energy recommendations may replace these estimates in the clinical setting. However, these estimates of TEE are not as reliable as those values obtained by more accurate research methods (eg, doubly labeled water).[81] Finally, it should be remembered that all estimates are guidelines for the initiation of nutritional therapy. Adjustments in the nutritional regimen are made over time based on objective measures, such as weight gain, laboratory data, and medical condition.

DRIs also provide updated protein recommendations (see Appendix II; also see Chapter 6, "Macronutrient Requirements for Growth: Protein and Amino Acids"). An adequate intake for protein in infants 0 to 6 months is based on the mean protein intake of healthy breast-fed infants.[82] Nitrogen intake, nitrogen balance (the minimum protein intake necessary to maintain nitrogen balance), rates of protein deposition, and efficiency of protein use all influence protein requirements. For individuals 7 months through 18 years of age, the protein recommendations are based on a combination of these factors, plus a safety factor to account for individual variation.[75] The DRIs provide protein recommendations (g/kg/d) by age from birth to 8 years and by age and sex starting from 9 years. Individualized needs can be estimated by multiplying the age/sex appropriate g protein/kg/d by the body weight. As previously noted, DRIs may be further individualized based on the child's nutritional, medical, and growth needs and should be adjusted over time based on clinical status and response to nutritional intervention.

CONCLUSION

In pediatric care, infancy, childhood, and adolescence are recognized as unique phases because adequate nutrition must support both usual nutrient requirements and nutrients needed for optimal growth and development. However, nutritional status depends in part on current and past illnesses, and a child's response to illness is affected by his or her nutritional status. Thus, understanding and addressing the nutritional status of a hospitalized child are important components of clinical care. No single measure provides an adequate assessment of nutrition status. A nutritional assessment often includes the input of many members of the health care team. This chapter provides the factors to consider in the nutritional assessment and monitoring of a hospitalized child. Initial nutritional goals are adjusted over time as the child's medical and nutrition status change to provide optimal care.

REFERENCES

1. Baker JP, Detsky AS, Wesson DE, et al. Nutritional assessment: A comparison of clinical judgement and objective measurements. N Engl J Med 1982;306:969–72.
2. Maka DA, Murphy LK. Drug–nutrient interactions: A review. AACN Clin Issues 2000;11:580–9.
3. American Academy of Pediatrics. Recommendations for preventative pediatric healthcare. Pediatric 2006;105:645–6.
4. Hubbard VA, Hubbard LR. Clinical assessment of nutritional status. In: Walker WA, Watkins JB, editors. Nutrition in Pediatrics: Basic Science and Clinical Applications, 2nd edition. Hamilton, ON: BC Decker; 1997, p. 7–28.
5. Gibson R. In: Principles of Nutritional Assessment, 2nd Edition. New York: Oxford University Press, 2005: 41–64.
6. Ziegler P, Briefel R, Clusen N, et al. Feeding Infants and Toddlers Study (FITS): development of the FITS survey in comparison to other dietary survey methods. J Am Diet Assoc 2006;106:S12–27.
7. Dwyer JT. Nutritional status: Dietary assessment. In: Encyclopedia of human nutrition. Sadler MJ, Strain JJ, Caballero B, editors. San Diego, CA: Academic Press; 1999, p. 1347–57.
8. Gordon C, Chumlea W, Roch A. In: Lohman T, Roche A, Martorell R, editors. Anthropometric Standardization Reference Manual. Champaign, IL: Human Kinetics Books, 1988:3–8.
9. Zemel B. In: Altschuler S, Liacouras C, editors. In: Pediatric Gastroenterology. London: Churchill Livingstone, 1998: 597–606.
10. WHO Expert Committee. Physical status: The use and interpretation of anthropometry. WHO Technical Report Series, WHO 854. Geneva: WHO; 1995.
11. Spender QW, Cronk CE, Charney EB, et al. Assessment of linear growth of children with cerebral palsy: Use of alternative measures to height or length. Dev Med Child Neurol 1989;31:206–14.
12. Stallings V, Zemel B.: Nutritional assessment of the disabled child. Sullivan P, Rosenbloom L, editors. In: Clinics in Developmental Medicine. London: MacKeith Press, 1996:62–76.
13. Martin A, Carter J, Hendy K, et al. In: Lohman T, Roche A, Martorell R, editors. Anthropometric Standardization Reference Manual. Champaign, IL: Human Kinetics Books, 1988:9–26.
14. Callaway C, Chumlea W, Bouchard C. In: Lohman T, Roche A, Martorell R, editors. Anthropometric Standardization Reference Manual. Champaign, IL: Human Kinetics Books, 1988:39–54.
15. American Academy of Pediatrics, Committee on Nutrition. In: Kleinman R, editors. Pediatric Nutrition Handbook. 5th edition Chicago: American Academy of Pediatrics, 2004:23–54.
16. Lubchenco LO, Hansman C, Dressler M, et al. Intrauterine growth as estimated from liveborn birth weight data at 24 to 42 weeks of gestation. Pediatrics 1963;32:793–800.
17. Lubchenco LO, Hansman C, Boyd E. Intrauterine growth in length and head circumference as estimated from live births at gestational ages from 26 to 42 weeks. Pediatrics 1966;37:403–8.
18. Babson SG, Benda GI. Growth graphs for the clinical assessment of infants of varying gestational age. J Pediatr 1976;89:814–20.
19. Alexander GR, Himes JH, Kaufman RB, et al. A United States national reference for fetal growth. Obstet Gynecol 1996;87:163–8.
20. Kramer MS, Platt RW, Wen SW, et al. A new and improved population-based Canadian reference for birth weight for gestational age. Pediatrics 2001;108:E35.
21. Fenton TR. A new growth chart for preterm babies: Babson and Benda's chart updated with recent data and a new format. BMC Pediatr 2003;3:13.
22. Kuczmarski RJ, Ogden CL, Grummer-Strawn LM, et al. CDC growth charts: United States. Adv Data 2000;1–27.
23. Enhancing the outcomes of low-birth-weight, premature infants. A multisite, randomized trial. The Infant Health and Development Program. JAMA 1990;263:3035–42.
24. Casey PH, Kraemer HC, Bernbaum J, et al. Growth status and growth rates of a varied sample of low birth weight, preterm infants: A longitudinal cohort from birth to three years of age. J Pediatr 1991;119:599–605.
25. Guo SS, Wholihan K, Roche AF, et al. Weight-for-length reference data for preterm, low-birth-weight infants. Arch Pediatr Adolesc Med 1996;150:964–70.
26. Guo SS, Roche AF, Chumlea WC, et al. Growth in weight, recumbent length, and head circumference for preterm lowbirthweight infants during the first three years of life using gestation-adjusted ages. Early Hum Dev 1997;47:305–25.
27. Ehrenkranz RA, Younes N, Lemons JA, et al. Longitudinal growth of hospitalized very low birth weight infants. Pediatrics 1999;104:280–9.

28. Hamill PV, Drizd TA, Johnson CL, et al. NCHS growth curves for children birth-18 years. United States. Vital Health Stat 11 1977;i-74.
29. de Onis M. WHO Child Growth Standards: Length/Height-for-Age, Weight-for-Age, Weight-for-Length, Weight-for-Height and Body Mass Index-for-Age: Methods and Development. Geneva: WHO; 2006.
30. de Onis M, Garza C, Onyango AW, et al. Comparison of the WHO child growth standards and the CDC 2000 growth charts. J Nutr 2007;137:144–8.
31. Baumgartner RN, Roche AF, Himes JH. Incremental growth tables: Supplementary to previously published charts. Am J Clin Nutr 1986;43:711–22.
32. Guo SM, Roche AF, Fomon SJ, et al. Reference data on gains in weight and length during the first two years of life. J Pediatr 1991;119:355–62.
33. Roche AF, Himes JH. Incremental growth charts. Am J Clin Nutr 1980;33:2041–52.
34. Roche AF, Mukherjee D, Guo SM, et al. Head circumference reference data: Birth to 18 years. Pediatrics 1987;79:706–12.
35. Roche AF, Guo S, Moore WM. Weight and recumbent length from 1 to 12 mo of age: Reference data for 1-mo increments. Am J Clin Nutr 1989;49:599–607.
36. Tanner JM, Davies PS. Clinical longitudinal standards for height and height velocity for North American children. J Pediatr 1985;107:317–29.
37. Cronk C, Crocker AC, Pueschel SM, et al. Growth charts for children with Down syndrome: 1 month to 18 years of age. Pediatrics 1988;81:102–10.
38. Cronk CE. Growth of children with Down's syndrome: Birth to age 3 years. Pediatrics 1978;61:564–8.
39. Himes JH, Roche AF, Thissen D, et al. Parent-specific adjustments for evaluation of recumbent length and stature of children. Pediatrics 1985;75:304–13.
40. Hamill PV, Drizd TA, Johnson CL, et al. Physical growth: National Center for Health Statistics Percentiles. Am J Clin Nutr 1979;32:607–29.
41. Mascarenhas MR, Zemel B, Stallings VA. Nutritional assessment in pediatrics. Nutrition 1998;14:105–15.
42. Kuczmarski RJ, Flegal KM. Criteria for definition of overweight in transition: Background and recommendations for the United States. Am J Clin Nutr 2000;72:1074–81.
43. Barlow SE, Dietz WH. Obesity evaluation and treatment: Expert committee recommendations. The Maternal and Child Health Bureau, Health Resources and Services Administration and the Department of Health and Human Services. Pediatrics 1998;102:E29.
44. Cole TJ, Bellizzi MC, Flegal KM, et al. Establishing a standard definition for child overweight and obesity worldwide: International survey. BMJ 2000;320:1240–3.
45. Mei Z, Grummer-Strawn LM, Pietrobelli A, et al. Validity of body mass index compared with other body-composition screening indexes for the assessment of body fatness in children and adolescents. Am J Clin Nutr 2002;75:978–85.
46. Bellizzi MC, Dietz WH. Workshop on childhood obesity: Summary of the discussion. Am J Clin Nutr 1999;70:173S–5S.
47. Hoffman DJ, Sawaya AL, Martins PA, et al. Comparison of techniques to evaluate adiposity in stunted and nonstunted children. Pediatrics 2006;117:e725–e32.
48. Eckhardt CL, Adair LS, Caballero B, et al. Estimating body fat from anthropometry and isotopic dilution: A four-country comparison. Obes Res 2003;11:1553–62.
49. Zhang Z, Lai HJ. Comparison of the use of body mass index percentiles and percentage of ideal body weight to screen for malnutrition in children with cystic fibrosis. Am J Clin Nutr 2004;80:982–91.
50. Harrison G, Buskirk E, Carter J. In: Lohman T, Roche A, Martorell R, editors. Anthropometric Standardization Reference Manual. Champaign, IL: Human Kinetics Books, 1988:55–70.
51. Frisancho AR. New norms of upper limb fat and muscle areas for assessment of nutritional status. Am J Clin Nutr 1981;34:2540–5.
52. Ponder SW. Clinical use of bone densitometry in children: Are we ready yet? Clin Pediatr (Phila) 1995;34:237–40.
53. NIH. Osteoporosis prevention, diagnosis, and therapy. NIH consensus statements 2002. URL: http://consensus.nih.gov/cons111/111_intro.htm
54. Leonard MB, Zemel BS. Current concepts in pediatric bone disease. Pediatr Clin North Am 2002;49:143–73.
55. Zemel BS, Petit M. Evaluation. In: Sawyer A, Baker JP, Fung E, editors. Current Clinical Practice: Bone Densitomerty in Growing Patients: Guidelines for Clinical Practice. Totowa, NJ: Humana Press Inc.; 2006, p. 115–25.
56. Olsen IE, Ittenbach RF, Rovner AJ, et al. Deficits in size-adjusted bone mass in children with Alagille syndrome. J Pediatr Gastroenterol Nutr 2005;40:76–82.
57. Molgaard C, Thomsen BL, Prentice A, et al. Whole body bone mineral content in healthy children and adolescents. Arch Dis Child 1997;76:9–15.
58. Leonard MB, Shults J, Elliott DM, et al. Interpretation of whole body dual energy X-ray absorptiometry measures in children: Comparison with peripheral quantitative computed tomography. Bone 2004;34:1044–52.
59. Burnham JM, Shults J, Semeao E, et al. Whole body BMC in pediatric Crohn disease: Independent effects of altered growth, maturation, and body composition. J Bone Miner Res 2004;19:1961–8.
60. Horlick M, Lappe JM, Gilsanz V, et al. The bone mineral density in childhood study (BMDCS): Baseline results for 1554 healthy pediatric volunteers. J Bone Min Res 2004; 19:S14.
61. Stallings V. Bone densitometry. Altschuler s, Liacouras C, editors. In: Clinical Pediatric Gastroenterology. 1st edition. Philadelphia, PA: Churchill Livingstone, 1998:613–9.
62. Fields DA, Goran MI, McCrory MA. Body-composition assessment via air-displacement plethysmography in adults and children: A review. Am J Clin Nutr 2002;75:453–67.
63. Urlando A, Dempster P, Aitkens S. A new air displacement plethysmograph for the measurement of body composition in infants. Pediatr Res 2003;53:486–92.
64. Ittenbach RF, Buison AM, Stallings VA, et al. Statistical validation of air-displacement plethysmography for body composition assessment in children. Ann Hum Biol 2006;33:187–201.
65. Tanner JM. Growth at adolescence. 2nd edition. Oxford, England: Blackwell Scientific Publications, 1962.
66. Duke P, Litt I, Gross R. Adolescents' self assessment of sexual maturation. Pediatric 1980;66:918–20.
67. Morris N, Udry J. Validation of self administered instrument to assess stage of adolescent development. J Youth Adolesc 1980;9:271–80.
68. Neinstein L. Adolescent self assessment of sexual maturation: Reassessment and evaluation in a mixed ethnic urban population. Clin Pediatr (Phila) 1982;21:482–4.
69. Schall J, Semeao E, Stallings V, et al. Self assessment of sexual maturity status in children with Crohn's disease. J Pediatr 2002;141:223–9.
70. Greulich W, Pyle S. Radiographic atlas of skeletal development of the hand and wrist. 2nd edition. Standford, CA: Standford University Press; 1959.
71. Tanner JM, Healy M, Goldstein H, et al. Assessment of Skeletal Maturity and Prediction of Adult Height TW3 Method. London: WB Saunders; 2001.
72. Tanner JM. Foetus into Man: Physical Growth from Conception to Maturity. Cambridge, MA: Harvard University Press; 1978.
73. Subcommittee on the tenth edition of the RDA's fanbcolsNRC. Summary: Recommended Dietary Allowances. Washington, DC: National Academy Press; 1989, p. 1–9.
74. Institute of Medicine. Introduction to dietary reference intakes. In: Otten J, Hellwig J, Meyers L, editors. Dietary Reference Intakes: The Essential Guide to Nutrient Requirements. Washington, DC: The National Academies Press; 2006, p. 5–17.
75. Institute of Medicine. Dietary Reference Intakes for Energy, Carbohydrate, Fiber, Fat, Fatty Acids, Cholesterol, Protein, and Amino Acids. Washington, DC: National Academies Press, 2002.
76. Food and Nutrition Board. Dietary Reference Intakes for Energy, Carbohydrate, Fiber, Fat, Fatty Acids, Cholesterol, Protein, and Amino Acids. Washington, DC: National Academy Press, 2002.
77. FAO/WHO/UNU Expert Consultation. Energy and protein requirements. WHO Technical Report Series. WHO 724. Geneva: WHO; 1985.
78. Sentongo TA, Tershakovec AM, Mascarenhas MR, et al. Resting energy expenditure and prediction equations in young children with failure to thrive. J Pediatr 2000;136:345–50.
79. Mascarenhas MR, Tershakovec AM, Stallings VA. Parenteral and enteral nutrition. In: Wyllie R, Hyams JS, editors. Pediatric Gastrointestinal Disease. Philadelphia: WB Saunders; 1999. p. 741–57.
80. Stallings V. Resting energy expenditure. In: Altschuler S, Liacouras C, editors. Pediatric Gastroenterology. London: Churchill Livingstone; 1998, p. 607–11.
81. Das S, Roberts S. Energy metabolism. In: present knowledge in nutrition. 8th edition. Washington, DC: ILSI Press, 2001: 3–12.
82. Institute of Medicine. Energy. In: Dietary Reference Intakes for Energy, Carbohydrate, Fiber, Fat, Fatty Acids, Cholesterol, Protein, and Amino Acids. Washington, DC: National Academy Press, 2002;5:5–114.

3

Laboratory Assessment of Nutritional Status

Melissa Wright, RD, LDN
Clifford W. Lo, MD, MPH, ScD

Pediatric nutrition assessment involves the integration of various parameters gathered by the clinician. Anthropometrics, dietary and medical history, clinical and physical assessment, and laboratory values provide essential information to evaluate the adequacy of a patient's diet, detect nutritional deficiencies, and monitor the effect of treatment.[1] Laboratory values can provide baseline data from which to monitor response to nutritional interventions, as well as allow detection of underlying causes of malnutrition, such as inadequate dietary intake, malabsorption, increased nutrient requirements, or excretion of nutrients. These tests can also provide an objective measure of depleted tissue stores before they result in functional nutrient pool deficiencies, and can also be used to determine biochemical levels of nutrients, their metabolites, or dependent enzyme activities that often go undetected by clinical or other methods.

Despite the availability of biochemical and immunologic assays, there are many barriers limiting nutrition assessment using laboratory parameters. No battery of standard, readily available, inexpensive tests has been universally accepted to evaluate various nutrients, due mainly to overly specific nutritional laboratory tests. Measurements of a certain nutrient will likely fluctuate depending on the body pool or other nutrient deficiencies. In addition, medications, diseases, stress, and environmental conditions can all result in skewed laboratory values. Clinicians must also consider that specimens may be contaminated or be collected under less than ideal conditions, leading to inaccurate values.[2]

ANALYSIS IN BLOOD

One of the major underlying difficulties of laboratory blood analysis is that most nutrients are not distributed evenly in the body and are not confined to one body pool. Thus, a single determination of blood, urine, or even tissue concentrations of these nutrients does not always provide a reliable indication of distribution or functional metabolic significance. Amounts of a nutrient in plasma might form only a very small percentage of whole-body stores and could be unrelated to tissue levels. Plasma levels can be regulated so that normal levels are maintained in spite of a severe tissue deficiency. For example, plasma calcium comprises less than 2% of whole-body calcium, and there is an even smaller percentage in the functional form of ionized calcium. Regulated by hormones, plasma calcium levels can be in the normal range even in the presence of severe bone calcium depletion (rickets).

Thus, plasma or serum levels of nutrients might not always be reliable indicators of nutritional status. Although relevant tissues can sometimes be difficult to obtain for biopsy (eg, liver, bone, brain, or muscle), some nutrients (such as vitamin C) can be better assessed by measuring their levels in whole blood, red cells, or leukocytes because these are also centers of metabolic activity. Even more relevant are functional assays of the activity in red cells of certain enzymes that are dependent on a particular nutrient. Good examples of these include transketolase activity for thiamin, glutathione reductase for riboflavin, transaminase for pyridoxine, and glutathione peroxidase for selenium.

ANALYSIS IN HAIR AND NAILS

Because the measurement of vitamin and trace minerals in hair and nail clippings reflects deposition of stores over the long term rather than recent dietary intake, it has been mainly used in research settings. Despite the apparent easy availability of tissue samples, collection procedures remain problematic because of contamination by external agents (eg, cosmetics, shampoos, forceps, collection vials) and selection of appropriate specimens (telogen hairs). Many studies continue to address the effect of contamination on the accuracy of measurement and the appropriateness of the use of these samples for nutritional assessment.[3,4]

ANALYSIS IN URINE

Nutrients can be metabolized into inactive (or active) forms that cannot be directly assayed. Most nutrients are eventually excreted in the urine, and many methods involve measuring levels of nutrients or their metabolites in the urine, which can be decreased in deficiency states. Some examples of these metabolites are 2-methyl nicotinamide from niacin and 4-pyridoxic acid from pyridoxine (vitamin B_6). On the other hand, there might be increased urine excretion of metabolic products that accumulate because of a specific nutrient deficiency; for example, methylmalonic acid in vitamin B_{12} deficiency and formiminoglutamic acid in folate deficiency. Urine excretion of metabolites can also be measured after specific "loading" of a nutrient to determine relative depletion, as in the tryptophan load test for pyridoxine deficiency and tyrosine load test for vitamin C deficiency. The problem with urine collections is that excretion from the bladder varies during the day, and concentrations are less reliable than cumulative daily total amounts. Ideally, a 24-hour urine collection should be used for assessment. Shorter sampling times have been studied for their accuracy when compared with 24-hour collections.[5,6]

METHODS OF ANALYSIS

Many nutrients are present in plasma in extremely low trace concentrations—in the nanogram to picogram per milliliter range. This has necessitated the development of extremely sophisticated assays, some of which are quite expensive. In many cases, these new techniques have replaced even more expensive bioassays, such as those still in use for biotin and pantothenic acid. The advent of multichannel sequential autoanalyzers has been a positive development in providing rapid, inexpensive analysis of a battery of enzymes and electrolytes in a small amount of serum, but they have not been specifically applied to nutritional assessment.

Emission flame photometry is a readily available method for analysis of major minerals, such as sodium, potassium, chloride, and calcium. Somewhat more involved, atomic absorption spectroscopy has now become the preferred method of analysis of many trace elements, such as zinc and copper. The fat-soluble vitamins (A, D, E, and K) and their metabolites can be measured by high-performance liquid chromatography.[7] Other techniques include radioimmunoassay, gas chromatography, thin-layer chromatography, and mass spectrometry.[8] The use of stable isotopes has led researchers to a better understanding of nutrition and metabolism. For example, much of the knowledge of neonatal nutrition has come from studies using stable isotopes.[9,10] Large-scale group or community studies most often use isotope studies for their populations. Routine use of stable isotopes in a clinical setting may be less feasible due to issues of logistics and expense.[11–13]

Table 1 Laboratory Tests for Nutritional Assessment

Nutrient	Initial Screening	Secondary Monitoring	Special Investigations
General status	Hemoglobin, hematocrit	Respiratory quotient	Total body K, total body N, indirect calorimetry
Protein	S albumin, S total protein, U protein (dipstick)	S transferrin, prealbumin, S retinol-binding protein, creatinine height index	U hydroxyproline index; S amino acid profiles, indices; nitrogen balance; stable isotope studies
Fat		S triglycerides, S cholesterol	S lipoprotein electrophoresis, triene/tetraene ratio
Carbohydrate	S glucose, U sugar (dipstick)	GTT, lactose, sucrose tolerance tests	Breath hydrogen test
Vitamins			
A		S retinol, S carotene	S retinol-binding protein, dark adaptation test
C		S ascorbate	WBC ascorbate, blood ascorbate, tyrosine load test
D		S 25-(OH)-D; S calcium, phosphorus; S alkaline phosphatase; bone radiograph	S 1,25-$(OH)_2$-D (HPLC), S vitamin D_2 (HPLC), S PTH (RIA)
E		S tocopherol	RBC hemolysis test, tocopherol transport capacity
K		Prothrombin time	Clotting time, S vitamin K (HPLC)
Thiamin		RBC transketolase activity	24-h U thiamin, TPP stimulation test
Riboflavin		RBC glutathione reductase activity	24-h U riboflavin, blood pyruvate
Niacin		Whole blood NAD	24-h U 2-Me nicotinamide, U 2-pyridone
B_6		S vitamin B_6, S pyridoxal phosphate	EGOT or EGPT index, U vitamin B_6, U 4-pyridoxic acid, tryptophan load test
B_{12}	Hemoglobin, RBC indices, RBC morphology	S vitamin B_{12}	U methylmalonic acid, RBC vitamin B_{12}, Schilling test
Folate	Hemoglobin, hematocrit, RBC indices, RBC morphology	S folate	U FIGLU, RBC folate
Pantothenate			S pantothenate, 24-h U pantothenate
Biotin			Whole blood biotin, 24-h U biotin
Minerals			
Calcium		S calcium, bone radiographs	Bone densitometry, calcium balance, S PTH
Phosphorus		S phosphorus	
Magnesium		S magnesium	
Iron	Hemoglobin, hematocrit, RBC indices, RBC morphology	S iron, S ferritin, S iron-binding capacity, S transferrin saturation	Marrow iron, free RBC protoporphyrin
Zinc		S zinc	RBC zinc, WBC zinc, salivary zinc, hair zinc, zinc isotope turnover, S alkaline phosphatase
Copper		S copper, S ceruloplasmin	RBC copper, 24-h U copper, hair copper, RBC superoxide dismutase, radiocopper turnover
Iodine		S thyroxine, S TSH	
Selenium		RBC selenium, RBC glutathione peroxidase	

EGOT = erythrocyte glutamic-oxaloacetic transaminase; EGPT = erythrocyte glutamic-pyruvic transaminase; FIGLU = formiminoglutamic acid; GTT = glucose tolerance test; HPLC = high-performance liquid chromatography; NAD = nicotinamide adenine dinucleotide; NBT = nitroblue tetrazolium; P = plasma; PTH = parathyroid hormone; RBC = red blood cell (leukocyte); RIA = radioimmunoassay; S = serum; TPP = thiamin pyrophosphate; TSH = thyroid-stimulating hormone; U = urine; WBC = white blood cell (leukocyte).

VITAMIN AND MINERAL ASSESSMENT

With more than 40 essential nutrients to measure, including 13 vitamins and at least 14 trace elements, plus an inexhaustible list of related metabolites, enzymes, hormones, and functional parameters, no battery of laboratory tests can hope to provide a complete comprehensive assessment of all nutrients. Even if this were possible, complete biochemical "normality" would not guarantee adequate health or nutrition, nor would immediate corrections necessarily be desirable in patients who have adapted to their nutritional state. For many nutrients, it is not clear that published normal biochemical values represent ideal levels. There are many genetic, racial, and regional differences in nutrient levels, some of which could represent chronic deficiency in the majority of the population. Iron status can be suboptimal in a large proportion of menstruating women, for example. Age and sex differences in normal levels must also be considered.[14–17] Indeed, the definition of *ideal* could be different to different evaluators. To a surgeon, ideal nutrition could mean lack of postoperative morbidity. To an epidemiologist, it might mean absence of chronic disease. To a pediatrician, it might mean adequate growth and development.

Determining the most useful laboratory values is an ongoing process. The ideal nutritional assessment test has yet to be developed. As proposed by Goldsmith, the ideal test would have a short half-life, have rapid response to improved nutritional intake, reflect moderate decreases in intake early, indicate current nutritional status, reflect the degree of deficit, and be unaffected by non-nutritional factors.[18] Laboratory assessment of nutritional status should not be an indiscriminate application of all possible tests. Rather, it should involve intelligent selection of appropriate tests in conjunction with dietary, anthropometric, and clinical information and consider availability, cost, predictive value, sensitivity, specificity, reliability, and validity.

Although assays for specific vitamins and minerals are covered in other chapters, Table 1 lists most of the readily available tests of nutritional status and their relative level of applicability. Generally accepted normal levels are listed in Table 2. In addition to the now-classic reference works of Sauberlich and colleagues[19] and Jelliffe and Jelliffe,[20] several reviews and symposia should be consulted for further details and values.[21–33]

ANALYSIS OF ENERGY IN SPECIFIC NUTRIENTS

Although energy in the body is stored mainly as fat (approximately 100,000 kcal in the average adult), most usual diets supply most of this energy as carbohydrate.[34] Analysis of foods in the bomb calorimeter to measure energy intake exactly was pioneered by Atwater and Benedict in the early 1900s. Direct calorimetry precisely determines energy expenditures as metabolic heat production (*M*) by measuring work performed (*W*); heat loss by evaporation (*E*), radiation (*R*), conduction (*K*), and convection (*C*); and body temperature changes (*S*)[35]:

$$M = S + R + C + K + E + W$$

Table 2 Pediatric Reference Intervals

Nutrient (Units)	Age of Subject	Male	Female
Serum albumin (g/dL)	0–5 d (<2.5 kg)	2.0–3.6	2.0–3.6
	0–5 d (>2.5 kg)	2.6–3.6	2.6–3.6
	1–3 yr	3.4–4.2	3.4–4.2
	4–6 yr	3.5–5.2	3.5–5.2
	7–19 yr	3.7–5.6	3.7–5.6
Serum prealbumin (mg/dL)	0–4 d	7.3–14.4	7.3–14.4
	1 mo–4 yr	6.7–17.1	6.7–17.1
	5–11 yr	9.1–22.0	9.1–22.0
	12–20 yr	12.4–30.2	12.4–30.2
Plasma folic acid (nmol/L)	0–1 yr	16.3–50.8	14.3–51.5
	2–3 yr	5.7–34	3.9–35.6
	4–6 yr	1.1–29.4	6.1–31.9
	7–9 yr	5.2–27	5.4–30.4
	10–12 yr	3.4–24.5	2.3–23.1
	13–18 yr	2.7–19.9	2.7–16.3
Serum iron (μg/dL)	1–30 d	32–112	29–127
	31–365 d	27–109	25–126
	1–3 yr	29–91	25–101
	4–6 yr	25–115	28–93
	7–9 yr	27–96	30–104
	10–12 yr	28–112	32–104
	13–15 yr	26–110	30–109
	16–18 yr	27–138	33–102
Plasma transferrin saturation	1–5 yr	0.07–0.44	0.07–0.44
	6–9 yr	0.17–0.42	0.17–0.42
	10–14 yr	0.11–0.36	0.11–0.36
	14–19 yr	0.06–0.33	0.06–0.33
Retinol binding protein (mg/dL)	0–5 d	0.8–4.5	0.8–4.5
	1–5 yr	1.0–7.6	1.0–7.6
	6–9 yr	2.0–7.8	2.0–7.8
	10–13 yr	1.3–9.9	1.3–9.9
	14–19 yr	3.0–9.2	3.0–9.2
	Term neonates (>37 wk)	1.02–3.14	1.02–3.14
	Preterm neonates (<36.6 wk)	0.72–2.88	0.72–2.88
Plasma/serum vitamin A (μg/dL)	1– 6 yr	20–43	20–43
	7–12 yr	20–49	20–49
	13–19 yr	26–72	26–72
	Term infants (>37 wk)	18–50	18–50
	Preterm infants (<36.6 wk)	13–46	13–46
Plasma vitamin B_{12} (pmol/L)	0–1 yr	216–891	168–1117
	2–3 yr	195–897	307–892
	4–6 yr	181–795	231–1038
	7–9 yr	200–863	182–866
	10–12 yr	135–803	145–752
	13–18 yr	158–638	134–605
Serum 25-hydroxy vitamin D (μg/L)[†]	1–30 d Summer	20.0–44.0	20.0–44.0
	1–30 d Winter	20.0–38.0	20.0–42.0
	1 mo–<1 yr Summer	26.0–48.0	23.0–62.0
	1 mo–<1 yr Winter	20.0–68.0	20.0–48.0
	1–3 yr Summer	20.0–60.0	20.0–62.0
	1–3 yr Winter	20.0–51.0	20.0–53.0
	4–12 yr Summer	20.0–49.0	20.0–48.0
	4–12 yr Winter	20.0–47.0	20.0–40.0
	13–18 yr Summer	20.0–41.0	20.0–38.0
	13–18 yr Winter	20.0–39.0	20.0–28.0
Plasma/serum vitamin E (μg/dL)	Premature	0.5–3.5	0.5–3.5
	Full term	1.0–3.5	1.0–3.5
	2–5 mo	2.0–6.0	2.0–6.0
	6–24 mo	3.5–8.0	3.5–8.0
	2–12 yr	5.5–9.0	5.5–9.0
Serum zinc (μg/dL)	0–5 d	65–140	65–140
	1–5 yr	67–118	67–118
	6–9 yr	77–107	77–107
	10–14 yr	76–101	79–118
	15–19 yr	64–104	60–101

(Continued)

Table 2 Pediatric Reference Intervals *(Continued)*

Nutrient (Units)	Age of Subject	Male	Female
Serum calcium (mg/dL)	0–7 d	7.3–11.4	7.5–11.3
	8–30 d	8.6–11.7	8.4–11.9
	31–90 d	8.5–11.3	8.0–11.1
	91–180 d	8.3–11.4	7.7–11.5
	181–365 d	7.7–11.0	7.8–11.1
	1–3 yr	8.8–10.6	8.4–10.6
	4–6 yr	8.8–10.6	8.5–10.6
	7–9 yr	8.7–10.3	8.6–10.2
	10–12 yr	8.7–10.2	8.6–10.2
	13–15 yr	8.5–10.2	8.4–10.0
	16–18 yr	8.4–10.3	8.6–9.8
Plasma magnesium (mg/dL)	Premature 0–6 d	1.6–2.7	1.6–2.7
	Newborns 0–6 d	1.2–2.6	1.2–2.6
	Premature 7–30 d	1.8–2.4	1.8–2.4
	Newborns 7–30 d	1.6–2.4	1.6–2.4
	1 mo–1 yr	1.6–2.6	1.6–2.6
	1–2 yr	1.6–2.6	1.6–2.6
	2–6 yr	1.5–2.4	1.5–2.4
	6–10 yr	1.6–2.3	1.6–2.3
	10–14 yr	1.6–2.2	1.6–2.2
	14 yr+	1.5–2.3	1.5–2.3
Plasma/serum phosphorus (mg/dL)	1–30 d	3.9–6.9	4.3–7.7
	31–365 d	3.5–6.6	3.7–6.5
	1–3 yr	3.1–6.0	3.4–6.0
	4–6 yr	3.3–5.6	3.2–5.5
	7–9 yr	3.0–5.4	3.1–5.5
	10–12 yr	3.2–5.7	3.3–5.3
	13–15 yr	2.9–5.1	2.8–4.8
	16–18 yr	2.7–4.9	2.5–4.8
Selenium (μg/dL)	3–5 yr	2.0–12.4	2.0–12.4
	6–8 yr	1.6–12.0	1.6–12.0
	9–11 yr	2.4–13.5	2.4–13.5
	12–13 yr	4.0–10.7	4.0–10.7
	14–16 yr	4.0–10.7	4.0–10.7
Carnitine (total) (μmol/L)	1–12 mo	15–39	15–39
	1–7 yr	18–37	18–37
	7–15 yr	31–43	31–43
Copper (μg/dL)	0–5 d	9.0–46	9.0–46
	1–5 yr	80–150	80–150
	6–9 yr	84–136	84–136
	10–14 yr	80–121	80–120
	15–19 yr	64–171	72–160
Total plasma homocysteine (μmol/L)	2 mo–10 yr	3.3–8.3	3.3–8.3
	11–15 yr	4.7–10.3	4.7–10.3
	16–18 yr	4.7–11.3	4.7–11.3
Hematocrit (%)	1–3 d	36.4–47.4	36.5–47.7
	4–7 d	35.9–46.6	36.1–44.0
	8–14 d	34.4–45.4	36.6–43.2
	15–30 d	33.6–41.0	34.1–41.8
	31–60 d	33.6–41.0	34.1–41.8
	61–180 d	30.5–37.7	30.5–38.6
	0.5–<2 yr	30.5–37.7	30.5–38.6
	2–<6 yr	31.5–36.8	31.8–37.0
	6–<12 yr	31.5–38.0	32.3–38.3
	12–<18 yr	31.4–41.0	32.1–38.7
	≥18 yr	33.0–43.4	31.7–39.1
Hemoglobin (g/dL)	1–3 d	12.5–16.6	12.7–16.4
	4–7 d	12.5–16.3	12.6–15.3
	8–14 d	11.9–15.7	12.7–14.9
	15–30 d	11.6–14.2	11.6–14.3
	31–60 d	10.2–12.7	11.1–13.7
	61–180 d	10.5–13.0	10.7–13.4
	0.5–<2 yr	10.4–12.5	10.8–12.6
	2–<6 yr	11.0–12.8	11.1–12.9
	6–<12 yr	11.0–13.3	11.3–13.4
	12–<18 yr	11.0–14.3	11.3–13.4
	≥18 yr	11.4–15.1	10.9–13.4

Table 2 Pediatric Reference Intervals *(Continued)*

Nutrient (Units)	Age of Subject	Male	Female
Mean corpuscular volume (μm³)	1–3 d	94.0–106.3	89.7–105.4
	4–7 d	87.1–96.5	86.5–93.8
	8–14 d	87.1–94.8	87.4–92.2
	15–30 d	88.0–95.2	88.4–93.3
	31–60 d	86.5–92.1	85.7–91.6
	61–180 d	79.6–86.3	82.0–87.0
	0.5–<2 yr	75.6–83.1	76.6–83.2
	2–<6 yr	76.8–83.3	77.7–84.1
	6–<12 yr	78.2–83.9	79.5–85.2
	12–<18 yr	80.6–86.6	82.1–87.7
	≥18 yr	83.5–90.2	82.7–89.4

*Adapted from Pediatric Reference Intervals 170.
†Although there is no consensus on optimal 25-hydroxy vitamin D levels, many experts define deficiency as a serum level less than 20–30 ng/mL. Holick MF. Vitamin D deficiency. N Engl J Med 2007;357(3):266–81.

This requires complete thermal isolation in a chamber or suit and is available only in a few research centers.

Indirect calorimetry bases energy expenditure on oxygen consumption (21.14 kJ/L of oxygen consumed), which can be somewhat more easily obtained by collection and analysis of inspired and expired air. Although many assumptions and calculations must be made, relatively accurate estimates of energy expenditure can be made with portable collection bags and gas analyzers within a few minutes using the Haldane transformation equation[36,37]:

$$O_2 \text{ consumed} = \frac{(V_{\text{air exp}} \times FN_{2\text{ exp}} \times FO_{2\text{ insp}}) - (V_{\text{air exp}} \times FO_2)_{\text{exp}}}{FN_{2\text{ insp}}}$$

where $V_{\text{air exp}}$ = volume of inspired air; $FN_{2\text{ exp}}$ = fraction of inspired oxygen; $FO_{2\text{ exp}}$ = fraction of expired oxygen; and $FN_{2\text{ insp}}$ = fraction of inspired nitrogen.[38]

Thus,

$$O_2 \text{ consumed} = V_{\text{air exp}} \frac{((FN_{2\text{ exp}} \times 0.2093) - FO_{2\text{ exp}})}{0.7094}$$

and adjusting for protein catabolism by the Weir equation[39,40]:

$$\text{MEE (kcal)} = 3.94 \times VO_2 + 1.06\ VCO_2 - 2.17 \times \text{UUN}$$

or as modified by Cunningham[41]:

$$\text{MEE (kcal)} = 3.76 \times VO_2 + 1.25 \times VCO_2 - 1.09 \times \text{UUN}$$

Measurement of carbon dioxide consumption divided by oxygen consumption yields the respiratory quotient (RQ), which can give an indication of the relative source of metabolic fuel, carbohydrates giving an RQ of 1.0 and fats decreasing it toward 0.7 [42]:

$$RQ = VCO_2/VO_2$$

Collection and analysis of expired carbon dioxide and oxygen intake require expensive instruments and are still subject to wide variation, depending on clinical and environmental conditions. Studies of indirect calorimetry continue to prove its usefulness in measuring resting energy expenditure (REE).[43,44] Unfortunately, indirect calorimetry is not always available to the clinician, and predicting energy needs falls to the use of equations.

If indirect calorimetry is not available, an estimate of basal metabolic rate (BMR) can be obtained by a number of equations, all widely researched in comparison to indirect calorimetry. The most widely known and, until the past few decades, the most widely used of these equations is the Harris–Benedict equation.[42] It should be noted that mistakes in transcribing the constant coefficient (ie, 655 for females and 66 for males) frequently lead to inaccurate estimates.[45,46] The Harris–Benedict equation was developed using information gathered on healthy individuals. The majority of research was done on the adult population. It is therefore difficult to justify its use on critically ill or hospitalized patients, especially in pediatrics.[47] A number of newer equations have been developed that can be used to determine energy needs in pediatrics and in a critical care setting.[48]

In 1985, a Food and Agricultural Organization/World Health Organization (FAO/WHO) committee established new predictive equations for estimating energy requirements.[49] Subsequent review and evaluation by Schofield led to equations that more closely relate to values obtained by indirect calorimetry, when factors are used for activity, stress, and disease state (Table 3).[50,51] Other predictive equations that have been proposed have been unable to relate as closely to measured energy requirements. Efforts to study predictive equations that will adequately assess energy requirements have only reinforced the fact that indirect calorimetry is the most accurate tool.[52–60]

In normal states, REE is about 10% above BMR, but this does not take into account additional requirements such as postoperative stress, burns, infection, or disease states, which can vary as much as 50% above or below BMR. Originally, calculations of BMR and REE were common for evaluation of thyroid function; their use today has shifted to research in obesity and in critically ill patients requiring nutritional support. Generally, critically ill patients require up to one and a half times their REE to prevent protein breakdown for gluconeogenesis. Precise measurements of individual energy requirements allow tailoring of nutritional support to prevent lean body mass breakdown without needlessly increasing oxygen consumption (which can compromise respiratory status) or fat deposition.

Finally, studies of energy metabolism over longer periods in subjects performing a variety of activities have used the doubly labeled water method.[61–64] Water enriched with the stable isotopes deuterium and ^{18}O ($^2H^2$ ^{18}O) is administered in a single oral or intravenous dose and several blood or urine samples are obtained over the next 5 to 14 days. Because ^{18}O is excreted as both urinary water and respiratory carbon dioxide, but deuterium is excreted only as water, the different rates of excretion can be measured by mass spectrometry and can be used to calculate metabolic rate. Although they are useful in validating long-term energy needs compared to reports of dietary

Table 3 Equations for Estimating Resting Energy Expenditure in Children

Harris–Benedict
Men: 66.5 (13.8 × W) + (5 × H) − (6.8 × A)
Women: 655 + (9.6 × W) + (1.8 × H) − (4 × A)
Infants: 22.10 + (31.05 × W) + (11.6 × H)
World Health Organization
Males
0–3 yr: (60.9 × W) − 54
3–10 yr: (22.7 × W) + 495
10–18 yr: (17.5 × W) + 651
Females
0–3 yr: (61 × W) − 51
3–10 yr: (22.5 × W) + 499
10–18 yr: (12.2 × W) + 746
Schofield
Males
0–3 yr: (0.167 × W) + (15.174 × H) − 617.6
3–10 yr: (19.59 × W) + (1.303 × H) + 414.9
10–18 yr: (16.25 × W) + (1.372 × H) + 515.5
Females
0–3 yr: (16.252 × W) + (10.232 × H) − 413.5
3–10 yr: (16.969 × W) + (1.618 × H) + 371.2
10–18 yr: (8.365 × W) + (4.65 × H) + 200.0

A = ages; H = height (cm); W = weight (kg).

intake,[65–67] their clinical use in the acute care setting is difficult because of the time and expense involved in stable isotope enrichment and mass spectrometry.

PROTEIN

The assessment of protein nutrition has presented one of the most important yet most problematic questions in the history of nutrition. Widespread protein-energy malnutrition worldwide has fueled interest in determining protein status and requirements, especially in children.[68] Many methods have been devised for measuring protein use, but the central problem of protein turnover remains. Approximately 15% of the body mass consists of protein stored in the liver, muscles, intestines, and other tissues. This, however, is in dynamic equilibrium with the much smaller percentage of body protein carried as plasma amino acids. Concentrations of plasma proteins or amino acids do not necessarily represent their relative concentrations in tissue storage pools.[69–71]

Attempts to measure the flux between these metabolic and storage pools using labeled amino acids generally assume a steady state in which protein synthesis equals protein breakdown. Although radioisotopes were previously used to trace amino acid flux between protein pools, more recent studies have employed non-radioactive, stable isotopes such as ^{13}C leucine and ^{15}N glycine. Because they require complicated mathematical calculations and mass spectrometer analysis, stable isotope infusions have generally been limited so far to research applications.[72,73] Thus, analysis of plasma proteins or amino acid levels cannot always be depended on to give a direct reflection of whole-body protein status. Of the thousands of plasma proteins, relatively few have been shown to have direct clinical significance as tests of health or nutritional status.[74] The future of protein analysis could lie in microassay chip technology now being developed for genetic analysis. Although the focus of this technology is currently on genetics and disease, it could be of use by clinicians for protein assessment.

Serum Albumin

Total serum proteins can be separated into albumins and globulins by electrophoresis. Because gamma-globulins can be increased in infection or malignancy, serum albumin levels are generally a better test of protein status than is total serum protein. Serum albumin levels have been one of the most popular measures of protein-energy malnutrition, and very low concentrations are a hallmark of kwashiorkor. Although albumin remains widely used as a marker of nutritional status, the clinician must take into account multiple other factors affecting the result. Albumin concentrations can be normal in mild or even severe marasmus, despite markedly reduced muscle mass. Conversely, serum albumin concentrations can also be affected by other disease states (eg, rapid blood loss, protein-losing enteropathy), stress, surgery, fluid shifts, and even postural changes. Albumin turnover is fairly slow, with a half-life of about 20 days. Therefore, serum concentrations do not reflect recent dietary intake; albumin levels might not be reduced even after 3 weeks on a protein-free diet.[75–79]

Other Serum Proteins and Enzymes

Other transport proteins, such as thyroxine-binding prealbumin (transthyretin),[80] retinol-binding protein,[81] transferrin,[82] and ferritin,[83] have been proposed as better markers of protein malnutrition because of their shorter half-lives, but they can also be affected by caloric restriction, iron deficiency, or infection, as well as protein deficiency.[84] Prealbumin is secreted by the liver in a complex containing retinol, retinol-binding protein, and thyroxine (T_4) and is thus also known as transthyretin. Although vitamin A deficiency can affect secretion of retinol-binding protein, it does not affect plasma concentrations of prealbumin.[85–89] Ferritin is an acute-phase reactant and can be elevated in liver disease or various inflammatory states.

Other plasma proteins that have been proposed as markers of nutritional status include fibronectin[90] and insulin-like growth factor-1 (IGF-1).[91,92] IGF-1 and IGF-1–binding proteins have both been widely studied for their connection with nutritional status.[93,94] Studies have shown that levels of both IGF-I and IGF-1–binding proteins are affected when calories or protein are restricted.[95,96] IGF-I and IGF-binding proteins might not have the same disadvantages as other proteins when used for assessment. Both values appear to be sensitive indicators in an acute setting to changes in nutritional status.[97,98]

Concentrations of various enzymes in plasma have been widely used in diagnosis of many disease states but, for that very reason, are less specific for protein deficiency. Plasma concentrations of pseudocholinesterase, alkaline phosphatase, amylase, and lipase are reported to be reduced in kwashiorkor, whereas lactic dehydrogenase, isocitrate dehydrogenase, and transaminase are increased. In children, elevated plasma ribonuclease activity can be increased in even mild to moderate malnutrition; comparison of plasma and urine activities can distinguish between moderate and severe malnutrition.[99,100]

Attempts have been made to use plasma amino acid profiles to assess nutritional status. Because concentrations of amino acids are not regulated and do not directly reflect tissue uptake and flux, use in clinical settings has not been widely received. Amino acid values are also affected by infection, injury, and other stressors.[101]

Urinary Protein Excretion

Another approach to the assessment of protein status uses urinary excretion of protein breakdown substances. Creatinine is a degradation product of muscle creatine, and urinary excretion of creatinine has been used since 1905 as a measure of lean body mass. The creatinine height index compares urinary creatinine excretion over 24 hours to a control value and has been widely used as a measure of protein depletion in kwashiorkor and marasmus.[102]

Other urinary excretion ratios using creatinine as a standard, such as the urea-creatinine ratio, the sulfur creatinine ratio, and the urinary hydroxyproline index, have been investigated but tend to reflect recent dietary protein intake rather than long-term nutritional status. Furthermore, these methods all require a 24-hour urine sample to minimize daily fluctuations in urine excretion, and this might not always be easy to obtain. Efforts to short-cut this difficulty have been frustrated by the variability of spot urine creatinine excretion.[103]

Nitrogen Balance Studies

Nitrogen balance studies can be useful in assessing individual protein status, although traditionally they have been used more in controlled metabolic research studies to determine protein requirements in populations or food protein quality. Nitrogen balance measurements can give a direct short-term comparison of dietary nitrogen intake versus fecal and urine excretion.[104] Nitrogen retention is calculated by subtracting fecal and urine nitrogen from oral intake:

$$\text{N retention} = \text{N intake} - \text{fecal N} - \text{urine N}$$

Ideally, balance studies should be performed for several days on a constant protein intake in steady-state conditions. Nitrogen intake can be estimated by dividing dietary protein intake (in grams) by 6.25. Nitrogen output is best analyzed by the rather time-consuming Kjeldahl method of sulfuric acid distillation but can also be estimated in adults by urine urea nitrogen,[105] using an estimate of 4 g/d for stool and skin losses, although these are likely much less in children:

$$\text{N retention} = (\text{protein intake}/6.25) - \text{urine urea N} - 4$$

Although nitrogen balance studies are used often in a clinical setting, they should not be used as the only means of assessing protein balance.[106–109]

LIPIDS

Plasma Lipids and Lipoproteins

Assessment of the fat status of individuals is complicated by similar considerations of storage and metabolic pools. Although fat stores in the body represent a considerable reserve of energy, only a small percentage of this fat is present in the plasma as free fatty acids. Additionally, much of the free fatty acids and triglycerides in the plasma are derived from endogenous synthesis rather than from recent dietary intake. Triglycerides are transported in the blood along with cholesterol and proteins as lipoproteins. These can be separated by ultracentrifugation or electrophoresis as very-low-density lipoprotein, low-density lipoprotein (LDL), and high-density lipoprotein (HDL).[110–111]

Whereas elevated total plasma cholesterol and LDL cholesterol levels are associated with atherosclerosis,[112] higher HDL levels have proven protective.[113] Studies of plasma lipids in adults have demonstrated links between multiple risk factors and cardiovascular disease.[114,115] Risk factors include age, sex, history of hypertension, smoking, diabetes, high LDL levels, and low HDL levels. Various criteria have been developed, such as the Adult Treatment Panel III guidelines, to provide clinicians with recommendations for assessment of cardiovascular risk. Family history and various diseases also affect cholesterol levels and do not necessarily reflect nutritional deficiency or excess.[116] While increased homocysteine levels correlate with the risk of cardiovascular disease in epidemiologic studies, the use of lowering homocysteine levels by supplementation of folate and B vitamins is controversial.[117] Studies in children are few, and recommendations for appropriate levels in the very young have not been assessed.[118–120]

Essential Fatty Acid Deficiency

Although nutritional fat deficiencies are rare, a greater appreciation of essential fatty acid deficiency has occurred in association with a syndrome of dermatitis, poor growth, and degenerative changes in several tissues.[121,122]

Certain fatty acids cannot be synthesized in the body but must be supplied in the diet. These include linoleic and alpha-linolenic acid. They are important as precursors for cholesterol, prostaglandins, and cell membranes.[123]

This requirement comprises 1 to 2% of total caloric intake, but even this might not be provided if a patient is receiving total parenteral nutrition without periodic intravenous fat supplements.[124] Essential fatty acid deficiency can be assessed by elevation of the triene-tetraene ratio because nonessential eicosatrienoic acid (20:3, a triene) levels rise, whereas arachidonic acid (20:4, a tetraene) levels fall. There has been a recent report of typical essential fatty acid deficiency symptoms occurring when linoleic acid, but not linolenic acid, was supplied for several months.[125]

Body Composition and Obesity

Obesity is less often assessed by biochemical parameters than by anthropometric measurements because most techniques for determining total body fat are practical only for research purposes. Potassium is distributed fairly evenly in fat-free tissue and contains a small percentage of the natural radioisotope ^{40}K. Very sensitive gamma counters can thus detect the amount of radioactive potassium in lean body mass, which can be subtracted from the total body mass to determine total body fat.[126,127] Because adipose tissue is very low in water content, total body fat can also be estimated by dilution of injected tritium, deuterium, or stable ^{18}O in the total body water compartment and subtracting that measurement from total body mass. Alternatively, determination of body density by plethysmography or immersion in water can differentiate between a relative amount of fat (with a lower specific gravity of 0.9) versus other tissues.[128]

Recent availability of dual photon absorptiometers, usually used to measure bone density, has led to their being adapted for body composition measurements because lean body tissue and fat can be differentiated and quantitated with a high degree of precision.[129,130]

Bioelectric impedance has been developed as a quick, inexpensive, and noninvasive measurement of lean body mass, which conducts electrical charge better than fat. However, measurements can be affected by changes in tissue fluid content, such as edema or dehydration.[131–135] Body composition is reviewed in more detail in Chapter 4, "Body Composition and Growth."

CARBOHYDRATES

Because serum glucose concentrations are regulated by insulin and other factors, they do not directly reflect nutritional stores or requirements.[136,137] Alterations in serum glucose concentrations are thus more likely to be the result of impaired regulatory mechanisms (eg, in diabetes mellitus) than of nutritional deficiencies. Rarely, hypoglycemia can be the result of lack of carbohydrate substrate, as in neonatal hypoglycemia, childhood ketotic hypoglycemia, or glycogen synthetase deficiency.[138,139] However, hypoglycemia is too often diagnosed in otherwise healthy persons on the basis of a borderline serum glucose concentration, either fasting or after a glucose tolerance test, and this should not be considered a nutritional disease.

Glucose tolerance tests and other oral carbohydrate tolerance tests (lactose, sucrose, xylose) have also been used to assess carbohydrate malabsorption, although breath hydrogen testing is superior for this purpose.[140,141] If an oral dose of carbohydrate is malabsorbed, it will pass into the colon, where bacteria will metabolize it to hydrogen. The hydrogen, which is not produced elsewhere in the body, is excreted in the breath, where it can be collected and measured by gas chromatography. Stable isotopes are used to study glucose metabolism but are better suited for research purposes and large populations than for clinical assessment.[142] See Chapter 61 "Carbohydrate Absorption and Malabsorption" for more details.

IMMUNE STATUS

Although not always sufficiently appreciated, interactions between nutritional status and infections have been amply demonstrated for some time. Not only do infections adversely affect nutritional status, but malnutrition also predisposes the patient to a host of infections: parasitic, viral, bacterial, and fungal.[143] Investigations by Chandra and Kumari[144,145] and others have elucidated some of the immune dysfunctions that accompany protein-calorie malnutrition and specific nutrient deficiencies[146] and mediate impaired resistance to infection (Table 4). Conversely, immunologic assays have been proposed as functional tests of nutritional status, tests that reflect the functional ability of the individual to resist infection, instead of mere static measurements of a single nutrient.[147,148]

Immune responses can be divided into three categories: (1) cellular, principally involving T lymphocytes; (2) humoral, including serum and secretory antibodies; and (3) nonspecific, including phagocytosis, complement, and mucosal immunity. Protein-energy malnutrition affects immune responses in all three of these areas but has been most often associated with profound defects in cell-mediated immunity.[149] Skin tests for a number of antigens, such as *Monilia* (*Candida*), streptokinase-streptodornase, *Trichophyton*, and mumps are normally positive (>5 mm induration after 72 hours) if there has been prior exposure to these antigens in the environment. However, there is a consistent loss of this cutaneous delayed-type hypersensitivity in moderate to severe protein-calorie malnutrition, and skin tests have been used as a sensitive indicator of functional malnutrition in field surveys as well as in hospital settings.[150] Although they do not require blood samples, skin tests do have the disadvantage that they cannot be read until 48 to 72 hours after taking the sample. If common recall antigens do not provoke any response, deliberate contact sensitization with dinitrochlorobenzene and subsequent rechallenge can be performed.[151]

Decreased cell-mediated immunity in malnutrition is also manifest as a decrease in lymphoid tissue, including thymus, tonsils, lymph nodes, and peripheral lymphocytes.[152] A quick estimate of the total lymphocyte count (TLC) can be easily obtained by multiplying the white cell count (WBC) by the percentage of lymphocytes seen on the peripheral smear:

$$\text{TLC} = \text{WBC} \times \%\ \text{lymphocytes}$$

A decrease in the total lymphocyte count to less than 1,500/mm^3 is seen in some, but not all, malnourished patients, although many other conditions can cause lymphopenia as well. Nonspecific transformation of lymphocytes into blast forms by phytohemagglutinin and pokeweed mitogen in the lymphocyte stimulation test is occasionally impaired in severe malnutrition,[153] but this is not a consistent observation.

B lymphocyte response in malnutrition is less affected, and quantitative serum immunoglobulins can be elevated, although this finding could be attributable to constant low-grade infection.[154,155] The complement cascade is important in cytolytic responses, and levels of all complement proteins,

Table 4 Immunologic Defects in Nutrient Deficiency

Immune Defect	Associated Nutrient Deficiency
Lymphocytes	
↓ Transferrin receptor metabolism	Selenium, vitamin E
↓ Skin test reactivity	Protein energy malnutrition (PEM)
T cells	
Thymic involution	PEM, zinc, magnesium
↓ Thymic export of T cells	PEM
↓ Cytotoxicity	Zinc, iron, PEM
↓ Th1 cytokin production	Zinc, selenium, iron, PEM
↓ Proliferative response	Zinc, selenium, vitamin A, PEM
↓ CD4/CD8 ratio	Betacarotene, vitamin A, PEM
↓ Th2 cytokine response	Vitamin A
T-cell apoptosis	Zinc, vitamin C
B-cell system	
↓ T-cell-dependent B-cell response	Zinc, PEM
↓ Antibody response to immunization	Vitamin A, zinc, PEM
↓ Human milk IgA antibodies	PEM
↑ IgA1, IgA2	PEM
↓ Bone marrow B-cell precursors	PEM, Zinc
Monocytes	
↑ PGE_2 production	Vitamin E
Innate immune function	
↓ Leukocyte phagocytosis	Vitamin C, copper, PEM
↓ C3 complement	PEM
↑ C4 complement	PEM
Natural killer cells	
↓ Cytotoxicity	Zinc, selenium, vitamins A and D, PEM
↓ Numbers	
Hematopoietic system	
Lymphopenia	Vitamin A
Neutropenia	Copper
Anemia	Vitamin E, riboflavin, pyridoxine, vitamin B_{12}, folic acid, iron, copper, PEM

Adapted from reference 171.
PGE_2 = prostaglandin E_2.

except C4, are markedly decreased in protein-energy malnutrition. The most commonly available assays for complement function are C3 and CH50 (50% hemolysis).[156,157] Finally, phagocyte function can be impaired in malnutrition, with decreased leukocyte chemotaxis and decreased intracellular bacterial killing, although these phenomena might be more attributable to infection than to malnutrition per se.[158,159] Leukocyte mobility and chemotaxis can be measured in vivo with a Rebuck skin window or in vitro in a Boyden chamber after separation of leukocytes. The nitroblue tetrazolium dye test measures reduced nicotinamide-adenine dinucleotide phosphate (NADPH) oxidase activity, which accompanies bacterial killing. Specific nutrient deficiencies also cause immune system dysfunction, notably iron, zinc, vitamin A, vitamin B12, pyridoxine, and folate deficiency.

APPLICATIONS

Nutritional Field Surveys

In nutritional field surveys, large numbers of relatively healthy people are sampled to determine the prevalence of malnutrition in the population. Because samples are usually collected by mobile field units removed from central laboratories, problems such as refrigeration, centrifugation, and timing put severe restraints on the types of assays possible. Twenty-four-hour urine collections are usually not practical, and reliance must be placed on spot urine samples. Blood samples are generally limited to what can be obtained from one venipuncture, and invasive tests are usually out of the question. In surveys of young children in developing countries, even venipuncture can be difficult, and laboratory tests are often limited to a fingerstick hematocrit and blood smear.

Careful selection of tests is of utmost importance to minimize needless duplication of information and to emphasize nutrients that are most likely to be deficient in the populations sampled. Standardization of collection, analysis, and reporting procedures must be maintained, and samples are generally transported to a central laboratory for processing. Some of the most elaborate nutritional surveys undertaken were the Ten-State Nutrition Survey (1968–1970) and its successors, the National Health and Nutrition Examination Surveys (NHANES). Results from the Third NHANES (1988–1994) continue to be studied and reported. Some of the biochemical tests used in these surveys are listed in Table 5.[160–162]

HOSPITAL MALNUTRITION

Although most of the classic epidemic vitamin deficiency diseases are now rarely seen in the United States, malnutrition in hospitalized patients is still a major problem. Until recently, nutritional assessment of hospitalized patients was rarely systematically or even routinely performed. Increasing attention has been paid to the widespread malnutrition detected by anthropometric and laboratory tests in acute care hospitals.[163] Hendricks and colleagues, using anthropometrics, laboratory assessment, and clinical nutrition assessment, repeated a study on the prevalence of malnutrition in a children's hospital.[164] Although a decrease in malnutrition was found, malnutrition was still prevalent in patients with chronic medical conditions, in children less than 2 years of age, and in patients older than 18 years. Although the need for nutritional assessment has been realized, both adult and pediatric patients still appear at risk for malnutrition, especially in a hospital setting. A Subjective Global Assessment (SGA) has been widely used to assess the nutritional status of adults.[165–168] Recent studies have successfully applied the SGA to the pediatric population and/or adapted the SGA to test its validity in the pediatric population with promising results.[169] See Chapter 44 "Nutrition Assessment of the Hospitalized Patient" for more details (Table 6).

CONCLUSIONS AND RECOMMENDATIONS

Numerous laboratory tests are available for the assessment of nutritional status. Many methods have been devised for quantitation of different proteins, lipids, vitamins, and minerals in the serum, urine, and other body fluids. Unfortunately, no one test or battery of tests gives a completely satisfactory picture of the global nutritional state of the individual. Most common, inexpensive, easily available tests are not sensitive enough to detect early malnutrition before it becomes clinically significant. Conversely, most assays tend to be too specific to reflect abnormalities in a broad range of nutrients. Although laboratory assessment has the advantage of providing reproducible, quantitative data, it is not always possible to determine tissue stores or functional reserve from a single serum or urine

Table 5 Laboratory Tests of Nutritional Status Employed in the Health and Nutrition Examination Surveys

Hemoglobin
Hematocrit
Serum iron
Serum iron-binding capacity
Blood folacin
Total serum protein
Serum albumin
Serum vitamin C
Plasma carotene
Plasma vitamin A
Urinary creatinine
Urinary thiamin
Urinary riboflavin
Urinary iodine

Table 6 Initial Screening Tests for Nutritional Assessment

Dietary assessment
24-h recall or
Typical day recall or
72-h diary or
Food frequency questionnaire
Anthropometric assessment
Height and height-for-age percentiles
Weight and weight-for-age percentiles, weight-for-height percentiles
Triceps skinfolds and arm circumference
Laboratory assessment
Complete blood count, including hemoglobin, hematocrit, WBC and differential, RBC smear
Serum albumin (or prealbumin or retinol-binding-protein), total protein
Serum electrolytes: sodium, potassium, chloride, bicarbonate
Renal function tests: blood urea nitrogen, creatinine
Serum glucose, triglycerides (fasting)
Serum cholesterol, HDL cholesterol, LDL cholesterol
Serum calcium, phosphorus, magnesium
Liver function tests: alanine aminotransferase, bilirubin
Urinalysis (dipstick)
Clinical assessment
Clinical history
Subjective global assessment
Physical examination

HDL = high-density lipoprotein; LDL = low-density lipoprotein; RBC = red blood cell; WBC = white blood cell.

sample. Many tests require timed collections, complicated analytic methods, and expensive instruments and are more suited for specific research investigations than for clinical screening. Recent efforts to develop a simple, streamlined battery of tests to detect hospital malnutrition have focused on the prognostic value of tests that predict clinical complications. Although no standard formula has achieved wide use, most include measurements of protein nutrition (serum albumin) and immune status (skin tests or lymphocyte count). However, these quick estimations might not have better predictive value than a global clinical assessment. Thus, laboratory assessment of nutritional status requires an intelligent selection of tests to fit the clinical situation. It should augment the dietary, clinical, and anthropometric data that should also be gathered and evaluated. Used in this way, laboratory data will allow better quantification, reproducibility, and objectivity in the assessment of nutritional status.

REFERENCES

1. Zemel BS, Riley EM, Stallings VA. Evaluation of methodology for nutritional assessment in children: Anthropometrics, body composition, and energy expenditure. Annu Rev Nutr 1997;17:211–35.
2. Gidden F, Shenkin A. Laboratory support of the clinical nutrition service. Clin Chem Lab Med 2000;38:693–714.
3. Contiero E, Folin M. Trace element nutritional status: Use of hair as a diagnostic tool. Biol Trace Elem Res 1994;40:151–60.
4. Folin M, Contiero E, Vaselli GM. Trace element determination in humans: The use of blood and hair. Biol Trace Elem Res 1991;31:147–58.
5. Lopez AM, Wolsdorf J, Raszynski A, et al. Estimation of nitrogen balance based on six hour urine collection in infants. JPEN J Parenter Enteral Nutr 1986;10:517–18.
6. Boehm G, Weiner M, Schmidt C, et al. Usefulness of short term urine collection in nutritional monitoring of low birth weight infants. Acta Paediatr 1998;87:339–43.
7. Hartwick RA, Brown PR. The use of high pressure liquid chromatography in clinical chemistry and biomedical research. Adv Clin Chem 1980;21:25–99.
8. Crews HM, Ducros V, Eagles J, et al. Mass spectrometric methods for studying nutrient mineral and trace element absorption and metabolism in humans using stable isotopes. Analyst 1994;119:2491 514.
9. Yudkoff M, Nissim I. Stable isotopes as metabolic probes for nutritional studies in neonates. Clin Perinatol 1995;22:97–109.
10. Wolfe RR. Radioactive and stable isotope tracers in biomedicine. In: Principles and Practice of Kinetic Analysis. New York: Wiley-Liss; 1992.
11. Abrams SA. Clinical studies of mineral metals in children using stable isotopes. J Pediatr Gastroenterol Nutr 1994;19:151–63.
12. Hambidge KM, Krebs NF, Miller L. Evaluation of zinc metabolism with use of stable isotope techniques: Implications for the assessment of zinc status. Am J Clin Nutr 1998;68:410S–13S.
13. Abrams SA. Using stable isotopes to assess mineral absorption and utilization by children. Am J Clin Nutr 1999;70:955–64.
14. Jacob RA, Milne DB. Biochemical assessment of vitamins and trace metals. Clin Lab Med 1993;13:371–85.
15. Solomons N. Assessment of nutritional status: Functional indicators of pediatric nutriture. Pediatr Clin North Am 1985;32:319–34.
16. Louw JA, Werbreck A, et al. Blood vitamin concentrations during the acute phase response. Crit Care Med 1992;20:934–41.
17. Mitchell CO, Lipschitz DA. The effect of age and sex on routinely used measurements to assess the nutritional status of hospitalized patients. Am J Clin Nutr 1982;36:340–9.
18. Goldsmith B. Nutritional assessment in pediatric patients: How can the laboratory help? Pediatr Pathol Lab Med 1996;16:1–7.
19. Sauberlich HE, Dowdy RP, Skala JH. Laboratory tests for the assessment of nutritional status. Boca Raton, FL: CRC Press; 1999.
20. Jelliffe DB, Jelliffe EFP. Community nutritional assessment. New York: Oxford University Press; 1989.
21. Lee RD, Nieman DC. Nutritional assessment. Madison, WI: Brown & Benchmark; 1993.
22. Benjamin DR. Laboratory tests and nutritional assessment. Pediatr Clin North Am 1989;36:139–61.
23. Pesce AJ, Kaplan LA, editors. Methods in Clinical Chemistry. St Louis, Mo: CV Mosby; 1987.
24. Anonymous. Nutrition monitoring and nutrition status assessment. J Nutr 1990;120:431–53.
25. McMahon MM, Bistrian BR. The physiology of nutritional assessment and therapy in protein-calorie malnutrition. Dis Mon 1990;36:373–417.
26. Labbe RF, editor. Symposium on laboratory assessment of nutritional status. Clin Lab Med 1981;1:603.
27. Selberg O, Sel S. The adjunctive value of routine biochemistry in nutritional assessment of hospitalized patients. Clin Nutr 2001;20:477–85.
28. Bernstein LH. Utilizing laboratory parameters to monitor the effectiveness of nutritional support. Nutrition 1994;10:58–60.
29. Holick MF. Vitamin D deficiency. N Engl J Med 2007;357:266–81.
30. Tanumihardjo SA. Assessing vitamin A status: Past, present, and future. J Nutr 2004;134:290S–293S. Review
31. Blanck HM, Bowman BA, Cooper GR, et al. Laboratory issues: Use of nutrition biomarkers. J Nutr 2003;133:888X–894S. Review.
32. Potischman N. Biologic and methodologic issues for nutritional biomarkers. J Nutr 2003;133:875–880S. Review.
33. Sarhill N, Mahmoud FA, Christie R, Tahir A. Assessment of nutritional status and fluid deficits in advanced cancer. Am J Hosp Palliat Care 2003;20:465–73. Review.
34. Lebenthal E, Hatch TF, Lee PC. Carbohydrates in pediatric nutrition—consumption, digestibility, and disease. Adv Pediatr 1981;28:99–139.
35. Jequier E. Studies with direct calorimetry in humans: Thermal body insulation and thermoregulatory responses during exercise. In: Kinney J, editor. Assessment of Energy Metabolism in Health and Disease, Report of the First Ross Conference on Medical Research. Columbus, OH: Ross Laboratories; 1980.
36. Stolwijk JAJ. Partitional calorimetry. In: Kinney J, editor. Assessment of Energy Metabolism in Health and Disease, Report of the First Ross Conference on Medical Research. Columbus, OH: Ross Laboratories; 1980.
37. Johnson RE. Techniques for measuring gas exchange. In: Kinney J, editor. Assessment of Energy Metabolism in Health and Disease, Report of the First Ross Conference on Medical Research. Columbus, OH: Ross Laboratories; 1980.
38. Haugen HA, Chan LN, Li F. Indirect calorimetry: A practical guide for clinicians. Nutr Clin Pract 2007;22:377–88.
39. Buskirk ER, Mendez J. Energy: Calorie requirements. In: Alfin-Slater RB, Kritchevsky D, editors. Human nutrition: A comprehensive treatise. Vol. 3A. New York: Plenum Press; 1980.
40. Weir JB. New methods for calculating metabolic rate with special reference to protein metabolism. Nutrition 1990;6:213–21.
41. Cunningham JJ. Calculation of energy expenditure from indirect calorimetry: Assessment of the Weir equation. Nutrition 1990;6:222–3.
42. Harris JA, Benedict FG. Standard basal metabolism constants for physiologists and clinicians. A biometric study of basal metabolism in man. Washington, DC: Carnegie Institute of Washington; 1919. Publication No.: 279.
43. McClave S, Snider H, Ireton-Jones C. Can we justify continued interest in indirect calorimetry? Nutr Clin Pract 2002;17:133–6.
44. Firouzbakhsh S, Mathis RK, Dorchester WL, et al. Measured REE in children. J Pediatr Gastroenterol Nutr 1993;16:136–42.
45. Van Way CW. Variability of the Harris–Benedict equation in recently published textbooks. JPEN J Parenter Enteral Nutr 1992;16:566–7.
46. Garrel DR, Jobin N, DeJonge LH, et al. Should we still use the HB equations? Nutr Clin Pract 1996;119:99–103.
47. Frankenfield DC, Mirth ER, Rowe WA. The Harris Benedict studies of human metabolism: History and limitations. J Am Diet Assoc 1998;98:439–51.
48. Hardy-Framson CM, Leleiko NS, et al. Energy expenditure in critically ill children. Pediatr Crit Care Med 2007;8:264–7.
49. World Health Organization. Energy and protein requirements: Report of joint FAO/WHO/UNU expert consultation. Geneva: WHO; 1985. WHO Technical Report Series No.: 724.
50. Schofield C. Predicting basal metabolic rate: New standards and review of previous work. Hum Nutr Clin Nutr 1985;39:5–42.
51. Stallings VA, Fung EB. Clinical nutrition assessment of infants and children. In: Shils ME, Olson J, Shike M, et al, editors. Modern Nutrition in Health and Disease, 9th edition. Baltimore (MD): Williams & Wilkins; 1999. p. 885–93.
52. Hardy CS, Dwyer J, Snelling L, et al. Pitfalls in predicting resting energy requirements in critically ill children: A comparison of predictive methods to indirect calorimetry. Nutr Clin Pract 2002;17:182–9.
53. Thomson MA, Bucolo S, Quirk P, et al. Measured vs predicted REE in infants: A need for reappraisal. J Pediatr 1995;126:21–7.
54. Kaplan AS, Zemel BS, Neiswender KM, Stallings VA. Resting energy expenditure in clinical pediatrics: Measured vs prediction equations. J Pediatr 1995;127:200–5.

55. Coss-Bu JA, Jefferson LS, Walding LS, et al. Resting energy expenditure in children in a pediatric intensive care unit: Comparison of Harris Benedict and Talbot predictions with indirect calorimetry values. Am J Clin Nutr 1998;67:74–80.
56. Finan K, Larson DE, Goran MI. Cross validation of prediction equations for resting energy expenditure in young healthy children. J Am Diet Assoc 1997;97:140–5.
57. White MS, Shepherd RW, McEniery JA, et al. Energy expenditure in 100 ventilated critically ill children. Crit Care Med 2000;28:2307–12.
58. Wells JC. Energy metabolism in infants and children. Nutrition 1998;14:817–20.
59. Flancbaum L, Choban PS, et al. Comparison of indirect calorimetry, the Fick method, and prediction equations in estimating the energy requirements of critically ill patients. Am J Clin Nutr 1999;69:461–6.
60. Bines JE, Truby HD. Measurement of resting energy expenditure in infants. J Paediatr Child Health 2004;40:380–3.
61. Schoeller DA, VanSanten E. Measurement of energy expenditure in humans by doubly labeled water method. J Appl Physiol 1982;53:955–9.
62. Schoeller DA. Recent advances from the application of doubly labeled water to measurement of human energy expenditure. J Nutr 1999;129:1765–8.
63. Jensen CL, Butte NF, Wong WW, et al. Determining energy expenditure in preterm infants: Comparison of doubly labeled water method and indirect calorimetry. Am J Physiol 1992;263:R685–92.
64. Westerterp KR, Lefeber HN, Sulkers EJ, et al. Comparison of short term indirect calorimetry and doubly labeled water method for the assessment of energy expenditure in preterm infants. Biol Neonate 1991;60:75–82.
65. Roberts SB, Coward WA, Schlingenseipen KH, et al. Comparison of the doubly labeled water method with indirect calorimetry and a nutrient balance study for simultaneous determinations of energy expenditure, water intake, and metabolisable energy intake in preterm infants. Am J Clin Nutr 1986;44:315–22.
66. Jones PJ, Winthrop AL, Schoeller DA, et al. Validation of doubly labeled water for assessing energy expenditure in infants. Pediatr Res 1987;21:242–6.
67. Katz DP, Suchner U, Askanazi J. New horizons in nutritional biochemistry and metabolism. Nutrition 1992;8:366.
68. Waterlow JC. Protein-energy malnutrition. London: Edward Arnold; 1992.
69. Torun B, Chew F. Protein-energy malnutrition. In: Shils ME, Olson J, Shike M, et al, editors. Modern Nutrition in Health and Disease. 9th edition. Baltimore, MD: Williams & Wilkins; 1999. p. 963–88.
70. Garlick PJ. Protein turnover in the whole animal and specific tissues. In: Florkin M, Neuberger A, van Deenen LM, editors. Protein Metabolism. Amsterdam: Elsevier-North Holland; 1980.
71. Shenkin A, Cederblad G, Elia M, et al. Laboratory assessment of protein energy status. J Int Fed Clin Chem 1996;9:58–61.
72. Young VR, Bier DM. Stable isotopes (^{13}C and ^{15}N) in the study of human protein and amino acid metabolism and requirements. In: Beers RF, Bassett EG, editors. Nutritional factors: Modulating effects on metabolic processes. New York: Raven Press; 1981.
73. Waterlow JC, Garlick PJ, Millward DJ. Protein turnover in mammalian tissues and in the whole body. Amsterdam: Elsevier-North Holland; 1978.
74. Killingsworth LM. Plasma protein patterns in health and disease. CRC Crit Rev Clin Lab Sci 1979;11:1–30.
75. Spiekerman AM. Proteins used in nutritional assessment. Clin Lab Med 1993;13:353–69.
76. Boosalis MG, Ott L, Levine AS, et al. Relationship of visceral protein to nutritional status in chronic and acute stress. Crit Care Med 1989;17:741–7.
77. Lacy JA. Albumin overview: Use as a nutritional marker and therapeutic intervention. Crit Care Nurs 1991;11:46–9.
78. Doweiko JP, Nompleggi DJ. The role of albumin in human physiology and pathophysiology, part III: Albumin and disease states. JPEN J Parenter Enteral Nutr 1991;15:476–83.
79. Mascarenhas MR, Zemel B, Stallings VA. Nutritional assessment in pediatrics. Nutrition 1998;14:105–15.
80. Ingenbleek Y, Young V. Transthyretin (prealbumin) in health and disease: Nutritional implications. Annu Rev Nutr 1994;14:495–533.
81. Winkler MF, Gerrior SA, Pomp A, et al. JE. Use of retinol binding protein and prealbumin as indicators of the response to nutrition therapy. J Am Diet Assoc 1989;89:684–7.
82. Roza A, Tuitt D, Shizgal H. Transferrin–a poor measure of nutritional status. JPEN J Parenter Enteral Nutr 1984;8:523–8.
83. Cook JD, Skikne BS. Serum ferritin: A possible model for the assessment of nutrient stores. Am J Clin Nutr 1982;35:1180–5.
84. Gibson RS. Principles of Nutritional Assessment. New York: Oxford Press; 1990.
85. Sawicky CP, Nippo J, Winkler MF, et al. Adequate energy intake and improved prealbumin concentration as indicators of the response to total parenteral nutrition. J Am Diet Assoc 1992;92:1266–8.
86. Chwals WJ. Serum visceral protein levels reflect protein-calorie repletion in neonates recovering from major surgery. J Pediatr Surg 1992;27:317–21.
87. Bernstein L, Pleban W. Prealbumin in nutrition evaluation. Nutrition 1996;12:255–9.
88. Beck FK, Rosenthal TC. Prealbumin: A marker for nutritional evaluation. Am Fam Physician 2002;65:1575–8.
89. Fletcher JP, Little JM, Guest PK. A comparison of serum transferrin and serum prealbumin as nutritional parameters. JPEN J Parenter Enteral Nutr 1987;11:144–8.
90. McKone TK, Davis AT, Dean RE. Fibronectin, a new nutritional parameter. Am Surg 1985;6:336–9.
91. Unterman TG, Vazquez RM, Slas AJ, et al. Nutrition and somatomedin XIII. Usefulness of somatomedin-C in nutritional assessment. Am J Med 1985;78:228–34.
92. Clemmons DR, Underwood LE, Dickerson RN, et al. Use of plasma somatomedin C/insulin like growth factor I measurements to monitor the response to nutritional repletion in malnourished patients. Am J Clin Nutr 1985;41:191–8.
93. Thissen JP, Ketelslegers JM, Underwood LE. Nutritional regulation of the insulin-like growth factors. Endocr Rev 1994;15:80–101.
94. Holly JM, Hughes SC. Measuring insulin like growth factors: Why, where and how. J Endocrinol 1994;140:257–63.
95. Smith WJ, Underwood LE, Clemmons DR. Effects of caloric or protein restriction on insulin-like growth factor I and insulin-like growth factor binding proteins in children and adults. J Clin Endocrinol Metab 1995;80:443–9.
96. Donahue SP, Phillips LS. Response of IGF-1 to nutritional support in malnourished hospital patients: A possible indicator of short term changes in nutritional status. Am J Clin Nutr 1989;50:962–9.
97. Smith WJ, Underwood LE, Keyes L, et al. Use of insulin-like growth factor I and insulin-like growth factor binding protein measurements to monitor feeding of premature infants. J Clin Endocrinol Metab 1997;82:3982–8.
98. Burgess EJ. Insulin like growth factor 1: A valid nutritional indicator during parenteral feeding of patients suffering from an acute phase response. Ann Clin Biochem 1992;29:137–44.
99. Carpentier YA, Barthel J, Bruyns J. Plasma protein concentration in nutritional assessment. Proc Nutr Soc 1982;41:405–17.
100. Sigulem DM, Brasel JA, Velaso EG, et al. Plasma and urine ribonuclease as a measure of nutritional status in children. Am J Clin Nutr 1973;26:793–7.
101. Askanazi J, Michelsen CB, Carpentier YA. Sequential changes in muscle and plasma amino acids during injury, infection, and convalescence. Surg Forum 1979;30:90–2.
102. Viteri FE, Alvarado J. The creatinine height index: Its use in the estimation of the degree of protein depletion and repletion in protein calorie malnourished children. Pediatrics 1970;46:696–706.
103. Kesteloot H, Joossens JV. Relationship between dietary protein intake and serum urea, uric acid, and creatinine, and 24-hour urinary creatinine excretion: The BIRNH study. J Am Coll Nutr 1993;12:42–6.
104. Konstantinides FN. Nitrogen balance studies in clinical nutrition. Nutr Clin Pract 1992;7:231–8.
105. Blackburn GL, Bistrian BR, Maini BS, et al. Nutritional and metabolic assessment of the hospitalized patient. JPEN J Parenter Enteral Nutr 1977;1:11–22.
106. Burge JC, Choban P, McKnight T, et al. Urinary ammonia plus urinary urea nitrogen as an estimate of total urinary nitrogen in patients receiving parenteral nutrition support. JPEN J Parenter Enteral Nutr 1993;17:529–31.
107. Fuller NJ, Elia M. Inadequacy of urinary urea for estimating nitrogen balance. Ann Clin Biochem 1990;27:510–11.
108. Burgess EJ, Fleck A. Inadequacy of urinary urea for the estimation of nitrogen balance during total parenteral nutrition. Ann Clin Biochem 1990;27:163–4.
109. Konstantinides FN, Konstantinides NN, Li JC, et al. Urinary urea nitrogen: Too insensitive for calculating nitrogen balance studies in surgical clinical nutrition. JPEN J Parenter Enteral Nutr 1991;15:189–93.
110. Havel RJ. Classification of the hyperlipidemias. Annu Rev Med 1977;28:195–209.
111. Bachorik PS, Wood PDS. Laboratory considerations in the diagnosis and management of hyperlipoproteinemia. In: Rifkind BM, Levy RI, editors. Hyperlipidemia: Diagnosis and Therapy. New York: Grune & Stratton; 1977.
112. Hunninghake DB. Diagnosis and treatment of lipid disorders. Med Clin North Am 1994;78:247–57.
113. Gordon DJ, Probstfield JL, Garrison RJ, et al. High-density lipoprotein cholesterol and cardiovascular disease: Four prospective American studies. Circulation 1989;79:8–15.
114. Batiste MC, Schaefer EJ. Diagnosis and management of lipoprotein abnormalities. Nutr Clin Care 2002;5:115–23.
115. Schaefer EJ. Lipoproteins, nutrition, and heart disease. Am J Clin Nutr 2002;75:191–212.
116. Second Expert Panel on Detection, Evaluation, and Treatment of High Blood Cholesterol in Adults. First executive summary of National Cholesterol Education Program. JAMA 2001;285:2486–97.
117. Verhoef P. Homocysteine—An indicator of a healthy diet? Am J Clin Nutr 2007;85:1446–7.
118. Holmes KW, Kwiterovich PO. Treatment of dyslipidemia in children and adolescents. Curr Cardiol Rep 2005;7:445–56.
119. Tonstad S. Role of lipid-lowering pharmacotherapy in children. Paediatr Drugs 2000;2:11–22.
120. Bhatnagar D. Should pediatric patients with hyperlipidemia receive drug therapy? Pediatr Drugs 2002;4:223–30.
121. Holman RT. Essential fatty acid deficiency in humans. In: Galli C, Jacini G, Pecile A, editors. Dietary Lipids and Postnatal Development. New York: Raven Press; 1973.
122. Friedman Z. Essential fatty acids revisited. Am J Dis Child 1980;134:397–408.
123. Sardesai VM. The essential fatty acids. Nutr Clin Pract 1992;7:179–86.
124. Innis SM. Essential fatty acids in growth and development. Prog Lipid Res 1991;30:39–103.
125. Holman RT, Johnson SB, Mercuri O, et al. Essential fatty acid deficiency in malnourished children. Am J Clin Nutr 1981;34:1534–9.
126. Alcock NW. Laboratory tests for assessment of nutritional status. In: Shils ME, Olson J, Shike M, et al., editors. Modern Nutrition in Health and Disease, 9th edition. Baltimore, MD: Williams & Wilkins; 1999. p. 903–21.
127. Ellis KJ, Shypailo RJ. Whole body potassium measurements independent of body size. In: Ellis KJ, Eastman JD, editors. Human Body Composition: In Vivo Methods and Assessments. New York: Plenum Press; 1993. p. 371–5.
128. Heymsfield SB, Baumgartner RN, Pan SF, et al. Nutritional assessment of malnutrition by anthropometric. In: Shils ME, Olson J, Shike M, et al., editors. Modern Nutrition in Health and Disease, 9th edition. Baltimore, MD: Williams & Wilkins; 1999.
129. Brambilla P, Rolland-Cachera MFC, Testolin C, et al. Lean mass of children in various nutritional states: Comparison between DEXA and anthropometrics. Ann N Y Acad Sci 2000;904:433–6.
130. Gutin B, Litaker M, Islan S. Body composition measurement in 9–11 year old children by DEXA, skinfold thickness measurements and bioelectrical impedance analysis. Am J Clin Nutr 1996;63:287–92.
131. Schoeller DA. Bioelectrical impedance analysis: What does it measure? Ann N Y Acad Sci 2000;904:159–62.
132. Baumgartner RN, Chuntka WC, Roche AF. Bioelectrical impedance phase angle and body composition. Am J Clin Nutr 1988;48:16–23.
133. Kusher RD, Gudivaka R, Schoeller DA. Clinical characteristics influencing bioelectrical impedence analysis measurements. Am J Clin Nutr 1996;64:423S–7S.
134. Suprasongsin C, Kalhan S, Arslanian S, et al. Determination of body composition in children and adolescents: Validation of bioelectrical impedence with isotope dilution technique. J Pediatr Endocrinol Metab 1995;8:103–9.
135. Nagano M, Suita S, Yamanouchi T. The validity of bioelectrical impedence phase angle for nutritional assessment in children. J Pediatr Surg 2000;35:1035–9.
136. Newsholme EA. Carbohydrate metabolism in vivo: Regulation of the blood glucose level. Clin Endocrinol Metab 1976;5:543–78.
137. Levine R, Haft DE. Carbohydrate homeostasis. N Engl J Med 1970;283:175–83.
138. Pagliara AS, Karl IE, Haymond M, Kipnis DM. Hypoglycemia in infancy and childhood. J Pediatr 1973;82:558–77.
139. Kogut MD. Hypoglycemia: Pathogenesis, diagnosis and treatment. Curr Probl Pediatr 1974;4:1–59.
140. Lo CW, Carter EA, Walker AW. Breath tests: Principles, problems, and promise. Adv Pediatr 1983;29:105–27.
141. Levitt MD, Donaldson RM. Use of respiratory hydrogen (H_2) excretion to detect carbohydrate malabsorption. J Lab Clin Med 1970;75:937–45.
142. Bodamer OA, Halliday D. Uses of stable isotopes in clinical diagnosis and research in the pediatric population. Arch Dis Child 2001;84:444–8.
143. Scrimshaw NS, SanGiovanni JP. Synergism of nutrition, infection and immunity: An overview. Am J Clin Nutr 1997;66:464S–77S.
144. Chandra RK, Kumari S. Nutritional and immunity: An overview. J Nutr 1994;124:14335–55.

145. Chandra RK. Nutrition and the immune system: An introduction. Am J Clin Nutr 1997;66:460S–3S.
146. Chandra RK. Immunodeficiency in undernutrition and overnutrition. Nutr Rev 1981;39:225–31.
147. Chandra RK. Immunocompetence as a functional index of nutritional status. Br Med Bull 1981;37:89–94.
148. Schweigert FJ. Inflammation-induced changes in the nutritional biomarkers serum retinol and carotenoids. Curr Opin Clin Nutr Metab Care 2001;4:477–81.
149. Harbige LS. Nutrition and immunity with emphasis on infection and autoimmune disease. Nutr Health 1996;10:285–312.
150. Meakins JL, Pietsch JB, Bubenick O, et al. Delayed hypersensitivity: Indicator of acquired failure of host defenses in sepsis and trauma. Ann Surg 1977;186:241–50.
151. Bistrian BR, Blackburn GL, Scrimshaw NS, et al. Cellular immunity in semistarved states in hospitalized adults. Am J Clin Nutr 1975;28:1148–55.
152. Smythe PM, Brereton-Stiles GG, Grace HJ, et al. Thymolymphatic deficiency and depression of cell-mediated immunity in protein-calorie malnutrition. Lancet 1971;2:939–43.
153. Miller CL. Immunological assays as measurements of nutritional status: A review. JPEN J Parenter Enteral Nutr 1978;2:554–66.
154. Suskind R, Sirishinha S, Vithayasai V, et al. Immunoglobulins and antibody response in children with protein-calorie malnutrition. Am J Clin Nutr 1976;29:836–41.
155. Bell RG, Turner KJ, Suharjono S, et al. Serum and small intestinal immunoglobulin levels in undernourished children. Am J Clin Nutr 1976;29:392–7.
156. Sirisinha S, Edelman R, Suskind R, et al. Complement and C3-proactivator levels in children with protein-calorie malnutrition and effect of dietary treatment. Lancet 1973;1:1016–20.
157. Chandra RK. Serum complement and immunoconglutinin in malnutrition. Arch Dis Child 1975;50:225–9.
158. Bhaskaram P. Immunobiology of mild micronutrient deficiencies. Br J Nutr 2001;8:75–80.
159. Briefel RR. Assessment of the U.S. diet in national nutrition surveys: National collaborative efforts and NHANES. Am J Clin Nutr 1994;59:164S–7S.
160. US Department of Health, Education, and Welfare. Ten-State Nutrition Survey, 1968–1970. Atlanta, GA: The Centers for Disease Control and Prevention; 1970. DHEW Publication No.: (H5M) 72–8134.
161. Abraham S, Lowenstein FW, Johnson CL. Preliminary Findings of the First Health and Nutrition Examination Survey, United States, 1971–1972. Rockville, MD: National Center for Health Statistics; 1978.
162. US Department of Health and Human Services, National Center for Health Statistics, Centers for Disease Control and Prevention. Third National Health and Nutrition Examination, 1988–1994.
163. Hendrikse WH, Reilly JT. Malnutrition in a children's hospital. Clin Nutr 1997;16:13–18.
164. Hendricks KM, Duggan C, Gallagher U, et al. Malnutrition in hospitalized pediatric patients: Current prevalence. Arch Pediatr Adolesc Med 1995;149:1118–22.
165. Detsky AS, Baker JP, Mendelson RA, et al. Evaluating the accuracy of nutritional assessment techniques applied to hospitalized patients: Methodology and comparisons. JPEN J Parenter Enteral Nutr 1984;8:153–9.
166. Detsky AS, McLaughlin JR, Baker JP, et al. What is subjective global assessment of nutritional status? JPEN J Parenter Enteral Nutr 1987;11:8–13.
167. Hirsch S, DeObaldia N, Peterman M, et al. Subjective global assessment of nutritional status: Further validation. Nutrition 1991;7:35–7.
168. Secker DJ, Jeejeebhoy KN. Subjective global nutritional assessment for children. Am J Clin Nutr 2007;85:1083–9.
169. Underwood BA. Evaluating the nutritional status of individuals: A critique of approaches. Nutr Rev 1986;44:213–23.
170. Soldin SJ, Brugnara C, Wong EC, editors. Pediatric Reference Intervals, 6th edition. Philadelphia, PA: AACC; 2007.
171. Cunningham-Rundles S, McNeeley DF, Ananworanich J. In: Steihm ER, Ochs HD, Winkelstein JA, editors. Immunologic Disorders in Infants and Children, 5th edition. Philadelphia, PA: Elsevier Saunders; 2004. p. 766.

4

Body Composition and Growth

Lori J. Bechard, MEd, RD, LDN
Emily Wroe, BA
Kenneth Ellis, PhD

Measurement of body composition, in both clinical and research settings, has advanced the understanding of human energy metabolism by allowing the observer a closer look at physiologic changes seen during growth and disease. Growth is the maturation process characterized by change, compensation, and adaptation; it is genetically predetermined and substantially affected by hormonal, nutritional, and environmental factors. The size and shape of an individual are a result of the dynamic events preceding the time of assessment. Changes in the components of body mass are also reflective of these events, and may only be apparent by measurements of body composition, particularly when total body mass is constant.

Discovery of the importance of body composition changes in areas of acute, chronic, and preventive medicine has led to further study and refinement of the techniques used in measuring these changes. Nutritional status can no longer be based on height and weight alone. In many diseases, including protein-energy malnutrition, cancer, inflammatory bowel disease, chronic renal disease, and acquired immune deficiency syndrome, weight measurements can overestimate the nutritional well-being of the patient. In addition, it is possible to achieve an acceptable weight while preserving or enhancing excess body fat or body water, thus confounding the benefits of traditional nutritional rehabilitation. A closer look at body composition can elucidate the attenuation of lean body mass associated with disease, permitting a customized approach to nutritional management.

The study of body composition delineates and describes the effect of genetic, nutritional, and physical activity factors on fat, muscle, and bone development. It is important to identify the amount of each component as well as their rates of growth and their regional variations in an effort to define possible relationships to current and future health risks.[1,2] Changes in body compartments that occur during fetal life and through infancy, childhood, adolescence, adulthood, and aging are presented in the first part of the chapter. An emphasis is placed on the distribution of fluid, fat, muscle, and bone mass in the different stages of the life cycle during health and disease.

The measurement of body composition has become an important clinical tool in the monitoring of changes of fat and fat-free mass (FFM) during growth, athletic conditioning, and in the nutritional management of patients with acute or chronic illness. An understanding of the various methods and measurements of body composition is crucial in the interpretation of pediatric and nutrition literature. Each method explores body composition from a different perspective, studying the chemical components or taking advantage of certain physical principles. On the whole, the use of different methods in the same set of subjects has allowed the cross-validation of the various techniques and has permitted a more detailed understanding of body composition. A glossary of commonly used body composition terms is given in Table 1.

BODY COMPOSITION CHANGES DURING GROWTH

A schematic representation of the changes in body composition throughout life is shown in Figure 1. More specific details of the compositional variation during growth are presented in Table 2. Figure 2 depicts changes in body compartments during fetal development; this graph can be helpful when assessing the growth of a preterm infant.[3]

Changes in Body Fat Mass

Fat is the most variable of body components, ranging from about 5% to more than 50% of body weight; the normal range is narrower, between about 10 and 30%. During intrauterine life, the differentiation of fat starts in the second trimester of gestation, between about the fourteenth and twenty-fourth weeks of pregnancy. It becomes evident in the head (buccal pad area) and neck, progressing rapidly to the trunk, arms, and, finally, the lower limbs. At the beginning of the third trimester, at approximately the twenty-eighth week, adipose tissue is already present in the principal fat deposit areas. Therefore, it appears that the second trimester of pregnancy is a sensitive period for the development of fat tissue.[7] In addition, abnormalities in fat mass can be attributed to changes in maternal nutrition in late gestation, during the period of maximal fetal growth.[8]

The possibility that nutritional alterations at critical periods of development are the source of nutritional states such as adult obesity has been suggested by certain authors.[8–10] Follow-up studies[11] of infants exposed to famine prenatally or early in life and of infants of diabetic mothers[12] strongly suggest that prenatal and perinatal under- or overnutrition influences the development of fatness and its related diseases in later life. For example, infants of diabetic mothers have increased body fat compared with infants of women with normal glucose tolerance.[12] Altered maternal nutrition can also change the expression of appetite-regulating neuropeptides in the fetal brain, enhancing the later risk for obesity.[10] Increased birth weight and postnatal growth are

Table 1 Glossary of Body Composition Terms

Term	Definition
Fat mass	All ether-extractable lipids in the body, including nonessential lipids (~90%), triglycerides, and essential lipids
Essential lipid	Lipids in bone marrow, cell membranes, phospholipids in neurons
Adipose tissue	Fat (80 to 85%) and its supporting cellular and extracellular structures (2% protein and 13 to 18% water)
Lean body mass (LBM)	Body mass free from adipose tissue
Fat-free mass	Nonfat mass, with four major constituents: water, protein, glycogen, and mineral; equals LBM plus nonfat components of adipose tissue
Total body water (TBW)	Total water amount in the body
Intracellular water (ICW)	Water content of the cellular compartment
Extracellular water (ECW)	Nonmetabolizing fluid surrounding cells; distributed primarily in the plasma and interstitial fluid compartments
Body cell mass	Cellular components of the body
Extracellular solids	Extracellular chemical compounds distributed in organic (collagen, reticular, and elastic fibers) and nonorganic (bone minerals, bicarbonate, and citrate) material.
Bone mineral content (BMC)	Bone mineral content (g/cm), as measured by absorptiometric techniques
Bone mineral density (BMD)	Ratio of BMC to bone width (g/cm^2), as measured by absorptiometric techniques

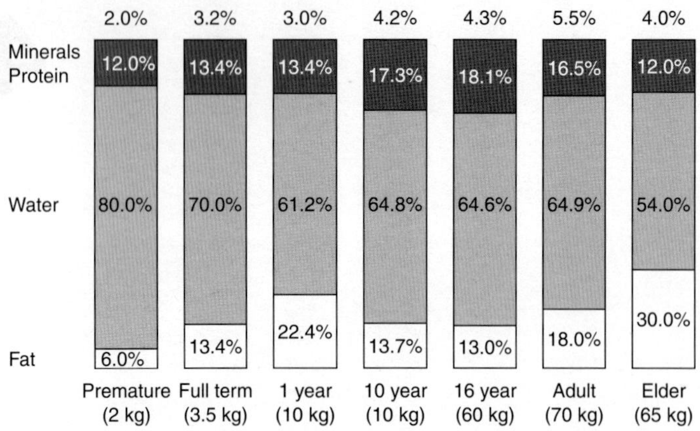

Figure 1 Changes in proportions of body composition with growth and aging.

positively correlated with lean body mass, an effect that can persist until later in life.[4,13] Increased birth weight is also positively correlated with body mass index (BMI) and inversely with central adiposity.[13,14] Therefore, low-birth-weight infants have higher percent body fat and less lean body mass, with an increased later risk for central obesity.[14,15] These data suggest that preventing growth failure in utero and in early life are important for body composition, and could have long-term consequences. See Chapter 27, "Fetal Infant and Childhood Growth and Diseases of Later Life," for more details.

Recent research also indicates that certain genes involved in embryonic development may play important roles in adipocyte development and fat distribution.[16] Even before birth, there appear to be regional differences in fat accumulation that could have important significance for the future. Cell characteristics and normal growth patterns differ from one fat depot to another. After birth, hormonal responsiveness of fat tissue varies according to its location.[7] It has also been suggested that the postnatal environment may be very influential in the development of obesity in later life; weight gain in the first week of life may be a critical determinant of adult obesity.

The infant in utero increases its fat content from 2.5% at 1 kg of weight to a fat mass of 13.7% for boys and 14.9% for girls in the full-term newborn.[4] From birth, the accumulation of fat progresses rapidly to peak at 29.1% in boys and 32.0% in girls at age 6 months,[6] probably owing to a high intake of energy and relatively little activity. An interesting finding in this area is that breast-fed infants have a different accumulation of fat than formula-fed infants do. Breast-fed infants have less fat, with the greatest differences evident between 9 and 15 months of age. Differences in body fat also depend on the proportion of protein and the type of fat contained in certain formulas. However, some studies have found that these differences do not persist after 1 year of life, and whether infant feeding mode affects body composition later in life is still unclear.[17] With increasing age, fat content drops, and the values fall to a minimum of 12.8% at 7 years in boys and 16.4% at 6 years in girls, with a discrete increase afterward, the "adiposity rebound,"[15] to 13.7% in boys and 19.4% in girls at the age of 10.[4]

Although there are sexual differences in body composition at birth or even sooner, the predominance of fatness in girls becomes remarkable during the adolescent years. In both sexes, puberty is characterized by substantial increases in both adipocyte size and total number and by a centripetal change in fat distribution, which is especially marked in males. In terms of fat percentage, males reach peak values during early adolescence and then show a decrease throughout adolescent growth, probably due to a rapid accumulation in lean body mass,[18] whereas females, after an initial decline, show a continuous increase in fat percentage throughout their eighteenth year. There are also significant gender differences in subcutaneous fat distribution, with a preponderance of adipose tissue in the upper part of the body (above the umbilicus) in males and in the lower part in females. This tendency for concentration of fat in the abdomen of males and the hips of females is seen at least as early as 4 years, with this sex difference in fat distribution becoming marked during adolescence. Some of this variation can be attributed to the effects of adrenal and ovarian hormones. In females, a significant secretion of estrogen and progesterone induces a slight increase in trochanteric adipocyte volume and number, whereas in males, the latter are significantly reduced by androgens.[7]

Table 2 Body Composition of Reference Children and Adolescents

			Percentage of Body Weight						
Age (y)	Length (cm)	Weight (kg)	Fat	Protein	Mineral	Carbohydrate	TBW	ECW	ICW
Boys									
Birth	51.6	3.5	13.7	12.9	3.2	0.5	69.6	42.5	27.0
0.5	67.9	8.04	29.1	10.9	2.4	0.5	57.2	32.9	24.3
1	76.1	10.03	25.6	12.3	2.7	0.5	59.0	31.6	27.4
1.5	82.6	11.43	24.5	12.9	3.0	0.5	59.1	30.1	29.4
2	87.6	12.46	25.4	13.5	3.1	0.5	58.1	26.6	30.7
5	109.9	18.7	14.6	15.8	3.7	0.5	65.4	30.0	35.4
10	137.5	31.4	13.7	16.8	4.1	0.5	64.8	26.7	38.0
12.5	153.0	42.3	16.3	16.4	4.1	0.6	62.7	26.4	36.4
15.5	171.5	59.5	13.0	17.4	4.5	0.6	64.6	25.8	38.8
18.5	177.0	69.9	12.9	17.7	4.8	0.7	64.1	24.7	39.4
Girls									
Birth	50.5	3.3	14.9	12.8	3.2	0.5	68.6	42.0	26.7
0.5	66.5	7.6	32.0	10.4	2.3	0.5	54.9	31.7	23.2
1	75.3	9.5	27.6	12.2	2.7	0.5	56.9	29.7	27.4
1.5	82.0	10.94	26.3	12.7	2.9	0.5	57.8	29.0	28.5
2	87.7	12.02	25.4	13.1	3.0	0.5	57.7	29.0	29.4
5	108.4	17.7	16.7	15.0	3.1	0.5	64.6	31.0	33.6
10	138.3	32.6	19.4	15.0	3.1	0.5	62.0	28.1	33.9
12.5	154.6	43.8	21.5	15.4	4.2	0.5	58.5	25.6	32.9
15.5	162.1	55.0	24.7	14.9	4.5	0.5	55.5	23.7	31.8
18.5	164.0	57.0	25.0	14.9	4.4	0.7	55.2	23.5	31.7

Adapted from references 4, 5, and 6.
ECW = extracellular water; ICW = intracellular water; TBW = total body water.

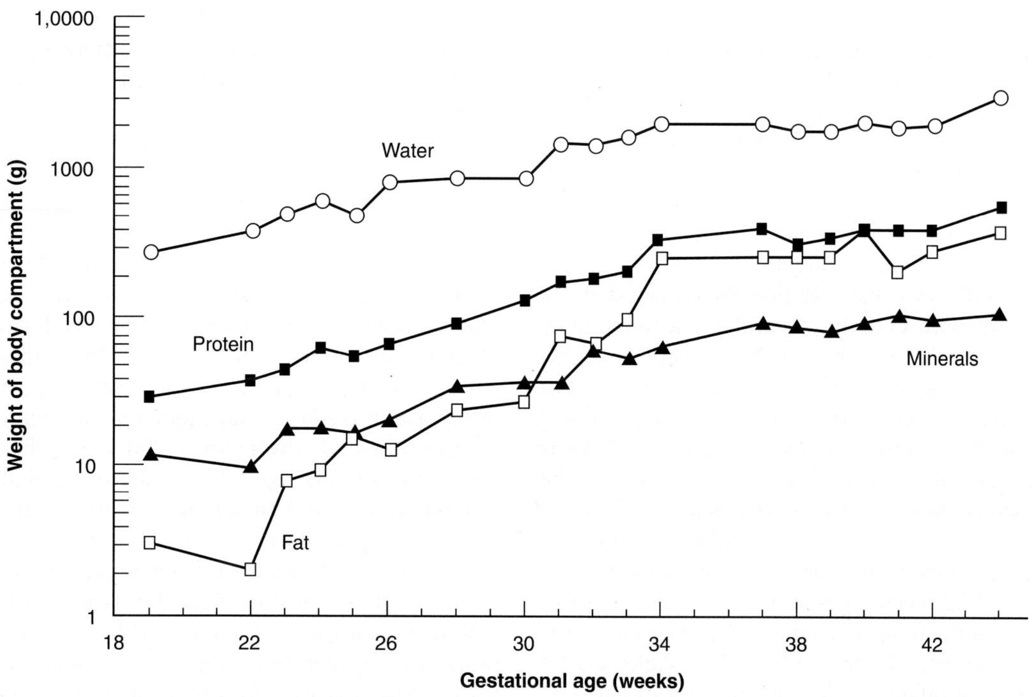

Figure 2 Changes in body composition during fetal development and early life. (Reproduced from reference 3.)

With aging, body fat in men slowly increases from about 18% in those 18 to 25 years of age to 36% in those 65 to 85 years old; in women, a gradual increase from 33 to 45% is found in similar age groups. In a multiethnic longitudinal study of Americans, percent fat mass in males increased from about 20 to 23% at age 18 years to about 25 to 27% at age 60 to 69 years. In females of the same ages, the increase was from about 31 to 33% to about 37 to 40%.[18] These larger means reflect the obesity epidemic. The preponderance of fat in females at all ages, especially in the lower part of the body, could be related to their capacity for childbearing as an adaptation mechanism for the preservation of the species. There is a need for important reserves for the fetus and newborn.[19] Nevertheless, in a minority of normal males and females, the adipose tissue distribution presents the sexual differentiation of the opposite sex.[19] In women with the android fat distribution, the risk factors for developing diabetes, hypertension, or hyperlipidemia are similar to those of men. In these women, there is no clear explanation for this different pattern of fat distribution, although it has been suggested that they might have an inherited increased sensitivity of their adipocytes to androgens and possibly to cortisol.[19]

Ethnic differences in fat accumulation during growth have been described. A study of White, African-American, and Hispanic girls reported a higher percentage of body fat in the Hispanic and African-American groups than in the White group when adjusted for body size. Bone mineral content and lean tissue mass were also greater in African-American girls than in White or Hispanic girls.[20] A similar study of multiethnic boys showed greater bone mineral content in the African-American children, but the highest percentage of body fat was found in the Hispanic group and the lowest body fat values were found in the African-American boys.[21] In another longitudinal study, no difference in total body fat was found across ethnic groups in males, but in females mean total body fat was highest in non-Hispanic African-American females, followed by Mexican-Americans and then non-Hispanic White females.[18] White children have a more peripheral distribution of body fat than Latin American, Japanese, or African-American children. African-American children tend to have a more centralized pattern. These ethnic differences are evident as early as the preschool period and continue throughout adolescence. The pattern of less peripheral fat has also been found in studies of children from several Latin American countries.[22] It could reflect genetic differences as well as different lifestyles and nutritional and health habits. Ethnic differences have also been found among Asian adolescents and adults. These studies suggest the need for ethnicity-specific references for body composition values.

The tracking of total body fat and fat distribution measurements has not been clearly demonstrated in children. Serial and repetitive measurements of body fat distribution might decrease intraindividual variation and improve reliability of tracking overtime. It appears that the majority of overweight 1-year-olds display normal levels of fatness as adolescents and adults and that whereas overweight in early childhood is not well correlated with adult obesity, overweight in later childhood and adolescence is.[23]

Long-term follow-up studies have found that truncal fat predominance and increased BMI in childhood were associated with an increased risk of central obesity in adulthood.[24] However, a longitudinal study of men and women followed from birth until age 43 found that for any given adult body size, those who had been lighter in childhood were more at risk for abdominal obesity, suggesting that insulin resistance may be linked to low weight in childhood.[25] Correlations have been shown between body fatness and risk factors for coronary heart disease and diabetes as early as 7 years of age.[26] Overweight in adolescent males has been associated with increased risk of mortality from all causes and from coronary heart disease after 55 years of follow-up.[27]

In addition to total body fat, the location of fat plays an important role in the risks of developing cardiovascular disease, diabetes, hypertension, gallbladder disease, stroke, and overall mortality. It appears that at least three principal components of body fat are associated with health outcome: total amount of fat expressed as a percentage of body weight, amount of subcutaneous truncal or abdominal fat, and quantity of visceral fat located within the intra-abdominal cavity.[28] Adult diabetogenic or atherogenic obesity tends to be more centripetal than peripheral, more the abdominal "apple" shape than the gluteofemoral "pear" shape, more intra-abdominal visceral than extra-abdominal subcutaneous, and more in the upper body than in the lower body; this holds true for both men and women with android distribution of fat.[19]

Risk factors for the development of obesity can be considered as either genetic or environmental from changes in diet, exercise, or lifestyle.[16] Some authors have reported a correlation between body fat and the amount of time spent watching television,[29] whereas others have not found this association.[30] Along with other benefits, regular exercise results in decreased body fat and increased bone mineralization and muscle mass.[31] In general, athletes have a lower percentage of body fat and greater lean body mass than their nonathletic peers. However, there is considerable variability among individuals and types of activities. Athletes participating in sports in which body weight is supported (eg, swimming, cycling, kayaking) or in which body weight is not translocated (eg, throwing, lifting) tend to have a higher percentage of body fat than athletes who participate in sports that require horizontal or vertical translation of body weight (eg, running, jumping). In sports in which weight is a factor, such as gymnastics, ballet, and wrestling, the effort to decrease body fat can affect performance and induce eating disorders. This phenomenon has occurred in both male and female athletes.[32] In obese adults, intensive and extensive aerobic exercise training can not only induce moderate to high fat losses but also reduce central subcutaneous fat, which is more noticeable in males.

The increased percentage of body fat seen in the elderly population is probably attributable to decreased physical activity. With aging, there is a decline in muscle strength and muscle mass that could be counteracted by regular physical exercise. The capacity to increase muscle mass and muscle strength is retained into old age. Physical training, especially resistance exercise of significant intensity, frequency, and duration, could retard the loss in muscle mass closely associated with bone mineral decline and increase in body fat. Hence, the associated abnormalities of diabetes, coronary heart disease, osteoporosis, and fractures could also be reduced.[33]

With some method of measuring body composition, the physician should assess the contribution of fat to the variation of body weight in order to make the appropriate recommendations concerning nutrition, exercise, or lifestyle to promote lifelong health.

Changes in Body Water

Water content is greatest during fetal life—about 88.6% of body weight at 24 weeks' gestation and approximately 75% at term. After birth, it drops rapidly and is about 60% at age 4 months. From then until adolescence, it ranges between 60 and 65%.[34] During the first years of life, the extracellular water (ECW) volume exceeds the intracellular water (ICW) volume, and with growth this relationship changes. The ratio of extracellular to intracellular fluid volume declines during growth. ICW initially is about 25 to 30% of body weight but by adolescence constitutes 35 to 40%, principally because the child's muscle mass increases. At the same time, ECW slowly drops from about 40% to approximately 20 to 25% of body weight.[34] In the elderly there is a decrease in total body water (TBW)[18] and an increase in the ratio of ECW to ICW, which can differ by race, with African-Americans showing the greatest relative increase in ECW.[35]

Small-for-gestational-age full-term and preterm infants have a greater proportion of body water at birth than do their appropriately grown peers, suggesting that fetal growth deficits in this population are not attributable to abnormalities in body water regulation.[36] In disease states such as malnutrition, there is an expansion of ECW; similar patterns have been observed after surgery, in patients with cancer, and in sepsis.[37] The ECW-to-ICW ratio appears to be an accurate predictor of clinical outcome and mortality,[37] and a strong correlation between ECW-to-ICW ratio changes and protein and energy intakes has been found. For this reason, the availability of these measurements could aid the clinician in monitoring nutritional rehabilitation in the acute care of critically ill patients.[37]

Changes in Body Mineral Content

Throughout life, bone is constantly being formed and resorbed. The process of bone modeling, characterized by changes in the shape of bones, takes place from birth until the cessation of longitudinal bone growth. Thereafter, bone tissue within the existing skeletal structure is continuously being formed and resorbed, through the remodeling process, with minimal change in bone volume.[38] The skeleton develops through infancy, childhood, and puberty, reaching maturity by late adolescence. The rate of bone modeling varies greatly during these different biologic stages. The skeletal mass of infants doubles during the first year of life, and approximately 37% of the total skeletal mass of adults is accumulated during adolescence.[39] The annual increment in bone mineral density (BMD) values is high during the first 3 years of life and decreases thereafter until puberty, as occurs with height growth velocity. During puberty, there is a 2-year peak of skeletal growth, during which adolescents accumulate over 25% of adult bone.[40] The adult reference man has a calcium content of 1.2 kg.[41]

Until 10 weeks' gestation, the human skeleton is composed entirely of cartilage, a tissue quite histologically and chemically distinct from cortical bone. At about 10 weeks, a primary center of ossification begins to develop in the shafts of long bones (eg, femur) and the collagen laid down is calcified by the deposition of mineral into it. The osseous tissue gradually extends along the shaft, replacing the cartilage and also forming the spongy trabecular bone of the metaphyses.[42] At around 22 weeks' gestation, cartilage comprises 42% of the total skeleton in the 500 g fetus; it is 33% in the full-term fetus.[43] The skeleton of a full-term infant contains about 30 g of calcium, most of which was deposited during the last trimester of intrauterine life.[38] Fetal intrauterine calcium accretion increases exponentially during the last trimester of pregnancy, from 130 mg/kg/d at 28 weeks' gestation to 150 mg/kg/d at 36 to 38 weeks' gestation.[43] These values are so high that human milk can supply to a premature infant only a fraction of the amounts needed to emulate the intrauterine accretion rate.[44] Insufficient intake of calcium and phosphate is the primary cause of osteopenia and rickets of prematurity.[45] In studies of premature infants when calcium and phosphate intake is increased by supplementing their mother's milk[46] or their formula, bone mineralization increases significantly, and can lead to normal bone mass at expected term.[47]

Absorptiometric techniques have permitted the study of bone mineralization measured as bone mineral content or BMD during growth. Intrauterine bone mineralization has been determined by measuring the BMD inappropriate for gestational age infants born at between 30 and 41 weeks' gestation[48] and between 22 and 42 weeks' gestation.[49] BMD and bone width at birth were found to correlate with gestational age and birth weight.[50] These values of BMD between 30 and 41 weeks' gestation have been used as reference curves[51] to compare various feeding regimens in the premature infant.

BMD increases over the first year of life, at a slower rate during the first 6 months, and varies with the type of feeding.[52] Higher BMD values have been found in supplemented breast-fed infants[46] or cow's milk formula-fed, full-term, and premature infants[53] when compared with those in unsupplemented breast-fed infants. In a study of preterm infants fed either preterm formula or fortified breast milk, no difference in bone mineralization and total bone mass was found among the two groups.[50] Lower values have been observed in infants receiving soy-based formula when compared with infants receiving cow's milk formula[54]; however, in later studies with soy formulas modified to improve the bioavailability of minerals, no differences in BMD were found when compared with cow's milk formula.[55] The long-term consequences of the differences in BMD with various types of feedings in early infancy are as yet unknown. One study found that bone mass accretion is less in infants fed human milk or low-mineral formula in the first 6 months of life, but those fed human milk had greater bone mass accretion in the second 6 months than those fed formula. By 1 year of age, there was no difference in bone mass among different feeding groups.[56] Similarly, no difference in BMD has been found in children of 4 years of age who were breast-fed versus those who were formula fed.[57] No gender or ethnicity differences in BMD content have been found in full-term or preterm newborns,[50] but in children up to 4 years, males have been found to have higher BMD regardless of feeding type.[57] After that, there is a wide variation in BMD as a function of age, gender, and ethnicity.[58–60] Some studies indicate that gender is more important than race in determining BMD.[59] Boys appear to have slightly higher BMD values in cortical bone than girls do,[58] and African-Americans have higher values than Whites.[61,62] With the onset of puberty, the difference between males and females increases significantly. Ethnic differences in BMD among Blacks, Whites, Lebanese, and Asians have also been reported in adolescents and adults.[58,62]

In the lumbar spine (predominantly trabecular bone), there is a gradual linear increase in BMD with age in both sexes before puberty, at approximately 9 to 10 years of age, followed by accelerated increments during puberty. Thereafter, BMD values are higher in girls, possibly because of earlier pubertal development, until the age of 15 years,[58] or until Tanner Stage IV[63] with marked slowing afterward. In girls, peak bone mass in the spine and femoral neck is probably achieved by 15 years of age, with the maximal peak mineralization velocity at 12.5 years.[40] In boys, the most rapid increase in axial BMD occurs at 14 years of age,[40] and peak bone mass is not achieved until the age of 17 or 18 years or Tanner Stage IV.[63] During puberty, skeletal bone mass reaches over 90% of its maximum, but does not peak until age 25 to 30.[64]

These absorptiometric data, showing the relatively greater importance in accumulating bone mass of early adolescence in girls compared with late adolescence, agree with studies done with other methods. Abrams, in a study of calcium kinetics in girls 4.9 to 16.7 year old using intravenous ^{42}Ca, found that calcium deposition and the size of the exchangeable pool in bone reached a maximum during early puberty and decreased in late puberty,[65] suggesting that the greatest period of calcium transfer to the bone is in the prepubertal and early pubertal periods. Because peak bone mass accumulation is achieved during adolescence, current recommendations for calcium nutrition reflect a greater requirement for these age groups (See Appendix II, "Nutritional

Requirements," for Dietary Reference Intakes). It has been suggested that prevention of osteoporosis consists primarily of maximizing peak bone mass during the years of growth and skeletal consolidation; however, there may be insufficient knowledge to link bone mineral status or growth rate in adolescents to long-term benefits in old age.[66]

Genetic factors are probably the strongest predictors of peak bone density. It has been suggested that genetics contribute 70 to 80% of the variance in bone mass, with the environment contributing the remaining 20 to 30%.[67] The influence of genetics is higher in premenopausal women,[68] and premenopausal daughters of postmenopausal women with osteoporosis have lower bone mass than other women of the same age.[69] Moreover, BMD correlates more closely in monozygotic than in dizygotic twins.[67,68]

Within the modifiable environmental factors, calcium intake could play a significant role in peak bone mass. For the growing individual, there is a significant positive relationship between calcium intake and retention. Variations in calcium nutrition early in life could account for as much as 5 to 10% of the difference in peak bone mass, and most older children and adolescents in the United States do not achieve the recommended intake of calcium, which is necessary for the development of peak bone mass and may be important in reducing the risk of fractures and osteoporosis later in life.[70] However, a firm link between bone mineral status in children and future fracture risk has yet to be established.[66] Finally, weight-bearing activity and physical exercise during childhood, adult life, and in the elderly have a positive impact on peak bone mass.

With this in mind, osteoporosis has become the domain of the pediatrician as the interplay of genetics, nutrition, and activity is better understood and preventive measures can be undertaken. There is an increasing prevalence of obesity in children, and children who are overweight could have an increased risk of fractures owing to lower BMD,[71] although some studies show no difference in bone mineral content between obese and lean children.[68] However, a higher proportion of lean body mass is associated with a higher BMD.[66] In practical terms, the pediatrician should encourage the attainment of normal body weight for height and the adequate intake of calcium during the first 3 years of life and also during the prepubertal and pubertal stages, when the highest rates of bone mineralization take place. Further research is needed to link bone density in young people to long-term fracture risk.[66]

Changes in Skeletal Muscle Mass

There is no definitive in vivo method of measuring total muscle mass. Neither total body potassium (TBK) nor total body nitrogen (TBN) can identify muscle cells specifically. However, because about 60% of TBK is found in skeletal muscle, accurate models to predict skeletal muscle mass have been developed using this strategy. Although two metabolic end products released from myocytes—creatinine and 3-methyl-histidine—have been used to estimate whole body muscle mass, their application is limited by the constraints stated in detail below.[72,73] However, in certain well-controlled conditions, they can give accurate results.[74]

Regional body muscle composition can be assessed by means of imaging techniques and also with absorptiometric techniques.[72] Accurate estimates of muscle mass can also be obtained with anthropometric measurements of midarm, midthigh, and midcalf circumferences, an inexpensive method useful in the field. However, the equations must be validated for specific study populations. This technique is particularly useful in the clinical setting when subjects can be followed overtime.

Skeletal muscle represents 22 to 25% (~850 g) of the mass of a newborn infant and approximately 30 to 45% (~28 kg) of the total body weight of an adult, although the range in values reported for the adult is highly variable. The skeletal muscle of a newborn contains 27% of TBN, 33% of TBK, and 28% of TBW.[41] The chemical change in the composition of skeletal muscle during early development is a decrease in the percentage of water and an increase in the protein concentration. As the fibers increase in number and size, the extracellular material, which makes up a large part of fetal skeletal muscle, is replaced by muscle fibers.[42] The muscle mass constitutes the largest part of the soft tissue mass, except in extremely obese individuals, in whom adipose tissue might predominate.[42] Depending on gender, age, and health status, between one-third and one-half of total body protein is within skeletal muscle.[72]

The process of growth of the total muscle mass is not uniform and develops slowly during childhood, with a growth spurt in the adolescent years, which is more intense and prolonged in boys than in girls.[41] The development of muscle mass is influenced by several factors, including age, sex, ethnicity, nutrition, hormonal and metabolic states, and exercise. Estimated muscle mass as a percentage of body weight increases from 42 to 54% in boys between 5 and 17 years of age. In girls, it increases from about 40 to 45% between 5 and 13 years of age, decreasing somewhat thereafter. This decrease is probably attributable to the relatively higher accumulation of fat in the adolescent female. At all ages from birth to adulthood, muscle mass predominates in males. After 60 years of age, after adjustment for height and weight, there is a substantial decrease in muscle mass.[58,75] This decrease is greater in men and in African-Americans. Low physical activity, tobacco smoking, and low testosterone are risk factors for sarcopenia in this population.[75] In a group of men and women over 64 years of age, sarcopenia was present in 22 to 27% of the individuals and increased with advancing age.[76]

This sarcopenia that occurs in the elderly could be delayed by regular exercise.[33] Physical activity should be promoted during the early periods of life to create positive habits that can continue thereafter, favoring the muscle, bone, and cardiovascular systems, to decrease the tendency toward obesity and sarcopenia.

Changes in Visceral Mass

Growth and development of the viscera are associated with the same changes in chemical composition as those seen in muscle mass, namely, a decrease in the proportion of water and an increase in the proportion of protein. Extracellular elements such as sodium and chloride decrease, whereas intracellular elements such as potassium and magnesium either remain the same or increase.

The brain grows rapidly from midgestation to 18 months after birth, when it reaches about 70% of its adult mass. Growth and development of the brain are characterized by a decrease in the percentage of water and an increase in protein, but the brain differs from most other tissues in that lipids form an integral part of the structure. Myelination begins before birth, but most of it takes place between birth and 3 years of age, when the brain is 80 to 90% of its mass at maturity. Up to the age of 3 years there is a considerable increase in the concentration of lipid, with a consequent decrease in the percentage of water. After 3 years, the changes in composition are relatively small.[42]

During the myelination period there is a rapid accumulation in the brain of the omega-3 and omega-6 long-chain polyunsaturated fatty acids (PUFAs)—docosahexaenoic acid (DHA; 22:6ω-3), arachidonic acid (AA; 20:4ω-6), and adrenic acid (22:4ω-6)—which are important structural components of the cell membrane phospholipids. The type of lipid that accumulates in the brain during these first few years is influenced by early nutrition and might have functional implications, especially related to visual maturation and cognitive development.[77] Preterm infants who receive formulas with a high linoleic to α-linolenic acid ratio and practically devoid of longer chain PUFAs show a marked decrease in the DHA-to-AA ratio in brain and retina.[78] On the other hand, human milk contains enough precursors and long-chain PUFAs to fulfill the infant's requirements for brain growth.[79] These factors have led to the study and development of infant formulas containing DHA and AA, which have been successful in approaching the fatty acid accretion pattern of breast-fed infants in babies who are fed with these formulas.[77]

The other major organs—liver, kidney, lung, heart, skin, and spleen—also change in chemical composition in the same way, with a decrease in the proportion of water and an increase in protein. The kidney has more sodium and less potassium at each age than muscle or liver does.

In the skin, the protein increases, but it also changes in type: In the fetus, less than 20% by mass is collagen; the rest is mainly elastin. By term, the collagen represents 63% and in the adult 90%.[42] Finally, the immune system is also an important component of the body's lean nonmuscle compartment; lymphocytes alone account for

Table 3 Contributions of Organs and Major Tissues to Body Weight

	Percentage of Body Weight			
Organ or Tissue	Fetus (20 to 24 wk)	Full-Term Newborn	Adult Male	Adult Female
Skeletal muscle	25.0	25.0	40.0	29.3
Skeleton	22.0	18.0	17.1	17.1
Skin	13.0	15.0	3.7	3.1
Liver	4.0	5.0	2.6	2.4
Brain	13.0	13.0	2.0	2.1
Lungs	3.3	1.5	1.4	1.4
Kidneys	3.1	1.6	0.4	0.5
Heart	0.6	0.5	0.5	0.4
Spleen	–	0.2	0.3	0.3

Adapted from reference 42.

approximately 2% of total body weight and 8% of fat-free solid in the adult. The status of the immune system is intimately related to body composition via the known effects of cytokines on muscle protein metabolism.[80]

The proportion of body weight contributed by major organs and tissues is presented in Table 3. At any age, muscle, skeleton, skin, liver, and brain account for more than 70% of body mass. With increasing age, some organs, such as liver, spleen, and kidneys, appear to atrophy, whereas hypertrophy is common in others, such as prostate, lungs, and heart.[81]

General Changes in Fat-Free Mass

Fat-free body mass increases rapidly during the late fetal and newborn period, followed by a rapid deceleration between the first and third years of life. Afterward, growth velocity slows until about 10 years of age, when the adolescent growth spurt is initiated. During the first years of life, there is a slight predominance of FFM in males. This difference between the sexes becomes more pronounced during the adolescent period. FFM in boys increases rapidly between 12 and 15 years of age and continues to age 18, while that of girls increases steadily until about 15 years of age, and then remains constant.[82,83] The pattern of growth in FFM is correlated with changes in height.[41] At the other end of the life cycle, aging is marked by a progressive loss of lean body mass, especially skeletal muscle and bone mass.[33]

Achieving Chemical Maturity

Most healthy young adults have achieved chemical stability of their FFM. This concept of chemical maturity was introduced by Moulton in 1923. Realizing the chemical changes that occur during growth, he found that the body composition of most species approached that of the adult when puberty was reached.[31] At this point, FFM becomes relatively constant, with a water content between 72 and 74%, a protein content of approximately 19%, a potassium content of 60 to 70 mmoles/kg of body weight in men and 50 to 60 mmoles/kg of body weight in women, and a mineral content of 6.8%.[31,84] The completion of chemical maturation is also reflected in the stabilization of various constants relating one component of body composition to another, such as potassium to nitrogen and ECW to ICW, and intracellular potassium concentration.[34] Because conditions such as pregnancy, aging, disease, nutritional status, and genetics can affect an individual's FFM composition, the usefulness of these constants is debatable.

Changes in the FFM of body compartments as a function of age are shown in Figure 3. Variation in chemical maturity during growth is greater than the changes associated with aging. During growth, chemical maturity occurs at different stages for different constituents of FFM. Muscles, visceral tissues, and bone all reach chemical maturity at different rates. For example, bone mineral maturation appears not to occur until the third decade of life. Body potassium, mainly reflecting increases in muscle mass, increases gradually from birth to 20 years of age in males and from birth to 15 to 18 years of age in females. Differences in peak muscle mass as it relates to timing of puberty are apparent between genders and among ethnicities.[83] Body potassium also declines in parallel with muscle mass in aging[41] (Figure 3A). The FFM of children contains relatively more water than that of adults. The hydration constant of FFM ranges from 80% in the newborn to 75% in early puberty and 73% in adults (Figure 3B). Protein content increases from about 15% at birth to about 19.5% in boys and 18.7% in girls at age 10 years.[11] Approximately 0.5% of body weight (0.6% of FFM) is carbohydrate. Bone mineral content rises during childhood and especially in adolescence. It gradually increases from 3.7% of FFM in infants to 5.2% in the prepubescent male, 6.2% in the postpubescent male at around 15.5 years of age, and then reaches 6.8% in the adult.[31] Bone gain continues during the third decade of life and then plateaus. Bone loss begins in the fourth or fifth decade of life, varying from one skeletal site to another and between sexes (Figure 3C).

The relative content of water, protein, and minerals determines the density of the FFM. During growth, as water content decreases and protein and mineral content rise, there is an increase in body density. Water and bone mineral are the principal factors in the change in density of the FFM, water because it is the largest constituent of the FFM and bone mineral because its density is very high, at 3.0 g/cm^3. With aging there is a decline in body density[86] (Figure 3D). Consequently, body composition in children is not correctly estimated if adult constants are used.

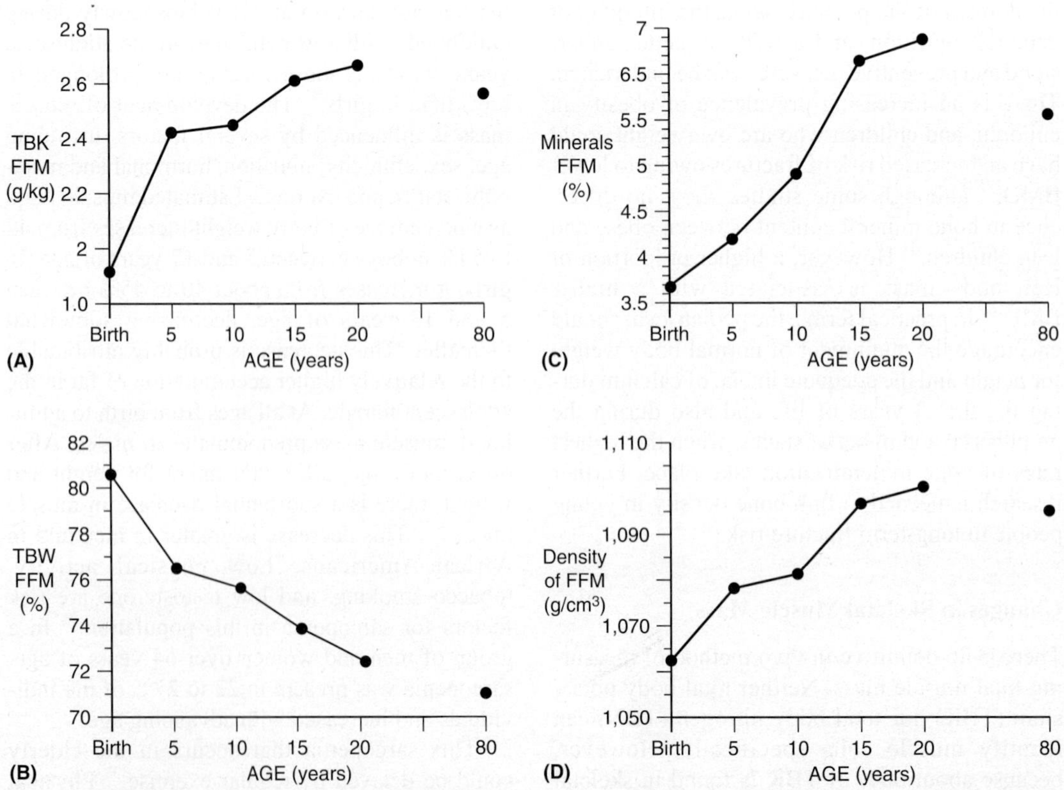

Figure 3 Changes in fat-free mass (FFM) body composition as a function of age. (A) Total body potassium (TBK) in relation to FFM. (B) Total body water (TBW) in relation to FFM. (C) Mineral content in relation to FFM. (D) Density of the FFM. (Adapted from references 4, 5, 31, and 85.)

For example, fat is underestimated when calculated on the basis of TBW and overestimated when calculated on the basis of TBK or body density.[84] Constants adjusted for age and gender during childhood and adolescence have been developed for FFM constituents,[31] making it possible to compare body composition by age, gender, and ethnic group.[83]

Changes in Linear Growth

Height velocity reaches its peak of 10 to 12 cm/mo between 16 and 30 weeks' gestation and decreases to 3 cm/mo (36 cm/yr) at birth. The postnatal curve is signaled by a deceleration in linear growth to 15 cm/yr at the end of the first year, 9 cm/yr at the end of the second year, and 8 cm/yr at the end of the third year. Between the ages of 4 and 5 years, it is 6.5 cm/yr, and from then to the time of puberty the growth velocity per year stabilizes to approximately 5 to 6 cm/yr.

Girls of Anglo-Saxon descent start the pubertal growth spurt at about 12 years of age, with a peak height velocity of 9 cm/yr. Boys start the growth spurt at about 14 years of age, with a peak velocity of 10 cm/yr. Total increments in stature after peak height velocity are slightly larger in males than in females. The annual increments decrease significantly after peak height velocity is achieved.[87] In the Fels longitudinal study, adult stature was reached at an average age of 21.2 years for males and 17.3 years for females. In girls, growth in stature continued at a slower rate for almost 5 years after menarche.[87]

Changes in height gain are linked to pubertal status. The age at which puberty occurs is significantly influenced by gender and ethnicity. Body composition changes are better related to physiologic age than to chronologic age. Children who begin their adolescent growth spurt earlier tend to be taller and heavier than those who are less mature at the same age.[82] Maximal stature has also been shown to vary by ethnicity, with African-American and European-American boys growing significantly taller than Mexican-American boys.[83] An index of sexual maturity, for example, Tanner staging, is an important component of growth assessment in children, particularly during the pubertal age period.

Changes with Weight Loss or Weight Gain

At birth, normal weight velocity is approximately 7 to 9 kg/yr; it decreases to 3.5 kg/yr at the end of the first year and 2.5 kg/yr at the end of the second year and then remains fairly stable at around 2 kg/yr until puberty. Weight changes unrelated to normal growth are almost always comprised of both FFM and fat. The contribution of each body component to the total weight change is related to the causative factors. In the circumstances of weight reduction, both fat mass and FFM are diminished. For instance, purposeful weight reduction produces comparable losses of both fat and protein stores.[88] While often a good indicator of excessive weight gain, changes in BMI may not accurately reflect changes in body composition, particularly in those with lower BMI.[89] Malnourished children can continue to show aberrations in body composition even after regaining weight.[90]

The situation is similar for individuals who gain significant amounts of body weight in response to excessive intake. The composition of the weight gain is both fat and FFM, though short-term weight gain is associated with proportionately greater increases in fat mass.[91] In obese subjects, weight gain is between 20 and 30% FFM. In subjects of normal or low weight, such as malnourished children, premature infants, or patients with anorexia nervosa, the proportion of weight gained as FFM is larger, around 60 to 75%, depending on the individual and type of diet. The excess weight of obese children is composed of FFM, fat mass, and mineral, in a continuous relationship with body weight. A propensity for greater fat mass accumulation in the trunk and greater mineral accumulation in the leg has been observed with regional measurements of body fat.[92] An exception to this trend may be small for gestational age infants, who, following catch-up weight gain, tend to have greater adiposity and abdominal fat than appropriate for gestational age infants.[93] These features may be linked to long-term risks for central adiposity and insulin resistance later in life.

Changes in Body Composition During Malnutrition and Disease

Malnutrition and disease can cause body composition alterations beyond those expected from underfeeding. Moreover, many of the methods used in measuring body composition changes assume the conditions of a healthy body that are generally not present in these children. For example, electrolyte derangement and altered body water distribution related to a disease or condition can invalidate the results of some techniques.[94,95] Disease-induced malnutrition can produce body compositional changes distinct from those caused by food deprivation alone. Changes in body compartments may be masked by overall weight normalcy.

Children with severe protein-energy malnutrition generally have increased TBW in relation to body weight. ECW as a percentage of TBW is also increased. These changes are indicative of severe losses of cell mass and body fat. The cells retract and lose potassium, magnesium, and phosphorus. Total body sodium is increased both extracellularly and intracellularly. The extracellular increase of sodium is generally less than the increase in ECW. This results in hyponatremia with a relative increase in total body sodium. TBK is decreased, although serum potassium levels are usually normal. Deficiencies in magnesium, calcium, phosphorus, and trace elements (zinc, copper, selenium, and chromium) with bone demineralization have also been reported. Total body protein is depleted. There is a marked loss of muscle mass, primarily as a result of a decrease in cell size rather than cell number. If the energy imbalance continues, the result is slowing or cessation in linear growth and stunting. Alterations in ECW, sodium, and potassium should be taken into account in the early management of children with acute malnutrition. The process of recovery should start carefully and slowly by correcting the water and electrolyte derangement to avoid dangers associated with refeeding syndrome, particularly heart failure[96] (see Chapter 13, "Protein-Energy Malnutrition: Pathophysiology, Clinical Consequences, and Treatment," for details).

In protein deprivation, there is a loss in fat mass and ICW. The body cell mass diminishes, at the expense, especially, of muscle and visceral protein, with a relative preservation of subcutaneous fat. The ICW decreases. There is expansion of the extracellular compartment with edema and hypoproteinemia. As the process develops, it becomes manifest with marked losses in muscle mass and an increase in ECW. The effect of this progression can obscure the severity of the malnutrition if body weight alone is used to assess the child.

Children with chronic diseases exhibit changes in body composition. These changes may be iatrogenic, caused by treatment for the underlying disease (eg, steroid-associated osteopenia). Typically, lean mass is compromised during the most acute phase of illness, while a combination of lean and fat mass depletion is observed in less serious chronic conditions. Cancer, Crohn's disease, and cystic fibrosis are among the diseases where body composition abnormalities have been described. Children in remission from cancer have a greater fat mass percentage than controls,[97,98] even when body weight is the same or less than age-matched controls.[99] Similarly, children with Crohn's disease have reduced lean body mass, compared to controls, without significant concomitant reductions in fat mass. Lean body mass is inversely correlated with disease severity.[100] Cystic fibrosis is associated with deficits in lean body mass, fat mass, and BMD, and negative relationships of body composition parameters with disease severity.[101] Lower FFM and higher fat mass was observed in a large group of patients at hospital admission, compared to a similar group of healthy controls. This suggests that abnormalities in body composition are widespread in disease, and could be linked to patient outcome.[102]

BODY COMPOSITION MODELS

Traditionally, body compartments have been divided into fat mass and FFM. The fat mass includes all ether-extractable lipids in the body. The FFM has four major constituents: water, protein, glycogen, and minerals. Adipose tissue includes the fat and its supporting cellular and extracellular structures. Lean body mass refers to the part of the body free of adipose tissue, whereas FFM consists of lean body mass plus the nonfat components of adipose tissue. In very obese individuals, the excess adipose tissue can increase FFM without increasing lean body mass. Therefore, because lean body mass and FFM are not synonyms, it is most accurate to use the terms fat mass and FFM in the two-compartment model of body composition.

Several methods of body composition measurement rely on the two-compartment model of fat mass and FFM, each assumed to be in constant composition. In general, these methods first measure one constituent of the FFM, such as density, water, or potassium. Then they assume that the concentration of that constituent of the FFM is a known constant and that the other components of the FFM also maintain a relatively constant composition to calculate the total FFM. FFM is then subtracted from body weight to calculate fat mass. The two-compartment model continues to be widely used, mainly because of the simplicity of its interpretation. Both of the assumptions noted above, however, are questionable because the FFM changes with a variety of conditions.[31,80,103,104] To address this problem, multicompartment models of body composition assessment have been developed in which more than one constituent of the FFM of each subject is measured.[105]

Multicompartment Models

Recent advances in methodology have allowed the measurement of several body compartments to overcome the limitations of many assumptions. As a result, body composition analysis has evolved from the traditional two-compartment system of fat and FFM to models based on four or more body-weight fractions. Now body composition in humans can be studied using several models at different levels of complexity (Figure 4)[3,85,106]: (1) atomic, (2) molecular, (3) cellular, (4) functional, and (5) whole body. The direct or indirect methods used to measure components at the five levels are presented in Table 4. Several of these methods are reviewed later.

Atomic Level. In the human body, there are approximately 50 different elements, but just 6 (oxygen, carbon, hydrogen, nitrogen, calcium, and phosphorus) account for more than 98% of body weight. Oxygen constitutes more than 60% of total body mass. The remaining 44 elements make up less than 2% of body weight.[106] Traditionally, elemental analysis of humans was possible only in cadavers, which was confounded by the possible alterations caused by disease and death. The availability of whole-body counting and neutron activation analysis (NAA), combined with a measurement of TBW, allows the measure of eight elements directly (hydrogen, carbon, nitrogen, calcium, phosphorus, sodium, potassium, and chlorine). This information is used to calculate the body content of three more elements (oxygen, magnesium, and sulfur). There are consequently 11 body components determined at the atomic level; these comprise at least 99% of body weight in living humans.[85,107] Equations have been developed using atomic components to calculate higher levels of body composition (Table 4).

Molecular Level. The molecular model of body composition is usually based on three main chemical groups: water, mineral, and organic.[105] The minerals are further separated into bone mineral and soft tissue components, and the organics are mainly defined by protein and fat components. Therefore, body weight = lipid mass (fat) + total body protein + bone mineral + soft tissue mineral + TBW.[3,105]

At this level, TBW by isotope dilution and bone mineral by whole-body dual-energy X-ray absorptiometry (DXA) can be determined directly.[106] The remaining components must be estimated indirectly. For example, protein can be determined from TBN by making two assumptions: that all body nitrogen is in protein and that 16% of protein is nitrogen.[106,107] Total body fat can be calculated by subtracting the nonlipid carbon from total body carbon and then converting this into fat, assuming that triglyceride is 77.4%

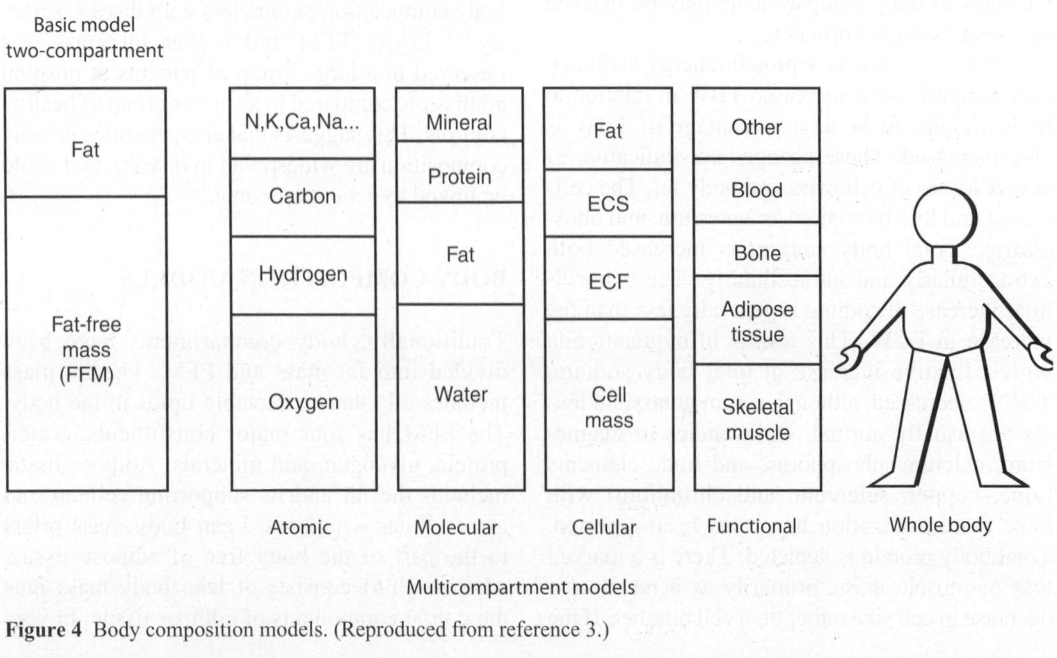

Figure 4 Body composition models. (Reproduced from reference 3.)

Table 4 Equations and Methods for Measuring Body Composition by Level

Atomic level	
Na, Cl, Ca, N, C, P	Neutron activation analysis
K	^{40}K counting
H_2O	Isotope dilution
Body weight = TBO + TBC + TBH + TBN + TBCa + TBP + TBK + TBCl + TBNa + TBMg + · · ·	
Molecular level	
Fat	Carbon in fat*/0.774
TBW	Isotope dilution
Total body protein	TBN × 6.25
Bone mineral	TBCa/0.364
	DXA
Soft tissue mineral	
K	TBK
Mg	TBK × 0.06
$H_2PO_4^-$	TBK × 1.7
Na	TBNa
Cl	TBCl
HCO_3^-	TBCl × 0.43
Body weight = lipid mass + total body water + total body protein + bone mineral + soft tissue mineral	
Cellular level	
Body cell mass	0.00833 × TBK
ECW	Isotope dilution
	Bioelectrical impedance analysis
Extracellular solids	TBNa + TBCl + $TBHCO_3$ + TBCa
	TBCa/0.177
Fat	Carbon in fat*/0.774
Body weight = body cell mass + extracellular water (ECW) + extracellular solids + fat	
Functional level	
Adipose tissue	DXA
	CT
	MRI
	Ultrasound
	Infrared interactance
	Anthropometry
Skeletal muscle	0.0196 × TBK − 0.0261 × TBN
Bone	TBCa
	DXA
	Quantitative CT
Other tissues	DXA
	CT
	MRI
	Ultrasound
Body weight = adipose tissue + skeletal muscle + bone + other tissues	
Whole body level	
	Anthropometry
	Densitometry
	Total body electrical conductivity
	Bioelectrical impedance analysis

Data from references 3, 106, and 107.
*Carbon in fat = TBC − [(3.37 × TBN) + (0.052 × TBCa) + (0.085 × TBCl)].

carbon.[108] Bone mineral can also be calculated from total body calcium. An important aspect of these estimates drawn from elements is that no known age dependencies are recognized. The main assumption is that the proportions of carbon, nitrogen, and calcium are known and constant within lipid, protein, and bone mineral, respectively.

Cellular Level. At the cellular level, the body is divided into four main compartments: cells, extracellular fluid, extracellular solids, and fat. Body cell mass reflects the cellular components of the body. The extracellular fluid is the fluid surrounding the cells. Extracellular solids consist of organic and inorganic chemical compounds. The organic extracellular solids include collagen, reticular, and elastic fibers. The inorganic extracellular solids represent the total body bone mineral (primarily calcium, phosphorus, and oxygen) and other inorganic components such as bicarbonate, citrate, magnesium, and sodium.[106]

At this level, the volume of extracellular fluid and its plasma subcompartment can be quantified directly by dilution methods. Body cell mass can be estimated by the difference between TBW and ECW or by the measurement of TBK. Extracellular solids can be estimated from elements measured by NAA.[106,107]

Functional Level. The fourth level of complexity comprises tissues, organs, and systems. Three specific tissues are particularly important in body composition studies: bone, adipose tissue, and muscle, which together comprise approximately 75% of body weight.[106]

The direct methods used to estimate the major compartments at this level are the imaging techniques, such as computed tomography (CT), nuclear magnetic resonance imaging (MRI), and ultrasonography. They can directly determine the regional and total body adipose tissue, skeletal muscle, liver, kidney, and spleen volumes. Brain volume can also be evaluated by CT, and heart mass can be estimated by echocardiography. DXA can be used to estimate fat tissue, bone, and skeletal muscle mass. Measurement of TBK, nitrogen, and calcium by NAA allows the indirect estimation of skeletal muscle mass and bone mass.

Whole Body Level. The whole body level of body composition measurement concerns body size, shape, and exterior and physical characteristics.[106] The techniques used in their estimation are mainly anthropometry and densitometry. Anthropometric evaluations, although less accurate, are simpler and easier to perform than are some of the measurements at the other four levels. Thus, the anthropometric techniques are often well suited for large-scale studies or for field work. Air displacement plethysmography, a densitometric method, can be used with children 5 years and older, in place of underwater weighing for determining body volume. It is important to recognize, in general, that changes in regional distribution are not measurable at this level.

BODY COMPOSITION MEASUREMENT METHODS

A number of methods have been developed for measurement of the composition of the human body. Each of these methods provides some type of information that is assumed to be related, directly or indirectly, to one or more of the various components of the different body composition models described in the previous section. In some cases, these models are method driven, meaning that to use that particular model, a specific measurement method must be used. Clearly, a multicompartment model would be the most informative, but these more advanced models also tend to require a combination of several methods. Also, whether the information is to be used at the population level, such as in epidemiological or field studies, or for the assessment of an individual, such as in a clinical setting, can also strongly influence the choice of models and methods.

Once a measurement is performed, the measured parameters have to be translated to their corresponding body composition value(s), which usually requires several assumptions.[3,109] For adults, the translation from the measured value to a body composition value often assumes a relatively constant relationship, with occasional minor adjustments for age, sex, and ethnicity. For infants and children, these relationships are not always as stable, and can be easily perturbed during periods of rapid growth and sexual maturation. Of the various methods described in this section, only a few research centers can perform all of the assays. The information obtained from a combination of these assays, however, provides our best estimates of body composition and often serve as the basis for calibration of less sophisticated techniques. In most cases, only one of the methods is available to the investigator or clinician.

Anthropometric-Based Techniques

The measurement of body weight is probably the most basic of anthropometric measurement of the human body. This measurement requires a minimum of equipment, can be obtained relatively quickly, and as frequently as needed. Height or stature may be the second most measured parameter. These measurements are routinely used in anthropological and epidemiological studies, as part of public health surveys, and are commonly obtained as part of routine clinical exams. Often, the classification of subjects vulnerable to under- or overnutrition is based on these measurements alone. In recent years, the BMI (BMI = body weight/stature^2) has been promoted as an international standard for obesity status in children.[109,110]

Clearly auxology has contributed significantly to our understanding of the general patterns of physical change of the body with growth and development. Many anthropometric-based measurements have been proposed for assessing body composition.[111] Whenever one of these indices has been directly compared with a more direct measure of body composition, the correlations have usually reached significance on a population basis. For the individual, however, these indices tend to be less reliable, except possibly for extreme outliers in the population. Although BMI appears to have the best validity on a population basis of all the different weight-and-height indices,[112] its sensitivity and specificity for the individual is limited.[113] Standardized BMI curves for children (Appendix I, "Nutritional Assessment") are available from the US Centers for Disease Control and Prevention. Use of this index alone is quickly becoming a routine part of health screening programs, including those in schools.

The measurement of the subcutaneous fat layer using skinfold thickness is an anthropometric technique that has been used for many years. This technique is based on the assumption that the thicknesses of the fat layers below the skin are proportional to the total amount of fat in the body. In practice, skinfold thickness needs to be measured at standardized regions and by experienced examiners using calipers (Harpenden, Holtain, or Lange) of known quality.[111] The triceps has been the site most frequently selected, but no single body region appears to be consistently representative of the whole subcutaneous fat layer, much less the total fat mass. A number of different prediction equations have been published, some using the same measurement sites. To learn more on this topic, we would direct the reader to the literature for the use of skinfold measurements.[114,115]

Alternate techniques, without the use of calipers, have been developed for the measurement of the subcutaneous fat layer. These techniques are based on the differences in the absorbance and reflectance properties of skin, fat, and lean tissue at different wavelengths.[73,116] The thickness of the overlaying skin layer has minimal effect, and the measurements have acceptable reproducibility. These techniques are well tolerated by the subject being examined, and provide an alternative to skinfold measurement. However, many of the same limitations as with skinfold measurements apply, namely extrapolation to total body fat content. Only a limited number of studies in different age groups have reported using this technology.[117–119] These techniques may be more useful for monitoring intrasubject changes than for intersubject comparisons. Also, there are no studies where it has been used in conjunction with a more direct method for measuring total body fat. Further studies are needed to better determine the full potential for this technology.

In Vivo Chemical Analyses

Historically, analytical chemical analyses of tissues are the quantitative basis for human body composition, and have contributed to our understanding the metabolic function of tissues. The advancement of modern physics lead to the development of nondestructive nuclear-based assays of tissue samples, which was later transferred to direct in vivo analyses in the 1970s.[120] The method, called NAA, is based on the principle that when atoms are exposed to neutrons, there is a finite probability that some of the neutrons will interact with the nucleus of atoms, resulting in the production of gamma rays that are characteristic of the interactions. These gamma rays can be produced during the time of the neutron interaction, or observed for several minutes following the exposure to a low-intensity beam of neutrons. For body composition measurements, the gamma rays are detected external to the body.[120,121] Using this approach, the total body content of calcium, sodium, chlorine, phosphorus, and nitrogen has been measured in adults and children.[122,123] If the gamma rays emitted during the irradiation can be measured, then the body content of carbon, oxygen, hydrogen, and nitrogen can also be determined.[121] This elemental information can be combined to derive the direct in vivo chemical model, or converted to estimates of body protein, water, fat, and bone mass.

Body Potassium Measurement. A very small fraction (~0.012%) of all potassium atoms found in nature are radioactive. This isotope, called ^{40}K, decays emitting high-energy gamma rays (1.46 MeV) about 11% of the time. At this energy, about half of the gamma rays produced within the human body will escape and can be detected external to the body. To improve the precision of this measurement, the detectors must be shielded to reduce background interference from gamma rays originating from other radioactive sources in the environment. This type of instrument is called a whole-body counter.[121] The availability of stable electronics, high-efficiency detectors, and PC-based analyzers has significantly decreased the cost of this technology. When properly calibrated, the whole-body counting procedure can produce an accurate and precise measure of TBK, which is directly related to body cell mass, the actively metabolizing tissues in the body.[41] Since most of TBK is in the ICW volume at a relatively constant concentration, this measurement has also been used to estimate the ICW volume.[121] TBK is no longer recommended as a measure of the FFM, because it may not accurately reflect changes in the ECW compartment, which also contributes to total FFM. The most recent application of TBK is for modeling of total body protein mass in adults and children.[124]

Body Water Measurements

Isotope Dilution Methods. Body water is the major component of the FFM, and is also the major contributor to body weight, with the exception of fat for extremely obese subjects. Hence the measurement of TBW may give one of the most reliable estimates of FFM, and when coupled with body weight, an estimate of body fat mass. The most common procedure used for the measurement of TBW is the tracer dilution technique, using water labeled with nonradioactive isotopes. Two body fluid samples (blood, urine, and/or saliva) are needed, one at baseline before administration of the oral tracer dose and one several hours later. Both deuterium and ^{18}O-enriched water are used, with the quantitative assays based on mass spectroscopy and infrared absorbance.[125] For research studies, the fluid samples are processed and usually frozen for later analysis. In the clinical setting, this approach would not be practical if there is an immediate need for this information. Also, if there is a need for repeat assays, they need to be sufficiently separated in time, in order for the earlier tracer to clear the body and not interfere with the subsequent measurement. Partly for these reasons, alternative methods such as bioelectrical impedance have been developed for the assessment of body water.

In a normally hydrated state, the ratio of TBW to FFM is assumed relatively constant for the individual. On average, this ratio is typically 0.732 for healthy adults and adolescents. The ratio is much higher at birth (~0.83) and decreases during early childhood (Figure 3B). Therefore, to estimate fat as the difference between body weight and FFM, age- and gender-specific adjustments for the hydration ratio of FFM should be used.[31]

The extracellular component of body water can also be determined using nonradioactive dilution methods. Bromide is the most commonly used tracer, and its concentration in blood or saliva is analyzed using either HPLC or X-ray florescence.[3] For infants, a sucrose tracer has also been used.[126] When these assays are obtained in conjunction with the TBW measurement, the difference between TBW and ECW can be used to indirectly estimate ICW volume. Again, repeat measurements are limited by the amount of time needed for the earlier tracer to clear the body. Partly for these reasons, methods based on bioelectrical impedance have also been developed for the assessment of extracellular body water volume.

Bioelectrical Methods. In electrical terms, impedance is a measure of the frequency-dependent opposition of a conductor to the flow of an alternating electric current.[73] Because the body's fluids contain electrolytes, and the lean tissues in the body contain virtually all of body water, these tissues can conduct an electrical current. This is the core basis for the bioelectric impedance analysis (BIA) methods used to measure body composition in humans. How these tissues conduct a current is also dependent on the capacitance properties of the cells. At lower frequencies (<10 kHz), membranes of cells are assumed to act like capacitors and not allow current to pass through the cells. At high frequencies (>500 kHz), the capacitance properties of cells are significantly diminished, and the current is now assumed to also pass through cells. That is, at low frequency the current passes mainly through the extracellular fluid volume, while at high frequency the electric current passes through all lean tissues or the TBW compartment. Since fat is a poor conductor of electricity at any frequency, a measurement of the body's impedance or resistance should be indirectly related to the body's TBW or FFM.

Most BIA measurements are made at a single frequency (50 kHz), while some instruments can make measurements at multiple frequencies.[127] The short-term precision of BIA measurements for an individual is good, but the accuracy of its translation to body composition values continues to be questioned in some studies.[128–130] One factor that appears to account for some of these inconsistencies is the difference in body shapes among individuals of the same stature. In the simplest electrical model, the circuit's impedance value is also affected by the assumed shape (geometry) of the conductor. In the case of the human body, where the electrodes are typically placed near the wrist and foot on one side of the body, the smaller cross-sectional areas of the arm and leg contribute the most to the resistance value. Also, a number of different BIA prediction equations for FFM, TBW, and ECW have been published, but with limited agreement among the predicted values for an individual.[3,120] Altered states of hydration including an abnormal intracellular-to-extracellular fluid ratio can quickly affect the single-frequency BIA-based estimates of body composition. The single-frequency BIA method, however, continues to be a popular choice in many research studies. Recently, advanced models for the multifrequency method have been reported.[131,132] The accuracy of the predicted body composition values still need to be independently verified with the more established methods and models.[106,107,120]

The BIA methods are based on the measurement of the body's resistance to the passage of an alternating electrical current through the body. However, if the body is placed within an external electromagnetic field, these same tissues will also interact with that external field. This is the basis for the total body electrical conductivity measurement of body composition.[133] This method was developed in the 1980s, but with the exception of a few centers, is no longer being used today.

The attractiveness of all of the bioelectrical methods is that they can be performed relatively quickly, require minimal cooperation on the part of the subject, the size of the BIA instruments make them portable, and their cost is relatively low compared with other techniques. The short-term precision of the measurements has been shown to be good; however, the accuracy of the measurements may limit its use to population studies.[3,129,130]

Densitometry Methods

Whole-Body Density Measurements. To measure the density of the whole body, one needs to know the weight and volume of the body. Body weight can easily be measured with high precision with a scale. Body volume, on the other hand, is more difficult to measure in order to attain the precision needed for body composition assessment of the individual. The classical method has been underwater weighing, which requires the subject to be weighted while totally submerged underwater and with as much air as possible exhaled from the lungs.[41] By comparing the subject's weight in air and underwater, the volume of water displaced is the same as the subject's body volume. Body density is defined as body weight divided by body volume. An object's weight is equal to the sum of its parts, and an object's volume is equal to the sum of the volumes of its parts. If the object is composed of two parts (eg, fat and FFM), and the density of each is known, then the weight and volume equations can be rearranged to calculate the mass of either part.[125] This is the basic principle of all methods that calculated body composition based on body density. The underwater weighing technique is one of three methods that have been developed to measure body volume. For many investigators, the underwater weighing method has been considered the "gold standard" measurement. All of the volume measurement techniques, however, have limitations, that if not adjusted for, can result in significantly inaccurate estimates of body composition. These include correction for residual lung volume, and the assumed density of the skeletal component of FFM.[125] When the method is used in older children, age- and gender-adjusted density values for the FFM must be used.[31] It is not feasible to use the underwater method in infants and younger children, nor in many hospitalized patients.

The development of air-displacement plethysmography has provided an alternative approach to the measurement of body volume.[134,135] In this case, the body displaces a volume of air inside a closed chamber to determine body volume. Corrections for lung volume are still needed, along with adjustments for the adiabatic effects of the skin.[136] Once body volume is obtained, the same calculations used in underwater weighting apply. At present, only one commercial instrument (BOD POD™, Life Measurement, Concord, CA) is available. Its performance has been shown to be in good agreement with underwater weighing for adults and children.[134,135]

An infant-sized air-displacement plethysmograph (PEA POD™, Life Measurement, Concord, CA) has also been developed.[137] Body composition results in healthy infants for this instrument were in good agreement with those obtained using the deuterium dilution method and a four-compartment body composition model as references.[138,139] Further testing, however, is needed for preterm infants and in sick infants where there may be significant alteration of normal hydration.

Dual-Energy X-Ray Absorptiometry. This technology originated with the use of a collimated radioactive source placed next to the lower arm, and counting the number of transmitted photons on the opposite side with a shielded detector.[3,120] Differences in the transmitted signal are related to the relative density and chemical makeup of the tissues in the path of photon beam. In the mid-1990s, the radioactive sources were replaced with X-rays sources, different types of detectors were used, and measurements were made at two energies.[140] The subject is exposed for a brief period to a relatively weak beam of X-rays. The exposure levels are classified as a minimum risk, and are comparable to other background sources of radiation exposure one encounters daily.[3,120] DXA or DEXA has emerged as a principal method for measuring bone mineral and body composition at all ages. It has high precision for bone mineral measurements in adults and older children, and has become the de facto standard for assessing bone status.[120] DXA measurements have been obtained in a number of studies of infants and children.[20,21,140,142] Body composition results for children obtained with the original adult software and pencil-beam instruments were inaccurate.[143] The newer fan-beam DXA instruments are being provided with software for specific use in pediatric populations. The newer values for bone are different when compared with the older software, especially for children below 40 kg body weight.[144] Similarly, differences can also be expected for the estimates of fat and lean tissues. The accuracy of DXA for use in infants has been questioned by others.[144,145]

It should be noted that DXA provides only a two-dimensional image of the region that is scanned. Therefore, true bone density (g/cm^3) is not obtained, and only bone mineral areal density (g/cm^2) can be calculated.[3,120,140] To measure true bone density, a quantitative three-dimensional imaging method is needed. A technique called peripheral quantitative computed tomography has been developed for this purpose. It has been used to measure the trabecular and cortical regions in the radius and tibia, and pediatric reference ranges are available.[146,147] Another feature of this technique is that the cross-sectional geometry of the bone can be measured.

Body Imaging Techniques

The most recent advances in measurement methods of body composition have been the use of imaging techniques.[148] Both CT and MRI have been used. Both methods can provide accurate reconstructed three-dimensional images of the body. An advantage for CT is that true density (g/cm^3) information is obtained, while its major limitation is that ionizing radiation is used. MRI, on the other hand, uses no ionizing radiation, but its information is more qualitative when compared with CT. A CT scan typically takes only a few seconds to complete, whereas an MRI scan can take considerably longer, although the newer MRI instruments have reduced these differences. The strength of the CT and MRI techniques is that organ-specific information can be obtained; however, if the focus is only on changes in the total body, alternate magnetic-based techniques can be considered.[149] To date, most of the emphasis using CT and MRI has been on the measurement of the subcutaneous and visceral components of abdominal adiposity.[148,150,151] Whole-body MRI can also be used with infants to monitor changes in body composition during early life.[152]

CONCLUSIONS

Energy homeostasis is known to be important to human health, and lean body mass is the major predictor of energy expenditure. Thus, assessment of body composition is an important aspect of understanding energy requirements during health and disease.[153] Body composition changes during normal growth, and also during unexpected changes in body size. Chemical maturity occurs at different stages for the various constituents of FFM. Fat mass varies greatly during the life cycle, depending on heredity, nutrition, lifestyle, and health status.

Body weight alone cannot be used as an acceptable measure of nutritional efficacy or status. The elaboration of growth standards in terms of body composition in childhood and adolescence, and in relation to sexual maturation, could allow the recognition of abnormalities in specific body components in disorders affecting growth and puberty; it could also allow recognition of the moment when a differing pattern of distribution or accretion appears in relation to age, gender, ethnicity, or illness.

The evaluation of body fat with some body composition method should allow the pediatrician to define deviations in body weight and to act in the prevention or treatment of early obesity. In this sense, the beneficial role of exercise and the negative roles of sedentarism must be emphasized. The possibility of critical periods for fat accretion and an understanding of the long-term consequences of different body fat distributions might have important implications in the nutritional management and long-term health outcome of children and adolescents.

As new and more accurate methods emerge, and with the combination of different methods in the multicompartment model, the values for the reference fetus, child, or adolescent might be more precisely defined by state-of-the-art techniques. Age, gender, and ethnicity standards will allow the use of less expensive, surrogate field methods suitable for office practice and for population studies. The ideal field method should be inexpensive, easy to use, reliable, noninvasive, portable, validated, and calibrated. The clinician has a variety of options in the body composition assessment armamentarium. Limitations and assumptions of the selected method should always be considered in the final interpretation.

ACKNOWLEDGMENT

This chapter is a revised and updated version of the previous chapter by Bechard LJ, Puig M. Body composition and growth. In Walker WA, Watkins JB, Duggan C, editors. Nutrition in Pediatrics: Basic Science and Clinical Applications, 3rd edition. BC Decker, Inc.; 2003.

REFERENCES

1. Rogers IS, Ness AR, Steer CD, et al. Associations of size at birth and dual-energy X-ray absorptiometry measures of lean and fat mass at 9 to 10 y of age. Am J Clin Nutr 2006;84:739–47.
2. Wells JCK, Fewtrell MS. Measuring body composition. Arch Dis Child 2006;91:612–7.

3. Ellis KJ. Human body composition: In vivo methods. Physiol Rev 2000;80:649–80.
4. Fomon SJ, Haschke F, Ziegler EE, Nelson SE. Body composition of reference children from birth to age 10 years. Am J Clin Nutr 1982;35:1169–75.
5. Haschke F. Body composition of adolescent males. Part I. Total body water in normal adolescent males. Part II. Body composition of the male reference adolescent. Acta Paediatr Scand Suppl 1983;307:1–23.
6. Butte NF, Hopkinson JM, Wong WW, et al. Body composition during the first 2 years of life: An updated reference. Pediatr Res 2000;47:578–85.
7. Poissonnet CM, Burdi AR, Garn SM. The chronology of adipose tissue appearance and distribution in the human fetus. Early Hum Dev 1984;10:1–11.
8. Budge H, Gnanalingham MG, Gardner DS, et al. Maternal nutritional programming of fetal adipose tissue development: Long-term consequences for later obesity. Birth Defects Res C Embryo Today 2005;75:193–9.
9. Euser AM, Finken MJ, Keijzer-Veen MG, et al. Associations between prenatal and infancy weight gain and BMI, fat mass, and fat distribution in young adulthood: A prospective cohort study in males and females born very preterm. Am J Clin Nutr 2005;81:480–7.
10. McMillen IC, Muhlhausler BS, Duffield JA, Yuen BS. Prenatal programming of postnatal obesity: Fetal nutrition and the regulation of leptin synthesis and secretion before birth. Proc Nutr Soc 2004;63:405–12.
11. Ravelli GP, Stein ZA, Susser MW. Obesity in young men after famine exposure in utero and early infancy. N Engl J Med 1976;295:349–53.
12. Catalano PM, Thomas A, Huston-Presley L, Amini SB. Increased fetal adiposity: A very sensitive marker of abnormal in utero development. Am J Obstet Gynecol 2003;189: 1698–704.
13. Rogers I. The influence of birthweight and intrauterine environment on adiposity and fat distribution in later life. Int J Obes Relat Metab Disord 2003;27:755–77.
14. Oken E, Gillman MW. Fetal origins of obesity. Obes Res 2003;11:496–506.
15. Rolland-Cachera MF, Deheeger M, Guilloud-Bataille M, et al. Tracking the development of adiposity from one month of age to adulthood. Ann Hum Biol 1987;14:219–29.
16. Gesta S, Bluher M, Yamamoto Y, et al. Evidence for a role of developmental genes in the origin of obesity and body fat distribution. Proc Natl Acad Sci U S A 2006;103:6676–81.
17. Butte NF, Wong WW, Hopkinson JM, et al. Infant feeding mode affects early growth and body composition. Pediatrics 2000;106:1355–66.
18. Chumlea WC, Guo SS, Kuczmarski RJ, et al. Body composition estimates from NHANES III bioelectrical impedance data. Int J Obes Relat Metab Disord 2002;26:1596–609.
19. Vague J, Vague P, Jubelin J, Barre A. Fat distribution, obesities and health: Evolution of concepts. In: Bouchard C, Johnston FE, editors. Fat Distribution During Growth and Later Health Outcomes. Current Topics in Nutrition and Disease, Volume 17. New York: Alan R. Liss; 1988. p. 9–41.
20. Ellis KJ, Abrams SA, Wong WW. Body composition of a young, multiethnic female population. Am J Clin Nutr 1997;65:724–31.
21. Ellis KJ. Body composition of a young, multiethnic, male population. Am J Clin Nutr 1997;66:1323–31.
22. Lopez-Blanco M, Hernandez-Valera Y, Landaeta-Jimenez M, Henriquez-Perez G. Crecimiento y nutricion en la region Latinoamericana. An Venez Nutr 1993;6:47–90.
23. Whitaker RC, Wright JA, Pepe MS, et al. Predicting obesity in young adulthood from childhood and parental obesity. N Engl J Med 1997;337:869–73.
24. Rolland-Cachera MF, Bellisle F, Deheeger M, et al. Influence of body fat distribution during childhood on body fat distribution in adulthood: A two-decade follow-up study. Int J Obes 1990;14:473–81.
25. Kuh D, Hardy R, Chaturvedi N, Wadsworth ME. Birth weight, childhood growth and abdominal obesity in adult life. Int J Obes Relat Metab Disord 2002;26:40–7.
26. Gutin B, Islam S, Manos T, et al. Relation of percentage of body fat and maximal aerobic capacity to risk factors for atherosclerosis and diabetes in black and white seven- to eleven-year-old children. J Pediatr 1994;125:847–52.
27. Must A, Jacques PF, Dallal GE, et al. Long-term morbidity and mortality of overweight adolescents: A follow-up of the Harvard Growth Study of 1922 to 1935. N Engl J Med 1992;327:1350–5.
28. Despres JP. Is visceral obesity the cause of the metabolic syndrome? Ann Med 2006;38:52–63.
29. Dennison BA, Erb TA, Jenkins PL. Television viewing and television in bedroom associated with overweight risk among low-income preschool children. Pediatrics 2002;109:1028–35.
30. Burdette HL, Whitaker RC. A national study of neighborhood safety, outdoor play, television viewing, and obesity in preschool children. Pediatrics 2005;116:657–62.
31. Lohman TG. Applicability of body composition techniques and constants for children and youths. Exerc Sport Sci Rev 1986;14:325–57.
32. Sabatini S. The female athlete triad. Am J Med Sci 2001;322:193–5.
33. Evans WJ, Campbell WW. Sarcopenia and age-related changes in body composition and functional capacity. J Nutr 1993;123:465–8.
34. Spady DW. Normal body composition of infants and children. In: Klish WJ, Kretchmer N, editors. Body Composition Measurements in Infants and Children. Report of the 98th Ross Conference on Pediatric Research. Columbus, OH: Ross Laboratories; 1989. p. 67–73.
35. Silva AM, Wang J, Pierson RN, Jr, et al. Extracellular water: Greater expansion with age in African Americans. J Appl Physiol 2005;99:261–67.
36. Hartnoll G, Betremieux P, Modi N. Body water content of extremely preterm infants at birth. Arch Dis Child Fetal Neonatal Ed 2000;83:F56–9.
37. Robert S, Zarowitz BJ, Hyzy R, et al. Bioelectrical impedance assessment of nutritional status in critically ill patients. Am J Clin Nutr 1993;57:840–4.
38. Matkovic V, Ilich JZ. Calcium requirements for growth: Are current recommendations adequate? Nutr Rev 1993;51:171–80.
39. Matkovic V. Calcium intake and peak bone mass. N Engl J Med 1992;327:119–20.
40. Whiting SJ, Vatanparast H, Baxter-Jones A, et al. Factors that affect bone mineral accrual in the adolescent growth spurt. J Nutr 2004;134:696S–700S.
41. Forbes GB. Human Body Composition: Growth, Aging, Nutrition and Activity. New York: Springer-Verlag; 1987.
42. White DR, Widdowson EM, Woodar HQ, Dickerson JW. The composition of body tissues (II): Fetus to young adult. Br J Radiol 1991;64:149–59.
43. Chan GM, Mileur L, Hansen JW. Calcium and phosphorus requirements in bone mineralization of preterm infants. J Pediatr 1988;113:225–9.
44. Forbes GB. Some remarks on bone mineralization. J Pediatr 1988;113:167–71.
45 Steichen JJ, Gratton TL, Tsang RC. Osteopenia of prematurity: The cause and possible treatment. J Pediatr 1980;96:528–34.
46. Greer FR, McCormick A. Improved bone mineralization and growth in premature infants fed fortified own mother's milk. J Pediatr 1988;112:961–9.
47. Lapillonne A, Salle BL, Glorieux FH, Claris O. Bone mineralization and growth are enhanced in preterm infants fed an isocaloric, nutrient-enriched preterm formula through term. Am J Clin Nutr 2004;80:1595–603.
48. Minton SD, Steichen JJ, Tsang RC. Bone mineral content in term and preterm appropriate-for-gestational-age infants. J Pediatr 1979;95:1037–42.
49. Greer FR, Lane J, Weiner S, Mazess RB. An accurate and reproducible absorptiometric technique for determining bone mineral content in newborn infants. Pediatr Res 1983;17:259–62.
50. De Schepper J, Cools F, Vandenplas Y, Louis O. Whole body bone mineral content is similar at discharge from the hospital in premature infants receiving fortified breast milk or preterm formula. J Pediatr Gastroenterol Nutr 2005;41:230–34.
51. Mimouni F, Tsang RC. Bone mineral content: Data analysis. J Pediatr 1988;113:178–80.
52. Hillman LS. Bone mineral content in term infants fed human milk, cow milk-based formula, or soy-based formula. J Pediatr 1988;113:208–12.
53. Abrams SA, Schanler RJ, Garza C. Bone mineralization in former very low birth weight infants fed either human milk or commercial formula. J Pediatr 1988;112:956–60.
54. Steichen JJ, Tsang RC. Bone mineralization and growth in term infants fed soy-based or cow milk-based formula. J Pediatr 1987;110:687–92.
55. Mimouni F, Campaigne B, Neylan M, Tsang RC. Bone mineralization in the first year of life in infants fed human milk, cow-milk formula, or soy-based formula. J Pediatr 1993;122:348–54.
56. Specker BL, Beck A, Kalkwarf H, Ho M. Randomized trial of varying mineral intake on total body bone mineral accretion during the first year of life. Pediatrics 1997;99:E12.
57. Young RJ, Antonson DL, Ferguson PW, et al. Neonatal and infant feeding: Effect on bone density at 4 years. J Pediatr Gastroenterol Nutr 2005;41:88–93.
58. Arabi A, Nabulsi M, Maalouf J, et al. Bone mineral density by age, gender, pubertal stages, and socioeconomic status in healthy Lebanese children and adolescents. Bone 2004;35:1169–79.
59. Taaffe DR, Cauley JA, Danielson M, et al. Race and sex effects on the association between muscle strength, soft tissue, and bone mineral density in healthy elders: The Health, Aging, and Body Composition Study. J Bone Miner Res 2001;16:1343–52.
60. Chan GM. Dietary calcium and bone mineral status of children and adolescents. Am J Dis Child 1991;145:631–34.
61. Vidulich L, Norris SA, Cameron N, Pettifor JM. Differences in bone size and bone mass between black and white 10-year-old South African children. Osteoporos Int 2006;17:433–40.
62. Bachrach LK, Hastie T, Wang MC, et al. Bone mineral acquisition in healthy Asian, Hispanic, black, and Caucasian youth: A longitudinal study. J Clin Endocrinol Metab 1999;84:4702–12.
63. Yilmaz D, Ersoy B, Bilgin E, et al. Bone mineral density in girls and boys at different pubertal stages: Relation with gonadal steroids, bone formation markers, and growth parameters. J Bone Miner Metab 2005;23:476–82.
64. Abrams SA. Normal acquisition and loss of bone mass. Horm Res 2003;60:71–6.
65. Abrams SA. Pubertal changes in calcium kinetics in girls assessed using 42Ca. Pediatr Res 1993;34:455–9.
66. Prentice A. Diet, nutrition and the prevention of osteoporosis. Public Health Nutr 2004;7:227–43.
67. Harris M, Nguyen TV, Howard GM, et al. Genetic and environmental correlations between bone formation and bone mineral density: A twin study. Bone 1998;22: 141–5.
68. Hunter DJ, de Lange M, Andrew T, et al. Genetic variation in bone mineral density and calcaneal ultrasound: A study of the influence of menopause using female twins. Osteoporos Int 2001;12:406–11.
69. Seeman E, Hopper JL, Bach LA, et al. Reduced bone mass in daughters of women with osteoporosis. N Engl J Med 1989;320:554–8.
70. Greer FR, Krebs NF. Optimizing bone health and calcium intakes of infants, children, and adolescents. Pediatrics 2006;117:578–85.
71. Goulding A, Taylor RW, Jones IE, et al. Overweight and obese children have low bone mass and area for their weight. Int J Obes Relat Metab Disord 2000;24:627–32.
72. Heymsfield SB, Smith R, Aulet M, et al. Appendicular skeletal muscle mass: Measurement by dual-photon absorptiometry. Am J Clin Nutr 1990;52:214–8.
73. Lukaski HC. Methods for the assessment of human body composition: Traditional and new. Am J Clin Nutr 1987;46:537–56.
74. Poortmans JR, Boisseau N, Moraine JJ, et al. Estimation of total-body skeletal muscle mass in children and adolescents. Med Sci Sports Exerc 2005;37:316–22.
75. Szulc P, Duboeuf F, Marchand F, Delmas PD. Hormonal and lifestyle determinants of appendicular skeletal muscle mass in men: The MINOS study. Am J Clin Nutr 2004;80:496–503.
76. Iannuzzi-Sucich M, Prestwood KM, Kenny AM. Prevalence of sarcopenia and predictors of skeletal muscle mass in healthy, older men and women. J Gerontol A Biol Sci Med Sci 2002;57:M772–7.
77. Fleith M, Clandinin MT. Dietary PUFA for preterm and term infants: Review of clinical studies. Crit Rev Food Sci Nutr 2005;45:205–29.
78. Martinez M. Tissue levels of polyunsaturated fatty acids during early human development. J Pediatr 1992;120:S129–38.
79. Innis SM. Human milk and formula fatty acids. J Pediatr 1992;120:S56–61.
80. Roubenoff R. Hormones, cytokines and body composition: Can lessons from illness be applied to aging? J Nutr 1993;123:469–73.
81. St-Onge MP. Relationship between body composition changes and changes in physical function and metabolic risk factors in aging. Curr Opin Clin Nutr Metab Care 2005;8:523–8.
82. Siervogel RM, Demerath EW, Schubert C, et al. Puberty and body composition. Horm Res 2003;60:36–45.
83. Ellis KJ, Shypailo RJ, Abrams SA, Wong WW. The reference child and adolescent models of body composition. A contemporary comparison. Ann N Y Acad Sci 2000;904:374–82.
84. Rolland-Cachera MF. Body composition during adolescence: Methods, limitations and determinants. Horm Res 1993;39:25–40.
85. Heymsfield SB, Wang J, Lichtman S, et al. Body composition in elderly subjects: A critical appraisal of clinical methodology. Am J Clin Nutr 1989;50:1167–75; discussion 1231–5.
86. Heymsfield SB, Wang Z, Baumgartner RN, et al. Body composition and aging: A study by in vivo neutron activation analysis. J Nutr 1993;123:432–7.

87. Roche AF. Growth, Maturation and Body Composition. The Fels Longitudinal Study 1929–1991. Cambridge: Cambridge University Press; 1992.
88. Nicholls D, Wells JC, Singhal A, Stanhope R. Body composition in early onset eating disorders. Eur J Clin Nutr 2002;56:857–65.
89. Demerath EW, Schubert CM, Maynard LM, et al. Do changes in body mass index percentile reflect changes in body composition in children? Data from the Fels Longitudinal Study. Pediatrics 2006;117:e487–95.
90. Scalfi L, Polito A, Bianchi L, et al. Body composition changes in patients with anorexia nervosa after complete weight recovery. Eur J Clin Nutr 2002;56:15–20.
91. Kyle UG, Zhang FF, Morabia A, Pichard C. Longitudinal study of body composition changes associated with weight change and physical activity. Nutrition 2006;22:1103–11.
92. Wells JC, Fewtrell MS, Williams JE, et al. Body composition in normal weight, overweight and obese children: Matched case-control analyses of total and regional tissue masses, and body composition trends in relation to relative weight. Int J Obes (Lond) 2006;30:1506–13.
93. Ibanez L, Ong K, Dunger DB, de Zegher F. Early development of adiposity and insulin resistance after catch-up weight gain in small-for-gestational-age children. J Clin Endocrinol Metab 2006;91:2153–8.
94. Warner JT, Evans WD, Webb DK, Gregory JW. Pitfalls in the assessment of body composition in survivors of acute lymphoblastic leukaemia. Arch Dis Child 2004;89:64–8.
95. Wells JC. Body composition in childhood: Effects of normal growth and disease. Proc Nutr Soc 2003;62:521–8.
96. Crook MA, Hally V, Panteli JV. The importance of the refeeding syndrome. Nutrition 2001;17:632–7.
97. Murphy AJ, Wells JC, Williams JE, et al. Body composition in children in remission from acute lymphoblastic leukemia. Am J Clin Nutr 2006;83:70–4.
98. Nysom K, Holm K, Michaelsen KF, et al. Degree of fatness after treatment for acute lymphoblastic leukemia in childhood. J Clin Endocrinol Metab 1999;84:4591–6; erratum appears in J Clin Endocrinol Metab 2001;86:1758.
99. Nysom K, Holm K, Michaelsen KF, et al. Degree of fatness after allogeneic BMT for childhood leukaemia or lymphoma. Bone Marrow Transplant 2001;27:817–20.
100. Burnham JM, Shults J, Semeao E, et al. Body-composition alterations consistent with cachexia in children and young adults with Crohn disease. Am J Clin Nutr 2005;82:413–20.
101. Bianchi ML, Romano G, Saraifoger S, et al. BMD and body composition in children and young patients affected by cystic fibrosis. J Bone Miner Res 2006;21:388–96.
102. Kyle UG, Morabia A, Slosman DO, et al. Contribution of body composition to nutritional assessment at hospital admission in 995 patients: A controlled population study. Br J Nutr 2001;86:725–31.
103. Hergenroeder AC, Klish WJ. Body composition in adolescent athletes. Pediatr Clin North Am 1990;37:1057–83.
104. Kuczmarski RJ. Need for body composition information in elderly subjects. Am J Clin Nutr 1989;50:1150–7; discussion 1231–5.
105. Heymsfield SB, Waki M. Body composition in humans: advances in the development of multicompartment chemical models. Nutr Rev 1991;49:97–108.
106. Wang ZM, Pierson RN, Jr, Heymsfield SB. The five-level model: A new approach to organizing body-composition research. Am J Clin Nutr 1992;56:19–28.
107. Heymsfield SB, Waki M, Kehayias J, et al. Chemical and elemental analysis of humans in vivo using improved body composition models. Am J Physiol 1991;261:E190–8.
108. Kehayias JJ, Heymsfield SB, LoMonte AF, et al. In vivo determination of body fat by measuring total body carbon. Am J Clin Nutr 1991;53:1339–44.
109. Cole TJ, Faith MS, Pietrobelli A, Heo M. What is the best measure of adiposity change in growing children: BMI, BMI %, BMI z-score or BMI centile? Eur J Clin Nutr 2005;59:419–25.
110. Dietz WH, Bellizzi MC. Introduction: The use of body mass index to assess obesity in children. Am J Clin Nutr 1999;70:123S–5S.
111. Lohman TG, Roche AF, Martorell R. Anthropometric Standardization Reference Manual. Champaign, IL: Human Kinetics Books; 1988.
112. Mei Z, Grummer-Strawn LM, Pietrobelli A, et al. Validity of body mass index compared with other body-composition screening indexes for the assessment of body fatness in children and adolescents. Am J Clin Nutr 2002;75:978–85.
113. Ellis KJ, Abrams SA, Wong WW. Monitoring childhood obesity: Assessment of the weight/height index. Am J Epidemiol 1999;150:939–46.
114. Chumlea WC, Baumgartner RN. Status of anthropometry and body composition data in elderly subjects. Am J Clin Nutr 1989;50:1158–66; discussion 1231–5.
115. Chumlea WC, Guo SS, Kuczmarski RJ, et al. Reliability for anthropometric measurements in the Hispanic Health and Nutrition Examination Survey (HHANES 1982–1984). Am J Clin Nutr 1990;51:902S–7S.
116. Moller R, Tafeit E, Smolle KH, et al. Estimating percentage total body fat and determining subcutaneous adipose tissue distribution with a new noninvasive optical device LIPOMETER. Am J Human Biol 2000;12:221–30.
117. Fuller NJ, Dewit O, Wells JC. The potential of near infrared interactance for predicting body composition in children. Eur J Clin Nutr 2001;55:967–72.
118. Jurimae T, Sudi K, Payerl D, et al. Relationships between bioelectric impedance and subcutaneous adipose tissue thickness measured by LIPOMETER and skinfold calipers in children. Eur J Appl Physiol 2003;90:178–84.
119. Kabir N, Forsum E. Estimation of total body fat and subcutaneous adipose tissue in full-term infants less than 3 months old. Pediatr Res 1993;34:448–54.
120. Mattsson S, Thomas BJ. Development of methods for body composition studies. Phys Med Biol 2006;51:R203–28.
121. Ellis KJ. Whole-body counting and neutron activation analysis. In: Heymsfield SB, Lohman TG, Wang ZM, Going SB, editors. Human Body Composition, 2nd edition. Champaign, IL: Human Kinetics; 2005. p. 51–62.
122. Ellis KJ. Reference man and woman more fully characterized. Variations on the basis of body size, age, sex, and race. Biol Trace Elem Res 1990;26–7:385–400.
123. Ellis KJ, Shypailo RJ, Hergenroeder A, et al. Total body calcium and bone mineral content: Comparison of dual-energy X-ray absorptiometry with neutron activation analysis. J Bone Miner Res 1996;11:843–8.
124. Wang Z, Heshka S, Wang J, Heymsfield SB. Total body protein mass: Validation of total body potassium prediction model in children and adolescents. J Nutr 2006;136:1032–6.
125. Schoeller DA. Hydrometry. In: Heymsfield SB, Lohman TG, Wang ZM, Going SB, editors. Human Body Composition, 2nd edition. Champaign, IL: Human Kinetics; 2005. p. 35–50.
126. Bauer K, Bovermann G, Roithmaier A, et al. Body composition, nutrition, and fluid balance during the first two weeks of life in preterm neonates weighing less than 1500 grams. J Pediatr 1991;118:615–20.
127. Segal KR, Burastero S, Chun A, et al. Estimation of extracellular and total body water by multiple-frequency bioelectrical-impedance measurement. Am J Clin Nutr 1991;54:26–9.
128. Mast M, Sonnichsen A, Langnase K, et al. Inconsistencies in bioelectrical impedance and anthropometric measurements of fat mass in a field study of prepubertal children. Br J Nutr 2002;87:163–75.
129. Coppini LZ, Waitzberg DL, Campos AC. Limitations and validation of bioelectrical impedance analysis in morbidly obese patients. Curr Opin Clin Nutr Metab Care 2005;8:329–32.
130. Gelbrich G, Reich A, Muller G, Kiess W. Knowing more by fewer measurements: About the (In)ability of bioelectric impedance to enhance obesity research in children. J Pediatr Endocrinol Metab 2005;18:265–73.
131. Kraemer M. A new model for the determination of fluid status and body composition from bioimpedance measurements. Physiol Meas 2006;27:901–19.
132. Moissl UM, Wabel P, Chamney PW, et al. Body fluid volume determination via body composition spectroscopy in health and disease. Physiol Meas 2006;27:921–33.
133. Fiorotto M. Application of the TOBEC measurement for determining fat and fat-free mass of the human infant. In: Klish WJ, Kretchmer N, editors. Body Composition Measurements in Infants and Children. Report of the 98th Ross Conference on Pediatric Research. Columbus, OH: Ross Laboratories; 1989. p. 57–64.
134. Fields DA, Goran MI, McCrory MA. Body-composition assessment via air-displacement plethysmography in adults and children: A review. Am J Clin Nutr 2002;75:453–67.
135. Wells JC, Fuller NJ. Precision of measurement and body size in whole-body air-displacement plethysmography. Int J Obes Relat Metab Disord 2001;25:1161–7.
136. Dempster P, Aitkens S. A new air displacement method for the determination of human body composition. Med Sci Sports Exerc 1995;27:1692–7.
137. Urlando A, Dempster P, Aitkens S. A new air displacement plethysmograph for the measurement of body composition in infants. Pediatr Res 2003;53:486–92.
138. Ellis KJ, Yao M, Shypailo RJ, et al. Body composition assessment in infancy: Air-displacement plethysmography versus a four-compartment criterion model. Am J Clin Nutr 2007; 85:90–5.
139. Ma G, Yao M, Liu Y, et al. Validation of a new pediatric air-displacement plethysmograph for assessing body composition in infants. Am J Clin Nutr 2004;79:653–60.
140. Mazess RB, Barden HS, Bisek JP, Hanson J. Dual-energy X-ray absorptiometry for total-body and regional bone-mineral and soft-tissue composition. Am J Clin Nutr 1990;51:1106–12.
141. Venkataraman PS, Ahluwalia BW. Total bone mineral content and body composition by X-ray densitometry in newborns. Pediatrics 1992;90:767–70.
142. Venkataraman PS, Duke JC. Bone mineral content of healthy, full-term neonates. Effect of race, gender, and maternal cigarette smoking. Am J Dis Child 1991;145:1310–12.
143. Laskey MA, Prentice A. Comparison of adult and paediatric spine and whole body software for the Lunar dual energy X-ray absorptiometer. Br J Radiol 1999;72:967–76.
144. Koo WW, Hammami M, Shypailo RJ, Ellis KJ. Bone and body composition measurements of small subjects: discrepancies from software for fan-beam dual energy X-ray absorptiometry. J Am Coll Nutr 2004;23:647–50.
145. Hammami M, Walters JC, Hockman EM, Koo WW. Disproportionate alterations in body composition of large for gestational age neonates. J Pediatr 2001;138:817–21.
146. Moyer-Mileur L, Xie B, Ball S, et al. Predictors of bone mass by peripheral quantitative computed tomography in early adolescent girls. J Clin Densitom 2001;4:313–23.
147. Schoenau E, Neu CM, Rauch F, Manz F. Gender-specific pubertal changes in volumetric cortical bone mineral density at the proximal radius. Bone 2002;31:110–3.
148. Fuller MF, Fowler PA, McNeill G, Foster MA. Imaging techniques for the assessment of body composition. J Nutr 1994;124:1546S–50S.
149. Ellis KJ, Shypailo RJ, Taicher Z. Body composition analysis using quantitative magnetic resonance (QMR). Obes Res, in press.
150. Kvist H, Chowdhury B, Grangard U, et al. Total and visceral adipose-tissue volumes derived from measurements with computed tomography in adult men and women: Predictive equations. Am J Clin Nutr 1988;48:1351–61.
151. Seidell JC, Bakker CJ, van der Kooy K. Imaging techniques for measuring adipose-tissue distribution-a comparison between computed tomography and 1.5-T magnetic resonance. Am J Clin Nutr 1990;51:953–7.
152. Olhager E, Flinke E, Hannerstad U, Forsum E. Studies on human body composition during the first 4 months of life using magnetic resonance imaging and isotope dilution. Pediatr Res 2003;54:906–12.
153. Zakeri I, Puyau MR, Adolph AL, et al. Normalization of energy expenditure data for differences in body mass or composition in children and adolescents. J Nutr 2006;136:1371–6.

5

Macronutrient Requirements for Growth: Carbohydrates

David B. Rhoads, PhD
Lynne L. Levitsky, MD

WHAT ARE CARBOHYDRATES?

Carbohydrates, or saccharides, are composed of carbon, hydrogen, and oxygen in a 1:2:1 ratio. They are the principal source of energy in most human diets and are largely derived from plant tissues. Milk is another significant source of carbohydrate. The lactose content of human milk is a little over 7% on average and provides approximately 40% of its calories. Milk from dairy cows is approximately 5% lactose, providing 30% of total calories. The monosaccharide glucose is the primary source of energy and carbon for most cells and an obligatory energy source for the brain, formed elements of blood, and the kidney cortex. Because many carbohydrates are easily digested and readily converted to glucose, they are important in human nutrition. Carbohydrates are also essential components of many biomolecules, including nucleic acids, glycoproteins, glycolipids, hormones, and several signaling molecules. The specific carbohydrate compounds required for these metabolic processes are often synthesized de novo. The ability to produce necessary sugars and derivatives endogenously, with ascorbic acid (vitamin C) as the notable exception, permits survival on carbohydrate-free diets or during limited fasting.

Carbohydrate Chemistry

A monosaccharide, or single-sugar unit, contains three to seven carbons in a linear chain with a general chemical formula of $C_nH_{2n}O_n$ (n = 3 to 7). Three common hexoses (n = 6) are shown in Figure 1A. Each monosaccharide has one carbonyl group (C=O) located at the terminal carbon C_1, as in glucose or galactose, or C_2, as in fructose. Hydration of sugars in solution fosters the formation of cyclic structures in either of two orientations (α or β; Figure 1B). Sugar amines are formed by condensation of ammonia with a hydroxyl moiety; uronic acids (eg, glucuronic acid) are formed by oxidation of the hydroxymethyl moiety; and sugar alcohols like sorbitol are formed by reduction of the C=O group to a hydroxyl moiety, usually by an aldoreductase enzyme. The three corresponding derivatives of glucose are shown in Figure 1C. Higher order structures of covalently linked monosaccharides are formed by condensation (removal of water) and are grouped by the number of subunits: disaccharide (2), oligosaccharide (3 to 10), or polysaccharide (>10). Common disaccharides are shown in Figure 1D.

Carbohydrates in Foods

Mono- and disaccharides, collectively labeled "simple sugars," are abundant in fruits, vegetables, grains, and milk. Complex carbohydrates (oligo- and polysaccharides), composed of monosaccharides and sugar derivatives in various combinations, are also prevalent in plants. Food sources for these carbohydrates are given in Table 1. Starches are complex carbohydrates

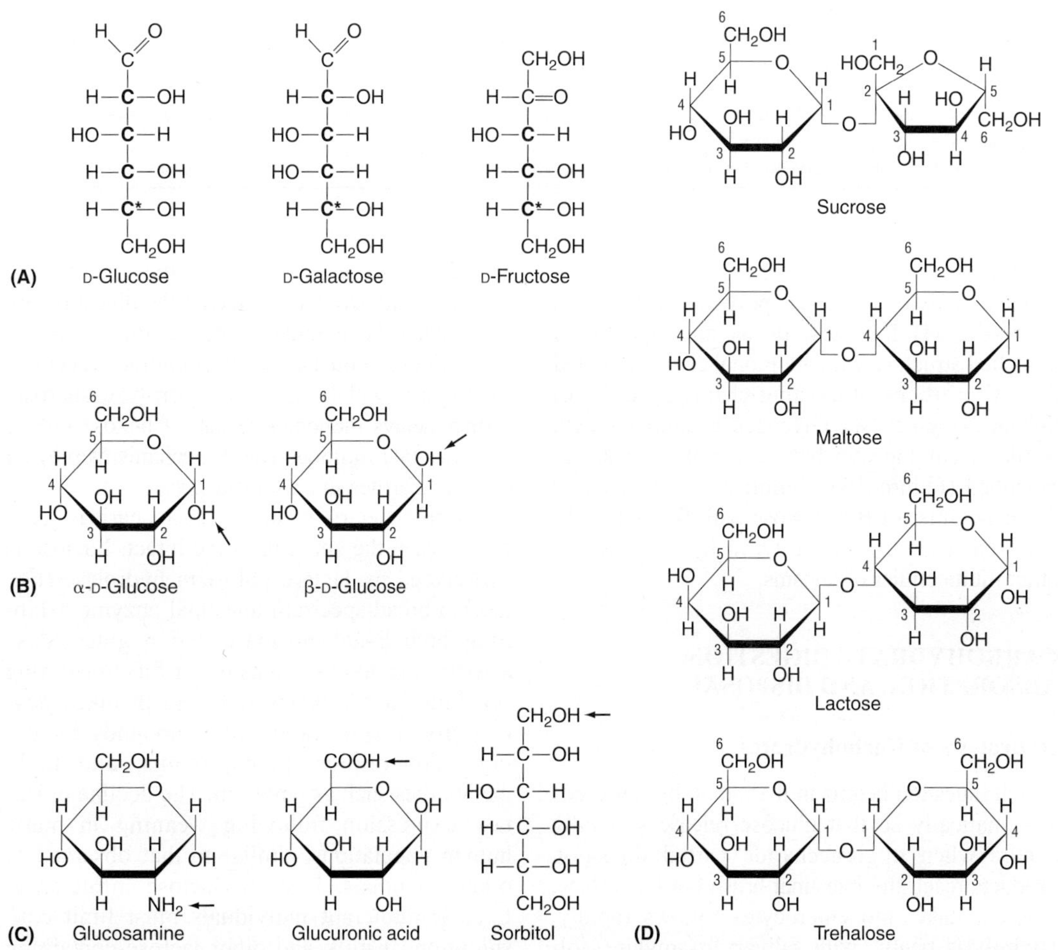

Figure 1 Simple sugars. **(A)** *Structures of three common hexoses.* D-Glucose, D-galactose, and D-fructose are shown as linear structures. The tetrahedral bonding geometry of carbon creates several possible spatial arrangements, leading to multiple molecular structures. By convention, different sugars are distinguished by the orientations of asymmetric carbons (bold) with the carbon farthest from the C=O group (asterisk) establishing the dextro- or levo- "handedness" (*d* vs. *l*; most natural sugars are *d*). **(B)** *Cyclic structures of D-glucose in solution.* Hydration of hexoses in solution fosters bonding of the C=O carbon to the C_5 oxygen, forming a cyclic structure that constrains C_6 and the resultant C_1 hydroxyl group to opposite sides (α form) or the same side (β form) of the ring. The arrow indicates the hydroxyl group that differentiates α and β forms. **(C)** *Glucose derivatives.* Arrows indicate the modified groups. Sorbitol, also called glucitol, cannot circularize. **(D)** *Structures of three common disaccharides.* A disaccharide bond involves the C_1 (or C_2) hydroxyl of at least one subunit. The form (α/β) and number of this carbon are used to identify the bond. In sucrose and maltose, the C_1 of α-D-glucose is linked to either the C_2 of fructose [α(1→2)] or the C_4 of another glucose [α(1→4)], respectively, making both α-glucosides. In lactose, the C_1 of β-D-galactose is linked to the C_4 of glucose [β(1→4)], making this sugar a β-galactoside. Linkage via a C=O carbon locks the monosaccharide into its cyclic form. Trehalose is a disaccharide composed of two glucose subunits like maltose, but linked via the C_1 carbons of each (α,α-1,1-glucosyl-glucoside).

Table 1 Classification of Carbohydrates

Class	Type/Name	Examples (Notes)	Source(s)
Monosaccharides	Aldohexoses	Glucose, galactose, mannose	Fruits, vegetables, etc
	Ketohexoses	Fructose (levulose), sorbose	Fruits, vegetables, etc
	Aldopentoses	Ribose (nucleic acids), L-arabinose (microbes, fibers), xylose (hemicellulose)	Various
	Ketopentoses	Ribulose, xylulose	Metabolic intermediates
	Tetrose	Erythrose	Microbes
	Triose	Glycerose	Synthetic
Disaccharides	Hexoses	Sucrose, lactose (only milk), maltose, trehalose	Fruits, vegetables, etc
	Isomaltose	$Glucose_2$, $\alpha(1\rightarrow6)$-linked	Partial starch digestion
Trisaccharides	Maltotriose	$Glucose_3$, $\alpha(1\rightarrow4)$-linked	Partial starch digestion
	Raffinose	Galactose-fructose-glucose	Legumes, cruciforms, grains
Oligosaccharides	α-Limit dextrins	Glucose polymers with both $\alpha(1\rightarrow4)$ and $\alpha(1\rightarrow6)$ linkages	Partial starch digestion
	Stachyose	Tetrasaccharide: $galactose_2$-glucose-fructose	Legumes
	Inulins	Fructans: $\beta(2\rightarrow1)$-linked fructose polymer (≈30 to 35 per molecule); soluble fiber*	Roots, rhizomes
Polysaccharides	Starch (plant)	Amylose: $\alpha(1\rightarrow4)$-linked glucose; amylopectin: also contains $\alpha(1\rightarrow6)$ branches	Seeds, grains
	Starch (animal)	Glycogen: $\alpha(1\rightarrow4)$-linked glucose backbone with profuse $\alpha(1\rightarrow6)$ branches	Liver, meat (muscle)
	Pectins	Galacturonan: galacturonic acid with rhamnose† at branches; soluble fiber	Fruits, potatoes
	Cellulose	Linear $\beta(1\rightarrow4)$-linked glucose polymer (7,000 to 15,000 per molecule); insoluble fiber	Cell walls of plants
	Hemicellulose	Amorphous heteropolymer: glucose + other subunits‡ (≈200/molecule); insoluble fiber	Cell walls of plants
	Hydrocolloids§	Carrageenan, agar (seaweed), gelatin (bovine, etc.), pomace (apple); soluble fiber	Various
Sugar alcohols	Hexitol (C-6)	Glucitol (sorbitol; also present stone fruits, eg, peaches), mannitol, galactitol	Food additives
	Pentitol (C-5)	Xylitol (sweet, well-adsorbed, low-energy yield)	Birch bark, food additive
	Dihexitols	Maltitol, lactitol	Food additives
	Carbocyclic	Inositol‖ ($C_6H_{12}O_6$)	Meat, liver

*Soluble fiber is digestible by colon microbiota.

†Rhamnose is an L-6-deoxyhexose ($C_6H_{12}O_5$), also found in plant glycosides.

‡Hemicellulose also contains xylose (second most abundant subunit), mannose, rhamnose, galactose, mannuronic acid, and galacturonic acid.

§Not all hydrocolloids are carbohydrates.

‖Inositol can be considered a member of the B complex vitamin group. Inositol is not an essential nutrient because humans can synthesize it.

composed solely of glucose. Plant starch occurs either as amylose, a linear polysaccharide chain with $\alpha(1\rightarrow4)$ linkages, or as amylopectin, a branched structure with additional chains initiated from C_6 carbons of existing chains by $\alpha(1\rightarrow6)$ linkages (Figure 2A). Glycogen is animal starch, similar to amylopectin, but much more extensively branched (Figure 2B). Cellulose is a nonstarch, linear polymer of β-D-glucose with $\beta(1\rightarrow4)$ linkages that cannot be hydrolyzed by humans and other multicellular organisms.

CARBOHYDRATE DIGESTION, ABSORPTION, AND DISPOSAL

Hydrolysis of Carbohydrates

Starch digestion begins in the mouth but proceeds systematically so that glucose release generally occurs when oligosaccharide partial digestion products reach the intestinal brush border surface, where uptake into enterocytes follows rapidly. Hydrolysis begins with salivary α-amylase, followed by pancreatic α-amylase delivered to the chyme entering the duodenum. Both enzymes are α-glycosidases active only on internal $\alpha(1\rightarrow4)$ bonds and release maltose, maltotriose (trisaccharide), and α-limit dextrins, oligosaccharides that contain $\alpha(1\rightarrow6)$ bonds. Intestinal hydrolysis is performed by 4-glycoside hydrolases localized to the apical (luminal) membranes of enterocytes.[1] Glucose monomers are released by the α-glycosidases maltase-glucoamylase, active on $\alpha(1\rightarrow4)$ linkages, and sucrase-isomaltase, also active on $\alpha(1\rightarrow6)$ linkages. Spatial restriction of these reactions to the absorptive surface moderates the increase in osmotic load from polysaccharide digestion by minimizing the luminal residence time of monosaccharides. Product feedback inhibition of sucrase-isomaltase, which can also hydrolyze sucrose, further delays monomer release if hexose uptake becomes rate limiting. These mechanisms prevent osmotic diarrhea in most instances.

Simple sugars, including disaccharides, generally reach the small intestine intact. Lactose is hydrolyzed by lactase phlorizin hydrolase (lactase), a broad-spectrum intestinal enzyme exhibiting both β-galactosidase and α-glucosidase activities. In addition to its major function during suckling, lactase releases α- and β-linked hexoses from a wide variety of compounds, including sphingolipids, glycoproteins, and mold metabolites such as phlorizin. The decline in lactase expression following weaning in many human populations, similar to that observed in other mammals, leads to lactose intolerance. Lactose-intolerant individuals must limit consumption of milk and other lactose-containing foods to avoid bloating and/or diarrhea from metabolism of the unabsorbed sugars by colon microbes. Maintenance of high lactase expression in populations such as those originating from Northern Europe permits continued consumption of dairy products. The fourth intestinal glycoside hydrolase is trehalase, which cleaves trehalose.

Although the human intestine is known to express only these glycoside hydrolases noted above, their multiple overlapping specificities likely account for the quantitative absorption of many ingested carbohydrates. Most can hydrolyze more than one type of glycosidic linkage and full substrate ranges have not been exhaustively characterized. Nevertheless, humans do lack intestinal enzymes for some glycosides routinely encountered in the diet including the mannosides and polymannans (polymannose-containing glycans) present in many plants, fungi, and animals. None of the human mannosidases are intestinal. Mannosidases secreted by commensal bacteria in the distal gut permit bacterial fermentation and assimilation.[2]

Hexose Transport

Transport of glucose and other monosaccharides, polar molecules that do not readily permeate lipid bilayers, is accomplished by integral membrane solute carrier proteins (transporters).[3] Hexose transporters fall into two classes differing in energy dependence: (1) Na^+-coupled glucose cotransporters (Na^+/glucose cotransporters; SGLTs) that couple glucose uptake to the inwardly directed electrochemical Na^+ gradient,[4] and (2) facilitated glucose transporters (GLUTs) that permit passive hexose movements in response to concentration gradients (Table 2).[5] The two classes are structurally similar but share little sequence homology. Each group contains over 10 members differing in specificity for hexoses or other compounds, tissue localization and regulation, and evolutionary conservation. Only a few of the hexose transporters are directly involved in carbohydrate absorption and disposal. Facilitated GLUTs are found in most if not all cells. The inherent bidirectional activity of GLUTs permits

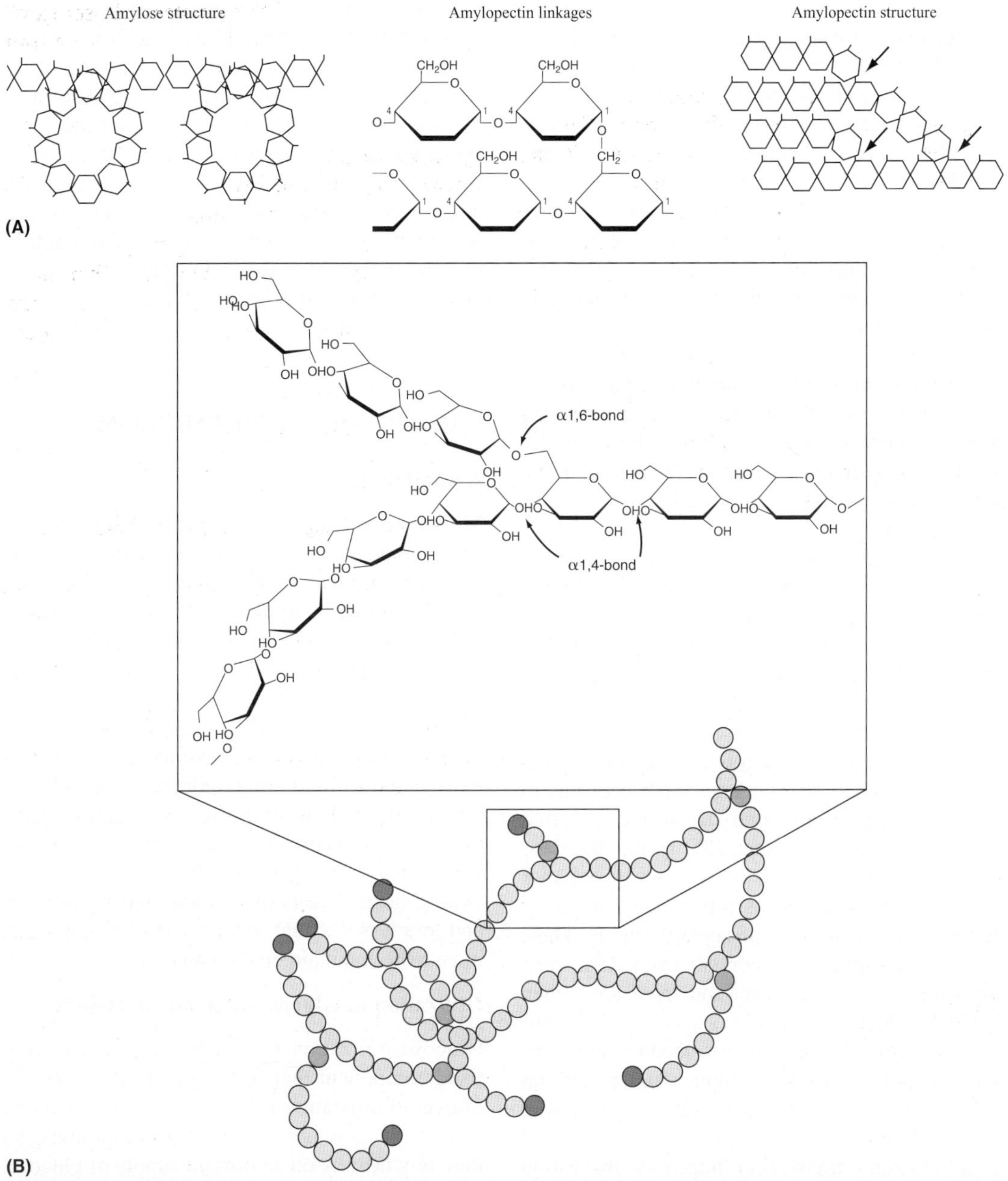

Figure 2 Starches. **(A)** *Plant starches.* Left: Amylose is a linear chain of α(1→4) linked glucose residues, schematically depicted in the typical helical structure found in foods. Center: Amylopectin has a branched structure, formed by initiating new chains from internal glucose subunits via α(1→6) linkages. Right: Amylopectin is depicted schematically to shown multiple branches (arrows). **(B)** *Animal starch.* Glycogen is similar to amylopectin with both α(1→4) and α(1→6) linkages (gray and green, respectively), but much more highly branched.

either uptake or release, depending on cell type and/or glucogenic status. In contrast, SGLTs are generally restricted to polarized epithelial cells of absorptive tissues, such as the small intestinal mucosa and renal proximal tubules. In these epithelia, cotransporters are localized to the apical, brush border membrane where substrate(s) can be extracted from the lumen. Some SGLTs are found in liver, heart, trachea, thymus, and other tissues, but the functional significance of these cotransporters is not fully understood. SVCT1, a Na^+-dependent cotransporter homologous to the SGLTs, is responsible for intestinal vitamin C absorption.[6] Other pathways,[7] including unidentified transporters and potential sugar sensors,[8] may also contribute to absorption of various dietary sugars (see Table 2).

Transepithelial hexose transport is possible because absorptive cells express one or more GLUT, generally localized to the basolateral membrane, in addition to an SGLT. In response to the electrochemical Na^+ gradient generated by the basolateral Na^+/K^+-ATPase, SGLT-mediated accumulation of glucose (or other hexose) creates a concentration gradient that drives GLUT-mediated transport across the basolateral membrane into the bloodstream. The high-affinity SGLT1 is the main intestinal cotransporter and is responsible for uptake of glucose, galactose, and a few other sugars. GLUT2, with a relatively wide substrate range, permits release of many absorbed hexoses. The combined activities of SGLT1 and the Na^+/K^+-ATPase also contribute significantly to fluid absorption.[9] Glucose/galactose movement in conjunction with basolateral Na^+ extraction creates an osmotic gradient that drives water (in excess of 250 water molecules/hexose molecule) through both SGLT1 and aquaporin water channels. This flux further creates a "solvent drag" that induces absorption of additional solutes. For instance, fructose uptake occurs by this mechanism via GLUT5, atypically located on enterocyte brush borders.[10] Indeed, SGLT1 activity appears instrumental because fructose released from sucrose is absorbed more efficiently than fructose delivered alone.[11]

Carbohydrates and Gut Peptide Hormones

Secretion of several gut hormones is linked to ingestion of carbohydrate. The interplay between carbohydrate absorption, intake, and utilization, in part controlled by these hormones, helps to tightly regulate levels of circulating blood glucose. Peptide hormones are secreted by the gastrointestinal tract, as well as brain, endocrine pancreas, and adipocytes, in anticipation of a meal and following ingestion.[12,13] These hormones serve to integrate intestinal functions with other tissues and physiological processes. Ghrelin, a growth hormone secretagogue, is released before meals largely by the gastric fundus, but also from the entire intestine.[14] Ghrelin is orexigenic (increases appetite) via receptors in the brain and its secretion is inhibited by ingestion of carbohydrates. The stomach and intestines secrete cholecystokinin in response to many nutrients and fibers, but not glucose. Cholecystokinin produces satiety and moderates postprandial glycemic excursions by slowing gastric emptying and potentiating amino acid–induced insulin release.[15,16] The proglucagon gene encodes the 158–amino-acid glucagon preprotein, which is processed by tissue-specific convertases (peptidases) in the intestinal tract, endocrine pancreas, and brain to yield several mature hormones.[17] The glucagon-like peptides GLP-1 and GLP-2 and oxyntomodulin are secreted by enteroendocrine cells of the distal gut (ileum and colon) in response to meals containing carbohydrates and/or fats.[18] GLP-1 slows gastric emptying, increases satiety, and enhances glucose-stimulated insulin release by β cells. GLP-2 is a potent trophic factor in the gut, but does not appear to affect insulin secretion or glucose homeostasis.[13] Oxyntomodulin has effects similar to GLP-1, in part by interaction with the same receptor.[19] Oxyntomodulin reduces food intake in humans[20,21] but the details of this action are not fully resolved. Peptide YY is secreted from the distal gut in response to ingestion of carbohydrate as well as other macronutrients and delays gastric emptying, among other effects.[19] Like oxyntomodulin, peptide YY administration acutely reduces food intake in humans, but its physiological role appears to be postponement of subsequent meals.[19] Gastric inhibitory peptide is secreted by the stomach and small intestine in response to many nutrients, but specifically to SGLT1 substrates.[22,23] Gastric inhibitory peptide and GLP-1 both enhance glucose-stimulated insulin release as well as promote β-cell proliferation, survival, and function.[13] Somatostatin is also secreted in response to carbohydrate and other macronutrients and appears to provide counterregulatory restraint for many meal-induced peptide hormones.[24] Many aspects of gastrointestinal endocrinology are still controversial or unresolved. Complicating factors in characterizing the actions of GI hormones include secretion of some by more than one tissue, local as well as systemic targets, and receptor affinities that overlap or depend on processing.

Carbohydrate Disposal

Carbohydrate disposal is largely orchestrated by the pancreatic islet hormones insulin and glucagon. The liver, muscle, and adipocytes are responsible for clearing most of the postprandial hexose load. Hepatocytes express GLUT2, GLUT5, and SGLT4 as well as GLUT8 and GLUT10, both of which also transport galactose. The combination could be necessary to accommodate the range of sugars encountered in the diet in addition to those produced by hepatocytes. The rates and direction of glucose transport by hepatocytes are established by the rates of glycogen synthesis compared with gluconeogenesis (new glucose production), which in turn are regulated by insulin and glucagon. Insulin stimulates glycogen synthase, driving the production of glycogen and increasing glucose transport into hepatocytes, while glucagon stimulates gluconeogenesis from three carbon precursors, and decreases glucose transport into the liver. Liver GLUTs are not regulated by insulin or glucagon. In contrast, the glucose transporter GLUT4 controls insulin-stimulated glucose transport into myocytes and adipocytes. Stimulation of insulin receptors initiates translocation of GLUT4 from intracellular vesicles to the plasma membrane where they enhance postprandial glucose clearance.[25,26] Basal glucose uptake between meals is maintained by GLUT1, the prototypic erythrocyte GLUT.[27,28] Other transporters about which less is known may also contribute to glucose disposal (Table 2).

FIBER AND INDIGESTIBLE CARBOHYDRATE

Dietary fiber, consisting of nonstarch polysaccharides, indigestible starches, and some noncarbohydrate macromolecules, remains undigested on reaching the colon. Nonstarch polysaccharides like cellulose escape digestion because humans lack the necessary hydrolytic enzymes. Other β-glucans as well as pectins, chitins, and various oligosaccharides also evade digestion partially or completely because their linkages or subunits fall outside the specificities of intestinal glycosidases. Examples include the fructose–fructose linkages in inulin, α-galactoside linkages in pectin, and the various subunits in hemicellulose. Nonpolysaccharide fiber consists of lignins (phenolic polymers) and waxes (aliphatic compounds). These, along with cellulose and hemicellulose, are classified as insoluble fiber that remains intact in the colon, contributing to bulk and softening stool by attracting water. Soluble fiber includes those carbohydrates that can be fermented in the colon, such as the pectins and hydrocolloids found in fruit pulp.

In principle, starch is completely digestible by humans, particularly when cooked. Hydration during cooking gelatinizes starch, essentially assuring its digestibility. However, some starches evade hydration due to incomplete release during processing or their physical state. In addition, cooking itself can render starch indigestible. Residual undigested starch is referred to as resistant starch[29] (RS) and is categorized according to its source: RS1 is enclosed starch due to partial milling of seeds and grains; RS2 is ungelatinized crystalline granules, such as that found in bananas and potatoes; and RS3 is retrograded amylose, formed by dehydration of cooked starch. Thus, pasta has a higher fiber content from RS1 when prepared with whole wheat and from RS3 when cooked al dente.

The term functional fiber is used to characterize the portion of total fiber with beneficial effects. Fiber contributes to satiety by adding bulk and delaying gastric emptying.[30] Increased small intestinal transit time improves absorption efficiency while moderating spikes in nutrient influx. Fiber conversely reduces colonic transit time, which likely reduces cancer risk by minimizing exposure to carcinogenic food constituents and metabolites. Soluble fiber entering the colon is metabolized to a greater or lesser extent by resident microbiota. These bacteria perform several beneficial functions: (1) production of fermentation metabolites that enhance absorption of essential minerals, such as magnesium[31]; (2) synthesis of micronutrients, such as vitamin K_2 (menaquinone)[32]; and (3) exclusion of pathogenic bacteria via niche habitation.[33] Excreted short-chain fatty acids have been suggested to contribute to energy harvest.[34] On the other hand, phytate-containing fiber is well known to antagonize uptake of some nutrients, such as iron and calcium.[35]

Table 2 Transporters Involved in Carbohydrate Absorption and Disposal

Class	Name	Substrate	Tissue(s)
Na^+-coupled cotransporters	SGLT1	Glucose, galactose	Small intestine, kidney (heart, trachea)
	SGLT3	Na^+ (H^+); glucose-coupled	Small intestine, etc (glucose sensor)
	SGLT4	Mannose	Small intestine, kidney, liver, lung, brain
	SVCT1	L-Ascorbic acid (vitamin C)	Small intestine (kidney, liver, others)
Facilitated transporters	GLUT1	Glucose	Widespread
	GLUT2	Several	Small intestine, liver
	GLUT3	Glc, gal, mannose, xylose	Brain (neurons, capillaries)
	GLUT4*	Glucose, *N*-acetyl-glcNH$_4$	Muscle, adipocytes
	GLUT5	Fructose	Intestine, liver, kidney, spermatocytes
	GLUT8*	Glucose, fructose, galactose	Testis, brain, liver, brown adipose, others
	GLUT10	Glucose, galactose	Heart, lung, brain, liver
	GLUT11	Glucose, fructose	Heart, muscle
	GLUT12	Orphan (substrate not known)	Heart, prostate, skeletal muscle

*GLUT4 and GLUT8 are insulin responsive. (Insulin stimulation induces relocation of transporters to the plasma membrane from intracellular vesicles.)

CARBOHYDRATE METABOLISM

Assimilation

Most ingested sugars are rapidly phosphorylated and converted to glucose-6-phosphate (G6P) by the liver. Further metabolism includes glycolysis, storage (glycogen, lipids), anabolism (synthesis of amino acids and other compounds), and dephosphorylation for export. Hepatic glycogenesis proceeds both from phosphorylated glucose and from resynthesized three-carbon compounds. Much of the remaining glucose is converted to glycogen in muscle and to lipids in adipocytes. The kidneys, brain, and small intestine also store small amounts of glycogen. These glycogen stores are rapidly depleted by glycogenolysis in the fasting state. During fasting, rates of gluconeogenesis in liver, and to a lesser extent kidney and small intestine, increase to maintain euglycemia.

Utilization in Glucose-Dependent Tissues

Glucose utilization by the brain is a relatively fixed component that forms a significant portion of overall utilization in the resting state. Neurons store little glycogen or energy compounds, so they rely heavily on a constant supply of glucose. Utilization of energy and oxygen by the brain increases markedly with neural stimulation. Glucose is transported across the blood–brain barrier by GLUT1 and into brain cells by GLUT3. Complete oxidation of one glucose molecule to carbon dioxide and water produces up to 38 molecules of ATP. Anaerobic glycolysis, on the other hand, yields only two molecules of ATP. Therefore complete glucose oxidation is a most important energy source for human metabolism. Newborns have brains that are approximately 10% of body weight and utilize 6 to 8 mg glucose/kg body weight/min. This rate decreases to 2 to 4 mg/kg/min in older children and plateaus at approximately 2 mg/kg/min in adults, correlating with the decrease in the proportion of brain to body weight. A lactate "shuttle" between astrocytes and neurons has been hypothesized and experimentally verified.[36,37] It is likely that astrocytes release lactate to neurons for complete oxidation and energy utilization.[38] When plasma glucose is limited, monocarboxylic acids (lactate, pyruvate, acetoacetate, and β-hydroxybutyrate) can partially fulfill brain energy needs. Specific monocarboxylic acid transporters permit uptake of these compounds across the blood–brain barrier and into neurons and glia.[39] Although compounds like ketone bodies cannot generate as much ATP as glucose, they also seem to be neuroprotective at least in part by increasing the energy generated during ATP hydrolysis. During prolonged fasting, brain glucose utilization may drop to half of control values.[40] Energy deprivation within the brain is equivalent to oxygen deprivation and has global effects on cellular metabolism, leading to the release of excitatory neurotransmitters which spread through the ventricular system, leaving a periventricular pattern of cell damage.

Most other tissues, including muscle, fat, and the splanchnic bed, readily use noncarbohydrate energy sources (fatty acids and ketones), when limited glucose supplies are depleted and do not rely on carbohydrate for continuing energy needs. The renal cortex and blood cells obligatorily require small amounts of glucose for oxidative metabolism.

Utilization in Macromolecules

Sugars and sugar derivatives are incorporated into a wide variety of macromolecules, which impact growth directly and indirectly through effects on collagen synthesis, cellular replication, and glycohormones that regulate growth. The pentose ribose is a constituent of ATP and GTP, high-energy triphosphates used to store oxidative energy in chemical bonds for use in biosynthetic and biomechanical processes. The phosphodiester backbones of RNA and DNA contain ribose and 2-deoxyribose, respectively. In some signaling pathways, cyclase enzymes convert the triphosphates ATP and GTP into their respective cyclic monophosphate derivatives cAMP and cGMP by bonding the α-phosphate to the C_2 hydroxyl group of ribose.[41,42] Glycoproteins are proteins to which sugars and derivatives are attached; these include glucose, galactose, mannose, fucose, *N*-acetylglucosamine, *N*-acetylgalactosamine, and sialic acid (*N*-acetylneuraminic acid). Glycoproteins tend to be membrane proteins or secreted proteins, but some cytoplasmic and nuclear proteins are also glycosylated.[43] Glycosylated hormones, as well as binding proteins important in their action, include thyroid-stimulating hormone, follicle-stimulating hormone, and growth hormone–binding proteins. *N*-linked glycosylation is important in maturation of glycoproteins within the Golgi apparatus, the endoplasmic reticulum, and ultimate trafficking into or through membranes.[44]

Some glycoproteins have structural functions, altering the behaviors, for instance, of cartilage, based upon proteoglycan content and aggregation.[45] Glycolipids also can function as recognition motifs on cell surfaces. A notable example is the ABO blood group of antigens. Type O is a glycolipid containing fucose, two galactose subunits, and an *N*-acetylglucosamine; addition of *N*-acetylgalactosamine creates type A, while addition of another galactose creates type B. Sugars are found in various signaling molecules. All can be synthesized from amino acids and/or lipids when insufficient in the diet: Examples include posttranslational modifications of molecules important in the immune response.[46] Moreover, intracellular signaling by nuclear and cytosolic proteins is modified by O-linked glycosylation pathways.[47,48]

RECOMMENDATIONS FOR CARBOHYDRATE INTAKE

Energy Needs

The ultimate fate of most absorbed carbohydrates is usage for energy. As such, their energy content is an important consideration in establishing values for adequate intake (AI) and the recommended daily allowance (RDA). The Food and Nutrition Board of the Institute of Medicine estimates that infants utilize approximately 115 kcal/kg/d up to 6 months and approximately 105 kcal/kg/d from 6 to 12 months. (one kilocalorie is the energy necessary to raise the temperature of 1,000 g H_2O from 0 to 1°C, or 4.184 kJ.) This translates to 800 to 1,200 kcal/d in 1-year-olds, depending on gender and size. By puberty, the range is 1,500 to over 3,000 kcal/d. With a fuel value of 4 kcal/g for carbohydrates, 50% of energy needs could be provided by approximately 50 g carbohydrates in newborns and 200 to 400 g in adolescents.

The dietary carbohydrate intake compatible with optimal health in infants, children, and adults is not known. Thus, adequate carbohydrate intake for children has not been established. In children who nurse, the approximately 74 g/L of lactose in human milk provides a daily carbohydrate supply ranging from about 60 g in newborns to 95 g in 7- to 12-month-olds. These amounts fall close to 50% of energy requirements. After 1 year, AI is estimated at 100 g/d to fulfill brain energy needs, regardless of age or gender. (Calculated AI is higher for pregnant and nursing women.) The RDA is set at 130 g/d to provide a 30% safety factor.

The Dietary Reference Intakes for macronutrients of the Food and Nutrition Board suggests a target of 45 to 65% of calories from carbohydrate at all stages of life. The target for protein intake increases slightly with age and conversely decreases for fats. Studies in infants have documented that there is no major adverse effect of formula diets containing as little as 30% of total energy as carbohydrate. For infants older than 6 months, carbohydrate intake is based on a combination of human milk or formula and supplementary foods of United States Department of Agriculture (USDA). These data are based upon the Third National Health and Nutrition Examination Survey.

Growth and development proceed normally as long as total calories, protein, fat, and micronutrients are adequate. Ketogenic diets, used to ameliorate severe seizure disorders, are compatible with relatively normal growth and development in children past the toddler age, if caloric intake is adequate.[49,50] Ketone bodies are thought to be anticonvulsant.[51] However, glucose utilization by the brain may drop to ≤20% of normal with carbohydrate deprivation to induce ketogenesis (or with starvation). Under these conditions, gluconeogenesis provides the requisite glucose for glucose-dependent tissues, utilizing amino acids from protein breakdown and glycerol from lipolysis. Approximately 1.0 g of glucose can be derived from 1.8 g of protein or 1.0 g of glycerol.

Carbohydrate Quality

The high proportion of carbohydrate-containing foods in many diets raises their importance as sources of vitamins and minerals. Fortification and improved processes in industrialized countries partially circumvent micronutrient losses in the food supply. However, the increasing use of refined sugars and degerminated grain starch (white flour) presents a challenge in maintenance of nutritional adequacy. The sources of energy in the US infant and toddler diet have been examined epidemiologically and there is concern that juices and fruit-flavored drinks make up the second and third most important sources of carbohydrate energy in the diet after breast milk, formula, and cow milk.[52] Consumption of added sugars may reduce the intake of protein as well as essential micronutrients such as vitamins A, C, B_6, and B_{12}.[53] In addition, the increase in carbohydrate intake has been epidemiologically associated with rising rates of obesity.[54] Increased use of fructose is also of concern because of its preferential incorporation into lipids.[55]

Plasma glucose levels typically increase transiently after consuming carbohydrates. Normal glucose tolerance is operationally defined as the ability to dispose of a bolus of ingested glucose within 2 hours as judged by return of plasma level to baseline (≤120 mg/dL). The hyperglycemic excursion is quantified as the average glucose concentration over this interval and foods have been classified based on the excursion induced. This measurement is termed the "glycemic index,"[56] formally the ratio of the excursion following consumption of a portion of food containing 100 g carbohydrate versus 100 g of glucose (or 100 g of carbohydrate in white bread). These values have been periodically tabulated.[57] The corresponding hyperglycemic impact of a given food is the "glycemic load."[58] While there is some disagreement regarding the practicality and efficacy of designing diets around their glycemic load, studies have generally supported the notion that low-glycemic diets reduce stress on pancreatic β cells, improve glycemic control, reduce plasma lipids, and reduce the risk of diabetes and coronary heart disease.[56]

Low-glycemic diets are generally also higher in fiber. Epidemiological studies have revealed a consistent association between increased dietary fiber and decreased risk for constipation, obesity, and bowel cancer.[59] While many sources of fiber also contain phytic acid (inositol hexaphosphoric acid, a phosphate-storage molecule in plants) that interferes with mineral absorption, the presence of soluble fiber has been found to promote mineral absorption in the colon.[60] Maternal milk is assumed to be an optimum source of infant nutrition. Therefore an RDA for fiber in the first year of life has not been set. Beyond that, AI is estimated at 19 g/d through age 3 years, 25 g/d for ages 4 to 8 years, and 26 and 31 g/d through age 13 for females and males, respectively. Intake of dietary fiber in children estimated from the Third National Health and Nutrition Examination Survey data was 10 g/d in 2- to 5-year-olds, increasing to approximately 13 g/d in older children and adolescents. Improvement in availability and utilization of foods containing fiber should enhance population health.

Dietary Supplements

Dietary supplements relevant to carbohydrate digestion include probiotics,[61] prebiotics,[62] and other sugar derivatives. Probiotics are microbial supplements ingested to modify the colonic bacterial composition with the intention of improving health and well-being. Often, the microbes used are similar or identical to those found in fermented foods, such as the lactic acid bacteria of yogurt. There is some evidence that prebiotics reduce the risk of colon cancer.[63] Prebiotics are natural or synthetic compounds, such as lactitol, that foster the growth or metabolism of specific populations of colon bacteria. Often sugar alcohols such as sorbitol or xylitol are also added to foods as texturizing agents, in part because they provide sweetness with less energy yield than glucose. Finally, several carbohydrate substances have been promoted as supplements from small to supraphysiological doses for their therapeutic potential. However, definitive evidence for actual value, as in the case of glucosamine for osteoarthritis, remains weak.[64]

Disorders Involving Carbohydrates

Malabsorption of several dietary carbohydrates is caused by mutations in genes coding for proteins involved in their absorption. As with lactose intolerance, a deficiency in a necessary hydrolase or transporter leads to gastrointestinal discomfort and diarrhea (see Chapter 61, "Carbohydrate Absorption and Malabsorption"). For instance, glucose–galactose malabsorption is an autosomal recessive disorder due to mutation in the gene for SGLT1.[65] In general, symptoms abate or resolve altogether once the offending SGLT1 substrates are eliminated from the diet. Even asymptomatic carbohydrate malabsorption may lead to significant nutrient losses as well as increases in daily energy expenditure.[66]

Rare disorders of carbohydrate metabolism cover a wide spectrum and include glycogen-storage diseases, galactosemia, and protein glycosylation disorders. These diverse conditions lead to failure to thrive and grow, as well as other symptomatology dependent upon the nature of the genetic defect.

Abnormalities in circulating blood glucose levels may be a result of some these rare disorders, or more common ones. Hypoglycemia is a surrogate marker for brain energy insufficiency. It is difficult to determine the precise serum glucose level that will cause transient or permanent central nervous system damage because measurements of peripheral serum glucose may not accurately reflect the glucose and alternative energy substrates available to neuronal cells. However, circulating serum glucose values of 60 mg/dL or less in children over the age of a year are usually associated with autonomic and central nervous system symptoms of hypoglycemia. Hypoglycemia results from an imbalance of glucose utilization over glucose production and/or carbohydrate intake. It may be a result of increased carbohydrate utilization because of decreased availability of lipid for energy needs, decreased gluconeogenesis, or inappropriately elevated insulin levels leading to increased carbohydrate storage and utilization without increased production.

Hyperglycemia, or elevated blood glucose, in contrast, is the result of greater glucose intake or production than utilization. Severe hyperglycemia, or diabetes, has been defined epidemiologically as a fasting blood glucose greater than 126 mg/dL, or an abnormal response to an oral glucose-tolerance test. It can result from insulin deficiency or severe insulin resistance. Persistent hyperglycemia often reflects decreased utilization of carbohydrates and other substrates and will be associated with weight loss and poor growth. Chronically elevated blood glucose levels also lead to a group of related pathologic events that cause damage to nerves, kidneys, blood vessels, and other body tissues. Hyperglycemia leads to generation of reactive oxygen species, oxidative DNA damage, and an enhanced inflammatory response.[67–69] Nonenzymatic glycation, a process which facilitates cell damage and alterations in collagen matrix through production of advanced glycation end products, occurs more rapidly when circulating glucose levels are above normal. Hyperglycemia also accelerates intracellular conversion of glucose to the sugar alcohol sorbitol, which cannot cross plasma membranes. Neural damage and an increased risk of cataract are attributed in part to osmotically induced cell injury.[70,71]

SUMMARY

A wide range of carbohydrate intake levels are compatible with normal growth, development, and activity. Numerous regulatory mechanisms assure that in normal individuals carbohydrate availability from exogenous and endogenous sources will be appropriately balanced for metabolic need.

Recommended carbohydrate intakes of approximately 50% of caloric need are based on few experimental prospective studies, but reflect general experience. Nonetheless, the quality of dietary carbohydrate is clearly important for AI of micronutrients and also plays an important role in weight maintenance, lipid metabolism, and general health.

REFERENCES

1. Gudmand-Hoyer E, Skovbjerg H. Disaccharide digestion and maldigestion. Scand J Gastroenterol Suppl 1996;216:111–21.
2. Sonnenburg ED, Sonnenburg JL, Manchester JK, et al. A hybrid two-component system protein of a prominent human gut symbiont couples glycan sensing in vivo to carbohydrate metabolism. Proc Natl Acad Sci U S A 2006;103:8834–9.
3. Hediger MA, Rhoads DB. Molecular physiology of sodium-glucose cotransporters. Physiol Rev 1994;74:993–1026.
4. Wright EM, Turk E. The sodium/glucose cotransport family SLC5. Pflugers Arch 2004;447:510–8.
5. Uldry M, Thorens B. The SLC2 family of facilitated hexose and polyol transporters. Pflugers Arch 2004;447:480–9.
6. Tsukaguchi H, Tokui T, Mackenzie B, et al. A family of mammalian Na^+-dependent L-ascorbic acid transporters. Nature 1999;399:70–5.
7. Tazawa S, Yamato T, Fujikura H, et al. SLC5A9/SGLT4, a new Na^+-dependent glucose transporter, is an essential transporter for mannose, 1,5-anhydro-D-glucitol, and fructose. Life Sci 2005;76:1039–50.
8. Diez-Sampedro A, Hirayama BA, Osswald C, et al. A glucose sensor hiding in a family of transporters. Proc Natl Acad Sci U S A 2003;100:11753–8.
9. Zeuthen T, Meinild AK, Loo DD, et al. Isotonic transport by the Na^+-glucose cotransporter SGLT1 from humans and rabbit. J Physiol 2001;531:631–44.
10. Ferraris RP. Dietary and developmental regulation of intestinal sugar transport. Biochem J 2001;360:265–76.
11. Riby JE, Fujisawa T, Kretchmer N. Fructose absorption. Am J Clin Nutr 1993;58:748S–53S.
12. Heijboer AC, Pijl H, Van den Hoek AM, et al. Gut-brain axis: Regulation of glucose metabolism. J Neuroendocrinol 2006;18:883–94.
13. Drucker DJ. The role of gut hormones in glucose homeostasis. J Clin Invest 2007;117:24–32.
14. Cummings DE, Overduin J. Gastrointestinal regulation of food intake. J Clin Invest 2007;117:13–23.
15. Liddle RA, Rushakoff RJ, Morita ET, et al. Physiological role for cholecystokinin in reducing postprandial hyperglycemia in humans. J Clin Invest 1988;81:1675–81.
16. Rushakoff RJ, Goldfine ID, Carter JD, Liddle RA. Physiological concentrations of cholecystokinin stimulate amino acid-induced insulin release in humans. J Clin Endocrinol Metab 1987;65:395–401.
17. Drucker DJ. Glucagon-like peptides: regulators of cell proliferation, differentiation, and apoptosis. Mol Endocrinol 2003;17:161–71.
18. Holst JJ. Enteroglucagon. Annu Rev Physiol 1997;59:257–71.
19. Murphy KG, Dhillo WS, Bloom SR. Gut peptides in the regulation of food intake and energy homeostasis. Endocr Rev 2006;27:719–27.
20. Cohen MA, Ellis SM, Le Roux CW, et al. Oxyntomodulin suppresses appetite and reduces food intake in humans. J Clin Endocrinol Metab 2003;88:4696–701.
21. Wynne K, Park AJ, Small CJ, et al. Subcutaneous oxyntomodulin reduces body weight in overweight and obese subjects: A double-blind, randomized, controlled trial. Diabetes 2005;54:2390–5.
22. Morgan LM, Wright JW, Marks V. The effect of oral galactose on GIP and insulin secretion in man. Diabetologia 1979;16:235–9.
23. Ganda OP, Soeldner JS, Gleason RE, et al. Metabolic effects of glucose, mannose, galactose, and fructose in man. J Clin Endocrinol Metab 1979;49:616–22.
24. Schusdziarra V, Schmid R. Physiological and pathophysiological aspects of somatostatin. Scand J Gastroenterol Suppl 1986;119:29–41.
25. Cushman SW, Wardzala LJ. Potential mechanism of insulin action on glucose transport in the isolated rat adipose cell: Apparent translocation of intracellular transport systems to the plasma membrane. J Biol Chem 1980;255:4758–62.
26. Suzuki K, Kono T. Evidence that insulin causes translocation of glucose transport activity to the plasma membrane from an intracellular storage site. Proc Natl Acad Sci U S A 1980;77:2542–5.
27. Kasahara M, Hinkle PC. Reconstitution of D-glucose transport catalyzed by a protein fraction from human erythrocytes in sonicated liposomes. Proc Natl Acad Sci U S A 1976;73:396–400.
28. Mueckler M, Caruso C, Baldwin SA, et al. Sequence and structure of a human glucose transporter. Science 1985;229:941–5.
29. Champ MM, Molis C, Flourie B, et al. Small-intestinal digestion of partially resistant cornstarch in healthy subjects. Am J Clin Nutr 1998;68:705–10.
30. Pereira MA, Ludwig DS. Dietary fiber and body-weight regulation. Observations and mechanisms. Pediatr Clin North Am 2001;48:969–80.
31. Coudray C, Demigne C, Rayssiguier Y. Effects of dietary fibers on magnesium absorption in animals and humans. J Nutr 2003;133:1–4.

32. Suttie JW. The importance of menaquinones in human nutrition. Annu Rev Nutr1995;15:399–417.
33. Fletcher CM, Coyne MJ, Bentley DL, et al. Phase-variable expression of a family of glycoproteins imparts a dynamic surface to a symbiont in its human intestinal ecosystem. Proc Natl Acad Sci U S A 2007;104:2413–8.
34. McBurney MI, Sauer WC. Fiber and large bowel energy absorption: Validation of the integrated ileostomy-fermentation model using pigs. J Nutr 1993;123:721–7.
35. Zhou JR, Erdman JW, Jr. Phytic acid in health and disease. Crit Rev Food Sci Nutr 1995;35:495–508.
36. Pellerin L, Magistretti PJ. Glutamate uptake into astrocytes stimulates aerobic glycolysis: A mechanism coupling neuronal activity to glucose utilization. Proc Natl Acad Sci U S A 1994;91:10625–9.
37. Kasischke KA, Vishwasrao HD, Fisher PJ, et al. Neural activity triggers neuronal oxidative metabolism followed by astrocytic glycolysis. Science 204;305:99–103.
38. Aubert A, Costalat R, Magistretti PJ, Pellerin L. Brain lactate kinetics: Modeling evidence for neuronal lactate uptake upon activation. Proc Natl Acad Sci U S A 2005;102:16448–53.
39. Pierre K, Pellerin L. Monocarboxylate transporters in the central nervous system: Distribution, regulation and function. J Neurochem 2005;94:1–14.
40. Redies C, Hoffer LJ, Beil C, et al. Generalized decrease in brain glucose metabolism during fasting in humans studied by PET. Am J Physiol 1989;256:E805–10.
41. Gilman AG. G proteins: Transducers of receptor-generated signals. Annu Rev Biochem 1987;56:615–49.
42. Montminy M. Transcriptional regulation by cyclic AMP. Annu Rev Biochem 1997;66:807–22.
43. Helenius A, Aebi M. Intracellular functions of N-linked glycans. Science 2001;291:2364–9.
44. Helenius A, Aebi M. Roles of N-linked glycans in the endoplasmic reticulum. Annu Rev Biochem 2004;73:1019–49.
45. Roughley PJ. The structure and function of cartilage proteoglycans. Eur Cell Mater 2006;12:92–101.
46. Rudd PM, Elliott T, Cresswell P, et al. Glycosylation and the immune system. Science 2001;291:2370–6.
47. Wells L, Vosseller K, Hart GW. Glycosylation of nucleocytoplasmic proteins: signal transduction and O-GlcNAc. Science 2001;291:2376–8.
48. Zachara NE, Hart GW. Cell signaling, the essential role of O-GlcNAc! Biochim Biophys Acta 2006;1761:599–617.
49. Vining EP, Pyzik P, McGrogan J, et al. Growth of children on the ketogenic diet. Dev Med Child Neurol 2002;44:796–802.
50. Liu YM, Williams S, Basualdo-Hammond C, et al. A prospective study: Growth and nutritional status of children treated with the ketogenic diet. J Am Diet Assoc 2003;103:707–12.
51. Hartman AL, Vining EP. Clinical aspects of the ketogenic diet. Epilepsia 2007;48:31–4252.
52. Fox MK, Reidy K, Novak T, Ziegler P. Sources of energy and nutrients in the diets of infants and toddlers. J Am Diet Assoc 2006;106:S28–42.
53. Bhargava A, Amialchuk A. Added sugars displaced the use of vital nutrients in the National Food Stamp Program Survey. J Nutr 2007;137:453–60.
54. Griel AE, Ruder EH, Kris-Etherton PM. The changing roles of dietary carbohydrates: From simple to complex. Arterioscler Thromb Vasc Biol 2006;26:1958–65.
55. Basciano H, Federico L, Adeli K. Fructose, insulin resistance, and metabolic dyslipidemia. Nutr Metab (Lond) 2005; 2:5.
56. Jenkins DJ, Kendall CW, Augustin LS, et al. Glycemic index: Overview of implications in health and disease. Am J Clin Nutr 2002;76:266S–73S.
57. Foster-Powell K, Holt SH, Brand-Miller JC. International table of glycemic index and glycemic load values: 2002. Am J Clin Nutr 2002;76:5–56.
58. Cordain L, Eaton SB, Sebastian A, et al. Origins and evolution of the Western diet: Health implications for the 21st century. Am J Clin Nutr 2005;81:341–54.
59. Anderson JW, Randles KM, Kendall CW, Jenkins DJ. Carbohydrate and fiber recommendations for individuals with diabetes: A quantitative assessment and meta-analysis of the evidence. J Am Coll Nutr 2004;23:5–17.
60. Greger JL. Nondigestible carbohydrates and mineral bioavailability. J Nutr 1999;129:1434S-5S61.
61. Fuller R. Probiotics in man and animals. J Appl Bacteriol 1989;66:365–78.
62. Macfarlane GT, Cummings JH. Probiotics and prebiotics: Can regulating the activities of intestinal bacteria benefit health? BMJ 1999;318:999–1003.
63. Commane D, Hughes R, Shortt C, Rowland I. The potential mechanisms involved in the anti-carcinogenic action of probiotics. Mutat Res 2005;591:276–89.
64. Clegg DO, Reda DJ, Harris CL, et al. Glucosamine, chondroitin sulfate, and the two in combination for painful knee osteoarthritis. N Engl J Med 2006;354:795–808.
65. Martin MG, Turk E, Lostao MP, et al. Defects in Na+/glucose cotransporter (SGLT1) trafficking and function cause glucose-galactose malabsorption. Nat Genet 1996;12:216–20.
66. Valois S, Rising R, Duro D, et al. Carbohydrate malabsorption may increase daily energy requirements in infants. Nutrition 2003;19:832–6.
67. Evans JL, Goldfine ID, Maddux BA, Grodsky GM. Oxidative stress and stress-activated signaling pathways: A unifying hypothesis of type 2 diabetes. Endocr Rev 2002;23:599–622.
68. Yan SF, Yan SD, Herold K, et al. Receptor for advanced glycation end products and the cardiovascular complications of diabetes and beyond: Lessons from ageing. Endocrinol Metab Clin North Am 2006;35:511–24.
69. Song F, Jia W, Yao Y, et al. Oxidative stress, antioxidant status and DNA damage in patients with impaired glucose regulation and newly-diagnosed Type II diabetes. Clin Sci (Lond) 2007;112:599–606.
70. Chung SS, Ho EC, Lam KS, Chung SK. Contribution of polyol pathway to diabetes-induced oxidative stress. J Am Soc Nephrol 2003;14:S233–6.
71. Dagher Z, Park YS, Asnaghi V, et al. Studies of rat and human retinas predict a role for the polyol pathway in human diabetic retinopathy. Diabetes 2004;53:2404–11.

6

Macronutrient Requirement for Growth: Protein/Amino Acid

Rachel M. Roth, MD
Leticia Castillo, MD

This chapter will provide an overview of the current state of knowledge of protein and amino acid requirement in children. The special protein and amino acid needs of premature infants are reviewed in Chapter 34, "The Low-Birth-Weight Infant: Outpatient Care."

Nitrogen utilization and therefore amino acid and protein requirements are critical in maintaining whole body homeostasis. Loss of more than 30% of body proteins results in death.[1] Amino acid utilization is needed for tissue formation and multiple physiologic functions.[2] Therefore, maintenance of whole body nitrogen stores is critical to survival. Proteins are the major functional and structural component of cells, enzymes, membrane transporters, intracellular matrices, etc. All these components are essential for life. Hence, an adequate provision of dietary protein is essential to maintain cellular integrity and function.

Proteins are made of carbon, oxygen, hydrogen, and a smaller proportion are also made also sulfur. But the chemical characteristic of proteins is their amino nitrogen group. Proteins are macromolecules consisting of long chain of amino acid subunits. The sequence of amino acids in the chain is known as the primary structure. Proteins fold into a definite three-dimensional structure. Their exact shape depends on their function and interaction with other molecules.

After ingestion of a protein meal, proteins are denatured by the acid in the stomach; they are cleaved by pepsin into smaller peptides. In the small intestine the denatured proteins and peptides are hydrolyzed by a variety of pancreatic enzymes, including trypsin, chymotrypsins, elastases, and carboxypeptidases. The mixture of free amino acids and small peptides is transported into the mucosal cells by specific carrier systems. Following intracellular hydrolysis, the free amino acids are secreted into the portal blood by other specific carrier systems, or they are further metabolized within the intestine itself. Absorbed amino acids pass into the liver where a fraction is taken up and utilized. This process is known as first-pass disappearance or splanchnic uptake. Therefore, less than 100% of the amino acids removed from the intestinal lumen reach the systemic circulation. The amino acid fraction that disappears in the splanchnic area differs among the different amino acids. The remainder amino acid fraction passes through the systemic circulation to be utilized by the whole body economy.[3] The utilization efficiency of most dietary proteins, or capacity to integrate into body proteins, is about 90%.[4] Protein losses in the intestine account for 25% of the obligatory nitrogen losses,[5] such as intestinal cell turnover, secretion of mucin, and enzymes. Protein is also lost by skin, urine, and hair. There is controversy in regard to the contribution of indispensable amino acids by the intestinal bacteria with conflicting data in favor of and against a significant contribution by the intestinal bacterial to the amino acid pool.[6–8]

Protein synthesis and degradation are balanced during steady state. Both increase during conditions of stress, but degradation offsets synthesis, resulting in a negative balance. Protein degradation occurs by a lysosomal or ubiquitin-proteasome–dependent mechanism.[9]

AMINO ACIDS

The amino acids that are incorporated into mammalian protein are α–amino acids, with the exception of proline, which is an α–amino acid. This means that they have a carboxyl group, an amino nitrogen group, and a side chain attached to a central α-carbon (Table 1). The structure of the side chains determines the functional differences among amino acids. Amino acids are provided in the diet or they can be synthesized from a carbon and nitrogen source. Amino acids are catabolized by removal of the nitrogen group through the process of transamination, which results in formation of other amino acids (alanine, pyruvate, aspartate, and glutamine) or by the process of deamination, which results in the formation of ammonia. Therefore, the nitrogen removed from any amino acid can be directed toward ammonia and aspartate, which are the precursors of urea. Urea synthesis takes place in the liver. Other organs like the intestine and kidney contain an incomplete set of urea cycle enzymes. Urea is released into the circulation by the liver and transported to the kidneys, where it is excreted in the urine. Therefore, nitrogen excretion occurs mainly as urea excretion. However, ammonium ions are also excreted and this contributes to the maintenance of acid–base balance.

The carbon moiety of the amino acids is catabolized by oxidation through the tricarboxylic acid (TCA) pathway of glucose oxidation. Some amino acids enter the TCA cycle as ketoacid analogs and others have specific degradation pathways which produce intermediates that are metabolized in the TCA cycle. The carbon skeleton of amino acids is also available for biosynthesis of glucose and fat. If the carbon skeleton enters as acetyl-CoA then fat or ketone bodies are formed. Other carbon skeletons from amino acids can be utilized for gluconeogenesis, hence, the classic division of amino acids in ketogenic or glucogenic, although some amino acids can give rise to both ketones and glucose.

Classification

Classification of amino acids was initially based on the classic studies of Rose and coworkers.[11–15] These studies were based on the qualitative significance of each amino acid in human nutrition. Rose defined amino acids as essential or nonessential based on their capacity to maintain nitrogen balance in young men (Table 2). Holt,[16] Snyderman,[17–26] and Fomon[27] extended Rose's studies to the pediatric population. In their studies they demonstrated that only the "essential" amino acids were needed to maintain growth in young infants and therefore conformed according to the original definition of "essentiality of amino acids."

Through the following decades it became evident that Rose's classification was limited and that a distinction between essential and nonessential amino acids was complex and could not be defined based solely on the nutritional criteria of maintenance of nitrogen balance or growth.[29] For example, histidine, an nonessential amino acid in the rat that was considered nonessential in humans in the original Rose classification, has been proven to be essential in health and disease, and was included as an essential amino acid by the Food Agricultural Organization/World Health Organization/United Nations University (FAO/WHO/UNU) expert report in 1985.[28]

Over the past decades the concept of essentiality based on maintenance of growth or of nitrogen equilibrium has been revisited and, with contributions by Mitchell,[30] Laidlaw,[31] Young,[32] Chipponi,[33] Reeds,[34] and others,[35] the concept of amino acid essentially has changed. Mitchell[30] considered a more dynamic concept of "essentiality" based on the ratio of supply to demand, rather than on the

Table 1 Amino Acid Structure

Name	Abbreviation	Formula
Aliphatic side chains		
Glycine	Gly	$H-CH(NH_2)-COOH$
Alanine	Ala	$CH_3-CH(NH_2)-COOH$
*Valine**	Val	$(CH_3)_2CH-CH(NH_2)-COOH$
*Leucine**	Leu	$(CH_3)_2CH-CH_2-CH(NH_2)-COOH$
*Isoleucine**	Ile	$CH_3-CH_2(CH_3)CH-CH(NH_2)-COOH$
Aromatic side chains		
Phenylalanine	Phe	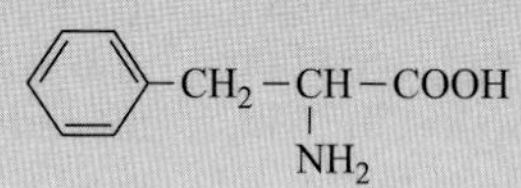
Tyrosine	Tyr	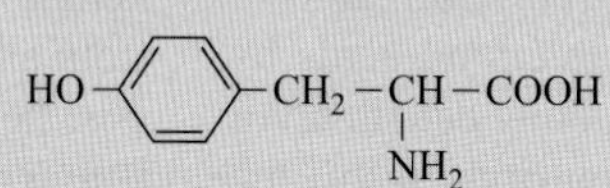
Tryptophan	Trp	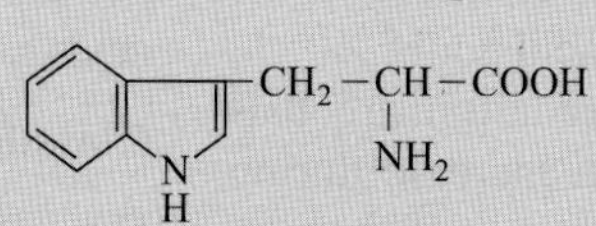
Hydroxyl groups in side chains		
Serine	Ser	$CH_2(OH)-CH(NH_2)-COOH$
Threonine	Thr	$CH_2-CH(OH)-CH(NH_2)-COOH$
Sulfur-containing side chains		
Cystine†	Cys	$HS-CH_2-CH(NH_2)-COOH$
Methionine	Met	$CH_3-S-CH_2-CH_2-CH(NH_2)-COOH$
Amino acids		
Proline‡	Pro	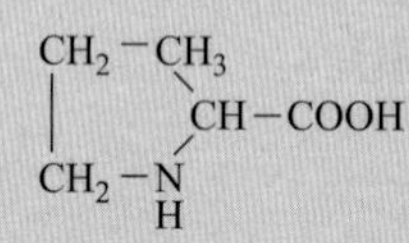
Acidic side chains and their amides		
Glutamic acid	Glu	$HOOC-CH_2-CH_2-CH(NH_2)-COOH$
Glutamine	Gln	$H_2N-C(=O)-CH_2-CH_2-CH(NH_2)-COOH$
Aspartic acid	Asp	$HOOC-CH_2-CH(NH_2)-COOH$
Asparagine	Asn	$H_2N-C(=O)-CH_2-CH(NH_2)-COOH$
Basic side chains		
Lysine	Lys	$H_2N-CH_2-CH_2-CH_2-CH_2-CH(NH_2)-COOH$
Arginine	Arg	$H_2N-C(=NH)-NH-CH_2-CH_2-CH_2-CH(NH_2)-COOH$
Histidine	His	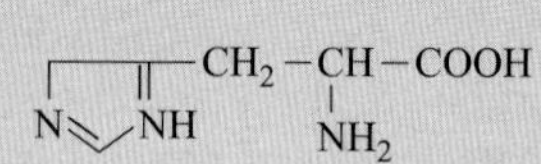

From reference 10.
*Leucine, valine, and isoleucine are known as the branch chain amino acids.
†Cysteine is found as a dimer, linked through the sulfur atoms by oxidation.
‡Proline is strictly an imino acid rather than amino acid.

maintenance of nitrogen balance or growth. The term "conditionally indispensable" has been used to refer to those nonessential or dispensable amino acids that become essential or indispensable under pathophysiologic conditions.[33] Because the carbon skeleton of the amino acid is the moiety that determines its nutritional indispensability, some classification of amino acids has been based on the ability to synthesize and/or aminate the carbon skeleton[34] In metabolic terms, the amino acids that are generally considered to be nutritionally essential contain specific chemical structures, the synthesis of which cannot be catalyzed by mammalian enzymes,[34] such as the branch aliphatic side chain of leucine, isoleucine, or valine; the primary amine of lysine; the secondary alcohol of threonine; the secondary thiol of methionine; the indol ring of tryptophan; the aromatic ring of phenylalanine; or the imidazol ring of histidine.[36] Table 2 summarizes the classic nutritional classification of amino acids and Table 3 shows an updated classification of amino acids.

Table 2 Amino Acid Classification by the FAO/WHO/UNU Expert Report, 1985[28]

Essential	Nonessential
Lysine	Glycine
Tryptophan	Alanine
Threonine	Serine
Isoleucine	Cystine
Leucine	Tyrosine
Methionine	Aspartic acid
Phenylalanine	Glutamic acid
Valine	Proline
Histidine	Hydroxyproline
	Arginine

It is important, however, to remember that an amino acid classification should not be based solely on nutritional (growth and maintenance), metabolic (de novo synthesis, tissue utilization, and catabolism), or chemical aspects of the amino acids, but also, and perhaps most importantly, on the maintenance of amino acid function. Some amino acids that would be considered truly dispensable in nutritional, metabolic, and chemical terms are utilized as precursors of other amino acids that maintain important physiologic functions, such as glutamate and serine, which serve, respectively, as precursors of glutamine and cystathionine. Other dispensable amino acids like alanine and aspartate contribute to physiologic and pathophysiologic events.[37,38] The involvement of amino acids in physiologic and metabolic functions is extensive and a partial description is shown in Table 4.

Protein and Amino Acid Homeostasis

The distribution of protein among the different organs varies with developmental age. Children have, proportionally, a larger amount of visceral (liver, kidney, brain, heart, and lung) protein than in the skeletal muscle, while in adults protein

Table 3 Nutritional Classification of Amino Acids

Indispensable	(a) Carbon skeleton cannot be synthesized
	(b) Rate limiting enzymes of catabolism regulated in relation to adequacy of intake and tissue supply
Conditionally indispensable	(a) Indispensable amino acid is a precursor (ie, phenylalanine-tyrosine)
	(b) Synthesis and degradation are modulated by dietary supply (ie, arginine, glycine)
	(c) Stressful states cause tissue depletion where rates of synthesis are insufficient to meet the increased rate of metabolic demand (proline, glutamine, arginine, glycine, taurine) or match the catabolic rate
Dispensable	(a) Rate of synthesis is not downregulated by intake of amino acid; metabolism largely a function of metabolic status of major energy-yielding substrates and/or overall nutritional status (alanine, glutamate, aspartate)

From reference 32.

Table 4 Involvement of Amino Acids in Physiologic and Metabolic Function

System	Function	Product	Precursor
Intestine	Energy generation	ATP	Glu, Asp, glutamine
	Proliferation	Nucleic acids	Glutamine, Gly, Asp
	Protection	Glutathione	Gys, Glu, Gly
		Nitric oxide	Arg
		Mucins	Thr, Cys, Ser, Pro
Skeletal muscle	Energy generation	Creatine	Gly, Arg, Met
	Peroxidative protection	Taurine (?)	Cys
Nervous system	Transmitter synthesis	Adrenergic	Phe
		Serotinergic	Try
		Glutaminergic	Glu
		Glycinergic	Gly
		Nitric oxide	Arg
	Peroxidative protection	Taurine (?)	Cys
Immune system	Lymphocyte proliferation	(?)	Glutamine, Arg, Asp
	Peroxidative protection	Glutathione	Cys, Glu, Gly
Cardiovascular	Blood pressure regulation	Nitric oxide	Arg
	Peroxidative protection (?)	Red cell glutathione	Cys, Glu, Gly

From reference 33.

constitutes about 15% of their weight.[10] During starvation or low protein intake, visceral protein is mobilized. This is called the "labile protein content." However, these "reserves" account only for 1% of total body protein.[39] During disease states muscle becomes the main contributor to protein loss.[40]

Body proteins are in a continuous dynamic state of synthesis and catabolism (Figure 1). Under physiologic conditions the amino acids released by protein breakdown are reused for protein synthesis. Protein turnover under these conditions is increased.

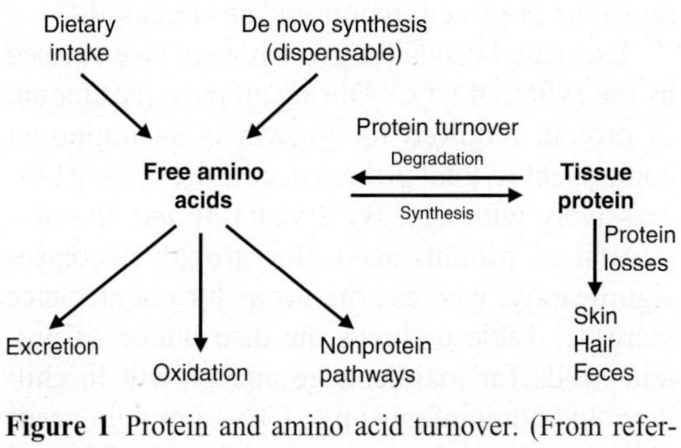

Figure 1 Protein and amino acid turnover. (From reference 10.)

Adequate nitrogen (protein) intake is essential for growth, development, and function. However, estimating "adequate" protein or specific amino acid requirement for the pediatric population is a complex and challenging endeavor.[10,28,29,41] First, the pediatric population constitutes a dynamic group, involving different clusters of individuals from newborn to adolescence. The pediatric population shows marked differences among the age groups regarding weight, rate of growth, hormonal milieu, activity, and other factors that may affect nutritional and metabolic status. Second, dietary recommendations for macro- and micronutrients among the different pediatric groups have been largely based on limited and inadequate data.[10,28,42–52] Because of ethical constraints that prevent the use of healthy children for more invasive research studies, data in the pediatric population are based on nitrogen balance studies obtained from children recovering from malnutrition.[47,48,51] Hence, pediatric data are rather limited. Third, with new knowledge emerging on nonnutritional function of nutrients, such as induction of gene expression[52] and nutritional rescue of metabolic conditions such as prevention of neural tube defects[53–55] or correction of hyperhomocysteinemia with folic acid[56] as well as the physiological and pharmacological properties of amino acids, the concept of amino acid requirement has changed from the traditional nutritional criteria based on growth or weight maintenance, to a broader functional outcome. Therefore, "adequacy" of nutritional support is ill defined and conditional to the end goals to be achieved. Based on this new knowledge about nonnutritional functions of amino acids,[34,36] a key question regarding nutritional adequacy is "what is the objective to be achieved?" Is the objective to promote growth and weight maintenance? To maintain nonnutritional functions? To prevent pathophysiologic events? To act as pharmacological agent(s)? To induce gene expression? Or for nutritional rescue? These important questions are just beginning to be explored and will be better answered in the future.

Estimates of Protein Requirements

Protein requirement is defined as "the true biological need for protein or amino acids," the lowest intake that will maintain functional needs of the individual.[10] However, since there is variation among individuals in regard to protein needs, the mean requirement has been taken as the starting point.[10,28] The Food and Nutrition Board from the Institute of Medicine, National Academy of Sciences reviewed values for the intake of nutrients.[10] The recommended dietary allowance (RDA) refers to the level of average daily dietary nutrient intake sufficient to meet the nutrient requirements of nearly all (97 to 98%) healthy individuals in a particular life stage and gender group. When RDA cannot be estimated, adequate intake is recommended, and it refers to the average daily intake level based on observed or experimentally determined approximations or estimates of nutrient intake by a group(s) of apparently healthy people that are assumed to be adequate.[10] The tolerable upper intake level is the highest average daily nutrient intake level that is likely to pose no risk of adverse health effects to almost all individuals in the general population.[10] Estimated average requirement refers to the average daily nutrient intake level estimated to meet the requirement of half the healthy individuals in a particular life stage and gender group.[10] The "safe level of intake" is defined as the amount that will meet or exceed the requirements of practically all individuals in a population, which is generally calculated as the mean requirement +2 standard deviations of the requirement.[28,41]

Dietary protein requirements involve two components: (1) total nitrogen for synthesis of the nutritionally dispensable and conditionally indispensable amino acids and for synthesis of other nitrogen-containing compounds with relevant physiologic functions, and (2) to provide for the nutritionally indispensable amino acids, which cannot be synthesized by human tissues to maintain metabolic needs and therefore, must be supplied by an exogenous source.[34,36]

The classical nitrogen balance studies by Rose[11–15] and others[45,46,51] have been used for estimation of protein and amino acid requirements in older children and adults. Nitrogen balance techniques have been significantly criticized for the difficulty in obtaining complete collections and measuring all routes of nitrogen loss (sweat, nitrate production, gaseous nitrogen, etc). Furthermore, nitrogen balance techniques do not provide information regarding the dynamic status of amino acid metabolism.[51] However, although there is a great deal of criticism for using nitrogen balance studies to estimate protein requirements, currently there are no alternative data available to estimate maintenance nitrogen needs of infants.[10,28,29,41]

Infants 0 to 6 Months of Age. In early infancy (age 0 to 6 months), the 1985 FAO/WHO/UNU considered that the protein intake of breast-fed infants constitutes the gold standard. This is based on the evolutionary assumption that breast milk is best suited to maintain the nutritional needs of the infant.[28] This approach assumes protein efficiency (weight gain per gram of protein consumed) of 90%, given the high biologic value of the protein consumed. Therefore, the protein needs of an infant would be met if energy needs are met and the food providing the energy contains protein in quantity and quality equivalent to that of breast milk.[10,28,41]

The Food and Nutrition Board has recommended an intake of 9.1 g/d or 1.52 g/kg/d of protein intake in infants age 0 to 6 months.[10] This was based on the average volume of milk intake, which was estimated to be 0.78 L/d and an average protein content in human milk of 11.7 g/L.

In 1996 the International Dietary Energy Consultancy Group (IDECG)[41] reevaluated the rationale used to determine the 1985 FAO/WHO/UNU recommendations for infants and children,[28] and concluded that the 1985 FAO/WHO/UNU expert report overestimated protein requirements during infancy by about 27 to 35%.

These overestimates were felt to be due to a number of factors. In infants from birth to 6 months, the revision yielded new data estimates on the intake of breast milk, the content of protein nitrogen and nonprotein nitrogen, and the efficiency of retention of nonprotein nitrogen (which the IDEC group postulated to be 46 to 61% in comparison to the assumed value of 100% used by the 1985 FAO/WHO/UNU). The 1996 IDECG also used body weights from breast-fed babies, rather than those of bottle-fed babies.[41]

In regard to estimates on the intake of breast milk, in the 1985 FAO/WHO/UNU expert report,[28] the average intake of breast-fed infants was assumed to approximate the mean requirement, which is defined as the amount of protein needed for growth in 50% of the children. However, this approach was flawed, since it automatically defined half of breast-fed infants as having deficient intakes[41]; therefore, mean intakes of breast milk do not equal requirement. The epidemiological probability approach indicated that at 3 to 4 months the nitrogen requirement is less than 170 mg/kg/d, whereas the mean nitrogen intake is about 231 mg/kg/d. Likewise, milk intake in the FAO/WHO/UNU report was not corrected for insensible water loss.[28] The IDECG revision was based on more extensive data on exclusively breast-fed infants until 6 months of age, correction for insensible water loss was made, and nonprotein nitrogen was taken into account.[41]

The protein content of human milk and utilization of nonprotein nitrogen was also revisited by IDECG.[41] The decline in protein content during the course of lactation was taken into account, as well as the ratio of whey:caseine in human milk throughout lactation. An important consideration in the assessment of the amount of protein available for tissue accretion and function (the biological value of a protein) is the relative amount of nonprotein nitrogen. The average nonprotein nitrogen of mature human milk has been estimated to be 26% of the total nitrogen content. The major nonprotein nitrogen compounds in human milk are amino acids, creatinine, urea, creatine, and uric acid. Of this nonprotein fraction it has been estimated that 27% of it, or about 7% of total nitrogen, is available for protein synthesis[10,41]

The proportion of nonprotein nitrogen in human milk was considered by the 1996 IDECG revision of protein requirements.[41] Table 5 shows the revised IDECG estimates on average intake of protein in breast-fed infants 0 to 6 months of age, and they are compared to the 1985 FAO/WHO/UNU expert report.[28] It is important to point out that average intake of protein in breast-fed infants does not necessarily translate into requirements. This table shows that the estimated protein intake in infancy is lower than the estimates by the 1985 FAO/WHO/UNU report when adjusted by the nonprotein nitrogen fraction. Also it is important to remember that protein concentration in milk decreases between 1 and 2 months. Decrease in protein milk concentration was not accounted for by the 1985 FAO/WHO/UNU report. Therefore, the 1996 IDECG values are 10 to 26% lower than the 1985 FAO/WHO/UNU estimates, assuming that at least 46% of the nonprotein nitrogen in human milk can be utilized.[28,41]

Infants, Children, and Adolescents. For infants older than 6 months and for children and adolescents, a factorial approach was used by the 1985 FAO/WHO/UNU expert report.[28] This approach takes into account (1) maintenance for obligatory losses, which is estimated by regression analysis of the relationship between nitrogen intake and nitrogen balance; (2) measurement of the rates of protein deposition, which are derived from body composition analysis; and (3) estimates of the efficiency of protein utilization, which is derived from the slope of the line relating intake and balance.

The factorial method is summarized as follows:

Mean dietary protein requirement = maintenance + protein accretion associated with growth × 100/utilization efficiency

Under this concept, the need of total protein and/or a particular amino acid for growth is equal to the rate of protein deposition and/or the content of that particular amino acid to the protein being deposited.[28,32,41] However, a problem with this approach is that the relation between protein intake and nitrogen retention is not linear; thus, the efficiency of nitrogen retention is less as zero balance point is approached.[51]

In the factorial approach used by the 1985 FAO/WHO/UNU the maintenance requirement at 6 months was taken to be 120 mg N/kg/d declining to 103 mg N/kg/d by age 18 months. A growth component was estimated and to which a 50% addition was made to provide a margin of safety, because growth rates vary from day to day and because protein is not "stored" when there is a relative excess intake. The fractional efficiency of nitrogen utilization from high-quality protein sources for both maintenance and growth was taken to be 0.7 and the coefficient of variation (CV) for maintenance and growth was taken to be 12.5 and 35%, respectively, for purposes of calculating the total CV and a recommended safe protein intake level.[28] The total CV was estimated as follows:

$$CV_{total} = (M \times CV_m)^2 + (G \times CV_g)^2/(M + G),$$

where M equals maintenance and G equals growth.

The requirements estimated by the 1985 FAO/WHO/UNU used the above described data and assumptions to reach their recommendations. The data and assumptions have been since revisited and with accrual or newer and more updated information, some modifications to recommended protein intakes in children have been proposed.

The 1996 IDECG concluded that the recommendations of the 1985 FAO/WHO/UNU overestimated protein requirements in childhood by 17 to 20%.[41]

For infants older than 6 months and young children, the 1996 IDECG revisited the factorial approach used by the 1985 FAO/WHO/UNU. The maintenance requirement of nitrogen estimated to be 120 mg/kg/d used by FAO/WHO/UNU was revised down to 90 mg/kg/d. The 1996 IDECG estimated maintenance nitrogen needs in infants and children, obtained from a series of nitrogen balance studies,[41,44–51] whereas the 1985 FAO/WHO/UNU had used only one study of nitrogen balance in children 9 to 17 months and other studies in older children, but none in children less than 12 months of age.[28] Based on these revisions, the 1996 IDECG derived new values of estimated basal and/or maintenance nitrogen needs in infants and children, which were found to be 82 to 93 mg N/kg/d. A value of 90 mg N/kg/d was used for the factorial model, in which the revisions of protein requirements are based.[41]

Estimated needs for growth were also revised by the 1996 IDECG.[41] During infancy, the amount of protein required for growth is an important component of total protein needs, decreasing progressively with age. By 2 years of age, the proportion of protein needs for growth decreases significantly, whereas the needs for maintenance increase. Table 6 shows the distribution of protein needs for maintenance and growth in children. In young infants up to 64% of protein needs will be utilized for growth, while after 2 years,

Table 5 1996 IDECG Revised Estimates on Average Protein Intake in Breast-Fed Infants 0 to 6 Months of Age and the Intakes Estimated by the 1985 FAO/WHO/UNU Expert Report

Age (Mo)	1985 FAO/WHO/UNU* "Crude Protein" (g/kg/d)	1996 IDECG† "Adjusted Protein" (g/kg/d)
0 to 1	2.46	1.95 to 2.04
2	1.93	1.41 to 1.48
3	1.74	1.19 to 1.25
4	1.49	1.11 to 1.16
6	—	1.05 to 1.11

*From 1985 FAO/WHO/UNU 1985.[28]
†From 1996 IDECG reference.[41] Exclusively breast-fed infants. Nitrogen intake includes nonprotein nitrogen (NPN). Adjusted protein intake is based on milk protein concentration plus 41 to 61% of the NPN (protein = 6.25 × nitrogen).

protein needs for growth account only for 11% of total protein needs. Therefore, after 2 years of age the utilization of nitrogen needs in terms of growth and maintenance are very similar to those of the adult population.[28,41,51]

Intraindividual day-to-day variation in the rate of growth and therefore in the need for protein to maintain that growth was estimated to about 50% by the 1985 FAO/WHO/UNU on the premises that there is no storage capacity for amino acids and therefore it would be necessary to allow for extra demand on the days of rapid growth.[28] There is no evidence to support a 50% day-to-day variation in the rate of growth, and therefore the 1996 IDECG discarded the 50% augmentation.[41]

The retention efficiency value or efficiency in conversion from dietary protein to body protein was left unchanged at 0.7. Based on available data it is presumed that efficiency is the same for maintenance than for growth. Efficiency is calculated as nitrogen retained divided by nitrogen intake and obligatory losses are subtracted.[41]

The coefficients of variance (CV) for the interindividual variability of the average requirement estimates for maintenance and growth of infant were also revised by 1996 IDECG. The average requirement estimates need to be modified based on the extent of interindividual variability. Therefore accurate estimation of CV is important. The 12.5% CV used by the 1985 FAO/WHO/UNU was obtained from short-term nitrogen balance studies in adults, and it was assumed to be the same in the pediatric population. Interindividual variability in growth was estimated to yield a CV of 35%. However, the CV for growth depends on the interval of measurement. The CV will be lower if the interval is longer. Although an arbitrary interval of 3 months was used by the 1996 IDECG, it yielded a more reliable CV.[41]

In summary the 1996 IDECG revision of the 1985 FAO/WHO/UNU report[28] found the following: (1) For infants 0 to 6 months the estimates of protein requirement were based on breast milk intake data. Intake is not equivalent to requirement and adjustment for nonprotein nitrogen yielded a lower estimate of protein requirement. (2) For infants >6 months and children a modified factorial approach estimating lower maintenance nitrogen needs of about 90 mg/kg/d, removing a 50% safety margin for intraindividual variation in growth and estimating interindividual variation in growth at a different interval yield lower estimates of protein requirements.

The current RDAs from the Food and Nutrition Board[10] are based on the factorial approach used in the 1985 WHO/FAO/UNU report[28] and on more recent data collected over the past decade.[57–62] However, the Food and Nutrition Board stated that "the use of nitrogen balance should no longer be regarded as the gold standard for the assessment of the adequacy of protein intake and alternative means should be sought."[10] It is expected that a new FAO/WHO/UNU will convene in the future and that the observations from the 1985 FAO/WHO/UNU report will be revisited. Table 7 shows the estimates of protein intake recommended by the Food and Nutrition Board.

Other Approaches Used in the Estimation of Protein Requirements in Infants

Protein requirements in infants have also been determined by a direct experimental approach, utilizing plasma amino acid and urea nitrogen concentrations as rough indicators of the balance between intake and utilization.[10,28,41] Postprandial plasma amino acid concentrations are indicative of protein turnover; this is influx into the amino acid pool from protein breakdown, synthesis, and dietary intake and outflow from the plasma pool via catabolism and excretion (Figure 1). An "operational" approach involving protein:energy ratios (P:E) has also been used to estimate protein requirements.[41] The protein requirements per unit of energy intake decrease rapidly in the first several months of life.[28,41,60] The P:E for 3 to 6 months and 6 to 9 months have been described as 1.5 and 1.4 g protein/100 kcal, respectively.[23,36]

The use of P:E requires estimating the ratio of the safe level for protein to the mean requirement for energy at each age.[10,46,63,64]

Other Factors That Influence Protein Requirements

Other factors such as intakes of other nutrients, protein digestibility, amino acid content of proteins, and protein quality will influence protein requirements.[10,28,41,51]

Vitamin B_6 is intimately linked to protein metabolism and high protein intakes will require higher intake of vitamin B_6.[65]

To estimate digestibility, it is required to measure dietary and fecal nitrogen loss associated with a given protein source. The derivation of the fecal index used in the estimate of "apparent protein digestibility" involves the calculation of a percentage of intake based on the subtraction of the fecal nitrogen output from the dietary nitrogen ingested. However, the input from the metabolism of endogenous proteins is not taken into account by this approach.[10,41,66,67] Hence,

$$\text{Apparent protein digestibility (\%)} = \frac{N_{\text{intake}} - \text{fecal } N \text{ output on test diet} \times 100}{N_{\text{intake}}}$$

$$\text{True protein digestibility (\%)} = \frac{N_{\text{intake}} - \text{fecal } N \text{ output on test diet} - \text{fecal } N \text{ output on nonprotein diet}}{N_{\text{intake}}}$$

True protein digestibility has been established mainly in rat models for a variety of proteins.[10,41]

The content and metabolic availability of individual indispensable amino acids are important variables affecting the nutritional value of a protein food. If the content of a single dispensable amino acid is less than the individual's requirement, the utilization of other amino acids will be limited. Therefore, normal rates of protein synthesis will be affected even if the total intake level of nitrogen (protein) is adequate. The "limiting amino acid" determines the nutritional value of the total protein in the diet.[68–70] For example, a larger intake of soy protein is required to maintain balance. But this difference is eliminated if sulfur amino acids are supplemented. Therefore, sulfur amino acids are the "limiting amino acid" in soy protein intake.[10] Lysine is the most limiting indispensable amino acid in diets based on cereal proteins.[32,69]

Protein quality refers to the amino acid pattern of food proteins that efficiently will meet both the nitrogen and indispensable amino acid requirements of the individual. The amino acid requirement or "scoring" pattern is based on estimated average requirements for the individual indispensable amino acids and on total protein requirement. Therefore, nitrogen × 6.25 estimates

Table 6 Protein Needs for Growth and Maintenance in Children of Different Ages

Age	Protein Gain (g/kg/d)	Maintenance (g/kg/d)	Maintenance/Total (%)	Growth/Total (%)
0 to 1 mo	1.00	0.56	36	64
1 to 3 mo	0.57	0.56	50	50
3 to 6 mo	0.30	0.56	65	35
6 to 12 mo	0.18	0.56	76	24
1 to 2 yr	0.11	0.56	89	11
1 to 2 yr	0.11	0.56	89	11
2 to 5 yr	0.07	·0.56	89	11

Maintenance assumed to be 90 mg/kg/d.
Modified from reference 41.

Table 7 Mean Daily Rates of Protein Deposition and Factorial Model Calculations of Mean Requirements for Protein

Age (yr)	Girls Protein Deposition (mg/kg/d)	Mean Requirement (g/kg/d)	Boys Protein Deposition (mg/kg/d)	Mean Requirement (g/kg/d)
0.75	232	1.09	252	1.12
1	189	1.01	160	0.96
1.5	119	0.89	114	0.88
2	83	0.83	88	0.84
3	54	0.78	57	0.78
1 to 3	111	0.88	105	0.87
4	48	0.77	44	0.76
5	44	0.76	40	0.76
6	48	0.77	42	0.76
7	46	0.76	46	0.76
8	42	0.76	51	0.77
4 to 8	46	0.76	45	0.76
9	48	0.77	55	0.78
10	36	0.74	51	0.77
11	35	0.75	48	0.77
12	39	0.75	48	0.77
13	29	0.74	41	0.76
9 to 13	37	0.75	49	0.77
14	23	0.73	38	0.75
15	19	0.72	34	0.74
16	8	0.70	28	0.73
17	0	0.69	19	0.72
18	0	0.69	6	0.70
14 to 18	10	0.71	25	0.73

From reference 10.

the weight ratio of protein to the nitrogen content in foods. It is assumed that in average nitrogen accounts for 16% by weight of mixed proteins. The protein: nitrogen ratio for whole milk is 5.62; for egg 5.38, and for soy milk 6.07.[10] Table 8 shows the proposed amino acid scoring pattern in infants and in children 1 year or older. There is no difference between preschool children and adults. Therefore the scoring pattern remains the same after 1 year of age.[10]

The 1989 FAO/WHO expert consultation on protein quality has established standards for many protein sources, such as egg protein (97%), soy flour (86%), and wheat (96%).[70]

Table 8 Food and Nutrition Board Amino Acid Scoring Pattern in Infants and in Children ≥1 Year of Age and in All Other Older Age Groups

Amino Acid	Infants* mg/g protein	All Other Groups† mg/g protein	All Other Groups† mg/g N
Histidine	23	18	114
Isoleucine	57	25	156
Leucine	101	55	341
Lysine	69	51	320
Methionine + cysteine	38	25	156
Phenylalanine + tyrosine	87	47	291
Threonine	47	27	170
Tryptophan	18	7	43
Valine	56	32	199

Modified for reference 10.
*Pattern based on amino acid composition of breast milk.
†Pattern derived form estimated average requirement for amino acid divided by estimated amino acid requirement for protein according to age.

Animal sources of protein provide all nine indispensable amino acids and for this reason are referred to as "complete proteins," whereas "incomplete" proteins are found in plants, grains, and vegetables and tend to be deficient in one or more of the indispensable amino acids.

The protein digestibility–corrected amino acid score (PDCASS) has been proposed for the assessment of protein quality.[4,70–72] The PDCASS is obtained by comparing the concentration of a "limiting" amino acid in the food protein source to that of a standard, such as egg protein, and multiplying by the true digestibility.[72] It is expressed as the percentage of the same limiting amino acid in the referenced amino acid pattern.[71] This assessment of protein quality is however limited. Some investigators[71] have considered the use of ileal rather than fecal digestibility for inclusion in the scoring procedure and to determine if total dietary nitrogen digestibility represents a valid indicator of the bioavailability of the individual amino acid. It has been suggested by the same authors[73] that the deposition of nitrogen during the prandial phase would constitute a critical factor in the determination of food protein quality, and this may be used to assess significant differences among dietary protein sources.

Amino Acid Requirements

The complexity of estimating individual amino acid requirement was described earlier in this chapter. Traditionally, amino acid requirement had been based on nutritional utilization: growth and maintenance, with protein deposition being the predominant influence. The composition of the indispensable amino acids in body proteins of immature mammals is similar. Therefore, the composition of body protein through different species is very similar. Hence, the relative needs of each indispensable amino acid (mg amino acids/g total amino acid) for growth will be the same across species.[28] The amino acid requirements for the support of protein deposition in the human will differ from other mammals only to the extent of the difference in growth rates between species.[41] Furthermore, even in young children, the major demand on amino acid requirement is for maintenance, rather than growth. Young and coworkers estimated that for a 2-year-old child, maintenance accounts for 80 to 90% of the total protein requirement,[51] and this is in agreement with data published by Millward who suggested a value of 85%.[74] Given that in humans, the obligatory amino acid needs for protein deposition are a minor fraction of the total amino acid requirement,[10,41] the greater demand for amino acid requirement will depend on amino acid utilization for maintenance.

The amino acid needs for maintenance have been the objective of much controversy.[8,28,32,68,73–76] It has been proposed by Reeds and coworkers that nitrogen requirement for maintenance may depend on (1) continuous loss in the intestine, (2) maintenance of key metabolites derived from amino acids, and (3) maintenance of pathways that use amino acids involved in host defense and nucleotide synthesis.[36,76] It has been observed that amino acids are consumed in physiologic functions that are not directly related to protein metabolism[36] and it is important now to quantify the effect of metabolic pathways on the needs for their precursor amino acids. Lyons and colleagues observed that in septic children receiving limited nutritional support, the rates of synthesis of glutathione were decreased by 60%.[77] Glutathione is a major antioxidant and its synthesis depends on the availability of cysteine. These findings suggest that under pathophysiologic conditions, requirements of some amino acids may need to be revised based on functional rather than nutritional terms.

Specific nutritional amino acid requirement has been determined by nitrogen or amino acid carbon balance. Nitrogen balance obtained from the early studies of several investigators,[16–27,45,47–49] and carbon balance studies obtained in adults and sick children more recently with stable isotopic techniques.[78–80]

Infants up to 6 Months of Age. In infants from birth to 6 months, the requirements for indispensable amino acids were reported by the 1985 in the FAO/WHO/UNU expert report.[28] These recommendations were obtained by using the intakes of cow's milk or breast milk that supported satisfactory growth. These estimates are unchanged from the FAO's 1971 report.[29] The 1996 IDECG used a factorial approach to estimate amino acid intakes in infants from 0 to 6 months of age.[41] The amino acid needs for growth were calculated using data from Fomon and colleagues,[57] based on the daily increment

Table 9 Estimated Average Requirement (EAR) and Recommended Dietary Allowance (RDA) for Amino Acids at Different Ages

Age and Gender Amino Acid	Maintenance (mg/kg/d)	Amino Acid Deposition (mg/kg/d)	Total EAR (mg/kg/d)	RDA (mg/kg/d)
7 to 12 mo, boys, girls				
Histidine	11	7	22	32
Isoleucine	15	9	30	43
Leucine	34	18	65	93
Lysine	31	18	62	89
Methionine + cysteine	15	9	30	43
Phenylalanine + tyrosine	27	18	58	84
Threonine	16	10	34	49
Tryptophan	4	3	9	13
Valine	19	12	39	58
1 to 3 yr, boys, girls				
Histidine	11	3	16	21
Isoleucine	15	4	12	28
Leucine	34	8	48	63
Lysine	31	8	45	58
Methionine + cysteine	15	4	22	28
Phenylalanine + tyrosine	27	8	41	54
Threonine	16	5	24	32
Tryptophan	4	1	6	8
Valine	19	5	28	37
4 to 8 yr, boys, girls				
Histidine	11	1	13	16
Isoleucine	15	2	18	22
Leucine	34	4	40	49
Lysine	31	3	37	46
Methionine + cysteine	15	2	18	22
Phenylalanine + tyrosine	27	3	33	41
Threonine	16	2	19	24
Tryptophan	4	1	5	6
Valine	19	2	23	28
9 to 13 yr, boys				
Histidine	11	1	13	17
Isoleucine	15	2	18	22
Leucine	34	4	40	49
Lysine	31	4	37	46
Methionine + cysteine	15	2	18	22
Phenylalanine + tyrosine	27	4	33	41
Threonine	16	2	19	24
Tryptophan	4	1	5	6
Valine	19	2	23	28
9 to 13 yr, girls				
Histidine	11	1	12	15
Isoleucine	15	1	17	21
Leucine	34	2	38	47
Lysine	31	2	35	43
Methionine + cysteine	15	1	17	21
Phenylalanine + tyrosine	27	2	31	38
Threonine	16	1	18	22
Tryptophan	4	<0.5	5	6
Valine	19	2	22	27
14 to 18 yr, boys				
Histidine	11	1	12	15
Isoleucine	15	1	17	21
Leucine	34	2	38	47
Lysine	31	2	35	43
Methionine + cysteine	15	1	17	21
Phenylalanine + tyrosine	27	2	31	38
Threonine	16	1	18	22
Tryptophan	4	<0.5	5	6
Valine	19	1	22	27
9 to 13 yr, girls				
Histidine	11	<0.5	12	14
Isoleucine	15	<0.5	16	19
Leucine	34	1	35	44
Lysine	31	1	32	40
Methionine + cysteine	15	<0.5	16	19
Phenylalanine + tyrosine	27	1	28	35
Threonine	16	<0.5	17	21
Tryptophan	4	<0.5	4	5
Valine	19	1	20	24

Modified from reference 10.

in body protein of breast-fed infants, and the amino acid pattern of whole body protein. Maintenance protein was calculated as follows: (1) by using the value of 120 mg N/kg/d and (2) by using nitrogen requirement from balance studies, but normalized to metabolic body size (0.75). The factorial approach gave lower estimates for essential amino acids in the 3- to 6-month group. However, given the significance of nonnutritional functions of amino acids and because the functional implications of amino acids in breast milk have not been fully understood, it appeared safer to continue to support the 1971 estimates, and no revision was proposed by 1996 IDECG.[41]

The recommended adequate intakes for infants 0 to 6 months estimated by the Food and Nutrition Board for infants 0 to 6 months is based on the 1985 FAO/WHO/UNU,[28] methods using average volume of milk intake of 0.78 L/d and the mean indispensable amino acid content of human milk. The recommended values are similar to those recommended by the 1985 FAO/WHO/UNU. Table 9 shows the estimated average requirement and RDA for amino acids at different ages by the Food and Nutrition Board.

Children and Adolescents. For preschool children amino acid requirements are based on nitrogen balance studies conducted at the Institute of Nutrition for Central America and Panama, Guatemala.[10,28,41,51] The data were presented only in summary form at a conference proceedings.[51] For older children the requirements from the 1971 FAO/WHO report were upheld. These data were obtained from studies conducted by Nakagawa in the 1960s in Japan,[49] but reexamined by the National Research Council, Washington DC, National Academy of Sciences.[50] Because of significant methodological limitations the data from the nitrogen balance studies were not used to determine requirements of indispensable amino acids in children 7 months through 18 years. Instead, the factorial approach has been used by the 1996 IDECG,[41] Millward,[74] Young,[51] and the Food and Nutrition Board[10] to estimate indispensable amino acid requirements. The values obtained are similar but slightly lower than the estimates of the 1985 FAO/WHO/UNU expert report.[28]

These recommendations are based in part on the 1985 FAO/WHO/UNU[28] and on other data. There is great need for further studies on the protein and amino acid requirements of children, for nutritional and functional outcomes.

Other Methods for Estimating Individual Amino Acid Requirement

Isotopic studies for quantitative estimates of amino acid requirements and for determination of the efficiency of dietary protein utilization

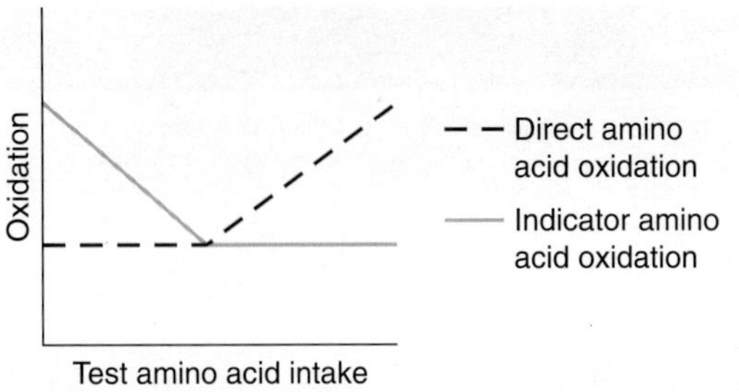

Figure 2 Direct amino acid oxidation and indicator amino acid oxidation and balance techniques for determination of amino acid requirements.

in meeting these requirements are based on various approaches: (1) bolus or continuous infusion of amino acid tracers and (2) ingestion of single amino acid–labeled protein or uniformly labeled protein.[10,80]

Amino Acid Oxidation and Balance (Obligatory Oxidative Losses Ool Technique). In this method the amino acid test of interest is given at graded levels of intake to subjects and measurement of the carbon oxidation of single indispensable amino acids is taken as indicator of the adequacy of the test amino acid.[81] This method is based on the concept that the nutritional indispensability of an amino acid is due to the inability to synthesize its carbon skeleton. Therefore, if the test amino acid is labeled with ^{13}C, the production of $^{13}CO_2$ in breath is assumed to accurately reflect the irreversible oxidative loss of the test amino acid. When this method is used at progressively lower levels of test amino acid intake, a minimum level or "break point" in the relation between the carbon catabolism, as estimated from the $^{13}CO_2$ in breath, and the test amino acid intake could be established. The break point is indicative of the relationship between the carbon catabolism of the amino acid and its intake (Figure 2). It is assumed that below the requirement, the test amino acid will be conserved and the rates of oxidation will be low and constant, but once the requirement is exceeded, the oxidation of the test amino acid will increase. Therefore, nutritional requirement will be established at the "break point" level.[82–84]

Noninvasive Indicator Amino Acid Oxidation (IAAO). This noninvasive method is based on the measurement of the oxidation of an indicator amino acid (^{13}C phenylalanine or ^{13}C lysine), which falls to a "break point" when the amino acid test requirement is achieved (Figure 2). It uses no adaptation to the test level of amino acid intake, an oral indicator amino acid tracer is used, and urine collections are obtained for isotopic enrichment, provided that no D-amino acid is present in the infusate.[85] Branched chain amino acid requirements were determined in five healthy children age 6 to 10 years, by this noninvasive method.[86]

The mean requirement was 147 mg/kg/d and the safe level of intake was 192 mg/kg/d. These values are 48% higher than the DRI recommendations of 99 mg/kg/d. Moreover, total sulfur amino acid requirements were also determined with this method in six preadolescent children. Mean requirement in this age group was 12.9 mg/kg/d and the safe level of intake was 17.2 mg/kg/d. These values were 22% lower than the DRI recommendations, but were similar to adult values of 12.6 mg/kg/d.[87]

Methionine requirements were estimated in healthy adolescents age 13 to 17 years by Gordon and coworkers[88] using the IAAO and balance technique (IAAOB). This technique has been used in healthy adults for estimation of amino acid requirements. This method shows methionine requirements of 25 mg/kg/d in the healthy adolescents, which are higher than DRI values of 17.2 mg/kg/d and than values of 12.9 mg/kg/d obtained by the noninvasive IAAO technique, but closer to values of 27 mg/kg/d reported by Nakagawa and obtained by nitrogen balance technique.[89]

Twenty-Four-Hour Indicator Amino Acid Oxidation and Balance Technique. Amino acid balance studies carried over a period of 24 hours have been obtained for leucine,[87] phenylalanine,[90] lysine[91] and threonine.[92] This approach provides a more accurate estimate of amino acid needs. However, tracer intake over the 24-hour period has been considered a drawback.

All these methods have drawbacks and strengths. The noninvasive IAAO technique uses another essential amino acid as the tracer (lysine, leucine, or phenylalanine in the presence of an excess of tyrosine), based on the principle that the tracer amino acid is independent of the changes in graded levels of intake of the test amino acid. As there is no storage of amino acids, the essential indicator amino acid is utilized for protein synthesis or oxidation, depending on the intake of the indispensable test amino acid. The precursor pool for oxidation does not increase, given that the test amino acid is different from the amino acid tracer given.[85] Adaptation to adequate protein and energy intake is conducted for 2 days, but there is no adaptation to the test amino acid, and the test level of intake is given only during the tracer study. Seven levels of test amino acid, three below and three above the target level, are given in order to obtain a "break point" between the level of amino acid intake and the rates of IAAO. The isotope tracer is hourly provided by the oral route, with the meals. Breath and urine samples are obtained every 30 minutes over 5 hours for measurement of breath $^{13}CO_2$ and urinary enrichment of the isotope tracer given. This method investigates only the fed state. The fasting state is not probed. The oral tracer study is repeated seven times at seven different levels of amino acid test intake in the same subject. Two-phase linear regression analysis is applied to obtain the "break point" between the different levels of test amino acid intake, and the rates of oxidation of the indicator amino acid. This break point is indicative of the test amino acid requirement (Figure 2). With this noninvasive method determination phenylalanine requirement in children with phenylketonuria[93] and branched chain and sulfur amino acid requirements in school age healthy children.[86]

There has been controversy in regard to the need for and the length of an adaptation period.[68,75,85,94] The proponents of a longer adaptation period state that it takes several days to adapt to dietary changes in nitrogen intake.[68] Therefore, a dietary adaptation period to the test level of amino acid intake had been considered essential.[10,68] In contrast, supporters of the short noninvasive IAAO method[85] point out that adaptation occurs at the acyl-*t*-RNA level, which adapts in less than 4 hours. Most studies aimed at exploring dietary adaptation have been conducted in animal studies.[95]

In one human study,[96] it was concluded that there was no difference in phenylalanine oxidation or flux between two adaptation levels or the length of adaptation. However, no study on amino acid requirement has been conducted using different adaptation periods in the same group of individuals. Hence, the issue of adaptation has not been settled.

Achieving isotopic steady state with oral tracer administration can be challenging because of variable gastric emptying and absorption rates may result in peaks and valleys in the isotopic enrichment, and a greater difficulty in establishing steady state. Likewise urinary enrichment may not be as accurate as plasma enrichment. Furthermore, this technique may be difficult to implement in pathophysiologic states where gastrointestinal and renal dysfunction may preclude its use.

The more invasive 24-hour IAAO and balance (24-h IAAOB) technique has been used for determination of amino acid requirements in healthy and malnourished adults[91,92,97,98] to obtain a more accurate determination of amino acid requirement. With the 24-hour IAAOB technique, an adaptation period of 5 to 7 days to each of seven test levels of amino acid intake is given, followed by a 24-hour, primed, constant, 12-hour fast, and 12-hour fed intravenous infusion of an indicator tracer amino acid. Breath and blood samples for $^{13}CO_2$ and plasma isotopic enrichment of the indicator amino acid are obtained every 30 minutes throughout the study. Hence, seven test levels of amino acid intake and seven 24-hour tracer infusions are conducted in each subject. This technique investigates both the fasting and fed metabolic states. Hence, a 24-hour amino acid balance can be obtained. Under these principles, the requirements of lysine,[99,100] methionine,[101] and threonine[92] in well-nourished and malnourished[93] adults have been determined. Although the 24-hour IAAOB is invasive and difficult to conduct, it is considered the "gold standard" by the Institute of Medicine.[10] These are the most reliable data on quantitative estimates of amino acid requirement in adults.

The 24-hour IAAOB method is more difficult to implement in children and modifications of this method have been applied by shortening the length of the adaptation period and the duration of the tracer infusion while maintaining the intravenous tracer and blood sampling.[88]

Amino Acid Supplementation

It has been proposed that supplementation with some amino acids may improve specific physiologic or pathophysiological conditions.[102–104] However, there are no dose-response human studies and currently only a few controlled randomized control trials have been conducted. Because of the lack of evidence, at this point dietary supplementation with a particular amino acid for improvement of a functional outcome remains to be established.

Amino Acid Toxicity

The risk of harmful interactions elicited by pharmacological doses of single amino acid supplements may be significant. In addition, supplement purity is a major concern. Hence, to date, there is controversy about single amino acid supplementation.

The safe upper level of intake is defined as the maximum level of habitual intake from all sources of a nutrient or related substance, which is judged to be unlikely to lead to adverse effects in humans.[105] Because of the higher risk of adverse effects, the safe upper level or tolerable upper level of intake is not desirable. There are limited data on amino acid toxicity in humans, and more extensive data in animal models.

In regard to branched chain amino acids, and despite the role of these amino acids in protein synthesis, there is no consensus on its use in pathophysiological conditions.[106] Sulfur amino acids exert beneficial effects through their role as precursor of glutathione, DNA methylation reactions, and synthesis of important substrates, such as creatine, choline, etc. Sulfur amino acids also increase high-density lipoprotein and decrease very low density lipoprotein.[107] However, methionine supplementation can be associated with increased homocysteine, a marker of cardiovascular risk and promoter of oxidative injury.[108] A large intake of methionine has been associated with fatalities in the pediatric[109] and adult populations.[110] Toxicity of sulfur amino acids can be significant and supplementation is not indicated. However, supplementation with *N*-acetyl cysteine appears promising in conditions of oxidative injury[111] and deserves further consideration.

CONCLUSION

In summary, the current recommendations for amino acid intakes are based on limited data. There is great need for further investigation on nutritional and functional requirements of amino acids and their safe upper levels of intake. Amino acid metabolism and requirements under pathophysiological conditions by the enteral and parenteral routes need to be further studied. The effect of developmental influences on the interactions between amino acids and energy (glucose and fat) metabolism needs to be closely explored. An exciting area of future development is focused on the physiological roles of D-amino acids.

REFERENCES

1. Haymond MW. Nutritional and metabolic endpoints. J Nutr 1999;129:273S–8S.
2. Imura K, Okada A. Amino acid metabolism in pediatric patients. Nutrition 1998;14:143–8.
3. Fouillet H, Bos C, Gaudichon C, Tome D. Approaches to quantifying protein metabolism in response to nutrient ingestion. J Nutr 2002;132:3208S–18S.
4. Tome D, Bos C. Dietary protein and nitrogen utilization. J Nutr 2000;130:1868S–73S.
5. Fuller MF, Reeds PJ. Nitrogen cycling in the gut. Annu Rev Nutr 1998;18:385–411.
6. Metges CC. Contribution of microbial amino acids to amino acid homeostasis of the host. J Nutr 2000;130:1857S–64S.
7. Metges CC, El Khoury AE, Henneman L. Availability of intestinal microbial lysine for whole body lysine homeostasis in human subjects. Am J Physiol 1999;277:E597–607.
8. Millward DJ, Rivers JP. The nutritional role of indispensable amino acids and the metabolic basis for their requirements. Eur J Clin Nutr 1988;42:367–93.
9. Ciechanover A, DiGiuseppe JA, Bercovich B, et al. Degradation of nuclear oncoproteins by the ubiquitin system in vitro. Proc Natl Acad Sci U S A 1991;88:139–43.
10. Institute of Medicine, Dietary Reference Intakes for Energy Carbohydrate Fiber Fat Fatty Acids Cholesterol Protein and Amino Acids. Washington, DC: National Academy of Sciences; 2002.
11. Rose WC. Amino acid requirements of man. Fed Proc. 1949;8:546–52.
12. Rose WC, Johnson JJ, Haines WJ. The amino acid requirements of man. I. The role of valine and methionine. J Biol Chem 1950;182:541–56.
13. Rose WC, Haines WJ, Warner DT. The amino acid requirements of man. V. The role of lysine, arginine, and tryptophan. J Biol Chem 1954;206:421–30.
14. Rose WC, Wixom RL, Lockhart HB, Lambert GF. The amino acid requirements of man. XV. The valine requirement; summary and final observations. J Biol Chem 1955;217:987–95.
15. Rose WC. The amino acid requirements of adult man. Nutr Abstr Rev Ser Hum Exp 1957;27:631–47.
16. Holt LE, Jr, Snyderman SE. Protein and amino acid requirements of infants and children. Nutr Abstr Rev 1965;35: 1–13.
17. Snyderman SE, Boyer A, Norton PM, et al. The essential amino acid requirements of infants. X. Methionine. Am J Clin Nutr 1964;15:322–30.
18. Snyderman SE, Pratt EL, Cheung MW, et al. The phenylalanine requirement of the normal infant. J Nutr 1955;56:253–63.
19. Snyderman SE, Holt LE, Jr, Smellie F, et al. The essential amino acid requirements of infants: Valine. Am J Dis Child 1959;97:186–91.
20. Snyderman SE, Boyer A, Norton PM, et al. The essential amino acid requirements of infants: Tryptophan. Am J Clin Nutr 1961;15:313–21.
21. Snyderman SE, Norton PM, Fowler DI, Holt LE, Jr. The essential amino acid requirements of infants: Lysine. AMA J Dis Child 1959;97:175–85.
22. Snyderman SE, Boyer A, Roitman E, et al. The histidine requirement of the infant. Pediatrics 1963;31:786–801.
23. Snyderman SE, Boyer A, Norton PM, et al. The essential amino acid requirements of infants. IX Isoleceucine. Am J Clin Nutr 1964;15:313–21.
24. Snyderman SE, Boyer A, Kogut MD, Holt LE, Jr. The protein requirement of the premature infant. I. The effect of protein intake on the retention of nitrogen. J Pediatr 1969;74:872–80.
25. Snyderman SE, Holt LE, Jr, Norton PM, Phansalkar SV. Protein requirement of the premature infant. II. Influence of protein intake on free amino acid content of plasma and red blood cells. Am J Clin Nutr 1970;23:890–5.
26. Phansalkar SV, Norton PM, Holt LE, Jr, Snyderman SE. Amino acid interrelationships: The effect of a load of leucine on the metabolism of isoleucine. Proc Soc Exp Biol Med 1970;134:262–3.
27. Fomon SJ. Requirements and recommended dietary intakes of protein during infancy. Pediatr Res 1991;30:391–5.
28. FAO/WHO/UNU. Energy and protein requirements: Reports of a Joint FAO/WHO/UNU Expert. Geneva: WHO; 1985.
29. FAO/WHO. Energy and protein requirements: Report of a joint FAO/WHO add hoc expert committee. FAO Nutrition Meetings Report Series, No 52. Geneva: WHO; 1971.
30. Mitchell HH. Comparative Nutrition of Man and Domestic Animals, Volume 1, 1st edition. New York: Academic Press; 1962. pp. 166–72.
31. Laidlaw SA, Kopple JD. Newer concepts of the indispensable amino acids. Am J Clin Nutr 1987;46:593–605.
32. Young VR, El Khoury AE. The notion of the nutritional essentiality of amino acids, revisited, with a note on the indispensable amino acid requirements in adults. In: Cynober LA, editor. Amino Acid Metabolism and Therapy in Health and Nutritional Disease. New York: CRC Press; 1995. p. 191–232.
33. Chipponi JX, Bleier JC, Santi MT, Rudman D. Deficiencies of essential and conditionally essential nutrients. Am J Clin Nutr 1982;35:1112–6.
34. Reeds PJ, Biolo G. Non-protein roles of amino acids: An emerging aspect of nutrient requirements. Curr Opin Clin Nutr Metab Care 2002;5:43–5.
35. Jackson AA. Amino acids: Essential and non-essential? Lancet 1983;1:1034–7.
36. Reeds PJ. Dispensable and indispensable amino acids for humans. J Nutr 2000;130:1835S–40S.
37. Skolnick P. Modulation of glutamate receptors: Strategies for the development of novel antidepressants. Amino Acids 2002;23:153–9.
38. Tsai G, Coyle JT. N-acetylaspartate in neuropsychiatric disorders. Prog Neurobiol 1995;46:531–40.
39. Young VR, Hussein MA, Scrimshaw NS. Estimate of loss of labile body nitrogen during acute protein deprivation in young adults. Nature 1968;218:568–9.
40. Hansen RD, Raja C, Allen BJ. Total body protein in chronic diseases and in aging. Ann N Y Acad Sci 2000;904:345–52.
41. Dewey KG, Beaton G, Fjeld C, et al. Protein requirements of infants and children. Eur J Clin Nutr 1996;50:S119–47.
42. Fomon SJ, Ziegler EE, Nelson SE, Edwards BB. Requirement for sulfur-containing amino acids in infancy. J Nutr 1986;116:1405–22.
43. Dewey KG. Protein and amino acids. Pediatrics 2000;106:1292.
44. Snyderman SE, Holt LE, Jr, Dancis J, et al. "Unessential" nitrogen: A limiting factor for human growth. J Nutr 1962;78:57–72.
45. Huang PC, Lin CP, Hsu JY. Protein requirements of normal infants at the age of about 1 year: Maintenance nitrogen requirements and obligatory nitrogen losses. J Nutr 1980;110:1727–35.
46. Torum B, Young VR, Rand WM. Obligatory nitrogen losses and factorial calculations of protein requirements of pre-school children. In: Torum B, Young VR, Rand WM, editors. Protein-Energy Requirements of Developing Countries: Evaluation of New Data. Tokyo, Japan: United Nations University; 2007. p. 159–63.
47. Intengan CL, Roxas BV, Loyola A, Carlos E. Protein requirements of Philipino children 20 to 29 months old consuming local diets. In: Torum EB, Young VR, Rand WM, editors. Protein-Energy Requirements of Developing Countries: Evaluation of New Data. Tokyo, Japan: United Nations University; 2007. p. 159–63.
48. Egana JI, Fuentes A, Uauy R. Protein needs of Chilean fed milk and soy protein isolates. In: Torum EB, Young VR, Rand WM, editors. Protein-Energy Requirements of Developing Countries: Evaluation of New Data. Tokyo, Japan: United Nations University; 1984. 249–57.
49. Nakagawa I, Takahashi T, Suzuki T, Kobayashi K. Amino acid requirements of children: Nitrogen balance at the minimal level of essential amino acids. J Nutr 1964;83:115–8.
50. National Research Council. Improvement of Protein Nutriture. Washington, DC: National Academy of Sciences; 1974
51. Young VR, Borgonha S. Nitrogen and amino acid requirements: The Massachusetts Institute of Technology amino acid requirement pattern. J Nutr 2000;130:1841S–9S.
52. Imagawa S, Tarumoto T, Suzuki N, et al. L-arginine rescues decreased erythropoietin gene expression by stimulating GATA-2 with L-NMMA. Kidney Int 2002;61:396–404.
53. Zhao R, Russell RG, Wang Y, et al. Rescue of embryonic lethality in reduced folate carrier-deficient mice by maternal folic acid supplementation reveals early neonatal failure of hematopoietic organs. J Biol Chem 2001;276:10224–8.
54. Rosenquist TH, Finnell RH. Genes, folate and homocysteine in embryonic development. Proc Nutr Soc 2001;60:53–61.
55. van der Put NM, Blom HJ. Neural tube defects and a disturbed folate dependent homocysteine metabolism. Eur J Obstet Gynecol Reprod Biol 2000;92:57–61.
56. Mayer O, Filipovsky J, Hromadka M, et al. Treatment of hyperhomocysteinemia with folic acid: Effects on homocysteine levels, coagulation status, and oxidative stress markers. J Cardiovasc Pharmacol 2002;39:851–7.
57. Fomon SJ, Haschke F, Ziegler EE, Nelson SE. Body composition of reference children from birth to age 10 years. Am J Clin Nutr 1982;35:1169–75.
58. Heird WC. Interpretation of the plasma amino acid pattern of low birth weight infants. Nutrition 1989;5:145–6.
59. Rand WM, Young VR. Statistical analysis of nitrogen balance data with reference to the lysine requirement in adults. J Nutr 1999;129:1920–6.
60. Clugston G, Dewey KG, Fjeld C, et al. Report of the working group on protein and amino acid requirements. Eur J Clin Nutr 1996;50:S193–5.
61. Butte NF, Hopkinson JM, Wong WW, et al. Body composition during the first 2 years of life: An updated reference. Pediatr Res 2000;47:578–85.

62. Ellis KJ, Shypailo RJ, Abrams SA, Wong WW. The reference child and adolescent models of body composition. A contemporary comparison. Ann N Y Acad Sci 2000;904:374–82.
63. Waterlow JC. Protein-energy interrelationships during rapid growth. In: Scrimshaw NS, Scurch B, editors. Protein-Energy Interactions. Proceedings of an IDECG workshop, Waterville Valley NH, October 1991. Lausanne, Switzerland: IDECG; 2007.
64. Jackson AA. Critique of protein-energy interactions in vivo: Urea kinetics. In: NS Scrimshaw and B Scurch, editors. Protein-Energy Interactions. Proceedings of an IDECG workshop, Waterville Valley NH, October 1991. Lausanne, Switzerland; IDECG. p. 63–80.
65. Miller LT, Leklem JE, Shultz TD. The effect of dietary protein on the metabolism of vitamin B-6 in humans. J Nutr 1985;115:1663–72.
66. Fomon SJ, Ziegler EE, Nelson SE, Frantz JA. What is the safe protein-energy ratio for infant formulas? Am J Clin Nutr 1995;62:358–63.
67. Fomon SJ, Demaeyer EM, Owen GM. Urinary and fecal excretion of endogenous nitrogen by infants and children. J Nutr 1965;85:235–46.
68. Young VR, El Khoury AE. Can amino acid requirements for nutritional maintenance in adult humans be approximated from the amino acid composition of body mixed proteins? Proc Natl Acad Sci U S A 1995;92:300–4.
69. Young VR, Pellett PL. Current concepts concerning indispensable amino acid needs in adults and their implications for international nutrition planning. Food Nutr Bull 1990;289–300.
70. FAO/WHO/UNU Expert Consultation. Energy and protein requirement. WHO Technical Report Series, no. 721. Geneva: WHO, 1985.
71. Darragh AJ, Hodgkinson SM. Quantifying the digestibility of dietary protein. J Nutr 2000;130:1850S–6S.
72. Reeds P, Schaafsma G, Tome D, Young VR. Summary of the workshop on criteria and significance of dietary protein sources in humans. J Nutr 2000;1874S–6S.
73. Millward DJ. Amino acid requirements in man. Am J Clin Nutr 1990;492–3.
74. Millward DJ. The nutritional value of plant-based diets in relation to human amino acid and protein requirements. Proc Nutr Soc 1999;58:249–60.
75. Millward DJ. Human amino acid requirements. J Nutr 1997;127:1842–6.
76. Reeds PJ, Hutchens TW. Protein requirements: From nitrogen balance to functional impact. J Nutr 1994;124:1754S–64S.
77. Lyons J, Rauh-Pfeiffer A, Ming-Yu Y, et al. Cysteine metabolism and whole blood glutathione synthesis in septic pediatric patients. Crit Care Med 2001;29:870–7.
78. Kriengsinyos W, Wykes LJ, Ball RO, Pencharz PB. Oral and intravenous tracer protocols of the indicator amino acid oxidation method provide the same estimate of the lysine requirement in healthy men. J Nutr 2002;132:2251–7.
79. Bross R, Ball RO, Clarke JT, Pencharz PB. Tyrosine requirements in children with classical PKU determined by indicator amino acid oxidation. Am J Physiol Endocrinol Metab 2000;278:E195–201.
80. Young VR. 2001 W.O. Atwater Memorial Lecture and the 2001 ASNS President's lecture. Human nutrient requirements: The challenge of the post-genome era. Am J Nutr 2002;132:621–9.
81. Young VR, Bier DM, Pellett PL. A theoretical basis for increasing current estimates of the amino acid requirements in adult man, with experimental support. Am J Clin Nutr 1989;50:80–92.
82. Raguso CA, Pereira P, Young VR. A tracer investigation of obligatory oxidative amino acid losses in healthy, young adults. Am J Clin Nutr 1999;70:474–83.
83. El Khoury AE, Fukagawa N, Sanchez M, et al. The 24-h pattern and rate of leucine oxidation, with particular reference to tracer estimates of leucine requirements in healthy adults. Am J Clin Nutr 1994;1012–20
84. Basile-Filho A, Beaumier L, El Khoury AE, et al. Twenty-four-hour L-[1-(13)C]tyrosine and L-[3,3-(2)H2]phenylalanine oral tracer studies at generous, intermediate, and low phenylalanine intakes to estimate aromatic amino acid requirements in adults. Am J Clin Nutr 1998;67:640–59.
85. Pencharz PB, Ball RO. Different approaches to define individual amino acid requirements. Annu Rev Nutr 2003;23:101–16.
86. Mager DR, Wykes LJ, Ball RO, Pencharz PB. Branched-chain amino acid requirements in school-aged children determined by indicator amino acid oxidation (IAAO). J Nutr 2003;133:3540–5.
87. Kurpad AV, Raj T, El Khoury A, et al. Daily requirement for and splanchnic uptake of leucine in healthy adult Indians. Am J Clin Nutr 2001;74:747–55.
88. Gordon WE, Sy J, Zurakowski D, et al. Methionine requirements in healthy adolescents. FASEB J 2007;21:838.
89. Nakagawa I, Takahashi T, Suzi T. Amino acid requirements of children: Minimal needs of lysine and methionine based on nitrogen balance method. J Nutr 1961;74:401–7.
90. Kurpad AV, Regan MM, Raj TD, et al. The daily phenylalanine requirement of healthy Indian adults. Am J Clin Nutr 2006;83:1331–6.
91. Kurpad AV, El Khoury AE, Beaumier L, et al. An initial assessment, using 24-h [13C]leucine kinetics, of the lysine requirement of healthy adult Indian subjects. Am J Clin Nutr 1998;67:58–66.
92. Borgonha S, Regan MM, Oh SH, et al. Threonine requirement of healthy adults, derived with a 24-h indicator amino acid balance technique. Am J Clin Nutr 2002;75:698–704.
93. Courtney-Martin G, Bross R, Raffi M, et al. Phenylalanine requirement in children with classical PKU determined by indicator amino acid oxidation. Am J Physiol Endocrinol Metab 2002;283:E1249–56.
94. Millward DJ. Metabolic demands for amino acids and the human dietary requirement: Millward and Rivers (1988) revisited. J Nutr 1998;128:2563S–76S.
95. Moehn S, Bertolo RF, Pencharz PB, Ball RO. Indicator amino acid oxidation responds rapidly to changes in lysine or protein intake in growing and adult pigs. J Nutr 2004;134:836–41.
96. Zello GA, Pencharz PB, Ball RO. Phenylalanine flux, oxidation, and conversion to tyrosine in humans studied with L- [1-13C]phenylalanine. Am J Physiol 1990;259: E835–43.
97. Kurpad AV, Raj T, Regan MM, et al. Threonine requirements of healthy Indian men, measured by a 24-h indicator amino acid oxidation and balance technique. Am J Clin Nutr 2002;76:789–97.
98. Kurpad AV, Regan MM, Raj T, et al. Lysine requirements of chronically undernourished adult Indian men, measured by a 24-h indicator amino acid oxidation and balance technique. Am J Clin Nutr 2003;77:101–8.
99. Kurpad AV, Raj T, El-Khoury A, et al. Lysine requirements of healthy adult Indian subjects receiving long-term feeding, measured with a 24-h indicator amino acid oxidation and balance technique. Am J Clin Nutr 2002;76:404–12.
100. Kurpad AV, Raj T, El Khoury A, et al. Lysine requirements of healthy adult Indian subjects, measured by an indicator amino acid balance technique. Am J Clin Nutr 2001;73:900–7.
101. Kurpad AV, Regan MM, Varalakshmi S, et al. Daily methionine requirements of healthy Indian men, measured by a 24-h indicator amino acid oxidation and balance technique. Am J Clin Nutr 2003;77:1198–205.
102. Ball PA, Hardy G. Glutamine in pediatrics: Where next? Nutrition 2002;18:451–4.
103. Badaloo A, Reid M, Forrester T, et al. Cysteine supplementation improves the erythrocyte glutathione synthesis rate in children with severe edematous malnutrition. Am J Clin Nutr 2002;76:646–52.
104. Amin HJ, Zamora SA, McMillan DD, et al. Arginine supplementation prevents necrotizing enterocolitis in the premature infant. J Pediatr 2002;140:425–31.
105. Munro IC, Renwick AG. The 5th workshop on the assessment of adequate intake of dietary amino acids: General discussion 2. J Nutr 2006;136:1755S–7S.
106. Cynober L, Harris RA. Symposium on branched-chain amino acids: Conference summary. J Nutr 2006;136:333S–6S.
107. Oda H. Functions of sulfur-containing amino acids in lipid metabolism. J Nutr 2006;136:1666S–9S
108. Cattaneo M. Hyperhomocysteinemia: An important risk factor for cardiovascular disease? Potentially, yes. J Thromb Haemost 2003;1:1878–9
109. Mudd SH, Braverman N, Pomper M, et al. Infantile hypermethioninemia and hyperhomocysteinemia due to high methionine intake: A diagnostic trap. Mol Genet Metab 2003;79:6–16.
110. Cottington EM, LaMantia C, Stabler SP, et al. Adverse event associated with methionine loading test: A case report. Arterioscler Thromb Vasc Biol 2002;22:1046–50.
111. van de Poll MC, Dejong CH, Soeters PB. Adequate range for sulfur-containing amino acids and biomarkers for their excess: Lessons from enteral and parenteral nutrition. J Nutr 2006;136:1694S–700S.

7

Macronutrient Requirements for Growth: Fats and Fatty Acids

Kathrin Krohn, MD
Hans Demmelmair, PhD
Berthold Koletzko, MD

INTRODUCTION

An adequate fat intake is essential for growth and development of infants and children. Dietary fat provides a large portion of energy and is the source of lipid-soluble vitamins and essential polyunsaturated fatty acids (PUFAs). The composition of dietary fat influences lipid absorption, metabolism, and tissue deposition, and thereby growth and body composition.

Fats or lipids can be defined as substances that have no or very limited solubility in water, but are soluble in organic solvents (eg, chloroform, hexane). Most of our dietary fats are triglycerides formed by three fatty acids esterified to a glycerol backbone. Vegetable oils, for example, consist almost entirely of triglycerides. Physicochemical properties of triglycerides (eg, the melting point of a fat) are determined by the composition of their fatty acids. Watery foods may contain triglycerides either as a separate lipid layer (eg, lipid droplets on a clear soup) or as an emulsion (eg, milk or intravenous lipid emulsion). Emulsification is facilitated by amphipathic lipids that contain both hydrophobic parts, which associate with neutral lipids, as well as hydrophilic components, which interact with polar molecules such as water. Amphipathic lipids include phospholipids, monoglycerides, unesterified cholesterol and plant sterols, and lipid-soluble vitamins bound to hydrophilic groups such as vitamin E acetate (tocopherol acetate). In contrast, cholesterol esters (esterified with a long-chain fatty acid) and vitamin A esters such as retinol palmitate are nonpolar.

FAT DIGESTION

Fat digestion and absorption involve

1. intraluminal solubilization and hydrolysis of lipids;
2. the subsequent intestinal absorption of hydrolyzed fatty acids and monoacylglycerols, reesterification of fatty acids, and secretion into the lymphatics in chylomicrons, or release of unesterified fatty acids into the portal venous system; and
3. uptake of the unesterified fatty acid or chylomicron triacylglycerols into the tissues.

Triacylglycerols (triglycerides) represent the major portion of dietary lipids and are hydrolyzed in the gut by intestinal lipases. The digestion process begins in the stomach and continues throughout the intestinal tract. The major proportion of fat is hydrolyzed in the duodenum, but initial partial hydrolysis in the stomach may be critically important to increase efficiency of pancreatic lipase.[1,2] About 10 to 30% of dietary fat is hydrolyzed in the stomach.[3] The rate of hydrolysis may be influenced by the initial droplet size in the stomach. A fine emulsion results in a higher degree of lipolysis compared to a coarse mixed emulsion.[4] This may not have major consequences for normal digestion since the capacity for hydrolysis is high, but it may become important in fat malassimilation, for example, due to exocrine pancreatic insufficiency and with tube feeding.[3]

Gastric lipase has an acidic pH optimum. When exposed to pancreatic proteases (trypsin, chymotrypsin) it is rapidly inactivated. In healthy individuals, gastric lipase may not be important in intraduodenal fat digestion. However, in patients with pancreatic insufficiency, such as cystic fibrosis patients, the low intraluminal concentrations of pancreatic proteases and acidic pH may favor its function.[5]

Gastric lipase has a functional specificity for the *sn*-3 ester bond of triacylglycerols and gives rise to free fatty acids and *sn*-1,2-diglycerides. Monoglycerides and free fatty acids enter the duodenum and stimulate the release of cholecystokinin in the duodenum. This in turn stimulates the release of biliary secretions and pancreatic enzymes. Digestion products are emulsified by bile salts, thereby increasing the available surface. Free fatty acids, which are released by gastric lipase, induce the binding between the colipase–lipase complex and fat globules.[6] Colipase-dependent lipase has a specificity for *sn*-1,3 ester bonds to give rise to *sn*-2-monoglycerides and free fatty acids. The level of enzyme secreted into the intestinal lumen changes with age. The level of colipase-dependent lipase secreted in adults is estimated to be 1,000-fold in excess of what would be necessary to hydrolyze the dietary fat ingested daily. However, in neonates postprandial luminal levels are much lower, since the pancreas is not fully developed after birth.[5] In addition to a low activity of colipase-dependent pancreatic lipase, neonates have a limited bile salt pool, and low intraluminal bile salt concentrations.

In infants fed human milk, hydrolysis of triacylglycerols results from the combined action of bile salt–stimulated lipase, which is produced in the mammary gland and secreted into the milk and the endogenous intestinal lipases. Bile salt–stimulated lipase hydrolyzes triacylglycerols at all three ester bonds resulting in the formation of free fatty acids and glycerol,[3] and is present in milk from about 26 weeks' gestation.[6,7]

FAT ABSORPTION

Unsaturated fatty acids are more readily absorbed than saturated fatty acids.[8] The preferential absorption of unsaturated fatty acids may be facilitated by better solubilization by bile salts, greater gastric lipolysis, preferential binding to intracellular fatty acid–binding protein, and subsequent reesterification or a decreased tendency to form soaps.[8–10]

Fat absorption is modulated by the chain length and degree of unsaturation of the fatty acids. High proportions of monounsaturated oleic acid (18:1) and polyunsaturated linoleic acid (18:2n-6) from vegetable oil triacylglycerols are absorbed (<90%).[11] In contrast, absorption of the saturated fatty acids myristic acid (14:0), palmitic acid (16:0), and stearic acid (18:0) is lower and decreases with increasing fatty acid chain length.

Absorption of saturated fatty acids depends on the position of the fatty acid in the triacylglycerol molecule.[12] In human milk, palmitic acid is the predominating saturated fatty acid. Most human milk palmitic acid is present at the *sn*-2 position of the triacylglycerol molecule.[13] Formula milks contain smaller quantities of palmitic acid compared to human milk, but the saturated fatty acids from the originating vegetable oils are largely esterified at the outer sn-1,3 positions of

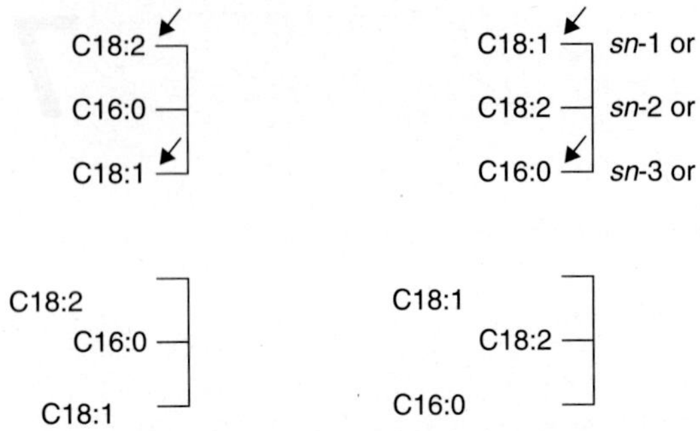

Figure 1 Intestinal lipases preferentailly hydrolyse triglyceride fatty acids in the *sn*-1 and *sn*-3 positions. Human milk lipids, lard, and some specifically structured lipids contain the saturated palmitic acid (C16:0) predominantly in the *sn*-2 position (left panel). Hydrolysis of these substrates produces most C16:0 as a monoglyceride, which is rather well water soluble and absorbed to a large extent. In contrast, saturated fatty acids in vegetable oils are more or less randomly esterified to the different positions of the molecule, and a greater proportion of C16:0 is liberated as a hydrophobic free fatty acid, which tends to bind to cations (soap formation) resulting in a poor absorption both of fat and of calcium. Benficial effects of structured lipids with saturated fatty acids in the *sn*-2 position both on fat and mineral absorption have been shown in infants.

the triacylglycerol molecule.[14] The lipolytic enzymes gastric and colipase-dependent lipases cleave fatty acids preferentially in *sn*-1 and *sn*-3 positions (Figure 1). Whereas 2-monoglyceride of palmitic acid is readily absorbed, free palmitic acid and palmitic acid in the *sn*-1 and *sn*-3 position of monoglycerides are not.[15] Therefore, infants fed formula milks with palmitic acid in these positions may be more likely to excrete more soaps and pass firmer stools than breast-fed infants.[16,17]

Soaps result from binding of free fatty acids released by lipolysis of triacylglycerols from the *sn*-1 and *sn*-3 position and calcium, resulting in reduced fat and mineral absorption.[18] However, the clinical significance in healthy infants is unclear. The difference in fat absorption may easily be compensated by the infants' ability to adapt the amount of milk consumed daily.[19]

Predominantly *sn*-2 monoacylglycerides are absorbed and the fatty acids are preserved in this position during the absorption process.[20] In contrast, fatty acids originating from the *sn*-1,3 positions are randomly reesterified during triacylglycerol resynthesis via the monoacylglycerol pathway. Following reassembly, the triacylglycerols are secreted as components of chylomicrons.

Medium-chain triacylglycerols (MCTs) contain predominantly saturated fatty acids with 8 and 10 carbon atoms. MCT have high water solubility and are rapidly cleaved by lipases and readily absorbed even in the presence of low amounts of intraluminal bile salts and pancreatic lipases.[21] MCT are used in low-birth-weight infant formulas to increase fat absorption. Preterm infant formulas in the USA contain up to 50% and in Europe up to 40% of total fat as MCT. Proposed advantage of MCT when compared to long-chain triacylglycerols (LCTs) with saturated fatty acids in low-birth-weight infant formulas include rapid, portal venous transport of the albumin-bound medium-chain fatty acids (MCFAs) to the liver, carnitine-independent transport into the mitochondria, and subsequent oxidation that is more rapid than for longer chain fatty acids. However, the energy content of MCT is about 16% lower than that of LCT (Figure 2). Therefore, a benefit of providing MCT rather than LCT with respect to increased energy absorption and supply can only be expected in subjects with a very severe degree of fat malassimilation, such as children with severe cholestasis, whereas most patients will not achieve an enhanced energy absorption with the use of MCT. Indeed, a Cochrane review did not demonstrate an advantage of preterm infant formulas containing high amounts of MCT (40% or more) versus formulas with low amounts of MCT (20% or less) with respect to weight gain achieved.[22] In patients with short-bowel syndrome, MCT are used to improve fat absorption.[23] In adult short-bowel patients the colon has been suggested as a digestive organ for medium-chain fat, probably absorbed as MCFA.[24] However, the available data on clinical effects achieved are limited.

TRANSPORT OF LIPIDS

Some lipids are transported predominantly via the portal vein whereas others are preferentially transported via the lymphatic system. The route of transport is generally related to chain length, to the level of unsaturation, and to the structure of the dietary lipid. Chain length is not the only but the most important factor affecting portal transport of fatty acids.[3]

MCT may be incorporated directly into mucosal cells and hydrolyzed. Liberated MCFA are then transported bound to albumin predominantly via the portal system. However, the separation of MCFA to be transported as unesterified, albumin-bound fatty acids via the portal venous route, and of fatty acids of carbon chain length 14 and longer to be transported in chylomicron triacylglycerols via the lymphatic system, is not complete. Physiologically significant amounts of saturated and unsaturated fatty acids, including linoleic acid (18:2n-6) and α-linolenic acid (18:3n-3), are transported via the portal pathway,[25] while MCFA are found in chylomicron triacylglycerols.

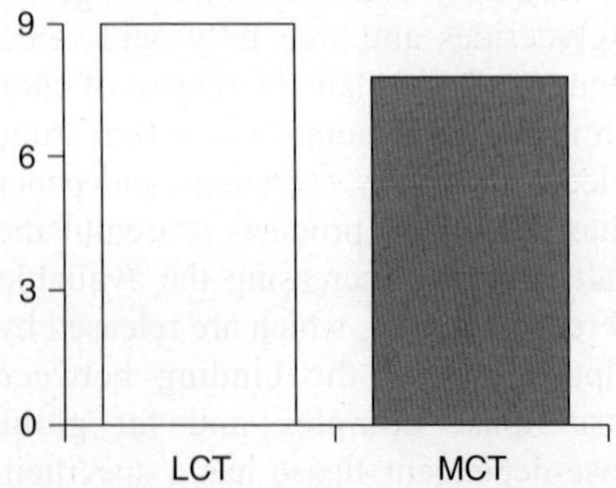

Figure 2 The energy content (kcal/g fat) of medium-chain triacylglycerols (MCTs) is about 16% lower than that of long-chain triacylglycerols (LCTs). Therefore, an increased energy absorption by the use of MCT can only be expected in subjects with very severe fat malassimilation, such as children with severe cholestasis.

ASSEMBLY OF LIPOPROTEINS

In the enterocyte, absorbed lipids are packed into lipoproteins, which enable transport in the aqueous environment. The major lipoproteins secreted by the intestine are chylomicrons and very low density lipoprotein (VLDL). Chylomicrons contain triacylglycerols, cholesterol ester, free cholesterol, and phospholipids.[3] They are secreted in the small intestine after a meal to transport lipids.[26] VLDL-sized particles are formed in intestinal cells during fasting.[3] The intestinal lipoproteins are secreted into the lymphatic system and enter the bloodstream via the thoracic duct.

Triacylglycerol constituents of intestinal chylomicrons and hepatic VLDL are hydrolyzed by lipoprotein lipase released from adipose tissue, muscle, and possibly other tissues to the capillary endothelium.

TOTAL DIETARY FAT INTAKE IN INFANTS

Dietary fat is essential for growth and development. It provides a source of energy that covers the needs for energy expenditure, fat oxidation, and fat deposition during growth. However, there is limited evidence on acceptable ranges of dietary fat intake in infants.[27]

With an energy content of about 9 kcal/kg, LCTs contain more than twice the energy per weight of carbohydrates or proteins. Growing infants have a very high energy requirement estimated to be about 120 kcal/kg/d during the first month of life and close to 100 kcal/kg/d during the rest of the first year of life.[28] The deposition of fat in healthy infants is very high. About 90% of the total energy deposited in growing tissues during the first six months of life consists of fat.[29] During the first two months of life, about 25% of dietary energy supply is deposited as fat, which rapidly decreases to less than 5% after 6 months.[28]

While lipids can be synthesized de novo from carbohydrates or proteins,[30] the capacity for endogenous net lipogenesis is limited and only nonessential fatty acids can be formed. Additionally energy would be lost in the process, because the synthesis of fatty acids from glucose consumes about 25% of the energy content of glucose invested. On the other hand, fat deposition from dietary fat requires only about 1 to 4% of the energy provided by the fat.[31]

In studies supplying isoenergetic diets with different fat contents a higher body weight and fat gain was achieved with lower energy expenditure in groups with higher fat intake.[32,33] Energy expenditure was also reduced in parenterally fed infants by providing lipids in addition to glucose.[30]

The Committee on Nutrition of the European Society for Pediatric Gastroenterology, Hepatology and Nutrition (ESPGHAN) recommended a total fat intake of about 40 to 50–55% of energy intake for young infants.[34] Similarly, a recent global expert committee concluded that fat supply with infant formulas should be in the range of 4.4 to 6.0 g/100 kcal,[35] which is equivalent to about 40 to 54% of energy content and similar to values found typically in human milk.[36] This recommendation was adopted by the reporting to the Codex Alimentarius Committee on Nutrition and Foods for Special Dietary Uses of the Food and Agriculture Organization of the United Nations and the World Health Organization. It is global standard for infant formulas.[37]

Energy needs per kg body weight and the proportion of dietary energy deposited as fat decrease rapidly in the first months of life.[28] Therefore, in the second half of the first year lower dietary fat intakes can meet the needs for growth. In a randomized intervention study in Finland, infants receiving a mean dietary fat intake of about 28% of energy from the age of 6 months onward showed normal growth and long-term development.[38]

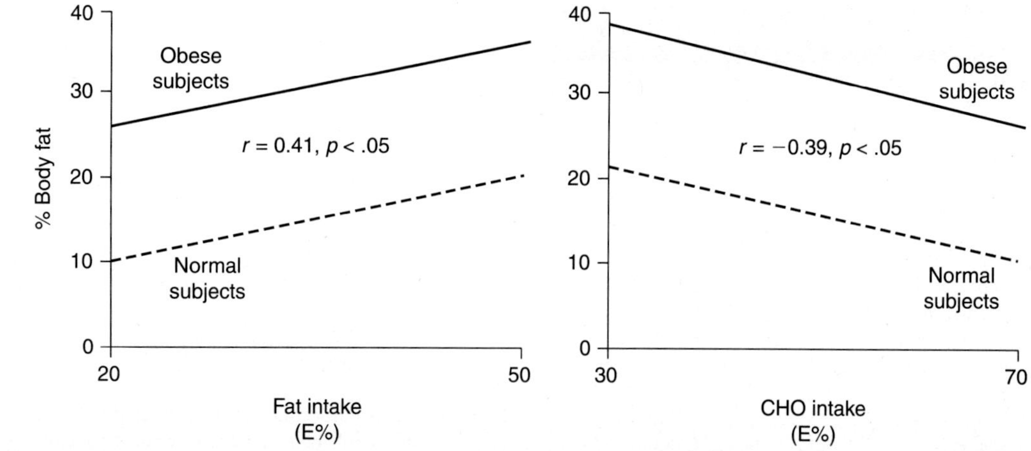

Figure 3 The percentage of dietary energy contributed by fat is positively correlated to body fat content in both obese and normal school age children, whereas the percentage contribution of carbohydrates (CHO) to energy intake is inversely related to body fat content. (Drawn from data of reference 41)

DIETARY FAT INTAKE IN CHILDREN

Similar to infants, also for children there is no firm evidence on which to set lower and upper limits of advisable lipid intakes. Both excessive and low supply of dietary lipids may be associated with adverse effects.

In populations of children and adolescents, the prevalence of obesity increases with a higher dietary fat intake (Figure 3).[39–41] This can be explained at least in part by the higher energy density (kcal/g) of foods with high fat contents, as compared to carbohydrate-rich foods, and the fact that a higher dietary energy density is associated with a higher total energy intake in populations.[42] Therefore, moderation of total dietary fat intake is an important strategy contributing to obesity prevention in populations, both in adults and in children. Moreover, concentrations of plasma total and low-density lipoprotein (LDL)-cholesterol increase with high intakes of saturated and *trans* unsaturated fatty acids,[43] which is considered as a risk factor for vascular lipid deposition and the occurrence of early vascular lesions.[44] Consequently, low intakes of saturated and *trans* unsaturated fatty acids are recommended to reduce the long-term risk of heart disease[45] (Table 1), and some have specifically advised that saturated and *trans* fatty acid intake should not exceed 10 and 1% of energy intake, respectively.[46] While there is some concern that the advice to markedly lower fat intake, for example as part of dietary treatment of hypercholesterolemia, might cause adverse effects on child growth, observational studies did not report adverse effects of low-fat diets on growth and biochemical measures of nutritional status.[47–49] One study in 663 children with hypercholesterolemia with a reduced fat intake in the intervention group (28,6% vs 33% in the usual care group) did not demonstrate a correlation of percentage of dietary energy intake as fat to weight, height, body mass index, and skinfold thickness.[50] However, other studies reported impaired growth in children with hypercholesterolemia treated with a low-fat diet.[51,52] Modification of the quality of dietary fat intake rather than a reduction of the quantity of fat intake, which has beneficial effects on plasma lipoprotein concentrations, is possible without any adverse effects on child growth.[53]

Table 1 Recommendations of the ESPGHAN Committee on Nutrition on Average Dietary Intakes for Children from the Age of 2 to 3 Years Onwards and for Adolescents Aiming at Prevention of Coronary Heart Disease in Later Life[45]

Saturated fatty acids	≤About 8 to 12% of energy
trans-Fatty acids	Low intake
Polyunsaturated fatty acids	About 6 to 10% of energy
Monounsaturated fatty acids	No limitation
Cholesterol	≤About 300 mg/d
Antioxidative vitamins	Generous intake desirable
Sodium chloride	Low intake desirable
Complex carbohydrates	Generous intake desirable
Total fat intake	About 30 to 35% of energy (as one approach to limit saturated and *trans*-fatty acid intake)

It is unclear whether the adverse effects on growth and weight gain observed in some studies with a reduced fat intake are attributable to a low energy intake rather than to the low fat intake per se. Diets with a low fat intake tend to have a lower energy density that may reduce total energy intake and thereby reduce weight gain and eventually length gain.

It is controversial to which extent fat-reduced diets may be associated with biologically significant reductions of the intakes of lipid-soluble vitamins and micronutrients. Some studies showed low intakes of vitamins and micronutrients, accompanied by lower energy intake,[47,54] whereas others did not find a compromise of the intake of these nutrients associated with reduced fat intake.[48,55,56]

Recommendations by the American Academy of Pediatrics[57] and the Committee on Nutrition of the ESPGHAN[45] advise an average fat intake of about 30% of energy intake (Table 1), which allows normal growth and development of healthy children and on a population basis can contribute to risk reduction for overweight and dyslipidemia.

FATTY ACIDS

The fatty acids esterified into lipids comprise the major component of fats in the diet and in the body, and they play a key role in modulating the physicochemical, metabolic, and functional properties of lipids. Fatty acids are conventionally classified according to their chain length as short-chain fatty acids (chain length < 8 carbon atoms), medium- (8 to 11), intermediate-(12 to 15 carbons), and long-chain fatty acids (≥16). Short formulas are used to describe fatty acids, which indicate the number of carbon atoms and double bonds as well as the position of the terminal double bond (Table 2). The chain length of a fatty acid is the major determinant of melting point, energy content (kcal/g), the degree of solubility in polar (eg, water) and nonpolar solvents (eg, hexane), and hence the efficacy of absorption in relation to the availability of conjugated bile salts in the intestinal lumen, as well as metabolic properties such as effects on lipoprotein metabolism, oxidative degradation, and tissue fat deposition. Fatty acid properties also depend on the number, type, and position of double bonds of which there may be none (saturated fatty acids), one (monounsaturated), or two or more (polyunsaturated) (Figure 4).

The position of double bonds in the fatty acid molecule is described by the distance to the terminal methyl group, that is, the omega-end of the fatty acid (Figure 4). This terminal part of the fatty acid molecule is little changed in human metabolism, because fatty acids are activated by reacting with coenzyme A at the carboxyl end. Therefore, enzyme-mediated biochemical reactions such as chain elongation, chain shortening

Table 2 Biologically Important Fatty Acids

Name	Short Formula
Saturated fatty acids	
Acetic acid	C2:0
Propionic acid	C3:0
Butyric acid	C4:0
Caproic acid	C6:0
Caprylic acid	C8:0
Capric acid	C10:0
Lauric acid	C12:0
Myristic acid	C14:0
Pentadecanoic acid	C15:0
Palmitic acid	C16:0
Margaric acid	C17:0
Stearic acid	C18:0
Arachidic acid	C20:0
Behenic acid	C22:0
Lignoceric acid	C24:0
cis-Monounsaturated fatty acids	
Palmitoleic acid	C16:1n-7
Oleic acid	C18:1n-9
Vaccenic acid	C18:1n-11
Essential fatty acids	
Linoleic acid (LA)	C18:2n-6
α-Linolenic acid (ALA)	C18:3n-3
γ-Linolenic acid	C18:3n-6
Dihomo γ-linolenic acid	C20:3n-6
Arachidonic acid (AA)	C20:4n-6
Eicosapentaenoic acid	C20:5n-3
Docosahexaenoic acid (DHA), cervonic acid	C22:6n-3
trans-Fatty acids	
Elaidic acid	C18:1n-9t
trans-Vaccenic acid	C18:1n-11t
Linolelaidic acid	C18:2n-6t
Conjugated linoleic acids (CLA)	C18:2-9c11t, C18:2-10t, 12c, and others

Short formulas are used to describe the number of carbon (C) atoms, the number of double bonds, the omega-position of the last double bond (n-x) and the double bond configuration in *cis* (c) or *trans* (t) position.

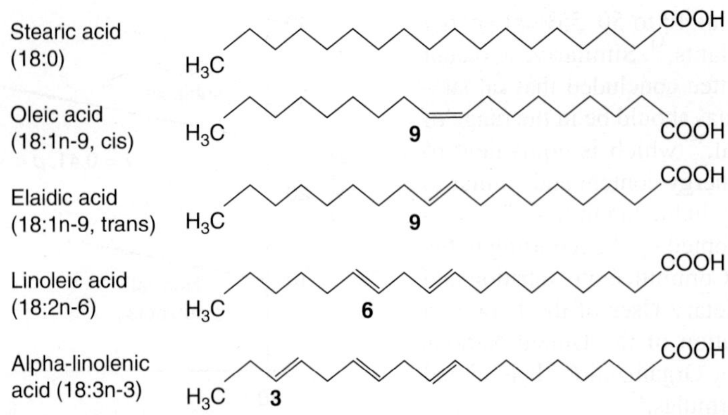

Figure 4 Structural formula of the saturated fatty acid stearic acid (18.0), the *cis*-monounsaturated fatty acid oleic acid (18:1n-9, one double bond located 9 carbon atoms from the methyl end of the molecule), the *trans*-monounsaturated fatty acid elaidic acid (18:1n-9, *trans*, one *trans*-double bond located 9 carbon atoms from the methyl end of the molecule), the n-6 polyunsaturated fatty acid linoleic acid (C18:2n-6; n-6 fatty acid with the terminal double bond located 6 carbon atoms from the methyl end of the molecule), and the n-3 polyunsaturated fatty acid α-linolenic acid (18:3n-3; n-3 fatty acid with the terminal double bond 3 carbon atoms from the methyl end).

by β-oxidation, or the introduction of new double bonds occur at the carboxyl end of the molecule. In contrast, the omega end of a fatty acid is usually unchanged in intermediary metabolism, unless the fatty acid is completely oxidized to carbon dioxide. Since humans and other higher organisms cannot introduce double bonds in the n-6 or n-3 positions, n-6 PUFA (eg, linoleic acid) and n-3 PUFA (eg, α-linolenic acid) are essential nutrients that must be provided with the enteral or parenteral substrate supply.

There are two isomeric forms of double bonds, *cis* and *trans* (Figure 4). Plant and mammalian cells introduce almost entirely *cis*-configurated double bonds into fatty acids, in which both parts of the adjoining carbon chain point to the same direction of the double bond and, therefore, the molecule is bent and becomes more flexible and fluid. *Trans*-isomeric fatty acids are formed primarily by rumen bacteria (in the forestomach of cows, goats, and sheep) and by technical fat hydrogenation.[58] *Trans*-fatty acids have a straight carbon chain, with a tertiary structure similar to saturated fatty acids (Figure 4), and they have higher melting points and less fluidity at body temperature than their respective *cis*-isomers. *Trans*-fatty acids may exert adverse effects on lipoprotein and essential fatty acid metabolism as well as fetal growth.[53,59–62] Therefore, the intake of dietary *trans*-fatty acids from foods produced with partially hydrogenated fats, French fries and other deep fried foods, baked goods with hydrogenated fats, and other foods high in *trans*-fatty acids should be limited.

Positional and *trans*-isomers of linoleic acid in which the double bonds are conjugated are called conjugated linoleic acids (CLAs). CLAs are formed primarily by biohydrogenation in ruminants. CLAs, in Western diet are predominantly supplied with cows' milk and cheese. CLA contents in bovine milk are in the order of about 1 to 2% of total fatty acids, with higher amounts resulting from barn feeding in the winter than from pasture feeding in the summer. Human milk contents depend on maternal dietary intake primarily from dairy products and reach a mean of about 0.4% CLA in human milk, with considerable intra- and interindividual variation.[63] CLA was found to be a high-affinity ligand and activator of the peroxisome proliferator–activated receptor-alpha and appears to have marked effects on lipid and energy metabolism. Studies in different species of experimental animals show that the consumption of CLA leads to a reduced energy intake, increased metabolic rate, and loss of fat and total body weight. In addition, these studies show that CLA also reduces the plasma concentrations of total and LDL cholesterol, has an anti-inflammatory effect, and can inhibit the development of mammary, skin, and prostatic cancers. While mixtures of CLA isomers as supplements or CLA-enriched products are widely marketed for human consumption, only few studies in healthy humans with relatively small sample sizes have been published so far. A recent systematic review concluded that there is not enough evidence yet to show that CLA has an effect on weight and body composition in humans, while some of these studies have observed that the administration of various CLA isomers has adverse effects on lipid profile with a decrease of high-density lipoprotein cholesterol concentration and increased Lp(a) levels, glucose metabolism, lipid oxidation, inflammation, or endothelial function.[64] Therefore, long-term randomized clinical trials with placebo controls are needed with sufficient power to evaluate the efficacy and safety of CLA isomers in humans before its use in human beings can be recommended.

ESSENTIAL FATTY ACIDS

Saturated fatty acids and unsaturated fatty acids of the n-9 and n-7 series can be synthesized de novo from acetyl coenzyme A. In contrast, humans cannot introduce double bonds in the n-6 or n-3 positions; therefore, n-6 PUFAs (linoleic acid and metabolites) and n-3 PUFA (α-linolenic acid and metabolites) are essential nutrients that must be provided with the enteral or parenteral substrate supply. An inadequate dietary supply of linoleic acid induces a specific deficiency syndrome with a dry, scaly dermatitis, and a variety of other signs and symptoms (Table 3). Linoleic acid deficiency has been observed mostly in infants, and a few adult patients on glucose-based, lipid-free parenteral nutrition. Infants are at a far higher risk of

Table 3 Signs and Symptoms of Essential Fatty Acid Deficiency

- Scaly, hyperkeratotic dermatitis
- Loss of hair
- Growth faltering
- Reduced utilization of dietary energy
- Reduced nitrogen retention
- Increased susceptibility to infection
- Disturbed wound healing
- Fatty liver, hepatomegaly, increased levels of ALAT* and ASAT†
- Anemia
- Thrombopenia, reduced platelet aggregation

*ALAT, Alanine Amino Transferase.† ASAT, Aspartate Amino Transferase.

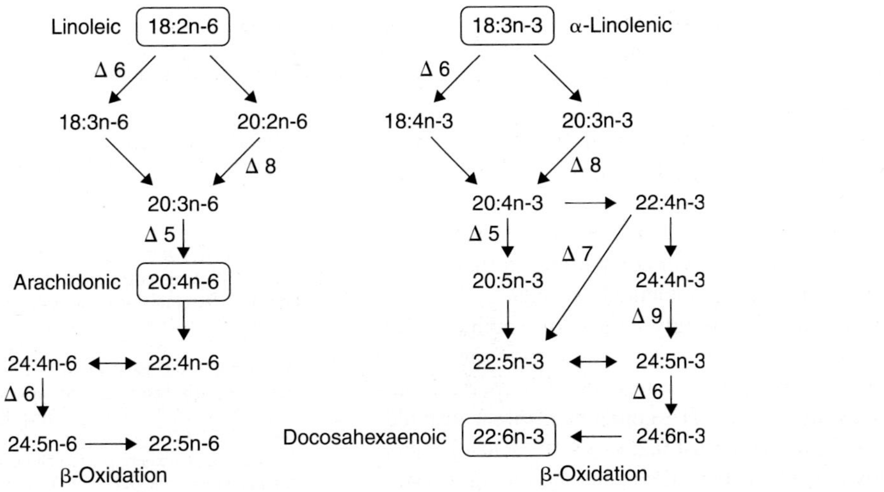

Figure 5 Pathways for the enzymatic conversion of the essential fatty acids linoleic acid (18:2n-6) and α-linolenic acid (18:3n-3) to long-chain polyunsaturated fatty acids (LC-PUFA).

deficiency because of higher requirements for PUFAs due to their rapid growth rate, while their body stores are very limited. Deficiency of n-3 fatty acids both in animals and in a limited number of human subjects on long-term tube feeding without adequate n-3 PUFA supply was reported to induce alterations of visual and neural functions.

The n-6 and n-3 fatty acids are not interconvertible, and they have different functions. Conversion of the dietary precursor essential fatty acids linoleic acid (18:2n-6) and α-linolenic acid (18:3n-3) occurs by alternating desaturation (insertion of double bonds) and elongation (addition of two carbon units) of the carbon chain (Figure 5) to highly unsaturated, long-chain polyunsaturated fatty acids (LC-PUFAs) with 20 and 22 carbon atoms and 3 to 6 double bonds. The LC-PUFA arachidonic acid (20:4n-6; AA) and docosahexaenoic acid (22:6n-3; DHA) are of particular metabolic importance in infant growth and development.

PERINATAL SUPPLY OF LONG-CHAIN POLYUNSATURATED FATTY ACIDS

There is accumulating evidence for an important functional role of the perinatal LC-PUFA supply and metabolism on early nervous system development.[65] LC-PUFAs, especially AA (20:4n-6) and DHA (22:6n-3), are preferentially deposited in relatively high concentrations in developing neural cells during the perinatal brain growth spurt. In humans, most brain LC-PUFAs are accumulated during the phase of rapid brain growth in the last trimester of gestation and the first two years after birth. The importance of brain DHA accumulation is mainly related to its roles in maintaining neurological and visual development; decreases in brain and retina DHA result in altered visual acuity, disturbed electroretinographic measurements, and learning impairment in various species. AA is a major component of structural phospholipids and serves as precursor for eicosanoids, which play important roles in cell division, signal transduction, and many other physiologic processes. The pathways to form DHA from the precursor essential fatty acid α-linolenic acid exist in humans (Figure 5), and the formation of LC-PUFA from the essential fatty acid precursors has been demonstrated even in newborn infants,[66] but the rate of essential fatty acid conversion is very low. However, the relative conversion of α-linolenic acid to n-3 LC-PUFA appears to be greater in women than in men, which may contribute to meeting the demands of the fetus and the breast-fed neonate for DHA and hence represent a protective mechanism. However, most evidence indicates that the overall contribution of α-linolenic acid to DHA is very limited.[67] Moreover, recent data indicate a considerable interindividual variation in the ability to convert the precursor α-linolenic acid to n-3 LC-PUFA, related to common polymorphisms in the human delta-5 and delta-6 desaturase genes *FADS1* and *FADS2*.[68] In nonhuman primates, the supply of preformed dietary DHA is about an order of magnitude more efficient as a source for the neonatal brain accretion of DHA than is α-linolenic acid.[69] Therefore, adequate supplies of preformed n-3 LC-PUFA, and in particular DHA, during perinatal development appear important for maintaining optimal tissue function.[70]

PLACENTAL FATTY ACID TRANSFER

Numerous studies reported significant differences between the fatty acid composition of maternal plasma lipids at the time of delivery and cord plasma lipids. Percentages of saturated and monounsaturated fatty acids are very similar between maternal plasma phospholipids and cord blood phospholipids, but in cord blood the parent essential fatty acid levels are significantly lower whereas the LC-PUFA metabolites are clearly higher.[71] These observations point to a preferential transfer of LC-PUFA by the placenta. Using stable isotope-labeled fatty acids we investigated the placental transfer in vivo in humans.[72] Palmitic-, oleic-, linoleic-, and DHAs labeled with the natural carbon variant ^{13}C were administered orally 4 hours before elective caesarean section to pregnant women. Tracer concentration was analyzed hourly in maternal blood samples until delivery, in cord blood and in placental tissue.[72] The ratios between enrichments in placental tissue and in maternal plasma were similar for the saturated palmitic acid, the monounsaturated oleic acid, and the parent essential fatty acid linoleic acid, but it was clearly higher for DHA pointing to a preferential DHA transfer across the placenta (Figure 6). It can be deduced that incorporation of DHA into placental tissue is three to seven times more intensive than for the other studied fatty acids.

The placental transfer of fatty acids is a complex process. Fatty acids bind to membrane proteins and cytoplasmatic transport proteins.[73] The placenta takes up circulating nonesterified fatty acids (NEFA) as well as NEFA released from maternal circulating lipids by placental lipases and in addition human placental tissue expresses receptors to VLDL, LDL, and high-density lipoproteins,[74] which can provide fatty acids to the placenta for transfer once they are released by intracellular lipases. NEFAs may enter placental tissue both through passive diffusion and by carrier protein–mediated transport. This facilitated transport mechanism seems to involve plasma membrane fatty acid–binding protein (FABPpm/GOT2), fatty acid translocase (FAT/CD36), fatty acid transport proteins (FATPs), and fatty acid–binding proteins (FABPs).[75] It was proposed that a further FABP located exclusively on the maternal-facing membranes, placental plasma membrane fatty acid–binding protein (p-FABPpm), is also involved in the preferential uptake of LC-PUFA by trophoplast cells,[73] but definitive evidence on the possible structure and function of p-FABPpm must await analysis of its complete amino acid and/or cDNA sequence. Several FABPs are involved in their transfer to the fetal circulation; for

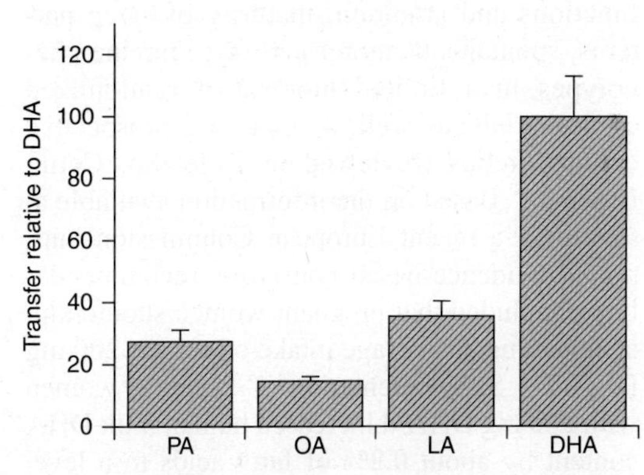

Figure 6 Ratio of fatty acid enrichments in placenta over maternal plasma in women with an elective cesarean section who received an oral dose of fatty acids labeled with the natural stable isotope carbon 13 at 4 hours prior to child birth. The relative incorporation of palmitic acid (PA), oleic acid (OA), and linoleic acid (LA) into placenta lipids is similar, whereas maternal–placental transfer of docosahexaenoic acid (DHA) is significantly higher. Results (M ± SEM) are expressed as percentage of DHA incorporation.

example, heart-FABP, liver-FABP, and adipose tissue-FABP have been identified in placenta.[76] The expression of the fatty acid transfer proteins FATP-1 and FATP-4 are correlated with placenta phospholipid DHA contents, which seems to indicate that they play a key role in facilitating preferential DHA transport from the mother to the fetus.[75] The presence of such an active and preferential maternofetal DHA transfer supports the hypothesis that fetal DHA supply is of biological importance.

DHA SUPPLY TO PREGNANT AND BREAST-FEEDING WOMEN

Enhanced maternal dietary intakes of DHA increase fetal supply and lead to higher DHA concentrations in cord blood.[77] The effects of supplementing pregnant women with n-3 LC-PUFA from fish oil or DHA-rich single-cell oils on pregnancy outcomes have been evaluated in a number of randomized controlled clinical trials, which provided daily DHA intakes from 150 to 200 mg up to about 1,200 mg/d, or up to 2.7 g total n-3 LC-PUFA/d. Systematic evaluation of these studies in recent meta-analyses revealed that n-3 LC-PUFA prolonged gestation by a mean of 1.6 or 2.6 days in two independent analyses, respectively, accompanied by a slight increase of birth weight by a mean 47 or 54 g, respectively.[78,79] Moreover, the supply of n-3 LC-PUFA reduced the risk of early preterm birth before 34 weeks of gestation by 31% in all pregnancies and by 61% in high-risk pregnancies.[79,80] Except for some reported discomfort associated with the intake of omega-3 oil capsules, such as belching and unpleasant taste, no adverse effects were detected up to the highest intake of 2.7 g total n-3 LC-PUFA/d tested in randomized controlled trials in pregnancy. A higher DHA supply to the fetus during pregnancy and to the infant after birth was associated with beneficial effects on the development of visual acuity, cognitive functions and attention, maturity of sleep patterns, spontaneous motor activity, immune phenotypes in a limited number of randomized clinical trials, as well as in several prospective cohort studies (reviewed in Koletzko, Cetin, Brenna).[70] Based on the information available at this time, a recent European Commission–supported evidence-based consensus recommendation concluded that pregnant women should aim at achieving an average intake of at least 200 mg DHA/d.[70] Supplementation of lactating women with 200 mg DHA/d increased human milk DHA content by about 0.2% of fatty acids to a level considered desirable for infant outcomes. Therefore, an average dietary intake of at least 200 mg DHA/d appears to be also adequate during lactation. An intake equivalent to 200 mg DHA/d is usually achieved by one to two meals of ocean fish per week, which includes fatty fish. This level of fish intake usually does not lead to an unacceptable daily intake of environmental pollutants.[70,81,82]

LC-PUFA SUPPLY TO INFANTS

Breast-fed infants are provided with a dietary source of the LC-PUFA AA and DHA.[83] A systematic review of effects of LC-PUFA supplementation of infant formulas on infant weight gain, based on original data analysis, indicates that the addition of DHA and AA to infant formula supports growth comparable to that seen in infants fed unsupplemented formula.[84] The available evidence strongly indicated benefits of adding both DHA and AA to infant formula that has been supported by international expert recommendations.[35,85] DHA contents in infant formulas should reach at least 0.2% of fatty acids, because lower contents have not been convincingly shown to provide benefits, and should not exceed 0.5% of fatty acids, because higher levels have not been systematically evaluated.[35] The amounts of added AA should at least be equal to those of added DHA, and the amount of EPA added should not exceed the amount of added DHA. It appears advisable that dietary sources of LC-PUFA are also provided after the first six months of life because effects of LC-PUFA status on indicators of neural function have been demonstrated in older infants and in children,[86–89] but the optimal intake levels have not been determined.

CONCLUDING REMARKS

Plenty of evidence has accumulated to show that the quantity and quality of dietary fat intake is of major importance for child growth and long-term health, including the modulation of risk of obesity, type 2 diabetes, and cardiovascular disease, visual, cognitive, and neuromotor development, as well as immune response, and risk of allergy and autoimmune diseases. Enormous methodological progress enables future research to further explore lipid supply and metabolism as well as its effects at the molecular level, and to identify the effects of interindividual genetic variation on the relationship between fat intake and health outcomes. Eventually, new scientific information should lead us to provide better advice on optimal lipid supplies to infants and children, both in health and in disease.

ACKNOWLEDGMENTS

The work of the authors is financially supported by the Commission of the European Communities, specific RTD Program "Quality of Life and Management of Living Resources," within the Fifth Framework Programme, research grants no. QLRT-2001-00389 and QLK1-CT-2002-30582, and the Sixth Framework Programme, contract no. 007036. This manuscript does not necessarily reflect the views of the commission and in no way anticipates the future policy in this area. BK is the recipient of a Freedom to Discover Award of the Bristol Myers Squibb Foundation, New York, NY, USA.

REFERENCES

1. Armand M, Hamosh M, Mehta NR, et al. Effect of human milk or formula on gastric function and fat digestion in the premature infant. Pediatr Res 1996;40:429–37.
2. Bernback S, Blackberg L, Hernell O. Fatty acids generated by gastric lipase promote human milk triacylglycerol digestion by pancreatic colipase-dependent lipase. Biochim Biophys Acta 1989;1001:286–93.
3. Mu H, Hoy CE. The digestion of dietary triacylglycerols. Prog Lipid Res 2004;43:105–33.
4. Armand M, Pasquier B, André M, et al. Digestion and absorption of 2 fat emulsions with different droplet sizes in the human digestive tract. Am J Clin Nutr 1999;70:1096–1106.
5. Hernell O, Blackberg L. Molecular aspects of fat digestion in the newborn. Acta Paediatr Suppl 1994;405:65–9.
6. Hernell O, Blackberg L, Bernback S. Digestion of human milk fat in early infancy. Acta Paediatr Scand Suppl 1989;351:57–62.
7. Bernback S, Blackberg L, Hernell O. The complete digestion of human milk triacylglycerol in vitro requires gastric lipase, pancreatic colipase-dependent lipase, and bile salt-stimulated lipase. J Clin Invest 1990;85:1221–6.
8. Ling SC, Weaver LT. The fate of fat in the infant´s colon. Q J Med 1997;90:553–5.
9. Ockner RK, Pittmann JP, Yager JL. Differences in the intestinal absorption of saturated and unsaturated long chain fatty acid. Gastroenterology 1972;62:981–92.
10. Hamosh M, Bitman J, Liao TH, et al. Gastric lipolysis and fat absorption in preterm infants: Effect of medium-chain triglyceride or long-chain triglyceride-containing formulas. Pediatrics 1989;83:86–92.
11. Chappell JE, Clandinin MT, Kearney-Volpe C, et al. Fatty acid balance studies in premature infants fed human milk or formula: Effect of calcium supplementation. J Pediatr 1986;108:439–47.
12. Mattson FH, Volpenhein RA. Rearrangment of glyceride fatty acids during digestion and absorption. J Biol Chem 1962;237:53–5.
13. Sauerwald TU, Demmelmair H, Koletzko B. Polyunsaturated fatty acid supply with human milk. Lipids 2001;36:991–6.
14. Carnielli VP, Luijendijk IH, Van Goudoever JB, et al. Structural position and amount of palmitic acid in infant formulas: Effects on fat, fatty acid, and mineral balance. J Pediatr Gastroenterol Nutr 1996;23:553–60.
15. Motil KJ. Fat and calcium absorption in infancy revisited. J Am Coll Nutr 1998;17:303–5.
16. Weaver LT, Ewing G, Taylor LC. The bowel habit of milk-fed infants. J Pediatr Gastroenterol Nutr 1988;7:568–71.
17. Qinlan PT, Lockton S, Irwin J, Lucas AL. The relationship between stool hardness and stool composition in breast- and formula-fed infants. J Pediatr Gastroenterol Nutr 1995;20:81–90.
18. Lien EL. The role of fatty acid composition and positional distribution in fat absorption in infants. J Pediatr 1994;125: S62–8.
19. Nelson SE, Frantz JA, Ziegler EE. Absorption of fat and calcium by infants fed a milk-based formula containing palm olein. J Am Coll Nutr 1998;17:303–5.
20. Innis SM, Dyer R, Nelson CM. Evidence that palmitic acid is absorbed as sn-2 monoacylglycerol from human milk by breast-fed infants. Lipids 1994;29:541–5.
21. Bach AC, Babayan VK. Medium-chain triglycerides: An update. Am J Clin Nutr 1982;36:950–62.
22. Klenoff-Brumberg HL, Genen LH. High versus low medium chain triglyceride content of formula for promoting short term growth of preterm infants. Cochrane Database Syst Rev 2003;CD002777.
23. Goulet O. Lipid requirements in infants with digestive diseases with references to short bowel syndrome. Eur J Med Res 1997;2:79–83.
24. Jeppesen PB, Mortensen PB. The influence of a preserved colon on the absorption of medium chain fat in patients with small bowel resection. Gut 1998;43:478–83.
25. Mc Donald GB, Weidman M. Partitioning of polar fatty acids into lymph and portal vein after intestinal absorption in the rat. Q J Exp Physiol 1987;72:153–9.
26. Hayashi H, Fujimoto K, Cardelli JA, et al. Fat feeding increases size, but not number, of chylomicrons produced by small intestine. Am J Physiol 1990;259:709–19.
27. Bier DM, Brosnan JT, Flatt JP, et al. Report of the IDECG Working Group on lower and upper limits of carbohydrate and fat intake. International Dietary Energy Consultative Group. Eur J Clin Nutr 1999;53:S177–8.
28. Koletzko B. Response to and range of acceptable fat intakes in infants and children. Eur J Clin Nutr 1999;53:S78–3.
29. Ziegler EE, Fomon SJ. Methods in infant nutrition research: Balance and growth studies. Acta Paediatr Scand Suppl 1982;299:90–6.

30. Van Aerde JE, Sauer PJ, Pencharz PB, et al. Effect of replacing glucose with lipid on the energy metabolism of newborn infants. Clin Sci (Lond) 1989;76:581–88.
31. Flatt JP. The difference in the storage capacities for carbohydrate and for fat, and its implications in the regulation of body weight. Ann N Y Acad Sci 1987;499:104–23.
32. Van Aerde JE, Sauer PJ, Pencharz PB, et al. Metabolic consequences of increasing energy intake by adding lipid to parenteral nutrition in full-term infants. Am J Clin Nutr 1994;59:659–62.
33. Dauncey MJ, Bingham SA. Dependence of 24h energy expenditure in man on the composition of the nutrient intake. Br J Nutr 1983;50:1–13.
34. Aggett PJ, Haschke F, Heine W, et al. Comment on the content and composition of lipids in infant formulas. ESPGAN Committee on Nutrition. Acta Paediatr Scand 1991;80:887–96.
35. Koletzko B, Baker S, Cleghorn G, et al. Global standard for the composition of infant formula: Recommendations of an ESPGHAN coordinated international expert group. J Pediatr Gastroenterol Nutr 2005;41:584–99.
36. Koletzko B, Rodriguez-Palmero M, Demmelmair H, et al. Physiological aspects of human milk lipids. Early Hum Dev 2001;65:S3–18.
37. Codex Alimentarius Commission. Joint FAO/WHO food standard programme. Report of the 28th session of the Codex Committee on Nutrition and Foods for Special Dietary Uses. Alinorm 2007;07/30/26.
38. Talvia S, Lagstrom H, Rasanen M, et al. A randomized intervention since infancy to reduce intake of saturated fat: Calorie (energy) and nutrient intakes up to the age of 10 years in the Special Turku Coronary Risk Factor Intervention Project. Arch Pediatr Adolesc Med 2004;158:41–7.
39. Ortega RM, Requejo AM, Andrés P, et al. Relationship between diet composition and body mass index in a group of Spanish adolescents. Br J Nutr 1995;74:765–73.
40. Tucker LA, Seljaas GT, Hager RL. Body fat percentage of children varies according to their diet composition. J Am Diet Assoc 1997;97:981–6.
41. Gazzaniga JM, Burns TL. Relationship between diet composition and body fatness, with adjustment for resting energy expenditure and physical activity, in preadolescent children. Am J Clin Nutr 1993;58:21–8.
42. Prentice AM, Jebb SA. Fast foods, energy density and obesity: A possible mechanistic link. Obes Rev 2003;4:187–94.
43. Svahn JC, Feldl F, Raiha NC, et al. Fatty acid content of plasma lipid fractions, blood lipids, and apolipoproteins in children fed milk products containing different quantity and quality of fat. J Pediatr Gastroenterol Nutr 2000;31:152–61.
44. Strong JP, Malcom GT, Newman WP, Oalmann MC. Early lesions of atherosclerosi in childhood and youth: Natural history and risk factors. J Am Coll Nutr 1992;11:51S–4S.
45. Aggett PJ, Haschke F, Heine W, et al. Committee report: Childhood diet and prevention of coronary heart disease. ESPAGN Committee on Nutrition. European Society of Pediatric Gastroenterology and Nutrition. J Pediatr Gastroenterol Nutr 1994;19:261–9.
46. Woodside JV, Kromhout D. Fatty acids and CHD. Proc Nutr Soc 2005;64:554–64.
47. Nicklas TA, Webber LS, Koschak M, Berenson GS. Nutrient adequancy of low fat intakes for children: The Bogalusa Heart Study. Pediatrics 1992;89:221–8.
48. Boulton TJ, Magarey AM. Effects of differences in dietary fat on growth, energy and nutrient intake from infancy to eight years of age. Acta Paediatr 1995;84:146–50.
49. Shea S, Basch CE, Stein AD, et al. Is there a relationship between dietary fat and stature or growth in children three to five years of age? Pediatrics 1993;92:579–86.
50. Obarzanek E, Hunsberger SA, Van Horn L, et al. Safety of a fat-reduced diet: The Dietary Intervention Study in Children (DISC). Pediatrics 1997;100:51–9.
51. Hansen D, Michaelsen KF, Skovby F. Growth during treatment of familial hypercholesterolemia. Acta Paediatr 1992;81:1023–25.
52. Lifshitz F, Moses N. Growth failure. A complication of dietary treatment of hypercholesterolemia. Am J Dis Child 1989;143:537–42.
53. Koletzko B. *Trans* fatty acids may impair biosynthesis of long-chain polyunsaturates and growth in man. Acta Paediatr 1992;81:302–6.
54. Vobecky JS, Vobecky J, Normand L. Risk and benefit of low fat intake in childhood. Ann Nutr Metab 1995;39:124–33.
55. Tonstad S, Sivertsen M. Relation between dietary fat and energy and micronutrient intakes. Arch Dis Child 1997;76:416–20.
56. Copperman N, Schebendach J, Arden MR, Jacobson MS. Nutrient quality of fat- and cholesterol-modified diets of children with hyperlipidemia. Arch Pediatr Adolesc Med 1995;149:333–6.
57. American Academy of Pediatrics: Committee on Nutrition. Cholesterol in Childhood. Pediatrics 1998;101:141–7.
58. Koletzko B. Potential adverse effects of *trans* fatty acids in infants and children. Eur J Med Res 1995;1:123–5.
59. Koletzko B, Decsi T. Metabolic aspects of *trans* fatty acids. Clin Nutr 1997;16:229–37.
60. Stender S, Dyerberg J, Holmer G, et al. The influence of *trans* fatty acids on health: A report from the Danish Nutrition Council. Clin Sci (Lond) 1995;88:375–92.
61. Carlson SE, Clandinin MT, Cook HW, et al. *trans* Fatty acids: Infant and fetal development. Am J Clin Nutr 1997;66:715S–36S.
62. Hunter JE. Dietary *trans* fatty acids: Review of recent human studies and food industry responses. Lipids 2006;41:967–92.
63. Precht D, Molkentin J. C18:1, C18:2 and C18:3 *trans* and *cis* fatty acid isomers including conjugated *cis* delta 9, *trans* delta 11 linoleic acid (CLA) as well as total fat composition of German human milk lipids. Nahrung 1999;43:233–44.
64. Salas-Salvado J, Marquez-Sandoval F, Bullo M. Conjugated linoleic acid intake in humans: A systematic review focusing on its effect on body composition, glucose, and lipid metabolism. Crit Rev Food Sci Nutr 2006;46:479–88.
65. Koletzko B, Larque E, Demmelmair H. Placental transfer of long-chain polyunsaturated fatty acids (LC-PUFA). J Perinat Med 2007;35:S5–S11.
66. Demmelmair H, v.Schenck U, Behrendt E, et al. Estimation of arachidonic acid synthesis in full term neonates using natural variation of ^{13}C content. J Pediatr Gastroenterol Nutr 1995;21:31–6.
67. Uauy R, Dangour AD. Nutrition in brain development and aging: Role of essential fatty acids. Nutr Rev 2006;64: S24–S33.
68. Schaeffer L, Gohlke H, Muller M, et al. Common genetic variants of the FADS1 FADS2 gene cluster and their reconstructed haplotypes are associated with the fatty acid composition in phospholipids. Hum Mol Genet 2006;15:1745–56.
69. Greiner RC, Winter J, Nathanielsz PW, Brenna JT. Brain docosahexaenoate accretion in fetal baboons: Bioequivalence of dietary alpha-linolenic and docosahexaenoic acids. Pediatr Res 1997;42:826–34.
70. Koletzko B, Cetin I, Brenna JT. Dietary fat intakes for pregnant and lactating women. Br J Nutr 2007;98(5):873–77.
71. Berghaus TM, Demmelmair H, Koletzko B. Fatty acid composition of lipid classes in maternal and cord plasma at birth. Eur J Pediatr 1998;157:763–8.
72. Larque E, Demmelmair H, Berger B, et al. In vivo investigation of the placental transfer of (13)C-labeled fatty acids in humans. J Lipid Res 2003;44:49–55.
73. Dutta-Roy AK. Transport mechanisms for long-chain polyunsaturated fatty acids in the human placenta. Am J Clin Nutr 2000;71:315S–22S.
74. Wadsack C, Tabano S, Maier A, et al. Intrauterine growth restriction is associated with alterations in placental lipoprotein receptors and maternal lipoprotein composition. Am J Physiol Endocrinol Metab 2007;292:E476–84.
75. Larque E, Krauss-Etschmann S, Campoy C, et al. Docosahexaenoic acid supply in pregnancy affects placental expression of fatty acid transport proteins. Am J Clin Nutr 2006;84:853–61.
76. Larque E, Demmelmair H, Klingler M, et al. Expression pattern of fatty acid transport protein-1 (FATP-1), FATP-4 and heart-fatty acid binding protein (H-FABP) genes in human term placenta. Early Hum Dev 2006;82:697–701.
77. Krauss-Etschmann S, Shadid R, Campoy C, et al. Effects of fish-oil and folate supplementation of pregnant women on maternal and fetal plasma concentrations of docosahexaenoic acid and eicosapentaenoic acid: A European randomized multicenter trial. Am J Clin Nutr 2007;85:1392–400.
78. Szajewska H, Horvath A, Koletzko B. Effect of n-3 long-chain polyunsaturated fatty acid supplementation of women with low-risk pregnancies on pregnancy outcomes and growth measures at birth: A meta-analysis of randomized controlled trials. Am J Clin Nutr 2006;83:1337–44.
79. Makrides M, Duley L, Olsen SF. Marine oil, and other prostaglandin precursor, supplementation for pregnancy uncomplicated by pre-eclampsia or intrauterine growth restriction. Cochrane Database Syst Rev 2006;3:CD003402.
80. Horvath A, Koletzko B, Szajewska H. Effect of supplementation of women in high-risk pregnancies with long-chain polyunsaturated fatty acids on pregnancy outcomes and growth measures at birth: A meta-analysis of randomized controlled trials. Br J Nutr 2007;98:253–9.
81. European Food Safety Authority. Opinion of the Scientific Panel on Contaminants in the Food Chain on a request from the commission related to mercury and methylmercury in food (request no. EFSA-Q-2003-030, adopted on 24 February 2004). EFSA J 2007;34:1–14.
82. European Food Safety Authority. Opinion of the Scientific Panel on contaminants in the food chain on a request from the European Parliament related to the safety assessment of wild and farmed fish (question no. EFSA-Q-2004-22, adopted on 22 June 2005). EFSA J 2007;236:1–118.
83. Yuhas R, Pramuk K, Lien EL. Human milk fatty acid composition from nine countries varies most in DHA. Lipids 2006;41:851–8.
84. Makrides M, Gibson RA, Udell T, Ried K. Supplementation of infant formula with long-chain polyunsaturated fatty acids does not influence the growth of term infants. Am J Clin Nutr 2005;81:1094–101.
85. Koletzko B, Agostoni C, Carlson SE, et al. Long chain polyunsaturated fatty acids (LC-PUFA) and perinatal development. Acta Paediatr 2001;90:460–4.
86. Agostoni C, Massetto N, Biasucci G, et al. Effects of long-chain polyunsaturated fatty acid supplementation on fatty acid status and visual function in treated children with hyperphenylalaninemia. J Pediatr 2000;137:504–9.
87. Beblo S, Reinhardt H, Muntau AC, et al. Fish oil supplementation improves visual evoked potentials in children with phenylketonuria. Neurology 2001;57:1488–91.
88. Hoffman DR, Birch EE, Castaneda YS, et al. Visual function in breast-fed term infants weaned to formula with or without long-chain polyunsaturates at 4 to 6 months: A randomized clinical trial. J Pediatr 2003;142:669–77.
89. Beblo S, Reinhardt H, Demmelmair H, et al. Effect of fish oil supplementation on fatty acid status, coordination, and fine motor skills in children with phenylketonuria. J Pediatr 2007;150:479–84.

8

Trace Elements

Nancy F. Krebs, MD, MS
K. Michael Hambidge, MD, ScD

More than 99.7% of the body weight is accounted for by 11 elements, termed the major elements (Table 1). The remainder of the body weight consists of approximately 25 trace elements, each of which contributes less than 0.01% to the body weight. Of these, a mammalian nutritional requirement has been established for iron, iodine, zinc, copper, chromium, selenium, molybdenum, manganese, cobalt, nickel, vanadium, silicon, arsenic, boron, and fluoride. Although it is reasonable to assume that the trace elements required by humans are similar to those required by other mammalian species, currently, a human nutritional requirement is accepted only for iron, iodine, zinc, copper, chromium, selenium, molybdenum, manganese, and cobalt (as vitamin B_{12}). Because of its beneficial effects in the prevention of dental caries, fluoride is also included in this list.

BIOLOGIC ROLES

Many enzyme systems depend on one or more specific trace elements, either as key components of metalloenzymes or as catalysts of metal ion–activated enzymes. The roles of metal ions in metalloenzymes may be structural, that is, maintaining the conformation of the protein, catalytic, or both. Iron, copper, zinc, molybdenum, selenium, and manganese have been identified as constituents of specific enzymes. Certain trace elements are of fundamental importance in the structure or metabolic activity of other compounds, including hemoglobin (iron), nucleic acids (multiple trace elements), transcription factor proteins (zinc), and vitamin B_{12} (cobalt).

Table 1 Elements with a Role in Human Physiology
Trace Elements

Major Elements	Recognized	Probable
Carbon (C)	Iron (Fe)	Nickel (Ni)
Hydrogen (H)	Iodine (I)	Vanadium (V)
Nitrogen (N)	Zinc (Zn)	Silicon (Si)
Oxygen (O)	Copper (Cu)	Arsenic (As)
Sodium (Na)	Chromium (Cr)	Boron (B)
Potassium (K)	Selenium (Se)	
Phosphorus (P)	Molybdenum (Mo)	
Sulfur (S)	Manganese (Mn)	
Chloride (Cl^-)	Cobalt (Co)	
Calcium (Ca)	Fluoride (F^-)	
Magnesium (Mg)		

The roles of iodine in thyroxine (T_4) and triiodothyronine (T_3), zinc in steroid hormone receptors, and chromium in facilitating the action of insulin are examples of the importance of trace elements in the activity of certain hormones. The dependence of many vital metabolic processes on trace elements confers a physiologic importance on these micronutrients that is analogous to that of vitamins and is out of proportion to their small contribution to body weight. Although considerable progress has been achieved in determining the functions of several trace elements, little is yet known about the biochemistry of others.

DOSE RESPONSE

An elementary but important concept is that the biologic effect of any trace element depends on the dose or, more specifically, on the level of intake and on tissue concentrations (Figure 1). For each element, there is an optimal range of intake, the magnitude of which varies considerably between different elements and depends on a number of factors, including the efficiency of homeostatic mechanisms. Obviously, if intakes are sufficiently high, any element will prove toxic. In the case of nonessential elements (eg, mercury), harmful effects can result only from toxic levels of intake. However, in the case of the "essential" trace elements, problems may result from intakes that are too low as well as too high. In animal husbandry, the economic importance of trace deficiency states has been recognized for many years.[1] However, in human nutrition, only iron and iodine deficiencies were recognized prior to the 1960s, and it is only more recently that a broader concept of trace element nutrition has started to develop with the recognition of zinc, copper, chromium, selenium, molybdenum, and possibly manganese deficiency states in humans. Likewise, greater appreciation has emerged for potential adverse effects of very high intakes, for example, from copper contamination of drinking water.

ETIOLOGY OF HUMAN TRACE DEFICIENCY STATES

The last several decades have been notable not only for the number of new trace elements implicated in deficiency disease but, perhaps more surprisingly, for the wide variety of different factors that have been discovered to play a role in the etiology of these deficiency states (Table 2). These include inherited or acquired alterations in metabolism and other special circumstances leading to increased nutritional requirements as well as factors that contribute to inadequate intakes of one or more of the trace elements.

Notable examples of the inborn errors of trace element metabolism are represented by acrodermatitis enteropathica (AE) and "Menke steely hair syndrome" (MSHS), which are genetic defects in zinc absorption and copper trafficking, respectively.[3,4] Although these entities are rare and not strictly nutritional deficiency diseases, some of them are important in a nutritional context because of the insight they provide into the clinical and metabolic effects of severe nutritional deficiencies. Moreover, in some instances, manipulation of dietary intake has remarkable therapeutic benefits. Both of these points are well illustrated by AE, which is discussed below. Although unresponsive to dietary supplements, Menkes is attributable in part to a de facto deficiency of copper in certain tissues and subcellular sites, resulting from deranged copper transport, including out of the enterocyte.

Diseases that cause intestinal malabsorption of fat and other nutrients may also lead to trace element deficiencies.[5] Excessive losses of trace elements occur in certain diseases through the kidneys, gastrointestinal tract, sweat, exudates, or

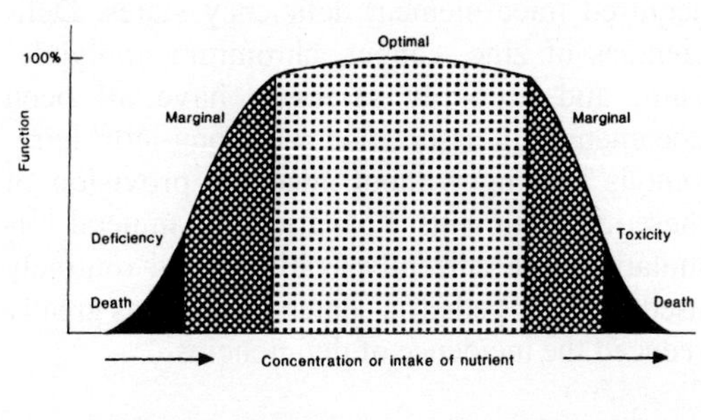

Figure 1 Dependence of biologic function on tissue concentration or intake of a nutrient. (Reproduced from reference 3.)

Table 2 Etiology of Trace Mineral Deficiencies

Etiology	Trace Elements*
Inadequate intake	
No special circumstances required but risk increased during infancy and pregnancy	Fe, Zn
Losses during food processing, including preparation of "humanized" infant milk formulas	Zn, Cr, Cu, Se
Poor bioavailability	Fe, Zn
Local deficiencies in geochemical environment	I, Se
In association with protein-energy malnutrition	Zn, Cu, Cr
Synthetic diets, including intravenous feeding	Zn, Cu, Cr, Se, Mo
Other circumstances	
Prematurity	Fe, Cu, Zn
Diseases and other unusual circumstances	Zn, Cu, Cr causing impaired intestinal absorption or excessive losses of trace elements
Inborn errors of trace element metabolism	Zn, Cu, Mo

*Elements given are notable examples, but not necessarily a complete list.

hemorrhage. Low blood plasma concentrations of specific trace elements can occur in certain disease states in association with the redistribution of these elements within the body. For example, movement of zinc and iron from the plasma to the liver occurs in stress situations, including infectious diseases. Correction of hypozincemia in these circumstances may be contraindicated, although the host response may depend on the specific cause of the stress.

The premature infant with very low birth weight provides a unique nutritional challenge that includes the provision of adequate trace elements.[6,7] Some elements, notably copper, iron, and possibly zinc, are stored extensively by the fetus during the last trimester. These stores, which are available to the term infant in early postnatal life, are diminished in the premature infant. Immaturity of intestinal absorption mechanisms and relatively high losses of endogenous zinc have been reported. These problems are aggravated further by the high nutritional requirements that are imposed by the rapid growth of the premature infant after the early postnatal period. Nutritional requirements may also be relatively high during periods of rapid growth in the term infant and in later childhood, as well as during pregnancy and lactation.

Although nutritional requirements for trace elements are small and these nutrients are ubiquitous in the environment, the quantities present in food and water are usually correspondingly low. Hence, contrary to earlier concepts, it is not surprising that humans are at risk from nutritional deficiencies of the trace elements. Iron deficiency, although outside the scope of this chapter, remains one of the most common human nutritional disorders. Other trace deficiencies occur in more restricted geographic locations owing to localized deficiencies in soils, plants, or water. The classic example of a geographic deficiency is that of endemic goiter, and low body content of selenium is observed in some countries, for example, New Zealand, whereas marked selenium depletion and deficiency occurs in large areas of China. Diets deficient in energy and other nutrients may also contain inadequate quantities of trace elements. Thus, deficiencies of zinc, copper, and chromium have been documented in association with protein-energy malnutrition.

Variations in bioavailability are a major factor in determining the adequacy of dietary intake of some of the trace elements. This also applies especially to the infant because of its dependence on one major food staple. Thus, if the milk or milk substitute that provides most or all of the nutrients consumed by the infant is low in available trace elements, there is no chance that this deficit will be compensated for by a more favorable supply in other food items. Although our understanding of this complex subject is far from complete, it is known that human milk confers important advantages with respect to the bioavailability of iron and zinc. Although not proven, it seems probable that this may also be true of other trace elements. As a corollary, the trace element concentrations in breast milk should be considered as a minimum guideline for corresponding concentrations in infant milk formulas, and higher concentrations of at least some elements, including iron and zinc, are necessary in the latter. However, indiscriminate supplementation may have adverse consequences, especially through undesirable interactions with other trace elements. Additional research directed at mineral–mineral interactions is needed to determine optimal fortification levels in foods and formulas.

The use of synthetic diets in medical practice, including those used in intravenous feeding, has provided some of the most dramatic examples of acquired trace element deficiency states. Deficiencies of zinc, copper, chromium, molybdenum, and probably selenium have all been documented in association with long-term intravenous feeding without adequate provision of these micronutrients. Pediatric trace mineral formulations are currently available and routinely used in major pediatric centers, which has greatly reduced the incidence of deficiencies.

NUTRITIONAL REQUIREMENTS

The evolving nutritional importance of trace elements has been recognized by the publication of guidelines, including those of the Food and Nutrition Board of the National Academy of Sciences (see Appendix II, "Nutritional Requirements").[8] A formal recommended dietary allowance (RDA) has been established for copper, iodine, iron, molybdenum, selenium, and zinc. An adequate intake (AI) has been set for chromium and manganese, which reflects the more limited data available on which to base an estimated average requirement (EAR). Information is limited on the quantities of some of these elements in individual food items, which limits the application of these guidelines by nutritionists and other health professionals. There are theoretic advantages to defining recommendations for such elements as zinc according to the bioavailability from different diets, as has been done by the World Health Organization (WHO),[9] but caution is warranted when currently available data are not adequate to support precise tailoring of such recommendations. A specific point that merits emphasis is that intakes below the recommended levels are not necessarily inadequate. In particular, it is wrong to conclude that human milk is deficient in a specific trace element because it provides relatively low quantities of that element.

Guidelines have also been published for intravenous administration of trace elements to children who have to be maintained with total intravenous nutrition (Table 3).[10] Intravenous requirements for zinc vary according to the extent of ongoing losses, especially from the gastrointestinal tract. Hence, it is desirable to monitor zinc status at regular intervals.

LABORATORY ANALYSES AND THE DETECTION OF TRACE ELEMENT DEFICIENCY STATES

Fundamental advances in analytic instrumentation, especially the advent and progressive refinement of atomic absorption spectrophotometry, have facilitated the quantitative measurement of trace elements that are present in the parts-per-billion as well as parts-per-million concentration

Table 3 Guidelines for Maintenance Intravenous Administration of Trace Elements during Parenteral Nutrition

Trace Element	Maintenance Requirement (μg/kg/d)
Zinc	100*
Copper	20
Chromium	0.2
Manganese	1
Selenium	2
Iodine	1

*Requirements for zinc may be much greater in patients who continue to excrete excessive quantities of zinc; also, in premature infants, 300 μg/kg/d should be administered.

ranges. Yet formidable analytic difficulties remain. For example, accurate measurement of chromium, which now appears to be present in blood plasma, urine, and milk in only parts-per-trillion concentrations, is extraordinarily difficult. Even for relatively simple measurements, such as those of zinc in plasma or serum, substantial interlaboratory differences in analytic results continue to be evident, and it is ideal that each laboratory establish its own normal range. Even when analytic data are accurate, interpretation is frequently problematic. Plasma concentrations of zinc, for example, may be depressed for reasons other than a nutritional deficiency and thus may fail to provide a sufficiently sensitive or reliable guide to body status. Established physiologic indices, such as the measurement of the activity of an enzyme that depends on a specific trace element, are generally unavailable. The depression of glutathione peroxidase (GPx) activity in selenium deficiency states is one exception, but the clinical significance of this observation remains uncertain. Overall, laboratory indices for detection of "newer" trace element deficiencies are not as dependable as those available for the detection of iron deficiency. Hence, for research purposes, more cumbersome approaches are necessary to confirm the suspicion of a specific deficiency, including especially the effects of supplementation on specific physiologic parameters and functional outcomes under carefully controlled conditions. Meanwhile, the health professional needs to be aware of the circumstances in which there is a risk of specific trace element deficiencies and of the clinical features that may be attributable to such a deficiency.

Hair analyses merit special mention because of their widespread misuse and the unsubstantiated claims for this diagnostic tool. Currently, the value of chemical analyses of hair in clinical practice is extremely limited.[11] Because of the inherent difficulties in interpretation of analytic data, it is unlikely that future research will lead to more useful clinical applications of hair analyses. Multielement hair analyses continue to be available commercially, often accompanied by interpretations of questionable validity, and the results merit caution and additional confirmatory evidence prior to therapeutic interventions.

ZINC

A nutritional requirement for zinc was first recognized in microorganisms in 1869, in plants in 1914, and in mammals in 1934.[1] In 1954, zinc deficiency was shown to be the cause of porcine parakeratosis. The first of the zinc metalloenzymes to be identified was carbonic anhydrase in 1940. Subsequently, over 100 zinc metalloenzymes have been identified, including at least one in every major enzyme classification. Understanding of the role of zinc in cell growth and differentiation took a major step forward with recognition of "zinc fingers" as the most frequent DNA-binding motif for transcription factor proteins.[12] The first reports of human zinc deficiency attributable to dietary factors emerged in the Middle East in the early 1960s in relation to the syndrome of adolescent nutritional dwarfism.[13] In the 1990s, the importance of zinc deficiency on childhood morbidity and mortality in the developing world was documented by a number of carefully conducted, large-scale, randomized, controlled supplementation trials in vulnerable populations.[14,15]

Table 4 Clinical Features of Zinc Deficiency*

Decrease in growth velocity
Impaired appetite and decreased food intake
Diarrhea
Increased susceptibility to infection with associated abnormalities of the immune system
Acro-orificial skin lesions; other epithelial lesions, including glossitis, alopecia, nail dystrophy, and hair loss
Behavioral abnormalities, including impairment of hedonic tone delayed sexual maturation and impotence
Eye lesions, including photophobia and lack of dark adaptation delayed healing of wounds, burns, and decubitus ulcers
Hypogeusia or dysgeusia
Low birth weight
Prematurity

*Features are dependent on severity of deficiency and other factors.

CLINICAL FEATURES OF ZINC DEFICIENCY

The clinical features of human zinc deficiency range from a life-threatening disease state, characterized by acro-orificial skin rashes, diarrhea, growth arrest, anorexia, depressed mood, and increased susceptibility to infection, to a mild impairment of growth velocity, often accompanied by other problems, including poor appetite (Table 4). In addition to the severity of the zinc depletion, the clinical sequelae appear to depend on other factors, including the speed of onset and associated clinical and dietary factors such as protein-energy malnutrition.

Decreased growth velocity or growth arrest is a consistent and early result of even mild zinc deficiency in young experimental animals and in infants, children, and adolescents. In severe acute zinc-deficiency states (eg, AE), there is an abrupt cessation of weight gain when the skin rash becomes manifest, and "catch-up" growth occurs when adequate zinc supplements are administered.[16] A meta-analysis of trials in prepubertal children that met strict criteria indicated that supplementation was associated with significant responses in both height and weight increments. Responses were strongest in those initially underweight and in children >6 months of age with evidence of stunting.[16a] These collective results suggest that zinc deficiency is a common cause of retarded growth velocity in the developing world. Zinc deficiency has also been linked to poor growth in association with certain diseases, including cystic fibrosis and sickle cell anemia.[17–19,20]

Anorexia is an early manifestation of zinc deficiency in experimental animals. Although this has long been recognized as a feature of AE and is also noted in association with milder zinc-deficiency syndromes, it has been difficult to acquire objective evidence of a direct cause-and-effect relationship in humans. However, a significant effect of zinc supplementation on food intake has been observed in some double-blind, controlled studies.[21,22]

Diarrhea is one of the hallmark features of the early descriptions of AE and occurs in a high percentage of cases of severe zinc deficiency. There is growing evidence that zinc deficiency contributes to the incidence, severity, and duration of acute infectious and persistent diarrhea in infants and young children in the developing world. On the basis of pooled analysis of zinc supplementation trials, a substantial reduction in the rate of treatment failure or death in children given zinc supplements has been estimated.[23] Diarrhea can itself also contribute to zinc deficiency because of the losses of endogenous zinc in diarrheal fluids. Thus, requirements for zinc are likely to be greater in the presence of diarrhea. In recognition of the beneficial effects of zinc supplementation and the high prevalence of marginal zinc status in young children in international settings, WHO and UNICEF have recommended routine administration of zinc supplements along with fluid replacement and continued feeding in all episodes of acute diarrhea.[24]

The skin lesions of severe acute zinc-deficiency syndromes have a characteristic distribution, primarily at the extremities and adjacent to the body orifices (Figure 2). However, lesions do occur elsewhere and may become generalized.

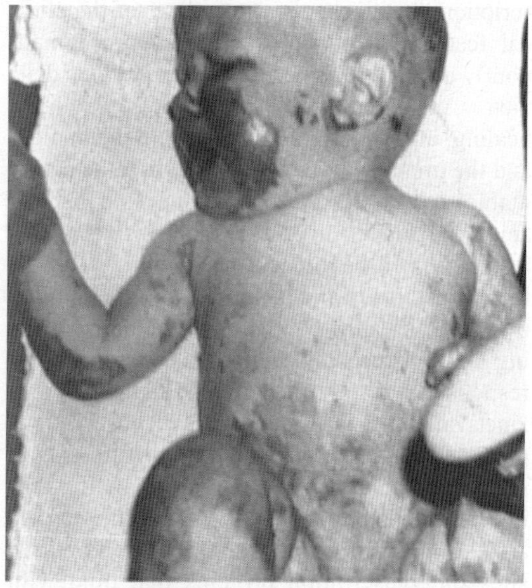

Figure 2 The acute skin lesions of acrodermatitis enteropathica are demonstrated in this 10-month-old infant. (Reproduced from reference 25.)

Most commonly, the rashes are erythematous, vesiculobullous, and pustular. Secondary infection is common, especially with staphylococci or *Candida*. In AE, the skin lesions typically occur in early infancy, although they are often delayed until after weaning if the infant is breast-fed. Other epidermal lesions include gingivitis, dermatitis, glossitis, conjunctivitis, blepharitis, alopecia, and, in chronic cases, nail dystrophies.

Behavioral abnormalities are a notable feature of severe zinc-deficiency states. Irritability, lethargy, and depression occur typically in conjunction with the skin rash of severe zinc deficiency. Hedonic tone and motivation to engage in the environment improve dramatically after the commencement of zinc therapy.[26] Cognitive development is impaired in young zinc-deficient animals, and there is evidence that the same applies in the human.[27]

Frequent bacterial and monilial infections, associated with abnormalities of the immune system, contribute to the progressive and often fatal course that characterizes untreated AE. Abnormalities of the immune system also occur in less severe zinc-deficiency states. Zinc supplementation of malnourished pre-school-aged children was associated with a significant reduction in anergic/hypoergic children, and a significantly greater rise in lymphocyte subsets.[28] Compared with studies of zinc and diarrhea, there are fewer trials examining the effects of zinc on the incidence of pneumonia, but the results of a pooled analysis suggest a 41% lower rate of pneumonia in zinc-supplemented children.[14] Although exact mechanisms have not been characterized, the general conclusion is that such findings suggest correction of a preexisting zinc deficiency, rather than a pharmacologic effect of the zinc supplements.

BIOCHEMICAL CORRELATES

Although there is now extensive knowledge about the biochemistry of zinc, especially its role in a wide range of enzyme systems and in gene transcription, the biochemical correlates of the clinical features of human zinc deficiency remain poorly defined. Many of the features of zinc deficiency, including growth retardation, poor wound healing, and abnormalities of fetal development and the immune system, are thought to be attributable, at least in part, to disturbances in nucleic acid metabolism and protein synthesis. Its role as a stabilizer of the molecular structure of subcellular constituents and membranes is exemplified by the observation of altered membrane signaling and postreceptor events that coordinate the response to insulin-like growth factor 1 when zinc availability is limited.[29,30] Such observations provide another plausible link to the growth retardation and impaired immune function during zinc deficiency. The so-called zinc fingers are the most common motif for the repetitive sites on transcription proteins that bind with DNA to initiate transcription.[12] Through this mechanism, which can be compromised by zinc restriction, zinc has an extraordinarily important role in gene expression. Additionally, several of the enzymes involved in nucleic acid synthesis are zinc dependent, including DNA and RNA polymerases, reverse transcriptase, and thymidine kinase, the activity of which is known to be reduced in human zinc deficiency.

Zinc is critical for normal immune function and interacts with several components of the immune system, ranging from the skin and its barrier function to aspects of both cellular and, to a lesser extent humeral, immunity. In vitro studies emphasize the responsiveness of some components to zinc concentrations, with both deficiency and supraphysiologic levels leading to impaired immune function. As a highly proliferative organ, the immune system strongly depends on an adequate zinc supply. Reviews address in vitro and in vivo studies of the role of zinc in normal immune function and the impact of zinc deficiency on common childhood illnesses.[31,32]

The importance of zinc to normal function of the central nervous system, including as a prominent neurosecretory product in the cerebrocortex and in its role in modulation of cortical excitability, has recently been reviewed.[33,34]

ETIOLOGIC FACTORS IN ZINC DEFICIENCY

The prototype of the severest forms of human zinc deficiency is provided by AE, a rare autosomal recessively inherited disorder. The phenotypic expression of this disease is attributable entirely to a severe zinc-deficiency state. Although total body zinc is not greatly reduced in AE, plasma zinc concentrations are typically extremely low. Before the beneficial effects of zinc therapy were recognized, this was a severe, progressive, and often fatal disease. The zinc deficiency results from a partial block in the intestinal absorption of this trace metal owing to mutations in the *SLC39A4* gene, also known as the *ZIP4* gene. The gene codes for hZip4, a transmembrane, histidine-rich protein, a member of the ZIP family of metal ion transporters, which functions in zinc uptake. The gene is expressed abundantly throughout the intestine, and accumulates at the apical surface of the enterocyte.[35] Clinical diagnosis by mutation analysis is now possible, although not yet routinely available.[36]

There have been numerous reports of similar severe zinc-deficiency states in breast-fed infants, especially those delivered prematurely. Several of these cases have been attributable to an inability of the mother's mammary gland to secrete normal quantities of zinc into the milk despite an otherwise apparently normal maternal zinc status. The specific mutation or mutations of zinc transporters localized to the mammary gland, responsible for this condition in humans, is an area of active research.[37,38] This mutation is characterized by normal zinc status in the mother, but markedly low milk zinc concentrations (~25% of normal for stage of lactation), resulting in severe zinc deficiency in the exclusively breast-fed infant. Supplemental zinc to the infant easily treats the infant's deficiency, as there is no absorptive defect in the infant. The prevalence of this defect is unknown, but clinical impression is that it is not rare.

Zinc deficiency has been well documented in premature and low-birth-weight infants if supplemental zinc is not provided. Contributory factors may include immaturity of the gastrointestinal homeostatic processes, including both absorption of exogenous zinc and conservation of endogenous zinc, relatively high urine losses, and relatively high zinc requirements when rapid postnatal growth commences. Fortification of human milk and use of fortified formulas designed to meet the needs of premature infants have been associated with positive net absorption and retention of zinc.[39] The results of zinc supplementation trials in low-birth-weight infants in developing countries have resulted in a striking reduction in morbidity and mortality, illustrating the apparent vulnerability of these infants to zinc deficiency without a generous dietary intake.[40,41] Findings of reduced zinc pool sizes at birth in small—compared to appropriate—for gestational age infants further supports this vulnerability.[41]

A wide variety of etiologic factors may contribute to more moderate and mild zinc-deficiency states. An "absolute" dietary deficiency is considered less common than relative deficiency owing to reliance on dietary sources of poor bioavailability. Older breast-fed infants are susceptible to mild zinc deficiency because of the low zinc concentrations in human milk after 6 months. Deficiency has been documented in infants in developing countries, where a combination of complementary foods with low zinc content and/or bioavailability and a high infectious burden likely contribute to the risk of deficiency.[22] As phytate intakes are high in many developing countries owing to dependence on plant staples such as maize, wheat, or legumes, there is particular concern about the adequacy of zinc intake in infants and young children in these settings.[43] Even in Western cultures, the traditional progression from iron-fortified infant cereals to fruits and vegetables, with relatively late introduction of meats, may pose a risk for mild zinc deficiency in older breast-fed infants.[44,45]

The risk of zinc deficiency is enhanced in certain disease states owing to malabsorption of zinc or excessive losses. Fat malabsorption or intestinal inflammation may impair zinc absorption and enhance losses of intestinal endogenous zinc, as in regional enteritis, celiac disease, and cystic fibrosis.[18,46] Excessive urinary losses of zinc occur in liver disease,[47] diabetes mellitus, sickle cell disease,[20] nephrosis, and catabolic conditions.[5] A number of chelating agents, diuretics, and other drugs can also cause excessive zinc excretion. More extensive data are needed to determine whether such clinical conditions pose a significant risk to zinc status.

DIAGNOSIS OF ZINC DEFICIENCY

The characteristic distribution of the skin lesions facilitates the clinical diagnosis of severe zinc-deficiency states. Unfortunately, however, the clinical features of more moderate and mild zinc-deficient states are nonspecific. Hypozincemia is not a consistent feature of mild chronic zinc-deficiency states. Currently, laboratory parameters are of only limited value in the confirmation of zinc deficiency. Plasma zinc concentrations are markedly depressed (<40 μg/dL) in the severest deficiency states, and moderate hypozincemia (40 to 60 μg/dL) occurs in more moderate zinc-deficiency states. However, plasma zinc levels are also depressed to this extent with the effects of various stresses, including infections, which result in hepatic sequestration of circulating body zinc. Interleukin-6 and other cytokines are responsible for the decline in plasma zinc associated with infections. Underlying zinc deficiency can obviously coexist with acute infection, and thus consideration of the benefit of zinc supplements should be given in settings of high risk of nutritional zinc deficiency.[48] Fasting is associated with higher plasma zinc levels, and the effects of meals result in progressively lower concentrations over the course of a day. Interlaboratory differences in normal ranges make it necessary to use local normal ranges for reference purposes. An analysis of national data for children under 10 year suggested a lower cutoff of 65 mg/dL for morning nonfasting sampling, and 57 mg/dL for afternoon sampling.[49] Serum zinc levels have been reported to be higher than plasma zinc levels; this is attributable to a delay in separation from red cells. Erythrocyte zinc is little affected by zinc deficiency and is not a sensitive index, and leukocyte zinc concentrations as an index of status have not withstood the test of time. Urine excretion rates are diminished in severe zinc deficiency, but this is also not a sufficiently sensitive assay. Unfortunately, no blood zinc fraction has been identified that will provide a good measure of zinc status or that is comparable to serum ferritin levels in the assessment of iron status. Serum alkaline phosphatase activity is depressed in moderate-to-severe zinc deficiency states and increases with zinc supplementation in cases of more moderate zinc-deficiency. However, this assay is not a sufficiently specific diagnostic tool used alone. Because of the limitations of currently available laboratory indices in the detection of mild zinc-deficiency states, the most reliable approach remains the demonstration of a functional response to a trial of zinc supplementation under adequately controlled conditions.

TREATMENT OF ZINC DEFICIENCY

AE can be treated effectively with 40 to 50 mg/d of elemental zinc administered as the sulfate, gluconate, or other salt. Requirements in infants and toddlers with AE may be considerably less (eg, 20 to 30 mg/d). Most other milder cases of zinc deficiency can be treated effectively with zinc, 1 mg elemental zinc/kg body wt/d, typically up to a maximum of 20 mg zinc/d. Somewhat larger quantities may be required in the presence of excessive ongoing losses or malabsorption. In severe zinc deficiency in premature breast-fed infants, temporary zinc supplements are necessary until other sources of zinc are added to the diet. One milligram of elemental zinc is equivalent to 4.4 mg of $ZnSO_4$ $7H_2O$; 7 mg of zinc gluconate; and 2.8 mg of zinc acetate (anhydrous).

Maintenance intravenous requirements for adults are approximately 2 mg and in infants 100 μg/kg body wt/d. In premature infants, 300 μg/kg body wt/d has been recommended.[10] Ongoing losses through the gastrointestinal tract owing, for example, to intractable diarrhea may substantially increase the intravenous requirement. For intravenous administration, zinc chloride is frequently used; 1 mg zinc is equivalent to 2.1 mg $ZnCl_2$.

TOXICITY

Acute toxicity is rare but can occur, for example, from the ingestion of large quantities of pharmacologic preparations of zinc or from the consumption of acidic drinks from galvanized cans. Symptoms are usually limited to diarrhea and vomiting, but there may be severe lethargy. Toxicity has also resulted from storage of dialysis water in a galvanized tank. Administration of zinc in quantities of 50 mg/d to adults can cause anemia owing to copper deficiency (see below) and may depress plasma high-density lipoprotein cholesterol levels.

ABSORPTION AND METABOLISM

The gastrointestinal tract, specifically the small intestine and the pancreas, have the major role in maintaining whole-body Zn homeostasis.[5] Over 20 zinc transporters have been identified in these organs, with the ZnT family generally functioning as zinc exporters and the ZIP family functioning in zinc uptake into the cytoplasm. Gene expression of the transporters is a major component of homeostatic regulation, including regulation of zinc absorption via the small intestine and excreting zinc via both the pancreas and the small intestine. As described above, the synthesis of a cellular localization of hZip4, the transporter that is defective in AE, responds to zinc depletion of the host.[50] Alterations of expression of individual transporters, which have been reported in animal models of zinc deficiency, however, do not yet fully explain the observations at the whole-body level made in humans.

Of note, studies in humans applying stable isotope techniques indicate that the quantity of zinc ingested, rather than host zinc status, is the principal factor triggering regulation of expression of the transporters involved with zinc absorption into and through the enterocyte.[5] Zinc absorption into and through the enterocyte is known to be a saturable transport process.[51] Fractional absorption, therefore, declines with increasing Zn intake and vice versa. Regulation of the quantity of endogenous Zn excreted has a major role in maintaining whole-body Zn homeostasis in most circumstances, and does appear to be influenced by host zinc status.

Fractional absorption of zinc averages about 60% when ingested in solution in water but is usually only in the range of 20 to 40% from composite meals or infant formulas. Fractional absorption of zinc from human milk approaches that of zinc absorption when taken with water alone.[52] This favorable bioavailability is undoubtedly in part owing to the relatively modest concentration of zinc in human milk. On the other hand, fractional absorption is depressed by certain dietary constituents, notably phytate (inositol hexaphosphate). The intestine is the major route for excretion of endogenous zinc, and conservation of intestinal endogenous zinc appears to be critical in maintaining or restoring zinc balance.[5,53] The ability of the intestine to conserve endogenous zinc may be impaired by a high intake of phytate from plant foods and by malabsorption, including cystic fibrosis.[18,54]

About 10% of total body zinc, 100 to 200 mg in adults, intermixes with circulating plasma zinc within 2 days.[55] This zinc is thought to be of special physiologic importance to many of the zinc-dependent metabolic processes in the body, and it is also this zinc that is vulnerable to dietary zinc restriction. This is likely to explain why symptoms of zinc deficiency occur with very little change in total body zinc. It has been found that the quantity of readily exchangeable zinc has a strong positive correlation with dietary zinc and an even stronger correlation with quantity of zinc absorbed.[5,53] A substantial part of this rapidly exchanging zinc is located in the liver.

In the systemic circulation, approximately 75% of the plasma zinc is loosely bound to albumin, and most of the remainder is tightly bound to α_2-macroglobulin. The normal zinc concentration in plasma averages about 0.85 μg/mL (13 μmol/L), with a range from 0.70 to 1.00 μg/mL. The zinc concentration in erythrocytes, most of which is incorporated in carbonic anhydrase, is approximately 12 μg/g wet weight. Leukocyte zinc concentrations are higher, with mean literature values of about 100 μg/10^{10} cells. The highest known zinc concentrations are in certain regions of the eye, including the retina. Bone, prostate, and hair all have concentrations near 100 μg/g or even greater. Muscle, liver, and kidney contain about 50 μg/g. The total body zinc content of an adult has been calculated to be about 2 g.[1]

DIETARY REQUIREMENTS

The results of recent studies of breast-fed and formula-fed infants using zinc stable isotope techniques allow reasonably accurate factorial estimates of zinc requirements. In fully breast-fed infants receiving mature human milk, conservation of endogenous zinc is critical to maintaining positive net absorption and averages approximately 50 μg zinc/kg body wt/d.[52] Because the amount of endogenous fecal zinc is positively correlated with dietary zinc intake and absorbed zinc, this figure is considerably higher in formula-fed infants receiving zinc-fortified formulas.[56,57] Allowing 10 μg zinc/kg body wt/day for urine, sweat, and integumental losses, total calculated minimal endogenous loss is 60 μg zinc/kg body wt/d. With an average fractional absorption of approximately 0.5, this figure translates into a dietary zinc requirement of approximately 150 μg zinc/kg/d. Actual zinc intake of breast-fed infants varies considerably over the first three months of life as milk zinc concentrations decline. Mean intakes at 5 months of age have been found to be close to this projected dietary requirement. Retention required for normal growth is approximately 20 μg zinc/g new tissue. In the young infant, the growth requirement may therefore reach 600 μg zinc (ie, approximately 150 μg zinc/kg body wt/d) or more per day, but part of this may be met by hepatic stores acquired in utero.[7,42] The physiologic requirement, the amount of zinc that must be absorbed to match endogenous losses and the zinc retained for new tissue synthesis, has been estimated to be 0.84 mg/d for infants 7 to 12 month of age.[8] Factorial estimations are higher for rapidly growing premature infants, for malnourished infants during the "catch-up" growth phase, and to compensate for unusual endogenous losses that occur, for example, with diarrhea and malabsorption.

The AI of 2 mg zinc/d for 0 to 6 months is based on the zinc intake of exclusively breast-fed infants at approximately 2 months of age (Appendix II, "Nutritional Requirements"). This does not imply that lower zinc intakes of exclusively breast-fed infants at 4 to 6 months are inadequate. EARs and RDAs for older infants and children have been calculated by extrapolation from factorial data for infants, as described above.[8] The tolerable upper intake levels (ULs) failed to take into account the fact that many North American infants and young children who are not exclusively breast-fed consume substantially more zinc than the ULs, with no detectable evidence of any harm.[58]

ZINC IN FOODS

The highest concentrations of zinc are found generally in cellular animal products, especially meats; whole grains, nuts, and legumes also contain substantial quantities of zinc, but this is less likely to be bioavailable owing to phytic acid. The zinc content and bioavailability of typical complementary foods for the older breast-fed infant vary widely both in developed and developing countries.[43,45] As noted above, unfortified plant food sources of zinc are often inadequate to meet the needs of the older infant and toddler. Several ready-to-eat breakfast cereals and some infant cereals in the United States are now fortified with zinc as well as iron and other micronutrients. The zinc content of human milk declines by severalfold from colostrum to mature milk. Concentrations seem to be minimally influenced by maternal zinc intake.[45] Infant formulas and a wide range of special formulas are now routinely zinc supplemented/fortified. An overview of the zinc and copper content of major food items is given in Table 5.

COPPER

Copper-dependent redox reactions developed very early in the evolutionary process. Because the earth's atmosphere changed from a reducing to an oxidizing environment, copper, together with iron, has been involved at the active sites of respiratory proteins. Recognition of copper as an essential trace mineral for humans followed demonstration of a role in treatment of some cases of hypochromic anemia in infants. Copper deficiency has subsequently been identified in several special circumstances, but its frequency and the extent of its clinical importance in some conditions remain unclear, for example, in the very low birth weight premature infant.

Although beyond the scope of this chapter, an introduction to copper would not be complete without reference to two inborn errors of copper metabolism, which have attracted more clinical interest than has dietary copper deficiency. The central role of copper in the pathophysiology of Wilson's disease was recognized in 1945 and of MSHS, or now termed simply Menkes disease, in 1962. The research stimulated by these inborn errors of copper metabolism has led to a clearer understanding of normal human copper metabolism. It is now recognized that these two conditions represent disruption of copper transport across cell membranes. The two homologous cation-transporting P-type adenosine triphosphatases (ATPases), the Menkes P-type ATPase (MNK protein, ATP7A) and Wilson ATPase (Wilson protein, ATP7B), are the gene products primarily responsible for cellular copper homeostasis. The MNK functions in copper trafficking to the secretory pathway for efflux from cells

Table 5 Trace Element Content of Common Foods

Item	Zinc (mg/100 g)	Copper (mg/100 g)
Meat group		
Regular ground beef	4.4	0.06
Round steak	5.8	0.05
Beef liver	5.1	4.6
Chicken—drumstick, fried	2.7	0.01
Pork chop	2.4	0.01
Bologna, all meat	1.8	0.02
Hot dog, all meat	1.6	0.08
Fish group		
Oyster, raw, Atlantic	74.7	3.62
Perch fillet	1.0	0.21
Tuna—in oil, drained, solids	1.1	0.01
Dairy and egg group		
Whole milk	0.4	0.005
Cheddar cheese	3.1	0.11
American cheese	3.0	0.11
Ice cream, vanilla	1.06	0.005
Eggs, hard-boiled	1.0	0.05
Infant formula	0.5	0.06
Nuts and legumes		
Common beans, cooked (red, kidney, pinto)	0.6	0.25
Peanut butter	2.9	0.61
Roasted peanuts	3.0	0.43
Bread and cereal group		
Whole wheat bread	1.0	0.17
Graham crackers	1.1	0.04
Corn flakes	0.3	0.02
Oatmeal, cooked	0.5	0.02
Macaroni, cooked	0.5	0.02
Rice	0.4	0.02
Vegetable and fruit group		
Green beans, canned	0.3	0.02–0.04
Potatoes, boiled	0.3	0.10
Potato chips	0.8	0.29
Lettuce	0.4	0.04
Apple	0.05	0.01
Banana	0.2	0.11
Orange juice	0.02	0.008

including enterocytes. In Menkes syndrome, there is reduced copper absorption and placental copper transport, resulting in reduced availability of the mineral to peripheral organs and tissues. Although the pathophysiology of MSHS is complex, at least some of the principal clinical features can be attributed to a de facto severe copper-deficiency state, including in the brain. The WND P-type ATPase also functions in copper trafficking to secrete excess copper into the biliary canalicular system. In Wilson's disease, mutations of the Wilson ATPase results in copper accumulation, especially in the liver, brain, and cornea.[59] Hence, recognition of the role of disordered copper metabolism in these diseases has helped to improve our understanding of the effects of severe human copper deficiency and of copper toxicity.[60,61]

CLINICAL FEATURES OF COPPER DEFICIENCY

The principal features of copper deficiency are hypocupremia, a hypochromic, normocytic anemia that is unresponsive to iron therapy, neutropenia, and osteoporosis. The bone marrow shows megaloblastic changes and vacuolization of the erythroid series. Iron deposits may be seen by electron microscopy in mitochondria and in some of the cytoplasmic vacuoles in red blood cell precursors. Maturation arrest of the granulocytic series may be evident. Iron stores in the intestinal mucosa, reticuloendothelial system, and liver cells are increased. The anemia is initially hypoferremic but later becomes hyperferremic because of the decreased uptake of transferrin-bound iron by the developing erythrocytes. Early radiologic findings are osteoporosis of the metaphyses and epiphyses and retarded bone age. Typical findings in the established case are increased density of the provisional zone of calcification and cupping with sickle-shaped spurs in the metaphyseal region.[62] Other skeletal abnormalities include periosteal layering and submetaphyseal and rib fractures.

Other clinical findings have been observed in association with copper deficiency, including pallor, decreased pigmentation of skin and hair, prominent superficial veins, skin lesions similar to those of seborrheic dermatitis, cardiac hypertrophy, and hepatosplenomegaly. Features suggestive of central nervous system involvement are hypotonia, lack of interest in outside surroundings, psychomotor retardation, ataxia, apparent lack of visual responses, and apneic episodes. Demyelination and myeloneuropathy have been reported in case reports of adults with hypocupremia, in one case with overuse of zinc supplements and in another with an apparent zinc-overload syndrome without clear exposure to excessive zinc.[63,64] In Menkes, there is severe and eventually fatal central nervous system involvement owing to disordered copper metabolism within the brain cells, which probably results in localized intracellular deficiencies at physiologically important subcellular sites. Other features attributable to copper deficiency in this complex entity include the hair changes, which are reminiscent of the wool of copper-deficient sheep and which led to the initial recognition of the role of disordered copper metabolism, hypothermia, and evidence of defective elastin and collagen formation.

BIOCHEMISTRY AND BIOCHEMICAL CORRELATES

Copper is an essential component of several oxidase enzymes, the reduced activity of which can explain many of the features of copper deficiency. Cytochrome oxidase is the terminal enzyme in the electron transport chain and catalyzes the oxidation of reduced cytochrome-*c* by molecular oxygen, which is itself reduced to water. This enzyme, which is necessary for normal cellular respiration, has been shown to be markedly reduced in the brains of copper-deficient lambs suffering from swayback. Reduced activity of this enzyme may be responsible for certain other features of copper deficiency, for example, the hypothermia that occurs in Menkes disease.

More than 90% of the circulating copper in plasma is tightly and specifically bound to ceruloplasmin, a glycoprotein that contains six copper atoms per molecule. The functions of this protein, which was first identified in 1948, have been and continue to be the focus of considerable interest and controversy. Roles in copper metabolism include copper transport, mobilization of iron for transfer in the plasma, and regulation of the biogenic amines.[65] Ceruloplasmin (ferroxidase I) exhibits enzymatic ferroxidase activity and is necessary for the oxidation of ferrous iron stored in the liver and bone marrow to ferric iron. This is an essential step in the release of iron from body stores and its attachment to transferrin for transport to developing erythrocytes in the bone marrow. Aceruloplasminemia, an autosomal recessive condition in humans, does not produce obvious disordered copper metabolism but results in iron accumulation in tissues.[65] Depressed activity of the ferroxidase role of ceruloplasmin is likely to be related to the hypoferremic, hypochromic anemia of copper deficiency. However, there are, in addition, abnormalities of iron metabolism within the erythroid cell line, and it appears that intracellular transport of iron is defective, so that, despite an abnormal accumulation of iron, there is a lack of iron availability for normal heme synthesis in the mitochondria.[65] The pathologic mechanisms for the neutropenia remain unexplained.

The bone lesions of copper deficiency are attributable, at least in part, to a lack of copper-dependent lysyl oxidase, which acts on lysine and hydroxylysine side chains of collagen and elastin, and is required in the cross-linking of these connective tissue components. These defects are responsible for the gross structural defects seen in arteries and veins in copper-deficient animals and in MSHS.

Among other copper-containing oxidases is tyrosinase, which catalyzes the first two steps in the oxidation of tyrosine to melanin. Lack of pigmentation is a prominent feature of copper deficiency in some species but is only mild in human copper deficiency. Copper proteins previously given other names such as cerebrocuprein, hepatocuprein, and erythrocuprein are now known to be superoxide dismutase, which catalyzes the dismutation of superoxide free radical ions.

Another copper-containing enzyme is superoxide dismutase, which catalyzes the dismutation of superoxide free radical ions and protects against oxidative damage. Detoxification of dangerous free radicals within the cell is of the greatest importance, but little is known about the activity of this enzyme in human copper-deficiency states and what role decreased activity may play in the pathophysiology of copper deficiency.

ETIOLOGIC FACTORS IN COPPER DEFICIENCY

The first cases of human copper deficiency were reported in infants and children in Peru who were recovering from protein-energy malnutrition. Prior to their initial hospitalization, the infants had long histories of inadequate nutrition, which consisted mainly of diluted milk. Cow's milk is a relatively poor dietary source of copper, and copper deficiency has been reported in otherwise healthy infants whose diets have consisted primarily of unmodified cow's milk.[66] Copper deficiency in association with malnutrition is probably not uncommon. For example, copper supplementation was associated with improved growth rates in copper-deficient Chilean infants recovering from malnutrition.[67]

The term infant accumulates substantial hepatic stores of copper, which is attached to metallothionein during the last 3 months of gestation. These stores are released postnatally and are thought to ensure protection of the young infant against copper deficiency. Very low birth weight infants born prematurely do not have the benefit of these stores and have very little copper at birth. Although premature infants are at risk for copper deficiency, positive copper balance is apparently achieved in early postnatal life in premature infants with current fortification of human milk and formulas, although the adequacy of retention is not yet clear.[7] The copper content of unmodified cow's milk is usually lower than that of human milk, and levels may be further decreased during processing. Other causes of human copper deficiency include intestinal malabsorption syndromes, chronic diarrhea, and chelation therapy. High intakes of zinc and possibly iron can precipitate a deficiency of copper.[68]

DIAGNOSIS OF COPPER DEFICIENCY

Both plasma copper and ceruloplasmin levels are depressed in copper-deficiency states. Unfortunately, these parameters are also influenced by other factors, some of which are likely to be operative when the possibility of copper deficiency is considered. Ceruloplasmin synthesis is limited in the liver of the term neonate, and neither serum copper nor ceruloplasmin concentrations reach adult levels until at least 1 month of age. In the very low birth weight infant, copper concentrations are even lower, averaging about 0.30 to 0.40 μg/mL, and do not start to increase until 41 weeks of gestational age.[69] It has been suggested that concentrations lower than 0.25 μg/mL may be abnormal in the young preterm infant and may be associated with neutropenia. However, the interpretation and value of the data on serum copper levels prior to 40 to 44 weeks of gestational age remain uncertain. By 6 months of postnatal age, serum copper and ceruloplasmin concentrations are similar to, or higher than, adult levels.[70]

Ceruloplasmin synthesis in the liver may be reduced in protein-energy malnutrition, and protein-losing enteropathy is associated with losses of ceruloplasmin. Hypocupremia is also a feature of both Wilson's disease and Menkes disease. Copper deficiency can also be difficult to confirm by laboratory assays when there is an increase in synthesis of ceruloplasmin, which is regarded as an acute-phase reactant and is elevated in response to inflammatory stimuli. Hence, hypercupremia occurs, for example, in association with infections, in the postoperative period, and in patients with neoplasms. Several hormones cause hypercupremia, most notably estrogens, and levels are increased substantially throughout pregnancy and for several weeks postpartum. Hypercupremia also occurs in obstructive liver disease owing to failure of the normal biliary excretory mechanisms.

Erythrocyte superoxide dismutase has been investigated as an index of copper status and has been reported to be an early indicator of disturbed copper metabolism. Its activity seems to be stable across age and sex categories and with hormonal therapy.[71] Significantly lower erythrocyte superoxide dismutase activities were reported in preterm infants supplemented with iron from approximately 4 weeks through 20 weeks postnatal age, but there was no effect on plasma copper or zinc concentrations, hematologic indices, or growth parameters.[68] Recently, another *copper* transporter, *copper chaperone for SOD1 (CCS)* has been proposed to be more sensitive to changes in copper status, but this test has not yet been evaluated as a clinical marker.[72]

Radiologically, separation of the epiphyses, an absence of metaphyseal fraying, and the increased density of the provisional zone of calcification may all help to distinguish copper deficiency from rickets. In contrast to scurvy, copper deficiency does not produce either a lucent line beneath the increased density of the provisional zone of calcification or a "corner sign," nor does it cause hemorrhages.

The diagnosis of copper deficiency should be considered in the presence of suggestive etiologic circumstances, particularly when there is a hypochromic anemia unresponsive to iron therapy. One case series also documented improvement in erythropoietin-resistant anemia in adult hemodialysis patients after correction of copper deficiency.[73] If the anemia is accompanied by neutropenia and osteoporosis, together with low ceruloplasmin or plasma copper levels, the diagnosis becomes likely. Confirmation will be provided by a prompt response to copper therapy with a reticulocytosis and increases in circulating neutrophils and in ceruloplasmin or plasma copper levels.

TREATMENT OF COPPER DEFICIENCY

Nutritional copper deficiency in infants has been treated successfully with 2 to 3 mg/d of copper sulfate as a 1% solution, which provides 400 to 600 μg of copper. Maintenance requirements for copper during intravenous nutrition are 0.5 to 1.0 mg/d for adults; as little as 20 μg/kg/d appears to be adequate for infants.[10] Although higher quantities may be required to achieve a positive balance, there is concern that the immature liver of the premature infant may be prone to cholestasis and thus to hepatotoxicity from intravenous copper.

TOXICITY

Copper toxicity has resulted from the accidental or deliberate ingestion of excess copper, hemodialysis with copper-contaminated solutions, and absorption of topically administered copper salts. Acute poisoning by the oral route causes a metallic taste, nausea, epigastric pain, green-blue vomitus, and diarrhea. Jaundice and hepatomegaly may occur 2 to 3 days later. Laboratory parameters are indicative of hepatic injury, and there is histologic evidence of centrilobular necrosis and biliary stasis. Jaundice may also result from intravascular hemolysis caused by free copper ions, which also cause hematuria and a direct renal tubular toxic effect, leading to oliguria and anuria. Copper salts may have a cardiotoxic effect, which is responsible for the hypotonia and coma seen in severe cases. Chronic copper poisoning is a rare entity that has been associated with drinking water with a high copper content. Indian childhood cirrhosis, a hereditary disease associated with greatly increased hepatic copper concentration, is manifest in conjunction with high copper intakes, such as with copper-contaminated animal milk introduced at an early age.[74]

Acrodynia and cirrhosis have both been attributed to chronic copper poisoning. A concentration of 2 mg/L in potable water has been recommended as safe for infants without causing gastrointestinal symptoms,[75] and this level has been provisionally endorsed by WHO.[76] However, higher levels (8 mg/L) in drinking water have not been associated with apparent toxicity. The daily recommended intakes (DRIs) set a UL for copper at 10 mg/d.[8]

ABSORPTION AND METABOLISM

Approximately 35% of ingested copper is absorbed in the stomach and upper small intestine. The percentage of absorption is inversely related to the quantity ingested and is increased in copper-deficiency states. The percentage of absorption also depends on the dietary form and on other dietary constituents. Studies using stable isotopes demonstrated a 40% absorption of copper in formula-fed premature infants, whereas absorption from human milk was approximately 70%. Studies in animal models have reported a range of copper absorption from infant formula, from 25 to 70%.[7] Zinc, iron, cadmium, calcium, sulfate, and molybdenum will interfere with copper absorption if given in sufficient quantities. In contrast to other trace elements, cellulose and phytate have not been found to have marked effects on copper absorption.

Absorbed copper passes through the portal circulation attached to albumin and is taken up by the hepatocytes. Copper may then be used by the hepatocytes for the synthesis of cuproproteins, especially ceruloplasmin, which is released 3 days later into the systemic circulation. Excess copper is excreted by the bile. Ceruloplasmin copper accounts for 90 to 95% of the circulating copper in plasma. The highest copper concentrations are found in the liver, brain, heart, and kidneys. Because of their large mass, bone and muscle contain 50% of the body copper, whereas the liver contains only 10%. The liver of full-term infants contains 200 to 400 μg of copper/g of dry weight, which is 10 to 20 times the adult concentration (12 to 48 μg/g of dry weight). Forty percent of neonatal hepatic copper occurs in the lysosomes attached to metallothionein. In contrast to liver copper, brain copper increases twofold from birth to adulthood. The highest concentrations are in the locus ceruleus of the brainstem and in the cortical gray matter. In erythrocytes, the copper concentration is similar to that of normal plasma (75 to 120 μg/dL). This copper concentration remains stable; 60% is associated with superoxide dismutase. The total copper content of an adult man is approximately 75 mg.

DIETARY REQUIREMENTS

Earlier, minimal estimates of copper requirements for older children and adults were 2 mg/d, and most diets were thought to contain at least this quantity. The most recent EAR, based on studies in normal adults under experimental depletion conditions, was set at 700 μg/d for adult men and women. The RDA was set at 900 μg/d.[8] Most recent national survey data indicate that median copper intakes for men and women are 1.0 to 1.6 mg/d. Six RDAs were established for children by extrapolation from the adult EAR; these are given in Appendix II.

The young term infant is protected from copper deficiency by hepatic stores accumulated in utero. Moreover, the term infant usually achieves a positive copper balance by 1 week of age or a little later. The Food and Nutrition Board established an AI of copper of 200 μg/d (30 μg/kg/d) for infants 0 to 6 months of age and 220 μg/d

(24 μg/kg/d) for infants 7 to 12 months.[8] The estimated dietary requirement of the very low birth weight premature infant is approximately 100 μg/kg/d of copper.[7]

FOOD SOURCES

The richest sources of copper are oysters, followed by nuts, liver, kidney, corn oil, margarine, and dry legumes (Table 5). The contribution of drinking water to the total copper intake varies with the type of piping and the hardness of the water. Information on the copper content of food items remains inadequate for optimal calculations of dietary intakes.

Infant formulas in North America now contain a minimum of 60 μg/100 kcal of copper, and those designed specifically for the premature infant contain substantially higher quantities, with a recommended range of 100 to 250 μg/100 kcal.[7] However, on a worldwide basis, there is still considerable variation in the copper content of infant formulas, and some contain higher quantities. Unprocessed cow's milk contains about 150 μg/L of copper, which is lower than that usually found in human milk (200 to 600 μg/L of copper) at any stage of lactation.[77]

SELENIUM

Interest in the toxicity of selenium in mammals developed in the 1930s with the discovery of both acute and chronic forms of selenosis among grazing animals in Nebraska and Wyoming. The proved toxicity of selenium in animal husbandry in "natural" circumstances (in seleniferous areas) has resulted in extreme and only partially justified caution in adding selenium supplements to diets that are low in selenium. A beneficial role for selenium was not demonstrated until 1957, when selenium supplements were found to protect against liver necrosis in rats fed certain diets. The following year, selenium deficiency was shown to cause naturally occurring muscular dystrophy in lambs and calves, a problem that occurs in many areas of the world. The early nutritional studies indicated that there was a close association between selenium and vitamin E. In 1973, selenium was shown to be an integral component of glutathione peroxidase (GPx), an enzyme that destroys hydroperoxides. Although numerous other selenoproteins have been identified, the functions of many of these proteins are not well characterized. The selenoproteins iodothyronine deiodinases (ID) (Types I–III) catalyze deiodination of thyroxine, triiodothyronine, and reverse triiodothyronine, and as such play an active role in regulation of active hormone triiodothyronine. Experimentally, selenium restriction has been shown to cause hypothyroidism. The thioredoxin reductases, selenoprotein P, and selenoprotein W all are involved in oxidant defense systems.

Although low selenium states have been recognized in certain populations, notably in New Zealand, for many years, it was not until the 1970s, when a geochemical deficiency of selenium in a large area of China was recognized as the major etiologic factor in Keshan disease (KD), that the clinical importance of human selenium deficiency was unequivocally demonstrated. Geochemical depletion of both selenium and iodine occurs when surface soils are depleted by erosion and glacial washout, resulting in both plant and animal foods from such areas contain relatively low amounts of both trace elements. Individual cases of selenium-related cardiomyopathy, as well as skeletal myopathies, have since been identified in North America and elsewhere, and less well-characterized milder selenium deficiency syndromes have also been reported.[78] An RDA for selenium was included for the first time in the tenth edition of the RDAs published by the National Academy of Sciences, and this has recently been revised.[79]

CLINICAL FEATURES AND ETIOLOGY OF SELENIUM DEFICIENCY

KD is an endemic cardiomyopathy affecting children and women of childbearing age. The disease, named for a county in northeastern China, has a clear-cut geographic distribution in a broad area of China from the northeast to the southwest, an area in which the selenium content of food staples has been shown to be exceptionally low.[80] A series of controlled selenium supplementation studies was associated with an 80% reduction in the incidence of KD, whereas the mortality of identified cases was only 1% of that of untreated children.[81] Some of the etiologic circumstances of KD have not been explained clearly. The seasonal and annual fluctuations in KD have raised the possibility of an interaction between nutritional state and an infectious etiology. The recognition that selenium deficiency increases the cardiovirulence of coxsackievirus in animal models by changing the viral genome sequence is particularly intriguing.[82] Further supportive evidence is the isolation of coxsackievirus from patients with KD in the selenium-deficient area of China, although not all serotypes are equally pathogenic.[83] More studies will be required to determine whether the observations in animal models are relevant to humans with KD. However, the permissive role of selenium deficiency and the public health benefits of selenium supplementation in prevention of KD have been established convincingly.

The main pathologic feature of KD consists of multiple focal areas of myocardial necrosis. Presentation may be acute, with heart failure, arrhythmias, and cardiogenic shock, or chronic, with cardiomegaly with or without congestive failure. Electrocardiographic features include low-voltage ST–T wave changes, right bundle branch block, or complete atrioventricular block. Serum selenium levels in KD are extremely low, typically less than 10 μg/L. Other laboratory indices are correspondingly low. Long-term total parenteral nutrition devoid of selenium supplements can also cause severe selenium deficiency with cardiomyopathy or skeletal myopathy.[84,85]

Kashin–Beck disease (KBD), a degenerative osteoarthropathy named for two investigators who studied patients in Siberia in the nineteenth century, has a geographic distribution similar to that of KD within China. KBD is an endemic osteoarthropathy involving children aged 5 to 13 years, and typically is endemic in selenium- and iodine-deficient geographic areas, including in China and central Africa. The disease is characterized pathologically by degeneration and necrosis of multiple articular cartilages and growth plates, causing enlargement especially of fingers, toes, and knees and shortened extremities. Disabilities are typically permanent. Millions of people are likely to be affected with KBD. The relationship between selenium deficiency and KBD is unclear. Evidence from epidemiologic studies suggests that selenium and iodine deficiencies may interact to cause the condition. In Tibet, a comparison of those with and without KBD showed selenium deficiency in both groups, but iodine deficiency, was more severe in those with KBD.[80] A randomized controlled trial of selenium supplementation, initiated after correction of iodine deficiency, in Tibetan children with KBD resulted in no effect on KBD, growth, or thyroid function. The authors concluded that correction of iodine deficiency was more efficacious than treatment of selenium deficiency for KBD.[86]

Current understanding of the changes in thyroid hormone metabolism with selenium deficiency has resulted principally from animal studies, including especially knockout mouse models. That an adequate selenium supply is essential for normal thyroid hormone biosynthesis is supported by observations in a range of human populations. For example, in goitrous children, the severity of selenium deficiency predicted the response to iodine supplementation, with respect to both reduction in thyroid size and improved biochemical measures of thyroid function.[78] Impaired T_4 conversion to T_3 and low regulation of T_3 production have been reported in children with phenylketonuria who were fed a phenylalanine-restricted diet that was also low in selenium,[87] but this has not been found consistently in children with phenylketonuria, even those with evidence of selenium deficiency and compromised antioxidant status.[88]

Moderately depressed levels of erythrocyte GPx activity, hair selenium, serum selenium, or blood selenium have been found in association with protein-energy malnutrition in developing countries and in low-birth-weight infants.[7] One report found significantly lower selenium levels in Malawian children with kwashiorkor who had congestive heart failure compared with those who did not develop this complication.[89] The clinical significance of these low selenium states remains unresolved. Milder degrees of selenium depletion, notably those associated with low dietary levels in New Zealand and certain other geographic areas, have not been associated with adverse clinical consequences. There have been case reports of children on long-term parenteral nutrition or synthetic oral diets without selenium supplements who had macrocytosis and loss of hair pigment, both of which normalized following selenium supplementation.[90]

Interest in selenium in adult and pediatric patients with HIV has been prompted by observations suggesting an ameliorating role in the pathophysiologic processes of this infection. The effects may be mediated by its antioxidant effects, especially via glutathione peroxidase (GPx), and possibly via inhibition of viral replication.[91] In a large cohort study in Tanzania in children born to HIV-positive mothers, plasma selenium levels were inversely associated with risk of all-cause mortality.[92] Interpretation of these findings is complicated by the likelihood of coexistence of multiple nutritional deficiencies and by the fact that plasma selenium is impacted by acute inflammation.

BIOCHEMISTRY AND METABOLISM

Several selenium proteins have been identified; two of these have clearly established physiologic roles: glutathione peroxidase and ID. Selenium is an essential component of cellular GPx, its plasma homologue, and the membrane-bound phospholipid-hydroperoxide GPx. Glutathione peroxidase uses two molecules of reduced glutathione to reduce hydrogen peroxide and convert it into two molecules of water. This enzyme also catalyzes the reduction of fatty acid hydroperoxides to hydroxy acids in the tissues and thus helps to protect the lipids in cell membranes from peroxidation. GPx is present in a wide variety of tissues and accounts for 90% of the selenium in erythrocytes. Messenger RNA levels of liver GPx decrease with dietary selenium restriction.

ID I has been identified as a selenoenzyme. This enzyme catalyzes the conversion of T_4 to T_3 in the liver and other tissues. Selenium, as selenocysteine, is an integral component of ID, and its expression is influenced by dietary selenium. This enzyme provides the link between iodine and selenium because both are involved in thyroid hormone production.

Absorption of selenium depends to some extent on its chemical form. Selenomethionine is better absorbed than inorganic forms of selenium. Intestinal absorption of food selenium is as high as 80%. Selenium homeostasis in the rat is controlled by the kidney, and the principal route of excretion in humans is the urine. The highest concentrations in the body are found in liver, tooth enamel, and nails. In the body, selenium is intimately associated with specific proteins, especially as selenocysteine. More than 80% of the selenium in the rat is present as selenocysteine.

DIAGNOSIS AND TREATMENT OF SELENIUM DEFICIENCY

Selenium depletion is associated with low levels of selenium in whole blood, plasma, and hair and low-erythrocyte GPx activity. Typical clinical assessment is achieved with plasma selenium concentrations; the 5th and 95th percentile range from the Third National Health and Nutrition Examination Survey (NHANES) was 100 to 154 μg/L (1.27 to 1.95 μmol/L). Plasma selenium concentrations less than 50 μg/L have been reported in healthy adults from low selenium areas. Selenium levels are low in young infants and gradually increase to adult values over a period of months. A strong positive correlation between erythrocyte GPx activity and whole blood selenium levels has been found in some populations. However, it is not yet clear how well these indicators may correlate with clinical features of selenium deficiency.[79]

The optimal treatment for selenium deficiency has not been determined. Currently, there are no clear-cut indications for oral selenium therapy apart from the prevention of KD, for which a weekly supplement of 500 μg in younger children and 1,000 μg in older children appears to suffice. On a daily basis, these quantities are somewhat above the RDA recommended by the Food and Nutrition Board.[79]

Selenium supplements should be added routinely to intravenous infusates, at least for those patients who receive a substantial portion of their nutrient intakes by the intravenous route for more than 2 weeks. The dose recommended is 2 μg/kg body wt/d.[10]

TOXICITY

Although excess selenium can cause undesirable consequences in agriculture, chronic selenium toxicity does not appear to be a problem in humans. Blood selenium levels are elevated in children living in seleniferous areas of Venezuela, but the only clinical findings were the somewhat poorly defined ones of nausea and pathologic nails. Loss of hair, brittleness of fingernails, garlic odor, a higher incidence of dental caries, and increased fatigue and irritability were reported to be signs of selenosis in an early survey of residents of South Dakota, where selenium toxicity occurred in farm animals. Urinary selenium excretion was elevated in these people.

Acute selenium poisoning is rare in humans but has been reported as a result of self-administration of selenium supplements. The outcome of acute toxicity appears to depend on both the amount ingested and the type of selenium compound. Acute ingestion of sodium selenite caused garlic odor on the breath and diarrhea in several cases. Evidence of mild, temporary liver damage and cardiac abnormality was seen in one case, but there were no permanent sequelae.

The highest selenium concentration observed in human milk in the United States, 60 μg/L, was used as the basis for the "no observed adverse effect level" in the 2000 DRIs,[79] and the DRI upper limit was set at 45 μg/d (7 μg/kg) for term infants 0 to 6 months. This amount was used parenterally in a supplementation trial of very low birth weight infants until the infants advanced to enteral feeds, at which time they received ~5 μg/kg until 36 weeks postmenstrual age, with no apparent adverse effects.[93]

DIETARY REQUIREMENTS

Dietary surveys of selenium intake in endemic and adjacent nonendemic KD areas have led to the conclusion that selenium requirements for adult Chinese men and women are 19 and 13 μg/d, respectively. This is the quantity calculated to be necessary to prevent KD. RDAs in this country have been set at 55 μg selenium/d for adult men and women.[79]

An AI was established for infants in 2000, recommending 15 μg/d (2.1 μg/kg/d) for infants up to 6 months of age, based on a mean selenium concentration of 18 μg/L in human milk and an average intake of 780 mL/d. The AI for older infants and young children (7 to 36 months) is 20 μg/d, for older children (4 to 8 years) 30 μg/d, and for adolescents 40 to 55 μg/d.[79] These recommendations have been extrapolated from adults with a generous addition for growth; actual requirements are substantially less. The intake of formula-fed infants prior to weaning has generally been 4 to 5 μg selenium/d in this country. Although higher intakes are desirable, there is no evidence that any harmful effects have resulted from this relatively low selenium intake.

FOOD SOURCES

The selenium content of human milk depends on maternal dietary selenium intake. Extremely low values, that is, less than 3 μg selenium/L, have been reported from areas where KD is endemic.[7] Concentrations between 5 and 10 μg selenium/L have been reported from other countries where maternal selenium intake is relatively low (eg, New Zealand, Finland, and Poland).[94] In the United States, the mean value for the selenium content of human milk is approximately 18 μg selenium/L.[7]

The selenium content of cow's milk is generally lower than that of human milk in this country. The selenium content is reduced in the preparation of cow's milk–based infant formulas. The minimum for standard infant formulas was recommended to be 1.5 μg/100 kcal.[95] Whether the low plasma selenium and GPx levels in low-birth-weight infants are increased by providing generous selenium supplementation of formulas has been controversial, and feeding regimens that have provided amounts adequate to increase biochemical markers of selenium status in low-birth-weight infants have not demonstrated clear clinical benefit. Nevertheless, premature infants are born with strikingly low serum selenium levels and GPx, and, without supplementation, these levels decline further.[93,96] An expert panel recently recommended a minimum concentration in formulas for preterm infants of 1.8 μg/100 kcal and a maximum of 5.0 μg/100 kcal, while acknowledging that it was unknown whether the lower amount would be adequate or optimal for preterm low-birth-weight infants.[7]

As noted above, concentrations of selenium in foods vary with geographic region and soil content. Generally, seafood (approximately 0.5 μg/g), kidney, liver, and meat (approximately 0.2 μg/g) are the best sources of selenium. Whole grains are also generally good sources of selenium, provided that the soils in which they are grown are not low in selenium. Vegetables and fruits, with the exception of garlic, provide little. Daily intake in North America has been reported to range from 60 to 220 μg/d, but in New Zealand, intake is only 6 to 35 μg/d.

CHROMIUM

A role for chromium in mammalian physiology was indicated first in 1959, when it was reported that trace amounts of this element are necessary for normal glucose tolerance in the rat. Subsequent research suggested that chromium acted as a cofactor for insulin. These observations stimulated considerable interest in a possible role for chromium deficiency in the high incidence of impaired glucose tolerance in industrialized societies. Progress has been hampered, however, by a lack of laboratory indices of chromium status that would be of the greatest value in identifying appropriate subjects to include in clinical trials of chromium supplementation.

CLINICAL FEATURES AND ETIOLOGY OF CHROMIUM DEFICIENCY

Experimental chromium deficiency in several animal species has been reported to result in impaired glucose tolerance in the presence of normal concentrations of circulating insulin. Features of chromium deficiency have been reported to include impaired glucose tolerance with relative insulin resistance and peripheral and/or central neuropathy. Weight loss and poor childhood growth have also been reported.

In the pediatric age range, chromium supplementation studies have been undertaken in infants and young children suffering from protein-energy malnutrition. The results of these studies, which involved the use of a single oral dose of 250 μg trivalent chromium, suggested that chromium deficiency may be one factor responsible for the impaired glucose tolerance that occurs in association with severe generalized malnutrition. Chromium deficiency has been reported to complicate protein-energy malnutrition in some but not all geographic areas. Lack of controls in some studies and limited subject numbers hamper definitive interpretation of these data.

Several trials of chromium supplementation have been reported in adults, including elderly subjects.[97] Most of these trials have been small. Subjects have included noninsulin-dependent diabetic patients and otherwise normal subjects with evidence of impaired glucose tolerance. Supplements have always been trivalent chromium, on some occasions as an inorganic salt and on others as brewer's yeast or in other forms that are thought to have favorable absorption. In several studies, chromium supplementation has been associated with improved glucose tolerance in more than 50% of the chromium-supplemented subjects. Other apparent effects noted in some studies include a decrease in insulin response to an oral glucose load, a decrease in total blood lipids, and an increase in high-density lipoprotein cholesterol. A meta-analysis of chromium supplementation trials reported for healthy individuals and in those with glucose intolerance or type 2 diabetes found no effect of chromium on glucose or insulin concentrations in nondiabetic subjects, whereas the results from trials in diabetic subjects were inconclusive.[98]

Chromium deficiency has also been reported in patients receiving long-term parenteral nutrition without supplementation. Clinical features attributed to the chromium deficiency were weight loss, peripheral neuropathy, and encephalopathy. An abnormally low removal rate of intravenous glucose and an abnormally low respiratory quotient indicating difficulty in metabolizing glucose for energy, dependence on exogenous insulin, and abnormalities of nitrogen and lipid metabolism all responded rapidly to intravenous chromium.[8]

BIOCHEMICAL CORRELATES

Although chromium may have several physiologic roles, for example, in nucleic acid metabolism, the role that has received most attention is its action as a cofactor for insulin. Experimental evidence is consistent with the hypothesis that chromium acts as a cofactor for insulin at the site of peripheral insulin receptors. Specifically, it has been hypothesized that a chromium-binding oligopeptide, termed chromodulin, facilitates the attachment of insulin to its receptors both at the cell membrane and intracellularly, and activates the insulin receptor kinase activity. Chromium may have to be in the trivalent ion form (Cr^{3+}) to be biologically active.[99] The biologic role of chromium as a cofactor for insulin requires further clarification and confirmation.

DIAGNOSIS OF CHROMIUM DEFICIENCY

The lack of established laboratory assays is especially evident for chromium, and deficiency states can be confirmed currently only by means of careful monitoring of the effects of chromium supplementation under controlled conditions. Normal values in such samples as blood plasma and urine have had a disconcerting tendency to fall as analytic techniques improve so that they remain near the detection limits of the equipment available at any particular time. Currently, normal levels for plasma chromium, for example, are considered to be only about 0.1 parts per billion (100 pg/mL). This means that it continues to be extraordinarily difficult to measure low values accurately. An additional difficulty in interpretation results from uncertainties about the physiologic meaning of low chromium levels. For example, it is thought that solitary plasma chromium levels do not reflect body chromium status but only recent intake. However, low plasma chromium levels have been reported in chromium-deficient subjects, in pregnant women, and in association with experimental infections that cause impaired glucose tolerance.[8] There have been conflicting reports about a measurable increase in plasma chromium in response to a glucose load. At best, this is a tedious and difficult test for assessing chromium status. Absence of detectable plasma chromium "response" has been reported in some diabetic patients, including gestational diabetic patients, and in some elderly people. An inverse correlation has been reported between the postprandial increase in plasma chromium and fasting blood glucose. Hair analyses provide only a crude index of chromium status. Theoretically, urine chromium levels, perhaps including measurement of the increase in urine excretion following a glucose load, should provide a useful index of chromium status. To date, however, this approach has not proved to have any conclusive value. Excessive urine chromium losses have been noted in diabetic patients, and it has been suggested that the low chromium content of adult American tissues could result from excessive urine losses triggered by a diet high in sucrose. Confirmation of excessive chromium losses during the consumption of such diets is lacking. In summary, chromium measurements in tissue and body fluids are of no proven value in the diagnosis of chromium deficiency even if adequate laboratory facilities are available.

TREATMENT OF CHROMIUM DEFICIENCY

Suspected chromium deficiency states can be treated with 200 μg of trivalent chromium daily for several weeks or months in adults. In malnourished children, a single dose of Cr^{3+} 250 μg has been effective. Current recommendations for chromium during parenteral nutrition are 10 to 15 μg/d for adults or 0.1 to 0.2 μg/kg body wt/d for infants and young children. Levels considerably lower than this are probably adequate and may be preferable.

TOXICITY

Trivalent chromium has a low toxicity, and there are no reports of toxicity from oral administration. The minimum lethal dose of intravenous chromium as chromic chloride in mice is 800 mg/kg. Hexavalent chromium is more toxic, but 100 parts per million in drinking water can be tolerated by animals for many years. Chromate is a local irritant and is a cause of acute and chronic disease of the respiratory system, including bronchogenic carcinoma in workers in the chromate industry.

Plasma chromium concentrations have been reported to be elevated in patients receiving total parenteral nutrition, including standard quantities of intravenous chromium, who develop evidence of renal disease.[100] Chronic interstitial nephritis has been associated with ingestion of chromium picolinate as a dietary supplement.[101,102] It has been suggested that the renal disease is a result of chromium toxicity, although animal studies have not confirmed such toxicity.[103] It is also possible that the elevated plasma chromium levels are secondary to impaired chromium excretion via the kidneys. It appears prudent to reduce or withhold intravenous chromium supplements in the presence of renal disease.

ABSORPTION/METABOLISM

Inorganic trivalent chromium is absorbed poorly. Absorption of ^{51}Cr-labeled chromium chloride is limited to approximately 0.5%. A larger percentage of chromium is thought to be absorbed from organic chromium complexes found, for example, in brewer's yeast. Chromium picolinate has been marketed aggressively with claims that it is well absorbed and has some special beneficial metabolic effects, but documentation of these claims is poor. It is thought that the liver may be the site of a specific pool of biologically active chromium and that GTF chromium is released from this pool in response to a glucose load. This response may be mediated by the response of endogenous insulin. GTF has been reported to be the only form in which chromium can cross the placenta to the fetus. The major excretory route for chromium is through the kidney, and the urine contains at least 80% of excreted chromium. The total body chromium content of adults has been estimated to be about 6 mg.

DIETARY REQUIREMENTS AND FOOD SOURCES

Dietary chromium intakes for adults in the United States range from 25 μg/d for women to 50 μg chromium/d for men. The estimated AI for dietary chromium intake for adults set by the Food and Nutrition Board is 35 μg/d for men and 25 μg/d for women.[8] The AI recommended for infants 0 to 6 months is 0.2 μg/d and 5.5 μg/d for infants 7 to 12 months. The large increase in the second half of the first year of life reflects the contribution of complementary foods. The AIs for children and adolescents range from 11 to 35 μg/d.[8]

The mean chromium concentration of breast milk is approximately 0.25 μg/L.[104] Hence, the intake of the breast-fed infant would be about 0.2 μg/d. The bioavailability of this chromium may be high by comparison with that of other trace elements, but this has not been determined. Concentrations of chromium in cow's milk and infant formulas have been reported to be higher than those in human milk.[95]

Spices, brewer's yeast, liver, and kidney are especially good sources of chromium, but only small quantities are present in fish, vegetables, and fruit. Major losses of chromium have been reported during milling of wheat and refining of sugar, but stainless steel cooking containers may add to the chromium intake. Calculations of chromium in food have undoubtedly varied, depending on methods of sample preparation and analyses. Moreover, absolute quantities may not be as important as the form in which the chromium is present in foods.

MANGANESE

A nutritional requirement for manganese has been established in a wide variety of organisms and was first shown to be "essential" for animals in 1931. Interest was stimulated by the discovery in the 1930s that two economically important diseases of poultry, perosis and chondrodystrophy, were caused by manganese deficiency. There are now extensive data on animal requirements, but knowledge of human manganese requirements and status is much more limited.[8]

One probable case of human manganese deficiency has been reported in a subject who was receiving an experimental synthetic diet that was retrospectively found to be low in manganese, providing only 350 μg/d of manganese for 3 months. Features attributed to manganese deficiency were hypocholesterolemia, depressed levels of clotting proteins in the plasma, weight loss, and slow growth of hair and nails. Low serum manganese levels have been reported in some diabetic and in epileptic children, and a negative manganese balance has been observed in children with pancreatic insufficiency. The clinical significance of any of these observations remains obscure, and no cases of nonexperimentally induced manganese deficiency have been reported. Experimental manganese depletion in animal models affects cartilage and bone structure and neurologic function and is associated with stunted growth and ataxia in newborns. Deficiency was also associated with lipid accumulation in liver and kidney and with hypocholesterolemia, a finding also observed in humans.

The low manganese concentrations found in blood plasma (approximately 1 ng/mL) and, until recently, the difficulty of obtaining accurate analyses have hindered progress in our understanding of manganese status in humans. Erythrocyte, plasma, and serum manganese concentrations demonstrate an age-dependent pattern, with the highest levels observed in young infants. Blood concentrations increase during pregnancy, which apparently result in high manganese concentrations in the fetus. Infants born prematurely have higher blood levels than term infants, and these relatively high levels persist for several weeks postnatally.[6]

Biochemically, manganese is required for the synthesis of mucopolysaccharides through the manganese-dependent enzymes polymerase and galactotransferase. Reduced activity of these enzymes, resulting in impaired mucopolysaccharide synthesis, accounts for the extensive skeletal abnormalities and the ataxia owing to impaired otolith synthesis that are seen in animals with manganese deficiency. Pyruvate carboxylase is a manganese metalloenzyme, and manganese is a potent, although not necessarily specific, promoter of oxidative phosphorylation. Peptidases, manganese superoxide dismutase, succinic dehydrogenase, and arginase appear to be manganese-dependent enzymes.

Adults absorb less than 5% of an ingested dose of ^{54}Mn.[75] Only half of this amount is retained 10 days later, but retention of the ingested dose at 10 days is 8% in the newborn and 16% in the premature infant. Breast-fed infants maintain positive balance on much lower manganese intakes than formula-fed infants. The higher retention of infants, especially those born prematurely, may reflect higher absorption efficiency but may also reflect less efficient excretory mechanisms. Manganese absorption is enhanced by iron deficiency, but the long-term effects on retention are less clear. Neither the effects in infants of feeding iron-fortified formula on achieving optimal manganese status nor of iron deficiency on predisposing to manganese toxicity are well understood. The emerging understanding of shared transport of manganese and iron in the brain and the potential for neurotoxicity highlight the potential importance of the interaction between these elements. Manganese is excreted almost entirely through the bile, and urine losses are small.[75]

Chronic manganese toxicity, owing principally to inhalation from occupational exposure and from excessive parenterally administered manganese, causes extrapyramidal neurologic disease similar to Parkinson's disease, Alzheimer's disease, and Huntington's disease. Such neurologic symptoms are associated with neuronal death in the globus pallidus and basal ganglia regions that are rich in dopamine. Pilot data in children from the vicinity of a hazardous waste site indicated an inverse relationship between hair concentrations of manganese and arsenic and intelligence scores and memory tests.[76] Cholestatic liver disease, including that associated with total parenteral nutrition, has been associated with manganese accumulation in the liver and brain.[75] Manganese, as well as copper, should be reduced or withheld from parenteral nutrition patients with cholestatic liver disease, and iron deficiency should also be avoided if possible.

Adults are in positive manganese balance with an intake of 2.5 mg/d, but intakes of 0.7 mg/d result in negative balance. Human milk contains only 3 to 4 μg/L of manganese.[7] Hence, it appears that the requirements of young infants are extremely small. The DRI AI level for healthy 0- to 6-month old infants was set at 3 μg/d (0.4 μg/kg), based on the mean manganese intake of exclusively breast-fed infants.[8] Formula-fed infants ingest much more manganese than breast-fed infants, with cow milk based formulas containing approximately a 10-fold greater content compared to human milk, and soy formulas being approximately 10-fold greater than cow milk formulas.[95,75] Although the toxicity of manganese administered by the oral route appears to be low and a wide range of intakes has appeared to tolerated without any clinical problems, recent reports in animal models have reported altered neurobehavioral measures in animals fed soy formula or given manganese supplementation.[105,106] Nuts and unrefined grains are rich sources of manganese, whereas animal products and seafood are relatively low in this trace element.

FLUORIDE

Fluoride has both beneficial (prevention of dental caries) and toxic (fluorosis) effects on teeth, with a small margin between intakes that are beneficial and those that are toxic.

Fluoride has proved to have beneficial cariostatic properties during tooth development and, for this reason, is generally accepted as a necessary micronutrient. Other beneficial properties, for example, in ameliorating osteoporosis and protecting against arterial calcification, have not been substantiated convincingly.

PREVENTION OF DENTAL CARIES

Fluoride is effective in preventing dental caries. The principal means by which this protection is conferred is via a local effect at thc tooth surface. Fluoride decreases demineralization of the enamel when the pH of the dental plaque is low owing to the action of oral bacteria on fermentable carbohydrates. Fluoride also accelerates remineralization when the pH rises.[107] In addition, fluoride appears to decrease production of organic acids from fermentable carbohydrates on the teeth. The fluoride concentration in saliva and in dental plaque fluid necessary to achieve effects is only 0.1 part per million.[108] The systemic effect of fluoride on teeth prior to eruption appears to be small, although some protection may be conferred by incorporation of fluoride into enamel crystals during tooth development.

Prior to the widespread use of fluoridated dentifrices, lifelong use of a water supply containing 1 part per million fluoride resulted in a 50 to 60% decrease in the prevalence of dental caries in permanent teeth. The beneficial effect on primary teeth was only slightly less. With the current widespread use of fluoridated dentifrices, the benefits of a fluoridated water supply have a somewhat decreased impact in the prevention of dental caries. Systematic reviews have confirmed the beneficial effects of topical fluoride (toothpaste, mouthrinses, varnishes, and gels) on prevention of dental caries in children and adolescents.[109]

Near-maximal protective effect is achieved with a fluoride concentration of 1 part per million in the drinking water. The beneficial effects are likely to be greatest among children from low-income families, whose use of fluoridated dentifrices is more restricted.

FLUOROSIS

Dental fluorosis is characterized by undermineralization of the surface and subsurface enamel, resulting in increased porosity. This is a developmental abnormality affecting both primary and permanent teeth.[110] Although the mechanism is not fully understood, fluoride appears to damage the ameloblasts that produce the enamel. The enamel appears opaque. Visible changes range from barely discernible fine white lines across the teeth to entirely chalky-white teeth. The outer enamel may break apart, and the exposed subsurface then becomes discolored.

The incidence of fluorosis has a linear relationship to calculated fluoride intake per unit body weight. This relationship is evident even at levels of fluoride intake that approach zero. The infant is thought to be especially susceptible to the effects of fluoride, with fluorosis resulting once the fluoride intake has reached a level of 40 to 100 μg/kg/d. The incidence of fluorosis, especially that of a mild degree, appears to have increased recently in communities with and without fluoridated water.[110] The teeth of greatest cosmetic concern are the permanent incisors and cuspids. Enamel formation in these teeth begins at 3 months and is completed by 7 years.

INTAKE OF FLUORIDE BY INFANTS

The fluoride content of breast milk is uniformly low whatever the maternal intake of this trace element.[111] Remarkably, the incidence of dental caries is relatively low in children who have been breast-fed as infants. Fluorosis is uncommon in children who have been breast-fed as infants. The intake of fluoride from unmodified cow's milk is also low, although not as low as from human milk. Fluoride concentrations approximate 40 and 60 μg/L, respectively. The fluoride intake from formula tends to be higher and potentially in a range that can cause fluorosis, even though the fluoride content of water used in the manufacture of infant formulas has been restricted since 1978 and even when dried formulas are made up with water of relatively low fluoride content. For example, the calculated intake of fluoride of a young infant receiving 150 mL formula/kg body wt/d, prepared by mixing powdered milk-based formula (fluoride content = 690 μg/L) with water containing only 200 μg fluoride/L, is 41 μg/kg/d. Ready-to-feed formulas contain <20 μg fluoride/L.[7] The fluoride content of bottled distilled water is low, but this does not apply to all bottled waters. Weaning foods may also provide significant quantities of fluoride, especially fruit juices, cereals, and poultry products.

Overall, the fluoride intake of young infants is less than it was two decades ago because of a decrease in fluoride content of formulas and because of the increased incidence of breast-feeding. On the other hand, the intake of older infants tends to be higher because of the progressive substitution of infant formulas for whole cow's milk at this age. Older infants may also start to use fluoridated dentifrices. Small children ingest most of this dentifrice, and the fluoride is subsequently absorbed. The AI for 0 to 6 months is 10 μg/d (1.4 μg/kg/d).[112] The American Academy of Pediatric Dentistry and the American Academy of Pediatrics recommend no fluoride supplementation for infants under 6 months of age. For older infants and children from 6 months to 3 years for whom the community water supply is less than 0.3 parts per million, a supplement of 250 μg/d is recommended. These recommendations and a broad discussion of use of fluoride to prevent and control dental caries have recently been published.[110]

IODINE

The clinical importance of adequate iodine intake has, like that of iron, been recognized for many years. Iodine was used in the treatment of goiter in the early years of the nineteenth century, and the major role of iodine deficiency in the etiology of endemic goiter was confirmed early in the twentieth century when the prophylactic value of iodine was demonstrated in Ohio schools. The early recognition of the nutritional role of this trace element can be attributed to the specific nature of the clinical features of iodine deficiency, the relative simplicity of measuring iodine in foods and other biologic samples, and the high concentration of iodine in one specific organ, the thyroid gland. Sixty percent of T_4 by weight is iodine, and the biologic importance of iodine is related entirely to its role in the thyroid hormones.[113]

Iodine deficiency disorders remain a global problem, despite aggressive prophylactic measures, and are the most prevalent cause of brain damage. WHO estimates that there may be nearly a billion people affected by iodine deficiency disorders, and as much as one-half of the world's population is at risk. Endemic goiter now occurs mainly in developing countries, typically mountainous areas such as the Andes and Himalayas and the mountainous chain extending through Southeast Asia and the South Pacific. Iodine deficiency also remains a problem in certain parts of Africa. Endemic goiter also persists in the Alps and in several Western and mid-European countries.[113]

The extreme result of hypothyroidism and iodine deficiency during development is cretinism. Two types of cretinism are described, neurologic and myxedematous, both of which exhibit severe mental retardation. The neurologic type prevails in most regions and is characterized by severe mental retardation, deaf mutism, spastic diplegia, and strabismus. The cretin appears normal at birth but is obviously retarded by 6 months of age. There is a characteristic vacant face with a large protruding tongue. The head appears large, and a lordosis is usually prominent. Clinical evidence of hypothyroidism is usually absent. The neurologic damage does not appear to be attributable to maternal or fetal hypothyroidism; there has been speculation that it may be owing to the direct effects of fetal iodine deficiency or to an imbalance between serum T_4 and T_3. In iodine deficiency, T_4 decreases, but T_3 remains normal or even elevated. The myxedematous type of cretin predominantly has the signs of congenital hypothyroidism but typically has only modest enlargement of the thyroid gland. This type, may result from a combination of a dietary goitrogen, and iodine deficiency, possibly complicated by coexisting selenium deficiency. This type predominates in some Central African countries. Endemic cretinism is not a distinct entity in a region of endemic goiter but rather the severe end of a spectrum of neurologic damage.[113]

In mildly iodine-deficient areas, goiters (enlargement of the thyroid gland owing to iodine deficiency) may not occur until adolescence or during pregnancy. These goiters disappear in adult males, but in women they become large. Degenerative changes then occur, and myxedema or, paradoxically, sometimes thyrotoxicosis, may follow. Milder cognitive and neuromuscular impairment owing to chronic iodine deficiency is much more common.

Early in the twentieth century, prophylaxis with iodized salt proved to be highly effective in North America. Although sporadic goiters still occur, these are apparently attributable primarily to unidentified goitrogens. Bread, water, milk, and chocolate are other vehicles that have been used to provide supplemental iodine. In areas of endemic goiter, intramuscular depot injections of 5 mL of iodized oil, providing 400 μg/mL of iodine, have also been used extensively. With the relatively high iodide concentrations now found in foods, especially milk, and the nationwide food distribution system in the United States, iodized salt is no longer considered to be necessary. In contrast, WHO and other international agencies have spearheaded national salt iodization programs in developing countries to eliminate the full spectrum of iodine deficiency disorders. In the 1990s, the number of countries with iodization programs doubled from 46 to 93, and there has been an accompanying improvement in the iodine status of these populations. Sustainability of these programs has been a challenge, however, resulting in persistence of widespread iodine deficiency.

Measurement of iodine excretion in casual or spot urine samples provides an excellent index of recent iodine intake and is a useful assay for assessing community iodide status. Urinary iodine concentrations <50 μg/L indicate moderate to severe deficiency; 100 to 199 μg/L indicates normal iodine status; >200 μg/L indicates more than adequate; and >300 μg/L indicates possible excess.[113] Once iodine deficiency is established, T_4 levels will be decreased (normal range equals 0.8 to 2.4 ng/dL). Thyroid size and thyroid-stimulating hormone and thyroglobulin concentrations reflect chronic iodine deficiency disorders.

With the increasing levels of iodide in the US food supply, the risk of iodide toxicity is currently of greater concern than that of iodide deficiency. More cases of goiter in this country are currently attributable to excess rather than to a lack of iodide. The effects of excessive iodide intake include thyroiditis, goiter, hypothyroidism, and hyperthyroidism.[113] Large intakes in adults may cause toxicity, especially in those who have previously had chronic iodine deficiency, which somewhat paradoxically predisposes to toxicity. A large prospective study of adults in China, which examined three distinct geographic areas with different levels of iodine intake, reported significantly higher risk of hypothyroidism and autoimmune thyroiditis in subjects with more than adequate or excessive iodine intake. Adverse effects were greatest in those who had previously been mildly deficient and subsequently increased iodine intake to greater than AI.[114]

Cow's milk is a major dietary source of iodide in the United States, one that has increased in recent years. This has resulted not only from use of iodized salt in the dairy industry but also from the use of iodates as sanitizers, especially in teat dips. Iodide concentrations in human milk are also relatively high in this country (ie, 140 to 180 μg iodide/L), much higher than the concentration in other countries.[8] The recommended range for term infant formulas is 53 to 230 μg iodide/L[95]; the comparable recommendation for preterm formulas is 48 to 280 μg iodide/L.[7] Fish is notable among other foods as naturally rich in iodide. Iodide in water does not usually contribute more than 10% of intake.

The adult EAR of iodide is 95 μg/d or approximately 1 μg iodide/kg body wt/d; the RDA is 150 μg/d.[8] AIs for infants are 110 μg/d before the age of 6 months and 130 μg/d in older infants.[8] The UL for adults is 1,100 μg iodide/d; ULs for children are provided in the Appendix.[8] These intake recommendations are generous. Some centers do not add iodide to intravenous nutrition because of that already present as contamination, including that derived from iodates used to clean tube connections. We recommend providing 1 μg iodide/kg body wt/d in case these alternative sources are not always effective. This low dose carries no risk of toxicity.

CONCLUSION

Recognition of the practical importance of the trace elements in human nutrition has progressed substantially within the past few years. Concurrently, there have been exciting advances in understanding of the biology, especially the molecular/subcellular biology of these micronutrients. Recent advances have been most notable for zinc, both in terms of basic biology and global public health. Identification of "new" biologic roles for selenium and increasing respect for its importance for human health serve as a reminder that knowledge of less prominent trace elements is likely far from complete. Although, globally, issues of trace element deficiencies pose major public health challenges, there are also issues of overabundance owing especially to food fortification programs. The latter tend to underscore the importance of both vigilance toward and further research on interactions and other possible adverse effects.

REFERENCES

1. Hambidge KM, Casey CE, Krebs NF. Zinc. In: Mertz W, editor. Trace Elements in Human and Animal Nutrition, Volume 2. Florida: Academic Press; 1986. p. 1–137.
2. Dufner-Beattie J, Wang F, Kuo YM, et al. The acrodermatitis enteropathica gene *ZIP4* encodes a tissue-specific, zinc-regulated zinc transporter in mice. J Biol Chem 2003;278:33474–81.
3. Mertz W. The essential trace elements. Science 1981;213:1332–8.
4. Kaler SG. Diagnosis and therapy of Menkes syndrome, a genetic form of copper deficiency. Am J Clin Nutr 1998;67:1029S–34S.
5. Krebs NF, Hambidge KM. Zinc metabolism and homeostasis: The application of tracer techniques to human zinc physiology. Biometals 2001;14:397–412.
6. Hambidge KM, Krebs NF. Zinc in the fetus and the neonate. In: Polin RA, Fox WW, Abman SH, editors. Fetal and Neonatal Physiology, Volume 1, 3rd edition. Philadelphia: Saunders; 2003. p. 342–347.
7. Klein CJ. Nutrient requirements for preterm infant formulas. J Nutr 2002;132:1395S–1577S.
8. Food and Nutrition Board, Institute of Medicine. Dietary Reference Intakes for Vitamin A, Vitamin K, Boron, Chromium, Copper, Iodine, Iron, Manganese, Molybdenum, Nickel, Silicon, Vanadium and Zinc. Washington, DC: National Academy Press; 2001.
9. World Health Organization. Trace Elements in Human Nutrition and Health. Geneva: WHO; 1996.
10. Greene HL, Hambidge KM, Schanler R, Tsang RC. Guidelines for the use of vitamins, trace elements, calcium, magnesium, and phosphorus in infants and children receiving total parenteral nutrition: Report of the Subcommittee on Pediatric Parenteral Nutrient Requirements from the Committee on Clinical Practice Issues of the American Society for Clinical Nutrition. Am J Clin Nutr 1988;48:1324–42; errata appear in Am J Clin Nutr 1989;49:1332 and 1989;50:560.
11. Hambidge KM. Hair analyses: Worthless for vitamins, limited for minerals. Am J Clin Nutr 1982;36:943–9.
12. Andrews GK. Cellular zinc sensors: MTF-1 regulation of gene expression. Biometals 2001;14:223–37.
13. Prasad AS, Miale A, Farid Z, et al. Zinc metabolism in patients with the syndrome of iron deficiency anemia, hepatosplenomegaly, dwarfism and hypogonadism. J Lab Clin 1963;61:537–49.
14. Bhutta ZA, Black RE, Brown KH, et al. Prevention of diarrhea and pneumonia by zinc supplementation in children in developing countries: Pooled analysis of randomized controlled trials. J Pediatr 1999;135:689–97.
15. Black RE. Zinc deficiency, infectious disease and mortality in the developing world. J Nutr 2003;133:1485S–9S.
16. Sehgal VN, Jain S. Acrodermatitis enteropathica. Clin Dermatol 2000;18:745–8.
16a. Brown KH, Peerson JM, Rivera J, et al. Effect of supplemental zinc on the growth and serum of prepubertal children: a meta-analysis of randomized controlled trials. Am J Clin Nutr 2002;75:1062–71.
17. Krebs NF, Sontag M, Accurso FJ, Hambidge KM. Low plasma zinc concentrations in young infants with cystic fibrosis. J Pediatr 1998;133:761–4.
18. Krebs NF, Westcott JE, Arnold TD, et al. Abnormalities in zinc homeostasis in young infants with cystic fibrosis. Pediatr Res 2000;48:256–61.
19. Patrizi A, Bianchi F, Neri I, Specchia F. Acrodermatitis enteropathica-like eruption: A sign of malabsorption in cystic fibrosis. Pediatr Dermatol 2003;20:187–8.
20. Zemel BS, Kawchak DA, Fung EB, et al. Effect of zinc supplementation on growth and body composition in children with sickle cell disease. Am J Clin Nutr 2002;75:300–7.
21. Krebs NF, Hambidge KM, Walravens PA. Increased food intake of young children receiving a zinc supplement. Am J Dis Child 1984;138:270–3.
22. Umeta M, West CE, Haidar J, et al. Zinc supplementation and stunted infants in Ethiopia: A randomised controlled trial. Lancet 2000;355:2021–6.

23. Bhutta ZA, Bird SM, Black RE, et al. Therapeutic effects of oral zinc in acute and persistent diarrhea in children in developing countries: Pooled analysis of randomized controlled trials. Am J Clin Nutr 2000;72:1516–22.
24. WHO U. WHO-UNICEF Joint Statement on the Clinical Management of Acute Diarrhea. Geneva: World Health Assembly; 2004.
25. Hambidge KM, Nichols PL, Jr, editors. Zinc and Copper in Clinical Medicine. Jamaica, NY: Spectrum Publications; 1978.
26. Walravens PA, Van Doorninck WJ, Hambidge KM. Metals and mental function [letter]. J Pediatr 1978;93:535.
27. Black MM. Micronutrient deficiencies and cognitive functioning. J Nutr 2003;133:3927S–31S.
28. Sazawal S, Jalla S, Mazumder S, et al. Effect of zinc supplementation on cell-mediated immunity and lymphocyte subsets in preschool children. Indian Pediatr 1997;34:589–97.
29. MacDonald RS. The role of zinc in growth and cell proliferation. J Nutr 2000;130:1500S–8S.
30. Hall AG, Kelleher SL, Lonnerdal B, Philipps AF. A graded model of dietary zinc deficiency: Effects on growth, insulin-like growth factor-I, and the glucose/insulin axis in weanling rats. J Pediatr Gastroenterol Nutr 2005;41:72–80.
31. Fraker PJ, King LE. Reprogramming of the immune system during zinc deficiency. Annu Rev Nutr 2004;24:277–98.
32. Cuevas LE, Koyanagi A. Zinc and infection: A review. Ann Trop Paediatr 2005;25:149–60.
33. Takeda A. Zinc homeostasis and functions of zinc in the brain. Biometals 2001;14:343–51.
34. Frederickson CJ, Koh JY, Bush AI. The neurobiology of zinc in health and disease. Nat Rev Neurosci 2005;6:449–62.
35. Wang F, Kim BE, Dufner-Beattie J, et al. Acrodermatitis enteropathica mutations affect transport activity, localization and zinc-responsive trafficking of the mouse ZIP4 zinc transporter. Hum Mol Genet 2004;13:563–71.
36. Lehnert T, Kury S, Burk G, et al. Acrodermatitis enteropathica (AE) is caused by mutations in the zinc transporter gene *SLC39A4*. Klin Padiatr 2006;218:221–3.
37. Michalczyk A, Varigos G, Catto-Smith A, et al. Analysis of zinc transporter, hZnT4 (Slc30A4), gene expression in a mammary gland disorder leading to reduced zinc secretion into milk. Hum Genet 2003;113:202–10.
38. Kelleher SL, Lonnerdal B. Molecular regulation of milk trace mineral homeostasis. Mol Aspects Med 2005;26:328–39.
39. Jalla S, Krebs NF, Rodden D, Hambidge KM. Zinc homeostasis in premature infants does not differ between those fed preterm formula or fortified human milk. Pediatr Res 2004;56:615–20.
40. Sazawal S, Black RE, Menon VP, et al. Zinc supplementation in infants born small for gestational age reduces mortality: A prospective, randomized, controlled trial. Pediatrics 2001;108:1280–6.
41. Sur D, Gupta DN, Mondal SK, et al. Impact of zinc supplementation on diarrheal morbidity and growth pattern of low birth weight infants in Kolkata, India: A randomized, double-blind, placebo-controlled, community-based study. Pediatrics 2003;112:1327–32.
42. Krebs NF, Westcott JL, Rodden DJ, et al. Exchangeable zinc pool size at birth is smaller in small-for-gestational-age than in appropriate-for-gestational-age preterm infants. Am J Clin Nutr 2006;84:1340–3.
43. Gibson RS, Ferguson EL, Lehrfeld J. Complementary foods for infant feeding in developing countries: Their nutrient adequacy and improvement. Eur J Clin Nutr 1998;52:764–70.
44. Krebs NF, Westcott JE, Butler N, et al. Meat as a first complementary food for breastfed infants: Feasibility and impact on zinc intake and status. J Pediatr Gastroenterol Nutr 2006;42:207–14.
45. Krebs NF, Hambidge KM. Complementary feeding: Clinically relevant factors affecting timing and composition. Am J Clin Nutr 2007;85:639S-645S.
46. Easley D, Krebs N, Jefferson M, et al. Effect of pancreatic enzymes on zinc absorption in cystic fibrosis. J Pediatr Gastroenterol Nutr 1998;26:136–9.
47. Narkewicz MR, Krebs N, Karrer F, et al. Correction of hypozincemia following liver transplantation in children is associated with reduced urinary zinc loss. Hepatology 1999;29:830–3.
48. Duggan C, MacLeod WB, Krebs NF, et al. Plasma zinc concentrations are depressed during the acute phase response in children with falciparum malaria. J Nutr 2005;135:802–7.
49. Hotz C, Peerson JM, Brown KH. Suggested lower cutoffs of serum zinc concentrations for assessing zinc status: Reanalysis of the second National Health and Nutrition Examination Survey data (1976–1980). Am J Clin Nutr 2003;78:756–64.
50. Liuzzi JP, Bobo JA, Lichten LA, et al. Responsive transporter genes within the murine intestinal-pancreatic axis form a basis of zinc homeostasis. Proc Natl Acad Sci U S A 2004;101:14355–60.
51. Hambidge KM, Miller LV, Tran CD, Krebs NF. Measurements of zinc absorption: Application and interpretation in studies designed to improve human zinc nutriture. Int J Vitam Nutr Res 2005;75:385–93.
52. Krebs NF, Reidinger CJ, Miller LV, Hambidge KM. Zinc homeostasis in breast-fed infants. Pediatr Res 1996;39:661–5.
53. Sian L, Mingyan X, Miller LV, et al. Zinc absorption and intestinal losses of endogenous zinc in young Chinese women with marginal zinc intakes. Am J Clin Nutr 1996;63:348–53.
54. Manary MJ, Hotz C, Krebs NF, et al. Zinc homeostasis in Malawian children consuming a high-phytate, maize- based diet. Am J Clin Nutr 2002;75:1057–61.
55. Miller LV, Hambidge KM, Naake VL, et al. Size of the zinc pools that exchange rapidly with plasma zinc in humans: Alternative techniques for measuring and relation to dietary zinc intake. J Nutr 1994;124:268–76.
56. Krebs N, Reidinger CJ, Miller LV, Borschel M. Zinc homeostasis in normal infants fed a casein hydrolysate formula. J Pediatr Gastro Nutr 2000;30:29–33.
57. Ziegler EE, Serfass RE, Nelson SE, et al. Effect of low zinc intake on absorption and excretion of zinc by infants studied with 70Zn as extrinsic tag. J Nutr 1989;119:1647–53.
58. Arsenault JE, Brown KH. Zinc intake of US preschool children exceeds new dietary reference intakes. Am J Clin Nutr 2003;78:1011–7.
59. Ferenci P. Pathophysiology and clinical features of Wilson disease. Metab Brain Dis 2004;19:229–39.
60. Daniel KG, Harbach RH, Guida WC, Dou QP. Copper storage diseases: Menkes, Wilsons, and cancer. Front Biosci 2004;9:2652–62.
61. Olivares M, Araya M, Uauy R. Copper homeostasis in infant nutrition: Deficit and excess. J Pediatr Gastroenterol Nutr 2000;31:102–11.
62. Grunebaum M, Horodniceanu C, Steinherz R. The radiographic manifestations of bone changes in copper deficiency. Pediatr Radiol 1980;9:101–4.
63. Hedera P, Fink JK, Bockenstedt PL, Brewer GJ. Myelopolyneuropathy and pancytopenia due to copper deficiency and high zinc levels of unknown origin: Further support for existence of a new zinc overload syndrome. Arch Neurol 2003;60:1303–6.
64. Rowin J, Lewis SL. Copper deficiency myeloneuropathy and pancytopenia secondary to overuse of zinc supplementation. J Neurol Neurosurg Psychiatry 2005;76:750–1.
65. Hellman NE, Gitlin JD. Ceruloplasmin metabolism and function. Annu Rev Nutr 2002;22:439–58.
66. Levy Y, Zeharia A, Grunebaum M, Nitzan M, Steinherz R. Copper deficiency in infants fed cow milk. J Pediatr 1985;106:786–8.
67. Castillo-Duran C, Uauy R. Copper deficiency impairs growth of infants recovering from malnutrition. Am J Clin Nutr 1988;47:710–4.
68. Barclay SM, Aggett PJ, Lloyd DJ, Duffty P. Reduced erythrocyte superoxide dismutase activity in low birth weight infants given iron supplements. Pediatr Res 1991;29:297–301.
69. Hillman LS. Serial serum copper concentrations in premature and SGA infants during the first 3 months of life. J Pediatr 1981;98:305–8.
70. Salmenpera L, Siimes MA, Nanto V, Perheentupa J. Copper supplementation: Failure to increase plasma copper and ceruloplasmin concentrations in healthy infants. Am J Clin Nutr 1989;50:843–7.
71. Milne DB. Copper intake and assessment of copper status. Am J Clin Nutr 1998;67:1041S–5S.
72. Bertinato J, Iskandar M, L'Abbe MR. Copper deficiency induces the upregulation of the copper chaperone for Cu/Zn superoxide dismutase in weanling male rats. J Nutr 2003;133:28–31.
73. Higuchi T, Matsukawa Y, Okada K, et al. Correction of copper deficiency improves erythropoietin unresponsiveness in hemodialysis patients with anemia. Intern Med 2006;45:271–3.
74. Tanner MS. Role of copper in Indian childhood cirrhosis. Am J Clin Nutr 1998;67:1074S–81S.
75. Aschner JL, Aschner M. Nutritional aspects of manganese homeostasis. Mol Aspects Med 2005;26:353–62.
76. Wright RO, Amarasiriwardena C, Woolf AD, et al. Neuropsychological correlates of hair arsenic, manganese, and cadmium levels in school-age children residing near a hazardous waste site. Neurotoxicology 2006;27:210–6.
77. Salmenpera L, Perheentupa J, Pakarinen P, Siimes MA. Cu nutrition in infants during prolonged exclusive breast-feeding: Low intake but rising serum concentrations of Cu and ceruloplasmin. Am J Clin Nutr 1986;43:251–7.
78. Zimmermann MB, Kohrle J. The impact of iron and selenium deficiencies on iodine and thyroid metabolism: Biochemistry and relevance to public health. Thyroid 2002;12:867–78.
79. Food and Nutrition Board, Institute of Medicine. Dietary Reference Intakes for Vitamin C, Vitamin E, Selenium, and Carotenoids. Washington, DC: National Academy Press; 2000.
80. Moreno-Reyes R, Suetens C, Mathieu F, et al. Kashin-Beck osteoarthropathy in rural Tibet in relation to selenium and iodine status. N Engl J Med 1998;339:1112–0.
81. Keshan Disease Research Group. Observations of effects of sodium selenite in prevention of Keshan disease. Chin Med J (Engl) 1979;92:471–6.
82. Beck MA, Shi Q, Morris VC, Levander OA. Rapid genomic evolution of a non-virulent coxsackievirus B3 in selenium-deficient mice results in selection of identical virulent isolates. Nat Med 1995;1:433–6.
83. Peng T, Li Y, Yang Y, et al. Characterization of enterovirus isolates from patients with heart muscle disease in a selenium-deficient area of China. J Clin Microbiol 2000;38:3538–43.
84. Yusuf SW, Rehman Q, Casscells W. Cardiomyopathy in association with selenium deficiency: A case report. JPEN J Parenter Enteral Nutr 2002;26:63–6.
85. Brown MR, Cohen HJ, Lyons JM, et al. Proximal muscle weakness and selenium deficiency associated with long term parenteral nutrition. Am J Clin Nutr 1986;43:549–54.
86. Moreno-Reyes R, Mathieu F, Boelaert M, et al. Selenium and iodine supplementation of rural Tibetan children affected by Kashin-Beck osteoarthropathy. Am J Clin Nutr 2003;78:137–44.
87. Jochum F, Terwolbeck K, Meinhold H, et al. Effects of a low selenium state in patients with phenylketonuria. Acta Paediatr 1997;86:775–7.
88. van Bakel MM, Printzen G, Wermuth B, Wiesmann UN. Antioxidant and thyroid hormone status in selenium-deficient phenylketonuric and hyperphenylalaninemic patients. Am J Clin Nutr 2000;72:976–81.
89. Manary MJ, MacPherson GD, McArdle F, et al. Selenium status, kwashiorkor and congestive heart failure. Acta Paediatr 2001;90:950–2.
90. Yannicelli S, Hambidge KM, Picciano MF. Decreased selenium intake and low plasma selenium concentrations leading to clinical symptoms in a child with propionic acidaemia. J Inherit Metab Dis 1992;15:261–8.
91. Ogunro PS, Ogungbamigbe TO, Elemie PO, et al. Plasma Selenium Concentration and Glutathione Peroxidase Activity in HIV-1/AIDS Infected Patients: A Correlation with the Disease Progression. Niger Postgrad Med J 2006;13:1–5.
92. Kupka R, Msamanga GI, Spiegelman D, et al. Selenium levels in relation to morbidity and mortality among children born to HIV-infected mothers. Eur J Clin Nutr 2005;59:1250–8.
93. Darlow BA, Winterbourn CC, Inder TE, et al. The effect of selenium supplementation on outcome in very low birth weight infants: A randomized controlled trial. The New Zealand Neonatal Study Group. J Pediatr 2000;136:473–80.
94. Zachara BA, Pilecki A. Selenium concentration in the milk of breast-feeding mothers and its geographic distribution. Environ Health Perspect 2000;108:1043–6.
95. Raiten DJ, Talbot JM, Waters JH Assessment of nutrient requirements for infant formulas J Nutr 1998;128:2059S–294S.
96. Darlow BA, Inder TE, Graham PJ, et al. The relationship of selenium status to respiratory outcome in the very low birth weight infant. Pediatrics 1995;96:314–9.
97. Anderson RA. Chromium as an essential nutrient for humans. Regul Toxicol Pharmacol 1997;26:S35–41.
98. Althuis MD, Jordan NE, Ludington EA, Wittes JT. Glucose and insulin responses to dietary chromium supplements: A meta-analysis. Am J Clin Nutr 2002;76:148–55.
99. Vincent JB. Recent advances in the nutritional biochemistry of trivalent chromium. Proc Nutr Soc 2004;63:41–7.
100. Moukarzel AA, Song MK, Buchman AL, et al. Excessive chromium intake in children receiving total parenteral nutrition. Lancet 1992;339:385–8.
101. Cerulli J, Grabe DW, Gauthier I, et al. Chromium picolinate toxicity. Ann Pharmacother 1998;32:428–31.
102. Wasser WG, Feldman NS, D'Agati VD. Chronic renal failure after ingestion of over-the-counter chromium picolinate. Ann Intern Med 1997;126:410.
103. Anderson RA, Bryden NA, Polansky MM. Lack of toxicity of chromium chloride and chromium picolinate in rats. J Am Coll Nutr 1997;16:273–9.
104. Anderson RA, Bryden NA, Patterson KY, et al. Breast milk chromium and its association with chromium intake, chromium excretion, and serum chromium. Am J Clin Nutr 1993;57:519–23.
105. Golub MS, Hogrefe CE, Germann SL, et al. Neurobehavioral evaluation of rhesus monkey infants fed cow's milk formula, soy formula, or soy formula with added manganese. Neurotoxicol Teratol 2005;27:615–27.

106. Tran TT, Chowanadisai W, Crinella FM, et al. Effect of high dietary manganese intake of neonatal rats on tissue mineral accumulation, striatal dopamine levels, and neurodevelopmental status. Neurotoxicology 2002;23:635–43.
107. Ten Cate JM. In vitro studies on the effects of fluoride on de- and remineralization. J Dent Res 1990;69:614–9; discussion 634–16.
108. Dawes C, Weatherell JA. Kinetics of fluoride in the oral fluids. J Dent Res 1990;69:638–44; discussion 682–33.
109. Marinho VC, Higgins JP, Logan S, Sheiham A. Topical fluoride (toothpastes, mouthrinses, gels or varnishes) for preventing dental caries in children and adolescents. Cochrane Database Syst Rev 2003(4):CD002782.
110. Centers for Disease Control and Prevention. Recommendations for using fluoride to prevent and control dental caries in the United States. Centers for Disease Control and Prevention. MMWR Recomm Rep 2001;50:1–42.
111. Esala S, Vuori E, Helle A. Effect of maternal fluorine intake on breast milk fluorine content. Br J Nutr 1982;48:201–4.
112. Food and Nutrition Board, National Reseach Council. Dietary Reference Intakes for Calcium, Phosphorus, Magnesium, Vitamin D, and Flouride. Washington, DC: National Academy Press; 1997.
113. Dunn J. Iodine. In: Shils ME SM, Ross AC, Caballero B, Cousins RJ, editors. Modern Nutrition in Health and Disease, 10th edition. Baltimore, MD: Lippincott Williams and Wilkins; 2006.
114. Teng W, Shan Z, Teng X, et al. Effect of iodine intake on thyroid diseases in China. N Engl J Med 2006;354:2783–93.

9

Iron

A.Z. Khambalia, MSc
S.H. Zlotkin, MD, PhD, FRCPC

With the exception of certain members of the bacterial genera, iron is an essential nutrient for all living organisms. Iron is a versatile and highly reactive group VIII transition metal with electrons distributed throughout five 3d orbitals.[1] Depending on the chemical environment iron can exist in several oxidation states (between −2 and +6). At physiological oxygen concentrations iron exists in its stable ferric (Fe^{3+}) state for most of its biological complexes. Ferrous (Fe^{2+}) iron is used in transmembrane transport of iron, deposition of iron in the storage protein and synthesis of heme.[2]

The only stable iron states in the aqueous environment of the human body and in food are ferric and ferrous iron. The human body contains 2 to 4 g of elemental iron, most of which is in the hemoglobin (Hb) of erythrocytes.[3] Over 65% of body iron is present in the Hb, up to 10% is found in myoglobin, and approximately 1 to 5% is present as part of enzymes.[4]

Iron is vital for metabolic processes such as oxygen transport, DNA synthesis, and electron transport. Tissue oxygenation is iron's key function. Oxygen is bound to an iron-containing porphyrin ring, either as part of the prosthetic group of Hb within erythrocytes or as part of myoglobin located within the cytoplasm of muscle cells.[5] Some critical proteins and enzymes that have iron as a component or cofactor include Hb, myoglobin, catalase, xanthine oxidase, aconitase, reduced nicotinamide adenine dinucleotide, ribonucleotide reductase, peroxidases, and cytochrome oxidase.

Iron's role in electron transport and reversible ligand binding is accredited to its ability to interconvert between oxidation states and achieve various redox potentials during electrochemical reactions. Heme is contained in the active sites of cytochromes that serve as electron carriers within the cell, in iron–sulfur proteins (flavoproteins, heme-flavoproteins) required for the first reaction in the electron transport chain, and in hydrogen peroxidases (eg, catalase and peroxidase).[1] The cytochrome P450 family of enzymes located in microsomal membranes of liver and intestinal mucosal cells also contain heme. Cytochrome P450 is involved in detoxification of foreign substances in the liver and synthesis of steroid hormones and bile acids.

ABSORPTION

Iron absorption occurs in the proximal duodenum and involves a sequence of events: (1) reduction, (2) apical uptake, (3) intracellular storage or trafficking, and (4) basolateral release. Clinical disorders that affect iron absorption include malabsorption syndromes such as steatorrhea and tropical sprue.

Reduction

Most inorganic iron in the diet is in the oxidized or ferric form. Before iron can be taken up by the intestinal epithelial cells or enterocytes, iron must first be reduced from its ferric to ferrous form in the luminal brush border of the enterocyte (Figure 1).[6] A strong candidate for the brush border ferrireductase is duodenal cytochrome *b*.[7] Ferrous iron is more readily absorbed than ferric iron due to higher solubility in the proximal small intestine. Iron reduction is facilitated by the acidic milieu of the gastric content and the meal composition.[8]

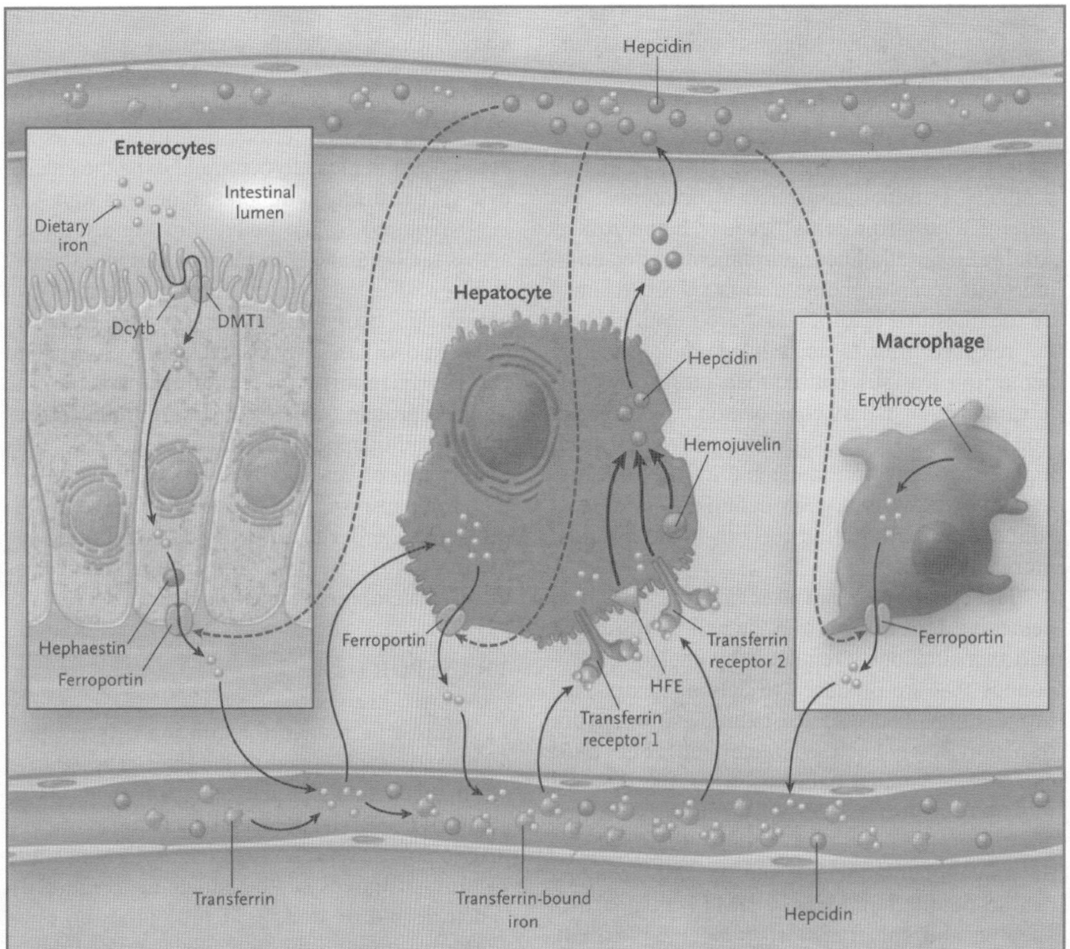

Interplay of Key Proteins in Iron Homeostasis.
In the duodenal enterocyte, dietary iron is reduced to the ferrous state by duodenal ferric reductase (Dcytb), transported into the cell by divalent metal transporter 1 (DMT1), and released by way of ferroportin into the circulation. Hephaestin facilitates enterocyte iron release. Hepatocytes take up iron from the circulation either as free iron or transferrin-bound iron (through transferrin receptor 1 and transferrin receptor 2). Transferrin receptor 2 may serve as a sensor of circulating transferrin-bound iron, thereby influencing expression of the iron regulatory hormone hepcidin. The hepcidin response is also modulated by HFE and hemojuvelin. Hepcidin is secreted into the circulation, where it downregulates the ferroportin-mediated release of iron from enterocytes, macrophages, and hepatocytes (dashed lines).

Figure 1 Interplay of key proteins in iron homeostasis. (Source: Reference 6.)

Apical Uptake

In order to reach the plasma, iron must pass from the gut through the apical (lumenal) and basolateral (serosal) membranes of the enterocyte.[9] Absorptive cells located in the crypts of the duodenum are organized as finger-like villous structures to increase surface area. Beginning as stem cells, these absorptive cells proliferate and migrate out of the crypt and up to the villus over a period of several days.[10] During migration the cells differentiate and perform their functions.[11]

During the intestinal phase of digestion iron is present in the lumen as either heme or nonheme iron. Nonheme iron that is liberated by gastric and pancreatic proteases becomes bound to intraluminal molecules. These iron-binding proteins prevent nonheme iron from being readily oxidized from ferrous to ferric iron in the alkaline environment and rendered insoluble and biologically unavailable.

The pathway by which heme iron is absorbed is less well defined than that of inorganic iron.[9] A specific duodenal receptor/transporter for heme has not yet been elucidated in humans.[6] Heme iron is released from proteins such as Hb and myoglobin in the lumen of the stomach and small intestine.[9] Although the chemical form of the resulting "free" heme has not been well defined, it is likely to be stabilized by various dietary constituents, including Hb degradation products. Luminal absorption of heme does not require binding proteins because heme iron is soluble in an alkaline environment. After binding to its receptor, heme iron is absorbed intact by the intestinal enterocytes.[12] Iron from heme is not released prior to its cellular uptake, making heme iron less susceptible than inorganic heme to variations in dietary composition.[13] The percent iron absorption from heme iron is 5- to 10-folds higher than that from nonheme iron. Most studies have shown that iron deficiency is able to stimulate the absorption of both heme iron and inorganic iron.[13]

The enterocyte's apical membrane transports heme and ferrous iron into the cell.[14] Iron transport is meticulously regulated by chelating compounds that are produced to detoxify extra- and intracellular iron.[9] At least three pathways for transport have been characterized. The most extensively studied pathway is via the divalent metal transporter, DMT1 (formerly called Nramp2 or DCT1).[15] DMT1 transfers iron across the apical membrane and into the cell through a proton-coupled process.[15] DMT1 is not iron specific and can transport manganese, cobalt, copper, zinc, cadmium, and lead. DMT1 expression is regulated by body iron stores, but it may also be susceptible to dietary iron or a posttranslational mechanism.[11]

Intracellular Storage or Trafficking

Once iron has been absorbed by enterocytes it is bound by, as of yet unidentified, chaperones. Inside the absorptive enterocyte, iron can either be stored as ferritin or transferred across the basolateral membrane into the circulation where it will be bound to apoferritin.[14] Proteins related to iron metabolism on the basolateral membrane of the precursor and mature enterocyte either sense body iron stores or facilitate regulated iron transport into the plasma. These proteins include the transferrin (Tf) receptor–hereditary hemochromatosis protein (HFE) complex, the basolateral iron transporter and the ceruloplasmin homologue, hephaestin.[11] Iron that remains in the form of ferritin as the enterocyte completes its life cycle will be sloughed off with the senescent cell and exit the body through the gastrointestinal tract (Figure 1). This maturation process takes approximately 3 to 5 days.[16]

Basolateral Release

The pathways by which inorganic and heme iron are taken up from the intestinal lumen by the enterocytes vary; however, it has been proposed that their basolateral export from enterocytes, that is, the step involving hepaestin and IREG1, is common to iron from both sources (Figure 1). The basolateral membrane mediates the transfer of iron from the intestinal epithelial cells to the rest of the body.[11] Once inside the epithelial cell heme is either split into ferrous iron and bilirubin by heme oxygenase or transported as the intact porphyrin ring.[13] The released ferrous iron likely enters the pool of iron in the enterocyte and exits the enterocyte via a pathway common to inorganic iron.[17]

If required by the body, iron rapidly moves across the basolateral membrane and into the circulation. The major molecule that carries iron across the basolateral membrane is ferroportin (also known as IREG1, MTP1).[9] Similar to DMT1, ferroportin is a multitransmembrane segment protein, which appears to prefer ferrous iron. A multicopper ferroxidase, hephaestin, acts in a way, as of yet unknown, to facilitate basolateral iron transport.[1] Hephaestin may serve to oxidize iron in order to allow binding of iron to the plasma iron carrier, Tf.[18] Once iron transverses the basolateral membrane it is bound to Tf.

TRANSPORT

Tf is a plasma protein for iron ion delivery predominantly synthesized in the liver. The 80 kDa serum iron–binding protein reversibly binds to two atoms of iron.[4] The polypeptide chain is arranged in two lobes, representing the N-terminal and C-terminal halves of the molecule (Figure 2). When devoid of iron, a Tf lobe takes an open conformation with the domains separated. Once iron is bound, the domains undergo a rigid rotation to enclose their iron-binding site, thereby guarding bound iron from hydrolysis and too facile release. Tf can acquire iron from dietary absorption or from heme that has been degraded by the phagocytosis of senescent red blood cells.

High-affinity binding of iron to Tf at physiological pH is required to prevent the toxic effect of iron ions, making it difficult to develop iron chelators that compete with Tf for iron binding.[19]

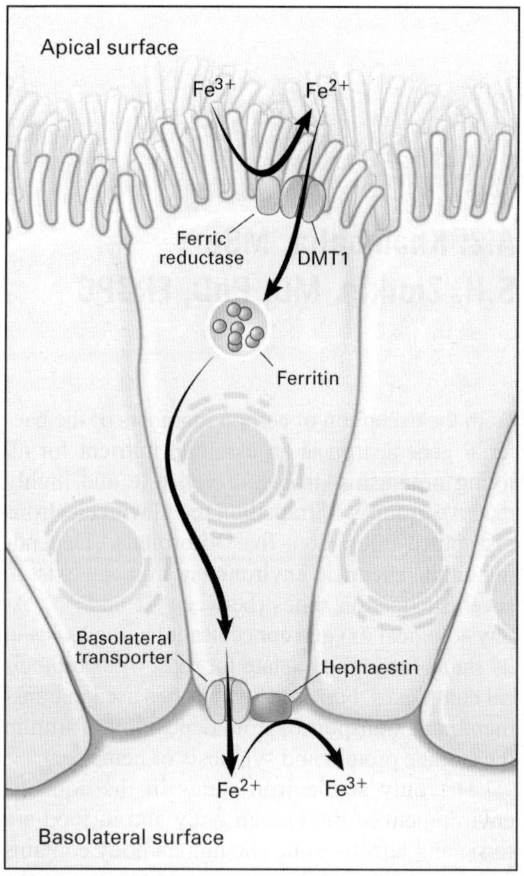

Figure 2 Schematic diagram of iron uptake into cells via the transferrin receptor. (Source: Reference 15.)

Normally all nonheme iron in the circulation is bound to Tf. However, approximately only 30% of Tf binding sites are occupied, so most of the protein is free of iron. Normal individuals never have full saturation of all Tf iron–binding sites, thus providing a safety margin to accommodate fluctuation of iron levels from dietary and environmental changes.[2] Complete saturation is only seen in pathological states such as hemochromatosis and transfusional iron overload. Transferrin receptors (TfRs) are able to distinguish between iron-free and iron-loaded Tf, ensuring cells do not waste efforts taking up the former.

TfRs are firmly anchored in cell membranes, with the major portion of the protein being external to the cell.[1] The density of surface TfRs on a given cell is proportional to the cell's iron requirements. In most tissues, however, the receptor number falls sharply as the cell matures. Two exceptions are placental cells and erythroid precursors—both rapidly dividing cells where large amounts of iron are required throughout the life span.

Tf–iron complexes attach to TfRs on the cell surface. The entire complex of Tf–iron and TfR are invaginated by part of the cell wall to form a vacuole. The complex is internalized by receptor-mediated endocytosis into clathrin-coated endosomes.[16] The pH in endosomal compartments are rapidly lowered through the action of an ATP-dependent proton pump.[4] The acidic milieu facilitates conformational changes in the Tf and TfR proteins.[18] Iron is released from the complex and reduced to its ferrous form. Iron is then transported across the endosomal membrane into the cytoplasm by divalent metal transporter 1 (DMT1, previously known as Nramp2, DCT1). The TfR–Tf complex returns to the cell surface where the physiological pH causes Tf to be released and recycled into the circulation.[9]

Most of the iron entering the plasma via Tf is provided from body sites where Hb destruction and degradation of ferritin and hemosiderin occur. Phagocytes of the reticuloendothelial system degrade Hb. In humans the average life span of an erythrocyte is 120 days.[1] At the end of their functional lifetime, erythrocytes undergo changes in the structure of their membrane, causing them to be recognized as sensescent cells.[1] Senescent red blood cells are taken up by macrophages and phagocytosed in the spleen, bone marrow (reticuloendothelial cell macrophages), and liver (Kupffer cells) (Figure 3). This internal erythroid circuit removes and replaces 0.66% of the body's total iron content each day.[1] By degrading Hb in senescent erythrocytes and loading ferric iron onto Tf for delivery to cells, these macrophages provide most of the body's usable iron. The daily requirement for the erythron alone is 20 mg of iron and yet only 1 to 2 mg of iron normally enters the body each day through the intestine.[15]

The heme portion of Hb is catabolized by hemoxygenase to biliverdin and subsequently, bilirubin.[18] Bilirubin is secreted into the bile for excretion from the body. Hemopexin and haptoglobin sequester serum or Hb from lysed cells, which is then transported to the marrow for erythropoiesis, incorporation into iron-dependent enzymes or as storage.[16] The mechanism for iron egress from the macrophage is unknown but is thought to involve ferroportin with the aid of the ferroxidase ceruloplasmin. The amount of iron that is recycled from effete red cells and returned to plasma Tf approximates the amount of iron needed for the synthesis of new erythrocytes.[18]

STORAGE

When intracellular iron exceeds cellular requirements, excess iron is kept in storage. All cells are capable of storing iron; however, principal storage sites in humans are the liver, spleen, and bone marrow.[2] The concentration of storage iron in the body varies by gender and iron status.

Iron is stored in the form of ferritin or hemosiderin. Ferritin is comprised of 24 similar polypeptide subunits that form a cage isolating iron from the cellular milieu. Ferritin exists in at least two different isoforms (H and L).[2] The relative proportions of the two subunits vary by tissue type and development. The H form is predominant in the heart, whereas the L form is predominate in the liver. Hemosiderin is an ill-defined water-soluble degradation product of ferritin that appears to result from incomplete lysomal processing.[2] The type of iron stored in hemosiderin is less chemically reactive than what is found in ferritin and potentially less available for mobilization.[1]

The liver contains about 60% of the ferritin in the body with the remaining amount present in muscle tissues and cells of the reticuloenthelial system. Macrophages act as a storage depot for iron recovered from effete erythrocytes or from medicinal forms of iron administered by injection. Their storage capacity is evident when tissues from patients with transfusional iron overload are stained for iron; large amounts of iron accumulate in macrophages before deposition in parenchymal cells becomes apparent.[18]

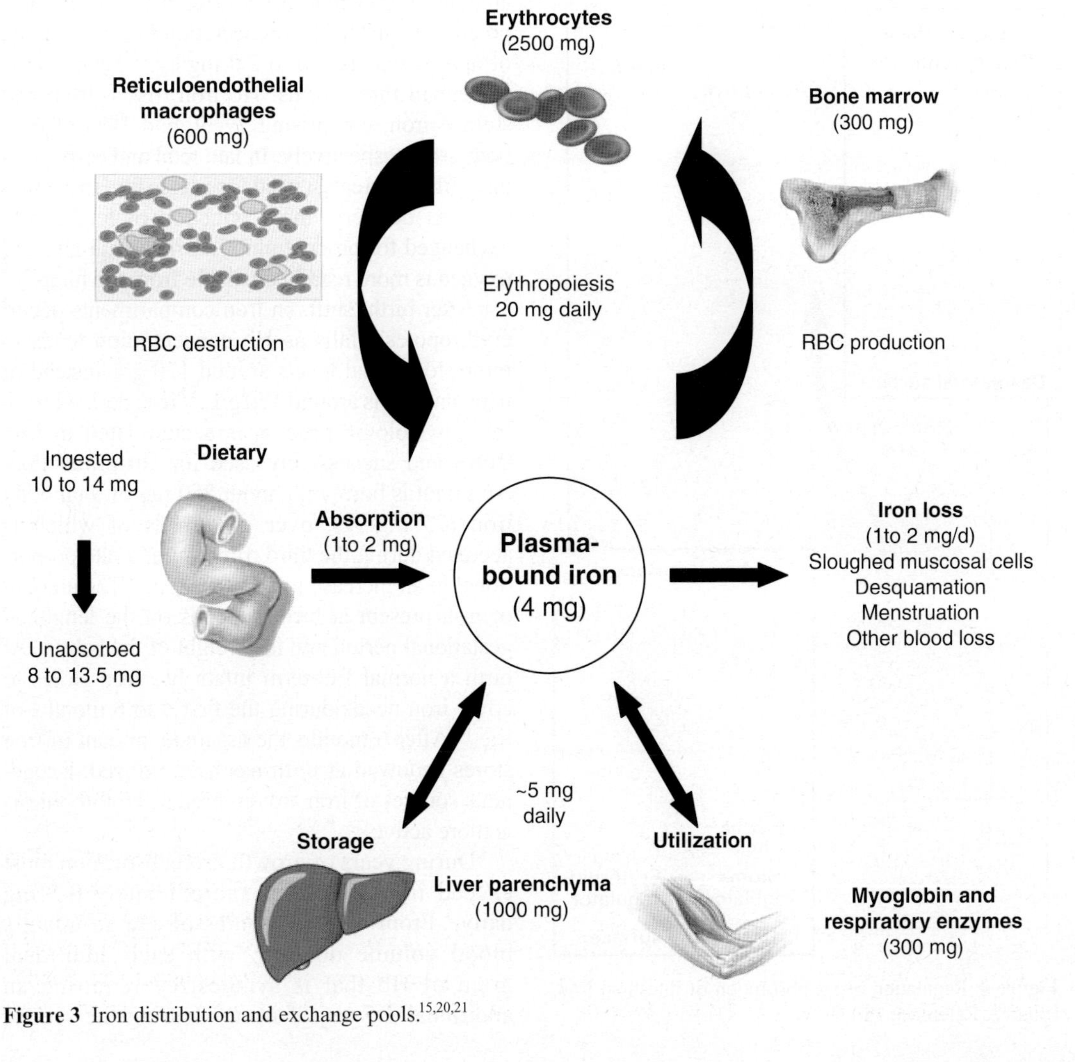

Figure 3 Iron distribution and exchange pools.[15,20,21]

EXCRETION

Iron in the human body is highly conserved. Only a small amount of iron is lost each day (Figure 3). Daily basal losses are limited to 0.90 to 1.02 mg/d in nonmenstruating women.[20] The majority of iron is lost in feces (derived from shed enterocytes, extravasated red blood cells, and biliary heme breakdown products that are poorly absorbed), with losses from the urine, gastrointestinal tract, and skin amounting to 0.08, 0.6, 0.2 to 0.3 mg/d, respectively.[1]

The amount of iron lost during menstruation is variable. The mean loss is estimated to be between 0.6 and 0.7 mg/d, which translates into a loss of 17.5 mg iron per period.[22] However, basal losses have been reported to decline to about 0.5 mg/d in an iron-deficient state and increase to about 2 mg/d during iron overload.[23] Nonphysiologic causes of iron losses include bleeding from gastrointestinal ulcers, intestinal parasites, cow's milk feeding to infants, aspirin, nonsteroidal antiinflammatory drugs or corticosteroid administration, or hemorrhage induced by surgery or injury.[3]

HOMEOSTASIS

Because humans lack a physiological pathway for iron excretion, the amount of iron in the body is determined by the regulation of iron absorption in the proximal small intestine.[19] Several processes have been found to influence the rate of iron absorption, including diet, body iron stores, marrow erythropoietic activity, blood Hb concentration, blood oxygen content, and the presence of systemic inflammation.[6] Iron absorption decreases in the presence of iron overload and inflammation and increases in response to iron deficiency, accelerated erythropoiesis, and hypoxia.[6] Some of these processes are interrelated and may occur simultaneously.

Regulatory mechanisms exist for a single cell; intracellular iron homeostasis involves the regulation of protein synthesis and action related to iron acquisition, utilization, and storage. Much of this process is regulated at the gene level by iron. Messenger RNAs (mRNA) for ferritin H and L subunits, TfR, DMT1, and ferroportin have stem loop structures called iron-responsive elements (IREs).[2]

IREs are located in the 3′ or 5′ untranslated region of key mRNA.[11] IREs regulate proteins involved in iron metabolism at the posttranscriptional level by interacting with iron-responsive proteins.[16] Iron-responsive proteins are RNA-binding proteins with specific sequences and structures that are found in the cytosol of all mammalian tissues.[14]

Humoral regulatory mechanisms for iron absorption include the dietary regulator, the stores regulator, and the erythropoietic regulator. Absorption of intestinal iron can be modulated by the amount of iron recently consumed. Absorptive enterocytes are resistant to acquiring additional iron several days after a dietary bolus.[15] This phenomenon is commonly referred to as the "mucosal block" theory. The hypothesis is that the amount of iron that is absorbed is dependent on previous exposure of the gastrointestinal tract to iron.[10] It is postulated that multipotent precursor cells in the epithelial layer of the duodenum act as sensors of body iron needs. Iron levels are programmed by enterocytes in the crypt, thus modulating iron absorption at the villus.[16] Upon differentiation new proteins required for iron absorption, storage, and export are expressed in the enterocyte. The lag period between injection of iron and change in iron absorption is thought to represent the time taken for cell differentiation and migration. Downregulation of iron absorption after oral loading has also been observed in the presence of systemic iron deficiency.[8]

The stores regulator senses iron levels but instead of responding to dietary iron appears to respond to total body iron.[15] After ingestion of foods or iron supplements, higher nonheme iron absorption occurs when stores are depleted and lower absorption occurs when stores are replete or enlarged.[10,24] An inverse linear relationship has been described between iron absorption and serum ferritin (a measure of iron stores). It has been suggested that once iron stores are replete there is a "set point" or steady state above which they do not further increase iron absorption. This predetermined "set point" for iron stores is believed to vary between individuals.

The erythropoietic regulator has been postulated to modulate iron absorption in response to acute marrow iron needs.[19] It is thought that this mechanism senses ineffective erythropoiesis such as occurs in congential disorders of red cell maturation (ie, thalassemia, sideroblastic anemia). Anemic states that stimulate iron absorption, such as thalassemia syndromes, congenital dyserythropoietic anemias, and sideroblastic anemias all involve destruction of erythroid cells near the site of their development, within the bone marrow. Anemias that are characterized by peripheral destruction of red cells, such as sickle cell anemia, hereditary spherocytosis, and autoimmune hemolytic anemia, do not cause increases in iron absorption leading to the speculation that another component of erythropoiesis other than its rate must explain the absorptive response.[25]

The discovery of the iron regulatory hormone hepcidin supports the liver's central role in determining the amount of iron that is absorbed by the gut and released from storage sites.[26] It has long been known that the liver is the major depot for iron; hepatocytes are the first cells in the body to have access to absorbed iron entering the portal circulation from the gut.[27] Iron can enter hepatocytes via receptor-mediated endocytosis of diferric TfR or as non-TfR–bound iron.[15] However, the liver's direct role in modulating iron absorption has only recently become evident from studies on hepcidin, a small antimicrobial peptide that is secreted by hepatocytes into the circulation.

Hepcidin (also called HAMP) is a 25-amino acid peptide that is primarily produced by the liver. It is secreted into plasma, and is cleared by the kidneys.[18] Hepcidin acts as an inhibitor of iron absorption and iron release. Important cellular targets for hepcidin are the villus enterocyte, the reticuloendothelial macrophage, and the hepatocyte (Figure 4). Hepcidin modulates the ferroportin-mediated release of cellular iron by binding to ferroportin and causing it to be degraded.[26] Decreased functional activity of ferroportin causes a decrease in basolateral iron transfer in the enterocyte and a decrease in iron export from reticuloendothelial macrophages and hepatocytes (increase in stored iron).[26]

The production of hepcidin is inversely related to iron stores, erythropoietic activity, Hb, oxygen content, and inflammation.[26] Hepcidin expression is decreased when body iron requirements are high, such as when iron stores decrease, during iron deficiency, accelerated erythropoiesis, and hypoxia.[27] Increased levels of hepcidin are observed in nongenetic iron overload and inflammation.[18] While it is clear that hepcidin is a strong negative regulator of iron absorption, there is much to be learned regarding the mechanisms by which the liver senses body iron status and erythropoietic demand.[17]

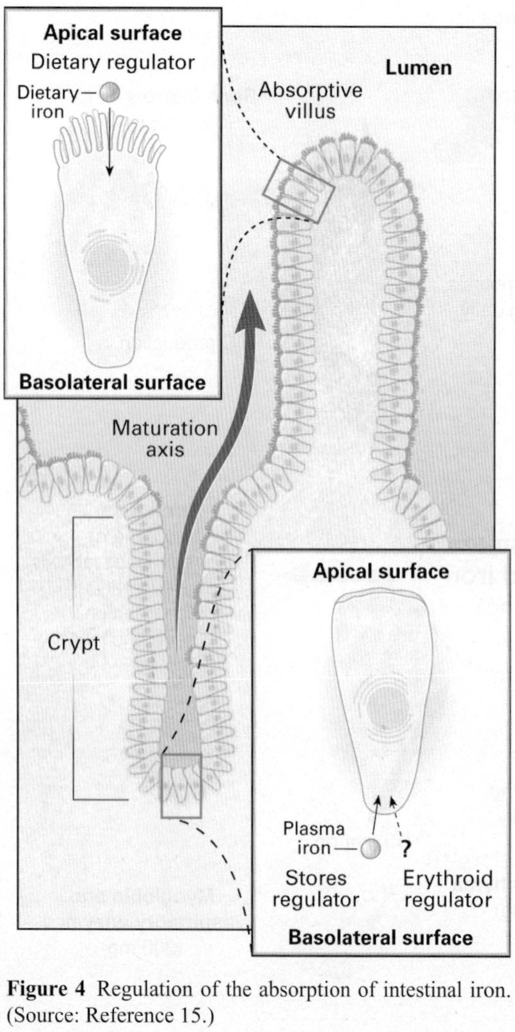

Figure 4 Regulation of the absorption of intestinal iron. (Source: Reference 15.)

IRON REQUIREMENTS

Iron requirements are high during periods of rapid growth such as the first years of life, adolescence, and pregnancy. During infancy, the amount of iron needed for growth is so great that the abundant iron stores present at birth are usually exhausted by 4 to 6 months of age. After the first year of life, adolescence is the second most critical period of physical growth in the life cycle. During pregnancy iron requirements rise significantly due to increased red cell mass, the expansion of plasma volume, and growth of the fetal-placental unit.[28]

INFANCY

Fetal Hb has a high affinity for oxygen, thereby giving the fetus precedence for oxygen over the mother at the placental interface.[19] Delivery of oxygen from fetal Hb to tissues is lowered. Consequently, the fetus needs more Hb to deliver a certain amount of oxygen to tissues (regulated by erythropoietin). Daily fetal iron accretion occurs at a rate of approximately 1.6 to 2.0 mg/kg.[29] Fetal iron is present in three forms: Hb iron, tissue iron, and storage iron, comprising 77, 9, and 14% of total body iron, respectively. In late fetal and early postnatal life the greatest need for iron is for Hb synthesis.[30] At delivery, the production of fetal Hb is exchanged for production of normal adult Hb, and oxygen is more readily available from the lungs.[19]

After birth, shifts in iron compartments occur; erythropoiesis falls as Hb concentration tends to return to normal levels around 120 g/L instead of neonatal levels around 170 g/L.[30] Iron derived from this physiologic process is accumulated in iron stores and successively used for Hb production. An infant is born with about 250 mg of total body iron (75 mg/kg), over two-thirds of which is accreted during the third trimester at a rate proportional to an increase in body weight.[29] The amount of iron present at birth depends on the length of gestational period and the weight of the baby.[31] At birth a normal full-term infant has iron stores to cover iron needs during the first 4 to 6 months of life.[12] After 6 months the assumed amount of iron stores endowed at birth has been utilized. Exogenous sources of iron are required as erythropoiesis is more active.

During years of growth, iron absorption must exceed iron losses by approximately 0.5 mg daily.[5] From 4 to 12 months of age an infant's blood volume doubles, with each additional gram of Hb that is synthesized requiring an additional 3.5 mg of iron.[29] During the second half of infancy exogenous iron requirements rapidly increase to concentrations that are higher than any other time in life on a body weight basis.[8] It is only after approximately 2 years of life that iron requirements begin to be reduced.[19]

Adolescence

During adolescence iron requirements nearly double in both boys and girls as a result of the expansion of the total blood volume and the increase in lean body mass.[32] Estimates of physiological iron requirements during the adolescent period have been computed using a factorial method of iron components (basal losses, menstrual losses, and accretion).[33] Preadolescent levels of overall iron requirements (0.7 to 0.9 mg Fe/d) increase to as much as 2.2 mg Fe/d.[34,35]

Female adolescents require an additional amount of iron to account for iron losses during menses. Menstrual losses may increase daily requirements to as much as 2.1 mg/d in girls at the 75th percentile of blood loss.[32] Among 14-year-old girls, median iron requirements can be 30% higher than for their mothers.[35] Iron requirements may increase further in heavily menstruating young women.

PREGNANCY

Pregnancy is associated with an increased red cell mass, plasma volume expansion, and growth in the fetal-placental unit, all of which contribute to a significant increase in iron requirements. The additional iron requirement for pregnancy (3 to 4 mg/d) is substantial and it is estimated that fewer than 50% of women have adequate iron stores to meet this additional need.[28] Furthermore, iron requirements are not distributed equally over the duration of pregnancy. Requirements are low in the first trimester (due to the absence of menstrual iron losses and the negligible needs of fetus) but rise to between 4 and 6 mg in the second and third trimesters, respectively.[36] During the last 6 to 8 weeks of pregnancy requirements may reach as much as 10 mg/d.[19]

By the end of pregnancy, approximately 1,200 mg of iron is required, either from body iron stores or from the diet.[37] The average requirement for a menstruating woman for the same period of time is roughly 400 mg. In order to accommodate this increased requirement of 800 mg and avoid a negative iron balance the average woman must absorb 500 mg (2 mg/d) more iron than she required while menstruating.[37]

In most cases, dietary intakes alone are insufficient to meet the requirements of pregnancy, especially in the latter part of pregnancy.[37] It is, therefore, estimated that a female needs 500 mg of stored iron to cover iron requirements during pregnancy.[19] A woman who routinely eats a diet high in bioavailable iron and enters pregnancy with sufficient iron stores will likely meet her requirements.[36] However, a higher amount of stored iron is needed when the diet is less than optimal.[19]

DIETARY SOURCES OF IRON

A normal diet contains approximately 13 to 18 mg of iron per day, of which only 1 mg of iron per day is needed in healthy persons to replace basal iron losses.[16] While many foods are good sources of iron, some are limited by the bioavailability of iron. Iron-rich foods include cocoa, liver, kidney, dried fish, shell-fish, sesame seed, soy flour, and pulses.[38] Foods with low-iron content include milk, cheese, sugar, sweets, jams, and unfortified milled cereals (Table 1).

There are two forms of iron in the diet—inorganic iron and heme iron. Heme iron is present in the Hb and myoglobin of animal tissues and is thus mainly associated with meat, poultry, and fish intake.[40] Heme iron may contribute up to 50% of the iron that actually enters the body.[30] In a single meal 5 to 35% of heme iron is absorbed.[13] Studies using radiolabeled heme or Hb have established that the intestinal absorption of heme is far more efficient than inorganic iron.[12] Heme iron is well absorbed regardless of meal composition with the exception of meat and calcium. Meat has been shown to enhance heme iron absorption.[41] Calcium is the only dietary factor known to negatively influence the absorption of heme iron and does so to the same extent that it influences nonheme iron.[42]

Inorganic iron, predominantly found in components of plant origin, is the most prevalent form of dietary iron.[43] Inorganic iron accounts for 80 to 90% of the iron in a standard diet.[1] Nonheme iron is generally poorly absorbed and greatly influenced by enhancing or inhibiting substances (Figure 5).[38] Meat, fish, amino acids, and organic acids (ie, ascorbic acid, lactic acid, citric acid, and malic acid) promote nonheme iron absorption.[43,44] These nonheme iron enhancers form soluble complexes with iron at low gastric pH levels and prevent the formation of insoluble hydroxides at the higher pH of small intestine.[30] Phenols, calcium, and phytates that are present in cereals and legumes impair nonheme iron absorption.[30] Phenolic compounds, which bear catechol or galloyl groups, have iron-binding properties.[38] Tea, coffee, cocoa, red wine, many vegetables (such as spinach), grains, herbs, and spices (such as oregano and cinnamon) contain phenolic compounds. Vitamin A may be capable of preventing the inhibiting effect of polyphenols on iron absorption.[38] Phytates are a storage form of phosphates and minerals in cereals, seeds, nuts, vegetables, and fruit. Bran, oats, and fiber-rich foods are rich in phytates. The effect of phytates is counteracted by ascorbic acid, meat, fish, and poultry.[38]

ASSESSMENT OF IRON STATUS

The most important clinical clue of moderate to severe chronic iron deficiency in adults is chronic fatigue. Other features include pallor of the skin and of the conjunctiva, stomatitis, ice eating (pagophagia), leg cramping, koilonychia, glossitis, gastric atrophy, and dysphagia.[45] It is also possible that some individuals with iron deficiency may not experience any symptoms.[1] Since clinical signs of anemia are not specific, it is recommended that biochemical tests be used to determine iron deficiency and its magnitude.[46]

Among the wide variety of laboratory methods that are available to assess iron status

Table 1 Iron Content of Various Foods[39]

Food	One Serving	Iron Content (mg)
Clam, mixed species, canned, drained solids	3 oz	23.8
Cereals, ready-to-eat, General Mills, Cherrios	1 cup	10.3
Soybeans, mature cooked, boiled, without salt	1 cup	8.84
Cereals, ready-to-eat, Kellogs, corn flakes	1 cup	8.12
Infant cereals, including rice, oats, mixed cereals	15 g	7.10
Lentils, mature seeds, cooked, boiled, without salt	1 cup	6.59
Chickpeas, matured seeds, cooked, boiled, without salt	1 cup	4.74
Rice, white, long-grained, parboiled, enriched, cooked	1 cup	3.17
Peas, edible-podded, boiled, drained, without salt	1 cup	3.15
Infant formula–with iron, ready-to-feed	240 mL	2.90
Sardine, Atlantic, canned in oil, drained solids with bone	3 oz	2.48
Chicken liver, cooked, simmered	1 liver	2.28
Potatoes, baked, flesh and skin, without salt	1 potato	2.18
Beef, 75% lean/25% fat, cooked, broiled	3 oz	2.01
Almonds	1 oz (24 nuts)	1.22
Tuna, light, canned in oil, drained solids	3 oz	1.18
Bread, whole, commercially prepared	1 slice	0.93
Egg, whole, raw, fresh	1 large	0.92
Blueberries, raw	1 cup	0.89
Rice, brown, long-grained, cooked	1 cup	0.82
Spinach, raw	1 cup	0.81
Broccoli, raw	1 cup	0.64
Bread, white, commercially prepared	1 slice	0.73
Infant formula–low iron, ready-to-feed	240 mL	0.30
Cheese, cheddar	1 oz	0.19
Apples, raw, with skin	1 apple	0.17
Milk, cow, whole, 3.25% milkfat	1 cup	0.07

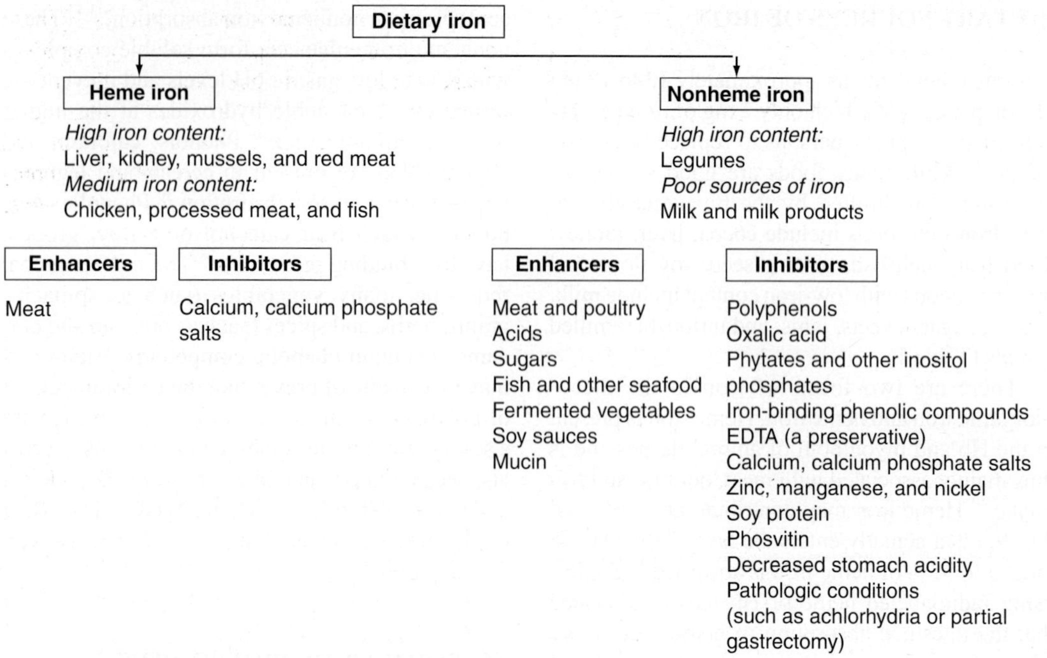

Figure 5 Factors affecting dietary iron absorption.

(ie, hematocrit, Hb, mean cell volume, erythrocyte mean index, free erythrocyte protoporphyrin, serum iron, total iron-binding capacity, serum Tf, Tf saturation, serum ferritin, and serum TfR), there is no one single test that is ideal. Diminished stainable iron in a bone marrow aspirate is generally accepted to be the reference standard for iron status.[47] However, the method is invasive, costly, and subject to variable interpretation.[48]

Rather than using a single measurement, a valid assessment of iron status is best characterized by multiple indices.[49] Presently, there is no consensus on the best definition of iron deficiency using multiple measures. In the United States, two combinations of multiple indices were used to assess low iron status and anemia in the National Health and Nutrition Examination Surveys II and III.[50,51] One included serum ferritin, Tf saturation, and FEP. The other method involved MCV, Tf saturation, and FEP.

Selecting the most appropriate combination of iron status indicators depends on the study objectives and the health of the study population.[47,52] Features of the more commonly accepted diagnostic indices are summarized in Tables 2 and 3. For a detailed review, see Gibson.[53]

HEMOGLOBIN

Hb measures the presence of anemia. While it is the most widely used screening tool for iron deficiency, Hb determination has serious limitations when relied upon as the only laboratory measurement because of its low specificity and sensitivity.[45] When used alone Hb concentration does not distinguish between anemia due to iron deficiency and that due to infection (eg, malaria, HIV), other micronutrient deficiencies (eg, folate, vitamin B_{12}, vitamin A), or other disease states (eg, sickle cell disease, thalassemia). Furthermore, the wide range of values in normal subjects means that Hb values overlap considerably between normal and iron-deficient anemic individuals.[19] Affected by diurnal variations, Hb values in the evening tend to be lower than values in the morning by up to 10 g/L.[53]

As with any other parameter, it is essential to interpret Hb concentration according to age-specific and sex-specific reference standards. In infants, reference values for iron status variables including Hb have not been well developed and may not be accurate since they are based on extrapolation of data from older age groups . The cutoff for anemia at sea level recommended by the WHO for infants 6 months to 5 years of age is 110 g/L. This cutoff concentration is based on studies in young children and has been extrapolated to cover infancy because of lack of more appropriate data.[53] However, several studies have indicated that this concentration may be too high.[8] Furthermore, there is growing opinion that the normative Hb distribution curve is not the same throughout the world.[56]

FERRITIN

Serum and erythrocyte ferritin concentrations reflect the level of storage iron.[12] Serum measurements are simpler and are the more common of the two tests.[48] Having been found to be directly proportional to the abundance of storage iron in normal subjects, serum ferritin concentration is used as a sensitive and specific index for iron deficiency. When used in combination with the measurement of Hb, serum ferritin distinguishes between the anemias of chronic disease and iron deficiency.

A low serum ferritin concentration is usually interpreted as depleted iron stores, but does not necessarily indicate systemic iron deficiency. Adequate iron for erythropoiesis can be maintained even in the presence of low stores, as occurs in frequent blood donors.[48] Once iron

Table 2 Cutoff Points by Age Used to Identify Abnormal Values of Iron Status Measures

Iron Measure	Age (yr)	Abnormal Values
Hemoglobin (g/L)*,†	0.5 to 5	<110
	5 to 11	<115
	12 to 15 (females)	<119
	12 to 15 (males)	<126
	16 to 19 (females)	<120
	16 to 19 (males)	<136
	Pregnant women	<110
Hematocrit*	0.5 to 5	<0.33
	5 to 11	<0.34
	12 to 13	<0.36
	Pregnant women	<0.33
Mean cell volume (fL)‡	1 to 3	<77
	3 to 5	<79
	6 to 11	<80
	11 to 14	<82
	15 to 74	<85
Serum ferritin (μg/L)†	1 to 25	<10
	6 to 16	<12
Transferrin Ssaturation (%)†	1 to 2	<10
	3 to 5	<12
	6 to 11	<14
	12 to 15	<14
	≥16	<15
Erythrocyte Protoporphrin (μmol/L RBCs)†	1 to 2	>1.42 (80 μg/dL RBCs)
	3 to 5	>1.24 (70 μg/dL RBCs)
	6 to 11	>1.24
	12 to 15	>1.24
	≥16	>1.24

*See reference 54.
†See reference 51.
‡See reference 55.

Table 3 Biochemical Indices for Measuring Iron Status

Indicator	Measurement	Advantages and Disadvantages	Factors That Affect Measurement
Bone marrow examination	Performed to judge the amount of hemosiderin in the reticulum cells; absence of stainable reticular iron is characteristic of latent iron deficiency; quantity of visible hemosiderin after staining with potassium ferrocyanide correlates well with the concentration of nonheme iron	Advantages High specificity for storage iron assessment Disadvantages Invasive technique; subjective nature (result depends on the skill of the investigator); requires a sufficient amount of available marrow stroma and a meticulous staining technique. Invasive and often painful. Not appropriate for children.	
Hemoglobin (Hb)	Hb is the protein molecule within red blood cells that carries oxygen; decreased concentration of Hb measures presence of anemia; most widely used test for IDA	Advantages Inexpensive; universally available Disadvantages Low sensitivity; low specificity	Diurnal variation, age, sex, race, pregnancy, high altitudes, other micronutrient deficiencies, parasitic infections, disease states
Hematocrit	Ratio of the volume of packed red blood cells to the total blood volume; indicator of the concentration of RBCs in the blood and impaired Hb formation; in presence of anemia decrease in red blood cells is observed	Advantages Inexpensive; requires a small sample volume; relatively fast analysis Disadvantages Sensitive to changes in plasma volume, as well as red cell volume; difficult to standardize because it is a calculated parameter	Measurement errors (poorly packed iron-deficient cells, improper mixing of blood because of intermittent blood flow, excessive anticoagulant in collection tube); elevated white blood cell counts; vitamin B_{12} deficiency, bleeding, kidney disease, cirrhosis of the liver, and malignancies; pregnancy
Mean cell volume (MCV)	Average volume of a red cell; calculated by dividing hematocrit (volume fraction) by red blood cell count (10^2/L)	Advantages Inexpensive; fairly specific indicator of iron deficiency once thalassemia and the anemia of chronic disease have been excluded	Chronic inflammation, certain hemoglobinopathies, lead poisoning, age, race
Mean cell Hb concentration (MCHC)	The average amount of Hb in the average red cell; determined by dividing Hb (g/L) by hematocrit (volume fraction)	Advantages Widely available; well established Disadvantages Late indicator; low specificity	Age
Red cell distribution width (RDW)	A measurement of the variability of red cell size; calculated by multiplying the standard deviation of mean cell volume by 100 and then dividing the product by the mean cell volum	Advantages More sensitive than serum iron, transferring (Tf) saturation, or serum ferritin level Disadvantages Low specificity; worthwhile when used in combination with other paramters	Age, micronutrient deficiencies, hemoglobinopathies
Serum iron	In fasting state serum iron levels reflect transit iron going from reticuloendothethlial system to the bone marrow	Advantages Sensitive to the stage of mild iron deficiency Disadvantages Wide diurnal variations; low specificity	Diurnal variation, age, sex, inflammation, chronic neoplastic diseases, blood loss or donation, pregnancy, with chronic infections, shock, pyrexia, rheumatoid arthritis, and malignancy
Total iron-binding concentration (TIBC)	Measures the extent to which iron-binding sites in the serum can be saturated; an indirect measurement of the amount of Tf in the blood	Disadvantages Low specificity; to properly understand a value for TIBC, one must also know the serum iron, the percent Tf saturation	Sex, age, oral contraceptives, infection, inflammation, chronic neoplastic diseases, liver disease
Tf saturation	Ratio of serum iron to iron-binding capacity; calculated by dividing serum iron (μmol/L) by TIBC (μmol/L) and multiplying the product by 100 to obtain a percentage	Advantages Most accurate indicator of iron supply to the bone marrow Disadvantages Wide diurnal variation and low specificity	Diurnal variation; oral contraceptives, infection, inflammation, chronic neoplastic diseases
Ferritin	Serum or plasma iron concentration reflects total amount of storage iron	Advantages Reliable and sensitive parameter for iron stores in healthy subjects; high specificity for iron deficiency Disadvantages Does not indicate the severity of the iron deficiency due to higher assay variability; acute phase reactant	Diurnal effect is minimal, age, sex, race, inflammatory diseases, infections, certain neoplastic diseases, and liver disorders
Zinc protoporphyrin (ZnPP); free erythrocyte protoporphyrin (FEP)	Zinc protoporphyrin is a product of disordered heme biosynthesis; about 90% of protoporphyrin in red blood cells is ZPP, while the remainder is present as FEP (not bound to zinc); testing method for ZPP measures both substances, and the results may be reported as either ZPP or FEP; elevated in the more advanced stage of iron-deficient erythropoiesis	Advantages Stability within the individual; easily measured using a hematofluorometer (which only a couple of drops of blood and minimal technical experience) Disadvantages Skin contamination may lead to false elevations; both test and blood lead values are needed for full evaluation; fluorescent substances in plasma may interfere with hematofluorometer results	Raised levels of EP found in subjects with lead poisoning and acquired defects in Hb synthesis

(Continued)

Table 3 Biochemical Indices for Measuring Iron Status *(Continued)*

Indicator	Measurement	Advantages and Disadvantages	Factors That Affect Measurement
Soluble transferrin receptor (sTfR)	Transferrin receptors (TfRs) are found on cell membranes and allow iron-bound Tf to enter the cell; an increase in serum receptor levels is seen in patients with iron-deficient erythropoiesis or iron-deficiency anemia	Advantages Remains normal in patients with acute or chronic inflammation or liver disease; effective in distinguishing iron-deficiency anemia from anemia of chronic disease Disadvantages Lack of standardization for assay and reference values; expensive assay cost	Hematologic disorders associated with expansion of erythroid marrow

stores have been completely exhausted, the concentration of serum ferritin no longer reflects the severity of iron deficiency. The absence of iron stores may not be associated with any adverse functional implications and should therefore only be regarded as a risk factor for the development of iron-deficiency anemia (IDA).[19]

The most important limitation of ferritin is its acute-phase response, which can mask an otherwise iron-depletion state in clinical conditions such as infection, inflammation, and malignancy.[48] To overcome this limitation, simultaneous measurement of a biomarker of the acute-phase response such as C-reactive protein and screening for the presence of malaria parasites should be conducted.[19]

The cutoff value for serum ferritin indicating depleted iron stores that is most commonly used is 12 μg/L; however, the appropriate cutoff value that is indicative of depleted iron stores in neonates and infants, with their rapidly changing erythropoietic activity, is still under discussion.[48] Current WHO cutoffs, including those for serum ferritin, are based on populations with an unknown prevalence of infection. Research in Honduras and Sweden established cutoffs at 9 μg/L at 6 months of age and at 5 μg/L at 9 months of age to define depleted iron stores. Some authors use the cutoff of 10 μg/L for infants and young children, which is based on the distribution of serum ferritin concentrations in a large survey in the United States (NHANES III), in which the fifth percentile indicated abnormal values.[8]

TRANFERRIN RECEPTOR

Soluble TfR (sTfR), a critical iron-binding protein in iron metabolism, has only recently been added to the available screening tests for iron deficiency. Using sensitive immunological assays, Kohgo et al (1986) were the first to detect small amounts of a TfR-like protein in human serum.[57] The TfR reflects the degree of deficiency in functional iron after iron stores have been depleted.[48] Inclusion of serum TfR in the determination of iron status is recommended because it can distinguish anemia of chronic disease from IDA in the presence of chronic infection or inflammation.[19] This noteworthy advantage contrasts with other biochemical tests for iron status, which are influenced by anemia of chronic disease. It should be emphasized that the sTfR cannot be used in isolation of other laboratory measurements to identify IDA in anemic patients, because it is also elevated in hematologic disorders associated with expansion of the erythroid marrow.[58]

Certain conditions affecting erythropoiesis such as hematological disorders (eg, sickle cell anemia, autoimmune hemolytic anemia, thalassemia) and nutritional deficiencies other than iron (eg, folate, vitamin B_{12}) may confound the diagnosis of iron deficiency since they have been demonstrated to raise sTfR concentration.[58] Hemolysis associated with malaria may elevate sTfR concentration and confuse the detection of iron deficiency, although the magnitude of this effect remains unknown.

A major laboratory issue that remains unsolved is the lack of proper standardization for the sTfR assay: There are several commercial assays available for sTfR, but no common reference material.[59] Over the past decade, a number of laboratories have developed different assays for measuring sTfR concentration and have explored its normal range. The normal range for sTfR reported in the literature varies considerably.[48] To date, there are no standards for measuring sTfR. The ratio of soluble transferrin receptor (sTfR) to serum ferritin (R/F ratio) has been shown to perform well in estimating body iron stores.[59] Further research is needed regarding age-appropriate cutoffs and the standardization of laboratory techniques such as the use of anticoagulant, blood collection methods, time delay between blood collection and centrifugation, incubation time, and the extent to which samples have to be diluted.[59]

IRON DEFICIENCY

In the World Health Report 2002 ("Reducing Risks, Promoting Healthy Life") nutritional iron deficiency was identified as one of the 10 leading risk factors for disease, disability, and death in the world today, with an impact greater than that of either zinc or vitamin A deficiency.[60] An estimated 2 billion people are affected, most of whom live in developing countries.[61]

While it is well recognized that iron deficiency is the single most common nutritional disorder worldwide and the leading cause of anemia during infancy, childhood, and pregnancy,[62] obtaining accurate estimates of its prevalence has proven to be a challenging task. Lack of national data and a single, inexpensive, and easy to use indicator of iron status are just two of the many hurtles in assessing the prevalence of iron deficiency and its anemia.[63]

In 1985, DeMaeyer and Adiels-Tegman published a landmark paper in which they compiled global data from large studies.[64] The data presented in that paper has constituted the core database for global prevalence estimates of anemia and IDA. Nutritional anemia was considered to be a large component of global anemia prevalence, and iron deficiency was considered the most common cause of nutritional anemia.[64] IDA was determined to be the most prevalent nutritional deficiency in the world affecting about 25% of all infants, especially in developing countries.[64] In the United States, data from the National Health and Nutrition Examination Survey III (1988 to 1994) found the prevalence of iron deficiency to be 9% in toddlers aged 1 to 2 years, 9% in adolescent females, and 11% in women.[51]

DEFINITION

Broadly defined, iron deficiency is a condition in which there is a lack of cellular iron to tissues.[28] Iron deficiency represents a spectrum of mild to severe forms characterized by the presence or absence of physiological, biochemical, hematological, and functional changes. Therefore, various definitions of iron deficiency have been formulated. The development of IDA is commonly thought of as a progression of three successive stages.[65]

The first-stage iron depletion (ID) is characterized by a mobilization of storage iron. A fall in serum iron reflects the progressive reduction of storage iron in the liver; however, the supply of iron to the functional compartment remains uncompromised. Levels of transport iron and Hb remain normal.

The second-stage iron-deficient erythropoiesis (IDE) involves a decrease in transport iron resulting in low levels of serum ferritin and serum Tf saturation and elevated levels of serum-TfR and free erythrocyte protoporphyrin (FEP).[66] This stage is commonly referred to as iron deficiency without anemia. The iron supply required for full maturation of erythropoietic cells is markedly reduced; however, mature red blood cells stay unaffected. Hb concentrations usually remain within in the normal range, although they may decrease slightly. Unlike IDA, in which iron stores are totally absent, IDE can occur with normal or increased amounts of storage iron resulting from the impaired release of iron to the plasma from the storage iron compartment.[45]

IDA is the third and final stage. IDA develops when the supply of transport iron decreases to the point where Hb synthesis is restricted. During this stage iron stores are exhausted, circulating levels of iron are declining, and microcytic, hypochromic anemia is evident. A restricted supply of iron to the bone marrow causes a reduction in the concentration of Hb in the red blood cells and an observable decline in hematocrit and red cell indices.

ETIOLOGY

The etiology of iron deficiency can be categorized into either physiological or pathological causes.[45] Physiological causes relate to a disparity between iron requirements, and the maximum absorption of iron from the diet.[67] Nutritional iron deficiency, a term that has been widely used to describe conditions where the diet cannot cover physiologic iron requirements is the most common cause of iron deficiency worldwide.[45] Segments of the population at risk for not meeting high iron requirements during periods of rapid growth include infants, adolescents, and childbearing females.[45] Impaired absorption of iron can occur in patients with achlorhydria and who have undergone gastric surgery. Gluten enteropathy is also associated with IDA, especially in young patients.[40]

Pathological iron deficiency results from excessive blood loss, which usually occurs in the GI tract.[45] In clinical practice a diagnosis of iron deficiency includes a search for pathologic causes of blood loss (eg, tumors in the gastrointestinal tract or uterus, especially if uterine bleedings have increased or changed in regularity). Blood loss can occur from chronic use of aspirin or other nonsteroidal antiinflammatory drugs or parasitic infestations (ie, hookworm).[40]

RISK FACTORS

Iron deficiency can arise from several risk factors, alone or in combination. Examples from the range of possible risk factors include (1) inadequate iron supply, (2) increased iron requirements imposed by growth, and (3) increased iron losses (Table 4).

Table 4 Main Factors Negatively Influencing Iron Balance According to Life Stage

Birth	Infancy	Childhood and Adolescence
Before birth	0 to 6 months	Antacid therapy
Maternal iron deficiency	Low/depleted body iron stores	Low dietary iron supply
Intrauterine growth retardation	Rapid weight gain	Low dietary iron availability
At birth	Blood loss due to frequent sampling	Intense physical activity
Low body iron stores at birth	Blood loss due to cow milk feeding	Adolescent pregnancy
Early onset of postnatal erythropoiesis	6 to 12 mo	Loss or dysfunction of absorptive enterocytes
Rapid postnatal catch-up growth	Low/depleted iron stores	Bowel resection
Low birth weight	Rapid weight gain	Celiac disease
Premature birth	Blood loss due to cow milk feeding	Intrinsic enterocyte defects
Fetal-maternal hemorrhage	Low dietary iron supply	Gastrointestinal blood loss: epistaxis, varices, gastritis, ulcer, tumor, Meckel's diverticulum, parasitosis, vascular malformations, inflammatory bowel disease, diverticulosis, hemorrhoids, menorrhagia, cancer, chronic infection, pulmonary hemosiderosis, trauma, excessive phlebotomy, large vascular malformations
Perinatal hemorrhage	Low dietary iron availability	
Twin-to-twin transfusion	Prolonged exclusive breast-feeding	
Umbilical cord preclamping	Frequent infections	
Phlebotomy losses		
Restrictive RBC transfusion practice		
Recombinant erythropoietin administration (preterm infants)		

Inadequate iron supply can be the consequence of low iron stores or low iron in the diet. At birth, low iron stores can result from low birth weight, perinatal bleeding, early clamping of umbilical cord, and maternal iron deficiency. Low birth weight influences iron stores in a linear proportion; a newborn weighing 1,500 has roughly half the iron content of a 3,000 g well-grown term newborn.[30] The preterm infants (born before 32 weeks' gestation) encounter low body iron stores because they miss out on the accretion of iron during last trimester of pregnancy.[29] In addition, preterm infants are at increased risk of iron deficiency from postnatal practices such as uncompensated phlebotomy losses, administration of recombinant human erythropoietin (rhEpo), and inadequate iron supplementation.[29] The timing of the clamping of the umbilical cord at delivery has been shown to impact the amount of blood transferred to the infant.[68] The timing of umbilical cord clamping depends on whether the cord is clamped early (less than a minute), intermediately (one to three minutes), or late (after pulsations cease). For example, if the cord is not cut until pulsations cease, the infants will receive a 20 to 30 mL/kg body weight transfusion, which is the equivalent to approximately 30 to 35 mg of additional iron.[68] To put this amount of iron into perspective, this is the equivalent to the amount of iron in 100 L of human milk.[68]

Maternal iron deficiency has been shown to affect infant iron stores and iron status. It was previously held that infants acted as parasites with respect to sequestering iron from their mother in utero. However, current evidence suggests that maternal iron stores over a wide range determine iron stores in the neonate [69–73] and that even moderate degrees of maternal ID (Hb 85 to 100 g/L) may result in lower body iron stores during infancy in the offspring.[74] In developing countries, maternal ID (Hb < 85 g/L) affects 30 to 50% of pregnancies and is arguably the most common cause of perinatal iron deficiency.[29]

Nutritional iron deficiency results from reduced dietary iron and/or low bioavailability of dietary iron. Despite the high bioavailability of the iron in human milk, human milk contains very little iron; thus, iron stores in the exclusively breast-fed infant will ultimately be depleted after 6 months of age.[75] If human milk remains the only food source, IDA will ultimately develop. The choice of complementary foods will markedly influence the risk of iron deficiency and anemia. Unfortunately, in developing countries typical home-prepared grain or rice-based complementary foods are poor sources of iron and may contain phytic acid, which is a potent inhibitor of iron absorption. For example, per 100 g, unfortified rice-based complementary foods contain 1 mg of iron and maize and wheat-based complementary foods contain 0.8 mg of iron.[76]

Adolescents at risk for nutritional iron deficiency include those on a restrictive diet, suffering from an unhealthy body image or practicing vegetarianism (restrictive intake of heme iron sources).[75] Many adolescent girls inadvertently limit iron intake by trying to control their weight or by passing through temporary periods of vegetarianism because of concerns for animal welfare.[77] Women who conceive during or shortly after adolescence are at increased risk for entering pregnancy with low or absent iron stores and subsequently developing iron deficiency during pregnancy.[37] The available data on iron intake in adolescents suggest that adolescent girls are unlikely to acquire substantial iron stores during this time period because intakes may average as little as 10 to 11 mg iron/d.[37] The bioavailability from diets in developing and industrialized countries indicates that a negative iron balance is likely in many female populations.

An important and common risk factor for ID is increased iron requirements imposed by growth. During the first 2 years of life, infants require relatively large amounts of iron due to their high growth rate. On average, during the first year of life, the birth weight and blood volume of the full-term, normal-birth-weight infant will triple.[78] In the postnatal period preterm infants are at risk of ID because of rapid growth rates, uncompensated iron losses from phlebotomy, and low nascent iron stores.[30] Other periods of high iron requirements include the growth spurt during adolescence and pregnancy. Iron requirements during adolescent pregnancies are particularly high because girls in their teens may not have reached their full growth.[12]

Iron deficiency can also result from increased iron losses. In young women of childbearing age menstrual blood loss (both "heaviness" and duration) can be a major determinant of iron status.[79] In infants, causes of considerable iron loss include blood sampling, birth weight, initial Hb concentration, the total amount of blood transfused, and weight-gain rate.[30] Since the majority of fetal iron is present as Hb, any blood loss that lowers neonatal Hb concentration (including twin-to-twin transfusion and fetal-maternal hemorrhage, perinatal hemorrhage, considerable blood draws after birth) will have an impact on iron balance.[30] Gastrointestinal bleeding is a common cause of increased iron loss in infancy. Gastrointestinal bleeding can result from food allergies, repeated episodes of acute diarrhea, or *Helicobacter pylori* infections.[62] In tropical areas, gastrointestinal bleeding may be due to infestation with parasites such as hookworm and hemoglobinuria due to malaria.[80] Occult gastrointestinal bleeding among formula-fed infants because of cow's milk protein sensitization or among healthy infants owing to feeding with fresh cow's milk commonly results in negative iron balance in the first year of life.[30] The precise cause of blood loss is not well understood but is likely to be an allergic-type reaction between aprotein in cow's milk and enterocytes of the GI tract.[33] Increased fecal blood loss in response to cow's milk is more common among infants who were breast-fed early in life than in infants who were never breast-fed.[30] Earlier exposure to cow's milk proteins may sensitize infants who are predisposed to allergy.[81]

CONSEQUENCES OF IRON DEFICIENCY

Clinical sequelae of iron deficiency include impaired cognitive performance, anemia, poor immune function, and decreased work performance.[82] In children, numerous studies have consistently demonstrated that even moderate anemia (Hb < 100 g/L) is associated with depressed mental and motor development in children.[83–85] Although the mechanism whereby iron influences development is not fully understood, older research identified the role of iron in central nervous system neurotransmitter function, and more recent work has shown that brain iron is essential for normal myelinization.[86–88]

Longitudinal studies have indicated that children who were anemic in early childhood continue to have poor cognitive and motor development and depressed school achievement into middle childhood.[85] For anemic children less than 2 years of age, there is no good evidence from randomized controlled trials that iron treatment helps their cognitive and motor development.[83] For children above 2 years of age, short-term treatment is associated with improvement in cognition but not in school achievement.

The study of cognitive function and iron status has been extended to older children and adolescents. In a randomized controlled trial, adolescent girls with depleted iron stores who received iron supplements improved their scores on a test of memory and verbal learning compared with the placebo-treated group.[89] Another large study in preadolescents and adolescents described an association between iron status and standardized mathematics scores.[90] Those with IDA or iron deficiency without anemia were 2.3 and 2.4 times more likely to have low mathematics scores than those with no iron deficiency. The authors of this report suggested that screening for iron deficiency might be warranted for all children and adolescents.

During pregnancy, the negative implications of anemia caused by iron deficiency alone or in combination with other factors, for example, folate deficiency, vitamin A deficiency, and malaria, include increased risk of preterm delivery and infant low birth weight (LBW).[91–94] There is some evidence to suggest an association between a higher risk of maternal mortality and severe anemia.[74,95] However, data were predominantly retrospective observations of maternal Hb concentrations at, or close to, delivery and subsequent mortality.[74] Furthermore, the iron deficiency component of this relationship is unknown.[80] Mechanisms by which IDA could increase maternal mortality needs to be elucidated.

Increased risk of maternal mortality has also been shown in women with severe anemia.[95] Children born to adolescent mothers are more likely to be of poor health and have a higher likelihood of infant mortality.[95] Concern for the health of young mothers and their infants has led to suggestions that adolescence may be an ideal time to optimize iron status and prevent iron deficiency during pregnancy.[96]

Rapid expansion of maternal blood volume and red cell mass during pregnancy and placental and fetal growth leave many women, even in developed countries, with low iron stores and tissue iron deficiency at parturition.[97] The consequences of poor maternal iron status postpartum is increasingly being recognized as a nonbenign condition, shown to be related to maternal fatigue, depression, and ability to care and nurture offspring.[98–100]

PREVENTION

In light of accumulating evidence regarding the adverse effects of IDA on maternal and infant outcomes, prevention rather than treatment is highly recommended. If implemented successfully, there are three interventions that are likely to prevent anemia. These include dietary diversification to foods with more bioavailable iron, fortification of foods targeted to full-term infants and children, and iron supplementation.

DIET

For infants 0 to 6 months, it is assumed that iron provided by human milk is adequate to meet iron needs of infants exclusively fed human milk from birth through 6 months.[101,102] Milk iron composition is unaffected by maternal iron intake or status.[103] While human milk iron content is low (0.2 to 0.4 mg/L), it is highly bioavailable (45 to 100%) compared to infant formula (10%).[30,33] Since the average iron concentration in human milk is 0.35 mg/L, the adequate intake level is 0.27 mg/d (0.78 L/d × 0.35 mg/L).[33] However, even after taking a high estimate of iron absorption from human milk (50%) into consideration and assuming an iron intake of 0.075 mg/kg/d from human milk, it is estimated that term infants will absorb less than 0.04 mg/kg/d.[104] Since this iron intake is less than the amount required for growth, storage iron will be depended upon until dietary iron increases. After 6 months of age, the introduction of iron-fortified cereals may support normal iron status; therefore, it is recommended that iron-fortified formulas and cereals be introduced once exclusive breast-feeding has stopped. The iron content of preterm milk is approximately 0.5 mg/L.[29] Because preterm infants are at high risk for iron deficiency, the major contributing factor being the lack of iron accretion during the last trimester, preterm infants exclusively fed human milk are recommended to take 2 to 4 mg/kg per day of elemental iron supplementation from 2 to 12 months.[105,106]

In contrast to human milk, cow's milk iron is low in both concentration (around 0.4 mg/L) and bioavailability, because of the high calcium and phosphorus and low ascorbic acid content of cow's milk.[30] Cow's milk and cow's milk formulas unfortified with iron cannot supply the infant with sufficient amounts of iron to maintain an optimal iron balance during the first 6 months of life.[30] Introduction of cow's milk is not recommended for ingestion by infants until 9 months of age according to the Canadian Pediatrics Society, or 12 months of age according to the American Academy of Pediatrics (AAP).[101,107]

The WHO (2000) recommends introducing iron-rich complementary foods at 6 months of age to meet iron needs.[108] For infants over the age of 6 months dietary diversification is recommended as an intervention strategy for preventing iron deficiency. Dietary diversification involves promotion of a diet with a wider variety of naturally iron-containing foods, especially red meat, poultry, fish, and food rich in vitamin C. The selection of weaning foods determines in large part whether an infant will be at risk of developing iron deficiency and associated anemia.[109] Typical homemade complementary foods used in developing countries are poor sources of bioavailable iron and, thus, are inadequate to meet infants' high iron requirements for rapid growth and blood volume expansion.[110]

Estimates for dietary iron requirements for infants over the age of 6 months are feasible and desirable to model using the factorial components of absorbed iron requirements. Two major factors were taken into consideration when determining the iron requirements. The first was the iron need of the individual and the second was the bioavailability of iron in the diet. Four major components of iron need were assessed for infants aged 7 to 12 months and children aged 1 to 8 years: obligatory fecal, urinary, and dermal losses; the increase in Hb mass; the increase in tissue iron; and the increase in storage iron. It was noted that building a small reserve is seen as important in very young children. The type of iron, heme or nonheme, and other dietary factors influence iron bioavailability in the diet. The diets of infants contain little meat and are therefore low in heme iron. Because their diets are high in cereals and vegetables, the diets were considered to have a medium iron bioavailability of 10%.[75] The bioavailability of iron in diets of children over the age of 1 year was determined to be 18%.[75] The recommended dietary allowance for iron (mg/d) is 11 (6 to 12 months), 7 (1 to 3 years), and 10 (4 to 8 years) (Table 5).

The estimated adequate requirement for children and adolescents ages 9 through 18 years was determined by factorial modeling of the median components of iron requirements.[33] The physiological processes associated with puberty that have a major impact on iron requirements are the growth spurt in both sexes, menarche in girls, and the major increase in Hb concentrations in boys. Total iron requirements for adolescent boys are computed from increased iron requirements required for the expansion of the total blood volume and the increase in the lean body mass. The increase in mean total iron requirements may exceed 1.8 mg/d or more than double those requirements of preadolescent males.[32] Iron requirements for adolescent girls include the amount of iron lost in menses beyond the growth requirements. In female adolescents, the recommended dietary allowance (RDA) increases from 8 mg Fe/d for those 9 to 13 years of age to 15 mg Fe/d for those 14 to 18 years of age (Table 5).

Table 5 Recommended Dietary Allowance (RDA) of Iron for Both Sexes from Birth to 18 Years[33]

Age	RDA for Total Iron Intake (mg/d)
0 to 6 mo	0.27
6 to 12 mo	11
1 to 3 yr	7
4 to 8 yr	10
9 to 13 yr	8
14 to 18 yr	11 for boys; 15 for girls
Pregnancy	27
Breast-feeding mothers under the age of 19 yr	10

FORTIFICATION

There are three types of fortification strategies: mass fortification, open market fortification, and targeted fortification. Mass fortification refers to the addition of micronutrients to foods consumed by all or most of the population. Mass fortification is regulated by the government. Wheat flour has been fortified in Canada, the United Kingdom, and the United States since the 1940s. National fortification programs were also in place in Denmark until 1987 and in Sweden until 1994.[111] Wheat is the cereal flour that is fortified most often, but several countries—particularly in Central and South America—also have programs for iron fortification of maize flour.[111] In developing countries mass fortification programs of fish sauce (in Thailand and Vietnam), sugar (in Guatemala), curry powder (in South Africa), and soy sauce (in China) have shown improved iron status.[111]

Open market fortification refers to the initiative of a food manufacturer to fortify one or more products with the aim of improving both public health and product profitability. Open market fortification of several processed foods, particularly breakfast cereals, is widely practiced, primarily in industrialized countries. Fortification of staple foods is likely to increase iron intake for those who eat the most (ie, adult males). However, infants and children who have a limited capacity to eat large quantities of food are not likely to benefit significantly from this strategy.

Targeted fortification (eg, infant formula and infant cereals) describes the specifically directed fortification of foods consumed by high-risk groups. Targeted fortification provides an excellent source of iron to those who need it the most. Infant cereals, for example, typically contain 7.1 mg of iron per 15 g serving, and breakfast cereals for children contain over 4 mg of iron per 30 g serving.[44] A single 30 g serving of these "ready-to-eat" cereals provides 60% of the RDA for children aged between 1 and 3 years, 45% of the RDA for children aged 4 to 8 years, and 75% for boys and girls aged 9 to 13 years. For adolescents, especially those who are restricting their total food intake or who are vegetarians, the use of iron-fortified breakfast cereals that typically contain 4 to 8 mg/iron per serving is an excellent way to prevent anemia. In fact, ready-to-eat cereals are among the top contributors to iron, folate, vitamin A and C, and zinc intakes.[112]

The AAP and Canadian Paediatric Society (1991) reviewed the role of commercial formulas in infant feeding and concluded that infants who are not, or only partially, fed human milk should receive an iron-fortified formula. The AAP recommends 2 to 4 mg/kg of iron per day up to a maximum of 15 mg/d of iron per day by the time the infant is 2 months old.[101] This may be offered as an iron-fortified formula or iron supplement. Iron-fortified formula will provide approximately 2 mg/kg/d if the infant's energy intake from formula is adequate. Most infants, including very low birth weight (VLBW) infants, should be offered formulas with iron at the time formula is introduced.

Term infants who are exclusively breast-fed do not need supplemental iron until they are 6 months of age. If solid foods are introduced earlier, they should contain an adequate amount of iron. After 6 months of age, breast-fed infants should receive extra iron in the form of iron-fortified infant cereals and other iron-rich foods. These infants should be offered an iron-fortified infant formula after they have been weaned from breast milk. Term infants who are not breast-fed should be given an iron-fortified infant formula from birth. Studies are still under way to determine the optimal iron content of these formulas, and further studies are encouraged. Until the results are known, the use of currently available iron-fortified formulas seems appropriate.

For premature infants, an iron supplement should be started by at least 8 weeks of age and continued until the first birthday.[105,106] Iron-fortified formula for bottle-fed infants or commercial iron drops for breast-fed infants are the recommended source of supplemental iron. Iron concentrations of iron-fortified formulas range from 10 to 12 mg/L in the United States and between 4 and 7 mg/L in Europe.[141] The dose, route, and commencement of supplementation to prevent ID in preterm infants is incompletely understood and hotly debated.[29]

IRON SUPPLEMENTS

Another approach for preventing or treating iron deficiency is through supplementation of individuals or communities at risk. This approach would be implemented for the treatment of individuals with anemia or in situations where at-risk communities of infants and young children do not have ready access to targeted iron-fortified foods. Global guidelines for iron supplementation have been published by the Nutritional Anemia Consultative Group/World Health Organization/UNICEF.[113] For children 6 to 24 months of age 12.5 mg/d of iron is recommended, in tandem with 50 μg/d of folic acid until 12 months of age. Recommendations for children and adolescents are as follows: 20 to 30 mg/d for children 2 to 5 years old; 30 to 60 mg/d for children 6 to 11 years old; 60 mg/d for adolescents and adults (plus 400 μg/d of folic acid for childbearing aged females); 60 mg/d in addition to 400 μg/d of folic acid for pregnant women, continuing for 3 months of lactation where anemia prevalence is high (>40%).

The most common form of iron in iron tablets is ferrous sulfate; however, fumarate and gluconate are also used. Infants are most commonly supplemented with a liquid formulation. When a soluble form of iron (such as ferrous sulfate or fumarate) is ingested in the proper dose, this intervention is efficacious. However, adherence to long-term ingestion of oral iron drops is often poor because of the unpleasant metallic taste of drops; drops can stain a baby's teeth unless wiped off immediately after use, and if the dose is high, the infant may complain of abdominal discomfort.

In many women, it is uncertain whether diet alone can provide the additional iron needs of pregnancy.[114] The need for iron supplementation during pregnancy is actively debated.[115–117] Most studies in pregnant women supplemented with iron show a change in total blood volume of $<45\%$, with an increase in plasma volume of $<50\%$ and an increase in red blood cell mass of $<35\%$.[36] While controlled trials of iron supplementation during pregnancy have consistently demonstrated positive effects on maternal iron status at delivery, the impact of iron supplementation in reducing factors that are associated with maternal anemia, that is, increased risk of preterm delivery and infant LBW, is less clear.[92]

A Cochrane systematic review on iron supplementation during pregnancy concluded that there were insufficient data on which to draw conclusions on the effects of iron supplementation during pregnancy, beneficial or harmful, on outcomes for the mother or her offspring.[118] However, two large double-blinded, placebo-controlled randomized trials conducted in Nepal have since found a significant impact of early iron supplementation during pregnancy on LBW, as defined as $<2{,}500$ g.[119–121]

Currently, iron supplements are almost universally prescribed for pregnant women. In developed countries, pregnant women are recommended to take 27 mg of iron daily.[33] For iron supplementation programs where anemia prevalence is high, the International Nutritional Anemia Consultative Group has recently changed its recommendation from 120 to 60 mg/d. However, if duration of iron supplementation during pregnancy is short, or if anemia is present, 120 mg/d is still recommended. The administration of iron supplements weekly instead of daily in humans (in which gut mucosal turnover occurs every 5 to 6 days) is being actively investigated as a viable means of controlling iron deficiency in populations, including pregnant women.[37]

When considering iron supplements, attention should be paid to possible interactions between iron and nutrients. Iron deficiency impairs vitamin A and iodine metabolism and may hinder the effectiveness of interventions aimed at improving these deficiencies.[122] A direct relationship has been found between Hb and serum retinol concentrations.[123] Dietary deficiencies of vitamin A and iron frequently coexist in developing countries and vitamin A deficiency appears to affect iron transport and red blood cell production.[123] Effects have not been demonstrated in vitamin A–sufficient subjects.[123] Studies in anemic children and pregnant women in regions with endemic vitamin A deficiency have shown improved iron status post vitamin A supplementation.[62] Due to the anti-infective properties of vitamin A, it has been suggested that the benefits of vitamin A on iron status may be a result of reduced level of infection.[62]

Some concern has been raised regarding the potential adverse effects of food iron supplements on zinc nutrition. While reduced absorption of one of the metals may occur when solutions of inorganic iron and zinc are administered, there appears to be little support for a significant effect when the metals are given with food in doses that are considered optimal for fortification.[123]

The interaction between iron and infection has been a continuing debate, largely due to associations between iron treatment and exacerbations of infection, in particular malaria.[124] A review of 13 randomized controlled trials determined that the known benefits of iron supplementation likely outweighs the risk of adverse effects in regions where malaria is endemic.[125] However, the results of two large-scale randomized controlled trials designed to evaluate the impact of iron and zinc supplementation on mortality and morbidity in young children found that iron supplementation may be associated with adverse effects in areas where malaria transmission is high.[126,127] Following these two trials, recommendations were made to target supplementation of iron and folic acid to children who are anemic or iron deficient and to provide children with concurrent protection from malaria and other infectious diseases.[128,129] To date no studies of oral iron supplementation have shown deleterious effects in nonmalarious or low-transmission malaria regions.[124,127,129]

IRON OVERLOAD

Iron toxicity is related to the generation of free radicals. Normally enzymes such as superoxide dismutase, glutathione peroxidase, and catalase metabolize and neutralize free radicals. Free iron has the ability to generate oxidative radicals that damage lipids, proteins, and DNA. Normal and pathological cellular processes produce superoxide (O_2^-) and hydrogen peroxide (H_2O_2) by-products. The redox capabilities of iron underlie its toxicity. The one-electron reduction of dioxygen by Fe^{2+} results in superoxide formation, which in turn, leads to the well-known Haber–Fenton sequence generating hydroxyl radical OH^{-2}:

$$Fe^{2+} + O_2 \rightarrow Fe^{3+} + O_2^-$$
$$2O_2^- + 2H^+ \rightarrow H_2O_2 + O_2$$
$$Fe^{2+} + H_2O \rightarrow OH^{\cdot} + OH^- + Fe^{3+}$$

The hydroxyl radical ($HO^{\cdot}$), perhaps the most powerful oxidant encountered in biological systems, can inactivate enzymes, cause DNA strand breaks, depolymerize polysaccharides, and initiate chain-propagating lipid peroxidation.[130]

The body's innate mechanisms for preventing tissue damage from free radical formation are to keep iron chelated during most absorption and distribution phases, keep iron in a trivalent redox state, and to store iron as ferritin.[5] Tissue iron loading occurs in two characteristic patterns. One type of tissue iron loading occurs when the amount of available plasma iron exceeds the iron-binding capacity of Tf, thus requiring parenchymal cells of liver to avidly take up iron. As iron overload progresses, iron is accumulated in cardiac myocytes, pancreatic acinar cells, and other cells of the body.[15] A different pattern of tissue iron loading occurs when iron overload results from increased catabolism of erythrocytes, such as is often the case in patients with repeat blood transfusions. Iron first accumulates in reticuloendothelial macrophages and only later deposits in parenchymal cells. Parenchymal iron loading leads to tissue damage and fibrosis. The reticuloendothelial system is generally a safe sink for iron because reticuloendothelial macrophages sequester iron and attenuate its activity.

EXCESS IRON INTAKE

There is no evidence that large iron stores provide a benefit to the individual. Although there is concern that high daily intake of iron may cause decreased absorption of competing minerals, prooxidant effects, and aggravating symptoms in diseases in which iron absorption is increased,[8] there are no clinical studies that have demonstrated negative prooxidant effects of iron in healthy term infants. The decision to select 60 mg/d as the lowest observed adverse effect level (LOAEL) was based on a study that found a significantly increased risk of constipation, higher rates of gastric pain and diarrhea, and more total gastrointestinal symptoms (nausea, gastric pain, constipation, and diarrhea) compared to placebo.[131]

IRON POISONING

Well-described cases of iron poisoning first appeared in publication in the 1940s and 1950s.[132] Classic animal experiments were conducted in the 1950s and 1960s and the chelator deferoxamine, used as an antidote for iron poisoning, was introduced in the 1960s. Almost all deaths from iron poisonings are in children under 3 years of age, resulting from ingestion of adult iron preparations (30 to 40 pills). However, deaths after exposure to as few as 5 pills have been reported.[133] Despite a vast number of exposures to iron-containing products, deaths rarely occur.[132] Hospitalization due to iron poisoning is an infrequent occurrence; the hospitalization rate among children aged 0 to 4 years has been estimated at 8.7 per 100,000 children.[134–136]

It is currently unknown how the highly regulated process of iron absorption is affected during iron overdose.[137] Rapid absorption occurs through intact intestinal mucosa. In volunteer studies, a peak serum iron is observed

Table 6 Stages of Acute Iron Toxicity[132]

Stage 1: Local gastrointestinal (GI) effects	Usually occurs within several hours
	Nausea, vomiting, diarrhea
	GI bleeding may lead to hematemesis or blood diarrhea
Stage II: Quiescent phase	Resolution of GI symptoms
	Rarely seen today because children presenting with Stage I would receive fluid resuscitation and chelation therapy
Stage III: Systemic toxicity	Hypovolemic shock and acidosis
	Hypoperfusion- pallor, cold extremities, tachycardia, and tachypnea
	Hypotension may be a late finding
	Myocardial dysfunction may be seen in severe iron poisoning
Stage IV: Recovery	Begins after initiation of fluid and antidotal therapy
Stage V: Gastrointestinal obstruction	Gastric and pyloric strictures (frequently require surgical therapy)
	May occur 2 to 8 wk after initial injury

within several hours of ingestion of supratherapeutic oral doses.[132] The clinical manifestations of iron poisoning occur in progressive stages (Table 6). Clinical management of iron poisoning includes clinical evaluation, fluid resuscitation, laboratory evaluation, abdominal radiograph, chelation therapy, and gastrointestinal decontamination.[132]

GENETIC DISORDERS OF IRON OVERLOAD

Hemochromatosis refers to the accumulation of iron in tissue. Since the late nineteenth century hemochromatosis has been recognized as a distinct clinical syndrome.[138] In the 1930s a genetic predisposition for the disease was discovered; a single gene defect was found that leads to an inborn error of iron metabolism.[15] In 1976, a French physician named Marcel Simon and colleagues found that the genetic predisposition to hemochromatosis was closely linked to the human major histocompatibility complex.[3] This finding led to the positional cloning of the hemochromatosis gene 20 years later.[3] Since the discovery of the *HFE* gene, hematochromosis conditions have been classified as primary (genetic) hemochromatosis and secondary hemochromatosis.[16]

Hereditary hemochromatosis (HH) is an autosomal recessive trait most commonly seen in people of Northern European descent.[139] Several mutations of the *HFE* gene have been described. Two main point mutations are either homozygotes for a gene designated C282Y (tyrosine, Y, substitution for a cysteine, C, mutation at position 282) or heterozygotes with C282Y/H63D (aspartic acid for histidine).[15]

Compared to normal individuals, patients with HH absorb two to three times as much dietary iron.[15] The consequences of HH are severe; iron deposits first in hepatocytes and then in other parenchymal cells, including heart, pancreas, and adrenals.[140] Excess iron in affected tissues catalyzes oxidative damage, resulting in cirrhosis, hepatoma, cardiomyopathy, diabetes, hypogonadism, and arthritis.[140] Because iron accumulation occurs gradually, the effects of the disease remain undetected until middle age or later.[15] In middle age, patients often present with diabetes from iron damage to islet calls and skin pigmentation from increased corticotrophin secretion (ATCH) secondary to adrenal insufficiency. These features are often accompanied by liver and gonadal dysfunction. One of the dilemmas of HH is that only half of patients with genetic mutations for HH show evidence of iron overload.[16] Population screening for HH has not been supported, because the penetrance is very low.[138] Previous diagnosis depended on analysis of iron by liver biopsy, an expensive procedure not without risk; however, genetic testing has recently become available.[140] The most efficient approach to diagnose patients suspected to have the disease is to measure the serum Tf saturation and ferritin levels.[138]

Not all patients with familial hemochromatosis disorders have mutations in the *HFE* gene. A subgroup of patients with non-HFE hemochromatosis that are genetically predisposed to severe iron loading during the first three decades of life are those with juvenile hemochromatosis (Table 7). These patients develop iron overload in the same tissue patterns as patients with classical HFE-associated hemochromatosis but at an accelerated rate.[3] Another disorder not associated with mutations in *HFE* is neonatal hemochromatosis (Table 7). Characterized by siderotic liver failure in newborn infants, iron overload occurs in the myocardium and in pancreatic acinar cells.[3] It is not clear whether the disease occurs as a result of iron loading or some other insult to developing hepatocytes. While medical therapies have not proven to be effective, the lives of some patients have been prolonged after liver transplantation.[3]

There is a distinct iron overload disorder in sub-Saharan Africa. Previously termed "Bantu siderosis," African overload affects up to 10% of some rural populations.[15] African iron overload results from a predisposition to iron loading that is exacerbated by excessive intakes of dietary iron. Iron overload was observed in Africans who drank a traditional beer brewed in nongalvanized steel drums. However, since serious iron overload does not develop in all beer drinkers and not all patients with iron overload consume excessive amounts of beer, it is postulated that a currently unidentified gene may confer susceptibility to the disorder. African overload is not due to mutations in the *HFE* gene and is not linked to the HLA locus.[15] Moreover, the pattern of iron disposition differs from that seen in HH. In African iron overload, marked iron loading occurs in hepatocytes and in hepatic Kuffer cells.

The aim of treatment of iron storage diseases is to remove excess iron from the body. In patients with one of the forms of primary hemochromatosis (ie, HH) removal of excess iron is best achieved by phlebotomy.[138] Treatment of secondary hemochromatosis consists of administration of iron-chelating agents.[138]

SUMMARY

The primary role of iron, an essential nutrient for living organisms, is tissue oxygenation. The amount of iron in the body is determined by the regulation of iron absorption in the proximal small intestine. The rate of iron absorption is influenced by the diet, body iron stores, marrow erythropoietic activity, blood Hb concentration, blood oxygen content, and the presence of systemic inflammation. The most prevalent iron disorder is iron deficiency. Negative iron balance can occur from consuming a diet low in bioavailable iron, during periods of rapid growth (ie, infancy, adolescence, and pregnancy), from malabsorption secondary to pathological conditions associated with the proximal small bowel (eg, gluten-induced enteropathy) or excessive blood loss.

Iron deficiency has been identified as one of the ten leading risk factors for disease, disability, and death in the world today and the leading cause of anemia during infancy, childhood, and pregnancy. Consequences of iron deficiency include poor immune function and decreased work performance. In children, moderate anemia has been associated with depressed mental and motor development. Anemia during pregnancy has been associated with increased risk of preterm delivery and infant LBW. Preventive strategies for iron deficiency include dietary diversification of foods with more bioavailable iron, fortification (commercial or in the home) of foods targeted to full-term infants and children, and iron supplementation.

Iron deficiency remains the most prevalent nutritional disorder in the world especially among children and pregnant women in developing countries. Further research is needed to elucidate the pathophysiological mechanisms of iron absorption and body iron homeostasis and to develop specific and sensitive measures for detecting iron deficiency in large-scale studies. In order to increase the effectiveness of public health prevention and treatment strategies further efforts need to be made toward developing products which improve compliance, and toward improving health service delivery and partnerships between the public and private sectors.

Table 7 Diseases of Iron Metabolism

Disorder	Etiology	Characterization
Neonatal hemochromatosis	Uncertain if fibrosis is from iron overload or whether fibrosis leads to iron accumulation in remaining hepatocytes and shunting of iron to other tissues	Usually diagnosed at autopsy. Hepatic iron staining with variable total iron stores, liver fibrosis, and bile duct proliferation. Iron deposits also found in heart, kidney, pancreas, and mucosal salivary glands. The reticuloendothelial system relatively spared from iron overload. At birth liver already heavily fibrotic
Juvenile hemochromatosis	Autosomal recessive. Gene has been mapped to chromosome I; however, exact location of gene and its functional gene product are still being investigated	Phenotypically similar to HH. Onset is earlier than HH. Patients have hypogonadism, joint pain, and unexplained stomach pain and die of cardiac dysfunction
African iron overload (also termed Bantu siderosis)	Hypothesized to be related to increased dietary intake from using iron pots to dominant inheritance of an uncharacterized defect or to increased beer from nongalvanized iron brew pots	Liver macrophages and hepatocytes show increased iron loading, suggesting a defect in iron recirculation
Sideroblastic anemias	Involves first step of heme synthesis (catabolized by erythroid aminolevulinic acid-e-ALAS) and the last step of loading iron into the protoporphyrin ring	Accumulation of mitochrondrial iron, along with anemia
X-linked sideroblastic anemia	Missense mutation of the gene on the X chromosome for e-ALAS causes iron to accumulate in the mitochondria of developing red blood cells	Prevents red blood cells from making sufficient Hb. Signs and symptoms usually begin during the first three decades of life. Characteristic features include pale skin, fatigue, dizziness, and an enlarged spleen and liver. Heart disease, liver damage, and kidney failure are severe medical problems that can result from these increased levels of iron
X-linked sideroblastic anemia with ataxia	Mutation in the ATP-binding cassette 7 gene (ABC7) on the X chromosome	Distinct form of X-linked iron overload. Associated with onset of nonprogressive ataxia by early childhood. Anemia is microcytic and hypochromic
Pearson's syndrome	Maternal inheritance pointed to mutation in mitochrondrial DNA, with chromosomal deletions commonly described	Vacuolization of marrow precursors and exocrine pancreatic dysfunction. Anemia is diagnosed before 1 year of age with macrocytic red cells and low neutrophil and platelet counts. Patients are short and have malabsorption
Friedreich ataxia	Autosomal recessive disorder	Degeneration of the central and peripheral nervous system, cardiomyopathy, and diabetes. Iron accumulation has been detected in heart myocytes. Deficiency in protein fraxetin also observed. Reduced levels of fraxetin may lead to mitochondrial respiratory failure and cellular damage and death
Hallervorden–Spatz syndrome	Family studies reveal a linkage to chromosome 20	Iron accumulation is limited to central nervous system, especially the basal ganglia. Clinical signs include dystonia, rigidity, and dementia
Aceruloplasminemia	Several mutations in the ceruloplasmin gene on the short arm of chromosome 3 have been discovered in affected families	Iron accumulation is observed in the spleen, heart, kidney, thyroid, and retina

REFERENCES

1. Beard JL, Dawson H, Pinero DJ. Iron metabolism: A comprehensive review. Nutr Rev 1996;54:295–317.
2. Aisen P, Enns C, Wesslin-Resnick M. Chemistry and biology of eukaryotic iron metabolism. Int J Biochem Cell Biol 2001;33:940–59.
3. Andrews NC. Iron metabolism: Iron deficiency and iron overload. Annu Rev Genom Hum Genet 2000;1:75–98.
4. Wessling-Resnick M. Iron transport. Annu Rev Nutr 2000;20:129–51.
5. Conrad ME, Umbreit JM. Iron absorption and transport—An update. Am J Hematol 2000;64:287–98.
6. Fleming RE. Advances in understanding the molecular basis for the regulation of dietary iron absorption. Curr Opin Gastroenterol 2005;21:201–6.
7. McKie AT, Barrow D, Latunde-Dada GO, et al. An iron-regulated ferric reductase associated with the absorption of dietary iron. Science 2001;291:1755–9.
8. Aggett P, Agosttoni C, Axelsson I, et al. Iron metabolism and requirements in early childhood: Do we know enough? A commentary by the ESPGHAN Committee on Nutrition. J Pediatr Gastroenterol Nutr 2002;34:337–45.
9. Andrews NC, Fleming MD, Gunshin H. Iron transport across biologic membranes. Nutr Rev 1999;57:114–23.
10. Frazer DM, Anderson GJ. The orchestration of body iron intake: How and where do enterocytes receive their cues? Blood Cells Mol Dis 2003;30:288–97.
11. Roy CN, Enns CA. Iron homeostasis: New tales from the crypt. Blood 2000;96:4020–7.
12. Hallberg L, Hulthen L. Perspectives on iron absorption. Blood Cells Mol Dis 2002;29:562–73.
13. Anderson GJ, Frazer DM, McKie AT, et al. Mechanisms of haem and non-heme iron absorption: Lessons from inherited disorders of iron metabolism. BioMetals 2005;18:339–48.
14. Schneider BD, Leipold EA. Regulation of mammalian iron homeostasis. Curr Opin Clin Nutr Metab Care 2000;3:267–73.
15. Andrews NC. Disorders of iron metabolism. N Eng J Med 1999;341:1986–96.
16. Hagar W, Theil WC, Vichinsky EP. Diseases of iron metabolism. Pediatr Clin N Am 2002;49:893–909.
17. Miret S, Simpson RJ, McKie AT. Physiology and molecular biology of dietary iron absorption. Annu Rev Nutr 2003;23:283–301.
18. Andrews NC. Molecular control of iron metabolism. Best Pract Res Clin Haematol 2005;18:159–69.
19. Hallberg L. Perspectives on nutritional iron deficiency. Annu Rev Nutr 2001;21:1–21.
20. Bothwell TH, Cook CR, Cook J, Finch CE. Iron Metabolism in Man. Oxford, England: Blackwell Scientific; 1979.
21. Conrad ME, Umbreit JM. A concise review: Iron absorption—the mucin-mobilferrin-integrin pathway. A competitive pathway for metal absorption. Am J Hematol 1993;42:67–73.
22. Hallberg L, Hulthen L, Bentgsson C, et al. Iron balance in menstruating women. Eur J Clin Nutr 1995;49:200–7.
23. Green R, Charlton RW, Seftel H, et al. Body iron excretion in man: A collaborative study. Am J Med 1968;45:336–53.
24. Tondeur MC, Schauer CS, Christofides AL, et al. Determination of iron absorption from intrinsically labeled microencapsulated ferrous fumarate (sprinkles) in infants with different iron and hematologic status by using a dual-stable-isotope method. Am J Clin Nutr 2004;80:1436–44.
25. Finch C. Regulators of iron balance in humans. Blood 1994;84:1697–702.
26. Fleming RE, Bacon BR. Orchestration of iron homeostasis. N Eng J Med 2005;352:1741–4.
27. Frazer DM, Anderson GJ. Iron imports.I. Intestinal iron absorption and its regulation. Am J Physiol Gastrointest Liver Physiol 2005;289:631–5.
28. Thornburg KL, Jacobson SL, Giraud GD, Morton MJ. Hemodynamic changes in pregnancy. Semin Perinatol 2000;24:11–4.
29. Rao R, Georgieff MK. Perinatal aspects of iron metabolism. Acta Paediatr Suppl 2002;438:124–9.
30. Faldella G, Corvaglia L, Lanari M, Salvioli GP. Iron balance and iron nutrition in infancy. Acta Paediatr 2003;441:82–5.
31. Zlotkin S. Clinical nutrition: 8. The role of nutrition in the prevention of iron deficiency anemia in infants, children and adolescents. CMAJ 2003;168:59–63.
32. Beard JL. Iron requirements in adolescent females. J Nutr 2000;130:437S–9S.
33. National Research Council Food and Nutrition Board. Dietary reference intakes for vitamin A, vitamin K, arsenic, boron, chromium, copper, iodine, iron, manganese, molybdenum, nickel, silicon, vanadium, and zinc. Washington, DC: National Academy Press; 2001.
34. Fairweather-Tait S. Iron requirements and prevalence of iron deficiency in adolescents. An overview. In: Hallberg L, editor. Iron Nutrition in Health and Disease. London, UK: John Libbey & Co; 1996. p. 137–48.
35. Rossander-Hulthen L, Hallberg L. Prevalence of iron deficiency in adolescents. In: Hallberg L, editor. Iron Nutrition in Health and Disease. London: Libbey; 1996. p. 149–56.

36. Bothwell TH. Iron requirements in pregnancy and strategies to meet them. Am J Clin Nutr 2000;72:257S–64S.
37. Tapiero T, Gate L, Tew KD. Iron: Deficiencies and requirements. Biomed Pharmacother 2001;55:324–32.
38. Zijp IM, Korver O, Tijburg LB. Effect of tea and other dietary factors on iron absorption. Crit Rev Food Sci Nutr 2000;40:371–98.
39. United States Department of Agriculture. Nutrient Database for Standard Reference: Release 14. Beltsville, MD: Nutrient Data Laboratory, Human Nutrition Research Center of the Agricultural Research Service (ARS); 2001.
40. World Health Organization. Iron. In: Report of a joint FAO/WHO expert consultation, editor. Human Vitamin and Mineral Requirements. Bangkok, Thailand: FAO and WHO; 2002.
41. Hallberg L, Bjorn-Rasmussen E, Howard L, Rossander L. Dietary heme iron absorption. A discussion of possible mechanisms for the absorption-promoting effect of meat and for the regulation of iron absorption. Scand J Gastroenterol 1979;7:769–79.
42. Harris SS. The effect of calcium consumption on iron absorption and iron status. Nutr Clin Care 2002;5:231–5.
43. Teucher B, Olivares M, Cori H. Enhancers of iron absorption: Ascorbic acid and other organic acids. Nutr Res 2004;74:403–19.
44. Hallberg L, Brune M, Rossander L. Effect of ascorbic acid on iron absorption from different types of meals. Studies with ascorbic-acid-rich foods and synthetic ascorbic acid given in different amounts with different meals. Hum Nutr Appl Nutr 1986;40:97–113.
45. Cook JD. Diagnosis and management of iron deficiency anemia. Best Pract Res Clin Haematol 2006;18:319–32.
46. DeMaeyer EM, Dallman PR, Gurney JM, et al. Preventing and Controlling Iron Deficiency Anemia Through Primary Health Care: A Guide for Health Administrators and Programme Managers. Geneva: WHO; 1989.
47. Umbreit J. Iron Deficiency: A concise review. Am J Hematol 2005;78:225–31.
48. Labbe RF, Dewanji A. Iron assessment tests: Transferrin receptor vis-a`-vis zinc protoporphyrin. Clin Biochem 2004;37:165–74.
49. Cook JD, Skikne BS, Baynes RD. Screening strategies for nutritional iron deficiency. In: Fomon SJ, Zlotkin S, editors. Nutritional Anemias. New York: Nestle, Vevey/Raven Press; 1992. p. 168.
50. Assessment of the Iron Nutritional Status of the U.S. Population Based Data Collected in the Second National Health and Nutrition Examination Survey, 1976–1980. Bethesda, MD: Life Sciences Research Office, Federation of the American Societies for Experimental Biology; 1984.
51. Looker AC, Dallman PR, Carroll MD, et al. Prevalence of iron deficiency in the United States. JAMA 1997;277:973–6.
52. Sharma N, Butterworth J, Cooper BT, et al. The emerging role of the liver in iron metabolism. Am J Gastroenterol 2005;100:201–6.
53. Gibson RS. Assessment of Iron Status. In: Gibson RS, editor. Principles of Nutritional Assessment. New York: Oxford University Press; 2005. p. 443–76.
54. Guidelines for the Use of Iron Supplements to Prevent and Treat Iron Deficiency Anemia: International Nutritional Anemia Consultative Group (INACG), World Health Organization (WHO), United Nations CHildren's Fund (UNICEF). Washington, DC: International Life Sciences Institute Press; 1998.
55. Dallman PR, Looker AC, Johnson SL, Carroll M. Influence of age on laboratory criteria for the diagnosis of iron deficiency anemia and iron deficiency in infants and children. In: Hallberg L, Asp N-G, editors. Iron Nutrition in Health and Disease. London, UK: John Libbey & Co; 1996, p. 65–74.
56. Stoltzfus RJ. Defining iron deficiency anemia in public health terms: A time for reflection. J Nutr 2001;565S–7S.
57. Kohgo Y, Nishisato T, Kondo H. Circulating transferrin receptor in human serum. Br J Haematol 1986;64:277–81.
58. Cook JD. The measurement of serum transferrin receptor. Am J Med Sci 1999;318:269–76. Review.
59. Brugnara C. Iron deficiency and erythropoiesis: New diagnostic approaches. Clin Chem 2003;49:1573–8.
60. The World Health Organization. Reducing Risks, Promoting Healthy Life. Geneva: WHO; 2002.
61. Sub-Committee on Nutrition (ACC/SCN). United Nations. Fourth Report on The World Nutrition Situation; 2000.
62. Olivares M, Walter T, Hertrampf E, Pizzaro F. Anemia and iron deficiency in children. Br Med Bull 1999;55:534–43.
63. Florentino RF, Guirriec RM. Prevalence of nutritional anemia in infancy and childhood with emphasis on developing countries. In: Stekel A, editor. Iron Nutrition in Infancy and Childhood. New York: Nestle, Vevey/Raven Press; 1984. p. 61–72.
64. DeMaeyer EM, Adiels-Tegman M. The prevalence of anemia in the world. World Health Stat Q 1985;38:302–16.
65. Panagiotou JP, Douros K. Clinicolaboratory findings and treatment of iron-deficiency anemia in childhood. Pediatr Hematol Oncol 2004;21:519–32.
66. Cook JD, Finch CA. Assessing iron status of a population. Am J Clin Nutr 1979;32:2115–9.
67. Yip R. The challenge of improving iron nutrition: Limitations and potentials of major intervention approaches. Eur J Clin Nutr 1997;51:516–24.
68. Mercer J, Nelson C, Skovgaard R. Umbilical cord clamping: Beliefs and practices of American nurse-midwives. Clin Pract Exch 2000;45:58–66.
69 Halvorsen S. Iron balance between mother and infant during pregnancy and breastfeeding. Acta Paediatr 2000;89:625–7.
70. Choi JW, Kim CS, Pai SH. Erythropoietic activity and soluble transferrin receptor level in neonates and maternal blood. Acta Paediatr 2000;89:675–9.
71. Singla PN, Gupta VJ, Agarwal KN. Storage iron in human foetal organs. Acta Paediatr Scand 1985;74:701–6.
72. Singla PN, Tyagi M, Hankar R, et al. Fetal iron status in maternal anemia. Acta Paediatr 1996;85:1327–30.
73. Gaspar MJ, Ortega RM, Moreiras O. Relationship between iron status in pregnant women and their new-born infants. Acta Obstet Gynecol Scand 1993;72:534–7.
74. Allen LH. Anemia and iron deficiency: Effects on pregnancy outcome. Am J Clin Nutr 2000;71:1280S–4S.
75. Zlotkin S. Strategies for the prevention of iron deficiency anemia in infants and children. Heinz Infant Nutrition Institute 2003;20:1–4.
76. Gibson RS, Ferguson EL, Lehrfeld J. Complementary foods for infants feeding in developing countries: Their nutrient adequacy and improvement. Eur J Clin Nutr 1998;52:764–70.
77. Wharton BA. Iron deficiency in children: Detection and prevention. Br J Haematol 1999;106:270–80.
78. Zlotkin S. Iron deficiency in Canadian children? Implications and prevention. Can J Pediatr 1993;18–23.
79. Gibson RS, Health ALM, Ferguson EL. Risk of suboptimal iron and zinc nutriture among adolescent girls in Australia and New Zealand: Causes, consequences and solutions. Asia Pacific J Clin Nutr 2002;11:S543–S52.
80. Brabin BJ. The role of malaria in nutritional anemias. In: Fomon SJ, Zlotkin S, editors. Nutritional Anemias. New York: Nestle, Vevey/Raven Press; 2006. p. 65–77.
81. Jarvinen KM, Suomalainen H. Development of cow's milk allergy in breast-fed infants. Clin Exp Allergy 2001;31:978–87.
82. Scholl TO. Iron status during pregnancy: Setting the stage for mother and infant. Am J Clin Nutr 2005;81:1218S–22S.
83. Grantham-McGregor S, Ani C. A review of studies on the effect of iron deificiency on cognitive development in children. J Nutr 2001;131:649S–68S.
84. Pollitt E. Iron deficiency and cognitive function. Ann Rev Nutr 1993;13:521–37.
85. Lozoff B, Jimenez MD, Hagen J, et al. Poorer behavioural and developmental outcome more than 10 years of treatment for iron deficiency in infancy. Pediatrics 2000;105:E51.
86. Youdin MBH. Neuropharmacological and neurobiochemical aspects of iron deficiency. In: Dobbing J, editor. Brain, Behaviour and Iron in the Infant Diet. London: Springer-Verlag; 1990. p. 83–106.
87. Roncagliolo M, Garrido M, Walter T, et al. Evidence of altered central nervous system development in infants with iron deficiency anemia at 6 mo: Delayed maturation of auditory brainstem responses. Am J Clin Nutr 1998;68:683–90.
88. Angulo-Kinzler RM, Peirano P, Lin E, et al. Spontaneous motor activity in human infants with iron deficiency anemia. Early Hum Dev 2002;66:67–79.
89. Bruner AB, Joffe A, Duggan AK, et al. Randomized study of cognitive effects of iron supplementation in non-anaemic iron-deficient adolescent girls. Lancet 1996;348:992–6.
90. Halterman JS, Kaczorowski JM, Aligne A, et al. Iron deficiency and cognitive achievement among school-aged children and adolescents in the United States. Pediatrics 2001;107:1381–6.
91. Yip R. Significance of an abnormally low or high hemoglobin concentration during pregnancy: Special consideration of iron nutrition. Am J Clin Nutr 2000;72:272S–9S.
92. Scholl TO, Reilly T. Anemia, iron and pregnancy outcome. J Nutr 2000;130:443S–7S.
93. Xiong X, Buekens P, Alexander S, et al. Anemia during pregnancy and birth outcome: A meta-analysis. Am J Perinatol 2000;17:137–46.
94. Steer PJ. Maternal hemoglobin concentration and birth weight. Am J Clin Nutr 2000;71:1288S–97S.
95. Brabin BJ, Hakimi M, Pelletier D. An analysis of anemia and pregnancy-related maternal mortality. J Nutr 2001;131:604S–14S.
96. Kurz KM, Galloway R. Improving adolescent iron status before childbearing. J Nutr 2000;130:437S–9S.
97. Picciano MF. Pregnancy and lactation: Physiological adjustments, nutritional requirements and the role of dietary supplements. J Nutr 2003;133:1997S–2002S.
98. Ross SD, Fahrbach K, Frame D, et al. The effect of anemia treatment on selected health related quality life domains: A systematic review. Clin Ther 2003;25:1786–1805.
99. Beard JL, Hendricks MK, Perez EM, et al. Maternal iron deficiency anemia affects postpartum emotions and cognition. J Nutr 2005;135:267–72.
100. Perez EM, Hendricks MK, Beard JL, et al. Mother-infant interactions and infant development are altered by maternal iron deficiency anemia. J Nutr 2005;135:850–5.
101. American Academy of Pediatrics. American Academy of Pediatrics Committee on Nutrition: The use of whole cow's milk in infancy. Pediatrics 1992;89:1105–9.
102. World Health Organization. The optimal duration of exclusive breastfeeding. Report of an Expert Consultation. WHO/FCH/CAH/01.24. Geneva: WHO; 2001.
103. Vuori E, Makinen SM, Kara R, Kuitunen P. The effects of the dietary intakes of copper, iron manganese, and zinc on the trace element content of human milk. Am J Clin Nutr 1980;33:227–31.
104. Griffin IJ, Abrams SA. Iron and breastfeeding. Pediatr Clin N Am 2001;48:401–13.
105. American Academy of Pediatrics Committee on Nutrition. Nutritional needs of low-birth-weight infants. Pediatrics 1985;58:765–8.
106. European Society of Paediatric Gastroenterology and Nutrition CoN. Nutrition needs of the preterm infant: Scientific basis and practical guidelines. Acta Paediatr Scand 1987;336:1–14.
107. Canadian Paediatric Society (CPS) Nutrition Committee. Meeting the iron needs of infants and young children: An update. CMAJ 1991;144:1451–4.
108. World Health Organization. Malnutrition: The Global Picture. Geneva: WHO; 2000.
109. Dallman PR. Iron deficiency in the weanling: A nutritional problem on the way to resolution. Acta Paediatr Scand 1986;323:59–67.
110. Wharf SG, Fox TE, Fairweather-Tait SJ, Cook JD. Factors affecting iron stores in infants 4–18 months of age. Eur J Clin Nutr 1997;51:504–9.
111. Lynch SR. The impact of iron fortification on nutritional anemia. Best Pract Res Clin Haematol 2005;18:333–46.
112. Subar AF, Krebs-Smith SM, Cook A, Kahle LL. Dietary sources of nutrients among US children, 1989–91. Pediatrics 1998;102:913–23.
113. International Nutritional Anemia Consultative Group. Guidelines for the Use of Iron Supplements to Prevent and Treat Iron Deficiency Anemia. Geneva: WHO; 1998.
114. Allen LH. Pregnancy and iron deficiency: Unresolved issues. Nutr Rev 1997;55:91–101.
115. Beard JL. Weekly iron intervention: The case for intermittent iron supplementation. Am J Clin Nutr 1998;68:209–12.
116. Hallberg L. Daily iron supplementation: Why it is necessary. Am J Clin Nutr 1998;68:213–7.
117. Viteri FE. Iron supplementation for the control of iron deficiency in populations at risk. Nutr Rev 1997;55: 195–209.
118. Mohamed K. Iron supplementation in pregnancy. Cochrane Database Systematic Review 2000;CD000117.
119. Christian P, Shrestha SR, LeClerq SC, et al. Supplementation with micronutrients in addition to iron and folic acid does not further improve the hematologic status of pregnant women in rural Nepal. J Nutr 2003;133:3492–8.
120. Christian P, Khatry SK, Katz J, et al. Effects of alternative maternal micronutrient supplements on low birth weight in rural Nepal: Double blind randomised community trial. BMJ 2003;326:571–4.
121. Osrin D, Vaidya A, Shrestha Y, et al. Effects of antenatal multiple micronutrient supplementation on birthweight and gestational duration in Nepal: Double-blind, randomized controlled trial. Lancet 2005;365:955–62.
122. Allen LH. Iron supplements: Scientific issues concerning efficacy and implications for research and programs. J Nutr 2002;132:813S–9S.
123. Lynch SR. Interaction of iron with other nutrients. Nutr Rev 1997;55:102–10.
124. Oppenheimer SJ. Iron and its relation to immunity and infectious disease. J Nutr 2001;131:616S–35S.
125. International Nutritional Anemia Consultative Group. Safety of iron supplementation programs in malaria-endemic regions. Washington, DC: ILSI Press; 2001.
126. Sazawal Z, Black RE, Ramsan M, et al. Effects of routine prophylactic supplementation with iron and folic acid on admission to hospital and mortality in preschool children in a high malaria transmission setting: Community-based, randomised, placebo-controlled trial. Lancet 2006;367:133–43.

127. Tielsch JM, Katry S, Stoltzfus RJ, et al. Effect of routine prophylactic supplementation with iron and folic acid on preschool child mortality in southern Nepal: Community-based, cluster-randomised, placebo-controlled trial. Lancet 2006;367:144–52.
128. World Health Organization. Iron Supplementation of Young Children in Regions Where Malaria Transmission is Intense and Infectious Disease Highly Prevalent. Geneva: WHO; 2004.
129. English M, Snow RW. Iron and folic acid supplementation and malaria risk. Lancet 2006;367:90–1.
130. McCord JM. Iron, free radicals, and oxidative injury. Semin Hematol 1998;35:5–12.
131. Fryman E, Bystrom M, Jansson U, et al. Side effects of iron supplements in blood donors: Superior tolerance of heme iron. J Lab Clin Med 1994;123:561–4.
132. Fine JS. Iron poisoning. Curr.Probl.Pediatr 2000;30:71–90.
133. Anonymous. Toddler deaths resulting from ingestion of iron supplements. Los Angeles, 1992–1993. MMWR Morb Mort Wkly Rep 1993;42:111–3.
134. Fazen LE, Lovejoy FH, Crone RK. Acute poisoning in a children's hospital: A 2-year experience. Pediatrics 1986;77:144–51.
135. Ferguson J, Sellar C, Goldace MJ. Some epidemiological observations on medicinal and non-medicinal poisoning in preschool children. J Epidemiol Community Health 1992;44:207–10.
136. Trinkoff AM, Baker SP. Poisoning hospitalizations and deaths from solids and liquids among children and teenagers. Am J Public Health 1986;76:657–60.
137. Tenenbein M. Toxicokinetics and toxicodynamics of iron poisoning. Toxicol Lett 1998;102:653–6.
138. Beutler E, Hoffbrand V, Cook JD. Iron deficiency and iron overload. Hematology Am Soc Hematol Educ Program 2003;40–61.
139. Yen AW, Fancher TL, Bowlus CL. Revisiting hereditary hemochromatosis: Current concepts and progress. Am J Med 2006;119:391–9.
140. Whitlock EP, Garlitz BA, Harris EL, et al. Screening for hereditary hemochromatosis: A systematic review for the U.S. Preventive Services Task Force. Ann Intern Med 2006;145:209–23.
141. American Academy of Pediatrics Committee on Nutrition. Iron fortification of infant formulas. Pediatrics 1999;104:119–23.

10

Vitamins

Roland Kupka, ScD
Eduardo Villamor, MD, DrPH
Wafaie Fawzi, MD, DrPH

INTRODUCTION

Since ancient times, diet has been used to prevent and treat ailments like night blindness, pellagra, scurvy, and rickets. However, it was not until the end of the nineteenth century that specific compounds in foodstuffs, beyond the three major sources of energy and building units (carbohydrates, fats, and proteins), began to be identified as responsible for vital functions in animals. The term "vitamine" was coined by Casimir Funk in 1911 to describe an antineuritic water-soluble compound discovered in rice bran that was initially believed to consist of an "amine" structure.[1] This compound, thiamine, would be identified as a "vitamin" later, together with other vital compounds of varied chemical structures that were discovered in the early twentieth century.

Traditionally, vitamins have been classified according to their hydrophilic potential as fat-soluble (hydrophobic): A, D, E, and K; and water-soluble: C, thiamin (B_1), riboflavin (B_2), niacin, pyridoxine (B_6), folate, cobalamin (B_{12}), biotin, and pantothenic acid. In this chapter we present a brief discussion on each vitamin, emphasizing the basic chemistry, physiology, and current epidemiological knowledge with special focus on issues pertaining to child health. A summary of information on the clinical examination of nutritional deficiencies and excesses, as well as on important food sources of vitamins, is provided in Table A-9 in Appendix I. The reader is referred to Chapter 11, "Dietary Reference Intakes," for a discussion on current US dietary reference intakes set forth by the Food and Nutrition Board of the Institute of Medicine (IOM) and to Table II-1 in Appendix II for a listing of recommended vitamin intakes.

VITAMIN A

History, Structure, and Metabolism

The importance of a substance present in certain foods for the treatment of night blindness was already known in ancient Egypt. The Greek physician Hippocrates (460 to 327 BC) recommended the intake of "raw beef liver, soaked in honey, once or twice by mouth" for the treatment of "nyctalopia," or the total inability to see in darkness.[2] However, it was only in the late nineteenth and early twentieth centuries when the biochemistry of this compound was clarified. In 1881, Nicholai Lunin reported that mice could not survive on a purified diet of fats, carbohydrates, proteins, and salts alone, but survival was more likely when whole milk was added.[3] Similar findings led Sir Frederick Gowland Hopkins to postulate in 1906 the existence of "unsuspected dietetic factors" that were necessary for life and growth.[4] For this he was awarded the Nobel Prize in 1929. A fat-soluble factor was isolated from egg yolk in 1909 by Wilhelm Stepp[5]; the same factor isolated from alfalfa leaves, liver, kidney, or butter fat was independently shown to promote growth in rats by Elmer V. McCollum,[6,7] and Thomas Osborne, and Lafayette Mendel in 1913,[8,9] and was dubbed "fat-soluble factor A." The factor was finally named vitamin A in 1920.[10] Before the discovery of vitamin A, various carotenoid pigments had been described in the nineteenth century. They were later found to be precursors of vitamin A,[11] and the structure of β-carotene, the major provitamin A carotenoid, was disclosed by Paul Karrer in 1930.[12] He won the Nobel Prize in 1937.

The term vitamin A groups a number of retinoid compounds with the biological activity of all-*trans*-retinol. Retinoids usually consist of four isoprenoid units with five conjugated carbon–carbon double bonds.[13] 11-*cis*-retinal is the oxidation product of retinol primarily involved in visual functions. Retinal can be further oxidized to retinoic acid, which possesses growth but not visual or reproductive functions. Retinyl palmitate, an ester, is the principal storage form of vitamin A. More than 600 carotenoids have been identified in nature, but only about 50 have the unsubstituted β-ionone ring that guarantees vitamin A activity. As opposed to retinol, most carotenoids have antioxidant properties due to their long chain of conjugated double bonds.

Vitamin A is usually ingested as retinyl palmitate from animal sources, and as carotenoids from plants and animal tissue. In the stomach, retinol and carotenoids are released from protein by proteolysis and then aggregate with lipids and pass into the upper part of the small intestine. Bile salts stimulate pancreatic lipase and esterases that hydrolyze retinyl esters to retinol in enterocytes. Retinol subsequently binds to the cellular retinol-binding protein CRBP(II). Carotenoids, on the other hand, pass into the mucosal cells unaltered, and are cleaved by a 15 to 15′-oxygenase into retinal, which also binds to CRPB(II). Retinal reductase and lecithin-retinol, acyltransferase recognize the CRPB(II) complexes and synthesize retinol which is then packed into chylomicrons before entering the circulation via the lymphatic system.[14] Triacylglycerol is hydrolyzed from circulating chylomicrons by plasma lipoprotein lipase to form chylomicron remnants. These remnants deliver retinol to the liver, where it is taken up by hepatocytes through high-affinity receptors of apolipoproteins E and B48. In hepatic lysosomes, an acidic hydrolase releases retinol to bind with apo-CRBP. At least three pathways could follow after this CRBP–retinol complex is formed: (1) synthesis of CRBP–retinal through retinol dehydrogenase and later retinal through retinal dehydrogenase, (2) retinol esterification mediated by lecithin-retinol acyltransferase, and (3) rapid mobilization of retinol catalyzed by the bile salt-independent reductase.[14]

From the hepatocyte, vitamin A can be locally transported to fat-storing stellate cells. Plasma concentrations of unbound retinol-binding protein RBP (also known as apo-RBP) regulate the mobilization of retinol from the liver. Increased concentrations of apo-RBP signal stellate cells to release retinyl esters for deesterification to retinol. The retinol bound to RBP (also known as holo-RBP) is secreted in plasma together with transthyretin, a tetramer that minimizes the loss of RBP in urine. The complex is then distributed to peripheral tissues or recycled back to the liver in a tightly regulated system that allows retinol molecules to recirculate more than seven times before final excretion. In the retina, holo-RBP binds to membrane receptors for internalization by endocytosis. These receptors have been also found in skin, placenta, and the blood–testes and blood-brain barriers.[15] However, they are not present in lung, kidney, or muscle. It is possible that in these and other organs retinol is taken up directly by lipid membranes on a receptor-independent fashion.

Bioconversion of carotenoids is inversely regulated by vitamin A status[16]; this offers a potential explanation to the lack of toxic effects even at extremely elevated intake of carotenoids. The bioavailability of vitamin A and carotenoids is influenced by the integrity of the intestinal mucosa and the intake of other nutrients.[17] Factors that increase bioavailability include the presence of fat, protein, vitamin E, zinc, and possibly iron; cooking; and processing. Dietary fiber from highly methoxylated pectins reduces absorption of carotenoids.[18] During the first 6 months of life, the most important sources of vitamin A for the infant are breastmilk and vitamin A available from the infant's own liver stores. The concentration of vitamin A in breastmilk is dependent on the mother's vitamin A status, so that the infant's vitamin A status may be compromised if the mother's vitamin A status is inadequate.[19] After 6 months of age, complementary foods increase in importance to meet the infant's vitamin A requirements. Among US children aged 2 to 18 years, ready-to-eat cereals and milk supply more than 40% of vitamin A intakes.[20]

Traditionally, the vitamin A activity of β-carotene has been expressed as retinol equivalents (REs). However, recent data indicate that the vitamin A activities of purified β-carotene in oil as well as dietary β-carotene are lower than what had previously been assumed. For this reason, the contribution of β-carotene, and in fact also of other provitamin A carotenoids, to dietary vitamin A intakes had been overestimated. To take into account the new data, requirements for vitamin A are now expressed as retinol activity equivalents (RAEs), rather than REs. While the RE for dietary β-carotene was 6 μg, the RAE for dietary β-carotene is 12 μg, indicating that 12 μg (instead of 6 μg) of β-carotene needs to be consumed to yield 1 μg of available retinol. The corresponding RAE for β-carotene and β-cryptoxanthin is 24 μg.[21]

Functions

Vitamin A exhibits an overarching function in gene expression that affects various physiological processes. In the form of its metabolite all-*trans* retinoic acid, vitamin A is a ligand for a family of nuclear receptors known as retinoic acid receptors, whereas another metabolite, 9-*cis* retinoic acid, activates retinoic acid receptors and retinoid X receptors. These receptors form heterodimers and bind to genes in regulatory regions known as retinoic acid response elements. The regulation of gene induction by retinoic acid can be further modulated by a large number of transcriptional mediators and repressors that include hormonal receptors.

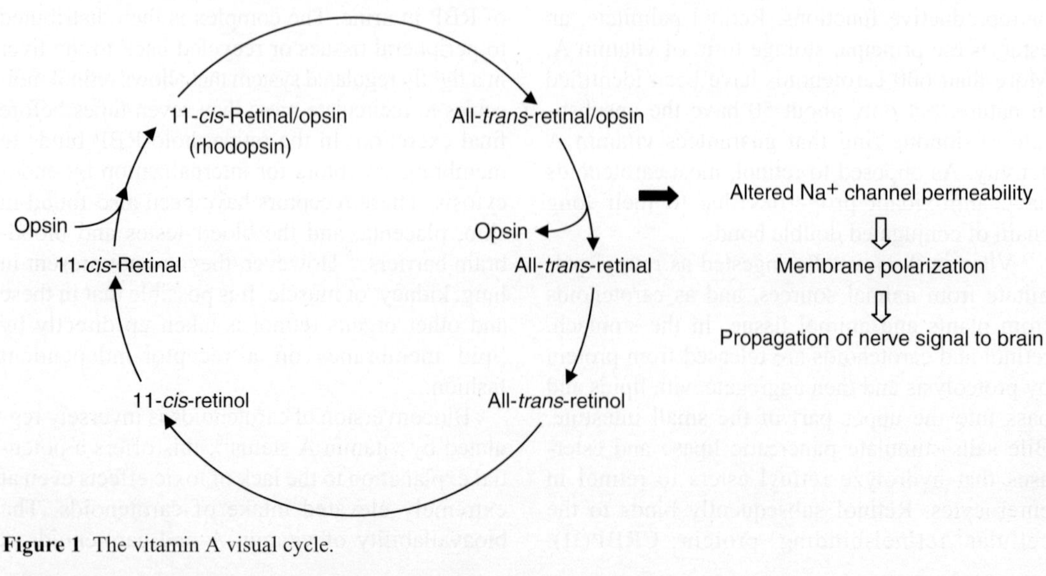

Figure 1 The vitamin A visual cycle.

Specific physiological functions exhibited by vitamin A include vision, immunity, cell differentiation, and growth. The visual role of vitamin A occurs in the rod cells of the eye and enables sight in dim-light conditions. In this biochemical process, all-*trans*-retinol undergoes isomerization and oxidation to yield the light-sensitive molecule 11-*cis*-retinal. The 11-*cis*-retinal molecule binds to opsin to form rhodopsin. As rhodopsin absorbs light, 11-*cis*-retinal changes to all-*trans*-retinal, causing it to dissociate from opsin. As all-*trans*-retinal is released, opsin undergoes a conformational change, which induces an alteration in permeability to cations, increased polarization of the membrane, and generation of a nerve impulse. Rhodopsin can be regenerated, which completes the vitamin A–dependent visual cycle (Figure 1).[22]

The role of vitamin A in immunity has recently been summarized[23] and seems to be mediated mainly through the acid metabolites of the vitamin, all-*trans* retinoic acid, and 9-*cis* retinoic acid.[24] At the level of mucosal immunity, vitamin A deficiency (VAD) is related to alterations in the integrity of ocular, respiratory, gastrointestinal (GI), and genitourinary epithelia. These alterations include replacement of normal ciliated and mucus-producing cells by keratinized epithelium. Keratinization and mucin production may be additionally regulated by vitamin A at the transcriptional level. Local secretion of humoral immune factors such as secretory IgA and lactoferrin may also be impaired by VAD.

Retinoids influence the differentiation of white cell lines in the bone marrow, as well as the function of circulating immune cells. Phagocytosis, chemotaxis, and production of free radicals carried out by neutrophils are altered in vitamin A–deficient animals, as well as the number and cytotoxic activity of natural killer cells. Retinoic acid enhances various functions of mononuclear cells in vitro, such as phagocytic activity of macrophages and release of tumor necrosis factor-α, interleukin 1 (IL-1), transforming growth factor-β, and expression of immunoglobulin receptors by monocytes that modulate proliferation of B lymphocytes. It also increases the capacity of Langerhans cells to present antigens to T lymphocytes in the skin.

Vitamin A appears to influence the antigen-specific proliferation of T lymphocytes. In animals, VAD impairs cytotoxic T lymphocyte activity. The growth and differentiation of B lymphocytes into immunoglobulin-producing cells also requires retinol, possibly through the induction of cytokine secretion by T helper lymphocytes. The antibody response against T cell–dependent antigens is usually impaired by VAD in animals, particularly during infections that would normally induce a T helper type-2 like response. In this case, instead of high production of IgG, IL-4, IL-5, and IL-10, a Th1 response seems to be favored with low antibody production and increased levels of IL-2 and interferon-γ. During infections that predominantly stimulate a Th1 immune response, it has also been suggested that VAD further upregulates such a response. Only a few studies have directly addressed the impact of vitamin A supplementation in humans on indicators of the immune function. The protective effect of vitamin A supplementation against infant morbidity and mortality is attributed to the vitamin's vital role in sustaining and enhancing the immune response at various levels.

A range of trials has examined the effect of vitamin A supplementation on mortality among children older than 6 months who live in developing countries. In two trials, vitamin A supplements had no effect on mortality, while a beneficial effect ranging from 19 to 54% was observed in the remaining studies. The pooled effect from eight clinical trials was estimated to be around 30%.[25] The effect varied with the dosage and frequency of administration; small weekly or daily doses were associated with a 42% mortality reduction, whereas large spaced doses (every 4 to 6 months) with a 19% risk decline. The effect also seemed greater among children ≤1 year old and was more strongly protective against death from diarrheal disease. More recent studies suggest that vitamin A supplements also prevent mortality due to HIV disease among children without access to antiretroviral therapy.[26,27] The effect of supplementation among infants <6 months is not clear. Administration of vitamin A to newborns resulted in a mortality reduction in one trial,[28] but three other trials found no effect.[29–31] Vitamin A supplements do not appear to reduce pneumonia recovery rates[32] or mortality due to respiratory infections among children.[33] Variation in the effect of vitamin A supplements across populations can be attributed to setting-specific conditions such as the presence of concomitant nutrient deficiencies that affect the absorption and utilization of vitamin A, the prevalence of infectious diseases, and the underlying severity of VAD in the population.

The effect of vitamin A on the incidence and severity of infections has been assessed in several community- and hospital-based trials. There is a clear benefit of vitamin A supplementation among children hospitalized with measles; the average mortality risk reduction is estimated to be 60%.[25] The effect is larger in children with measles pneumonia, and among infants compared with older children. Also, vitamin A reduces the risk of acquiring pneumonia in children with uncomplicated measles.[34] Children with measles and diarrhea who received vitamin A recovered more rapidly from the diarrheal episode.[35] Based on the beneficial effects of vitamin A for recovery from measles disease, the American Academy of Pediatrics (AAP) recommends vitamin A supplementation for children aged 6 months to 2 years who are hospitalized with measles and children older than 6 months with measles and additional risk factors for VAD.[36] Children 1 year of age and older should receive 200,000 IU (60,000 μg) retinol by mouth, while children aged 6 months to 1 year should receive 100,000 IU (30,000 μg) retinol.

Vitamin A also appears to have a beneficial effect on the incidence and severity of certain types of diarrhea. Several community-based studies demonstrated reductions in diarrhea-specific mortality[37] and number of severe diarrheal episodes,[38,39] including acute watery diarrhea.[27] Among hospitalized children in Bangladesh, vitamin A supplementation reduced diarrheal symptoms caused by shigellosis[40] but not symptoms related to rotavirus and enterotoxigenic *Escherichia coli* infections.[41] A study from Mexico among children aged 6 to 15 months also demonstrated pathogen-dependent effects of vitamin A on diarrheal outcomes,[42] possibly due to differences in the mucosal immune response.[43]

Vitamin A supplements may increase the occurrence of cough and other signs of respiratory infection, but such symptoms may be due to an improved inflammatory response induced by vitamin A therapy.[44,45] Some data suggest that vitamin A supplementation may reduce the occurrence and severity of malaria in children.[46] In observational studies on the role of vitamin A in mother-to-child transmission of HIV, low retinol levels were associated with increased risk of transmission, suggesting that vitamin A supplementation may be beneficial. However, evidence from clinical trials showed either no effect of vitamin A supplements or a detrimental effect.[47]

Vitamin A was discovered as a growth-promoting factor[6,7]; in the 1930s, growth arrest, particularly on weight gain, was demonstrated in vitamin A–depleted rats.[48] However, the role of vitamin A in growth and body composition of humans is less clear. Positive relationships between vitamin A status and growth have been reported from observational studies, particularly in malnourished populations. Children with ocular signs of severe VAD, including night blindness and xerophthalmia, are usually stunted[49]; however, at subclinical stages of VAD other determinants of poor linear growth might be important.[50] High dietary β-carotene and total vitamin A intake have been positively related to linear growth in children 2 to 19 years[51] and 6 to 72[52] respectively. However, these observational studies are limited by potential confounding by other nutrient deficiencies and infection. Various randomized clinical trials of vitamin A supplementation in children, conducted in Asia and Africa, showed an overall lack of effect on weight or height gains.[53–58] However, when the effect was examined in subgroups of children, vitamin A supplements were found to selectively improve the growth pattern of children at higher risk of VAD as reflected in their age above 2 years,[59,60] poor breast-feeding status,[57,61] low seasonal availability of vitamin A–rich foods,[62] and low serum vitamin A levels.[61,62] Lately, vitamin A supplementation has been related to large improvements in growth among children suffering from debilitating infectious diseases including HIV, malaria, and persistent diarrhea.[63]

Vitamin A functions in the normal metabolism of iron and research indicates that VAD is a risk factor for iron-deficiency anemia.[64,65] Vitamin A enhances the growth and differentiation of erythrocyte progenitor cells, aids in the mobilization of iron stores from tissues, and improves resistance to infections, all of which prevent the development of anemia.[66] The trace element zinc plays a role in the absorption, transport, and utilization of vitamin A.[67] Zinc supplements have been shown to restore vision under dim-light conditions, which suggests an interaction between zinc status and vitamin A–related functions.[68]

Retinol dosages ≥150,000 μg among adults, and lower dosages among children proportional to body weight, induce transient toxic effects that include nausea, vomiting, headache, increased cerebrospinal fluid pressure, vertigo, blurred vision, and muscular incoordination. Chronic exposure to retinol at dosages of approximately 6,000 μg/d or higher have also been associated with bulging fontanel among infants.[21] Using this data and applying a large safety margin, the IOM recommends that children from 0 to 36 months should have preformed retinol intakes from dietary and supplemental sources below 600 μg/d.[21] However, it has been pointed out that this estimate may be overly conservative, given that 25 to 30% of young children, as assessed by the Continuing Survey of Food Intakes by Individuals, have intakes above that level without evidence of adverse effects.[69] Women of childbearing age should be advised against consuming more than 2,800 to 3,000 μg/d of retinol to lower the risk of teratogenicity.[21]

VITAMIN D

History, Structure, and Metabolism

Rickets, a disorder due to vitamin D deficiency, has afflicted humanity since Neanderthal times some 200,000 years ago. Nevertheless, it was described scientifically not until the seventeenth century. In 1919, Sir Edward Mellanby linked rickets to a nutritional deficit by feeding dogs a synthetic diet and by showing that it could be prevented with the administration of cod liver or butter.[70] This led him to propose that the dietary factor responsible for rickets was vitamin A. In 1922, Elmer McCollum distinguished the antirachitic from the antixerophthalmic factors in diet because the former did not lose its properties after intense heating and aeration, and called it vitamin D.[71] Also in 1919, Huldschinsky had shown that rickets could be cured with exposure to ultraviolet (UV) rays, but the realization that there was a relationship between the UV and dietary actions against rickets occurred only later when Goldblatt and Soames demonstrated that irradiation of food could also cure rickets,[72] and when Hess and Weinstock showed that UV irradiation induced the formation of an antirachitic factor in the skin.[73]

Vitamin D designates a group of compounds derived from the cyclopentanoperhydrophenanthrene molecule, which have antirachitic activity.[74] All these substances have a conjugated triene system of double bonds. The two most abundant forms of the vitamin are D_3 and D_2. Vitamin D_3 is also called cholecalciferol and is produced in the skin from 7-dehydrocholesterol, by solar radiation. Vitamin D_2, or ergocalciferol, is derived industrially from ergosterol, a plant steroid. Given that vitamin D can be produced by the human body, there is no dietary requirement for the vitamin as long as access to sunlight is available. For these reasons, vitamin D does not strictly fulfill the definition of a vitamin, and based on its various metabolic functions, the active metabolite 1,25-dihydroxycholecalciferol ($1\alpha,25(OH)_2D_3$) is classified as a steroid hormone.[75]

Absorption of vitamin D from the diet is relatively low, as only about 50% of dietary vitamin is absorbed. The major source of the vitamin in humans is from photochemical conversion of 7-dehydrocholesterol to previtamin D in the skin, and posterior isomerization to vitamin D (Figure 2). Vitamin D then passes to the systemic circulation bound to its transporter, the vitamin D–binding protein (DBP). Vitamin D–binding protein, carries most biological forms and metabolites of the vitamin. Vitamin D is taken up rapidly by the liver but it is not preferentially stored there.[74] The highest concentrations of vitamin D are found in blood, although adipose and muscle tissue in humans are also major storage sites.[77] During deprivation, turnover from these sites is slow, and the supply of vitamin D to peripheral organs can be sustained for a period of time.

Vitamin D_3 does not have known biological functions, as it must first be hydroxylated to $25(OH)D_3$ in the liver. $25(OH)D_3$ is the most abundant circulating form of the vitamin, and is a good proxy of vitamin D_3 status. It is transported to the proximal tubules of the kidney, where a 1-hydroxylase converts it into $1\alpha,25(OH)_2D_3$. This hydroxylase is considered the most important regulatory mechanism of the vitamin D endocrine system,[74] and its activity is regulated by the concentration of $1\alpha,25(OH)_2D_3$,

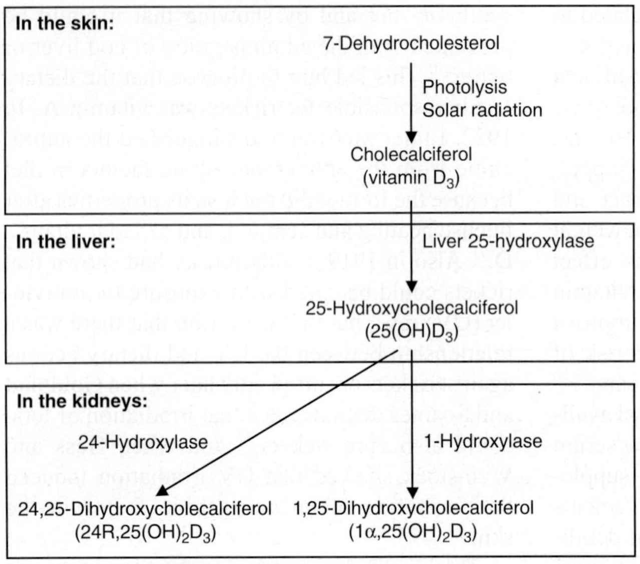

Figure 2 Vitamin D metabolism.

parathyroid hormone (PTH), calcium, and phosphate. The second hydroxylated metabolite of D_3 produced in the kidney is $24R,25(OH)_2D_3$. Although this metabolite may play unique roles in vitamin D functions such as regulating PTH and bone mineralization, it is likely that both $25(OH)_2D_3$ and $24R,25(OH)_2D_3$ are required. Vitamin D is mostly excreted in bile through catabolic pathways that are not well understood yet. Only small amounts of the vitamin are recovered during enterohepatic circulation.[78] Some water-soluble metabolites of vitamin D, especially calcitroic acid (1α-hydroxy-23 carboxy-24,25,26,27-tetranorvitamin D_3), are also excreted in urine.[79]

Functions

Vitamin D has a well-described role in bone health and calcium and phosphorous homeostasis. It also regulates genes that function in immune responses as well as cellular growth, differentiation, and apoptosis.[80] As part of its steroid form $1\alpha,25(OH)_2D_3$, vitamin D is biologically active by rapidly activating several signal transduction pathways through the membrane receptor VDR_{mem} as well as by regulating gene transcription through its nuclear receptor VDR_{nuc}.[81]

The rapid, nongenomic physiological responses triggered by the interaction of $1\alpha,25(OH)_2D_3$ with the membrane receptor VDR_{mem} include the stimulation of Ca^{2+} absorption in the intestine (transcaltachia), opening of Ca^{2+} and Cl^- channels, activation of protein kinase C and mitogen-activated kinase, Ca^{2+} entry in skeletal muscle cells, and Ca^{2+} uptake by osteoblasts.[81]

The mechanisms involving gene transcription are initiated when $1\alpha,25(OH)_2D_3$ binds in target organs to its nuclear receptor, VDR_{nuc}, which has domains also found in other steroid hormone receptors. After binding, VDR forms a heterodimer with retinoid X receptor and later, the complex interacts with the vitamin D response element in the transcription control region of target genes. These activated promoter genes may also bind to coactivator proteins such as TATA, TBP, and TFIIB, and the resulting transcriptional complex is then able to modulate DNA transcription.[82] Of the more than 60 genes regulated by $1\alpha,25(OH)_2D_3$, the gene linked to the induction of the calcium-binding protein calbindin D is one of the most important ones, as it is directly related to many of the known physiological functions of vitamin D.[74]

Regulation of mineral homeostasis is the classical function attributed to vitamin D. This process occurs at various target organs. In the intestine, $1\alpha,25(OH)_2D_3$ induces the transport of calcium and phosphate from lumen to plasma, possibly by activating calbindin, and also through changes in the membrane composition of the brush border cells.[83] In the kidney, $1\alpha,25(OH)_2D_3$ downregulates $25(OH)D_3$-1α-hydroxylase, thus controlling its own production.[84] $1\alpha,25(OH)_2D_3$ also stimulates the activity of $25(OH)D_3$-24-hydroxylase.

In bone, $1\alpha,25(OH)_2D_3$ and PTH mobilize monocytic stem cells to become mature osteoclasts, which mobilize calcium stores from bone. Thus, vitamin D stimulates bone resorption and is thus important for maintaining constant serum calcium concentrations independent of calcium intake. $1\alpha,25(OH)_2D_3$ may promote bone growth and mineralization through its effect on increasing intestinal calcium absorption, and perhaps also by promoting differentiation of growth plate cells via chondrocyte membrane receptors and augmenting osteoblast proliferation and calcium uptake.[85]

In skeletal muscle, vitamin D may be an important stimulant of calcium release during hypocalcemia. Myopathy frequently accompanies bone diseases related to vitamin D deficiency. In the skin, $1\alpha,25(OH)_2D_3$ appears to foster differentiation of keratinocytes, and protects them from UV stress.[86] Some types of psoriasis can improve with the topical application of vitamin D analogs.[87] Pancreatic β-cells respond to vitamin D with insulin secretion and vitamin D deficiency is accompanied with impaired insulin production.[88] Some studies suggest that high doses of vitamin D may decrease the risk of type 1 diabetes in children.[89]

Various actions of vitamin D on the immune system have been reported. Immune cells such as T and B lymphocytes, monocytes, and dendritic cells may be dependent on vitamin D as they contain VDR_{nuc}.[90–94] However, the relation between vitamin D status and host defense is not well characterized. Recent data indicate that vitamin D deficiency may depress innate immunity and predispose to microbial infections.[95] Furthermore, there is evidence that vitamin D downregulates Th1 immune responses, which may explain why vitamin D suppresses various autoimmune diseases and prolongs allograft survival. Conversely, vitamin D upregulates Th2 immune responses that protect against extracellular pathogens but that also drive the development of allergies and asthma.[96] Thus, there is concern that children who are exposed to vitamin D early in life may have an increased risk of developing allergies in later life.[97,98]

Poor maternal vitamin D status impairs fetal vitamin D accretion during pregnancy and further compromises child vitamin D status because of reduced vitamin D concentrations in breastmilk.[99] However, regular small exposure to sunlight can offset low dietary intakes of vitamin D, but is less effective among dark-skinned groups.[100,101] According to revised 2003 AAP guidelines, 200 IU supplemental vitamin D should be provided to (1) all breast-fed infants beginning during the first 2 months of life, unless they are also receiving at least 500 mL vitamin D–fortified formula or milk per day; (2) all non–breast-fed infants who are ingesting less than 500 mL of vitamin D–fortified formula or milk per day; and (3) children and adolescents who lack regular sunlight exposure, do not ingest at least 500 mL vitamin D–fortified milk per day, or are not taking a daily multivitamin supplement with at least 200 IU vitamin D.[102] It has also been argued that dietary reference intakes set by IOM in 1997 need to be revised upward as new knowledge on vitamin D requirements has accumulated since their issue.[103]

The 1997 IOM report outlines that toxicity symptoms may occur after vitamin intakes above 1,000 IU/d among infants and above 2,000 IU/d among children and adults. Symptoms are generally mediated by hypercalcemia and show clinically as polyuria, polydipsia, hypercalcuria, calcification of soft tissues, and central nervous system impairments.[104] However, more recent evidence indicates that these tolerable upper intake levels (ULs) (see Chapter 11, "Dietary Reference Intakes," for more information) may be too conservative, as higher dosages have been used without signs of adverse effects.[103]

VITAMIN E

History, Structure, and Metabolism

Vitamin E was discovered by Herbert Bishop and Katherine Evans in 1922 as a fat-soluble compound in wheat and lettuce that was necessary to avoid fetal death in rats.[105] The vitamin was shown to be essential among humans not until the late 1960s, when its deficiency was linked to hemolytic anemia among premature infants.[106] The potential protective role of vitamin E as an antioxidant against chronic and degenerative illness is currently an active field of research.

Natural vitamin E occurs in the form of eight different isomers, four tocopherols and four tocotrienols. A chromanol ring is common to all isomers, but while tocopherols have a saturated phytyl tail, tocotrienols have an unsaturated tail. Based on the number of methyl groups on the chromanol ring, the isomers are grouped into α-, β-, γ-, and δ-forms of tocopherol and tocotrienol. Recent evidence indicates that the various isomers of vitamin E are not interconvertible in humans and that they have different metabolic functions. Only certain forms of α-tocopherol are maintained in the plasma and are thus considered to be the active forms that are relevant to establish nutritional requirements. These active forms are the *2R*-stereoisomers of α-tocopherol (classified as *RRR*-, *RSR*-, *RRS*-, and *RSS*-α-tocopherol), while the *2S*-stereoisomeric forms (*SRR*-, *SSR*-, *SRS*-, and *SSS*-α-tocopherol) are not maintained in plasma and are thus not considered active. Synthetic forms of vitamin E are a mixture of all eight α-tocopherol stereoisomers (prefixed "*all-rac*-," for all-racemic), while only the *RRR*-stereoisomer occurs in food.[21]

After ingestion, all forms of vitamin E combine with bile salts and pancreatic secretions in the intestinal lumen, form micelles, and are taken up into enterocytes.[107] Absorption of all forms of vitamin E is low but appears to be inversely related to intake. It is also reduced by long-chain polyunsaturated fatty acids but increased by medium-chain triglycerides.[108] At the enterocyte, all forms of vitamin E are incorporated into chylomicrons and enter the circulation via the lymphatic system. As a result of chylomicron catabolism, vitamin E is distributed to tissues by means of circulating lipoproteins. Chylomicron remnants that contain the remainders of newly absorbed vitamin E are taken up by the liver. A selection process occurs in the liver, as *RRR*-α-tocopherol, the active form of α-tocopherol, is preferentially resecreted into nascent very low density lipoproteins (VLDLs) by α-tocopherol transfer protein and recirculated through the body.[109] During the conversion of VLDL to form low-density lipoprotein (LDL), some α-tocopherol is transferred to HDLs, which transport it to all of the circulating lipoproteins. The α-tocopherol remaining in LDL enters the cells of peripheral tissues through the LDL receptor pathway.[110] The metabolic products of α-tocopherol after oxidation are dimers and trimers, as well as tocopheryl chromanoxy radicals that can be reverted to tocopherol by reducing agents such as vitamin C and glutathione. Subsequent oxidation of the tocopheroxyl radical produces tocopheryl quinone that, after reduction, can be excreted in the feces, or converted into tocopheronic acid by side-chain oxidation and excreted in urine as glucuronate conjugates.[108] Other nonoxidation metabolites of the tocopherol phytyl tail are excreted in urine. These include 2,5,7,8-tetramethyl-2-(2′-carboxyethyl)-6-hydroxychroman, or α-CEHC, and γ-CEHC. High amounts of supplemental vitamin E result in increases in urinary α-CEHC concentrations.[111] Due to the low bioavailability of ingested vitamin E, large amounts of the vitamin are excreted in feces. Absorbed forms of the vitamin that are in excess of requirements are excreted unchanged in bile.

Functions

Vitamin E deficiency in animal models results most commonly in necrotizing myopathy, but may also lead to encephalomalacia, exudative diathesis, and embryonic degeneration. Deficiency symptoms also appear to depend on the status of other nutrients like selenium and some amino acids.[112] In humans, vitamin E deficiency due to a poor diet is rare. However, it may occur among premature infants and secondary to pathologies causing fat malabsorption, such as abetalipoproteinemia, cystic fibrosis, and cholestatic disease. Neurological alterations are the most common manifestation of vitamin E deficiency in humans.[113]

The specific mechanisms of vitamin E deficiency syndromes are not clearly understood. However, it is accepted that the most important function of vitamin E is protection against tissue damage caused by lipid peroxidation.[114] Primordial free radicals (eg, superoxide) can originate from normal metabolism and through the effect of toxins. These free radicals may contribute to the formation of lipid free radicals when conjugated with polyunsaturated fatty acids. The lipid radicals undergo a propagation sequence whose final products are lipid hydroperoxides (LOOH), which enter an autoxidative chain sequence until two radicals combine in a 2-electron bond. Vitamin E prevents autoxidation in at least two steps: (1) it traps peroxyl radicals; thus, a stable LOOH molecule is formed with a vitamin E radical subproduct; and (2) this vitamin E radical can still bind to another lipid radical. It is estimated that one tocopherol molecule is enough to protect 100 polyunsaturated fatty acid molecules from autoxidation.[115] Some functions of vitamin E are strongly dependent on interactions with other nutrients. The antioxidant efficacy of tocopherol is enhanced by the presence of other antioxidant systems. The glutathione peroxidase system is selenium dependent, and may explain the fact that selenium reduces the severity of vitamin E deficiency and that both may act synergistically against oxidative stress.[116] Vitamin C (ascorbic acid) appears to reduce the vitamin E requirement by regenerating tocopherol after oxidation.[117] β-carotene may also be a coadjuvant of vitamin E in its membrane antioxidant functions; on the other hand, vitamin E increases the lymphatic uptake of β-carotene and its conversion to retinol.[118] High intakes of polyunsaturated fatty acids increase vitamin E requirements but the extent remains unclear.[107]

Vitamin E may have functions unrelated to its antioxidant role, but it is generally difficult to rule out pathways that are regulated by oxidative stress. Tocopherol may be an important structural part of cell membranes that contributes to stability and permeability.[119] It regulates the synthesis of xanthine oxidase, an important enzyme in the conversion of purine bases to uric acid,[120] and modulates the activity of microsomal oxidases, protein kinases, and proliferation of smooth-muscle[121] and endothelial[122] cells. α-Tocopherol decreases the genetic expression of important regulatory receptors, the collagenase and scavenger receptor (SR-A and CD36), and upregulates the expression of connective tissue growth factor.[123] Vitamin E has positive effects on the immune function at various levels. It inhibits the activity of cyclooxygenase in macrophages, thus decreasing the production of proinflammatory prostaglandins like PGE-2[124]; it also increases the mitogenic activity of T cells and the production of IL-2[125] and interferon-γ.[126] Vitamin E has anti-DNA mutagenic damage properties,[127] and downregulates the generation of hydrogen peroxide in the mitochondria.[128] These mechanisms may explain the protective effects of vitamin E against upper respiratory infection[129] and degenerative pathologies such as certain cancers,[130] cardiovascular disease,[131,132] and Alzheimer's disease.[133]

There is no evidence that toxic amounts of vitamin E can be ingested from food alone. However, supplemental intakes of vitamin E should not exceed 1,000 mg among adults to prevent hemorrhagic toxicity and diminished blood coagulation among individuals who are on anticoagulant therapy or who are vitamin K deficient.[21] Lower ULs have been defined for children older than 1 year to safeguard against potential toxic effects. For infants, the IOM has not determined a UL, given that there is a paucity of data and given that food should be the only source of the vitamin for infants. While supplemental vitamin E may lower the risk of retinopathy of prematurity, there are no convincing data to suggest that supplemental vitamin E reduces the occurrence of bronchopulmonary dysplasia or intraventricular hemorrhage. According to the AAP, large parenteral doses of vitamin E in preterm infants, which elevate serum levels >40 μg/mL, are contraindicated, as they may increase the risk of bacterial and fungal sepsis.[134] The IOM recommends that premature infants should not ingest more than 21 mg of α-tocopherol to prevent hemorrhagic toxicity.[107]

VITAMIN K

History, Structure, and Metabolism

In 1929, Henrik Dam described a bleeding condition in chicks fed diets formulated to investigate cholesterol metabolism.[135] He suggested the existence of a new vitamin in 1935 after this fat-soluble compound effectively prevented the bleeding condition in chicks.[136] In 1939, a research group led by Doisy attributed its chemical and physical properties to a substituted 1,4-naphthoquinone.[137] Dam and Doisy jointly received the Nobel prize for medicine in 1943 for the discovery of the vitamin and for the elucidation of the chemical structure.

Vitamin K is a fat-soluble vitamin that consists of a family of compounds with a common 2-methyl-1,4-naphthoquinone ring structure. The vitamin K found in plants is phylloquinone, or vitamin K_1, and represents the major dietary form of vitamin K. Bacteria synthesize multiple forms of menaquinones, or vitamin K_2. While phylloquinone has a phytyl side chain, menaquinones have unsaturated isoprenyl side chains of varying lengths. The parent 2-methyl-1,4-naphthoquinone ring structure, also referred to as menadione or vitamin K_3, does not occur in nature, but can be alkylated to menaquinone-4 (MK-4); hence, menadione can be considered as provitamin K.

Vitamin K is absorbed from the first half of the small intestine with fat as part of micelles that form in the presence of pancreatic enzymes and bile salts. Absorption of pharmacologic preparations of phylloquinone in adult humans is about 80%, but it is significantly lower from food sources.[138] Whereas cooking and preparation do not appear to affect the bioavailability of vitamin K, the presence of fat may increase its absorption by a factor of 3.[139] After lymphatic absorption, phylloquinone is taken up by the liver from chylomicron remnants through apolipoprotein E receptors. There is no known carrier protein and phylloquinone is principally transported with triacylglycerol-rich lipoproteins.[140] Little is known on menaquinone transport or clearance from the circulation. Vitamin K is principally stored in the liver, and menaquinones account for about 90% of hepatic vitamin K stores, while phylloquinone accounts for the remainder. Nevertheless, vitamin K is also found at relatively high concentrations in trabecular and cortical bone, as well as in heart, pancreas, brain, and kidney.[140]

At birth, liver menaquinone levels are either absent or extremely low and build up slowly during the first weeks of life. This build up has been attributed to the intestinal colonization of menaquinone-producing bacteria.[141] However, there is still uncertainty about the bioavailability of bacteria-produced menaquinones.[142] Despite their presence in the liver and plasma, bacteria-produced menaquinones may only contribute little to satisfying human vitamin K requirements. This is based on the observation that dietary restriction of vitamin K leads to vitamin K insufficiency among otherwise health subjects. In line with this, phylloquinone concentrations in serum or plasma range from 0.3 to 3.0 nmol/L and are therefore much lower than those of other fat-soluble vitamins.[143] While it is known that menaquinones circulate at physiologically significant amounts, reference ranges have not been established.[143] The excretion of the vitamin occurs in the feces via bile, and to a lesser degree in urine.[144]

Functions

Vitamin K functions as a coenzyme in the carboxylation of glutamic acid to form γ-carboxyglutamic acid (Gla), which is an essential component of a large number of proteins in vertebrates and invertebrates. This reaction occurs at the luminal surface of the endoplasmic reticulum. After carboxylation, vitamin K is oxidized to vitamin K 2,3-epoxide, which can be successively recycled to quinine and hydroquinone in reactions catalyzed by dithiol-dependent reductases. These reductases can be inhibited by coumarinic drugs such as warfarin, which explains their anticoagulant effects. Undercarboxylated proteins, which have a decreased affinity for calcium, have historically been referred to as proteins induced by vitamin K absence or antagonism, or PIVKAs. Undercarboxylated prothrombin, also known as PIVKA-II, is a sensitive marker of subclinical vitamin K deficiency.[141]

The metabolic functions of vitamin K are best described with regard to blood coagulation. Initially, the hemorrhagic condition due to dietary vitamin K deficiency was related to a decrease in prothrombin, or clotting factor II, activity. Further research identified clotting factors VII, IX, and X. In the coagulation cascade, factors VII and IX activate factor X through the extrinsic and intrinsic pathways, respectively, while factor X activates the synthesis of prothrombin from thrombin. The vitamin K–dependent proteins C, S, and Z act as anticoagulants in hemostasis, rather than as procoagulants. All are synthesized in the liver and contain 10 to 13 Gla residues that facilitate calcium-mediated binding to membrane phospholipids in platelets and endothelial cells.[140]

Vitamin K is important for bone health as a cofactor for the bone Gla proteins osteocalcin, protein S, and matrix Gla protein (MGP). Osteocalcin, also known as bone Gla protein, is produced in osteoblasts and odontoblasts and binds to hydroxyapatite crystals through its three Gla residues. The percentage of undercarboxylated osteocalcin (%ucOC) is a sensitive marker of vitamin K status, and better vitamin K status, as evidenced by high plasma phylloquinone and low %ucOC, was associated with decreased bone turnover among healthy US girls.[145] In turn, supplementation with vitamin K_2 may maintain bone mineral density and prevent fractures among osteoporotic patients.[146] Protein S deficiency has been associated with osteopenia and osteonecrosis but its exact role in bone metabolism remains unknown.[147] While MGP is expressed in various soft tissues and cell types, it normally accumulates only in the extracellular matrix of bone and calcified cartilage. It inhibits cartilage formation in bone, as illustrated by experiments with mice that developed osteopenia when lacking MGP.[148] MGP may inhibit calcification by binding calcium in nucleating hydroxyapatite to inhibit crystal growth.[149] Alternatively, MGP may regulate osteogenesis by binding to BMP-2, one of the bone morphogenic proteins.[150]

The role of MGP in calcification is also relevant for cardiovascular health, as MGP deficiency in mice induces severe arterial calcification, leading to aortic rupture.[148] In line with this evidence from animal experiments, low vitamin K intake among women is associated with calcification of the abdominal aorta.[151] Protein S may also be relevant for cardiovascular health by facilitating the vascular repair process.[152]

There is emerging evidence that vitamin K protects brain sphingolipids, which are important lipid-signaling molecules that participate in motor and cognitive behavior.[153] The myelin-rich regions in the brain have high concentrations of MK-4, which is produced by a tissue-specific conversion from phylloquinone.[154] MK-4 and phylloquinone prevent oxidative stress and may thus slow the age-related decline in motor and cognitive behavior.[153] Even though Gas6 and, to a lesser extent, protein S, are present in the brain, it is not clear whether these vitamin K–dependent proteins play a role in these mechanisms.[140] Vitamin K deficiency may also be relevant for the development of other diseases, such as cancer,[155] glomerular kidney disease,[156] and hepatitis C.[157]

Among adults, signs of vitamin K deficiency, such as abnormal hemostatic control, are extremely uncommon. However, conditions leading to fat malabsorption may predispose to vitamin K deficiency, as may the use of megadoses of vitamin E.[140] In contrast to the general adult population, infants are at risk for vitamin K deficiency, as the vitamin is poorly transported across the placenta and breastmilk intake may be insufficient to meet requirements. Vitamin K deficiency among infants leads to an insufficient production of clotting factors in the liver and a subsequent bleeding syndrome originally known as hemorrhagic disease of the newborn, but now known as vitamin K–deficiency bleeding (VKDB) in infancy.[158] The early form of the disorder, which is defined as vitamin K–deficient bleeding within the first 24 hours of life, is rare but may be fatal because of bleeding from intracranial, intrathoracic, intra-abdominal, and GI sites. The classical form of VKDB occurs between days 2 and 7 of life and since the bleeding is typically restricted to the GI tract, umbilicus, skin, nose, or site of circumcision, the mortality rate from classical VKDB in the developed world is very low. Late VKDB peaks between weeks 3 and 8, but may occur as late as 6 months. It generally occurs among exclusively breast-fed infants, but may also occur among infants who have malabsorption due to liver disease, cystic fibrosis, or short-bowel syndrome. The disorder is often marked by acute intracranial hemorrhage and thus accompanied by high rates of neurological handicaps or death.[141]

To prevent VKDB, the AAP recommends that vitamin K_1 should be administered to all newborns as a single, intramuscular dose of 0.5 to 1 mg. While oral forms have been in use to prevent VKDB, the recommendations outline that further research is necessary to determine the efficacy, safety, and bioavailability of such oral formulations. Furthermore, families should be counseled on the risks of late VKDB due to inadequate oral vitamin K prophylaxis, especially among exclusively breast-fed children.[159] Research conducted in the UK in the 1990s related intramuscular vitamin K with an increased risk of childhood cancer, especially leukemia.[160,161] However, these findings have not been replicated in other studies[162] and a single, intramuscular dose of vitamin K thus remains the recommended prevention strategy for VKDB in the United States.[159]

High dietary intakes of vitamin K decrease the therapeutic effectiveness of anticoagulant medications such as warfarin. Therefore, dietary and supplementation habits should not be altered once the anticoagulant dose has been established. There is no evidence that high intakes of phylloquinone or menaquinones from food or supplements lead to adverse effects among persons who are not on anticoagulant therapy.[163]

VITAMIN C

History, Structure, and Metabolism

Medical writings from ancient Egyptians, Greeks, and Romans described a syndrome that was probably scurvy, the disease associated with vitamin C deficiency. The first modern accounts of scurvy appear in the sailing logs of the Portuguese and Spanish marine expeditions of the early sixteenth century.[164] During Vasco da Gama's expedition to the Cape of Good Hope, intake of oranges was associated with relief from apparent symptoms of scurvy. However, this practice did not become popular knowledge and it was only in 1747, when James Lind conducted his famous clinical trial on board of the British vessel Salisbury, that the dietary origin of scurvy was completely proven. It took the British navy another 50 years to routinely provide lemon juice to its sailors.[165] In 1932, research groups led by Albert Szent-Gyoergyi[166,167] and Charles Glen King[168] isolated and identified vitamin C. Shortly thereafter, Norman Haworth determined the structure of ascorbic acid and synthesized the vitamin.[169,170] For their groundbreaking work on vitamin C, Szent-Gyoergyi and Haworth received the Nobel Prize in 1937.

Vitamin C has been defined as a redox system composed of L-ascorbic acid, monodehydro-L-ascorbic acid (a free radical), and oxidized ascorbate (dehydro-L-ascorbic acid, or DHA). Chemically, ascorbic acid is composed of a 6-carbon γ-lactone. Except in guinea pigs, bats, and primates including humans, most animals can synthesize ascorbic acid from glucose via the hexuronic acid pathway. Humans lack L-gluconolactone oxidase, an enzyme necessary for the synthesis of ascorbic acid, and depend completely on the diet for the supply of vitamin C. After ingestion, ascorbic acid is absorbed in the small intestine, preferentially in the distal segment, through a sodium-dependent mechanism that is saturable and dose dependent. Glucose can inhibit this mechanism.[171] At higher GI concentrations, ascorbic acid is also absorbed by passive diffusion. While between 70 and 90% of ascorbic acid is absorbed when the vitamin is consumed at usual dietary intake levels (30 to 180 mg/d), absorption falls to below 50% when intake levels exceed 1 g/d.[172] The bioavailability from foods is similar to that from synthetic sources.[173]

Once absorbed, the vitamin moves to the systemic circulation via facilitated diffusion. It is oxidized to DHA, which is the form of the vitamin that enters cellular membranes. Once in the cell, it is again reduced to ascorbate by glutathione-dependent mechanisms. Owing to this recycling mechanism, relatively low amounts of the vitamin are lost through catabolism. However, if the mechanism is compromised, such as among diabetics,[174] smokers,[175] and patients with the glucose transporter protein syndrome, DHA is degraded to oxalic acid and excreted in urine.[176] Renal excretion of vitamin C increases proportionally with higher intake levels and reaches 100% after about 500 mg of an injected dose.[177]

Functions

Vitamin C is a water-soluble nutrient that functions biochemically as a cofactor for enzymes required for hydroxylation reactions. As a reducing agent, vitamin C also has important antioxidant roles that are not mediated by enzymes.

The vitamin C–dependent enzymes prolyl-4-hydroxylase, prolyl-3-hydroxylase, and lysyl-hydroxylase are required for the hydroxylation of lysine and proline residues in the synthesis of collagen. In the absence of this hydroxylation step, precursor molecules of collagen are unable to fold into their final triple helical structure, which leads to the accumulation of nonhelical trimers. This leads to a weakening of collagen-rich tissues, which explains many of the symptoms of scurvy, including gum bleeding, bruising, and inadequate repair of damaged tissue. Vitamin C is also a cofactor for 6-*N*-trimethyl-L-lysine hydroxylase and γ-butyrobetaine, two enzymes involved in the synthesis of carnitine. Carnitine deficiency and decreased oxidation of fatty acids in muscle may also be responsible for the muscular weakness characteristic of scurvy. Vitamin C is a cofactor of dopamine-β hydroxylase in the synthesis of norepinephrine and epinephrine, and peptidylglycine α-amidating monooxygenase in the activation of hormones and neurotransmitters. As part of 4-hydroxyphenylpyruvatedioxygenase, vitamin C functions in tyrosine metabolism.[178]

Ascorbic acid has strong antioxidant properties by scavenging reactive oxygen species. It thus neutralizes phagocyte-derived oxidants and protects plasma lipids, lipid membranes, and ocular tissue from oxidative damage.[179] The antioxidant properties of ascorbic acid suggest that the vitamin may have protective properties against degenerative diseases such as atherosclerosis and cancer. Large supplemental doses of vitamin C have been related to decreased LDL peroxidation and improved vasomotor function in humans.[180,181] In a study among hyperlipidemic children, antioxidant therapy with vitamins C (500 mg/d) and E (400 IU/d) restored endothelial function.[182] Furthermore, low plasma vitamin C concentrations have been linked to an increased risk of myocardial infarction[183] and accelerated progression of *Helicobacter pylori* infection to gastric dysplasia or gastric cancer.[184] However, a protective effect of vitamin C against mortality from coronary heart disease or the incidence of cancers of the digestive tract has yet to be demonstrated in clinical trials.

There is evidence to suggest that vitamin C is related to several aspects of the immune function. Ascorbic acid supplementation improves neutrophil chemotaxis. However, it does not appear to enhance bactericidal activity or lymphocyte proliferation. Vitamin C destroys histamine, and it has been suggested that this antihistaminic effect may be responsible for the reduction in the severity of cold symptoms that is observed among supplemented patients.[185]

In vitro assays indicate a possible antiviral role of the vitamin. It inhibits intracellular replication of HIV in chronically infected lymphocytes, and inhibits the reverse transcriptase enzyme.[186] In humans, local application of ascorbic acid on *Herpes simplex* lesions reduces viral shedding, and accelerates the disappearance of the lesions.[187]

Vitamin C interacts with other nutrients in vivo. Ascorbic acid positively interacts with the endogenous antioxidant glutathione and may contribute to antioxidant protection by maintaining glutathione in its reduced form. Vitamin C may regenerate α-tocopherol and reduce the intestinal absorption of copper, but these interactions have not been well characterized in humans.[188] The interaction between vitamin C and iron absorption is better known. Vitamin C reduces ferric iron found in dietary nonheme iron to the more absorbable ferrous iron form, and may impair the formation of unavailable iron complexes with ligands normally present in the GI lumen.[189] Dietary vitamin C intakes between 20 and 75 mg have been shown to augment nonheme iron absorption two to threefold from test meals.[178] Nevertheless, adding vitamin C to meals for extended periods of time has not improved body iron status among populations at risk for iron deficiency.[190,191]

Vitamin C deficiency among infants manifests itself as infantile scurvy in the form of bone abnormalities, hemorrhage symptoms, and anemia. However, vitamin C deficiency is unlikely to occur when infants are exclusively breast-fed during the first 6 months of life or when fortified infant formulas are used.[21]

The risk of adverse effects due to vitamin C ingested through food is extremely low. However, people with hemochromatosis, glucose-6-phosphate dehydrogenase deficiency, and renal disorders may be more susceptible to adverse effects of the vitamin, and are thus recommended to avoid ingesting levels in excess of the recommended dietary allowance. Among healthy adults, excess intake through supplements

(>3,000 mg/d) has been associated with mild adverse effects, such as osmotic diarrhea and intestinal discomfort. To prevent vitamin C–related adverse effects, healthy adults should not consume vitamin C at levels above the UL set at 2,000 mg/d; taking into account their lower body weight, ULs are lower for children.[21]

THIAMIN

History, Structure, and Metabolism

Descriptions of beriberi or *kakke*, the disease caused by thiamin deficiency, appeared in Chinese medical manuscripts more than four millennia ago. The prevalence of this polyneuritic paralysis had been traditionally higher in far east societies with high consumption of rice, than in the rest of the world. However, it increased in Europe during the nineteenth century, with the advent of highly efficient polishing rice mills that remove the aleurone layer of thiamin-rich cells, between the germ and the endosperm.[192] The first reference to a potential nutritional cause of beriberi appeared in 1884 when a Japanese surgeon, Takaki, showed that the prevalence of the disease in the navy could be reduced by feeding sailors meat, wheat, and milk instead of their usual diet, which consisted of polished rice and dried fish.[193] In 1890, a Dutch physician working in Java, Christian Eijkman, documented polyneuritis in chicken caused by a diet of polished rice and proposed that an antitoxin should be present in the bran. In 1901, Gerrit Grijns found that the antineuritic factor in rice bran was water soluble, and Casimir Funk coined the term "vitamine" in 1911, to refer to this compound.[1] Frazier and Stanton successfully used extracts of rice polishing to cure beriberi in humans in 1909 to 1915, and Roger Williams elucidated the structure of the vitamin in 1936.[194]

Thiamin, also called vitamin B_1, vitamin F, and aneurine, consists of a pyrimidine nucleus and a thiazole ring linked by a methylene bridge. The natural form of the vitamin is a base, and the commercial form is usually a chloride hydrochloride salt.

After ingestion, thiamin is absorbed preferentially in the proximal small intestine by an active, saturable, and energy-dependent transport; at high luminal concentrations, it is also absorbed by passive diffusion.[195] Only a small amount of high doses of thiamin is absorbed. Thiamin is phosphorylated at the brush border of intestinal epithelial cells but is converted back to free thiamin before being transported across the basolateral surface for delivery into the circulation.[192] The vitamin is transported by both erythrocytes and plasma and is distributed relatively evenly in tissues, but higher concentrations are found in liver and kidney.[196] Nervous tissue has lower concentrations but it can conserve thiamin levels more effectively than other tissues.[197] Urinary thiamin excretion increases rapidly when tissue levels are elevated and decreases when tissue levels are depleted to conserve vitamin status.[198] Nevertheless, tissue thiamin depletion occurs relatively rapidly under low dietary intake.

Functions

In the form of thiamin pyrophosphate, the coenzymatic and most abundant form of the vitamin in tissues, thiamin functions as cofactor in the metabolism of carbohydrates and branched-chain amino acids. These biochemical reactions involve active aldehyde transfers and can be grouped into the oxidative decarboxylation of α-keto acids and the transketolase reaction.

The oxidative decarboxylation of α-keto acids includes (1) oxidative decarboxylation of pyruvic acid, the first step in the conversion of pyruvate to acetyl coenzyme A (CoA) in the mitochondria; (2) oxidative decarboxylation of α-ketoglutaric acid, a step within the tricarboxylic acid cycle in which α-ketoglutarate is converted into succinyl CoA; and (3) oxidative decarboxylation of the branched-chain α-keto acids α-ketoisocaproate, α-keto-β-methylvalerate, and α-ketoisovalerate, to produce isovaleryl CoA, α-methylbutyryl CoA, and isobutyryl CoA, respectively, in high energy-generating pathways. The transketolase reaction occurs in the cytosol as part of the pentose phosphate pathway and is important for the biosynthesis of fatty acids and pentoses. Recent research indicates that thiamin pyrophosphate is also a cofactor in the β-oxidation of 3-methyl-substituted fatty acids such as phytanic acid.[199]

Owing to the high number of thiamine-dependent enzymes, thiamine deficiency is associated with a wide range of cellular impairments. Studies in animals suggest that maternal thiamin deficiency impairs brain lipogenesis[200] and the development of enzymes involved in brain energy metabolism.[201] Maternal thiamin deficiency may increase the risk of intrauterine growth retardation,[202] and in conjunction with niacin and pyridoxine deficiencies it may increase the risk of oral facial clefts.[203]

Among adults, thiamin deficiency can occur as a consequence of low dietary thiamin intake accompanied by high intake of carbohydrate from milled rice. Thiamin depletion is also related to chronic alcoholism and the consumption of fermented raw fish, betel nuts, and fermented tea leaves. Thiamin deficiency continues to be an important nutritional problem in emergency settings such as refugee camps.[204,205] The deficiency may be manifest itself as dry beriberi, wet beriberi, or the Wernicke–Korsakoff syndrome. Dry beriberi is a chronic, generally nonfatal condition characterized by peripheral neuropathy with sensory, motor, and autonomic compromises, predominantly of the distal segments of the limbs. Wet beriberi is associated with signs of congestive heart failure and may be rapidly fatal. Wernicke's disease is an encephalopathy of acute onset characterized by ataxia of gait and paralysis of eye movements, usually accompanied by the Korsakoff psychosis, which consists of amnesia and other mental alterations. Chronic alcohol abuse is a major factor in the etiology of this syndrome.[192]

Infantile beriberi may be found in children 2 to 3 months of age, whose mothers have low thiamin concentrations in breastmilk. It may present as four forms.[206] The cardiac or acute fulminating form is characterized by the rapid appearance of beriberi signs such as loud piercing cry, cyanosis, dyspnea, vomiting, tachycardia, and cardiomegaly; the prognosis is fatal unless thiamin is administered. The aphonic form is characterized by the child's voice tone, which may vary from hoarseness to total aphonia due to paralysis of phonation nerves. The pseudomeningitic form presents with normal cerebrospinal fluid and with neurological abnormalities that may include vomiting, nystagmus, purposeless movement of the extremities, and convulsion. In the mixed form, any combination of the cardiac, aphonic, or pseudomeningitic forms can be present.[206]

Nationwide shortages of intravenous multivitamins used in US hospitals and home-healthcare agencies led to the development of acute thiamin deficiency among several patients receiving total parenteral nutrition in the years 1989 and 1996. The chief deficiency symptom in these patients was severe lactic acidosis, based on impairment in the oxidation of α-keto acids. Patients who received treatment with parenteral thiamin showed rapid clinical improvements.[207,208] In 2003, a defective soy-based infant formula caused an outbreak of thiamine deficiency among Israeli infants.[209] Cases were treated with intramuscular doses of thiamin (50 mg/d) for 2 weeks, resulting in rapid clinical improvements without side effects.

There are no reports of toxicity from excess thiamin intake from food or supplements, presumably due to low absorption efficiency of intakes >5 mg and rapid urinary excretion when tissue levels are elevated.[21]

RIBOFLAVIN

History, Structure, and Metabolism

Riboflavin, or vitamin B_2, was discovered as a fluorescent "yellow growth factor" in the heat-stable fraction of antipellagra extracts found by McCollum and collaborators. It was synthesized by Kuhn [210] and Karrer in 1935,[211] and its structure was elucidated by Warburg and Christian in 1938.[212]

All riboflavin-related compounds have an isoalloxazine ring. Riboflavin itself does not have significant physiological functions, but it is the substrate for the coenzymes flavin mononucleotide (FMN), and flavin adenine dinucleotide (FAD). The former contains a phosphate group, and the latter is formed by a combination of FMN with adenosine 5′-triphosphate in the presence of FAD pyrophosphorylase. FAD can be further metabolized and bound covalently to proteins. Riboflavin is very sensitive to UV radiation, and can be destroyed during phototherapy of neonatal jaundice.[213] Most of the riboflavin in food is present as FAD, and smaller amounts are present as the free form and as FMN.

After ingestion, the riboflavin coenzyme derivatives are hydrolyzed to riboflavin in the brush border of enterocytes and absorbed in the proximal small intestine by an active, saturable, and carrier-mediated transport system.[214] At high intakes, small amounts of passive absorption may also occur. The rate of absorption is proportional up to intakes of about 30 mg contained in a meal but decreases sharply after higher intakes.[215,216] In enterocytes, free riboflavin undergoes an adenosine 5′-triphosphate–dependent phosphorylation to form FMN, most of which is further converted to FAD by an FAD-dependent synthetase. To allow transport across the basolateral membrane, nonspecific phosphatases act on intracellular flavins, so that riboflavin enters the blood as the free form or as FMN.[217] In the blood, riboflavin is transported mainly bound to immunoglobulins and to a lesser degree to albumin.[218] The vitamin is converted to its coenzymatic forms in the cytoplasm of many tissues, especially in the small intestine, liver, heart, and kidney.[219] In tissues, the coenzyme forms are generally bound to enzymes, which is a way to trap riboflavin in cells, as the coenzyme forms would otherwise be hydrolyzed to the free forms, which diffuses from cells and is excreted.[217] Alcohol interferes with digestion and absorption, and some psychotropic, chemotherapeutic, and antimalaric medications, which inhibit the conversion of riboflavin into its coenzyme forms.[220] Excretion of riboflavin occurs in urine, predominantly as free riboflavin.

Functions

As an integral component of the flavoproteins FMN and FAD, riboflavin is important for various redox reactions. Due to the coenzymatic activity of FAD in the respiratory chain, riboflavin plays a key role in energy production. FAD is required for the regeneration of glutathione in the glutathione peroxidase antioxidant system, which protects tissues against lipid peroxidation. Therefore, antioxidant defense may be compromised during riboflavin deficiency. Riboflavin enzymes are also involved in the metabolism of drugs, lipids, and several nutrients.[198,220] FAD is important for folate and vitamin B_{12} metabolism, as it is a cofactor for the enzyme 5,10-methylenetetrahydrofolate reductase, which catalyzes the conversion of methylene tetrahydrofolate to methyl tetrahydrofolate. The latter is required for the remethylation of homocysteine to methionine. In the metabolism of vitamin B_6, FMN is required for the conversion of pyridoxal-5-phosphate, while in niacin metabolism, the FAD-dependent kynurenine hydroxylase is needed for the conversion of tryptophan to niacin.[198] Riboflavin deficiency may also impair iron absorption.[221,222]

Several signs and symptoms have been related to riboflavin deficiency in humans, including stomatitis, glossitis, dermatitis, keratitis, anemia, and neurological dysfunction. Riboflavin deficiency may increase the risk of cancers at certain sites, such as the esophagus[223] and cervix.[224] Riboflavin nutritional status may also be relevant for cardiovascular health. It may limit tissue damage associated with ischemia reperfusion due to its antioxidant function[225,226] and may prevent cardiovascular disease by lowering homocysteine concentrations.[227] Further research is warranted to confirm the role of riboflavin in cancer and cardiovascular disease.[217]

The effect of pharmacologic doses of riboflavin over extended periods of time has not been examined, but the evidence to date indicates that high intakes do not lead to adverse effects, presumably due to limited GI absorption and rapid urinary excretion of the vitamin.

NIACIN

History, Structure, and Metabolism

Pellagra, the manifestation of niacin deficiency in humans, was first described in 1735 in Spain as a disease primarily affecting the very poor. The disorder was soon recognized throughout southern and eastern Europe as well as Egypt, where corn became the major food crop. The disease was also common in the United States in the early twentieth century, where it affected hundreds of thousands of people, with up to 7,000 reported annual deaths.[228] Nicotinic acid, one of two chemical forms of niacin, was first isolated in 1867 and work initiated by Goldberger in 1914 showed that pellagra was a nutritional deficiency disease. In 1937, nicotinic acid was shown to cure the manifestation of pellagra in dogs[229] and humans.[230]

The term niacin refers to nicotinic acid (pyridine-3-carboxylic acid), nicotinamide (nicotinic acid amide), and functional nicotinamide derivatives. Nicotinamide can be formed from nicotinic acid in the body.

Nicotinic acid and nicotinamide are absorbed in the stomach and small intestine. At physiological concentrations, niacin is absorbed in the stomach and intestine by pH-dependent facilitated diffusion, while passive diffusion predominates at higher concentrations.[231] Nicotinamide adenine dinucleotide (NAD) and nicotinamide adenine dinucleotide phosphate (NADP), the major forms of niacin in food, are converted by enzymatic action in the gut mucosa to nicotinamide.[232] In the blood, nicotinamide constitutes the major form of vitamin and serves in the tissue synthesis of NAD when needed. However, both NAD and NADP can be synthesized in all tissues of the body from nicotinic acid or nicotinamide. Niacin is unique among the B vitamins in that it can be synthesized from a precursor molecule. The essential amino acid tryptophan can be converted to NAD via the formation of quinolinic acid and nicotinic acid ribonucleotide. It has been estimated that 60 mg of dietary tryptophan yields 1 mg niacin,[233] but the conversion may be inhibited by deficiencies in other nutrients and by certain disease states, as explained in the next section. Excess niacin is excreted in the urine, mainly in the forms of N^1-methylnicotinamide and 2-pyridone.[234]

Functions

The metabolically active forms of niacin are NAD and NADP, whose nicotinamide moiety serves as an electron carrier or hydrogen donor in numerous redox reactions that are essential in carbohydrate, lipid, and amino acid metabolism. The NAD coenzyme generally functions as an electron acceptor in catabolic reactions that produce energy (eg, the citric acid cycle). It also serves as the substrate for enzymes in nonredox pathways that cleave the β-*N*-glycosylic bond of NAD to free nicotinamide and catalyze the transfer of ADP-ribose. These nonredox pathways may modulate or regulate DNA and genome fidelity, and inflammatory and immune responses. Through these actions, niacin nutritional status may affect the progression of chronic diseases such as cancer, diabetes, and dementia.[235] NADP participates in reductive biosynthetic pathways involving fatty acid and cholesterol synthesis. It functions with NAD as a cohydrogenase in the pentose phosphate pathway in the oxidation of glucose 6-phosphate to ribose 5-phosphate.[235]

The classical symptoms of the niacin-deficiency disease pellagra can be summarized as dermatitis, diarrhea, dementia, and potentially death (often called "the four Ds"). Pellagra develops when dietary niacin and tryptophan are insufficient to meet niacin requirements. Human experiments indicate that pellagra could develop after 50 to 60 days on a corn diet, which is low in both bioavailable niacin and tryptophan. Other dietary factors may contribute to the development of pellagra by inhibiting the conversion of tryptophan to niacin. They are excessive intake of the amino acid leucine and inadequate intakes of iron, riboflavin, or vitamin B_6. Pellagra-like symptoms in humans have also been reported after prolonged isoniazid treatment, during malignant carcinoid syndrome, and in Hartnup's disease. On the other hand, there is evidence that the conversion of tryptophan to niacin is augmented considerably among pregnant women and women taking oral contraceptives.[236]

Pharmacologic doses of nicotinic acid (but not nicotinamide) in the range of 1.5 to 4 g/d have proven effective at reducing the risk of atherosclerotic heart disease.[237] This risk reduction is brought about by an improvement in the blood lipid profiles of at-risk patients, such as reductions of total cholesterol, LDLs, and triglycerides, and increases of high-density lipoproteins.[237]

The first adverse effect of excess pharmacologic niacin intakes is flushing, while higher intakes may lead to liver toxicity, impaired glucose tolerance, as well as nausea and vomiting. For children younger than 1 year, no UL has been defined due to a lack of data and suggestions that intakes should occur from food alone. For older children, ULs were defined based on adult data on flushing and subsequent adjustments based on body weight.[21] However, it has been argued that data on flushing is not relevant for children, so that there is little data to support a UL for children.[69]

VITAMIN B_6

History, Structure, and Metabolism

Vitamin B_6 was discovered by Paul Gyoergy in 1934 during investigations on the etiology of the niacin-deficiency disease pellagra.[238] In 1939, Harris and Folkers elucidated the structure of pyridoxine and accomplished its synthesis.[239–241] Five years later, they were able to confirm that pyridoxal and pyridoxamine were the other free forms of vitamin B_6 in nature.[242]

The term vitamin B_6 encompasses a group of compounds that are metabolically interchangeable and that, in their free form, are named pyridoxine (an alcohol), pyridoxal (an aldehyde), and pyridoxamine (an amine). These forms also exist in their respective 5′-phosphates pyridoxine phosphate (PNP), pyridoxal phosphate (PLP), and pyridoxamine phosphate (PMP) forms. The major forms of vitamin B_6 in animal foods are PLP and PMP, while pyridoxine and PNP predominate in plant-derived foods.

Vitamin B_6 is absorbed by passive diffusion in the small intestine and bioavailability is approximately 75%. Since only free forms of the vitamin can enter the intestinal mucosa, the phosphate ester forms of the vitamin first have to be hydrolyzed to yield the free absorbable forms. These are taken up by the liver and converted to their respective 5′-phosphates by pyridoxal kinase. Phosphorylation of free forms of the vitamin also occurs in many other tissues. About three quarters of the body's vitamin B_6 pool is present in muscle. This pool is resistant to depletion even after prolonged intake of a vitamin B_6–deficient diet, which indicates that muscle vitamin B_6 is not a storage form of the vitamin that can be drawn upon in times of inadequate vitamin B_6 intakes.[243] Catabolism of vitamin B_6 occurs mostly in the liver and excretion of the vitamin occurs in the urine, predominantly as 4-pyridoxic acid.[244]

Functions

Vitamin B_6 functions as a coenzyme, usually in the form of PLP, for more than 100 enzymes. PLP facilitates the transfer of amino groups and is thus critical for the production of nonessential amino acids. For example, PLP is a cofactor for the enzyme glutamate-oxaloacetate aminotransferase, which catalyzes the formation of aspartic acid from glutamate. As a cofactor for kynureninase, PLP facilitates the conversion of the amino acid tryptophan to active niacin and the decarboxylation of precursor amino acids to generate several neurotransmitters, such as serotonin, taurine, dopamine, norepinephrine, histamine, and γ-aminobutyric acid.[245] In the transsulfuration pathway from homocysteine to cysteine, PLP acts in concert with cystathione synthase to convert homocysteine to cystathione. In carbohydrate metabolism, PLP functions in the production of glucose 1-phosphate from glycogen, while in lipid metabolism, it functions in the production of carnitine and phospholipids. Lastly, PLP catalyzes the formation of δ-aminolevulinate required for heme synthesis.[219,246]

Vitamin B_6 deficiency is first evidenced by decreases in plasma PLP levels and lowered amount of the excretory product 4-pyridoxic acid in the urine. Continued vitamin B_6 deficiency leads to seborrheic dermatitis and decreased synthesis of neurotransmitters, resulting in depression, confusion, and abnormal brain wave patterns as indicated by abnormal electroencephalograms. Infants fed vitamin B_6–deficient formula are also at risk of developing convulsions.[247] Vitamin B_6 deficiency may depress humoral and cell-mediated immunity, presumably due to an impairment in the production of one-carbon units necessary for nucleic acid synthesis.[245] Impairments of heme synthesis may lead to hypochromic microcytic anemia. By impairing homocysteine metabolism, vitamin B_6 has been implicated in the development of coronary heart disease.[248]

Levels of vitamin B_6 in breastmilk are dependent on maternal intakes of the vitamin and there is evidence that lactating mothers who consume inadequate levels of vitamin B_6 pass on deficient amounts of the vitamin to the infant.[249] Vitamin B_6 deficiency in humans most commonly occurs in the elderly, in alcoholics, in individuals consuming drugs that interact with vitamin B_6 such as penicillamine, isoniazid, and L-3,4-dihydroxyphenylalanine, and in several inborn errors in vitamin B_6 function. Impairments resulting from genetic conditions have been shown to respond to high doses of supplemental vitamin B_6.[250]

Supplemental intakes of vitamin B_6 of 2,000 mg/d or more, which are used to treat conditions such as carpal tunnel syndrome, painful neuropathies, seizures, premenstrual syndrome, asthma, and sickle cell disease, may lead to adverse effects in the form of sensory neuropathy and dermatological lesions among adults. To safeguard against toxic effects of vitamin B_6, it is recommended that adults should not consume >100 mg/d. While healthy infants do not appear to require supplemental vitamin B_6, ULs have been set for children aged 1 to 18 years that are based on extrapolations from the adult UL.[21]

FOLATE

History, Structure, and Metabolism

In 1931, Lucy Wills described clinical folate deficiency as a tropical "macrocytic anemia" that was distinct from the signs of the vitamin B_{12}–deficiency disease pernicious anemia.[251] The condition could be cured by a yeast extract, from which folate was identified as the corrective substance several years later. Folate was extracted from spinach leaves in 1941 by Mitchell, Snell, and Williams and named after the latin word *folium* (leaf).[252] In recent years, folate has received considerable attention in the prevention of cardiovascular disease, cancer, and neural tube defects (NTDs).[253]

Folate is a generic term for a family of compounds that have nutritional properties of the simplest form of the vitamin, folic acid. Folic acid (pteroylglutamic acid) consists of a pteridine bicyclic ring system linked to *p*-aminobenzoic acid, which is connected by a peptide bond to glutamic acid. Folic acid is the chemical form used in synthetic folate supplements but it does not occur in appreciable amounts in foods. Rather, most folates in nature occur as polyglutamates, with 5 to 8 glutamate residues joined to the first glutamate. Next to modifications in the length of the glutamate chain, the vitamin may be modified by reduction of the pteridine ring system to generate dihydrofolic acid and tetrahydrofolic acid (THF). The N-5 and N-10 positions of THF, either individually or in concert, can carry 1-C units including methyl ($-CH_3$), formyl (–HCO), methylene ($-CH_2$), formyl (–CH=O), or formimino (–CH=NH) groups.

Folylpolyglutamates contained in foods need to undergo hydrolysis to be absorbed. In the enterocyte, the membrane-bound enzyme γ-glutamyl hydrolase catalyzes the hydrolysis of folylpolyglutamates to folylmonoglutamates. Transport across the brush border membrane of folylmonoglutamates occurs by a pH-dependent mechanism whose carrier has only recently been identified.[254,255] In the plasma, 5-methyl-THF-monoglutamate is the predominant form of the vitamin and the majority of it is associated with protein. After cellular uptake, folylmonoglutamates are converted back to folylpolyglutamates to retain the vitamin in the cell, to strengthen the binding of the vitamin to folate-dependent enzymes, and to allow for channeling reactions to occur. Excess folate is excreted in the form of cleavage products in the urine. Fecal losses of folate occur as well but are difficult to quantify.

Functions

Folate, in the form of its primary coenzyme THF, serves in the transfer of 1-C compounds needed in the metabolism of amino and nucleic acids (Figure 3). In the metabolism of amino acids, serine can transfer a methylene group to THF, to form glycine and 5,10-Methylene-THF. The latter can be reduced to 5-methyl-THF, which is the methyl donor in the synthesis of methionine from homocysteine and which may be important in sustaining sufficient methionine pools for *S*-adenosylmethionine. The methyl donation of *S*-adenosylmethionine is involved in more than a hundred physiological reactions, such as in the methylation of DNA, RNA, and membrane phospholipids. 5,10-Methylene-THF can also donate a methyl group for the formation of the pyrimidine thymidylate, a necessary precursor of DNA synthesis and erythrocyte formation. The enzyme C1-THF synthetase converts 5,10-methylene THF to 10-formyl THF, which is necessary for the de novo synthesis of the purines adenine and guanine.

The first manifestation of folate deficiency is a decline in serum folate levels, occurring approximately after 2 weeks of consumption of a folate-deficient diet. Hyperpigmentation of

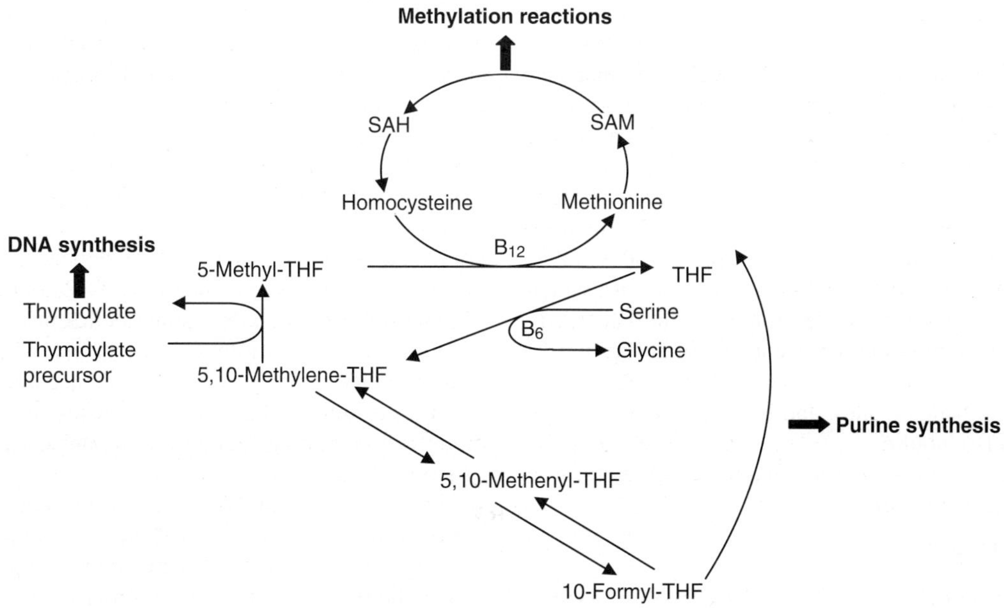

Figure 3 Summary diagram of folate metabolism.

neutrophils and a rise in homocysteine levels can be noted, while abnormally nucleated erythrocytes start to appear in the bone marrow. If folate deficiency continues, megaloblastic anemia can occur. Due to the rapidly dividing nature of cells lining the GI tract and the unmet need for folate for DNA synthesis, GI symptoms may result from folate deficiency. Elevated plasma homocysteine concentrations may occur during folate deficiency and have been associated with increased risk of ischemic heart disease and stroke in adult life.[256] Folate supplementation reduces homocysteine levels,[257] and research is under way to examine the effect of folate supplementation on cardiovascular disease. Poor folate status has been associated with increased risk of cancer, especially colon cancer, possibly due to abnormal synthesis and methylation of DNA.[258] Furthermore, folate deficiency has been linked to abnormal mental function, but more research is needed to substantiate this association.[259]

Adequate folate status early in pregnancy greatly decreases the risk of NTDs, the most common major congenital abnormality in many countries.[260] For this reason, folic acid has been added to enriched grains and mixed food items containing these grains in the United States since 1998 at levels of 0.14 mg/100 g flour.[261] Fortified grains have thus become a good source of folate and there is evidence that the folate status of the general population has increased as a result of this fortification program.[262] Women of child bearing age are advised to consume 400 μg folic acid daily from fortified foods, supplements, or both to reduce the risk of NTDs. This amount should be consumed in addition to folate from a varied diet.[219,263]

The growth of the fetus and related tissues increase folate requirements during pregnancy. Folate secreted in milk also increases maternal requirements during lactation. Folate deficiency during infancy may result from inadequate intakes of the vitamin, such as in infants fed on goat's milk, which is a poor source of folate. Deficiencies may also occur due to impaired absorption of the vitamin and after intake of a range of medications, including methotrexate, anticonvulsants, and anticancer drugs that have antifolate activity.

Deficiencies in either folate or vitamin B_{12} lead to megaloblastic anemia due to a lack of adequate 5,10-methylenetetrahydrofolate,[264] but only vitamin B_{12} deficiency also leads to neurological complications.[265,266] There is concern that excessive intakes of folate may obscure or delay the diagnosis of vitamin B_{12} deficiency, especially among older adults with atrophic gastritis and those who follow a vegan diet or who suffer from pernicious anemia and bacterial overgrowth in the gut. The recommended ULs for folate proposed by the IOM attempt to safeguard against the masking of vitamin B_{12}.[267] Since vitamin B_{12} deficiency may be uncommon in children other than those exclusively breast-fed from vegan mothers or those with GI pathologies, the ULs established for children may be conservative.[69,268]

VITAMIN B_{12}

History, Structure, and Metabolism

The symptoms of the main vitamin B_{12}–deficiency disorder, pernicious anemia, were first described in the midnineteenth century by Thomas Addison. In 1926, Minot and Murphy showed that large quantities of liver normalized the hematological symptoms of pernicious anemia.[269] In 1948, the vitamin was isolated in the crystalline form from liver by Folkers[270] and Smith.[271]

Vitamin B_{12} is a large molecule similar to porphyrin that has a complex ring structure (corrin ring). At its center, it possesses a cobalt molecule. Its chemical name is cobalamin and it is solely synthesized by microorganisms. Supplemental forms of vitamin B_{12} are generally in the form of cyanocobalamin but hydroxocobalamin has also been used.

Absorption of vitamin B_{12} takes place at receptor sites in the distal ileum. To aid this process, parietal cells of the gastric mucosa secrete intrinsic factor, which is a highly specific glycoprotein for the vitamin. In plasma, vitamin B_{12} is associated with the plasma-binding proteins transcobalamin (TC) I, II, or III. While TCI transports about 80% of vitamin B_{12} in plasma, TCII is the protein that delivers the vitamin to tissues.[272] Cellular uptake of the TCII–B_{12} complex proceeds via receptor-mediated endocytosis and the vitamin is subsequently released in the lysosome. Vitamin B_{12} is readily converted to the two active coenzyme forms methylcobalamin and 5-deoxyadenosylcobalamin. Vitamin B_{12} is stored in the liver and among healthy omnivores, stores amount to about 2 to 3 mg.[273]

Fecal losses are the main route of excretion for vitamin B_{12}. Losses through the biliary route are minimal as the vitamin is reabsorbed during enterohepatic circulation. Greater fecal losses occur from desquamated cells, gastric and intestinal secretions, vitamin B_{12} derived from colonic bacteria, and unabsorbed vitamin B_{12} from food. Fecal losses are proportional to stores. At very high plasma concentrations, such as after injections of the vitamin, urinary excretion also occurs.[267]

Functions

Vitamin B_{12} functions as part of the coenzymes methylcobalamin, the main coenzymatic form in plasma, and 5-adenosylcobalamin, found in the liver, most body tissues, and foods. Vitamin B_{12} deficiency impairs normal hematological, neurological, and GI function.

In methyl transfer reactions and the synthesis of purines and DNA, the function of vitamin B_{12} is closely related to that of folate.[264] Methylcobalamin is required by methionine synthase for the methyl transfer from 5-methyl-tetrahydrofolate to homocysteine, to yield the end products methionine and tetrahydrofolate (THF) (Figure 3). In the absence of vitamin B_{12}, folate becomes trapped in its inactive form 5-methyl-tetrahydrofolate, DNA synthesis is impaired, and megaloblastic anemia develops. The hematologic features of this type of anemia are indistinguishable from those of folate deficiency.[274]

As part of 5-adenosylcobalamin, vitamin B_{12} is required for the enzyme L-methylmalonyl-CoA mutase to convert L-methylmalonyl-CoA to succinyl-CoA in an isomerization reaction. Lack of production of succinyl-CoA due to vitamin B_{12} deficiency is unlikely to have serious metabolic consequences, as succinyl-CoA is abundantly derived from fats and carbohydrates. However, accumulation of L-methylmalonyl-CoA in the cell can lead to increased production of odd-chain and branched-chain fatty acids through a sequence of reactions. These fatty acids may be abnormally incorporated into nerve cell membranes and they may account for neurological symptoms due to degeneration of myelin nerve sheaths.[265,266] Such neurological symptoms may include tingling and numbness sensations in the extremities, motor disturbances, and cognitive changes such as loss of concentration and dementia. In extreme cases, the degeneration of peripheral nerves may progress to irreversible paralysis. Neurological complications may in some cases present without hematological symptoms. In fact, there is evidence of an inverse association between the prominence of neurological complications and the severity of anemia; that is, more prominent neurological complications tend to occur in individuals who are less anemic.[265,275] As described in the section on folate found in this chapter, folate deficiency does not induce neurological complications.

GI impairments due to vitamin B_{12} deficiency include atrophic glossitis, papillary atrophy of the tongue, appetite loss, flatulence, and constipation. Among children, vitamin B_{12} deficiency has been associated with irritability, anorexia, failure to thrive, developmental delays, and poor brain growth.[276]

Foods of animal origin are the best naturally occurring sources of vitamin B_{12} and those who follow a vegan diet are therefore at risk for vitamin B_{12} deficiency. Vegan mothers may also have depressed vitamin B_{12} in their breastmilk and are thus advised to supplement their infants from birth with vitamin B_{12} at the level of the adequate intake.[267] Generally, however, vitamin B_{12} deficiency is due to poor absorption and less as a result of inadequate intake. Infants and children with diseases or resection of the terminal ileum (eg, Crohn's disease, short-bowel syndrome) are at risk of vitamin B_{12} deficiency. Malabsorption can also be due to pernicious anemia, a chronic atrophic gastritis that is characterized by the presence of autoantibodies to parietal cells, which causes loss of these intrinsic factor–producing cells. Autoantibodies to intrinsic factor have also been demonstrated.[277] Pernicious anemia in children is generally the result of a genetically determined defect in secretion of intrinsic factor or the secretion of a defective intrinsic factor.[278,279] The vitamin deficiency can be corrected by large monthly injections of vitamin B_{12}.

There is no evidence of adverse effects of vitamin B_{12} obtained from foods or supplements. As a result, ULs have not been defined for vitamin B_{12}.[267]

BIOTIN

History, Structure, and Metabolism

Using feeding studies with dried egg white, Boas first described in 1927 that mammals require the water-soluble vitamin biotin.[280] Koegl and Toennis isolated the vitamin from egg yolk in 1932[281] and the chemical structure was elucidated by du Vigneaud and colleagues in 1942.[282] One year later, Harris and colleagues accomplished the chemical synthesis of biotin.[283]

Biotin is an imidazole derivative with chemical structure $C_{10}H_{16}N_2O_3S_1$. The vitamin is widely distributed in foods, mostly bound to protein. Digestion of dietary protein releases biotinyl peptides and intestinal biotinidases further hydrolyze biotinyl peptides to biotin.[284] At low luminal biotin concentrations, the vitamin is absorbed by a sodium-dependent saturable mechanism that uses the sodium-dependent multivitamin transporter, which binds biotin, pantothenic acid, and lipoic acid with similar affinity.[285] At high luminal biotin concentrations, a nonsaturable process dominates.[286] The bioavailability of biotin from food and supplements is close to 100% but is impaired by the consumption of raw eggs, which contain the heat labile protein avidin that tightly binds to biotin and prevents biotin absorption.[287] Biotin is transported by biotidinase, which has two biotin-bending sites, and by albumin, α-globulin, and β-globulin.[286–288] The vitamin is stored in the liver[289] and is excreted mainly in urine and to a lesser degree in bile.[290]

Functions

Biotin has long been known to function as a coenzyme in bicarbonate-dependent carboxylation reactions in energy metabolism, fatty acid synthesis, and amino acid metabolism.[291] More recently, novel roles for biotin in cell signaling, epigenetic control of gene expression, and chromatin structure have also been discovered.[292]

Biotin serves as a covalently bound coenzyme for four carboxylases. As part of pyruvate carboxylase, biotin aids in gluconeogenesis and replenishment of oxaloacetate for the citric acid cycle. As part of propionyl-CoA carboxylase, it catalyzes a crucial step in the metabolism of cholesterol, odd-chain fatty acids, and the amino acids isoleucine, valine, methionine, and threonine. In conjunction with acetyl-CoA carboxylase, biotin catalyzes the production of malonyl-CoA necessary for fatty acid synthesis, and with β-methylcrotonyl-CoA carboxylase, the vitamin metabolizes the amino acid leucine.[287]

Recent research indicates that biotin is covalently bound to DNA-binding proteins called histones, which play an important role in the folding of DNA into chromatin. The modification of histones due to the attachment of biotin may be relevant for gene silencing, cell proliferation, and the cellular response to DNA damage.[292]

Human biotin deficiency has been noted among persons on biotin-free total parenteral nutrition and among persons who consume large amounts of raw eggs over extended periods of time. The first manifestation of biotin deficiency is a depressed biotin level in urine. Subsequently, the following clinical signs may develop: dermatitis, conjunctivitis, alopecia, and central nervous system abnormalities such as depression, lethargy, hallucinations, and parathesia of the extremities. Among infants, deficiency symptoms occur after 3 to 6 months on biotin-free total parenteral nutrition, which is earlier than among adults, possibly because of increased biotin requirements due to growth. Biotin deficiency among infants leads to neurological disorders such as hypotonia, lethargy, development delays, and a peculiar withdrawn behavior.[21,286]

Biotin deficiency may also be due to genetic defects. Infants with a genetic defect in the enzyme biotinidase fail to recycle biotin and lose large amounts of biotin metabolites in the urine. Symptoms generally occur after the first week of life but before age and include poor feeding, vomiting, rash around eyes, nose, and mouth, and neurological symptoms such as muscle pain, lethargy, and numbness. Biotinidase deficiency is rare with an incidence of about 1 in 120,000.[293] Genetic defects may also induce deficiencies in individual and multiple carboxylases, which cause biotin-deficiency symptoms and accumulation of substrates. Pharmacologic doses of oral biotin restore normal function in the presence of genetic defects.[294]

There are no reports of adverse effects due to high doses of biotin. Even doses as high as 200 mg given orally and 20 mg given intravenously did not lead to toxicity symptoms.[286,295]

PANTOTHENIC ACID

History, structure, and metabolism

Pantothenic acid was discovered as a growth factor for yeast and certain bacteria by Roger J. Williams in 1933.[296] Elvehjem and Jukes showed in 1939 that pantothenic acid was required for growth and prevented dermatitis in chickens.[297,298] Williams established the structure of the vitamin in 1940.[299]

The chemical structure of pantothenic acid consists of β-alanine and a dihydroxy acid called pantoic acid joined by an amide link. In food, the vitamin is present as CoA or as 4′-phosphopantetheine (Ppant). Hydrolysis of CoA and Ppant in the intestinal lumen renders pantothenic acid readily absorbable.[300] The vitamin is absorbed in the small intestine by active, saturable transport at low concentrations and passive transport at higher concentrations.[301] After absorption, the vitamin is transported in the bloodstream to various tissues where the enzyme pantothenate kinase regulates the synthesis of CoA from pantothenic acid. Synthesis of the cofactor Ppant proceeds without direct involvement of pantothenic acid, as the reaction proceeds from CoA as substrate. Excretion of the vitamin occurs in the urine, primarily as pantothenic acid.[302]

Functions

Pantothenic acid serves as the substrate for the synthesis of CoA and acyl carrier protein, which play important roles in the metabolism of carbohydrates, proteins, and fats. As part of CoA, pantothenic acid functions in the transfer of acetyl and acyl groups in many vital reactions. These include reactions related to the citric acid cycle and the acetylation of sugars and proteins. As part of acyl carrier protein, pantothenic acid functions in the synthesis of fatty acids.

A variety of health claims have been made for pantothenic acid. As summarized by Miller et al,[302] these include potential effects on lowering cholesterol, enhanced athletic performance, and benefits for rheumatoid arthritis, wound healing, and lupus erythematosus. While pantothenic acid supplementation may have some benefit for these conditions, more research is needed before specific recommendations can be made.[302]

Pantothenic acid deficiency in humans is rare. Manifestations of deficiency may include neurological symptoms such as listlessness, fatigue, headaches, tingling sensations in arms and legs, and GI symptoms such as vomiting, abdominal cramps, and flatulence. Historically, it has been implicated in the "burning feet" syndrome, a condition noted among malnourished prisoners of war during World War II. Experimental states of pantothenic acid deficiency have been induced by feeding volunteers synthetic diets devoid of pantothenic acid or by administering pantothenic acid antagonists.[303,304] There is no data on potential toxic effects of pantothenic acid in animals or humans.

REFERENCES

1. Rosenfeld R. Vitamine—vitamin. The early years of discovery. Clin Chem 1997;43:680–5.
2. Wolf G. A history of vitamin A and retinoids. FASEB J 1996;10:1102–7.
3. Lunin G. Ueber die bedeutung der anorganischen salze bei der ernährung des thieres. Zeitschr Physiol Chem 1881;5:31–9.
4. Hopkins FG. The analyst and the medical man. Analyst 1906;31:385–404.
5. Stepp W. Experiments on feeding with lipoid-free food. Biochemistry 1909;22:452–60.
6. McCollum E, Davis M. The necessity of certain lipids in the diet during growth. J Biol Chem 1913;15:167–75.
7. McCollum EV, Davis M. The essential factors in the diet during growth. J Biol Chem 1915;23:231–54.
8. Osborne TB, Mendel LB. The relation of growth to the chemical constituents of the diet. J Biol Chem 1913;15:311–26.
9. Osborne TB, Mendel LB. The influence of cod liver oil and some other fats on growth. J Biol Chem 1914;17:401–8.
10. Drummond JC. The nomenclature of the so-called accessory food factors (vitamins). Biochem J 1920;14:660.
11. Moore T. The relation of carotene to vitamin A. Lancet 1929;2:380–1.
12. Karrer P, Helfenstein A, Wehrli H, Wettstein A. Pflanzenfarbstoffe. XXV. Über die konstitution des lycopins und carotins. Helv Chim Acta 1930;13:1084–99.
13. Solomons NW. Vitamin A and carotenoids. In: Bowman BA, Russell RM, editors. Present Knowledge in Nutrition, 8th edition. Washington, DC: International Life Sciences Institute; 2001. p. 127–45.
14. Napoli JL. A gene knockout corroborates the integral function of cellular retinol-binding protein in retinol metabolism. Nutr Rev 2000;50:230–5.
15. Blomhoff R. Transport and metabolism of vitamin A. Nutr Rev 1994;52:13–23.
16. van Vliet T, van Vlissingen MF, van Schaik F, van den Berg H. ß-carotene absorption and cleavage in rats is affected by the vitamin A concentration of the diet. J Nutr 1996;126:2555–6.
17. Fawzi WW. Environmental factors that impact the efficacy of vitamin A supplements among children. Environ Nutr Interact 1997;1:299–333.
18. Erdman JW, Fahey GC, White CB. Effects of purified dietary fiber sources on ß-carotene utilization by the chick. J Nutr 1986;116:2415–23.
19. Underwood BA. Maternal vitamin A status and its importance in infancy and early childhood. Am J Clin Nutr 1994;59:517S–22S.
20. Subar AF, Krebs-Smith SM, Cook A, Kahle LL. Dietary sources of nutrients among US children, 1989–1991. Pediatrics 1998;102:913–23.
21. Otten JJ HJ, Meyers LD, editors. Dietary reference intakes: The essential guide to nutrient requirements. Washington, DC: National Academies Press; 2006.
22. Wolf G. The discovery of the visual function of vitamin A. J Nutr 2001;131:1647–50.
23. Villamor E, Fawzi WW. Effects of vitamin A supplementation on immune responses and correlation with clinical outcomes. Clin Microbiol Rev 2005;18:446–64.
24. Semba RD. The role of vitamin A and related retinoids in immune function. Nutr Rev 1998;56:S38–48.
25. Fawzi W, Chalmers T, Herrera M, Mosteller F. Vitamin A supplementation and child mortality: A meta-analysis. JAMA 1993;269:898–903.
26. Semba RD, Ndugwa C, Perry RT, et al. Effect of periodic vitamin A supplementation on mortality and morbidity of human immunodeficiency virus-infected children in Uganda: A controlled clinical trial. Nutrition 2005;21:25–31.
27. Fawzi W, Mbise R, Spiegelman D, et al. Vitamin A supplements and diarrheal and respiratory infections among children in Dar es Salaam, Tanzania. J Pediatr 1999;137:660–7.
28. Humphrey J, Agoestina T, Wu L, et al. Impact of neonatal vitamin A supplementation on infant morbidity and mortality. J Pediatr 1996;128:489–96.
29. Malaba LC, Iliff PJ, Nathoo KJ, et al. Effect of postpartum maternal or neonatal vitamin A supplementation on infant mortality among infants born to HIV-negative mothers in Zimbabwe. Am J Clin Nutr 2005;81:454–60.
30. West KP, Jr, Katz J, Shrestha SR, et al. Mortality of infants <6 mo of age supplemented with vitamin A: A randomized, double-masked trial in Nepal. Am J Clin Nutr 1995;62:143–8.
31. WHO/CHD Immunization-Linked Vitamin A Supplementation Study Group. Randomized trial to assess benefits and safety of vitamin A supplementation linked to immunization in early infancy. Lancet 1998;352:1257–63.
32. Brown N, Roberts C. Vitamin A for acute respiratory infection in developing countries: A meta-analysis. Acta Paediatr 2004;93:1437–42.
33. The Vitamin A and Pneumonia Working Group. Potential interventions for the prevention of childhood pneumonia in developing countries: A meta-analysis of data from field trials to assess the impact of vitamin A supplementation on pneumonia morbidity and mortality. Bull World Health Organ 1995;73:609–19.
34. Rosales F, Kjolhede C, Goodman S. Efficacy of a single oral dose of 200,000 IU of oil-soluble vitamin A in measles-associated morbidity. Am J Epidemiol 1996;143:413–22.
35. Ogaro F, Orinda V, Onyango F, Black R. Effect of vitamin A on diarrheal and respiratory complications of measles. Trop Geogr Med 1993;45:283–6.
36. American Academy of Pediatrics Committee on Infectious Diseases. Vitamin A treatment of measles. Pediatrics 1993;91:1014–5.
37. Ghana VAST Study Team. Vitamin A supplementation in northern Ghana: Effects on clinic attendances, hospital admissions, and child mortality. Lancet 1993;342:7–12.
38. Barreto M, Santos L, Assis A, et al. Effect of vitamin A supplementation on diarrhoea and acute lower respiratory tract infections in young children in Brazil. Lancet 1994;344:228–31.
39. Bhandari N, Bhan M, Sazawal S. Impact of massive dose of vitamin A given to preschool children with acute diarrhoea on subsequent respiratory and diarrhoeal morbidity. BMJ 1994;309:1404–7.
40. Hossain S, Biswas R, Kabir I, et al. Single dose vitamin A treatment in acute shigellosis in Bangladesh children: Randomised double blind controlled trial. BMJ 1998;316:422–6.
41. Henning B, Stewart K, Zaman K, et al. Lack of therapeutic efficacy of vitamin A for non-cholera, watery diarrhoea in Bangladeshi children. Eur J Clin Nutr 1992;46:437–43.
42. Long KZ, Santos JI, Rosado JL, et al. Impact of vitamin A on selected gastrointestinal pathogen infections and associated diarrheal episodes among children in Mexico City, Mexico. J Infect Dis 2006;194:1217–25.
43. Long KZ, Estrada-Garcia T, Rosado JL, et al. The effect of vitamin A supplementation on the intestinal immune response in Mexican children is modified by pathogen infections and diarrhea. J Nutr 2006;136:1365–70.
44. Dibley MJ, Sadjimin T, Kjolhede CL, Moulton LH. Vitamin A supplementation fails to reduce incidence of acute respiratory illness and diarrhea in preschool-age Indonesian children. J Nutr 1996;126:434–42.
45. Sempertegui F, Estrella B, Camaniero V, et al. The beneficial effects of weekly low-dose vitamin A supplementation on acute lower respiratory infections and diarrhea in Ecuadorian children. Pediatrics 1999;104:e1.
46. Shankar AH, Genton B, Semba RD, et al. Effect of vitamin A supplementation on morbidity due to Plasmodium falciparum in young children in Papua New Guinea: A randomised trial. Lancet 1999;354:203–9.
47. Wiysonge CS, Shey MS, Sterne JA, Brocklehurst P. Vitamin A supplementation for reducing the risk of mother-to-child transmission of HIV infection. Cochrane Database Syst Rev 2005;CD003648.
48. Orr JB, Richards MB. Growth and vitamin A deficiency. Biochem J 1934;28:1259–73.
49. Sommer A. Nutritional Blindness: Xerophthalmia and Keratomalacia. New York: Oxford University Press; 1982.
50. Sommer A, West KP. Vitamin A Deficiency. Health, Survival and Vision. New York: Oxford University Press; 1996.
51. Graham GG, Creed HM, MacLean WCJ, et al. Determinants of growth among poor children: Nutrient intake-achieved growth relationships. Am J Clin Nutr 1981;34:539–54.
52. Fawzi WW, Herrera MG, Willett WC, et al. Dietary vitamin A intake in relation to child growth. Epidemiology 1997;8:402–7.
53. Rahmathullah L, Underwood BA, Thulasiraj RD, Milton RC. Diarrhea, respiratory infections, and growth are not affected by a weekly low-dose vitamin A supplement: A masked, controlled field trial in children in southern India. Am J Clin Nutr 1991;54:568–77.
54. Lie C, Ying C, En-Lin W, et al. Impact of large dose vitamin A supplementation on childhood diarrhea, respiratory disease and growth. Eur J Clin Nutr 1993;47:88–9.
55. Ramakrishnan U, Latham M, Abel R. Vitamin A supplementation does not improve growth of preschool children: A randomized, double-blind field trial in South India. J Nutr 1995;125:202–11.
56. Kirkwood BR, Ross DA, Arthur P, et al. Effect of vitamin A supplementation on the growth of young children in northern Ghana. Am J Clin Nutr 1996;63:773–81.
57. Fawzi WW, Herrera MG, Willett WC, et al. The effect of vitamin A supplementation on the growth of preschool children in the Sudan. Am J Public Health 1997;87:1359–62.
58. West KP, LeClerq SC, Shrestha SR, et al. Effects of vitamin A on growth of vitamin A-deficient children: Field studies in Nepal. J Nutr 1997;127:1957–65.
59. West KPJ, Djunaedi E, Pandji A, et al. Vitamin A supplementation and growth: A randomized community trial. Am J Clin Nutr 1988;48:1257–64.
60. Muhilal, Permeisih D, Idjradinata YR, et al. Vitamin A-fortified monosodium glutamate and health, growth, and survival of children: A controlled field trial. Am J Clin Nutr 1988;48:1271–6.
61. Hadi H, Stoltzfus RJ, Dibley MJ, et al. Vitamin A supplementation selectively improves the linear growth of Indonesian preschool children: Results from a randomized controlled trial. Am J Clin Nutr 2000;71:507–13.
62. Bahl R, Bhandari N, Taneja S, Bhan MK. The impact of vitamin A supplementation on physical growth of children is dependent on season. Eur J Clin Nutr 1997;51:26–9.
63. Villamor E, Mbise R, Spiegelman D, et al. Vitamin A supplements ameliorate the adverse effect of HIV-1, malaria, and diarrheal infections on child growth. Pediatrics 2002;109:E6.
64. Bloem MW, Wedel M, van Agtmaal EJ, et al. Vitamin A intervention: Short-term effects of a single, oral, massive dose on iron metabolism. Am J Clin Nutr 1990;51:76–9.
65. Mejia LA, Chew F. Hematological effect of supplementing anemic children with vitamin A alone and in combination with iron. Am J Clin Nutr 1988;48:595–600.
66. Semba RD, Bloem MW. The anemia of vitamin A deficiency: Epidemiology and pathogenesis. Eur J Clin Nutr 2002;56:271–81.
67. Christian P, West KP, Jr. Interactions between zinc and vitamin A: An update. Am J Clin Nutr 1998;68:435S–41S.
68. Udomkesmalee E, Dhanamitta S, Sirisinha S, et al. Effect of vitamin A and zinc supplementation on the nutriture of children in Northeast Thailand. Am J Clin Nutr 1992;56:50–7.
69. Zlotkin S. A critical assessment of the upper intake levels for infants and children. J Nutr 2006;136:502S–6S.
70. Mellanby E, Cantab MD. Experimental investigation on rickets. Lancet 1919;196:407–12.
71. McCollum EV, Simmonds N, Becker JE, Shipley PG. Studies on experimental rickets. XXI. An experimental demonstration of the existence of a vitamin which promotes calcium deposition. J Biol Chem 1922;53:293–312.
72. Goldblatt H, Soames KM. A study of rats on a normal diet irradiated daily by the mercury vapor quartz lamp or kept in darkness. Biochem J 1923;17:294–7.
73. Hess AF, Weinstock M. The antirachitic value of irradiated cholesterol and phytosterol. J Biol Chem 1925;63:305–9.
74. Collins ED, Norman AW. Vitamin D. In: Rucker R, Suttie JW, McCormick DB, Machlin LJ, editors. Handbook of Vitamins, 3rd edition. New York: Marcel Dekker; 2001. p. 59–98.
75. Bouillon R, Okamura WH, Norman AW. Structure-function relationships in the vitamin D endocrine system. Endocr Rev 1995;16:200–57.
76. Otterbein LR, Cosio C, Graceffa P, Dominguez R. Crystal structures of the vitamin D-binding protein and its complex with actin: Structural basis of the actin-scavenger system. Proc Natl Acad Sci U S A 2002;99:8003–8.

77. Mawer EB, Backhouse J, Holman CA, et al. The distribution and storage of vitamin D and its metabolites in human tissues. Clin Sci 1972;43:413–31.
78. Fraser DR. The physiological economy of vitamin D. Lancet 1983;1:969–72.
79. Reddy GS, Tserng KY. Calcitroic acid, end product of renal metabolism of 1,25-dihydroxyvitamin D_3 through C-24 oxidation pathway. Biochemistry 1989;28:1763–9.
80. Omdahl JL, Morris HA, May BK. Hydroxylase enzymes of the vitamin D pathway: Expression, function, and regulation. Annu Rev Nutr 2002;22:139–66.
81. Norman AW, Henry HH. Vitamin D. In: Bowman BA, Russell RM, editors. Present Knowledge in Nutrition, Volume 1, 9th edition. Washington, DC: International Life Sciences Institute; 2006. p. 198–210.
82. Haussler MR, Whitfield GK, Haussler CA, et al. The nuclear vitamin D receptor: Biological and molecular regulatory properties revealed. J Bone Miner Res 1998;13:325–49.
83. Brown AJ, Finch J, Slatopolsky E. Differential effects of 19-nor-1,25-dihydroxyvitamin D(2) and 1,25-dihydroxyvitamin D(3) on intestinal calcium and phosphate transport. J Lab Clin Med 2002;139:279–84.
84. Beckman MJ, DeLuca HF. Regulation of renal vitamin D receptor is an important determinant of 1alpha,25-dihydroxyvitamin D(3) levels in vivo. Arch Biochem Biophys 2002;401:44–52.
85. Schwartz Z, Sylvia VL, Larsson D, et al. 1alpha,25(OH)2D3 regulates chondrocyte matrix vesicle protein kinase C (PKC) directly via G-protein-dependent mechanisms and indirectly via incorporation of PKC during matrix vesicle biogenesis. J Biol Chem 2002;277:11828–37.
86. Ravid A, Rubinstein E, Gamady A, et al. Vitamin D inhibits the activation of stress-activated protein kinases by physiological and environmental stresses in keratinocytes. J Endocrinol 2002;173:525–32.
87. Lambert J, Trompke C. Tacalcitol ointment for long-term control of chronic plaque psoriasis in dermatological practice. Dermatology 2002;204:321–4.
88. Ogunkolade BW, Boucher BJ, Prahl JM, et al. Vitamin D receptor (VDR) mRNA and VDR protein levels in relation to vitamin D status, insulin secretory capacity, and VDR genotype in Bangladeshi Asians. Diabetes 2002;51:2294–300.
89. Harris S. Can vitamin D supplementation in infancy prevent type 1 diabetes? Nutr Rev 2002;60:118–21.
90. Bhalla AK, Amento EP, Clemens TL, et al. Specific high-affinity receptors for 1,25-dihydroxyvitamin D3 in human peripheral blood mononuclear cells: Presence in monocytes and induction in T lymphocytes following activation. J Clin Endocrinol Metab 1983;57:1308–10.
91. Provvedini DM, Tsoukas CD, Deftos LJ, Manolagas SC. 1,25-dihydroxyvitamin D3 receptors in human leukocytes. Science 1983;221:1181–3.
92. Reinhardt TA, Horst RL, Littledike ET, Beitz DC. 1,25-Dihydroxyvitamin D3 receptor in bovine thymus gland. Biochem Biophys Res Commun 1982;106:1012–8.
93. Morgan JW, Morgan DM, Lasky SR, et al. Requirements for induction of vitamin D-mediated gene regulation in normal human B lymphocytes. J Immunol 1996;157:2900–8.
94. Brennan A, Katz DR, Nunn JD, et al. Dendritic cells from human tissues express receptors for the immunoregulatory vitamin D3 metabolite, dihydroxycholecalciferol. Immunology 1987;61:457–61.
95. Liu PT, Stenger S, Li H, et al. Toll-like receptor triggering of a vitamin D-mediated human antimicrobial response. Science 2006;311:1770–3.
96. Cantorna MT, Zhu Y, Froicu M, Wittke A. Vitamin D status, 1,25-dihydroxyvitamin D3, and the immune system. Am J Clin Nutr 2004;80:1717S–20S.
97. Wjst M, Dold S. Genes, factor X, and allergens: What causes allergic diseases? Allergy 1999;54:757–9.
98. Hypponen E, Sovio U, Wjst M, et al. Infant vitamin D supplementation and allergic conditions in adulthood: Northern Finland birth cohort 1966. Ann N Y Acad Sci 2004;1037:84–95.
99. Zeghoud F, Vervel C, Guillozo H, et al. Subclinical vitamin D deficiency in neonates: Definition and response to vitamin D supplements. Am J Clin Nutr 1997;65:771–8.
100. Clemens TL, Adams JS, Henderson SL, Holick MF. Increased skin pigment reduces the capacity of skin to synthesise vitamin D3. Lancet 1982;1:74–6.
101. Nesby-O'Dell S, Scanlon KS, Cogswell ME, et al. Hypovitaminosis D prevalence and determinants among African American and white women of reproductive age: Third National Health and Nutrition Examination Survey, 1988–1994. Am J Clin Nutr 2002;76:187–92.
102. Gartner LM, Greer FR. Prevention of rickets and vitamin D deficiency: New guidelines for vitamin D intake. Pediatrics 2003;111:908–10.
103. Weaver CM, Fleet JC. Vitamin D requirements: Current and future. Am J Clin Nutr 2004;80:1735S–9S.
104. Food and Nutrition Board. Dietary Reference Intakes for Calcium, Phosphorus, Magnesium, Vitamin D, and Fluoride. Washington, DC: National Academy Press; 1997. p. 250–87.
105. Evans HM, Bishop KS. On the existence of a hitherto unrecognized dietary factor essential for reproduction. Science 1922;56:650–651.
106. Oski FA, Barness LA. Vitamin E deficiency: A previously unrecognized cause of hemolytic anemia in the premature infant. J Pediatr 1967;70:211–20.
107. Food and Nutrition Board. Dietary Reference Intakes for Vitamin C, Vitamin E, Selenium, and Carotenoids. Washington, DC: National Academy Press; 2000. p. 186–283.
108. Chow CK. Vitamin E. In: Rucker R, Suttie JW, McCormick DB, Machlin LJ, editors. Handbook of Vitamins, 3rd edition. New York: Marcel Dekker; 2001. p. 167–97.
109. Kayden HJ, Traber MG. Absorption, lipoprotein transport, and regulation of plasma concentrations of vitamin E in humans. J Lipid Res 1993;34:343–58.
110. Traber MG. Vitamin E. In: Bowman BA, Russell RM, editors. Present Knowledge in Nutrition, Volume 1, 9th edition. Washington, DC: International Life Sciences Institute; 2006. p. 211–9.
111. Schultz M, Leist M, Petrzika M, et al. Novel urinary metabolite of α -tocopherol, 2,5,7,8-tetramethyl-2-(2'-carboxyethyl)-6-hydroxychroman, as an indicator of an adequate vitamin E supply? Am J Clin Nutr 1995;62:1527S–34S.
112. Chow CK. Vitamin E. In: Rucker R, Suttie JW, McCormick DB, Machlin LJ, editors. Handbook of Vitamins, 3rd edition. New York: Marcel Dekker; 2001.
113. Sokol RJ. Vitamin E deficiency and neurological disease. Annu Rev Nutr 1988;8:351–73.
114. Chow CK. Vitamin E and oxidative stress. Free Rad Biol Med 1991:215–32.
115. Pryor WA. Vitamin E. In: Bowman BA, Russel RM, editors. Present Knowledge in Nutrition, 8th edition. Washington, DC: International Life Sciences Institute; 2001. p. 156–63.
116. Noaman E, Zahran AM, Kamal AM, Omran MF. Vitamin E and selenium administration as a modulator of antioxidant defense system: Biochemical assessment and modification. Biol Trace Elem Res 2002;86:55–64.
117. Chan AC, Tran K, Raynor T, et al. Regeneration of vitamin E in human platelets. J Biol Chem 1991;266:17290–5.
118. Wang XD, Marini RP, Rebuterne X, et al. Vitamin E enhances the lymphatic transport of beta-carotene and its conversion to vitamin A in the ferret. Gastroenterology 1995;108:719–26.
119. Urano S, Inomori Y, Sugawara T, et al. Vitamin E: Inhibition of retinol-induced hemolysis and membrane-stabilizing behavior. J Biol Chem 1992;15:18365–70.
120. Catignani GL, Chytil F, Darby WJ. Vitamin E deficiency: Immunochemical evidence for increased accumulation of liver xanthine oxidase. Proc Natl Acad Sci U S A 1974;71:1966–8.
121. Tasinato A, Boscoboinik D, Bartoli GM, et al. d-Alpha tocopherol inhibition of vascular smooth muscle cell proliferation occurs at physiological concentrations, correlates with protein kinase c inhibition, and is independent of its antioxidant properties. Proc Natl Acad Sci U S A 1995;92:12190–4.
122. Tang FY, Meydani M. Green tea catechins and vitamin E inhibit angiogenesis of human microvascular endothelial cells through suppression of IL-8 production. Nutr Cancer 2001;41:119–25.
123. Azzi A, Ricciarelli R, Zingg JM. Non-antioxidant molecular functions of alpha tocopherol (vitamin E). FEBS Lett 2002;519:8–10.
124. Beharka AA, Wu D, Serafini M, Meydani SN. Mechanism of vitamin E inhibition of cyclooxygenase activity in macrophages from old mice: Role of peroxynitrite. Free Radic Biol Med 2002;32:503–11.
125. Adolfsson O, Huber BT, Meydani SN. Vitamin E-enhanced IL-2 production in old mice: Naive but not memory T cells show increased cell division cycling and IL-2-producing capacity. J Immunol 2001;167:3809–17.
126. Han SN, Wu D, Ha WK, et al. Vitamin E supplementation increases T helper 1 cytokine production in old mice infected with influenza virus. Immunology 2000;100:487–93.
127. Claycombe KJ, Meydani SN. Vitamin E and genome stability. Mutat Res 2001;475:37–44.
128. Chow CK, Ibrahim W, Wei W, Chan AC. Vitamin E regulates mitochondrial hydrogen peroxide generation. Free Rad Biol Med 1999;27:580–7.
129. Meydani SN, Leka LS, Fine BC, et al. Vitamin E and respiratory tract infections in elderly nursing home residents: A randomized controlled trial. JAMA 2004;292:828–36.
130. Fairfield KM, Fletcher RH. Vitamins for chronic disease prevention in adults: Scientific review. JAMA 2002;287:3116–26.
131. Stephens NG, Parsons A, Schofield PM, et al. Randomised controlled trial of vitamin E in patients with coronary disease: Cambridge Heart Antioxidant Study (CHAOS). Lancet 1996;347:781–6.
132. Rimm EB, Stampfer MJ, Ascherio A, et al. Vitamin E consumption and the risk of coronary heart disease in men. N Engl J Med 1993;328:1450–6.
133. Engelhart MJ, Geerlings MI, Ruitenberg A, et al. Dietary intake of antioxidants and risk of Alzheimer disease. JAMA 2002;287:3223–9.
134. American Academy of Pediatrics. Pediatric Nutrition Handbook. Elk Grove Village, IL: American Academy of Pediatrics; 2004. p. 350.
135. Dam H. Cholesterinstoffwechsel in Huehnereiern und Huehnchen. Biochem Z 1929;215:475–92.
136. Dam H. The antihemorrhagic vitamin of the chick. Occurrence and chemical nature. Nature 1935;135:652–653.
137. MacCorquodale DW, Cheney LC, Binkley SB, et al. The constitution and synthesis of vitamin K1. J Biol Chem 1939;131:357–70.
138. Garber AK, Binkley NC, Krueger DC, Suttie JW. Comparison of phylloquinone bioavailability from food sources or a supplement in human subjects. J Nutr 1999;129:1201–3.
139. Gijsbers BLMG, Jie KS, Vermeer C. Effect of food composition on vitamin K absorption in human volunteers. Br J Nutr 1996;76:223–9.
140. Ferland G. Vitamin K. In: Bowman BA, Russell RM, editors. Present Knowledge in Nutrition, Volume 1, 9th edition. Washington, DC: International Life Sciences Institute; 2006. p. 220–32.
141. Shearer MJ, Zhang HF. Early infant vitamin K deficiency: Extent, health consequences and approaches to prophylaxis. In: Delanghe FM, West KP, Jr, editors. Micronutrient Deficiencies in the First Months of Life, Volume 52. Vevey, Switzerland: Nestle; 2003. p. 181–208.
142. Conly JM, Stein KE. The absorption and bioactivity of bacterially synthesized menaquinones. Clin Invest Med 1993;16:45–57.
143. Suttie JW. The importance of menaquinones in human nutrition. Annu Rev Nutr 1995;15:399–417.
144. Shearer MJ, McBurney A, Barkhan P. Studies on the absorption and metabolism of phylloquinone (vitamin K1) in man. Vitam Horm 1974;32:513–42.
145. Kalkwarf HJ, Khoury JC, Bean J, Elliot JG. Vitamin K, bone turnover, and bone mass in girls. Am J Clin Nutr 2004;80:1075–80.
146. Shiraki M, Shiraki Y, Aoki C, Miura M. Vitamin K2 (menatetrenone) effectively prevents fractures and sustains lumbar bone mineral density in osteoporosis. J Bone Miner Res 2000;15:515–21.
147. Pierre-Jacques H, Glueck CJ, Mont MA, Hungerford DS. Familial heterozygous protein-S deficiency in a patient who had multifocal osteonecrosis. A case report. J Bone Joint Surg Am 1997;79:1079–84.
148. Luo G, Ducy P, McKee MD, et al. Spontaneous calcification of arteries and cartilage in mice lacking matrix GLA protein. Nature 1997;386:78–81.
149. Price PA, Faus SA, Williamson MK. Warfarin causes rapid calcification of the elastic lamellae in rat arteries and heart valves. Arterioscler Thromb Vasc Biol 1998;18:1400–7.
150. Bostrom K, Tsao D, Shen S, et al. Matrix GLA protein modulates differentiation induced by bone morphogenetic protein-2 in C3H10T1/2 cells. J Biol Chem 2001;276:14044–52.
151. Jie KSG, Bots ML, Vermeer C, et al. Vitamin K intake and osteocalcin levels in women with and without aortic atherosclerosis: A population-based study. Atherosclerosis 1995;116:117–23.
152. Shearer MJ. The roles of vitamins D and K in bone health and osteoporosis prevention. Proc Nutr Soc 1997;56:915–37.
153. Denisova NA, Booth SL. Vitamin K and sphingolipid metabolism: Evidence to date. Nutr Rev 2005;63:111–21.
154. Thijssen HH, Drittij-Reijnders MJ. Vitamin K status in human tissues: Tissue-specific accumulation of phylloquinone and menaquinone-4. Br J Nutr 1996;75:121–7.
155. Lamson DW, Plaza SM. The anticancer effects of vitamin K. Altern Med Rev 2003;8:303–18.
156. Yanagita M. The role of the vitamin K-dependent growth factor Gas6 in glomerular pathophysiology. Curr Opin Nephrol Hypertens 2004;13:465–70.
157. Habu D, Shiomi S, Tamori A, et al. Role of vitamin K2 in the development of hepatocellular carcinoma in women with viral cirrhosis of the liver. JAMA 2004;292:358–61.
158. Sutor AH, von Kries R, Cornelissen EA, et al. Vitamin K deficiency bleeding (VKDB) in infancy. ISTH Pediatric/Perinatal Subcommittee. International Society on Thrombosis and Haemostasis. Thromb Haemost 1999;81:456–61.

159. American Academy of Pediatrics Committee on Fetus and Newborn. Controversies concerning vitamin K and the newborn. Pediatrics 2003;112:191–2.
160. Golding J, Greenwood R, Birmingham K, Mott M. Childhood cancer, intramuscular vitamin K, and pethidine given during labour. BMJ 1992;305:341–6.
161. Golding J, Paterson M, Kinlen LJ. Factors associated with childhood cancer in a national cohort study. Br J Cancer 1990;62:304–8.
162. Fear NT, Roman E, Ansell P, et al. Vitamin K and childhood cancer: A report from the United Kingdom Childhood Cancer Study. Br J Cancer 2003;89:1228–31.
163. Food and Nutrition Board. Dietary Reference Intakes for Vitamin A, Vitamin K, Arsenic, Boron, Chromium, Copper, Iodine, Iron, Manganese, Molybdenum, Nickel, Silicon, Vanadium, and Zinc. Washington, DC: National Academy Press; 2000. p. 162–96.
164. Carpenter KJ. The History of Scurvy and Vitamin C. Cambridge: Cambridge University Press; 1986.
165. Rajakumar K. Infantile scurvy: A historical perspective. Pediatrics 2001;108:e76.
166. Svirbely JL, Szent-Gyoergyi A. Hexuronic acid as the antiscorbutic factor. Nature 1932;129:576.
167. Svirbely JL, Szent-Gyoergyi A. The chemical nature of vitamin C. Biochem J 1932;26:865–70.
168. Waugh NA, King CG. Isolation and identification of vitamin C. Biol Chem 1932;97:325–31.
169. Haworth WN, Hirst EL, Zilva SS. Physiological activity of synthetic ascorbic acid. J Chem Soc 1934;ii:1155–6.
170. Haworth WN, Hirst EL. Synthesis of ascorbic acid. Chem Ind (London) 1933;52:645–6.
171. Malo C, Wilson JX. Glucose modulates vitamin C transport in adult human small intestinal brush border membrane vesicles. J Nutr 2000;130:63–9.
172. Kallner A, Hartmann D, Hornig D. Steady-state turnover and body pool of ascorbic acid in man. Am J Clin Nutr 1979;32:530–9.
173. Mangels AR, Block G, Frey CM, et al. The bioavailability to humans of ascorbic acid from oranges, orange juice and cooked broccoli is similar to that of synthetic ascorbic acid. J Nutr 1993;123:1054–61.
174. Sinclair AJ, Girling AJ, Gray L, et al. Disturbed handling of ascorbic acid in diabetic patients with and without microangiopathy during high dose ascorbate supplementation. Diabetologia 1991;34:171–5.
175. Maranzana A, Mehlhorn RJ. Loss of glutathione, ascorbate recycling, and free radical scavenging in human erythrocytes exposed to filtered cigarette smoke. Arch Biochem Biophys 1998;350:169–82.
176. Klepper J, Vera JC, De Vivo DC. Deficient transport of dehydroascorbic acid in the glucose transporter protein syndrome. Ann Neurol 1998;44:286–7.
177. Levine M, Conry-Cantilena C, Wang Y, et al. Vitamin C pharmacokinetics in healthy volunteers: Evidence for a recommended dietary allowance. Proc Natl Acad Sci U S A 1996;93:3704–9.
178. Johnston CS. Vitamin C. In: Bowman BA, Russel RM, editors. Present Knowledge in Nutrition, Vol 1, 9th edition. Washington, DC: International Life Sciences Institute; 2006. p. 233–41.
179. Gibson RS. Assessment of vitamin C status. In: Gibson RS, editor. Principles of Nutritional Assessment, 2nd edition. New York: Oxford University Press; 2005. p. 529–44.
180. Sakuma N, Yoshikawa M, Hibino A, et al. Ascorbic acid protects against peroxidative modification of low-density lipoprotein, maintaining its recognition by LDL receptors. J Nutr Sci Vitaminol (Tokyo) 2001;47:28–31.
181. Kugiyama K, Motoyama T, Hirashima O, et al. Vitamin C attenuates abnormal vasomotor reactivity in spasm coronary arteries in patients with coronary spastic angina. J Am Coll Cardiol 1998;32:103–9.
182. Engler MM, Engler MB, Malloy MJ, et al. Antioxidant vitamins C and E improve endothelial function in children with hyperlipidemia: Endothelial Assessment of Risk from Lipids in Youth (EARLY) Trial. Circulation 2003;108:1059–63.
183. Nyyssonen K, Parviainen MT, Salonen R, et al. Vitamin C deficiency and risk of myocardial infarction: Prospective population study of men from eastern Finland. BMJ 1997;314:634–8.
184. You WC, Zhang L, Gail MH, et al. Gastric dysplasia and gastric cancer: Helicobacter pylori, serum vitamin C, and other risk factors. J Natl Cancer Inst 2000;92:1607–12.
185. Douglas RM, Hemila A, Chalker E, et al. Vitamin C for preventing and treating the common cold. Cochrane Database Syst Rev 2004;CD000980.
186. Harakeh S, Jariwalla RJ. Comparative study of the anti-HIV activities of ascorbate and thiol- containing reducing agents in chronically HIV-infected cells. Am J Clin Nutr 1991;54:1231S–5S.
187. Hamuy R, Berman B. Treatment of Herpes simplex virus infections with topical antiviral agents. Eur J Dermatol 1998;8:310–9.
188. Food and Nutrition Board. Dietary Reference Intakes for Vitamin C, Vitamin E, Selenium, and Carotenoids. Washington, DC: National Academy Press; 2000. p. 95–185.
189. Hallberg L, Brune M, Rossander-Hulthen L. Is there a physiological role of vitamin C in iron absorption? Ann N Y Acad Sci 1987;498:324–32.
190. Hunt JR, Gallagher SK, Johnson LK. Effect of ascorbic acid on apparent iron absorption by women with low iron stores. Am J Clin Nutr 1994;59:1381–5.
191. Garcia OP, Diaz M, Rosado JL, Allen LH. Ascorbic acid from lime juice does not improve the iron status of iron-deficient women in rural Mexico. Am J Clin Nutr 2003;78:267–73.
192. Bates CJ. Thiamin. In: Bowman BA, Russell RM, editors. Present Knowledge in Nutrition, Vol 1, 9th edition. Washington, DC: International Life Sciences Institute; 2006. p. 242–9.
193. Carpenter KJ. Beriberi, White Rice, and Vitamin B. A Disease, a Cause, and a Cure. Berkeley, CA: University of California Press; 2000.
194. Williams RR. Structure of vitamin B1. J Am Chem Soc 1936;58:1063–4.
195. Hoyumpa AM, Jr, Strickland R, Sheehan JJ, et al. Dual system of intestinal thiamine transport in humans. J Lab Clin Med 1982;99:701–8.
196. Hammarstrom L, Ullberg S, Neujahr H. Autoradiographic studies on 35S-thiamine distribution in mice. Acta Pharmacol Toxicol (Copenh) 1966;24:24–32.
197. Spector R. Thiamine homeostasis in the central nervous system. In: Sable HZ, Gubler CJ, editors. Thiamine: Twenty Years of Progress, Volume 378. New York: New York Academy of Sciences; 1982. p. 344–54.
198. Gibson RS. Assessment of the status of thiamin, riboflavin, and niacin. In: Gibson RS, editor. Principles of Nutritional Assessment, 2nd edition. New York: Oxford University Press; 2005. p. 545–74.
199. Casteels M, Foulon V, Mannaerts GP, Van Veldhoven PP. Alpha-oxidation of 3-methyl-substituted fatty acids and its thiamine dependence. Eur J Biochem 2003;270: 1619–27.
200. Trostler N, Sklan D. Lipogenesis in the brain of thiamine-deficient rat pups. J Nutr Sci Vitaminol (Tokyo) 1978;24:105–11.
201. Fournier H, Butterworth RF. Effects of maternal thiamine deficiency on the development of thiamine-dependent enzymes in regions of the rat brain. Neurochem Int 1989;15:439–44.
202. Heinze T, Weber W. Determination of thiamine (vitamin B2) in maternal blood during normal pregnancies and pregnancies with intrauterine growth retardation. Z Ernahrungswiss 1990;29:39–46.
203. Krapels IP, van Rooij IA, Ocke MC, et al. Maternal dietary B vitamin intake, other than folate, and the association with orofacial cleft in the offspring. Eur J Nutr 2004;43:7–14.
204. Butterworth RF. Maternal thiamine deficiency: Still a problem in some world communities. Am J Clin Nutr 2001;74:712–3.
205. McGready R, Simpson JA, Cho T, et al. Postpartum thiamine deficiency in a Karen displaced population. Am J Clin Nutr 2001;74:808–13.
206. Tanphaichitr V. Thiamine. In: Rucker R, Suttie JW, McCormick DB, Machlin LJ, editors. Handbook of Vitamins. New York: Marcel Dekker; 2001. p. 275–316.
207. Centers for Disease Control and Prevention. Deaths associated with thiamine-deficient total parenteral nutrition. MMWR 1989;38:43–6.
208. Centers for Disease Control and Prevention. Lactic acidosis traced to thiamine deficiency related to nationwide shortage of multivitamins for total parenteral nutrition-United States, 1997. MMWR 1997;46:523–8.
209. Fattal-Valevski A, Kesler A, Sela BA, et al. Outbreak of life-threatening thiamine deficiency in infants in Israel caused by a defective soy-based formula. Pediatrics 2005;115:e233–8.
210. Kuhn R, Reinemund K, Weygand F, Stroebele R. Ueber die synthese des lactoflavins. Ber Deutsch Chem Gesells 1935;68:1765–74.
211. Karrer P, Scopp K, Benz F. Synthesis of flavins IV. Helv Chim Acta 1935;18:426.
212. Warburg O, Christian W. Co-ferment der d-aminosaeure-deaminase. Biochem Z 1938;295:261.
213. Shumyantseva VV, Bulko TV, Schmid RD, Archakov AI. Photochemical properties of a riboflavins/cytochrome P450 2B4 complex. Biosens Bioelectron 2002;17:233–8.
214. Jusko WJ, Levy G. Absorption, metabolism, and excretion of riboflavin-5'-phosphate in man. J Pharm Sci 1967;56:58–62.
215. McCormick DB. Two interconnected B vitamins: Riboflavin and pyridoxine. Physiol Rev 1989;69:1170–98.
216. Zempleni J, Galloway JR, McCormick DB. Pharmacokinetics of orally and intravenously administered riboflavin in healthy humans. Am J Clin Nutr 1996;63:54–66.
217. Powers HJ. Riboflavin (vitamin B-2) and health. Am J Clin Nutr 2003;77:1352–60.
218. Innis WSA, McCormick DB, Merril AH. Variations in riboflavin binding by human plasma: Identification of immunoglobulins as the major proteins responsible. Biochem Med 1985;34:151–65.
219. Food and Nutrition Board. Dietary Reference Intakes for Thiamin, Riboflavin, Niacin, Vitamin B6, Folate, Vitamin B12, Pantothenic Acid, Biotin, and Choline. Washington, DC: National Academy Press, 1998. p. 87–122.
220. Rivlin RS. Riboflavin. In: Bowman BA, Russell RM, editors. Present Knowledge in Nutrition, Vol 1, 9th edition. Washington, DC: International Life Sciences Institute; 2006. p. 250–68.
221. Powers HJ, Wright AJ, Fairweather-Tait SJ. The effect of riboflavin deficiency in rats on the absorption and distribution of iron. Br J Nutr 1988;59:381–7.
222. Powers HJ, Weaver LT, Austin S, et al. Riboflavin deficiency in the rat: Effects on iron utilization and loss. Br J Nutr 1991;65:487–96.
223. van Rensburg SJ. Epidemiologic and dietary evidence for a specific nutritional predisposition to esophageal cancer. J Natl Cancer Inst 1981;67:243–51.
224. Liu T, Soong SJ, Wilson NP, et al. A case control study of nutritional factors and cervical dysplasia. Cancer Epidemiol Biomarkers Prev 1993;2:525–30.
225. Hultquist DE, Xu F, Quandt KS, et al. Evidence that NADPH-dependent methemoglobin reductase and administered riboflavin protect tissues from oxidative injury. Am J Hematol 1993;42:13–8.
226. Mack CP, Hultquist DE, Shlafer M. Myocardial flavin reductase and riboflavin: A potential role in decreasing reoxygenation injury. Biochem Biophys Res Commun 1995;212:35–40.
227. Stampfer MJ, Malinow MR, Willett WC, et al. A prospective study of plasma homocyst(e)ine and risk of myocardial infarction in US physicians. JAMA 1992;268:877–81.
228. Park YK, Sempos CT, Barton CN, et al. Effectiveness of food fortification in the United States: The case of pellagra. Am J Public Health 2000;90:727–38.
229. Elvehjem CA, Madden RJ, Strong FM, Woolley DW. Relation of nicotinic acid and nicotinic acid amide to canine black tongue. Am Chem Soc 1937;59:1767–68.
230. Spies TD. The response of pellagrins to nicotinic acid. Lancet 1938;i:252–53.
231. Bechgaard H, Jespersen S. GI absorption of niacin in humans. J Pharm Sci 1977;66:871–2.
232. Henderson LM, Gross CJ. Metabolism of niacin and niacinamide in perfused rat intestine. J Nutr 1979;109:654–62.
233. Horwitt MK, Harper AE, Henderson LM. Niacin-tryptophan relationships for evaluating niacin equivalents. Am J Clin Nutr 1981;34:423–7.
234. Mrochek JE, Jolley RL, Young DS, Turner WJ. Metabolic response of humans to ingestion of nicotinic acid and nicotinamide. Clin Chem 1976;22:1821–7.
235. Jacob RA. Niacin. In: Bowman BA, Russell RM, editors. Present Knowledge in Nutrition, Vol 1, 9th edition. Washington, DC: International Life Sciences Institute; 2006. p. 260–8.
236. Rose DP, Braidman IP. Excretion of tryptophan metabolites as affected by pregnancy, contraceptive steroids, and steroid hormones. Am J Clin Nutr 1971;24:673–83.
237. Crouse JR, 3rd. New developments in the use of niacin for treatment of hyperlipidemia: New considerations in the use of an old drug. Coron Artery Dis 1996;7:321–6.
238. Gyoergy P. Vitamin B2 and the pellagra-like dermatitis of rats. Nature 1934;133:498–9.
239. Harris SA, Stiller ET, Folkers K. Structure of vitamin B6. II. J Am Chem Soc 1939;61:1242–4.
240. Harris SA, Folkers K. Synthesis of vitamin B6. I. J Am Chem Soc 1939;61:1245–7.
241. Harris SA, Folkers K. Synthesis of vitamin B6. II. J Am Chem Soc 1939;61:3307–10.
242. Harris SA, Heyl D, Folkers K. The vitamin B6 group. The structure and synthesis of pyridoxamine and pyridoxal. J Am Chem Soc 1944;66:2088–92.
243. Coburn SP, Ziegler PJ, Costill DL, et al. Response of vitamin B-6 content of muscle to changes in vitamin B-6 intake in men. Am J Clin Nutr 1991;53:1436–42.
244. Merrill AH, Jr, Henderson JM, Wang E, et al. Metabolism of vitamin B-6 by human liver. J Nutr 1984;114:1664–74.
245. Gibson RS. Assessment of vitamin B6 status. In: Principles of Nutritional Assessment, 2nd edition. New York: Oxford University Press; 2005. p. 575–94.
246. Food and Nutrition Board. Dietary Reference Intakes for Thiamin, Riboflavin, Niacin, Vitamin B6, Folate, Vitamin

B_{12}, Pantothenic Acid, Biotin, and Choline. Washington, DC: National Academy Press; 1998. p. 150–96.
247. Coursin D. Convulsive seizures in infants with pyridoxine-deficient diet. JAMA 1954;154:406–8.
248. Selhub J, Jacques PF, Bostom AG, et al. Association between plasma homocysteine concentrations and extracranial carotid-artery stenosis. N Engl J Med 1995;332:286–91.
249. Kang-Yoon SA, Kirksey A, Giacoia GP, West KD. Vitamin B-6 adequacy in neonatal nutrition: Associations with preterm delivery, type of feeding, and vitamin B-6 supplementation. Am J Clin Nutr 1995;62:932–42.
250. Rosenberg L. Vitamin-responsive inherited diseases affecting the nervous system. In: Bowman B, Russell R, editors. Research Publication of the Association of Nervous and Mental Disorders, Volume 53. New York: Raven Press; 1974.
251. Wills L. Treatment of "pernicious anaemia of pregnancy" and "tropical anaemia" with special reference to yeast extract as a curative agent. BMJ 1931;1:1059–64.
252. Mitchell HK, Snell EE, Williams RJ. The concentration of "folic acid". J Am Chem Soc 1941;63:2284.
253. Pietrzik K, Bronstrup A. Folate in preventive medicine: A new role in cardiovascular disease, neural tube defects and cancer. Ann Nutr Metab 1997;41:331–43.
254. Selhub J, Rosenberg IH. Folate transport in isolated brush border membrane vesicles from rat intestine. J Biol Chem 1981;256:4489–93.
255. Qiu A, Jansen M, Sakaris A, et al. Identification of an intestinal folate transporter and the molecular basis for hereditary folate malabsorption. Cell 2006;127:917–28.
256. Wald DS, Law M, Morris JK. Homocysteine and cardiovascular disease: evidence on causality from a meta-analysis. BMJ 2002;325:1202.
257. Brattstrom LE, Israelsson B, Jeppsson JO, Hultberg BL. Folic acid-an innocuous means to reduce plasma homocysteine. Scand J Clin Lab Invest 1988;48:215–21.
258. Choi SW, Mason JB. Folate and carcinogenesis: An integrated scheme. J Nutr 2000;130:129–32.
259. Joyal CC, Lalonde R, Vikis-Freibergs V, Botez MI. Are age-related behavioral disorders improved by folate administration? Exp Aging Res 1993;19:367–76.
260. Willett W. Nutritional Epidemiology, 2nd editon. New York: Oxford University Press; 1998. p. 467–83.
261. FDA. Food standards; amendment of standards of identity for enriched grain products to require addition of folic acid, final rule. Fed Regist 1996;61:8781–97.
262. Jacques PF, Selhub J, Bostom AG, et al. The effect of folic acid fortification on plasma folate and total homocysteine concentrations. N Engl J Med 1999;340:1449–54.
263. Food and Nutrition Board. Dietary Reference Intakes for Thiamin, Riboflavin, Niacin, Vitamin B6, Folate, Vitamin B12, Pantothenic Acid, Biotin, and Choline. Washington, DC: National Academy Press; 1998. p. 196–304.
264. Chanarin I, Deacon R, Lumb M, Perry J. Cobalamin-folate interrelations. Blood Rev 1989;3:211–15.
265. Healton EB, Savage DG, Brust JC, et al. Neurologic aspects of cobalamin deficiency. Medicine (Baltimore) 1991;70:229–45.
266. Lindenbaum J, Healton EB, Savage DG, et al. Neuropsychiatric disorders caused by cobalamin deficiency in the absence of anemia or macrocytosis. N Engl J Med 1988;318:1720–8.
267. Food and Nutrition Board. Dietary Reference Intakes for Thiamin, Riboflavin, Niacin, Vitamin B6, Folate, Vitamin B12, Pantothenic Acid, Biotin, and Choline. Washington, DC: National Academy Press; 1998. p. 306–56.
268. Rasmussen SA, Fernhoff PM, Scanlon KS. Vitamin B12 deficiency in children and adolescents. J Pediatr 2001;138:10–7.
269. Minot GR, Murphy WP. Response of reticulocytes to liver therapy: Particularly in pernicious anemia. Am J Med Sci 1928;175:581–99.
270. Rickes EL, Brink NG, Koniuszy FR, et al. Crystalline vitamin B12. Science 1948;107:396–7.
271. Smith EL. Purification of antipernicious anaemia factors from liver. Nature 1948;161:638–9.
272. Seetharam B, Alpers DH. Absorption and transport of cobalamin (vitamin B12). Annu Rev Nutr 1982;2:343–69.
273. Gibson RS. Assessment of folate and vitamin B12 status. In: Gibson RS, editor. Principles of Nutritional Assessment, 2nd edition. New York: Oxford University Press; 2005. p. 595–640.
274. Stabler SP. Vitamin B12. In: Bowman BA, Russell RM, editors. Present Knowledge in Nutrition, Vol 1, 9th edition. Washington, DC: International Life Sciences Institute; 2006. p. 302–13.
275. Savage D, Gangaidzo I, Lindenbaum J, et al. Vitamin B12 deficiency is the primary cause of megaloblastic anaemia in Zimbabwe. Br J Haematol 1994;86:844–50.
276. Graham SM, Arvela OM, Wise GA. Long-term neurologic consequences of nutritional vitamin B12 deficiency in infants. J Pediatr 1992;121:710–4.
277. Toh BH, van Driel IR, Gleeson PA. Pernicious anemia. N Engl J Med 1997;337:1441–8.
278. Katz M, Lee SK, Cooper BA. Vitamin B12 malabsorption due to a biologically inert intrinsic factor. N Engl J Med 1972;287:425–9.
279. McIntyre O, Sullivan L, Jeffries G, Silver R. Pernicious anemia in childhood. N Engl J Med 1965;272:981–6.
280. Boas MA. The effect of desiccation upon the nutritive properties of egg-white. Biochem J 1927;21:712–24.
281. Koegl F, Toennis B. Darstellung von krystallisiertem biotin aus eigelb. Z Physiol Chem 1932;242:43–73.
282. du Vigneaud V, Melville DB, Folkers K, et al. The structure of biotin: A study of desthiobiotin. J Biol Chem 1942;146:475–85.
283. Harris SA, Wolf DE, Mozingo R, Folkers K. Synthetic biotin. Science 1943;97:447–8.
284. Wolf B, Grier RE, Secor McVoy JR, Heard GS. Biotinidase deficiency: A novel vitamin recycling defect. J Inherit Metab Dis 1985;8:53–8.
285. Prasad PD, Wang H, Kekuda R, et al. Cloning and functional expression of a cDNA encoding a mammalian sodium-dependent vitamin transporter mediating the uptake of pantothenate, biotin, and lipoate. J Biol Chem 1998;273:7501–6.
286. Mock DM. Biotin. In: Ziegler EE, Filer LJ, editors. Present Knowledge in Nutrition, 7th edition. Washington, DC: International Life Sciences Institute; 1996. p. 220–35.
287. Camporeale G, Zempleni J. Biotin. In: Bowman BA, Russell RM, editors. Present Knowledge in Nutrition, Vol 1, 9th edition. Washington, DC: International Life Sciences Institute; 2006. p. 314–26.
288. Hendricks KM, Duggan C, Gallagher L, et al. Malnutrition in hospitalized pediatric patients. Current prevalence. Arch Pediatr Adolesc Med 1995;149:1118–22.
289. Petrelli F, Moretti P, Paparelli M. Intracellular distribution of biotin-14COOH in rat liver. Mol Biol Rep 1979;4:247–52.
290. Zempleni J, Green GM, Spannagel AW, Mock DM. Biliary excretion of biotin and biotin metabolites is quantitatively minor in rats and pigs. J Nutr 1997;127:1496–500.
291. Knowles JR. The mechanism of biotin-dependent enzymes. Annu Rev Biochem 1989;58:195–221.
292. Zempleni J. Uptake, localization, and noncarboxylase roles of biotin. Annu Rev Nutr 2005;25:175–96.
293. Wolf B. Worldwide survey of neonatal screening for biotinidase deficiency. J Inherit Metab Dis 1991;14:923–7.
294. Wolf B, Feldman GL. The biotin-dependent carboxylase deficiencies. Am J Hum Genet 1982;34:699–716.
295. Food and Nutrition Board. Dietary Reference Intakes for Thiamin, Riboflavin, Niacin, Vitamin B6, Folate, Vitamin B12, Pantothenic Acid, Biotin, and Choline. Washington, DC: National Academy Press; 1998. p. 374–89.
296. Williams RJ, Lyman CM, Goodyear GH, et al. "Pantothenic acid", a growth determinant of universal biological occurrence. J Am Chem Soc 1933;55:2912–27.
297. Wooley DA, Waisman HA, Elvehjem CA. Nature and partial synthesis of the chick antidermatitis factor. J Am Chem Soc 1939;61:977–8.
298. Jukes TH. The pantothenic acid requirements of the chick. J Biol Chem 1939;129:225–31.
299. Williams RJ, Majors RT. The structure of pantothenic acid. Science 1940;91:246–8.
300. Shibata K, Gross CJ, Henderson LM. Hydrolysis and absorption of pantothenate and its coenzymes in the rat small intestine. J Nutr 1983;113:2107–15.
301. Fenstermacher DK, Rose RC. Absorption of pantothenic acid in rat and chick intestine. Am J Physiol 1986;250:G155–60.
302. Miller JW, Rogers LM, Rucker RB. Pantothenic Acid. In: Bowman BA, Russell RM, editors. Present Knowledge in Nutrition, Volume 1, 9th edition. Washington, DC: International Life Sciences Institute; 2006. p. 327–39.
303. Fry PC, Fox HM, Tao HG. Metabolic response to a pantothenic acid deficient diet in humans. J Nutr Sci Vitaminol 1976;22:339–46.
304. Hodges R, Bean W, Ohlson M, Bleiler R. Human pantothenic acid deficiency produced by omega-methyl pantothenic acid. J Clin Invest 1959;38:1421–5.

Dietary Reference Intakes

Alice H. Lichtenstein, DSc
Stephen R. Daniels, MD, PhD

INTRODUCTION

The dietary reference intakes (DRIs) are a set of recommendations intended to provide guidance in evaluating nutrient intakes and planning meals on the basis of nutrient adequacy.[1] In contrast to their predecessor, recommended dietary allowances (RDAs) last published in 1989, the DRIs differ in two ways; the emphasis was shifted from preventing nutrient deficiencies to reducing chronic disease risk and guidance was provided for maximum upper levels at which no adverse health outcomes would be expected, termed tolerable upper intake levels (ULs).

The DRIs were established during the mid 1990s to the early 2000s by a series of committees which included both American and Canadian members under the auspices of the Food and Nutrition Board, Institute of Medicine, the National Academies of Science, in collaboration with Heath Canada. Separate committees were established for the following subcategories of nutrients; calcium, phosphorus, magnesium, vitamin D, and fluoride[2]; thiamin, riboflavin, niacin, vitamin B_6, folate, vitamin B_{12}, pantothenic acid, biotin, and choline[3]; vitamin C, vitamin E, selenium, and carotenoids[4]; vitamin A, vitamin K, arsenic, boron, chromium, copper, iodine, iron, manganese, molybdenum, nickel, silicon, vanadium, and zinc[5]; energy, carbohydrate, fiber, fat, fatty acids, cholesterol, protein, and amino acids1; and water, potassium, sodium, chloride, and sulfate.[6]

Depending on the available data for each nutrient, their DRIs are composed of estimated average requirements (EARs) and recommended dietary allowances (RDAs) or, when inadequate data were available, adequate intakes (AIs), and UL.[7] In the case of macronutrients, there is an additional category of recommendations, acceptable macronutrient distribution ranges (AMDRs).[1] This category was established because the evidence indicated that for energy containing nutrients optimal health outcomes were observed over a range of intakes. Table 1 provides summary definitions for these terms as established by the Food and Nutrition Board.[8]

BASIS FOR ESTABLISHING DRI VALUES

In formulating the DRIs, data were drawn primarily from peer reviewed publications. In some cases, the basis on which the reference values were derived was scanty, especially for the younger age categories. In those cases, with the exception of birth through 1 year of age, the reference values were extrapolated from adult data. The actual criteria on which nutrient adequacy were based, by necessity, varied among nutrients and from age group to age group, and are documented in detail, in each of the DRI committee reports.[1–6]

The DRI values are presented for the following age categories; 0 to 6 months, 7 to 12 months, 1 to 3 years, 4 to 8 years, 9 to 13 years, 14 to 18 years, 19 to 30 years, 31 to 50 years, and greater than 70 years. This chapter will be restricted to recommendations for categories up to and including age 18 years.

In general, recommendations for infants aged 0 to 6 months are based on average consumption from human milk, and 7 to 12 months on average consumption from human milk and complementary foods. For subsequent age groups sources of data, depending on the specific nutrient, included mean national intake data (continuing survey of food intake by individuals) and amounts shown to provide the greatest protection against a specified chronic disease or deficiency state. Also taken into consideration was whether the recommendations provided for adequate levels of energy to meet expenditure plus energy deposition and maintenance of nitrogen equilibrium plus protein deposition. Criteria used to assess adequacy can differ for individuals at different stages in the life cycle.

Table 1 Dietary Reference Intakes

Estimated average requirements (*EARs*): The average daily nutrient intake level estimated to meet the requirements of half the healthy individuals in a particular life stage and gender group.

Recommended dietary allowance (*RDA*): The average daily nutrient intake level sufficient to meet the nutrient requirements of nearly all (97 to 98%) healthy individuals in a particular life stage and gender group.

Adequate intake (*AI*): A recommended average daily nutrient intake level based on observed or experimentally determined approximations or estimates of nutrient intake by a group (or groups) of apparently healthy people that are assumed to be adequate—used when an RDA cannot be determined.

Tolerable upper intake level (*UL*): The highest average daily nutrient intake level likely to pose no risk of adverse health effects to almost all individuals in the general population. As intake increases above the UL, the potential risk of adverse effects increases.

Acceptable macronutrient distribution ranges (*AMDR*): The intakes that are associated with reduced risk of chronic disease, intakes at which essential dietary nutrients can be consumed at sufficient levels and intakes based on adequate energy intake and physical activity to maintain energy balance.

Adapted from reference 8.

DIETARY REFERENCE INTAKES

Estimated Average Requirement

EAR is the daily value that is estimated to meet the requirement, defined by a predetermined indicator or criterion of adequacy, of half the healthy population of individuals represented by each age and sex group. The underlying assumption is that the distribution of actual requirements in a population is normally distributed. The EAR value is dependent on the indicator used to assess nutrient adequacy. The primary use of EAR values is to establish RDA values.

Recommended Dietary Allowance

RDA is the daily value that is estimated to meet the requirement, defined by a predetermined indicator or criterion of adequacy, of 97 to 98% or nearly all of the healthy population of individuals represented by each age and sex group. By definition, the RDA value is calculated by summing the EAR and two standard deviations of the EAR if there are adequate data on which to calculate the variance. In cases where there are inadequate data with which to calculate the standard deviation of the EAR, the variance is assumed to be 10% of the EAR and the RDA is calculated by summing the EAR and twice 10% of the EAR. The primary use of RDA values is as a goal for daily intake by individuals. For nutrients where there were inadequate data on which to calculate EAR and RDA values for children, the numbers were extrapolations from adult data.

Adequate Intake

AI is the daily value that is estimated from actual intake data of healthy people when there are inadequate data with which to calculate an EAR.

Table 2 Dietary Reference Intakes (DRIs): Acceptable Macronutrient Distribution Ranges (Food and Nutrition Board, Institute of Medicine, National Academies)

	Range (Percent of Energy)	
Macronutrient	Children, 1–3 yr	Children, 4–18 yr
Fat	30–40	25–35
n-6 polyunsaturated fatty acids* (linoleic acid)	5–10	5–10
n-3 polyunsaturated fatty acids (α-linolenic acid)	0.6–1.2	0.6–1.2
Carbohydrate	45–65	45–65
Protein	5–20	10–30

Adapted from reference 1.
*Approximately 10% of the total can come from longer-chain *n*-3 or *n*-6 fatty acids.

The AI values are expected to meet or exceed the amounts needed to maintain a defined nutritional state or criterion of adequacy in essentially all members of a specific age and sex group. Hence, the AI values may exceed the EAR values. The AIs are intended to be used similarly to the RDAs. Nonetheless, the level of certainty for AI values is less than that for RDA values. Both the RDA and AI are used as goals for nutrient adequacy.

Acceptable Macronutrient Distribution Range

AMDR is the range of intakes at which macronutrients can be consumed that is associated with reduced risk of chronic disease (Table 2). The AMDRs are based on energy intake and physical activity levels that will maintain energy balance. Ranges were established because of the interrelated nature of the macronutrients. The recommendations are expressed as percent of energy intake because their intake should be determined by total energy needs. For the most part, the criteria used for assessing macronutrient adequacy were the range associated with reduced risk of chronic disease and to permit sufficient intakes of essential nutrients. In some cases subclasses of the macronutrients, for which specific functions independent of meeting energy needs were identified, additional criteria were used to establish either ERA or AI values. Examples of this approach include omega-3 fatty acids and indispensable amino acids.

Tolerable Upper Limit

The UL is the daily value that is estimated to be the highest level likely to pose no risk of adverse health effects for most people. The word "tolerable" was chosen as a qualifier for "upper levels" specifically to avoid implying that the upper levels are preferable or beneficial, especially compared to the RDAs or AIs. UL values were determined using risk assessment methodology. ULs are a new category of recommendations and were added because of the concern that widespread and chronic fortification of foods and common use of dietary supplements can result in intake levels considerably higher than that attainable with a mixed diet and may result in adverse health outcomes.

The relationship among the EAR, RDA, and UL values is depicted in Figure 1. Intakes between the RDA and UL values are assumed to be optimal because the risk of inadequacy and excess are both estimated to be close to zero.

INTENDED USES OF THE DRIS

The major uses of the DRIs as defined by the Food and Nutrition Board include determining nutrient adequacy and planning diets of both individuals and groups of individuals (Table 3). They serve as the nutrition basis for all federal Nutrition programs and are used to set dietary values (DVs) for Food and Drug Administration's mandated nutrition labeling of packaged foods.

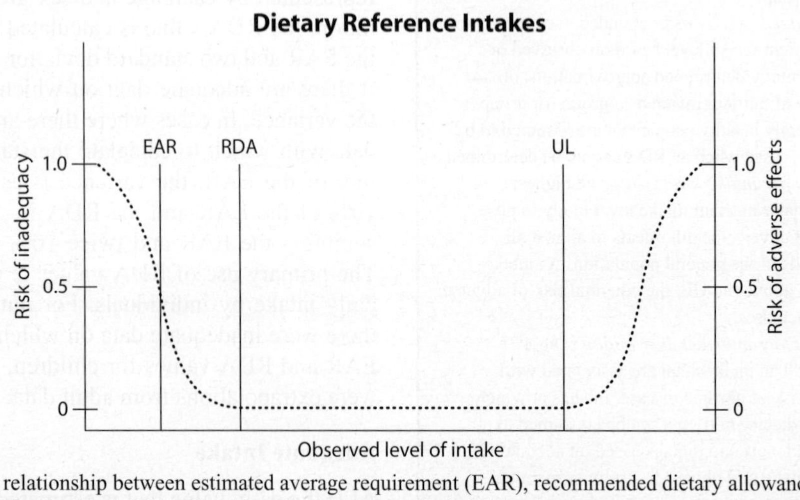

Figure 1 The relationship between estimated average requirement (EAR), recommended dietary allowance (RDA), and tolerable upper intake level (UL). The risk of inadequate intake is 50% at the EAR, 2 to 3% at the RDA, and close to 0% at the UL. Risks of adverse effects are close to 0% at the UL but increase with increasing intake. (Reproduced with permission from the Institute of Medicine.[2])

DRI LIFE STAGE GROUPS RELEVANT TO THE PEDIATRIC POPULATION

Infancy

DRI values are provided for two 6-month-age groups during the first year of life, 0 to 6 months and 7 months to 1 year. Recommendations are based on the assumption that the infants are full-term, born to healthy and well nourished women, and are exclusively fed human milk. Ethical considerations preclude the experimental determination of EAR values for infants. For this reason all the recommended values for these age categories are AIs. They are derived from average composition of an average volume of milk consumed by the specific age group. Because the recommendations are based on AIs, the values may exceed the EAR values. It is important to note that the decision of the Food and Nutrition Board to base the AIs on human milk is consistent with the recommendation of the American Academy of Pediatrics and the Canadian Paediatric Society, both of which state that exclusive breastfeeding is the preferred method of feeding for normal full-term infants for the first 4 to 6 months of life.

Zero to Six Months

For the first 6 months of life, food intake relative to body weight is for the most part constant. As an infant grows, their food intake will increase. The mean intake of a nutrient is calculated based on the average concentration of the nutrient from 2 to 6 months of lactation and an average volume of milk (780 mL/d). It is also assumed that infants will have adequate access to human milk and can thus increase their intake to meet their requirements for growth and maintenance.

Seven to Twelve Months

For the second 6 months of life, the assumption is that growth velocity slows and daily nutrient needs on a body weight basis will be lower. Taken into consideration is that the infant will be gradually weaned and a mixed diet including solid foods will be introduced. It was likewise assumed on the basis of available data that nutrient needs do not change markedly during this time period.

Toddlers: Ages 1 to 3 Years

For ages 1 to 3 years, the assumption is that growth velocity in height is greater than other age periods after infancy. From a practical perspective the Food and Nutrition Board also took into consideration that after age 4 years children tend to transition into daycare and school systems; hence, the source and exposure to food frequently change around 4 years of age. It is noteworthy that data for individual nutrients are relatively scarce for this age category and many values were extrapolated.

Early Childhood: Ages 4 to 8 Years

For ages 4 to 8 years, the assumption is that continued changes in growth velocity and endocrine

Table 3 Uses of DRIs for Assessing Intakes of Individuals and Groups

For an Individual	For a Group
EAR: Use to examine the probability that usual intake is inadequate	EAR: Use to estimate the prevalence of inadequate intakes within a group
RDA: Usual intake this level has a low probability of inadequacy	RDA: Do not use to assess intakes of groups
AI: Usual intake at or above this level has a low probability of inadequacy	AI: Mean usual intake at or above this level implies a low prevalence of inadequate intakes*
UL: Usual intake above this level may place an individual at risk of adverse effects from excessive nutrient intake	UL: Use to estimate the percentage of the population at potential risk of adverse effects from excessive nutrient intake

EAR: estimated average requirement, RDA: recommended dietary allowance, AI: adequate intake, UL: tolerable upper intake level.
Adapted from reference 8.
*When the AI for a nutrient is not based on mean intakes of healthy populations, this assessment is made with less confidence.

status separate it from the younger and older age categories. Although limited, the Food and Nutrition Board determined there were more data to define EARs and AIs values for this than for the prior age category. The DRIs for ages 4 to 8 years form the basis of many school feeding programs.

Puberty/Adolescence: Ages 9 to 13 Years and Ages 14 to 18 Years

The distinction between ages 9 to 13 years and 14 to 18 years was made on the basis of multiple developmental criteria. For girls the criteria were increased estrogen secretion physically marked by breast development and onset of the growth spurt. For boys the criteria were initiation of testicular development and onset of the growth spurt. In general, the growth spurt in boys begins about 2 years later than in girls. For this reason sex specific recommendations are made starting with these age categories.

TYPES OF DATA USED TO FORMULATE THE DRIS

The type of data used to formulate the DRIs varies from age group to age group and nutrient to nutrient, especially between energy containing and non-energy containing nutrients. Nevertheless, there are certain common features. The primary source of the data used to formulate the DRI values is clinical, dose–response, balance, depletion-repletion, observational, and case-controlled studies.

On the basis of a review of the available data, the possible criteria of nutrient adequacy were identified by each committee for each individual nutrient. The collective scientific judgment of the committee members was then used to select the indicator criterion to determine whether the available data would allow for the establishment of an EAR or AI value. The criterion differed among nutrients and in many cases differed by life stage group. The evaluation and decision were documented for each nutrient by the committee members and was included in the individual reports. Factors that went into the decisions were strength of the data, consistency and preponderance of the data, and degree of concordance among epidemiological, clinical, and laboratory findings.

The following factors were taken into consideration when assessing the available data; strength of association (usually expressed as relative risk); dose–response relationship; temporally correct association (with exposure preceding the onset of disease); consistency of association; specificity of association; and biological plausibility.

RECOMMENDED DIETARY ALLOWANCES AND ADEQUATE INTAKES FOR INFANTS, CHILDREN, AND ADOLESCENTS

Summarized in Appendix II, "Nutritional Requirements," are the vitamin and elements, the water, fiber, and macronutrients (carbohydrate, fat and protein, linoleic acid, and alpha-linolenic acid, RDA and AI values for infants, children, and adolescents. Note that it is the intent that these numbers be targets. Actual intakes should be averaged over a number of days to assess adequacy. More detailed information for all age groups can be obtained from the Food and Nutrition Boards website http://www.iom.edu/?id=21377.

Summarized in Appendix II, "Nutritional Requirements," are the AMDRs for the macronutrients (fat, carbohydrate, and protein) and *n*-6 and *n*-3 fatty acids. The later subcategories of the macronutrient fat was created because these fatty acids are essential, that is, humans cannot make them in adequate amounts to support growth, development, and maintenance. For those nutrients, age specific recommendations are made for fewer categories for individuals below the age of 18 years; children aged 1 to 3 years and 4 to 18 years, due to limited data indicating unique needs within each grouping.

Summarized in Table 4 are additional macronutrient recommendations for non-essential dietary components: cholesterol, *trans* fatty acids, saturated fatty acids, and added sugars. These non-essential dietary components are ubiquitous in the food supply and intakes and have been associated with increased risk of chronic diseases.[9] These are general recommendations across all age and sex categories.

TOLERABLE UPPER INTAKE LEVELS

Summarized in Appendix II, "Nutritional Requirements," are the UL for those nutrients for which values have been established. The dearth of data for some nutrients precluded establishing UL values. It is important to keep in mind that the UL can only be used to assess the likelihood that an individual may be at risk for adverse effects, not that they actually will be at risk. As indicated, these values represent upper limits at which no adverse effects are likely to occur, not optimal intakes.

SELECTED NUTRIENT FUNCTIONS AND MAJOR FOOD SOURCES FOR VITAMINS AND ELEMENTS

Summarized in Appendix I, "Nutritional Assessment," and Table 5 are nutrient functions and major sources in the US and Canadian food supply. The wide range of foods noted among the nutrients is reflective of natural occurrence and mandatory federal guidelines for fortification. For example, there is a limited number of naturally occurring food sources of vitamin D. For this reason the federal government has mandated that all fluid milk be fortified with vitamin D. Fluid milk was chosen because of the unique needs of growing children and adolescents for this nutrient and historically the habitual food intake patterns of these age groups. As the intake of milk declines in these age groups, alternate approaches may be needed to ensure AI of this essential nutrient.[10]

With the increasing trend for widespread fortification of the food supply, issues related to potential intakes approaching the UL values need to be followed.[11] In some cases the consumption of fortified foods can be passive, in some cases intentional. In both cases nontraditional sources of vitamins and elements will alter total intake. This general issue came to light when it was reported that long-term intake of a diet high in retinol, independent of dietary supplements, was associated with the risk of osteoporotic hip fractures in women.[12] Better nation wide monitoring tools, especially for children, are necessary.

Table 4 Dietary Reference Intakes (DRIs): Additional Macronutrient Recommendations (Food and Nutrition Board, Institute of Medicine, National Academies)

Macronutrient	Recommendation
Dietary cholesterol	As low as possible while consuming a nutritionally adequate diet
Trans fatty acids	As low as possible while consuming a nutritionally adequate diet
Saturated fatty acids	As low as possible while consuming a nutritionally adequate diet
Added sugars	Limit to no more than 25% of total energy

Adapted from reference 1.

Table 5 Dietary Reference Intakes: Macronutrients

Nutrient	Function	Selected Food Sources
Carbohydrate—total digestible	RDA based on its role as the primary energy source for the brain; AMDR based on its role as a source of kilocalories to maintain body weight	Starch and sugar are the major types of carbohydrates. Grains and vegetables (corn, pasta, rice, potatoes, breads) are sources of starch. Natural sugars are found in fruits and juices. Sources of added sugars are soft drinks, candy, fruit drinks, and desserts
Total fiber	Improves laxation, reduces risk of coronary heart disease, assists in maintaining normal blood glucose levels	Includes dietary fiber naturally present in grains (such as found in oats, wheat, or unmilled rice) and functional fiber synthesized or isolated from plants or animals and shown to be of benefit to health
Total fat	Energy source and when found in foods, is a source of *n*–6 and *n*–3 polyunsaturated fatty acids. Its presence in the diet increases absorption of fat soluble vitamins and precursors such as vitamin A and provitamin A carotenoids	Butter, margarine, vegetable oils, whole milk, visible fat on meat, and poultry products, invisible fat in fish, shellfish, some plant products such as seeds and nuts, and bakery products
n-6 polyunsaturated fatty acids (linoleic acid)	Essential component of structural membrane lipids, involved with cell signaling, and precursor of eicosanoids. Required for normal skin function	Nuts, seeds, and vegetable oils such as soybean, safflower, and corn oil
n-3 polyunsaturated fatty acids (α-linoleic acid)	Involved with neurological development and growth. Precursor of eicosanoids	Vegetable oils such as soybean, canola, and flax seed oil, fish oils, fatty fish, with smaller amounts in meats and eggs
Saturated and *trans* fatty acids, and cholesterol	No required role for these nutrients other than as energy sources was identified; the body can synthesize its needs for saturated fatty acids and cholesterol from other sources	Saturated fatty acids are present in animal fats (meat fats and butter fat), and coconut and palm kernel oils. Sources of cholesterol include liver, eggs, and foods that contain eggs such as cheesecake and custard pies. Sources of *trans* fatty acids include sticking margarines and foods containing hydrogenated or partially-hydrogenated vegetable shortenings
Protein and amino acids	Serves as the major structural component of all cells in the body, and functions as enzymes, in membranes, as transport carriers, and as some hormones. During digestions and absorption dietary proteins are broken down to amino acids, which become the building blocks of these structural compounds. Nine of the amino acids must be provided in the diet; these are termed indispensable amino acids. The body can make the other amino acids needed to synthesize structures form other amino acids	Proteins from animal sources, such as meat, poultry, fish, eggs, milk, cheese, and yogurt, provide all nine indispensable amino acids in adequate amounts, and for this reason are considered "complete proteins." Proteins from plants, legumes, grains, nuts, seeds, and vegetables tend to be deficient in one or more of the indispensable amino acids and are called "incomplete proteins." Vegan diets adequate in total protein content can be "complete" by combining sources of incomplete proteins which lack different indispensable amino acids

Source: Dietary Reference Intakes for Energy, Carbohydrates, Fiber, Fat, Fatty Acids, Cholesterol, Protein, and Amino Acids (2002/2005). This report may be accessed via www.nap.edu. Adapted from reference 8.

DIETARY GUIDELINES FOR AMERICANS

In addition to the DRIs, the Department of Agriculture, the US Departments of Health and Human Services and Agriculture jointly issue Dietary Guidelines for Americans (http://www.health.gov/dietaryguidelines/dga2005/document/). The guidance is organized around ten chapters. They include Background and Purpose of the Dietary Guidelines for Americans; Adequate Nutrients Within Calorie Needs; Weight, Physical Activity; Food Groups To Encourage; Fats; Carbohydrates; Sodium and Potassium; and Alcoholic Beverages and Food Safety. Key Recommendations are provided to summarize and focus the information in terms of actionable items. The US Dietary Guidelines are reviewed and revised on the basis of the most recent scientific evidence every 5 years.

The intent of the Dietary Guidelines is to summarize and synthesize current knowledge in the area of nutrition with the intent of providing straightforward recommendations on food choices to promote health and decrease chronic disease risk. The Dietary Guidelines are intended for the entire US population. More specific recommendations, termed "Key Recommendations for Specific Population Groups," are provided when the scientific evidence supports additional specificity. Those that pertain to infants, children, and adolescents are shown in Table 6.

PRACTICAL ASPECTS OF ADEQUATE DIETARY INTAKE IN CHILDREN AND ADOLESCENTS

The DRI values are a helpful tool with which to evaluate whether individuals or groups are taking in adequate levels of nutrients to ensure appropriate growth and development throughout childhood and adolescence. An understanding

Table 6 US Dietary Guidelines for Americans, 2005—Key Recommendations for Children

Overweight children—Reduce the rate of body weight gain while allowing growth and development. Consult a healthcare provider before placing a child on a weight-reduction diet.
Children and adolescents—Engage in at least 60 minutes of physical activity on most, preferably all, days of the week.
Children and adolescents—Consume whole-grain products often; at least half the grains should be whole grains. Children 2 to 8 years should consume 2 cups/d of fat-free or low-fat milk or equivalent milk products. Children 9 years of age and older should consume 3 cups/d of fat-free or low-fat milk or equivalent products.
Children and adolescents—Keep total fat intake between 30 to 35% of calories for children 2 to 3 years of age and between 25 to 35% of calories for children and adolescents 4 to 18 years of age, with most fats coming from sources of polyunsaturated and monounsaturated fatty acids, such as fish, nuts and vegetable oils.
Infants and young children—Do not eat or drink raw (unpasteurized) milk or any products made from unpasteurized milk, raw or partially cooked eggs or foods containing raw eggs, raw or undercooked meat and poultry, raw or undercooked fish or shellfish, unpasteurized juices, and raw sprouts.

of DRI values and the Dietary Guidelines can help pediatricians and other pediatric health professionals guide families in developing appropriate dietary patterns. Unfortunately, this may not be enough as parents, caregivers, and children are making dietary choices in a challenging food environment where some types of foods are highly promoted and advertised while other foods, more consistent with the guidance provided by the Dietary Guidelines, are not. Additional concerns include the cost of more nutrient dense relative to less dense foods,[13] the availability of foods in schools, and after school programs and difficulty with portion sizes and packaging which are not designed for meeting dietary requirements of children.

The DRI values and Dietary Guidelines were designed in part to recognize issues of growth and development as well as the contribution of diet to the development of chronic disease risk. This relationship is increasingly true in the pediatric age range where the prevalence of obesity is increasing along with the more frequent development of type 2 diabetes and other risk factors for future cardiovascular disease.[14] Thus, the practical implementation of developing dietary patterns in children that will meet the age appropriate DRI intake levels without exceeding energy requirements is critical. There are age-specific issues regarding the implementation of DRIs that must be considered.

Newborns

The American Academy of Pediatrics has recommended breastfeeding as the best strategy for feeding newborns. Human breast milk is the reference against which other forms of infant feedings must be judged.[15] Breast milk is relatively high in saturated fat and cholesterol and is low in sodium. The American Academy of Pediatrics has encouraged breastfeeding exclusively, if possible, for the first 4 to 6 months of life.[16] Breast milk appears to be uniquely tailored to meet nutritional needs over the first 6 months of life. The composition of breast milk changes over time to meet these needs.[15] Babies appear to digest breast milk more easily than formula[17] and babies who were breastfed appear to adapt more readily to new foods when solids are introduced.[18] Nevertheless, some mothers find exclusive breastfeeding for the first 6 months difficult. For these mothers, commercial formula or a combination of breast milk and the gradual introduction of solid foods provides an appropriate alternative.

Age 6 Months to 6 Years

This age range is when children adopt eating patterns that are more similar to adults. The transition period toward solid foods provides a unique and important opportunity for parents to develop healthful eating patterns in their children. However, in the later part of this period it is also a time when children begin to be influenced by other aspects of the food environment such as eating patterns in peers, food advertising, and the availability of foods at home. Food consumption data indicate that infants and young children are exposed to a wide variety of foods that are high in saturated fat and sugars.[19] These foods and drinks include fruit juice, sweetened beverages, snack foods, and French fries. For children 1 to 4 years of age, current intakes may exceed calorie and other requirements by 30% or more.[20]

It is important that parents introduce more healthful foods during this age period. This includes the introduction of fresh fruits and vegetables, whole grain products, fish, and, after age 2 years, low-fat dairy products. Parents should avoid introducing foods with lower nutritional value and should recognize that new foods may need to be introduced repeatedly before their ultimate acceptance by young children. This may require as many as 10 repetitions to establish acceptance and taste preference.[21,22] During this period of time, as with older children, parents should be mindful of their attitudes and behavior toward food and eating because in many cases they will be reflected in their children's behaviour.[23,24]

Parents should use this time to establish healthy eating patterns and as much as possible choose and maintain on a regular basis consistent times for meals. Self-regulation of the amount of food a child consumes serves to allow them to develop appropriate cues for satiety, a behavior that should be encouraged.[25] Parents can help to manage this by providing appropriate portion sizes for the age of the child. Likewise it is important for parents to recognize that the amount of food eaten at any one time will vary from meal to meal and day to day, and to allow their children to adapt to internal clues. In addition, parents should be aware of and, when appropriate, limit snacking and other food intake that may be related to boredom or other cues rather than hunger.[23] It is important to establish healthy eating patterns early in young children.

Age 7 to 12 Years

During this age range eating outside the home, at school, aftercare programs, friends' houses, and quick-serve establishments, becomes a greater part of the daily pattern. Schools and other venues have become an increasingly difficult part of the food environment for children due to the availability of competitive foods and drinks which are high in calories. Fortunately, there are strong and consistent efforts to improve school menus, especially those available to children.

Although establishing good habits for food choices prior to the onset of school can be challenging, maintaining these habits as children get older and more independent is ever more complex due to peer pressure and other factors external to the home environment. These include increased exposure to food advertising and the introduction of fad diets.

Parents must continue to equip children and early adolescents with strategies to maintain healthful dietary patterns. Pediatricians and other pediatric health professionals can also help by emphasizing these issues as part of routine health maintenance. Parents and health professionals can also be important advocates for children and for appropriate diet at their schools and other organized programs (eg, sports teams, after school activities). Parents can work with those involved in providing meals and snacks to assess and improve the food environment. They can also encourage school systems to include more age-appropriate educational programs regarding diet for children. The objective should be to make more healthful foods and drinks available and to adopt local marketing strategies to encourage students to make more appropriate food choices.

Adolescents

Adolescence may be a particularly vulnerable period for diet. Because of accelerated growth and maturation, nutritional needs change during adolescence. The increased caloric need may stimulate appetite. These factors combined with a difficult food environment and peer factors may lead to less healthful choices.

In this age range food choices and purchases are increasingly made outside of parental control. Current data suggest adolescents have increased intake of fast food including pizza, hamburgers, and French fries, as well as increased consumption of sweetened, high calorie beverages.[26] These foods and drinks tend to displace the recommended fruits, vegetables, low fat dairy, whole grains, lean meats, and fish. This dietary pattern leads to excess intake of saturated fat, *trans* fatty acids, sugar, and insufficient intake of some micronutrients such as calcium, iron, zinc, and potassium. In addition, intake of vitamins A, D, C, and folic acid intake may be low.[26,27]

Parents and pediatric health professionals can have an important impact on the dietary intake of adolescents. Interactions with adolescents must take into account their increasing independence and must recognize that they will ultimately be making their food choices with less and less outside influence. Recommendations and counseling must be individualized to account for different household and lifestyle situations. In addition, the food environment at home and the role-modeling of parents' choices remain important. The family remains an important influence for many adolescents.

It is clear that many factors influence the food selection of children and their families. These issues must be recognized and considered in attempts to guide children and adolescents to appropriate foods choices which then result in meeting the DRIs for energy, macronutrients, and micronutrients. Better strategies need to be developed to accomplish this goal.

CONCLUSIONS

The DRIs are a set of recommendations intended to provide guidance in evaluating nutrient intakes and planning meals on the basis of nutrient adequacy. They are nutrient, not food based recommendations. The emphasis on the development of the DRIs was on reducing chronic disease risk. Depending on the available data for each nutrient, their DRIs are comprised of EAR and RDA or when inadequate data is available AI, and UL. In the case of macronutrients, there is an additional category of recommendations, AMDR. Within the category of infants to adolescents, DRI values have been established for the following age categories; 0 to 6 months, 7 to 12 months, 1 to 3 years, 4 to 8 years, 9 to 13 years, and 14 to 18 years. When assessing the available data the following were taken into consideration: strength of association (usually expressed as relative risk), dose–response relationship, temporally correct association (with exposure preceding the onset of disease), consistency of association, specificity of association, and biological plausibility. For full-term infants born to healthy mothers, it is expected that all nutrient needs will be met by exclusive breastfeeding for the first 4 to 6 months of life. For the second 6 months of life, the expectation is that nutrient needs will be met by a transition from breast milk to a mixed diet which includes solid foods. As children get older, the assumption was made that an increasing amount of food will be consumed outside the home, and, as the child becomes more independent, that they will be determining more and more of these food choices. Inherent in the ability of children and adults to meet their nutrient requirements is the need to make wise food choices. It is important for parents, health care professions, daycare providers, and schools to education children in the area of food and nutrition. This includes making healthy food choices available and encouraging children to take advantage of these options. In addition, it is important for adults to serve as positive role models for children in terms of behavior and attitudes about food and nutrition.

REFERENCES

1. IOM. Dietary Reference Intakes. Energy, Carbohydrate, Fiber, Fat, Fatty Acids, Cholesterol, Protein and Amino Acids. Washington, DC: National Academy of Sciences; 2002.
2. IOM. Dietary Reference Intakes. Calcium, Phosphorus, Magnesium, Vitamin D, and Fluoride. Washington, DC: National Academy of Sciences; 1997.
3. IOM. Dietary Reference Intakes. Thiamin, Riboflavin, Niacin, Vitamin B6, Folate, Vitamin B12, Pantothenic Acid, Biotin and Choline. Preventing Childhood Obesity: Health in the Balance. Washington, DC: National Academy of Sciences; 1998.
4. IOM. Dietary Reference Intakes. Vitamin C, Vitamin E, Selenium and Carotenoids. Washington, DC: National Academy of Sciences; 2000.
5. IOM. Dietary Reference Intakes. Vitamin A, Vitamin K, Arsenic, Boron, Chromium, Copper, Iodine, Iron, Manganese, Molybdenum, Nickel, Silicon, Vanadium and Zinc. Washington, DC: National Academy of Sciences; 2001.
6. IOM. Dietary Reference Intakes. Water, Potassium, Sodium, Chloride and Sulfate. Washington, DC: National Academy of Sciences; 2005.
7. IOM. How Should the Recommended Dietary Allowances be Revised? Washington, DC: National Academy of Sciences; 1994.
8. IOM. Dieary Reference Intakes. The Essential Guide to Nutrient Requirements. Washington, DC: National Academy of Sciences; 2006.
9. Lichtenstein AH, Appel LJ, Brands M, et al. Diet and lifestyle recommendations revision 2006: A scientific statement from the American Heart Association Nutrition Committee. Circulation 2006;114:82–96.
10. Nielsen SJ, Popkin BM. Changes in beverage intake between 1977 and 2001. Am J Prev Med 2004;27:205–10; erratum appears in Am J Prev Med 2005;28:413.
11. Lichtenstein AH, Russell RM. Essential nutrients: Food or supplements? Where should the emphasis be? JAMA 2005;294:351–8.
12. Feskanich D, Singh V, Willett WC, et al. Vitamin A intake and hip fractures among postmenopausal women. JAMA 2002;287:47–54.
13. Andrieu E, Darmon N, Drewnowski A. Low-cost diets: More energy, fewer nutrients. Eur J Clin Nutr 2006;60:434–6.
14. IOM. Preventing Childhood Obesity: Health in the Balance. Preventing Childhood Obesity: Health in the Balance. Washington, DC: National Academy of Sciences; 2005.
15. Gartner LM, Morton J, Lawrence RA, et al. American Academy of Pediatrics Section on B. Breastfeeding and the use of human milk. Pediatrics 2005;115:496–506.
16. Kramer MS, Kakuma R. The optimal duration of exclusive breastfeeding: A systematic review. Adv Exp Med Biol 2004;554:63–77.
17. Hamosh M. The milky way: From mammary gland to milk to newborn—Macy-Gyorgy Award presentation (1999). Adv Exp Med Biol 2002;503:17–25.
18. Mennella JA, Griffin CE, Beauchamp GK. Flavor programming during infancy. Pediatrics 2004;113:840–5.
19. Fox MK, Pac S, Devaney B, et al. Feeding infants and toddlers study: What foods are infants and toddlers eating? J Am Diet Assoc 2004;104:s22–30.
20. Devaney B, Ziegler P, Pac S, et al. Nutrient intakes of infants and toddlers. J Am Diet Assoc 2004;104:s14–21.
21. Addessi E, Galloway AT, Visalberghi E, et al. Specific social influences on the acceptance of novel foods in 2–5-year-old children. Appetite. 2005;45:264–71.
22. Sullivan SA, Birch LL. Infant dietary experience and acceptance of solid foods. Pediatrics 1994;93:271–7.
23. Francis LA, Birch LL. Does eating during television viewing affect preschool children's intake? J Am Diet Assoc 2006;106:598–600.
24. Faith MS, Scanlon KS, Birch LL, et al. Parent-child feeding strategies and their relationships to child eating and weight status. Obes Res 2004;12:1711–22.
25. Birch LL, Fisher JO. Development of eating behaviors among children and adolescents. Pediatrics 1998;101:539–49.
26. Putnam J, Allshouse J, Kantor LS. U.S. per capita food supply trends: More calories, refined carbohydrates, and fats. Food Rev 2002;25:2–15.
27. Bowman SA, Gortmaker SL, Ebbeling CB, et al. Effects of fast-food consumption on energy intake and diet quality among children in a national household survey. Pediatrics 2004;113:112–8.

12

International Nutrition

Benjamin Caballero, MD, PhD

While the study of global health has traditionally been of particular interest to those working in international health agencies or in developing countries, today's world makes it essential for all health professionals to understand the global forces shaping people's health. The AIDS epidemic, the emergence of new communicable diseases, and the global epidemic of obesity are examples of major domestic public health issues closely linked to the global situation. In addition, the dramatic expansion in travel and communications and the globalization of the economy are weakening cultural and geographic barriers and exposing a variety of populations to similar dietary and lifestyle factors affecting risk of disease. In this chapter, we focus on global factors affecting child survival, growth, and well-being.

CHILD MORTALITY AND SURVIVAL: GLOBAL TRENDS

Over 10 million children die each year, the majority of them in developing countries. A child born in the less developed world today has a life expectancy of 52 years. Major threats to survival are poverty, war, and HIV/AIDS.[1] In relative terms, children are more exposed to poverty because they constitute a much larger proportion of the population in poorer than in richer countries. While in industrialized countries children <18 years represent 21% of the total population, they constitute 49% of the population of the least developed countries. Similarly, 16% of children in poorest countries are <5 years of age, compared with only 6% in developed countries.[2]

Children in the poorest countries have a significantly higher risk of dying before the age of 5 years. Income inequality, that is, the range between the top and bottom quartile of income distribution, is one key predictor of child mortality risk, and closely tracks disparities in mortality. For example, in Latin America, the region with the highest household income inequality in the world, Peruvian children living in the lower 20% of income are five times more likely to die before the age of 5 years than those in the upper 20%.[2] The geographic distribution of world child deaths is shown in Figure 1.

Mortality is the end result of a complex interaction of health, nutritional, and environmental factors, but it is generally acknowledged that prior nutritional status and current dietary intake are key factors,[4–6] particularly breast-feeding duration and timing of introduction of complementary foods.[7–9] Other determinants include access and utilization to prenatal care,

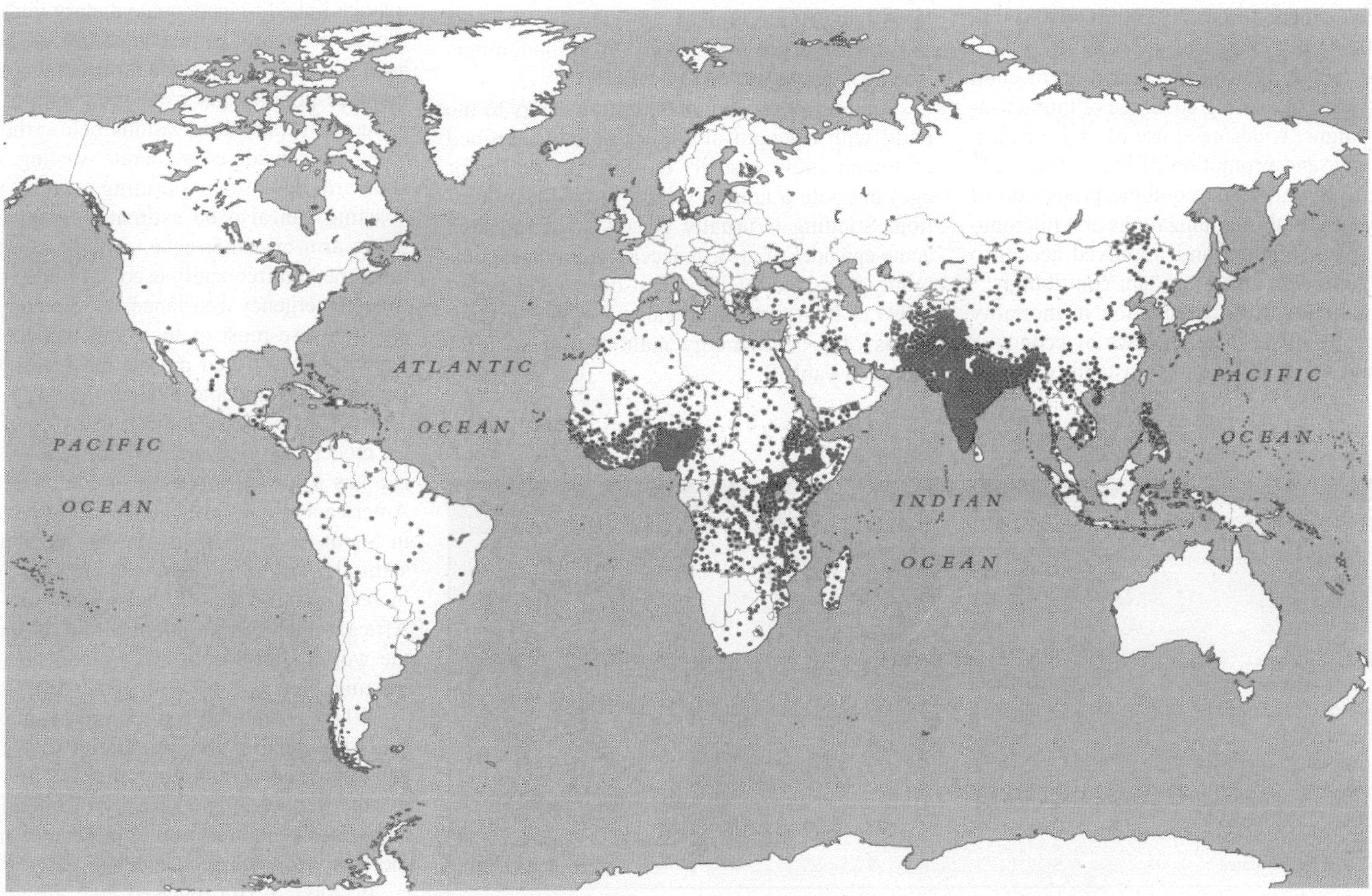

Figure 1 Geographic distribution of global child deaths. Each dot represents 5,000 deaths. (Reproduced with permission from reference 3.)

Table 1 Global Trends in Childhood Mortality Rates, 1990 and 2004

	Under-5 Mortality Rate*		Infant Mortality Rate† (Under 1)	
	1990	2004	1990	2004
World	95	79	65	54
Industrialized countries	10	6	9	5
Developing countries	105	87	72	59
Least developed countries	182	155	115	98
Sub-Saharan Africa	188	171	112	102
Middle East and North Africa	81	56	59	44
South Asia	129	92	89	67
East Asia and Pacific	58	36	43	29
Latin America and Caribbean	54	31	43	26
CEE/CIS and Baltic States	54	38	44	32

Source: UNICEF.[2]
CEE = central eastern Europe; CIS = Commonwealth of Independent States.
*Per 1,000 live births.
†Per 1,000 live births, at exactly one year of age.

immunizations, maternal education, and access to electricity.

The major causes of death in children <5 years are pneumonia (19%), diarrhea (13%), and malaria (9%). Neonatal deaths of different causes constitute over 40% of the total death in children under 5 years. Child mortality rates continue to decline in almost all regions of the world. Figures for world regions as defined by the United Nations are presented in Table 1.[2,4,5] In spite of this overall trend, there are substantial disparities among countries: almost half of all child deaths occur in only six countries, and the gap between mortality rates in developed countries and in the poorest regions has widened from 20-fold in 1990 to 29-fold in 2000.[3]

Major factors driving the reduction in child mortality were increasing coverage of immunization campaigns, widespread use of oral rehydration therapy, and promotion of breast-feeding.[10] Integrated programs that combine promotion of breast-feeding with immunizations and micronutrient supplementation, and improved access to prenatal care were also important contributors.[11] However, trends toward reduction in mortality were partially offset in some cases by economic decline and social and political instability.[4,12]

Nutrition, Growth, and Mortality

Undernutrition (low body weight) is associated with as much as 60% of deaths during the first 5 years of life. In the developing world, underweight and micronutrient deficiencies (such as vitamin A and zinc) are major contributors to the high mortality rates from diseases such as pneumonia, malaria, diarrhea, and measles. About one of every four children under 5 years of age in the developing world have a weight deficit (underweight), totaling around 146 million children.[1] About half of these children are in only three countries: India, Bangladesh, and Pakistan. Boys and girls are similarly affected, but children in rural areas are more likely to be undernourished compared with urban children.

Stunting or chronic malnutrition refers to the child with a length or stature below a defined minimum cutoff (usually the fifth percentile for age) but with a normal weight-to-height proportion. Stunting is usually the result of repeated acute episodes of growth deceleration, most commonly related to infectious episodes.[13–15] Current (1999 to 2004) data on prevalence of the different forms of protein-energy malnutrition are presented in Table 2.

Over the past two decades, a consistent decline in stunting has been documented. In 1980, 41% of children under 5 years of age had some degree of growth retardation for their age. By 2005, estimates put that figure at 32%, still leaving about 192 million children with inadequate growth.[10]

The geographic distribution of stunting is far from uniform. While one-third of children in the developing world are currently defined as stunted, 70% of these children live in Asia (61% of the total number reside in South Asia), 26% in Africa, and the remaining 4% in Latin America and the Caribbean. Similarly, while the overall trend is in decline, a slight increasing trend (of about 0.08%/yr) is observed in sub-Saharan Africa.[10] Table 2 depicts trends in stunting in UN regions from 1980 through 2005.[1,16]

Several studies have demonstrated an inverse correlation between stunting, cognitive, and physical development in young children, and consequently lower intelligence levels in older children, and functional impairment in adulthood, in terms of both intellectual and physical aspects, impairing work capacity. Stunting also increases obstetric risk in women, and also has a transgenerational effect leading to the perpetuation of suboptimal growth in the population as a whole.[17]

Wasting, usually measured by weight-for-height, is an indicator of acute malnutrition. A low weight-for-height can occur in a previously healthy child, but more commonly it affects populations of children who are already suffering from chronic malnutrition (stunting). Acute weight loss may be linked to inadequate dietary intake due to illness, or simply to unavailability of food, such as in natural or man-made disasters that suddenly displace populations from their natural habitat. Values 2 standard deviations below the median value are considered moderate wasting, with <3 standard deviations defining severe wasting. Wasting can also be estimated using the mid-upper arm circumference, a more rapid assessment method frequently used in refugee camps to triage emergency assistance.[18,19] Severely wasted children lose most of their subcutaneous fat, as well as some of their muscle mass, resulting in a very low mid-upper arm circumference.

Recent global data indicate that 10% of children are moderately to severely wasted (Table 2). Wasting has a low-to-moderate prevalence in Latin America and the Caribbean, and high prevalence in South Asia. In Africa prevalence shows substantial variability across countries, with an increasing trend from West to East. Sub-Saharan Africa, which has the highest rate of stunting in the world, shows only low-to-moderate rates of wasting.[16]

Whereas stunting has long-term implications for adult health and productivity, wasting is closely linked to child mortality.[20,21] By increasing the frequency and severity of infectious diseases, acute malnutrition significantly increases mortality from communicable diseases.[22–24]

In 2006, WHO released new growth curves for the assessment of child growth derived from

Table 2 Current Prevalence of Low Birth Weight and Malnutrition

	Percentage of Infants With Low Birth Weight	Percentage of Under-5 with Moderate or Severe		
		Underweight	Wasting	Stunting
World	16	26	10	31
Industrialized countries	7	—	—	—
Developing countries	17	27	10	31
Least developed countries	19	36	10	42
Sub-Saharan Africa	14	28	9	38
Middle East and North Africa	15	14	6	21
South Asia	31	46	14	44
East Asia and Pacific	7	15	—	19
Latin America and Caribbean	9	7	2	16
CEE/CIS and Baltic States	9	5	3	14

Source: UNICEF.[2]

the Multicenter Growth Reference Study conducted between 1997 and 2003. Detailed anthropometric measurements were obtained from infants from Brazil, Ghana, India, Norway, Oman, and the United States who were exclusively breast-fed for at least 4 months, partially breast-fed for at least 12 months, and whose mothers did not smoke cigarettes. These curves, included in Appendix I, "Nutritional Assessment" are designed to be the international standard for growth between birth and age 5, as well as to establish the breast-fed infant as the normative model for growth and development. See Chapter 2, "Clinical Assessment of Nutritional Status" for more details about these and other growth curves.

Fetal Growth and Birth Weight

Twenty-one of the twenty-five million low-birth-weight (LBW: <2500 g) infants born every year are in the developing world. Birth weight is a potent indicator of infant growth, response to environmental stimuli, and ultimately to infant survival. LBW infants have a 10-fold higher risk of neonatal mortality compared with newborns weighing 3 to 3.5 kg.[21,25] The prevalence of LBW in the developing world ranges from 9% in Latin America to 31% in South Asia.[2] Rates for each world region are shown in Table 2. Whereas prematurity is the main contributor to LBW in the developed world, the vast majority of LBW infants in developing countries are small for gestational age, reflecting intrauterine growth retardation (IUGR). The more common type of IUGR in the developing world is symmetric IUGR, indicating a sustained energy restriction throughout pregnancy. Hypoglycemia, hyperviscosity, hypothermia, perinatal asphyxia, and aspiration are more frequent in the wasted neonate. These findings persist despite correction for both birth weight and gestational age.[26]

In the developing world, maternal prepregnancy weight is strongly correlated with birth weight. A low prepregnancy body mass index is associated with higher morbidity and mortality for both mother and fetus.[23] Thus, there is an intergenerational effect of stunting, since stunted girls reaching their reproductive age will have an increased risk of producing low-birth-weight babies. Maternal behaviors and cultural factors determining level of physical activity and food intake also influence energy balance during pregnancy.[23]

In addition to dietary energy, micronutrient deficiencies can significantly affect fetal growth, as well as impact on obstetric mortality. Vitamin A deficiency appears to have a significant effect on maternal mortality, as suggested by studies in Nepal where vitamin A supplementation reduced mortality by 30%.[27] Other studies in Nepal by the same researchers reported that prenatal folic acid and iron supplementation had modest positive effects on birth weight.[28] There is increasing interest on the role of zinc deficiency on gestational outcomes. While most studies have failed to document a clear beneficial effect of zinc supplementation on birth weight, significant effects have been reported for fetal neurobehavioral development.[29,30] Additional maternal factors increasing the risk of LBW are low maternal age (<18 years), chronic infections, such as malaria, gastrointestinal parasites, STDs, first time births, the latter also seen in the industrialized world.[25]

The implications of IUGR extend beyond those of anthropometrics and growth. Studies in the developing world have reported lower Bayley scores and lower mental development index scores in low-birth-weight infants. These findings, however, are associated with environmental factors as well, such as standard of living, housing, and parental education. The trends in these studies would suggest that cognitive development and deficits change over time, and many of the conclusions drawn are dependant at the age at which they are actually followed up, and may actually be transient.[31–33]

The Guatemala longitudinal study[15] documented some degree of catch-up growth of infants with IUGR during the first 2 years of life, with subsequent stabilization at the centiles achieved by that age. Body weight and height deficits in 17- to 19-year-olds were evident, averaging 5 kg and 5 cm below non-IUGR children.[34,35]

Prevention of IUGR in developing countries has centered on improving nutritional status of women of reproductive age, providing access to prenatal care, malaria prevention and treatment, tetanus immunization, and reduction of tobacco exposure.[36–38]

THE INTERACTION OF NUTRITION AND INFECTION

The vicious circle of protein-energy malnutrition, impaired immune response, increased infections, and decreased food intake has been well recognized since the seminal work of Scrimshaw et al.[39] Malnutrition affects most of the host defense systems against infection, including epithelial and mucosal integrity, mucociliary clearance, gastric acid production, immunoglobulin synthesis, and lymphocyte differentiation.[24,40] Micronutrient deficiencies, particularly of vitamin A and zinc, also result in severe impairment of host resistance mechanisms. The role of vitamin A on the immune system and on infectious disease morbidity and mortality has been extensively studied.[41,42] The evidence from field trials led to the widespread policy of administering vitamin A as part of the acute infection management of children at risk of hypovitaminosis A. The role of zinc deficiency on susceptibility to infection and the efficacy of supplementation to reduce infection morbidity and mortality was explored in several field trials,[43,44] showing that zinc supplementation significantly reduces the incidence of pneumonia and diarrhea, with a modest but significant effect on mortality as well.

The cumulative effect of mild but repeated infectious episodes on child growth has been well documented in a variety of settings in the developing world[13,45–48]; Figure 2 depicts the growth pattern of a child in the village of Santa Maria Cauque, Guatemala. Decreased dietary intake due to anorexia or withholding of food by caregivers, excess nutrient losses, and increased nutrient requirements are the usual mechanisms by which infection aggravates nutritional status. In addition, the immune response to infection induces a catabolic state that may persist beyond the clinical course of the infectious episode, as shown by the pioneering studies of

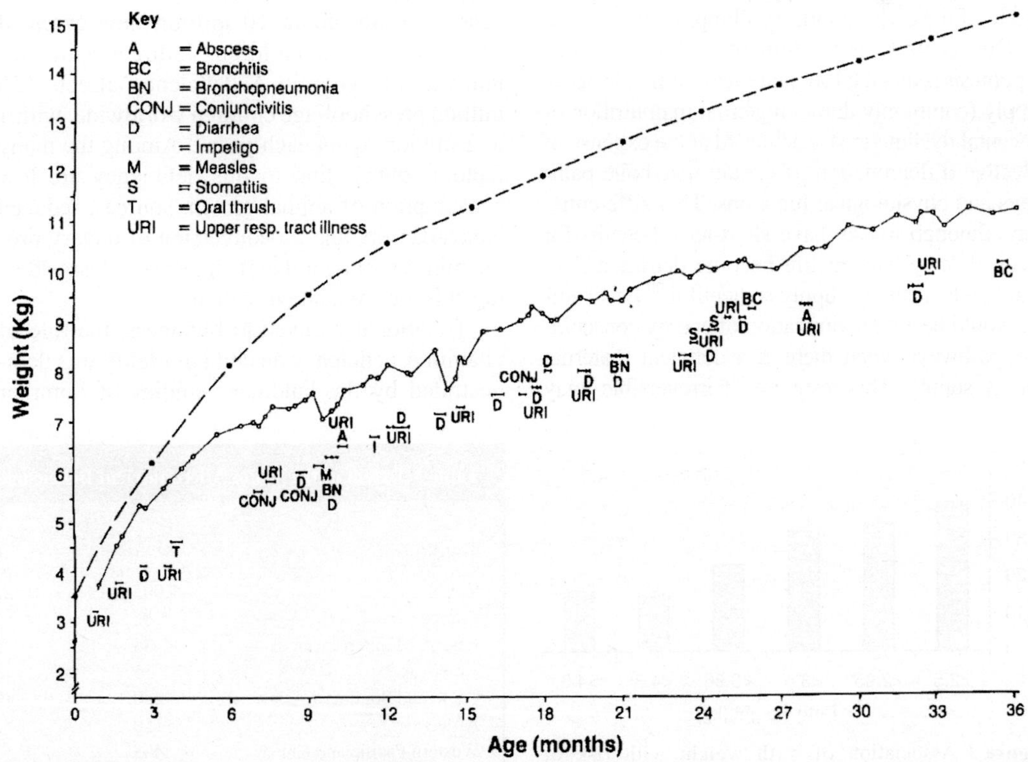

Figure 2 The impact of repeated infections on growth of a child in rural Guatemala. The solid line represents the weight of the child; the broken line is the 50th percentile of reference weight standards (INCAP, 1956). Horizontal lines above disease codes indicate duration of each infectious episode. (Reproduced with permission from reference 13.)

Beisel et al.[40] A novel mechanism for the nutrition–infection interaction was described in mice, consisting on mutation of the viral genome by selenium deficiency in the host, resulting in enhanced or newly acquired virulence.[49]

The vicious circle of infection-impaired nutrition–infection results in a significantly higher morbidity and mortality when an infection affects a malnourished host. This increase in mortality is more or less proportional to the severity of the underlying protein-energy malnutrition. It is estimated that an impaired nutritional status contributes to 56% of deaths due to infectious diseases in children.[22]

EARLY GROWTH PATTERNS AND ADULT DISEASES

The long-term effects of early nutritional experiences have received increasing attention since the emergence of the so-called Barker hypothesis (also known as the "fetal origins" hypothesis), linking prenatal undernutrition to risk for chronic diseases in adulthood.[50] This phenomenon was first documented by Widdowson, who showed that a short-term food restriction in rats had dramatically different effect depending on when it occurred in the life cycle of the animal. An early restriction caused a permanent change in food intake and thus in growth rate, whereas a restriction after weaning was quickly compensated by transient overeating and catch-up growth. There is now a consistent body of evidence, both from descriptive epidemiological studies and from biological experiments, documenting the impact of early growth and metabolic differentiation on long-term risk of disease.[50–58] Figure 3 depicts the association between birth weight and risk of type 2 diabetes as shown in one of the early reports by Phipps et al.[59]

One central proposition of the fetal origins hypothesis is that fetal adaptation to a limited energy supply (commonly due to maternal malnutrition or placental dysfunction) is achieved at the expense of selective differentiation of certain metabolic pathways and physiological functions. This differentiation, although it may have short-term benefits for survival, may later in life become detrimental to health, when energy supply is plentiful.[60] An example would be the maximization of energy conservation pathways when there is a deficient maternal energy supply. This response, if irreversible, may result in an increased risk of obesity later in life, particularly in face of unrestricted dietary energy availability.[57,61–65] Similar explanations have been put forth to explain hypertension risk based on restricted placental blood flow, and diabetes risk based on impaired glucose supply.[55,66–70]

Some evidence points to type and timing of feeding during the first 12 months of life as another important factor impacting on chronic disease risk in the adult. Of particular interest is the role of breast-feeding. Overall, published studies suggest a modest protective effect of breast-feeding against adult obesity.[71–73] For further discussion of these concepts, please see Chapter 27, "Human Growth and Disease in Later Life."

MICRONUTRIENT MALNUTRITION

Single- and multiple-nutrient deficiencies are widespread, affecting over 2 billion persons worldwide, mostly but not only in developing countries. Iron deficiency is considered the most prevalent single-nutrient deficiency, affecting more than 1 billion persons, followed by hypovitaminosis A and iodine. The global prevalence of deficiencies for vitamin A, iodine, and iron is presented in Table 3. There are less data on the global prevalence of zinc, calcium, and folate deficiencies, but most estimates consider deficiency of these nutrients more widespread than recognized earlier. Infectious diseases are an important contributor to micronutrient deficiencies. They increase gastrointestinal losses and may impair effective utilization of dietary sources as well. Conversely, micronutrient deficiencies may increase susceptibility to infection, as noted above.[31,74]

Vitamin A deficiency is one of the major single-nutrient deficiencies in the world. Every year there are about 10 million new cases of xerophthalmia in children. Indirect estimates indicate that vitamin A deficiency affects 130 million preschool-age children worldwide, with 1 to 2 million dying each year.[41] Among the many factors contributing to this deficiency are low consumption of animal protein sources, reduced bioavailability and bioconversion of dietary provitamin A (beta-carotene), and excess losses during episodes of acute infection.

Traditionally linked to blindness, the role of vitamin A deficiency on child mortality was demonstrated by the landmark studies of Sommer et al[75–79] in the early 1980s, showing that a single large dose of vitamin A resulted in a 30% reduction in child mortality. Numerous subsequent trials in different countries have confirmed those findings, yielding on average a reduction of about 20% in mortality.[80] Supplementation is now national policy in most countries with endemic hypovitaminosis A. The effect of vitamin A on mortality is likely due to its positive effects on integrity of epithelia, cell differentiation, and the immune system, thus reducing the severity of many infectious diseases, particularly gastrointestinal and respiratory.[78,81]

It has been postulated that micronutrient content of breast milk is dependent on maternal intake for some micronutrients, but independent for others. Vitamins A and B complex and iodine are expressed in lower concentrations in the case of relative maternal deficiency, but increase in response to maternal supplementation. Vitamin D, folate, zinc, iron, and calcium are maintained at relatively stable concentrations in breast milk, even in maternal deficiency states.

Multiple-nutrient deficiency is receiving increasing attention, particularly during reproductive age. The role of folic acid on pregnancy is well recognized in developed countries, but there is less information for developing countries, where populations are likely to present folic acid deficiency combined with other micronutrient deficiencies. Recently completed field trials have yielded rather disappointing results on the impact of prenatal supplementation with multiple micronutrients on infant mortality[27] and birth weight,[28] indicating that they are not more effective than folic acid plus iron only. A trend toward higher maternal mortality in the group receiving multivitamin minerals needs further evaluation. It was suggested that an enhanced fetal growth and birth size might increase obstetric risk in a chronically undernourished mother.[82]

Combating Micronutrient Malnutrition

Based on the evidence from numerous field trials showing significant benefits from micronutrient supplementation, several countries have implemented regional or national supplement distribution programs. While the supplement themselves are usually inexpensive, the logistics of mass distribution (transportation, coverage, etc) are complex and difficult to sustain over time.[83,84] Distribution

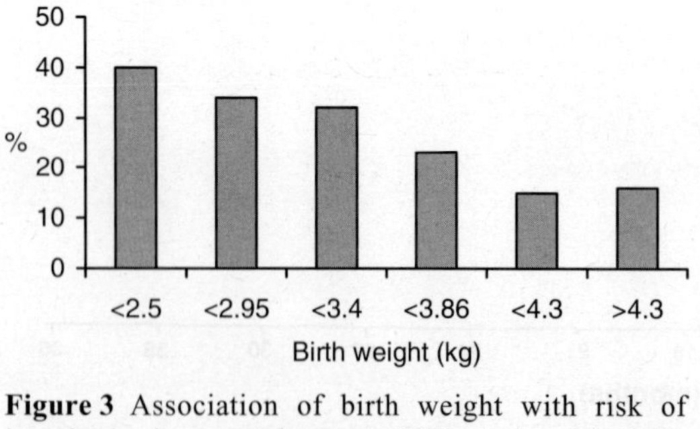

Figure 3 Association of birth weight with risk of impaired glucose tolerance (IGT) and noninsulin-dependent diabetes (NIDD) in adulthood. (Adapted from reference 59.)

Table 3 Extent of the Major Micronutrient Deficiencies in Different World Regions (in Millions of Persons)

Region	Iodine		Vitamin A		
	At Risk	Affected	At Risk	Affected	Iron*
World	1,005	225	190	13.8	2,150
Europe	82	14	—	—	27
Eastern Mediterranean	33	12	13	1.0	149
Americas	55	30	2	0.1	94
South and Southeast Asia	280	100	138	10.0	616
Africa	150	39	18	1.3	206
Western Pacific and China	405	30	19	1.4	1,058

Source: WHO.[4]
*With and without anemia

programs, therefore, are considered an interim response to endemic deficiencies, with the ultimate goal of ensuring adequate intake through locally available foods, with or without fortification. Nevertheless, given the complexity of factors affecting food availability and intake in different populations, it is likely that micronutrient supplementation will continue to be a cost-effective option for the immediate future.

Food fortification is a powerful approach to combat micronutrient malnutrition. Although its implementation and sustainability is more complex than for supplement distribution, it can take advantage of the market forces and food distribution channels, requiring little direct involvement from the target population. The requirements for a successful fortification program have been well defined.[84] A number of countries have implemented fortification programs with varied degree of success. Salt iodization has reduced the incidence and prevalence of iodine-deficiency–related diseases, including cognitive and mental impairment, growth failure, and cretinism on a global scale. Similarly, folic acid fortification had a significant impact on the prevalence of neural tube defects.

Agricultural policies can provide incentive to rotate crops and to enhance the diversity and yield of foods grown and available. Agricultural technology, selective crop breeding, and transfer of technology may aid in increasing the micronutrient content of particular foods. Subsidization of certain seed types and of fertilizers may aid in encouraging the horticulture of certain crops as well. Finally, sustainability will ultimately depend on progress in educating consumers and on the overall behavioral change of the population.

THE NUTRITION TRANSITION

The dramatic advances in communications and transportation and the globalization of economic markets are promoting rapid changes in diet and lifestyle in developing countries. This phenomenon, often termed the nutrition transition, is a key factor in the changing disease patterns for developing countries. Projections from data for the past decade indicate that by the year 2020, chronic, noncommunicable diseases will account for 70% of the disease burden in these transitional countries.[85] This in turn will impose tremendous demands on the health care system of these countries, currently geared predominantly toward maternal and child care. A detailed analysis of the nutrition transition can be found elsewhere.[86]

Urbanization, which occurs at a faster pace in the developing world, is having a profound effect on dietary patterns and lifestyle. The UN predicts that almost 90% of the projected population growth for the next 20 years will occur in urban areas of the developing world (Figure 4). Thus, the absolute number of persons whose diet and lifestyle will be modulated by the urban environment will increase dramatically.

The urban environment has important effects on dietary and lifestyle patterns. Consumption of

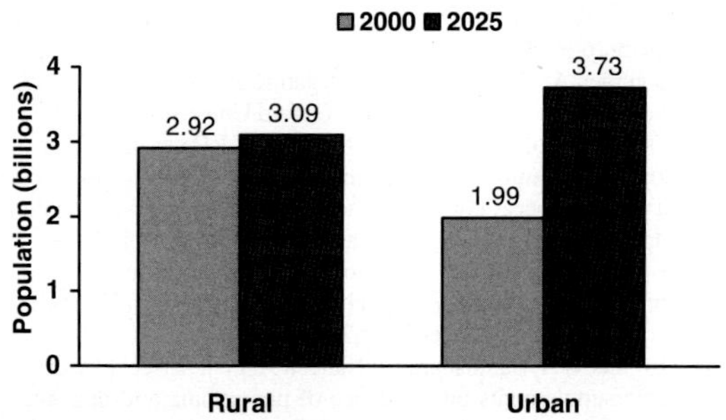

Figure 4 Actual and projected population growth, 2000 and 2025. Relative population increases in urban and rural areas. (Data from the UN Population Council.)

processed foods, usually of higher fat content, and total dietary energy intake tends to increase.[87] Urban families become dependent on the cash food market, which exhibit high price elasticity, thus having the potential for driving food choices in low-income populations.[88] Daily energy expenditure in the urban setting is usually substantially lower than in rural areas. The intense physical labor of rural work in the fields is replaced by sedentary, low-energy work of service jobs or automated manufacturing.[88,89] Television viewing is also a well-documented factor in increasing physical inactivity in adults and adolescents. The combined effect of an increased energy intake and a reduced energy output is weight gain and obesity. In addition, sedentary lifestyle per se carries an increased risk for cardiovascular diseases.[90] The impact of urban dwelling on obesity prevalence has been documented for several regions in the developing world. Childhood obesity has increased steadily in developed and developing countries. A recent global assessment by Wang and Lobstein predicts that by the year 2010 obesity rates will reach over 20% in China, India, and countries in East Asia.[91] In countries of intermediate development (with a GNP of ~$2,000/yr) a phenomenon called "dual burden" of disease is emerging, in which under- and overnutrition can be present in the same household, usually an underweight child with overweight adults.[92] This suggests that, as the economic growth of a country advances, obesity risk tends to switch from the upper to the lower socioeconomic groups, which also continue to have substantial rates of undernutrition. The association between under-and overweight is obviously complex, and is affected by a number of factors such as urbanization, demographic profile, and others.[93]

CONFRONTING THE CHALLENGE OF THE NUTRITION TRANSITION

The World Health Organization has recognized diet- and lifestyle-related chronic diseases as a strategic challenge for world health, and has defined a blueprint for action at the global and local level.[94] Several countries have begun to consider the long-term implications of their socioeconomic changes on the health of their population as well. Local and national initiatives to improve dietary patterns and increase physical activity have been proposed or implemented.[95,96] Other countries like China are testing regional programs to promote healthy eating and lifestyle, particularly in the urban population. There are some comprehensive experiences in preventive interventions in developed countries, which can provide insight into effective approaches. Among these the Karelia study is well recognized as a successful model of integration of public and private efforts to use market forces, the media, and consumer education to improve dietary patterns.[97]

CONCLUSIONS

This chapter has summarized current global trends in child survival and health, emphasizing their close links with nutritional status. In spite of the overall positive trends in child survival, child mortality is still unacceptably high in many parts of the world, and the gap between the lower and higher mortality countries has widened substantially over the past decade. In 2000, world leaders agreed on the Millennium Development Goals, which calls for halving the prevalence of child mortality by 2015. Projections from current data indicate that many developing countries will not reach that target until 2030 and beyond. This means that by 2015, still 8.7 million children will die before age 5.

To the challenge of undernutrition is now added the burden of chronic, noncommunicable diseases that are increasing at alarming rate in countries of intermediate development. Confronting this chronic disease epidemic will pose an enormous burden on the health case system. In spite of these challenges, the success of several programs aimed at reducing malnutrition, controlling micronutrient deficiencies, improving food security, and expanding immunization coverage is encouraging. Community involvement, empowerment of women, recognition of unique local social, cultural, and economic conditions, all seem to be key ingredients for success.

REFERENCES

1. UNICEF. Progress for Children: A Report Card on Nutrition. New York: UNICEF; 2006.
2. UNICEF. The State of the World's Children 2006. New York: UNICEF; 2006.
3. Black RE, Morris SS, Bryce J. Where and why are 10 million children dying every year? Lancet 2003;361:2226–34.
4. UNICEF. The State of the World's Children 2002: Official Summary. Geneva: UNICEF.
5. WHO. The World Health Report 2000—Health Systems: Improving Performance. Geneva: WHO; 2000.
6. Rutstein SO. Factors associated with trends in infant and child mortality in developing countries during the 1990s. Bull World Health Organ 2000;78:1256–70.
7. Brown KH, Sharma S. Complementary feeding of infants and young children. Indian Pediatr 1999;36:547–54.
8. Betran AP, de Onis M, Lauer JA, Villar J. Ecological study of effect of breast feeding on infant mortality in Latin America. BMJ 2001;323:303–6.
9. Ahmad OB, Lopez AD, Inoue M. The decline in child mortality: A reappraisal. Bull World Health Organ 2000;78:1175–91.
10. de Onis M, Frongillo EA, Blossner M. Is malnutrition declining? An analysis of changes in levels of child malnutrition since 1980. Bull World Health Organ 2000;78:1222–33.
11. Kulier R, de Onis M, Gulmezoglu AM, Villar J. Nutritional interventions for the prevention of maternal morbidity. Int J Gynaecol Obstet 1998;63:231–46.

12. Hobcraft JN, McDonald JW, Rutstein SO. Socio-economic factors in infant and child mortality: A cross-national comparison. Popul Stud (Camb) 1984;38:193–223.
13. Mata L. The Children of Santa Maria Cauque: A Prospective Field Study of Health and Growth. Cambridge, MA: MIT Press; 1978.
14. Mata L, Simhon A, Urrutia JJ, Kronmal RA. Natural-history of rotavirus infection in the children of Santa-Maria-Cauque. Prog Food Nutr Sci 1983;7:167–77.
15. Martorell R. Results and implications of the INCAP follow-up study. J Nutr 1995;125:1127S–38S.
16. WHO. World Health Statistics 2006. Available at http://www.who.int/evidence. Accessed on 18 December, 2006.
17. Ramakrishnan U, Martorell R, Schroeder DG, Flores R. Role of intergenerational effects on linear growth. J Nutr 1999;129:544S–9S.
18. WHO Expert Committee on Physical Status. Infants and Children. Physical Status: The Use and Interpretation of Anthopometry. Geneva: WHO; 1995. p. 161–255.
19. WHO Expert Committee on Physical Status. Technical Framework. Physical Status: The Use and Interpretation of Anthopometry. Geneva: WHO; 1995. p. 4–33.
20. de Onis M. Measuring nutritional status in relation to mortality. Bull World Health Organ 2000;78:1271–4.
21. Pelletier DL. The relationship between child anthropometry and mortality in developing-countries—implications for policy, programs and future-research. J Nutr 1994;124:S2047–81.
22. Pelletier D, Frongillo E, Schroeder D, Habicht JP. Estimating the contribution of malnutrition to child-mortality in developing-countries. FASEB J 1994;8:A155.
23. ACC/SCN. Fourth Report on The World Nutrition Situation: Nutrition Throughout the Life Cycle. Geneva: WHO/IFPRI; 2000.
24. Rice AL, Sacco L, Hyder A, Black RE. Malnutrition as an underlying cause of childhood deaths associated with infectious diseases in developing countries. Bull World Health Organ 2000;78:1207–21.
25. ACC/SCN: Low birth weight. Nutrition policy paper no. 18, World Health Organization, Geneva, 2000.
26. Caulfield LE, Haas JD, Belizan JM, et al. Differences in early postnatal morbidity risk by pattern of fetal growth in Argentina. Paediatr Perinat Epidemiol 1991;5:263–75.
27. Christian P, West KP, Khatry SK, et al. Effects of maternal micronutrient supplementation on fetal loss and infant mortality: A cluster-randomized trial in Nepal. Am J Clin Nutr 2003;78:1194–202.
28. Christian P, Khatry SK, Katz J, et al. Effects of alternative maternal micronutrient supplements on low birth weight in rural Nepal: Double blind randomised community trial. BMJ 2003;326:571–6.
29. Caulfield LE, Zavaleta N, Shankar AH, Merialdi M. Potential contribution of maternal zinc supplementation during pregnancy to maternal and child survival. Am J Clin Nutr 1998;68:499S–508S.
30. Merialdi M, Caulfield LE, Zavaleta N, et al. Adding zinc to prenatal iron and folate tablets improves fetal neurobehavioral development. Am J Obstet Gynecol 1999;180:483–90.
31. Black RE, Sazawal S. Zinc and childhood infectious disease morbidity and mortality. Br J Nutr 2001;85:S125–9.
32. Goldenberg R, Hack M, Grantham M, Schurch B. Report of the IDECG/IUNS working group on IUGR effects on neurological, sensory, cognitive, and behavioral function. Eur J Clin Nutr 1998;52:S100–1.
33. Hack M. Effects of intrauterine growth retardation on mental performance and behavior, outcomes during adolescence and adulthood. Eur J Clin Nutr 1998;52:S65–71.
34. Haas JD, Murdoch S, Rivera J, Martorell R. Early nutrition and later physical work capacity. Nutr Rev 1996;54:S41–8.
35. Martorell R, Ramakrishnan U, Schroeder DG, et al. Intrauterine growth retardation, body size, body composition and physical performance in adolescence. Eur J Clin Nutr 1998;52:S43–52.
36. de Onis M, Villar J, Gulmezoglu M. Nutritional interventions to prevent intrauterine growth retardation: Evidence from randomized controlled trials. Eur J Clin Nutr 1998;52:S83–93.
37. Gulmezoglu M, de Onis M, Villar J. Effectiveness of interventions to prevent or treat impaired fetal growth. Obstet Gynecol Surv 1997;52:139–49.
38. Kafatos AG, Vlachonikolis IG, Codrington CA. Nutrition during pregnancy. The effects of an educational intervention program in Greece. Am J Clin Nutr 1989;50:970–9.
39. Scrimshaw NS, Taylor CE, Gordon JE. Interactions of nutrition and infection. Monogr Ser World Health Organ 1968;57:3–329.
40. Beisel WR. Metabolic response to infection. Annu Rev Med 1975;26:9–20.
41. Sommer A, West Keith P, Jr. Vitamin A Deficiency: Health, Survival and Vision. New York: Oxford University Press; 1996.
42. Deloria-Knoll M, Steinhoff M, Semba RD, et al. Effect of zinc and vitamin A supplementation on antibody responses to a pneumococcal conjugate vaccine in HIV-positive injection drug users: A randomized trial. Vaccine 2006;24:1670–9.
43. Brooks WA, Yunus M, Santosham M, et al. Zinc for severe pneumonia in very young children: Double-blind placebo-controlled trial. Lancet 2004;363:1683–8.
44. Brooks WA, Santosham M, Naheed A, et al. Effect of weekly zinc supplements on incidence of pneumonia and diarrhoea in children younger than 2 years in an urban, low-income population in Bangladesh: Randomised controlled trial. Lancet 2005;366:999–1004.
45. Martorell R, Yarbrough C, Yarbrough S, Klein RE. The impact of ordinary illnesses on the dietary intakes of malnourished children. Am J Clin Nutr 1980;33:345–50.
46. Poskitt EM, Cole TJ, Whitehead RG. Less diarrhoea but no change in growth: 15 years' data from three Gambian villages. Arch Dis Child 1999;80:115–9.
47. Lamb WH, Foord FA, Lamb CM, Whitehead RG. Changes in maternal and child mortality rates in three isolated Gambian villages over ten years. Lancet 1984;2:912–4.
48. Whitehead RG, Coward WA, Lunn PG, Rutishauser I. A comparison of the pathogenesis of protein-energy malnutrition in Uganda and the Gambia. Trans R Soc Trop Med Hyg 1977;71:189–95.
49. Beck MA, Levander OA. Host nutritional status and its effect on a viral pathogen. J Infect Dis 2000;182:S93–6.
50. Barker DJ. Fetal growth and adult disease. Br J Obstet Gynaecol 1992;99:275–6.
51. Burke JP, Williams K, Gaskill SP, et al. Rapid rise in the incidence of type 2 diabetes from 1987 to 1996: Results from the San Antonio Heart Study. Arch Intern Med 1999;159:1450–6.
52. Haffner SM, Stern MP, Mitchell BD, Hazuda HP. Predictors of obesity in Mexican Americans. Am J Clin Nutr 1991;53:1571S–6S.
53. Menard SW, Park MK, Scholfield J. The San Antonio Biethnic children's blood pressure study: Anthropometric findings. Clin Excell Nurse Pract 1999;3:19–27.
54. Jones AP, Simson EL, Friedman MI. Gestational undernutrition and the development of obesity in rats. J Nutr 1984;114:1484–92.
55. Barker DJ, Gluckman PD, Godfrey KM, et al. Fetal nutrition and cardiovascular disease in adult life. Lancet 1993;341:938–41.
56. Valdez R, Gonzalez-Villalpando C, Mitchell BD, et al. Differential impact of obesity in related populations. Obes Res 1995;3:223S–32S.
57. Martorell R, Stein AD, Schroeder DG. Early nutrition and later adiposity. J Nutr 2001;131:874S–80S.
58. Barker DJ, Forsen T, Uutela A, et al. Size at birth and resilience to effects of poor living conditions in adult life: Longitudinal study. BMJ 2001;323:1273–6.
59. Phipps K, Barker DJ, Hales CN, et al. Fetal growth and impaired glucose tolerance in men and women. Diabetologia 1993;36:225–8.
60. Godfrey KM, Barker DJ. Fetal nutrition and adult disease. Am J Clin Nutr 2000;71:1344S–52S.
61. Ravelli AC, Der Meulen JH, Osmond C, et al. Obesity at the age of 50 y in men and women exposed to famine prenatally. Am J Clin Nutr 1999;70:811–6.
62. Ravelli GP, Stein ZA, Susser MW. Obesity in young men after famine exposure in utero and early infancy. N Engl J Med 1976;295:349–53.
63. Roseboom TJ, Der Meulen JH, Ravelli AC, et al. Effects of prenatal exposure to the Dutch famine on adult disease in later life: An overview. Twin Res 2001;4:293–8.
64. Schroeder DG, Martorell R, Rivera J, et al. Age-differences in the impact of supplement on growth. FASEB J 1993;7:A283.
65. Caballero B. Obesity as a consequence of undernutrition. J Pediatr 2006;149:S97–9.
66. Eriksson J, Forsen T, Tuomilehto J, et al. Fetal and childhood growth and hypertension in adult life. Hypertension 2000;36:790–4.
67. Eriksson J, Forsen T, Tuomilehto J, et al. Size at birth, childhood growth and obesity in adult life. Int J Obes 2001;25:735–40.
68. Eriksson JG, Forsen T, Tuomilehto J, et al. Size at birth, growth in childhood and future risk of type 2 diabetes. Diabetes 1999;48:A72.
69. Eriksson JG, Forsen T, Tuomilehto J, et al. Catch-up growth in childhood and death from coronary heart disease: Longitudinal study. BMJ 1999;318:427–31.
70. Eriksson JG, Forsen T, Tuomilehto J, et al. Early growth and coronary heart disease in later life: Longitudinal study. BMJ 2001;322:949–53.
71. Pettitt DJ, Forman MR, Hanson RL, et al. Breastfeeding and incidence of non-insulin-dependent diabetes mellitus in Pima Indians. Lancet 1997;350:166–8.
72. von Kries R, Koletzko B, Sauerwald T, et al. Breast feeding and obesity: Cross sectional study. BMJ 1999;319:147–50.
73. Dewey KG. Is breastfeeding protective against child obesity? J Hum Lact 2003;19:9–18.
74. Semba RD, Tang AM. Micronutrients and the pathogenesis of human immunodeficiency virus infection. Br J Nutr 1999;81:181–9.
75. Sommer A, Tarwotjo I, Hussaini G, Susanto D. Increased mortality in children with mild vitamin A deficiency. Lancet 1983;2:585–8.
76. Sommer A. Mortality associated with mild, untreated xerophthalmia. Trans Am Ophthalmol Soc 1983;81:825–53.
77. Sommer A, Tarwotjo I, Djunaedi E, et al. Impact of vitamin A supplementation on childhood mortality. A randomised controlled community trial. Lancet 1986;1:1169–73.
78. Sommer A, West KP. Vitamin A and childhood mortality. Lancet 1991;337:925.
79. West KP, Jr, Katz J, Shrestha SR, et al. Mortality of infants <6 mo of age supplemented with vitamin A: A randomized, double-masked trial in Nepal. Am J Clin Nutr 1995;62:143–8.
80. Beaton, GH, Martorell, R, Aronson KJ, et al. Effectiveness of Vitamin A Supplemenation in the Control of Young Child Morbidity & Mortality in Developing Countries. ACC/SCN State-of-the-Art Series Nutrition Policy Discussion Paper 13. Toronto, Ontario, Canada: United Nations; 1993.
81. Troen G, Eskild W, Fromm SH, et al. Vitamin A-sensitive tissues in transgenic mice expressing high levels of human cellular retinol-binding protein type I are not altered phenotypically. J Nutr 1999;129:1621–7.
82. Katz J, Christian P, Dominici F, Zeger SL. Treatment effects of maternal micronutrient supplementation vary by percentiles of the birth weight distribution in rural Nepal. J Nutr 2006;136:1389–94.
83. The International Bank for Reconstruction and Development. Enriching Lives: Overcoming Vitamin and Mineral Malnutrition in Developing Countries. Washington, DC: The World Bank; 1994.
84. Institute of Medicine. Prevention of Micronutrient Deficiencies: Tools for Policy Makers and Public Health Workers. Washington, DC: National Academy Press; 1998.
85. Murray CJL, Lopez AD. The Global Burden of Disease. Cambridge, MA: Harvard University Press; 1996.
86. Hamadani JD, Fuchs GJ, Osendarp SJ, et al. Zinc supplementation during pregnancy and effects on mental development and behaviour of infants: A follow-up study. Lancet 2002;360:290–4.
87. Drewnowski A, Popkin BM. The nutrition transition: New trends in the global diet. Nutr Rev 1997;55:31–43.
88. Popkin BM. The nutrition transition and obesity in the developing world. J Nutr 2001;131:871S–3S.
89. Martorell R, Khan LK, Hughes ML, Grummer-Strawn LM. Obesity in Latin American women and children. J Nutr 1998;128:1464–73.
90. Caballero B. Obesity in developing countries: Biological and ecological factors. J Nutr 2001;131:866S–70S.
91. Wang Y, Lobstein T. Worldwide trends in childhood overweight and obesity. Int J Pediatr Obes 2006;1:11–25.
92. Caballero B. A nutrition paradox: Underweight and obesity in developing countries. N Engl J Med 2005;352:1514–6.
93. Duran P, Caballero B, de Onis M. The association between stunting and overweight in Latin American and Caribbean preschool children. Food Nutr Bull 2006;27:300–5.
94. WHO/FAO. Diet, Nutrition and the Prevention of Chronic Diseases. Geneva: WHO; 2003.
95. Matsudo V, Matsudo S, Andrade D, et al. Promotion of physical activity in a developing country: The Agita Sao Paulo experience. Public Health Nutr 2002;5:253–61.
96. WHO and NPH. Physical Activity and Health (PAH): Components of WHO Strategic Plan (2002–2003). Geneva: Department of NCD Prevention and Health promotion (NPH). Geneva: WHO; 2002.
97. Puska P, Tuomilehto J, Nissinen A, et al. The North Karelia project: 15 years of community-based prevention of coronary heart disease. Ann Med 1989;21:169–73.

13

Protein-Energy Malnutrition: Pathophysiology, Clinical Consequences, and Treatment

Mary E. Penny, MA, MB, ChB, MRCP

The number of children affected by and the long-term consequences of malnutrition place it among the greatest public health problems facing the world today. The World Health Organization (WHO) estimates that malnutrition contributes to 54% of child mortality worldwide.[1–4] Even mild degrees of malnutrition double the risk of mortality[2,3] for both respiratory and diarrheal disease mortality[4] and malaria,[5] but this risk is greatly increased in more severe degrees of malnutrition.[2,3] Severe malnutrition, also called protein-energy malnutrition (PEM), is eminently treatable, but, sadly, this is an area where the gap between existing knowledge of successful practice and the reality of the management of most malnourished children is abysmal. Recent reports illustrate how the adoption of improved management can drastically reduce mortality even in resource-restricted circumstances.[6] The global importance of malnutrition and the long-term consequences are dealt with in Chapter 12, "International Nutrition." The public health significance, as discussed in Chapter 14, "Childhood Malnutrition: Prevention and Control at the National Level," emphasizes the necessity for the combination of policies designed to prevent malnutrition with programs to treat children with existing malnutrition. These authors describe the success in Chile of such an approach. Malnutrition is not only a problem of developing countries. Failure to recognize malnutrition may also contribute to increased morbidity and mortality in other conditions seen in developed countries such as congenital heart disease[7] and cystic fibrosis.[8] This chapter deals with the clinical management of severe malnutrition and attempts to show how an understanding of the pathophysiology provides a basis for the treatment of the severely malnourished child. The multiple factors that contribute to the development of malnutrition are detailed elsewhere; this chapter is principally concerned with severe PEM as a clinical entity because the failure to recognize the special needs of these children contributes to the high mortality.[9]

DEFINITIONS OF MALNUTRITION

Malnutrition has many causes. In any individual, inadequate food intake, infections, psychosocial deprivation, the environment, and perhaps genetic variability contribute. The clinical manifestations in the child depend on the duration and degree of shortfall in dietary intake, the quality of the diet, host factors such as age, and the interplay with infection.

The first step in the diagnosis of malnutrition is nutrition assessment. This is an essential part of any clinical pediatric evaluation and is discussed in detail in Chapter 2, "Clinical Assessment of Nutritional Status." Repeated nutritional assessments of all ill children are important to prevent the insidious onset of malnutrition, which may hinder recovery. Adequate growth is an indication of health and recovery. For the individual child, the most important information is gained from serial measurements of the child's growth, and this provides essential information for diagnosing cause and guiding treatment. The importance of using this often available but overlooked information cannot be overstated.

Although measurements of height and weight are the usual mainstays of diagnosis, additional information on body composition can be obtained from skinfold thickness and other more sophisticated methods. Biochemical and hematologic tests may also be useful, especially in monitoring progress. PEM is often associated with micronutrient deficiency, and examination should include a specific search for Bitot's spots or xerophthalmia, manifestations of vitamin A deficiency,[10] and signs of other micronutrient deficiencies.

Sole reliance on weight and length or height can lead to failure to recognize kwashiorkor and an underestimation of the severity of the malnutrition in these children. The scheme recommended by WHO (Table 1) has the merit of distinguishing these two entities and is useful in clinical practice.[11] Figure 1 illustrates a child with marasmus and shows the characteristic muscle wasting particularly evident in the buttocks, the pinched face, and anxious demeanor. Figure 2 shows the same child on recovery.

Figure 3 illustrates a child with kwashiorkor. Symmetric edema is evident, especially in the lower limbs. The hair is sparse, and the flaky paint rash is seen on the buttocks, legs, and arms. Figure 4 shows the typical bilateral symmetric edema of the legs.

Marasmus is generally thought to be the result of a cumulative, usually slow, inadequate energy and protein intake. The child's metabolism has adapted, producing changes that prolong survival and protect essential visceral and brain function. This is the type of PEM traditionally seen in famine, food restriction, or anorexia. Kwashiorkor is also a severe form of malnutrition. The etiology is not well understood, but the long-held view that protein deficiency in the face of adequate energy intake causes kwashiorkor cannot explain all of the evidence. Observed findings are more in keeping with an interaction between

Table 1 Classification of Moderate and Severe Malnutrition

	Moderate Malnutrition	Severe Malnutrition
Symmetric edema?	No	Yes edematous malnutrition or kwashiorkor
Weight for age		
SD score	−2 to −3	<−3 severe wasting
% Median	70 to 79	<70 or marasmus
Length for age		
SD score	−2 to −3	<−3 severe stunting
% Median	85 to 89	<85

Adapted from reference 11.

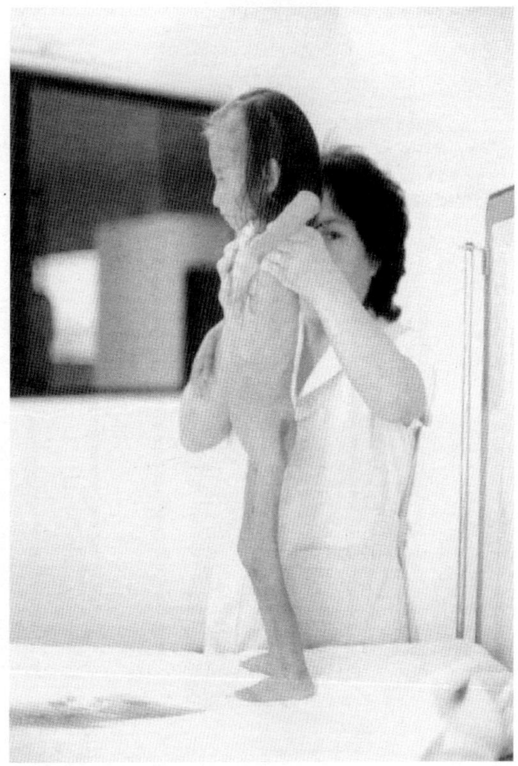

Figure 1 Child with marasmus.

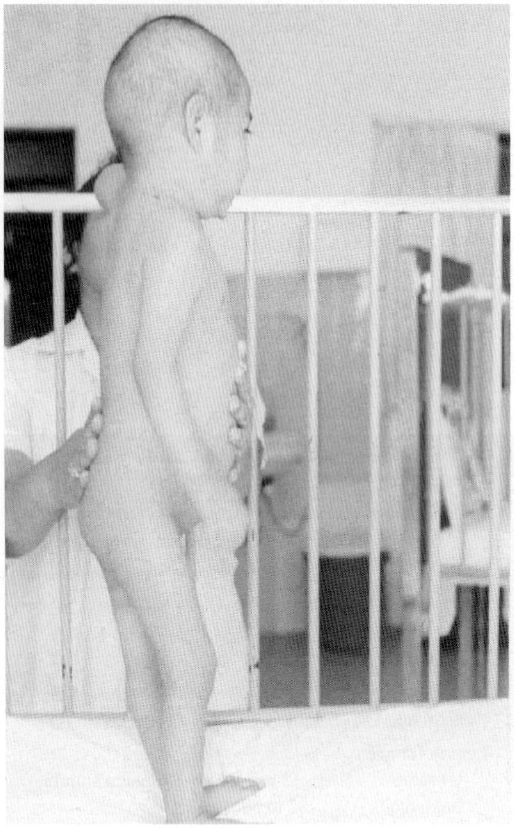

Figure 2 Same child as shown in Figure 1, on recovery.

nutritional deficits and the response to injury, infection, and oxidative stress. Marasmus and kwashiorkor commonly coexist, and although a simple unified approach to clinical management can be applied successfully to both conditions,[11] the two are clinically distinct entities.

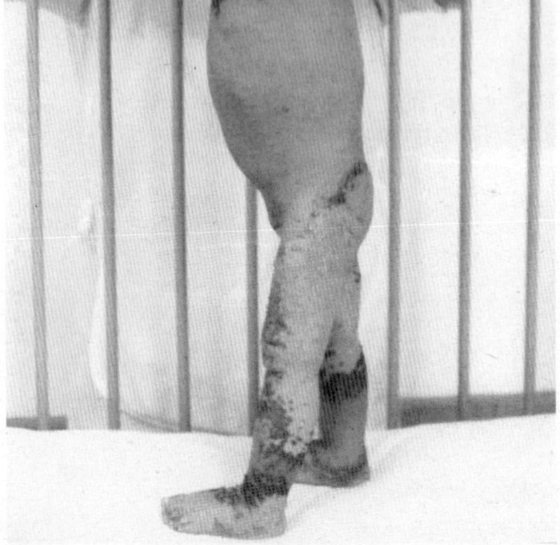

Figure 3 Child with kwashiokor.

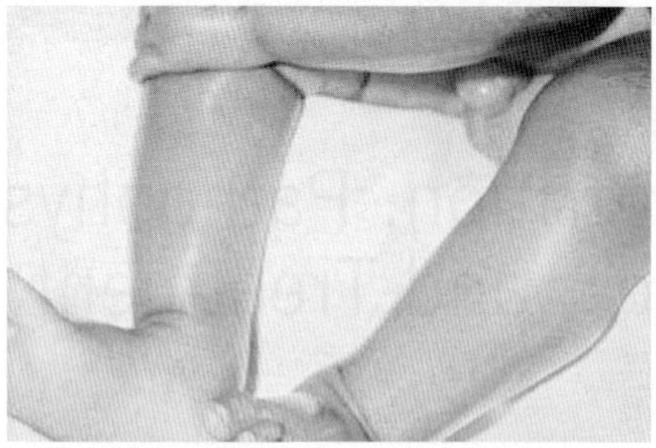

Figure 4 Lower limbs of a child with kwashiorkor.

PATHOPHYSIOLOGY

Metabolic Responses to Inadequate Energy Intake

PEM is the result of a chronic and cumulative failure to meet physiologic energy and nutrient requirements.[12] The manifestations of this process depend on different factors: age, concomitant infection, prior nutritional state, and the nature of the dietary restriction, to name four. Both the early classic experimental studies of food energy deprivation and starvation in animals and humans and studies of severely malnourished children on admission and during recovery have contributed to our understanding, although the situation is complicated by the multifactorial causes of malnutrition in most children. A detailed description is beyond the scope of this chapter, but the interested reader is referred to excellent reviews.[13,14]

In the absence of infection, fasting results in an initial depletion of fat stores and then glycogen stores mediated by metabolic and endocrine changes that have the common goal of preserving vital functions, allowing the animal or human to survive until dietary energy can be restored. Early changes include a reduction in activity that conserves energy expenditure.[15] Growth is slowed, reducing the energy need to maintain this, and changes occur in body composition. Metabolic rate expressed in relation to height or lean body mass decreases.[14] Brain and viscera are relatively preserved (Figure 5),[16] resulting in the body composition typical of marasmic children.[17] There is an increase in total-body water, which is mainly extracellular but may also be intracellular.[12,13,18]

These metabolic adjustments to starvation are mediated, at least in part, by hormones. Cortisol concentration rises but remains responsive to stress.[17,19] Insulin secretion falls, and there is a reduction in plasma insulin levels, a reduced response to glucose, and peripheral insulin resistance.[20,21] Growth hormone is generally high, and the normal suppression by glucose load is lost, although exceptions occur in marasmus.[22] There is low activity of insulin-like growth factor 1, the metabolic effector of the growth promoting effect of growth hormone.[17] The net effects of these hormonal changes are mobilization of fat, degradation of muscle protein, and reduction in basal metabolic rate. Increased aldosterone contributes to potassium loss already compromised by the effects of energy restriction and reduced adenosine triphosphate synthesis on the sodium pump.[23]

Adaptation to Reduced Protein Intake

During protein deprivation, skeletal muscle is lost as structural protein is recycled to conserve essential enzymes and provide energy for metabolic processes. There is both a fall in muscle protein synthesis and an increase in breakdown, which provides essential amino acids to the liver for protein synthesis and gluconeogenesis.[17] Within the liver, there is a shift in the rates of synthesis of different proteins; synthesis of albumin, transferrin, and apolipoprotein B are decreased, but the synthesis of other proteins is maintained.[24]

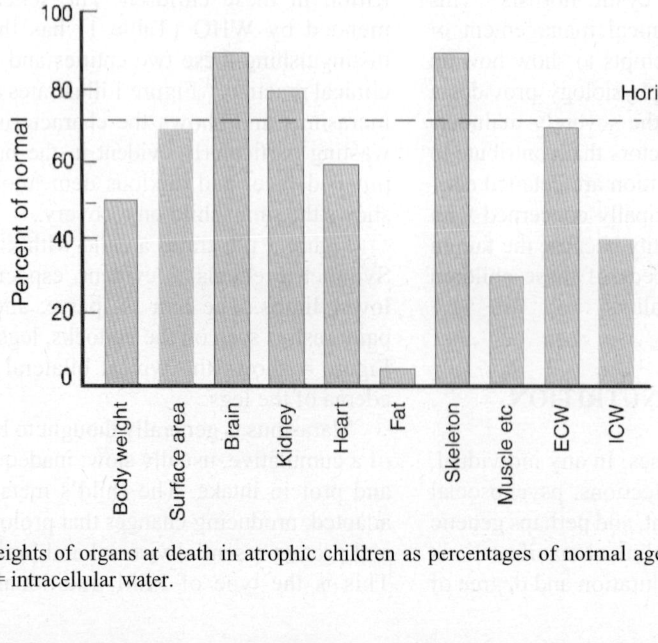

Figure 5 Weights of organs at death in atrophic children as percentages of normal age controls. ECW = extracellular water; ICW = intracellular water.

Changes in Electrolytes

Changes in chemical composition of the body that occur during malnutrition have important consequences for treatment. Sodium, potassium, and phosphate merit special mention, but changes in other electrolytes, such as magnesium and calcium, are probably important but have been less studied.

The vast proportion of total-body potassium is intracellular, in contrast to sodium, which is actively removed from cells by the sodium pump. In both marasmus and kwashiorkor, sodium retention occurs, resulting in an increase in whole-body sodium, even though serum levels may be low, reflecting an increase in extracellular water. There is a decrease in total-body potassium,[25] although serum potassium may remain normal. Alleyne and colleagues described how potassium kinetics are altered during recovery.[26]

There was an initial acute repletion of potassium when hypokalemia and whole-body deficiency improved, followed by a longer phase of cell membrane recovery and reestablishment of the normal Na/K gradients. A third phase occurred when rapid growth of skeletal muscle increased potassium requirements.[27,28] Nichols and colleagues calculated from balance studies that 7.0 mmol/kg body weight of potassium was needed in the first week or acute phase of recovery, an amount similar to the level of supplement giving best results in a clinical trial in Malawi.[29,30]

The inconsistencies between serum and total-body potassium are explained by events at the cell membrane. In marasmus, there is a decrease in the activity of the ouabain-sensitive energy-dependent sodium pump, resulting in increased intracellular sodium and reduced potassium.[31] Different mechanisms operate in kwashiorkor, in which there is an increase in cell membrane leakiness.

Different mechanisms operate in kwashiorkor sodium, responding to the electrolyte gradient, enters the cell, stimulating increased activity of the sodium pump but not enough to prevent Na increase and K loss.[31,32] Similar differences between marasmus and kwashiorkor were reported by Kaplay in India.[33] Forrester and colleagues found that these electrolyte changes could be reproduced in in vitro erythrocytes if glutathione was artificially reduced, resembling the situation in kwashiorkor.[34] Increased intracellular sodium is accompanied by increased cell water, which may be one of the explanations for edema in kwashiorkor.[35] Hypoinsulinemia is implicated in this process.[36] These electrolyte changes are the basis for the recommendations of dietary restriction of sodium, the use of low-sodium oral rehydration solutions (ORSs), and potassium supplementation in all severely malnourished children.

Hypophosphatemia has been shown to occur in malnourished children and is associated with high mortality. In a South African study, 10 of 60 patients died, all but one with very low serum phosphate.[37] The lowest levels of serum phosphate were associated with diarrhea and dehydration. A more recent study from Malawi supports the association of hypophosphatemia and increased mortality.[38] However, it is difficult to distinguish the effects of low phosphate from hypokalemia, which also causes hypotonia and sudden death. In Jamaica, serum phosphate levels were generally higher than those recorded in Africa and although these correlated with edema, hypophosphatemia was not associated with mortality. Repletion, even on a milk diet, took 2 to 3 weeks.[39] In India, severe hypophosphatemia was not observed.[40]

Interaction with Infection

Infection and nutrition are mutually interlocked in a vicious cycle that operates at many levels, from social cultural interrelations to intracellular metabolism. Environmental conditions that give rise to inadequate energy and protein intakes are also associated with conditions in which bacterial and other microbial contamination is often rife.[41] In addition, in famine or poverty, children's diets tend to consist largely of carbohydrate staples with little or no animal products or fat.[42] Animal products such as red meat, poultry, offal, fish, milk, and eggs are important bioavailable sources of minerals and other micronutrients that have an essential role in combating infections.[43] Fat, needed to provide essential fatty acid (EFA) and facilitate the absorption of fat-soluble vitamins such as E, D, and A, which also protect against infections, is also often low in these diets.

During infection, there are metabolic changes that concentrate body energy resources on production of acute phase proteins in the liver and are often the opposite of those seen in starvation.[44] The production of acute-phase proteins and the metabolic consequences of infection are mediated by protein cytokines, lipid-derived factors that include prostaglandins, leukotrienes, and platelet activation factor. Endocrine changes also play a role; the concentration of catabolic hormones such as glucocorticoids, glucagons, and epinephrine increases. The cytokine interleukin (IL)-6 increases norepinephrine, cortisol, and glucagon and is the main stimulus for the mobilization of acute-phase proteins in the liver. Cytokines also enhance the effect of stress-related hormones on the production of acute-phase proteins.[45] Because of the interaction between food restriction and infection in the pathogenesis of malnutrition, any integrated approach to explaining the pathophysiology has to take both into account. The differences between kwashiorkor and marasmus may be partially explained by an increased shift toward the metabolic consequences of infection in children with kwashiorkor. In addition, preceding nutritional status may modify the metabolic effects of infection. An example is the increased rate of breakdown and synthesis of protein in response to infection in children with marasmus but not those with kwashiorkor[46] and the slower recovery from infectious diarrhea.

CYTOKINES

Cytokines and the Response to Infection

Because of the fundamental role of cytokines in infection and the interaction with malnutrition, a brief summary of their action is necessary. For more detail, readers are referred to more complete reviews.[45,47,48] Cytokines are small, nonstructural proteins that can be produced by nearly all nucleated cells in very small amounts, have local and systemic effects, and are involved in the primary response to infection. Synthesis of cytokines is rapidly induced in response to infection, trauma, ischemia, and other events. Cytokines are also involved in mediating the changes in protein metabolism and muscle function that accompany infections, fasting, and cancer cachexia. The family of tumor necrosis factors (TNFs), IL-1, and IL-6 are all proinflammatory cytokines. The proinflammatory cytokines mediate the local inflammatory response, which includes local heat, redness, pain, swelling, and systemic effects such as fever and anorexia. To avoid self-injury during the inflammatory response, the induction and synthesis of cytokines are controlled in a complex interactive process full of checks and balances. This tightly controlled system is disturbed in malnutrition. Clinically, children with severe malnutrition often have a reduced inflammatory reaction and blunted febrile response[49] and some studies have reported reduced levels of in vitro production of IL-1 and TNF by circulating monocytes in malnutrition.[50,51] Other studies have reported high concentrations of TNFα in the sera of non infected malnourished children[52] and Azavedo et al. report[53] high levels of TNFα production with increased sensitivity to very low concentration of LPS (the lipopolysaccharide of bacterial membranes) in children not currently infected. This study suggest that, in a similar way to well nourished children, the immune cells of marasmic children are able to mount a cytokine response involving of IL-6 and TNFα and this occurs in response to acute infection.[49] It is less clear to what extent this occurs in vivo and how to interpret these results in the context of the malnourished child's reduced acute phase response and the blunted clinical expression of the inflammatory response.

ACUTE-PHASE PROTEINS

Acute-Phase Proteins

Cytokines modulate the production of acute-phase proteins. C-reactive protein, alpha-1-antitrypsin, alpha-macroglobulin, and fibrinogen are examples of positive acute-phase proteins, so called because their synthesis by the liver increases in response to stresses, including infection.[44] Serum concentration of the so-called negative acute-phase proteins (albumin, prealbumin, fibronectin, retinol binding protein) is reduced in children with malnutrition[51,54] despite an overall net increase in hepatic protein synthesis. Low levels of fibronectin have been reported to be a useful early indicator of malnutrion.[55] Positive acute-phase proteins are an essential part of the defense against infections, but uncontrolled inflammation has been linked to adverse consequences, for instance, in inflammatory bowel disease, rheumatoid arthritis, and perhaps kwashiorkor. Studies are complicated by the coexistence of infection and malnutrition and the limitations of interpreting serum levels, which represent a balance between synthesis and catabolism. Studies in Ghana on children without sign of infection found raised concentrations of C-reactive protein in kwashiorkor and to a lesser extent in marasmus.[56] Alpha-1 acid glycoprotein levels were raised in kwashiorkor in Thai children.[54] On the other hand, Ekanem and colleagues,[57] studying children, 75% of whom had kwashiorkor, documented only slight increases in C-reactive protein in children without infection and large increases in infected children, indicating apparent preservation of the acute-phase response to infection in this population of children. This is in contrast to findings in Jamaica[58] of normal levels of C-reactive protein and serum amyloid A with a blunted response in the expected acute-phase response to diphtheria-pertussis-tetanus vaccination. Elegant studies in Jamaica and in Malawi using stable isotope labelled leucine, in marasmatic children, with infections showed that that there was an increase in some acute phase proteins (C-reactive protein, haptoglobin, alpha-1 acid glycoprotein, and alpha 1 antitrypsin) in response to infection but this response was attenuated despite preservation of the cytokine response. The increase in plasma levels of acute-phase proteins was attributable to a reduction in catabolism rather than an increase in synthesis of the proteins, in contrast to the situation in normally nourished infected children.[59] Plasma fibrinogen, which is normally increased in response to infection, showed no response in these children. A recent study from Malawi[60] suggests that the reduced acute phase protein response might be modulated by the protein content of the diet. A diet with higher protein from egg white and additional tryptophan, the rate limiting amino acid for acute phase protein synthesis resulted in an increase in serum concentrations of six acute phase proteins. The clinical consequences of this promising advance have not yet been determined.

The consequence of a reduced inflammatory response to infections has important clinical repercussions both because the usual manifestations of infection may be absent in PEM making diagnosis difficult and because the mortality from infection is greatly increased. Further studies are needed to understand the different changes which occur in the response to infection and most importantly the way in which dietary management may counteract these changes.

Kwashiorkor

Kwashiorkor has historically been attributed to a diet lacking in protein, and the edema was thought to be explained by low albumin. In consequence, children were treated with high-protein diets. However, several observations cast doubt on this hypothesis.[61] Kwashiorkor often follows infections such as measles and dysentery and has been reported in breast-fed babies, who presumably are ensured adequate protein intake, and children in the same community on very similar diets may develop kwashiorkor or marasmus. Edema has been shown to improve independently of albumin.[62] Golden demonstrated that recovery was possible with relatively low-protein diets and was dependent on energy intake and not protein.[63] It seems unlikely that simple protein deficiency is the cause of kwashiorkor.

Free Radicals

Excess free radical production has been suggested as the fundamental explanation of the clinical findings in kwashiorkor.[64] The acute inflammatory cells that form the first line of defense against infections respond with a respiratory burst during which free radicals are produced. This response to infection or cell injury relies on these free radicals for the destruction of bacteria. The free radicals are characterized by one or more unpaired electrons, which makes them highly reactive and unstable.[65] Reactive oxygen species include oxygen radicals such as singlet oxygen and nonradicals such as hydrogen peroxide; reactive nitrogen species include nitric oxide. The most potent free radicals include the hydroxyl radical and iron free radicals, which occur when unbound iron is present during free radical production. Free radicals are produced in normal metabolism, and a certain level of these radicals is required for normal functioning. However, this amount is kept to a minimum by a number of scavenging mechanisms, which detoxify the radicals. Free radical production is increased by stresses, which include inflammation, infections, and environmental stresses.[66] Oxidative stress is a process in which the normal balance between prooxidants and antioxidants is shifted toward the oxidant side, resulting in an increase in free radicals that cause biologic damage.[67] Increased oxidative stress has been demonstrated in kwashiorkor.[68] The damage caused by free radicals includes disrupting enzymes and nucleic acids and the peroxidation of lipoproteins and EFAs in cell membranes by hydrogen peroxide. Dietary antioxidants protect from oxidant damage either directly by scavenging free radicals or because they are required for enzymes, which neutralize free radicals such as superoxide dismutase (copper, zinc dependent) or glutathione peroxidase (selenium dependent) and catalase. Many studies show low concentrations of antioxidants in the serum and red cells of children with malnutrition, especially kwashiorkor.[68–70] Blood cell concentrations of glutathione, vitamin E, and the vitamin E to cholesterol ratio are reduced,[52] resulting in diminished resistance to oxidative stress. The hypothesis proposes that the balance between production and quenching of free radicals is perturbed in kwashiorkor, resulting in oxidative stress. This is attributable to low levels of dietary antioxidants, with possibly increased free radicals as a consequence of the disturbance in the acute-phase response to infections and other environmental stresses. However, a recent placebo controlled trial designed to test the dietary antioxidant deficiency hypothesis gave daily supplementation of an antioxidant mixture of riboflavin, vitamin E, selenium and N-acetylcysteine for 20 weeks to children in Malawi but failed to prevent the occurrence of kwashiorkor.[71] Essential fatty acids were not included in the supplement.

Lipid Metabolism, Polyunsaturated Fatty Acids, and Free Radicals

Recent research investigating the role of lipids in malnutrition lends support to the theory of oxidant stress as a cause of kwashiorkor. It has long been known that there are changes in the lipid profile of red cell membranes and plasma in malnutrition.[72–74] Recent interest has focused on these EFAs and their metabolites as these have protean functions, which include maintaining the integrity of cell membranes and involvement in the synthesis of immunologically active elements such as prostaglandins and leukotrienes.[75] A low proportion of arachidonic acid, one of the EFAs, in the lipid profile of cell membranes and low concentrations in the plasma of children with severe malnutrition have been reported.[76] These changes in EFAs are not owing to dietary deficiency alone and are more likely a result of shifts in the metabolism of these EFAs. In particular, desaturation, which is subject to endocrine influence, is reduced, and low desaturase activity has been reported in PEM.[77] There may also be peroxidative degradation of EFAs in cell membranes. Levels of antioxidants are consistently reduced in PEM, and this increases the peroxidation of membrane long-chain polyunsaturated fatty acids (PUFAs).[78,79]

Leukotrienes are a family of mediators involved in the inflammatory response. The EFA arachidonic acid mentioned above is a precursor of the leukotrienes. Glutathione is also needed for the synthesis of leukotrienes from arachidonic acids, and several studies have documented low levels of whole-blood glutathione and low urinary excretion in kwashiorkor and marasmus patients,[70,80,81] suggesting that synthesis of the leukotrienes might be compromised in severe malnutrition. However, it seems that different leukotrienes are affected in different ways because concentrations of the cysteinyl leukotrienes LTE4 and LTC4, which mediate vascular damage and edema, have been found to be increased in the red cells of children with kwashiorkor but not marasmus, whereas LTB4, which stimulates chemotaxis, was much reduced.[82] Cysteine supplementation improved the erythrocyte synthesis rate in children with kwashiorkor.[83]

The changes in sodium and potassium fluxes across cell membranes characteristic of kwashiorkor may also be explained in this model of reduced antioxidants. In an in vitro model, red cells depleted of glutathione showed increased leakiness to sodium and potassium, mimicking the findings seen in kwashiorkor.[70] The active transport of sodium out of the cell was increased but could not compensate for the increased permeability, resulting in the low K, high Na typical of malnutrition.

In summary, much remains to be learned about the pathophysiology of kwashiorkor. At present, it seems that the syndrome results from the interplay of nutrient deprivation and infectious or environmental stresses, which leads to a disturbed balance in the normal physiologic response to these insults. The syndrome may be predisposed by a specific pattern of nutrient deficiencies, which include protein, antioxidants, trace elements, sulfur amino acids, and probably others. In kwashiorkor, there is evidence of low antioxidants and increased oxidative stress, resulting in changes of free radical damage, increased sodium/K flux across membranes, triglyceride accumulation in the liver, low albumin, changes in n-6 PUFAs, and altered leukotriene production.

The role, cause, or effect of changes in the acute-phase reaction, including the cytokine inflammatory response, remains to be elucidated.

Alternative theories to explain kwashiorkor have not been supported by more recent evidence. The postulated association with the hepatic toxin aflatoxin may be an example of one environmental trigger with a role in some geographic areas where fungal contamination of staple foods is common,[84] but this hypothesis has not been supported by absence of aflatoxins in liver samples from kwashiorkor, even in areas where aflatoxins are common.[57]

Changes in Organs and Systems in Malnutrition

In addition to the myriad cellular manifestations of PEM, widespread alterations in organ and system function occur, many of which are relevant to clinical management.

Endocrine System. Endocrine changes mediate the metabolic adaptation to starvation and have been mentioned above. These changes have important consequences on the clinical management of severely malnourished child. Pancreatic atrophy is a common finding in marasmus,[85] and the consistent findings in severe malnutrition of a reduction in serum insulin levels and impaired insulin response to a glucose load, glucagons, and arginine[12,20] explain the vulnerability of the child to delays in starting feeding and the need for frequent small feeds. Hypokalemia contributes to this effect,[86] hence the importance of potassium supplements. There is also a reduction in insulin receptor affinity.[21] These hormonal effects rapidly reverse on refeeding, with weight gain.[87]

Studies in malnutrition have generally reported raised concentrations of growth hormone on admission,[22] but these concentrations reduce in those gaining weight on dietary treatment. Cortisol concentrations rise, especially in kwashiorkor, and the circadian rhythm is abolished, but the response to adrenocorticotropic hormone is preserved.[12,88] Cortisol levels also rise with infection; 80% of children with kwashiorkor showed a rise in cortisol in response to infection compared with only 50% of those with marasmus.[12]

This reduced response in marasmus may explain why these children are so susceptible to hypoglycemia. High levels of adrenaline are reported early in hospitalization, especially in kwashiorkor.[12] Both the plasma concentration and the secretion rate of aldosterone are high.[23]

Thyroid gland function is altered in malnutrition.[89,90] During nutrition deprivation, at first thyroxine (T4) increases, but as malnutrition becomes more severe, and especially if kwashiorkor develops, total T4 decreases. There is also a decrease in thyroid binding proteins, but this does not account for all of the reduction in T4 and suggests a primary effect on synthesis.[91] Increased thyroid-stimulating hormone secretion heralds recovery.[92] There is also a reduction in deiodination of T4 to triiodothyronine (T3), resulting in reduced T3.

Immune System. Children with severe malnutrition are very susceptible to infection, especially with gram-negative organisms, and deaths are often attributable to sepsis. The subject has been extensively reviewed[93–97] and is dealt with in more detail in Chapter 23, “Malnutrition and Host Defenses.” In summary, there are profound changes in cell-mediated immunity, the complement system, and function of polymorphonuclear cells and fewer reported effects on humoral immunity.

Cell-Mediated Immunity. Cell-mediated immunity is altered in severe malnutrition.[95] The thymus, necessary for normal differentiation of T cells, is consistently reduced in size,[98] and the production of thymic hormones is reduced.[96,97] Evidence of T-cell functional impairment also comes from the observation of reduced cutaneous tests to recalled antigens, for instance, the tuberculin test[99]; however, studies differ in reports of numbers of circulating T cells and the ratio and effect on T-cell subsets. In general, it appears that T4 cells are relatively reduced, and T8 cells are affected to a lesser degree. At the gastrointestinal level, atrophy of gut-associated lymphoid aggregates as a prominent feature of malnutrition has been reported.[100]

Humoral Immunity. Immune globulin production by B cells has been reported to be normal or raised,[95] and immunoglobulin (Ig)G seroconversion in response to several vaccines is preserved.[101] Increased IgA has been reported, but there was a reduced response of secretory IgA in nasopharyngeal secretions to measles vaccine,[102] and children with severe malnutrition in Brazil were found to have lower secretory IgA in urine, which increased on rehabilitation.[103] The complement system shows consistent abnormalities with decreased C3 level.[104,105] This seems to be related to protein metabolism.[56] Some studies report particularly low concentrations of C3 in kwashiorkor. However, Ekanem and colleagues found that C3 levels, although low, rose significantly in the presence of infection.[57] C4 levels seem to be increased or unaffected by nutritional status. Other potentially important disturbances in the immune system include impaired phagocytic activity by polymorphonuclear cells.[94] The consequence of these various effects is a reduced capacity of the malnourished child to respond to and combat infections, leading to an increased risk of sepsis, one of the main reasons for mortality in malnourished children.

Liver. In the liver, there is a shift from the production of carrier proteins and a relative increase in the production of acute inflammatory proteins, indices of response to injury or infection. This is particularly marked in kwashiorkor. The liver in kwashiorkor is often enlarged and shows a fatty infiltrate owing to accumulation of triglycerides.[106,107] These changes improve on clinical recovery, and there is no evidence that kwashiorkor per se results in long-term liver damage or cirrhosis.[108]

Cardiac System. Cardiac output is reduced in children with acute PEM compared with cardiac output on recovery.[17] Cardiac muscle, however, shows only nonspecific changes, and muscle contractility is normal. Sinus bradycardia may be present, as well as mild hypotension. Concomitant deficiencies such as hypokalemia, anemia, and vitamin deficiencies may affect the heart. Pericardial effusion may be present in edematous malnutrition. During recovery, the heart size increases rapidly owing to chamber enlargement, and left ventricle musculature increases in proportion to increasing weight.[109] However, if dietary repletion is rapid, especially if there is also a high sodium load, heart failure may develop and sudden death occur. Prompt action to reduce hyperalimentation, restrict sodium intake, and administer diuretics can reverse the heart failure, but because this condition may not be recognized or is confused with sepsis, this complication is responsible for unnecessary deaths. This cardiac pathology is not considered primary to the heart but is more probably part of the refeeding syndrome described later.[17,109]

Respiratory System. The reduction in muscle mass that occurs in severe malnutrition affects respiratory muscle, including the diaphragm; this leads to reduced muscular function, which influences vital capacity and maximal inspiration and inspiratory pressures.[110] This weakness may be exacerbated by electrolyte abnormalities such as low phosphate[111] and hypokalemia. The ventilatory response to hypoxia is blunted, but not the response to hypercapnia.[112] Despite these alterations, tachypnea and subcostal retraction remain useful signs in diagnosing pneumonia in malnutrition.[113]

Gastrointestinal Tract. Diarrhea and malnutrition often occur together. Malnutrition increases the risk of more prolonged episodes of diarrhea,[114] and the combination of persistent diarrhea (more than 14 days of diarrhea) and malnutrition carries an especially high mortality.[115] Diarrhea and malnutrition so often coexist that it is difficult to determine the extent to which each contributes to pathology. Nevertheless, both animal and human studies suggest that severe malnutrition per se affects the intestinal tract with reduced gastric acid production, thinning of the small intestinal mucosa, and flattening or disappearance of the villi with relative sparing of the crypts.[17,116] There is increased cellularity of the lamina propria, especially in children with kwashiorkor.[116] These anatomic changes are reflected in impaired mucosal function, increased permeability as demonstrated by the double sugar technique,[117,118] and malabsorption as shown by nutrient absorption studies.[119] The mucosa seems to be particularly affected in kwashiorkor. In children with PEM in Malawi, kwashiorkor was associated with abnormal intestinal permeability results, and persistent diarrhea was not an independent risk factor for altered permeability.[118] Loss of the villous architecture of the small intestine for any reason reduces disaccharide activity because the disaccharides, especially lactase, are found at the villous tips. Thus, lactose malabsorption is a common finding in PEM.[120]

Fat malabsorption is also seen in both persistent diarrhea[121] and PEM.[122] As well as the mucosal changes, bacterial overgrowth in the upper small intestine has been described in PEM and may lead to bile salt deconjugation, further impairing fat absorption.[123]

On the other hand, the human intestine has a remarkable reserve capacity, and the clinical consequences of the demonstrated pathology need to be put into context. In the first place, the intestinal mucosa receives nutrients directly from the lumen, and enteral feeding is necessary for recuperation of intestinal health. We now know that even the damaged intestine benefits from food. Even in the face of malabsorption, diets can be designed to capitalize on remaining function. Carbohydrates are well absorbed in the small intestine until disaccharidase capacity is overwhelmed, at which point, the unabsorbed sugars cause osmotic diarrhea and the risk of dehydration. Presenting a mixture of different carbohydrates in small frequent feeds in presentations with relatively slow gastric emptying, such as milk, allows even lactose to be tolerated. Studies in children with persistent diarrhea, many of whom were malnourished, demonstrated that locally prepared diets with less than 3 g/kg body wt/d as lactose were well tolerated and led to prompt recovery.[124] In contrast to carbohydrate, fractional fat absorption remains constant over a wide range of intake,[125] so more fat in the diet results in more fat absorbed, and in practice, the increased fat loss is of little clinical consequence.[122] This is of considerable practical importance because the high energy density of fat means that more calories can be given in smaller volume, which is essential when feeding PEM children, who are usually anorexic. Although we lack randomized clinical controlled trials of early feeding in PEM, such as those that provided conclusive evidence for continued feeding in acute diarrhea,[126] cumulated experience demonstrates the success of this strategy. Early initiation of oral feeding was one of the major management changes associated with the introduction of a specific protocol for PEM in Bangladesh that halved mortality. Specifically, deaths from hypoglycemia were reduced.[6] Further aspects of gut function are discussed in Chapter 22, "Immunophysiology and Nutrition of the Gut."

Hematology: Anemia. Anemia is common in severe malnutrition and may be attributable either to iron deficiency and/or reduced red cell production in adaptation to a smaller lean body mass.[127] Despite the fact that most children will have been consuming a diet deficient in bioavailable iron, in kwashiorkor, there is elevated hepatic iron, and bone marrow iron shows stainable iron in half of children. This is an unusual finding in marasmus.[128] Iron is tightly bound to proteins during storage and transport to prevent free iron forming the extremely damaging hydroxyl radical. In kwashiorkor, the reduced plasma levels of transferrin mean that iron binding capacity is reduced and the concentration of free iron may increase.[129] Low serum transferrin has been associated with an increased risk of mortality in hospitalized children with PEM.[130,131] It has been suggested that free iron causes or contributes to the etiology of kwashiorkor,[131,132] although not all children with kwashiorkor have raised indices of free iron. Children with PEM absorb oral iron and this is the preferred route.[133] The homeostatic control of intestinal iron absorption is maintained in children with kwashiorkor and those with high serum ferritin and high percent saturation of transferrin absorb less oral iron than those with low serum ferritins.[134] The iron issue is important not only because of its possible role in the etiology of kwashiorkor but also because iron supplements might actually increase mortality in acute PEM. Smith and colleagues, in a small nonrandomized study in Nigeria, found higher mortality; 10 of 31 children given iron supplements at admission of day 3 died compared with 2 of 12 nonsupplemented children.[135] Whatever the role of iron supplements during the acute phase of malnutrition, during recovery, with its accompanying increase in lean body and red cell mass, iron is required, and stores are quickly exhausted so that classic iron deficiency features occur.[136] Iron supplements should be given during this stage.

Little is known about the relative role of other micronutrient deficiencies in contributing to the anemia of malnutrition. In studies in South Africa and Egypt, there was no evidence of vitamin B_{12} deficiency, but serum folic acid levels were low.[137,138] In Cairo, low serum folate levels correlated with megaloblastic findings on bone marrow and with improvement in these parameters following treatment with injected folic acid, but in South Africa, serum folate was unrelated to hemoglobin levels, which improved without folic acid supplements. Copper, riboflavin, and vitamin E deficiencies may contribute to the anemia of PEM. Nutritional anemias are reviewed in chapter.[62]

Skin, Hair, and Teeth. In marasmus, the dry wrinkled loose skin is a result of almost total loss of subcutaneous fat. This leads to a relative increase in surface area, reduced protection from ambient temperature, and therefore increased susceptibility to hypothermia. Hair is thin, grows slowly, and falls out readily, and on microscopy, there is a lack of hair root bulbs and a shift to the resting state of hair growth.[139] In kwashiorkor, skin changes may be florid and show the characteristic signs described earlier, or they may be absent. Some changes are similar to those seen in acrodermatitis enteropathica,[140] and improvement may occur with zinc ointments, suggesting that concomitant zinc deficiency may be implicated.[141] Other nutrient deficiencies, such as EFA deficiency, the B vitamins, and amino acid deficiencies, also cause skin changes and may contribute. Hair is also affected; depigmentation is a classic sign. Hair follicles show fewer and abnormal growing bulbs, showing atrophy and shaft constriction with depletion of pigment.[139]

Even a single episode of prolonged malnutrition in the first year of life delays primary dentition and is associated with higher prevalence of primary dentition caries and possibly also permanent dentition caries.[142,143]

Brain Function and Development. Most child malnutrition occurs at a time of rapid development, so any insult at this time may have far-reaching consequences. In addition to primary effects on neuronal tissue, there may be secondary effects owing to anemia, micronutrient deficiencies, apathy, and reduced activity. The environment in which most malnourished children live often fails to provide the stimulation and support that the developing child needs to realize his or her potential. The clinically recovered child usually returns to this same environment, thus making it difficult to determine the impact of malnutrition per se on longterm development. Early studies comparing the outcome of children recovered from severe malnutrition who either returned home or were adopted into families with more resources suggested that environmental influences outweighed the sequelae of the malnutrition.[144] The randomized trials conducted by Grantham-McGregor in Jamaica and others have contributed greatly to our understanding of the importance of stimulation as well as dietary therapy in reversing developmental delay.[145,146] This important subject is further addressed in Chapter 24, "Neuropsychological Development."

Bones. Children with severe malnutrition often remain stunted after recovery. Branca and colleagues used pyridinoline and deoxypyridinoline, cross-linking amino acids of collagen that are excreted in the urine in proportion to skeletal turnover, to study bone turnover in severe malnutrition.[147] They found low rates of bone turnover during the acute phase of malnutrition and much higher levels during recovery. Age, severity of wasting on admission, and crosslink excretion accounted for 44% of the variability in height velocity during recovery.[147–149] Bone demineralization has also been reported and may be attributable to phosphate deficiency.[150] Bone changes typical of copper deficiency may also be present as well as scurvy caused by vitamin C

Table 2 Factors to Consider when Admitting Children with Protein-Energy Malnutrition

Child factors	
Severity of the malnutrition	The more severe the malnutrition, the greater the need for specialized refeeding, monitoring, and intervention to treat complications such as infection, electrolyte abnormalities, hypothermia, and hypoglycemia.
Edema	Children with edematous malnutrition may not appear to be ill and do not induce the same shock horror response as a child with marasmus. Their edematous weight masks the severity of their condition.
Presence of infection	Malnourished children should be regarded as immunodeficient so that infections are more likely to need parenteral antibiotic treatment and close monitoring, which is difficult to do at home. Persistent diarrhea may present special problems and usually quickly improves with a clean diet and appropriate therapy in hospital.[119]
Presence of other conditions	Malnutrition is not always a consequence of primary energy and protein deprivation. The presence of other conditions such as congenital heart disease, cystic fibrosis, and tuberculosis may determine where these children will be best managed. Therapeutic malnutrition units may not be best able to cope with these pediatric emergencies.
Family circumstances	
Social circumstances	The ability of carers to follow treatment schedules at home, who looks after the child, conflicting work and other family constraints on outpatient attendance, nearness to health facilities, availability of backup services and nutritional support in the community are all factors to be taken into consideration.
Previous treatment	Previous attempts at treatment should be taken into account. A child who is worsening despite being in an outpatient or community care program should not have to wait to reach a specific degree of severity to be admitted once the alternatives have failed.
Home social circumstances	These include the nearness to health facilities able to deal with emergencies or monitor the child and the presence of community support with or without food supplements. Children treated in well-organized programs may avoid hospitalization, although there needs to be provision for those who deteriorate, and this may occur suddenly and catastrophically.
Economic considerations	Inevitably, economic considerations will influence decisions and sadly often are the deciding factor, although not in the interest of the child. However, it is very important that health professionals do not add to financial burden with unnecessary tests that do not change management or expensive versions of medicines or medicines of no proven efficacy that compete in the household budget for the food that the child needs or dissuade parents from seeking help for their children.
Hospital facilities	
Infection risk	Children with severe malnutrition are vulnerable. If admission to hospital means being on a general ward with children with measles and diarrhea, then they may be safer at home, despite the severity of their condition. Obviously, the best option is to provide isolation facilities and hand washing, but this may not always be the case in practice.
Feeding arrangements	Children with malnutrition require frequent feeding. Emergency departments may not have provisions for feeding; even on the ward, provision of food may depend on parents, and this may present an additional complication for caretakers if their time is split between home and hospital. Families may have to buy or prepare the food for their child.

deficiency. Vitamin D deficiency which causes rickets and osteomalacia, deserves special mention. Once a common condition, rickets almost disappeared with the widespread consumption of vitamin D fortified milk, but it is now being reported more frequently and subclinical vitamin D deficiency is thought to be common,[151] and Vitamin D is known to be essential for B and T cell function,[152] especially phagocytosis.[153] Children with rickets are at greater risk of pneumonia[154] and recent studies have shown an association between asymptomatic low concentrations of serum 25-hydroxyvitamin D3 (25OHD3) and lower respiratory tract infections.[155] Low concentrations of 25OHD3 have also reported to increase risk of tuberculosis especially in those with certain polymorphisms of the Vitamin D receptor.[156] In addition there is evidence that vitamin D deficiency in childhood is associated with increased risk of chronic diseases such as type 1 diabetes and some cancers in adults.[151] Although little studied, malnourished children may be at increased risk of vitamin D deficiency because of low dietary calcium and vitamin D intakes, including insufficient vitamin D in breastmilk, low dietary fat and perhaps less sun exposure if they are frequently ill and more likely to be indoors.

Clinical Management

Treatment regimens for the clinical management of severe malnutrition have been developed by a limited number of specialist centers across the world. These regimens tend to be experience rather than evidence based, and there is a need for clinical trials to clarify many different management issues. Nevertheless, the WHO, in consultation with experts from many parts of the world, has formulated recommendations, and this clear, didactic protocol is now available for centers wherever malnourished children are treated.[11] The following discussion of management adheres in general to the WHO guidelines.

Clinical Assessment and Triage

When malnourished children first present, health personnel are usually faced with a question about whether hospitalization is advisable. This is often a tricky decision and deserves some discussion. Risk factors for mortality in a series of studies include severity of malnutrition, young age, pneumonia, severe diarrhea (more than six stools a day, dehydration),signs of sepsis, hypothermia, fever, and electrolyte abnormalities.[157–159] Children with these risk factors should be admitted urgently. Table 2 lists factors to be taken into consideration when deciding on admission.

Hospital Versus Community Rehabilitation

Hospitalization is usually required for the severely ill child with PEM, but once the acute conditions have been treated, other alternatives include rehabilitation centers or community care. Increasingly community care is being shown to be feasible especially when ready to use therapeutic food which provides high calorie density with essential micronutrients in a convenient low contamination preparation is available.[160] The importance of local support and intensive nutrition education was demonstrated in a study in Bangladesh where community nutrition promotors working within an intergrated nutrition project were able to rehabilitate children with moderate malnutrition even without food supplements.[161]

Phases of Treatment

The child admitted with PEM should be treated according to a locally developed protocol based on the WHO guidelines. The use of such protocols has been shown to reduce mortality.[6] The management of malnutrition is a team activity, and all staff who come into contact with the child or the child's caretaker in any way should be aware of the management plan.

Treatment can be divided into three phases:

1. The initial or acute phase (2 to 10 days) when the child is being treated for complications such as dehydration, hypoglycemia, and infections. Dietary therapy starts.
2. The second phase of recovery or rehabilitation (2 to 6 weeks) when the child will increase dietary intake and gain weight.
3. The follow-up phase (6 to 26 weeks), which may be after discharge.

Phase 1: Examination and Emergency Treatment. A full clinical history should be obtained; symptoms suggestive of infection and diarrhea are particularly relevant. Birth history is important because low birth weight may explain the infant's low weight, and it is essential to review any growth data that may be available. A developmental history and past medical problems may reveal concomitant conditions that cause or contribute to the malnutrition. Most children will have been chronically ill, and information on medication and therapies, including traditional healers, may be relevant. It will be essential to have information on the child's diet history, including breast-feeding, family diet, food constraints, and access to food programs, as well as a full social and family history, but this information may be better obtained once the acute phase is completed and is part of building up a relationship with the family. A detailed clinical examination is essential, but care should be taken not to stress the patient and to protect him or her from cold. Table 3 shows some signs and symptoms of particular importance and their management.

Management of Diarrhea and Dehydration. The principles of management, rehydration, and continued feeding are no different in the malnourished child. (See Chapter 57, "Diarrheal Diseases"). Signs of dehydration and their management are shown in Table 4. Particular attention has to be paid to the volume of fluid given and electrolyte management.

Most children with dehydration can be managed with oral rehydration therapy. In moderate dehydration (WHO plan B), 70 to 100 mL/kg of ORS should be given over 8 to 12 hours, starting frequently (5 mL/kg every 30 minutes). Lower osmolarity ORS has been shown to give better results than the old standard ORS[165] although if available ReSoMal is the recommended option (Table 5) as it contains additional minerals. However only one clinical trial has evaluated ReSoMal. ReSoMal was compared with standard WHO formula ORS. ReSoMal resulted in less hypokalemia but was associated with severe hyponatremia especially in children with high purging rates.[166] In such children, for instance those with cholera, standard WHO ORS with added potassium should be used. The child's clinical state should be monitored at least hourly. If vomiting occurs, then rehydration can be detained 30 to 60 minutes and then resumed. If the child refuses to drink or becomes very tired by the effort of drinking, a nasogastric tube should be used. If the child drinks avidly, then only small amounts should be offered by spoon, never by bottle, as taking a large amount at a time may provoke vomiting. If the child does not show signs of recovery (improved general condition, passing urine), consider sepsis. If diarrhea is ongoing, estimate diarrhea losses and increase the rehydration fluid volume accordingly. A diarrheal stool in a child less than 2 years can be estimated as 50 to 100 mL and 100 to 200 mL in an older child or in very severe diarrhea. Once the child has clinically recovered and signs of dehydration have improved, the child can be started on diet, even though the programmed amount of ORS has not yet been completed or diarrhea continues. Alternate ORS and diet.

Intravenous Therapy. Intravenous infusions should be avoided as far as possible. If unavoidable, for instance in shock, the volume of intravenous therapy should be kept to a minimum, and particular attention should be paid to protecting the site of intravenous access from infection. If antibiotics are to be given intravenously, a heparinized cannula, rather than a continuous infusion, is safer to avoid fluid overload. It may be difficult to establish venous access in malnourished children, especially those with edema, but prolonged attempts and "cut-downs" performed without anesthesia and with little attention to sterility place the malnourished child at risk of hypoglycemia, hypothermia, sepsis, and stress, which increase mortality. Sometimes an intravenous line is started because it is a "routine in all sick children" or "in case it is needed later." Such practices should be avoided in children with PEM. The only absolute indications are circulatory collapse caused by severe dehydration or septic shock. In this case, solutions with low sodium, such as half-strength Darrow's solution, Ringer's lactate, or half-normal 0.45% saline, all with 5% glucose, should be used. Potassium chloride should be added to provide 20 mmol/L, infused at 15 mL/kg/h, preferably using a programmable pump. The child's hydration status, pulse, and respiratory rate should be reviewed at least hourly. If the child was dehydrated, improvement should be obvious; if not, septic shock is likely, and parenteral antibiotics should be started, if not already given, and blood transfusion considered. If blood is not available, plasma is an alternative. Transfusion should be given slowly (10 mg/kg over 3 hours) with close monitoring of jugular veins and respiration rate as malnourished children are at high risk of congestive heart failure. Diuretics such as furosemide 1 mg/kg may be given if there is any suggestion of heart failure.

Parasites and Gut Flora. Parasites should be treated if identified in the stools. If *Giardia* lamblia is present, metronidazole is recommended. A lower than usual dose, metronidazole 12.0 mg/kg/d, has been suggested on the basis of pharmacokinetic studies.[167] Bacterial contamination of the small intestine has been described in children with PEM, but the functional significance of this is not clear.[168] Children admitted to the hospital from highly contaminated home environments were found to have bacterial contamination of duodenal fluid regardless of nutritional or diarrheal status.[169] The bacterial flora reduced within days of eating a clean diet and without antibiotic therapy.[121] The need to treat all children with PEM for bacterial overgrowth remains controversial, and randomized controlled trials are needed.

General Care of the Malnourished Child. Sadly, the mortality rate for children hospitalized for severe malnutrition is often high,[9,170–173] and some of these deaths are a consequence of hospital practices, such as long waits without food, indiscriminate use of intravenous fluids, and the dangers of admission to a high-risk environment. Adoption of recommended guidelines and the use of protocols that facilitate a team approach have resulted in spectacular reductions in mortality rates.[6] An important aspect of these improvements is the organization of services with a view to preventing complications. Early deaths, within the first day, are often attributable to hypoglycemia and/or failure to recognize and treat infections adequately. Later deaths may be owing to overwhelming infections, but sudden unexpected deaths after a few days may be caused by cardiac failure associated with the refeeding syndrome.

Prevention of Hypoglycemia. It is important to give thought to how to prevent hypoglycemia. Travel to the hospital and waits to be seen in the emergency or outpatient department can place the child at risk, and this may be exacerbated by hospital policies such as "nil by mouth" until the child is reviewed and reluctance to start any "treatment" until experts are consulted or test results are available. Mothers should be encouraged to breast-feed their babies while waiting, and a triage system that quickly identifies children with severe malnutrition and directs them into a protocol providing immediate feeding will reduce the risk of hypoglycemia and the attendant mortality. Frequent feeds every 2 to 4 hours are needed at first.

Nighttime, when staffing levels are reduced, often provides a challenge, and health facilities should have a plan to cope with this. This might involve having prepared diets or ingredients always available in the emergency department or on the ward and using nasogastric tube feeds if staff or family is not available for the time-consuming process of encouraging the malnourished child to eat frequent feeds. Monitoring is very important. If the mother is accompanying the child, she should have access to refreshments; otherwise, she may be tempted to share the child's ration.

Prevention of Hypothermia. Children with PEM, especially those with marasmus, have less insulating fat and a relatively large surface area, so that body temperature tends to reflect ambient temperature, and they are very vulnerable to hypothermia.[174,175] Prevention requires planning to avoid having the child unclothed for long periods, for instance, while having radiographs or during medical examination, and providing an ambient temperature that is warm, 25° to 30°C, and without draughts. Washing should be kept to a minimum, and the child should be dried and wrapped immediately. At night, temperatures often fall, so additional precautions may be necessary.

Dietary Management. Dietary therapy must be started rapidly, and is best accomplished with a protocol. The health care professional should specify dietary therapy when the child is first seen. The exact diet to be used will

Table 3 Identification and Management of Complications of Protein-Energy Malnutrition

Sign or Symptom	Findings	Management
Edema	Usually symmetric and positional; pretibial edema may be evident only on pressing on the shin with a finger and looking for the indentation. The presence of edema also means that gross weight underestimates the child's degree of malnutrition.	Edema indicates kwashiorkor and is an indication of severity. Dietary guidelines for kwashiorkor should be applied.
Odd facies, palmar creases, heart murmurs, cyanosis, signs of congenital abnormalities	Chromosomal and congenital disorders may contribute to malnutrition.	These children should receive the same treatment for their malnutrition, but concomitant conditions will affect outcome and long-term management. .
Developmental assessment	An adequate developmental assessment is not possible in a sick or malnourished child, but signs such as increased tone and contractures may point to cerebral palsy and degenerative neurologic disorders may be discernable.	Stimulation is important to recovery of malnourished children. Gentle massage and talking to the child should be encouraged from admission.
Infection	Malnourished children may not mount a full-blown inflammatory response to infection, so signs may be attenuated and diagnostic tests misleading. The febrile response is reduced.[162]	WHO recommends starting all children with severe malnutrition on a broad-spectrum antibiotic such as cotromoxazole (sulfamethoxazole 20 mg plus trimethoprim 4 mg)/kg 2 × daily even in the absence of signs of infection.
Sepsis	Difficult to distinguish from dehydration. Recent apathy, reduced level of consciousness, jaundice, abdominal distention (babies), fever or hypothermia, hypoglycemia, petechiae, and poor peripheral perfusion are all indicators of possible sepsis.	If there is any doubt, the child should be treated as septic and intravenous antibiotics used. These should be broad- spectrum and cover gram-negative bacteria. Combinations of aminoglycosides such as gentamicin (7.5 mg/kg IM daily) with ampicillin (50 mg/kg 6 hourly) or amoxicillin or third-generation cephalosporins such as ceftriaxone are recommended.
Focal infections	Pneumonia is very common,[163] but cough may be absent. Tachypnea and subcostal recession are preserved. In otitis media, the tympanum may not appear red, and infections may present with perforation and otic discharge. Urine should be examined for urinary tract infections, but false positives owing to dehydration mean that it is better to obtain nonurgent samples after rehydration. The skin should be carefully examined all over.	Infections should be treated as in well-nourished children, using appropriate antibiotics preferably based on local sensitivity patterns. Because of the depressed immunity, disturbed gut function, which might reduce absorption of oral preparations,[164] and limited muscle bulk for frequent intramuscular injection, intravenous antibiotics should be used for all serious infections.
HIV/AIDs	In many parts of the world, a large proportion of children presenting with severe malnutrition will have HIV/AIDS.	The same management principles apply and the malnutrition should be treated actively. Improving the malnutrition will improve the child's quality of life.
Tuberculosis	Clinical manifestations may be absent. Radiographic changes may be seen only when the child starts to recover from malnutrition. Tuberculin skin tests are usually negative.[99] A positive family history should be sought.	Tuberculosis therapy should be started once tracheal aspirate or gastric cultures have been collected. A trial of therapy is sometimes needed in children in whom there is a suspicion of tuberculosis.
Diarrhea and dehydration	Diarrhea is common, and signs of dehydration should be sought (see Table 4).	Diarrhea is not a contraindication to starting diet. Dehydration should be managed as indicated below.
Electrolyte disorders	All malnourished children should be considered to have sodium retention and potassium depletion. Measurement of serum electrolytes is useful to guide management, but low serum sodium is not an indication for administering sodium. Children with kwashiorkor may urinate infrequently and in small volume; neither this nor normal serum potassium should deter the administration of potassium supplements. Hypotonia may be a manifestation of hypokalemia.	Severely malnourished children are best managed with relatively low sodium oral rehydration solutions. The old standard WHO oral rehydration solution (90 mmol sodium) is not recommended. A solution with 60 mmol sodium was found to be superior and to speed recovery.[165] WHO recommends ReSoMal (see Table 5), but if not available, the new standard 75 mmol oral rehydration solution could be used. Potassium at 40 mmol/L is recommended. Treatment schedules are given below.
Hypoglycemia	Blood sugar <54 mg/dL or 3 mmol/L. Floppiness, unresponsiveness, hypothermia, convulsions, and coma are signs of hypoglycemia. If the child is convulsing, hypoglycemia should be assumed and treatment started empirically even before procedures such as lumbar puncture to exclude meningitis.	If the child is conscious, oral glucose (50 mL of 10% solution) may be given, by nasogastric tube if necessary. Follow with milk or diet as soon as possible. If in coma, an intravenous infusion of 10% glucose (5 mL/kg) should be given and followed by oral glucose or diet. Children with hypoglycemia should be considered septic and treated with antibiotics.
Hypothermia	Rectal temperature is more accurate, and, ideally, a low reading thermometer should be available. Rectal temperature <35.5°C is diagnostic. Axillary temperature, <35°C is suggestive.	The child should be warmed gradually either by wrapping in blankets, warming the room, or using the skin to skin kangaroo technique. If the child is hypothermic, assume sepsis.
Anemia	Malnourished children are often anemic, but in nonmalarial areas, severe anemia, <8 g/dL, should not be assumed owing to nutritional deficiency, and other reasons should be sought.	Intestinal parasites, especially hookworm, may be present and should be treated. Anemia is usually chronic and only needs immediate treatment if there are signs of cardiac failure or hemoglobin <5 g/dL. In this case, transfusion should be given with great care as discussed with intravenous therapy.

Table 4 Signs of Dehydration and Interpretation in Severe Malnutrition

Sign	Mild or Absent Plan A	Moderate Plan B	Severe (with shock) Plan C	Comment
Conscious level	Normal/alert	Agitated/irritable	Lethargic/ comatose	Agitation is typical. Infection and hypoglycemia also give lethargy
Eyes	Normal	Sunken	Very sunken	Ask mother about eyes
Tears	Present	Absent	Absent	Tears often absent
Buccal mucosa	Moist	Dry	Very dry	Mouth breathing may cause dryness
Skin pinch	Returns quickly	Returns slowly <2 s	Returns very slowly >2 see	More difficult in PEM
Thirst	Drinks normally	Drinks avidly	Unable to drink	If avid, useful

PEM = protein-energy malnutrition.

Table 5 Composition of Oral Rehydration Salts for Severely Malnourished Children (ReSoMal)

Component	Concentration (mmol/L)
Glucose	125
Sodium	45
Potassium	40
Chloride	70
Citrate	7
Magnesium	3
Zinc	0.3
Copper	0.045
Osmolarity	300

Adapted from reference 11.

depend on local circumstances. In some cases, it may be easiest to have infant formula available when the diet kitchen or daytime nursing is not available, even though it is too expensive to continue. When families are expected to provide food for patients, a special diet will need to be prescribed and made available until family food can take over. This might be the WHO-recommended F75 and F100 (Table 6), which have been designed and tested in malnutrition treatment centers.[11] The F75 is designed for the initial phase and F100 for the rehabilitation phase, but many centers use F100 from the start, especially in marasmic children. Alternative local diets have been used successfully; an example used at the Instituto de Investigacion Nutricional, Lima, is given in Table 7. Whatever diet is chosen, this should have an energy density of 75 to 100 kcal/100 mL, the osmolarity should be lower than 350 to 400 mOsmol/L,[170] and 6 to 12% of the calories should come from protein[176,177] and at least some of this from an animal source (milk, chicken meat, or egg). Techniques such as fermentation and the combination of complementary vegetable proteins can improve the protein quality and may add valuable vitamins.[178] Although diets based on vegetable protein have been used successfully, nitrogen retention is usually less than that seen with milk diets (Table 8).[179,180] At least 50% or more of calories can come from fat; higher fat results in higher overall energy absorption.[181] Diets should be liquid if nasogastric tube feeding is to be used; they should not thicken on standing, a problem of higher proportions of carbohydrate, and they should be palatable. Amylase rich flour has been used successfully to reduce viscocity and increase dietary intakes and acceptance in malnourished children Bangladesh,[182] Malt is an alternative. Sodium should not exceed 2 mmol/kg/d, and potassium should be added to give 5 to 7 mmol/kg/d. Additional vitamins and minerals should be added to provide one to two times the daily requirement. A local vitamin supplement can be used, but it is often harder to find a mineral source, and WHO provides a recipe for a mineral mix that can be made in a local pharmacy or biochemistry department.[11] An exciting advance is the development of ready to feed therapeutic foods high-fat solid rehabilitation diets resistant to bacterial contamination and with excellent preservation of micronutrients.[183,184]

Children should receive 80 to 100 kcal/kg/d; <80 kcal/kg is insufficient to maintain metabolic needs, and >100 kcal may put the child at risk of the refeeding syndrome discussed below. Feeds should be given every 2 to 4 hours at first. The amount actually consumed should be monitored by direct observation. Continuing or developing diarrhea does not necessarily mean that the diet should be changed. Only if diarrhea becomes worse, for instance more than six voluminous liquid stools per day, or dehydration occurs is it necessary to change to a low lactose diet with the same calorie content. Oral rehydration fluid should be given between meals to compensate for stool losses. An algorithm illustrating the dietary management in the acute phase is shown in Figure 6.

Breast-fed Children. The mothers of breast-fed children should be encouraged to nurse as breast milk continues to provide important nutritional support even through the second year of life.[42] Breast-feeding should be encouraged in the hospital whenever the child is strong enough to suck; if possible, breast milk may be extracted to add to the diet, and this may help the mother feel involved and important.

Younger exclusively breast-fed babies may occasionally present with PEM, and it is not reasonable to assume that a baby who has become severely malnourished on the breast will improve if no action is taken. These babies need additional food. Improving breast-feeding technique and relactation may be tried to increase breast milk supply once the baby is improving but are not suitable for the initial phase of management. For babies under 4 months of age, a modified cow's milk formula is the recommended food; for infants older than 4 months, a cereal milk diet can be given. The youngest babies present a problem when infant formulas are beyond the resources of parents or the hospital, but priority should be given to obtaining milk formula for babies under 4 months. Complementing with another woman's breast milk is possible only if a safe sterile supply is available.

Table 6 Preparation of F75 and F100 Diets

Ingredients	Energy 0.75 kcal/cc	1 kcal/cc
Dried skimmed milk (g)	25	80
Sugar (g)	70	50
Cereal flour (g)	35	—
Vegetable oil (g)	27	60
Mineral mix (mL)	20	20
Vitamin mix (mg)	140	140
Water to total volume (cc)	1,000	1,000

Adapted from reference 11.

Table 7 Preparation of Rice Milk Diet

Ingredients	Energy 1 kcal/cc		Household Measures for 100 cc
Full-fat dried milk (g)	76	7.6	5 heaped spoonfuls
Rice (g)	74	7.4	5 heaped spoonfuls
Vegetable oil (cc)	33	3.3	1 oz or measure with syringe
Sugar (g)	27	2.7	2 heaped spoonfuls
potassium chloride 20% solution	9	0.9	Measure with syringe
Water to total volume (cc)	1,000	100	—

Diet used at the Instituto de Investigacion Nutricional, Lima.

Table 8 Composition of Mineral Mix Solution

Substance	Amount
Potassium chloride	89.5 g
Tripotassium citrate	32.4 g
Magnesium chloride ($MgCl_2 \cdot 6\ H_2O$)	30.5 g
Zinc acetate	3.3 g
Copper sulfate	0.56 g
Sodium selenate*	10 mg
Potassium iodide*	5 mg
Water to make	1,000 mL

Adapted from reference 11.
*If it is not possible to weigh very small amounts accurately, this substance may be omitted.

Mineral and Vitamin Supplements. Micronutrient deficiencies are common in malnutrition. Regardless of signs of vitamin A deficiency, this should be assumed and retinol palmitate given orally on

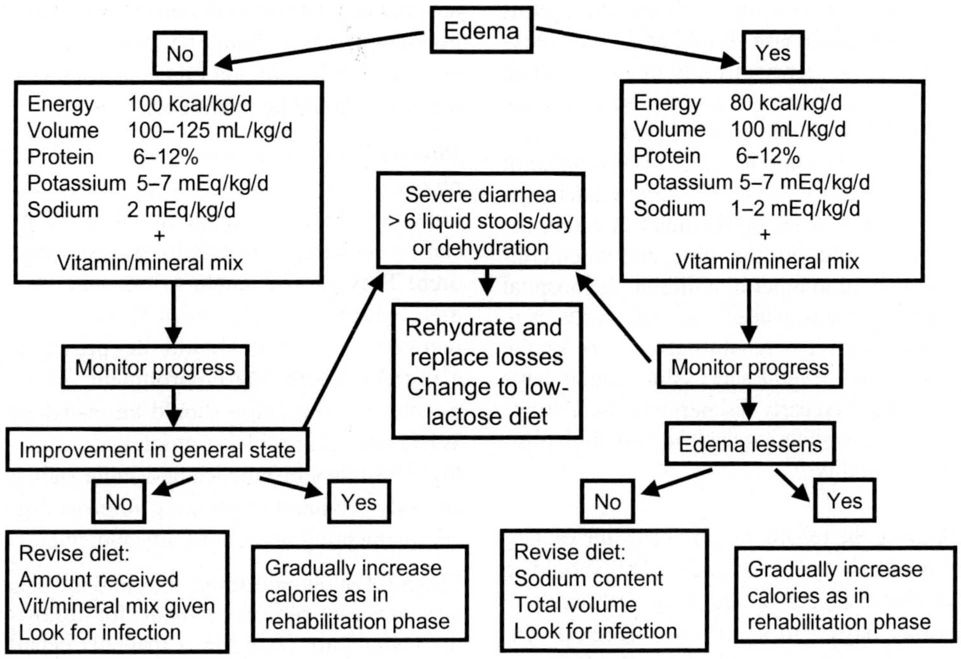

Figure 6 Phase 1: Nutritional Management.

admission, 50,000 IU for children <6 months age, 100,000 IU for children age 6 to 12 months, and 200,000 IU for older children. A repeat dose should be given the next day and a third dose after 2 weeks or on discharge, whichever is sooner. A single oral dose of 5 mg folic acid on admission is recommended followed by 1 mg daily. Other vitamins and minerals are best given with the diet or as a daily supplement during recovery.

Zinc supplementation of malnourished children has been shown to improve weight gain[185,186] and improve immunologic outcomes, and 1 mL/kg/d of a 1.5% zinc acetate solution daily is recommended. Care should be taken not to provide too much zinc as mortality was increased in Bangladeshi children receiving 6 mg elemental zinc/kg/d.[187]

Copper deficiency has been reported in malnourished children,[188] and copper sulfate should be added to the diet if not included in the mineral mix.

Iron supplements are not recommended during the acute phase because of the risk of producing iron free radicals, as described earlier in the chapter.[130] However, iron supplements are essential once growth and rehabilitation start and muscle and blood are being synthesized.[189] Ferrous sulfate or fumarate syrup may be given 4 mg elemental iron/kg body wt.[190] As mentioned earlier, electrolyte disturbance is part of the pathophysiology of malnutrition. A triad of interrelated electrolyte deficiencies, potassium, magnesium, and phosphate, occurs. Deficiency of these elements may become especially critical once treatment is instigated and recovery starts. Potassium should be added to the diet to ensure a total of at least 5 mmol/kg/d or more. Magnesium is needed for potassium to enter cells, and magnesium supplements should be added to the diet and, if possible, mineral ORS used (ReSoMal). If not given in the diet or ORS on the first day, an alternative is to give magnesium sulfate 50% solution, 0.3 mL/kg intramuscularly (maximum 2 mL) once, and then include it in the diet. Hypophosphatemia is associated with increased risk of dying and should be included in the diet. Milk provides an excellent source.

Children with rickets should be treated with a single intramuscular dose of 600,000 IU of vitamin D as ergocalciferol or cholecalciferol repeated at 12 weeks plus calcium supplements providing 1 g calcium as calcium carbonate or lactate daily for 12 weeks. The combination of vitamin D and calcium is more effective than vitamin D alone.[191] Children <12 months should receive half the dose of vitamin D and calcium. Malnourished children, especially those who are predominately breastfed are at risk of vitamin D deficiency. Even children in sunny climates may not get enough exposure to sunlight because of cultural considerations or of the adverse effects of the sun and diets are often low in calcium. Dairy foods to provide calcium should be included in the diet, and Vitamin D supplements (400 IU daily)[192] as cholecalciferol or ergocalciferol should be provided, cod liver oil may be a practical alternative.

Refeeding Syndrome. The refeeding syndrome is a potentially lethal complication of an increase in calorie intake following starvation. Sudden onset of lethal cardiac failure occurring during refeeding was first reported in the classic studies of experimental starvation in adults in Minnesota and later in starved Japanese prisoners of war, the survivors of concentration camps, and following the wartime famine in the Netherlands, when, following starvation, there was sudden access to unlimited food.[193,194] This syndrome also occurs in severely malnourished children and may be responsible for considerable mortality, although the precise incidence is difficult to know as, clinically, the syndrome may be difficult to distinguish from pneumonia and sepsis deaths. Sudden death shortly after refeeding has started in a child who seemed to be doing well is suspicious. The syndrome also occurs with parenteral and enteral feeding.

When glucose becomes available during refeeding, gluconeogenesis is inhibited, and there is a rise in plasma glucose and insulin excretion. Rebound hyperglycemia may occur with polyuria and dehydration. There is a flux of glucose, potassium, magnesium, and phosphate into cells, which may result in rapid lowering of serum levels. The sudden reduction of serum levels of these three electrolytes is thought to explain most of the consequences of the refeeding syndrome. Phosphate depletion results in anorexia, adverse neuromuscular effects (eg, diaphragmatic weakness and respiratory insufficiency), and a reduction in myocardial contractility.[195] Cell membrane electrolyte fluxes are perturbed, and there is an intracellular accumulation of calcium, sodium chloride, and water, which may result in edema and is probably one of the mechanisms that explain recurring edema when children with kwashiorkor are refed too rapidly. There is also a derangement of phospholipids in cell membranes.[196] When refeeding with high-carbohydrate diets occurs, there is an increased need for phosphate for phosphorylation and protein synthesis and a shift of available phosphate into cells. Although hypophosphatemia was thought to be the main cause of the refeeding syndrome, the clinical effects of potassium and magnesium deficiency are similar, and it is likely that all three electrolyte disturbances contribute to a certain extent. Thiamin deficiency may also be important and has been reported in refeeding alcoholics and following starvation treatment of obesity. Its role in the refeeding of malnourished infants is not known. Thiamin is an essential cofactor for various enzymes, and carbohydrate refeeding causes increased thiamin use.

The key to prevention of the refeeding syndrome is the avoidance of rapid refeeding, especially with high-carbohydrate diets, whether intravenous or enteral, and the replenishment with potassium, magnesium, and phosphate and restricted sodium intake. The safest way to correct phosphate deficiency is with milk diets because oral phosphate salts are laxatives and may well exacerbate diarrhea. Milk is also useful as a good source of magnesium, as well as protein and energy, but needs to be mixed with a cereal, such as rice, or sugar to reduce the sodium, protein, and lactose load. If intravenous treatment is unavoidable and oral feeding is delayed, phosphate can be given intravenously with care and should be included in parenteral feeding regimens. If children are dehydrated, magnesium and potassium can be added to oral rehydration therapy as in the ReSoMal recommended by WHO. Vitamins, including thiamin, should be added to the diet from the start. The reader is referred to several reviews of this subject.[194,197,198]

Skin and Eye Care. The skin lesions of kwashiorkor improve with dietary therapy but, in the initial phase, may become infected and are a potential source of pathogens causing sepsis. Care should be taken to avoid pressure on affected areas and the skin should be kept clean and dry; 1% potassium permanganate solution may be applied to the worst areas. If possible, the perineum and buttocks should be left uncovered and carefully cleaned and dried immediately after defecation. Special care should be taken of the eyes of children with signs of vitamin A deficiency (xerophthalmia). Retinol supplements should be given immediately in the same doses noted above,[10,190] and the eyes should be protected with pads soaked in saline. Atropine and antibiotic eye drops should be applied at least four times daily until there is no sign of inflammation.[10,190]

Phase 2: Rehabilitation. The initial phase of management lasts while metabolic and electrolyte abnormalities are corrected and infections treated. This phase may last from 1 to 7 days, sometimes longer, if infection is difficult to treat and edema slow to resolve. The recognition of recovery is subjective but usually obvious to staff. There is a general improvement in the child's condition. The return of appetite, reduction in apathy, and return of smiling are encouraging signs indicating improvement. Weight gain may not occur at this stage, and in kwashiorkor, there is usually a brisk weight loss as edema disappears. If the child does not seem to be recovering and edema continues without obvious cause, suspect occult infection, for instance, tuberculosis, inadequate potassium repletion, and phosphate deficiency. An algorithm for the dietary management of the child during this phase is shown in Figure 7.

If the child shows signs of improvement, the rehabilitation phase can start. In this phase, emphasis is on intensive feeding to restore lost weight and emotional and physical stimulation to optimize recovery. For long-term successful recovery and to prevent relapse, the clinical unit needs to work closely with the family during this phase. Ideally, this phase should be 2 to 6 weeks to give the child, especially his or her immune system, the best chance to recover before being challenged by the home environment. A reasonable goal is for the child to reach –1 SD (90%) of the median weight for length[199] before discharge. In some settings, it is very difficult to retain the child in the hospital for this time, and when children are exposed to other ill children, the hospital may not be the safest place.[200] An alternative is to seek out or establish rehabilitation care in the community, and several successful models have been reported. Too early discharge in the absence of follow-up rehabilitation leads to very high post-discharge mortality.[201]

Diet. During the rehabilitation phase, the dietary calorie intake should be increased. This should be gradual, for instance, an additional 25 kcal/kg/d every other day,[176] to avoid the refeeding syndrome and should be guided by the child's appetite and general condition. Diets are calculated based on body weight, so correction will need to be made for the child's changing weight. Most children will reach intakes of between 150 and 250 kcal/kg/d, and rapid weight gain at this stage is desirable as it is associated with the same body composition as lower weight gains.[202] The same diet started in the initial phase may be continued; if F75 was used, then F100 should be substituted. Readers are referred to a review of the criteria for rehabilitation diets and guidance on practical aspects.[176,203,204] At first, it is useful to continue a set diet as it is easier to calculate intakes, but as the child improves, the diet should be varied, and the child should be encouraged to eat a variety of locally available solid foods. Wherever possible, mothers not only should be taught about diets based on nutrient-dense local weaning foods but should prepare and feed these preparations in the hospital or rehabilitation unit. During this phase, iron supplements should be started at 3 to 4 mg elemental iron/kg/d and other micronutrient supplements should be continued.

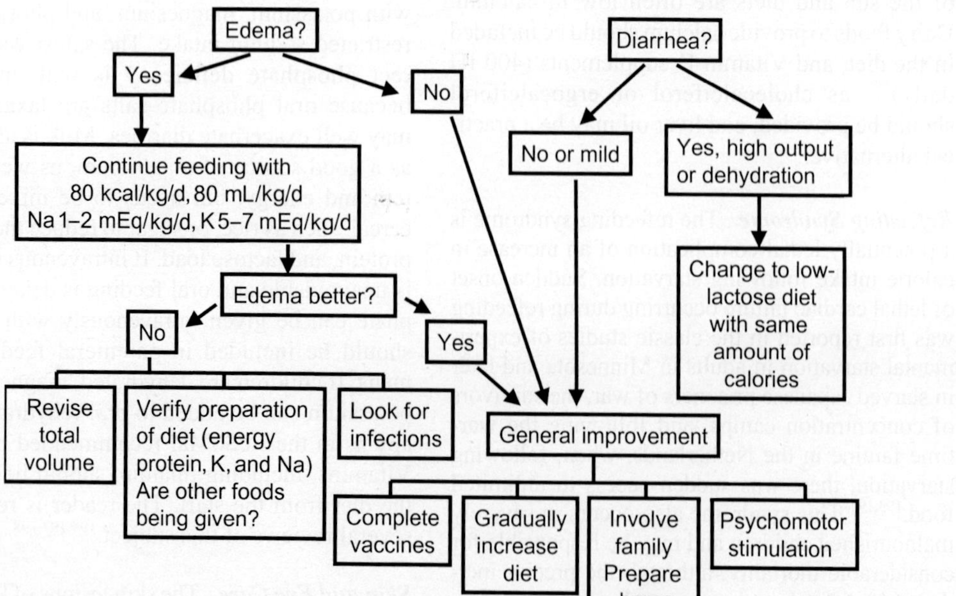

Figure 7 Rehabilitation phase.

Physical and Emotional Stimulation. Early physical and emotional stimulation are very important. Even during the initial phase, mothers can be encouraged to talk to and hold their children. They can be taught to massage their children, which has been shown to increase growth recovery. Children should de provided with a visually interesting environment. As soon as possible, play therapy should be instigated. The WHO manual provides examples of easy-to-make toys.[11] Studies in Jamaica and India showed that an early stimulation program improved growth, complementing micronutrient supplements.[145,146]

Phase 3: Follow-up Before the child is discharged, arrangements should be made for follow-up in the community or in the outpatients department. Recently recovered malnourished children often relapse, and children have a high mortality rate after discharge.[201] Families should have easy and rapid access to medical care, ideally on the unit where the child is known. The choice of follow-up, like the length of hospital stay, will depend on the availability of services. The availability of a well-designed follow-up program can make all the difference to subsequent risk of dying.[205] Studies following children treated for severe malnutrition have shown variable recovery of nutritional status and intellectual development.[206,207] Sustained recovery of nutritional status is possible, although stunting usually remains.[208] Growth following rehabilitation depends on the favorable home circumstances.[144] When family circumstances remain unchanged, the outlook is poor.[209] A study in Lima comparing children returning home with those who had to be adopted and were integrated into families with few resource constraints showed both the importance of follow-up care but also the potential for recovery of these children.[144] Children should be followed up for at least 6 months to ensure successful rehabilitation.

CONCLUSIONS

The last few years have brought exciting advances in management of severe malnutrition. Lessons learned in the past are now being applied in hospitals and rehabilitation centers all over the world, although much more needs to be done to ensure that this information reaches and changes practice in all of the situations in which severe PEM is treated. Greater understanding of the pathophysiology of PEM has contributed to more rational therapy, and some clinical trials of therapies, new diet possibilities, and management strategies are being reported. Nevertheless, there is a great need for more research. The pathophysiology of kwashiorkor is still unclear, and the complicated interplay between infection and nutrition in PEM and its consequences are not resolved. Many of the recommendations for management have never been properly assessed.

The long-term goal, of course, is to prevent PEM. Some aspects could be relatively easily achieved. Medical practices, for instance, that deprive children of food while they are ill, especially with diarrhea, have been unequivocally shown to be unnecessary and harmful, but the use of diluted diets or "resting the gut" continue. Attention is now being given to early enteral feeding of critically ill children, which reduces malnutrition and mortality.[210] Great strides have been made in understanding the importance of exclusive breast-feeding and the requirements for adequate complementary feeding practices, but much work is still needed to change complementary feeding practices in many countries and overcome the restraints on food security. Changing child care practices is never easy but a recent randomized trial showed that nutrition education through the health services was able to prevent stunting in poor periurban population in Peru[211] and an intensive education program in the community was also successful in preventing malnutrition in Bangladesh[166] Infections, which are very common among the most deprived populations, contribute to malnutrition. Whereas children with access to sufficient food of high nutritional value experience only transient effects, those on marginal diets are caught in a cycle of infection, exacerbating malnutrition and vice versa. Interventions that reduce the burden of disease will reduce malnutrition in these populations. Measles was once a common precursor to kwashiorkor and severe vitamin A deficiency but, with vaccination, has now disappeared in many countries.[212] Other vaccines against diarrheal diseases could make important contributions. Severe PEM is an entirely preventable disease, but it will continue to kill and contribute to the deaths of millions of children while war and natural and man-made disasters continue to affect large parts of the world.

REFERENCES

1. Pelletier DL, Frongillo EAJ, Schroeder DG, et al. A methodology for estimating the contribution of malnutrition to child mortality in developing countries. J Nutr 1994;124:2106–22.
2. Schroeder DG, Brown KH. Nutritional status as a predictor of child survival: Summarizing the association and quantifying its global impact. Bull World Health Organ 1994;72:569–79.
3. Bryce J, Boschi-Pinto C, Shibuya K, et el. WHO estimates of the causes of death in children. Lancet 2005;365 1147–52.
4. Caulfield LE, de Onis M, Blossner M, et al. Undernutrition as an underlying cause of child deaths associated with diarrhea, pneumonia, malaria, and measles. Am J clin Nutr 2004;80:193–8.
5. Olumese PE, Sodeinde O, Ademowo OG, et al. Protein energy malnutrition and cerebral malaria in Nigerian children. J Trop Pediatr 1997;43:217–9.
6. Ahmed T, Ali M, Ullah MM, et al. Mortality in severely malnourished children with diarrhoea and use of a standardized management protocol. Lancet 1999;353: 1919–22.
7. Venugopalan P, Akinbami FO, Al-Hinai KM, et al. Malnutrition in children with congenital heart defects. Saudi Med J 2001;22:964–7.
8. Sharma R, Florea VG, Bolger AP, et al. Wasting as an independent predictor of mortality in patients with cystic fibrosis.Thorax 2001;56:746–50.
9. Schofield C, Ashworth A. Why have mortality rates for severe malnutrition remained so high? Bull World Health Organ 1996;74:223–9.
10. WHO/UNICEF/IVACG Task Force. Vitamin A Supplements: A Guide to Their Use in the Prevention and Treatment of Vitamin A Deficiency and Xerophthalmia. Geneva: WHO; 1997.
11. World Health Organization. Management of Severe Malnutrition: A Manual for Physician and Other Senior Health Workers. Geneva: WHO; 1999.
12. Frenk S. Metabolic adaptation in protein energy malnutrition. J Am Coll Nutr 1986;5:371–81.
13. Waterlow JC. The nature and significance of nutritional adaptation. Eur J Clin Nutr 1999;53:S2–5.
14. Shetty PS. Adaptation to low energy intakes: The response and limits to low intake in infants, children and adults. Eur J Clin Nutr 1999;53:S14–33.
15. Gorsky RD, Galloway DH. Activity pattern changes with decrease in food energy intake. Hum Biol 1983;55:577–86.
16. Kerpal-Fronius E, Frank K. Einige Besonderheiten de Korperzusammensetzung und Wasserverteilung bei Sauglinsatrophie. Ann Paediatr 1949;173:321–30.
17. Waterlow JS. Protein-Energy Malnutrition. Sevenoaks, UK: Edward Arnold; 1992.
18. Garrow JS, Fletcher K, Halliday D. Body composition in severe infantile malnutrition. J Clin Invest 1965;44:417–25.
19. Frenk S, Luengas J, Junco E. Cortisol sangúineo en la desnutrición protéica-energetica grave. Arch Invest Med Mex 1975;6:397–402.
20. Coward WA, Lunn PG. The biochemistry and physiology of kwashiorkor and marasmus. Br Med Bull 1981;37:19–24.
21. Payne-Robinson HM, Coore HG, Golden MH, et al. Changes in red cell insulin receptors during recovery from severe malnutrition. Eur J Clin Nutr 1990;44:803–12.
22. Brasel J. Endocrine adaptation to malnutrition. Pediatr Res 1980;14:1299–303.
23. Beitins IZ, Graham GG, Kowarski A, et al. Adrenal function in normal infants and in marasmus and kwashiorkor: Plasma aldosterone concentration and aldosterone secretion rate. J Pediatr 1974;87:444–51.
24. James WPT. Protein synthesis and breakdown and amino acid catabolism in protein-calorie malnutrition. Proc Nutr Soc 1972;31:225–31.
25. Garrow JS. Total body potassium in kwashiorkor and marasmus. Lancet 1965;2:455–8.
26. Alleyne GAO, Millward DJ, Scullard GH. Total body potassium, muscle electrolytes and glycogen in malnourished children. J Pediatr 1970;76:75–81.
27. Alleyne GAO. Studies on total potassium in malnourished infants: Factors affecting potassium repletion. Br J Nutr 1970;24:205–12.
28. Mann MD, Bowie MD, Hansen JDL. Total body potassium and serum electrolyte concentrations in protein energy malnutrition. S Afr Med J 1975;49:613–5.
29. Nichols BL, Alvarado J, Rodriguez J. Therapeutic implications of electrolyte, water and nitrogen losses during recovery from protein-energy malnutrition. J Pediatr 1974;84:759–68.
30. Manary MJ, Brewster DR. Potassium supplementation in kwashiorkor. J Pediatr Gastroenterol Nutr 1997;24:194–201.
31. Patrick J, Golden MHB. Leukocyte electrolytes and sodium transport in protein energy malnutrition. Am J Clin Nutr 1977;30:1478–81.
32. Willis JS, Golden MH. Active and passive transport of sodium and potassium ions in erythrocytes of severely malnourished Jamaican children. Eur J Clin Nutr 1988;42:635–45.
33. Kaplay SS. Erythrocyte membrane Na+ and K+ activated adenosine triphophatase in protein-calorie malnutrition. Am J Clin Nutr 1978;31:579–84.
34. Forrester T, Golden M, Brand S, et al. Reduction in vitro of red cell glutathione reproduces defects of cellular sodium transport seen in oedematous malnutrition. Eur J Clin Nutr 1990;44:363–9.
35. Patrick J. Oedema in protein energy malnutrition: The role of the sodium pump. Proc Nutr Soc 1979;38:61–79.
36. Soliman AT, Alsalmi I, Asfour M. Hypoinsulinaemia has an important role in the development of oedema and hepatomegaly during malnutrition. J Trop Pediatr 1996;42:297–9.
37. Freiman I, Pettifor JM, Gopal MM. Serum phosphorus in protein energy malnutrition. J Pediatr Gastr Nutr 1982;1:547–50.
38. Manary MJ, Hart CA, Whyte MP. Severe hypophosphatemia in children with kwashiorkor is associated with increased mortality. J Pediatr 1998;133:789–91.
39. Waterlow JC, Golden MHN. Serum inorganic phosphate in protein energy malnutrition. Eur J Clin Nutr 1994;48: 503–6.
40. Kalra K, Mital VP, Pal R, et al. Serum electrolyte studies in malnutrition. Indian Pediatr 1975;12:1135–40.
41. Motarjemi Y, Kaferstein F, Moy G, et al. Contaminated weaning foods: A major risk factor for diarrhoea and associated malnutrition. Bull World Health Organ 1993;71:79–92.
42. World Health Organization. Complementary Feeding of Young Children in Developing Countries: A Review of Current Scientific Knowledge. Geneva: WHO; 1998.
43. Bhan MK, Sommerfelt H, Strand T. Micronutrient deficiency in children. Br J Nutr 2001;85:S199–203.
44. Beisel WR. Herman Award Lecture. Infection-induced malnutrition—from cholera to cytokines. Am J Clin Nutr 1995;62:813–9.
45. Woolf N. Cell, Tissue and Disease: The Basis of Pathology. London: WB Saunders; 2000.
46. Manary MJ, Broadhead RL, Yarasheski KE. Whole-body protein kinetics in marasmus and kwashiorkor during acute infection. Am J Clin Nutr 1998;67:1205–9.
47. Abbas AK, Lichtman AH, Pober JS. Cellular and Molecular Immunology, 3rd edition. Philadelphia: WB Saunders; 1997.
48. Remick DG, Friedland JS. Cytokines in Health and Disease, 2nd edition. New York: Marcel Dekker; 1997.
49. Manary MJ, Yarasheski KE, Berger R, et al. Whole body leucine kinetics and the acute phase response during acute infection in marasmic Malawian children. Ped Res 2004;55:940–6.
50. Muñoz C, Aréval M, López M, et al. Impaired interleukin-1 and tumor necrosis factor production in protein-calorie malnutrition. Nutr Res 1994;14:347–52.
51. Doherty JF, Golden MHN, Remick DG, et al. Production of interleukin-6 and tumour necrosis factor-α in vitro is reduced in whole blood of severely malnourished children. Clin Sci 1994;86:347–51.
52. Sauerwein RW, Mulder JA, Mulder L, et al. Inflammatory mediators in children with protein-energy malnutrition. Am J Clin Nutr 1997;65:1534–9.
53. Azavedo ZMA, Luz RA, Victal SH, et al. Increased production of tumor necrosis factor-α in whole blood cultures from children with primary malnutrition. Braz J Med Biol Res 2005;38:171–83.
54. Schelp FP, Migasena P, Pongpaew P, et al. Serum proteinase inhibitors and other serum proteins in protein-energy malnutrition. Br J Nutr 1977;38:31–8.
55. Hassanein el-SA, Assem HM, Rezk MM, et al. Study of plasma albumin, transferrin, and fibronectin in children with mild to moderate protein-energy malnutrition. J Trop Pediatr 1998;44:362–5.
56. Rikimaru T, Taniguchi K, Yartey JE, et al. Humoral and cell mediated immunity in malnourished children in Ghana. Eur J Clin Nutr 1998;52:344–50.
57. Ekanem EE, Umotong AB, Raykundalia C, et al. Serum C reactive protein and C3 complement protein levels in severely malnourished Nigerian children with and without bacterial infections. Acta Paediatr 1997;86:1317–20.
58. Doherty JF, Golden MH, Raynes JG, et al. Acute-phase protein response is impaired in severely malnourished children. Clin Sci (Lond) 1993;84:169–75.
59. Morlese JF, Forrester T, Jahoor F. Acute-phase protein response to infection in severe malnutrition. Am J Physiol 1998;275:E112–7.
60. Manary MJ, Yarasheski KE, Smith S, et al. Protein quantity, not quality, accelerates whole-body leucine kinetics and the acute-phase response during acute infection in marasmic Malawian children. Br J Nutr 2004;92:589–95.
61. Golden MH. Oedematous malnutrition. Br Med Bull 1998;54:433–44.
62. Golden MHN, Golden BE, Jackson AA. Albumin and nutritional oedema. Lancet 1980;i:114–6.
63. Golden MH. Protein deficiency, energy deficiency, and the oedema of malnutrition. Lancet 1982;i:1261–5.
64. Golden MH, Ramdath D. Free radicals in the pathogenesis of kwashiorkor. Proc Nutr Soc 1987;46:53–68.
65. Majno G, Joris I. Cells, Tissues and Disease. Principles of General Pathology. Cambridge, MA: Blackwell Science; 1996.
66. Gutteridge JM, Halliwell B. Free radicals and antioxidants in the year 2000. Ann NY Acad Sci 2000;899:136–47.
67. Evans PS, Halliwell B. Micronutrients: Oxidant/antioxidant stress. Br J Nutr 2001;85:s67–74.
68. Manary MJ, Leeuwenburgh C, Heinecke JW. Increased oxidative stress in kwashiorkor. J Pediatr 2000;137:421–4.
69. Ashour MN, Salem SI, El-Gadban HM, et al. Antioxidant status in children with protein-energy malnutrition (PEM) living in Cairo, Egypt. Eur J Clin Nutr 1999;53:669–73.
70. Forrester T, Golden M, Brand S, et al. Reduction in vitro of red cell glutathione reproduces defects of cellular sodium transport seen in oedematous malnutrition. Eur J Clin Nutr 1990;44:363–9.
71. Ciliberto H, Ciliberto M, Briend A, et al. Antioxidant supplementation for the prevention of kwashiorkor in Malawian children: Randomized, double-blind, placebo controlled trial. BMJ 2005;330:E1109.
72. Decsi T, Koletzko B. Effect of protein energy malnutrition and human immunodeficiency virus-1 infection on essential fatty acid metabolism in children. Nutrition 2000;E16:447–53.

73. Franco VH, Hotta JK, Jorge SM, et al. Plasma fatty acids in children with grade III protein-energy malnutrition in its different clinical forms: Marasmus, marasmic kwashiorkor, and kwashiorkor. J Trop Pediatr 1999;45:71–5.
74. Leichsenring M, Sutterlin N, Less S, et al. Polyunsaturated fatty acids in erythrocyte and plasma lipids of children with severe protein-energy malnutrition. Acta Paediatr 1995;84:516–20.
75. Sammon AM. Dietary linoleic acid, immune inhibition and disease. Postgrad Med J 1999;75:129–32.
76. Houssaini FZ, Foulon T, Iraqi MR, et al. Lipids, lipoproteins, and fatty acids during infantile marasmus in the Fes area of Morocco. Biomed Pharmacother 1999;53:278–83.
77. Holman RT, Johnson SB, Mercuri O, et al. Essential fatty acid deficiency in malnourished children. Am J Clin Nutr 1981;34:1534–9.
78. Lenhartz H, Ndasi R, Anninos A, et al. The clinical manifestation of the kwashiorkor syndrome is related to increased lipid peroxidation. J Pediatr 1998;132:879–81.
79. Okunade WG, Olorunsogo OO. Effect of reactive oxygen species on the erythrocyte calcium-pump function in protein-energy malnutrition. Biosci Rep 1992;12:433–43.
80. Mayatepek E, Becker K, Gana L, et al. Leukotrienes in the pathophysiology of kwashiorkor. Lancet 1993;342:958–60.
81. Jackson AA. Blood glutathione in severe malnutrition in childhood. Trans R Soc Trop Med Hyg 1986;80:911–3.
82. Reid M, Badaloo A, Forrester T, et al. In vivo rates of erythrocyte glutathione synthesis in children with severe protein-energy malnutrition. Am J Physiol Endocrinol Metab 2000;278:E405–12.
83. Badaloo A, Reid M, Forrester T, et al. Cysteine supplementation improved the erythrocyte synthesis rate in children with severe edematous malnutrition. Am J Clin Nutr 2002;76:646–52.
84. Hendrickse RG. Of sick turkeys, kwashiorkor, malaria, perinatal mortality, heroin addicts and food poisoning: Research on the influence of aflatoxins on child health in the tropics. Ann J Trop Med Parasitol 1997;91:787–93.
85. Brooks SE, Golden MH. The exocrine pancreas in kwashiorkor and marasmus. Light and electron microscopy. West Indian Med J 1992;41:56–60.
86. Mann MD, Becker DJ, Pimstone BL, et al. Potassium supplementation, serum immunoreactive insulin concentrations and glucose tolerance in protein-energy malnutrition. Br J Nutr 1975;33:55–61.
87. Payne Robinson HM, Cocks T, Kerr D, et al. Hormonal control of weight gain in infants recovering from protein energy malnutrition. I. The effect of insulin and metabolic rate. Pediatr Res 1980;14:28–33.
88. Alleyne GAO, Young VH. Adrenocortical function in children with severe protein-calorie malnutrition. Clin Sci 1967;33:189–200.
89. Das BK, Panda BK, Dhingra R, et al. Thyroid hormone studies in protein-energy malnutrition. J Trop Pediatr 1999;45:375–6.
90. Orbak Z, Akin Y, Varoglu E, et al. Serum thyroid hormone and thyroid gland weight measurements in protein energy malnutrition. J Pediatr Endocrinol Metab 1998;11:719–24.
91. Onuora C, Maharajan G, Singh A, et al. Thyroid status in various degrees of protein-calorie malnutrition in children. Clin Endocrinol 1983;18:87–93.
92. Kalk WJ, Hofman KJ, Smit AM, et al. Thyroid hormone and carrier protein interrelationships in children recovering from kwashiorkor. Am J Clin Nutr 1986;43:406–13.
93. Chandra RK. Golan memorial lecture. Nutritional regulation of immunity and infection: From epidemiology to phenomenology to clinical practice. J Pediatr Gastroenterol Nutr 1986;5:844–52.
94. Chandra RK, Kumari S. Nutrition and immunity: An overview. J Nutr 1994;124:1433S–5S.
95. Rikimaru T, Taniguchi K, Yartey JE, et al. Humoral and cell mediated immunity in malnourished children in Ghana. Eur J Clin Nutr 1998;52:344–50.
96. Chevalier P, Sevilla R, Zalles L, et al. Immuno-nutritional recovery of children with severe malnutrition. Sante 1996;6:201–8.
97. McMurray DN. Cell mediated immunity in nutritional deficiency. Prog Food Nutr Sci 1984;8:193–228.
98. Golden MHN, Jackson AA, Golden BE. Effect of zinc on thymus of recently malnourished children. Lancet 1977;ii:1057–9.
99. Harland PSEG. Tuberculin reactions in malnourished children. Lancet 1965;ii:719–21.
100. Chandra RK, Wadhwa M. Nutrition modulation of intestinal mucosal immunity. Immunol Invest 1989;18:119–26.
101. El-Gamal Y, Aly RH, Hossny E, et al. Response of Egyptian infants with protein-calorie malnutrition to hepatitis B vaccination. J Trop Pediatr 1996;42:144–5.
102. Chandra RK. Reduced secretory antibody response to live attenuated measles and polio virus vaccines in malnourished children. BMJ 1975;2:583–5.
103. Teodosio MR, Oliveira EC. Urinary secretory IgA after nutritional rehabilitation. Braz J Med Biol Res 1999;32:421–6.
104. McMurray DN, Watson RR, Reyes MA. Effect of renutrition on humoral and cell mediated immunity in severely malnourished children. Am J Clin Nutr 1981;34:2117–26.
105. Suskind R, Edelman R, Kukapongs P, et al. Complement activity in children with protein-calorie malnutrition. Am J Clin Nutr 1976;29:1089–92.
106. McLaren DS, Faris R, Zekian B. The liver during recovery from protein-calorie malnutrition. J Trop Med Hyg 1968;71:271–81.
107. Doherty JF, Adam EJ, Griffin GE, et al. Ultrasonographic assessment of the extent of hepatic steatosis in severe malnutrition. Arch Dis Child 1992;67:1348–52.
108. Cook GC, Hutt MSR. The liver after kwashiorkor. BMJ 1967;3:454–57.
109. Chaithiraphan S. The heart in protein-energy malnutrition. J Med Assoc Thai 1986;69:170–7.
110. Ghignone M, Quintin L. Malnutrition and respiratory function. Int Anaesthesiol Clin 1986;24:65–74.
111. Aubier M, Murciano D, Lecocguic Y, et al. Effect of hypophosphatemia on diaphragmatic contractility in patients with acute respiratory failure. N Engl J Med 1985;313:420–4.
112. Doekel RC, Zwillich CW, Scoggin CH, et al. Clinical semi-starvation: Depression of hypoxic ventilatory response. N Engl J Med 1976;295:358–61.
113. Cherian T, Steinhoff MC, Simoes EA, et al. Clinical signs of lower respiratory infections in malnourished infants and children. Pediatr Infect Dis J 1997;16:490–4.
114. Black RE, Brown KH, Becker S. Malnutrition is a determining factor in diarrhea duration, but not incidence, among young children in a longitudinal study in rural Bangladesh. Am J Clin Nutr 1984;37:87–94.
115. Bhandari N, Bhan MK, Sazawal S. Importance of persistent diarrhea in childhood mortality. Acta Paediatr Suppl 1992;381:3–6.
116. Brunser O. Effect of malnutrition on intestinal structure and function in children. Clin Gastroenterol 1977;2:341–53.
117. Behrens RH, Lunn PG, Northrop CA, et al. Factors affecting the integrity of the intestinal mucosa of Gambian children. Am J Clin Nutr 1987;45:1433–41.
118. Brewster DR, Manary MJ, Menzies IS, et al. Intestinal permeability in kwashiorkor. Arch Dis Child 1997;76:236–41.
119. James WPT. Effect of protein calorie malnutrition on intestinal absorption. Ann NY Acad Sci 1971;176:244–61.
120. James WPT. Sugar absorption and intestinal motility in children when malnourished and after treatment. Clin Sci 1970;39:305–18.
121. Penny ME. The role of the duodenal microflora as a determinant of persistent diarrhoea. Acta Pediatr Suppl 1992;381:114–20.
122. Arora NK, Anand NK, Bhan MK, et al. Nutrient absorption from a fat-enriched diet in young malnourished children: A randomised controlled trial. Acta Paediatr 1998;87:143–8.
123. Viteri FE, Schneider R. Gastrointestinal alterations in proteincalorie malnutrition. Med Clin North Am 1974;58:1487–505.
124. International Working Group on Persistent Diarrhoea. Evaluation of an algorithm for the treatment of persistent diarrhoea: A multicentre study. Bull World Health Organ 1996;74:479–89.
125. Holt E, Tidwell HC, Kirk CM, et al. Studies in fat metabolism.1: Fat absorption in normal infants. J Pediatr 1935;6:428–80.
126. Brown KH, Gastañaduy AS, Saavedra JM, et al. Effect of continued oral feeding on clinical and nutritional outcomes of acute diarrhea in children. J Pediatr 1988;112:191–200.
127. McKenzie D, Freidman R, Katz S, et al. Erythropoietin levels in anemia in kwashiorkor. S Afr Med J 1977;4:1044–6.
128. Sive AA, Dempster WS, Rosseau S, et al. Bone marrow and chelatable iron in patients with protein energy malnutrition. S Afr Med J 1996;86:1410–3.
129. Dempster WS, Sive AA, Rosseau S, et al. Misplaced iron in kwashiorkor. Eur J Clin Nutr 1995;49:208–10.
130. Ramdath DD, Golden MHN. Non-haematological aspects of iron nutrition. Nutr Res Rev 1989;2:29–50.
131. Reddy S, Adcock KJ, Adeshina H, et al. Immunity, transferrin, and survival in kwashiorkor. BMJ 1970;4:268–70.
132. Sive AA, Dempster WS, Malan H, et al. Plasma free iron: A possible cause of oedema in kwashiorkor. Arch Dis Child 1997;76:54–6.
133. Massa E, Maclean WC, Jr, de Romaña GL, et al. Oral iron absorption in infantile protein-energy malnutrition. J Pediatr 1978;93:10–9.
134. Caballero B, Solomons NW, Batres R, et al. Homeostatic mechanisms in the utilization of exogenous iron in children recovering from severe malnutrition. J Pediatr Gastroenterol Nutr 1985;4:97–102.
135. Smith IF, Taiwo O, Golden MH. Plant protein rehabilitation diets and iron supplementation of the protein-energy malnourished child. Eur J Clin Nutr 1989;43:763–8.
136. El Shobaki FA, El Howary MFS, Morcos SR, et al. Iron metabolism in Egyptian infants with protein-calorie deficiency. Br J Nutr 1972;28:81–9.
137. Adams EB, Scragg JN, Naidoo BT, et al. Observations on the aetiology and treatment of anaemia in kwashiorkor. BMJ 1967;3:451–4.
138. Halsted CH, Sourial N, Guindi S, et al. Anemia of kwashiorkor in Cairo: Deficiencies of protein, iron and folic acid. Am J Clin Nutr 1969;22:1371–82.
139. McLaren DS. Skin in protein energy malnutrition. Arch Dermatol 1987;123:1674–6a.
140. Maverakis E, Fung MA, Lynch PJ, et al. Acrodermatitis enteropathica and an overview of zinc metabolism. J AM Acad Dermatol 2007;56:116–24.
141. Golden MHN, Golden BE, Jackson AA. Skin breakdown in kwashiorkor responds to zinc. Lancet 1980;1:1256.
142. Alvarez JO, Eguren JC, Caceda J, et al. The effect of nutritional status on the age distribution of dental caries in the primary teeth. J Dent Res 1990;69:1564–66.
143. Alvarez JO, Caceda J, Woolley TW, et al. A longitudinal study of dental caries in the primary teeth of children who suffered from infant malnutrition. J Dent Res 1993;1573–6.
144. Graham GG, Adrianzen TB. Growth, inheritance and environment. Pediatr Res 1971;5:691–7.
145. Grantham-McGregor SM. The effect of malnutrition on mental development. In: Waterlow JS, editor. Protein-Energy Malnutrition. Sevenoaks, UK: Edward Arnold; 1992. p. 344–60.
146. Elizabeth KE, Sathy N. The role of developmental stimulation in nutritional rehabilitation. Indian Pediatr 1997;34:681–95.
147. Branca F, Robins SP, Ferro-Luzzi, et al. Bone turnover in malnourished children. Lancet 1992;340:1493–6.
148. Himes JH. Bone growth and development in protein-calorie malnutrition. World Rev Nutr Diet 1978;28:143–87.
149. Walker SP, Golden MHN. Growth in length of children recovering from severe malnutritrion. Eur J Clin Nutr 1988;42:395–404.
150. Ndiaye B, Lemonnier D, Sall MG, et al. Serum osteocalcin regulation in protein-energy malnourished children. Pediatr Res 1995;37:606–10.
151. Holick MF. Resurrection of vitamin D deficiency and rickets. J Clin Investig 2006;116:2062–72.
152. Lemire JM, Adams JS, Kermani-Arab V, et al. 1,25-Dihydroxyvitamin D3 suppresses human T helper/inducer lymphocyte activity in vitro. J Immunol 1985;134:3032–5.
153. Stroder J, Kasal P. Evaluation of phagocytosis in rickets. Acta Paediatr Scand 1970;59:288–92.
154. Muhe L, Lulseged S, Mason KE, et al. Case control study of the role of nutritional rickets in the risk of developing pneumonia in Ethiopian children. Lancet 1997;349:1801–4.
155. Wayse V, Yousafzai A, Mogale K, et al. Association of subclinical vitamin D deficiency with severe acute lower respiratory infection in Indian children under 5y. Eur J Clin Nutr 2004;58:563–7.
156. Wilkinson RJ, Llewelyn M, Toossi Z, et al. Influence of vitamin D deficiency and vitamin D receptor polymorphisms on tuberculosis among Gujarati Asians in west London: A case control study. Lancet 2000;355:618–21.
157. Gernaat HBPE, Dechering WHJC, Voorhoeve HWA. Mortality in severe protein energy malnutrition at Nchelenge, Zambia. J Trop Pediatr 1998;44:211–7.
158. Ahmed T, Begum B, Badiuzzaman, et al. Management of severe malnutrition and diarrhea. Indian J Pediatr 2001;68:45–51.
159. Brewster DR, Manary MJ, Graham SM. Case management of kwashiorkor: An intervention project at seven nutrition rehabilitation centres in Malawi. Eur J Clin Nutr 1997;51:139–47.
160. Ciliberto MA, Sandige H, Ndekha MJ, et al. Comparison of home-based therapy with ready to use therapeutic food with standard therapy in the treatment of malnourished Malawian children: A controlled randomized effectiveness trial. Am J clin Nutr 2005;81:864–70.
161. Roy SK, Fuchs GJ, Mahmud Z, et al. Intensive nutrition education with or without supplementary feeding improves the nutritional status of moderately-malnourished children in Bangladesh. J Health Popul Nutr 2005;23:320–30.
162. Doherty JF, Golden MHN, Griffin GE, et al. Febrile response in malnutrition. West Indian Med J 1989;38:209–12.

163. Wafula EM, Ngamau DW, Onyango FE, et al. X-ray diagnosable pneumonia in children with severe malnutrition at Kenyatta.East Afr Med J 1998;75:567–71.
164. Bolme P, Eriksson M, Paalzow L, et al. Malnutrition and pharmacokinetics of penicillin in Ethiopian children. Pharmacol Toxicol 1995;76:259–62.
165. Duggan C, Fontaine O, Pierce NF, et al. Scientific rationale for a change in the composition of oral rehydration solution. JAMA 2004; 291:2628–31.
166. Alam NH, Hamadan JD, Dewan N, et al. Efficacy and safety of a modified oral rehydration solution (ReSoMal) in the treatment of severely malnourished children with watery diarrhea. J Pediatr 2003;143:614–9.
167. Lares-Asseff I, Cravioto J, Santiago P, et al. A new dosing regime for metronidazole in malnourished children. Scand J Infect Dis 1993;25:115–21.
168. Riordan SM, Bolin TD. Malnutrition in the developing and developed world. Is small intestinal bacterial colonization important? Scand J Gastroenterol Suppl 1995;208:53–7.
169. Penny ME, Paredes P, Brown KH, et al. Lack of a role of the duodenal flora in pathogenesis of persistent diarrhea and diarrhea-related malabsorption in Peruvian children. Pediatr Infect Dis J 1990;97:479–87.
170. De Monte CM, Ashworth A, Sa ML, et al. Effectiveness of nutrition centres in Ceara State, northeastern Brazil. Rev Panam Salud Publica 1998;4:375–82.
171. Puoane T, Sanders D, Chopra M, et al. Evaluating the clinical management of severely malnourished children—a study of two rural district hospitals. S Afr Med J 2001;91:137–41.
172. Tolboom JJM, Ralitapole-Maruping AP, Kabir H, et al. Severe protein energy malnutrition in Lesotho, death and survival in hospital, clinical findings. Trop Geogr Med 1986;38:351–8.
173. Gernaat HBPE, Dechering WHJC, Voorhoeve HWA. Mortality in severe protein-energy malnutrition at Nchelenge, Zambia. J Trop Pediatr 1998;44:211–7.
174. Brooke OG. The influence of malnutrition on the body temperature of children. BMJ 1972;1:331–3.
175. Brook OG, Harris M, Salvosa CB. The response of malnourished babies to cold. J Physiol 1973;233:75–91.
176. Brown KH. Appropriate diets for the rehabilitation of malnourished children in the community setting. Acta Pediatr Scand Suppl 1991;374:151–9.
177. Thomas M, Anand NK, Gupta S. Evaluation of different regimes of management in malnourished children. Indian Pediatr 1977;14:725–30.
178. Kalavi FNM, Muroki NM, Omwega AM, et al. Effect of tempe-yellow maize porridge and milk yellow-maize porridge on growth rate, diarrhoea, and duration of rehabilitation of malnourished children. East Afr Med J 1996;73:427–31.
179. Brewster DR, Manary MJ, Menzies IS, et al. Comparison of milk and maize based diets in kwashiorkor. Arch Dis Child 1997;76:242–8.
180. Hansen JDL, Schendel HE, Wilkins JA, et al. Nitrogen metabolism in children with kwashiorkor receiving milk and vegetable diets. Pediatrics 1960;25:258–82.
181. Holt LE, Tidwell HC, Kirk CM, et al. Studies in fat metabolism. I. Fat absorption in normal infants. J Pediatr 1935;6:427–80.
182. Hossain MI, Wahed MA, Ahmed S. Increased food intake after the addition of amylase-rich flour to supplementary food for malnourished children in rural communities of Bangladesh. Food Nutr Bull 2005;26:323–9.
183. Briend A. Highly nutrient-dense spreads: A new approach to delivering multiple micronutrients to high-risk groups. Br J Nutr 2001;85:S175–9.
184. Manary MJ, Ndkeha MJ, Ashorn P, et al. Home based therapy for severe malnutrition with ready-to-use food. Arch Dis Child 2004;89:557–61.
185. Golden MHN, Golden BE. Trace elements: Potential importance in human nutrition, with particular reference to zinc and vanadium. Br Med Bull 1981;37:31–6.
186. Khanum S, Alam AN, Anwar I, et al. Effect of zinc supplementation on the dietary intake and weight gain of Bangladeshi children recovering from protein-energy malnutrition. Eur J Clin Nutr 1988;42:709–14.
187. Doherty C, Sarkar K, Shakur S, et al. Zinc supplementation and severe malnutrition—higher dosage regimes associated with increased mortality but not through the precipitation of copper deficiency. J Pediatr Gastroenterol Nutr 1998;26:589.
188. Cordano A, Baertl JM, Graham GG. Copper deficiency in infancy. Pediatrics 1964;34:324–36.
189. Macdougall LG, Moodley G, Eyberg C, et al. Mechanisms of anemia in protein-energy malnutrition in Johannesburg. Am J Clin Nutr 1982;35:229–35.
190. World Health Organization/UNICEF. Management of the Child with a Serious Infection or Severe Malnutrition. Geneva: WHO; 2000.
191. Thacher TD, Fischer PR, Pettiflor JM, et al. A comparison of calcium, vitamin D, or both for nutritional rickets in Nigerian Children. NEJM 1999;341:563–8.
192. Gartner LM, Greer FR. Prevention of rickets and vitamin D deficiency: New guidelines for vitamin D intake. Pediatrics 2003;111:908–10.
193. Keys A, Brozek J, Henschel A, et al. The Biology of Human Starvation, Vols 1 and 2. Minneapolis: University of Minnesota Press; 1950.
194. Solomon SM, Kirby DF. The refeeding syndrome: A review. JPEN J Parenter Enteral Nutr 1990;14:90–7.
195. Kreusser W, Vetter H, Mittmann H, et al. Cardiac function and metabolism in phosphate depleted dogs—effects of hormone stimulation. Adv Exp Med Biol 1982;151:251–8.
196. Håglin L. Hypophosphataemia in anorexia nervosa. Postgrad Med J 2001;77:305–11.
197. Crook MA, Hally V, Panteli JV. The importance of the refeeding syndrome. Nutrition 2001;17:632–7.
198. Melchior J-C. Les complications de la re-nutrition. Ann Med Interne 2000;151:635–43.
199. National Center for Health Statistics. Growth Charts United States, HRA 76-1120.25.3. Rockville Pike, MD: Public Health Service, Health Resources Administration; 1976.
200. Parent F, Coppieters Y. Assessment of hospital morbidity, mortality, and cost effectiveness of a nutrition program for children under 5 years of age in Pala, Chad. J Trop Pediatr 2000;46:252–4.
201. Sadre M, Donozo G, Hedayat H. The fate of the hospitalized malnourished child in Iran. Environ Child Health 1973;29–31.
202. Fjeld CR, Schoeller DA, Brown KH. Body composition of children recovering from severe protein-energy malnutrition at two rates of catch-up growth. Am J Clin Nutr 1989;50:1266–75.
203. Ashworth A, Jackson A, Khanum S, et al. C. Ten steps to recovery. Child Health Dialogue 1996;3–4:10–12.
204. Ashworth A. Practical aspects of dietary management during rehabilitation from severe protein-energy malnutrition. J Hum Nutr 1980;34:360–9.
205. Pecoul B, Soutif C, Hounkpevi M, et al. Efficacy of a therapeutic feeding centre evaluated during hospitalisation and a follow-up period, Tahoua, Niger, 1987–1988. Ann Trop Paediatr 1992;12:47–54.
206. Stoch MB, Smythe PM. 15 year development study on effects of severe undernutrition during infancy on subsequent physical growth and intellectual functioning. Arch Dis Child 1976;51:327–36.
207. Winick M. Long term effects of kwashiorkor. J Pediatr Gastroenterol Nutr 1987;6:833–40.
208. Banurpurmath CR, Prasad SM, Banurpurmath S, et al. Follow-up studies of survivors of severe protein-energy malnutrition. Indian Pediatr 1999;36:139–43.
209. Hennart P, Beghin D, Bossuyt M. Long-term follow-up of severe protein-energy malnutrition in Eastern Zaire. J Trop Pediatr 1987;33:10–2.
210. Briassoulis G, Zavras N, Hatzis T. Malnutrition, nutritional indices, and early enteral feeding in critically ill children. Nutrition 2001;17:548–57.
211. Penny ME, Creed-Kanashiro HM, Robert RC, et al. Effectiveness of an educational intervention delivered through the health services to improve nutrition in young children: A cluster-randomised controlled trial. Lancet 2005;365:1863–72.
212. CDC. Progress in reducing global measles deaths: 1999–2004. MMWR 2006;55:247–9.

Childhood Malnutrition: Prevention and Control at the National Level

Gerardo Weisstaub, MD, MSc
Magdalena Araya, MD, PhD
Ann Hill, PhD
Ricardo Uauy, MD, PhD

NUTRITION A KEY FACTOR FOR HUMAN AND SOCIAL DEVELOPMENT

The nutritional status of children is directly related to their health condition and both in turn are key determinants of the human and social development of communities around the world. Improvement of nutrition and health increase the chances of child survival and is a precondition for economic development. UNICEF has proposed a conceptual model to understand the causation of malnutrition beyond the obvious immediate determinants (Figure 1). Undoubtedly the basic determinants relate to the social, economic, cultural, and political structure of society. These define what resources are controlled by individual families including access to information and education, household food security, care of women and children, access to health and healthy environment. It is within this context that children have inadequate access to food in terms of quantity and quality; in addition, infection will further compromise nutrition by augmenting nutrient losses and increasing nutrient needs.

Nutrition has been considered a basic human right and expressly recognized by international human rights covenants since 1924,[1] yet this right is commonly the subject of political demagogy rather than being actively upheld, respected, protected, and promoted. The relationship between poverty and malnutrition has been well established in both directions, that is how poverty conditions nutritional status and vice versa. Moreover, the correlation is by no means linear. There are multiple examples that illustrate how nutrition can improve despite economic limitations. Economic development is by no means sufficient to improve nutrition, especially in countries where wealth is concentrated in a few hands. The UN Human development index illustrates how nutrition and health can be dissociated with economic status.[2] For example, Indonesia has a higher per caput gross national product (GNP) than China, but malnutrition is presently rare in the latter whereas it is frequent in the former. Brazil has experienced significant economic growth over the past decade but malnutrition in children less than 6 years of age remains high. Recent analysis of trends reveals significant reductions in malnutrition assessed by underweight or stunted linear growth except in sub-Saharan Africa and Central America. These regions have experienced protracted civil wars and more recently that African region has been stricken by HIV/AIDS and its consequences. On the contrary, Latin America and the Caribbean combined have reduced malnutrition to about a third of the 1970 figure despite the unchanged proportion of families living in poverty (Figure 2).[3] This concept should be stressed since health professionals frequently work under the assumption that nothing can be done in terms of prevention and control of protein energy malnutrition (PEM) unless social conditions change and poverty reduction is achieved. Undoubtedly both should proceed in tandem, since improved nutrition will contribute to socio-economic improvement.

WHO, UNICEF, and other International Organizations concerned with malnutrition have recognized for several decades the role of malnutrition in defining infant mortality. The immediate cause of death may be diarrhea or pneumonia but the risk of dying from these conditions is increased by manifold by severe and moderate malnutrition. The work of Puffer and Serrano in the Americas, and more recently Pelletier and Habitch working with data from Africa and Asia have documented with precision the contribution of malnutrition to infant mortality.[4,5] The conclusion reached by both is that over half of all infant death is determined by malnutrition. UNICEF in its annual World Children Report states "malnutrition is directly related to over half of all infant deaths that occur worldwide."[1] Chapter 12 "International Nutrition" discusses nutrition and infection interactions and the contribution of malnutrition to infant death as a crucial underlying factor.

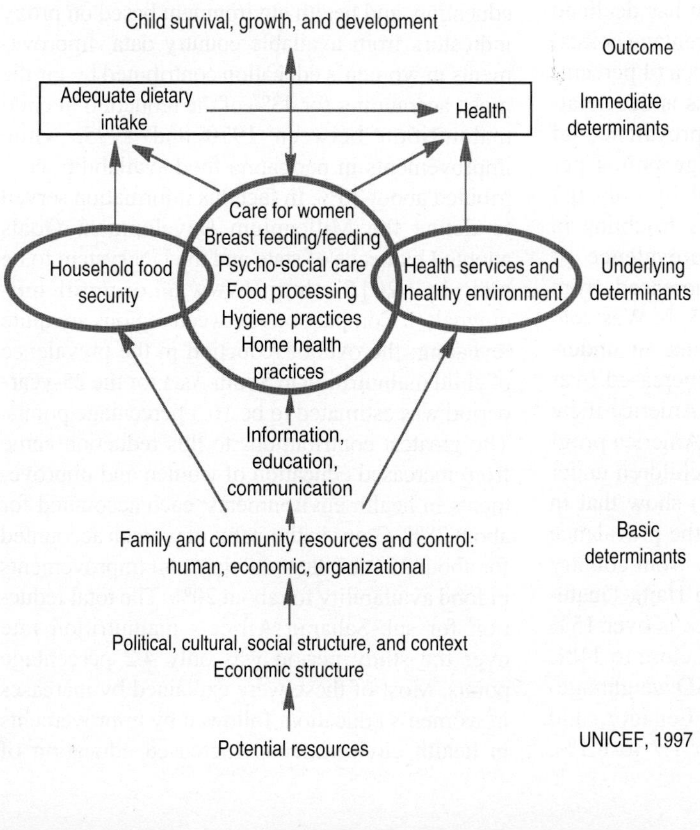

Figure 1 Conceptual model of child development useful in the analysis prevention and control of malnutrition. (Adapted from ACC/SCN Commission on the Nutrition Challengers of the XXI Century.)

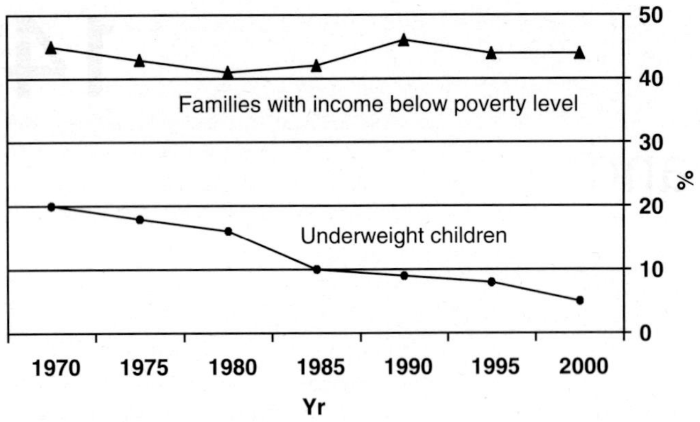

Figure 2 Child undernutrition in Latin America and the Caribbean: trends, reasons, and lessons. Over the past 30 years, population under poverty line has remained stable, but malnutrition has declined significantly.

MALNUTRITION AS A GLOBAL PUBLIC HEALTH PROBLEM

Weight, height, and head circumference measurements have been widely used as indicators of nutritional adequacy. Selection of the indicator to be used influences the magnitude of the prevalence calculated. Weight for age is a sensitive but not very specific indicator of malnutrition since it may overlook stunting. Thus, children may be underweight for age but of normal or even overweight for height. Height for age is the most demanding indicator of nutritional adequacy since it implies adequate weight for age and appropriate weight for height.

Malnutrition as a public health problem is assessed based on growth indices relative to those derived form a standard population. Yet, most growth standards describe what may be considered normal growth based on values obtained in a given normative population. Normal is derived from statistical normalcy, rather than based on specific health and/or quality of life outcomes related to a set of growth parameters. For example the 1979 National Center for Health Statistics (NCHS) growth reference standard, used as the basis for the former WHO international standards for infants 0 to 36 months derived from children growing in a relatively affluent, predominantly artificially fed, rural community from Yellow Springs Ohio over 30 years ago.[6] New growth standards have been developed by WHO/UNU based on the growth of more than 8,000 healthy infants and children (from middle income, nonsmoking, and well-educated mothers from Brazil, Norway, India, Ghana, USA, and Oman), who are exclusively breast-fed for 4 to 6 months and given appropriate complementary foods after weaning. The resulting charts indicate that infants fed according to present WHO recommendations and living in appropriate conditions gain weight less rapidly than the NCHS median reference value, particularly after 4 to 6 months, while their length is slightly greater. The consequences of applying the new charts as shown by de Onis (http://www.who.int/childgrowth/en/) are lower rates of undernutrition after the first 6 months of life and higher rates of overweight and obesity, with slightly higher prevalences of stunting than observed with the old WHO standards.[7] This new reference provides a scientifically reliable descriptor of physiologic growth and a powerful tool for advocacy in support of good health and nutrition.[8] Another objective of the new reference is to support, based on actual evidence, the concept that human growth during the first year of life is very similar across groups of children of different ethnic backgrounds. This confirms that existing differences in growth across countries are predominantly environmentally derived and can be narrowed over time. The new reference supports the right of all children to grow equally well and demands that society provides an environment that does not restrict growth. (see also Chapter 2, "Clinical Assessment of Nutritional Status," for a discussion of the new WHO growth curves).

The evolution in prevalence of underweight and stunting reveals significant reductions for most countries over the past two decades, yet the rate of progress (0.5%/yr) is insufficient to achieve the stated goal of the world summit for children. While the prevalence of malnutrition in developing countries as a whole fell from 46.5 to 31% between 1970 and 1995, about 15 percentage points in all for this 25 year period, progress in reducing malnutrition has varied greatly from one region to another. Malnutrition has declined the fastest in South Asia (by 23 percentage points) and the slowest in sub-Saharan Africa (4 percentage points), but the rate of progress is decelerating. During 1970 to 1985 the prevalence of malnutrition fell by 0.8 percentage points per year; during 1985 to 1995, it fell by only 0.3 points. The situation is particularly troubling in sub-Saharan Africa where the prevalence of underweight children actually increased from almost 29% in 1990 to 31% in 1995. In West and East African regions the prevalence in underweight and stunting has actually increased over the past three decades. In Central America there is no improvement while in South America progress has been significant. Data on children under 6 years of age by UNICEF (2005) show that in Latin America and the Caribbean the prevalence of low weight/age (<-2 SD) vary from country to country (from 0.7 to 22.7%). In Haiti, Guatemala, and Honduras this prevalence is over 15% and in Ecuador and El Salvador is close to 11%. As for severe malnutrition (<-3 SD weight/age) in Haiti, Guatemala, Honduras, Ecuador, and Bolivia the prevalence vary from 1.7 to 8.1%. Even under ideal conditions it is hard to obtain drops in prevalence greater than 2 to 3% per year on weight related indicators while drops in stunting prevalence of 1 to 2% per year are the maximum that can be observed. Independent of the improvement of national figures, severe malnutrition including edematous forms can still be detected in hospital settings in some regions of the world.[9]

Since 1970, the prevalence of underweight children has decreased in 35 developing countries, held steady in 15, and increased in 12, with most of the countries with increases in sub-Saharan Africa.[10]

The causes behind the insufficient progress are multiple and complex in their interactions. Political strife, government unresponsive to the needs of the community, stagnant economies, low status of women and unequal rights, poor education and inadequate access to health, poor sanitation and unclean water, high prevalence of infections and low birth weight interact in determining poor post natal growth and high rates of malnutrition.[11] Since most of these factors are interrelated, it becomes virtually impossible to isolate their effects from retrospective trend data or regression models. Decreases in the prevalence of malnutrition have been described in relation to improvements in household food security, supply of clean water and environmental sanitation, education of women, early treatment of diarrhea with oral rehydration solutions in the community, early treatment of respiratory infections, promotion of breast feeding, appropriate complementary feeding, immunization, growth monitoring, and surveillance for early identification of malnutrition

Smith and Haddad have attempted to explain the key factors responsible for the different rate of progress across regions of the world (see Figure 3).[12] They examined the contribution of national food supply, women's status, women's education, and health environment based on proxy indicators from available country data. Improvements in women's education contributed by far the most, accounting for 43% of the reduction in child malnutrition between 1970 and 1995, while improvements in per capita food availability contributed about 26%. In fact this information served to define the Millennium Development Goals adopted by heads of state and the UN system to be met by 2015 (http://www.un.org/millenniumgoals/). Comparisons between regions are quite revealing; the overall reduction in the prevalence of child malnutrition in South Asia for the 25-year-period was estimated to be 16.5 percentage points. The greatest contributions to this reduction came from increased education of women and improvements in health environments; each accounted for about 28%. Gains in the status of women accounted for about 25% of the reduction, and improvements in food availability for about 20%. The total reduction for sub-Saharan Africa's malnutrition rate over the study period was only 4.2 percentage points. Most of these were explained by increases in women's education, followed by improvements in health environments. Increased education of

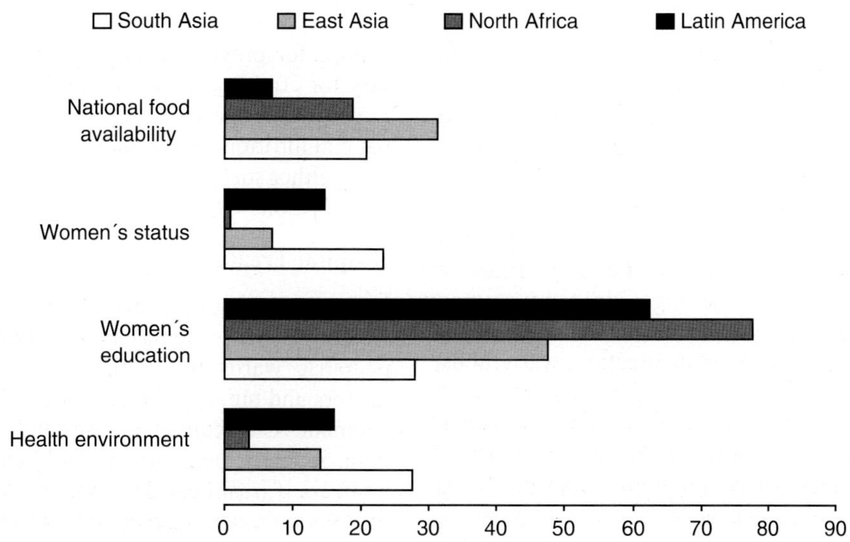

Figure 3 Estimated contributions of underling determinant variables.

women made strong contributions in all periods except for the late 1980s, when enrollments actually declined. Improvements in health environments have made their greatest contribution after 1985. Women's relative status as evidence by gender differences in life expectancy has continually declined in the region since the 1970s, most precipitously after 1985. The consequence has been a recent worsening in prevalence of child malnutrition in the region. Changes in food availabilities have played a large role in both directions. Substantial improvements in the late 1980s and early 1990s were outweighed by deteriorations during the 1970 to 1985 period.

Latin American and the Caribbean experienced an estimated 11-percentage-point reduction in child malnutrition over the study period, most of which took place during 1970 to 1980. Since then, reductions in child malnutrition have continued at a much slower pace. Like the other regions, the greatest contribution comes from women's education, which explained 62% of the improvement whereas the contribution of environmental health to this improvement has steadily declined. Strong improvements in the status of women in the 1970s were followed by very small improvements in the 1980s. Food availability improved in the 1970s, but declined slightly in the early 1980s.

Prevention and control of infections are clearly a critical aspect of malnutrition reduction efforts. As documented in Chapter 12, "International Nutrition," and Chapter 13, "Protein-Energy Malnutrition: Pathophysiology, Clinical Consequences and Treatment," infection has a definite adverse effect on nutritional status, while malnutrition compromises the host defenses and immune responses increasing case fatality and disease susceptibility.[13] Relative risk of death from infection is directly correlated with severity of malnutrition: relative risk 8.7 [95% CI 5.5 to 13.7] for severe PEM, 4.2 (95% CI 3.1 to 5.5) for moderate PEM and 2.0 (95% CI 1.7 to 2.4) for mild PEM.[14] Yet, since the severely malnourished represent a small proportion of total population, most malnutrition related death are accounted by moderate malnourished individuals. It has been estimated that close to 80% of all malnutrition infection related death are attributable to moderate and mild malnutrition. Despite the obvious public health implications in terms of preventing death, given the high mortality of the severely malnourished, the cost effectiveness of PEM treatment is greater than that of controlling moderate malnutrition.

The adequacy of breast feeding and weaning foods also plays a key role in malnutrition prevalence, especially after 6 months of life. In most countries where malnutrition prevails the time of onset is after 6 months, this is when breast milk is insufficient to meet the infant needs and also a time when mothers have increased competition for their time/dedication to the infant. This is coupled by inadequate, low energy density, low nutrient density weaning foods. Under these conditions, feeding frequency and added starch or oil to increase energy density becomes crucial to prevent malnutrition.[15] A study in Bangladesh examined the role of education during the weaning period demonstrating that education on complementary feeding given to mothers was effective in enhancing weight gain despite the fact that no foods were actually provided. The authors suggest the educational efforts on what constitutes adequate complementary feeding and on how to prevent microbial contamination of weaning foods are important as malnutrition prevention strategies.[16]

There are no easy answers or a magic "silver bullet" in combating malnutrition, several options can be suggested based on the success and accomplishments of some countries in malnutrition reduction. In most cases poverty reduction efforts need to go hand in hand, but should not be considered a precondition for success. Suggesting that poverty reduction is a precondition for success is simply not realistic since malnutrition is not only a determinant but also a consequence of poverty. Thus, the efforts should not be postponed until major political or economic events improve the economic condition of the poor since reducing malnutrition contributes by itself to poverty reduction. The notion of human capital as a major determinant of economic growth has been recognized globally with the award of two Nobel prizes in economics over the past decade.[17]

A strategy for action, based on what has worked in different settings around the world (Costa Rica, Thailand, Cuba, Chile, Kerala–India, amongst others), is proposed in Figure 4. This serves to analyze the necessary interactions amongst the key social actors required for successful implementation of malnutrition control and prevention programs. The basic and critical component is social mobilization to establish the demands for action from the political actors; this process should lead to community actions as well as responses by government. A responsive government is one that responds to community demands; this requires some degree of participation by society in government, ideally but not necessarily a government by the people, from the people, and for the people. Communities that are so empowered and able to participate in the political process will be successful in demanding appropriate actions from governments. Malnutrition needs to become unacceptable to society in order to trigger the level of action required to address the issue frontally. What does it take to trigger this process? In most cases, proactive academics and/or NGOs that have a strong voice, independent from government have catalyzed the process and led the way. "Political will" does not come easy nor it is generated from within; professionals, academics, NGOs, community leaders, and the press should act in concert to elicit action. The role of the press in generating public awareness and communicating public concern of malnutrition as a key restriction for national development is crucial. Recruiting and training select journalists will serve to generate widespread recognition of the problem and make people aware that the solutions are credible and feasible by illustrating what has worked elsewhere. Academics and professionals should propose the necessary actions that are required to implement effective programs to control and prevent malnutrition, ideally based on technical consensus rather than political considerations. They should promote a critical review of policy options based on what may work in a given setting; international organizations can assist in reaching a technical consensus by providing evidence and expert advice

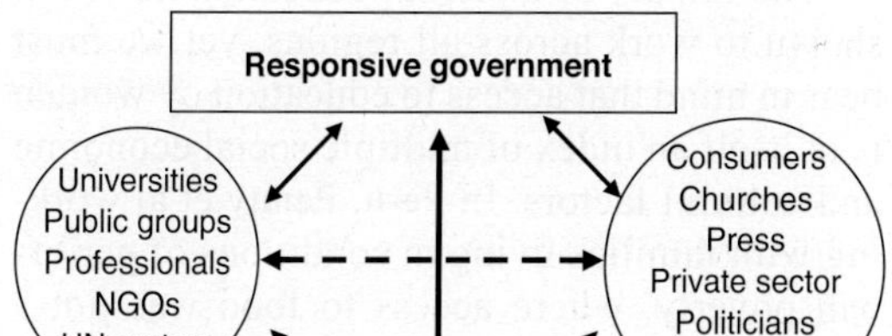

Figure 4 Networks and malnutrition. See text for details on dynamic interactions between stakeholders. NGO = non governmental organization.

on successful examples of malnutrition reduction. The private industrial or business sector is usually a latecomer in this scene. Yet, public private partnerships are a must for sustainable programs since industry is a key partner in the implementation of programs; for example in nutrient supplementation, fortification, and other food based strategies.[18] By the end of the day, unless we activate the political process and include industry we get no action.

Governments must be committed to generate the necessary actions to solve malnutrition as a public health problem. Governments are usually restricted in meeting social demands by the available monetary resources and are not willing to commit funds unless they see a clear return on investment. Thus, it is crucial to clearly present the cost benefit analysis of various programs for nutrition improvement. Moreover, if the community is truly aware and the issue has become a political priority, there may be a clear political benefit as well as an economic gain in terms of human capital formation. The involvement of the press in facilitating social communications is important in open societies. For example, the cost of providing half of all critical micronutrient needs per person per day for a year by fortifying a staple food has been estimated to be less than a dollar per year; this is less than a pack of cigarettes in most countries. The World Bank has estimated the cost benefit ratio of micronutrient fortification to be at least 17:1. On a relative basis not all programs are equal in terms of cost benefit or cost effectiveness, thus the tools of economic assessment should be used in defining policy options. As previously discussed (Figure 4), the mix of policies that will work differs in various settings. Working through networks is particularly helpful in countries where human and material resources are limiting, the potential for complementarity and synergy between groups should be exploited. However, there are multiple preconditions to operate successful networks. Groups must share clearly stated objectives, common short and mid term objectives, participants must share decision-making, activities must have continuity and be sustained. It is also helpful to geographically map where the problems are and where agencies are located and programs are in place in order to improve resource utilization.

The impact of maternal education has been shown to work across all regions, yet we must bear in mind that access to education by women is in itself an index of multiple social economic and cultural factors. In Peru, Penny et al working with families living in conditions of periurban poverty, where access to food was not a limiting factor, demonstrated that nutrition education, delivered through preexisting health services, significantly decreased the prevalence of stunting in young children by 11 points.[19] In our experience in Bolivia we have come to realize that understanding the cultural representations of the mother, the family, and the health team is fundamental to interpret health behaviors that otherwise appear irrational and incomprehensible

Nutrition and food policies should be integrated in the context of national development strategies. Nutritional problems are determined by economic and labor policies, health and education sector policies as well as welfare policies. The integrated approach may be more difficult to implement in most settings, since government structures are sectorial, yet harmonization of policies is a must to avoid duplication, wasteful use of resources and overburden personnel budgets.[20] Cost effectiveness evaluation of programs should be included at the outset in the present climate of fiscal policies. Today, program sustainability in a world of competing interests will progressively depend on the capacity to demonstrate cost effectiveness over time. Technical considerations should prevail over political interest in defining what should be done, because this is the best way to optimize chances of success. This is true at all levels, national and international programs are not always guided by best technical advice but many times, respond to politically motivated actions.

The emerging orientation to guide nutrition and food policy by the ethical dimension and human rights concern can no longer be ignored. In a world of plenty malnutrition can no longer be justified as a problem of the poor or a problems that affects others but not us. Globalization should be not only about business and trade; but mostly about how we as humans face a common future. We cannot afford to have over a third of the people in the planet under conditions of poverty and malnutrition. Pediatricians should be concerned with the status of children worldwide. As we are convinced that our research should not ignore that we are citizens of a common planet, our advocacy and our research should not only serve those around us but children around the world. Funding for applied research in nutrition and health of children should be as important as the present emphasis given to protection from bioterrorism and the war on terrorist activity worldwide. Providing for a better future for children across the world will do more for peace than the massive bombings that have recently taken place. Controlling and preventing malnutrition should top the list.

POTENTIAL STRATEGIES FOR THE TREATMENT AND CONTROL OF SEVERE AND MODERATE MALNUTRITION

First, we should clearly establish that prevention and treatment of malnutrition are complementary. Although the adage "prevention is better than cure" is a public health imperative, it cannot be used to withhold treatment from those already affected by malnutrition. Both strategies must work in tandem to avoid malnutrition from occurring and to recuperate those who are moderately or severely malnourished and at risk of death and/or severe disability. Although the actions for prevention differ from those necessary for effective treatment, they should be seen as part of the spectrum of efforts needed to combat malnutrition. What can we learn from experience, either success or failure, in the treatment of malnutrition?

Hospital Treatment

Even though severe malnutrition (ie, severe wasting and/or edema) is commonly seen in pediatric wards in developing countries, few doctors and nurses have been trained in its management. Consequently case-fatality rates are high. Severely malnourished children die in large numbers if treatment does not take into account the physiological and metabolic changes that arise during reductive adaptation.[21] (For details of treatment see Chapter 13, "Protein Energy Malnutrition: Pathophysiology, Clinical Consequences and Treatment"). One way to try to prevent children dying during treatment is to provide case-management guidelines. WHO first produced such guidelines in 1981. These encapsulated the basic principles of care that are still recognized today, namely stabilization with small frequent feeds day and night, rehydration with low-sodium fluids, provision of potassium, magnesium, and micronutrients, and antibiotics for all children as infections are often silent, followed by rehabilitation with a high-energy, high-protein diet to rebuild wasted tissues. With advances in knowledge, notably the importance of withholding iron during the stabilization phase and providing zinc and other trace nutrients and psychosocial stimulation, WHO updated the guidelines in 1999,[22,23] and developed a training course.[24] Where the guidelines have been fully implemented, deaths among hospitalized severely malnourished children have fallen dramatically; for example, case-fatality rates of 30 to 45% have fallen to <10%.[25]

In some hospitals, staff have accessed the WHO guidelines and implemented them with no outside help, and the improvements in the children's rates of recovery and survival have led to the guidelines becoming hospital policy. In other hospitals, training courses have been the trigger for change. There are also examples, however, where training courses have led only to a transient or partial adoption of improved practices. The reasons are varied and include high staff turnover and lack of motivation. Factors that favor adoption of improved practices and sustainability are:-

- A functioning health system, and basic resources
- Leadership, mentoring, and managerial support
- In-service education so that everyone is confident about what to do
- Induction of new staff
- Supervision of junior staff and carers
- Regular audit and feedback, and discussion of critical incidents and lessons learned
- Good teamwork.

A major hindrance to reducing case-fatality rates is that treatment of severe malnutrition is not included in many medical and nursing curricula. The consequence of this omission is illustrated by experiences in a South African hospital where the case fatality rate increased from 18 to 38% with the arrival of newly qualified doctors who had no specific training in the management of severe malnutrition. The sudden rise in case-fatality coincided with lower prescribing of potassium (13% vs 77%), antibiotics with gram-negative cover (13% vs 46%), and vitamin A (76% vs 91%).[26] In many hospitals in developing countries, severely malnourished children comprise the majority of pediatric deaths, so it is imperative to train young doctors and nurses to care for these children correctly. This will require recognition of the importance of malnutrition in clinical practice, establishing a severe malnutrition ward or "corner" where correct treatment is provided day and night, having adequate supplies, and having ward and emergency staff trained in malnutrition case-management.

Community-Based Treatment

Some of the lowest case-fatality rates for severe malnutrition are to be found in humanitarian emergencies where well-trained staff systematically follows treatment protocols. When thousands of families congregate in crowded camps the risk of disease increases so, as far as possible, case-management should be provided in their communities.[27,28] Community outreach workers screen children for wasting and edema. A mid-upper arm circumference of <110 mm is used to assess wasting in those aged 6 months to 5 years. Children identified as having mild/moderate edema or are wasted, but have a good appetite and are alert and appear clinically well, are treated at home with ready-to-use therapeutic food (RUTF). Only those who have poor appetite or are ill, or have severe edema, or edema plus wasting, are referred for inpatient care.[29]

The components of community-based care include:

- Community sensitization and active case-finding to identify malnourished children early, before their condition deteriorates
- Community mobilization to improve access to care and achieve high coverage
- Treatment of moderately malnourished cases
- Treatment of severely malnourished children with good appetite and who are clinically well (uncomplicated severe malnutrition).

Carers are instructed how to manage their child's recovery at home. Antibiotics, antihelminthics, vitamin A, and RUTF are provided. The child's progress is monitored every week for programs implemented in an emergency context, or every 2 weeks in nonemergency settings. In 21 programs in Malawi, Ethiopia, and Sudan, more than 22,000 children have been treated in this way, with a case-fatality rate of 4.8% and coverage rates of more than 70%.[30]

Where an effective system of community-based care is in place, children requiring inpatient management can be discharged after completion of the stabilization phase and their rehabilitation completed at home with supervision by a trained health worker at a health post, or health centre, or by home visits where these are feasible.[31] Treatment in the community can:

- Benefit children by reducing their exposure to hospital-acquired infections
- Benefit families by reducing the time carers spend away from home and the risk of possible neglect of siblings
- Benefit families by reducing the opportunity costs associated with hospital treatment
- Act as a catalyst for strengthening nutrition activities within clinics for treatment and prevention of malnutrition
- Lead to community action to prevent malnutrition.

Rehabilitation at home can be achieved by provision of RUTF or by families using their own resources to make specific mixtures of family foods. High energy intakes (>150 kcal/kg/d), high protein intakes (4 to 5 g/kg/d), and provision of micronutrients are essential for rapid weight gain. Protein and energy intakes should be adjusted according to rate of growth and stage of recovery. RUTFs are specially designed for home-feeding in the rehabilitation phase: they contain electrolytes, minerals, and vitamins and have low water content so pathogens cannot grow in them.

Advantages of well-run, effective community-based programs are that:

- Timely action should reduce the number of cases requiring inpatient treatment
- The rehabilitation phase can be completed in the community rather than in hospital, which should reduce length of stay
- Discharged children can be provided with continuity of care
- Treatment is more cost-effective.

Early discharge must always be linked with effective follow-up, but at present there are many countries where this is nonexistent. Hospitals with a policy of early discharge and no system of follow-up are usually unaware of high rates of postdischarge mortality. Failure of children to appear at outpatient clinics is easily misinterpreted as parental irresponsibility, rather than to child death.

Nutrition Rehabilitation Centers and Day-Care Centers

There is a long tradition of treatment of moderate and severe cases of malnutrition in residential or day-care nutrition centers, but their low coverage and high opportunity cost make these the least favoured option in many settings. Nevertheless, such centers could be a "half-way-house" between hospital and home. For example, attendance for 1 week could achieve rapid weight gain and provide practical education sessions for mothers and carers and precede rehabilitation at home. Center staff could monitor progress during home rehabilitation through home visits and/or having children return to the center for assessment. Centers could also receive moderately wasted children and treat uncomplicated severe malnutrition. In urban areas with high numbers of severely malnourished children, well-resourced nutrition centers could be alternatives to hospital admission if staff is sufficiently trained. The centers should be integrated into the child health services and could be attached to a clinic.

Factors for successful rehabilitation. Successful programs share several features:

- All follow the basic principles of treatment of severe malnutrition (ie, high-energy, high-protein intakes in the rehabilitation phase along with potassium, magnesium, minerals, and vitamins)
- All provide frequent meals (at least 5), comprising specific food mixtures that families can afford, or RUTF
- Those not giving RUTF make considerable efforts to teach mothers about child feeding in a memorable way, using a variety of teaching methods and providing opportunities for mothers to practise preparing children's meals
- Most address the wider social, economic and health issues that face poor families: some integrate rehabilitation with poverty alleviation activities
- All have motivated and carefully trained staff.

The advantages and disadvantages of (1) residential and day-care nutrition centers, (2) home rehabilitation with no free food given, and (3) home rehabilitation with RUTF are summarized in Table 1.

Each option has advantages and disadvantages: some options may be better suited to particular contexts, such as urban families, mothers working for a wage, or food insecure communities. Health system infrastructure, accessibility, and staff competencies must also be taken into account. For successful rehabilitation, the system chosen should:

- Achieve intakes that will promote catch-up growth and improve immune function
- Provide timely treatment of infections and close monitoring of progress.

Ideally the system should integrate both the treatment and prevention of malnutrition.

Khanum and Ashworth compared the cost-effectiveness of three treatment modalities in 437 severely malnourished Bangladeshi children aged 12 to 60 months. The children were allocated either to (1) inpatient treatment, (2) day-care treatment, or (3) 1 week of day-care followed by home care. The three groups were comparable at admission: most (98%) had edema and the mean weight-for-height was

Table 1 Characteristics of Different Treatment Modalities for Malnutrition: Advantages and Disadvantages According Need

Advantages	Disadvantages
At home with RUTF	
• Independent of home resources • RUTF contains electrolytes and micronutrients; needs no cooking or refrigeration • Liked by carers/children: few defaulters • Can achieve high coverage, rapid scaling-up • Responsive to fluctuating numbers • Avoids need for formative research as to which home foods to promote • Avoids need for intensive teaching of carers on what to give	• Little opportunity to learn about good child feeding practices and malnutrition prevention • Need clinic/health post nearby for monitoring progress etc • Need efficient transport and distribution networks • Need quality control measures if RUTF is locally made
At home using own resources	
• Cost-effective • Liked by carers: few defaulters • Teaches mothers about child feeding • Potential to prevent malnutrition in the long term by learning to make good food mixtures and feed frequently and responsively • Potential ripple effect • Responsive to fluctuating numbers	• Families must have food resources • Carer must be at home full-time • Need formative research to develop educational messages • Need clinic/health post nearby to monitor progress and provide timely treatment when ill • Need to provide micronutrient supplements • Need motivated staff; good communicators
Residential or day-care nutrition centers	
• Supervised feeding with high chance of success • Opportunity for teaching mothers • Potential for preventing malnutrition in the long term • Circumvents poor primary health care system	• Need high malnutrition prevalence, or a center attached to a clinic • High institutional cost if "stand-alone" • Burdensome to carers, with risk of defaulting • Low coverage

RUTF = ready to use therapeutic feeding.

<70%. The costs to reach the target of 80% weight-for-height were compared. The days required to reach the target in the three groups were 18, 23, and 35 days respectively. Although the home-treated group took the longest time, it was the most cost-effective treatment. The respective costs expressed in US$ were $156, 59, and 29 per treated child. Mortality was equally low (<5%) in all three groups (Figure 5). Home treatment was the option most preferred by parents: day-care was the least preferred option.[32,33]

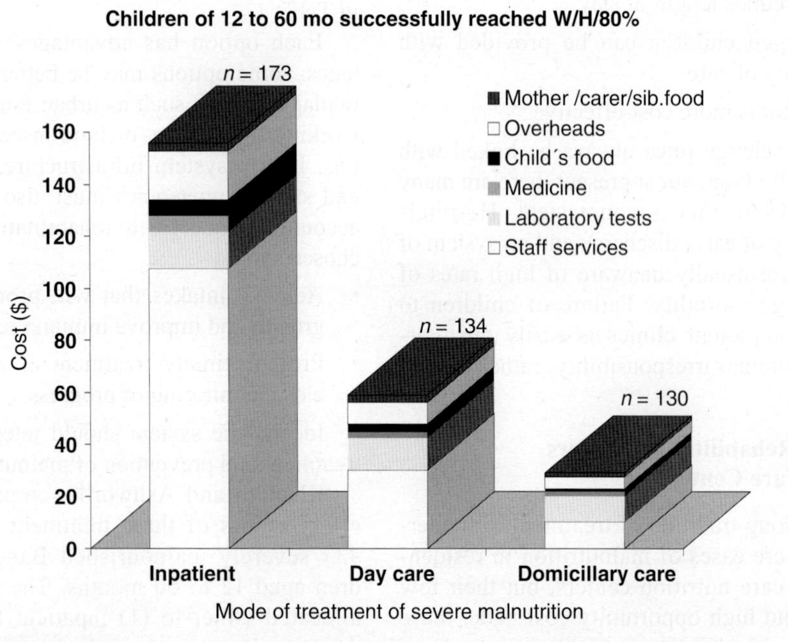

Figure 5 Cost-effective treatment in severe malnutrition. Children were allocated to hospitalization (n = 173), day care nutrition recovery center (n = 134), and ambulatory treatment (n = 130). All achieved a similar degree of recovery (weigth for heigth 80% of Word Health Organization Standard). Cost is expressed in US dollars per treated child for treatment to reach the goal.

IMPLEMENTATION OF PROGRAMS TO PREVENT AND REDUCE MALNUTRITION AT THE NATIONAL LEVEL: THE EXPERIENCE OF CHILE

We need to examine not only the specific actions to treat severely and moderately malnourished children to understand how Chile succeeded in reducing malnutrition, but also assess the multiple programs that acted in synergy to achieve this goal. A key component was the primary health infrastructure with wide coverage and the human/material resources necessary for effective action. The capacity to identify and refer the severely malnourished to nutrition recovery centers when appropriate is vital for success. A nutrition recovery program focused on treatment of the severely malnourished working in isolation will have a little or no impact unless it is coordinated with an effective primary and secondary prevention program working through the primary health system.[34]

Chile stands out among countries of Latin America and the Caribbean for the notable improvement of its health and nutrition situation, particularly in pregnant women and young children. This improvement has been achieved progressively and continuously through comprehensive health, nutrition, sanitation, education, and reproductive health strategies initiated in the 1940s. Results came 30 to 40 years later but much earlier than the considerable economic progress experienced by the country during recent decades. A key element in the success of the Chilean experience has been the uninterrupted application of programs defined based on technically consensus independent of major political, social, and economic changes. The programs remained in place and were even expanded in periods of social instability, radical political changes, and serious economic crisis. Only recently, poverty reduction has contributed to improved food security and to the improvement of the quality of life of low-income groups.

The achievements obtained in children's health can be appreciated in the declining rates of infant mortality, mortality due to acute diarrhea and to bronchopneumonia. Infant mortality dropped by approximately 90%, and mortality due to respiratory infections and acute diarrhea by over 95%. Between 1940 and 1960, total infant mortality was reduced in Chile from 193 to 120 per thousand live births. From 1960 to 1990 it fell to 17 per thousand and over the past decade it dropped to around 10 per thousand. See Table 2 for degree of achievements of 2000 goals for nutrition of children and women, note the virtual eradication of malnutrition and the rise of obesity as the major diet and nutrition related public health problem.[35,36]

A key strategic factor in the development of nutritional programs in Chile has been the emphasis placed on the political dimension of nutritional problems. Nutrition of the population, and especially its more vulnerable sectors, has been at the center of the political debate for the past 40 or 50 years. It has been transformed

Table 2 Degree of Achievement of Nutritional Goals Chile 2000 to 2005

Indicator (%)	Base 87–89 (%)	Goal 2000 (%)	2005* (%)
Pregnant women with low W/H	25	15	12
Anemia in infants	30	10	3
Anemia in pregnant women	25	10	25
Newborn with low birth weight	6.9	6.0	5.0
Newborn with insufficient weight	21	15	12.5
Breastfeeding exclusively to 4 mo	44	80	60
Breastfeeding to 12 mo	20	35	34
Student gr. 1 elem. with height <−1 SD	33	20	10.4
Under 6 yr old with W/A <−2 SD	2.2	2.0	0.8
Food insecure households	35	20	14
Indigent population	18	15	5
Obesity in preschool children	4.6	3	14
Obesity in children entering school	6.5	4.5	19.5
Obesity in pregnant women	12	8	36

Source: Plan Nacional de la Infancia, UNICEF 1994.
*Latest figures Ministry of Health Chile 2001.

into a key indicator to assess social justice and equal opportunity for all. The 1970 Presidential election campaign is a good example of this. All three main candidates to the Presidency (one representing the conservative right, a second representing the center left Christian Democratic, and the third representing the Socialist left) proposed the eradication of malnutrition as a key target of their respective future governments. Salvador Allende, the socialist candidate was elected on that occasion with the promise of providing half a liter of milk per day to every child up to 15 years of age in the country.

The community demanded access to health and food, not only to meet this basic need but as a fundamental human right. The process initiated by academic researchers led to policy development and implementation of nutritional programs. The expansion of these programs became part of the social demands made by the population to the governments, and those politicians that satisfied these demands of providing more food to the economically vulnerable groups were elected and maintained in office.

Community organizations, political parties, the Catholic Church, concerned academics, labor unions as well as multiple social organizations played key roles in demanding action. Most of the nutrition programs were eventually built into the law specifying universal coverage and the respective yearly budget allocations. Any changes to the supplementary feeding programs have always been undertaken with extreme caution by governments, since they are reluctant to take risks on a matter of such high political sensitivity.[35,36]

The National Supplementary Feeding Program (PNAC) is the main nutritional program for the prevention and control of malnutrition. It consists of the distribution of milk and other food products free of charge to children less than 6 years of age, pregnant women, and breast-feeding mothers, with the sole condition of complying with the scheduled out patient visits and preventive health actions determined by the Ministry of Health. In its present form, PNAC began operating in 1954 for the purpose of protecting and improving the nutritional state of pregnant women and children. Until 1974 it provided milk with variable fat content as the sole product. During the period from 1974 to 1981, studies were conducted with various milk-cereal blends for children after 2 years of age, in an effort to reduce cost and to prevent the dilution of the product within the family. This alternative based on milk/wheat blends fortified with micronutrients has remained in place till now. All products are distributed in water-soluble dry powder form (except rice which is given to families with greater need). PNAC's coverage was extended to all children under 14 for a brief period (1971 to 1973), to return later to its original target population.[37]

Between 1975 and 1993, when the criterion for diagnosing "malnutrition" was based on weight for age below 1 SD of the median for age and gender, using as Standard of Reference described by M. Sempé, the preschool population was under control at the primary health care units of the National System of Health Services and was equivalent to close to 75% of the total population of children under 6 in the country. These standard and diagnosis criteria were maintained over a period of almost 20 years, which made easy to appreciate the rapid reduction of malnutrition in this population.[38]

The National Nursery Schools Council (JUNJI), just like National Council for Students Assistance and Scholarships (JUNAEB), is an autonomous public Corporation created by law in 1971 that is functionally dependent on the Ministry of Education. JUNJI plans, promotes, coordinates, provides incentives, and supervises the organization and functioning of day care centers which, as the name implies, provide day care for preschool children until they are old enough to start attending elementary education. JUNJI coordinates and supervises preschool education in the context of integral attention of preschool-age children. Together with food and education in accordance with the child's age, this program also provides social assistance to the family when required.

The programs of food and social assistance to school children were initiated in 1929 by the Student Assistance and Scholarships Committees, which operated at the municipal level with local financing and some resources from the central government. In 1952, the Ministry of Education assumed, at the central level, the administration of these programs. This situation continued until 1964 when this and other responsibilities were handed over to an autonomous public corporation created by law for that purpose: the JUNAEB.

Conceived as a state assistance organization to support the work of the Ministry of Education, JUNAEB works on the basis of integral assistance, for the purposes of providing maximum support to poor students, not only in terms of nutrition but also through programs of health, housing, educational recreation, scholarships, etc.

JUNAEB provides orientation, plans, and coordinates the execution of these social and economic assistance programs directed to students at the preschool, elementary, and high school level, in order to make effective the equal opportunities in education. Program activities are aimed at providing incentives for incorporation and permanence in the educational system, preventing school desertion, and improving academic results of children in municipal and subsidized private schools. The school feeding program (PAE) take up most of the institution's resources.

In 1951 fortification of wheat flour with B complex vitamins was established for the purpose of "improving the nutritional situation of the Chilean population." The only product available for this fortification contained iron and calcium, in addition to thiamin, riboflavin, and niacin. Iron was added in low concentration and, due to the presence of calcium and the type of compounds used, it was probably poorly absorbed. In 1967, regulations on iron fortification were amended, making the process much more effective from a nutritional point of view. Even now, bread made from wheat flour is the main source of calories in the Chilean diet. The main source of calories in the lowest income quintile is wheat flower (bread and pasta) about 40% while in the highest income group only 20% is obtained from wheat. Quality control carried out by the Ministry of Health serves to monitor the iron content in flour samples obtained in a regular and random manner in the mills. A study on iron content in bread obtained at commercial bakeries indicates that 87% of bakeries in the Metropolitan Region use flour with iron. Although it has been impossible to fully assess the efficacy of the fortification program, its impact has produced a change in the prevalence rates of iron deficiency anemia. Bread alone supplies 0.36 mg/d in children 2 to 6 years of age and almost 1 mg/d in adolescents.[39] In fact, anemia problem has virtually disappeared in school children (7% in 1974 to less than 1% in 1994) and adolescents (5 to 1%).

The first law that established mandatory iodination of salt was passed in 1959, and the Food Sanitary Regulations of 1960 determined the obligation of salt fortification. This measure did not really become effective until 1982 when the same Regulations, in a new version, allowed the existence of both iodized and noniodized salt in the market. In 1989, the Ministry of Health declared that edible salt must contain iodine added in the form of sodium or potassium iodates or iodides, in concentration of 100 ppm. One single producer supplies approximately 90% of the edible salt market and has managed to maintain a good level of iodination for the salt that is consumed. As a result, endemic goiter has been eradicated as a public health problem. A study conducted in 1994 in four surveillance areas showed that less than 10% of school children between 6 and 16 years of age had goiter. When present, it is type I-a with high levels of urinary iodine. At present, an inter-sector commission, with the participation of PAHO, UNICEF, the salt industry and the Ministry of Health, work to safeguard this achievement and are making efforts to amend the regulations currently in force, which establish extremely high levels of fortification (100 ppm) in the finished product.[40,41]

National Program of Nutrition Recovery Centers (CNRCs). Severe malnutrition of the marasmic type was concentrated, in 1975, on children under 12 months of age. In fact, among the cases of severe malnutrition that were admitted to hospital, 76% were under 6 months of age. The population of these children, estimated at that time at around 15,000 at the national level, had an important effect on child mortality rates and overburdened pediatric hospital services, where their mortality, due to concurrent infections, was extremely high. Belonging, in general, to homes in extreme poverty, the severely malnourished infants that survived their hospital stay were discharged only partially recovered, or even with yet greater nutritional deterioration, to return their homes where the existing poverty and marginality conditions determined their death or re-admittance to hospital very shortly thereafter.

For the purpose of putting an end to this problem, in 1975 the Chilean Nutrition Foundation (CONIN) was created, a private nonprofit foundation that established throughout the country a system of 33 closed nutrition recovery centers (CNRC) with 1,400 beds destined to the integral treatment of children with severe malnutrition. This treatment includes as basic elements: pediatric and nutritional attention; psychomotor, social, and emotional stimulation of the child; the incorporation of the mother to the child's recovery process; and integral child care training for the mother. At the same time, efforts are made to improve the socioeconomic situation of the family as well as the conditions existing at home.

The CNRCs are directed by a pediatrician in collaboration with a professional team made up of nurse, nutritionist, social worker, child care worker, nurse's aids, and a variable number of volunteer workers. At the central level, CONIN provides support on technical aspects of the program through pediatricians with experience in public health and nutrition, psychologists and physical therapies that monitor the psychomotor stimulation program, and a social assistance and training unit that designs strategies for education and social reinsertion of the mothers and family group of the children under treatment.

The CONIN program is to a great extent financed with funds provided by the Ministry of Health on the basis of annual projections of treatments. CONIN, through various mechanisms, generates supplementary resources. Volunteer workers play an important role in the institution, participating both in the care of the children and in the search for resources to assist the family group. In this task, CONIN centers generally count on the support of local governments.[34]

The program applied by CONIN has been successful. The reduction of malnutrition has led to the closing of many CNRCs, with only 12 remaining throughout the country. Of these, only some maintain their original objectives, although the children being treated today are, almost exclusively, suffering from moderate malnutrition due to social deprivation and/or maternal neglect. Some other centers have destined their beds to reinforcement of the work of the Ministry of Justice with minors under socially deprived environment or due to maternal neglect. As primary malnutrition subsided, five of the existing centers are now concentrating their effort to the study and treatment of children with secondary malnutrition.

SELECTING THE BEST APPROACH TO TREAT SEVERELY MALNOURISHED CHILDREN

The selection of treatment modality for malnourished children starts by defining the severity of the malnutrition. Gomez in the late 1940s proposed the first classification of PEM based on weight expressed as a percentage of normal value for age, despite the limitations of this expression it is still used by many because of its simplicity. First degree or mild PEM is defined as between 75 to 90% of norm, second degree or moderate 60 to 75%, and third degree or severe as <60% of expected for age.[42] Bengoa with his functional classification in the mid 1950s established treatment modalities based on the Gomez criteria, indicating that those with first degree should be treated in the primary health or outpatient health clinic by providing education and dietary advice; those with second degree should be treated in the day care nutrition recovery center using complementary foods in addition to education. Finally, third degree PEM should be treated in the hospital. To a great extent with the caveats described in the corresponding sections, the Bengoa approach remains valid.[20] Hospitalization should last for strictly the minimal time required to treat complications and stabilize the patient, then feed nutrient and energy dense foods as tolerated. Closed nutritional recovery centers should be reserved to situations where PEM is highly prevalent, particularly in young infants and family conditions do not permit recovery at the home. The choice of treatment modality should also consider parental choice, cost effectiveness of treatment under real life situations, access to primary health care system, availability of health infrastructure, social support system available in the community, maternal education and overall condition, and psychosocial interactions within the family. See Chapter 13, "Protein Energy Malnutrition: Pathophysiology, Clinical Consequences and Treatment."

The main barriers or impediments in control and treatment of malnutrition relate to the multiple conditioning factors presented earlier. Translating theoretical concepts into practices that lead to improved nutrition and health of children is also a challenge. Treatment norms and preventive strategies may be well known but they are harder to establish as standards of practice. In addition, physicians commonly depart from rules to demonstrate their autonomy and status, or challenge specific aspects of the norm based on anecdotal personal experience rather than on firm evidence. Health professionals often consider malnutrition as an unavoidable consequence of poverty, thus may accept it as a social problem outside the health realm. The common acceptance of malnutrition by communities and the political leadership as a chronic unsolvable problem inherent to social structure for ages leads to passive acceptance and inaction. Physicians often define health expenditure priorities, particularly by those with greater financial status such as surgeons and internists; they choose based on what is more attractive for medicine per se, rather than basing decisions on objective measures of impact on burden of death and disease. Physicians are more interested and have greater incentives in providing individual health care rather than addressing public health problems.

The organizational environment is also an important barrier, physician lead administration usually centered on medical interest rather than on patients needs. Moreover, other health professionals are seen as subservient to the physician rather than team members with equal participation. Physicians in general have limited skills for networking and to develop partnerships, they are poorly trained for teamwork; they associate success with individual recognition rather than group effort. These traits can prevent physicians from leading multiprofessional multidisciplinary teams such as those needed to address malnutrition effectively. Promoting new attitudes and skills, training for team work, active listening, and defining funding priorities based on public health needs of the community are mandatory to establish effective malnutrition prevention and treatment programs.

FACTORS THAT CAN EXPLAIN THE EFFECT OF NUTRITION PROGRAMS IN RISING OBESITY TRENDS

The transit from undernutrition to good nutrition often leads to increasing rates of overweight and obesity, as observed in Table 2. Countries may reach the goals linked to reduced undernutrition but at the same time have rising prevalence of obesity and related chronic disease.[43] In order to prevent this from occurring, PEM prevention programs should include from the outset the need to consider obesity prevention strategies. For example, there is a need to monitor not only of weight-for-age, but also of length-for-age as well as weight-for-length. The use of combined indicators should permit identification of the stunted overweight or obese child. Beneficiaries should not be selected based solely on socioeconomic conditions, but on true assessment of nutritional status. Stunted children of low weight-for-age but normal weight-for-length should not be given excess energy, since this will lead to obesity. The quality of the foods provided is crucial in preschool and school feeding programs; fruits and vegetables should be included in the diet of children to provide micronutrients and prevent energy excesses. Obesity prevention requires optimizing linear growth and lean tissue mass gain; thus micronutrients and quality of the protein source are important.

PEM prevention programs need periodic evaluation, including targeting of beneficiaries, definition of real needs, and impact on obesity. Food products may need to be modified in urban settings. For example, in situations where stunting and obesity coexist, providing Fe and Zn fortified skimmed milk in preschool feeding programs, rather than full-fat products, is highly recommended.

Programs should be redesigned on the basis of actual need, considering the rapid transition of most urban communities in developing countries. Planners should consider the assessment of physical activity; if low, increased activity should be promoted. Food programs designed to combat PEM may become outdated as rapid improvements in socioeconomic and environmental conditions occur. Slashing social benefits without redirecting them is always unpopular. Policy makers can prevent this reaction by reallocating these funds to alternative social programs that enhance the quality of life of the poor. Thus, the changes will not be seen as taking away benefits from the poor, but rather as responding to a new situation where other needs become more relevant. Ideally the right to food should be upheld by providing access to safe and nutritious foods, based on what people can buy or grow for themselves.[44]

CONCLUSIONS

Presently the world produces enough food to feed the 6 billion inhabitants of the planet. Food production has increased by 25% over the past decade reaching a daily availability of 2,750 cal and 76 g of protein per person.[10] Yet, undernutrition affects close to a billion people, stunting and underweight affects close to 180 million children under 5 years of age, especially in South Asia and sub-Saharan Africa. The overall trend is toward a small decrease in the proportion of undernourished children with a minute decrease in the absolute number. Unfortunately the goal established by the UN for year 2000 two decades ago to reduce malnutrition by 50% was not met. The present level of progress (0.72% per year) is only half of the 1.5% decrease required to reach this goal in the next 20 years. Moreover some regions like sub-Saharan Africa show a rising prevalence of malnutrition. This situation is worse in countries affected by civil strife and draught, where death of children during famine is 20 to 40 times greater than those found in the general population. We can firmly state that malnutrition and growth failure of children remain an issue, which affects not only survival but also the quality of life of children in many parts of the world. Prevention is the best form of treatment. There is no doubt that sufficient knowledge exists to treat and prevent primary malnutrition in virtually all children. The condition should be considered a preventable disease, but its eradication requires full commitment by society to assign a high priority to the well-being of children. Changing the social, economic, and political forces that condition abnormal growth and development in PEM goes beyond the realm of specific medical action but concerted participation of physicians as advocates for children in the political process. Placing demands on political leaders is essential to assure that children from the time of conception throughout their various development stages are provided adequate nutrition to allow for the full expression of their genetic potential. Acceptance of this basic premise by the community is essential before appropriate prevention strategies can be successfully undertaken.[3]

Treatment of childhood malnutrition initiated as a response to a basic humanitarian duty to prevent death during the first half of the past century remains a problem in many regions of the developing world. Presently the mandate is based on the right to adequate food and nutrition for all children as part of the global human and social development agenda. National and International Nutrition and Food Programs developed over the past 50 years have been implemented as integral components of broader strategies of primary health care and education, oriented toward preventing deaths and improving quality of life of low socioeconomic groups. Pediatricians worldwide should also be aware of malnutrition as a conditioning factor delaying recovery from illness and as a major determinant of the quality of life of children with chronic disease.[3]

The key for effective malnutrition prevention is integrating, health care, household food security, and care as proposed by the UNICEF model presented at the outset. The following are some of the components of malnutrition primary prevention programs that have been developed and tested over past decades throughout the world in a variety of political and social settings:

1. Promote early contact between mother and infant to improve chance for successful breast feeding. Establish hospital and other health routines that support breast feeding while in the maternity ward and later, successful early bonding and documented breast feeding is vital. Support breast feeding by health team and by legal framework that promotes, protects, and sustains the right of working women to practice it.
2. Monitor growth and development with adequate standards (present standards are being revised based on present recommended feeding modes). Intervene only when appropriate to prevent malnutrition and specific micronutrient deficits. Mothers should be familiar with growth monitoring cards and be ready to take appropriate actions when growth faltering occurs. The degree of actions taken by the community will depend on the strength of the primary health care.
3. Introduce appropriate micronutrient rich complementary foods and supplements at 6 months of age. If complementary foods are needed earlier, consider the risks associated with interference of breast feeding. Ideally these should be based on local foods that are accessible to the population. Micronutrient will be required in most cases, new developments include fortification at the household level either with tablets, sauces or sprinkles. Food donations should be incorporated into existing programs and not be dependent on whether surplus exists in industrialized countries. Occasional food donations no matter how well meaning can have adverse consequences in the long term when they disappear.
4. Identify infants at risk for malnutrition and growth failure based on biological and social risk factors. Provide adequate social and medical support for families with children at risk. Early identification should be based on community surveillance not only of growth but of caring practices and of critical food insecurity. Early interventions at this level are significantly more cost effective. This area is presently receiving insufficient attention despite being at the core of the problem.
5. Educate parents and adolescent girls (who will be mothers) on how to promote growth and development through appropriate home environment, care, and stimulation. Verbal and cognitive stimulation for malnourished children results in higher growth rates than for children without such stimulation. Interactions with parents, caregivers, and other children are essential for the young child and these interactions can be improved by education of parents and other caregivers. Care initiatives should go beyond focusing on individual practices and behaviors to bring in dimensions of care for the family and the community.
6. Provide universal coverage of children to basic health care services, full coverage for all children with immunizations to prevent infectious disease, and avoid their adverse effects on nutritional status and provide early diagnosis and treatment of diarrheal disease at the

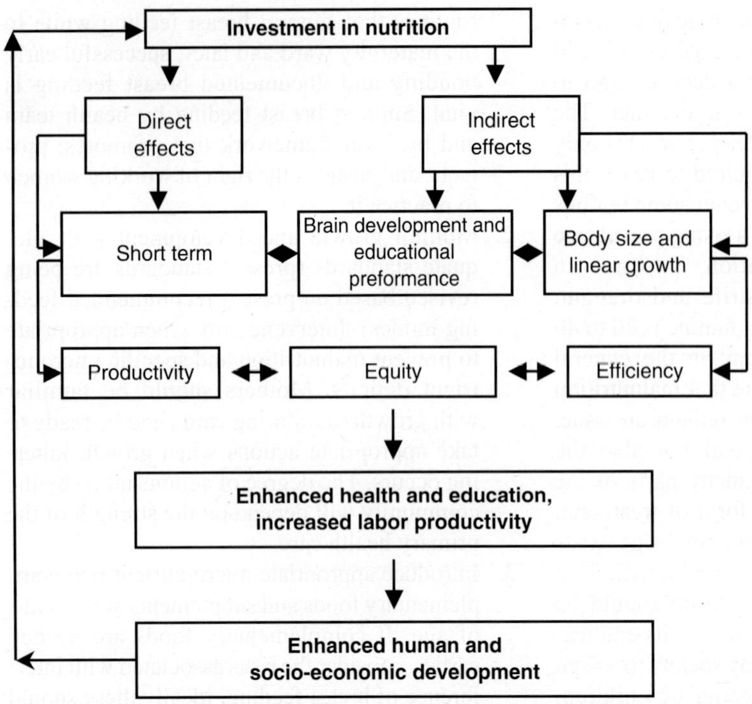

Figure 6 Model to explain how investment in nutrition contributes to economic growth and national development. Short-term improvement in food intake is coupled to better linear growth and enhanced mental development. These translate into better health, decreased infectious morbidity and mortality, enhanced educational performance, and increased capacity for physical work. These interactions in the appropriate social and political conditions lead to increased efficiency, productivity and increased equity. The product of the investment is better health, education and productivity; thus generating economic growth and greater human and social development. This virtuous cycle is closed as more investment in nutritional improvement takes place.

community level using oral rehydration. Linking this effort to the community based surveillance for effective prevention and control of mild and moderate PEM. Depending on what is available in the country the approach may not require expensive infrastructure but rather be community based and sustained.

Treating hundreds or thousands of affected children will not solve the problem of malnutrition as a global public health problem. Unless society at large confronts this issue in its full dimension the problem will continue. Access to adequate amount and quality of food represent a basic human right and is a necessary precondition for health. In turn good nutrition and health are prerequisites for human, social, and economic development (Figure 6). Physicians and especially pediatricians should not be passive bystanders but rather be activists in this process. Reducing malnutrition of infants and young children means a brighter future for all humankind.

REFERENCES

1. UNICEF. The State of the World's Children 1998. New York: Oxford University Press; 1998.
2. UNDP. Human Development Report. York, NY: UN Nations Development Program New; 1998.
3. ACC/SCN Commission on the nutrition challenges of the XXI century. Food Nutr Bull 2000;21:1–88.
4. Puffer RC, Serrano CV. Patterns of mortality in childhood. Scientific Publication No. 262. Washintong, DC: PAHO; 1973.
5. Pelletier D, Frongillo E, Schroeder DG, Habitcht JP. A methodology for estimating the contribution of malnutrition to child mortality in developing countries. J Nutr 1994;124:2106S–22S.
6. NCHS Growth Curves. DHEW Publication N (PHS) 1979;Series 11-N: 78–1650.
7. Onis M, Garza C, Onyango AW, Borghi E. Comparison of the WHO Child Growth Standards and the CDC 2000 Growth Charts. J Nutr 2007;137:144–8.
8. Kramer MS, Kakuma R. The Optimal Duration of Exclusive Breastfeeding: A Systematic Review. Geneva: WHO; 2001. Available at: http://www.who.int./inf-pr-2001/en/note2001-07.html.
9. Weisstaub G, Soria R, Araya M. Improving quality of care for severe malnutrition [letter]. Lancet 2004;363:2090.
10. ACC/SCN. Fourth Report on The World Nutrition Situation: Nutrition Throughout the Life Cycle. Geneva: WHO/IFPRI; 2000.
11. de Onis M, Frongillo EA, Blossner M. Is malnutrition declining? An analysis of changes in levels of child malnutrition since 1980. Bull World Health Organ 2000;78:1222–33.
12. Smith CL, Haddad L, editors. IFPRI Explaining Child Malnutrition in Developing Countries: A Cross-Country Analysis. Washington DC: IFPRI; 2000.
13. Rice AL, Sacco L, Hyder A, Black R. Malnutrition as an underlying cause of childhood deaths associated with infectious diseases in developing countries. Bull World Health Organ 2000;78:1207–21.
14. Caulfield LE, de Onis M, Blössner M, Black RE. Undernutrition as an underlying cause of child deaths associated with diarrhea, pneumonia, malaria, and measles Am J Clin Nutr 2004;80:193–8.
15. Brown KH, Lutter CK. Potential role of processed complementary foods in the improvement of early childhood nutrition in Latin America. Food Nutr Bull 2000;21:5–11.
16. Brown LV, Zeitlin MF, Peterson KE, et al. Evaluation of the impact of weaning food messages on infant feeding practices and child growth in rural Bangladesh. Am J Clin Nutr 1992;56:994–1003.
17. Fogel RW. Economic growth, population theory, and physiology: The bearıng of long term processes on the making of economic policy. Am Econ Rev 1984;84:369–94.
18. Uauy R, Hertrampf E, Reddy M. Iron fortification of foods: Overcoming technical and practical barriers. J Nutr 2002;132:849S–52S.
19. Penny ME, Creed-Kanashiro HM, Robert RC, et al. Effectiveness of an educational intervention delivered through the health services to improve nutrition in young children: A cluster-randomised controlled trial. Lancet 2005;365:1863–72.
20. James WPT, Norum K, Smitasiri S, it al. Ending malnutrition by 2020: An agenda for change in the millennium. Food Nutr Bull 2000;21:1–88.
21. Schofield C, Ashworth A. Why have mortality rates for severe malnutrition remained so high? Bull World Health Organ 1996;74:223–9.
22. World Health Organization. Management of Severe Malnutrition: A Manual for Physicians and Other Senior Health Workers. Geneva: WHO; 1999. Available at: http://whqlibdoc.who.int/hq/1999/a57361.pdf.
23. Ashworth A, Khanum S, Jackson A, Schofield C. Guidelines for the Inpatient Treatment of Severely Malnourished Children. Geneva: WHO; 2003. Available at: http://whqlibdoc.who.int/publications/2003/9241546093.pdf.
24. World Health Organization. Training Course on the Management of Severe Malnutrition. WHO/NHD/02.4(P)1. Geneva: WHO; 2002.
25. Jackson AA, Ashworth A, Khanum S. Improving child survival: Malnutrition Task Force and the paediatrician's responsibility. Arch Dis Child 2006;91:706–10.
26. Ashworth A, Chopra M, MeCoy D, et al. WHO guidelines for management of severe malnutrition in rural South African hospitals: Effect on case fatality and the influence of operational factors. Lancet 2004;363:1110–5.
27. Collins S. Changing the way we address severe malnutrition during famine. Lancet 2001;358:498–501.
28. Collins S. Community-Based Therapeutic Care. A New Paradigm for Selective Feeding in Nutritional Crises. Overseas Development Institute, London: Humanitarian Practice Network; 2004.
29. Collins S, Sadler K, Dent N, et al. Key issues in the success of community-based management of severe malnutrition. Food Nutr Bull 2006;27:S49–82.
30. Collins S, Dent N, Binns P, et al. Management of severe acute malnutrition in children. Lancet 2006;368:1992–2000.
31. Ashworth A. Efficacy and effectiveness of community-based treatment of severe malnutrition. Food Nutr Bull 2006;27: S24–48.
32. Khanum S, Ashworth A, Huttly SRA. Controlled trial of three approaches to the treatment of severe malnutrition. Lancet 1994;344:1728–32.
33. Ashworth A, Khanum S. Cost-effective treatment for severely malnourished children: What is the best approach? Health Policy Plan 1997;12:115–21.
34. Monckeberg F, Riumallo J. Nutrition recovery centers: The Chilien experience. In: Underwood B, editor. Nutrition Intervention Strategies in National Development. New York: Academic Press; 1983. p. 189–99.
35. Uauy-Dagach R. The practice of clinical nutrition in a developing nation. J Nutr 1994;124:1449S–54S.
36. Albala C, Vio F, Kain J, Uauy R. Nutrition transition in Latin America: The case of Chile. Nutr Rev 2001;59:170–6.
37. FAO-Perfiles Nutricionales por países. Chile, octubre 2001. Available at: ftp://ftp.fao.org/es/esn/nutrition/ncp/chimap.pdf. Accessed on: January 16, 2007.
38. Sempé P, Sempé M, Padrón G. Croissance et maduration osseuse. Paris: Theraplix; 1971.
39. Walter T, Hertrampf E, Olivares M, Pizarro F. Fortification. In: Ramakrisshnan U, editor. Nutritional Anemias, Series in Modern Nutrition. Boca Raton, FL: CRC Press; 2001. p. 153–83.
40. Riumalló J. Situación de la Yodación en Chile. Informe Técnico. Unidad de Nutrición, Ministerio de Salud, Chile; 1995.
41. Muzzo, S. Situación de la Nutrición en Yodo en Escolares de Cuatro Zonas Censoras. Informe a UNICEF; 1994.
42. Gómez F, Ramos Galvan R, Frenk S, et al. Mortalidad asociada a la malnutrición de segundo y tercer grado. Bull World Health Organ 2000;78:1275–80.
43. Uauy R, Albala C, Kain J. Obesity trends in Latin America: Transiting from under- to overweight. J Nutr 2001;131: 893S–9S.
44. Uauy R, Kain J. The epidemiological transition: Need to incorporate obesity prevention into nutrition programs. Public Health Nutr 2002;5:223–9.

Community Nutrition and Its Impact on Children: Industrialized Countries

Johanna Dwyer, DSc, RD
Melanie A. Stuart, MS, RD
Kristy Hendricks, DSc, RD

If the future of a society is to be shaped by its children, then a strong national commitment is needed to develop their bodies, minds, and spirits. Good nutrition plays a role in growth, development and later health, prevention, control and treatment of disease, and improvement of quality of life. Community efforts are key to making this happen.

REASONS FOR CONCERN

Nutrition is an important component of health care for infants, children, and adolescents. Infants grow rapidly and have requirements for protein, energy, and other essential nutrients that are higher per unit of body weight than at any other time in childhood, making them vulnerable to dietary deficiencies and growth failure. Dietary habits of toddlers and preschoolers are important in shaping their later health and may play a role in increasing or decreasing obesity, blood pressure, serum cholesterol, and dental caries later in life. Adolescence, a time of emotional, physical, social, biologic, and educational transitions, is a period with particular susceptibility to weight concerns, eating disorders, alcohol abuse, and other poor dietary habits. Children with special health care needs at all ages, because of a variety of disabilities, handicaps, and chronic illnesses and conditions they may have, often need special complex and involved care and require particular attention to enable them to achieve their maximum potential.

Eating patterns begin to develop early in childhood and can profoundly affect health throughout life. In childhood, the immediate effects of improper diet are most apparent in such conditions as failure to thrive, obesity, the dietary deficiency diseases, and fetal alcohol effects. Later, chronic degenerative disease risks increase. The leading causes of death and disability for adults today include cancer, heart disease, stroke, osteoporosis, and alcoholism. Each involves risks associated with dietary patterns, as well as other preventable factors. Programs for the family and community must be designed to accommodate all of these diet-related problems.

COMMUNITY NUTRITION AND CHILDREN TODAY

The current status of some key national indicators of child well-being in the United States today has recently been summarized.[1] In the year 2004, there were 73 million children under age 18 in the United States, about 25% of the population, down from the peak of 36% in 1964 at the end of the baby boom. America's children are racially and ethnically diverse. In 2005, 60% of US children were white nonHispanic, 20% were white Hispanic, 15% were black nonHispanic, 4% were Asian or Pacific Islanders, and 1% were American Indians and Native Americans. In that same year, 67% of children under 18 lived in a family with two married parents; most of the others lived with their mothers. From birth to kindergarten age, fully 61% of children received child care on a regular basis from a caretaker who was not their parent.

For many socioeconomic and health indicators, gains have been impressive over the past decade. For example, with respect to poverty, the rate for children living with their families is now 17%, which is lower than it has been for decades. In 2004, 19% lived in households reporting any level of food insecurity, rates that were lower than in prior years. However, problems still exist. For example, children in families below the poverty line are much more likely to experience food insecurity and hunger than their peers in families above the poverty line. According to the Healthy Eating Index in 2000, 27% of children 2 to 5 years had "good" scores, whereas only about 15% of those 6 to 9 years of age did. Children in families living in poverty were less likely than those from higher-income families to have a dietary pattern rated as "good." They also tended to be in poorer health than their more affluent counterparts. Therefore, many health and nutritional problems remain. Ways of ameliorating them by community-wide interventions are the focus of this chapter.

As a nation, we have made great strides in nutrition over the past century. The situation today differs dramatically from that in 1900, when dietary deficiency disease and undernutrition were the major problems.[2] Then, undernutrition and food insecurity were major societal problems. Now although there are still some individuals who suffer from these problems. there are new faces to malnutrition. Overnutrition and obesity are increasing; 18% of children aged 6 to 17 years were overweight in 2003 to 2004. Sometimes overweight coexists in the same individuals who suffer from other dietary deficiencies. Although malnutrition, starvation, and dietary deficiency diseases will probably continue to be problems in some areas in the United States in the future, more prevalent nutrition problems involving overconsumption and imbalances in the types and amounts of food consumed and excesses of certain nutrients are also challenges, particularly in an environment of physical inactivity.[2] Obesity is a prevalent and growing problem.[3] Social and economic changes, such as altered family structures with more single parents, increasing ethnic diversity, a predominantly urban maternal and child population, high rates of poverty among children and their families, and more eating outside of the home, are some key variables in explaining the new forms of malnutrition we see today.[4]

THE FUTURE

There will be more children and a greater percentage of children in the population by the year 2010 than there are today.[1] For this reason alone, continued efforts to improve child health at the community level are necessary. Whether America's children will be healthier than ever before in the future will depend on sustained efforts on the part of parents and caretakers as well as the larger community. Systems for tracking health promotion and disease prevention objectives that include nutrition and other aspects of child and family health are now available that permit us to monitor our progress and to make corrections to improve health when they are necessary.

DEFINITIONS

Public Health

Public health is "the science and art of preventing disease, prolonging life, and promoting health and efficiency through organized community effort, so organizing these benefits as to enable every citizen to realize his birthright of health and longevity."[5] The goal of public health is to attain the highest level of physical, mental, and social well-being and longevity consistent with available knowledge and resources at a given time and place.[6] It accomplishes these objectives by focusing on the community or on large population groups rather than on individuals, on planning and monitoring rather than on delivering services.

Community Nutrition

Communities are groups of individuals or families living in a defined geographic area who live and work together, hold similar values, are influenced by the same environment, and share a number of common concerns. An understanding of the influences of society and of the community is necessary for planning effective nutrition interventions. Community nutrition applies scientific knowledge in food, nutrition, and health to a specific group of people to improve their health and welfare. To be successful, it must take into consideration the wide range of societal influences and constraints.

The community nutritionist must take into account an individual's cultural eating habits, ethnic background, income, health history, clinical assessment, dietary intake, and use of community nutrition programs to screen, assess needs, and intervene effectively.

The objectives of community nutrition are to promote health; prevent nutrient deficiencies, excesses, and imbalances; prevent diet-related diseases or conditions; and rehabilitate those suffering from nutrition-related problems. This is done by promoting healthful eating habits, ensuring access to food, and integrating nutrition into primary, secondary, and tertiary health care services.[2] Thus, it represents the traditional public health concerns (such as mass prevention and intervention measures) as well as a personal health services focus to ensure that high-risk, high-priority children especially receive health and other services they need. In this respect, community nutrition represents a fusion of both the personal health service's focus on individuals and the public health focus on the entire population.

GOALS OF COMMUNITY NUTRITION

The US Department of Health and Human Services' (DHHS) Healthy People 2010 plan singles out nutrition as essential to promote optimal health and prevent disease and provides nutrition goals for children and adolescents, which are listed in Table 1.[7] The midcourse review is now in process, but it is already obvious that some objectives, especially those related to overweight, are not being met. This chapter focuses on needs and meeting these goals at the community level.

Table 1 Healthy People 2010 Nutrition-Related Goals for Children and Adolescents

Increase abstinence from alcohol use by pregnant women
Increase to at least 80% those women of childbearing age who take a vitamin with the recommended 0.4 mg folic acid daily
Reduce low birth weight to no more than 5% of live births and very low birth weight to 1% or less
Increase to 75% mothers who breast-feed their babies in the early postpartum period, to at least 50% those who breast-feed until their infants are 6 mo old, and to at least 25% those who breast-feed until their infants are 1 yr old
Reduce growth retardation among low-income children aged 5 and younger to 5% or less
Reduce to 5% or less the prevalence of overweight and obesity (defined as at or above the sex- and age-specific 95th percentile of BMI from the NCHS/CDC growth charts) in children aged 6–11 and adolescents 12–19 yr
In those 2 years of age and older, increase to at least
75% those who meet the dietary guidelines' average daily goal of no more than 30% of calories from fat
75% those who meet the dietary guidelines' average daily goal of less than 10% of calories from saturated fat
75% those who meet the dietary guidelines' minimum average daily goal of at least five servings of vegetables and fruits
80% those who meet the dietary guidelines' minimum average daily goal of at least six servings of grain products
90% those who meet dietary recommendations for calcium
65% those who meet the daily value of 2,400 mg or less of sodium consistent with the dietary guidelines
Reduce iron deficiency to 5% or less among children 1–2 yr, to less than 1% among children 3–4 yr
Increase the proportion of children and adolescents 6–19 yr whose intake of meals and snacks at school from all sources contributes proportionally to good overall dietary quality
Increase the proportion of the nation's public and private elementary schools that teach all essential nutrition education topics to their students in at least three different grades and the proportion of middle/junior high and high schools that teach all essential nutrition education topics in at least one required course
Increase the prevalence of food security among US households to at least 94% of all households

Adapted from US Department of Health and Human Services.
BMI = body mass index; CDC = Centers for Disease Control and Prevention; NCHS = National Center for Health Statistics.

The goals of child nutrition programs are to optimize growth and decrease the risk of all diet-related diseases. Strategies to accomplish the goals in the community must include consideration of the child's family; the efforts of the child, the family, and many members of the health care team; and contributions by institutions as well as economic resources in the health, food, education, and welfare sectors of the community. A supportive physical environment is also important.

In the community setting, strategies should focus on health promotion, early intervention, and prevention of diet-related diseases in groups of children and their families. In addition, community-level efforts must focus on ensuring that preventive and curative health services are in place.

Federal and state governments have been committed to promoting child health since early in this century.[8] However, the many programs they have instituted are useless unless communities make them available and families take advantage of them. Both states and communities exhibit considerable variation in the extent to which they provide supportive services and extra funds for reaching nutrition objectives. Detailed advice is available for discovering and mobilizing community nutrition resources.[9]

In the clinical setting, community nutrition-related strategies should focus on providing anticipatory guidance, preventive activities, and control of clinical problems involving both primary and secondary malnutrition in all children but particularly in high-risk children.

All health care team members need to understand the importance of community nutrition, know what programs are (or should be) available, know how to obtain them for patients and clients, and know how to advocate their extension. Otherwise, those who provide direct care to children may fail to meet all of their nutrition needs.

HISTORY OF COMMUNITY NUTRITION AND HEALTH

Only in the twentieth century did the federal government begin to play a role in ensuring and safeguarding the health of American children. The Children's Bureau was established in the Department of Labor in 1912 to "investigate and report ... upon all matters pertaining to the welfare of children and child life among all classes of our people."[8] It was the forerunner of efforts now centered in the Maternal and Child Health Bureau of the DHHS. The first federal grants-in-aid to the states for planning to improve infant and maternal health were authorized by the Sheppard-Towner Act of 1921. This legislation was first administered by the Children's Bureau in the Labor Department, but since the 1960s, the US Public Health Service in the DHHS has administered such programs.

Title V of the Social Security Act of 1935 initiated the federal and state partnership for maternal and child health that served as the major impetus for the development of public health nutrition services for mothers and children. The states used these federal funds for planning and developing a wide range of programs to improve the health of mothers and children. In 1981, Title V changed with the creation of the Maternal and Child Health Service Block Grant, which provided monies with fewer specific requirements and more state discretion within the general realm of maternal and child health needs. Fifty-nine states and jurisdictions now receive funding. The federal government also provides small amounts of federal set-aside funds to support special projects of regional or national significance. Other categorical programs for specific purposes are funded from the DHHS, the US Department of Agriculture (USDA), and other branches of government. With these funds and their own matching resources, the states provide a variety of services. However, access to health care remains an unresolved issue today.[10,11] Lack of access to medical nutrition therapy and other health services is a major problem for children who have health problems that cannot be solved by community nutrition or public health efforts. Community efforts supplement, but are not substitutes for, individual health services.[12]

Today more than 2,000 public health nutritionists are employed in federal, state, and local public health agencies. They also serve as members of health care teams, where they have the responsibility of assessing community nutrition needs as well as planning and directing programs of nutrition services for individuals. Many other health professionals, including over 60,000 registered dietitians, devote some of their time and effort beyond the scope of individual counseling to community programs and also play a role in ensuring that community nutrition needs are met.

NUTRITION SCREENING, ASSESSMENT, AND INTERVENTION

Nutrition screening, assessment, and intervention are important at both the level of the individual patient and that of population groups. A systematic approach and an integrated structure for screening, assessing, and intervening are needed to deal with nutrition problems in both health and social service settings.[13] The approach is summarized in Table 2. Details on how nutrition screening and assessment apply to individuals are provided elsewhere in this book.

The first step in developing an appropriate care plan for a community is nutrition screening of the entire maternal and child population to identify major problems. This may involve examination of relevant statistics and resources of actual surveys. Next, the specific subpopulation of interest must be considered. Screening aims both to increase nutrition awareness among communities, families, and health professionals and to identify factors increasing nutritional risks in target groups. In the community nutrition context, the screening process might involve review of health indicators, such as the prevalence of low birth weight, with further delineation of high-risk groups using income, ethnicity, age, and other characteristics of parents or infants. Those groups who are found to be at risk are then further assessed.

The second step in care planning is a comprehensive nutritional assessment of the community in which the children live. Nutrition screening and assessment should be used in an effort to find groups at especially high nutritional risk. Some nutritional issues can be easily assessed and remedied by the health and social service systems. Others require further medical or social assessment before the causes of the malnutrition can be assessed. The process of setting priorities for intervention among the groups found to be in need of services and allocating resources appropriately to these efforts depends on the individual initiative and political will of the group's providers.

The final step in care planning is intervention, which may be at either the individual or the community level. This may involve nutritional measures such as food or counseling or other interventions that improve nutritional status more indirectly, such as oral health, pharmacy, social, and mental health services. The ultimate goal is to prevent, control, or ameliorate nutrition-related problems. The end result should always be to improve or ameliorate children's health.

NUTRITIONAL MONITORING AND SURVEILLANCE AT THE STATE AND NATIONAL LEVELS

Monitoring and surveillance are analogous to repeated screening and evaluation efforts at the individual level. Monitoring is the periodic measurement of factors that indicate that changes in nutritional status have occurred. It applies to specific individuals, communities, and the general population. Surveillance is the continuous and regular collection of data that are compiled to detect warning signs of problems at the community level early enough to provide feedback for health care team members.

The purpose of monitoring and surveillance is to provide continuous, reliable information on a community's nutritional status and the factors that influence it to find ways to improve it.

National nutrition monitoring involves measurement of health status, food supply, food consumption and composition, and dietary knowledge and attitudes.[13,15] At the federal level today, nutrition monitoring and surveillance are conducted by several different government agencies. Within the DHHS, the National Center for Health Statistics of the Centers for Disease Control and Prevention (CDC) conducts the National Health and Nutrition Examination Survey (NHANES). NHANES is a periodic,

Table 2 Pediatric Nutrition Screening, Assessment, and Intervention in the Community

Screen for risk: identify individuals and groups in the community needing further assessment for potential health problems with nutritional implications	Look for the following *"DETERMINE"* risk factors: *D*isease *E*ating disorders *T*ooth decay *E*conomic hardship *R*educed nutrition education *M*ulticultural issues *I*nadequate food intake *N*utrient deficiencies *E*levated or reduced body weight
Screen and assess community resources	Determine whether nutrition resources are adequate, which groups are at high risk, and extent to which community nutrition needs are being met by existing programs. Tools include demographics, socioeconomic stratification, health statistics, local health resources, cultural factors, housing, food supply, child nutrition programs, social welfare programs, education, occupational data, etc
Assess child: confirm that diet-related problems are present and whether growth and nutrition are inadequate owing to dietary deficiency, excess, or imbalance or secondary to disease	Follow the *ABCDEF*s of assessing nutritional status: *A*nthropometrics: height, weight, triceps skinfold, arm circumference *B*iochemical: hemoglobin/hematocrit, albumin, transferrin *C*linical: skin, tongue, hair *D*ietary intake: by 24-h recall *E*mpathy *F*unctional status at all levels: physical, mental, emotional
Intervene at individual and community levels	identify and use community and individual health care resources, using the mnemonic SOMe Meds and Nutrition: *S*ocial services *O*ral health *M*ental health *Med*ical care and medications *Nutrition* counseling, education, and support

Adapted from references 13 and 14.

population-based survey providing national data on specific health status measures, including dietary intake, eating habits, and biochemical and anthropometric indices related to nutrition. NHANES is now continuously in the field. The NHANES data provide useful benchmarks for the health of these groups. However, the number of children and adolescents surveyed is small, and not all relevant problems can be examined in each survey. Therefore, occasionally, special surveys have been conducted that oversample these groups.

In 1999, the USDA's CSFII (Continuous Survey of Food Intake of Individuals) was merged with the NHANES. Both the USDA and the CDC's National Center for Health Statistics now partner on the dietary portion of the survey, which is called "What We Eat in America." The combined survey has been conducted each year since then and recent results are available at http://www.cdc.gov/nchs/nhanes.htm.

The USDA monitors food security in the United States through an annual survey of 40,000 US households conducted as a supplement to the US Census Bureau's nationally representative Current Population Survey. The most recent food security survey revealed that 89% of US households were food secure. The remaining 11% were food insecure; at some time during the prior year, these households were uncertain about having or were unable to acquire enough food to meet the basic needs of all house-hold members because they had insufficient money or other resources.[15] Single mothers with children had the highest levels of food stress. Minority group black and Hispanic households also had rates of food insecurity and hunger above the national average.

The USDA also provides funds for grants and contracts to universities and nonprofit organizations to perform analysis and research in support of improving food consumption practices. These include rating food intakes of various portions of the population from national survey data using the Healthy Eating Index,[16] which is currently available at http://www.cnpp.usda.gov/Publications/HEI/healthyeatingindex2005factsheet.pdf. Also program-specific analyses, such as studies of the National School Lunch and Breakfast Programs are available.[17]

Many other publications on these and other programs are available at http://www.ers.usda.gov.

The CDC of the DHHS conducts ongoing state-based nutritional monitoring activities. The database consists of data collected on children and pregnant women enrolled in health department clinics, the special supplemental nutrition program for women, infants, and children (WIC), and the Head Start programs at the state and local levels. Programs include the pediatric nutrition surveillance system, the pregnancy surveillance system, and the severe pediatric undernutrition surveillance systems. These surveys are not necessarily representative of the entire population but provide much useful data on groups at special risk.[18]

DIVISION OF LABOR: MANAGEMENT OF COMMUNITY NUTRITION SERVICES

The management process consists of planning, organizing, implementing, directing, controlling, and monitoring. The dynamic aspects of the process of community nutrition service management are illustrated in Figure 1 and occur on two levels. First, there is program management at the indirect service level, which includes macrolevel planning, administration, supervision, consultation, and training, as well as screening and assessment of problems at the community level. Program management and evaluation efforts generally occur at this level. Second, direct service delivery may be provided to both groups and individuals, and this includes screening, assessment, intervention, and follow up. Both levels must focus on the child and his or her family if the programs are ultimately to be effective.

Planning

Planning is a process of devising a course of action to reduce uncertainty and to anticipate and initiate change. Community nutrition planning involves analyzing subjective and objective data, writing mission statements, setting goals and objectives, and activating means of achieving objectives. Nutrition planning is influenced by the internal culture and capabilities of each organization involved, as well as by the public agenda, state of scientific knowledge, wants and needs of the families, and advocacy of experts, parents, and professional groups.

Community nutritionists should participate in the planning processes of the agency, study the agency or community health plans, know those who participate in the planning group, get involved, and involve others. Planning goes beyond administrators, leaders, and program managers and should include those who will be responsible for implementation and those who will be recipients of services.[20]

Planning for high-priority nutrition problems can be aided by forming alliances with related constituencies in the service network. Some examples are collaborative planning by nutrition service providers, advocates, and patients. This sort of collaboration may build political support and bridge organizational and ideological boundaries, identify mutual goals, and build cohesion and capacity to act together if potential

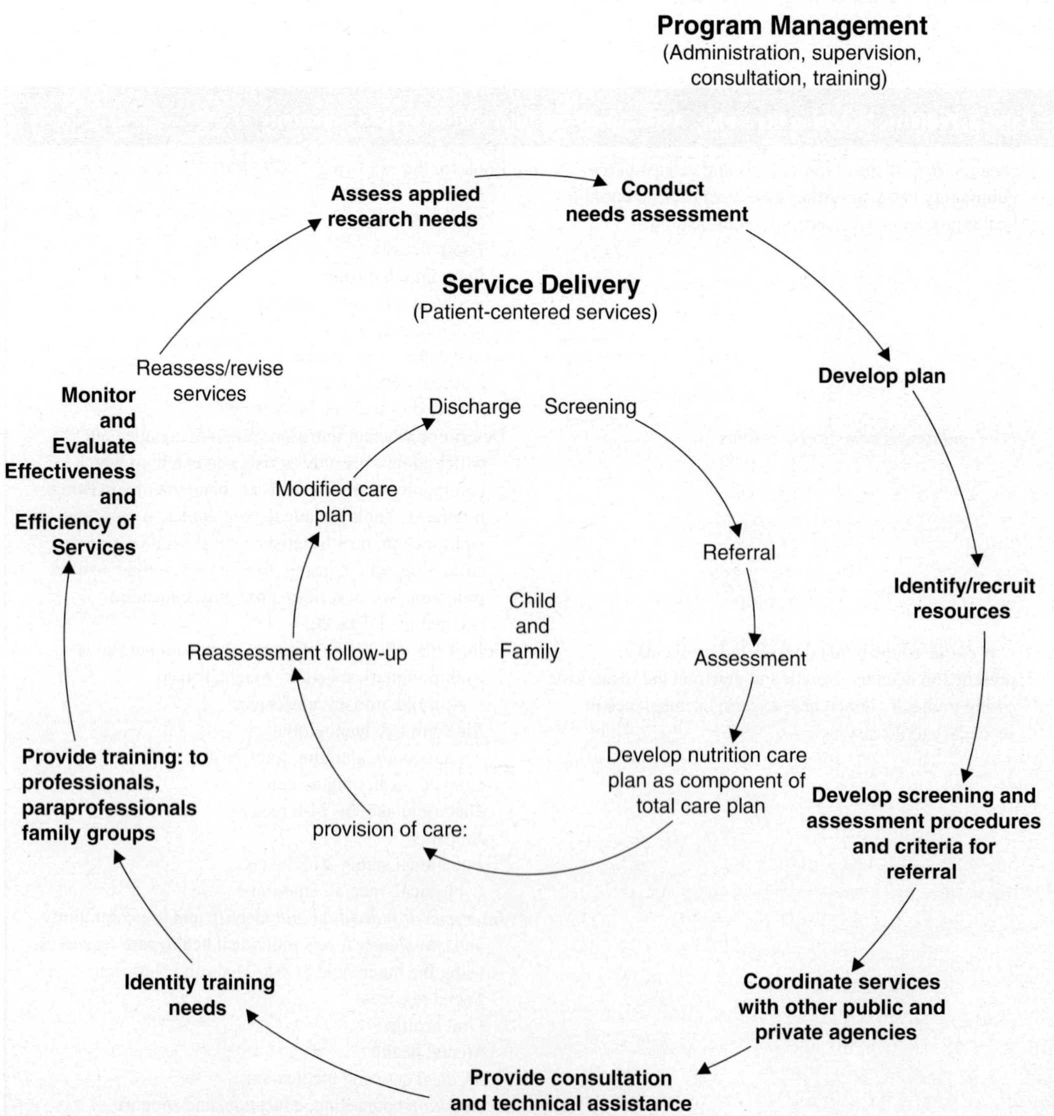

Figure 1 System for nutrition services. (Adapted from reference 19.)

adversaries are approached, co-opted, and included in the process. In some instances, it may assist in making difficult decisions about using limited resources.

Implementing

Planning identifies what to do. Implementation begins the process of doing. Effective community nutrition program implementation requires administrative support (budget, staff, space, equipment); commitment of staff to program goals, objectives, and interventions; and support and respect of a target population who is also convinced of the benefits of the program and willing to commit time and effort to participate.

Screening and assessment at the community level are the responsibilities of the community nutritionist, who ensures that systems are in place in community programs and encourages their institution in personal health services. Nutrition screening and assessment also occur at the direct service delivery level, where they are usually administered by health or social welfare care team members such as dietitians, physicians, nurses, social workers, and physical therapists.

The role of the community nutritionist in implementing programs varies. Depending on the health and nutritional problems found, children and/or families are referred to different community and personal health services for interventions including nutritional counseling, food, welfare education, and health programs or to private physicians.

Monitoring and Evaluation

Community nutrition program implementation must be systematically monitored by the collection and analysis of appropriate data to provide the continuous feedback needed to assess performance. Evaluation involves the systematic measurement of results by comparing the data collected with preestablished standards or controls to decide whether to continue, expand, redesign, or terminate the program.

Monitoring must also be accomplished at both direct and indirect service levels. At the direct personal health service delivery level, the health care team evaluates program impact on a population or community by observing improvements in health. At the indirect level, the management of the community nutrition program may also evaluate effectiveness, efficiency, and cost through cost-effectiveness analysis to determine whether the program's benefits are sufficient to offset its cost. One current effort of this type is the Preventive Health Services Task Force. Its publications on health services that are viewed as effective are increasingly being used as a guide for services.[21]

Another key document for monitoring progress at the community level is the tracking system for the Healthy People 2010 objectives.[22]

CURRENT NUTRITIONAL STATUS OF INFANTS, CHILDREN, AND ADOLESCENTS

This section summarizes the major problems of different age groups today and some diet-related risk factors. It provides recommendations needing incorporation in both community nutrition programs and personal health and social services for children.

Some nutrition problems such as iron deficiency anemia, growth retardation, dental caries, obesity, and possibly diet-related decreased resistance to infection affect some children at all ages and are matters of concern across the entire developmental period.[23] Others, as described below, affect specific age groups.

Pregnant Women and Infants

Community concern about good nutrition should start before birth. Nutritional needs in pregnancy and lactation at both the individual and community levels have recently been summarized.[23–25] High-risk women who are poor need to be enrolled in the WIC and provided with nutrition counseling, food education, and other specialized health services.

Adequate nutrition is vital for premature, small-for-date, and other low-birth-weight infants who are at risk of developmental disadvantage. (See other chapters in this volume for more details.) Early intervention programs to encourage and promote good nutrition among those infants most in need are of particular concern.

The March of Dimes recently published a report that summarizes interventions that are needed to deal with the new faces of nutritional problems that confront Americans today, particularly those that affect those in the childbearing years.[26] These include not only undernutrition and food insecurity but also nutritional imbalances and excesses. The report emphasizes prevention, not only in one-on-one health visits but also by social marketing and health communications to create healthier environments in the larger community. The importance of prevention particularly targeting childhood and preconceptional females is highlighted. Some of the key recommendations of the report that have implications for community nutrition include the following:

Early Nutrition Matters. Attending to early nutrition of infants and children under 2 years is critical. Steps include promoting and supporting exclusive breast-feeding for 6 months and continued breast-feeding with complementary foods up to 12 months of age or longer. The special needs of nutritionally at-risk infants, including preterm and/or low-birth-weight infants, must be ensured. Promotion and support of programs to ensure adequate intakes in pregnant and lactating mothers and the introduction of safe, nutritionally adequate, and developmentally appropriate complementary foods are needed.

Healthy Weight Matters. It is important to increase awareness of healthy weight throughout the life cycle to improve health, including good pregnancy outcomes. Those who are at risk of pregnancy with body mass indices under 18.5 or over 25 should reduce them to more healthful levels. Increasing the average age at first pregnancy will permit full maturation before childbearing. Women who are pregnant need assistance to gain a healthful amount of weight during pregnancy and also may need help in achieving a healthy weight after birth.

Nutritious, Safe Food, and Diet Quality Matter. Food-based dietary guidelines must address the nutritional requirements of periconceptional, pregnant, and lactating women and very young children. When it is not possible to meet all of their needs through available food sources, including fortified foods, appropriate specific vitamin, and mineral supplements for women of childbearing age, infants, and young children should be provided.

Nutrition is especially critical in the first year of life.[27] Nutrient needs are high because growth and development are more rapid in infancy than at any other time after birth. Weight usually triples and height doubles in the first year. Approximately a third of calories consumed is used for growth during the first 4 months. This rapid growth in the healthy term infant during the first 4 months of life requires more energy, protein, and other essential nutrients per unit of body weight than at any other time in infancy or childhood. Feeding nourishing foods to infants promotes adequate growth and good health.

The gastrointestinal tract of the newborn infant is well developed but immature. All of the secretions of the digestive tract contain enzymes especially suited to the digestion of human milk. The ability to handle foods other than human milk or formula depends on the physiologic development of the infant. Thus, it is important to encourage breast-feeding and to feed infants age-appropriate foods selected on the basis of their developmental readiness.[27] Not only will this help to prevent complications, it will also help to build positive attitudes about food and eating.

Attention to feeding the appropriate type and amount of food is essential. All parents and caretakers need appropriate advice and guidance. For the poor at high risk, WIC, which provides food, health services, and education, may be in order. For the ill, Title V and Medicaid-supported health services, as well as special services for those with especially severe handicapping conditions, may be in order.

Some of the common nutritional and health problems and related risk factors in infants that need attention by community nutritionists are summarized in Table 3. Table 4 provides recommendations for promoting good nutritional status during this period.

Table 3 Current Nutritional Issues and Recommendations for Infants

Current Health Problems	Related Nutrition Risk Factors
Growth retardation, underweight	Dietary inadequacies, low birth weight, inappropriate introduction of foods
Dental caries	Excessive, frequent consumption of sweets that are retained in the mouth, baby bottle toothdecay, lack of fluoride
Iron deficiency anemia	Early introduction of cow's milk, malnutrition, inadequate dietary iron intake
Other nutrient deficiencies	Inadequate intake of certain nutrients, lack of appropriate supplements
Infections	Malnutrition, lack of breast-feeding

What Needs to Be Done?

- Improve nutrition training of health professionals
- Increase nutrition counseling and education of parents and caretakers
- Strengthen breast-feeding support
- Develop nutrition and feeding guidelines for agencies responsible for the administration of health, social welfare, and related program services
- Enhance the research base for current issues in infant nutrition
- Prevent or treat inappropriate weight gain

Table 4 Recommendations for Enhancing the Nutritional Status of Infants

Early Infancy (0–6 mo)

- Breast-feed until 4–6 mo of age
- If breast milk is not provided, feed with a hygienic, nutritionally adequate source of heat-treated for mula until 4–6 mo of age
- Supplement with vitamin D and iron if the infant is solely breast-fed for the first 6 mo of life or if these are not provided in formula
- Supplement with fluoride if the water or formula is devoid in the nutrient
- Avoid unsuitable feedings (solids, cow's milk, and skim milk) under 6 mo of age and encourage breast-feeding and adequate supplementation
- Ensure that the infant receives enough food by monitoring growth
- Use proper feeding techniques to avoid gas, aspiration, and other problems
- Delay introduction of solid foods until age 5–6 mo, when the infant is developmentally ready to deal with them
- Avoid foods commonly causing allergies, intolerances, or hypersensitivities
- Ensure that water intakes are adequate
- If family resources are inadequate, obtain assistance from federally sponsored food programs for infants and children
- Obtain relevant anticipatory guidance on feeding and health

Later Infancy (6–12 mo)

- Use iron-fortified formulas, iron supplements, and iron-fortified cereals
- Ensure a gradual transition to family diets rather than attempting to wean suddenly
- Introduce solid foods sequentially after 4–6 mo when the child is developmentally ready and needs supplementary feedings
- Take common problems in stride. Temporary refusals of solid foods at weaning and failures to switch over from pureed or baby foods to foods that must be chewed are normal setbacks
- Consult health providers if feeding problems persist
- Encourage self-feeding
- Realize that some decrease in appetite in late infancy is to be expected as growth slows and that it is no cause for alarm
- Avoid struggles and battles of will with the child about food
- Keep environments safe (especially with respect to lead and common household chemicals, which are poisonous) and begin to teach child to shun mouthing and eating nonfood objects
- Begin oral hygiene measures

Preschool and School-Aged Children

Table 5 outlines some of the current nutritional concerns and Table 6 provides recommendations on promoting good nutrition after infancy in the preschool and school years.

In late infancy, children begin to learn to feed themselves independently. They progress from eating with their hands to using utensils. Children need to be independent and able to try new skills to help them develop positive attitudes about food and eating.

Children's growth rates slow considerably after the first year of age, resulting in decreased appetite and food intake. This normal phenomenon is often mistaken for poor appetite, although it is not. In spite of the slower growth rates, appropriate nutrition is vital to provide needed nutrients and energy to maintain resistance to infections, materials needed to build new tissues as growth proceeds, and adequate nutrient stores.

Good nutrition is important to sustain growth and permit development. It is especially important in the weaning period to prevent the risks of iron deficiency anemia, dental caries, and obesity and diet-related risks that may contribute to later hyperlipidemia and hypertension.

Obesity is increasing in Americans, with estimates of obesity in 10 to 30% of school-aged children.[28,29] Therefore, attention to nutrition must not be neglected in the preschool, primary, and middle school years. In 2001, the US surgeon general called for immediate action on obesity, particularly in children and adolescents.[30] Today 13% of children and adolescents are overweight, and these figures among adolescents have tripled since 1980. Also, associated conditions such as asthma and type 2 diabetes are rising among children, and diet-related chronic disease risks linked to obesity are also on the rise. Minorities and low-income families often are particularly afflicted. Therefore, there is a need for immediate action. The National Institutes of Health have produced many useful materials that are on line to help that can be accessed at http://wecan.nhlbi.nih.gov, and additional publications are available at the CDC's Division of Nutrition and Physical Activity (access at http://www.cdc.gov/nccdphp/dnpa/publications. Strategies that communities can use in helping to address overweight and obesity especially in children and adolescents involve "*CARE*": communication of the problem and steps to correct it, actions, research, and evaluation. These action options include the following:

Physical Activity. Require daily, quality physical education at all school grades. Today only about one in three teenagers nationwide take part in some form of physical education, and about half play on at least one sports team. It is also important to provide safe and accessible facilities for the recreation of people of all ages. Community facilities should be available for physical activity

Table 5 Current Nutritional Issues and Recommendations for Children

Current Health Problems	Related Nutrition Risk Factor
Obesity	Caloric consumption exceeds caloric need
Failure to thrive	Dietary inadequacies
Iron deficiency anemia	Malnutrition, inadequate dietary iron intake
Dental caries	Excessive, frequent consumption of foods high in sugar and starch with poor oral hygiene
High blood pressure	Overweight, high sodium intake
High blood cholesterol	Excessive intakes of saturated fat trans-fat and cholesterol

What needs to be done?

- Achieve adequate nutrition services in daycare programs and early childhood education (head start)
- Increase participation in and coverage of child nutrition programs (school lunch and breakfast)
- Increase parent and community nutrition education
- Improve nutrition training of health professionals
- Enhance the research base to answer existing questions in child nutrition
- Change policy to integrate nutrition services into all aspects of child health care

Table 6 Recommendations for Enhancing Nutritional Status in Children

Preschool years
Ensure that levels of physical activity and rest suffice to maintain normal growth and development and a good appetite
Provide nutritious food in the home and in other settings in which the child eats to encourage good food choices
Teach the child to choose and eat nutritious foods for meals and snacks
Avoid sugary starchy snacks that are retained in the mouth and encourage oral hygiene practices to promote good dental health
Foster appropriate eating behaviors by providing suitable role models, by permitting the child to choose food portions, by giving some latitude in food preferences, by exposing him or her to new foods, by fostering table manners appropriate to his or her developmental level, and by keeping meals as times for social interchange
Recognize and deal with feeding problems early before they become well established
Handle struggles over food reasonably to avoid the development of feeding problems
Feed and hydrate children appropriately during illness
Help the child grow out of fatness by encouraging physical activity
Ensure that iron needs are met by wise food choices
Ensure that the child learns to distinguish food and nonfood objects
School years
Monitor growth in height to ensure that nutritional status is satisfactory
Provide good examples and guidance to instill healthful habits and attitudes about foods and eating
Establish consistent guidelines and follow them to ensure that the child's diet is nutritionally adequate
Promote eating and physical activity habits that will foster normal body fatness
If excessive fatness is a problem, encourage child to increase physical activity and help him or her to cut energy intakes slightly so that the child can grow out of his or her fatness
Ensure that diet-related risks of dental caries are minimized
Help the child to distinguish between reliable sources of information on food choices and promotional messages, which may be unreliable
Ensure dietary moderation with respect to dietary fat, cholesterol, sugar, and sodium
Ensure that diets are adequate in fiber
Ensure that iron needs are met by wise food choices

for all people, including on the weekends, and there should be more opportunities for physical activity at work sites. At the same time, it is important to reduce the time people spend in watching television and in other sedentary behaviors. In 1999, 43% of high school students reported watching two or more hours of television a day.

Food Options. Ensure the availability of more food options that are low in saturated fat and calories, as well as fruits, vegetables, whole grains, and low-fat or nonfat dairy products, on school campuses and at school events. It is important to enforce existing USDA regulations that prohibit serving foods of minimal nutritional value during mealtimes in school food-service areas, including vending machines. MyPyramid.gov Web site provides a special food guide for children with smaller portions called MyPyramid for Kids.

Communications. Change the perception of obesity so that health, and not simply personal appearance, becomes the chief concern. This means providing appropriate education in schools and communities and training of health professionals about healthful eating habits and regular physical activity, based on the dietary guidelines for Americans, for people of all ages.

Growth Monitoring. New growth charts are now available for children and adolescents to evaluate their size and growth.[30,31] They need to be used on a continuing basis, and can be accessed at http://www.cdc.gov/nchs/about/major/nhanes/rowthcharts/htm.

Adolescents

Puberty is a unique and complex developmental period marking the transition from childhood to adulthood. It is accompanied by a series of physical, physiologic, biochemical, hormonal, social, and psychological changes. Adolescence is a nutritionally vulnerable period for several reasons. A dramatic increase in physical growth occurs during puberty. The growth spurt is highly sensitive to nutrient deprivation. Inadequate nutrition during this time may delay or stunt linear growth.[32] Alterations in body composition in puberty and during the consolidation that occurs in later adolescence, as maturity is reached, increase nutrient and energy needs. During the second decade of life, children gain about 20% of their adult height and 50% of their adult weight.[33] After puberty, although linear growth ceases, changes continue until maturity is reached.

The larger body requires increased amounts of nutrients. Calcium is a nutrient of particular concern because bone growth and bone mass accumulate rapidly during this time of life. Osteoporosis is a disease that afflicts mostly the elderly, but just as is the case with atherosclerosis, its seeds are sown in childhood. One of the most effective ways to prevent osteoporosis is to build a strong, dense skeleton during the growing years to act as a reserve later in life. Moreover, changes in individual behaviors and lifestyle preferences in younger children may last through adolescence and into adulthood, again contributing a lifetime of optimal bone health. Increasing attention is being paid to school programs that will increase bone accretion and muscular strength in children starting in early elementary school, aged 5 to 7 years of age, and continuing into adolescence. The interventions now being tested include weight-loading physical activity and calcium-rich snacks for children as well as age-appropriate, behaviorally focused active learning to promote skill building and self-competence while building bone quality and bone strength.

Growing independence, the need for peer acceptability, concern with appearance, and active lifestyles of adolescents often affect eating habits, food choices, nutrient intake, and thus nutrition status. Adolescents are seeking to establish their identity and are susceptible to peer pressure and mass media. They are also preoccupied with physical appearance and body shape and size. Desires to be lean and to have an attractive body, societal pressures, and an abundance of food in the environment can lead to inappropriate weight reduction, dietary aberrations, and nutrient deficiencies.[34] Chronic dieters are at high risk for inadequate diets. In adolescent females, such behavior may lead to eating disorders, such as anorexia nervosa and bulimia nervosa.[35,36]

Common nutritional problems in adolescents are provided in Table 7. They include obesity,

Table 7 Current Nutritional Issues and Recommendations for Adolescents

Current health problems	*Related nutrition risk factors*
Hypertension	Overweight, excessive sodium intake, low potassium intake
Underweight	Undernutrition, anorexia nervosa, bulimia nervosa
Obesity	Caloric consumption exceeds caloric need, sedentary lifestyle
Dental caries	Excessive, frequent consumption of sugary starchy foods that are retained in the mouth, lack of oral hygiene
Iron deficiency anemia	Malnutrition, inadequate dietary iron intake, pregnancy without iron supplementation
Elevated serum cholesterol	Excessive saturated fat and cholesterol intake
Nutrient deficiencies	Inadequate nutrient intakes, extended periods of dieting
Eating disorders	Societal pressure to be thin, peer pressure, diet fads
Alcohol abuse	Underage alcohol use

What needs to be done?

- Include nutrition in comprehensive health education in schools
- Develop national guidelines for school-based nutrition education programs
- Increase nutrition education to parents and communities
- Increase School Lunch and Breakfast participation
- Improve training and continuing education for all health care providers in the area of nutrition
- Integrate nutrition screening, education, and intervention services into health services aimed at teenagers
- Expand school-based health clinics especially for teenagers who have no primary physician
- Expand research on nutritional needs of adolescents

hyperlipidemia, dental caries, and hypertension.[37,38] These problems of dietary imbalance and excesses may coexist with undernutrition with respect to iron, energy, and other nutrients in some individuals. Dietary factors increasing the later risk for chronic diseases such as osteoporosis (inadequate intakes of calcium and vitamin D), heart disease (excessive intake of saturated fat and cholesterol, low-intake of fiber), and some types of cancer may be present.[38] Table 8 provides recommendations to enhance nutritional status during adolescence.

Pregnancy and lactation in adolescence also increase nutrition risk because the young female needs a supply of nutrients to support her own growth as well as the growth of the fetus and nutrition of the suckling infant.[39] Nutritional needs of pregnancy and lactation are discussed else where in this book.

NUTRITION FOR CHILDREN WITH SPECIAL NEEDS

Some of the most common nutritional issues of children with special needs are outlined in Table 9. Children with special health care needs make up approximately 10 to 20% of the pediatric population, depending on the definition used.[40] The term special needs describes a group of infants, children, and youth with or at risk for physical or developmental disability or with a chronic medical condition caused by or associated with genetic/metabolic disorders, birth defects, prematurity, trauma, or infection (including HIV infection). They present a particular challenge to community nutritionists today because many special needs children who were formerly institutionalized now dwell with their families in the community.

Table 10 provides some recommendations for enhancing the nutritional status of special needs children. Some of the nutrition needs of children with special health care needs are unique (eg, the child with a metabolic disorder controllable only by diet), but in most aspects, their nutritional needs are similar to those of other children. The "special needs" child in the family is first of all a child who has the same nutrient needs for optimal health, growth, and development as any other child. Superimposed on these needs, however, may be multiple risks, ranging from social/environmental factors, such as decreased access to food because of limited finances, to factors involving disorders, such as feeding problems or the need for chronic medication.[41] These factors may place a child at risk for inadequate nutrient intake, impaired nutrient absorption or use, or increased nutrient excretion. Such insults, if they are severe and/or prolonged, and especially if they occur early in life, can have lasting effects on the child's growth and cognitive development. Various handicapping conditions have different nutrition-related problems and needs.[42]

These are represented schematically in Figure 2 and are discussed in more detail in another chapter.

An amendment (PL 99-457) to the Federal Education for the Handicapped Act gives nutrition professionals the opportunity to have a voice in establishing nutrition policy and standards of care for young handicapped and high-risk children. Preventive services now extend to children as young as 3 years of age, and Part H of the law provides financial incentives for states to provide services to children with special health care needs from birth to 2 years of age. Nutrition should be included in these services.

EXISTING PROGRAMS

Federal Programs

Either the USDA or the DHHS administers most federally funded food and/or nutrition programs for mothers and children. The programs are administered on the state level by the Department of Welfare, Department of Education, or Department of Health depending on their particular focus. One type of federal support is through benefits or cash assistance that goes directly to eligible recipients (such as the Food Stamp program, which provides food vouchers, or the School

Table 8 Recommendations for Enhancing Nutritional Status in Adolescents

- Maintain desirable weights. Avoid obesity and eating disorders by developing healthful attitudes toward food, appropriate energy intakes, and a physically active lifestyle, including both aerobic and strength-building exercise
- Abstain from self-induced vomiting, bulimia, and laxative abuse
- Eat a variety of foods to ensure dietary sufficiency of protective nutrients, including protein, vitamin, minerals, and fiber
- Avoid dietary imbalances, stressing moderation with respect to fat, saturated fat, cholesterol, sugars, and salt by moderation in intakes of foods high in these and low in protective nutrients
- Find ways to eat that fulfill the teenager's individual needs, philosophies, wants, and schedules without doing violence to nutritional status
- Identify and alter eating habits that are not conducive to good nutrition, including long-standing poor dietary intakes, irregular or unplanned food intakes, and excessive intakes of fat, cholesterol, sodium, sugar, and alcohol
  - Avoid alcohol use
- Provide assistance for special problems such as teenage pregnancy, diets for competitive athletes, diets for those with allergies and disease
- Ensure adequate intakes of calcium and vitamin D to maximize bone density

Table 9 Current Nutritional Issues and Recommendations for Children with Special Needs

Current Health Problems	Related Nutrition Risk Factors
Growth retardation, underweight	Increased needs; inadequate intake caused by mechanical difficulties with chewing, swallowing, or feeding oneself; malabsorption
Obesity	Reduced resting metabolism, decreased energy expenditure, excessive calorie intake
Gastrointestinal complications	Diet not adequate in fiber and water
Nutrient deficiencies	Inadequate intake of certain nutrients, lack of supplementation, increased needs, drug–nutrient interactions
Infections	Malnutrition

What needs to be done?

- Ensure that community programs for special needs children are in place to screen and assess nutrition problems
- Implement use of standardized screening and referral tools for service providers
- Improve nutrition training of health professionals
- Increase nutrition counseling and education for families
- Develop nutrition and feeding guidelines for agencies responsible for the administration of health, social welfare, and related program services
- Enhance the research base for current issues in nutrition for children with special needs

Table 10 Recommendations for Enhancing Nutritional Status in Children with Special Needs

- Recognize that expectations for growth may be different; use appropriate standards when available
- Provide adequate nutrition to achieve optimal growth potential
- Consider the extra or lessened energy needs owing to the child's condition and adjust intake accordingly
- Use vitamin and mineral supplements if directed by physician
- Frequently evaluate adequacy of child's diet
- Ensure adequate intake of fluid and fiber
- Consult an interdisciplinary team and develop a care plan that includes realistic expectations regarding the child's potential, under-standing of feeding skill progression and recognition of developmental readiness for next steps, and enrolment in early intervention programs as needed
- If warranted, adjust feign positioning to allow for adequate food intake, use appropriate nipples and feeding devices for children unable to use standard equipment, and adjust pace of feeding appropriately
- Determine family's need for food assistance, support with home and money management, diet information, and emotional support

DISORDER	PREVALENCE ESTIMATES PER 1,000 (AND RANGE)	EXAMPLE OF NUTRITION PROBLEMS AND FACTORS CONTRIBUTING TO HIGH NUTRITIONAL RISK — Child-related: Altered nutrient needs	Altered energy needs/intake	Problems with oral cavity	Nutrient deficiencies	Constipation/diarrhea	Poor appetite	Delayed feeding skills	Malabsorption	Nutrient-drug interactions	Maladaptive behaviors	Lack of knowledge	Caregiver-related: Difficulty understanding diet	Does not limit intake	Inappropriate feeding practices
Asthma Moderate to Severe	38 (20–53) 10 (8–15)		•		•		•			•					
Visual Impairment Impaired Visual Acuity Blind	30 (20–35) 20 0.6 (0.5–1)							•			•				
Mental Retardation	25 (20–30)		•	•		•		•			•				•
Hearing Impairment Deafness	16 0.1 (0.6–1.5)														
Congenital Heart Disease Severe Congenital Disease	7 (2–7) 0.5	•	•		•		•		•	•		•			
Seizure Disorder	3.5 (2.6–4.6)	•								•		•			
Cerebral Palsy	2.5 (1.4-5.1)		•	•	•	•	•	•		•		•		•	•
Arthritis	2.2 (1–3)	•	•									•			
Paralysis	2.1 (2–2.3)		•			•		•			•	•		•	
Diabetes Mellitus	1.8 (1.2–2.0)											•	•	•	
Cleft Lip/Palate	1.5 (1.3–2.0)		•	•				•				•			•
Down Syndrome	1.1		•	•		•		•			•	•		•	•
Sickle Cell Disease	< 1.0	•			•										
Neural Tube Defect	< 1.0		•			•				•				•	
Autism	< 1.0						•			•	•				•
Cystic Fibrosis	< 1.0	•	•		•	•	•		•	•		•	•	•	•
Hemophilia	< 1.0														
Acute Lymphocytic Leukemia	< 1.0	•	•		•	•	•			•					
Phenylketonuria	< 1.0	•			•							•	•	•	
Chronic Renal Failure	< 1.0	•	•		•	•	•			•		•	•		
Bronchopulmonary Dysplasia	< 1.0	•	•		•			•		•					
AIDS	< 1.0	•	•	•	•	•	•	•	•	•		•			
Gastrointestinal Disorders	< 1.0	•			•	•	•		•						

Figure 2 Prevalence of certain chronic conditions with associated nutrition-related problems.

Lunch program, which provides inexpensive or free meals). Another type is in-kind services [such as the USDA's Expanded Food and Nutrition Education Program (EFNEP), which provides nutrition education to low-income families].

Means-tested programs require assessment of means or income before one qualifies for them. They are special cash or in-kind services targeted to provide a safety net to protect children in low-income families. Eligibility for such programs, such as Food Stamps, Medicaid, general relief payments, funded child health services, or free school lunch and breakfast, is assessed by review of family incomes. These programs are valuable contributions for maintaining or improving the nutritional status of low-income families. Such families may have limited access or resources available to buy food, and those who are particularly vulnerable from the physiologic standpoint include infants, young children, and pregnant and lactating women.

Community nutrition services for families and children are also available as part of other health and social services, such as intensive infant care programs, services for handicapped children, dental health programs, family planning service, school health, and teenage pregnancy/parenting programs.

The federal government also provides grants for planning and service provisions to states for program development to provide food assistance, nutrition education, and counseling to eligible families at the local level through health centers, school systems, and community action agencies.

Health care providers need to know about the many food and nutrition programs available in their local areas and how and when to refer their patients to them.

USDA Programs. The USDA provides various public health programs at the community level. These include Food Stamps, School Lunch and Breakfast, Special Milk Program for Children, Child Care Food Program, Summer Food Service Program for Children, WIC, EFNEP, and Commodity Supplemental Food Program (CSFP). These programs served an estimated one in six Americans at some point during 2002, with all food programs totaling almost $38 billion.[43] Food pantries and soup kitchens are also available for some families that lack food. Surplus foods, both dry and perishable, are distributed to food pantries and soup kitchens. Table 11 presents a summary of current expenditures on these programs.

Food Stamp Program ***What It Is*** This is the largest and most far-reaching food assistance program for low-income families in the United States to help them buy the food they need for a nutritionally adequate diet. The amount provided is based on the USDA's Thrifty Food Plan, a market basket of suggested amounts of food that make up a nutritious diet and that can be purchased at a relatively low cost. The federal government pays for all benefits issued through the program and shares administrative costs with the states. Puerto Rico, American Samoa, and the Marianas receive cash grants instead under the Nutrition Assistance Program that permits them to provide food assistance programs for their low-income residents. Food Stamps is a means-tested entitlement program; any household that meets program eligibility requirements may receive them. Households participating in the program actually receive their benefits by an electronic benefits transfer card system rather than by stamps or coupons, as in days gone by. Benefits can be used to buy food but not alcohol, tobacco, or nonfood items such as soap or paper supplies. Nationally, the majority of all Food Stamp recipients are children, and the preponderance of Food Stamp benefits is paid to families with children.

Who Qualifies. For families with children, the principal eligibility requirement is that gross household income is below 130% of the federal poverty level and that net income, after various deductions, is at or below 100% of the poverty level. The value of a household's assets (eg, cash on hand, checking or savings accounts, stocks and bonds, recreational boats and vehicles, some cars, and land that is owned but not inhabited by the household) is also accounted for in determining eligibility.

Table 11 Food Assistance Program Expenditures, USDA, 2001

Program Costs, Food Assistance Program	2006 (Million Dollars)
Food stamp–related programs	32,806
Food stamp program	
Nutrition assistance programs	
Child nutrition programs	
National school lunch program	8,152
School breakfast program	2,031
Child and adult care food program	2,149
Summer food service program	273
Special milk program	15
Supplemental food programs	
WIC	5,088
Commodity supplement food program	131
Food donation programs	
Food distribution on Indian reservations	74
Disaster feeding program	7
Emergency food assistance Program TEFAP	2,980
Charitable institutions and summer camps	3

Adapted from reference 43.
WIC = Special Supplemental Nutrition Program for Women, Infants, and Children.

How to Enroll. Contact the state or local welfare office and obtain an application.

Child Care Food Program ***What It Is.*** This program provides cash reimbursement and/or commodities for the provision of meals and snacks to institutions such as child care centers and family and group daycare homes providing nonresidential child care to children from low-income families. This program funds the meals provided in Head Start. This is not an entitlement program. Subsidies are provided for two meals and one snack per day for children less than 12 years old. Meals must meet USDA-specified requirements. Family or group daycare homes are paid a fixed reimbursement, depending on the type of meals served. Daycare centers are reimbursed for meals at rates depending on the type of meal and eligibility of children for free, reduced-price, or paid meals.

Who Qualifies. Institutions eligible to participate include child care centers, settlement houses, neighbor-hood and Head Start centers, and institutions providing day care for the handicapped and their families or group daycare homes. Private daycare centers can participate only when at least 25% of their enrolled children are from low-income families receiving benefits through Title XX of the Social Services Act.

How to Enroll. Contact the local school authority or child care center.

School Lunch and School Breakfast Programs ***What They Are.*** Over 90% of all schools in the United States participate in the National School Lunch Program. They receive cash assistance to help purchase food and pay labor costs as well as direct donations of agricultural food commodities. Participating schools must agree to serve meals at a reduced price or free to children who are unable to pay the locally established full price. The federal reimbursement level is such that all meals fed to children receive some subsidies, but they are largest for the poorest children, who receive meals free. To receive a free or reduced-price meal, means tests are required. Each year, the Secretary of Agriculture issues uniform national standards for free and reduced-price eligibility based on national poverty guidelines.

To ensure that the nutrition goals of the program are met, minimum meal pattern requirements are specified, and the USDA periodically updates these. The lunch is designed to provide about one-third of the recommended dietary allowances for age and the breakfast about one-fourth. Recent regulatory changes have provided for more flexibility in the quantities and types of foods offered in the meal pattern; for example, skimmed milk, unflavored low-fat milk, flavored whole milk, or buttermilk can be offered as a choice for those who do not wish regular whole milk. Children can now choose three of the five meal components for lunch, and the school will still be reimbursed for the whole price of the meal. This provision of offering instead of simply serving all meal components is designed to cut down on waste.

Who Qualifies. Any public or nonprofit private school of high school grade or under is eligible. Public and licensed nonprofit private residential child care institutions such as orphanages, homes for retarded children, juvenile detention centers, and temporary shelters for run-away children also are eligible.

How to Enroll. Contact the local school authority.

Special Milk Program for Children ***What It Is.*** This program reduces the cost of each half-pint of milk served to children by providing for cash reimbursement at an annually adjusted rate to public and nonprofit schools, child care centers, summer camps, and similar institutions that do not participate in any other federally assisted nutrition program. Participants can choose to provide milk free or at low cost to all children or may elect to serve free milk to children whose families are below 130% of poverty.

Who Qualifies. This program is available only to institutions that do not participate in the National School Lunch, School Breakfast, or Commodity Programs.

How to Enroll. Contact the local school authority.

Summer Food Service Program for Children ***What It Is.*** This program provides nutritious meals for preschool and school-aged children under 18 years of age in recreation centers or summer camps, during vacations in areas operating under a continuous school calendar, or in areas with poor economic conditions. Meals are served free and must meet the minimum standards established by the USDA.

Who Qualifies. Sponsors of the program must be public or private-nonprofit school food authorities; state, local municipal, or county governments; or public, private-nonprofit residential summer camps. The programs must be in areas where at least half of the children are from households with incomes at or below 185% of federal poverty guidelines; there is no income test for eligibility in these low-income areas, and any child in the program may participate. Other programs that contain at least half of children from families at or below 185% of the federal poverty guidelines may also provide food to all children in the program. Individual children in these programs may participate without regard to their family's income, and they may receive as many as two meals and two snacks per day. The USDA reimburses sponsors of the program.

How to Enroll. Contact the local school authority.

WIC ***What It Is.*** Since its inception in 1972, the WIC program grew from $20 million to more than $5.1 billion yearly in authorized funds. The USDA provides annual cash grants to state health departments or comparable agencies on the basis of a formula that considers food costs and administrative costs. The program is very large, but it is not an entitlement program; rather, it is a grant program with funding limits that are set annually. Participation is an option for states and localities, but today it is available in virtually all parts of the country.

The WIC program differs from all other federal food assistance programs in its close association with health care services and inclusion of food, health, and nutrition education services together.[45,46] These services are defined as ongoing, routine pediatric and obstetric care. Health care itself, other than screening and limited assessment and care provided by WIC, must be supported by state, local public and private-nonprofit health or human service agencies as well as the private sector. The amount and kind of health services provided to WIC recipients vary from state to state and locally.

The benefits of the program include vouchers for the purchase of specific foods tailored to the dietary needs of infants, children, and pregnant or postpartum women. Physicians or health professionals may also prescribe special infant formulas and certain medical foods for WIC participants with special medical conditions. In addition to food, WIC also provides referrals to health and social services, including prenatal care, and nutrition counseling and education sessions. In addition, many pregnant women gain initial access to prenatal care via their WIC screening. Efforts are made to adapt the education activities to the individual participant's nutritional needs, cultural preferences, and education levels. Approximately 75% of the current participants are children ranging in age from newborn to 5 years.

Who Qualifies. Low-income pregnant and postpartum women, lactating mothers, infants, and children up to 5 years old who are determined to be at nutritional risk by a health professional are eligible if they fall below 185% of federal poverty guidelines. The criteria for nutritional risk include dietary risk, anthropometric risk (eg, overweight, underweight), biochemical risk (eg, low hematocrit), and medical risk (eg, diabetes mellitus) and other factors such as homelessness. A priority system is in place that categorizes participants on the basis of severity of potential effects and outcomes so that those at highest risk are served first. Participants must be recertified every 6 months to continue receiving benefits.

How to Enroll. To obtain WIC benefits, an individual must apply at a WIC clinic.

Commodity Supplemental Food Program ***What It Is.*** This program provides nutritious supplemental foods at no cost to infants and children up to their sixth birthday and to pregnant and postpartum women who are at or below 185% of the federal poverty level who are not served by WIC. The program provides food packages that are tailored to the needs of participants.

Who Qualifies. Those below 185% of federal poverty levels who are not served by WIC qualify. States can require that participants be nutritionally at risk to qualify for the program. It operates in parts of 18 states and the District of Columbia.

EFNEP ***What It Is.*** This program provides instruction in basic food and nutrition-related topics to low-income families and individuals and is operated through the state Cooperative Extension Service. It is not an entitlement program. Its aim is to develop understanding and awareness through a variety of methods, including direct teaching by nutrition assistants in existing groups (such as employment and training programs and shelters for homeless families), cluster groups consisting of two to five participants, one-on-one home visits, mailings, telephone, and mass media efforts. EFNEP teaches participants how to plan for daily food needs; prepare nutritious, low-cost meals that meet the daily recommended dietary allowances of nutrients; select and buy food economically; and effectively use other supplemental programs available, such as Food Stamps, WIC, School Meal Programs, and CSFP.

Who Qualifies. Families with children under 19 years of age, pregnant women, and individuals who are responsible for purchasing and preparing foods (such as special needs adults, teens living independently) are eligible. To qualify, applicants must have income at or below 185% of federal poverty guidelines and be at nutritional risk as determined by an EFNEP nutritionist.

How to Enroll. Call the national EFNEP office at 202-720-8855. A coordinator will refer the applicant to an EFNEP office in his or her area.

CSFP *What It Is* This in-kind program provides food and is available at local option in several states. Providing commodity supplemental foods and nutrition education to participants, the CSFP is designed to supplement their diets with nutritious foods. The foods supplied by CSFP are different from WIC foods in their variety (ie, they consist of canned meat or poultry and canned vegetables). CSFP distributes food rather than vouchers for redemption at the grocery store. Also, the provision of health care to recipients is encouraged but not mandated, unless it was already in existence prior to 1978. Simultaneous participation in WIC and CSFP is prohibited. The supplemental foods (usually surplus agricultural commodities) are distributed to state agencies, Indian tribes, or groups responsible for administering the program. Each state selects local, private, nonprofit agencies to administer the program at the local level. Local agencies determine the eligibility of applicants, distribute the supplemental foods, and provide nutrition education. Federal funds provide for some of the administrative costs such as outreach, warehousing of food, and transportation to obtain food if necessary.

Who Qualifies. Low-income pregnant, lactating, and postpartum women, infants, and children to age 6 years are eligible.

How to Enroll. Contact state or local public or private-nonprofit health agencies.

Food Distribution Program on Indian Reservations *What It Is.* This program provides commodities to low-income households on participating reservations and to Native American families living in designated areas near reservations. This is an alternative to the Food Stamp program for American Indians who do not have easy access to food stores. Participants receive a monthly food package containing a variety of foods to meet their health needs and preferences.

Who Qualifies. Program eligibility is based on a person's household income, assets, and residence on or near a reservation.

The Emergency Food Assistance Program (TEFAP) *What It Is.* First started as a way to reduce inventories and storage costs of surplus commodities by distributing them to needy households, it now also includes funds appropriated by Congress to purchase additional commodities. The USDA buys the food, processes and packages it, and ships it to the states based on a formula that takes into account the number of people below the poverty level and the number unemployed.

Who Qualifies. States set their own eligibility criteria and select emergency feeding organizations such as soup kitchens, food recovery organizations, and food banks to distribute the food.

Charitable Institutions and Summer Camp Food Distribution Program *What It Is.* The USDA donates food to nonprofit charitable institutions serving meals on a regular basis to summer camps for children, orphanages, soup kitchens, temporary shelters, and church-operated community kitchens for the homeless. The amount of food donated depends on the amount of surplus and price support commodities that are available.

Who Qualifies. Institutions participating in the Summer Food Service Program are not eligible.

DHHS. The DHHS provides a wide variety of public health programs at the community level, as well as payments for health services. The public health programs include the Head Start and Early Intervention (EI) programs and the Aid to Families with Dependent Children (AFDC) program. In addition, limited monies are provided for nutrition services such as assessment and counseling. Title V of the Social Security Act of 1935 authorized grants to states to plan for provision of comprehensive health services to mothers and children. In subsequent years, funding of categorical programs provided monies for planning and provision of special services, such as lead poisoning prevention, services for handicapped children, and family planning. Monies for planning such programs are provided from federal funds by the DHHS. Demonstration grant funds have also been available on an increasingly limited basis over the past few decades for high-risk communities and groups. The comprehensive services include medical and dental care, nursing, nutrition, and social work.

Head Start *What It Is.* This program is particularly well known for its multifaceted approach to child health and development, including social and educational development. Administered by DHHS and funded directly to local agencies, Head Start provides low-income preschoolers and their families with day care, access to medical care and social services, and nutrition services, including meals, nutrition education, and staff training.[47]

Head Start programs are funded through grants from the Administration for Children, Youth and Families regional offices and the Native American Migrant Program branches. These grants are awarded to a variety of local public agencies, private-nonprofit organizations, and public school systems. The program is very large but not an entitlement. It is at the discretion of states and localities and serves primarily children from poor families.

Head Start programs serve a multiracial, multiethnic group of low-income children and families. Each program must offer four major components: education, social services, parent involvement, and health services. With the goal of meeting each child's individual needs, the program offers a wide variety of learning experiences aimed at fostering intellectual, social, and emotional growth. Head Start also aims to meet the ethnic and cultural characteristics of the communities served.

Head Start's nutrition program is part of the health component offered and provides nutritious meals from the Child Care Food Program, as well as nutrition education for children, staff, and parents.

Who Qualifies. To be eligible for Head Start, a child must be between 3 and 5 years of age and come from a low-income family whose total annual income does not exceed 100% of the federal poverty guideline or who is receiving public assistance from programs such as AFDC or Supplemental Security Income.

How to Enroll. Contact the Head Start Bureau, which is located in the Administration for Children, Youth and Families, Office of Human Development Services, DHHS.

Head Start for Children with Special Needs *What It Is.* Head Start is the largest provider in this country of services for preschool children with handicapping conditions.

Who Qualifies. It is mandated to serve preschool children who have a broad range of handicaps. Children with severe or multiple handicaps present additional challenges to Head Start staff in the planning and provision of individual services. Program requirements call for individualized plans for special education, treatment, and related services for all handicapped children served by Head Start. These plans must be based on the child's specific handicapping conditions, as well as the unique needs arising from those conditions.

How to Enroll. Contact the Head Start Bureau, which is located in the Administration for Children, Youth and Families, Office of Human Development Services, DHHS.

Early Intervention Programs and Services *What It Is and Who Qualifies.* EI programs and services for infants, toddlers, and their families have existed in many areas of the United States for more than 25 years. These services are organized to address the developmental needs of young children between birth and 3 years of age who may be at risk for poor developmental outcome because of an identified disability or because of biologic or environmental risk factors.48,49 Although all of these programs share the common goal of optimal infant development, they approach it in different ways. That is why collaboration is essential in the development of an Individual Family Service Plan (IFSP), which addresses all of the child's needs that must be met for the child's potential to be reached. Some EI programs are home-based models, others are center-based models, and others are a combination of those two approaches. Intervention programs also differ with respect to their program philosophy and goals, the population that is served, team composition, program content, and program evaluation. Services are generally multidisciplinary, in recognition of the interrelationship of development in various domains, and may include input by developmental educators, occupational and physical therapists, speech pathologists, psychologists, nurses, dietitians, and social workers.

Federal law significantly influences the development of EI programs. The most applicable law, enacted in 1986, is Title I, Part H, Handicapped Infants and Toddlers, of PL 99-457, Education of the Handicapped Amendments of 1986. That law extends public education to children 3 years old and older and provides incentives to states to serve children with special needs from birth onward. It includes nutrition as one of eight disciplines to be included on the team providing services to these handicapped infants and their families.

Part H of PL 99-457 requires that services designed for children from birth through 36 months meet their developmental needs. It mandates psychological services, parent and family training and counseling, transition services, diagnostic medical services, case management, and health services that will enable the child to benefit from other early interventions. The eight disciplines specified by PL 99-457 include special education, nursing, nutrition, psychology, physical therapy, occupational therapy, speech-language pathology, and social work. This law provides great opportunities for nutrition intervention in preschool children with handicapping conditions and their families. To date, however, most states have done little to develop community-wide networks to provide EI services that include nutrition.

How to Enroll. Contact the state Maternal and Child Health Department.

Personal Responsibility and Work Opportunity Reconciliation Act *What It Is.* In 1996, under the Personal Responsibility and Work Opportunity Reconciliation Act, the basic cash assistance program AFDC was eliminated and replaced with Temporary Assistance for Needy Families.[50] The 1996 welfare legislation provides block grants to states for time-limited cash assistance and made other program changes (Food Stamps, Supplemental Security Income for children and others). How these programs develop will have a profound effect on families living in poverty in the United States and the potential to significantly impact the nutritional status of children. The overall effects of welfare reform on child health and nutrition need to be closely monitored.

Who Qualifies. States have much more control over the money block granted including time limits, sanctions, and categorical restrictions. Although there are advantages to this (flexibility), there are no assurances that the funds will be spent where most needed, and the program may lack focus.

How to Enroll. Contact the local Department of Public Health in the area the individual lives in.

State and Local Programs

There is a great deal of variability between states and localities in the extent to which they supplement federal nutrition funds or provide additional in-kind resources, such as health services. These variations make it essential for community nutritionists to know the specifics of state and local programs in their areas.

WEB-BASED RESOURCES FOR COMMUNITY NUTRITION

The DHHS has developed a number of Web-based resources that may be helpful in planning community nutrition efforts. Many nutrition resources not specified below are listed at this Web site: http://www.nutrition.gov. The gateway to reliable consumer health information on the Internet is provided at http://www.healthfinder.gov. Healthy People 2010–related materials include a general description of the initiative at http://www.health.gov/healthypeople, a community-planning guide using Healthy People 2010, entitled *Healthy People in Healthy Communities*, at http://www.health.gov/healthypeople/ publications/HealthyCommunities2001. Information on temporary assistance for needy families is available at http://www.neighborhoodlaw.org/ aprimer.htm. A "toolkit" for planning at the state level is at this Web site: http://www.health.gov/healthypeople/state/toolkit. The CDC's planned approach to community health is provided at http://www.cdc.gov/nccdphp/patch/index.htm.

Several Web sites focus on physical activity and health. These include the surgeon general's report on this topic at http://www.cdc.gov/nccdphp/sgr/sgr.htm. The President's Council on Physical Fitness and Sports is available at http://www.fitness.gov. Tips for promoting better health for young people through physical activity and sports are provided at http://www.cdc.gov/nccdphp/dash/presphysactrpt/index.htm. For obesity prevention see http://www.cdc.gov/VERB.

The USDA provides several Web sites to improve access to Food Stamp and food program-related nutrition resources for assisting community nutrition efforts.

All USDA Web sites are available at the National Agricultural Library's homepage: http:/www.nal.usda.gov. Some specific Web sites include the following:

- ***The Food and Nutrition Information*** Center is a large, Web-based information center backed up with trained nutritionists who can help in locating information and borrowing additional resources from the collection of the National Agricultural Library. Access it at http://www.nal.usda.gov/fnic.
- ***The Food Stamp Nutrition Connection*** has a training center with a collection of social marketing and programming resources on Food Stamps, a resource library providing ready-to-use educational materials, information on hot topics, contacts at the state and national levels, and program facts. These are available at http://www.nal.usda.gov/foodstamp.
- The ***WIC*** program has a Web site that summarizes recent studies on WIC and provides other educational materials. It is located at http://www.fns. usda.gov/oae/menu/published/wic/wic.htm.
- A special Web site for ***child care nutrition*** resources focuses on food programs for children in child care. It is located at www.nal.usda.gov/childcare.
- ***The Healthy School Meals Resource System*** is a searchable Web site that provides information to persons working in USDA's child nutrition programs. It includes materials to assist nutrition educators both in the classroom and in the school cafeteria. Access it at http://www.schoolmeals.usda.gov/8001.
- ***The Dietary Guidelines for Americans*** are available on the Web http://www.health.gov/dietaryguidelines.; Possible implications for US agriculture are provided at www.ers.usda.gov/publications/err31.

LESSONS LEARNED FROM COMMUNITY NUTRITION EFFORTS

Community Investments in Child Health and Nutrition Make Sense

As early as the fourth century BC, the philosopher Plato stressed the importance of investing in children from an early age. Several millennia later, numerous studies confirm Plato's suppositions about the importance of investing in our children.[51] For example, supplementing the diets of pregnant women and infants and immunizing children against early childhood diseases save lives and improve health. It is to be hoped that, in the future, programs such as Head Start, EI, and WIC, with demonstrated success in strengthening the bodies and minds of children, will reach more of their target populations. Also, special attention must be paid to nutrition for children with special needs and other chronic health problems. Current programs do not cover them adequately.

Table 11 shows current federal spending for a number of key health and food programs involving children.

Community Health and Children's Health Care Must be Equal Partners

Community health and nutrition efforts expand the traditional focus of direct health services. Both are necessary to ensure child and family health. Also, broader economic factors that affect food insecurity must be dealt with.[52] The distinctions between traditional public health and personal health services are slowly blurring in this country. In the future, community nutrition concerns will need to be incorporated into both systems. There is the danger that nutrition will "fall through the cracks" because there are other pressing needs. Thus, it behooves all of those who are interested in the health of children to pay attention to ensuring that federal, state, and local governments employ nutritionists to look after community needs in nutrition. These professionals must work with others in health, welfare, education, and food agencies in the public and private sectors to ensure that all children are well nourished. At the same time, dietary concerns must be increasingly incorporated into personal health services. Only when these steps are taken will community nutrition realize its potential to have a positive impact on children.

Child Nutrition and Physical Activity are Inextricably Linked, Like Siamese Twins

Both physical activity and sound nutrition in the community help to keep children healthy and ready to learn and also prevent later chronic disease risk.[53] Long-term community efforts at the school, family, and individual levels are necessary to yield the benefits of lower health risks over the long term. Community leaders, experts in health and education, and parents themselves must be involved in school-based and other prevention-oriented programs.

School-Based Programs Offer Much Potential for Health Promotion and Primary Prevention of Diet- and Physical Activity-Related Risk Factors if Supplemented by Parent, Family, and Community-Wide Efforts

School-based programs are excellent sites for these efforts. However, changes in the curriculum alone are not sufficient to bring about alterations in risk factors for cardiovascular disease or obesity; changes in school meals and alterations in physical education programs are also needed. More attention to physical training components that increase strength may be important in preventing later osteoporosis risk. Thus, multiple risk factors need to be targeted. Also, community efforts to reinforce these efforts are needed.[54]

In addition to school-based efforts, family and community efforts are also required. Children do not spend all of their waking hours in school. The microenvironment of the family is an important milieu for enhancing and carrying forward school-based health promotion and physical education efforts. The macroenvironment of schools and of the community must also be conducive to healthy lifestyles.

Healthful Eating Patterns for the Whole Family are Critical

Foods must be eaten to be nutritious, and overall diets are the most important. Children and their families eat foods, not individual nutrients. There is often a gap in teaching about the merits and demerits of individual foods, and broader guidance on healthful diets or eating patterns is needed. Existing scientific evidence shows that overall eating patterns and diets and not consumption of individual foods or nutrients are most closely linked to positive effects on health. Therefore, families need information about healthful, enjoyable eating patterns that provide a broad, food-based context for healthful eating and about healthful physical activity and exercise patterns. When needs cannot be met by food-based solutions alone, supplementation with vitamins and minerals may be considered.[55,56]

Information on Healthful Eating and Physical Activity Must be Communicated More Effectively at the Community Level

Consumers and policy makers must view the dietary guidelines for Americans and other nutrition education guidance and programs as acceptable and actionable as well as authoritative if they are to be used. The dietary guidelines,[57] the USDA's Food Group Pyramid,[58] the Healthy Eating Pyramid for children (which is based on the dietary reference intakes and the dietary guidelines), food labels, and health claims provide such guidance to the community.[59] Information about them needs to be communicated, coordinated, and harmonized to facilitate food purchases and consumption decisions, and diet-related efforts must be accompanied and reinforced by physical activity programs. This challenge is one that food producers, marketers, public policy makers, and educators face together. Intervention strategies from the social and behavioral sciences may be helpful in tailoring messages to our diverse population.[60,61]

CONCLUSION

Community efforts in this country are in line with those of the overarching goals of the World Health Organization's Health for All campaign in the twenty-first century to increase healthy life expectancy, ensure universal access to quality health care, and achieve greater equality in health status within and among countries.[62]

REFERENCES

1. Federal Interagency Forum on Child and Family Statistics. America's Children in Brief: Key National Indicators of Well Being 2006, Washington, DC: US Government Printing Office; 2006. Available at http//www.childstats.gov.
2. Frazao E. America's Eating Habits: Changes and Consequences. Agriculture Information Bulletin No. 750. Washington, DC: Economic Research Service, US Department of Agriculture; 1999.
3. Goran MI, Sothern MS, editors. Handbook of Pediatric Obesity. CRC Taylor and Frances: Boca Raton; 2006.
4. Rogers CC. A look at America's children and their families. Food Rev 2001;4:2–7.
5. Winslow CEA. The field of public health. Mod Med 1920;2:183–95.
6. Kaufman M. Understanding public health. In: Kaufman M, editor. Nutrition in Public Health. Rockville, MD: Aspen; 1990. p. 3–13.
7. US Department of Health and Human Services, Public Health Service. Healthy People 2010 Objectives: National Health Promotion and Disease Prevention Objectives. Washington, DC: US Government Printing Office; 2000.
8. Egan MC, Oglesby AC. Nutrition services in the maternal and child health program: A historical perspective. In: Sharbaugh CO, Egan MC, editors. Call to Action-Better Nutrition for Mothers, Children, and Families. Washington, DC: National Center for Education in Maternal and Child Health; 1991. p. 73–92.
9. Wolfe WS, Bremner B, Ferris-Morris M. Monitoring the Nutrition of Your Community: A "How-To" Manual. New York: Division of Nutritional Sciences, Cornell University; 1992.
10. Board on Children Youth and Families, and Institute of Medicine Childrens' Health. The Nation's Wealth: Assessing and Improving Child Health. Washington, DC: National Academy Press; 2004.
11. Committee on Consequences of Uninsurance. Health Insurance is a Family Matter. Washington, DC: National Academy Press; 2002.
12. Isaacs SL, Knickman JR, editors. To Improve Health and Health Care 2001. Princeton, NJ: Robert Wood Johnson Foundation; 2001.
13. Gallagher-Allred C. Implementing Nutrition Screening and Intervention Strategies. Washington, DC: The Nutrition Screening Initiative; 1993.
14. Dwyer JT. Strategies to detect and prevent malnutrition in the elderly: The Nutrition Screening Initiative. Prepared for Lugano Forum; 1994; 29:15–24.
15. Nord M, Andrews M, Carlson S. Household Food Security in the United States, 2005. Springfield, VA: Economic Research Service, US Department of Agriculture. Available at www.ers.usda.gov/publications/err29.
16. Bowman SA, Lino M, Gerrior SA, et al. The healthy eating index 1994–96. Fam Econ Nutr Rev 1998;11:2–14. See updates at http://www.cnpp.usda.gov/HealthyEatingIndex.htm.
17. Fox MK, Crepinsek MK, Connor P, et al. School Nutrition Dietary Assessment Study II. A Report Completed by Abt Associates Inc. for the US Department of Agriculture, Food and Nutrition Service, January 2001. Boston: Abt Associates; 2001.
18. Fanelli-Kuczmarski M, Kuczmarski RJ. Nutrition monitoring in the United States. In: Shils ME, Olson JA, Shike M, Ross AC, editors. Modern Nutrition in Health and Disease, 9th edition. Baltimore: Williams & Wilkins; 1999. p. 1743–55.
19. Baer MT, editor. Nutrition Services for Children with Handicaps: A Manual for State Title V Programs. Los Angeles: University Affiliated Program, Center for Child Development and Developmental Disorders. Los Angeles, CA: University of California & Los Angeles;1982.
20. Owen AL, Roth-Yousy L, Splett PL. Planning and decision making. In: Frankle RT, Owen AL, editors. Nutrition in the Community. St. Louis: Mosby-Year Book; 1993. p. 357–95.
21. US Preventive Services Task Force. Guide to Clinical Preventive Services 2006: Recommendations of the US Preventive Services Task Force. Washington: Agency for Healthcare Research and Quality, US Department of Health and Human Services; 2006. Available at http://www.ahrq.gov/clinic/pocketgd.pdf.
22. US Department of Health and Human Services. Health Resources and Services Administration, Maternal and Child Health Bureau Child Health USA 2005. Rockville, MD: US Department of Health and Human Services; 2005.
23. US Department of Health and Human Services. Tracking Healthy People 2010. Washington, DC: US Government Printing Office; November 2000.
24. Maternal and Child Health Bureau, HRSA, Public Health Service, US Department of Health and Human Services. Update for Nutrition During Pregnancy and Lactation: An Implementation Guide. Arlington, VA: National Center for Education in Maternal and Child Health; 1998.
25. Allen LH. Pregnancy and lactation. In: Bowman BA, Russell RM, editors. Present Knowledge in Nutrition, 8th edition. Washington, DC: ILSI Press; 2001. p. 403–15.
26. March of Dimes Task Force on Nutrition and Optimal Human Development. Nutrition Today Matters Tomorrow. Wilkes Barre, PA: March of Dimes Fulfillment Center; 2002.
27. Heird WC. Nutritional requirements during infancy. In: Bowman BA, Russell RM, editors. Present Knowledge in Nutrition, 8th edition. Washington, DC: ILSI Press; 2001.p. 416–25.
28. Mokdad AH, Bowman BA, Ford ES, et al. The ongoing epidemics of obesity and diabetes in the US. JAMA 2001;286:1195–1200. Updates posted at http://www.cdc.gov/nccdphp/dnpa/obesity
29. US Department of Health and Human Services. The Surgeon General's Call to Action to Prevent and Decrease Overweight and Obesity 2001. Rockville, MD: Office of the Surgeon General, Public Health Service, US Department of Health and Human Services; 2001.
30. Kuczmarski RJ, Ogden CL, Grummer-Strawn LM, et al. CDC Growth Charts: United States Advance Data From Vital and Health Statistics No. 314 June 8, 2000 (revised). Hyattsville, MD: National Center for Health Statistics; 2000.

31. Kuczmarski RJ, Ogden CL, Guo SS, et al. 2000 CDC Growth Charts for the United States. Methods and Development, Vital Health Statistics 11 (246). DHHS Publication No. (PHS) 2002–1696. Hyattsville, MD: National Center for Health Statistics; 2002.
32. Mascarenhas MR, Zemel BS, Tershakovec AM, et al. Adolescence. In: Bowman BA, Russell RM, editors. Present Knowledge in Nutrition, 8th edition. Washington, DC: ILSI Press; 2001. p. 426–38.
33. Mitchell J. Nutritional Issues in Adolescent Health. Rockville, MD: US Department of Health and Human Services; 1988.
34. Meredith CN, Frontera WR. Adolescent fitness. In: Nussbaum MP, Dwyer JT, editors. Adolescent Medicine—State of the Art Reviews: Adolescent Nutrition and Eating Disorders. Philadelphia: Hanley & Belfus; 1992. p. 391–404.
35. Huse DM, Lucas AR. Behavioral disorders affecting food intake: Anorexia nervosa, bulimia nervosa, and other psychiatric conditions. In: Shils ME, Olson JA, Shike M, Ross AC, editors. Modern Nutrition in Health and Disease, 9th edition. Baltimore: Williams & Wilkins; 1999. p. 1513–22.
36. Fairburn CG, Brownell KD, editors. Eating Disorders and Obesity: A Comprehensive Handbook, 2nd edition. New York: Guilford Press; 2002.
37. Bandini LG. Obesity in the adolescent. In: Nussbaum MP, Dwyer JT, editors. Adolescent Medicine-State of the Art Reviews: Adolescent Nutrition and Eating Disorders. Philadelphia: Hanley & Belfus; 1992. p. 459–71.
38. Dwyer JT. Nutrition and the adolescent. In: Suskind RM, Lewinter-Suskind L, editors. Textbook of Pediatric Nutrition, 2nd edition. New York: Raven Press; 1993. p. 257–64.
39. Worthington-Roberts BS, Mitchell Rees J. The pregnant adolescent: Special concerns. In: Worthington-Roberts BS, Williams SR, editors. Nutrition in Pregnancy and Lactation, 6th edition. Boston: WCB McGraw-Hill; 1997. p. 292–317.
40. American Dietetic Association. Position of the American Dietetic Association: Nutrition services for children with special needs. J Am Diet Assoc 1989;89:1133–7.
41. Taylor Baer M, Farnan S, Mauer AM. Children with special health care needs. In: Sharbaugh CO, Egan MC, editors. Call to Action—Better Nutrition for Mothers, Children, and families. Washington, DC: National Center for Education in Maternal and Child Health; 1991. p. 191–208.
42. Rokusek C, Prendergast A, Walberg-Ekvall S. Nutrition in community-based programs and nutrition resources. In: Walberg-Ekvall S, editor. Pediatric Nutrition in Chronic Disease and Developmental Disorders: Prevention, Assessment, and Treatment. New York: Oxford University Press; 1993. p. 77–84.
43. Oliveira V. Food assistance expenditures increase in 2001. Food Rev 2002;25:45–52.
44. USDA Food and Nutrition Service, Key data, 2006. Available at http://www.fns.usda.gov/pd/ann8ual.htm. Accessed December 20, 2006.
45. Institute of Medicine. WIC Nutrition Risk Criteria: A Scientific Assessment. Washington, DC: National Academy Press; 1996.
46. Institute of Medicine. Dietary Risk Assessment in the WIC Program. Washington, DC: National Academy Press; 2002.
47. Stubbs PE. Head start. In: Wallace HM, Ryan GM, Oglesby AC, editors. Maternal and Child Health Practices, 3rd edition. Oak-land, CA: Third Party Publishing Co; 1988. p. 455–62.
48. Schuman A, Benham R. Early childhood intervention: A nation-wide resource. Semin Pediatr Gastroenterol Nutr 1993;4:8–11.
49. Taft Bayerl C, Ries JD, Bettencourt MF, et al. Nutritional issues of children in early intervention programs: Primary care team approach. Semin Pediatr Gastroenterol Nutr1993;4:11–5.
50. Duncan GJ, Brooks-Gunn J. Family poverty, welfare reform and child development. Child Dev 2000;71:188–96.
51. Healy T, Cote S, Helliwell JF, et al. The Well Being of the Nation: The Role of Human and Social Capital. Paris: Organization for Economic Cooperation and Development; 2001.
52. Pelletier DL, Olson CM, Frongillo EA. Food insecurity, hunger and undernutrition. In: Bowman BA, Russell RM, editors. Present Knowledge in Nutrition, 8th edition. Washington, DC: ILSI Press; 2001. p. 701–15.
53. National Center for Chronic Disease Prevention and Health Promotion. Physical Activity and Health: A Report of the Surgeon General. Atlanta: US Department of Health and Human Services, Centers for Disease Control and Prevention, National Center for Chronic Disease Prevention and Health Promotion; 1996.
54. Institute of Medicine. Schools and Health: Our Nation's Investment. Washington DC: National Academy Press; 1997.
55. Baranowksi T. Families and health action. In: Gochman DS, editor. Handbook of Health Behavior Research, Vol IV: Relevance for Professionals and Issues for the Future. New York: Plenum Press; 2004. p. 179–206.
56. Baranowski T, Hearn M. Families and health behavior change. In: Gochman DS, editor. Handbook of Health Behavior Research, Vol IV: Relevance for Professionals and Issues for the Future. New York: Plenum Press;2004. p. 303–23.
57. US Department of Agriculture, US Department of Health and Human Services. Nutrition and Your Health: Dietary Guide-lines for Americans, 6th edition. Washington, DC: US Department of Agriculture; 2005.
58. US Department of Agriculture. My Pyramid. DC: US Department of Agriculture, Food Nutrition and Consumer Services, Center for Nutrition Policy and Promotion; 2005.
59. Murphy SP. Nutrition guidelines to maintain health. In: Coulston AM, Rock CL, Monsen ER. Nutrition in the Prevention and Treatment of Disease. San Diego: Academic Press; 2001. p. 753–72.
60. Institute of Medicine. Promoting Health: Intervention Strategies From Social and Behavioral Research. Washington, DC: National Academy Press; 2000.
61. Institute of Medicine. Speaking of Health: Assessing Health Communication Strategies for Diverse Populations. Washington, DC: National Academy Press; 2001.
62. Health for All in the Twenty-First Century. Geneva: World Health Organization. Geneva: WHO; 1998.

APPENDIX: GUIDE TO ADDITIONAL READINGS IN COMMUNITY NUTRITION PROGRAMS AND SERVICES FOR CHILDREN AND ADOLESCENTS

1. Sulz HA, Young KM. Health Care USA, 4th edition, Understanding Its Organization and Delivery. Sudbury, MA: Jones and Bqrtlett Publishers; 2004.
2. Shi L, Singh DA. Delivering Health Care in America: A Systems Approach. Sudbury, MA: Jones and Bartlett; 2004.
3. Mathematika Policy Institute. Hunger In America 2006. NJ: Mathematika Policy Research Institute Princeton; 2006.
4. Eaton DK, Kann L, Kinchen S, et al. Youth risk behvioe surveillance: United States 2005. MMWR 2005;55:1–23.
5. Fox MK, Hamilton W, Lin BH. Effects of Food Assistance and Nutrition Programs on Nutrition and Health, Vol 4, Executive Summary of the Literature Review US Department of Agriculture, Economic Research Service, Food Assistance and Nutrition Research Report, 19–4. Washington: USDA; 2004.
6. FITS (a supplement discussing weaning and toddler nutrition) Supplement 1. J Am Diet Assoc 2006;106: S5–149.
7. Centers for Disease Control and Prevention. Report of the task force on community preventive services: Public health strategies for preventing and controlling overweight and obesity in school and worksite ettings. Morb Mortal Wkly Rep 2005;54:1–8.
8. USDHHS, Agency for Health Care Research and Quality. The Guide to Clinical Preventive Services: Recommendations of the US Preventive Services Task Force, AHRQ Pub No. 06–0588; Atlanta, GA, 2006.
9. USDHHS. 4th Report on the Diagnosis, Evaluation and Treatment of High Blood Pressure in Children and Adolescents, NIH Pub No. 05–5267; Bethesda, MD, 2005.
10. Guide to Community Preventive Services: Evidence-Based Recommendations to Improve Community Health. Available at www.thecommunityguide.org.
11. Goals in Action: School Health Index Centers for Disease Control and Prevention. Available at http://www.cdc.gov.goals.
12. Pennington J. Nutrition monitoring in the United States. In: Berdanier C, Dwyer JT, editors. CRC Handbook on Food and Nutrition. Boca Raton, FL: CRC; in press.
13. Position of the American Dietetic Association. Child and adolescent food and nutrition programs. J Am Diet Assoc 2006;106:1467–75.
14. Position of the American Dietetic Association. Individual, family, school and community based interventions for pediatric overweight. J Am Diet Assoc 2006;106:925–45.
15. Position of the American Dietetic Association. Local support for nutrition integrity in schools. J Am Diet Assoc 2006;106:122–33.
16. Position of the American Dietetic Association. Benchmarks for nutrition programs in child care settings. J Amer Diet Assoc 2005;105:979–86.
17. Position of the American Dietetic Association. Dietary guidance for healthy children ages 2–11 years. J Amer Diet Assoc 2004;104:660–77.
18. Position of the American Dietetic Association, Society for Nutrition Education, and American School Food Service Association. Nutrition services: An essential component of comprehensive school health programs. J Nutr Educ Behav 2003;35:57–67.
19. Centers for Disease Control and Prevention, US Department of Health and Human Services. The CDC has developed many excellent resources for promoting physical activity and healthy eating in schools at these sites: http://store.tcpress.com/0807737135.shtml#364; http://www.cdc.gov/healthyyouth/SHI; http://www.nasbe.org/HealthySchools/States/State–Policy.asp; and http://www.fns.usda.gov/tn/Healthy/wellnesspolicy.html.
20. US Department of Health and Human Services. Using What Works: Adapting evidence-based programs to fit your needs. US Department of Health and Human Services, National Cancer Institute, National Institutes of Health. NIH Pub No. 06:5874; Bethesda, MD, 2006.
21. Goran MI, Southern MS. Handbook of Pediatric Obesity: Etiology, Pathophysiology and Prevention. Boca Raton, FL: CRC Taylor and Francis; 2006.
22. Food and Nutrition Board, Institute of Medicine. Progress in Preventing Child Obesity: How do We Measure up? Washington: National Academy Press; 2006.
23. Rolfes SR, DeBruyne LK, Whitney EN. Life Span Nutrition: Conception Through Life, 2nd edition. New York: West Wadsworth; 1999.
24. Feld LG, Hyams JS. Childhood obesity. Consens Pediatr 2004;1:1–36.
25. Kessler DB, Baker SS, Silverman LA, editors. Growth assessment and growth failure. Consens Pediatr 2004;1:1–28.
26. Martin J, Conklin MT. Managing Child Nutrition Programs: Leadership for Excellence. Gaithersburg, MD: Aspen Publishers; 1999.
27. Kleinman R, editor. Pediatric Nutrition Handbook, 5th edition. Elk Grove, IL: American Academy of Pediatrics; 2004.
28. Hendricks KM, Duggan C, Walker A. Manual of Pediatric Nutrition, 3rd edition. Hamilton: BC Decker; 2000.
29. Food and Nutrition Board. Dietary Reference Intakes: Essential Guide to Nutrient Requirements. Washington: National Academy Press; 2006
30. Marabou Symposium. Nutrition and human development. Nutr Rev 2006;64:S1–88.

Nutritional Epidemiology

Carine M. Lenders, MD, MS
Walter C. Willett, MD, DrPH

Nutritional epidemiology is the study of relationships between diet and disease. Although the effects of nutritional deficiencies have been recognized for centuries, the chemical structures of compounds responsible for these deficiencies have been determined only this past century. Globally, the four most commonly recognized deficiencies in children include protein-calorie malnutrition and iron, iodine, and vitamin A deficiencies. The importance of folate deficiency has also become apparent in the past two decades. Interventions have evolved beyond the treatment of deficiencies to the reduction of disease risk (eg, food fortification with iodine, iron, and folate; zinc and vitamin A supplementation programs; and breast-feeding campaigns). More recently, the relationship between nutrition and disease has been expanded from that of deficiency to that of excess; the concept of *nutrition transition* has been developed. Countries undergoing modernization and westernization are faced with diseases associated with both under- and overnutrition. Globally, overnutrition and related complications have become the most important nutritional problem.

In contrast to those of most adults, children's needs vary with time as they grow and mature; therefore, assessment of pediatric diet, nutrition, and associated diseases is more challenging than that of adults. The dietary choices of children depend on their food preferences and on parental choice and control, food availability and cost, peer pressure, and advertising. Young children's ability to report their dietary intake is limited; thus, dietary assessment often requires a surrogate reporter. Despite these differences in approaches to assessment, current national surveys conducted in the United States have shown overall similar dietary trends in adults and children aged 2 to 18 years.

The development of techniques to assess diet and breast-feeding, the refinement of anthropometric methods, and the identification of biochemical indicators of diet (biomarkers) specific to population groups have greatly facilitated the field of nutritional epidemiology. Information from basic research has been used at the population level, and new questions in epidemiologic studies have been brought to the laboratory bench and the clinical setting. Methods used to investigate the relationships among diet, nutrition, and diseases include descriptive, analytic, and experimental studies. The development of hypotheses often comes from ecologic observations, and prevalence rates and diet–biochemical relationships are typically based on cross-sectional studies. The assessment of etiologic relationships is usually performed using case-control studies and prospective studies, which are typically expensive and of long duration. Each type of study has its own benefits and pitfalls. Although the best evidence for causation comes from experimental studies such as randomized, double-blind trials, in many situations it is not feasible to randomly assign subjects to diet for long periods of time.

In this updated overview of nutritional epidemiology, we briefly describe issues and approaches for assessing dietary intake and nutritional status, the application of different study designs, and considerations in the analysis and interpretation of data. Because of its vital importance to child health, we use the relationship between folate intake and incidence of neural tube defects (NTDs) to illustrate various approaches in nutritional epidemiology.

ASSESSMENT OF DIETARY INTAKE

Diet exposure can be measured either in terms of foods or as nutrient and nonnutrient components. The power to detect an association between diet and disease is usually greater when using nutrients (from all foods) rather than one food or food group to represent diet, and interpretation of associations is easier to explain biologically. However, food analyses are used frequently because people eat foods, not nutrients, and food can reflect the combined effects of multiple nutrients and differences in bioavailability of nutrients. Each dietary representation has its benefits and weaknesses, and the use of both methods provides the greatest insight.

An association between a food and disease can lead to the identification of a substance that is responsible for disease or its prevention. A classic example is that of scurvy. As recorded by Hippocrates, symptoms of scurvy were already recognized in ancient Egypt, Greece, and Rome. Later, a tree extract provided by North American natives cured scurvy among members of an expedition led by Cartier in the sixteenth century. Lind, in his *Treatise of the Scurvy* (1753),[1] documented that lemons and oranges also cured subjects with scurvy. However, the relationship between scurvy and vitamin C deficiency was made much later. Celiac disease provides another example.[2] Although descriptions of symptoms compatible with celiac disease were recorded in antiquity, Samuel Gee (1888) defined the classic symptoms of celiac disease in the mid-nineteenth century. These symptoms included chronic diarrhea, abdominal distention, and poor weight gain several months after the introduction of solid foods. The relationship between certain types of cereals and celiac disease was determined when the typical symptoms of pediatric celiac disease disappeared during the food shortages of World War II and relapsed after cereal supplies were restored.[3] Gluten, the major component of cereal proteins, was implicated.[4]

Intake of nutrients or foods is typically interrelated, which can result in difficulties in interpreting findings. For example, an inverse relationship exists between dietary fat and fiber intake among children.[5] Therefore, associations between food and disease could be attributable to foods either high in fiber or low in fat, or both. Sometimes multivariate analysis can be used to disentangle these associations. To minimize interrelations, investigators sometimes use food groups or account for the contributions of nutrient intake from various food groups.

Also, "pattern analysis,"[6] based on factor or cluster analysis, groups together subjects with similar intakes of food. These patterns can then be evaluated in relation to disease risk.

DIETARY ASSESSMENT METHODS

Methods to measure dietary intake include 24-hour recall, food records, food frequency questionnaires (FFQs), diet histories, and observation (Table 1). New tools, including short questionnaires, interactive software, and picture cards, are being developed to target specific nutrients (eg, calcium) and foods (eg, fruits and vegetables) and specific populations.[7] Other methods are being developed to assess healthful and unhealthful food and eating behaviors in 9- to 14-years-old children.[8,9] The validity and the reliability of dietary intake methods among 2- to 18-year-old children and adolescents from industrialized countries have been reviewed elsewhere.[7,10–12] Most validation studies have used observation, diet records, or repeated 24-hour recalls as reference standards. Assuming energy balance, the doubly labeled water method is considered the best method for validation of energy intake using traditional dietary assessment methods.

The doubly labeled water method is the first truly noninvasive means to measure total daily energy expenditure accurately in free-living humans and is based on measurement of CO_2 using

Table 1 Advantages and Disadvantages of Dietary Assessment Methods

Method	Recording Time	Period	Interviewer Training	Subject Literacy	Affects Diet Intake	Memory	Subject Burden	Food Description	Automated Procedure	Budget
Recall	Short	Defined	High	No	No	Yes	No	Yes	Yes	Expensive
Food record	Defined	Defined	High	Yes	Yes	No	Yes	Yes	Yes	Expensive
Food frequency	Short	Long	None	Yes	No	Yes	Yes	No (ranks)	Yes	Relatively inexpensive
	—	—	—	—	—	—	—		—	
Histories	Long	Imprecise	High	No	No	Yes	Yes	Yes	No	Expensive
Observation	Long	Defined	High	No	No	No	No	Yes	No	Expensive

a nonradioactive isotope. The technique was introduced in the 1950s, but applications started being made among adults in the 1980s. The total energy expenditure obtained from the doubly labeled water method can be accurate,[13] but large interlaboratory variability has been found in a blinded evaluation of multiple laboratories.[14] Also, the reproducibility of this method at an interval of several months or more has not been evaluated in free-living populations of children. Overall, food records and recalls are more accurate than other dietary assessment methods in school-age children.[7] Studies also show that most dietary assessment methods provide better estimates for the composition of the diet—after adjusting for energy intake—rather than absolute intake of nutrients or energy and for a group rather than individuals.[15,16] As a measure of validity, correlation coefficients above .5 between a new method and a standard method, such as many days of food records, are recommended for nutrients of interest in epidemiological studies.

24-Hour Recall

The 24-hour recall method is based on an interview, typically conducted by a trained dietary interviewer. It provides appropriate mean estimations for groups but not for individuals because of large day-to-day variation in individual intakes. Surrogate reporters are required for children who are young (preteen),[12,17] mentally retarded, or too sick to respond by themselves. Reporting problems can arise if parents spend less time with their children, for example, when they work outside of the household or have a large family.[16]

Twenty-four-hour recalls by children aged 2 to 18 years, or by surrogate reporters, have been compared to reference standards (observations, food records, and food chemical analysis) and summarized elsewhere.[11] In their review, McPherson and colleagues showed correlation coefficients (*r* values) of .2 to .9 for energy intake and .4 to .6 for most nutrients compared with the standard methods.[11] The correlation coefficients for nutrients improved after adjusting for energy intake. Compared with the standard method, recalls tended to either over- or underestimate energy intake.[11] The extent of underreporting was greater in adolescents than in all other age groups[18,19] and among girls participating in a dietary intervention compared to control.[20] Food eaten varied from 68 to 84% when diet recall was compared with the validation standard.[11] The validity of the dietary recall improved when individual meals were compared rather than using 24-hour periods[11] and when school-age children (8 to 10 years old) were trained to record their food intake using diet records and then asked to recall their 24-hour food intakes using the diet records as memory prompts during interviews.[21] Baxter and colleagues found that the accuracy of dietary recall did not vary with gender or ethnicity.[22]

The number of days for which dietary recording is necessary to accurately identify specific nutrient intakes in children has been calculated by determining the day-to-day intraindividual variation in dietary intake data for infants 4 to 6 months of age[23] and preschool children.[24] Quandt obtained dietary information using 24-hour recall among 28 mothers for their infants' diets on four random days over approximately 1 month.[23] In contrast to what is the case with adults, investigators found no effect of day of the week on nutrient variation in this age group. Interindividual variation exceeded intraindividual variation for all nutrients except vitamin C.

Stein and colleagues measured intraindividual day-to-day variation and tracking of nutrient intakes in a longitudinal study of 181 preschool children (93% Hispanic) aged 45 to 60 months recruited through a hospital-based pediatrics practice in New York.[24] In that study, 24-hour dietary recalls were administered four times in the first year and three times in the third year to children's mothers. Although the reliability of estimates (intraclass correlation coefficients) of energy and nine nutrients obtained from a single administration of the dietary recall ranged from .15 to .38, the authors were able to show substantial tracking of underlying diets among preschool children over a 19-month period, despite day-to-day variation.

Fisher and colleagues showed that body weight also influenced the accuracy of dietary reports made by children and their parents in a sample of 146 children aged 4 to 11 years using the doubly labeled water method to validate the energy intake measured using 24-hour recalls.[25]

Food Record

The food record method consists of a detailed diary of foods consumed over one or more days.[26] It provides appropriate mean values for groups but not for individuals, unless the number of days is substantial. The information is collected at the time of consumption so that memory is not a limitation. However, assessment is imprecise when dining out and can interfere with dietary intake. McPherson and colleagues pointed out that there were no specific validation studies of portion size collection and none of the studies reviewed presented results on validity in reporting food items.[11] Underreporting in children's adult-assisted food records increased with age (9 to 12 years old) when energy expenditure was measured with doubly labeled water. In that study, the investigators found differences in reporting by race but not by gender. African-American children were significantly more likely to underreport energy intake than were white children.

Black and colleagues studied the day-to-day variation in energy intake of 48 breast-fed infants using 4-day diet records at monthly intervals from age 1.5 to 7.5 months and of 37 fully weaned infants studied at 10, 12, 15, and 18 months of age.[27] Dietary variation was lowest in fully breast-fed infants, increased as solids were introduced, and approached values found for adults in the 18-month-old infants. Nelson and colleagues showed that with the exception of ascorbic acid, intakes were lowest in the youngest age groups (less than 36 months of age) and rose through childhood to peak in adolescence and young adulthood.[28] In contrast to the homogeneity of the intragroup coefficient of variation (CV_w) of specific nutrients among children and adults, the intergroup coefficient of variation (CV_b) varied largely by age group and gender, resulting in variance ratios that were relatively low for toddlers, high for children aged 5 to 17 years, and intermediate for adults. The lower toddler's variance ratios are best explained by their ability to adjust their energy intake at successive meals resulting in relatively constant within-subject daily energy intake.[29] Nelson and colleagues found that up to 4 years of age, 7 days were adequate to estimate all macronutrients except type of fat.[28] For animal protein, the number of days required to achieve a level of accuracy of ranking at and above .9 was 18 days (Table 2).

As determined by the doubly labeled water method, underreporting of energy intakes on children's assisted food records increased with age.[11,30] Using that same reference method, other investigators have also shown that estimations by food record can be made at the group, but not at individual level. O'Connor compared measurements of energy intake from diet records and total energy expenditure using the doubly labeled water method in 47 children aged

Table 2 Number of Days Dietary Records are Required for a Correlation Coefficient of .9 between Observed and True Intakes

	Days for Children 1 to 4 Years Old	Days for Boys 5 to 15 Years Old	Days for Girls 5 to 15 Years Old
Protein	5	6	15
Animal protein	6	7	18
Fat	7	8	12
Saturated	8	6	12
Polyunsaturated	15	18	28
Monounsaturated	11	9	14
Cholesterol	27	18	21
Carbohydrate	6	10	9
Folate	6	9	22

Adapted from reference 28.

6 to 9 years.[31] Although the mean energy intake and the total energy expenditure were not significantly different, the authors showed no significant correlation between energy intake and total energy expenditure. Findings of this study confirm the notion that energy intake assessed by diet records is not representative of total energy expenditure at the individual level but that 3-day-food records could be used to estimate energy intake at the population level. Even longer periods of dietary records (eg, 7 days) compared to the doubly labeled water method can underestimate energy intake, especially in overweight adolescents.[32]

Food Frequency Questionnaire

In contrast to food records and 24-hour recalls, FFQs are relatively inexpensive and aim to represent long-term intake. The food frequency method relies on a food list, and participants are asked to report the frequency of consumption of each food item; the design of these questionnaires is described in detail elsewhere.[12,16] FFQs can be used to rank respondents by levels of intake. The period of time covered by the FFQ can be weeks, months, or years, and the questionnaires can be classified as quantitative (ie, food models shown for usual portion size), semiquantitative (ie, standard serving size used), or nonquantitative (only frequency assessed). Overestimation of intakes of energy and other nutrients was observed in studies using a validation standard (diet record or repeated 24-hour recall) when adults' rather than children's portion size were used in children studies.[11]

When multiple 24-hour recalls, rather than just one, were used as the validation standard, investigators observed similar estimates for energy intake obtained with the 24-hour recalls and the FFQ, referred to as the Youth-Adolescent Food Frequency Questionnaire.[12] In that study, further adjustment for intraindividual variation in recalls improved the nutrient correlation coefficients. Inner-city sixth and seventh grade students demonstrated the ability to provide valid estimates of intake of calories and a variety of nutrients over 1 year. However, children in the fourth and fifth grades in inner-city schools experienced difficulties in completing the same FFQ.[33] This finding shows that surrogates are needed in older children from disadvantaged populations. A FFQ for low-income, 1- to 3-years-old Hispanic, African-American, and white children who attended the WIC program, was recently found to have excellent reliability and acceptable validity.[34] Blum and colleagues also validated the use of a shortened version of the Youth-Adolescent FFQ in Caucasian and Native American children ages 1 to 5 years, with a parent or guardian filling out the questionnaire.[35] The average correlation was similar to that found in validation studies among adolescents and adults. Finally, the use of a 124-item FFQ has been found to be a reasonably valid method to capture adolescent diet recalled by young adults.[36]

In contrast to the accuracy of repeated 24-hour recalls[37] and weighed diet records,[19] when the doubly labeled water method was used as a standard, energy intake was overestimated by 50% in infants when FFQs were used.[38] Using the same doubly labeled water method as a standard in a group of older children (9 to 16 years old), energy intake obtained from the Youth-Adolescent FFQ was underestimated. However, the authors showed that despite a wide range of variability in reporting accuracy across adiposity status and gender, this method estimated the mean energy intake of a group with appropriate accuracy.[39]

Diet History

Diet history provides information on typical meals, food intakes, and preparation of food using a questionnaire, an interview, or both. This method is more qualitative than FFQs; the interview can take between 1 and 2 hours. Studies in children have shown overestimation of nutrients and energy intakes in the first interview compared with overestimations in subsequent interviews.[40] In addition, Livingstone and colleagues validated the energy intake assessed by *7-day* weighted food records and diet histories with that obtained using the doubly labeled water method in 78 subjects aged 3 to 18 years.[19] Food records underestimated energy intake, whereas diet histories tended to overestimate energy intake in most age groups if it is assumed that the results from the doubly labeled water method were without error.[14]

Observation

Trained personnel can observe patients in a variety of settings, especially schools. Food intake can be measured once or multiple times. The method is intrusive and is impractical in large studies. However, this method is often used as a validation standard for school-age children and is reliable.[41]

SPECIAL CASE FOR DIETARY ASSESSMENT: BREAST-FEEDING

Studies relating breast-feeding to illness are difficult to evaluate because of the use of a variety of definitions for breast-feeding,[42,43] selection bias,[44,45] confounding,[46] and reverse causality.[45] As reviewed below, a few studies have addressed the reproducibility and validity of breast-feeding assessment methods. Several techniques have been used to evaluate the intake of breast milk among breast-feeding children. The doubly labeled water method is considered the gold standard for evaluating energy intake in breast-fed children.[47] Other techniques include test weighing and the evaluation of the duration and frequency of breast-feeding using observation, recall, and record studies.

Doubly Labeled Water Technique

The use of doubly labeled water has been validated against periodic open circuit respiratory gas exchange in infants.[48] Prentice and colleagues first showed that the energy requirements of infants were lower than recommended intakes, based on the combination of energy deposited during growth and total energy expenditure obtained by the doubly labeled water technique in 355 healthy infants aged up to 3 years.[50] Butte and colleagues conducted a validation study of conventional weighing techniques to estimate milk intake in breast-fed and formula-fed infants using the doubly labeled water method.[48] They found a mean difference between methods of 14% (106 g/d) in breast-fed infants and 8% (70 g/d) in formula-fed infants. Based on this method, these researchers also showed that energy requirements of infants and toddlers were 80% of current recommendations and were lower in breast-fed than in formula-fed infants. As a result new recommendations for energy intake have been decreased in infancy and early childhood and recommendations for physical activity have been provided.[49]

Test-Weighing Techniques

Conventional test-weighing techniques include weighing either infants or mothers before and after a known or unknown amount of breast milk intake. Brown and colleagues conducted validation studies of different test-weighing techniques among 64 infants before and after the consumption of a known amount of milk.[51] The measured bottle weight corresponded to 94.9 ± 13.2% of the estimated change in weight of the infant. These techniques allowed good estimates of breast milk consumption to be made, noting that the average amount of breast milk received declined with time from 632 g/d for the 5 to 12 month olds to 368 g/d for the 24 to 30 month olds.[52] Because of the intrusive nature of test weighing, it generally will not be directly useful in epidemiologic studies, but it could serve as a standard in validation studies of other methods.

Observation, Recalls, and Questionnaires

Piwoz and colleagues conducted a validation study of breast-feeding recall using observation as the reference standard.[53] He obtained 1,574 single-day dietary intakes (12-hour observations plus 12-hour recall) and mothers' monthly reports of usual feeding practices. They demonstrated that single-day studies produced a different view of feeding practices compared to the mothers' reports. Exclusive breast-feeding was observed 25% more frequently among infants younger than 4 months than was self-reported. In contrast, self-reported formula consumption was 30% more frequent compared to observation data. Differences between reported and observed practices were related to mothers' age and education, number of children younger than 5 years in the home, and infant age and disease on the observation day. The investigators concluded that consumption of breast milk or formula during the past 24 hours should not be used alone as the basis for classifying infant feeding practices in surveys.

Infant breast-feeding assessment tool, the mother baby assessment tool, and the LATCH assessment tool were evaluated for reliability (6 months) and validity using videotapes of breast-feeding sessions.[54] Using food records and FFQs, the relative agreement for the frequency of breast milk and study formula consumption was found to be very good.[55,56]

Most epidemiologic studies have used recalled or observed data to provide information on breast-feeding. Investigators have used information on the duration, frequency, and minutes of breast-feeding rather than test-weighting or isotopic methods to evaluate the relationship between breast-feeding and outcome (ie, growth and disease), and some, but not all, studies have gathered information on additional sources of foods besides breast-feeding. For example, Zeitlin and Ahmed examined the relationship among breast-feeding, total energy intake, and growth of infants in Bangladesh using observation (minutes of breast-feeding) and 24-hour recall to estimate breast milk and other food intake in infants and children aged 5 to 23 months.[57] Beaudry and colleagues used a self-administered standardized questionnaire mailed to every mother 1 week before infants reached 6 months of age to evaluate past breast-feeding and weaning behaviors.[58] Recently, Vähätalo and colleagues found that a dietary interview method including a short FFQ was useful for ranking infant subjects according to the consumption frequency of breast milk and infant(study formula, as well the amount of formula used.[59] However, the amounts of study formula were overestimated by the dietary interview as compared with two 48-h recalls.[59] Types of questions asked during the interview are reported by the authors in the methods section and the FFQ used in that study can be found in the appendix of that article. Finally, some authors have previously suggested that clarification of the intensity and duration of breast-feeding might help detect dose-response effects of breast-feeding.[43]

ASSESSMENT OF GROWTH AND BODY COMPOSITION

The focus of many studies in nutritional epidemiology is body weight, but recent techniques have evolved to better characterize changes in body weight in terms of body composition. Chapter 4, "Body Composition and Growth," describes the theory and practice of many of these techniques, as well as what is known about developmental changes in body composition. Recently, air displacement plethysmography has been shown to be a promising practical method compared to underwater densitometry, dual-energy X-ray absorptiometry (DXA) scan, skinfolds, and deuterium[60–62] to evaluate fat and nonfat compartments,[63–66] even among infants.[67]

Because nutritional epidemiologic studies in pediatrics often employ a variety of body composition techniques, the relationships among them are of interest Densitometry is typically considered the gold standard for a two-compartment model of fat and nonfatty tissue in adults and depends on measurements of total body density. Despite the lack of data on fat and fat-free mass densities in children,[68] densitometry has been compared with anthropometric measurements involving weight, height, and skinfold thickness measurements (Table 3). Likewise, anthropometric data based on weight and height indices have been compared with skinfold thickness measurements (Table 4).

Data on weight and height were also compared more recently not only to measurement of skinfold thickness but also to DXA among children aged 2 to 19 years.[77] Compared to weight for height and the Rohrer's index (Wt/Ht^3), the Quetelet index, or body mass index (BMI; Wt/Ht^2), was identified as the better predictor of overweight (but not underweight) when average skinfold thickness measurements were used as standard. BMI was also shown to perform better than the Rohrer index when the standard for percent body fat or total fat mass was estimated using DXA in children aged 3 to 19 years. No differences were found between BMI and weight for height in detecting overweight or underweight.

As described in Table 5, anthropometric measurements are most useful in large-scale studies. A recent study of bioelectrical impedance analysis (BIA) and BMI in adults[80] suggested that BIA was not superior to BMI as a predictor of overall adiposity. Likewise, Eisenman and colleagues found that BIA had limited utility in estimating body composition in their validation study among 3- to 8-year-old children (age of adiposity rebound) using anthropometry (BMI, waist circumference, and skinfolds), BIA, and DXA scan.[81] Recommendations from these studies are to use BMI, skinfolds, and waist circumference measurements in epidemiological studies.

Although BMI does not directly measure body fat, it is typically used to evaluate adiposity in adults and has been recognized as a useful predictor of adiposity in children and adolescents, which, in turn, also predicts risks for present or future medical complications of obesity.[82] The weight indices are considered adequate when the correlation with percent body fat is high and the correlation with height is low. Although there is no perfect weight index of over- and underweight—irrespective of height and width—BMI turned out to be a reasonable index from childhood to adulthood.[77] Transformation of weight and height is also discussed in Gasser and colleagues' review.[83] Frontini and colleagues further demonstrated that the association of weight-to-height index was not superior to BMI as an indicator of adiposity compared to skinfold thickness measurements as reference standards and related cardiovascular risk factors during childhood in the Bogalusa study.[76]

Self-reported weight and height among adults is frequently used in nutritional epidemiology. In contrast to the findings in adult studies, results from adolescents aged 12 to 17 years in the third national health and nutrition examination survey (NHANES III) showed that self-reported weights were missing in 40% of 12 year olds and 25% of 13 year olds. Based on their findings, the investigators did not recommend the use of self-reported weight and height as proxy measures of weight and height among adolescents aged less than 14 years.[84] In contrast to these findings, Strauss considered that the available self-reported weights and heights among 12 to 16 year olds in NHANES III were reliable (n = 1,657 of 1,932).[85] In that study, correlations between self-reported weight and actual weight ranged between .87 and .94, depending on gender or race. In a recent study of 72 overweight and obese children and adolescents 8–18 years old, self assessment of weight, height, and sexual maturation were not found to be valid proxy measures for a physician's assessment, although the reproducibility of self report of height and weight was good or excellent.[86] The renewed interest in body composition, combined with the awareness of the growing obesity epidemic, has resulted in the need for improved reference data for body composition (see Chapter 55, "Cancer Treatment").

BIOMARKERS OF DIETARY INTAKE

Biochemical indicators (biomarkers) of dietary intake—blood, urine, stool, and tissue nutrients—can reflect nutrient intake. Biomarkers are important in epidemiology because they can be used as surrogates for dietary intake when the nutrient content in a food varies greatly. They can also be useful as determinants of disease, even if they reflect intake poorly; serum cholesterol provides a good example. Biomarkers can also be used to validate nutrient intake assessed by dietary assessment methods. When biomarkers need to represent the intake of a specific nutrient in an epidemiologic study, the most important requirements are its sensitivity to changes in dietary intake and its ability to reflect the cumulative average intake over an extended period of time.[16]

Sensitivity of a Biomarker

The sensitivity of a biomarker depends on how well the biomarker reflects true nutrient intake, which can vary with the chemical form of the nutrient. For example, the bioavailability is lower for dietary folate than for supplemental folate, so serum levels will differ with the form of folate.

Table 3 Correlations between Anthropometric Measurements and Total Body Densitometry

Author(s)	Sample	Weight	Height	Weight/Height	Weight/Height^2	Weight/Height^3	Triceps Skinfold	Subscapular Skinfold
Parizkova*[69]	N = 62 white girls 12 to 16 yr	—	—	—	—	—	−.74	−.80
Seltzer et al.†[70]	N = 32 obese white girls 12 to 18 yr	−.53	−.23	—	—	—	−.69	−.59
Young et al.‡[71]	N = 102 white girls 9 to 16 yr	−.36	—	—	—	—	−.73	—
	N = 41 prepubertal	−.75	—	—	—	—	−.82	—
	N = 15 pubertal	−.69	—	—	—	—	−.78	—
	N = 46 postpubertal	−.42	—	—	—	—	−.70	—
Harsha et al.[72]	White, 6 to 16 yr; N = 79 boys,	−.17/−.52	.31/.03	—	—	—	−.76/−.75	
	n = 64 girls						−.75/−.80	
	Black, 6 to 16 yr; n = 49 boys,	−.36/−.59	.25/.14	—	—	—	−.82/−.82	
	n = 50 girls						−.75/−.87	
	N = 242 boys and girls 6 to 16 yr	−.32	.18	—	—	—	−.81	−.76
Roche et al.[73]	N = 68 boys, n = 49 girls 6 to 12 yr	.74/.74	—	.75/.62	.90/.84	.66/.55	.81/.74	.84/.80
	N = 63 boys, n = 81 girls 13 to 17 yr	.65/.88	—	.91/.87	.88/.89	.91/.82	.93/.86	.94/.87
Maynard et al.[74]	N = 35 boys, n = 39 girls 8 yr	—	.27/.34	—	.93/.67	—	—	—
	N = 49 boys, n = 56 girls 9 yr	—	.27/.46	—	.86/.74	—	—	—
	N = 79 boys, n = 63 girls 10 yr	—	.46/.43	—	.90/.79	—	—	—
	N = 90 boys, n = 79 girls 11 yr	—	.51/.42	—	.94/.78	—	—	—
	N = 103 boys, n = 86 girls 12 yr	—	.44/.28	—	.90/.85	—	—	—
	N = 103 boys, n = 81 girls 13 yr	—	.39/.39	—	.89/.82	—	—	—
	N = 101 boys, n = 74 girls 14 yr	—	.30/.16	—	.86/.84	—	—	—
	N = 94 boys, n = 80 girls 15 yr	—	.13/.01	—	.83/.88	—	—	—
	N = 91 boys, n = 87 girls 16 yr	—	.22/.19	—	.83/.85	—	—	—
	N = 90 boys, n = 83 girls 17 yr	—	−.09/.7	—	.90/.90	—	—	—
	N = 100 boys, n = 85 girls 18 yr	—	.03/.11	—	.84/.85	—	—	—

Of note, the correlation coefficients between predictors of adiposity and total body densitometry tend to be positive when authors have transformed body density measurements using an equation to estimate fat (as in Maynard or Roche) but tend to be negative when using direct measurements of hydrodensitometry (as in Horsha). In the Bogalusa study, the authors used W/H^p rather than W/H^3. They calculated the optimal "p" for each category of gender, race, and age because they wanted to obtain an index that was independent of H during growth and early life development [log(W) = a + p log(H) + e].

*The relationship between body density and triceps skinfold for the nonobese adolescents was [body density = 1.128 − 78 log triceps skinfold].

†Arm circumference had the highest correlation with both weight (r = .90) and bone density (r = .63). The authors showed body densities for their subjects similar to those shown by previous authors estimated from skinfold thickness measures [body density = 1.1516 − .09256 log triceps skinfold] and comparable to real body density measurements.

‡Total skinfolds provided (at least 12 sites from the chin to the knee). Overall, correlation for triceps was .79 and .72 for subscapular.

Table 4 Correlations of Body Mass Indices with Skinfold Thickness Measures in Large Studies

Study	Sample	Skinfold Thickness	W/H	W/H^2	W/H^3
Forsyth County study[75]	N = 832 5 to 12 yr boys	Triceps	.72	.81	.81
	N = 835 5 to 12 yr girls		.73	.80	.64
	N = 66 boys/n = 80 girls 5 yr		—	.24/.68	—
	N = 98 boys/n = 86 girls 6 yr		—	.53/.71	—
	N = 107 boys/n = 121 girls 7 yr		—	.67/.66	—
	N = 110 boys/n = 116 girls 8 yr		—	.79/.75	—
	N = 137 boys/n = 144 girls 9 yr		—	.78/.84	—
	N = 110 boys/n = 88 girls 10 yr		—	.82/.81	—
	N = 89 boys/n = 83 girls 11 yr		—	.89/.86	—
	N = 115 boys/n = 118 girls 12 yr		—	.79/.81	—
Bogalusa study[76]	N = 821 white boys 4 to 5 yr	Triceps/subscapular	—	.53/.52	.53/.51
	N = 523 black boys 4 to 5ry		—	.50/.44	.51/.44
	N = 838 white girls 4 to 5 yr		—	.61/.71	.60/.67
	N = 499 black girls 4 to 5 yr		—	.63/.60	.63/.56
	N = 1570 white boys 12 to 13 yr		—	.72/.86	.76/.81
	N = 925 black boys 12 to 13 yr		—	.64/.81	.67/.71
	N = 1462 white girls 12 to 13 yr		—	.81/.84	.77/.82
	N = 821 black girls 12 to 13 yr		—	.83/.84	.81/.81
NHANES (III)[77]	Boys/girls 2 to 5 yr	Average triceps and subscapular	.67/.73	.68/.71	.61/.66
	Boys/girls 6 to 11 yr		.79/.82	.81/.85	.77/.82
	Boys/girls 12 to 19 yr		.79/.83	.81/.85	.79/.84

Serum sodium is an example of a biochemical measure biomarker that is not sensitive to intake because it is tightly regulated to remain within a specific range. The 24-hour urinary measurement of 3-methylhistidine is an example of a good biomarker for animal protein intake (r = .77).[87]

Period Covered by a Biomarker

Studies of chronic diseases require biomarkers that are less susceptible to short-term fluctuations. For example, serum folate is sensitive to changes in intake and modestly sensitive to temporary changes in folate metabolism. Data from the Framingham study demonstrated a strong inverse correlation between plasma homocysteine and folate intake over long periods, assessed using FFQs.[88] Another example is that of plasma amino acids. There is evidence that plasma amino acids are indicators of

Table 5 Characteristics of Body Composition Measurements in Children

Characteristics	Weight	BMI	Skinfold	Conduction*	Densitometry	Isotopes†	Radiology‡
Advantages							
Convenient	Excellent	Excellent	Very good	Good	No	No	No
Reproducible	Excellent	Excellent	Very good	Good	Very good	Very good	Very good
Fast	Excellent	Excellent	Very good	Relatively	No	No	No
Expensive	No	No	No	No	Yes	Yes	Yes
Correlates with morbidity	Excellent	Excellent	Excellent	Good	Good	Good	Excellent
Large studies	Good	Good	Good	Good	Not good	Not good	Not good
Standard	Excellent	Excellent	Excellent	Good	Very good	Very good	Very good (some lack)
Disadvantages							
Correlates with Height	Highly	Not highly	Not highly	No	No	No	No
Assess fat distribution	Poorly	Poorly	Excellent	Poorly	Poor	Poor	Excellent
Equations	No	No	Many	Many	Many	Many	Many
Training	Some	Some	High	High	Very high	Very high	Very high
Radiation	No	No	No	No	No	No	Yes (CT)

Adapted from references 78 and 79.

*Conduction studies such as bioelectrical impedance, total-body electrical conductivity.

†Isotope studies such as ^{40}K, doubly labeled water.

‡Radiology studies such as computed tomography (CT) scan, magnetic resonance imaging, and ultrasonography.

dietary amino acids if they are measured within 2 hours of a protein meal.[89] Plasma amino acid measurements in the postabsorptive state (at least 8 hours without food consumption) are an indicator of dietary intake of amino acids when similar protein meals have been consumed for at least 2 weeks.[90] Although, red blood cells membrane fatty acids were not found to be reliable as an independent measure of compliance for dietary saturated fatty acids intake in short-term studies,[91] red cell levels of the monounsaturated fatty acid, oleic acid, and the polyunsaturated fatty acids ecosapentanoic acid (EPA) and decosahexanoic acid (DHA) were more useful biomarkers during short term intervention trials. Cholesterol ester appears to be the most suitable serum fraction to assess short-term dietary compliance.[92]

Source of Biomarker Measurements

Sources of biomarkers in humans include direct measurements of nutrients, enzyme activity, products of the metabolic pathway, and challenge (tolerance) tests. The biomarker can be measured directly in body fluids or tissues such as plasma, serum, erythrocytes, adipose tissue, muscle, urine, stool, hair, and nails. For example, mean population intakes of iodine and sodium can be estimated by casual urine samples.[93] Another example is that of dietary fatty acids. Using dietary intake from 200 FFQs as well as tissue, whole blood, and plasma levels of fatty acids, the correlation coefficient for alpha-linolenic acid and linoleic acid was .38 and .43 between diet and whole blood, .51 and .52 between diet and adipose tissue, and .39 and .41 between diet and plasma. In this study, for alpha-linolenic and linoleic acid, high correlations were observed between whole-blood and adipose tissue ($r = .59$ and $r = .67$) and between whole blood and plasma ($r = .96$ and $r = .88$).[94] Enzyme activity can be used to evaluate specific dietary nutrients (eg, alkaline phosphatase for zinc, glutathione peroxidase for selenium, and erythrocyte transketolase for thiamin).

Plasma homocysteine is a sensitive, but not a specific, marker of folate, and 25-dihydroxy vitamin D is a good marker for vitamin D deficiency. Although serum ferritin is a sensitive test of iron status and continues to be the leading single determination for individual iron status, it is not recommended in inflammatory states because it is an acute-phase reactant. Serum transferrin receptor is a promising alternative because it is more specific than ferritin. Another example of a nutrient that can be confounded by inflammation is serum betacarotene.[95] Finally, byproducts of nutrients can be related to disease, such as protein carbonyl content, which is the most widely used marker of oxidative modification of proteins.[96]

Factors Influencing Biomarker Measurements

The relationship between dietary nutrients and biomarkers can be influenced by sample collection, storage techniques, seasonal timing, time of day, study design, contamination (eg, zinc collected in ethylenediaminetetraacetic acid tubes), stability, storage temperature, and freeze–thaw cycles, as well as level of quality control.[16]

Biomarkers to Validate Dietary Assessment Methods

Biomarkers can be useful for validating other methods of dietary assessment such as FFQs, diet records, or recalls.[94,97–101] A major advantage is that the source of error in the biochemical measurement and intake assessment should be independent. For example, good correlations between folate intake and serum or red cell folic acid provided important documentation about the assessment of dietary folate, despite concerns about bioavailability and stability in food processing.

TRACKING DIETARY INTAKE

For adults, year-to-year dietary intakes, assessed by FFQs, show correlations of .6 to .7,[16] with decreasing correlations over longer intervals,[102] but diet tracking varies according to age category among children. Although parents have a dramatic influence on their children's dietary intakes, young children's preferences are not necessarily similar to those of their parents; however, as children grow older, their preferences become more similar.[103] Energy-density manipulation studies show that children are able to adjust their daily energy intake when they focus on their own hunger and satiety cues rather than on their parents asking them to "clean their plates."[103]

There was substantial tracking of underlying diets in a study of preschool children (45 to 60 months old) over a 19-month period.[24] After correction for intraindividual variation, the correlations ranged between .2 and .6. The correlation between nutrient intake at age 2 and at age 4 was examined in the Bogalusa study cohort of children aged 6 months to 4 years.[104] Total protein, animal protein, total sugar, sucrose, starch, total fat, saturated fatty acids, polyunsaturated fatty acids, and cholesterol showed correlations of .5 to .6 in children aged 2 years compared with children aged 4 years. At 2 years of age, 47 to 65% of children in the top tertile for total fat, saturated fat, and cholesterol intake remained in the top tertile by age 4.

Tracking of diets has also been studied in older children and adolescents. Tracking of fruit and vegetable intakes (food records) among children in third grade showed correlations of .4 to .5 ovr 2 years.[105] Calcium and dairy intake (diet histories) from adolescence into adulthood (13 to 27 years old) showed a correlation of .4.[106] Using three 24-hour recalls per survey, a longitudinal study of 984 children aged 6 to 13 years tracked nutrient intakes over a 6-year period in China.[107] The authors concluded that even under conditions of rapid socioeconomic change, children were likely to maintain their dietary intake patterns from childhood into adolescence. The correlations between dietary intakes measured at a 6-year interval ranged between .28 and .51 for macronutrients and major food groups (vegetable and fruit, meat, and edible oils).

Results from a recently published longitudinal English study of 198 participants with two 3-day food diaries collected in 1980 and 2000 (at ages 12 and 33 years) showed that adolescent food intake was correlated with that in adulthood, but it was not a strong predictor. Dietary changes were influenced by variables including gender, location and socioeconomic status.[108] However these results could also reflect longitudinal societal changes over time. As an example, trends in food consumption patterns of 1,584 10-year-old children at seven separate cross-sectional surveys (65% Euro American, 35% African-American) changed over time (1973 to 1994).[109]

TRACKING OF NUTRIENTS AND BIOMARKERS

Using 3-day dietary records, participants in the Penn State young women's health study showed weaker tracking of nutrients over a 6-year period among subjects who were 12 years of age at initiation of the study until they reached 18 years.[108] Although the year-to-year correlation coefficient for body weight over the 6-year period of that study was .9, rank and correlation analyses showed low tracking among nutrients examined (fat, sugar, iron, and vitamin C). Another longitudinal study of tracking between 13 and 33 years of age in Amsterdam showed that tracking of nutrient intakes showed relatively low but significant stability coefficients for all macro- and micronutrients (.28 to .52).[110] Overall, most nutrient tracking studies have shown that patterns of dietary intake are already present by 2 years of age. Although tracking varies with age, most studies show a low to modest correlation over time. Possible reasons for conflicting results of tracking could include study design, age groups under study, dietary instrument used to assess diet, socioeconomic background, and prevalence of overweight, among others.

Studies of tracking of diet and disease using biomarkers in pediatrics are few, except for those of cardiovascular disease. One example is that of diet and cardiovascular disease risk factors in the Bogalusa study, carried out in Louisiana.[111] Dietary cholesterol changes correlated significantly with serum total cholesterol changes (r = .42) and low-density lipoprotein cholesterol (r = .50) from 6 months to 4 years of age. The correlation between dietary intake and subscapular skinfold thickness measurements was .3 to .4 for total protein, total fat, starch, and energy.[111,112] In another longitudinal study from birth to 5 years of age, tracking of serum cholesterol was similar to that in older children and adolescents once the weaning process was completed.[113] The composition of fatty acids in blood has been shown to reflect the quality of dietary fat. Therefore, the long-term stability (tracking) of the serum (and hence dietary) fatty acid composition of serum cholesteryl ester fatty acids was analyzed in a randomly selected population sample of 1,029 Finnish boys and girls aged 3, 6, 9, 12, 15, and 18 years and again 3 years later. The correlations were high for all fatty acids; both linoleate and arachidonate had correlations of .6.[114]

EVALUATION OF DIET–DISEASE RELATIONSHIPS

The ability to detect an association between a dietary variable and disease requires adequate interindividual variation in that dietary factor.[16,115] This implies that the likelihood of detecting a risk associated with a specific food or nutrient among homogeneous populations who are characterized by little variation in the food or nutrient studied will be low. Dietary intake can vary with cultural background (eg, among religious groups), type of foods consumed (eg, vegetarianism), type of soil (eg, soil with little selenium or iodine), food preparation (eg, manioc with cyanide), and disease state (eg, lactose intolerance, heart disease). The detection of an association between food and disease or nutrient and disease can also be limited by errors in measuring dietary intake. Variation in diet over time can be considered to be an error if long-term average intake for an individual is etiologically important. Specific data collection and statistical procedures can be applied to minimize the effects of error.

Adjustment for Energy Intake

The major components of energy intake have been reviewed elsewhere[16,116] and include body size, growth, physical activity and fidgeting, and metabolic efficiency. Most of the variation in energy intake among subjects is attributable to differences in body size and physical activity. Although metabolic efficiency and fidgeting also vary among subjects, they are not measured in nutritional epidemiology because of the lack of practical measures. In addition, a large proportion of the variation in nutrient intake is attributable to total energy intake. Adjusting for total energy intake can be viewed as a measure of nutrient composition rather than as a measure of absolute intake. Even though the association between nutrients and predictors of total energy intake is complex, failure to adjust for energy intake can result in misleading conclusions. Thus, and for the same reasons that animal studies of nutrient effects are conducted under isocaloric conditions, taking total energy intake into consideration when evaluating the relationships between diet and disease is usually important. An exception could be when the outcome being evaluated is growth or weight gain. Because adjusting for total energy is important in nutritional epidemiology, especially when energy intake is related to disease, models have been proposed and are reviewed elsewhere (Table 6).[16,117]

Table 6 Possible Models That Account for Total Energy Intake in Epidemiologic Studies

Residual model
Disease = nutrient residual
Disease = nutrient residual + calories
Standard multivariate model
Disease = calories + nutrient
Energy partition model
Disease = $\text{calories}_{(\text{nutrient})}^{*}$ + $\text{calories}_{(\text{other})}^{\dagger}$
Multivariate nutrient density model
Disease = (nutrient/calories) + calories

Adapted from reference 16.

*$\text{Calories}_{(\text{nutrient})}$ corresponds to caloric intake from a specific nutrient.

†$\text{Calories}_{(\text{other})}$ corresponds to calories from other nutrients than those under study.

Residual Model. Nutrient residuals are computed using a regression model with the absolute nutrient as the dependent variable and calories as the independent variable and then entered into a regression model with disease as the dependent variable. This model is comparable to isocaloric metabolic studies, in which total energy intake is constant, except for the modification in one nutrient. In the case of macronutrient calories, this model can also be viewed as the caloric substitution of one macronutrient for a similar number of calories from other sources.

To make the interpretation of actual nutrient intake easier, a constant (typically the mean nutrient intake of the study population) is added to the residual values, which have a mean of zero and include negative values. When total energy intake is an important predictor of disease, total energy intake is added to the model, which already includes the nutrient-adjusted variable, as summarized in the second equation in the first model in Table 6. However, the magnitude of the relationship between total energy intake and disease can vary among studies because the contribution of foods to total energy intake can be different.

Standard Multivariate Model. In the standard multivariate model, both absolute nutrient intake and calories are considered independent variables in a regression model. Although the nutrient is adjusted for total energy intake in this model, the meaning has changed to calories independent of the nutrient. If we consider that total energy intake includes only protein, fat, and carbohydrate calories and the nutrient studied is protein, then energy intake corresponds to carbohydrate and fat calories. Although the meaning of total energy intake has changed, the coefficient of the nutrient studied is the same as that of the second residual model presented in Table 6. Some authors have concerns about this type of model, in which variables can be strongly correlated. McGee and colleagues have shown that results can vary widely when using highly correlated variables.[118] They suggest that variables with coefficient correlations of approximately 0.6 should not be included in the same model.

Energy Partition Model. The energy partition model is very different from the two preceding models. This is not an isocaloric model. Using the same example of total energy intake being equivalent to calories from protein, carbohydrate, and fat, this model implies that we examine the relationship between disease and increasing amount of protein in the diet, while keeping term for other calories (including fat and carbohydrate) constant. Therefore, the relationship between nutrient and disease can still be confounded by total energy intake and could erroneously indicate an effect of protein on disease.

Multivariate Nutrient Density Model. In the multivariate nutrient density model, the nutrient density is calculated as the nutrient divided by the total energy intake in a regression model, in which a term for calories is added as a second independent variable. This is an isocaloric model. This model can be interpreted as the relationship between the nutrient composition of the diet with disease when total energy intake is constant. Because nutrient densities are not highly correlated with total energy intake, the calories will retain their meaning of total energy intake.

Unlike in the residual model with calories and the standard multivariate model, in which the effect of the nutrient is considered similar in subjects consuming high- or low-energy diets, the nutrient density model can be useful when body size (and therefore total energy intake) varies widely among subjects. However, nutrient densities can result in an erroneous relationship. For example, when a nutrient has a weak correlation with total energy intake or a low variability and is subsequently divided by total energy intake, the nutrient can become highly correlated to total energy intake. Therefore, dividing by another variable does not necessarily mean that its effect is removed. As for absolute nutrient, nutrient densities can result in erroneous conclusions when total energy intake is associated with disease. Given the inclusion of the inverse of total energy intake in nutrient densities, nutrient densities tend to be associated with disease in the direction opposite that of total energy intake.

It is clear from this discussion that the interpretation of energy intake depends on the other variables added in the models. Therefore, the addition of predictors of energy intake to a model will also modify its interpretation. For example, if we assume energy balance, the interpretation of total energy intake in a model in which physical activity and body size were included would be that of metabolic efficiency. In another example, when residuals of weight on height (remove the effect of height on weight) and residuals of height on weight (remove the effect of weight on height) are included in a model with energy intake, height represents lean body mass, weight represents fat, and energy intake represents both physical activity and metabolic efficiency.[16]

The relationships between dietary intake and disease are complex. Although the interpretation of energy intake varies with the analytic method, the association between absolute nutrient intakes and disease should take into account total energy intake because the observed association can simply reflect that of total energy intake and disease. The presentation of various analytic approaches could further strengthen the findings of an association between diet and disease.

Type of Studies

The case of the relationship between folate deficiency and NTDs will be used to illustrate the contribution of a variety of study designs to the determination of a causal relationship between nutrient intake and an important health outcome. In addition, this example shows how the knowledge of a relationship between a nutrient and an outcome might not be sufficient to develop prevention interventions. Finally, it also demonstrates the value of nutritional epidemiology in establishing and evaluating public health policies.

Descriptive Epidemiology. The description of variation in rates of disease among different populations and locations, and over time, is generally called descriptive epidemiology. An environmental role in the development of NTDs was suspected from ecologic (differences in rates among geographic areas) and migration studies. The frequency of NTDs was higher in the northern United Kingdom and decreased when populations moved from high-prevalence areas in the United Kingdom to the United States. High prevalence of NTDs seemed to plague disadvantaged populations. For example, an epidemic of NTDs was observed during the Great Depression in Boston.[119] Another example comes from the decreasing rates of NTDs in Ireland over one decade concurrent with the use of fortified breakfast cereals.[120]

Clinical Observations and Intervention Studies. Clinical observations often provide important leads for further study. The finding of a relationship between socioeconomic background and NTDs resulted in a study of mother's and children's folate status in the United Kingdom. Smithells and colleagues performed blood tests to study micronutrients and found that folate, among others, was low among mothers whose infants had NTDs.[121] It was also observed that drugs interfering with folate metabolism were associated with the risk of NTDs.[122]

Risk of recurrence was examined in a nonrandomized prevention trial of multivitamin and mineral supplementation in England and suggested a beneficial effect of supplementation.[123,124] Supplementation started at entry to prenatal care for all women. Women who received supplements before 6 weeks of gestation (which corresponds to the cutoff point for neural tube closure) were further compared with women who received supplements later. Other smaller intervention studies showed nonsignificant lower risk of NTDs among supplemented women. Overall, intervention studies showed a fourfold decrease in risk of NTDs among women taking a multivitamin, but the studies have been criticized because many of the data were from nonrandomized trials.

Case-Control and Cohort Studies of Vitamin Supplements. In case-control studies, previous diet or use of supplements by cases (or, in this example, mother of the case) is compared with that of controls. In cohort studies, nutrient data are collected before the occurrence or recurrence of disease; thus, these studies tend to take longer and are more expensive. However, cohort studies are less subject to methodological bias.

Only four studies examined folate intake from the diet; others used information on supplements containing folic acid. Mulinare and colleagues used a birth defects registry to identify children born with NTDs and retrospectively asked about periconceptional multivitamin use (a period of up to 14 years before the interview).[125] The risk of NTDs was approximately 60% lower for women who reported taking supplements. In contrast, Mills and colleagues did not find a significant relationship between folate and NTDs.[126] Shaw and colleagues found a similar reduction in NTD risk when folate supplementation was started after 3 months of gestation, raising concerns about the causality between folate and NTDs.[127] Milunsky and colleagues conducted a prospective cohort study of multivitamin use and NTDs by telephoning mothers at the end of the first trimester of pregnancy to inquire about the type of supplement taken.[128] Findings showed a strong inverse relationship between multivitamin intake during the first 6 weeks of pregnancy and protection against NTDs.

In summary, all case-control and cohort studies except one supported a protective effect of periconceptional multivitamin use. It was unlikely that results observed in most studies were attributable solely to chance because of the variety of design and the choice of controls. However, confounding factors could have led to these findings. For example, NTDs occurred more often in populations of lower socioeconomic background, so that, in principle, socioeconomic background could have been a confounding factor. Also, the association between folate and NTDs might have been attributable to other vitamins in the multivitamin preparation.

Case-Control and Cohort Studies of Serum Folate. Daly and colleagues collected blood samples prospectively from more than 50,000 women attending their first antenatal clinic in Dublin maternity hospitals from 1986 to 1990.[129] They used a nested case-control design (sample from all cases and a matched sample of mothers who did not develop an NTD pregnancy) comparing early pregnancy blood folate concentrations in 81 women with pregnancies subsequently affected by NTDs and in a systematic sample of 247 control pregnancies. Folate levels were found to be lower for mothers who later had children who developed NTDs. The same authors found that a woman's risk of having a child with an NTD was associated with early pregnancy red cell folate concentrations in a continuous dose–response relationship.[129] However, in the absence of double-blind randomization, the social and reproductive differences between mothers who took the supplement and those who were considered part of the control group (mothers received supplements after the periconceptional period or refused to take the supplement) led to uncertainty as to the significance of the results.

Randomized Trials. The evidence for the relationship between folate intake and NTDs from randomized trials comes from two studies. One was on the *recurrence* of NTDs (history of previous pregnancy resulting in an NTD) conducted by the Medical Research Council Vitamin Study Research Group. This was a randomized trial conducted in five European countries, Israel, and Canada.[130] The other trial was on the *occurrence* of NTDs (first pregnancy resulting in an NTD), conducted in Hungary.[131] In the Medical Research Council study of recurrence, women were randomized in a 2 × 2 factorial design to 4 mg of folate versus placebo or to other vitamins typically contained in multivitamins versus placebo. The trial was stopped early because of the findings of a 72% protection rate for folate. The Hungarian study used a multivitamin with trace elements and folate versus trace elements and vitamin C. This trial was also stopped because of a high occurrence of NTDs in the placebo group.

Implications. The findings from these studies led to policy responses that were controversial and unclear. A variety of strategies could have been used to improve the folate status of the population: (1) increase intakes of foods rich in folate, (2) recommend routine use of supplements, or (3) suggest the fortification of foods.

Although increasing intakes of fruits and vegetables rich in folate would be beneficial in many respects, its effect on occurrence of disease would be minimal. Not only would large amounts of folate be necessary to increase plasma levels, but national programs to increase fruit and vegetable intake have not been particularly successful in the past. In addition, the bioavailability of folate in foods is not as good as that of supplemental folate.[132] Cuskelly and colleagues conducted a randomized trial of strategies to provide a daily intake of 0.4 mg of folate through either supplementation, food fortification, free provision of folate-rich foods, or dietary advice regarding folate-rich foods compared with a control group over a 3-month period.[133] Concentration of folate in red cells increased significantly only in the groups receiving folate supplements or folate-fortified foods. This study reinforces the concern of the effectiveness of dietary interventions in view of social and economic barriers.

The strategy that consisted of recommending folate supplementation to women during their reproductive years was supported by most epidemiologic studies and was endorsed by the Centers for Disease Control and Prevention in 1992. The Centers for Disease Control and Prevention recommended the use of 0.4 mg of folate daily in women who planned a pregnancy and 4 mg for those who had a history of NTD pregnancies. Although multivitamin consumption was affordable for most, the timing of supplementation and compliance were of concern. Many institutions supported the notion of informing women about folate supplementation; failure to provide this information was considered negligent. Targeting supplementation to a population at risk was difficult because there were no clear affordable screening tools available to identify subjects at risk and the population as a whole seemed to be at risk, based on Daly and colleagues' study.[129]

Finally, the strategy of fortifying the food supply had been used long before with success in many countries (eg, with iron and iodine). Fortification of the food supply would have an impact on the entire population and would not require ongoing educational campaigns. Nevertheless, the level of fortification and the type of foods to be fortified were the center of intense debate. The main concern was the masking of vitamin B12 deficiency. However, given that about 25% of the population of the United States consumed multivitamins with 0.4 mg of folate, the rare report of neurologic complications associated with vitamin B_{12} was reassuring. Nevertheless, the US Food and Drug Administration considered that levels of folate consumption from food and supplements above 1 mg of folate daily were concerning.

Although flour was a good candidate for fortification because it is consumed by most subjects in the population, the amount of consumption varies in the population. Therefore, simulations of food fortification of specific foods were performed by artificially increasing the folate content of products made of flour in existing food intake databases. Results from these simulations showed that folate intakes higher than 0.4 mg would have to be tolerated to increase folate intake of the entire population. Using this method, Oakley and colleagues showed that fortification with 0.35 mg of folate in 100 g of flour would increase the average intake by 0.25 mg, but 30% of women would still have a total folate intake below the recommended 0.4 mg and 15% of the women would have an intake above 1 mg/d (for most multivitamin users). Fortification with 0.14 mg of folate in 100 g of flour would result in an average increase of only 0.1 mg/d.[134] The US Food and Drug Administration recommended the use of 0.14 mg of folate in 100 g of flour; this was implemented in 1998. Since then, fortification of flour became mandatory in the United States, Canada and Chile which, substantially improved folate and homocysteine status while NTDs rates fell by between 31% and 78%.[135] However, the fortification of flour is considered suboptimal to prevent spina bifida and the debate continues.[136] Tragically, recommendations alone in other countries such as in France, did not influence trends in NTD.[137]

The demonstration that folic acid plays a major role in the prevention of *recurrence and occurrence* of NTDs stimulated further research on the possible mechanisms underlying the relationship and a possible nutrient–gene relationship. The association of a polymorphism in a folic acid metabolizing gene with the risk of NTD strongly supports the role of folate in the etiology of NTDs and could indicate a group with a higher folate requirement. A polymorphism in the 5,10-methylenetetrahydrofolate reductase gene is associated with a reduction of activity of that specific enzyme. An increase in the prevalence of this polymorphism was observed in infants born with NTDs and in their parents compared with controls.[138] The possible role of vitamin B_{12} in NTDs is still unclear, as reviewed elsewhere.[139–141]

Findings on folate and the risk of NTDs have given credibility to the search for other examples in which suboptimal intakes of nutrients could lead to high risk of chronic disease. The case of folate and NTDs was resolved in a relatively short time, in part because of the short interval (first 6 weeks of pregnancy) of exposure during which a nutritional imbalance could result in detrimental effects. In addition, the period between exposure and outcome was relatively short, the exposure could be evaluated by dietary assessment techniques and biomarkers, safe randomized trials could be conducted, and the strength of the relationship was large. Although a causal relationship is typically based on randomized clinical trials, the case of folate and NTDs suggests that a combination of study approaches can provide sufficient evidence when randomized studies cannot be easily performed.

SUMMARY

Nutrition epidemiology has been highly successful in identifying the responsible factors in many diseases, including scurvy, pellagra, blindness, and spina bifida. Nutritional epidemiology can potentially contribute substantially to our understanding of diseases in children and to the relationship between diet during childhood and risk of chronic diseases and cancer. The latency period between dietary exposure and disease can be years rather than weeks. Support for the long-term effects of diet comes from studies of diabetes and cardiovascular disorders[142] that led to the Barker hypothesis of fetal origin of chronic disease, as well as from studies of cancer.[143] A variety of approaches will provide the best evidence on these relationships, particularly when used in conjunction with clinical, biochemical, and molecular data.

REFERENCES

1. Lind J. A Treatise on Scurvy. London: A. Millar; 1753.
2. Farrell RJ, Kelly CP. Current concepts: Celiac sprue. N Engl J Med 2002;346:17180–8.
3. Dicke WK. Investigation of the Harmful Effects of Certain Types of Cereals on Patients With Coeliac Disease [Doctoral Thesis]. Utrecht, The Netherlands: University of Utrecht; 1950.
4. Dicke WK, Weijers HA, Van de Kramer JH. The presence in wheat of a factor having a deleterious effect in cases of celiac disease. Acta Paediatr 1953;42:34–6.
5. Nicklas TA, Myers L, Berenson GS. Dietary fiber intake of children: The Bogalusa Heart Study. Pediatrics 1995;96:988–94.
6. Jacobson HN, Stanton JL. Pattern analysis in nutrition research. Clin Nutr 1996;5:249–53.
7. Rockett HR, Berkey CS, Colditz GA. Evaluation of dietary assessment instruments in adolescents. Curr Opin Clin Nutr Metab Care 2003;6:557–62.
8. Feskanich D, Rockett HR, Colditz GA. Modifying the Healthy Eating Index to assess diet quality in children and adolescents. J Am Diet Assoc 2004;104:1375–83.
9. Isasi CR, Soroudi N, Wylie-Rosett J. Youth WAVE Screener: Addressing weight-related behaviors with school-age children. Diabetes Educ 2006;32:415–22.
10. Serdula MK, Alexander MP, Scanlon KS, Bowman BA. What are preschoolers eating. A review of dietary assessment. Annu Rev Nutr. 2001;21:475–98.
11. McPherson RS, Hoelscher DM, Alexander M, et al. Dietary assessment methods among school-aged children: Validity and reliability. Prev Med 2000;31:S11–33.
12. Rockett HR, Colditz GA. Assessing diets of children and adolescents. Am J Clin Nutr 1997;65:1116S–22S.
13. Schoeller DA. Recent advances from application of doubly labeled water to measurement of human energy expenditure. J Nutr 1999;129:1765–8.

14. Roberts SB, Dietz W, Sharp T, et al. Multiple laboratory comparison of the doubly labeled water technique. Obes Res 1995;3:3–13.
15. Willett W. Invited commentary: A further look at dietary questionnaire validation Am J Epidemiol 2001;154:1100–2.
16. Willett W. Nutrition Epidemiology. Oxford, UK: Oxford University Press; 1998.
17. Baxter SD, Thompson WO, Litaker MS, et al. Low accuracy and low consistency of fourth-graders' school breakfast and school lunch recalls. J Am Diet Assoc 2002;102:386–95.
18. Bandini LG, Schoeller HN, Cyr HN, et al. Validity of reported energy intake in obese and non-obese adolescents. Am J Clin Nutr 1990;52:421–5.
19. Livingstone MBE, Prentice AM, Coward WA, et al. Validation of estimates of energy intake by weighed dietary record and diet history in children and adolescents. Am J Clin Nutr 1992;56:29–35.
20. Harnack L, Himes JH, Anliker J, et al. Intervention-related bias in reporting of food intake by fifth-grade children participating in an obesity prevention study. Am J Epidemiol 2004;160:1117–21.
21. Weber JL, Lytle L, Gittelsohn J, et al. Validity of self-reported dietary intake at school meals by American Indian children: The pathways study. J Am Diet Assoc 2004;104:746–52.
22. Baxter SD, Thompson WO, Davis HC, et al. Impact of gender, ethnicity, meal component, and time interval between eating and reporting on accuracy of fourth-graders' self-reports of school lunch. J Am Diet Assoc 1997;97:1293–8.
23. Quandt SA. Variation in nutrient intake of infants and its implications for collecting reliable dietary intake data. Am J Phys Anthropol 1987;73:515–23.
24. Stein AD, Shea S, Basch CE, et al. Variability and tracking of nutrient intakes of preschool children based on multiple administrations of the 24-hour dietary recall. Am J Epidemiol 1991;134:1427–37.
25. Fisher JO, Johnson RK, Lindquist C, et al. Influence of body composition on the accuracy of reported energy intake in children. Obes Res 2000;8:597–603.
26. Thompson FE, Byers T. Dietary assessment resource manual. J Nutr 1994;124:2245S–317S.
27. Black AE, Cole TJ, Wiles SJ, et al. Daily variation in food intake of infants from 2 to 18 months. Hum Nutr Appl Nutr 1983;37:448–58.
28. Nelson M, Black AE, Morris JA, et al. Between- and within-subject variation in nutrient intake from infancy to old age: Estimating the number of days required to rank dietary intakes with desired precision. Am J Clin Nutr 1989;50:155–67.
29. Birch LL, Johnson SL, Andresen G, et al. The variability of young children's energy intake. NEJM 1991;324:232–5.
30. Champagne CM, Baker NB, DeLany JP, et al. Assessment of energy intake underreporting by doubly labeled water and observations on reported nutrients intakes in children. J Am Diet Assoc 1998;98:426–30.
31. O'Connor J, Ball EJ, Steinbeck KS, et al. Comparison of total energy expenditure and energy intake in children aged 6–9 y. Am J Clin Nutr 2001;74:643–9.
32. Bratteby LE, Sandhagen B, Fan H, et al. Total energy expenditure and physical activity as assessed by the doubly labeled water method in Swedish adolescents in whom energy intake was underestimated by 7-d diet records. Am J Clin Nutr 1998;67:905–11.
33. Field AE, Peterson KE, Gortmaker SL, et al. Reproducibility and validity of a food frequency questionnaire among fourth to seventh grade inner-city school children: Implications of age and day-to-day variation in dietary intake. Public Health Nutr 1999;2:293–300.
34. Klohe DM, Clarke KK, George GC, et al. Relative validity and reliability of a food frequency questionnaire for a triethnic population of 1-year-old to 3-year-old children from low-income families. JADA 2005;105:727–34.
35. Blum RE, Wei EK, Rockett HR, et al. Validation of a food frequency questionnaire in Native American and Caucasian children 1 to 5 years of age. Matern Child Health J 1999;3:167–72.
36. Maruti SS, Feskanich D, Rockett HR, et al. Validation of adolescent diet recalled by adults. Epidemiology 2006;17:226–9.
37. Johnson RK, Driscoll P, Goran MI. Cross-calibration of energy intake by 24-hour recall against total energy expenditure by doubly labeled water in young children. J Am Diet Assoc 1996;96:1140–4.
38. Kaskoun MC, Johnson R, Goran MI. Comparison of energy intake by food frequency questionnaire with total energy expenditure by doubly labeled water in young children. Am J Clin Nutr 1994;60:43–7.
39. Perks SM, Roemmich JN, Sandow-Pajewski M, et al. Alterations in growth and body composition during puberty. iv. Energy intake estimated by the youth-adolescent food-frequency questionnaire: Validation by the doubly labeled water method. Am J Clin Nutr 2000;72:1455–60.
40. Thompson FE, Byers T. Dietary assessment resource manual. J Nutr 1994;124:2245S–317S.
41. Simons-Morton BG, Forthofer R, Huang IW, et al. Reliability of direct observation of school-children's consumption of bag lunches. J Am Diet Assoc 1992;92:219–21.
42. Raisler J, Alexander C, O' Campo P. Breastfeeding and infant illness: A dose-response relationship? Am J Public Health 1999;89:25–30.
43. Jain A, Concat J, Leventhal JM. How good is the evidence linking breastfeeding and intelligence? Pediatrics 2002;109:1044–53.
44. Habicht JP, DaVanzo J, Butz WP. Does breastfeeding really save lives, or are apparent benefits due to biases? Am J Epidemiol 1986;123:279–90.
45. Anandaiah R, Choe MK. Are the WHO/UNICEF guidelines on breastfeeding appropriate for India? National Family Health Survey Bulletin 2000;16:1–4. International Institute for Population Sciences, Mumbai, India and the East-West Center, Honolulu, HI. Last accessed September 11, 2007 at www.eastwestcenter.org/res_ph.asp.
46. Fawzi WW, Herrera MG, Nestel P, et al. A longitudinal study of prolonged breastfeeding in relation to child undernutrition. Int J Epidemiol 1998;27:255–60.
47. Butte NF, Wong WW, Hopkinson JM, et al. Energy requirements derived from total energy expenditure and energy deposition during the first 2 y of life. Am J Clin Nutr 2000;72:1558–69.
48. Jones PJ, Winthrop AL, Schoeller DA, et al. Validation of doubly labeled water for assessing energy expenditure in infants. Pediatr Res 1987;21:242–6.
49. Brooks GA, Butte NF, Rand WM, et al. Chronicle of the Institute of Medicine physical activity recommendation: How a physical activity recommendation came to be among dietary recommendations. Am J Clin Nutr 2004;79:921S–30S.
50. Prentice AM, Lucas A, Vasquez-Velasquez L, et al. Are current dietary guidelines for young children a prescription for overfeeding? Lancet 1988;ii:1066–9.
51. Brown KH, Black RE, Becker S, et al. Consumption of foods and nutrients by weanlings in rural Bangladesh. Am J Clin Nutr 1982;36:878–89.
52. Brown KH, Black RE, Becker S. Seasonal changes in nutritional status and the prevalence of malnutrition in a longitudinal study of young children in rural Bangladesh. Am J Clin Nutr 1982;36:303–13.
53. Piwoz EG, Creed de Kanashiro H, Lopez de Romana G, et al. Potential for misclassification of infants' usual feeding practices using 24-hour dietary assessment methods. J Nutr 1995;125:57–65.
54. Riordan JM, Koehn M. Reliability and validity testing of three breastfeeding assessment tools. J Obstet Gynecol Neonatal Nurs 1997;26:181–7.
55. Andersen LF, Lande B, Arsky GH, et al. Validation of a semi-quantitative food-frequency questionnaire used among 12-month-old Norwegian infants. Eur J Clin Nutr 2003;57:881–88.
56. Marshall TA, Eichenberger Gilmore JM, Broffitt B, et al. Relative validation of a beverage frequency questionnaire in children ages 6 months through 5 years using 3-day food and beverage diaries. JADA 2003;103:714–20.
57. Zeitlin MF, Ahmed NU. Nutritional correlates of frequency and length of breastfeeds in rural Bangladesh. Early Hum Dev 1995;41:97–110.
58. Beaudry M, Dufour R, Marcoux S. Relation between infant feeding and infections during the first six months of life. J Pediatr 1995;126:191–7.
59. Vahatalo L, Barlund S, Hannila ML, et al. Relative validity of a dietary interview for assessing infant diet and compliance in a dietary intervention trial. Matern Child Nutr 2006;2:181–7.
60. Elberg J, McDuffie JR, Sebring NG, et al. Comparison of methods to assess change in children's body composition. Am J Clin Nutr 2004;80:64–9.
61. Fields DA, Goran MI, McCrory MA. Body-composition assessment via air-displacement plethysmography in adults and children: A review. Am J Clin Nutr 2002;75:453–67.
62. McCrory MA, Gomez TD, Bernauer EM, et al. Evaluation of a new air displacement plethysmograph for measuring human body composition. Med Sci Sports Exerc 1995;27:1686–91.
63. Buchholz AC, Majchrzak KM, Chen KY, et al. Use of air displacement plethysmography in the determination of percentage of fat mass in african-american children. Pediatr Res 2004;56:47–54.
64. Ginde SR, Geliebter A, Rubiano F, et al. Air displacement plethysmography: Validation in overweight and obese subjects. Obes Res 2005;13:1232–7.
65. Gately PJ, Radley D, Cooke CB, et al. Comparison of body composition methods in overweight and obese children. J Appl Physiol 2003;95:2039–46.
66. Ittenbach RF, Buison AM, Stallings VA, et al. Statistical validation of air-displacement plethysmography for body composition assessment in children. Ann Hum Biol 2006;33:187–201.
67. Ma G, Yao M, Liu Y, et al. Validation of a new pediatric air-displacement plethysmograph for assessing body composition in infants. Am J Clin Nutr 2004;79:653–60.
68. Lohman TG. Applicability of body composition techniques and constants for children and youths. Exerc Sports Sci Rev 1986;14:325–57.
69. Parizkova J. Total body fat and skinfold thickness in children. Metabolism 1961;10:794–807.
70. Seltzer CC, Goldman RF, Mayer J. The triceps skinfold as a predictive measure of bone density and body fat in obese adolescent girls. Pediatrics; 1965;36:212–8.
71. Young CM, Sipin SS, Roe DA. Body composition of preadolescent and adolescent girls. J Am Diet Assoc 1968:67:25–31.
72. Harsha DW, Frerichs RR, Berenson GS. Densitometry and anthropometry of black and white children. Hum Biol 1978;50:261–80.
73. Roche AF, Siervogel RM, Chumlea C, et al. Grading body fatness from limited anthropometric data. Am J Clin Nutr 1981;34:2231–8.
74. Maynard LM, Wisemandle W, Roche AF, et al. Childhood body composition in relation to body mass index. Pediatrics 2001;107:344–50.
75. Michielutte R, Diseker RA, Corbett WT, et al. The relationship between weight-height indices and the triceps skinfold measure among children age 5 to 12. Am J Public Health 1984;74:604–6.
76. Frontini MG, Bao W, Elkasabany A, et al. Comparison of weight-for-height indices as a measure of adiposity and cardiovascular risk from childhood to young adulthood: The Bogalusa heart study. J Clin Epidemiol 2002;54:817–22.
77. Mei Z, Grummer-Strawn LM, Pietrobelli A, et al. Validity of body mass index compared with other body-composition screening indexes for the assessment of body fatness in children and adolescents. Am J Clin Nutr 2002;75:978–85.
78. Ellis KJ. Human body composition: In vivo methods. Physiol Rev 2000;80:649–80.
79. American Academy of Pediatrics, Nutrition Committee. Obesity in children. Pediatric Nutrition Handbook. Elk Grove Village, IL: AAP; 1998. p. 423–58.
80. Willett K, Jiang R, Lenart E, et al. Comparison of bioelectrical impedance and BMI in predicting obesity-related medical conditions. Obesity (Silver Spring) 2006;14:480–90.
81. Eisenmann JC, Heelan KA, Welk GJ. Assessing body composition among 3- to 8-year-old children: Anthropometry, BIA, and DXA. Obes Res 2004;12:1633–40.
82. Dietz WH, Robinson TN. Use of the body mass index (BMI) as a measure of overweight in children and adolescents. J Pediatr 1998;132:191–3.
83. Gasser T, Ziegler P, Seifert B, et al. Measures of body mass and of obesity from infancy to adulthood and their appropriate transformation. Ann Hum Biol 1994;21:111–25.
84. Himes JH, Faricy A. Validity and reliability of self-reported stature and weight of US adolescents. Am J Hum Biol 2001;13:255–60.
85. Strauss RS. Comparison of measured and self-reported weight and height in a cross-sectional sample of young adolescents. Int J Obes Relat Metab Disord 1999;23:904–8.
86. Lee K, Valeria B, Kochman C, et al. Self-assessment of height, weight, and sexual maturation: Validity in overweight children and adolescents. J Adolese Health 2002;39:346–52.
87. McKeown-Eyssen GE, Yeung KS, Bright-See E. Assessment of past diet in epidemiologic studies. Am J Epidemiol 1986;124:94–103.
88. Rader JI. Folic acid fortification, folate status and plasma homocysteine. J Nutr 2002;132:2466S–70S.
89. Bounous G, Kongshavn PAL. Influence of protein type in nutritionally adequate diets on the development of immunity. In: Friedman M, editor. Absorption and Utilization of Amino Acids, Vol II. Boca Raton, FL: CRC Press; 1989. p. 219–33.
90. Sanchez A, Hubbard R. Dietary protein modulation of serum cholesterol: The amino acid connection. In: Friedman M, editor. Absorption and Utilization of Amino Acids, Vol II. Boca Raton, FL: CRC Press; 1989. p. 247–73.
91. Poppitt SD, Kilmartin P, Butler P, et al. Assessment of erythrocyte phospholipid fatty acid composition as a biomarker for dietary MUFA, PUFA or saturated fatty acid intake in a controlled cross-over intervention trial. Lipids Health Dis 2005;4:30.
92. Baylin A, Campos H. The use of fatty acid biomarkers to reflect dietary intake. Curr Opin Lipidol 2006;17:22–7.
93. Ovesen L, Boeing H. The use of biomarkers in multicentric studies with particular consideration of iodine, sodium, iron, folate and vitamin D. Eur J Clin Nutr 2002;56:S12–7.
94. Baylin A, Kim MK, Donovan-Palmer A, et al. Fasting whole blood as a biomarker of essential fatty acid intake in epidemiologic studies: Comparison with adipose tissue and plasma. Am J Epidemiol 2005;162:373–81.
95. Erlinger TP, Guallar E, Miller ER, 3rd, et al. Relationship between systemic markers of inflammation and serum beta-carotene levels. Arch Intern Med 2001;161:1903–8.
96. Chevion M, Berenshtein E, Stadtman ER. Human studies related to protein oxidation: Protein carbonyl content as a marker of damage. Free Radic Res 2000;33:S99–108.

97. Tasevska N, Runswick SA, Bingham SA. Urinary potassium is as reliable as urinary nitrogen for use as a recovery biomarker in dietary studies of free living individuals. J Nutr 2006;136:1334–40.
98. Weinstein SJ, Vogt TM, Gerrior SA, Healthy Eating Index scores are associated with blood nutrient concentrations in the third National Health And Nutrition Examination Survey. JADA 2004;104:576–84.
99. Neuhouser ML, Patterson RE, King IB, et al. Selected nutritional biomarkers predict diet quality. Public Health Nutr 2003;6:703–9.
100. Hambidge M. Biomarkers of trace mineral intake and status. J Nutr 2003;133:948S–955S.
101. Shai I, Rosner BA, Shahar DR, et al. Dietary evaluation and attenuation of relative risk: Multiple comparisons between blood and urinary biomarkers, food frequency, and 24-hour recall questionnaires: The DEARR Study. J Nutr 2005;135:573–9.
102. Byers TE, Rosenthal RI, Marshall JR, et al. Dietary history from the distant past: A methodological study. Nutr Cancer 1983;5:69–77.
103. Birch LL, Krahnstoever Davidson K. Family environmental factors influencing the developing behavioral controls of food intake and childhood overweight. Pediatr Clin North Am 2001;48:893–907.
104. Nicklas TA, Webber LS, Berenson GS. Studies of consistency of dietary intake during the first four years of life in a prospective analysis: Bogalusa heart study. J Am Coll Nutr 1991;10:234–41.
105. Resnicow K, Smith M, Baranowski T, et al. Two-year tracking of children's fruit and vegetable intake. J Am Diet Assoc 1998;98:785–9.
106. Welten DC, Kemper HC, Post GB, et al. Longitudinal development and tracking of calcium and dairy intake from teenager to adult. Eur J Clin Nutr 199;51:612–8.
107. Wang Y, Bentley ME, Zhai F, et al. Tracking of dietary intake patterns of Chinese from childhood to adolescence over a six-year follow-up period. J Nutr 2002;132:430–8.
108. Cusatis DC, Chinchilli VM, Johnson-Rollings N, et al. Longitudinal nutrient intake patterns of US adolescent women: The Penn State Young Women's Health Study. J Adolesc Health 2000;26:194–204.
109. Nicklas TA, Elkasabany A, Srinivasan SR, et al. Trends in nutrient intake of 10-year-old children over two decades (1973–1994): The Bogalusa Heart Study. Am J Epidemiol 2001;153:969–77.
110. Lake AA, Mathers JC, Rugg-Gunn AJ, et al. Longitudinal change in food habits between adolescence (11–12 years) and adulthood (32–33 years): The ASH30 Study. J Public Health (Oxford) 2006;28:10–6.
111. Berenson GS, Srinivasan SR, Nicklas TA. Atherosclerosis: A nutritional disease of childhood. Am J Cardiol 1998;82:22T–9T.
112. Nicklas TA, Farris RP, Smoak CG, et al. Dietary factors relate to cardiovascular risk factors in early life. Bogalusa heart study. Arteriosclerosis 1988;8:193–9.
113. Kallio MJ, Salmenpera L, Siimes MA, et al. Tracking of serum cholesterol and lipoprotein levels from the first year of life. Pediatrics 1993;91:949–54.
114. Moilanen T, Viikari J, Rasanen L, et al. Three-year tracking of serum fatty acids in Finnish boys and girls. Atherosclerosis 1987;67:191–7.
115. Kushi LH. Gaps in epidemiologic research methods: Design considerations for studies that use food-frequency questionnaires. Am J Clin Nutr 1994;59:180S–4S.
116. Goran MI, Treuth MS. Energy expenditure, physical activity, and obesity in children. Pediatr Clin North Am 2001;48:931–53.
117. Willett WC, Howe GR, Kushi LH. Adjustment for total energy intake in epidemiologic studies [discussion 1229S–31S]. Am J Clin Nutr 1997;65:1220S–8S.
118. McGee DL, Reed DM, Yano K. The result of logistic analysis when the variables are highly correlated: An empirical example using diet and coronary heart disease incidence. J Chron Dis 1984;37:713–9.
119. MacMahon B, Yen S. Unrecognized epidemic of anencephaly and spina bifida. Lancet 1971;i:31–3.
120. Kirke PN, Molloy AM, Daly LE, et al. Maternal folate and vitamin B12 are independent risk factors for neural tube defects. Q J Med 1993;86:703–8.
121. Smithells RW, Sheppard S, Schorah CJ. Vitamin deficiencies and neural tube defects. Arch Dis Child 1976;51:944–50.
122. Rhoads GG, Mills JL. The role of the case-control study in evaluating health interventions. Vitamin supplementation and neural tube defects. Am J Epidemiol 1984;120:803–8.
123. Smithells RW, Sheppard S, Schorah CJ, et al. Possible prevention of neural-tube defects by periconceptional vitamin supplementation. Lancet 1980;1:339–40.
124. Smithells RW, Sheppard S, Schorah CJ, et al. Apparent prevention of neural tube defects by periconceptional vitamin supplementation. Arch Dis Child 1981;56:911–8.
125. Mulinare J, Cordero JF, Erikson JD, et al. Periconceptional use of multivitamins and the occurrence of neural tube defects. JAMA 1988;260:3141–5.
126. Mills JL, Rhoads GG, Simpson JL. The absence of a relationship between the periconceptional use of vitamins and neural tube defects. N Engl J Med 1989;321:430–5.
127. Shaw GM, Schaffer D, Velie EM, et al. Periconceptual vitamin use, dietary folate and the occurrence of neural tube defects in California. Epidemiology 1995;6:219–26.
128. Milunsky A, Jick H, Jick SS, et al. Multivitamin/folic acid supplementation in early pregnancy reduces the prevalence of neural tube defects. JAMA 1989;262:2847–52.
129. Daly LE, Kirke PN, Molloy A, et al. Folate levels and neural tube defects: Implications for prevention. JAMA 1995;274:1698–702.
130. Medical Research Council Vitamin Study Research Group (MRCVSRG). Prevention of neural tube defects: Results of the MRCVS. Lancet 1991;338:131–7.
131. Czeizel AE, Dudas I. Prevention of the first occurrence of neural tube defects by conpericonceptual vitamin supplementation. N Engl J Med 1992;327:1832–5.
132. Gregory JF. The bioavailibility of folate. In: Bailey LB, editor. Folate in Health and Disease. New York: Marcel Dekker; 1995. p. 195–235.
133. Cuskelly GJ, McNulty H, Scott JM. Effect of increasing dietary folate on red-cell folate: Implications for prevention of neural tube defects. Lancet 1996;347:657–9.
134. Oakley GP, Adams MJ, Dickinson CM. Urgent need to increase folic acid for everyone, now. J Nutr 1996;126:751S–5S.
135. Eichholzer M, Tonz O, Zimmermann R. Folic acid: A public-health challenge. Lancet 2006;367:1352–61.
136. Brent RL, Oakley GP, Jr. The food and drug administration must require the addition of more folic acid in "enriched" flour and other grains. Pediatrics 2005;116:753–5.
137. Stoll C, Alembik Y, Dott B. Are the recommendations on the prevention of neural tube defects working? Eur J Med Genet 2006;49:461–5.
138. Van der Put NM, Steegers-Theunissen RP, Frost P, et al. Mutated methylenetetrahydrofolate reductase as a risk factors for spina bifida. Lancet 1995;346:1070–1.
139. Wald NJ, Hackshaw AK, Stone R, et al. Blood folate and vitamin B_{12} in relation to neural tube defects. Br J Obstet Gynaecol 1996;103:319–24.
140. Groenen PM, van Rooij IA, Peer PG, et al. Marginal maternal vitamin B_{12} status increases the risk of offspring with spina bifida. Am J Obstet Gynecol 2004;191:11–7.
141. Suárez L, Hendricks K, Felkner M, et al. Maternal serum B_{12} levels and risk for neural tube defects in a Texas-Mexico border population. Ann Epidemiol 2003;13:81–8.
142. Hales CN, Barker DJP. Type 2 (non-insulin-dependent) diabetes mellitus: The thrifty phenotype hypothesis. Diabetologia 1992;35:595–601.
143. Hunter DJ, Willett WC. Nutrition and breast cancer. Cancer Causes Control 1996;7:56–68.

17

Food Safety

Catherine E. Woteki, PhD, RD
Brian D. Kineman, MS

Safe food and water supplies are prerequisites for good nutrition and the overall health of a population, especially for infants and children whose immune systems are immature and therefore more vulnerable to foodborne infections. Foodborne hazards encompass microbiologic, chemical, and physical agents that can cause injury and disease when ingested. Microbiologic agents include pathogens and parasites that are either present in food when purchased or introduced into food by cross-contamination during preparation or eating. Chemical hazards are substances that are naturally occurring toxicants or that are introduced into food intentionally (such as pesticide residues or food-coloring or -preserving additives) or through environmental contamination. Physical hazards include pebbles, glass, metal, wood, or plastic shards that can cause physical injury or choking when ingested. Infants and young children are among the most vulnerable to foodborne infections because of their lower body weight and immature immune systems. A dose of foodborne pathogen that may cause no illness or only mild illness in an adult can cause severe illness in a young child. Therefore, extra care needs to be taken in preparing food for young children to minimize the chance of cross-contamination.

FOODBORNE DISEASE

The terms "foodborne disease or illness" and "food poisoning" are often used interchangeably to describe general symptoms associated with consuming a contaminated food. Specifically, food poisoning refers to all forms of serious injury from gastroenteritis, whereas foodborne disease can be more broadly interpreted as encompassing all injury or illness associated with eating foods contaminated with pathogenic chemical or physical agents. In addition, the term foodborne disease can include all chronic sequelae, such as arthritis, associated with foodborne pathogens. Agents of foodborne illness can be classified into one of three categories: biologic, chemical, or physical. Biologic pathogens include bacteria, fungi, parasites, viruses, and prions. Pathogenic chemical agents linked to foodborne illness include pesticides, herbicides, naturally occurring toxins produced by bacteria or mushrooms, mycotoxins produced by fungi, radioisotopes, and toxic heavy metals, such as copper, arsenic, and zinc. Glass, dirt, rocks, and plastic are examples of physical agents that can be introduced into the food supply and, when ingested, cause injury. Some agents associated with foodborne illness, notably bacteria and fungi, are capable of rapidly multiplying and producing toxins in foods. Foods, on the other hand, merely serve as vehicles of infection for viruses and parasites. This chapter focuses on some of the key agents associated with foodborne illness and provides background information on how to protect infants and children from foodborne illness. Only the most serious or common agents associated with foodborne illness in children are profiled, including a general description of the agent, high-risk foods, modes of transmission, and notable symptoms of illness, including incubation periods (time between consumption of agent and onset of illness) and, where relevant, infectious dose (the amount generally required to cause illness in a "healthy" individual) and recent outbreaks, to further illustrate the nature of the agent being discussed.

BACTERIAL FOODBORNE PATHOGENS

Bacteria are small, single-celled organisms that possess no distinct nucleus. They are probably the most adaptable organisms on earth and are known to exist in all environments—in the air, in soil, and on rocky surfaces. Bacteria can be found in extreme climates, from the Arctic cold to the scorching temperatures of geysers, and have evolved to survive and thrive at high acid and high salt concentrations. Many environmental bacteria form spores—resistant, dormant structures within the cell—that protect the organism from adverse conditions, such as when adequate nutrition or moisture is lacking. Such bacteria are capable of staying in a dormant state for a couple of months, until optimal conditions are restored. With such abilities to adapt to various stresses and the capability of thriving in practically all environments, it is no wonder that bacteria exist in a wide variety of foods. Bacteria are classified on the bases of shape [spherical (cocci), rod (bacilli), or spiral], group orientation (some bacteria such as *Bacillus* sp are noted for lining up into "chains," for instance), oxygen tolerance (aerobe, microaerobe, facultative anaerobe, and anaerobe), cell wall structure (gram positive or gram negative), the capability to form spores, motility (possession of a flagellum), ability to ferment different sugars, and the presence of certain surface antigens, to name just a few characteristics. Most of these organisms exist as free living, but a few have ecologic niches in the external, mucosal, and other surfaces of humans and other creatures. Bacteria, for the most part, are harmless and perform beneficial roles to the environment and their human or animal host. A tiny minority, however, possess certain characteristics, such as the ability to produce toxins, that give them the capacity to threaten their host. Over 200 different species are considered to be pathogenic toward humans, many of which are associated with foodborne illness. The Centers for Disease Control and Prevention recently estimated the number of foodborne illnesses associated with various pathogens.[1] The top seven bacteria in the analysis, including estimated foodborne illness and hospitalizations, are listed in Table 1. A brief review of some of these bacterial pathogens, as well as additional agents that are responsible for foodborne illness in children, is explored in this section. Emphasis is placed on

Table 1 Estimated Number of Foodborne Illnesses and Foodborne Hospitalizations from Seven Bacterial Pathogens

	Estimated Foodborne Bacteria Illnesses	Estimated Foodborne Hospitalizations
Campylobacter spp	1,963,141	10,539
Salmonella, nontyphoidal	1,341,873	15,608
Clostridium perfringens	248,520	41
Staphylococcus food poisoning	185,060	1,753
Shigella spp	89,648	1,246
Yersinia enterocolitica	86,731	1,105
Escherichia coli O157:H7	62,458	1,843

Adapted from Mead PS et al.[1]

organisms with higher rates of hospitalization, not necessarily those associated with higher estimated rates of illness.

Campylobacter jejuni

Campylobacteriosis is the leading cause of diarrhea in the developed world, with the number of cases exceeding those of salmonellosis and shigellosis.[2] *Compylobacter jejuni*, the bacterial agent responsible for the illness, is a gram-negative, slender, curved rod. It grows under microaerophilic conditions (in an atmosphere of approximately 5% oxygen) and has the unusual property of having an optimal temperature for growth of 42°C instead of the more typical 37°C, which is associated with most human pathogens. *C. jejuni* is found in the normal gastrointestinal and genitourinary flora of many animals, including sheep, cattle, chickens, wild birds, and domestic dogs. *C. jejuni*, when ingested, colonizes the intestinal mucosa, but the exact mechanism behind its pathogenesis has yet to be fully elucidated. It is postulated that gastrointestinal illness from *C. jejuni* infection results from toxin production and bacterial invasion and proliferation with the intestinal mucosa.[3] The infectious dose, as indicated by volunteer human feeding studies, appears to be very low—around 100 organisms.[4] Onset of illness typically occurs 2 to 5 days after consumption, with symptoms consisting of severe abdominal pain, fever, and bloody diarrhea with nausea; vomiting is not commonly associated with *C. jejuni* food poisoning. Symptoms are usually self-limiting, lasting for several days to more than 1 week. *C. jejuni*, in extreme cases, can result in acute and chronic sequelae such as bacteremia, urinary tract infection, meningitis, endocarditis, peritonitis, and reactive arthritis. *C. jejuni* has also been linked to being the potential cause of Guillain–Barré syndrome, an autoimmune disorder of the peripheral nervous system, which is characterized by limb paralysis. *C. jejuni* is the most common microorganism identified in patients with Guillain–Barré syndrome.[5] Nevertheless, fatalities from *C. jejuni* are very rare. Because a number of animals serve as reservoirs for *C. jejuni*, many foods can be associated with *C. jejuni* contamination. Undercooked meat and chicken are typical sources of *C. jejuni* infection. Unpasteurized milk and nonchlorinated water can also harbor the organism. *C. jejuni* is very susceptible to heat and low pH, so typical cooking temperatures and acid washes, when applied properly, can kill the organism. But, owing to its low infectious dose, it is still a very difficult organism to control.

Cross-contamination during food processing in the factory or food preparation in the kitchen can be a real problem with any organism with such a potent pathogenicity. *C. jejuni* accounts for a large number of sporadic cases of illness throughout the summer months; large outbreaks are rare. Most outbreaks are attributed to the consumption of contaminated milk. One such outbreak occurred in 1986, when 172 students at an elementary school were infected from improperly pasteurized milk. The dairy supplying milk to the school did not vat pasteurize the milk at a high enough temperature or for the required length of time.[4]

Salmonella spp

Salmonella spp are gram-negative, facultative anaerobic, non-spore-forming bacilli that are widely distributed in nature. They reside in the intestinal tracts of animals and humans. The bacteria are excreted in the feces, where they can contaminate virtually any object that comes into contact with the feces. Over 2,000 distinct antigenic variants of *Salmonella* have been identified based on analysis of cell wall, capsular, and flagellar antigens. Human infection is linked to only a few of these serotypes, however. The symptom of illness greatly depends on the type of *Salmonella* involved. *S. typhi* is the most serious of the *Salmonella* spp, being the agent responsible for enteric (typhoid) fever. *S. typhi* can penetrate the intestine and enter the bloodstream. There the organism has the ability to evade the initial immune response by entering macrophages and multiplying. Illness occurs 7 to 28 days after exposure, with symptoms that include high fever, headache, vomiting, and diarrhea. Symptoms of nontyphoid salmonellosis are similar to those associated with enteric fever, only milder. The bacteria, following ingestion, pass through the stomach and adhere to the epithelial cells lining the small intestine, causing inflammation. Ingestion of 10,000 or more bacilli is required to cause illness in healthy individuals; in children and immunocompromised individuals, the required dose is much smaller.[4] Clinical manifestations of salmonellosis, following a broad incubation period of 6 to 72 hours, include nausea and vomiting followed by nonbloody diarrhea and abdominal cramps. Diarrhea persists as the major symptom for 3 to 4 days. The illness is usually self-limiting after about 7 days. Occasionally, the microorganisms can enter the blood and cause sepsis. Once in the bloodstream, the bacteria can cause a number of problems by invading tissue. Arthritis, aneurisms, and meningitis are just a few of the chronic sequelae that can result from salmonellosis. Raw meats, fish, poultry, eggs, and milk and dairy products are the typical risk foods for *Salmonella* spp contamination. Outbreaks associated with orange juice, tomatoes, cantaloupe, cilantro, and alfalfa sprouts have also been reported.[6–10] Thorough cooking of foods can control the organism because they are susceptible to heat (71.7°C for 15 seconds has been shown to be effective in destroying the bacteria). *Salmonella* spp are also susceptible to acidic conditions (pH 4.0) but are resistant to both freezing and drying.[11] *Salmonella* spp account for a large number of reported outbreaks. A large salmonellosis outbreak in the US history, involving 16,284 confirmed cases, occurred in 1985. The cause of the outbreak was believed to be pasteurized milk, which had been cross-contaminated with raw milk.[12] The largest US outbreak of salmonellosis occurred in 1994 when 224,000 people, nationwide, became ill from ice cream contaminated with *S. enteritidis.*[13] Surprisingly, the cause was not linked to an egg product in the ice cream but resulted from an unsanitized truck in which some of the product had been transported. The truck had previously hauled nonpasteurized liquid eggs containing the pathogen.

Escherichia coli

Of all of the members of the family Enterobacteriaceae, *Escherichia coli* is the largest colonizer of the intestine of humans and animals. *E. coli* probably holds the honor of being the most feared bacterial pathogen among the general public owing to recent dramatic reports of outbreaks associated with *E. coli* O157:H7. Most strains of *E. coli* perform a beneficial role for the host, aiding in the digestion of foods, the destruction of other pathogenic bacteria, and the production of vitamins. However, a few strains are capable of producing harmful toxins that can cause a variety of conditions, ranging from mild diarrhea to death. *E. coli* is a gram-negative, rod-shaped organism. It is classified as a facultative anaerobe and is a typical coliforman enteric bacterium that ferments lactose to acid end products. Transmission of the bacteria occurs through fecal contamination. In nature, the organism can survive readily with minimum nutrients. *E. coli* can also colonize the skin as well as the female genital tract. Pathogenic *E. coli* that causes gastroenteritis is classified in accordance with its virulence properties. The four types of diarrhea causing *E. coli* are enterohemorrhagic, enteroinvasive (EIEC), enteropathogenic (EPEC), and enterotoxigenic (ETEC). EIEC, as the name implies, invades and proliferates within epithelial cells of the intestine, causing a mild form of bacillary dysentery. ETEC adheres to the mucous layer of the small intestine and produces toxins that result in watery diarrhea. EIEC and ETEC are uncommon agents of foodborne illness in developed nations; therefore, they will not be discussed in any more detail in this section. EPEC is a very common cause of infant diarrhea. EPEC cells form small clumps by binding tightly to the enterocytes of the small intestine, causing the lining cells to disrupt. Resulting symptoms can include bloody or watery diarrhea. The infectious dose for infants is believed to be very low, although no exact figures are reported. In healthy adults, a dose of 10^6 cells is probably required for associated illness to occur.[4] Enterohemorrhagic includes *E. coli* O157:H7, a recent emerging pathogen that was identified in 1982 as the cause of two major outbreaks of hemolytic colitis in Oregon and Michigan attributed to hamburgers.[14] *E. coli* O157:H7 produces a very powerful toxin similar to the one associated with *Shigella dysenteriae,* a bacterium that causes a severe form of bacteria dysentery. The incubation period is somewhere in the range of 3 to 9 days. Characteristic symptoms of infection include intense abdominal pain and nonbloody diarrhea, which progresses within 1 to 2 days to bloody diarrhea that can become quite severe. Vomiting and low-grade fever can occur as well. Illness usually persists for about 8 days and then subsides. *E. coli* O157:H7 is also a major cause of renal failure [hemolytic uremic syndrome (HUS)] in humans and the leading cause in children.[15] About 10% of cases progress into HUS.[16] The infective dose of *E. coli* O157:H7 is unknown but is believed to be very low—less than 10 organisms.[4] The majority of reported *E. coli* O157:H7 outbreaks are linked to undercooked ground beef, but associations with raw milk, vegetables (including sprouts), cheese, water, juice, and fruit have been reported. Many foods can account for EPEC illness. As with *E. coli* O157:H7, raw beef and chicken are the primary risk foods. More importantly, contaminated water is probably the number one vehicle for EPEC transmission. *E. coli* O157:H7 is sensitive to heat (grows poorly at 45°C) but has an unusual resistance to acid. Studies have demonstrated that the organism can survive in apple cider with a pH of 3.6.[17,18] There are numerous reports in recent years of outbreaks associated with *E. coli* O157:H7. The largest outbreak in the United States occurred in 1993 throughout the Pacific Northwest (Washington, Idaho, California, and Nevada).[19] In all, over 700 cases were confirmed; 178 people were hospitalized and four children died. Contaminated hamburgers from a fast-food chain were determined to be the cause of the outbreak. The largest outbreak in world history occurred in 1996 in Japan.[20] Radish sprouts contaminated with the organism were responsible for over 10,000 illnesses, a vast number of them being school-aged children. Unpasteurized, commercially sold apple juice was the source of an unusual 1996 outbreak in the United States. The reported median age of the 45 victims was 5 years, with 12 persons being diagnosed with HUS.[21] Fecal to oral transmission is also a common cause of outbreaks with *E. coli* O157:H7. This is especially true for daycare centers. An example of this was reported in Minnesota, where 68 cases of *E. coli* O157:H7 infection were identified over an 18-month period, involving nine daycare facilities.[22] In addition, younger children have been reported to shed the organisms for longer periods after resolution of symptoms compared with adults, which makes the risk factor of daycare centers even greater than once suspected.[23] *E. coli* O157:H7 transmission via the fecal-oral route can also occur by swimming in contaminated waters, as was demonstrated in an outbreak involving 12 individuals, ages 2 to 12 years, in 1995.[24]

Listeria monocytogenes

To avoid the possible misconception that only gram-negative bacteria are responsible for foodborne illness, *Listeria monocytogenes* is a small, gram-positive bacillus that is also a very important foodborne pathogen. It is found everywhere in nature—in the soil and water, for example. The bacterium also colonizes the intestine of humans and animals, primarily ruminants (ie, cattle, sheep, goats, deer, and elk). It is one of the few environmental gram-positive bacilli that do not form spores. Owing to its omnipresence, foods can easily become contaminated with *L. monocytogenes* through fecal or environmental transmission.

Listeriosis rarely occurs in healthy adults; however, it is a grave threat to the immunocompromised populations (human immunodeficiency virus [HIV]-positive individuals, patients subjected to chemotherapy, etc), the elderly, infants, and pregnant women. The symptoms of listeriosis are highly variable, depending on the host and particular strain of infection. In healthy individuals, symptoms are typically very mild and go unnoticed. As an opportunistic infection, symptoms may include nausea, vomiting, and abdominal pain, followed by fever. Pregnant women may also suffer flulike symptoms. The onset of illness, like the symptoms, varies greatly, spanning from as short as 1 day to as long as 3 weeks after consumption. The very serious clinical features of listeriosis include meningitis, septicemia, and encephalitis. Listeriosis in pregnant women can lead to spontaneous abortion or stillbirth. Additionally, mothers can contaminate the skin and respiratory tract of their newborns by transmitting the organism from their gastrointestinal tract and perianal region if they are carriers. The infectious dose of *L. monocytogenes* is unknown, but in susceptible people, fewer than 1,000 organisms can probably cause disease.[4] *L. monocytogenes* produces a hemolysin that, in conjunction with other factors, allows the organism to evade macrophages. In this respect, the organism is able to spread, avoiding much of the immune response. This is the reason that the strength of the immune system is extremely crucial in the ability of the body to adequately defend against the organism. Beef, pork, ready-to-eat foods, soft cheeses, foods purchased at delicatessen counters, milk, poultry, fruits, and vegetables are all examples of reported sources of contamination.[25,26] *L. monocytogenes* is extremely hardy for an organism that does not form spores. The organism has the ability to grow at refrigeration temperatures (3°C) and is resistant to acid pH and salt treatments that are often used to ensure food safety. However, cooking or pasteurizing foods can effectively eliminate the risk of foodborne listeriosis in foods that can be cooked.[27] Listeriosis occurs sporadically, but, from time to time, outbreaks of *L. monocytogenes* do occur, associated most typically with contaminated cheese or milk. Southern California was the scene of a mass outbreak in 1995, in which 142 people became ill from consuming Mexican-style soft cheese contaminated with *L. monocytogenes.*[28] There were 48 deaths, of which 10 were neonatal and 20 fetal. Hot dogs and delicatessen meats contaminated with a rare strain of *L. monocytogenes* were the culprits in a large multistate outbreak in late 1998 and early 1999 that resulted in 20 deaths.[29] Chocolate milk, contaminated from a tank drain at the dairy, was the vehicle of *Listeria* transmission at a picnic in Illinois, which resulted in 45 cases.[30]

Clostridium perfringens

Clostridium perfringens is a large, anaerobic, spore-forming, gram-positive rod that is widely distributed in nature, residing in the soil. The organism can be harbored in the intestine of humans and many animals, where it is passed in the feces. *C. perfringens* is the agent responsible for a common form of food poisoning as well as gas gangrene, anaerobic puerperal sepsis, and anaerobic cellulites. Food poisoning resulting from *C. perfringens* is typically a mild illness. The illness has an incubation period of 8 to 24 hours, followed by nausea, abdominal pain, and diarrhea. Fever is not associated with illness; vomiting is rare. The illness usually self-resolves within 24 hours. In fact, the illness is often mistaken for a case of the "24-hour stomach flu." The infectious dose required for onset of associated symptoms is quite large—10^8 vegetative cells.[4] After ingestion, the bacteria release an endotoxin into the upper gastrointestinal tract, which is responsible for the clinical manifestations of infection. The spores of *C. perfringens* are very resistant to heat, being able to withstand temperatures of 100°C for more than 1 hour. Foods associated with *C. perfringens* illness include meats, meat products, and gravy. Outbreaks associated with *C. perfringens* are very common, even though many cases go undetected or unreported, owing to the mild symptoms associated with the illness. Two outbreaks of *C. perfringens* following St. Patrick's Day meals occurred in 1993.[31] Over 200 people became ill in two states after consuming contaminated corned beef. In one state, the delicatessen that had served the meat initially boiled it for 3 hours and allowed it to cool to room temperature before refrigeration. The corned beef was then heated to 120°F (48.8°C), sliced, and served to the public. Some amount of the product, which was made for catering, was allowed to stand at room temperature for several hours before serving. It was recommended by the state health department, after the outbreak, that the meat, not served directly after cooking, be divided into small pieces, placed in shallow pans, and chilled rapidly on ice before refrigeration. Before reserving, it was further recommended that the meat be rapidly heated so that the internal temperature of the meat would reach at least 165°F (74°C). An unusual outbreak occurred in 1990 at a conference for cake decorators.[32] Thirty-two of the forty-two attendees became ill after consuming contaminated minestrone soup. The soup, which consisted of chicken, fresh vegetables, canned tomatoes, chicken base, navy beans, and peas, was heated under boiling (a temperature too low to destroy vegetative cells). Also, it was determined that the chicken stock used in the soup was not chilled before preparation and the leftover soup was held at room temperature for too long before reheating.

Clostridium botulinum

Clostridium botulinum is a gram-positive, anaerobic, endospore-forming bacillus that is widely found in the soil. *C. botulinum* produces seven different types of a very potent toxin, referred to as types A, B, C, D, E, F, and G. Humans are susceptible to types A, B, and E and animals to types C and D. Because of its potency, botulinum toxin is an agent associated with biologic warfare because only a few nanograms of it can cause death. The toxins produced by *C. botulinum* are responsible for causing three types of botulism: foodborne, infant, and wound. Wound botulism is quite rare and occurs when the organism is introduced into the body through a wound. Foodborne botulism results from the ingestion of the toxin through a food source. Symptoms for foodborne botulism begin to develop between 12 and 36 hours after the toxin is introduced into the body. The botulism toxin works by binding to the neuromuscular junction of nerves, preventing the release of acetylcholine, which results in muscle paralysis. Dizziness, weakness of limbs, blurred vision, general fatigue, and difficulty in swallowing are all early characteristics of infection. Vomiting, nausea, and diarrhea may also occur but usually are not accompanied by fever. Antitoxin serums and respiratory support systems are often required for treatment in more severe cases. Death is usually caused by paralysis of the diaphragm, leading to asphyxiation. Infant botulism occurs when the ingested spores of *C. botulinum* germinate and colonize the child's gastrointestinal tract. The defining symptom of infant botulism is a severe loss of head control. Other symptoms include constipation, weakness, and poor feeding. Most cases require mechanical ventilation. A 12-year case study at one tertiary-care hospital revealed that 68% of its infant patients were mechanically ventilated during the course of their illness.[33]

Any food that has a low acidity and salt concentration and supports an anaerobic environment for the organism is a high-risk food. Foods that are sources of foodborne botulism include canned and bottled foods (especially home-canned foods) and foods that are submerged in oil or fat. Honey is the primary food of concern for infant botulism. It is reported that 25% of honey products have been found to contain spores.[34] Although *C. botulinum* spores are very resistant to heat, the toxin itself is very susceptible to heat. Certain processing conditions have to be met to ensure safety from botulism, especially in the canning industry. Food processors exploit the fact that the organism is very sensitive to acidic conditions to achieve this. *C. botulinum* is not capable of producing the toxin in such conditions. Because of dramatic changes in food safety practices in the canning industry, outbreaks of foodborne botulism are not as common as they once were. When they do occur, it is usually the result of an isolated flaw in production, such as a leak in a can. Occasionally, ethnic foods cause an outbreak of foodborne botulism. Eight individuals in the United States and Israel became ill after eating a salted fish known as *ribyetz,* a Russian food, contaminated with type E botulism.[35] Infant botulism occurs sporadically. A typical case resulting from the consumption of honey contaminated with spores is described in a recent report in which an 11-week-old child was admitted to a hospital with infant botulism: "The child was initially admitted with the sole symptom of vomiting. Soon she progressively became weak and noticeably floppy in appearance. She had poor head control, decreased limb tone, and a 'frog-like' leg posture. The baby required intubation and artificial ventilation for 18 days. She was treated with cefotaxime and ampicillin for 48 hours and was discharged after 33 days. She was readmitted after 4 days owing to respiratory difficulty. After another stay of 12 days, this time not requiring respiratory assistance, she was discharged. A history examination revealed that the mother had dipped the infant's pacifier in commercial honey."[36]

OTHER BACTERIAL FOODBORNE PATHOGENS

There are numerous bacterial agents that are capable of contaminating our food system and causing some form of illness. The focus of this chapter does not allow for full coverage of all of the important agents; a clinical microbiology text could easily do more justice to the subject. Instead, the brief profiles are included as a quick reference point for a more detailed study. Some of the other microorganisms that are frequently associated with foodborne illness include *Shigella* sp, a group of bacteria that consists of some strains that produce toxins similar to *E. coli* O157:H7, and *Yersinia enterocolitica,* an organism whose infection can produce intense abdominal pain, similar to appendicitis. *B. cereus* and *Staphylococcus aureus* are both gram-positive, toxin-producing bacteria that can contaminate food. The toxin associated with *B. cereus,* a common soil bacterium, produces symptoms almost identical to that of *C. perfringens* infection. *S. aureus* is a bacteria that is harbored in the nose and throat and on the hair and skin of humans, which links the organism to a number of foods. Its toxin is fairly potent and results in a quick onset of illness, with symptoms that include abdominal cramping, nausea, and vomiting.

VIRAL FOODBORNE PATHOGENS

Foodborne viruses infect through ingestion and are passed through the feces. With very few known exceptions, transmission of viruses occurs via the fecal-oral route or through contaminated water or food. Viruses are thought to be the major causes of unexplained foodborne outbreaks because, unlike bacteria, very few specific foodborne viruses have been identified. Children are a high-risk group for foodborne viral infections because many such illnesses are associated with schools and daycare centers.

Rotavirus

Rotavirus is the most common diarrheal pathogen in the world and infects an estimated 2.7 million children in the United States each year.[37] The *Rotavirus* virus particle is a spherical, "wheel-shaped" structure (65 to 75 nm in diameter) that contains a genome consisting of 11 segments of double-stranded RNA, surrounded by a double-shelled outer capsid. Different serogroups of the virus exist, based on the variety of antigens present on the outer capsid. Transmission of the virus occurs via the fecal-oral route.

The majority of infections are asymptomatic in neonates and adults.[38] Onset of symptomatic illness occurs 1 to 3 days after ingestion of the virus particles, with the initial symptom of vomiting followed, within hours, by watery diarrhea that is characterized by brown, copious stools. Low-grade fever may also be present. In severe cases, the diarrhea becomes clear. The illness is usually self-limiting, with vomiting lasting for 1 to 3 days and diarrhea for 5 to 8 days. Death rarely occurs, but when it does, it is typically in the elderly and infant populations. The virus is especially contagious because so few particles are required for infection (10 to 100), yet so many are excreted in the feces (up to 1,000 particles/mL feces).[4]

Foods that are eaten raw such as salads and fruits can serve as good vehicles for the virus. The virus is fairly resistant to low pH and low temperature (it can survive at a pH of 2.8 and a temperature of 4°C for 3 days) but is susceptible to heat; a temperature of 60°C for 10 minutes will destroy it.[39] Thorough cooking and reheating of potentially contaminated foods should be effective in eliminating the virus. The peak time of year for infections is in the winter months, probably because this is when people are in close proximity to each other, allowing for the easy transmission of the organism. Group A *Rotavirus*, although it is the most important serotype of *Rotavirus*, is rarely associated with foodborne or waterborne outbreaks. Group B *Rotavirus* has been found only in China, and group C *Rotavirus* is rarely detected owing to a lack of adequate diagnostic methods.[40]

Hepatitis A

The hepatitis A virus is an unenveloped, small molecule (27 nm diameter) that consists of a single strand of RNA surrounded by a protein capsid. There are at least five different hepatitis viruses, of which hepatitis A and E are associated with foodborne illness. Hepatitis A and E are transmitted through the fecal-oral route. Hepatitis E infection is usually acquired from contaminated water, whereas A is commonly transmitted through food and water. The hepatitis A virus replicates in the gut mucosa and spreads to the liver. Necrosis of the liver parenchymal cells is the determining factor in the severity of the disease. Infection is associated with a very long incubation period (14 to 40 days). Symptoms at the onset include fever, nausea, abdominal pain, and anorexia, followed in several days by jaundice. The infectious dose is believed to be in the range of 10 to 100 particles.[4] Age and previous exposure are important factors on the infection-to-disease ratio. This is one of the rare pathogens in which adults are at greater risk of suffering clinical disease from the infection than children. Once infected, most people develop a lifelong immunity to the virus. Currently, no treatment exists for hepatitis A infection, but, owing to the mild nature of the illness, adequate nutrition and rest are sufficient. A number of foods can be contaminated by the virus—lettuce, delicatessen meats, fruits, juices, milk, vegetables, raw seafood, and iced tea—because the virus is stable at cold temperatures (−20°C) and low pH. Outbreaks are usually associated with conditions of crowding such as hospitals, restaurants, and schools. In 1997, frozen strawberries, imported from Mexico, were responsible for an outbreak in three different school districts in Calhoun County, Michigan.[41]

Norwalk Virus

The Norwalk virus is the leading reported cause of viral gastroenteritis in adults and older children in the United States and the most commonly identified cause of illness, along with *Salmonella*, in school-related outbreaks.[42,43] A member of the Calicivirus family of viruses, Norwalk virus particles are 27 to 38 nm in diameter and consist of a single positive strain of RNA. The organism is transmitted from person to person through the fecal-oral route. Infection has an incubation period of 10 to 51 hours. Symptoms are very similar to *Rotavirus*, consisting of vomiting, nausea, abdominal pain, and diarrhea. The nature of the illness is mild and self-resolves in about 1 to 2 days. The inoculation dose is unknown but believed to be very small. Norwalk virus is very hardy and can remain active after exposure to acid (pH 2.7) and heat (60 minutes at 60°C).[44] Foods that have been reported in outbreaks include salads, fruits, eggs, coleslaw, and raw shellfish. Outbreaks are usually associated with public food facilities, such as cafeterias and restaurants. An example of this occurred recently at a Texas university, where 23 students were treated for acute gastroenteritis at a local hospital. Reverse transcriptase polymerase chain reaction methods were employed to determine that the vehicle was delicatessen-served foods, at the university cafeteria, which were contaminated with the Norwalk-like virus.[45] A food handler denied having the illness but quit her job instead of submitting a stool specimen for confirmation.

PARASITES

In developed nations, foodborne parasitic infection is not a common problem. Globally, however, the burden of such infection is tremendous. The two parasites discussed in detail in this section, *Cryptosporidium parvum* and *Toxoplasma gondii*, are protozoa. Other protozoa that are significant foodborne pathogens include *Entamoeba histolytica*, which causes amebic dysentery, and *Giardia lamblia.*

Both of these organisms are transmitted in a very similar manner, through fecally contaminated water or food, and cause illness when an individual consumes cysts that contain the organism larvae. There are several helminths that are associated with foodborne disease because they use an animal as a host during some stage of their life cycle. Tapeworms, flukes, and roundworms are different groups of helminths that are of concern to human health and are notable for being associated with eating raw or undercooked meats and fish.

Cryptosporidium parvum

C. parvum is a protozoan that accounts for a significant number of diarrheal illnesses in children. The life cycle of the organism consists of an egg (cysts), which is ingested by a human or an animal. Sporozoites are released from the cysts in the small intestine. Several stages of the life cycle occur in the cell membrane of the small intestine, where the organism reproduces, before new cysts are shed in the feces. Transmission of the cysts to humans can occur through contaminated food, water, animals, or other humans. In individuals with healthy immune systems, symptoms include severe, watery diarrhea that can last 2 to 14 days and can result in dehydration. The infection dose is very low, about 10 organisms.[4] Onset of illness occurs 1 to 2 weeks after exposure. *C. parvum* is also a very important opportunistic pathogen. Illness from *C. parvum* infection in the immunocompromised host can result in severe, prolonged diarrhea that can lead to death. Because the cysts are transmitted through fecal contamination, virtually all foods can be potential sources of contamination. Oocysts are susceptible to freezing and high temperatures. For this reason, foods that are considered low risk include frozen, pasteurized, or processed canned foods. Large outbreaks are usually associated with contaminated water. The largest outbreak of cryptosporidiosis in US history occurred in Milwaukee, Wisconsin, in 1993 in which 403,000 people contracted the illness from a contaminated public water supply.[46]

Daycare centers are very common settings for cryptosporidiosis outbreaks, where diaper changing close to food preparation areas can contaminate food or formula. An outbreak at a daycare center was reported in Georgia in 1989, and stool samples from 39 children and three staff members were found to contain the organism.[47] Diarrhea in some children resolved only to reappear again later on, indicating the potential for reinfection under conditions of poor hygiene.

Toxoplasma gondii

T. gondii is an opportunistic pathogen and a concern for pregnant women. It is a two-host parasite that uses the domestic cat as the definitive host and warm-blooded mammals as intermediate hosts. Humans can become infected with the organism either by ingesting sporulated oocyst in contaminated meat or water or by consuming cysts in undercooked, contaminated meats. Domestic cats pass unsporulated oocysts in their feces, which can be easily introduced into a food or water source through fecal contamination. The rate of placental transmission is reported to be between 17 and 25%, although infection of the fetus occurs only if the woman has no prior exposure to the organism.[48] When this occurs, abortion and stillbirth can result. An estimated 1 child per 1,000 to 10,000 is born with toxoplasmosis each year in the United States.[49] In healthy adults, *T. gondii* infections are often asymptomatic. Antibody data suggest that 30 to 60% of the US adult population has been infected with the organism at one point or another.[48] In liveborn children with toxoplasmosis, symptoms may not appear for months or years later and may result in such chronic sequelae as epilepsy, palsies, slight deafness, and retardation.[50] Ocular toxoplasmosis occurs when cysts rupture in the retina of the eye, resulting in vision impairment. A number of meats can be associated with *T. gondii* contamination, including pork, lamb, and beef. The biggest risk factor, however, is the presence of cats in the household. Pregnant women should avoid contact with cat feces and soil and wash their hands before eating and after handling raw meat.[48] Cooking meat at a temperature of 61°C or higher for at least 3.6 minutes has been demonstrated to be sufficient in inactivating cysts.[51]

To date, no outbreaks of toxoplasmosis have been reported in the United States. Occasional small outbreaks occur worldwide. Two separate outbreaks of human toxoplasmosis occurred in Korea in late 1994 and early 1995.[52] All three infected individuals in the first incident suffered vision loss and all five in the second one had lymphadenopathy. In both cases, eating undercooked pork was linked to infection.

FUNGI

Fungi are a broad class of microorganisms that require organic compounds for energy and carbon. They share the characteristic of being eukaryotes that possess an outer cell wall. Fungi exist everywhere in nature, and some are parasites on humans and animals. For the most part, they perform a beneficial role by contributing to the decomposition of matter and recycling of nutrients. A small number cause illness in humans, however. Of the over 100,000 species of fungi that exist, only about 100 have been identified as being pathogenic toward humans.[53] The fungi kingdom consists of molds and yeasts. Yeasts are nonfilamentous, unicellular organisms, whereas molds are multicellular and have hyphae (long filaments of cells joined together). Several species of yeast, such as *Candida albicans* and *Cryptococcus neoformans*, are pathogenic in humans and account for a considerable number of illnesses among the immunocompromised. Although yeast can cause spoilage in foods, only molds produce toxins that result in foodborne illness. These mycotoxins, as a general rule, are extremely resistant to high temperatures; they cannot be destroyed by merely cooking food, in other words. However, measures can be taken to avoid fungal contamination of foods. Certain foods, such as grains and plant products, are high risk for mold contamination because of frequent environmental exposure. Aflatoxin, one of the most familiar mycotoxins associated with foods, is discussed in brief as an example of the risk associated with mold contaminations and preventive measures that can be taken.

Aflatoxin

Aflatoxins are secondary metabolites produced by certain strains of *Aspergillus* (*A. flavus* and *A. parasiticus*). *Aspergillus* spp are fast-growing molds that can be found everywhere. The major aflatoxins of concern to humans are aflatoxins B1, B2, G1, and G2. The B and G letters refer to the colors produced (blue or green) under ultraviolet light and the numbers 1 and 2 refer to their separation patterns on thin-layer liquid chromatography plates.[54] Acute toxicity from aflatoxin exposure is quite rare. Of more concern are the potential long-term effects of low-level consumption: necrosis, cirrhosis, and carcinoma of the liver in animals and humans.[54] Reports have also indicated that exposure may play some role in mental retardation development.[55] *A. flavus* is one of the most common mold contaminants in peanuts, oilseeds, and corn. Cereals and spices are also associated foods, but aflatoxin production in these is rare and the result of poor drying, handling, or storage.[54] Aflatoxin can also be found in milk as the result of cows eating moldy corn. Relative humidities of 88 to 94% and storage at temperatures between 25 and 30°C provide optimal conditions for *A. flavus* growth.[56] Although the toxin is resistant to heat, reduction of oxygen through packaging can inhibit aflatoxin production. Also, caffeine has been shown to be effective in inhibiting the growth and mycotoxin production from *Aspergillus* spp.[56] Outbreaks of aflatoxin poisoning are very rare in developed countries but do occasionally occur worldwide. A tragic incident was recently reported in Malaysia, where 13 children died from acute hepatic encephalopathy as the result of consuming noodles that contained high levels of aflatoxin.[57] In all, 17 were infected. Initial symptoms reported included vomiting, hematemesis, seizures, diarrhea, fever, and abdominal pain. All of the victims were reported to have liver dysfunction.

CHEMICAL CONTAMINANTS

Children today are exposed to nearly 15,000 synthetic chemicals, with the potential toxicity of more than half of these being untested.[58] Many of these chemicals are dispersed widely in the environment and contaminate much of our food supply. In addition to these synthetic chemicals, children can be exposed through food ingestion to the toxic effects of a vast number of natural elements, including heavy metals and toxins produced by fish. Nearly all of the synthetic chemicals that were produced within the last 50 years pose food safety risks and include pesticides, industrial chemicals and by-products, and food additives. Synthetic and naturally occurring toxic chemicals can account for a variety of disorders and diseases. Excessive exposure to some of these agents has been linked to neurotoxicity, growth retardation, sexual and endocrine disorders, and cancer, to name a few.[58] Children are especially vulnerable to the potential threat posed by environmental contaminants because, pound for pound, they consume more food and drink more water than adults do and their metabolic pathways are immature.[59]

Pesticides

Pesticides have proven to be of value to society by increasing crop yields, improving the quality of fruits, and controlling insects and rodents in the household. Persistent organic pollutants (fat-soluble chemicals that degrade slowly) accumulate in the environment and pose a threat to health, especially children.

There are several different types of pesticides, including insecticides, herbicides, fungicides, wood preservatives, rodenticides, and insect repellents. Many different categories of chemical structures exist for each of these different types of pesticides. Organophosphates and carbamates are discussed in more detail here because they are the compounds that most commonly cause systemic illness.[60] Organophosphates and carbamates are toxic compounds and include many insecticides used today.[61] Both of these compounds inhibit the breakdown of the enzyme neurotransmitter acetylcholinesterase. This inhibition results in overstimulation of certain parts of the nervous system that contain acetylcholine.[62] Acute symptoms may appear within 4 hours of exposure and can include headache, dizziness, nausea, and abdominal pain initially. Blurred vision, anxiety, confusion, vertigo, convulsions, and possibly coma may result from the nerve stimulatory effects of the compounds.[63] Poisoning from both compounds exhibits similar symptoms, but carbamate insecticide poisoning is more reversible; therefore, it is considered less severe than poisoning from organophosphates.[60] Symptoms from carbamate poisoning may last for only 6 to 8 hours. Aldicarb is a specific example of a pesticide that is an important threat to children because it can be found in various vegetables and fruits, such as bananas. Some bananas have aldicarb levels that are reported to be 10 times greater than the legal limit established by the Environmental Protection Agency (EPA).[64] Aldicarb is a carbamate insecticide that is used on a variety of crops, including citrus fruits, nuts, potatoes, and ornamental plants. It is applied to the soil and is absorbed by the root system of the plant; therefore, residues can contaminate the edible portion of food crops.[64] Like other carbamate pesticides, toxicity is associated with acetylcholinesterase inhibition. When ingested, aldicarb is absorbed through the gut and is distributed throughout the body. Symptoms from aldicarb poisoning vary depending on the dosage and age of the individual and can include skeletal muscle weakness, diarrhea, excessive sweating, nausea, vomiting, nonreactive contracted pupils, blurred vision, dyspnea, and muscle convulsions.[65] The EPA has placed aldicarb in its highest acute toxicity category.[66] Various outbreaks and incidents of aldicarb poisoning have been reported. Documented ingestion of the pesticide has been linked to suicide attempts and from consuming cucumbers.[67,68] The largest foodborne outbreak associated with a pesticide was the result of aldicarb-contaminated watermelons.[69] In 1985, 1,373 people throughout the states of Oregon, Washington, and California reportedly became ill from consuming the contaminated watermelons.

Polychlorinated Biphenyls

Polychlorinated biphenyls (PCBs) are a family of compounds that are nonvolatile, hydrophobic oils that were extensively used by industry from the 1930s through the 1970s as hydraulic fluids, plasticizers, adhesives, fire retardants, wax extenders, lubricants, and inks, among many other things.[70] Even though PCBs are no longer used today—production was banned by the Toxic Substances Act of 1977—much of what was produced remains in the environment.[63] PCBs are a common food contaminant, especially in fish. These compounds are a special concern because they cannot be metabolized or excreted from the body (except through breast milk); therefore, even a little exposure can accumulate to significant amounts over time. The pathology behind the toxic effects of PCBs is not understood. Symptoms from acute exposure of the compounds can include diarrhea and chloracne, a specific skin reaction associated with cyclic halogenated compounds that is characteristically similar to acne vulgaris except that cysts tend to be more severe and inflammation less prominent.[70] Prenatal exposure, through the cord blood, can occur.[63] Long-term effects from such exposure are debatable, but compelling evidence suggests that it can be quite damaging. An extensive study conducted on Michigan children whose mothers consumed fish from Lake Michigan revealed that elevated cord serum PCB levels correlated with lower birth weights and a reduction in head circumference and gestational age. These same children at the age of 4 had lower body weights and poorer short-term memory compared with other children.[71] A follow-up study on Japanese children who suffered during a massive epidemic from cooking oil contaminated with PCBs in 1968 found that the children 9 years later showed apathy, lethargy, soft neurologic signs, and growth deficiency.[72] A similar study, following a 1979 outbreak in Taiwan, reported that the children several years later showed an average reduction of five to eight points on standard IQ scales, short stature, and hyperactive behavior.[72] During the 1968 epidemic in Japan, one of the children was stillborn, which suggests that high levels of prenatal exposure can prove fatal as well. Breast milk can be a significant source of infant exposure to PCBs. However, studies suggest that the chemical levels of breast milk do not pose a significant threat to the health of infants.[73] The American Academy of Pediatrics, after considering this topic, still recommends breast-feeding.[63] PCBs are unavoidable contaminants found in fatty foods, such as meat, fish, milk, and milk products. The US Food and Drug Administration (FDA) established tolerances for PCB levels in these foods. Milk, eggs, other dairy products, poultry, fish, shellfish, and infant foods are required to contain less than 0.2 to 3 parts of PCBs per million parts of food.[74]

Mercury

Inorganic and organic mercury are toxic to humans, but organic mercury (in the form of methylmercury) is associated with ingestion more than inorganic mercury. Inorganic mercury salts are poorly absorbed after ingestion; dermal exposure is more toxic. In contrast, nearly 100% of methylmercury is absorbed after ingestion.[63] Inorganic mercury in lakes and streams can be converted into organic mercury by bacteria and enter the food supply.[75] Methylmercury is consumed primarily through eating fish because all fish are contaminated to some extent with the compound.[76] About 95% of methylmercury that is ingested is absorbed in the gastrointestinal tract and is rapidly distributed to all tissues.[77] It can pass easily into the nervous system, where it irreversibly damages the cells of the granular layer in the cerebellum, the cerebral cortex, and the calcarine cortex. Methylmercury crosses the placental barrier and accumulates in the fetal brain and blood.[78] The latent period for mercury poisoning can be very long—several weeks to months to years. Clinical manifestations that result from long-term methylmercury poisoning can include paresthesia of the mouth, lips, tongue, hands, feet, fingers, and toes; constriction of visual fields; hearing difficulty; speech disorders; weakness and fatigue; memory loss; emotional instability; ataxia; coma; and, in the most extreme cases, death.[78] To limit consumption of methylmercury, avoid eating large, long-lived fish that feed on other fish because they accumulate higher mercury levels than other fish. Examples of such fish would include shark, swordfish, king mackerel, and tilefish. Pregnant women are advised to limit consumption to 12 oz/wk of cooked fish.[79]

PHYSICAL CONTAMINANTS

Objects from the environment (pebbles, twigs, etc) and production equipment (shards of metal, plastic, glass, etc) occasionally contaminate food products. Every year, numerous recalls occur as the result of such findings in commercial food products.[80–84] Occasionally, ingestion of objects in food can cause lacerations of the mouth and digestive tract and occasionally broken teeth. Most are passed harmlessly in the feces. With children, it is probably best to closely examine foods for any evidence of foreign objects and avoid foods with damaged packaging.

FOOD SAFETY PRACTICES IN THE HOME ENVIRONMENT

So what can parents or child care providers do to prevent foodborne illness in infants and children? A wealth of information devoted to educating the general public on food safety issues can be located throughout the Internet and on bookshelves. Reliable sources of publications include government agencies (such as the Department of Agriculture Food Safety Inspection Service, the FDA, or the Centers for Disease Control and Prevention), international organizations devoted to health issues such as the World Health Organization, or professional and scientific societies such as the American Academy of Pediatrics and the American Society for Microbiology.

Unfortunately, the general public remains unaware of some fundamental knowledge and simple steps to be taken to prevent foodborne illnesses. For instance, a national survey in 1993 revealed that consumers falsely believe that foodborne illness is a minor sickness and that such illnesses usually result from eating a contaminated food at a restaurant.[85] Table 2 summarizes the recommendations of several reliable organizations.[86–90] Although some of this advice seems obvious and merely common sense, it is warranted to briefly discuss it in more detail because the general public is not fully aware of these basic concepts.

Cook Foods Properly

Probably the best defense mechanism against foodborne illness is heat. All foods should be thoroughly defrosted before cooking. It is important to cook foods until steaming hot throughout, making sure that the internal portions of meat are not left merely warm; a minimum internal temperature of 160°F should be reached for beef, 180°F for poultry, 160°F for pork, and 145°F for seafood. Thermometers should be used to determine that hamburgers have reached an internal temperature of 160°F to ensure that *E. coli* O157:H7 is killed. Microwave ovens need to be used with extreme caution because they do not uniformly heat foods. In addition, high salt concentrations in foods suppress microwave heating.[91] When heating foods in microwave ovens, make sure to use appropriate containers recommended by the manufacturer of the unit. To ensure that foods are heated uniformly in microwave ovens, avoid salting foods before they go into the microwave and occasionally mix the foods when heating.

Properly Store Cooked Foods

It is important to properly store foods before and after they are cooked. When serving infants, serve cooked foods immediately after preparation and avoid, if at all possible, storing leftovers altogether. If foods are stored, keep the foods at either cold temperatures (below 45°F) or at high temperatures (above 140°F). Remember, some organisms, most notably *L. monocytogenes*, can survive in the cold environment of the refrigerator; therefore, always reheat foods before serving to a temperature of at least 74°C (165°F). Always refrigerate leftover foods immediately and reserve within 3 days unless the foods are frozen completely. Make a habit of checking the temperature on your refrigerator and freezer. Refrigerators should operate at a temperature range of 40 to 42°F and freezers should be kept at a temperature of 0°F.

Be Cautious of Raw Foods

Raw foods provide very attractive vehicles for a number of microorganisms and should be handled with care. Avoid cross-contaminating raw foods with cooked foods. For instance, avoid having cooked foods or foods that will be served raw coming into any contact with utensils, dishes, or cutting boards that were previously in contact with raw meats or seafood. It is important to separate raw food items from other foods in the grocery cart and bag as well. Avoid serving raw meats, raw unpasteurized milk, or cheese made from raw milk. Also, avoid items that contain raw eggs, such as home-made ice cream or mayonnaise; *Salmonella* can be harbored in uncooked whole eggs.

Clean Hands Are Essential

Proper hand washing technique is paramount to ensuring food safety in the home. Most people are under the mistaken impression that splashing the hands with running faucet water and patting them dry with a towel is the required approach to achieving sanitized hands. When washing your hands, always use warm, running water and soap. Rub the hands together until a soapy lather develops and continue for at least 20 seconds. Rinse your hands and dry with a clean towel. Always wash your hands before preparing food, after handling raw meat and poultry, and after any interruption, such as going to the restroom, coming into contact with pets, or changing diapers.

Use Clean Equipment

A clean kitchen with clean appliances is also an essential requirement for food safety. A seemingly clean kitchen may not actually be so. A study of 14 households revealed that the sites in the households that were contaminated with the most fecal bacteria were the sponge/dishcloths in the kitchen and the kitchen sink drain area; the areas that had the lowest contamination were the bathroom countertops and the toilet seats.[92] The point is that if dirty dishcloths are used to clean dishes and surface areas in the kitchen, the work is done in vain. Change hand and dish towels frequently and use hot soapy water or a disinfectant solution when cleaning kitchen surface areas.

Table 2 Guidelines for Food Safety

Agency/Organization	Cook Foods Properly	Properly Store Cooked Foods	Be Cautious of Raw Foods	Clean Hands Are Essential for Food Safety	Food Safety Also Means Using Clean, Proper Equipment	Other Advice
World Health Organization[86]	All foods must be cooked at minimum temperature of 70°C	Keep cool (below 10°C). When served again, heat to at least 70°C	Do not cross-contaminate cooked foods with raw foods. Hands and utensils should be washed after coming into contact with raw foods	Wash hands thoroughly before preparing food and after every interruption (ie, changing baby, using toilet, coming into contact with animals, etc)	Avoid feeding infants with a bottle. It is usually difficult to get bottles and teats completely clean. Cups, spoons, dishes, and utensils should be washed thoroughly	Water used in preparing food should be bottled unless the food is adequately cooked
American Academy of Pediatrics[87]	Cook all foods thoroughly. Use a meat thermometer for large items like roasts or turkeys and cut into pieces to see if it is done	Do not let prepared foods stay at room temperature for more than 2 h. Freeze immediately if stored. When reheating, cover and reheat thoroughly	Wash hands and all surfaces that have come into contact with raw meat with hot, sudsy water. Do not serve raw meat. Do not use raw milk or cheese made from raw milk	Always wash hands before preparing meals and after going to the bathroom or changing your baby's diaper	Carefully examine any canned food for signs of bacterial contamination. Look for cracked jars, loose lids, and swollen cans or lids	Do not give honey to a baby under 1 yr of age. Buy all meats and seafoods from a reputable supplier
Centers for Disease Control and Prevention[88]	Make sure that all meats, especially poultry and hamburger, are cooked completely	Foods should be kept at 40°F or colder or at 140°F or warmer. Leftovers should be refrigerated immediately	No foods containing raw eggs should be served, including home-made ice cream with raw eggs	Use proper hand washing techniques. Do not handle food if you change diapers. In this case, proper hand washing is essential	Use only approved food equipment (check local child care licensing regulations). Only use cutting boards that can be disinfectd (made of nonporous materials such as glass, Formica, or plastic)	Do not prepare or serve food if you have diarrhea. Supervise meal and snack times to make sure that children do not share plates, utensils, or food
Food Safety Inspection Service[89]	Cook ground meats to 100°F, ground poultry to 165°F, and all fresh pork to 160°F. Whole poultry should reach 180°F	Discard any food left out at room temperature for more than 2 h (1 h if above 90°F). Place food into shallow container and immediately freeze. Use cooked leftovers within 4 d	Separate raw meat from other foods in grocery cart and refrigerator. Always wash hands and utensils with hot, soapy water after they have come into contact with raw foods. Never serve food on a plate that previously held raw foods	Wash your hands with hot, soapy water before and after handling food	Keep sponges and dishcloths clean. These items can harbor bacteria	When packing a lunch, keep hot foods hot and cold foods cold. A thermos or an ice pack will help. Keep lunch in coolest place possible; never leave in direct sun
Food and Drug Administration[90]	Cook beef at 71°C (160°F), poultry at 82°C (180°F), and seafood at 63°C (145°F) for 15 s	Cooked foods should not be left out more than 2 h. Refrigerate leftovers as quickly as possible. Use within 3 d. Reheat foods to at least 74°C (165°F)	Always wash boards after exposure to raw meat. Keep raw foods from other foods	Wash hands with warm water and soap for at least 20 s. Hot water that is comfortable for hands is not hot enough to kill bacteria. Always use soap	Use only hard wood or nonporous cutting boards. Always use clean utensils. Wash the lids of canned foods before opening. Clean blade of can opener before use	Do not serve juice or cider if you cannot determine if it has been pasteurized

Also, do not soak dishes in water without detergent. Use only hard wood or nonporous cutting boards because these surfaces can be disinfected. Other important advice includes always washing fruits and vegetables before serving. With infants, peel the fruit or vegetable if possible. Avoid serving honey to children under the age of 1 year owing to the risk of infant botulism. In group settings with children, such as daycare centers or schools, make sure that children do not share foods and that diaper-changing areas are located away from food preparation areas. Avoid serving apple cider or unpasteurized fruit juices to children; *E. coli* O157:H7 can grow at a pH less than 4.0, meaning that it can survive in apple cider and unpasteurized juices.[93] If you cannot determine if a juice product has been pasteurized, avoid it. Make sure that you store all food items away from garbage, pesticides, disinfecting agents, or other chemicals. Finally, clean water is an essential prerequisite for food safety. Ice made from unsafe water is unsafe itself.

Traveling

Food safety is very important to consider when traveling with children. When traveling on the road with food for longer than 30 minutes, always place items in a cooler with ice or freezer packs. Meat and poultry should be packed while frozen and kept separate from other items. When hiking or camping, do not drink from streams or rivers, instead, pack bottled drinks, especially water. Do not eat anything that sits at ambient temperatures for too long. When traveling in developing nations, pack or order bottled drinks, such as water or carbonated sodas. If such items are not available, boil water and let it cool before consumption. This applies to unpasteurized milk also. In areas of poor sanitation, bottled or boiled water should be used to brush teeth. Peel fruits and vegetables before eating them. If this is not possible, cook the foods first. Raw foods should be avoided because they pose a heavy risk of contamination. Foods that have been cooked and are still hot can be considered safe. Seafood in certain tropical areas of the world can be unsafe, even when cooked, owing to the presence of toxins. This especially applies to fishes that are caught on tropical reefs. Traveler's diarrhea can be a real problem when traveling in developing regions. The illness is not associated with any particular pathogen and usually is self-limiting after a few days. Sometimes the illness can be severe, however, if dehydration occurs. Pack oral rehydration solution when traveling with infants or young children. These items can usually be located at most pharmacies. If diarrhea occurs, drink more fluids, such as bottled water, fruit juice, or soup; avoid dairy products. In the case of mild dehydration, the oral rehydration solution should be used. The solution should be prepared as instructed on the package. Parents should be counseled to seek medical assistance about treatment of diarrhea in children and infants. It is recommended that children or persons with serious infection should not be administered antidiarrheal medications, such as Lomotil(TM), for instance. If bloody diarrhea, dehydration, fever in excess of 102°F, or persistent vomiting occurs, seek medical help immediately.

Food Safety Applied to Each Stage of Childhood

Until this point, food safety issues have been discussed in general terms, without any real consideration of the different stages of child development, but some concerns are different for each stage of childhood feeding. Steps for ensuring food safety for children at the age of 3 years and up are very similar to those of adults. Food safety for the infant is addressed in further detail owing to a few unique considerations for each stage. Breast-feeding is widely recommended over formula feeding, despite the presence of chemical residues, such as DDT (dichlorodiphenyltrichloroethane) and PCBs.[94] This is because human milk provides hormones, enzymes, and immunoglobulins that simply cannot be replicated in infant formula.[95] The advantages of breast milk far exceed the minimum hazards that it poses. Local health departments provide advice specific to pediatricians when local food habits may put breast-fed infants at risk. When formula is administered to a child, special care needs to be taken to follow label instructions. Most liquid formula should be fed directly and not diluted. Liquid formulas labeled as ready-to-use should be fed directly and not diluted, while concentrated liquid formulas should be prepared as directed on their labels. It is recommended that powder formulas be prepared fresh for each meal and all remaining formula, following feeding, be discarded and not used for future meals.[96] Powder formulas should not be reconstituted using boiling water or heated following reconstitution.[96] The FDA withdrew an earlier recommendation to use boiling water in reconstituting powder formula, due to the possible loss of heat-sensitive nutrients, changes in the physical characteristics of some formulas, the inability to ensure adequate destruction of Enterobacter sakazakii, and safety concerns.[97] In addition to using sterile water, sterile equipment (bottles, nipples, utensils used in the preparation procedure, etc) is extremely important. Honey, syrups, raw eggs, or unpasteurized milk should never be added to formula. Formula should be refrigerated properly and not stand at room temperature too long. Refrigerated formula should be used within 24 hours after preparation or discarded. Microwave ovens should not be used to heat formulas.[98] Finally, home-made infant formulas should be avoided.[99] Introducing solid foods to the young child's diet requires some additional care. Prepare fresh fruits by scrubbing and peeling them. All bones, skin, gristle, and fat should be removed from meats. Make sure that all foods are cooked thoroughly and prepared using clean equipment and utensils. As mentioned before, avoid cross-contaminating raw foods with cooked foods and never serve unpasteurized juices or ciders. Store-bought baby foods can be considered to be safe because federal standards are stricter for processed foods. In such foods, residue levels of pesticides are generally lower. Some manufacturers of baby foods voluntarily make their products free of all pesticides.[63] Do not let baby foods sit out at room temperature for more than 2 hours and refrigerate as soon as possible. Always seal foods in clean containers tightly when storing them. Cooked vegetables or fruits should be served within 3 days and raw fruits and meats within 24 hours. The same care for food safety in hospitals must be maintained.[100]

Other Factors That Influence Food Safety

Geography influences the safety of some foods. The Great Lake basin, for example, is contaminated with a wide array of chemical contaminants, including PCBs, DTT, and hexachlorethane, to name a few.[101] Consuming fish from these waters poses an increased risk, and advisory messages are periodically issued warning pregnant women and other vulnerable groups about these risks. Likewise, the Hudson River is known to be contaminated with PCBs owing to old industrial facilities along the river that still leak up to 3 ounces of PCBs each day.[102] The EPA has measured PCB levels as high as 41 ppm in fish caught in the Upper Hudson River.[102] Even though commercial fishing has been banned in the area, people still consume fish that is caught in the contaminated waters. Also, people residing in countries bordering the Gulf of Mexico are at a higher risk of consuming food or drinking water contaminated with *Vibrio* bacteria, one species of which, *Vibrio cholerae,* is the agent that causes cholera.[103] Certain ethnic food practices, lifestyles, and feeding habits can result in increased risk of foodborne illness. As part of the traditional Eskimo diet, for example, salmon heads, salmon eggs, whale muktuk, and seal flippers are placed in a shallow wood or animal skin and covered with moss underground, which ferments the food. This tradition has resulted in outbreaks of botulism.[104]

FOOD SAFETY TECHNOLOGY

The US food supply is one of the safest in the world, largely attributable to the work of the government and the food industry. Food processors have a wide array of techniques to use to help reduce the threat of microbial contamination of their products. A variety of physical methods of food preservation are currently used in the industry, including freeze drying, ohmic heating (electrical heating), pasteurization (a mild form of heating that minimizes damage to food but helps destroy 99 to 99.9% of bacterial cells), high hydrostatic pressure preservation, and electric and magnetic field effects, to name only a few examples. Chemical preservatives and antimicrobial compounds are added to foods to help retard microbial growth or kill microorganisms. One of the most promising recent techniques in food technology is the use of irradiation to reduce the risk of foodborne illness. Food irradiation (sometimes called cold pasteurization) employs ionizing radiation at doses sufficient to damage the DNA of bacterial cells, destroying them in the process. Irradiation of foods is a safe process and does not induce additional radioactivity into foods.[105] Irradiation can be performed after foods are packaged, preventing additional handling. Currently, it is used on spices and certain imported fruits and vegetables and is approved for use in raw poultry and meats. Finally, a mention must be made of the importance of the Hazard Analysis Critical Control Point System (HACCP), which has revolutionized food safety during the past 20 years. HACCP provides a systematic, structured approach to food safety. The principles behind the system can be adopted and followed by any sector of the food industry to help design programs to assist in the production of safer products. The basic idea behind the system is examining all steps of a production process, identifying places in which problems are likely to occur, and developing measures to address these potential hazards. HACCP systems are required for all meat, poultry, and seafood processors. Currently, the FDA[106] is phasing in requirements for HACCP systems to be in place for fruit juice processors as well. Even though the food industry does a great deal to improve the quality and safety of its food products, the threat of foodborne illness is still very present. It is essential that the general public become more educated about food safety.

REFERENCES

1. Mead PS, Slutsker L, Dietz V, et al. Food-related illness and death in the United States. Emerg Infect Dis 1999;5:607–25.
2. Altekruse SF, Stern NJ, Fields PI, Swerdlow DL. *Campylobacter jejuni*—an emerging foodborne pathogen. Emerg Infect Dis 1999;5:28–35.
3. Park SF. The physiology of *Campylobacter* species and its relevance to their role as foodborne pathogens. Int J Food Microbiol 2002;74:177–88.
4. US Food and Drug Administration. Bad bug book. Available at: http://www.cfsan.fda.gov. Accessed November 21, 2002.
5. Blaser MJ, Allos BM, Lang D. Development of Guillain–Barre syndrome following *Campylobacter* infection. J Infect Dis 1997;176:S91.
6. Cook KA, Dobbs TE, Hiady G, et al. Outbreak of *Salmonella* serotype Harford infections associated with unpasteurized orange juice. JAMA 1998;280:1504–9.
7. Cummings K, Barrett E, Mohle-Boetani JC, et al. A multistate outbreak of *Salmonella enterica* serotype Baildon associated with domestic raw tomatoes. Emerg Infect Dis 2001;7:1046–8.

8. Mohle-Boetani JC, Reporter R, Werner SB, et al. An outbreak of *Salmonella* serogroup saphra due to cantaloupes from Mexico. J Infect Dis 1999;180:1361–4.
9. Campbell JV, Mohle-Boetani J, Reporter R, et al. An outbreak of *Salmonella* serotype thompson associated with fresh cilantro. J Infect Dis 2001;183:984–7.
10. Mahon BE, Ponka A, Hall WN. An international outbreak of *Salmonella* infections caused by alfalfa sprouts grown from contaminated seeds. J Infect Dis 1997;175:876–82.
11. Baird-Parker AC. Foodborne salmonellosis. Lancet 1990;336:1231–4.
12. Ryan CA, Nickels MK, Hargrett-Bean NT, et al. Massive outbreak of antimicrobial-resistant salmonellosis traced to pasteurized milk. JAMA 1987;258:3269–74.
13. Hennessy TW, Hedberg CW, Slutsker L, et al. A national outbreak of *Salmonella enteritidis* infections from ice cream. N Engl J Med 1996;334:1281–6.
14. Riley LW, Remis RS, Helgerson SD, et al. Hemorrhagic colitis associated with a rare *Escherichia coli* serotype. N Engl J Med 1983;30:681–5.
15. Boyce TG, Swedlow DL, Griffin PM. *Escherichia coli* O157:H7 and the hemolytic-uremic syndrome. N Engl J Med 1995;333:364–8.
16. Featherstone C. *Escherichia coli* O157:H7: Superbug or mere sensation? Lancet 1997;349:930.
17. Juneja VK, Snyder OP, Marmer BS. Thermal destruction of *Escherichia* O157:H7 in beef and chicken: Determination of *D*- and *z*- values. Int J Food Microbiol 1997;35:231–7.
18. Zhao T, Doyle MP, Besser RE. Fate of enterohemorrhagic *Escherichia coli* O157:H7 in apple cider with and without preservatives. Appl Environ Microbiol 1993;59:2526–30.
19. Bell BP, Goldoft M, Griffin PM, et al. A multistate outbreak of *Escherichia coli* O157:H7-associated bloody diarrhea and hemolytic uremic syndrome from hamburgers. JAMA 1994;272:1349–53.
20. Watanabe Y, Ozasa K, Mermin JH, et al. Factory outbreak of *Escherichia coli* O157:H7 infection in Japan. Emerg Infect Dis 1999;5:424–8.
21. Centers for Disease Control and Prevention. Outbreak of *Escherichia coli* O157:H7 infections associated with drinking unpasteurized commercial apple juice—British Columbia, California, Colorado, and Washington, October 1996. MMWR Morb Mortal Wkly Rep 1996;45:975.
22. Belongia EA, Osterholm MT, Soler JT, et al. Transmission of *Escherichia coli* O157:H7 infection in Minnesota child daycare facilities. JAMA 1993;269:883–8.
23. Swerdlow DL, Griffen PM. Duration of faecal shedding of *Escherichia coli* O157:H7 among children in day-care centres. Lancet 1997;349:745–6.
24. Centers for Disease Control and Prevention. Lake-associated outbreak of *Escherichia coli* O157:H7-Illinois, 1995. MMWR Morb Mortal Wkly Rep 1995;45:437–9.
25. Schuchat A, Deaver KA, Wenger JD, et al. Role of foods in sporadic listeriosis: I. Case-control study of dietary risk factors. JAMA 1992;267:2041–5.
26. Pinner RW, Schuchat A, Swaminathan B, et al. Role of foods in sporadic listeriosis: II. Microbiologic and epidemiologic investigation. JAMA 1992;267:2046–50.
27. Schlech WF. Foodborne listeriosis. Clin Infect Dis 2000;31:770–5.
28. Linnin MJ, Mascola L, Lou XD, et al. Epidemic listeriosis associated with Mexican-style cheese. N Engl J Med 1988;319:823–8.
29. Centers for Disease Control and Prevention. Update: Multistate outbreak of listeriosis. MMWR Morb Mortal Wkly Rep 1999;47:1117–8.
30. Dalton CB, Austin CC, Sobel J, et al. An outbreak of gastroenteritis and fever due to *Listeria monocytogenes* in milk. N Engl J Med 1997;336:100–5.
31. Centers of Disease Control and Prevention. *Clostridium perfringens* gastroenteritis associated with corned beef served at St. Patrick's Day meals—Ohio and Virginia, 1993. MMWR Morb Mortal Wkly Rep 1994;43:137–44.
32. Roach RL, Sienko DG. *Clostridium perfringens* outbreak associated with minestrone soup. Am J Epidemiol 1992;136:1288–91.
33. Schreiner MS, Field E, Ruddy R. Infant botulism: A review of 12 years experience at the children's hospital of Philadelphia. Pediatrics 1991;87:159–65.
34. Cox N, Hinkle R. Infant botulism. Am Fam Physician 2002;65:1388–92.
35. Centers for Disease Control and Prevention. International outbreak of type E botulism associated with ungutted, salted whitefish. MMWR Morb Mortal Wkly Rep 1987;36:812–3.
36. McMaster P, Piper S, Schell D, et al. Instructive case: A taste for honey. J Paediatr Child Health 2000;36:596–7.
37. Parashar UD, Holmann RC, Clarke MJ, et al. Hospitalizations associated with rotavirus diarrhea in the United States, 1993 through 1995: Surveillance based on the new ICD-9-CM rotavirus specific diagnostic code. J Infect Dis 1998;177:7–13.
38. Bishop RF, Barnes GL, Cipricin E, Lund JS. Clinical immunity after neonatal rotavirus infection: A prospective longitudinal study in young children. N Engl J Med 1983;309:72–6.
39. O'Mahony J, O'Donoghue M, Morgan JG, Hill C. Rotavirus survival and stability in foods as determined by an optimized plaque assay procedure. Int J Food Microbiol 2000;61:177–85.
40. Svensson L. Diagnosis of foodborne viral infections in patients. Int J Food Microbiol 2000;59:117–26.
41. US Department of Health and Human Services. Release no. 0100.97. Hepatitis an outbreak in Michigan schools. April 2, 1997. Available at: http://www.usda.gov/news/releases/1997/04/0100. Accessed November 21, 2002.
42. Glass RI, Noel J, Ando T, et al. The epidemiology of enteric caliciviruses from humans: A reassessment using new diagnostics. J Infect Dis 2000:181:S254–61.
43. General Accounting Office. Food safety: Continued vigilance needed to ensure safety of school meals. GAO-02-669T. April 30, 2002. Available at: http:www.gao.gov/new.items/do266qt.pdf. Accessed April 15, 2006.
44. Dolin R, Blacklow NR, DuPont H, et al. Biological properties of Norwalk agent of acute infectious nonbacterial gastroenteritis. Proc Soc Exp Biol Med 1972;140:578–83.
45. Daniels HA, Bergmire-Sweat DA, Schwab KJ, et al. A foodborne outbreak of gastroenteritis associated with Norwalk-like viruses: First molecular traceback to deli sandwiches contaminated during preparation. J Infect Dis 2000;181:1467–70.
46. MacKenzie WR, Hoxie NJ, Proctor ME. A massive outbreak in Milwaukee of *Cryptosporidium* infection transmitted through the public water supply. N Engl J Med 1994;331:161–7.
47. Tangermann RH, Gordon S, Wiesner P, Kreckman L. An outbreak of cryptosporidiosis in a day-care center in Georgia. Am J Epidemiol 1991;133:471–6.
48. Frenkel JK. Toxoplasmosis in human beings. J Am Vet Assoc 1990;196:240–8.
49. Roberts T, Frenkel JK. Estimating income losses and other preventable costs caused by congenital toxoplasmosis in people in the United States. JAMA 1990;196:249–56.
50. Guerina NG, Hsu HW, Meissner HC, et al. Neonatal serologic screening and early treatment for congenital *Toxoplasma gondii* infection. N Engl J Med 1994;330:1858–63.
51. Dubey JP, Kotula AW, Sharar A, et al. Effect of high temperature on infectivity of *Toxoplasma gondii* cysts in pork. J Parasitol 1990;76:201–4.
52. Choi W, Nam H, Kwak H, et al. Foodborne outbreaks of human toxoplasmosis. J Infect Dis 1997;175:1280–2.
53. Tortora GJ, Funke BR, Case CL. Microbiology: An Introduction, 4th edition. Menlo Park, CA: Benjamin/Cummings; 1992.
54. Doyle MP, Beuchat LR, Montville TJ. Food microbiology: Fundamentals and frontiers. Washington, DC: ASM Press; 1997.
55. Caster WO, Burton TA, Irvin TR, Tanner MA. Dietary aflatoxins, intelligence, and school performance in southern Georgia. Int J Vitam Nutr Res 1986;56:291–5.
56. Hui YH, Kitts D, Stanfield PS. Foodborne Disease Handbook, Volume 4: Seafood and Environmental Toxins. New York: Marcel Dekker; 2001.
57. Lye MS, Ghazali AA, Mohan J, et al. An outbreak of acute hepatic encephalopathy due to severe aflatoxicosis in Malaysia. Am J Trop Med Hyg 1995;53:68–72.
58. Landrigan PJ, Carlson JE, Bearer CF, et al. Children's health and the environment: A new agenda for prevention research. Environ Health Perspect 1998;106:787–94.
59. National Research Council. Environmental Neurotoxicology. Washington, DC: National Academy Press; 1992.
60. O'Malley M. Clinical evaluation of pesticide exposure and poisonings. Lancet 1997;349:1161–6.
61. National Research Council. Pesticides in the Diets of Infants and Children. Washington, DC: National Academy Press; 1993.
62. Zwiener RJ, Ginsburg CM. Organophosphate and carbamate poisoning in infants and children. Pediatrics 1988;81:121–6.
63. Committee on Environmental Health. Handbook of Pediatric Environmental Health. Elk Grove Village, IL: American Academy of Pediatrics; 1999.
64. Goldman LR, Beller M, Jackson RJ. Aldicarb food poisonings in California, 1985–1988: Toxicity estimates for humans. Arch Environ Health 1990;45:141–7.
65. Risher JF, Mink FL, Stara JF. The toxicologic effects of the carbamate insecticide aldicarb in mammals: A review. Environ Health Perspect 1987;72:267–81.
66. Centers for Disease Control and Prevention. Aldicarb as a cause of food poisoning—Louisiana, 1998. MMWR Morb Mortal Wkly Rep 1999;48:269–71.
67. Centers for Disease Control and Prevention. Poisonings associated with illegal use of aldicarb as a rodenticide—New York City, 1994–1997. MMWR Morb Mortal Wkly Rep 1997;46:961–3.
68. Goes EA, Savage EP, Gibbons G, et al. Suspected foodborne carbamate pesticide intoxications associated with ingestion of hydroponic cucumbers. Am J Epidemiol 1980;111:254–60.
69. Green MA, Heumann MA, Wehr M, et al. An outbreak of watermelon-borne pesticide toxicity. Am J Public Health 1987;77:1431–4.
70. Wexler P. Encyclopedia of Toxicology. San Diego, CA: Academic Press; 1998.
71. Rice DC. Neurotoxicity of lead, methylmercury, and PBCs in relation to the Great Lakes. Environ Health Perspect 1995;103:71–87.
72. Rogan WJ. Environmental poisoning of children—lessons from the past. Environ Health Perspect 1995;103:19–23.
73. Rogan WJ, Gladen BC, McKinney JD, et al. Polychlorinated biphenyls (PCBs) and dichlorodiphenyl dicholorethene (DDE) in human milk: Effects on growth, morbidity, and duration of lactation. Am J Public Health 1987;77:1294–7.
74. Agency for Toxic Substances and Disease Registry. Polychlorinated biphenyls (PCBs). Case no.: 1336-36-3, September 1997. Available at: http://atsdr1.atsdr.cdc.gov:8080/tfacts17.html. Accessed November 21, 2002.
75. World Health Organization. Environmental Health Criteria 101: Methylmercury. Geneva: WHO; 1990.
76. Davidson PW, Myers GJ, Cox C, et al. Effects of prenatal andpostnatal methylmercury exposure from fish consumption on neurodevelopment. JAMA 1998;280:701–7.
77. Clarkson TW. The three modern faces of mercury. Environ Health Perspect 2002;110:11–23.
78. Arena JM. Poisoning: Toxicology Symptoms and Treatments, 4th edition. Springfield, IL: Charles C. Thomas; 1979.
79. Food and Drug Administration. Consumer advisory: An important message for pregnant women and women of childbearing age who may become pregnant about the risks of mercury in fish. March 2001. Available at: http://vm.cfsan.fda.gov/~dms/admehg.html. Accessed November 21, 2002.
80. Food Safety Inspection Service. Class I recall: Ohio firm recalls ham products for possible contamination with nonfood foreign material. Recall release: FSIS-RC-01-087. December 29, 2001. Available at: http://www.fsis.usda.gov/OA/recalls/prelease/pr087-2001.htm. Accessed November 21, 2002.
81. Food Safety Inspection Service. Class I recall: Maryland firm recalls chicken for possible contamination with metal. Recall release: FSIS-RC-02-020. February 28, 2002. Available at: http://www.fsis.usda.gov/OA/recalls/prelease/pr020-2002.htm. Accessed November 21, 2002.
82. Food Safety Inspection Service. Class I recall: Illinois firm recalls bratwurst for possible contamination with plastic. Recall release: FSIS-RC-035-2002. April 26,2002. Available at: http://www.fsis.usda.gov/OA/recalls/prelease/pr035-2002.htm. Accessed November 21, 2002.
83. Food Safety Inspection Service. Class II recall: Arkansas firm recalls chili tortilla product for possible contamination with plastic. Recall release: FSIS-RC-037-2002. May 1, 2002. Available at: http://www.fsis.usda.gov/OA/recalls/prelease/pr037-2002.htm. Accessed November 21, 2002.
84. Food Safety Inspection Service. Class I recall: Ohio firm recalls chicken nuggets for possible contamination with plastic. Recall release: FSIS-RC-01-073. December 17, 2001. Available at: http://www.fsis.usda.gov/OA/recalls/prelease/pr073-2001.htm. Accessed November 21, 2002.
85. Fein SB, Lin CT, Levy AS. Foodborne illness: Perceptions, experience and preventive behaviors in the United States. J Food Protect 1995;58:1405–11.
86. World Health Organization. Basic principles for the preparation of safe food for infants and young children. Available at: http://www.who.int/fsf/brochure/basic.pdf. Accessed November 21, 2002.
87. American Academy of Pediatrics. Caring for your baby and young child: Birth to age 5. New York: Bantam Books; 1998.
88. Centers for Disease Control and Prevention. The ABC's of Safe and Healthy Child Care. Washington, DC: Department of Health and Human Services; 1996.
89. Food Safety Inspection Service. Available at: http://www.fsis.usda.gov/index.htm. Accessed November 21, 2002.
90. Food and Drug Administration. Available at: http://www.fda.gov/. Accessed November 21, 2002.
91. Dealler SF, Lacey RW. Superficial microwave heating. Nature 1990;344:496.
92. Rusin P, Orosz-Coughlin P, Gerba C. Reduction of faecal coliform, coliform and heterotrophic plate count bacteria in the household kitchen and bathroom by disinfection with hypochlorite cleaners. J Appl Microbiol 1988;85:819–28.

93. Koodie L, Dhople AM. Acid tolerance of *Escherichia coli* O157:H7 and its survival in apple juice. Microbios 2001;104:167–75.
94. Rogan WJ. Pollutants in breast milk. Arch Pediatr Adolesc Med 1996;150:981–90.
95. Food and Drug Administration. Infant formula: Second best but good enough. FDA Consumer [Serial online] 1996. Available at: http://www.cfsan.fda.gov/~dms/fdacinf.html. Accessed November 21, 2002.
96. European Society for Paediatric Gastroenterology, Hepatology and Nutrition (ESPGHAN). Preparation and Handling of Powdered Infant Formula: A Commentary by the ESPGHAN Committee on Nutrition. JPGN 2004;39:320–22.
97. Food and Drug Administration, Center for Food Safety and Applied Nutrition. Office of Nutritional Products, Labeling and Dietary Supplements. Health professionals letter on Enterobacter sakazakki infections associated with use of powdered (dry) infant formulas in neonatal intensive care units. April 11, 2002; revised October 10, 2002. http://www.cfsan.fda.gov/~dms/inf-ltr3.html.Accessed September 2, 2007.
98. Robbins ST, Beker LT, editors. Infant Feedings: Guidelines for preparation of formula and breast milk in health care facilities. American Dietetic Association. 2004.
99. Food and Drug Administration. Overview of infant formulas. Available at: http://www.cfsan.fda/gov/~dms/ds-inf.html. Accessed November 21, 2002.
100. Buccheri C, Casuccio A, Giammanco S, et al. Food safety in hospital: Knowledge, attitudes and practices of nursing staff at two hospitals. In Sicily, Italy. BMC Health Serv Res 2007; 7:45.
101. Foster WG. The reproductive toxicology of Great Lakes contaminants. Environ Health Perspect 1995;103:63–7.
102. Claudio L. The Hudson: A river runs through an environmental controversy. Environ Health Perspect 2002;110: A184–7.
103. Levine WC, Griffin PM, Gulf Coast Working Group. *Vibrio* infections on the Gulf Coast: Results of first year of regional surveillance. J Infect Dis 1993;167:479–83.
104. Wainwright RB, Heyward WL, Middaugh JP, et al. Foodborne botulism in Alaska, 1947–1985: Epidemiology and clinical findings. J Infect Dis 1988;157:1158–62.
105. Shea KM. Technical report: Irradiation of food. Pediatrics 2000;106:1505–9.
106. Connor JA. Making sense of the food and drug administration. Semin Pediatri Surg 2006;15:293–301.

Drug Therapy and Role of Nutrition

Kathleen M. Gura, PharmD, BCNSP, FASHP
Lingtak-Neander Chan, PharmD, BCNSP

The nutritional status of patients and the constituents of their diet can significantly impact a drug's pharmacokinetic and pharmacodynamic properties.[1] These can affect the absorption, distribution, metabolism, transport, and excretion of drugs. Body weight and/or surface area are also important determinants of proper dosages, and abnormal body composition may impact proper drug dosing. Various nutritional components can impact gastrointestinal (GI) motility, blood flow rates, gastric secretions, and enzymatic activity, ultimately affecting drug metabolism and disposition. These interactions, however, are highly variable, complex, and often difficult to predict. Susceptibility to drug-induced nutrient deficiency appears to be greater during periods of increased requirements (ie, during growth, pregnancy, and lactation). When developing a therapeutic plan for the pediatric patient, it is important that practitioners consider the interactions that occur between nutritional status, age, disease state, and drug action. This chapter discusses the developmental changes that occur in the pharmacokinetics and pharmacodynamics of drugs and presents a discussion on the impact of nutrition on these factors. By definition, pharmacokinetics is the action of drugs in the body over a period of time, including the processes of absorption, distribution in tissues, metabolism, and elimination. This contrasts with pharmacodynamics, which is the study of the biochemical and physiologic effects of drugs and the mechanisms of their actions, including the correlation of actions and effects of drugs with their chemical structure, as well as the effects on the actions of another drug or nutrient. Figure 1 provides an example of the age-dependent variation in pharmacokinetic and pharmacodynamic properties. It should be remembered, however, that in the pediatric patient, in addition to true pharmacokinetic and pharmacodynamic differences, some alterations in drug response may be due to perception as medications are often not adequately studied in children of different ages and different disease states. Thus, there may be difficulties in assessing small but significant differences in medication response because limitations associated with conventional outcome measures.

DEVELOPMENTAL CHANGES IN BODY COMPOSITION

Unlike the adult, the pediatric patient is undergoing tremendous growth and development. Children should not be thought of as "little adults" because there are a number of developmental aspects that must be considered when approaching pediatric therapeutics. In fact, during the first decade of life, growth is erratic and does not follow a linear path, thus making simplified dosing approaches inappropriate.[3] Drug–receptor interactions, ontogenetic changes in receptor number, receptor affinity, receptor–effector coupling, and receptor modulation and regulation change as the child grows.[4] Moreover, during infancy and childhood, the proportions of body weight contributed by fat, protein, intracellular water, and extracellular water change dramatically. In the full-term neonate, total body water comprises approximately 70 to 80% of body weight.[5] By age 5 months, this decreases to 60%. From infancy to young adulthood, extracellular water decreases, although the percentage of total body water does not change significantly. In addition, neonates have reduced muscle mass, lower concentrations of albumin, and less intracellular fluid than adults.[6] The change in body water content may significantly affect the volume of distribution of drugs, especially those that are highly hydrophilic. Changes in serum protein (eg, albumin) may alter the free concentration of certain drugs and thus change the patient's pharmacodynamic response. During the second year of life, fat mass is reduced with a corresponding increase in protein mass. For additional information, refer to chapter which reviews the differences in body composition in premature infants, neonates, and adults.

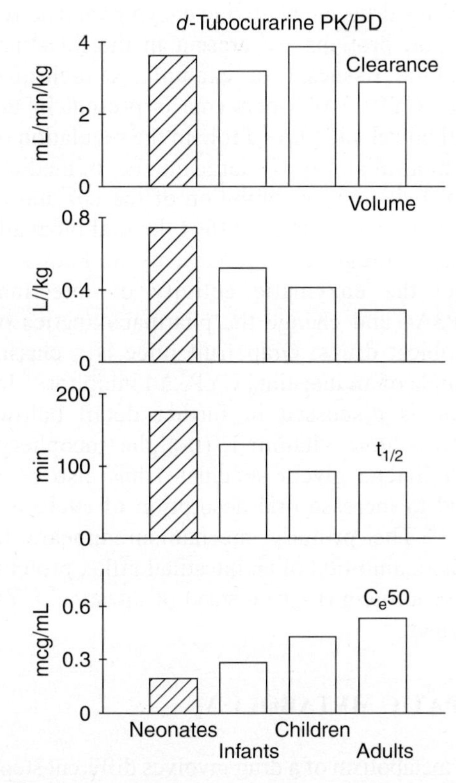

Figure 1 Age-dependent variability in the pharmacodynamic and pharmacokinetic properties of *d*-tubocurarine. In this example, neonates require significantly lower plasma concentrations of *d*-tubocurarine to achieve 50% paralysis in comparison to older children and adults, suggesting that neonates have increased receptor sensitivity. The larger volume of distribution in the neonate may also account for the prolonged half-life, although plasma clearance is comparable in all four age groups. (Adapted from reference 2.)

As the child grows, there is a corresponding change in liver and kidney size, with each organ reaching maximum relative size for weight in the 1- to 2-year-old child, when the capacity for drug metabolism and elimination is high.[4] For example, in the term infant, the glomerular filtration rate (GFR) is approximately 2 to 4 mL/min/1.73 m^2, whereas a premature infant may be as low as 0.6 to 0.8 mL/min/1.73 m^2 and adult values are achieved within the first 8 to 12 months of life.[3] In the infant and young child, body surface area is greatest relative to body mass in comparison with the older child or young adult. As a percentage of adult norms, intestinal length in infants and children exceeds other anthropometric measurements.[3] Furthermore, the absorptive surface of small intestine is proportionately greater, whereas GI transit time is shorter.

During adolescence, there is an approximately 25% increase in height, whereas weight nearly doubles.[4] In prepubertal males and females, lean body mass, skeletal mass, and body fat per unit body weight are similar, but, by maturity, women have twice as much fat relative to total body weight in comparison with adult men.

FACTORS THAT IMPACT DRUG KINETICS

The aforementioned differences in body composition in the pediatric population are an important consideration when determining the pharmacokinetics of a given medication (Table 1). Nutrients and drugs delivered via the GI tract need to go through an absorption phase prior to reaching the systemic circulation and the sites of action.

Table 1 Factors Associated with Differences in Pharmacokinetic/Pharmacodynamic Parameters in Neonates versus Adults
Altered receptor sensitivity
Enhanced intramuscular absorption
Greater blood–brain barrier permeability
Hepatic enzyme immaturity /limited enzyme capacity
Higher gastric pH
Immature renal function
Increased percutaneous absorption
Larger liver/body weight ratio
Limited protein binding capacity
Reduced fat mass
Slower GI absorption/increased gastric emptying time

Absorption from the GI lumen into the hepatic portal vein and subsequently to the systemic circulation is a series of complex processes including the dissolution of the solid dosage form, passing of the chyme along the GI tract (ie, gastric emptying and intestinal transit), passive diffusion, active transport, and presystemic metabolism of the compounds. Each of these processes alone may affect the pharmacokinetics of the drug.

GASTRIC EMPTYING AND INTESTINAL TRANSIT

The oral route continues to be the most widely used route of administration in the pediatric patient. As a result, intraluminal pH in different areas of the GI tract can impact medication stability and extent of drug absorption. Neonates typically have a higher gastric pH (greater than 4) and thus acid labile drugs such as penicillin G are more bioavailable and lower doses can be used, whereas weakly acidic drugs such as phenobarbital require much larger oral doses to reach therapeutic levels.[3] With the exception of a few acidic drugs (eg, aspirin), maximal absorption of most drugs and nutrients takes place in the small bowel. Therefore, gastric emptying and intestinal transit time have a significant impact on the rate and magnitude of the oral absorption of the drugs and certain nutrients.

Gastric emptying time changes in early postnatal life and is likely one of the many explanations for erratic drug absorption rate and oral bioavailability in infants and young children.[7] During infancy, the rate of drug absorption is slower than in older children. As the intestinal tract matures, antral contractions improve and with it a marked increase in gastric emptying. Similarly, intestinal motor activity increases in amplitude and frequency as well as duration of contractions.[3] In addition, gastric acid secretion is low in infants and does not reach the normal adult gastric pH until 3 to 7 years of age.[7]

The lack of developed physiologic regulation of GI motility and gastric acidity during infancy and early childhood suggests that the oral route may not be a reliable route for optimal drug delivery. For instance, delayed absorption and/or decreased bioavailability have been observed for acetaminophen, phenytoin, and phenobarbital in young children.[8]

As the child continues to grow, GI motility increases by both neuronal and hormonal input.[9] Vagal stimulation increases upper gastric contraction and decreases pyloric sphincter and duodenal contractions. As a result, gastric emptying is promoted and the time it takes for the drug or nutrient to reach the small intestine is shortened. For drugs that are absorbed in the small intestine, this action can result in shortening the time of reaching peak plasma concentration and may promote faster onset of drug action. In addition, because of the decrease in intestinal motility, more complete absorption of the drug may be achieved. Anticholinergic drugs (eg, sedative antihistamines, phenothiazines, tricyclic antidepressants) can reverse these trends by counteracting the effect of the vagus nerve.

PRESYSTEMIC CLEARANCE

Presystemic clearance, also known as first-pass effect, refers to the removal of orally ingested compounds prior to reaching the systemic circulation. Presystemic effect occurs primarily in the intestine and the liver, whereas the stomach has only a minor role.[10] Type III alcohol dehydrogenase, for example, is present in the gastric mucosa and is responsible for the activation of some biogenic amines and steroids.

Many drug-metabolizing enzymes and active transport proteins are present in the intestinal epithelial tissues. For example, cytochrome P450 (CYP) 3A4 isoenzyme is present in the small bowel and plays a role in the regulation of oral bioavailability of a large number of medications. Induction or inhibition of the enzyme in the gut by nutrients can affect the oral bioavailability of drugs. Certain nutrients are known to affect the enzymatic activity of intestinal CYP3A4 and change the pharmacokinetics of the object drugs. Grapefruit juice is a classic example of an intestinal CYP3A4 inhibitor.[10] Its action is discussed in further detail below. Water-soluble vitamin E (D-alpha–tocopheryl polyethylene glycol succinate) has also been found to increase oral absorption of cyclosporine.[11] The primary mechanism appears to involve inhibition of an intestinal efflux protein, P-glycoprotein (P-gp) instead of intestinal CYP enzymes.[12]

HEPATIC METABOLISM

The metabolism of a drug involves different steps once it has been absorbed from the GI tract. As drugs are metabolized, they first undergo biotransformation (ie, phase I metabolism), which results in the formation of a more polar compound by oxidation, reduction, hydroxylation, etc. This results in either an activation of the drug or a deactivation. The second phase (ie, phase II reaction) is a synthetic process, involving conjugation of the polar compound with endogenous molecules such as glucuronic acid, sulfate, glutathione, glycine, and acetate, resulting in a more hydrophilic compound that is more suitable for excretion into bile or urine.[13] It is important to point out that some drugs do not have to go through phase I metabolism prior to undergoing phase II metabolism. Lorazepam, for example, undergoes phase II metabolism (glucuronidation) by UDP-glucuronosyltransferase (UGT) 2B7 without any phase I reaction involved. The resultant conjugated metabolite is then excreted renally. An enzyme system responsible for the metabolism of most nutrients and drugs is the CYP enzyme superfamily, principally located in the endoplasmic reticulum of the hepatocytes and enterocytes, which is somewhat unique in its ability to use a wide range of substrates.

The maturation of phase I and phase II enzymes varies among individuals. Limited studies suggest that fetal and neonatal CYP, the most important phase I enzyme in metabolizing drugs and biogenic amines and steroids, has about 50 to 70% of the adults' activity and continues to mature throughout childhood. Altough some children may have fully matured CYP enzyme activities as early as 6 months of age, it may take up to 12 months for others.[7] For example, the serum half-life of theophylline, a bronchodilator primarily metabolized by CYP1A2 and CYP3A4, is significantly longer in neonates and younger infants than in adults. Similarly, N-demethylation of diazepam, a CYP2C19-mediated pathway, is also significantly slower in infants. There is no well-documented dietary factor known to promote the maturation of these enzymes during the prenatal period and infancy.

RECTAL ADMINISTRATION

Rectal route of drug administration is an alternative way of drug delivery when the enteral route is not preferable. Unlike the small bowel venous mesentery, the rectal capillary blood supply collects blood directly into the inferior vena cava instead of the hepatic portal vein. Although certain phase II enzymes are present in the colon (eg, UGT1A9), there is no strong evidence to suggest the presence of drug-metabolizing enzyme in the rectum.[14] Hence, presystemic metabolism of the administered drug is prevented. Therefore, compared with oral administration, the relative bioavailability of the drug is usually higher with rectal administration.[15] Drugs that are more commonly delivered rectally in children include anticonvulsants (eg, diazepam), antiemetics (eg, trimethylbenzamide), and sedative agents (eg, chloral hydrate).

DRUG AND NUTRIENT TRANSPORT SYSTEM

Intestinal transport molecules facilitate the absorption of drugs or nutrients.[16] In addition, some transporters efflux molecules already absorbed in the cytoplasm of the enterocyte back into the intestinal lumen, thus decreasing the bioavailability of certain compounds. This is believed to be an intrinsic protective mechanism by the host to minimize xenobiotic exposure. P-gp is a representative of this type of efflux system.[17] P-gp belongs to the family of adenosine triphosphate-binding cassette transporters and is an efflux widely distributed in normal tissues, including the intestinal epithelium, renal tubule, liver, and blood–brain barrier. Although no formal studies have been published, nutrients may interact with drugs by either inhibiting or inducing P-gp.

CYP3A4 and P-gp are the two most important limiting factors in regulating the oral bioavailability of drugs.[18] For instance, cyclosporine is a known substrate for both CYP3A4 and P-gp. After oral administration, absorption of cyclosporine across the epithelium in the small intestine is limited by P-gp efflux and prehepatic CYP3A4 metabolism. The P-gp-mediated efflux of cyclosporine from the intestinal cell back into the lumen enables the CYP3A4 enzymes another opportunity to metabolize the drug when it again enters the enterocyte. These mechanisms explain why the oral bioavailability remains poor despite improvement of its formulation to microemulsion.[19] When cyclosporine is coadministered with a CYP3A4 and P-gp inhibitor, such as ketoconazole, erythromycin, or diltiazem, significantly higher maximum blood cyclosporine concentration is observed, indicating an increase in absolute oral bioavailability. Oral bioavailability can be increased by over 40% with concomitant administration of water-soluble vitamin E.[11] The mechanism is mediated through intestinal P-gp inhibition by the formulation. It appears that polyethylene glycol, the surfactant incorporated in the liquid formation, instead of vitamin E is the inhibitor of P-gp.[12,20]

BINDING INTERACTIONS BETWEEN FEEDINGS AND DRUGS REVISITED

Feeding and food intake are common causes of drug–nutrient interactions. Enteral feeding is the preferred method of providing nutrition support and also allows easy access for administering drugs to patients who are unable to swallow. However, enteral feeding formulas have been implicated in a number of drug–nutrient interactions.[21] Moreover, in children with chronic medical conditions receiving tube feedings, nutrient deficiencies are also a concern because multiple medications and complicated feeding regimens can result in a decrease intake due to feedings being held or due to drug interactions.[22] For example, the oral absorption of warfarin, tetracycline, fluoroquinolone antibiotics, and phenytoin is decreased with concomitant enteral feeding.[23,24] Possible explanations include a decrease in the anticoagulant effect of warfarin caused by increased vitamin K absorption from the enteral formulas or binding of warfarin by a protein component of the enteral formula.[23] It has also been reported that the acidic nature of most enteral formulas alters the solubility of phenytoin. Phenytoin, a weak acid, is not readily absorbed in acidic conditions and absorption is optimal when it is given in the ionized state. Furthermore, when phenytoin is given with nasogastric feeds, it may become bound to the tubing when it is nonionized in a low pH environment.[25] Drug–nutrient interaction through chelation of divalent and trivalent cations has also been proposed (eg, enteral feeding formulas or dairy products interact with fluoroquinolones).[19] A case of scurvy was reported in a child who received long-term enteral tube feedings using a commercial product. Scurvy occurred owing to the degradation of the ascorbic acid in the formula due to prolonged storage after mixing and from the addition of an iron supplement that further catalyzed the reaction.[26]

Unlike medications given via the oral route, whenever a medication is delivered via feeding tube, tube placement and device characteristics must also be considered. Medications may adhere to the sides of the feeding tube, and thus not be delivered to the patient, or may obstruct the tube in the case of an oral solid not properly pulverized and diluted prior to administration. In some instances, medications are best absorbed in the "fasted" state, requiring that feedings be held so as to optimize absorption. Intragastric administration of a medication may delay gastric emptying rates. Medication administration to patients with jejunostomy, nasojejunal, or nasoduodenal-feeding tubes present an additional challenge as these devices bypass the stomach where medications are dissolved and diluted with gastric contents. Due to the narrow bore of the devices and direct administration of medication into the small intestine, liquid medications must be used. Several factors must be considered, however, including the osmolality of the drug, its viscosity, and particle size. Medications that are hypertonic and not diluted prior to administration into the small bowel can result in dumping. The osmolality of stomach secretions is approximately 300 mOsm/kg and many liquid medications exceed this value significantly, resulting in an osmotic induced diarrhea if given in its undiluted stated. Whenever a hypertonic medication is given undiluted, gastric emptying rates are altered and there is a flux of water and electrolytes into the small bowel and the absorptive capacity of the small bowel is overwhelmed. Proper dilution of the medication can prevent this flux and improved medication as well as nutrient absorption. Moreover, if the feeding tube does terminate in the jejunum, pH is an important consideration. Enteric-coated products such as lansoprazole and omeprazole need to be dissolved in an alkaline vehicle prior to administration into the jejunum.

EFFECTS OF MALNUTRITION ON DRUG KINETICS

It has become increasingly recognized that nutritional status is capable of modifying the pharmacologic effect of a medication. Both malnutrition and obesity can substantially alter drug pharmacokinetics and pharmacologic responses by causing functional and structural alterations in organs that directly affect drug disposition.[27] These changes can affect the absorption, distribution, metabolism, and elimination of a medication that can ultimately affect the therapeutic or toxic response of the drug. Moreover, interindividual and intraindividual variations in the pharmacokinetic responses to a medication can further complicate interpreting the actual impact of altered nutritional status on drug disposition. The variation can be 3- to over 20-fold, depending on genetic (eg, genetic polymorphism) and environmental factors, patient variables, and underlying disease.[27] Pediatric patients, of course, have a higher incidence of undernutrition.

The pathologic changes seen in malnutrition can impact the pharmacokinetics of drugs in all phases of disposition within the body, suggesting that the degree of malnutrition can determine the body's response to a particular drug. Physiologic changes of protein-energy malnutrition (PEM) may result in alterations in the absorptive capacity of the GI tract, body fluid status, cardiac output, GFR, and plasma protein concentrations, as well as hormonal and metabolic changes. Therapeutic drug levels may be altered as a result of malnutrition-associated tissue receptor alterations.[28] It is conceivable that the risk of toxicities owing to a drug or its metabolites is greater in malnourished patients, with a subsequent risk of morbidity or mortality. This suggests that close drug therapy monitoring and modification of dosage in malnourished patients are imperative. Drugs with narrow therapeutic indices or narrow dose–response curves (ie, phenytoin, theophylline) are particularly susceptible as even small changes in absorption can become significant.

Relatively little is known about the handling of drugs in malnourished children despite the fact that the combination of malnutrition and accompanying disease (typically infection) in need of treatment is a common pediatric problem in many parts of the word. It is possible that the high morbidity of mortality so characteristic of malnutrition may be enhanced by adverse drug reactions.[29]

ABSORPTION

Little research has been done on the effect of malnutrition on drug absorption. O'Doherty and colleagues observed that phenytoin absorption was slow and erratic in PEM, although the peak concentration and time to reach peak concentration did not differ significantly from controls.[30] Mehta and colleagues reported similar findings with acetaminophen disposition in children suffering from PEM.[31] Like O'Doherty and colleagues, they observed that the absorption rate constant was not altered in malnutrition. This contrasts with work by Raghuram and colleagues indicating that tetracycline absorption was significantly reduced in subjects with malnutrition and pellagra but not in patients with vitamin B complex deficiency or in patients with severe anemia.[32]

DISTRIBUTION

Only free, unbound drug molecules are pharmacologically active. Because the amount of serum protein changes over the first few years of life, the pharmacokinetics and pharmacodynamics of a drug may change. The important serum proteins that bind to drug molecules and biogenic amines and lipids include albumin, alpha 1-acid glycoprotein, sex-hormone-binding proteins, and lipoproteins. These changes in circulating plasma proteins can impact the distribution of highly bound drugs. In neonates and young infants, a reduction in total plasma proteins can result in the availability of active drug due to an increase in the free fraction of drug.[3] The serum concentration of alpha 1-acid glycoprotein is lower in children. On the other hand, the concentrations of certain fetal serum proteins are higher in infants and may lead to relatively unique pharmacokinetic changes in this population. For example, in neonates, the presence of fetal albumin is associated with reduced binding capacity to weak acids and, this, along with a corresponding increase in bilirubin and free fatty acids, resulting in a high free fraction of highly protein bound drugs such as phenytoin.[3]

Drugs can be distributed into various body compartments such as the intracellular fluids, extravascular space, lean body tissue, and adipose tissue. Alterations in body composition, particularly the presence of edema, can influence the plasma clearance of drug by changing the medication's volume of distribution.[33] Many medications, once in the systemic circulation, become bound to plasma protein, such as albumin, globulins, and lipoproteins. These binding proteins play an important role in the intravascular transport of the drugs to the target organs. In the bloodstream, drugs that are not bound to plasma proteins are free and are able to exert their pharmacologic response. Malnutrition can alter the rate of tissue protein synthesis as well as the concentration of plasma proteins. The extent of drug-protein binding depends on the concentration of plasma bind proteins as well as the physicochemical properties of the medication. In malnutrition, albumin and lipoprotein synthesis are reduced, whereas globulin and α1-acid glycoprotein synthesis are increased.[19] Drugs extensively bound to α1-acid glycoprotein, such as propranolol, have a decreased percentage of drug unbound in malnutrition, resulting in a lesser amount of active drug available to exert a therapeutic response. Other drugs, such as metronidazole, have no significant change in volume of distribution between malnourished and well-fed children.[34]

METABOLISM

In chronic starvation, the body is able to adapt and alter various processes to protect or maintain enzyme activities.[35] In fact, in chronic starvation, enzyme activity may even increase. Endocrine tissue is typically affected in semistarvation as many hormones serve as substrates for drug-metabolizing enzymes.[36] For example, elevations in free cortisol are often seen in malnutrition that may enhance the metabolism of contraceptive steroids in malnourished women, thus increasing the risk of contraceptive failure in that population.[37]

CLEARANCE

Hepatic clearance of drugs may be affected by several major physiologic changes that occur during malnutrition. Protein deprivation or malnutrition may result in a reduction in cardiac function with a subsequent decreased perfusion of the liver and kidneys.[38] Typically, hepatic drug clearance is determined by three independent factors: hepatic blood flow, the amount of free fraction of the drug in blood, and hepatic clearance of the unbound drug. Diminished hepatic blood flow can reduce the clearance of drugs with high extraction ratios (ie, those in which hepatic clearance of the unbound drug depends on hepatic blood flow but not on changes in protein binding). Presystemic metabolism can become altered. Increases in the unbound fraction of a drug owing to hypoalbuminemia provide more available drug for metabolism, resulting in lower serum concentrations.[38]

The kidney is extensively involved in drug elimination. Renal elimination includes the processes of glomerular filtration, active tubular secretion, and passive tubular excretion. Drugs or their metabolites that are primarily filtered and excreted renally may be affected by nutritional status. Dietary protein increases renal blood flow, GFR, and renal tubular function.[39] Severe PEM is associated with decreased GFR and renal blood flow.[40] When renal perfusion is reduced, less drug is available to be filtered by the tubules. However, because plasma protein binding is also reduced, more free drug becomes available for renal excretion, thus further reducing plasma drug concentrations. Medications that have decreased renal elimination in severely malnourished patients include penicillins, tetracyclines, cefoxitin, aminoglycosides, and methotrexate.[27]

Refeeding an undernourished patient can often increase the systemic clearance of a medication, necessitating a dosage adjustment to maintain efficacy. For example, with theophylline, the volume of distribution decreases and the rate of elimination gradually increases in malnourished patients given a dextrose-based parenteral nutrition (PN) solution for at least 2 days.[41] The protein component of enteral or PN, however, appears to be the major macronutrient enhancing systemic clearance of affected drugs in patients transitioned from the "unfed" to the "fed" state. Lares-Asseff and associates confirmed these findings in their study investigating the pharmacokinetics of metronidazole in severely malnourished children.[34] Based on the clearance data, they recommended that the daily maintenance doses for pediatric patients with severe malnutrition should be 60% less of the usual pediatric dose to achieve and maintain a therapeutic plasma concentration of metronidazole.

DRUGS IN KWASHIORKOR

Kwashiorkor is associated with edema resulting from increases in total body water, extracellular fluid volume, and plasma volume along with a decrease in intracellular water.[42] Lares-Asseff and colleagues studied the effects of nutritional status of children with autoimmune disease on the disposition of acetylsalicylic acid and its metabolites.[43] They concluded that a decrease in the hydrolysis and oxidative reaction of the metabolic pathway of acetylsalicylic acid and its metabolites occurs in children with PEM with juvenile rheumatoid arthritis. This suggests that the hepatic elimination of salicylates may be altered by disorders of nutritional state.[44]

Based on these and other studies, it is thought that low protein intake results in a negative nitrogen balance that decreases drug metabolism, whereas drug metabolism in patients receiving adequate total calories but with less than optimal protein intake is not significantly impacted.[45]

DRUGS IN MARASMUS

Unlike kwashiorkor, marasmus can be considered as an adaptation to an insufficient energy intake. There is decreased total body water, reduced intracellular water, increased extracellular fluid, and increased plasma volume.[27] Gentamicin, which distributes predominantly to extracellular fluids, has an increased volume of distribution in malnourished patients compared with well-nourished patients.[46] Antipyrine, a drug model commonly used as an index of hepatic drug-metabolizing capacity, distributes primarily in total body water and has been shown to have no variation in the apparent volume of distribution in malnourished children.[47] Likewise, in patients treated with metronidazole, a medication that also has a large volume of distribution, no difference in volume of distribution was observed between malnourished and nutritionally rehabilitated children.[34] A pharmacokinetic study by Treluyer and colleagues focused on the impact of human global PEM on quinine metabolism.[48] In that study, they reported that the metabolism of quinine is increased in children with global malnutrition, suggesting that the dosing interval in these children be reduced to obtain the same therapeutic quinine levels as seen in well-nourished children.

In summary, normal or increased drug metabolism occurs in mild to moderate cases of malnutrition, whereas decreased metabolism is seen in severe cases of malnutrition. Given the unique needs of the malnourished ill child special guidelines have been created for the use of antimicrobial agents.[49]

OBESITY

Obesity (ie, BMI >95th percentile for age and sex) results in altered body composition in which there is both an increased proportion and absolute amount of adipose tissue as well as an increase in lean body mass, blood volume, cardiac output, and organ size.[50] In children, obesity can result in an expansion of blood volume, resulting in increased stroke volume and cardiac output. Increased abdominal fat can also lead to increased intraabdominal pressure and impact gastric emptying.[51] Drug distribution depends on body composition and may be altered in obese patients. Absorption of drugs evaluated to date appears to be unchanged owing to obesity; however, the data are very limited.[52] Severely obese patients who have undergone bariatric surgery for weight loss are more likely to experience altered drug absorption that may affect the clinical responses to therapy. Generally speaking, malabsorption of drugs is more likely to occur with the primary malabsorptive procedures such as jejunoileal bypass and pancreatobiliary diversion. A commonly performed surgical procedure for weight loss is the Roux-en-Y gastric bypass, which is a primary restrictive procedure with mild malabsorptive component. The impact of Roux-en-Y gastric bypass on pharmacokinetics has not been investigated systematically.

The lipophilicity of a drug determines the extent to which obesity influences the volume of distribution and ultimately whether dosing should be based on actual or adjusted body weight. Highly lipophilic drugs, such as lidocaine, thiopental, phenytoin, verapamil, and most benzodiazepines, have an increased volume of distribution in severely obese patients.[50] Modest increases in volume of distribution have also been reported for aminoglycosides, heparin, ibuprofen, methylxanthines, prednisolone, and vancomycin, suggesting that an adjusted body weight rather than actual body weight (ABW) be used to avoid toxicity.[52] However, the most accurate approach to adjust for the excess body mass is unknown and appears to be different depending on the characteristics of individual compounds. Therapeutic drug monitoring is recommended when applicable to optimize therapy.

Although the protein binding of acidic drugs is unchanged, the free fraction of basic drugs may be decreased.[52] Similarly, changes in hepatic drug clearance are variable. Phase 1 reactions and phase I acetylation appear to be unaffected by obesity, but the phase II glucuronidation and sulfonation pathways are enhanced. Obesity may also affect systemic clearance of highly extracted drugs such as aminoglycosides and unmetabolized procainamide.[52] Both glomerular filtration and tubular secretion also appear to be increased.[32] Renal clearance of drug that mediated by both glomerular filtration and active secretion, such as digoxin and cimetidine, are relatively unchanged in obesity.[52]

Aminoglycosides are distributed within the extracellular fluid compartment. Early dosing recommendations suggested that initial dosing be based on ideal body weight (IBW) as it was thought that the drug distributed only into lean body mass. Schwartz and colleagues, however, have since determined that when the volume of distribution is corrected for total body weight, it is significantly smaller when compared with normal-weight subjects.[53] The distribution of aminoglycosides into excess body weight is estimated to be about 40% of that distributed into ideal body tissue. The authors concluded that initial dosing of aminoglycosides in obese patients be determined by adding 40% of the excess weight to the patient's IBW, with subsequent dosage adjustments based on serum drug levels and clinical status.

Example: For a 7-year-old child, 41 kg, 135 cm, gentamicin, 2.5 mg/kg/dose intravenously every 8 hours, is ordered:

1. Determine IBW[14]

$$IBW = \frac{ht^2 \times 1.65}{1000} = IBW \text{ kg, height cm}$$

$$IBW = \frac{135^2 \times 1.65}{1000} = 30 \text{ kg}$$

2. Determine dosing weight (DW): DW = IBW + (ABW−IBW) × 0.4 DW is in kg, ABW is in kg

$$DW = 30 \text{ kg} + (41-30) \times 0.4 \; DW = 34.4 \text{ kg}$$

3. Calculate gentamicin dose using DW: mg/kg/dose × DW = dose in mg 2.5 mg/kg/dose × 34.4 kg = 86 mg intravenously every 8 hours

A similar controversy exists for optimizing theophylline dosing in obese patients and whether actual or IBW should be used to calculate the initial theophylline loading dose. This is attributable to conflicting data suggesting that variations in distribution volume may be the result of differences in the degrees of obesity within study populations.[55] Visram and colleagues suggested that the differences in theophylline volume of distribution based on IBW and ABW increases as the degree of obesity increases.[55] They recommended that theophylline dosing in patients with mild to moderate obesity be based on ABW but that IBW be used when initiating therapy in severely or morbidly obese patients.

Hepatic drug metabolism may also be altered in patients with nonalcoholic steatohepatitis (NASH),[34] including enhanced glucuronidation and sulfonation, causing a faster drug excretion compared with normal-weight subjects.[52] CYP2E1 expression and activities are increased in obese patients with nonalcoholic fatty liver disease, including NASH.[56] Compounds that are metabolized by CYP2E1 include fatty acids, ketones, and ethanol. It appears that the presence of an increase amount of fatty acids, such as in the case of NASH, leads to an induction of this enzyme. The metabolic pathways of fatty acids and other xenobiotics may lead to the release of free radicals, which can cause lipid peroxidation and liver injury, including mitochondrial damage. These changes are partially responsible for the hepatic inflammation and fibrosis sometimes observed in patients with NASH.[57] Patients with fatty liver may also be more susceptible to the toxic effects of drugs owing to impaired metabolism.[58]

EFFECT OF DIETARY MANIPULATION ON DRUG KINETICS

Several dietary factors can alter the rate of drug metabolism. Model drugs, such as antipyrine, theophylline, and acetaminophen, have often been used in these studies. Both food and fluids can alter the rate and extent of drug absorption. These alternations in response may occur as a result of influences on gastric pH, gastric emptying time, intestinal motility, and mesenteric and hepatic portal blood flow or biliary flow, or the activities of the enzymes and transport proteins in the gut.[59] Direct physicochemical interactions with dietary components can also alter the absorption of susceptible agents.[60] Interactions such as the binding of the medication with metal ions, solubilization of the drug in dietary fat, or adsorption of the drug to insoluble dietary components may occur.[61]

Dietary changes can alter the expression and activity of hepatic drug-metabolizing enzymes.[62] This can lead to alteration in the systemic elimination kinetics of medications metabolized by these enzymes; however, the impact of this change is typically minimal.[62] The rate of drug metabolism can be accelerated by drugs themselves or by a variety of dietary factors, such as protein supplementation or inclusion of cruciferous vegetables or charcoal-broiled meats in the diet.[63] It has also been reported that charcoal-broiled beef induces the metabolism of antipyrine and theophylline, reducing the half-lives of these drugs by 20%.[64] These effects were related to hepatic enzymatic induction caused by charcoal-broiled beef that contains large quantities of polycyclic aromatic hydrocarbons (PAHs).[65] PAHs are potent inducers of CYP1A2, the primary metabolizing enzyme for theophylline and antipyrine. Conversely, low-protein, high-carbohydrate diets, and various vitamin and mineral deficiencies can reduce levels of drug-metabolizing enzymes and consequently the rate of drug metabolism so that the serum drug concentrations decline much more slowly, resulting in increased drug potency.[63]

In general, when orally administered medications are taken with meals, the rate rather than the extent of absorption is more significantly affected. Food affects drug absorption by enhancing gastric blood flow in conjunction with delayed gastric emptying. Food can increase, decrease, or have no effect on the absolute systemic availability of a medication.[66] Concomitant food ingestion reduces the absorption of drugs such as ampicillin, penicillin, and isoniazid.[27] Conversely, food may actually enhance the absorption of other

Table 2 Medications Whose Absorption Is Affected by Food

Drug Absorption Reduced/Delayed by Food	Drug Absorption Enhanced by Food
Ampicillin	Atovaquone
Aspirin	Carbamazepine
Atenolol	Chlorothiazide
Azithromycin	Cefuroxime
Captopril	Clofazimine
Cefaclor	Diazepam
Cefixime	Erythromycin estolate
Cephalexin	Erythromycin ethyl succinate
Ciprofloxacin	Ganciclovir
Didanosine	Griseofulvin
Doxycycline	Hydralazine
Dirithromycin	Hydrochlorothiazide
Erythromycin stearate	Itraconazole
Famciclovir	Ketoconazole
Indinavir	Lithium
Isoniazid	Lovastatin
Loratidine	Methylphenidate
Naficillin	Metoprolol
Penicillin G or V	Nelfinavir
Phenobarbital	Nitrofurantoin
Phenytoin	Propanolol
Rifampin	Propoxyphene
Sucralfate	Ritonavir
Tetracycline	Saquinavir
Thioridazine	Spironolactone
Zafirlukast	

Adapted from reference 67.

medications, including diazepam, lithium, carbamazepine, and griseofulvin. Table 2 lists medications whose absorption is altered by food. In most cases, changing the rate of absorption of a drug alone without affecting the total amount absorbed should not affect its efficacy.

The composition of the meal will alter splanchnic blood flow. Blood flow can be doubled by a high-protein liquid meal and slightly reduced by a liquid glucose meal.[68] The significance of this effect on splanchnic flow is important for those medications with high hepatic extraction.[61] Continued meal intake, especially food with high fat content, will also slow the rate of gastric emptying, which may subsequently cause a delay in drug absorption from the GI tract. Changes in gastric emptying are related not only to the physicochemical properties of the drug but also to the type of meal itself. Hot meals, highly viscous solutions, or those rich in fat have the most significant affect in slowing down gut motility.[61] Melander and colleagues reviewed the impact of food on the presystemic clearance of drugs.[69] They observed that meals commonly enhanced presystemic clearance of lipophilic basic drugs (eg, propranolol, amitriptyline) but rarely altered the clearance of drugs that were lipophilic acids (eg, salicylic acid, penicillin). Alternatively, food may reduce presystemic clearance of some lipophilic basic drugs via transient, complex effects on splanchnic-hepatic blood flow. Furthermore, repeated intake of specific nutrients (eg, protein) and food contaminants (eg, benzopyrene) can enhance presystemic drug clearance by enzyme induction.

In some instances, dietary manipulation can act as a therapeutic strategy. Nutt and colleagues reported that large neutral amino acids and the medication levodopa compete for transport from the plasma to the brain and may be partly responsible for the "on-off" phenomenon often seen in patients treated with levodopa for Parkinson's disease.[70] By reducing protein intake, patients who failed to respond to a dosage adjustment in their levodopa may see clinical improvement.

IMPACT OF SPECIFIC NUTRIENTS ON DRUG KINETICS

Until recently, most practitioners dismissed the possibility that dietary substances could significantly alter medication response by affecting intestinal transporter and metabolizing enzymes. This is based on the commonly believed misconception that the absorption of most drugs is a passive process and that the role of the intestine in drug elimination is minimal.[62] Since the report of the interaction between grapefruit juice and several medications was described, this premise has changed, and the role of the diet on drug performance is being reevaluated.[71]

CARBOHYDRATES

The impact of carbohydrates on drug metabolism is conflicting. It is known that high-carbohydrate diets may induce the expression of several glycolytic and lipogenic hepatic enzymes.[72] but some suggest that carbohydrates have little impact on drug metabolism.[73] Kappas and colleagues, however, noted that antipyrine and theophylline metabolism decreased in carbohydrate-supplemented diets but increased in the protein-enriched diet, suggesting that carbohydrates and protein have opposite effects on oxidative drug metabolism.[63] Although many medications are often given to children in a sugar syrup, little research has been done on its effect on disposition and action. Animal studies by Sonawane and colleagues suggested that dietary carbohydrates and fat may significantly influence the hepatic drug-metabolizing enzymes.[74] It has been hypothesized that these changes may occur owing to alteration in the phospholipid composition of endoplasmic reticulum or by limiting the supply of cofactor(s) necessary for optimal functioning of CYP and UGT.

PROTEIN

Several investigators have reported that medications that undergo extensive first-pass effect, such as propranolol, metoprolol, and lidocaine, can have enhanced bioavailability after a high-protein meal owing to enhanced hepatic blood flow. High-extraction drugs can then rapidly pass through the liver, allowing higher drug concen-trations in the systemic circulation.[62,69] A decrease in dietary protein depresses creatinine clearance and renal plasma flow.[75] Specific dietary proteins can also impact a response to a medication. One of the classic examples is that of the monoamine oxidase inhibitor (MAO-I) drug class and the amino acid tyramine that is contained in aged cheeses, pickled/smoked meats, fermented foods, and red wines. Tyramine is an indirect sympathomimetic amine that releases norepinephrine from the adrenergic neurons, causing a significant pressor response. Typically, tyramine is metabolized by the enzyme monoamine oxidase before any significant increases in blood pressure are seen. If the enzyme is blocked, however, severe and potentially fatal rises in blood pressure can occur when tyramine-rich foods are ingested. Although MAO-Is are not used routinely as antidepressants, other medications, such as the oxazolidinone antibiotic, linezolid, also have MAO-I properties and patients should avoid ingesting large amounts of tyramine while being treated with this antibiotic.[76]

Dietary protein also affects the renal tubular transport of certain compounds, although the mechanism by which this occurs is still not understood. The binding of dietary proteins to a drug may underscore changes in bioavailability after a protein meal. For example increases in both the maximum concentration (Cmax) and area under the curve (AUC) are seen in patients receiving gabapentin. This enhanced absorption was attributed to trans-simulation, a carrier-mediated process in which increased intestinal luminal amino acid concentrations result in an upregulation and/or increased activity of the L-amino acid transporter.[77]

DIETARY FAT

Lipids are an essential part of cell membrane structure and are involved in many of the normal enzymatic activities located within the cell membrane.[73] Diets that are deficient in fat or essential fatty acids decrease the activity of the enzyme systems responsible for the metabolism of nutrients.[78] Plasma free fatty acid levels become elevated after consumption of a high-fat meal, increasing the potential to become bound to plasma albumin, and subsequently displace albumin bound drugs, increasing the risk of drug toxicity.[73] Dietary fats along with food-stimulated secretions (eg, bile salts) may facilitate the solubilization and dispersion of lipophilic compounds. This may contribute to a reduction in the extent of first past metabolism due to enhanced splanchnic blood flow.[79] Ingestion of diets high in fat has been associated with the induction of CYP2E1. The extent to which this enzyme is upregulated is dependent upon the type of fat. Polyunsaturated fats such as corn and menhaden oils appear to have the greatest influence in comparison to lard or olive oils. This can result in enhanced peroxidation of the polyunsaturated fatty acid substrates and contribute to free radical production.[80] The rate of gastric emptying is also influenced by the fat content of a meal. Fat retards gastric emptying to a greater degree than does protein or carbohydrate.[81]

The effect of dietary fat on drug absorption, however, depends upon the route of the drug absorption, either portal or lymphatic. For medications absorbed via the lymphatic route, dietary fat enhances the absorption of the dissolved drug, whereas poorly bioavailable lipophilic drugs absorbed by the portal route have their absorption enhanced by improved drug dissolution. Conversely, lipophilic medications that have good bioavailability will less likely to be impacted by a high-fat meal. Moreover, hydrophilic medications are not impacted significantly when coadministered with fatty meals.[82]

The impact of food on the absorption of cyclosporine is controversial. There are conflicting reports stating that food impairs, enhances, or does not affect cyclosporine compared with the fasting state.[83] Similarly, high-fat meals may affect sirolimus bioavailability. When taken with a high-fat meal, the rate of sirolimus absorption is slower and results in a greater AUC in comparison to when taken in the fasted state. This contrasts with tacrolimus in which a 71% mean decrease in Cmax and a 39% mean decrease in AUC was seen immediately following its administration after a high-fat meal relative to when the same dose was given in the fasted state.[84]

The antiviral agent zidovudine is also impacted by dietary fat. When administered orally, its absorption is reduced when the drug is taken with a high-fat meal in comparison with when taken in the fasted state.[85] It is recommended that zidovudine be taken on an empty stomach to achieve peak serum concentrations.

MINERALS

In most instances, mineral deficiencies (ie, zinc, iodine, magnesium, and potassium) have been associated with a decrease in drug oxidation and drug clearance.[86] Low dietary intake of iron, however, has been associated with an increase in some mixed function oxidase system (MFOS) functions and a decrease in other degradative activities, the reasons for which are not fully apparent.

VEGETABLES

Diets rich in vegetables and fruit may also impact the response to medications. Both serve as sources of trace minerals that are contained in metalloenzymes, including several antioxidants. Many plants contain flavonoids, isothiocyanates, and allyl sulfides that are potent modulators of the cytochrome monoxygenase system.[87]

Phyotochemicals are linked with the modulation of a variety of metabolic pathways. The most frequently sources include cruciferous vegetables, citrus juices, and spices. Dietary supplements and herbs are also associated with this category. There are five major families of phytochemicals: carotinoids (eg, beta carotene, lycopene), alkaloids, phenolics (include flavonoids, coumarins, tannins), nitrogen compounds, and sulfur compounds (eg, isothiocyanates, allylic sulfur).[88] Recent research has focused on how vegetables and fruits can influence a variety of enzymatic pathways. Typically induction of these enzyme systems is rapid and plateaus within 5 days of continued daily ingestions of the food with the enzyme inducing capacity.[88]

Cruciferous vegetables, including brussels sprouts, cabbage, turnips, broccoli, cauliflower, and spinach, contain indols that induce aryl-hydrocarbon hydroxylase enzyme activity as well as the conjugation of phenacetin and acetaminophen.[89,90] In one study, patients fed a diet of brussels sprouts and cabbage had a 50% lower serum phenacetin level in comparison with the same subjects fed a control diet that contained none of the enzyme-inducing vegetables.[90] A later study investigated the effects of cruciferous vegetables on acetaminophen conjugation.[89] The researchers found that the test diet of cruciferous vegetables enhanced acetaminophen glucuronide conjugation as evidenced by a 16% decrease in the AUC, a 17% increase in metabolic clearance, and an increased plasma acetaminophen glucuronide-to-acetaminophen ratio.

Cruciferous vegetables are not the only plants that can impact drug response. Potatoes, tomatoes, and eggplant contain natural insecticide compounds called solanaceous glycoalkaloids that even in small amounts may greatly slow the metabolism of muscle relaxants and anesthetic agents such as suxamethonium, mivacurium, and cocaine. Cooking does not reduce them and they may remain in the body for several days after ingestion. Solanaceous glycoalkaloids inhibit butyryl cholinesterase, which breaks down many anesthetic agents, and cetylcholinesterase, which breaks down acetylcholine. When these enzymes are inhibited, patients receiving medications metabolized by them may take longer to recover from anesthesia.[91]

GRAPEFRUIT JUICE AND DRUG INTERACTIONS

Bailey and his colleagues discovered that grapefruit juice, which was used as a taste-masking agent for alcohol, caused a two- to threefold increase in oral absorption of the calcium channel blocker felodipine.[92] This finding has subsequently led to the intensive investigation of grapefruit juice and drug interactions. This interaction is the classic example of drug–nutrient interaction exclusively caused by inhibition of intestinal CYP3A4. Oral absorption pharmacokinetic studies of CYP3A4 substrates, such as cyclosporine or felodipine, consistently showed that grapefruit juice increased the oral bioavailability of these agents. Interestingly, the plasma half-lives of most of the drugs studied were not affected, suggesting that the systemic clearance or hepatic metabolism of these drugs was unchanged by grapefruit juice. It was later determined that this interaction occurs in the enterocytes but not in the hepatocytes. Furthermore, Lown and his colleagues showed that repeated consumption of grapefruit juice inhibits not only the intestinal CYP3A4 activity but also the expression of this gene in the enterocytes.[10] As grapefruit juice inhibits intestinal CYP3A4 expression and thus decreases the presystemic metabolism of certain drugs, the bioavailability of the affected agents will remain increased until the expression of the CYP3A4 gene returns to baseline. This suggests that mere separation of the administration time between grapefruit juice and the potential interacting drugs cannot prevent this interaction. Rather than reduce the dose of the affected drugs to avoid toxicity, patients should be advised to avoid grapefruit juice. In some centers, grapefruit juice has been removed from the institutional formulary to minimize the risk of this interaction.

HIGH-FIBER DIETS

Dietary fiber and other bulk-forming compounds may interfere with the GI absorption of a medication.[93] The bioavailability of digoxin is reduced significantly when given with a fiber-rich meal, with almost half of the dose sequestered in or bound to the fiber.[94] Similar effects have been reported with lithium salts and lovastatin.[95] Stewart reported that several patients with recurrent major depression who had been successfully treated with tricyclic antidepressants became refractory to treatment after beginning a high-fiber diet.[96] Nutrient absorption can also be negatively impacted in the presence of a high-fiber diet. Zinc absorption in the intestine is reduced by the binding of zinc to a number of materials, including phytate, which is found in high-fiber diets.[97]

COOKING METHODS

Drug metabolism can also be enhanced by the ingestion of charcoal-broiled beef. Patients fed such a diet saw a significant drop in serum phenacetin levels in comparison to the same subjects fed a control diet. It has also been reported that charcoal-broiled beef induced the metabolism of antipyrine and theophylline, reducing the half-lives of these drugs by 20%.[98] It has been postulated that these effects were related to the large quantities PAHs present in charcoal-broiled beef.

VEGETARIANISM

Drug metabolism among vegetarians will vary dramatically depending on the protein intake. Most research has focused on Asian vegetarians in which the half-lives of drugs that underwent significant hepatic metabolism (antipyrine, acetaminophen, phenacetin) were significantly longer than in nonvegetarians.[99] When similar studies were conducted in white vegetarians, they found no significant difference in half-life between the vegetarians and nonvegetarians.[100] Protein quality may contribute to these findings as the authors found that protein intake between the white vegetarians and the nonvegetarians was similar.

Vegetarian diets are also associated with lower circulating concentrations of sex steroids hormones, increased fecal excretion of estrogens and different hormonal profiles in comparison to individuals consuming an omnivorous diet.[101] Vegetable intake may influence total body estrogen load via the modulation of CYP enzymes involved in estrogen metabolism. CYP13C, found in cruciferous vegetables, can increase estrogen hydroxylation.[102]

VERY LOW CALORIE DIETS

In diets involving severe protein-energy restriction, such as extreme slimming diets, the metabolism of drugs may be affected in one of two ways. First, tissue protein is catabolized and used as an energy source, thus reducing the availability of amino acids for protein synthesis, which in turn reduces the amount of enzymes available for drug metabolism. Second, endogenous substrates derived from carbohydrate and protein such as glucuronide, sulfate, and glycine could also compete for the tissue needs for these nutrients and that of the drug metabolism/detoxification.[103] Eating habits, especially among dieters that omits or severely restrict whole categories of foods, have a negative impact on micronutrient status. Diets that eliminate all animal foods provide almost no cyanocobalamin and have been associated with other vitamin deficiencies including vitamin C. Moreover, skipping meals and fad diets to lose weight frequently compromise micronutrient intake. It should be routinely assumed that it is extremely difficult to meet all the requirements at intakes of less than 1,200 calories per day. An analysis of 11 published weight loss diets showed that none provided 100% of the US recommended dietary allowance for representative vitamins.[103]

In a review by Anderson, the author suggests that the metabolic improvements seen after obese patients receive very low calorie diets are not different from those obtained by equally large weight loses promoted by other methods.[104] Patients with very low calorie diet weight loss have improved hyperinsulinism as a result of a reduction in basal insulin production as well as enhanced hepatic insulin extraction. Moreover, it is thought the weight loss through very low calorie diet lowers the hepatic glucuronidation of drugs leading to higher plasma concentrations of the affected drugs.[105] Despite this, however, the fatty liver may still be more susceptible to drug toxicity.[106] For example, several reports in have suggested that caloric restriction may contribute to acetaminophen hepatotoxicity by altering drug metabolism although under controlled conditions, Schenker and colleagues so no impact on food restriction of acetaminophen metabolism.[107]

OTHER DIETARY RESTRICTIONS

In addition to caloric restriction, restriction of other dietary components can also impact drug response. In patients who have sodium restricted diets, there is an increased risk of acute renal failure if these same patients are given concomitant angiotensin-converting enzyme inhibitors or nonsteroidal antiinflammatory agents. There is enhanced nephrotoxicity in patients who are sodium depleted and are given cyclosporine or tacrolimus. Sodium restriction can also increase the renal tubular absorption of lithium, leading to toxicity. Patients receiving aminoglycosides, amphotericin, cisplatin, or radiocontrast media in conjunction with a low-sodium diet have an increased risk for hemodynamic nephrotoxic and ischemic acute renal failure. For reasons still not known, the efficacy of calcium channel blockers is reduced in patients on a sodium-restricted diet.[108]

IMPACT OF BEVERAGE TYPE ON DRUG BIOAVAILABILITY

To most practitioners, the term beverage refers to any drinkable liquid other than plain water. They are typically classified as caffeinated, alcoholic, milk-based, mineral waters, or fruit/vegetables juices.[109] Depending upon the type of fluid taken with a medication, drug absorption may be affected. Mixing drugs with fruit juices or other beverages to mask their taste may impact absorption due to changes in gastric pH. Dairy products decrease the absorption of tetracyclines and reduce their bioavailability due to the formation of insoluble chelates between the drug and the calcium present in the beverage. Similar decreases in bioavailability were noted when fluoride tablets are taken with milk. Tannins present in teas may impair iron absorption. Alcoholic beverages reduce the absorption of folic acid, cyanocobalamin, and magnesium. Soft drinks, such as colas, may decrease drug absorption for a variety of reasons. The phosphoric acid and sugar present in these drinks can slow gastric emptying and the tendency to serve them chilled may also reduce the rate of blood flow within the intestines. Moreover, the carbonation may increase mixing and possibly motility. Interestingly, the acidic pH of cola beverages can be used to optimize clinical responses of both ketoconazole and itraconazole in patients with gastric hypochlorhydria, such those patients with AIDS gastropathy.[109] The effects of grapefruit juice on drug disposition are discussed separately.

PARENTERAL NUTRITION

Lack of oral nutrient intake during PN leads to mucosal atrophy of the bowel along with a reduction in gastric biliary, pancreatic, and intestinal secretions.[110] Bacterial overgrowth can result in a progressive decline in intestinal function owing to impaired motility and depressed enzyme activity. This may alter the rate and extent of absorption of specific nutrients as well as various drugs. Decreases in nutrient absorption include fat, iron, peptides, and vitamins A and B_{12} as well as drugs such as chloramphenicol, chloroquine, tetracycline, and rifampin.[38]

PN has been observed to decrease hepatic drug and xenobiotic metabolism in animals and humans.[111,112] Drug metabolism may be altered due to jejunal and ileal mucosal hypoplasia and hypofunction as parenterally administered nutrients bypass the intestine. Studies using antipyrine as a marker have shown that PN regimens containing amino acids have higher antipyrine clearance than regimens consisting mainly of dextrose.[111] Burgess and colleagues investigated the response of PN regimens on antipyrine clearance.[112] Patients receiving a postoperative 2,000 kcal PN regimen providing all nonprotein calories as dextrose showed a 34% reduction of mean antipyrine clearance after 7 days of total parenteral nutrition compared with unfed controls. This effect was seen also in patients receiving a 1,600 kcal dextrose-based regimen Moreover, patients receiving a 2,000 kcal PN regimen in which 500 kcal were provided as lipid, mean antipyrine clearance was not significantly different from that of the unfed control group. This study suggested that hepatic CYP1A activity might be affected by different total parenteral nutrition regimens.

EFFECTS OF DRUGS ON NUTRIENT STATUS

Drugs can alter the use of many nutrients by a variety of mechanisms, both specific and nonspecific. Malabsorption syndromes may occur from direct toxic effects of the medication to the intestinal mucosa, inhibition of enzymes, binding of bile and fatty acids, alteration of dietary ions, or alteration of GI pH. Indirect, nonspecific effects of a drug may manifest themselves as a decrease in appetite, ultimately leading to a decrease in food intake.

Although the concept of drug–nutrient interactions is not a new one, only recently has it reached the forefront in the medical world. Malnutrition, as well as the composition of the diet, can affect the disposition of a medication's half-life.[113] In addition to traditional dietary components, nonnutrient ingredients, such as food additives, preservatives, antioxidants, sweeteners, flavoring, and coloring agents, can interact with a medication. Natural products, such as plant food groups, contain alkaloids, flavonoids, and other compounds; can behave in the body in the same manner that a drug would; and, consequently, can be involved in a variety of interactions and are potentially toxic if they are consumed or accumulate in the body.[114] Drug–nutrient interactions are typically defined as situations that result from chemical, physical, physiologic, or pathophysiologic relationships between nutrients and drugs.[115] Infants and adolescents, like the elderly, are at particular risk for drug–nutrient interactions. Several factors may influence the possible interactions: first, their nutrient needs are typically higher; second, the systems for detoxification of nutrients may be incomplete; and third, adolescents (especially females) tend to restrict their diets and thus are unable to meet the actual recommended intakes for a variety of micronutrients.[116] Furthermore, the minimum dietary requirement may be insufficient when a patient is under psychological and pathologic stresses, as in the case of pregnancy or athletic training. In pathologic states, the requirement for some micronutrients may be increased.

Drugs may potentially cause vitamin deficiency ranging from subclinical deficiency to clinical intensity of the interaction may in many cases depend on the nutritional status of the patient. Patients with borderline intake of vitamins or those in poor nutritional health appear to be at greater risk of developing symptomatic vitamin deficiency states. Other factors include the type of drug treatment, dose, and duration of therapy, as well as the age of the patient. For example, individuals on a normal diet rarely become vitamin K deficient, although malnourished patients, regardless of cause, often have moderate or significant deficiency, often with prolonged bleeding times.[116,117] Cohen and colleagues reported that hospitalized patients may become vitamin K deficient within 7 to 10 days after admission, with those at greatest risk being those who were previously malnourished and had received antibiotics for seven or more days.[118] Adolescents, due to periods of rapid growth, are particularly sensitive to micronutrient status. Even a typical diet may not meet their high nutrient demands necessary for growth. Intake of folate and vitamin A tend to be less than optimal.[103]

ABSORPTION OF NUTRIENTS

There are also many secondary mechanisms that can interfere with nutrient absorption. Medications may alter gastric or intestinal secretion, pancreatic exocrine function, or hepatic bile secretion. For example, H_2 antagonists and proton pump inhibitors inhibit gastric acid production. Chronic use of these medications can significantly decrease the absorption of vitamin B_{12}.[116]

The direct systemic effect of a drug on one nutrient may have secondary effects on another nutrient. Isoniazid and cimetidine inhibit the hydroxylation of vitamin D in the liver and kidney, and phenytoin and phenobarbital promote the breakdown of vitamin D metabolites, each resulting in a functional deficiency of vitamin D and secondary impairment of calcium absorption.[119] Neomycin, colchicine, and para-aminosalicylic acid may damage intestinal mucosa and destroy intestinal villi and microvilli, resulting in an inhibition of brush border enzymes and intestinal transport systems.[120] Nonsteroidal anti-inflammatory agents can cause multiple small hemorrhages of the intestinal mucosa leading to iron deficiency anemia and decreased absorption of vitamin C.[121] Folic acid deficiency and macrocytic anemia can occur in patients on chronic aspirin therapy, especially if their diet is low in dietary sources of folate.[94]

Laxative abuse has also been implicated with malabsorption of vitamin D and calcium. Use of irritant laxatives, such as phenolphthalein and bisacodyl, may damage intestinal epithelial cells and impair colonic reabsorption, resulting in steatorrhea, protein-losing enteropathy, and decreased absorption of glucose, potassium, calcium, and vitamin D.[122] Other stool regimen medications, such as docusate, alter electrolyte transport and can cause hypomagnesemia owing to GI losses and failure of colonic reabsorption.[123] Orally ingested mineral oil can coat ingested food particles along with the surface of the intestines. This forms a mechanical barrier to the digestion and absorption of nutrients. Mineral oil also increases gastric motility, which reduces the time required to adequately absorb ingested nutrients.[124] Furthermore, studies have shown that mineral oil, especially when taken at mealtime or during the postprandial absorptive period of optimal nutrient absorption, can reduce the absorption of vitamin D.[124]

Alterations in vitamin and mineral absorption can also occur owing to chelation or precipitation with a medication. Cholestyramine, a basic anion-exchange resin, binds bile salts and impairs the absorption of fat-soluble vitamins, vitamin B_{12}, folic acid, and the minerals calcium, iron, and zinc.[125] Aluminum hydroxide and magnesium hydroxide-containing antacids may form nonabsorbable phosphates in the gut lumen, resulting in hypophosphatemia along with anorexia and secondary syndromes of hypomagnesemia and osteomalacia.[119]

Alteration in GI pH may also cause drug-induced malabsorption. Drugs that increase gastric pH (eg, H_2 antagonists) can also decrease the breakdown of fat necessary to complex with calcium, thus reducing gut absorption.[126] Antacids can also reduce the bioavailability of riboflavin and folic acid as well as copper and iron, all of which depend on a low pH.[127] In some cases, the effect of drugs on nutrient malabsorption may be indirect. Proton-pump inhibitors (eg, omeprazole, lansoprazole) suppress gastric acid release and induce a mild achlohydric state. The decrease in gastric pH leads reduces the amount of cobalamin liberated from diet. This, in turn, limits the binding of cobalamin to intrinsic factor. Chronic use of this class of drugs may lead to malabsorption of cobalamin in some patients. Vitamin supplementation may be necessary to minimize the risk of developing anemia.[128]

METABOLISM OF NUTRIENTS

Drugs may affect nutrient metabolism by several methods. They may inhibit the essential intermediary metabolism of a nutrient, usually a vitamin, or promote the catabolism of the nutrient. Medications with these properties may be used therapeutically, as in the case of coumarin anticoagulants or methotrexate. In other cases, this may be an unwanted side effect, as in the case of pyridoxine antagonism seen in isoniazid and hydralazine use. Isoniazid and hydralazine can result in pyridoxine deficiency by the inhibition of pyridoxal kinase. Both compounds deplete pyridoxine stores and consequently the neurotransmitter gamma-aminobutyric acid, resulting in seizures. Administration of pyridoxine in cases of isoniazid overdose eliminates seizures and metabolic acidosis, which often occur.[129]

Many medications induce drug metabolism enzymes. This results in greater activity of these enzymes, increasing the demand for their vitamin cofactor, and, with chronic drug therapy and marginal nutrient intakes, can precipitate signs of deficiency of several vitamins, especially folic acid. Triamterene can inhibit dihydrofolate reductase, resulting in megaloblastosis.[130] The 3-hydroxy-3-methylglutaryl coenzyme A reductase inhibitor class of antihyperlipidemic agents (ie, statins) can lower plasma concentration of endogenous ubiquinone (coenzyme Q), a cellular antioxidant.[131]

Patients receiving chronic anticonvulsant therapy are at particular risk of developing metabolic bone disease as a result of these types of reactions.[132] Several mechanisms have been suggested. One suggests that drugs such as phenytoin, a microsomal enzyme inducer, stimulate the catabolism of vitamin D to produce an inactive metabolite.[133] Another theory suggests that phenytoin, alone or in combination with phenobarbital, interferes with vitamin K metabolism, with a corresponding elevation in serum osteocalcin levels without α-carboxyglutamate (Gla) residues, resulting in metabolic bone disease because osteocalcin-containing Gla residue is necessary for normal bone mineralization.[134]

Patients treated with cephalosporin antibiotics may develop hemorrhagic states owing to drug-induced vitamin K deficiency.[135] It is thought that these antibiotics block the vitamin K reductase, which is necessary for vitamin K activation.[136] They may also block carboxylation of vitamin K-dependent peptides to yield Gla residues that are required for calcium binding in the conversion of vitamin K-dependent proenzymes to their active state, which are needed in the coagulation cascade.[136]

Some drugs have been linked with subnormal serum folate levels, probably owing to weakly bound folate to serum proteins that can be easily displaced by drugs.[137] The mechanism for this interaction has yet to be described, but it appears that there is a decrease in serum binding of methyltetrahydrofolate caused by the drug itself or one of its metabolites.[138]

Folate deficiency secondary to long-term phenytoin therapy is a common occurrence; approximately 75% of patients taking anticonvulsants have low serum folic acid levels.[139] Progression to megaloblastic anemia is relatively rare, however.[140] Supplementation of folic acid with as little as 1 mg/d may lead to a significant decrease in serum phenytoin concentrations in 15 to 50% of the patients.[141] Although the exact mechanism is unknown, pharmacokinetic analysis of phenytoin suggests that folic acid may increase the affinity of the metabolic enzyme(s) involved in the elimination of the phenytoin without causing overall enzymatic induction.[141,142] To avoid potential folate deficiency and subsequent fluctuations in serum phenytoin levels, practitioners should routinely supplement all patients with folate when phenytoin therapy is initiated.[141]

Like phenytoin, sulfasalazine, an anti-inflammatory agent used to treat Crohn's disease and juvenile rheumatoid arthritis, is one of the leading causes of drug-induced folic acid deficiency in children.[142] Megaloblastic anemia, caused by folate deficiency, has been reported in patients receiving high doses of sulfasalazine for prolonged periods.[143]

Aspirin has also been linked with folate deficiency. Serum folate levels are known to be low in many patients with rheumatoid arthritis.[116] It is thought that aspirin alters the transport of folate by competing for binding sites on serum proteins.

Methotrexate, a chemotherapeutic agent that is also used to treat psoriasis, rheumatoid arthritis, and Crohn's disease, limits the availability of methyl groups derived from one-carbon metabolism by inhibiting competitively a key enzyme in the intracellular folate metabolism.[144] Methotrexate functions as an antimetabolite, reversibly inhibiting dihydrofolatereductase.

Valproic acid (VPA), an antiepileptic agent, has been associated with folate deficiency. Like other agents, the mechanism is not fully understood; however, it is thought that VPA causes an alteration in the methionine cycle.[145] This results in an elevation of tetrahydrofolate levels and a reduction of both formulated forms of folate. This could also explain VPA's role as a teratogen.[146] In addition, it has been established that VPA may induce L-carnitine deficiency. Patients who develop VPA-induced carnitine deficiency typically experience hyperammonemia syndrome with no other abnormality in the liver function tests. If diagnosed early, the clinical presentation, which includes altered mental status or encephalopathy, can be reversed by L-carnitine supplementation.[147]

DRUG EFFECTS ON NUTRIENT TRANSPORT

There are several mechanisms by which a drug can impact nutrient transport and then lead to nutritional deficiency. A nutrient can become displaced from plasma protein binding sites by a medication, leading to an increase in the renal excretion of the nutrient, or a drug may compete with a nutrient such that intracellular use of the nutrient is impaired.[148] This may occur when folate stores become depleted in patients receiving therapeutic doses of aspirin.[148]

EXCRETION

Thiamin deficiency can occur in patients treated with chronic loop diuretic therapy. Seligmann and colleagues reported that patients with congestive heart failure treated with long-term furosemide therapy had increased urinary excretion of thiamin, leading to frank deficiency over time that may have contributed to poor cardiac performance.[149] Similar findings were reported by Brady and colleagues, who observed laboratory evidence of thiamin deficiency in congestive heart failure patients being treated with loop diuretics on a chronic basis.[150]

DRUG-INDUCED FLUID AND ELECTROLYTE IMBALANCE

Several widely used medications can affect electrolyte balance, as summarized in Table 3. Sodium balance is altered by thiazide diuretics and the neuroleptic carbamazepine.[151,152] Patients treated long-term with carbamazepine have been reported to develop the syndrome of inappropriate antidiuretic hormone, resulting in hyponatremia and water retention.[152] In those patients, hyponatremia develops owing to the enhanced renal conservation of water. Similarly, patients receiving excessive diuretic therapy with fluid loss replaced with excessive water are prone to developing syndrome of inappropriate antidiuretic hormone.[151] Conversely, certain medications can cause hypernatremia as a result of water loss and subsequent dehydration. Hypernatremia, secondary to excessive lactulose therapy for hepatic encephalopathy or constipation, is a common drug-induced cause of this disorder.[153]

Renal wasting of potassium, resulting in hypokalemia, has been associated with thiazide and loop diuretics, corticosteroids, amphotericin B, and antipseudomonal penicillins.[35] Insulin and inhaled β2-agonists (eg, albuterol) can cause a shift of potassium from the extracellular to the intracellular spaces.

Potassium-sparing diuretics (eg, spironolactone), angiotensin-converting enzyme inhibitors (eg, enalapril), heparin, and trimethoprim can cause hyperkalemia.[154] A variety of mechanisms are involved. Trimethoprim has weak diuretic properties with potassium-sparing activity.[155] Heparin can suppress aldosterone, leading to sodium wasting and potassium retention. Patients with renal insufficiency or diabetes mellitus appear to be more susceptible to heparin-induced hyperkalemia.[156]

The impact of medications on phosphorus balance is important in patients receiving nutritional support as the synthesis of new cells increases the need for phosphorus. Patients already at risk for refeeding syndrome are particularly susceptible to the effects of drugs known to decrease available phosphorus stores.[157] Drugs such as antacids and sulcralfate can alter the absorption of phosphorus from the GI tract by binding to dietary phosphate, thus preventing its absorption. Conversely, patients with renal dysfunction are at risk for development of hyperphosphatemia owing to the inherent phosphate content present in the phospholipid emulsifiers in intravenous fat emulsion or clindamycin phosphate injection.[157]

As previously discussed, medications such as isoniazid and cimetidine can inhibit the hepatic and/or renal hydroxylation of vitamin D, leading to impaired calcium absorption.[158] Odes and colleagues concluded that even short-term therapy with cimetidine altered vitamin D metabolism in humans.[158] The researchers came to this conclusion after studying 25-hydroxyvitamin D_3 levels for 30 days in patients treated with cimetidine.

Chronic corticosteroid use can cause a net negative calcium balance and increased bone resorption owing to suppressed intestinal absorption of calcium in conjunction with increased renal calcium and phosphate excretion and a subsequent decrease in renal tubular calcium resorption, resulting in bone osteopenia.[119,159] Even frequent use of inhaled steroids has been associated with this response.[160]

Hypomagnesemia as a result of renal wasting can occur in patients treated with loop diuretics, thiazide diuretics, amphotericin B, aminoglycosides, cisplatin, or cyclosporine. Cisplatin-induced hypomagnesemia is dose and duration dependent.[161] Cisplatin induces hypomagnesemia by reducing magnesium reabsorption in the ascending loop of Henle and the distal tubule.[162] Forastiere and colleagues reported that the total exposure of free platinum contributes to direct injury and renal toxicity.[163] Carboplatin, an antineoplastic with a chemical structure similar to cisplatin, has been reported to have a lower incidence of hypomagnesemia.[164]

Renal wasting of magnesium is also common in patients on prolonged courses of high doses of aminoglycosides.[119,165] Aminoglycosides can inhibit the proximal tubular transport of magnesium in the kidney, predisposing patients with already low intakes of magnesium to hypomagnesemia.[165]

If left untreated, hypomagnesemia will ultimately lead to hypocalcemia. Magnesium deficiency can induce a transient hypoparathyroidism by reducing the secretion of parathyroid hormone (PTH) and a blunted PTH response. This results in an inhibition of the hypocalcemic feedback loop.[161] Other agents, such as aluminum salts, also suppress PTH secretion, resulting in hypocalcemia. Treatment for hypocalcemia induced by hypomagnesemia involves correcting the hypomagnesemia first and then managing the magnesium losses. In some cases, calcium supplementation may be unnecessary.[161]

TRACE ELEMENTS

Zinc is essential for the function of hundreds of enzymes such as dehydrogenases, aldolases, and peptidases and is involved in a variety of metabolic processes.[166] The formation and activation of zinc-dependent enzymes are regulated by zinc tissue levels.[167] Zinc metalloenzymes are responsible for structural integrity at the cellular level and for the regulation of various aspects of RNA and DNA metabolism.[167] Zinc deficiency limits the activity of these enzymes, resulting in decreased cell replication and tissue growth and repair.

Table 3 Examples of Drug–Nutrient Interactions

Medication/Drug Class	Nutrient	Interaction
Albuterol	Glucose	Hyperglycemia (in diabetics)
Aminoglycosides	Potassium, magnesium, sodium, calcium	Increased urinary excretion of potassium and magnesium, may also deplete sodium and calcium
Amphotericin	Magnesium, potassium, sodium	Electrolyte wasting
Aspirin	Folic acid	Decreased serum folate levels
Calcium carbonate	Iron	Decreased iron absorption
Captopril	Potassium	May cause hyperkalemia
Chloramphenicol	Protein, riboflavin B_6 B_{12}	Decreased protein synthesis
Cholestyramine	Fat, MCT, vitamins A, D, E, K, B_{12}, folate, calcium, glucose, xylose	Decreased absorption
Cimetidine	Vitamin B_{12}	Depletion of B_{12} stores
Cisplatin	Magnesium	Magnesium depletion
Corticosteroids	Glucose	Hyperglycemia
Digoxin	Bran, fiber, calcium, magnesium, potassium	Decrease drug absorption; arrhythmias hypomagnesemia or hypokalemia may enhance toxic effect of digoxin; arrhythmias
Ethambutol	Copper, zinc	Copper and zinc depletion
Fluconazole	Potassium	Hypokalemia
Fluorouracil	Thiamine	Inhibits conversion of thiamine to thiamine pyrophosphatase; increase thiamine requirements
Foscarnet	Calcium, magnesium, phosphorus, potassium	Electrolyte wasting
Furazolidine	Tyramine-rich foods	Increased risk of hypertensive effects if used chronically or at high doses with tyramine-rich foods
Furosemide	Calcium, magnesium, potassium, sodium	Electrolyte depletion
Gemfibrozil	Vitamin E, ubiquinone	Decreased absorption
Insulin	Dextrose	Increased insulin requirements
H-2 antagonists (cimetidine, ranitidine, famotidine)	Vitamin B_{12}, Zinc	Depletion of B_{12} stores. May deplete zinc
Isoniazid	Pyridoxine, tyrosine-rich foods, histamine-rich foods, tyramine-rich foods	Vitamin B6 antagonism blocks conversion of tyrosine to niacin. May cause headaches, itching, redness, chills, hypotension. Isoniazid has some MAO-I activity, tyramine-rich foods may cause hypertensive crisis
Linezolid	Tyramine-rich foods	Linezolid has some MAO-I properties, tyramine rich foods may cause hypertensive crisis
Lithium	Sodium	Increased sodium intake decreases lithium's effectiveness; decreased sodium intake may increase lithium toxicity
Methotrexate	Folic acid	Methotrexate may cause folate deficiency; folate supplementation may decrease methotrexate effects
Mineral oil	Fat soluble vitamins	Decreased absorption of fat soluble vitamins with chronic use
Neomycin	Fat soluble vitamins, MCT, B_{12}, sodium, glucose, lactose, sucrose, xylose	Impaired absorption
Nonsteroidal anti-inflammatory agents	Potassium	Hyperkalemia in patients with renal disease or receiving potassium supplements or potassium sparing diuretics
Orlistat	Vitamin E	Reduced vitamin E absorption
Oral contraceptives	Ascorbic acid, folic acid, pyridoxine	Ascorbic acid, folic acid, and vitamin B_6 requirements increased
para-Aminosalicylic acid (PAS)	B_{12}, folate, calcium, iron, magnesium	Decreased absorption of B_{12}, folate, calcium, iron, magnesium
Penicillamine	Acidic foods/beverages	Decreased penicillamine absorption/inactivation
Penicillin	Acidic foods/beverages	Penicillin inactivation
Phenobarbital	Ascorbic acid vitamin D	Decreased ascorbic acid absorption Interferes with vitamin D metabolism
Phenytoin	Folic acid pyridoxine vitamin D	High-dose folic acid may antagonize phenytoin effects; phenytoin may cause folate deficiency resulting in megaloblastic anemia May antagonize phenytoin Interferes with vitamin D metabolism
Primidone	Folic acid	May cause folic acid deficiency leading to megaloblastic anemia
Proton pump inhibitors	Iron B_{12}	Decreased absorption
Pyrimethamine	Folic acid	Decreased serum folate levels
Spironolactone	Sodium, potassium	May cause hyponatremia May cause hyperkalemia
Sulfasalazine	Folic acid	Inhibits the absorption of folic acid
Terbutaline	Glucose	Hyperglycemia (in diabetics)
Theophylline	Caffeine, carbohydrates, charcoal-broiled meat protein	Increases theophylline side effects. Decreased carbohydrate intake may decrease plasma half-life of theophylline. May decrease theophylline half-life. Increased protein intake may decrease plasma half-life of theophylline
Thiazide diuretics	Magnesium, potassium, sodium	Increased electrolyte wasting
Triamterene	Folic acid	May cause folic acid depletion
Trimethoprim	Folic acid	May cause folic acid depletion
Valproic acid	Carnitine	May cause carnitine deficiency with hyperammonemia
Warfarin	Vitamin K, onions, garlic, vitamin E	May inhibit warfarin response; increase dose needed. Excessive amounts may increase the fibrinolytic activity of warfarin. May enhance anticoagulant effect of warfarin
Zidovudine	Carnitine, folic acid	May cause carnitine deficiency. May cause megaloblastic anemia
Zonisamide	Biotin, vitamin B_1, vitamin B_2, niacin, pyridoxine, vitamin B_{12}, vitamin K	May deplete stores.

Table 4 Medications That Alter Glucose Metabolism/Response

Medication/Drug Class	Response
Acritretin	Hyperglycemia
Amprenavir	Hyperglycemia
Arginine	Hyperglycemia
Corticosteroids	Hyperglycemia
Cyproheptadine	Hyperglycemia
Diazoxide	Hyperglycemia
Diuretics	Hyperglycemia
Epinephrine	Hyperglycemia
Fosphenytoin	Hypoglycemia
Glucagon	Hyperglycemia
Glycerol	Hyperglycemia
Indinavir	Hyperglycemia
L-asparaginase	Hyperglycemia
Megestrol	Hyperglycemia
Nelfinavir	Hyperglycemia
Nicotinic acid	Hyperglycemia
Oral contraceptives	Hyperglycemia
Octreotide	Hyper/hypoglycemia
Penacillamine	Hypoglycemia
Pentamidine	Hyper/hypoglycemia
Phenytoin	Hyperglycemia
Quinine	Hypoglycemia
Ritonavir	Hyperglycemia
Saquinavir	Hyperglycemia
Sertraline	Hyperglycemia
Tacrolimus	Hyperglycemia

Zinc interacts with several other nutrients. At supplemental doses, zinc may impair copper absorption.[168] Zinc deficiency can also negatively impact vitamin A metabolism by impairing the mobilization of retinol from the liver and altering retinal visual pigment metabolism, which may contribute to the night blindness seen in zinc deficiency.[169] It is thought that zinc deficiency may result in abnormal dark adaptation and/or age-related macular degeneration.[170]

Patients receiving PN are at risk for developing zinc deficiency. Zinc balance during PN depends on the infusion of zinc in amounts sufficient to offset urinary and GI losses that occur independent of zinc intake.[171] Premature infants receiving PN will experience a progressive decline in plasma zinc levels despite 14 days of continuous treatment, reflecting their high metabolic demands.[171]

GLUCOSE

Patients with diabetes mellitus or others with insulin resistance (eg, severe infections, catabolic stress) are susceptible to the effects of medications known to impact glucose metabolism. Thiazide diuretics, corticosteroids, and cyclosporine have all been associated with inducing hyperglycemia in susceptible patients.[172] Hyperglycemia occurs in approximately 20% of patients treated with pentamidine.[173] Moreover, protease inhibitors have been recognized as a cause of hyperglycemia.[174] The long-acting somatostatin analog octreotide has been shown to inhibit insulin secretion and may result in a transient deterioration in glucose tolerance on initiation of therapy.[175] In most cases, alteration of carbohydrate metabolism does not appear to be a problem. Table 4 lists some of the more common medications that alter glucose metabolism or response.

Hypoglycemia is the most common metabolic abnormality associated with pentamidine therapy.[176] The mechanism responsible for this adverse effect may involve a direct cytolytic effect on pancreatic beta cells, resulting in insulin release and hypoglycemia and a subsequent insulin deficiency owing to loss of beta cell function.[177] Eventually, however, pentamidine-induced pancreatic beta cell damage may lead to insulin deficiency and result in hyperglycemia, although this is considerably less frequent than hypoglycemia.[177]

Drugs or foods that have the ability to induce a rapid release of insulin can increase the risk of hypoglycemia, especially if taken with alcohol. Beta-blockers such as propranolol can inhibit glycogenolysis and, during periods of vigorous exercise, induce hypoglycemia.[178]

FAT

With increased awareness of lipid abnormalities and coronary artery disease, drug-induced lipoprotein abnormalities must be considered; especially in patients in whom no other causes of dyslipidemia exist. Some of the most common causes of secondary dyslipidemia are medications. When a drug is used for a short period only, practitioners need to be aware of the effects on the patient's lipoprotein profile versus the chance that an underlying dyslipidemia has been exacerbated. Drugs used chronically may be more problematic as they may predispose the patient to atherosclerosis.[179] Table 5 lists medications associated with dyslipidemia.

Protease inhibitors interfere with some proteins involved in fat metabolism (ie, cytoplasmic retinoic acid–binding protein type 1).[180] Protease-inhibitor binding to low-density lipoprotein (LDL) receptor-related proteins (LRPs) impair hepatic chylomicron uptake and triglyceride clearance by the endothelial LRP–lipoprotein lipase complex. The resulting hyperlipidemia contributes to central fat deposition and insulin resistance.[180] It is also thought that protease inhibitors may also disrupt steroid hormone production, leading to lipodystrophy.[181] See Chapter 49, "Pediatric HIV Infection" for a full discussion of HIV lipodystrophy.

L-Asparaginase has been reported to cause abnormalities in lipid metabolism, ranging from hypocholesterolemia and hypotriglyceridemia to hypercholesterolemia and hypertriglyceridemia. Parsons and colleagues suggested that this alteration in lipid metabolism is caused by structural

Table 5 Medications Associated with Dyslipidemia

Medication	Total Lipids	Total Cholesterol	Triglycerides	Low-Density Lipoprotein	High-Density Lipoprotein	Very Low Density Lipoprotein
Abacavir			↑			
Amiodarone		↑	↑			
Amprenavir		↑	↑			
Anabolic steroids				↑	↓	
Beta-blockers			↑			
Calcitriol		↑				
Cholestyramine			↑			
Cyclosporine	↑	↑	↑	↑		
Dexrazoxane			↑			
Didanosine			↑			
Disopyramide		↑	↑			
Efavirenz		↑	↑		↑	
Enoxaparin	↑					
Ergocalciferol		↑				
Estrogen			↑			
Fluconazole		↑	↑			
Glucocorticoids	↑	↑	↑	↑	↓	↑
Interferons			↑			↑
Isotretinoin		↑	↑		↑	
Itraconazole			↑			
L-asparaginase			↑			
Miconazole (IV)	↑	↑				
Mycophenolate		↑				
Nelfinavir	↑					
Paclitaxel			↑			
Phenothiazines						
Progestins			~	↑	↓	↓
Propofol	↑					
Retinoids (vitamin A)			↑	↑	↓	↑
Risperidone			↑			
Ritonavir		↑	↑			
Sertraline		↑	↑	↑		Possible ↑
Tacrolimus				↑		↑
Valproic acid						↑

changes in the high-density lipoprotein (HDL) particles from higher to lower density that is reflected in an altered ratio of lipid to protein.[182] The authors suggested that prior to the initiation of L-asparaginase therapy, HDL-cholesterol particles are protein rich but gradually become lipid rich because of an asparaginase-associated reduction in protein synthesis. They also concluded that modifications in asparaginase therapy are not necessary; however, close monitoring is recommended for patients whose triglyceride levels exceed 2,000 mg/dL when the risk of pancreatitis is increased.

In addition to asparaginase-associated lipid abnormalities, patients being treated for acute lymphoblastic leukemia often receive corticosteroids that may alter lipid and lipoprotein metabolism by increasing hepatic cholesterol synthesis.[182] Corticosteroids increase the frequency of hypercholesterolemia and hypertriglyceridemia with elevations in LDL and HDL levels, often in a dose-related manner.[179] Females appear to be more susceptible than males to these changes. Switching to alternate-day therapy may reduce lipoprotein levels in some patients.[179]

Orally administered estrogens decrease serum LDL and increase serum HDL levels in a dose-related manner.[179] Moreover, these agents are known to increase serum triglyceride levels by 30 to 87%.[179] It has been suggested that low-dose estrogens be used to minimize elevations in triglyceride levels without compromising their favorable impact on LDL and HDL levels.[179] Interestingly, other routes of estrogen administration (topical, intradermal, intramuscular) tend not to have as pronounced an effect on lipoproteins, perhaps because these routes bypass first-pass metabolism through the liver, thus having a smaller impact on hepatic protein synthesis.[179,183] Progestins, often used in combination with estrogens in various oral contraceptive products, can also affect lipoprotein levels. Generally, progestins elevate LDL levels and decrease triglyceride, HDL, and very low density lipoprotein levels, correlating with the androgenic activity associated with specific progestins.[179] Newer low-dose triphasic oral contraceptives (eg, ethinyl estradiol-levonorgestrel, ethinyl estradiol-norethindrone) do not have any appreciable alterations in lipid profiles or at best mild increases in serum cholesterol, LDL, and triglycerides.[183]

Like estrogens, anabolic steroids can also cause profound, dose-related effects on lipoprotein metabolism. Reductions in HDL levels in conjunction with an elevation in LDL levels are often seen in patients using these agents.[179] The exact mechanism has not yet been defined, but caution is advised in using these agents in patients prone to dyslipidemia or atherosclerosis.

GASTROINTESTINAL ADVERSE EFFECTS

Many medications can adversely affect the function of the GI tract. Most are minor and resolved over time without any specific intervention. Others, however, can be significant and resulting in severe GI illness (eg, esophagitis, colitis) that can negatively impact the tolerance to an oral or tube fed diet. Drug induced esophagitis can occur with doxycycline capsules, iron sulfate tablets, extended release potassium chloride tablets, and tetracycline.[184] Typically, this occurs in adolescents who drink inadequate amounts of fluid with their medications, or patients with left atrial enlargement or cardiomegaly as the heart impinges on the esophagus, thus increasing the transit time of the medication in the esophagus. Switching to a liquid medication or administering the problematic drug with plenty of water often helps alleviate the situation.

DRUGS AND APPETITE

Impairment of nutritional status owing to drug use often results in drug-induced nutritional deficiencies in those cases in which the medication results in appetite suppression and decreased food intake. Often these signs and symptoms of nutrient deficiencies are nonspecific and may mimic those of other diseases and conditions.

Drugs can reduce food intake through a variety of mechanisms. Drugs that affect appetite (Table 6) may do so by either a central or peripheral effect, including loss of appetite, inducing sedation, or evoking adverse response when food is ingested.[185] The primary effect typically centers around appetite suppression, a centrally acting mechanism that includes the catecholaminergic (eg, dextroamphetamine), dopaminergic (eg, levodopa), serotoninergic (eg, fenfluramine), and endorphin (eg, naloxone) modulators, which may all act to suppress appetite.[186] Peripherally acting mechanisms that can indirectly suppress appetite include those agents that inhibit gastric emptying (eg, levodopa) or bulking agents (eg, methylcellulose).

Table 6 Drugs That Affect Appetite

Drugs That Decrease Appetite	Drugs That Stimulate Appetite
Aluminum hydroxide	Benzodiazepines
Amphetamines	Clemastine
Cisplatin	Cyproheptadine HCl
Cholestyramine	Dronabinol
Dactinomycin	Glucocorticoids
Digoxin	Insulin
Ethambutol	Lithium
Furosemide	Megestrol acetate
Griseofulvin	Oral contraceptives
Hydralazine	Phenothiazines
Hydroxychloroquine	Tricyclic antidepressants
Hydroxyurea	
Itraconazole	
Lamivudine	
Methenamine	
Methotrexate	
Methylcellulose	
Mineral oil	
Nitrofurantoin	
Penicillamine	
Sibutramine	
Spironolactone	
Sulfasalazine	
Thiazide diuretics	
Topiramate	

Adapted from reference 67.

A secondary response may also occur when an adverse response to food caused by the drug results in a loss of appetite. The emetic center, located within the brainstem, is easily stimulated by the action of many drugs. These include drugs that cause nausea and vomiting (eg, digoxintoxic dose), drugs causing a loss of taste (eg, penicillamine), drugs causing stomatitis (eg, fluorouracil), and hepatoxic agents (eg, alcohol).[185]

Another way in which medications can cause anorexia is through depletion of various nutrients. High-doses of aluminum- or magnesium-containing antacids can result in phosphate depletion, leading to muscle weakness and anorexia.[187] Similarly, loop diuretics can lead to depletion of sodium, potassium, and magnesium, which can result in anorexia.[188] Drugs known to deplete folate, such as phenytoin, sulfasalazine, and trimethoprim, can result in weight loss and anorexia.[189] Penicillamine, which induces zinc depletion, can lead to diminished taste acuity and possibly decreased food intake.[190] Ironically, even a nutrient can induce anorexia. Belle and Halpern reported that patients taking relatively large doses of niacin for hyperlipidemia experienced GI symptoms that resulted in poor appetite and moderate weight loss.[191]

Zinc supplements have been used to treat drug-induced hypogeusia with mixed results. Although zinc supplementation has been used successfully to manage hypogeusia in patients undergoing dialysis, Dahl and colleagues did not see similar findings when patients with acetazolamide-induced taste disturbances were given zinc supplements.[192]

In some cases, weight gain may be an undesirable side effect of a medication. Antiepileptic drugs, both old and new, have weight changes associated with their use. Antiepileptic drugs associated with marked weight gain include carbamazepine, gabapentin, VPA and vigabatrin. Lamotrigine and levetiracetam are both considered weight-neutral, whereas felbamate and topiramate have been associated with significant weight loss.[193]

APPETITE ENHANCERS

Appetite enhancers are useful in reversing the anorexia of disease, in particular cancer cachexia and HIV wasting. Several medications are frequently used, although none have yet become a standard of therapy.

The appetite-boosting properties of corticosteroids have been well established.[194] Their impact on weight gain seems to be short term, however. Moertel and colleagues suggested that patients treated with dexamethasone saw appetite improvement after 2 weeks of treatment, but the effect disappeared by week 4.[195] Some attribute the improved appetite to the mood-enhancing properties of steroids rather than a specific effect on appetite.[196] The antihistamine cyproheptadine has become one of the most commonly used appetite stimulants in pediatric patients, particularly those with anorexia nervosa. It is a potent serotonin antagonist. By decreasing brain serotonin levels, appetite is enhanced and food intake is increased, resulting in weight gain.[197] Megestrol acetate is a drug with antiestrogen properties whose original indication was in the treatment of breast cancer. It was one of the first drugs used to treat HIV wasting. It is a powerful appetite stimulant, and weight gain seen with its use is substantial, although it tends to be mostly fat, with minimal increases in lean body mass.[198] Megestrol also lowers testosterone levels in males, which may explain its minimal increases in lean body mass. Adrenal suppression has also been reported with long-term megestrol use; thus, abrupt discontinuation should be avoided.[199] Megestrol acetate also has been used to stimulate appetite and promote weight gain in a limited number of patients with cachexia associated with neoplastic disease. Although the exact mechanism of action has not been determined, it has been suggested that megestrol and/or its metabolites may, either directly or indirectly, stimulate appetite, resulting in weight gain, or may alter metabolic pathways by interfering with the production or response of mediators such as cachectin, a hormone that inhibits adipocyte lipogenic enzymes.[200]

Dronabinol is a derivative of marijuana that is primarily used in pediatric patients as an antiemetic but has some use in treating anorexia, primarily in HIV wasting.[201] Like megestrol, it can stimulate appetite as well as interest in food. Its effects on mental status, however, limit its usefulness.

Because cytokine effects on appetite can contribute to the anorexia of disease, anticytokine monoclonal antibodies and receptor antagonists may have a role in inhibiting cytokine action.[202] Some agents, such as the corticosteroids, inhibit the transcription of interleukin-1, tumor necrosis factor, and other cytokineses. Other agents appear to act by binding a mitogen-activating protein kinase necessary for the translation of messenger RNAs.[202] Fish oil supplements that are rich in omega-3 fatty acids decrease the anorectic effect of interleukin-1 and tumor necrosis factor.[203] Unfortunately, the fishy taste associated with these supplements makes them a less than desirable option.

APPETITE SUPPRESSANTS

Although, for long-term success, weight loss takes a great deal of self-control to resist the many internal and external cues to eat, appetite suppressants can augment weight loss by reducing the hunger drive, thereby assisting the patient to adhere to a restricted caloric diet.[204] The major class of drugs currently in use for the adjunctive treatment is the centrally acting appetite suppressants. This class is further subdivided into those that act on the noradrenergic nervous system and those that act on the serotoninergic nervous system.

Given their high potential for abuse and numerous side effects, the noradrenergic agents (eg, dextroamphetamine) are no longer routinely used in weight loss management unless other therapies have been proven ineffective. These agents block the reuptake of dopamine and norepinephrine from the synapse, thus increasing the amount available in the cerebral cortex and reticular activating system.[204]

The neurotransmitter serotonin is responsible for appetite suppression and satiation. Serotonin, as part of a complex negative feedback loop, accumulates in certain areas of the brain in response to feeding.[204] Fenfluramine, dexfenfluramine, and fluoxetine inhibit serotonin reuptake at presynaptic spaces. They have few central stimulatory effects.

Other agents that have the potential to cause anorexia and may have a potential role in weight loss management are the thermogenic drugs.[205] These include endogenous hormones (ie, insulin, thyroid hormone) and sympathomimetic agents with alpha- or beta-adrenergic properties.[205] Currently, exogenous thyroid has no role in obesity management owing to its adverse effects on protein breakdown, cardiovascular complications, and bone mineralization.[206]

VITAMIN AND MINERAL SUPPLEMENTATION/ HPERVITAMINOSIS

Megavitamin therapy has been advocated in the treatment of various disease states, including schizophrenia, cancer, and the common cold.[207] A megadose is generally considered to be 10 or more times the recommended dietary allowance.[208] Although excess water-soluble vitamins are excreted and usually cause few problems, side effects have been reported in cases of excessively high doses.[209] Dietary supplementation can also impact response to medications. If used carelessly, vitamin and mineral supplementation alone or as part of a fad diet can potentiate or exacerbate nutrient–nutrient interactions, as summarized in Tables 7 and 8.

Drug-metabolizing enzyme systems have been shown to be highly dependent on vitamin C status. Houston and colleagues showed that normal individuals receiving supplemental ascorbic acid had a substantial increase in antipyrine clearance, whereas Beatie and Sherlock reported that vitamin C deficiency was partly responsible for impaired drug clearance in patients with liver disease.[210] When ascorbic acid is taken in excessive amounts, enzyme saturation occurs, and the vitamin acts as a chemical and enters into nonenzymatic reactions.[211] Ascorbic acid is a strong reducing agent and is able to impact other dietary components as well as alter drug disposition.[211] Ironically, scurvy, the main deficiency state associated with inadequate dietary intake of ascorbic acid, a relatively rare condition today, can occur in infants born to mothers taking large doses of vitamin C.[211] Both the mother and fetus increase their metabolic destruction of ascorbic acid after maternal ingestion of large doses of ascorbic acid. At birth, any dietary ascorbic acid ingested by the infant is degraded rapidly, leading to a deficiency state. Reports of acute scurvy have been reported in infants breast-fed by mothers who had ingested more than 400 mg vitamin C daily during pregnancy.[212] A similar situation can occur in adults

Table 7 Examples of Nutrient–Nutrient Interactions

Nutrient	Interaction
Calcium	High calcium intake interferes with manganese, phosphorus, and iron absorption. Calcium absorption is potentiated by vitamin D, reduced by dietary oxalates. Excessive protein intake may increase calcium losses
Chromium	A high-sugar diet may increase urinary chromium losses
Copper	High intake may impair zinc absorption
Cysteine	May chelate with copper in parenteral nutrition solutions
Iron	Iron salts might decrease gastrointestinal zinc resorption; impairs manganese absorption Soy products, including soy-based infant formula, significantly reduce absorption of iron vitamin C enhances absorption of iron Calcium salts may reduce iron absorption vitamin A deficiency increases liver storage of iron
Magnesium	High magnesium intake may impair calcium absorption, decreases phosphorus absorption
Manganese	Calcium and iron salts decrease manganese absorption zinc enhances manganese absorption
Phosphorus	High intake decreases magnesium absorption
Thiamine	High carbohydrate diet or intravenous dextrose may increase thiamine requirement
Zinc	High zinc intake may impair copper absorption. Zinc may increase manganese absorption Iron salts may impair zinc absorption
Vitamin A	Megadoses may interfere with iron, iodine, copper, calcium absorption; can also interfere with absorption of ascorbic acid, vitamin K, vitamin E, and vitamin D
Vitamin C	Increases iron absorption, impairs copper absorption, interferes with cyanocobalamin absorption
Vitamin D	Reduced intake impairs calcium and phosphorus absorption and utilization
Vitamin E	Inhibits the reticulocyte and hemoglobin response to iron

Table 8 Examples of Vitamin–Drug Interactions

Nutrient	Medication	Interaction
Ascorbic acid (vitamin C)	Coumarin anticoagulants, gentamicin, iron salts, oral contraceptives, tricyclic antidepressants	Shortens prothrombin time, may antagonize warfarin response; acidifies urine, decreases efficacy of gentamicin; increased iron absorption; intermittent use may cause contraceptive failure; megadoses (>2 g/d) may reduce therapeutic response of tricyclic antidepressants
Folic acid	Phenytoin, pyrimethamine	Reduces phenytoin bioavailability, may antagonize anticonvulsant action of phenytoin; reduces pyrimethamine efficacy
Niacin	Adrenergic blockers, aspirin, HMG-CoA reductase inhibitors ("statins"), isoniazid	Enhances vasodilation, may cause orthostatic hypotension aspirin decreases flushing seen with niacin use; increased risk of statin-associated myopathy/rhabdomyolysis with concurrent use; increased niacin requirement seen with isoniazid use
Pyridoxine (vitamin B_6)	Barbiturates, levodopa, phenytoin	Reduced barbiturate response, reduces levodopa response; megadoses may impair phenytoin effect, cause decrease in phenytoin levels
Vitamin A	Aluminum hydroxide, coumarin anticoagulants, isotretinoin, oral contraceptives	Reduced vitamin A absorption; megadoses of vitamin A can enhance anticoagulant response, increase risk of bleeding; isotretinoin competes with vitamin A; increases serum vitamin A levels
Vitamin D	Digoxin	Vitamin D may cause hypercalcemia, leading to arrhythmias
Vitamin E	Coumarin anticoagulants, vitamin A, iron salts	Potentiates anticoagulant response; increases serum vitamin A levels; inhibits the reticulocyte and hemoglobin response to iron therapy
Vitamin K	Coumarin anticoagulants	Antagonizes anticoagulant response

Adapted from reference 67.

dependent on large doses of vitamin C. Therefore, it is recommended that patients receiving megadoses of vitamin C not be abruptly stopped but rather tapered by 10 to 20% until discontinued or on maintenance doses. Other complications associated with megadoses of ascorbic acid include vitamin B_{12} deficiency. Herbert and Jacob reported that even ascorbic doses as little as 250 mg may destroy up to 81% of cyanocobalamin in a moderate vitamin B_{12}-containing meal and up to 25% in a vitamin B_{12}-rich meal.[213] To blunt the intensity of this interaction, the authors suggested that ascorbic acid be taken two or more hours after meals. Oxalate stones may occur in susceptible patients receiving doses of greater than 4 g/d of ascorbic acid. Auer and colleagues reported that a hematuria and calcium oxalate dihydrate crystal formation in a 25-year-old male 8 days after ingesting 4 g of ascorbic acid daily resolved 5 days after discontinuing ascorbic acid supplementation.[214]

The daily consumption of vitamin B_6 (pyridoxine) in doses of 50 to 500 mg is not unusual given the currently available strengths of over-the-counter products. High-doses, however, may have a toxic action on the nervous system.[215] Sensory neuropathies have been reported in adults who received daily doses of 2 g of pyridoxine over a 4-month period or as soon as 2 months when daily doses of 5 g were ingested.

Megadoses of folic acid given to patients on long-term phenytoin therapy exhibit seizures and electroencephalogram abnormalities.[216] It appears that folic acid supplementation increases phenytoin liver metabolism; studies suggest increased phenytoin parahydroxylation and another suggests increased O-methylation of the catechol metabolite.[217] Another study concluded that folic acid does not stimulate phenytoin metabolism, but rather it changes the rates of elimination.[218]

Trace elements such as manganese can also impact the absorption of other nutrients such as iron. In patients with iron deficiency, there is a greater absorption of manganese. When iron supplementation occurs, there is a corresponding decrease in the amount of manganese absorbed with a greater amount appearing in the feces. This interaction appears to be due to competition for similar binding and absorption sites of (nonheme) iron and manganese.[219]

Hypervitaminosis A and D has been described in children, but the occurrence is rare.[220,221] Both are life threatening on an acute basis; vitamin A may cause increased intracranial pressure, whereas vitamin D may cause fatal hypercalcemia. Infants and young children are especially susceptible to excessive doses of vitamin A. Acute toxicity has been reported in infants receiving doses of 50,000 to 100,000 µg (166,666 to 333,333 IU) retinol as palmitate. Individual variation is significant, however. Field studies have used periodic massive doses of vitamin A, with thousands of 1- to 6-year-old children receiving 200,000 IU of retinyl palmitate (60,000 µg retinol), with approximately 1% exhibiting signs of intolerance that disappeared within hours of administration.[222] Chronic toxicity seen in infants and young children usually results from daily doses of 10,000 to 50,000 µg (33,333 to 166,666 IU) for several months.[223] Symptoms gradually disappear on discontinuation. The American Academy of Pediatrics recommends that daily vitamin A supplementation of more than 3,000 µg (10,000 IU) for young children be used under medical supervision.[224]

In typical doses, vitamin D is used to prevent and treat rickets.[225] Serious poisoning can occur with excessive doses. Sustained daily intake of as little as 1,800 IU in children has been reported as toxic.[226] Excessive vitamin D leads to increased absorption of calcium from the GI tract and enhanced bone resorption, with a subsequent loss of renal concentrating ability. Children typically will present with anorexia, vomiting, polyuria, or irritability associated with the increased serum calcium concentrations.[227] It should be noted, however, that very high doses of vitamin D have been effective in some patients with hereditary vitamin D–resistant rickets.[228] Hereditary vitamin D–resistant ricket accompanied by alopecia reflects a more severe form of vitamin D receptor resistance and is rarely responsive to vitamin D. Initial ergocalciferol therapy for children with vitamin D–resistant rickets is 1,000 to 2,000 µg/d (40,000 to 80,000 U) with phosphate supplement. The daily dose is increased at 3- to 4-month intervals in 250 to 500 µg (10,000 to 20,000 U) increments.[229]

In 1992, an outbreak of hypercalcemia owing to vitamin D intoxication was noted. In the case series, eight patients suffered vitamin D toxicity that was traced to excessive amounts of the vitamin in milk produced by a single dairy.[230] These were the first reported cases of hypervitaminosis D from commercial food products in the United States since fortification became commonplace in the 1930s. A second study summarized the findings of an analysis of 42 containers of milk and 10 cans of infant formulas from supermarkets in five states.[231] Nearly two-thirds of the milk container samples had less than 80% of the stated amount, whereas 4 of the 42 samples had over 120% of the labeled vitamin D content. The 10 infant formulas tested had vitamin D levels ranging from 111 IU/100 kcal to 250 IU/100 kcal, exceeding the maximum permitted by the US Food and Drug Administration regulation of 100 IU/100 kcal. Food and Drug Administration-compliant studies on both dairy products and infant formulas compiled over a 10-year period also showed some variance in vitamin D levels but not to the extent that would constitute a health risk.[232]

Vitamin K-rich foods (ie, green leafy vegetables, cabbage, broccoli), when intake is irregular, can alter response to anticoagulants such as warfarin. When ingested in high amounts, these foods can be associated with anticoagulant failure, resulting in the need for higher doses. Similarly, when patients who have been stable on warfarin suddenly decrease their intake of these vitamin K-rich foods, they can put themselves at risk for bleeding because they are suddenly receiving too large a warfarin dose. Warfarin creates a partial deficiency of the active form of vitamin K involved in the post-translational modification factors (II, VII, IX, X, and proteins C and S).[233] Other sources of vitamin K, such as intravenous fat emulsions that are prepared from soybean or safflower and soybean oils, contain phytosterols that contain vitamin K.[234] Warfarin resistance has been reported in patients taking warfarin who also received intravenous fat emulsions.[234] This interaction presumably occurs because of the vitamin K content of the intravenous fat emulsion. Frequent monitoring of the international normalized ratio and warfarin dosage adjustments are imperative in these patients.

CONCLUSION

The human diet is highly heterogeneous in its composition, method of preparation, quantity, and time of consumption. Consequently, drug kinetics as a result of diet varies widely in subjects based on age, gender, culture, and economic status. Even within the same individual, seasonal variations will occur that impact dietary habits and ultimately drug-related effects. Although each factor may play a small role by itself, a much larger synergistic effect could occur when combined with other dietary factors, as well as genetic and environmental factors.

REFERENCES

1. Waler-Sack I, Klotz U. Influence of diet and nutritional status on drug metabolism. Clin Pharmacokinet 1996;31:47–64.
2. Fisher DM, O'Keeffe C, Stanski DR, et al. Pharmacokinetics and pharmacodynamics of *d*-tubocurarine in infants, children, and adults. Anesthesiology 1982;57:203–8.
3. Kearns GL, Abdel-Rahman SM, Alander SW, et al. Developmental pharmacology-drug disposition, action, and therapy in infants and children. N Engl J Med 2003;349:1157–67.
4. Yaffee SJ, Sonawane BR. Drug therapy and the role of nutrition. In: Walker WA, Watkins JB, editors. Nutrition in Pediatrics, 2nd edition. Hamilton, ON: BC Decker; 1997. p. 320–34.
5. Skaer TL. Dosing considerations in the pediatric patient. Clin Ther 1991;13:526–44.
6. Soldin OP, Soldin SJ. Review: Therapeutic drug monitoring in pediatrics. Ther Drug Monit 2002;24:1–8.
7. Stewart CF, Hampton EM. Effect of maturation on drug disposition in pediatric patients. Clin Pharm 1987;6:548–64.
8. Loebstein R, Koren G. Clinical pharmacology and therapeutic drug monitoring in neonates and children. Pediatr Rev 1998;19:423–8.
9. Berseth CL. Gastrointestinal motility in the neonate. Clin Perinatol 1996;23:179–90.
10. Lown KS, Bailey DG, Fontana RJ, et al. Grapefruit juice increases felodipine oral availability in humans by decreasing intestinal CYP3A protein expression. J Clin Invest 1997;99:2545–53.
11. Pan S, Lopez RR, Sher LS, et al. Enhanced oral cyclosporine absorption with water-soluble vitamin E after liver transplantation. Pharmacotherapy 1996;16:59–65.
12. Chan L, Humma LM, Schriever CA, et al. Vitamin E formulation affects digoxin absorption by inhibiting P-glycoprotein (P-gp) in humans [abstract]. Clin Pharmacol Ther 2004;75:95.
13. Guengerich FR. Influence of nutrients and other dietary materials on cytochrome P450 enzymes. Am J Clin Nutr 1995;61:651S–8S.
14. Strassburg CP, Strassburg A, Kneip S, et al. Developmental aspects of human hepatic drug glucuronidation in young children and adults. Gut 2002;50:259–65.
15. van Hoogdalem E, de Boer AG, Breimer DD. Pharmacokinetics of rectal drug administration, part I. General considerations and clinical applications of centrally acting drugs. Clin Pharmacokinet 1991;21:11–26.
16. Reuss L. One-hundred years of inquiry: The mechanism of glucose absorption in the intestine. Annu Rev Physiol 2000;62:939–46.
17. Kim RB. Drugs as P-glycoprotein substrates, inhibitors, and inducers. Drug Metab Rev 2002;34:47–54.
18. Ito K, Kusuhara H, Sugiyama Y. Effects of intestinal CYP3A4 and P-glycoprotein on oral drug absorptiontheoretical approach. Pharm Res 1999;16:225–31.
19. Chan L-N. Drug–nutrient interactions in transplant recipients. JPEN J Parenter Enteral Nutr 2001;25:132–41.
20. Collnot EM, Baldes C, Wempe MF, et al. Influence of vitamin E TPGS poly(ethylene glycol) chain length on apical efflux transporters in Caco-2 cell monolayers. J Control Release 2006;111:35–40.
21. Singh BN. Effects of food on clinical pharmacokinetics. Clin Pharmacokinet 1999;37:213–55.
22. Skelton JA, Havens PL, Werlin SL. Nutrient deficiencies in tube-fed children. Clin Pediatr (Phil) 2006;45:37–41.
23. Penod LE, Allen JB, Cabacungan LR. Warfarin resistance and enteral feedings: 2 case reports and a supporting in vitro study. Arch Phys Med Rehabil 2001;82:1270–3.
24. An Yeung SCS, Ensom MHH. Phenytoin and enteral feedings: Does evidence support an interaction? Ann Pharmacother 2000;34:896–905.
25. Fleisher D., Sheth N, Kou JH. Phenytoin interaction with enteral feedings administered through nasogastric tubes. JPEN J Parenter Enteral Nutr 1990;14:513–6.
26. Gorman SR, Armstrong G, Allen KR, et al. Scarcity in the midst of plenty: Enteral tube feeding complicated by scurvy. J Pediatr Gastroenterol Nutr 2002;35:93–5.
27. Mayhew SL, Christensen ML. Pharmacokinetic alterations in malnutrition and obesity. Hosp Pharm 1993;28:836–7.
28. Mehta S. Drug disposition in children with protein energy malnutrition. J Pediatr Gastroenterol Nutr 1983;2:407–17.
29. Erikson M, Catz C, Yaffe S. Effect of weanling malnutrition upon hepatic drug metabolism. Biol Neonate 1975;27:339–51.
30. O'Doherty DS, O'Malley WE, Denckla MB. Oral absorption of diphenylhydantoin as measured by gas liquid chromatography. Trans Am Neurol Assoc 1969;94:318–9.
31. Mehta S, Nain CK, Yadav D, et al. Disposition of acetaminophen in children with protein calorie malnutrition. Int J Clin Pharmacol Ther Toxicol 1985;23:311–5.
32. Raghuram TC, Krishnaswamy K. Tetracycline absorption in malnutrition. Drug Nutr Interact 1981;1:23–9.
33. Salako LA, Sowun A, Akibami FO. Pharmacokinetics of quinine in African children suffering from kwashiorkor. Br J Clin Pharmacol 1989;28:197–201.
34. Lares-Asseff I, Cravioto J, Santigo P, Perex-Ortiz B. Pharmacokinetics of metronidazole in severely malnourished and nutritionally rehabilitated children. Clin Pharmacol Ther 1992;51:42–50.
35. Krishnaswamy K. Nutrients/non-nutrients and drug metabolism. Drug Nutr Interact 1985;4:235–47.
36. Fishman J, Bradlow HL. Effect of malnutrition on the metabolism of sex hormones in man. Clin Pharmacol Ther 1977;22:721–7.
37. Prasad KVS, Rao BSN, Sivakumar B, et al. Pharmacokinetics of norethinodrone in Indian women. Contraception 1979;20:77–90.
38. Boudreaux JP, Hayes DH, Mizrahi S, et al. Use of water-soluble E to enhance cyclosporine absorption in children after liver transplant. Transplant Proc 1993;25:1975.
39. Park GD, Spector R, Kitt TM. Effect of dietary protein on renal tubular clearance of drugs in humans. Clin Pharmacokinet 1989;17:441–51
40. Alleyne GA. The effect of severe protein calorie malnutrition on renal function of Jamaican children. Pediatrics 1967;39:400–11.
41. Cuddy PG, Bealer JF, Lyman EL, Pemberton B. Theophylline disposition following parenteral feeding of malnourished patients. Ann Pharmacother 1993;28:836–7.
42. Brinksman GI, Bowie MD, Friis-Hansen B, Hansen JDL. Body water composition in kwashiorkor before and after loss of edema. Pediatrics 1965;36:94–103.
43. Lares-Asseff I, Flores-Perez J, Juarez-Olguin H, et al. Influence of nutritional status on the pharmacokinetics of acetylsalicylic acid and its metabolites in children with autoimmune disease. Am J Clin Nutr 1999;69:318–24.
44. Johansson V, Portinsson S, Akesson A, et al. Nutritional status in girls with juvenile chronic arthritis. Hum Nutr Clin Nutr 1986;40:57–67.
45. Feldman CH, Huthinson VE, Pigpenger CE, et al. Effect of dietary protein and carbohydrate on theophylline metabolism in children. Pediatrics 1980;66:956–62.
46. Zarowtiz B, Pilla A, Popovich J. Expended gentamicin volume of distribution in patients with indicators of malnutrition. Clin Pharm 1990;9:40–4.
47. Naran RK, Mehta S, Mathur BS. Pharmacokinetics study of antipyrine in malnourished children. Am J Clin Nutr 1977;30:1979–82.
48. Treluyer JM, Roux A, Mugnier C, et al. Metabolism of quinine in children with global malnutrition. Pediatr Res 1996;40:558–63.
49. World Health Organization. Management of Severe Malnutrition: A Manual for Physicians and Other Senior Health Workers. Geneva: WHO; 1999.
50. Abernathy DR, Greenblatt DJ. Drug disposition in obesehumans: An update. Clin Pharmacokinet 1986;11:199–213.
51. Strauss SG, Lynn AM, Bratton SL, Nespeca MK. Ventilatory response to CO_2 in children with obstructive sleep apnea from adenotonsillar hypertrophy. Anesth Analg 1999;89:328–32.
52. Blouin RA, Kolpek JH, Mann HJ. Influences of obesity on drug disposition. Clin Pharm 1987;6:706–14.
53. Schwartz SN, Pazin GJ, Lyon JA, Ho M. A controlled investigation of the pharmacokinetics of gentamicin and tobramycin in obese patients. J Infect Dis 1978;138:499–505.
54. Traub SL, Johnson CE. Comparison of methods of estimating creatinine clearance in children. Am J Hosp Pharm 1980;37:195–201.
55. Visram N, Friesen EG, Jamali F. Theophylline loading dose in obese patients. Clin Pharm 1987;6:188–9.
56. Emery MG, Fisher JM, Chien JY, et al. CYP2E1 activity before and after weight loss in morbidly obese subjects with nonalcoholic fatty liver disease. Hepatology. 2003;38:428–35.
57. Lieber CS. CYP2E1: From ASH to NASH. Hepatol Res 2004;28:1–11.
58. Corcoran GB, Salazar DE. Obesity as a risk factor in drug-induced organ injury. IV. Increased gentamycin nephrotoxicity in the obese overfed rat. J Pharmacol Exp Ther 1989;248:17–22.
59. Evans AM. Influence of dietary components on the gastrointestinal metabolism and transport of drugs. Ther Drug Monit 2000;22:131–6.
60. Fleisher D, Li C, Zhou Y, et al. Drug, meal and formulation inter-actions influencing drug absorption after oral administration. Clinical implications. Clin Pharmacokinet 1999;36:233–54.
61. Vessell ES. Complex effects of diet on drug disposition. Clin Pharmacol Ther 1984;36:285–96.
62. Ioannides C. Effect of diet and nutrition on the expression of cytochrome P450. Xenobiotica 1999;29:109–54.
63. Kappas A, Anderson KE, Conney AH, et al. Influence of dietary protein and carbohydrate on antipyrine and theophylline metabolism in man. Clin Pharmacol Ther 1976;20:643–53.
64. Kappas A, Alvares AP, Anderson KE, et al. Effect of charcoal broiled beef on antipyrine and theophylline metabolism. Clin Pharmacol Ther 1978;23:445–50.
65. Conney AH. Pharmacological implications of microsomal enzyme induction. Pharmacol Res 1967;19:317–66.
66. Welling PG, Lyons LL, Craig WA, Trochta GA. Influence of diet and fluid on bioavailability of theophylline. Clin PharmacolTher 1975;17:475–80.
67. Gura KM. Drug-nutrient interactions. In: Hendricks KM, Duggan C, editors. Manual of Pediatric Nutrition, 4th edition. Hamilton, ON: BC Decker; 2005.
68. Schwartz JG, McMahan CA, Green GM, Phillips WT. Gastric emptying in Mexican Americans compared to non-Hispanic whites. Dig Dis Sci 1995;40:624–30.
69. Melander A, Danielson K, Schersten B, Wahlin E. Enhancement of the bioavailability of propranolol and metoprolol by food. Clin Pharmcol Ther 1977;22:108–12.
70. Nutt JG, Woodward WR, Hammerstad JP, et al. The "on-off" phenomenon in Parkinson's disease. Relation to levodopa absorption and transport. N Engl J Med 1984;310:483–8.
71. Bailey DG, Spence JD, Munoz C, et al. Interaction of citrus juices with felodipine and nifedipine. Lancet 1991;337:268–9.
72. Corthesy-Theulaz I, den Dunnen JT, Ferre P, et al. Nutrigenomics: The impact of biomics technology on nutrition research. Ann Nutr Metab 2005;49:355–65.
73. Williams L, David JA, Lowenthal DT. The influence of food on the absorption and metabolism of drugs. Med Clin North Am 1993;77:815–29.
74. Sonawane BR, Coates PN, Yaffe SJ, et al. Influence of dietary carbohydrates (alpha-saccharides) on hepatic drug metabolism in male rats. Drug Nutr Interact 1983;2:7–16.
75. Anderson KE. Influences on diet and nutrition on clinical pharmacokinetics. 1988;14:325–46.
76. Cantarini MV, Painter CJ, Gilmore EM, et al. Effect of oral linezolid on thepressor response to intravenous tyramine. Br J Cln Pharmacol 2004;58:470–5.
77. Singh BN. Effects of food on clinical pharmacokinetics. Clin Pharmacokinet 1999;37:213–55.
78. Guengerich FB. Effects of nutritive factors on metabolic processes involving bioactivation and detoxification of chemicals. Annu Rev Nutr 1984;4:207–31.
79. Zimmerman JJ, Ferron GM, Lim HK, Parker V. The effect of a high-fat meal on the oral bioavailability of the immunosuppressant sirolimus (rapamycin). J Clin Pharmacol 1999;39:1155–61.
80. Murray M. Altered CYP expression and function in response to dietary factors: Potential roles in disease pathogenesis. Curr Drug Metab 2006;7:67–81.

81. Singh BN. Effects of food on clinical pharmacokinetics. Clin Pharmacokinet 1999;37:213–55.
82. Zhi J, Rakhit A, Patel IH. Effects of dietary fat on drug absorption. Clin Pharmacol Ther 1995;58:487–91.
83. Tan KKC, Trull AK, Uttridge JA, et al. Effect of dietary fat on the pharmacokinetics and pharmacodynamics of cyclosporine in kidney transplant recipients. Clin Pharmacol Ther 1995;57:425–33.
84. Zimmerman JJ, Ferron GM, Lim HK, Parker V. The effect of a high-fat meal on the oral bioavailability of the immunosuppressant sirolimus (rapamycin). J Clin Pharmacol 1999;39:1155–61.
85. Unadkat JD, Collier AC, Crosby SS, et al. Pharmacokinetics of oral zidovudine (azidothymidine) in paients with AIDS when administered with and without a high fat meal. AIDS 1990;4:229–32.
86. Bidlack WR, Brown RC, Mohan C. Nutritional parameters that alter hepatic drug metabolism, conjugation, and toxicity.Fed Proc 1986;45:142–8.
87. Lampe JW. Health effects of vegetables and fruit: Assessing mechanisms of action in human experimental studies. Am J Clin Nutr 1999;70:475S–90S.
88. Sreerama L, Hedge MW, Sladek NE. Identification of a class 3 aldehyde dehydrogenase in human saliva and increased levels of this enzyme, glutathione S-transferases, and DT-diaphorase in the saliva of subjects who continually ingest large quantities of coffee or broccoli. Clin Cancer Res 1995;1:1153–63.
89. Pantuck EJ, Pantuck CB, Anderson KE, et al. Effect of brussels sprouts and cabbage on drug conjugation. Clin Pharmaco Ther 1984;35:161–9.
90. Pantuck EJ, Pantuck CB, Garland WA, et al. Stimulatory effect of brussels sprouts and cabbage on human drug metabolism. Clin Pharmacol Ther 1979;25:88–95.
91. Tanne JH. Food and drugs alter response to anaesthesia. BMJ 1998 24;317:1102.
92. Bailey DG, Spence JD, Edgar B, et al. Ethanol enhances the hemodynamic effects of felodipine. Clin Invest Med 1989;12:357–62.
93. D'Arcy PF. Nutrient-drug interactions. Adverse Drug React Toxicol Rev 1995;14:233–54.
94. Zvaifler NJ, Rath CE. Interrelationship of rheumatoid arthritis, folic acid, and aspirin. Blood 1971;38:405–16.
95. Richter WO, Jacob BG, Schwandt P. Interaction between fibre and lovastatin. Lancet 1991;338:706.
96. Stewart DE. High-fiber diet and serum tricyclic antidepressant levels. J Clin Psychopharmacol 1992;12:438–40.
97. Champagne ET. Low gastric hydrochloric acid secretion and mineral bioavailability. Adv Exp Med Biol 1989;249:173–84.
98. Kappas A, Alvares AP, Anderson KE, et al. Effect of charcoal broiled beef on antipyrine and theophylline metabolism. Clin Pharmacol Ther 1978;23:445–50.
99. Muclow JC, Caraher MT, Henderson DB, Rawlins MB. The effect of individual dietary constituents on antipyrine clearance in Asian immigrants. Br J Clin Pharmacol 1979;7:416–7.
100. Brodie MJ, Boobis AR, Toverud EL, et al. Drug metabolism in white vegetarians. Br J Clin Pharmacol 1980;9:523–5.
101. Rose DP. Dietary fiber, phytoestrogens, and breast cancer. Nutrition 1992;8:47–51.
102. Michnovicz JJ, Bradlow HL. Induction of estradiol metabolism by dietary indole-3-carbinol in humans. J Natl Cancer Inst 1990;82:947–9.
103. Alonso-Aperte E, Varela-Moreiras G. Drugs-nutrient interactions: A potential problem during adolescence. Eur J Clin Nutr 2000;54:S69–74.
104. Anderson KE. Influences of diet and nutrition on clinical pharmacokinetics. Clin Pharmacokinet. 1988;14:325–46.
105. Sonne J, Dragsted J, Loft S, et al. Influence of a very low calorie diet on the clearance of oxazepam and antipyrine in man. Eur J Clin Pharmacol 1989;36:407–9.
106. Corcoran GB, Salazar DE. Obesity as a risk factor in drug-induced organ injury. IV. Increased gentamicin nephrotoxicity in the obese overfed rat. J Pharmacol Exp Ther 1989;248:17–22.
107. Schenker S, Speeg KV Jr, Perez A, Finch J. The effects of food restriction in man on hepatic metabolism of acetaminophen. Clin Nutr 2001;20:145–50.
108. Bennett WM. Drug interactions and consequences of sodium restriction. Am J Clin Nutr 1997;65:678S–81S.
109. Singh BN. Effects of food on clinical pharmacokinetics. Clin Pharmacokinet. 1999;37:213–55.
110. Bistiran BR, Blackburn G, Vitalie J, et al. Prevalence of malnutrition in general medical patients. JAMA 1976;235:1567–70.
111. Pantuck EJ, Pantuck CB, Weissman C, et al. Effects of parenteral nutritional regimens on oxidative drug metabolism. Anesthesiology 1984;60:534–6.
112. Burgess P, Hall RI, Bateman DN, Johnston ID. The effect of total parenteral nutrition on hepatic drug oxidation. JPEN J Parenter Enteral Nutr 1987;11:540–3.
113. Knapp HR. Nutrient-drug interactions. In: Ziegler EF, Filer LJ, editors. Present Knowledge in Nutrition. Washington, DC: ILSI Pres; 1996. p. 540–6.
114. Roe DA. Drug-folate interrelationships: Historical aspects and current concerns. In: Picciano MF, Stokstad ELP, Gregory JF III, editors. Folic acid metabolism in health and disease, New York: Wiley-Liss; 1990. p. 91–120.
115. Chan L-N. Redefining drug–nutrient interactions. Nutr Clin Pract 2000;15:249–52.
116. Alonso-Aperte E, Varela-Moreiras G. Drugs–nutrient interactions: A potential problem during adolescence. Eur J Clin Nutr 2000;54:S69–74.
117. Streiff RR. Anemia and nutritional deficiency in the acutely ill hospitalized patients. Med Clin North Am 1993;77:911–8.
118. Cohen H, Scott D, Mackis IJ, et al. The development of hypoprothrombinema following antibiotic therapy in malnourished patients with low serum vitamin K levels. Br J Haematol 1988;68:63–6.
119. Gura KM, Couris RR. Drug-induced bone disease. US Pharmacist 2002;27:HS43–57
120. Dobbins WO, 3rd, Herrero BA, Mansbach CM. Morphologic alterations associated with neomycin induced malabsorption. Am J Med Sci 1968;255:63–77.
121. Black DA, Fraser CM. Iron deficiency anaemia and aspirin use in old age. Br J Gen Pract 1999;49:729–30.
122. Tolstoi LG. Nutritional problems related to stimulant laxative abuse. Hosp Pharm 1988;23:564–73.
123. Schindler AM. Isolated neonatal hypomagnesaemia associated with maternal overuse of stool softener [letter]. Lancet 1984;ii:822.
124. Clark JH, Russell GJ, Fitzgerald JF, et al. Serum beta-carotene, retinol, and alpha-tocopherol levels during mineral oil therapy for constipation. Am J Dis Child 1987;141:1210–2.
125. Thomas FB, McCullough FS, Greenberger NJ. Inhibition of the intestinal absorption of inorganic and hemoglobin iron by cholestyramine. J Lab Clin Med 1971;78:70–80.
126. Aou S, Ma J, Shiramine K, Hori T. The stomach is the etiologic organ for immobilization-induced hypocalcemia in rats. Am J Physiol 1993;265:376–9.
127. Walan A, Strom M. Metabolic consequences of reduced gastric acidity. Scand J Gastroenterol Suppl 1985;111:24–30.
128. Ruscin JM, Page RL, 2nd, Valuck RJ. Vitamin B(12) deficiency associated with histamine(2)-receptor antagonists and a proton-pump inhibitor. Ann Pharmacother. 2002;36:812–6.
129. Romero JA, Kuczler FJ, Jr. Isoniazid overdose: Recognition and management. Am Fam Physician 1998;57:749–52.
130. Corcino J, Waxman S, Herbert V. Mechanism of triamtereneinduced megaloblastosis. Ann Intern Med 1970;73:419.
131. Palomaki A, Malminiemi K, Solakivi T, Malminiemi O. Ubiquinone supplementation during lovastatin treatment: Effect on LDL oxidation ex vivo. J Lipid Res 1998;39:1430–7.
132. Williams C, Netzloff M, Folkerts L, et al. Vitamin D metabolism and anticonvulsant therapy: Effect of sunshine on incidence of osteomalacia. South Med J 1984;77:834–6.
133. Hahn TJ, Avioli LV. Anticonvulsant-drug-induced mineral disorders. In: Roe DA, Campbell TC, editors. Drugs and Nutrients: The Interactive Effects, New York: Marcel Dekker; 1984.
134. Keith DA, Gundbeg CM, Japour A, et al. Vitamin K-dependent protein and anticonvulsant medication. Clin Pharmacol Ther 1983;34:529–32.
135. Reddy J, Bailey RR. Vitamin K deficiency developing in patients with renal failure, treated with cephalosporin antibiotics. N Z Med J 1980;92:378–9.
136. New example of vitamin K-drug interactin [editiorial] Nutr Rev 1984;42:161–3.
137. Lambie DG, Johnson RH. Drugs and folate metabolism. Drugs 185;30:145–55.
138. Labadarios D. The effect of chronic drug administration on folate status and drug toxicity. In: Parks DV, Ioannides C, Walker R, editors. Food, Nutrition and Chemical Toxicity. London: Smith-Gordon; 1993
139. Mallek HM, Nakamoto T. Dilantin and folic acid status. Clinical implications for the periodontist. J Periodontol 1981;52:255–9.
140. Rivey MP, Schottelius DD, Berg MJ. Phenytoin-folic acid: A review. Drug Intell Clin Pharm 1984;18:292–301.
141. Lewis DP, Van Dyke DC, Wilhite LA, et al. Phenytoin-folic acid interaction. Ann Pharmacother 1995;29:726–35.
142. Seligmann H, Potasman I, Weller B, et al. Phenytoin-folic acid interaction: A lesson to be learned. Clin Neuropharmacol 1999;22:268–72.
143. Hoshino J, Sugawara K, Ishikawa S, et al. A case of ulcerative colitis with folate deficient megaloblastic anemia induced by sulfasalazine. Nippon Shokakibyo Gakkai Zasshi 1999;96:840–5.
144. Selhub J, Seyoum E, Pomfret EA, Zeisel SH. Effects of choline deficiency and methotrexate treatment upon liver folate content and distribution. Cancer Res 1991;51:16–21.
145. Wegner C, Nau H. Alteration of embryonic folate metabolism by valproic acid during organogenesis: Implications for mechanism of teratogenesis. Neurology 1992;42:17–24.
146. Ubed N, Alonso E, Martin-Rodriguez JC, et al. Valproic induced developmental modifications may be partially prevented by coadministration of folinic acid and S-adenosylmethionine. Int J Dev Biol 1996;40:291S–2S.
147. Ohtani Y, Endo F, Matsuda I. Carnitine deficiency with hyperammonemia associated with valproic acid therapy. J Pediatr 1982;101:782–5.
148. Branda RF, Nelson NL. Inhibition of 5-methyltetrahydrolic acid transport by amphipathic drugs. Drug Nutr Interact 1981;1:45–53.
149. Seligmann H, Halkin H, Rauchefleisch S, et al. Thiamine deficiency in patients with congestive heart failure receiving long-term furosemide therapy: A pilot study. Am J Med 1991;91:151–5.
150. Brady JA, Rock CL, Horneffer MR. Thiamine status, diuretic medications, and the management of congestive heart failure. J Am Diet Assoc 1995;95:541–4.
151. Sonneblick M, Friedlander Y, Rosin AJ. Diuretic-induced severe hyponatremia. Review and analysis of 129 reported patients. Chest 1993;103:601–6.
152. Lahr MB. Hyponatremia during carbamazepine therapy. Clin Pharmacol Ther 1985;37:693–6.
153. Nelson DC, McGrew WR, Hoyumpa AM. Hypernatremia and lactulose therapy. JAMA 1983;249:1295–8.
154. Tolstoi LG. Drug-induced hyperkalemia. Hosp Pharm 1996;31:221–8.
155. Velazquez H, Perazella MA, Wright FR, Ellison DH. Renal mechanism of trimethoprim-induced hyperkalemia. Ann Intern Med 1993;119:296–301.
156. Oster JR, Singer I, Fishman LM. Heparin-induced aldosterone suppression and hyperkalemia. Am J Med 1995;98:575–86.
157. Brown GR, Greenwood JK. Drug- and nutrition-induced hypophosphatemia: Mechanisms and relevance in the critically ill. Ann Pharmacother 1994;28:626–32.
158. Odes HS, Fraser GM, Krugliak P, et al. Effect of cimetidine on hepatic vitamin D metabolism in humans. Digestion 1990;20:251–62.
159. LoCascio V, Bonucci E, Imbinbo B, et al. Bone loss in response to long term glucocorticoid therapy. Bone Miner 1990;8:39–51.
160. Isreal E, Banerjee TR, Fitzmaurice GM, et al. Effects of inhaled glucocorticoids on bone density in premenopausal women. N Engl J Med 2001;345:941–7.
161. al-Ghamdi SM, Cameron EC, Sutton RA. Magnesium deficiency: Pathophysiologic and clinical overview. Am J Kidney Dis 1994;24:737–52.
162. Maviachak V, Coppin CM, Wong NL, et al. Renal magnesium wasting and hypocalcemia in chronic cis-platinum nephropathy in man. Clin Sci 1988;75:203–7.
163. Forastiere AA, Belliveau JF, Goren MP, et al. Pharmacokinetic and toxicity evaluation of five-day evaluation of five day continuous infusion versus intermittent bolus cisdiamminedichloroplatinum III) in head and neck cancer patients. Cancer Res 1988;48:3869–74.
164. Ferra C. Berlanga JJ, Gallardo D, et al. Mitoxantreone, etoposide, carboplatinum and Ara-C combination therapy in refractory and relapsed acute leukemia. Leuk Lymphoma 2000;39:583–90.
165. Shetty AK, Rogers NI, Mannick EE, Aviles DH. Syndrome of hypokalemic metabolic alkalosis and hypomagnesemia associated with gentamicin therapy: Case reports. Clin Pediatr 2000;39:529–33.
166. Arlette JP. Zinc and the skin. Pediatr Clin North Am 1983;30:583–96.
167. Prasad AS. Clinical, biochemical and pharmacological role of zinc. Annu Rev Pharmacol Toxicol 1979;2:393–426.
168. Prasad AS, Brewer GJ, Schoomaker EB, et al. Hypocupremia induced by zinc therapy in adults. JAMA 1978;240:2166–8.
169. Solomons NW. Zinc and copper in human nutrition: Nutrition in the 1980's: Constraints on our knowledge. New York: Alan R. Liss; 1981.
170. Ugarte M, Osborne NN. Zinc in the retina. Prog Neurobiol 2001;64:219–49.
171. Michie DD, Wirth FH. Plasma zinc levels in premature infants receiving parenteral nutrition. J Pediatr 1978;92:798–800.
172. Pandit MK, Burke J, Gustafson AB, et al. Drug-induced disorders of glucose tolerance. Ann Intern Med 1993;118: 529–39.
173. Shopbell JM, Hopkins B, Shronts EP. Nutritional screening and assessment. In: Gotschlich MM, editor. ASPEN core curriculum. Dubuque, IA: Kendall/Hunt; 2001. p. 107–40.
174. Kaufman MG, Simionatto C. A review of protease inhibitor-induced hyperglycemia. Pharmacotherapy 1999;19:114–7.
175. Plewe G, Beyer J, Krause U, et al. Long-acting and selective suppression of growth hormone secretion b somatostatin analogue SMS 201–995 in acromegaly. Lancet 1984;ii:782–4.

176. O'Brien JG, Dong BJ, Coleman RL, et al. A 5-year retrospective review of adverse drug reactions and their risk factors in human immunodeficiency virus-infected patients who were receiving intravenous pentamidine therapy for pneumocystis carinii pneumonia. Clin Infect Dis 1997;24:854–9.
177. Coyle P, Carr AD, Depczynski BB, et al. Diabetes mellitus associated with pentamidine use in HIV-infected patients. Med J Aust 1996;165:587–8.
178. Mills GA, Horn JR. Beta-blockers and glucose control. Drug Intell Clin Pharm 1985;19:246–51.
179. Henkin J, Como JA, Oberman A. Secondary dyslipidemia: Inadvertent effects of drugs in clinical practice. JAMA 1992;267:961–8.
180. Korach M, Leclercq P, Peronnet F, Leverve X. Metabolic response to a C-glucose load in human immunodeficiency virus patients before and after antiprotease therapy. Metab Clin Exp 2002;51:307–13.
181. Jain RG, Furfine ES, Pedneault L, et al. Metabolic complications associated with antiretroviral therapy. Antiviral Res 2001;51:151–77.
182. Parsons SK, Skapek S, Neufeld EJ, et al. Asparaginase-associated lipid abnormalities in children with acute lymphoblastic leukemia. Blood 1997;89:1886–95.
183. Baker VL. Alternatives to oral estrogen replacement. Transdermal patches, percutaneous gels, vaginal creams and rings, implants, other methods of delivery. Obstet Gynecol Clin North Am 1994;21:271–97.
184. Bonavina L, Demeester TR, McChesney L, et al. Drug-induced esophageal strictures. Ann Surg 1987;206:173–83.
185. Welling PG. Effects of food on drug absorption. Annu Rev Nutr 1996;16:383–415.
186. Leong RW, Chan FK. Drug–induced side effects affecting the gastrointestinal tract. Expert Opin Drug Sat 2006;5:585–92.
187. Herzog P, Holtermuller KH. Antacid therapy—changes in mineral metabolism. Scand J Gastroenterol Suppl 1982;75:56–62.
188. Kinzie BJ. Management of the syndrome of inappropriate secretion of antidiuretic hormone. Clin Pharm 1987;6:625–33.
189. Dreizen S, McCredie KB, Keating MJ, Andersson BS. Nutritional deficiencies in patients receiving cancer chemotherapy. Postgrad Med 1990;87:163–7.
190. Knudsen L, Weismann K. Taste dysfunction and changes in zinc and copper metabolism during penicillamine therapy for generalized scleroderma. Acta Med Scand 1978;204:75–9.
191. Belle M, Halpern MM. Oral nicotinic acid for hyperlipidemia with emphasis on side effects. Am J Cardiol 1985;2:449–52.
192. Heyneman CA. Zinc deficiency and taste disorders. Ann Pharmacother 1996;30:186–7.
193. Sheth RD, Gidal BE. Optimizing epilepsy management in teenagers. J Child Neurol. 2006;21:273–9
194. Wilcox JC, Car J, Shaw J, et al. Prednisolone as an appetite stimulant in patients with cancer. BMJ 1984;288:27.
195. Moertel CG, Schutt AJ, Reitemeier RJ, Hahn RG. Corticosteroid therapy of preterminal gastrointestinal cancer. Cancer 1974;33:1607–9.
196. Bruera E, Roca E, Cedaro L, et al. Action of oral methylprednisolone in terminal cancer patients: A prospective randomized double-blind study. Cancer Treat Rep 1985;69:751–4.
197. Nobel RE. Effect of cyproheptadine on appetite and weight gain in adults. JAMA 1969;209:2054–5.
198. Oster MH. Megestrol acetate in patients with AIDS and cachexia. Ann Intern Med 1994;121:400–8.
199. Leinung MC, Liporace R, Miller CH. Induction of adrenal suppression by megestrol acetate in patients with AIDS. Ann Intern Med 1995;122:843–5.
200. McCarthy HD, Crowder RE, Dryden S, et al. Megestrol acetate stimulates food and water intake in the rat: Effects on regional hypothalamic neuropeptide-y concentration. Eur J Pharmacol 1994;265:99–102.
201. Plasse TF, Gorter RW, Krasnow SH, et al. Recent clinical experience with dronabinol. Pharmacol Biochem Behav 1991;40:695–700.
202. Hellerstein MK, Meydani SN, Meydani M, et al. Interleukin-1-induced anorexia in the rat. Influence of prostaglandins. J Clin Invest 1989;84:228–35.
203. Mulrooney HM, Grimble RF. Influence of butter and of corn, coconut and fish oils on the effect of recombinant human tumour necrosis factor alpha in rats. Clin Sci 1993;84:105–7.
204. Silverstone T, Goodalle E. Centrally acting anorectic drugs: A clinical perspective. Am J Clin Nutr 1992;55:211S–4S.
205. Landsberg L, Young JB. Sympathoadrenal activity and obesity: Physiological rationale for the use of adrenergic thermogenic drugs. Int J Obes Relat Metab Disord 1993;17:S29–34.
206. Uzzan B, Campos J, Cucherat M, et al. Effects on bone mass of long term treatment with thyroid hormones: A metaanalysis. J Clin Endocrinol Metab 1996;81:4278–89.
207. Ban TA. Pharmacotherapy of schizophrenia with special reference to megavitamin therapy. Can J Psychiatr Nurs 1973;14:6–9.
208. Dipalma JR. Vitamin toxicity. Am Fam Physician 1978;18:106–9.
209. On the toxicity of water-soluble vitamins. Nutr Rev 1984;42:265–7.
210. Beattie AD, Sherlock S. Ascorbic acid deficiency in liver disease. Gut 1976;17:571–5.
211. Herbert VD. Megavitamin therapy. J Am Pharm Assoc 1977;17:764–6.
212. Cochrane W. Overnutrition in prenatal and neonatal life. Can Med Assoc J 1965;93:893–9.
213. Herbert V, Jacob E. Destruction of vitamin B_{12} by ascorbic acid. JAMA 1974;230:241–2.
214. Auer BK, Auer D, Rodgers AL. Relative hyperoxaluria, crystalluria and haematuria after megadose ingestion of vitamin C. Eur J Clin Invest 1998;28:695–700.
215. Schaumburg H, Kaplan J, Winderbank A, et al. Sensory neuropathy from pyridoxine abuse. N Engl J Med 1983;309:445–8.
216. Ch'ien LT, Krumdieck CL, Scott CW, Jr, Butterworth CE, Jr. Harmful effect of megadoses of vitamins: Electroencephalogram abnormalities and seizures induced by intravenous folate in drug-treated epileptics. Am J Clin Nutr 1975;28:51–8.
217. Makki KA, Perucca E, Richens A. Stimulation of drug metabolism by folate replacement in folate-deficient epileptic patients. Br J Clin Pharmacol 1980;9:304–5.
218. Andreason PB, Hansen JM, Skovsted L, et al. Folic acid and the half-life of diphenylhydantoin in man. Acta Neurol Scand 1971;47:117–9.
219. Rodriguez-Matas MC, Campos MS, Lopez-Aliaga I, et al. Iron-manganese interactions in the evolution of iron deficiency. Ann Nutr Metab 1998;42:96–109.
220. Nako Y, Fukushima N, Tomomasa T, et al. Hypervitaminosis D after prolonged feeding with a premature formula. Pediatrics 1993;92:862–4.
221. Gamble JG, Ip SC. Hypervitaminosis A in a child from mega dosing. J Pediatr Orthoped 1985;5:219–21.
222. Arroyave G, Bauemfeind JC, Olson JA, Underwood BA. Selection of intervention strategies. In: Guidelines for the eradication of vitamin A deficiency and xeropthalmia. Report of the International Vitamin A Consultative Group. Washington, DC: The Nutrition Foundation; 1976. p. 1–8.
223. Jeghers H, Marro H, Hypervitaminosis A. Its broadening spectrum. Am J Clin Nutr 1958;6:335–72.
224. Yaffe SJ, Filer LJ, Jr. Use and abuse of vitamin A. Pediatrics 1971;48:655–6.
225. Chesney RW. Requirement and upper limits of vitamin D intake in the term neonate, infant and older child. J Pediatr 1990;116:19–66.
226. Haddad JG. Vitamin D solar rays, the Milky Way or both? N Engl J Med 1992;326:1213–5.
227. British Pediatric Association. Hypercalcemia in infants and vitamin D. BMJ 1956;2:149–55.
228. Malloy PJ, Pike JW, Feldman D. The vitamin D receptor and the syndrome of hereditary 1,25-dihydroxyvitamin D-resistant rickets. Endocrine Rev 1999;20:156–88.
229. Taketomo CK, Hodding JH, Kraus DM. Pediatric Dosage Hand Book, 8th edition. Cleveland, OH: Lexi-Comp Inc. Hudson (Cleveland); 2001.
230. Blank S, Scanolon KS, Sinks TH, Falk H. An outbreak of hypervitaminosis D associated with overfortification of milk from a home-delivery dairy. Am J Public Health 1995;85:656–9.
231. Jacobus CH, Holick MF, Shao Q, et al. Hypervitaminosis D associated with drinking milk.N Engl J Med 1992;326:1173–7.
232. US Food and Drug Administration, Center for Food Safety and Applied Nutrition. Washington, Mailgram, May 4, 1992.
233. Stirling Y. Warfarin-induced changes in procoagulant and anticoagulant proteins. Blood Coagul Fibrinolysis 1995;6:361–73.
234. Lutomski DM, Palascak JE, Bower RH. Warfarin resistance associated with intravenous lipid administration. JPEN J Parenter Enteral Nutr 1987;11:316–8.

II PHYSIOLOGY AND PATHOPHYSIOLOGY

19 Nutrition and Gene Expression

Mona Bajaj-Elliott, BSc, PhD
Ian R. Sanderson, MD, MSc, MRCP

Altering the expression of genes has become a rapidly evolving area of research in medicine. The realization that gene expression is important in a wide range of diseases, and not just in inherited disease, has resulted in recognition of the whole field of gene expression as one that may bring new therapeutic options. Although more recent attention has focused on the benefits of altering gene expression by inserting new genetic material into cells by a variety of vectors, the expression of genes can also be altered by other means, most notably by changing the molecular environment that cells inhabit. Utilizing the natural responses of a cell to changes in its surroundings offers a new and amenable way to alter the expression of its genes. Many ways of altering these surroundings can be proposed, but no single act alters the environment of the cells of the body more than the ingestion of food. Thus, the future of nutrition as a therapeutic tool may lie in its potential for influencing gene regulation. This chapter will examine this emerging field and will lay down some concepts that may prove useful in establishing the scientific basis from which future treatments may develop.

The survival of a child to reproductive age and beyond requires an ability to respond to external demands. Every organ in the body is attuned to this need. Many organ systems have two levels of response to external changes. There is a rapid response, often occurring within seconds of a new stimulus, for example, contraction of muscle fibers following a neuronal impulse or the breakdown of glycogen by the liver during hypoglycemia. Such responses do not involve changes in gene expression. The cells maintain themselves in a state of readiness, responding rapidly to external stimuli by altering protein/ion activity. Behind this immediate response, there lie other slower, but more lasting, responses that require genetic control. For example, exercise on a regular basis not only leads to muscle mass increase, but change in activity of the attendant enzymes that serve the increased metabolic need also occurs. Similarly, regular exposure of the liver to drugs induces the expression of enzymes that catalyze their breakdown.

There are few external stimuli on a child more important than his or her nutritional environment. The metabolic processes underlying the rapid response of cells to nutritional variations have long been documented in humans and other mammals.[1] However, the mechanisms whereby gene expression changes in response to nutritional stimuli is still poorly understood in humans or indeed in any multiorgan animal. This is, at first, surprising because in bacteria, the study of nutritional changes led to our understanding of some of the most fundamental mechanisms of gene expression. The elucidation of the induction of proteins that transport and hydrolyze lactose (the *lac* operon) after adding lactose to bacterial culture media[2] was the first examination of any form of gene regulation. These observations spawned an explosion of research in other regulatory genes in bacteria and in unicellular, eukaryotic organisms such as yeast. The upregulation of the bacterial genes that handle tryptophan when this amino acid is scarce (the *trp* operon) has become another well-understood example of nutrient–gene interaction.[3]

Progress in the study of nutrient–gene interaction in eukaryotic cells has been slower for two main reasons. First, the molecular mechanisms controlling gene expression are more complex than in bacteria, and second, it is more difficult to identify the metabolites of nutrients that may be responsible for inducing such changes. This review will therefore cover some of the major advances in the study of nutrition and gene expression in the human and, where necessary, in other mammals. Nutritional changes ultimately impinge on most cells in the body; however, it is the epithelium of the gastrointestinal (GI) tract that first encounters any variation in nutrient intake. Much of this chapter will therefore concentrate on how nutritional factors can alter the expression of genes in intestinal epithelial cells. The relevance of nutrient–gene interactions to human physiology will also be stressed. Finally, because manipulating nutritional intake may be a way of treating disease in children, the review will discuss nutritional therapy in childhood in the light of its effects on gene expression.

PHYSIOLOGIC IMPORTANCE OF NUTRITIONAL REGULATION IN GENE EXPRESSION

The effect of nutrients on gene expression may have different implications in different individual situations (Table 1). First, genes may be upregulated to better utilize the supply of a particular nutrient when it is scarce. Transporters of nutrients and the enzymes that metabolize them are examples of proteins that may be induced by nutrients. Second, the expression of genes required for the storage of a particular nutrient may be altered according to that nutrient's abundance. Third, nutrients regulate the secretion of hormones that control the homeostasis of metabolic processes. For example, insulin synthesis increases after increased carbohydrate intake to maintain glucose homeostasis. Finally, food is part of our external environment and, as such, represents a challenge to the cells that come into intimate contact with it. This challenge is met in the main body by the epithelial cell lining of the GI tract.[4] The ability of these cells to alter the expression of their genes with changes in food intake is one of the ways by which the intestinal epithelium senses and modulates the intestinal environment.

Table 1 Physiologic Importance of Nutritional Regulation of Gene Expression

To satisfy the nutritional needs of an organ
To manage storage fuels required by other organs
Production of hormones essential to whole body metabolism
Direct interaction with the body's external environment along the GI tract

Certain fundamental characteristics are found in the mechanisms that underlie each of these different aspects of nutrient–gene interactions. They include (Figure 1) a specific interaction between the cell and a particular nutrient (sensing) and a pathway by which such an interaction may translate into alterations in gene expression (signal transduction). We have little understanding of these mechanisms at present. However, some aspects of the molecular biology of these two functions will be examined later in this chapter.

Genes Controlling the Nutritional Requirements of Individual Organ Systems

Survival of cells depends on their ability to extract nutrients and other essential molecules from their surroundings, and they synthesize proteins specifically for this purpose. Broadly speaking, two categories of genes are involved: those genes that express proteins that transport nutrients across cell membranes and those genes that express enzymes that metabolize nutrients. In

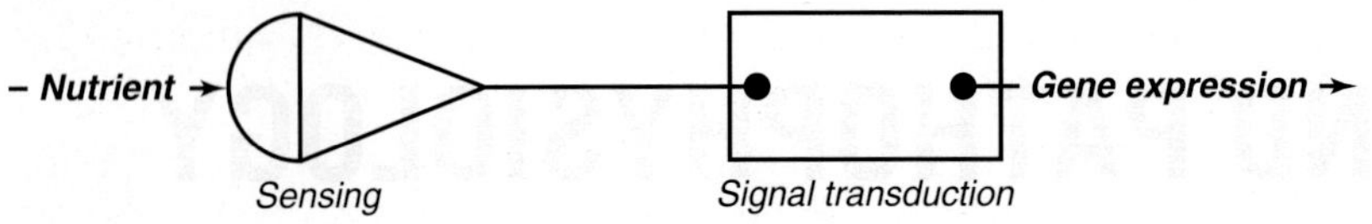

Figure 1 The regulation of gene expression by nutrients requires two generic mechanisms. First, molecules (either receptors or enzymes) within the cell must recognize the nutrient. Second, this interaction must initiate a sequence of events that ultimately alters the transcription or translation of genes. These functions of sensing and signal transduction have been depicted in this diagram using electronic symbols.

both cases, genes are regulated purely to satisfy the requirements of an organ system. This form of gene regulation is similar in concept to the regulatory genes of bacteria like the *trp* operon.[3] The cells are changing their phenotype to their own advantage, rather than to suit the needs of the body as a whole.

A good model of how cells may respond to their nutritional environment for their own needs is the utilization of glutamine by skeletal muscle.[5] Glutamine availability modulates muscle turnover, and glutamine is an important source of amino nitrogen for muscle cells.[6] Glutamine and glutamate are transported into cells by sodium-coupled transporters. For experimental purposes, rat skeletal muscle can be grown as primary cell cultures. These cells exhibit an upregulation in intracellular transport of both glutamine and glutamate when they are deprived of an exogenous glutamine supply.[7–9] In addition, the activity of glutamine synthetase (GS) simultaneously increases. This enzyme catalyzes the addition of an amino group to the carboxyl moiety of the glutamate molecule to form glutamine. Two different nutrients, glutamine and glutamate, can therefore ultimately satisfy the glutamine requirements of the muscle cell through separate pathways, each of which is under genetic control. This system exemplifies how different nutrients can cross-stimulate the expression of a related set of proteins: Removal of glutamine or glutamate from the cell medium results in an enhancement of the transport of both amino acids. Not only does lack of glutamine and glutamate enhance the expression of their own transport proteins, but deprivation of either substrate also upregulates the transporter of the other.[8] A study of the kinetics of transport[9] demonstrated that withdrawal of glutamine (or glutamate) enhanced the maximum rate at which the amino acid is transported into the cell (V_{max}), without altering the affinity of the transporter for its amino acid. This suggests that deprivation resulted in an increase in the production of the number of transporters available. The time required to double the V_{max} was 4 hours. This fact, taken together with the observation that the induction of both glutamate and glutamine transporters was lost when glutamine was withdrawn in the presence of actinomycin D (inhibitor of RNA synthesis), indicates that their regulation is mediated through the initiation of transcription.

In recent years there has been an explosion in our understanding of the physiology of glutamine transporter systems.[10] At least four distinct families have been identified to date, which include the Na^+-dependent glutamine transporter, system N (SN1), system A (ATA1 and ATA2), system ASC/B, and system y (+)L, the latter encoding for Na^+-independent glutamine transporter genes.[11,12] Molecular characterization of these systems suggest specific roles in glutamine efflux and uptake[12]; however, the exact mechanism(s) by which transport regulates gene expression remain unclear.

In vivo, glutamine homeostasis is to a large extent determined by the activities of GS and glutaminase.[13] Both enzymes exhibit regulation of gene expression at both transcriptional and post-transcriptional levels. During stress and sepsis, glutamine production is enhanced primarily due to greater GS activity in the skeletal muscle.[14] Beneficial effects of glutamine during sepsis include amelioration of endotoxin-induced chemokine production, a process that is associated with signal transducer of activator of transcription-4 (STAT-4) transcription activity.[15]

Although glutamine regulates the expression of health-promoting proteins in the gut epithelia,[16] overall the glutamate/glutamine circuit constitutes only a minor part of nutrient homeostasis in vivo. Glucose, on the other hand, is central to human metabolism. Glucose, galactose, and fructose are the major dietary saccharides and the derangement of glucose handling in diabetes mellitus constitutes the most common condition requiring nutritional advice. Intensive research in the last two decades has revealed the great complexity involved in glucose transport. Glucose is transported into enterocytes primarily by the sodium–glucose cotransporter (SGLT-1). Two Na^+ ions must first bind to the transporter and then one molecule of glucose or galactose may be actively transported into the cell. To date, 11 members of the SGLT-1 family in humans have been identified on the basis of sequence homology within the human genome.[17] Efforts to curb the ever-burgeoning epidemics of diabetes and obesity have made dietary manipulation and therefore the SGLT family is an attractive therapeutic target.[18] One must also not forget that oral rehydration therapy (ORT) developed to treat diarrheal dehydration is intimately linked with carbohydrate digestion. The therapy relies on the ability of SGLT-1 to cotransport water without affecting Na^+ or glucose uptake. In addition to SGLT proteins, facilitative diffusion glucose transporter (GLUT) proteins catalyze glucose transport into cells. Several mammalian GLUT proteins have been identified, each a separate gene product with unique properties.[19] GLUT-1, -3, and -4 can transport glucose and galactose but not fructose, GLUT-2 can transport all three, whereas GLUT-5 and -7 recognize fructose.[19–21] The GLUT family can be divided into three groups: class I (the previously known glucose transporters GLUT1-4), class II (GLUT-5, -7, -9, and -11), and class III (GLUT-6, -8, -10, and -12 and the myo-inositol transporter HMIT1). The various members exhibit both tissue and subcellular specificity, which most likely represents another level of regulation. (See reference 22 for a recent review.) Analysis of GLUT protein levels in patients with non–insulin-dependent diabetes mellitus revealed a four- to fivefold induction in SGLT-1, GLUT-2, and GLUT-5 protein levels, highlighting dysregulation in monosaccharide transport.[23] Identity of mechanism(s) by which these essential dietary carbohydrates directly affect their own uptake (via availability of GLUT and SGLT proteins) is most urgent if we are to understand the marked increase in the incidence of childhood obesity and diabetes facing the developed world.[22,24]

Genes Regulating the Storage of Nutrients

The storage of nutrients is essential to provide energy in times of fasting, and the mechanisms that control this function must be regulated by nutrient intake to be effective. The two most important organs involved in nutrient storage are the liver and adipose tissue. Both cell types transport glucose and other nutrients and convert them into fat; in the case of the liver, glucose is also converted to glycogen. Insulin is the major hormone that promotes glucose utilization and induces storage. Its sensitive response to dietary intake complicates the study of the direct effects of nutrients on genes that regulate storage. The direct effects of glucose, in particular, on the expression of transporters and metabolic enzymes have to be dissected from the effects of insulin on these same genes. (The action of hormones, such as insulin, on target organs is beyond the scope of this review, but it is well covered by a number of excellent articles within the field of endocrinology.)[25,26] Experiments performed in vivo make the distinction between the direct effects of nutrients and those mediated through hormonal changes difficult to achieve.

The molecular mechanism(s) by which glucose directly modulates the transcriptional regulation of lipogenic enzymes was until recently poorly understood. In 2001 Kawaguchi and coworkers identified a hepatic transcription factor carbohydrate response element-binding protein (ChREBP), which is regulated at two different levels: nuclear entry and DNA-binding via phosphorylation events mediated by glucose and cyclic adenosine monophosphate (cAMP).[27,28] Earlier studies investigating the direct contribution of glucose toward increased nutrient storage in the liver have focused on the three main control points of glucose metabolism before it enters the mitochondrion as pyruvate. These are the enzymes glucokinase (GK),

6-phosphofructokinase (PFK), and L-type pyruvate kinase (PK). Fructose is also metabolized to pyruvate, bypassing the first two enzymes. PK is therefore a regulatory enzyme in the metabolism of both monosaccharides. The transcription factor ChREBP was purified by its ability to bind to the glucose–carbohydrate response elements present in the PK promoter sequence.[27]

Both in vitro and in vivo studies have identified a second critical transcription factor, sterol regulatory element-binding protein (SREBP) in insulin-mediated transcriptional control of genes involved in glucose, fatty acid, and triglyceride metabolism.[29] The involvement of at least two transcription factors (ChREBP and SREBP) for optimum lipogenesis may reflect the degree of molecular complexity required for coordinated integration of hormonal and nutritional signals in regulating energy requirements of a cell.[30] More recent studies have identified TFE3/Foxo1 and SREBP-1c to reciprocally regulate insulin sensitivity in the liver.[31]

Insulin has a major effect on the activity of the three glycolytic enzymes via transcriptional and/or posttranslational modifications. GK mRNA expression is induced by insulin via an insulin receptor substrate (IRS)-1-phosphatidylinositol–3(PI3)-kinase–dependent pathway.[32] PI3-kinase and p44/p42 mitogen-activated protein kinase (MAPK) activities play a role in the transient activation of PK by insulin.[33] However, glucose itself independently alters the expression of PK by increasing the transcription of its mRNA.[34] Glucose similarly enhances the expression of fatty acid synthetase (FAS), a key enzyme in lipogenesis. GK regulates the flow of substrate to PK. Because GK requires insulin for its activity, it has been difficult to study the independent effects of glucose and its metabolites on PK expression. Nevertheless, two separate approaches directly demonstrate the effects of glucose on PK expression. The first approach was to demonstrate that the effects of insulin on transcription of PK mRNA was glucose dependent, thus identifying glucose as a separate variable.[35] The second approach examined a particular hepatoma cell clone (mhAT3F), whose GK (which is insulin dependent) had been replaced through spontaneous mutation by hexokinase (which is not insulin dependent). This allowed the effects of PK to be examined in the absence of insulin.[36] Several signaling pathways that may play a key role in glucose-dependent *L-PK* gene transcription are now known (for reviews, see references 31 and 37). The glucose response elements (GREs) in the promoter region of the *L-PK* gene interact directly or indirectly with various families of transcription factors, including the Sp1 family and the upstream stimulatory factors (USFs).[38] The complex interactions between the various factors (UFSs, chicken ovalbumin upstream promoter transcription factor II [COUP-TF II], and ChREBP) is likely to act as a "glucose-sensing" mechanism, allowing the cell to respond appropriately to continuous variation in its nutritional status.[31,37]

Nutrient Stimulation of Hormone Secretion

Insulin. In children, hormones are secreted into the circulation in response to nutritional stimulation for two main reasons: (a) to effectively store nutrients in appropriate storage compartments, and (b) to signal to tissues that substrate for growth is available, thus coordinating cellular manifestations of growth (cell proliferation, differentiation, and controlled cell death) with the influx of nutrients. These two actions are mutually compatible, and a number of hormones and growth factors serve both functions to varying degrees. Insulin, for example, is mainly a storage hormone, but it is also able to stimulate growth; the increased weight of babies born to diabetic mothers is due to increased fetal insulin acting as a growth hormone (GH). Similarly, factors primarily responsible for growth, such as insulin-like growth factor 1 (IGF-1), which mediates many of the actions of GH, are able to vary the rate of glucose uptake into cells.

The secretion of insulin by the pancreatic islets is tightly controlled by glucose concentrations in the blood. Alterations in gene expression play no part in these rapid responses to glucose. Regulatory proteins within islet cells are ready to respond to increases in glucose. Release of insulin from storage granules occur following calcium influx, which in turn is probably induced by minor increases in ATP from the metabolism of glucose and other nutrients. Circulating hormones also affect insulin release. The quick-acting mechanisms that do not involve control lie beyond the scope of this review. Again, the reader is referred to several excellent reviews on the subject.[39–41]

In addition to these rapid responses, glucose also exerts a more lasting effect on insulin production through increased translation and transcription of the insulin gene. This allows a child to adapt to longer periods of starvation or carbohydrate repletion. Glucose enhances the rate of translation of proinsulin mRNA to protein by three methods.[42] It increases the transfer of initiated insulin mRNA from free to membrane-bound ribosome. It also decreases the rate of pausing of the proinsulin mRNA as it passes along the ribosome. Lastly, glucose directly stimulates the cellular machinery involved in the elongation of proteins in pancreatic islet cells.[43,44] Long-term changes in insulin production are also mediated by transcription. Rats fasted over 4 days have low insulin mRNA concentrations, which return to normal on refeeding.[45,46] These changes control the ability of the pancreas to secrete insulin during dietary manipulations, and they enable the islet cell to adapt to long-term dietary changes.

In addition to whole animal studies, pancreatic islet cell preparations have also been used to study how glucose alters insulin expression. Interesting information regarding signal transduction from nutrients to the initiation of transcription has been gleaned from this system (to be discussed). The studies on insulin expression complement those on the role of glucose in PK and FAS expression.

IGF-1 and IGF-Binding Proteins. Although we do not fully understand the mechanisms whereby children whose nutritional intake is reduced beyond a certain point stop growing, it is certainly true that nutrient intake has a significant effect on final adult height. This is common knowledge in developed countries with large immigrant populations from the developing world. The children in the immigrant communities grow up to be taller on average than their parents, whose childhoods may have been spent in lands where food was less abundant. Poor linear growth also occurs in childhood diseases such as cystic fibrosis (CF). In inflammatory diseases, such as Crohn's disease (CD) or juvenile rheumatoid arthritis, the characteristic rate of growth may, in part, be related to poor nutritional intake,[47,48] as well as to the direct effects of intestinal inflammation.[49,50]

IGF-1 and -2 are a family of polypeptide growth factors whose functions include mediation of GH action, stimulation of insulin activity, and autocrine regulators of cellular proliferation.[51,52] IGF-1 has been shown to be a key player in regulating organ and body growth during post-natal development both in rodents and in humans.[53] There is now compelling evidence that IGF-1 secretion may be the point at which regulation of growth is controlled both in health and in disease.[54,55] Although IGF is an important modulator of GH action, GH itself does not correlate with depressed linear growth under nutritional restriction[56] or in children with active inflammation.[57] Alterations in tissue responses to GH may therefore mediate the effects of nutrition on growth. This has resulted in two separate lines of investigation:

1. The effect of nutritional alterations on expression of the GH receptor.[58,59]
2. The study of nutritional factors on IGF-1 and -2 secretion in association with secretion of IGF-binding proteins (IGFBPs).

Nutritional status is a major determinant of IGF-1 mRNA expression in liver and nonhepatic tissues. Fasting, caloric restriction animal model studies all show a decrease in circulatory IGF-1 levels,[60] although circulating levels of GH remain elevated. Although fasting reduces the binding of GH to its receptor,[61] downregulation of the GH receptor does not occur with dietary restriction,[62] and it is believed that neither of the above are principal causes of reduced IGF-1. Further, administration of IGF-1, but not GH, stimulates mucosal hyperplasia in surgically stressed rats with intestinal atrophy induced by hypocaloric total parenteral nutrition.[63] Low protein intake studies in a liver-specific IGF-1–deficient mouse model led to a decrease in nonhepatic IGF-1 secretion into the circulation, with an increase in GH levels. Increased IGFBP-3 mRNA was also observed, which supports the hypothesis that the binding protein may contribute to greater sequestration of locally synthesized IGF-1.[64] These studies support the view that the splenic GH/IGF-1 axis responds to nutritional stress to maintain tissue homeostasis.

Regulation of IGF mRNA expression is complex. The rat *IGF-1* gene contains six exons spanning 100 kb of DNA. Exons 1 and 2 encode alternative amino terminal sequences of the IGF-1 protein. The gene has two distinct promoter regions upstream of exons 1 and 2, which can be separately activated.[65] After transcription, alternative splicing results in further heterogeneity of the IGF-1 mRNA. Furthermore, there are two different terminal poly-A addition sequences in exon 6, adding to the general complexity. However, these myriad possibilities result in only three different-sized mRNA transcripts: a 3.8 kb, a 4.2 kb, and an 8 kb transcript. The importance of these different mRNAs to IGF-1 production and to growth awaits further investigation, but they are of interest because several studies have demonstrated that different forms of malnutrition affect the transcripts differently.[51,52,66] Total energy restriction induces a coordinate decrease in all three forms of mRNA. In contrast, protein restriction results in a profound decrease in the 8 kb fragment with less effect on the two smaller fragments.[51,66] These observations open up two questions of further interest: (1) How do different nutrients differentially affect gene expression in a particular family of genes? (2) How do these differences in gene expression translate into differences in a child's final phenotype? We will be returning to similar questions when we consider the small intestinal epithelium, where nutritional variations are greater than those seen in the circulation. Corresponding changes in IGF-1 have been seen in childhood illness. IGF-1 concentration correlates with increased intake and subsequent growth of children with CD, whereas growth has no correlation with GH production.[52,57] Children with CF frequently manifest hormonal abnormalities that may contribute to malnutrition. Interestingly in a study by Bucuvalas et al no effect of exogenous IGF-1 on linear growth in prepubertal children with CF was found, although an increase in glucose/insulin ratio was observed.[67]

In extracellular fluids, IGF-1 is bound to IGFBPs, of which six have been cloned and characterized.[51,52] IGFBP-3 is the main carrier of IGF-1 and in the presence of an acid-labile subunit, a bio-inactive ternary complex is maintained during circulation. The complex allows greater control on IGF-1 bioavailability.[68] IGFBP-3 may also modulate IGF-1–stimulated DNA synthesis.[69] The biological function of each binding protein is under intense investigation.[70] Protection from the hypoglycemic effects of IGF-1 has also been suggested as a function. Nutritional factors alter the circulating levels of IGFBPs. There is an inverse correlation of the expression of binding proteins with that of IGF-1. Protein restriction results in an increase of IGFBP-1, which falls on refeeding. However, IGFBP-1 is sensitive to insulin, and it is not clear how nutrients in the liver alter their expression directly.

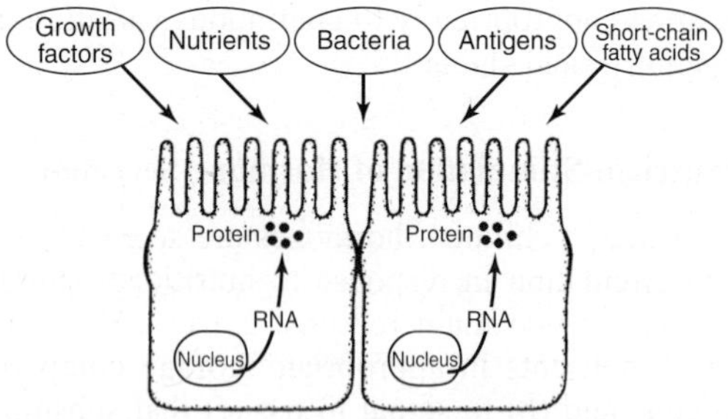

Figure 2 The luminal factors that influence gene expression in the enterocyte. Factors can affect individual genes or they may influence enterocyte differentiation and new cell lineages.

Interestingly, IGFBPs are predominantly secreted by Kupffer cells,[71] unlike IGF-1, which is synthesized by hepatocytes. The difference between these two cell types in terms of their location and their expression of surface receptors could allow for subtle regulation of IGF action in the face of nutrients and other factors in the circulation, such as cytokines.

Effect of Intestinal Contents on Genes in the Epithelium

The GI tract is the only part of the body that normally comes into contact with nutrients before they are absorbed. The GI tract is therefore exposed to a wider variety of nutrient molecules than any other organ of the body. The picture is further complicated because the lumen of the intestine is not a direct reflection of the food ingested. It also contains bacteria and their by-products and factors secreted into lumen in response to the ingestion of food (Figure 2). The study of nutrient effects on the enterocyte should therefore consider how changes in diet may affect the area around the apical aspect of a particular epithelial cell. The dissociation between nutrients ingested and the changes observed in the bowel lumen becomes greater the further one proceeds down the GI tract. The contents of the distal colon are completely different from food, although even here they are affected to some extent by dietary intake. This relationship between ingested nutrients and the local environment of the lumen is a separate issue from the interaction of that local environment with genes in the enterocyte.

It has been traditional to assume that the expression of genes in the small intestinal epithelium is preprogrammed and that their expression is not influenced by events in the lumen of the intestine. However, this view may be incomplete. An alteration in epithelial cell phenotype secondary to nutritional factors would have three possible advantages (Table 2). First, the intestine could adapt to absorb nutrients more effectively if specific digestive enzymes and transporters of the epithelium were upregulated by the repeated intake of a particular nutrient. Second, as all mammals are fed from mother's milk, the opportunity exists for breast milk to influence the development of the epithelium through actions of its own constituents. Third, if the genes affected in the epithelium were immunologically important, the intestinal epithelium could influence mucosal immune responses by signaling information to the mucosal immune system and beyond through changes in the expression of epithelial cell genes. Each of these areas is likely to represent important physiologic mechanisms that have implications for child health.

Table 2 Relevance of Dietary Regulation of Enterocyte Gene Expression

Intestinal adaptation
Influence of maternal breast milk
Signaling from lumen to mucosal immune system

Polarity of Epithelia

The cell types that we have discussed earlier in this chapter do not depend on a separation of functions to different cellular poles. For example, the pancreatic islet receives signals from the entry of glucose at any point on the plasma membrane, and as far as we can judge, the insulin response is not affected by the site of glucose entry. Insulin can also be released in any direction, eventually diffusing into the circulation. Cells that form epithelia are different in that they exhibit polarity. This separation between the apical side (bordering the lumen in the case of the intestinal epithelium) and the basolateral side is central to epithelial activity. This property is well recognized in the field of intestinal transport. Ions,[72] small molecules,[22,73] and macromolecules[74] are all transported differently across the apical membrane than across the basolateral membrane (Figure 3). It is the polarity of the epithelium that gives direction to the movement of these substances across the epithelium into or out of the body. But this property must also be considered when one is examining all aspects of intestinal epithelial cell function. Polarity is also of fundamental relevance in the study of nutrient–gene interactions in the intestinal epithelium. The polarity of the epithelial cell distinguishes the two major mechanisms by which nutrients (and other luminal factors) affect genes: (1) a direct effect on enterocytes and (2) an indirect effect mediated through hormones, growth factors, and cytokines (Figure 3). As with the effects

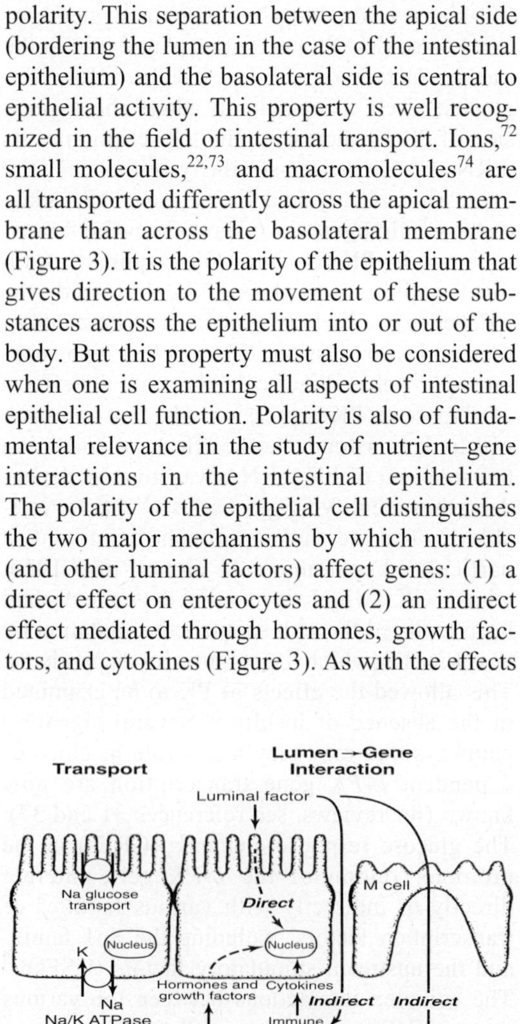

Figure 3 Dietary changes may affect gene expression directly (being mediated through the apical membrane) or indirectly (through the basolateral membrane).

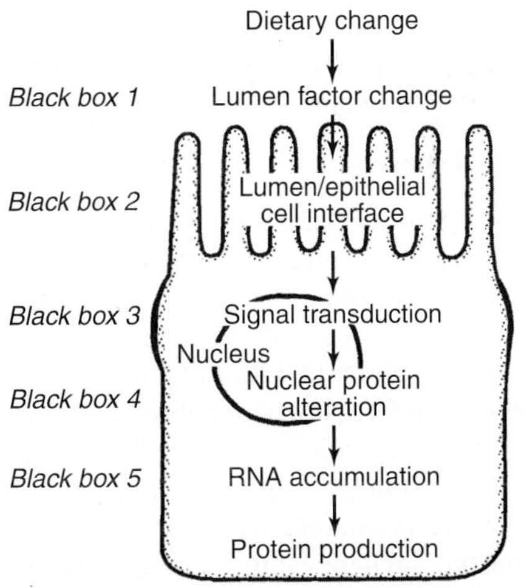

Figure 4 The pathway connecting dietary alterations to changes in gene expression is not well understood. It is likely that the pathway is mediated by a series of steps that, at present, we can regard only as black boxes. Different luminal events will influence gene expression through different series of black boxes.

of insulin on target tissues, the mechanism(s) of action of cytokines and growth factors on the epithelium is beyond the scope of this chapter. The reader is again referred to excellent reviews on how epithelial cell expression can be regulated by a multitude of agents.[22,75,76]

The apical membrane mediates the direct effects of luminal factors on the epithelium. The functions of nutrient recognition (sensing) and signal transduction (see Figure 1) will therefore lie between the apical membrane and the apparatus of gene expression. The exact molecular mechanisms involved require further investigation. For purposes of investigation they can be considered as a series of black boxes connecting the lumen and gene expression (Figure 4). These black boxes contain the mechanisms that regulate gene expression and constitute the way by which molecules in the lumen "cross-talk" with the nucleus of the enterocyte. Figure 4 depicts the pathway linking single factors in the lumen to the expression of a single cell in a single gene. This is, of course, a gross oversimplification. As we have mentioned, an alteration in diet may alter different factors at the cell surface, and any one of these factors may have an effect on several different genes through different pathways (Figure 5). In addition, method(s) by which a particular protein may be expressed is not necessarily always due to the induction of a single gene in cells along the crypt–villus axis.[22,77] It can also be due to changes in the state of differentiation of the cells in the epithelium, the expression of a particular gene being just one component of that change. Lastly, alterations in luminal contents may not necessarily affect epithelial cells that are already formed along the epithelium, but instead result in the generation of new lineages of cells that express the gene arising from the crypt.[77] In this case, the mechanisms linking the lumen to gene expression would lie in the stem cell at the base of the crypt, rather than in the individual enterocyte itself.

Adaptation of Enterocytes to the Nutritional Environment

The efficient utilization of food requires digestion, followed by absorption of digestion products and their release into the circulation. Adaptation is, by definition, the upregulation of one or all of these functions in the presence of a relevant nutrient. Adaptive mechanisms are more likely to be associated with foods whose intake varies between different individuals. The similarity here with prokaryotic cells is clear. Bacterial gene regulation was discovered in the study of enzymes that metabolized nutrients whose abundance varied widely in the environment, like lactose or tryptophan. For children, of course, there are many foods whose abundance can vary, but to illustrate this section we have chosen two: sucrose and dietary fat. These two examples demonstrate different aspects of adaptation: Digestion and absorption of sucrose is controlled entirely by the enterocyte itself; in contrast, fat digestion is primarily controlled by enzymes secreted from the pancreas and gastric glands.

Sucrose Intake. The intake of sucrose can vary greatly between individual human beings. This is especially true when one compares individuals from different times in history. Until the industrial revolution, sucrose was present in the diet only when brought from the East as part of the spice trade, and its availability was limited. The introduction of plantations in the Caribbean in the eighteenth century, coupled with the industrial process of refining, resulted in an explosion of sucrose intake. In England in 1700, the estimated per capita daily consumption in adults was 4.5 g, rising to 37 g in 1800. By 1968 it had reached 140 g daily, which is around 15% of the total energy derived from food.[78] Sucrose is digested by the epithelial cell brush border, where it is hydrolyzed to fructose and glucose by sucrase isomaltase (SI). Fructose is absorbed by the carrier GLUT family members[22] and glucose by the specific sodium-dependent glucose transporter. Both sugars exit the cell through the basolateral membrane by facilitated diffusion via GLUT-2. The upregulation of any of these proteins by

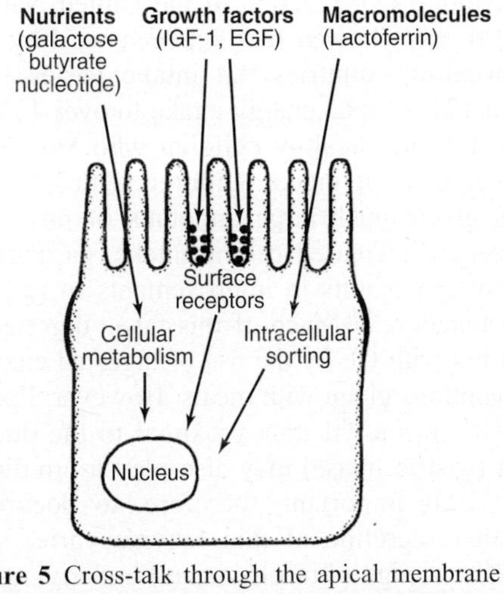

Figure 5 Cross-talk through the apical membrane will depend on the particular signal involved. EGF = epidermal growth factor; IGF = insulin-like growth factor.

their substrate would constitute a nutrient–gene interaction.[22,79]

The brush-border disaccharidases represent the final step in the digestion of carbohydrates.[80] Their activity can affect the glycemic response to oral carbohydrate.[81] More importantly, low levels of hydrolase activity in the face of carbohydrate in the intestine result in osmotic diarrhea.[82] A mechanism whereby expression of these enzymes could be linked to sugar intake would therefore have clear benefits. SI is one of three β-glucosidases (together with maltase and trehalase). The remaining disaccharidase, lactase, is a β-galactosidase. Sucrase is anchored to the microvillus membrane of the enterocyte by the isomaltase subunit of the SI protein.[22,83] Both subunits are synthesized as a single protein that is later cleaved.

The regulation of the induction of sucrase is not simple. The timing of its appearance during ontogeny in rodents was elegantly shown to be independent of luminal contents.[84] When the investigators transplanted isografts into animals 5 days younger than the donors, sucrase appeared earlier in the transplanted intestine than in the host. Therefore, luminal factors in this case did not induce sucrase nor did circulating factors in the host (whose intestine would have been susceptible to them). This evidence suggests that sucrase is controlled by an internal biologic clock within the intestine itself. However, luminal contents can have a marked effect on the activity of sucrase, which is separate from this internal mechanism: (1) early feeding with sucrose will induce precocious sucrase induction in rodents[82]; (2) reduction of carbohydrate intake results in a reduction of sucrase activity even when caloric intake is unchanged[85]; (3) feeding with glucose instead of sucrose reduces brush-border hydrolase activity[86]; and (4) refeeding sucrose after a period of abstinence leads to rapid recrudescence of the hydrolase activity.[87] Increase in sucrose from 2 to 55% of total energy intake has differing effects on the enterocyte depending on its location in the small intestine; that is, sucrase activity increases in the duodenum and upper jejunum, but not in more distal segments.[88] Further, cells from the midvillus of the proximal intestine show the greatest alterations, with lesser increases in the villus tip and crypt–villus junction.

The control of sucrase activity is complex and depends on events within the enterocyte in addition to external influences. Sucrase activity depends mainly on events in the sucrase promoter since expression of GH mirrors that of sucrase in transgenic animals containing a sucrase promoter–GH construct.[89] The expression of sucrase may therefore reflect nuclear protein–promoter interactions.[90] Evolutionarily conserved *cis*-acting elements in the promoter region have been found to interact specifically with transcription factors such as GATA-4 and caudal-related homeodomain (Cdx) proteins.[91–93] Further combinatorial interactions between hepatocyte nuclear factor 1α (HNF-1α) protein, GATA-4, and Cdx-2 may play a critical role in the temporal and spatial regulation of the SI gene expression during postnatal development.[92,93] Posttranscriptional events may also likely to influence enzymatic activity; for example, reduction in lactase activity following weaning does not necessarily correlate with lactase mRNA, but may be regulated during translation.[94]

Glucose Transporter Expression. Glucose enters the epithelial cell by active transport via a sodium-coupled glucose transporter, SGLT-1.[22,95] SGLTs represent part of a family of proteins that carry nutrients into the cell across concentration gradients. SGLT-1 is located in the brush border or apical surface of the enterocyte and along with Na^+ transports glucose and galactose into the cytosol. GLUT-2 is basolateral and transports glucose, galactose, and fructose (transported in from the lumen via GLUT-5) from the cytosol into circulation.

Direct transport studies undertaken before the identification of sodium-dependent transporters showed that glucose uptake increased with glucose feeding.[96] This increase was not due to changes in the affinity of glucose to the enterocyte (K_m), but due to an increase in the uptake (V_{max}), indicating an increase in the production of proteins that transport glucose. It is now well established that dietary sugars regulate the activity and the expression of intestinal SGLT-1. Structurally, an intact mucosa is necessary for rapid upregulation of glucose transporters by luminal glucose.[97] Modulation of SGLT-I expression by dietary carbohydrate has also been observed in the human intestine.[17,22,95] Mechanisms involved in the regulation of glucose transport are complex and have been difficult to characterize, as two distinct timescales of dietary carbohydrate exposure are now known to play a role.[98] Glucose transporters can respond within an hour to glucose[97] and also exhibit distinct changes in gene expression over a period of 1 to 3 days to a high-carbohydrate diet.[99] Intestinal glucose transport is also subject to diurnal changes, adding further complexity to the system. The increase in glucose transporters in response to dietary changes is analogous to the acquisition in bacteria of enzymes and transporters that are induced by lactose (*lac* operon). There are, however, notable differences between induction of enzymes and transporters in bacteria and those seen in the mammalian intestine. First, the activity of transporters in bacteria increases by 100- to 1000-fold, whereas the nutrient transporters in mammals show smaller variation with diet. For example, feeding mice with diets containing high levels of either D-glucose or nonmetabolizable analogs of D-glucose led to only a two- to threefold increase in SGLT-1 activity.[100,101] Second, in bacteria, the cell that receives the stimulus is the same cell that exhibits alterations in gene expression. In mammalian intestine, this appears not to be the case with the glucose transporter.[102,103] Sequential elution of different fractions of epithelial cells was used to distinguish different cells along the crypt–villus axis of mice.[104] Increase in carbohydrate intake resulted in enhanced expression of the glucose transporter (as measured by phlorhizin binding). Importantly, changes were observed in the crypts before they were seen in the villi. Similarly, when carbohydrate was stopped, it was in the crypts that the reduction in transporter was first observed. Thus crypt cells respond to changes in diet before villus cells, indicating that the changes in the expression of the glucose transporter were effected by new cell lineages from stem cells. It is the stem cell producing the new cell lineage that therefore must contain the machinery for detection of carbohydrate. The resulting cell population that ascends along the crypt–villus axis expresses this change. This separates carbohydrate detection temporally and spatially from glucose transporter expression. It is not known whether other genes in the intestine follow a similar pattern. Identification of molecular mechanisms underlying carbohydrate detection and signal transduction are currently under active investigation in several laboratories[105,106] (see Figure 1).

Sucrose induces an increase in the enzyme (SI) that hydrolyzes it and in SGLT-1 that allows a greater influx into the enterocyte across a concentration gradient. This absorptive system is central to the efficacy of oral rehydration solution in the treatment of gastroenteritis and cholera.[22] The greater the number of transporters, the more sodium and fluid that can be transported into a child during dehydration. Upregulation of SGLT-1 has therefore a potential therapeutic role in alleviating the loss of sodium and fluid with glucose solutions. An understanding of the mechanisms regulating this process would define to what extent and over what time period sodium and fluid transport could be maximized in children with gastroenteritis.

Intake of Dietary Fat. The intake of fat as a component of total energy varies considerably between different children. Fat consumption has been increasing in children from developed countries and has accelerated over the last 100 years. Contemporary comparison of fat intake between nations now shows large variations. For example, Perissé et al reviewed countries for the Food and Agriculture Organization of the United Nations (FAO), and showed that between wealthy and nonwealthy countries, fat intake varies from about 12% of total energy intake to over 40%.[107] It is not only healthy children who have seen a change in fat intake; children with CF have been given much larger amounts of fats. This is because increased calorie intake, particularly that of fat, results in improvements in respiratory function.[108] Much of this fat is digested in children with CF by the use of ingested enzyme preparations given with meals. However, lipases secreted in the GI tract proximal to the duodenum (gastric lipase) may also play a prominent role. It is important, therefore, to document whether secretion of this enzyme varies with fat. Knowledge of mechanism(s) underlying this possible adaptive effect may lead to therapeutic optimization of enzyme production and better utilization of fat in children who are continually under threat of malnutrition.

Gastric Lipase

Gastric lipase accelerates the digestion of triglycerides in human milk,[109] by releasing free fatty acids which enhance pancreatic lipase and colipase activities. The actions of gastric lipase are magnified in children with little pancreatic lipase activity, as in CF. Newborn babies also have relatively low pancreatic lipase activity[110,111] and the relative importance of gastric lipase is exaggerated in the premature neonate.[112,113] There are significant biochemical differences between pancreatic and gastric lipase, most significant of which is the difference in pH required for maximal activity.[114,115] In addition, gastric lipase activity requires no bile salt or colipase. In the human, the gastric mucosa secretes all the preduodenal lipase.[116,117] In the rodent, the tongue is the most significant source, and here the equivalent enzyme is termed lingual lipase. There may also be some lingual production in the preterm human infant because lipase activity has been detected in esophageal pouches of infants with esophageal atresia with no communication to the stomach.[113] The rabbit predominantly secretes its preduodenal lipase from the gastric mucosa, making the rabbit a more appropriate model than the rodent in which to study the effect of dietary influence on this enzyme.

Gastric lipase activity is more susceptible than pancreatic lipase to dietary changes. Increasing the dietary fat intake in rabbits from 2.7 to 6.0% for 2 weeks was sufficient to induce a 100% increase in gastric lipase activity.[118] This increase had no effect on pancreatic lipase production. Indeed, pancreatic lipase activity was enhanced only when the fat intake was increased to 12% of diet and then the increase was only modest, a 10% increase in pancreatic lipase activity. Studies in adult human volunteers have shown similar data with a doubling (5.7 to 9.95 U/mL) of gastric lipase after changing from a low-fat to a high-fat diet.[119] The mechanisms that detect the amount of fat intake (see Figure 1) need further examination, but triglyceride composition had no effect on the adaptive response in the rabbit.[118] This implicates a metabolite of fatty acid breakdown, which is not specific for either saturated or unsaturated fatty acids, as the cellular agent that initiates changes in gene expression. The signal may not have to come directly from the lumen of the GI tract, because there is preliminary evidence, in neonates at least, indicating that increasing lipid intake parenterally results in enhanced gastric lipase activity. This suggests that signals from the serosal side of the epithelial cell may be possible in this case.

Gastric lipase is therefore under the control of dietary signals. Although we do not at present understand the mechanisms that underlie this phenomenon, their elucidation may eventually allow us to manipulate gastric lipase expression when it is clinically important, as in the nutrition of CF patients and in the oral intake of the newborn.

Fatty Acid Uptake. Fatty acid uptake in the GI tract is facilitated by the presence of fatty acid transporter proteins (FATPs) with intestinal FATP-4 attracting considerable attention.[120] FATP-4 is expressed in significant amounts in enterocytes and recent studies highlight FATP-4 localization to the endoplasmic reticulum (ER). Further, FATP-4 exhibits catalytic function with the ability to esterify fatty acids.[121] Whether FATP-4 can function both as a transporter and as an enzyme requires further clarification. Despite extensive research our understanding of how various lipids migrate from the site of absorption to the ER where complex lipid biosynthesis takes place remains unclear. Fatty acid–binding proteins (FAPBs) have been implicated in this action. Ex vivo model studies of fetal jejunum explants implicate FABP-2 polymorphism to specifically influence small intestinal lipid absorption with minimal effect on glucose uptake or metabolism.[122] Epidemiological analyses of polymorphisms at codon 54(A/T) in *FABP-2* gene suggest that this variant may play a role in cardiovascular pathogenesis in the presence of insulin-resistance syndrome or hypertriglyceridemia.[123]

Further studies are required to clarify the potential role of these transporters in health and disease. A third fatty acid transporter (FAT; CD36) located mainly at the apical surface of the villus epithelia has been implicated in fatty acid uptake and in the pathogenesis of insulin resistance.[124] However, in a separate study CD36 knockout mice were shown to absorb triacylglycerol and fatty acid, as well as wild-type litter mates.[125] Although evidence suggests that CD36 plays a role in fatty acid uptake in adipose tissue,[126] muscle, and heart,[127] its role in the small intestine remains unclear.

Breast Milk and Gene Expression

Nutrition and protection of the infant are the primary roles of breast-feeding, and the nutritional and immunologic properties of breast milk are reviewed in other chapters of this book. Nevertheless, the cells of the GI tract are the first cells of the child to encounter breast milk, and it is not fanciful to suppose that breast milk may influence the development of these cells. A number of factors in milk can affect the expression of genes in the intestinal epithelium, particularly those genes that are associated with enterocyte differentiation. Growth factors vascular endothelial growth factor (VEGF),[128] epidermal growth factor (EGF),[129] and hepatocyte growth factor (HGF) are found in breast milk[130] and enhance brush-border enzyme activity and cell proliferation. Although the exact effect of EGF in breast milk on the development of the intestinal epithelium depends on the age of the subject, its effect on enterocyte growth and development is not surprising. Less expected, perhaps, is the demonstration that other breast milk components such as nucleotides also affect the same cellular processes.[131,132] Although the list of constituents in breast milk that may affect expression of genes in the intestinal epithelium is ever increasing (references 133 and 134 are recommended for recent update), due to space constraint we describe below our current understanding of the role of one critical milk component, that is, the role of lactoferrin in modulating intestinal homeostasis.

Lactoferrin. Lactoferrin, an 80 kDa iron-binding glycoprotein of the transferrin family, is a major component of mammalian colostrum and milk.[135] Lactoferrin is also found in mucosal secretions, neutrophil granules, and plasma, concentrations in the latter being relatively low.[136,137] Lactoferrin has bactericidal properties and is a source of iron in breast-fed infants. The protein has been found to have diverse biological functions, including facilitating iron absorption,[138] host defense,[139] regulation of cell proliferation and differentiation, modulating the immune system, and embryonic development.[140,141]

Specific binding sites for lactoferrin have been observed in activated human blood lymphocytes,[142] liver cells,[143] and cells lining the GI tract.[144] Lactoferrin receptor has been detected in intestinal brush-border membrane vesicles prepared from the human fetus,[145] rhesus monkey,[146] rabbit,[147] and mice.[148] Lactoferrin is relatively resistant to proteolytic degradation.[149] Intact protein with iron-binding capacity has been detected in murine fecal samples[150] and in urine samples from human infants.[151] The stability of the intact protein through transit in the gut suggests that it has the potential of interacting directly with the intestinal epithelium. The lactoferrin protein consists of a bactericidal domain (lactoferricin), which can be generated in vitro by pepsin digestion.[152] An understanding of the actions of lactoferrin at the molecular level is particularly relevant as some artificial milk formulas now contain added bovine lactoferrin. Its major role is thought to be delivery of iron to the intestinal epithelium.[153] The number of lactoferrin-binding sites increases in cultured epithelial cells when depleted of iron,[154] resulting in a specific increase of iron transport into enterocytes. The actions of lactoferrin are therefore interconnected with the actions of iron. Iron has well-characterized effects on the translation of ferritin and transferrin mRNA,[155] but its effect on gene expression in the enterocyte is less well understood and is currently an active area of investigation.[156,157]

Although lactoferrin increases the bioavailability of iron in the neonatal intestine, studies suggest that lactoferrin may also act as a proliferative factor in a variety of cell types, including human lymphocytes,[158] murine osteoblasts,[159] and Caco-2 cells, a colonic adenocarcinoma cell line.[160] The effect of lactoferrin on the expression of brush-border enzymes has also been examined. In tissue culture experiments, the effect of lactoferrin on sucrase, lactase, and alkaline phosphatase-specific activities was found to be dependent upon protein concentration[160] and on the degree of iron saturation.[161]

There is a school of thought that proposes that the main function of lactoferrin in vivo is not to transport iron into the epithelium, but to scavenge iron (and possible other substances) in the intestinal lumen. This unbound iron might otherwise cause free radical–mediated damage to sensitive tissues.[162] Accordingly, lactoferrin would have no direct effect on the intestinal epithelium, and only indirectly interact with it through the sequestration of other substances in the lumen. These luminal factors, if left free in solution, may have an impact on enterocyte gene expression. An example of this is lactoferrin's binding to lipopolysaccharide,[163] a major component of bacterial cell walls, thereby modulating the effect of this moiety on the epithelium. However, a purely luminal role for lactoferrin is difficult to reconcile with the identification of specific receptors for lactoferrin on the surface of the small intestinal brush-border membrane.[147] Initially, the binding of lactoferrin to brush borders was explained on the assumption that lactoferrin was binding to transferrin receptors,[164] but the use of rhesus monkeys has made possible an examination of the specificity of lactoferrin binding to its receptor.[146] Binding was specific and time dependent and reached saturation; monkey and human lactoferrin effectively inhibited the binding of rhesus lactoferrin at 50-fold excess, while a similar excess of bovine lactoferrin or human transferrin had no effect on binding. These results taken together are good evidence for a specific lactoferrin receptor. Any direct effect of lactoferrin on gene expression should be transmitted through this receptor, and its analysis may therefore give clues as to how lactoferrin might do this. Human[165] and porcine[166] intestinal lactoferrin receptors have been cloned and further studies are likely to highlight molecular interactions critical for the activation of this ligand–receptor complex.

Signaling from the Intestinal Lumen to the Mucosal Immune System

The function of the small intestinal epithelium is to absorb nutrients from the environment while providing a barrier to the external world.[4] The barrier is not complete, as the intestine allows macromolecules to be sampled and actively absorb nutrients. The success of the intestine in achieving the balance between these competing aims was the critical step in the evolution of multiorgan animals. The ability of the intestine to monitor the environment is a key element in this process, in which the mucosal immune system plays an important part. Curiously, however, the possibility that epithelium may respond to luminal factors (and signal their presence to the mucosal immune system) has been substantially ignored. The epithelium has mainly been regarded as a passive barrier with points of selective filtration (Figure 6A), surveillance of the luminal contents occurring after this filtration has taken place.

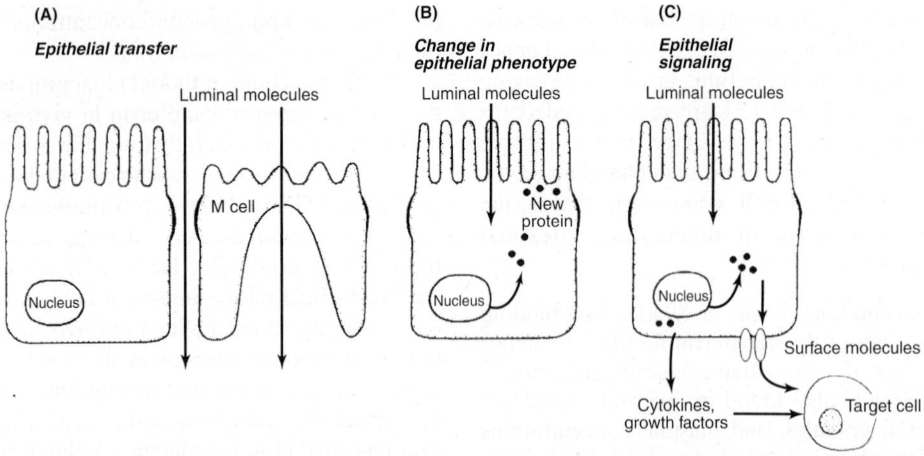

Figure 6 Possible interactions of molecules from the intestinal lumen with the epithelium. Traditionally, the epithelium has been seen as a selective barrier to molecules, admitting those required for energy intake or immunosurveillance and excluding others (A). However, nutrients can alter the phenotype of the epithelium to adapt to changing nutritional needs (B). When changes in the intestinal lumen induce new proteins that interact with mucosal immune cells, the epithelium can act as a membrane signaling information from the lumen to the immune system (C).

Earlier in this chapter we examined genes whose activity is restricted to the confines of the epithelial cell monolayer of the intestine (Figure 6B). Nutrient transporters and disaccharidases all contribute to the actions of the epithelium. When genes within the enterocyte express proteins whose actions occur away from the epithelium, such as cytokines and growth factors, the relevance of luminal factors on enterocyte gene expression becomes different. In this new situation (Figure 6C), the epithelium acts as a mediator between the luminal contents of the intestine and target cells beyond the epithelial barrier. Such cells include immunocytes from the mucosa, with the potential for additional cells being recruited from the circulation. The small intestinal epithelium is now recognized to be a part of the mucosal immune system.[4,167–169] For example, it expresses innate host pattern recognition receptors, such as Toll-like receptors and nucleotide oligomerization domain proteins, which are involved in microbial detection.[170] Dysregulated activation of bacteria-driven epithelial inflammatory processes is kept under tight control by a spectrum of negative regulators who collectively ensure maintenance of intestinal homeostasis.[171,172] It is the breakdown of these cellular processes that is now known to contribute to disease pathogenesis in inflammatory bowel disease(s).[76,173] The epithelial cell also expresses proteins that may interact with immunocytes within the intestine. These include surface molecules such as class II major histocompatibilty complex[75] and secretory chemokines[174] and cytokines[167] that may directly alter immune responses. The epithelium also expresses families of growth factors and their binding proteins, which may affect the proliferation of immune cells. It may also itself directly present antigen to T cells.[175] The molecular mechanisms governing the expression of these genes have features in common with other enterocyte genes that respond to nutrients and factors in the lumen. For example, the epithelial cell must recognize (or "sense") the nutrient or other luminal factor(s), and mechanism(s) must then "transduce" this recognition into molecular changes that can directly alter gene expression (see Figures 1 and 4).[176] The main difference in molecular terms from the adaptive response described earlier (Figure 6B) is that the resultant proteins escape from the compass of the epithelium and interact with receptors on target cells (Figure 6C).

Signaling, by transducing molecular interactions with the epithelium into secretion of messenger proteins, allows luminal factors to influence immune responses while maintaining full epithelial barrier integrity (Figure 6C). Although the absorption of luminal factors (Figure 6A) is an important method by which the mucosal immune system surveys the intestinal lumen,[4] it requires the entry of molecules through the epithelial barrier. This provides a potential source for invasion by pathogens. The poliovirus, for example, enters by this means, exploiting the normal uptake of macromolecules. The ability of the epithelium to signal information to the mucosal immune system without the need for a physical pathway from the lumen to the serosal surface offers obvious advantages in terms of epithelial protection.

The notion of epithelial signaling (Figure 6C) implies that the epithelium can modulate the level of immune activity in the mucosal immune system according to the environment of the intestinal lumen. Mucosal immune responses play a large part in GI inflammatory diseases, particularly CD, ulcerative colitis, and celiac disease. The milieu of the intestinal lumen could therefore be manipulated for therapeutic purposes, by alterations in diet.

Genes of Immunologic Importance in the Intestinal Epithelium. An increasing list of immunologically active proteins is now known to be synthesized by the intestinal epithelium (Table 3),[177–180] and these originally were thought to be produced only by other cell types. Human diseases are associated with the increased production of some of these proteins in the circulation and in the GI tract. Emerging data from our and other laboratories show that the expression of these proteins in the epithelium is influenced by dietary factors.

Cytokines. An interesting example of one of many cytokines secreted by the epithelium is interleukin 8 (IL-8). This protein is small (8 kDa) and has a long half-life in vivo relative to other cytokines, making it a feasible candidate for long-lasting control over mucosal immune responses. IL-8 is a member of a superfamily of cytokines, "the chemokines," which have chemotactic properties, recruiting as well as activating a number of immunologic cell types. It is a potent chemotactic factor for neutrophils and T lymphocytes and may be important in recruiting them to the GI tract. Invasion by neutrophils is a hallmark of inflammatory bowel disease (greater influx in ulcerative colitis compared to CD), a condition in which IL-8 production is enhanced.[181,182] IL-8 also stimulates the release of superoxide radical in neutrophils as well as other potential mediators of damage in intestinal inflammation. Furthermore, it increases the permeability of vascular endothelium to albumin resulting in tissue edema. IL-8 production in intestinal epithelial cells has

Table 3 Immunologically Relevant Genes Expressed by Intestinal Epithelial Cells

Gene	Experimental System	Reference
Chemokines		
IL-8	Primary human ileal and colonic epithelia	177
ENA-78	Primary human colonic epithelia and cell lines	178
IP-10, MIG	Human epithelial cell lines	179
IL-1R antagonist	Primary human ileal and colonic epithelia	177
CCL28	Primary human colonic epithelium and cell lines	180
Cytokines		
GM-CSF, TNF-α	Colon carcinoma cell lines	167
Ant-microbial peptides	Primary human colonocytes and cell lines	192, 193
Acute-phase respondents	Colon carcinoma cell lines	167
Surface molecules		
Class II	Sections of murine small intestine	201
MHC Invariant chain	Primary mouse epithelial cells, IEC-6 cells	202
Growth factors		
IGF-I	Colon carcinoma cell lines	75, 184, 208
IGFBPs	Colon carcinoma cell lines	207

IGF = insulin-like growth factor; IGFBP = insulin-like growth factor binding protein; IL = interleukin; MHC = major histocompatibility complex; MIP = macrophage inflammatory protein.

been documented in response to bacterial invasion[167] and by other agents, including phorbol-12-myristate-13-acetate (PMA) and IL-1. Studies from our laboratory have shown unequivocally that the surface epithelium and its products can orchestrate the mucosal immune system of the gut. Macrophage inflammatory protein 2 (MIP-2) (mouse chemokine similar to human IL-8) transgenic mice were generated where the chemokine expression was confined to the small intestinal and colonic epithelium by the use of fatty acid–binding protein promoter.[174] The epithelium from the first generation of the founder showed effects on both neutrophil and lymphocyte recruitment. In the small intestine where the FABPI promoter is active neutrophil, recruitment (myleoperoxidase activity as the indicator) was significantly greater. In the distal colon where the promoter is inactive there was no effect. These studies clearly show that the epithelium can, through the release of chemokines, alter the mucosal immune function in vivo.

Further analysis of the immune system demonstrated that the small intestine has increased lymphocyte infiltration, in addition to the presence of increased neutrophils. Lymphocyte numbers in the lamina propria are significantly increased ($P < .05$), and there was also a doubling of the number of intraepithelial (IEL) lymphocytes. The increase in IELs was due to an increase in both αβ and γδ lymphocyte populations. Interestingly, these cells express CXCR2, the receptor for MIP-2. These studies highlight the potential recruitment capacity of a single chemotactic activity; the in vivo situation, however, is likely to be more complex with simultaneous alteration of various immune regulators.

Increasing evidence suggests that expression of various epithelial-derived immune regulatory molecules is altered by dietary factors.[4,75,176] *n*-Butyrate is a short-chain fatty acid produced by the metabolism of normal intestinal bacteria whose levels in the intestine vary with diet.[183] Newborn babies have very low butyrate levels in either the small or large intestine. However butyrate levels increase with time, reaching adult levels by 2 years of age.[184] It has long been known that infants fed casein-based formulas[185] produce large amounts of butyric acid and propionic acid in the stool, whereas the predominant fatty acid in breast-fed infants is acetic acid. Furthermore, the bacterial flora (*Lactobacillus*) responsible for high acetate/butyrate production is inhibited by casein.[185] In addition, the amount of butyrate produced in the stool is altered by the type of fiber consumed in the diet.[186] Butyrate levels depend on the type of bacteria in the gut and how much substrate is available for butyrate production. Butyrate levels therefore reflect events in the intestinal lumen, and we hypothesized that their concentrations may alter cell signaling. We therefore examined its effects on IL-8 and *MCP-1* gene and protein expression.[187] We found that butyrate increased IL-8 secretion in enterocytes while simultaneously downregulated another chemotactic cytokine, macrophage chemotactic protein 1 (MCP-1).[187] More recent studies suggest that butyrate can also modulate pathogen-driven epithelial inflammatory responses.[188] Studies from our laboratory have defined a role for butyrate-induced histone acetylation in the regulation of chemokine gene expression.[189] Unlike IL-8, which attracts neutrophils, MCP-1 attracts macrophages and monocytes. It is constitutively secreted by the intestinal epithelium,[190] whereas IL-8 is not. These observations are consistent with events in the whole intestine in vivo where, in healthy tissue, neutrophils are absent and macrophages abound. With increasing butyrate levels, IL-8 secretion is induced but MCP-1 production is depressed. Such "chemokine switching" in response to butyrate may well alter the population of immune cells in the lamina propria. Thus, butyrate may affect both the number and types of cells in inflamed tissue through changes in chemokine production of epithelium during inflammation.

Antimicrobial Peptides. In the last decade a new family of endogenous epithelial cell–derived antimicrobial peptides has been identified. (For detailed reviews, see references 168, 191, and 192.) To date, mRNA expression of members of two families, the β-defensin and cathlecidin (LL-37), has been observed in enterocytes. (The expression of α-defensins is confined only to Paneth cells.) Several studies have shown dynamic changes in the expression of these peptides during infectious and inflammatory episodes implicating them in the front line of host defense in the GI tract.[193–196]

Class II Major Histocompatibility Complex and Invariant Chain Expression. The initiation of an immune response to protein antigen normally requires the help of T lymphocytes. Activation of T cells in turn depends on the processing and presentation of peptides by an antigen-presenting cell (APC).[197] Class II MHC heterodimers (Ia in the rodent) are the molecules that present the processed exogenous antigen to the T-cell receptor. In addition to classic APCs (dendritic cells, macrophages, and B lymphocytes), a number of cell types express class II MHC (Ia antigen) including intestinal epithelial cells and may function as APCs. In recent years, several studies have noted that both the small intestinal and colonic epithelium may function as an APC.[198,199] The requirement for cell viability and an intact cytoskeleton suggests pinocytosis as a major mechanism for active antigen uptake by intestinal epithelial cells; however, passive diffusion and adsorption may also contribute to the process. Processing and presentation of exogenous antigen requires an additional protein, the invariant chain (Ii).[200] Diet has a marked effect on the expression of class II MHC and its associated invariant (Ii) chain in the mouse intestinal epithelium. The expression of class II MHC and Ii mRNA is developmentally regulated[201] in the epithelium (unlike its expression in the lamina propria, where it is expressed from before birth). In addition, the timing of expression can be altered by delaying the age of weaning from mother's milk to normal chow.[202] Expression of class II MHC and Ii chain is apparent 3 to

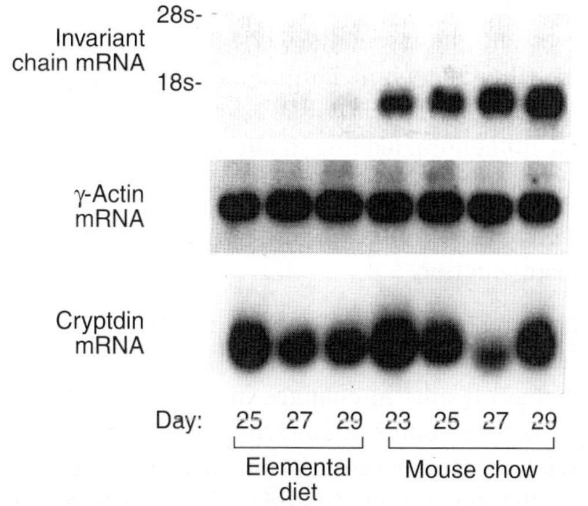

Figure 7 Dietary factors alter the expression of class II MHC and invariant chain expression in intestinal epithelial cells. Figure shows Northern blot of ribonucleic from epithelial cells taken from individual mice of a single split litter weaned at day 17 onto elemental diet or Purina mouse chow. The blot was probed with invariant chain complementary deoxyribonucleic acid (cDNA) and autoradiographed for 48 hours. Mice were examined at days 23, 25, 27, and 29. Blots were also probed with γ-actin and cryptdin cDNA to verify uniformity of enterocyte extraction mRNA = messenger ribonucleic acid. (Reproduced from Sanderson et al[201]).

4 days after weaning on chow. However, weaning onto an elemental diet (which contains chemically synthesized amino acids, simple sugars, and fats) did not induce the expression of class II MHC or invariant chain (Figure 7). Thus the expression of these genes in the intestinal epithelium is influenced by dietary manipulation in vivo. The fact that elemental diets used in these experiments were the same as those administered therapeutically in CD lends support to the idea that alterations in gene expression may by a significant tool in the treatment of disease (see below).

Insulin-Like Growth Factor–Binding Proteins. Immune responses depend not only on the activation of T cells, but also on the ability of these T cells to proliferate. Earlier sections of this chapter described the importance of IGF-1 on growth. However, IGF-1 is also an agent that affects cells of the immune system. IGF-1 exerts a range of effects on T-cell physiology.[203] The growth factor induces a marked increase in the gene and protein expression of both CD25 and IL-2 and modulates T-cell proliferation via both autocrine and paracrine mechanisms.[204] Treatment of adult mice with recombinant human IGF-1 induces striking modifications in lymphocyte number and function.[205] Fourteen days of treatment with IGF resulted in increases in both $CD4^+$ T cells and splenic B cells. Mitogenic responses of T and B cells were also enhanced, demonstrating that IGF-1 increases lymphocyte numbers and activity. As discussed earlier, IGFBPs modulate the actions of IGF-1. Because cultured intestinal epithelial cells[206,207] secrete IGFBPs, it is possible that the epithelium can influence the proliferation of activated lymphocytes by this means. Furthermore, studies have shown that nutritional factors affect the production of IGFBPs in cell lines in vitro.[208] Therefore, not only may nutritional factors influence IGF/IGFBP secretion by the liver into the circulation, resulting in changes in growth of the whole individual, but nutrients may also affect the IGF/IGFBP system in the intestinal epithelium, leading to alterations in the proliferation of the local immune system.

Nutrient Recognition and Signal Transduction

The mechanisms whereby a nutrient (or other factor in the intestinal lumen altered by dietary change) results in changes in RNA transcription are not well understood (see Figure 1). It is likely that increases in transcription are the consequence of alterations in the binding of nuclear transcription and accessory factors to the promoter of a particular gene, but the steps by which a cell recognizes a change in that nutrient will differ for every nutrient examined, so too will the mechanisms that transduce this signal into alterations of nuclear protein binding. In the enterocyte we have seen the variety of mechanisms that might occur simply by appreciating the many factors that may alter when the diet is changed (see Figure 2). Different theoretic mechanisms of interaction exist between the lumen and epithelial cells. These mechanisms differ, depending on the exact luminal factor involved (see Figure 5). Small nutrients such as butyrate or galactose are likely to enter the cell and affect gene expression through their respective metabolic pathways. Growth factors and lactoferrin involve specific receptors on the surface of the epithelium, and large proteins may enter the cell and alter gene expression as they are sorted. Some complex entities may affect more than one pathway. Bacteria for instance may interact through all three pathways: they could influence enterocyte metabolism; they may produce factors or components of their cell walls (e.g., endotoxin), which may interact with surface receptors; and the macromolecules from which they are composed may enter enterocyte compartments and be sorted inside the cell. Each pathway may influence aspects of nuclear function. In addition, indirect actions of cytokines produced from immune cells may also play a role.

Although sensing and signal transduction mechanisms (see Figure 1) in the epithelium require further investigation, there are some data on the mechanisms by which glucose regulates the expression of PK (in the liver) and insulin (in pancreatic islet cells). Three key questions relate to the effect of glucose on the expression of these two proteins: (1) What are the glucose metabolites that set in train the effects on transcription? (2) How is binding of nuclear proteins to gene promoter elements induced? (3) What is the sequence of DNA in the promoter that confers glucose sensitivity on the gene in question (the so-called nutrient response element)?

In practice, this last question is the easiest to answer because DNA sequences can be easily manipulated in the laboratory. Promoters linked to reporter genes allow researchers to directly measure promoter activity. This was first examined in the *PK* gene in response to glucose. The actual sequence in the PK promoter was determined by mutational analysis of the promoter and its effects on reporter activity. The GREs in the *PK* gene and in the insulin 1 gene were discovered by this means. To determine the GRE in the *PK* gene promoter, promoter DNA sequences were transiently transfected into hepatocytes in culture[209,210] and were also examined in transgenic mice.[211] Mutations induced into the DNA demonstrated a GRE occurring twice in the PK promoter. This motif is known as an E box because of its resemblance to a similar sequence in a promoter of the adenovirus, which had been given this name. This same DNA sequence also occurs in other genes that regulate glucose metabolism, most notably the *FAS* gene, whose protein product catalyzes one of the later steps in the conversion of carbohydrate to fat, and one that is upregulated when glucose is abundant in the diet.

The rat insulin gene also contains an E box, which is termed the Far element. Paradoxically, this element does not confer glucose sensitivity to the insulin gene. This attribute is conferred by a sequence 10 bases away termed the FLAT element. We now understand some of the features of the signal transduction from nutrient to nuclear function in the insulin gene. MacFarlane et al[212] identified a nuclear factor, insulin upstream factor 1 (IUF-1), which binds to the insulin promoter. IUF-1 binding was examined in vitro by assessing the degree of binding of nuclear extracts from cultured islet cells to radiolabeled promoter DNA. There was a high degree of IUF-1 binding in cells incubated with 20 mmol/L glucose, but this was abolished in cells incubated in 3 mmol/L glucose. In addition, this protein–DNA binding depended on the phosphorylation of IUF-1. Phosphorylation therefore alters a factor in the initiation of transcription of at least one glucose-sensitive gene. It is particularly interesting that phosphorylation is the signal that transduces glucose intake to induce insulin transcription, because it is also phosphorylation that directly affects the activity of enzymes in the Embden–Meyerhoff pathway. Thus, in this system phosphorylation acts as a common transduction mechanism, responsible for both the quick and slow responses to glucose uptake.

The metabolites derived from nutrients responsible for the change in nutrient gene expression have not been elucidated in any system. Glucose-6-phosphate may possibly be the metabolite that activates the GRE in the *FAS*[213] and *PK* genes. This was demonstrated by comparing the effects of the two glucose analogs, 2-deoxyglucose (2dG) and 3-*O*-methyl glucose (3OMeG). Neither analog can be metabolized. However, 2dG can be phosphorylated, but not 3OMeG; 2dG stimulated transcription, but 3OMeG did not. Therefore, only the phosphorylated sugar was able to stimulate the transduction mechanisms that resulted in transcription, which it did without further metabolism. Whether this phosphate bond provides the energy to phosphorylate a nuclear factor to bind to DNA is not known, but it is an interesting possibility.

CLINICAL AND THERAPEUTIC IMPLICATIONS OF NUTRIENT–GENE INTERACTIONS

The role of diet on fetal[214] and adult[215] health is an area attracting considerable attention from medical scientists and the general public. However, the relationship between dietary factors and the health of most organs has been difficult to examine, other than by using epidemiology.[215] Occasionally, data have emerged suggesting that particular diets benefit certain disease states. For example, renal failure was shown to be less progressive in rats whose protein intake had been restricted,[216] but even this has been difficult to substantiate in children.[217] Furthermore, it is not easy to see how the protein load has its effect. We have no knowledge of which cell types in the kidney may be affected, let alone how their phenotype may be altered by protein intake. On the other hand, in the small intestine, the relation between diet and GI function is clearer.

In clinical practice, one of the most substantial changes in the content of the intestine occurs before and after parenteral nutrition. The effects of such changes have profound consequences for the small intestinal epithelium in human subjects (see Figure 6B). Intestinal brush-border hydrolase activity is diminished during parenteral feeding.[218] Moreover, the ability of the mucosa to form a barrier is compromised. Moore et al studied 74 patients who had suffered abdominal trauma randomized to receive either enteral or parenteral nutrition.[219] Those fed parenterally had more episodes of infective complications (pneumonia and abdominal abscesses) than those fed enterally. Calorie and nitrogen intake was equivalent in the two groups. As it is thought that the main source of sepsis following trauma is the GI tract, this study suggests that enteral feeding directly affects the ability of the injured patient to contain bacteria within the GI lumen.

The effect of parenteral nutrition on the morphology of the intestine in animals has long been known.[220] Considerable attention has been paid to the question of which enteral components are responsible for maintaining normal bowel morphology and function. No clear answer has yet emerged. For example, Spector et al observed that luminal infusions of both 30% dextrose and 5% amino acids were effective in restoring intestinal weight, protein content, and DNA content after a period of intravenous alimentation.[221] Amino acids were more potent on a weight-for-weight basis or on a molar basis than dextrose. Changes in the intestine seen in animals fed via parenteral nutrition have been compared with the changes seen during weaning.[87] Intestinal length, mucosal mass, DNA, protein, and disaccharidase activities were significantly lower in animals sustained by intravenous nutrition when compared to normally weaned controls. However, restoration of luminal feeding resulted in a return to normal of the intestine in the total parenteral nutrition–fed group.

There are now many reports of the relationship of intestinal function to parenteral nutrition.[222,223] However, a study of the interaction between luminal content and the molecular control of intestinal cell function is just the beginning, and this relationship is likely to provide the key to our understanding of how enteral feeds maintain a healthy epithelium.

It is also likely that epithelial signaling (see Figure 6C) may have important therapeutic implications for diseased intestine. First, the contents of the intestinal lumen are directly amenable to therapeutic manipulation, whereas the environment that surrounds other, more internal, organs is maintained in strict homeostasis by a plethora of mechanisms. Second, although we do not know exactly how the local environment surrounding the epithelial cell is changed by diet (see Figure 2), dietary manipulations are an important aspect of management of GI disease states.

The activity of CD is greatly influenced by altering the contents of the intestinal lumen. Inflammation subsides in patients that are fed parenterally and receive no oral nutrients[224] and in those receiving elemental diets.[225,226] These chemically defined diets induce remission as effectively as high-dose oral corticosteroids in both adults[226] and children.[227,228] The return of inflammatory changes to normal in the intestine has been documented indirectly by the use of markers of intestinal permeability,[229,230] scanning of labeled neutrophils,[231] endoscopic examination,[232] and quantifying protein metabolism.[233]

It has been hypothesized that a reduction in antigen load in the intestine may underlie the efficacy of elemental diets in CD[227] in a fashion similar to that in cow's milk–sensitive enteropathy and celiac disease. However, the switch from normal diet to an elemental diet alters many constituents of the intestinal milieu apart from food antigens (see Figure 2). In particular, bacterial populations (and therefore bacterial products) are profoundly altered by dietary alteration. Moreover, giving whole protein in the form of liquid diets (polymeric diets) is also an effective treatment for CD.[232] Removal of protein antigen is therefore not essential for the efficacy of the formula diet. It is more likely that the diets are altering many factors in the local environment of the intestinal lumen (see Figure 2). The concept of genes in the epithelium signaling events to the mucosal immune system is a first step to understanding the basis of how such events may occur because it seeks to identify molecular pathways from the intestinal lumen, through enterocytes to the mucosal immune system and other target cells beyond the epithelium. Certainly, this would be in keeping with data presented earlier (see Figure 7), showing that class II MHC and invariant chain expression in the epithelium are related to dietary factors. There was no expression in epithelial cells of the mice weaned onto an elemental diet[202] and this diet was the same as that used in the treatment of CD. Genes other than class II MHC, with common promoter elements, may also be altered by similar maneuvers, and may be important in regulating intestinal inflammation.

CONCLUSIONS AND SPECULATION

Certain concepts have been laid down in this chapter that can be used as the basis for examining how dietary factors may affect the expression of genes in various cell types including the intestinal epithelium. The essential components for an effective transition between nutrient and gene expression in cells have been documented. These components (see Figure 1) comprise a system of recognizing changes in factors as they interact with a cell (sensing) and a mechanism of converting these external molecule–cellular molecule interactions into changes in gene expression (signal transduction). It is not yet understood how these mechanisms integrate to yield tissue homeostasis. This chapter has presented evidence that nutritional factors do indeed alter gene expression in cells, but it is likely that different molecular species are sensed by completely different mechanisms. In the case of the epithelial cell (see Figure 5) these sensing mechanisms can be at the cell surface or part of the internal mechanisms of the cell. It is also possible that special receptors exist on the surface of the cell and detect more complex external molecules, such as large proteins and oligosaccharides. The apical surface of mucosal epithelial cells expresses a number of molecules belonging to the immunoglobulin superfamily whose expression can also be modulated by nutrition.[234] The function of many members remains unclear; however, one family member ICAM-1 allows rhinovirus attachment.[235] As the primary function of these molecules on the mucosal surface cannot be to serve as a conduit for viral infection, it is tempting to suggest that they and other similar molecules might play a role in the immunosurveillance of macromolecules in the GI tract. Signaling through these molecules would require alterations in epithelial cell gene expression for this surveillance to be transmitted to the mucosal immune system. If antigens are recognized by epithelial cells of the GI tract, it is possible that this information is correlated with information garnered from the previous penetration of similar antigens across the epithelium.[74]

Finally, this field of nutrient–gene interaction may have important therapeutic implications; the ability of the epithelium to interact with other immune cells makes it an active member of normal human defense.[179,199,236] This physiologic role may allow it to influence inflammatory reactions in pathologic situations. The opportunity exists through dietary means to manipulate the constituents of the lumen of the intestine by opening up a new vista for treatment of human disease. Genetic expression is now regarded as a central feature of human disease states, particularly those in which certain genes are defective. However, genetic influences also affect a much wider variety of diseases than those that are due to simple inherited gene mutations. The possibility that expression of genes can be modulated by means other than insertion of new DNA should be added to the armamentarium of the medical community. An understanding of how dietary factors may alter gene expression is an early step in this direction.

This work was supported by NIH grants DK07703, DK40561, and DK47753 and a grant from the Crohn's and Colitis Foundation of America.

REFERENCES

1. Newsholme EA, Start C. Regulation in Metabolism. London: Wiley; 1973.
2. Dickson R, Abelson J, Barnes W, Reznikoff W. Genetic regulation: The lac control region. Science 1975;187:27–35.
3. Platt T. Regulation of gene expression in the tryptophan operon of *Escherichia coli*. In: Miller JH, Reznikoff WS, editors. The Operon. New York: Cold Spring Harbor Laboratory; 1978. p. 213–302.
4. Sanderson IR, Walker WA. Mucosal barrier. In: Ogra R, Mestecky J, McGhee J, et al, editors. Handbook of Mucosal Immunology, 2nd edition. San Diego, CA: Academic Press; 1999. p. 5–17.
5. Rennie MJ, MacLennan PA, Hundal HS, et al. Skeletal muscle glutamine transport, intramuscular glutamine concentration and muscle protein turnover. Metabolism 1989;38:47–51.
6. Feng B, Shiber SK, Max SR. Glutamine regulates glutamine synthetase expression in skeletal muscle cells in culture. J Cell Physiol 1990;145:376–80.
7. Durschlag RP, Smith RL. Regulation of glutamine production by skeletal muscle cells in culture. Am J Physiol 1985;248:C442–8.
8. Tadros LB, Willhoft NM, Taylor PM, Rennie MJ. Effects of glutamine deprivation on glutamine transport and synthesis in primary tissue culture of rat skeletal muscle. Am J Physiol 1993;265:E935–42.
9. Low SY, Rennie MJ, Taylor PM. Sodium-dependent glutamate transport in cultured rat myotubes increases after glutamine deprivation. FASEB J 1994;8:127–31.
10. Bode BP. Recent molecular advances in mammalian glutamine transporters. J Nutr 2001;131:2475S–87S.
11. Chaudhry FA, Reimer RJ, Krizaj D, et al. Molecular analysis of system N suggests novel physiological roles in nitrogen metabolism and synaptic transmission. Cell 1999;99:769–80.
12. Chaudhry FA, Reimer RJ, Edwards RH. The glutamine commute: Take the N line and transfer to the A. J Cell Biol 2002;157:349–55.
13. Labow BI, Souba WW, Abcouwer SF. Mechanisms governing the expression of the enzymes of glutamine metabolism-glutaminase and glutamine synthetase. J Nutr 2001;131:2467S–74S.
14. Karinch AM, Pan M, Lin CM, et al. Glutamine metabolism in spesis and infection. J Nutr 2001;131:2535S–8S.
15. Liboni K, Li N, Neu J. Mechanism of glutamine-mediated amerlioration of lipopolysacchride-induced IL-8 production in Caco-2 cells. Cytokine 2004;26:57–65.
16. Lenartes K, Mariman E, Bouwman F, et al. Glutamine regulates the expression of proteins with a potential health-promoting effect in human intestinal Caco-2 cells. Proteomics 2006;6:2454–64.
17. Wright EM, Martin MG, Turk E. Intestinal absorption in health and disease–sugars. Best Pract Res Clin Gastroenterol 2003;17:943–56.
18. Voss AA, Diez-Sampedro A, Hirayama BA, et al. Imino sugars are potent agonists of the human glucose sensor SGLT3. Mol Pharmacol 2007;71:628–34.
19. Joost HG, Thorens B. The extended GLUT-family of sugar/pylol transport facilitators: Nomenclature, sequence characteristics, and potential function of its novel members. Mol Membr Biol 2001;18:247–56.
20. Rogers S, Macheda ML, Docherty SE, et al. Identification of a novel glucose transporter-like protein-GLUT 12. Am J Physiol Endocrinol Metab 2002;283:E733–8.
21. Manolescu A, Salas-burgos AM, Fischbarg J, et al. Identification of a hydrophobic residue as a key determinant of fructose transport by the facultative hexose transporter SLC2A7 (GLUT 7). J Biol Chem 2005;280:42978–83.
22. Drozdowski LA, Thomson ABR. Intestinal sugar transport. World J Gastroenterol 2006;12:1657–70.

23. Dyer J, Wood IS, Palejwala A, et al. Expression of monosaccharide transporters in intestine of diabetic humans. Am J Physiol 2002;282:G241–8.
24. Stuart CA, Howell ME, Yin D. Over-expression of GLUT5 in diabetic muscle is reversed by pioglitazone. Diabetes Care 2007;30:925–31.
25. Shoelson SE, Lee J, Goldfine AB. Inflammation and insulin resistance. J Clin Invest 2006;116:1793–801.
26. Shoelson SE, Herrero L, Naaz A. Obesity, inflammation and insulin resistance. Gastroenterology 2007;132:2169–80.
27. Kawaguchi T, Takenoshita M, Kabashima T, Uyeda K. Glucose and cAMP regulate the L-type pyruvate kinase gene by phosphorylation/dephosphorylation of the carbohydrate response element-binding protein. Proc Natl Acad Sci U S A 2001;98:13710–15.
28. Uyeda K, Yamashita H, Kawaguchi T. Carbohydrate responsive element-binding protein (ChREBP): A key regulator of glucose metabolism and fat storage. Biochem Pharmacol 2002;63:2075–7080.
29. Stoeckman AK, Towle HC. The role of SREBP-1c in nutritional regulation of lipogenic enzyme gene expression. J Biol Chem 2002;277:27029–35.
30. Dentin R, Pegorier JP, Benhamed F, et al. Hepatic glucokinase is required for the synergistic action of ChREBP and SREBP-1c on glycolytic and lipogenic gene expression. J Biol Chem 2004;279:20314–26.
31. Shimano H. SREBP-1c and TFE3, energy transcription factors that regulate hepatic insulin signalling. J Mol Med. 2007;85:437–44.
32. Matsummoto M, Ogawa W, Teshigawara K, et al. Role of the insulin receptor substrate 1 and phosphotidylinositol-3-kinase signalling pathway in insulin-induced expression of sterol regulatory element binding protein 1c and glucokinase genes in rat hepatocytes. Diabetes 2002;51:1672–80.
33. Carrillo JJ, Ibares B, Esteban-Gamboa A, Feliu JE. Involvement of both phosphatidyl 3-kinase and p44/p42 mitogen-activated protein kinase pathways in the short-term regulation of pyruvate kinase L by insulin. Endocrinology 2001; 142:1057–64.
34. Vaulont S, Vassaur-Cognet M, Kahn A. Glucose regulation of gene transcription. J Biol Chem 2000;275:31555–8.
35. Decaux JF, Marcillat O, Pichard AL, et al. Glucose-dependent and -independent effect of insulin on gene expression. J Biol Chem 1991;266:3432–8.
36. Lefrancois-Martinez A-M, Diaz-Guerra M-JM, Vallet V, et al. Glucose-dependent regulation of the L-pyruvate kinase gene in a hepatoma cell line is independent of insulin and cyclic AMP. FASEB J 1994;8:89–96.
37. Billin AN, Ayer DE. The Mlx network: Evidence for a parallel Max-like transcriptional network that regulates energy metabolism. Curr Top Microbiol Immunol 2006;302:255–78.
38. Yamada K, Tanaka T, Miyamoto K, Noguchi T. Sp family members and nuclear factor-Y cooperatively stimulate transcription from the rat pyruvate kinase gene distal promoter region via their direct interactions. J Biol Chem 2000;275:18129–33.
39. Gunawardana SC, Rocheleau JV, Head WS. Mechanism of time dependent potentiation of insulin release: Involvement of nitric oxide synthase. Diabetes 2006;55:1029–33.
40. Schumann DM, Maedler K, Franklin I. The Fas pathway is involved in pancreatic beta-cell secretory function. Proc Natl Acad Sci U S A 2007;104:2861–6.
41. MacDonald PE, Rorsman P. The ins and outs of secretion from pancreatic beta cells: Control of single vesicle exo and endocytosis. Physiology 2007;22:113–21.
42. Welsh M, Schrerberg N, Gilmore R, Steiner DF. Translational control of insulin biosynthesis. Evidence for regulation of elongation, inititiation and signal-recognition-particle-mediated translational arrest by glucose. Biochem J 1986;235:13590–4.
43. Guest PC, Baileys EM, Rutherford NG, Hutton JC. Insulin secretory granule biogensis: Co-ordinate regulation of the biosynthesis of the majority of constituent protein. Biochem J 1991;274:431–7.
44. Nishio Y, Aiello LP, King GL. Glucose induced genes in bovine aortic smooth muscle cells identified by mRNA differential display. FASEB J 1994;8:103–6.
45. Giddings SJ, Chirgwin J, Permutt MA. Effects of fasting and refeeding on preproinsulin messenger RNA. J Clin Invest 1981;67:952–60.
46. Giddings SJ, Chirgwin J, Permutt MA. Effects of glucose on proinsulin messenger RNA in rats *in vivo*. Diabetes 1982;31:624–9.
47. Kirschner BS. Nutritional consequences of inflammatory bowel disease on growth. J Am Coll Nutr 1988;7:301–8.
48. Kanof ME, Lake AM, Bayless TM. Decreased height velocity in children and adolescents before the diagnosis of Crohn's disease. Gastroenterology 1988;95:1523–7.
49. Corkins MR, Gohil AD, Fitzgerald JF. The insulin-like growth factor axis in children with inflammatory bowel disease. J Pediatr Gastroenterol Nutr 2003;36:228–34.
50. Sawczenko A, Azooz O, Paraszczuk J, et al. Intestinal inflammation-induced growth retardation acts through IL-6 in rats and depends on the -174 IL-6 G/C polymorphism in children. Proc Natl Acad Sci U S A 2005;102:13260–5.
51. Theiss AL, Furchtman S, Lund PK. Growth factors in inflammatory bowel disease: The actions and interactions of growth hormone and insulin-like growth factor-1. Inflamm Bowel Dis 2004;10:871–80.
52. Clark RP, Schuenke M, Keeton SM, et al. Effect of growth hormone and insulin-like growth factor-1 on muscle in mouse models of human growth disorders. Horm Res 2006;66:26–34.
53. Fant ME, Weisoly D. Insulin and insulin-like growth factors in human development: Implications for the perinatal period. Semin Perinatol 2001;6:426–35.
54. Cianfarani S, Liguori A, Germani D. IGF-1 and IGFBP-3 assessment in the management of childhood onset of growth hormone deficiency. Endocr Rev 2005;9:66–75.
55. Ekstrom K, Salemyr J, Zachrisson I, et al. Normalisation of IGF1/IGFBP axis by sustained nightly insulinisation in type 1 diabetes. Diabetes Care 2007;30:1357–63.
56. Vance ML, Herman ML, Thorner MO. Growth hormone and nutrition. Horm Res 1992;38:85–8.
57. Farthing MJ, Campbell CA, Walker-Smith J, et al. Nocturnal growth hormone and gonadotrophin secretion in growth retarded children with Crohn's disease. Gut 1981;22:933–8.
58. Dauncey MJ, Burton KA, White P, et al. Nutritional regulation of growth hormone receptor gene expression. FASEB J 1994;8:81–8.
59. Katsumata M, Cattaneo D, White P, et al. Growth hormone receptor gene expression in porcine skeletal and cardiac muscles is selectively upregulated by postnatal undernutrition. J Nutr 2000;130:2482–8.
60. Frystyk J, Delhanty PJD, Skjaerbaek C, Baxter RC. Changes in the circulating IGF system during short term fasting and refeeding in rats. Am J Physiol 1999;277:245–52.
61. Maes M, Underwood LE, Ketelslegers JM. Plasma somatomedin-C in fasted and refed rats: Close relationship with changes in liver somatogenic but not lactogenic binding sites. J Endocrinol 1983;97:243–52.
62. Thissen JP, Triest S, Maes M, et al. The decreased plasma concentration of insulin-like growth factor-1 in protein-restricted rats is not due to decreased numbers of growth hormone receptors on isolated hepatocytes. J Endocrinol 1990;124:159–65.
63. Peterson CA, Gillingham MB, Mohapatra NK, et al. Enterotrophic effect of insulin-like growth factor 1 but not growth hormone and localised expression of insulin-like growth factor 1, insulin-like growth factor binding protein-3 and –5 mRNAs in jejunum of paraenterally fed rats. J Parenter Enteral Nutr 2000;5:288–95.
64. Naranjo WM, Yakar S, Sanchez-Gomez M, et al. Protein calorie restriction affects non-hepatic IGF-1 production in lymphoid system: Studies using the liver specific IGF-1 gene knock-out mouse model. Endocrinology 2002;143:2233–41.
65. Alfieri CM, Evans-Anderson HJ, Yutzey RE. Developmental regulation of the mouse IGF-1 exon 1 promoter region by calcineurin activation of NFAT in skeletal muscle. Am J Physiol Cell Physiol 2007;292:C1887–94.
66. Zhang J, Whitehead RE, Underwood LE. Effect of fasting on insulin-like growth factor (IGF)-IA and IGF-IB messsenger ribonuceic acids and prehormones in rat liver. Endocrinology 1997;138:3112–8.
67. Bucuvalas JC, Chernausek SD, Alfaro MP, et al. Effect of insulin-like growth factor-1 treatment in children with cystic fibrosis. J Pediatr Gastroenterol Nutr 2001;33:576–58.
68. Martin JI, Baxter RC. Insulin-like growth factor binding protein-3: Biochemistry and physiology. Growth Regul 1992;2:88–99.
69. Conover CA. Potentiation of insulin-like growth factor (IGF) action by IGF-binding protein-3: Studies of underlying mechanism. Endocrinology 1992;130:3191–9.
70. Silha JV, Murphy LJ. Insulin-like growth factor binding proteins in development. Adv Exp Med Biol 2005;567:55–89.
71. Villafuerte BC, Koop BL, Pao CI, et al. Coculture of primary rat hepatocytes and nonparenchymal cells permits expression of insulin-like growth factor binding protein-3 *in vitro*. Endocrinology 1994;134:2044–50.
72. Chang EB, Rao MC. Intestinal water and electrolyte transport. In: Johnson LR, editor. Physiology of the Gastrointestinal Tract, 3rd edition. New York: Raven Press; 1994. p. 2027–81.
73. Sanderson IR, Parsons DS. Influence of vascular flow on amino acid transport across the frog small intestine. J Physiol 1980;309:447–60.
74. Sanderson IR, Walker WA. Uptake and transport of macromolecules by the intestine: Possible role in clinical disorders (an update). Gastroenterology 1993;104:622–39.
75. Sanderson IR, Croft NM. The antiinflammatory effects of enteral nutrition. J Parenter Enteral Nutr 2005;29:S134–8.
76. Xavier RJ, Podolsky DK. Unravelling the pathogenesis of inflammatory bowel disease. Nature 2007;448:427–34.
77. Kapoor A, Joyce Li H, Leiter AB. Intestinal development: The many faces of Wnt signalling. Gastroenterol 2007;133:710–2.
78. Cox TM. Aldolase B and fructose intolerance. FASEB J 1994;8:62–71.
79. Le Gall M, Tobin V, Stolarczyk E, et al. Sugar sensing by enterocytes combines polarity, membrane-bound detectors and sugar metabolism. J Cell Physiol 2007;213:834–43.
80. Sibley E. Carbohydrate intolerance. Curr Opin Gastroenterol 2004;20:162–7.
81. Robinson J, Heineke EW, Belgovic ME. Quantitative relationship between intestinal sucrase inhibition and reduction of the glycemic response to sucrose in rats. J Nutr 1990;120:105–11.
82. Goda T, Yamada K, Bustamante S, et al. Precocious increase of sucrase activity by carbohydrates in the small intestine of suckling rats. I. Significance of the stress effect of sugar-induced diarrhea. J Pediatr Gastroenterol Nutr 1985;4:468–75.
83. Hunziker W, Spiess M, Semenza G, Lodish HF. The sucrase-isomaltase-complex: Primary structure, membrane-orientation, and evolution of a stalked, intrinsic brush border protein. Cell 1986;46:227–32.
84. Yeh KY, Holt PR. Ontogenic timing mechanism initiates the expression of rat intestinal sucrase activity. Gastroenterology 1986;90:520–6.
85. Rosamond WD, Savaiano DA. Maintenance of sucrase activity in rat small intestine: Influence of diet and age. Dig Dis Sci 1988;33:1397–402.
86. Alpers DH, Gerber JE. Monosaccharide inhibition of human intestinal lactase. J Lab Clin Med 1971;78:265–74.
87. Castillo RO, Feng JJ, Stevenson DK, Kwong LK. Altered maturation of small intestinal function in the absence of intraluminal nutrients: Rapid normalization with refeeding. Am J Clin Nutr 1991;53:558–61.
88. Ferraris RP, Villenas SA, Diamond J. Regulation of brush border enzyme activities and enterocyte migration rates in mouse small intestine. Am J Physiol 1992;262:G1047–59.
89. Markowitz A, Birkenmeier E, Traber PG. The 5'-flank of the human sucrase isomaltose (SI) gene directs intestine-specific transcription in transgenic mice. Gastroenterology 1991;102:A285.
90. Traber PG, Wu GD, Want W. Novel DNA-binding proteins regulate intestine-specific transcription of the sucrase-isomaltose gene. Mol Cell Biol 1992;12:3614–27.
91. Bourdeau F, Zhu Y, Traber PG. Sucrase-isomaltase gene transcription requires the hepatocyte nuclear factor-1 (HNF-1) regulatory element and is regulated by the ratio of HNF-1 alpha/HNF-1 beta. J Biol Chem 2001;276:32122–8.
92. Boudreau FB, Rings EH, Van Wering HM, et al. Hepatocyte-nuclear-factor-1 (HNF-1 alpha), GATA-4 and caudal-related homeodomain protein Cdx2 functionally interact to modulate intestinal gene transcription: Implication for the developmental regulation of the sucrase-isomaltase gene. J Biol Chem 2002;277:31909–17.
93. Bosse T, Fialkovich JJ, Piaseckyj CM, et al. GATA-4 and HNF-1 alpha are partially required for the expression of specific intestinal genes during development. Am J Physiol Gastrointest Liver Physiol 2007;292:G1302–4.
94. Freund JN, Deluc I, Raul F. Lactase expression is controlled differently in the jejunum and ileum during development in rat. Gastroenterology 1990;100:388–94.
95. Wright EM, Hirayama BA, Loo DF. Active sugar transport in health and disease. J Intern Med 2007;261:32–43.
96. Kotler DP, Levine GM, Shiau YF. Effects of nutrients, endogenous secretions, and fasting on *in vitro* glucose uptake. Am J Physiol 1980;238:G219–27.
97. Sharp PA, Debnam ES, Srai SK. Rapid enhancement of brush border glucose uptake after exposure of rat jejunal mucosa to glucose. Gut 1996;39:545–50.
98. Ferraris RP. Dietary and developmental regulation of intestinal sugar transport. Biochem J 2001;360:265–76.
99. Ferraris RP, Diamond JM. Crypt/villus site of substrate-dependent regulation of mouse intestinal glucose transporters. Proc Natl Acad Sci U S A 1993;90:5868–72.
100. Solberg DH, Diamond JM. Comparison of different dietary sugars as inducers of intestinal sugar transporters. Am J Physiol 1987;252:G574–84.
101. Ferraris RP, Diamond JM. Specific regulation of intestinal nutrient transporters by their dietary substrates. Ann Rev Physiol 1989;51:125–41.
102. Ferraris RP, Diamond J. Crypt-villus site of glucose transporter induction by dietary carbohydrate in mouse intestine. Am J Physiol 1992;262:G1069–73.
103. Shirazi-Beechey SP. Intestinal sodium-dependent D-glucose co-transporter: Dietary regulation. Proc Nutr Soc 1996;55:167–78.

104. Ferraris R, Villenas SA, Hirayama BA, Diamond J. Effect of diet on glucose transporter site density along the intestinal crypt-villus axis. Am J Physiol 1992;262:G1060–8.
105. Hu Z, Yang Y, Graham WV, et al. MAPAPK-2 is a critical signalling intermediate in NH3 activation followign Na^+ glucose transport. J Biol Chem 2006;281:24247–53.
106. Yu LC, Turner JR, Buret AG. LPS/CD14 activation triggers SGLT-1 mediated glucose uptake and cell rescue in intestinal epithelial cells via early apoptotic signals upstream of caspase 3. Exp Cell Res 2006;312:3276–86.
107. Perissé J, Sizaret F, François P. FAO Nutr Newslett 1969;7:1–9.
108. Sheppard RW, Holt TL, Thomas BJ, et al. Nutritional rehabilitation in cystic fibrosis, controlled studies of effect on nutritional growth retardation, body protein turnover and course of pulmonary disease. J Pediatr 1986;109:788–94
109. Bernback S, Blackberg L, Hernell O. Fatty acids generated by gastric lipase promote human milk triacylglycerol digestion by pancreatic colipase-dependent lipase. Biochim Biophys Acta 1989;1001:286–93.
110. Fredickson B, Olivecrona T. Decrease of lipase and esterase activities in intestinal contents of newborn infants during test meals. Pediatr Res 1978;12:631–4.
111. Dipalma J, Kirk CL, Hamosh M, et al. Lipase and pepsin activity in the gastric mucosa of infants, children and adults. Gastroenterology 1991;101:116–21.
112. Hamosh M, Scanlon JW, Ganot D, et al. Fat digestion in the newborn: Characterization of lipase in gastric aspirates of premature and term infants. J Clin Invest 1981;67:838–46.
113. Lee PC, Borysewicz R, Struve M, et al. Development of lipolytic activity in gastric aspirates from premature infants. J Pediatr Gastroenterol Nutr 1993;17:291–7.
114. Miled N, Canaan S, Dupuis L, et al. Digestive lipases: From three-dimensional structure to physiology. Biochimie 2000;82:973–86.
115. Armand M. Lipases and lipolysis in the human digestive tract: Where do we stand? Curr Opin Nutr Metab Care 2007;10:156–64.
116. Moreau H, Luagier R, Gargouri Y, et al. Human preduodenal lipase is entirely of gastric fundic origin. Gastroenterology 1988;95:1221–6.
117. Abrams CK, Hamosh M, Lee TC, et al. Gastric lipase: Localization in the human stomach. Gastroenterology 1988;95:1460–8.
118. Borel P, Armand M, Senft M, et al. Gastric lipase: Evidence of an adaptive response to dietary fat in the rabbit. Gastroenterology 1991;100:1582–9.
119. Armand M, Hamosh M, DiPalma JS, et al. Human gastric lipase expression is affected by dietary fat. Pediatr Res 1995;37:119A.
120. Tso P, Nauli A, Lo C-M. Enterocyte fatty acid uptake and intestinal fatty acid-binding protein. Biochem Soc Trans 2004;32:75–8.
121. Milger K, Harrmann T, Becker C, et al. Cellular uptake of fatty acids driven by ER-localised acyl-CoA synthetase FATP4. J Cell Sci 2006;119:4687–88.
122. Levy E, Menard D, Delvin E, et al. The polymorphism at codon 54 of the FABP2 gene increases fat absoprtion in human intestinal explants. J Biol Chem 2001;276:39679–84.
123. Stan S, Lambert M, Delvin E, et al. Intestinal fatty acid binding protein and microsomal triglyceride transfer protein polymorphisms in French-Canadian youth. J Lipid Res 2005;46:320–7.
124. Hajri T, Xia Han X, Bonen A, Abumrad NA. Defective fatty acid uptake modulates insulin responsiveness and metabolic responses to diet in CD36-null mice. J Clin Invest 2002;109:1381–9.
125. Goudriaan JR, Dahlmans VE, Febbraio M, et al. Intestinal lipid absoprtion is not affected in CD36 deficient mice. Mol Cell Biochem 2002;239:199–202.
126. Hajri T, Hall AM, Jensen DR, et al. CD36-facilitated fatty acid uptake inhibits leptin production and signalling in adipose tissue. Diabetes 2007; 7:1872–80.
127. Yasunaga T, Koga S, Ikeda S, et al. Cluster differentiation-36 deficiency type 1 and acute coronary syndrome without major cardiovascular risk factors: Case report. Circ J 2007;71:166–9.
128. Siafakas CG, Anatolitou F, Fusunyan RD, et al. Vascular endothelial growth factor (VEGF) is present in human breast milk and its receptor is present on intestinal epithelial cells. Paediatr Res 1999;45:652–7.
129. Playford RJ, MacDonald CE, Johnson WS. Colostrum and milk-derived peptide growth factors for the treatment of gastrointestinal disorders. Am J Clin Nutr 2000;72:5–14.
130. Kobata R, Tsukahara H, Ohshima Y, et al. High levels of growth factors in human breast milk. Early Hum Dev; in press.
131. He Y, Chu SH, Walker WA. Nucleotide supplements alter proliferation and differentiation of cultured human (Caco-2) and rat (IEC-6) intestinal epithelial cells. J Nutr 1993;123:1017–27.
132. Sanderson IR, He Y. Nucleotide uptake and metabolism by intestinal epithelial cells in tissue culture. J Nutr 1994;124:131S–7S.
133. Schack-Nielsen L, Michaelsen KF. Breast feeding and future health. Curr Opin Clin Nutr Metab Care 2006;9:289–96.
134. Schack-Nielsen L, Michaelsen KF. Advances in our understanding of the biology of human milk and its effects on the offspring. J Nutr 2007;137:503S–10S.
135. Masson PL, Heremans JF. Lactoferrin in milk from different species. Comp Biochem Physiol 1971;39B:119–29.
136. Masson PL, Heremans JF, Schonne E. Lactoferrin, an iron-binding protein in neutrophilic leukocytes. J Exp Med 1969;130:643–58.
137. Bennett RM, Eddie-Quartey AC, Holt PJL. Lactoferrin: An iron-binding protein in synovial fluid. Arthritis Rheum 1973;16:186–90.
138. Domellof M. Iron requirements, absoprtion and metabolism in infancy and childhood. Curr Opin Clin Nutr Metab Care 2007;10:329–35.
139. Weinberg ED. Antibiotic properties and applications of lactoferrin. Curr Pharm Des 2007;13:801–11.
140. Baker EN. Lactoferrin: A multi-tasking protein par excellence. Cell Mol Life Sci 2005;62:2529–30.
141. Legrand D, Elass E, Carpentier M, Mazurier J. Interaction of lactoferrin with cells involved in immune function. Biochem Cell Biol 2006;84:282–90.
142. Mincheva-Nilsson L, Hammarstom S, Hammarstom ML. Activated human gamma delta T cells express functional lactoferrin receptors. Infect Immun 1997;46:609–18.
143. McAbee DD, Bennatt DJ, Ling YY. Identification and analysis of a Ca^{2+} dependent lactoferrin receptor in liver. Lactoferrin binds to the asialoglycoprotein receptor in a galactose-independent manner. Adv Exp Med Biol 1998;443:113–21.
144. Lonnerdal B. Lactoferrin binding to its intestinal receptor. Adv Exp Med Biol 1991; 310:145–50.
145. Kawakami H, Lonnerdal B. Isolation and function of a receptor for human lactoferrin in human fetal intestinal brush-border membranes. Am J Physiol 1991;261:G841–6.
146. Davidson LA, Lonnerdal B. Specific binding of lactoferrin to brush-border membrane: Ontogeny and effect of glycan chain. Am J Physiol 1988;254:G580–5.
147. Mazurier J, Montreuil J, Spik G. Visualization of lactotransferrin brush-border receptors by ligand-blotting. Biochem Biophys Acta 1985;821:453–60.
148. Hu W-L, Mazurier J, Sawatzki G, et al. Lactotransferrin receptor of mouse small-intestinal brush border. Binding characteristics of membrane-bound and Triton X-100-solubilized forms. Biochem J 1988;249:435–41.
149. Britton JR, Koldovsky O. Gastric luminal digestion of lactoferrin and transferrin by preterm infants. Early Hum Dev 1989;19:127–35.
150. Kuwata H, Yip TT, Yamauchi K, et al. The survival of ingested lactoferrin in the gastrointestinal tract of adult mice. Biochem J 1998;334:321–3.
151. Hutchens TW, Henry JF, Yip TT. Structurally intact forms of maternal lactoferrin purified from urine of preterm infants fed human milk. Proc Natl Acad Sci U S A 1991;88:2994–8.
152. Strom M, Haug B, Rekdal Y, et al. Important structural features of 15-residue lactoferricin derivatives and methods for improvement of antimicrobial actvitiy. Biochem Cell Biol 2002;80:67–74.
153. Lopez V, Suzuki YA, Lonnerdal B. Ontogenic changes in lactoferrin receptor and DMTI in mouse small intestine: Implications for iron absorption during early life. Biochem Cell Biol 2006;84:337–44.
154. Mikogami T, Marianne T, Spik G. Effect of intracellular iron depletion by picolinic acid on expression of the lactoferrin receptor in the human colon carcinoma cell subclone HT29-18-C_1. Biochem J 1995;308:391–7.
155. Klausner RD, Rouault TA, Harford JB. Regulating the fate of mRNA: The control of cellular iron metabolism. Cell 1993;72:19–28.
156. Mulligan P, White NR, Monteleone G, et al. Breast milk lactoferrin regulates gene expression by binding bacterial CpG motifs but not genomic DNA promoters in model intestinal cells. Pediatr Res 2006;59:656–61.
157. Wakabayashi H, Takakura N, Yamauchi K, Tamura Y. Modulation of immunity related gene expression in small intestines of mice by oral administration of lactoferrin. Clin Vaccine Immunol 2006;13:239–45.
158. Zimecki M, Stepnaik D, Szynol A, Kruzel ML. Lactoferrin regulates proliferative response of human peripheral blood mononuclear cells to phytohemagglutinin and mixed lymphocyte reaction. Arch Immunol Ther Exp 2001;49:147–54.
159. Naot D, Grey A, Reid IR, Cornish J. Lactoferrin—A novel bone growth factor. Clin Med Res 2005;3:93–101.
160. Buccigrossi V, de Marco G, Bruzzese E, et al. Lactoferrin induces concentration dependent functional modulation of intestinal proliferation and differentiation. Pediatr Res 2007;61:410–4.
161. Oguchi S, Walker WA, Sanderson IR. Iron saturation alters the effect of lactoferrin on the proliferation and differentiation of human enterocytes (Caco-2) cells. Biol Neonate 1995;67:330–9.
162. Sharp P, Srai SK. Molecular mechanisms involved in intestinal iron absorption. World J Gastroenterol 2007;13:4716–24.
163. Miyazawa K, Mantel C, Lu L, et al. Lactoferrin-lipopolysaccharide interactions. Effect on lactoferrin binding to monocyte/macrophage-differentiated HL-60 cells. J Immunol 1991;146:723–9.
164. Kawakami H, Dosako S, Lonnerdal B. Iron uptake form transferrin in human fetal intestinal brush-border membrane vesicles. Am J Physiol 1990;261:G535–41.
165. Suzuki YA, Lopez V, Lonnerdal B. Mammalian lactoferrin receptors: Structure and function. Cell Mol Life Sci 2005;62:2650–75.
166. Liao Y, Lopez V, Shafizadeh TB, et al. Cloning of a pig homologue of the human lactoferrin receptor: Expression and localisation during intestinal maturation in piglets. Comp Biochem Physiol A Mol Integr Physiol 2007;148:584–90.
167. Kagnoff MF, Eckmann L. Epithelial cells as sensors for microbial infection. J Clin Invest 1997;100:6–10.
168. Dommett R, Zilbauer M, George JT, Bajaj-Elliott M. Innate immune defence in the gastrointestinal tract. Mol Immunol 2005;42:903–13.
169. Clavel T, Haller D. Molecular interactions between bacteria, epithelium and the mucosal immune system in the intestinal tract: Implications for chronic inflammation. Curr Issues Intest Microbiol 2007;8:25–43.
170. Mitchell JA, Paul-Clark MJ, Clarke GW, et al. Critical role of toll-like receptors and nucleotide oligomerisation domain in the regulation of health and disease. J Endocrinol 2007;193:323–30.
171. Naik S, Kelly EJ, Meijer L, et al. Absence of Toll-like receptor 4 explains endotoxin hyporesponsiveness in human intestinal epithelium. J Pediatr Gastroenterol Nutr 2001;32:449–53.
172. Shibolet O, Podolsky DK. TLRs in the Gut. Negative regulation of Toll like receptors and intestinal homestasis: Addition by substraction. Am J Physiol Gastrointest liver Physiol 2007;292:G1469–73.
173. Strober W, Fuss I, Mannon P. The fundamnetal basis of inflammatory bowel disease. J Clin Invest 1007;117:514–21.
174. Ohtsuka Y, Lee J, Stamm DS, Sanderson IR. MIP-2 secreted by epithelial cells increases neutrophil and lymphocyte recruitement in the mouse intestine. Gut 2001;49:526–33.
175. Westendorf AM, Bruder D, Hansen W, Buer J. Intestinal epithelial antigen induces CD4+ Tcell regulatory phenotype in a transgenic autoimmune model. Ann N Y Acad Sci 2006;1072:401–6.
176. Sanderson IR. Dietary regulation of genes expressed in the developing intestinal epithelium. Am J Clin Nutr 1998;68:999–1005.
177. Diag R, Rogler G, Aschenbrenner E, et al. Human intestinal epithelial cells secrete interkeukin-1 receptor antagonist and interleukin 8 but not interleukin 1 or interleukin 6. Gut 2000;46(3):50–8.
178. Keates S, Keates AC, Mizoguchi E, et al. Enterocytes are the primary source of chemokine ENA-78 in normal colon and ulcerative colitis. Am J Physiol1997;273(1):G75–82.
179. Shibahara T, Wilcox JN, Couse T, et al. Characterisation of epithelial chemoattractants for human intestinal intraepithelial lymphocytes. Gastroenterol 2001;120(1):60–70.
180. Ogawa H, limura M, Eckmann L, et al. Regulated production of the chemokine CCL28 in human colon epthelium. Am J Physiol Gastroinest Liver Physiol 2004;287(5):G1062–9.
181. Marks DJ, Harbord MW, MacAllister R, et al. Defective acute inflammation in Crohn's disease: A clinical investigation. Lancet 2006;367:668–78.
182. Kayo S, Ikura Y, Suekane T, et al. Close association between activated platelets and neutrophils in the active phase of ulcerative colitis in humans. Inflamm Bowel Dis 2006;12:727–35.
183. Flint HJ, Duncan SH, Scott KP, Louis P. Interactions and competition between the microbial community of the human colon: Links between diet and health. Environ Microbiol 2007;9:1101–11.
184. Sanderson IR, Naik S. Dietary regulation of gene expression. Ann rev Nutr 2000;20:311–38.
185. Bullen CL, Tearle PV, Stewart MG. The effect of "humanised" milks and supplemented breast feeding on the faecal flora of infants. J Med Microbiol 1977;10:403–13.
186. Weaver GA, Krause JA, Miller TL, Wolin MJ. Cornstarch fermentation by the colonic microbial community yields more butyrate than does cabbage fiber fermentation. Am J Clin Nutr 1992;55:70–7.
187. Fusunyan RD, Ohno Y, MacDermott RP, Sanderson IR. Short-chain fatty acids enhance interleukin-8 by Caco-2 cells. Gastroenterology 1995;108:A726.
188. Weng M, Walker WA, Sanderson IR. Butyrate regulates the expression of pathogen-triggered IL-8 in intestinal epithelia. Pediatr Res; in press.

189. Fusunyan RD, Quinn JJ, Fujimoto M, et al. Butyrate switches the pattern of chemokine secretion by intestinal epithelial cells through histone acetylation. Mol Med 1999;5:631–40.
190. Reinecker HC, Loh EY, Ringler DJ, et al. Monocyte-chemoattractant protein 1 gene expression in intestinal epithelial cells and inflammatory bowel disease mucosa. Gastroenterology 1995;108:40–50.
191. Salzman NH, Underwood MA, Bevins CL. Paneth cells, defensins and the commensal microbiota: A hypothesis on interplay at the intestinal mucosa. Semin Immunol 2007;19:70–83.
192. Wehkamp J, Schmid M, Stange EF. Defensins and other antimicrobial peptides in inflammatory bowel disease. Curr Opin Gastroenterol 2007;23:370–8.
193. Islam D, Bandholtz L, Nilsson J, et al. Dpownregulation of bactericidal peptides in enteric infections; a novel immune escape mechanism with bacterial DNA as a potential regulator. Nat Med 2001;7:180–5.
194. Bajaj-Elliott M, Fedeli P, Smith GV, et al. Modulation of host antimicrobial peptides (-defensin 1 and 2) expression during gastritis. Gut 2002;51:356–61.
195. Nuding S, Fellerman K, Wehkamp J, Stange EF. Reduced mucosal antimicrobial activity in Crohn's disease of the colon. Gut 2007;56:1240–7.
196. Wehkamp J, Wang G, Kubler I, et al. The Paneth cell alpha defensin deficiency in ileal Crohn's disease is linked to Wnt/TCF-4. J Immunol 2007;179:3109–18.
197. Gutcher I, Becher B. APC-derived cytokines and T cell polarization in autoimmune inflammation. J Clin Invest 2007;117:1119–27.
198. Mayer L, Blumberg RS. Antigen presenting cells: Epithelial cells. In: Orga PL, Mestecky J, Lamm ME, editors. Mucosal Immunology, 2nd edition. San Diego, CA: Academic Press; 1999. p. 365–79.
199. Telega GW, Baumgart DC, Carding SR. Uptake and presentation of antigen to T cells by primary colonic epithelial cells in normal and diseased states. Gastroenterology 2000;119:1548–59.
200. Stockinger B, Pessara U, In RH, et al. A role of Ia-associated invariant chains in antigen processing and presentation. Cell 1989;56:683–9.
201. Sanderson IR, Ouellette AJ, Carter EA, Harmatz PR. Ontogeny of class II MHC mRNA in the mouse small intestinal epithelium. Mol Immunol 1992;29:1257–63.
202. Sanderson IR, Ouellette AJ, Carter EA, Harmatz PR. Ontogeny of Ia messenger RNA in the mouse intestinal epithelium is modulated by age of weaning and diet. Gastroenterology 1993;105:974–80.
203. Wolf SE, Woodside KJ, Ramirez RJ, et al. Insulin-like growth factor 1/insulin-like growth factor protein 3 alters lymphocyte resposiveness follwign severe burn. J Surg Res 2004;117:251–61.
204. Brocardo MG, Schillaci R, Galeano A, et al. Early effects of insulin-like growth factor-1 in activated human lymphocytes. J Leukoc Biol 2001;70:297–305.
205. Clark R, Strasser J, McCabe S, et al. Insulin-like growth-factor stimulation of lymphocytes. J Clin Invest 1993;92:540–8.
206. Oguchi S, Walker WA, Sanderson IR. Profile of IGF-binding proteins secreted by human intestinal epithelial cells changes with differentiation. Am J Physiol 1994;267:G843–50.
207. Oguchi S, Walker WA, Sanderson IR. Insulin-like growth factor binding protein profile secreted by human intestinal epithelial cells varies with polarity. Biochem Biophys Res Commun 1993;196:789–93.
208. Nishimura A, Martinez O, Oguchi S, et al. Profile of IGF-binding proteins secreted by intestinal epithelial cells changes with difference nutrients. Gastroenterology 1995;108:A742.
209. Diaz-Guerra MJ, Bergort MO, Martinez A, et al. Functional characterization of the L-type pyruvate kinase gene glucose response complex. Mol Cell Biol 1993;13:7725–33.
210. Liu Z, Thompson KS, Towle HC. Carbohydrate regulation of the rat L-type pyruvate kinase gene requires two nuclear factors: LF-A1 and a member of the c-myc family. J Biol Chem 1993;268:12787–95.
211. Cuif MH, Porteau A, Kahn A, Vaulot S. Exploration of a liver-specific glucose/insulin-responsive promoter in transgenic mice. J Biol Chem 1993;268:13769–72.
212. MacFarlane WM, Read ML, Gilligan M, et al. Glucose modulates the binding activity of the beta-cell transcription factor IUF1 in a phosphorylation-dependent manner. Biochem J 1994;303:625–31.
213. Foufelle F, Gouhot B, Pegorier JP, et al. Glucose stimulation of lipogenic enzyme gene expression in cultured white adipose tissue. J Biol Chem 1992;267:20543–6.
214. Derbyshire E. A review of maternal nutrition and fetal gene expression. Br J Nurs 2007;16:820–2.
215. Willett WC. Diet and health: What should we eat? Science 1994;264:532–7.
216. Hostetter TH, Meyer TW, Rennke HG, Brenner BM. Chronic effects of dietary protein on renal structure and function in the rat with intact and reduced renal mass. Kidney Int 1986;30:509–17.
217. Heycock GB. Renal disease. In: McLaren DS, Burman DS, Belton AR, Williams AF, editors. Textbook of Paediatric Nutrition, 3rd edition. Edinburgh: Churchill-Livingston; 1991. p. 237–56.
218. Guedon C, Schmitz J, Lerebours E, et al. Decreased brush border hydrolase activities without gross morphologic changes in human intestinal mucosal after prolonged total parenteral nutrition of adults. Gastroenterology 1986;90:373–8.
219. Moore FA, Moore EE, Jones TN, et al. TEN versus TPN following major abdominal trauma reduced septic morbidity. J Trauma 1989;29:916–22.
220. Feldman EJ, Dowling RH, McNaughton J, Peters TJ. Effects of oral versus intravenous nutrition on intestinal adaptation after small bowel resection in the dog. Gastroenterology 1976;70:712–9.
221. Spector MH, Levine GM, Deren JL. Direct and indirect effects of dextrose and amino acids on gut mass. Gastroenterology 1977;72:706–10.
222. Baker SS, Baker RD. Enteric versus Parenteral Feeding and Mucosal Function. Immunophysiology of the Gut. San Diego, CA: Academic Press; 1993. p. 401–14.
223. Liu X, Nelson DW, Holst JJ, Ney DM. Synergitic effect of supplemental enteral nutrients and exogenous glucagon-like peptide 2 on intestinal adaptation in a rat model of short bowel syndrome. Am J Clin Nutr 2006;84:1142–50.
224. Rombeau JL, Afonso JJ. Clinical and scientific basis for nutritional support of patients with inflammatory bowel disease. In: MacDermott RP, Stenson WF, editors. Inflammatory Bowel Disease. New York: Elsevier; 1992. p. 525–53.
225. Sanderson IR, Walker-Smith JA. Enteral feeding. In: McLaren DS, Burman D, Belton NF, Williams AF, editors. Textbook of Paediatric Nutrition,. 3rd edition. Edinburgh: Churchill-Livingston; 1991. p. 321–36.
226. O'Morain C, Segal M, Levi AJ. Elemental diet in acute Crohn's disease: A controlled trial. BMJ 1984;288:1859–62.
227. Sanderson IR, Udeen S, Davies PSW, et al. Remission induced by an elemental diet in small bowel Crohn's disease. Arch Dis Child 1987;62:123–7.
228. Thomas AG, Taylor F, Miller V. Dietary intake and nutritional treatment in childhood Crohn's disease. J Pediatr Gastroenterol Nutr 1993;17:75–81.
229. Sanderson IR, Boulton P, Menzies I, Walker-Smith JA. Improvement of abnormal lactulose rhamnose permeability ratio in active small bowel Crohn's disease by an elemental diet. Gut 1987;28:1073–6.
230. Teahon K, Smethurst P, Pearson M, et al. The effect of elemental diet on intestinal permeability and inflammation in Crohn's disease. Gastroenterology 1991;110:84–9.
231. Nicholls S, Domizio P, Williams CB, et al. Cyclosporin as initial treatment for Crohn's disease. Arch Dis Child 1994;71:243–7.
232. Ruuska T, Savilahti E, Maki M, et al. Exclusive whole protein enteral diet versus prednisolone in the treatment of acute Crohn's disease in children. J Pediatr Gastroenterol Nutr 1994;19:175–80.
233. Steiner SJ, Pfefferkorn MD, Fitzgerald JF, Denne SC. Protein and energy metabolism response to the initial dose of infliximab in children with Crohn's disease. Inflamm Bowel Dis 2007;13:737–44.
234. Sano Y, Gomez FE, Kang W, et al. Intestinal polymorphic immunoglobulin receptor is affected by type and route of nutirtion. J Parenter Enteral Nutr 2007;31:351–7.
235. Staunton DE, Merluzzi VJ, Rothlein R, et al. A cell adhesion molecule, ICAM-1, is the major surface receptor for rhinoviruses. Cell 1989;56:849–53.
236. Pollok RC, Farthing MJG, Bajaj-Elliott M, et al. Interferon-gamma induces enterocyte resistence against infection by the intracellular pathogen *Cryptosporidium parvum*. Gastroenterology 2001;120:99–107.

20

Nutrition and the Humoral Regulation of Growth

William E. Russell, MD
J. Marc Rhoads, MD

Hormones and nutrients interact to influence growth at all levels of biologic organization. Growth is often loosely defined to include all aspects of somatic enlargement and maturation. The principal impact of malnutrition on the growing child is to diminish or reverse weight gain. When malnutrition is of sufficient duration or intensity, statural growth is retarded, although under some unusual circumstances, malnutrition may selectively impair linear growth without a preceding or concomitant loss in weight.[1] The manifestations of malnutrition effects on growth are often subtle, frequently masquerading as social, ethnic, or racial characteristics. In a study of ethnically homogeneous conscripts in the Polish army, Bielicki and colleagues found that young men from large families, from the countryside, and from lower socioeconomic classes were smaller than their counterparts from smaller, urban, and more privileged families.[2] These authors concluded that the negative impact of these variables on stature could all be attributed to suboptimal nutrition. On a large scale, the effect of malnutrition is often so striking as to produce major population differences in stature that appear to be genetic. For instance, prior to World War II, native Japanese were smaller than Americans of European ancestry and smaller than Japanese-Americans raised in the United States.[3] However, with the significant nutritional improvements that took place in Japan following World War II, these differences vanished.[4]

NUTRIENTS, HORMONES, AND GROWTH

Hormones and Growth Factors

Hormones are generally defined as the secretions of glands that specialize in their production; classic hormones, acting through an endocrine mode of regulation, therefore require conveyance through the circulation to alter the function of distant tissues. Their concentrations and association with binding proteins can be readily measured in the blood and other body fluids. Regulation occurs not only through changes in the concentration of the hormone, but also in the numbers and cellular distribution of their peripheral receptors and in the systems of second messengers within the target cells that convey these signals to the genome or other cellular compartment. Each of these steps can be regulated by developmental programs and by the local milieu of nutrients and other hormones.

The body-wide endocrine system, however, is also an integrating system that is superimposed upon multiple local regulatory systems that employ *paracrine* modes of regulation.[5] Paracrine control refers to the release by cells of soluble messengers that act upon neighboring cells of another type. A circulation is not required because only physical proximity and the presence of receptors are required for effect. In 1980, Sporn and Todaro added the concept of *autocrine* control to include the substances that cells secrete to regulate their own growth.[6] Although autocrine control was initially thought to be a mode of growth control for neoplastic cells exclusively, autocrine control also characterizes the growth and function of many normal cells. Examples of autocrine control include the release of epidermal growth factor (EGF) by ulcerated gastrointestinal mucosa and release of transforming growth factor-alpha by normal intestinal epithelial cells.[7] As a consequence of the narrow range of action within the extracellular space of autocrine and paracrine growth factors, their roles in cellular regulation are much more difficult to document in clinical situations. It has recently emerged that proteolytic events at the cell surface are critical regulators of the accessibility of autocrine and paracrine factors to their receptors.[8] Multiple proteases associated with extracellular matrix or cell membranes are known to solubilize and activate growth factors from their cell surface anchored, but biologically inactive, precursors.

It has been proposed that growth factors can exert biologic actions without release into the extracellular space. *Juxtacrine* control refers to the actions of growth factors that remain anchored to the plasma membranes of the cells that produced them; cell-to-cell contact brings them into contact with receptor-bearing target cells.[9] Finally, some growth-regulatory molecules can activate receptors on intracellular membranes including those in the cytoplasm, the nucleus, nucleolus, or mitochondrion, a mode of action called *intracrine* control.[10] In some instances, intracrine factors originate within their target cell and in other instances they are internalized from the extracellular space. Intracrine action appears to be critical for the regulation of the chicken ovalbumin gene.[11] In conjunction with the neuroendocrine mode of regulation, which makes use of axons to direct regulatory neurotransmitters to their target cells, the multiple systems of cellular regulation provide a diversity of regulatory options, each of which has relevance to an understanding of nutritional influences on growth. The characteristics of endocrine, paracrine, autocrine, juxtacrine, intracrine, and neuroendocrine modes of regulation are summarized in Table 1.

In addition to the protein and steroid molecules that comprise the classic hormones of the endocrine system, locally acting substances, often designated "growth factors" are the principal

Table 1 Modes of Cellular Regulation

Mode	Agent	Source	Vehicle	Target	Modulators
Endocrine	Hormone	Gland	Circulation	Heterologous tissue	Neurons Hormones Growth factors
Paracrine	Growth factor	Local site	Diffusion	Heterologous cell	Hormones Growth factors
Autocrine	Growth factor	Local site	Diffusion	Autologous cell	Hormones Growth factors
Juxtacrine	Growth factor precursor	Local site	Cell contact	Adjacent cell	Proteases
Intracrine	Hormone Growth factor Nutrient	Intracellular	Cytoplasm	Intracellular receptor	?
Neuroendocrine	Neurotransmitter Growth factor	Neuron	Axon	Heterologous tissue	Hormones Growth factors Neurons

agents of the paracrine, autocrine, juxtacrine, and intracrine systems.[12] The distinction between hormones and growth factors is generally a functional one. There are instances in which a substance may be released from a gland into the circulation to act as a hormone at a distant site, whereas within a highly specialized tissue the same substance might be locally secreted as a growth factor to influence the function of adjacent cells. In many instances, nature has retained the basic structure of successful regulatory molecules and, through a divergent evolution, has created new uses for them. The structural homology of insulin and the insulin-like growth factors, which are discussed later in this chapter, illustrates how a substance with predominantly nutrient-transporting properties, which is found in even primitive unicellular organisms, has evolved to regulate highly differentiated functions.

Nutrients and the Growth of Cells

Holley was among the first to propose that the intracellular availability of nutrients is the ultimate regulator of cell growth.[13,14] He postulated that when cellular nutrition is adequate, mammalian cells require no additional extrinsic growth-promoting substances, and that hormones and growth factors regulate tissue growth ultimately by altering the availability of nutrients. In the laboratory, the growth of cells and tissues clearly requires the proper combinations of hormones and growth factors in addition to an adequate supply of nutrients. There is ample evidence that growth factors and hormones influence the transport and utilization of nutrients by cells.[15–19]

Hormones and nutrients interact in a delicate balance: hormones alter the nutritional requirements of cells, and conversely, nutrients alter cellular hormonal requirements. McKeehan and McKeehan found that cultured human lung fibroblasts require lower concentrations of various minerals and substrates in the culture medium as the concentration of serum growth factors is increased.[20,21] Conversely, they found that adequate concentrations of nutrients reduce the need for growth factors, an interaction that has been systematically probed.[22,23]

Although adequate supplies of nutrients are necessary to allow full manifestations of the effects signaled by hormones and growth factors, hormones influence cell growth by mechanisms other than changing their cellular nutritional status. Thyroid and steroid hormones, for example, can change cell function by directly influencing the transcription of target genes in the nucleus, although adequate "nutrition" in the form of high-energy phosphates and other low–molecular-weight substrates is required for full manifestation of the signal. In contrast, most polypeptide hormones and growth factors bind to cell-surface receptors, and their ability to influence the genome requires the initiation of a cascade of reactions that involve lipids, proteins, and ions as second messengers. Specific micronutrients, such as glutamine, allow the amplification of growth factor signaling, and individually activate intracellular signaling kinases (eg, mitogen activated protein kinases) in intestinal and liver cells.[24,25] Furthermore, there are amino acid response elements in the promoter of nutritionally important genes. One gene regulated by amino acid deprivation and the endoplasmic reticulin stress response is asparagine synthetase. Asparagine synthetase is recognized as a target of antileukemic chemotherapy and is essential for maintenance of cell viability.[26]

Nutrients and the Growth of Tissues

The study of cellular proliferation in the laboratory culture dish can provide information on the hormonal and nutritional needs of dividing cells, but the growth and development of the organism as a whole require that the enlargement and maturation of each tissue occur at appropriate rate and in proper sequence.[27] As they can influence nutrient requirements of individual cells, hormones can also affect the nutrient needs of complex tissues as well as the supply of nutrients in the fluid milieu in which they are bathed. The effects of a given hormone on its various target tissues can be quite different: catabolic in one tissue, anabolic in another (Table 2). These effects are generally not without coordination, as catabolism in one tissue can serve to increase the supply of nutrients to another tissue that is rendered anabolic by the same hormone. For example, under normal circumstances, anabolic hormones increase the protein content of both viscera and muscles.[28] In the nutrient-deficient state, however, anabolic agents such as growth hormone (GH) and androgens continue to preferentially support carcass protein (muscle) synthesis even at the expense of visceral protein. Androgens, for instance, diminish the rate of muscle breakdown in fasted guinea pigs, while accelerating the loss of protein from the liver.[29] Similarly, the weight loss of food-restricted swine can be reduced by the administration of GH, but the effect is to preferentially retain muscle mass, while depleting body fat.[30] Similar effects are seen in humans (see below) and have led to abuse of GH by competitive athletes. Conversely, an important adaptive response to long-standing malnutrition is a generalized inhibition of anabolic systems, such as those involving GH and androgens, in order to conserve essential body compartments.

Although anabolic hormones preferentially preserve muscle mass when nutrients are in short supply, catabolic hormones serve to protect the viscera. Brief exposure of rats to glucocorticoids or to thyroxine increases the protein and glycogen content of the liver, whereas the protein content of muscle is depleted.[28] These effects are direct ones on hepatic uptake and synthetic processes and not merely the result of increased substrate availability from the carcass.[35] Even a prolonged exposure to glucocorticoids, which depletes both viscera and muscle, reduces visceral mass proportionally less than muscle.

Table 2 Actions of Hormones on Body Compartments

Hormone	Protein	Carbohydrate	Fat
Glucocorticoid	Breakdown in muscle, synthesis in viscera	Permissive for gluconeogenesis, glycogen synthesis	Redistribution
Insulin	Synthesis in muscle and liver	Glycogen synthesis in liver, glycolysis	Lipogenesis, inhibits lipolysis
Growth hormone	Synthesis in muscle	Insulin-like effects (acute), insulin antagonistic (chronic)	Lipolysis, inhibits lipogenesis
Thyroid hormone	Synthesis in liver, breakdown in muscle	Glycogenolysis, gluconeogenesis	Lipolysis
Androgen	Synthesis in muscle and viscera	Increased insulin sensitivity[31,32]	Redistribution[33]

Adapted from reference 34.

Critical Periods in Tissue Growth

The ability of tissues to recover from a nutritional insult varies greatly at different times during development. The study of normal tissue growth has provided a model of normal tissue development that has been used to analyze the variable effects of malnutrition at different developmental stages. As the organ or tissue approaches its predetermined complement of cells, the organ grows by increasing both its cell number and the size of each cell. When the adult complement of cells is attained, cell division ceases and tissue growth results totally from enlargement of existing cells.[36] Between these two periods, tissue growth appeared to result from both cellular hyperplasia and hypertrophy.

Widdowson and McCance performed studies on growing animals that clearly established the existence of critical periods of sensitivity to the effects of malnutrition.[37–39] They manipulated the litter size and therefore the milk supply of rat pups during suckling and observed their subsequent growth. Rats that were nutritionally deprived during this period were small, and their growth could not be restored by institution of normal food intake.[40] The mechanism for this runting appears to be an irreversible effect of undernutrition on the number of cells. Similar mechanisms are likely to operate in some forms intrauterine growth retardation in children, although the irreversibility of the growth deficit has come into question. About 85% of infants born small for gestational age (SGA) will exhibit catch-up growth in the first 2 to 3 years of life, but a small group has a high risk of short stature in adult life. It has been demonstrated that irrespective of basal GH secretory status, GH treatment can accelerate growth in SGA children, and lead to normalization of adult stature.[41]

Winick and Noble provided further evidence that the nutritional state of the neonatal period influences cell proliferation and consequently determines the ultimate size of the animal and its organs.[42] Food restriction in the first 21 days of life produced a subnormal complement of cells in most tissues. However, the size of the cells was normal. Adequate nutrition after weaning could not restore normal growth, presumably because of an irreplaceable deficit of cells. Food restriction between 21 and 42 days resulted in a comparable stunting of growth in most tissues, but the brain and lung were able to resume normal growth with the restoration of proper nourishment. In these tissues, the total adult cell number had already been attained, and malnutrition produced a reversible decrease in cell size. When malnutrition was induced between 65 and 86 days, almost all organs underwent a reversible decrease in cell size only.

Growing tissues are as sensitive to an excess of nutrients as to a shortage. When rat litter sizes were reduced to provide supranormal nutrition, the offspring were larger than normal and were found to have hypercellular organs.[43]

As it has evolved from studies such as these, the critical period hypothesis proposes that abnormal nutrition, either excessive or deficient, during the phase of tissue growth by cellular proliferation, can increase or decrease the ultimate size of a tissue by enhancing or impairing cell division. These effects are irreversible because they bring the tissue into the phase of growth by cellular hypertrophy with an abnormal number of cells or abnormal organization. When nutritional surfeit or deficit occurs after establishment of the adult complement of cells, the net effect is a change in cell volume, but not in cell number, and is reversible by normalization of the nutrient supply. Because tissues mature at different rates, the long-term effects of nutritional variations occur most prominently in those tissues that are at a susceptible developmental period.[44] An important example of this principle of "programming" following an insult at a critical, sensitive period of early life is that mothers who are malnourished during pregnancy often have infants with intrauterine growth retardation, subsequent growth retardation, and ultimately with disproportionately high rates of coronary heart disease, high blood pressure, and high cholesterol, during adult life.[45] Intrauterine growth retardation in girls has recently been linked to the development of hyperandrogenism, insulin resistance, and ovulatory dysfunction in adolescent years.[46–48]

Catch-Up Growth

Parents often want an estimate of their child's ultimate height. Mid-parental height combined with an assessment of skeletal maturity, or "bone age", is widely used to predict adult height and is probably its single best predictor.[49–52] However, in situations where the parents are either unusually short or unusually tall, the child can be relatively less short or tall, respectively—an observation called "regression to the median."[53]

Children have the remarkable capacity to accelerate their growth when recovering from a growth-impairing influence such as malnutrition or disease. At the complex level of organization that is required for statural growth, the ability of nutritionally deprived cells and tissues to be restored to functional health is reflected in the phenomenon of "catch-up growth," a term used by Prader and colleagues.[54] Subsequently, "catch-down" was coined to refer to the complementary process that follows removal of growth-accelerating influences, such as occurs with suppression of precocious puberty, restriction of food in obesity, or cessation of GH therapy in hypopituitary children.

Even under the most favorable circumstances, the accretion of height does not occur at a fixed rate, but is developmentally regulated. Gender-specific, nutritional, and—in some cultures—seasonal influences are also superimposed. The period of most rapid postnatal growth in children occurs in the first months of life, when length increases by 14 to 22 cm/yr. By the second birthday, the mean growth velocity has slowed to about 8 cm/yr, and to about 5 cm/yr just before puberty. Then, under the influence of sex steroids (but involving the coordinated actions of GH, insulin-like growth factors [IGFs], thyroid hormones, and others), growth velocity nearly doubles before statural growth ceases, as the epiphyses close.

After the second year of life and continuing throughout childhood, growth velocity is modulated to maintain stature at a constant position relative to the general population. The height percentile attained by about 2 years of age is maintained faithfully throughout childhood and correlates well with the height percentile in adulthood.[55] Statural growth along a predetermined percentile on a growth chart is often called *canalization*. Growth-retarding or growth-accelerating processes disrupt canalization and growth curves cross channels. With amelioration of the abnormal condition, a compensatory acceleration or deceleration occurs to restore the original growth channel (Figure 1).

In the first 2 years of life, catch-up growth can be a normal adaptation in children whose birth size is at variance with their genetic potential. Although statural growth from age 2 to adulthood is primarily controlled by genetic influences, the determinants of body size during fetal life are largely determined by maternal and nutritional influences. The interval between birth and roughly 2 years of age is a preprogrammed period of catch-up or catch-down growth and is characterized by a shift of growth channels as maternal influences give way to genetically determined forces. It is essential for the clinician to be aware of these forces during this period because genetically programmed changes in growth velocity can be misconstrued as manifestations of disease.[56]

From a practical standpoint, for catch-up growth to be complete, the insult must be limited in duration and must not occur during certain vul-

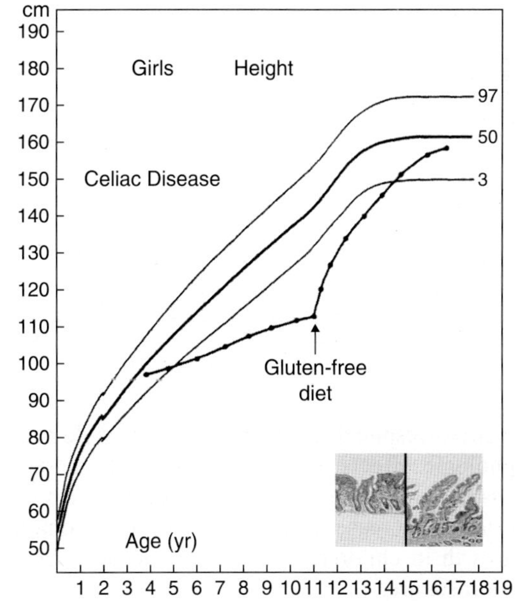

Figure 1 Catch-up growth in a girl with celiac disease. After 8 years of growth failure, she was placed on a gluten-free diet and exhibited striking catch-up growth. Note return to previous growth percentiles. (Courtesy JM Tanner) Inset. Left: duodenal biopsy showing stunted villi. Right: return to normal histology after gluten-free diet.

nerable periods. Williams and coworkers noted that the degree of catch-up growth is generally muted if it begins when growth is normally decelerating.[57,58] Based on observations in birds and mammals, Wilson proposed that catch-up growth potential is modified by the nature of the insult, its severity, its duration, and the developmental state of the animal at the onset of the insult. For example, it had been assumed that GH deficiency and hypothyroidism were two conditions with the potential for essentially complete catch-up. However, the catch-up potential of hypothyroid children is diminished in proportion to the duration of the hypothyroidism before treatment.[59] The subjects studied had been hypothyroid for approximately 5 years and had deficits from their predicted heights of 25 cm at the onset of therapy; however, at the conclusion of therapy an average deficit of 7 cm remained (Figure 2). The magnitude of deficit between final height and predicted height was in proportion to the duration of hypothyroidism before treatment began. Similar conclusions resulted from studies of children with GH deficiency of long duration before treatment.[60] Incomplete catch-up growth has also been documented in children with acute nutritional insults, such as diarrhea, when they are superimposed on a background of chronic malnutrition.[61,62]

In addition to its duration, the specific nature of the insult may be important in determining the extent of catch-up because some growth-arresting conditions appear to cause irreversible changes. Mosier found that cortisone-treated rats failed to regain normal body size after cessation of treatment, whereas rats that were comparably stunted by fasting resumed normal growth when refed.[63] Cartilage from the steroid-treated rats had increased numbers of dead and dying cells, altered cell morphology, and alterations in the

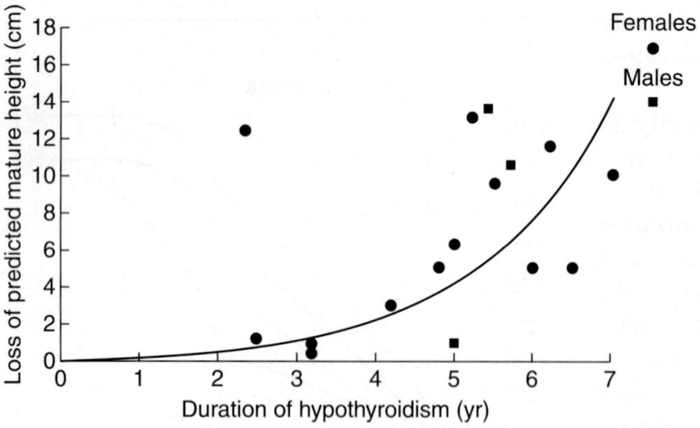

Figure 2 Loss of catch-up potential with long-standing hypothyroidism. Relationship between loss in adult height and duration of hypothyroidism before treatment in children. Loss of predicted height is predicted height at time of diagnosis minus actual mature height. Duration of hypothyroidism is chronologic age minus bone age at diagnosis. (Adapted from reference 59.)

matrix. Despite these seemingly irreversible morphologic effects on chondrocytes, GH therapy has been shown to reverse many of the catabolic effects, increase anabolic ones, and promote growth in children with glucocorticoid-induced short stature.[64]

It has been suggested that the catch-up growth of recovery from malnutrition in some experimental conditions is associated with an increase in the efficiency of energy utilization.[65] Fasted rats are capable of a fivefold increase in energy utilization efficiency for weight gain during recovery, perhaps by decreased thermogenesis.[66] The situation may be different in humans: children recovering from malnutrition often have increased appetite and caloric intake, suggesting to others that energy utilization is not efficient.[67] Some marasmic children do not begin to gain weight until 3 to 5 weeks of refeeding, despite an intake of more than 130 kcal/kg/d.[68] (Mary Penny chapter in this textbook). In fact, once the infant is resuscitated with respect to fluid balance, infection therapy, glucose control, and temperature control, they usually require between 150 to 220 kcal/kg/d in order to gain weight.[69]

Implied in the concept of catch-up or catch-down growth is an ability of the organism to constantly monitor its size and determine the extent of deviation from the intended size; to alter its velocity when unrestrained from the growth-perturbing influence; and finally, to again modulate its altered velocity to prevent overshooting or undershooting the channel.[70–73] Wilson stressed the theoretical importance of distinguishing between *catch-up* growth and *compensatory* growth.[73] He recognized that the former involved growth to attain a projected (and moving) statural target, while the latter involved the growth of a tissue or organ to restore actual lost mass as in the regeneration of liver following a partial hepatectomy.[74]

Two divergent, but not necessarily exclusive, models have been put forward to explain the ability of the organism to monitor body size and initiate catch up. Tanner postulated the existence of a "sizostat" in the central nervous system (CNS) that maintained communication with the peripheral tissues.[75] Along the same lines, Leibel proposed that the concentration of a circulating hormone, such as insulin (or its ratio to other hormones or metabolites), might reflect the size of a body compartment, such as the adipose mass, by monitoring the number of insulin receptors on adipocytes.[76] With the isolation of leptin, the data that support a neuroendocrine control of *weight regulation* have been far stronger than that of a neuroendocrine control of statural catch-up. For example, in order to initiate catch-up growth in conditions of malnutrition, the child must attain a body weight that is 85% of the normal weight for height.[77] The interactions between adipose mass and the CNS are discussed in the section on Reproductive Function in Malnutrition.

In contrast to a neuroendocrine mechanism of catch-up growth, Baron and colleagues focused on the growth plate as the key tissue in catch-up growth.[78] Their data showed that a unilateral growth-suppressing influence, accomplished by transient administration of glucocorticoids to a single growth plate, was accompanied by catch-up growth acceleration at that growth plate only, not systemically.[79] Although their model does not preclude the involvement of systemic hormones and the CNS, they proposed that growth-inhibiting conditions decrease proliferation of growth plate stem cells, thus conserving their proliferative potential. Catch-up growth results from a putative clock, or time tally to use Tanner's term, within the stem cell compartment.

Although it is likely that both systemic (neuroendocrine and endocrine) and local (paracrine, autocrine, and juxtacrine) signals will be implicated as critical regulators of the proliferation that occurs during catch-up or catch-down growth, there is little evidence to date that hormones and growth factors are significant mediators of the catch-up phenomenon. These data are extensively reviewed in reference 77.

GROWTH HORMONE, INSULIN-LIKE GROWTH FACTORS, AND INSULIN

Normal Growth

Growth Hormone and IGFs in Normal Growth. GH or somatotropin is essential for normal, balanced somatic growth from childhood to normal adult stature. GH deficient children are not only short but have profound deficits in lean body mass and excess adipose tissue in addition to abnormalities in glucose homeostasis. The mechanism by which this process is regulated is incompletely understood, especially in the fetus. The actions of GH involve a complex interaction among GH genes, GH receptors, IGFs or somatomedins, IGF receptors, and IGF-binding proteins (IGF-BPs). In addition, the GH-IGF axis is entwined in a regulatory web that is strongly modulated by nutritional signals.

IGFs and the Somatomedin Hypothesis. With the advent of techniques for the culture of tissues and cells in the laboratory almost 50 years ago, it became evident that few of the biochemical events that had been attributed to GH *in vivo* could be reproduced in isolated tissues. These included effects on chondrocyte proliferation and sulfate incorporation into glycosaminoglycans of growth plate cartilage. These observations led Salmon and Daughaday to propose the "somatomedin hypothesis": that the growth-promoting effects of GH are not direct ones on its target tissues, but result indirectly from the actions of a "mediator" substance under GH control.[80] Reviewed in reference 81, initially called sulfation factor or thymidine factor, based on the assay system used to detect its presence, it was later determined that these two biological activities resided in the same molecule, which was renamed somatomedin.[82] Other somatomedin species were initially proposed, but somatomedin-C (Sm-C) was determined to be the GH mediator present in serum.

IGFs were purified in parallel, but independent, studies to characterize the source of the insulin-like biological activity of serum, only a small part of which derives from insulin itself. Two molecules were identified, IGF-I and IGF-II, the amino acid sequences of which were found to be remarkably similar to proinsulin.[83,84] Sm-C is identical to IGF-I, and current convention prefers the IGF terminology, although a number of IGF-I assays available from clinical reference laboratories retain the Sm-C designation. The properties of IGF-I and IGF-II are contrasted in Table 3. Although the current nomenclature has the disadvantage of dissociating the IGFs from their regulatory link with GH, it does more firmly root these substances in the realm of nutritional control.

Initial iterations of the somatomedin hypothesis were inspired by endocrine models of growth control: liver was found to be a major producer of somatomedin activity and the paradigm that evolved had the liver functioning as an endocrine gland under the control of pituitary GH to secrete somatomedins whose ultimate target tissue was the growth plate. To further support an endocrine model, IGFs were found to feed back to the pituitary and inhibit the release of GH.

However, in the 1980s it became clear that multiple tissues express mRNA for IGFs and are involved in IGF production.[85,86] Most compelling was the observation that IGF-1 mRNA is expressed in perichondrium and periosteum, suggesting that local production of IGFs in the epiphysis might account for the growth stimulating effects of GH. Indeed, Isaksson had shown that GH elicits an increase in both IGF-I mRNA and protein in rat epiphyses.[87] Based on analogy to the work of Greene and colleagues[88] on the role of GH in the differentiation of adipocytes, Isaakson

Table 3 Insulin-Like Growth Factors

Property	IGF-I	IGF-II
Synonyms	Somatomedin C, basic somatomedin	Multiplication stimulating activity (MSA), neutral somatomedin
Chromosome location	12	11
Molecular weight	7,649	7,471
Serum concentration	193 ± 58 ng/mL	647 ± 126 ng/mL
GH dependence of serum concentration	+++	+
Insulin-like actions	+	+++
Mitogenicity in cultured cells	+++	+
Developmental role	Postnatal	Fetal
Sensitivity to undernutrition	+++	+/−

GH = growth hormone.

and colleagues proposed that GH stimulates the differentiation of chondrocytes in the germinal zone of the growth plate; once the stem cells become chondrocytes, their proliferation would result from local (autocrine/paracrine) production of IGF-1.[87] However, inconsistencies remain among the data: GH- or GHR-deficient mice and humans have no paucity of differentiated chondrocytes, and growth plate chondrocytes can proliferate normally without IGF-1 (reviewed in reference 81). Nonetheless, the consensus is that locally generated IGFs in the epiphysis are the critical regulators of linear growth.

The weakness of the original somatomedin hypothesis was most clearly illustrated by the creation of a liver-specific knockout of the *IGF-1* gene. Using Cre/loxP technology, Le Roith and colleagues produced mice with hepatic IGF-1 mRNA levels reduced to less than 1% of normal, resulting in a 75% reduction in serum IGF-1.[89,90] Nonetheless, these mice lacking hepatic IGF-1 grew normally, and "there were no phenotypic distinctions between the liver-specific *IGF-1* gene-deleted animals and their wild-type littermates."[81] While these studies do not confirm that *bone-derived* IGFs are the critical determinants of linear growth, they do support the contention that circulating IGFs are not critical to skeletal growth. As expected based on their markedly reduced serum IGF-1 levels, the liver-specific IGF-1 knockout animals had elevated concentrations of GH, leading LeRoith to speculate that the major role of circulating IGF-1 might be to modulate GH secretion.

IGF-Binding Proteins. In contrast to GH, which circulates in association with a fragment of the GH receptor called the GH-binding protein (GH-BP), IGF concentrations in blood are maintained at relatively stable levels by serum binding proteins that markedly delay IGF clearance. IGF binding in serum and other fluids resides in six different molecules, collectively known as the IGF-BPs. The IGF-BPs are summarized in Table 4. (Reviewed in reference 91) The major IGF binding complex in serum consists of IGF-BP3 in association with the acid-labile subunit (ALS). IGF-BP5 can also interact with ALS and IGFs in the serum. Circulating IGF-BP3 concentrations, like those of IGF-I, are GH dependent. It is now clear that many, if not all, of the so-called somatomedin inhibitors identified in early bioassays of somatomedin activity, especially in conditions of malnutrition and disease, were actually IGF-BPs.

Table 4 Insulin-Like Growth Factor-Binding Proteins

Property	BP-1	BP-2	BP-3	BP-4	BP-5	BP-6
Molecular weight	25,000	33,000	54,000	24,000	31,000	30,000
Chromosome location	7	2	7	17	5	12
Serum concentration (nM)	0.8–2.8	6.1–18.3	60.170	Present		Present
Tissue localization	Serum, amniotic fluid, kidney, reproductive tissues	Serum, CSF	Serum	Serum, CNS	Placenta, kidney, bone, thyroid	Serum, CSF
Regulation by GH	↓___	↓___	↑↑___			↑___
Regulation by insulin	↓↓___	↓___				
Proposed function	Transport of IGFs from vascular space; immediate early gene	Transport of IGFs from vascular space	Major component of 150 kDa serum IGF complex intravascular reservoir	Blocks IGF action in cells	Potentiates IGF action in cells	

CNS = central nervous system; CSF = cerebrospinal fluid; IGF = insulin-like growth factor.

All six proteins have higher affinity for both IGF-I and IGF-II than do IGF receptors. IGF-BPs were initially proposed to function as IGF-sequestering agents, thus limiting the concentration of free IGFs. However, IGF-BPs modify IGF actions in a variety of ways; they transport IGFs across vessel walls and capillary membranes, they regulate the concentration of IGFs in the vicinities of specific tissues and cell types, they control IGF interaction with cell-surface IGF receptors, and at least three of these molecules (IGF-BP1, BP3, and BP5) can augment IGF action. Baxter has proposed that a binary complex of a single IGF-BP and IGF-I, which can leave the circulation rapidly, facilitating access of IGFs to their receptors, whereas a ternary complex consisting of IGF, IGF-BP3 (or BP5), and ALS cannot cross the endothelial barrier and remains in the circulation to sequester free IGF-I.[91] The implications of this on nutritional regulation of IGF action are discussed below. As noted in Table 4, serum concentrations of the three principal IGF-BPs are profoundly influenced by nutritional signals (mediated by insulin) and by GH. IGF binding and action can also be modulated by posttranslational modifications of the IGF-BPs such as phosphorylation, proteolysis, and matrix association.[92] Three of the IGF-BPs appear to be able to influence cell function independent of their role as an IGF-BP. For example, IGF-BP3 can inhibit proliferation in cells that have no IGF receptors.[93] Specific cell surface receptors for the IGF-BPs have been proposed, and IGF-BP3 may have direct effects in the nucleus by interacting with the retinoid X receptor α, RXRα.[94]

Growth Hormone, IGF, and IGF-Binding Protein Genes. In humans, GH is encoded within a cluster of five structurally similar genes on the long arm of chromosome 17.[95] These genes include the so-called normal GH gene (*GH-N* or *GH-A*), a variant GH gene (*GH-V* or *GH-B*), and three genes for placental lactogen (chorionic somatomammotropin). Only *GH-N* is translated into GH in the pituitary gland, and the other four genes of the family are expressed in placenta. Two distinct forms of GH result from differential splicing of the mRNA that is transcribed from the *GH-N* gene. The predominant product is a single chain of 191 amino acids with a molecular weight of 22 kDa. The product of alternate splicing of the *GH-N* gene is 20 kDa GH, which results from a deletion of 15 amino acids and comprises about 10% of circulating GH. Clear evidence for a differential regulation of the secretion of these two GHs is lacking, although they may differ in some of their biologic actions.

Each of the IGFs is encoded by a separate gene, although alternative splicing of each of the genes and other posttranscriptional modifications result in multiple IGF mRNA species. The extent

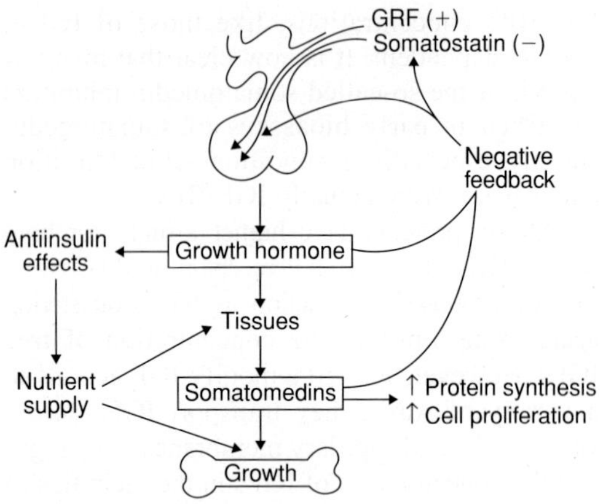

Figure 3 The growth hormone–somatomedin axis. (+) stimulatory action; (−) inhibitory action.

to which the modification of IGF gene transcripts is important in the regulation of IGF action is unclear. The IGF-BPs as well arise from a gene superfamily that includes proteins whose function and relationship to IGF physiology are as yet undetermined.[96]

The Growth Hormone-Insulin-Like Growth Factor Axis: Physiologic Regulation. Pituitary GH release is regulated by two principal hypothalamic peptides, one stimulatory (GH-releasing factor, GRF or GHRH) and one inhibitory (somatostatin, SRIF) (Figure 3). Blood concentrations and patterns of GH secretion result from an interplay between these two substances on the somatotropes of the anterior pituitary. The hypothalamus receives rich innervation from higher centers in the brain, providing a mechanism by which even emotional influences can alter GH secretion (see discussion of "psychosocial dwarfism" later in this chapter). However, other modulating influences on GH release have been identified. Both free fatty acids and the orexigenic (appetite-stimulating) neuropeptide Y are known to directly inhibit GH secretion, while the fat-derived hormone, leptin (see below) stimulates GH release, perhaps by inhibiting secretion of neuropeptide Y.[97–101] Very recently ghrelin has come to the fore as a potent regulator of GH secretion, food intake, and fat mass. Ghrelin levels surge before every meal, and ghrelin injections rapidly stimulate food intake. Levels are very high in ravenous Parder-willi patients and are low after gastric bypass.[102] Investigators studying a family of synthetic GH-releasing peptides, the GHRPs,[103] identified a novel CNS receptor for these peptides and then identified ghrelin as its natural ligand. Ghrelin is produced by hypothalamic neurons and by a highly specialized population of endocrine cells in the fundus of the stomach, where its secretion is suppressed by food intake. The model that is emerging ties stomach-produced ghrelin to the nocturnal stimulation of GH secretion, while hypothalamic ghrelin regulates food intake.[104]

Peripherally produced IGFs feed back to inhibit GH secretion by the pituitary. IGF-I can stimulate the secretion of somatostatin by the hypothalamus[105] and may also directly inhibit GH synthesis.[106] It remains to be clarified whether IGFs of peripheral or hypothalamic origin are responsible for the inhibition of GH secretion, but the observations previously cited of enhanced GH secretion in the liver of the IGF-I knockout mouse suggest that circulating IGF-I is a prime regulator of GH secretion.[89]

In response to GH, but modified by other hormones and most critically by nutritional factors, multiple tissues in the body synthesize and secrete IGFs. Although the liver is the major producer of circulating IGFs, its primacy in the GH-IGF axis has been supplanted. Multiple cell types in virtually every tissue examined from both fetus and adult can synthesize IGFs. Thus a model of IGF action has evolved that is primarily a paracrine one in which IGFs are produced in multiple tissues and act upon target cells in the vicinity of the producing cells. Thus the function of the large quantities of circulating IGFs is not clear, but they may be more important for their insulin-like effects on metabolism than on their mitogenic effects.

Growth Hormone and IGF Concentrations in Blood. Although it was believed that GH circulates in the blood free of binding proteins, it is now recognized that between 25% and 35% of circulating GH is loosely complexed to a 60 kDa glycoprotein referred to as the GH-BP.[107] This protein is identical to the extracellular domain of the GH receptor, but it is unclear whether in humans GH-BP arises from alternative splicing of the GH receptor mRNA, as it does in the rat, or is shed from cell surface receptors by peptidases. Changes in serum concentrations of GH-BP reflect changes in the number of cell-surface GH receptors.[108] In contrast to the prolonged half-life of IGFs bound to the IBF-BPs (more than 12 hours), the plasma half-life of GH is about 20 minutes. Clinically, IGF-I concentrations in blood have been shown to reliably mirror the total GH secretory activity. Thus, in older children and adults who are well nourished and do not have hypothyroidism, serum IGF-I measurements are more useful than random measurements of GH in diagnosing conditions of GH deficiency (hypopituitarism) and excess (gigantism or acromegaly). The marked influence of nutritional status on IGF production is discussed later in this chapter.

GH secretion in humans is highly episodic. Blood concentrations are generally low or undetectable for much of the day and are interrupted by burst of secretion that results in high concentrations for roughly 90 minutes before returning to the low baseline. This pattern is developmentally regulated.[109] The number and amplitude of secretory episodes are small in young children. Under the influence of gonadal steroids, both the frequency and amplitude increase dramatically and reach their highest levels during puberty, especially during sleep; they then gradually decline over the ensuing decades.

The combined concentration of IGF proteins in the blood is on the order of 750 μg/L or 100 nM. Although GH remains the predominant regulator of IGF production and IGF-BPs, which are the principal regulators of bioavailable IGFs, a number of other hormones influence IGF-I concentrations in blood. IGF-I is low or nonexistent in fetal life, when IFG-II appears to be the predominant somatomedin. During fetal life, placental lactogen or the product of the *GH-V* gene is likely to be the major regulator of somatomedin production.[110] Prolactin, another GH-like hormone, can also stimulate the production of IGFs in cultured cells and probably in clinical conditions of prolactin excess. Blood levels of the IGFs remain low during infancy and early childhood but rise dramatically at puberty in response to increases in GH secretory activity. In addition, IGF-I concentrations are low in patients with hypothyroidism.[111]

Direct versus Indirect Actions of Growth Hormone: A Unifying Hypothesis? GH initiates a signal by binding to specific receptors on the surface of target cells. A single GH molecule contains two separate receptor-binding domains, which facilitate the formation of receptor homodimers upon GH binding.[112] Receptor dimerization is a feature common to a number of growth factor receptors and appears to be a prerequisite for signaling. When activated by ligand, the GH receptor dimerizes and associates with Janus Kinase 2 (JAK2). JAK2 then phosphorylates a family of proteins called signal transducers and activators of transcription (STATs). STAT proteins directly bind to DNA and directly regulate gene transcription. STAT target genes include those that encode a negative regulatory protein called suppressor of cytokine signaling-3 (SOCS-3).

The sequence of GH-initiated signaling events often extends to intracellular pathways that are activated or modulated by other hormones or growth factors, leading to complex intracellular interactions and diverse, but coordinated physiologic events. Among the targets of the activated GH receptors are insulin receptor substrate-1 (IRS-1) and IRS-2, which in turn recruit phosphatidylinositol-3 kinase (PI3-kinase) to the IRS-proteins. Activated PI3-kinase activates protein kinase B (PKB)/Akt, which in turn activates glucose transporters (GLUT4) and increases cellular glucose uptake. PKB/Akt can also activate phosphodiesterase 3B, which lowers cellular concentrations of cAMP, resulting in decreased phosphorylation of the hormone sensitive lipase and inhibition of lipolysis. (Reviewed in references 81 and 113)

The actions of GH in vivo have been categorized as either indirect (IGF-mediated) or direct ones. The direct actions vary significantly depending on the duration of exposure. After short-term administration to GH-deficient individuals or to isolated GH-sensitive tissues in culture, GH has effects very much like those of insulin. They are rapid in onset, transient in duration, and not mediated through the actions of IGFs. They include the stimulation of glucose and amino acid transport and protein synthesis. GH also has inductive effects on a number of enzymes. In patients with gastrointestinal and pancreatic disease who are taking parenteral nutrition (PN), administration of GH is associated with an increase in protein, potassium, and phosphorus balance.[114]

Chronic GH administration, in contrast, results in biochemical actions that appear antagonistic to insulin; blood sugar rises and fat mobilization and fatty acid oxidation occur. In fact, release of GH is one of the stress responses that the body uses to maintain euglycemia, while individuals with GH-secreting tumors can develop frank diabetes mellitus. About 3% of athletes take GH, often combining it with anabolic steroids. There is no conclusive evidence that GH enhances athletic performance, and an excess can cause acromegaly, myopathy, and hypertension. However, it does produce perceptible fluid shifts and reduced subcutaneous fat, resulting in a more "toned" appearance.[115]

The origins of these paradoxical "direct" GH actions are not clear but may reside in the structure of the GH molecule itself. The 20-kDa variant has been reported to have only one-fifth the insulin-like activity of the 22-kDa GH molecule, while retaining normal growth-promoting and diabetogenic activity.[116,117] However, analysis of the biologic activities of both the 22-kDa and 20-kDa GH molecules in transgenic mice demonstrated largely overlapping activities with regard to linear growth and carbohydrate metabolism.[118]

The concept that IGFs can mediate the actions of GH in promoting linear growth has been validated by a number of studies that show that IGF-I injections increase tibial width and costal cartilage DNA synthesis in hypophysectomized rats to an extent that is comparable to that in GH-treated controls. In human newborn infants, umbilical cord plasma levels of IGF-1 and leptin (see below) show a strong positive correlation with increasing birth weight and birth length.[119] Both IGF-1 and leptin, which is secreted by both adipocytes and placenta, are important for fetal growth. The ability of IGF-I to stimulate linear growth in the absence of GH is strongly supported by studies demonstrating overgrowth in transgenic mice overexpressing IGF-I and in IGF-I treated humans with Laron-type dwarfism, a condition that results from the hereditary absence of GH receptors.

IGF-I, IGF-II, and a truncated form of IGF-I, in addition to EGF, are also present in colostrum and in breast milk.[120] Importantly, intestinal IGFs are also locally produced by the mesenchymal cells within the lamina propria. Milk-derived IGFs appear to act on cells in the gut and do not have direct effects on somatic growth. However, by improving bowel function, they may increase nutrient absorption, thereby promoting somatic growth. The trophic effects of IGFs have generally been observed in the distal bowel (ileum) more than jejunum. In the piglet intestine, oral rhIGF-1 increased small intestinal weight, protein and DNA content, and jejunal and ileal villus height.[121] Additionally, oral rhIGF-1 has been shown to increase intestinal sodium absorption and the maximal rate of glucose and alanine absorption in newborn piglets.[122]

When intestinal cells are studied, IGFs are well-known stimulators of cell proliferation[123] but also are potent stimulators of cell migration, a mechanism central to the healing of ulcers, villus damage in viral enteritis, and other lesions. The mechanism by which migration/restitution is stimulated appears to be dependent on protein kinase C.[124] However, other signaling pathways are activated by IGF-1, including the PI3-kinase pathway, c-Jun nuclear kinase, and mitogen-activated protein kinases.[125] Consequently, growth factors have been extensively investigated as therapeutic agents to enhance gut integrity and facilitate repair.

Orally administered growth factors have been found to exert trophic effects to the intestinal mucosa in experimental rotavirus enteritis and in rats with short bowel syndrome.[126,127] In two studies, the combination of the primary metabolic fuel of the intestine, glutamine, with either systemic GH or IGF-I resulted in a synergistic trophic response.[128,129] A synergistic trophic response of glutamine with transforming growth factor-alpha was seen after ischemia/reperfusion injury of the porcine intestine.[130]

In viral enteritis, exogenous growth factors have enhanced mucosal mass without reducing diarrheal output or increasing specific activities of jejunal disaccharidase enzymes.[126,131] In short bowel syndrome and ischemic bowel disease, growth factors and the trophic amino acid L-glutamine have been shown to have synergistic effects.[132,133] These effects have not been translated into clinical therapy for diarrheal diseases to date.

Another disease for which enteral growth factor therapy has begun to be studied is short bowel syndrome. In this condition, which is the leading cause of intestinal failure in newborns, the infant's bowel length limits absorption, leading to a prolonged dependence on PN, which, in turn, can result in end-stage liver disease. In several studies, Donovan and colleagues treated malnourished newborn piglets (given 80% of required calories via PN) with enteral IGF-I.[134] They found that enteral IGF-I improved intestinal morphology and markedly increased disaccharidase activity in parenterally fed piglets when compared to those given partial enteral nutrition alone. The mechanism by which lactase activity in the mucosa was so markedly increased appeared to be posttranslational in nature.[135]

Some notable differences between GH and IGF-1 responses in the gut have further strengthened the concept that GH has both direct and IGF-mediated actions.[136] Transgenic mice overexpressing GH and IGF-1 have increased body weight, as well as increased small bowel length and mass. However, GH had more profound effects on body mass compared to IGF-1 (60% vs 23% increase), while IGF-1 had much greater effects on bowel length (44% vs 20% increase). IGF-1 but not GH overexpression increases intestinal crypt cell proliferation while reducing crypt cell apoptosis. In further support, murine knockout models of IGF-1, the GH receptor, or both show that both factors have major independent effects on somatic growth (30–50%), while lack of functional expression of both growth factors profoundly affects growth. *Igf-1/ghr* double knockouts reach only 17% of the expected adult body weight.[137]

Insulin in Normal Growth. The prominent influence of insulin on normal growth is best illustrated in disorders at the extremes of altered insulin secretion. Especially in the fetus, hyperinsulinemia produces somatic overgrowth. Hyperinsulinemic infants born to poorly controlled diabetic mothers or infants with hyperinsulinism of infancy[138] exhibit visceromegaly, increased body fat, and increased length. Conversely, the hypoinsulinemic infant born with severe insulin resistance or pancreatic agenesis is small and depleted in body fat.[139] In postnatal life, poorly controlled diabetes mellitus can be associated with a striking growth failure, the so-called Mauriac syndrome.[140] The growth-promoting actions of insulin both in prenatal and postnatal life are complex and likely to result from both direct, largely metabolic, effects mediated through the insulin receptor and indirect, predominantly mitogenic effects mediated through the structurally homologous IGF-I receptor. Insulin mediates the feeding-stimulated enhancement of muscle and skin protein synthesis, but insulin is not related to feeding-induced stimulation of protein synthesis in the viscera.[141]

Insulin Receptor-Mediated Actions of Insulin. High-affinity insulin receptors mediate the rapid biologic actions of insulin in stimulating the cellular transport of substrates and in the induction of enzymes that promote glycogen and fat synthesis and that inhibit gluconeogenesis, lipolysis, and ketogenesis.

An indirect consequence of insulin action appears to be the stimulation of IGF production. A number of clinical studies have shown that the depressed IGF concentration associated with poorly controlled diabetes mellitus can be returned to normal with insulin therapy.[142] Insulin appears to directly stimulate IGF production in whole liver, liver slices, or cultured hepatocytes.[143] Additionally, insulin may regulate IGF production by influencing the number of GH receptors on important IGF-producing tissues. In poorly controlled diabetes mellitus, there is a dramatic reduction in the number of somatogenic GH binding sites in liver. These can be restored to normal with insulin therapy.[144]

IGF Receptor-Mediated Actions of Insulin. In a few cell types, such as hepatocytes, certain teratocarcinoma cells, and mammary tumor cells, insulin appears to be directly mitogenic by binding to its own receptor at physiologic concentrations. However, some of the growth-promoting actions of insulin can be attributed to activation of IGF receptors. There are two principal IGF receptors, type I and type II. The insulin receptor and the IGF-I receptor are homologous "heterotetramers," consisting of two α and β subunits. The binding of insulin or IGFs to their respective α subunits activates a tyrosine kinase on the cytoplasmic portion of their respective β subunits. This kinase, in turn, transphosphorylates tyrosines on the adjacent β subunit and on other cytoplasmic substrates that are essential for the actions of both insulin and IGF-I.[145] Both IGF-I and IGF-II can bind to and activate the insulin receptor, although with much lower affinity than insulin.

Crossover of IGF and insulin actions also occurs when type I IGF receptors are activated by insulin. Although type I receptors preferentially bind IGF-I, they can be activated by 10- to 100-fold excess concentrations of insulin, conditions that are achieved in some cases of hyperinsulinism, such as insulin-resistant states. Another level of overlap between IGF-I and insulin action is suggested by the finding that a single α, β subunit of the insulin receptor can associate with an α, β subunit of the type I IGF receptor, forming a hybrid tetramer.[146]

The IGF-II receptor is more enigmatic.[147] It preferentially binds IGF-II over IGF-I but is also the receptor that (at a different binding site) shuttles mannose-6-phosphate-containing extracellular proteins into lysosomes. The type II receptor does not contain an intracellular tyrosine kinase domain, and its role (if any) in intracellular signaling is unclear. Most of the actions of IGF-II are thought to be mediated through the type IGF-I or insulin receptors. IGF-II receptors do not bind insulin, but physiologic concentrations of insulin dramatically upregulate the number of these receptors on adipocytes.[148]

Insulin Synergy with Other Growth Factors. One further mechanism by which insulin appears to influence cellular growth is to alter the cellular requirements for mitogenic signals from other growth factors. As discussed previously regarding the interactions of nutrients and hormones, growth factor signals frequently converge on common pathways within a cell so that low concentrations of two growth factors can amplify the actions of one another. In cultured hepatocytes, insulin can potentiate the mitogenic signal of EGF or of vasopressin,[149] and in the well-studied BALB/c 3T3 fibroblast, the presence of insulin or IGF-I strongly modulates the mitogenic actions of EGF and platelet-derived growth factor.

Malnutrition

Growth Hormone in Malnutrition

Serum Growth Hormone Levels in Malnutrition. In humans, experimental fasting and malnutrition generally result in elevated serum concentrations of GH. Studies of malnourished populations in different parts of the world have often led to conflicting conclusions, in part from differing criteria for malnutrition, from the inaccuracies inherent in characterizing complex GH secretory patterns from a single blood sample, and perhaps to some extent from confounding features such as infection.[150] The normal physiology of nutrient regulation of GH secretion is also complex; amino acids such as arginine stimulate GH release, whereas carbohydrates and fatty acids inhibit GH secretion. Clinical malnutrition results from a combination of dietary deficiencies that could be expected to have variable effects on GH release.

Table 5 Enhanced Pulsatility of Growth Hormone Release in Fasting

Measure of Pulsatility	Day 0	Day 1	Day 5
GH peaks (number/24 h)	5.8 ± 0.7	7.3 ± 0.6*	9.9 ± 0.7*
GH peak amplitude (ng/mL)	5.9 ± 1.1	13.1 ± 1.2*	12.3 ± 1.6*
24-hour IGHC (μg/mL/min)	2.8 ± 0.5	7.8 ± 1.1**	8.8 ± 0.8**

Adapted from reference 151.
GH = growth hormone; IGHC = 24-hour integrated GH concentration.
Frequent venous sampling of six adult male subjects was performed during a control fed day (day 0) and during the first (day 1) and fifth (day 5) days of a fast.
*$p < .005$, compared with day 0; **$p > .0009$.

Recently, attention has turned to the effects of fasting on the pattern of GH release from the pituitary. As previously described, GH secretion in humans is episodic, and measurement of GH concentrations on random blood samples, as is typical of field studies, might be expected to give inconsistent results. Ho and coworkers performed frequent blood sampling (every 20 minutes) of fasted volunteers and uncovered an inherent pulsatility in GH secretion in humans that appears to be suppressed in the fed state, perhaps by the negative feedback of IGFs.[151] Over the course of a 5-day fast, those authors measured significant increases in GH pulse frequency, maximal pulse amplitude, and 24-hour integrated concentration (Table 5). These changes coincided with a decline in concentrations of IGF-I and glucose and a rise in those of free fatty acids and acetoacetate. Subsequent studies led those authors to conclude that fasting-induced enhancement of GH secretion is mediated by an increase in GH-releasing hormone pulsatility and a decrease in somatostatin release.[152]

Serum GH concentrations are elevated in children with both kwashiorkor and marasmus,[153–157] but do not allow distinction between the two. Becker and associates observed the magnitude of GH elevation to be inversely related to the severity of protein malnutrition, as judged by the serum albumin concentration.[153] In their subjects, GH concentrations fell after feeding a protein-rich diet for 36 to 72 hours. The critical role of protein in the refeeding diet was also demonstrated by Pimstone and colleagues,[157] who found that refeeding with a high-carbohydrate, protein-free diet does not normalize GH concentrations. When caloric deprivation predominates, the GH response appears to be variable; some groups have reported depressed GH concentrations and others have reported elevations.[158,159] In short-term malnutrition, the adaptive benefits of elevated GH concentrations are suggested by the known direct effects of GH to increase gluconeogenesis, lipolysis, and fatty acid oxidation. Elevated GH concentrations might be expected to increase glucose production initially, while shifting the organism to a lipolytic, protein-sparing state.

Although short-term protein-calorie malnutrition is associated with elevated GH concentrations, long-standing malnutrition results in depressed GH secretion. Beas and coworkers described a group of infants with low concentrations not only of GH but also of adrenal and thyroid hormones,[160] suggesting generalized pituitary hypofunction. An adaptive function of a hypopituitary state in reducing metabolic activity had previously been proposed by Mulinos and Pomerantz,[161] who likened the malnourished state to a "pseudohypophysectomy."

Clinical Uses of Growth Hormone in Disease States. GH signaling (as measured by IGF-1 concentrations) is reduced in many conditions, including malnutrition, Prader-Willi syndrome,[162] thalassemia major,[163] type I diabetes,[164] leukemia,[165] and premature osteoporosis.[166] Also, Laron dwarfism, which results from inactivating mutations in the GH receptor, is characterized by dramatically reduced IGF-1 concentrations.[167] The adaptive changes in GH release that accompany malnutrition have prompted a number of studies on the possible uses of GH in promoting anabolism during recovery from operation or injury. Clemmons and coworkers determined the effects of GH injections on obese individuals subjected to hypocaloric diets.[168] Although dietary restriction produced comparable weight loss in subjects receiving GH and those receiving placebo, those treated with GH (0.1 mg/kg every 48 hours) had a significantly lower daily nitrogen deficit than controls. Similar findings were reported by Manson and Wilmore,[169] who administered GH to volunteers receiving hypocaloric PN (Figure 4). GH therapy decreased the rate of weight loss and increased nitrogen retention. In parenterally nourished patients recovering from gastrointestinal surgery, GH administration has resulted in sustained nitrogen retention,[170,171]

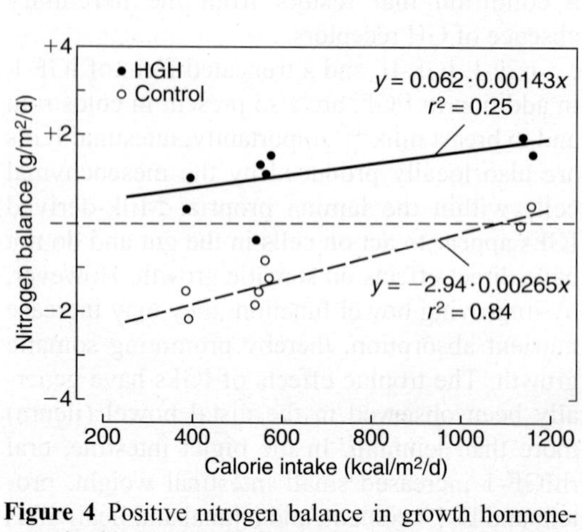

Figure 4 Positive nitrogen balance in growth hormone-treated subjects at all levels of hypocaloric calorie provision. Eight male subjects were exposed to various levels of hypocaloric intravenous feeding. Only adequate energy intake resulted in positive nitrogen balance in the controls (*open circles*) whereas growth hormone-treated subjects (*closed circles*) were in positive nitrogen balance at all levels of energy intake. (Adapted from reference 169.)

suggesting a possible role for this agent in promoting recovery from a variety of catabolic states.

Unfortunately, a series of investigations in critically ill adults with multi-organ system failure in several placebo-controlled, masked trials found that high-dose recombinant human GH treatment produced a twofold increase in mortality, increased the length of stay in-hospital, and prolonged the duration of mechanical ventilation.[172] However, similar doses of GH administered to critically ill children with extensive body burns did not increase morbidity or mortality and reduced intravenous albumin and calcium requirements, compared to placebo-treated children. There were increased hyperglycemic episodes and insulin requirements in the treated group, although these were not considered dangerous.[173]

In an animal model of colitis (interleukin-10 knockout mouse), GH injections decreased disease activity, increased weight gain, and reduced apoptosis in the colon. The improvement was mediated by upregulation of a protein called SHP-2, which in turn reduced STAT-3 (see above) activation, while increasing the antiapoptotic protein bcl-2.[174] Similarly, administration or overexpression of IGF-1 reduced inflammation and fibrosis in experimental ileo-colitis[175] and in toxic hepatitis.[176]

In humans with several gastroenterological conditions, exogenous GH administration has been shown to have beneficial effects. In cystic fibrosis, GH treatment improved growth rate (linear and ponderal) and—by as yet undetermined mechanisms—reduced pulmonary exacerbations.[177,178] In adults with Crohn's disease, a preliminary placebo-controlled trial of GH therapy for 4 months significantly improved the disease activity index score.[179] In children, inflammatory bowel disease activity was not influenced, but a 4-month treatment with GH enhanced the lean body mass, decreased the fat mass, and enhanced linear growth velocity.[180]

Substantial world-wide experimental support has emerged for GH treatment of infants born SGA, a condition also called intrauterine growth retardation, or IUGR. This condition, highly prevalent in developing countries, is associated with low body fat at birth, low IGF-1 levels up to age 2, and subsequently abnormal catch-up growth characterized by increased adiposity, insulin resistance, and low-grade inflammation.[181] IUGR therefore is associated with subsequently high rates of coronary heart disease, high blood pressure, diabetes, and high cholesterol.[182] Treatment of children manifesting IUGR with daily GH shots increased linear growth velocity in many studies, while delaying the onset of puberty and exhibiting few if any side effects.[183,184–187] However, treatment for years was required, higher doses were more effective, and younger children (3 to 5 years old) were more responsive to treatment.[188] Of major concern is the global scope of this problem with IUGR, however, because IUGR affects 20% of children in Malawi[189] and 25% of children in Pakistan.[190] Clearly, ethical problems will arise as to which children can be treated with this expensive and long-term therapy.

Table 6 Effects of Undernutrition on the GH-IGF Axis

Increased GH secretion
GH resistance in peripheral tissues
Decreased GH receptor mRNA
Decreased GH binding
Diminished postreceptor signaling (P)
Decreased somatomedin bioactivity
Decreased IGF-I production
Decreased IGF-I gene transcription
Diminished IGF-I mRNA stability (P)
Diminished IGF-I mRNA translation (P)
Normal IGF-II production
Increased IGF-BP-1 production
Decreased IGF-BP-3 production (P)
Increased IGF-I clearance
Increased IGF inhibitor production
Decreased tissue sensitivity to IGF-I

(P) indicates features more typical of protein deprivation or chronic malnutrition than of fasting.
GH = growth hormone; IGF = insulin-like growth factor; IGF-BP = insulin-like growth factor binding protein; mRNA = messenger ribonucleic acid.

IGFs in Malnutrition

IGF Bioactivity, IGF Inhibitors, and IGF-Binding Proteins. Despite elevated GH levels in fasting or short-term malnutrition, the production of IGF-I is dramatically reduced in malnutrition. Studies using somatomedin bioassays were the first to indicate that serum IGF bioactivity falls with malnutrition. More recent data using highly specific radioimmunoassays indicate that the depressed bioactivity of serum from fasted or malnourished individuals results from a dramatic fall in IGF-I concentrations, minimal if any change in IGF-II concentrations,[191] and changes in IGF-BPs (Table 6).

Measuring serum somatomedin bioactivity in a sulfation factor assay, Grant and associates were among the first to show a nutritional influence on somatomedin activity[192]; they found low levels in the serum of malnourished South African children despite elevated GH concentrations. Those authors found both hormones to return toward normal by the ninth day of refeeding. Similar results using somatomedin bioassays were forthcoming from other malnourished populations,[193] including malnourished Thai[194] and Nigerian[195] infants and children and patients with celiac disease[196] and anorexia nervosa.[197]

Bioassays of IGF activity in blood, although relatively nonspecific as to which of the two IGFs is being measured, allow the detection of physiologically important IGF inhibitors in serum. Much of the older data on somatomedin inhibitors can be attributed to changes in the concentration of known IGF-BPs. Increased concentrations of inhibitors have been found in the serum of malnourished children and hypopituitary adults[193,198,199] and in serum from starved, hypophysectomized, or diabetic rats.[200,201] Salmon and colleagues partially purified a 27 to 40 kDa, heat-labile inhibitor from fasted rat serum.[202] Recent studies have suggested that this inhibitor may be the serum-binding protein, IGF-BP-1[203] (see Table 4). Serum concentrations of BP-1 almost double with fasting and decrease after meals.[204] In addition, they are elevated in diabetes,[205] consonant with the proposed role of insulin in the regulation of BP-1 production. Phillips and associates have shown that concurrent with the fall in IGF activity of rat serum during fasting, total IGF inhibitor activity rises.[206] The IGF inhibitory activity of serum appears to be more nutritionally sensitive than the IGF activity itself. After 6 hours of refeeding, the IGF inhibitor activity had fallen significantly, but there was little change in IGF activity; both returned to normal with continued refeeding.

IGF-I and IGF-II in Malnutrition. As measured by specific radioimmunoassays, IGF-I concentrations drop dramatically with fasting in adult volunteers,[207] while those of IGF-II do not.[191] Clemmons found that fasting of overweight adult volunteers for 10 days produced a drop of IGF-I concentrations to hypopituitary levels; refeeding produced a return toward normal[207] (Figure 5). The decline in serum IGF-I correlated with nitrogen balance. In some physiologic circumstances, however, the fall in serum IGF-I concentrations becomes dissociated from the changes in nitrogen

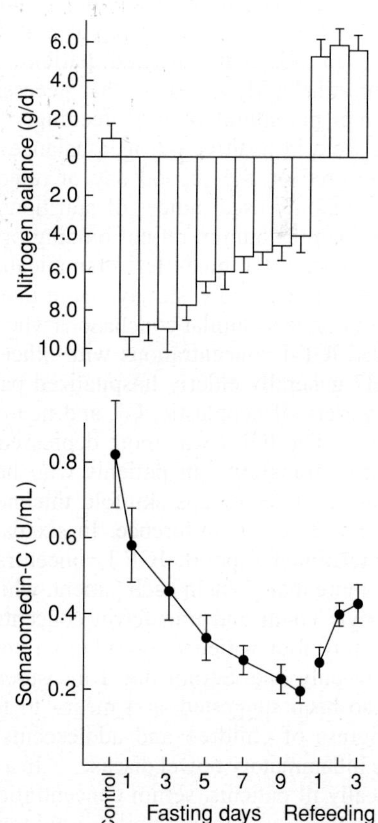

Figure 5 The effects of fasting on plasma somatomedin-C (IGF-I) and nitrogen balance. The subjects were seven males 20 to 70% above ideal body weight. During the control period, they were fed a 1,500 kcal diet for 3 days. Between days 4 and 13 they fasted, receiving only water, vitamins, and potassium chloride. Refeeding consisted of resumption of the control diet. Each point is the mean ± SEM. (Adapted from reference 207.)

balance. Smith and coworkers studied six conditioned athletes and concluded that strenuous exercise, which produces negative caloric balance, causes as much of a fall in serum IGF-I as does comparable caloric restriction without exercise, but a much lower nitrogen loss.[208]

In contrast to the apparent insensitivity of serum IGF-II to fasting in adults,[191] Soliman and associates have documented depressed IGF-II concentrations in children with severe marasmus and marasmic kwashiorkor.[209] These returned to normal with refeeding. The magnitude of IGF-II depression was not nearly as great as that of IGF-I, and the IGF-II concentrations in sera of children who were underweight or had only kwashiorkor were not depressed. Thus, severe or long-lasting malnutrition in children may eventually depress IGF-II production, although IGF-I remains the more acutely sensitive to malnutrition. In addition, IGF-1 levels may reflect imbalanced or abnormal nutrition. For example, infants with short bowel syndrome maintained on PN who developed liver disease had low levels of IGF-1.[210]

Serum IGF-I as an Index of Nutritional Status. The striking correlation between (as yet unidentified) aspects of nutritional status and serum IGF-I concentrations has led some investigators to suggest that the latter might provide a highly sensitive and quantitative way of following nutritional status. Clemmons and colleagues found that IGF-I increased by 170% over 10 days in six malnourished patients with gastrointestinal (GI) disorders that necessitated either total parenteral or tube feedings.[211] All patients were in positive nitrogen balance when first measured on the second day of refeeding. Other commonly used indices of nutritional status, such as prealbumin, retinol binding protein, and transferring, fell much less dramatically and normalized much more slowly. Unterman and coworkers came to similar conclusions when they compared IGF-I concentrations with other indices in 37 generally elderly hospitalized patients with a variety of neoplastic, GI, and neurologic diseases.[212] The IGF-I was more depressed than albumin or transferrin in patients who had no reduction in either triceps skinfold thickness or mid-arm muscle circumference. In six patients given nutritional support, IGF-I concentrations rose by more than 70% in each patient, while the lymphocyte count and transferrin concentration rose in only four patients and albumin concentration in only one. Serum IGF-I measurements have also been suggested as a means to follow the progress of children and adolescents with chronic inflammatory bowel disease.[213] In a study of critically ill patients, serum concentrations of prealbumin, retinol binding protein, and transferrin levels were strongly correlated with levels of IGF-I, IGF-II, IGF-BP3, and ALS.[214]

Mechanisms of IGF Regulation by Nutrients. A number of studies have attempted to determine the specific components of the refeeding diet that regulate IGF-I production in recovery from an acute fast. When normal-weight human volunteers were fasted for 5 days and then refed with a normal diet, a diet that was isocaloric but protein deficient, or a diet deficient in both protein and calories, Isley and associates concluded that intake of adequate quantities of both protein and calories is critical for the restoration of IGF-I after a fast.[215] Animal studies have indicated that the roles played by protein and calorie intake in regulating serum IGF-I concentrations may be developmentally influenced. Prewitt and coworkers placed 3-week-old rats on diets in which the protein content was varied (5, 10, or 15% lactalbumin) at one of three levels of energy intake (100, 75, or 50% ad libitum).[216] After 2 weeks, protein intake played the major role in regulating IGF-I concentrations, whereas after 9 weeks, both protein and caloric intake were important.

The malnourished state is one of resistance to the effects of GH. As noted previously, GH secretion increases in the fasted state, while serum concentrations of IGF-I fall. Merimee and colleagues found that GH administered to fasted, GH-deficient subjects induced a minimal increase in serum IGF-I concentrations in comparison with the 10-fold increase GH induced in normally fed, GH-deficient subjects. Studies in fasted[217–219] and diabetic[219] rats have correlated the fall in serum IGF-I concentrations with a decline in the number of hepatic GH receptors, suggesting that a primary effect of malnutrition, perhaps mediated by decreased insulin concentrations, is to decrease GH receptors and consequently IGF-I production. Indeed, fasting results in decreased GH receptor mRNA in the liver.[220,221] The situation may differ in protein-deprived rats, in whom a postreceptor defect in GH action has been suggested.[148] The net result of fasting is a decrease in the concentrations of IGF-I mRNA in the liver and other tissues.[220] This results from decreased transcription of the *IGF-I* gene, although the effects of protein deprivation may further influence IGF-I mRNA stability and also decrease the translation of IGF-I mRNA into peptide.[222]

The fasted or malnourished state is also one of resistance to the action of IGF-I. Thissen and associates showed that, in contrast with normally fed, hypophysectomized rats, an infusion of recombinant IGF-I into protein-restricted rats did not stimulate an increase in weight gain or linear growth, despite restoring normal serum concentrations.[223] Somewhat surprisingly, this nutritionally induced IGF-I resistance does not result from a decrease in IGF-I receptors at target tissues; instead, most tissues show increased IGF-I binding.[224]

IGF-BPs in Malnutrition. Among the IGF-BPs, BP3 is unique in its diurnal rhythm that appears to be regulated by food intake. IGF-BP1 is rapidly suppressed following a meal, and it acutely rises in response to hyperglycemia. In this context, IGF-BP1 may serve as a glucose counter-regulatory hormone by further depressing free IGF concentrations in the hypoglycemic state. In addition to its regulation by nutrients, IGF-BP1 is stimulated by glucocorticoids and by cytokines such as TNFα and various interleukins. Nutritional status appears to also influence the phosphorylation status of IGF-BP1. Baxter has postulated that increases in IGF-BP-2, BP-4, and BP-6 during acute illness could serve to redistribute IGFs from ternary complexes in the serum to binary complexes in the extracellular space and make them more available to the tissues.[91]

Insulin in Malnutrition. With fasting or protein-calorie malnutrition, plasma insulin concentrations are reduced, although in some instances high and normal levels have been reported.[209] Some of these discrepancies might be explained by the observations of Lunn and associates that in kwashiorkor there is an early phase of hyperinsulinism that is followed by insulinopenia.[155] Diminished insulin release results in impaired tolerance to glucose or an amino acid load.[225] Pimstone and coworkers noted that the insulin response to oral glucose is abnormal in malnourished children but that intravenous glucose elicits a normal response,[226] suggesting that deficiencies of the so-called "incretins" may be important in determining the response to malnutrition. Those authors also demonstrated that the impaired insulin response to a glucose load in kwashiorkor could be ameliorated by the addition of potassium to the diet. The relationship of malnutrition and diabetes mellitus has been reviewed by Rao,[227] who concluded that a malnourished condition can influence the diabetogenicity of other agents, including dietary toxins, drugs, and viruses, but does not directly cause diabetes. Additionally, an initial presentation with malnutrition, dehydration, and hypoglycemia ($<$40 mg/dL) has been associated with a high mortality ($>$40%) for children with diarrheal dehydration.[228]

Psychosocial Growth Failure. The interactions of nutritional and hormonal influences have been extensively studied in cases of "psychosocial growth failure" or "deprivation dwarfism," terms used to describe the growth failure that can accompany severe emotional deprivation. Early in this century, it was recognized that emotional deprivation could be associated with growth retardation in institutionalized children.[229] Subsequent studies revealed that such children need not be in an institutional setting and that an impoverished emotional environment in the home is sufficient. Affected children have a voracious appetite with bizarre eating and drinking behavior such as foraging, drinking from the toilet bowl, and gorging. In addition, delayed speech, foul-smelling stools, a protuberant abdomen, and characteristic neurological postures have been described.[229,230]

Patton and Gardner speculated that emotional deprivation could produce growth retardation in a variety of ways, including failure of the care giver to provide adequate nutrition, depression-induced anorexia in response to the emotional environment, altered gastrointestinal function, or changes in metabolism.[231] Considerable attention has been paid to whether the growth failure and endocrine-metabolic changes of psychosocial dwarfism are the result of emotional deprivation alone or are secondary to impaired caloric intake.

A large body of evidence suggests that a hypopituitary state can develop in some children with emotional deprivation. Talbot found significant malnutrition in a group of 51 children with growth failure of no identifiable etiology and postulated that they might have "functional hypopituitarism" as a means of adapting to limited caloric intake.[132] Twenty years later, Powell and colleagues studied emotionally deprived children and demonstrated diminished reserves of adrenocorticatropic hormone (ACTH) and GH, which were normalized when the affected children were removed from their adverse surroundings.[233,234] The authors found little evidence of caloric deprivation in their patients and suggested that psychic factors caused their hypopituitarism. Miller and colleagues demonstrated a loss of GH secretory episodes during a 6-hour period of blood sampling in four children with psychosocial deprivation.[135] In one child, GH secretion normalized after hospitalization and rehabilitation. Despite the apparent state of GH deficiency, attempts to induce growth in such children by administration of GH have been unsuccessful.[236,237]

Psychological factors were also invoked by Widdowson to explain her observations on the growth of children in two German orphanages after World War II.[238] Orphans under the care of a stern and forbidding supervisor who chose meal times to rebuke the children gained weight at about one-third the rate of children at another, more hospitable orphanage despite comparable food intake. When the supervisor of the first orphanage was transferred to the second, the pattern reversed, and the new children under her care gained weight poorly.

A counter theme to the hypothesis of a strictly emotional etiology of psychosocial growth failure has been the suggestion that underfeeding by care givers is the primary cause of growth failure in these children. From their studies on emotionally deprived infants between 3 and 24 months of age, Whitten and colleagues observed dramatic weight gain in 11 of 13 children when the infants were given adequate nutrition in a hospital setting designed to reproduce the impoverished emotional ambience of their homes.[239] During a control period in which these children were fed equal amounts of food but also given a high level of mothering care, their weight gain was no greater. Other studies have found elevated fasting levels of GH in a number of infants and children with emotional deprivation, leading to the speculation that these infants suffered from food deprivation as well as emotional deprivation.[240]

Contemporary dietary and health misconceptions have created a modern-day version of the growth-retarded child from a turn-of-the-century foundling house or war orphanage. Pugliese and colleagues described a group of 14 adolescents who presented with short stature and malnutrition from self-imposed caloric restriction.[241] These children showed no evidence of overt psychiatric disease or anorexia nervosa but had restricted their food intake from a fear of obesity. Similar findings were reported in a group of younger children, 7 to 22 months of age, who presented with nutritional failure to thrive secondary to parental restriction of food arising from a fear of obesity, cardiovascular disease, or unhealthy eating habits.[242]

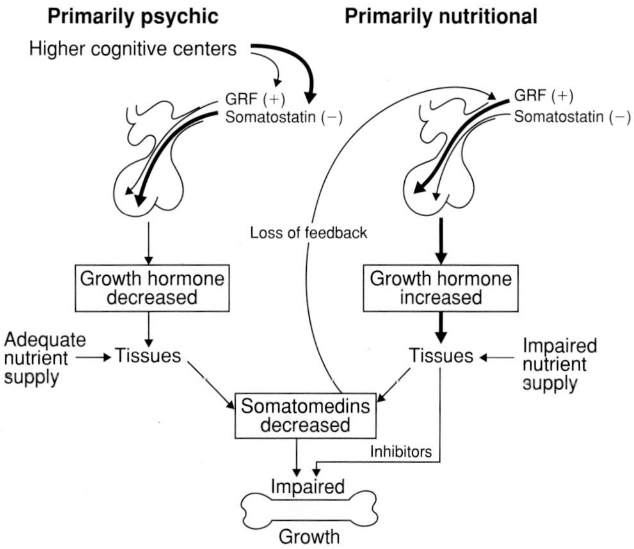

Figure 6 Psychosocial growth failure. Two possible mechanisms of psychosocial growth failure are proposed: primarily psychic (neuroendocrine) and nutritional. Under largely psychological influences, pituitary growth hormone secretion is diminished in the face of normal nutrition (*left*). When undernutrition predominates, the endocrine changes observed are adaptive ones (*right*). Somatomedin production is reduced, IGF-binding proteins are increased, and growth hormone secretion is increased.

It is reasonable to propose from these somewhat disparate observations that the mechanisms involved in the growth failure associated with emotional deprivation form a spectrum (Figure 6). At one extreme are children in whom growth failure is nutritional in origin, whether from limited access to food, from emotionally induced anorexia, or from altered gastrointestinal function. In these children, endocrine alterations are adaptive and occur in response to malnutrition. At the other extreme of the spectrum are those children whose hormonal and metabolic alterations are emotionally induced. The growth failure of these children is probably mediated by hormone deficiencies rather than by inadequate nutrition. It would appear that many of the children with clinical features of psychosocial growth failure combine features of both extremes of the spectrum.

THYROID HORMONES

Thyroid Hormones and Normal Growth

The actions of the thyroid hormones, like those of insulin, can be broadly separated into directly metabolic ones and those that result from thyroid induction of other genes that regulate cell growth and function. Increased oxygen consumption, heat production, and accelerated metabolism constitute the allergenic effects of the thyroid hormones.[243] The mechanism by which thyroid hormones affect these actions is not clearly understood. Thyroid hormone signaling increases basal thermogenesis by increasing ATP turnover and decreasing the efficiency of ATP synthesis. Decreased efficiency of ATP utilization has been linked to the generation of a proton leak across the inner mitochondrial membrane.[244] Unlike peptide hormones, which bind to cell membrane receptors and regulate cell function and gene transcription via second messengers, thyroid hormone receptors exist in the cytoplasm and directly regulate the transcription of other genes by binding to regulatory regions of DNA in the genome.[245] Many of the developmental effects of the thyroid hormones may result from induction of the genes for other hormones and growth factors, such as epidermal and nerve growth factors.[246]

Thyroxine (T_4) is the major hormone secreted by the thyroid, but it is deiodinated at its outer ring to produce triiodothyronine (T_3), which is the metabolically active hormone (Figure 7). Deiodination occurs both in the thyroid gland and at peripheral sites such as liver, kidney, and brain. Thyroxine may also be deiodinated at its inner ring to form reverse T_3 (rT_3), which is metabolically inactive. Regulation of the relative activity of the inner and outer ring deiodinases to vary the concentrations of T_3 and rT_3 is a major control point in the thyroid economy. Thyroxine release from the thyroid is stimulated by thyroid-stimulating hormone (TSH, thyrotropin), which in turn is released from the anterior pituitary under the influence of the hypothalamic modulator, thyrotropin-releasing hormone (TRH). Perhaps in conjunction with T_4, T_3 feeds back to inhibit TSH secretion.

The influence of thyroid hormones on growth occurs at many levels. Within the cell, they have profound effects on metabolic processes, including the induction of mitochondrial enzymes and an increase in Na, K-ATPase activity. Thyroid hormones influence the GH-IGF axis, as evidenced by the fact that hypothyroid rats have a diminished pituitary content of GH, low circulating GH levels, and depressed IGF levels.[246–249] T_3 has been shown to stimulate transcription of the GH gene.[250] In contrast to animal models, hypothyroid children do not consistently demonstrate subnormal GH release.[111,251,252] Furthermore, the growth-retarding effects of hypothyroidism in rats are not reversed by GH treatment. In addition to a GH-mediated influence on IGF secretion, thyroid hormones augment IGF-I actions on cartilage growth,[252] and their absence is evident at the growth plate cartilage by altered morphology.[253] In addition, some thyroid hormone actions on growth plate chondrocytes appear to be IGF-mediated, as the mitogenic actions of T_3 on cartilage growth can be blocked with an antibody to IGF-I. In contrast, the effects of T_3 on cartilage morphology and functional maturation do not appear to be IGF-mediated, direct ones.[254]

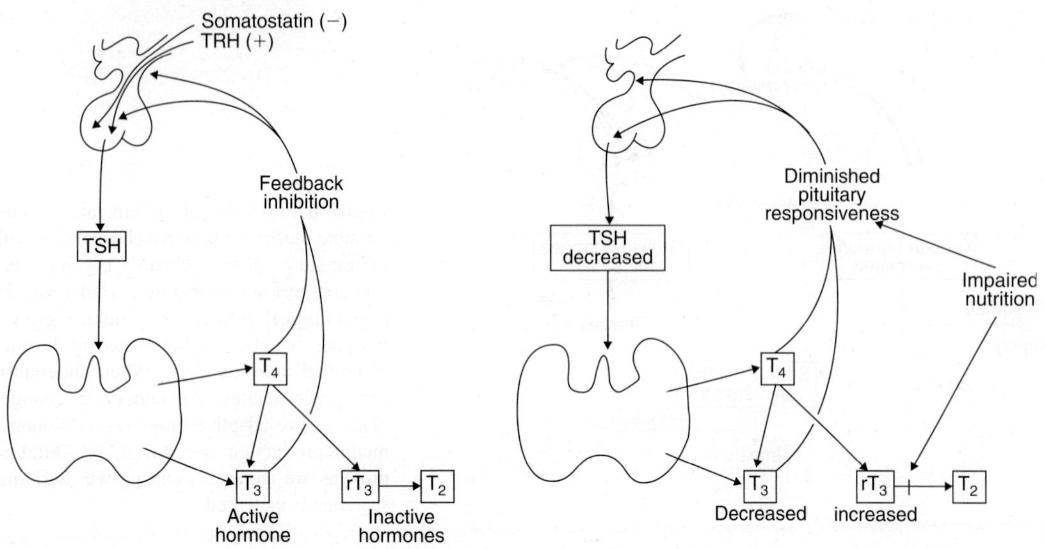

Figure 7 The pituitary–thyroid axis. (A) When nutrition is normal, thyroxine (T_4) is converted primarily to the calorigenic hormone triiodothyronine (T_3) in the thyroid and peripheral tissues. Levels of the inactive hormones reverse T_3 (rT_3) and T_2 are relatively low. (B) After fasting, reverse T_3 concentrations rise primarily because of decreased degradation to T_2, and to some extent through preferential conversion of T_4 to rT_3. Fasting also diminishes the pituitary responsiveness to hypothalamic factors. Thyroid stimulating hormone (TSH) levels do not rise as in other forms of hypothyroidism. (+) stimulatory action; (−) inhibitory action.

Thyroid Hormones and Malnutrition

Fasting and malnutrition induce a hypothyroid-like state characterized by a diminished rate of T3 production and, consequently, a depressed heart rate and basal metabolic rate, as well as a diminished loss of nitrogen.[160,255,256] Similarly, bradycardia is a feature of anorexia nervosa. Concomitant with the fall in T_3 in malnutrition is a depression of sympathetic nervous system activity, as measured by norepinephrine secretion.[257] Within 48 hours of a fast, T_3 concentrations fall into the hypothyroid range while concentrations of T_4 change little, and those of rT_3, the inactive metabolite of T_4, rise (Figure 7). These changes result from a starvation-induced inhibition of the deiodination of T_4 to T_3, while the serum half-life of rT_3 is prolonged by preventing its deiodination to T_2. In addition, malnutrition also results in a diminished synthesis of the plasma thyroid-binding proteins, also leading to depressed thyroid hormone levels.

The low levels of thyroid hormones in the undernourished state are likely to be an adaptive mechanism meant to diminish the extent of catabolism. Danforth and Burger have shown that when T_3 is administered to fasting subjects sufficient to maintain T_3 levels in the normal range, nitrogen losses are accentuated.[244] Despite a low serum T_3, TSH secretion is not increased in fasting, and the TSH response to TRH is either normal or somewhat blunted.[256,258] The condition of depressed levels of metabolically active thyroid hormones without elevation in TSH in malnutrition or illness has often been called the "euthyroid sick syndrome" or "nonthyroidal illness syndrome," and recent developments in the field have cautiously supported the administration of thyroid hormones to individuals in this physiologic state.[259,260]

The depressed T_3 levels of the fasted state can be corrected by refeeding as little as 100 kcal of carbohydrate, whereas the protein or fat content of the diet does not significantly affect the recovery of T_3.[261] As little as 50 g of carbohydrate will prevent the effect of dietary restriction on serum T_3 levels.[87] As in those subjected to acute starvation, chronically malnourished children and adults have depressed serum T_3 and elevated rT_3 concentrations. However, the TSH concentrations are either normal or elevated in chronic malnutrition, and the TSH response to TRH is exaggerated.[156,215,262]

CORTISOL AND SEX STEROIDS

Cortisol in Intestinal Maturation

Development of critical intestinal absorptive transporters and digestive enzymes is a prelude to somatic growth. There is a striking maturation of absorptive function of the intestine following birth, with ample evidence to suggest that glucocorticoids regulate the process. Most of the data on the regulation of gut maturation have been derived from studies in rats and other small mammals. Coincident with the period of weaning and, consequently, a decreasing reliance on lactose and other milk sugars for nourishment, there is a fall in the high activity of lactase in the small intestine and a rise in the activity of intestinal sucrase, maltase, and pancreatic amylase.[263] In addition, there is a loss of the mechanisms by which the ileal and jejunal mucosa take up macromolecules and transport immunoglobulins. Delay of weaning has no significant effect on the timing of these changes. In contrast, deprivation of pituitary hormones by hypophysectomy in the newborn period elicits a marked delay.[264,265] These observations have led to studies of the role of pituitary-derived or pituitary-regulated hormones in the maturation of gut function.

The experimental data support roles for both glucocorticoids and thyroid hormones in intestinal maturation. Coincident with the enzymatic changes in the rat gut at the end of the second week of life, there is a prominent rise in circulating corticosterone. Breast milk might provide an additional source of glucocorticoids.[266] Glucocorticoid administration to preweanlings results in early maturation of intestinal enzymes such as sucrase[263] and of pancreatic amylase, bile acid synthesis, and transport phenomena such as bile salt absorption.[267] The dependence on glucocorticoids is not absolute; however, as adrenalectomy on day 9 of life does not prevent the appearance of sucrase or delay the maturation of sucrase to adult levels of activity.[263] A comparable role for thyroid hormones has also been suggested, although it appears that the ability of thyroxine to induce maturation of the intestinal enzymes requires the presence of intact adrenal glands. Administration of thyroxine to rats results in increased blood concentrations of corticosterone. Thus, the observed effects of thyroxine may be through induction of glucocorticoids.[263]

Cortisol in Malnutrition

Reflecting the metabolic stress, malnutrition in humans and laboratory animals results in elevated cortisol concentrations, with an abolition of the normal diurnal rhythm and a slowed clearance of exogenous cortisol.[268] Fasting also depresses production of cortisol-binding proteins, resulting in a further elevation of free glucocorticoids.[269] Despite the glucocorticoid excess, the adrenal glands remain suppressible with dexamethasone and responsive to ACTH in the malnourished state.

A prominent metabolic effect of cortisol is the diversion of substrates to the liver for protein synthesis. Rao and coworkers have demonstrated that infants with marasmus have higher cortisol levels than do infants with kwashiorkor and that the response of cortisol to ACTH is better preserved in marasmus.[270] Those authors postulated that the development of kwashiorkor is coincident with failure of the adrenal gland to secrete adequate cortisol to maintain normal protein levels. In rats, the biochemical manifestations of kwashiorkor resulting from a low-protein diet can be reversed by glucocorticoids.[271] As previously indicated, glucocorticoids have a deleterious effect on cartilage growth and act as IGF antagonists in somatomedin bioassays. In his studies on malnourished Nigerian children, Smith postulated that elevated cortisol, acting as an inhibitor of IGF action at the epiphyses was a major contributor to the poor growth of his subjects.[195]

Reproductive Function in Malnutrition

The potent gonadal steroids testosterone and estradiol are primarily responsible for the establishment of reproductive fitness. Other, weaker androgenic hormones, however, which are produced by the gonads and adrenal glands of both sexes, are important in the maintenance of normal anabolism. These include androstenedione, dehydroepiandrosterone, and its metabolite dehydroepiandrosterone-sulfate. Whereas reproductive functions are expendable and potentially damaging during times of nutrient deficit, considerable attention has been paid to the importance of weaker androgenic hormones, or anabolic steroids, as possible therapeutic agents for the recovery from catabolic states.

In malnourished adults, hypogonadism often develops, and the secretion of sex steroids by the gonads decreases; in malnourished children, the onset of puberty is delayed.[272] Men suffering from chronic protein-calorie malnutrition often experience gonadal failure. In adults, nutrients appear to influence reproduction at both the hypothalamic and gonadal levels. In a group of Indian men suffering from malnutrition, Smith and colleagues found low-plasma testosterone and elevated gonadotropins, indicating impaired testicular function.[273] During recovery, these men continued to have elevated levels of luteinizing hormone and a subnormal release of testosterone to chorionic gonadotropin (hCG). In contrast, Klibanski found evidence for hypothalamic hypofunction when mildly obese men were fasted for 10 days.[274]

In addition to the effects of malnutrition in delaying puberty, a number of studies on young athletes have suggested a connection between body composition and reproductive fitness. In young female athletes and dancers who train extensively before puberty, menarche can be delayed by several years.[275] In some instances, the delay in menarche can be related directly to the duration of training prior to menarche: 5 months for every year of training.[276] These observations led Frisch and McArthur to propose that normal menstrual function depends on the attainment of at least 22% body fat.[277] This model assumed that some aspect of body fat content signals permission for the secretion of gonadotropic hormones to trigger menstruation. The identification of leptin as the adipocyte-derived product of the ob gene, has shed some light on the relationship between body fat and puberty. Leptin levels in the blood increase with adiposity. Leptin receptors have been identified in the anterior pituitary and gonads, and leptin accelerates the pulsatility of gonadotropin releasing hormone as well as being critical for the synthesis of adrenal androgens (reviewed in reference 278).

Anabolic Steroids as Therapeutic Agents in Catabolic Disease

Despite all attempts, it has been impossible to synthesize steroids with anabolic actions that are divorced from their androgenic (masculinizing) ones. Coupled with their anabolic effects, these hormones also have behavioral effects such as increased aggressiveness and an enhanced appetite. Like all androgens, synthetic anabolic steroids suppress gonadotropin production and result in a lipogenic profile of cholesterol metabolism. High doses can alter liver function and result in hepatocellular carcinoma. Anabolic agents have been shown to decrease nitrogen loss after minor surgery,[279] but have had no consistent effect on weight gain in geriatric patients[280] or in patients with chronic renal failure.[281]

There has been considerable popular attention in recent years to the use of anabolic steroids to increase performance in bodybuilding and other sports. Well-controlled studies in adult male athletes are few, and the results are conflicting.[282] Those whose performance stands to benefit the most from increased androgenic activity are those who produce relatively low levels of androgens endogenously: females, prepubertal children, and adolescents. These are the groups in whom additional adverse effects such as virilization, balding, sexual precocity, and premature closure of the epiphyses would be the most damaging. At this time, there appears to be no clear role for anabolic agents in the treatment of catabolic states. Their use in augmenting athletic performance entails significant medical risk.

SUMMARY AND CONCLUSIONS

The humoral controls on growth are highly sensitive to the nutritional milieu and are programmed to alter and even abort the body's developmental scheme as required during conditions of nutritional want or excess. The specific components of the diet that are monitored by the various nutritionally sensitive endocrine systems are still not known, although our understanding is growing as to how nutrients can alter the expression of specific genes that encode key regulatory hormones, growth factors, and enzymes. Nonetheless, a careful assessment of physical growth and maturation can serve as a sensitive and accurate index of nutritional status and disease, both for individuals and for whole populations.

The capacity of the growing organism to accommodate changes in the availability of nutrients by slowing or halting growth is a generally reversible process (catch-up), designed to permit adaptation to a changing nutrient supply. However, the ability to resume normal growth after the correction of metabolic insults is dependent on the nature of the insult, its duration, and the developmental phase of the organism during which it occurs. The damage incurred during certain susceptible periods of growth may be irreversible, perhaps owing to a reduction in the number or critical organization of the cells that make up key tissues. The mechanisms by which a tissue or organism can monitor its own size and correct discrepancies with its "intended" size are unknown. They probably involve coordination between mechanisms for catch-up that are extant in individual tissues and regulatory centers in the CNS; classic hormones probably do not play a key regulatory role.

Recent years have brought the discovery of new hormone systems with close ties to the nutritional status of the organism. The discoveries of leptin, an appetite suppressant produced by adipose tissue, and ghrelin, an appetite stimulant produced in the alimentary tract, shed new light on how the body monitors its nutritional status. Other adipocyte-secreted substances such as Acrp30 and resistin may contribute to the insulin resistant state of obesity. We have an abundance of candidate molecules to begin to elucidate the mechanisms involved in obesity and diabetes and to suggest therapeutic strategies against these disorders.

From our current vantage point, the metabolic changes of undernutrition are adaptive ones, designed to ensure survival until adequate reserves exist to permit growth and reproduction again. In some instances, however, morbidity may actually result from maladaptive endocrine changes. The development of kwashiorkor, for example, may result when the adrenal gland is no longer able to maintain adequate production of glucocorticoid hormones to facilitate withdrawal of proteins from structural stores, such as muscle.

A better understanding of the normal regulation of hormones and growth factors in conditions of altered nutrition has suggested new diagnostic and therapeutic approaches. Blood levels of IGF-I or some of its binding proteins may provide a more sensitive means of assessing nutritional status than many other currently employed tests. Administration of GH to individuals in catabolic states may hasten their recovery. Studies of anabolic steroid hormones in catabolic states have generally not been promising.

The future challenge is to better delineate the full spectrum of humoral and neuroendocrine changes that accompany nutritional alterations and to define those components of "nutrition" that are the actual signals that can regulate the production and actions of hormones and growth factors. The accelerated rate at which "new" hormone systems have been discovered illustrates the fact that we have not yet identified all of the relevant humoral control systems, let alone understand them. The characterization of genes identified by the Human Genome Project and the advent of new technologies such as proteomic analysis may allow us to finally identify all of the critical components of the interface between nutrition and cellular control. At this time, the measurement of growth factors, their receptors, and their downstream signaling events within tissues is an invasive proposition and of little clinical practicality. When the physiology of these substances is better understood, however, the promise for therapeutic intervention will be great.

REFERENCES

1. Trowbridge FL, Marks JS, deRomana GL, et al. Body composition of Peruvian children with short stature and high weight-for-height. II. Implications for the interpretation of weight-for-height as an indicator of nutritional status. Am J Clin Nutr 1987;46:411–8.
2. Bielicki T, Szczotka H, Charzewski J. The influence of three socio-economic factors on body height in Polish military conscripts. Hum Biol 1981;53:543–55.
3. Greulich WW. A comparison of the physical growth and development of American-born and native Japanese children. Am J Phys Anthropol 1957;15:489–515.
4. Greulich WW. Some secular changes in the growth of American-born and native Japanese children. Am J Phys Anthropol 1976;45:553–68.
5. Feyrter F. Uber die Peripheren Endokrinen (Parakrinen) Drusen des Menschen. Wein: W Maudrich; 1953.

6. Sporn MB, Todaro GJ. Autocrine secretion and malignant transformation of cells. N Engl J Med 1980;303:878–80.
7. Barnard JA, Beauchamp RD, Russell WE, et al. Epidermal growth factor-related peptides and their relevance to gastrointestinal pathophysiology. Gastroenterology 1995;108:564–80.
8. Werb Z. ECM and cell surface proteolysis: Regulating cellular ecology. Cell 1997;91:439–42.
9. Anklessaria P, Teixido J, Laiho M, et al. Cell–cell adhesion mediated by binding of membrane anchored transforming growth factor alpha to epidermal growth factor receptors promotes cell proliferation. Proc Natl Acad Sci U S A 1990;87:3289–93.
10. Re RN. The origins of intracrine hormone action. Am J Med Sci 2002;323:43–8.
11. O'Malley BW. Did eucaryotic steroid receptors evolve from intracrine gene regulators? Endocrinology 1989;125:1119–20.
12. Russell WE, Van Wyk JJ. Peptide growth factors. In: DeGroot LJ, editor. Endocrinology, 3rd edition. Philadelphia: WB Saunders; 1995. p. 2590–623.
13. Holley RW. A unifying hypothesis concerning the nature of malignant growth. Proc Natl Acad Sci U S A 1972;69: 2840–1.
14. Holley RW. Control of growth of mammalian cells in culture. Nature 1975;258:487–90.
15. Barnes D, Sato G. Serum free cell culture: A unifying approach. Cell 1980;22:649–55.
16. Barsh GS, Cunningham DD. Nutrient uptake and control of animal cell proliferation. J Supramol Struct 1977;7:61–77.
17. Eagle H. Metabolic controls in cultured mammalian cells. Science 1965;148:42–51.
18. Gospodarowicz D, Moran JS. Growth factors in mammalian cell culture. Ann Rev Biochem 1976;45:531–58.
19. Temin HM, Pierson HM, Dulak NC. The role of serum in the control of multiplication of avian and mammalian cells in culture. In: Rothblat GH, Cristofalo JJ, editors. Growth, Nutrition and Metbolism of Cells in Culture. New York: Academic; 1972. p. 1.
20. McKeehan WL, McKeehan KA. Serum factors modify the cellular requirement for Ca^{2+}, K^{+}, Mg^{2+}, phosphate ions, and 2-oxycarboxylic acids for multiplication of normal human fibroblasts. Proc Natl Acad Sci U S A 1980;77:3417–21.
21. McKeehan WL, McKeehan KA. Extracellular regulation of fibroblast multiplication: A direct kinetic approach to analysis of role of low-molecular-weight nutrients and serum growth factors. J Supramol Struct 1981;15:83–110.
22. Rizzino A, Rizzino H, Sato G. Defined media and the determination of nutritional and hormonal requirements of mammalian cells in culture. Nutr Rev 1979;37:369–78.
23. Wu R, Sato GH. Replacement of serum in cell culture by hormones: A study of hormonal regulation of cell growth and specific gene expression. J Toxicol Environ Health 1978;4:427–48.
24. Rhoads M. Glutamine signaling in intestinal cells. JPEN J Parenter Enteral Nutr 1999;23:S38–40.
25. Haussinger D, Graf D, Weiergraber OH. Glutamine and cell signaling in liver. J Nutr 2001;131:2509S–14S.
26. Barbosa-Tessman IP, Chen C, Zhong C, et al. Activation of the human asparagine synthetase gene by the amino acid response and the endoplasmic reticulum stress response pathways occurs by common genomic elements. J Biol Chem 2000;275:26976–85.
27. Palsson H. Conformation and body composition. In: Hammond J, editor. Progress in the Physiology of Farm Animals. London: Butterworths; 1955. p. 430–542.
28. Munro HN. General aspects of the regulation of protein metabolism by diet and by hormones. In: Munro HN, Allison JB, editors. Mammalian Protein Metabolism. New York: Academic; 1964. p. 381–481.
29. Kochakian CD, Tillotson C, Austin J. A comparison of the effect of inanition, castration and testosterone on the muscles of the male guinea pig. Endocrinology 1957;60:144.
30. Machlin LJ. Effect of porcine growth hormone on growth and carcass composition of the pig. J Anim Sci 1972;35:794–800.
31. Marin P, Krotkiewski M, Bjorntorp P. Androgen treatment of middle-aged, obese men: Effects on metabolism, muscle and adipose tissues. Eur J Med 1992;1:329–36.
32. Marin P, Holmang S, Jonsson L, et al. The effects of testosterone treatment on body composition and metabolism in middle-aged obese men. Int J Obes Relat Metab Disord 1992;16:991–7.
33. Jensen MD. Androgen effect on body composition and fat metabolism. Mayo Clin Proc 2000;75:S65–8.
34. Eisenstein AP, Singh SP. Hormonal control of nutrient metabolism. In: Goodheart RS, Shils ME, editors. Modern Nutrition in Health and Disease, 6th edition. Philadelphia: Lea & Febiger; 1980.
35. Sokoloff L, Kauffman S. Thyroxine stimulation of amino acid incorporation into protein. J Biol Chem 1961;236: 795–803.
36. Enesco M, Leblond CP. Increase in cell number as a factor in the growth of the organs and tissues of the young male rat. J Embryol Exp Morhpol 1962;10:530–64.
37. McCance RA. Critical periods of growth. Proc Nutr Soc 1976;35:309–13.
38. Widdowson EM, McCance RA. Some effects of accelerating growth: I. General somatic development. Proc R Soc Lond (Biol) 1960;152:188–206.
39. Widdowson EM, McCance RA. A review: New thoughts on growth. Pediatr Res 1975;9:154–6.
40. Widdowson EM, McCance RA. The effect of finite periods of undernutrition at different ages on the composition and subsequent development of the rat. Proc R Soc Lond (Biol) 1963;158:329–42.
41. van Pareren Y, Mulder P, Houdijk M, et al. Adult Height after long-term, continuous growth hormone (GH) treatment in short children born small for gestational age: Results of a randomized, double-blind, dose-response GH trial. J Clin Endocrinol Metab 2003;88:3584–90.
42. Winick M, Noble A. Cellular response in rats during malnutrition at various ages. J Nutr 1966;89:300–6.
43. Winick M, Noble A. Cellular response with increased feeding in neonatal rats. J Nutr 1967;91:179–182.
44. Winick M, Brasel JA. Nutrition and cell growth. In:Goodhart RS, Shils ME, editors. Modern Nutrition in Health and Disease. Philadelphia: Lea & Febiger; 1980. p. 592–607.
45. Godfrey KM, Barker DJ. Fetal programming and adult health. Public Health Nutr 2001;4:611–24.
46. Ibanez L, Potau N, Marcos MV, et al. Exaggerated adrenarche and hyperinsulinism in adolescent girls born small for gestational age. J Clin Endocrinol Metab 1999;84:4739–41.
47. Ibanez L, Potau N, Enriquez G, et al. Reduced uterine and ovarian size in adolescent girls born small for gestational age. Pediatr Res 2000;47:575–7.
48. Ibanez L, Potau N, Ferrer A, et al. Reduced ovulation rate in adolescent girls born small for gestational age. J Clin Endocrinol Metab 2002;87:3391–3.
49. Abitbol C, Chan JC, Trachtman H, et al. Growth in children with moderate renal insufficiency: Measurement, evaluation, and treatment. J Pediatr 1996;129:s3–8.
50. Posada ME, Ruben M, Esquivel M. On growth of children: Effect of some socioeconomic and genetic factors. Acta Paediatr Hung 1987;28:37–43.
51. Karlberg J, Lawrence C, bertsson-Wikland K. Prediction of final height in short, normal and tall children. Acta Paediatr Suppl 1994;406:3–9.
52. Gohlke BC, Stanhope R. Final height in psychosocial short stature: Is there complete catch-up? Acta Paediatr 2002;91:961–5.
53. Wright CM, Cheetham TD. The strengths and limitations of parental heights as a predictor of attained height. Arch Dis Child 1999;81:257–60.
54. Prader A, Tanner JM, von Harnack GA. Catch-up growth following illness or starvation: An example of developmental canalization in man. J Pediatr 1963;62:646–59.
55. Tanner JM. Growth at Adolescence, 2nd edition. Oxford: Blackwell Scientific Publishers; 1962.
56. Smith DW, Truog W, Rogers JE, et al. Shifting linear growth during infancy: Illustrations of genetic factors in growth from fetal life through infancy. J Pediatr 1976;89:225–30.
57. Williams JPG, Hughes PCR. Catch-up growth in rats undernourished for different periods during the suckling period. Growth 1975;39:179–93.
58. Williams JPG, Tanner JM, Hughes PCR. Catch-up growth in male rats after growth retardation during the suckling period. Pediatr Res 1974;8:149–56.
59. Rivkees SA, Bode HH, Crawford JD. Long-term growth in juvenile acquired hypothyroidism. N Engl J Med 1988;318:599–602.
60. Burns EC, Tanner JM, Preece MA, et al. Final height and pubertal development in 155 children with idiopathic growth hormone deficiency treated for between 2 and 15 years with growth hormone. Eur J Pediatr 1981;137:155–64.
61. Guerrant RL, Schorling JB, McAuliffe JF, et al. Diarrhea as a cause and an effect of malnutrition; diarrhea prevents catch-up growth and malnutrition increases diarrhea frequency and duration. Am J Trop Med Hyg 1992;47:28–35.
62. Golden MH. Is complete catch-up possible for stunted malnourished children? Eur J Clin Nutr 1994;48:58–70.
63. Mosier HD. Failure of compensatory (catch-up) growth in the rat. Pediatr Res 1971;5:59–63.
64. Allen DB, Julius JR, Breen TJ, et al. Treatment of glucocorticoid-induced growth suppression with growth hormone. J Clin Endocrinol Metab 1998;83 2824–8.
65. Ashworth A. Growth rates in children recovering from protein-calorie malnutrition. Br J Nutr 1969;23:835–45.
66. Bjorntorp P, Yang MU. Refeeding after fasting in the rat: Effects on body composition and food efficiency. Am J Clin Nutr 1982;36:444–9.
67. Krieger I, Whitten CF. Energy metabolism in infants with growth failure due to maternal deprivation, undernutrition or causes unknown. J Pediatr 1969;75:374–9.
68. Correlation between weight increase and caloric intake in infants with severe marasmic malnutrition. 26th annual meeting of the Society for Pediatric Research; Atlantic City, NJ: 1966.
69. WHO. Management of severe malnutrition: A manual for physicians and other senior health workers. Geneva: WHO; 2006.
70. Forbes GB. A note on the mathematics of "catch-up" growth. Pediatr Res 1974;8:929–31.
71. Mosier HD. Catch-up and proportionate growth. Med Clin North Am 1978;62:337–50.
72. Tanner JM. Catch-up growth in man. Br Med Bull 1981;37:233–8.
73. Williams JPG. Catch-up growth. J Embryol Exp Morhpol 1981;65:89–101.
74. Fausto N. Campbell JS, Riehle KJ. Liver regeneration. Hepatology 2006;43:S45–53.
75. Tanner JM. The regulation of human growth. Child Dev 1963;34:817–47.
76. Leibel RL. A biologic radar system for the assessment of body mass: The model of a geometry sensitive endocrine system is presented. J Theor Biol 1977;66:297–306.
77. Gafni RI, Baron J. Catch-up growth: Possible mechanisms. Pediatr Nephrol 2000;14:616–19.
78. Baron J, Klein KO, Colli MJ, et al. Catch-up growth after glucocorticoid excess: A mechanism intrinsic to th growth plate. Endocrinology 1994;135:1367–71.
79. Kay's SK, Hindmarsh PC. Catch-up growth: An overview. Pediatric Endocrinology Reviews 2006;3:365–78.
80. Salmon WD, Jr, Daughaday WH. A hormonally controlled serum factor which stimulates sulfate incorporation by cartilage in vitro. J Lab Clin Med 1957;49:825–6.
81. Le Roith D, Bondy C, Yakar S, et al. The somatomedin hypothesis: 2001. Endocr Rev 2001;22:53–74.
82. Daughaday WH, Hall K, Raben MS, et al. Somatomedin: Proposed designation for sulphation factor. Nature 1972;235:107.
83. Rinderknecht E, Humbel RE. The amino acid sequence of human insulin-like growth factor I and its structural homology with proinsulin. J Biol Chem 1978;253:2769–76.
84. Zapf J, Schmid CH, Froesch ER. Biological and immunological properties of insulin-like growth factors (IGF) I and II. Clin Endocrinol Metab 1984;13:3–30.
85. D'Ercole AJ, Applewhite GT, Underwood LE. Evidence that somatomedin is synthesized by multiple tissues in the fetus. Dev Biol 1980;75:315–28.
86. Lowe WT, Lasky SR, LeRoith D, et al. Distribution and regulation of rat insulin-like growth factor I messenger ribonucleic acids encoding alternative carboxy-terminal E-peptides: Evidence for differential processing and regulation in liver. Mol Endocrinol 1988;2:528–35.
87. Isaksson O, Lindahl A, Nilsson A, et al. Mechanism of the stimulatory effect of growth hormone on longitudinal bone growth. Endocr Rev 1987;8:426–38.
88. Green H, Morikawa M, Nixon T. A dual effector theory of growth hormone action. Differentiation 1985;29:195–8.
89. Yakar S, Liu JL, Stannard B, et al. Normal growth and development in the absence of hepatic insulin-like growth factor I. Proc Natl Acad Sci U S A 1999;96:7324–9.
90. Sjogren K, Liu JL, Blad K, et al. Liver-derived insulin-like growth factor I (IGF-I) is the principal source of IGF-I in blood but is not required for postnatal body growth in mice. Proc Natl Acad Sci U S A 1999;96:7088–92.
91. Duan C, Xu Q. Roles of insulin-like growth factor (IGF) binding proteins in regulating IGF activity. Gen and Comp Endocrinol 2005;142:44–52.
92. Jones JI, Gockerman A, Busby WJ, et al. Insulin-like growth factor binding protein 1 stimulates cell migration and binds to the alpha 5 beta 1 integrin by means of its Arg-Gly-Asp sequence. Proc Natl Acad Sci U S A 1993;90:10553–7.
93. Valentinis B, Bhala A, DeAngelis T, et al. The human insulin-like growth factor (IGF) binding protein-3 inhibits the growth of fibroblasts with a targeted disruption of the IGF-I receptor gene. Mol Endocrinol 1995;9:361–7.
94. Lee KW, Cohen P. Nuclear effects: Unexpected intracellular actions o insulin-like growth factor binding protein-3. J Endocrinol 2002;175:33–40.
95. Miller WL, Eberhardt NL. Structure and evolution of the growth hormone gene family. Endocr Rev 1983;4:97–130.
96. Hwa V, Oh Y, Rosenfeld RG. The insulin-like growth factor binding protein (IGFBP) superfamily. Endocr Rev 1999;20:761–87.
97. Muggeo M, Tiengo A, Fedele D, et al. The influence of plasma triglycerides on human growth hormone response to arginine and insulin: A study in hyperlipidemics and normal subjects. Horm Metab Res 1975;7:367–74.

98. Carro E, Senaris R, Considine RV, et al. Regulation of in vivo growth hormone secretion by leptin. Endocrinology 1997;138:2203–6.
99. Tannenbaum GS, Gurd W, Lapointe M. Leptin is a potent stimulator of spontaneous pulsatile growth hormone (GH) secretion and the GH response to GH-releasing hormone. Endocrinology 1998;139:3871–5.
100. Vuagnat BA, Pierroz DD, Laloui M, et al. Evidence for a leptin-neuropeptide Y axis for the regulation of growth hormone secretion in the rat. Neuroendocrinology 1998;67:291–300.
101. Chan YY, Steiner RA, Clifton DK. Regulation of hypothalamic neuropeptide-Y neurons by growth hormone in the rat. Endocrinology 1996;137:2109–12.
102. Cummings DE. Ghrelin and the short- and long-term regulation of appetite and body weight. Physiol Behav 2006;89:71–84.
103. Ghigo E, Arvat E, Gianotti L, et al. Growth hormone-releasing activity of hexarelin, a new synthetic hexapeptide, after intravenous, subcutaneous, intranasal, and oral administration in man. J Clin Endocrinol Metab 1994;78:693–8.
104. Bowers CY. Unnatural growth hormone-releasing peptide begets natural ghrelin. J Clin Endocrinol Metab 2001;86:1464–9.
105. Berelowitz M, et al. Somatomedin-C mediates growth hormone negative feedback by effects on both the hypothalamus and the pituitary. Science 1981;212:1279.
106. Brazeau P, Guillemin R, Ling N, et al. Inhibition by somatomedin of growth hormone secretion stimulated by hypothalamic growth hormone releasing factor (somatocrinin, GRF), or the synthetic peptide hpGRF. CR Acad Sci 1982;iii:651–4.
107. Herington AC, Ymer S, Stevenson J. Identification and characterization of specific binding proteins for growth hormone in normal human sera. J Clin Invest 1986;77:1817–23.
108. Daughaday WH, Trivedi B, Andrews BA. The ontogeny of serum GH binding protein in man: A possible indicator of hepatic GH receptor development. J Clin Endocrinol Metab 1987;65:1072–4.
109. Finklestein JW, Roffwarg HP, Boyar RM, et al. Age-related changes in the twenty-four hour spontaneous secretion of growth hormone. J Clin Endocrinol Metab 1972;35:665–70.
110. Frankenne F, Rentier-Delrue F, Scippo ML, et al. Expression of the growth hormone variant gene in human placenta. J Clin Endocrinol Metab 1987;64:635–7.
111. Chernausek SD, Underwood LE, Utiger RD, et al. Growth hormone secretion and plasma somatomedin-C in primary hypothyroidism. Clin Endocrinol 1983;19:337–44.
112. Cunningham BC, Ultsch M, DeVos AM, et al. Dimerization of the extracellular domain of the human growth hormone receptor: Crystal structure of the complex. Science 1991;254:821–5.
113. Ridderstrale M. Signaling mechanism for the insulin-like effects of growth hormone-another example of a classical hormonal negative feedback loop. Curr Drug Targets Immune Endocr Metab Disord 2005;5:79–92.
114. Ziegler TR, Rombeau JL, Young LS, et al. Recombinant human growth hormone enhances the metabolic efficacy of parenteral nutrition: A double-blind, randomized controlled study. J Clin Endocrinol Metab 1992;74:865–73.
115. Calfee R, Fadale P. Popular ergogenic drugs and supplements in young athletes. Pediatrics 2006;117:e577–89.
116. Smal J, Closset J, Hennen G, et al. The receptor binding properties of the 20K variant of human growth hormone explain its discrepant insulin-like and growth promoting activities. Biochem Biophys Res Comm 1986;134:159–165.
117. Kostyo JL, Cameron DM, Olson KC, et al. Biosynthetic 20-kilodalton methionyl-human growth hormone has diabetogenic and insulin-like activities. Proc Natl Acad Sci U S A 1985;82:4250–3.
118. Stewart TA, Clift S, Pitts-Meek S, et al. An evaluation of the functions of the 22-kilodalton (kDa), the 20-kDa, and the N-terminal polypeptide forms of human growth hormone using transgenic mice. Endocrinology 1992;130:405–14.
119. Vatten LJ, Nilsen ST, Odegard RA, et al. Insulin-like growth factor I and leptin in umbilical cord plasma and infant birth size at term. Pediatrics 2002;109:1131–5.
120. Francis GL, Upton FM, Ballard FJ, et al. Insulin-like growth factors 1 and 2 in bovine colostrum. Sequences and biological activities compared with those of a potent truncated form. Biochem J 1988;251:95–103.
121. Burrin DG, Wester TJ, Davis TA, et al. Orally administered IGF-I increases intestinal mucosal growth in formula-fed neonatal pigs. Am J Physiol 1996;270:R1085–91.
122. Alexander AN, Carey HV. Insulin-like growth factor-I stimulates Na^+-dependent glutamine absorption in piglet enterocytes. Dig Dis Sci 2002;47:1129–34.
123. Simmons JG, Pucilowska JB, Lund PK. Autocrine and paracrine actions of intestinal fibroblast-derived insulin-like growth factors. Am J Physiol 1999;276:G817–27.
124. Andre F, Rigot V, Remacle-Bonnet M, et al. Protein kinases C-gamma and -delta are involved in insulin-like growth factor I-induced migration of colonic epithelial cells. Gastroenterology 1999;116:64–77.
125. Kuemmerle JF, Bushman TL. IGF-I stimulates intestinal muscle cell growth by activating distinct PI 3-kinase and MAP kinase pathways. Am J Physiol 1998;275:G151–8.
126. Zijlstra RT, Odle J, Hall WF, et al. Effect of orally administered epidermal growth factor on intestinal recovery of neonatal pigs infected with rotavirus. J Pediatr Gastroenterol Nutr 1994;19:382–90.
127. Gillingham MB, Dahly EM, Carey HV, et al. Differential jejunal and colonic adaptation due to resection and IGF-I in parenterally fed rats. Am J Physiol Gastrointest Liver Physiol 2000;278:G700–9.
128. Gu Y, Wu ZH, Xie JX, et al. Effects of growth hormone (rhGH) and glutamine supplemented parenteral nutrition on intestinal adaptation in short bowel rats. Clin Nutr 2001;20:159–66.
129. Ziegler TR, Mantell MP, Chow JC, et al. Gut adaptation and the insulin-like growth factor system: Regulation by glutamine and IGF-I administration. Am J Physiol 1996;271: G866–75.
130. Blikslager AT, Rhoads JM, Bristol DG, et al. Glutamine and transforming growth factor-alpha stimulate extracellular regulated kinases and enhance recovery of villous surface area in porcine ischemic-injured intestine. Surgery 1999;125:186–94.
131. Rhoads JM, Ulshen MH, Keku EO, et al. Oral transforming growth factor-alpha enhances jejunal mucosal recovery and electrical resistance in piglet rotavirus enteritis. Pediatr Res 1995;38:173–81.
132. Ziegler TR, Mantell MP, Chow JC, et al. Gut adaptation and the insulin-like growth factor system: Regulation by glutamine and IGF-I administration. Am J Physiol 1996;271:G866–75.
133. Ahdieh N, Blikslager AT, Bhat BG, et al. L-glutamine and transforming growth factor-alpha enhance recovery of monoacylglycerol acyltransferase and diacylglycerol acyltransferase activity in porcine postischemic ileum. Pediatr Res 1998;43:227–33.
134. Park YK, Monaco MH, Donovan SM. Enteral insulin-like growth factor-I augments intestinal disaccharidase activity in piglets receiving total parenteral nutrition. J Pediatr Gastroenterol Nutr 1999;29:198–206.
135. Park YK, Dudley MA, Burrin DG, et al. Intestinal protein and LPH synthesis in parenterally fed piglets receiving partial enteral nutrition and enteral insulinlike growth factor 1. J Pediatr Gastroenterol Nutr 2001;33:189–95.
136. Lund PK. Molecular basis of intestinal adaptation: The role of the insulin-like growth factor system. Ann N Y Acad Sci 1998;859:18–36.
137. Butler AA, Yakar S, LeRoith D. Insulin-like growth factor-I: Compartmentalization within the somatotropic axis? News Physiol Sci 2002;17:82–5.
138. Glaser B, Phillip M, Carmi R, et al. Persistent hyperinsulinemic hypoglycemia of infancy ("nesidioblastosis"): Autosomal recessive inheritance in 7 pedigrees. Am J Med Genet 1990;37:511–5.
139. Hill DJ, Milner RDG. Insulin as a growth factor. Pediatr Res 1985;19:879–86.
140. Lee RGL, Bode HH. Stunted growth and hepatomegaly in diabetes mellitus. J Pediatr 1977;91:82–4.
141. Davis TA, Fiorotto ML, Beckett PR, et al. Differential effects of insulin on peripheral and visceral tissue protein synthesis in neonatal pigs. Am J Physiol Endocrinol Metab 2001;280:E770–9.
142. Amiel SA, Sherwin RS, Hintz RL, et al. Effect of diabetes and its control on insulin-like growth factors in the young subject with type I diabetes. Diabetes 1984;33:1175–9.
143. Binoux M, Lassarre C, Jardoudin N. Somatomedin production by rat liver in organ culture: III. Studies on the release of insulin-like growth factor and its carrier protein measured by radioligand assays. Acta Endocr (Copenh) 1982;99:422–30.
144. Maes M, Ketelslegers JM, Underwood LE. Low plasma somatomedin-C in streptozotocin-induced diabetes mellitus. Diabetes 1983;32:1060–9.
145. Myers MJ, Wang LM, Sun XJ, et al. Role of IRS-1-GRB-2 complexes in insulin signaling. Mol Cell Biol 1994;14:3577–87.
146. Moxham CP, Duronio V, Jacobs S. Insulin-like growth factor-1 receptor beta-subunit heterogeneity: Evidence for hybrid tetramers composed of insulin-like growth factor 1 and insulin heterodimers. J Biol Chem 1989;264:13228–44.
147. Roth RA. Structure of the receptor for insulin-like growth factor II: The puzzle amplified. Science 1988;239:1269–71.
148. Rechler MM, Nissley SP. The nature and regulation of the receptors for insulin-like growth factors. Ann Rev Physiol 1985;47:425–42.
149. McGowan JA, Strain AJ, Bucher NLR. DNA synthesis in primary cultures of adult rat hepatocytes in a defined medium: Effects of epidermal growth factor, insulin, glucagon and cyclic-AMP. J Cell Physiol 1981;108:353–63.
150. Whitehead RG, Rowland MGM, Cole TJ. Infection, nutrition and growth in a rural African environment. Proc Nutr Soc 1976;35:369–75.
151. Ho KY, Veldhuis JD, Jphnson ML, et al. Fasting enhances growth hormone secretion and amplifies the complex rhythms of growth hormone secretion in man. J Clin Invest 1988;81:968–75.
152. Hartman ML, Veldhuis JD, Johnson ML, et al. Augmented growth hormone (GH) secretory burst frequency and amplitude mediate enhanced GH secretion during a two-day fast in normal men. J Clin Endocrinol Metab 1992;74:757–65.
153. Becker DJ, Pimstone BL, Hansen JDL, et al. Serum albumin and growth hormone relationships in kwashiorkor and the nephrotic syndrome. J Lab Clin Med 1971;78:865–71.
154. Coward WA, Lunn PG. The biochemistry and physiology of kwashiorkor and marasmus. Br Med Bull 1981;37:19–24.
155. Lunn PG, Whitehead RG, May RW, et al. Progressive changes in serum cortisol, insulin and growth hormone concentrations and their relationship to the distorted amino acid pattern during the development of kwashiorkor. Br J Nutr 1973;29:399–422.
156. Parra A. Insulin-growth hormone adaptations in marasmus and kwashiorkor as seen in Mexico. In: Gardner LI, Amacher P, editors. Endocrine Aspects of Malnutrition: Marasmus, Kwashiorkor and Psychosocial Deprivation. Santa Ynez, CA: The Kroc Foundation; 1973. p. 31–43.
157. Pimstone BL, Barbezat G, Jansen JDL, et al. Studies on growth hormone secretion in protein-calorie malnutrition. Clin Nutr 1973;21:482–7.
158. Beas F, Muzzo S. Growth Hormone and Malnutrition: The Chilean Experience. Santa Ynez, CA: The Kroc Foundation; 1973.
159. Robinson H, Cocks T, Kerr D, et al. Fasting and postprandial levels of plasma insulin and growth hormone in malnourished Jamaican children, during catch-up growth and after complete recovery. In: Gardner LI, Amacher P, editors. Endocrine Aspects of Malnutrition: Marasmus, Kwashiorkor and Psychosocial Deprivation. Santa Ynez, CA: The Kroc Foundation; 1973. p. 45–72.
160. Beas F, Monckeberg F, Horwitz I, et al. The responses of the thyroid gland to thyroid-stimulating hormone (TSH) in infants with malnutrition. Pediatrics 1966;38:1003–8.
161. Mulinos MG, Pomerantz L. Pseudo-hypophysectomy: A condition resembling hypophysectomy produced by malnutrition. J Nutr 1940;19:493–504.
162. Miller J, Silverstein J, Shuster J, et al. Short-term effects of growth hormone on sleep abnormalities in Prader-Willi syndrome. J Clin Endocrinol Metab 2006;91:413–7.
163. Low LC. Growth of children with beta-thalassemia major. Indian J Pediatr 2005;72:159–64.
164. Bideci A, Camurdan MO, Cinaz P, et al. Ghrelin, IGF-I and IGFBP-3 levels in children with type 1 diabetes mellitus. J Pediatr Endocrinol Metab 2005;18:1433–9.
165. Krawczuk-Rybak M, Muszynska-Roslan K, Kitszel A, et al. Relationship between insulin-like growth factors (IGF-I and IGF-II), IGF-binding proteins (IGFBP-3, IGFBP-2), leptin and anthropometric parameters (height, body mass index) during antileukaemic treatment in children. Rocz Akad Med Bialymst 2005;50:208–11.
166. Rusinska A, Chlebna-Sokol D. Insulin-like growth factor-I and mineral metabolism markers in children with idiopathic decrease in bone mass. Clin Chim Acta 2006;366:257–63.
167. Laron Z, Ginsberg S, Lilos P, et al. Long-term IGF-I treatment of children with Laron syndrome increases adiposity. Growth Horm IGF Res 2006;16:61–4.
168. Clemmons DR, Snyder DK, Williams R, et al. Growth hormone administration conserves lean body mass during dietary restriction in obese subjects. J Clin Endocrinol Metab 1987;64:878–83.
169. Manson JM, Wilmore DW. Positive nitrogen balance with human growth hormone and hypocaloric intravenous feeding. Surgery 1986;100:188–97.
170. Mode A, Norstedt G, Simic B, et al. Continuous infusion of growth hormone feminizes hepatic steroid metabolism in the rat. Endocrinology 1981;108:2103–8.
171. Ziegler TR, Young LS, Manson JM, et al. Metabolic effects of recombinant human growth hormone in patients receiving parenteral nutrition. Ann Surg 1988;208:6–16.
172. Ruokonen E, Takala J. Dangers of growth hormone therapy in critically ill patients. Ann Med 2000;32:317–22.
173. Ramirez RJ, Wolf SE, Barrow RE, et al. Growth hormone treatment in pediatric burns: A safe therapeutic approach. Ann Surg 1998;228:439–48.

174. Han X, Sosnowska D, Bonkowski EL, et al. Growth hormone inhibits signal transducer and activator of transcription 3 activation and reduces disease activity in murine colitis. Gastroenterology 2005;129:185–203.
175. Theiss AL, Fuller CR, Simmons JG, et al. Growth hormone reduces the severity of fibrosis associated with chronic intestinal inflammation. Gastroenterology 2005;129:204–19.
176. Sanz S, Pucilowska JB, Liu S, et al. Expression of insulin-like growth factor I by activated hepatic stellate cells reduces fibrogenesis and enhances regeneration after liver injury. Gut 2005;54:134–41.
177. Hardin DS, Ellis KJ, Dyson M, et al. Growth hormone improves clinical status in prepubertal children with cystic fibrosis: Results of a randomized controlled trial. J Pediatr 2001;139:636–42.
178. Taylor AM, Thomson A, Bruce-Morgan C, et al. The relationship between insulin, IGF-I and weight gain in cystic fibrosis. Clin Endocrinol 1999;51:659–65.
179. Slonim AE, Bulone L, Damore MB, et al. A preliminary study of growth hormone therapy for Crohn's disease. N Engl J Med 2000;342:1633–7.
180. Mauras N, George D, Evans J, et al. Growth hormone has anabolic effects in glucocorticosteroid-dependent children with inflammatory bowel disease: A pilot study. Metabolism 2002;51:127–35.
181. Ibanez L, Ong K, Dunger DB, et al. Early development of adiposity and insulin resistance after catch-up weight gain in small-for-gestational-age children. J Clin Endocrinol Metab 2006;91:2153–8.
182. Godfrey KM, Barker DJ. Fetal nutrition and adult disease. Am J Clin Nutr 2000;71:1344S–52S.
183. de Zegher F, bertsson-Wikland K, Wilton P, et al. Growth hormone treatment of short children born small for gestational age: Metanalysis of four independent, randomized, controlled, multicentre studies. Acta Paediatr Suppl 1996;417:27–31.
184. de Zegher F, bertsson-Wikland K, Wollmann HA, et al. Growth hormone treatment of short children born small for gestational age: Growth responses with continuous and discontinuous regimens over 6 years. J Clin Endocrinol Metab 2000;85:2816–21.
185. Bundak R, Darendeliler F, Gunoz H, et al. Growth hormone treatment in short children with intrauterine growth retardation. J Pediatr Endocrinol 2001;14:313–8.
186. Boguszewski M, bertsson-Wikland K, Aronsson S, et al. Growth hormone treatment of short children born small-for-gestational-age: The Nordic Multicentre Trial. Acta Paediatr 1998;87:257–63.
187. Rekers-Mombarg LT, Kamp GA, Massa GG, et al. Influence of growth hormone treatment on pubertal timing and pubertal growth in children with idiopathic short stature. Dutch Growth Hormone Working Group. J Pediatr Endocrinol 1999;12:611–22.
188. de Zegher F, Butenandt O, Chatelain P, et al. Growth hormone treatment of short children born small for gestational age: Reappraisal of the rate of bone maturation over 2 years and metanalysis of height gain over 4 years. Acta Paediatr Suppl 1997;423:207–12.
189. Verhoeff FH, Brabin BJ, van Buuren S, et al. An analysis of intra-uterine growth retardation in rural Malawi. Eur J Clin Nutr 2001;55:682–9.
190. Shamim A, Khan HO, Rana JS, et al. Intrauterine growth restriction: A perspective for Pakistan. JPMA J Pak Med Assoc 1999;49:82–5.
191. Davenport ML, Svoboda ME, Koerber KL, et al. Serum concentrations of insulin-like growth factor II are not changed by short-term fasting and refeeding. J Clin Endocrinol Metab 1988;67:1231–6.
192. Grant DB, Hambley J, Becker DJ, et al. Reduced sulphation factor in undernourished children. Arch Dis Child 1973;48:596.
193. Van den Brande JL, Du Caju MVL. Plasma somatomedin activity in children with growth disturbance. In: Raiti S, editor. Advances in Human Growth Hormone Research. Washington, DC: U.S. Government Printing Office; 1974. p. 98–115.
194. Hintz RL, Suskind R, Amatayakul K, et al. Plasma somatomedin and growth hormone values in children with protein-calorie malnutrition. J Pediatr 1978;92:153-6.
195. Smith IF. Blood plasma levels of cortisol, insulin, growth hormone and somatomedin in children with marasmus, kwashiorkor and intermediate forms of protein-energy malnutrition. Proc Soc Exp Biol Med 1981;167:607-11.
196. Lecornu M, David L, Francois R. Low somatomedin activity in celiac disease. Helv Paediatr Acta 1978;33:509-16.
197. Rappaport R, Prevot C, Czernichow P. Somatomedin activity and growth hormone secretion. I. Changes related to body weight in anorexia nervosa. Acta Paediatr Scand 1980;69:37–41.
198. Ashton IK, Franics MJO. An assay for plasma somatomedin: 3H thymidine incorporation by isolated rabbit chondrocytes. J Endocrinol 1977;74:205–12.
199. Van den Brande JL. Further observations on plasma somatomedin activity in children. Adv Metab 1975;8:171–82.
200. Phillips LS, Young HS. Nutrition and somatomedin. II. Serum somatomedin activity and cartilage growth activity in streptozotocin-diabetic rats. Diabetes 1976;25:516–27.
201. Salmon WD. Interaction of somatomedin and a peptide inhibitor of serum of hypophysectomized and starved, pituitary-intact rats. Adv Metab 1975;8:183–99.
202. Salmon WD, Holladay LA, Burkhalter VJ. Partial characterization of somatomedin inhibitor in starved rat serum. Endocrinology 1983;112:360–70.
203. Graubert MD, Goldstein S, Phillips LS. Nutrition and somatomedin. XXVII. Total and free IGF-I and IGF binding proteins in rats with streptozotocin-induced diabetes. Diabetes 1991;40:959–65.
204. Busby WH, Snyder DK, Clemmons DR. Radioimmunoassay of a 26,000-dalton plasma insulin-like growth factor-binding protein: Control by nutritional variables. J Clin Endocrinol Metab 1988;67:1225–30.
205. Unterman TG, Patel K, Mahathre VK, et al. Regulation of low molecular weight insulin-like growth factor binding proteins in experimental diabetes mellitus. Endocrinology 1990;126:2614–24.
206. Phillips LS, Goldstein S, Gavin JI. Nutrition and somatomedin. XVI. Somatomedins and somatomedin inhibitors in fasted and refed rats. Metabolism 1988;37:209–16.
207. Clemmons DR, Klibanski A, Ridgeway EC, et al. Reduction of plasma immunoreactive somatomedin-C during fasting in humans. J Clin Endocrinol Metab 1981;53:1247–50.
208. Smith AT, Clemmons DR, Underwood LE, et al. The effect of exercise on plasma somatomedin-C/insulin-like growth factor I concentrations. Metabolism 1987;36:533–7.
209. Soliman AT, Gassan AEHI, Aref MK, et al. Serum insulin-like growth factors I and II concentrations and growth hormone and insulin responses to arginine infusion in children with protein-calorie malnutrition before and after nutritional rehabilitation. Pediatr Res 1986;20:1122–30.
210. Nucci AM, Reyes J, Yaworski JA, et al. Serum growth factors and growth indices pre- and post-pediatric intestinal transplantation. J Pediatr Surg 2003;38:1043–7.
211. Clemmons DR, Underwood LE, Dickerson RN, et al. Use of plasma somatomedin-C/insulin-like growth factor I measurements to monitor the response to nutritional repletion in malnourished patients. Am J Clin Nutr 1985;41:191–8.
212. Unterman TG, Vasquez RM, Slas AJ, et al. Nutrition and somatomedin. XIII. Usefulness of somatomedin-C in nutritional assessment. Am J Med 1985;78:228–34.
213. Kirschner BS, Sutton MM. Somatomedin-C levels in growth-impaired children and adolescents with chronic inflammatory bowel disease. Gastroenterology 1986;91:830–6.
214. Baxter RC, Hawker FH, To C, et al. Thirty-day monitoring of insulin-like growth factors and their binding proteins in intensive care unit patients. Growth Horm IGF Res 1998;8:455–63.
215. Isley WL, Underwood LE, Clemmons DR. Dietary components that regulate serum somatomedin-C concentrations in humans. J Clin Invest 1983;71:175.
216. Prewitt TE, D'Ercole AJ, Switzer BR, Van Wyk JJ. Relationship of serum immunoreactive somatomedin-C to dietary protein and energy in growing rats. J Nutr 1982;112:144.
217. Baxter RC, Bryson JM, Turtle JR. The effect of fasting on liver receptors for prolactin and growth hormone. Metabolism 1981;30:1086–90.
218. Postel-Vinay MC, Cohen-Tanugi E, Charrier J. Growth hormone receptors in rat liver membranes: Effect of fasting and refeeding, and correlation with plasma somatomedin activity. Mol Cell Endocrinol 1982;28:657–69.
219. Maes M, Underwood LE, Ketelslegers JM. Plasma somatomedin-C in fasted and refed rats: Close relationship with changes in liver somatogenic but not lactogenic binding sites. J Endocrinol 1983;97:243–52.
220. Bornfeldt KE, Arnqvist HJ, Enberg B, et al. Regulation of insulin-like growth factor-I and growth hormone receptor gene expression by diabetes and nutritional state in rat tissues. J Endocrinol 1986;122:651–6.
221. Straus DS, Takemoto CD. Effect of fasting on insulin-like growth factor-I and growth hormone receptor mRNA levels and IGF-I gene transcription in rat liver. Mol Endocrinol 1991;4:91–100.
222. Thissen JP, Triest S, Moats-Staats BM, et al. Evidence that pretranslational and translational defects decrease serum IGF-I concentrations during dietary protein energy restriction. Endocrinology 1991;129:429–35.
223. Thissen JP, Ketelslegers JM, Underwood LE. Nutritional regulation of the insulin-like growth factors. Endocr Rev 1994;15:80–101.
224. Lowe WT, Adamo M, Werner H, et al. Regulation by fasting of rat insulin-like growth factor I and its receptor. Effects on gene expression and binding. J Clin Invest 1989;84:619–26.
225. Cahill GF. Hormone fuel interrelationships during fasting. J Clin Invest 1966;45:1751.
226. Pimstone BL, Becker DJ, Weinkove C, et al. Insulin secretion in protein-calorie malnutrition. In: Gardner LI, Amacher P, editors. Endocrine Aspects of Malnutrition: Marasmus, Kwashiorkor and Psychosocial Deprivation. Santa Ynez, CA: The Kroc Foundaton; 1973. p. 289–305.
227. Rao RH. Diabetes in the undernourished: Coincidence or consequence? Endocrinology 1988;9:67–87.
228. Bennish ML, Azad AK, Rahman O, et al. Hypoglycemia during diarrhea in childhood. Prevalence, pathophysiology, and outcome. N Engl J Med 1990;322:1357–63.
229. Goldbloom RB. Failure to thrive. Pediatr Clin North Am 1982;29:151–166.
230. Powell GF, Brasel JA, Blizzard RM. Emotional deprivation and growth retardation simulating idiopathic hypopituitarism. I. Clinical evaluation of the syndrome. N Engl J Med 1967;276:1271–87.
231. Patton RG, Gardner LI. Deprivation dwarfism (psychosocial deprivation): Disordered family environment as a cause of so-called idiopathic hypopituitarism. In: Gardner LI, editor. Endocrine and Genetic Diseases of Childhood and Adolescence. Philadelphia: WB Saunders; 1975. p. 85–9.
232. Talbot NB. Dwarfism in healthy children: Its possible relation to emotional, nutritional and endocrine disturbances. N Engl J Med 1947;236:783–93.
233. Powell GF, Brasel JA, Raiti S, et al. Emotional deprivation and growth retardation simulating idiopathic hypopituitarism: II. Endocrinologic evaluation of the syndrome. N Engl J Med 1967;276:1279–83.
234. Powell GF, Hopwood NJ, Barratt ES. Growth hormone studies before and during catch-up growth in a child with emotional deprivation and short stature. J Clin Endocrinol Metab 1973;37:674–9.
235. Miller JD, Tannenbaum GS, Colle E, et al. Daytime pulsatile growth hormone secretion during childhood and adolescence. J Clin Endocrinol Metab 1982;55:989–93.
236. Frasier SD, Rallisen ML. Growth retardation and emotional deprivation: Relative resistance to treatment with human growth hormone. J Pediatr 1946;80:603.
237. Tanner JM, Whitehouse RH, Hughes PCR, et al. The effects of human growth hormone treatment for 1 to 7 years on growth of 100 children with growth hormone deficiency, low birth weight, inherited smallness, Turner's syndrome and other complaints. Arch Dis Child 1971;46:745.
238. Widdowson EM. Mental contentment and physical growth. Lancet 1951;1:1316–8.
239. Whitten CR, Pettit MG, Fishoff J. Evidence that growth failure from maternal deprivation is secondary to undereating. JAMA 1969;209:1675–82.
240. Krieger I, Mellinger RC. Pituitary function in the deprivation syndrome. J Pediatr 1971;79:216–25.
241. Pugliese MT, Lifshitz F, Grad G, et al. Fear of obesity: A cause of short stature and delayed puberty. N Engl J Med 1983;309:513–8.
242. Pugliese MT, Weyman-Daum M, Moses N, et al. Parental health beliefs as a cause of nonorganic failure to thrive. Pediatrics 1987;80:175–82.
243. Bernal J, Refetoff S. The actions of thyroid hormone. Clin Endocrinol 1977;7:227–49.
244. Silva JE. The thermogenetic effect of thyroid hormone and its clinical implications. Ann Int Med. 2003;139:205–13.
245. Evans RM. The steroid and thyroid hormone receptor superfamily. Science 1988;240:889–95.
246. Fisher DA, Hoath S, Lakshmanan J. The thyroid hormone effects on growth and development may be mediated by growth factors. Endocr Exp 1982;16:259–271.
247. Burstein PJ, Draznin B, Johnson DJ, et al. The effect of hypothyroidism on growth, serum growth hormone, the growth hormone-dependent somatomedin, insulin-like growth factor, and its carrier protein in rats. Endocrinology 1979;104:1107.
248. Coiro U. Effect of hypothyroidism and thyroxine replacement on growth hormone in the rat. Endocrinology 1979;105:641–6.
249. Urist MR, DeLang RJ, Finerman GAM. Bone cell differentiation and growth factors. Science 1983;220:680.
250. Wegnez M, Schachter BS, Baxter JD, et al. Hormone regulation of growth hormone messenger RNA. DNA 1982;1:145–53.
251. Root AW, Rosenfield RL, Bongiovanni AM, et al. The plasma growth hormone response to insulin-induced hypoglycemia in children with retardation of growth. Pediatrics 1967;39:844.
252. Froesch ER. Nonsuppressible insulin-like activity and thyroid hormones: Major pituitary-dependent sulfation factors for chick embryo cartilage. Proc Natl Acad Sci U S A 1976;73:2904–8.

253. Dearden LC, Espinosa T. Comparison of mineralization of the tibial epiphyseal plate in immature rats following treatment with cortisone, propylthiouracil or after fasting. Calcif Tissue Res 1974;15:93–110.
254. Burch WM, Van Wyk JJ. Triiodothyronine stimulates cartilage growth and maturation by different mechanisms. Am J Physiol (Endocr Metab 15) 1987;252:E176–82.
255. Jung RT, Shetty PS, James WPT. The effect of refeeding after semistarvation on catecholamine and thyroid metabolism. Int J Obes 1980;4:95–100.
256. Vagnati L, Finley RJ, Hagg S, et al. Protein conservation during prolonged fast: A function of triiodothyronine levels. Trans Assoc Am Physiol 1978;91:169–79.
257. O'Dea K, Esler M, Leonard P, et al. Noradrenaline turnover during under- and overeating in normal weight subjects. Metabolism 1982;31:896–9.
258. O'Brian JT. Thyroid hormone homeostasis in states of relative caloric deprivation. Metabolism 1980;29:721–9.
259. Wartofsky L, Burman KD. Alterations in thyroid function in patients with systemic illness: The "euthyroid sick syndrome". Endocr Rev 1982;3:164–217.
260. Nicoloff JT, LoPresti JS. Nonthyroidal illnesses. In: DeGroot LJ, editor. Endocrinology, 3rd edition. Philadelphia: WB Saunders; 1995. p. 665–75.
261. DeGroot LJ. Non-thyroidal illness syndrome is a manifestation of hypothalamic-pituitary dysfunction, and in view of current evidence, should be treated with appropriate replacement therapies. Crit Care Clin 2006; 22:57–86.
262. Rastogi GK, Sawhney RC, Panda NC, et al. Thyroid hormone levels in adult protein calorie malnutrition (PCM). Horm Metab Res 1974;6:528–9.
263. Henning SJ. Ontogeny of enzymes in the small intestine. Ann Rev Physiol 1985;47:231–45.
264. Yeh KY, Moog F. Development of the small intestine in the hypophysectomized rat. II. Influence of cortisone, thyroxine, growth hormone, and prolactin. Dev Biol 1975;47:173–84.
265. Moog F, Yeh KY. Pinocytosis persists in the ileum of hypophysectomized rats unless closure is induced by thyroxine or cortisone. Dev Biol 1979;69:159–69.
266. Yeh KY. Corticosterone concentrations in the serum and milk of lactating rats: Parallel changes after induced stress. Endocrinology 1984;115:1364–70.
267. Little JM, Lester R. Ontogenesis of intestinal bile salt absorption in the neonatal rat. Am J Physiol (Gastrointest Liver Physiol) 1983;239:G319–23.
268. Alleyne GAO, Young VH. Adrenocortical function in children with severe protein-calorie malnutrition. Clin Sci 1967;33:189–200.
269. Leonard PJ, MacWilliam KW. The binding of aldosterone in the serum in kwashiorkor. Am J Clin Nutr 1965;16:360.
270. Rao KSJ, Srikantia SG, Gopalan C. Plasma cortisol levels in protein-calorie malnutrition. Arch Dis Child 1968;43:365–7.
271. Lunn PG, Whitehead RG, Baker BA, et al. The effect of cortisone acetate on the course of development of experimental protein-energy malnutrition in rats. Br J Nutr 1976;36:537–50.
272. Eveleth PB, Tanner JM. Worldwide Variation in Human Growth. Cambridge: Cambridge University Press; 1976.
273. Smith SR. The pituitary-gonadal axis in men with protein-calorie malnutrition. J Clin Endocr Metab 1975;41:60–9.
274. Klibanski A. Reproductive function during fasting in men. J Clin Endocr Metab 1981;53:258–63.
275. Warren MP. The effects of exercise on pubertal progression and reproductive function in girls. J Clin Endocr Metab 1980;51:1150.
276. Frisch RE, Gotz-Welbergen AV, McArthur JW, et al. Delayed menarche and amenorrhea of college athletes in relation to age of onset of training. JAMA 1981;246:1559.
277. Frisch RE, McArthur JW. Menstrual cycles: Fatness as a determinant of minimum weight for height necessary for their maintenance or onset. Science 1974;185:949.
278. Shalitin S, Phillip M. Role of obesity and leptin in the puberal process and puberal growth-a review. Int J Obes Relat Metab Disord: J Int Assoc Study Obes 2003;27:869–74.
279. Tweedle D, Walton C, Johnston IDA. The effect of an anabolic steroid on postoperative nitrogen balance. Br J Clin Pract 1972;27:130–2.
280. Watson RN, Bradley MH, Callahan R, et al. A six month evaluation of an anabolic drug, norethandrolone, in underweight persons. Am J Med 1959;26:238–42.
281. Thaysen JH. Anabolic steroids in the treatment of renal failure. In: Gross F, editor. Protein Metabolism. Berlin: Springer-Verlag; 1962. p. 450–78.
282. Wilson JD. Androgen abuse by athletes. Endocr Rev 1988;9:181–99.

21

Gastrointestinal Development: Implications for Infant Feeding

Josef Neu, MD
Martha Douglas-Escobar, MD

The field of gastrointestinal (GI) development has been advancing at a rapid pace in the past 30 years.[1] The level of GI maturity of an individual infant is a major determinant of whether the infant will be able to meet nutritional needs by sole use of the GI tract or if parenteral means will be necessary. The GI tract is not only an organ for digestion and absorption of nutrients; it also performs major endocrine, neural, and immunologic functions. In this chapter, anatomic, functional, and biochemical development will be described and related to means by which enteral nutrition can be used to optimize health and prevent disease. The focus of this chapter will be on neonatal period.

ANATOMIC DEVELOPMENT

The intestine undergoes tremendous growth during fetal life. It elongates 1,000-fold from 5 to 40 weeks. The length doubles in the last 15 weeks of gestation, reaching a mean length at birth of 275 cm. In the small intestine, finger-like projections, the villi, are already formed at 16 weeks of gestation. In the large intestine, villi are also present, but these partially regress at around 29 weeks of gestation. Microvilli begin to cover the apical surface of the small intestinal epithelium so that by adulthood, the intestinal surface provides the largest interface between the outside environment and the internal milieu (approximately 2,000,000 cm^2, which is about the size of a tennis court).

There are numerous cell types in the small intestine. These include the intestinal absorptive epithelium, Paneth cells (involved in secretion of defensins and other peptides implicated in the innate immunity), Goblet cells (involved in the secretion of the mucous lining the intestine), and other cell types involved in the intestinal neuroendocrine and immune systems. After intestinal epithelial cells undergo mitotic division in the crypt, they migrate up the villus, where they undergo differentiation and become actively absorbing cells and then after apoptosis become sloughed into the intestinal lumen. There is only one population of cells that migrate deeper into the crypt and these are the Paneth cells. Specific issues regarding these cell types will be discussed later in this chapter.

DEVELOPMENT OF MECHANICAL FUNCTION

Readiness to feed by mouth is a major developmental milestone for the premature neonate. Mechanical function of the GI tract, the major determinant of this readiness, includes suck–swallow coordination, gastroesophageal sphincter tone, gastric emptying, and intestinal motility. These will be discussed separately even though they function along a continuum in the GI tract to propel food to areas where digestive absorptive functions occur.

Suck–Swallow Coordination

Very premature infants prior to about 32 weeks' gestation have a suck–swallow pattern that differs from that of the more term infant.[2] The very preterm infant is not able to coordinate sucking activities during the swallowing process. Furthermore, preterm infants swallow preferentially at different phases of respiration than those of their full-term counterparts[2] and this results in an inefficient and potentially dangerous pattern that may result in aspiration of gastric contents into the trachea and lungs if these infants are fed by mouth. Thus, most of the very low birth weight (VLBW) infants are tube fed. Feeding directly into the stomach and/or intestine by gastric and transpyloric feeding, respectively, bypasses the immature suck–swallow coordination in these infants, but remains subject to other immaturities such as gastroesophageal reflux (GER), poor gastric emptying, and immature small intestinal motility. When transitioning to nipple feeding with a bottle, use of nipples that offer relatively high resistance to flow may be helpful in preventing a rate of intake higher than the infant's immature suck–swallow respiration pattern can manage.

Gastroesophageal Junction and Gastroesophageal Reflux

Ganglia are present in the esophagus at 5 weeks' gestation and complete their migration to the rectum by 24 weeks' gestation. Despite this, the esophagus of the premature infant demonstrates slower propagation velocities and contraction duration that is more prolonged than in the older child. At about 28 weeks' gestation, the lower esophageal sphincter resting pressure is only 4 mm Hg, but it increases to adult values (18 mm Hg) by term.[3] Dramatic increases in GER have been seen after diaper changes, an intervention that results in increased intra-abdominal pressure.[4] Although GER occurs commonly in premature infants, as do chronic lung disease, apnea, and bradycardia, it remains unclear whether a cause–effect relationship exists between these problems, and is a highly debated issue. The prevalence of actual gastroesophageal reflux disease is still also a debatable issue. At this juncture, most of the techniques to determine reflux have relied on acid measurement techniques, but it is known that reflux does not need to be acid to cause reflex apnea. Since apnea is a major problem encountered in the neonatal intensive care unit (NICU), if a cause–effect relationship exists and is present in a significant number of infants, pharmacologic (antireflux medications) or feeding technique–related (thickening, positioning, type of nipple) therapies could have a major impact on treatment and/or prevention of apnea and bradycardia. Studies employing newer techniques of measuring reflux based on nonacid measurements, for example, impedance, may yield important new information in this area. Although the short-term problems associated with GER remain an area of major interest, the recent suggestion that GER in low birth-weight infants may play a role in the development of adenocarcinoma of the esophagus when these children reach late adulthood is intriguing.[5]

Gastric Emptying

Gastric emptying is slower in premature than in term infants[6,7] and leads to a greater residual volume of gastric contents; thus, it is closely tied to the problem of GER. Infants between 32 and 39 weeks' gestation provided with progressive increments of caloric density decreased the rate of gastric emptying.[8] Changes in osmolality from 279 to 448 mOsm/kg do not significantly alter the rates of gastric emptying of isocaloric formulas.[8] These are potentially intriguing findings in that the fetus normally swallows significant amounts of low-caloric-density amniotic fluid (up to about 450 mL/d) during the last trimester of pregnancy,[9] but has difficulty tolerating higher caloric density formula and even breast milk postnatally when born prematurely. In adults, the rate of gastric emptying is controlled by feedback from the small and large intestine. Stimulation of duodenal receptors by acid, fat, carbohydrates, tryptophan, or increasing osmolality decreases rates of gastric emptying.[8] Very little information on the ability of duodenal feedback to control the rate of gastric emptying in the VLBW infants between 25 and 32 weeks' gestation is available. However, providing a formulation that is low in some of the agents (high carbohydrate, lipid, etc) that slow gastric emptying may be one technique to improve tolerance in terms of gastric emptying and also not to overwhelm the more distal intestinal tract motility and digestive absorptive functions. Several studies suggest that therapeutic agents that increase gastric emptying rates in children and adults are also effective in premature infants. Randomized trials of erythromycin are mixed but some suggest improvement in feeding tolerance without significant complications.[10–12] Metoclopramide also increases gastric emptying rate in preterm and term infants[13] but it is somewhat difficult to monitor side effects (extrapyramidal movement disorders or tardive dyskinesias) of this agent in this age group. Cisapride, in one small trial, did not increase gastric emptying rates in preterm infants.[14] However the efficacy and safety of this agent would need to be studied in larger randomized trials. Cisapride is currently not available in the US market because of concerns related to cardiac arrhythmias.[15] Nasojejunal (transpyloric) feeding bypasses the immature gastric emptying and is often employed to decrease the likelihood of reflux-related aspiration and apnea, but there are little data to support the efficacy of this technique in decreasing morbidity.

Intestinal Motility

The small bowel motility patterns are poorly developed before 28 weeks' gestation. Gastroanal transit ranges from 8 to 96 hours in premature infants as compared with 4 to 12 hours in adults. Berseth et al[16] in studies of small intestine showed disorganized motility patterns between 27 and 30 weeks' gestation, which progress to a more mature pattern so that migrating myoelectric complexes are present at 33 to 34 weeks' gestation. In preterm infants, the motilin receptor is not present until 32 weeks' gestation, and the cyclic release of motilin is not present. Despite this, several of the studies of the motilin agonist erythromycin[11,12] have demonstrated improved feeding tolerance. Whether erythromycin might act through mechanisms not related to motilin agonists remains speculative. Minimal enteral feedings also increase motility and this will be discussed later in this chapter.

DEVELOPMENT OF DIGESTIVE–ABSORPTIVE FUNCTION

Protein Digestion

Our knowledge of digestive–absorptive processes has increased significantly in the past three decades. Hydrolysis of protein begins in the acid environment of the stomach and proceeds distally in the intestine through the action of various proteases. Gastric acid secretion is limited in VLBW infants. In the first 24 to 48 hours after birth, intragastric pH remains at about 5.5 to 7 (whereas the gastric pH in normal children and adults is 2 to 3) and is relatively resistant to pentagastrin. However, both basal and pentagastrin-stimulated acid secretion doubles from the first to fourth week of postnatal life in preterm infants.[17] Gastric acid serves as a barrier to microorganisms. This is an important consideration when using H2 blockers because decrease in gastric acid production may lead to a higher load of bacteria in the more distal regions of the intestine.[18] Several studies have now supported that critically ill patients treated with H2 blockers have a higher incidence of nosocomial sepsis[19] and one recent study suggests a greater incidence of necrotizing enterocolitis (NEC) with the use of H2 blockers.[20]

The pancreatic protease digestive cascade is catalyzed by food-stimulated secretion of enterokinase from the upper small intestinal epithelium. Enterokinase catalyzes the activation of trypsinogen to trypsin, which in turn activates several other inactive zymogens into proteases. Active luminal enterokinase is detectable at 24 weeks' gestation but its activity level is relatively low and reaches only 25% adult activity at term.[21] This may limit protein digestion and may be responsible for an increased capability of larger antigens and/or microorganisms to pass into the intestine without breakdown by luminal enzymes. After luminal digestion, small peptides and amino acids are absorbed and transported to the villus capillaries. The absorptive proteases are usually present and fully active before 24 weeks' gestation and should not be limiting.[22] This would suggest that hydrolyzed protein would be better tolerated. Indeed, one study demonstrated more rapid establishment of full enteral feeding with a hydrolyzed protein formula compared to a nonhydrolyzed protein formula.[23] Nevertheless, these studies did not utilize a human milk–fed control group. In other studies, human milk was much better tolerated than formulas.[24] Before initiating use of a hydrolyzed formula for the premature it is important to remember that many hydrolyzed protein formulas are not nutritionally formulated for the premature infant.

Lipid Digestion and Absorption

Lipid makes up about 50% of the nonprotein energy content of human milk and formulas. However, both term and preterm infants have pancreatic insufficiency when compared to older children and adults and this may result in malabsorption of certain types of lipids.

The digestion of lipid can be split into phases.[25] The luminal phase of lipid digestion involves lipase deesterification of triglycerides to 3-monoglycerides and free fatty acids, and bile acid–mediated micellar solubilization. Several lipases participate in the fat digestion, including the lipase found in human milk (bile salt–stimulated lipase), lingual, gastric, pancreatic, and epithelial lipases. Human milk has a lipase (absent in cow's milk and formulas) that becomes active in the small intestine lumen only in the presence of bile acids.[25] Lingual lipase is secreted by glands at the base of the tongue and is involved in gastric lipid hydrolysis. Other lipases involved in lipid hydrolysis are produced in the stomach; others are secreted from the pancreas. Bile acids synthesized in the liver are critical to efficient fat digestion and absorption. VLBW infants have a lower duodenal concentration of bile acids due to lower synthesis and ileal reabsorption of bile.[26,27] Therefore a lower micellar solubilization leads to lower lipid absorption. Long-chain fatty acids but not medium-chain fatty acids depend on bile acids for solubilization and thus are the most susceptible to inefficient absorption. Despite this limitation, meta-analysis of studies comparing medium-chain triglycerides (MCTs) to long-chain triglycerides feeding do not show clear benefits in terms of weight gain.[28]

The next phases, lipid absorption and assimilation, include the permeation of fatty acids and 2-monoglycerides from the lumen into the cell, intracellular reesterification, chylomicron formation, and transport to the chylomicrons from the cell into the circulation. After luminal digestion, fatty acids and monoglycerides approximate the absorptive surface, and enter the intracellular milieu by processes that are not yet well understood. After entry into the cell, MCTs undergo a relatively simple process of assimilation where they do not undergo reesterification and chylomicron formation, as do the long-chain lipids. MCTs are taken directly into the portal venous system whereas chylomicrons formed from long-chain fats enter the lymphatics. Table 1 summarizes some[29] of these differences. In conditions where the lymphatics are obstructed (eg, chylous ascites), MCT-predominant formula is thus recommended (rather than long-chain triglyceride-predominant formula).

Lipid requirements are limited[29] to the 18-carbon essential fatty acids (linoleic or linolenic acid). However, there is considerable interest and debate about the capability of neonates, especially prematures, to convert the dietary essential fatty acids (linoleic and linolenic) into longer chain fatty acids (with 20 or more carbons) using desaturase and elongase enzymatic pathways. The end

Table 1 Comparison of Short-, Medium-, and Long-Chain Fatty Acid Digestion and Assimilation

Overview of Fatty Acid Uptake
• Short- and medium-chain fatty acids – Enter portal blood directly from enterocytes – Bound to albumin in blood as Albumin–Free Fatty Acids (FFA) complex – Oxidized in liver or elongated and used for triglyceride formation • Long-chain fatty acids – Form chylomicrons in intestinal cell – Drain into the lymphatics via the lacteal – Enter bloodstream at the thoracic duct upstream from liver – Slow entry into the blood

result is the formation of the long-chain polyunsaturated fatty acids (LCPUFAs),[30] which are critical in the formation of eicosanoids and structural components of the central nervous system. Preformed LCPUFAs are found in relatively high concentrations in human milk but are not found in commercial intravenous lipid preparations or, until recently, most neonatal formulas. A meta-analysis and systematic review of data from premature and term infants indicate advantages of docosahexaenoic acid (DHA, an omega-3-LCPUFA)–supplemented formulas over unsupplemented formulas in both behavioral- and electrophysiological-based measurements of visual acuity.[31,32] Although there is a suggestion from recent research that there may be some benefit to VLBW infants, whether addition of these to formulas results in improvement in cognitive neurodevelopment remains the subject of current investigation.[30] Nevertheless, while on minimal enteral feeding and/or parenteral nutrition (PN), premature infants receive very little, if any, preformed omega-3-LCPUFAs, a deficiency of which is likely to have detrimental consequences in both nervous tissue formation and inflammatory responses.

Most of the lipids from the formulas or intravenous lipids are derived from vegetable oil (rich in omega-6- but not omega-3-LCPUFAs). Therefore, the majority of essential fatty acids provided to neonates are derived from the omega-6 family (linoleic acid). Numerous studies have demonstrated that products derived from the omega-6 fatty acids (2-series prostaglandins) have a greater inflammatory effect than those derived from the omega-3 fatty acids (3-series prostaglandins).[33] Although there is a considerable amount of information in adults about the omega-3 fatty acids ameliorating inflammation, that is, rheumatoid arthritis, coronary artery disease, and other conditions, very little information exists in human neonates. One study in a rat model of NEC suggests a decrease in NEC with omega-3 fatty acid supplementation.[34] Whether providing more omega-3 lipids would decrease NEC, chronic lung disease, or neurological problems related to inflammation in human infants remain intriguing possibilities that require additional investigation.

CARBOHYDRATE DIGESTION AND ABSORPTION

Carbohydrates ingested by neonates are either natural lactose (the primary carbohydrate in most human and mammalian milks) or in the form of glucose polymers, sucrose, or hydrolyzed starches. Pancreatic amylase, which cleaves internal one to four glucose bonds to maltose, maltotriose, limit dextrin, and glucose, is a major enzyme that hydrolyzes starches. Pancreatic secretion is poorly developed in the first several months of life; therefore, at least this mode of starch hydrolysis could serve as a limiting factor and leave a lot of undigested starch in the intestine. Experimental studies suggest that glucose polymers (18 to 29 glucose units) can be hydrolyzed by salivary amylases, but this digestion still falls substantially short of that accomplished by usual concentrations of pancreatic amylase.[35] Many infant formulas including those used for preterm infants contain corn syrup solids or tapioca, which are partially hydrolyzed starches. The more extensively the starch is hydrolyzed, the less reliance is placed on an immature digestive capability, but the greater the osmolality (and risk of hyperosmolar diarrhea and/or intestinal inflammation). Maturation of mechanisms for carbohydrate absorption occurs in a defined sequence during human fetal development.[22,29,36,37] The intestinal epithelial absorptive enzymes, lactase, sucrase, maltase, isomaltase, and glucoamylase are at mature levels in the term newborn.[21] In the preterm infant, sucrase, maltase, and isomaltase are usually near fully active, but lactase activity, which increases markedly from 24 to 40 weeks, may be low depending upon gestational age.[21] Despite these developmental patterns, clinical lactose intolerance is uncommon. Postnatal adaptive responses to ingested carbohydrates lead to competent carbohydrate utilization.[38] Furthermore, there is a colonic salvage of nonabsorbed carbohydrates The colonic microbiota ferment the nonabsorbed carbohydrates to hydrogen gas and short-chain fatty acids (SCFAs, which are easily absorbed).[36]

Feeding and composition of the feeding has been shown to affect the development of intestinal lactase activity.[38] Preterm infants who received early enteral feedings had greater lactase activity at 10 and 28 days of age (by 100 and 60%, respectively) than a control group that had feedings initiated later (standard time of initiation of feedings). At 10 days of age lactase activity was also greater in human milk–versus formula-fed infants. The time required achieving full enteral feedings, the number of abnormal abdominal X-ray examinations, and the total numbers of abdominal X-ray examinations were inversely related to lactase activity. It was concluded that early feeding increases intestinal lactase activity in preterm infants. Lactase activity is a marker of intestinal maturity and may influence clinical outcomes.

The presence of a high lactose concentration in human milk thus should not be a contraindication for its use in the VLBW infant. Feedings for VLBW infants are rarely initiated at levels intended to meet the infants' entire nutritional requirements and are usually advanced slowly. The rationale for using a lactose-free formula instead of human milk or even a commercial lactose-containing formula is weak and may theoretically be harmful. Slow initiation of enteral feedings is unlikely to exceed the lactose hydrolytic and salvage capability of the small and large intestine. This is especially unlikely when the quantity fed is less than 50% of the caloric requirement provided via the GI tract (unless the infant's bowel has been radically shortened by surgery). Human milk also contains several lactose-derived oligosaccharides and other glycoconjugates that may play an important immunologic role.

Studies examining the crypt to villus gradient of intestinal carbohydrase activities demonstrate that the majority of lactase activity is found at the mid-to-upper villus, whereas sucrase, maltase, and glucoamylase are concentrated at the midvillus region.[39,40] This is likely to be pertinent to intestinal injury and villus damage. Lactase is usually the first enzyme to be lost and the last to be fully regenerated after injury. Congenital lactase deficiency is extremely rare. A large proportion of the world's population develops lactose intolerance in the first few years of life because of a decline in lactase activity, but further discussion of this phenomenon and its clinical implications is beyond the scope of this chapter.

INNATE DEFENSE AND BARRIER FUNCTION DEVELOPMENT

The GI tract presents the largest surface area of the body to which antigens and microbes are exposed. The intestine must therefore have intricate mechanisms to allow entry of nutrients and other beneficial molecules while preventing potentially harmful microbes and other agents from gaining entry into the inner milieu. Shortly after birth, the establishment of an intestinal bacterial community is very important for maintenance of normal homeostasis. The VLBW infant in the NICU is presented with special challenges. Several factors lead to a hostile GI environment that predisposes the infant to disease. These include the introduction of feeding tubes into the stomach or more distal intestine, the routine use of broad-spectrum antibiotics that select for resistant pathogens that thrive in the unusual microbial environment of the NICU, intrinsic immaturities of the infant GI tract, and the lack of adequate enteral nutrition. Thus, combining total parenteral nutrition (TPN), the lack of enteral nutrition, and the introduction of a hostile microbiota into an immature GI tract offers a fertile environment for initiation of various forms of morbidity related to intestine-derived systemic inflammation and perhaps even programming of pathologic immune responses that leads to lifelong consequences.

Intestinal defenses may be broadly divided into innate and adaptive categories. The importance of the innate system is that it constitutes the first line of host defense. Each of the components of the innate system acts in concert to maintain mucosal integrity in the intestine. Several of these components are presented here.

Breast Milk

Breast milk is an integral component of innate defense for the neonate because numerous components of breast milk are known to be protective to the infant. These include immunoglobulins, lactoferrin, lysozyme, glycoconjugates, oligosaccharides, and various types of white blood cells. Antibodies in human milk reflect the antigenic repertoire of the mother's intestine and respiratory tract. Colonization of the lactating mother's intestine with specific strains of *Escherichia coli* results in the appearance of corresponding antibodies in the mother's milk.[41] This effect is achieved by seeding-primed plasma cells to the breast tissue. Thus the repertoire of antibacterial, antiviral, antifungal, and antifood antibodies in human milk is considerable. It varies from mother to mother and is determined by the antigens ingested and inhaled by her infant.[42] Thus, if the same bacteria colonize the mother and infant, and if there is close contact, the mother can produce specific antibodies that can protect the infant through her milk. This comprises the so-called enteromammary system.[43] Furthermore, mother's milk is colonized by bacteria that may play a positive role and act as a natural "probiotic."[44] Oligosaccharides in mother's milk may act as nutrients for beneficial commensal bacteria (a "prebiotic" role) and fermentation of these oligosaccharides and lactose in mother's milk may lead to the production of SCFAs that play a "postbiotic" role, especially butyrate, which can be effective as a major fuel for colonocytes, an antiapoptotic, proproliferative agent, that may also aid in the strengthening of intercellular tight junctions,[45] and also stimulate the synthesis of glucagon-like-peptide 2, a hormone that is highly trophic for the intestine.[46] Human milk contains high levels of interleukin 10 (IL-10) and transforming growth factor beta, which are anti-inflammatory and serve to modulate otherwise uncontrolled propagation of intestinal inflammation.[47]

Gastric Acid and Pancreaticobiliary Secretions

Gastric acid and pancreaticobiliary secretions decrease the load of viable microorganisms as well as intact dietary protein antigens that reach the small intestine.[48] Pancreatic insufficiency can last through the first year of life.[49] Lack of stimulation of gastric acid and pancreaticobiliary secretions can adversely affect the intestine by allowing a greater bacterial and/or antigenic load to pass to the distal intestine. Proteolysis will destroy the structure of antigens, thereby destroying the epitopes for immunologic recognition.[50] Studies by Walker et al[51] demonstrated an increase in bovine serum albumin in the intestine of rats given bicarbonate at the same time they were fed with bovine serum albumin. This is important because many VLBW infants are not provided nutrients by the enteral route for the first several days of life, thereby having minimal intestinal protease and acid stimulation, with resultant high gastric pH. These same infants are often given H2-blocking agents routinely often for poorly defined reasons in order to decrease gastric acid secretion. The breakdown of intact protein molecules, bacteria, and other microbes may therefore be less. The detrimental effect of this practice is evidenced by the greater incidence of hospital-acquired sepsis and even NEC seen in infants who receive H2-blocking agents.[20,52] Studies in newborn rats have also demonstrated that use of H2 blockers leads to greater bacterial translocation.[18]

SURFACE EPITHELIUM

Intestinal Absorptive Epithelium

The absorptive lining epithelium of the primitive intestine is initially stratified but becomes a single layer of columnar cells at the end of the first trimester. The intestinal epithelial enterocyte derives from the same undifferentiated stem cell that gives rise to columnar absorptive epithelium, mucus-producing goblet cells, and Paneth and M cells in the intestine.[53] The function of these cells beyond nutrient absorption is well recognized and some of their major roles include bacterial mucosal cross-talk and innate barrier function.

Goblet Cells

These are specialized mucus-secretory cells found throughout the intestine. Goblet cells mature from the base of the crypt (proliferative zone) and migrate along the crypt–villus axis. After 5 to 7 days they reach the tip of the villi and are exfoliated (by a particular programmed cell death called "anoikis"). They secrete mucus/mucin, which is very important in the nonspecific protection of the gut lining. Intestinal mucus is a complex gel that covers the surface of the villous epithelium and contributes significantly to cytoprotection at the same time that it offers many ecological advantages for the microbiota. It is composed primarily of water and electrolytes but also contains mucins, glycoproteins, immunoglobulins, glycolipids, and albumin.[54] Bioactive factors such as lactoferrin, lysozyme, and glycolipids from breast milk may also be contained within the surface mucus gel.[55] Mucus is secreted into the lumen of the intestine from storage vacuoles in goblet cells that are interspersed among enterocytes along the villus–crypt axis. Mucous gels containing foreign dietary antigens and pathogenic bacteria are sufficiently stable to keep their contents trapped. The intestine is capable of responding to a threatening insult by the rapid outpouring of mucin and at the same time, resident microbiota can induce an increase in the production of mucins. The mechanism of this response is not well understood. Mucins may be classified according to their structure as gel forming, soluble, and membrane bound. Mucins develop binding sites for lectins, selectins, adhesion molecules, growth factors, cytokines, and chemokines, suggesting that they are implicated in cellular signaling. Mucins lower the diffusion of large molecules (which limit the antigenic load exposure) but allow the passage of small nutrient molecules.

Marked changes in their composition occur during development. Mucin from small intestine of newborn rats contains more protein than does the adult rat intestine.[56] Carbohydrate composition also changes; the newborn has less fucose and *N*-acetyl-cysteine than does the mucin from adults. Levels of mucin in the small intestine decrease in experimental protein-calorie undernutrition, which could reduce the GI protection during the perinatal period.[57] Lower amounts of mucin caused by malnutrition could affect the normal protective function of mucin, particularly in the perinatal period. Certain nutrients such as threonine have a major effect on mucin production[58] and need to be considered in the nutrition of critically ill individuals.

Paneth Cells

Paneth cells represent one of the four major epithelial cell lineages in the small intestine and are the only lineages that migrate downward into the crypt base after originating in the crypt stem cell region. The location of Paneth cells adjacent to crypt stem cells house suggests that they play a critical role in defending epithelial cell renewal. In response to pathogen attack, the Paneth cells secrete a wide spectrum of antimicrobial peptides (AMPs) against gram-negative and gram-positive bacteria, fungi, protozoa, and viruses. The AMPs are able to kill the pathogens by different mechanisms. They are able to attach to and insert into microbial membrane bilayers to form pores, reduce the synthesis of cell wall and nucleic acid, and inhibit enzymatic activity. Some of the major enteric pathogens have developed resistances to AMPs as a way to evade innate mucosal defenses.

One of the main group of AMPs secreted by Paneth cells are alpha-defensins, also known as cryptdins.[59] These peptides have hydrophobic and positively charged domains that can interact with phospholipids in cell membranes. This structure allows defensins to form pores that disrupt bacterial membrane function, leading to cell killing. Paneth cells are stimulated to secrete defensins when exposed to bacteria (both gram-positive and gram-negative types) or other bacterial products such bacterial products as lipopolysaccharide (LPS). Alteration of AMPs released from the Paneth cell is detrimental to host defense against *E. coli* infection in the neonatal small intestine. In addition to defensins, Paneth cells secrete lysozyme and phospholipase A2, both of which have clear antimicrobial activity. This battery of secretory molecules gives Paneth cells a potent arsenal against a broad spectrum of agents, including bacteria, fungi, and even some enveloped viruses.

M Cells

M cells in the intestine do not have well-developed microvilli and allow macromolecular transport, whereas the absorptive enterocyte has better developed microvilli. M cells occur only in the follicle-associated epithelia that overlie organized mucosa-associated lymphoid tissues.[60] They are specialized for delivering foreign antigens and microorganisms to organized lymphoid tissues within the mucosa of the small and large intestines. They are thought to play a major role in specific immunity to luminal antigens. Their relationship to disease in the human neonate remains to be established.

Interepithelial Junctions

Special mechanisms are required to allow passage of certain substances between intestinal epithelial cells and prevention of passage by other substance. Special junctions and interdigitations join the intestinal epithelial cells as seen in Figure 1A and B. The tight junction (zonula occludens) is the most apical component of the junctional complex and serves as the permeability barrier between the external and internal milieus of the body. The tight junction completely encircles the apical end of absorptive cells as a belt-like band. Several transmembrane proteins and proteins on the cytosolic leaflet are a part of the tight junction. These include the claudins and occludin protein families. Interactions of some of these proteins with the actin cytoskeleton are a major determinant of tight junction structure and play a role in the regulation of tight junction assembly.[61] Just below the tight junction, the adhesion junction (zonula adherens) is connected to actin filaments in the cytoplasm and anchors each cell to adjacent cells. Below this, the desmosome (macula adherens) functions in a similar manner to the zonula adherens. The relationship between density of zonula occludens strands and epithelial resistance has been demonstrated in cell culture studies.[62] These junctions allow for physiologic passage of fluids, electrolytes, and small macromolecules up to 11 amino acids long,[63] but larger proteins may not pass this route under physiologic conditions. However, pathologic insults may alter these junctions so that they allow abnormal passage of particles. Additionally, these intercellular junctions are exquisitely sensitive to modulation by small molecules. SCFAs produced by bacterial fermentation such as butyrate have been shown to enhance restoration of mucosal barrier function after injury.[64] Administration of glutamine, an amino acid known to be conditionally essential during critical illness, can also prevent the disruption of tight junctions and subsequent increased paracellular permeability induced by a variety of insults.[65,66] Our ability to manipulate these junctions may be key for prevention of several diseases that are autoimmune in nature and may at least partially relate to "a leaky gut" in its pathogenesis.[67] Figure 2 illustrates some of these diseases.

Epithelial Turnover and Restitution

It is unclear whether the infant can respond to injury to the same extent as the adult. In nonhuman mammals, the intestinal epithelial turnover in the infant is much slower (4 to 5 days) in the infant than in the adult (2 days).[69] If the turnover in human neonates is longer than the adult as in other mammals, this may be significant in that regeneration of injured mucosa in the infant will be much slower than the adult. In addition, environmental factors may contribute to poor restitution in intestinal epithelial cells after injury. In an animal model of NEC, it was determined that intestinal restitution was significantly impaired compared to control animals.[70] The mechanism of this effect was evaluated in vitro with rat crypt cells (IEC-6), which were shown to undergo significant inhibition of restitution after exposure to LPS.[70] Glutamine has been demonstrated to prevent cytokine-mediated apoptosis in human colonic cells.[71] Another amino acid, arginine, also induced intestinal epithelial migration, but through the mammalian target of rapamycin (mTOR) pathway.[72] The role of these amino acids in counteracting intestinal stresses and insults deserve further investigation.

THE INTESTINAL ECOSYSTEM AND MICROBIOTA

It is clear that there is a close interplay between the major cell types lining the intestine, nutrients, and the microbiota, which are all constituents of the intestinal ecosystem. Reduction of normal commensal bacteria in the context of infection or after antibiotic treatment may interfere with nutrient availability and impair beneficial stimulation of the GI immune response. Similarly, a lack of enteral nutrients for both the host and the microbiota may also result in detrimental consequences.

We are beginning to appreciate the profound changes that occur in the intestinal ecosystem when young mammals are weaned form their mother's milk. An example of such a change that normally occurs is in the angiogenins, potent AMPs released from the Paneth cells of the crypt.[73] In mice raised in a conventional environment, angiogenin mRNA expression is markedly

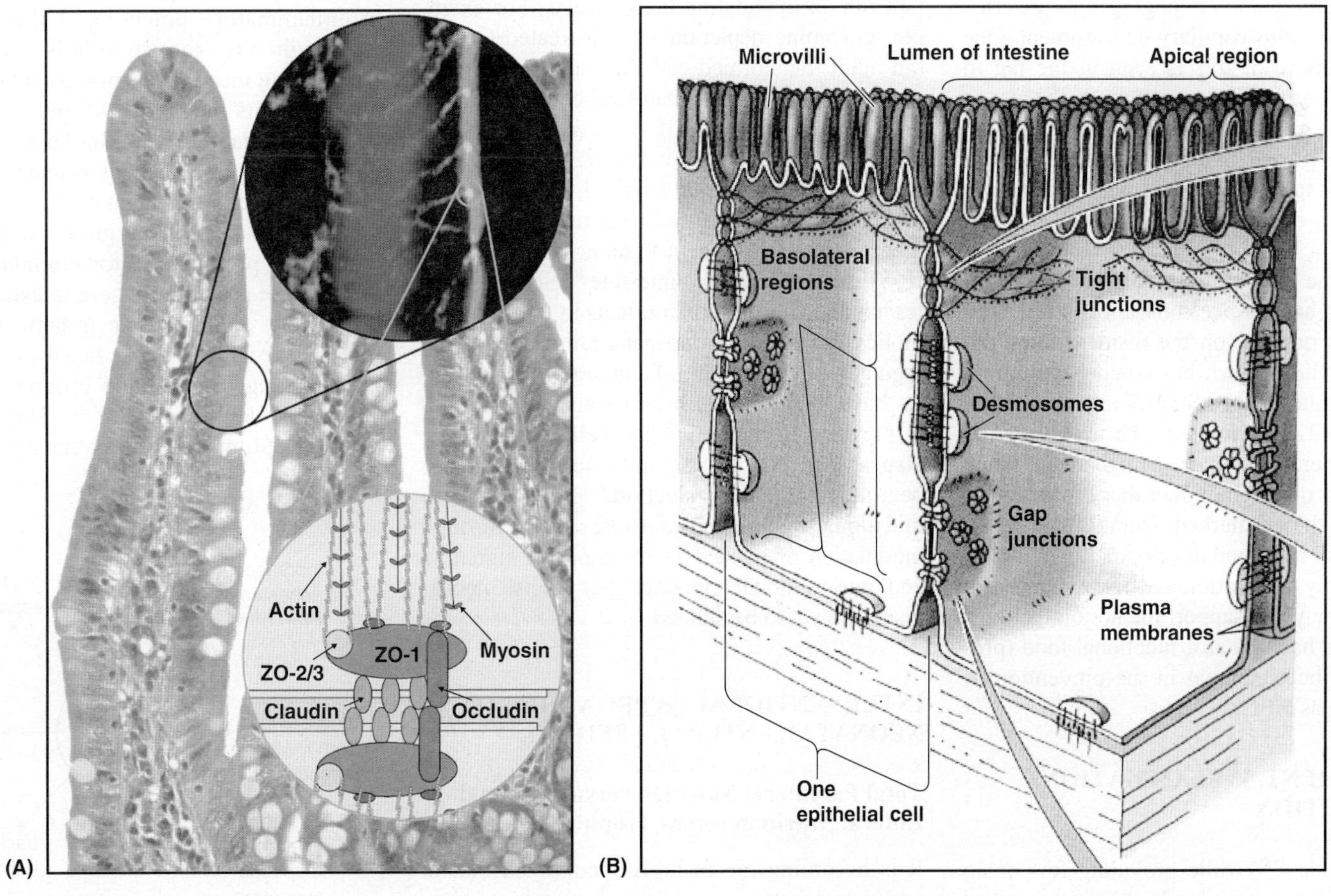

Figure 1 **(A)** Intestinal villi with immunofluorescence of tight junction proteins. (With permission from reference 68.) **(B)** Relation of tight junctions to the other junctional complexes.

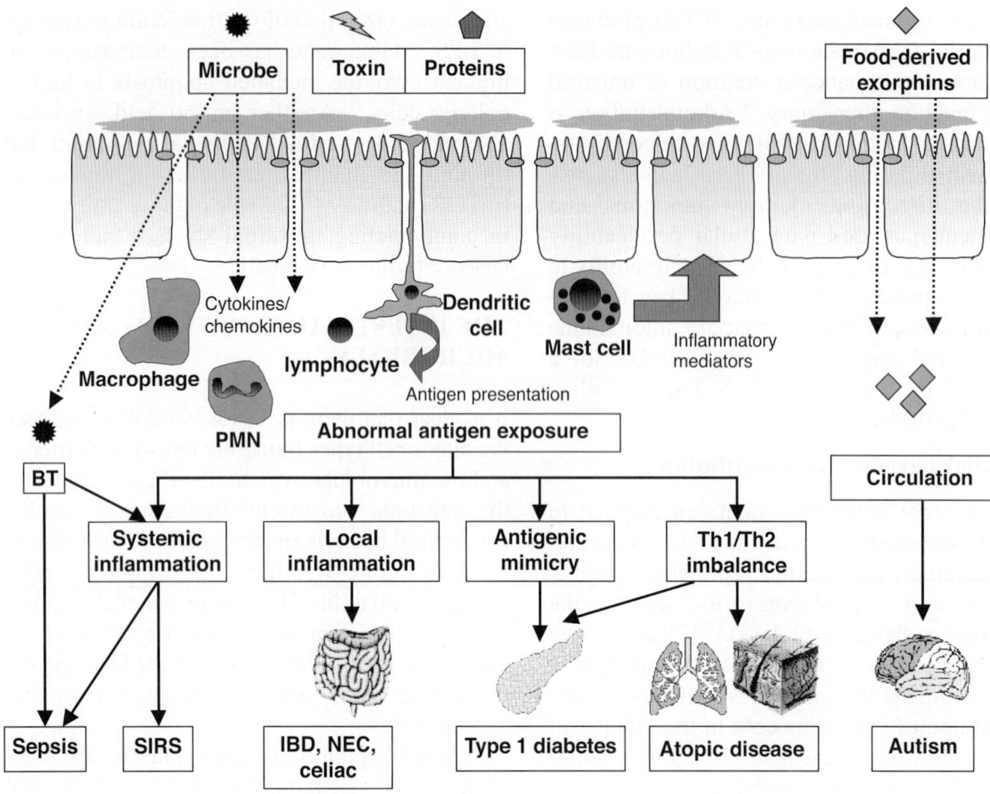

Figure 2 Problems associated with a "leaky gut." (Reprinted with permission from reference 67.)

increased at the time of weaning from mother's milk to an adult diet. This change occurs to a much lesser degree in germ-free mice.[74] It is also thought that commensal bacteria, through "cross-talk," and the production of angiogenins are critical for normal villus capillary development. One dramatic example of this is seen in the lag in development of the villus capillaries in the mouse small intestine grown in a germ-free environment versus normal growth in an environment containing normal mixed flora or even only one species of commensal bacterium (*Bacteroides thetaiotaomicron*).[75]

Most of the premature infants in NICUs are treated with broad-spectrum antibiotics. The effect of this practice on the resident intestinal microbiota is not known but could have potentially detrimental effects. Studies in rodents have shown marked alterations in the ability of the intestine to tolerate otherwise benign insults when the intestine is depleted of microbes[76,77] and other studies have shown marked alterations in genes responsible for intestinal development after treatment with only one antibiotic.[78] Several studies in the past few years support the notion that providing certain bacteria as a functional food (probiotics) may be beneficial in the prevention of diseases such as NEC.

DEVELOPMENT, INFLAMMATION, AND NUTRITION

The reliance on PN while providing few or no enteral nutrients may be highly detrimental because it promotes intestinal inflammation, atrophy, and sepsis, as seen in Figure 3. The role of enteral nutrients in the prevention of the intestine-derived inflammatory response syndrome is becoming increasingly recognized.[79] Certain individual nutrients may play an important role in modulating these effects. For example, glutamine depletion in LPS-treated Caco-2 (an adult transformed cell line) and, even more dramatically, in H4 (human fetal cells), results in marked upregulation of IL-8 production.[80] Similarly, in infant rats fed a commercial diet by gastrostomy and stimulated with LPS, glutamine decreases chemokine-induced neutrophil chemoattractant (the rodent counterpart of human IL-8) production in the intestine.[81] Several studies have suggested similar effects in vitro for probiotics, but studies in neonatal animals showing regulation of intestinal inflammation by probiotics have only recently been published.[82] Studies in human intestinal epithelial cell cultures have also shown that human milk suppresses IL-1 beta-induced IL-8 production.[83] Many of these nutritional agents appear to be acting through modulation of nuclear factor kappa B signaling and transcriptional regulation, but precise mechanisms are yet to be defined.

INTERVENTIONAL APPROACHES TO NEONATAL ENTERAL FEEDING

Total Parenteral Nutrition versus Minimal Enteral Nutrition versus Trophic Feeding

It is becoming increasingly recognized that in addition to immaturity of the neonatal intestine, a lack of enteral nutrients when receiving TPN contributes to mucosal breakdown, bacterial translocation, and an increased propensity to systemic inflammation[79] (see Figure 3). The preterm, especially the VLBW preterm, infant frequently is also highly stressed because of respiratory insufficiency, thermoregulation, and other challenges. Protein requirements are frequently not met in these infants. The trend in the past decade has been to provide greater amino acids by the parenteral route[84] in the acute phase of illness in the first weeks after birth and then to transition to human milk or formula by the enteral route. Although a step in the right direction for improved nutrition, this is likely to be suboptimal: If these infants receive any enteral nutrition at all in the first weeks of life, it is usually in the form of "minimal enteral nutrition." Despite often being termed "trophic nutrition" it is unlikely that minimal enteral (roughly defined as an amount of nutrition that does not meet the nutritional requirements for growth but confers some benefit, and is usually less than 20% of the total nutritional requirements provided for at least 5 days) along with PN is adequate to provide a significant trophic effect on the intestine or whether it actually enhances barrier function.[85] However, it is clear that the use of TPN is significantly associated with hospital-acquired sepsis,[86] which is increasingly thought to have its origin in translocation of intestinal bacteria[87] and intestinal inflammation. Studies in animals support that provision of enteral nutrients can reverse the effects of PN-associated translocation of intestinal bacteria as well as the exquisite proinflammatory potential of the intestines.[88] Although the recent trends toward early increases in intravenous protein intake may provide benefits in terms of protein synthesis, decreased catabolism, and perhaps even somatic growth, there are questions whether this practice provides benefits for maintenance of the GI barrier function and optimal growth of the GI tract, which is a prerequisite for modulation of several disease processes where intestine-mediated breakdown and systemic inflammation play a role. These include NEC, hepatic inflammation, chronic lung disease, and progression of periventricular leukomalacia.[89–91] There is a great need for optimization of an enteral formulation

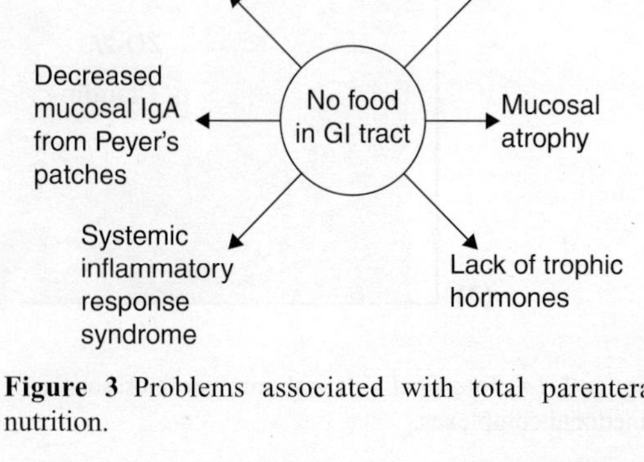

Figure 3 Problems associated with total parenteral nutrition.

that can be safely used in critically ill infants as an adjunct to minimal enteral nutrition shortly after birth that will decrease the need for PN.

Minimal Enteral Nutrition

Considerable emphasis has been placed on nutrition of the low-birth-weight infant after the period of critical illness. Until recently there were very few systematic studies on how to best nourish the infant during the period of critical illness while on mechanical ventilation and when the infant is likely to be the most catabolic in the first 2 to 3 weeks of life. This is a period of extremely high vulnerability and time of high nutrient requirement. A lack of essential nutrients during this time may result in significant short-term morbidity as well as life-long consequences.

When and how quickly should we advance enteral feedings? Because of individual characteristics of each patient, one feeding protocol or guideline cannot be used for all infants. From the available studies, minimal enteral feedings should be instituted within the first days of life. There is no clear evidence that the concomitant use of umbilical catheters, continuous positive airway pressure (CPAP), mechanical ventilation, indomethacin, or the presence of apneic and bradycardic episodes preclude the use of minimal enteral nutrition because of an increased risk of NEC.

When we decide on feeding strategies for premature infants, it is important to remember that infants given early minimal enteral nutrition have faster maturation of motor patterns and release of GI hormones than infants given no enteral feedings. Early fed infants have less feeding intolerance, establish oral feedings sooner, and do not differ in their incidence of NEC. In addition to timing of the feedings, the manner in which the feeding is provided may also be important.[92] Motor responses appear to be less intense on the more diluted formulas. The amount of volume does not appear to have a benefit in maturing motor function. Motor responses are equally intense whether feedings are instilled intragastrically or transpylorically. They are similar whether feedings are given chilled, at room temperature, or warmed to body temperature. When infants are fed a slow infusion over 120 minutes, they display an intense fed response that is accompanied by brisk gastric emptying. However, when the same volume is fed over 15 minutes, duodenal motor responses are far less intense and are accompanied by delayed gastric emptying. Because two-thirds of all preterm infants display an immature duodenal fed pattern that is accompanied by delayed gastric emptying, many preterm infants may not be as physiologically prepared to process bolus feedings as well as slow infusion feedings from the viewpoint of motor activity. A suggested scheme for initiation of minimal enteral feedings in VLBW infants is illustrated in Figure 4.

Some Future Directions

The fetus receives about 450 mL/d of amniotic fluid through the GI tract during the last trimester of pregnancy,[9] whereas the most enteral volume supplied to premature infants during the first weeks of life is what has been termed “minimal enteral nutrition,” and usually constitutes approximately 5 to 10% of the volume that would go through the intestine per day in utero. This suggests that the postnatal immature GI tract actually might be able to tolerate more volume than what is commonly provided, but in a different form than the nutrient-dense preparations currently provided. Compositional differences such as osmolality and lipid composition, which act as stimuli to decrease motility, are likely to slow gastric emptying and intestinal motility, critical factors in tolerance to enteral feeding.

There are several individual nutrients that could be utilized to enhance intestinal growth and function. Here, we will discuss a few of them, enteral protein, glutamine (GLN), long-chain omega-3 PUFAs and SCFAs.

Protein

Since protein is the major macronutrient required for growth, it is likely that protein (amino acids) provided via the parenteral versus the enteral route does *not* provide the intestine with an equivalent amount of trophic stimulation for intestinal growth. In a study using an infant canine model, it was demonstrated that approximately 40% of the intake required for normal growth needs to be supplied by the enteral route before a trophic effect on the mucosa occurs.[85,93] This intestinal trophism is most likely derived from protein rather than lipid or carbohydrate. Mucosal growth and prevention of atrophy are critical because they relate to several functional capabilities including digestion and absorption, bacterial, or antigenic translocation and the capability for luminal microorganisms and/or toxins to incite an inflammatory response causing pathology such as NEC or systemic inflammation.

Glutamine

Most NICUs do not routinely supplement critically ill premature babies with the amount of GLN they would be receiving had they remained in utero. A comprehensive review of GLN action is beyond the scope of this chapter. A significant period of enteral nutrition *and* GLN deprivation experienced by the majority of VLBW infants is a likely contributor to the lack of intestinal mucosal integrity and exquisite susceptibility to intestinal injury.

Despite several studies over the past decade that demonstrate efficacy and safety of GLN supplementation in highly stressed, critically ill patients' babies born prematurely receive very little, if any, GLN during this highly vulnerable period because they rarely reach full enteral feedings (which contain GLN) for weeks and because GLN is absent in routinely used intravenous solutions. Early studies of enteral GLN supplementation in VLBW infants demonstrated a decrease in hospital-acquired sepsis along with a decrease in the stimulation of CD16 and HLA DR markers on peripheral blood lymphocyte populations, consistent with decreased stimulation of the inflammatory response secondary to decreased translocation of proinflammatory antigens.[94] A recently completed multicenter trial of enteral GLN supplementation in 649 VLBW infants showed significant improvement in intestinal function and a decrease in Grades 3 and 4 intraventricular hemorrhages or periventricular leukomalacia in survivors.[95] An additional, more recent study, using enteral GLN supplementation, showed a beneficial effect on hospital-acquired sepsis.[96] One large study of intravenous GLN supplementation in neonates, however, did not show benefit.[97] Better targeting of patient subgroups, dosages, route, and timing of administration will be necessary to fully evaluate the presence

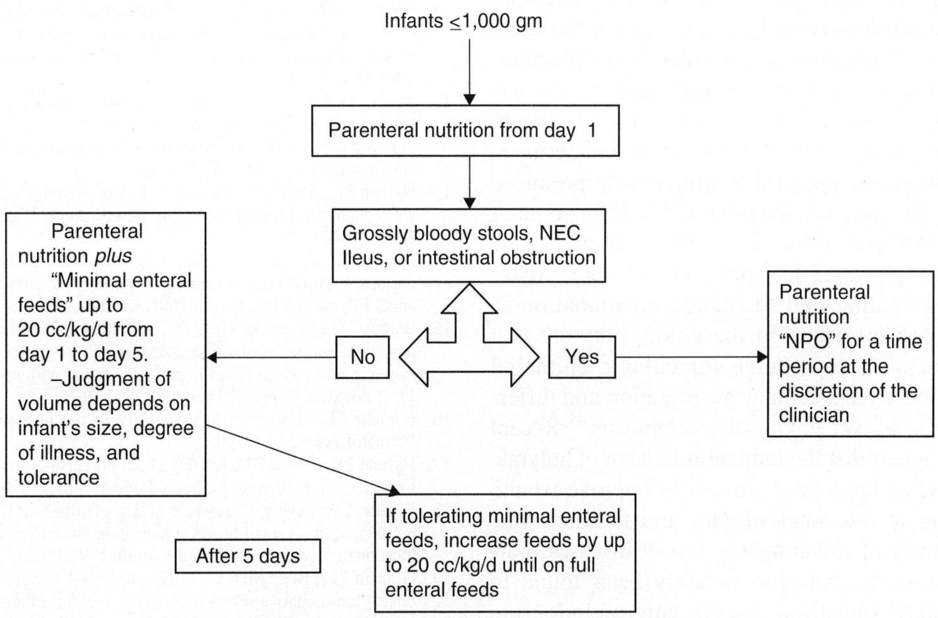

Figure 4 Suggested scheme for minimal enteral feedings in very low birth weight infants.

or absence of beneficial effects.[98] An example of such a group could be infants born to mothers with chorioamnionitis or other inflammatory conditions.

Omega-3 Fatty Acids

An important change to the composition of infant formula in the past several years has been the addition of LCPUFAs. The key LCPUFAs added have been DHA (22:6n–3) and arachidonic acid (AA, 20:4n–6). Both DHA and AA are found in human milk, and infants fed unsupplemented formulas have lower concentrations of DHA and AA in their plasma and erythrocytes than do infants who are breast-fed or fed supplemented formulas. It is also recognized that DHA and AA are integral structural components of all cells and may, therefore, have other health effects. Despite the voluminous information pertaining to potential benefits of the omega-3 LCPUFAS in both premature and term infants, the VLBW infant in the NICU receives only minimal quantities through the enteral route when receiving minimal enteral nutrition or parenteral route in the form of intravenous lipids, which are largely composed of the proinflammatory omega-6 fatty acids. Omega-3 LCPUFAs from fish oils and seed extracts decrease the production of inflammatory eicosanoids and cytokines. They act both directly, by replacing AA as an eicosanoid substrate and by inhibiting AA metabolism, and indirectly, by altering the expression of inflammatory genes through effects on transcription factor activation.[99] Thus omega-3 LCPUFAs are potentially useful anti-inflammatory agents and studies are needed to determine whether they would benefit patients, especially high-risk neonates.

Short-Chain Fatty Acids

SCFAs especially butyrate play central metabolic roles in maintaining the mucosal barrier in the gut. These SCFAs are a product of bacterial metabolism of carbohydrates, and may be responsible for the several of the beneficial effects of commensal bacteria or probiotics.[45] They can therefore be considered as "postbiotics." There is currently major controversy pertaining to the use of probiotics for premature infants, partially based on safety concerns in providing live bacteria to immunocompromised hosts. Butyrate has the potential to offer some of the benefits of probiotic bacteria without the side effects. Butyrate has been shown to increase wound healing and to reduce inflammation in the small intestine. In the colon, butyrate is a dominant energy source for colonic epithelial cells and affects cellular proliferation and differentiation by yet unknown mechanisms.[45] Recent data suggest that the luminal provision of butyrate may be an appropriate means to improve wound healing in intestinal surgery and to ameliorate symptoms of inflammatory bowel diseases. Furthermore, butyrate has recently been found to stimulate intestinal L-cell enteroedndocrine production of glucagon-like peptide-2, a highly intestinotrophic peptide.[46,100] Very little research has been done on the effects of butyrate as a nutrient for the developing intestine.[45]

SUMMARY

Several aspects of anatomic, physiologic, and biochemical development of the GI tract have been presented in this chapter. The importance of the GI tract beyond the classic paradigm of digestion and absorption of nutrients for optimization of growth should be evident. It should also be clear that the GI tract should be provided with luminal nutrients whenever possible. The developing GI tract has needs that cannot be met by merely nourishing the prematurely born infant similar to a term infant, or the way the fetus is nourished in utero. Optimization of nutrition for these infants based on the level of intestinal maturity continues to provide us with challenges with major implications for health during the lifetime of the individual.

REFERENCES

1. Montgomery RK, Mulberg AE, Grand RJ. Development of the human gastrointestinal tract: Twenty years of progress. Gastroenterology 1999;116:702–31.
2. Lau C, Smith EO, Schanler RJ. Coordination of suck-swallow and swallow respiration in preterm infants. Acta Paediatr Jpn 2003;92:721–7.
3. Jadcherla SR. Gastroesophageal reflux in the neonate. Clin Perinatol 2002;29:135–58.
4. Newell SJ, Booth IW, Morgan ME, et al. Gastro-oesophageal reflux in preterm infants. Arch Dis Child 1989;64:780–6.
5. Kaijser M, Akre O, Cnattingius S, Ekbom A. Preterm birth, low birth weight, and risk for esophageal adenocarcinoma. Gastroenterology 2005;128:607–9.
6. Cavell B. Gastric emptying in infants fed human milk or infant formula. Acta Paediatr Scand 1981;70:639–41.
7. Cavell B. Reservoir and emptying function of the stomach of the premature infant. Acta Paediatr Scand Suppl 1982;296:60–1.
8. Lebenthal E, Siegel M. Understanding gastric emptying: Implications for feeding the healthy and compromised infant. J Pediatr Gastroenterol Nutr 1985;4:1–3.
9. Pritchard JA. Fetal swallowing and amniotic fluid volume. Obstet Gynecol 1966;28:606–10.
10. Patole S, Rao S, Doherty D. Erythromycin as a prokinetic agent in preterm neonates: A systematic review. Arch Dis Child Fetal Neonatal Ed 2005;90:301–6.
11. Ng PC, So K, Fung KS, et al. Randomised controlled study of oral erythromycin for treatment of gastrointestinal dysmotility in preterm infants. Arch Dis Child Fetal Neonatal Ed 2001;84:F177–82.
12. Ng SC, Gomez JM, Rajadurai VS, et al. Establishing enteral feeding in preterm infants with feeding intolerance: A randomized controlled study of low-dose erythromycin. J Pediatr Gastroenterol Nutr 2003;37:554–8.
13. Hyman PE, Abrams C, Dubois A. Effect of metoclopramide and bethanechol on gastric emptying in infants. Pediatr Res 1985;19:1029–32.
14. Barnett CP, Omari T, Davidson GP, et al. Effect of cisapride on gastric emptying in premature infants with feed intolerance. J Paediatr Child Health 2001;37:559–63.
15. Barbey JT, Lazzara R, Zipes DP. Spontaneous adverse event reports of serious ventricular arrhythmias, QT prolongation, syncope, and sudden death in patients treated with cisapride. J Cardiovasc Pharmacol Ther 2002;7:65–76.
16. Berseth CL. Gastrointestinal motility in the neonate. Clin Perinatol 1996;23:179–90.
17. Hyman PE, Clarke DD, Everett SL, et al. Gastric acid secretory function in preterm infants. J Pediatr 1985;106:467–71.
18. Basaran UN, Celayir S, Eray N, et al. The effect of an H2-receptor antagonist on small-bowel colonization and bacterial translocation in newborn rats. Pediatr Surg Int 1998;13:118–20.
19. Graham PLr, Begg MD, Larson E, et al. Risk factors for late onset gram-negative sepsis in low birth weight infants hospitalized in the neonatal intensive care unit. Pediatr Infect Dis J 2006;25:113–7.
20. Guillet R, Stoll BJ, Cotten CM, et al. Association of H2-blocker therapy and higher incidence of necrotizing enterocolitis in very low birth weight infants. Pediatrics 2006;117:e137–42.
21. Antonowicz I, Lebenthal E. Developmental pattern of small intestinal enterokinase and disaccharidase activities in the human fetus. Gastroenterology 1977;72:1299–303.
22. Lebenthal E, Lee PC, Heitlinger LA. Impact of development of the gastrointestinal tract on infant feeding. J Pediatr 1983;102:1–9.
23. Mihatsch WA, Franz AR, Hogel J, Pohlandt F. Hydrolyzed protein accelerates feeding advancement in very low birth weight infants. Pediatrics 2002;110:1199–203.
24. Schanler RJ. The use of human milk for premature infants. Pediatr Clin North Am 2001;48:207–19.
25. Hamosh M. Digestion in the newborn. Clin Perinatol 1996;23:191–209.
26. Balistreri WF. Immaturity of hepatic excretory function and the ontogeny of bile acid metabolism. J Pediatr Gastroenterol Nutr 1983;2:S207–14.
27. Boehm G, Braun W, Moro G, Minoli I. Bile acid concentrations in serum and duodenal aspirates of healthy preterm infants: Effects of gestational and postnatal age. Biol Neonate 1997;71:207–14.
28. Klenoff-Brumberg HL, Genen LH. High versus low medium chain triglyceride content of formula for promoting short term growth of preterm infants. Cochrane Database Syst Rev 2003;CD002777.
29. Neu J, Koldovsky O. Nutrient absorption in the preterm neonate. Clin Perinatol 1996;23:229–43.
30. Georgieff MK, Innis SM. Controversial nutrients that potentially affect preterm neurodevelopment: Essential fatty acids and iron. Pediatr Res 2005;57:99R–103R.
31. SanGiovanni JP, Parra-Cabrera S, Colditz GA, et al. Meta-analysis of dietary essential fatty acids and long-chain polyunsaturated fatty acids as they relate to visual resolution acuity in healthy preterm infants. Pediatrics 2000;105:1292–8.
32. Morale SE HD, Castaneda YS, Wheaton DH, et al. Duration of long-chain polyunsaturated fatty acids availability in the diet and visual acuity. Early Hum Dev 2005;81:197–203.
33. Calder PC. Can n-3 polyunsaturated fatty acids be used as immunomodulatory agents? Biochem Soc Trans 1996;24:211–20.
34. Caplan MS, Russell T, Xiao Y, et al. Effect of polyunsaturated fatty acid (pufa) supplementation on intestinal inflammation and necrotizing enterocolitis (nec) in a neonatal rat model. Pediatr Res 2001;49:647–52.
35. Murray RD, Kerzner B, Sloan HR, et al. The contribution of salivary amylase to glucose polymer hydrolysis in premature infants. Pediatr Res 1986;20:186–91.
36. Kien CL. Digestion, absorption, and fermentation of carbohydrates in the newborn. Clin Perinatol 1996;23:211–28.
37. Neu J. Functional development of the fetal gastrointestinal tract. Semin Perinatol 1989;13:224–35.
38. Shulman RJ, Schanler RJ, Lau C, et al. Early feeding, feeding tolerance, and lactase activity in preterm infants. J Pediatr 1998;133:645–9.
39. Kim YS, Perdomo J, Ochoa P, Isaacs RA. Regional and cellular localization of glycosyltransferases in rat small intestine: Changes in enzymes with differentiation of intestinal epithelial cells. Biochim Biophys Acta 1975;391:39–50.
40. Boyle JT, Celano P, Koldovsky O. Demonstration of a difference in expression of maximal lactase and sucrase activity along the villus in the adult rat jejunum. Gastroenterology 1980;79:503–7.
41. Mellander L, Carlsson B, Jalil F, et al. Secretory IgA antibody response against *Escherichia coli* antigens in infants in relation to exposure. J Pediatr 1985;107:430–3.
42. Goldblum RM, Ahlstedt S, Carlsson B. Antibody forming cells in human colostrum after oral immunisation. Nature 1975;257:797–9.
43. Kleinman RE, Walker WA. The enteromammary immune system: An important new concept in breast milk host defense. Dig Dis Sci 1979;24:876–82.
44. Martin R, Olivares M, Marin ML, et al. Probiotic potential of 3 Lactobacilli strains isolated from breast milk. J Hum Lact 2005;21:8–17.
45. Scheppach W, Weiler F. The butyrate story: Old wine in new bottles? Curr Opin Clin Nutr Metab Care 2004;7:563–7.
46. Bartholome A, Albin D, Baker D, et al. Supplementation of total parenteral nutrition with butyrate acutely increases structural aspects of intestinal adaptation after an 80% jejunoileal resection in neonatal piglets. JPEN J Parenter Enteral Nutr 2004;28:210–22.
47. Fituch CC, Palkowetz KH, Goldman AS, Schanler RJ. Concentrations of IL-10 in preterm human milk and in milk from mothers of infants with necrotizing enterocolitis. Acta Paediatr 2004;93:1496–500.

48. Dinsmore JE, Jackson RJ, Smith SD. The protective role of gastric acidity in neonatal bacterial translocation. J Pediatr Surg 1997;32:1014–6.
49. Lebenthal E, Lee PC. Development of functional response in human exocrine pancreas. Pediatrics 1980;66:556–60.
50. Rubinstein E, Mark Z, Haspel J, et al. Antibacterial activity of the pancreatic fluid. Gastroenterology 1985;88:927–32.
51. Walker WA, Wu M, Isselbacher KJ, Bloch KJ. Intestinal uptake of macromolecules. IV. The effect of pancreatic duct ligation on the breakdown of antigen and antigen-antibody complexes on the intestinal surface. Gastroenterology 1975;69:1223–9.
52. Beck-Sague CM, Azimi P, Fonseca SN, et al. Bloodstream infections in neonatal intensive care unit patients: Results of a multicenter study. Pediatr Infect Dis J 1994;13:1110–6.
53. Cheng H, Leblond CP. Origin, differentiation and renewal of the four main epithelial cell types in the mouse small intrestine. I. Columnar cell. II. Mucus cell. III. Entero-endocrine cells. IV. Paneth cells. Am J Anat 1974;141:461–536.
54. Laboisse CL. Structure of gastrointestial mucins: Searching for the rosetta stone. Biochimie 1986;68:611–7.
55. Clamp JR, Creeth JM. Some non-mucin components of mucus and theri possible biologic roles. Ciba Foundation Symposium 1984;109:121–36.
56. Shub MD, Pang KY, Swann DA, Walker WA. Age-related changes in chemical composition and physical properties of mucus glycoproteins from rat small intestine. Biochem J 1983;215:405–11.
57. Sherman P, Forstner J, Roomi N, et al. Mucin depletion in the intestine of malnourished rats. Am J Physiol 1985;284: G418–23.
58. Faure M, Moennoz D, Montigon F, et al. Dietary threonine restriction specifically reduces intestinal mucin synthesis in rats. J Nutr 2005;135:486–91.
59. Bevins CL. Paneth cell defensins: Key effector molecules of innate immunity. Biochem Soc Trans 2006;34:263–6.
60. Gebert A, Rothkotter HJ, Pabst R. M cells in Peyer/s patches of the intestine. Int Rev Cytol 1996;167:91–159.
61. Denker BM, Nigam SK. Molecular structure and assembly of the tight junction. Am J Physiol 1998;274:F1–9.
62. Madara JL. Occludin junction structure-function relationships in a cultured epithelial monolayer. J Cell Biol 1985;101:2124–33.
63. Atsook K, Madara JL. An oligopeptide permeates intestinal tight junctions at glucose-elicited dilatations: Implications for oligopeptide absorption. Gastroenterology 1991;100:719–24.
64. Venkatraman A, Ramakrishna BS, Pulimood AB. Butyrate hastens restoration of barrier function after thermal and detergent injury to rat distal colon in vitro. Scand J Gastroenterol 1999;34:1087–92.
65. Li N, Lewis P, Samuelson D, et al. Glutamine regulates Caco-2 cell tight junction proteins. Am J Physiol Gastrointest Liver Physiol 2004;287:G726–33.
66. Seth A, Basuroy S, Sheth P, Rao RK. L-Glutamine ameliorates acetaldehyde-induced increase in paracellular permeability in Caco-2 cell monolayer. Am J Physiol Gastrointest Liver Physiol 2004;287:G510–7.
67. Liu Z, Li N, Neu J. Tight junctions, leaky intestines, and pediatric diseases. Acta Paediatr 2005;94:386–93.
68. Clayburgh DR, Shen L, Turner JR, et al. A porous defense: The leaky epithelial barrier in intestinal disease. Lab Invest 2004;84:282–91.
69. Koldovsky O, Sunshine P, Kretchmer N. Cellular migration of intestinal epithelia in suckling and weaned rats. Nature 1966;212:1389–90.
70. Cetin S, Ford HR, Sysko LR, et al. Endotoxin inhibits intestinal epithelial restitution through activation of Rho-GTPase and increased focal adhesions. J Biol Chem 2004;279: 24592–600.
71. Evans ME, Jones DP, Ziegler TR. Glutamine prevents cytokine-induced apoptosis in human colonic epithelial cells. J Nutr 2003;133:3065–71.
72. Rhoads JM, Niu X, Odle J, Graves LM. Role of mTOR signaling in intestinal cell migration. Am J Physiol Gastrointest Liver Physiol 2006;291:6510–7.
73. Hooper LV, Stappenbeck TS, Hong CV, Gordon J. Angiogenins: A new class of microbicidal proteins involved in innate immunity. Nat Immunol 2003;4:269–73.
74. Hooper LV. Bacterial contributions to mammalian gut development. Trends Microbiol 2004;12:129–34.
75. Stappenbeck TS, Hooper LV, Gordon JI. Developmental regulation of intestinal angiogenesis by indigenous microbes via Paneth cells. Proc Natl Acad Sci U S A 2002;99:15451–5.
76. Rakoff-Nahoum S, Paglino J, Eslami-Varzaneh F, et al. Recognition of commensal microflora by toll-like receptors is required for intestinal homeostasis. Cell 2004;118:229–41.
77. Madara J. Building an intestine-architectural contributions of commensal bacteria. N Engl J Med 2004;351:1685–6.
78. Schumann A, Nutten S, Donnicola D, et al. Neonatal antibiotic treatment alters gastrointestinal tract developmental gene expression and intestinal barrier transcriptome 10.1152/physiolgenomics.00057.2005. Physiol Genomics 2005;23:235–45.
79. Kudsk KA. Current aspects of mucosal immunology and its influence by nutrition. Am J Surg 2002;183:390–8.
80. Liboni K, Li N, Neu J. Mechanism of glutamine-mediated amelioration of lipopolysaccharide-induced IL-8 production in Caco-2 cells. Cytokine 2004;26:57–65.
81. Li N, Liboni K, Fang MZ, et al. Glutamine decreases lipopolysaccharide-induced intestinal inflammation in infant rats. Am J Physiol Gastrointest Liver Physiol 2004;286:G914–21.
82. Zhang L, Li N, des Robert C, et al. Lactobacillus rhamnosus GG decreases lipopolysaccharide-induced systemic inflammation in a gastrostomy-fed infant rat model. J Pediatr Gastroenterol Nutr 2006;42:545–52.
83. Minekawa R, Takeda T, Sakata M, et al. Human breast milk suppresses the transcriptional regulation of IL-1beta-induced NF-kappaB signaling in human intestinal cells. Am J Physiol Cell Physiol 2004;287:C1404–11.
84. Thureen PJ, Melara D, Fennessey PV, Hay WWJ. Effect of low versus high intravenous amino acid intake on very low birth weight infants in the early neonatal period. Pediatr Res 2003;53:24–32.
85. Niinikoski H, Stoll B, Guan X, et al. Onset of small intestinal atrophy is associated with reduced intestinal blood flow in TPN-fed neonatal piglets. J Nutr 2004;134:1467–74.
86. Stoll BJ, Hansen N, Fanaroff AA, et al. Late-onset sepsis in very low birth weight neonates: The experience of the NICHD Neonatal Research Network. Pediatrics 2002;110:285–91.
87. Alverdy JC, Laughlin RS, Wu L. Influence of the critically ill state on host-pathogen interactions within the intestine: Gut-derived sepsis redefined. Crit Care Med 2003;31:598–607.
88. Wildhaber BE, Yang H, Spencer AU, et al. Lack of enteral nutrition—effects on the intestinal immune system. J Surg Res 2005;123:8–16.
89. Harris MC, D'Angio CT, Gallagher PR, et al. Cytokine elaboration in critically ill infants with bacterial sepsis, necrotizing entercolitis, or sepsis syndrome: Correlation with clinical parameters of inflammation and mortality. J Pediatr 2005;147:462–8.
90. Speer CP. Pre- and postnatal inflammatory mechanisms in chronic lung disease of preterm infants. Paediatr Respir Rev 2004;5:S241–4.
91. Volpe JJ. Neurobiology of periventricular leukomalacia in the premature infant. Pediatr Res 2001;50:553–62.
92. Berseth CL, Bisquera JA, Paje VU. Prolonging small feeding volumes early in life decreases the incidence of necrotizing enterocolitis in very low birth weight infants. Pediatrics 2003;111:529–34.
93. Owens L, Burrin DG, Berseth CL. Minimal enteral feeding induces maturation of intestinal motor function but not mucosal growth in neonatal dogs. J Nutr 2002;132:2717–22.
94. Neu J, Roig JC, Meetze WH, et al. Enteral glutamine supplementation for very low birth weight infants decreases morbidity. J Pediatr 1997;131:691–9.
95. Vaughn P, Thomas P, Clark R, Neu J. Enteral glutamine supplementation and morbidity in low birthweight infants. J Pediatr 2003;142:662–8.
96. van den Berg A, van Elburg RM, Westerbeek EA, et al. Glutamine-enriched enteral nutrition in very-low-birth-weight infants and effects on feeding tolerance and infectious morbidity: A randomized controlled trial. Am J Clin Nutr 2005;81:1397–404.
97. Poindexter BB, Ehrenkranz RA, Stoll BJ, et al. Effect of parenteral glutamine supplementation on plasma amino acid concentrations in extremely low-birth-weight infants. Am J Clin Nutr 2003;77:737–43.
98. Neu J. Glutamine supplements in premature infants: Why and how. J Pediatr Gastroenterol Nutr 2003;37:533–5.
99. Calder PC. Polyunsaturated fatty acids and inflammation. Biochem Soc Trans 2005;33:423–7.
100. Tappenden KA, Albin DM, Bartholome AL, Mangian HF. Glucagon-like peptide-2 and short-chain fatty acids: A new twist to an old story. J Nutr 2003;133:3717–20.

22

Immunophysiology and Nutrition of the Gut

Samuli Rautava, MD, PhD
W. Allan Walker, MD

INTRODUCTION

The intestinal surface comes into contact with a continuous flux of a vast variety of antigens. The primary function of the intestinal mucosa is absorption of nutrients. This function necessitates the transport of molecules across a single layer of epithelial cells and distinguishes the intestinal mucosa functionally from that of the respiratory or genitourinary tracts. The intestinal immune system must be able to recognize potential pathogens and inhibit their adherence and invasion by protective immune exclusion or inflammatory responsiveness while allowing uptake and transport of dietary compounds and certain intact macromolecules (eg, growth factors and maternal immunoglobulins in breast milk) without inappropriate and detrimental immune reactions. Appreciation of this intricate balance is paramount to our understanding of intestinal immunophysiology.

The intestinal immune system has unique have evolved to fulfill the dual task of immune defense and tolerance. An overview of the intestinal immune system with emphasis on immune responses directed toward dietary antigens is provided in the first half of this chapter. The establishment and maintenance of nonresponsiveness or tolerance to dietary and commensal microbial antigens is the result of active and coordinated immune responses which mature postnatally upon contact with foreign antigens, particularly colonizing bacteria. The indigenous intestinal microbiota is established during the same period and commensal bacteria have a profound impact on the structural and functional maturation of the gut. Indeed, the intestinal microbiota may be considered an essential component of the intestinal immune system (Figure 1).

The second half of this chapter is dedicated to the effects of nutritional factors to gut immune physiology. Malnutrition is still a major threat to infant and child health in large portions of the world. The effects of protein and energy malnutrition as well as the lack of certain individual nutrients on gut immunophysiology are overviewed in this chapter but discussed in detail in Chapter 8, "Trace Elements," Chapter 9, "Iron," Chapter 10, "Vitamins," and Chapter 13, "Protein-Energy Malnutrition: Pathophysiology, Clinical Consequences, and Treatment." The increasing evidence from clinical and experimental studies indicating that the route of nutrition, that is, enteral versus parenteral nutrition, affects intestinal immune functions and therefore child health is then discussed. In the final paragraphs, an overview of novel nutritional approaches aiming to enhance intestinal and systemic immune functions, namely probiotics and prebiotics, is given.

IMMUNE MONITORING OF INTESTINAL ANTIGENS

The Intestinal Immune System

The intestinal immune system must be able to recognize potential pathogens and launch protective immune responses in order to avoid invasion by microbes. The innate immune system consists of evolutionarily conserved immune defense mechanisms which provide the host with immediate antimicrobial protection. These include soluble factors such as lysozyme, peroxidase, and lactoferrin as well as phagocytic immune cells, most importantly macrophages and neutrophilic granulocytes. Pattern-recognition receptors (PRRs) such as cell membrane–bound Toll-like receptors (TLRs) and cytosolic nucleotide-binding oligomerization domain (NOD) molecules identify specific molecular patterns characteristic to microbes and initiate rapid innate immune responses. The common characteristic of innate immune responsiveness is generally thought to be the lack of immune memory; that is, innate responses remain unaltered upon reencounter with the same antigen.[1] However, it is also well established that exposure to microbial antigens can increase or decrease the expression of PRRs in vitro and in vivo.[2,3] Moreover, the innate immune system controls adaptive immune responses through PRR signaling and activation of antigen-presenting cells (APCs).[4,5]

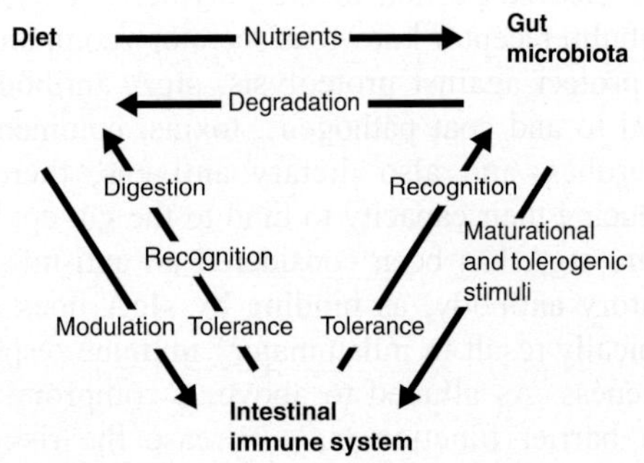

Figure 1 The interaction between diet, the indigenous intestinal microbiota, and the intestinal immune system.

Adaptive or acquired immune responses are by definition characterized by antigen-specific immune memory. Induction of adaptive immunity is considerably slower than that of innate immunity but upon subsequent challenge with the same antigen a prompt and powerful specific immune protective response is elicited. Adaptive immunity is characteristic of vertebrate animals and its evolutionary development intriguingly coincides with the appearance of other important structural and functional organ changes including the appearance of the lower jaw.[6] In addition to its role in defense against potential pathogens, immunological memory is essential for avoiding inappropriate inflammatory reactions against dietary antigens and commensal microbes. It may therefore be suggested that intestinal immunophysiology necessitated the development of an adaptive immune system and, indeed, the intestinal immune system comprises intraepithelial lymphocytes and organized gut-associated lymphoid tissues is the largest lymphoid organ in the body. The functions of the intestinal adaptive immune system range from production and secretion of polymeric immunoglobulin IgA antibodies in the gut lumen to induction of protective immune responses which may then be elicited locally, systemically, or at other mucosal effector sites such as the mammary gland.

Intestinal Mucosal Barrier

The intestinal immune system must be able to monitor luminal antigens in order to prevent potential pathogens from adhering and invading the epithelium and to neutralize microbial toxins. Immunophysiologic factors that restrict mucosal colonization by pathogens, prevent foreign noxious antigens and pathogens from penetrating the mucosa, and regulate antigen-specific immune responses are collectively referred to as the intestinal mucosal barrier (Figure 2).[7] To carry out the primary function of nutrient uptake in the gut, however, these protective mechanisms must also allow the controlled entry of certain antigens. Permeability of the gut barrier is increased during the neonatal period, which may have a physiologic role in allowing the uptake of growth factors and maternal IgG antibodies from breast

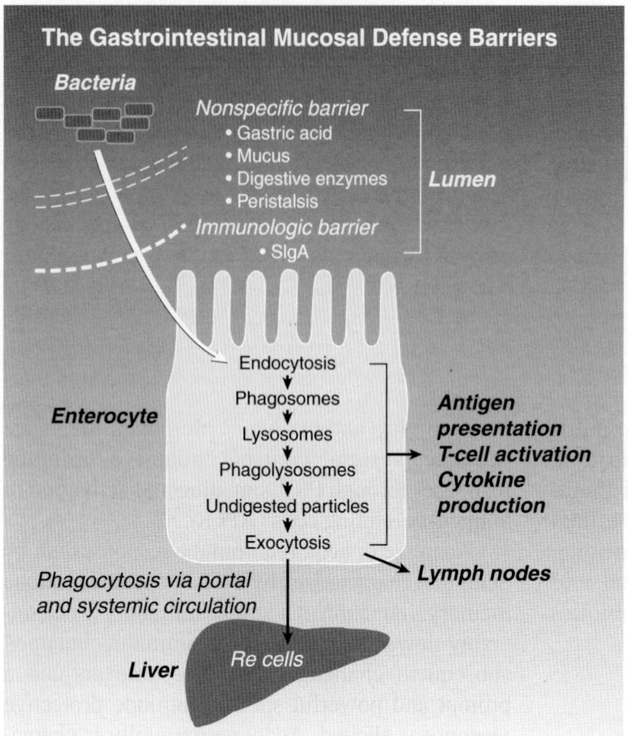

Figure 2 The intestinal mucosal barrier selectively restricts mucosal pathogen colonization and invasion and prevents foreign antigens from penetrating the mucosa. While nutrients such as glucose and amino acids are absorbed through the apical cell membrane and traverse the enterocyte to exit at the basolateral membrane, macromolecules may bind to specific receptors on the enterocyte and then be engulfed by the cell in membrane-bound vesicles invaginating from the apical cell membrane. The endocytosed antigens may then be directed to lysosomes and destroyed or released on the basolateral border of the enterocyte as in the case of maternal IgG antibodies and growth factors from breast milk. Moreover, presentation of intact antigens to T lymphocytes of the adaptive immune system is necessary for the induction of protective sIgA production and the establishment of oral tolerance. SIgA = secretory immunoglobulin A.

milk. On the other hand, this relative intestinal permeability may render the neonate susceptible to pathogen invasion and allergen sensitization. A compromised gut barrier function is also characteristic of pathological conditions such as necrotizing enterocolitis (NEC) and inflammatory bowel disease (IBD).[8,9]

External Mucosal Barrier. The intestinal mucosal barrier may be considered to be composed of four major components (Table 1). It should be born in mind, however, that these components are structurally and functionally interrelated and thus this division is merely an arbitrary conceptual aid. The first line of mucosal defense limits the amount of antigen coming into contact with the epithelial surface and consists of luminal factors including gastric acid and digestive enzymes, nonspecific antimicrobial substances and IgA antibodies secreted into the lumen, and an intestinal mucus layer coating the mucosal surface. The acidic environment of the stomach and upper duodenum is lethal to many ingested pathogenic bacteria and may affect proteolysis of antigens by digestive enzymes and hence reduce availability of intact antigens for uptake. In addition, intestinal epithelial cells have interestingly been observed to create an acidic microclimate on their apical surface.[10] Digestive enzymes by definition cleave intraluminal antigens and as a consequence have a profound impact on their immunogenic properties, thus reducing the antigenic load. Intestinal immune cells secrete a number of nonspecific humoral defense factors including lysozyme, lactoferrin, peroxidase, defensins, and trefoil peptides which exhibit a variety of antimicrobial activities.

Table 1 Components of the Intestinal Mucosal Barrier

1. External barrier
• Gastric acid
• Digestive enzymes
• Nonspecific antimicrobial factors (eg, lysozyme, lactoferrin, peroxidase, defensins)
• Secretory IgA
• Intestinal mucus
• Peristalsis
2. Epithelial layer
• Microvilli
• Plasma membrane
• Tight junctions
• Innate immune receptors
• Intraepithelial immune cells
3. Intestinal lymphoid tissue
• Uptake and presentation of antigens
• Induction of secretory IgA production
• Local and systemic inflammatory responses
• Maintenance of tolerance
4. Indigenous intestinal microbiota
• Degradation of luminal antigens
• Inhibition of colonization and adherence of pathogens
• Stimulation of the intestinal immune system

Secretory (s)IgA is a dimeric mucosal antibody produced by plasma cells in the lamina propria and transported across the epithelial layer bound to a polymeric immunoglobulin receptor. Dimeric IgA is secreted in the gut lumen bound to a cleaved portion of the polymeric immunoglobulin receptor known as secretory component to protect against proteolysis. sIgA antibodies bind to and coat pathogens, toxins, commensal microbes, and also dietary antigens, thereby reducing their capacity to bind to the gut epithelium. sIgA has been considered an anti-inflammatory antibody, as binding by sIgA does not typically result in inflammatory immune responsiveness. As alluded to above, a compromised gut barrier function may increase the risk of sensitization to dietary antigens and prior exposure to dietary antigens has been reported to reduce uptake of intact food proteins as a result of induction of sIgA.[11] As an example of this function, IgA-deficient individuals have a heightened frequency of food allergy.[12] The role of sIgA in immune responses toward dietary antigens remains elusive, however, as healthy individuals have little or no food-specific intestinal IgA antibodies.[13]

The epithelial surface of the gastrointestinal tract is lined with a mucus coat composed of a mixture of mucin glycoproteins which vary greatly in both molecular weight (ranging from one to several million daltons) and carbohydrate side chains attached to the mucin protein skeleton.[14] The thick mucus coat of the stomach protects the underlying mucosa from gastric acid damage. In addition, mucus viscidity and sIgA antibodies within the mucus layer trap particles including toxins and pathogenic bacteria. Intestinal epithelial cells, particularly goblet cells, continuously produce mucin molecules and the entrapped particles are expelled by gut peristalsis with shed mucus.

The Intestinal Epithelium and Innate Immune Responses. Epithelial cells lining the surface of the body form a protective physical barrier against the external environment. The intestinal epithelium, however, must simultaneously be able to selectively absorb nutrients and therefore the epithelium in the alimentary tract (with the exception of the oral cavity, esophagus, and rectum) consists of a single layer of cells. The majority of the cells in the epithelial monolayer consist of polarized absorptive cells referred to as enterocytes. The apical surface of enterocytes is covered with negatively charged protrusions or microvilli, 100 μm in diameter. There are approximately 40 microvilli per 5 μm in the intestinal epithelium of children.[15] The lipid bilayer microvillus membrane and the dense microvilli with the overlying glycocalyx formed by membrane-bound glycoproteins constitute a significant barrier to antigen entry. Paracellular antigen penetration is prevented by tight junctions between apical surfaces of enterocytes. The permeability of tight junctions may be modified by cytokines, such as tumor necrosis factor (TNF)-α and transforming growth factor (TGF)-β, or substances secreted by pathogens.[16,17]

Intestinal epithelial cells express a number of PRRs to recognize microorganism-associated molecular patterns (MAMPs). MAMPs are present on both commensal and pathogenic microbes and required for their survival and therefore evolutionarily highly conserved.[18] These conserved microbial structures include unmethylated CpG motifs characteristic of bacterial DNA, virus-derived single-stranded RNA, bacterial flagellin, and bacterial cell wall compounds such as lipoteichoic acid, muramyl dipeptide, peptidoglycan, and lipopolysaccharide.[4,18,19] In contrast, with the exception of nucleic acids, MAMPs are not expressed by the host. Intestinal PRRs and their ligands are presented in Table 2.

The most extensively investigated epithelial PRRs to date are TLRs. Thus far, 10 individual TLRs (TLR1-10) have been identified in humans

Table 2 Intestinal Pathogen Recognition Receptors and Their Known Ligands

Receptor	Ligand
TLR1	Lipopeptides
TLR2	Lipopeptides and lipoteichoic acid of gram-positive bacteria
TLR3	Viral dsRNA, viral sense ssRNA
TLR4	LPS
+CD14	
+MD-2	
TLR5	Bacterial flagellin
TLR6	Lipoteichoic acid
TLR8	Viral antisense ssRNA
TLR9	CpG DNA
NOD1	Diaminopimelic acid of peptidoglycan
NOD2	Muramyl dipeptide

CD-cluster of differentiation; CpGDNA-unmethylated cytosine-guanine–rich deoxyribonucleic acid; dsRNA-double-stranded ribonucleic acid; LPS-lipopolysaccharide; MD-2-myeloid differentiation protein-2; MyD88-myeloid differentiation primary-response protein 88; NOD-nucleotide-binding oligomerization domain; ssRNA-single-stranded ribonucleic acid; TLR-Toll-like receptor.

and TLR2-6 and TLR9 have been detected on human intestinal epithelial cells.[18,20–23] In addition, TLR1-6, TLR8, and TLR9 messenger RNAs are expressed by human intestinal epithelial cells.[24] TLRs are also present on intestinal macrophages and dendritic cells (DCs).[23,25] Structurally, TLRs are transmembrane proteins with a short transmembrane region.[18,26] The extracellular domain of TLRs includes a leucine-rich repeat region with divergent ligand-binding properties. The intracellular domain contains a structure common to TLR and the interleukin (IL)-1 receptor family referred to as the Toll/interleukin 1 receptor (TIR). The TIR domain is essential for initiation of TLR signaling, which may lead to activation of a number of transcription factors and, consequently, the induction of a variety of immune response genes. The type of immune activation induced via different TLRs is dependent on the cofactors and adaptor proteins involved in signal transduction. Antigen binding by all known TLRs is capable of activating the myeloid differentiation primary-response protein 88 (MyD88)-dependent pathway, which involves activation of members of interleukin 1 receptor–associated kinase family and leads to expression of inflammatory genes through activation of a number of transcription factors including nuclear factor κB (NF-κB) and activator protein 1.[26] In addition to MyD88 activation, at least four alternate TLR signaling pathways involving the adaptor proteins Mal/TIRAP, TRIF/TICAM-1, TRAM/Tirp/TICAM-2, or SARM have been identified.[27] Recognition of pathogens by TLRs thus rapidly initiates protective immune responses. Interestingly, however, inflammatory immune responsiveness against harmless indigenous microbes binding to TLRs appears to be prevented by sophisticated mechanisms involving the IL-1 receptor associated kinase activation suppressor Toll-interacting protein and NF-κB agonist peroxisome proliferators–activated receptor γ (PPARγ).[24] Other inhibitors of TLR signal transduction include single immunoglobulin IL-1R–related protein, suppressor of cytokine signaling, the zinc finger protein A20, and the cytokines TGF-β and IL-10.[28]

Two PRRs in the NOD family, NOD1 and NOD2 [also known as caspase activation and recruitment domain (CARD)4 and CARD15, respectively], of cytosolic receptors have recently been investigated with regard to their role in regulation of intestinal immunology. Both NOD1 and NOD2 bind to bacterial cell wall structures. The specific ligands are γ-D-glutamyl-meso-diamino-pimelic acid of gram-negative bacteria for NOD1 and muramyl dipeptide for NOD2.[29,30] Ligand binding to NOD1 or NOD2 leads to NF-κB activation via the Rip2/RICK/CARDIAK serine-threonine kinase but the details of the signaling pathway still remain elusive.[31]

Indigenous Intestinal Microbiota. The human gastrointestinal tract harbors an enormous quantity of indigenous microbes. The number of prokaryotic cells in the intestine has been estimated to be 10^{14}, the vast majority of which are found in the colon. These microbes belong to more than 500 culturable species and through the emergence of culture-independent molecular identification techniques the number of microbial species constituting the gut microbiota has been suggested to exceed 1,000. This complex ecosystem of microbes is referred to as the intestinal microbiota. Colonization of a sterile gastrointestinal tract commences at birth and proceeds in a stepwise and systematic fashion. Maternal intestinal and vaginal microbiota provide the first bacterial inoculum to the newborn and hence facultative gram-positive cocci (staphylococci, streptococci, and enterococci) and enterobacteria are the first bacteria to colonize the intestine. Consequently, gut microbiota composition in infants born by caesarian section differs significantly from that of vaginally born infants.[32] This has been suggested to partially explain the heightened risk of atopic disease and sensitization to dietary antigens in infants born by caesarian section.[33] Early nutrition has a profound impact on the composition of the infant's gut microbiota. In particular, breast-feeding promotes the growth of bifidobacteria, which become the predominant microbiota species in breast-fed infants.[34] After weaning the gut microbiota composition of infants resembles that of adults.

Intestinal microbes have been shown to be necessary for normal morphological and immunological maturation of the gut in experimental studies conducted using germ-free animals.[35] Germ-free mice exhibit impaired sIgA production.[36] Moreover, specific strains of intestinal microbiota have been shown to modulate the expression of host genes involved in a variety of intestinal functions including nutrient absorption, metabolism, mucosal barrier function, and intestinal maturation.[37] It has recently been reported that defective immune maturation in germ-free mice could be corrected by colonization with *Bacteroides fragilis,* a member of murine indigenous intestinal microbiota.[38]

As discussed above, PRRs of the intestinal immune system recognize MAMPs present on both pathogens and indigenous intestinal microbes. Interestingly, however, pathogen recognition by TLRs leads to inflammatory responsiveness mediated by the NF-κB pathway, whereas nonpathogenic intestinal microbes have been observed to suppress the same pathway.[19,39] There are also data indicating that intestinal epithelial cells cultured in vitro are unresponsive to TLR ligands on indigenous intestinal microbes.[22] Monocolonization of germ-free rats with the commensal *Bifidobacterium lactis* has been shown to transiently activate the NF-κB pathway via TLR2 signaling but this activation does not result in tissue damage.[40] Moreover, recognition of commensal bacteria through TLRs appears to be necessary for protection against epithelial injury, as mice deficient in TLR2, TLR4, or MyD88, a downstream TLR signaling molecule, exhibit increased morbidity and mortality from chemically induced colitis.[41] It has recently been shown that while intestinal macrophages rapidly kill commensal bacteria that penetrate the surface epithelial layer, intestinal DC may retain live bacteria intracellularly and induce protective sIgA production in the mesenteric lymph nodes without systemic immune activation.[42]

Indigenous microbes contribute to intestinal barrier function by degrading intraluminal antigens and by inhibiting adherence and colonization by pathogenic microbes. Antigen transport across the intestinal epithelium is increased in the absence of intestinal microbes in experimental animals. The immunomodulatory consequences of luminal antigen degradation by microbial proteases are demonstrated by in vitro experiments in which lymphocyte proliferation and production of IL-4 were suppressed by cow's milk casein hydrolyzed with enzymes derived from lactobacilli.[43,44]

Antigen Presentation and Induction of Adaptive Immunity in the Gut-Associated Lymphoid Tissue. Despite the effects of degradation by digestive enzymes of the host or indigenous microbes and coating with antigen-specific sIgA antibodies in the gut lumen discussed above, a nonnegligible amount of immunologically intact macromolecules reaches the intestinal surface. Intestinal adaptive immune responses against ingested antigens are orchestrated by T lymphocytes of gut-associated lymphoid tissue (GALT). Instead of being an anatomically well-defined lymphoid organ, GALT is composed of a complex network of immune cells distributed within the intestine as isolated intraepithelial and lamina propria lymphocytes or organized lymphoid structures such as Peyer's patches (PPs) and lymphoid follicles in the small intestine and colon. PPs located in the small intestinal submucosa are thought to be the principal induction site of intestinal adaptive immunity. The PP is covered with specialized epithelium referred to as follicle-associated epithelium characterized by the presence of microfold (M) cells which lack protective microvilli and thick mucus.[45] M cells are so named because of their basolateral surface, which has pockets enfolding lymphocytes, DCs, and macrophages. It is believed that antigens are not degraded by M cells but delivered intact to be processed by the underlying APCs. Recently, signaling through TLRs has been shown to regulate the functions of the follicle-associated epithelium, as TLR2 activation was observed to enhance transepithelial transport of antigens by M cells.[46]

Intestinal DCs are professional APCs which express microbial peptides bound to class II major histocompatibility (MHC) molecules on their surface and activate T-cell responses after having migrated to mesenteric lymph nodes. DCs residing in M-cell pockets ingest and sample antigens passing through M cells. In addition, there are data to suggest that DCs may monitor the intestinal content by extending dendrites into the gut lumen after opening tight junctions.[47] Activation, maturation, and trafficking of intestinal DCs are dependent on microbial stimulation through TLRs and DCs, in turn, play a pivotal role in determining the type of adaptive immune responses to be launched (Figure 3).[48]

Based on cytokine production patterns, adaptive immune responses may be divided into cross-regulatory Th1 and Th2 subsets. Th1 cells are characterized by secretion of IFN-γ, IL-2, and TNF-α, with little or no IL-4, IL-5, IL-9, or IL-13, and orchestrate immune defense against intracellular pathogens. Th2 cells, on the other hand, secrete IL-4, IL-5, IL-6, IL-9, IL-10, and IL-13, but not IFN-γ or TNF-α, and are implicated in humoral responses, especially those of the IgE class, and are involved in defense against helminthic infections. Both Th1- and Th2-type responses have been implicated in the pathogenesis of human disease.[49] Inflammatory immune reactions driven by Th1-type responses are encountered in many autoimmune states whereas Th2-type responsiveness is central in the pathogenesis of allergic disorders. In particular, Th2-skewed immune responsiveness has been detected in individuals with food allergy.[50]

There are limited data regarding the type of T-cell responsiveness preferentially elicited toward dietary antigens in the intestine. An early study conducted using a mouse model suggested that PP T-cell responses are preferentially of the Th2 type with pronounced IL-5 production.[51] Subsequent studies on human subjects, however, have shown that human PP T cells spontaneously produce considerable amounts of the Th1 cytokine IFN-γ.[52] Moreover, PP T cells have been reported to respond to stimulation with cow's milk antigens by production of IL-12 and expansion of $CD4^+CD25^+$ T cells.[53] Th1 and Th2 cells develop from naïve $CD4^+$ T cells which become polarized under the influence of genetic and microenvironmental factors and there is a cross-regulatory balance early in adaptive responses with Th1 cytokines inhibiting Th2 responses and vice versa.[54] IL-12 and IFN-γ thus promote further Th1 polarization and it is therefore likely that human PP T-cell responses toward dietary antigens in nonallergic individuals are preferentially of the Th1 type, even though food-antigen–specific effector T cells are usually not found in the intestinal mucosa.[50] Food proteins per se appear to affect the maturation of the intestinal immune system since animals receiving a protein-free diet, albeit not malnourished, display defective Th1 responsiveness and limited production of IgA and IgG antibodies.[55]

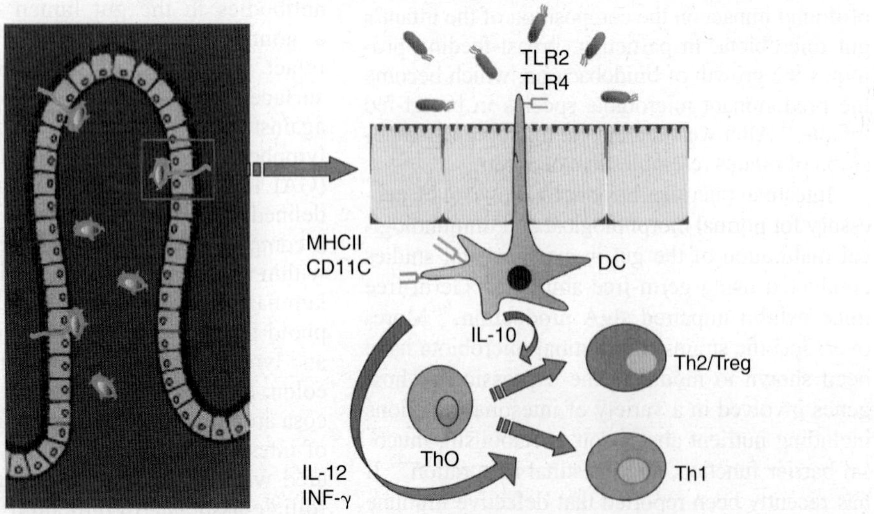

Figure 3 Recognition of luminal antigens by dendritic cells (DCs) and induction of adaptive immune responses. Intestinal DCs expressing CD11c sample luminal contents by extending dendrites expressing Toll-like receptors through tight junctions and then present microbial peptides bound to class II major histocompatibility molecules to naïve T cells. This antigen presentation by DCs plays a decisive role in determining the type of adaptive immune responses to be launched. Intestinal DCs producing IL-10 promote the development of T helper (Th)2 cells or regulatory T cells, whereas Th1 polarization develops in the presence of IL-12 and IFN-γ. CD = cluster of differentiation; IFN-γ = interferon-γ; IL = interleukin.

Establishment and Maintenance of Immune Tolerance to Dietary Antigens

Specific immune functions have developed to prevent inappropriate and potentially detrimental inflammatory reactions against food antigens. These functions as a whole and the resulting apparent nonresponsiveness are referred to as oral tolerance. An intricate network of regulatory immune responses has developed in the gut to orchestrate the establishment and maintenance of oral tolerance which is induced by small amounts of antigens crossing the mucosal surface in immunologically intact form. The active nature of immune tolerance is underscored in a definition suggested by Weiner according to which tolerance is defined as "any mechanism by which a potentially injurious immune response is prevented, suppressed, or shifted to a noninjurious class of immune response."[56]

In experimental studies, oral tolerance has successfully been induced against antigens as diverse as heavy metals, heterologous red blood cells, allogeneic leukocytes, extracts of pollen and other aeroallergens, inactivated viruses and bacteria, and a large variety of proteins.[57] In addition, the host is tolerant to its indigenous microbiota. Abrogation of oral tolerance to dietary antigens results in food allergy whereas inappropriate inflammatory immune responsiveness against indigenous intestinal microbiota has been described in IBD.[58] Several studies indicate that oral tolerance cannot be induced in germ-free animals.[59] Sudo and colleagues have elegantly demonstrated that mice raised in germ-free conditions exhibit impaired development of the intestinal immune system and defective oral tolerance formation with an excessive Th2-type immune responsiveness.[60] Reconstitution of the intestinal microbiota with bifidobacteria in these animals restored the ability to establish oral tolerance in the neonatal period but not at a later age. In a similar fashion, oral administration of lipopolysaccharide has been reported to induce tolerance in germ-free mice.[61] Recent advances in understanding innate immunity suggest that the modulation of tolerance might be mediated via DCs or directly through TLRs on regulatory $CD4^+CD25^+$ T cells.[62,63] In accord with this observation, indigenous microbes have been reported to be necessary for the induction of regulatory T cells (T_{reg}s).[64]

T-Cell Deletion and Anergy. Ingestion of large doses of antigen may lead to inactivation of antigen-specific T cells. There are experimental data to suggest that feeding large quantities of antigen lead to clonal deletion of T cells but the significance of this phenomenon in oral tolerance is not clear.[65] T-cell anergy refers to a state of antigen-specific hyporesponsiveness characterized by an inability to produce IL-2 resulting from priming with the same antigen. Stimulation of the T-cell receptor in the absence of proinflammatory costimulatory molecules on the APC or costimulatory signaling through the cytotoxic T-lymphocyte-associated protein (CTLA)-4 on T cells leads to T-cell anergy.[66] Anergic T cells may in some instances act as T_{reg}s and therefore T-cell anergy and T_{reg} function may be regarded as two aspects of the same cell rather than distinct mechanisms of tolerance.[57,59]

Active Immunosuppression by Regulatory T cells. Distinct regulatory mechanisms mediated by regulatory T-cell subsets including gut-derived Th3 and T regulatory 1 cells and thymus-derived or peripherally induced $CD4^+CD25^+$ T cells, modulate adaptive Th1 and Th2 responses.[67] Th3 and T regulatory 1 cells are thought to exert their effects through production of the cytokines TGF-β and IL-10, respectively, while $CD4^+CD25^+$ T cells mainly act through contact-dependent mechanisms involving CTLA-4 and membrane-bound TGF-β.[67–69]

However, both the nomenclature and the functional or developmental interrelations of these regulatory T-cell populations are still somewhat unclear.

Oral administration of antigen leads to the generation of TGF-β-secreting Th3 cells in both animal models and human subjects.[70,71] TGF-β induces the development of $CD4^+CD25^+$ T cells through the transcription factor FOXP3.[72] Antigen feeding has been shown to lead to the induction of $CD4^+CD25^+$ T cells in the GALT and the number of $CD4^+CD25^+$ T cells expressing FOXP3 and CTLA-4 is increased in PPs after oral exposure to antigen.[73–75] There are a number of studies indicating that T_{reg}s are implicated in clinical food allergy and development of tolerance in human subjects. Infantile food allergy may be considered a manifestation of a primary failure to establish oral tolerance. A defect in regulatory adaptive immune responses in food allergy is suggested by a report according to which cow's milk–specific T-cell clones isolated from peripheral blood of children with cow's milk allergy (CMA) exhibit diminished IL-10 production compared to those from tolerant children.[76] In addition, the number of TGF-β-producing T cells has been reported to be reduced in the intestinal epithelium and lamina propria of children with food allergy.[77] Interestingly, the development of tolerance in children with CMA is associated with the appearance of circulating allergen-responsive $CD4^+CD25^+$ T cells.[78] Nonetheless, $CD4^+CD25^+$ T cells appear to be present and functional in adult patients with CMA.[79]

IMMUNOMODULATORY FACTORS IN NUTRITION

Nutrition and nutrients have diverse effects on host immunophysiology. During the first months of life, when the immune system still lacks mature competence and oral tolerance and the intestinal microbiota are first established, breast milk provides the infant with both passive immunoprotection in the form of soluble antimicrobial molecules and maturational signals including growth factors and cytokines. Lack of proper nutrition affects host immunophysiology and these effects contribute to the morbidity and mortality caused by malnutrition. A number of nutrients, including vitamins, iron, zinc, and other trace elements, glutamine and other amino acids, and certain lipids influence immune functions by mechanisms beyond correction of dietary deficiencies.

Breast Milk

Breast milk provides the newborn infant with optimal nutrition for growth and development and immunoprotection during a critical period when the neonatal immune defenses are still immature. Infectious disease is a major threat to the neonate and the leading cause of infant mortality in many areas of the world. It is well established that breast-feeding protects the infant from infectious disease. This protective effect is mediated by a number of passive antimicrobial factors, including lysozyme, lactoferrin, peroxidase, defensins, cathelicidin, sIgA, TLRs with soluble CD14, and oligosaccharides which are discussed in detail in Chapter 31, "Protective Properties of Human Milk," of this volume. The protection provided by breast milk is crucial in developing countries, where breast-feeding also reduces the infant's need to consume potentially contaminated water. In addition to passive immunoprotection, breast milk contains factors which contribute to immune maturation by stimulating the intestinal immune system either directly or via modulating the indigenous intestinal microbiota.

The role of breast milk in reducing the risk of NEC in premature neonates is well established.[80] This effect may partially be mediated by TGF-β, which is present in colostrum in significant amounts. TGF-β has been shown to attenuate intestinal epithelial cell inflammatory responses associated with the development of NEC.[81] Increased gut permeability during the first days of life may increase the risk of NEC. Breast-feeding has been shown to improve the intestinal barrier in the neonatal period as assessed by the absorption of macromolecules in a rabbit model and TGF-β is known to enhance intestinal repair.[82,83]

The long-term immunological consequences of breast-feeding have most thoroughly been investigated in the context of immunologically mediated diseases such as asthma and atopic disease. The epidemiological data on the subject are somewhat discrepant, which may be explained by differences in breast milk composition between individuals which in turn may partially result from hereditary factors predisposing to atopic disease. Nonetheless, a report from a prospective birth cohort study of more than 2,000 children in Australia indicates that the duration of exclusive breast-feeding is associated with a reduced risk of asthma and atopic sensitization.[84] The exact mechanisms through which breast milk enhances immune maturation and thereby protects from the development of immunopathology in infants are not well characterized. It has been demonstrated, however, that low breast milk concentrations of TGF-β or n-3 fatty acids are associated with increased risk of subsequent development of atopic disease.[85,86]

Aberrant Nutritional States and Immune Function

Malnutrition. Malnutrition is still a major burden to child health in large areas of the world. Insufficient intake of energy and protein is often accompanied by deficiency of a variety of vitamins, minerals, and other factors related to host immunophysiology. Indeed, malnutrition is the most common cause of immunodeficiency in children. Long-term deficiency of energy, protein, vitamins, and minerals results in marasmus or nonedematous malnutrition whereas more acute malnutrition, induced by, for example, infection, often leads to an edematous state of malnutrition referred to as kwashiorkor. A combination of the aforementioned states may also be encountered.

The immunological consequences of malnutrition have been investigated in experimental animal models. In addition to reducing growth, energy malnutrition has been observed to result in aberrant intestinal mucin production and severe protein deficiency leads to a drastic decline in intestinal sIgA production in rats.[87,88] According to recent reports, acute malnutrition increases serum concentrations of the regulatory cytokines IL-10 and TGF-β1 as well as IgE and IgG1 antibodies in mice.[89,90]

Children with severe protein and energy malnutrition exhibit pathological small intestinal architecture characterized by villous atrophy.[91,92] Importantly, increased intestinal permeability as assessed using the lactulose–mannose test has been reported even in malnourished individuals without histological intestinal abnormality.[93] The significance of this phenomenon remains to be elucidated but it may be hypothesized that abrogation of the gut barrier may provide a route of entry for pathogens and thus contribute to the heightened risk of infectious disease in malnourished children. The effects of malnutrition on host defense are discussed in detail in Chapter 23, "Malnutrition and Host Defenses." Infection and malnutrition may have overlapping effects on gut immune function in the same individual. However, malnourished children suffering from infections have been observed to have decreased numbers of circulating $CD45^+RO^+$ memory T cells as compared to well-nourished children with similar infections.[94]

In a study conducted by Campbell and colleagues, small bowel biopsies were obtained from 38 Gambian children in different nutritional states and compared to biopsies from 19 children from Britain.[95] Interestingly, all Gambian children regardless of nutritional status exhibited signs of chronic cell-mediated enteropathy with increased intestinal permeability, villous atrophy, crypt hyperplasia, and intraepithelial lymphocytosis characterized by infiltration by $CD25^+$ cells. Malnutrition was associated with reduced numbers of intestinal T and B cells. Moreover, the expression of TGF-β in the intestinal mucosa decreased progressively with a worsening nutritional state suggesting impaired immunoregulation as a result of protein-energy malnutrition.

Total Parenteral Nutrition. Parenteral nutrition is a crucial element in the care of severely ill neonates, infants, and children, as discussed in detail in Chapter 69, "Parenteral Nutrition," but it is also associated with increased risk of infectious complications. While risks related to central venous catheters are likely to explain increased morbidity to some extent, it is also well established that total parenteral nutrition (TPN) may lead to atrophy of intestinal villi and lamina propria, epithelial cell apoptosis, and increased intestinal permeability.[96,97] In addition, a significant reduction in the number of lymphocytes in PPs and the lamina propria as well as intraepithelial lymphocytes is seen as a result of TPN in mice.[98] Both B- and T-cell numbers and lamina propria $CD4^+$ T cells in particular appear to be affected by the lack of enteral nutrition.[99,100] There are data to suggest that the mucosal atrophy resulting from TPN may be reduced by using TPN supplemented with short-chain fatty acids (SCFAs) or glutamine.[101,102] The importance of enteral nutrition or antigenic stimulation to both intestinal microbiota and gut immunophysiology is demonstrated by studies indicating that TPN results in a reduction of both aerobic and anaerobic indigenous bacteria and decreased intestinal concentrations of IgA, IL-4, and IL-10.[100,103,104]

Selected Nutrients

Trace Elements. Zinc is a micronutrient essential to intestinal health. Children suffering from acrodermatitis enteropathica, a condition characterized by severe zinc deficiency resulting from a genetic defect in intestinal zinc transport, manifest with chronic diarrhea and dermatitis.[105] Dietary zinc deficiency leads to increased epithelial permeability due to decreased tight function integrity in the rat intestine.[106] In humans, zinc deficiency has been reported to be associated with increased susceptibility to infections, which suggests a role for zinc in immunophysiology.[107] Indeed, zinc has been observed to be involved in a number of immune functions including T-cell responses and production of antibodies and cytokines.[108,109] Zinc deficiency leads to decreased NF-κB activity and loss of precursor T and B cells in the bone marrow which in turn results in lymphopenia and thymic atrophy.[109,110]

Based on the role of zinc in immunophysiology, it has been hypothesized that zinc supplementation may improve host immunity and that these beneficial effects might extend beyond correcting deficient dietary zinc intake. Zinc supplementation has been shown to accelerate mucosal regeneration, increase intestinal brush border enzymes and secretory antibody concentrations, and enhance cellular immunity.[111] Nonetheless, the role of zinc supplementation in clinical practice has not yet been established. In the developing world, zinc supplementation during diarrheal disease has been reported to reduce the duration and severity of diarrhea and enhance catch-up growth.[112] Contrary to previous studies, however, a recent report from a trial conducted in India failed to show improved recovery from pneumonia by zinc supplementation in hospitalized children less than 2 years of age.[113] Zinc supplementation did not affect growth, development, or infection risk in term breast-fed infants in a study carried out in the United States.[114]

Dietary deficiencies in copper or iron are associated with increased susceptibility to infections.[115,116] Copper deficiency is associated with impaired cell-mediated immunity characterized by defective macrophage activation and cytokine production.[115] Iron deficiency on the other hand has been observed to impair T-cell function and IL-1 production.[117,118] Dietary copper deficiency in infants and children is rare. In contrast, deficiency in iron is not uncommon and it is therefore noteworthy that excessive iron intake, which may result from inappropriate supplementation, may also increase the risk of infectious disease.[119]

Glutamine and Arginine. The nonessential amino acid glutamine influences host immune functions and is critical during catabolic stress.[120] Glutamine is an important nutrient to both enterocytes and immune cells and depletion of glutamine leads to intestinal mucosal damage and atrophy in experimental animals.[121] In human intestinal tissue cultures, glutamine has been reported to reduce the production of the inflammatory cytokines IL-6 and IL-8.[122] There a data to suggest that this reduction in intestinal inflammatory responsiveness is mediated by inhibition of IκBα ubiquitination.[123] As alluded to above, glutamine supplementation has been reported to reverse a number of detrimental consequences of TPN: Experimental animals receiving glutamine-supplemented TPN exhibit improved integrity of the intestinal barrier as well as less impaired IgA and cytokine responses compared to animals receiving conventional TPN.[124–126]

In clinical trials, glutamine-supplemented TPN has been demonstrated to decrease the risk of infectious complications in critically ill patients and after bone-marrow transplantation.[127,128] Two randomized trials with relatively small numbers of subjects have suggested that enteral glutamine supplementation might reduce the risk of septicemia in very low birth weight neonates.[129,130] However, a multicenter trial with 649 very low birth weight neonates found no differences in the occurrence of verified or suspected sepsis in infants receiving enteral glutamine or placebo, nor did parenteral glutamine supplementation reduce mortality in a study of more than 1,400 extremely low birth weight infants.[131,132]

Arginine is a nonessential amino acid which is known to modulate immunophysiology by enhancing proliferation and cytotoxicity of lymphocytes.[133] In an animal model of septic peritonitis, enteral but not parenteral arginine supplementation prior to the onset of disease resulted in significantly improved intestinal immune responses by enhancing IgA and IL-10 secretion.[134] The clinical effects of arginine supplementation are as of present difficult to assess because most trials with nutritional intervention include arginine in combination with other immunomodulatory nutrients. Early enteral nutrition with arginine, fiber, and antioxidant supplementation reduced the risk of catheter-related sepsis but did not reduce mortality in critically ill patients in a Spanish multicenter study.[135] These data are consistent with a meta-analysis of 22 clinical trials, which concluded that commercial nutrition products with high arginine contents are associated with reduced infectious morbidity but do not affect overall mortality.[136]

Vitamins. Vitamin A is required for optimal mucosal immune function. Vitamin A deficiency has been shown to lead to compromised gut barrier function with impaired sIgA and mucus production and increased bacterial translocation.[137–139] The reduced IgA production may in part be explained by data according to which the number of IL-4 and IL-5 producing T cells which induce humoral responses is reduced in the intestine of vitamin A–deficient mice.[140,141] Correcting the deficiency with vitamin A supplementation has been shown to restore both IgA concentrations and mucosal integrity.[141,142]

Children deficient in vitamin A exhibit heightened risk for infections in the gastrointestinal and respiratory tracts. An impressive 20 to 50% reduction in childhood mortality has been reported from developing countries after implementation of large-scale vitamin A supplementation programs.[143] Nonetheless, recent meta-analyses of clinical trials assessing the effects of vitamin A supplementation on infectious disease morbidity or mortality have yielded somewhat contradictory results: One meta-analysis of randomized clinical trials concluded that vitamin A supplementation resulted in a 30% reduction in infant and child mortality whereas three other meta-analyses have failed to find significant reduction in either morbidity or mortality in diarrheal disease or pneumonia.[144–147] There are no convincing data to suggest that vitamin A supplementation beyond correcting a state of deficiency is associated with beneficial enhancement of immune functions.

In addition to its role in maintaining calcium balance, vitamin D has a number of immune regulatory properties. The active form of vitamin D, 1,25-dihydroxyvitamin D_3, modulates Th1 and Th2 cell responses and there are experimental data which indicate that suppression of Th1 responsiveness by vitamin D may ameliorate Th1-mediated autoimmune disease[148] Vitamin D deficiency is associated with increased susceptibility to respiratory tract infections in children and it also appears to be linked to the development of immune-mediated diseases such as IBD.[148,149] However, especially bearing in mind the potential toxicity of vitamin D, there are no data to imply benefit of vitamin D supplementation beyond correcting dietary deficiency.

Vitamin E (α-tocopherol) is a fat-soluble vitamin which scavenges free oxygen radicals. Oral supplementation of a water-soluble vitamin E derivative has been shown to limit chemically induced colitis in rats.[150] In addition, dietary vitamin E has immunomodulatory properties beyond its antioxidant function including effects on lymphocytes and antibody and cytokine production.[151] Vitamin E has been demonstrated to suppress Th2 cytokine responses and IgE production in a murine asthma model.[152] However, supplementation with vitamin E has not been of benefit to patients with allergic rhinitis or asthma in clinical trials.[153,154]

Vitamin C (ascorbic acid) has antioxidant and immunomodulatory effects. Consequently, vitamin C supplementation is widely used to prevent and treat viral infections of the respiratory tract. According to a meta-analysis of clinical trials, however, vitamin C supplementation does not reduce the incidence of common colds in the general population but may reduce the risk of colds in people exposed to heavy physical or cold stress.[155] In addition, a small but consistent beneficial effect on the duration and severity of cold episodes was detectable in individuals using regular vitamin C prophylaxis but the clinical significance of this effect is questionable. Currently existing data do not support the use of vitamin C supplements to enhance immune functions in non-vitamin C–deficient individuals.

Fatty Acids. Fatty acids have a wide array of immunomodulatory effects. Fatty acids from diet and cellular lipids are precursors for a number of immune molecules referred to as eicosanoids, which include prostaglandins, thromboxanes, and leukotrienes.[156] In addition, fatty acids and their metabolites can influence immune cell gene expression by activating PPAR nuclear transcription factors.[157] Polyunsaturated fatty acids (PUFAs) and SCFAs have been most extensively studied with regard to their effects on host immunophysiology.

Both n-3 and n-6 PUFAs bind to PPARs.[158] A diet rich in n-6 PUFA has been reported to increase blood mononuclear cell mitogenic responses, as well as IL-1β and TNF production in vitro, while n-3 PUFA diet was associated with a decrease in the production of these inflammatory cytokines.[159] However, subsequent studies have provided discrepant data regarding the anti-inflammatory effects of n-3 PUFA and the issue is in need of further clarification. In rats, dietary linoleic acid, eicosapentaenoic acid, and docosahexaenoic acid (DHA) inhibit lymphocyte proliferation.[160,161] Eicosapentaenoic acid has also been reported to suppress APC function by reducing the expression of MHC II molecules.[162] SCFAs, on the other hand, have been associated with increased intestinal IL-1β and IL-6 responses in rats receiving TPN.[163] Whether dietary intake of PUFAs above current recommendations offers additional health benefits remains to be elucidated.

FUTURE DIRECTIONS: DIETARY INTERVENTIONS AIMED TO INFLUENCE INTESTINAL IMMUNOPHYSIOLOGY

Probiotics

Probiotics are live microorganisms, which when administered in adequate amounts confer a health benefit to the host.[164] Probiotic effects include degradation of dietary antigens, promotion of mucosal barrier functions, inhibition of mucosal pathogen adherence, and interaction with the innate and adaptive immune systems of the host.[165] In addition to several identified potential targets for probiotic intervention, results from experimental studies and clinical trials suggest future indications for their therapeutic use.

Probiotics may be of benefit in reducing the risk and treatment of infectious disease as a result of the ability to promote mucosal barrier functions, inhibit mucosal pathogen adherence, and modulate host immunophysiology.[165] Two independent meta-analyses of double-blind, placebo-controlled clinical trials have concluded that probiotics are effective in treatment of acute infectious diarrhoea in infants and children.[166,167] According to a recent meta-analysis, probiotics are also effective in reducing the risk of antibiotic-associated diarrhea in children.[168] In addition, there are clinical trials to suggest that *Lactobacillus* GG may also reduce the risk of acute infantile diarrhea in different settings, including nosocomial spread of infection and undernourished children in the developing world.[169,170] The data on the effects of probiotics with regard to respiratory tract infections are more limited. The combination of the probiotics *B. lactis* Bb-12 and *L. reuteri* was not effective in reducing the risk of respiratory tract infections during a 12-week period in a double-blind, placebo-controlled study of 201 infants.[171] A modest reduction in the severity of respiratory tract infections and absence from daycare without significant reduction in the occurrence of infections has been reported using milk supplemented with *L.* GG.[172]

Alterations in the intestinal microbiota composition in infancy precede the development of atopic disease suggesting a causal link between indigenous gut bacteria and the atopic phenotype.[165] Probiotic bacteria have a number of immunological effects which may contribute to reducing the risk and treatment of allergic disease. In experimental studies, probiotics have been observed to suppress IgE responses and Th2 cytokine production and induce T_{reg}s.[165,173] Supplementation with *L.* GG during late pregnancy and lactation has been reported to induce anti-inflammatory mucosal immune responses indicated by an increase in the concentration of TGF-β2 in breast milk.[174] *L.* GG and *B. lactis* Bb-12 supplementation commenced at the time of weaning has been reported to result in increased mucosal cow's milk–specific IgA production and increased serum concentrations of soluble CD14 in infants.[3] Administration of *L. acidophilus,* however, had no effect on cytokine production patterns during the first 6 months of life in a recent study of 230 infants.[175]

Several probiotic strains of lactobacilli have been reported to be effective in the treatment of atopic dermatitis in infants and children, and hypoallergic formula supplemented with *L.* GG has been shown to alleviate symptoms and the intestinal inflammation in infants with CMA and atopic dermatitis.[165] *L.* GG has also shown promising potential in reducing the risk of atopic dermatitis in infants at high hereditary risk for atopic disease. In a double-blind, placebo-controlled clinical trial of 159 pregnant women *L.* GG was administered 2 to 4 weeks prior to expected delivery and the probiotics were subsequently administered to either the breast-feeding mother or the infant until the age of 6 months.[176] Probiotic supplementation reduced the risk of atopic dermatitis in these high-risk infants from 46 to 23% during the first 2 years of life and this protective effect has subsequently been reported to extend to the age of 4 years.[177] These results need to be confirmed by larger studies before practical recommendations on the use of probiotics in prevention or treatment of atopic disease can be given.

The pathogenesis of NEC, albeit largely not yet clarified, involves increased gut permeability combined with enteral feeding and altered intestinal microbiota composition.[178,179] Consequently, probiotics might be suggested to reduce the risk of developing NEC by promoting gut barrier function and inhibiting colonization by potentially pathogenic bacteria. A significant reduction in NEC occurrence has been reported from a neonatal intensive care unit in Colombia after supplementation of infants in the unit with the probiotics *L. acidophilus* and *B. infantis* was commenced.[180] Subsequently, two randomized, placebo-controlled trials using different probiotic combinations have also found significantly reduced incidence of NEC compared to placebo whereas in one multicenter study *L.* GG offered no beneficial effect on the incidence of NEC, bacterial sepsis, or urinary tract infections.[181–183]

IBD is characterized by mucosal inflammation as a result of detrimental immune reactivity toward indigenous intestinal microbes. Thus modulating the composition of either intestinal microbiota or mucosal immune responses by probiotics might provide a means to treat or even prevent IBD. *L.* GG has been shown to enhance intestinal IgA production in patients with Crohn's disease.[184] A probiotic strain of *E. coli* is effective in maintaining remission in patients with UC and the probiotic combination VSL#3 (containing *L. casei, L. plantarum, L. acidophilus, L. delbrueckii* subsp. *bulgaricus, B. longum, B. breve, B. infantis,* and *Streptococcus salivarius subsp. thermophilus*) has recently been shown to induce remission in mild-to-moderate UC.[185,186] VSL#3 has also been demonstrated to be effective in prevention of acute pouchitis, a nonspecific inflammation of the ileal reservoir.[187] Furthermore, VSL#3 reduces the risk of recurrence of chronic pouchitis.[188,189] These beneficial effects might be the result of induction of tolerogenic immune responses as administration of VSL#3 resulted in a significant increase in IL-10 in biopsies from patients with pouchitis.[190]

Prebiotics

Nondigestible food ingredients that beneficially affect the host by selectively stimulating the growth or activity of intestinal bacteria and thus promote host health are referred to as prebiotics.[191] The most commonly used prebiotics include lactulose, inulin, and oligosaccharides such as fructo-oligosaccharides (FOSs) and galacto-oligosaccharides (GOSs). The effects of prebiotic oligosaccharides in promoting bifidobacteria in the intestinal microbiota of infants have been demonstrated in a number of double-blind, placebo-controlled trials.[192–195] In addition to the stimulating effect on the growth of bifidobacteria, infant formula supplemented with GOS and FOS has been reported to result in intestinal microbial metabolic activity closer to that observed in breast-fed infants compared to infants fed unsupplemented formula.[195] Interestingly, prebiotics may also modulate nutrient intake as demonstrated by a study according to which administration of an inulin-type fructan to adolescents significantly increased calcium absorption and bone mineralization during pubertal growth.[196]

There are limited published data regarding the immunological effects of prebiotics to date. No immunological effects, including no changes in serum immunoglobulin or sIgA concentrations or IL-4 and IFN-γ secretion by monocytes in vitro, were detected in a study assessing the effects of a mixture of prebiotic raftilose and raftiline in elderly people.[197] Infant cereal supplemented with FOS appeared to have no effect of *Haemophilus influenzae* B vaccination responses nor did it reduce the risk of diarrheal disease in a study conducted in Peru.[198] Given the epidemiological link between intestinal microbiota composition and the development of atopic disease, prebiotics have been hypothesized to be of benefit in reducing the risk and treatment of atopic disorders. Recently surfaced data from a randomized, double-blind, placebo-controlled trial of 259 infants indeed indicate that hypoallergic formula supplemented with GOS/FOS may reduce the risk of atopic dermatitis in high-risk infants.[199] In addition, prebiotics have been reported to improve the skin condition of children with atopic dermatitis.[200] These data regarding reducing the risk or treatment of atopic disease are preliminary and need to be confirmed by future trials.

CONCLUSIONS

In this chapter, an overview of the interactions between dietary factors, the intestinal immune system, and the indigenous gut microbiota in health and disease has been provided. Nutrients affect mucosal and systemic immune functions and the gut microbiota. General malnutrition or lack of certain nutrients may result in immunodeficiency predisposing to infectious disease. Indigenous intestinal microbes process dietary antigens and contribute to gut immune homeostasis by excluding pathogens and providing maturational and modulatory stimuli. The intestinal immune system constantly monitors intestinal antigens. Protective immune defenses are launched against potential pathogens, while a number of active processes ensure tolerance toward dietary antigens and the microbiota. Abrogation of this tolerance may result in food hypersensitivity reactions or IBD. Recent advances in understanding the mechanistic basis of these interactions provide means to design specific interventions to restore intestinal homeostasis by supplementation of immunomodulatory nutrients or pre- or probiotics. It is to be hoped that these novel therapeutic and preventive modalities will be refined by basic research on more detailed mechanisms on the molecular level and coordinated rigorously conducted clinical trials in the coming years.

REFERENCES

1. Delves PJ, Roitt IM. The immune system: First of two parts. N Engl J Med 2000;343:37–49.
2. Lauener RP, Birchler T, Adamski J, et al. Expression of CD14 and Toll-like receptor 2 in farmers' and non-farmers' children. Lancet 2002;360:465–6.
3. Rautava S, Arvilommi H, Isolauri E. Specific probiotics in enhancing maturation of IgA responses in formula-fed infants. Pediatr Res 2006;60:221–4.
4. Schnare M, Barton GM, Holt AC, et al. Toll-like receptors control activation of adaptive immune responses. Nat Immunol 2001;2:947–50.
5. Pasare C, Medzhitov R. Toll pathway-dependent blockade of CD4+CD25+ T cell-mediated suppression by dendritic cells. Science 2003;299:1033–6.
6. MacDonald T, Miller R. Phylogeny of the gut-associated lymphoid tissue (GALT). In: Mestecky J, Lamm M, Strober W, Bienenstock J, McGhee J, Mayer L, editors. Mucosal Immunology, 3rd edition. Boston: Elsevier Academic Press; 2005. p. 323–34.
7. Sanderson IR, Walker WA. Uptake and transport of macromolecules by the intestine: Possible role in clinical disorders (an update). Gastroenterology 1993;104:622–39.
8. Malin M, Isolauri E, Pikkarainen P, et al. Enhanced absorption of macromolecules: A secondary factor in Crohn's disease. Dig Dis Sci 1996;41:1423–8.
9. Israel EJ. Neonatal necrotizing enterocolitis, a disease of the immature intestinal mucosal barrier. Acta Paediatr Suppl 1994;396:27–32.
10. Rechkemmer G, Wahl M, Kuschinsky W, von Engelhardt W. pH-microclimate at the luminal surface of the intestinal mucosa of guinea pig and rat. Pflugers Arch 1986;407:33–40.
11. Walker WA, Isselbacher KJ, Bloch KJ. Intestinal uptake of macromolecules: Effect of oral immunization. Science 1972;177:608–10.
12. Gryboski JD, Kocoshis S. Immunoglobulin deficiency in gastrointestinal allergies. J Clin Gastroenterol 1980;2:71–6.
13. O'Mahony S, Arranz E, Barton JR, Ferguson A. Dissociation between systemic and mucosal humoral immune responses in coeliac disease. Gut 1991;32:29–35.
14. Cone R. Mucus. In: Mestecky J, Lamm M, Strober W, Bienenstock J, McGhee J, Mayer L, editors. Mucosal Immunology, 3rd edition. Boston: Elsevier Academic Press; 2005. p. 49–72.
15. Phillips AD, France NE, Walker-Smith JA. The structure of the enterocyte in relation to its position on the villus in childhood: An electron microscopical study. Histopathology 1979;3:117–30.
16. Diebel LN, Liberati DM, Baylor AE, III, et al. The pivotal role of tumor necrosis factor-alpha in signaling apoptosis in intestinal epithelial cells under shock conditions. J Trauma 2005;58:995–1001.
17. Planchon SM, Martins CA, Guerrant RL, Roche JK. Regulation of intestinal epithelial barrier function by TGF-beta 1: Evidence for its role in abrogating the effect of a T cell cytokine. J Immunol 199415;153:5730–9.
18. Kaisho T, Akira S. Toll-like receptor function and signaling. J Allergy Clin Immunol 2006;117:979–87.
19. Zhang G, Ghosh S. Toll-like receptor-mediated NF-kappaB activation: A phylogenetically conserved paradigm in innate immunity. J Clin Invest 2001;107:13–9.
20. Cario E, Rosenberg IM, Brandwein SL, et al. Lipopolysaccharide activates distinct signaling pathways in intestinal epithelial cell lines expressing Toll-like receptors. J Immunol 2000;164:966–72.
21. Takeshita F, Leifer CA, Gursel I, et al. Cutting edge: Role of Toll-like receptor 9 in CpG DNA-induced activation of human cells. J Immunol 2001;167:3555–8.
22. Melmed G, Thomas LS, Lee N, et al. Human intestinal epithelial cells are broadly unresponsive to Toll-like receptor 2-dependent bacterial ligands: Implications for host-microbial interactions in the gut. J Immunol 2003;170:1406–15.
23. Hausmann M, Kiessling S, Mestermann S, et al. Toll-like receptors 2 and 4 are up-regulated during intestinal inflammation. Gastroenterology 2002;122:1987–2000.
24. Otte JM, Cario E, Podolsky DK. Mechanisms of cross hyporesponsiveness to Toll-like receptor bacterial ligands in intestinal epithelial cells. Gastroenterology 2004;126:1054–70.
25. Hart AL, Al-Hassi HO, Rigby RJ, et al. Characteristics of intestinal dendritic cells in inflammatory bowel diseases. Gastroenterology 2005;129:50–65.
26. Cario E. Bacterial interactions with cells of the intestinal mucosa: Toll-like receptors and NOD2. Gut 2005;54:1182–93.
27. O'Neill LA, Fitzgerald KA, Bowie AG. The Toll-IL-1 receptor adaptor family grows to five members. Trends Immunol 2003;24:286–90.
28. Haller D, Jobin C. Interaction between resident luminal bacteria and the host: Can a healthy relationship turn sour? J Pediatr Gastroenterol Nutr 2004;38:123–36.
29. Inohara N, Ogura Y, Fontalba A, et al. Host recognition of bacterial muramyl dipeptide mediated through NOD2. Implications for Crohn's disease. J Biol Chem 200321;278:5509–12.
30. Girardin SE, Boneca IG, Carneiro LA, et al. Nod1 detects a unique muropeptide from gram-negative bacterial peptidoglycan. Science 2003;300:1584–7.
31. Chin AI, Dempsey PW, Bruhn K, et al. Involvement of receptor-interacting protein 2 in innate and adaptive immune responses. Nature 2002;416:190–4.
32. Gronlund MM, Lehtonen OP, Eerola E, Kero P. Fecal microflora in healthy infants born by different methods of delivery: Permanent changes in intestinal flora after cesarean delivery. J Pediatr Gastroenterol Nutr 1999;28:19–25.
33. Negele K, Heinrich J, Borte M, et al. Mode of delivery and development of atopic disease during the first 2 years of life. Pediatr Allergy Immunol 2004;15:48–54.
34. Harmsen HJ, Wildeboer-Veloo AC, Raangs GC, et al. Analysis of intestinal flora development in breast-fed and formula-fed infants by using molecular identification and detection methods. J Pediatr Gastroenterol Nutr 2000;30:61–7.
35. Hooper LV. Bacterial contributions to mammalian gut development. Trends Microbiol 2004;12:129–34.
36. Macpherson AJ, Harris NL. Interactions between commensal intestinal bacteria and the immune system. Nat Rev Immunol 2004;4:478–85.
37. Hooper LV, Wong MH, Thelin A, et al. Molecular analysis of commensal host-microbial relationships in the intestine. Science 2001;291:881–4.
38. Mazmanian SK, Liu CH, Tzianabos AO, Kasper DL. An immunomodulatory molecule of symbiotic bacteria directs maturation of the host immune system. Cell 2005;122:107–18.
39. Neish AS, Gewirtz AT, Zeng H, et al. Prokaryotic regulation of epithelial responses by inhibition of IkappaB-alpha ubiquitination. Science 2000;289:1560–3.
40. Ruiz PA, Hoffmann M, Szcesny S, et al. Innate mechanisms for Bifidobacterium lactic to activate transient pro-inflammatory host responses in intestinal epithelial cells after the colonization of germ-free rats. Immunology 2005;115:441–50.
41. Rakoff-Nahoum S, Paglino J, Eslami-Varzaneh F, et al. Recognition of commensal microflora by toll-like receptors is required for intestinal homeostasis. Cell 2004;118:229–41.
42. Macpherson AJ, Uhr T. Induction of protective IgA by intestinal dendritic cells carrying commensal bacteria. Science 2004;303:1662–5.
43. Sutas Y, Hurme M, Isolauri E. Down-regulation of anti-CD3 antibody-induced IL-4 production by bovine caseins hydrolysed with Lactobacillus GG-derived enzymes. Scand J Immunol 1996;43:687–9.
44. Sutas Y, Soppi E, Korhonen H, et al. Suppression of lymphocyte proliferation in vitro by bovine caseins hydrolyzed with Lactobacillus casei GG-derived enzymes. J Allergy Clin Immunol 1996;98:216–24.
45. Mowat AM. Anatomical basis of tolerance and immunity to intestinal antigens. Nat Rev Immunol 2003;3:331–41.
46. Chabot S, Wagner JS, Farrant S, et al. TLRs regulate the gatekeeping functions of the intestinal follicle-associated epithelium. J Immunol 2006;176:4275–83.
47. Rescigno M, Urbano M, Valzasina B, et al. Dendritic cells express tight junction proteins and penetrate gut epithelial monolayers to sample bacteria. Nat Immunol 2001;2:361–7.
48. Niess JH, Reinecker HC. Dendritic cells: The commanders-in-chief of mucosal immune defenses. Curr Opin Gastroenterol 2006;22:354–60.
49. Romagnani S. Th1 and Th2 in human diseases. Clin Immunol Immunopathol 1996;80:225–35.
50. Beyer K, Castro R, Birnbaum A, et al. Human milk-specific mucosal lymphocytes of the gastrointestinal tract display a TH2 cytokine profile. J Allergy Clin Immunol 2002;109:707–13.
51. Xu-Amano J, Aicher WK, Taguchi T, et al. Selective induction of Th2 cells in murine Peyer's patches by oral immunization. Int Immunol 1992;4:433–45.
52. Monteleone G, Holloway J, Salvati VM, et al. Activated STAT4 and a functional role for IL-12 in human Peyer's patches. J Immunol 2003;170:300–7.
53. Nagata S, McKenzie C, Pender SL, et al. Human Peyer's patch T cells are sensitized to dietary antigen and display a Th cell type 1 cytokine profile. J Immunol 2000;165:5315–21.
54. Delves PJ, Roitt IM. The immune system: Second of two parts. N Engl J Med 2000;343:108–17.
55. Menezes Jda S, Mucida DS, Cara DC, et al. Stimulation by food proteins plays a critical role in the maturation of the immune system. Int Immunol 2003;15:447–55.
56. Weiner HL. Oral tolerance: Immune mechanisms and the generation of Th3-type TGF-beta-secreting regulatory cells. Microbes Infect 2001;3:947–54.
57. Mowat AM, Faria AMC, Weiner HL. Oral tolerance: Physiologic basis and clinical applications. In: Mestecky J, Lamm ME, Strober W, Bienenstock J, McGhee JR, Mayer L, editors. Mucosal Immunology, 3rd edition. Boston: Elsevier Academic Press; 2005. p. 487–537.
58. Duchmann R, Kaiser I, Hermann E, et al. Tolerance exists towards resident intestinal flora but is broken in active inflammatory bowel disease (IBD). Clin Exp Immunol 1995;102:448–55.
59. Iweala OI, Nagler CR. Immune privilege in the gut: The establishment and maintenance of non-responsiveness to dietary antigens and commensal flora. Immunol Rev 2006;213:82–100.
60. Sudo N, Sawamura S, Tanaka K, et al. The requirement of intestinal bacterial flora for the development of an IgE production system fully susceptible to oral tolerance induction. J Immunol 1997;159:1739–45.
61. Wannemuehler MJ, Kiyono H, Babb JL, et al. Lipopolysaccharide (LPS) regulation of the immune response: LPS converts germfree mice to sensitivity to oral tolerance induction. J Immunol 1982;129:959–65.
62. Moseman EA, Liang X, Dawson AJ, et al. Human plasmacytoid dendritic cells activated by CpG oligodeoxynucleotides induce the generation of CD4+CD25+ regulatory T cells. J Immunol 2004;173:4433–42.

63. Zanin-Zhorov A, Cahalon L, Tal G, et al. Heat shock protein 60 enhances CD4+ CD25+ regulatory T cell function via innate TLR2 signaling. J Clin Invest 2006;116:2022–32.
64. Strauch UG, Obermeier F, Grunwald N, et al. Influence of intestinal bacteria on induction of regulatory T cells: Lessons from a transfer model of colitis. Gut 2005;54:1546–52.
65. Chen Y, Inobe J, Marks R, et al. Peripheral deletion of antigen-reactive T cells in oral tolerance. Nature 1995;376:177–80.
66. Schwartz RH. T cell anergy. Annu Rev Immunol 2003;21:305–34.
67. Umetsu DT, Akbari O, Dekruyff RH. Regulatory T cells control the development of allergic disease and asthma [quiz 8]. J Allergy Clin Immunol 2003;112:480–7.
68. Nakamura K, Kitani A, Fuss I, et al. TGF-beta 1 plays an important role in the mechanism of CD4+CD25+ regulatory T cell activity in both humans and mice. J Immunol 2004;172:834–42.
69. Oida T, Xu L, Weiner HL, et al. TGF-beta-mediated suppression by CD4+CD25+ T cells is facilitated by CTLA-4 signaling. J Immunol 2006;177:2331–9.
70. Chen Y, Inobe J, Kuchroo VK, et al. Oral tolerance in myelin basic protein T-cell receptor transgenic mice: Suppression of autoimmune encephalomyelitis and dose-dependent induction of regulatory cells. Proc Natl Acad Sci U S A 1996;93:388–91.
71. Fukaura H, Kent SC, Pietrusewicz MJ, et al. Induction of circulating myelin basic protein and proteolipid protein-specific transforming growth factor-beta1-secreting Th3 T cells by oral administration of myelin in multiple sclerosis patients. J Clin Invest 1996;98:70–7.
72. Chen W, Jin W, Hardegen N, et al. Conversion of peripheral CD4+CD25− naive T cells to CD4+CD25+ regulatory T cells by TGF-beta induction of transcription factor Foxp3. J Exp Med 2003;198:1875–86.
73. Hauet-Broere F, Unger WW, Garssen J, et al. Functional CD25- and CD25+ mucosal regulatory T cells are induced in gut-draining lymphoid tissue within 48 h after oral antigen application. Eur J Immunol 2003;33:2801–10.
74. Zhang X, Izikson L, Liu L, Weiner HL. Activation of CD25(+)CD4(+) regulatory T cells by oral antigen administration. J Immunol 2001;167:4245–53.
75. Nagatani K, Sagawa K, Komagata Y, Yamamoto K. Peyer's patch dendritic cells capturing oral antigen interact with antigen-specific T cells and induce gut-homing CD4(+)CD25(+) regulatory T cells in Peyer's patches. Ann N Y Acad Sci 2004;1029:366–70.
76. Tiemessen MM, Van Ieperen-Van Dijk AG, Bruijnzeel-Koomen CA, et al. Cow's milk-specific T-cell reactivity of children with and without persistent cow's milk allergy: Key role for IL-10. J Allergy Clin Immunol 2004;113:932–9.
77. Perez-Machado MA, Ashwood P, Thomson MA, et al. Reduced transforming growth factor-beta1-producing T cells in the duodenal mucosa of children with food allergy. Eur J Immunol 2003;33:2307–15.
78. Karlsson MR, Rugtveit J, Brandtzaeg P. Allergen-responsive CD4+CD25+ regulatory T cells in children who have outgrown cow's milk allergy. J Exp Med 2004;199:1679–88.
79. Tiemessen MM, Van Hoffen E, Knulst AC, et al. CD4 CD25 regulatory T cells are not functionally impaired in adult patients with IgE-mediated cow's milk allergy. J Allergy Clin Immunol 2002;110:934–6.
80. Updegrove K. Necrotizing enterocolitis: The evidence for use of human milk in prevention and treatment. J Hum Lact 2004;20:335–9.
81. Claud EC, Savidge T, Walker WA. Modulation of human intestinal epithelial cell IL-8 secretion by human milk factors. Pediatr Res 2003;53:419–25.
82. Bernt KM, Walker WA. Human milk as a carrier of biochemical messages. Acta Paediatr Suppl 1999;88:27–41.
83. Udall JN, Colony P, Fritze L, et al. Development of gastrointestinal mucosal barrier. II. The effect of natural versus artificial feeding on intestinal permeability to macromolecules. Pediatr Res 1981;15:245–9.
84. Oddy WH, Sherriff JL, de Klerk NH, et al. The relation of breastfeeding and body mass index to asthma and atopy in children: A prospective cohort study to age 6 years. Am J Public Health 2004;94:1531–7.
85. Kalliomaki M, Ouwehand A, Arvilommi H, et al. Transforming growth factor-beta in breast milk: A potential regulator of atopic disease at an early age. J Allergy Clin Immunol 1999;104:1251–7.
86. Hoppu U, Rinne M, Lampi AM, Isolauri E. Breast milk fatty acid composition is associated with development of atopic dermatitis in the infant. J Pediatr Gastroenterol Nutr 2005;41:335–8.
87. Sherman P, Forstner J, Roomi N, et al. Mucin depletion in the intestine of malnourished rats. Am J Physiol 1985;248: G418–23.
88. Sullivan DA, Vaerman JP, Soo C. Influence of severe protein malnutrition on rat lacrimal, salivary and gastrointestinal immune expression during development, adulthood and ageing. Immunology 1993;78:308–17.
89. Hillyer L, Dao B, Niemiec P, et al. Elevated bioactivity of the tolerogenic cytokines, interleukin-10 and transforming growth factor-beta, in the blood of acutely malnourished weanling mice. Exp Biol Med (Maywood) 2006;231:1439–47.
90. Neyestani TR, Woodward B. Blood concentrations of Th2-type immunoglobulins are selectively increased in weanling mice subjected to acute malnutrition. Exp Biol Med (Maywood) 2005;230:128–34.
91. Stanfield JP, Hutt MS, Tunnicliffe R. Intestinal biopsy in kwashiorkor. Lancet 1965;2:519–23.
92. Schneider RE, Viteri FE. Morphological aspects of the duodenojejunal mucosa in protein-calorie malnourished children and during recovery. Am J Clin Nutr 1972;25:1092–102.
93. Welsh FK, Farmery SM, MacLennan K, et al. Gut barrier function in malnourished patients. Gut 1998;42:396–401.
94. Najera O, Gonzalez C, Toledo G, et al. CD45RA and CD45RO isoforms in infected malnourished and infected well-nourished children. Clin Exp Immunol 2001;126:461–5.
95. Campbell DI, Murch SH, Elia M, et al. Chronic T cell-mediated enteropathy in rural west African children: Relationship with nutritional status and small bowel function. Pediatr Res 2003;54:306–11.
96. Rossi TM, Lee PC, Young C, Tjota A. Small intestinal mucosa changes, including epithelial cell proliferative activity, of children receiving total parenteral nutrition (TPN). Dig Dis Sci 1993;38:1608–13.
97. Sun X, Spencer AU, Yang H, Haxhija EQ, Teitelbaum DH. Impact of caloric intake on parenteral nutrition-associated intestinal morphology and mucosal barrier function. JPEN J Parenter Enteral Nutr 2006;30:474–9.
98. Kiristioglu I, Antony P, Fan Y, et al. Total parenteral nutrition-associated changes in mouse intestinal intraepithelial lymphocytes. Dig Dis Sci 2002;47:1147–57.
99. King BK, Li J, Kudsk KA. A temporal study of TPN-induced changes in gut-associated lymphoid tissue and mucosal immunity. Arch Surg 1997;132:1303–9.
100. Li J, Kudsk KA, Gocinski B, et al. Effects of parenteral and enteral nutrition on gut-associated lymphoid tissue [discussion-2]. J Trauma 1995;39:44–51.
101. Koruda MJ, Rolandelli RH, Settle RG, et al. Effect of parenteral nutrition supplemented with short-chain fatty acids on adaptation to massive small bowel resection. Gastroenterology 1988;95:715–20.
102. O'Dwyer ST, Smith RJ, Hwang TL, Wilmore DW. Maintenance of small bowel mucosa with glutamine-enriched parenteral nutrition. JPEN J Parenter Enteral Nutr 1989;13:579–85.
103. Schneider SM, Le Gall P, Girard-Pipau F, et al. Total artificial nutrition is associated with major changes in the fecal flora. Eur J Nutr 2000;39:248–55.
104. Fukatsu K, Kudsk KA, Zarzaur BL, et al. TPN decreases IL-4 and IL-10 mRNA expression in lipopolysaccharide stimulated intestinal lamina propria cells but glutamine supplementation preserves the expression. Shock 2001;15:318–22.
105. -Riveros C, Franca LF, Alves AC, Sanches JA, Jr. Acrodermatitis enteropathica: Case report and review of the literature. Pediatr Dermatol 2002;19:426–31.
106. Moran JR, Lewis JC. The effects of severe zinc deficiency on intestinal permeability: An ultrastructural study. Pediatr Res 1985;19:968–73.
107. Prasad AS, Miale A, Jr, Farid Z, et al. Zinc metabolism in patients with the syndrome of iron deficiency anemia, hepatosplenomegaly, dwarfism, and hypogonadism. J Lab Clin Med 1963;61:537–49.
108. Shi HN, Scott ME, Stevenson MM, Koski KG. Zinc deficiency impairs T cell function in mice with primary infection of Heligmosomoides polygyrus (Nematoda). Parasite Immunol 1994;16:339–50.
109. Fraker PJ, King LE, Laakko T, Vollmer TL. The dynamic link between the integrity of the immune system and zinc status. J Nutr 2000;130:1399S–406S.
110. Prasad AS. Effects of zinc deficiency on Th1 and Th2 cytokine shifts. J Infect Dis 2000;182:S62–8.
111. Folwaczny C. Zinc and diarrhea in infants. J Trace Elem Med Biol 1997;11:116–22.
112. Sazawal S, Black RE, Bhan MK, et al. Zinc supplementation in young children with acute diarrhea in India. N Engl J Med 1995;333:839–44.
113. Bose A, Coles CL, Gunavathi, John H, et al. Efficacy of zinc in the treatment of severe pneumonia in hospitalized children <2 y old. Am J Clin Nutr 2006;83:1089–96.
114. Heinig MJ, Brown KH, Lonnerdal B, Dewey KG. Zinc supplementation does not affect growth, morbidity, or motor development of US term breastfed infants at 4–10 mo of age. Am J Clin Nutr 2006;84:594–601.
115. Prohaska JR, Lukasewycz OA. Effects of copper deficiency on the immune system. Adv Exp Med Biol 1990;262:123–43.
116. Bondestam M, Foucard T, Gebre-Medhin M. Subclinical trace element deficiency in children with undue susceptibility to infections. Acta Paediatr Scand 1985;74:515–20.
117. Krantman HJ, Young SR, Ank BJ, et al. Immune function in pure iron deficiency. Am J Dis Child 1982;136:840–4.
118. Helyar L, Sherman AR. Iron deficiency and interleukin 1 production by rat leukocytes. Am J Clin Nutr 1987;46:346–52.
119. Murray MJ, Murray AB, Murray MB, Murray CJ. The adverse effect of iron repletion on the course of certain infections. BMJ 1978;2:1113–5.
120. McNurlan MA, Garlick PJ. Protein and amino acids in nutritional support. Crit Care Clin 1995;11:635–50.
121. Baskerville A, Hambleton P, Benbough JE. Pathological features of glutaminase toxicity. Br J Exp Pathol 1980;61:132–8.
122. Coeffier M, Miralles-Barrachina O, Le Pessot F, et al. Influence of glutamine on cytokine production by human gut in vitro. Cytokine 2001;13:148–54.
123. Hubert-Buron A, Leblond J, Jacquot A, et al. Glutamine pretreatment reduces IL-8 production in human intestinal epithelial cells by limiting IkappaBalpha ubiquitination. J Nutr 2006;136:1461–5.
124. Li J, Kudsk KA, Janu P, Renegar KB. Effect of glutamine-enriched total parenteral nutrition on small intestinal gut-associated lymphoid tissue and upper respiratory tract immunity. Surgery 1997;121:542–9.
125. Kudsk KA, Wu Y, Fukatsu K, et al. Glutamine-enriched total parenteral nutrition maintains intestinal interleukin-4 and mucosal immunoglobulin A levels [discussion 4–5]. JPEN J Parenter Enteral Nutr 2000;24:270–4.
126. Khan J, Iiboshi Y, Cui L, et al. Alanyl-glutamine-supplemented parenteral nutrition increases luminal mucus gel and decreases permeability in the rat small intestine. JPEN J Parenter Enteral Nutr 1999;23:24–31.
127. Dechelotte P, Hasselmann M, Cynober L, et al. L-alanyl-L-glutamine dipeptide-supplemented total parenteral nutrition reduces infectious complications and glucose intolerance in critically ill patients: The French controlled, randomized, double-blind, multicenter study. Crit Care Med 2006;34:598–604.
128. Ziegler TR, Young LS, Benfell K, et al. Clinical and metabolic efficacy of glutamine-supplemented parenteral nutrition after bone marrow transplantation: A randomized, double-blind, controlled study. Ann Intern Med 1992 ;116:821–8.
129. Neu J, Roig JC, Meetze WH, et al. Enteral glutamine supplementation for very low birth weight infants decreases morbidity. J Pediatr 1997;131:691–9.
130. van den Berg A, van Elburg RM, Teerlink T, et al. A randomized controlled trial of enteral glutamine supplementation in very low birth weight infants: Plasma amino acid concentrations. J Pediatr Gastroenterol Nutr 2005;41:66–71.
131. Vaughn P, Thomas P, Clark R, Neu J. Enteral glutamine supplementation and morbidity in low birth weight infants. J Pediatr 2003;142:662–8.
132. Poindexter BB, Ehrenkranz RA, Stoll BJ, et al. Effect of parenteral glutamine supplementation on plasma amino acid concentrations in extremely low-birth-weight infants. Am J Clin Nutr 2003;77:737–43.
133. Suchner U, Heyland DK, Peter K. Immune-modulatory actions of arginine in the critically ill. Br J Nutr 2002;87:S121–32.
134. Shang HF, Wang YY, Lai YN, et al. Effects of arginine supplementation on mucosal immunity in rats with septic peritonitis. Clin Nutr 2004;23:561–9.
135. Caparros T, Lopez J, Grau T. Early enteral nutrition in critically ill patients with a high-protein diet enriched with arginine, fiber, and antioxidants compared with a standard high-protein diet. The effect on nosocomial infections and outcome [discussion-9]. JPEN J Parenter Enteral Nutr 2001;25:299–308.
136. Heyland DK, Novak F, Drover JW, et al. Should immunonutrition become routine in critically ill patients? A systematic review of the evidence. JAMA 2001;286:944–53.
137. Wiedermann U, Hanson LA, Holmgren J, et al. Impaired mucosal antibody response to cholera toxin in vitamin A-deficient rats immunized with oral cholera vaccine. Infect Immun 1993;61:3952–7.
138. Stephensen CB. Vitamin A, infection, and immune function. Annu Rev Nutr 2001;21:167–92.
139. Wiedermann U, Hanson LA, Bremell T, et al. Increased translocation of *Escherichia coli* and development of arthritis in vitamin A-deficient rats. Infect Immun 1995;63:3062–8.
140. Carman JA, Smith SM, Hayes CE. Characterization of a helper T lymphocyte defect in vitamin A-deficient mice. J Immunol 1989;142:388–93.
141. Nikawa T, Odahara K, Koizumi H, et al. Vitamin A prevents the decline in immunoglobulin A and Th2 cytokine levels in small intestinal mucosa of protein-malnourished mice. J Nutr 1999;129:934–41.
142. Thurnham DI, Northrop-Clewes CA, McCullough FS, et al. Innate immunity, gut integrity, and vitamin A in Gambian and Indian infants. J Infect Dis 2000;182:S23–8.

143. Humphrey JH, West KP, Jr, Sommer A. Vitamin A deficiency and attributable mortality among under-5-year-olds. Bull World Health Organ 1992;70225–32.
144. Fawzi WW, Chalmers TC, Herrera MG, Mosteller F. Vitamin A supplementation and child mortality: A meta-analysis. JAMA 1993;269:898–903.
145. Grotto I, Mimouni M, Gdalevich M, Mimouni D. Vitamin A supplementation and childhood morbidity from diarrhea and respiratory infections: A meta-analysis. J Pediatr 2003;142:297–304.
146. Brown N, Roberts C. Vitamin A for acute respiratory infection in developing countries: A meta-analysis. Acta Paediatr 2004;93:1437–42.
147. Ni J, Wei J, Wu T. Vitamin A for non-measles pneumonia in children. Cochrane Database Syst Rev 2005;CD003700.
148. Cantorna MT, Zhu Y, Froicu M, Wittke A. Vitamin D status, 1,25-dihydroxyvitamin D3, and the immune system. Am J Clin Nutr 2004;80:1717S–20S.
149. Wayse V, Yousafzai A, Mogale K, Filteau S. Association of subclinical vitamin D deficiency with severe acute lower respiratory infection in Indian children under 5 y. Eur J Clin Nutr 2004;58:563–7.
150. Isozaki Y, Yoshida N, Kuroda M, et al. Effect of a novel water-soluble vitamin E derivative as a cure for TNBS-induced colitis in rats. Int J Mol Med 2006;17:497–502.
151. Gu JY, Wakizono Y, Sunada Y, et al. Dietary effect of tocopherols and tocotrienols on the immune function of spleen and mesenteric lymph node lymphocytes in Brown Norway rats. Biosci Biotechnol Biochem 1999;63:1697–702.
152. Okamoto N, Murata T, Tamai H, et al. Effects of alpha tocopherol and probucol supplements on allergen-induced airway inflammation and hyperresponsiveness in a mouse model of allergic asthma. Int Arch Allergy Immunol 2006;141:172–80.
153. Velazquez BB, Jauregui-Renaud K, Banuelos Arias Adel C, et al. Vitamin E effects on nasal symptoms and serum specific IgE levels in patients with perennial allergic rhinitis. Ann Allergy Asthma Immunol 2006;96:45–50.
154. Pearson PJ, Lewis SA, Britton J, Fogarty A. Vitamin E supplements in asthma: A parallel group randomised placebo controlled trial. Thorax 2004;59:652–6.
155. Douglas RM, Hemila H, D'Souza R, et al. Vitamin C for preventing and treating the common cold. Cochrane Database Syst Rev 2004;CD000980.
156. Fritsche K. Fatty acids as modulators of the immune response. Annu Rev Nutr 2006;26:45–73.
157. Kliewer SA, Sundseth SS, Jones SA, et al. Fatty acids and eicosanoids regulate gene expression through direct interactions with peroxisome proliferator-activated receptors alpha and gamma. Proc Natl Acad Sci U S A 1997;94:4318–23.
158. Xu HE, Lambert MH, Montana VG, et al. Molecular recognition of fatty acids by peroxisome proliferator-activated receptors. Mol Cell 1999;3:397–403.
159. Meydani SN, Lichtenstein AH, Cornwall S, et al. Immunologic effects of national cholesterol education panel step-2 diets with and without fish-derived N-3 fatty acid enrichment. J Clin Invest 1993;92:105–13.
160. Jeffery NM, Cortina M, Newsholme EA, Calder PC. Effects of variations in the proportions of saturated, monounsaturated and polyunsaturated fatty acids in the rat diet on spleen lymphocyte functions. Br J Nutr 1997;77:805–23.
161. Jeffery NM, Newsholme EA, Calder PC. Level of polyunsaturated fatty acids and the n-6 to n-3 polyunsaturated fatty acid ratio in the rat diet alter serum lipid levels and lymphocyte functions. Prostaglandins Leukot Essent Fatty Acids 1997;57:149–60.
162. Hughes DA, Pinder AC. n-3 polyunsaturated fatty acids inhibit the antigen-presenting function of human monocytes. Am J Clin Nutr 2000;71:357S–60S.
163. Milo LA, Reardon KA, Tappenden KA. Effects of short-chain fatty acid-supplemented total parenteral nutrition on intestinal pro-inflammatory cytokine abundance. Dig Dis Sci 2002;47:2049–55.
164. Reid G, Sanders ME, Gaskins HR, et al. New scientific paradigms for probiotics and prebiotics. J Clin Gastroenterol 2003;37:105–18.
165. Rautava S, Kalliomaki M, Isolauri E. New therapeutic strategy for combating the increasing burden of allergic disease: Probiotics-A Nutrition, Allergy, Mucosal Immunology and Intestinal Microbiota (NAMI) Research Group report. J Allergy Clin Immunol 2005;116:31–7.
166. Szajewska H, Mrukowicz JZ. Probiotics in the treatment and prevention of acute infectious diarrhea in infants and children: A systematic review of published randomized, double-blind, placebo-controlled trials. J Pediatr Gastroenterol Nutr 2001;33:S17–25.
167. Van Niel CW, Feudtner C, Garrison MM, Christakis DA. Lactobacillus therapy for acute infectious diarrhea in children: A meta-analysis. Pediatrics 2002;109:678–84.
168. Szajewska H, Ruszczynski M, Radzikowski A. Probiotics in the prevention of antibiotic-associated diarrhea in children: A meta-analysis of randomized controlled trials. J Pediatr 2006;149:367–72.
169. Szajewska H, Kotowska M, Mrukowicz JZ, et al. Efficacy of Lactobacillus GG in prevention of nosocomial diarrhea in infants. J Pediatr 2001;138:361–5.
170. Oberhelman RA, Gilman RH, Sheen P, et al. A placebo-controlled trial of Lactobacillus GG to prevent diarrhea in undernourished Peruvian children. J Pediatr 1999;134:15–20.
171. Weizman Z, Asli G, Alsheikh A. Effect of a probiotic infant formula on infections in child care centers: Comparison of two probiotic agents. Pediatrics 2005;115:5–9.
172. Hatakka K, Savilahti E, Ponka A, et al. Effect of long term consumption of probiotic milk on infections in children attending day care centres: Double blind, randomised trial. BMJ 2001;322:1327.
173. Di Giacinto C, Marinaro M, Sanchez M, et al. Probiotics ameliorate recurrent Th1-mediated murine colitis by inducing IL-10 and IL-10-dependent TGF-beta-bearing regulatory cells. J Immunol 2005;174:3237–46.
174. Rautava S, Kalliomaki M, Isolauri E. Probiotics during pregnancy and breast-feeding might confer immunomodulatory protection against atopic disease in the infant. J Allergy Clin Immunol 2002;109:119–21.
175. Taylor AL, Hale J, Wiltschut J, et al. Effects of probiotic supplementation for the first 6 months of life on allergen- and vaccine-specific immune responses. Clin Exp Allergy 2006;36:1227–35.
176. Kalliomaki M, Salminen S, Arvilommi H, et al. Probiotics in primary prevention of atopic disease: A randomised placebo-controlled trial. Lancet 2001;357:1076–9.
177. Kalliomaki M, Salminen S, Poussa T, et al. Probiotics and prevention of atopic disease: 4-year follow-up of a randomised placebo-controlled trial. Lancet 2003;361:1869–71.
178. Fell JM. Neonatal inflammatory intestinal diseases: Necrotising enterocolitis and allergic colitis. Early Hum Dev 2005;81:117–22.
179. Bennet R, Eriksson M, Nord CE, Zetterstrom R. Fecal bacterial microflora of newborn infants during intensive care management and treatment with five antibiotic regimens. Pediatr Infect Dis 1986;5:533–9.
180. Hoyos AB. Reduced incidence of necrotizing enterocolitis associated with enteral administration of Lactobacillus acidophilus and Bifidobacterium infantis to neonates in an intensive care unit. Int J Infect Dis 1999;3:197–202.
181. Bin-Nun A, Bromiker R, Wilschanski M, et al. Oral probiotics prevent necrotizing enterocolitis in very low birth weight neonates. J Pediatr 2005;147:192–6.
182. Lin HC, Su BH, Chen AC, et al. Oral probiotics reduce the incidence and severity of necrotizing enterocolitis in very low birth weight infants. Pediatrics 2005;115:1–4.
183. Dani C, Biadaioli R, Bertini G, et al. Probiotics feeding in prevention of urinary tract infection, bacterial sepsis and necrotizing enterocolitis in preterm infants. A prospective double-blind study. Biol Neonate 2002;82:103–8.
184. Malin M, Suomalainen H, Saxelin M, Isolauri E. Promotion of IgA immune response in patients with Crohn's disease by oral bacteriotherapy with Lactobacillus GG. Ann Nutr Metab 1996;40:137–45.
185. Rembacken BJ, Snelling AM, Hawkey PM, et al. Non-pathogenic Escherichia coli versus mesalazine for the treatment of ulcerative colitis: A randomised trial. Lancet 1999;354:635–9.
186. Bibiloni R, Fedorak RN, Tannock GW, et al. VSL#3 probiotic-mixture induces remission in patients with active ulcerative colitis. Am J Gastroenterol 2005;100:1539–46.
187. Gionchetti P, Rizzello F, Helwig U, et al. Prophylaxis of pouchitis onset with probiotic therapy: A double-blind, placebo-controlled trial. Gastroenterology 2003;124:1202–9.
188. Gionchetti P, Rizzello F, Venturi A, et al. Oral bacteriotherapy as maintenance treatment in patients with chronic pouchitis: A double-blind, placebo-controlled trial. Gastroenterology 2000;119:305–9.
189. Mimura T, Rizzello F, Helwig U, et al. Once daily high dose probiotic therapy (VSL#3) for maintaining remission in recurrent or refractory pouchitis. Gut 2004;53:108–14.
190. Ulisse S, Gionchetti P, D'Alo S, et al. Expression of cytokines, inducible nitric oxide synthase, and matrix metalloproteinases in pouchitis: Effects of probiotic treatment. Am J Gastroenterol 2001;96:2691–9.
191. Gibson GR, Roberfroid MB. Dietary modulation of the human colonic microbiota: Introducing the concept of prebiotics. J Nutr 1995;125:1401–12.
192. Moro GE, Mosca F, Miniello V, et al. Effects of a new mixture of prebiotics on faecal flora and stools in term infants. Acta Paediatr Suppl 2003;91:77–9.
193. Schmelzle H, Wirth S, Skopnik H, et al. Randomized double-blind study of the nutritional efficacy and bifidogenicity of a new infant formula containing partially hydrolyzed protein, a high beta-palmitic acid level, and nondigestible oligosaccharides. J Pediatr Gastroenterol Nutr 2003;36:343–51.
194. Knol J, Boehm G, Lidestri M, et al. Increase of faecal bifidobacteria due to dietary oligosaccharides induces a reduction of clinically relevant pathogen germs in the faeces of formula-fed preterm infants. Acta Paediatr Suppl 2005;94:31–3.
195. Knol J, Scholtens P, Kafka C, et al. Colon microflora in infants fed formula with galacto- and fructo-oligosaccharides: More like breast-fed infants. J Pediatr Gastroenterol Nutr 2005;40:36–42.
196. Abrams SA, Griffin IJ, Hawthorne KM, et al. A combination of prebiotic short and long-chain inulin-type fructans enhances calcium absorption and bone mineralization in young adolescents. Am J Clin Nutr 2005;82:471–6.
197. Bunout D, Hirsch S, Pia de la Maza M, et al. Effects of prebiotics on the immune response to vaccination in the elderly. JPEN J Parenter Enteral Nutr 2002;26:372–6.
198. Duggan C, Penny ME, Hibberd P, et al. Oligofructose-supplemented infant cereal: 2 randomized, blinded, community-based trials in Peruvian infants. Am J Clin Nutr 2003;77:937–42.
199. Moro G, Arslanoglu S, Stahl B, et al. A mixture of prebiotic oligosaccharides reduces the incidence of atopic dermatitis during the first six months of age. Arch Dis Child 2006;91:814–9.
200. Passeron T, Lacour JP, Fontas E, Ortonne JP. Prebiotics and synbiotics: Two promising approaches for the treatment of atopic dermatitis in children above 2 years. Allergy 2006;61:431–7.

23

Malnutrition and Host Defense

Susanna Cunningham-Rundles, PhD
Aeri Moon, MD
David F. McNeeley, MD, MPHTM

This at least I clearly know: that bread has different effects in the human body according as it is fine or coarse, made of wheat winnowed or unwinnowed, mixed with much or little water, kneed much or not at all, baked thoroughly or underbaked—and a thousand other differences besides. If one fails to consider these points or having considered does not understand them, how can he know anything about human disease?

—Hippocrates, 460–377 BC,[1]

INTRODUCTION

The vital importance of nutrition in host defense has been recognized since the time of Hippocrates,[1] well before the appearance of the germ theory of infection in the nineteenth century.[2] Although traceable in origin to Metchnikoff[3] and the cell theory, immunology in its present form emerged in the 1960s,[4] when the morbidity of protein-calorie malnutrition (PCM) in children was also first characterized as a "thymolymphatic deficiency."[5] This concept is valid today.[6] Furthermore, there are indications that lesser degrees of perinatal nutrient insufficiency lead to reduced thymic function and reduced response to polysaccharide immunization in later life.[7,8] The central mechanism of nutrient interaction in the thymus involves zinc deficiency,[9,10] and this is directly associated with decreased host defense.[11] The effects of zinc deficiency are mediated by altered hematopoiesis and involve endocrine and neuroendocrine as well as immune mediators.[12] The selective sensitivity of the thymus to nutritional injury is specifically important to the formative phases of the fetal and neonatal immune system. Programmed involution of the thymus develops gradually over the first decades of life and has been viewed as the inevitable cause of human immune senescence.[13] Recent studies show that functionally active peripheral perivascular space thymic components predominate in adult life, and that regulatory alterations in neuroendocrine-thymus interactions rather than simple loss of thymic tissue mediate reduced T cell function.[13,14] Reduced zinc bioavailablity may be the key to loss of thymic function,[15] and supplementation may be effective in improving related immune responses.[16,17]

Innate immune signal transduction pathways are now appreciated as major regulators of adaptive immunity.[18] In the absence of memory T cells, neonates rely on the developing innate immune system. Recognition of microbes through common pathogen associated molecular patterns by the Toll-like receptor (TLR) system, begins at birth with colonization of the gastrointestinal tract and the priming of immune response through nutrient intake and bacterial cross talk.[19] The weaker response of neonatal monocytes and macrophages to multiple TLR ligands correlates with increased risk of infection.[20] Nutrients and growth factors present in human milk are critical regulators for the development of this system.[21,22] Nutrients also regulate functions of the complement system, and specialized natural killer (NK) cell receptors that distinguish "nonself," "missing-self," and "induced-self" and the TLR system.[23–25] Some edible plant products such as tea, mushrooms, and apples express alkylamines that are recognized by human gamma delta T cells as conserved molecular patterns shared by microbes and this can trigger immune response.[26]

Micronutrients have an important function in protection and restoration of cells and tissues after oxidant-mediated tissue injury, which normally occurs during host defense against infectious agents.[27] The cost of immune activation alone has been shown experimentally to have a measurable effect on survival.[28] Nutrient requirements for immune response or maintenance of host defense physiology may vary with stage of development, during the acute phase of infection or recovery from injury or surgical intervention. Glutamine, arginine, zinc, and vitamin A have been identified as conditional essential dietary nutrients or functional foods, required for immune recovery in selected settings.[29,30] Glutamine supplementation can reduce intestinal permeability and systemic infections in adults[31] and prevented sepsis when given before infection in a rat model of sepsis.[32] However, a trial of enteral supplementation to extremely low-birth-weight babies, who are glutamine deficient, did not reduce incidence of late onset sepsis or mortality.[33] More studies are needed to evaluate potential use in this setting.

Investigation of nutrient immune interaction is increasingly focused on genetic regulation.[34–36] Emerging studies show that genes regulating zinc metabolism affect signal transduction pathways especially those influencing immune response, responses to stress and redox imbalance, growth, and energy utilization.[37] The effects of nutrient level, deficiency or excess, on intestinal gene expression appear to correlate with disease expression as well as with changes in metabolism.[38,39] The discovery that host polymorphisms in the vitamin D receptor regulate immune response to mycobacteria and Hepatitis B[40,41] suggests that other host gene variants controlling nutrient metabolism may also affect response to endemic pathogens due to selection pressure. Dietary deprivation of a single nutrient can affect tissue expression of both genes directly associated with the deficiency and those regulating other nutrients that affect transport or redox balance as shown by the interaction of iron deficiency and copper genes.[39] Experimental malnutrition in the mouse illustrates the complexity of signaling effects. The early effect of multinutrient deprivation was to depress necrosis factor (NF) kappa B activity, which led to lower tumor necrosis factor-alpha (TNF-alpha) proinflammatory cytokine production and then to reduced levels of nitric oxide (NO). Low levels of NO then eliminated the negative feedback signal to NF kappa B activity leading to increased transcription activity in the later phase.[42] Knowledge concerning how nutrients can modify specific stages of the cytokine response program is relevant for the rational design of future supplementation trials.

The effect of malnutrition on clinical infection is to increase severity and morbidity.[43] The mechanisms include both modulation of specific cytokine responses and the overall cytokine pattern. Malnutrition is associated with impaired cytokine response to antigen[44] and increased levels of circulating proinflammatory cytokines.[45] The acute phase response to infection is blunted in malnutrition.[46] Infection in chronically malnourished children is associated with an increased cortisol response and greater loss of amino acids.[47] Concurrent infection also complicates the evaluation of malnutrition since transient losses of micronutrients may mimic a true deficiency.[48] Infants appear to have an intrinsically weaker ability to produce a compensatory anti-inflammatory response and therefore may be especially sensitive to the combination of infections and nutrient deficiency.[49] Some of the observed effects of malnutrition involve reactivation of opportunistic

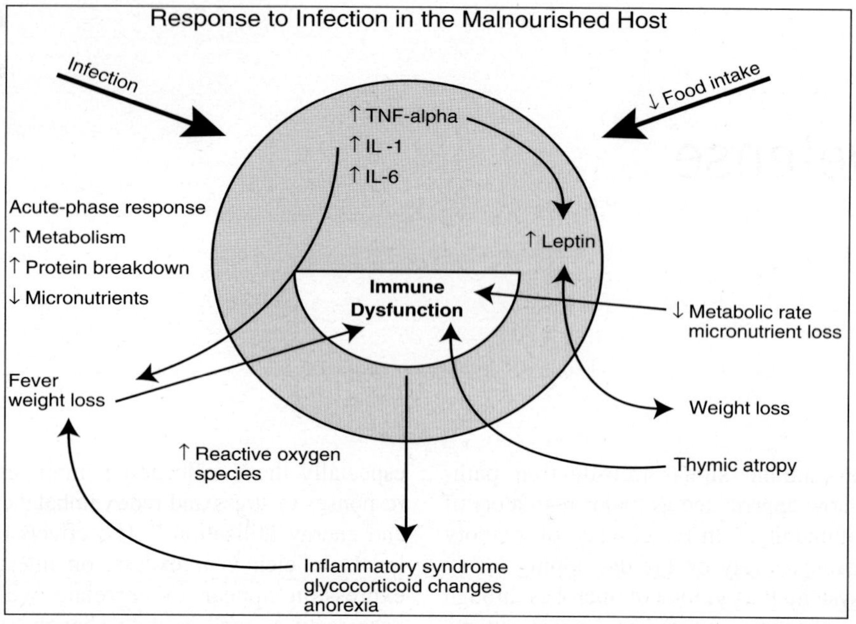

Figure 1 Illustrates some of the key interactions that lead to altered immune response in the malnourished host during infectious exposure. IL = intereleukin; TNF = tumor necrosis factor.

infections leading to altered activation of the acute phase response as illustrated in Figure 1. Examples include the effects of malnutrition on chronic infections such as *Mycobacterium tuberculosis* (TB), the human immunodeficiency virus type 1 (HIV-1) infection, and hepatitis.[41,50–53] Nutrients can have direct actions on specific immune cells and pathways or affect many different types of cells[54] (see Figure 2). Mechanisms of nutrient action may vary according to setting, concentration, and valid assessment requires appropriate methodology.[55–57] The impact of supplementation is also affected by conditions in the host.[58] Correlations that are observed in the compromised host may not hold true in the healthy host.

PCM nutrient deficiency occurring in children in the absence of contributing clinical cause is usually the result of poverty, lack of adequate supply, or other environmental factors.[59] Rare innate occurrences include the genetic defect of zinc metabolism, Acrodermatitis enteropathica (AE),[60] and defects of copper in Menkes or Wilson's disease.[61] However, deficient intake of essential nutrient requirements may easily be caused by altered metabolism in association with an underlying congenital condition, or acute illness and this impairs or worsens host response to emergent pathogens. Although malnutrition is often considered as mainly an issue for underdeveloped countries, suboptimal nutrition is common in children throughout the world, and is a significant cause of susceptibility to infection.[62] The changing social conditions of childhood, increasingly fragmented family life, and global infections have shifted the responsibility for children's health to the community. Professional knowledge of how nutrients may affect the development of immune response will have greater critical importance for preventive efforts to support future host defense against both old and emerging new pathogens.

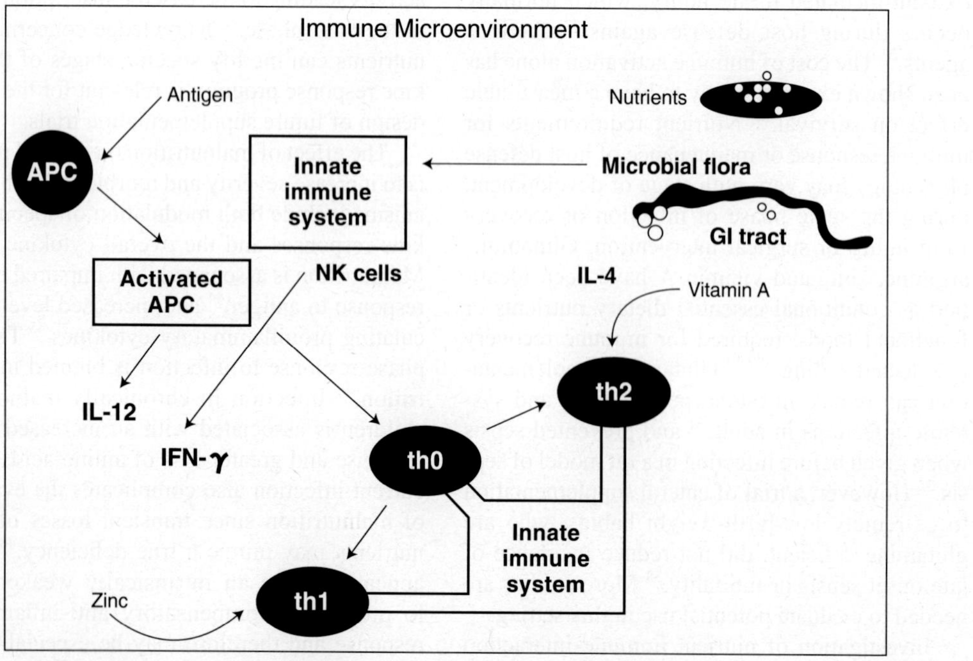

Figure 2 Indicates the role of nutrients in how the microenvironment influences the production of cytokines by the adaptive immune system. APC = antigen-presenting cell; GI = gastrointestinal; IFN = interferon; IL = interleukin; NK = natural killer; Th = T helper.

THE MICROENVIRONMENT AND MUCOSAL IMMUNE RESPONSE

The effect of nutrients on host response is pathogen specific and is affected by site of action, for example, the gastrointestinal associated lymphoid tract (GALT), thymus, spleen, regional lymph nodes, or immune cells of the circulating blood and upon the presence of infection or other immunogens. Thus experimental zinc deficiency in human volunteers decreased T-helper type 1 (Th1) production of Interleukin-2 (IL-2) and interferon gamma (IFN gamma), but had no effect on IL-4 response of peripheral blood mononuclear cells.[9] In contrast, zinc deficiency in nematode infected mice caused enhanced parasite survival in association with decreased T-helper type 2 (Th2) IL-4 responses in the GALT.[63] Differentiation of immune cell function and cell–cell interactions are critically determined by the local immune microenvironment and the presence of specialized immune cells, which may be tissue specific such as the adaptive intraepithelial lymphocytes in the intestinal tract, products such as mucus, and soluble mediators such as cytokines, interferons, lysozymes, and defensins. Studies in a mouse model of visceral leishmaniasis have shown that malnutrition promoted visceralization through loss of lymph node barrier function after *Leishmania donovani* infection. This was caused by excessive production of prostaglandin E_2, decreased levels of IL-10 and NO.[64] The effect of diet on mucosal integrity is a key measure of effective nutritional rehabilitation in infants. Protein deficiency predisposes both to skin and mucosal atrophy and compromises barrier function. As shown by a comparative study of maize-soy-egg to the standard milk diet in the treatment of kwashiorkor, milk had a better effect on reducing intestinal permeability as shown by the lactulose–rhamnose test. Despite the greater frequency of diarrhea, milk treatment was associated with reduced sepsis and improved survival.[65]

Chemotaxis, phagocytosis, and microbial killing mechanisms become impaired in malnutrition causing susceptibility to infections. The mechanisms involve reduced production of key mediators including complement C3, leukotrienes, cathelicidin antimicrobial peptide, and leptin.[66–69] The activities of many innate immune cells including neutrophils, monocytes, macrophages, dendritic, and NK cells are susceptible to altered nutrient levels.[70–72] Deficiencies can be particularly critical in the perinatal period as shown by the reduced level of NK cells in neonates born to mothers who were selenium deficient and the therapeutic effect of short-term renutrition in malnourished infants on defective neutrophil phagocytic activity.[73,74]

Vitamin A and vitamin D are critical regulators of mucosal immune function. Experimental vitamin A deficiency leads to functional disturbance of intestinal epithelium enzymes, diarrhea, and increased bacterial translocation in gnotobiotic rats.[75] Supplementation of vitamin A deficient measles patients lowered the risk of measles-related pneumonia.[76] In a study of vitamin A supplemented children infected with enteropathogenic *Escherichia coli* investigators observed reduced monocyte chemoattractant protein –1 levels compared with children in the placebo group consistent with an anti-inflammatory effect.[77] A recent study in mildly malnourished uninfected children, using the lactulose/mannitol test reported that intestinal barrier function was inversely correlated with serum retinol concentrations.[78] Retinoic acid, the vitamin A metabolite, is an inducer for the gut-homing specificity of T cells that enhances the expression of the integrin alpha4beta7 and CCR9 on T cells upon activation.[79] Retinoic acid has also been shown to synergize with GALT-DC-derived IL-6 or IL-5 to induce IgA secretion.[80] Since impaired gut immune response in early infancy may contribute to the development of atopic sensitization, Pesonen and colleagues looked for an association between plasma retinol concentrations and the subsequent development of allergic symptoms in healthy infants. They found that retinol concentration at 2 months correlated inversely with positive skin prick test at 5 and 20 years, and with allergic symptoms at 20 years.[81]

Both experimental vitamin D deficiency and human vitamin D receptor polymorphisms are associated with inflammatory bowel disease.[82,83] Association between subclinical vitamin D deficiency and lower respiratory tract infections in young children has also been reported.[84] Reduced vitamin D status is associated with susceptibility to active *M. tuberculosis* infection. Recent studies have shown that TLR stimulation of human macrophages induces vitamin D-1-hydroxylase genes, leading to the conversion of 25(OH) D3 to active 1,25(OH) 2D3, expression of the vitamin D receptor, and leads to antimicrobial peptide gene expression, induction of cathelicidin, and killing of intracellular *M. tuberculosis.*[85] This mechanism is also important for resistance to *Pseudomonas aeruginosa*, an important pathogen in cystic fibrosis.[68,85]

Dietary nucleotides provide preformed purine and pyrimidine bases that can be used for nucleic acid synthesis and may provide a means to support growth of the gut in the premature infant through reduction of intestinal permeability and absorption of macromolecules by enhancing immune response.[86,87] Martinez-Augustin and colleagues have shown that IgG antibodies against the main antigenic proteins in cow's milk are generally higher when nucleotide supplementation is provided. This difference reached significance for antibody to beta-lactoglobulin at 30 days of life when gut closure had occurred.[88] Others have shown that supplementation enhanced infants' responses to polio vaccination[87] and that the immunophenotype of infants fed nucleotide supplemented formula tended to be more like those fed human milk.[86] A recent study has reported that formula-fed infants given nucleotide supplementation had significantly higher responses to tetanus toxoid compared to controls.[89] Others have speculated that the benefits of nucleotides on the gastrointestinal and immune systems in the premature infant are related to increased splanchnic blood flow and effects on gut-associated lymphoid tissues.[90]

Human milk provides bioavailable micronutrients such as zinc, cytokines, and growth factors that are important for development of the gastrointestinal tract, as well as a source of maternal antibodies for passive protection against microbes common to mother and infant.[91] Secretory IgA antibodies in milk reactive against antigens in the maternal gut are protective against gastrointestinal disease.[92] In addition, milk contains oligosaccharides and glycans that inhibit binding by specific enteric pathogens.[93] IgA antibodies in colostrum and human milk may also prevent antigen entry at the intestinal surface of the breast-fed infant. A low IgA content in maternal milk is associated with development of cow's milk allergy suggesting that low IgA in milk is associated with defective exclusion of food antigens.[94] The composition of milk differs in mothers of premature infants from those from mothers of full-term infants. Higher concentrations of epidermal growth factor and transforming growth factor-alpha which are trophic peptides that support recovery of injured gastrointestinal mucosa have been found in milk from mothers with extremely preterm babies.[95]

Maternal malnutrition is associated with decline in total milk IgA, C3, and C4 and lower thymic weight in infants.[96] Perinatal supplementation of malnourished mothers with vitamin A leads to higher levels in milk postpartum and decreased infections and morbidity in infants in the perinatal period.[97] Low levels of fatty acids, such as decosahexanoic acid in maternal milk correlate directly with low levels in malnourished children. Recent studies show that bioactive immune mediators in milk such as transforming growth factor-beta and soluble CD14 receptor (sCD14), the bacterial pattern recognition receptor, are key elements in regulating the development of neonatal immunity. Mammary epithelial cells produce sCD14 in response to lipopolysaccharide (LPS) or bacteria, which activates intestinal epithelial cell secretion of IL-8, TNF-alpha, and epithelial neutrophil activator.[98] Another study showed that supplementation with fish oil during pregnancy leads to increased omega-3 polyunsaturated fatty acid levels that correlate with increased IgA and sCD14 levels, suggesting a possible fundamental relationship between fatty acid status and mucosal immune function.[99]

HOST DEFENSE IN PROTEIN-CALORIE MALNUTRITION

PCM, sometimes termed protein-energy malnutrition, is the most common cause of secondary immune deficiency in the world because of wide spread chronic and seasonal food shortages, as well as chronic poverty, the deprivations of war, and maternal malnutrition.[100] PCM may involve energy deficiency, protein deficiency, and vitamin and mineral deprivation. If prolonged, PCM produces wasting and stunting. Protein insufficiency alone, with or without infection, causes edema associated with hepatomegaly from fatty infiltration of the liver. The clinical manifestations are related to type, severity, and duration of nutritional impairment and may be subclinical, reversible, or irreversible depending upon availability of treatment, presence of other diseases or complicating disorders, and the degree of damage. Classically, PCM is divided into two types—marasmus and kwashiorkor. Marasmus is caused by total calorie deficiency, and is characterized by chronic wasting and gross underweight. Kwashiorkor develops due to protein deficiency in the diet and causes moderate growth retardation. Children with kwashiorkor have a characteristic moon facies and altered hair and sad appearance.[59] Vitamin and mineral deficiencies are commonly found in both marasmus and kwashiorkor. The causes of protein deficiency include use of low-protein milk substitutes such as rice "milk," which contains no milk product and other substitute beverages.[101–103]

Malnutrition can be classified as either primary or secondary. Primary malnutrition is caused by inadequate calorie and nutrient intake. Although calorie intake is presumed to be adequate in developed countries, inadequate intake of micronutrients including vitamin A, E, calcium, iron, and zinc are actually fairly common among children under 10 years of age although often goes unrecognized especially in minority populations.[104] Primary malnutrition in infants can also occur through child neglect or accidental nutrient insufficiency.[105,106] Rarer causes of single nutrient deficiency include a primary genetic defect in the mother that impairs zinc transport from blood into breast milk and leads to secondary zinc deficiency in infancy[107] and inheritance of the autosomal recessive zinc transporter mutation AE in the infant.[108]

Primary malnutrition is associated with atrophy of lymphoid organs and profound immune malfunction leading to susceptibility to pathogens, reactivation of viral infections, and development of opportunistic infections. Malnutrition in the neonatal period and early childhood can lead to severe immune deficiency and high mortality. Although the effects can be broad, impaired T-cell responses secondary to effects on thymic architecture and function are the most common. The thymus is central to the development of controlled adaptive immunity in providing the microenvironment in which bone-marrow-derived progenitors undergo proliferation, T-cell receptor rearrangement, and thymocyte differentiation into mature T cells.[109] Congenital thymic absence, DiGeorge syndrome, is associated with recurrent infections, which can be fatal. Other developmental anomalies that stem from chromosome 22q11 deletions comprising the CATCH-22 (cardiac defects, abnormal facies, thymic hypoplasia, cleft palate, and hypocalcemia) group of disorders may also have clinically significant immune deficiency in association with reduced thymic function.[110] A zinc finger gene, *ZNF74*, has been identified in the commonly deleted region.[111] Nutritionally caused thymic involution is very similar to congenital thymic aplasia in terms of effects on immune function and host defense. Measurements of thymic size and the frequency of T-cell receptor excision circles indicate that both thymus size and function are sensitive to perinatal malnutrition.[8] A small thymus at birth in infants born in impoverished environment predicts an increase in risk of infection related mortality in infancy.[112] Seasonal variations in breast milk associated with food shortages leading to reduced levels of IL-7 is a possible mediator of these effects.[8]

Thymic atrophy caused by PCM is associated with hormonal imbalance, loss of leptin, and increase in serum glucocorticoid level. Leptin levels normally increase acutely during infection and inflammation,[113] but this does not occur in PCM. The reduction of serum leptin levels and insulin-like growth factor-1 in marasmus and kwashiorkor[114] may compromise response to infection. Loss of immune function in malnourished children correlates with low leptin levels, and refeeding leads to increase in leptin levels and immunological recovery.[115] Immune structure and function are more compromised in edematous PCM than in nonedematous PCM. Children who are malnourished mount a partial acute phase response to infection and this defect is more marked in children with kwashiorkor, the edematous form of PCM.[116] Differences have been observed at the level of specific protein pools suggesting that in kwashiorkor expansion of the haptoglobin pool was due to reduction in the rate of catabolism relative to the rate of synthesis. Infections are commonly found. For children living in a rural environment in a developed country, one study reported that one-third of all patients hospitalized for malnutrition had bacterial infections.[117] Host response to infection is also altered. Well-nourished children show a relative increase in B lymphocytes in response to bacterial infection, while B cell response was significantly reduced in malnourished children.[118] In general the humoral immune response is relatively preserved, although serum levels of IgA1, IgA2, and C4 tend to be higher than in normal children, serum level of C3 and the proportion of B cells are significantly lower.[119] IgE levels are lower even among asthmatic children.[120] Although response to vaccines is often effective,[121] there is reason for caution as relatively few studies have examined the potential long-term effects of neonatal nutrient deficiency.

Nutrient deficiencies may have an indelible effect during critical periods of early development by exerting an imprinting effect on the fundamental program of future development. This concept, advanced by Barker as "developmental origins of health and disease" hypothesis,[122] has been applied to nutritional status at birth by Dobbing[123] and to immune response.[7,124] Mc Dade and colleagues reported that adolescents who were small for gestational age at birth had lower thymopoietin levels when compared with adolescents who were appropriate for gestational age at birth. In both groups thymopoietin level during adolescence correlated with growth in length during the first year of life. In addition, the probability of mounting a positive antibody response for adolescents who were small for gestational age and also undernourished at the time of immunization was lower compared to adolescents who were appropriate for gestational age.[124] Moore and colleagues have reported similar findings in adults using the same purified Vi surface polysaccharide extracted from *Salmonella typhi*. Interestingly while they found a correlation for both IgG and IgM antibody response to Vi vaccine with birth weight, they did not find this for rabies or typhoid. The studies suggest that polysaccharide T independent immune response may be specifically compromised by fetal growth retardation.[8]

Secondary malnutrition can be caused by reduced intake of food, malabsorption, impaired nutrient utilization, and nutrient losses associated with chronic infection and many other clinical conditions as well. Examples include inflammatory bowel disorders, celiac disease, chronic anemia, renal disorders, and cystic fibrosis. In both primary and secondary malnutrition, understanding of the relevant genetic mechanisms can be helpful in approaching the clinical manifestations. Genetic mechanisms of malnutrition that affect susceptibility to infectious disease include mutations affecting metabolism of the trace elements zinc, iron, and copper, and several vitamins as well as those underlying complex, inherited disorders such as cystic fibrosis and celiac disease. Primary malnutrition impairs immunity impeding host response to infection, but these effects are reversible with nutrient repletion. However, calorie and nutritional supplement alone cannot resolve the secondary malnutrition with organic etiology.

Obesity is emerging as a malnutrition syndrome that develops when energy intake exceeds expenditure. Human obesity often becomes a permanent condition and appears to involve changes in the neural-endocrine network that regulates energy intake, expenditure, and storage[125] Leptin, the adipocyte-secreted hormone that regulates weight centrally and ghrelin, a gastrointestinal hormone regulating feeding and energy balance, are signals in this system. Leptin has cytokine-like activities and acts as a mediator for the interactions of nutritional status with neuroendocrine and immune responses. Leptin production increases acutely during infection perhaps in response to glucocorticoids and is higher in survivors of sepsis.[125,126] Leptin deficient mice show increased mortality from bacterial infections.[69] Congenital human leptin deficiency is a rare cause of severe early-onset obesity characterized by absence of leptin and carries a high risk of death due to infection in childhood.[127,128]

Obesity-prone individuals appear to have an inborn reduction in their catabolic responses to glucose, leptin, and insulin.[128,129] Elevated circulating leptin levels are characteristic in obesity and may contribute significantly to the reported low-grade systemic inflammation[128] and perhaps to the high incidence of atopy.[130] Generally the incidence and severity of specific types of infectious illnesses are higher in obese persons.[131] Weight loss in obesity is associated with improved immune function in vitro.[132] The genetic interactions between leptin and its receptor are affected by host polymorphisms, some of which are associated with increased BMI and may promote the immune dysfunction associated with obesity and risk of non-Hodgkin lymphoma as recently proposed.[133] A Common inherited IL-6 promoter polymorphism has been linked to increased serum leptin and increased BMI suggesting a functional relationship since IL-6 which increases acutely in infection also reduces fat mass.[134] Obesity may also involve altered metabolism secondary to changes in microflora. The gut microbiota as a whole is essential for production of short chain fatty acids from polysaccharides, and is a regulator of host metabolism through direct effects on fat storage.[135] A direct role for viral infection in obesity has also been proposed[136] and may operate through some of these mechanisms.

MICRONUTRIENTS AND IMMUNE FUNCTION

Selective micronutrient deficiencies can occur when food and calorie intake is adequate. Iron, copper, and zinc deficiencies are the most common. Results from a large double blind trial of fortified milk in preschool children showed that intervention was associated with reduced morbidity from diarrhea, respiratory infections, and other illnesses, as well as improved iron status and growth.[137] Selenium deficiency occurs in environments where selenium levels are low in the soil or where bioavailability is limited. As a constituent of selenoproteins, selenium is needed for the functioning of neutrophils, macrophages, NK cells, and T lymphocytes. Mild selenium deficiency is relatively widespread and appears to worsen viral infection.[138] Selenium and vitamin E deficiency in the mouse have been shown to promote the virulence of Coxsackie B3 virus and influenza by inducing genetic changes in the genomes of the viruses.[139] Selective micronutrient deficiency frequently occurs in patients with underlying systemic illnesses, chronic viral infection, and in low-birth-weight infants.[140,141] Low dietary intake of antioxidant nutrients can influence both response to infection or produce an inflammatory state that mimics infection. Nair

Table 1 Regulatory Effects of Micronutrients on Immune Response

Nutrient	Target cell	Effect	Mechanism
Zinc	T cell, NK cell, B cell	• Deficiency promotes infection, impairs immune response, ↓ hematopoiesis • Lymphopenia, dermatitis, enteritis • ↓ Thymic activity • ↓ Antioxidant enzyme activity	• Deficiency causes glucocorticoid mediated early T cell and B cell apoptosis • Required for thymic hormone function • Required for activity of >100 enzymes • Required for zinc finger dependent transcription factors
Iron	T cell, monocyte	• Iron deficiency causes ↓ neutrophil oxidative burst activity and ↓IgG4 levels • Anemia linked with mortality in HIV Iron excess causes infection in the genetically susceptible host	• Promotes Th-2 response, ROS production needed for intracellular killing; chronic ROS linked to immune dysfunction • Promotes bacterial growth, enhances HIV viral replication • Host polymorphisms, *HFE* gene affect regulate iron
Copper	Monocyte, T cell, neutrophil	• Deficiency leads to infections • Deficiency ↓ proliferation, phagocyte activity	• Modulation of MHC Class II expression • Affects selenoglutathione peroxidase activity • Reduces IL-2 response
Selenium	Monocyte	• Deficiency suppresses antigen presentation • Repletion ↑proliferation • Deficiency linked to ↑ HIV infection	• Antioxidant • Affects IL-2 response, regulates NF kappa B • May interact with viral genes
Vitamin A	T cell, NK cell, B cell	• Deficiency causes infections, mortality from infections, ↓ NK activity • Repletion improves gut integrity at weaning • Repletion reduces morbidity, mortality from infections	• Promotes Th-2 cytokine and IgA production • Inducer for gut-homing of T cells • IL-2 receptor beta, interferon regulatory factor, transcription factor mRNA • Affects IL-12 and IL-10 production
Vitamin C	Phagocyte	• Promotes phagocytic and NK activity • Reduces stress IL-6 response • Improves response to strep infection • Reduces growth of *Helicobacter pylori*	• Decreases monocyte response to LPS • Increases phagocytosis • Increases NK activity
Vitamin D, 1,25-dihydroxy-vitamin D3	T cell, B cell, monocyte, macrophage, dendritic cell	• Vitamin D3 affects differentiation, maturation, and function of cells	• Functions through a nuclear receptor, vitamin D receptor (VDR) which binds to response elements in target genes
		• Vitamin D3 suppresses autoimmune disease in animal models • Vitamin D deficiency promoted TB infection	• Affects differentiation of monocytes, dendritic cells • VDR polymorphisms regulate response to mycobacteria, hepatitis B, inflammatory bowel disease through TLR signaling
Vitamin E	T cell, B cell, monocyte	• ↑ Proliferative, IL-2 response in vitro • Improves skin test response • Deficiency may promote viral virulence	• Modulates cyclic AMP response element binding proteins • Affects prostaglandin production

and colleagues[142] observed that patients with gastritis had reduced alpha-tocopherol levels in serum and mucosa irrespective of *Helicobacter pylori* infections, whereas carotenoids and ascorbic acid levels were similar to controls. Inflammation induced by *H. pylori* infection, especially with the CagA positive strain, is associated with decreased gastric vitamin C into the gastric lumen in children.[143] Studies in mice show that vitamin C and the carotenoid, astaxanthin, show antimicrobial activity against *H. pylori* that appeared to be mediated by altered immune response characterized by a shift from a Th-1 type immune response to a mixed Th-1/ Th-2 response, which was dominated by IL-4 and IFN-gamma production.[144] Strains of *H. pylori* that were rendered more sensitive to antioxidants were less able to colonize the gastric mucosa suggesting that both antioxidant as well as immune mediated effects could be significant.[145]

Trace elements and vitamins perform antioxidant functions through participation in enzyme-catalyzed reactions. These reactions are essential to offset potential oxidative damage caused by free radical formation. Three antioxidant enzymes, the copper, zinc, and manganese superoxide dismutases, require trace metals for biological activity. In addition, micronutrients are pivotal regulators of cytokine production. Intracellular redox balance has a signaling role in immune cell development and function and the antioxidant effects of micronutrients regulate cytokine production.[146] Table 1 summarizes the role of key micronutrients in regulation of immune response. The implications and significance of these functions for the development of immune response to pathogens are outlined below:

Iron

The controversy about iron supplementation has continued over several decades because of concern that excess, or inappropriate timing of iron repletion, would promote bacterial growth. The current consensus is that iron supplementation has a high probability of adversely affecting outcome in individuals who present with concurrent infection or who carry genes predisposing to iron overload.[147] Iron overload secondary to blood transfusion is a serious complication of beta thalassemia that increases both risk and severity of infection.[148,149] Circulating levels of micronutrients (vitamins A and E, zinc, selenium, and copper) are lower in children with thalassemia maintained by red cell transfusion compared to age matched controls.[150] In hereditary hemochromatosis, a disorder of increased iron uptake, there is a paradoxical iron deficiency of macrophages, which may actually result in increased resistance to bacterial pathogens.[151] Iron chelation therapy in *Plasmodium falciparum* infection alleviates the clinical course of cerebral malaria in children. However, the basis of this appears to be enhanced generation of NO rather than reduced iron availability to the parasite.[152]

Iron deficiency anemia in children is associated with reduced neutrophil oxidative bust activity and reduced levels of IgG4.[70] Iron supplementation has a significant and positive effect on iron status in anemia secondary to malaria and no impact on the incidence of malarial infection.[153] Vegetarian diet and *H. pylori* infection can be causes of iron deficiency anemia.[154,155] Pangastritis is more common in children whose *H. pylori* infection is accompanied by anemia.[143] Experimental iron deficiency leads to upregulation of apical iron transport-related proteins, transferrin receptor and heme oxygenase, and copper loading genes, and decreased expression of genes involved in the oxidative stress response.[39]

Zinc

Zinc deficiency affects about one-third of the world's populations and is a frequent complication of PCM.[156] Zinc deficiency is also a significant complication of IgA deficiency, fetal alcohol syndrome, sickle cell disease, enteritis, celiac disease, and many forms of diarrhea.[7,157,158] Zinc deficiency presenting as dermatitis similar to AE can be a sign of cystic fibrosis.[159] Zinc is an essential cofactor for the activity of many enzymes including thymic hormone.[10] Deficiency leads to reduced Th-1 cytokines and thymic hormone activity[11,160,161] and to lymphopenia.[162] Zinc supplementation improves host defense in severely malnourished children.[163] Prolonged deficiency causes reprogramming of the immune system, beginning with activation of the HPA (hypothalamic pituitary axis) causing chronic production of glucocorticoids that accelerates apoptosis among early T and B cells.[12] Zinc deficiency induced in human volunteers led to decreased IFN-gamma and IL-2 production but not IL-4, IL-6, or IL-10.[9] Zinc inhibits LPS-induced TNF-alpha and IL-1-beta release from primary human monocytes by inhibiting the enzyme activity of phosphodiesterase leading to increasing intracellular cycic GPM (cGMP) (guanosine 3',5'-cyclic monophosphate) levels.[164] A recent study suggests that the enhancing effect of zinc on Th-1, cytokine response in cultured human peripheral blood cells, is mediated by NK cell upregulation and increased IFN-gamma production.[165] The implications for enhancement of immune response, for example, to vaccine, may be complex as shown by a recent study of response in children to subunit B cholera toxin. Although zinc supplementation enhanced vibriocidal antibody response, cholera toxin response was suppressed.[166]

The autosomal recessive genetic defect of zinc absorption, AE, presents in infancy as skin lesions, diarrhea, alopecia, and increased incidence of infections caused by severe immune deficiency.[60] Immune defects in AE range from severe thymic atrophy and profound lymphopenia to skin test anergy and loss of NK cell activity.[11] AE is centrally caused by mutations in SLC39A4, which encodes a ZIP zinc transporter protein. Increased zinc availability increases expression of zinc transporters and therefore patients with AE respond to increased zinc supplementation.[167] Differential mRNA display and cDNA array analysis have identified zinc-regulated genes. Dietary zinc intake, high or low, affected about 5% of genes in the monocytic/macrophage THP-1 cell line. Many needed for host defense were among those identified as zinc responsive, including cytokine receptor genes and genes associated with amplification of the Th1 immune response.[168] A recent study examined the effect of modest zinc supplementation in healthy volunteers on immune function. TNF-alpha and IL-1-beta expression were greater in activated monocytes and granulocytes, and IFN-gamma mRNA levels were higher in activated T lymphocytes compared to baseline.[169] Zinc-fortified formulas have been used to improve both linear growth and immunocompetence as shown by improved delayed type hypersensitivity, enhanced lymphoproliferative responses, and increased salivary IgA in severely malnourished infants.[170]

Copper

Copper and zinc deficiencies are common in children with hypoproteinemia and anemia and this leads to reduced antioxidant function as measured by Cu/Zn superoxide dismutase (SOD-1) activity.[171] Transgenic mice overexpressing SOD-1 demonstrate a significant increase in macrophage release of TNF-alpha and the metalloproteinases.[172] Zinc competes with copper for gastrointestinal uptake, and increased zinc intake can induce copper deficiency causing clinically significant neutropenia.[173] The IL-2 response is reduced in copper deficiency[174] and marginal copper deficiency may lead to immune dysfunction.[175] Serum copper or ceruloplasmin levels reflect the severity of malnutrition.[176]

Copper also interacts with iron since ceruloplasmin, which contains most of the plasma copper, is a ferroxidase. Ceruloplasmin facilitates release of tissue iron into plasma by oxidizing ferrous iron into ferric iron, which is then bound to transferrin for delivery to the bone marrow for hematopoiesis. Aceruloplasminemia is an inherited disorder of iron metabolism.[177] Copper transporting P-type ATPases, ATP7A, and ATP7B, maintain copper balance. Impaired intestinal transport of copper, resulting from mutations in the *ATP7A* gene, leads to Menkes disease. Defects in a similar gene, the copper transporting ATPase *ATP7B*, result in Wilson disease. This ATP7B transporter has two functions: transport of copper into the plasma protein ceruloplasmin, and elimination of copper through the bile.[178]

Selenium

Selenium is an important micronutrient for health[179] and is critical for antioxidant function acting via the selenium-dependent enzyme, glutathione peroxidase, to protect cellular membranes and organelles from peroxidative damage. Soil deficiencies of selenium and iodine are common in some countries such as New Zealand, Australia, Finland, and in parts of China.[180] Selenium deficiency can be a critical component of PCM and is linked with congestive heart failure in this setting.[181] Juvenile cardiomyopathy (Keshan) appears to involve both selenium deficiency and enteroviral infection. Experimental studies suggest that selenium deficiency enhances viral virulence.[182] Selenium has been used in vitro to correct membrane fluidity, IL-2 production, and IL-2R expression in patients with chronic hepatitis, which were significantly lower than controls.[53] Some studies have suggested that risk of cancer is increased in selenium deficiency.[183,184] Selenoproteins are an important component of the antioxidant host defense system affecting leukocyte and NK cell function.[185] Selenium is emerging as a critical micronutrient in host defense against viral infection since selenium deficiency is associated with progression in HIV disease and in viral shedding.[186,187]

Antioxidant Vitamins

The antioxidant vitamins, vitamin E, C, A, and the precursor of vitamin A, beta-carotene, are cofactors in immune response. Vitamin A (retinol) is a key micronutrient needed for resolution of infection. In environments with endemic low levels of vitamin A, supplementation significantly reduces childhood mortality.[188] Vitamin A has long been appreciated as a significant factor in the severity of infection such as measles, rotavirus diarrhea, and HIV in the malnourished host.[189,190] Reduced levels of serum trans-retinol are common in infants of HIV-1 infected mothers.[191] Xerophthalmia is associated with childhood infections such as measles, diarrhea, and respiratory tract infections among hospitalized children.[192] Respiratory infection and diarrhea can be signs of subclinical low levels of vitamin A.[193] Serum retinol and provitamin-A as well as carotenoid concentrations are lower in children with acute phase infections compared to healthy controls and correlate inversely with C-reactive protein suggesting decreased synthesis or increased utilization of these antioxidants in infection.[194] Low vitamin A levels are associated with the occurrence of chronic bacterial infections and splenomegaly as well as high neopterin levels in common variable immune deficiency or hypogammaglobulinemia.[195] Supplementation in vivo led to improved immune function in vitro.

Vitamin A deficiency impairs both Th1 and Th2 mediated immune responses, although Th2 responses seem to be principally affected.[196] Vitamin A deficiency at the time of antigen exposure induces secretion of T regulatory IL-10 and diminishes Th-1 memory cell response in the mouse.[197] Organized vitamin A supplementation in areas of endemic deficiency is beneficial for protection against diarrhea and acute respiratory infections.[198] The mechanism of vitamin A protection against morbidity of infections has not been clarified. To address this issue, a large study of children less than 2 years of age were followed in randomized, double-blind, placebo-controlled, vitamin A supplementation trial and IL-4, IL-6, IFN-gamma, and gastrointestinal pathogens were evaluated in stool. Vitamin A-supplemented children infected with enteropathogenic *E. coli* had reduced IL-4 and IFN-gamma levels but increased IL-4 levels when infected with *Ascaris lumbricoides*. IL-4 levels increased and IFN-gamma levels decreased among vitamin A-supplemented children with diarrhea compared with the placebo group. These findings suggest that the effects of vitamin A may depend on the infecting enteric pathogen and clinical stage.[199]

Vitamin E is a strong antioxidant that can support monocyte/macrophage-mediated response.[200,201] Vitamin E influences T cell function by down modulating prostaglandin E_2 in elderly subjects.[202] Current studies suggest that vitamin E deficiency may enhance virulence in viral infections.[139] Vitamin E supplementation enhances proliferative response in vitro[203] and improves IL-2 cytokine response.[204] Vitamin E deficiency causes reduced transferrin receptor internalization in the mouse, which suggests restriction of intracellular iron stores that would be needed for cellular function and proliferation.[205] A recent study has shown that antioxidant deficiency is common in a very large cohort of cystic fibrosis patients. Carotenoid and vitamin E deficiencies were found to occur early in the course of the disease and level of antioxidants decreased with bronchial infection.[206]

Vitamin C is a regulator of redox and metabolic checkpoints controlling activation and survival of immune cells. In vitro studies have shown that vitamin C selectively influences cytokine production in response to LPS by reducing the number of monocytes producing IL-6 and IL-2 without affecting IL-1 and IL-8.[207] Ascorbate regulates the phagocytic process by decreasing free radical production and thus potentially reduces the severity of the endotoxin response.[208] During stress exercise, contracting skeletal muscle is a major contributor to the exercise-induced increase of plasma IL-6; supplementation with vitamins C and E attenuates this response.[209] Vitamin C concentrations in the plasma and leukocytes decline during infections and stress. Supplementation with antioxidant vitamins including vitamin C has been shown to improve immune response to group A streptococcal infection compared to penicillin alone.[210] Supplementation may enhance phagocytosis and NK cell activity,[211] *H. pylori* infection is associated with a decrease in gastric juice ascorbic acid concentration; this effect is greater in children infected with the CagA-positive strain A.[143] Both vitamin C and astaxanthin, a carotenoid, show antimicrobial activity against *H. pylori* that may be mediated through immune mechanisms.[212]

MALNUTRITION AND CHRONIC INFECTION

Chronic infection commonly involves malabsorption and malnutrition that is associated with altered cytokine patterns affecting both regional and systemic immune response altering metabolism and growth. Although less prevalent in industrialized countries, chronic infections such as HIV and *M. tuberculosis* are significant problems in which host defense is affected by nutritional status. When recent immigrant populations are included, otherwise highly unusual parasitic infections must be considered as significant chronic infections in children living in developed countries.[213,214] In these infections, nutrient deficiencies are associated with reduced host defense. In contrast to studies in the mouse where short-term starvation induced hepatitis B viral replication,[215] dietary restriction of total calories, fat, iron, and protein in adult patients with chronic hepatitis C virus reduces serum alanine aminotransferase levels without adverse effect.[216]

HIV Infection

Malnutrition continues to be a significant problem in pediatric HIV infection. Studies show that micronutrient impairment is causally associated with the course of infection and progression of immune dysfunction.[217,218] Nutritional intervention may restore intestinal absorption and increase CD4 cell numbers.[219] Vitamin A deficiency is common in HIV infection and low maternal serum retinol level is a risk factor for mother-to-child transmission. Postpartum maternal and neonatal vitamin A supplementation of HIV-positive infants prolongs survival.[220] However, the same supplementation regimen increased progression to death for breast-fed children who were HIV negative at 6 weeks and infected through breast milk.[220] New studies have revealed a relationship between mannose-binding lectin (MBL) gene polymorphisms and response to vitamin A in HIV infection. MBL-2 allele variants are associated with deficiencies in innate immunity, which correlate with susceptibility to HIV infection. MBL is a component of the innate immune system that binds to carbohydrate ligands on the surface of many pathogens and activates the lectin pathway of the complement system. Study of HIV transmission in a supplementation study of vitamin A plus beta-carotene showed that infants with MBL-2 variants in the control arm showed increased maternal HIV transmission compared to the supplementation arm.[221] The study suggests that vitamin A plus beta-carotene corrected the effect of the MBL variant in increasing risk of HIV transmission. Selenium deficiency increases the virulence of HIV and enhances disease progression, whereas supplementation reduces high levels of IL-8 and TNF-alpha.[222] Lipodystrophy is an increasingly common complication of antiretroviral therapy for HIV infection that is prevalent in children. The lipodystrophy syndrome includes both fat accumulation and wasting, and is often accompanied by metabolic derangements in glucose and lipid metabolism.[223] Lipodystrophy appears to reflect a chronic mitochondrial toxicity that may be linked to HIV infection and L-carnitine deficiency.[224] L. carnitine is a non-essential micronutrient that regulates fatty acid transport into mitochondria and also modulates immune function and the effects of supplementation are currently being studied.

Tuberculosis

Generally declining rates of TB in industrialized countries have lead to less rigorous surveillance. However, TB is an important opportunistic pathogen that can lead to significant infection in persons with nutritional insufficiency such as anorexia nervosa[225] and is a major coinfection in HIV disease.[226] International adoptees are at high risk for TB and progression to active TB infection.[227] The natural history and clinical manifestations are different in children and are associated with the age at infection and the host immune status. Primary malnutrition increases the incidence and exacerbates clinical manifestations of TB infection. Experimental studies in the mouse have shown that PCM reduces production of IFN-gamma, TNF-alpha, and NO after infection leading to a decreased granulomatous reaction, higher lung bacillary load, and a more fatal TB course than in well nourished control mice, and that this could be reversed by restoring a diet with normal protein content.[228,229] Iron status is recognized as a potential cofactor in TB infection and progression since excess iron could enhance growth. Host polymorphisms in genes that regulate iron handling candidate genes, haptoglobin and natural- resistance-associated-macrophage protein-1, may be important discriminators for the pathogenesis of TB.[230] Selenium status also affects the pathogenesis of mycobacterial disease in adults with both HIV and TB infection.[231]

Vitamin D deficiency and vitamin D receptor polymorphisms are associated with an increased risk for TB infection.[232] In vitro studies show that 1,25-dihydroxyvitamin, the most active form of the vitamin, enhances mycobacterial killing by increasing NO production. Aerosol-challenge with *M. bovis* in the NO synthase 2 [NOS2(−/−)] deficient mouse leads to increased mycobacterial colonization and lesion formation compared to the wild-type mouse. Infected NOS2(−/−) mice developed severe necrotizing pyogranulomatous inflammation.[233] Lung colonization and lesion area of vitamin D deficient mice was greater compared to vitamin D replete mice, regardless of NOS2 phenotype demonstrating a fundamental role for vitamin D but also suggesting that vitamin D also has NO-independent effects. A role for the NO defense pathway human response to TB has been proposed.[234]

Endemic Infection

Parasitic infections cause malnutrition and impair host immune response, and are affected by host nutrition and immunity. Intestinal hookworm causes significant anemia.[235] Blood loss is directly proportional to the intensity of infection. Even a modest infection of *Necator americanus* can result in blood loss that exceeds physiologic daily requirements. Light infections of *Ancylostoma duodenale* may cause severe anemia in an infant that is difficult to correct with iron supplementation alone. Heavy infections with *Ascaris* may result in malabsorption, mild anemia, and wasting. The worm metabolizes vitamin A and heavy infections have been associated with vitamin A deficiency. Micronutrient deficiencies are common in parasitic infections.[236] Zinc deficiency impairs immune response to intestinal nematode infections at both systemic and intestinal level.[237] Infection also alters host nutritional since diarrhea promotes zinc loss. Giardiasis increases the serological levels of copper, while zinc and iron levels are decreased due to malabsorption.[238] CD4+ Th2 cells are critical for host protection while Th1 response actually inhibits protective immunity to nematode infection. IL-4, a Th2 cytokine, is required for protection and can also limit severity of infection. Protein malnutrition may increase the survival of nematode parasites by decreasing gut-associated IL-4 (Th-2) and increasing IFN-gamma (Th-1), leading to reduced intestinal and systemic Th-2 effector responses.[239]

One study of US immigrants reported that the most common pathogens were *Trichuris trichiura, Giardia lamblia,* and *A. lumbricoides. G. lamblia* was more prevalent in the younger than 5-year-old age group, and helminths were more prevalent in the 6- to 10-year-old age group. No helminths were found in immigrants who had been in the US for more than 3 years.

Infection caused by intestinal parasites irritates the GI tract, causes pain, anorexia, flatulence, tenderness, and affects the host nutrition directly as a result of inflammatory and noninflammatory diarrhea. Host response mechanisms include accelerated epithelial cell turnover.[240] Trace element deficiencies affect the host pathogen interaction. Examples include the exacerbating effect of selenium deficiency on *Trypanosoma cruzi,* which is responsible for Chagas disease.[241] Malnutrition can cause an imbalance in T cell subpopulations that may lead to a defective T cell maturation and a decreased specific anti-*Ascaris* IgE response and worsens infection with *A. lumbricoides*.[242] Malaria causes the most serious nutritional consequences of any major parasite. It infects the placenta and compromises blood flow to the fetus, causing low-birth-weight. It also causes PCM in pregnant and lactating women and young children. Anemia, recurrent fever with acute phase cytokine responses, vomiting, and anorexia all produce adverse nutritional consequences in an already fragile child or pregnant woman. Recent investigation suggests that micronutrients such as vitamin A, vitamin E, and zinc may improve the morbidity of malaria through immune modulation and alteration of oxidative stress.[243]

REFERENCES

1. Brock AJ. Greek Medicine. London and Toronto: J.M. Dent and Sons; 1927.
2. Garrison, FH. An Introduction to History of Medicine. Philadelphia, PA: W.B. Saunders and Sons; 1929. 413ff.
3. Metchnikoff E. Virchow Archiv 1899;96:177.
4. Moulin AM. Immunology old and new: The beginning and the end. In: Paulin MH, editor. Essays on the History of Immunology. Toronto: Wall and Thompson; 1989. p. 292–8.
5. Smythe PM, Schonland M, Brereton-Stiles GG, et al. Thymolymphatic deficiency and depression of cell-mediated immunity in protein-calorie malnutrition. Lancet 1971;2:939–43.
6. Prentice AM. The thymus: A barometer of malnutrition. Br J Nutr 1999;81:345–7.
7. McDade TW, Beck MA, Kuzawa CW, Adair LS. Prenatal undernutrition and postnatal growth are associated with adolescent thymic function. J Nutr 2001;131:1225–31.
8. Moore SE, Collinson AC, Tamba N'Gom P, et al. Early immunological development and mortality from infectious disease in later life. Proc Nutr Soc 2006;65:311–8.
9. Prasad AS. Effects of zinc deficiency on Th1 and Th2 cytokine shifts. J Infect Dis 2000;182:S62–8.
10. Dardenne M. Zinc and immune function. Eur J Clin Nutr 2002;56:S20–3.
11. Fraker PJ, King LE, Laakko T, Vollmer TL. The dynamic link between the integrity of the immune system and zinc status. J Nutr 2000;130:1399S–406S.
12. Fraker PJ, King LE. Reprogramming of the immune system during zinc deficiency. Annu Rev Nutr 2004;24:277–98.
13. Haynes BF, Markert ML, Sempowski GD, et al. The role of the thymus in immune reconstitution in aging, bone marrow transplantation, and HIV-1 infection. Annu Rev Immunol 2000;18:529–60.
14. Mocchegiani E, Santarelli L, Costarelli L, et al. Plasticity of neuroendocrine-thymus interactions during ontogeny and ageing: Role of zinc and arginine. Ageing Res Rev 2006;5:281–309.
15. Mocchegiani E, Muzzioli M, Giacconi R, et al. Metallothioneins/PARP-1/IL-6 interplay on natural killer cell activity in elderly: Parallelism with nonagenarians and old infected humans. Effect of zinc supply. Mech Ageing Dev 2003;124:459–68.
16. Saha AR, Hadden EM, Hadden JW. Zinc induces thymulin secretion from human thymic epithelial cells in vitro and augments splenocyte and thymocyte responses in vivo. Int J Immunopharmacol 1995;17:729–33.
17. Haase H, Mocchegiani E, Rink L. Correlation between zinc status and immune function in the elderly. Biogerontology 2006;7:421–8.
18. Hoebe K, Janssen E, Beutler B. The interface between innate and adaptive immunity. Nat Immunol 2004;5:971–4.
19. Walker WA. Role of nutrients and bacterial colonization in the development of intestinal host defense. J Pediatr Gastroenterol Nutr 2000;30:S2–7.
20. Marodi L. Innate cellular immune responses in newborns. Clin Immunol 2006;118:137–44.
21. LeBouder E, Rey-Nores JE, Raby AC, et al. Modulation of neonatal microbial recognition: TLR-mediated innate immune responses are specifically and differentially modulated by human milk. J Immunol 2006;176:3742–52.
22. Lee JY, Plakidas A, Lee WH, et al. Differential modulation of toll-like receptors by fatty acids: Preferential inhibition by n-3 polyunsaturated fatty acids. J Lipid Res 2003;44:479–86.
23. Bunout D, Barrera G, Hirsch S, et al. Effects of a nutritional supplement on the immune response and cytokine production in free-living Chilean elderly. JPEN J Parenter Enteral Nutr 2004;28:348–54.
24. Bussiere FI, Tridon A, Zimowska W, et al. Increase in complement component C3 is an early response to experimental magnesium deficiency in rats. Life Sci 2003;73:499–507.
25. Ekanem EE, Umotong AB, Raykundalia C, Catty D. Serum C-reactive protein and C3 complement protein levels in severely malnourished Nigerian children with and without bacterial infections. Acta Paediatr 1997;86:1317–20.
26. Kamath AB, Wang L, Das H, et al. Antigens in tea-beverage prime human Vgamma 2Vdelta 2 T cells in vitro and in vivo for memory and nonmemory antibacterial cytokine responses. Proc Natl Acad Sci U S A 2003;100:6009–14.
27. Erickson KL, Medina EA, Hubbard NE. Micronutrients and innate immunity. J Infect Dis 2000;182:S5–10.
28. Moret Y, Schmid-Hempel P. Survival for immunity: The price of immune system activation for bumblebee workers. Science 2000;290:1166–8.
29. Kudsk KA. Immunonutrition in surgery and critical care. Annu Rev Nutr 2006;26:463–79.
30. Ziegler TR, Evans ME, Fernandez-Estivariz C, Jones DP. Trophic and cytoprotective nutrition for intestinal adaptation, mucosal repair, and barrier function. Annu Rev Nutr 2003;23:229–61.
31. De-Souza DA, Greene LJ. Intestinal permeability and systemic infections in critically ill patients: Effect of glutamine. Crit Care Med 2005;33:1125–35.
32. Yeh SL, Lai YN, Shang HF, et al. Effects of glutamine supplementation on innate immune response in rats with gut-derived sepsis. Br J Nutr 2004;91:423–9.
33. Poindexter BB, Ehrenkranz RA, Stoll BJ, et al. Parenteral glutamine supplementation does not reduce the risk of mortality or late-onset sepsis in extremely low birth weight infants. Pediatrics 2004;113:1209–15.
34. Kapoor R, Huang YS. Gamma linolenic acid: An antiinflammatory omega-6 fatty acid. Curr Pharm Biotechnol 2006;7:531–4.
35. van Erk MJ, Blom WA, van Ommen B, Hendriks HF. High-protein and high-carbohydrate breakfasts differentially change the transcriptome of human blood cells. Am J Clin Nutr 2006;84:1233–41.
36. Gonzalez C, Gonzalez H, Rodriguez L, et al. Differential gene expression in lymphocytes from malnourished children. Cell Biol Int 2006;30:610–4.
37. Cousins RJ, Blanchard RK, Moore JB, et al. Regulation of zinc metabolism and genomic outcomes. J Nutr 2003;133:1521S–6S.
38. Sanderson IR, Naik S. Dietary regulation of intestinal gene expression. Annu Rev Nutr 2000;20:311–38.
39. Collins JF, Franck CA, Kowdley KV, Ghishan FK. Identification of differentially expressed genes in response to dietary iron deprivation in rat duodenum. Am J Physiol Gastrointest Liver Physiol 2005;288:G964–71.
40. Gelder CM, Hart KW, Williams OM, et al. Vitamin D receptor gene polymorphisms and susceptibility to Mycobacterium malmoense pulmonary disease. J Infect Dis 2000;181:2099–102.
41. Suneetha PV, Sarin SK, Goyal A, et al. Association between vitamin D receptor, CCR5, TNF-alpha and TNF-beta gene polymorphisms and HBV infection and severity of liver disease. J Hepatol 2006;44:856–63.
42. Anstead GM, Chandrasekar B, Zhang Q, Melby PC. Multinutrient undernutrition dysregulates the resident macrophage proinflammatory cytokine network, nuclear factor-kappaB activation, and nitric oxide production. J Leukoc Biol 2003;74:982–91.
43. Norton EB, Archibald LK, Nwanyanwu OC, et al. Clinical predictors of bloodstream infections and mortality in hospitalized Malawian children [discussion 151–5]. Pediatr Infect Dis J 2004;23:145–51.
44. Rodriguez L, Gonzalez C, Flores L, et al. Assessment by flow cytometry of cytokine production in malnourished children. Clin Diagn Lab Immunol 2005;12:502–7.
45. Dulger H, Arik M, Sekeroglu MR, et al. Pro-inflammatory cytokines in Turkish children with protein-energy malnutrition. Mediators Inflamm 2002;11:363–5.
46. Manary MJ, Yarasheski KE, Berger R, et al. Whole-body leucine kinetics and the acute phase response during acute infection in marasmic Malawian children. Pediatr Res 2004;55:940–6.
47. Phillips RS, Enwonwu CO, Okolo S, Hassan A. Metabolic effects of acute measles in chronically malnourished Nigerian children. J Nutr Biochem 2004;15:281–8.
48. Abraham K, Muller C, Gruters A, et al. Minimal inflammation, acute phase response and avoidance of misclassification of vitamin A and iron status in infants-importance of a high-sensitivity C-reactive protein (CRP) assay. Int J Vitam Nutr Res 2003;73:423–30.
49. Schultz C, Temming P, Bucsky P, et al. Immature anti-inflammatory response in neonates. Clin Exp Immunol 2004;135:130–6.
50. Ustianowski A, Shaffer R, Collin S, et al. Prevalence and associations of vitamin D deficiency in foreign-born persons with tuberculosis in London. J Infect 2005;50:432–7.
51. Singh M, Mynak ML, Kumar L, et al. Prevalence and risk factors for transmission of infection among children in household contact with adults having pulmonary tuberculosis. Arch Dis Child 2005;90:624–8.
52. Walker AS, Mulenga V, Sinyinza F, et al. Determinants of survival without antiretroviral therapy after infancy in HIV-1-infected Zambian children in the CHAP trial. J Acquir Immune Defic Syndr 2006;42:637–45.
53. He SX, Wu B, Chang XM, et al. Effects of selenium on peripheral blood mononuclear cell membrane fluidity, interleukin-2 production and interleukin-2 receptor expression in patients with chronic hepatitis. World J Gastroenterol 2004;10:3531–3.
54. Cunningham-Rundles S, McNeeley DF, Moon A. Mechanisms of nutrient modulation of the immune response. J Allergy Clin Immunol 2005;115:1119–28.
55. Cunningham-Rundles S. Evaluation of nutrient interaction in immune function. In: Calder PC, Field CJ, Gilled HS, editors. Nutrition and Immune Function. Oxon, UK: CABI; 2002. p. 21–39.
56. Cunningham-Rundles, S. Issues in the study of human immune function. In: Hughes DA, Darlington LG, Bendich A, editors. Dietary Enhancement of Human Immune Function. SCR Wallingford, Oxon, UK: Humana Press; 2003. p. 17–34.
57. Albers R, Bol M, Bleumink R, et al. Effects of supplementation with vitamins A, C, and E, selenium, and zinc on immune function in a murine sensitization model. Nutrition 2003;19:940–6.
58. Albert MJ, Qadri F, Wahed MA, et al. Supplementation with zinc, but not vitamin A, improves seroconversion to vibriocidal antibody in children given an oral cholera vaccine. J Infect Dis 2003;187:909–13.
59. Cunningham-Rundles S, McNeely D, Ananworanich JM. Immune response in malnutrition. In: Stiehm ER, Ochs HD, Winkelstein JA, editors. Immunologic Disorders in Infants and Children, 5th edition. Philadelphia, PA: Elsevier Saunders; 2004. p. 761–78.
60. Moynahan EJ. Letter: Acrodermatitis enteropathica: A lethal inherited human zinc-deficiency disorder. Lancet 1974;2:399–400.
61. Ferenci P, Caca K, Loudianos G, et al. Diagnosis and phenotypic classification of Wilson disease. Liver Int 2003;23:139–42.
62. Caballero B. Global patterns of child health: The role of nutrition. Ann Nutr Metab 2002;46:3–7.
63. Scott ME, Koski KG. Zinc deficiency impairs immune responses against parasitic nematode infections at intestinal and systemic sites. J Nutr 2000;130:1412S–20S.
64. Anstead GM, Chandrasekar B, Zhao W, et al. Malnutrition alters the innate immune response and increases early visceralization following Leishmania donovani infection. Infect Immun 2001;69:4709–18.
65. Brewster DR, Manary MJ, Menzies IS, et al. Comparison of milk and maize based diets in kwashiorkor. Arch Dis Child 1997;76:242–8.
66. Sakamoto M, Fujisawa Y, Nishioka K. Physiologic role of the complement system in host defense, disease, and malnutrition. Nutrition 1998;14:391–8.
67. Peters-Golden M, Canetti C, Mancuso P, Coffey MJ. Leukotrienes: Underappreciated mediators of innate immune responses. J Immunol 2005;174:589–94.
68. Wang TT, Nestel FP, Bourdeau V, et al. Cutting edge: 1,25-Dihydroxyvitamin D3 is a direct inducer of antimicrobial peptide gene expression. J Immunol 2004;173:2909–12.

69. Mancuso P, Gottschalk A, Phare SM, et al. Leptin-deficient mice exhibit impaired host defense in gram-negative pneumonia. J Immunol 2002;168:4018–24.
70. Ekiz C, Agaoglu L, Karakas Z, et al. The effect of iron deficiency anemia on the function of the immune system. Hematol J 2005;5:579–83.
71. Piemonti L, Monti P, Sironi M, et al. Vitamin D3 affects differentiation, maturation, and function of human monocyte-derived dendritic cells. J Immunol 2000;164:4443–51.
72. Coutant F, Agaugue S, Perrin-Cocon L, et al. Sensing environmental lipids by dendritic cell modulates its function. J Immunol 2004;172:54–60.
73. Dylewski ML, Mastro AM, Picciano MF. Maternal selenium nutrition and neonatal immune system development. Biol Neonate 2002;82:122–7.
74. Vasquez-Garibay E, Campollo-Rivas O, Romero-Velarde E, et al. Effect of renutrition on natural and cell-mediated immune response in infants with severe malnutrition. J Pediatr Gastroenterol Nutr 2002;34:296–301.
75. Kozakova H, Hanson LA, Stepankova R, et al. Vitamin A deficiency leads to severe functional disturbance of the intestinal epithelium enzymes associated with diarrhoea and increased bacterial translocation in gnotobiotic rats. Microbes Infect 2003;5:405–11.
76. Rosales FJ. Vitamin A supplementation of vitamin A deficient measles patients lowers the risk of measles-related pneumonia in Zambian children. J Nutr 2002;132:3700–3.
77. Long KZ, Santos JI, Estrada Garcia T, et al. Vitamin A supplementation reduces the monocyte chemoattractant protein-1 intestinal immune response of Mexican children. J Nutr 2006;136:2600–5.
78. Quadro L, Gamble MV, Vogel S, et al. Retinol and retinol-binding protein: Gut integrity and circulating immunoglobulins. J Infect Dis 2000;182:S97–102.
79. Iwata M, Hirakiyama A, Eshima Y, et al. Retinoic acid imprints gut-homing specificity on T cells. Immunity 2004;21:527–38.
80. Mora JR, Iwata M, Eksteen B, et al. Generation of gut-homing IgA-secreting B cells by intestinal dendritic cells. Science 2006;314:1157–60.
81. Pesonen M, Kallio MJ, Siimes MA, Ranki A. Retinol concentrations after birth are inversely associated with atopic manifestations in children and young adults. Clin Exp Allergy 2007;37:54–61.
82. Cantorna MT, Zhu Y, Froicu M, Wittke A. Vitamin D status, 1,25-dihydroxyvitamin D3, and the immune system. Am J Clin Nutr 2004;80:1717S–20S.
83. Simmons JD, Mullighan C, Welsh KI, Jewell DP. Vitamin D receptor gene polymorphism: Association with Crohn's disease susceptibility. Gut 2000;47:211–4.
84. Wayse V, Yousafzai A, Mogale K, Filteau S. Association of subclinical vitamin D deficiency with severe acute lower respiratory infection in Indian children under 5 y. Eur J Clin Nutr 2004;58:563–7.
85. Liu PT, Stenger S, Li H, et al. Toll-like receptor triggering of a vitamin D-mediated human antimicrobial response. Science 2006;311:1770–3.
86. Buck RH, Thomas DL, Winship TR, et al. Effect of dietary ribonucleotides on infant immune status. Part 2: Immune cell development. Pediatr Res 2004;56:891–900.
87. Schaller JP, Kuchan MJ, Thomas DL, et al. Effect of dietary ribonucleotides on infant immune status. Part 1: Humoral responses. Pediatr Res 2004;56:883–90.
88. Martinez-Augustin O, Boza JJ, Navarro J, et al. Dietary nucleotides may influence the humoral immunity in immunocompromised children. Nutrition 1997;13:465–9.
89. Hawkes JS, Gibson RA, Roberton D, Makrides M. Effect of dietary nucleotide supplementation on growth and immune function in term infants: A randomized controlled trial. Eur J Clin Nutr 2006;60:254–64.
90. Carver JD, Stromquist CI. Dietary nucleotides and preterm infant nutrition. J Perinatol 2006;26:443–4.
91. Walker WA. The dynamic effects of breastfeeding on intestinal development and host defense. Adv Exp Med Biol 2004;554:155–70.
92. Kelly D, Coutts AG. Early nutrition and the development of immune function in the neonate. Proc Nutr Soc 2000;59:177–85.
93. Newburg DS, Ruiz-Palacios GM, Morrow AL. Human milk glycans protect infants against enteric pathogens. Annu Rev Nutr 2005;25:37–58.
94. Jarvinen KM, Laine ST, Jarvenpaa AL, Suomalainen HK. Does low IgA in human milk predispose the infant to development of cow's milk allergy? Pediatr Res 2000;48:457–62.
95. Dvorak B, Fituch CC, Williams CS, et al. Increased epidermal growth factor levels in human milk of mothers with extremely premature infants. Pediatr Res 2003;54:15–9.
96. Collinson AC, Moore SE, Cole TJ, Prentice AM. Birth season and environmental influences on patterns of thymic growth in rural Gambian infants. Acta Paediatr 2003;92:1014–20.
97. Basu S, Sengupta B, Paladhi PK. Single megadose vitamin A supplementation of Indian mothers and morbidity in breastfed young infants. Postgrad Med J 2003;79:397–402.
98. Vidal K, Labeta MO, Schiffrin EJ, Donnet-Hughes A. Soluble CD14 in human breast milk and its role in innate immune responses. Acta Odontol Scand 2001;59:330–4.
99. Dunstan JA, Roper J, Mitoulas L, et al. The effect of supplementation with fish oil during pregnancy on breast milk immunoglobulin A, soluble CD14, cytokine levels and fatty acid composition. Clin Exp Allergy 2004;34:1237–42.
100. Accorsi S, Fabiani M, Nattabi B, et al. The disease profile of poverty: Morbidity and mortality in northern Uganda in the context of war, population displacement and HIV/AIDS. Trans R Soc Trop Med Hyg 2005;99:226–33.
101. Carvalho NF, Kenney RD, Carrington PH, Hall DE. Severe nutritional deficiencies in toddlers resulting from health food milk alternatives. Pediatrics 2001;107:E46.
102. Eastlack JP, Grande KK, Levy ML, Nigro JF. Dermatosis in a child with kwashiorkor secondary to food aversion. Pediatr Dermatol 1999;16:95–102.
103. Liu T, Howard RM, Mancini AJ, et al. Kwashiorkor in the United States: Fad diets, perceived and true milk allergy, and nutritional ignorance. Arch Dermatol 2001;137:630–6.
104. Ganji V, Hampl JS, Betts NM. Race-, gender- and age-specific differences in dietary micronutrient intakes of US children. Int J Food Sci Nutr 2003;54:485–90.
105. Fattal-Valevski A, Kesler A, Sela BA, et al. Outbreak of life-threatening thiamine deficiency in infants in Israel caused by a defective soy-based formula. Pediatrics 2005;115:e233–8.
106. Obladen M, Loui A, Kampmann W, Renz H. Zinc deficiency in rapidly growing preterm infants. Acta Paediatr 1998;87:685–91.
107. Kaur S, Thami GP, Kanwar AJ. Acrodermatitis enteropathica in a full-term breast-fed infant. Indian J Pediatr 2002;69:631–3.
108. Kury S, Kharfi M, Kamoun R, et al. Mutation spectrum of human SLC39A4 in a panel of patients with acrodermatitis enteropathica. Hum Mutat 2003;22:337–8.
109. Madhok AB, Chandrasekran A, Parnell V, et al. Levels of recent thymic emigrant cells decrease in children undergoing partial thymectomy during cardiac surgery. Clin Diagn Lab Immunol 2005;12:563–5.
110. Jawad AF, McDonald-Mcginn DM, Zackai E, Sullivan KE. Immunologic features of chromosome 22q11.2 deletion syndrome (DiGeorge syndrome/velocardiofacial syndrome). J Pediatr 2001;139:715–23.
111. Van Esch H, Groenen P, Nesbit MA, et al. GATA3 haplo-insufficiency causes human HDR syndrome. Nature 2000;406:419–22.
112. Aaby P, Marx C, Trautner S, et al. Thymus size at birth is associated with infant mortality: A community study from Guinea-Bissau. Acta Paediatr 2002;91:698–703.
113. Faggioni R, Feingold KR, Grunfeld C. Leptin regulation of the immune response and the immunodeficiency of malnutrition. FASEB J 2001;15:2565–71.
114. Savino W. The thymus gland is a target in malnutrition. Eur J Clin Nutr 2002;56:S46–9.
115. Palacio A, Lopez M, Perez-Bravo F, et al. Leptin levels are associated with immune response in malnourished infants. J Clin Endocrinol Metab 2002;87:3040–6.
116. Reid M, Badaloo A, Forrester T, et al. The acute-phase protein response to infection in edematous and nonedematous protein-energy malnutrition. Am J Clin Nutr 2002;76:1409–15.
117. Russell BJ, White AV, Newbury J, et al. Evaluation of hospitalisation for Indigenous children with malnutrition living in Central Australia. Aust J Rural Health 2004;12:187–91.
118. Najera O, Gonzalez C, Toledo G, et al. Flow cytometry study of lymphocyte subsets in malnourished and well-nourished children with bacterial infections. Clin Diagn Lab Immunol 2004;11:577–80.
119. Rikimaru T, Taniguchi K, Yartey JE, et al. Humoral and cell-mediated immunity in malnourished children in Ghana. Eur J Clin Nutr 1998;52:344–50.
120. Forte WC, Santos de Menezes MC, Horta C, Carneiro Leao Bach R. Serum IgE level in malnutrition. Allergol Immunopathol (Madr) 2003;31:83–6.
121. Moore SE, Goldblatt D, Bates CJ, Prentice AM. Impact of nutritional status on antibody responses to different vaccines in undernourished Gambian children. Acta Paediatr 2003;92:170–6.
122. Barker DJ. The developmental origins of chronic adult disease. Acta Paediatr Suppl 2004;93:26–33.
123. Dobbing J. Fetal nutrition and cardiovascular disease in adult life. Lancet 1993;341:1421–2.
124. McDade TW, Beck MA, Kuzawa C, Adair LS. Prenatal undernutrition, postnatal environments, and antibody response to vaccination in adolescence. Am J Clin Nutr 2001;74:543–8.
125. Dagogo-Jack S, Tykodi G, Umamaheswaran I. Inhibition of cortisol biosynthesis decreases circulating leptin levels in obese humans. J Clin Endocrinol Metab 2005;90:5333–5.
126. Bornstein SR, Licinio J, Tauchnitz R, et al. Plasma leptin levels are increased in survivors of acute sepsis: Associated loss of diurnal rhythm, in cortisol and leptin secretion. J Clin Endocrinol Metab 1998;83:280–3.
127. Gibson WT, Farooqi IS, Moreau M, et al. Congenital leptin deficiency due to homozygosity for the Delta133G mutation: Report of another case and evaluation of response to four years of leptin therapy. J Clin Endocrinol Metab 2004;89:4821–6.
128. Otero M, Lago R, Gomez R, et al. Towards a pro-inflammatory and immunomodulatory emerging role of leptin. Rheumatology 2006;45:944–50.
129. Levin BE. Factors promoting and ameliorating the development of obesity. Physiol Behav 2005;86:633–9.
130. Vieira VJ, Ronan AM, Windt MR, Tagliaferro AR. Elevated atopy in healthy obese women. Am J Clin Nutr 2005;82:504–9.
131. Falagas ME, Kompoti M. Obesity and infection. Lancet Infect Dis 2006;6:438–46.
132. Tanaka S, Inoue S, Isoda F, et al. Impaired immunity in obesity: Suppressed but reversible lymphocyte responsiveness. Int J Obes Relat Metab Disord 1993;17:631–6.
133. Skibola CF, Holly EA, Forrest MS, et al. Body mass index, leptin and leptin receptor polymorphisms, and non-hodgkin lymphoma. Cancer Epidemiol Biomarkers Prev 2004;13:779–86.
134. Wernstedt I, Eriksson AL, Berndtsson A, et al. A common polymorphism in the interleukin-6 gene promoter is associated with overweight. Int J Obes Relat Metab Disord 2004;28:1272–9.
135. Backhed F, Ding H, Wang T, et al. The gut microbiota as an environmental factor that regulates fat storage. Proc Natl Acad Sci U S A 2004;101:15718–23.
136. Dhurandhar NV. Contribution of pathogens in human obesity. Drug News Perspect 2004;17:307–13.
137. Juyal R, Osmamy M, Black RE, et al. Efficacy of micronutrient fortification of milk on morbidity in pre-school children and growth-a double blind randomised controlled trial. Asia Pac J Clin Nutr 2004;13:S44.
138. Lyons GH, Stangoulis JC, Graham RD. Exploiting micronutrient interaction to optimize biofortification programs: The case for inclusion of selenium and iodine in the HarvestPlus program. Nutr Rev 2004;62:247–52.
139. Beck MA, Williams-Toone D, Levander OA. Coxsackievirus B3-resistant mice become susceptible in Se/vitamin E deficiency. Free Radic Biol Med 2003;34:1263–70.
140. van den Broek N. Anaemia and micronutrient deficiencies. Br Med Bull 2003;67:149–60.
141. Klinger G, Shamir R, Singer P, et al. Parenteral selenium supplementation in extremely low birth weight infants: Inadequate dosage but no correlation with hypothyroidism. J Perinatol 1999;19:568–72.
142. Nair S, Norkus EP, Hertan H, Pitchumoni CS. Micronutrient antioxidants in gastric mucosa and serum in patients with gastritis and gastric ulcer: Does *Helicobacter pylori* infection affect the mucosal levels? J Clin Gastroenterol 2000;30:381–5.
143. Baysoy G, Ertem D, Ademoglu E, et al. Gastric histopathology, iron status and iron deficiency anemia in children with *Helicobacter pylori* infection. J Pediatr Gastroenterol Nutr 2004;38:146–51.
144. Bennedsen M, Wang X, Willen R, et al. Treatment of *H. pylori* infected mice with antioxidant astaxanthin reduces gastric inflammation, bacterial load and modulates cytokine release by splenocytes. Immunol Lett 1999;70:185–9.
145. Olczak AA, Seyler RW, Jr, Olson JW, Maier RJ. Association of *Helicobacter pylori* antioxidant activities with host colonization proficiency. Infect Immun 2003;71:580–3.
146. Goth SR, Chu RA, Gregg JP, et al. Uncoupling of ATP-mediated calcium signaling and dysregulated interleukin-6 secretion in dendritic cells by nanomolar thimerosal. Environ Health Perspect 2006;114:1083–91.
147. Brewster UC, Perazella MA. Intravenous iron and the risk of infection in end-stage renal disease patients. Semin Dial 2004;17:57–60.
148. Chung BH, Ha SY, Chan GC, et al. *Klebsiella* infection in patients with thalassemia. Clin Infect Dis 2003;36:575–9.
149. Cunningham-Rundles S, Giardina PJ, Grady RW, et al. Effect of transfusional iron overload on immune response. J Infect Dis 2000;182:S115–21.

150. Nasr MR, Ali S, Shaker M, Elgabry E. Antioxidant micronutrients in children with thalassaemia in Egypt. East Mediterr Health J 2002;8:490–5.
151. Moalem S, Weinberg ED, Percy ME. Hemochromatosis and the enigma of misplaced iron: Implications for infectious disease and survival. Biometals 2004;17:135–9.
152. Fritsche G, Larcher C, Schennach H, Weiss G. Regulatory interactions between iron and nitric oxide metabolism for immune defense against *Plasmodium falciparum* infection. J Infect Dis 2001;183:1388–94.
153. Berger J, Dyck JL, Galan P, et al. Effect of daily iron supplementation on iron status, cell-mediated immunity, and incidence of infections in 6–36 month old Togolese children. Eur J Clin Nutr 2000;54:29–35.
154. Sanders TA. Vegetarian diets and children. Pediatr Clin North Am 1995;42:955–65.
155. Mattsson N, Kilander A, Bjornsson E. *Helicobacter pylori* can in rare cases be the cause of iron and vitamin B12 deficiency. No increased risk of iron and vitamin B12 deficiency due to proton pump inhibitors. Lakartidningen 2004;101:2014–5.
156. Lopez A. Malnutrition and the burden of disease. Asia Pac J Clin Nutr 2004;13:S7.
157. Bhatnagar S, Natchu UC. Zinc in child health and disease. Indian J Pediatr 2004;71:991–5.
158. Bhaskaram P. Micronutrient malnutrition, infection, and immunity: An overview. Nutr Rev 2002;60:S40–5.
159. Crone J, Huber WD, Eichler I, Granditsch G. Acrodermatitis enteropathica-like eruption as the presenting sign of cystic fibrosis—case report and review of the literature. Eur J Pediatr 2002;161:475–8.
160. Mocchegiani E, Ciavattini A, Santarelli L, et al. Role of zinc and alpha2 macroglobulin on thymic endocrine activity and on peripheral immune efficiency (natural killer activity and interleukin 2) in cervical carcinoma. Br J Cancer 1999;79:244–50.
161. Fraker PJ. Roles for cell death in zinc deficiency. J Nutr 2005;135:359–62.
162. Fraker PJ, Lill-Elghanian DA. The many roles of apoptosis in immunity as modified by aging and nutritional status. J Nutr Health Aging 2004;8:56–63.
163. Raqib R, Roy SK, Rahman MJ, et al. Effect of zinc supplementation on immune and inflammatory responses in pediatric patients with shigellosis. Am J Clin Nutr 2004;79:444–50.
164. von Bulow V, Rink L, Haase H. Zinc-mediated inhibition of cyclic nucleotide phosphodiesterase activity and expression suppresses TNF-alpha and IL-1 beta production in monocytes by elevation of guanosine 3',5'-cyclic monophosphate. J Immunol 2005;175:4697–705.
165. Metz CH, Schroder AK, Overbeck S, et al. T-helper type 1 cytokine release is enhanced by in vitro zinc supplementation due to increased natural killer cells. Nutrition 2006.
166. Qadri F, Ahmed T, Wahed MA, et al. Suppressive effect of zinc on antibody response to cholera toxin in children given the killed, B subunit-whole cell, oral cholera vaccine. Vaccine 2004;22:416–21.
167. Kury S, Dreno B, Bezieau S, et al. Identification of *SLC39A4*, a gene involved in acrodermatitis enteropathica. Nat Genet 2002;31:239–40.
168. Cousins RJ, Blanchard RK, Popp MP, et al. A global view of the selectivity of zinc deprivation and excess on genes expressed in human THP-1 mononuclear cells. Proc Natl Acad Sci U S A 2003;100:6952–7.
169. Aydemir TB, Blanchard RK, Cousins RJ. Zinc supplementation of young men alters metallothionein, zinc transporter, and cytokine gene expression in leukocyte populations. Proc Natl Acad Sci U S A 2006;103:1699–704.
170. Schlesinger L, Arevalo M, Arredondo S, et al. Effect of a zinc-fortified formula on immunocompetence and growth of malnourished infants. Am J Clin Nutr 1992;56:491–8.
171. Thakur S, Gupta N, Kakkar P. Serum copper and zinc concentrations and their relation to superoxide dismutase in severe malnutrition. Eur J Pediatr 2004.
172. Marikovsky M, Ziv V, Nevo N, et al. Cu/Zn superoxide dismutase plays important role in immune response. J Immunol 2003;170:2993–3001.
173. Botash AS, Nasca J, Dubowy R, et al. Zinc-induced copper deficiency in an infant. Am J Dis Child 1992;146:709–11.
174. Percival SS. Copper and immunity. Am J Clin Nutr 1998;67:1064S–8S.
175. Bonham M, O'Connor JM, Hannigan BM, Strain JJ. The immune system as a physiological indicator of marginal copper status? Br J Nutr 2002;87:393–403.
176. Squali Houssaini FZ, Iraqi MR, Arnaud J, et al. Trace elements and protein-calorie malnutrition in the Fes area (Morocco). Biomed Pharmacother 1997;51:349–51.
177. Miyajima H, Takahashi Y, Kono S. Aceruloplasminemia, an inherited disorder of iron metabolism. Biometals 2003;16:205–13.
178. Cox DW, Moore SD. Copper transporting P-type ATPases and human disease. J Bioenerg Biomembr 2002;34:333–8.
179. Rayman MP. The importance of selenium to human health. Lancet 2000;356:233–41.
180. Thomson CD. Selenium and iodine intakes and status in New Zealand and Australia. Br J Nutr 2004;91:661–72.
181. Manar MJ, MacPherson GD, McArdle F, et al. Selenium status, kwashiorkor and congestive heart failure. Acta Paediatr 2001;90:950–2.
182. Beck MA, Levander OA, Handy J. Selenium deficiency and viral infection. J Nutr 2003;133:1463S–7S.
183. Salonen JT, Alfthan G, Huttunen JK, Puska P. Association between serum selenium and the risk of cancer. Am J Epidemiol 1984;120:342–9.
184. Virtamo J, Valkeila E, Alfthan G, et al. Serum selenium and risk of cancer. A prospective follow-up of nine years. Cancer 1987;60:145–8.
185. Ferencik M, Ebringer L. Modulatory effects of selenium and zinc on the immune system. Folia Microbiol (Praha) 2003;48:417–26.
186. Baum MK, Shor-Posner G, Lai S, et al. High risk of HIV-related mortality is associated with selenium deficiency. J Acquir Immune Defic Syndr Hum Retrovirol 1997;15:370–4.
187. Baeten JM, Mostad SB, Hughes MP, et al. Selenium deficiency is associated with shedding of HIV-1-infected cells in the female genital tract. J Acquir Immune Defic Syndr 2001;26:360–4.
188. Stephensen CB. Vitamin A, infection, and immune function. Annu Rev Nutr 2001;21:167–92.
189. Fawzi WW, Chalmers TC, Herrera MG, Mosteller F. Vitamin A supplementation and child mortality. A meta-analysis. JAMA 1993;269:898–903.
190. Sommer A, Davidson FR. Assessment and control of vitamin A deficiency: The Annecy Accords. J Nutr 2002;132:2845S–2850S.
191. Cunningham-Rundles S, Kim SH, Dnistrian A, et al. Micronutrient and cytokine interaction in congenital pediatric HIV infection. J Nutr 1996;126:2674S–2679S.
192. Al-Kubaisy W, Al-Rubaiy MG, Nassief HA. Xerophthalmia among hospitalized Iraqi children. East Mediterr Health J 2002;8:496–502.
193. Tan Z, Ma G, Lin L, et al. Prevalence of subclinical vitamin A deficiency and its affecting factors in 8669 children of China. Zhonghua Yu Fang Yi Xue Za Zhi 2002;36:161–3.
194. Cser MA, Majchrzak D, Rust P, et al. Serum carotenoid and retinol levels during childhood infections. Ann Nutr Metab 2004;48:156–62.
195. Aukrust P, Muller F, Ueland T, et al. Decreased vitamin A levels in common variable immunodeficiency: Vitamin A supplementation in vivo enhances immunoglobulin production and downregulates inflammatory responses. Eur J Clin Invest 2000;30:252–9.
196. Wieringa FT, Dijkhuizen MA, West CE, et al. Reduced production of immunoregulatory cytokines in vitamin A- and zinc-deficient Indonesian infants. Eur J Clin Nutr 2004;58:1498–504.
197. Stephensen CB, Jiang X, Freytag T. Vitamin A deficiency increases the in vivo development of IL-10-positive Th2 cells and decreases development of Th1 cells in mice. J Nutr 2004;134:2660–6.
198. Grubesic RB, Selwyn BJ. Vitamin A supplementation and health outcomes for children in Nepal. J Nurs Scholarsh 2003;35:15–20.
199. Long KZ, Estrada-Garcia T, Rosado JL, et al. The effect of vitamin A supplementation on the intestinal immune response in Mexican children is modified by pathogen infections and diarrhea. J Nutr 2006;136:1365–70.
200. Park OJ, Kim HY, Kim WK, et al. Effect of vitamin E supplementation on antioxidant defense systems and humoral immune responses in young, middle-aged and elderly Korean women. J Nutr Sci Vitaminol (Tokyo) 2003;49:94–9.
201. van Tits LJ, Demacker PN, de Graaf J, et al. Alpha-tocopherol supplementation decreases production of superoxide and cytokines by leukocytes ex vivo in both normolipidemic and hypertriglyceridemic individuals. Am J Clin Nutr 2000;71:458–64.
202. Wu D, Meydani SN. Mechanism of age-associated up-regulation in macrophage PGE2 synthesis. Brain Behav Immun 2004;18:487–94.
203. Lee CY, Man-Fan Wan J. Vitamin E supplementation improves cell-mediated immunity and oxidative stress of Asian men and women. J Nutr 2000;130:2932–7.
204. Malmberg KJ, Lenkei R, Petersson M, et al. A short-term dietary supplementation of high doses of vitamin E increases T helper 1 cytokine production in patients with advanced colorectal cancer. Clin Cancer Res 2002;8:1772–8.
205. Pighetti GM, Eskew ML, Reddy CC, Sordillo LM. Selenium and vitamin E deficiency impair transferrin receptor internalization but not IL-2, IL-2 receptor, or transferrin receptor expression. J Leukoc Biol 1998;63:131–7.
206. Lagrange-Puget M, Durieu I, Ecochard R, et al. Longitudinal study of oxidative status in 312 cystic fibrosis patients in stable state and during bronchial exacerbation. Pediatr Pulmonol 2004;38:43–9.
207. Hartel C, Strunk T, Bucsky P, Schultz C. Effects of vitamin C on intracytoplasmic cytokine production in human whole blood monocytes and lymphocytes. Cytokine 2004;27:101–6.
208. Victor VV, Guayerbas N, Puerto M, et al. Ascorbic acid modulates in vitro the function of macrophages from mice with endotoxic shock. Immunopharmacology 2000;46:89–101.
209. Fischer CP, Hiscock NJ, Penkowa M, et al. Supplementation with vitamins C and E inhibits the release of interleukin-6 from contracting human skeletal muscle. J Physiol 2004;558:633–45.
210. Ahmed J, Zaman MM, Ali SM. Immunological response to antioxidant vitamin supplementation in rural Bangladeshi school children with group A streptococcal infection. Asia Pac J Clin Nutr 2004;13:226–30.
211. Wintergerst ES, Maggini S, Hornig DH. Immune-enhancing role of vitamin C and zinc and effect on clinical conditions. Ann Nutr Metab 2006;50:85–94.
212. Akyon Y. Effect of antioxidants on the immune response of *Helicobacter pylori*. Clin Microbiol Infect 2002;8:438–41.
213. Schwarzwald H. Illnesses among recently immigrated children. Semin Pediatr Infect Dis 2005;16:78–83.
214. Salas SD, Heifetz R, Barrett-Connor E. Intestinal parasites in Central American immigrants in the United States. Arch Intern Med 1990;150:1514–6.
215. Shlomai A, Paran N, Shaul Y. PGC-1alpha controls hepatitis B virus through nutritional signals. Proc Natl Acad Sci U S A 2006;103:16003–8.
216. Iwasa M, Iwata K, Kaito M, et al. Efficacy of long-term dietary restriction of total calories, fat, iron, and protein in patients with chronic hepatitis C virus. Nutrition 2004;20:368–71.
217. van Lettow M, West CE, van der Meer JW, et al. Low plasma selenium concentrations, high plasma human immunodeficiency virus load and high interleukin-6 concentrations are risk factors associated with anemia in adults presenting with pulmonary tuberculosis in Zomba district, Malawi. Eur J Clin Nutr 2005;59:526–32.
218. Guarino A, Bruzzese E, De Marco G, Buccigrossi V. Management of gastrointestinal disorders in children with HIV infection. Paediatr Drugs 2004;6:347–62.
219. Guarino A, Spagnuolo MI, Giacomet V, et al. Effects of nutritional rehabilitation on intestinal function and on CD4 cell number in children with HIV. J Pediatr Gastroenterol Nutr 2002;34:366–71.
220. Humphrey JH, Iliff PJ, Marinda ET, et al. Effects of a single large dose of vitamin A, given during the postpartum period to HIV-positive women and their infants, on child HIV infection, HIV-free survival, and mortality. J Infect Dis 2006;193:860–71.
221. Kuhn L, Coutsoudis A, Trabattoni D, et al. Synergy between mannose-binding lectin gene polymorphisms and supplementation with vitamin A influences susceptibility to HIV infection in infants born to HIV-positive mothers. Am J Clin Nutr 2006;84:610–5.
222. Baum MK, Miguez-Burbano MJ, Campa A, Shor-Posner G. Selenium and interleukins in persons infected with human immunodeficiency virus type 1. J Infect Dis 2000;182:S69–73.
223. Ergun-Longmire B, Lin-Su K, Dunn AM, et al. Effects of protease inhibitors on glucose tolerance, lipid metabolism, and body composition in children and adolescents infected with human immunodeficiency virus. Endocr Pract 2006;12:514–21.
224. Day L, Shikuma C, Gerschenson M. Acetyl-L-carnitine for the treatment of HIV lipoatrophy. Ann N Y Acad Sci 2004;1033:139–46.
225. Hotta M, Nagashima E, Takagi S, et al. Two young female patients with anorexia nervosa complicated by Mycobacterium tuberculosis infection. Intern Med 2004;43:440–4.
226. Hesseling AC, Westra AE, Werschkull H, et al. Outcome of HIV infected children with culture confirmed tuberculosis. Arch Dis Child 2005;90:1171–4.
227. Miller LC. International adoption: Infectious diseases issues. Clin Infect Dis 2005;40:286–93.
228. Boelaert JR, Gordeuk VR. Protein energy malnutrition and risk of tuberculosis infection. Lancet 2002;360:1102.
229. Chan J, Tian Y, Tanaka KE, et al. Effects of protein calorie malnutrition on tuberculosis in mice. Proc Natl Acad Sci U S A 1996;93:14857–61.

230. McDermid JM, Prentice AM. Iron and infection: Effects of host iron status and the iron-regulatory genes haptoglobin and NRAMP1 (SLC11A1) on host-pathogen interactions in tuberculosis and HIV. Clin Sci (Lond) 2006;110:503–24.
231. Shor-Posner G, Miguez MJ, Pineda LM, et al. Impact of selenium status on the pathogenesis of mycobacterial disease in HIV-1-infected drug users during the era of highly active antiretroviral therapy. J Acquir Immune Defic Syndr 2002;29:169–73.
232. Wilkinson RJ, Llewelyn M, Toossi Z, et al. Influence of vitamin D deficiency and vitamin D receptor polymorphisms on tuberculosis among Gujarati Asians in west London: A case-control study. Lancet 2000;355:618–21.
233. Waters WR, Palmer MV, Nonnecke BJ, et al. Mycobacterium bovis infection of vitamin D-deficient NOS2–/–mice. Microb Pathog 2004;36:11–7.
234. Nathan C. Role of iNOS in human host defense. Science 2006;312:1874–5; author reply 1874–5.
235. Stoltzfus RJ, Chway HM, Montresor A, et al. Low dose daily iron supplementation improves iron status and appetite but not anemia, whereas quarterly anthelminthic treatment improves growth, appetite and anemia in Zanzibari preschool children. J Nutr 2004;134:348–56.
236. Hesham MS, Edariah AB, Norhayati M. Intestinal parasitic infections and micronutrient deficiency: A review. Med J Malaysia 2004;59:284–93.
237. Koski KG, Scott ME. Gastrointestinal nematodes, nutrition and immunity: Breaking the negative spiral. Annu Rev Nutr 2001;21:297–321.
238. Ertan P, Yereli K, Kurt O, et al. Serological levels of zinc, copper and iron elements among Giardia lamblia infected children in Turkey. Pediatr Int 2002;44:286–8.
239. Ing R, Su Z, Scott ME, Koski KG. Suppressed T helper 2 immunity and prolonged survival of a nematode parasite in protein-malnourished mice. Proc Natl Acad Sci U S A 2000;97:7078–83.
240. Cliffe LJ, Humphreys NE, Lane TE, et al. Accelerated intestinal epithelial cell turnover: A new mechanism of parasite expulsion. Science 2005;308:1463–5.
241. Rivera MT, De Souza AP, Araujo-Jorge TC, et al. Trace elements, innate immune response and parasites. Clin Chem Lab Med 2003;41:1020–5.
242. Hagel I, Lynch NR, Puccio F, et al. Defective regulation of the protective IgE response against intestinal helminth Ascaris lumbricoides in malnourished children. J Trop Pediatr 2003;49:136–42.
243. Nussenblatt V, Semba RD. Micronutrient malnutrition and the pathogenesis of malarial anemia. Acta Trop 2002;82:321–37.

24

Neuropsychological Development

Maureen M. Black, PhD
John P. Ackerman, PhD

Nutritional deprivation is a worldwide public health concern that can result in long-term deficits to children's growth and development. A recent series of papers in *The Lancet*[1–3] found that more than 200 million children under 5 years fail to reach their developmental potential because of poverty, poor health and nutrition (especially iodine and iron deficiency), and lack of early stimulation. These disadvantaged children are likely to experience neuropsychological problems, perform poorly in school and subsequently have low incomes, high fertility, and provide poor care for their children, thus contributing to the intergenerational transmission of poverty. However, early home- and center-based programs targeted toward young disadvantaged children throughout the world can disrupt the negative cycle and contribute to positive effects on children's neuropsychological development, academic performance, and life chances.[2]

This chapter examines the relationship between nutritional deficiencies and neuropsychological development in children. It reviews the history of research linking nutrition and children's development, methods used to study child development, and the evidence linking nutrition and child development, with an emphasis on micronutrient deficiencies and lead exposure. Finally, recommendations are made to reduce the burden that children experience from nutritional deficiencies.

HISTORICAL CONSIDERATIONS

The association between nutritional deprivation and child development has been a topic of interest for over 40 years. Initially, investigators focused on protein-energy malnutrition (PEM), caused by a lack of calories. During the acute phase of nutritional deprivation, children have been described as lethargic, apathetic, and inactive, with poor performance on measures of cognitive functioning.[4,5]

Most of the research in this area has addressed the long-term consequences associated with early nutritional deprivation. Guided by findings from animal research that nutritional deprivation can lead to structural and functional changes in the developing brain,[6] investigators have used a variety of standardized assessment tools, such as IQ tests or ratings of performance or social-emotional behavior, to determine whether nutritionally deprived children recover or experience long-term neurobehavioral consequences. Most investigators use case-control, retrospective designs to study children with a history of nutritional deprivation and compare their performance on tasks with the performance of adequately nourished children. Findings generally indicate long-lasting deficits in intelligence and school performance.[7]

Nutritional deprivation often occurs in the context of poverty. Although most investigators handled socioeconomic differences in study populations by recruiting comparison children from similar socioeconomic backgrounds, little attention has been directed to individual differences or how children's response to nutritional rehabilitation varies by environmental characteristics. Advances in the areas of growth, nutrition, animal research, behavioral neuroscience, and child development have influenced recent investigations of nutritional deprivation and child development.

Growth

In the absence of adequate nutrients, a young child's body conserves energy by limiting weight gain and then by limiting linear growth. Linear growth or length is influenced by genetic factors, environmental factors, and medical conditions. The National Center for Health Statistics (NCHS) has developed age- and gender-specific growth charts for health professionals to track children's length over time (see Appendix I, "Nutritional Assessment"). Length is converted to length-for-age, often expressed as a percentile. Children growing between the 5th and 95th percentiles are considered to be growing within normal limits.

Stunting, defined as length-for-age that is more than 2 SD below the NCHS or World Health Organization (WHO) International Growth Reference, serves as a general indicator of a child's nutritional status over long periods of time. Growth stunting is a gradual process that occurs in response to chronic biological insults, including malnutrition and infectious diseases, during periods of linear bone growth. It often begins in utero and extends through the first 2 years. Childhood stunting is closely associated with poverty and is often used as a population-based indicator to compare nutritional adequacy across countries. Without environmental changes, such as adoption, stunting can lead to a permanent reduction in growth. Unless puberty is delayed, thereby expending the growing period, children who experience stunting early in life may be shorter during childhood and adulthood than peers who had adequate early growth. Approximately one-third of the world's children experience nutritional deficiencies that are severe enough to interfere with their early growth.[8]

The WHO recently published new international growth references from the Multicountry Growth Reference Study, which examined how healthy children grow in homes that engage in health-promoting practices (breastfeeding and not smoking). Approximately 8,500 children from varying ethnic and cultural groups in six diverse countries (Brazil, Ghana, India, Norway, Oman, and the United States) participated in the study. Children were measured from birth through age 5 years. There was a strong similarity in linear growth across the six sites, providing evidence for the use of a single international growth standard and demonstrating that when children's health and environmental needs are met, growth is similar[9] (see Chapter 2, "Clinical Assessment of Nutritional Status," for discussion of these new growth curves).

Nutrition

In addition to PEM, which continues to be a prevalent problem, especially in low-income countries, recent evidence suggests that micronutrient deficiencies are a major impediment to children's development. Micronutrients represent small quantities of essential vitamins and minerals that promote healthy growth and development. Since they are not produced by the body, they must be acquired either through the diet, fortification, or supplementation. The relationship between micronutrient deficiency and early cognitive development has captured recent attention because micronutrients are related to specific physiological and neurological processes.[10]

Micronutrient deficiencies are a critical concern among children throughout the world. Iodine, iron, and zinc have been linked to cognitive processes in infants and young children and will be addressed in this review. Approximately 30% of the world's population live in iodine-deficient areas and 25% of the world's children under age 3 have iron-deficiency anemia (IDA), with higher rates in developing countries.[11] When iron deficiency without anemia is considered, rates are even higher.[12] Less is known about rates of zinc deficiency. Estimates from dietary intakes of children from developing countries suggest high rates of zinc deficiency among infants and toddlers,[13] and low zinc intake may be common among middle-class infants and toddlers in America.[14]

Animal Research

Animal models, primarily involving rats, have been widely utilized in research linking nutrition

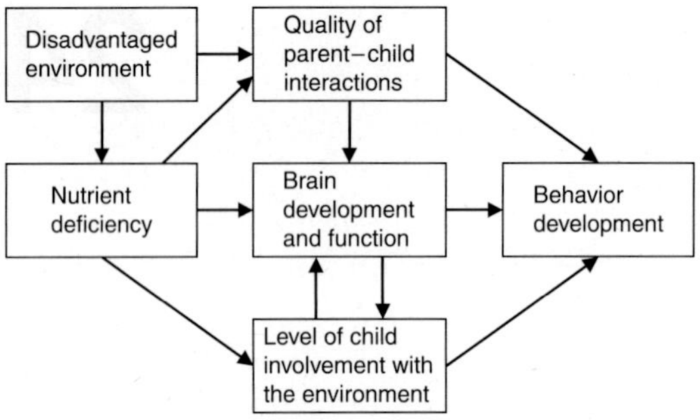

Figure 1 Association between nutritional deficiency and children's behavior and development. (Adapted from reference 17.)

to cognitive functioning. Much of the neurological development of rats occurs postnatally, enabling investigators to study the timing and chronicity of nutritional deprivation.[6] In the past, animal researchers often experienced difficulty disentangling the environmental and nutritional effects on young animals. Many of the techniques used to introduce nutritional deprivation (eg, increasing the number of infants for a mother to feed, decreasing access to the mother, feeding the mother an inadequate diet, ligating the mother's nipples) altered mother–pup interaction and the social environment, thus confounding the research. Through innovative designs, such as the introduction of artificial feeding, investigators were able to vary both nutritional intake and environmental stimulation.[15,16] These studies have found that animals who experience both nutritional and environmental deprivation tend to have worse performance than animals deprived in only one condition, suggesting that the environmental stimulation may moderate the adverse consequences of undernutrition.[15] Levitsky and Barnes described the process whereby nutritional deficiencies are partially mediated through caregiving behavior as functional isolation (Figure 1).[17] Thus, in addition to the direct effects of nutritional deprivation, undernourished animals who are unable to elicit environmental stimulation may also be denied the environmental enrichment that promotes development.

The recognition that the link between nutritional deprivation and intellectual performance depends on nonnutritional factors and can be influenced by environmental stimulation had an important impact on research involving nutritionally deprived children. It illustrated the necessity of incorporating caregiving variables, such as the quality of parent–child interaction, into models of child development, rather than merely controlling for socioeconomic differences.[18]

The timing of nutritional deprivation has been a particularly relevant question in animal research because early investigations were guided by the sensitive period hypothesis that developing organs deprived of essential nutrients would experience irreversible structural damage.[6] Although some changes induced by nutritional deprivation remain following rehabilitation, particularly related to myelin (the fatty substance that surrounds nerve cells and aids with transmission), neuronal mitrochondria, and neurotransmitter metabolism,[15] many structural changes can be reversed with nutritional rehabilitation.[19] Recent evidence suggests that there may be metabolic or neurochemical consequences of nutritional deprivation.[15]

In a review of 165 animal studies, there were inconsistent findings regarding long term consequences of nutritional deprivation on cognitive functioning. Following rehabilitation, nutritionally deprived animals were often compromised in their ability to run complex mazes, perform tasks requiring visual discrimination, and extinguish learned responses. Their cognitive flexibility appeared to be limited and they had a tendency to display perseverative responses.[15] However, rehabilitated animals were not impaired in all tasks (eg, spatial learning, active avoidance, and left/right discrimination) and, in some cases, achieved better performance than adequately nourished animals, particularly when performance was tied to a food reward.

Rehabilitated animals with a history of nutritional deprivation appear to be at risk for changes in their emotionality, motivation, anxiety, and cognitive flexibility, evidenced by behaviors such as increased spilling, hyperreactivity to unfamiliar stimuli, and increased aggression. These behaviors may interfere with performance on cognitive tasks. Levitsky and Strupp explain that early malnutrition may alter neurochemical–receptor systems and result in "a decreased ability of adrenergic receptors to exhibit down regulation" which may result in a "diminished ability to adapt to stressful situations."[17] Studies among stunted school-age children with an early history of undernutrition suggest that an altered stress response can result from inadequate nutritional intake, as indicated by elevated cortisol levels, heart rate, and urinary epinephrine.[20]

Behavioral Neuroscience

Recent advances in behavioral neuroscience have shown the important role that experiences have on brain development, particularly with respect to pruning, myelination, and synaptic formation.[21] Brain development begins prenatally and continues through school years (Figure 2).[22] It begins with the formation of brain cells, followed by cell migration and differentiation, and the development of synapses to enable cells to communicate with one another. Finally, the supportive tissue (myelin) is formed to protect the nerve cells and facilitate communication.[23]

The process of forming and eliminating synapses occurs throughout the developmental period and is influenced by individual experiences.[23] Greenough and colleagues[24,25] argue for the distinction between two types of experiences: experience-expectant and experience-dependent. Experience-expectant development refers to species-specific development, such as sensory and motor systems. The maturational influences that guide development are operationalized by experiences that are expected, such as adequate nutrients. Nutrients, like other experiences "influence the brain by causing chemical changes within cells that influence cell function and structure."[23]

In contrast, experience-dependent development occurs in the context of experiences that are unique to the individual. They enable individuals to adapt to specific cultures and the demands of their environment. When individuals are denied such experiences (eg, through sensory deficits or lack of nutrients), they may not develop the synapses necessary for optimal functioning. The structural changes in synaptic formation appear to be dependent on neurochemical–receptor systems that, in turn, are influenced by experiences as basic as caregiving.[23]

The timing of early developmental experiences has been a central issue in studying behavioral neuroscience. The critical or sensitive period hypothesis suggests that if an event, such as nutritional deprivation, occurs during a specified period of time, often during period of rapid development, it will have specific effects on the organism.[6] Developmental scientists often prefer the term "sensitive" period, rather than "critical" period because it more accurately captures the brain's plasticity throughout development.[26] In addition, since components of the central nervous system develop along differing schedules, it is likely that the sensitive periods of the components vary with respect to onset and duration.

Child Development

Child development is defined here as the orderly progression of skills that children acquire as they mature and adapt to their specific caregiving settings. Although there are universal aspects of child development, particularly early in life as children gain motor skills and learn to roll over, sit, stand, and walk, there are also individual differences in the acquisition of skills. In addition, there are culture-specific aspects of child development that depend on specific interactions that children have with their caregivers. For example, children learn to understand and speak the languages they hear in their household.

A transactional system approach provides a useful framework for understanding the link between nutrition and early child development because it emphasizes the interplay that occurs between children and their environment, mediated through relations with their caregivers (Figure 3).[18,27,28] A child's development is influenced by characteristics from the child (eg, nutritional status), from the caregiver (eg, maternal education), and from interactions between the child and caregiver (eg, reciprocity and clarity of communication during feeding). The process becomes clear when applied to problems associated with children's growth.

For example, a woman who is undernourished during her pregnancy and does not receive prenatal care is more likely to give birth to a child with low birthweight (LBW) (<2,500 g). In comparison with full-term infants, infants born with LBW are smaller and often have weaker cries and sucking skills.[29] These characteristics make infants

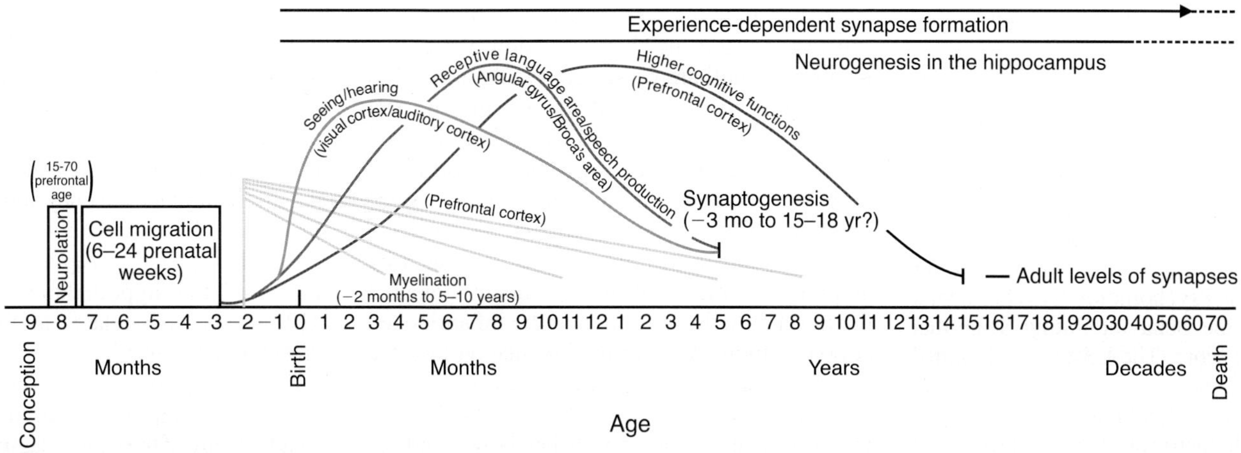

Figure 2 Human brain development. (Adapted from reference 22.)

with LBW more difficult to feed, particularly for mothers who are undernourished themselves. A cycle emerges whereby the small and weak infant is difficult to feed, does not grow well, may be vulnerable to illnesses, and lags behind in developmental skills. Mothers may feel frustrated and/or frightened by their infants who are small and sickly and may limit their caregiving to holding, rather than talking or encouraging exploration.[30] This process results in a negative cycle whereby infants do not elicit or receive the care and attention they need to promote optimal development. Intervention can occur at multiple points within the transactional system. For example, intervention could be directed to the infant with LBW, perhaps through nutritional and developmental intervention that might be available through community nutrition programs, or through early intervention programs. If the child's growth and development improve, the child will be more likely to elicit and receive age-appropriate care and interaction from the caregiver.

Intervention could also be directed toward the caregiver and the interaction between the caregiver and the child. Children's cues are analyzed to be sure the caregiver understands how the child expresses hunger or satiety, and caregivers learn how to read and respond to children's cues. There are several examples of successful randomized controlled trials that utilize components of the transactional system to promote the development of undernourished children.[31,32]

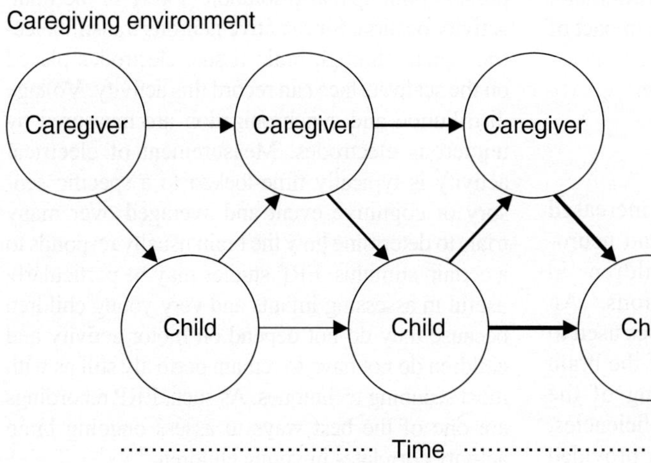

Figure 3 The transactional model.

Although most of the attention has been directed to the impact of inadequate nutritional and caregiving practices on children's nutritional status, children may influence caregiver behavior through their nutritional status, as predicted by the transactional system. Children with PEM have been described as negative, wary, and lethargic.[33] It is not surprising that during home observations, mothers of malnourished infants were less sensitive and responsive than mothers of healthy infants,[34] and tended to hold or carry them, rather than play with them.[30] Caregivers who treat their infants as though they are ill or unable to participate in age-appropriate activities may be inadvertently denying them opportunities for developmental stimulation and enrichment.

In one of the only studies to observe caregiver–child interaction prior to the child's becoming malnourished, investigators in Mexico reported that infants of mothers who lacked sensitivity and affection were more likely to become malnourished, compared to infants of more sensitive mothers.[35] In turn, after infants received nutritional supplements, their mothers were more engaged, both in caregiving and in enrichment activities, compared with mothers of nonsupplemented infants, suggesting that mothers respond to their infants' increased energy and activity.

Young children are dependent on interactions with their primary caretaker and are more active when their caregiver is present than absent.[36] As children grow physically and demonstrate more skills, their caregivers respond with expectations for increasingly complex behavior. For example, caregivers are likely to have higher expectations for a 3-year-old of average height who communicates in sentences, compared with a 3-year-old who is stunted and speaks in single words or brief phrases. In addition, children who are perceived by their caregivers as having easy or pleasant temperaments are more likely to elicit positive caregiving interactions; whereas caregivers tend to become less involved with children whom they perceive to be difficult.[37]

METHODOLOGY

Most research examining associations between early nutritional deprivation and subsequent intellectual skills has been retrospective and observational. The choice of an adequate control group has been challenging and many studies have not accounted for differences in environmental or caregiving factors that could contribute to differences in findings. This section examines the choice of outcome and predictor variables, and a consideration of environmental and caregiving variables that may confound findings.

Childhood Measures of Intelligence

The primary outcome measures used in studies of recovery from nutritional deprivation have been generalized tests of intelligence administered during the school-age years, such as the Wechsler Intelligence Scale for Children (WISC). The WISC is a standardized assessment that yields an intelligence quotient (IQ) that is stable over time and predicts both academic performance and occupational status.[38] Although many other factors contribute to academic performance and occupational success (eg, motivation), IQ is a useful indicator of successful rehabilitation.

Infant Measures of Intelligence

Infant intelligence is very difficult to measure. Not only is it challenging to ensure that infants are not hungry, tired, or irritable when testing is scheduled, but infancy is marked by rapidly changing skills with discontinuities in early development. In addition, generalized infant tests require the integration of multiple cognitive and noncognitive processes.

General Tests of Intelligence. Investigators have used either generalized tests of infant intelligence, such as the Bayley Scales of Infant Development (BSID), or specific information processing tests. The BSID is a well-standardized assessment that includes three scales: a Mental Scale that yields a Mental Developmental Index (MDI), a Motor Scale that yields a Psychomotor Developmental Index (PDI), and the Behavior Rating Scale that yields a percentile score. The BSID was designed to determine if infants were able to complete age-normed tasks, not to predict future functioning.[39] It has excellent psychometric properties, with internal consistencies measured by coefficient alphas ranging from 0.84 to 0.88, depending on the scale, and test-retest reliabilities at 12 months ranging from 0.77 to 0.90, depending on the scale. However, correlations from infant assessments administered prior to 18 to 24 months of age to later intellectual performance are notoriously low, lower than predictions from socioeconomic variables, such as maternal IQ or education.[40] In addition, correlations between scores from the Bayley Scales and specific information processing tests, such as visual habituation and attention to a novel stimulus, are low,[41] probably because the information processing tests are tapping specific areas and the BSID examines higher order functioning, thereby incorporating motivation, attention, and multiple cognitive processes. Beyond age 2, once infants gain the skills of symbol formation, predictability from infant assessments to subsequent intellectual performances increases dramatically.[40]

Specific Tests of Intelligence. Several specific information processing tests administered during infancy (eg, visual attention, learning, and memory) have been shown to be predictive of school-age intellectual performance.[42] The predictability from rate of habituation (number of trials to reach habituation) and response to novelty are higher than the predictability from generalized tests of infant intelligence, particularly when infants are assessed between 2 and 7 months of age. It is not clear why the associations are strongest during this period. The early infant information processing tests may measure speed of processing and/or the ability to inhibit attention to irrelevant stimuli. The drop in predictability after 7 months of age may be related to competing systems, such as sociability.

Habituation is a measurement of visual learning that has been widely used. It is measured by an infant's response to a repeating series of stimuli.[43] As the infant forms an internal representation of the stimulus, the intensity of the response decreases, resulting in a learning curve. Examiners may score the rate of the decline, the number of trials necessary to reach criterion, the duration of looking time prior to response decline, the pattern of the decline, and the infant's ability to recover and respond to a novel stimulus.[43] The psychometric properties of habituation measures, as indicated by test–retest reliability, are only modest.

The paired comparison test has been used to assess short- and long-term visual recognition memory.[43] It includes two phases: familiarization and test. During the familiarization phase, two identical stimuli are presented and the infant has an opportunity to view them. During the test phase, a familiar stimulus is paired with a novel stimulus. The observer notes the proportion of time the infant gazes at each stimulus. Since infants are likely to spend more time gazing at the novel stimulus, a novelty score is calculated by dividing the amount of time the infant looked at the novel stimulus by the time the infant looked at both stimuli. As with the habituation test, the psychometric properties are only modest.[43]

The Fagan test is the most widely used test of visual recognition memory. It has been standardized, published, and includes guidelines for training, administration, and scoring, with reference data.[44] However, only one indicator from the test has predictive validity, percentage of infant visual fixation to the novel stimulus averaged over all items.[44]

There are a number of other processing tests that can be administered during infancy, including focused attention (concentration devoted to processing information about an object),[45] cross-modal transfer (transfer of learning from one sensory modality to another),[46] and the A-not-B task (a Piagetian task that examines object permanence).[47] There has been limited use of infant information procedures with infants who experienced nutritional deprivation. For example, Rose[48] found that nutritionally deprived infants (5 to 12 months of age) from India had difficulty with two tasks related to cognitive processing—visual recognition memory and cross-modal transfer and Lozoff found differences in visual processing on the Fagan Test related to children's iron status.[49] Most investigators recommend that tasks be selected to assess specific processes and that multiple measures be used, beyond IQ, to gain a comprehensive understanding of how nutritional deprivation and recovery impact processing skills.[40,43]

Nutritional deprivation has a negative impact on motor development, leading investigators to examine how nutritional interventions affect motor development, measured by standardized tests, such as the Bayley Psychomotor Scale or the Alberta Infant Motor Scale; maternal reports of the acquisition of motor milestones; or observation. Although motor development promotes independence and potentially advances cognitive development by enabling children to explore their environment, there are no long-term evaluations of the impact of variations in early motor development on subsequent cognitive or academic performance.

Measures of Brain Function

In recent years there has been an increased emphasis on the neurophysiological and neuropsychological development of children in response to environmental conditions. An increase in the sophistication of measures used to assess the structure and functioning of the brain allows for an improved understanding of the developmental effects of nutritional deficiencies. Research in the nutrition sciences has provided evidence that optimal brain development during childhood relies on the intake of specific nutrients such as fatty acids, proteins, and carbohydrates. Specifically, lipids and proteins are needed for adequate cellmembrane formation, neurotransmitter release, and myelination which enhance neuronalefficiency and processing speed throughout the central nervous system. Carbohydrates also appear to play a key role in the regulation of the hypothalamic-pituitary-adrenal (HPA) axis as it relates to food intake under stressful conditions.[50]

The ability to assess the brain functioning of children has improved substantially in the past decade. Many of the neuroimaging techniques used previously had significant drawbacks that made working with children somewhat problematic. Computerized tomography (CT) assesses structural and density changes in the brain using X-rays. However, no functional data are obtained, and CT scans provide relatively gross anatomical information. Positron emission tomography (PET) provides additional information about alterations of regional blood flow in various anatomic structures by mapping how a radioactive isotope is metabolized by the brain. Although the side effects of CT and PET scans are minimal, both utilize small doses of radiation (through X-rays or radioactive substance) and, as such, are often limited to diagnostic procedures involving patients with known or suspected clinical problems. Less invasive measures are needed for clinical investigations. Additionally, both CT and PET lack a high degree of temporal resolution, meaning that it is difficult to determine how different events affect the brain in real time.

Other tools such as event-related potentials (ERP), functional magnetic resonance imaging (fMRI), diffusion tensor imaging (DTI), and magnetic resonance spectroscopy may be effective methods for determining associations between nutrition and brain functioning. Each assessment method possesses strengths that make it amenable to particular research questions regarding neurodevelopment.

Electrophysiological techniques involve the measurement of electric signals in the body and are generally superior to brain scanning techniques in terms of temporal resolution (*when* activity in the brain occurs in response to an event), but typically possess poor spatial resolution (*where* in the brain activity occurs). Since active neurons transmit electric signals through brain tissue, electrodes placed on the scalp surface can record this activity. Voltage distribution and synchronization are measured by numerous electrodes. Measurement of electrical activity is typically time-locked to a specific sensory or cognitive event and averaged over many trials to determine how the brain usually responds to a certain stimulus. ERP studies may be particularly useful in assessing infants and very young children because they do not depend on motor activity and children do not have to remain perfectly still as with most scanning techniques. As such, ERP recordings are one of the best ways to assess ongoing brain activity correlates in young children.[51]

fMRI is an alternative technique used to identify the location of neural activity. When a specific area of the brain is activated, blood flow to that area increases and oxygen is created. Because oxygenated and deoxygenated hemoglobin behave differently when pulsed with a magnetic field, this contrast in oxygen can be mapped onto consecutive "slices" of the brain. The MRI scanner determines the areas of greatest activation. The fMRI procedure has been used with adults to study the location of neural activity, and developmental scientists are beginning to use it with children. Using fMRI in combination with behavioral, cognitive, or neuropsychological assessments can further provide detailed information about which specific brain regions are activated in response to certain tasks. A limitation is that hemodynamic response is relatively slow (several seconds) in comparison to ERP techniques (milliseconds). Moreover, fMRI scanning requires the child to be still, making it appropriate only for children who can be trained to remain immobile. Additionally, the cost of fMRI is prohibitive for routine use.

DTI and magnetic resonance spectroscopy (MRS) represent more recent advances in neuroimaging that may be particularly relevant for research involving the neurodevelopmental effects of nutrition. DTI is a technique based on magnetic resonance imaging that produces functional images of the location, orientation, and activity of the brain's white-matter tracts. DTI reveals the integrity of white-matter tracts that link regions of the brain to each other by assessing water diffusion in the axons and their myelin sheaths.[52] Clinical research applications of DTI involve the localization of white-matter lesions and the assessment of the white-matter maturation in children.[53,54] A recent study demonstrated that deficiencies in nutrients such as iron or essential fatty acids can interfere with myelination in preterm infants.[55] DTI technology is likely to be increasingly utilized to determine associations between nutritional intake and the efficiency of axonal connections throughout the brain.

MRS goes beyond providing information about tissue water content and provides data regarding the chemical nature of a brain region distinguishing the properties of one area relative to those of surrounding areas. MRS can assess the concentration of common metabolites and biological compounds giving important information about glial processes, membrane phospholids, and high-energy phosphates.[56,57] Changes in these chemical compositions could be monitored following dietary supplementation throughout a child's postnatal development or after a period of nutritional deprivation.[51]

Stress and Neurodevelopmental Processes

As mentioned previously, nutritional deprivation frequently occurs in the context of poverty, highlighting the need to consider how contextual variables, including environmental stress and caregiving behavior, relate to brain development. Although brief periods of moderate stress allow children to develop appropriate stress responses,[23] evidence from animal and human studies suggests that exposure to high levels of stress early in life during periods of rapid brain development can lead to numerous physical and developmental problems.[58–61] Research with children who have been maltreated suggests that chronic and unpredictable stress can have lasting negative neurodevelopmental consequences[60] may undermine children's emotional and cognitive development, ultimately interfering with their academic achievement and social relationships.

The neurobiological mechanisms proposed to account for the cognitive deficits that occur in children with a history of malnutrition include deficits in the nutrients necessary for adequate physical growth and functioning as well as dysregulated HPA axis functioning.[20,62,63] The HPA system coordinates the stress response through multiple mechanisms resulting in the eventual release of glucocorticoids (cortisol) from the adrenal cortex. The brain is rich in receptors for cortisol with concentrations noted in the hippocampus and hypothalamus, prefrontal cortex, amygdala, and anterior cingulate gyrus. As excessive cortisol can impair brain regions housing cortisol receptors, intact HPA regulation is important for early development and ongoing maintenance of cortical systems involved with emotion, learning, memory and attention, and impulse control.[64–66]

In addition to an inadequate and/or inconsistent food supply, malnourished children often experience a lack of positive interactions with their primary caregivers. Effective caregivers play a critical role in helping children to modulate their emotional and physiological response to stressful events.[67] In the absence of positive interactions and stimulation, children may experience deficits in the development of their stress-sensitive regulatory systems. If they are also undernourished, they may be in a position of double jeopardy. An overexposure to stress in combination with disruptions in HPA-axis functioning may be harmful to children's neurodevelopment.[68] Heavily secreted neuroendocrine agents associated with chronic stress produce neurotoxic effects that may damage the developing brain, especially in areas rich in glucocorticoids such as the hippocampus, corpus callosum, and areas of the prefrontal cortex.[69] Elevated levels of catecholamines and cortisol can also lead to inadequate brain development through the mechanisms of accelerated loss of neurons,[70] delays in myelination,[71] abnormal pruning,[72] and the inhibition of neurogenesis.[73] Children who are repeatedly exposed to stress are at a higher risk for being chronically hyperaroused to aspects of their environment, with possible negative effects on their attention and executive cognitive processes.[74]

In summary, a nonresponsive caregiving environment may undermine children's neural development.[75] The combination of nutritional and caregiving risk factors early in life may place malnourished children at risk for negative cognitive outcomes, possibly mediated by poorly modulated stress reactivity.

Environmental and Caregiving Factors

Nutritional deficiencies often occur in a context of poverty among families who have few economic resources and limited education. Not only do many low-income families have restricted access to nutritionally healthy food, but mothers who are poorly educated are less likely to choose nutritionally appropriate foods for their children, compared with better educated mothers.[48] Thus, poverty and factors associated with poverty, such as low maternal education, may have a direct effect on children's development.

Caregivers contribute to their child's development through their care practices, such as providing food and basic care required by young children.[76] In the past, much attention regarding care practices was directed toward defining the quality and quantity of food that children require. However, recent evidence has demonstrated that care practices play a role in children's development that extends beyond the provision of food. Care practices include the relationships that caregivers form with their children during feeding and other daily activities.[23,76] Healthy care practices include behavior that is responsive to children's needs and is characterized by warmth and affection.[76]

LONG-TERM CONSEQUENCES OF EARLY NUTRITIONAL DEFICIENCIES

Information on the long-term consequences of early nutritional deficiencies is available from several natural experiments, including nutritionally deprived children adopted into middle class families or nutritional deficiencies occurring among children from middle class families caused by disasters or chronic illness. In addition, information is available from follow-up studies of children from low-income countries who experienced moderate to severe nutritional deprivation or children from middle-income countries who experienced mild nutritional deprivation. However, data on the long-term consequences of early nutritional deficiencies can be difficult to interpret because children who experience nutritional deficiencies are often raised in low-income families where they also experience environmental deficiencies.

Natural Experiments

Female orphans from Korea who varied in their nutritional status were adopted by middle-class American families, and tested during their school-age years. The children who had been undernourished early in life achieved scores in the normal range, but lower than those of better nourished Korean adoptees (Figure 4).[77] Although these findings demonstrate the impact of an enriched environment on children's intellectual skills, they also suggest that early nutritional deficiencies may limit children's ability to benefit from their environment.

The 1944 famine in Holland affected the entire population, regardless of economic standing.

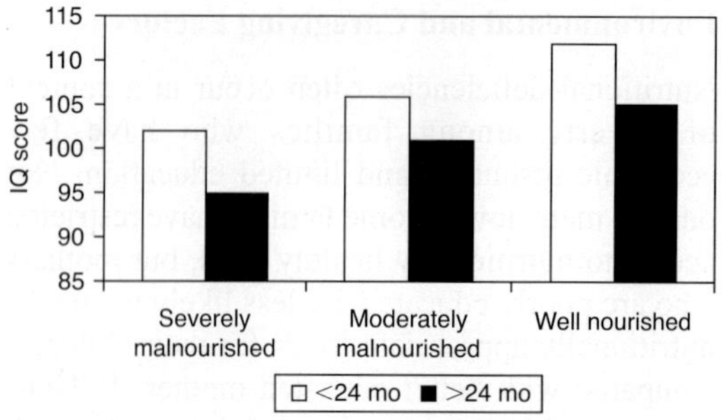

Figure 4 IQ scores among female Korean orphans varying by history of malnutrition and age of adoption.

When the youth were tested at 19 years of age as part of an army physical there was no long-term evidence of intellectual deficiencies, compared with scores from nonfamine years.[78] These findings suggest that environmental opportunities had overcome any deficiencies associated with the early nutritional deficiencies.

Children with chronic diseases, such as cystic fibrosis, are at risk for malnutrition due to malabsorption. Long-term consequences varied by family income. Among children from middle-income families, there were no differences in school-age intellectual scores, based on nutritional history.[79,80] In contrast, among children from low-income families, those with a history of nutritional deficiencies secondary to chronic disease had lower scores than those who had been hospitalized, but were well nourished. These studies illustrate the buffering effects of a nurturing environment on the intellectual performance of nutritionally deprived children.

Long-Term Consequences of Moderate to Severe Nutritional Deficiencies

Mounting evidence from Peru,[81] Jamaica,[4,82] the Phillipines,[83] Guatemala,[84] and Kenya[85] suggests that children who experienced nutritional deprivation severe enough to cause stunting early in life have cognitive deficits during school-age years that can interfere with successful academic performance. Early stunting undermines children's long-term performance and has been used as an indicator to estimate the number of children worldwide who do not reach their developmental potential.[1]

Long-Term Consequences of Mild Nutritional Deficiencies

Findings on the long-term consequences of children from middle-income countries diagnosed with failure to thrive (FTT) add to our information on nutritional deprivation and cognition. Although there are no agreed upon criteria for the diagnosis of FTT, the term is generally used to describe children under age three who have experienced a deceleration in growth over time, such that their weight-for-age or weight-for-height is below the 5th or 3rd percentile.[86] Children with FTT usually experience mild forms of deficiency, compared to children identified with nutritional deficiencies in low-income countries. During infancy and toddlerhood, the cognitive scores of children with FTT are lower than scores of comparison children with adequate growth, and often remain low through the preschool period.[87–89]

Previous follow-up studies among children hospitalized for FTT reported long-term deficits in cognitive, academic, and behavioral performance. However, recent follow-up studies of infants referred for FTT, but not hospitalized, report that by school-age, children with a history of FTT differ from children without a history of FTT by approximately 4 IQ points.[90–94] There is some evidence that children with a history of FTT experience more academic problems than adequately nourished peers.[92]

The studies showing no long-term cognitive deficiencies employed community samples of children,[90–94] whereas the studies suggesting that long-term cognition is affected included children with severe FTT, either hospitalized[95] or with chronic growth failure.[96,97]

The relationship between nutritional status and cognitive functioning is often mediated by family, environmental, and cultural variables,[87,98,99] making the family an ideal context for prevention of the negative consequences of FTT. Intervention studies among children with FTT highlight the importance of environmental enrichment. We conducted a randomized trial in which all infants received services through an interdisciplinary Growth and Nutrition Clinic, but experimental infants also received weekly home intervention targeted toward enhancing caregiver-child interactions.[87] After 1 year, infants who received the home intervention had a more child-centered home environment, better cognitive scores, and better expressive language scores, compared to infants who did not receive the home intervention. Two years after the intervention ended, infants who received the intervention had better motor scores only if their caregivers did not report symptoms of depression, anxiety, or hostility.[88] When the children were 8 years of age, children with a history of FTT who had not received the intervention were shorter, thinner, and had worse arithmetic scores than children with a history of adequate growth.[90] Children with a history of FTT who received the early intervention had intermediate scores and had fewer teacher-reported internalizing problems and better work habits than children with FTT who did not receive the intervention. There were no group differences in IQ, reading, or mother-reported behavior problems. Findings suggest that the early home-visiting intervention attenuated some of the negative effects of early FTT, possibly by promoting maternal sensitivity and helping children build strong work habits that enabled them to benefit from school.

INTERVENTION STUDIES

As illustrated by the transactional system, optimal child development depends not only on food quality and availability, but also on the care the family provides to the child, especially during the first few years of life.[23] Evaluations of psychosocial stimulation delivered to malnourished children provide evidence for the importance of caregiving environment in promoting development. In Jamaica, Grantham-McGregor and colleagues[31] demonstrated that stunted children who received either nutritional supplementation or psychosocial stimulation showed improved mental and motor development. The effects of the interventions were additive, children who received *both* supplementation and stimulation achieved mental and motor scores that approximated those of the nonstunted comparison group. Long-term follow-up demonstrated that although the benefits of the early interventions were still present, they were rather modest, suggesting some decay over time.[100] These findings are extremely encouraging because they demonstrate that not only can children benefit from environmental enrichment, but their benefits extend over time. They also suggest that enrichment should extend over the developmental period.

Studies from Cali and Bogota, Columbia also illustrate the importance of including both nutritional and psychological interventions.[101,102] In the Cali study, children who received both supplementation and stimulation had better psychological performance at age nine, compared with control group children.[103] In thc Bogota study, supplemented infants were more active than non-supplemented infants, and 3 years after the study ended, when the children were 6 years of age, those who received both supplementation and stimulation were taller.[102]

In a long-term evaluation of a community-based supplementation program in Guatemala, Pollitt and colleagues found that children who were supplemented early in life had a faster reaction time in information processing tests and higher scores on tests of knowledge, numeracy, reading, and vocabulary during adolescence, compared to children who did not receive the high-protein supplement.[104] Their analysis also demonstrated the importance of looking for moderator effects because in the villages that did not receive the supplement, they found the greatest benefits on academic performance among children from the poorest homes.[105]

MICRONUTRIENTS

Iodine Deficiency

Iodine deficiency is a major problem that affects children in areas where iodine is depleted from the soil, primarily mountainous regions, such as the Himalayas and the Andes, and flood plains.[106] A 1993 WHO report estimates that 1.6 billion people or 30% of the world's population live in iodine-deficient areas and are therefore at risk for iodine deficiency.[11]

Iodine is an essential component of at least two thyroid hormones that are necessary for skeletal growth and neurological development.[106] When iodine is deficient, hypothyroidism occurs, resulting in increased production of TSH, which stimulates production of thyroid hormones. The most common manifestation of iodine deficiency is goiter, which is an enlarged thyroid gland.[106]

When iodine deficiency occurs in utero, it leads to fetal hypothyroidism and irreversible neurological and cognitive deficits, manifested as cretinism. Neurological cretinism includes mental retardation, primitive reflexes, visual problems, facial deformities, stunted growth, and diplegia.[107] When iodine deficiency occurs postnatally, the child may experience thyroid failure that can lead to hypothyroidism. Observational studies that have compared children with and without a goiter have had mixed results; some have reported cognitive deficits among children with goiters and others have not. One explanation for the lack of clarity may be that differing levels of hypothyroidism can lead to a goiter.[106] In a meta-analysis of 18 observational studies that compared children based on whether they lived in an iodine-deficient area or not, children who lived in iodine-deficient areas had deficits in cognitive functioning.[108] In a well-controlled observational study in Bangladesh, investigators found that children with mild levels of hypothyroidism had deficits in spelling and reading, compared to healthy controls.[109] Although evidence from these studies is compelling, families who live in iodine-deficient areas are often more impoverished than families in areas where iodine is adequate.

Several randomized trials have been conducted to examine the impact of iodine supplementation on the cognitive performance of children in iodine-deficient areas. However, results have not been consistent. In a recent longitudinal follow-up of school-age children, all of whom received iodine, those who received iodine in utero prior to the third trimester had better scores on a measure of psychomotor performance than children who received iodine later in pregnancy or at age 2 years.[110] There was a similar trend when measures of cognitive performance were considered; however, the differences did not reach significance. Thus, the effects of postnatal iodine deficiency on children's cognitive performance are less clear than the effects of prenatal iodine deficiency. In addition, many of the studies have had methodological problems that interfere with interpretation.

Iron Deficiency

Iron deficiency is the most common nutritional deficiency in the world. UNICEF and WHO committees estimate that worldwide there are 2 billion individuals with anemia and up to 5 billion who are iron deficient.[12] The highest risk of iron deficiency occurs during times of rapid growth and nutritional demand, during infancy (ages 6 to 24 months), early childhood, adolescence, and pregnancy.

Iron is necessary for hemoglobin synthesis. Iron deficiency leads to reduced oxygen-carrying capacity and can impact immunity, growth, and development. Although iron status is often assessed by anemia (low blood hemoglobin concentration), only 50% of anemia is caused by iron deficiency.[111] Iron has multiple roles in neurotransmitter systems and may affect behavior through its effects on dopamine metabolism.[112] This is highly relevant to children's cognitive development as dopamine clearance has strong effects on attention, perception, memory, motivation, and motor control.[113]

A number of observational studies have found that children who experienced anemia early in life had low scores on tests of mental performance and were fearful, inattentive, and solemn with low levels of initiation and exploration.[114–116] Many children continued to demonstrate lower academic performance during their school-age years, even when the anemia had been treated. For example, Hurtado and colleagues examined the records of children who enrolled in the Special Supplemental Nutrition Program for Women, Infants, and Children prior to age 5.[117] Those who were anemic were more likely to experience academic problems at 10 years of age, compared to children who were not anemic on enrollment. Concurrent iron status is also related to academic performance, as demonstrated in an investigation from over 5,000 6- to 16-year-old children from NHANES III.[118] When standardized math test scores were examined controlling for background variables, children with iron deficiency with and without anemia had lower scores than children with normal iron status. These findings suggest that iron deficiency, even without anemia, may place children at risk for cognitive delays.

Among infants with poor iron status, most studies have reported that even after $\geq$ 3 months of iron therapy, children's development continued to be poor, compared with children with a history of adequate iron status. Several studies have followed children up to adolescence. A recent meta-analysis estimated IQ to be 1.73 points lower for each 10 g/L decrease in hemoglobin. A follow-up of Costa Rican adolescents who had been born at term and were free of health problems in infancy other than ID, showed persisting motor differences, more grade repetition, increased anxiety/depression, social problems, and inattention rated by parents and teachers, and a widening gap in cognitive scores to 19 years, despite iron therapy that corrected IDA in infancy.[119] In contrast, several recent randomized controlled trials of iron supplementation conducted in developing countries have shown improved motor and social-emotional development in infants who received iron.

IDA has been associated with poor and slow cognitive performance among college women[120] and with depression and parenting behavior characterized by low responsivity and controlling behavior.[121,122] Iron treatment improved the women's iron status, cognitive processing, depressive symptoms, and parenting behavior. Thus, IDA among children may impact their development directly and IDA among their caregivers may alter their caregiving environment.

Zinc Deficiency

Zinc is a trace mineral that is involved with DNA and RNA synthesis and the metabolism of proteins, carbohydrates, and fat. Findings on the cognitive effects from the zinc supplementation studies lack clarity.[123] Four published trials reported beneficial effects of zinc supplementation on children's activity, motor quality, or motor development[124–127]; one reported that zinc-supplemented infants were more cooperative,[128] three found no differences on mental development,[124,127,129] and one reported that supplemented children had slightly lower scores on mental development than comparison children.[129]

There have been at least three randomized trials of zinc supplementation measuring cognitive development among school-age children. A trial in Canada found no differences when children were tested with subscales from the Detroit Test of Learning Abilities.[130] However, trials in China and Mexican-American children from Texas have found that zinc-supplemented children demonstrated superior neuropsychological performance, particularly reasoning, when compared with controls.[131,132] More work is needed to replicate existing studies and clarify the effect of zinc supplementation on children's academic performance.

At least two studies have examined zinc supplementation in combination with iron supplementation. One found beneficial effects of the two micronutrients on infants' motor development and behavior[133] and the other did not.[134] However, there were no adverse effects of administering the two micronutrients together in a 1–1 molar ratio.

One study found beneficial effects of zinc supplementation on general infant development, but only in the context of psychosocial stimulation,[33] suggesting that the beneficial effects of the supplement may only be apparent in the context of a stimulating environment. Thus, more work is necessary to clarify the role of zinc in the context of other micronutrients and a stimulating environment.

EFFECTS OF LEAD EXPOSURE

Numerous studies have documented that lead exposure has a neurotoxic effect on infants and young children and is associated with impairments in intellectual and behavioral functioning.[135–137] Although significant progress has been made in reducing the average blood lead level in many parts of the world, lead remains a major cause of encephalopathy in children. Even in the absence of encephalopathy, lead poisoning contributes to permanent neuropsychological impairments including deficits in general intellectual functioning, ability to sustain attention on tasks, aspects of speech production and language comprehension, motor coordination, flexible problem-solving, and behavioral self-regulation. Several recent reviews that focused on the impact of low levels of lead exposure (blood lead levels $<$10 μ/dL) among children indicated that even low-level lead exposure can lead to a decline in IQ scores.[138,139] An international pooled analysis found a dose-response effect associated with the amount of lead found in children's blood.[139] An increase in blood lead levels from 2.4 to 10 μ/dL resulted in a 1.1 point decline in IQ, 10 to 20 μ/dL resulted in an additional 1.9 point decline, and for blood lead concentrations from 20 to 30 μ/dL, there was an additional 3.9 point decline in IQ scores (a total decrement of 6.9 IQ points for the 20 to 30 μ/dL group).

In general, the long-term effects of prenatal or postnatal lead exposure appear to be nonspecific, impacting multiple areas of the brain and making it difficult to pinpoint the specific neurodevelopmental mechanisms responsible for cognitive and behavioral changes in lead-exposed children. However, there is evidence that lead alters neuropsychological development by disrupting processes of neuronal migration, synaptogenesis, and myelination.[136] Many of the neurotoxic effects of lead can be traced to lead's ability to mimic or inhibit the action of calcium as a regulator of cell function.[140] As such, exposure to lead causes changes in how neurotransmitters are stored and released, which may cause an inhibition of synaptic growth and detract from the efficiency of the developing brain. Lead also disrupts the main structural components of the blood–brain barrier by damaging astrocytes and the endothelial microvasculature. This damage allows for the passage of certain molecules (eg, albumin) that are toxic and typically restricted by the blood–brain barrier.[140] Other researchers note that lead exposure alters second and third messenger activity,[141] which also interferes with cognitive efficiency.

Children are typically more vulnerable to lead exposure than adults because they are more likely to ingest lead, resulting in severe consequences. Hand-to-mouth activity and behaviors such as pica (which peaks at around 2 years of age) increase the likelihood of ingesting lead-contaminated substances.[138] The most common ways that children are exposed to lead are through the consumption of soil, lead-based paint, water from pipes with lead-soldered joints, and contaminants brought home from parents engaged in mining/industrial activities. Once ingested, lead may have a more deleterious effect on the developing central nervous system of children than on adults. Children's increased vulnerability to lead is attributable to several factors. First, a greater proportion of ingested lead is absorbed from the gastrointestinal tract of children than of adults. Second, a greater proportion of circulating lead crosses the blood–brain barrier in children, especially children under the age of five, than in adults.[136] Finally, the developing brain seems to be more vulnerable to the neurotoxic effects of lead than the mature brain. The neurotoxic effects of lead are particularly evident in the prefrontal cortex, the cerebellum, and the hippocampus.[141] Investigators speculate that because regions such as the prefrontal cortex are in a phase of rapid development during the first few years of life, they may be particularly susceptible to the harmful effects of neurotoxins. The vulnerability of the prefrontal cortex could also explain the consistent associations between elevated blood lead levels and poor performance on tasks involving sustained attention and executive functioning.[135,142,143]

SUMMARY

Most of the research examining the impact of nutritional deficiencies on children's intellectual development has hypothesized a direct effect, possibly through changes in neuroanatomy or neurotransmission. However, many studies have relied on general measures of intellectual skills and, as a result, little is known about specific processing changes related to nutritional deprivation.

It is also possible that behavior changes associated with nutritional deficiencies alter the caregiving that the child receives, thereby compromising the child's development even further. The result could be a child who experiences both the neurochemical changes that have been associated with nutritional deficiency, together with limited environmental enrichment. Future research should consider how the caregiving system is related to child development and whether it mediates the effects of nutritional deficiencies.

The findings linking nutritional deficiencies, especially micronutrient deficiencies, and child development point to the importance of effective prevention programs that begin prenatally or early in life and extend through the periods of vulnerability, which may include adolescence. Yet, there are many unanswered questions regarding nutritional deficiencies and child development that require further research, including the timing of the deficiency, the long-term consequences on academic achievement, the specific processes involved, and the impact of multiple nutrient deficiencies.

REFERENCES

1. Grantham-McGregor S, Cheung YB, Cueto S, et al. Over two hundred million children fail to reach their developmental potential in the first five years in developing countries. J Lancet 2007;369:60–70.
2. Engle PL, Black MM, Behrman JR, et al. Strategies to avoid the loss of developmental potential in more than 200 million children in the developing world. Lancet 2007;369:229–42.
3. Walker SP, Wachs TD, Meeks Gardner J, et al. Child development: Risk factors for adverse outcomes in developing countries. Lancet 2007;369:145–57.
4. Richardson SA, Birch HG, Grabie E, et al. The behavior of children in school who were severely malnourished in the first two years of life. J Health Soc Behav 1972;13:276–84.
5. Grantham-McGregor S, Stewart M, Powell C. Behaviour of severely malnourished children in a Jamaican hospital. Dev Med Child Neurol 1991;33:706–14.
6. Dobbing J. Vulnerable periods of brain development. In: Knight EK, editor. Lipids, Malnutrition and the Developing Brain. Amsterdam: North Holland; 1972. p. 9–29.
7. Grantham-McGregor S. A review of existing studies of the effect of severe malnutrition on mental development. J Nutr 1995;125:2223S–8S.
8. Bellamy C. The State of the World's Children, 2005. Childhood Under Threat. New York: UNICEF Publications; 2004.
9. WHO Multicentre Growth Reference Study Group. WHO child growth standards based on length/height, weight and age. Acta Paediatr 2006;95:76–85.
10. Grantham-McGregor S, Ani C. The role of micronutrients in psychomotor and cognitive development. Br Med Bull 1999;55:511–27.
11. WHO. Global prevalence of iodine deficiency disorders. Geneva, Switzerland: World Health Organization; 1993.
12. WHO. Maternal health and safe motherhood programmes. The prevalence of anemia in women: A tabulation of available information. Geneva, Switzerland: World Health Organization; 1992.
13. Hotz C, Brown KH. Identifying populations at risk of zinc deficiency: The use of supplementation trials. Nutr Rev 2001;59:80–4.
14. Skinner JD, Carruth BR, Houck KS, et al. Longitudinal study of nutrient and food intakes of infants aged 2 to 24 months. J Am Diet Assoc 1997;97:496–504.
15. Smart JL. Malnutrition, learning, and behavior: Recent advances in laboratory animal research. Washington, DC: Pan American Health Organization; 1998.
16. Tonkiss J, Smart JL, Massey RF. Effects of early life undernutrition in artificially-reared rats. 2. Subsequent behaviour. Physiol Behav 1987;41:555–62.
17. Levitsky DA, Barnes RH. Nutritional and environmental interactions in the behavioral development of the rat: Long-term effects. Science 1972;176:68–71.
18. Wachs T. Necessary but not sufficient. The respective roles of single and multiple influences on human development. Washington, DC: American Psychological Association 2000.
19. Levitsky DA, Strupp BJ. Malnutrition and the brain: Changing concepts, changing concerns. J Nutr 1995;125:2212S–20S.
20. Fernald LC, Grantham-McGregor SM. Stress response in school-age children who have been growth retarded since early childhood. Am J Clin Nutr 1998;68:691–8.
21. Nelson CA, Bloom FE. Child development and neuroscience. Child Dev 1997;68:970–87.
22. Nelson CA, Thompson RA. Developmental science and the media. Early brain development. Am Psychol 2001;56:5–15.
23. Shonkoff JP, Phillips DA. From Neurons to Neighborhoods: The Science of Early Childhood Development. Washington, DC: National Academy Press; 2000.
24. Greenough W. The Nature and Nurture of Behavior: Developmental Psychobiology. In: Freeman W, editor. San Francisco, CA: W.H. Freeman; 1973.
25. Klintsova AY, Greenough WT. Synaptic plasticity in cortical systems. Curr Opin Neurobiol 1999;9:203–8.
26. Bornstein MH. Sensitive periods in development: Structural characteristics and causal interpretations. Psychol Bull 1989;105:179–97.
27. Bronfenbrenner U, Ceci SJ. Nature-nurture reconceptualized in developmental perspective: A bioecological model. Psychol Rev 1994;101:568–86.
28. Sameroff A, Chandler M. Reproductive risk and the continuum of caretaking causality. In: Horowitz F, editor. Review of Child Development and Research. Chicago, IL: University of Chicago Press; 1975.
29. Hack M, Taylor HG. Perinatal brain injury in preterm infants and later neurobehavioral function. JAMA 2000;284:1973–4.
30. Graves PL. Nutrition, infant behavior, and maternal characteristics: A pilot study in West Bengal, India. Am J Clin Nutr 1976;29:305–19.
31. Grantham-McGregor SM, Powell CA, Walker SP, et al. Nutritional supplementation, psychosocial stimulation, and mental development of stunted children: The Jamaican Study. Lancet 1991;338:1–5.
32. Super C, Clement J, Vuori L, et al. Infant and caretaker behavior as mediators of nutritional and social interventions in the barrios of Bogota. In: Field T, Sostek, AM, Vietze, P, Leiderman, PH, editors. Culture and Early Interventions. Hillsdale, NJ: Erlbaum Associates; 1981. p. 171–88.
33. Meeks Gardner J, Grantham-McGregor SM, Chang SM, et al. Activity and behavioral development in stunted and nonstunted children and response to nutritional supplementation. Child Dev 1995;66:1785–97.
34. Valenzuela M. Maternal sensitivity in a developing society: The context of urban poverty and infant chronic undernutrition. Dev Psychol 1997;33:845–55.
35. Cravioto J, DeLicardie E. Mother-infant relationship prior to the development of clinically severe malnutrition in the child. In: White P, Selve N, editors. Proceedings of the Western Hemisphere Nutrition Congress IV. Boston, MA: Massachusetts Publishing Sciences Group; 1975. p. 126–37.
36. Routh D, Schroeder C, O'Tuama L. Development of activity level in children. Dev Psychol 1996;10:163–8.
37. Maccoby E, Snow N, Jacklin C. Children's disposition and mother-child interaction at 12 and 18 months. Dev Psychol 1984;20:459–72.
38. McCall R. Nature-nurture and the two realms of development: A proposed integration with respect to mental development. Child Dev 1981;52:1–12.
39. Black MM, Matula K. Essentials of Bayley Scales of Infant Development II Assessment. New York: John Wiley & Sons; 2000.
40. McCall R, Mash C. Long chain polyunsaturated fatty acids and the measurement and prediction of intelligence In: Dobbing J, editor. Developing Brain and Behaviour: The Role of Lipids in Infant Formula. New York: Academic Press; 1997. p. 295–338.
41. Lewis M, Brooks-Gunn J. Visual attention at three months as a predictor of cognitive functioning at two years of age. Intelligence 1981;5:131–40.
42. Bornstein MH, Sigman MD. Continuity in mental development from infancy. Child Dev 1986;57:251–74.

43. Columbo J. Individual differences in infant cognition: Methods, measures, and models In: Dobbing J, editor. Developing Brain and Behaviour: The Role of Lipids in Infant Formula. New York: Academic Press; 1997. p. 339–85.
44. Singer L. Methodological considerations in longitudinal studies of infant risk. In: Dobbing J, editor. Developing Brain and Behaviour: The Role of Lipids in Infant Formula. New York: Academic Press; 1997. p. 209–52.
45. Lawson K, Ruff H. Focused attention: Assessing a fundamental cognitive process in infancy In: Singer L, Zeskind P, editors. Biobehavioral Assessment of the Infant. New York: Guilford Press; 2001. p. 293–311.
46. Rose S, Orlin E. Visual information processing In: Singer L, Zeskind P, editors. Biobehavioral Assessment of the Infant. New York: Guilford Press; 2001. p. 274–92.
47. Noland J. The A-not-B task. In: Singer L, Zeskind P, editors. Biobehavioral Assessment of the Infant. New York: Guilford Press; 2001. p. 312–22.
48. Wachs T, McCabe G. Relation of maternal intelligence and schooling to offspring nutritional intake. Intl J Behav Dev 2001;25:444–9.
49. Lozoff B, De Andraca I, Castillo M, et al. Behavioral and developmental effects of preventing iron-deficiency anemia in healthy full-term infants. Pediatrics 2003;112:846–54.
50. Walker C-D. Nutritional aspects modulating brain development and the responses to stress in early neonatal life. Prog Neuropsychopharmacol Biol Psychiatry 2005;29:1249–63.
51. Thomas KM. Assessing brain development using neurophysiologic and behavioral measures. J Pediatr 2003;143: S46–53.
52. Poupon C, Mangin JF, Clark CA, et al. Toward inference of human brain connectivity from MR diffusion tensor data. Med Image Anal 2001;5:1–15.
53. Schmithorst VJ, Wilke M, Dardzinski BJ, et al. Correlation of white matter diffusivity and anisotropy with age during childhood and adolescence: A cross-sectional diffusion-tensor MR imaging study. Radiology 2002;222:212–8.
54. Klingberg TT, Vaidya CJ, Gabrieli JDE, et al. Myelination and organization of the frontal white matter in children: A diffusion tensor MRI study. NeuroReport 1999;10:2817–21.
55. Georgieff MK, Innis SM. Controversial nutrients that potentially affect preterm neurodevelopment: Essential fatty acids and iron. Pediatr Res 2005;57:99–103.
56. Urenjak J, Williams SR, Gadian DG, et al. Proton nuclear magnetic resonance spectroscopy unambiguously identifies different neural cell types. J Neurosci 1993;13:981–9.
57. Ross B, Michaelis T. Clinical applications of magnetic resonance spectroscopy. Magn Reson Q 1994;10:191–247.
58. Gunnar M, Quevedo K. The neurobiology of stress and development. Annu Rev Psychol 2007;58:145–73.
59. Suomi SJ. Developmental trajectories, early experiences, and community consequences: Lessons from studies with rhesus monkeys. New York: Guilford Press; 1999.
60. De Bellis MD, Keshavan MS, Shifflett H, et al. Brain structures in pediatric maltreatment-related posttraumatic stress disorder: A sociodemographically matched study. Biol Psychiatry 2002;52:1066–78.
61. Hart J, Gunnar M, Cicchetti D. Salivary cortisol in maltreated children: Evidence of relations between neuroendocrine activity and social competence. Dev Psychopathol 1995;7:11–26.
62. De Bellis MD. The psychobiology of neglect. Child Maltreat 2005;10:150–72.
63. Fernald LC, Grantham-McGregor SM, Manandhar DS, et al. Salivary cortisol and heart rate in stunted and nonstunted Nepalese school children. Eur J Clin Nutr 2003;57:1458–65.
64. Bremner JD, Vermetten E. Stress and development: Behavioral and biological consequences. Dev Psychopathol 2001;13:473–89.
65. Teicher MH, Andersen S, Polcari A, et al. Developmental neurobiology of childhood stress and trauma. Psychiatr Clin North Am 2002;25:397–426.
66. Van Voorhees E, Scarpa A. The effects of child maltreatment on the hypothalamic-pituitary-adrenal axis. Trauma Violence Abuse 2004;5:333–52.
67. Gunnar MR, Brodersen L, Krueger K, et al. Dampening of adrenocortical responses during infancy: Normative changes and individual differences. Child Dev 1996;67:877–89.
68. Perry BD. Childhood trauma, the neurobiology of adaptation, and 'use-dependent' development of the brain: How 'states' become 'traits'. Infant Ment Health J 1995;16:271–91.
69. Carrion VG, Weems CF, Eliez S, et al. Attenuation of frontal asymmetry in pediatric posttraumatic stress disorder. Biol Psychiatry 2001;50:943–51.
70. Sapolsky RM, Uno H, Rebert CS, et al. Hippocampal damage associated with prolonged glucocorticoid exposure in primates. J Neurosci 1990;10:2897–902.
71. Dunlop SA, Archer MA, Quinlivan JA, et al. Repeated prenatal corticosteroids delay myelination in the ovine central nervous system. J Matern Fetal Med 1997;6:309–13.
72. Todd RD. Neural development is regulated by classical neurotransmitters: Dopamine D2 receptor stimulation enhances neurite outgrowth. Biol Psychiatry 1992;31:794–807.
73. Tanapat P, Galea LA, Gould E. Stress inhibits the proliferation of granule cell precursors in the developing dentate gyrus. Int J Dev Neurosci 1998;16:235–9.
74. Perry BD. Neurobiological sequelae of childhood trauma: PTSD in children. In: Murburg M, editor. Catecholamine Function in Posttraumatic Stress Disorder: Emerging Concepts. Washington, DC: American Psychiatric Press; 1994. p. 233–55.
75. Pollak S, Cicchetti D, Klorman R. Stress, memory, and emotion: Developmental considerations from the study of child maltreatment. Dev Psychopathol 1998;10:811–28.
76. Engle PL, Bentley M, Pelto G. The role of care in nutrition programmes: Current research and a research agenda. Proc Nutr Soc 2000;59:25–35.
77. Winick M, Meyer KK, Harris RC. Malnutrition and environmental enrichment by early adoption. Science 1975;190:1173–5.
78. Stein Z, Susser M, Saenger G, et al. Nutrition and mental performance. Science 1972;178:708–13.
79. Beardslee W, Wolff P, Hurwitz I, et al. The effects of infantile malnutrition on behavioural development: A follow-up study. Am J Clin Nutr 1982;35:1437–41.
80. Lloyd-Still JD, Hurwitz I, Wolff PH, et al. Intellectual development after severe malnutrition in infancy. Pediatrics 1974;54:306–11.
81. Berkman DS, Lescano AG, Gilman RH, et al. Effects of stunting, diarrhoeal disease, and parasitic infection during infancy on cognition in late childhood: A follow-up study. Lancet 2002;359:564–71.
82. Walker SP, Grantham-Mcgregor SM, Powell CA, et al. Effects of growth restriction in early childhood on growth, IQ, and cognition at age 11 to 12 years and the benefits of nutritional supplementation and psychosocial stimulation. J Pediatr 2000;137:36–41.
83. Mendez MA, Adair LS. Severity and timing of stunting in the first two years of life affect performance on cognitive tests in late childhood. J Nutr 1999;129:1555–62.
84. Martorell R, Rivera J, Kaplowitz J, et al. Long term consequences of growth retardation during early childhood. In: Hernandez M, Argenta, J, editors. Human Growth: Basic and Clinical Aspects. Amsterdam: Elsevier; 1992. p. 143–9.
85. Neumann C, McDonald MA, Sigman M, et al. Relationships between morbidity and development in mildly to moderately malnourished Kenyan toddlers. Pediatrics 1991;88:934–42.
86. Wright CM. Identification and management of failure to thrive: A community perspective. Arch Dis Child 2000;82:5–9.
87. Black MM, Dubowitz H, Hutcheson J, et al. A randomized clinical trial of home intervention for children with failure to thrive. Pediatrics 1995;95:807–14.
88. Hutcheson JJ, Black MM, Talley M, et al. Risk status and home intervention among children with failure-to-thrive: Follow-up at age 4. J Pediatr Psychol 1997;22:651–68.
89. Singer LT, Fagan JF, 3rd. Cognitive development in the failure-to-thrive infant: A three-year longitudinal study. J Pediatr Psychol 1984;9:363–83.
90. Black MM, Dubowitz H, Krishnakumar A, et al. Early intervention and recovery among children with failure-to-thrive: Follow-up at age 8. Pediatrics 2007;120:59–69.
91. Boddy J, Skuse D, Andrews B. The developmental sequelae of nonorganic failure to thrive. J Child Psychol Psychiatry 2000;41:1003–14.
92. Drewett RF, Corbett SS, Wright CM. Cognitive and educational attainments at school age of children who failed to thrive in infancy: A population-based study. J Child Psychol Psychiatry 1999;40:551–61.
93. Kerr MA, Black MM, Krishnakumar A. Failure-to-thrive, maltreatment and the behavior and development of 6-year-old children from low-income, urban families: A cumulative risk model. Child Abuse Negl 2000;24:587–98.
94. Mackner LM, Black MM, Starr RH. Cognitive development of children in poverty with failure to thrive: A prospective study through age 6. J Child Psychol Psychiatry 2003;44:743–51.
95. Dowdney L, Skuse D, Morris K, et al. Short normal children and environmental disadvantage: A longitudinal study of growth and cognitive development from 4 to 11 years. J Child Psychol Psychiatry 1998;39:1017–29.
96. Oates RK, Peacock A, Forrest D. Long-term effects of nonorganic failure to thrive. Pediatrics 1985;75:36–40.
97. Drotar D. Sampling issues in research with nonorganic failure-to-thrive children. J Pediatr Psychol 1990;15: 255–72.
98. Drotar D, Eckerle D, Satola J, et al. Maternal interactional behavior with nonorganic failure-to-thrive infants: A case comparison study. Child Abuse Negl 1990;14:41–51.
99. Frank DA, Drotar D, Cook JT, et al. Failure to thrive. In: Reece RM, Ludwig S, editors. Child Abuse: Medical Diagnosis and Management. 2nd edition. Philadelphia, PA: Lea & Feiber; 2001. p. 307–38.
100. Grantham-McGregor S, Schofield W, Powell C. Development of severely malnourished children who received psychosocial stimulation: Six-year follow-up. Pediatrics 1987;79:247–54.
101. McKay H, Sinisterra L, McKay A, et al. Improving cognitive ability in chronically deprived children. Science 1978;200:270–8.
102. Super CM, Herrera MG, Mora JO. Long-term effects of food supplementation and psychosocial intervention on the physical growth of Colombian infants at risk of malnutrition. Child Dev 1990;61:29–49.
103. Sinisterra L, McKay H, McKay A, et al. Response of malnourished children to multidisciplinary intervention. In: Brozek J, editor. Behavioral Effects of Energy and Protein Deficits. Washington, DC: NIH Publication No. 79-1906 Government Printing Office; 1979.
104. Pollitt E, Gorman KS, Engle PL, et al. Early supplementary feeding and cognition: Effects over two decades. Monogr Soc Res Child Dev 1993;58:1–99; discussion 111-8.
105. Pollitt E, Gorman K, Engle P, et al. Nutrition in early life and the fulfillment of intellectual potential. In: Dunn J, editor. Iodine Deficiency—The Next Target for Elimination. J Nutr 1995; 25:1111S-8S. N Engl J Med 1995:267–8.
106. Delange F, de Benoist B, Pretell E, et al. Iodine deficiency in the world: Where do we stand at the turn of the century? Thyroid 2001;11:437–47.
107. Halpern J. The neuromotor deficit in endemic cretinism and its implications for the pathogenesis of the disorder In: Stanbury J, editor. The Damaged Brain of Iodine Deficiency. New York: Cognizant Communication; 1994. p. 15–24.
108. Bleichrodt N, Resing W. Measuring intelligence and learning potential in iodine-deficient and noniodine deficient populations. In: Stanbury JB, editor. The Damaged Brain of Iodine Deficiency. New York: Cognizant Communication; 1994. p. 27–36.
109. Huda SN, Grantham-McGregor SM, Rahman KM, et al. Biochemical hypothyroidism secondary to iodine deficiency is associated with poor school achievement and cognition in Bangladeshi children. J Nutr 1999;129: 980–7.
110. O'Donnell KJ, Rakeman MA, Zhi-Hong D, et al. Effects of iodine supplementation during pregnancy on child growth and development at school age. Dev Med Child Neurol 2002;44:76–81.
111. Yip R. Iron deficiency: Contemporary scientific issues and international programmatic approaches. J Nutr 1994;124:1479S–90S.
112. Beard JL. Iron biology in immune function, muscle metabolism and neuronal functioning. J Nutr 2001;131:568S–80.
113. Lozoff B. Iron deficiency and child development. Food Nutr Bull (in press).
114. Lozoff B, Klein NK, Prabucki KM. Iron-deficient anemic infants at play. J Dev Behav Pediatr 1986;7:152–8.
115. Lozoff B, Klein NK, Nelson EC, et al. Behavior of infants with iron-deficiency anemia. Child Dev 1998;69:24.
116. Honig AS, Oski FA. Solemnity: A clinical risk index for iron deficient infants. Early Child Dev Care 1984;16:69–83.
117. Hurtado EK, Claussen AH, Scott KG. Early childhood anemia and mild or moderate mental retardation. Am J Clin Nutr 1999;69:115–9.
118. Halterman JS, Kaczorowski JM, Aligne CA, et al. Iron deficiency and cognitive achievement among school-aged children and adolescents in the United States. Pediatrics 2001;107:1381–6.
119. Jimenez E, Smith JB, Lozoff B. Double burden of iron deficiency in infancy and low socioeconomic status: A longitudinal analysis of cognitive test scores to age 19 years. Arch Pediatr Adolesc Med 2006;160:1108–13.
120. Murray-Kolb LE, Beard JL. Iron treatment normalizes cognitive functioning in young women. Am J Clin Nutr 2007;85:778–87.
121. Perez EM, Hendricks MK, Beard JL, et al. Mother-infant interactions and infant development are altered by maternal Iron Deficiency Anemia. J Nutr 2005;135:850–5.
122. Beard JL, Hendricks MK, Perez EM, et al. Maternal iron deficiency anemia affects postpartum emotions and cognition. J Nutr 2005;135:267–72.
123. Black MM. Zinc deficiency and child development. Am J Clin Nutr 1998;68:464S–9.
124. Friel JK, Andrews WL, Matthew JD, et al. Zinc supplementation in very-low-birth-weight infants. J Pediatr Gastroenterol Nutr 1993;17:97–104.
125. Sazawal S, Bentley M, Black RE, et al. Effect of zinc supplementation on observed activity in low socioeconomic Indian preschool children. Pediatrics 1996;98:1132–7.

126. Bentley ME, Caulfield LE, Ram M, et al. Zinc supplementation affects the activity patterns of rural Guatemalan infants. J Nutr 1997;127:1333–8.
127. Castillo-Duran C, Perales CG, Hertrampf ED, et al. Effect of zinc supplementation on development and growth of Chilean infants. J Pediatr 2001;138:229–35.
128. Ashworth A, Morris SS, Lira PI, et al. Zinc supplementation, mental development and behaviour in low birth weight term infants in northeast Brazil. Eur J Clin Nutr 1998;52:223–7.
129. Hamadani JD, Fuchs GJ, Osendarp SJ, et al. Randomized controlled trial of the effect of zinc supplementation on the mental development of Bangladeshi infants. Am J Clin Nutr 2001;74:381–6.
130. Gibson RS, Vanderkooy PD, MacDonald AC, et al. A growth-limiting, mild zinc-deficiency syndrome in some southern Ontario boys with low height percentiles. Am J Clin Nutr 1989;49:1266–73.
131. Penland JG, Sandstead HH, Alcock NW, et al. A preliminary report: Effects of zinc and micronutrient repletion on growth and neuropsychological function of urban Chinese children. J Am Coll Nutr 1997;16:268–72.
132. Sandstead HH, Penland JG, Alcock NW, et al. Effects of repletion with zinc and other micronutrients on neuropsychologic performance and growth of Chinese children. Am J Clin Nutr 1998;68:470S–5S.
133. Black MM, Baqui AH, Zaman K, et al. Iron and zinc supplementation promote motor development and exploratory behavior among Bangladeshi infants. Am J Clin Nutr 2004;80:903–10.
134. Lind T, Lonnerdal B, Stenlund H, et al. A community-based randomized controlled trial of iron and zinc supplementation in Indonesian infants: Effects on growth and development. Am J Clin Nutr 2004;80:729–36.
135. Canfield RL, Gendle MH, Cory-Slechta DA. Impaired neuropsychological functioning in lead-exposed children. Dev Neuropsychol 2004;26:513–40.
136. Lidsky TI, Schneider JS. Lead neurotoxicity in children: Basic mechanisms and clinical correlates. Brain 2003;126:5–19.
137. Needlman HL, Riess JA, Tobin MJ, et al. Bone lead levels and delinquent behavior. JAMA 1996;275:363–9.
138. Koller K, Brown T, Spurgeon A, et al. Recent developments in low-level lead exposure and intellectual impairment in children. Environ Health Perspect 2004;112:987–94.
139. Lanphear BP, Hornung R, Khoury J, et al. Low-level environmental lead exposure and children's intellectual function: An international pooled analysis. Environ Health Perspect 2005;113:894–9.
140. Bressler JP, Goldstein GW. Mechanisms of lead neurotoxicity. Biochem Pharmacol 1991;41:479–84.
141. Finkelstein Y, Markowitz ME, Rosen JF. Low-level lead-induced neurotoxicity in children: An update on central nervous system effects. Brain Res Rev 1998;27:168–76.
142. Bellinger D, Hu H, Titlebaum L, et al. Attentional correlates of dentin and bone lead levels in adolescents. Arch Environ Health 1994;49:98–105.
143. Hunter J, Urbanowicz MA, Yule W, et al. Automated testing of reaction time and its association with lead in children. Int Arch Occup Environ Health 1985;57:27–34.

Nutrition and the Behavior of Children

Kathleen S. Gorman, PhD
Elizabeth Metallinos-Katsaras, PhD, RD

There is a widely held belief that there is a direct causal association between nutritional factors and children's behavior. While there is strong evidence to suggest behavioral effects of some nutrient deficiencies (ie, iron deficiency anemia), the evidence for other nutrient deficiencies is somewhat less clear. However, popular opinion seems to rely heavily on anecdotal data, which suggest that behavioral problems and poor academic achievements are the result of poor nutrition. Given the implications of such beliefs and the fact that many social programs have grown out of the theory that nutrition is a critical factor in children's development, it is important to thoroughly examine the available evidence.

Establishing a causal link between nutrition and behavior is complicated by the fact that malnutrition, and the associated nutritional deficiencies, rarely occurs in isolation. Even children who are mildly malnourished are likely to come from families or homes characterized by factors (eg, low levels of education and income) well known to pose risks to the optimal development of children (Figure 1). A major constraint of the ability to conduct high-quality research on these associations is that developmental processes and behavior are complex phenomena. Isolating individual nutrients and linking them specifically to a particular behavior within a design that takes into consideration the wide array of environmental confounds and covariates is extremely challenging. Although the role of the environment has long been recognized as an explanatory factor in the association between nutrition and development, only recently has the research attempted to build environmental variation into the designs and explore the interactions between nutrition and environmental variables.

In this chapter we examine the current evidence for the causal effects of nutrition on behavioral outcomes in children. In general, malnutrition refers to a condition that results from an "excess, imbalance, or deficit of nutrient availability in relation to tissue needs."[1] The literature on malnutrition comes primarily from low-income countries and provides evidence for the effects of nutrient restrictions on infant and child development, while the evidence for specific nutrient deficiencies and or nutrient properties comes from research on both well-nourished and malnourished populations. In addition, a growing body of literature has emerged on the effects of hunger and related nutritional insufficiencies among well-nourished populations. An additional body of literature explores how the ingestion of particular nutrients (or nonnutrient additives) may pose potential harm (or benefit) to individual development. This section on special topics, which considers the potential effects of presumed deficiencies as well as megadosages, includes sugar, multivitamins, and minerals, as well as brief attention to issues of food additives. This research is primarily focused on a narrow range of outcomes, including but not limited to Attention deficit disorder with hyperactivity (ADHD) and autism. The research on overnutrition and eating disorders is not reviewed here (see Part IV Obesity and Energy Balance as well as Chapter 64, "Adolescence: Healthy and Disordered Eating").

Behavior, as discussed in this chapter, refers to a variety of outcomes that have been studied in association with nutrition, including cognition, achievement, activity, and attention. The behavioral outcome examined varies depending on the type of nutritional input; for example, low-energy intake during gestation and infancy is often believed to affect overall cognitive function, whereas short-term hunger and intakes of specific nutrients (eg, sugar) are more often thought to affect attention and activity levels.[2]

Given the limitations of experimental research on malnutrition in human subjects, much of what is known about the causal effects of malnutrition on behavior comes from the animal literature. Early research noted that inadequate intake of nutrients results in changes in brain structure and size, and it was hypothesized that malnutrition during fetal development and periods of rapid brain growth directly impairs brain development.[3] This impaired brain growth was presumed to result in brain damage and subsequent mental retardation.

While it is well documented that malnutrition can affect brain development and structure, there is no clear consensus that such changes are permanent or that they necessarily result in functional consequences.[3,4] At the same time, advances in neuropsychobiology have identified more subtle alterations in function associated with nutritional deficiencies such as central nervous system (CNS) changes at the level of neuroanatomy and/or neurochemistry.[4] Furthermore, it has been hypothesized that many of the behavioral effects of malnutrition observed in animals (eg, increased emotionality) may be involved in the observed deficits in learning and cognition in humans as well.[5] The growing body of literature on the relationship between nutrition and brain development is reviewed elsewhere in this volume. (see Chapter 24, "Neurophyschological Development").

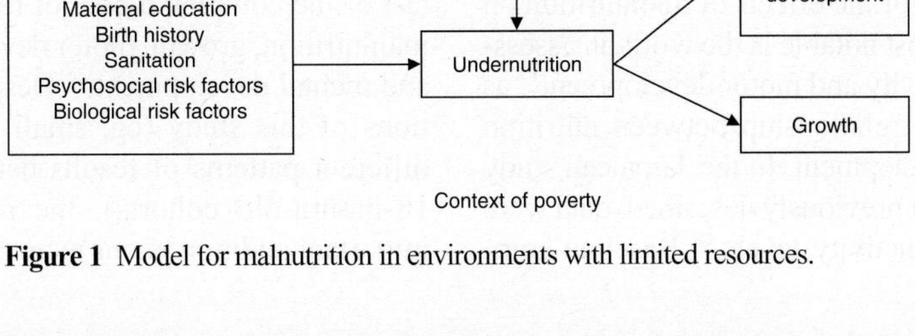

Figure 1 Model for malnutrition in environments with limited resources.

PROTEIN-ENERGY MALNUTRITION AND BEHAVIOR

Recent estimates (2006) suggest that 146 million children (27%) under the age of 5 suffer from malnutrition in the developing world.[6] Nutritional deficiencies are both less common and less severe in countries such as the United States. Nonetheless, data from the Pediatric Nutrition Surveillance System 2004[7] on low-income children and families who participate in federally funded programs [eg, special supplimental nutrition program for women, infants, and children (WIC)] show the prevalence of several nutritional indicators (ie, low height for age, low birth weight, and anemia) among children under 5 years of age to be elevated relative to that expected within the general population. Although the high prevalence of poor nutrition within this sample may reflect, in part, the successful targeting efforts of at-risk populations (eg, WIC gives preferential enrolment to high-nutritional-risk families), the evidence indicates that a large number of children in the United States are at elevated levels of health and nutritional risk. While there remains little doubt that severe levels of malnutrition adversely affect the psychomotor and cognitive development in children as well as long-term school learning and achievement,[3,8] of relevance here is the research on mild-to-moderate malnutrition.

Table 1 Summary of Early Experimental/Quasi-Experimental PEM Supplementation Studies

	Age of Subjects at Initiation	Supplemenatation Duration	Natrient Characteristics of Supplement: Kcal	Protein	Micronutrient	Control*	Educational Component	Outcomes
Guatemala, 1969–1977	Gestation –7	Gestation and 7 yr	X	X	X	Q†	C, MV	Composite infant scale, preschool battery, school, psychoeducational test
Jamaica	2 mo–2 yr	2 yr	X	X		N	X	Griffiths
Cali, 1971–1974	4 yr+	3 yr	X	X	X	N	X‡	Preschool battery, WISC
Bogotá	Gestation–6 mo	Gestation and 3 yr	X	X	X	N	X	Griffiths, Einstein
Indonesia	6–20 mo	3 mo	X	X		Q	N	Bayley
Taiwan	Maternal only	Gestation and lactation	X	X	X	Q	C, MV	Bayley, 5-yr-old IQ
New York City	Maternal only	Gestation	X	X	X		MV	Bayley, object permanence, play, habit/dishabit
Mexico		Maternal and 3 mo+	5 yr	X	X	X	N	Mother–infant contract activity, maternal care, and concern

Reproduced with permission from Gorman KS.[2]

*Supplement administered to control group: C = calorie; MV = multivitamin and mineral supplement; N = none.

†Consumption quantifiable.

‡Education not separate from nutritional intervention.

Bayley = Bayley Scales of Infant Development; Einstein = Einstein Measurement of Children's Cognitions; Griffiths = Griffiths Mental Development Scales; WISC = Wechsler Intelligence Scale for Children.

Most of the foundational studies were conducted in low-income countries during the 1960s and 1970s and tested the hypothesis that improved nutrition at different developmental periods was associated with improved cognitive performance.[2] In each study, children at nutritional risk were supplemented and compared with children who remained unsupplemented. Overall, a summary of the results suggests small, yet statistically significant, findings on a variety of outcomes (eg, mental and motor development, preschool cognitive function) (Table 1).[2]

During the 1980s, better designed studies and the use of improved statistical analyses strengthened the conclusions of a causal relation between nutrition and behavior.[2,9,10] In Jamaica, Grantham-McGregor and her colleagues[11] randomly assigned previously malnourished children, as defined by low height for age to one of four treatment groups: (1) food supplementation, (2) psychosocial stimulation, (3) supplementation and stimulation, and (4) control. The results showed significant and independent effects of both nutrition and stimulation on the Developmental Quotient of the Griffiths Mental Development Scales as compared to control subjects and an additive effect of the combined intervention. After 2 years of treatment, the combined intervention group scored significantly better than the other groups and similarly to a matched group of nonstunted children. The use of children with different nutritional histories and multiple treatment conditions in a randomized study highlights the significance of individual differences and potential interactive effects of interventions. However, follow-up of these children at 4 and 8 years posttreatment indicate few significant enduring effects of the nutritional intervention. In the first follow-up, the authors report benefits of psychosocial stimulation on cognitive performance and an interaction of the supplement with parental behavior.[12] Children whose mothers had higher vocabulary scores showed increased effects of nutritional supplementation on cognitive performance. By the time the children were about 12, only the effects of psychosocial stimulation remained.[13]

A follow-up of rural Guatemalan children who had been supplemented with either high-calorie/high-protein supplement or a low-calorie supplement throughout the first several years of life found significantly better performance on various measures of psychoeducational tests (eg, reading, numeracy, vocabulary, and general knowledge) in adolescents who were exposed to the high-calorie/high-protein supplement.[14] More important, the effects of the supplementation varied by levels of socioeconomic status (SES) and by schooling history. That is, subjects from the poorest families seemed to benefit the most from the supplementation and performed similarly to those from higher SES homes. In addition, children with more exposure to school (beyond 3 years) showed greater benefits of the supplementation than those with fewer years of schooling. Taken together, the results of these studies provide evidence for the effects of nutritional supplementation on cognitive development. Further, the results illustrate the potential for long-term effects and the role that the environment (ie, characteristics of families, home, school) plays in mediating such a relationship. Finally, the results highlight the significance of both the timing and the duration of the intervention, as well as the particular domains of cognition that may be linked to particular nutritional deficiencies.[14,15]

As a result, the focus of current research has been to attempt to elucidate the potential pathways that may account for the effects of malnutrition on behavior.[3,14–16] Most notable is the work on assessing the role of activity and motor development[17] as a mediator in the relationship between nutrition and cognitive development. In the Jamaican study of stunted children previously described, data were also collected on activity levels.[18] Baseline comparisons showed that stunted children were significantly less active than nonstunted children. However, there were no effects of supplementation on activity levels and activity was not found to mediate the relationship between supplementation and cognition. In contrast, data from an experimental study in Pangalengan, Indonesia,[19] provide some initial evidence on the complexity of developmental trajectories of malnourished children. Building on hypotheses developed from his work in Guatemala,[14,15] Pollitt and his colleagues explore the relationships between nutrition and growth, motor development, motor activity, parental behavior, affective behavior, and cognitive development.[17] In this study, two cohorts of infants (12 months, 18 months) were each randomly assigned to one of three types of supplements over the course of 12 months: high energy + micronutrients (E), low energy + micronutrients (M), low energy (S).[20] Data on a wide range of variables were collected periodically over the course of a year. In general, the results provide support for the benefits of high-energy supplement on a number of outcomes. Infants receiving the supplement (E) showed earlier acquisition of motor milestones, higher motor development scores, and increased duration of activity as compared to children receiving the low-energy supplement.[21,22] Furthermore, high-energy-supplemented children showed earlier acquisition of object concept, increased vocalizations, and earlier emotional maturity (decreased fussing) than their peers.[23] The effects of the micronutrient supplement were less clear, except in the case of children with iron-deficiency anemia (IDA).[24] This study represents the first empirical test of the complex model of relationships among malnutrition, growth, motor development, activity, and mental development.[25] Despite several limitations of this study (eg, small sample sizes, and different patterns of results between the 12- and 18-month-old cohorts), the results provide an important addition to our increasing understanding of the mechanisms underlying the relationship between malnutrition and behavior.

In contrast to large field studies described above, most of the recent research on malnutrition has shifted focus to examine specific nutrients and their potential interactions in relation to cognition and behavior with far fewer studies focusing solely on protein-energy malnutrition (PEM) (for exceptions see studies by Liu[26,27]). These nutrient-specific studies are addressed in subsequent sections.

BREAST MILK AND COGNITION

Although the benefits of breast-feeding on immune function, morbidity, growth, and infection are well established,[28,29] the evidence for its effects on mental development, particularly among healthy well-nourished infants, is less convincing.[30–32] Despite literally hundreds of studies attempting to establish a causal link, the research on the effects of breast milk on cognitive function is complicated by two main factors: the fact that mothers who choose to breast-feed vary in a number of ways from those who do not, and researcher's inability to randomly assign mothers to treatment groups.[32–35] Mothers who choose to breast-feed and mothers who bottle-feed have been reported to differ in age, socioeconomic status, education, and ego development,[33–36] all of which are factors also known to affect infant developmental outcomes. Research controlling for these variables has resulted in a reduction in the magnitude of associations between breast-feeding and mental development,[33,35–37] suggesting that these variables account for a significant portion of variation often attributed to breast milk. Furthermore, in some studies, the association between breast-feeding and cognition has been reduced to zero when maternal IQ and parenting skills were also factored in.[31] Hence, studies that purport to establish a relationship between breast-feeding and cognition without controlling for these variables may not be valid.

Despite these limitations, investigators have continued to design studies that attempt to address these methodological difficulties in a number of ways. Many studies focus on collecting data on as many additional covariates as possible, while others have used duration or exclusive/nonexclusive breast-feeding as the exposure variable despite the fact that both of these approaches continue to be confounded by self-selection bias inherent in breast-feeding behavior. In a recent meta-analysis of many of these studies, the authors identified 20 studies that met their initial criteria. (All studies had to include a comparison group, a cognitive outcome measure, and an assessment between infancy and adolescence.)[38] Results, based on comparisons between a smaller number of studies (11) determined to have included a sufficient numbers of covariates, indicated that after adjustment, breast-fed infants had significantly higher levels of cognitive function as compared to formula-fed infants. In addition, it was reported that the differences were consistent across a range of ages and were larger for studies with low-birth-weight (LBW) infants as compared to normal-birth-weight infants. However, others have criticized their conclusions based on a number of methodological limitations of the individual studies included in their analysis.[39,40]

In a similar attempt to evaluate the evidence, a critical evaluation of 24 studies[41] came to a different conclusion, suggesting that the evidence continues to be inconclusive regarding the effects of breast-feeding on cognitive development as compared to formula feeding. In this review, which required three methodological standards for inclusion (ie, clearly defined outcomes, specification of partial vs exclusive breast-feeding, and control of confounds), of the 24 studies initially selected, only 6 met the criteria sufficiently to be included in the analysis. Of these studies, 4 reported positive effects of breast-feeding on cognition. The authors argue that given the limited number of studies that met the criteria that it would be premature to conclude a significant effect of breast-feeding on infant cognition. More specifically, the review identified a number of difficulties of comparing across studies, and in particular the degree to which breast-feeding data can be classified (partial, exclusive, duration—sometimes as little as a few weeks, and the use of dichotomous variables). In a third review, again attempting to determine the link between breast-feeding and intelligence, the authors identified 40 studies, of which only 2 met their criteria for inclusion.[39] Similar to others, the authors conclude that despite the conclusion by a vast majority of studies of the link between breast-feeding and cognition, there is limited evidence from high-quality studies to support this conclusion.

The difficulty of studying this phenomenon cannot be understated and the methodological constraints pose significant challenges. In his review, Rey[40] notes several important limitations of existing research, including observational designs, limited data on confounds, precision in quantifying/classifying breast-feeding data, inclusion of varying levels of risk of infants (eg, premature, low birth weight, health full term), and theoretical issues relating to effects of the process of breast-feeding versus breast milk content. The review included a total of 35 studies, including 10 studies on LBW or SGA (small for gestational age). He concludes that there is limited evidence of cognitive benefits of breast-feeding among normal-weight infants, and considers the results of research on LBW populations separately.

Several authors have concluded that the benefits of breast-feeding to be more significant among LBW infants. Much of the focus of this research is based on evidence from a series of studies conducted in Great Britain, in which Lucas and colleagues attempted to control for many of these potentially confounding variables.[42–44] Most specifically, the studies are strengthened by the fact that all infants were fed by nasogastric tube, hence controlling for any potential behavioral differences associated with the act of breast-feeding. In a two-center study of preterm, low birth weight infants (<1,850 g), and infants of non-breast-feeding mothers were randomly assigned to a standard full term or a special preterm formula (designed to more closely mimic the properties of breast milk than standard formula), while infants whose mothers chose to provide breast milk were also randomly assigned to one of two supplemental formula groups for a period of 4 weeks. In this way, differences between breast milk and formula could be compared as well as differences in standard versus preterm formula. In an assessment of the infants at 18 months, comparisons between formula types demonstrated significant benefits of preterm as compared to term formula on the psychomotor development index (PDI) of Bayley.[42] Similarly, among infants receiving supplementary feeding in addition to breast milk, those who had received preterm formula scored higher on the social quotient from the Vineland than those receiving term formula. When subjects were combined, comparisons between term and preterm formula indicated advantages of preterm formula on the PDI and the Vineland social maturity scale.

In a follow-up at age 7, comparisons were made between infants of mothers who chose to provide breast milk and those who did not on the Wechsler Intelligence Scale for Children (revised for UK).[43,44] According to the authors, similar percentages of infants in each group had received the different types of formulas. Initial findings show a 10-point advantage on each of the IQ scales (verbal, performance, and overall IQ) for those in the breast milk group. In a subsequent analysis between formula groups,[44] the authors report that males showed a benefit of the preterm formula as compared to term formula on language development. There was an apparent dose response to the preterm formula, suggesting that the more formula ingested, the greater the developmental gains.

In a similarly designed, three-center study, results of comparisons between infants who were randomly assigned to either donor breast milk or preterm formula showed no significant differences.[45] Given the previously noted advantages of preterm formula over term formula,[42] the authors suggested that the lack of advantage of the preterm formula in this study pointed to advantages of specific properties of breast milk rather than the macronutrient content. In a nonrandomized comparison across the two different studies to further test this hypothesis, post hoc analyses showed benefits of banked donor breast milk as compared to term formula on motor but not mental development.[45] Based on the assumption that donor breast milk was considered by the authors to be most comparable to term formula at a macronutrient level, ongoing research has focused on examining specific properties of breast milk that may be related to neurodevelopment. More specifically, the results of these studies have advanced a number of theories regarding long-chain polyunsaturated fatty acids (LC-PUFAs), and their association with brain development.[46–49]

Illustrative is a recent review on Long Chain Polyunsaturated Fatty Acids (LC-PUFAs) that reported that breast-fed infants have higher plasma levels of LC-PUFAs than formula-fed infants.[50]

Two fatty acids are essential in humans because they cannot be synthesized. These are the n-3's and n-6's fatty acids, specifically alpha-linolenic and linoleic acids.[51] The primary role of alpha-linolenic acid is in the synthesis of eicosapentaenoic acid (EPA) and docosahexaenoic acid (DHA).[51] It is unknown to what extent the fetus and newborn (preterm or term) has the ability to convert alpha-linolenic to EPA and DHA.[51] These latter two fatty acids are purported to be important for the development of the CNS and vision[51] during gestation and early infancy.[51,52] In order to test the hypothesis that these LCFAs may be one of the underlying reasons for the developmental differences reported between breast-fed and formula-fed infants, two types of randomized controlled trials have been recently undertaken: randomized controlled trials of maternal supplementation of LCFAs during pregnancy and randomized controlled trials of infants beginning in early life. The studies that supplement formula with these LC-PUFAs, namely docasahexaenoic acid and arachidonic acid, in preterm infants, have shown some benefit of human milk or supplemented formula on visual function and visual acuity in comparison to unsupplemented formula. In contrast, studies of visual acuity in term infants have been inconsistent; some have shown effects of supplemented formula, while others have not.[50,53] The research on the effects of LC-PUCFAs on more general measures of cognitive and behavioral development in preterm or term infants is inconclusive.[50] One recent randomized controlled trial on preterm infants supplemented with DHA with or without arachidonic acid found that supplementation (with DHA or DHA + AA) was associated with higher scores on the Bayley's mental and psychomotor scales as compared to controls who did not receive the LCFA supplementation.[54] Among recent studies in term infants some have found benefits of supplementation (with DHA and AA) on mental development,[55] while others have found no association between supplementation and general cognitive and behavioral measures.[53,56] Recent randomized controlled trials of maternal supplementation with LCFAs have also yielded conflicting results, with some finding no effect of supplementation of DHA alone or in combination with arachidonic acid[57] and another reported a positive effect of cod liver oil (high in DHA and EPA) on mental development at 4 years of age.[52] An earlier study even suggested that there were adverse developmental effects of supplementing DHA alone (without arachidonic acid) during pregnancy.[58] Differences in the timing and composition of the supplement, the tests used, as well as potential confounders (ie, maternal smoking), may be at least in part responsible for the lack of agreement in the findings. In addition, the length of follow-up in most of these studies has been short, which makes it difficult to draw conclusions about long-term benefits of the LC- PUFAs.

Nonetheless, it is important to note that even if subsequent analyses uphold these findings of a causal association between breast milk properties (eg, LC-PUFAs) and cognitive development among at-risk infants, the issue of generalizability to term infants is unknown.

IRON-DEFICIENCY ANEMIA AND OTHER MICRONUTRIENT DEFICIENCIES

This section reviews the evidence for a causal association between micronutrient deficiencies and cognitive outcomes. The micronutrients most often linked to infant and child development include iodine, iron, zinc, and B_{12}. This focus on these micronutrients can be explained by the fact that they are those most likely to be deficient in infants and children and can be linked to physiological processes that are potentially related to development.[59] The difficulty of isolating the effects of specific nutrients is particularly challenging since the most significant contributors to dietary iron, zinc, and B_{12} are typically the same food sources, namely meat, poultry, and fish. Furthermore, children consuming diets lacking in these nutrients are often exposed to environmental factors (ie, poverty) that adversely affect development. This often undermines the certainty with which one can attribute cause and effect to these relationships.

A further difficulty of conducting research on the adverse effects of micronutrient deficiencies lies with their known effects on other health-related outcomes, which then precludes the withholding of treatment due to ethical considerations. This has led to treatment designs that do not include either a placebo group, or more frequently, prevention trials in which the subjects have not been diagnosed with a deficiency. In prevention trials, those at high risk for developing a deficiency are randomly assigned to a supplement or placebo and longitudinal assessments of outcomes are subsequently conducted with comparisons made between treated (presumably replete) and placebo (expected to demonstrate evidence of subsequent deficiency) groups. Prevention trials have the advantage of assessing effects of more mild levels of micronutrient deficiencies before they become moderate or severe. The underlying hypothesis being tested is whether a deficiency in the nutrient is what is causing the differences in developmental outcomes. While one limitation to a prevention trial is that some of those not supplemented will never develop a deficiency and thus, will dilute any significant effects of the supplement, they have the advantage of providing a more realistic estimate of effectiveness for use in public health interventions.

In the following sections, we summarize current knowledge about the effects of three major micronutrient deficiencies on behavior in children, iron, zinc, and iodine. B_{12} will not be addressed because there is a dearth of research on this topic in infants and children. Most of the research on B_{12} and cognition has been conducted in the elderly.[60]

Iron

Worldwide it is estimated that iron deficiency anemia (IDA) affects 2 billion people, mostly women and children.[61] Although the prevalence of IDA in the United States has declined between the 1988 to 1994 and 1999 to 2000 National Health and Nutrition Examination Survey III among the general population of infants, children, and adolescents, 7% of toddlers ages 1 to 2 years, 5% of preschoolers, and 9 to 16% of adolescent girls and women of childbearing age are iron deficient based on laboratory tests of iron status.[62] Moreover, the prevalence of iron deficiency varies by ethnicity and income status, with higher rates among Mexican American 1- to 2-year-olds (17%) and 3- to 4-year-olds (6%) and among low-income 1- to 2-year-olds (12%) and 3- to 4-year-olds (5%).[63] Thus, risk for iron deficiency anemia (IDA) continues to be high in the United States, particularly among infants and toddlers during a time considered sensitive for cognitive development. The elevated risk has provided the impetus for the infancy period being the most common target for investigations of the behavioral effects of IDA.

Numerous observational studies examining the association between IDA and cognition and/or achievement have found that these infants score lower on mental and motor development tests, explore their environment less, and induce less stimulating behaviors in their caretakers.[64–66] Children's achievement, among both preschool and school-age subjects, is poorer for formerly anemic children than nonanemic children.[64–68] The correlational design of these studies and the inability to control for the large number of social, health, and environmental risk factors that coexist with IDA has constrained the interpretation of such differences as being causal.

Randomized clinical trials (both prevention and treatment) provide the best evidence that IDA is at least in part a cause of the developmental and achievement gaps observed between IDA and nonanemic infants and children, although results have not always been consistent. In some treatment trials, IDA infants treated with iron scored significantly higher on developmental tests than IDA infants given a placebo.[69,70] The results of one iron supplementation trial (no placebo group) with long-term follow-up on infants with IDA reported that cognitive differences between previously IDA and nonanemic infants persisted throughout the preschool period,[66] childhood,[66] and adolescence,[71] while suggestive limitations in study design (ie, lack of a placebo group) preclude our attributing cause and effect to this relationship.

As a result of the ethical issues surrounding the inclusion of a IDA-placebo group, the use of prevention trials during prenatal and infant periods has been a more recent focus of the research in this area. Most have supplemented with iron alone and a few have examined effects of iron in combination with zinc.[59,72] As noted previously, one advantage to these studies is that they can better isolate effects of mild IDA and ID without anemia; this is particularly true for those studies which are conducted in healthy infants in industrialized countries.

Of the eight randomized controlled iron-deficiency prevention trials (two in combination with zinc) in children less than 3 years of age[59,72,73–78] that have been published in the past decade, one found no effect of iron supplementation on the cognitive outcomes assessed[75] and seven reported some beneficial effects on cognitive outcomes.[59,72–74,76–78] Of these seven, all included a global measure of development (eg, Bayley's or the Griffiths) as an outcome. Five demonstrated effects of iron supplementation on these global developmental outcomes (Bayley's or Griffiths)[59,72,74,76,78] and two did not. Of the five studies reporting significant effects of iron supplementation, four found effects on the psychomotor scores,[59,72,74,78] although one found effects of iron only when administered in combination with zinc.[59] Additionally, one found effects on the prevention of a decline in Griffiths developmental scores.[76] Most studies also included a variety of other outcome measures; significant effects of iron supplementation were noted in visual perceptual skills,[73] visual acuity,[78] information processing,[77] orientation engagement,[59] and indices of social behavior (eg, affect).[77]

The double blind randomized controlled prevention trial conducted by Friel[78] is particularly intriguing because it was conducted on healthy full-term Canadian infants ($n = 77$) who were successfully breast-fed at 1 month of age (ie, at the beginning of the study) and were not iron deficient or IDA at entry into the study. Breast-fed infants have had a relatively higher risk of IDA between 6 and 12 months of age.[78] Beginning at 1 month of age, infants were supplemented with 7.5 mg elemental iron or placebo until 6 months of age. At 13 months of age iron-supplemented infants scored significantly better on the Bayley's psychomotor developmental indices (mean scores 100 in iron-supplemented and 93 in the placebo groups) and had better visual acuity, although this was not statistically significant ($p = .07$) unless only compliers were included. The authors note that visual acuity is a sensitive marker of general neurodevelopmental status. Despite the limitation of a relatively high dropout rate that was nevertheless similar in iron-supplemented and placebo groups, these results suggest that early iron deficiency (even without anemia) may have neurodevelopmental effects.

Although fewer in number, studies on preschool and school-age children show an effect of IDA on measures of intelligence and other cognitive processes (eg, discrimination learning tasks, visual recall, selective attention).[79–84] Generally the studies on preschool and school-age children provide support for the adverse effects of iron deficiency on development even in apparently otherwise healthy children. Of the five treatment trials examining the effects of IDA on development among preschoolers,[81–85] three samples were drawn from populations in which undernutrition is common[81–83] and two were drawn from a generally well-nourished population.[80,84]

Among those conducted in samples drawn from undernourished populations, iron supplementation was associated with improvements in verbal and performance IQ,[82] discrimination,[81,83] and oddity learning.[83] Among those conducted among a well-nourished population, supplementation was associated with improvements in discrimination learning[80] and selective attention.[84]

Illustrative is a treatment trial conducted on a preschool sample drawn from a generally well-nourished population.[84] Within iron status groups (ie, IDA or "good iron status") children were randomly assigned to 15 mg elemental iron + multivitamins or multivitamins alone 5 days a week for 2 months while they were at daycare. Iron supplementation (as compared to the placebo) was associated with significant improvements in selective attention (ie, specificity, accuracy, and efficiency on a continuous performance test) but not on oddity learning tasks among those who were IDA but not among those who had good iron status.[84]

While the data on infants are compelling, to our knowledge, there has only been one randomized placebo-controlled trial on prenatal iron-supplementation (20 mg/d) of well-nourished pregnant women. In this study, no differences in mean IQ (Standford Binet) or IQ subscales between iron-supplemented and placebo children at 4 years of age were reported.[86]

In summary, the evidence from numerous studies supports the contention that iron deficiency anemia has an adverse effects on infant and child cognitive development and that this association is causal. The effects of iron supplementation have been observed on a wide range of outcomes from performance on global tests of intelligence to specific cognitive processes. The prevention trials provide evidence that less severe forms of iron deficiency may also have adverse effects on development. Although the research suggests that chronic IDA in infancy may be associated with irreversible physiological changes in the brain of animals, whether this translates into irreversible developmental effects in humans is still unknown. Two recent reviews have presented compelling arguments for the potential mechanisms by which IDA may alter brain or neural development and functioning.[71,87] Based on animal models the authors argue that iron deficiency particularly during "critical periods" may affect changes in the structure (eg, myelination) and function (eg, neurotransmission, particularly the dopaminergic system) of the CNS.[87] A true test of irreversibility would be exposure to a remediation program that would not only include nutritional adequacy but also enclude environmental conditions which strongly support and promote development. While there is still much research needed to further substantiate the levels of deficiency that may correspond to developmental effects and the extent to which effects are age specific, the wealth of well-designed studies conducted during the past 15 to 20 years point to the need for primary prevention of iron deficiency.

Zinc

Considerable attention has recently focused on the effects of zinc deficiency on behavior. The known effects of zinc deficiency on growth have lead researchers to hypothesize that there are effects on cognitive and behavioral development as well. Zinc deficiency is characterized by lethargy, apathy, and slow movement, all behaviors that closely parallel those described in other malnourished groups. In laboratory animals (eg, rhesus monkeys), zinc-deprived animals had lower activity levels, longer response times, poorer attention, and impaired success at learning tasks as compared to controls.[88,89] Studying the effects of zinc deficiency is more complicated than iron because there is no good measure of zinc status that could definitively identify those who are deficient; thus, most zinc supplementation research utilize prevention trials. Of zinc supplementation studies conducted on infants or toddlers at nutritional risk (LBW or from low-income countries) effects have been noted on motor development scores,[90] motor quality and mental developmental scores,[91] and activity.[92] However, in one recent supplementation study on Bangladeshi infants, supplementation with zinc from 1 to 5 months of age was associated with a significantly lower mental development score at 13 months.[93] The authors suggest that the adverse effect may have been due to an imbalance of nutrients because only zinc was supplemented in this generally undernourished group; for example, zinc competes with both iron and copper for absorption. Two additional randomized controlled trials, also in low-income countries (Bangladesh and Indonesia), addressed this issue by supplementing infants for 6 months (at 6 to 12 months of age) with iron and zinc (singly or together) to evaluate both the separate and joint effects of these nutrients.[59,72] The study on Bangladeshi infants demonstrated significant effects on a prevention of motor score decline between 6 to 12 months among the infants receiving both iron and zinc but not with the single nutrient supplements. In addition, children who received any of the treatment combinations (ie, zinc alone, iron alone, or zinc and iron) had higher scores on indices of exploratory behavior, which has been hypothesized as a potential mechanism for the decline in motor scores often observed in undernourished children.[59] In contrast, no effect of zinc either singly or in combination with iron on any developmental measure was reported in the Indonesian study.[72] The conflicting findings may be a function of the degree of severity of malnutrition among the two groups, although it is unclear why the more severely malnourished Bangladeshi infants would respond to a simple micronutrient supplement when the less severely malnourished infants from Indonesia did not. In fact, research on chronically and severely undernourished toddlers suggests that supplementation with multivitamins alone in comparison with multivitamins + energy is associated with poorer mental developmental trajectories between 12 and 18 months.[94]

Among school-age nutritionally at-risk children, one intervention study[95] reported a significant improvement in scores on several neuropsychological tests [ie, continuous performance task (CPT), oddity learning, tapping, tracking], while another[96] found a significant effect of zinc on reasoning (ie, fewer trials were needed to learn simple concepts). In the former study, it was unclear whether assignment to different intervention groups was random. Another study of stunted-school-age boys found no effect of zinc supplementation either on attention or on academic performance.[97]

Finally two randomized placebo-controlled prevention trials were conducted on pregnant women, one in a low-income country (Bangladesh) and the other among low-income African-American women in the United States.[98,99] One reported lower 13-month mental and motor scale scores in 13-month-old infants whose mothers were zinc supplemented prenatally compared to placebo,[98] while the other found no effect of prenatal zinc supplementation on developmental outcomes at age 5,[99] despite significant effects on head circumference. While the evidence is limited, these two studies of very different populations, with different follow-up periods, do not support any beneficial effect of zinc supplementation on developmental outcomes during the prenatal period.

In summary while there is some evidence that zinc deficiency may affect development and that zinc supplementation of infants and children at high risk for zinc deficiency may benefit developmental outcomes, recent studies showing potential adverse effects of prenatal and postnatal zinc supplementation on child development underscore the need to better understand nutrient interactions, and how supplementation may exacerbate coexisting micro- or macronutrient deficiencies. More randomized controlled trials are needed in human populations which are designed in order to address coexisting deficiencies and acknowledge the fact that micro- and macronutrients are required simultaneously; differing population specific nutrient needs may be the underlying reason conflicting results have been found.

Iodine

Worldwide iodine-deficiency disorders affect about 240 million people.[61] In addition to the fairly conclusive evidence on iron deficiency anemia, it is well established that maternal iodine deficiency results in cretinism, deafness, and poor motor and cognitive outcomes for the fetus.[100–104] Iodine supplementation prior to pregnancy or during the first trimester results in improved developmental outcomes.[102] Research on mild levels of iodine deficiency during pregnancy has been associated with delays in information processing and motor development in infants,[105] with some indication that environmental variables (eg, maternal education) may moderate the association. Recent research among well-nourished populations indicates that maternal hypothyroidism during pregnancy may be associated with measures of continuous performance task and word discrimination in school-age children,[106] although children born to mothers whose deficiency was treated, but who continued to show evidence of hypothyroidism, performed more similarly to matched controls than to their untreated peers. While the authors interpret the large discrepancies between the untreated group and the matched controls to hypothyroidism, the fact that those who were "inadequately" treated performed more like controls calls into question the causal link between iodine deficiency and the cognitive outcome. A randomized clinical trial of prepregnant women found that infants born to iodine-replete women scored significantly higher on measures of information processing as compared to placebo infants; no differences were reported between groups on either the mental development index (MDI) or the psycomotor development index (PDI).[107] Finally, the effects of iodine supplementation on cognitive development among children who display signs of iodine deficiency show mixed results.[108–110] A recently reported iodine supplementation trial of school children in Albania, with improved methodology, suggests that iodine supplementation of children with very high levels of iodine deficiency may result in improved cognitive functioning, most specifically in areas of speed and efficiency.[111] Further research on whether these effects are long lasting and whether or not they are observed among children with less significant levels of iodine deficiency is warranted.

In conclusion, the research strongly suggests that iodine deficiency affects children's development. While the evidence for iron deficiency also points to a causal association with development, particularly motor development, the research for zinc is less clear and more research is needed. Although science demands the isolation of one factor in order to examine whether that factor is associated with an outcome, studies in undernourished populations are challenging due to the multiple and differing nutrient deficiencies. Whether a deficiency affects development may depend on both the outcome under study, the nutrient in question, any other concurrent nutrient (macro or micro) deficiencies and the context (ie, environment) under which the child lives. Designing studies to address the complexity of child development is needed to further elucidate how and to what extent micronutrients affect development. Despite our attention to these three micronutrients, it is important to note that the number of nutrients with the potential to affect behavior is vast; our knowledge of the roles of specific nutrients is constantly being revised. For example, evidence from a correlational study has suggested that maternal vitamin B_6 status is associated with performance on neonatal assessments, maternal responsiveness, and infant development between 3 and 6 months.[112]

Food Insecurity and Hunger

In the preceding sections, the literature on malnutrition and specific nutrient deficiencies and their effects on cognition and behavior have been reviewed. In the introduction we note that while severe malnutrition is uncommon in the United States, inadequate nutrient intake and more mild forms of micronutrient deficiencies may be more common.

In the United States, an increasingly large segment of the population may be at risk for poor nutrition (both under and over) due to poverty and lack of resources. For example, in 2005, an estimated 13% of all people were living below the federal poverty level and almost one in five children were living in poverty.[113] Given that the poverty level ($16,600 for a family of three in 2006)[113] grossly underestimates the amount of money a family requires to meet its basic needs, the estimates of children living in households with inadequate access to good nutrition is likely much higher. Further, estimates of food security and a measure of one's ability to access adequate and nutritious food suggests that 11.4% of US households were food insecure. In addition, rates of food insecurity are markedly higher for households with young children (16.7% for children under 6), and children in female-headed households (30.8%).[114]

The ability to effectively measure food insecurity and hunger has long been debated, and the recent move by the federal government to replace the word "hunger" with the more quantifiable term "very low food security"[115] has met with skepticism. Nonetheless, a significant body of research has established strong associations between food insecurity, hunger, and a range of health, behavioral, and psychosocial outcomes[116–118] among otherwise well-nourished populations. Specifically, food insecurity among school-age children has been associated with impaired growth,[119] increased behavioral problems,[120] as well as lower achievement test scores and more grade repetitions.[121]

The potential mechanisms to account for such associations are hypothesized to result from either the effects of deficient dietary intake over time or the more immediate metabolic or hormonal short-term effects of reduced food intake on cognitive functions, including but not limited to memory and attentional processes.[122] Methodologically, the association is difficult to establish since hunger and food insecurity rarely occur in isolation but rather coexist with a number of factors (eg, poverty, low wages, lack of medical care, lack of social support) that put both adults and children at risk for poor outcomes.[123,124]

In general a number of different types of designs have been used to assess the effects of hunger on cognition. In the following sections, we review studies that broadly fall into two categories. The first refers specifically to whether the condition of hunger affects cognitive function, and the data come from a number of experimental or quasi-experimental studies that have measured children's response to fasting (eg, eating or not eating breakfast). The second refers to whether provision of food to children at nutritional risk can affect school performance and comes from food assistance and feeding programs that target low-income children in an attempt to reduce hunger and thereby improve school performance. In both types of studies reviewed, breakfast is the treatment variable. Breakfast has been shown to be a key component of a good diet by providing an important portion of the days' calories.[125,126] Its absence is considered to have potential adverse effects on learning and school performance. Various surveys of children's eating habits suggest that anywhere from 5 to 26% of school-age children frequently skip breakfast.[127,128]

Experimental Studies

Among the first type of studies, exploring the effects of fasting (or hunger) on cognition, a variety of designs have been used. In some studies, children serve as their own control and are measured under two experimental conditions (breakfast, BR and no breakfast, NBR).[129–134] In others, children are randomly assigned to either a BR or NBR condition.[132–138] Still others have used children's natural state (prior BR or NBR), and then randomly assigned to either treatment (ie, glucose) or a placebo condition.[136] The results of these studies are mixed and highlight many of the limitations of this research.

In a number of studies, the positive effects of breakfast on cognitive function and/or the negative effects of fasting have been reported but these effects are not always consistent. For example, in several studies an increase in errors on a matching familiar figures test (MFFT) was noted in the NBR condition (or a parallel decrease in errors with BR).[129,130,137] Similarly, slower word recall and spatial memory performance has also been reported to result from fasting,[136] although no differences were found on these same tasks in terms of errors between BR and NBR groups. Some studies have reported differences in memory, favoring the BR condition,[139] but others report no differences.[135] At least three studies have found positive effects of fasting on memory,[129] learning recall,[130] and math and MFFT performance.[133]

One of the potential mechanisms for the association between breakfast and cognition is the relation of glucose to brain function. It has been argued that because the brain has a high requirement for glucose relative to other organs,[140] the availability of glucose and the timing of its provision prior to cognitive tasks may be particularly critical. While some have reported a relationship between glucose tolerance and cognitive performance,[139,141] studies that did not control for prior breakfast consumption[142,143] or the nutritional content of the breakfast[144] limit the consistency of the findings. Interestingly, research using animal models finds a U-shaped relationship between blood glucose and memory; at both high and low doses of glucose, the ability to retain learned information is impaired.[145] While this type of relationship could account for the mixed findings, it is unclear whether this relationship would be replicated in children. Furthermore, a recent study found that individual differences in glycemic tolerance interacted with particular properties of the diet to affect performance on measures of memory, reaction times, and vigilance.[141] These findings highlight the need to consider individual characteristics as well as current and previous diet more carefully in future research.

Several investigators have hypothesized that fasting may have more detrimental effects on children who are either malnourished or previously malnourished. In studies that have examined the association between fasting and cognition among children at nutritional risk, the results suggest that previously malnourished children may be more responsive to the provision of breakfast, although these results were not consistent across all studies.[131,132] In one study, results showed no effects of fasting on tests of intelligence or vocabulary but significant effects of fasting on two cognitive tasks.[131] Boys at nutritional risk (low weight for height, low height for age) performed worse on a stimulus discrimination task and the Sternberg memory search under fasting conditions as compared to the breakfast condition. Similarly, results of two studies in Jamaica showed that missing breakfast resulted in lower test performance on verbal fluency and coding in children at nutritional risk (previously malnourished or stunted), as compared to nonstunted controls.[133] In a separate study, poorly nourished Jamaican children performed significantly better on tests of verbal fluency (but not, visual search, digit span, or speed of processing) after eating breakfast, as compared to well-nourished children.[134] However, as with the studies of well-nourished populations, the nonstunted controls' math performance and MFFT efficiency scores improved as a function of missing breakfast.[133] Finally, a study of school-age children in Chile compared the effects of breakfast or no breakfast on the cognitive performance of normal, wasted, and stunted children and found no significant differences on any of the cognitive tasks, although methodological considerations (only partially successful randomization) may have contributed to the results.[138]

SCHOOL-BASED PROGRAMS

A second area of study has focused on the effects of school-based feeding programs. One of the underlying assumptions of the school-based programs is that children who come to school hungry will have a more difficult time attending to the learning process.[122] With the introduction of federally funded nutrition assistance programs in the schools, and in particular, the school breakfast program, investigators have been able to use these interventions as an alternative model to assess the effects of breakfast on school performance as well as to evaluate the effectiveness of the investment.

Data from evaluations of school breakfast programs have provided support for their benefits.[126,146] In one study, data on achievement, absenteeism, and tardiness collected prior to the initiation of school breakfast program were compared with similar data after the school breakfast program. As compared to nonparticipants, children participating regularly in the school breakfast program showed significantly higher performance on the comprehensive test of basic skills (CTBs) and lower rates of absenteeism and tardiness. Most notably, even after controlling for a large number of potentially confounding variables (eg, sex, ethnicity, family size, income, pretest CTBs scores), the school breakfast program continued to show independent effects on the outcomes. One limitation of this study is that participation was voluntary, and this introduced a potential self-selection bias that could not be taken into account in the analyses.

In a two-state, three-school evaluation of the breakfast program, researchers found initial differences in academic performance between students with high participation in the school breakfast program (ie, those who typically ate school breakfast) as compared to those with lower participation rates[147] on a wide range of assessments including test scores, indicators of depression and anxiety, hyperactivity, and attendance. After introducing universal school breakfast (making the program free for all students in the school) program participation rates increased to 100%. The authors report that after 4 months of this breakfast program, students who frequently ate school breakfast showed improved rates of attendance and punctuality, decreased rates of psychosocial symptoms, and improved academic functioning (math grades) as compared to those who ate breakfast infrequently. While suggestive, multiple methodological problems (nonrandom design, small sample sizes, loss of subjects, and no control for usual breakfast consumption) prohibit the ability to establish any causal relationship between breakfast and student behavior, it is likely that children who chose to eat breakfast are significantly different in a number of ways from those who do not eat breakfast.

In another study, the effects of participation in the SBP on children's nutritional status as well as school performance was examined.[148] Prior to the onset of a universal school breakfast program (USBP) in which all children can participate at no cost, children were categorized based on their current nutritional status (based on dietary recall data). After 6 months of participation in the USBP, children whose nutritional status had improved were also more likely to attend school, participate in the breakfast program, and report less hunger. The changes in nutritional status were also associated with improvements in math and behavioral problem indicators. Despite small sample size and selective participation, the ability to link changes in nutritional intake to performance indicators is promising.

Data available from a limited number of studies in low-income countries also support these findings and suggest that children's performance[149,150] and attendance[132] improve with the introduction of a breakfast program, although based on the designs, these effects are likely the result of increased motivation rather than any specific nutritional effect.

In sum, despite the absence of strong support for a direct impact of school feeding programs on school performance, consideration of many of the methodological and evaluation designs is likely to lead to more robust findings.[151] It should not be surprising that program evaluations of school feeding programs have not yielded strong effects on learning, given the limitations of study designs available in school-based research, particularly since these programs often limit the ability to target those children at highest risk, who may also be the most likely to benefit the most from such programs. Further, future research should include study designs that consider how attendance, absenteeism, and participation may be mediating factors in the potential long-term effects of school feeding programs on school achievement.[126,146]

In conclusion, results from experimental research on short-term fasting and school feeding programs provide support for an association between hunger and behavior of children, despite the fact that many of the studies reviewed have methodological limitations (for recent reviews, see Rampersaud,[128] Granthan-McGregor[151]). In general, the research suggests that short-term hunger has effects on cognition, and specifically memory, while the evidence for other outcomes is less consistent.[128] Further, children at nutritional risk, at least in the short term, may be more likely to benefit from interventions such as school breakfast as compared to their healthy peers.[128,151] Finally, in order to further our understanding of the causal role of hunger on child behavior, future research will require longitudinal randomized designs, as well as consideration of a wide range of variables, including family background variables (eg, socioeconomic status), school level variables, individual level data (ie, child age, sex, and nutritional status), and more precise information on the treatment variable (ie, timing, nutritional content, and prior nutrient intakes).

SPECIAL TOPICS

This section addresses several other topics of current interest that do not fall strictly under the theoretical framework guiding the research presented in this chapter, namely, for two reasons. First, many of the topics included below address nutrients or substances that are not necessarily purported to be the cause of children's behavior. In addition, much of the research is conducted without any evidence of a nutrient deficiency. Unlike previous sections in which there was evidence that the study question addressed nutrient deficiencies as causes of behavioral outcomes, the following special topics are not grounded in any theory regarding nutrient inadequacies or excesses causing behavior changes. Many of these are either exploratory in nature (eg, multivitamin [MV] supplementation) or attempt to address popular belief (eg, sucrose).

Multivitamin and Mineral Supplementation

Over the past 25 years, a number of researchers have proposed a causal association between MV supplementation and performance on intelligence tests. The hypothesis driving much of this research is that a subset of the generally well-nourished population, despite the absence of any anthropometric, biochemical, or clinical signs of micronutrient deficiencies, may have compromised cognitive function due to marginal micronutrient status, even though there is no physiologic basis for such an effect in an adequately nourished population. A recent review argued that the first signs of a micronutrient deficiency may be psychological[152]; however, a causal association would need to have been demonstrated vis a vis repeated positive findings using internally valid study designs in order to support such a conclusion. While some studies have shown support for a causal association between MV/mineral supplementation and cognitive performance[153–157] others have not.[155,158,159] Given the implications that such an association would have for public health policy, it is important to closely scrutinize the evidence.

In order to test whether specific nutrients are causally related to behavioral outcomes, a rigorous model requires selecting samples that are deficient or replete in the nutrient in question (based on quantitative assessment of nutritional status), establishing an initial relationship between cognition and a deficiency in this nutrient, conducting a randomized placebo-controlled trial of supplementation of the nutrient that is deficient in both the replete and deficient groups, examining the differential effect of the supplement based on initial nutritional status, and accounting for any effect of study participation.[160] While this model has been utilized with relative success in the iron deficiency and cognition literature, it has not been used in other areas of nutrition and behavior research, most notably in the assessment of the relationship between multivitamin/mineral (MV/mineral) supplementation of generally well-nourished groups and cognitive performance.[154] It should be noted that one challenge to using this rigorous model is that unlike iron status, which is accurately assessed using a combination of biochemical indicators, some micronutrients do not have such biochemical (blood or urine) indicators which reflect status accurately.[161]

The evidence for the positive effects of MV/mineral comes from several studies in which healthy children have been mass supplemented. The length of supplementation has varied between 6 weeks and 12 months, and the levels of nutrients provided differed considerably within MV/mineral supplement (as low as 10% of RDA for iron in some supplements) and between studies (average levels ranged from 50 to 200% RDA). Although several early studies concluded that MV/mineral supplementation significantly improved nonverbal intelligence of preschoolers and school-age children,[155,156,162] a critical examination of the research reveals methodologic shortcomings that call the validity of these conclusions into question. For example, studies failed to document convincing evidence of a nutritional deficiency,[153–156,162] to control for confounding factors or bias that may have influenced the results,[153,156,162] and to provide a rationale for the nutrient composition of the supplementation.[153–156] Further, in some cases, the "effects" are the result of a negative effect of the placebo rather than improved performance resulting from supplementation.[155,156]

In addition to nonverbal IQ, other studies have examined MV effects on more specific cognitive processes. Two studies on university students reported statistically significant treatment effects on reaction time.[153,154] However, in one study, the effects were noted among females only[153] and were limited by a potential selection bias. (Only 61.4% of the original sample included in the final analysis.) In the second study, the treatment effect of a multivitamin supplement on reaction time was attributed to thiamine despite the fact that blood transketolase activation values (ie, an indication of thiamine status) did not indicate a thiamine deficiency.[154]

The results of the largest and most controversial of the mass supplementation studies of children showed a net gain of 3.5 IQ points among 401 children provided 100% recommended dietary allowances (RDA) of most micronutrients (compared to placebo); there were no effects in the groups supplemented with either 50% or 200% RDA.[156,162] Current knowledge of nutritional biochemistry makes a theoretical explanation of effects difficult. Furthermore, incomplete and incorrect presentation of data, errors in statistical analyses, the exclusion of 35% of the original sample due to their refusal to give blood, as well as evidence for less than ideal testing conditions for some of the tests [162–164] raise serious questions about the validity of the findings.

Three studies were conducted which attempted to address some of the limitations of previous studies by matching on baseline cognitive measures, and/or on anthropometric indicators of nutritional status, and/or assessing blind to treatment.[155,157,158] Two showed no effect of MV/mineral supplementation on nonverbal intelligence,[155,158] while one demonstrated a significant effect.[157] In the latter study, school-age children, 6 to 12 years of age ($n = 388$), completed a randomized double-blind placebo-controlled trial of a MV/mineral tablet; only 245 subjects were included in the final analyses due to an a priori decision to exclude data from six testers who did not meet specific criteria.[157] The duration of the intervention was 3 months, and randomization was stratified by preintervention nonverbal IQ, and by classroom. The MV/mineral tablet included between 50 and 67% of the RDA depending on the vitamin/mineral. Teachers distributed the tablets at the schools. At pretest there were no significant group differences in age, gender, race, grade, or primary language at baseline. At the posttest, both groups showed a mean IQ score gain with a statistically significant difference ($p < .038$) of 2.47 favoring the MV/mineral group. Subsequent analysis revealed that this difference was primarily due to a subset of the children whose increase in IQ score was greater than 15 points. Over a third of those randomized to MV (35%) exhibited such an increase as compared to only 21% of those given placebo ($p < .01$, Chi-square test). The authors contend that the significant increase among the MV group was likely due to improved nutrition among a subset of poorly nourished children despite a lack of any evidence to support this claim. The fact that 21% of the placebo group showed similarly large IQ improvements (>15 points) raises questions about the mechanisms that may account for the increase in the MV group.

A macroanalysis of 13 trials concluded that the improved performance on nonverbal IQ tests in favor of MV groups over controls was not due to chance ($p < .0002$).[159] In fact, when all the data were aggregated from these 13 studies, the author reports a net gain of 3.2 IQ points among those given MV/mineral. Despite statistical significance, a difference of this magnitude is of questionable applied significance.

In summary, available research does not support the contention that supplementation with MV/minerals improves intelligence test scores of the general pediatric population in which there is no evidence of a deficiency. One finding that was common to several of the studies is that a subset of those supplemented exhibit a large change in test scores. It may well be that a subset of children are deficient in a specific nutrient or nutrients and hence respond favorably to treatment. However, while the data supporting this hypothesis are intriguing, they are by no means conclusive. Another consideration is the fact none of the essential nutrients can be individually implicated. Indiscriminate supplementation of most essential vitamins and minerals is neither a feasible nor an acceptable public health practice.

In order to respond to these concerns, future research will need to use better designs that allow for a true test of the hypothesis. At a minimum, such studies should include (1) samples of deficient and nondeficient children, (2) multiple measures to assess nutritional status, (3) double-blind, randomized, placebo-controlled trials for both types of children, (4) randomization by initial nutritional status, and (5) assessment of both nutritional and cognitive outcomes.

MEGAVITAMIN/MEGAMINERAL THERAPY

Children with particular behavioral profiles, typically autism and attention deficit disorder with hyperactivity, have often been targeted for megavitamin or megamineral therapies. Although the theory is that these children are highly deficient in certain nutrients, there is rarely evidence that these nutrient deficiencies are causally related to the behavioral disorders. One consideration in both the evaluation of the research in this area and its application to clinical practice is the potential toxicity of specific micronutrients in large quantities.[165] Fat-soluble vitamins, particularly vitamin A, have shown toxic effects in large amounts, and although most water-soluble vitamins have been considered relatively safe, pyridoxine (B_6), a vitamin used frequently in megavitamin therapy, has produced ataxia and a severe sensory neuropathy in some individuals.[165] The basic assumption underlying this research is that the metabolic requirements of certain groups of children may be greater for certain nutrients, although biochemical evidence to support this contention is rarely available.

While the etiology of autism is unknown, it is believed to be driven primarily by genetic factors combined with a number of environmental contributors. There appears to be a legitimate reason to suspect that nutrition may contribute to autism symptoms based on a number of different factors, including the common gastrointestinal tract disturbances and allergies including specific reactivity to casein and gliadin often reported among children and adults with autism[166]; however, there is no evidence that nutrition is an underlying cause of autism. Two nutrients postulated to positively affect behaviors of children with autism are B_6 and magnesium. There is biochemical evidence that children with autism have a higher B_6 requirement.[167] Children with autism have been found to have significantly higher plasma B_6 than children without autism and this seems to be related to an impairment of pyridoxal kinase which converts pyridoxine to its cofactor, pyridoxal phosphate.[167] However, while numerous studies have been conducted on B_6 and magnesium supplementation in children with autism with many showing some beneficial effects,[167] most of them suffer from methodological limitations which limit the validity of these studies.[168] A recent Cochrane review[168] assessed the efficacy of B_6–Mg treatment of individuals with autism spectrum disorder for the following outcomes: social interaction, communication, and stereotypical behavioral performance. A total of 19 studies were identified; however, only 3 were considered to meet the standards of a high-quality research design in order to be included in the review. Serious methodological limitations included small sample sizes, nonrandomization, wide range of ages/symptoms/diagnoses among participants, and the short duration of the therapies. Two of these well-designed studies[169,170] demonstrated no significant difference by treatment condition (ie, B_6–magnesium or placebo) on any of the behaviors examined, although some nonsignificant differences between treated and placebo were noted (eg, compulsive behavior, teacher rating of hyperactivity). These favored the B_6–magnesium–treated group. One study found a significant effect of treatment on verbal IQ in favor of the B_6–magnesium-group.[168] The conclusions of the review however were that there was insufficient evidence to demonstrate efficacy of B_6–magnesium treatment.[168]

In a review of three well-controlled studies examining the effect of megavitamin supplementation on behavior in children with attention deficit hyperactivity disorder (ADHD), two showed no effect while one reported adverse effects of supplementation.[171] All of these studies employed a between-subjects analysis; that is, the response of the control group (those ADHD children on the placebo) was compared to that of the treatment group (those ADHD children given megavitamins), which the authors noted may not be sufficiently sensitive to detect effects of the supplement.[171] A fourth study assessed the impact of a megavitamin supplement (250 mg niacinamide, 250 mg ascorbic acid, 50 mg pyridoxine, 100 mg calcium pantothenate) on 12 children with ADHD, using a crossover design so that children would be exposed to both the vitamin and the placebo.[172] Unfortunately, because of parental refusals and one dropout, only seven subjects were included in the final analysis. Despite the small sample size, several significant effects emerged; however, the direction of effects was not consistent. Teachers' reports of conduct problems and parental reports of hyperactivity and learning problems significantly declined while subjects were on the placebo. At the same time, teachers' reports of both inattentive and passive behavior and mothers' reports of psychosomatic complaints significantly decreased during the megavitamin treatment. Furthermore, there were some reported side effects of the megavitamin preparation, such as nausea and vomiting. These inconsistent findings are particularly important since the sample consisted solely of children who had responded to an open trial of megavitamin therapy, which should have maximized the probability of finding effects.

In summary, it does not appear that megavitamin supplementation has a consistent positive impact on the behavior of autistic or hyperactive children. Although some studies have associated B_6–magnesium supplementation with improvements in behavior of autistic children, design limitations have constrained the ability to interpret these findings as being caused by the treatment. Well-controlled studies with larger sample sizes are urgently needed in order to adequately assess the effectiveness of B_6–magnesium supplementation as an intervention for autism before any recommendations can be made.[168] In addition, the available evidence does not support the contention that megavitamin supplementation of children with attention deficit disorder or hyperactivity improves behavior. Furthermore, the documentation of adverse side effects of such megavitamin preparations[172] points to prudence in the scope of clinical use of such regimens.

SUCROSE

There is a widely held belief by parents and teachers alike that sugar *causes* hyperactivity even in children who do not have ADHD. However, most of the purported evidence to support such an association is purely correlational. ADHD experts in fact characterize this belief as a myth.[173] This is based on the fact that most studies have reported no effect of sucrose on behavior[174,175] and others have reported effects in the opposite direction as those hypothesized, that is, a decrease in activity and an increase in drowsiness in children after sugar ingestion.[174–177]

One of the underlying assumptions of such research is that children with specific behavior problems such as attention deficit disorders (ADDs) and hyperactivity may be particularly sensitive to the effects of sugar. Despite this assumption, many studies have examined samples comprised primarily normally active (without attention deficit disorder or hyperactivity) children, while others have focused specifically on samples composed primarily of children diagnosed with ADD, with or without hyperactivity.

In six double-blind sucrose-challenge studies in normal children, two found no effects of sucrose on behavior,[175,178] two showed what might be considered positive effects,[174,177] and two others showed negative effects.[175,179]

Among the studies reporting adverse effects of sugar consumption, weaknesses in design may account for such findings. For example, in one study, after the high-sucrose challenge, girls (but not boys) made a greater number of errors on the paired associates task than when on the low-sucrose challenge; there were no differences between high sucrose and aspartate.[179] In addition, a global rating of children's behavior indicated that teachers perceived significantly greater activity in the high-sucrose versus low-sucrose challenge. There were no effects of the high-sucrose challenge on other cognitive measures, fidgeting, or the Abbreviated Conner's Teacher's Rating Scale (used to diagnose hyperactivity), of particular concern is that the significant differences were between high sucrose and low sucrose rather than the aspartate control, suggesting some mechanism other than sugar content (eg, perceived sweetness) as mediating the behavioral changes observed.

Studies that have examined the effects of sucrose on children diagnosed with ADD with or without hyperactivity have shown very little support[175,180,181] of a causal association. In a study of 7- to 10-year-old hyperactive boys, there was no effect of a sucrose challenge on performance on a sustained attention test (CPT), paired associate learning, matching familiar figures, fine or gross motor movements, or the draw-a-line slowly or draw-a-line fast tests.[175] Another study using hyperactive boys attending a day treatment program for hyperactive children[175] reported no differences in behaviors during recreational periods, academic performance, or teacher ratings based on sucrose challenge. In still another study that also used tests of attention among children with ADD, an oral 5-hour glucose-tolerance test found no effect of glucose on the CPT, although interestingly the catecholamine response to the glucose was significantly lower in those with ADD than in the control group.[180] Finally, the results of a thorough meta-analysis concludes that the available evidence does not support a relationship between sugar consumption and behavior or cognitive performance of children.[175] This conclusion is strengthened by the fact that only designs that met criteria of scientific rigor were included.

Despite all the research to the contrary, there has been an obvious resistance of parents and teachers to fully accept such a conclusion. Some of this may stem from expectancy and common association (ie, high sugar consumption corresponding to events which may in and of themselves cause excitement in children). The results of one study illustrated the effect of parental expectancy on behavioral ratings.[182] Boys who were 5 to 7 years of age and who were reported to be sugar sensitive took part in a challenge study. Although all children got a placebo (aspartame), half the mothers were told that their children were given a large dose of sugar and the other half were told that their children were given placebo. Mothers who were told that their sons received sugar rated their children as significantly more hyperactive than those who were told that their children were given a placebo. Videotapes failed to corroborate their perceptions.[182]

In summary, research from well-controlled studies, including multiple outcomes and comparisons, does not support a causal association between sucrose ingestion and children's behavior. These results are true for children diagnosed with ADD and/or hyperactivity and normally active children. Positive effects of elimination diets in treating ADD children may be due to the concurrent elimination of other substances such as caffeine or allergens and not the elimination of sucrose.[173,183] In addition, parental or teacher expectancy likely plays a role in reports of sugar sensitivity and in the perceived success of elimination diets. Whether a highly specific subgroup of children is sensitive to sucrose is still not supported by the bulk of the available research; however, this possibility cannot be definitely eliminated based on current research.

FOOD ADDITIVES

In addition to sugar, food additives have frequently been implicated as causes of children's behavioral problems, and specifically hyperactivity. While data from correlational studies and open trials, where normal diets are replaced with additive-free diets (the Feingold diet), have provided support for such an association, the evidence of a causal link is limited.[171] One of the major difficulties of such research is that neither the child nor the family is blinded to treatments involving changes in a child's diet. Furthermore, many other factors may also change with dietary manipulations, making it impossible to directly link food additives to behavioral change.

Two other types of studies offer a better test of the association between food additives and behavior: dietary studies and challenge studies. Dietary studies include two randomly assigned diets (one without additives and a placebo); in challenge studies, the subject is provided either a food with additives or an additive capsule after being on a nonadditive diet for a specified period of time. Of 11 studies using these two techniques in children diagnosed with hyperactivity to test for the effect of a single or a class of substances (ie, artificial colors), only three found an effect of the challenge on the child's behavior.[184] In those studies, two showed effects on teachers' ratings of child behavior.[184]

More recently, studies have employed a standardized technique of "double-blind placebo-controlled food challenge" (DBPCFC) to diagnose adverse food reactions.[185] This procedure includes an elimination diet and a subsequent reintroduction of the suspected food (or additive) and may also include allergy skin testing. Although a well-controlled design, this technique does not always allow the investigator to identify any one item or specific substance, but rather to identify a food or a class of foods to which the individual may be sensitive.

Three studies using this technique provide limited support for either specific food sensitivities of some children with ADD[186,187] and/or sensitivity to food additives, although effects were often seen in only a subgroup of children.[184] In one study[184] differences in energy intake between diets may have affected the behavioral effects attributed to food additives.

In summary, the available evidence does not support the notion that food additives adversely affect the behavior of hyperactive children. What does seem to be true, however, is that a small subset of hyperactive children may be particularly sensitive or allergic to some foods and/or food additives, and these children may benefit from a modified diet.[173]

REFERENCES

1. Dietz WH, Trowbridge FL. Symposium on the identification and prevalence of undernutrition in the United States: Introduction. Bethesda, MD: American Institute of Nutrition; 1990. p. 917–8.
2. Gorman KS. Malnutrition and cognitive development: Evidence from experimental/quasi-experimental studies among the mild-to-moderately malnourished. J Nutr 1995;125:2239S–44S.
3. Levitsky D, Strupp, B. Malnutrition and the brain: Changing concepts, changing concerns. J Nutr 1995;125:2212S–21S.
4. Roa R, Georgieff MK. Early nutrition and brain development. In: Nelson CA, editor. The Effects of Early Adversity on Neurobehavioral Development: The Minnesota Symposia on Child Psychology, Volume 31. Mahwah, NJ: Lawrence Erlbaum Associates; 2000. p. 1–30.
5. Strupp B, Levitsky D. Developmental psychobiology: Theoretical premises that help in the understanding of the effect of malnutrition on development. J Nutr 1995;125:2221S–32S.
6. UNICEF. Progress for children: A report card on nutrition. 2006;108:44–53. Available at: http://www.childinfo.org/areas/malnutrition/index.php. Accessed December 21, 2006.
7. US Department of Health and Human Services. Pediatric Nutrition Surveillance, 2004 Report, Atlanta, GA: Center for Disease Control and Prevention; 2006.
8. Grantham-McGregor S. A review of existing studies of the effect of severe malnutrition on mental development. J Nutr 1995;125:2223S–8S.
9. Husaini MA, Karyadi L, Husaini YK, et al. Developmental effects of short-term supplementary feeding in nutritionally-at-risk Indonesian infants. Am J Clin Nutr 1991;54:799–804.
10. Pollitt E, Watkins WE, Husaini MA. Three-month nutritional supplementation in Indonesian infants and toddlers benefits memory function 8 y later. Am J Clin Nutr 1997;66:1357–63.
11. Grantham-McGregor SM, Powell CM, Walker SP, Himes JH. Nutritional supplementation, psychosocial stimulation, and mental development of stunted children: The Jamaican study. Lancet 1991;338:1–5.
12. Grantham-McGregor SM, Walker SP, Chang SM, Powell CA. Effects of early childhood supplementation with and without stimulation on later development in stunted Jamaican children. Am J Clin Nutr 1997;66:247–53.
13. Walker SP, Grantham-McGregor SM, Powell CA, et al. Effects of growth restriction in early childhood on growth, IQ, and cognition at age 11 to 12 years and the benefits of nutritional supplementation and psychosocial stimulation. J Pediatr 2000;137:36–41.
14. Pollitt E, Gorman KS, Engle PL, et al. Early supplementary feeding and cognition. Monogr Soc Res Child Devel 1993;58:1–118.
15. Pollitt E, Golub M, Gorman K, et al. A reconceptualization of the effects of undernutrition on children's biological, psychosocial, and behavioral development. Soc Policy Rep 1996;X:1–21.
16. Wachs TD. Effects of mild to moderate malnutrition on human development: Correlational studies. Paper Prepared for the IDECG Task Force Meeting on the Effects of Protein-Energy Malnutrition on Cognitive Development. Davis, CA, December 6–10, 1993.
17. Walka H, Pollitt E. A preliminary test of a developmental model for the study of undernourished children in Indonesia. Eur J Clin Nutr 2000;54:S21–7.
18. Meeks Gardner JM, Grantham-McGregor SM, Chang SM, et al. Activity and behavioral development in stunted and nonstunted children and response to nutritional supplementation. Child Dev 1995;66:1785–97.
19. Pollitt E. A developmental view of the undernourished child: Background and purpose of the study in Pangalengan, Indonesia. Euro J Clin Nutr 2000;54:S2–10.
20. Pollitt E, Durnin JVGA, Husaini M, et al. Effects of an energy and micronutrient supplement on growth and development in undernourished children in Indonesia: Methods. Euro J Clin Nutr 2000;54:S16–20.
21. Jahari AB, Saco-Pollitt C, Husaini MA, et al. Effects of an energy and micronutrient supplement on motor development and motor activity in undernourished children in Indonesia. Eur J Clin Nutr 2000;54:S60–8.
22. Walka H, Triana N, Jahari AB, et al. Effects of an energy and micronutrient supplement on play behavior in undernourished children in Indonesia. Eur J Clin Nutr 2000;54:S91–106.
23. Pollitt E, Saco-Pollitt C, Jahari A, et al. Effects of an energy and micronutrient supplement on mental development and behavior under natural conditions in undernourished children in Indonesia. Eur J Clin Nutr 2000;54:S80–90.

24. Harahap H, Jahari AB, Husaini MA, et al. Effects of an energy and micronutrient supplement on iron deficiency anemia, physical activity and motor and mental development in undernourished children in Indonesia. Eur J Clin Nutr 2000;54:S114–9.
25. Pollitt E, Jahari A, Walka H. A developmental view of the effects of an energy and micronutrient supplement in undernourished children in Indonesia. Eur J Clin Nutr 2000;54:107–13.
26. Liu J, Raine A, Venables Pl, Mednick SA. Malnutrition at age 3 years and externalizing behavior problems at ages 8, 11, and 17 years. Am J Psychiatry 2004;161:2005–13.
27. Liu J, Raine A, Venables PH, et al. Malnutrition at age 3 years and low cognitive ability at age 11 years. Arch Pediatr Adolesc Med 2003;157:593–600.
28. Lucas A, Fewtrell MS, Davies PSW, et al. Breastfeeding and catch-up growth in infants born small for gestational age. Acta Paediatr 1997;86:564–9.
29. Rider E, Samuels R, Wilson K, Homer C. physical growth, infant nutrition, breastfeeding, and general nutrition. Curr Opin Pediatr 1996;8:293–7.
30. Jacobson SW. Assessment of long-chain polyunsaturated fatty acid nutritional supplementation on infant neurobehavioral development and visual acuity. Lipids 1999;34:151–60.
31. Jacobson SW, Chiodo LM, Jacobson JL. Breastfeeding effects on intelligence quotient in 4 and 11 year-old children. Pediatrics 1999;103:71–82.
32. Rogan WJ, Gladen BC. Breast-feeding and cognitive development. Early Hum Dev 1993;31:181–93.
33. Greene LC, Lucas A, Barbara E, et al. Relationship between early diet and subsequent cognitive performance during adolescence. Biochem Soc Trans 1995;23:376S.
34. Horwood J, Fergusson DM. Breastfeeding and later cognitive and academic outcomes. Pediatrics 1998;101:9–20.
35. Mortensen EL, Michaelsen KF, Sanders SA, Reinisch JM. The association between duration of breastfeeding and adult intelligence. JAMA 2002;287:2365–71.
36. Morrow-Tlucak M, Haude RH, Ernhart CB. Breastfeeding and cognitive development in the first 2 years of life. Soc Sci Med 1988;26:635–63.
37. Taylor B, Wadsworth J. Breast feeding and child development at five years. Dev Med Child Neurol 1984;26:73–80.
38. Anderson JW, Johnstone BM, Remley DT. Breast-feeding and cognitive development: A meta-analysis. Am J Clin Nutr 1999;70;525–35.
39. Jain A, Concato J, Leventhal JM. How good is the evidence linking breastfeeding and intelligence? Pediatrics 2002;109;1044–53.
40. Rey J. Breastfeeding and cognitive development. Acta Paediatr Suppl 2003; 442:11–8.
41. Drane DL, Logemann, JA. A Critical evaluation of the evidence on the association between type of infant feeding and cognitive development. Paediatr Perinat Epidemiol 2000;14:349–56.
42. Lucas A, Morley R, Cole TJ, et al. Early diet in preterm babies and developmental status at 18 months. Lancet 1990;335:1477–81.
43. Lucas A, Morley R, Cole TJ, et al. Breast milk and subsequent intelligence quotient in children born preterm. Lancet 1992;339:261–4.
44. Lucas A, Morley R, Cole TJ. Randomised trial of early diet in preterm babies and later intelligence quotient. BMJ 1998;317:1481–7.
45. Lucas A, Morley R, Cole TJ, Gore SM. A randomized multicentre study of human milk versus formula and later development in preterm infants. Arch Dis Child 1994;70:141–6.
46. Crawford MA. The role of essential fatty acids in neural development: Implications for perinatal nutrition. J Clin Nutr 1993;57:703S–10S.
47. Lucas A. Does early diet program future outcome? Acta Paediatr Scand 1990;365:58–67.
48. Kretchmer N, Beard JL, Carlson S. The role of nutrition in the development of normal cognition. Am J Clin Nutr 1996;63:997S–1001S.
49. Uauy R, de Andraca I. Human milk and breast feeding for optimal mental development. J Nutr 1995;125:2278S–80S.
50. Heird WC. The role of polyunsaturated fatty acids in term and preterm infants and breastfeeding mothers. Pediatr Clin North Am 2001;48:173–88.
51. Food and Nutrition Board, Institute of Medicine of the National Academies Committee on Dietary Reference Intakes. Dietary fats, total fats and fatty acids. In: Dietary Reference Intakes for Energy, Carbohydrate, Fiber, Fat, Fatty Acids, Cholesterol, Protein and Amino Acids. Washington, DC: National Academies Press; 2002. p. 422–541.
52. Helland IB, Smith L, Saarem K, et al. Maternal supplementation with very-long-chain n-3 fatty acids during pregnancy and lactation augments children's IQ at 4 years of age. Pediatrics 2003;111:39–44.
53. Auestad N, Scott DT, Janowsky JS, et al. Visual, cognitive, and language assessments at 39 months: A follow-up study of children fed formulas containing long-chain polyunsaturated fatty acids to 1 year of age. Pediatrics 2003;112:177–83.
54. Clandinn MT, Van Aerde JE, Merkel KL, et al. Growth and development of preterm infants fed infant formulas containing docosahexaenoic acid and arachidonic acid. J Pediatr 2005;146:461–8.
55. Birch E, Garfield S, Hoffnab DR, et al. A randomized controlled trial of early dietary supply of long chain polyunsaturated fatty acids and mental development in term infants. Dev Med Child Neurol 2000;42:174–81.
56. Auestad N, Halter R, Hall R, et al. Growth and development in term infants fed long-chain polyunsaturated fatty acids: a double-masked randomized, parallel, prospective, multivariate study. Pediatrics 2001;108:372–81.
57. Tofail F, Kabir I, Hamadini JD, et al. Supplementation of fish-oil and soy-oil during pregnancy and psychomotor development of infants. J Health Popul Nutr 2006;24: 48–56.
58. Scott DT, Janowsky JS, Carroll RE, et al. Formula supplementation with long-chain polyunsaturated fatty acids: Are there developmental benefits? Pediatrics 1998;102:59–61.
59. Black M, Baqui AH, Zaman BK, et al. Iron and zinc supplementation promote motor development and exploratory behavior among Bangladeshi infants. Am J Clin Nutr 2004;80:903–10.
60. Black M. Micronutrient deficiencies and cognitive functioning. J Nutr 2003;133:3927S–3931.
61. Diaz JR, de las Cagigas A, Rodriguez R. Micronutrient deficiencies in developing and affluent countries. Euro J Clin Nutr 2003;57:S70–2.
62. Centers for Disease Control and Prevention. Iron deficiency-United States, 1999-2000. MMRW 2002;51:897–899.
63. Schneider JM, Fujii JL, Lamp CL, et al. Anemia, iron deficiency, and iron deficiency anemia in 12-36-mo-old children from low-income families. Am J Clin Nutr 2005;82: 1269–75.
64. Grantham-McGregor S, Ani C. A review of studies on the effect of iron deficiency on cognitive development in children. J Nutr 2001;131:649S–68S.
65. Hurtado EK, Claussen AH, Scott KG. Early childhood anemia and mild or moderate mental retardation. Am J Clin Nutr 1999;69:115–9.
66. Lozoff B, Jimenez E, Hagen J, et al. Poorer behavioral and developmental outcome more than 10 years after treatment for iron deficiency in infancy. J Pediatr 2000;105:1–11.
67. Halterman JS, Kaczorowski M, Aligne A, et al. Iron deficiency and cognitive achievement among school-aged children and adolescents in the United States. Pediatrics 2001;107:1381–6.
68. Sungthong R, Mo-suam, Chongsuvivatwong V. Effects of haemoglobin and serum ferritin on cognitive function in school children. Asia Pacific J Clin Nutr 2002;11:117–22.
69. Idjradinata P, Pollitt E. Reversal of developmental delays in iron-deficient anaemic infants treated with iron. Lancet 1993;341:1–4.
70. Akman M, Cebecci D, Okur V, et al. The effects of iron deficiency on infants' developmental test performance. Acta Paediatr 2004;93:1391–6.
71. Lozoff B, Beard J, Connor J, et al. Long-lasting neural and behavioral effects of iron deficiency in infancy. Nutr Rev 2006;64:S34–43.
72. Lind T, Lonnerdal B, Stenlund H, et al. A community-based randomized controlled trial of iron and zinc supplementation in Indonesian infants: Effects on growth and development. Am J Clin Nutr 2004;80:729–36.
73. Lozoff B, Brittenham GM, Wolf AW, et al. Iron deficiency anemia and iron therapy effects on infant developmental test performance. Pediatrics 1987;79:981–95.
74. Moffatt MEK, Longstaffe S, Besant J, Dureski C. Prevention of iron deficiency and psychomotor decline in high-risk infants through use of iron-fortified infant formula: A randomized clinical trial. J Pediatr 1994;125:527–34.
75. Morley R, Abbott R, Fairweather T, et al. Iron fortified follow on formula from 9 to 18 months improves iron status but not development on growth: A randomised trial. Arch Dis Child 1999;81:247–52.
76. Williams J, Wolff A, Daly A, MacDonald A, Aukett A, Booth IW. Iron supplemented formula milk related to reduction in psychomotor decline in infants from inner city areas: randomised study. BMJ 1999;318:693–7.
77. Lozoff B, De Andraca I, Castillo M, et al. Behavioral and developmental effects of preventing iron-deficiency anemia in healthy full term infants. Pediatrics 2003:112:846–54.
78. Friel JK, Aziz K, Andrews W, et al. A double-masked, randomized control trial of iron supplementation in early infancy in healthy term breast-fed infants. J Pediatr 2003;143:582–6.
79. Bruner AB, Joffe A, Duggan AK, et al. Randomised study of cognitive effects of iron supplementation in non-anaemic iron-deficient adolescent girls. Lancet 1996;348:992–6.
80. Pollitt E, Leibel RL, Greenfield DB. Iron deficiency and cognitive test performance in preschool children. Nutr Behav 1983;1:137–46.
81. Pollitt E, Saco-Pollitt C, Leibel RL, Viteri FE. Iron deficiency and behavioral development in infants and preschool children. Am J Clin Nutr 1986;43:555–65.
82. Seshadri S, Gopaldas T. Impact of iron supplementation on cognitive functions in preschool and school-aged children: The Indian experience. Am J Clin Nutr 1989;50:675–81.
83. Soewondo W, Husaini M, Pollitt E. Effects of iron deficiency on attention and learning processes in preschool children: Bangdung Indonesia. Am J Clin Nutr 1989;50:667–73.
84. Metallinos-Katsaras E, Valassi-Adam I, Dewey KG, et al. Effect of iron supplementation on cognition on Greek preschoolers. Eur J Clin Nutr 2004;58:1532–42.
85. Pollitt E, Hathirat P, Kotchabhakdi NJ, et al. Iron deficiency and educational achievement in Thailand. Am J Clin Nutr 1989;50:687–97.
86. Zhou SJ, Gibson RA, Crowther CA, et al. Effect of iron supplementation during pregnancy on the intelligence quotient and behavior of children at 4 y of age: Long-term follow up of a randomized controlled trial. Am J Clin Nutr 2006;83:1112–7.
87. Beard J. Iron deficiency alters brain development and functioning. J Nutr 2003;133:1468S–72S.
88. Golub MS, Gershwin ME, Hurley LS, et al. Studies of marginal zinc deprivation in rhesus monkeys: Infant behavior. Am J Clin Nutr 1985;42:1229–39.
89. Golub MS, Takeuchi PT, Keen CL, et al. Activity and attention in zinc-deprived adolescent monkeys. Am J Clin Nutr 1996;64:908–15.
90. Black MM. Zinc deficiency and child development. Am J Clin Nutr 1998;68:464S–9S.
91. Castillo-Duran C, Perales CG, Herrampf Marin VB, et al. Effect of zinc supplementation on development and growth of Chilean infants. J Pediatr 2001;138:229–35.
92. Sazawal S, Bentley M, Black RE, et al. Effect of zinc supplementation on observed activity in low socioeconomic Indian preschool children. J Pediatr 1996;98:1132–7.
93. Hamadini JD, Fuchs GJ, Osendarp SJM, et al. Randomized controlled trial of the effect of zinc supplementation on the mental development of Bangladeshi infants. Am J Clin Nutr 2001;74:381–6.
94. Pollitt E, Jahari A, Husaini M, et al. Developmental trajectories of poorly nourished toddlers that received a micronutrient supplement with and without energy. J Nutr 2002;132:2617–25.
95. Penland JG, Sandstead HH, Alcock NW, et al. A preliminary report: Effects of zinc and micronutrient repletion on growth and neuropsychological function of urban Chinese children. J Am Coll Nutr 1997;16:268–72.
96. Penland JG. Behavioral data and methodology issues in studies of zinc nutrition in humans. J Nutr 2000;130:361S–4S.
97. Gibson RS, Smit Vanderkooy PD, MacDonald AC, et al. A growth-limiting, mild zinc-deficiency syndrome in some southern Ontario boys with low height percentiles. Am J Clin Nutr 1989;49:1266–73.
98. Hamadini JD, Fuchs GJ, Osendarp SJM, et al. Zinc supplementation during pregnancy and effects on mental development and behaviour of infants: A follow-up study. Lancet 2002;360:290–4.
99. Tamura T, Goldenberg R, Ramey SL, et al. Effect of zinc supplementation of pregnant women on the mental and psychomotor development of their children at 5 yr of age. Am J Clin Nutr 2003;77:1512–6.
100. Bleichrodt N, Garcia I, Rubio C, et al. Developmental disorders associated with severe iodine deficiency. In Hetzel BS, Dunn JT, Stanbury JB, editors. The Prevention and Control of Iodine Deficiency Disorders. Amsterdam: Elsevier Science Publishers; 1987. p. 65–84.
101. Boyages SC, Collins JK, Maberly GF, et al. Iodine deficiency impairs intellectual and neuromotor development in apparently normal persons: A study of rural inhabitants of north-central China. Med J Aust 1989;150:676–82.
102. Cao XY, Jiang XM, Dou ZH, et al. Timing of vulnerability of the brain to iodine deficiency in endemic cretinism. N Engl J Med 1994;331:1793–44.
103. Fierro-Benitez R. Long-term effects of correction of iodine deficiency on psychomotor and intellectual development. In: Dunn JT, Pretell EA, Daza CH, Viteri FE, editors. Towards the Eradication of Endemic Goiter, Cretinism, and Iodine Deficiency. Washington, DC: Pan American Health Organization (PAHO); 1986. p.182–200. PAHO Publication No.: 502.
104. Pharoah P, Connolly K, Ekins RP, Harding AG. Maternal thyroid hormone levels in pregnancy and the subsequent cognitive and motor performance of children. Clin Endocrinol 1984;21:265–70.

105. Choudhury N, Gorman, K. Subclinical prenatal iodine deficiency negatively affects infant development in Northern China. J. Nutr 2003;133:3162–5.
106. Haddow JE, Palomaki GE, Allan WC, et al. Maternal thyroid deficiency during pregnancy and subsequent neuropsychological development of the child. N Engl J Med 1999;341:549–55.
107. Gorman K, Choudhury N, Hongzhuan T, Watkins W. The effects of maternal iodine supplementation on indices of infant cognitive and behavioral development: Results of a clinical trial in Hunan Providence, PRC; in press.
108. Bautista A, Barker PA, Dunn JT, et al. The effects of oral iodized oil on intelligence, thyroid status, and somatic growth in school-aged children from an area of endemic goiter. Am J Clin Nutr 1982;35:127–34.
109. Shrestha RM. Effect of iodine and iron supplementation on physical, psychomotor and mental development in primary school children in Malawi. Doctoral dissertation. Wageningen Agricultural University: Wageningen, Netherlands; 1994.
110. Huda SN, Grantham-McGregor SM, Tomkins A. Cognitive and motor functions of iodine-deficient but euthyroid children in Bangladesh do not benefit from iodized poppy seed oil (Lipidol). J Nutr 2001;131:72–77.
111. Zimmerman MB, Connolly K, Bozo M, et al. Iodine supplementation improves cognition in iodine-deficient schoolchildren in Albania: A randomized, controlled, double-blind study. Am J Clin Nutr 2006;83:108–14.
112. McCullough AL, Kirksey A, Wachs TD, et al. Vitamin B_6 status of Egyptian mothers: Relation to infant behavior and maternal-infant interactions. Am J Clin Nutr 1990;51:1067–74.
113. US Department of Health & Human Services. The 2006 HHS Poverty Guidelines. Available at: http://aspe.hhs.gov/poverty/06poverty.shtml. Accessed December 21, 2006.
114. Nord M, Andrews M, Carlson S. Household Food Security in the United States, 2005. Washington, DC: Economic Research Service, US Department of Agriculture; 2006.
115. US Department of Agriculture. Food Security Measurements: Concepts and Definitions. Economic Food Security Briefing Room. Available at: http://www.ers.usda.gov/briefing/FoodSecurity. Accessed December 21, 2006.
116. Center on Hunger & Poverty. The Consequences of Hunger and Food Insecurity for Children: Evidence from Recent Scientific Studies. MA: Heller School for Social Policy and Management, Brandeis University; 2002.
117. Jyoti DF, Frongillo EA, Jones SJ. Food insecurity affects school children's academic performance, weight gain, and social skills. J Nutr 2005;135:2831–9.
118. Sullivan A, Choi E. Hunger and Food Insecurity in the 50 States: 1998–2000. Food Security Institute, Center on Hunger and Poverty, Brandeis University; 2002.
119. Casey PH, Szeto K, Lensing S, et al. Children in food-insufficient, low-income families: Prevalence, health, and nutrition status. Arch Pediatr Adolesc Med 2001;155:508–17.
120. Murphy MJ, Wehler CA, Pagano ME, et al. Relationship between hunger and psychosocial functioning in low-income American children. J Am Acad Child Adolesc Psychiatry 1998;37:163–70.
121. Alaimo K, Olson C, Frongillo E. Food insufficiency and American school aged children's cognitive, academic and psychosocial development. Pediatrics 2001;108:44–53.
122. Pollitt E. Does breakfast make a difference in school? J Am Diet Assoc 1995;95:1134–9.
123. Bronfenbrenner U, McClelland P, Wethington E, et al. The State of Americans: This Generation and the Next. New York, NY: The Free press; 1996.
124. Kim M, Ohls J, Cohen R. Hunger in America 2001: Local Report Prepared for Rhode Island Community Food Bank, Final Report. Mathematica Policy Research, Inc, Princeton, NJ: 2001.
125. Nicklas TA, Bao W, Webber LS, Berenson GS. Breakfast consumption affects adequacy of total daily intake in children. J Am Diet Assoc 1993;93:886–91.
126. Kennedy E, Davis C. US Department of Agriculture School Breakfast Program. Am J Clin Nutr 1998;67:798S–803S.
127. Sampson AE, Sujata D, Meyers AF, Houser R. The nutritional impact of breakfast consumption on the diets of inner-city African-American elementary school children. J Natl Med Assoc 1995;87:195–202.
128. Rampersaud GC, Pereira MA, Girard BL, et al. Breakfast habits, nutritional status, body weight, and academic performance in children and adolescents. J Am Diet Assoc 2005;105:743–60.
129. Pollitt E, Leibel RL, Greenfield D. Brief fasting, stress, and cognition in children. Am J Clin Nutr 1981;34:1526–33.
130. Pollitt E, Lewis NL, Garza C, Shulman RJ. Fasting and cognitive function. J Psychiatr Res 1982;83:169–74.
131. Cueto S, Jacoby E, Pollitt E. Breakfast prevents delay of attention and memory functions among nutritionally at-risk boys. J Appl Dev Psychol 1998;19:219–33.
132. Pollitt E, Jacoby ER, Cueto S. School breakfast and cognition among nutritionally at-risk children in the Peruvian Andes. Nutr Rev 1996;54:S22–6.
133. Simeon DT, Grantham-McGregor S. Effects of missing breakfast on the cognitive functions of school children of differing nutritional status. Am J Clin Nutr 1989;49:646–53.
134. Chandler AK, Walker SP, Connolly K, Grantham-McGregor S. School breakfast improves verbal fluency in undernourished Jamaican children. J Nutr 1995;125:894–900.
135. Cromer BA, Tarnowski KJ, Stein AM, et al. The School Breakfast program and cognition in adolescents. Dev Behav Pediatr 1990;11:295–300.
136. Benton D, Parker PY. Breakfast, blood glucose, and cognition. Am J Clin Nutr 1998;67:772S–8S.
137. Conners CK, Blouin AG. Nutritional effects on behavior of children. J Psychiatr Res 1982;83:17:193–201.
138. Lopez I, de Andraca I, Perales CG, et al. Breakfast omission and cognitive performance of normal, wasted and stunted schoolchildren. Eur J Clin Nutr 1993;47:533–42.
139. Donohoe RT, Benton D. Glucose tolerance predicts performance on test of memory and cognition. Physiol Behav 2000;71:394–401.
140. Benton D. The impact of the supply of glucose to the brain on mood and memory. Nutr Rev 2001;59:S20–1.
141. Nabb S, Benton D. The influence on cognition of the interaction between the macro-nutrient content of breakfast and glucose tolerance. Physiol Behav 2006;87:16–23.
142. Benton D, Owens DS, Parker PY. Blood glucose influences memory and attention in young adults. Neuropsychologia 1994;32:595–607.
143. Owens DS, Benton D. The impact of raising blood glucose on reaction times. Neuropsychobiology 1994;30:106–13.
144. Donohoe RT, Benton D. Cognitive functioning is susceptible to the level of blood glucose. Psychopharmacology 1999;145:378–85.
145. White JW, Wolraich M. Effect of sugar on behavior and mental performance. Am J Clin Nutr 1995;621:242S–9S.
146. Meyers AF, Sampson AE, Weitzman M, et al. School Breakfast program and school performance. Am J Dis Child 1989;143:1234–9.
147. Murphy MJ, Pagano ME, Nachmani J, et al. The relationship of school breakfast to psychosocial and academic functioning. Arch Pediatr Adolesc Med 1998;152:899–907.
148. Kleinman RE, Hall S, Green H, et al. Diet, breakfast, and academic performance in children. Ann Nutr Metab 2002;46:24–30.
149. Richter LM, Rose C, Griesel RD. Cognitive and behavioural effects of a school breakfast. S Afr Med J 1997;87:93–100.
150. Vera Noriega JA, Ibanez SED, Ramos MOP, et al. Evaluacion de los efectos de un programa de desayunos escolares en atencion y memoria. Arch Lat Am Nut 2000;50:35–41.
151. Grantham-McGregor S. Can the provision of breakfast benefit school performance? Food Nutr Bull 2005;26:S144–S158.
152. Benton D. Micro-nutrient supplementation and the intelligence of children. Neurosci Biobehav Rev 2002;25:297–309.
153. Benton D, Fordy J, Haller J. The impact of long-tern vitamin supplementation on cognitive functioning. Psychopharmacology 1995;117:298–305.
154. Benton D, Griffiths R, Haller J. Thiamine supplementation mood and cognitive functioning. Psychopharmacology 1997;129:66–71.
155. Nelson M. Vitamin and mineral supplementation and academic performance in schoolchildren. Proc Nutr Soc 1992;51:303–13.
156. Schoenthaler SJ, Amos SP, Eysenck HJ, et al. Controlled trial of vitamin-mineral supplementation: Effects on intelligence and performance. Person Indiv Diff 1990;12:351–2.
157. Schoenthaler SJ, Bier ID, Young K et al. The effect of vitamin-mineral supplementation on the intelligence of American schoolchildren: A randomized, double-blind placebo-controlled trial. J Altern Complement Med 2000;6:19–29.
158. Nelson M, Naismith D, Burley V, et al. Nutrient intakes, vitamin and mineral supplementation in British schoolchildren. Br J Nutr 1990;64:13–22.
159. Schoenthaler SJ, Bier ID. Vitamin-mineral intake and intelligence: A macrolevel analysis of randomized controlled trials. J Altern Complement Med 1999;5:125–34.
160. Fairchild MW, Hass JD, Habicht J-P. Iron deficiency and behavior: Criteria for testing causality. Am J Clin Nutr 1989;50:566–74.
161. Willett W. Biochemical indicators of dietary intake. In: Hunter D, editor. Nutritional Epidemiology. New York: Oxford University Press; 1998. p .174–243.
162. Peritz E. The Turlock vitamin-mineral supplementation trial: A statistical re-analysis. J Biosoc Sci 1994;26:155–64.
163. Blinkhorn S. A dose of vitamins and a pinch of salt. Nature 1991;350:13.
164. Pagliari CH. Effects of nutritional supplements on intelligence: Comment on paper by Schoenthaler et al. Person Indiv Diff 1991;14:491.
165. Food and Nutrition Board, Institute of Medicine of the National Academies Committee on Dietary Reference Intakes. Dietary Reference Intakes for Vitamin A, Vitamin K, Arsenic, Boron, Chromium, Copper, Iodine, Iron, Manganese, Molybdenum, Nickel, Silicon, Vanadium, and Zinc. Washington, DC: National Academies Press; 2001.
166. Clinical Nutrition Updates. Nutrition and autism, issue 241. Available at www.arborcom.com.
167. Adams JB, George F, Audhya T. Abnormally high plasma levels of vitamin B6 in children with autism not taking supplements compared to controls not taking supplements. J Alter Comp Med 2006;12:59–63.
168. Nye C, Brice A. Combined vitamin B6-magnesium treatment in autism spectrum disorder (review). Cochrane Collab 2006;2:1–15.
169. Findling RL, Maxwell K, Scotese-Wojtila L, et al. High-dose pyridoxine and magnesium administration in children with autistic disorder: An absence of salutary effects in a double-blind, placebo-controlled study. J Autism Dev Disord 1997;27:467–79.
170. Tolbert L, Haigler T, Waits MM, Dennis T. Brief report: Lack of response in an autistic population to a low dose clinical trial of pyridoxine plus magnesium. J Autism Dev Disord 1993;23:193–9.
171. Levitsky D, Strupp B. Nutrition and the behavior of children. In Walker WA, Watkins JB, editors. Nutrition in Pediatrics: Basic Science and Clinical Applications, 1st edition. Boston: Little, Brown; 1985. p. 357–72.
172. Haslam RHA. Is there a role for megavitamin therapy in the treatment of attention deficit hyperactivity disorder? Adv Neurol 1992;58:303–10.
173. Weyandt LL. An ADHD Primer, 2nd edition. Mahwah, NJ: Lawrence Erlbaum Association; 2006.
174. Wolraich ML, Lindgren SD, Stumbo PJ, et al. Effects of diets high in sucrose or aspartame on the behavior and cognitive performance of children. N Engl J Med 1994;330:301–7.
175. Wolraich ML, Wilson DB, White JW. The effect of sugar on behavior or cognition in children. JAMA 1995;274: 1617–21.
176. Rapoport JL. Diet and hyperactivity. Nutr Rev 1986;44: 158–62.
177. Saravis S, Schachar R, Zlotkin S, et al. Aspartame: Effects of learning, behavior, and mood. Pediatrics 1990;86:75–83.
178. Kruesi MJP, Rapoport JL, Cummings EM, et al. Effects of sugar and aspartame on aggression and activity in children. Am J Psychiatry 1987;144:1487–90.
179. Rosen LA, Bender ME, Sorrel S, et al. Effects of sugar (sucrose) on children's behavior. J Consult Clin Psychol 1988;56:583–9.
180. Girardi NL, Shaywitz SE, Shaywitz BA, et al. Blunted catecholamine responses after glucose ingestion in children with attention deficit disorder. Pediat Res 1995;38:539–42.
181. Wender EH, Solanto MV. Effects of sugar on aggressive and inattentive behavior in children with attention deficit disorder with hyperactivity and normal children. Pediatrics 1991;88:960–66.
182. Hoover DW, Milich R. Effects of sugar ingestion expectancies on mother-child interactions. J Abnorm Child Psychol 1994;22:501–15.
183. Kanerak R. Does sucrose or aspartame cause hyperactivity in children? Nutr Rev 1994;52:173–5.
184. Boris M, Mandel FS. Foods and additivies are common causes of the attention deficit hyperactive disorder in children. Ann Allergy 1993;72:462–8.
185. Bock SA, Sampson HA, Atkins FM, et al. Double-blind, placebo-controlled food challenge (DBPCFC) as an office procedure: A manual. J Allergy Clin Immunol 1988;82:986–97.
186. Carter CM, Urbanowicz M, Hemsley R, et al. Effects of a few food diets in attention deficit disorder. Arch Dis Child 1993;69:564–8.
187. Kaplan BJ, McNicol J, Conte RA, Moghadam HK. Dietary replacement in preschool-aged hyperactive boys. Pediatrics 1989;83:7–17.

III PERINATAL NUTRITION

26

Maternal Nutrition and Pregnancy Outcome

Theresa O. Scholl, PhD, MPH

Adverse pregnancy outcomes such as preterm delivery, intrauterine growth restriction, and low birth weight are increased two- to threefold among infants born to poor urban women from countries like the United States.[1] Other factors affecting outcome include inadequate gestational weight gain, inadequate prenatal care, smoking, drinking alcohol, and substance abuse.[2,3] A history of spontaneous abortion or other poor outcome in a prior pregnancy plays a role by increasing risk in the current pregnancy.[3] Poor maternal intake of micronutrients, iron, folic acid, calcium, and zinc in particular is also associated with an increased risk of adverse events in the course and outcome of pregnancy.[2] However, apart from rare occurrences, inadequate intake of a single nutrient does not occur in isolation. Unlike in animal studies that involve experimentally induced deficiencies of single nutrients, the link between maternal nutritional status and the course and outcome in human pregnancy is less secure. Apart from its immediate effects, maternal nutrition during pregnancy also has important implications for risk of chronic disease development in later life (see Chapter 25 "Nutrition and the Behaviour of Children").

IRON AND ANEMIA

Iron is essential for the formation of hemoglobin, which transports oxygen, and for the synthesis of enzymes that use oxygen to provide cellular energy. Iron deficiency is defined by three stages of increasing severity: depletion of iron stores (Stage 1), impaired hemoglobin production (Stage 2), and iron-deficiency anemia (IDA) (Stage 3). Anemia is an abnormally low concentration of hemoglobin (or hematocrit). Specific cut points have been formulated for its diagnosis by age and sex and by trimester during pregnancy.[2]

Supplementation with iron is recommended during pregnancy to meet the demands of both the mother and the rapidly growing fetus. Table 1 shows the intakes that are currently recommended by the Institute of Medicine for iron and other nutrients during pregnancy (online at http://www.nap.edu). Anemia (low hemoglobin levels) and IDA sometimes also serve as indicators of overall maternal nutritional status during pregnancy. When overall dietary intake is inadequate, risk of anemia is increased.[4–6]

Maternal anemia and hemoglobin (or hematocrit) concentration are linked with an increased risk of poor pregnancy outcome. Evidence suggests that anemia and iron deficiencies are associated with an increased risk of low-infant-birth weight, preterm delivery, and perinatal mortality.[8–13] The relationship between maternal hemoglobin and pregnancy outcome is U shaped, with "low" hemoglobin probably reflecting a mix of true and physiologic anemia and "high" hemoglobin reflecting hypovolemia—failure of the plasma volume to expand in association with maternal pathology—maternal hypertension, preeclampsia, or diabetes.[9,14] Poorly nourished animals have reduced plasma volume expansion during pregnancy, low cardiac output, lower uteroplacental blood flow, and reduced nutrient transmission to the fetus.[15] Thus, it is possible that hypovolemia has nutritional antecedents.

The increase in anemia during pregnancy is partly an artifact of maternal plasma volume expansion, a normal physiologic response to pregnancy.[16] Although the maternal red blood cell (RBC) mass also increases during gestation, its expansion and the expansion of the plasma volume occur at different times.[2,8] Consequently because the timing of delivery can vary, maternal anemia at delivery is subject to a time-of-sampling artifact that can distort the relation of anemia to pregnancy outcome.[8,13]

During the first and second trimesters, hemoglobin concentration declines, reaches a low point early in the third trimester, and rises thereafter. Depending on the stage of gestation when anemia is assessed, it can be difficult to separate truly anemic women from those whose anemia results from hemodilution. The best time to

Table 1 Dietary Reference Intakes or Adequate Intake and Upper Limit of Intake During Pregnancy

	Dietary Reference or Adequate Intake	Tolerable Upper Limit of Intake
Minerals		
Iron	27 mg[*]	45 mg
Zinc	12 mg,[†] 11 mg[‡]	34 mg,[†] 40 mg[‡]
Calcium	1,000 mg	2,500 mg
Phosphorus	700 mg	3,500 mg
Magnesium	400 mg,[†] 350 mg,[‡] 360 mg[§]	350 mg[‖]
Iodine	220 μg	900 μg,[†] 1,100 μg[‡]
Selenium	60 μg	400 μg
Copper	1.0 mg	10.0 g
Manganese	2.0 mg	9.0 mg,[†] 11.0 mg[‡]
Chromium	29 μg,[‡] 30 μg[‡]	Not set
Molybdenum	50 μg	1,700 μg,[†] 2,000 μg[‡]
Vitamins		
Folate	600 μg[#]	800 μg,[†,**] 1,000 μg[‡,**]
Thiamin	1.4 mg	Not set
Riboflavin	1.4 mg	Not set
Niacin	18 mg	30 mg,[†] 35 mg[‡]
Vitamin B_6	1.9 mg	80 mg,[†] 100 mg[‡]
Vitamin B_{12}	2.6 μg	Not set
Biotin	30 μg	Not set
Pantothenic acid	6 mg	Not set
Choline	450 mg	3,000 mg,[†] 3,500 mg[‡]
Vitamin A	750 μg,[†] 770 μg[‡]	2,800 μg,[†] 3,000 μg[‡]
Vitamin C	80 μg,[†] 85 mg[‡]	1,800 mg,[†] 2,000 mg[‡]
Vitamin D	5 μg	50 μg
Vitamin E	15 mg	800 mg,[†] 1,000 mg[‡]
Vitamin K	75 μg,[†] 90 μg[‡]	Not set

Adapted from reference 7.
[*]Often requires iron supplements.
[†]Pregnant women 14 to 18 years.
[‡]Pregnant women 19 to 30, 31 to 50 years.
[§]Pregnant women 31 to 50 years.
[‖]For magnesium supplements.
[#]Includes 400 μg synthetic folic acid.
[**]Synthetic folic acid.

detect risk associated with maternal anemia may be early in pregnancy before the plasma volume is fully expanded. This was originally examined in Camden separating anemia by time, that is, early (entry to prenatal car) and late (week 28) and etiology (IDA and other causes). Early in pregnancy there were clear differences in mean corpuscular volume (MCV) and diet in women with and without IDA that were absent or greatly diminished during the third trimester. IDA at entry was associated with greater than twofold increases in the risks of low-birth-weight and preterm delivery, while anemia from other causes was associated with a small but nonsignificant increase in risk. In the third trimester, risk of preterm delivery was reduced for women with IDA, and there was no increased risk for women with other anemias.[6,17] Consistent observations were made in women from Papua, New Guinea, where severe anemia (hemoglobin <80 g/L) that was attributable to iron deficiency and occurred early in pregnancy increased risk of low birth weight (sixfold) among primiparous women. [18] Risk was not increased with IDA at delivery.

The association of maternal anemia, based upon early pregnancy hemoglobin with preterm delivery and other poor outcomes, has been confirmed in studies from many countries in the developing world, including Nepal, Egypt, and China[19–21] and in the United States with data from Pregnancy Nutritional Surveillance conducted by the Centers for Disease Control.[22] The relationship now extends to the time before conception. Anemic Chinese textile workers who became pregnant had substantial higher (five- to sixfold) risks of infant low birth weight and fetal growth restriction and gave birth to infants with lower birth weights (−139 to −192 g). When anemia was attributable to iron deficiency, birth weight reduction was greater still amounting to a decrease of −242 g.[23] Thus, it seems reasonable to presume that some, but not all, maternal anemia is caused by the expansion of maternal plasma volume. At present, this state is poorly differentiated late in pregnancy but more readily distinguished before pregnancy or early in its course.

Maternal Anemia: Randomized Trials

Because most data on maternal anemia are observational, it is not certain that adverse outcomes could be prevented by supplementing pregnant women with iron. Observational data on anemia imply that supplementation should be started early in pregnancy, if not before, in order to prevent low-birth-weight and preterm delivery. If this is true, as an animal model suggests, then supplementation started after midpregnancy may be unlikely to reduce risk.[24]

A clinical trial was conducted in 275 nonanemic, iron-replete women enrolled at entry to care (<20 wk) and randomly assigned to supplemental iron (30 mg/d as ferrous sulphate) or placebo until week 28 gestation. [25] During the third trimester women who became iron deficient (low serum ferritin) were supplemented regardless of initial assignment. Prophylactic iron supplementation did not increase maternal iron status or reduce the frequency of anemia. However, after adjusting for pregravid weight and baseline serum ferritin concentration the proportion with absent iron stores and IDA at week 28 was significantly lower among the iron supplemented. Supplemented women had significantly longer gestations (+0.6 wk), higher infant birth weights (+206 g), and a reduced risk of low birth weight and preterm low birth weight. Risk of preterm delivery, reckoned solely from the mother's recall of her last menstrual period (LMP) was not altered.

Women residing in rural Nepal were randomly assigned by geographic sector of residence to one of five treatment arms early in pregnancy.[26] These included vitamin A (1,000 ug retinol equivalents), vitamin A plus folic acid (400 ug), and vitamin A plus folic acid plus iron (30 mg). The other arms added zinc (30 mg) or multiple micronutrients in addition to vitamin A. Gravidas receiving vitamin A and folate showed no reduction in the risk of low birth weight, whereas those receiving vitamin A with iron and folate had increased infant birth weight (+37 g) and a reduction of 14% in risk of low birth weight.

A trial of iron-replete women randomly assigned them to prenatal supplements with and without iron (ferrous sulfate 30 mg), also before 20 weeks' gestation, showed a positive effect. Infant birth weight was increased (+109 g), and risk of preterm delivery reduced by 85% (p = .05). Again, maternal measures of iron status were no different apart from the frequency of iron depletion (ferritin <20 ug/L) which was marginally lower (p = .08) among the iron supplemented.[27] A randomized trial done of nonanemic Australian women, starting before 20 weeks' gestation showed no improvement in birth weight or gestation for women assigned to supplemental iron (ferrous sulfate 20 mg). In contrast, maternal iron status improved with supplementation. In this instance fewer women assigned to iron had IDA (3% vs 11%) or iron deficiency (35% vs 58%).[28] It is unclear why the results of this trial differ from the two trials done in the US. The authors suggest that health outcomes associated with IDA are "more obvious" in populations with fewer healthy women or with a higher baseline risk of adverse outcomes. And it remains unclear why an iron supplement should have improved birth weight and gestation without also improving maternal anemia or iron deficiency.

Plausible biologic mechanisms underpinning the effect of iron status and supplementation in pregnancy include chronic hypoxia from anemia that initiates a stress response, with the release of placental corticotropin-releasing hormone (CRH) and an increase in fetal production of cortisol, increased oxidative stress among deficient women that damages the maternal-fetal unit, and reduced maternal immune function with increased risk of infection leading to preterm delivery and reduced fetal growth.[29] None of these have been explored in detail.

During pregnancy, low intakes of zinc and folate have been associated with IDA before or early in the course of pregnancy.[5,6] Recommendations for intake of these nutrients during pregnancy, along with information about the upper limit considered safe, are given in Table 1. Zinc is an element involved either directly as a metalloenzyme in the production of enzymes, which include DNA and ribonucleic acid polymerase, or as a catalyst in the synthesis of other enzymes.[2] Folic acid functions as a coenzyme in the transfer of single-carbon atoms from donors such as serine and histidine to intermediates in the synthesis of amino acids, purines, and thymidylic acid.[2] Although many other nutrients in addition to these two would be limited in a marginal maternal diet, inadequate intake of either zinc, folate, or both potentially leads to impaired cell division and alterations in protein synthesis. Such alterations are most notable and have the greatest potential to do harm during times of rapid tissue growth, such as pregnancy.

ZINC

Neggers and colleagues demonstrated a positive association between maternal serum zinc at 16 weeks' gestation and birth weight in a large population of low-income Alabama women.[30] Serum zinc in the lowest quartile was associated with an eightfold increase in risk of low birth weight, suggesting a threshold effect for circulating zinc levels during pregnancy. Kirksey and colleagues examined the relationship of maternal zinc nutriture to birth weight and found that plasma zinc concentrations in the second trimester, along with pregnancy weight at 3 months' gestation, formed the best predictor model of birth weight for these pregnancies, accounting for 39% of the variance.[31]

Scholl and colleagues examined dietary zinc intake in 818 Camden women and reported increased risks of complications and adverse pregnancy outcomes in association with low intakes of dietary zinc (6 mg/d or less).[5] These complications included decreased gestational weight gain and an increased risk of IDA at entry to care. Poor outcomes associated with low zinc intake included risk of low birth weight, preterm delivery, and very preterm delivery that were two to three times greater than in controls. In the presence of IDA, the risk of very preterm delivery was greater than fivefold higher. Others have also reported a positive relationship between low-serum zinc and reduced birth weight or an increased risk of low infant birth weight.[32–34] However, the finding of inverse relationships between maternal zinc levels and birth weight could also suggest greater fetal uptake of maternal zinc by larger infants.[35–37]

Tamura and colleagues used data from more than 3,400 gravidas to examine the relationship between pregnancy outcome and zinc in the first to early third trimesters.[38] They found no relationship between maternal plasma zinc and risk of fetal growth restriction, preterm delivery, or selected pregnancy complications and no significant correlation with birth weight or gestation duration.

However, women with plasma zinc below the median had been removed from the sample and enrolled in a clinical trial that demonstrated a positive effect of zinc on gestation duration and birth weight.[39] Thus, prescreening might have removed vulnerable women from the population at risk.

Because serum or plasma zinc represents less than 1% of the total body zinc pool, it might not be the most reliable indicator of zinc status. Meadows and colleagues were the first to demonstrate that both lower leukocyte zinc concentration in maternal serum and in cord blood were associated with impaired fetal growth.[40,41] No differences were noted between the mean leukocyte zinc concentrations of women delivering preterm appropriate for gestational age and normal-weight infants. Wells and colleagues also noted an association between maternal leukocyte zinc and lower birth weight.[42] Simmer and Thompson measured maternal concentrations of zinc in polymorphonuclear and mononuclear cells within 48 hours of delivery and found lower zinc levels associated with fetal growth retardation.[43] Adeniyi reported the opposite: Maternal leukocyte zinc and placental zinc concentrations were lower in preeclamptic women with normal-birth-weight infants compared with women delivering lower birth weight infants.[44]

Inconsistencies in the relationship of zinc and pregnancy outcome could arise from the fact that there is no agreed upon indicator of zinc status; maternal serum or plasma zinc might not reliably assess zinc nutritional status. Clinical trials of zinc supplementation have focused on entire groups of low-income women in which the mean zinc intake is low. These trials have also yielded equivocal results, perhaps because of an approach that selects a population, as opposed to individuals, at risk.

Two trials have shown effects that were conditional on maternal weight, that is, a lower rate of preterm delivery in zinc-supplemented women who were not overweight.[39,45] Cherry and colleagues reported a response to supplementation status for pregnant adolescents at less than 25 weeks' gestation.[45] Low-serum zinc concentrations were more common in underweight and multiparous women. The frequency of preterm delivery was less in the zinc-treated normal-weight women compared with the placebo group. Zinc treatment of underweight multiparous women was associated with a gestational age increase of nearly 3 weeks. Zinc supplementation was also associated with a reduced need for assisted respiration in newborns of normal-weight women.

The trial conducted by Goldenberg and colleagues took a more targeted approach and recruited women with plasma zinc levels below the median and randomly assigned them to zinc or placebo.[39] The analysis was stratified after the fact by body mass index (BMI) above or below 26 kg/m^2. Zinc supplementation was associated with longer gestation duration—by approximately half a week (p = .06)—and increased birth weight, mainly because of longer duration of gestation. Women with BMIs of less than 26 benefited most from zinc treatment, experiencing a 248 g increase in infant birth weight and a 0.7 cm increase in infant head circumference. Consistent with prior results, effects were increased for women with lower pregravid BMIs. In addition, Kynast and Saling found that zinc treatment between 20 and 34 weeks' gestation was associated with lower incidences of preterm labor, placental abruption, vaginal bleeding, fetal acidosis, and fetal growth retardation when zinc-supplemented gravidas were compared with control subjects.[46] Thus, there is some support for a positive effect of zinc on pregnancy outcome among poor women from the developed world and among women from countries where social factors are improving.[47]

In contrast, two recent trials from the developing world (Peru and Bangladesh), where one might suppose that zinc deficiency would be common, did not show this.[48,49] Nor did a clinical trial of HIV-infected pregnant women from Tanzania show increases in birth weight or gestation, or maternal CD4, CD8, or CD3 counts among the zinc supplemented.[50] The overall consensus from zinc supplementation trials in the developing world is that effects are rarely and not consistently observed.[51,52] However, preliminary data do suggest other reasons to supplement pregnant women with zinc to reduce risk of cleft/lip palate, improve neonatal immune status, and reduce infectious disease in the infant.[52]

Low-plasma zinc has a number of potential causes.[53] It is of interest that when Bangladeshi women were screened less than 4% had zinc levels at or below the median-plasma zinc used to enroll women from the United States in Goldenberg and colleagues' trial.[39,48] It is possible that maternal zinc status is affected by other factors—multiple nutritional deficiencies, interaction between the zinc supplement and other nutrients, the presence of maternal infections or gastrointestinal disorders—that reduce the bioavailability of zinc or otherwise limit fetal growth.[53,54] In theory, a low-plasma zinc might reflect a secondary zinc deficiency in response to a maternal stressor such as smoking, alcohol abuse, strenuous exercise, or a heavy work load. In the developing world, low-plasma zinc could result from reduced zinc absorption, due to high intakes of phytate, fiber, or calcium from a vegetarian diet.[54] Thus, despite evidence from zinc-deficient animals, there is no conclusive evidence that zinc supplementation improves the outcome of pregnancy in humans.

FOLIC ACID

Folate is critically important for development and is a cofactor for many essential cellular reactions, including the transfer of single-carbon units; it is required for cell division because of its role in DNA synthesis.[55,56] Folate is also a substrate for a variety of reactions that affect metabolism of several amino acids on the transmethylation and transsulfuration pathways. A central feature of fetal development is widespread and sustained cell division. Because of its role in nucleic acid synthesis, the need for folate increases during times of rapid tissue growth. During pregnancy, folate-dependent processes include increase in the RBC mass, enlargement of the uterus, and growth of the placenta and fetus.

It is recommended that pregnant women consume 600 μg folic acid per day, which includes 400 μg of synthetic folic acid from supplements or fortified cereals, to reduce risk of neural tube defects (see Table 1). Less than one-third of women in their reproductive years consume this amount.[57] Fortification of flour and cereal products in the United States with folic acid (since 1998) has been associated with a 19% decline in risk of live born infants with neural tube defects, along with changes in biomarkers of folate status, including increases in serum and RBC folate and a decline in homocysteine levels.[58,59]

Serum folate is a sensitive indicator of the folate available to replicating cells with high turnover rates, whereas RBC folate reflects folate status over preceding months. A metabolic effect of folate deficiency is an elevation of homocysteine.[60] Hyperhomocysteinemia can occur when dietary folate intake is low. In other cases, genetic factors and the interaction between genes and the environment increase the metabolic requirement for folate, increasing risk of spontaneous abortion and fetal growth restriction and decreasing gestation duration.[60]

More than three decades ago, Hibbard described an increased risk of placental abruption in gravidas with abnormal formiminoglutamic acid excretion and attributed it to a defect in folate metabolism.[61] Hyperhomocysteinemia, a risk factor for cardiovascular disease, is known to cause vascular damage.[60] About half of the pregnancies occurring in women with hereditary homocystinuria terminate in fetal demise.[56] High levels of homocysteine might also do injury in the course of pregnancy, increasing the risk of serious complications such as pregnancy-induced hypertension (PIH) and placental abruption.[62] Both are risk factors for adverse outcome, increasing intrauterine growth restriction and with it the possibility of preterm delivery, in particular, preterm delivery that is medically indicated.

The role of folic acid in DNA synthesis and cell replication suggests its potential to have an important effect on birth weight, gestation duration, or both. An absolute deficiency of folate—from a diet inadequate to meet the needs of pregnancy—in theory interferes with growth of the conceptus. The influence of dietary and circulating folate on preterm delivery and low infant birth weight was studied in 832 women from Camden, one of the poorest cities in the continental United States.[6] Low folate intake (<240 ng/d) was associated with a greater than threefold increase in the risk of low infant birth weight and preterm delivery, after controlling for maternal age, smoking, energy, and other confounding variables. Circulating folate at week 28 was also associated with risk; the adjusted odds for low birth weight increased by 1.5%, and preterm delivery increased by 1.6% per unit decrease in concentration. Later in Camden, the investigators described a nutrient–gene interaction between dietary folate intake and a deletion allele for dihydrofolate reductase (DHFR). DHFR is an enzyme that converts folic acid that is used in supplements to fortify the US food supply to the reduced folate forms used by cells. The deletion allele increased risk of preterm delivery threefold and when folate intake was also low (<400 ug/d) it was associated with low birth weight (eightfold increase) as well as preterm birth (fivefold increase).[63]

Although the effect of the DHFR deletion allele has not yet been replicated, the relation of poor folate nutritional status during pregnancy to birth weight and gestation was confirmed by two recent studies. Lower dietary folate intake (<500 ug/d) at 24 to 29 weeks' gestation was associated with approximately twofold increased risk of preterm delivery in women from North Carolina. Low levels of serum or RBC folate at the same gestation were each associated with increased risk of preterm birth.[64] In pregnant women from Newcastle on Tyne, RBC folate, measured early in gestation (11.5 ± 5 weeks), was modestly but positively related to infant birth weight adjusted for gestation duration and fetal gender.[65] Others have reported increased infant birth weight for mothers whose folate intake was high[66] and positive correlations between maternal serum and RBC folate with birth weight or gestation duration.[67–71]

Higher maternal homocysteine is associated with increased risk including complications of pregnancy like preeclampsia and fetal demise as well as fetal growth restriction.[72,73] Malinow assessed the influence of maternal homocysteine and serum folate at term (37 to 42 weeks) on infant birth weight and gestation duration in 35 healthy nulliparous.[74] Higher maternal homocysteine was associated with significantly lower infant birth weight and shorter gestation, whereas higher maternal folate correlated positively with increased birth weight (univariate analyses). Burke and colleagues, however, failed to detect differences in $N = 37$ women giving birth to growth-restricted infants.[75] Inadequate statistical power, along with the use of a less sensitive test (fasting vs postload homocysteine), posed limitations to this research.

Homocysteine levels measured in more than 5,800 women aged 40 to 42 were linked to past data on pregnancy outcome contained in Norwegian birth registries.[76] Higher homocysteine correlated with older age at delivery, higher cholesterol levels, less multivitamin use, and lifestyle factors (cigarette smoking and high coffee consumption). Women with high homocysteine were more likely to have had a past reproductive history that included preeclampsia, preterm delivery, low birth weight, or fetal growth restriction.

Two recent studies supported these adverse effects with measurements of homocysteine taken before or during pregnancy. In China, preconceptional levels of maternal homocysteine were associated with a fourfold increased risk of preterm delivery.[77] An evaluation in 93 Spanish women before and during pregnancy showed that homocysteine levels fell during the first and second trimesters, plateaued, and then increased between week 32 and delivery. Maternal and fetal levels of homocysteine were positively correlated ($r = .5$ to $r = .7$); levels were reduced by use of folate-containing vitamins. Birth weights of infants in the highest homocysteine tertiles before conception, at 8 weeks' gestation, and at delivery were approximately 200 g below those of women with lower levels of homocysteine.[78]

Unlike in observational studies, randomized trials of supplementation with folic acid have shown less uniform benefit. Fleming and colleagues enrolled 146 Australian women before midpregnancy (week 20) into a randomized trial with five arms:

1. Placebo
2. Folic acid (0.5 mg)
3. Iron sulfate (60 mg)
4. Iron in combination with low-dose folate (0.5 mg)
5. Iron combined with high-dose folate (5 mg)

A total of 89 women completed the study with sample sizes of 15 to 20 per group; there were no significant differences in placental weight, birth weight, or gestation duration among the groups.[79] Small sample size and associated statistical power would limit the ability to detect an effect of folate, if any.

Fletcher and colleagues conducted a randomized, controlled study comparing iron (200 mg ferrous sulfate) with iron with folate (5 mg). Supplements were administered to 643 London women at entry to care.[80] No significant differences in birth weight, gestation, or incidence of congenital defects were found.

Giles and colleagues performed a double-blind, randomized, controlled trial of 692 women in Melbourne, Australia, assigned to folate (5 mg/d) or placebo.[81] Four groups were stratified by gestation at entry from less than 10 weeks to greater than 30 weeks. Outcomes, examined in babies born alive and well, suggested small differences in birth weight and gestation among groups and in multiparas between the index and penultimate pregnancies. None, however, were statistically significant.

Baumslag and colleagues administered iron alone (200 mg) or in combination with folic acid (5 mg/d) or with folate and vitamin B_{12} (50 μg/d) to South African women who had been allocated to one of these three groups.[82] There was no effect of the folate among the White women who were studied, but among Bantu women, who subsisted primarily on maize porridge, the risk of bearing an infant of less than 1,870 g was reduced fourfold by folic acid supplementation.

Iyengar and Rajalakshmi allocated 500 poor Indian women alternately to either iron alone (60 mg as ferrous fumarate) or in combination with folate (500 μg/d). Of these, 239 delivered in hospital; 189 had data included in the analysis.[83] There was a significant difference between folate and iron supplementation, favoring folate in infant birth weight (+ 200 g) and placental weight (+61 g). Risk of low infant birth weight was nearly twice as high among iron-supplemented (34%) compared with folate-supplemented (18%) gravidas.

Rolschau and colleagues studied 40 Danish women, matched for age, parity, smoking, pregravid weight, and housing conditions and allocated them to iron (200 mg ferrous fumarate) plus multivitamins with and without folic acid (5 mg).[84] Among the folate-supplemented subjects, serum and RBC folate increased significantly, infant birth weight was greater by more than 400 g, and placental weight was higher by almost 50 g.

Blot and colleagues assigned 200 French women to iron (105 mg elemental iron) alone or in combination with folic acid (350 mg/d).[85] of these, 109 were reevaluated at delivery. Women treated with folate had higher serum and RBC folate at delivery. Gestation duration was increased among supplemented women (40.7 ± 1.2 vs 39.9 ± 1.2 weeks), as were birth weight (3,461 ± 430 g vs 3,303 ± 375 g) and placental weight (660 ± 130 g vs 604 ± 115 g). In this study, the main effect of folic acid was to extend gestation by nearly 1 week.

Czeizel and colleagues reported the effect of periconceptional supplementation (from more than 28 days before conception to second missed menstruation) with folate-containing multivitamins (0.8 mg folate) or trace minerals.[86–88] Thus, only the effect of periconceptional folic acid supplementation was addressed. In an analysis that included both singleton and multiple births, there was a small but statistically significant excess of low-birth-weight infants among the folic acid-supplemented. Supplementation with folate also increased rate of multiple births, and when the analysis was confined to singletons, the excess of low-birth-weight infants in the folate group was no longer statistically significant.

Since the effect of folic acid supplementation during the course of pregnancy was unclear, data from a large randomized trial conducted in Aberdeen 1966 to 1967 ($N = 2,928$) were reexamined. Supplementation was found to have no effect on mean birth weight, gestation at delivery, or placental weight. However when data were pooled with data from other trials, a high dose of folic acid (5 mg/d) was found to be associated with a small effect, a 37% reduction in risk of infant low birth weight.[89] This is consistent with another small effect based upon vital records. After folic acid fortification of the US food supply, rates of preterm delivery, very low birth weight, and low birth weight declined between 4 and 10% among California live born infants.[90]

In summary, although observational studies of folate and pregnancy suggest a potential benefit of folate supplementation during pregnancy—a decrease in serious complications and an improvement in birth weight and gestation—randomized trials imply that routine folate supplementation might have a small benefit at best for most pregnant women. Women who are at risk, either because of common genetic polymorphisms that alter folate metabolism or because of environmental factors associated with a diet low in folate, would seem to benefit the most.

MULTIVITAMIN AND MINERAL SUPPLEMENTS

In the United States, about one-quarter of women (26% of White women and 15.5% of Black women) in their reproductive years regularly take vitamin or mineral supplements.[91] In one study, 16% of low-income gravidas in Massachusetts took vitamins before pregnancy.[92] In Camden, New Jersey, 17% of low-income minority gravidas reported using supplements before they became pregnant.[93] Preconceptional supplement use was more likely to occur in women with a history of spontaneous abortion or other poor pregnancy outcome.

Information on recommended dietary intakes for pregnant women in the United States is given in Table 1. Use of prenatal vitamins by women from the United States and Europe before or during pregnancy is associated with reductions in the risk of preterm delivery, very preterm delivery, low infant birth weight, gestational hypertension, and preeclampsia.[93–97] Another study, which examined multivitamin use with data from the 1988 National Maternal and Infant Health Survey, reported no effect of multivitamin use on pregnancy outcomes, including preterm delivery.[98] However, conclusions are limited by the fact that the survey questionnaire was geared toward regular multivitamin use (3 d/wk or more) and did not differentiate women who used vitamins from those who did not.

In the developing world, pregnant women are often deficient in a wide variety of vitamins and minerals that have the potential to affect the course and outcome of pregnancy. Fawzi and colleagues examined the effect of supplementing more than 1,000 human immunodeficiency virus–positive (HIV+) women from Tanzania with multivitamins, vitamin A, and placebo in a double-blind, placebo-controlled trial.[99] Multivitamin supplementation decreased the risk of very preterm delivery (an approximately twofold reduction) along with decreasing risk of low infant birth weight and fetal growth restriction. The multivitamin supplement had the bonus of increasing CD4, CD8, and CD3 counts in the women. Another trial of multiple micronutrients, conducted in Zimbabwe included many HIV+ participants and showed a trend toward the positive. Multiple micronutrients increased birth weight (+50 g, $p = .08$), gestation duration (+0.3 week, $p = .06$), and head circumference (+0.2 cm, $p = .07$) compared to placebo.[100] Subsequent research suggested that multivitamin administration also reduced risk of maternal mortality and delayed the progression of HIV disease in pregnant women.[101]

Two clinical trials conducted in Nepal came to similar conclusions on effectiveness. In the cluster randomized trial described more fully in the section on iron, multiple micronutrient supplements had significant effects—birth weight was increased (+64 g) and infant low birth weight reduced (−14%) in comparison to controls receiving Vitamin A alone. These effects, however, were said to be comparable to those of iron–folate supplements, which yielded a 37 g increase in birth weight (NS) and 16% reduction in infant low birth weight.[26] In a subsequent trial, Nepalese women were supplemented with 15 micronutrients; an iron–folate regimen was utilized for comparison. Micronutrient supplementation increased birth weight (+77 g), reduced infant low birth weight (−25%), and had a marginal effect on preterm delivery (+0.2 week increase, $p = .12$).[102] However, when Mexican women were randomly assigned to multiple micronutrients or toiron (60 mg/d) there was no difference in birth weight or gestation duration for the group receiving micronutrients.[103] High maternal BMI (mean 24.3) and the prevalence of overweight (33%) may have buffered effects of the supplements.

An increasing number of individuals are using megadoses of vitamin or mineral supplements—5.5% in 1997, up from 2.4% in 1990.[104] Use of megadoses of nutritional supplements by pregnant women and their effect on the course and outcome of pregnancy have not been investigated. The upper limit of nutritional intake is the highest level considered safe for use. The recommendations of the Institute of Medicine for the upper limits of nutritional intake during pregnancy are given in Table 1.

HERBAL PRODUCTS

Herbal products are considered nutritional supplements. They are used during pregnancy primarily for relief of nausea and vomiting (eg, ginger, raspberry leaf, chamomile) and closer to term to ripen the cervix and to stimulate labor (eg, black cohosh, blue cohosh, raspberry leaf, castor oil, evening primrose oil).[105–108] Little is known of their safety and efficacy. There is a serious bias that is made when estimating how frequently herbal products are used. One cross-sectional survey of pregnant women from San Francisco reported a response rate of 24%, and surveys of nurse-midwives had response rates of 34 and 68%.[105,107,108] The largest survey to date was done by telephone and, although not limited to pregnant women, had an estimated response of 60%.[104] Because of failure to participate in such surveys is common, use of herbal preparations by pregnant women is probably different than much of the published literature suggests. Use of herbal products during pregnancy has been reported to range between 4 and 36% in English-speaking countries.[109–111]

Most herbal products are perceived as natural, with benign effects, and safe for use during pregnancy.[112] The problem is that most observational or randomized studies have small sample sizes with inadequate statistical power to detect adverse effects most of which are relatively uncommon. Case reports are often the only indicator of an adverse experience.[113–114] However, a few studies have suggested that use of certain commonly used herbal remedies during pregnancy may have untoward consequences. In Finland, glycyrrhizin (licorice) consumption is common. Glycyrrhizin inhibits the breakdown of cortisol by the placenta. A case-control study showed that women who had heavy consumption (>500 mg/wk) had a twofold increased risk of delivering preterm and a threefold increase of delivering very preterm (<34 weeks).[115] Likewise, a large study ($N = 14{,}551$) from Taiwan suggested that 16.9% of pregnant women with live born infants used herbal medicines during the first trimester.[116] Certain herbs used by 1% or more of the women including Huanglian (1.5%) and An-Tai-Yin (11.4%) were associated with seven- to eightfold increased risk of congenital defects of the central nervous system(CNS), musculoskeletal system, and eye. Ginseng, used by less than 1%, was associated with increased risks (CNS, musculoskeletal, and urogenital defects) but these were not statistically significant.

FISH OIL SUPPLEMENTS

Consumption of supplements that contain fish oil, as well as eating a diet rich in marine foods that contain omega-3 polyunsaturated fatty acids (n-3-PUFA), may be associated with longer gestation duration. Canadian Inuit with high n-3 PUFA intake have longer gestations (+5.4 days) and increased infant birth weights (+77 g).[117] The clinical trial conducted by the People's League of Health on London women on the eve of World War II suggested that supplementing a diet that was not markedly deficient with minerals, vitamins, and halibut oil extended gestation.[118] Fewer infants were born before the fortieth week of gestation to the supplemented women (20% among supplemented subjects vs 24% among the unsupplemented), although there was no difference in mean birth weight.

A trial of 533 Danish women who received, fish oil, olive oil, or no supplement by 30 weeks' gestation showed that women taking the fish oil supplement had longer average gestations (+4 days) and bore infants with higher average weights (+107 g), which was mostly attributable to the change in gestation.[119] The effect of fish oil was strongest for women with low fish consumption at entry to care and amounted to an increase of 7.4 days' gestation for this group. There was little effect of the supplement on women with high fish consumption at entry (–1.6 days). Thus, the hypothesized effect of omega-3 fatty acids on gestation appeared to have a threshold and to be specific to the initiation of idiopathic preterm labor.

A multicenter trial of high-risk women enrolled gravidas with a history of preterm delivery, fetal growth restriction, or preeclampsia. Some of the centers enrolled women with threatened preeclampsia or suspected fetal growth restriction. Women were randomized to either fish oil or olive oil. Fish oil reduced the recurrence risk of preterm delivery approximately twofold but did not alter the recurrence of the other poor pregnancy outcomes.[120] A clinical trial of a high-risk, low-income population that was primarily African-American showed that the consumption of eggs fortified with docosahexanoic acid late in second trimester increased gestation duration by 6 days on average.[121] However, a recent meta-analysis of several randomized trials suggested that while the effect of n-3 PUFAs on gestation duration was present it was weaker than this (+1.5 days).[122]

Conversely, results with fish oil supplements and fish intake have demonstrated some striking inconsistencies.[123] For example, birth weight and head circumference of infants born to healthy young Icelandic women with a BMI in the normal range were shown to increase with increasing fish intake. However, when fish oil was the source of the n-3 PUFA infant head circumference and birth length were significantly decreased.[124] And, in the United States increasing seafood intake and of marine n-3 PUFA supplement use both were associated with decreased infant birth weight and fetal growth, with no change in gestation duration or risk of preterm delivery.[125]

Finally, ecologic studies have indicated that the consumption of large quantities of fish during pregnancy is associated with lower blood pressure and thus, in theory, with a lower incidence of PIH. Consistent with this is the reduction in the incidence of preeclampsia as noted in the People's League of Health Study.[118] However, because of the multiple supplementation regimens, it could not be attributed to the use of the fish oil per se. A multicenter trial of fish oil supplements showed no effect on the risk of preeclampsia or on blood pressure reduction.[120]

CALCIUM

The skeleton acts as the calcium reservoir of the body (99% is stored there), and when dietary calcium intake is low or poorly absorbed, calcium is withdrawn from bone to support serum calcium homeostasis.[2] During pregnancy, retention of an estimated 30 g of calcium, most of which is transferred during the third trimester, is needed to mineralize the fetal skeleton.[2] Although it is often assumed that pregnancy, like lactation, might be a setting for bone mass loss because of this requirement, this might be buffered by a 60 to 70% enhancement in intestinal calcium absorption during pregnancy.[126] Although several studies have examined longitudinally the change in bone mass with pregnancy, only two have examined the influence of dietary calcium on bone mass as an independent variable.[127,128] Lamke and colleagues evaluated 14 mature pregnant women in the second trimester and postpartum and reported a significant decrease in trabecular bone and a small gain in cortical bone.[127] Christiansen and colleagues studied serial changes in radial bone mass in 13 Danish women during pregnancy and found no change.[128] These women were, however, ingesting an average of 650 mg/d in calcium supplements, apart from their diet. Sowers and colleagues found no change in femoral bone mineral density in 32 women, aged 20 to 40 years, with measurement prior to pregnancy and following delivery, compared with matched controls, but again the average calcium intake exceeded the recommended dietary allowance for both groups.[129] Drinkwater and Chestnut studied changes in bone mineral density (pregravid and 6-week postpartum) in 6 women who experienced pregnancy and 25 controls; mean calcium intake was high (>1,500 mg/d) in each group.[130] Despite this, pregnancy was associated with significant decrements in bone at the femoral neck and radial shaft; increased bone density was found for the tibia.

One reason for the limited number of subjects and studies during pregnancy is risk of radiation exposure, making ultrasonography desirable for measuring bone change during pregnancy. Several recent studies have measured change in either the os calcis or the phalanges, and all have reported significant decreases in ultrasonographic measures of bone density during pregnancy.[131–134] The largest of these, with a sample size of 250 gravidas, reported a quantitative ultrasonographic index 3.6% lower at 6-week postpartum than at entry.[131] Although the amount of bone lost was small, it is consistent with the fetal demand for calcium. In this study, there was no relationship between dietary calcium intake and bone loss. However, Aguado and colleagues detected an overall decrease in bone propagation (phalanges 2 to 5) as seen by ultrasonography during the second and third trimesters that was greater for gravidas with low dietary calcium intake (<1,000 mg/d). Decreases in maternal bone propagation were paralleled by increases in markers of bone turnover.[132]

Calcium intake, particularly during growth, could be an important determinant of bone mineralization and thus bone density.[135] Higher calcium intakes during childhood and adolescence are associated with higher bone mass at maturity.[136] Maternal growth and pregnancy often coincide, and approximately half of all pregnant teenagers continue to grow while pregnant.[137] Ultrasonographic bone measures of the os calcis during pregnancy showed that bone loss was greater for growing teenage gravidas (–5.5%) than for mature women (–1.9%).[131] In the case of pregnancy in a still-growing girl, calcium nutriture might be limited by maternal diet but simultaneously driven by the need to retain enough calcium to mineralize two skeletons.

Presumably, continued maternal growth could affect the risk of osteoporosis and osteoporotic fractures in later life, particularly if the maternal diet was deficient in calcium during childhood and adolescence. Iowa women with a first pregnancy before age 19 had, at maturity, a bone mass (measured at the middistal forearm) that was –0.52 standard deviation units (SDU) below that of other women.[138] Calcium consumption was also related to bone density (–0.68 SDU for lower intakes), and the joint effect for early pregnancy and lower calcium intake, assuming additivity, exceeded –1 SDU in bone mass. A longitudinal study from a third community carried out 5 years later also showed that bone mass was significantly reduced in those with a teenage birth.[139] A cross-sectional study by Fox and colleagues yielded similar results in perimenopausal women.[140]

Another approach has been to examine the cross-sectional relationship of parity to bone mineral density or risk of fracture. In general, cross-sectional studies of bone mass and parity, usually confined to mature white women, have shown increased bone mass, decreased fracture risk, or no effect of parity on bone mass.[141] Lower bone mineral density has been reported in parous minority women compared with controls of the same ethnic group. Goldsmith and Johnston reported lower radial bone densities in 52 parous Black women compared with Black nulliparous. Among Whites, parous women had a bone density 1% higher than nulliparous controls.[142] Carter and Haynes showed that lower bone density was present in adults with scoliosis.[143] Parous Black women were more likely to have scoliosis than were nonparous Blacks. However, parity does not measure the effects of pregnancy but the cumulative effect of the reproductive experience, along with antecedents and consequences. For example, a positive correlation between parity and bone density could reflect greater antecedent hormonal integrity and possibly increased body weight of women who bear children compared with women who are infertile. It is uncertain the extent to which small decrements in bone mass with parity among Black women reflect an overrepresentation of women with adolescent childbearing.

Maternal calcium metabolism is altered during pregnancy, and these alterations could be involved in the etiology of preeclampsia. During pregnancy, maternal serum calcium levels fall and urinary calcium excretion rises, whereas serum ionized calcium remains unchanged. Preeclampsia and gestational hypertension are marked by aberrations involving calcium: Affected women have hypocalciuria, low levels of ionized calcium, lower levels of 1,25-dihydroxyvitamin D, elevated levels of parathyroid hormone, and increased intracellular concentrations of calcium in erythrocytes, platelets, and lymphocytes.[144] Thus, preeclampsia could be a pathologic manifestation of a calcium-conserving mechanism. Calcium supplementation might reduce smooth muscle reactivity, including the reactivity of uterine and vascular smooth muscle by reducing parathyroid hormone and intracellular calcium levels.[145] On the other hand, disturbances in calcium metabolism could be a marker for preeclampsia, a response to an unknown and underlying metabolic perturbation.

Diets low in calcium, especially during pregnancy, have been associated with increased blood pressure levels through heightened smooth muscle reactivity (see Table 1 for recommended dietary intake of calcium and other nutrients during pregnancy). The pathogenesis of PIH may or may not involve calcium in the maternal diet. Belizan and Villar reported an inverse relationship between eclampsia and dietary calcium from ecologic-level data that showed countries where calcium intake was low had a higher frequency of eclampsia than countries where calcium intake was higher.[146] More recently, gestational hypertension (but not preeclampsia or eclampsia) and maximum diastolic pressure were found to be weakly correlated with low dietary calcium intakes.[147] Several smaller scale clinical trials have confirmed that calcium supplementation is associated with decreased blood pressure during pregnancy, consistent with reports of an inverse association between calcium and systolic blood pressure in nonpregnant subjects.[148–149]

A meta-analysis of 14 randomized, controlled trials of calcium supplementation involving more than 2,400 pregnant women showed statistically significant reductions in systolic and diastolic blood pressure with the administration of calcium salts (375 to 2,000 mg/d elemental calcium).[150] Risk of preeclampsia was reduced more than twofold among women supplemented with calcium during these trials. Duration of treatment ranged from 10 to 22 weeks, with most studies starting the supplement during the second trimester. Although differences in the risk of preeclampsia were significant in the aggregate, only two of the nine studies showed statistically significant differences.

A large, randomized, double-blind, placebo-controlled trial of 5,489 low-risk nulliparous women showed no effect of calcium supplementation.[151] Pregnant women were enrolled at centers throughout the United States and prescreened for compliance with supplement use and for conditions associated with abnormal calcium metabolism or increased risk of preeclampsia. Women were supplemented with 2 g of elemental calcium (or placebo) beginning at 13 to 21 weeks' gestation and continuing until they delivered. Calcium supplementation did not significantly reduce the risk of preeclampsia, gestational hypertension without preeclampsia (either mild or severe), or pregnancy-associated proteinuria without hypertension. Blood pressure was also unaffected. Between 20 and 40 weeks' gestation, systolic pressure was lower by 0.3 mm Hg and diastolic pressure was 0.03 mm Hg higher among the calcium-supplemented women; these small differences were not statistically significant. Likewise, risk did not differ when data were examined according to hypothesized moderating variables: quintile of dietary calcium intake at baseline, maternal age, urinary calcium excretion, or gestation at entry to the study. These results suggest no effect of calcium supplementation on preeclampsia; however, participants' dietary intake of calcium was high, averaging about 1,100 mg/d.[151]

Recently, an Australian trial of calcium supplementation in gravidas ($N = 456$) with dietary calcium intakes (median, 1,100 to 1,200 g/d), maternal characteristics, and pregnancy outcomes very similar to those in the US trial reported a positive effect of supplementation.[145] Calcium supplementation (1.8 g/d from week 24) resulted in a greater than twofold reduction in the risk of preeclampsia. Although the proportion of women with PIH, severe PIH, and severe preeclampsia was slightly less in the treatment group, differences from placebo were not statistically significant.

During pregnancy, an increased risk of PIH or preeclampsia associated with lower calcium intake could result in an increased risk of preterm delivery because an indicated preterm delivery is one method of reducing the maternal-fetal morbidity and mortality associated with preeclampsia and eclampsia. Consequently, supplementation with calcium during pregnancy could have a side effect of reduced preterm birth risk. Preeclampsia involves the failure to adequately perfuse many organs, including the placenta, and is also associated with fetal growth restriction and low infant birth weight (<2,500 g).

Two calcium supplementation trials among high-risk women showed promising results. In Ecuadorian women with low calcium intake, gestation duration increased by 1.8 weeks ($p < .01$) for the calcium-supplemented subjects ($n = 22$).[152,153] Among teenagers from Baltimore, the calcium-supplemented group had a lower incidence of preterm delivery compared with the placebo group.[148] Further, life-table analysis demonstrated an overall shift to a higher gestational age with calcium. Another randomized, controlled trial of supplementation of 260 pregnant Ecuadorian teenagers (age 17.5 years and less) with 2,000 mg/d elemental calcium increased gestation duration from 38.7 weeks (0.3 weeks) for placebo to 39.6 weeks (0.4 weeks) with calcium supplement. Risk of PIH was reduced by 80% in this trial with calcium supplementation.[154] Baseline dietary calcium intake was low and amounted to less than 50% of the recommended dietary allowance for pregnancy. The more recent clinical trial from Australia also showed a reduction in the risk of preterm delivery from 10% (placebo) to 4.4% (calcium supplemented) as well as for low birth weight (7.4% vs 2.6%).[145] There were also reductions in admissions for threatened preterm labor ($p = .03$) and in preterm premature rupture of membranes ($p = .08$) for gravidas assigned to calcium.

A large calcium supplementation trial of more than 1,000 women from Argentina, however, showed a decrease in the incidence of PIH but no effect on preeclampsia or on preterm delivery.[149] The meta-analysis cited above also showed no effect of calcium intake on preterm delivery or fetal growth restriction.[150] Likewise, the US clinical trial performed by Levine and colleagues, discussed above, also found no effect of calcium supplementation on obstetric outcomes, including preterm delivery, birth weight, low birth weight, or fetal growth restriction.[151]

It was thought that the ability of supplemental calcium to decrease the risk of preeclampsia might be confined to high-risk populations in which there was either a severe dietary restriction of calcium or a high demand for calcium as in adolescent pregnancy. A recent WHO trial involving more than 8,300 pregnant women from populations where dietary calcium intakes were low (<600 mg/d) supported the original ecologic observations made on eclampsia.[155] Calcium supplements (1.5 g/d) did indeed reduce the relative risk of eclampsia (by 47%), severe gestational hypertension (by 40%), severe preeclamptic complications (by 32%), the severe maternal morbidity and mortality index (by 25%) and neonatal mortality (by 43%). However, overall risk of preeclampsia was not lower on the calcium regimen than placebo (4.1% vs 4.5%). For women age 20 years or less, very preterm delivery (<32 weeks) was significantly reduced (by 56%) and preterm delivery showed a nonsignificant trend in the same direction. Thus while calcium supplementation did not prevent preeclampsia, among women from populations with a low calcium diet it had important effects—it reduced risks of eclampsia, neonatal mortality and, among the younger women, risk of very preterm delivery.

REFERENCES

1. Martin JA, Hamilton BE, Sutton PD, et al. Births: Final data for 2004, NVSR 55, No 1. Maryland: National Center for Health Statistics; 2006.
2. Institute of Medicine, Committee on Nutritional Status during Pregnancy and Lactation. Nutrition During Pregnancy. Washington, DC: National Academy Press; 1990.
3. Kramer MS. Determinants of low birth weight: Methodological assessment and meta-analysis. Bull World Health Org 1987;65:663–737.
4. Scholl TO, Hediger ML, Fischer RL, et al. Anemia vs iron deficiency: Increased risk of preterm delivery in a prospective study. Am J Clin Nutr 1992;55:985–8.
5. Scholl TO, Hediger ML, Schall JI, et al. Low zinc intake during pregnancy: Its association with preterm and very preterm delivery. Am J Epidemiol 1993;137:1115–24.
6. Scholl TO, Hediger ML, Schall JI, et al. Dietary and serum folate: Their influence on the outcome of pregnancy. Am J Clin Nutr 1996;63:520–5.
7. Institute of Medicine. Dietary Reference Intakes: The Essential Guide to Nutrient Requirements. Washington, DC: National Academy Press; 2006.
8. Klebanoff MA, Shiono PH, Berendes HW, et al. Facts and artifacts about anemia and preterm delivery. JAMA 1989;262:511–5.
9. Murphy JF, O'Riordan J, Newcombe RG, et al. Relation of haemoglobin levels in first and second trimesters to outcome of pregnancy. Lancet 1986;i:992–5.
10. Garn SM, Ridella SA, Petzoid AS, et al. Maternal hematologic levels and pregnancy outcomes. Semin Perinatol 1981;5:155–62.
11. Steer P, Alam MA, Wadsworth J, et al. Relationship between maternal haemoglobin concentration and birth weight in different ethnic groups. BMJ 1995;310:489–91.
12. Meis PJ, Michielutte R, Peters TJ, et al. Factors associated with preterm birth in Cardiff, Wales. Am J Obstet Gynecol 1995;173:590–6.
13. Klebanoff MA, Shiono PH, Selby JV, et al. Anemia and spontaneous preterm birth. Am J Obstet Gynecol 1991;164:59–63.
14. Lao TT, Chan LY, Tam K-F, et al. Maternal hemoglobin and risk of gestational diabetes mellitus in Chinese women. Obstet Gynecol 2002;99:807–12.
15. Rosso P, Salas SP. Mechanisms of fetal growth retardation in the underweight mother. Adv Exp Med Biol 1994;352:1–9.
16. Whittaker PG, Macphail S, Lind T. Serial hematologic changes and pregnancy outcome. Obstet Gynecol 1996;88:33–9.
17. Scholl TO, Hediger ML. Anemia and iron deficiency anemia, compilation of data on pregnancy outcome. Am J Clin Nutr 1994;59:492S–501S.
18. Brabin B, Ginny M, Supau J, et al. Consequences of maternal anaemia on outcome of pregnancy in malaria endemic area in Papua, New Guinea. Ann Trop Med Parasitol 1990;84:11–24.

19. Zhou LM, Yang WW, Hua JZ, et al. Relation of hemoglobin measured at different times in pregnancy to preterm birth and low birth weight in Shanghai, China. Am J Epidemiol 1998;148:998–1006.
20. Bondevik GT, Lie RT, Kvale G. Maternal hematological status and risk of low birth weight and preterm delivery in Nepal. Acta Obstet Gynecol Scand 2001;80:402–8.
21. Arafa M, Abou-Zied H, Attia AF, et al. Maternal haemoglobin and premature child delivery. East Mediterr Health J 1998;4:480–6.
22. Scanlon KS, Yip R, Schieve LA, et al. High and low hemoglobin levels during pregnancy: Differential risks for preterm birth and small for gestational age. Obstet Gynecol 2000;96:741–8.
23. Ronnenberg AG, Wood RJ, Wang X, et al. Preconception hemoglobin and ferritin concentrations are associated with pregnancy outcome in a prospective cohort of Chinese women. J Nutr 2004;134:2586–91.
24. Gambling L, Andersen HS, Czopek A, et al. Effect of timing of iron supplementation on maternal and neonatal growth and iron status of iron-deficient pregnant rats. J Physiol 2004;561:195–203.
25. Cogswell ME, Parvanta I, Ickes L, et al. Iron supplementation during pregnancy, anemia, and birth weight: A randomizes control trial. Am J Clin Nutr 2003;78:773–81.
26. Christian P, Khatry SK, Katz J, et al. Effects of alternative maternal micronutrient supplements on low birth weight in rural Nepal: A double blind randomized community trial. BMJ 2003;326:571–6.
27. Siega-Riz AM, Hartzema AG, TurnbullC, et al. The effects of prophylactic iron given in prenatal supplements on iron status and birth outcomes: A randomized controlled trial. Am J Obstet Gynecol 2006;194:512–9.
28. Makrides M, Crowther CA, Gibson RA, et al. Efficacy and tolerability of low-dose iron supplements during pregnancy: A randomized controlled trial. Am J Clin Nutr 2003;78:145–53.
29. Allen LH. Biological mechanisms that might underlie iron's effects on fetal growth and preterm birth. J Nutr 2001;131:581S–9S.
30. Neggers YH, Cutter GR, Acton RT, et al. A positive association between maternal serum zinc concentration and birth weight. Am J Clin Nutr 1990;51:678–84.
31. Kirksey A, Wachs T, Yunis F, et al. Relationship of maternal zinc nutriture to pregnancy outcome and infant development in an Egyptian village. Am J Clin Nutr 1994;60:782–92.
32. Jameson S. Variations in maternal serum zinc during pregnancy and correlation with congenital malformations, dysmaturity, and abnormal parturition. Acta Med Scand 1976;593:21–37.
33. Ghosh A, Fong LYY, Wan CW, et al. Zinc deficiency is not a cause for abortion, congential abnormality and small-for gestational age infant in Chinese women. Br J Obstet Gynaecol 1985;92:886–91.
34. Singh PP, Khushlani K, Veerwal PC, et al. Maternal hypozincemia and low birth weight infants. Clin Chem 1987;33:1950.
35. Metcoff J, Cottilo J, Crosby W, et al. Maternal nutrition and fetal outcome. Am J Clin Nutr 1981;34:708–21.
36. McMichael AJ, Dreosti IE, Gibson GT, et al. A prospective study of serial maternal serum zinc levels and pregnancy out-come. Early Hum Dev 1982;7:59–69.
37. Mukherjee MD, Sandstead HH, Ratnaparkhi MV, et al. Maternal zinc, iron, folic acid, and protein nutriture and outcome of human pregnancy. Am J Clin Nutr 1984;40:496–507.
38. Tamura T, Goldenberg RL, Johnston KE, et al. Maternal plasma zinc concentrations and pregnancy outcome. Am J Clin Nutr 2000;71:109–13.
39. Goldenberg R, Tamura T, Neggers Y, et al. The effects of zinc supplementation on pregnancy outcome. JAMA 1995;274:463–8.
40. Meadows N, Ruse W, Smith MF, et al. Zinc and small babies. Lancet 1981;ii:1135–7.
41. Meadows N, Ruse W, Keeling PWN, et al. Peripheral blood leucocyte zinc depletion in babies with intrauterine growth retardation. Arch Dis Child 1983;58:807–9.
42. Wells JL, James DK, Luxton R, et al. Maternal leucocyte zinc deficiency at start of third trimester as a predictor of fetal growth retardation. BMJ 1987;294:1054–7.
43. Simmer K, Thompson RPH. Maternal zinc and intrauterine growth retardation. Clin Sci 1985;68:395–9.
44. Adeniyi FA. The implications of hypozincemia in pregnancy. Acta Obstet Gynecol Scand 1987;66:579–82.
45. Cherry FF, Sandstead HH, Rohas P, et al. Adolescent pregnancy: Associations among body weight, zinc nutriture and pregnancy outcome. Am J Clin Nutr 1989;50:945–54.
46. Kynast G, Saling E. Effect of oral zinc application during pregnancy. Gynecol Obstet Invest 1986;21:117–23.
47. Castillo-Duran C, Weisstaub G. Zinc supplementation and growth of the fetus and low birth weight infant. J Nutr 2003;133:1494S–7S.
48. Osendarp SJM, van Raaiji JMA, Wahed MA, et al. A randomized, placebo controlled trial of the effect of zinc supplementation during pregnancy on pregnancy outcome in Bangladeshi urban poor. Am J Clin Nutr 2000;71:114–9.
49. Caufield LE, Zavaleta N, Figueroa A, et al. Maternal zinc supplementation does not affect size at birth or pregnancy out-come. J Nutr 1999;129:1563–8.
50. Fawzi WW, Villamor E, Msamanga GI, et al. Trial of zinc supplements in relation to pregnancy outcomes, hematologic indicators, and T cell counts among HIV-1-infected women in Tanzania. Am J Nutr Clin 2005;81:161–7.
51. Osendarp SJM, West CE, Black RE, et al. The need for maternal zinc supplementation in developing countries: An unresolved issue. J Nutr 2003;133:817S–27S.
52. Shah D, Sachdev HPS. Zinc deficiency in pregnancy and fetal outcome. Nutr Rev 2006;64:15–30.
53. Pilch SM, Senti FM, editors. Assessment of the Zinc Nutritional Status of the US Population. Bethesda, MD: Life Sciences Research Office, Federal American Society of Experimental Biology; 1984.
54. King JC. Determinants of maternal zinc status during pregnancy. Am J Clin Nutr 2000;71:1334S–43S.
55. Rosenblatt DS. Inherited disorders of folate transport and metabolism. In: Scriver CR, Beaudet AL, Sly WS, Valle D, editors. The Metabolic and Molecular Bases of Inherited Disease. New York: McGraw-Hill; 1995. p. 3111–28.
56. Mudd SH, Levy HL, Skovby F. Disorders of transsulfuration. In: Scriver CR, Beaudet AL, Sly WS, Valle D, editors. The Metabolic and Molecular Bases of Inherited Disease. New York: McGraw-Hill; 1995. p. 1279–327.
57 Sherwood KL, Houghton LH, Tarasuk V, et al. One-third of pregnant and lactating women may not be meeting their folate requirements from diet alone based on mandated levels of folate fortification. J Nutr 2006;136:2820–26.
58. Honein MA, Paulozzi LJ, Mathews TJ, et al. Impact of folic acid fortification on the US food supply on the occurrence of neural tube defects. JAMA 2001;285:2981–6.
59. Neuhouser ML, Beresford SAA. Folic acid: Are current fortification levels adequate? Nutrition 2001;17:868–72.
60. Tamura T, Picciate MF. Folate and human reproduction. Am J Clin Nutr 2006;83:993–1016.
61. Hibbard BM. The role of folic acid in pregnancy. J Obstet Gynaecol Br Commonwealth 1964;71:529–42.
62. Ray JG, Ladkin CA. Folic acid and homocysteine metabolic defects and the risk of placental abruption, preeclampsia and spontaneous pregnancy loss: A systematic review. Placenta 1999;20:519–29.
63. Johnson WG, Scholl TO, Spychala JR, et al. Common dihydrofolate reductase 19-base deletion allel: A novel risk factor for preterm delivery. Am J Clin Nutr 2005;81:664–8.
64. Siega-Riz AM, Savitz SA, Zeisel SH, et al. Second trimester folate status and preterm birth. Am J Obstet Gynecol 2004;191:1851–7.
65. Relton CL, Pearce MS, Parker L. The influence of erythrocyte folate and serum vitamin B_{12} status on birth weight. Br J Nutr 2005;93:593–9.
66. Neggers YH, Goldenberg RL, Tamura T, et al. The relationship between maternal dietary intake and infant birthweight. Acta Obstet Gynecol Scand 1997;165:71–5.
67. Frelut ML, deCourcy GP, Christides JP, et al. Relationship between maternal folate status and foetal hypotrophy in a population with a good socio-economical level. Int J Vitam Nutr Res 1995;65:267–71.
68. Ek J. Plasma and red cell folate in mothers and infants in normal pregnancies. Acta Obstet Gynecol Scand 1982;61:17–20.
69. Whiteside MG, Ungar B, Path MC, et al. Iron, folic acid and vitamin B12 levels in normal pregnancy, and their influence on birth-weight and the duration of pregnancy. Med J Aust 1968;1:338–42.
70. Tchernia G, Blot I, Rey A, et al. Maternal folate status, birthweight and gestational age. Dev Pharmacol Ther 1982;4:58–65.
71. Rondo PHC, Abbott R, Rodrigues LC, et al. Vitamin A, folate, and iron concentrations in cord and maternal blood of intra-uterine growth retarded and appropriate birth weight babies. Eur J Clin Nutr 1995;49:391–9.
72. deVries JIP, Huijgens PC, Blomberg BME, et al. Hyperhomocysteinemia and protein S deficiency. Br J Obstet Gynaecol 1997;104:1248–54.
73. Rajkovic A, Catalano PM, Malinow MR. Elevated homocyst(e)ine levels with preeclampsia. Obstet Gynecol 1997;90:168–71.
74. Malinow MR, Rajkovic A, Duell PB, et al. The relationship between maternal and neonatal umbilical cord plasma homocyst(e)ine suggests a potential role for maternal homocyst(e)ine in fetal metabolism. Am J Obstet Gynecol 1998;178:228–33.
75. Burke G, Robinson K, Refsum H, et al. Intrauterine growth retardation, perinatal death, and maternal homocysteine levels. N Engl J Med 1992;326:69–70.
76. Vollset SE, Refsum H, Emblem BM, et al. Plasma total homocysteine, pregnancy complications and adverse pregnancy outcomes: The Hordaland Homocysteine Study. Am J Clin Nutr 2001;71:962–8.
77. Ronnenberg AG, Goldman MB, Chen D, et al. Preconception Homocysteine and B vitamin status and birth outcomes in Chinese women. Am J Clin Nutr 2002;76:1385–91.
78. Murphy MM, Scott JM, Arija V, et el. Maternal homocysteine before conception and throughout pregnancy predicts fetal Homocysteine and birth weight. Clin Chem 2004;50:1406–12.
79. Fleming AF, Martin JD, Hahnel JR, et al. Effects of iron and folic acid antenatal supplements on maternal haematology and fetal wellbeing. Med J Aust 1974;2:429–36.
80. Fletcher J, Gurr A, Fellingham FR, et al. The value of folic acid supplements in pregnancy. J Obstet Gynaecol Br Commonwealth 1971;78:781–5.
81. Giles PFH, Harcourt AG, Whiteside MG. The effect of prescribing folic acid during pregnancy on birth-weight and duration of pregnancy. Med J Aust 1971;2:17–21.
82. Baumslag N, Edelstein T, Metz J. Reduction of incidence of pre-maturity by folic acid supplementation in pregnancy. BMJ 1970;1:16–7.
83. Iyengar L, Rajalakshmi K. Effect of folic acid supplement on birth weights of infants. Am J Obstet Gynecol 1975;122:332–6.
84. Rolschau J, Date J, Kristoffersen K. Folic acid supplement and intrauterine growth. Acta Obstet Gynecol Scand 1979;58:343–4.
85. Blot I, Papiernik E, Kaltwasser JP, et al. Influence of routine administration of folic acid and iron during pregnancy. Gynecol Obstet Invest 1981;12:294–304.
86. Czeizel AE, Dudas I, Metneki J. Pregnancy outcomes in a randomised controlled trial of periconceptional multivitamin supplementation. Arch Gynecol Obstet 1994;255:131–9.
87. Czeizel AE, Metneki J, Dudas I. The higher rate of multiple births after periconceptional multivitamin supplementation: An analysis of causes. Acta Genet Med Gemellol 1994;43:175–84.
88. Czeizel A. Controlled studies of multivitamin supplementation on pregnancy outcome. Ann N Y Acad Sci 1993;678:266–75.
89. Charles DHM, Ness AR, Campbell D, et al. Folic acid supplements in pregnancy and birth outcome: Re-analysis of a large randomized controlled trial and update of Cochrane review. Paediatr Perinat Epidemiol 2005;19:112–24.
90. Shaw GM, Carmichael SL, Nelson V, et al. Occurrence of low birthweight and preterm delivery among California infants before and after compulsory food fortification with folic acid. Public Health Rep 2004;119:170–3.
91. Block G, Cox C, Madans J, et al. Vitamin supplement use, by demographic characteristics. Am J Epidemiol 1988;127:297–309.
92. Suitor CW, Gardner JD. Supplement use among a culturally diverse group of low-income pregnant women. J Am Diet Assoc 1990;90:268–71.
93. Scholl TO, Hediger ML, Bendich A, et al. Use of multivitamin/mineral prenatal supplements: Influence on the outcome of pregnancy. Am J Epidemiol 1997;146:134–41.
94. Vahratian A, Siega-Riz AM, Savitz DA, et al. Multivitamin use and the risk of preterm birth. Am J Epidemiol 2004;16:886–92.
95. Hininger I, Favier M, Arnaud J, et al. Effects of a combined micronutrient supplementation on maternal biological status and newborn anthropometrics measurements: A randomized double-blind, placebo-controlled trial in apparently healthy pregnant women. Eur J Clin Nutr 2004;58:52–9.
96. Bodnar LM, Tang G, Ness RB, et al. Periconceptional multivitamin use reduces the risk of preeclampsia. Am J Epidemiol 2006;164:470–7.
97. Hernandez-Diaz S, Werler MM, Louik C, et al. Risk of gestational hypertension in relation to folic acid supplementation during pregnancy. Am J Epidemiol 2002;156:806–12.
98. Wu TJ, Buck G, Mendola P. Can regular multivitamin/mineral supplementation modify the relation between maternal smoking and select adverse birth outcomes? Epidemiology 1998;8:179–83.
99. Fawzi WW, Msamanga GI, Spiegelman D, et al. Randomized trial of effects of vitamin supplements on pregnancy outcomes and T cell counts in HIV-1-infected women in Tanzania. Lancet 1998;351:1477–82.
100. Friis H, Gomo E, Nyazema N, et al. Effect of multimicronutrient supplementation on gestational length and birth size: A randomized, placebo-controlled, double-blind effectiveness trial in Zimbabwe. Am J Clin Nutr 2004;80:178–84.

101. Fawzi WW, Msamanga GI, Spiegelman D, et al. A randomized trial of multivitamin supplements and HIV disease progression and mortality. N Engl J Med 2004;351:23–32.
102. Osrin D, Vaidya A, Shrestha Y, et al. Effects of antenatal multiple micronutrient supplementation on birthweight and gestational duration in Nepal: Double-blind, randomized controlled trial. Lancet 2005;365:955–62.
103. Ramakrishnan U, Gonzalez-Cossio T, Neufeld LM, et al. Multiple micronutrient supplementation during pregnancy does not lead to greater infant birth size than does iron-only supplementation: A randomized controlled trial in a semirural community in Mexico. Am J Clin Nutr 2003;77:720–5.
104. Eisenberg DM, Davis RB, Ettner SL, et al. Trends in alternative medicine use in the United States, 1990–1997. JAMA 1998:1569–75.
105. Tsui B, Dennehy CE, Tsourounis C. A survey of dietary supplement use during pregnancy at an academic medical center. Am J Obstet Gynecol 2001;185:433–7.
106. Murphy PA. Alternative therapies for nausea and vomiting of pregnancy. Obstet Gynecol 1998;91:149–55.
107. McFarlin BL, Gibson MH, O'Rear J, et al. A national survey of herbal preparation use by nurse-midwives for labor stimulation. J Nurse Midwifery 1999;44:205–16.
108. Allaire AD, Moos MK, Wells SR. Complementary and alternative medicine in pregnancy: A survey of North Carolina certified nurse-midwives. Obstet Gynecol 2000;95:19–23.
109. Forster DA, Denning A, Wills G, et al. Herbal medicine use during pregnancy in a group of Australian women. Available at: www.biomedcentral.com/1471–2393/6/21/prepub. Accessed June 19, 2006.
110. Refuerzo JS, Blackwell SC, Sokol RJ, et al. Use of over-the-counter medications and herbal remedies in pregnancy. Am J Perinatol 2005;22:321–4.
111. Maats FH, Crowther CA. Patterns of vitamin, mineral and herbal supplement use prior to and during pregnancy. Aust N Z J Obstet Gynaecol 2002;42:494–6.
112. Johns T, Sibeko L. Pregnancy outcome in women using herbal therapies. Birth Defects Res 2003;68:501–4.
113. Ernst E. Herbal medicinal products during pregnancy: Are they safe? BJOG 2002;190:227–35.
114. Marcus DM, Snodgrass WR. Do no harm: Avoidance of herbal medicines during pregnancy. Obstet Gynecol 2005;105:1119–22.
115. Strandberg TE, Andersson S, Jarvenpaa AL, et al. Preterm birth and licorice consumption during pregnancy. Am J Epidemiol 2002;156:803–5.
116. Chuang CH, Doyle P, Wang JD, et al. Herbal medicines used during the first trimester and major congenital malformations. Drug Safety 2006;29:537–48.
117. Lucas M, Dewailly E, Muckle G, et al. Gestational age and birthweight in relation to n-3 fatty acids among Inuit (Canada). Lipids 2004;39:617–26.
118. People's League of Health. Nutrition of expectant and nursing mothers. Lancet 1942;ii:10–12.
119. Olsen SF, Sorensen JD, Secher NJ, et al. Randomized controlled trial of effect of fish-oil supplementation on pregnancy duration. Lancet 1992;339:1003–7.
120. Olsen SF, Secher NJ, Tabor A, et al. Randomized clinical trials of fish oil supplementation in high-risk pregnancies. Br J Obstet Gynaecol 2000;107:382–95.
121. Smuts CM, Huang M, Mundy D, et al. A randomized trial of docosahexaenoic acid supplementation during the third trimester of pregnancy. Obstet Gynecol 2003;101:469–79.
122. Szajewska H, Horvath A, Koletzko B. Effect of n-3 long chain polyunsaturated fatty acid supplementation of women with low-risk pregnancies on pregnancy outcomes and growth measures at birth: A meta-analysis of randomized controlled trials. Am J Clin Nutr 2006;83:1337–44.
123. Jensen CL. Effects of n-3 fatty acids during pregnancy and lactation. Am J Clin Nutr 2006;83:1452S–7S.
124. Thorsdottir I, Birgisdottir BE, Halldorsdottir S, et al. Association of fish and fish liver oil intake in pregnancy with infant size at birth among women of normal weight before pregnancy in a fishing community. Am J Epidemiol 2004;160:460–5.
125. Oken E, Kleinman KP, Olsen SF, et al. Associations of seafood and elongated n-3 fatty acid intake with fetal growth and length of gestation: Results from a US pregnancy cohort. Am J Epidemiol 2004;160:774–83.
126. Kalkwarf HJ, Sprecker BL. Bone mineral changes during pregnancy and lactation. Endocrine 2002;17:49–53.
127. Lamke B, Brundin J, Moberg P. Changes of bone mineral content during pregnancy and lactation. Acta Obstet Gynecol Scand 1977;56:217–9.
128. Christiansen C, Rodbro P, Heinild B. Unchanged total body calcium in normal human pregnancy. Acta Obstet Gynecol Scand 1976;53:141–3.
129. Sowers MF, Crutchfield M, Jannausch M, et al. A prospective evaluation of bone mineral change in pregnancy. Obstet Gynecol 1991;77:841–5.
130. Drinkwater BL, Chestnut CH. Bone density changes during pregnancy and lactation in active women: A longitudinal study. Bone Miner 1991;14:153–60.
131. Sowers MF, Scholl TO, Harris L, et al. Bone loss in adolescent and adult pregnant women. Obstet Gynecol 2000;96:189–93.
132. Aguado F, Revilla M, Hernandez ER, et al. Ultrasonic bone velocity in pregnancy: A longitudinal study. Am J Obstet Gynecol 1998;1016–21.
133. Yamaga A, Taga M, Minaguchi H, et al. Changes in bone mass as determined by ultrasound and biochemical markers of bone turnover during pregnancy and puerperium: A longitudinal study. J Clin Endocrinol Metab 1996;81:752–6.
134. Gambacciani M, Spinetti A, Gallo R, et al. Ultrasound bone characteristics during normal pregnancy: Longitudinal and cross-sectional evaluation. Am J Obstet Gynecol 1995;173:890–3.
135. Matkovic V, Kostial K, Simonovic I, et al. Bone status and fracture rates in two regions of Yugoslavia. Am J Clin Nutr 1979;32:540–9.
136. Sandler RB, Slemenda CW, LaPorte RE, et al. Postmenopausal bone density and milk consumption in childhood and adolescence. Am J Clin Nutr 1985;42:270–4.
137. Scholl TO, Hediger ML, Schall JI. Maternal growth and fetal growth: Pregnancy course and outcome in the Camden Study. Ann N Y Acad Sci 1997;817:281–91.
138. Sowers MF, Wallace RB, Lemke JH. Correlates of forearm bone mass among women during maximal bone mineralization. Prev Med 1985;14:585–96.
139. Sowers MF, Clark K, Wallace R, et al. Prospective study of radial bone mineral density in a geographically defined population of postmenopausal women. Calcif Tissue Int 1991;48:232–9.
140. Fox KM, Magaziner J, Sherwin R, et al. Reproductive correlates of bone mass in elderly women. Study of osteoporotic fractures research group. J Bone Miner Res 1993;8:901-8.
141. Michaelsson K, Baron JA, Faramand BY, et al. Influence of parity and lactation on hip fracture risk. Am J Epidemiol 2001;153:166–72.
142. Goldsmith NF, Johnston JO. Bone mineral: Effects of oral contraceptives, pregnancy, and lactation. J Bone Joint Surg 1975;57:A657–68.
143. Carter OD, Haynes SG. Prevalence rates for scoliosis in U.S. adults: Results from the First National Health and Nutrition Examination Survey. Int J Epidemiol 1987;16:537–44.
144. Ohara N. Calcium metabolism in pregnancy: Disturbed calcium homeostasis in diabetic pregnancy and preeclampsia. Clin Exp Obstet Gynecol 2001;28:133–41.
145. Crowther CA, Hiller JE, Pridmore B, et al. Calcium supplementation in nulliparous women for the prevention of pregnancy-induced hypertension, preeclampsia and preterm birth: An Australian randomized trial. Aust N Z Obstet Gynecol 1999;39:12–8.
146. Belizan JM, Villar J. The relationship between calcium intake and edema-, proteinuria-, and hypertension-gestosis: An hypothesis. Am J Clin Nutr 1980;33:2202–10.
147. Marcoux S, Brisson J, Fabia J. Calcium intake from dairy products and supplements and the risks of preeclampsia and gestational hypertension. Am J Epidemiol 1991;33:1266–72.
148. Repke JT, Villar J. Pregnancy-induced hypertension and low birth weight: The role of calcium. Am J Clin Nutr 1991;54:237S–41S.
149. Belizan JM, Villar J, Gonzalez L, et al. Calcium supplementation to prevent hypertensive disorders of pregnancy. N Engl J Med 1991;325:1399–405.
150. Buchler HC, Guyatt GH, Cook RJ, et al. Effect of calcium supplementation on pregnancy-induced hypertension and preeclampsia. JAMA 1996;275:1113–7.
151. Levine RJ, Hauth JC, Curet LB, et al. Trial of calcium to prevent preeclampsia. N Engl J Med 1997;337:69–76.
152. Lopez-Jaramillo P, Narvaez M, Weigel RM, et al. Calcium supplementation reduces the risk of pregnancy-induced hyper-tension in an Andes population. Br J Obstet Gynaecol 1989;96:648–55.
153. Lopez-Jaramillo P, Narvaez M, Felix C, et al. Dietary calcium supplementation and prevention of pregnancy hypertension. Lancet 1990;335:293–5.
154. Lopez-Jaramillo P, Delgado F, Jacome P, et al. Calcium supplementation and the risk of preeclampsia in Ecuadorian pregnant teenagers. Obstet Gynecol 1997;90: 162–7.
155. Villar J, Abdel-Aleem H, Merialdi M, et al. World Health Organization randomized trial of calcium supplementation among low calcium intake pregnant women. Am J Obstet Gynecol 2006;194:639–49.

27

Human Growth and Disease in Later Life

David J.P. Barker, FRS

INTRODUCTION

Coronary heart disease and the related disorders, stroke, hypertension, and type 2 diabetes, are more common among people whose birthweights were toward the lower end of the normal range. The associations depend on lower birthweights in relation to the duration of gestation rather than the effects of premature birth. They are thought to be consequences of developmental plasticity, the phenomenon by which one genotype can give rise to a range of different physiological or morphological states in response to different environmental conditions during development. Impaired growth in infancy and rapid childhood weight gain exacerbate the effects of impaired prenatal growth. It seems likely that the placenta plays a central role in programming the baby, but as yet little is known about this. Common chronic diseases arise through a series of interactions between environmental influences and the pathways of growth and development that precede them.

There is now clear evidence that the pace and pathway of early growth is a major risk factor for the development of a group of chronic diseases that includes coronary heart disease (CHD) and type 2 diabetes, a disorder which predisposes to cardiovascular disease. This has led to a new "developmental" model for the disease.[1,2] The model proposes that nutrition during fetal life, infancy, and early childhood changes gene expression and thereby establishes functional capacity, metabolic competence, and responses to the later environment.[2,3]

To explore the developmental origins of chronic disease required studies of a kind that had not hitherto been carried out. It was necessary to identify groups of men and women now in middle or late life whose size at birth had been recorded at the time. Their birthweight could thereby be related to the later occurrence of CHD. In Hertfordshire, UK, from 1911 onwards, when women had their babies they were attended by a midwife, who recorded the birthweight. A health visitor went to the baby's home at intervals throughout infancy, and the weight at 1 year was recorded. Table 1 shows the findings in 10,636 men born between 1911 and 1930.[1,4] Hazard ratios for CHD fell with increasing birthweight. There were stronger trends with weight at 1 year. A subsequent study confirmed a similar trend with birthweight among women but no trend with weight at 1 year.[4] Table 2 shows findings for a sample of men who had glucose tolerance tests.[5]

The percentage with impaired glucose tolerance or type 2 diabetes fell steeply with increasing birthweight. The association between low birthweight and CHD has now been replicated among men and women in Europe, North America, and India.[6–12] Low birthweight has been shown to predict altered glucose tolerance in studies of men and women around the world.[13–17] The associations between low birthweight and later disease depend on slow fetal growth rather than premature birth.

Table 1 Hazard Ratios (95% Confidence Intervals) for Death from Coronary Heart Disease According to Weight at Birth and at Age 1 Year in 10,636 Men in Hertfordshire

Weight (lb)	Death from CHD: Before 65 yr	Death from CHD: All Ages
At birth		
≤5.5	1.50 (0.98-2.31)	1.37 (1.00–1.86)
–6.5	1.27 (0.89 to 1.83)	1.29 (1.01 to 1.66)
–7.5	1.17 (0.84 to 1.63)	1.14 (0.91 to 1.44)
–8.5	1.07 (0.77 to 1.49)	1.12 (0.89 to 1.40)
–9.5	0.96 (0.66 to 1.39)	0.97 (0.75 to 1.25)
>9.5	1.00	1.00
p for trend	.001	.005
Age 1 yr		
≤18	2.22 (1.33 to 3.73)	1.89 (1.34 to 2.66)
–20	1.80 (1.11 to 2.93)	1.58 (1.15 to 2.16)
–22	1.96 (1.23 to 3.12)	1.66 (1.23 to 2.25)
–24	1.52 (0.95 to 2.45)	1.36 (1.00 to 1.85)
–26	1.36 (0.82 to 2.26)	1.29 (0.93 to 1.78)
≥27	1.00	1.00
p for trend	<0.001	<0.001

BIOLOGICAL BASIS

Like other living creatures in their early life human beings are "plastic" and able to adapt to their environment. The development of the sweat glands provides a simple example of this. All humans have similar numbers of sweat glands at birth but none of them function. In the first 3 years after birth a proportion of the glands become functional, depending on the temperature to which the child is exposed. The hotter the conditions, the greater the number of sweat glands that are programmed to function. After 3 years the process is complete and the number of sweat glands is fixed. Thereafter, the child who has experienced hot conditions will be better equipped to adapt to similar conditions in later life, because people with more functioning sweat glands cool down faster.

Table 2 Percentage of Men Aged 64 Years with Impaired Glucose Tolerance or Diabetes according to Weight at Birth in 370 Men in Hertfordshire

Weight (lb)	% of Men with 2 h Glucose of ≥7.8 mmol/L	Odds Ratio (95% CI)*
≤5.5	40	6.6 (1.5 to 28)
–6.5	34	4.8 (1.3 to 17)
–7.5	31	4.6 (1.4 to 16)
–8.5	22	2.6 (0.8 to 8.9)
–9.5	13	1.4 (0.3 to 5.6)
>9.5	14	1.0
p for trend	<0.001	

*Adjusted for current body mass index.

This brief description encapsulates the essence of developmental plasticity: a critical period when a system is plastic and sensitive to the environment, followed by loss of plasticity and a fixed functional capacity. For most organs and systems the critical period occurs in utero. There are good reasons it may be advantageous in evolutionary terms for the body to remain plastic during development. It enables the production of phenotypes that are better matched to their environment than would be possible if the same phenotype was produced in all environments. Developmental plasticity is defined as the phenomenon by which one genotype can give rise to a range of different physiological or morphological states in response to different environmental conditions during development.[18] Plasticity during intrauterine life enables animals and humans to receive a "weather forecast" from their mothers that prepares them for the type of world in which they will have to live.[19] If the mother is poorly nourished, she signals to her unborn baby that the environment it is about to enter is likely to be harsh. The baby responds to these signals by adaptations, such as reduced body size and altered metabolism, which help it to survive a shortage of food after birth. In this way plasticity gives a species the ability to make short-term adaptations, within one generation, in addition to the long-term genetic adaptations that come from natural selection. Because, as Mellanby noted long ago, the ability of a human mother to nourish her baby is partly determined when she herself is in utero, and by her childhood growth, the human fetus is receiving a weather forecast based not only on conditions at the time of the pregnancy but on conditions a number of decades before.[3,20] This may be advantageous in populations that experience periodic food shortages.

Until recently we have overlooked a growing body of evidence that systems of the body that are closely related to adult disease, such as the regulation of blood pressure, are also plastic during early development. In animals it is surprisingly easy to produce lifelong changes in the blood pressure and metabolism of a fetus by minor modifications to the diet of the mother before and during pregnancy.[21,22.]

The different size of newborn human babies exemplifies plasticity. The growth of babies has to be constrained by the size of the mother, otherwise normal birth could not occur. Small women have small babies: in pregnancies after ovum donation they have small babies even if the woman donating the egg is large.[23] Babies may be small because their growth is constrained in this way or because they lack the nutrients for growth. As McCance wrote, "The size attained *in utero* depends on the services which the mother is able to supply. These are mainly food and accommodation.[24]" Research into the developmental origins of disease has focussed on the nutrient supply to the baby, while recognizing that other influences, such as hypoxia, stress, and maternal size also influence fetal growth. This focus on fetal nutrition was endorsed in a recent review.[25] The availability of nutrients to the fetus is influenced by the mother's nutrient stores and metabolism, as well as by her diet during pregnancy. In developing countries many babies are undernourished because their mothers are chronically malnourished. Despite current levels of nutrition in Western countries, the nutrition of many fetuses and infants remains suboptimal because the nutrients available are unbalanced or because their delivery is constrained by maternal metabolism. Globally, size at birth in relation to gestational age is a marker of fetal nutrition.[25]

A striking feature of the associations between birthweight and later disease is that they are graded, extending across the entire range of birthweights. This implies that what were regarded as normal variations in the delivery of nutrients to the human fetus have profound long-term effects on the health of the next generation.[3]

DEVELOPMENTAL ORIGINS HYPOTHESIS

The developmental origins hypothesis proposes that CHD, stroke, hypertension, and type 2 diabetes originate in developmental plasticity, in response to undernutrition during fetal life and infancy.[2,26] Why should fetal responses to undernutrition lead to disease in later life? The general answer is clear: "life history theory," which embraces all living things, states that during development increased allocation of energy to one trait, such as brain growth, necessarily reduces allocation to one or more other traits, such as tissue repair processes. Smaller babies, who have had a lesser allocation of energy, must incur higher costs and these, it seems, include disease in later life. A more specific answer to the question is that people who were small at birth are vulnerable to later disease through three kinds of process. First, they have less functional capacity in key organs, such as the kidney: one theory holds that hypertension is initiated by the reduced number of glomeruli found in people who were small at birth.[27] A second process is the setting of hormones and metabolism. An undernourished baby may establish a "thrifty" way of handling food. Insulin resistance, which is associated with low birthweight, may be viewed as persistence of a fetal response by which blood glucose concentrations were maintained for the benefit of the brain but at the expense of glucose transport into the muscles and muscle growth.[28]

A third link between low birthweight and later disease is that people who were small at birth are more vulnerable to adverse environmental influences in later life. Observations on animals show that the environment during development permanently changes not only the body's structure and function but also its responses to environmental influences encountered in later life.[19] Table 3 shows the effect of low income in adult life on CHD among men in Helsinki.[29] As expected, men who had a low taxable income had higher rates of the disease There is no agreed explanation for this but the association between poverty and CHD is a major component of the social inequalities in health in many western countries. Among the men in Helsinki the association was confined to men who had slow fetal growth and were thin at birth, defined by a ponderal index (birthweight/length^3) of less than 26 kg/m^3 (Table 3). Men who were not thin at birth showed no association of CHD with income, which implies that they were resilient to the effects of low income.

One explanation for these findings emphasizes the psychosocial consequences of a low position in the social hierarchy, as indicated by low income and social class, and suggests that perceptions of low social status and lack of success lead to changes in neuroendocrine pathways and hence to disease.[30] The findings in Helsinki seem consistent with this. People who were small at birth are known to have persisting alterations in responses to stress, including raised serum cortisol concentrations.[31] It is suggested that persisting small elevations of cortisol concentrations for many years may have effects similar to those seen when tumors lead to more sudden, large increases in glucocorticoid concentrations. People with Cushing's syndrome, the result of overactivity of the adrenal cortex, are insulin-resistant and have raised blood pressure, both of which predispose to CHD.

INFANT AND CHILDHOOD GROWTH AND CORONARY HEART DISEASE

Figure 1 shows the growth of 357 men who were either admitted to hospital with CHD or died from it.[32] They belong to a cohort of 4,630 men who were born in Helsinki. Their mean height, weight, and body mass index (BMI, weight/height^2) at each month from birth to 2 years of age, and at each year from 2 to 11 years of age, are expressed as standard deviations (z scores). The mean z score for the cohort is set at zero and a boy maintaining a steady position as tall or short, or fat or thin, in relation to other boys would follow a horizontal path in Figure 1. The mean body size of the boys who later had CHD was approximately 0.2 standard deviations below the average and they were thin. Between birth and 2 years of age, mean z scores for each measurement fell, so that at 2 years the boys were thin and short. After 2 years of age their z scores for BMI began to increase and continued to do so. In a simultaneous regression, both low BMI at 2 years of age and high BMI at 11 years of age were associated with later coronary events ($p < .001$ and $p = .05$ respectively). When BMI at birth was added to the model, the measurements of body size at each of the three ages were associated with later coronary events ($p = .04$ for low BMI at birth, $p = .001$ for low BMI at 2 years of age, and $p = .03$ for high BMI at 11 years of age).

As with the boys, the mean body size of the 87 girls who later had coronary events was below the average (Figure 1). They tended to be short at birth rather than thin, but their mean z scores for BMI fell progressively after birth so that, like the boys, they were thin at 2 years of age. After 4 years of age the z scores began to increase and continued to do so, reaching the average at

Table 3 Hazard Ratios (95% CI) for Coronary Heart Disease in 3,629 Men in Helsinki According to Ponderal Index at Birth (Birthweight/Length^3) and Household Income in Adult Life

Household Income in £/Yr	Ponderal Index ≤ 26.0 kg/m^3 (n = 1,475)	Ponderal Index > 26.0 kg/m^3 (n = 2,154)
>15,700	1.00	1.19 (0.65 to 2.19)
15,700	1.54 (0.83 to 2.87)	1.42 (0.78 to 2.57)
12,400	1.07 (0.51 to 2.22)	1.66 (0.90 to 3.07)
10,700	2.07 (1.13 to 3.79)	1.44 (0.79 to 2.62)
≤8,400	2.58 (1.45 to 4.60)	1.37 (0.75 to 2.51)
p for trend	<.001	.75

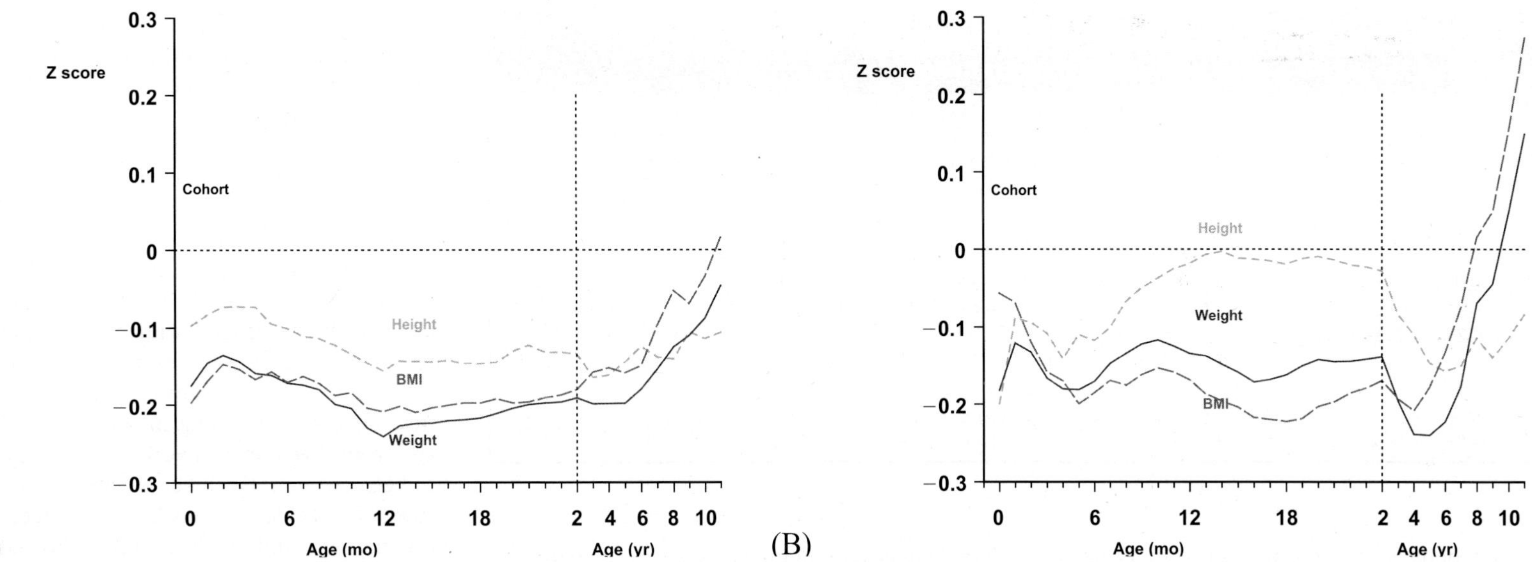

Figure 1 Mean *z* scores for height, weight, and body mass index in the first 11 years after birth among **(A)** boys and **(B)** girls who had coronary heart disease as adults. The mean values for all boys and all girls are set at zero, with deviations from the mean expressed as standard deviations (*z* scores).

approximately 8 years of age. Similarly to the boys, in a simultaneous regression body size at each of the three ages was associated with later coronary events ($p = .02$ for short length at birth, $p = .002$ for low BMI at 2 years of age, and $p = .02$ for high BMI at 11 years of age).

In Table 4 findings for boys and girls have been combined to show the simultaneous effect of birth weight and BMI at 2 years of age, divided into three, on hazard ratios for coronary events. The highest hazard ratios were among subjects with birthweights below 3.0 kg and BMIs at 2 years of age of 17 kg/m^2 or less. Table 5 shows the simultaneous effects of BMI at 2 and 11 years of age. The highest hazard ratios were among people with BMIs below 16 kg/m^2 at 2 years of age and above 17.5 kg/m^2 at 11 years of age. The hazard ratios in Tables 4 and 5 were a little changed if they were adjusted for socioeconomic status or income in adult life.

These observations demonstrate that CHD is independently associated with both prenatal and postnatal growth.[33] One explanation of the associations with small body size at birth and thinness at 2 years of age is that babies who are thin or short at birth and during infancy lack muscle, a deficiency that will persist into childhood as there is little cell replication in muscle after around 1 year of age.[34] Rapid weight gain in childhood may lead to a disproportionately high fat mass in relation to muscle mass. This could underlie the strong associations between low birthweight, low BMI at 2, and high BMI at 11 and later insulin resistance, which was found when 2,003 subjects in the Helsinki cohort were examined at the age of 62 years.[32]

The Helsinki study gives no support to the recent hypothesis that promoting early growth with high intake of nutrients in the first few months after birth will adversely affect cardiovascular health.[35] This hypothesis arose from studies of intermediary markers among young people born prematurely. In the Helsinki cohort at any birthweight and at any period up to 2 years of age, greater weight gain was associated with a lower incidence of CHD in later life.

Table 4 Hazard Ratios (95% Confidence Intervals) for Coronary Heart Disease According to Birthweight and Body Mass Index (BMI) at 2 Years of Age for Boys and Girls Combined

	BMI at Age 2 (kg/m^2)		
Birthweight (kg)	<16	16 to 17	>17
<3.0	1.9 (1.3 to 2.8)	1.9 (1.2 to 3.0)	1.3 (0.7 to 2.2)
3.0 to 3.5	1.5 (1.0 to 2.1)	1.6 (1.1 to 2.2)	1.2 (0.8 to 1.8)
>3.5	1.7 (1.2 to 2.5)	1.5 (1.1 to 2.2)	1.0

Table 5 Hazard Ratios (95% Confidence Intervals) for Coronary Heart Disease According to Body Mass Index (BMI) at 2 and 11 Years of Age for Boys and Girls Combined

	BMI at Age 11 (kg/m^2)		
BMI at Age 2 (kg/m^2)	<16	16 to 17.5	>17.5
<16	1.6 (0.8 to 3.3)	2.4 (1.2 to 4.9)	3.0 (1.4 to 6.3)
16 to 17	1.4 (0.7 to 3.1)	1.6 (0.8 to 3.3)	1.9 (0.9 to 3.9)
>17	1.0	1.3 (0.6 to 2.7)	1.1 (0.5 to 2.3)

TYPE 2 DIABETES AND HYPERTENSION

People who were small at birth remain biologically different to people who were larger, and these differences include an increased susceptibility to type 2 diabetes and hypertension. Table 6 shows odds ratios for these two disorders according to birthweight and fourths of BMI at age 11 years. The two disorders are associated with the same general pattern of growth as CHD.[26] Risk of disease falls with increasing birthweight and rises with increasing BMI.

Associations between low birthweight and type 2 diabetes shown in Table 2 have been found in other studies.[5,13–17] The association with hypertension has also been found elsewhere.[36] There is a substantial body of literature showing that birthweight is associated with differences in insulin sensitivity and blood pressure within the normal range.[5,13,17,37] These differences are found in children and adults but they tend to be small. A 1 kg difference in birthweight is associated with around 3 mm Hg difference in systolic pressure. The contrast between this small effect and the large effect on hypertension (see Table 6) suggests that lesions that accompany poor fetal growth and that tend to elevate blood pressure, and which may include a reduced number of glomeruli, have a small influence on blood pressure within the normal range because counter-regulatory mechanisms maintain normal blood pressure levels. As the lesions progress, however, possibly through hyperfiltration of the reduced number of glomeruli and consequent glomerulosclerosis, these mechanisms are no longer able to maintain homeostasis. This may initiate a cycle of rise in blood pressure resulting in further progression of the lesions and further rise in blood pressure.[27,38] Rapid increase in body size after birth may exacerbate glomerular injury because

Table 6 Odds Ratios (95% Confidence Intervals) for Type 2 Diabetes and Hypertension According to Birthweight and BMI at Age 11 Years Among 13,517 Men and Women in Helsinki

	BMI at Age 11 (kg/m^2)			
Birthweight (kg)	<15.7	−16.6	−17.6	>17.6
Type 2 diabetes (698 cases)				
<3.0	1.3 (0.6 to 2.8)	1.3 (0.6 to 2.8)	1.5 (0.7 to 3.4)	2.5 (1.2 to 5.5)
−3.5	1.0 (0.5 to 2.1)	1.0 (0.5 to 2.1)	1.5 (0.7 to 3.2)	1.7 (0.8 to 3.5)
−4.0	1.0 (0.5 to 2.2)	0.9 (0.4 to 1.9)	0.9 (0.4 to 2.0)	1.7 (0.8 to 3.6)
>4.0	1.0	1.1 (0.4 to 2.7)	0.7 (0.3 to 1.7)	1.2 (0.5 to 2.7)
Hypertension (2,997 cases)				
<3.0	2.0 (1.3 to 3.2)	1.9 (1.2 to 3.1)	1.9 (1.2 to 3.0)	2.3 (1.5 to 3.8)
−3.5	1.7 (1.1 to 2.6)	1.9 (1.2 to 2.9)	1.9 (1.2 to 3.0)	2.2 (1.4 to 3.4)
−4.0	1.7 (1.0 to 2.6)	1.7 (1.1 to 2.6)	1.5 (1.0 to 2.4)	1.9 (1.2 to 2.9)
>4.0	1.0	1.9 (1.1 to 3.1)	1.0 (0.6 to 1.7)	1.7 (1.1 to 2.8)

greater body size leads to increased excretory loads and glomerular hyperfiltration.[39] Direct evidence in support of this has come from a study of the kidneys of people killed in road accidents. Those being treated for hypertension had fewer, but larger, glomeruli.[40]

THE ROLE OF THE PLACENTA

Table 7 shows the systolic pressures of a group of men and women who were born at term.[41] They are grouped according to their birthweight and placental weight. As expected systolic pressures fall between those with low birthweight and high birthweight. In addition the pressures increase with increasing placental weight. People with a mean systolic pressure of 150 mm Hg or more, a level used to define hypertension, comprise a group who as babies were relatively small in relation to the size of their placentas. In Table 7 the fall in pressures of 10 mm Hg across the range of birthweight is statistically opposed by the rise of 12 mm Hg associated with increasing placental weight. These large trends are concealed when all pressures at a given birthweight are combined as in the right-hand column.

In studies of children and adults the association between placental enlargement and raised blood pressure has been inconsistent.[42] Animal studies offer a possible explanation of this. In sheep the placenta enlarges in response to moderate undernutrition in mid-pregnancy.[43] This is thought to be an adaptive response to extract more nutrients from the mother. It is not, however, a consistent response but occurs only in ewes that were well nourished when they conceived. In the Helsinki birth cohort people who had both hypertension and type 2 diabetes had slow placental weight at birth, whereas those with hypertension alone had large placental weight in relation to birthweight.[44] These statistically opposing trends may also explain why some studies have failed to find associations between placental weight and later blood pressure.

Animal studies show that the placenta is highly responsive to hypoxia and maternal undernutrition. The inconsistency of the epidemiological findings has led some researchers to discount its role in programming. This seems premature as placental biology suggests that it will play a central role, though one about which remarkably little is known.

PATHWAYS TO DISEASE

New studies, especially the Helsinki studies with their detailed information on child growth and socioeconomic circumstances, increasingly suggest that the pathogenesis of CHD and the disorders related to it depend on a series of interactions occurring at different stages of development. To begin with, the effects of the genes acquired at conception may be conditioned by the early environment. Table 8 is based on a study of 476 elderly people in Helsinki.[45] It shows mean fasting plasma insulin concentrations according to which of two polymorphisms of the peroxisome proliferators-activated receptor (PPAR)-γ gene was present. The Pro12Pro polymorphism is known to be associated with insulin resistance, indicated by elevated fasting plasma insulin concentrations. Table 8 shows, however, that this effect occurs only among men and women who had low birthweight. Conversely, low birthweight has been consistently linked to later insulin resistance,[28] but Table 8 shows that this effect occurs only among people with the Pro12Pro polymorphism. As birthweight serves as a marker of fetal nutrition,[25] this gene birthweight interaction may reflect a gene–nutrient interaction during development.

The effects of the intrauterine environment on later disease are conditioned not only by events at conception but also by events after birth. Table 6 shows how the effects are conditioned by childhood BMI. Table 3 shows that the effects of low ponderal index at birth are conditioned by living conditions in adult life. Table 9 shows how the

Table 7 Mean Systolic Blood Pressure (mmHg) of Men and Women Aged 50, Born after 38 Weeks Completed Weeks of Gestation, According to Placental Weight and Birthweight

	Placental Weight, lb (g)				
Birthweight, lb (kg)	≤1.0 (454)	−1.25 (568)	−1.5 (681)	>1.5 (681)	All
−6.5 (2.9)	149	152	151	167	152
−7.5 (3.4)	139	148	146	159	148
>7.5 (3.4)	131	143	148	153	149
All	144	148	148	156	149

Table 8 Mean Fasting Insulin Concentrations (pmol/L) in Elderly People in Helsinki According to Peroxisome Proliferators-Activated Receptor (PPAR)-γ Gene Polymorphism and Birthweight

	Birthweight (kg)			
	<3.0	3.0 to 3.5	>3.5	*p* for trend
Pro12Pro	84 (56)*	71 (161)	65 (107)	.003
Pro12Ala/Ala12Ala	60 (37)	60 (67)	65 (48)	.31
p for difference	.008	.02	.99	

*Figures in parentheses are numbers of subjects.

Table 9 Cumulative Incidence (%) of Hypertension According to Birthweight and Father's Social Class in 8,760 Men and Women in Helsinki

	Father's Social Class			
Birthweight (g)	Laborer	Lower Middle Class	Upper Middle Class	*p* for Trend
<3,000	22.2	20.2	10.5	.002
−3,500	18.8	15.2	10.6	<.001
−4,000	14.5	12.5	10.3	.04
>4,000	11.1	15.6	15.7	.11
p for trend	<.001	.05	.79	

effects of low birthweight on later hypertension are conditioned by living conditions in childhood, indicated by the occupational status of the father.[46] Among all the men and women, low birthweight was associated with an increased incidence of hypertension, as has been shown before.[36] This association, however, was present only among those who were born into families where the father was a laborer or of lower middle class.

It seems that the pathogenesis of cardiovascular disease and type 2 diabetes cannot be understood within a model in which risks associated with adverse influences at different stages of life add to each other. Rather, disease is the product of branching paths of development. The environment triggers the branchings. The pathways determine the vulnerability of each individual to what lies ahead.[39,47]

A clinical study of 2003 people within the Helsinki birth cohort showed that two different paths of fetal, infant, and childhood growth preceded the development of hypertension in adult life (unpublished). In one, which was associated with more severe hypertension in people who tended to be overweight, small body size at birth, and during infancy were followed by rapid weight gain, so that at age 11 years the children's body size was around the average. This is the same path of growth that led to insulin resistance and CHD (Figure 1) in the other path of growth, which was associated with less severe hypertension, slow linear growth in utero, and during infancy were followed by persisting small body size so that at age 11 years the children were short and thin. A similar path of growth leads to stroke.[48] One possible process underlying this is that slow growth is associated with impaired development of the cerebral vasculature during a period of rapid brain growth, and also with altered lever metabolism and the development of an atherogenic liver profile. The two different paths of growth may lead to hypertension through different biological mechanisms and may produce two groups of patients who respond differently to medication.

We are beginning to understand the processes through which different paths of development initiate hypertension.[39] The changes occur at different levels and include allocation of stem cells and alteration of gene expression in the embryo, changes in renal growth, and alteration in haemostatic set-points that control blood pressure. These changes can make the affected systems more vulnerable to disruptive influences in postnatal life, which include rapid weight gain, oxidative stress, environmental stress, and a high salt intake.

REFERENCES

1. Barker DJP, Osmond C, Winter PD, et al. Weight in infancy and death from ischaemic heart disease. Lancet 1989;2:577–80.
2. Barker DJP. Fetal origins of coronary heart disease. BMJ 1995;311:171–4.
3. Jackson AA. All that glitters. Br Nutr Found Nutr Bull 2000;25:11–24.
4. Osmond C, Barker DJP, Winter PD, et al. Early growth and death from cardiovascular disease in women. BMJ 1993;307:1519–24.
5. Hales CN, Barker DJP, Clark PMS, et al. Fetal and infant growth and impaired glucose tolerance at age 64. BMJ 1991;303:1019–22.
6. Frankel S, Elwood P, Sweetnam P, et al. Birthweight, body mass index in middle age, and incident coronary heart disease. Lancet 1996;348:1478–80.
7. Stein CE, Fall CHD, Kumaran K, et al. Fetal growth and coronary heart disease in South India. Lancet 1996;348:1269–73.
8. Rich-Edwards JW, Stampfer MJ, Manson JE, et al. Birth weight and risk of cardiovascular disease in a cohort of women followed up since 1976. BMJ 1997;315:396–400.
9. Forsén T, Eriksson JG, Tuomilehto J, et al. Mother's weight in pregnancy and coronary heart disease in a cohort of Finnish men: Follow up study. BMJ 1997;315:837–40.
10. Leon DA, Lithell HO, Vagero D, et al. Reduced fetal growth rate and increased risk of death from ischaemic heart disease: Cohort study of 15,000 Swedish men and women born 1915–29. BMJ 1998;317:241–5.
11. Forsén T, Eriksson JG, Tuomilehto J, et al. Growth in utero and during childhood among women who develop coronary heart disease: Longitudinal study. BMJ 1999;319:1403–7.
12. Forsén T, Osmond C, Eriksson JG, et al. Growth of girls who later develop coronary heart disease. Heart 2004;90:20–4.
13. Lithell HO, McKeigue PM, Berglund L, et al. Relation of size at birth to non-insulin dependent diabetes and insulin concentrations in men aged 50–60 years. BMJ 1996;312:406–10.
14. McCance DR, Pettitt DJ, Hanson RL, et al. Birth weight and non-insulin dependent diabetes: Thrifty genotype, thrifty phenotype, or surviving small baby genotype? BMJ 1994;308:942–5.
15. Forsén T, Eriksson J, Tuomilehto J, et al. The fetal and childhood growth of persons who develop type 2 diabetes. Ann Intern Med 2000;133:176–82.
16. Rich-Edwards JW, Colditz GA, Stampfer MJ, et al. Birthweight and the risk for type 2 diabetes mellitus in adult women. Ann Intern Med 1999;130:278–84.
17. Newsome CA, Shiell AW, Fall CHD, et al. Is birthweight related to later glucose and insulin metabolism? A systematic review. Diabet Med 2003;20:339–48.
18. West-Eberhard MJ. Phenotypic plasticity and the origins of diversity. Ann Rev Ecolo System 1989;20:249.
19. Bateson P, Martin P. Design for a Life: How Behaviour Develops. London: Jonathan Cape; 1999.
20. Mellanby E. Nutrition and child-bearing. Lancet 1933;2:1131–7.
21. Widdowson EM, McCance RA. The effect of finite periods of undernutrition at different ages on the composition and subsequent development of the rat. Proc R Soc Lond B 1963;158:329–42.
22. Kwong WY, Wild A, Roberts P, et al. Maternal undernutrition during the pre-implantation period of rat development causes blastocyst abnormalities and programming of postnatal hypertension. Development 2000;127: 4195–202.
23. Brooks AA, Johnson MR, Steer PJ, et al. Birth weight: Nature or nurture? Early Hum Dev 1995;42:29–35.
24. McCance RA. Food, growth and time. Lancet 1962;2:621–6.
25. Harding JE. The nutritional basis of the fetal origins of adult disease. Int J Epidemiol 2001;30:15–23.
26. Barker DJP, Eriksson JG, Forsén T, et al. Fetal origins of adult disease: Strength of effects and biological basis. Int J Epidemiol 2002;31:1235–39.
27. Brenner BM, Chertow GM. Congenital oligonephropathy: An inborn cause of adult hypertension and progressive renal injury? Curr Opin Nephrol Hypertens 1993;2:691–5.
28. Phillips DIW. Insulin resistance as a programmed response to fetal undernutrition. Diabetologia 1996;39:1119–22.
29. Barker DJP, Forsén T, Uutela A, et al. Size at birth and resilience to the effects of poor living conditions in adult life: Longitudinal study. BMJ 2001;323:1273–76.
30. Marmot M, Wilkinson RG. Psychosocial and material pathways in the relation between income and health: A response to Lynch et al. BMJ 2001;322:1233–6.
31. Phillips DIW, Walker BR, Reynolds RM, et al. Low birth weight predicts elevated plasma cortisol concentrations in adults from 3 populations. Hypertension 2000;35:1301–6.
32. Barker DJP, Osmond C, Forsén TJ, et al. Trajectories of growth among children who have coronary events as adults. N Engl J Med 2005;353:1802–9.
33. Dietz WH. Overweight in childhood and adolescence. N Engl J Med 2004;350:855–7.
34. Widdowson EM, Crabb DE, Milner RDG. Cellular development of some human organs before birth. Arch Dis Child 1972;47:652–5.
35. Singhal A, Lucas A. Early origins of cardiovascular disease: Is there a unifying hypothesis? Lancet 2004;363:1642–5.
36. Curhan GC, Chertow GM, Willett WC, et al. Birth weight and adult hypertension and obesity in women. Circulation 1996;94:1310–5.
37. Huxley RR, Shiell AW, Law CM. The role of size at birth and postnatal catch-up growth in determining systolic blood pressure: A systematic review of the literature. J Hypertens 2000;18:815–31.
38. Ingelfinger JR. Is microanatomy destiny? N Engl J Med 2003;348:99–100.
39. Barker DJP, Bagby S, Hanson M. Mechanisms of disease: in utero programming in the pathogenesis of hypertension. Nat Clin Pract Nephrol 2006;2:700–7.
40. Keller G, Zimmer G, Mall G, et al. Nephron number in patients with primary hypertension. N Engl J Med 2003;348:101–8.
41. Barker DJP, Bull AR, Osmond C, et al. Fetal and placental size and risk of hypertension in adult life. Br Med J 1990;301:259–62.
42. Whincup PH, Cook D, Papacosta O, et al. Birthweight and blood pressure: Cross-sectional and longitudinal relations in childhood. Br Med J 1995;311:773–6.
43. McCrabb GJ, Egan AR, Hosking BJ. Maternal undernutrition during mid-pregnancy in sheep; variable effects on placental growth. J Agric.Sci 1992;118:127–32.
44. Eriksson J, Forsen T, Tuomilheto J, et al. Fetal and childhood growth and hypertension in adult life. Hypertension 2000;36:790–4.
45. Eriksson JG, Lindi V, Uusitupa M, et al. The effects of the Pro12Ala polymorphism of the peroxisome proliferators-activated receptor-γ2 gene on insulin sensitivity and insulin metabolism interact with size at birth. Diabetes 2002;51:2321–4.
46. Barker DJP, Forsén T, Eriksson JG, et al. Growth and living conditions in childhood and hypertension in adult life: Longitudinal study. J Hypertens 2002;20:1951–6.
47. Barker DJP. Birthweight and hypertension. Hypertension 2006;48:357–8.
48. Osmond C, Kajantie E, Forsén T, et al. Infant growth and stroke in adult life: The Helsinki birth cohort. Stroke 2007;38:264–70.

28

Development of the Fetus: Carbohydrate and Lipid Metabolism

William W. Hay, Jr., MD

The rapid rates of metabolism and growth of the placenta and fetus require ready sources of carbon for energy production and deposition in energy stores (adipose tissue and glycogen) and structural tissues (proteins). Maternal plasma glucose provides most of the carbon for placental and fetal energy requirements. As much as 20 to 30% of the amino acids taken up by the fetus may be oxidized, however, providing most of the additional carbon necessary to meet the fetal requirements for oxidation. Glucose carbon also gets to the fetus as lactate that is produced in the placenta. Twenty to forty percent of glucose carbon is also deposited in growing body tissues; most of this goes to glycogen, some to protein, and some to adipose tissue. Lipid, on the other hand, appears to be directed primarily to growth, as there is little capacity to oxidize long-chain fatty acids in fetal tissues. Lipids account for fetal growth through the provision of essential fatty acids (EFAs) supplied to developing structural membranes. Fatty acids also account for fetal growth through adipose tissue development and growth.[1–5]

Based on experimental data from late-gestation fetal sheep, and estimated data from term human fetuses, it is possible to construct reasonable estimates for the rates of carbon supply to the fetus from glucose (including products of glucose metabolism in the placenta such as lactate and fructose) and amino acids, as well as for fatty acids, and to compare these rates with requirements for energy production and storage. Such estimates are shown in Table 1.[5–7]

Table 1 Nutrient Substrate Balance in Late Gestation Fetal Sheep and Humans

Carbon–Calorie Balance	Carbon (g/kg/d)	Calories (kcal/kg/d)
Requirement		
Accretion in carcass: non fat (sheep)	3.2	32
Accretion in carcass: non fat (human)	3.2	32
Accretion in carcass: fat (human)	3.5	33
Excretion as CO_2	4.4	0
Excretion as urea	0.2	2
Excretion as glutamate	0.3	2
Heat (measured as O_2 consumption)	0.0	50
Total		
Without fat (sheep)	8.1	86
With fat (human)	11.6	119
Uptake		
Amino acids (sheep and human)	3.9	45
Glucose (sheep)	2.4	17
Glucose (human)	3.7	26
Lactate (sheep)	1.4	14
Lactate (human)	1.7	21
Fructose (sheep)	1.0	7
Acetate (sheep)	0.2	3
Fatty Acids (human)	1.1–2.2	17–34
Total		
Sheep	8.9	86
Human	10.4–11.5	109–126

Adapted from references 5–7.

CARBOHYDRATES

Sources of Glucose for the Placenta and Fetus

Maternal Glucose Supply. Maternal plasma glucose provides all of the glucose for the placenta and fetus, except under relatively uncommon conditions of prolonged maternal hypoglycemia or fetal hypoxemia when the fetus can produce its own glucose by glycogenolysis or gluconeogenesis. The placenta can also use its own glycogen for glycolysis, but insufficient glucose-6-phosphatase has been found in the placenta for its glycogen to be available for production into the fetal circulation. Qualitative evidence demonstrating that maternal glucose is the sole source of glucose for the placenta and fetus under normal conditions comes from studies in which tracers of glucose that are infused into the mother have the same specific activity or enrichment (ratio of tracer glucose to unlabeled glucose) in blood sampled from the fetus, indicating no dilution of fetal glucose with glucose other than from the maternal circulation.[8,9] Quantitative evidence to support these observations has come from tracer studies in the fetal sheep during fed, normoglycemic conditions.[9–11] In these studies, net uptake of glucose by the fetus from the placenta equals fetal glucose utilization; that is, there is no source of glucose for fetal glucose utilization other than what comes from the mother by way of the placenta.

Fetal Glucose Production. Only after prolonged periods (several days) of decreased fetal glucose supply, producing sustained fetal hypoglycemia and hypoinsulinemia, does fetal glucose utilization exceed supply, demonstrating a new source of fetal glucose production.[12] A natural onset of fetal glucose production does tend to develop in late gestation.[13] Most species appear to have sufficient functional activities of hepatic gluconeogenic enzymes in late fetal life, except the rat, in which mitochondrial PEPCK (phosphoenolpyruvate carboxykinase) develops only after birth.[14] Thyroid hormone is also essential for glucogenesis, acting on both the hepatic glucogenic pathways and on the mechanisms activating glucogenesis. These thyroid effects include upregulation of catecholamine secretion and effects and increased or maintained concentrations of enzymes necessary for glucose production such as glucose-6-phosphatase, fructose diphosphatase, and alanine aminotransferase.[15]

In the case of selective hypoinsulinemia, produced for example by injection of streptozotocin, a drug that destroys the pancreatic insulin-producing β-cells,[16] or by fetal pancreatectomy,[17] fetal glucose concentration actually increases. At the same time, fetal glucose utilization rate remains near normal despite up to 70 to 80% reduction in glucose supplied by the placenta. Infusion of glucose into these animals increases glucose utilization rate but does not appear to decrease the rate of fetal glucose production. Only by reinfusion of insulin to normal or higher-than-normal levels can this glucose production by the fetus be diminished. Thus, fetal plasma insulin concentration appears to be a more important and more specific regulator of fetal glucose production than fetal glucose supply or concentration.

Fetal glucose production can also come from glycogenolysis. The principal source of fetal hepatic glycogen is fetal plasma glucose. Circulating lactate[14] and certain amino acids such as alanine,[18,19] serine,[20] and glutamine[21] can label fetal glycogen. In vivo and in vitro studies with magnetic resonance spectroscopy using ^{13}C-labeled glucose indicate that only about 10% of glycogen (at least in the fetal sheep) could come from nonglucose precursors, that is, by the indirect pathway of reverse glycolysis (DiGiacomo, Battaglia, Shapiro, Chang, and Hay, unpublished data). Glycogen accumulates progressively toward term in most organs.[22] Lung glycogen content decreases late in gestation, however, presumably as part of surfactant production, although this issue is controversial. Glycogenolysis in the fetus is rapidly activated by catecholamine infusion, glucagon injection, and hypoxemia/ischemia[23];

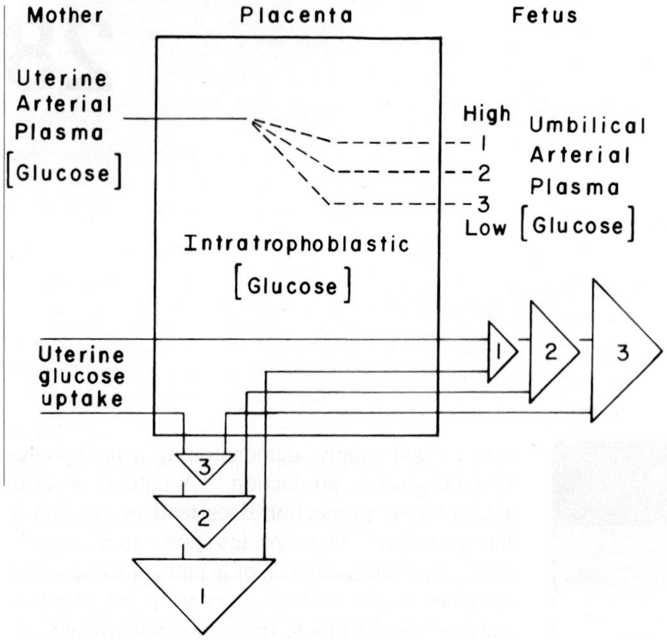

Figure 1 Schema of effects of fetal glucose concentration of placental glucose transfer to the fetus and uteroplacental glucose consumption, adapted from data in sheep. A decrease in fetal glucose concentration relative to maternal glucose concentration promotes maternal-to-fetal glucose transfer at the expense of uteroplacental glucose consumption. These findings demonstrate a reciprocal relationship between placental glucose transfer and uteroplacental glucose consumption that is determined by the fetal glucose concentration. (Reproduced with permission of the Nutrition Society.[2])

all of the enzymes necessary for glycogenolysis are present early in gestation.[24]

Mechanisms of Placental Glucose Uptake and Transport

A principal action of fetal glucose production, regardless of cause or mechanism, is to divert uterine glucose supply to the placenta. As shown in Figure 1, an increase in fetal glucose concentration that is independent of the maternal glucose concentration can separately regulate the partition of uterine glucose uptake into glucose transfer to the fetus and uteroplacental glucose consumption. This observation demonstrates complex regulation of glucose uptake, metabolism, and transfer to the fetus by the placenta.

Maternal Glucose Concentration. Glucose enters the placenta and fetus from the maternal circulation according to concentration-dependent mechanisms, making the maternal plasma glucose concentration the principal regulator of placental and fetal glucose supply.[25] Maternal glucose concentration tends to decrease slightly during the second half of gestation,[26] the balance of two opposing forces: (1) it tends to decrease from the increasing consumption of glucose by the growing placenta and fetus; (2) it tends to increase from the development of maternal insulin resistance and glucose intolerance caused by certain hormones (perhaps, eg, placental lactogen, progesterone, prolactin, estrogen, and glucocorticoids)[27] and certain competitive substrates (eg, fatty acids).[28] In women who develop overt diabetes mellitus with insulin resistance and glucose intolerance during late gestation, the insulin resistance appears to be the primary defect. Studies by Friedman and colleagues indicate that the mechanism for this insulin resistance involves alterations in the insulin signal transduction cascade independent of hormonal influence, as well as potentially significant effects of placental growth hormone.[29–31]

Placental Glucose Transporters. Glucose uptake and transport by the placenta are mediated by facilitative transporter proteins. Both glucose transporter-1 (Glut-1) (all species) and Glut-3 (human, rat, sheep) isoforms have been identified at both the maternal-facing microvillous trophoblast membrane and the fetal-facing basal trophoblast membrane,[32] although quantitative distribution has varied among studies and species.

Glut-4 has also been found in the human placenta, but there is no evidence that insulin signal transduction activates its translocation or increases glucose uptake. One recent study, however, showed increased glucose uptake in perfused human placentas from insulin-treated diabetic women; the mechanism for such an effect is not known.[33] In another study, JAr placental cells showed stimulation of mitogenesis via the MAPK (mitogen activated protein kinase) signaling pathway but did not show insulin stimulation of PI3-kinase-dependent PKB (protein kinase B) activation sufficient to stimulate glucose transport or glycogen synthesis, highlighting the placenta as a nonclassic target organ of insulin regulation of glucose metabolism.[34]

In the human placenta, Glut-1 is the principal transporter at the maternal-facing microvillous membrane while Glut-3 shows up more on the fetal-facing basal membrane or localized in extravillous trophoblast and villous cytotrophoblast cells.[35] Hahn and coworkers found that hyperglycemia downregulates the Glut-1 glucose transport system in term placental trophoblast studied in vitro by downregulating both Glut-1 protein concentration and translocating membrane Glut-1 protein to intracellular sites where they would be less or not effective in mediating glucose.[36] In contrast, Illsely and colleagues have suggested that hyperglycemia in diabetic pregnancies enhances fetal-glucose-stimulated insulin and (insulin-like growth factor) IGF-1 production, the latter acting to promote Glut-1 at the fetal-facing basal trophoblast membrane, thereby maintaining an increased placental glucose transport capacity.[37–39] To date, however, there is no in vivo evidence for this mechanism, except for increased fetal-facing basal membrane Glut-1 protein concentrations in placentas from diabetic pregnancies. Hyperglycemia itself also may promote further hyperglycemia in pregnancy. For example, pregnant women with gestational diabetes mellitus release greater amounts of tumor necrosis factor-alpha from both the placenta and maternal adipose tissue in response to high glucose. Tumor necrosis factor-alpha specifically interrupts the insulin signal transduction pathway leading to insulin resistance, glucose intolerance, and progression of hyperglycemia.[40,41] In other species, different patterns have been observed. For example, in the sheep, chronic hyperglycemia was associated with reduced Glut-1 and Glut-3 concentrations and with increased glucose uptake by the uteroplacenta from the mother. There was no change in fetal glucose uptake, however. In contrast, chronic hypoglycemia decreased placental Glut-1 concentrations but did not appear to change placental Glut-3 concentrations, although uterine, uteroplacental, and fetal glucose uptake rates were decreased.[42] Obviously, change in transporter expression can occur in response to changes in glycemia, particularly when the glycemic changes are chronic, but the impact of such changes on placental Glut expression are not necessarily directly related to placental glucose transport to the fetus, which appears to exert independent control over its rate of glucose uptake.

Nutritional patterns during gestation also affect the expression of placental glucose transporters. In sheep, for example, early gestational nutrient restriction decreases placental size but no change in placental weight-specific Glut-1 transporter abundance. When such sheep were refed later in gestation, placental mass and Glut-1 abundance both increased when fed to sufficiency but neither increased if the ewes were overfed.[43] Nutrient restriction studies in the rat have shown no change in placental Glut-1 expression, but did show reduced Glut-3 expression. However, there was no change in fetal glucose concentration.[44] An additional study compared rodent and ovine placental Glut-1 responses to changes in glucose.[45] In the rat, 6 days of sustained hyperglycemia caused no change in Glut-1 protein levels, whereas 3 days of IUGR with fetal hypoglycemia and ischemic hypoxia decreased Glut-1 levels by 50%. In pregnant sheep, maternal and fetal hyperglycemia caused an initial threefold increase in Glut-1 with a persistent decline over the next 2 to 3 weeks, whereas maternal and fetal hypoglycemia led to a 30 to 50% decline in placental Glut-1 levels. In a rat placental cell line, high glucose concentrations decreased Glut-1 concentrations, which was counteracted in part by exposure to low oxygen concentrations. Clearly there is considerable need for more research into the regulation of placental glucose transporter expression and related placental glucose uptake, metabolism, and transport to the fetus, since there are demonstrable differences among isoform specificity, time-dependency, and species.

The arrangement of glucose transporter proteins on both sides of the trophoblast allows bidirectional transport of glucose across both membranes, as well as the whole placenta.[46] Thus, placental glucose transfer to the fetus is regulated by the combined effects of the concentrations of glucose in the maternal and fetal plasma and the kinetic function of the glucose transporter proteins at both the maternal- and fetal-facing trophoblast membranes.[47]

Transplacental Glucose Concentration Gradient. Net transport of glucose from mother to fetus across the placenta requires a net maternal–fetal plasma glucose concentration gradient. In all species studied, including man, the fetal plasma glucose concentration has been observed to be significantly lower than that measured in a simultaneously obtained blood sample from the mother.[48] In addition, a significant linear relationship has been observed between the prevailing glucose concentration in the mother and that in the fetus.[11,49] This linear relationship between maternal and fetal glucose concentration covers the physiologic range of glycemia but has experimentally been seen during acute hyperglycemia induced by glucose infusion to the mother and during hypoglycemia induced by insulin infusion to the mother.[50]

Placental Glucose Consumption. The transplacental glucose concentration gradient is produced by both placental and fetal glucose consumption. The contribution by the placenta is large as the placenta is a highly metabolically active organ; in pregnant sheep near term, for example, the placenta can consume almost twice as much glucose as does the fetus, even though the placental/fetal weight ratio is only about 1:10.[51] Thus, a large part of uterine glucose uptake is consumed by placenta glucose metabolism, which contributes significantly to the physiologic hypoglycemia of the fetus and helps to establish the transplacental glucose concentration gradient; without placental glucose consumption, fetal arterial glucose concentration would be more than double.[25] Glucose utilization in the placenta also contributes to glycogen formation via glycogenin.[52] There is no evidence, however, that this glycogen serves other than local purposes, as the amount of glucose-6-phosphatase in the placenta appears insufficient to release enough glucose into the fetal circulation to account for any significant portion of fetal glucose utilization.[53]

Placental Glucose Transport Kinetics. The relationship between the rate of placental glucose transfer to the fetus and the maternal–fetal plasma glucose concentration gradient is complex. Placental and fetal glucose consumption rates vary independently of each other. Furthermore, in vivo studies in the pregnant sheep model have shown that the glucose transporter proteins at both maternal and fetal placental membranes demonstrate saturation kinetics[54,55] (Figure 2[56]). In these studies, glucose clamp experiments produced steady state net fluxes of glucose into and across the placenta and into the fetus at different concentrations of glucose in the maternal and fetal circulations. Uptake and net consumption of glucose by the uteroplacenta demonstrated saturation kinetics with a V_{max} of about 0.23 mmol/min. K_m (maternal arterial glucose concentration at $V_{max}/2$) and K_s (maternal arterial glucose concentration at which V_{max} is reached) were 2.8 mmol/L and 8.0 mmol/L, respectively, not significantly different from the same parameters for uterine glucose uptake. Similar results have been measured in a variety of in vitro perfusion experiments in human placentas, although V_{max} in the human placenta studied in vitro is severalfold higher than under normoglycemic conditions.

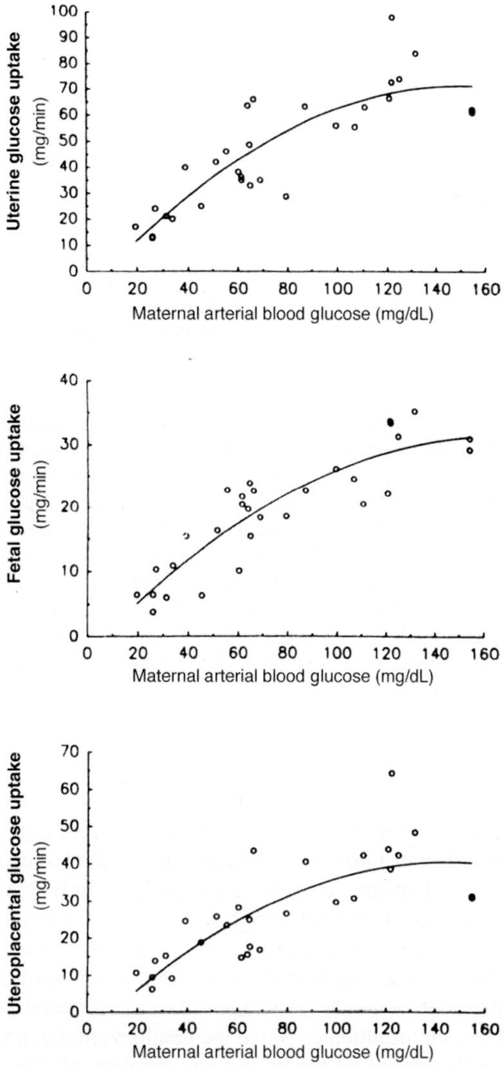

Figure 2 Relationship between maternal glucose concentration and the net uptake of glucose by the uterus, fetus, and uteroplacenta. Glucose was infused into pregnant sheep after an overnight fast to produce a large variety of maternal arterial blood glucose concentrations. Net glucose uptake rates by the uterus **(A)**, fetus **(B)**, and uteroplacenta **(C)** were quantified by the Fick principle. All three relationships show saturation kinetics with an approximate K_m value (a measure of the sensitivity of the transport processes to maternal glucose concentration) in the physiological range of maternal glucose concentration (about 50 to 60 mg/dL [2.8 to 3.3 mM]). These results show that maternal glucose concentration determines the entry of glucose into the uterus, uteroplacenta, and fetus. (Reproduced with permission of the Society for Experimental Biology and Medicine.[3])

Summary of Placental Glucose Uptake, Consumption, and Transport

Figure 3 summarizes the regulation and quantitative aspects of placental glucose uptake and transport. First, uterine, placental, and fetal glucose uptake are directly related to maternal glucose concentration (Figure 3, left panel).[56] Second, fetal glucose uptake is separately regulated by fetal glucose concentration by which a relatively lower glucose concentration in the fetus establishes a larger maternal–fetal glucose concentration gradient and thus increased transfer of glucose to the fetus (Figure 3, middle panel).[56] In contrast, at any maternal glucose concentration, placental glucose consumption is directly related to fetal arterial plasma glucose concentration (Figure 3, right panel).[47] In fact, the fetal side of the placenta has an eightfold greater capacity to take up glucose than the maternal side, so that changes in fetal glucose concentrations have a strong influence on placental glucose flux and metabolism.

Fetal Glucose Utilization

Kinetics of Glucose Utilization in the Fetus. Placental glucose transfer to the fetus is also due to the saturation of the capacity for glucose utilization in the fetus. This capacity itself is variable, as increased fetal glucose supply from the placenta and increased fetal plasma glucose concentration act to increase fetal insulin secretion. In turn, increased fetal insulin concentration augments fetal glucose utilization and plasma clearance, effectively limiting the increase in fetal glucose concentration as maternal glucose concentration and maternal-to-fetal glucose transfer increase.[16]

Effects of Fetal Plasma Glucose and Insulin on Fetal Glucose Metabolism. The rate of fetal glucose metabolism (total utilization as well as the rate of fetal glucose oxidation) depends directly on the simultaneous interaction of fetal plasma glucose and insulin concentrations (Tables 2 and 3). An example in near-term fetal sheep depicting the effect of glucose and insulin concentrations simultaneously on fetal glucose utilization, measured as glucose oxidation to CO_2, is shown in Figure 4.[57] Although both glucose and insulin act independently (ie, additively) to increase glucose utilization and oxidation in the fetus according to saturation kinetics, the relative proportion of glucose oxidized during short-term 3- to 4-hour studies (about 55% in fetal sheep) does not change significantly over the entire range of glucose utilized. Thus, the principal metabolic effect of insulin in the fetus is to increase the permeability of insulin-sensitive cells to glucose, enhancing glucose uptake and utilization in general, and oxidation of glucose in proportion to uptake and utilization, rather than to differentially affecting intracellular pathways of glucose metabolism. At least this is true on balance for the whole fetus; individual tissues and metabolic pathways may vary significantly in their responsiveness to insulin. Such a permissive role for insulin in fetal sheep is different from that in adult humans, in whom higher rates of glucose utilization are

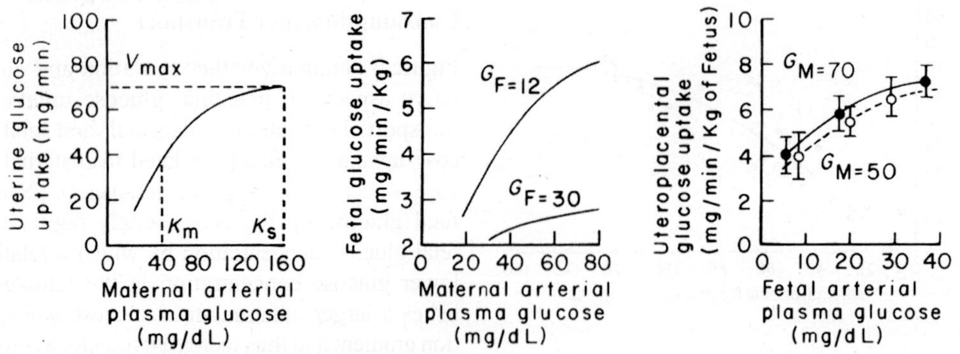

Figure 3 Left Panel: Net rate of glucose transfer into the uterus from the maternal plasma versus maternal plasma glucose concentration. V_{max} is the maximum rate that glucose can enter the uterus; K_m is one half of V_{max} and a measure of the sensitivity of uterine glucose uptake to maternal glucose concentration; K_s is the maternal glucose concentration at which V_{max} is reached. Middle panel: Net rate of glucose transfer into the fetus from uteroplacenta versus maternal plasma glucose concentration; a lower fetal glucose concentration relative to any maternal glucose concentration produces a greater maternal–fetal glucose concentration gradient and a higher rate of placental to fetal glucose transfer (upper curve versus lower curve). Right panel: Net rate of uteroplacental glucose consumption versus fetal plasma glucose concentration; at any maternal glucose concentration (data for maternal glucose concentrations of 50 and 70 mg/dL are shown), uteroplacental glucose consumption is directly related to fetal glucose concentration. These data show that maternal glucose concentration determines the rate of glucose entry into the uterus (and thus the fetus and placenta), but the rate of uteroplacental glucose consumption is regulated by the fetal glucose concentration. (Adapted from references 47 and 56.)

partitioned more into glucose storage (fat and glycogen) than into oxidation. The same may be true in the human fetus, which, like the human adult, has the capacity to synthesize fat to a greater extent than the leaner fetal sheep. In fetal sheep the disposition of nonoxidized glucose-carbon is less certain. Recent studies, however, have demonstrated significant contributions of glucose carbon to the formation of glycogen in the liver, heart, and lung, and a significant contribution to the carbon contained in amino acids and synthesized proteins (DiGiacomo, Carter, Battaglia, and Hay, 1990, unpublished data).

Glucose Transporters and Glucose Uptake and Metabolism in the Fetus. Glucose is transported into cells in the fetus, just as in the newborn and adult, by a family of structurally related membrane-spanning glycoproteins transporters.[58–61] Glut-1 is the predominant fetal glucose transporter isoform.[62–64] Glut-1 is found in abundance in most fetal tissues.[62,64,65] In contrast, tissue specific isoforms, such as the neuronal Glut-3 in brain,[66] Glut-2 in hepatocytes and pancreatic β-cells,[67] and Glut-4 in insulin-responsive tissues such as skeletal muscle, heart, and adipose tissue[68] are expressed in low amounts in fetal tissues compared with Glut-1.[66–68] Studies in the fetal sheep have demonstrated time-dependent universal suppression of fetal peripheral tissue Glut-1 and Glut-4 concentrations by chronic hyperglycemia.[65] These observations in the fetal sheep mimic results obtained in the rat fetus exposed to a maternal diabetic environment.[69] Since the results varied in the rat dependent on the timing and duration of exposure to hyperglycemia,[69,70] there obviously are independent effects of glucose and insulin on fetal glucose transporters, particularly Glut-1.

Both acute and chronic changes in fetal glucose and insulin concentrations have been studied in fetal sheep to address the interrelationships among absolute changes in glucose and insulin concentrations, duration of change in glucose and insulin concentrations, expression of glucose transporter concentrations, and glucose utilization rates in the fetus. In chronic studies lasting 2 to 4 weeks in late gestation, sustained hyperglycemia was associated with a progressive decrease to normal or subnormal insulin concentrations.[71] Under these conditions there was a transient increase in brain Glut-1 but not Glut-3 concentrations, and a progressive decline in liver and adipose tissue Glut-1 and myocardial and skeletal muscle Glut-1 and Glut-4.[69] Further studies showed that the chronic hyperglycemia and reduction in Glut-4 correlated with the development of insulin resistance.[72] Chronic hypoglycemia (produced by maternal insulin infusion) produced a decline in brain Glut-3, and increase in brain Glut-1, and a subsequent decline in liver Glut-1, but no significant change in insulin-sensitive myocardium, skeletal muscle, or adipose tissue Glut-1 or -4 concentrations.[69] These time-dependent and tissue- and isoform-specific changes in response to altered circulating glucose and/or insulin concentrations showed that cellular adaptations in Glut-1 and Glut-3 are geared toward protecting the fetus from perturbations in substrate availability, and the adaptations in Glut-4 are geared toward development of insulin resistance.

In acute studies, expressions of Glut-1, 3, and 4 were studied in response to 1, 2.5, and 24 hours of selective hyperglycemia or hyperinsulinemia.[73] Hyperglycemia initially increased fetal glucose utilization rate associated with an increase in Glut-1 and 3 isoforms that mediate basal glucose utilization, but no change in Glut-4 that mediates insulin action. Fetal glucose utilization rate subsequently returned to normal values by the end of 24 hours. These results contrast with the tissue-specific effects of selective hyperinsulinemia, which produced a sustained increase in fetal glucose utilization rate associated with a sustained increase in hepatic Glut-1 and a myocardial-specific emergence of mild insulin resistance associated with a downregulation of Glut-4. In skeletal muscle specifically, there was a lack of sustained temporal association between the increases in transporter proteins and glucose utilization rates.[74] This observation indicates that subcellular localization and activity of transporter or tissues other than skeletal muscle contribute to net fetal glucose utilization rate.

These observations support an immediate but transient cellular adaptation of augmented glucose uptake associated with a transient increase in Glut-1 concentration in response to an acute hyperglycemic perturbation in the intrauterine milieu. In contrast, alterations in the hormonal milieu (specifically of insulin) did not demonstrate any acute effects on the mechanisms underlying insulin-induced cellular glucose transport, except for a sustained increase in hepatic Glut-1 concentrations and an increase in skeletal muscle Glut-4 concentrations. Whether chronic hyperinsulinemia in the presence of hyperglycemia or euglycemia leads to adaptations of fetal ovine glucose transporter proteins toward enhancing or limiting intracellular substrate delivery remains unknown, as do the mechanisms, such as Glut gene transcription or translation and posttranslational protein stability, that underlie both acute and chronic

Table 2 What Glucose Does in the Fetus

Enters the fetus from the placenta according to the transplacental, maternal–fetal plasma glucose concentration gradient
Enters fetal tissues (via glucose transporters) according to saturation-limited (Michaelis–Menten) kinetics, independent of and additive to that of insulin (in fetal sheep)
Promotes its own oxidative and nonoxidative metabolism, to equal extents in fetal sheep, perhaps more to nonoxidative fat deposition in the human fetus
Increases fetal oxidation and oxygen consumption
Inhibits protein breakdown
Contributes most of the substrate for fetal glycogen formation
Increases insulin production and secretion
Maintains fetal growth

Table 3 What Insulin Does in the Fetus

Increases glucose uptake into insulin-sensitive (via Glut-4 transporters) tissues according to saturation-limited (Michaelis–Menten) kinetics, independent of and additive to that of glucose (in fetal sheep); perhaps more into adipose tissue in the human fetus
Increases plasma glucose clearance
Produces hypoglycemia
Increases the transplacental maternal–fetal glucose concentration gradient and thereby increases the transfer of glucose across the placenta and into the fetal plasma
Inhibits glucose production
Inhibits protein breakdown (most likely through increased glucose utilization)

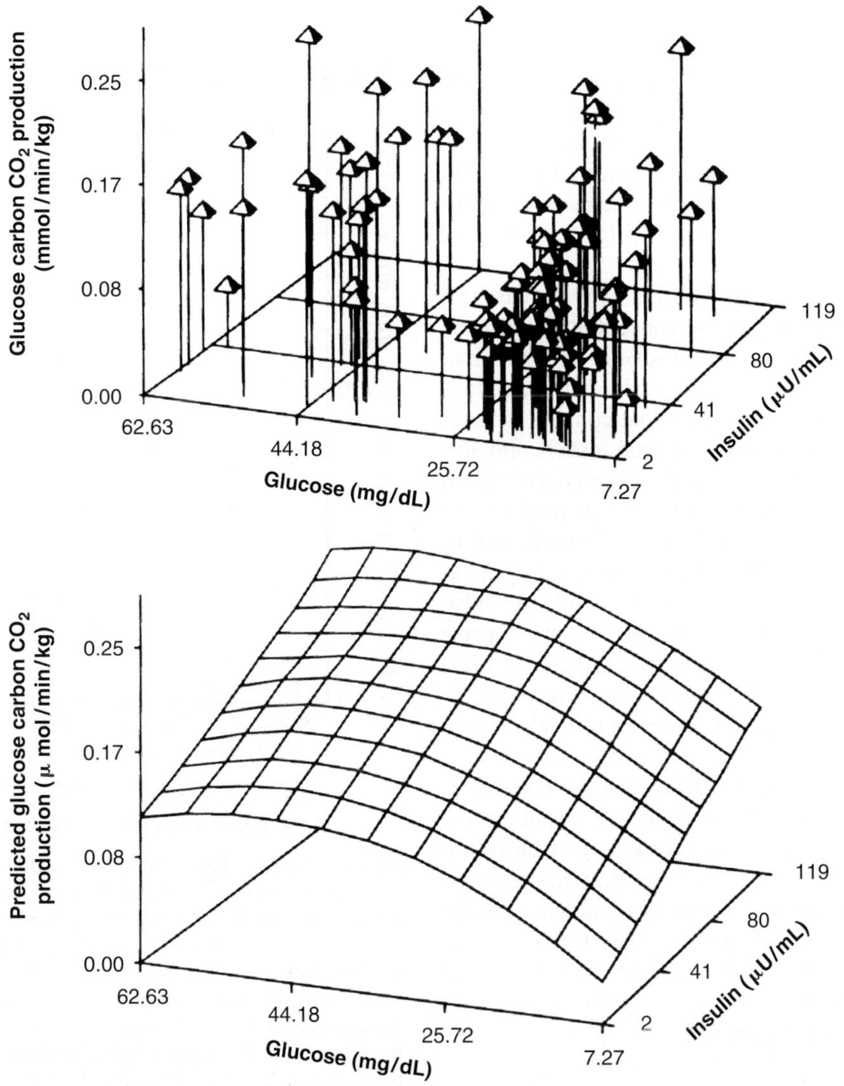

Figure 4 Data from fetal sheep showing the additive effects of plasma glucose and insulin concentrations on fetal glucose oxidation rate measured as CO_2 production rate. **(A)** Three-dimensional plot of individual values of the rate of glucose oxidation to CO_2 at different concentrations of glucose and insulin. **(B)** Predicted values of the rate of fetal glucose oxidation to CO_2 displayed as a three-dimensional glucose x insulin surface from the values in **(A)**. (Reproduced with permission of the American Journal of Physiology.[57])

adaptation to changes in circulating glucose and insulin concentrations.

Basal Insulin Concentration. The basal concentration of insulin in the fetus probably has a role in fetal glucose utilization, but direct evidence for this is not as convincing as the effect of hyperinsulinemia. For example, an acute decrease of fetal plasma insulin concentration with somatostatin infusion does not appear to affect fetal glucose concentration or glucose utilization.[75] In contrast, a chronic decrease of fetal plasma insulin concentration, either by pancreatectomy or streptozotocin injection into the fetus, reduces fetal growth[17,76] and decreases umbilical glucose uptake in relation to fetal hyperglycemia. The hyperglycemia results from decreased peripheral tissue insulin sensitivity and glucose utilization and from the release of insulin's normal inhibition of hepatic glucose production.

Interaction between Glucose and Alternative Carbon Substrates for Fetal Oxidative Metabolism. At markedly reduced rates of glucose supply to the fetus, fetal glucose utilization rate decreases proportionally.[47,56] Under such short-term conditions fetal oxygen consumption remains near normal,[57] indicating active reciprocal oxidation of other substrates, at least over the short term, such as glucose released from glycogen, lactate, amino acids, fatty acids, and ketoacids. Over longer periods (more than 3 weeks) of reduced glucose supply, fetal oxygen consumption tends to decrease by 25 to 30%; because the rate of fetal growth decreases at the same time and to the same extent as the decrease in oxygen consumption, the reduction in fetal oxygen consumption probably represents the oxidative requirements of the decreased protein synthetic activity.[76]

Fetal Glucose Utilization Rates. Quantitative aspects of fetal glucose utilization have been made in several large animal models. In most studies, fetal glucose is about 5 mg/min/kg fetal weight near term, down from values nearly twice as high in mid-gestation,[77] when fetal growth and metabolic rate are also as much as twice as great as they are closer to term. In man, based on the increase in total maternal glucose production in late gestation, fetoplacental glucose utilization is estimated to be about 5 to 6 mg/min/kg fetal weight.[8] This rate is similar to that measured in normal term infants.[78] Table 4 presents estimated utilization rates of glucose in several fetal organs and the remaining carcass of fetal sheep in late gestation. The fraction of glucose oxidized versus that entering tissue accretion pathways in these organs has not been determined, and the factors that regulate glucose uptake in specific organs remains poorly studied. Most organs appear dependent on plasma glucose concentration for their specific rate of glucose uptake, and certain organs such as skeletal muscle and probably the heart and liver are insulin-sensitive (at least in sheep studied in vivo).

Gestational Development of Placental Glucose Transport and Fetal Glucose Utilization. The fetus grows severalfold in size over the second half of gestation; so does its absolute rate of glucose utilization. Placental glucose transfer to the fetus, therefore, must increase to meet the increasing metabolic requirements for glucose of the larger, growing fetus. The increase in placental glucose transport occurs for two reasons: (1) the transplacental glucose concentration gradient increases as the fetal glucose concentration decreases relative to maternal glucose concentration (Figure 5, top panel); (2) the placental transport capacity itself increases (Figure 5, middle panel).[77]

Placental glucose transport capacity develops primarily by an increase in the total amount[79]

Table 4 Metabolic Rates in the Fetus That Account for Glucose Utilization (Based On Data in Fetal Sheep and Estimates for Human Fetuses for Brain)

	Glucose Utilization Rate (mg/min/kg fetus)	Percent of Total
Whole fetus (sheep, measured)	5.0	100
Whole fetus (human, estimated)	6.0–8.0	100
Brain (sheep, measured)	0.8	16
Brain (human, estimated)	4.0	50–67
Heart (sheep, measured)	0.65	13
Lungs (sheep, estimated)	0.1	2
Liver (sheep, measured)	0.1	2
Red blood cells (human, estimated)	0.1	2
Gut (sheep, estimated)		
Carcass/skeletal muscle (estimated, sheep)	3.25	65
Total of organs accounted for		
Sheep	5.0	100
Human	8.2	103–137

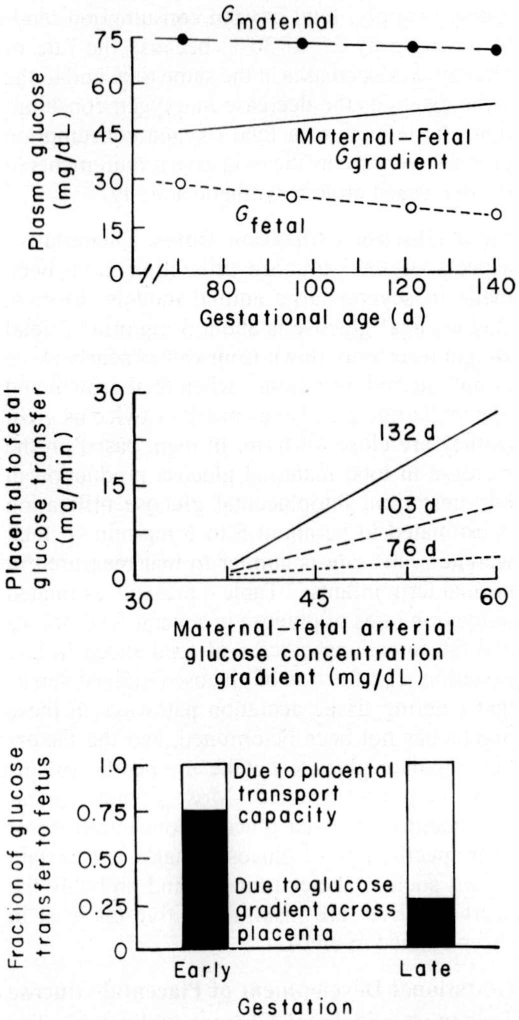

Figure 5 Upper panel: Plasma glucose concentration tends to decrease in fetal sheep (–O–) over the second half of gestation relative to the maternal plasma glucose concentration (–●–). This increases the maternal–fetal plasma glucose concentration gradient or the driving force for transplacental glucose transfer (—). Middle panel: Placental-to-fetal glucose transfer (PGT) increases about eightfold over this same period. This increase in transport largely reflects transport capacity, shown by the increasing slope of PGT as gestational age increases. Bottom panel: At mid gestation, most of PGT is due to the maternal–fetal glucose concentration gradient whereas by term, the placental transport capacity for glucose accounts for most of PGT (Adapted from reference 77).

rather than the affinity of the glucose transporters.[77] The number of glucose transporter proteins can increase by an increase in the trophoblast membrane surface area, an increase in the concentration of transporters per unit membrane area, or both. Although there is some evidence from in vitro studies that glucose concentration can regulate placental glucose transporter expression, either directly or through IGF-I action,[80] Glut-1 mRNA may vary independently of Glut-1 protein; for example, Glut-1 protein decreases over gestation in the rat, but it parallels Glut-1 protein in the sheep. There is no evidence, however, that such changes affect the actual rate or the capacity (maximal rate) of placental glucose transport. In fact, in vitro perfusion studies in human placentas and in vivo studies in humans and sheep indicate that placental glucose transport capacity is much greater than actual transport rates, indicating that small changes in placental glucose transporter content may have a little or no effect on the rate of placental glucose transport.[55,56] By late gestation, however, glucose transport capacity by the placenta has a dominant role in the regulation of glucose transport to the fetus (Figure 5, bottom panel).

Fetal glucose concentration may decrease relative to maternal glucose concentration over the second half of gestation for several reasons. First, fetal cellularity increases over this period, as does the fraction of body weight that consists of insulin sensitive tissues (eg, skeletal muscle and adipose tissue).[81] Second, fetal insulin concentration increases, developmentally and in response to glucose and other secretagogues.[82] Third, insulin-sensitive Glut-4 transporters on fetal skeletal muscle and adipose tissue cell membranes also increase over gestation, at least due to the increase in the relative body content of these insulin-sensitive tissues. The result is an increase in the effectiveness of insulin to promote fetal glucose utilization and glucose clearance, thereby reducing the relative fetal plasma glucose concentration. On balance, however, by late gestation, the increasing gradient of glucose concentration across the placenta contributes only limited control over placental transport of glucose to the fetus. The combination of these developmental processes and how they interact to promote net glucose transfer to the fetus by the placenta are summarized in Figure 6.[47]

Fetal Insulin Secretion

Many studies have addressed the onset and development of insulin secretion from the fetal pancreas. The fetal pancreas develops in the late first to early second trimester, producing measurable insulin concentrations by mid-gestation. As noted above, there is a gradual increase in basal insulin concentration and glucose- and arginine-induced insulin secretion toward term.[82] In the rat, very little insulin is secreted in the fetus,[83,84] while in the human fetus, which normally does not secrete much insulin,[85,86] sustained hyperglycemia in pregnant diabetics,[87] particularly when the hyperglycemia is pulsatile, produces considerable insulin. Fetal sheep are somewhere in between, showing downregulation of glucose-induced and basal insulin secretion in the presence of chronic, sustained, marked hyperglycemia as with the rat,[70] but increased insulin secretion with pulsatile hyperglycemia as in humans.[88] Hypoglycemia decreases basal and glucose-induced insulin secretion,[89] perhaps a fundamental aspect of how intrauterine growth restriction (IUGR) with fetal hypoglycemia decreases fetal pancreatic development and insulin secretion capacity. Clearly fetal insulin secretion responds variably to changes in glucose concentration that are dependent on the absolute change in glucose concentration, its magnitude, and its pattern.

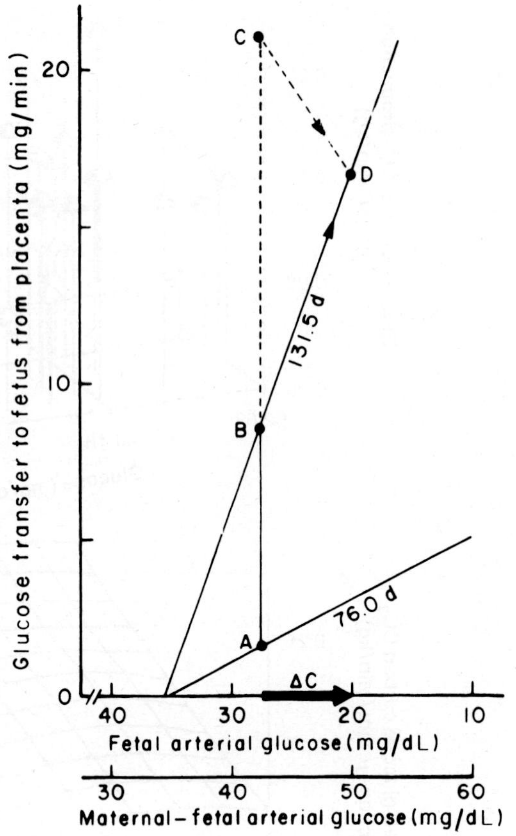

Figure 6 Graphic illustration of interrelationships among developmental changes in placental glucose transport capacity, fetal glucose demand, and fetal glucose concentration from mid- to late gestation in the sheep model. Placental glucose transfer capacity increases over gestation, shown by the increased slope of the 131.5-day gestational age line versus the slope of the mid-gestation, 76-day line, supplying more glucose to the fetus (A to B). Fetal growth demands more glucose; however, represented by point C. Additional glucose is provided by the simultaneous decrease in fetal glucose concentration relative to that of the mother which increases the transplacental glucose concentration gradient (the X-axis segment ΔC); although the fetal hypoglycemia increases fetal glucose uptake, it also tends to decrease the disposal of glucose into the fetal tissues from the fetal plasma. These opposing forces combine to produce the actual glucose supply to the fetus at point D. (Reproduced with permission of the American Physiological Society.[47])

Alternate Carbohydrates Produced in the Placenta

The fetal glucose/oxygen metabolic quotient is less than 1.0,[5] which means that glucose does not (in fact, could not) account for all of the carbon necessary for the rate of fetal oxidation. Furthermore, tracer studies in fetal sheep have shown that the fraction of fetal glucose utilization that does produce CO_2 is only about 0.5 to 0.6.[92] Thus, there remains a need for carbon substrates other than glucose to meet the oxidative requirements imposed by the fetal respiratory rate (VO_2 or net rate of oxygen consumption), even if all of the glucose consumed by the fetus were oxidized. To meet at least part of the need for other carbon substrates, the placenta plays an important role by metabolizing glucose to lactate (in most or all species) and fructose (in ruminants). Lactate and fructose are produced directly in relation to placental glucose supply.[90,91] Based on preliminary

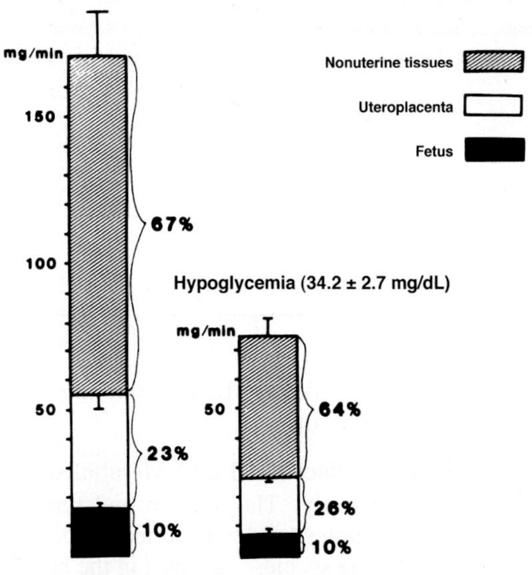

Figure 7 Fractional partition of maternal glucose production to nonuterine maternal tissues, uteroplacenta, and fetus in normoglycemic sheep (first column) and hypoglycemic sheep (second column) showing that short term there is no change in the relative proportions of glucose used by these three sets of tissues. Thus, fetal and placental glucose needs are dependent on the supply of glucose from the maternal plasma glucose pool; with maternal glucose deficiency, either the fetus must use its own sources of glucose (glycogenolysis or gluconeogenesis) or rely on other substrates such as amino acids for carbon balance. (Reproduced with permission of the American Physiological Society.[93])

observations, approximately 50 to 70% of uteroplacental glucose consumption goes to lactate (at low and high values, respectively, of maternal and fetal glucose concentrations and the rate of placental glucose consumption), and 3 to 5% goes to fructose under the same conditions. Lactate produced in the placenta enters both maternal and fetal circulations at about equal rates under normal conditions,[90] whereas fructose produced in the placenta only enters the fetal circulation.[91] At normal rates of lactate and fructose uptake by the fetus and their oxidation fractions in fetal tissues measured in late-gestation pregnant sheep,[92] these two substrates could supply carbon sufficient to account for another 20 to 30% of the carbon requirements for fetal oxygen consumption above that provided by glucose. Amino acids and perhaps fatty acids and ketoacids are the only other substrates available to make up the balance.

Adaptations to Changes in Glucose Supply

Hypoglycemia (Table 5). Short-term maternal hypoglycemia has been studied in the late-gestation pregnant sheep.[93] As shown in (Figure 7),[93] several days of fasting-induced hypoglycemia produce proportional reductions in glucose uptake by maternal nonuterine tissues, the fetus, and the uteroplacenta. Similar changes in glucose utilization by these tissues have been found with acute, several hour insulin-induced hypoglycemia.[56] At the same time, however, uteroplacental oxygen consumption rate does not change. Thus, even with hypoglycemic conditions, other substrates must substitute for glucose to maintain oxidative metabolism. Recent studies demonstrate that as glucose utilization by the placenta is decreased, so is uteroplacental production of lactate and fructose.[90,91] There is a little or no change in placental utilization of free fatty acids, ketoacids, or amino acids. Thus, uteroplacental oxygen consumption can be maintained by a balance in which a decreased supply of glucose to the fetus also results in a decreased production of exported products of glucose metabolism, allowing glucose carbon to be used preferentially for oxidative metabolism. This pattern is maintained with much longer periods of hypoglycemia, but two other adaptations develop under chronic conditions as well. First, fetal glucose production develops.[76] This increases the fetal glucose concentration relative to that of the mother and shifts the balance of glucose uptake by the uterus more to placental glucose consumption and less to glucose transfer to the fetus (see Figure 1). Fetal glucose production thus serves two purposes: (1) the maintenance of fetal glucose metabolism and (2) the diversion of diminished glucose supply to the uterus into placental metabolism.[94] Fetal glucose production, therefore, maintains the glucose metabolic requirements of the fetus and placenta without further drain on the diminished availability of glucose in the mother; this may represent a simple "survival" adaptation.

Table 5 Fetal Responses to Decreased Glucose Supply and Hypoglycemia

Acute
Decreased glucose uptake
Decreased insulin production and secretion
Hypoinsulinemia
Decreased glucose utilization
Increase in the rate of placental glucose transfer to the fetus as fetal hypoglycemia tends to increase the maternal–fetal glucose concentration gradient
Decreased placental lactate production
Decreased fetal lactate uptake and utilization
Substitution of other stubstrates to main oxidative metabolism
Chronic
Initial increase in fetal glucose production, then a return toward the normal condition of little or no fetal glucose production
Initial increase in amino acid oxidation, then a return to normal rates
Decreased insulin sensitivity
Increased ratio of fetal to maternal glucose concentration
Increased ratio of placental glucose consumption to placental glucose transfer
Acute: mild-moderate
Increased glucose uptake
Increased insulin production and secretion
Hyperinsulinemia
Increased glucose utilization
Increased fetal oxygen consumption
Mild arterial hypoxemia
Respiratory acidosis
Increased placental lactate production
Increased fetal lactate uptake and utilization
Acute: severe
Arterial hypoxemia
Hypoinsulinemia
Increased erythropoietin
Increased fetal oxygen consumption
Metabolic acidosis
Decreased placental perfusion
Fetal demise
Chronic
Decreased insulin secretion and/or synthesis
Decreased peripheral insulin sensitivity
Increased ratio of placental glucose consumption to placental glucose transfer

The second adaptation to chronic hypoglycemia in late gestation is a reduction in placental and fetal growth rates, resulting in lower fetal and placental weights.[76] Because placental glucose transfer capacity does not change at the same time, placental weight reduction, or failure to maintain weight, does not appear to include a reduction in placental membrane surface area or glucose transporter number or affinity. The advantage of a smaller placenta is not clear, but since the overall carbon balance in the placenta is maintained, it provides additional evidence that with chronic hypoglycemia and decreased placental glucose supply, placental glucose carbon is shunted to oxidative metabolism, that is, it is not shunted to nonoxidative processes such as the production of placental tissue and the production of normally exported products of placental glucose metabolism such as lactate and fructose. It is interesting to speculate that all of these adaptations take place to substitute reduced rates of fetal and placental growth for reduced substrate supply, thereby maintaining normal fetal and placental tissue-specific rates of metabolism, and preserving their function and viability without further demands on maternal metabolism.

Intrauterine Growth Restriction. IUGR is a unique example of how fetal glucose metabolism and its regulatory mechanisms adapt to glucose deficiency and hypoglycemia to maintain normal fetal glucose metabolism. Regardless of the model (Table 6),[95] when the fetus is deprived of glucose by placental insufficiency or maternal hypoglycemia, fetal weight-specific glucose utilization rate is not very much different from normal rates.[95]

This indicates that one of the mechanisms to enhance glucose uptake by the fetus from the placenta is the production of further hypoglycemia, thereby increasing the maternal–fetal glucose concentration gradient. To do this, there must be an increase in the fetal tissue capacity for glucose uptake and/or utilization. This could come about by increased concentrations and/or activity and/or plasma membrane localization of glucose transporters, increased insulin signal transduction and thereby effectiveness to promote Glut-4 (and perhaps Glut-1) translocation to the cell membrane, or mechanisms of insulin metabolism into oxidative and/or nonoxidative pathways. In both fetal sheep and fetal rats with IUGR, Glut-1 and Glut-4 concentrations in myocardium, adipose tissue, and skeletal muscle do not decrease with sustained hypoglycemia,[65,67,68] perhaps a positive adaptation to maintain glucose utilization despite hypoglycemia. It has not been determined if this maintenance of glucose transporter concentration is sufficient by itself to maintain fetal glucose utilization at normal rates. Future studies are necessary to sort

Table 6 Fetal Weights, Glucose Concentrations, and Glucose Uptake Rates in Four Ovine Models of Intrauterine Growth Restriction

	Adolescent		Heat-Stress		Caruncleclomy		Hypoglycemia	
Model	Control	Study	Control	Study	Control	Study	Control	Study
Fetal weight (g)	4,478	3,144**	3,112	1,645**	2,671	1,675**	3,500	2,700**
Fetal glucose (μmol/mL)	1.00	0.79#	1.17	0.74***	0.73	0.43***	1.14	0.67*
Fetal glucose uptake (μmol/min/kg)	34.9	30.0#	31.8	29.6	33.0	31.0	26.7	22.5*

Adapted from reference 95.
Data are means. *p* values determined by unpaired Student's *t* test comparing control with study animals within each model.
$^{\#}p < .06$; $^{*}p < .05$; $^{**}p < .01$; $^{***}p < .001$.

out this fascinating and complex adaptation to glucose deficiency among the many tissues in the fetus.

Hyperglycemia (Table 6). Acute maternal hyperglycemia produces an increase in uteroplacental glucose uptake with saturation kinetics that parallel those of the fetus. At the same time, uteroplacental oxygen consumption rate does not change;[56] thus, increasing amounts of glucose consumed by the placenta are shunted into nonoxidative pathways. These include increased rates of lactate and fructose production, as well as increased use of glucose carbon for placental tissue, particularly glycogen.

With chronic hyperglycemia in the mother, produced by glucose infusion or experimental diabetes, similar patterns of glucose metabolism in the placenta have been observed. Fetal adaptations produce other changes as well. For example, chronic fetal hyperglycemia in experimental animals, in response to chronic maternal hyperglycemia, eventually appears to downregulate fetal pancreatic insulin secretion.[96] This involves the basal rate of insulin secretion and also appears to later involve the secretion of insulin in response to acute hyperglycemia.[97] As a result of the relative decrease in circulating insulin concentrations in the presence of hyperglycemia, fetal hyperglycemia is exaggerated, shifting the increased rate of uterine glucose uptake more into uteroplacental glucose consumption. Oxidative metabolism, measured as the uteroplacental rate of oxygen consumption, still does not change. Thus, uteroplacental glucose metabolism increasingly enters nonoxidative pathways. The particular metabolic pathways of glucose carbon under these conditions have not been explored. Placental size is not dramatically increased, suggesting that export of placental glucose carbon into lactate and fructose and perhaps other products accounts for the balance of glucose carbon not used for oxidative metabolism. Of course, glucose carbon could substitute for the oxidation of carbon normally provided by other substrates, including ketoacids and fatty acids, but principally the amino acids. Normally, the glucose oxidation fraction in the placenta of sheep in late gestation, corrected for lactate carbon and fructose carbon export, is still only about 50%. Thus, half of placental oxidative metabolism must be supplied by other substrates. Some amino acids such as leucine and serine may be oxidized within the placenta directly as they are taken up from the maternal plasma and concentrated within the trophoblast cytosol. In contrast, glutamate is produced in the fetal liver from glutamine and then taken up by the placenta where as much as 70 to 80% is oxidized.[98] It is certainly possible, therefore, that under hyperglycemic conditions excess glucose carbon could substitute for carbon that is derived from amino acids, ketoacids, and fatty acids under normoglycemic conditions. Thus, there are clear interrelationships among a variety of carbon substrates that can act as sources of carbon for placental oxidative metabolism, and these interrelationships appear to be regulated by placental glucose supply.

Summary of Placental and Fetal Glucose Metabolism

Acute and chronic adaptations to extremes of changes in glucose supply to the placenta involve active and complex adjustments in the patterns of placental metabolism and growth. The one constant is placental oxidative metabolism, which, on a weight-specific basis, appears to be maintained in spite of major shifts in the relative supplies of substrate carbon and the rate of placental growth.

LIPIDS

Considerably less is known about placental lipid uptake, metabolism, and transfer to the fetus than is known for glucose, principally because most experimental animal models, especially the sheep, demonstrate little capacity for lipid uptake, metabolism, and transport by the placenta. Also, lipid transport by the human placenta has not been studied in vivo, and there is large variation in the data obtained from human placental tissue studied in vitro. Even so, the human placenta appears to have considerable capacity for lipid transfer. Transporters for specific fatty acids are primarily involved. More complex pathways include lipoprotein dissociation by placental lipoprotein lipase (LPL) activity (although the exact cellular source of LPL in the placenta remains in question), triglyceride uptake and metabolism (including metabolic pathways of oxidation, chain-lengthening, synthesis, and interconversion pathways), and release into the fetal plasma as free fatty acids or lipoproteins.[99]

Placental Lipid Uptake, Metabolism, and Transfer to the Fetus

Importance of Placental Lipid Metabolism to Fetal Lipid Supply. The amount and type of fatty acid or complex lipid transported by the placenta vary among species—greatest in the hemochorial placenta of the human, guinea pig, and rabbit, and least in the epitheliochorial placenta of the ruminant and the endotheliochorial placenta of the carnivores. Furthermore, it is interesting that fetal fat content at term among species varies reasonably directly with the lipid transport capacity of the placenta.[100] There are many lipid substances in the plasma that are transported across the placenta, which are essential for placental and fetal development even if they do not contribute to nutritional or energy metabolism. Also, brown fat is common to all fetuses; it is essential for postnatal thermogenesis, even if the neonate is not "fat" with white adipose tissue. Furthermore, many lipid substances entering the fetus are qualitatively different from those taken up by the uterus and uteroplacenta, implying active placental metabolism of individual lipid substances. Placental lipid metabolism, therefore, is qualitatively as well as, in some cases, quantitatively important for fetal development and growth, even if the fetus does not get very fat.

Placental Uptake, Synthesis, Metabolism, and Hydrolysis of Fatty Acids. A schema of lipid uptake, metabolism, and transport in the human placenta is shown in Figure 8.[4,99] After entering the placenta, fatty acids may be used for triglyceride synthesis, cholesterol esterification, membrane biosynthesis, direct transfer to the fetus, or oxidation. The most important factor that regulates the flux of lipid into the placenta and into the various pathways of transport and metabolism is the concentration of maternal plasma lipids, including free fatty acids (FFA) and triglycerides. For example, placental triglyceride content increases in women who are fasting, who deliver preterm infants, or who have diabetes mellitus—all conditions in which maternal plasma FFA concentrations are increased.

Placental tissue from different species has been shown to express LPL activity as well as phospholipase A_2.[101–108] Maternal plasma triglycerides are hydrolyzed by these enzymes and the released fatty acids are then taken up by the placenta. In the trophoblast cells, the fatty acids are then reesterified and further hydrolyzed, facilitating their diffusion into the fetal circulation. Cultured placental

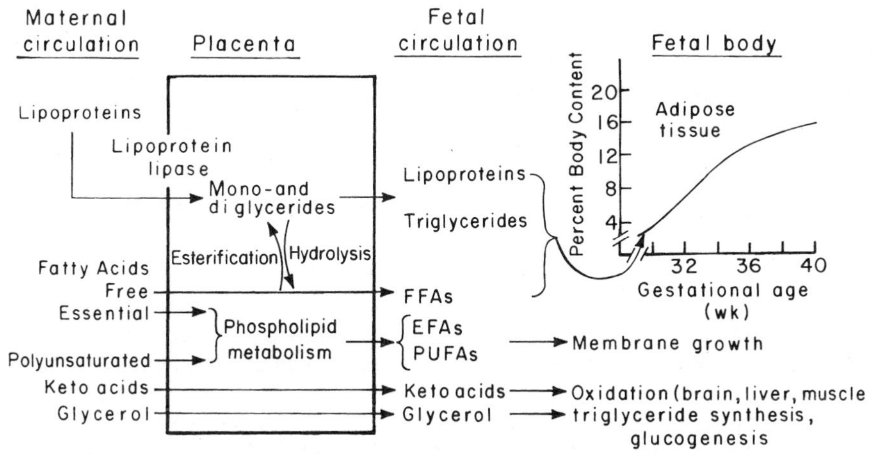

Figure 8 Schematic of placental–fetal interrelationships in humans for various aspects of placental lipid metabolism, fetal lipid uptake and metabolism, and fetal lipogenesis into adipose tissue. (Adapted from references 4 and 99.)

trophoblast cells have shown that esterified intracellular lipids provide a reservoir of fatty acids that can be released into the medium.[109]

All fatty acids cross lipid bilayers such as those in the syncytiotrophoblast by simple diffusion. Partition studies in pure phospholipid bilayers indicate that this diffusion is rapid, on the order of 20 to 30 milliseconds.[110] In addition fatty acid transport across membranes is facilitated by fatty acid binding proteins, which aid in intracellular channeling of fatty acids.[111–115] The main membrane associated fatty acid binding proteins are the plasma membrane fatty acid binding protein (FABPpm) and the fatty acid transfer proteins (FAT/CD36 and FATP).[111] These transfer proteins have been found on both the maternal facing microvillous and fetal facing basal membranes of the placental trophoblast, while a placenta-specific protein, p-FABPpm, has been found exclusively on the microvillous membrane.[116] p-FABPpm has a unique amino acid composition that enhances the binding affinity and capacity of this protein for arachidonic acid (AA) and docosahexaenoic acid (DHA) compared with LA and linoleic acids.[117–119] The syncytiotrophoblast also contains cytoplasmic binding proteins, which appear to act by removing fatty acids from the inner membrane and channeling them to their respective metabolic fates.[111,113,120]

Fatty acid transport into the fetal circulation is largely determined by the transplacental gradient of nonesterified fatty acids (NEFAs) relative to available circulating binding protein concentrations and the activity and availability of their binding sites. The concentration of NEFAs in the maternal plasma at term is about three times that in the fetal circulation, but the concentration of albumin, the primary carrier protein for NEFAs, is actually 10 to 20% higher in the fetal than the maternal circulation.[121] Thus the ratio of plasma NEFAs to albumin on the fetal side of the placenta is about 25% of that on the maternal side at term.[122] The higher concentration of NEFAs relative to available binding sites on albumin, α-fetoprotein, and other lipoproteins in the maternal compared to the fetal plasma is reflected in the concentration of unbound NEFAs, which is greater in the maternal (12 nM) than the fetal (9 nM) circulation.[123] Human cordocentesis data from 18 to 36 weeks indicate an exponential decrease in the concentration of NEFAs in the fetal circulation over this period,[124] presumably because of increasing use of fatty acids in the fetus for rapidly growing structures like the brain and adipose tissue.

Although most fatty acids appear to be transported by diffusion and direct carrier-mediated mechanisms, some studies suggest that chain-altering metabolism in intratrophoblast peroxisomes may lead to a greater transfer of medium-chain fatty acids into the fetal circulation.[125] This might be advantageous to fetal lipid metabolism, which appears to be limited in its capacity for oxidation of long-chain fats, an apparent result of low cytosolic and/or mitochondrial carnitine concentrations.[126] Fatty acids may also be esterified to di- and triglycerides and to phospholipids. These may be stored transiently or for the long term, or hydrolyzed by phospholipases and acylglycerol lipases to release fatty acids into the fetal circulation.

Additional evidence for the hypothesis that transient placental esterification of fatty acids occurs during transport of fatty acid by the placenta comes from measurements of activities of enzymes required for the isolation of glycerol-3-phosphate.[127] Such enzymes are located in the endoplasmic reticulum and have been identified in placental trophoblast cells. While enzymatic specific activity and total enzyme content do not necessarily reflect metabolic flux, the presence of these enzymes indicates that fatty acid esterification followed by hydrolysis is a reasonable hypothetical pathway for placental lipid metabolism and transport.

Fatty Acid Synthesis in the Placenta. Fatty acids are also synthesized in the placenta. Significant fatty acid synthesis has been measured in placental tissue and cultured trophoblast cells from human,[128] sheep,[129] and pig placentas.[130] Primarily long-chain fatty acids (oleic, palmitic, and palmitoleic acids) are formed.[131] Radiolabeled palmitate can be incorporated rapidly into triglycerides in human placental slices, and studies of human trophoblast cells in culture have shown that incubation with albumin-bound ^{14}C-oleate produces ^{14}C-labeled cellular triglycerides. Similar observations have been made in 21-day pregnant rats studied in vivo, showing incorporation of ^{14}C-palmitate into placental triglycerides and phospholipids.[132]

Lipoprotein Synthesis in the Placenta. There is conflicting evidence regarding the synthesis of lipoproteins by placental tissue and their use for transport of fatty acids to the fetal circulation. By day 21 of gestation in the rat, the placenta appears to synthesize apoprotein B which is normally an integral part of the major plasma lipoprotein carriers of triglycerides.[132] Such observations have not been made in the human placenta, which may secrete lipoproteins only during the early part of gestation, if at all.[133] Small amounts of low-density lipoprotein (LDL) and very low-density lipoprotein have been identified in human amniotic fluid, but their source has not been determined.[131]

Cholesterol Metabolism and Transfer by the Placenta. LDL cholesterol is taken up by endocytosis into trophoblast cells and degraded by lysozymes.[134] LDL cholesterol appears to be the major precursor for placental production of progesterone and estrogen. High-density lipoprotein cholesterol also contributes to placental progesterone production in cultured human trophoblast cells. Some of this cholesterol is transferred directly to the fetus, although the role of this transport is uncertain, given the large capacity and rate of cholesterol synthesis in the fetal liver.[135]

Nonessential Fetal Lipid Supply. The bulk of placental lipid transport is dependent on the maternal plasma fatty acid and lipid concentrations and the maternal–fetal plasma fatty acid concentration gradients. In humans, the concentrations of free fatty acids are higher in maternal blood than in fetal blood, and their concentrations are highly correlated. Under normal circumstances, the fetal/maternal ratio of free fatty acids is less than 0.5.[136] In humans, fetal patterns of **EFA**s and structural lipids correlate directly with the fatty acid/lipid composition of the maternal plasma (and, indirectly, the maternal diet).[54] This direct correlation may be unique to the human due to the high lipid transport capacity of the human placenta. Sheep, for example, transport very little total lipid across the placenta except for some long-chain **EFA**s, and the horse produces a lipid profile in the fetal plasma that is qualitatively and quantitatively different from the maternal plasma, perhaps the product of placental metabolism or different rates of transfer for different chain lengths of fatty acids.[137]

In the fetal plasma the fatty acids are bound to albumin and α-fetoprotein and transported to the liver where they are synthesized into triglycerides and released into the fetal circulation. Since maternal triglyceride concentration determines the activity of placental LPL and fatty acid transport across the placenta is concentration dependent, there is a direct relationship between maternal and fetal plasma triglyceride concentrations, even though there is no direct uptake and transfer of intact triglycerides by the placenta.

The fetal impact of maternal plasma FFA and lipid concentrations is also reflected in fetal lipid content and adipose tissue development. Fatter human fetuses develop in pregnant women who have higher plasma concentrations of fatty acids and other lipids. Experimentally, diabetic rats (induced by streptozotocin) have increased free fatty acids, and their fetuses have carcass and hepatic lipid contents that are increased twofold above normal.[138] Similarly, rabbits fed oil rich diets show increased neonatal adipose stores.[139] In humans, umbilical venous–arterial fatty acid concentration differences in cord blood samples show that the net flux of free fatty acids into the fetus from the maternal circulation can account for the fetal requirement of fatty acids during the end of pregnancy.[140] In contrast, the perfused human placenta may transfer fatty acids at a rate that can account for only about 20% of that required for the accumulation of fetal adipose tissue deposited during the third trimester.[141] Other estimates, based on fetal lipid accumulation as well as in vitro transfer experiments, estimate that as much as 50% of fetal fatty acid requirements are transferred across the human placenta[99]; similar estimates have been made in the rat using the incorporation of ^3H from ^3H_2O into fatty acids, indicating that fatty acids are derived about equally from the mother and from fetal fatty acid synthesis.[142] Estimates in the rabbit[143] and the monkey[144] indicate that in these species, placental fatty acid transfer across the placenta could account for all of fetal fat deposition in late gestation. Overall, therefore, it appears that there is a general relationship between the permeability of the placenta to lipids, especially fatty acids, and the adiposity of the fetus at term, with human fetuses developing the most fat (15 to 18% of body weight at term),[145] guinea pigs second at about 12%, and rabbits third at about 7% (Figure 9).

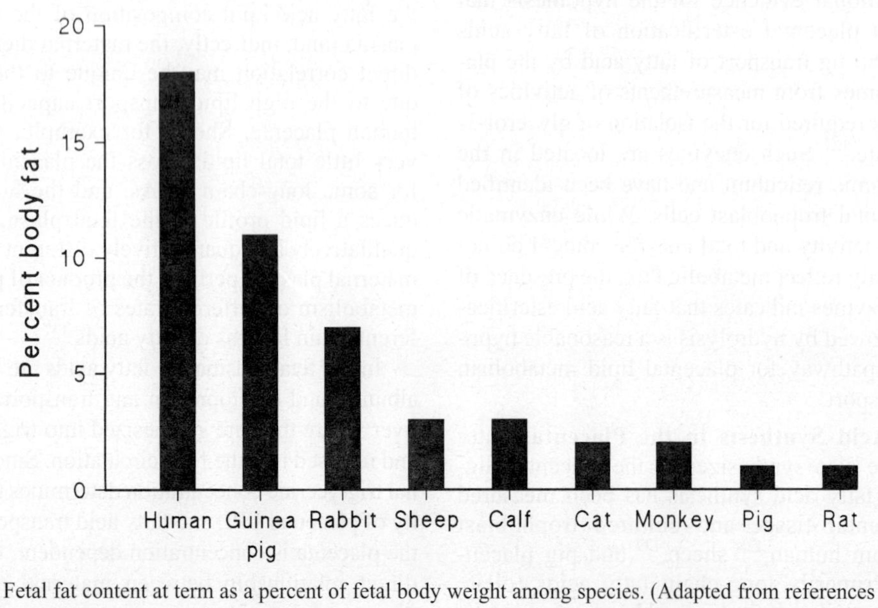

Figure 9 Fetal fat content at term as a percent of fetal body weight among species. (Adapted from references 2, 4, 5, 7, and 100.)

Availability of Essential Fatty Acids to the Fetus

Essential Fatty Acid Metabolism and Transfer by the Placenta. The supply of EFAs and long-chain polyunsaturated fatty acid (LCPUFA) is critical and central to the synthesis of structural lipids and hence to normal development of the fetus. Linoleic acid (18:2, ω-6) and α-linolenic acid (18:3, ω-3) are the only fatty acids known to be essential for complete nutrition and must be supplied in the diet. All of the ω-6 and ω-3 fatty acid structure acquired by the fetus must, therefore, come from the mother via the placenta, either in the form of these two EFAs or their LCPUFA derivatives of which AA (20:4, ω-6) and DHA (22:6, ω-3) are metabolically the most important.[146]

EFAs are readily transferred to the fetal plasma in all species studied so far. Cultured trophoblast cells incubated with ^{14}C-acetate do not label AA, however, and delta-5 and delta-6 desaturase activities in human placental microsomes are absent at least early in gestation,[147,148] consistent with the absence of measurable conversion of γ-linolenic acid to AA.[149] This emphasizes the requirement for direct transfer of the essential LCPUFAs to the fetus from the maternal plasma. In fact, higher concentrations of these EFAs are found in the fetus compared with the mother.[150–153] These results suggest that fetal AA is either transferred directly from the mother or has a higher biding capacity in the fetal plasma, but does not exclude the possibility that some might be synthesized from linoleic acid in the fetal liver. Although formation of AA and DHA from EFA precursors has been shown in term and preterm infants,[154–160] the degree to which the fetus is capable of fatty acid desaturation and elongation is not clear. Fetal baboons can synthesize both DHA (22:6, ω-3) and AA (20:4, ω-6) from their precursors, α-linolenic acid (18:3, ω-3) and linoleic acid (18:2, ω-6), respectively.[161,162] A low enzymatic activity of delta-5 desaturation has been proposed as one factor limiting AA synthesis,[163] and although high delta-5 and delta-6 desaturase activities in the liver of one 18 week and two 22 week fetuses,[147] which were close to those found in adult liver,[164] have been reported, human fetal liver desaturase-elongase chain reactions have not been clearly demonstrated in physiological conditions

Maternal Diet and Essential Fatty Acid Supply to the Fetus. In general, reduced maternal EFA nutrition has been correlated with reduced neonatal growth and head circumference in humans.[165] Significant linear correlations between the mother and fetus or newborn have been found for both LCPUFA and EFAs in healthy women eating normal, unsupplemented diets.[166–168] Parallel increases in plasma DHA in the mothers and newborns have also been found after fish-oil supplementation during pregnancy.[169,170] These observations show the importance of maternal dietary fatty acids to regulate the availability of LCPUFA to the fetus and newborn. In fact, because the developing fetus depends primarily on the maternal supply of EFAs, maternal dietary supplement with LCPUFA-rich oils during the last trimester of pregnancy to increase levels in neonates has been advised.[169,170] However, the competitive desaturation of the ω-3 and ω-6 series by Δ-6 and Δ-5 desaturases is of major significance because of their controlling role in the desaturating and elongating pathways of the parent EFAs.[171] Thus, excessive dietary intake of linolenic acid from vegetable oils, particularly safflower, sunflower, and corn oil, may inhibit Δ-6 desaturase and decrease the formation of DHA from α-linolenic acid. Similarly, AA formation is lower when excessive linolenic acid is provided, as seen in externally or parentally fed infants receiving corn or safflower oil as the predominant source of fatty.[172–175] Further, the inhibitory effect of eicosapentaenoic acid on Δ-5 desaturase activity has been considered responsible for the lower plasma AA found when fish oil, high in eicosapentanoic acid and DHA, is consumed.[171] Also, excessive fish oil intake can inhibit intake of linolenic acid from vegetable oils, particularly safflower, sunflower, and corn oil, and may inhibit Δ-6 desaturase activity and decrease AA levels.[176,177] The consumption of fish oils modifies membrane phospholipid composition, increasing eicosapentaenoic acid and DHA concentrations at the expense of AA content, and adverse effects of low AA concentration in serum and red blood cell phospholipids on growth during infancy have been observed.[178–180] AA status in preterm infants has also been correlated with their birth weight.[178,181,182] Foods containing lipid peroxides are potentially toxic, and the higher the content of LCPUFAs in the diet, the more likely peroxidation will occur.[183–185] Thus, excess intake of PUFA may reduce antioxidant capacity,[186] enhancing susceptibility to oxidative damage,[187] a condition that has been shown to be responsible for fetal damage during pregnancy in rats.[188–190]

Dietary olive oil appears to protect the LCPUFA series better than fish oil.[191] Olive oil also does not affect AA concentrations,[192–194] and is much more resistant to lipid peroxidation.[185,195,196] The effect of a diet supplemented with 10% fish oil versus the same amount of olive oil during pregnancy on the fatty acid profile and vitamin E concentration has been studied in the rat. A decrease in both AA and α-tocopherol concentrations as well as delayed postnatal development was found in the offspring of rats fed the fish oil-rich diet.[197] The study was extended to determine whether dietary supplementation with either vitamin E or y-linolenic acid (18:3, ω-6) as a precursor of AA could ameliorate these changes. AA concentrations and postnatal development indices, but not α-tocopherol concentrations, were improved when the fish-oil diet was supplemented with y-linolenic acid. In contrast, postnatal development indices were not improved when the fish oil-rich diet was supplemented with sufficient exogenous vitamin E to normalize α-tocopherol levels.[197] Thus although feeding a fish oil-rich diet during pregnancy and lactation decreased both α-tocopherol and AA concentrations, the latter deficiency rather than the former seemed to be responsible for delayed postnatal development of rat pups. In this same study, another group of pregnant and lactating rats fed the fish oil-rich diet received a supplement with AA instead of y-linolenic acid, and although both treatments restored brain phospholipid content and AA content in the pups, improvement in growth rate and neurodevelopment indexes was more efficient in the y-linolenic acid group. The only difference between the two groups was the absence of linolenic acid (18:2, ω-6) in brain phospholipids when rats were supplemented with AA, whereas it was present at a normal level in those supplemented with y-linolenic acid.[197] These findings agree with those previously in humans fed diets rich in AA in which the proportion of linolenic acid in plasma phospholipids decreased,[198] likely a consequence of replacing linolenic acid by AA in tissues.[199]

These observations in humans and experimental animals emphasize the exquisite sensitivity of endogenous LCPUFA metabolism to changes in maternal dietary fatty acid composition during perinatal development and the quite remarkable consequences to fetal and neonatal development. Since benefits and risks of modifying maternal fat intake in pregnancy and lactation are not yet completely established, and the safety of high intakes of LCPUFA during pregnancy is still unclear,[200–202] further studies are required before recommendations to increase LCPUFA intake in pregnancy can be made.

Placental Uptake, Metabolism, and Transfer of Essential Fatty Acids. Maternal plasma EFAs are the principal source of LCPUFAs to the fetus.[148,152,203] Cellular uptake of FFA occurs by facilitated transmembrane transport involving a FABPpm.[204–208] The preference for human placental transfer from the maternal to the fetal circulation has been reported to be DHA>α-linolenic>linoleic>oleic>AA.[209] AA, however, has the highest accumulation of all of these fatty acids in the placenta.[209] AA uptake by placental syncytiotrophoblast membranes is highly dependent on ATP and sodium,[210] implying an active transport mechanism for this fatty acid. Selective LCPUFA placental transfer is also due to trophoblast cellular metabolism; for example, a certain proportion of AA is converted to prostaglandins in the placenta.[148] Also a selective incorporation of certain fatty acids into phospholipids has been found in the ovine placenta[211] and selective placental trophoblast fatty acid oxidation[212] and lipid synthesis have been reported.[109,213,214]

Fetal Accumulation of Essential Fatty Acids

Intrauterine requirements for ω-6 and ω-3 fatty acids in the human fetus during the last trimester of fetal development through the early weeks of life have been estimated to be 400 and 50 mg/kg/d, respectively.[215,216] In tissues such as the brain, where lipids constitute about 50% dry weight, almost half of the total lipid content is composed of LCPUFA.[217] Both arachidonic and DHAs are readily incorporated into the structural lipids of the developing brain [218] where, besides their role in maintaining membrane fluidity, permeability, and conformation, they play an important functional role. For example, once released from phospholipids by the action of phospholipase A_2, AA is the main precursor for eicosanoids, prostaglandins, and leukotrienes,[219] and is essential for fetal and neonatal growth,[220] while DHA has a key role in the development of visual function.[150,221,222] Although the relative rates of desaturation by rat liver and brain differ between those of adult and 10-day-old animals,[223] the degree to which the human fetus is capable of desaturation and elongation is not clear. It is normally believed that the supply of EFAs and LCPUFA is critical and central to the synthesis of structural lipids and hence to normal fetal development.[151,154,224]

Fetal Lipid Metabolism: Utilization

Physiological changes that develop in the fetus in late gestation and increase nutrient utilization, such as the increase in plasma insulin concentration, act to enhance net maternal-to-fetal fatty acid and lipid transport by increasing fatty acid utilization in the fetus (largely to develop adipose tissue, it appears). Increased utilization of fatty acids by fetal tissues lowers fetal plasma fatty acid concentrations relative to those in the maternal plasma and increases the maternal-to-fetal fatty acid concentration gradients. For example, human maternal venous blood concentrations of fatty acids are directly related to the umbilical artery free fatty acid concentrations and the umbilical vein–artery concentration differences of free fatty acids.[145] Similar observations have been made in the rabbit[143] and the guinea pig,[225] including, in the latter, evidence that experimentally lowering the fetal fatty acid concentration relative to that in the maternal plasma independently increases fatty acid transfer across the placenta (using an in situ perfusion model). Even at the same concentrations, furthermore, naturally occurring or experimentally increased fetal plasma concentrations of albumin directly increase the transfer of fatty acids across the placenta; this observation is based on data from both in vitro perfused human placentas [226] and in situ perfused guinea pig placentas.[225] The effect of albumin seems to be one of simply providing increased esterification capacity in the fetal plasma to bind free fatty acids transferred directly across the placenta.

Whether the processes of fatty acid transfer to the fetus by the placenta and fatty acid incorporation into fetal tissues actually begin during gestation, and whether or not they occur with simultaneous development of placental fatty acid transporters and placental lipid metabolic capacity, remain to be determined, although human fetal fat accretion develops primarily in the third trimester.[7] During late gestation, maternal lipid metabolism changes to a catabolic state,[227] as shown by increased adipose tissue lipolysis and reduced uptake of circulating triglycerides.[228] The reduced uptake is the result of decreased adipose tissue LPL activity.[229] There is also an overproduction of triglyceride by the liver and enhanced absorption of dietary lipids. Together, these changes in maternal lipid metabolism produce increasing concentrations of nearly all types of circulating plasma lipids as late gestation proceeds, including free fatty acids, glycerol, and triglyceride-rich very low-density lipoprotein and chylomicron particles. When the pregnant mother is well fed, plasma concentrations of ketoacids (β-hydroxybutyrate and acetoacetate) are not increased, although during fasting, when the concentrations of these substrates do increase, they may also contribute significantly to the supply of nutrient substrates to the uteroplacenta and the fetus.

Fetal Leptin

Leptin mediates a multitude of biological actions in the adult, including regulation of weight by controlling hypothalamic mechanisms involved in food intake[230] and in regulating insulin secretion,[231,232] insulin action to promote peripheral glucose utilization,[233,234] and metabolic rate.[235,236] Emerging evidence supports roles for leptin in the fetus as well, including enhancement of growth.[237] Umbilical cord leptin concentrations correlate with birth weight,[238,239] being higher in macrosomic infants of diabetic mothers,[238] and lower in infants with IUGR,[239] indicating that the fetal metabolic and hormonal milieu independent of fetal fat content may regulate leptin synthesis and circulating concentrations. In fetal sheep, fetal white adipose tissue leptin mRNA amounts increase with fetal development and gestational age and with basal insulin concentrations.[240] Glucose infusions producing hyperglycemia and hyperinsulinemia and insulin infusions producing hyperinsulinemia alone also increased circulating leptin concentrations, showing that insulin itself can affect fetal leptin production, which thus may mediate at least some of insulin's influence on fetal growth.

Summary of Placental and Fetal Lipid Metabolism

The transport of fatty acids and other lipid substances across the placenta, and the deposition of lipids in adipose tissue, are late-gestation phenomena and highly species-specific. The human hemochorial placenta transfers the most lipid and produces the fattest of all land mammals at birth. EFA transport, however, occurs in all species and begins early in gestation, allowing membrane lipids, particularly those of neurons, to develop throughout gestation. At preterm birth, however, the human newborn is in a precarious balance with respect to lipid metabolism. Failure to provide sufficient nonprotein energy will lead to increased rates of lipolysis and fatty acid oxidation. This may or may not result in breakdown of membrane lipids for oxidation, but certainly it produces a metabolic situation in which EFAs will be oxidized along with other fatty acids to produce necessary energy in preference to membrane deposition. This could lead to deleterious alteration in the amount and structure of critical membrane development in the brain, leading potentially to abnormal neurological function and long-term outcome.[241]

ACKNOWLEDGEMENT

This work was supported in part by grants DK52138 and HD28794 (WW Hay Jr, Principal Investigator) from the National Institutes of Health.

REFERENCES

1. Hay WW, Jr. Placental nutrient metabolism and transfer. In: Herrera E, Knopp R, editors. Perinatal Biochemistry. Boca Raton, FL: CRC Press; 1992. p. 93–130.
2. Hay WW, Jr. Energy and substrate requirements of the placenta and fetus. Proc Nutr Soc 1991;50:321–36.
3. Hay WW, Jr, Wilkening RB. Metabolic activity of the placenta. In: Thorburn GD, Harding R, editors. Textbook of Fetal Physiology. Oxford: Oxford Medical Publications; 1994. p. 30–47.
4. Hay WW, Jr. Metabolic interrelationships of placenta and fetus. Placenta 1995;16:19–30.
5. Battaglia FC, Meschia G. An Introduction to Fetal Physiology. Orlando, FL: Academic Press; 1986.
6. Hay WW, Jr. Fetal requirements and placental transfer of nitrogenous compounds. In: Polin RA, Fox WW, editors. Fetal and Neonatal Physiology. Philadelphia, PA: WB Saunders; 1991. p. 431–42.
7. Sparks JW, Girard J, Battaglia FC. An estimate of the caloric requirements of the human fetus. Biol Neonate 1980;38:113–9.
8. Kalhan SC, D'Angelo LJ, Savin SM, Adam PAJ. Glucose production in pregnant women at term gestation. Sources of glucose for the human fetus. J Clin Invest 1979;63:388–94.
9. Hay WW, Jr, Sparks JW, Quissel BJ, et al. Simultaneous measurements of umbilical glucose uptake, fetal utilization rate, and fetal turnover rate of glucose. Am J Physiol 1981;240:E662–8.
10. Gleason CA, Rudolph AM. Gluconeogenesis by the fetal sheep liver in vivo. J Dev Physiol 1985;7:185–94.
11. Hay WW, Jr, Sparks JW, Wilkening RB, et al. Fetal glucose uptake and utilization as functions of maternal glucose concentration. Am J Physiol 1984;246:E237–42.
12. DiGiacomo JE, Hay WW, Jr. Regulation of placental glucose transfer and consumption by fetal glucose production. Pediatr Res 1989;25:429–34.
13. Fowden AL, Mundy L, Silver M. Developmental regulation of glucogenesis in the sheep fetus during late gestation. J Physiol 1991;508:937–47.
14. Girard J. Gluconeogenesis in late fetal and early neonatal life. Biol Neonate 1986;50:237–58.
15. Fowden AL, Mapstone J, Forhead AJ. Regulation of glucogenesis by thyroid hormone in fetal sheep during late gestation. J Endocrinol 2001;170:461–69.
16. Hay WW, Jr, Meznarich HK, Fowden AL. Effect of streptozotocin of rates of ovine fetal glucose utilization, oxidation and production in the sheep fetus. Metabolism 1988;38:30–7.
17. Fowden AL, Hay WW, Jr. The effects of pancreatectomy on the rates of glucose utilization, oxidation and production in the sheep fetus. Q J Exp Physiol 1988;73:973–84.
18. Schwartz AL, Rall TW. Hormonal regulation of incorporation of alanine-U-^{14}C into glucose in human fetal liver explants. Diabetes 1975;24:650–7.
19. Prior RL, Christenson RK. Gluconeogenesis from alanine in vivo by the ovine fetus and lamb. Am J Physiol 1977;233: E462–8.
20. Plas C, Forest N, Pringault E, Menuelle P. Contribution of glucose and gluconeogenic substrates to insulin-stimulated glycogen synthesis in cultured fetal hepatocytes. J Cell Physiol 1982;113:475–80.
21. Levitsky LL, Paton JB, Fisher DE. Precursors to glycogen in ovine fetuses. Am J Physiol 1988;255:E743–7.
22. Shelley HJ, Neligan GA. Neonatal hypoglycemia. Br Med Bull 1966;22:34–9.
23. Rudolph CD, Roman C, Rudolph AM. Effect of acute umbilical cord compression on hepatic carbohydrate metabolism in the fetal lamb. Pediatr Res 1989;25:228–33.
24. Greengard O. Enzymatic differentiation of human liver: Comparison with the rat model. Pediatr Res 1977;11:669–76.
25. Simmons MA, Battaglia FC, Meschia G. Placental transfer of glucose. J Dev Physiol 1979;1:227–43.
26. Gilbert M, Hay WW, Jr, Johnson RL, Battaglia FC. Some aspects of maternal metabolism throughout pregnancy in the conscious rabbit. Pediatr Res 1984;18:854–9.
27. Zorzano A, Palacín M, Testar X. Insulin resistance in pregnancy. In: Herrera E, Knapp RH, editors. Perinatal Biochemistry. Boca Raton, FL: CRC Press; 1992. p. 69–92.
28. Gilbert M, Pere MC, Baudelin A, Battaglia FC. Role of free fatty acids in hepatic insulin resistance during late pregnancy in conscious rabbits. Am J Physiol 1991;260: E938–45.
29. Catalano PM, Nizielski SE, Shao J, et al. Downregulated IRS-1 and PPARgamma in obese women with gestational diabetes: Relationship to FFA during pregnancy. Am J Physiol Endocrinol Metab 2002;282:E522–33.
30. Shao J, Yamashita H, Qiao L, et al. Phosphatidylinositol 3-kinase redistribution is associated with skeletal muscle insulin resistance in gestational diabetes mellitus. Diabetes 2002;51:19–29.
31. Barbour LA, Shao J, Qiao L, et al. Human placental growth hormone causes severe insulin resistance in transgenic mice. Am J Obstet Gynecol 2002;186:512–7.
32. Smith CH, Moe AJ, Ganapathy V. Nutrient transport pathways across the epithelium of the placenta. Ann Rev Nutr 1992;12:183–206.
33. Osmond DT, King RG, Brennecke SP, Gude NM. Placental glucose transport and utilization is altered in insulin-treated, gestational-diabetic patients. Diabetologia 2001;44:1133–9.
34. Boileau P, Cauzac M, Pereira MA, et al. Dissociation between insulin-mediated signaling pathways and biological effects in placental cells: Role of protein kinase B and MAPK phosphorylation. Endocrinology 2001;142: 3974–9.
35. Hahn D, Blaschitz A, Korgun ET, et al. From maternal glucose to fetal glycogen: Expression of key regulators in the human placenta. Mol Hum Reprod 2001;7:1173–8.
36. Hahn T, Hahn D, Blaschitz A, et al. Hyperglycemia-induced subcellular redistribution of GLUT1 glucose transporters in cultured human term placental trophoblast cells. Diabetologia 2000;43:173–80.
37. Illsley NP. Placental glucose transport in diabetic pregnancy. Clin Obstet Gynecol 2000;43:116–26.
38. Gaither K, Quraishi AN, Illsley NP. Diabetes alters the expression and activity of the human placental GLUT1 glucose transporter. J Clin Endocrinol Metab 1999;84:695–701.
39. Illsley NP, Sellers MC, Wright RL. Glycaemic regulation of glucose transporter expression and activity in the human placenta. Placenta 1998;19:517–24.
40. Coughlan MT, Oliva K, Georgiou HM, et al. Glucose-induced release of tumour necrosis factor-alpha from human placental and adipose tissues in gestational diabetes mellitus. Diabet Med 2001;18:921–7.
41. Kirwan JP, Hauguel-De Mouzon S, Lepercq J, et al. TNF-alpha is a predictor of insulin resistance in human pregnancy. Diabetes 2002;51:2207–13.
42. Das U, He J, Ehrhardt RA, et al. Time-dependent physiological regulation of ovine placental GLUT-3 glucose transporter protein. Am J Physiol Regul Integr Comp Physiol 2000;279:R2252–61.
43. Dandrea J, Wilson V, Gopalakrishnan G, et al. Maternal nutritional manipulation of placental growth and glucose transporter 1 (GLUT-1) abundance in sheep. Reproduction 2001;122:793–800.
44. Lesage J, Hahn D, Leonhardt M, et al. Maternal undernutrition during late gestation-induced intrauterine growth restriction in the rat is associated with impaired placental GLUT3 expression, but does not correlate with endogenous corticosterone levels. J Endocrinol 2002;174:37–43.
45. Das UG, Sadiq HF, Soares MJ, et al. Time-dependent physiological regulation of rodent and ovine placental glucose transporter (GLUT-1) protein. Am J Physiol Regul Integr Comp Physiol 1998;274:R339–47.
46. Hay WW, Jr, Sparks JW, Wilkening RB, et al. Fetal glucose uptake and utilization as functions of maternal glucose concentration. Am J Physiol 1984;246:E237–42.
47. Hay WW, Jr, Molina RD, DiGiacomo JE, Meschia G. Model of placental glucose consumption and transfer. Am J Physiol 1990;258:R569–77.
48. Kalhan S. Metabolism of glucose and methods of investigation in the fetus and newborn. In: Polin RA, Fox WW, editors. Fetal and Neonatal Physiology. Philadelphia, PA: WB Saunders; 1992. p. 357–72.
49. Whaley WH, Zuspan FP, Nelson GH. Correlation between maternal and fetal plasma levels of glucose and free fatty acids. Am J Obstet Gynecol 1966;94:419–21.
50. Coltart TM, Beard RW, Turner RC, Oakley NW. Blood glucose and insulin relationships in the human mother and fetus before onset of labor. Br Med J 1969;4:17–9.
51. Meschia G, Battaglia FC, Hay WW, Jr, Sparks JW. The utilization of substrates by the ovine placenta in vivo. Fed Proc 1980;9:245–9.
52. Hahn D, Blaschitz A, Korgun ET, et al. From maternal glucose to fetal glycogen: Expression of key regulators in the human placenta. Mol Hum Reprod 2001;7:1173–8.
53. Matsubara S, Takizawa T, Suzuki T, et al. Glucose-6-phosphate dehydrogenase is present in normal and pre-eclamptic placental trophoblasts: Ultrastructural enzyme-histochemical evidence. Placenta 2001;22; 90–5.
54. Johnson LW, Smith CH. Monosaccharide transport across microvillous membrane of human placenta. Am J Physiol 1980;238:C160–8.
55. Haugel S, Desnaizieres V, Challier JC. Glucose uptake, utilization, and transfer by the human placenta as functions of maternal glucose concentration. Pediatr Res 1986;20:269–73.
56. Hay WW, Jr, Meznarich HK. Effect of maternal glucose concentration on uteroplacental glucose consumption and transfer in pregnant sheep. Proc Soc Exp Biol Med 1988;190:63–9.
57. Hay WW, Jr, DiGiacomo JE, Meznarich HK, et al. Effects of glucose and insulin on fetal glucose oxidation and oxygen consumption. Am J Physiol 1989;256:E704–13.
58. Bell GI, Burant CF, Takeda J, Gould GW. Structure and function of mammalian facilitative sugar transporters. J Biol Chem 1993;268:19161–4.
59. Carayannopoulos MO, Chi MM-Y, Cui Y, et al. Glut 8 is a glucose transporter responsible for insulin-stimulated glucose uptake in blastocyst. Proc Natl Acad Sci U S A 2000;97:7313–8.
60. Devaskar SU, Mueckler M. The mammalian glucose transporters. Pediatr Res 1992;31:1–12.
61. Phay JE, Hussain HB, Moley JF. Cloning and expression analysis of a novel member of the facilitative glucose transporter family, SLC2A9 (GLUT9). Genomics 2000;66:217–20.
62. Ehrhardt RA, Bell AW. Developmental increases in glucose transporter concentration in the sheep placenta. Am J Physiol Regul Integr Comp Physiol 1997;273:R1132–41.
63. Hiraki Y, Rosen OM, Birnbaum MJ. Growth factors rapidly induce expression of the glucose transporter gene. J Biol Chem 1988;263:13655–62.
64. Werner H, Adamo M, Lowe WL, Jr, et al. Developmental regulation of the rat brain/Hep G2 glucose transporter gene expression. Mol Endocrinol 1989;3:273–9.
65. Das UG, Schroeder RE, Hay WW, Jr, Devaskar SU. Time-dependent and tissue-specific effects of circulating glucose on fetal ovine glucose transporters. AM J Physiol Regul Integr Comp Physiol 1999;276:R809–17.
66. Khan JY, Rajakumar RA, McKnight RA, et al. Developmental regulation of genes mediating murine brain glucose uptake. Am J Physiol Regul Integr Comp Physiol 1999;276: R892–900.
67. Sadiq HF, deMello DE, Devaskar SU. The effect of intrauterine growth restriction upon fetal and postnatal hepatic glucose transporter and glucokinase proteins. Pediatr Res 1998;43:91–100.
68. Sadiq HF, Das UG, Tracy TF, Devaskar SU. Intrauterine growth restriction differentially regulates perinatal brain and skeletal muscle glucose transporters. Brain Res 1999;823:96–103.
69. Schroeder RE, Doria-Medina CL, Das UG, et al. Effect of maternal diabetes upon fetal rat myocardial and skeletal muscle glucose transporters. Pediatr Res 1997;41:11–9.
70. Atkins V, Flozak AS, Ogata ES, Simmons RA. The effects of severe maternal diabetes on glucose transport in the fetal rat. Endocrinology 1994;135:409–15.

71. Carver TD, Anderson SM, Aldoretta PW, et al. Glucose suppression of insulin secretion in chronically hyperglycemic fetal sheep. Pediatr Res 1995;38:754–62.
72. Aldoretta PW, Hay WW, Jr. Chronic hyperglycemia induces insulin resistance and glucose intolerance in fetal sheep. Pediatr Res 2001;49:307A.
73. Anderson MS, Flowers-Ziegler J, Das UG, et al. Glucose transporter protein responses to selective hyperglycemia or hyperinsulinemia in fetal sheep. Am J Physiol Regul Integr Comp Physiol 2001;281:R1545–52.
74. Anderson MS, He J, Flowers-Ziegler J, et al. Effects of selective hyperglycemia and hyperinsulinemia on glucose transporters in fetal ovine skeletal muscle. Am J Physiol Regul Integr Comp Physiol 2001;281:R1256–63.
75. DiGiacomo JE, Hay WW, Jr. Effect of hypoinsulinemia and hyperglycemia on fetal glucose utilization and oxidation. Am J Physiol 1990;259:E506–12.
76. DiGiacomo JE, Hay WW, Jr. Fetal glucose metabolism and oxygen consumption during sustained maternal and fetal hypoglycemia. Metabolism 1990;39:193–202.
77. Molina RD, Meschia G, Battaglia FC, Hay WW, Jr. Maturation of placental glucose transfer capacity in the ovine pregnancy. Am J Physiol 1991;261:R697–704.
78. Kalhan SC, Savin SM, Adam PAJ. Measurement of glucose turnover in the human newborn with glucose-1-^{13}C. J Clin Endocrinol Metab 1976;43:704–7.
79. Ehrhardt RA, McNeill DM, Bell AW. Identification of and developmental increases in glucose transport protein in the sheep placenta [abstract 1024]. FASEB J 1994;8:A177.
80. Bassett NS, Currie MJ, Woodall SM, et al. The effect of maternal IGF-1 treatment on placental GLUT gene expression. Proceedings of Thorburn Symposium. Hamilton Island, Queensland, Australia, 1994. Program, Combined Meeting of the Australian and New Zealand Perinatal Societies, Auckland, NZ, April 2–5, 1995.
81. Bell AW, Battaglia FC, Meschia G. Relation between metabolic rate and body size in the ovine fetus. J Nutr 1987;117:1181–6.
82. Aldoretta PW, Carver TD, Hay WW, Jr. Maturation of glucose-stimulated insulin secretion in fetal sheep. Biol Neonate 1998;73: 375–86.
83. Rorsman P, Arkhammar P, Bokvist K, et al. Failure of glucose to elicit a normal secretory response in fetal pancreatic beta cells results from glucose insensitivity of the ATP-regulated K* channels. Proc Natl Acad Sci U S A 1989;86:4505–9.
84. Weinhaus AJ, Poronnik P, Cook DI, Tuch BE. Insulin secretagogues, but not glucose, stimulate an increase in $[Ca^{2+}]_i$ in the fetal rat βcell. Diabetes 1995;44:118–24.
85. Coltart TM, Beard RW, Turner RC, Oakley NW. Blood glucose and insulin relationships in the human mother and fetus before the onset of labour. Br Med J 1969;iv:17–9.
86. Milner RDG, Hales CN. Effect of intravenous glucose on concentration of insulin in maternal and umbilical-cord plasma. Br Med J 1965;i:284–6.
87. Obenshain SS, Adam PAJ, King KC, et al. Human fetal insulin response to sustained maternal hyperglycemia. New Engl J Med 1970;283:566–70.
88. Carver TD, Anderson SM, Aldoretta PW, Hay WW, Jr. Effect of low-level basal plus marked "pulsatile" hyperglycemia on insulin secretion in fetal sheep. Am J Physiol Endocrinol Metab 1996;271:E865–71.
89. Limesand SW, Hay WW, Jr. Adaptation of ovine fetal pancreatic insulin secretion to chronic hypoglycemia and euglycemic conditions. J Physiol 2003;547:95–105.
90. Sparks JW, Hay WW, Jr, Bonds D, et al. Simultaneous measurements of lactate turnover rate and umbilical lactate uptake in the fetal lamb. J Clin Invest 1982;70:179–92.
91. Meznarich HK, Hay WW, Jr, Sparks JW, et al. Fructose disposal and oxidation rates in the ovine fetus. Q J Exp Physiol 1987;72:617–25.
92. Hay WW, Jr, Meyers SA, Sparks JW, et al. Glucose and lactate oxidation rates in the fetal lamb. Proc Soc Exp Biol Med 1983;73:553–63.
93. Hay WW, Jr, Sparks JW, Wilkening RB, et al. Partition of maternal glucose production between conceptus and maternal tissues in sheep. Am J Physiol 1983;245:E347–50.
94. DiGiacomo JE, Hay WW, Jr. Regulation of placental glucose transfer and consumption by fetal glucose production. Pediatr Res 1989;25:429–34.
95. Wallace JM, Bourke DA, Aitken RP, et al. Blood flows and nutrient uptakes in growth-restricted pregnancies induced by overnourishing adolescent sheep. Am J Physiol Regul Integr Comp Physiol 2002;282:R1027–36.
96. Jackson BT, Cohn HE, Morrison SH, et al. Hypoxia-induced sympathetic inhibition of the fetal plasma insulin response to hyperglycemia. Diabetes 1993;42:1621–5.
97. Hay WW, Jr, Aldoretta PW, Carver TD. Glucose-Specific Suppression of Insulin Secretion and Glucose Utilization in Late-Gestation Fetal Sheep. Monduzzi Editore, Bologna: Acta Second World Congress of Perinatal Medicine; 1993. p. 835–9.
98. Moores RR, Jr, Vaughn PR, Battaglia FC, et al. Glutamate metabolism in fetus and placenta of late-gestation sheep. Am J Physiol 1994;267:R89–96.
99. Coleman RA. Placental metabolism and transport of lipid. Fed Proc 1986;45:2519–23.
100. Widdowson EM. Growth and composition of the human fetus and newborn. In: Assali NS, editor. Biology of Gestation, Volume 2. New York: Academic Press; 1968. p. 1–48.
101. Elphick MC, Hull D. Rabbit placental clearing-factor lipase and transfer to the foetus of fatty acids derived from triglycerides injected into the mother. J Physiol (Lond) 1977;273:475–87.
102. Rotherwell JE, Elphick MC. Lipoprotein lipase activity in human and guinea pig placenta. J Dev Physiol 1982;4: 153–9.
103. Bonet B, Brunzell JD, Gown AM, Knopp RH. Metabolism of very-low-density lipoprotein triglyceride by human placental cells: The role of lipoprotein lipase. Metabolism 1992;41:596–603.
104. Farrugia W, Aiken MA, van Dunne F, et al. Type II phospholipase A2 in human gestational tissues: Subcellular distribution of placental immuno- and catalytic activity. Biochim Biophys Acta 1993;1166:77–83.
105. Rice GE, Wong MH, Farrugia W, Scott KF. Contribution of type II phospholipase A2 to in vitro phospholipase A2 enzymatic activity in human term placenta. J Endocrinol 1998;157:25–31.
106. Biale Y. Lipolytic activity in the placentas of chronically deprived fetuses. Acta Obstet Gynecol Scand 1985;64:111–4.
107. Kaminsky S, D'Souza SW, Massey RF, et al. Effects of maternal undernutrition and uterine artery ligation on placental lipase activities in the rat. Biol Neonate 1991;60:201–6.
108. Mochizuki M, Morikawa H, Ohga Y, Tojo S. Lipolytic action of human chorionic somatomammotropin. Endocrinol Jpn 1975;22:123–9.
109. Coleman RA, Haynes EB. Synthesis and release of fatty acids by human trophoblast cells in culture. J Lipid Res 1987;28:1335–41.
110. Kamp F, Zakim D, Zhang FL, et al. Fatty-acid flip-flop in phospholipid-bilayers is extremely fast. Biochemistry 1995;34:11928–37.
111. Glatz JFC, vanderVusse GJ. Cellular fatty acid-binding proteins: Their function and physiological significance. Prog Lipid Res 1996;35:243–82.
112. Glatz JFC, vanNieuwenhoven FA, Luiken JJFP, et al. Role of membrane-associated and cytoplasmic fatty acid-binding proteins in cellular fatty acid metabolism. Prostaglandins Leukot Essent Fatty Acids 1997;57:373–8.
113. Glatz JFC, Luiken JJFP, vanNieuwenhoven FA, vanderVusse GJ. Molecular mechanism of cellular uptake and intracellular translocation of fatty acids. Prostaglandins Leukot Essent Fatty Acids 1997;57:3–9.
114. Veerkamp JH, Peeters RA, Maatman RG. Structural and functional features of different types of cytoplasmic fatty acid-binding proteins. Biochim Biophys Acta 1991;1081:1–24.
115. Veerkamp JH, van Moerkerk HTB, Zimmerman AW. Effect of fatty acid-binding proteins an intermembrane fatty acid transport—studies on different types and mutant proteins. Eur J Biochem 2000;267:5959–66.
116. Campbell FM, Bush PG, Veerkamp JH, Dutta-Roy AK. Detection and cellular localization of plasma membrane-associated and cytoplasmic fatty acid-binding proteins in human placenta. Placenta 1998;19:409–15.
117. Campbell FM, Dutta-Roy AK. Plasma membrane fatty acid binding protein (FABPpm) is exclusively located in the maternal facing membranes of the human placenta. FEBS Lett 1995;375:227–30.
118. Dutta-Roy AK. Transport mechanisms for long-chain polyunsaturated fatty acids in the human placenta. Am J Clin Nutr 2000;71:315S–22S.
119. Campbell FM, Gordon MJ, Dutta-Roy AK. Placental membrane fatty acid-binding protein preferentially binds arachidonic and docosahexaenoic acids. Life Sci 1998;63:235–40.
120. Veerkamp JH. Fatty-acid transport and fatty acid binding proteins. Proc Nutr Soc 1995;54:23–37.
121. Benassayag C, Mignot TM, Haourigui M, et al. High polyunsaturated fatty acid, thromboxane A2, and alpha-fetoprotein concentrations at the human feto-maternal interface. J Lipid Res 1997;38:276–86.
122. Benassayag C, Rigourd V, Mignot TM, et al. Does high polyunsaturated free fatty acid level at the feto maternal interface alter steroid hormone message during pregnancy? Prostaglandins Leukot Essent Fatty Acids 1999;60:393–9.
123. Patel MN, Kleinfeld AM, Richeiri GV, et al. Serum levels of unbound free fatty acids. I: Normative data in term newborn infants. J Am Coll Nutr 1997;16:81–4.
124. Economides DL, Crook D, Nicolaides KH. Investigation of hypertriglyceridemia in small for gestational age fetuses. Fetal Ther 1988;3:165–72.
125. Thomas CR, Evans JL, Buttriss C, Lowy C. Lipid chain length alterations during placental transfer in the guinea pig. J Dev Physiol 1985;7:305–11.
126. Schmidt-Sommerfeld E, Penn D, Sodha RJ, et al. Transfer and metabolism of carnitine and carnitine esters in the in vitro perfused human placenta. Pediatr Res 1985;19:700–6.
127. Szabo AG, De Lellis R, Grimaldi RD. Triglyceride synthesis by the human placenta. I. Incorporation of labeled palmitate into placental triglycerides. Am J Obstet Gynecol 1973;115:257–62.
128. Roux JF, Green R. Lipid metabolism by the human placenta. Obstet Gynecol 1968;29:446.
129. Christie WW, Noble RC. Fatty acid biosynthesis in sheep placenta and maternal and fetal adipose tissue. Biol Neonate 1982;42:79–86.
130. Martin RJ, Housman GJ. Placental development and fatty acid metabolism in pigs fed ad libitum or restricted during gestation. Proc Soc Exp Biol Med 1981;166:472–8.
131. Coleman RA, Haynes EB. Synthesis and release of fatty acids by human trophoblast cells in culture. J Lipid Res 1987;28:1335–41.
132. Hummel L, Schwartze A, Schirrmeister W, et al. Maternal plasma triglycerides as a source for fetal fatty acids. Acta Biol Med Germ 1976;35:1635–41.
133. Knopp RH, Warth MA, Charles D, et al. Lipoprotein metabolism in pregnancy, fat transport to the fetus, and the effects of diabetes. Biol Neonate 1986;50:297–317.
134. Winkel CA, Gilmore J, MacDonald PC, Simpson ER. Uptake and degradation of lipoproteins by human trophoblastic cells in primary culture. Endocrinology 1980;107:1892–8.
135. Lin DS, Pitkin RM, Connor WE. Placental transfer of cholesterol into the human fetus. J Obstet Gynecol 1977;128:735–9.
136. Feldman M, Van Aerde JE, Clandinin MT. Lipid accretion in the fetus and newborn. In: Polin RA, Fox WW, editors. Fetal and Neonatal Physiology. Philadelphia, PA: WB Saunders; 1992. p. 299–314.
137. Stammers JP, Hull D, Leadon DP, et al. Maternal and umbilical venous plasma lipid concentrations at delivery in the mare. Equine Vet J 1991;23:119–22.
138. Goldstein R, Levy E, Shafrir E. Increased maternal–fetal transport of fat in diabetes assessed by polyunsaturated fatty acid content in fetal lipids. Biol Neonate 1985;47:343–9.
139. Stammers JP, Elphic MC, Hull D. Effect of maternal diet during late pregnancy on fetal lipid stores in rabbits. J Dev Physiol 1983;5:395–404.
140. Elphick MC, Hull D, Sanders RR. Concentrations of free fatty acids in maternal and umbilical cord blood during elective cesarean section. Br J Obstet Gynaecol 1976;83:539–44.
141. Dancis J, Hansen V, Kayden JH, et al. Transfer across perfused human placenta. II. Free fatty acids. Pediatr Res 1973;7:192–7.
142. Hummel L, Simmermann T, Wagner H. Quantitative evaluation of the fetal fatty acid synthesis in the rat. Acta Biol Med Germ 1978;37:229–32.
143. Elphick MC, Hull D. The transfer of free fatty acids across the rabbit placenta. J Physiol (Lond) 1977;264:751–66.
144. Portman OW, Behrman RE, Soltys P. Transfer of free fatty acids across the primate placenta. Am J Physiol 1969;216:143–7.
145. Hay WW, Jr. Placental transport of nutrients to the fetus. Horm Res 1994;42:215–22.
146. Herrera E. Implications of dietary fatty acids during pregnancy on placental, fetal and postnatal development a review. Trophoblast Res 2002;16:S9–19.
147. Chambaz J, Ravel D, Manier MC, et al. Essential fatty acids interconversion in the human fetal liver. Biol Neonate 1985;47:136–40.
148. Hendrickse W, Stammers JP, Hull D. The transfer of free fatty acids across the human placenta. Br J Obstet Gynaecol 1985;92:945–53.
149. Booth C, Elphick MC, Hendrickse W, Hull D. Investigation of [14C]linoleicacid conversion into [14C]arachidonic acid and placental transfer of linoleic and palmitic acids across the perfused human placenta. J Dev Physiol 1981;3:177–89.
150. Innis SM, Nelson CM, Lwanga D, et al. Feeding formula without arachidonic acid or docosahexaenoic acid has no effect on preferential looking acuity or recognition memory in healthy full-term infants at 9 months of age. Am J Clin Nutr 1996;64:40–6.

151. Hornstra G, Al MDM, V Houwelingen AC, Foreman-van Drongelen MMHP. Essential fatty acids in pregnancy and early human development. Eur J Obstet Gynecol Reprod Biol 1995;61:57–62.
152. Coleman RA. The role of the placenta in lipid metabolism and transport. Semin Perinatal 1989;13:180–91.
153. Crawford MA, Doyle W, Drury P, et al. *n*-6 and *n*-3 fatty acids during early human development. J Intern Med 1989;225:159–69.
154. Clandinin MT, Chappell JE, Leong S, et al. Intrauterine fatty acid accretion rates in human brain: Implications for fatty acid requirements. Early Hum Dev 1980;4: 121–9.
155. Foreman-van Drongelen MMHP, Van Houwelingen AC, Kester ADM, et al. Long-chain polyunsaturated fatty acids in preterm infants, status at birth and its influence on postnatal levels. J Pediatr 1995;126:611–8.
156. Leaf AA, Leightfield MJ, Casteloe KL, Crawford MA. Longchain polyunsaturated fatty acids and fetal growth. Early Hum Dev 1992a;30:183–91.
157. Neuringer M, Connor WE. Omega-3 fatty acids in the brain and retina: Evidence of their essentiality. Nutr Rev 1986;44:285–94.
158. Sauerwald TU, Hachey DL, Jensen CL, et al. Intermediates in endogenous synthesis of C22:6_3 and C20:4_6 by term and preterm infants. Pediatr Res 1997;41:183–7.
159. Uauy R, Mena P, Wegher B, Nieto S, Salem N, Jr. Long chain polyunsaturated fatty acid formation in neonates: Effect of gestational age and intrauterine growth. Pediatr Res 2000;47:127–35.
160. Szitanyi P, Koletzko B, Mydlilova A, Demmelmair H. Metabolism of 13C-labeled linoleic acid in newborn infants during the first week of life. Pediatr Res 1999;45:669–73.
161. Su HM, Corso TN, Nathanielsz PW, Brenna JT. Linoleic acid kinetics and conversion to arachidonic acid in the pregnant and fetal baboon. J Lipid Res 1999;40:304–12.
162. Su HM, Huang MC, Saad NMR, et al. Fetal baboons convert 18:3n-3 to 22:6n-3 in vivo: A stable isotope tracer study. J Lipid Res 2001;581–6.
163. Demmelmair H, Baumheuer M, Koletzko B, et al. Metabolism of U-13C-labeled linoleic acid in lactating women. J Lipid Res 1998;39:1389–96.
164. De Gomez Dumm INT, Brenner RR. Oxidative desaturation of linolenic and stearic acids by human liver microsomes. Lipids 1975;10:315–7.
165. Jumpsen J, Van Aerde J, Clandinin MT. Fetal lipid requirements: Implications in fetal growth retardation. In: Battaglia FC, editor. Placental Function and Fetal Nutrition. Philadelphia, PA: Nesttec Ltd, Vevey/Lippincott-Raven Publ; 1997. p. 157–65.
166. Crastes de Paulet P, Sarda P, Boulot P, Crastes de Paulet A. Fatty acids blood composition in foetal and maternal plasma. In: Ghisolfi J, Putet G, editors. Essential, Fatty Acids and Infant Nutrition. Paris: John Libbey Eurotest; 1992. p. 65–77.
167. Al MDM, Hornstra G, Van der Schouw YT, et al. Biochemical EFA status of mothers and their neonates after normal pregnancy. Early Hum Dev 1990;24:239–48.
168. Matorras R, Perteagudo L, Sanjurjo P, Ruiz JI. Intake of long chain w3 polyunsaturated fatty acids during pregnancy and the influence of levels in the mother on newborn levels. Eur J Obstet Gynecol Reprod Biol 1999;83:179–84.
169. Van Houwelingen AC, Sorensen JD, Hornstra G, et al. Essential fatty acid status in neonates after fish-oil supplementation during late pregnancy. Br J Nutr 1995;74:723–31.
170. Connor WE, Lowensohn R, Hatcher L. Increased docosahexaenoic acid levels in human newborn infants by administration of sardines and fish oil during pregnancy. Lipids 1996;31:S183–7.
171. Uauy-Dagach R, Mena P. Nutritional role of omega-3 fatty acids during the perinatal period. Clin Perinatol 1995;22:157–75.
172. Brenner RR, Peluo RO. Regulation of unsaturated fatty acid biosynthesis. Biochim Biophys Acta 1969;176:471–9.
173. Innis SM. Essential fatty acids in growth and development. Prog Lipid Res 1991;30:39–103.
174. Simopoulos AP. ω-3 Fatty acids in health and disease and in growth and development. Am J Clin Nutr 1991;54:438–63.
175. Sprecher H. Metabolism of highly unsaturated *n*-3 and *n*-6 fatty acids. Biochim Biophys Acta Mol Cell Biol Lipids 2000;1486:219–31.
176. Garg ML, Thomson ABR, Clandinin MT. Interactions of saturated, *n*-6 and *n*-3 polyunsaturated fatty acids to modulate arachidonic acid metabolism. J Lipid Res 1990;31:271–7.
177. Raz A, Kamin-Belsky N, Przedecki F, Obukowicz MG. Fish oil inhibits delta6 desaturase activity in vivo: Utility in a dietary paradigm to obtain mice depleted of arachidonic acid. J Nutr Biochem 1997;8:558–65.
178. Koletzko B, Braun M. Arachidonic acid and early human growth: Is there a relation? Ann Nutr Metab 1991;35:128–31.
179. Carlson SE, Cooke RJ, Rhodes PG, et al. Long-term feeding of formulas high in linolenic acid and marine oil to very low birth weight infants: Phospholipid fatty acids. Pediatr Res 1991;30:404–12.
180. Carlson SE, Werkman SH, Pepples JM. Arachidonic acid status correlates with first year growth in preterm infants. Proc Natl Acad Sci U S A 1993;90:1073–7.
181. Leaf AA, Leighfield MJ, Costeloe KL, Crawford MA. Factors affecting long-chain polyunsaturated fatty acid composition of plasma choline phosphoglycerides in preterm infants. J Pediatr Gastroent Nutr 1992b;14: 300–8.
182. Woltil HA, Van Beusekom CM, Schaafsma A, et al. Long-chain polyunsaturated fatty acid status and early growth of low birth weight infants. Eur J Pediatr 1998;157: 146–52.
183. Halliwell B, Chirico S. Lipid peroxidation: Its mechanism, measurement, and significance. Am J Clin Nutr 1993;57:715S–25S.
184. Esterbauer H. Cytotoxicity and genotoxicity of lipid-oxidation products. Am J Clin Nutr 1993;57: 779S–86S.
185. Berry EM, Eisenberg S, Haratz D, et al. Effects of diets rich in monounsaturated fatty acids on plasma lipoproteins—the Jerusalem Nutrition Study: High MUFAs vs high PUFAs. Am J Clin Nutr 1991;53:899–907.
186. Cho S-H, Choi Y. Lipid peroxidation and antioxidant status is affected by different vitamin E levels when feeding fish oil. Lipids 1994;29:47–52.
187. Maziere C, Dantin F, Conte MA, et al. Polyunsaturated fatty acid enrichment enhances endothelial cell-induced low-density-lipoprotein peroxidation. Biochem J 1998;336: 57–62.
188. Viana M, Herrera E, Bonet B. Teratogenic effects of diabetes mellitus in the rat. Prevention by vitamin E. Diabetologia 1996;39:1041–6.
189. Siman CM, Eriksson UJ. Vitamin E decreases the occurrence of malformations in the offspring of diabetic rats. Diabetes 1997;46:1054–61.
190. Viana M, Aruoma OI, Herrera E, Bonet B. Oxidative damage in pregnant diabetic rats and their embryos. Free Rad Biol Med 2000;29:1115–21.
191. Navarro MD, Periago JL, Pita ML, Hortelano P. The *n*-3 polyunsaturated fatty acid levels in rat tissue lipids increase in response to dietary olive oil relative to sunflower oil. Lipids 1994;29:845–9.
192. Giron MD, Mataix FJ, Faus MJ, Suarez MD. Effect of long-term feeding olive and sunflower oils on fatty acid composition and desaturation activities of liver microsomes. Biochem Internat 1989;19:645–56.
193. Periago JL, Suarez MD, Pita ML. Effect of dietary olive oil, corn oil and medium-chain triglycerides on the lipid composition of rat red blood cell membranes. J Nutr 1990;120:986–94.
194. Rao CV, Zang E, Reddy B. Effect of high fat corn oil, olive oil and fish oil on phospholipid fatty acid composition in male F344 rats. Lipids 1993;28:441–7.
195. Scaccini C, Nardini M, D'Aquino M, et al. Effect of dietary oils on lipid peroxidation and on antioxidant parameters of rat plasma and lipoprotein fractions. J Lipid Res 1992;33:627–33.
196. Oztezcan S, Toker G, Uysal M. The susceptibility of plasma to lipid peroxidation in rats fed on diets supplemented with olive oil and sunflower seed oil. Biochem Arch 1996;12:13–8.
197. Amusquivar E, Ruperez FJ, Barbas C, Herrera E. Low arachidonic acid rather than α-tocopherol is responsible for the delayed postnatal development in offspring of rats fed fish oil instead of olive oil during pregnancy and lactation. J Nutr 2000;130:2855–65.
198. Sinclair AJ, Mann NJ. Short-term diets rich in arachidonic acid influence plasma phospholipid polyunsaturated fatty acid levels and prostacyclin and thromboxane production in humans. J Nutr 1996;126:1110S–4S.
199. Whelan J. Antagonistic effects of dietary arachidonic acid and *n*-3 polyunsaturated fatty acids. J Nutr 1996;126:1086S–91S.
200. Brown JE, Kahn ESB. Maternal nutrition and the outcome of pregnancy—a renaissance in research. Clin Perinatol 1997;24:433–49.
201. Eritsland J. Safety considerations of polyunsaturated fatty acids. Am J Clin Nutr 2000;71:197S–201S.
202. Lauritzen L, Hansen HS, Jorgensen MH, Michaelsen KF. The essentiality of long chain *n*-3 fatty acids in relation to development and function of the brain and retina. Prog Lipid Res 2001;40:1–94.
203. Benassayag C, Mignot TM, Haourigui M, et al. High polyunsaturated fatty acid, thromboxane A2, and alpha-fetoprotein concentrations at the human feto-maternal interface. J Lipid Res 1997;38:276–86.
204. Abumrad NA, Park JH, Park CR. Permeation of long-chain fatty acids into adipocytes. J Biol Chem 1984;259: 8954–3.
205. Goresky CA, Stremmel W, Rose CP, et al. The capillary transport system for free fatty acids in the heart. Circ Res 1994;74:1015–26.
206. Campbell FM, Gordon MJ, Dutta-Roy AK. Preferential uptake of long chain polyunsaturated fatty acids by isolated human placental membranes. Mol Cell Biochem 1996;155:77–83.
207. Campbell FM, Gordon MJ, Dutta-Roy AK. Plasma membrane fatty acid binding protein from human placenta: Identification and characterization. Biochem Biophys Res Commun 2000;209:1011–7.
208. Campbell FM, Clohessy AM, Gordon MJ, et al. Uptake of long chain fatty acids by human placental choriocarcinoma (BeWo) cells: Role of plasma membrane fatty acid binding protein. J Lipid Res 1997;38:2558–68.
209. Haggarty P, Page K, Abramovich DR, et al. Long-chain polyunsaturated fatty acid transport across the perfused human placenta. Placenta 1997;18:635–42.
210. Lafond J, Moukdar F, Rioux A, et al. Implication of ATP and sodium in arachidonic acid incorporation by placental syncytiotrophoblast brush border and basal plasma membranes in the human. Placenta 2000;21:661–9.
211. Zimmermann T, Hummel L, Mollr U, Kinzl U. Oxidation and synthesis of fatty acids in human and rat placental and fetal tissues. Biol Neonate 1979;36:109–12.
212. Robertson A, Sprecher H, Karp W. Oxidation of palmitate by human placental tissue slices. Phys Chem Phys 1971;3:293–301.
213. Tulenko TN, Rabinowitz JL. Fatty acid metabolism in human fetal placental vasculature. Am J Physiol 1981;240: E65–71.
214. Robertson A, Sprecher H. Human placental lipid metabolism. III. Synthesis and hydrolysis of phospholipids. Lipids 1967;2:403–5.
215. Clandinin MT, Chappell JE, Heim T, et al. Fatty acid utilization in perinatal de novo synthesis of tissues. Early Hum Dev 1981;5:355–66.
216. Van Aerde JE, Feldman M, Clandinin MT. Accretion of lipid in the fetus and newborn. In: Polin RA, Fox WW, editors. Fetal and Neonatal Physiology. Philadelphia, PA: W.B. Saunders Co; 1998. p. 458–77.
217. Gurr M. Fats. In: Garrow JS, James WPT, editors. Human Nutrition and Dietetics. Edinburgh: Churchill Livingstone; 1993. p. 77–102.
218. Crawford MA, Hassan AG, Williams G, Whitehouse WL. Essential fatty acids and fetal brain growth. Lancet I 1976:452–3.
219. Sellmayer A, Koletzko B. Long-chain polyunsaturated fatty acids and eicosanoids in infants Physiological and pathophysiological aspects and open questions. Lipids 1999;34:199–205.
220. Carlson SE, Cook RJ, Werkman SH, Tolley EA. First year growth of preterm infants fed standard compared to marine oil *n*-3 supplemented formula. Lipids 1992;27:901–7.
221. Birch E, Birch D, Ho.man D, et al. Breast-feeding and optimal visual development. J Pediatr Ophthalmol Strabismus 1993;30:33–8.
222. Carlson SE, Werkman SH, Rhodes PG, Tolley EA. Visual acuity development in healthy preterm infants: Effect of marine oil supplementation. Am J Clin Nutr 1993;58: 35–42.
223. Cook HW. Fatty acid desaturation and chain elongation in eucaryotes. In: Vance DE, Vance J, editors. Biochemistry of Lipids, Lipoproteins and Membranes. Amsterdam, The Netherlands: Elsevier; 1991. p. 141–69.
224. Leaf A, Gosbell A, McKenzie L, et al. Long chain polyunsaturated fatty acids and visual function in preterm infants. Early Hum Dev 1996;45:35–53.
225. Thomas CR, Lowy C. Placental transfer of free fatty acids: Factors affecting transfer across the guinea pig placenta. J Dev Physiol 1983;5:323–32.
226. Dancis J, Jansen V, Kayden JH, et al. Transfer across perfused human placenta. III. Effect of chain length on transfer of free fatty acids. Pediatr Res 1974;8:796–9.
227. Knopp RH, Herrera E, Freinkel N. Carbohydrate metabolism in pregnancy. VIII. Metabolism of adipose tissue isolated from fed and fasted pregnant rats during late gestation. J Clin Invest 1970;49:1438–46.
228. Herrera E, Gómez-Coronado D, Lascunción MA. Lipid metabolism in pregnancy. Biol Neonate 1987;51:70–7.
229. Herrera E, Lascunción MA, Gómez-Coronado D, et al. Role of lipoprotein lipase activity on lipoprotein metabolism and the fate of circulating triglycerides in pregnancy. Am J Obstet Gynecol 1988;158:1575–83.
230. Baskin DG, Latteman DF, Seeley RJ, et al. Insulin and leptin: Dual adiposity signals to the brain for the regulation of food intake and body weight. Brain Res 1999;848:114–23.
231. Ookuma M, Ookuma K, York DA. Effects of leptin on insulin secretion from isolated rat pancreatic islets. Diabetes 1998;47:219–23.

232. Zho AZ, Bornfeldt KE, Beavo JA. Leptin inhibits insulin secretion by activation of phosphodiesterase 3B. J Clin Invest 1998;102:869–73.
233. Minokoshi Y, Haque MS, Shimazu T. Microinjection of leptin into the ventromedial hypothalamus increases glucose uptake in peripheral tissues in rat. Diabetes 1999;48: 287–91.
234. Yaspelkis BB, Ansari L, Ramey EL, et al. Chronic leptin administration increases insulin-stimulated skeletal muscle glucose uptake and transport. Metabolism 1999;48:671–6.
235. Sivitz WI, Fink BD, Donohue PA. Fasting and leptin modulate adipose and muscle uncoupling protein: Divergent effects between messenger ribonucleic acid and protein expression. Endocrinology 1999;140:1511–9.
236. Wang T. Hartzell DL, Rose BS, et al. Metabolic responses to intracerebroventricular leptin and restricted feeding. Physiol Behav 1999;65:839–48.
237. Hoggard N. Hunter L, Lea RG, et al. Ontogeny of the expression of leptin and its receptor in the murine fetus and placenta. Br J Nutr 2000;83:317–26.
238. Ong KK, Ahmed ML, Sherrif A, et al. Cord blood leptin is associated with size at birth and predicts infancy weight gain in humans. J Clin Edocrinol Metab 1999;84: 1145–8.
239. Tarquini B, Tarquini R, Perfetto F, et al. Genetic and environmental influences on human cord blood leptin concentration. Pediatrics 1999;103:998–1006.
240. Devaskar SU, Anthony R, Hay WW, Jr. Ontogeny and insulin regulation of fetal ovine white adipose tissue leptin expression. Am J Physiol Regul Integr Comp Physiol 2002;282:R431–8.
241. Innis S. Benefits of early IV lipids for nutrition of ELBW(LBW infants. In: Hay WW, Jr, editor. Seminars in Neonatal Nutrition and Metabolism, Volume 3. Columbus, OH: Ross Laboratories; 1995. p. 1–3.

Amino Acid Nutrition In Utero: Placental Function and Metabolism

Timothy R.H. Regnault, PhD
Frederick C. Battaglia, MD

This chapter will review placental function and metabolism as it relates to the issue of fetal amino acid nutrition. The review will include information available in human pregnancy although, of necessity, most of the in vivo information has been collected in various animal species, and this, too, will be reviewed. In all mammalian species, the 20 amino acids of the genetic code are required for net protein accretion. The rate of protein accretion, which varies among mammals, is based primarily upon fetal growth rate. The nutritional supply of amino acids for growth is defined as the net umbilical uptake of amino acids, representing the net transfer from the placenta to the fetus, including backflux from the fetus to the placenta of essential and nonessential amino acids. In the ovine fetus, where these data are available, the quantity taken up by the fetus clearly exceeds requirements for growth,[1–4] and is associated with a high rate of fetal amino acid oxidation. In this review we aim to detail aspects of fetal amino acid requirements, placental transport, and metabolism of amino acids and highlight factors influencing these processes, such as fetal growth restriction (FGR). In addition, we will discuss umbilical uptake, interorgan cycling, and fetal and placental amino acid utilization including, specifically, fetal hepatic and hindlimb amino acid metabolism. In concluding this chapter, we will deal with the neonatal implications of fetal amino acid metabolism.

PLACENTAL DELIVERY OF FETAL AMINO ACID REQUIREMENTS

The primary source of nitrogen for the growing mammalian fetus is the circulating maternal free amino acid pool. In considering the primary role of the placenta in the delivery of amino acids to the fetus, it is important to consider the multiplicity of factors that may affect these overall delivery rates. Figure 1 presents in diagrammatic form the potential fate of an amino acid that has been transported across the plasma membrane of the microvillous maternal surface into the trophoblast cytosol, prior to its entry into the fetal circulation through the basal membrane. Pathway 1 represents the direct transplacental flux of an amino acid from the maternal circulation across the plasma membranes on the maternal and fetal surfaces of the trophoblast and into the fetal circulation. Pathway 2

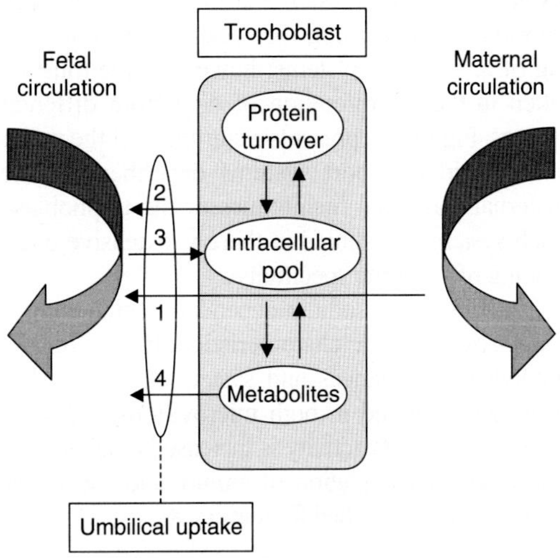

Figure 1 A diagrammatic representation of potential pathways for the delivery of an amino acid into the fetal circulation. (See text for full description of pathways.)

represents the delivery of an amino acid that has entered the intracellular pool via protein turnover within the trophoblast. Pathway 3 represents the backflux from the fetal circulation into the trophoblast of the same amino acid and pathway 4 refers to the transformation of the amino acid to a metabolite which can then enter the fetal circulation. The later example would be the transamination of leucine to ketoisocaproic acid, which can then be delivered to the fetus. The algebraic sum of these fluxes represents the net umbilical uptake, which is the nutritionally important measurement, because it represents the net supply of the amino acid delivered to the fetus. The relative importance of each of the pathways in determining the umbilical uptake differs among amino acids. Examples of amino acids that are utilized extensively within the placenta (such as glutamate) or are synthesized at a relatively high rate within the placenta (such as glycine) will be described in the following sections. There is already ample evidence to show that for different amino acids, one or another of these pathways may predominate.

It is becoming apparent that the fetus not only accrues nitrogen in the new tissues formed during growth, but also extensively metabolizes its nitrogen source by synthesizing, oxidizing, and transaminating amino acids.[5] The current estimate of ovine fetal uptake of nitrogen is approximately 0.9 gm/kg/d, which is approximately equal to the estimated fetal nitrogen requirement.[4] Therefore, the quantity of amino acids transported is sufficient to meet the current estimation of fetal nitrogen requirements. This estimation includes the fate of amino acids metabolized and excreted as ammonia or urea from the fetoplacental unit.[6–9] Other potential sources of nitrogen, such as intact proteins or peptides, which may be important in embryogenesis, do not appear to be required to meet fetal nitrogen needs.

Estimations of fetal protein synthetic rates have been performed in fetal sheep utilizing a variety of methodologies.[10–15] Leucine was used as a tracer amino acid in chronically catheterized fetal sheep to assess protein synthetic rates at different gestational ages.[12,15] These studies demonstrated that the absolute fractional protein synthetic rate (Ks) decreased from midgestation to term, and that this decrease was greater than that was seen in the fractional protein accretion rate. Figure 2 demonstrates the inverse relationship noted between the fetal K_s and fetal age. Therefore, protein breakdown, defined as the difference between protein accretion and synthesis, also appears to decrease in late

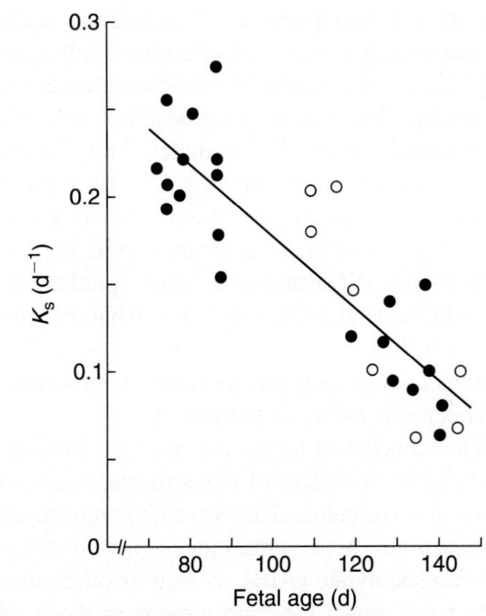

Figure 2 In chronically catheterized fetal sheep, the protein synthetic rate (K_s) was noted to decrease with fetal age. Protein synthetic rates were determined using [1-^{13}C-leucine (dots) and [U-^{14}C]-lysine (open circles). Regression line ($r = .87$) was drawn according to equation: $y = 0.39 - 0.021x$. (Adapted from reference 12.)

gestation. The higher protein synthetic rate of the midgestation fetus is proportional to the higher metabolic rate at that stage of gestation. Absolute fractional protein synthetic rate declines at a similar rate as fetal O_2 consumption (V_{O_2}), giving a relatively constant ratio of K_s/V_{O_2}.[12] Thus, protein synthesis per millimole of oxygen consumed is quite constant from midgestation until term.[12] Fetal metabolic studies have advanced our conceptual framework of the key factors that alter metabolic rate per kilogram of body weight during development.[12,13,16–18] Since many metabolic variables such as protein synthetic rate, lactate utilization rate, and urea production rate bear a relationship to metabolic rate, studies of the ontogenetic changes in fetal metabolic rate have helped to clarify the developmental changes in metabolic measurements such as the protein synthetic rate.[10,12,13,16]

PLACENTAL AMINO ACID TRANSPORT

In recent years, both in vivo[2,4,19–21] and in vitro[22–34] studies have brought out the complexity of the placenta as an organ for amino acid transport and metabolism. It is important to emphasize that unlike an organ such as the liver, the placenta must function as an organ of transport, delivering amino acids from the maternal circulation into the fetal circulation. The complexity of the organ stems not only from the different cell types required to affect such net transport, but also from the capacity of the placenta to metabolize or synthesize various amino acids. The human placenta has at least two cell types that are critically important in determining its overall transport characteristics: the trophoblast and the endothelium. In other species additional cell layers may be present, for example, in the epitheliochorial placenta of sheep and goats there is an endometrial cell layer as well.

The concentration of most amino acids, including some of the essentials, is higher in fetal than in maternal plasma,[2,4,35] consistent with a process of active transport of amino acids across the placenta. An increased fetal-to-maternal ratio of plasma amino acid concentrations has been documented for man,[36,37] primates,[38] rat,[39] guinea pig,[40–42] sheep,[1,2,4,21] and cow.[43] Although the fetal-to-maternal concentration ratio is greater than 1.0 for most amino acids measured, there are quantitative differences among species. For example, the fetal-to-maternal ratio in human whole blood for the cationic amino acids lysine and histidine is consistently greater than 1.0, whereas in the sheep, the ratio is less than 1.0.

This concept of active transport has been corroborated by a variety of experiments. Studies of placental tissue cultured in vitro with nonmetabolizable amino acid analogues, for example, α-aminoisobutyrate (AIB), as well as other amino acids, have shown the concentration of those substances intracellularly to be at a level several times greater than extracellular maternal concentration.[44–50] Placental tissues have also been found to have extremely high levels of the amino acids taurine, glutamate, and aspartate, as well as moderately high levels of alanine, glycine, serine, glutamine, and threonine [36,37] when compared to maternal or fetal concentrations. It should be emphasized that measurements of placental tissue amino acid concentrations have not been corrected for extracellular fluid content of the tissue. Therefore, the intracellular tissue concentrations are likely to be considerably higher than the values in the literature.

The uptake of amino acids occurs through active transport. Mammalian transport systems have been characterized over the years by such general properties as ion dependence, kinetics, substrate specificity, and regulation of activity and this has allowed the description of multiple transport systems for neutral, anionic, and cationic amino acids.[51–53] Studies in human and rat trophoblast have yielded much information concerning the location and functioning of amino acid systems; however, care must be taken in the interpretation of data from different species. Figure 3 represents a summary of the major amino acid transport systems described for the maternal and basal membranes of the trophoblast. Each system is distinct but there is extensive overlapping of substrate specificity.

System A is a sodium-dependent, unidirectional transporter with a characteristic affinity for *N*-methylated substances and system A activity has been demonstrated in both microvillous and basal membrane.[54–56] Its activity is increased as an adaptation to cellular depletion of amino acid substrates, similar to that described for system X_{AG}^-,[57,58] and its

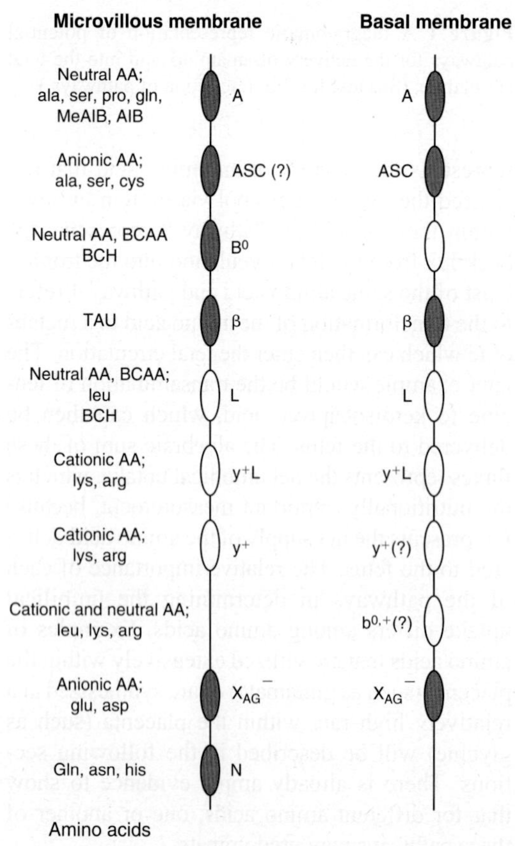

Figure 3 Schematic representation of the sodium-dependent (•) and sodium-independent (○) amino acid transport systems for both the microvillous (maternal) and basal (fetal) membranes of the trophoblast. Amino acid substrates are listed on the left and references on the right. AIB-α-Aminoisobutyric acid; BCH-2-Aminobicyclo-(2,2,1)-heptane-2-carboxylic acid; MeAIB-Methylaminoisobutyric acid.

mRNA appears to be regulated under hypoxia.[59] System ASC has been described for neutral amino acid transport, specifically alanine, serine, and cysteine, as well as for some anionic amino acids.[54,55,60,61] It is a sodium-dependent obligate exchanger localized at the basal membrane, though studies utilizing BeWo cells suggest that system ASC transporters may be present on the microvillous membranes as well, but after differentiation and syncytial formation such activity is lost.[62] A sodium-independent group of transporters (Asc), with similar transport characteristics,[63] has now been reported to exist in placental tissue.[64,65] In addition, the broad-scope sodium-dependent transporter B° is responsible for neutral amino acid transport including branched chain amino acids (BCAAs), and has been localized to the microvillous and basal membranes.[66–69] The β-amino acid taurine utilizes the β transport system. Studies have demonstrated that this β transport system is a sodium-dependent transporter found on both membranes,[70–75] though with a greatly reduced basal membrane activity compared to the microvillous membrane.[73]

System L (or l) transporters are sodium-independent exchange transporters and have been localized to both trophoblast membranes.[53,54,76] They play a major role in the transport of essential amino acids, having a high affinity for leucine and the other BCAAs.[77] The cationic amino acid transport system y^+L is considered as a low-capacity, high-affinity system which exchanges cationic amino acids for neutral amino acids and its activity is localized to both the microvillous membrane and the basal membrane.[78–81] A proposed hypothesis is that this transporter system in the basal membrane is the major supply route of cationic amino acids to the fetus through the uptake of neutral amino acids from fetal circulation in exchange for cationic amino acids from the placenta.[81] The sodium-independent, low-affinity, high-capacity y^+ transport system is a high-capacity system, which transports cationic amino acids such as arginine, lysine, and ornithine in a sodium-independent manner. It is considered to be the major cationic transport system in placental tissues,[81–83] and is localized to the microvillous membrane[78,81,84,85] and possibly to the basal membranes.[86] A role for the related $b^{o,+}$ system in placental tissues has been reported[84,86,87]; however, further vesicle studies suggest that there is no functional evidence for this system in either term microvillous or basal membrane[81] despite the observation of associated mRNA.[88]

The placenta takes up the anionic amino acids, glutamate, and aspartate from the maternal and fetal circulations, but does not actively transfer these amino acids from mother to fetus. Studies utilizing isolated human and rat placental membrane vesicles and immunohistochemical localization in human placenta have revealed the presence of a high-affinity transport system for aspartate and glutamate via the sodium-dependent X_{AG}^- system within both the microvillous and basal plasma membranes.[89–93] This system may mediate the concentrative uptake of anionic amino acids from the maternal and fetal circulations into the placenta. System N transports neutral amino acids, but differs from systems A and ASC in that it displays a preference for amino acids containing nitrogen-bearing side chains, transporting only glutamine, aspargine, and histidine.[77,94,95] System N activity was first found in the liver but has also been localized in the human placenta,[94] though some studies have failed to report placental mRNA [96] and others have attributed this system N–like transport activity, in the rat placenta, to a combination of system A, possibly system ASC, and $B^{o,+}$ and y^+L.[68]

PLACENTAL AMINO ACID TRANSPORTER PROTEINS

Historically, placental amino acid transport has been described in terms of transport systems based on competitive inhibition studies, though it is now becoming possible to move to a more precise description of the protein chemistry of the transporter system. The ability to clone, sequence, and study the expression of transporters has led to an explosion of data concerning the molecular basis of amino acid transport systems and their potential in vivo function.[63,88,97–99] It is now clear that some placental transporters exist as a monomeric protein, while other transport systems exist as heterodimeric complex.[99–101] Those monomeric transport systems induce amino acid uptake in a similar manner to the amino acid uptake associated with permeases described in microorganisms,[102–105] though the regulation of placental membrane acquisition of monomeric systems has not yet been studied. Heterodimeric systems involve the grouping together of two proteins to facilitate amino acid transport. In placental tissues, monomeric transport systems are believed to include y^+, ASC, A, and most likely the X_{AG}^- system,[88,106] while heterodimeric transport systems include system L, y^+L, and the Asc system.[65,88,107,108] Those systems that operate in a heterodimeric manner are generally made up of a common heavy chain, specifically one of the type II membrane glycoproteins, 4F2hc (comparable to the CD98 surface antigen, CD98hc),[109–111] the neutral and basic amino acid transport (NBAT, equivalent to rBAT or D2[112–115]) protein, or as yet undefined proteins,[64] which associate with one of a variety of light-chain transport proteins, providing a range of amino acid transport systems.[101,107,108,110,116] There is also evidence that these heavy chains may interact with themselves and each other to form homodimers and/or heterodimers before interacting with a specific light chain to induce activity.[81] A summary of the traditional transport systems and their heavy-and light-chain associations that have been reported in placental tissues and membranes is presented in Table 1.

The 4F2hc mRNA is ubiquitously expressed.[117] While 4F2hc is expressed in placental tissues throughout pregnancy, NBAT expression appears only in first and early second trimester placenta and is not present in term tissues.[81,118] During human and rat pregnancy, whole tissue studies have demonstrated 4F2hc predominantly in the microvillous membrane, with the content increasing as gestation advances.[81,111,118] However, 4F2hc has not been detected in the human basal membrane,[81,111] despite reports of 4F2hc mRNA in rat basal membrane preparations[118] and evidence that 4F2hc plays a role in basal membrane amino acid transport in other tissues, including the intestine and kidney.[115]

The glycosylated 4F2hc protein is composed of a single transmembrane region with a large C-terminal extracellular domain.[110,119,120] Since mammalian substrate transporters appear to have multiple transmembrane helices, it is unlikely that the 4F2hc protein is capable of inducing amino acid transport alone.[121] It is postulated that 4F2hc is in fact the modulator of heterodimeric transport systems and acts as a "guidance molecule," translocating the nonglycosylated light chains to the plasma membrane, after which disulfide linkage between 4F2hc and the light chain occurs.[101,122–124] The subcellular location of the light-chain proteins and their interaction with 4F2hc protein are not well defined. Presently, the model of interaction involves an intracellular pool of light chains that are available for incorporation with the membrane-bound heavy chain.[106,110] The movement is independent of the formation of the disulphide bonds, which suggests a noncovalent steric association.[124] An additional level of complexity in understanding these protein movements and interactions is presented when considering the controlling factors of transporter membrane localization. The PDZ-binding motif is known to be responsible for membrane localization of some membrane proteins and studies have demonstrated that many human amino acid transporters possess potential PDZ-binding motifs as reviewed.[88] Following membrane localization and if required light-chain and heavy-chain interaction, functional transport may then occur.[101,125,126] The expression of the heavy chain and not that of the light chains is best correlated with placental amino acid transport system activity.[106,110]

Table 1 The Placental Transport Systems and Associated Light Side Chains.*

Transporter System	Amino Acid Transporter Type	System Interaction	Heavy-Chain Protein	Light-Chain Protein	Gene
A	Neutral	Monomeric		ATA-1	*SLC38A1*
	Sodium dependent			ATA-2	*SLC38A2*
				ATA-3	*SLC38A4*
ASC	Neutral			ASCT-1	*SLC1A4*
	Sodium dependent				
B°	Neutral			ASCT-2	*SLC1A5*
	Sodium dependent				
$b^{o,+}$	Neutral	Heterodimeric	rBAT	$b^{o,+}$AT	*SLC7A9*
	Sodium independent				
β	Neutral	Monomeric		TAUT	*SLC6A6*
	Sodium dependent				
Asc	Neutral	Heterodimeric	4F2hc	Asc-1	*SLC7A10*
	Sodium independent		Unknown	Asc-2	*SLC7A12*
L	Ne utral	Heterodimeric	4F2hc	LAT-1	*SLC7A5*
	Sodium independent		4F2hc	LAT-2	SLC7A8
				LAT-3	*SLC43A1*
				LAT-4	*SLC43A2*
y^+L	Cationic	Heterodimeric	4F2hc	y^+LAT-1	*SLC7A7*
	Sodium independent			y^+LAT-2 (?)	*SLC7A6*
y^+	Cationic	Monomeric		CAT-1	*SLC7A1*
	Sodium independent			CAT-2B	*SLC7A2*
				CAT-4	*SLC7A4*
X_{AG}^-	Anionic			EAAT-1	*SLC1A3*
				EAAT-2	*SLC1A2*
				EAAT-3	*SLC1A1*

*Refer to text for light chain protein expanded Abbreviations.

Neutral Amino Acid Transporter Light-Chain Proteins

Currently, three subtypes of the amino acid system A have been cloned: amino acid transporter SNAT1 (SLC38A1), SNAT2 (SLC38A2), and SNAT4 (SLC38A4). The SNAT1 (ATA-1 or GlnT[127,128]) system has a limited tissue expression, being expressed predominantly in the human placenta and heart and is responsible for the transport of small short-chain neutral amino acids, such as alanine, serine, methionine, asparagine, and glutamine.[127] The functional characteristics of SNAT2 are similar to those of SNAT1, though found in a wider range of tissues, including the placenta.[127,129] Until recently SNAT4 appeared to have a unique tissue distribution predominantly in hepatic and skeletal muscle tissues.[130,131] Recent reports also place it in the placenta, in both human microvillous and basal membranes, being expressed from early pregnancy onward, similar to SNAT1 and SNAT2.[132]

The ASCT-1 (SLC1A4),[121] a component of the ASC transport system, has been localized to human placenta tissue, though its expression is very low.[133] Another component of the ASC system, ASCT-2, has also been cloned,[134] though this is thought to code protein related to the related transport family system B°. The B° is a sodium-dependent neutral amino acid transport system for which the related gene *ASCT2* (SLC1A5) is proposed to represent the B° system in the human placental choriocarcinoma cell line, JAR, and isolated human placental poly(A)$^+$ mRNA.[67,135]

The B title represents this system's broad substrate preference, and the capital status indicates its sodium dependence. The superscript ° defines it as accepting zwitterionic or neutral amino acids, which distinguishes it from the $B^{o,+}$ system which also accepts cationic amino acids.[67,136] These systems are differentiated from the $b^{o,+}$ system which also transports neutral and cationic amino acids, but in a sodium-independent manner. This latter system has been reported in basal membrane preparations,[86] though recently this localization has been questioned with its activity attributed instead to the y^+L system.[81] The β transporter for taurine has exhibited activity in placenta apical and basal placental preparations,[70–75,137] and this activity is associated with an mRNA encoding TAUT (SLC6A6), in placental cell lines and human placental poly(A)$^+$ mRNA.[137,138]

The sodium-independent transport of small neutral amino acids is carried out by the Asc system, composed of the proteins Asc-1 (SLC7A10) and Asc-2 (SLC7A12), both of which have been identified in placental mRNA.[64,65] Asc-1 forms a heterodimeric complex with 4F2hc (SLC3A2),[65] whereas Asc-2 appears to interact with a presently unknown heavy chain.[64]

Light-chain proteins also associate with 4F2hc to form the functional L transport system,[125,126] catalyzing the uptake of neutral amino acids in a sodium-independent manner. System L-amino acid transporter-1 LAT-1 (SLC7A5), LAT-2 (SLC7A8), LAT-3 (SLC43A1), and LAT-4 (SLC43A2) have all been reported in placental tissues.[106,107,111,117,126,139–144] The 4F2hc/LAT-1 transport activity displays a narrow specificity toward neutral amino acids, uninfluenced by pH, whereas 4F2hc/LAT-2 activity has a broad specificity and is stimulated by decreasing pH.[141] Immunological and functional studies suggest that at term, the light chain LAT-1 is located predominantly in the microvillous membrane and the syncytiotrophoblast layer of the villi.[63,111,142,145] Furthermore, the L transport system phenotype associated with that of the placental microvillous membrane is found to occur when the LAT-1 and not the LAT-2 catalytic subunit is coexpressed with the 4F2hc.[145] In a similar manner, human LAT-2 mRNA has been identified in the choriocarcinoma BeWo cell line and placental villous tissues[107,145] and its activity has been localized to the basal membrane[63,145] and not the microvillous membrane as is the case for LAT-1.[126,145,146] These studies suggest that the localization of system activity may be further defined through specific light-chain location. LAT-1 and LAT-2 function as classic obligatory exchangers, moving substrates in exchange for other amino acids,[147] and unaffected by hypoxia.[59] Two additional system L light chains, LAT-3 and LAT-4, have recently been reported in placental tissues. While transporting a restricted group of system L substrates (leucine, isoleucine, and phenylalanine) they appear to also differ from the traditional system L transport in that they do not appear to require the coexpression of 4F2hc and function as facilitative diffusion transporters.[143,144]

Cationic Transport System Light-Chain Proteins

Transport of cationic amino acids occurs predominantly through the y^+L and y^+ systems. Placental y^+L system activity is determined by which light-chain system y^+L-amino acid transporter-1 (y^+LAT-1, SLC7A7), or system y^+L-amino acid transporter-2 (y^+LAT-2, SLC7A6), forms a heterodimer with the membrane-bound 4F2hc. Human placental preparations contain y^+LAT-1 mRNA[108,116] and when this mRNA is coexpressed with 4F2hc in *Xenopus laevis* oocytes, amino acid uptake characteristics similar to that of system y^+L are displayed.[116] Presently, it is unclear if system y^+LAT light-chain proteins display a tissue distribution pattern similar to that displayed by the LAT proteins. However, this system appears to play an essential role in supplying cationic amino acids to the fetal circulation by exchanging cationic amino acids from within the trophoblast, for neutral amino acids such as glutamine and leucine from fetal circulation. This mode of operation provides a route of efflux, overcoming the outward positive potential difference across the trophoblast basal plasma membrane.[98] The related system y^+ activity is dependent only on the expression of monomeric proteins (or CAT gene products),[148] which unlike systems L and y^+L require expression of both a common heavy chain and a related light chain.[106,116,141] Currently there are three known mRNAs, which encode for proteins related to this cationic amino acid transport system in placental tissues, namely the cationic amino acid transporters CAT-1 (SLC7A1), CAT-2 (SLC7A2), and CAT-4 (SLC7A4).[81,82] This system activity has been reported on both membranes of the rat and human placenta,[79,80,84] with a higher uptake in the microvilli membranes compared with the basal membrane surface.[80] However, contrasting kinetic and substrate inhibition studies and reverse transcriptase (RT-PCR) studies localizing CAT-4 mRNA in human placental tissue suggest that y^+ activity is limited to the microvillous membrane and not the basal membrane.[81] Specifics of these differences are reviewed elsewhere.[88]

Anionic Transport System Light-Chain Proteins

Five cDNAs encoding proteins capable of mediating high-affinity sodium-coupled transport have been reported and three of these have been cloned from placenta tissue.[90,92] These placental proteins, excitatory amino acid transport (EAAT)-1 (GLAST1), EAAT-2 (GLT1), and EAAT-3 (EAAC1), are known to mediate placental sodium-dependent D-aspartate-inhibitable anionic amino acid transport or system X_{AG}^- activity.[90] All three forms have been detected in human placental tissue,[93,149,150] and in rat placenta tissues.[92,151] The regulation of these proteins appears to be under the control of growth hormone (GH) and insulin-like growth factor (IGF) family members[151] and upregulation of the system has been demonstrated through cell density and nutrient deprivation studies in muscle and placental cell lines.[57,92] These latter studies demonstrated that EAAT-1 and EAAT-3 play a key role in the basal anionic amino acid transfer, while EAAT-2 may be involved in conditions of amino acid depletion.[92]

Alterations in Amino Acid Transporter Proteins and Disease

The importance of the heavy- and light-chain proteins in placental amino acid transport and metabolism is highlighted by studies showing that alterations in 4F2hc and/or y^+LAT-1 expression may be responsible for lysinuric protein intolerance,[116,152] cystinuria,[153] alterations in maternal-to-placenta essential amino acid supply,[123,142] and maternal immune response failure during implantation.[154–156] The identification of individual transporter proteins in the trophoblast will be expanded considerably as sequence data for specific transporters permit rapid identification of other members of the same family of transporters. Thus, the information provided in Table 1 and Figure 3 should be regarded as an interim report in a rapidly changing field.

OTHER FACTORS REGULATING PLACENTAL AMINO ACID TRANSPORT

As pregnancy advances, the increasing nutrient demands of the developing conceptus must be met through an appropriate increase in placental nutrient transport. This enhanced performance is facilitated through alterations in placental perfusion and changes in membrane exchange surface area. Recent studies in human pregnancies have shown that umbilical blood flow increases during gestation in a pattern similar to fetal growth rate. The relationship between blood flow and body size is quite good, although not perfect. As shown in Figure 4, when blood flow is expressed per kilogram fetal weight, it falls slightly throughout gestation. This pattern of decline is similar to the changes in fetal heart rate in human pregnancies, which decreases as gestation advances. Heart rate is closely linked to metabolic rate. Thus, the changes in blood flow and in fetal metabolic rate appear to be reasonably well linked in human pregnancies. The decrease in umbilical blood flow per kilogram fetal weight in human pregnancies does not present a problem in terms of supplying amino acids

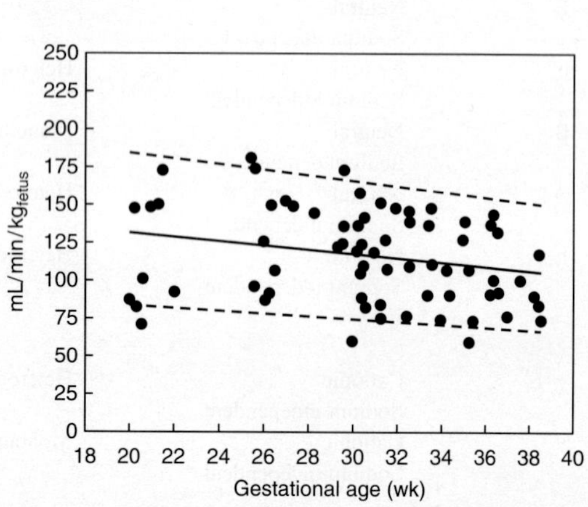

Figure 4 Umbilical vein blood flow per kilogram of fetal weight plotted against gestational age for human pregnancies. Slight linear decrease observed was not significant ($y = -1.3636x + 155.9964$). Both 5th and 95th percentiles are shown (dashed lines). (Adapted from reference 165.)

to the fetus as it grows. This is not the case, as changes in blood flow are compensated for by an increase in placental surface area, and presumably an increase in the number of membrane-bound transporters available for delivery of amino acids. Between the 16th week of pregnancy and term, human fetal weight increases approximately 20-fold, whereas the peripheral villous surface area increases only 9-fold.[157–160] More importantly, the multiplication factor of nine actually decreases in late gestation.[160] It should be emphasized, however, that there are only a few careful ontogenetic studies of how total surface area, including microvillous surface, changes over gestation.[160–163] The increase in total surface area of the placenta alone can not account for the exponential fetal growth occurring over this time period. These data suggest the total transport capacity of the trophoblast is likely to be determined by total villous surface area, placental permeability, the concentration of specific amino acid carrier proteins on the cell membrane surfaces, as well as the affinity characteristics of transporter proteins and the circulating amino acid concentrations at both the maternal and fetal surfaces. Indeed as gestation advances, the efficiency of the placenta as reported as fetal weight per 1 g of placenta increases.[164]

Accompanying the maturational changes in trophoblast surface area, amino acid transport systems are reported to have differing expression and transport parameters through gestation.[56,81,84,111,166,167] For example, in term placentae, L-arginine transport in microvillous membrane preparation is through both y^+ and y^+L systems, while in the basal membrane transport may be restricted to the y^+L system.[81] Furthermore, the functional properties of transport systems may also change as gestation advances. For example, first-trimester microvillous membrane has increased transport activity compared to term placental vesicles,[167] and 4F2hc protein levels differ between early/mid pregnancy and term placentae.[81,111] Early in gestation the K_m of the microvillous high-affinity system y^+L is significantly less than in term preparations.[81] Such studies highlight the complex interactions that occur between developing microvillous membrane and basal membrane, within the trophoblast and between the two circulations, to facilitate an increase in nutrient delivery to the growing fetus as gestation advances.

Placental tissue contains a number of hormone receptors (ie, for insulin, gonadotropins, growth factors, somatomedins, beta-adenergics, cholinergics, opiates). How hormones interact with the regulation of amino acid transport is incompletely understood at present. There is some evidence, however, that insulin infusion may enhance placental amino acid uptake, concentration, and transport to the fetus.[168,169] Karl and colleagues found that AIB uptake by cultured trophoblast cells was enhanced by insulin as well as by dexamethasone, glucagon, and 8-Br-cAMP.[168] They postulated that since trophoblasts are known to produce IGF-I, insulin may initially enhance AIB uptake via IGF-I. Insulin receptor concentrations were found to be markedly reduced in placentas from small for gestational age (SGA) infants, and AIB uptake was decreased in the cultures of these trophoblast cells.[168,170–172]

AMINO ACID TRANSPORT SYSTEMS AND FETAL GROWTH RESTRICTION

In clinical studies, the concentration of amino acids has been observed to be lower in the fetal and maternal plasma of pregnancies that were complicated by FGR[173–176] suggesting alterations in amino acid delivery. This depression in amino acid concentrations is true, regardless of whether fetal concentrations were determined at the time of delivery or many weeks prior to delivery. Additionally it has also been found that lower amino acid concentrations are found in FGR pregnancies even if the fetus had normal fetal heart rate and velocimetry measurements,[173,174] suggesting that this may antedate other clinical pathologic findings.[177] Studies in human FGR demonstrate that system A may be impaired.[178] An in vitro study utilizing microvillous membrane vesicles from the placentae of appropriate for gestational age and SGA babies demonstrated markedly lower activity (by 63%) of the A system transporters in the SGA compared to the appropriate for gestational age membrane vesicles,[170] suggesting a positive association between fetal growth and system A activity. Inhibition of system A transport in rat pregnancies has been associated with slight decreases in fetal weight, demonstrating a potential role for system A transport in maintaining normal fetal growth.[179] Of particular interest is that imprinted genes control the supply of nutrients to the fetus, and in the mouse, the *Slc38a4* gene has been shown to be imprinted. In studies utilizing the placental-specific *Igf2* transcript (P0) knockout to generate FGR, placental growth is compromised, though fetal demands are met presumably through an upregulation of transporter genes *Slc2a3* (glucose transporter) and the imprinted *Slc38a4*.[180,181] Interestingly when fetal demands for nutrients are removed through removal of the fetal *Igf2*, the upregulation does not occur, providing evidence of regulation of placental transport activity via fetal growth demand genes. Both the *Igf2* and the *Slc38a4* are paternally expressed and this interaction is seen as a display of paternally inherited genes maximizing extraction of maternal nutrients.[180]

In human FGR vesicle studies, TAUT protein expression is unaltered,[137] though the transport activity of this transporter is reduced.[73] It is important to emphasize that the vesicle studies have not taken into account the possibility of nonhomogeneity in the placenta for FGR pregnancies. There remains the very real possibility that the proportion of terminal villi to intermediate and stem villi are altered in FGR pregnancies and, depending on the distribution of any transporter, this maldevelopment could profoundly affect transport in vivo even without any changes in transporter expression or activity. In addition, studies inducing FGR through maternal protein deprivation in rats have demonstrated a downregulation of placental amino acid transport, specifically system A, and also systems X_{AG}^- and y^+.[85,85,182] Again one must be cautious in extrapolating such studies to humans since protein deprivation in the rat has a profound effect upon maternal plasma amino acid concentrations which is not found in human FGR pregnancies and amino acid accretion and utilization of a rat fetuses is much greater than the human fetus given the much faster growth rate of the rat fetus, up to 20 times faster near term. With regard to system X_{AG}^- transport, the basal membrane activity of EAAT-1 is reduced in a FGR rat model, which could impact placental glutamate uptake from the fetal circulation,[85] though in human studies, no differences were found in the distribution of the glutamate transporters between control and intrauterine growth restriction (IUGR) placentae.[93]

Microvillous membrane system y^+ and y^+L activity does not appear to be altered in human FGR,[80,183] though basal membrane transport of lysine is reduced as represented by reduced mediated lysine uptake and a reduced V_{max} for the y^+L system,[80] and in pregnancy, array data demonstrate upregulation of system y^+ components.[184] Reductions in the uptake of leucine in both microvillous and basal membrane preparations of FGR placentae highlight possible alterations in the L transport system.[80] These changes in basal membrane transport properties could be an important adaptive response by the trophoblast, limiting the backflux of amino acids from the fetal circulation to the placenta. In vivo studies of ovine FGR placental transport have indeed shown a reduced backflux of leucine and threonine from the fetal circulation to the placenta, suggesting that changes in basal membrane function may have occurred.[185,186] At steady state, the fetal-to-maternal enrichment ratio (F/M) of leucine in normal human pregnancies is approximately 0.8, a much higher ratio than the 0.4 ratio in sheep.[185,187] However, in both species, this ratio is significantly lower in FGR pregnancies. In the ovine FGR model, the reduction in F/M ratio was due to a significant reduction in transplacental leucine flux,[185] which is probably also the mechanism in human FGR pregnancies. Furthermore, the magnitude of the leucine ratio reduction correlates with a clinical classification of FGR severity based upon a completely different set of clinical data, namely fetal arterial velocimetry and fetal heart rate data.[177] In addition, recent clinical studies have shown that the leucine and phenylalanine (F/M) enrichment ratio is significantly lower in human FGR compared to normal pregnancies, and that vesicle transporter activity is also impaired.[80,187,188]

Finally, the observations of differences in amino acid transport activity in the FGR placenta highlight the important point that the activity of transport systems must be considered in conjunction with other contributors to amino acid flux. In studies comparing normal and FGR placentas there are reported reductions in total villous surface area,[161,163,189] suggesting that morphometric changes contribute to the overall reduction in placental amino acid transport capacity. Thus, at the present time, it appears that both reductions in surface area for exchange and reductions in specific transporter number and activities are the major factors contributing to the reduction in amino acid transport in FGR pregnancies.

MULTIPLE ROLES OF AMINO ACIDS

Since the first description of amino acids as important neuroexcitatory or neuroinhibitory compounds in the brain, it has become increasingly clear that amino acids serve important functions beyond that of components of proteins and/or as metabolic fuels for tissues. Even in the latter role, their importance had been underestimated by studies that examined the contribution of amino acids to total CO_2 production in the whole organism. It took some time to appreciate the fact that oxidation may be organ specific. Thus glutamate/glutamine oxidation by the small bowel may represent a relatively minor contribution to total CO_2 production in man, but may be crucial to meeting energy requirements of the gastrointestinal tract. The oxidation of glutamate appears to be important not only in the small bowel, but in the heart and in the placenta as well. Similarly, amino acids, whose intracellular concentrations may change rapidly, can play an important role as idiosmoles in regulating water balance across tissues.[190] The interorgan shuttling and interconversion of amino acids may also play an important role for purposes not directly related to providing carbon and nitrogen for growth or as metabolic fuels. Traditionally, we have come to appreciate the role of alanine and glutamine in shuttling carbon from skeletal muscle to the liver where it is used for glucose production. Recent studies have brought out the importance of glutamate cycling between the fetal liver and placenta.[191–193] Normally, in fetal life, there is no significant rate of gluconeogenesis in the fetal liver. This is useful to the fetus, for it permits the fetus to meet its glucose requirements by obtaining glucose from the maternal glucose pool via transplacental transport, but the large amount of carbon coming to the fetal liver would require oxidation if there was no alternative carbon released from the liver instead of glucose. In fetal life, glutamate serves this important function. The fetal liver releases a large amount of glutamate into the circulation, which reduces the fetal hepatic oxygen requirement for the metabolism of glutamate. The bulk of the hepatic-derived glutamate is taken up in a first-pass clearance by the placenta where it is used as a mitochondrial fuel.[194] In this sense, the placenta assists the liver by reducing its oxygen requirement significantly. Such interorgan transport and interconversion of nutrients may serve other functions as well. The placental oxidation of glutamate provides a source of reduced nicotinamideadenine dinucleotide phosphate (NADPH)[194–196] which can be used in steroidogenesis. The production of NADPH from glutamate oxidation in the placenta may also provide a link to sugar metabolism within the placenta. In ovine pregnancies it has been shown that normally there is a net production of sorbitol from glucose within the placenta. This step requires NADPH as a cofactor. There is no net production of inositol. However, in FGR ovine pregnancies, sorbitol production is curtailed and inositol production increased. This may be due to a limitation in the placental supply of NADPH in FGR pregnancies. These additional roles of interorgan shuttling between the fetal liver and placenta are also evident in serine and glycine metabolism.[197–200] Serine is another amino acid that is released from the fetal liver and is taken up from the fetal circulation into the placenta, where it is used for glycine production. This pathway provides a supply of methylene tetrahydrofolate within the placenta, as will be discussed later in this chapter. More recently, attention has focused on the role of the interconversion of arginine and citrulline in providing substrate for nitric oxide synthase leading to nitric oxide production, a potent vasodilator.[201] Other functions of nitric oxide as a signaling compound are being described.[183] Its role in regulating insulin release from beta cells is under investigation and may provide a link between amino acid metabolism and endocrine regulation of carbohydrate metabolism. The work in fetal metabolism has only served to further strengthen the concept that amino acids play multiple roles in the body and that their metabolism and utilization tend to be organ specific.

PLACENTAL AMINO ACID METABOLISM

The amino acid requirements of the placenta for energy and for protein accretion during its growth are not well known. The placenta contains enzymes related to carbohydrate and amino acid metabolism that give it the capacity to oxidize a number of amino acids as well as perform glycolysis, glycogenolysis and glycogen, protein, and fatty acid synthesis.[202,203] Four amino acids (alanine, glutamine, threonine, and serine) that are found in high concentrations in placental tissues and are known gluconeogenic precursors are transported by the three transport systems A, L, and ASC.[63,88,98,204] This could be a protective mechanism to ensure adequate fetal supply of these important amino acids. Preincubation of placental tissue for several hours in amino acid–free medium leads to an increased concentrating capacity of the placental tissues for AIB.[24,205] This increased concentrating capacity can be blocked by inhibitors of protein synthesis, indicating that the placental vesicles respond to hypoaminoacidemia by upregulation of the A system transporters. Far less is known about the placental vascular endothelium, though still in debate, it may share at least one characteristic with that of the cerebral circulation, namely the absence of system A transporter.[206] The metabolism of amino acids within the placenta during transport has not been well studied.

So far, amino acid oxidation by human placental mitochondria has been demonstrated for alanine, aspartate, glutamate, and glycine.[196] Given the data on the large uptake of glutamate by the placenta from the fetal circulation, it is likely that glutamate is the predominant amino acid functioning as a metabolic fuel for the placenta.[192] Placental metabolic requirements are very large. In vivo estimates of its oxygen consumption are approximately equal to those for the brain, and oxidation of amino acids is a major metabolic function of the brain and placenta.[207] In vivo there is a significant production and excretion of ammonia into both uterine and umbilical circulations by the ovine placenta.[7,8] The absolute rate of uteroplacental ammonia production, approximately 25 μmol/min in the ovine pregnancy at midgestation (73 to 97 days, term 147 ± 3 days), is approximately equal to that of the term placenta. Since in vitro data indicate that there is minimal urea cycle activity within the placenta,[208] this suggests that ammonia and not urea is the end product of amino acid deamination within the placenta. Some of the ammonia produced by the placenta is consumed by the fetal liver and, in fetal sheep near term, the uptake by the fetal liver is approximately 1.5 to 1.8 times that taken up by the umbilical circulation from the placenta.[7,8,208] This indicates that fetal tissues as well as the placenta produce ammonia and uptake of ammonia by the fetal liver undoubtedly contributes to its high rate of urea production.

In part, the ammonia production by the placenta is derived from the transamination of branched chain amino acids (BCAAs).[209] The activity of the branched chain aminotransferases is high in the placenta and since the activity of α-keto decarboxylases is low, it is clear that the α-ketoacids derived from the BCAA are not oxidized further. These α-ketoacids represent part of a group of compounds that are produced in the placenta and are delivered into both uterine and umbilical circulations. These compounds include ammonia, lactate, and one of the polyols, sorbitol (Figure 5). The placental production of glutamate as a consequence

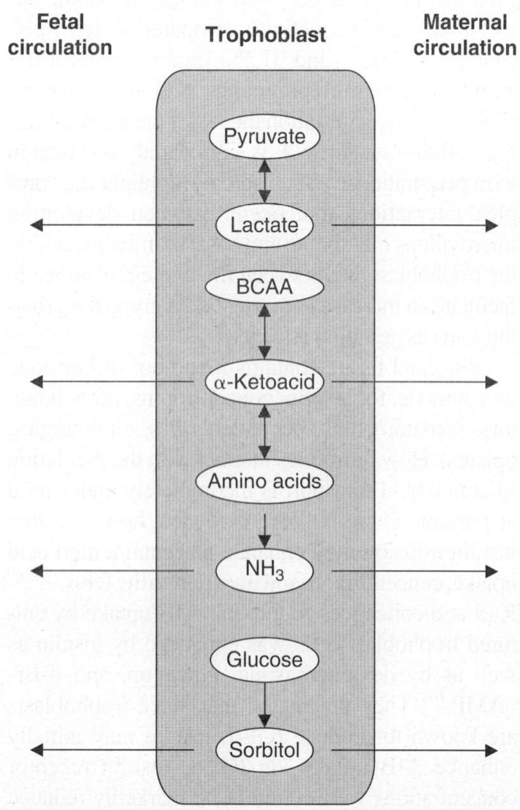

Figure 5 A schematic representation of some of the metabolites produced in the placenta which are then delivered into both the maternal and fetal circulations.

of transamination of a α-ketoglutarate from BCAA,[97] together with the placental uptake of fetal plasma glutamate at 4.8 μmol/min/kg fetus,[194] represent the two major influxes of glutamate into the ovine placenta. Although the ovine placenta contains the enzyme glutamine synthetase, only a small fraction of glutamate that is taken up by the placenta from fetal circulation is returned to the fetus as glutamine.[194,210] It is the oxidation of glutamate that appears to be the predominant pathway of placental glutamate disposal.

It is likely that placental ammonia production is not confined to the epitheliochorial placenta of the sheep. It has been described for the perfused human placenta and a net efflux of ammonia from the pregnant uterus into the maternal circulation has also been found in rabbits, guinea pigs, and sheep.[209,211–214] It is intriguing to speculate on the possible biologic significance of mammalian fetuses growing and developing in an environment of an elevated ammonia concentration. Ammonia can affect hepatic metabolism and may play a role in glial development and in the development of other tissues rich in glutamine synthetase. Ammonia is now one of a number of compounds which have been shown to be produced in the ovine trophoblast and delivered into both fetal and maternal circulation. The enzymes involved in these pathways have been found in the human trophoblast, although in most instances studies that document the production of these metabolites in human trophoblast in vivo are lacking.

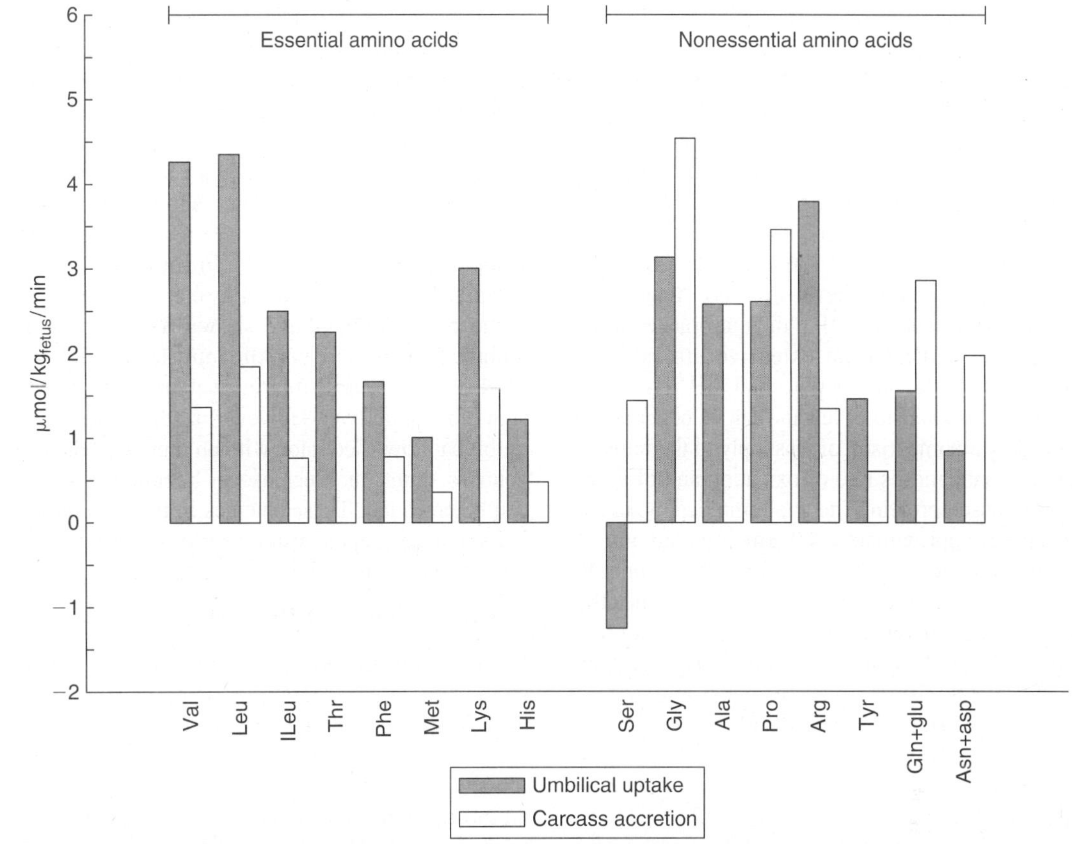

Figure 6 Comparison between mean umbilical uptakes and estimated normal fetal accretions of amino acids. For pairs of amino acids (glutamine + glutamate and asparagine + aspartate) individual accretion rates are not known. (Adapted from reference 215.)

UMBILICAL UPTAKE OF AMINO ACIDS

Measurements of unidirectional flux are currently available only for the ovine species and not for other mammalian species. A number of studies involving examination of the umbilical uptake of amino acids in chronic, unstressed sheep models have revealed that most amino acids (particularly the neutral amino acids) are delivered into the fetal circulation in amounts that exceed their net rates of accretion.[2,4,9,18,215] The most complete data on the uterine and umbilical uptakes of amino acids are presented in Figure 6.[215]

Several studies of the umbilical uptake of amino acids under normal conditions have shown that there is no measurable uptake of aspartate and, in fact, a significant net uptake from the fetal circulation into the placenta of serine and glutamate. Thus for these three amino acids, it is clear that fetal requirements must be met by production within fetal tissues. Stegink and colleagues infused labeled tracer isotopes of glutamate and aspartate into both fetal and maternal circulations of rhesus monkeys and found essentially no transfer of the compounds across the placenta.[216,217] Schneider and colleagues, utilizing an in vitro perfused human placenta preparation, found significant uptake of glutamate from the fluid perfusing the fetal side of the placenta rather than a net transfer of glutamate from the maternal to the fetal side.[218] Not surprisingly, since amino acid requirements and protein synthetic rates are linked to fetal metabolic rates, the umbilical uptake or dietary supply of amino acids per kilogram of fetal body weight is much higher in early gestation compared to term.[18] A key question in fetal nutrition is how maternal concentrations of amino acids are related to the umbilical uptake. This question is important because it would help to define the extent to which changes in maternal amino acid concentrations could impact the fetal delivery of amino acids. The question has been studied in both ovine pregnancies and human pregnancies by infusions of amino acids into the maternal circulation with measurements of their umbilical uptake. The relationship between maternal concentration and umbilical uptake is a complex one. In ovine studies, the flux from the maternal circulation to the fetal circulation is most rapid for five amino acids and for those five, differences in their fluxes are directly attributable to differences in their normal maternal plasma concentrations,[219] as shown in Figure 7. In human pregnancies, it is possible for most amino acids to increase the fetal delivery by increasing the maternal concentration.[214] This has been shown for both normal pregnancies and pregnancies complicated by FGR.[188] However, for some amino acids, this has not been possible when an infusion of many amino acids is given to the mother presumably due to competitive inhibition by other amino acids in the infusate.

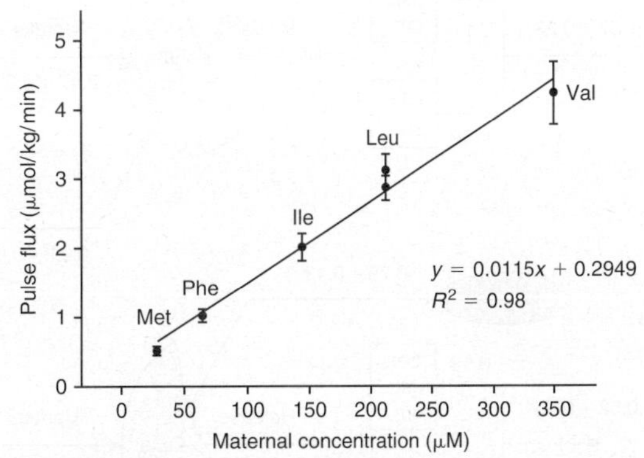

Figure 7 Pulse flux calculated over the first 10 minute after the bolus versus maternal plasma arterial concentration for the five essential amino acids that have high and similar pulse flux clearances. The two leucine data represent two separate studies. (Adapted from reference 219.)

It is clear that the umbilical uptake of amino acids cannot be considered solely a reflection of the amino acid supply derived from the maternal plasma pool via transplacental transport, but may also include a contribution derived from production within the placenta or release from placental protein breakdown. It is important to understand which amino acids are provided to the fetus primarily through placental production versus placental transport, because different forms of placental pathology may adversely affect the mode of delivery of those amino acids to the fetus.

FETAL AND PLACENTAL OXIDATION

The use of multiple-tracer methodology in animal models has allowed further elucidation of amino acid metabolism within the placenta and the fetus.

Fetal and placental metabolism of the essential amino acids leucine and threonine have been studied in some detail.[185,186,220] For leucine, Loy and colleagues[220] were the first to demonstrate that even for an essential amino acid there may be extensive catabolism both within the fetus and within the placenta. They found that 20 to 25% of the (1-^{14}C) leucine infused into the fetus could be accounted for as $^{14}CO_2$ produced by the fetus. Unlike glutamate, there was no measurable oxidation of leucine within the uteroplacental tissues. This indicated an extensive utilization of leucine as a fetal but not placental fuel. The extensive fetal catabolism of leucine can be better appreciated by a comparison of its supply to the fetus via the placenta and its rate of oxidation and of accretion in tissue protein. The total umbilical uptake of leucine is approximately 4.9 μmol/min/kg and net accretion of leucine in tissue proteins accounts for only 2.0 μmol/min/kg in late gestation. On the other hand, the rate of leucine oxidation is 2.8 μmol/min/kg or 57% of its uptake. Thus far, the fetal and placental metabolism of other essential amino acids has not been studied in such detail.

The oxidation rates in the fetus and/or placenta have been measured for leucine, lysine, threonine, alanine, glycine, serine, and glutamate,[185,18,194,219–222] and it is apparent that fetal oxidation of amino acids is not confined to the nonessential amino acids. In fact, it is an important safety feature for fetal nutrition that amino acids are provided in amounts which exceed their rates of accretion.[4,5] This mandates a fairly high oxidation rate for most amino acids including the essential amino acids. It is not surprising, therefore, that there is a relatively high rate of urea production by the fetus. This has been directly measured in the ovine fetus,[6] and estimated for the human fetus.[223]

In FGR, the oxidation of amino acids is decreased, sparing the amino acids for protein synthesis. The principal amino acid used as a metabolic fuel by the ovine placenta appears to be glutamate.[194] There are no data in other species, but an uptake of glutamate from the fetal plasma into the placenta has been shown for human pregnancies. This observation supports the idea that it probably plays a similar role for the human placenta.

FETAL HEPATIC CIRCULATION AND AMINO ACID METABOLISM

Probably no area of fetal physiology and metabolism has progressed more rapidly since the last edition of this book than fetal hepatic physiology. The advances are both in studies relating to the perfusion of the fetal liver and in studies of fetal hepatic metabolism of amino acids.

Fetal Hepatic Circulation

The umbilical vein carries the most oxygenated and nutrient-rich blood of the fetus and a large fraction of this blood perfuses the fetal liver. Thus, the fetal liver, in contrast to the postnatal liver, is a site of preferred oxygenation. It is a vitally important defense for the fetus during periods of chronic or acute hypoxia because it continues to take up lactate from the fetal circulation and release pyruvate. The pyruvate can then be metabolized by other fetal tissues. For human pregnancies, the percent of umbilical blood flow shunted away from the fetal liver through the ductus venosus has now been measured.[224–226] The shunt gradually decreases from 40 to 15% over a gestational age range from 20 weeks to term. In some FGR pregnancies, this shunt is significantly increased.[225,227,228] Since other studies have shown a reduction in umbilical blood flow per kilogram fetal weight in FGR pregnancies,[229] this in itself reduces perfusion of the fetal liver. However, if the reduction in umbilical flow is coupled with an increased ductus venosus shunt, the decrease in hepatic perfusion can be profound. These changes in the fetal circulation must be kept in mind in terms of its potential importance upon fetal hepatic metabolism.

Hepatic Amino Acid Metabolism

Fetal hepatic uptake of amino acids has been studied in late-gestation fetal lambs and fetal hepatic uptake and the umbilical uptake of amino acids have been compared. A large hepatic uptake of all the essential and most of the nonessential amino acids by both lobes of the fetal liver has been reported.[4] During normal fetal development there is no appreciable rate of fetal gluconeogenesis. This is understandable since fetal hepatic glucose production would be self-defeating for the fetus. It would increase plasma glucose concentration, which would reduce the transplacental glucose gradient leading to a reduced umbilical glucose uptake from the mother. The absence of fetal gluconeogenesis is not accompanied by a reduced amino acid uptake in the fetal circulation from the placenta,[191] as shown in Figure 8. There is a large uptake of amino acids including all of the gluconeogenic amino acids, as well as a large fetal uptake of lactate.[191] In fetal life, the carbon is released primarily as glutamate and pyruvate with a smaller contribution coming from the hepatic release of serine, ornithine, and aspartate. This is in contrast to what occurs in postnatal life, where the carbon from these amino acids is released from the liver solely as glucose.

The hepatic uptake of lactate and release of pyruvate are of special interest because of the importance of these compounds during fetal hypoxia. As mentioned earlier, the fetal liver is a site of preferred oxygenation because it is perfused with oxygen-rich umbilical venous blood. This is quite different from hepatic perfusion in postnatal life. The uptake of lactate and release of pyruvate continues under conditions of fetal hypoxia providing pyruvate which can be metabolized by nonhepatic tissues even under hypoxic conditions.[230]

The interorgan shuttling of the two amino acid pairs, glutamate and glutamine and serine and glycine, plays an important role in this overall carbon balance for the fetus. The release of glutamate, serine, and pyruvate effectively replaces the glucose carbon release characteristic of the liver in postnatal life. This is clearly brought out in Figure 8, which shows what happens when gluconeogenesis is triggered in the fetal liver by the infusion of glucagon.[191] With the advent of net glucose released from the liver, the efflux of glutamate, serine, and pyruvate is markedly reduced and the overall carbon balance is maintained. The exchange of glutamate and glutamine between the fetal liver and placenta does not represent a cycling of carbon between the two organs. Glutamate is largely oxidized in the placenta and in the fetus. The exchange of glutamate and glutamine changes quite markedly during parturition and during glucocorticoid or glucagon administration to the fetus.[192,193] Under these conditions, there is a decrease of fetal hepatic glutamate release which results in a decrease of placental glutamate uptake. What role these metabolic changes in the fetal liver play in parturition is not yet established. Studies have shown that FGR is also associated with changes in fetal and placental glutamate metabolism. Fetal plasma glutamate concentrations are significantly lower in ovine FGR pregnancies compared to normal pregnancies.[231]

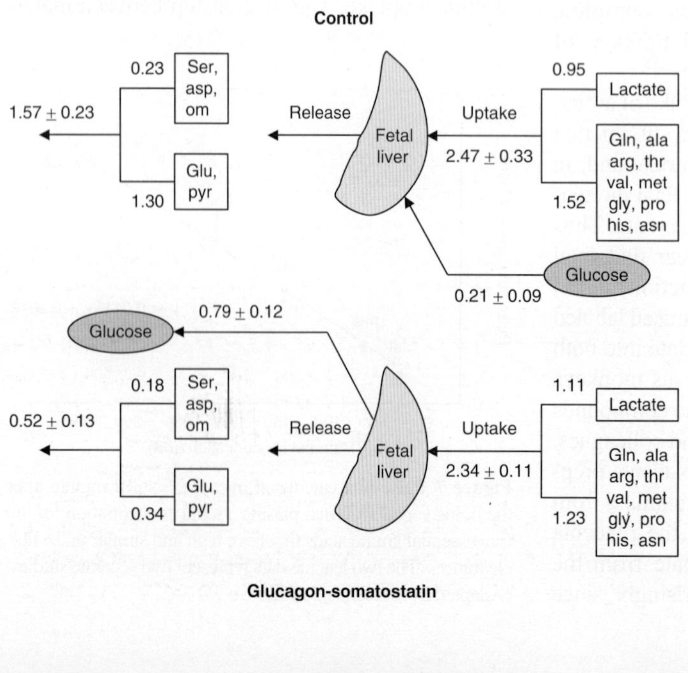

Figure 8 Fetal hepatic uptake and output of glucose carbon and glucogenic substrate carbon under normal physiologic conditions (control) and during a fetal glucagon somatostatin infusion. Each number represents a substrate carbon-to-oxygen uptake ratio. (Adapted from reference 191.)

Glycine and serine are another metabolically related pair of amino acids that demonstrate a similar pattern of release and uptake across the ovine fetal liver and placenta.[4,197,200,232] The fetal glycine oxidation rate is high and glycine is almost totally oxidized within the fetal liver. Fetal hepatic glycine oxidation and serine production from glycine are linked in the fetal liver by the enzyme systems glycine oxidase and serine hydroxymethyltransferase.[221,232,233] The combined action of these enzymes is the production of one mole of CO_2 and one mole of serine for every two moles of glycine consumed.[197,198] This is also true in adult tissues,[234,235] though adult liver is not normally a site of net serine release.[236]

Infusion of tracer serine into the fetus has demonstrated a rapid bidirectional transport of serine between the fetal blood and placenta, as well as placental conversion of fetal plasma serine to glycine.[198] In contrast to glycine oxidation, the bulk of fetal plasma serine oxidation occurs in extrahepatic tissues. Moores and colleagues[221] infused labeled serine into the maternal circulation of pregnant sheep and found that despite high maternal enrichments of serine, there was no fetal plasma enrichment evident. However, the infusion of maternal tracer serine did lead to the appearance of labeled glycine in the fetal circulation. Thus, placental glycine production utilizes serine derived from both the maternal and fetal circulations. This brings out the complexity of pathways by which an amino acid such as glycine is delivered to the fetus from the placenta. The pathway for glycine production from serine is thought to be via serine hydroxymethyltransferase, since ovine placental tissue is known to have moderately high activity for the mitochondrial isoform of this enzyme.[232] A by-product of placental glycine production via serine hydroxymethyltransferase is methylene tetrahydrofolate, which could be involved in a variety of methylation reactions within the placenta.[221,232] These examples of placental–fetal interorgan shuttling of amino acids, and particularly between the fetal liver and placenta, are now recognized to be an important and unique aspect of fetal metabolism.

FETAL HINDLIMB METABOLISM OF AMINO ACIDS

Several laboratories have studied the amino acid uptake by the fetal ovine hindlimb, as being representative of the fetal carcass/extrahepatic tissues. Its metabolism has been evaluated under normal, maternal fasting, and fetal euglycemic hyperinsulinemic states.[237,238] Under normal physiologic conditions, the hindlimb of a growing fetus shows a net uptake of both essential and nonessential amino acids from the fetal circulation.[238] This is in contrast to adult hindlimb studies that show a large output of alanine and glutamine.[239] It is theorized that the high amino acid uptake by the fetal hindlimb could be explained by the relatively high nitrogen accretion rate of the fetus.[238] There is a net uptake across the hindlimb of two amino acids that are not supplied by the placenta: glutamate and serine. It is estimated that the net fetal hepatic output could account for the combined uptake of glutamate by the placenta and the hindlimb.[238] Given the large uptake of alanine by the fetal liver, it is interesting that the fetal hindlimb shows no net release of alanine.

Theoretically, these amino acids could not be taken up by the fetal liver and be utilized for glucose production during a state of reduced umbilical glucose uptake (ie, maternal fasting).[240] Liechty and colleagues reported a relatively high activity for ketoacid carboxylase activity in fetal skeletal muscle.[241] In pregnant sheep, after fasting, there is an approximate fivefold increase in the utilization of glutamine and a twofold increase in the utilization of the BCAAs by the uteroplacental tissues, suggesting a possible interorgan cycle between hindlimb and placenta, with the hindlimb supplying glutamine during the maternal fasted state.[242] Under euglycemic, hyperinsulinemic conditions, fetal lambs were noted to have significantly decreased arterial concentrations of most amino acids, and significantly increased limb uptake of alanine, asparagine, glycine, isoleucine, methionine, and tyrosine and a decreased uptake of aspartate, but with no significant change in net total nitrogen uptake.[238] These studies show that the stimulation of alanine uptake by insulin is opposite to the effect of maternal fasting, suggesting that insulin or insulin-like growth factors may play a role in regulating an alanine exchange between fetal circulation and nonvisceral fetal tissues.[238]

NEONATAL IMPLICATIONS OF FETAL AMINO ACID SUPPLY AND METABOLISM

One may ask what studies of amino acid nutrition and metabolism during fetal life can contribute to our approach to optimal nutrition for very premature infants in a neonatal intensive care unit. First, it is important to recognize that normal fetal development and postnatal development are vastly different biologic states. Not only are there profound endocrine changes triggered by delivery and its associated separation from the placenta, but the interorgan cycling of amino acids between the fetal organs and placenta is abruptly terminated. However, certain principles of amino acid metabolism during early development still apply. To summarize, during fetal development, amino acids are taken up in amounts that exceed their requirements for growth. This leads to a high rate of amino acid oxidation and a relatively high rate of urea production. A second general characteristic is the absence of gluconeogenesis, which leads to a hepatic production and release of serine and glutamate. It is important to emphasize that the requirements of amino acids change quite markedly with increasing gestational age, and also upon whether there has been normal or abnormal fetal growth. In the normal term newborn, the rate of net protein accretion in utero is quite low, with fat accretion dominating growth. In FGR fetuses, there are changes in plasma amino acid concentrations reflecting the reduced placental supply. There may also be vascular changes which lead to hepatic injury.

The delivery of optimal nutrition to the small premature infant is a critical factor to its overall care. Very premature infants have been delivered before they have gone through the phase of in utero development associated with rapid accretion of fat depots and glycogen stores. Preterm infants are born at gestational ages associated with rapid accretion of protein in utero. This has led to a neonatal nutritional approach which emphasizes the early provision of amino acids to very preterm babies. It should be emphasized, however, that this makes an assumption of good liver perfusion and the absence of any prenatal liver injury. Neither of these conditions necessarily applies to an individual newborn in the immediate neonatal period. The best guideline for assessing the nutritional status of the low-birth-weight infant is not clear. However, one approach would include achieving a postnatal growth that approximates the in utero growth rate of a normal fetus.[243] By this guideline, the intrauterine accretion rate of amino acids becomes a reference point defining the minimal requirements in the neonatal period. As delineated in the previous discussion, the mammalian fetus utilizes the circulating maternal free amino acid pool as its primary nitrogen source for growth with certain conspicuous exceptions. Since amino acid oxidation is linked to hepatic gluconeogenesis in postnatal life and since gluconeogenesis is a requirement for postnatal adaptation, one would expect amino acid oxidation to be sustained during postnatal development, significantly increasing amino acid requirements. For the premature infant, the primary sources of nitrogen are obtained from a parenteral nutrition composition, human breast milk, or premature infant formulas. Current nutritional management for preterm and FGR infants aims at early provision of amino acids.

Recommendations for the quantity of protein delivery include 3.6 to 3.8 g/kg/d gross protein intake for the stable growing infant at <27 weeks gestation and $<1,000$ g, and 3.0 to 3.6 g/kg/d for the 1,000 to 1,750 g infant at 28- to 34-week gestation. Although the exact quantity is debated (ie, European guidelines versus American guidelines), it is generally accepted that the stable growing low-birth-weight infant requires, on the average, a parenteral amino acid intake of 3.0 g/kg/d to ensure accretion of nitrogen at the intrauterine rate of approximately 300 mg/kg/d. This amino acid intake plus an energy intake of 80 to 100 kcal/kg/d results in a weight gain that approximates the intrauterine rate of 15 gm/kg/d.[244] However, the studies of the fetal circulation in FGR pregnancies make it clear that the general recommendations should be used with caution in newborns of any weight or gestational age when there is evidence of circulatory compromise in utero. A high carbohydrate and relatively low nitrogen intake is prudent. Certainly, if a high nitrogen intake is given to such infants, there should be an assessment of ammonia and urea levels as well as measurement of amino acid concentrations to be sure the nitrogen load is not compromising the infant. This caution reflects the fact that there are still no ideal approaches to assess both the quality and the quantity of amino acids provided as protein in milk feedings to low-birth-weight infants. Breast milk provides a large array of compounds not included in formula feedings. Some of these compounds such as glycoproteins and peptides contain amino acids. However, owing to the instability of glutamine it is currently omitted from parenteral nutrition solutions and infant formulas. Glutamine has recently been found to be an important metabolic fuel for lymphocytes[245,246] and intestinal epithelial cells,[247] and is supplied to the fetus in large amounts throughout gestation.

It has already been demonstrated that formula-fed, very low birth weight infants, whose weight gain was comparable to that of a normal fetus, retained the same amount of protein (approximately 1.9 g/kg/d), but accumulated fat at approximately three times the rate of the fetus. This indicates that the body composition of the premature infant will differ from that of the comparable placentally nourished fetus.[248] How this will impact on long-term growth and neurodevelopment is unclear and a matter of much debate.[249–251]

As the complex interplay among fetus, placenta, and maternal dietary supply of amino acids becomes increasingly clear, it is hoped that this information can be used to understand more completely the remarkable process of fetal growth and maturation. This, in turn, will then be invaluable information in the further modification and design of feeding regimens for premature infants in order to optimize growth and long-term neurodevelopment.

REFERENCE

1. Young M, McFadyen I. Placental transfer and fetal uptake of amino acids in the pregnant ewe. J Perinat Med 1973;1:174–82.
2. Lemons JA, Adcock EW, Jones MDJ, et al. Umbilical uptake of amino acids in the unstressed fetal lamb. J Clin Invest 1976;58:1428–34.
3. Lemons JA, Schreiner RL. Amino acid metabolism in the ovine fetus. Am J Physiol 1983;244:E459–66.
4. Marconi AM, Battaglia FC, Meschia G, Sparks JW. A comparison of amino acid arteriovenous differences across the liver and placenta of the fetal lamb. Am J Physiol 1989;257: E909–15.
5. Lemons JA. Fetal-placental nitrogen metabolism. Semin Perinatol 1979;3:177–90.
6. Gresham EL, James EJ, Raye JR, et al. Production and excretion of urea by the fetal lamb. Pediatrics 1972;50:372–79.
7. Holzman IR, Lemons JA, Meschia G, Battaglia FC. Ammonia production by the pregnant uterus. Proc Soc Exp Biol Med 1977;156:27–30.
8. Holzman IR, Philipps AF, Battaglia FC. Glucose metabolism, lactate, and ammonia production by the human placenta in vitro. Pediatr Res 1979;13:117–20.
9. Lemons JA, Reyman D, Schreiner RL. Fetal and maternal amino acid concentrations during fasting in the ewe. J Pediatr Gastroenterol Nutr 1984;3:249–55.
10. Schaefer AL, Krishnamurti CR. Whole body and tissue fractional protein synthesis in the ovine fetus in utero. Br J Nutr 1984;52:359–69.
11. Noakes DE, Young M. Measurement of fetal tissue protein synthetic rate in the lamb in utero. Res Vet Sci 1981;31:336–41.
12. Kennaugh JM, Bell AW, Teng C, et al. Ontogenetic changes in the rates of protein synthesis and leucine oxidation during fetal life. Pediatr Res 1987;22:688–92.
13. Meier PR, Peterson RG, Bonds DR, et al. Rates of protein synthesis and turnover in fetal life. Am J Physiol 1981;240:E320–4.
14. Milley JR. Protein synthesis during hypoxia in fetal lambs. Am J Physiol 1987;252:E519–24.
15. van Veen LC, Teng C, Hay WW, Jr, et al. Leucine disposal and oxidation rates in the fetal lamb. Metab: Clin Exp 1987;36:48–53.
16. Bell AW, Kennaugh JM, Battaglia FC, et al. Metabolic and circulatory studies of fetal lamb at mid-gestation. Am J Physiol 1986;250:E538–44.
17. Bell AW, Battaglia FC, Meschia G. Relation between metabolic rate and body size on the ovine fetus. J Nutr 1987;117:1181–86.
18. Bell AW, Kennaugh JM, Battaglia FC, Meschia G. Uptake of amino acids and ammonia at mid-gestation by the fetal lamb. Q J Exp Physiol 1989;74:635–43.
19. Holzman IR, Lemons JA, Meschia G, Battaglia FC. Uterine uptake of amino acids and placental glutamine-glutmate balance in the pregnant ewe. J Dev Physiol 1979;1:137–49.
20. Battaglia FC, Meschia G. Fetal nutrition. Annu Rev Nutr 1988;8:43–61.
21. Morriss FH, Jr, Adcock EW, Paxson CLJ, Greeley WJ, Jr. Uterine uptake of amino acids throughout gestation in the unstressed ewe. Am J Obstet Gynecol 1979;135:601–08.
22. Sybulski S, Tremblay PC. Uptake and incorporation into protein of radioactive glycine by human placentas in vitro. Am J Obstet Gynecol 1967;97:1111–18.
23. Nesbitt RE, Jr, Rice PA, Rourke JE, et al. In vitro perfusion studies of the human placenta. A newly-designed apparatus for extracorporeal perfusion achieving dual closed circulation. Gynecol Invest 1970;1:185–203.
24. Smith CH, Adcock EW, Teasdale F, et al. Placental amino acid uptake: Tissue preparation, kinetics, and preincubation effect. Am J Physiol 1973;224:558–64.
25. Smith NC, Brush MG, Luckett S. Preparation of human placental villous surface membrane. Nature 1974;252:302–03.
26. Miller RK, Berndt WO. Characterization of neutral amino acid accumulation by human term placental slices. Am J Physiol 1974;227:1236–42.
27. Boyd CA, Lund EK. L-proline transport by brush border membrane vesicles prepared from human placenta. J Physiol 1981;315:9–19.
28. Bissonnette JM. Review article: Membrane vesicles from trophoblast cells as models for placental exchange studies. Placenta 1982;3:99–106.
29. Carstensen MH, Leichtweiss HP. L-alanine carriers at maternal and fetal surfaces of the guinea pig placenta trophoblast. Gynecol Obstet Invest 1986;22:172–85.
30. Zuckermann FA, Head JR. Isolation and characterization of trophoblast from murine placenta. Placenta 1986;7:349–64.
31. Schneider H, Proegler M, Sodha R, Dancis J. Asymmetrical transfer of alpha-aminoisobutyric acid (AIB), leucine and lysine across the in vitro perfused human placenta. Placenta 1987;8:141–51.
32. Karl PI, Chang B, Fisher SE. Calcium-sensitive uptake of amino acids by human placental slices. Pediatr Res 1988;23:9–13.
33. Yagel S, Casper RF, Powell W, et al. Characterization of pure human first-trimester cytotrophoblast cells in long-term culture: Growth pattern, markers, and hormone production. Am J Obstet Gynecol 1989;160:938–45.
34. Douglas GC, King BF. Differentiation of human trophoblast cells in vitro as revealed by immunocytochemical staining of desmoplakin and nuclei. J Cell Sci 1990;96:131–41.
35. Beckman DA, Pugarelli JE, Jensen M, et al. Sources of amino acids for protein synthesis during early organogenesis in the rat. I. Relative contributions of free amino acids and of proteins. Placenta 1990;11:109–21.
36. Montgomery D, Young M. The uptake of naturally occurring amino acids by the plasma membrane of the human placenta. Placenta 1982;3:13–20.
37. Philipps AF, Holzman IR, Teng C, Battaglia FC. Tissue concentrations of free amino acids in term human placentas. Am J Obstet Gynecol 1978;131:881–87.
38. Kerr GR. The free amino acids of serum during development of Macaca mulatta. II. During pregnancy and fetal life. Pediatr Res 1968;2:493–500.
39. Palou A, Arola L, Alemany M. Plasma amino acid concentrations in pregnant rats and in 21-day foetuses. Biochem J 1977;166:49–55.
40. Reynolds ML, Young M. The transfer of free alpha-amino nitrogen across the placental membrane in the guinea-pig. J Physiol 1971;214:583–97.
41. Hill PM, Young M. Net placental transfer of free amino acids against varying concentrations. J Physiol 1973;235:409–22.
42. Young M. Placental factors and fetal nutrition. Am J Clin Nutr 1981;34:738–43.
43. Ferrell CL, Ford SP. Blood flow steroid secretion and nutrient uptake of the gravid bovine uterus. J Anim Sci 1980;50:1113–21.
44. Dancis J, Money WL, Springer D, Levitz M. Transport of amino acids by placenta. Am J Obstet Gynecol 1968;101:820–29.
45. Battaglia FC, Meschia G. Principal substrates of fetal metabolism [review] [196 refs]. Physiol Rev 1978;58:499–527.
46. Gaull GE, Raiha NC, Saarikoski S, Sturman JA. Transfer of cyst(e)ine and methionine across the human placenta. Pediatr Res 1973;7:908–13.
47. Schneider H, Dancis J. Amino acid transport in human placental slices. Am J Obstet Gynecol 1974;120:1092–98.
48. Lines DR, Waisman HA. Placental transport of phenylalanine in the rat: Maternal and fetal metabolism. Proc Soc Exp Biol Med 1971;136:790–93.
49. Smith CH, Depper R. Placental amino acid uptake. II. Tissue preincubation, fluid distribution, and mechanisms of regulation. Pediatr Res 1974;8:697–703.
50. Wapnir RA, Dierks-Ventling C. Placental transfer of amino acids in the rat. II. Aromatic amino acids. Biol Neonate 1971;17:373–80.
51. Christensen HN. Role of amino acid transport and countertransport in nutrition and metabolism. Physiol Rev 1990;70:43–77.
52. Kilberg MS, Stevens BR, Novak DA. Recent advances in mammalian amino acid transport. Annu Rev Nutr 1993;13:137–65.
53. Ramamoorthy S, Leibach FH, Mahesh VB, Ganapathy V. Modulation of the activity of amino acid transport system L by phorbol esters and calmodulin antagonists in a human placental choriocarcinoma cell line. Biochim Biophys Acta 1992;1136:181–88.
54. Johnson LW, Smith CH. Neutral amino acid transport systems of microvillous membrane of human placenta. Am J Physiol 1988;254:C773–80.
55. Hoeltzli SD, Smith CH. Alanine transport systems in isolated basal plasma membrane of human placenta. Am J Physiol 1989;256:C630–7.
56. Novak DA, Beveridge MJ, Malandro M, Seo J. Ontogeny of amino acid transport system A in rat placenta. Placenta 1996;17:643–51.
57. Low SY, Rennie MJ, Taylor PM. Sodium-dependent glutamate transport in cultured rat myotubes increases after glutamine deprivation. FASEB J 1994;8:127–31.
58. Taylor PM, Kaur S, Mackenzie B, Peter GJ. Amino-acid-dependent modulation of amino acid transport in *Xenopus laevis* oocytes. J Exp Biol 1996;199:923–31.
59. Nelson DM, Smith SD, Furesz TC, et al. Hypoxia reduces expression and function of system A amino acid transporters in cultured term human trophoblasts. Am J Physiol Cell Physiol 2003;284:C310–5.
60. Kudo Y, Yamada K, Fujiwara A, Kawasaki T. Characterization of amino acid transport systems in human placental brush-border membrane vesicles. Biochim Biophys Acta 1987;904:309–18.
61. Karl PI, Teichberg S, Fisher SE. $Na(^{+})$-dependent amino acid uptake by human placental microvillous membrane vesicles: Importance of storage conditions and preservation of cytoskeletal elements. Placenta 1991;12:239–50.
62. Furesz TC, Smith CH, Moe AJ. ASC system activity is altered by development of cell polarity in trophoblast from human placenta. Am J Physiol 1993;265:C212–7.
63. Kudo Y, Boyd CA. Human placental amino acid transporter genes: Expression and function. Reproduction 2002;124:593–600.
64. Chairoungdua A, Kanai Y, Matsuo H, et al. Identification and characterization of a novel member of the heterodimeric amino acid transporter family presumed to be associated with an unknown heavy chain. J Biol Chem 2001;276:49390–99.
65. Fukasawa Y, Segawa H, Kim JY, et al. Identification and characterization of a $Na(^{+})$-independent neutral amino acid transporter that associates with the 4F2 heavy chain and exhibits substrate selectivity for small neutral D and L-amino acids. J Biol Chem 2000;275:9690–98.
66. Carbo N, Lopez-Soriano FJ, Argiles JM. Neutral amino acid transport in placental plasma membrane vesicles in the late pregnant rat. Evidence for a B0-like transport system. Eur J Obstet Gynecol Reprod Biol 1997;71:85–90.
67. Kekuda R, Prasad PD, Fei YJ, et al. Cloning of the sodium-dependent, broad-scope, neutral amino acid transporter Bo from a human placental choriocarcinoma cell line. J Biol Chem 1996;271:18657–61.
68. Novak DA, Beveridge MJ. Glutamine transport in human and rat placenta. Placenta 1997;18:379–86.
69. Torres-Zamorano V, Leibach FH, Ganapathy V. Sodium-dependent homo and hetero-exchange of neutral amino acids mediated by the amino acid transporter ATB degree. Biochem Biophys Res Commun 1998;245:824–29.
70. Karl PI, Fisher SE. Taurine transport by microvillous membrane vesicles and the perfused cotyledon of the human placenta. Am J Physiol 1990;258:C443–51.
71. Miyamoto Y, Balkovetz DF, Leibach FH, et al. Na^{+} + Cl^{-} -gradient-driven, high-affinity, uphill transport of taurine in human placental brush-border membrane vesicles. FEBS Lett 1988;231:263–67.
72. Moyer MS, Insler N, Dumaswala R. The role of chloride in taurine transport across the human placental brush-border membrane. Biochim Biophys Acta 1992;1109:74–80.

73. Norberg S, Powell TL, Jansson T. Intrauterine growth restriction is associated with a reduced activity of placental taurine transporters. Pediatr Res 1998;44:233–38.
74. Kulanthaivel P, Leibach FH, Mahesh VB, Ganapathy V. Tyrosine residues are essential for the activity of the human placental taurine transporter. Biochim Biophys Acta 1989;985:139–46.
75. Kulanthaivel P, Cool DR, Ramamoorthy S, et al. Transport of taurine and its regulation by protein kinase C in the JAR human placental choriocarcinoma cell line. Biochem J 1991;277:53–8.
76. Ganapathy ME, Leibach FH, Mahesh VB, et al. Characterization of tryptophan transport in human placental brush-border membrane vesicles. Biochem J 1986;238:201–08.
77. Yudilevich D, Sweiry J. Transport of amino acids in the placenta. Biochim Biophys Acta 1985;822:169–201.
78. Eleno N, Deves R, Boyd CA. Membrane potential dependence of the kinetics of cationic amino acid transport systems in human placenta. J Physiol 1994;479:291–300.
79. Furesz TC, Moe AJ, Smith CH. Lysine uptake by human placental microvillous membrane: Comparison of system y^+ with basal membrane. Am J Physiol 1995;268:C755–61.
80. Jansson T, Scholtbach V, Powell TL. Placental transport of leucine and lysine is reduced in intrauterine growth restriction. Pediatr Res 1998;44:532–37.
81. Ayuk PT, Sibley C, Donnai P, et al. Development and polarization of cationic amino acid transporters and regulators in the human placenta. Am J Physiol 2000;278:c1162–71.
82. Kamath SG, Furesz TC, Way BA, Smith CH. Identification of three cationic amino acid transporters in placental trophoblast: Cloning, expression, and characterization of hCAT-1. J Membr Biol 1999;171:55–62.
83. Malandro MS, Beveridge MJ, Kilberg MS, Novak DA. Effect of low-protein diet-induced intrauterine growth retardation on rat placental amino acid transport. Am J Physiol 1996;271:C295–C303.
84. Malandro MS, Beveridge MJ, Kilberg MS, Novak DA. Ontogeny of cationic amino acid transport systems in rat placenta. Am J Physiol 1994;267:C804–11.
85. Malandro MS, Beveridge MJ, Novak DA, Kilberg MS. Rat placental amino acid transport after protein-deprivation-induced intrauterine growth retardation. Biochem Soc Trans 1996;24:839–43.
86. Furesz TC, Moe AJ, Smith CH. Two cationic amino acid transport systems in human placental basal plasma membranes. Am J Physiol 1991;261:C246–52.
87. Furesz T, Smith C. Identification of two leucine-sensitive lysine transport activities in human placental basal membrane. Placenta 1997;18:649–55.
88. Cariappa R, Heath-Monnig E, Smith CH. Isoforms of amino acid transporters in placental syncytiotrophoblast: Plasma membrane localization and potential role in maternal (fetal transport. Placenta 2003;24:713–26.
89. Hoeltzli SD, Kelley LK, Moe AJ, Smith CH. Anionic amino acid transport systems in isolated basal plasma membrane of human placenta. Am J Physiol 1990;259:C47–55.
90. Matthews JC, Beveridge MJ, Malandro MS, et al. Activity and protein localization of multiple glutamate transporters in gestation day 14 vs. day 20 rat placenta. Am J Physiol 1998;274:C603–14.
91. Moe AJ, Smith CH. Anionic amino acid uptake by microvillous membrane vesicles from human placenta. Am J Physiol 1989;257:C1005–11.
92. Novak D, Quiggle F, Artime C, Beveridge M. Regulation of glutamate transport and transport proteins in a placental cell line. Am J Physiol Cell Physiol 2001;281:C1014–22.
93. Noorlander CW, de Graan PN, Nikkels PG, et al. Distribution of glutamate transporters in the human placenta. Placenta 2004;25:489–95.
94. Karl PI, Tkaczevski H, Fisher SE. Characteristics of histidine uptake by human placental microvillous membrane vesicles. Pediatr Res 1989;25:19–26.
95. Kilberg MS, Handlogten ME, Christensen HN. Characteristics of an amino acid transport system in rat liver for glutamine, asparagine, histidine, and closely related analogs. J Biol Chem 1980;255:4011–19.
96. Nakanishi T, Kekuda R, Fei YJ, et al. Cloning and functional characterization of a new subtype of the amino acid transport system. Nortn. Am J Physiol Cell Physiol 2001;281:C1757–68.
97. Battaorth a FC, Regnault TR. Placental transport and metabolism of amino acids. Placenta 2001;22:145–61.
98. Jansson T. Amino acid transporters in the human placenta. Pediatr Res 2001;49:141–47.
99. Palacin M, Estevez R, Bertran J, Zorzano A. Molecular biology of mammalian plasma membrane amino acid transporters. Physiol Rev 1998;78:969–1054.
100. Palacin M. A new family of proteins (rBAT and 4F2hc) involved in cationic and zwitterionic amino acid transport: A tale of two proteins in search of a transport function. J Exp Biol 1994;196:123–37.
101. Estevez R, Camps M, Rojas AM, et al. The amino acid transport system y^+L(4F2hc is a heteromultimeric complex. FASEB J 1998;12:1319–29.
102. Horak J. Amino acid transport in eucaryotic microorganisms. Biochim Biophys Acta 1986;864:223–56.
103. Sophianopoulou V, Diallinas G. Amino acid transporters of lower eukaryotes: Regulation, structure and topogenesis. FEMS Microbiol Rev 1995;16:53–75.
104. Martinez P, Ljungdahl PO. The SHR3 homologue from S. pombe demonstrates a conserved function of ER packaging chaperones. J Cell Sci 2000;113:4351–62.
105. Ljungdahl PO, Gimeno CJ, Styles CA, Fink GR. SHR3: A novel component of the secretory pathway specifically required for localization of amino acid permeases in yeast. Cell 1992;71:463–78.
106. Kudo Y, Boyd CA. Heterodimeric amino acid transporters: Expression of heavy but not light chains of CD98 correlates with induction of amino acid transport systems in human placental trophoblast. J Physiol 2000;523:13–8.
107. Pineda M, Fernandez E, Torrents D, et al. Identification of a membrane protein, LAT-2, that Co-expresses with 4F2 heavy chain, an L-type amino acid transport activity with broad specificity for small and large zwitterionic amino acids. J Biol Chem 1999;274:19738–44.
108. Pfeiffer R, Rossier G, Spindler B, et al. Amino acid transport of y^+L-type by heterodimers of 4F2hc/CD98 and members of the glycoprotein-associated amino acid transporter family. EMBO J 1999;18:49–57.
109. Bertran J, Magagnin S, Werner A, et al. Stimulation of system $y(^+)$-like amino acid transport by the heavy chain of human 4F2 surface antigen in *Xenopus laevis* oocytes. Proc Natl Acad Sci U S A 1992;89:5606–10.
110. Mastroberardino L, Spindler B, Pfeiffer R, et al. Amino-acid transport by heterodimers of 4F2hc/CD98 and members of a permease family. Nature 1998;395:288–91.
111. Okamoto Y, Sakata M, Ogura K, et al. Expression and regulation of 4F2hc and hLAT1 in human trophoblasts. Am J Physiol Cell Physiol 2002;282:C196–C204.
112. Bertran J, Werner A, Chillaron J, et al. Expression cloning of a human renal cDNA that induces high affinity transport of L-cystine shared with dibasic amino acids in Xenopus oocytes. J Biol Chem 1993;268:14842–49.
113. Wells RG, Hediger MA. Cloning of a rat kidney cDNA that stimulates dibasic and neutral amino acid transport and has sequence similarity to glucosidases. Proc Natl Acad Sci U S A 1992;89:5596–600.
114. Markovich D, Stange G, Bertran J, et al. Two mRNA transcripts (rBAT-1 and rBAT-2) are involved in system $b^{o,(+)-}$ related amino acid transport. J Biol Chem 1993;268:1362–67.
115. Yao SY, Muzyka WR, Elliott JF, et al. Cloning and functional expression of a cDNA from rat jejunal epithelium encoding a protein (4F2hc) with system y^+L amino acid transport activity. Biochem J 1998;330:745–52.
116. Torrents D, Estevez R, Pineda M, et al. Identification and characterization of a membrane protein (y^+L amino acid transporter-1) that associates with 4F2hc to encode the amino acid transport activity y^+L. A candidate gene for lysinuric protein intolerance. J Biol Chem 1998;273:32437–45.
117. Segawa H, Fukasawa Y, Miyamoto K, et al. Identification and functional characterization of a Na^+-independent neutral amino acid transporter with broad substrate selectivity. J Biol Chem 1999;274:19745–51.
118. Novak DA, Matthews JC, Beveridge MJ, et al. Demonstration of system y^+L activity on the basal plasma membrane surface of rat placenta and developmentally regulated expression of 4F2HC mRNA. Placenta 1997;18:643–48.
119. Teixeira S, Di Grandi S, Kuhn LC. Primary structure of the human 4F2 antigen heavy chain predicts a transmembrane protein with a cytoplasmic NH2 terminus. J Biol Chem 1987;262:9574–80.
120. Quackenbush E, Clabby M, Gottesdiener KM, et al. Molecular cloning of complementary DNAs encoding the heavy chain of the human 4F2 cell-surface antigen: A type II membrane glycoprotein involved in normal and neoplastic cell growth. PNAS 1987;84:6526–30.
121. McGivan JD, Pastor-Anglada M. Regulatory and molecular aspects of mammalian amino acid transport. Biochem J 1994;299:321–34.
122. Wells RG, Lee WS, Kanai Y, et al. The 4F2 antigen heavy chain induces uptake of neutral and dibasic amino acids in Xenopus oocytes. J Biol Chem 1992;267:15285–88.
123. Wang Y, Tate SS. Oligomeric structure of a renal cystine transporter: Implications in cystinuria. FEBS Lett 1995;368:389–92.
124. Nakamura E, Sato M, Yang H, et al. 4F2 (CD98) heavy chain is associated covalently with an amino acid transporter and controls intracellular trafficking and membrane topology of 4F2 heterodimer. J Biol Chem 1999;274:3009–16.
125. Fei YJ, Prasad PD, Leibach FH, Ganapathy V. The amino acid transport system y^+L induced in *Xenopus laevis* oocytes by human choriocarcinoma cell (JAR) mRNA is functionally related to the heavy chain of the 4F2 cell surface antigen. Biochemistry 1995;34:8744–51.
126. Prasad PD, Wang H, Huang W, et al. Human LAT1, a subunit of system L amino acid transporter: Molecular cloning and transport function. Biochem Biophys Res Commun 1999;255:283–88.
127. Wang H, Huang W, Sugawara M, et al. Cloning and functional expression of ATA1, a subtype of amino acid transporter A, from human placenta. Biochem Biophys Res Commun 2000;273:1175–79.
128. Varoqui H, Zhu H, Yao D, et al. Cloning and functional identification of a neuronal glutamine transporter. J Biol Chem 2000;275:4049–54.
129. Hatanaka T, Huang W, Wang H, et al. Primary structure, functional characteristics and tissue expression pattern of human ATA2, a subtype of amino acid transport system A. Biochim Biophys Acta 2000;1467:1–6.
130. Sugawara M, Nakanishi T, Fei YJ, et al. Cloning of an amino acid transporter with functional characteristics and tissue expression pattern identical to that of system A. J Biol Chem 2000;275:16473–77.
131. Sugawara M, Nakanishi T, Fei YJ, et al. Structure and function of ATA3, a new subtype of amino acid transport system A, primarily expressed in the liver and skeletal muscle. Biochim Biophys Acta 2000;1509:7–13.
132. Desforges M, Lacey HA, Glazier JD, et al. The SNAT4 isoform of the system A amino acid transporter is expressed in human placenta. Am J Physiol Cell Physiol 2005;00258.
133. Shafqat S, Tamarappoo BK, Kilberg MS, et al. Cloning and expression of a novel $Na(^+)$-dependent neutral amino acid transporter structurally related to mammalian $Na+$(glutamate cotransporters. J Biol Chem 1993;268:15351–55.
134. Utsunomiya-Tate N, Endou H, Kanai Y. Cloning and functional characterization of a system ASC-like Na^+-dependent neutral amino acid transporter. J Biol Chem 1996;271:14883–90.
135. Torres-Zamorano V, Kekuda R, Leibach FH, Ganapathy V. Tyrosine phosphorylation-and epidermal growth factor-dependent regulation of the sodium-coupled amino acid transporter B^o in the human placental choriocarcinoma cell line JAR. Biochim Biophys Acta 1997;1356:258–70.
136. Van Winkle LJ, Christensen HN, Campione AL. Na^+-dependent transport of basic, zwitterionic, and bicyclic amino acids by a broad-scope system in mouse blastocysts. J Biol Chem 1985;260:12118–23.
137. Roos S, Powell TL, Jansson T. The human placental taurine transporter in uncomplicated and IUGR pregnancies: Cellular localization, protein expression and regulation. Am J Physiol Regul Integr Comp Physiol 2004;287(4):886-93.
138. Ramamoorthy S, Leibach FH, Mahesh VB, et al. Functional characterization and chromosomal localization of a cloned taurine transporter from human placenta. Biochem J 1994;300:893–900.
139. Kanai Y, Segawa H, Miyamoto K, et al. Expression cloning and characterization of a transporter for large neutral amino acids activated by the heavy chain of 4F2 antigen (CD98). J Biol Chem 1998;273:23629–32.
140. Rossier G, Meier C, Bauch C, et al. LAT2, a new basolateral 4F2hc(CD98-associated amino acid transporter of kidney and intestine. J Biol Chem 1999;274:34948–54.
141. Rajan DP, Kekuda R, Huang W, et al. Cloning and functional characterization of a Na^+-independent, broad-specific neutral amino acid transporter from mammalian intestine. Biochim Biophys Acta 2000;1463:6–14.
142. Ritchie JW, Taylor PM. Role of the system L permease LAT1 in amino acid and iodothyronine transport in placenta. Biochem J 2001;356:719–25.
143. Bodoy S, Martin L, Zorzano A, et al. Identification of LAT4, a novel amino acid transporter with system L activity. J Biol Chem 2005;280:12002–11.
144. Babu E, Kanai Y, Chairoungdua A, et al. Identification of a novel system L amino acid transporter structurally distinct from heterodimeric amino acid transporters. J Biol Chem 2003;278:43838–45.
145. Kudo Y, Boyd CA. Characterisation of L-tryptophan transporters in human placenta: A comparison of brush border and basal membrane vesicles. J Physiol 2001;531:405–16.
146. Deves R, Boyd CA. Surface antigen CD98/4F2): Not a single membrane protein, but a family of proteins with multiple functions. J Membr Biol 2000;173:165–77.
147. Broer S. Adaptation of plasma membrane amino acid transport mechanisms to physiological demands. Pflugers Archiv Eur J Physiol 2002;444:457–66.

148. Closs EI, Graf P, Habermeier A, et al. Human cationic amino acid transporters hCAT-1, hCAT-2A, and hCAT-2B: Three related carriers with distinct transport properties. Biochemistry 1997;36:6462–68.
149. Fairman WA, Vandenberg RJ, Arriza JL, et al. An excitatory amino-acid transporter with properties of a ligand-gated chloride channel. Nature 1995;375:599–603.
150. Nakayama T, Kawakami H, Tanaka K, Nakamura S. Expression of three glutamate transporter subtype mRNAs in human brain regions and peripheral tissues. Mol Brain Res 1996;36:189–92.
151. Matthews JC, Beveridge MJ, Dialynas E, et al. Placental anionic and cationic amino acid transporter expression in growth hormone overexpressing and null IGF-II or null IGF-I receptor mice. Placenta 1999;20:639–50.
152. Borsani G, Bassi MT, Sperandeo MP, et al. SLC7A7, encoding a putative permease-related protein, is mutated in patients with lysinuric protein intolerance. Nat Genet 1999;21:297–301.
153. Rosenberg LE, Downing S, Durant JL, Segal S. Cystinuria: Biochemical evidence for three genetically distinct diseases. J Clin Invest 1966;45:365–71.
154. Munn DH, Shafizadeh E, Attwood JT, et al. Inhibition of T cell proliferation by macrophage tryptophan catabolism. J Exp Med 1999;189:1363–72.
155. Kudo Y, Boyd CA, Sargent IL, Redman CW. Tryptophan degradation by human placental indoleamine 2,3-dioxygenase regulates lymphocyte proliferation. J Physiol 2001;535:207–15.
156. Kudo Y, Boyd CA. The role of L-tryptophan transport in L-tryptophan degradation by indoleamine 2,3-dioxygenase in human placental explants. J Physiol 2001;531:417–23.
157. Baur R. Morphometry of the placental exchange area. Adv Anat Embryol Cell Biol 1977;53:3–65.
158. Teasdale F. Gestational changes in the functional structure of the human placenta in relation to fetal growth: A morphometric study. Am J Obstet Gynecol 1980;137:560–68.
159. Teasdale F. Morphometric evaluation. Contrib Gynecol Obstet 1982;9:17–28.
160. Teasdale F, Jean-Jacques G. Morphometric evaluation of the microvillous surface enlargement factor in the human placenta from mid-gestation to term. Placenta 1985;6:375–81.
161. Mayhew TM, Manwani R, Ohadike C, et al. The placenta in pre-eclampsia and intrauterine growth restriction: Studies on exchange surface areas, diffusion distances and villous membrane diffusive conductances. Placenta 2007;28:233–8.
162. Teasdale F. Histomorphometry of the human placenta in pre-eclampsia associated with severe intrauterine growth retardation. Placenta 1987;8:119–28.
163. Woods DL, Rip MR. Placental villous surface area of light-for-dates infants at term. Early Hum Dev 1987;15:113–17.
164. Boyd JD, Hamilton WJ. The Human Placenta. Cambridge: Heffer and Sons; 1970.
165. Barbera A, Galan HL, Ferrazzi E, et al. Relationship of umbilical vein blood flow to growth parameters in the human fetus. Am J Obstet Gynecol 1999;181:174–9.
166. Mahendran D, Donnai P, Glazier JD, et al. Amino acid (system A) transporter activity in microvillous membrane vesicles from the placentas of appropriate and small for gestational age babies. Pediatr Res 1993;34:661–5.
167. Mahendran D, Byrne S, Donnai P, et al. Na+ transport, H^+ concentration gradient dissipation, and system A amino acid transporter activity in purified microvillous plasma membrane isolated from first-trimester human placenta: Comparison with the term microvillous membrane. Am J Obstet Gynecol 1994;171:1534–40.
168. Karl P, Alpy K, Fisher S. Amino acid transport by the cultured human placental trophoblast: Effect of insulin on AIB transport. Am J Phys 1992;262:C834–9.
169. Greenberg RE, Wogenrich FJ, Garcia P, Johnson J. Fetal insulin increases placental amino acid transport. Clin Res 1989;37:178.
170. Dicke JM, Henderson GI. Placental amino acid uptake in normal and complicated pregnancies. Am J Med Sci 1988;295:223–7.
171. Potau N, Riudor E, Ballabriga A. Insulin receptors in human placenta in relation to fetal weight and gestational age. Pediatr Res 1981;15:798–802.
172. Wang CY, Daimon M, Shen SJ, et al. Insulin-like growth factor-I messenger ribonucleic acid in the developing human placenta and in term placenta of diabetics. Mol Endocrinol 1988;2:217–29.
173. Cetin I, Marconi AM, Bozzetti P, et al. Umbilical amino acid concentrations in appropriate and small for gestational age infants: A biochemical difference present in utero. Am J Obstet Gynecol 1988;158:120–6.
174. Cetin I, Corbetta C, Sereni LP, et al. Umbilical amino acid concentrations in normal and growth-retarded fetuses sampled in utero by cordocentesis. Am J Obstet Gynecol 1990;162:253–61.
175. Cetin I, Marconi AM, Corbetta C, et al. Fetal amino acids in normal pregnancies and in pregnancies complicated by intrauterine growth retardation. Early Hum Dev 1992;29:183–6.
176. Economides DL, Nicolaides KH, Gahl WA, . Plasma amino acids in appropriate and small-for-gestational-age fetuses. Am J Obstet Gynecol 1989;161:1219–27.
177. Pardi G, Cetin I, Marconi AM, et al. Diagnostic value of blood sampling in fetuses with growth retardation. N Engl J Med 1993;328:692–6.
178. Glazier JD, Cetin I, Perugino G, et al. Association between the activity of the system A amino acid transporter in the microvillous plasma membrane of the human placenta and severity of fetal compromise in intrauterine growth restriction. Pediatr Res 1997;42:514–19.
179. Cramer S, Beveridge M, Kilberg M, Novak D. Physiological importance of system A-mediated amino acid transport to rat fetal development. Am J Physiol Cell Physiol 2002;282:C153–60.
180. Constancia M, Angiolini E, Sandovici I, et al. Adaptation of nutrient supply to fetal demand in the mouse involves interaction between the Igf2 gene and placental transporter systems. Proc Natl Acad Sci U S A 2005;102:19219–24.
181. Constancia M, Hemberger M, Hughes J, et al. Placental-specific IGF-II is a major modulator of placental and fetal growth. Nature 2002;417:945–48.
182. Rosso P. Maternal-fetal exchange during protein malnutrition in the rat. Placental transfer of glucose and a nonmetabolizable glucose analog. J Nutr 1977;107:20006–10.
183. Ayuk PT, Theophanous D, D'Souza SW, et al. L-Arginine transport by the microvillous plasma membrane of the syncytiotrophoblast from human placenta in relation to nitric oxide production: Effects of getation, preclampsia, and intrauterine growth restriction. J Clin Endocrinol Metab 2002;87:747–51.
184. McMinn J, Wei M, Schupf N, et al. Unbalanced placental expression of imprinted genes in human intrauterine growth restriction. Placenta 2006;27:540–49.
185. Ross JC, Fennessey PV, Wilkening RB, et al. Placental transport and fetal utilization of leucine in a model of fetal growth retardation. Am J Physiol 1996;270:E491–503.
186. Anderson AH, Fennessey PV, Meschia G, et al. Placental transport of threonine and its utilization in the normal and growth-restricted fetus. Am J Physiol 1997;272:E892–900.
187. Marconi AM, Paolini CL, Stramare L, et al. Steady state maternal-fetal leucine enrichments in normal and intrauterine growth-restricted pregnancies. Pediatr Res 1999;46:114–9.
188. Paolini CL, Marconi AM, Ronzoni S, et al. Placental transport of leucine, phenylalanine, glycine, and proline in intrauterine growth-restricted pregnancies. J Clin Endocrinol Metab 2001;86:5427–32.
189. Woods DL, Malan AF, Heese HD. Placental size of small-for-gestational-age infants at term. Early Hum Dev 1982;7:11–5.
190. Trachtman H, Barbour R, Sturman JA, Finberg L. Taurine and osmoregulation: Taurine is a cerebral osmoprotective molecule in chronic hypernatremic dehydration. Pediatr Res 1988;23:35–9.
191. Teng C, Battaglia FC, Meschia G, et al. Fetal hepatic and umbilical uptakes of glucogenic substrates during a glucagon-somatostatin infusion. Am J Physiol Endocrinol Metab 2002;282:E542–50.
192. Timmerman M, Teng C, Wilkening RB, et al. Effect of dexamethasone on fetal hepatic glutamine-glutamate exchange. Am J Physiol Endocrinol Metab 2000;278:E839–45.
193. Timmerman M, Teng C, Wilkening RB, et al. Net amino acid flux across the fetal liver and placenta during spontaneous ovine parturition. Biol Neonate 2001;79:54–60.
194. Moores RRJ, Vaughn PR, Battaglia FC, et al. Glutamate metabolism in fetus and placenta of late-gestation sheep. Am J Physiol 1994;267:R89–96.
195. Makarewicz W, Swierczynski J. Phosphate-dependent glutaminase in the human term placental mitochondria. Biochem Med Metab Biol 1988;39:273–8.
196. Robertson AF, Karp WB, Johnsson J. Human placental amino acid oxidation. Biol Neonate 1972;30:142–4.
197. Cetin I, Fennessey PV, Quick ANJ, et al. Glycine turnover and oxidation and hepatic serine synthesis from glycine in fetal lambs. Am J Physiol 1991;260:E371–8.
198. Cetin I, Fennessey PV, Sparks JW, et al. Fetal serine fluxes across fetal liver, hindlimb, and placenta in late gestation. Am J Physiol 1992;263:E786–93.
199. Narkewicz MR, Thureen PJ, Sauls SD, et al. Serine and glycine metabolism in hepatocytes from mid gestation fetal lambs. Pediatr Res 1996;39:1085–90.
200. Narkewicz MR, Jones G, Morales D. Serine and glycine transport in fetal ovine hepatocytes. Biochim Biophys Acta 2000;1474:41–6.
201. Schmidt HH, Warner TD, Ishii K, et al. Insulin secretion from pancreatic B cells caused by L-arginine-derived nitrogen oxides. Science 1992;255:721–3.
202. Diamant YZ, Mayorek N, Neumann S, Shafrir E. Enzymes of glucose and fatty acid metabolism in early and term human placenta. Am J Obstet Gynecol 1975;121:58–61.
203. Gustke HH, Kowalewski S. Glycolytic enzymes in the normal human term placenta. Enzyme 1975;19:154–64.
204. Regnault TRH, de Vrijer B, Battaglia FC. Transport and metabolism of amino acids in placenta. Endocrine 2002;19:23–41.
205. Gusseck DJ, Yuen P, Longo LD. Amino acid transport in placental slices. Mechanism of increased accumulation by prolonged incubation. Biochim Biophys Acta 1975;401:278–84.
206. Mann GE, Pearson JD, Sheriff CJ, Toothill VJ. Expression of amino acid transport systems in cultured human umbilical vein endothelial cells. J Physiol 1989;410:325–39.
207. Meschia G, Battaglia FC, Hay WW, Sparks JW. Utilization of substrates by the ovine placenta in vivo. Fed Proc 1980;39:245–9.
208. Edwards EM, Rattenbury J, Varnam GC, et al. Enzyme activities in the sheep placenta during the last three months of pregnancy. Biochim Biophys Acta 1977;497:133–43.
209. Jozwik M, Teng C, Meschia G, Battaglia FC. Contribution of branched-chain amino acids to uteroplacental ammonia production in sheep. Biol Reprod 1999;61:792–6.
210. Pell JM, Jeacock MK, Shepherd DA. Glutamate and glutamine metabolism in the ovine placenta. J Agric Sci 1983;101:275–81.
211. Johnson RL, Gilbert M, Block SM, Battaglia FC. Uterine metabolism of the pregnant rabbit under chronic steady-state conditions. Am J Obstet Gynecol 1986;154:1146–51.
212. Battaglia FC, Meschia G. An Introduction to Fetal Physiology. Orlando, FL: Academic Press, Inc; 1986. p. 1–51.
213. Kodama I. Studies on ammonia metabolism of placenta. Nippon Sanka Fujinka Gakkai Zasshi Acta Obstetrica et Gynaecologica Japonica 1972;24:155–64.
214. Jozwik M, Teng C, Battaglia FC, Meschia G. Fetal supply of amino acids and amino nitrogen after maternal infusion of amino acids in pregnant sheep. Am J Obstet Gynecol 1999;180:447–53.
215. Chung M, Teng C, Timmerman M, et al. Production and utilization of amino acids by ovine placenta in vivo. Am J Physiol 1998;274:E13–22.
216. Stegink LD, Reynolds WA, Filer LJ, Jr, et al. Monosodium glutamate metabolism in the neonatal monkey. Am J Physiol 1975;229:246–50.
217. Stegink LD, Pitkin RM, Reynolds WA, et al. Placental transfer of glutamate and its metabolites in the primate. American J Obstet Gynecol 1975;122:70–8.
218. Schneider H, Mohlen K, Challier J, Dancis J. Transfer of glutamic acid across the human placenta perfused in vitro. Br J Obstet Gynaecol 1979;86:299–306.
219. Paolini CL, Meschia G, Fennessey PV, et al. An in vivo study of ovine placental transport of essential amino acids. Am J Physiol Endocrinol Metab 2001;280:E31–9.
220. Loy GL, Quick ANJ, Battaglia FC, et al. Measurement of leucine and alpha-ketoisocaproic acid fluxes in the fetal(placental unit. J Chromatogr 1991;562:169–74.
221. Moores RRJ, Rietberg CC, Battaglia FC, et al. Metabolism and transport of maternal serine by the ovine placenta: Glycine production and absence of serine transport into the fetus. Pediatr Res 1993;33:590–4.
222. Timmerman M, Chung M, Wilkening RB, et al. Relationship of fetal alanine uptake and placental alanine metabolism to maternal plasma alanine concentration. Am J Physiol 1998;275:E942–50.
223. Gresham EL, Simons PS, Battaglia FC. Maternal-fetal urea concentration difference in man: Metabolic significance. J Pediatr 1971;79:809–11.
224. Bellotti M, Pennati G, Pardi G, Fumero R. Dilatation of the ductus venosus in human fetuses: Ultrasonographic evidence and mathematical modeling. Am J Physiol 1998;275:H1759–67.
225. Bellotti M, Pennati G, De Gasperi C, et al. Role of ductus venosus in distribution of umbilical blood flow in human fetuses during second half of pregnancy. Am J Physiol Heart Circ Physiol 2000;279:H1256–63.
226. Kiserud T, Stratford L, Hanson MA. Umbilical flow distribution to the liver and the ductus venosus: An in vitro investigation of the fluid dynamic mechanisms in the fetal sheep. Am J Obstet Gynecol 1997;177:86–90.
227. Baschat AA, Harman CR. Venous Doppler in the assessment of fetal cardiovascular status. Curr Opin Obstet Gynecol 2006;18:156–63.
228. Kiserud T. Liver length in the small-for-gestational-age fetus and ductus venosus flow. Am J Obstet Gynecol 2000;182:252–53.
229. Ferrazzi E, Rigano S, Bozzo M, et al. Umbilical vein blood flow in growth-restricted fetuses. Ultrasound Obstet Gynecol 2000;16:432–8.
230. Holcomb RG, Wilkening RB. Hepatic metabolism during acute hypoxia in fetal lambs. Pediatr Res 1998;43:49A.

231. Regnault TRH, de Vrijer B, Trembler KA. The umbilical uptake of glutamate in IUGR pregnancies. J Perinat Med 2001;29:546.
232. Narkewicz MR, Moores RR, Jr, Battaglia FC, Frerman FF. Ontogeny of serine hydroxymethyltransferase isoenzymes in fetal sheep liver, kidney, and placenta. Mol Genet Metab 1999;68:473–80.
233. Moores RRJ, Carter BS, Meschia G, et al. Placental and fetal serine fluxes at midgestation in the fetal lamb. Am J Physiol 1994;267:E150–5.
234. Jois M, Hall B, Fewer K, Brosnan JT. Regulation of hepatic glycine catabolism by glucagon. J Biol Chem 1989;264:3347–51.
235. Jois M, Ewart HS, Brosnan JT. Regulation of glycine catabolism in rat liver mitochondria. Biochem J 1992;283:435–9.
236. Ewart HS, Jois M, Brosnan JT. Rapid stimulation of the hepatic glycine-cleavage system in rats fed on a single high-protein meal. Biochem J 1992;283:441–7.
237. Lemons JA, Liechty EA. Nitrogen flux across ovine maternal and fetal hindquarters during fasting. J Dev Physiol 1987;9:151–8.
238. Wilkening RB, Boyle DW, Teng C, et al. Amino acid uptake by the fetal ovine hindlimb under normal and euglycemic hyperinsulinemic states. Am J Physiol 1994;266: E72–8.
239. Ballard FJ, Filsell OH, Jarrett IG. Amino acid uptake and output by the sheep hind limb. Metab: Clin Exp 1976;25:415–8.
240. Hay WW, Jr, Sparks JW, Quissell BJ, et al. Simultaneous measurements of umbilical uptake, fetal utilization rate, and fetal turnover rate of glucose. Am J Physiol 1981;240: E662–8.
241. Liechty EA, Barone S, Nutt M. Effect of maternal fasting on ovine fetal and maternal branched-chain amino acid transaminase activities. Biol Neonate 1987;52: 166–73.
242. Smeaton TC, Owens JA, Kind KL, Robinson JS. The placenta releases branched-chain keto acids into the umbilical and uterine circulations in the pregnant sheep. J Dev Physiol 1989;12:95–9.
243. American Academy of Pediatrics Committee on Nutrition. Nutritional needs of low-birth-weight infants. Pediatrics 1985;75:976–86.
244. Zlotkin SH, Bryan MH, Anderson GH. Intravenous nitrogen and energy intakes required to duplicate in utero nitrogen accretion in prematurely born human infants. J Pediatr 1981;99:115–20.
245. Parry-Billings M, Evans J, Calder PC, Newsholme EA. Does glutamine contribute to immunosuppression after major burns? Lancet 1990;336:523–5.
246. Newsholme EA, Crabtree B, Ardawi MS. Glutamine metabolism in lymphocytes: Its biochemical, physiological and clinical importance. Q J Exp Physiol 1985;70:473–89.
247. Souba WW, Klimberg VS, Hautamaki RD, et al. Oral glutamine reduces bacterial translocation following abdominal radiation. J Surg Res 1990;48:1–5.
248. Reichman B, Chessex P, Putet G, et al. Diet, fat accretion, and growth in premature infants. N Engl J Med 1981;305:1495–500.
249. Barker D, Osmond C, Simmonds S, Wield G. The relation of small head circumference and thinness at birth to death from cardiovascular disease in adult life. B M J 1993;306:422–6.
250. Eriksson UJ. Lifelong consequences of metabolic adaptations in utero? Diabetologia 1996;39:1123–5.
251. McMillen IC, Adams MB, Ross JT, et al. Fetal growth restriction: Adaptations and consequences. Reproduction 2001;122:195–204.

30

Human Milk: Nutritional Properties

Sharon M. Donovan, PhD, RD

HEALTH BENEFITS OF HUMAN MILK FOR THE INFANT

Human milk provides nutrients with high bioavailability and in sufficient qualities to support the needs of the rapidly growing human infant.[1,2] As such, the recommended dietary intakes for infants in the first 6 months of life are based on the nutrient analysis of human milk and average volumes of milk consumption by healthy, full-term, exclusively breast fed infants.[3] The specific nutrient requirements of the term infant are discussed further in Chapter 35, "The Term Infant." Human milk is also recommended for the preterm, low-birth-weight infant due to the associations between human milk feeding and reduced incidence of necrotizing enterocolitis[4] and improved IQ scores.[5] However, the nutrient content of either term or preterm human milk is insufficient to meet the needs of infants <1,500 g and should be supplemented with a human milk fortifier for optimal nutrition.[4] The specific nutrient requirements of the low-birth-weight infant are presented in Chapter 33, "The Low-Birth-Weight Infant: Inpatient Care," and Chapter 34, "The Low-Birth-Weight Infant: Outpatient Care."

In addition, human milk contains bioactive factors whose functions extend beyond providing essential nutrients and energy and appear to facilitate the optimal transition of the infant from intra- to extrauterine life.[1,6,7] Components in human milk actively protect the infant from pathogenic infection and facilitate the establishment of the microbiota, the latter of which is required to activate the mucosal immune system.[8,9] Indeed, clinical and epidemiological data provide strong evidence that human milk feeding decreases the incidence and/or severity of diarrhea,[10,11] respiratory[11] and urinary[12] tract infections, otitis media,[10,13] and necrotizing enterocolitis.[4] This protection likely is mediated through the immunoprotective proteins, lipids, and carbohydrates (oligosaccharides) in human milk that exert antibacterial and antiviral activities[7–9] (see Chapter 31, "Protective Properties of Human Milk," for additional discussion of protective properties of human milk).

Additionally, there is evidence that breast-feeding confers longer term risk reduction for autoimmune diseases. Exposure to beneficial components in human milk that promote the development of the immune system and/or a lack of exposure to stimuli that would trigger an inappropriate immunologic response in genetically predisposed individuals have been proposed as mechanisms underlying the reduced risk of developing autoimmune diseases,[14] although the relative contributions of these two effects are unknown. Breast-feeding is associated with lower risk of Celiac disease,[15] insulin-dependent diabetes mellitus,[16] and asthma.[17] Evidence for prevention of atopy[18,19] and inflammatory bowel diseases is less conclusive,[20,21] and further research in needed to elucidate the interaction between the infant's genetic predisposition and breast-feeding in modulating the risk of these diseases. As dietary antigens cross the placenta, as well as pass into human milk, many pediatricians recommend maternal antigen avoidance during pregnancy and/or lactation as a strategy to prevent or treat atopic diseases in children at high risk for developing atopic diseases. A systematic review of the randomized or quasi-randomized trials found that antigen avoidance during pregnancy did not substantially reduce the risk of the child developing atopy and may adversely affect maternal and fetal nutritional status and, thus, is not recommended.[22] Antigen-avoidance diets during lactation may prevent the development and/or severity of atopic eczema in the infant; however, Kramer and Kakuma concluded that larger trials are needed in this area.[22]

In addition, breast-feeding is associated with higher IQ scores[6,23–25] compared to formula feeding. Breast-feeding for more than 4 to 6 months was associated with a 3- to 6-point augmentation in the IQ scores of 2-year-old or 6- to 8-year-old children, even after adjusting for confounding factors (socioeconomic status, parental IQ, etc).[23] The greatest benefit was gained by preterm versus term infants,[23–25] particularly those who received human milk for at least 6 months.[24] In one study, duration of breast-feeding, the infant's gestational week, and maternal milk docosahexaenoic acid to arachidonic acid (DHA/AA) ratio yielded a three-factor model that explained 76% of the variation in total IQ ($p < .001$).[25]

Lastly, recent epidemiologic studies support an inverse relationship between breast-feeding and the risk of pediatric overweight[26–28] and the development of type 2 diabetes in later life.[29] Breast-feeding for >4 months is associated with an approximately 20 to 25% reduction in the risk of pediatric overweight,[26–28] but duration of breast-feeding showed a dose–response relationship among non-Hispanic whites.[26] An additive interaction was observed between maternal pre-pregnancy body mass index (BMI) and breast-feeding, in that 2- to 14-year-old children of obese mothers (BMI ≥ 30) who were never breast-fed had a 6.1-fold greater risk (95% confidence interval 2.8, 13.1) of being overweight (BMI ≥ 95th percentile) than children of normal-weight mothers who were breast-fed.[27] However, among women who chose to breast-feed, maternal overweight (BMI ≥ 25) or diabetes did not attenuate the protective effect of breast-feeding against the development of overweight in 9- to 14-year-olds.[28] Taken together, these latter two studies provide compelling justification to promote breast-feeding in all mothers, particularly those with high BMI. However, several recent studies suggest that overweight women experienced delayed initiation of lactation and may require additional measures of lactation support.[30,31] Additional information on breast-feeding can be found in Chapter 32, "Approach to Breast-Feeding." A recent review of seven studies encompassing nearly 77,000 subjects reported a 39% reduced risk of developing type 2 diabetes (95% confidence interval 0.44, 0.85) in infants who were breast-fed.[29] Breast-fed infants also had lower blood glucose and serum insulin concentrations in infancy and marginally lower insulin concentrations in adulthood.[29]

POLICY RECOMMENDATIONS AND BREAST-FEEDING TRENDS

Breast-feeding is the preferred form of nutrition for the human infant and is recommended by national and international health organizations and pediatric societies, including the American Academy of Pediatrics (AAP),[1] the United States Department of Health and Human Services,[32,33] and the World Health Organization (WHO).[34,35] The WHO and AAP recommend exclusive breast-feeding for the first 6 months of life.[1,34] The AAP further recommends that breast-feeding continue for at least the first year of life and beyond for as long as mutually desired by the mother and child, with the addition of complementary foods at 6 months of age.[1] The timing and composition of complementary feeding are discussed further in Chapter 36, "Complementary Feeding."

Two separate, large surveys have reported that breast-feeding rates have risen over the past decade and, in 2001, more than two-thirds of infants received some human milk in the first year of life.[36,37] Rates of breast-feeding initiation and persistence at 6 months of age increased across all socioeconomic groups between 1996 and 2001.[35] Breast-feeding initiation rates (~69%)[36,37] were near the Surgeon General's Healthy People 2010 goal of 75%[32] and it was estimated that if breast-feeding were to continue to increase at the current rate (~2%/year), in-hospital breast-feeding in the United States should meet or exceed the Healthy People 2010 goal.[36] However, breast-feeding rates at 6 and 12 months postpartum were lower than the Healthy People 2010 goals of 50 and 25%, respectively,[36,37] and these goals will likely not be met in all subgroups in the population if current trends persist.[36] Maternal age, education, race/ethnicity, income, geographic location, and participation in the Special Supplemental Nutrition Program for Women, Infants and Children (WIC) affected breast-feeding rates, with rates being highest for white non-Hispanic, older, college-educated mothers.[36–38] From 1978 to 2003, breast-feeding initiation among WIC participants was nearly 25% lower than non-WIC participants, and at 6 months postpartum, mothers not enrolled in WIC were more than twice as likely to breast-feed than were WIC participants.[38] Thus, for Healthy People 2010 goals to be achieved, effective strategies must be developed to promote breast-feeding in young, less educated mothers and those participating in WIC.[36–38]

ASSESSING THE GROWTH OF BREAST-FED INFANTS

It has been recognized for over 20 years that the patterns of linear growth and weight gain differ between breast-fed and formula-fed infants[39] or infants who are breast-fed for short duration versus longer term exclusive breast-feeding.[34,40] When the weights and lengths of exclusively breast-fed infants are recorded on National Center for Health Statistics (NCHS) reference growth curves, rapid growth is observed relative to the standards during the first 3 months of age, with a slight decline in weight-for-age Z scores between 3 and 12 months of age.[34,39,40] Similarly, length for age Z scores of exclusively breast-fed infants plotted on NCHS reference curves begin to decline by 6 months, but catch up with the reference by 12 months of age, such that breast-fed infants are typically leaner than formula-fed infants at 1 year of age.[34,39,40] Importantly, head circumference did not differ between breast-fed and formula-fed infants,[39] and breast-fed infants experienced lower morbidity and achieved normal developmental milestones during the first year of life.[10,34] Thus, the pattern of growth of breast-fed infants is not associated with any adverse clinical outcomes and should not be interpreted as growth faltering or as a need for supplemental formula or complementary foods.[1,10,34]

The NCHS reference growth charts were published in 1977, based on growth data collected predominantly from Caucasian, formula-fed infants.[40] Therefore, in 2000, the Centers for Disease Control and Prevention (CDC) published revised versions of the 1977 NCHS growth charts using data obtained from the National Health and Nutrition Examination Surveys.[41] The CDC growth charts incorporate anthropometric data from both breast- and formula-fed infants and are more representative of the current racial and ethnic demographics in the United States. The growth charts are available on the Internet as high-quality PDF documents (http://www.cdc.gov/growthcharts)[41] as well as in Appendix I.

The WHO adopted the NCHS growth curves and, currently, 100 countries are using these standards.[42] However, because of the biologic and technical limitations of these growth standards, new international growth standards recently were released by the WHO to "document how children should grow in all countries, rather than describing how they grew at a particular time and place"[42] as well as in Appendix I. The WHO standards were generated from anthropometric data collected from about 8,500 children in Brazil, Ghana, India, Norway, Oman, and the United States through the WHO Multicenter Growth Reference Study.[43] The results of this study were published in April 2006 as a supplement to *Acta Paediatrica*[43] and the growth standards are available on the Internet (http://www.who.int/childgrowth/standards/en). The WHO standards are based on healthy, breast-fed infants and provide a better tool for monitoring the growth of breast-fed infants than the NCHS curves.[43,44] The WHO standards also demonstrate that children worldwide who are raised in healthy environments, according to international feeding recommendations, exhibit similar patterns of growth.[44] Using the WHO standards, *healthy* breast-fed infants tracked along the mean weight-for-age Z scores, whereas these same infants appeared to falter relative to the NCHS reference at 2 months and after.[44] However, for undernourished infants, the prevalence of wasting (–2 standard deviations Z score) or severe wasting (–3 standard deviations Z score) were 2.5 and 3.5 times higher using the WHO standards than estimates based on the NCHS references during the first 6 months of life, which could have significant implications for international child health programs.[44]

In summary, several growth charts currently are available. The CDC growth charts are more representative of current demographics in the United States than the NCSH standards and include data from both breast-fed and formula-fed infants in the data set. The WHO international growth standards are based on exclusively breast-fed infants and represent the growth patterns of infants following current AAP and WHO recommendations.[1] Whichever growth charts a practitioner chooses to use, it should be kept in mind that growth charts are tools that contribute to forming an overall clinical impression of the child and should not be used as a sole diagnostic instrument.

MILK PRODUCTION

The lactation cycle consists of four phases, mammogenesis, lactogenesis, galactopoiesis, and involution, which is further discussed in Chapter 32, "Approach to Breast-Feeding." Lactogenesis is associated with the expression of lactation-specific genes in mammary secretory epithelial cells and is divided into two stages.[45,46] Lactogenesis I occurs during pregnancy and represents the initiation of the unique synthesis capacity of the mammary gland.[35,46] Lactogenesis II occurs close to birth and is associated with a drop in circulating progesterone concentrations, the initiation of copious milk secretion, and marked changes in milk composition.[46] The onset of lactogenesis II typically occurs between 30 and 40 h postpartum in mothers delivering at term[45]; however, premature delivery,[46,47] cesarean delivery,[48,49] endocrine disturbances,[46] and insulin-dependent diabetes mellitus[46] have been reported to suppress or delay lactogenesis II and detrimentally impact the successful establishment of lactation.

Even among highly educated, motivated women who delivered at term, nearly 50% of mothers experienced suboptimal breast-feeding behaviors (SIBB) on the day of delivery, which declined to 22 and 14% by days 3 and 7 postpartum.[48] Primiparity, Cesarean section, prolonged stage II labor (>1 hour), birth medications, and infant status at birth were associated with SIBB, suggesting that birth-related events can detrimentally impact the initiation of lactation.[49] Flat or inverted nipples, the use of nonhuman milk fluids within the first 48 h postpartum and pacifier use were also risk factors for SIBB.[49] Thus, lactation success can be improved by proactively addressing modifiable factors during delivery and the early postpartum period, and all breast-feeding mothers should be evaluated for SIBB at 72 to 96 h postpartum.[48] Dewey and col leagues also identified high maternal BMI (>27) as a risk factor for SIBB.[48] Subsequent studies confirmed that prepregnancy BMI was negatively associated with the onset of lactogenesis II[29] and overweight or obese mothers breast-fed their infants for a shorter duration than normal-weight women.[31] There may be a physiological basis for the lower lactation success in that overweight and obese women had a reduced prolactin response to suckling in the first week postpartum.[31]

The volume of human milk produced can be assessed by "test weighing" a breast-feeding infant before and after each feeding for a 12- or 24-hour period, or by the deuterium oxide dilution method.[34] A systematic review of 22 studies found that mean human milk intake of exclusively breast-fed infants increased approximately 20 to 30 g/month from 699 g/d at 1 month, to 731, 751, 780, 796, and 854 g/d at months 2 to 6, respectively.[34] Kent and colleagues monitored 775 breast-feeding episodes of infants aged 1 to 6 months and assessed milk production by test weighing and the extent of breast emptying by milk fat content.[50] In that study, infants nursed on average 11 ± 3 times/d (range 6–18), with an interfeeding interval of 138 ± 43 min (range 4–658 min) and 64% of infants breast-fed 1 to 3 times per night.[50] There were no differences in breast-feeding frequency with age or gender; however, the volume per feeding increased with age and was greater in male than female infants.[50] Infants consumed 76.0 ± 12.6 g milk (range 0 to 240 g) per feeding and overall 24-hour milk production was 788 ± 169 g/d (range 440–1,365 g/d).[50] Consistent with previous studies,[51] they found that milk production differed between breasts, with the right breast producing on average nearly 90 g/d more than the left breast (443 g/d vs 356 g/d).[50] Interestingly, for 53% of the breast-feeding episodes, the contents of one breast were sufficient to satisfy the infant for at least 1 hour and, on average, only 67.3 ± 7.8% (range 0–100%) of the available milk in the breast was removed at each feeding.[44] These data suggested that both breasts do not need to be offered at each feeding episode, nor does a breast need to be fully drained at every feeding to maintain adequate milk production.[50] The authors concluded that breast-feeding mothers should be encouraged to "feed their infants on demand rather than conform to average recommendations that may not be appropriate for that mother-infant dyad."[50]

DYNAMIC NATURE OF HUMAN MILK COMPOSITION

The nutrient composition of human milk is dynamic and changes in response to mammary gland physiology (lactogenesis, involution) and, for some nutrients, maternal diet.[51–54] Milk composition also differs between mothers who deliver prematurely and those at term,[53,54] which, in part, may reflect the degree of mammary gland maturation at delivery. Breast-feeding is a normal stage in the reproductive life of a woman, where just as in all the other stages of life, a lactating mother's diet needs to be healthy, balanced, and adequate, taking into consideration any specific medical conditions. Breast-feeding mothers should be encouraged to consume the recommended dietary allowances for all essential nutrients; however, in the case of inadequate intake, some nutrients, such as energy stores, such as body fat, calcium, and iron may be mobilized from maternal stores. Many of the ingredients in human milk are present in constant proportions for all breast-feeding mothers and at every feed, whereas others may vary as a result of the maternal diet (Table 1). While the amount and composition of carbohydrate and protein remain relatively constant in mature human milk, the composition of fat is highly variable and is affected within hours and to a large extent by maternal nutrition intake. Therefore, inadequate maternal intake of long-chain polyunsaturated fatty acids, or excessive consumption of *trans* fatty acids, will result in breast milk with a less than optimal fatty acid composition for neonatal development. The vitamin content of human milk depends on the mother's vitamin status; when maternal intake of specific vitamins is chronically low, these vitamins in turn are found in low levels in the milk. Vitamin supplementation raises vitamin concentrations in milk. Water-soluble vitamins in milk are generally more responsive to maternal dietary intake than fat-soluble ones. Concentrations of calcium, iron, and zinc in milk seem to be independent of maternal nutrition. Concentrations of manganese, iodine, and selenium depend on maternal nutrition. How stage of lactation and maternal diet impact the content and composition of individual classes of nutrients will be discussed in depth in subsequent sections of this chapter.

Table 1 Overview of the Influence of Maternal Diet on Milk Composition

Little or no effect of maternal diet
Lactose concentration
Macromineral concentration (calcium, phosphorus, magnesium, etc)
Some trace elements (iron, zinc, copper, etc)
Electrolytes (sodium, potassium, chloride)
Minimal effect, except under cases of severe undernutrition
Protein concentration and composition
Nonprotein nitrogen concentration and composition
Influenced by maternal diet
Fatty acid content and composition
Long-chain polyunsaturated fatty acids
trans Fatty acids
Manganese, iodine, and selenium concentration
Water-soluble vitamin concentration (ascorbic acid, folate, vitamin B_{12}, niacin, etc)
Fat-soluble vitamin concentration (vitamins A, D, E, and K)

In general, the composition of human milk varies throughout the course of lactation.[50–54] The first milk produced, or colostrum, persists from birth to 5 days postpartum. *Colostrum* is a low-fat, high-protein fluid that is rich in immune-protective components. The milk produced over the next 9 days is termed *transitional milk* and is most variable in its composition as women transition at different rates from lactogenesis II to galactopoiesis.[34] Typically, by 15 days postpartum, *mature* human milk is produced, and its composition is relatively stable until weaning.[34,52–54] At weaning, minor changes in milk protein, lactose, chloride, and sodium concentrations were observed when milk volume declined to less than 400 mL/d.[39] While considerable information is available regarding changes in human milk composition in early lactation[52–54] or at weaning,[45] less is known about the effect of sustained extended lactation (>6–12 mo) on the nutrient content of human milk, particularly for micronutrients.[55] Kara and colleagues reported that, zinc, calcium, and vitamins B_6 and C tended to decrease between 7 and 25 months postpartum, whereas folate concentrations remained constant and only magnesium levels decreased after 18 months of lactation.[55] These decreases in milk nutrient content between 7 and 25 months of lactation may have little nutritional significance for the infant as the mean number of breast-feedings per day declined from six to two or three over this period of time[55] and infants' diets at this age include other foods.

In addition, milk composition changes markedly within a single feeding. The first milk (fore-milk) released by the mammary gland is low in fat and the fat content increases throughout the feeding and is highest in the hind-milk.[44,53] A comparison of paired fore- and hind-milk samples collected from the same mother showed protein and lactose content to be similar, whereas the fat content of hind-milk was two- to threefold higher and provided approximately 25 to 35 kcal/100 mL more energy than fore-milk.[53] These normal variations in human milk composition must be taken into account when obtaining samples for compositional analysis. The most accurate values will be obtained when the complete contents of the breast are expressed and mixed prior to obtaining a sample for analysis.

BIOCHEMICAL COMPOSITION

Nutrients in human milk are contained in discrete compartments that reflect their chemical characteristics as well as their processing and packaging during milk synthesis. Most water-soluble nutrients are present in the aqueous phase (whey), which represents the largest compartment of human milk.[52] Casein proteins are present in milk as a colloidal dispersion and fats and fat-soluble components are present in an emulsion of milk-fat globules surrounded by a milk-fat globule membrane.[52] The physical compartmentalization of nutrients in human milk differs from infant formulas and likely contributes to the dissimilarities in nutrient bioavailability between the two fluids.

Mature human milk is approximately 88% water, with a specific gravity of 1.030. The osmolarity of human milk is approximately 286 mOsm/L, compared with 185 to 374 mOsm/L in infant formulas.[56] There is no evidence that healthy appropriate-weight[57] or low-birth-weight[58] infants require additional water, even in hot climates. The total solids in human milk are approximately 122 g/L, of which 70 g/L is carbohydrate, 40 g/L is fat, 10 g/L is protein, and 2 g/L is mineral ash.[2,52] In comparison, bovine milk contains three times more protein (35 g/L) and mineral ash (7 g/L), less lactose (9 g/L), and similar amounts of total solids (128 g/L), fat (37 g/L), and water (87%).[2,52]

Energy Content

The energy content of human milk can be directly measured by bomb calorimetry or approximated from the protein, carbohydrate, and fat content of milk multiplied by their Atwater values.[59] Typically, mature human milk contains between 2,730 and 2,940 kJ/L or 650 and 700 kcal/L (Table 2).[52,59] The energy content of colostrum

Table 2 Energy and Macronutrient Composition of Colostrum and Mature Human Milk*†‡

Constituent (per L)	Colostrum	Mature Milk
Energy (kJ)†	2,431	2,835
Total carbohydrate (g)	50–70	70–85
Lactose (g)	30–50	67–70
Oligosaccharides (g)	22–24	5–15
Glucose (g)	0.2–1.0	0.2–0.3
Total lipid (g)	15–20	35–48
Triglyceride (g)	14.5–19.5	34–47
Fatty acids (g)	13–17	30–42
Cholesterol (g)	0.2–0.3	0.1–0.2
Cholesteryl esters (g)	0.05	0.01
Phospholipids and sphingolipids (g)	N.R.‡	0.25–0.30
Total nitrogen (g)	3.0	1.9
Nonprotein nitrogen (g)	0.5	0.45
Protein nitrogen (g)	2.5	1.45
Total protein (g)	15–20	8–11
Casein (g)	*3.8*	*3–5*
β-casein (g)	2.6	3–4
κ-casein (g)	1.2	1–2
Whey proteins (g)	*11–15*	*5–6*
α-lactalbumin (g)	3.6	2–3
IgM (g)	0.02	0.01
IgG (g)	0.01	0.05
Lactoferrin (g)	3.5	1–3
Lysozyme (g)	0.1–0.2	0.1
Secretory IgA (g)	2.0	0.5–1.0
Serum albumin (g)	0.4	0.3

*Mean values adapted from references 2, 52, 62, and 72–75.
†1 kJ = 0.2389 kcal.
‡Data not reported.

(days 2–7 postpartum; 571 ± 80 kcal/L) and transitional (days 8–20 postpartum; 629 ± 76 kcal/L) human milk is lower than mature milk (≥21 days postpartum; 642 ± 36 kcal/L).[59] Milk caloric density, calculated as the sum of the energy provided by each macronutrient, was 6 to 10% higher than that obtained by bomb calorimetry of the same milk samples, suggesting that the former method may overestimate the energy content of human milk.[59] In addition, it is important to keep in mind that some human milk proteins[60] and oligosaccharides[61] are resistant to digestion in the neonatal gastrointestinal tract. Therefore, bomb calorimetry may also overestimate the bioavailable energy content of human milk.

Carbohydrate

The predominant macronutrient present in human milk is carbohydrate in the form of lactose and oligosaccharides.[52,62] Lactose, the disaccharide of glucose and galactose, is readily digested by nearly all infants, whereas oligosaccharides are nondigestible and play a number of functional roles in host defense.[62]

Lactose and Glucose. After water, lactose is the most prevalent nutrient in human milk, with an average concentration of 70 g/L (67–76 g/L) in mature human milk (Table 2).[52] The lactose content of colostrum is lower than mature milk,[63] although colostrum is rich in oligosaccharides.[62] All oligosaccharides contain lactose at their reducing end[62]; therefore, the amount of free lactose in human milk may be overestimated if the analytical method used to quantify lactose cleaves the lactose from oligosaccharides. Lactose is the major osmole in human milk and its concentration is positively correlated with milk yield. The concentrations of lactose and α-lactalbumin (α-LA) in milk also are positively correlated, because lactose is synthesized by the actions of α-LA and galactosyltransferase.[64] Lactose is one of the most stable constituents in human milk and varies little once lactation is established.[53,55,63] Human milk contains very low levels of free glucose[63,65] (Table 2) and other glucose metabolites,[65] which are likely of little nutritional significance to the infant. Glucose concentrations were not higher in the milk of insulin-dependent diabetic mothers.[40,65] Glucose level normally rises in milk with the onset of lactogenesis II[40]; however, this rise was delayed by 1 to 4 days in insulin-dependent diabetic mothers, associated with compromised initiation of lactation.[40,65]

Oligosaccharides. Human milk is unique in that it contains a diverse array of highly complex oligosaccharides, which comprise the third largest component in human milk.[2,62] Oligosaccharide concentrations in human colostrum and mature milk are 22 to 24 g/L and 12 to 14 g/L, respectively (Table 2).[62] Over 200 separate forms of acidic or neutral oligosaccharides have been described in human milk, and their composition is influenced by maternal genetics.[62,66] Oligosaccharides are formed by the elongation of lactose with galactose or *N*-acetylglucosamine to form the two core neutral oligosaccharides, lacto-*N*-tetraose and lacto-*N*-neotetraose, respectively.[66] More complex oligosaccharides then are formed by the addition of fucose and sialic acids,[66] the latter of which are a subset of the nine-carbon sugar, neuraminic acid.[67] The *N*-acetylated form, *N*-acetylneuraminic acid, is the most predominant form and the only one found in humans.[68]

Many neutral oligosaccharides in human milk contain fucose on the nonreducing end.[62,66] These oligosaccharides are synthesized by one of three fucosyltransferases that are not uniformly distributed in the population.[62,66] The "secretor" or "nonsecretor" status of a mother is characterized by the presence of fucosyltransferase II activity; which catalyzes synthesis of α-1,2-fucosylated (3'-FL) oligosaccharides.[66,69] The other fucosylated oligosaccharides include the 3'-FL derivatives, which are synthesized by several fucosyltransferases, and difucosyllactose, which contains both α-1,2 and α-1,3 linages.[66]

Obermeier and colleagues orally administered ^{13}C-galactose to lactating women to assess the degree of utilization of dietary carbohydrates for lactose and oligosaccharide synthesis.[69] Approximately 7% of the oral dose (2 g) of ^{13}C-galactose was incorporated in lactose and neutral oligosaccha rides within 8 h and isotopically labeled lactose, 2'-FL, lacto-*N*-tetraose, fucosyllacto-*N*-tetraose, and difucosyllactose were detectable in the urine of their nursing infants.[69] Oligosaccharides are resistant to hydrolysis in the neonatal small intestine[61] and have the potential to exert widespread beneficial effects on neonatal intestinal health and host defense.[62,70,71] A complete discussion of human milk oligosaccharides and their mechanisms of action are presented in Chapter 31, "Protective Properties of Human Milk."

Fat

Fat is the second most prevalent class of macronutrients, averaging 15 to 20 g/L in colostrum and 35 to 48 g/L in mature milk, and represents approximately 45 to 55% of the energy content of human milk.[52,72–74] Triglycerides account for nearly all of the fat in human milk (97.5–98%), with small amounts of phospholipids and sphingolipids (0.7%) and cholesterol (0.5%) (Table 2).[52,72–74] Triglycerides are synthesized within mammary epithelial cells from glycerol and fatty acids that are either synthesized within the mammary gland or extracted from the maternal circulation through the action of lipoprotein lipase.[75,76] Maternal plasma lipids are the major source of longer chain (>16 carbon atoms) fatty acids in human milk, whereas saturated fatty acids (10–14 carbon atoms) are synthesized de novo within the mammary gland and their proportion increases in women consuming high-carbohydrate or low-fat diets.[75] Maternal diet contributes approximately 30% of the long-chain fatty acids (16:0, 18:0, 18:1n9, and 18:2), whereas maternal adipose tissue likely contributes the majority of the remaining 70%, including the long-chain polyunsaturated fatty acids (LCPUFAs).[75,76]

Within the mammary epithelial cell, milk fat is packaged with other lipophilic compounds and secreted into milk as milk fat globules, which average in size from 1 to 10 μm.[77] Each globule is surrounded by a bipolar milk fat globule membrane (MFGM) that is derived from the mammary apical plasma and mature Golgi vesicle membranes.[72,77] The MFGM emulsifies the milk fat and contains a number of bioactive lipids, proteins, and carbohydrates, including lactadherin and MUC1, which may play a role in host defense.[78]

Fatty Acid Composition. Fatty acids esterified to triglycerides account for 88% of the fat; very little nonesterified fatty acids are present in human milk.[52,72–74] Approximately 43% of fatty acids are saturated, 35% are *cis*-monounsaturated, 1 to 7% are *trans*-monounsaturated, and 20% are polyunsaturated fatty acids (19% n-6 and 1% n-3),[79] although these values can be markedly influenced by maternal diet[52,74,80] and, to a lesser degree, by stage of lactation.[74,79,81] For example, the amount of linoleic acid can vary from 1 to 45% of total fatty acids in milk.[52,73] Although 160 different fatty acids have been identified in human milk, predominant are the palmitic ($C_{16:0}$; 22%), stearic ($C_{18:0}$; 7%), oleic ($C_{18:1n\text{-}9}$; 34%), and linoleic ($C_{18:2}$; 8%) acids (Table 3).[52,73,74,79–82] Fat digestion and absorption from human milk is more

Table 3 Major Fatty Acids in Colostrum and Mature Human Milk*

Fatty Acids (% by wt of total fatty acids)	Colostrum	Mature Milk
Saturated	40	45 (32–52)
$C_{8:0}$	0.10–0.30	0.10–0.24
$C_{10:0}$	0.50–0.75	0.9–1.3
$C_{12:0}$	4.0–4.4	5.0–6.8
$C_{14:0}$	6.6–7.6	7.0–8.3
$C_{16:0}$	20–25	15–29
$C_{18:0}$	7.0–7.2	6.6–7.5
$C_{20:0}$	0.20–0.30	0.22–0.41
$C_{22:0}$	0.10–0.40	0.10–0.40
$C_{24:0}$	0.10–0.40	0.10–0.40
Cis-monounsaturated	40	40 (30–50)
$C_{14:1n\text{-}5}$	0.3	0.3
$C_{16:1n\text{-}9}$	0.4	0.4
$C_{16:1n\text{-}7}$	3.0	2.2–3.5
$C_{18:1n\text{-}9}$	33	30–34
$C_{18:1n\text{-}7}$	2.0	1.9
$C_{20:1n\text{-}11}$	0.20	0.15
$C_{20:1n\text{-}9}$	0.45	0.39
$C_{22:1n\text{-}9}$	0.04	0.02–0.06
$C_{24:1n\text{-}9}$	0.10–0.40	0.10–0.40
Trans-monounsaturated	7.0	(2.5–13.8)
$C_{16:1n\text{-}9t}$	N.R.†	0.24–0.53
$C_{18:1n\text{-}5t}$	N.R.	0.0–0.04
$C_{18:1n\text{-}6t}$	N.R.	0.0 0.06
$C_{18:1n\text{-}7+8t}$	N.R.	0.10–1.3
$C_{18:1n\text{-}9t}$	N.R.	0.17–1.7
$C_{18:1n\text{-}10t}$	N.R.	0.31–3.3
$C_{18:1n\text{-}11t}$	N.R.	0.28–3.0
$C_{18:1n\text{-}12t}$	N.R.	0.27–5.7
$C_{18:1n\text{-}13t}$	N.R.	0.0–2.7
$C_{18:1n\text{-}14t}$	N.R.	0.0–0.32
$C_{18:1n\text{-}15t}$	N.R.	0.0–0.15
$C_{18:1n\text{-}16t}$	N.R.	0.02–0.76
Total polyunsaturated	12.0	14.0 (11–27)
n-3 series	*2.0*	*1.5–1.8*
$C_{18:3}$	0.7	1.2
$C_{20:4}$	0.16	0.12
$C_{22:5}$	.0.27	0.13
$C_{22:6}$	0.5	0.2
n-6 series	*9.0*	*11.0*
$C_{18:2}$	7.0	8.0
$C_{18:3}$	0.06	0.10
$C_{20:2}$	0.75	0.20–0.55
$C_{20:3}$	0.57	0.25–0.45
C20.4	*0.7*	*0.34–0.45*
$C_{22.4}$	0.28	0.04–0.10
$C_{22.5}$	0.05	0.02
CLA isomers	*0.40–0.50*	*0.45–0.55*
$C_{18:2n\text{-}9c,11t}$	0.25	0.43
$C_{18:2n\text{-}9c,12t}$	0.05	0.06
$C_{18:2n\text{-}10t,12c}$	0.02	0.01
$C_{18:2n\text{-}11c,13t}$	0.04	0.05
$C_{18:2n\text{-}11c,13c}$	0.02	0.03

*Mean values (range) adapted from references 79 to 83 and 86 to 89.
†Data not reported.

efficient than from formula. One mechanism may be the presence of bile salt–stimulated lipase (BSSL) in human milk, which is complementary to pancreatic lipase.[72] Another potential explanation is that human milk triglycerides contain palmitic acid primarily in the sn-2 position, whereas infant formula fat blends contain palmitic acid primarily in the sn-1 and sn-3 positions.[72,81] Pancreatic lipase selectively hydrolyzes triglycerides in the sn-1 and -3 positions, producing two free fatty acids and a monoglyceride. Human infants efficiently absorb the 2-monopalmitin, produced from human milk fat digestion, whereas free palmitate may form soaps with calcium and be lost in the feces.[81]

Human milk contains relatively low concentrations of short-chain fatty acids (C_4–C_8), but significant amounts of the n-3 and n-6 LCPUFA arachidonic acid (AA, C20:4n6) and docosahexaenoic acid (DHA, C20:4n6) (Table 3).[52,72–74,79–82] The AA content of human milk averages 0.3 to 0.6 wt% and is relatively constant worldwide. In contrast, the DHA content of human milk can vary sixfold (<0.1–1.0 wt%) and reflects maternal DHA intake.[72,82] Recently, the LCPUFA content of milk produced by mothers delivering prematurely was shown to be greater than that in milk produced by mothers delivering at term[83]; however, this has not been a consistent observation.[72] The LCPUFA levels in neonatal plasma, erythrocyte membranes, and neural and retinal tissues is determined primarily by their dietary intake.[82,84] Beneficial effects of dietary AA and DHA intake on visual and cognitive development[25] of preterm and, to a lesser degree, term infants have been demonstrated, and LCPUFAs are now routinely supplemented to preterm and most term infant formulas.[82,84]

The *trans* fatty acid content of human milk also is influenced by material diet.[85–87] The main source of *trans* fatty acids in the diet are partially hydrogenated fats; *trans* fatty acids can comprise up to 60% of the fatty acids in shortenings and food sources made with shortenings. *Trans* fatty acids represent approximately 7.7% of the fatty acid intake (2.5% of energy) of lactating women, and the primary dietary sources are bakery products and breads (32%), snacks (15%), fast foods (11%), and margarines and shortenings (11%).[88] Human milk *trans* fatty acid content varies worldwide, ranging from 0.2 to 0.8% in milk samples from China and Africa to 7 wt% in the milk of North American mothers.[87–89] High concentrations of *trans* fatty acids in human milk are of potential concern as they may adversely affect the growth and development of infants by interfering with n-3 and n-6 fatty acid metabolism or by altering membrane fatty acid composition.[85,88] Indeed, milk *trans* fatty acids are inversely associated with milk linoleic and α-linolenic acids.[88] Furthermore, *trans* fatty acid, linoleic acid, α-linolenic acid, AA, and DHA concentrations in milk were directly related to their concentrations in the plasma of breast-fed infants.[88] Thus, it is warranted to recommend that lactating women reduce their *trans* fatty acid consumption. The inclusion of *trans* fatty acid content on food labels was associated with a decline in milk *trans* fatty acid content in Canadian mothers and a reduction in exposure of infants from 2.0 mg/kg/d in 1998 to 1.3 mg/kg/d in 2005, suggesting that increased consumer awareness of food sources of *trans* fatty acids has reduced their intake and subsequent secretion into milk.[88]

Dairy products and the meat of ruminant animals also are sources of *trans* fatty acids that are produced by biohydrogenation of fatty acids in the rumen.[86,89] Dairy products typically contain 2 to 5% *trans* fatty acids, primarily as conjugated isomers of linoleic acid.[89] Conjugated linoleic acids (CLAs) constitute a group of structurally related fatty acids with 18 carbon atoms and two conjugated double bonds. The most abundant naturally occurring CLA in the human diet and human milk is rumenic acid ($18{:}2_{c9t11}$) (Table 3).[89] Rumenic acid is produced in the bovine and human mammary gland via the desaturation of vaccenic acid ($18{:}2_{t11}$) by d-9 desaturase.[89] Other forms of CLA, such as $18{:}2_{t10c12}$, are found in dietary supplements and in low levels in human milk (Table 3).[89] In dairy cattle, $18{:}2_{t10c12}$ reduced milk fat content by 17 to 35% by reducing de novo fat synthesis in the mammary gland.[90] Similarly, milk fat content was reduced by 25% in lactating women after consuming a CLA supplement for 5 days.[91] Thus, nursing mothers should be cautioned against consuming CLA supplements.[91]

Sterols. Milk sterols are composed of 90% cholesterol and 8.6% desmosterol, with negligible quantities of phytosterols.[72,73] The cholesterol content of human milk declines from approximately 300 to 350 mg/L in colostrum to 100 to 200 mg/L in mature milk, and concentrations are correlated with milk fat content.[72,73] Approximately 10 to 15% of the cholesterol is present as cholesteryl esters, which, similarly, decline from 50 to 10 mg/L from colostrum to mature human milk.[92] Interestingly, unsaturated fatty acids are preferentially esterified to cholesterol (73 wt% of the fatty acids in cholesteryl esters).[92] Linoleic acid represented 31% of the fatty acids esterified to cholesterol versus 13% of the total fatty acids in milk.[92] Breast-fed infants consume approximately fourfold more cholesterol per day than adults (4.3 vs 25 mg/kg body weight) and have higher circulating cholesterol concentrations than infants fed formula devoid of cholesterol.[72,82]

Phospholipids and Sphingolipids. Phospholipids are dipolar lipids that are present as a component of the MFGM. Their concentration in milk is approximately 250 mg/L, or 0.6 g/100 g lipid.[72,73] The principal classes of phospholipids are sphingomyelin, phosphatidylcholine, phosphatidylethanolamine, phosphatidylserine, and phosphatidylinositol.[72,73] Choline, which can be synthesized from phosphatidylcholine and sphingomyelin, is a major constituent of cell membranes in neural tissues and is essential for the formation of acetylcholine.[93,94] Recent studies have demonstrated a key role for prenatal and early postnatal choline intake for optimal hippocampal development and memory.[94] Human infants excrete large amounts of betaine, a product of choline oxidation, regardless of choline intake, suggesting an obligatory choline requirement.[93] Although infant formulas contain choline, the concentration may not be sufficient to meet the increased demand of the human infant.[93] In contrast, human milk choline concentration doubles between colostrum and mature milk and appears to be sufficient to account for betaine excretion in full-term infants.[93] Additionally, human milk contains several classes of sphingolipids and glycolipids, including gangliosides.[72,73,95] Gangliosides may play a role in host defense by binding cholera and other toxins,[96] and in neural development.[97] Analysis of neural tissue obtained postmortem from infants who had died of sudden infant death syndrome demonstrated greater ganglioside and glycoprotein sialic acid concentrations in the brain frontal cortex of breast-fed infants compared with formula-fed infants, suggesting increased synaptogenesis and differences in neurodevelopment.[97]

Protein and Nonprotein Nitrogen

Human milk nitrogen content declines from colostrum (3.0 g/L) to mature milk (1.9 g/L) (Table 2). The nitrogen component of human milk is composed of whey and casein proteins and a diverse class of over 200 nonprotein nitrogen (NPN) components.[2,98,99] Approximately 25% of the nitrogen in human milk is NPN; thus, human milk protein content is most accurately determined as (total nitrogen – NPN) × 6.25. Using this approach, the protein content of human colostrum and mature milk averages approximately 15 to 20 g/L and 9 to 10 g/L, respectively.[2,98,100] The protein content of mature human milk is markedly lower than cow's milk (35 g/L) and cow's milk–based (13–15 g/L) or soy protein–based infant formulas (18–20 g/L).[98] Formulas not only contain more total protein than human milk but also contain a different pattern of amino acids.[101] Infants fed cow's milk–based formulas typically have higher urea N and amino acids, except taurine and cystine, than breast-fed infants.[101]

Protein. Human milk contains a heterogeneous mixture of proteins (casein and whey) and peptides. The protein content and composition of human milk undergoes dramatic changes during the course of lactation, which are matched to the developmental needs of the infant.[98,101] For example, colostrum is whey-predominant (90:10 whey/casein ratio) and contains higher concentrations of growth factors[102] and immune protective proteins, including sIgA, lactoferrin, and lysozyme, than mature milk.[101] As lactation progresses, the concentrations of growth factors and antimicrobial proteins decrease and casein, which predominantly serves as a source of amino acids, increases, resulting in a whey/casein ratio of approximately 60:40 in mature human milk.[2,98,100] The milk produced by mothers delivering preterm is higher in total protein and some differences in the casein and whey protein content compared to term human milk have been reported.[53,98]

Casein. There are four major families of casein proteins: α-casein, β-casein, γ-casein, and κ-casein.[2,97,99] Human milk is relatively low in casein (3–5 g/L) compared to bovine milk (26 g/L) and the forms of casein differ between the two species (Table 2).[98] The main caseins in human milk are β-casein (3–5 g/L) and κ-casein (1–3 g/L).[98] α-Casein, the predominant casein in bovine milk, is absent from human milk.[2,98] Casein proteins are high in proline and low in cystine and undergo extensive posttranslational phosphorylation and glycosylation.[98] Human milk κ-casein is highly glycosylated (40% carbohydrate) versus bovine κ-casein (10% carbohydrate).[98] Casein proteins precipitate at pH 4.6 and will form a "curd" in the infant's stomach. Human milk caseins tend to form looser micelles and softer curds, making them more easily digestible by carboxypeptidase. A number of peptides are formed during the proteolytic degradation of casein that have been proposed to regulate intestinal motility (opioid-like compounds) or enhance calcium absorption (phosphopeptides).[103]

Whey. Whey is the fluid remaining following precipitation of casein micelles. In human milk, whey proteins account for 60 to 70% of the total proteins versus 20% in bovine milk.[98] Human milk whey contains a variety of proteins, some of which are milk-specific and synthesized by the mammary gland (eg, α-LA) and others which are extracted from the maternal circulation (eg, serum albumin) (Table 2). α-Lactalbumin is the predominant whey protein in human milk (28% of total human milk protein and 40% of whey protein), whereas β-lactoglobulin is the primary whey protein in bovine milk and infant formulas and is absent from human milk.[100,104] A number of beneficial physiologic functions have been ascribed to α-LA for the mother and the infant.[100,104] Within the mammary gland, α-LA participates in lactose synthesis and, as the major osmole in milk, facilitates milk production and secretion.[64,104] For the infant, α-LA provides a well-balanced supply of essential amino acids and may enhance mineral and trace element absorption.[100,104] During α-LA digestion, peptides that have immunostimulatory and antibacterial properties appear to be transiently formed.[104,105] Furthermore, a novel folding variant of multimeric α-LA, termed HAMLET (human α-lactalbumin made lethal to tumor cells), recently has been discovered that specifically enhances apoptosis of tumor cells.[105] The formation of HAMLET requires partial unfolding of the protein, and its antitumor activity requires binding of oleic acid ($C_{18:1}$) to the protein as a cofactor.[105] HAMLET has been proposed potentially to impact intestinal mucosal cell turnover; however, there is no evidence to date that it is formed in the gastrointestinal tracts of human infants.[104] Although α-LA comprises only 2 to 3% of the protein in bovine milk, bovine α-LA-enriched whey sources are commercially available and currently are being used to produce infant formulas with higher α-LA content that have high protein quality.[106]

Functional Roles of Milk Proteins. In addition to serving as a source of amino acids, broader physiologic and immunologic roles of human milk proteins have been identified that provide nutritional and developmental benefits to the neonate.[7,100,104] For example, human milk proteins bind essential nutrients present in milk, which may enhance their bioavailability either through improved solubility or via direct interaction with receptors lining the gastrointestinal tract. Examples include haptocorrin and vitamin B_{12}, folate-binding protein and folate, and the binding of minerals and trace elements to β-casein, α-LA, lactoferrin, and α-glycomacropeptide.[7,100,104]

As previously discussed, another key function of human milk proteins centers on host defense, which occurs through antimicrobial protection, stimulation of immunocompetence, and promotion of the establishment of a beneficial microbiota.[8,9] Roles for sIgA, lactoferrin, lactoperoxidase, and lysozyme in neonatal host defense have long been appreciated[8,100]; however, recent investigations have added new proteins to the cadre of human immunoprotective components, including haptocorrin[107] and κ-casein.[108] In addition, proteolytic products of milk proteins recently have been shown to exert bioactivities distinct from the intact proteins, contributing to the complexity of the potential interactions between milk components and the infant. For example, antimicrobial peptides were produced following an in vitro digestion of lactoferrin[109] and α-LA,[110] and bifidogenic peptides were produced from lactoferrin and secretory component.[111] The multifunctional roles of proteins such as α-LA and lactoferrin and the potential for their proteolytic products to exert bioactive functions within the neonatal gastrointestinal tract illustrate the complexity of human milk protein bioactivity.[7,100,104]

Hormones and Growth Factors. Hormones and growth factors constitute another class of bioactive proteins and peptides in milk.[7,102,112] Insulin-like growth factor I, epidermal growth factor, and transforming growth factor α and β are among the most well studied.[7,102,113] Cell culture and animal models show that growth factors can initiate cellular growth and expression of differentiated function, and that they are important in adaptation and repair following injury.[7,102,113] There is evidence that orally administered recombinant growth factors survive digestion and exert biological effects within the neonatal gastrointestinal tract.[7,102,113,114] However, most studies investigating growth factors have applied supraphysiological doses, and there is little clinical data to support a direct role of any growth factor *at the concentrations normally present in human milk* on neonatal intestinal development.

Enzymes. A variety of enzymes are present in human milk that influences the digestion of other milk components. Bile salt–stimulated lipase improves the digestion and absorption of lipids and lipid-soluble vitamins,[115] whereas protease inhibitors, such as α_1-antitrypsin and antichymotrypsin, limit the digestion of some milk proteins.[116] This latter function may be critical to preserving the physiologic functions of the nutrient-binding and immunologic proteins within the neonatal gastrointestinal tract. Indeed, intact human proteins are present in the feces of both term and preterm infants.[60]

Nonprotein Nitrogen. Approximately 20% of the nitrogen in human milk is present as nonprotein nitrogen (NPN), which is considerably higher than that in bovine milk (5%).[52,98,99,117] The NPN content of infant formulas is variable and is influenced by whether the whey protein concentrate was prepared by electrodialysis or ultrafiltration, the latter of which removes more NPN components.[117] The NPN components are characterized as less than 10,000 mol wt nitrogen-containing compounds. The NPN in human milk comprises a heterogeneous group of more than 200 compounds, including urea, free amino acids, such as taurine and glutamine, small peptides, including many growth factors, amino sugars, nucleic acids, polyamines, nucleotides, and carnitine.[52,99] A number of these compounds have physiological roles in the infant and were found to be lower in the plasma of formula-fed versus breast-fed infants, which led to their addition to infant formulas, including taurine and carnitine in the 1980s and, most recently, nucleotides. Urea N accounts for approximately 50% of the NPN in human milk[99,117] and appears to be utilized to synthesize nonessential amino acids. Heine and colleagues estimated that 2 to 3.6% of serum proteins are synthesized from urea nitrogen,[118] and 10 to 40% of the ^{15}N from an oral dose of $^{15}N,^{15}N$-urea was retained by preterm infants.[119] Thus, while NPN is not included in the protein fraction of human milk, it may contribute to the pool of available nitrogen for protein synthesis by the infant.

Vitamins

Human milk contains all the essential water- and fat-soluble vitamins and their content can be influenced by maternal diet.[120–124] Allen proposed that "maternal micronutrient status in the periconceptional period, and throughout pregnancy and lactation, should be viewed as a continuum; too often, these three stages are treated and discussed separately from both a scientific and a public health perspective."[120] Healthy breast-fed infants of well-nourished mothers are at low risk for vitamin deficiencies and the need for vitamin supplementation is rare, with a few exceptions where milk concentrations may be inadequate. Examples include vitamin B_{12} in milk of vegan mothers, vitamin D in milk produced by mothers with insufficient dietary intake or sun exposure, and vitamin K in most mothers.[125] Vitamin D and K deficiencies have been described in breast-fed infants, and these are the only two vitamins for which supplementation for the breast-fed infant is recommended by the AAP.[126,127] These will be discussed in greater detail below.

Fat-Soluble Vitamins. Most fat-soluble vitamins are delivered to the infant within the milk fat globule membrane, and their absorption is enhanced by BSSL in milk.[115] An exception is vitamin D, which is found in the whey bound to vitamin D–binding proteins.

Retinoids and Carotenoids. Retinoids and carotenoids comprise a group of closely related compounds that have vitamin A activity (eg, retinol), can be converted to vitamin A (eg, β-carotene, α-carotene, β-cryptoxanthin), or do not have pro–vitamin A activity but have other physiological functions in the body (eg, lutein, zeaxanthin, lycopene).[128,129] For example, lutein and zeaxanthin are the only dietary carotenoids present in macular pigment and may protect photoreceptors against light-initiated oxidative damage.[128] Colostrum and breast milk are rich in retinoids, principally as retinol esters (Table 4).[128–132] Retinol ester is the principal form of vitamin A in human milk. Its concentration is influenced by maternal diet and varies about twofold across eight countries.[129] Milk retinol concentration in term human milk declines as lactation progresses; however, this trend has not been observed in preterm human milk, and the absolute concentrations were higher in transitional and mature preterm than term milk.[130] Human milk contains approximately 1.8 μmol/L total carotenoids, with the pro–vitamin A carotenoids (α-carotene, β-carotene, β-cryptoxanthine) accounting for 50% of the carotenoids.[129] In general, the carotenoid content declines from colostrum to mature milk, but the magnitude of decrease was influenced by the polarity of the carotenoids, with the most polar carotenoids exhibiting the smallest decrease.[131,132] Thus, colostrum had a higher proportion of less polar carotenoids (eg, β-carotene), whereas mature milk contained more lutein and zeaxanthin.[130] Lietz and colleagues demonstrated that human milk α- and β-carotene content could be increased by dietary supplementation, without decreasing milk lutein or zeaxanthin content.[128] They also showed that the concentrations of hydrocarbon carotenoids (α- and β-carotene) were greater in maternal plasma than milk, whereas the opposite was true for xanthophylls (lutein or zeaxanthin), suggesting regulated uptake and transport of polar carotenoids into milk.[128]

Vitamin D. Unlike the other fat-soluble vitamins, vitamin D is present in whey attached to plasma or cytosolic vitamin D–binding proteins.[52] The principal form of vitamin D is 25-OH vitamin D and its content is influenced by maternal diet

Table 4 Vitamin Composition of Human Milk*

Constituent (per L)	Colostrum	Mature Milk
Fat-soluble vitamins		
Vitamin A and carotenoids		
Retinol esters (μmol)	1.45–2.0	1.22
Total carotenoids (μmol)	5.35	1.8–3.0
α-Carotene (μmol)	0.17	0.02–0.03
β-Carotene (μmol)	0.42	0.04–0.07
β-Cryptoxanthin (μmol)	0.23	0.03–0.06
Lutein/zeaxanthin (μmol)	0.2	0.04–0.10
Lycopene (μmol)	0.51	0.02–0.06
Vitamin D_3 (cholecalciferol) (μg)	0.1–0.3	0.1–1.0
Vitamin E		
α-tocopherol (mg)	15	3–5
γ-tocopherol (mg)	1.5	1.0
Vitamin K		
Phylloquinone, K_1 (μg)	1.8–2.3	1.5–3.0
Menaquinone, K_2 (μg)	2.4–2.6	1.2–2.0
Water-soluble vitamins		
Ascorbic Acid (mg)	80–100	40–100
Biotin (μg)	4.5	5–9
Vitamin B_{12} (μg)	1.2–1.5	0.5–0.8
Folate (μg)	5–10	50–100
Niacin (mg)	0.5	1.5–2.0
Pantothenic Acid (mg)	2.5	2.0–2.5
Pyridoxine, B_6 (μg)	20–40	90–300
Riboflavin, B_2 (μg)	500	300–400
Thiamin, B_1 (μg)	20	160–210

*Mean values adapted from references 52, 72, 125, 130, 135, 138–140, 147, and 148.

and sun exposure.[52,72,126] Endogenous vitamin D synthesis is detrimentally impacted by darker skin pigmentation and other factors that reduce skin UVB exposure, including winter season, environmental pollution, use of sunscreens, and lifestyle or cultural practices that limit sunlight exposure.[126] Greer and colleagues showed that milk vitamin D content could be increased tenfold by 1.5 MED (minimal erythemal dose of total body UVB exposure), which is approximately 90 s of irradiation in Caucasians.[132]

Exclusively breast-fed infants can obtain vitamin D from human milk, by endogenous synthesis from sunlight exposure, or by mobilizing vitamin D stored during gestation. However, vitamin D stores of infants are rapidly depleted, even in infants born to mothers with normal vitamin D status and after 2 months of age, infants are dependent upon exogenous sources of vitamin D.[126] Human milk typically contains 1 μg or 40 IU/L or less of vitamin D (Table 4), which is insufficient to meet the current vitamin D recommendation of 200 IU/day for infants.[126] Furthermore, the AAP recommends that infants less than 6 months of age be kept out of direct sunlight and that protective clothing, as well as sunscreen, should be used.[133] To reduce the risk of rickets, the AAP currently recommends a daily supplement of 200 IU for all breast-fed infants and for non–breast-fed infants receiving less than 500 mL/day of vitamin D–supplemented formula.[126]

Vitamin E and Coenzyme Q10. Analogous to vitamin A, the term *vitamin E* describes a family of closely related compounds (α-, β-, and γ-tocopherol) that function as antioxidants in cell membranes by scavenging free radicals. Human milk contains α- and γ-tocopherol, but insignificant levels of β-tocopherol.[131] The α- and γ-tocopherol content of colostrum is greater than that of mature milk (Table 4).[131] In addition, the α- and γ-tocopherol content of preterm human milk is greater than milk from mothers delivering at term.[131] Infants appear to differentially utilize natural and synthetic forms of vitamin E,[134] but both human milk and formula contain sufficient vitamin E to meet requirements and prevent significant lipid peroxidation,[135] even in preterm infants who are exposed to greater oxidative stress than term infants.

Recently, coenzyme Q10, a lipophilic antioxidant, has been reported in term and preterm human milk[136,137] and the coenzyme Q10, α- and γ-tocopherol concentrations were directly correlated with the antioxidant capacity of the milk.[137] Compared to term human milk, the coenzyme Q10 content was lower in colostrum (0.50 vs 0.81 μmol/L) and transitional (0.45 vs 0.75 μmol/L) milk from mothers delivering preterm.[137] In term human milk, coenzyme Q10 content declined from colostrum (0.80 μmol/L) to transitional (0.57 μmol/L) and mature milk (0.44 μmol/L) samples, which was more evident when expressed on the basis of milk lipid content, or 137, 86, and 67 μmol/mol cholesterol, respectively.[136]

Vitamin K. Vitamin K (phylloquinone) is a necessary cofactor for the vitamin K–dependent carboxylase, which catalyzes the formation of γ-carboxyglutamic acid (Gla). The formation of Gla residues creates calcium-binding sites that are necessary for the function of proteins such as prothrombin and other coagulation factors. Vitamin K is not readily transported across the placenta; thus, vitamin K deficiency can cause unexpected bleeding in the first week of life.[127] The AAP currently recommends that a single, intramuscular dose of vitamin K (0.5–1.0 mg) be given to all newborns to prevent vitamin K deficiency bleeding.[127]

Human milk contains both forms of vitamin K, phylloquinone (K_1) and menaquinones (K_2), in approximately equal concentrations.[138] Overall, a weak relationship has been noted between maternal dietary phylloquinone intake and milk phylloquinone content; however, the vitamin K content and composition can be impacted by maternal diet and supplement use.[122,138] Maternal supplementation with a pharmacological dose of 5 mg phylloquinone per day increased its concentration in milk and in the serum of breast-feeding infants.[122] Recently, Kojima and colleagues[138] identified two menaquinones, menaquinone-4 (MK-4) and menaquinone-7 (MK-7) in the milk of Japanese women. Menaquinone-4 is synthesized by bacteria and is associated with maternal intake of fermented soybeans, whereas MK-4 (menatetrenone) is widely available in Japan as a dietary supplement.[138] Prophylactic vitamin K administration is particularly important for exclusively breast-fed infants because human milk vitamin K (phylloquinone) concentrations (typically 1–3 μg/L) (Table 4) are insufficient to meet the recommended intake of 2 μg/day for infants.[127] In addition, *bifidobacteria*, which are more predominant in breast- than formula-fed infants, do not synthesize vitamin K, and the vitamin K content in the stool of breast-fed infants was insignificant compared to formula-fed infants.[139]

Water-Soluble Vitamins. The concentrations of water-soluble vitamins in human milk are influenced by maternal nutritional intake and supplementation will increase milk vitamin content to a plateau concentration.[123,140] The thiamin and riboflavin contents of human milk typically are sufficient to meet the needs of the exclusively breast-fed infant, but vitamin B_6, vitamin B_{12}, and folate may be low in milk produced by mothers from lower socioeconomic groups.[123] Although supplementation may be beneficial for women with poor dietary intake, only niacin and vitamin B_{12} can be increased further in milk when the mother's vitamin status is adequate.[52,72,140]

Vitamin C. The concentration of ascorbic acid in human milk can range from 40 to 100 mg/L in well-nourished women, and within an individual mother the concentration decreases from colostrum to mature milk (Table 4).[52,72,140] Low maternal intake lowers milk ascorbic acid content. For example, mean human milk ascorbic acid was 50% lower in the milk of African (31 mg/L) versus European (63 mg/L) women.[141] Furthermore, the response to a high dose of ascorbic acid supplementation (1,000 mg/d for 10 days) was modest in European women (60–70 mg/L) in contrast with the threefold increase in mean human milk ascorbic acid content (19–60 mg/L) in African women,[141] suggesting that human milk ascorbic acid content is regulated. In African women, an intake of one serving of orange juice per week had no significant effect, whereas three or five servings per week (100 mg ascorbic acid per serving) for 6 weeks doubled mean human milk ascorbic acid content from 16 to 32 mg/L.[141] Human milk ascorbic acid is sufficient to meet the needs of exclusively breast-fed infants and no supplementation is recommended.[125]

Thiamine. The thiamine content of colostrum is low (20 μg/L), but increases to 160 to 200 μg/L in mature milk and this amount can be further increased with maternal supplementation (Table 4). The thiamine intake of breast-fed infants is lower than the recommended dietary allowance (RDA); however, the intake appears adequate to meet their needs and infantile beriberi is rare in the United States.[142] Other than ensuring adequate maternal thiamine intake, supplementation of the infant is not recommended.[124,125]

Riboflavin. The riboflavin content of colostrum is high and decreases to 400 to 600 μg/L in mature human milk (Table 4). In well-nourished women, riboflavin is only increased by pharmacological intakes (>3 times the RDA).[52,124] The riboflavin intake of breast-fed infants is adequate and no supplementation of infants is needed.[125]

Niacin. The niacin content of colostrum is approximately 0.5 mg/L and 1.5 to 2.0 mg/L in mature milk (Table 4). The content in milk can be increased to as high as 6.0 mg/L by maternal intake.[52,140] In addition, niacin can be synthesized from excess dietary tryptophan, which contributes to the milk niacin content.[52,140] Niacin supplementation is not recommended for exclusively breast-fed infants.[125]

Vitamin B_6. The vitamin B_6 content of colostrum is low and increases to 90 to 310 μg/L in mature milk (Table 4).[52,125] Vitamin B_6 in human milk of well-nourished women is adequate for the exclusively breast-fed infant[125]; however, low maternal intake can reduce milk B_6 content.[123]

Folate and Vitamin B_{12}. The folate content of human milk increases from 5 to 10 μg/L in colostrum to 50 to 100 μg/L in mature milk.[123] It was estimated that one-third of pregnant and lactating women are not meeting their folate requirement by diet alone, even after the mandatory supplementation of folate to enriched flour, pasta, and grains in North America in 1998.[143] However, folate deficiency has not been reported in breast-fed infants and supplements are not recommended for the infant.[125]

The content of vitamin B_{12} in human milk decreases from colostrum (~1.2 μg/L) to mature milk (~0.5 μg/L).[125,140] Infants of well-nourished mothers with adequate vitamin B_{12} intake do not require supplementation. However, the vitamin B_{12} content of milk of vegan mothers can be insufficient to meet the needs of the exclusively breast-fed infant and deficiencies have been reported.[144] In addition, maternal gastric bypass surgery can place the mother and infant at risk for B_{12} deficiency.[145] Thus, in some clinical situations, supplements of vitamin B_{12} are warranted for the mother or infant.[125]

Biotin and Pantothenic Acid. The biotin content of colostrum is approximately 4.5 μg/L and its concentration increases to 5 to 9 μg/L in mature milk (Table 4).[146,147] However, mature milk biotin does not reach a stable plateau and varies substantially between mothers (0–27 μg/L) (Table 4).[147] The concentration of pantothenic acid in human milk is 2.0 to 2.5 mg/L (Table 4).[148] There were no differences in milk pantothenic acid concentration between 2 weeks and 4 months postpartum, but its concentration was responsive to maternal dietary intake.[148] Pantothenic acid was also higher in preterm (3.5 mg/L) versus term (2.5 mg/L) human milk.[148]

In summary, in well-nourished women, human milk contains all essential vitamins at adequate concentrations to meet the needs of the exclusively breast-fed infant. Two exceptions are vitamins D and K, but deficiencies can be avoided by adequate maternal dietary and maternal sun exposure, in the case of vitamin D, and prophylactic vitamin K injection at birth. Mothers following restricted diets or those with previous gastric bypass surgery are at risk for low milk vitamin B_{12} content and should be encouraged to take supplemental vitamin B_{12}. As the content of all fat- and water-soluble vitamins in human milk is influenced by maternal intake, it may be prudent to encourage all lactating mothers to consider a daily multivitamin supplement to ensure adequate milk nutrition content.[120]

Macro- and Microminerals

Over 20 macro- and microminerals have been identified in human milk and, in general, their content changes over the course of lactation, with most declining from colostrum to mature milk.[149–151] In direct contrast to vitamins, mineral concentrations in milk generally do not correlate to maternal serum or typical dietary intake[152] and do not respond to supplementation.[153] Mineral transport into milk is tightly regulated by the mammary gland.[154] Specific micromineral (Cu, Zn, and Fe) transporters have been identified and their molecular and hormonal regulation are under study.[154] The absolute concentrations of most macro- and microminerals are lower in human milk than bovine milk or infant formulas[150,151]; however, they are characterized by enhanced bioavailability.[155] Thus, the mineral requirements of exclusively breast-fed term infants can be met for the first 6 months of life.[52,155]

Macrominerals. The major macrominerals in milk include calcium, magnesium, phosphorus, sodium, potassium, and chloride (Table 5).[52,72,150] Some minerals, such as sodium and potassium, are totally soluble in water and found primarily in whey. In contrast, calcium forms complexes with phosphate and casein. Therefore, approximately 85% is found in the whey and 15% associated with casein micelles in calcium–phosphate linkages.[72,156]

Calcium, Magnesium, and Phosphorus. Calcium content of colostrum (300–350 mg/L) is greater than human mature milk (200–250 mg/L) (Table 5),[149,150] but both are markedly lower than that present in bovine milk (1,200–1,350 mg/L).[149] Once lactation is established (3–26 weeks postpartum), the calcium and magnesium content of human milk is relatively stable, whereas the phosphorus content of human milk declines by approximately 40%.[157] Calcium bioavailability is high from human milk, due in part to the calcium-to-phosphorus ratio of 2:1, and the levels of calcium, phosphorus, and magnesium in human milk are adequate to meet the needs of the term human infant.[52] However, calcium supplements should be provided to all preterm infants to prevent rickets and hypocalcemic tetany.[5]

Sodium, Potassium, and Chloride. The concentrations of electrolytes in milk are influenced by an electrochemical gradient in the mammary secretory cells, which is established by the passage of water.[52] In early lactation, changes in the concentrations of lactose, sodium, and chloride signal closure of paracellular pathways between the mammary epithelial cells at 1 to 2 days postpartum.[46] Overall, the concentrations of sodium, potassium, and chloride are lower in mature milk than colostrum, but the magnitude of difference is greater for potassium and chloride (60–70% lower) than sodium (30–35% lower).

Microminerals. The predominant microminerals, or trace elements, in human milk include iron, copper, and zinc, as well as manganese, selenium, chromium, fluoride, iodine, and boron (Table 5).[52,73,149,151] The concentrations of trace elements in human milk are low; however, their bioavailability is much higher than from bovine milk or infant formula.[155] The presence of lactoferrin in human milk has been proposed to facilitate iron and manganese uptake via an intestinal receptor for this protein.[155] Furthermore, high concentrations of ascorbic acid and citrate also may facilitate the uptake of trace elements from human milk, while a high concentration of casein in cow's milk and cow's milk formulas may limit trace element absorption from these diets.[155] The physical distribution of trace elements differs between human and cow milk, which also may influence their bioavailability.[156] For example, 24% of the iron, 44% of the copper, and 84% of the zinc is bound to casein in bovine milk, whereas comparable values for human milk are 9, 7, and 8%, respectively, and most of these trace elements are found in the whey.[155] A significant proportion of the iron in both bovine (14%) and human (33%) milk is associated with the outer MFGM.[156]

Table 5 Macromineral and Micromineral Composition of Human Milk*

Constituent (per L)	Colostrum	Mature Milk
Macrominerals		
Calcium (mg)	250	200–250
Chloride (mg)	600–800	400–450
Magnesium (mg)	30–35	30–35
Phosphorus (mg)	120–160	120–140
Potassium (mg)	600–700	400–550
Sodium (mg)	300–400	150–250
Microminerals		
Boron (μg)	30	28
Chromium (μg)	17	25–75
Copper (mg)	0.5–0.8	0.1–0.3
Fluoride (μg)	5–20	4–15
Iodine (μg)	40–50	140–150
Iron (mg)	0.5–1.0	0.3–0.75
Manganese (μg)	5–12	3–4
Selenium (μg)	235–32	10–25
Zinc (mg)	5–12	1–3

*Mean values adapted from references 52, 72, 149–151, and 156–161.

Iron, Zinc, Copper, and Manganese. The iron concentration in human milk averages 0.5 to 1.0 mg/L in colostrum and 0.35 to 0.70 mg/L in mature milk (Table 5).[149,157] The bioavailability of iron from human milk is high (20–50%) relative to infant formulas (4–7%).[155] Exclusively breast-fed infants generally do not need iron supplements prior to 6 months of age, at which time the AAP recommends the gradual introduction of iron-enriched solid foods.[1] Infants who have low iron stores or anemia may require iron supplementation prior to 6 months of age to avoid iron-deficiency anemia.[1] However, trace elements that share absorptive pathways compete for uptake, and excessive iron supplementation may create imbalances in the ratios between trace elements (Fe/Zn, Zn/Cu, Fe/Mn) and impair trace element absorption.[155] The zinc concentration of human milk rapidly declines from 5 to 12 mg/L in colostrum to 1 to 3 mg/L in mature milk.[149,157] Similarly to iron, the bioavailability of zinc from human milk (60%) is greater than from formula (~30%).[155] Following a similar trend to iron and zinc, the copper content of human colostrum and milk declines from colostrum (0.5–0.8 mg/L) to mature milk (0.1–0.3 mg/L).[158] Copper absorption is similar from human milk (25%) and cow's milk–based infant formula (23%); however, the copper concentrations in formula are double that of human milk, suggesting the potential for excess copper intake in formula-fed infants.[158] Similar to the other trace elements, the manganese content of human milk (3–4 μg/L) is lower than colostrum (5–12 μg/L)[149,157] and its bioavailability from human milk is greater than from infant formula.[155]

Selenium, Iodine, and Fluoride. The selenium, fluoride, and iodine contents of human milk vary worldwide. Mean selenium concentrations in colostrum and milk are 33 to 40 μg/L and 8 to 12 μg/L, respectively (Table 5).[149,157] Maternal selenium status has a strong influence on milk selenium content and a multicountry comparison showed that levels in milk from the Philippines was much higher than milk from Swedish or Hungarian mothers.[149] Likewise, milk fluoride was reported to vary from 7 to 118 μg/L in samples collected worldwide, but does not appear to be affected by stage of lactation.[149] In many countries, fluoride is supplemented to the water supply. Esala and colleagues compared milk samples collected from mothers living in two areas having an average of 0.2 and 1.7 mg fluoride/L in the drinking water.[159] The fluoride content of breast milk in the high-fluoride areas (10.9 μg/L; range 4.5–50.7 μg/L) was statistically significantly higher than the low-fluoride areas (7.0 μg/L; range 4.3–14.0 μg/L), respectively.[159] To avoid fluorosis, the AAP recommends that fluoride not be administered to infants during the first 6 months after birth, whether they are breast- or formula-fed.[1] During the period from 6 months to 3 years of age, breast-fed infants (and formula-fed infants) require fluoride supplementation, only if the water supply is severely deficient in fluoride (<0.3 mg/L).[1] Lastly, milk iodine content varies widely by geographic location and maternal intake and iodized salt and seafood are primary dietary sources. Overall, iodine content in human milk has been reported in the range of 33 to 348 μg/L.[149,160] In Germany, the mean iodine content of human milk has doubled in recent years, suggesting greater maternal dietary intake; however, a one-time supplement of 175 μg did not impact milk iodine content.[160]

In summary, milk mineral content, with the exception of selenium, iodine, and fluoride, is not significantly influenced by maternal diet. In well-nourished women, human milk contains all essential macro- and microminerals at adequate concentrations to meet the needs of the exclusively breast-fed infant for the first 6 months and life and supplements are not recommended under normal circumstances.

DRUGS, ENVIRONMENTAL CONTAMINANTS, AND VIRUSES IN HUMAN MILK

The presence in breast milk of environmental chemicals that may disrupt the nervous, endocrine, and reproductive systems of humans has gained increased attention from regulatory agencies and groups advocating women's and children's health.[162–166] Environmental chemicals in milk encompass substances that are introduced from food, pharmaceuticals, or exposure to environmental contaminants.[162–165] Although scientific evidence to date indicates that the advantages of breast-feeding outweigh any risks from contaminants, it is important to identify contaminant trends, locate disproportionately exposed populations, and take public health measures to decrease and eliminate chemical pollutants from mother's milk.[164] This is particularly important, as human milk often serves as the sole source of nutrition for the breast-fed infant and, owing to the rapid mental and physical changes that are taking place, infants may be more susceptible than adults to adverse effects resulting from chemical exposures.[164,165]

Pharmaceuticals and Drugs

Most women require drug therapy in the early postpartum period to treat chronic or acute medical conditions, and it has been reported that 90% of women take some form of medication in their first week postpartum.[167] Mothers are often concerned about the potential risk to their nursing infant from drugs introduced through milk.[162,166,167] Nearly a quarter of breast-feeding mothers who were prescribed an antibiotic either stopped breast-feeding or did not take the medication.[167] Analysis of risk to the infant must take into account how much of the drug is excreted into milk and whether that level of exposure poses a risk of adverse effects to the infant. Factors affecting the transfer of compounds into milk include the following: the pKa of the compound, its lipid solubility, the presence of maternal plasma protein binding, and its molecular weight.[162] In general, small (less than 200 Da), ionized, lipid-soluble compounds will appear in milk within 1 hour after maternal ingestion and the maternal plasma-to-milk ratio of the drug will be close to 1.[162] For most drugs, the plasma-to-milk ratio is less than 1, whereas 25% have ratios close to 1 and 15% have ratios of 2 or more, indicating that they are concentrated in milk.[167] For many years, the plasma-to-milk ratio was used as a proxy for neonatal exposure along with the amount of milk ingested (150 mL/kg/d); however, this does not take into account the drug clearance rate by the infant, which is as important as the concentration in milk.[167] Unfortunately, for most drugs the clearance rate by the infant is unknown. For most drugs, the dose below which there is no potential for clinical effect in the infant is unknown. Therefore, a drug has been arbitrarily defined as safe if the dose delivered in the breast milk is less than 10% of the therapeutic dose.[167] Data collected from over 800 infants who were exposed to various drugs though breast milk suggest that clinically important adverse effects were rare, although 10% of mothers reported minor effects that did not require medical attention.[168] The current AAP statement concerning the transfer of drugs and chemicals into milk supports the safe use of drugs for maternal therapy in almost all cases.[166] However, cases of significant infant toxicity exist, supporting the need for a case-by-case risk assessment to be made before the mother initiates breast-feeding or drug therapy.[167] In general, drugs of abuse, antineoplastics, some anticonvulsants, ergot alkaloids, and radioisotopes should not be taken, and levels of amiodarone, cyclosporine, and lithium should be monitored (Table 6).[167,168] In summary, only a few drugs pose clinically significant risk to infants. However, to make an informed decision, it is critical that appropriate and the most up-to-date sources be consulted when making recommendations to patients. In cases where a contraindicated drug is medically required for a breast-feeding mother, milk production can be maintained by pumping extra breast milk prior to initiating the therapy, frozen and fed to the infant. During the therapy, mothers can express and discard the milk until the level of excretion into milk is safe for the infant. Readers are referred to the AAP statement and other recent reviews for specific recommendations for the clinical management of breast-feeding mothers when medical treatment is necessary, including the use of radioisotopes.[166,157]

Table 6 Drugs with Reported Toxicity to Breast-Fed Infants.*

Antineoplastics and immune suppressants
β–Blockers
Ergot alkaloids
Gold salts
Iodine
Lithium carbonate
Radioisotopes
Drugs of abuse (cocaine and others)
Nonmedicinal substances (ethanol, caffeine, nicotine)

*Adapted from references 166 and 167.

Environmental Contaminants

Decades of inadequately controlled pollution of the environment by persistent, bioaccumulative, and toxic (PBT) chemicals has resulted in the contamination of human milk by polychlorinated biphenyls (PCBs), dichloro-diphenyl-trichloroethane (DDT) and its metabolites, dioxins, dibenzofurans, polybrominated-diphenyl-ethers (PBDEs), and heavy metals.[162,163] Women may be exposed to lipophilic chemicals from various sources including air, food, water, and occupational and household environments. These compounds are encountered to varying extents among women in industrially developed as well as in developing nations.[162,163] Some of the highest levels of contaminants are seen among women in agricultural areas of the developing world that are extensively treated with pesticides and among women in remote areas, such as the Canadian Inuit, who eat species high on the marine food chain that accumulate heavy burdens of PBT chemicals.[163,165]

Lipophilic chemicals are stored and accumulated over time in body fat and are mobilized into milk during lactation. Generally, chemicals enter breast milk by passive transfer from plasma, and their concentration in milk is proportional to their solubility and lipophilicity. Twenty percent or more of maternal body burden of some persistent pollutants, such as PCBs, can be transferred during 6 months of lactation.[162] The levels of PBTs in human milk increase with the age of the mother, decline over the course of lactation and with each successive lactation.[164] However, studies of infants exposed to environmental chemicals in human milk have, for the most part, not shown adverse health effects to the nursing infant.[164] Thus, while more research is needed, current scientific evidence does not support altering the global public health recommendation of exclusive breast-feeding for 6 months followed by continued breast-feeding, up to 2 years of age or beyond.[32–34,164,165]

Human Immunodeficiency Virus Type 1

Transmission of human immunodeficiency virus type 1 (HIV-1) through breast-feeding has been conclusively demonstrated.[169] Therefore, to avoid mother-to-child transmission, the AAP and CDC recommend complete avoidance of breast-feeding by HIV-1–infected mothers in the United States.[169]

OVERALL SUMMARY AND CONCLUSIONS

Breast-feeding is the optimal form of nutrition for the human infant and has numerous nutritional advantages over infant formula. In addition, human milk confers short- and long-term health protection against infection and may have life-long consequences for metabolism and chronic disease incidence. All mothers should be strongly encouraged by health care providers to breast-feed their infants, and medical and societal programs should be established to support exclusive breast-feeding from the first 6 months of life, including ensuring that all hospitals become "Baby Friendly."[170]

REFERENCES

1. American Academy of Pediatrics, Section on Breastfeeding. Breastfeeding and the use of human milk. Pediatrics 2005;115:496–506.
2. Kunz C, Rodriguez-Palermo M, Koletzko B, Jensen R. Nutritional and biochemical properties on human milk, Part I: General aspects, proteins and carbohydrates. Clin Perinatol 1999;26:307–33.
3. Yates AA. Dietary reference intakes: Concepts and approaches underlying protein and energy requirements. Nestle Nutr Workshop Ser Pediatr Program 2006;58:79–90.
4. Schanler RJ, Shulman RJ, Lau C. Feeding strategies for premature infants: Beneficial outcomes of feeding fortified human milk versus preterm formula. Pediatrics 1999;103:1150–7.
5. Smith MM, Durkin M, Hinton VJ, et al. Influence of breastfeeding on cognitive outcomes at age 6–8: Follow up of very low birthweight infants. Am J Epidemiol 2003;158:1075–82.
6. Oddy WH. The impact of breastmilk on infant and child health. Breastfeed Rev 2002;10:5–18.
7. Donovan SM. Role of human milk components in gastrointestinal development: Current knowledge and future needs. J Pediatr 2006;149:49–61.
8. Field CJ. The immunological components of human milk and their effect on immune development in infants. J Nutr 2005;135:1–4.
9. Walker WA. The dynamic effects of breastfeeding on intestinal development and host defense. Adv Exp Med Biol 2004;554:155–70.
10. Dewey KG, Heinig MJ, Nommsen-Rivers LA. Differences in morbidity between breast-fed and formula-fed infants. J Pediatr 1995;126:696–702.
11. Lopez-Alarcon M, Villalpando S, Fajardo A. Breast-feeding lowers the frequency and duration of acute respiratory infection and diarrhea in infants under six months of age. J Nutr 1997;127:436–43.
12. Marild S, Hansson S, Jodal U, et al. Protective effect of breastfeeding against urinary tract infection. Acta Paediatr 2004;93:164–8.
13. Duncan B, Ey J, Holberg CJ, et al. Exclusive breast-feeding for at least 4 months protects against otitis media. Pediatrics 1993;91:867–72.
14. Kostraba JN, Cruickshanks KJ, Lawler-Heavner J, et al. Early exposure to cow's milk and solid foods in infancy, genetic predisposition, and the risk of IDDM. Diabetes 1993;42:288–95.
15. Greco L, Auricchio S, Mayer M, Grimaldi M. Case control study on nutritional risk factors in celiac disease. J Pediatr Gastroenterol Nutr 1988;7:395–9.
16. Sadauskaite-Kuehne V, Ludvigsson J, Padaiga Z, et al. Longer breastfeeding is an independent protective factor against development of type 1 diabetes mellitus in childhood. Diabetes Metab Res Rev 2004;20:150–7.
17. Chulada PC, Arbes SJ, Dunson D, Zeldin DC. Breastfeeding and the prevalence of asthma and wheeze in children: Analyses from the Third National Health and Nutrition Examination Survey, 1988–1994. J Allergy Clin Immunol 2003;111:328–36.
18. van Odijk J, Kull I, Borres MP, et al. Breastfeeding and allergic disease: A multidisciplinary review of the literature (1966–2001) on the mode of early feeding in infancy and its impact on later atopic manifestations. Allergy 2003;58:833–43.
19. Pesonen M, Kallio MJ, Ranki A, Siimes MA. Prolonged exclusive breastfeeding is associated with increased atopic dermatitis: A prospective follow-up study of unselected healthy newborns from birth to age 20 years. Clin Exp Allergy 2006;36:1011–8.
20. Klement E, Cohen RV, Boxman J, et al. Breastfeeding and risk of inflammatory bowel disease: A systematic review with meta-analysis. Am J Clin Nutr 2004;80:1342–52.
21. Baron S, Turck D, Leplat C, et al. Environmental risk factors in paediatric inflammatory bowel diseases: A population based case control study. Gut 2005;54:357–63.
22. Kramer MS, Kakuma R. Maternal dietary antigen avoidance during pregnancy or lactation, or both, for preventing or treating atopic disease in the child. Cochrane Database Syst Rev 2006;3:CD000133.
23. Gomez-Sanchiz M, Canete R, Rodero I, et al. Influence of breast-feeding and parental intelligence on cognitive development in the 24-month-old child. Clin Pediatr (Phila) 2004;43:753–61.
24. Rao MR, Hediger ML, Levine RJ, et al. Effect of breastfeeding on cognitive development of infants born small for gestational age. Acta Paediatr 2002;91:267–74.
25. Gustafsson PA, Duchen K, Birberg U, Karlsson T. Breastfeeding, very long polyunsaturated fatty acids (PUFA) and IQ at 6 1/2 years of age. Acta Paediatr 2004;93:1280–7.
26. Grummer-Strawn LM, Mei Z. Does breastfeeding protect against pediatric overweight? Analysis of longitudinal data from the Centers for Disease Control and Prevention Pediatric Nutrition Surveillance System. Pediatrics 2004;113:e81–6.
27. Li C, Kaur H, Choi WS, et al. Additive interactions of maternal prepregnancy BMI and breast-feeding on childhood overweight. Obes Res 2005;13:362–71.
28. Mayer-Davis EJ, Rifas-Shiman SL, Zhou L, et al. Breast-feeding and risk for childhood obesity: Does maternal diabetes and obesity status matter? Diabetes Care 2006;29:2231–7.
29. Owen CG, Martin RM, Whincup PE, et al. Does breastfeeding influence risk of type 2 diabetes in later life? A quantitative analysis of published evidence. Am J Clin Nutr 2006;84:1043–54.
30. Oddy WH, Li J, Landsborough L, et al. The association of maternal overweight and obesity with breastfeeding duration. J Pediatr 2006;149:185–91.
31. Rasmussen KM, Kjolhede CL. Prepregnant overweight and obesity diminish the prolactin response to suckling in the first week postpartum. Pediatrics 2004;113:e465–71.
32. US Department of Health and Human Services. Healthy People 2010: Conference Edition, Volumes I and II. Washington, DC: US Department of Health and Human Services, Public Health Service, Office of the Assistant Secretary for Health; 2000. p. 47–8.
33. US Department of Health and Human Services. HHS Blueprint for Action on Breastfeeding. Washington, DC: US Department of Health and Human Services, Public Health Service, Office on Women's Health; 2000.
34. Kramer MS, Kakuma R. The optimal duration of exclusive breastfeeding: A systematic review. Geneva, World Health Organization, document WHO/NHD/01.08-WHO/FCH/CAH/01.23; 2002.
35. Kramer MS, Kakuma R. The optimal duration of exclusive breastfeeding: a systematic review. Adv Exp Med Biol 2004;554:63–77.
36. Ryan AS, Wenjun Z, Acosta A. Breastfeeding continues to increase into the new millennium. Pediatrics 2002;110:1103–9.
37. Li R, Darling N, Maurice E, et al. Breastfeeding rates in the United States by characteristics of the child, mother, or family: The 2002 National Immunization Survey. Pediatrics 2005;115:e31–7.
38. Ryan AS, Zhou W. Lower breastfeeding rates persist among the Special Supplemental Nutrition Program for Women, Infants and Children participants, 1978–2003. Pediatrics 2006;117:1136–46.
39. Heinig MJ, Nommsen LA, Peerson JM, et al. Intake and growth of breast-fed infants and formula-fed infants in relation to the timing of introduction of complementary foods: The DARLING study. Davis Area Research on Lactation, Infant Nutrition and Growth. Acta Paediatr 1993;82:999–1006.
40. Kramer MS, Guo T, Platt RW, et al. Breastfeeding and infant growth: Biology or bias? Pediatrics 2002;110:343–7.
41. Kuczmarski RJ, Ogden C, Grummer-Strawn LM, et al. CDC Growth Charts: United States. NCHS Advance Data Report No. 314. Hyattsville, MD: US Department of Health and Human Services; 2000.
42. Garza C, de Onis M, for the WHO Multicenter Growth Reference Study Group. Rationale for developing a new international growth reference. Food Nutr Bull 2004;25:S5–14.
43. World Health Organization Multicenter Growth Reference Study Group. WHO child growth standards. Acta Paediatr Suppl 2006;450:1–101.
44. de Onis M, Onyango AW, Borghi E, et al. Comparison of the World Health Organization (WHO) child growth standards and the National Center for Health Statistics/WHO international growth reference: Implications for child health programs. Pub Health Nutr 2006;9:924–47.
45. Neville MC, Allen JC, Archer PC, et al. Studies in human lactation: Milk volume and nutrient composition during weaning and lactogenesis. Am J Clin Nutr 1991;54:81–92.
46. Hartmann PE, Cregan M. Lactogenesis and the effects of insulin-dependent diabetes mellitus and prematurity. J Nutr 2001;131:3016S–20S.
47. Cregan MD, De Melio TR, Kershaw D, et al. Initiation of lactation in women after preterm delivery. Acta Obstet Gynecol Scand 2002;81:870–7 .
48. Dewey KG, Nommsen-Rivers LA, Heinig MJ, Cohen RJ. Risk factors for suboptimal infant breastfeeding behavior, delayed onset of lactation, and excess neonatal weight loss. Pediatrics 2003;112:607–19.
49. Chapman DJ, Young S, Ferris AM, Perez-Escamilla R. Impact of breast pumping on lactogenesis stage II after cesarean delivery: A randomized clinical trial. Pediatrics 2001;107:e94.
50. Kent JC, Mitoulas LR, Cregan MD, et al. Volume and frequency of breastfeedings and fat content of breastmilk throughout the day. Pediatrics 2006;117:e387–95.
51. Mitoulas LR, Kent JC, Cox DB. Variation in fat, lactose and protein content in human milk over 24 h and throughout the first year of lactation. Br J Nutr 2002;88:29–37.
52. Picciano MF. Nutrient composition of human milk. Pediatr Clin North Am 2001;48:53–67.
53. Saarela T, Kokkonen J, Koivisto M. Macronutrient and energy contents of human milk fractions during the first six months of lactation. Acta Paediatr 2005;94:1176–81.
54. Velona T, Abbiati L, Beretta B, et al. Protein profiles in breast milk from mothers delivering term and preterm babies. Pediatr Res 1999;45:658–63.
55. Karra MV, Udipi SA, Kirksey A, Roepke JL. Changes in specific nutrients in breast milk during extended lactation. Am J Clin Nutr 1986;43:495–503.
56. Paxson CL, Adcock EW, Morriss FH. Osmolalities of infant formulas. Am J Dis Child 1977;131:139–41.
57. Ashraf RN, Jalil F, Aperia A, Lindblad BS. Additional water is not needed for healthy breast-fed babies in a hot climate. Acta Paediatr 1993;82:1007–11.
58. Cohen RJ, Brown KH, Rivera LL, Dewey KG. Exclusively breastfed, low birthweight infants do not need supplemental water. Acta Paediatr 2000;89:550–2.
59. Hosoi S, Honma K, Daimatsu T, et al. Lower energy content of milk than calculated using conversion factors. Pediatr Int 2005;47:7–9.
60. Davidson LA, Donovan SM, Lönnerdal B, Atkinson SA. Excretion of human milk proteins by term and premature infants. In: Atkinson SA, Lönnerdal B, editors. Protein and Non-Protein Nitrogen in Human Milk. Boca Raton, FL: CRC Press; 1989. p. 161–72.
61. Gnoth MJ, Kunz C, Kinne-Saffran E, Rudloff S. Human milk oligosaccharides are minimally digested in vitro. J Nutr 2000;130:3014–20.
62. Kunz C, Rudloff S, Baier W, et al. Oligosaccharides in human milk: Structural, functional, and metabolic aspects. Annu Rev Nutr 2000;20:699–722.
63. Coppa GV, Gabrielli O, Pierani P, et al. Changes in carbohydrate composition in human milk over 4 months of lactation. Pediatrics 1993;91:637–41.
64. Brew K, Hill RL. Lactose biosynthesis. Rev Phys Biochem Pharmacol 1975;72:105–58.

65. Arthur PG, Kent JC, Hartmann PE. Metabolites of lactose synthesis in milk of diabetic and nondiabetic women during lactogenesis II. J Pediatr Gastroenterol Nutr 1994;19:100–8.
66. Emey RM, Malone WT, Skelding MB, et al. Variability of human milk neutral oligosaccharides in a diverse population. J Pediatr Gastroenterol Nutr 2000;30:181–92.
67. Traving C, Schauer R. Structure, function and metabolism of sialic acids. Cell Mol Life Sci 1998;54:1330–49.
68. Wang B, Brand-Miller J, McVeagh P, Petocz P. The concentration and distribution of sialic acid in human milk vs. infant formulas. Am J Clin Nutr 2001;4:510–5.
69. Obermeier S, Rudloff S, Pohlentz G, et al. Secretion of ^{13}C-labelled oligosaccharides into human milk and urine after an oral [^{13}C]-galactose load. Isotopes Environ Health Stud 1999;35:119–25.
70. Newburg DS, Ruiz-Palacios G, Morrow AL. Human milk glycans protect infants against enteric pathogens. Annu Rev Nutr 2005;25:37–58.
71. Newburg DS. Do the binding properties of oligosaccharides in milk protect human infants from gastrointestinal bacteria? J Nutr 1997;127:980S–4S.
72. Rodriguez-Palmero M, Koletzko B, Kunz C, Jensen R. Nutritional and biochemical properties of human milk, II: Lipids, micronutrients, and bioactive factors. Clin Perinatol 1999;26:335–59.
73. Jensen RG. The lipids in human milk. Prog Lipid Res 1996;35:53–92.
74. Agostoni C, Marangoni F, Lammardo AM, et al. Long-chain polyunsaturated fatty acid concentrations in human hindmilk are constant throughout 12 months of lactation. Adv Exp Med Biol 2001;501:157–61.
75. Thompson BJ, Smith S. Biosynthesis of fatty acids by lactating human breast epithelial cells: An evaluation of the contribution to the overall composition of human milk fat. Pediatr Res 1985;19:139–43.
76. Demmelmair H, Baumheuer M, Koletzko B, et al. Metabolism of U^{13}C-labeled linoleic acid in lactating women. J Lipid Res 1998;39:1389–96.
77. Michalsky MC, Briard V, Michel F, et al. Size distribution of fat globules in human colostrum, breast milk, and infant formula. J Dairy Sci 2005;88:1927–40.
78. Hamosh M, Peterson JA, Henderson TR, et al. Protective function of human milk: The milk fat globule membrane. Semin Perinatol 1999;23:242–9.
79. Minda H, Kovács A, Funke S, et al. Changes in the fatty acid composition of human milk during the first month of lactation: A day-to-day approach in the first week. Ann Nutr Metab 2004;48:202–9.
80. Torres AG, Ney JG, Meneses F, Trugo NM. Polyunsaturated fatty acids and conjugated linoleic acid isomers in breast milk are associated with plasma non-esterified and erythrocyte membrane fatty acid composition in lactating women. Br J Nutr 2006;95:517–24.
81. Straarup EM, Lauritzen L, Faerk J, et al. The sterospecific triacylglycerol structures and fatty acids profiles of human milk and infant formulas. J Pediatr Gastroenterol Nutr 2006;42:293–9.
82. Desci T, Fekete M, Koletzko B. Plasma lipid and apolipoprotein concentrations in full term infants fed formula supplemented with long-chain polyunsaturated fatty acid and cholesterol. Eur J Pediatr 1997;156:397–400.
83. Kovács A, Funke S, Marosvölgyi T, et al. Fatty acids in early human milk after preterm and full-term delivery. J Pediatr Gastroenterol Nutr 2005;41:454–9.
84. Fleith M, Clandinin MT. Dietary PUFA for preterm and term infants: Review of clinical studies. Crit Rev Food Sci Nutr 2005;45:205–9.
85. Desci T. Nutritional relevance of trans isomeric fatty acid in human milk. Acta Pediatr 2003;156:1369–71.
86. Mosley EE, Wright AL, McGuire MK, McGuire MA. trans Fatty acids in milk produced by women in the United States. Am J Clin Nutr 2005;82:1292–7.
87. Friesen R, Innis SM. Trans fatty acids in human milk in Canada declined with the introduction of trans fat food labelling. J Nutr 2006;126:2558–61.
88. Innis SM, King DJ. *trans* Fatty acids in human milk are inversely associated with concentrations of all-cis n-6 and n-3 fatty acids and determine trans, but not n-6 and n-3, fatty acids in plasma lipids of breastfed infants. Am J Clin Nutr 1999;70:383–90.
89. Mosley EE, McGuire MK, Williams JE, McGuire MA. Cis-9, trans-11 conjugated linoleic acid is synthesized from vaccenic acid in lactating women. J Nutr 2006;136:2297–301.
90. Peterson DG, Matitashvili EA, Bauman DE. Diet-induced milk fat depression in dairy cows results in increased trans-10, cis-12 CLA in milk fat and coordinate suppression of mRNA abundance for mammary enzymes involved in milk fat synthesis. J Nutr 2003;133:3098–102.
91. Masters N, McGuire MA, Beerman KA, et al. Maternal supplementation with CLA decreases milk fat in humans. J Lipids 2002;37:133–8.
92. Bitman J, Wood DL, Mehta MR, et al. Comparison of cholesteryl ester composition of human milk from preterm and term mothers. J Pediatr Gastroent Nutr 1986;5:780–6.
93. Holmes-McNary M, Snodgrass GJAI, Zeisel SH. Changes in choline content of human breast milk in the first 3 weeks after birth. Eur J Pediatr 2000;159:198–204.
94. Zeisel SH. The fetal origins of memory: The role of dietary choline in optimal brain development. J Pediatr 2006;149:131–6.
95. Pan XL, Izumi T. Variation of the ganglioside compositions of human milk, cow's milk and infant formulas. Early Hum Dev 2000;57:25–31.
96. Laegreid A, Otnaess AB, Fuglesang J. Human and bovine milk: Comparison of ganglioside composition and enterotoxin-inhibitory activity. Pediatr Res 1986;20:416–21.
97. Wang B, McVeagh P, Petrocz P, Brand-Miller J. Brain ganglioside and glycoprotein sialic acid in breastfed compared with formula-fed infants. Am J Clin Nutr 2003;78:1024–9.
98. Rudloff S, Kunz C. Protein and nonprotein nitrogen components in human milk, bovine milk and infant formula: Quantitative and qualitative aspects in infant nutrition. J Pediatr Gastroent Nutr 1997;24:328–44.
99. Carlson SE. Human milk nonprotein nitrogen: Occurrence and possible functions. Adv Pediatr 1985;32:43–70.
100. Lönnerdal B. Nutritional and physiologic significance of human milk proteins. Am J Clin Nutr 2003:77:1537S–43S.
101. Karlsland Akeson PM, Axelsson IE, Raiha NC. Protein and amino acid metabolism in three- to twelve-month-old infants fed human milk or formulas with varying protein concentrations. J Pediatr Gastroenterol Nutr 1998;26:297–304.
102. Donovan SM and Odle J. Growth factors in milk as mediators of infant development. In: Olson RE, Bier DM, McCormick DB, editors. Annual Reviews of Nutrition. Vol 14. Palo Alto: Annual Reviews Inc; 1994. p. 147–67.
103. Ferranti P, Traisci MC, Picariello G, et al. Casein proteolysis in human milk: Tracing the pattern of casein breakdown and the formation of potential bioactive peptides. J Dairy Res 2004;71:74–87.
104. Lönnerdal B, Lien EL. Nutritional and physiologic significance of alpha-lactalbumin in infants. Nutr Rev 2003;61:295–305.
105. Håkansson A, Andreasson J, Zhivotovsky B, et al. Multimeric-lactalbumin from human milk induces apoptosis through a direct effect on cell nuclei. Exp Cell Res 1999;246:451–60.
106. Lien EL, Davis A, and Multi-center Study Group. Growth and safety in term infants fed reduced protein formula with added bovine alpha-lactalbumin. J Pediatr Gastroenterol Nutr 2004;38:170–6.
107. Adkins Y, Lönnerdal B. Potential host-defense role of human milk vitamin B-12-binding protein, haptocorrin, in the gastrointestinal tract of breastfed infants, as assessed with porcine haptocorrin in vitro. Am J Clin Nutr 2003;77:1234–40.
108. Strömqvist M, Falk P, Bergström S, et al. Human milk κ-casein and inhibition of *Helicobacter pylori* adhesion to human gastric mucosa. J Pediatr Gastroenterol Nutr 1995;21:288–96.
109. Tomita M, Bellamy W, Takase M, et al. Potent antibacterial peptides generate by digestion of bovine lactoferrin. J Dairy Sci 1991;74:4137–42.
110. Pelligrini A, Thomas U, Bramaz N, et al. Isolation and identification of three bactericidal domains in the bovine α-lactalbumin molecule. Biochem Biophys Acta 1999;1426:439–48.
111. Liepke C, Adermann K, Raida M, et al. Human milk provides peptides highly stimulating the growth of bifidobacteria. Eur J Biochem 2002;269:712–8.
112. Koldovsky O. The potential physiological significance of milk-borne hormonally active substances for the neonate. J Mammary Gland Biol Neoplasia 1996;1:317–23.
113. Howarth GS, Shoubridge CA. Enhancement of intestinal growth and repair by growth factors. Curr Opin Pharmacol 2001;1:568–74.
114. Houle VM, Laswell SC, Freund GG, Dudley MA, Donovan SM. Investigation of three doses of oral insulin-like growth factor-I on jejunal lactase phlorizin hydrolase activity and gene expression and enterocyte proliferation and migration in piglets. Pediatr Res 2000;48:497–503.
115. Hernell O, Bläckberg L. Digestion of human milk lipids: Physiologic significance of sn-2monoacylglycerol hydrolysis by bile-salt stimulated lipase. Pediatr Res 1983;16:882–5.
116. Lindberg T, Ohlsson K, Weström B. Protease inhibitors and their relation to proteases in human milk. Pediatr Res 1982;16:479–83.
117. Donovan SM, Lönnerdal B. Non-protein nitrogen and true protein in infant formulas. Acta Paediatr Scand 1989;78:497–504.
118. Heine W, Tiess M, Wutzke K. 15N tracer investigations of the physiological availability of urea nitrogen in mother's milk. Acta Paediatr Scand 1986;75:439–43.
119. Donovan SM, Lönnerdal B, Atkinson SA. Bioavailability of urea nitrogen for the low birthweight infant. Acta Paediatr Scand 1990;79:899–905.
120. Allen LH. Multiple micronutrients in pregnancy and lactation: An overview. Am J Clin Nutr 2005;81:1206S–12S.
121. Olafsdottir AS, Wagner KH, Thorsdottir I, Elmadfa I. Fat soluble vitamins in the maternal diet, influence of cod liver oil supplementation and impact of the maternal diet on human milk composition. Ann Nutr Metab 2001;45:265–72.
122. Greer FR, Marshall SP, Foley AL, et al. Improving the vitamin K status of breastfeeding infants with maternal vitamin K supplementations. Pediatrics 1997;99:88–92.
123. Sneed SM, Zane C, Thomas MR. The effects of ascorbic acid, vitamin B_6, vitamin B_{12}, and folic acid supplementation on the breast milk and maternal nutritional status and of low-income socioeconomic lactating women. Am J Clin Nutr 1981;34:1338–46.
124. Nail PA, Thomas MR, Eakins R. The effect of thiamine and riboflavin supplementation on the level of those vitamins in breastmilk and urine. Am J Clin Nutr 1980;33:198–204.
125. Greer FR. Do breastfed infants need supplemental vitamins? Pediatr Clin North Am 2001;48:415–23.
126. American Academy of Pediatrics, Section on Breastfeeding and Committee on Nutrition. Prevention of rickets and vitamin D deficiency: New guidelines for vitamin D intake. Pediatrics 2003;111:908–10.
127. American Academy of Pediatrics, Committee on Fetus and Newborn. Controversies concerning vitamin K and the newborn. Pediatrics 2003;112:191–2.
128. Lietz G, Mulokozi G, Henry JCK, Tomkins AM. Xanthophyll and hydrocarbon carotenoid patterns differ in plasma and breast milk of women supplemented with red palm oil during pregnancy and lactation. J Nutr 2006;136:1821–7.
129. Canfield LM, Clandinin MT, Davies DP, et al. Multinational study of major breast milk carotenoids of healthy mothers. Eur J Nutr 2003;42:133–41.
130. Macias C, Schweigert FJ. Changes in the concentration of carotenoids, vitamin A, alpha-tocopherol and total lipids in human milk throughout early lactation. Ann Nutr Metab 2001;45:82–5.
131. Chappell JE, Francis T, Clandinin MT. Vitamin A and E content of human milk at early stages of lactation. Early Hum Dev 1985;11:157–67.
132. Greer FR, Hollis BW, Cripps D. The effects of ultraviolet B irradiation on the vitamin D content of human milk. J Pediatr 1984;105:431–3.
133. American Academy of Pediatrics, Committee on Environmental Health. Ultraviolet light: A hazard to children. Pediatrics 1999;114:328–33.
134. Stone WL, LeClair I, Ponder T, et al. Infants discriminate between natural and synthetic vitamin E. Am J Clin Nutr 2003;77:899–906.
135. Korchazhkina O, Jones E, Czauderna M, Spencer SA. Effects of exclusive formula or breastmilk feeding on oxidative stress in healthy preterm infants. Arch Dis Child 2006;91:329–9.
136. Niklowitz P, Menke T, Giffei J, Andler W. Coenzyme Q10 in maternal plasma and milk throughout early lactation. Biofactors 2005;25:67–72.
137. Quiles JL, Ochoa JJ, Ramirez-Tortosa MC, et al. Coenzyme Q concentration and total antioxidant capacity of human milk at different stages of lactation in mothers of preterm and full-term infants. Free Radic Res 2006;40:199–206.
138. Kojima T, Asoh M, Yamawaki N, et al. Vitamin K concentrations in the maternal milk of Japanese women. Acta Paediatr 2004;93:457–63.
139. Greer FR, Mummah-Schendel L, Marshall S, Suttie JW. Vitamin K_1 and K_2 in the newborn. J Pediatr 1988;81:137–40.
140. Picciano MF. Water-soluble vitamins in human milk. In Jensen RG, editors. The Handbook of Milk Composition. San Diego: Academic Press; 1995. p. 675–87.
141. Daneel-Otterbech S, Davidsson L, Hurrell R. Ascorbic acid supplementation and regular consumption of fresh orange juice increase the ascorbic acid content of human milk: Studies in European and African lactating women. Am J Clin Nutr 2005;81:1088–93.
142. Debuse PJ. Shoshin beriberi in an infant of a thiamine-deficient mother. Acta Paediatr 1992;81:723–4.
143. Sherwood KL, Houghton LA, Tarasuk V, O'Connor DL. One-third of pregnant and lactating women may not be meeting their folate requirements from diet alone based on mandated levels of folic acid fortification. J Nutr 2006;136:2820–6.

144. Weiss R, Fogelman Y, Bennett M. Severe vitamin B_{12} deficiency in an infant associated with a maternal deficiency and a strict vegetarian diet. J Pediatr Hematol Oncol 2004;26:270–1.
145. Grange DK, Finlay JL. Nutritional vitamin B_{12} deficiency in a breastfed infant following maternal gastric bypass. Pediatr Hematol Oncol 1994;11:311–8.
146. Salmenpera L, Perheentupa J, Pispa JP, Siimes MA. Biotin concentrations in maternal plasma and milk during prolonged lactation. Int J Vitam Nutr Res 1985;55:281–5.
147. Mock DM, Mock NI, Dankle JA. Secretory patterns of biotin in milk. J Nutr 1992;122:546–52.
148. Song WO, Chan GM, Wyse BW, Hansen RG. Effect of pantothenic acid status on the content of the vitamin in human milk. Am J Clin Nutr 1984;40:317–24.
149. Parr RM, DaMaeyer EM, Iyengar VG, et al. Minor and trace elements in human milk from Guatemala, Hungary, Nigeria, Philippines, Sweden and Zaire. Results from a WHO/IAEA joint project. Biol Trace Elem Res 1991;29:51–75.
150. Atkinson SA, Alston-Mills B, Lönnerdal B, et al. Major minerals and ionic constituents in human and bovine milk. In: Jensen RG, editor. The Handbook of Milk Composition. San Diego: Academic Press; 1995. p. 593–621.
151. Casey CE, Smith A, Zhang P. Microminerals in human and animal milks. In: Jensen RG, editor. The Handbook of Milk Composition. San Diego: Academic Press; 1995. p. 622–74.
152. Domellof M, Lönnerdal B, Dewey KG, et al. Iron, zinc and copper concentrations in breast milk are independent of maternal mineral status. Am J Clin Nutr 2004;79:111–5.
153. Chierici R, Sacccomandi D, Vigi V. Dietary supplements for the lactating mother: Influence on the trace element content of milk. Acta Paediatr Scand 1999;88:7–13.
154. Kelleher SL, Lönnerdal B. Molecular regulation of milk trace mineral homeostasis. Mol Aspects Med 2005;26:328–39.
155. Lönnerdal B. Trace element absorption in infants as a foundation to setting upper limits for trace elements in infant formulas. J Nutr 1989;119:1839–44.
156. Fransson GB, Lönnerdal B. Distribution of trace elements and minerals in human and cow's milk. Pediatr Res 1983;17:912–5.
157. Krachler M, Li FS, Rossipal E, Irgolic KJ. Changes in the concentrations of trace elements in human milk during lactation. J Trace Elem Med Biol 1998;12:171–81.
158. Lönnerdal B. Copper nutrition during infancy and childhood. Am J Clin Nutr 1998;67:1046S–53S.
159. Esala S, Vuori E, Helle A. Effect of maternal fluorine intake on breast milk fluorine content. Br J Nutr 1982;48:201–4.
160. Bader N, Moller U, Leiterer M, et al. Pilot study: Tendency of increasing iodine content in human milk and cow's milk. Exp Clin Endocrinol Diabetes 2005;113:8–12.
161. Hunt CD, Butte NF, Johnson LK. Boron concentrations in milk from mothers of exclusively breast-fed healthy full-term infants are stable during the first four months of lactation. J Nutr 2005;135:2383–6.
162. LaKind JS, Wilkins AA, Berlin CM, Jr. Environmental chemicals in human milk: A review of levels, infant exposures and health, and guidance for future research. Toxicol Appl Pharmacol 2004;198:184–208.
163. Massart F, Harrell JC, Federico G, Saggese G. Human breast milk and xenoestrogen exposure: A possible impact on human health. J Perinatol 2005;25:282–8.
164. Landrigan PJ, Sonawane B, Mattison D, et al. Chemical contaminants in breast milk and their impacts on children's health: An overview. Environ Health Perspect 2002;110:313–5.
165. Pronczuk J, Akre J, Moy G, Vallenas C. Global perspectives in breast milk contamination: Infectious and toxic hazards. Environ Health Perspect 2002;110:349–51.
166. American Academy of Pediatrics, Committee on Drugs. The transfer of drugs and other chemicals into human milk. Pediatrics 2001;108:776–89.
167. Ito S, Lee A. Drug excretion into breast milk—an overview. Adv Drug Deliv Rev 2003;55:617–27.
168. Ito S, Blajchman A, Stephenson M, et al. Prospective follow-up of adverse reactions in breast-fed infants exposed to maternal medication. Am J Obstet Gynecol 1993;168;1393–9.
169. American Academy of Pediatrics, Committee on Pediatric AIDS. Human milk, breastfeeding, and transmission of human immunodeficiency virus type 1 in the United States. Pediatrics 2003:112:1196–203.
170. World Health Organization. Protecting, Promoting and Supporting Breastfeeding: The Special Role of Maternity Services, a Joint WHO/UNICEF Statement. Geneva, Switzerland: WHO; 1989.

Protective Properties of Human Milk

Anne Donnet-Hughes, PhD
Eduardo J. Schiffrin, MD, PhD
W. Allan Walker, MD

Human breast milk is an undeniably unique, natural source of nutrition for the human infant. However, in addition to the nutritive value it imparts, breast milk and breast-feeding are well recognized to protect against gastrointestinal infections, diarrheal diseases, and respiratory infections.[1] Such protective effects have been variously ascribed to the presence in milk of maternal leukocytes, immunoglobulins, growth factors, and immune factors. While some of these components interact directly with bacterial cells, others mediate their effects by promoting proliferation, maturation, and activation of neonatal cells and by ensuring homeostasis. The net result is an enhanced protection of the immature intestine against colonization and invasion by pathogenic bacteria.

Much of the immunologic benefit of breast milk previously described in reviews of the subject has been attributed to the passive protection that it provides.[2] It is apparent that although breast milk supplies a combination of protective factors, functional redundancy is not rare. Not only do several factors exhibit the same biological function, a single molecule can have a range of biological activities. This complexity and the change in the concentration of specific components as lactation proceeds are testimony to a dynamic biological fluid, the complete function of which has still to be fully appreciated. Indeed, there is now evidence to suggest that protective effects of breast milk extend beyond the neonatal period and can influence the development of pathologic diseases later in life.[3] This is further support for a more intimate association between the maternally derived milk factors and the neonatal immune system beyond that required to prevent pathogen colonization and infection.

The mechanisms underlying the long-lasting benefits of breast milk are likely to be multifarious. However, at least two different and partially overlapping processes are probably involved. First, breast milk factors, in shaping the composition of the neonatal microbiota, indirectly influence immune system development and response. Second, breast milk directly "educates" the neonatal immune system to react with appropriate innate or adaptive immune responses upon microbial and antigenic challenge. Indeed, there is increasing evidence to suggest that upon exposure to antigen, breast milk educates the neonatal immune system in the decisions to be made.

Breast milk contains a myriad of factors that, qualitatively or quantitatively, may modulate how neonatal cells perceive microbial components or respond to microbes with which they come in contact. Examples are immunoglobulins, glycoproteins, and glycolipids, which interfere with bacterial binding to epithelial cells, and oligosaccharides and antimicrobial peptides, which encourage the preponderance of particular microbial species.

It has also been suggested that the latter is achieved via breast milk–derived bacteria that ultimately colonize the neonatal gut.[4] However, an emerging concept is that breast milk influences the neonatal immune system's perception of "danger." To do so, some milk molecules may actually facilitate the intestinal response to specific microbial motifs by activating intracellular signaling pathways such as that of nuclear factor (NF)-κB, a major regulator of the inflammatory response. At first, this might appear to contradict the recognized anti-inflammatory effect of breast milk. However, the present chapter will elaborate further on breast milk factors that modulate the neonate's perception of danger signals in the absence of exaggerated inflammation. More specifically, it will address those factors that promote a beneficial microbial flora either directly or indirectly via education of neonatal cells. Moreover, it will challenge the theory that milk is strictly anti-inflammatory by proposing novel mechanisms by which the mother already educates her infant in the immediate postnatal period.

THE BASIS OF INNATE AND ADAPTIVE IMMUNE RESPONSES IN THE INTESTINE

The intestine is the largest immune apparatus in the body and, as such, the immunological events taking place in its tissues have a major impact on the overall immune status of the host. The development and effectiveness of this system is influenced by a number of cellular elements and luminal antigens that include but are not limited to epithelial and immune sentinel cells in the mucosal tissue and dietary antigen, immunomodulatory factors, and a substantial, heterogenous inoculum of microbial motifs in the lumen.[5] A prerequisite for a healthy intestine is an immune system that can differentiate these luminal antigens and initiate a protective response to "danger signals" while remaining tolerant to nonthreatening microbes, dietary antigens, and endogenous host cells and molecules.[6,7]

The single layer of epithelial cells overlying the lamina propria and lymphoid follicles of the intestine is in direct contact with luminal contents and functions as an early warning system of impending microbial attack. Any delay in response to real threat could seriously compromise the host; thus, an alert is triggered by all organisms. However, the magnitude and precise nature of the response are determined by the characteristics of the microbe. Broadly speaking, nonpathogens mount limited responses with a transient innate component[8] that might explain the low level of physiological inflammation observed in the intestine. In contrast, pathogens induce rapid and more vigorous responses that are accompanied by some tissue damage.[6] In each case, both innate and adaptive immune processes are engaged. Thus, the host reaction can be considered as a stratified response whose primary tier is triggered by most bacteria and is proinflammatory, but whose second level of activation involves an assembly of gene products that are defined by the virulence traits of the organism.[9] However, the nature of the response is also governed by the level of maturation and activation of immune sentinel cells. Upon antigenic challenge, pattern recognition receptors (PRRs), such as the Toll-like receptor (TLR) family of proteins, empower these cells to recognize and interact with a number of microbial components and endogenous host proteins[6,7] and to relate cellular signals needed for appropriate action. Several members of the TLR family, capable of recognizing single or multiple microbial motifs, have been identified (Table 1). Their expression can be inducible or constitutive and is dependent on cell type and intestinal location.[10] Nucleotide-binding oligomerization domain (NOD) 1 and NOD2 are a structurally distinct family of intracellular PRRs that are expressed in intestinal epithelial cells (IECs), Paneth cells,[11] in macrophages, T and B cells, and dendritic cells (DCs).[12] These PRRs have been less studied and, to date, the only known ligands for NOD1 and NOD2 are, respectively, the gram-negative peptidoglycan (PGN) derivative γ-D-glutamyl-*meso*-diamino-pimelic acid and muramyl dipeptide.[10]

Table 1 Recognition of Bacterial and Viral Motifs by Human Toll-Like Receptors

Microbial Components: Bacterial (b) and Viral (v)	Host TLR Molecules	Main Cellular Compartment*
Triacyl lipopeptides (b)	TLR1 / TLR2	Plasma membrane
Proteoglycan, porins, lipomamnan, lipoarabinomannan (b)	TLR2	Plasma membrane
Hemagglutinin protein (v)	TLR2	Plasma membrane and intracellular
dsRNA (v)	TLR3	Intracellular
Lipopolysaccharide (b)	TLR4	Plasma membrane
Envelope proteins (v)	TLR4	Plasma membrane
Flagellin (b)	TLR5	Plasma membrane
Diacyl lipopeptides, lipotheichoic acid (b)	TLR6 / TLR2	Plasma membrane
ssRNA (v)	TLR7 and TLR8	Intracellular
CpG-DNA (b)	TLR9	Intracellular
DNA (v)	TLR9	Intracellular

*Epithelial and immune cells.

NEONATAL INTESTINAL IMMUNITY AND THE DEVELOPMENT OF THE MICROBIOTA

The neonatal intestine is sterile at birth but is immediately exposed, not only to potential pathogens but to a multitude of nonpathogenic organisms, some of which ultimately form the commensal microbiota. This potentially hazardous process is nevertheless vital for the development and maturation of the intestinal immune system.[13] Indeed, the hygiene hypothesis, proposed to explain the rise in atopic diseases, suggests that early in life, microbial antigens interacting with the innate immune system tip adaptive immune responses toward a T helper (Th)-1, and away from a Th2, response. A recent adaptation of this hypothesis proposes that instead of priming immune activation, such microbial stimulation primes immunoregulation via T regulatory (T_{reg}) cells and regulatory antigen presenting cells.[14]

During the first days of life, the intestinal microbiota undergoes major compositional changes until a steady state is reached around weaning.[15] The mode of delivery, the gestational age, hospitalization and length of hospital stay, the use of antibiotics, as well as the type of nutrition all have some bearing on the composition of the neonatal microbiota.[16] Bifidobacteria, lactobacilli, streptococci, staphylococci, *Bacteroides* species, and *Escherichia coli* are present in the newborn fecal matter[17] but while bifidobacteria has a net predominance in the stools of breast-fed infants, enterobacteria, coliforrms, and clostridia reach high levels almost equivalent to those of bifidobacteria in the stools of the formula fed.[18] The number and type of bacteria competing for an intestinal habitat, as well as the high density of microbial antigens and molecular motifs, may be contributory factors in a variety of immune and inflammatory neonatal conditions such as necrotizing enterocolitis (NEC) and gut-derived sepsis. It has been postulated that in human newborns, particularly preterm infants, an inappropriate inflammatory reaction to intestinal microorganisms is a causative factor for NEC.[19] Furthermore, overgrowth of abnormal bacterial flora can cause septicemia in human newborns receiving enteral nutrition.[20] Importantly, breast milk protects against bacterial translocation in neonatal animals and against septicemia and NEC in premature human infants.[21,22]

For successful colonization, healthy immune status and a beneficial relationship with the microbiota throughout life, the most elementary immunoregulatory mechanisms must already exist in the neonatal intestine at birth. Certainly, some immune instruction already begins prenatally and depends on the thymus for the generation of self-tolerant effector and regulatory T cells.[23] Immature T cells interact with thymic epithelial cells in a vital process that ensures the maturation, differentiation, and selection processes of the mature T cell pool.[24] These prenatal events explain the central features of adaptive immunity already present at birth. However, while it is important to restrict antigen exposure in utero for fetal survival, it leads to deficits in adaptive immunity in the newborn period.

Although the innate response is not considered to require previous immunological experience to be activated, the sophisticated control mechanisms operating in the adult intestine are not expected of the naïve neonatal immune system, particularly if one considers that the same host receptors recognize both pathogens and nonpathogens.[25] Indeed, the increased susceptibility of neonates to infection and certain allergens suggests that the capacity to handle antigenic challenge is not inherent but develops over time and/or through education and experience. In the immediate postnatal period, the cellular composition of the microbiota is highly variable as many organisms vie to colonize the mucosa. This physiological process can trigger an inflammatory response not only in the gut but also systemically owing to the high permeability of the neonatal intestine.[26] Remarkably, detrimental inflammatory reactions do not normally occur and immune homeostasis prevails. Possible explanations are a low expression of TLR2 and TLR4 on IECs and lamina propria cells[25] and/or limited cellular signaling following engagement with nonpathgens.[27] However, the greater incidence of infections, inflammation, and allergy in formula-fed infants compared to breastfed infants suggests that breast milk is a source of protective regulatory factors.

MILK FACTORS DEFINING THE INTESTINAL MICROBIOTA AND THE ORGANISMS THAT INTERACTS WITH THE NEONATAL IMMUNE SYSTEM

Closer scrutiny of the interplay among specific milk molecules, microbes, and the mucosal immune system is beginning to unravel some of the intricacies of breast milk protection. It is becoming apparent that exogenous factors in milk play a regulatory, or even an educational, role in the underlying immune processes. Simplistically, soluble factors in breast milk can prevent microbial antigens, pathogenic or not, from reaching the cells in host tissues (Table 2). Through their bacteriostatic or bactericidal action, some of these factors define the nature of microbial antigens that succeed in interacting with the intestinal immune system. The most recent research now suggests that breast milk permits, and indeed

Table 2 Human Milk Factors That Define the Intestinal Microbiota

Oligosaccharides and glycoconjugates	Receptor analogues that inhibit binding of pathogens and their toxins to epithelial cells
	Bifidogenic effect
Mucin 1	Inhibits binding of *S*-fimbriated *E. coli* and rotavirus to epithelial cells
Lactadherin	Inhibits binding of rotavirus to epithelial cells
Defensins and cathelicidins	Bacterial killing via membrane disruption
Lactoferrin	Bacterial killing by lactoferricin peptide
	Bacteriostatic activity by binding ferric iron
	Bifidogenic effect
Lysozyme	Bacterial killing via membrane disruption
Secretory IgA	Inhibits binding of pathogens to the intestinal mucosa
	Facilitates biofilm formation by the normal flora
	Bifidogenic effect of secretory component
α-Lactalbumin	Antibacterial peptides
Fatty acids	Antibacterial activity

encourages, interaction between particular microbial motifs and this immune system but curbs any energetic innate reaction. In so doing, breast milk cultivates a healthy relationship between the neonatal immune system and the various bacterial communities that constitute the permanent microbiota of the gut.

Antimicrobial Human Milk Oligosaccharides and Glycoconjugates

Human milk oligosaccharides (HMOs) are synthesized by specific mammary gland glycosyltransferases, which sequentially add fucose, galactose, *N*-acetylglucosamine, and sialic acid to lactose. The large number of oligosaccharides present in human milk decrease in concentration with increased lactation[28] length and are key elements in preventing bacterial adherence to, and colonization of, the neonatal stomach and small bowel.[29] This is achieved by molecular mimicry. Different pathogens, such as *Streptococcus pneumoniae*, *E. coli*, *Campylobacter jejuni*, *Listeria monocytogenes*, *Shigella*, *Salmonella*, and *Vibrio cholera*, initiate the infectious process by adhering, via carbohydrate-binding proteins, to oligosaccharides expressed on epithelial cell membranes.[30] In vitro, epidemio logical and clinical studies[31] suggest that HMOs protect against infection by serving as soluble ligands for the virulence factors of adhesion, the specificity of the effects being determined by the chemical nature of the HMO. However, HMOs may also mediate their protective effects by modifying the composition of the glycocalyx or the expression of glycoproteins on the epithelial surface.[32] Together, these mechanisms suppress colonization by harmful microorganisms. The impact in shaping the commensal microbiota has not been addressed but is implied by the observation that breast-fed infants harbor less P-fimbriated *E. coli* than type 1 fimbriated *E. coli*, and are thereby less likely to suffer from urinary infections.[33]

The milk fat globule membrane glycoproteins, mucin (MUC)-1 and lactadherin, inhibit rotavirus replication and prevent experimental gastroenteritis through their sialic acid residues.[34] Milk MUC1 has also been shown to inhibit the adhesion of S-fimbriated *E. coli* to epithelial cells in vitro.[35] Several other glycoconjugates of human milk are now known and include the ganglioside GM1, which binds to cholera toxin and labile toxins of *E. coli* and *C. jejuni*; the neutral glycolipid globotriosyl ceramide, which binds to toxins of *Shigella* and *E. coli*; a mannosylated glycoprotein that inhibits binding of some strains of *E. coli* to human intestinal epithelium; and finally, glycosaminoglycans, which inhibit binding of the outer membrane protein of the AIDS virus to CD4 T cells.[36]

Antimicrobial Proteins and Peptides

Antimicrobial proteins and peptides (AMPs) are key effectors of the innate immune response. They are expressed by circulating cells and epithelial cells and mediate their effect by disrupting microbial membranes. They have broad-spectrum antibiotic activity against bacteria, viruses, yeast, and fungi and thereby modulate the composition of the intestinal microbiota and confer protection against environmental and pathogenic organisms. Numerous peptides and proteins with antimicrobial activity have been described in humans, but they differ in their tissue localization, regulation, and additional biological activities.[37] Important classes are the cationic α- and β-defensins and the cathelicidins, which protect against bacterial colonization of gut, lung, and skin epithelia.

While α-defensins are constitutively expressed in human neutrophils and Paneth cells of the small intestinal crypts, β-defensins are expressed predominantly in the epithelial cells of the gastrointestinal tract, and cathelicidin (LL-37/hCAP18) is expressed by neutrophils and mast cells, as well as by differentiated epithelial cells in the colon and stomach and in Brunner's glands of the duodenum.[37] Paneth cells are considered particularly important in antibacterial defense since they secrete other antimicrobial peptides such as lysozyme and secretory phospholipase A2. Both the numbers of Paneth cells and the expression of antimicrobial peptides are developmentally regulated and can already be detected in human fetal intestine at 24 weeks' gestation.[38] However, the human newborn has fewer numbers of Paneth cells and less antimicrobial peptides than adults.

The importance of Paneth cells and their expression of antimicrobial peptides in neonatal defence are suggested by animal studies demonstrating increased susceptibility to infection in animals following ablation of the Paneth cell population.[39] Furthermore, the absence of lysozyme in the Paneth cells of preterm and term infants with NEC supports a causative link between Paneth cell secretion of antimicrobial peptides and NEC.[40] The presence of an exogenous source of antimicrobial peptides in human breast milk may therefore compensate for the deficit in Paneth cells and antimicrobial peptides observed in the immature neonatal intestine. Certainly, lysozyme, defensins, and cathelicidin are produced by mammary gland epithelial cells and milk cells, are present in milk in significant concentrations throughout lactation, and have demonstrable antimicrobial activity against a range of organisms.[41–43]

Lactoferrin is a major protein of breast milk that is present throughout lactation and has multiple biological effects. By virtue of its iron-binding properties, lactoferrin has been proposed to play a role in iron uptake by the intestinal mucosa and to act as a bacteriostatic agent by withholding iron from iron-requiring bacteria.[44] An antimicrobial effect of lactoferrin, independent of the degree of iron saturation, has also been described[45] and may be due to the generation of the bactericidal peptide, lactoferricin, during digestion.[46] However, lactoferrin is relatively stable in the neonatal intestine and can be found intact or partially hydrolysed in the feces of suckling but not formula-fed infants.[47] In vitro studies have also demonstrated antifungal[48] and antiviral effects of lactoferrin.[49]

Growth Factors for the Commensal Microbiota

Breast milk may directly influence the composition of the neonatal microbiota other than by antimicrobial activity. For example, it also contains a variety of factors that promote the growth of beneficial bacteria. The majority of studies examining such factors have focused on HMO. These are resistant to gastrointestinal digestion and arrive in the colon in an intact form where they serve as nutrients for colonic bacteria and preferentially support the growth of bifidobacteria.[50] However, lactoferrin has also been shown to promote growth of *Bifidobacterium* and *Lactobacillus* species.[51] Moreover, peptides generated from lactoferrin and from the secretory component of sIgA have also been shown to be bifidogenic.[52]

Immunoglobulins

Although intestinal lymphoid structures are present at birth, immunoglobulin-producing B cells are not fully operational for several weeks.[53] This delay in B cell activation causes a deficit in secretory IgA (sIgA) production and reduced protection of the neonatal intestinal mucosa.[54] However, microbial stimulation leads to an active B cell population by 1 month postpartum. These B cells become plasma cells that produce polymeric IgM and, most frequently, dimeric IgA, which are transported through the epithelium by polymeric immunoglobulin receptors.[55]

In the early newborn period, breast milk–derived antibodies compensate for the deficit in neonatal production. These milk antibodies are produced in the mammary gland by B lymphoblasts that have trafficked from gastrointestinal and bronchial lymphoid tissues in the mother.[56] The dominant immunoglobulin in milk is sIgA, which protects neonatal mucosal surfaces by agglutinating and immobilizing different pathogens.[57] The repertoire of milk antibody specificity is governed by the infectious agents to which the mother has been exposed[58] and can be directed against both enteric and respiratory pathogens, including viruses.[59] Concentrations of sIgA are higher in the feces of breast-fed infants than in those of formula-fed infants[60] and may reflect the capacity of milk sIgA to resist gastrointestinal digestion. By a mechanism known as "immune exclusion," sIgA binds and agglutinates pathogens and thereby, prevents their adhesion to the intestinal epithelium and facilitates their elimination by peristalsis.[61] However, although many bacteria in the intestinal microbiota are also coated with sIgA, they are not permanently removed from the intestine.[62] The reasons for this apparent inconsistency are not known but could be related to the type and specificity of the antibody in each case. In addition, sIgA may also facilitate biofilm formation by the normal flora in the large bowel, a process that may aid in the development of the normal flora and attenuate growth of pathogenic microorganisms.[63]

IMMUNOMODULATORY ACTIVITIES OF BREAST MILK DURING NEONATAL INTESTINAL COLONIZATION

Protection and education of offspring are integral parts of evolutionary success, and breast milk composition has adapted to meet these requirements. However, while the passive protection afforded by breast milk is well recognized, the manner by which it educates the neonatal immune system is less obvious. Through their immunomodulatory activity, milk growth factors and cytokines may affect neonatal immune development, but arguably, the finest education is achieved through experience. To this end, milk limits but does not completely veto bacterial interaction with the intestinal immune system. Indeed, such interactions are important for postnatal maturation of intestinal immunity,[13] and any delay to this maturation, such as that caused by reduced microbial stimulation, may increase susceptibility to allergic disease.[14] The following sections discuss how milk may modulate microbial interactions with receptors on host cells thereby encouraging cellular activation to particular microbial motifs but preventing crude, exaggerated inflammatory responses that may occur more readily in immature cells.

PRR–Bacteria Interactions in the Presence of Breast Milk

Lipopolysaccharide of gram-negative bacteria is a potent stimulator of the innate immune response, but it requires several host humoral and cell-surface proteins to mediate its effects. These include the acute-phase lipopolysaccharide (LPS)-binding protein (LBP), and the glycoproteins CD14, TLR4, and myeloid differentiation protein–2 (MD-2).[64] Cellular activation begins when LPS binds to LBP, which subsequently accelerates LPS binding to CD14 on the cell surface[65] However, LPS is then transferred from the CD14–LBP complex to a cell-surface TLR4–MD-2 complex, which transduces intracellular signaling.[66] In contrast, cellular activation by the lipoteichoic acid (LTA) of gram-positive bacteria involves LBP-, CD14-, and TLR2-mediated signals.[67]

TLRs belong to a superfamily called the TLR/IL-1R whose members have a Toll/IL-1 receptor (TIR) domain.[68] Upon ligand binding to TLRs, this cytoplasmic domain activates a cascade of adapter signaling molecules that include myeloid differentiation marker (MyD88), IL-1 receptor–activated kinase (IRAK), and tumor necrosis factor receptor–associated factor (TRAF)-6. Their sequential recruitment leads to activation of NF-κB and mitogen-activated protein kinases[69] and induction of an inflammatory response.

Human breast milk contains high levels of soluble forms of CD14 (sCD14)[70,71] and TLR2,[72] which with lactoferrin may modulate TLR signaling (Table 3). Depending on its concentration and environment, sCD14 can activate or inhibit responses to LPS by respectively transferring LPS to[73] or diverting LPS from[74] membrane CD14 (mCD14). Furthermore, sCD14 can transfer LPS directly to the TLR4–MD2 receptor complex in cells that lack mCD14, such as endothelial and epithelial cells.[75] It is feasible therefore that the ambivalent nature of sCD14 allows physiological activation of cells for homeostasis but prevents exaggerated inflammation during infection or sepsis. Further assurance may be provided by additional milk proteins that bind sCD14 and lessen sCD14–LPS or sCD14-bacterial lipoprotein (BLP)-mediated cell activation. An example of the former is the antimicrobial protein lactoferrin that binds specifically and with high affinity to the lipid A region of LPS[76] as well as to sCD14 and the sCD14–LPS complex.[77] The more recently discovered sTLR2 also decreases in concentration over the lactation period and, by binding to sCD14 in milk, has been postulated to moderate responses to BLP.[72]

Thus, some receptors in cell-surface TLR complexes exist as soluble forms in milk and act as decoy receptors for microbial motifs (Table 3). Still other proteins found in milk, such as IL-10 and transforming growth factor (TGF)-β, at constant levels throughout the first months of lactation,[59] may modify TLR-mediated responses by regulating the expression of the various proteins in the TLR receptor complex. In this respect, IL-10 increases the expression of CD14 on monocytes[78] but does not alter their expression of TLR4.[79] In contrast, TGF-β downregulates the expression of CD14 on macrophages.[80] Importantly, TGF-β null mice have increased TLR4 expression[81] and inflammatory lesions in multiple tissues.[82]

Cellular Reactivity to Bacteria in the Presence of Breast Milk

The predominant production of Th2 cytokines in fetal and neonatal life is a key element in depressing innate immune responses in the newborn[83] This deficiency results in impaired LPS-induced production of the proinflammatory, Th1-polarizing cytokines tumor necrosis factor (TNF)-α, interferon (IFN)-γ,[84] and IL-12[85] by neonatal mononuclear cells. An increased ratio of IL-6/TNF-α further polarizes toward a Th2 response.[86] Deficits in TLR4 and TLR2 expression may explain this.[85]

A similar deficit may exist in intestinal epithelium. It has been postulated that hyporeactivity to the microbiota is due to low expression of TLR2 and TLR4[87,88] and no expression of MD2[88] on IECs. In contrast to neonatal mononuclear cells and adult IECs, human fetal enterocytes express TLR2 and TLR4 and are hyperresponsive to LPS.[89,90] This hyperreactivity may also depend on a lower expression of the inhibitory intracellular molecule I-κBα, which binds NF-κB and retains it in the cytosol.[89]

An animal model suggests that an interaction between luminal microbes and aberrantly overexpressed TLR4 on neonatal IECs underlies the development of NEC.[91] Thus, increased TLR expression on human fetal enterocytes could explain the increased susceptiblity of premature infants to NEC. Although studies in mice suggest that the TLR expression and responsiveness of IECs diminish shortly after birth,[92] this apparent physiological window of hyperreactivity may compromise newborns. Nevertheless, a transient activation of IECs, with IκB-α phosphorylation and subsequent NF-κB nuclear translocation, may be required for subsequent postnatal tolerance to endotoxin.[92] Indeed, continuous activation in the presence of bacterial ligands is then thought to downregulate TLR expression on IECs,[88] perhaps via shedding of the receptors.[72] It is relevant that TLR4 expression gradually decreases on the intestinal epithelium of mother-fed newborns in an animal model of NEC.[91]

Remarkably, the presence of soluble PRRs and their partners in breast milk may participate in both the transient activation of innate immunity and in its subsequent downregulation. Certainly, milk sCD14 mediates the production of proinflammatory cytokines IL-8 and TNF-α and of the chemokine ENA-78 by IECs exposed to LPS[70] and the production of IL-8 in monocytes and DCs exposed to LPS.[70,93] At first glance, it is difficult to reconcile why high levels of sCD14 in breast milk, in the presence of an important bacterial inoculum, do not lead to excessive

Table 3 Human Milk Factors That Modulate Responses to Bacteria

Soluble CD14	Transfers lipopolysaccharide and lipoteichoic acid to Toll-like receptor (TLR) receptor complexes or to lipoproteins Modulates TLR signaling Proinflammatory
Soluble TLR2	Modulates TLR signalling Anti-inflammatory
Lactoferrin	Modulates TLR signalling Anti-inflammatory
Interleukin 10	Increases expression of CD14 Anti-inflammatory
Transforming growth factor β	Decreases expression of CD14 and TLR4 Anti-inflammatory
Osteoprotegerin	Anti-inflammatory
β-Defensin 2	Activates dendritic cells and induces Th1 immune responses via TLR4

inflammation in the intestine. One possible explanation is that strong activation leads to shedding of the TLR involved in the response.[72] However, it is also possible that other proteins in milk refine the response by interacting with sCD14 or sCD14 complexes as described earlier. An example is lactoferrin, which in addition to downregulating LPS-induced production of proinflammatory cytokines via NF-κB,[94] also inhibits sCD14–LPS-induced expression of IL-8 by human endothelial cells[95] as well as their increased expression of adhesion molecules, E-selectin and intercellular adhesion molecule (ICAM)-1.[77]

It is also noteworthy that the TLR2 ligand LTA does not stimulate proinflammatory cytokine production by IECs in the presence of milk, but rather inhibits sCD14-mediated LPS effects.[96] This observation suggests that gram-positive bacteria, via their LTA, may moderate cellular reactivity to LPS. However, more recent work has shown that sTLR2 in human milk can bind sCD14 and that sTLR2 can inhibit monocyte production of IL-8 and TNF-α in response to synthetic BLP.[72]

It is now known that multiple rounds of NF-κB activation are necessary in a first instance for immune defence and thereafter for resolution of inflammation and tissue repair[97] and that the latter is achieved through IKK-α inhibition of NF-κB.[98] It is becoming apparent that breast milk has evolved to provide molecules that act at several levels of this process. First, it permits the neonate to mount a limited response to the microbial "danger" signal by promoting the production of proinflammatory cytokines. Thereafter, it may activate a second set of genes that may be part of a negative feedback mechanism.[93]

Perhaps as a precautionary measure, breast milk already provides anti-inflammatory factors and antimicrobial peptides whose expression in the neonatal mucosa would otherwise require additional NF-κB activation (Table 3).[99,100] In agreement with this, a certain ambivalency is seen with some milk factors such as TGF-β,[101] sCD14,[73] and the antimicrobial factors lactoferrin and lysozyme,[102] which have the capacity to activate and inhibit NF-κ activation depending on concentration and cellular environment.

The TRAF6 signal transducer of the TLR/IL-1R superfamily is also important for signaling of the receptor activator of NF-κB (RANK) and its ligand (RANKL),[103,104] both of which are key regulators of lymph node formation and T cell–DC crosstalk.[105] Osteoprotegerin (OPG), a natural, soluble decoy receptor for RANKL, is expressed by human mammary gland and breast milk cells, is present in human breast milk for at least the first 6 months postpartum and can be detected in the serum of neonatal animals after gavage.[106] OPG is also expressed by IECs and is upregulated in the tissues of inflammatory bowel disease patients.[107] This increased production may be a protective responsive since OPG has been demonstrated in animal models of colitis, to inhibit intestinal inflammation by reducing DC numbers.[108] Interestingly, mice lacking OPG produce lower levels of proinflammatory cytokines after LPS injection.[109]

Maternal milk also inhibits IL-1β–induced NF-κB signaling in human IECs in vitro,[110] perhaps due to the presence of the IL-1 receptor antagonist (IL-1ra) whose levels persist throughout lactation.[59,111] Certainly, both human milk and an infant formula supplemented with human IL-1ra, have anti-inflammatory effects on chemically induced colitis in rats.[112] Soluble TNF-α receptor[111,113] and IL-10[114] in milk may behave in a similar manner.

As well as being a fuel for bacteria, HMO may also keep the reactivity of the neonatal immune response in check. They can interfere in protein–carbohydrate interactions such as those mediated by selectins and can inhibit formation of platelet–neutrophil complexes and the subsequent transmigration of neutrophils through activated endothelium at sites of inflammation.[50]

Linking Innate and Adaptive Immunity

Besides alerting the immune system of danger signals in the lumen, the innate system activates and coordinates adaptive immunity. DCs are at the heart of the decision-making processes and through the expression of TLRs determine the outcome of the primary response.[115] Following TLR engagement, DCs traffic to lymphoid organs upregulates expression of major histocompatibility complex and costimulatory molecules and acquires the capacity to prime naïve T cells, which then develop into Th1, Th2, or T_{reg} effector cells. Th1 cells produce IFN-γ and TNF-β and activate cell-mediated immunity, while Th2 cells favor humoral responses by secreting IL-4, IL-5, and IL-13 and by promoting B cell isotype switching to IgG1, IgA, and IgE or T_{reg} cells.[116] T_{reg} cells, which mediate their effects via secretion of IL-10 or TGF-β, are thought to prevent autoimmune responses by specifically suppressing activation and proliferation of CD4 and CD8 effector T cells.[115]

Neonates are susceptible to microbial infection and mount poor adaptive immune responses. The reasons for this are multifactorial and may include a lack of memory B and T cells and reduced T cell responses,[117] reduced numbers[118] and maturation[119] of DCs, a high proportion of T_{reg} cells but with naïve phenotype, and a bias toward Th2 immune responses.[83] However, specific TLR stimulation can overcome some of these defects[119,120] and may inhibit the development of Th2 responses.[120]

Breast-fed infants are less prone to develop asthma, atopic dermatitis, eczema, and allergy than formula-fed infants.[59] Some studies have reported a correlation between the development of these diseases and the concentration of milk molecules sCD14, TGF-β, and sIgA.[121,122] Mechanistic studies certainly support a regulatory role for milk molecules in adaptive immunity and in correcting imbalances in Th1 and Th2 responses. For example, sCD14 mediates LPS-induced TNF-α, IL-6, IL-8, and IL-12 release by DCs as well as their expression of costimulatory molecules.[123] Furthermore, it acts directly on activated human T cells to inhibit IL-2 production and cell proliferation, as well as the production of another Th1-like cytokine, IFN-γ, and a Th2-like cytokine, IL-4.[124] Direct interaction of sCD14 with B cells, resulting in higher levels of IgG1 and marked inhibition of IgE production, has also been observed.[125] Consistent with these observations, administration of milk sCD14 to neonatal mice enhances antibody secretion.[71]

TGF-β is a multifunctional cytokine that inhibits the development of exaggerated responses to self or nonharmful antigens without compromising immune responses to pathogens.[101] It controls the initiation and resolution of inflammation through the regulation and survival of multiple cell types, including lymphocytes, NK cells, DCs and macrophages, mast cells, and granulocytes[101] and influences IgA production by B cells.[126] Indeed, a correlation has been observed between TGF-β levels in milk and newborn serum levels of IgA.[127] Furthermore, given orally to allergic neonatal animals, TGF-β downregulates the antigen-specific IgG1 and total IgE levels, inhibits mucosal mast cell activation, and increases the expression of the Th1 cytokines, IL-18, IL-12, and IFN-γ.[128]

Several in vitro and in vivo studies have now demonstrated a role for lactoferrin in T cell differentiation (reviewed in reference 129) and the capacity of orally administered lactoferrin to correct the Th1/Th2 cytokine imbalance in both Th1 and Th2 models of disease.

Studies in OPG null mice have shown that OPG regulates B cell maturation and the development of efficient antibody responses.[130] Furthermore, OPG is a survival factor for DCs but can reduce DC numbers in animal models of colitis.[131] It is also noteworthy that Peyer's patch DCs express RANK and that treatment with antagonists of RANKL enhances the induction of tolerogenic immune responses.[132] It is feasible therefore that the high levels of OPG in milk may mediate similar effects.

HMO, specifically the Lewis X component, can interact with DCs via the cell-surface molecule dendritic cell–specific intercellular adhesion molecule-grabbing nonintegrin (DC-SIGN).[133] DC-SIGN is implicated in various functions, mainly related to pathogen recognition and antigen processing and presentation to $CD4^+$ lymphocytes,[133] and can function both as an adhesion receptor and as a phagocytic pathogen-recognition receptor, similar to the Toll-like receptors.[134] Although likely, more studies are required to determine whether HMO interference with the interaction of DC-$CD4^+$ cell interactions renders the newborn host tolerant to components of the microbiota.

Role of Milk Leukocytes in Immune Education

Many viable cells are present in human milk but their concentration declines during lactation.[135] The cell populations present include granulocytes, macrophages, and lymphocytes, which are predominantly T cells. A significant proportion of $CD8^+$ T cells with an effector memory phenotype are constantly present in human milk and may be important in the control of viral passage from mother to infant .[136] Recent work demonstrating that $CD14^+$ milk mononuclear cells in milk express HLA-DR, CD86, CD83, and DC-specific ICAM-3–grabbing nonintegrin suggests that these cells are partially differentiated DCs.[137] They are a source of some of the soluble factors found in milk such as sCD14,[70,71] OPG,[106] as well as several cytokines and chemokines.[59] There is some evidence that the neutrophils and macrophages in milk are phagocytic[138,139] and that upon ingestion they induce a respiratory burst.[140]

The milk leukocytes seem capable of surviving gastrointestinal transport, penetrating the neonatal intestinal barrier and migrating to the mesenteric lymph nodes.[141] In addition to maternal eukaryotic cells, there is accumulating evidence that bacteria of maternal origin are transmitted to the infant via the colostrum and milk.[4,142] Most of these organisms arise from the mother's skin but certain milk species may colonize the neonatal intestine. Interestingly, bacteria considered intrinsic to human milk are associated with mononuclear cells and perhaps cells with an immature DC phenotype.[143] It has previously been shown that milk leukocytes are cells that have migrated from the gut- and bronchial-associated lymphoid tissue to the lactating mammary gland via the lymphatics and the circulation.[56,59,144] It now appears that such migrating cells also transport bacterial and their genetic material.[143] The role of these cells in the neonate is not known but they may represent an inoculum for the development of the microbiota and/or be a way to educate the neonatal immune system.

Other Protective Factors in Milk

Additional immunomodulatory factors in milk may regulate innate and/or adaptive immune responses. These include the antimicrobial β-defensin 2,[145] which induces cytokines and chemokines, is chemotactic for DCs, and uses TLR4 to activate DCs and induce Th1 immune responses (reviewed in reference 146). Numerous cytokines and chemokines, such as IL-1β, IL-6, and TNF-α, monocyte colony stimulating factor, monocyte chemotactic protein 1, IL-8, and RANTES,[59] as well as fatty acids[147] have also been described.

α-Lactalbumin is a major milk protein in all mammals. Its digestion provides a source of biologically important amino acids, antimicrobial peptides, and an immunomodulatory peptide that enhances macrophage phagocytic activity.[148] In addition, a unique form of α-lactalbumin in human milk can induce apoptosis.[149]

Milk is also a rich source of hormones and growth factors that may aid in nutrient transport and the growth and differentiation of neonatal tissues.[59,150]

CONCLUSION

Breast milk provides a well-recognized passive protection against pathogens in the neonatal period. However, recently discovered functions suggest that protection extends beyond the newborn period. The cocktail of biologically active factors that milk provides targets neonatal innate and adaptive immune responses at multiple levels. Milk's primordial task is to alert the innate arm of potential danger. To do so, it supplies molecules that actively promote a proinflammatory primary response upon exposure to antigens or microbial components. However, as a pivotal link between innate and adaptive immunity, it ultimately instructs the neonatal immune system to remain tolerant to nonthreatening antigens and components of the commensal microbiota but to eliminate potential pathogens. To achieve this, it already provides a variety of anti-inflammatory factors that would otherwise imply further activation of neonatal cells. These additional factors fine-tune the type and level of reactivity. Differences between breast-fed and formula-fed infants suggest that in some infant formulas, certain elements needed for the control of these processes are lacking and the infant is more susceptible to antigenic challenge.

REFERENCES

1. American Academy of Pediatrics. Breastfeeding and the use of human milk. Work Group on Breastfeeding. Pediatrics 1997;100:1035–9.
2. Hanson LA. Breastfeeding provides passive and likely long-lasting active immunity. Ann Allergy Asthma Immunol 1998;81:523–33.
3. Jackson KM, Nazar AM. Breastfeeding, the immune response, and long-term health. J Am Osteopath Assoc 2006;106:203–7.
4. Martin R, Langa S, Reviriego C, et al. Human milk is a source of lactic acid bacteria for the infant gut. J Pediatr 2003;143:754–8.
5. Macdonald TT, Monteleone G. Immunity, inflammation, and allergy in the gut. Science 2005;307:1920–5.
6. Matzinger P. The danger model: A renewed sense of self. Science 2002;296:301–5.
7. Janeway CA, Medzhitov R. Innate immune recognition. Annu Rev Immunol 2002;20:197–216.
8. Haller D, Bode C, Hammes WP, et al. Non pathogenic bacteria elicit a differential cytokine response by intestinal epithelial cell/leukocyte co-cultures. Gut 2000;47:79–87.
9. Jenner RG, Young RA. Insights into host responses against pathogens from transcriptional profiling. Nat Rev Micorbiol 2005;3:281–94.
10. Cario E. Bacterial interactions with cells of the intestinal mucosa: Toll-like receptors and NOD2. Gut 2005;54:1182–93.
11. Lala S, Ogura Y, Osborne C, et al. Crohn's disease and the NOD2 gene: A role for paneth cells. Gastroenterology 2003;125:47–57.
12. Pauleau AL, Murray PJ. Role of nod2 in the response of macrophages to toll-like receptor agonists. Mol Cell Biol 2003;23:7531–9.
13. Cebra JJ. Influences of microbiota on intestinal immune system development. Am J Clin Nutr 1999;69:1046S–51S.
14. Rook GA, Brunet LR. Microbes, immunoregulation, and the gut. Gut 2005;54:317–20.
15. Bäckhed F, Ley RE, Sonnenbur JL, et al. Host-bacterial mutualism in the human intestine. Science 2005;307:1915–20.
16. Penders J, Thijs C, Stelma FF, et al. Factors influencing the composition of the intestinal microbiota in early infancy. 2006;118:511–21.
17. Rotimi VO, Duerden BI. The development of the bacterial flora in normal neonates. J Med Microbiol 1981;14:51–62.
18. Balmer SE, Wharton BA. Diet and faecal flora in the newborn: Breast milk and infant formula. Arch Dis Child 1989;64:1672–7.
19. Caplan MS, MacKendrick W. Necrotizing enterocolitis: A review of pathogenetic mechanisms and implications for prevention. Pediatr Pathol 1993;13:357–69.
20. van Saene HK, Taylor N, Donnell SC, et al. Gut overgrowth with abnormal flora: The missing link in parenteral nutrition–related sepsis in surgical neonates. Eur J Clin Nutr 2003;57:548–53.
21. Steinwender G, Schimpl G, Sixl B, et al. Effect of early nutritional deprivation and diet on translocation of bacteria from the gastrointestinal tract in the newborn rat. Pediatr Res 1996;39:415-20.
22. Ronnestad A, Abrahamsen TG, Medbo S, et al. Septicemia in the first week of life in a Norwegian national cohort of extremely premature infants. Pediatrics 2005;115:e262–8.
23. Bleul CC, Corbeaux T, Reuter A, et al. Formation of a functional thymus initiated by a postnatal epithelial progenitor cell. Nature 2006;441:992–6.
24. Derbinski J, Gäbler J, Bros B, et al. Promiscuous gene expression in thymic epithelial cells is regulated at multiple levels. J Exp Med 2005;202:33–45.
25. Cario E, Podolsky DK. Intestinal epithelial TOLLerance versus inTOLLerance of commensals. Mol Immunol 2005;42:887–93.
26. Walker WA. Gastrointestinal host defence: Importance of gut closure in control of macromolecular transport. Ciba Found Symp 1979;70:201–19.
27. Kelly D, Conway S, Aminov R. Commensal gut bacteria: Mechanisms of immune modulation. Trends Immunol 2005;26:326–33.
28. Coppa GV, Pierani P, Zampini L, et al. Oligosaccharides in human milk during different phases of lactation. Acta Paediatr 1999;88:89–94.
29. Kunz C, Rudloff S, Baier W, et al. Oligosaccharides in human milk: Structural, functional, and metabolic aspects. Annu Rev Nutr 2000;20:699–722.
30. Sharon N. Carbohydrate-lectin interactions in infectious diseases. Adv Exp Med Biol 1996;408:1–8.
31. Newburg DS. Oligosaccharides in human milk and bacterial colonization. J Pediatr Gastroenterol Nutr 2000;30:S8–S17.
32. Angeloni S, Rider JL, Kusy N, et al. Glycoprofiling with micro-array of glycoconjugates and lectins. Glycobiology 2005;15:31–41.
33. Wold AE, Adlerberth I. Breast feeding and the intestinal microflora of the infant—Implications for protection against infectious diseases. Adv Exp Med Biol 2000;478:77–93.
34. Yolken RH, Peterson JA, Vonderfecht SL, et al. Human milk mucin inhibits rotavirus replication and prevents experimental gastroenteritis. J Clin Invest 1992;90:1984–91.
35. Schroten H, Hanisch FG, Plogmann R, et al. Inhibition of adhesion of S-fimbriated *Escherichia coli* to buccal epithelial cells by human milk fat globule membrane components: A novel aspect of the protective function of mucins in the nonimmunoglobulin fraction. Infect Immun 1992;60:2893–9.
36. Dai D, Nanthkumar NN, Newburg DS, Walker WA. Role of oligosaccharides and glycoconjugates in intestinal host defense. J Pediatr Gastroenterol Nutr 2000;30: S23–S33.
37. Eckmann L. Defence molecules in intestinal innate immunity against bacterial infections. Curr Opin Gastroenterol 2005;21:147–51.
38. Mallow EB, Harris A, Salzman N, et al. Human enteric defensins. Gene structure and developmental expression. J Biol Chem 1996;271:4038–45.
39. Sherman MP, Bennett SH, Hwang FF, et al. Paneth cells and antibacterial host defense in neonatal small intestine. Infect Immun 2005;73:6143–6.
40. Coutinho HB, da Mota HC, Coutinho VB, et al. Absence of lysozyme (muramidase) in the intestinal Paneth cells of newborn infants with necrotising enterocolitis. J Clin Pathol 1998;51:512–4.
41. Murakami M, Dorschner RA, Stern LJ, et al. Expression and secretion of cathelicidin antimicrobial peptides in murine mammary glands and human milk. Pediatr Res 2005;57:10–15.
42. Blau H, Passwell JH, Levanon M, et al. Studies on human milk macrophages: Effect of activation on phagocytosis and secretion of prostaglandin E2 and lysozyme. Pediatr Res 1983;17:241–5.
43. Jia HP, Starner T, Ackermann M, et al. Abundant human beta-defensin-1 expression in milk and mammary gland epithelium. J Pediatr 2001;138:109–12.
44. Lonnerdal B, Iyer S. Lactoferrin: Molecular structure and biological function. Annu Rev Nutr 1995;15:93–110.
45. Arnold RR, Brewer M, Gauthier JJ. Bactericidal activity of human lactoferrin: Sensitivity of a variety of microorganisms. Infect Immun 1980;28:893–8.
46. Yamauchi K, Tomita M, Giehl TJ, Ellison RT, III. Antibacterial activity of lactoferrin and a pepsin-derived lactoferrin peptide fragment. Infect Immun 1993;61:719–28.
47. Goldman AS, Garza C, Schanler RJ, Goldblum RM. Molecular forms of lactoferrin in stool and urine from infants fed human milk. Pediatr Res 1990;27:252–5.
48. Andersson Y, Lindquist S, Lagerqvist C, Hernell O. Lactoferrin is responsible for the fungistatic effect of human milk. Early Hum Dev 2000;59:95–105.

49. Portelli J, Gordon A, May JT. Effect of compounds with antibacterial activities in human milk on respiratory syncytial virus and cytomegalovirus in vitro. J Med Microbiol 1998;47:1015–8.
50. Bode L. Recent advances on structure, metabolism, and function of human milk oligosaccharides. J Nutr 2006;136:2127–30.
51. Kim WS, Ohashi M, Tanaka T, et al. Growth-promoting effects of lactoferrin on *L. acidophilus* and *Bifidobacterium* spp. Biometals 2004;17:279–83.
52. Liepke C, Adermann K, Raida M, et al. Human milk provides peptides highly stimulating the growth of bifidobacteria. Eur J Biochem 2002;269:712–8.
53. Brandtzaeg P, Nilssen DE, Rognum TO, Thrane PS. Ontogeny of the mucosal immune system and IgA deficiency. Gastroenterol Clin North Am 1991;20:397–439.
54. MacDonald TT. Development of mucosal immune function in man: potential for GI disease states. Acta Paediatr Jpn 1994;36:532–6.
55. Mostov KE, Friedlander M, Blobel G. The receptor for transepithelial transport of IgA and IgM contains multiple immunoglobulin-like domains. Nature 1984;308:37–43.
56. Roux ME, McWilliams M, Phillips-Quagliata JM, et al. Origin of IgA-secreting plasma cells in the mammary gland. J Exp Med 1977;146:1311–22.
57. Wright AL, Bauer M, Naylor A, et al. Increasing breastfeeding rates to reduce infant illness at the community level. Pediatrics 1998;101:837–44.
58. Brandtzaeg P. Mucosal immunity: Integration between mother and the breast-fed infant. Vaccine 2003;21:3382–8.
59. Lawrence RM. Host-resistance factors and immunologic significance of human milk. In: Lawrence RA, Lawrence RM, editors. Breastfeeding. A Guide for the Medical Profession. Mosby, PA: Elsevier; 2005. Chapter 5, p. 171–214.
60. Schanler RJ, Goldblum RM, Garza C, Goldman AS. Enhanced fecal excretion of selected immune factors in very low birth weight infants fed fortified human milk. Pediatr Res 1986;20:711–5.
61. Lamm ME. Interaction of antigens and antibodies at mucosal surfaces. Annu Rev Microbiol 1997;51:311–40.
62. van der Waaij LA, Limburg PC, Mesander G, van der Waaij D. In vivo IgA coating of anaerobic bacteria in human faeces. Gut 1996;38:348–54.
63. Bollinger RR, Everett ML, Palestrant D, et al. Human secretory immunoglobulin A may contribute to biofilm formation in the gut. Immunology 2003;109:580–7.
64. Aderem A, Ulevitch RJ. Toll-like receptors in the induction of the innate immune response. Nature 2000;406:782–7.
65. Hailman E, Lichenstein HS, Wurfel MM, et al. Lipopolysaccharide (LPS)-binding protein accelerates the binding of LPS to CD14. J Exp Med 1994;179:269–77.
66. da Silva Correia J, Soldau K, Christen U, et al. Lipopolysaccharide is in close proximity to each of the proteins in its membrane receptor complex. Transfer from CD14 to TLR4 and MD-2. J Biol Chem 2001;276:21129–35.
67. Schroder NW, Morath S, Alexander C, et al. Lipoteichoic acid (LTA) of *Streptococcus pneumoniae* and *Staphylococcus aureus* activates immune cells via Toll-like receptor (TLR)-2, lipopolysaccharide-binding protein (LBP), and CD14, whereas TLR-4 and MD-2 are not involved. J Biol Chem 2003;278:15587–94.
68. O'Neill LA. Signal transduction pathways activated by the IL-1 receptor/toll-like receptor superfamily. Curr Top Microbiol Immunol 2002;270:47–61.
69. O'Neill LA, Dunne A, Edjeback M, et al. Mal and MyD88: Adapter proteins involved in signal transduction by Toll-like receptors. J Endotoxin Res 2003;9:55–9.
70. Labéta MO, Vidal K, Rey Nores JE, et al. Innate recognition of bacteria in human milk is mediated by a milk derived highly expressed pattern recognition receptor, soluble CD14. J Exp Med 2000;191:1807–12.
71. Filipp D, Alizadeh-Khiavi K, Richardson C, et al. Soluble CD14 enriched in colostrum and milk induces B cell growth and differentiation. Proc Natl Acad Sci U S A 2001;98:603–8.
72. LeBoulder E, Rey Nores JE, Rushmere NK, et al. Soluble forms of toll-like receptor (TLR)2 capable of modulating TLR2 signaling are present in human plasma and breast milk. J Immunol 2003;171:6680–9.
73. Kitchens RL, Thompson PA. Modulatory effects of sCD14 and LBP on LPS-host cell interactions. J Endotoxin Res 2005;11:225–59.
74. Hailman E, Vasselon T, Kelley M, et al. Stimulation of macrophages and neutrophils by complexes of lipopolysaccharide and soluble CD14. J Immunol 1996;156:4384–90.
75. Pugin J, Schurer-Maly CC, Leturcq D, et al. Lipopolysaccharide activation of human endothelial and epithelial cells is mediated by lipopolysaccharide-binding protein and soluble CD14. Proc Natl Acad Sci U S A 1993;90:2744–8.
76. Appelmelk BJ, An YQ, Geerts M, et al. Lactoferrin is a lipid A-binding protein. Infect Immun 1994;62:2628–32.
77. Baveye S, Elass E, Fernig DG, et al. Human lactoferrin interacts with soluble CD14 and inhibits expression of endothelial adhesion molecules, E-selectin and ICAM-1, induced by the CD14-lipopolysaccharide complex. Infect Immun 2000;68:6519–25.
78. Rahimi AA, Gee K, Mishra S, et al. STAT-1 mediates the stimulatory effect of IL-10 on CD14 expression in human monocytic cells. J Immunol 2005;174:7823–32.
79. Moreno C, Merino J, Vazquez B, et al. Anti-inflammatory cytokines induce lipopolysaccharide tolerance in human monocytes without modifying toll-like receptor 4 membrane expression. Scand J Immunol 2004;59:553–8.
80. Imai K, Takeshita A, Hanazawa S. Transforming growth factor-beta inhibits lipopolysaccharide-stimulated expression of inflammatory cytokines in mouse macrophages through downregulation of activation protein 1 and CD14 receptor expression. Infect Immun 2000;68:2418–23.
81. McCartney-Francis N, Jin W, Wahl SM. Aberrant Toll receptor expression and endotoxin hypersensitivity in mice lacking a functional TGF-beta 1 signaling pathway. J Immunol 2004;172:3814–21.
82. Kulkarni AB, Huh CG, Becker D, et al. Transforming growth factor beta 1 null mutation in mice causes excessive inflammatory response and early death. Proc Natl Acad Sci U S A 1993;90:770–4.
83. Marodi L. Innate cellular immune responses in newborns. Clin Immunol 2006;118:137–44.
84. Levy O. Innate immunity of the human newborn: Distinct cytokine responses to LPS and other Toll-like receptor agonists. J Endotoxin Res 2005;11:113–6.
85. Chelvarajan RL, Collins SM, Doubinskaia IE, et al. Defective macrophage function in neonates and its impact on unresponsiveness of neonates to polysaccharide antigens. J Leukoc Biol 2004;75:982–94.
86. Angelone DF, Wessels MR, Coughlin M, et al. Innate immunity of the human newborn is polarized toward a high ratio of IL-6/TNF-alpha production in vitro and in vivo. Pediatr Res 2006;60:205–9.
87. Otte JM, Cario E, Podolsky DK. Mechanisms of cross hyporesponsiveness to Toll-like receptor bacterial ligands in intestinal epithelial cells. Gastroenterology 2004;126:1054–70.
88. Abreu MT, Vora P, Faure E, et al. Decreased expression of Toll-like receptor 4 and MD-2 correlates with intestinal epithelial cell protection against dysregulated pro-inflammatory gene expression in response to bacterial lipopolysaccharide. J Immunol 2001;167:1609–16.
89. Claud EC, Lu L, Anton PM, et al. Developmentally regulated I_B expression in intestinal epithelium and susceptibility to flagellin-induced inflammation. Proc Natl Acad Sci 2004;101:7404–8.
90. Fusunyan R D, Nanthakumar NN, Baldeon ME, Walker WA. Evidence for an innate immune response in the immature human intestine: Toll-like receptors on fetal enterocytes. Pediatr Res 2001;49:589–93.
91. Jilling T, Simon D, Lu J, et al. The roles of bacteria and TLR4 in rat and murine models of necrotizing enterocolitis. J Immunol 2006;177:3273–82.
92. Lotz M, Gütle D, Walther S, et al. Postnatal acquisition of endotoxin tolerance in intestinal epithelial cells. J Exp Med 2006;203:937–84.
93. LeBouder E, Rey-Nores JE, Raby AC, et al. Modulation of neonatal microbial recognition: TLR-mediated innate immune responses are specifically and differentially modulated by human milk. J Immunol 2006;176:3742–52.
94. Haversen L, Ohlsson BG, Hahn-Zoric M, et al. Lactoferrin down-regulates the LPS-induced cytokine production in monocytic cells via NF-kappa B. Cell Immunol 2002;220:83–95.
95. Elass E, Masson M, Mazurier J, Legrand D. Lactoferrin inhibits the lipopolysaccharide-induced expression and proteoglycan-binding ability of interleukin-8 in human endothelial cells. Infect Immun 2002;70:1860–6.
96. Vidal K, Donnet-Hughes A, Granato D. Lipoteichoic acids from *Lactobacillus johnsonii* strain La1 and *Lactobacillus acidophilus* strain La10 antagonize the responsiveness of human intestinal epithelial HT29 cells to lipopolysaccharide and gram-negative bacteria. Infect Immun 2002;70:2057–64.
97. Lawrence T, Gilroy DW, Colville-Nash PR, Willoughby DA. Possible new role for NF-kappaB in the resolution of inflammation. Nat Med 2001;7:1291–7.
98. Lawrence T, Bebien M, Liu GY, et al. IKKalpha limits macrophage NF-kappaB activation and contributes to the resolution of inflammation. Nature 2005;434:1138–43.
99. Vora P, Youdim A, Thomas LS, et al. Beta-defensin-2 expression is regulated by TLR signaling in intestinal epithelial cells. J Immunol 2004;173:5398–405.
100. Lee KY, Ito K, Hayashi R, et al. NF-kappaB and activator protein 1 response elements and the role of histone modifications in IL-1beta-induced TGF-beta1 gene transcription. J Immunol 2006;176:603–15.
101. Li MO, Wan YY, Sanjabi S, et al. Transforming growth factor-beta regulation of immune responses. Annu Rev Immunol 2006;24:99–146.
102. Edde L, Hipolito RB, Hwang FF, et al. Lactoferrin protects neonatal rats from gut-related systemic infection. Am J Physiol Gastrointestinol Liver Physiol 2001;281: G1140–50.
103. Wong BR, Besser D, Kim N, et al. TRANCE, a TNF family member, activates Akt/PKB through a signaling complex involving TRAF6 and c-Src. Mol Cell 1999;4:1041–9.
104. Wong BR, Josien R, Lee SY, et al. The TRAF family of signal transducers mediates NF-kappaB activation by the TRANCE receptor. J Biol Chem 1998;273:28355–9.
105. Jones DH, Kong YY, Penninger JM. Role of RANKL and RANK in bone loss and arthritis. Ann Rheum Dis 2002;61: ii32–9.
106. Vidal K, van den Broek P, Forget F, Donnet-Hughes A. Osteoprotegerin in human milk: A potential role in the regulation of bone metabolism and immune development. Pediatr Res 2004;55:1001–8.
107. Vidal K, Serrant P, Schlosser B, et al. Osteoprotegerin production by human intestinal epithelial cells: A potential regulator of mucosal immune responses. Am J Physiol Gastrointestinol Liver Physiol 2004;287:G836–44.
108. Ashcroft AJ, Cruickshank SM, Croucher PI, et al. Colonic dendritic cells, intestinal inflammation, and T cell-mediated bone destruction are modulated by recombinant osteoprotegerin. Immunity 2003;19:849–61.
109. Maruyama K, Takada Y, Ray N, et al. Receptor activator of NF-kappa B ligand and osteoprotegerin regulate proinflammatory cytokine production in mice. J Immunol 2006;177:3799–805.
110. Minekawa R, Takeda T, Sakata M, et al. Human breast milk suppresses the transcriptional regulation of IL-1beta-induced NF-kappaB signaling in human intestinal cells. Am J Physiol Cell Physiol 2004;287:C1404–11.
111. Buescher ES, Malinowska I. Soluble receptors and cytokine antagonists in human milk. Pediatr Res 1996;40:839–44.
112. Grazioso CF, Werner AL, Alling DW, et al. Antiinflammatory effects of human milk on chemically induced colitis in rats. Pediatr Res 1997;42:639–43.
113. Buescher ES, McWilliams-Koeppen P. Soluble tumor necrosis factor-alpha (TNF-alpha) receptors in human colostrum and milk bind to TNF-alpha and neutralize TNF-alpha bioactivity. Pediatr Res 1998;44:37–42.
114. Fituch CC, Palkowetz KH, Goldman AS, et al. Concentrations of IL-10 in preterm human milk and in milk from mothers of infants with necrotizing enterocolitis. Acta Paediatr 2004;93:1496–1500.
115. Mazzoni A, Segal DM. Controlling the Toll road to dendritic cell polarization. J Leukoc Biol 2004;75:721–30.
116. Murphy KM, Reiner SL. The lineage decisions of helper T cells. Nat Rev Immunol 2002;2:933–44.
117. Siegrist CA. Vaccination in the neonatal period and early infancy. Int Rev Immunol 2000;19:195–219.
118. Kadowaki N, Liu YJ. Natural type I interferon-producing cells as a link between innate and adaptive Immunity. Hum Immunol 2002;63:1126–32.
119. Gold MC, Donnelly E, Cook MS, et al. Purified neonatal plasmacytoid dendritic cells overcome intrinsic maturation defect with TLR agonist stimulation. Pediatr Res 2006;60:34–37.
120. Andersson AC, Seppala U, Rudin A. Activation of human neonatal monocyte-derived dendritic cells by lipopolysaccharide down-regulates birch allergen-induced Th2 differentiation. Eur J Immunol 2004;34:3516–24.
121. Jones CA, Holloway JA, Popplewell EJ, et al. Reduced soluble CD14 levels in amniotic fluid and breast milk are associated with the subsequent development of atopy, eczema, or both. J Allergy Clin Immunol 2002;109:858–66.
122. Savilahti E, Siltanen M, Kajosaari M, et al. IgA antibodies, TGF-beta1 and -beta2, and soluble CD14 in the colostrum and development of atopy by age 4. Pediatr Res 2005;58:1300–5.
123. Verhasselt V, Buelens C, Willems F, et al. Bacterial lipopolysaccharide stimulates the production of cytokines and the expression of costimulatory molecules by human peripheral blood dendritic cells: Evidence for a soluble CD14-dependent pathway. J Immunol 1997;158:2919–25.
124. Rey Nores JE, Bensussan A, Vita N, et al. Soluble CD14 acts as a negative regulator of human T cell activation and function. Eur J Immunol 1999;29:265–76.
125. Arias MA, Rey Nores JE, Vita N, et al. Cutting edge: Human B cell function is regulated by interaction with soluble CD14: Opposite effects on IgG1 and IgE production. J Immunol 2000;164:3480–6.

126. van Ginkel FW, Wahl SM, Kearney JF, et al. Partial IgA-deficiency with increased Th-2 type cytokines in TGF-[beta]1 knockout mice. J Immunol 1999;163:1951–7.
127. Ogawa J, Sasahara A, Yoshida T, et al. Role of transforming growth factor-beta in breast milk for initiation of IgA production in newborn infants. Early Hum Dev 2004;77:67–75.
128. Penttila I. Effects of transforming growth factor-beta and formula feeding on systemic immune responses to dietary beta-lactoglobulin in allergy-prone rats. Pediatr Res 2006;59:650–5.
129. Fischer R, Debbabi H, Dubarry M, et al. Regulation of physiological and pathological Th1 and Th2 responses by lactoferrin. Biochem Cell Biol 2006;84:303–11.
130. Yun TJ, Tallquist MD, Aicher A, et al. Osteoprotegerin, a crucial regulator of bone metabolism, also regulates B cell development and function. J Immunol 2001;166:1482–9.
131. Ashcroft AJ, Cruickshank SM, Croucher PI, et al. Colonic dendritic cells, intestinal inflammation, and T cell-mediated bone destruction are modulated by recombinant osteoprotegerin. Immunity 2003;19:849–61.
132. Williamson E, Bilsborough JM, Viney JL. Regulation of mucosal dendritic cell function by receptor activator of NF-kappa B (RANK)/RANK ligand interactions: Impact on tolerance induction. J Immunol 2002;169:3606–12.
133. Naarding MA, Ludwig IS, Groot F, et al. Lewis X component in human milk binds DC-SIGN and inhibits HIV-1 transfer to $CD4^+$ T lymphocytes. J Clin Invest 2005;115:3256–64.
134. Cambi A, Figdor CG. Dual function of C-type lectin-like receptors in the immune system. Curr Opin Cell Biol 2003;15:539–46.
135. Pittard WB, III, Geddes M, Pepkowitz SH, Carr R. The immunologic composition of neonatal milk: Cellular components. Clin Immunol Immunopathol 1988;46:294–8.
136. Sabbaj S, Ghosh MK, Edwards BH, et al. Breast milk-derived antigen-specific $CD8^+$ T cells: An extralymphoid effector memory cell population in humans. J Immunol 2005;174:2951–6.
137. Ichikawa M, Sugita M, Takahashi M, et al. Breast milk macrophages spontaneously produce granulocyte-macrophage colony-stimulating factor and differentiate into dendritic cells in the presence of exogenous interleukin-4 alone. Immunology 2003;108:189–95.
138. Ho PC, Lawton JW. Human colostral cells: Phagocytosis and killing of *E. coli* and *C. albicans*. J Pediatr 1978;93:910–5.
139. Hughes A, Brock JH, Parrott DM, Cockburn F. The interaction of infant formula with macrophages: Effect on phagocytic activity, relationship to expression of class II MHC antigen and survival of orally administered macrophages in the neonatal gut. Immunology 1988;64:213–8.
140. Adam R, Kuczera F, Kohler H, Schroten H. Superoxide anion generation in human milk macrophages: Opsonin-dependent versus opsonin-independent stimulation compared with blood monocytes. Pediatr Res 2001;49:435–9.
141. Goldman AS. Evolution of the mammary gland defense system and ontogeny of the immune system. J Mammary Gland Biol Neoplasia 2002;7:277–89.
142. Moughan PJ, Birtles MJ, Cranwell PD, et al. The piglet as a model animal for studying aspects of digestion and absorption in milk-fed human infants. Nutritional triggers for health and disease. World Rev Nutr Diet 1992;67:40–113.
143. Perez PF, Doré J, Leclerc M, et al. Bacterial imprinting of the neonatal immune system: Lessons from maternal cells? Pediatrics 2007;119:e724–32.
144. Goldman AS, Goldblum RM. Transfer of maternal leukocytes to the infant by human milk. Curr Top Microbiol Immunol 1997;222:205–13.
145. Armogida SA, Yannaras NM, Melton AL, Srivastava MD. Identification and quantification of innate immune system mediators in human breast milk. Allergy Asthma Proc 2004;25:297–304.
146. Oppenheim JJ, Biragyn A, Kwak LW, Yang D. Roles of antimicrobial peptides such as defensins in innate and adaptive immunity. Ann Rheum Dis 2003;62:ii17–21.
147. Calder PC, Krauss-Etschmann S, de Jong EC, et al. Early nutrition and immunity — progress and perspectives. Br J Nutr 2006;96:774–90.
148. Lonnerdal B, Lien EL. Nutritional and physiologic significance of alpha-lactalbumin in infants. Nutr Rev 2003;61:295–305.
149. Gustafsson L, Hallgren O, Mossberg AK, et al. HAMLET kills tumor cells by apoptosis: Structure, cellular mechanisms, and therapy. J Nutr 2005;135:1299–303.
150. Grosvenor CE, Picciano MF, Baumrucker CR. Hormones and growth factors in milk. Endocr Rev 1993;14:710–28.

Approach to Breast-feeding

Ruth Lawrence, MD
Robert M. Lawrence, MD

"Babies were born to be breast-fed" is the tagline for the national campaign to promote breast-feeding.[1]

The health goals of our nation include a statement regarding breast-feeding. By the year 2010, 75% of women will leave the hospital breast-feeding, at least 50% will continue to breast-feed for at least 6 months, and at 12 months at least 25% will still be breast-feeding. The goal particularly addresses high-risk women, those from minority, low-income, and undereducated groups.[2]

The Institute of Medicine issued a report on nutrition during lactation as part of a review of nutrition in the perinatal period that stated that breast-feeding was ideal for all infants under ordinary circumstances.[3] It further stated that even women without perfect diets could produce good milk and nourish their young well.[3] Professional medical associations such as the American Academy of Pediatrics,[4] the American College of Obstetrics and Gynecology, and the Academy of Family Practice have developed policies encouraging universal breast-feeding. The World Health Organization and United Nations International Children's Emergency Fund (UNICEF) have taken very strong positions in support of worldwide breast-feeding, including the development of the Baby Friendly Hospital Initiative.[5,6]

Human milk is specifically designed for the needs of the human infant. Its nutritional advantages have been noted to be especially important for brain growth.[7–9] In the first year of life, the brain of the human infant doubles in size.[10] The myelinization of nerves is equally important and occurs extensively in the first year of life. Taurine, cholesterol, and omega fatty acids are essential to brain growth and are uniquely present in human milk.[11]

The presence of dozens of active enzymes, the immunologic properties, infection protection properties, and allergy protection are some of the compelling reasons breast-feeding is superior for human infants.[12–15]

The number of women who elect to breast-feed has continued to increase, and the renaissance of breast-feeding is well established.[16,17] It is important for the clinician to be knowledgeable about the value of human milk, the advantages of breast-feeding, the clinical management of lactation, and the diagnosis and treatment of problems.[18] The current scientific literature provides a large resource of information on these topics, which will be summarized here.

ANATOMY AND PHYSIOLOGY

Lactation is the completion of the normal reproductive cycle. It is a physiologic process triggered by the termination of pregnancy, but anticipated both anatomically and physiologically from early development.[11]

The breast bud is present at birth in both sexes, but remains dormant until early pubescence, when growth is stimulated by the increase in estrogen and progesterone in the female.[19,20] The ductal system proliferates and the breast matures. This maturation continues with stimulus from each menstrual cycle until age 25. When growth stabilizes, further proliferation does not occur until pregnancy intervenes (Figure 1).

Changes in circulating hormones result in profound changes in the ductular–lobular–alveolar growth during pregnancy.[21] There is marked increase in ductular sprouting, branching, and lobular formation evoked by luteal and placental hormones (Figure 2). Placental lactogen, prolactin, and chorionic gonadotropin have been identified as contributors to the accelerated growth.

From the third month of gestation, secretory material resembling colostrum appears in the alveoli. By the second trimester, placental lactogen begins to stimulate the production of colostrum so that a woman delivering immaturely as early as 16 weeks may secrete colostrum although her baby is not viable. Until delivery, the production of milk is suppressed by prolactin-inhibiting hormone produced by the placenta. Progesterone produced by the placenta has been recognized as important in blocking milk production in pregnancy. At delivery, the withdrawal of placental and luteal sex hormones and the infant's sucking result in the loss of the inhibiting hormones and the stimulation of prolactin-releasing factors.[22]

The initiation of milk secretion at delivery and the continued production of milk occur because the breast has developed extensively throughout pregnancy.[11] The ductal system has arborized to form an extended network of collecting ducts. The alveoli are richly lined with epithelial cells varying from flat to low columnar in shape, all capable of producing milk. Some cells protrude into the lumen of the alveoli; others are short and smooth. The lumen of the alveolus is crowded with fine granular material and lipid droplets (Figure 3). The division and differentiation of the mammary epithelial cells and presecretory alveolar cells into secretory milk-releasing alveolar cells completes the preparation for milk production. The biosynthesis of milk involves this cellular site, where the metabolic processes occur. There are stem cells and highly differentiated secretory alveolar cells at the terminal ducts. The stem cells are stimulated by growth hormone and insulin, which is synergized by prolactin to stimulate the cells to secretory activity. The breast acts in response to the interactions of the pituitary, thyroid, pancreatic, adrenal, and ovarian hormones (Figure 4).

The process of milk synthesis involves apocrine secretion for the de novo production of fat and protein and the merocrine secretion of lactose synthesized from glucose.[19] Ions diffuse across the membrane and, in some cases, are actively transported. The primary alveolar milk is then diluted within the lumen to be isotonic with plasma by water that diffuses from extracellular fluid.[22,23] The pathways for milk synthesis and secretion into the mammary alveolus include[22] (1) exocytosis of protein and lactose, (2) formation of the milk fat globule, (3) secretion of ions and water, (4) pinocytosis–exocytosis of immunoglobulins, and (5) the paracellular pathway (Figure 5).

Because lactation is anticipated, the body prepares the breast during pregnancy and also develops additional nutritional maternal stores that will be needed during lactation, in the form of 6 to 8 pounds of body weight apart from the uterus and its contents. When lactation begins, there is a redistribution of blood supply from the uterus to the breast, where there is an increased demand for nutrients and an increased metabolic rate to accommodate the demands of milk production. The mammary gland may have to produce milk at the expense of other organs if stores are inadequate. There are cardiovascular adjustments as mammary blood flow increases. The mammary blood flow, cardiac output, and milk secretion are suckling dependent. In addition, suckling induces the release of anterior pituitary hormones, prolactin and oxytocin, which act directly on the breast tissue and on the uterus.[22]

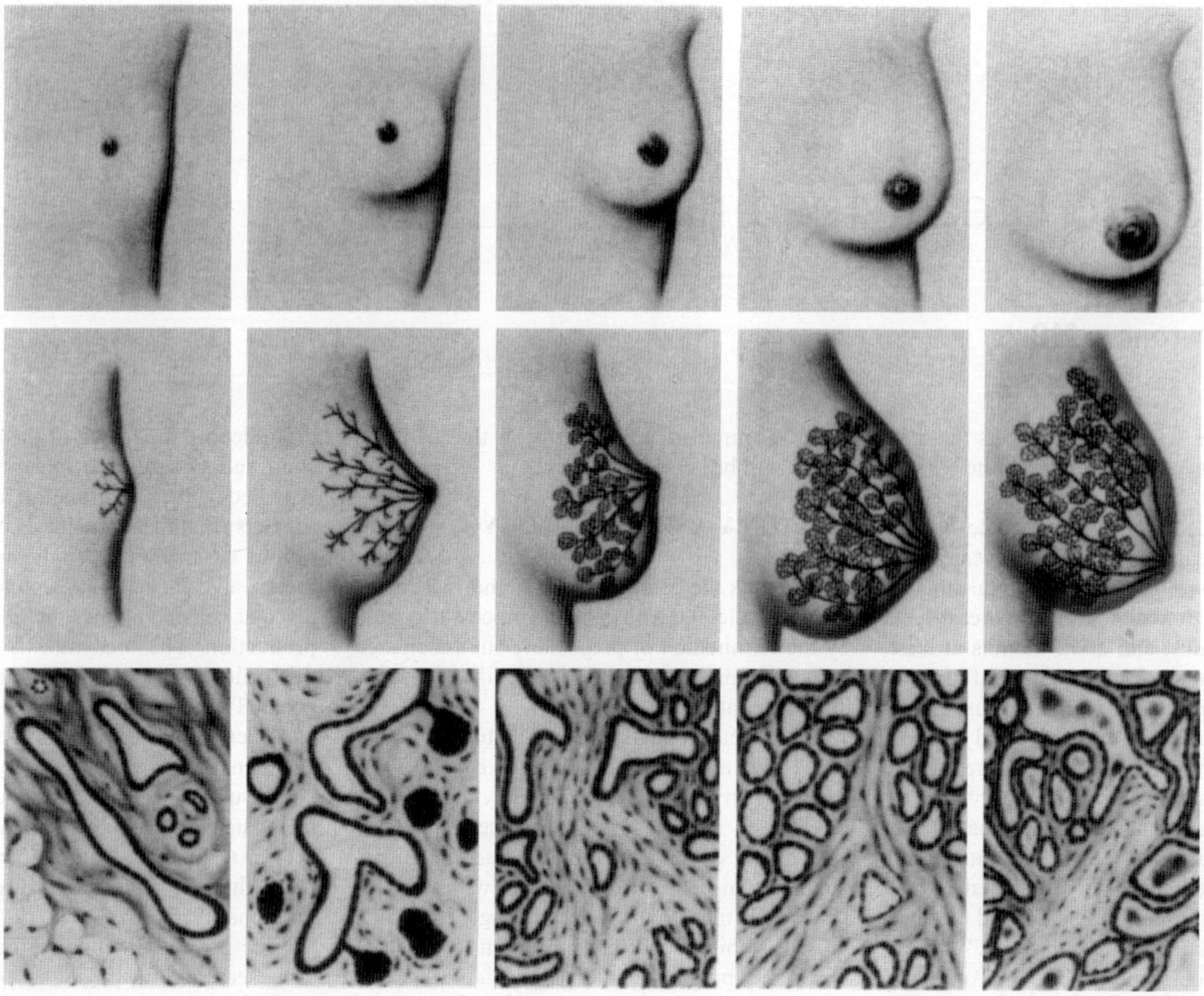

Figure 1 Female breast from infancy to lactation with corresponding cross-section and duct structure. *A, B, C,* Gradual development of well-differentiated ductular and peripheral lobular-alveolar system. *D,* Ductular sprouting and intensified peripheral lobular-alveolar development in pregnancy Glandular luminal cells begin actively synthesizing milk fat and proteins near term. Only small amounts are released into lumen *E,* With postpartum withdrawal of luteal and placental sex steroids and placental lactogen, prolactin is able to induce full secretory activity of alveolar cells and release of milk into alveoli and smaller ducts. Reproduced with permission from Lawrence RA and Lawrence RM.[10]

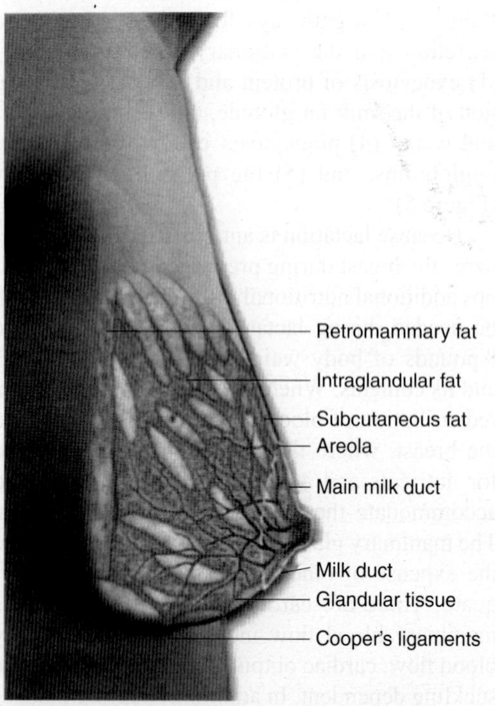

Figure 2 Morphology of mature breast with dissection to reveal mammary fat and duct system. Reproduced with permission from Lawrence RA and Lawrence RM.[10]

In addition to glandular preparation, the nipple and areola are also preparing for lactation. There is an increase in vascularization. The Montgomery glands, which are sebaceous glands on the areolae circling the nipple, become enlarged and begin to secrete a substance that lubricates and protects the areola and nipple during pregnancy and lactation.[11]

The use of ultrasound imagery[24–28] to examine the working of the human breast has replaced some beliefs about the anatomy that were originally derived from the dissection of formalin-prepared specimens in 1840.[29] Imaging the actively secreting breast has revealed that only about 9 to 12 (range 4–18) ducts are at the base of the nipple, not 15 to 25, as originally believed. The ducts were measured to be 1.9 ± 0.6 mm (1.0–4.4 mm) in diameter. The number of ducts and their diameter did not correlate with nipple size or radius of the areolae or actual milk production. The amount of glandular tissue in the lactating breast was about 64% (range 45–83%) of the breast tissue, and the fatty tissue only accounted for 38% (16–51%). There was no correlation

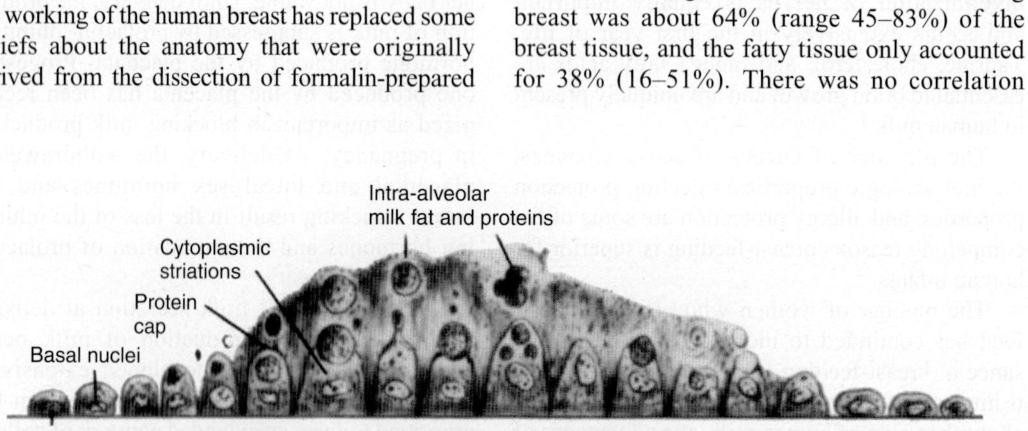

Figure 3 Cycle of secretory cells from resting stage to secretion and return to resting stage. Reproduced with permission from Lawrence RA and Lawrence RM.[10]

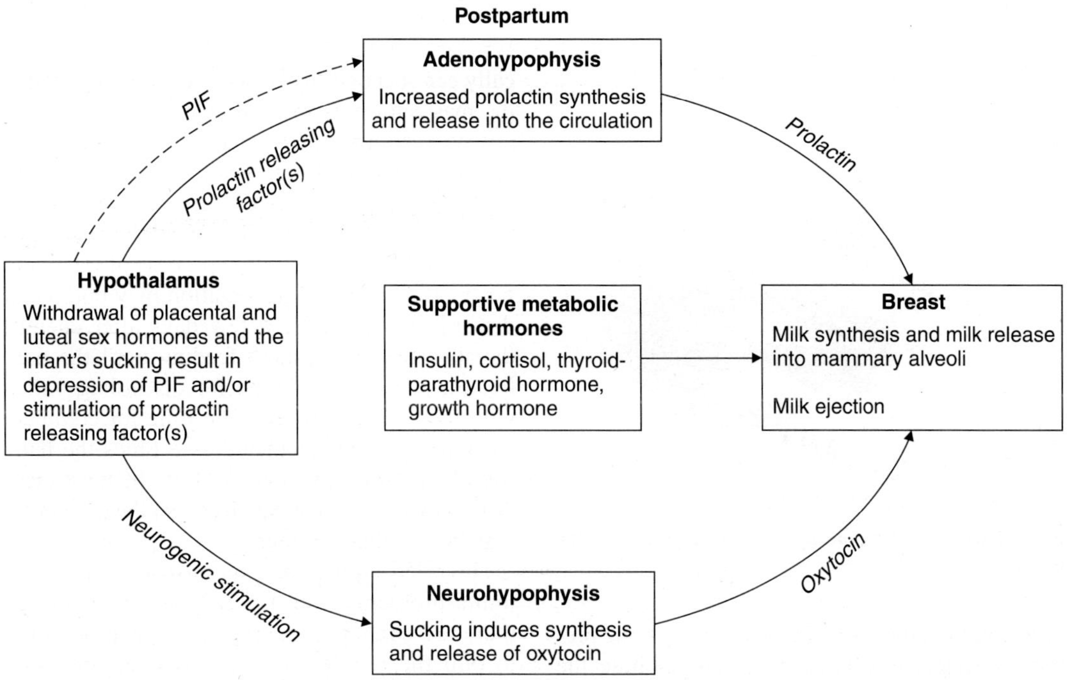

Figure 4 Hormonal preparation of breast postpartum for lactation. Reproduced with permission from Lawrence RA and Lawrence RM.[10]

between milk production and the amount of glandular tissue as measured by ultrasound[24,25] (Figure 3). The nipple has many sensory nerve fibers but the areola does not: an important fact in terms of comfort for the mother while nursing.[26] The response to tactile sensation of the nipple increases dramatically at delivery as an adaptation for lactation that enhances the nervous response to suckling by the infant (Figure 6).

INITIATION OF MILK SECRETION

Withdrawal of placental and luteal sex hormones and stimulation of prolactin-releasing factor result in the increased prolactin synthesis by the adenohypophysis, which stimulates milk synthesis in the mammary alveoli. The release of milk from the alveolar collecting ductules depends on the ejection or let-down reflex (Figure 6). The let-down reflex is a simple arc that is initiated by the suckling of the infant.[30] This suckling stimulates the mechanoreceptors in the nipple and areola that send stimuli along nerve pathways to the hypothalamus, which stimulates the posterior pituitary to release oxytocin.[31,32] Oxytocin, which is carried via the bloodstream to the breast and uterus,[33,34] stimulates the myoepithelial cells that envelop the secretory alveoli and the collecting ductules in the breast to contract, ejecting milk through the ductule. The oxytocin also stimulates the myoepithelial cells in the uterus to contract, causing the "after pains" a mother associates with lactation. Physiologically, this uterine contraction enhances the uterine postpartum involution, so that the uterus of the lactating woman returns to normal more quickly postpartum. Oxytocin release can also be stimulated by seeing or hearing the infant; thus a woman notices that her milk begins to drip when she sees her infant.[34] Prolactin, however, is only released when the breast is stimulated by suckling or pumping.

Prolactin, which is also released from the hypothalamus during sucking, stimulates the production of milk.[30] Prolactin levels during early lactation are increased 10 to 20 times greater than normal. The technology required to obtain prolactin levels has been available for clinical investigation, but the role of prolactin in the volume of milk produced is still not clearly defined. It is clear, however, that the surge in prolactin to about twice the baseline levels is critical to the successful production of an adequate supply of milk. When evaluating prolactin during lactation, a sample of blood is drawn at baseline and then a second sample is drawn after 10 minutes of breast-feeding or pumping with an electric pump.[11] The baseline should be above normal range for the laboratory and poststimulus should be increased to almost double baseline.

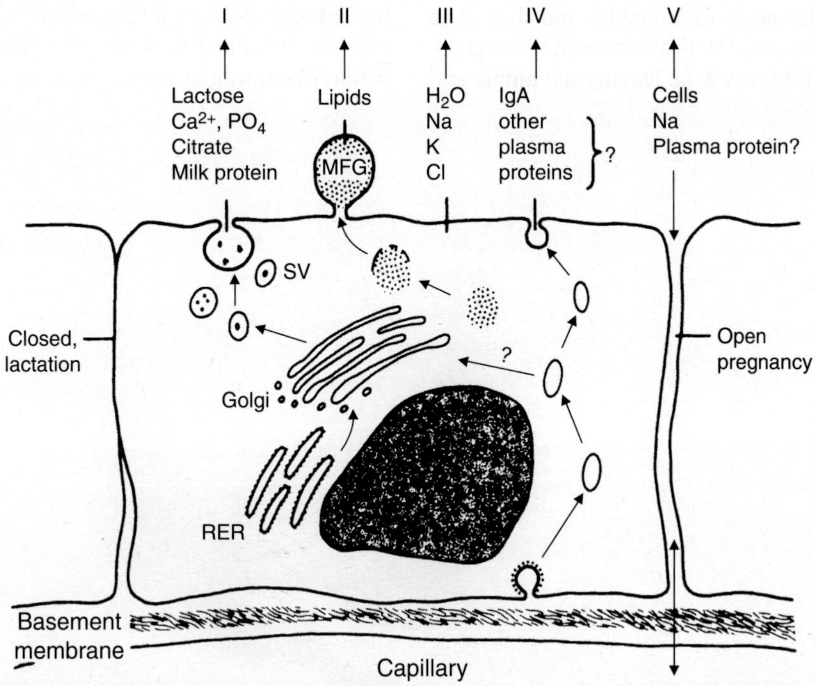

Figure 5 The pathways for milk synthesis and secretion in the mammary alveolus. (II) Exocytosis of milk protein and lactose in Golgi-derived secretory vesicles. (III) Secretion of ions and water across the apical membrane. (IV) Pinocytosis-exocytosis of immunoglobulins. (V) The paracellular pathway of plasma components and leukocytes. MFG = milk fat globule; RER = rough endoplasmic reticulum; SV = secretory vesicle. Adapted from Neville MC.[18] Reproduced with permission from Lawrence RA and Lawrence RM.[10]

PRENATAL CONSIDERATIONS

Although the breast prepares for lactation independent of the mother's decision to breast-feed, it is important to introduce the question of feeding the infant as soon as possible during pregnancy so that the mother can make an informed choice on behalf of her baby.[31] Although it has been suggested that well-educated mothers have made up their minds about how they will feed their infants long before conception occurs, there are many women who need to be informed about breast-feeding and need to receive reinforcement from their physician.[31] Many women, especially primiparas, will need considerable assistance to lactate successfully. The significant benefits of human milk to the human infant have already been reviewed in previous chapters. The psychological benefits are equally as important to both mother and child.[32]

The nutritional benefits of human milk, although legion, can in part be substituted with a modern prepared formula, but the infection protection, immunologic properties, and the psychological benefits of human milk cannot be

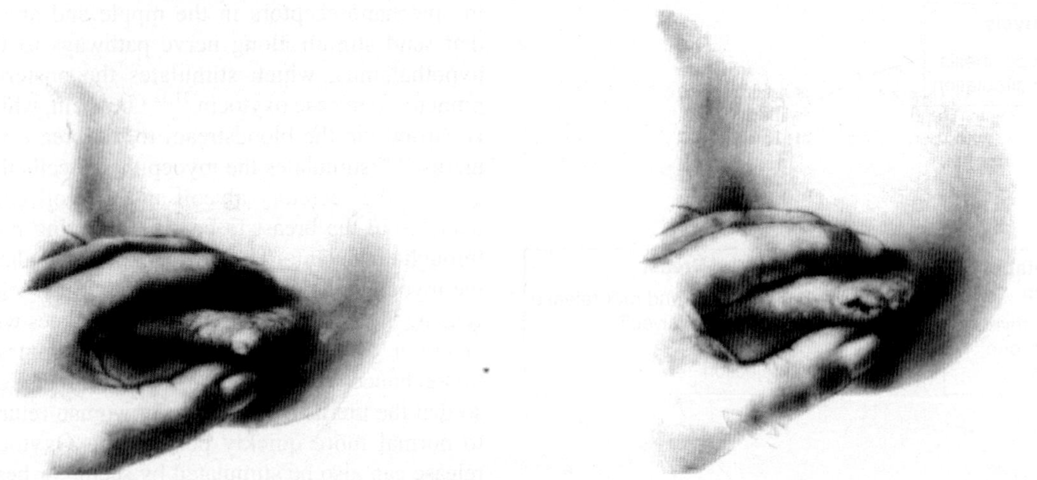

Figure 6 (A) Normal nipple everts with gentle pressure. (B) Inverted or tied nipple inverts with gentle pressure. Reproduced with permission from Lawrence RA and Lawrence RM.[10]

duplicated.[14,15] In the mid–twentieth century, when bottle feeding was rampant, the single, clear, unchallenged advantage to breast-feeding that was articulated was the special interrelationship between the mother and her baby.[32] The key elements of attachment are said to include early contact, closeness, eye-to-eye contact, smell, and body warmth. Breast-feeding includes these naturally. A woman has a surge of oxytocin and prolactin during each feeding, which has been demonstrated biologically to stimulate mothering behavior.[33,34]

When a mother wishes to be free of the responsibility of breast-feeding, it is often so that she will not be tied down, will not always have to be available, and can have others feed the infant, thus depriving the infant of this special frequent closeness with the mother.

Preparation of the Breasts

Nature prepares the breasts. It is not necessary to manipulate the breasts and nipples prenatally in preparation in the normal woman. Part of the prenatal physical examination should include the breasts with respect to lactation so that any anatomic variations that may interfere with lactation can be discussed.[31] The size of the breast is not related to lactation success and is not a measure of glandular potential.[28] Women who have had benign cysts removed can still nurse successfully. Augmentation mammoplasty does not usually interfere with lactation if the nipple and duct system have been left intact, that is, the nipple has not been realigned and the implant is placed under the breast tissue on the chest wall. Unless the implant has ruptured and has caused scarring, lactation should be successful. When breast size has been surgically diminished by reduction mammoplasty, the duct system may have been interrupted if the nipple was completely removed and replaced central to the remaining tissue. This may make lactation improbable, and this issue should be discussed with the operating surgeon. If the procedure was done leaving the nipple and areola on a pedicle, lactation may be successful. Women who have had one breast removed surgically can successfully breast-feed, although when the mastectomy is for malignant disease, it may not be recommended because of the potential effect of continued high levels of sex steroids in the system if pregnancy occurs within 5 years of treatment. It should be discussed with the oncologist. Women who are in the process of treatment for breast cancer during lactation may pump and discard their milk for a few days after chemotherapy and then resume feeding until the next treatment. Length of time for discarding varies with the drug employed. The time for complete clearance can be calculated as 5 times the half-life of the drug involved.[11] Many of the cancer drugs have very short half-lives, so the disruption may be less than 24 hours.

Inverted nipples are the most common anatomic problem identified (Figure 7). Although there are stretching exercises that can be done, to pull the nipple out, exercises require time, considerable dedication, and a commitment on the part of the mother to this daily manipulation. Some mothers find nipple exercises distasteful. Nipple stimulus prenatally may trigger uterine contractions and premature labor. Another method of treatment for inverted nipples is wearing specially designed plastic shells inside the normal brassiere daily during the last 6 weeks of pregnancy, beginning with a few minutes a day and increasing time worn to 8 to 10 hours after about 2 weeks. The continued gentle pressure on the areola, stretching the fibrous tissue, will evert the nipple through the central hole. After delivery, these shells can be worn between feedings (but not during) until the eversion is firmly established postpartum and the nipple is easily grasped by the infant. A controlled study by Alexander and colleagues found that the technique was not very effective and it often discouraged some women from even

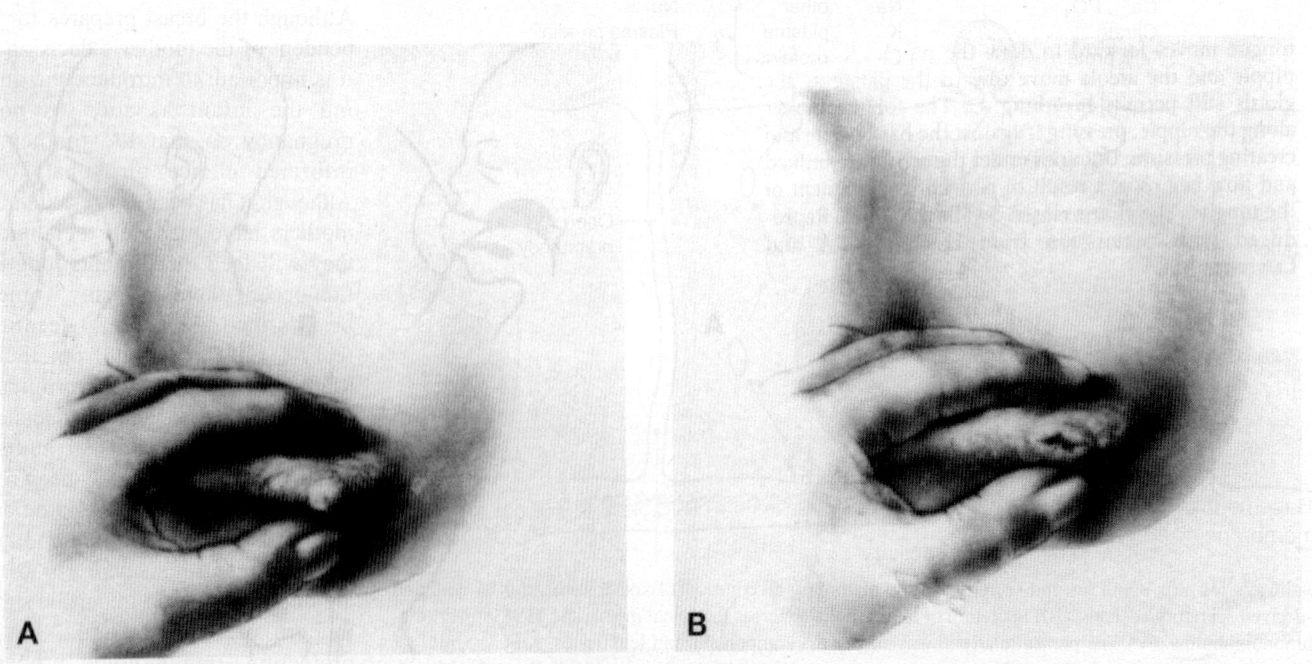

Figure 7 Breast shell in place inside a brassiere to evert the nipple. Reproduced with permission from Lawrence RA and Lawrence RM.[10]

initiating breast-feeding.[35] Inverted or small nipples may best be everted by using a good hand pump or an electric pump just prior to putting the infant in position to latch on for a feeding in the first few days postpartum. Usually, the nipple will remain erect without pumping after a week of these efforts. In subsequent pregnancies, the nipples are more everted probably due to the stretching of the fibers that were tying the nipple down initially.

Only gentle face soap and clear water are needed for breast care. No ointments or lotions are advised prophylactically as they irritate the skin and plug the natural pores, inhibiting the natural secretions. The sebaceous secretions of the glands of Montgomery on the areola are intended to lubricate the areola and nipple. Buffing the tissues briskly with a turkish towel or a toothbrush is neither necessary nor recommended. In a very dry climate where skin dryness is a problem, a bland ointment such as a vitamin A and D ointment or purified lanolin might be prescribed in some cases.

Removing colostrum in the last few weeks of pregnancy by manual expression is not recommended as it may irritate the tissues and cause an early mastitis. Because the colostrum is discarded, it wastes a very valuable commodity, which should be left for the infant. Such manipulation of the breast may also stimulate premature contractions of the uterus. Prior to delivery, the mother should purchase and bring to the hospital a well-constructed nursing brassiere to support the breasts, especially as the milk first comes in. This will alleviate the feeling of heaviness and engorgement. Many women wear a nursing brassiere night and day, especially in the first few weeks postpartum.

A new mother may find it helpful to attend breast-feeding classes prenatally and actually see an infant at the breast before she delivers if she is totally unfamiliar with breast-feeding.[36] Many childbirth classes include breast-feeding in the curriculum. If not, the physician may wish to have the office staff provide that educational service or refer the patient to a community breast-feeding support group, such as La Leche League.

Initiating Lactation: The First Feed

As soon after birth as possible, preferably within the first hour of life, the infant should be breast-fed.[5,6] Once the infant is stable, with the airway clear and respirations established, he can be offered the breast with the mother lying on her side facing the infant, who is also lying on his side. The infant should be held close to the breast. The areola will be soft and compressible. If the mother strokes the infant's lower lip with the nipple, he will quickly root, open the mouth wide, grasp the nipple and areola, and begin to suckle. The nipple and areola elongate to form a teat as they are drawn into the mouth. The infant should grasp well beyond the nipple so as to compress the areola and ductules, which lie under the areola (Figures 8 and 9). Because nipple size and areola size vary, the infant may not be able to get the entire areola into the mouth. Even at the first feeding, the infant will receive colostrum. The mother should be further instructed in the art of positioning herself comfortably and supporting her breast with her hand. Changing her position at different feedings allows the infant to grasp from different angles.[18,36,37] This will rotate the point of greatest suckling pressure and will evenly distribute the suckling pressure over the entire areola. After the first feed, a mother may lie down or sit up as she chooses. If the nipple is tender, the baby can be held on the right breast as if he were nursing on the left side, that is, facing the mother's right side with feet to her right (or the reverse on the left breast, with the infant facing the mother's left side). The key to correct positioning is having the infant face the breast. The infant can be brought close by moving the mother's arm that is holding the infant and not by pushing the infant's head toward the breast. Pushing the head toward the breast causes the infant to arch back away from the breast, which is the natural arching reflex. This results when the back of the head is held. This appears to the mother as if the infant is rejecting the breast.

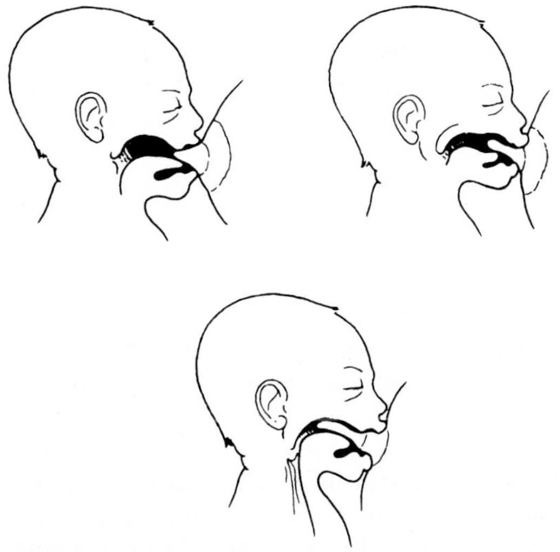

Figure 8 (A) As the infant grasps the breast, the tongue moves forward to draw the nipple in. (B) The nipple and the areola move toward the palate as the glottis still permits breathing. (C) The tongue moves along the nipple, pressing it against the hard palate and creating pressure, Ductules under the areola are milked and flow begins as a result of peristaltic movement of the tongue. The glottis closes. Swallow follows. Reproduced with permission from Lawrence RA and Lawrence RM.[10]

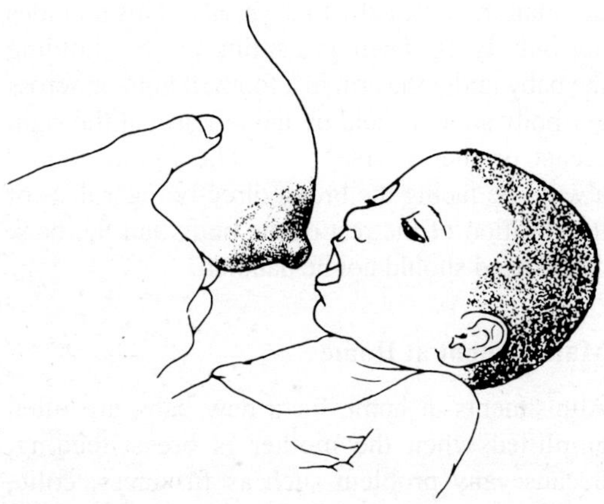

Figure 9 Latching on. In response to stimulating the infant's lower lip with the nipple, the mouth opens wide. Reproduced with permission from Lawerence RA and Lawerence RM.[10]

Initially, a mother may offer both breasts at each feeding to stimulate each breast as often as possible during the first weeks. The infant, however, should nurse long enough on the first side to receive the hind milk, that is, over 5 minutes. In reality, he may drift off to sleep before being switched to the second side. At the next feeding, he should be offered the other breast first. This will balance the stimulus and, thus, milk production. The infant should nurse every time he awakens and is alert and hungry, which may be as frequently as every 2 hours. Intervals between feedings should not be greater than 4 to 5 hours in the beginning when frequent stimulus is critical to establishing a good milk supply. If the infant sleeps 6 hours, he should be awakened in the first few weeks of life. Having the mother and baby cared for in close proximity as in rooming-in or by mother–baby nursing staff assignments will facilitate frequent appropriate feeding and will enhance milk production. In programs where infants are fed more than six times daily (average 10–12 times), the length of each feeding tends to be shorter. With frequent feeding, there is better milk production, less weight loss, earlier regain of birth weight, and less neonatal jaundice.[38–42] This increase in feeding frequency has not been associated with an increase in sore nipples. Sore nipples are associated with inappropriate positioning at the breast. Care should be taken not to overwhelm the mother with many suggestions for different positions, alternate hand grips, and other angles for the infant. She should find a simple way that works before leaving the hospital. If there is a problem, then different approaches can be suggested. The infant should feed when hungry with no rules for timing or intervals. Crying is a late sign of hunger. Every mother should be observed feeding her baby by a skilled observer before discharge.

Healthy mothers and their infants are being discharged in 48 hours or less in sharp contrast to the 4- to 5-day stay of the past. Mothers with cesarean sections may leave in 36 hours. Having a helpless newborn totally dependent on a mother is an awesome, frightening, and sometimes discouraging responsibility. The mother is no longer an independent person. This responsibility may be overwhelming unless care is taken to "mother the mother," because our culture does not automatically provide maternal support.[43] In fact, our culture programs a superwoman concept in which the new mother must return to her other household chores unless the health professional intervenes. Adequate rest should be prescribed. Discussing the joint responsibilities of parenthood with both parents may facilitate a smoother transition from the sheltered hospital environment to home. Early discharge home also places a responsibility on the physician to see the breast-fed infant in the first week of life at home. Provision for weight checks and assessment of jaundice should involve a home visit or an office visit within 2 days of discharge.[4,41] Many offices have a nurse practitioner skilled in newborn care and breast-feeding who provides this service.

Nourishment for the lactating woman should make sense, but nurturance while providing these nutrients is equally important. Raphael has expressed it as the need for a *doula,* which is taken from the Greek language to mean "a helpful friend from across the street."[43] It means that someone must care for the mother, support her efforts to breast-feed, and make her feel confident in her ability to mother her infant.

Supplementation with Milk or Water

Careful study of weight loss in breast-fed and formula-fed infants in the first days of life indicates that the breast-fed baby does not lose more weight than the formula fed baby when breast-feeding is adequately assisted. Furthermore, infants who are fed frequently at the breast in the first few days begin to gain weight at least by the fourth day. Studies correlating the method of feeding with the level of bilirubin show no significant difference between breast-feeding and formula feeding.[40–42] Studies comparing frequency of feeding in the breast-feeding group show that infants who are fed seven or more times per day have significantly lower bilirubin levels than those fed six or less times per day. Findings were independent of the total number of minutes per day spent nursing.[39,40] In terms of lactation physiology, the breast produces milk in response to suckling and the removal of milk by suckling or pumping. The greatest volume of milk is obtained in the first 5 to 10 minutes at each breast. If the infant feeds more frequently, he receives more milk, and the breast produces more in response. Animal studies by Gartner and Herschel suggest a relationship between elevated bilirubin levels and starvation.[41] Weight loss of greater than 5% requires evaluation of the breast-feeding, as does unexplained hyperbilirubinemia.[4,38]

If, on the other hand, the influence of giving water or milk supplements to babies who are breast-fed is scrutinized, it is noted that supplementation, especially with water, is associated with increased weight loss and increased bilirubin levels in the first few days of life.[39–41,44] If the influence of water or milk supplements on babies who are breast-fed is investigated from the standpoint of successful establishment of lactation, length of breast-feeding, and reasons for early weaning, it is also noted to be negative. Mothers who add supplements have more difficulty establishing a good milk supply, are more apt to wean early, and give "insufficient milk" as a reason for weaning. Supplements interfere with successful lactation.[45]

In the first few weeks of lactation, it is important to encourage a feeding program that meets the infant's needs, that is, providing feeding when the infant is awake and hungry (so-called demand or on-request feeding). This may be 12 to 16 times per day. Most babies have a period of a few hours when they want to nurse every hour and that is appropriate for several feedings. There is, however, a relationship between the fatigue and stamina of the mother that has to be balanced against the true needs of the infant. A fussy breast-fed infant who has been well fed may need to be comforted by someone else. This is an important role for the father. Lactating women may not be able to comfort their own infants without offering the breast because the infant smells the milk and will root even though he is well fed. This sometimes leads to incessant nonnutritive suckling, which may be a drain on the mother's energy resources and traumatic to the nipple. Nonnutritive comforting is a significant need of most infants and can be provided by the father.

An additional side effect of supplementation is the use of a bottle and a rubber nipple, which may lead to nipple confusion on the part of the newborn.[46] The sucking mechanism utilized at the breast is the sucking reflex present at birth. The infant will have much of the areola in the mouth, compressing it against the hard palate as it elongates into a teat, maintaining the seal with the gum and lips. The tongue undulates with a peristaltic motion that also triggers the swallow and initiates peristalsis in the esophagus and the stomach. The nipple is a passive passageway for the milk to exit. When a bottle is used, the infant's jaws do little but hold the nipple in place. There is little undulating of the tongue, and milk flows easily with a little suction created by the seal. The tongue may even be thrust upward to control the flow from the unyielding rubber nipple. Because this is a different position and action, some babies are confused by switching back and forth between breast and bottle, especially in the first few weeks or when the infant is slightly premature. When the tongue thrusting of bottle-feeding is used with the breast, it pushes the human nipple out of the mouth.

The position a mother assumes while nursing should be comfortable and relaxing for her. A rocking chair is often the best for the sitting position. It is recommended that a mother may increase her comfort if she varies the hold and orientation of the baby to the breast. This includes not only lying down and sitting up, but holding the baby under the arm in a football hold or across her body so he is held by the left arm at the right breast or the reverse.[11,37,47] The infant should always be facing the breast directly regardless of the position of the rest of the body and the back of the head should not be handled.

Management at Home

Adjustments at home for a new baby are often amplified when the mother is breast-feeding, because any problem such as fussiness, colic, wakefulness, or night feedings are assumed by the mother to be due to a problem with breast-feeding. Instilling confidence in the mother's ability to care for and nourish her infant is important. Closer surveillance by the physician in the first few days, however, is necessary to be certain that the new inexperienced mother does not interpret long sleeping periods with little feeding as adequate for proper growth. Successful breast-feeding results in fewer problems and illnesses later. Review of weight status, number of wet diapers (at least six per day), stool pattern (at least three per day in the first month), and feeding pattern is a further check on successful lactation. When a breast-fed infant does not stop losing weight by 5 days, does not produce a stool every day, does not void adequately, or does not regain birth weight by 14 days, aggressive intervention is indicated. The physician needs to evaluate infant and the breast-feeding.[47]

Maternal Nutrition

The nursing mother should have a nutrition check to confirm her appropriate food intake. A lactating woman should have 500 extra calories over the pre-pregnancy baseline, 20 extra grams of protein, and a balanced diet. Mothers who are concerned about losing weight should be counseled to consume no less than 1,800 kcal per day and to consume adequate vitamins and minerals.[3,48] Maternal weight loss after the initial drop should not exceed 1 to 1.5 kg per month in the first 6 months of lactation. The most important dietary increase is calcium and phosphorus, to a total of 1,200 mg per day.[49] The neonatal calcium–phosphorus requirement exceeds that of the fetus in the last trimester of pregnancy. Dairy products are the best source, but if these products are not tolerated by the mother, she needs to seek out additional sources in dark green vegetables, nuts, legumes, and certain dried fruits. Dark-green leafy vegetables such as kale, cabbage, collards, and turnip greens contain readily available calcium, whereas the calcium in spinach, swiss chard, and beet greens is bound to oxalic acid and is unabsorbable.[3,48] The amount of calcium in the diet will not influence the amount in the milk, but a deficiency will lead to leaching from maternal bone and significant osteoporosis. A lactating woman does not need added iron for milk but will need to replace stores lost in pregnancy and parturition. A balanced diet should provide all other nutrients. The quality of the milk day by day is balanced by intake and stores (Figure 10).

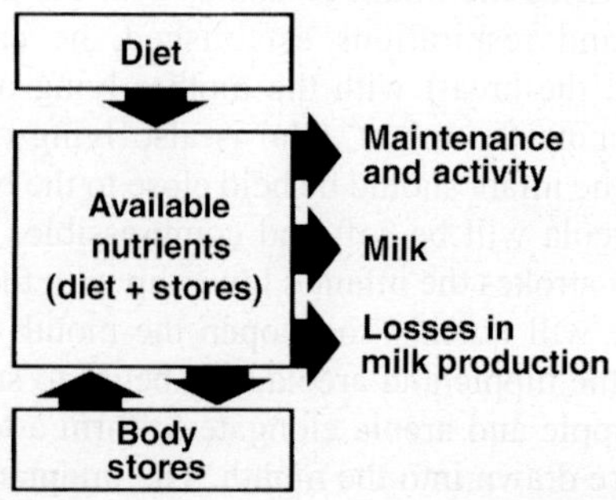

Figure 10 Energy use in lactation, showing availability of body stores and dietary sources. Reproduced with permission from Lawrence RA and Lawrence RM.[10]

Table 1 Herbal Teas

Ingredient	Botanical Source	Pharmacologic Principle	Use	Effects
African yohimbe bark, yohimbe	*Corynanthe yohimbe*	Yohimbine	Smoke or drink as stimulant	Mild hallucinogen
Catnip	*Nepeta cataria*	Nepetalactone	Smoke or drink as marijuana substitute	Mild hallucinogen
Gordolobo yerbal	*Senecio douglassi*	Pyrrolizidine alkaloids	Drink	Sore throat therapy, ? tranquilizer
Hops	*Humulus lupulus*	Lupuline	Smoke or drink as sedative and marijuana substitute	? None
Kavakava	*Piper methysticum*	Yangonin, pyrones	Smoke or drink as marijuana substitute	Mild hallucinogen
Kola nut	*Cola* spp.	Caffeine, theobromine, kolanin	Smoke, drink, or take as capsules as stimulant	Stimulant
Lobelia	*Lobelia inflata*	Lobeline	Smoke or drink as marijuana substitute	Mild euphoriant
Mandrake	*Mandragora officinarum*	Scopolamine, hyoscyamine	Drink as hallucinogen	Hallucinogen
Mate	*Ilex paraguayensis*	Caffeine	Drink as stimulant	Stimulant
Mormon tea	*Ephedra nevadensis*	Ephedrine	Drink as stimulant	Stimulant
Nutmeg	*Myristica fragrans*	Myristicin	Drink as hallucinogen	Hallucinogen
Passion flower	*Passiflora incarnata*	Harmine alkaloids	Smoke, drink, or take as capsules as marijuana	Mild stimulant
Periwinkle	*Catharanthus roseus*	Indole alkaloids	Smoke or drink as euphoriant	Hallucinogen
Snakeroot	*Rauwolfia serpentina*	Reserpine	Smoke or drink as tobacco substitute	Tranquilizer
Thorn apple	*Datura stramonium*	Atropine, scopolamine	Smoke or drink as tobacco substitute or hallucinogen	Strong hallucinogen
Valerian	*Valeriana officinalis*	Chatinine, velerine alkaloids	Drink or take as capsules as tranquilizer	Tranquilizer
Wormwood	*Artemisia absinthium*	Absinthe	Smoke or drink as relaxant	Narcotic-analgesic

Adapted from reference 44. Reproduced with permission from reference 10.

The strict vegetarian is in jeopardy, however, of causing B_{12} deficiency in her offspring, unless she takes supplements, because B_{12} is not found in nature except in animal protein.

The lactating woman does have increased needs for fluids and thus increased thirst. If a woman selects beverages that contain caffeine or other active pharmacologic principles, it could affect the infant. Beverages that either contain no caffeine or have been decaffeinated are appropriate. With the increasing interest in herbal teas, attention should be given to the content of such teas.[50] A partial list of products is shown in Table 1. Many teas contain very potent glucosides having pharmacologic properties, others are benign and a few even nutritious, such as rose hips, which contain vitamin C.

Documenting the consumption of herbal teas by the mother or given to the infant directly should be part of the medical history. Some herbs are reputed to enhance lactation such as fenugreek. The required dose is large and soon the milk and all secretions and the infant smell like maple syrup. It helps some women but not all. There can be a cross allergy to peanuts and chickpeas that may cause colic in the infant. Comfrey has been widely used in midwifery and in lactation but is banned in many countries. The FDA has also issued a warning as its use can cause veno-occlusive disease and even be fatal, especially in infants.[51]

STAGES OF BREAST-FEEDING

Adaptation

Initially, there is a period of adjustment and adaptation as the mother and baby settle into a reciprocal relationship of supply-and-demand. The infant can be exclusively nourished at the breast for the first 6 months of life. During that time there may be gradual changes in the feeding pattern as the infant matures and sleeps longer between feedings and also spends more time awake and socializing. Growth spurts are accompanied by a temporary increase in feeding frequency. This may alarm the mother if she has not been alerted to this possibility. Periods of stress or illness in the infant may be marked with temporarily increased suckling, especially nonnutritive suckling for comfort. Human milk meets all the nutrient needs of the infant for the first 6 months except for a select group of women who live in cold climates with little sunshine, have dark pigmented skin, wear occlusive clothing, or use sunscreen frequently, who may be vitamin D deficient.[52] Concern about widespread vitamin D deficiency has resulted in reconsideration of vitamin D requirements. Recommendations from the Centers for Disease Control and Prevention suggest supplementing the infants with 400 units vitamin D daily by mouth with a vitamin D–only preparation for breast-fed infants.[53] Very-low-birth-weight infants may need iron. Healthy exclusively breast-fed infants do not need iron for the first 6 months of life. When weaning foods are added in the second 6 months, they should be iron containing, such as iron-supplemented cereal.[54]

Adding Solid Foods

The infant ideally is exclusively breast-fed for the first 6 months. The single nutrient needed to add to solid foods in an exclusively breast-fed infant is the need for additional dietary iron; thus introduction of iron-fortified weaning foods at around 6 months is recommended, although the exact age is poorly defined.[54] At about 6 months of age, it is appropriate to begin the addition of solid foods to the infant's diet for nutritional reasons (see Chapter 28, "The Low Birth Weight Infant"). Learning to take solid foods is also an important developmental milestone that involves a new use of tongue, jaw, and lips—a use that differs from suckling.[55] Beginning to take fluids from a cup is also a developmental task that should be learned around 7 months of age. The infant who is exclusively breast-fed to this point needs to explore these activities and develop these skills just as a bottle-fed infant would. The fluids can be water, juice, or pumped breast milk. If a mother continues to provide her milk, there is no need to introduce formula. Cow's milk when the infant is under 1 year of age is not recommended.

Weaning

To wean is "to transfer the young of any animal from dependence on its mother's milk to another form of nourishment" or "to estrange from former habits or associations" according to the dictionary.[56] The weaning process takes many forms, depending on the mother's schedule and beliefs and the needs of the infant. Some women plan to breast-feed for only a few months "to give the baby a good start"; other mothers wean as soon as solid foods can be started, and some continue to offer the breast for several years, even during a subsequent pregnancy and while feeding a new baby. The appropriate time for weaning should be based on nutritional and psychological needs and developmental milestones. Feeding is an important social as well as nutritional encounter, and eating solids and drinking from a cup are important social accomplishments. This does not mean the infant is taken completely off the breast. In practice, the mother is usually the instigator of weaning. The process ideally is gradual, replacing one feeding at a time with solids and the introduction of a bottle or cup, depending on the infant's age and stage of development. After the adjustment has been made to substitute one feeding, a second feeding is replaced, usually at the opposite time of day. The process is continued until there is only one nursing at night and one in the morning. These two feedings may be maintained for many months or gradually discontinued over weeks. A mother may be able to express milk from the breast for weeks after the final feeding. An infant who has not weaned by 18 to 24 months usually does spontaneously wean until 4 or 5 years of age.[11]

Emergency weaning because of a crisis such as illness or separation may be stormy for the dyad. The infant may reject the bottle and refuse all nourishment at first. The mother who abruptly weans may experience severe engorgement, pain, and systemic symptoms attributed to the resorption of milk, referred to as "milk fever." Emergency weaning is facilitated by the assistance of another adult who can initiate the new feeding method and is patient and understanding with the child. Cup feeding with a small medicine cup may be a helpful alternative.

Breast-Feeding and the Return to Work

Returning to work has been cited by epidemiologists as a major hurdle in the initiation and duration of breast-feeding.[57,58] Because they need to return to work or to school, women often think it is best not to start. Before the industrial revolution, all women worked on the farm or in a cottage industry, keeping their children with them. In developing countries today, women carry their infants with them to feed them whenever necessary while working. It was the industrial revolution that separated home and work and made parenting a separate role for women.

More women are employed today outside the home than ever before.[59] Women with children under 6 years of age are the fastest-growing segment of the female workforce in 2000 (64.4% of women with a child under 6 years old). Even more startling are the number of working mothers with children under 3 years of age (60.7%).[60] Of the women who work during pregnancy, over 50% plan to return to work by 3 months postpartum. These dramatic statistics make it clear that the decision about infant feeding is an important part of this issue.[61] Child care also presents another consideration for the women who may well have to choose day care or some form of child care that means her infant will be in close contact with other children. In modern pediatrics, "Day Care Syndrome" is real. It is the increase in number of infections, especially diarrhea, respiratory illness, and otitis media experienced by young infants in day care.

The data are clear that breast-feeding impacts these figures. These illness data predominantly represent bottle-fed infants. A quantitative study has shown that extending breast-feeding from 4 months of age to 6 months decreases the risk of respiratory infection including pneumonia and otitis media even further.[12] The protective properties in human milk (Chapter 30, "Human Milk: Nutritional Properties") are even more important for the child exposed to other children early in life while mother works or attends school. A comparison of mothers' absenteeism showed that those who were breast-feeding had reduced absenteeism.[62] Looking at illness rates of children whose mothers work, 75% of children who were bottle-fed were ill and only 25% of those breast-fed had any illness.

The feeding pattern for mothers who work: Ideally, the mother does not return to work for at least 6 weeks so she is able to establish her milk supply before having to add work to her schedule. Mother will have to decide how she will cope.[63] If her job permits her to visit her child several times a day, then she can just feed the infant at the usual times. An employer who has a day care center on the premises makes such an arrangement possible. Professional women who control their own schedules (lawyers, doctors, consultants) may be able to keep the infant on the premises under the care of a baby attendant and feed on demand. For most women, however, their jobs are more rigid and they may have to settle for an opportunity to pump their milk every 3 or 4 hours on lunch or coffee breaks and store the milk in a cooler to take home for the next day's feedings. Most women practice pumping at home several weeks ahead of time and store up a supply of milk in the freezer so they do not run out.

Employers such as hospitals, health departments, and family-friendly industries like Amoco Chicago, Dow Chemical of Midland, Michigan, and the Los Angeles Department of Water and Power, to name a few, have been recognized for their support of "Healthy Mothers and Healthy Babies" and their accommodations for nursing mothers. They provide a room to pump, electric pumps, refrigerators, and in some cases lactation consultants to assist with any breast-feeding issues. This support improves the incidence and duration of breast-feeding for the working woman.[63]

Pumping and Storing Milk

If the employer does not provide pumps, a mother should obtain a pump by either renting or purchasing several weeks in advance of the return to work. All pumps are not equal.[64,65] There are, however, several brands of good portable electric pumps that provide disposable attachments for those parts that contact the breast and the milk. Attachments that allow pumping both sides simultaneously save time and for some women stimulate more milk release. Other women find double pumping overwhelming and choose to do one side at a time. Hand (manual) pumps are good for stimulating milk release and relieving engorgement but not for large-volume pumping for most women. Many hospitals have lactation consultants on staff and a shop or service that rents pumps and sells other breast-feeding devices such as breast pads and storage bottles. Information about local resources should be available on the postpartum floor. If not, a mother can call La Leche League International, 1-800-LALECHE (1-800-525-3243) for a local contact person. After each pumping session, the disposable flanges, tubing, and bottles used for pumping should be rinsed with cool water first and then washed in warm soapy water and thoroughly rinsed and air dried. After rinsing with cold water to remove the milk, the equipment may also be washed in an electric dishwasher.

The pumped milk should be placed in a glass bottle or a firm plastic polypropylene nursing bottle that can be capped with an airtight seal without a nipple, and then used to feed the infant later. Polyethylene bags are adequate for term baby use. Storage temperatures and times have been carefully studied.[64] The container, which should be labeled with name, date, and time, should be placed in a refrigerator immediately or in a cooling bag or container with freezer packs if at work or school, where there is no refrigerator. It is safe in a cooler bag as long as the packs remain cold (24 hours). Upon arrival home, the bottles should be placed in the refrigerator if it will be used within 3 days or in the freezer if stored for later use. When milk is pumped at home, it can be placed in the refrigerator (4°C) immediately and kept for 5 days. Actually, when there is no alternative or a bottle has been inadvertently left out, milk can be kept in a sterile container at room temperature for 8 hours and then used immediately or refrigerated for a day.[11]

If milk is placed in the freezer of the refrigerator that has a separate door, it can be stored for 3 months if it is placed in the back to avoid thawing and freezing when the door is opened. If milk is placed in a deep freeze (−20°C), it can be kept for 6 months, and if at −70°C, it is good for a year or longer.[59,63,65] The impact of freezing on the milk is minimal, destroying only the cells and their function. The effect of refrigeration is also minimal, decreasing the cells and some of their function. Nutrients are unchanged Preserving nutrition. Storing mother's milk for her own infant does not require pasteurization. Providing donor milk to another infant does require pasteurization by regulation owing to the increase in risk of infection in the present environment. Pasteurization does affect some properties, destroying cells and decreasing lipase activity and some other enzymes (see Table 2).[59,66]

Day Care for the Breast-Feeding Infant

In choosing a day care service, care should be taken to ensure that breast-feeding and breast

Table 2 Storage and Use of Pumped Milk for Healthy Term Infants

Place	Length of Time
Refrigerator (4°C)	5 d at home; 3 d in day care
Freezer section (separate door) refrigerator (−20°C)	3 mo
Deep freeze (manual defrost) (−20°C)	6 mo
Commercial deep freeze (−70°C)	1 y
Sterile container at room temperature (23°C) (not ideal but milk need not be discarded)	8 h
Stored in cooler bag with frozen packs (as long as packs are still cold)	Less than 24 h
Thawed, previously frozen in refrigerator	24 h

milk are welcome. When taking an infant to day care, a mother may wish to nurse the infant just before she leaves her child or she may wish to nurse the infant at day care when she has a break from work. Further, she may wish to feed the child before she sets out for home with the infant in the afternoon. There needs to be a place to sit quietly with the infant out of the mainstream of activity. The staff should be prepared to make these accommodations and delay a feeding if mother is going to arrive shortly.

The mother will probably wish to provide her stored breast milk for her infant to receive during the day. It is not necessary for the caretaker to wear gloves to handle the milk or feed the infant. It is, however, appropriate to wear gloves to change any babies' diaper. If the milk was frozen, it can be thawed in the refrigerator at day care or thawed by swirling in a container of warm water. It should not be warmed in the microwave because of possible hot spots and scalding the infant. Microwaving interferes with the anti-infective properties as well as decreasing the vitamin C content. If the infant does not empty the container, it can be refrigerated and fed later unless it has been microwaved.[11] This is not true of formula but the protective factors in human milk will keep the bacterial count down. The day care attendants should save the containers for reuse by the mother. Thawed breast milk can be maintained in the refrigerator for 24 hours.

The milk containers should be carefully labeled with name and date of collection. The attendant should carefully confirm the name on the container before feeding. Mishaps of giving the wrong milk to the wrong infant do occur. It should be reported to both families and the day care's medical consultant with an incident report. There are no reported cases of injury following such an event.

FAILURE TO THRIVE WHILE BREAST-FEEDING

Paralleling the increasing incidence of breast-feeding, there has been an increase in the number of clinical reports, including one in the *Wall Street Journal,* describing a few cases of failure to thrive while breast-feeding.[24,44,67,68] The *New York Times* followed the dramatic story of a teenage mother prosecuted for the death of her 8-week-old breast-fed son from starvation. The event followed a series of misadventures and refusal to see the child at a Medicaid clinic.[70] The majority of these cases have reflected a lack of clinical knowledge on the part of the professionals regarding the basic physiology of lactation and a general failure of the health care system to provide an appropriate safety net for new and inexperienced mothers following the current early-postpartum discharge practices (hospital stay (≤2 days). As cost drives the health care system to earlier and earlier discharge, the risk of infant problems increases since lactation will not be well established prior to discharge.[71,72] The American

Table 3 Differential Diagnosis in Poor Weight Gain

Slow Gainer	Failure to Thrive
Alert, healthy appearance	Apathetic or crying
Good muscle tone	Poor tone
Good skin turgor	Poor turgor
At least 6 wet diapers daily	Few wet diapers
Pale unconcentrated urine	"Strong" urine
Stools frequent and seedy (or, if infrequent, large and soft)	Stools infrequent and scanty
8 or more nursings daily lasting 15–20 min	Fewer than 8 feedings, often brief
Well-established let-down reflex	No signs of functioning let-down reflex
Weight gain consistent but slow	Weight erratic (loss may occur)

Reproduced with permission from reference 10.

Academy of Pediatrics has recommended that infants be seen by the pediatrician within a week of discharge but in 2 days if breast-fed.[4]

Failure to thrive in children has been thoroughly reviewed in Chapter 43, "Failure to Thrive: Malnutrition in the Pediatric Outpatient Setting" however, there are some critical differential factors when the infant is breast-fed. Most cases of significant failure to thrive in the breast-fed infant manifest themselves in the first few weeks or months of life. There is also an important distinction between failure to thrive and the slow-gaining breast-fed infant.[45,69] The weight curve of an adequately nourished breast-fed infant from birth may well include a weight loss of 6 to 8% and the regain of birth weight at 10 to 14 days in contrast to the formula-fed infant, who may lose only 3 to 4% of birth weight and quickly regain birth weight by 5 to 7 days, often beginning on a path to obesity.

The critical clinical distinctions between failure to thrive and slow gaining are enumerated in Table 3. The salient points include the slow increase in weight compared to the erratic gaining and losing pattern in failure to thrive. The slow-gaining infant is alert and active, with good skin turgor and muscle tone. It feeds frequently night and day, wets many diapers with pale dilute urine, and has a normal stool pattern. The infant looks scrawny but well.[69]

Because it sleeps long periods between feeds, the failure-to-thrive infant may be mistakenly considered satisfied when actually he has starvation inanition. The infant often fed poorly in the first few days or for various other reasons does not stimulate good milk production. Since breast milk production depends on supply-and-demand phenomenon, when the infant sucks weakly, he receives little milk, and thus remains weak from some degree of starvation. This infant also has few wet diapers, the urine is concentrated and described as "strong" by the mother. There are few and small stools, often the green mucus of starvation. The tone and turgor are poor, the cry is weak and infrequent, and the infant looks sick. This may well be a medical emergency requiring hospitalization. The feeding pattern should be evaluated, especially focusing on the length of time spent at the first breast during a feeding to be sure it is long enough to allow the high-fat hind milk to be obtained. Sometimes the pattern of slow gaining can be reversed by limiting a feeding to a single breast to ensure high-fat, high-calorie feeds.[73] Switching back and forth between breasts several times during a feeding does not increase milk supply and can reduce the amount of high-calorie fat provided.

The diagnostic work-up of these phenomena requires the same clinical assessment that is appropriate when the infant is not breast-fed and for this, the reader is referred to Chapter 43, "Failure to Thrive: Malnutrition in the Pediatric Outpatient Setting." Since the breast-feeding infant is part of a synchronous dyad, there are additional considerations in the differential diagnosis.[11] A suggested schema for identifying the cause of the problem is presented in Figure 11.

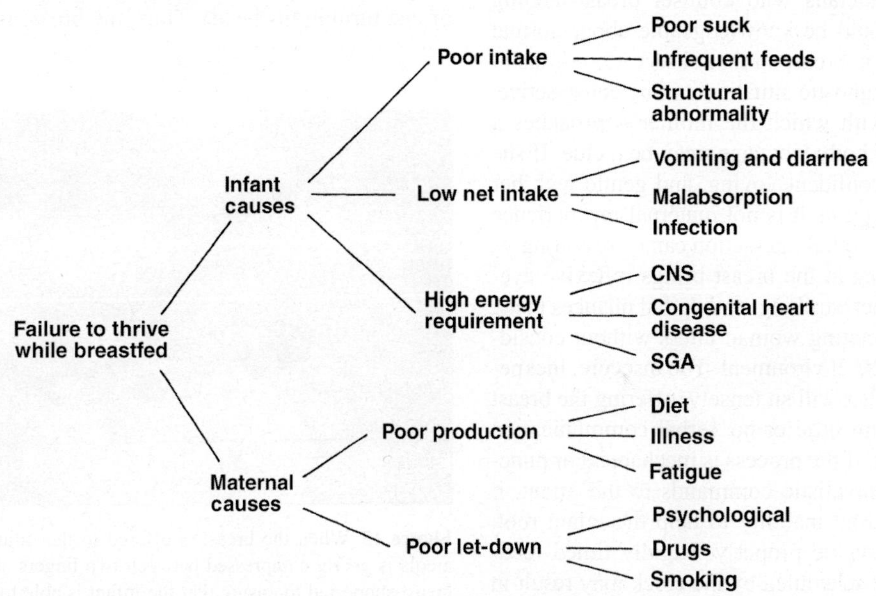

Figure 11 Diagnostic flow chart for failure to thrive. Reproduced with permission from Lawrence RA and Lawrence RM.[10] CNS = central nervous system; SGA = small for gestational age.

The clinician should take a history oriented to the process of lactation. This history should include additional parameters that affect the success of the breast-feeding dyad, such as the mother's perinatal history, general health, diet, habits, psychosocial state, social support system, and the attitudes of the father and family about breast-feeding. Parameters unique to the breast-fed infant include any anatomic or physiologic conditions that would interfere with sucking, which is a critical link in the milk production process.

Difficulties with sucking include anatomic abnormalities that result in mechanical interference with sucking such as cleft lip, cleft palate, hypoplasia of the jaw, macroglossia, ankyloglossia (tongue "tie") and tumors or cysts of the oropharynx. These abnormalities can be identified by physical examination, which includes observation of the infant's suck. There may be neurologic interference, resulting in a diminished or absent suck. Events at birth, such as maternal anesthesia or analgesia and fetal anoxia or hypoxia, may contribute to poor suckling in the immediate neonatal period and failure to provide adequate stimulus to the breast to initiate lactation. The ensuing lack of nutrition for the infant leads to hypometabolism and continued lack of vigor. Congenital cardiac anomalies may present in this manner. Other causes of neurologic deficit in sucking include trisomy 13 to 15, trisomy 21, and neuromuscular syndromes such as Werdnig-Hoffmann, neonatal myasthenia gravis, and congenital muscular dystrophy. Hypothyroidism, prematurity, and congenital intrauterine viral infections contribute to poor suck and lack of vigor. The greatest number of infants, however, are entirely normal but have not had sufficient assistance in establishing the proper grasp of the breast, and possibly have been further confused by being given a bottle supplement, which continues to confound their learning experience.[46] In addition to examining the infant and the maternal breast, the clinician should observe the feeding dynamics.[71,72]

All physicians who counsel breast-feeding mothers should be knowledgeable about normal sucking at the breast so that observation of lactation in a diagnostic situation can be constructive. The style with which the mother approaches a feeding, her body language, may be a clue. If she is relaxed, confident, loving, and gentle with her infant, it suggests it is not maternal inexperience at fault. Her verbal interaction can be revealing. A baby suckling at the breast brings reflexive eye-to-eye contact, stroking, and verbal nuances that a seasoned lactating woman utters without consideration for the environment. The insecure, inexperienced mother will sit tensely, offering the breast gingerly, with little or no verbal communication to the infant. If the process is mechanical or punctuated by unrealistic commands to the infant, it may suggest an inability to help the infant root, grasp, and suckle properly. Rigidly timed feedings that are scheduled by the clock may result in poor milk production. The treatment rests with frequent on-request feedings that fit the infant's biologic rhythms. Suggesting a quiet room, a rocking chair, soft music, or a relaxing beverage for the mother may all improve the situation.

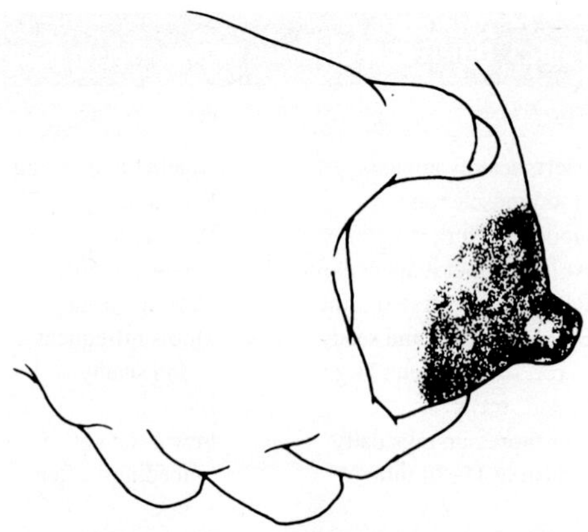

Figure 12 Palmar grasp (C-hold). When the palm and fingers cup the breast with support and the thumb rests lightly above the areola, the nipple projects straight ahead or slightly downward (correct). Reproduced with permission from Lawrence RA and Lawrence RM.[10]

The behavior of the infant when offered the breast may indicate an infant with a suckling disorder, not associated with any other neurologic symptom or long-range problem. Sucking inadequately at the breast can be altered so the infant learns the technique. The infant is identified when it is noted the infant cannot maintain the breast in the mouth unless his mother holds it there. In other words, when she takes her hand away, the breast falls away. A normal infant sucks without help from his mother's hands if the grip is proper and the seal is adequate. When the infant does begin to suck when the breast is held in position, the suck may be a flutter or ineffective tongue actions. This may be improved by having the mother hold the breast between thumb and index finger, with fingers under the breast (palmar hold) (Figure 12) rather than with areolar compressed between the middle and index finger (scissor hold) (Figure 13). The infant's position should be adjusted so his body is turned toward the mother's body (instead of just turning his head). Thus, the breast is centered toward the infant, and this position will improve the effectiveness of the infant's efforts. The mother may have to continue to hold the breast in place for weeks until the infant perfects his technique. The mother may also have to pull his lower lip down to keep infant from drawing the lip into the mouth and moving it along the lower surface breast. The lip should be held as part of the seal holding the breast in place and permitting development of some negative sucking pressure. If the mother stimulates the rooting reflex by stroking the center of the lower lip, the infant will open wide and draw the nipple and areola into the mouth to form a teat.

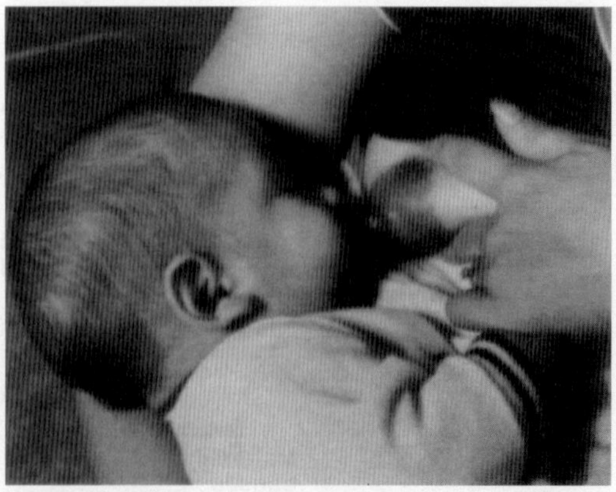

Figure 13 When the breast is offered to the infant, the areola is gently compressed between two fingers and the breast supported to ensure that the infant is able to grasp the areola adequately. Reproduced with permission from Lawrence RA and Lawrence RM.[10]

While the infant is learning to suckle properly, it is urgent to avoid introduction of a rubber nipple on a bottle or a pacifier.[71,72] This poses a problem if adequate nutrition is critical and the mother's supply needs to be stimulated to be adequate. A trial of frequent feeds, waking the infant every 2 hours, may suffice. Extra calories may be offered by medicine cup or Haberman feeder. When the failure to thrive has reached critical starvation, a more aggressive approach is mandatory. If hospitalization is necessary, intravenous therapy to treat dehydration may also be necessary. Hypernatremia and hypochloremia have been described, and a complete work-up, including pH, electrolytes, blood urea nitrogen, and creatinine are essential.[23,44,47,74,75] While the infant receives intravenous therapy, the mother should be assisted to pump frequently to develop and increase her milk supply. When it is safe to begin oral feedings, the infant should be exclusively breast-fed as far as sucking is concerned, and additional nourishment should be provided by intravenous line, gastric tube, or medicine cup. Thus, the infant avoids the introduction of a bottle. When the crisis has abated and full breast-feeding is appropriate but the milk production is still inadequate, the use of a nursing supplementer (Lact-Aid) may be useful. This device permits the uninterrupted nursing at the breast while supplementary nourishment is provided via a fine capillary tube that runs along the breast into the infant's mouth (Figure 14). The tube brings the supplementary fluid from a reservoir plastic bag that hangs around the mother's neck. The system is carefully engineered. It provides fluid only when the baby sucks; thus, it coordinates with the infant's swallowing mechanism. It is not a siphon or a pump. When used to help establish or increase milk production as with a premature infant first going to breast, the infant is usually weaned from the supplementer within 1 or 2 weeks by providing smaller and smaller volumes of supplement as maternal production increases. The supplementing device may make the critical difference when the degree of starvation is great and lactation is being preserved. It is important to point out that all too often the infant is quickly weaned to a bottle without any effort to solve the underlying lactation problem, which is unfortunate (Figures 14 and 15).

In rare cases of failure to thrive while breast-feeding, the underlying cause is actually metabolic

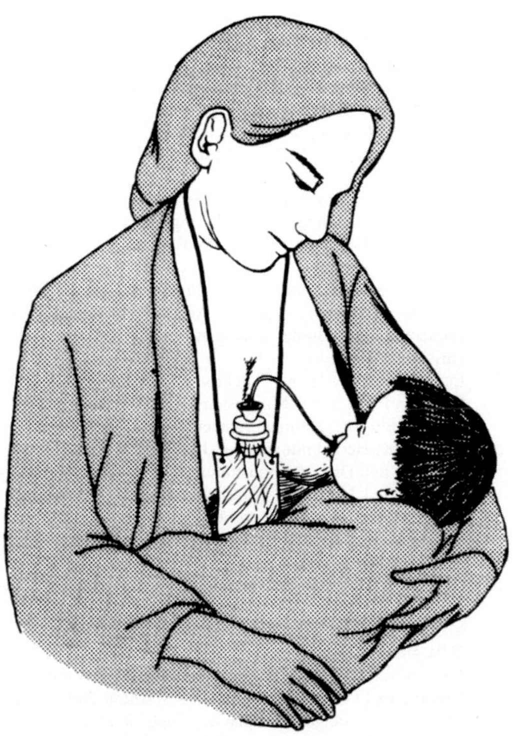

Figure 14 Lact-Aid Nursing Trainer System (Lact-Aid International, Inc.). Reproduced with permission from Lawrence RA and Lawrence RM.[10]

and the infant does even less well on formula prepared from cow's milk or soy protein. In that case, it is quite possible to have the mother re-lactate. It is an art practiced in most cultures over the centuries and resorted to when the biologic mother became ill or died and another female (often the grandmother) had to assume the nourishment of the baby. In the case of premature weaning there has already been the biologic stimulus of pregnancy and early lactation so reinstituting the milk supply occurs more easily. The lactation supplementer may be of great value in this situation, as the infant can return to the breast and be nourished with donor human milk while the mother builds up her own supply (see Figure 15).

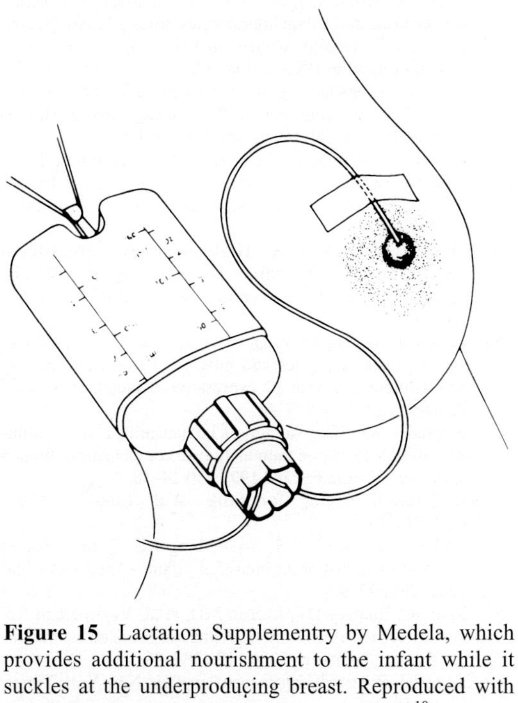

Figure 15 Lactation Supplementry by Medela, which provides additional nourishment to the infant while it suckles at the underproduçing breast. Reproduced with permission from Lawrence RA Lawrence RM.[10]

Maternal Causes of Failure to Thrive

Poor milk production may be the cause of the failure. This is usually characterized by an alert, active infant who cries hungrily and is very demanding but never satisfied. This baby demands attention and is usually seen by the physician because of his dissatisfaction. The quiet, sleepy, starved baby gets into serious trouble before he is discovered because his sleeping is interpreted as satiation. It is rare in the United States that diet is the true cause of insufficient milk although it is appropriate to evaluate the mother's diet and make recommendations for increases or adjustments where needed (see Figure 10).[76] An additional 600 kcal or a minimum of 1,800 kcal per day, a balance of foods with 20 g extra protein and 400 mg extra calcium, is minimal for every mother. Many mothers feel better taking Brewer's yeast. "Mothering the mother" by caring about her diet may have a positive effect. However, the major factor in poor production is fatigue. It is the single most important element in milk production. The present-day "super-mom" model that has been developed by women may be the actual destructive element. A postpartum woman needs rest to recover whether she nurses or not. When she is also nourishing an infant she needs more rest. This is often neglected when the infant needs care every 3 to 4 hours around the clock, and only the mother is involved in the feeding of the infant. When her physician suggests that the mother needs to reorder her priorities and schedule naps for herself, it may be the necessary official approval she needs to do so. A mother may need to be told it is not only okay but it is necessary for her to take care of herself in order to provide for her baby. The physician may need to prescribe rest as well as nourishment.

There is a small number of women who are unable to make sufficient milk. Some of these women have inadequate glandular tissue. Markedly asymmetric breasts, conical shaped breasts, and extremely small ones may be in this category. Even extremely large breasts are occasionally nonfunctional. Failure of the breasts to change and enlarge during pregnancy and/or failure of the breasts to become engorged immediately postpartum are signs of inadequately functioning tissue. These signs prenatally should alert the medical team to extra vigilance as lactation is initiated.

Failure to Let Down Milk

A woman may make milk abundantly but be unable to release it. As the practitioner observes the lactation process, evidence of successful let-down should be sought. If the sucking is interrupted by breaking the suction (by putting a finger in the corner of the infant's mouth), milk should continue to flow in a steady drip if not a stream.

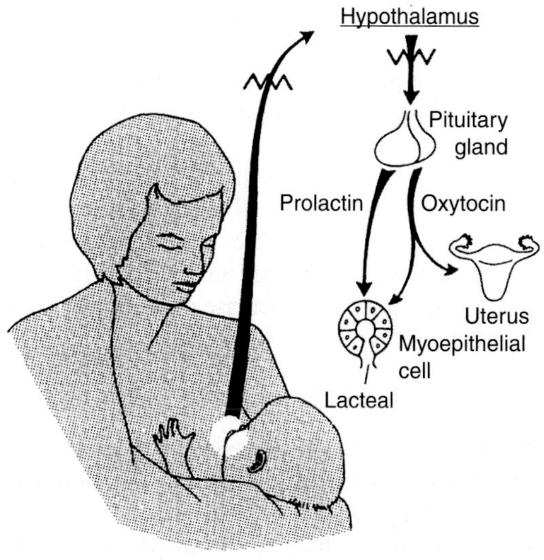

Figure 16 Ejection reflex are. When suckling the breast, the infant stimulates mechanoreceptors in the nipple and areola that send a stimulus along nerve pathways to the hypothalamus, which stimulates the posterior pituitary to release oxytocin. It is carried via the bloodstream to the breast and uterus. Oxytocin stimulates myoepithelial cells in the breast to contract and eject milk from the alveolus. It is secreted by the anterior pituitary gland in response to suckling. Stress such as pain and anxiety can inhibit the let-down reflex. The sight or cry of an infant can stimulate it. Reproduced with permission from Lawrence RA and Lawrence RM.[10]

Although many women describe a tingling and turgescence when the milk lets down, it is possible to have an effective ejection reflex without these sensations. As indicated in Figure 16, it is possible for pain or stress to interfere with let-down. If mother has sore nipples or the infant has an improper grasp at the breast, the pain may interfere with let-down.[30] If the adjustments and remedial actions to avoid stress and enhance confidence do not result in a change in the release of milk, it may be necessary to temporarily provide the oxytocin needed for the let-down arc.[11] Synthetic oxytocin can be prepared by the pharmacist as a nasal spray for home use utilizing the injectable oxytocin. It is packaged in a 5- to 10-mL nasal dropper bottles. It contains 10 USP units (IU) per milliliter of oxytocin, a polypeptide hormone of the posterior pituitary gland. A prescription is required. It is destroyed in the gastrointestinal tract; therefore, it must be used nasally on the mucous membranes, where it is rapidly absorbed. Four to six drops into one nostril followed by having the infant suckle within 2 to 3 minutes is sufficient. This is repeated using the second nares if the infant is switched to the second breast. This may also be used when using a breast pump and collecting for an infant who cannot nurse directly as in the case of a premature baby. Usually, it is only necessary to use the medication for a few days as the natural process will take over.

A rare finding in lactation failure is the lack of a prolactin surge when the breast is stimulated by the suckling or pumping. The prolactin should double over baseline upon suckling. If prolactin levels are obtained, the samples should be carefully timed so that the baseline sample is drawn from a heparin lock after the mother has recovered from the needle stick. Then she should feed the infant or pump her breasts for 10 minutes, and a second sample should be drawn. The percentage increase in prolactin over baseline should approach 50%. The baseline should be above normal for the laboratory. Replacement prolactin is not clinically available although prolactin stimulation with fenugreek or meclopromide or other galactogues may increase milk supply while the treatment is continued.[11]

Knowing When to Discontinue Breast-feeding

Although breast-feeding provides species-specific nourishment, infection protection, immunologic protection, and psychological benefits for both mother and baby, there are times when it should be discontinued. The role of the physician is a delicate one, one in which true support of breast-feeding is necessary for credibility. On the other hand, the physician must recognize when other alternatives are medically preferable. The mother will need help in accepting this. Having to wean prematurely or before the planned date is not to be construed as maternal failure. It is still possible to nurture the infant, to be a good mother, and to have a good mother–infant relationship, even though the mother may no longer be able to breast-feed.

The indications for premature weaning are rare but include severe illness in the mother, severe galactosemia in the infant, and a few maternal drugs such as therapeutic doses of radioactive pharmaceuticals.[11,77]

REFERENCES

1. US Department of Health & Human Services. Public Service Campaign to Promote Breastfeeding Awareness Launched: Emphasizes "Babies Were Born To Be Breastfed." Ad Council, http://www.hhs.gov/news, June 4, 2004.
2. US Department of Health & Human Services. Healthy People 2010. Conference edition, 2 volumes. Washington, DC; January 2000.
3. Committee on Nutrition During Lactation. Report: Nutrition During Lactation, Food and Nutrition Board, Institute of Medicine, National Academy of Sciences, National Academy Press, Washington, DC, 1991.
4. American Academy of Pediatrics, Committee on Breastfeeding. Breastfeeding and the use of human milk. Pediatrics 2005;115:496–506.
5. World Health Organization, Family and Reproductive Health, Division of Child Health and Development: Evidence for the Ten Steps to Successful Breastfeeding. Publication No. WHO/CHD/98.9. Geneva: WHO; 1998.
6. World Health Organization. Protecting, Promoting and Supporting Breastfeeding: The Special Role of Maternity Services. A joint WHO/UNICEF statement. Geneva, WHO; 1989.
7. Horwood LJ, Fergusson DM. Breastfeeding and later cognitive and academic outcomes. Pediatrics 1998;101:91–7.
8. Rogan WJ, Gladen BC. Breastfeeding and Cognitive Development. Early Human Dev 1993;31:181–93.
9. Temboury MC, Otero A, Polanco I, et al. Influence of breastfeeding on infant's intellectual development. J Pediatr Gastroenterology Nutr 1994;28:32–6.
10. Lawrence RA. A review of the medical benefits and contraindications to breastfeeding in the United States. Maternal and Child Health Technical Information Bulletin. Arlington, VA: National Center for Education in Maternal Child Health; 1997.
11. Lawrence RA, Lawrence RM. Breastfeeding: A Guide for the Medical Profession. 6th edition. St. Louis, MO: Mosby; 2005.
12. Chantry CJ, Howard CR, Auinger P. Full breastfeeding duration and associated decrease in respiratory tract infection in U.S. children. Pediatrics 2006;117:425–32.
13. Davis MK. Breastfeeding and chronic disease in childhood and adolescence. In: Schanler RJ, editor. Breastfeeding, Part I: The Evidence for Breastfeeding. Pediatr Clin North Am 2001;48:125–41.
14. Hanson LA. Human milk and host defense: Immediate and long term effects. Acta Paediatr (Suppl) 1999;88:42–46.
15. Wilson A, Stewart Forsyth J, Greene S, et al. Relation of infant diet to childhood health: Seven year follow up at a cohort of children in Dundee infant feeding study. BMJ 1998;316:21–5.
16. Abbott Laboratories, Ross Products Division. Mothers Survey: breastfeeding trends through 2003. Available at: www.ross.com.
17. Ryan AS, Wenjun Z, Acosta A. Breastfeeding continues to increase into the new millennium. Pediatrics 2006;110:1103–9.
18. Chandran L, Gelfer P. Breastfeeding: The essential principles. Pediatr Rev 2006;27:409–17.
19. Neville MC. The physiological basis of milk secretion, Part I: Basic physiology. Ann NY Acad Sci 1990;586:1–11.
20. Vorherr H. The Breast—Morphology, Physiology, and Lactation. New York: Academic; 1974.
21. Neville MC. Physiology and endocrine changes underlying human lactogenesis II. J Nutr 2001;131:3005S–8S.
22. Neville MC, Morton J, Umemura S. Lactogenesis: Transition from pregnancy to lactation. In: Schanler RJ, editor. Breastfeeding, Part I: The Evidence for Breastfeeding. Pediatr Clin North Am 2001;48:35–52.
23. Asnes RS, et al. The dietary chloride deficiency syndrome occurring in a breastfed infant. J Pediatr 1982;100:923–4.
24. Ramsay DT, Kent JC, Hartmann RL, Hartmann PE. Anatomy of the lactating human breast redefined with ultrasound imaging. J Anatomy 2005;206:525–35.
25. Ramsay DT, Mitoulas LR, Kent JC, et al. Milk flow rates can be used to identify and investigate milk ejection in women expressing breast milk using an electric breast pump. Breastfeed Med 2006;1:14–23.
26. Love SM, Barsky SH. Anatomy of the nipple and breast ducts revised. Cancer 2004;101:1947–57.
27. Mendelson EB. The Breast. In: Rumack CM, Wilson SR, Charboreau JW, editors. Diagnostic Ultrasound. 2nd edition. St. Louis, MO: Mosby.
28. Ramsay DT, Kent JC, Owens RA, Hartmann PE. Ultrasound imaging of milk ejection in the breast of lactating women. Pediatrics 2004;113:361–7.
29. Cooper AP. Anatomy of the Breast. Longman, Orme, Green, Browne and Longmans, 1840.
30. Newton M, Newton NR. The let-down reflex in human lactation. J Pediatr 1948;33:698–704.
31. Winikoff B, Baer EC. The obstetrician's opportunity: Translating "breast is best" from theory to practice. Am J Obstet Gynecol 1980;138:105–17.
32. Newton NR. Psychologic differences between breast and bottle feeding. Am J Clin Nutr 1971;24:993–1004.
33. Uvnas-Moberg K, Eriksson M. Breastfeeding: Physiological, endocrine and behavioral adaptations caused by oxytocin and local neurogenic activity in the nipple and mammary gland. Acta Paediatr 1996:85:525–30.
34. Moberg, KU. The Oxytocin Factor: Tapping the Hormone of Calm, Love and Healing. Cambridge: Da Capo Press; 2003.
35. Alexander JM, Grant AM, Campbell MJ. Randomized controlled trial of breast shells and Hoffman's exercises for inverted and non-protractile nipples. Br Med J 1992;304:1030–2.
36. Slusser W, Powers NG. Breastfeeding update 1: Immunology, nutrition, and advocacy. Pediatr Rev 1997;17:111–9.
37. Powers NG, Slusser W. Breastfeeding update 2: Clinical lactation management. Pediatr Rev 1997;18:147–61.
38. AAP Subcommittee on Hyperbilirubinemia. Management of hyperbilirubinemia in the newborn infant 35 or more weeks of gestation. Pediatrics 2004;114(1):297–316.
39. DeCarvalho M, Hall M, Harvey D. Effects of water supplementation on physiological jaundice in breastfed babies. Arch Dis Child 1981;56:568–9.
40. DeCarvalho M, Klaus MH, Merkatz RB. Frequency of breastfeeding and serum bilirubin concentration. Am J Dis Child 1982;136:737–8.
41. Gartner LM, Herschel M. Jaundice and breastfeeding. In: Schanler RJ, editor. Breastfeeding, Part II: The Management of Breastfeeding. Pediatr Clin North Am 2001;48:389–99.
42. Hansen TW. Bilirubin production, breast-feeding and neonatal jaundice. Acta Paediatr 2001;90(7):716–7.
43. Raphael D. The Tender Gift: Breastfeeding. New York: Schocken Books; 1976.
44. Gilmore HE, Rowland TN. Critical malnutrition in breastfed infants: Three case reports. Am J Dis Child 1978;132:885–7.
45. Powers N. Slow weight gain and low milk supply in the breastfeeding dyad. Perinatology 1999;26:399–430.
46. Neifert MR, Lawrence R, Seacat J. Nipple confusion: Toward a formal definition. J Pediatr 1995;126(Suppl):125–29.
47. Neifert MR. Prevention of breastfeeding tragedies. In: Schanler RJ, editor. Breastfeeding, Part II: The Management of Breastfeeding. Pediatr Clin North Am 2001;48:273–97.
48. Committee on Nutrition During Pregnancy and Lactation, Institute of Medicine, National Academy of Sciences. An Implementation Guide. Washington, DC: National Academy Press; 1992.
49. Institute of Medicine. Dietary Reference Intakes for Calcium, Phosphorus, Magnesium, Vitamin D and Fluoride. Washington, DC: National Academy Press; 1999.
50. Siegel, RK. Herbal intoxication. JAMA 1976;236:473–6.
51. US Food and Drug Administration, Center for Food Safety and Applied Nutrition. FDA advises dietary supplement manufacturers to remove comfrey products from the market. Available at: www.cfsan.fda.gov/~dms/supplmnt.html. Accessed July 6, 2001.
52. Greer FA. Do breastfed infants need supplemental vitamins? In: Schanler RJ, editor. Breastfeeding, Part II: The Management of Breastfeeding. Pediatr Clin North Am 2001;48:415–23.
53. Centers for Disease Control and Prevention. Vitamin D Expert Panel Final Report, Scanlon KS, editor; 2002. Available at: www.cdc.gov/nccdphp/dnpa/nutrition.htm.
54. Griffin IJ, Abrams SA. Iron and breastfeeding. In: Schanler RJ, editor. Breastfeeding, Part II: The Management of Breastfeeding. Pediatr Clin North Am 2001;48:401–14.
55. World Health Organization. Global strategy for infant and young child feeding: The optimal duration of breastfeeding. In: 54th World Health Assembly, May 1, 2001. Available at: http://www.who.int/child-adolescent-health/New_Publications/NUTRITION/gs_iycf.pdf. Accessed August 3, 2006.
56. The World Encyclopedia Americana, Funk & Wagnalls Standard Dictionary. Vol. 2. New York: Funk & Wagnalls; 1960.
57. Fein SB, Roe B. The effect of work status on initiation and duration of breastfeeding. Am J Public Health 1998;88:1042–6.
58. United States Breastfeeding Committee. Workplace Breastfeeding Support. Raleigh, NC: United States Breastfeeding Committee; 2002.
59. Lawrence RA. Milk banking: The influence of storage procedures and subsequent processing on immunological components of human milk. In: Draper HH, Woodward W, editors. Advances in Nutritional Research. New York: Kluwer Academic/Plenum Publishers; 2001. p. 389–404.
60. US Department of Labor. Facts on women workers. Available at: www.bls.gov.
61. Cohen R, Mrtek MB, Mrtek RG. Comparison of maternal absenteeism and infant illness rates among breast-feeding and formula-feeding women in two corporations. Am J Health Promotion 1995;10:148–53.
62. Meek JY. Breastfeeding in the work place. In: Schanler RJ, editor. Breastfeeding, Part II: The Management of Breastfeeding. Pediatr Clin North Am 2001;48:461–74.
63. Cohen R, Mrtek MB. The impact of two corporate lactation programs on the incidence and duration of breastfeeding by employed mothers. Am J Health Promotion 1994;6:436–41.
64. Slusser W, Frantz K. High-technology breastfeeding. In: Schanler RJ, editor. Breastfeeding, Part II: The Management of Breastfeeding. Pediatr Clin North Am 2001;48:505–16.
65. Zinaman M, Hughes V, Queenan J, et al. Acute prolactin and oxytocin responses and milk yield to infant suckling and artificial methods of expression in lactating women. Pediatrics 1992;89:437–40.
66. Lawrence RA. The storage of human milk and the influence of procedures on immunological components of human milk. Acta Paediatr Scand 1999;430:14–18.
67. Helliker K. Dying for Milk. Wall Street J 1994; CCXXIV:15.
68. Roddey OF, Martin ES, Swetenburg RL. Critical weight loss and malnutrition in breastfed infants. Am J Dis Child 1981;135:597–9.
69. Kent JC, Ramsey DT, Cregan MD, et al. Volume and frequency of breastfeeds and fat content of breastmilk throughout the day. Pediatrics 2006;117:e387–95.
70. Editorial. Breastfeeding as manslaughter. New York Times, March 18, 1999.

71. Howard CR, Howard FM, Lanphear B, et al. The effects of early pacifier use on breastfeeding duration. Pediatrics 1999;103:e33.
72. Righard L. Are breastfeeding problems related to incorrect breastfeeding technique and use of pacifiers and bottles? Birth 1998;25:40–44.
73. Woolridge MW, Ingram JC, Baum JD. Do changes in pattern of breast usage alter the baby's nutrient intake? Lancet 1990;336:395–7.
74. Anand SK, Sandborg C, Robinson RG, Lieberman, E. Neonatal hypernatremia associated with elevated sodium concentration of breast milk. J Pediatr 1980;96:66–8.
75. Rowland TW, Zori RT, LaFleur MD, Reiter EO. Maintenance and hypernatremic dehydration in breastfed infants. JAMA 1982;247:1016–7.
76. USDA/DHHS. US Dietary Guidelines for Americans, 2002.
77. American Academy of Pediatrics Committee on Drugs. Drugs in breastmilk. Pediatrics 2001;108:776.
78. Huggins K. The Nursing Mother's Companion, Revised Edition. The Harvard Common Press, Harvard and Boston, Massachusetts, 2005.
79. Meek JY (Ed). The New Mother's Guide to Breastfeeding. AAP Section on Breastfeeding. Bantam Books, 2005.

The Low-Birth-Weight Infant: Inpatient Care

Richard J. Schanler, MD
Diane Anderson, PhD, RD

INTRODUCTION

In the neonatal period, low-birth-weight (LBW) infants have greater nutritional needs to achieve optimal growth than at any time in their life. Many LBW infants either are born at the beginning of the third trimester of pregnancy or are products of pregnancies complicated by diminished uterine blood flow. These circumstances result in decreased nutrient deposition in the fetus. Thus, many LBW infants are growth restricted at birth.[1] In addition, their medical condition postnatally may contribute to increased nutrient needs. Impediments to growth include the stress of common pathophysiologic events (hypotension, hypoxia, acidosis, infection, surgical intervention) and their therapies (corticosteroids), as well as physiologic immaturity (decreased gastrointestinal motility and enzyme immaturity).[1] There also is a fear that aggressive feeding may produce pathology (feeding intolerance, necrotizing enterocolitis) and that some nutritional regimens may produce toxic effects on organ development. Lastly, despite well-intended efforts, many infants are discharged from the NICU with significant cumulative deficits in energy and protein.[2] In fact, more infants fall below the 10th percentile at discharge than at birth.[3] Thus, intense support is needed to prevent and correct deficits and enable appropriate growth.

Special considerations regarding nutrient needs of LBW infants begin at birth. Because of limited body stores, increased expenditure, severity of illness, and/ or immaturity, enteral feedings often are precluded immediately after birth and a regimen of total parenteral nutrition (PN) is initiated, consisting of intravenous glucose, amino acids, electrolytes, vitamins, and lipid. Subsequently, minimal enteral nutrition is added in the form of small, priming quantities of milk. As the infant matures physiologically and the medical condition stabilizes, PN is slowly replaced with enteral nutrition. This chapter describes the nutritional needs and goals for LBW infants. Both parenteral and enteral nutritional needs will be addressed (Tables 1 and 2).

GOALS FOR NUTRIENT INTAKES

The nutritional reference standard for the term newborn is the exclusively breastfed infant. A similar standard is not available for LBW infants. Instead, the reference standard for the LBW infant is the estimated intrauterine nutrient accretion rate at corresponding stages during the last trimester of pregnancy. We use the data on the nutrient composition of the fetus derived from chemical analyses of fetal cadavers to determine the net deposition or retention of particular nutrients during the last trimester of pregnancy.[4,5] From analyses of smoothed curves, these data have been computed on a daily basis per kilogram body weight (Table 3). Although the original data were derived from fetal carcass analyses, the data for several minerals have been corroborated by noninvasive neutron activation techniques.[6]

The intrauterine accretion data provide a reference for nutrient deposition. To determine the advisable intake needed for a particular nutrient, we use the factorial approach.[7,8] This method includes a summation of the quantity of the nutrient deposited and an estimate of nutrient losses (Table 4). For infants receiving PN the advisable intake includes estimates of nutrient deposition, cutaneous and urinary losses, and an additional allowance to account for variability. For enteral

Table 1 Parenteral and Enteral Fluid, Energy, and Nutrient Intakes for Stable, Growing VLBW Infants[245]

Component (Units)	Unit/kg/d (Except as Noted)	
	Parenteral	Enteral
Water (mL)	120–160	135–190
Energy (kcal)	90–100	110–130
Protein (g)	3.2–3.8	3.4–4.2
Fat (g)	3–4	5.3–7.2
Carbohydrate (g)	9.7–15	7–17
Linoleic acid (mg)	340–800	600–1440
Vitamin A (IU)	700–1500	700–1500
Vitamin D (IU)	40–160	150–400
Vitamin E (IU)	2.8–3.5	6–12
Vitamin K (μg)	10	8–10
Thiamin (vitamin B_1) (μg)	200–350	180–240
Riboflavin (vitamin B_2) (μg)	150–200	250–360
Pyridoxine (vitamin B_6) (μg)	150–200	150–210
Vitamin B_{12} (μg)	0.3	0.3
Niacin (mg)	4–6.8	3.6–4.8
Folic acid (μg)	56	25–50
Sodium (mg)	69–115	69–115
Potassium (mg)	78–117	78–117
Chloride (mg)	107–249	107–249
Calcium (mg)	60–80	100–220
Phosphorus (mg)	45–60	60–140
Magnesium (mg)	4.3–7.2	7.9–15
Iron (mg)	0.1–0.2	2–4
Zinc (μg)	400	1,000–3,000
Copper (μg)	20	120–150
Chromium (μg)	0.05–0.3	0.1–2.25
Manganese (μg)	1	0.7–7.5
Selenium (μg)	1.5–4.5	1.3–4.5
Carnitine (mg)	~3	~3

Vitamin K, 0.5–1.0 mg given at birth. The following conversion factors are used: Ca, 40 mg = 1 mmol = 2 mEq; P, 31 mg = 1 mmol; Mg, 24 mg = 1 mmol = 2 mEq; Na, 23 mg = 1 mmol = 1 mEq; K, 39 mg = 1 mmol = 1 mEq; Cl, 35 mg = 1 mmol = 1 mEq; Vitamin A, 1 μg retinol = 3.33 IU vitamin A = 6 μg β-carotene = 1.83 μg retinyl palmitate = 1 retinol equivalent (RE); Vitamin E, 1 mg tocopherol = 1 IU vitamin E; Vitamin D, 1 μg vitamin D (cholecalciferol) = 40 IU vitamin D (cholecalciferol); Niacin, 1 mg niacin = 1 niacin equivalent (NE) = 60 mg tryptophan.

Table 2 Minimum and Maximum Nutrient Contents for Enteral Products for LBW Infants, LSRO[8]

Component (Units)	Minimum	Maximum
Energy (kcal/100 mL)	67	94
Protein (g/100 kcal)	2.5	3.6
Fat (g/100 kcal)	4.4	5.7
Carbohydrate (g/100 kcal)	9.6	12.5
Sodium (mg/100 kcal)	39	63
Potassium (mg/100 kcal)	60	160
Chloride (mg/100 kcal)	60	160
Calcium (mg/100 kcal)	123	185
Phosphorus (mg/100 kcal)	82	109
Magnesium (mg/100 kcal)	6.8	17
Iron (mg/100 kcal)	1.7	3.0
Zinc (μg/100 kcal)	1100	1500
Copper (μg/100 kcal)	100	250
Manganese (μg/100 kcal)	6.3	25.0
Selenium (μg/100 kcal)	1.8	5.0
Vitamin A (μg /100 kcal)	204	380
Vitamin D (IU/100 kcal)	75	270
Vitamin E (IU/100 kcal)	2	8
Vitamin K (μg/100 kcal)	4	25
Thiamin (μg/100 kcal)	30	250
Riboflavin (μg/100 kcal)	80	620
Pyridoxine (μg/100 kcal)	30	250
Vitamin B_{12} (μg/100 kcal)	0.08	0.7
Niacin (mg/100 kcal)	0.55	5.0
Folic acid (μg/100 kcal)	30	45

LSRO = Life Sciences Research Office, American Society for Nutrition.

nutrition, the factorial approach is amended to account also for the bioavailability of the particular nutrient. For example, the average calcium absorption from preterm formulas is approximately 50%. To provide a best estimate for calcium intake, we use the factorial approach (Table 4).

ENERGY

Based on a series of observations, the daily energy need for the growing LBW infant has been summarized (Table 5).[9] The values are not absolute. The range in resting energy expenditure has been reported from 49 to 60 kcal/kg/d at 8 to 63 days postnatal age.[10] When nourished parenterally, the LBW infant has less fecal energy loss, generally fewer episodes of cold stress, and somewhat less activity, so that the actual energy needs for growth are lowered to approximately 80 to 100 kcal/kg/d.

Table 3 Estimated Intrauterine Nutrient Accretion Rates[4,5]

Nutrient*	Unit/kg/d
Calcium (mg)	105
Copper (μg)	50
Magnesium (mg)	2.7
Nitrogen (mg)	325
Phosphorus (mg)	70
Potassium (mmol)	0.7
Sodium (mmol)	1.2
Zinc (μg)	240

*Values averaged from last trimester, adjusted for body weight. These values represent tissue deposition.

In circumstances of chronic disease, such as bronchopulmonary dysplasia, the resting energy expenditure rises significantly.[11,12] Total energy needs in LBW infants with bronchopulmonary dysplasia are increased because of greater energy expenditure, activity, and possibly fecal energy losses. It is not surprising to find that these infants require 150 kcal/kg/d to achieve weight gain.

The distribution of nonprotein calories, the quantity of calories derived from fat and from carbohydrate, should be considered. A balanced distribution between calories derived from glucose and fat is appropriate to avoid potential effects on respiratory metabolism, especially in infants who are ill, requiring respiratory support or receiving PN. Most milks for LBW infants have a balance in nonprotein calories, approximately 40 to 45% each from fat and carbohydrate. Imbalances in calories arise with PN. A distribution of calories favoring glucose (therefore, low fat), or a surplus of glucose calories such that glucose is converted to fat, will increase the production of carbon dioxide, increase the partial pressure of carbon dioxide, increase alveolar minute ventilation, raise the respiratory quotient, and may increase the oxygen consumption.[13,14] In addition, a balanced distribution of glucose-lipid calories favors protein accretion while glucose-only solutions are associated with protein oxidation.[15] Daily monitoring of the intakes for all energy sources in PN is essential to ensure a relatively balanced distribution of calories derived from glucose and fat. One example of the computation of calorie distribution is provided in Table 6.

Table 4 Computation of Net Enteral and/or Parenteral Nutrient Need Based on the Factorial Approach Using Data from Rates of Fetal Nutrient Accretion[5,33,229]

Net fetal Ca deposition	= 105 mg/kg/d
Postnatal urinary losses	= 5 mg/kg/d
Postnatal cutaneous losses	= 2 mg/kg/d
Subtotal (parenteral need)	= 112 mg/kg/d
Net absorption (%)	= 50%
Total (enteral need)	= 224 mg/kg/d

Table 5 Estimation of the Energy Requirements for LBW Infants[246]

	Average Estimate, kcal/kg/d
Energy expended	40–60
Resting metabolic rate	40–50*
Activity	0–5*
Thermoregulation	0–5*
Synthesis	15†
Energy stored	20–30†
Energy excreted	15
Energy intake	90–120

*Energy for maintenance.
†Energy cost of growth.

PARENTERAL NUTRITION

There are several reasons why the LBW infant should receive PN as soon as practical. They are born with limited nutrient stores, may have increased energy expenditure and severity of illness, and because of their immaturity, enteral feedings often are precluded immediately after birth. Thus, a regimen of PN is initiated, consisting of intravenous glucose, amino acids, electrolytes, vitamins, and lipid.

Glucose

The LBW infant requires a high glucose infusion rate (approximately 5–8 mg/kg/min) to meet their needs because of their diminished stores, higher energy expenditure, and relatively greater brain-to-body weight ratio, compared with the term newborn (3–5 mg/kg/min). Although in the first days after birth, the LBW infant's minimal metabolic rate is low, approximately 30 kcal/kg/d, their needs rise by the end of the first week.[9] As their clinical condition may preclude enteral nutrition directly after birth, PN can provide adequate glucose to prevent hypoglycemia. The extremely LBW infant, however, may develop hyperglycemia. Several reasons have been given for the hyperglycemia: ineffective insulin secretion and end-organ sensitivity, decreased intracellular transporters, elevated catecholamines and glucocorticoids, and as a response to a high glucose infusion rate. There is a concern that hyperglycemia increases morbidity in the extremely LBW infant.[16] Some clinicians have advocated the use of insulin therapy, but no threshold glucose concentration for treatment has been adopted. There

Table 6 Suggested Goal for Distribution of Energy Sources in Parenteral Nutrition Solutions for LBW Infants

	Concentration (%)	g/kg/d	kcal/kg/d	% kcal
@135 mL/kg/d				
Glucose	12.5	16.9	57.5	57
Amino acids	2.5	3.4	13.6	13
@15 mL/kg/d				
Lipid	20	3.0	30	30

Assume total fluid intake is 150 mL/kg/d and total calorie intake is 101 kcal/kg/d.

is a suggestion that insulin therapy may promote an anabolic response and enhance growth, as well as preventing hyperkalemia and hyperosmolality.[17] Moreover, insulin use is problematic as the protein adheres to infusion tubing and so the dose is difficult to quantitate. Investigators found no anabolic effect of insulin therapy, and also suggested that such therapy is detrimental in extremely LBW infants receiving glucose at high infusion rates because it contributed to metabolic (lactic) acidosis.[18] As extremely LBW infants have been shown to manifest gluconeogenesis, an alternative strategy to prevent hyperglycemia is early PN (see later, section "Early Initiation of Amino Acids"). Amino acids and lipid contribute substrates for gluconeogenesis, enabling lower glucose infusion rates to be achieved.[19]

Amino Acids

The essential amino acids include isoleucine, leucine, lysine, methionine, phenylalanine, threonine, tryptophan, and valine. For the LBW infant, several investigators also consider arginine, cysteine, glutamine, glycine, histidine, taurine, and tyrosine to be conditionally essential amino acids.[20] The content of specific amino acids also varies among the representative preparations. For example, tyrosine and cysteine are not present in all preparations, principally because of difficulties in solubility.[20–22] Taurine and glutamic acid are not present in all solutions.[20,23] Because of the high proportion of essential and conditionally essential amino acids, commensurate with the initiation of PN in the first days after birth, a previously elevated blood urea nitrogen (BUN) may decline more rapidly.[24]

Although several amino acid solutions are available for PN, the percentage of essential/total amino acids is variable: 53% TrophAmine (B. Braun), 53% PremaSol (Baxter), 48% Primene (Baxter), 48% FreAmine III (B.Braun), 46% Aminosyn PF (Hospira), 45% Clinisol (Baxter), and 40% Travasol (Baxter). Comparison of amino acid contents suggests that TrophAmine, and the nearly identical PremaSol, approach target amino acid needs for LBW infants based on best approximations.[25]

It is known that there is a direct relationship between the quantity of nitrogen (amino acids) provided in PN and nitrogen balance or retention.[26,27] It is also known that specific amino acids may affect nitrogen balance, a fact that has been useful in determining the essentiality of particular amino acids. Malloy[28] observed that the addition of cysteine hydrochloride to PN increased plasma free and total cyst(e)ine and urinary cyst(e)ine concentrations. One study, however, was unable to demonstrate a significant effect of increasing cysteine intake on nitrogen balance or weight gain.[29] Nevertheless, in a study using stable isotope methodology, Rivera[30] demonstrated that cysteine positively affected nitrogen balance and weight gain in extremely LBW infants. Cysteine also serves as a precursor of glutathione. In vitro studies suggest that, even in LBW infants, cysteine is an ideal substrate for glutathione production.[31] Because cysteine hydrochloride is not stable, it must be added to PN solutions daily. The addition of cysteine hydrochloride lowers the pH of the mixture, which serves to augment the solubility of calcium and phosphorus.[32] Thus, cysteine hydrochloride is added to PN solutions, not only to meet cysteine needs and to enhance glutathione synthesis, but also because it allows for greater intakes of calcium and phosphorus salts. Occasionally, the use of cysteine hydrochloride results in a mild metabolic acidosis so acetate should be the anion added preferentially[33,34]

Glutathione is the major intracellular antioxidant and its primary function is to protect the cell against free-radical damage (eg, from peroxides). The liver synthesizes glutathione from cysteine, glutamine, and glycine. Not only is cysteine considered rate-limiting for glutathione synthesis, but lack of glutamine may also affect the rate of glutathione production.[35] Glutamine is abundant in muscle and plasma. It has a role in intestinal cell growth, a particularly important concern in parenterally nourished infants when the gastrointestinal tract is not being used. Plasma glutathione concentrations increase when glutamine is added to PN solutions.[35] In extremely LBW infants, one study reported a shorter time to full feedings, fewer days of PN, and less need for prolonged mechanical ventilation with the addition of glutamine to PN.[36] A large, multicenter randomized trial, however, failed to identify a benefit of parenteral glutamine supplementation with respect to growth, protein synthesis, or host defense.[37] Routine PN solutions do not contain significant quantities of glutamine. Current formulations of the amino acid are not stable for prolonged periods in PN mixtures necessitating daily preparation.

Nitrogen retention can be augmented either by providing the best mixture of essential/nonessential amino acids, increasing the nitrogen intake, or within a narrow range by increasing the energy intake (approximately 50–90 kcal/kg/d).[26] The positive relationship between energy intake and nitrogen balance for any given nitrogen intake is linear within the usual intakes of nitrogen and energy. Nitrogen balance (retention) increases markedly as energy intake is increased from 50 to 90 kcal/kg/d at the same nitrogen intake.[26,38] Understanding these principles is important when intakes of nitrogen are limited or when energy intakes are not optimized within this range.

The use of TrophAmine and FreAmine III has been evaluated in LBW infants of 32 weeks' gestation.[39] The group receiving TrophAmine had significantly greater gain in body weight and net nitrogen balance than the group receiving FreAmine III. It appears that the plasma amino acid pattern is directly related to the composition of the parenteral amino acid solution.[40] Because it was developed to ensure optimal levels, plasma amino acid patterns in LBW infants receiving TrophAmine appear to be more "balanced" than plasma amino acid patterns of other formulations.[20,25,39,41] Thus, the importance of selecting the optimal mixture cannot be underestimated.

Serial balance studies were conducted for 3 weeks in a longitudinal study of PN (using TrophAmine 2.2% at 130 mL/kg/d [2.9 g/kg/d] and Intralipid 20% at 20 mL/kg/d [4.0 g/kg/d]) in LBW infants.[33] Significant positive relationships were observed between nitrogen retention and intake. On the basis of those relationships, Table 7 depicts the amino acid concentration and intake

Table 7 Suggested Intakes of Parenteral Nutrients for LBW Infants Based on Regression Equations When PN Is Administered at 130 mL/kg/d[33]

Component	Unit/kg/d	Unit/L	Molar Unit/kg/d	Molar Unit/L
Amino acids*	3.0 g	24 g	–	–
Calcium	120 mg	920 mg	3.0 mmol	23 mmol
Copper	64 μg	500 μg	1.0 μmol	8 μmol
Magnesium	9.6 mg	72 mg	0.4 mmol	3 mmol
Phosphorus	87 mg	650 mg	2.8 mmol	21 mmol
Potassium	100 mg	800 mg	2.6 mmol	20 mmol
Sodium†	175 mg	1300 mg	7.5 mmol	58 mmol
Zinc	350 μg	2700 μg	5.4 μmol	42 μmol

*Assumes TrophAmine (B. Braun) as source.
†Derived from actual sodium intake from all sources, including medications.
Computations based on intake of 130 mL/kg/d.

Table 8 Early, Immediate Parenteral Nutrition for LBW Infants[121]

Component	Quantity	Approximate Intake (unit/kg/d)
Water	100 mL	10
Amino acids	2.5 g/100 mL	2.5 g
Glucose	5–10 g/100 mL	5–10 g
Calcium gluconate	500–650 mg/100 mL	500–650 mg
MVI-Pediatric	2 mL/kg/d	2 mL
Heparin	1 unit/mL	100 units
Lipid (by separate infusion)	5 mL/kg/d	1 g
Water		100 + 5 = 105 mL

Note: Contains no electrolytes, phosphorus, magnesium, trace elements, or cysteine. Monitor glucose to determine whether to increase glucose infusion rate, and monitor electrolytes, phosphorus, and magnesium to determine when these are to be added. When phosphorus is added, ensure that cysteine has been added so that solubility of minerals is optimized.

needed to meet the intrauterine accretion rate for nitrogen. These and other investigations suggest that an amino acid intake of approximately 3 to 3.5 g/kg/d is appropriate for LBW infants receiving PN.[8,20,33] Indeed, a review of amino acid intakes in the first weeks after birth suggested that intakes greater than or equivalent to 4 g/kg/d were tolerated without adverse effects, and associated with lower rates of subsequent bronchopulmonary dysplasia, compared to intakes of approximately 3 g/kg/d.[42]

Early Initiation of Amino Acids

The use of a combined glucose and amino acid source for PN should be initiated soon after birth (Table 8).[24,43] The provision of this combination of nutritional support reverses the negative nitrogen balance attributed to a constant urinary nitrogen loss, equivalent to a loss of protein of 1 g/kg/d,[24,33,43,44] and increases the serum concentration of essential amino acids[24,45] and the rate of protein synthesis.[30,43,46] An amino acid intake of 3 g/kg/d was associated with a significantly more positive nitrogen balance and greater plasma insulin concentrations without significant effects on BUN or glucose concentrations when started 24 h after birth in extremely LBW infants.[47] Improved outcomes are observed if 2.4 g/kg/d of amino acids are initiated within 2 hours of birth compared with a slower daily increment of amino acids.[48,49] Use of those amino acid intakes along with intravenous lipid (2 g/kg/d) and low glucose infusion rates (as low as 4.5 g/kg/d) maintains blood glucose values in the normal range even in extremely LBW infants.[19] Thus, even the extremely LBW infant manifests gluconeogenesis by utilizing amino acid and lipid precursors. It can be reasoned from these data that the incidence of hyperglycemia, a problem common to extremely LBW infants, may be lessened following higher amino acid intakes.

Long-term follow-up studies of extremely LBW infants (average birth weight 800 g, gestational age 26 weeks) suggest that by 36 weeks postmenstrual age significant benefits to growth are observed for infants given early amino acid infusions compared to late initiation of PN.[50] Improved results for head growth are sustained for at least 18 months corrected age.[50]

Intravenous Lipid Emulsions

Essential fatty acids, linoleic acid (18:2ω6) and linolenic acid (18:3ω3), cannot be synthesized and thus need to be provided to the LBW infant (Table 9). Without provision of these fatty acids, essential fatty acid deficiency, characterized by dermatitis, thrombocytopenia, infection, and failure to thrive, may manifest in the first week after birth. Classically, essential fatty acid deficiency is assessed by measuring the plasma triene/tetraene ratio. As a deficient intake results in decreased arachidonic acid (tetraene, 20:4ω6) relative to a normal triene (20:3ω9) ratio, an abnormal state is characterized by a triene/tetraene ratio greater than 0.2 to 0.4. Small amounts of essential fatty acid (~4% of total calories or 0.5 g/kg/d) are required to prevent essential fatty acid deficiency.

Intravenous lipid emulsions containing combinations of soybean oil and/or safflower oil with glycerin and egg yolk phospholipids as emulsifiers given along with the PN regimen in the first few days will prevent essential fatty acid deficiency,[51,52] provide needed energy for tissue healing and growth, and equalize the distribution of nonprotein calories (Tables 1 and 6). Intravenous lipid emulsion has been used in sick LBW infants beginning on the day of birth without short-term adverse effects.[53] Intravenous lipid reportedly protects the lung from oxygen toxicity by increasing the content of polyunsaturated fatty acids in the lung.[54] This finding may be especially important in ventilator-dependent LBW infants. Indeed, a review of early use of intravenous lipid identified no adverse effects on growth, lung disease, or overall morbidity when compared with later use of intravenous lipid infusion.[55]

The concentration of the lipid emulsion (10% vs 20%) affects the infant's tolerance of the lipid preparation. Despite similar or even greater doses of lipid, there is better tolerance of the 20% versus 10% intravenous lipid solution. LBW infants receiving the 20% solution at the same or even greater lipid intakes had lower serum concentrations of triglycerides, cholesterol, and phospholipids than similar infants receiving the 10% solution.[56,57] Given the same dose of lipid, the greater volume required for the 10% solution contributes more phospholipid, cholesterol, and liposomes, which accumulate to form lipoprotein X. Lipoprotein X particles compete with lipoprotein lipase to reduce the clearing of triglycerides.[20,56,57] Thus, regardless of the dose of lipid or the age of the infant, LBW infants should receive the 20% solution.

The method of lipid infusion also affects triglyceride clearance. Intermittent infusion may produce higher serum triglyceride concentrations than continuous infusion (over a 24-h interval) of the same dose.[58] The use of intermittent infusions and lipid-free intervals do not appear to be justified in routine circumstances.[59,60] Indeed, deleterious effects on pulmonary function have

Table 9 Intravenous Lipid Emulsions for LBW Infants Compared with a Novel Lipid Emulsion[69,247]

	Intralipid (Baxter Healthcare/Fresenius Kabi)	Liposyn II (Hospira)	Liposyn III (Hospira)	Omegaven (Fresenius AG)*
Concentrations	10%, 20%, 30%	10%, 20%	10%, 20%, 30%	10%
Oil source	Soybean 100%	Soybean 50% Safflower 50%	Soybean 100%	Fish 100%
Fatty acids (%)				
Linoleic	44–62	66	55	0.1–0.7
Linolenic	4–11	4	8	0.2
Palmitic	7–14	9	11	0.25–1.0
Oleic	19–30	18	22	0.6–1.3
Stearic	1.4–5.5	3.4	4	0.05–0.2
EPA	0	0	0	1.25–2.82
DHA	0	0	0	1.44–3.09
Egg yolk phospholipids (%)	1.2	1.2	1.2, 1.2, 1.8	1.2
Glycerin (%)	2.25, 2.25, 1.7	2.5	2.5	2.5
Energy density (kcal/mL)	1.1, 2.0, 3.0	1.1, 2.0	1.1, 2.0, 2.9	1.1
Osmolarity (mosm/L)	260, 260, 200	276, 258	284, 292, 293	308–376†

*Not available in the United States.
†mOsm/kg.

been demonstrated in adults who received large bolus doses of intravenous lipid, resulting in markedly elevated (>300 mg/dL) plasma triglyceride concentrations.[61] For any given dose of lipid, triglyceride concentrations in LBW infants are more elevated at 1 week postnatal age than 2 to 3 weeks postnatal age.[62] Most authorities suggest using plasma triglyceride concentrations to monitor lipid tolerance. A plasma triglyceride concentration >150 mg/dL usually is avoided. Plasma free fatty acid concentrations provide a more direct measure of lipid tolerance. Because of the complexity of the assay, however, this method is not performed routinely.

There have been some concerns regarding the worsening of pulmonary function and the potential for oxidant toxicity as a result of the use of intravenous lipid.[63-65] In vitro studies suggest that the formation of hydroperoxides in the lipid emulsion may be deleterious to lung function.[66] Clinical studies, however, do not indicate an increased risk from the administration of intravenous lipid emulsions.[55] Indeed, the concern actually may focus on the lack of appropriate antioxidants to protect the infant.[67] The use of intravenous lipid emulsion, even when administered within 12 hours of birth, was not associated with either an increase in oxygen requirement or the development of chronic respiratory disease, in infants who were extremely LBW.[65] Infants who have clinical sepsis may be intolerant of their lipid infusion as manifest by elevated triglyceride concentrations.[68] A triglyceride concentration should be measured in such infants and, if elevated greater than approximately 150 mg/dL, the infusion adjusted. In general, however, the benefits of intravenous lipid as an energy source, as a contributor to the balance of nonprotein calories, and in the prevention of essential fatty acid deficiency, outweigh the potential risks.

Newer intravenous fat emulsions are appearing (Table 9). One product (Omegaven, Fresenius Kabi AG, Bad Homburg, Germany) contains long-chain polyunsaturated fatty acids (DHA, docosahexaenoic acid, and EPA, eicosapentaenoic acid) and has been associated with reversing the progression of cholestasis seen with prolonged PN exposure.[69] It is hypothesized that ω6 fatty acids and plant phytosterols contained in soybean-based lipid emulsions, may be proinflammatory and contribute to liver injury.[69] Other lipid emulsion sources (olive and safflower) with less soybean components are not as readily available in the United States. The fish oil emulsion (Table 9) has sufficient very long chain fatty acids to prevent essential fatty acid deficiency and also EPA, which may reduce triglyceride production in the liver.[69] Further research in this new area is warranted.

Intravenous Carnitine

Carnitine is one of several conditionally essential nutrients. Carnitine, present in all milks fed to infants but not included in usual PN mixtures, has a role in fatty acid transport into the mitochondria, fatty acid oxidation, and ketogenesis. Supplementation of PN with L-carnitine (8–10 mg/kg/d) results in greater plasma total and acylcarnitine concentrations in premature infants compared with infants not receiving carnitine-supplemented PN.[70,71] Study infants who were supplemented with carnitine also appeared to have greater fatty acid oxidation as evidenced by increased ketone production.[71] Supplementation with high doses of carnitine (48 mg/kg/d), however, results in a slower weight gain and an anomalous increase in protein oxidation.[65] Carnitine supplementation, in general, is not associated with improvements in weight gain or in amelioration of apnea.[72,73] Thus, if used because of no enteral intake for a prolonged interval of more than 2 weeks, parenteral carnitine intakes in doses of 10 to 20 mg/kg/d may be used until any milk is provided.

Minerals: Calcium, Phosphorus, and Magnesium

The LBW infant is prone to several clinical conditions that cause or result in abnormalities in mineral metabolism, for example, hypocalcemia, hyperphosphatemia, hypermagnesemia. These conditions may affect the provision of PN. In the fetus, calcium (Ca) is transported actively from the mother, under the influence of parathyroid hormone-releasing peptide (PTHrP). Most transplacental transfer of Ca occurs in the last trimester. Postnatally, serum Ca declines and the LBW infant may not have compensatory mechanisms to increase serum Ca. Parathyroid hormone response to hypocalcemia appears to be blunted and some investigators report elevated calcitonin levels in LBW infants. Thus, Ca must be provided in the early postnatal period to prevent, and to treat, hypocalcemia. Because there is a transient period of oliguria and renal insufficiency, postnatal serum phosphorus (P) values occasionally may be elevated in some LBW infants. Yet, with renal maturation, serum P concentrations decline. Therefore, phosphorus must be provided in parenteral nutrition solutions. Ca and P must be provided together for optimal bone deposition; without P, bone Ca deposition is blunted, and hypercalcemia and hypophosphatemia will be manifest. Hypermagnesemia in LBW infants is not an uncommon finding following maternal magnesium therapy. However, once serum magnesium (Mg) concentrations normalize, parenteral Mg should be provided.

Inadequate intakes of Ca and P results in the spectrum of bone undermineralization, osteopenia of prematurity, rickets, and fractures in LBW infants.[74,75] Osteopenia may potentiate chronic lung disease because undermineralization affects chest wall stability. An increasingly more compliant chest wall leads to atelectatic changes in the lung.[76] Phosphorus deficiency has been associated with diaphragmatic paralysis and respiratory failure in adults.[77] Ca and P deficiency also result in hypercalciuria and, in combination with the use of diuretics, may result in nephrocalcinosis.[78,79]

Although the direct relationship between intake and net retention aids in determining optimal intakes of these minerals, intakes are limited by the solubility of Ca and P in solution. Careful attention to pH, amino acid concentration and source, and temperature must be given so as to provide a recommendation for the appropriate quantity of Ca and P in PN.[80,81] To optimize solubility further, during preparation of PN, the phosphorus is added first and the calcium is added in the last step.

Proportional increases in elemental Ca and P, up to 76 and 45 mg/kg/d, respectively, are retained by the infant.[81] Prestridge[82] demonstrated increased net retention, without increased urinary losses, when Ca intakes were increased from 60 to 80 mg/kg/d and P intakes were increased from 55 to 80 mg/kg/d, respectively. The effects of the greater Ca and P intakes also were manifest by increased bone mineral content during and well beyond the 3-week PN study interval.[82]

Daily intakes of Ca and P can be increased if each is delivered separately.[83] However, alternate-day infusion methods result in hypercalciuria and hypercalcemia when P is omitted, and hyperphosphaturia and hyperphosphatemia when Ca is omitted. The two minerals, therefore, must be delivered together for deposition into bone. Indeed, abnormal serum Ca and P concentrations are observed when one of the two minerals is omitted in the PN solution. If P is omitted from PN, the resulting biochemical pattern is observed: hypophosphatemia, hypophosphaturia, hypercalcemia, and hypercalciuria. Small changes in the molar ratio of Ca to P, however, may be necessary to normalize abnormal blood levels.

The optimal molar ratio of Ca to P in PN for LBW infants is generally ≥1:1.[75,84] Molar ratios <1:1 result in elevated urinary P and serum P concentrations, suggestive of inadequate P utilization because of inadequate Ca intake.[82] However, it appears that the absolute quantity of Ca and P is more important than the ratio. If the quantity is limited, the ratio will affect net retention as much as an increase in the intake of the two minerals. Table 7 depicts the intake required to achieve the intrauterine accretion rate for Ca, P, and Mg. However, as mentioned earlier, solubility issues prevent the achievement of these intakes with current formulations. A plan for Ca and P concentrations in PN is found in Table 10. Note that recommendations for Ca and P are dependent upon the quantity of amino acids in the solution.

Early, immediate provision of PN solutions are provided to LBW infants. In addition to glucose, amino acids, lipid, and calcium are added to prevent and/or treat hypocalcemia. Generally, doses of elemental Ca of 25 to 75 mg/kg/d are used.[85] Phosphorus may not be needed in the first 1 or 2 days, until the serum P normalizes (Table 8).

The parenteral intakes of Mg needed to meet intrauterine accretion rates were derived in a longitudinal study evaluating serial Mg balance studies using TrophAmine 2.2% (130 mL/kg/d) and Intralipid 20% (20 mL/kg/d).[33,82] As elevated serum Mg concentrations and net retention were

Table 10 Calcium, Phosphorus, and Magnesium in PN[33,84,185]

	Term Infants Usual Short-Term	Premature Infants Usual Short-Term	All Infants Long-Term Use	All Infants Special Circumstances
Calcium	1.2 (48)*	1.5 (60)	1.75 (70)	2.0 (80)
Phosphorus	1.2 (37)	1.5 (47)	1.75 (54)	2.0 (62)
Magnesium	0.21 (5)	0.25 (6)	0.25 (6)	0.25 (6)

*mmol (mg)/dL.
Short-term: assumes PN with ≥ 2.4% amino acids + cysteine.; Long-term: assumes PN with >2.5% amino acids + cysteine. Special: assumes PN with >3% amino acids + cysteine.

observed with intakes of 12 mg/kg/d, the linear relationship between intake and net retention suggested that a lower parenteral Mg intake was appropriate (Table 7). That intake derived for Mg is easily attainable (Table 10).

Electrolytes

Serum sodium (Na) is a useful indicator of hydration in LBW infants. Sodium needs in the early days postnatally may be determined by the serum Na. The usual parenteral needs for Na and potassium (K) are determined in each clinical circumstance, with a range of intakes recommended (Tables 1 and 2). Serial balance studies were conducted for 3 weeks in a study of PN (using TrophAmine 2.2% at 130 mL/kg/d and Intralipid 20% at 20 mL/kg/d) in LBW infants.[33] It was also noted that the majority of the Na intake was derived from common medications received by the LBW infant.[86] Significant relationships were determined between specific nutrient intake and net retention for Na and K. Thus, a derived intake for these electrolytes takes into account all potential sources for Na and K (Table 7).

A relative degree of acidosis, manifest by a low serum bicarbonate concentration and a borderline low serum pH, also may occur with PN. The LBW infant has decreased renal reabsorption of bicarbonate. Moreover, the use of amino acid solutions with low pH (generally 5.5–6.5), and the use of cysteine hydrochloride, further reduce the pH.[20] The addition of acetate to the solution, as either the Na or K salt, has been reported to correct the acidosis. The small quantity of acetate, 1 to 2 mEq/kg/d, has not been observed to affect the solubility of the minerals in PN solutions containing TrophAmine and cysteine hydrochloride.[34]

Trace Elements

Suggested parenteral intakes of copper (Cu) and zinc (Zn) for LBW infants have been evaluated from serial balance studies (using TrophAmine 2.2% at 130 mL/kg/d and Intralipid 20% at 20 mL/kg/d) conducted during the first 3 weeks postnatally.[33] Net retention and urinary excretion did not increase over the 3 weeks of study, suggesting that the elements were utilized by the infant during the early weeks postnatally. As intakes were correlated with net retention, the estimated intake needed to meet the intrauterine accretion rate was determined (Table 7). Estimated parenteral intakes of Zn have been reported, which are in a similar range of 350 to 450 μg/kg/d.[84,87] A greater dose may be indicated in LBW infants with ongoing intestinal losses of Zn.[88] Estimated parenteral intakes of Cu were similar to those reported by Zlotkin[87] and slightly greater than those reported by Greene.[84] Differences in recommendations may arise due to the various sources of amino acids used and medical conditions of the infants studied (Table 11).

An estimate of Zn status can be obtained from serum Zn concentrations, which range between 70 and 120 μg/dL in adults. Severe Zn deficiency generally is associated with plasma zinc concentrations below 20 to 30 μg/dL.[84] Copper status is more difficult to define with serum indices.[89] Plasma Cu and ceruloplasmin concentrations increase with postmenstrual age.[84] At 30 weeks, plasma Cu concentrations are 35 μg/dL and at 40 weeks are between 50 and 60 μg/dL. Copper needs are increased in cases of excess biliary losses and in patients with jejunostomies. It is important to recognize that impaired biliary secretion, however, will lead to a buildup of Cu. Therefore, it is advised that Cu intakes be reduced in patients with impaired biliary excretion, such as that which occurs in cholestatic syndromes.[84] To prevent copper deficiency in infants with cholestasis, some clinicians provide parenteral copper once or twice per week.

Selenium (Se) is a component of glutathione peroxidase and its absence from long-term PN solutions results in a deficiency of the element.[90–92] A review of parenteral Se intakes suggests that intakes of 1.5 to 7 μg/kg/d were associated with significant reductions in neonatal sepsis compared with no Se in PN.[93] Approximately 75% of an absorbed dose is excreted by the kidney, so Se intake should be reduced in patients with impaired renal function. The suggested parenteral intake is 2 μg/kg/d (Table 11).[84]

Recommendations for manganese (Mn) intakes are not clearly defined (Table 11).[84] The ratio of Mn to Zn in the available trace element solution used for LBW infants provides a greater intake of Mn than presumed to be needed. Mn excretion is diminished markedly in cholestatic syndromes. The use of Mn in cholestatic disease should be avoided, or reduced.

Chromium (Cr) needs may be associated with insulin activity at the receptor level.[84] Cr deficiency, therefore, may result in impaired glucose tolerance. High doses of Cr may accumulate in the body.[94] A recommended intake of approximately 0.3 μg/kg/d appears to be appropriate (Table 11).

Some clinicians recommend that multiple trace element solutions be used only after 2 to 4 weeks of age, with the exception of zinc which should be started immediately.[84]

Vitamin A

Vitamin A has diverse functions, being essential for vision, growth, reproduction, cell differentiation, and immunocompetency.[95] Retinol is the

Table 11 Suggested Preparation of PN Solution for LBW Infants[248]

Component	Concentration/Additive	Intake
Glucose	12.5%	(Glucose = 16 g/kg/d)
Amino acids*	2.4%	(Amino acids = 3.1 g/kg/d)
Cysteine-HCl	30 mg/g amino acids	
NaCl	2.6 mmol = 2.6 mEq	(Na = 3.4 mmol/kg/d)
KCl	0–0.2 mmol (mEq)	(Total K = 3.1–3.8 mmol/kg/d)
K_2PO_4–$KHPO_4$†	1.5–2.0 mmol P	(P = 2.0–2.6 mmol/kg/d)
Ca gluconate‡	1.5–2.0 mmol Ca	(Ca = 2.0–2.6 mmol/kg/d)
$MgSO_4$	0.25 mmol = 0.5 mEq	(Mg = 0.3 mmol/kg/d)
MVI-Pediatric§	40% of vial (2 mL/kg/d)	
MTE-4‖	0.2 mL/kg/d	(Zn, Cu, Mn, Cr, Se)
Zn	200 μg/kg/d	(Total Zn = 200 μg/kg/d)
Selenium	2 μg/kg/d	(Cu = 20 μg/kg/d)
		(Mn = 5 μg/kg/d)
		(Cr = 0.4 μg/kg/d)
		(Se = 2 μg/kg/d)
Total Zn = 200 + 200 = 400 μg/kg/d		
Heparin	1 unit/mL	
Intralipid 20%#	5–20 mL/kg/d	
Total fluid	150 mL/kg/d	

*TrophAmine (B. Braun).
†Monobasic-dibasic phosphate contains 1.4 mmol K/mmol P or 1.3 mmol Na/mmol P, depending upon the preparation used. Use the higher P concentration for PN duration >2 weeks.
‡Use the higher concentration for PN duration >2 weeks. Add last in the preparation of PN.
§MVI-Pediatric, Mayne Pharma (USA), Inc, Paramus, NJ.
‖MTE-4, American Regent, Inc., Shirley, NY.
#Begin lipid at 1 g/kg/d and increase stepwise to 3-4 g/kg/d.

Table 12 Suggested Intakes of Vitamins for LBW Infants Receiving PN[84,248]

Vitamin	Current Suggestion* (unit/kg/d)	Best Estimate for New Formulation (unit/kg/d)	Maximum Not to Exceed Term Infant (unit/d)
Fat-soluble vitamins			
A (μg)†	280	500	700
E (mg)‡	2.8	2.8	7
K (μg)	80	80	200
D (μg)§	4	4	10
Water-soluble vitamins			
C, Ascorbic acid (mg)	32	25	80
B_1, Thiamin (mg)	0.48	0.35	1.2
B_2, Riboflavin (mg)	0.56	0.15	1.4
B_6, Pyridoxine (mg)	0.40	0.18	1.0
Niacin (mg)	6.8	6.8	17
Pantothenate (mg)	2	2	5
Biotin (μg)	8	6	20
Folate (μg)	56	56	140
Vitamin B_{12} (μg)	0.40	0.30	1.0

*Practical approach using 40% of a vial of MVI-Pediatric (Mayne Pharma (USA), Inc., Paramus, NJ) per kg body weight or 2 mL/kg/d.[84] Infuvite Pediatric (Sandoz Canada Inc., Boucherville, Quebec, Canada) has composition similar to MVI-Pediatric, with the following exceptions (per 5 mL): aluminum (4.2 vs 0.2 μg) and polysorbate 20 vs 0.8 mg), infuvite vs. 0.8 mg), in infuvite vs. MVI-Pediatric, respectively.

†1 μg retinol = 3.33 IU vitamin A = 6 μg β-carotene = 1.83 μg retinyl palmitate = 1 retinol equivalent (RE).

‡1 mg α-ocopherol = 1 IU vitamin E.

§1 μg vitamin D (cholecalciferol) = 40 IU vitamin D (cholecalciferol).

dietary component present as retinyl esters (palmitate, stearate) in animal sources, and carotene is the vitamin A precursor of plant origin. The amount of vitamin A in the diet is quantitated as retinol equivalents (RE): 1 RE equals 1 μg all-*trans* retinol or 3.33 IU vitamin A; 6 μg β-carotene equals 1 μg retinol (Table 12).

Carotene and retinyl esters are converted to retinol in the proximal small intestine. Retinol is absorbed into intestinal cells, esterified, and incorporated into chylomicrons that are transported via the lymphatics to the circulation, and eventually taken up by the liver. In the liver, the vitamin is esterified and stored as retinyl palmitate.[95] Retinol is mobilized from the liver to the circulation bound with retinol-binding protein (RBP) and transthyretin. More than one-third (37%) of LBW infants were found to have hepatic vitamin stores <20 μg/g, signifying deficiency, while more than three-fourths (76%) had stores of <40 μg/g.[96] Vitamin A also is stored in the lung and may be involved in growth and differentiation of the lung. Therefore, LBW infants may be vitamin A deprived and their lungs susceptible to the effects of this deficiency.[96]

Photodegradation of retinol occurs when milk or an intravenous solution is exposed to light during continuous infusions, so increased light exposure should be avoided.[97,98] In addition, between 30 and 75% of the original retinol is lost by adsorption to the tubing before it reaches the infant. Greater plasma retinol concentrations occur when the vitamin is mixed with intravenous lipid emulsion or with the use of retinyl esters.[99,100] Plasma vitamin A concentrations in LBW infants receiving PN are low. When receiving 455 μg/d, there is no change in plasma vitamin concentrations over baseline.

Infants developing bronchopulmonary dysplasia (BPD) are reported to have lower plasma vitamin A concentrations at 4, 14, 21, and 28 days of age compared with infants not developing BPD.[101] Randomized controlled trials of vitamin A supplementation in LBW infants susceptible to BPD have been reported.[102] In a randomized comparison of vitamin A intakes from all sources over the first month, an intake of 510 μg/kg/d was associated with less plasma vitamin A deficiency and less BPD than control infants receiving 130 μg/kg/d. Vitamin A—supplemented infants also had less airway infection and retinopathy of prematurity than control infants.[96]

Not all randomized studies observe a significant effect of vitamin A supplementation on BPD outcomes.[103] However, a meta-analysis suggests that supplementation with vitamin A is associated with a modest reduction in oxygen requirement at 36 weeks postmenstrual age (summary relative risk = 0.85 [95% confidence interval 0.73–0.98]), and a trend toward a reduction in retinopathy of prematurity.[102] Despite high vitamin A intakes in a large multicenter study, 24% of the supplemented group had plasma concentrations <20 μg/dL. The authors concluded that because of the modest decrease in chronic lung disease, the safety, lack of toxicity, and low cost, further investigations using higher doses of the vitamin were warranted.[104] Guidelines should be adopted and parenteral preparations reformulated to provide intakes that approximate 500 μg/kg/d for vitamin A, initiated within the first 12 hours after birth.[84]

Vitamin E

Vitamin E functions in humans as a biological antioxidant: a free-radical scavenger that inhibits the naturally occurring peroxidation of polyunsaturated fatty acids, components of the lipid layer of cell membranes.[105]

Daily parenteral administration of 2.1 mg is associated with normal plasma vitamin E concentrations by 48 hours.[106] Mixing the vitamin E dose with intravenous lipid increases plasma vitamin E concentrations. Early use of PN-containing multivitamins is effective in raising plasma vitamin E concentrations to physiologic ranges within the first 24 hours.[107] Current PN regimens recommend vitamin E intakes of 2.8 mg/kg/d (40% of a vial of MVI-Pediatric, Mayne Pharma Inc, Paramus, NJ) for infants weighing below 2.5 kg and 7 mg/d (1 vial of MVI-Pediatric) for infants weighing greater than 2.5 kg.[84]

Data from older randomized trials in LBW infants suggest that there may be a relationship between pharmacologic doses of vitamin E and the entities of retinopathy of prematurity (ROP), bronchopulmonary dysplasia, and intraventricular hemorrhage. The incidence of severe ROP (Stage 3+) was 2.4% with vitamin E-supplementation and 5.3% in the control group, a modest effect despite pharmacologic doses of the vitamin.[108–111] Despite initial studies demonstrating a modest effect on the reduction of BPD, pharmacologic vitamin E supplementation has not been demonstrated to reduce the severity of the disease.[112–114] In older studies, if vitamin E was given within 12 hours of birth, a reduction in the incidence and severity of IVH was observed.[115,116] Studies demonstrating an effect of intramuscular vitamin E on IVH have suggested a target plasma concentration >1.0 mg/dL by 24 hours and >2 mg/dL at 3 days.[117] Those plasma vitamin E concentrations can be achieved with PN-containing multivitamins if initiated soon after birth (Tables 8 and 12). Guidelines should be adopted and PN preparations reformulated to provide intakes that approximate 3 mg/kg/d for vitamin E, which should be initiated soon after birth.

Water-Soluble Vitamins

Current formulations generally provide more water-soluble vitamins than are needed by LBW infants. Plasma ascorbate (vitamin C) and vitamin B_2 (riboflavin) concentrations reportedly were elevated in LBW infants receiving PN.[99,118,119] The elevated riboflavin concentrations appear paradoxical in view of the known degradation of the vitamin under continuous infusion and nursery lighting conditions. Thus, significantly lower doses of some of the water-soluble vitamins are indicated (Table 12). When used in a dose of 2 mL/kg/d (40% of the vial M.V.I.-Pediatric), no deficiencies of thiamin or riboflavin were detected, and plasma concentrations of folate and B_{12} indicated sufficient status.[120]

Summary of Parenteral Nutrient Needs

Parenteral nutrient needs consider the needs for growth and greater energy expenditure and potential for nutrient losses as a result of illness. LBW infants receiving PN should have biochemical monitoring to avoid excesses or deficiencies of particular nutrients (Table 13). Complications related to PN therapy are recognized and will be described in Chapter 69, "Parenteral Nutrition." Early, immediate use of parenteral nutrition is

Table 13 Biochemical Monitoring for LBW Infants Receiving PN[248]

Energy	Urine glucose, serum triglycerides
Protein	BUN
Minerals	Ca, P, Mg, Na, K, Cl, CO_2, alkaline phosphatase activity
Other	Creatinine, conjugated bilirubin, ALT, trace element concentrations

Table 14 Advantages of Gastrointestinal Priming

Shortens time to regain birth weight
Improves feeding tolerance
Reduces duration of parenteral nutrition
Enhances enzyme maturation
Reduces intestinal permeability
Improves GI motility
Matures hormone responses
Improves mineral absorption, mineralization
Lowers incidence of cholestasis
Reduces duration of phototherapy
Earlier use of mother's milk
Mothers begin milk expression earlier
Infants receive more mother's milk
Psychological advantage for mothers
Safety

important to prevent deficiencies in LBW infants (Table 8). A general protocol for routine PN has been devised (Table 11).[121]

GASTROINTESTINAL PRIMING

The lack of enteral nutrients poses several problems for the development of the intestinal tract. The absence of enteral nutrients is associated with diminished intestinal size and weight, atrophy of intestinal mucosa, delayed maturation of intestinal enzymes, and increases in permeability and bacterial translocation.[122,123] A lack of enteral nutrients also affects intestinal motility, perfusion, and responses to gastrointestinal trophic hormones.[124] The hormonal response to feeding premature infants has been evaluated by measuring the plasma concentrations of selected gastrointestinal trophic hormones in response to milk feeding during the first week after birth.[125] Significant hormone surges are noted after milk feeding but no response is observed in absence of feeding. The responses to feeding are observed both in healthy premature infants as well as those with respiratory distress. Most surges in hormone concentrations occur after feeding small quantities of milk, approximately 24 mL.[125]

The above observations prompted prospective randomized clinical studies of small volumes of milk as early minimal enteral nutrition, or gastrointestinal priming, in premature infants. When studied in the first or second week after birth, infants given "early" priming feedings had a better feeding tolerance when feedings were advanced, required a shorter duration of parenteral nutrition, and had a lower incidence of conjugated hyperbilirubinemia compared with similar infants given only parenteral nutrition during the same interval (Table 14).[126,127] Probably because of better tolerance to feeding, premature infants receiving the trophic feedings had greater cumulative milk intakes, which was associated with lower serum alkaline phosphatase activity.[126] The lower alkaline phosphatase activity, primarily of bone origin, was observed for 14 weeks, well beyond the initial intervention in the first week. Significant stimulation of gastrointestinal hormones, such as gastrin and GIP, also were reported following the early feeding of small quantities of milk.[128] Intestinal motility patterns matured more rapidly and intestinal transit time was not as lengthened in premature infants receiving early enteral feeding.[129,130] Subsequent investigations demonstrated that trophic feeding was associated with greater absorption of Ca and P, greater lactase activity, greater bone mineral content, and a reduced intestinal permeability.[130-133] Although the benefits of GI priming vary among studies, no study has reported any adverse effects of such a protocol (Table 14). The meta-analysis of gastrointestinal priming studies indicated that its use was associated with a shorter time to full feeding, fewer days when feedings were held, and a shorter duration of hospitalization, but no increase in the incidence of necrotizing enterocolitis.[134]

Noteworthy in the studies of minimal enteral nutrition is that the subject population consisted of premature infants selected because they had the greatest risk of feeding intolerance and necrotizing enterocolitis. For example, feedings were administered during mechanical ventilation and while umbilical arterial and venous catheters were in place.[126,127,135] The infants also had the usual morbidities of patent ductus arteriosus, intraventricular hemorrhage, and systemic hypotension. These data suggest that by the end of the first week after birth, in the absence of major cardiovascular instability (severe acidosis, hypotension, hypoxemia), the intestinal tract of the premature infant can be primed with small volumes of milk.

One study was appropriately designed to extend the minimal enteral nutrition observations to a protocol of early advancement of enteral feedings.[136] At the discretion of the attending physician, infants less than 32 weeks' gestation were assigned randomly to trophic feeding of 20 mL/kg/d versus a protocol of advancing feedings by 20 mL/kg/d for a 10-day interval. The study was stopped after enrollment of 141 infants because of a significantly greater incidence of NEC in the advancing group compared with the trophic feeding group. It is difficult to conclude causality as there were a number of issues with the study, including no differences in death between groups and a shorter hospital stay and more rapid attainment of full oral feeding in the advancing group compared with the trophic feeding group. Further study is warranted.

Thus, for extremely LBW infants who are ill, trophic feeding of small volumes (10–20 mL/kg/d) should be initiated in the first few days after birth and continue for approximately 3 to 7 days before advancement of feeding.[130] The decision for advancement of feedings, however, is made after clinical feeding tolerance is proven and clinical stability is achieved.

ENTERAL NUTRITION

Protein

Milk Composition. In the first few weeks after birth, the protein content of milk from mothers who deliver premature infants (preterm milk) is greater than term milk, the milk obtained from women delivering term infants.[137] The protein content in both milks declines, such that beyond 2 weeks it levels off to what we call mature milk (Table 15). Human milk contains 70% whey and 30% casein whereas bovine milk contains 18% whey and 82% casein. The whey fraction of milk consists of soluble proteins that are digested more easily. The quality of protein (eg, the proportion of whey and casein) in human milk is particularly suitable for the premature infant. A whey- and/or casein-dominant commercial formula, therefore, refers to these proportions of bovine milk. Human milk and then whey-dominant bovine milk, in that order, promote more rapid gastric emptying than casein-dominant milk.[138] Elevated concentrations of potentially toxic amino acids (phenylalanine, methionine, and tyrosine) are reported in premature infants fed formulas with high casein contents.[139,140] Hepatic enzyme immaturity may explain the higher plasma amino acid concentrations. Because we infer that elevations of particular amino acids may be toxic to brain development, there may be a concern when feeding premature infants a casein-dominant milk, especially at a high protein intake.

The compositions of the whey fractions of human and bovine milks differ significantly. The major human whey protein is α-lactalbumin, a nutritional protein for the infant and a component of mammary gland lactose synthesis. Lactoferrin, lysozyme, and secretory immunoglobulin A (sIgA) are specific human whey proteins that are particularly resistant to hydrolysis and, as such, line the gastrointestinal tract to play a primary role in host defense.[141] These proteins, therefore, may be suitable for the premature infant who is exposed to multiple pathogens in the nursery environment. The three host defense proteins are present only in trace quantities in bovine milk. The major whey protein in bovine milk is β-lactoglobulin, the protein associated with bovine milk protein allergy and colic.[142]

The major amino acid for the fetus and in human milk is glutamine, which is not found in commercial formula because of problems with stability of the free amino acid. Glutamine, however, is an important amino acid for cell growth, specifically intestinal epithelial growth, has a role in immune function, and is a precursor in glutathione synthesis. When commercial formula was supplemented with glutamine, one study found that premature infants had better feeding tolerance and a significantly lower incidence of sepsis than

Table 15 Nutrient Composition of Human Milk and Selected Fortified Human Milk[175,249–252]

Component (Units)	Human Milk (1 wk)	Mature Preterm Human Milk (1 mo)	Mature Preterm Human Milk + Human Milk Fortifier
Volume (mL)	100	100	100
Energy (kcal)	67	69	83
Protein (g)	2.4	1.5	2.5–2.6
Whey/casein (%)	70/30	70/30	70/30
Fat (g)	3.8	3.6	4.0–4.6
MCT (%)	2	2	11–17
Carbohydrate (g)	6.1	6.7	7.1–8.5
Lactose (%)	100	100	80–85
Calcium (mg)	25	29	119–146
Phosphorus (mg)	14	9.3	59–76
Magnesium (mg)	3.1	2.4	3.4–9.4
Sodium (mEq; mmol)	2.2	0.9	1.6
Potassium (mEq; mmol)	1.8	1.3	2–2.9
Chloride (mEq; mmol)	2.6	1.5	1.9–2.6
Zinc (μg)	500	215	935–1215
Copper (μg)	80	51	95–221
Vitamin A (IU)	560	227	847–1177
Vitamin D (IU)	4	1.2	122–151
Vitamin E (mg)	1.0	0.3	3.5–4.9

Enfamil Human Milk Fortifier (Mead Johnson Nutritionals, Evansville, IN); Similac Human Milk Fortifier (Ross Laboratories, Columbus, OH); 4 packets + 100 mL Mature Preterm Human Milk.

infants fed unsupplemented formula.[143] However, subsequent studies have not confirmed an effect of enteral glutamine on infection in this population.[144,145] It remains to be determined whether this amino acid should be supplied if human milk is not fed.

Protein Needs. The quantity and quality of protein needed for premature infants have been investigated.[146] Formulas providing protein intakes of 2.25 and 4.50 g/kg/d as either whey- or casein-dominant preparations were compared with pasteurized human milk with a protein intake of approximately 1.6 g/kg/d. Although absolute growth rates reportedly were similar during the in-hospital study, hospital duration was longer for the infants fed human milk, suggesting a slower rate of weight gain than infants fed formula.[139,140] Those infants receiving protein intakes of 4.5 g/kg/d, as well as infants given casein-dominant milk, had more abnormalities in plasma amino acids and protein indices of nutritional status (elevated blood concentrations of urea nitrogen and ammonia, acidosis, lethargy, and fever) indicative of excess protein intake.[147] Although generally considered excessive protein intake, 4.5 g/kg/d were provided with a relatively low intake of energy (115 kcal/kg/d) and minerals. Some investigators comment that energy and mineral intakes may have limited the ability to utilize the protein, and that such intakes may be appropriate if the total diet is adjusted.

The appropriate intake of protein for LBW infants has been defined further from evaluations of weight gain, nitrogen retention, and serum biochemical indicators of protein nutritional status.[148,149] Protein intakes of 2.2 and 2.8 g/kg/d resulted in lower serum biochemical indicators of protein status, weight gain, and nitrogen retention, while a protein intake of 3.8 g/kg/d appeared somewhat excessive. Therefore, the investigators concluded that protein intakes of approximately 3.5 g/kg/d at 120 kcal/kg/d seem appropriate for the otherwise healthy LBW infant.[148]

An alternate way to compute the protein needs of the premature infant is to use the factorial approach to add the needs for tissue deposition, derived from intrauterine accretion rates of 1.8 to 2.2 g/kg/d, to the postnatal losses of protein from the skin (approximately 0.2 g/kg/d) and the urine (1.0 g/kg/d). As approximately 85% of the protein is absorbed, the calculated enteral protein intake is 3.2–4.0 g/kg/d.[8] A range of protein intakes are found if all products available are considered (Table 16). However, the above computations provide the basis on which to select appropriate products designed for LBW infants: fortified human milk and preterm formula.

The above studies were conducted using formulations with whole or intact protein. Although fetal nitrogen uptake is composed primarily of amino acids, no data suggest that postnatal formulations include hydrolyzed proteins or free amino acids. Whey-dominant protein formulations are well-absorbed, and the provision of hydrolyzed protein formulations, usually casein-derived, for the otherwise healthy premature infant are not indicated (Tables 16 to 18).

Protein needs should be considered in conjunction with energy. Protein synthesis requires energy. If energy intake is inadequate, protein synthesis may be depressed and amino acid oxidation increase.[150] Protein retention, or balance, generally is a function of protein intake if energy intake is adequate.[26] Greater protein intakes are more of a risk if energy intake is limited.[151]

Human Milk Protein Needs. The aforementioned studies demonstrated that the lowest

Table 16 Nutrient Composition of Fortified Human Milk, Preterm Formula, Postdischarge Formula, and Term Formula

Component (Units)	Fortified Human Milk	Preterm Formula	Postdischarge Formula	Term Formula
Volume (mL)	100	100	100	100
Energy (kcal)	83	81	73	67
Protein (g)	2.5–2.6	2.4	2.0–2.1	1.4–1.5
Whey/casein (%)	70/30	60/40	60/40, 50/50	100/0, 60/40, 48/52
Protein calories (%)	12	12	11	8–9
Fat (g)	4.0–4.6	4.1–4.4	3.9–4.1	3.4–3.7
MCT (%)	11–17	40–50	20–25	0
Fat calories (%)	43–50	44–47	47–49	46–49
Carbohydrate (g)	7.1–8.5	8.4–9.0	7.5–7.6	7.3–7.5
Lactose (%)	80–85	40–50	40–50	70–100
CHO calories (%)	34–41	41–44	40–42	43–45
Calcium (mg)	119–146	134–146	78–88	43–53
Phosphorus (mg)	59–76	65–81	46–48	24–29
Magnesium (mg)	3.4–9.4	7.3–9.7	5.9–6.7	4.0–5.4
Sodium (mEq; mmol)	1.6	1.5–2.0	1.1	0.7–0.8
Potassium (mEq; mmol)	2.0–2.9	2.0–2.7	2.0–2.7	1.8–1.9
Chloride (mEq; mmol)	1.9–2.6	1.9–2.0	1.6	1.2
Zinc (μg)	935–1,215	1200	913	500–670
Copper (μg)	95–221	100–200	88	50–61
Vitamin A (IU)	847–1,177	1000	329–342	200
Vitamin D (IU)	122–151	120–194	52–58	40
Vitamin E (mg)	3.5–4.9	3.2–5.1	2.7–2.9	1.0–1.3
Osmolality (mOsm/L)	325–385	280–300	250–260	250–300
Potential renal solute load (mOsm)	22–23	22–23	18.1–18.7	12.7–13.1

FHM: Enfamil Human Milk Fortifier (Mead Johnson Nutritionals, Evansville, IN) and Similac Human Milk Fortifier (Ross Laboratories, Columbus, OH), 4 packets + 100 mL Mature Preterm Human Milk; Preterm: Similac Special Care Advance with iron (Ross) and Enfamil Lipil Premature Formula with iron (Mead Johnson); Postdischarge: NeoSure Advance (Ross) and EnfaCare Lipil (Mead Johnson); Term: Enfamil Lipil with iron (Mead Johnson), Good Start Supreme (Nestle), Similac Advance with iron (Ross).

Table 17 Comparison of Selected Fortifiers for Human Milk (Prepared per 100 mL Preterm Human Milk)

Component (Units)	Preterm HM	Enfamil HMF	Similac HMF	Aptamil	S-26	FM85
Energy (kcal)	69	83	83	84	84	86
Fat (g)	3.6	4.6	4	3.6	3.8	3.6
Carbohydrate (g)	6.7	7.1	8.5	9.7	9.1	10
Protein (g)	1.5	2.6	2.5	2.3	2.5	2.5
Calcium (mg)	29	119	146	94	119	104
Phosphorus (mg)	9.3	59	76	54	55	54
Magnesium (mg)	2.4	3.4	9.4	8.4	5.4	4.8
Sodium (mEq)	9	1.6	1.6	1.8	1.7	1.8
Zinc (μg)	215	935	1215	615	345	1015
Copper (μg)	51	95	221	81	51	91
Vitamins	Yes	Multi	Multi	Multi	Multi	Multi

Preterm HM = Preterm Mature Human Milk (Table 16); Enfamil HMF = Enfamil Human Milk Fortifier (Mead Johnson Nutritionals, Evansville, IN); Similac HMF = Similac Human Milk Fortifier (Ross Laboratories, Columbus, OH); Aptamil = Aptamil Human Milk Fortifier (Milupa, Friedrichsdorf, Germany); S-26 = S-26 Human Milk Fortifier Wyeth Nutritionals International, Philadelphia, PA); FM85 = FM85 Human Milk Fortifier (Nestle, Vevey, Switzerland); Multi = Added multivitamins: A, D, E, K, B_1, B_2, B_6, C, Niacin, Folate, B_{12}, pantothenate, biotin.

plasma concentrations of amino acids, albumin, and urea nitrogen, and the slowest rates of weight gain were found in the human milk–fed premature infants.[146,152] These observations suggest that after the first 2 weeks of lactation, the human milk–fed LBW infant receives a lower protein intake, which may lead to protein deficiency. To meet protein needs, the human milk–fed premature infant needs a protein supplement (Table 15). The protein contents of mature human milk and fortified human milk are 1.0 and 2.2 g/dL, respectively, and preterm formula is 2.2 g/dL. Growth rates and serum protein and urea nitrogen concentrations in premature infants increase when human milk is fortified with protein to achieve a protein intake of at least 3 to 3.5 g/kg/d.[153] This range of protein intake is adequate assuming that no protein deficit has arisen as a result of a prolonged or deficient parenteral nutrition phase. For this reason, greater intakes of protein may be necessary for premature infants to allow for catch-up protein nutritional support. Thus, intakes of approximately 4.0 g/kg/d, with adequate intakes of energy and minerals, often may be indicated.

Fat

Human Milk Lipid Composition. The lipid system in human milk is structured in a way that facilitates fat digestion and absorption. There is an organized human milk fat globule containing an outer protein coat and an inner lipid core. The pattern of fatty acids (high in palmitic 16:0, oleic 18:1, linoleic 18:2ω6, and linolenic 18:3ω3), their distribution on the triglyceride molecule (16:0 at the 2-position of the molecule), and the presence of bile salt–stimulated lipase characterize the lipid system in human milk.[154] Because the lipase is heat-labile, the superior fat absorption from human milk is reported only when unprocessed milk is fed.[154]

The most variable nutrient component in human milk is fat, the major energy source, comprising nearly 50% of the calories. The fat content of human milk varies among women, changes during the day, rises slightly during lactation, and increases dramatically within a single milk expression.[155] The variability in total fat content is unrelated to maternal dietary fat intake. Because it is not homogenized, upon standing, the fat separates out of human milk. The separated fat may adhere to collection containers, feeding tubes, and syringes. The loss of fat, therefore, robs the premature infant of needed energy. The greatest losses of fat occur from continuous milk infusion systems. Care should be taken when using the continuous milk infusion system to ensure the inclusion of only a short length of tubing. If the system contains a cassette interface, much of the fat will be lost when the tubing system is changed. Milk infusion systems that use a syringe and small infusion pump, where the syringe is oriented upright, will allow more complete delivery of fat.[156] Fat loss was reduced from 48% to less than 8% with the change in methods of continuous infusion.

Manufacturers of infant formulas modify their fat blends to mimic the fat absorption from human milk. This accounts for the differences in the constituent fatty acids between human milk and cow's milk–based formulas. Generally, commercial formulations have a greater quantity of medium-chain-length fatty acids (MCFA) to compensate for the absence of lipase and the unique structure of triglycerides in human milk.[154,157] In human milk, saturated fatty acids, particularly palmitic acid, is esterified in the 2-position of the triglyceride molecule. The end product of digestion of the triglyceride is a 2-monoglyceride and minimal free fatty acid. The 2-monoglyceride is absorbed to a greater degree than the free fatty acid. This is important because free palmitic acid has a great tendency to bind with minerals to form soaps. In that case, both fat and mineral absorption would be limited. Thus, the overall structure of human milk is designed to provide optimal fat and mineral absorption.

Hindmilk. The variability in the fat content of human milk may be made advantageous for the premature infant. Most milk transfer during a feeding occurs in 10 to 15 minutes, but continued serial milk expressions yield a low volume with a high fat content (hindmilk) than the earlier foremilk. The fat content of hindmilk may be 1.5- to 3-fold greater than that of foremilk. The use of hindmilk in selected cases may provide the premature infant with additional energy.

Table 18 Comparison of Preterm Formula, Casein Hydrolysate Formulas, and Amino Acid–Based Formulas per 100 mL

Component (Units)	Preterm Formula, 24 kcal	Pregestimil, 20 kcal	Pregestimil, 24 kcal	Elecare, 20 kcal	Elecare, 24 kcal	Neocate, 20 kcal	Neocate, 24 kcal
Energy (kcal)	81	67	81	67	81	67	81
Protein (g)	2.4	1.9	2.2	2	2.4	2.1	2.5
Whey/casein (%)	60/40	0/100 casein hydrolysate	0/100 casein hydrolysate	Free L–amino acids	Free L–amino acids	Free L–amino acids	Free L–amino acids
Protein calories (%)	12	11.2	11.2	12.1	12	12.4	12.3
Fat (g)	4.1–4.4	3.7	4.4	3.2	3.9	3	3.7
MCT (%)	40–50	55	55	33	33	5	5
Fat calories (%)	44–47	50.4	50.4	42.9	42.8	40.5	40.6
Carbohydrate (g)	8.4–9	6.8	8.1	7.2	8.7	7.9	9.5
Lactose (%)	40–50	0	0	0	0	0	0
CHO calories (%)	41–44	40.8	40.8	42.8	42.7	46.8	46.9
Calcium (mg)	134–146	77	91	73	88	84	101
Phosphorus (mg)	65–81	50	60	55	66	63	76
Magnesium (mg)	7.3–9.7	8	9.5	5.4	6.5	8.4	10.1
Sodium (mEq; mmol)	1.5–2	1.4	1.6	1.3	1.6	1.1	1.3
Potassium (mEq; mmol)	2.0–2.7	1.9	2.2	2.6	3.1	2.7	3.2
Chloride (mEq; mmol)	1.9–2.0	1.6	1.9	1.2	1.4	1.5	1.8
Zinc (μg)	1200	730	870	740	890	1,120	1,350
Copper (μg)	100–200	73	87	85	102	84	101
Vitamin A (IU)	1000	253	302	185	222	277	332
Vitamin D (IU)	120–194	33	40	28	34	41	49
Vitamin E (mg)	3.2–5.1	2.5	3.0	1.4	1.7	0.8	0.9
Osmolality (mOsm/L)	280–300	280	330	335	422	375	479
Potential renal solute load	22–23	17.1	20.4	18.4	22.2	19.3	23

Preterm: Similac Special Care Advance (Ross Laboratories) and Enfamil Premature Lipil (Mead Johnson Nutritionals); Pregestimil (Mead Johnson Nutritionals); Elecare (Ross Laboratories); Neocate (Nutricia North America).

Fractionation of each milk expression into two portions, foremilk and hindmilk, is practical if mothers' milk production is greater than needed by her infant. The additional fat, and therefore, energy intake from hindmilk has been shown to improve the body weight gain in premature infants.[158] Examination of the composition of foremilk and hindmilk indicates similar contents of nitrogen, calcium, phosphorus, sodium, and potassium, and approximately 5% lower copper and zinc concentrations in hindmilk.

The differences between foremilk and hindmilk also should be considered in terms of the distribution of calories. Fat and protein comprised 42 and 12% of calories in foremilk and 55 and 9% of calories in hindmilk, respectively. Theoretically, the long-term feeding of hindmilk could exert a negative effect on protein status. A greater proportion of protein calories (10–12%) is recommended for premature infants. Usual commercial human milk fortifiers (Tables 15 and 17), when mixed with hindmilk, raise the proportion of protein calories in hindmilk to approximately 12%. The use of hindmilk, therefore, can be recommended for premature infants whose rate of weight gain is low (below 15 g/kg/d).

Essential Fatty Acids. The essential fatty acids, linoleic and linolenic, are present in ample quantities in human milk and commercial formula. Without an adequate intake of these fatty acids, essential fatty acid deficiency (thrombocytopenia, dermatitis, increased infections, and delayed growth) develops in one week. Approximately 0.5 g/kg/d (~4% of total energy intake) of essential fatty acids will prevent the deficiency.[52] Derivatives of linoleic and linolenic acids are arachidonic acid (20:4ω6) and docosahexaenoic acid (22:6ω3). The very long-chain polyunsaturated fatty acids (LCPUFA), which are found in human but not bovine milk, are components of phospholipids found in brain, retina, and red blood cell membranes.[159,160] Arachidonic and docosahexaenoic acids functionally have been associated with body growth, vision, and cognition.[160,161] In addition, the fatty acids are integral parts of prostaglandin metabolism. When their diet was supplemented with LCPUFA, formula-fed premature infants had red blood cell concentrations of 22:6ω3 that parallel those of similar infants fed human milk.[159] Follow-up studies of such supplemented infants suggest improvements in visual acuity and short-term neurodevelopmental measures compared with unsupplemented infants, but of similar magnitude to infants fed human milk.[161–163] The consensus is that premature infants should receive LCPUFAs either via human milk or supplemented formula.

Medium-Chain Fatty Acids. The proportion of MCFA, here defined as carbon length 6:0 to 12:0, is below 12% of total fatty acids in human milk, but approaches 50% in preterm formulas (Table 16). MCFA are not essential fatty acids. Previous reports suggested that MCFA were absorbed passively and to a greater extent than long-chain fatty acids (LCFA), and affected growth and mineral absorption positively.[164,165] Subsequent studies comparing premature infants receiving MCFA (42 vs 7% of total fatty acids) in a crossover design found no differences in either the absorption of fat or weight gain.[166] Similarly, no differences in nitrogen retention, weight gain, and energy digestibility, expenditure, and storage were found in premature infants participating in a randomized, crossover study of formulas with MCFA at 46 versus 4%.[167] Other reports also confirm the lack of effect of MCFA on weight gain and mineral absorption compared with exclusive LCFA diets.[168] When used in a high proportion, MCFA may be incompletely oxidized, and contribute to increased urinary dicarboxylic acid excretion and metabolic inefficiency compared with LCFA.[169,170] When added exogenously to milk, MCFA have been reported to adhere to feeding tubes and diminish fat delivery to the infant.[171] Thus, there are no compelling data to suggest that a high proportion of MCFA is needed for preterm formulas. Indeed, formulas containing a very high proportion of MCFA (>80%) may produce essential fatty acid deficiency if fed for a prolonged period of time.

Carnitine

Carnitine is synthesized from lysine and methionine and serves as an important effector of fatty acid oxidation in the mitochondria. The provision of carnitine in the diet results in improved fatty acid oxidation.[71] Human milk contains abundant carnitine and all infant formulas are supplemented with carnitine.

Carbohydrate

The carbohydrate fraction of human milk is composed of lactose (90–95%) and oligosaccharides (5–10%). The lactose content of human milk rises from 55 g/L in colostrum to 70 g/L in mature milk. Although studies in term infants demonstrate a small proportion of lactose in the feces, the presence of lactose is assumed to be a normal physiological effect of feeding human milk. A softer stool consistency, more nonpathogenic bacterial fecal flora, and improved absorption of minerals have been attributed to the presence of small quantities of unabsorbed lactose in feces.[172] Dietary lactose also has been associated with increased mineral absorption.[173] Theoretical concerns that lactose may not be digested adequately by premature infants less than 34 weeks postmenstrual age may be unfounded as clinical studies indicate that they tolerate the feeding of lactose-containing milk. Premature infants absorb >90% of the lactose in human milk.[174] The feeding of milk, and, in particular human milk, in premature infants stimulates intestinal lactase activity compared with no feeding or formula feeding.[131] Thus, early feeding of human milk also may be beneficial to promote better lactose utilization.

Because of conflicting data regarding lactose utilization by premature infants, and as a result of attempts to reduce the osmolality of the milk, preterm formulas contain a large proportion of carbohydrate as corn syrup solids (glucose polymers).[173] The usual lactose/glucose polymer mixture is 50:50. Glucose polymers are well absorbed by premature infants.

Calcium and Phosphorus

Calcium and phosphorus are primary components of the skeleton, accounting for 99 and 85%, respectively, of bone mass. The goal for premature infant nutrition is to achieve a bone mineralization pattern similar to the fetus and to avoid osteopenia and fractures. Preterm human milk contains approximately 250 and 140 mg/L, respectively, of Ca and P.[175] In contrast, the Ca and P content of enteral products designed for premature infants in the United States is significantly greater (Tables 15–17). In human milk, Ca and P exist in ionized and complexed forms, which are easily absorbed. The salts in commercial formulas, however, are relatively insoluble. Thus, in the design of commercial formulas, greater quantities of these minerals are added to compensate for their poorer bioavailability. However, distinct from the term infant, the premature infant requires significantly greater quantities of Ca and P than can be provided in human milk.

For the human milk–fed premature infant, Ca and P intakes are deficient throughout lactation and far below those necessary to achieve respective intrauterine accretion rates.[176] Skeletal radiographs may reveal poor bone mineralization, rickets, and fractures in the premature infant fed unsupplemented human milk.[177] Deficient intakes of Ca and P are associated with biochemical markers, such as low serum and urine P concentrations, elevated serum alkaline phosphatase activity, and elevated serum and urine Ca concentrations.[178] Usually, serum P concentrations are the best indicator of Ca and P status in human milk-fed premature infants.[179] Prolonged deficiency of these minerals tends to stimulate bone resorption to normalize serum Ca concentrations. This bone activity often is correlated with elevated serum alkaline phosphatase activity. It has been reported that the majority of premature infants having an elevated serum alkaline phosphatase activity were those fed human milk.[180] Moreover, follow-up of the same infants at 9 and 18 months noted that linear growth was significantly lower in the group that had the higher serum activity of alkaline phosphatase in the neonatal period.[180] A high alkaline phosphatase value in the neonatal period is a negative predictor of height in 9- to 12-year-old adolescents.[181]

The supplementation of human milk with both Ca and P not only improves the net retention of both minerals, but also improves bone mineral content.[182,183] Current management of human milk–fed premature infants emphasizes the need for supplements of both Ca and P.[184] A linear relationship exists between Ca (or P) intake and net retention in enterally fed premature infants.[185] Premature infants receiving unfortified human milk never achieve intrauterine accretion rates for Ca and P. Intakes of Ca and P of approximately

200 and 100 mg/kg/d, respectively, can be achieved with the use of specialized human milk fortifiers and preterm formulas, thus making it possible to meet intrauterine estimates (Tables 15 to 17). However, term infant formulas and specialized (not "preterm") formulas provide inadequate quantities of Ca and P to meet the needs of growing premature infants (Tables 16 and 18). Several factors affect the absorption of Ca and P, including postnatal age and intake of Ca, P, lactose, fat, and vitamin D. Vitamin D, however, is responsible for only a small component of Ca absorption in premature infants.[186]

The time to supply sufficient Ca and P stores for premature infants is during the initial hospitalization, before their discharge and the beginning of exclusive breastfeeding. However, because of prolonged parenteral nutrition and the inability to provide "catch-up" quantities of Ca and P in milks, some infants may benefit from additional Ca and P after hospital discharge.

Magnesium

Approximately 60% of body magnesium is in bone. Preterm human milk contains approximately 30 mg/L of magnesium.[175] The absorption of Mg is significantly greater in unfortified human milk (73%) compared with formula (48%).[185] Net Mg retention in human milk–fed premature infants meets intrauterine estimates. Thus, the data from balance studies and biochemical monitoring suggest that Mg supplements are not needed for premature infants fed human milk.[187] Similar studies in premature infants fed preterm formulas indicate that, despite lower absorption compared with human milk, intrauterine estimates for Mg accretion are surpassed.

TRACE ELEMENTS

Zinc

Several factors affect the zinc needs for the enterally fed premature infant. Fetal accretion of zinc is approximately 0.85 mg/kg/d.[4] Growth is a major determinant of zinc needs. The major excretory route is via the gastrointestinal tract. Infants with large gastrointestinal fluid losses may become zinc deficient. Premature infants receiving pooled pasteurized human milk (Zn intake approximately 0.7 mg/kg/d) are in negative zinc balance for 60 days postnatally and never meet the intrauterine accretion rate.[188] In contrast, intakes of 1.8 to 2 mg/kg/d are associated with net retention of Zn that surpasses intrauterine accretion rates.[189–191] The classical signs of zinc deficiency include an erythematous skin rash involving perioral, perineal, and facial areas, as well as the extremities.[150] Although there are limitations to the assay, plasma zinc values <50 μg/dL are highly suggestive of deficiency.[150] A very low serum alkaline phosphatase activity, a zinc-dependent enzyme, also is suggestive of deficiency. Symptomatic Zn deficiency in unsupplemented human milk–fed premature infants occurs as lactation advances.[192,193]

Copper

There are no universally accepted methods to assess copper status clinically. Balance study data only provide an estimate of copper retention at one point in time. Premature infants receiving pooled pasteurized human milk (copper intakes approximately 85 μg/kg/d) are in negative Cu balance for 30 days postnatally and never meet the intrauterine accretion rate.[188] Fortified human milk provides a Cu intake of as much as 180 μg/kg/d and balance study data surpass intrauterine accretion rates.[191] Copper retention is quite variable from formula providing intakes of 200 to 300 μg/kg/d.[189,191] Symptoms of copper deficiency include osteopenia, neutropenia, and hypochromic anemia. As copper is excreted in bile, cases of severe cholestasis warrant limiting copper intakes.

Iron

The iron needs of the premature infant are determined by birth weight, initial hemoglobin, rate of growth, and magnitude of iron loss and/or transfused blood.[150] There are three phases of postnatal iron metabolism. In the first phase, there is decreased erythropoiesis. The hemoglobin concentration declines to a nadir, "physiologic anemia of prematurity," which is at approximately 2 to 3 months postnatal age. In the second phase, the hemoglobin rises as active red cell production is occurring. This phase needs iron. The third phase is an exhaustion of iron stores, or "late anemia of prematurity," observed if iron supplementation is inadequate.[150]

The concentration of iron in human milk declines through lactation, from approximately 0.6 mg/L at 2 weeks to 0.3 mg/L after 5 months of lactation.[194] The absorption of Fe is affected adversely by blood transfusion.[195] Premature infants fed human milk are in negative Fe balance which, if not transfused, corrects with Fe supplements.[195] Iron absorption also appears to be facilitated by a modest degree of anemia.[196] Thus, the usual recommendations for premature infants suggest delaying Fe supplementation until 2 to 3 months postnatal age, a time when hemoglobin concentrations are at a nadir.[197] However, the provision of small doses of Fe at 2 mg/kg/d beginning 2 weeks postnatally has been demonstrated, in the absence of blood transfusions, to prevent the development of Fe deficiency at 3 months postnatal age.[197] When recombinant erythropoietin for the treatment of anemia of prematurity is used, higher doses of Fe are needed, in the range of 6 mg/kg/d, to support the more rapid rate of erythropoiesis.[198] Generally, ferrous sulfate (25 mg/mL, 2 mg/kg/d) drops are used in human milk–fed premature infants beginning soon after the achievement of complete enteral feedings. Formula-fed premature infants should receive iron-fortified formula from the onset of milk feeding.

Sodium and Potassium

Premature infants generally need more sodium per unit body weight than term infants.[150] This is due to immature renal Na conservation mechanisms. Sodium wasting is inversely related to gestational age. A comparison of Na intakes of 2.9 and 1.6 mEq (mmol)/kg/d in premature infants suggested that the former intake provided more appropriate serum sodium concentrations.[199] Hyponatremia also may occur in premature infants primarily fed human milk because the sodium content of preterm milk continues to decline through lactation.[199] The need for these electrolytes may increase during or after diuretic usage.

Vitamins

The fat-soluble vitamins, A, D, E, and K, are stored in the body and large doses may result in toxicity. Water-soluble vitamins, thiamin, riboflavin, niacin, vitamin B_6, folate, vitamin B_{12}, pantothenic acid, biotin, and vitamin C, are not stored in the body and excess intakes are excreted in the urine or bile (vitamin B_{12}). The intake of water-soluble vitamins, therefore, should be at frequent intervals to avoid deficiency states. Vitamin A and riboflavin concentrations decline in human milk under conditions of light exposure and after passage through feeding tubes.[98] As a consequence of exposure to air, ascorbic acid concentrations are lower in pooled human milk.[200] Supplementary vitamins are provided in human milk fortifiers and in preterm formulas. There is no indication for additional multivitamin supplements for infants receiving adequate intakes of fortified human milk, preterm formula, or enriched formula. Once the premature infant transitions to unfortified human milk or standard formula, a multivitamin supplement should be added. The supplemental vitamins should be continued until the infant is consuming 300 kcal/d or weighs more than 2.5 kg.[201]

HUMAN MILK

The American Academy of Pediatrics acknowledges that human milk also is beneficial in the management of premature infants. The beneficial effects generally relate to improvements in host defenses, digestion and absorption of nutrients, gastrointestinal function, neurodevelopment, and maternal psychological well-being. However, the special needs of the premature infant that arise as a result of metabolic and gastrointestinal immaturity, immunologic compromise, and associated medical conditions, must be considered so that adequate nutrition can be provided to meet the needs for intrauterine rates of growth and nutrient accretion. Human milk is capable of satisfying most of the needs of premature infants if careful attention is given to nutritional status.

Benefits of Human Milk

The use of human milk in NICUs is a result of the profound effects of human milk on host defense and neurodevelopmental outcome. Clinical studies in nurseries throughout the world have suggested a decrease in the rate of a variety of infections, including sepsis, necrotizing enterocolitis, and urinary tract infection, in premature infants fed human milk compared with the feeding of formula.[191,202–205]

Necrotizing enterocolitis, the devastating acute intestinal inflammatory disease in premature infants, appears less frequently when the prior diet is human milk compared with formula. A large, nonrandomized study of hospitalized premature infants reported that the incidence of necrotizing enterocolitis was significantly lower in infants fed human milk, either exclusively or partially, compared with infants fed formula.[206] That study reported clinical cases as well as cases confirmed at surgery or autopsy. When compared with exclusive human milk feeding (mother's own milk or donor human milk), the receipt of only formula was associated with a 6.5-fold increase (95% confidence interval 1.9–22, $p < .001$) in confirmed cases of NEC. A significant 3-fold increase in NEC also was seen when a diet of exclusive formula feeding was compared with formula used as a supplement to human milk (confidence interval for confirmed cases 1.4–6.5, $p < .005$). Late-onset sepsis and/or NEC were of greater incidence in infants receiving preterm formula, but if infants received a combination of mother's milk and preterm formula they had the highest risk of sepsis and/or NEC.[191] The latter study identified a dose of human milk, > 50 mL/kg/d, that potentially might be protective. This dose of mother's milk also was shown to protect against late-onset sepsis in a 4-week study of premature infants when compared with average daily doses of 1 to 24 and 25 to 49 mL/kg.[207] These data provide some encouragement for the potential prevention of necrotizing enterocolitis.

Specific factors such as sIgA, lactoferrin, lysozyme, oligosaccharides, cytokines (such as IL-10), enzymes (such as acetylhydrolase), growth factors (such as epidermal growth factor), and cellular components may affect the host defense of the premature infant. One of the major protective effects of human milk on the recipient infant operates through the enteromammary immune system. It is reasonable to expect that exposure of the mother to the environment of the neonatal nursery through skin-to-skin contact with her premature infant may be advantageous to the infant. In this manner, mothers potentially might be "induced" to make specific antibodies against the nosocomial pathogens in the nursery environment.

The NICU diet may affect long-term neurodevelopmental outcomes in premature infants. An 8-year follow-up of 300 premature infants (approximately 1.4 kg and 31 weeks' gestation at birth) observed that when factors affecting intelligence quotient (social class, maternal education, infant gender, and duration of mechanical ventilation) were considered in a regression model, the receipt of breast milk in the NICU was associated with an eight-point advantage, slightly more than one standard deviation of the mean.[208] A cohort of adolescents were followed since their NICU stay as premature infants and significant cognitive and psychomotor benefits were ascribed to the feeding of human milk.[209–211] A large multicenter follow-up study of more than 1,000 extremely LBW infants who had extensive nutritional data collected during their hospitalization was conducted to determine the relationship between human milk intake in-hospital and neurodevelopmental outcome at 18 to 22 months of age[212]. Neonatal birth weight, gestational age, intraventricular hemorrhage status, sepsis, bronchopulmonary dysplasia, and hospital stay were similar between those never receiving (25% of cohort) and those who received human milk (75% of cohort) during their hospitalization. There were differences in socioeconomic variables, race and ethnicity, educational attainment, and parity between groups. When adjusted for these variables as well as biological confounders, there were significantly positive effects for human milk intake on mental and motor development. The magnitude of the effect was greatest in the highest quintile (>80%), which averaged 110 mL/kg/d. The impact of feeding 100 mL/kg/d of human milk was an increase in Bayley Mental Development Index (MDI) of 5 points (1/3 of an SD), an increase in Psychomotor Development Index of 6 points, and a decrease in rehospitalization rate by 6%.[212] Others have reported that even the 5-point difference on the MDI would have a significantly meaningful effect on the outcome of ELBW infants.[213]

Limitations in the Use of Unfortified Human Milk

A major impediment in advocating human milk for premature infants is the difficulty many mothers experience in providing sufficient quantities of milk. Several explanations have been given for the low milk production, including biological immaturity of the mammary gland, maternal stress and/or illness, and difficulty maintaining a supply without a suckling infant. Another reason of concern is that nutrient intake is limited by milk volume restrictions imposed on premature infants because they cannot feed ad libitum and also because their medical condition warrants fluid restriction.

The most compelling reason for concern is that nutrient intake is inadequate to meet the very great needs of the premature infant. Unfortified human milk may not supply sufficient quantities of nutrients for several reasons. Because of differences in the methods of milk expression and storage, the feeding of "spot" samples (individual samples of expressed milk from one or both breasts or milk partially expressed from one breast), the use of feeding tubes, and the differences in length of lactation, there is a large variation in the macronutrient composition of human milk used in feeding premature infants. Much of the variation in energy content, for example, is a result of differences in fat content of the unfortified milk (2.2–4.7 g/dL).

There also are significant declines in the contents of protein and sodium through lactation.[214] The content of other nutrients (calcium, phosphorus) is too low the meet the great needs of the premature infant. In addition, technical reasons associated with the collection, storage, and delivery of milk to the infant also result in a decreased quantity of available nutrients (fat, vitamin C, vitamin A, riboflavin). Thus, the exclusive feeding of unfortified human milk in very LBW infants, generally infants with birth weights less than 1500 g, has been associated with poorer rates of growth and nutritional deficits, during and beyond the period of hospitalization.[152,174,178,215,216]

Human Milk Fortification

Growth and nutrient deficits in the premature infant can be corrected with the addition to human milk of multinutrient nutrient supplements, or fortifiers.[153,183,217,218] Mineral supplementation normalizes biochemical indices, improves linear growth, and increases bone mineralization during and beyond the neonatal period.[184,219,220] Protein and energy supplementation are associated with improved rates of weight gain and indices of protein nutritional status: blood urea nitrogen, serum albumin, transthyretin.[152,153]

Current practice suggests the use of multinutrient fortification of human milk. Nutritional outcomes of feeding fortified human milk in the United States indicate that premature infants receive less volume, but greater intakes, of protein and minerals, and experience greater gain in weight and increment in linear growth than infants fed unfortified human milk exclusively.[187,191,218,221] Balance study data indicate that the use of fortified human milk results in net nutrient retention that approaches or is greater than expected intrauterine rates of accretion. Fat absorption, however, with the use of some fortifiers has been lower than expected.[184,222] Fat absorption potentially may be augmented by newer human milk fortifiers that contain fat.[223,224]

Questions have been raised as to whether the addition of bovine-derived human milk fortifiers affects feeding tolerance in premature infants. Gastric residual volumes often are used to assess feeding tolerance. When compared throughout hospitalization, the use of fortified human milk was not associated with feeding intolerance, as manifest by abdominal distention, vomiting, changes in stool frequency, or volume of gastric aspirate when compared with control-supplemented human milk.[221] Comparisons with preterm formula also have been made and no major differences in feeding tolerance has been attributed to human milk fortification.[191,225]

A major concern with human milk fortification is that the added nutrients may affect the complex system of host defense. The effects of nutrient fortification on some of the general host defense properties of the milk have been evaluated.[226] Fortification did not affect the concentration of IgA. Bacterial colony counts do not increase with 24 hours of refrigerator storage of fortified human milk. Despite extensive nutrient fortification of human milk, LBW infants have reduced rates of infection while fed fortified human milk.[191,204,221,227]

Comparison of Human Milk Fortifiers

Human milk fortifiers are designed to be mixed with human milk. A variety of fortifiers is available globally, but few head-to-head comparisons have been published. Most fortifiers are powdered nutrient preparations that contain protein, carbohydrate, calcium, phosphorus, magnesium, and sodium; the contents of zinc, copper, and vitamins are variable (Table 17). Inherent in the design is the adequacy of mothers' milk production to meet the needs of the infant. The use of pasteurized donor human milk has not been advocated routinely because of concerns with contamination, lack of sufficient supply, and cost. One study in extremely LBW infants did not find any benefit to receipt of pasteurized donor milk compared with preterm formula.[228]

One study examined the nutrient adequacy of a liquid human milk fortifier mixing a preterm formula 1:1 with human milk.[229] Nitrogen, energy, calcium, and phosphorus retentions were below intrauterine rates of accretion. More beneficial outcomes may be observed if preterm formula is alternately fed with fortified mother's milk.

FEEDING TOLERANCE

The ability to tolerate enteral feedings is a major problem for premature infants. Moreover, the infants' tolerance of enteral feeding is a primary concern of neonatologists because it affects their decision to initiate, advance, and discontinue feedings. Because of these concerns, feeding intolerance may be a major factor affecting the duration of hospitalization. The fetus experiences swallowing of amniotic fluid from early gestation, but, postnatally, many premature neonates do not appear to share as "simple" a tolerance for enteral fluid, even dilute fluid mixtures. Several factors affect how feedings are tolerated: immature intestinal motility and digestive enzymes, too rapid or large volume of feeding, and infant medical complications.

Despite its importance, there are no universally agreed upon criteria to judge feeding tolerance in premature infants. Clinical criteria of feeding tolerance (Table 19) generally include physical examination findings of abdominal distention and abdominal tenderness, presence or absence and quality of bowel sounds, and signs of residual gastric fluid aspirated from the feeding tube just prior to the next feeding, emesis, and changes in stool output.[230] There are associated signs that occasionally suggest intolerance to a feeding. These associated signs include increased episodes of apnea and bradycardia, diminished oxygen saturation (desaturation events), and lethargy.

The gastric residual volume, usually measured prior to the next feeding, is an indication of milk remaining in the stomach several hours after a feeding.[231] The gastric residual volume indicates the rapidity of gastric emptying and appears to be a final common pathway, such that changes in the clinical examination may result in decreases in gastric emptying. The nonspecific nature of this assessment is that changes in the clinical examination may or may not be related to intestinal pathology. Gastric residual volume has been quantitated on the basis of body weight (eg, an abnormal sign being >2 mL/kg per feeding), or on the volume of feeding (eg, >50% of 3 hours of feeding).[130] Some premature infants have measurable gastric residual volumes before every feeding, while others never have any measurable volume. In the latter infants, therefore, any small change might indicate a change in the feeding tolerance. Furthermore, it would be expected that gastric residual volume would be difficult to interpret in infants receiving continuous gastric milk infusions. Such is not always true, as these infants generally empty their stomachs rapidly and should still be evaluated every 2 to 4 hours in a similar manner as infants fed by the intermittent bolus technique.[130]

Table 19 Selected Indices to Assess Feeding Tolerance in LBW Infants

Abdominal distention
With visible bowel loops
Without visible bowel loops
Abdominal tenderness
Emesis
Gastric residual volume
>2 mL/kg
>50% of 3 h of feeding
Any change from previous pattern
Gastric residual characteristics
Green, bilious
Red, blood-tinged
Stool output
Increase frequency
Decreased frequency
Feeding withheld
Document reasons feedings withheld
Assess number of feedings held
Clinical condition
Any worsening in previous medical condition

The quality of the gastric residual also has been discussed as a tool to determine feeding tolerance. Gastric residuals that are green, or bilious, could indicate intestinal obstruction, but more often indicate overdistention of the stomach and retrograde reflux of bile into the stomach. A blood-tinged residual could indicate an inflammatory process, but may indicate residual swallowed blood from delivery or postnatal manipulations or slight mucosal irritation from the indwelling gastric tube.

Unfortunately, the aforementioned criteria have little prognostic significance. Infants having more gastric residuals and emesis episodes were just as likely to reach the milestone of full enteral tube-feeding than infants not having any increases in these measurements.[225]

Most clinicians use the pattern of the above criteria, as opposed to a single measurement, as an aid to determine feeding status. Several instances will occur where infants' feedings are held because of one or more of the above signs. Often a single feeding is discarded. Careful assessment and examination prior to the next feeding generally aid the decision to continue feedings. If one feeding is held, further enteral feeding can be considered if the physical examination permits. Too often feedings are held for prolonged periods of time, which can extend dependence on parenteral nutrition and length of stay.

The evaluation of the infant with a large gastric residual, for example, would include the following considerations. Has the medical condition worsened, such that gastric emptying is delayed due to systemic disease? Is the infant's feeding tube in the correct location? If the feeding tube is high in the esophagus or of too small a caliber, then swallowed air may not be evacuated. Large amounts of swallowed air may cause gastric overdistention and displace milk, resulting in emesis and/or large residuals. Body positioning also may play a role. Gastric emptying in some infants is improved by their being in the prone position or in the right lateral decubitus position as compared with the supine position. At times, intolerance is corrected by lowering milk intake somewhat.

FEEDING METHODS

Tube feeding is an essential tool in enteral nutrition because the premature infant may be unable to suck and/or coordinate suck-swallow-breathe. There are a variety of methods for tube feeding, continuous or intermittent bolus, and a number of approaches, orogastric, nasogastric, transpyloric, or gastrostomy. The selection of practice relates to the duration of the proposed therapy: premature infants eventually will suckle, so a temporary oro(naso)gastric tube is used; infants with major congenital anomalies may require a semipermanent gastrostomy.

The bolus feeding method mimics the normal adult feed-fast routine and has greater hormonal responses than continuous infusions.[232] The bolus technique does not require an infusion pump. Differences between continuous and intermittent bolus methods have been evaluated. Premature infants had more feeding intolerance and a slower rate of weight gain with continuous infusion compared with the bolus technique.[130] Intermittent bolus tube feeding results in shorter time to full feeding.[233] Neither method enhanced nutrient absorption.

Occasionally, intolerance is observed in the bolus-fed premature infant. In some instances, duodenal motility decreases following the bolus feeding.[234] A bolus feeding given over a longer time interval, such as 30 minutes to 120 minutes, results in a return of motility and improved tolerance. The continuous infusion technique has been associated with increased nutrient absorption in infants with gastrointestinal disease.[235] It seems prudent to use this method in infants who have had intestinal surgery. In some infants with persistent gastric residuals or emesis in absence of obvious intestinal pathology, the use of transpyloric feeding has been successful, although no beneficial contemporary studies have been published.[236] Owing to limited compliance of the small intestine, continuous feedings are indicated for infants receiving milk via a transpyloric tube.

FEEDING ISSUES

Enteral feeding and concomitant use of an umbilical arterial catheter has been a subject of much concern. However, most infants had an indwelling umbilical arterial catheter in the recent studies of gastrointestinal priming and no untoward events were reported.[126,130] Infants were no more likely to develop intolerance or necrotizing enterocolitis if they received enteral feedings while they had an umbilical arterial catheter in place than if they received enteral feeding 24 hours after the catheter was removed.[135] Moreover, fewer evaluations for sepsis and less usage of central venous catheters were observed in the group receiving feeding while the catheter was in place. Thus, there appears to be no increased risk of enteral feeding while an umbilical arterial catheter is in place, as long as the catheter is functioning optimally.

The use of diluted milks has been suggested for feeding premature infants. In one study, however, intestinal motility responses to feeding were initiated earlier and persisted longer following the use of full-strength formula compared with one-third and two-third dilutions of the formula.[237] The use of water for enteral feeding also has been shown not to affect intestinal motility as compared with milk.[238] Thus, initiating feedings with full-strength milk appears to be tolerated and appropriate.

The advancement of daily feeding volumes also has been investigated, especially with respect to the development of necrotizing enterocolitis. When compared with matched case–controls, infants with NEC were more likely to have received enteral nutrition with daily intakes >20 mL/kg, averaging 46 mL/kg.[239] One study compared the morbidity of LBW infants whose daily increments in feeding volume was 15 or 35 mL/kg/d.[240] The infants whose feedings were advanced rapidly had a shorter duration of time to achieve full tube feeding and regain birth weight, and no difference in morbidity, than infants whose feedings were advanced slowly.

NUTRITIONAL ASSESSMENT

Neonatal nutritional assessment requires both knowledge of nutritional biochemistry and neonatal medical conditions. A nutrition protocol for the NICU is important to provide staff and clinicians with evidence-based policies. Implementation of such protocols has been found to reduce morbidity in the NICU.[241] The neonatal dietitian is a key person to provide input, on a daily basis, that is compatible with the medical condition of the infant.[242]

The nutritional status of the premature infant is monitored by daily assessments of fluid and energy intake and serial evaluations of the rate of growth in weight, length, and head circumference (Table 20). Growth parameters are plotted on graph paper or a specific chart for current premature infants' growth. See Appendix I: Nutritional Assessment for growth charts of premature infants. The charts are helpful, but equally important is the computation of the weekly rate of growth (Table 21).[243] Once the infant reaches 2.5 kg, a daily weight gain of 20 to 30 g/d is appropriate.

Table 20 Nutritional Assessment of the Enterally Fed LBW Infant

Fluid intake (mL/kg/d)	Daily
Parenteral intake	
Enteral intake	
Nutrient intake (unit/kg/d)	Daily
Energy intake (kcal)	
Protein intake (g)	
Specific nutrient (unit)	
Anthropometry	
Body weight (g)	Same time each day
Length (cm)	Weekly
Head circumference (cm)	Weekly
Biochemical monitoring	
Hemoglobin, hematocrit	Weekly
Reticulocyte count	Weekly
Serum electrolytes	Weekly ×2, then q 2 wk*
Calcium, phosphorus	Weekly ×2, then q 2 wk
Alkaline phosphatase	Weekly ×2, then q 2 wk
BUN	Weekly ×2, then q 2 wk†

*If infant receiving human milk or diuretics.
†Add albumin and/or prealbumin if abnormal.

The nutritional status of the premature infant also is monitored by serial evaluations of biochemical indices. These assessments include serum Ca, P, and alkaline phosphatase activity to assess bone mineral status, and albumin and urea nitrogen to assess protein status. If more specific indices of protein status are needed, as in the case where additional protein supplementation is used, the serum prealbumin (transthyretin) is measured before and 1 week after the supplementation. Serum sodium, chloride, and bicarbonate are evaluated in infants receiving diuretics, those whose intakes are limited, or those with slow growth. The hemoglobin and reticulocyte count are monitored to assess anemia. Specific determinations of plasma zinc and copper are not routinely useful, but zinc may be measured in infants with unusual losses, such as after gastrointestinal surgery and from enterostomies. The pattern of changes in biochemical indices may be more reflective of nutritional status than isolated values. Occasionally, renal ultrasound to determine the presence of nephrocalcinosis and wrist X-ray to identify rickets are warranted.

Table 21 Growth Guidelines for LBW Infants In-Hospital

Weight gain	>15 g/kg/d for infants <2.0 kg >20 g/d for infants >2.0 kg
Length gain	0.7–1.0 cm/wk
Head circumference gain	0.7–1.0 cm/wk

SUMMARY OF NUTRITIONAL SUPPORT

A comprehensive nutrition pathway for LBW infants has been described. The approach is multifaceted, beginning with intravenous total parenteral nutrition, transitioning via trophic feeding to enteral nutrition, and continuing to full enteral feeding and hospital discharge. This approach does not increase the risks already associated with LBW infants. Indeed, the use of an aggressive approach to nutritional support has resulted in improved growth, with fewer infants falling below the 10th percentile in standard growth charts.[50,244] While improvements are found in growth, no increase in sepsis or necrotizing enterocolitis are associated with the more aggressive approach to nutritional support.[244]

REFERENCES

1. Hay WW, Jr, Lucas A, Heird WC, et al. Workshop summary: Nutrition of the extremely low birth weight infant. Pediatrics 1999;104:1360–8.
2. Embleton NE, Pang N, Cooke RJ. Postnatal malnutrition and growth retardation: An inevitable consequence of current recommendations in preterm infants? Pediatrics 2004;107:270–3.
3. Cazacu A, Fraley JK, Schanler RJ. We are inadequately nourishing healthy low birth weight infants. Pediatr Res 2001;49:343A.
4. Widdowson EM. Importance of nutrition in development, with special reference to feeding low-birth-weight infants. In: Sauls HS, Bachhuber WL, Lewis LA, editors. Meeting Nutritional Goals for Low-Birth-Weight Infants. Columbus: Ross Laboratories; 1982. p. 4–11.
5. Ziegler EE, O'Donnell AM, Nelson SE, Fomon SJ. Body composition of the reference fetus. Growth 1976;40:329–41.
6. Ellis KJ, Shypailo RJ, Schanler RJ, Langston C. Body elemental composition of the neonate: New reference data. Am J Hum Biol 1993;5:323–30.
7. Ziegler EE, Biga RL, Fomon SJ. Nutritional requirements of the premature infant. In: Suskind RM, editor. Textbook of Pediatric Nutrition. New York: Raven; 1981. p. 29–39.
8. Klein CJ. Nutrient requirements for preterm infant formulas. J Nutr 2002;132:1395S–577.
9. Sinclair JC. Metabolic rate and body size of the newborn. Clin Obstet Gynecol 1971;14:840–54.
10. Sinclair JC. Energy balance of the newborn. In: Sinclair JC, editor. Temperature Regulation and Energy Metabolism in the Newborn. New York: Grune & Stratton; 1978. p. 187–204.
11. Weinstein MR, Oh W. Oxygen consumption in infants with bronchopulmonary dysplasia. J Pediatr 1981;99:958–93.
12. Yunis KA, Oh W. Effects of intravenous glucose loading on oxygen consumption, carbon dioxide production, and resting energy expenditure in infants with bronchopulmonary dysplasia. J Pediatr 1989;115:127–32.
13. Bresson JL, Bader B, Rocchiccioli F, et al. Protein-metabolism kinetics and energy-substrate utilization in infants fed parenteral solutions with different glucose-fat ratios. Am J Clin Nutr 1991;54:370–6.
14. Piedboeuf B, Chessex P, Hazan J, et al. Total parenteral nutrition in the newborn infant: Energy substrates and respiratory gas exchange. J Pediatr 1991;118:97–102.
15. Salas-Salvadó J, Molina J, Figueras J, et al. Effect of the quality of infused energy on substrate utilization in the newborn receiving total parenteral nutrition. Pediatr Res 1993;33:112–7.
16. Hays SP, Smith EO, Sunehag AL. Hyperglycemia is a risk factor for early death and morbidity in extremely low birth-weight infants. Pediatrics 2006;118:1811–8.
17. Collins JW, Jr, Hoppe M, Brown K, et al. A controlled trial of insulin infusion and parenteral nutrition in extremely low birth weight infants with glucose intolerance. J Pediatr 1991;118:921–7.
18. Poindexter BB, Karn CA, Denne SC. Exogenous insulin reduces proteolysis and protein synthesis in extremely low birth weight infants. J Pediatr 1998;132:948–53.
19. Sunehag AL, Haymond MW, Schanler RJ, et al. Gluconeogenesis in very low birth weight infants receiving total parenteral nutrition. Diabetes 1999;48:791–800.

20. Mitton SG. Amino acids and lipid in total parenteral nutrition for the newborn. J Pediatr Gastroenterol Nutr 1994;18:25–31.
21. Roberts SA, Ball RO, Filler RM, et al. Phenylalanine and tyrosine metabolism in neonates receiving parenteral nutrition differing in pattern of amino acids. Pediatr Res 1998;44:907–14.
22. van Goudoever JB, Sulkers EJ, Timmerman M, et al. Amino acid solutions for premature neonates during the first week of life: The role of *N*-Acetyl-L-Cysteine and *N*-Acetyl-L-Tyrosine. J Parenter Enteral Nutr 1994;18:404–8.
23. Zelikovic I, Chesney RW, Friedman AL, Ahlfors CE. Taurine depletion in very low birth weight infants receiving prolonged total parenteral nutrition: Role of renal immaturity. J Pediatr 1990;116:301–6.
24. van Goudoever JB, Collen T, Wattimena JDL, et al. Immediate commencement of amino acid supplementation in preterm infants: Effect on serum amino acid concentrations and protein kinetics on the first day of life. J Pediatr 1995;127:458–65.
25. Heird WC, Dell RB, Helms RA, et al. Amino acid mixture designed to maintain normal plasma amino acid patterns in infants and children requiring parenteral nutrition. Pediatrics 1987;80:401–8.
26. Zlotkin SH, Bryan MH, Anderson GH. Intravenous nitrogen and energy intakes required to duplicate in utero nitrogen accretion in prematurely born human infants. J Pediatr 1981;99:115–20.
27. Malloy MH, Rassin DK, Richardson CJ. Total parenteral nutrition in sick preterm infants: Effects of cysteine supplementation with nitrogen intakes of 240 and 400 mg/kg/day. J Pediatr Gastroenterol Nutr 1984;3:239–44.
28. Malloy MH, Rassin DK, Richardson CJ. Cyst(e)ine measurements during total parenteral nutrition. Am J Clin Nutr 1983;37:188–91.
29. Zlotkin SH, Bryan MH, Anderson GH. Cysteine supplementation to cysteine-free intravenous feeding regimens in newborn infants. Am J Clin Nutr 1981;34:914–23.
30. Rivera A, Bell EF, Bier DM. Effect of intravenous amino acids on protein metabolism of preterm infants during the first three days of life. Pediatr Res 1993;33:106–11.
31. Viña J, Vento M, García-Sala F, et al. L-Cysteine and glutathione metabolism are impaired in premature infants due to cystathionase deficiency. Am J Clin Nutr 1995;61:1067–9.
32. Dunham B, Marcuard S, Khazanie PG, et al. The solubility of calcium and phosphorus in neonatal total parenteral nutrition solutions. J Parenter Enteral Nutr 1991;15:608–11.
33. Schanler RJ, Shulman RJ, Prestridge LL. Parenteral nutrient needs of very low birth weight infants. J Pediatr 1994;125:961–8.
34. Laine L, Shulman RJ, Pitre D, et al. Cysteine usage increases the need for acetate in neonates who receive total parenteral nutrition. Am J Clin Nutr 1991;54:565–7.
35. Denno R, Rounds JD, Faris R, et al. Glutamine-enriched total parenteral nutrition enhances plasma glutathione in the resting state. J Surg Res 1996;61:35–8.
36. Lacey JM, Crouch JB, Benfell K, et al. The effects of glutamine-supplemented parenteral nutrition in premature infants. J Parenter Enteral Nutr 1996;20:74–80.
37. Poindexter BB, Ehrenkranz RA, Stoll BJ, et al. Parenteral glutamine supplementation does not reduce the risk of mortality or late-onset sepsis in extremely low birth weight infants. Pediatrics 2004;113:1209–15.
38. Pierro A, Carnielli V, Filler RM, et al. Characteristics of protein sparing effect of total parenteral nutrition in the surgical infant. J Pediatr Surg 1988;23:538–42.
39. Helms RA, Christensen ML, Mauer EC, Storm MC. Comparison of a pediatric versus standard amino acid formulation in preterm neonates requiring parenteral nutrition. J Pediatr 1987;110:466–70.
40. Chessex P, Zebiche H, Pineault M, et al. Effect of amino acid composition of parenteral solutions on nitrogen retention and metabolic response in low birth weight infants. J Pediatr 1985;106:111–7.
41. Heird WC, Hay W, Helms RA, et al. Pediatric parenteral amino acid mixture in low birth weight infants. Pediatrics 1988;81:41–50.
42. Porcelli PJ, Sisk PM. Increased parenteral amino acid administration to extremely low-birth-weight infants during early postnatal life. J Pediatr Gastroenterol Nutr 2002;34:174–9.
43. van Lingen RA, van Goudoever JB, Luijendijk IH, Wattimena JLD. Effects of early amino acid administration during total parenteral nutrition on protein metabolism in pre-term infants. Clin Sci 1992;82:199–203.
44. Anderson TL, Muttart CR, Bieber MA, et al. A controlled trial of glucose versus glucose and amino acids in premature infants. J Pediatr 1979;94:947–51.
45. Rivera A, Bell EF, Stegink LD, Ziegler EE. Plasma amino acid profiles during the first three days of life in infants with respiratory distress syndrome: Effect of parenteral amino acid supplementation. J Pediatr 1989;115:465–8.
46. Van Den Akker CHP, Te Braake FWJ, Wattimena JDL, et al. Effects of early amino acid administration on leucine and glucose kinetics in premature infants. Pediatr Res 2006;59:732–5.
47. Thureen PJ, Melara D, Fennessey PV, Hay WW, Jr. Effect of low versus high intravenous amino acid intake on very low birth weight infants in the early neonatal period. Pediatr Res 2003;53:24–32.
48. Te Braake FWJ, Van Den Akker CHP, Wattimena JDL, van Goudoever JB. Amino acid administration to premature infants directly after birth. J Pediatr 2005;147:457–61.
49. Poindexter BB. Early amino acid administration for premature infants. J Pediatr 2005;147:420–1.
50. Poindexter BB, Langer JC, Dusick AM, Ehrenkranz RA. Early provision of parenteral amino acids in extremely low birth weight infants: Relation to growth and neurodevelopmental outcome. J Pediatr 2006;148:300–5.
51. Friedman Z, Danon A, Stahlman MT, Oates JA. Rapid onset of essential fatty acid deficiency in the newborn. Pediatrics 1976;58:640–54.
52. Gutcher GR, Farrell PM. Intravenous infusion of lipid for the prevention of essential fatty acid deficiency in premature infants. Am J Clin Nutr 1991;54:1024–8.
53. Gilbertson N, Kovar IZ, Cox DJ, et al. Introduction of intravenous lipid administration on the first day of life in the very low birth weight neonate. J Pediatr 1991;119:615–23.
54. Sosenko IRS, Innis SM, Frank L. Intralipid increases lung polyunsaturated fatty acids and protects newborn rats from oxygen toxicity. Pediatr Res 1991;30:413–7.
55. Simmer K, Rao SC. Early introduction of lipids to parenterally-fed preterm infants. Cochrane Database Syst Rev 2005.
56. Haumont D, Deckelbaum RJ, Richelle M, et al. Plasma lipid and plasma lipoprotein concentrations in low birth weight infants given parenteral nutrition with twenty or ten percent lipid emulsion. J Pediatr 1989;115:787–93.
57. Haumont D, Richelle M, Deckelbaum RJ, et al. Effect of liposomal content of lipid emulsions on plasma lipid concentrations in low birth weight infants receiving parenteral nutrition. J Pediatr 1992;121:759–763X.
58. Kao LC, Cheng MH, Warburton D. Triglycerides, free fatty acids, free fatty acids/albumin molar ratio, and cholesterol levels in serum of neonates receiving long-term lipid infusions: Controlled trial of continuous and intermittent regimens. J Pediatr 1984;104:429–35.
59. Brans YW, Dutton EB, Andrew DS, et al. Fat emulsion tolerance in very low birth weight neonates: Effect on diffusion of oxygen in the lungs and on blood pH. Pediatrics 1986;78:79–84.
60. Spear ML, Stahl GE, Hamosh M, et al. Effect of heparin dose and infusion rate on lipid clearance and bilirubin binding in premature infants receiving intravenous fat emulsions. J Pediatr 1988;112:94–8.
61. Greene HL, Hazlett D, Demaree R. Relationship between intralipid-induced hyperlipemia and pulmonary function. Am J Clin Nutr 1976;29:127–35.
62. Pereira GR, Fox WW, Stanley CA, et al. Decreased oxygenation and hyperlipemia during intravenous fat infusions in premature infants. Pediatrics 1980;66:26–30.
63. Hammerman C, Aramburo MJ. Decreased lipid intake reduces morbidity in sick premature neonates. J Pediatr 1988;113:1083–8.
64. Pitkanen O, Hallman M, Andersson S. Generation of free radicals in lipid emulsion used in parenteral nutrition. Pediatr Res 1991;29:56–9.
65. Sosenko IRS, Rodriguez-Pierce M, Bancalari E. Effect of early initiation of intravenous lipid administration on the incidence and severity of chronic lung disease in premature infants. J Pediatr 1993;123:975–82.
66. Helbock HJ, Motchnik PA, Ames BN. Toxic hydroperoxides in intravenous lipid emulsions used in preterm infants. Pediatrics 1993;91:83–7.
67. Inder TE, Graham P, Sanderson K, Taylor BJ. Lipid peroxidation as a measure of oxygen free radical damage in the very low birth weight infant. Arch Dis Child 1994;70:F107–11.
68. Park W, Paust H, Schroder H. Lipid infusion in premature infants suffering from sepsis. J Parenter Enteral Nutr 1984;8:290–2.
69. Gura KM, Duggan CP, Collier SB, et al. Reversal of parenteral nutrition-associated liver disease in two infants with short bowel syndrome using parenteral fish oil: Implications for future management. Pediatrics 2006;118:197–201.
70. Schmidt-Sommerfeld E, Penn D, Wolf H. Carnitine deficiency in premature infants receiving total parenteral nutrition: Effect of L-carnitine supplementation. J Pediatr 1983;102:931–5.
71. Bonner CM, DeBrie KL, Hug G, et al. Effects of parenteral L-carnitine supplementation on fat metabolism and nutrition in premature neonates. J Pediatr 1995;126:287–92.
72. Pande S, Brion LP, Campbell DE, et al. Lack of effect of L-carnitine supplementation on weight gain in very preterm infants. J Perinatal 2005;25:470–7.
73. Kumar M, Kabra NS, Paes B. Role of carnitine supplementation in apnea of prematurity: A systematic review. J Perinatol 2004;24:158–63.
74. MacMahon P, Blair ME, Treweeke P, Kovar IZ. Association of mineral composition of neonatal intravenous feeding solutions and metabolic bone disease of prematurity. Arch Dis Child 1989;64:489–93.
75. Koo WWK. Parenteral nutrition-related bone disease. J Parenter Enteral Nutr 1992;16:386–94.
76. Glasgow JFT, Thomas PS. Rachitic respiratory distress in small preterm infants. Arch Dis Child 1977;5:268–73.
77. Aubier M, Murciano D, Lecocguic Y, et al. Effect of hypophosphatemia on diaphragmatic contractility in patients with acute respiratory failure. N Engl J Med 1985;313:420–49.
78. Atkinson SA, Shah JK, McGee C, Steele BT. Mineral excretion in premature infants receiving various diuretic therapies. J Pediatr 1988;113:540–5.
79. Stafstrom CE, Gilmore HE, Kurtin PS. Nephrocalcinosis complicating medical treatment of posthemorrhagic hydrocephalus. Pediatr Neurol 1992;8:179–82.
80. Fitzgerald KA, MacKay MW. Calcium and phosphate solubility in neonatal parenteral nutrient solutions containing TrophAmine. Am J Hosp Pharm 1986;43:88–93.
81. Pelegano JF, Rowe JC, Carey DE, et al. Simultaneous infusion of calcium and phosphorus in parenteral nutrition for premature infants: Use of the physiologic calcium/phosphorus ratio. J Pediatr 1989;114:115–9.
82. Prestridge LL, Schanler RJ, Shulman RJ, et al. Effect of parenteral calcium and phosphorus therapy on mineral retention and bone mineral content in very low birth weight infants. J Pediatr 1993;122:761–8.
83. Hoehn GJ, Carey DE, Rowe JC, et al. Alternate day infusion of calcium and phosphorus in very low birth weight infants: Wasting of the infused mineral. J Pediatr Gastroenterol Nutr 1987;6:752–7.
84. Greene HL, Hambidge KM, Schanler RJ, Tsang RC. Guidelines for the use of vitamins, trace elements, calcium, magnesium, and phosphorus in infants and children receiving total parenteral nutrition: Report of the Subcommittee on Pediatric Parenteral Nutrient Requirements from the Committee on Clinical Practice Issues of The American Society for Clinical Nutrition. Am J Clin Nutr 1988;48:1324–42.
85. Koo WWK, Tsang RC. Calcium, magnesium, phosphorus, and vitamin D. In: Tsang RC, Lucas A, Uauy R, Zlotkin S, editors. Nutritional Needs of the Preterm Infant: Scientific Basis and Practical Guidelines. Baltimore: Williams & Wilkins; 1993. p. 135–56.
86. Bhatia J. Fluid and electrolyte management in the very low birth weight neonate. J Perinatol 2006;26:19–21.
87. Zlotkin SH, Buchanan BE. Meeting zinc and copper intake requirements in the parenterally fed preterm and fullterm infant. J Pediatr 1983;103:441–6.
88. Shulman RJ. Zinc and copper balance studies in infants receiving total parenteral nutrition. Am J Clin Nutr 1989;49:879–83.
89. Sutton AM, Harvie A, Cockburn F, et al. Copper deficiency in the preterm infant of very low birthweight. Arch Dis Child 1985;60:644–51.
90. Lockitch G, Jacobson B, Quigley G, et al. Selenium deficiency in low birth weight neonates: An unrecognized problem. J Pediatr 1989;114:865–70.
91. Kien CL, Ganther HE. Manifestations of chronic selenium deficiency in a child receiving total parenteral nutrition. Am J Clin Nutr 1983;37:319–28.
92. Van Caillie-Bertrand MV, Degenhart HJ, Fernandes J. Selenium status of infants on nutritional support. Acta Paediatr Scand 1984;73:816–9.
93. Darlow BA, Austin NC. Selenium supplementation to prevent short-term morbidity in preterm neonates. Cochrane Database Syst Rev 2003.
94. Bougle D, Bureau F, Deschrevel G, et al. Chromium and parenteral nutrition in children. J Pediatr Gastroenterol Nutr 1993;17:72–4.
95. Greer FR, Zachman RD. Neonatal vitamin metabolism: Fat soluble. In: Cowett RM, editor. Principles of Perinatal-Neonatal Metabolism. New York: Springer-Verlag; 1999. p. 943–75.
96. Shenai JP. Vitamin A. In: Tsang RC, Lucas A, Uauy R, Zlotkin S, editors. Nutritional Needs of the Preterm Infant. Baltimore: Williams & Wilkins; 1993. p. 87–100.
97. Zachman RD. Retinol (vitamin A) and the neonate: Special problems of the human premature infant. Am J Clin Nutr 1989;50:413–24.
98. Bates CJ, Liu DS, Fuller NJ, Lucas A. Susceptibility of riboflavin and vitamin A in breast milk to photodegradation and

its implications for the use of banked breast milk in infant feeding. Acta Paediatr Scand 1985;74:40–4.
99. Baeckert PA, Greene HL, Fritz I. Vitamin concentrations in very low birth weight infants given vitamins intravenously in a lipid emulsion: Measurement of vitamins A, D, and E and riboflavin. Pediatrics 1988;113:1057–65.
100. Porcelli PJ, Greene HL, Adcock EW. Retinol (vitamin A) and riboflavin (vitamin B_2) administration and metabolism in very low birth weight infants. Semin Perinatol 1992;16:170–80.
101. Shenai JP, Chytil F, Stahlman MT. Vitamin A status of neonates with bronchopulmonary dysplasia. Pediatr Res 1985;19:185–8.
102. Darlow BA, Graham PJ. Vitamin A supplementation for preventing morbidity and mortality in very low birth weight infants (Cochrane Review). The Cochrane Library 2002.
103. Pearson E, Bose C, Snidow T, et al. Trial of vitamin A supplementation in very low birth weight infants at risk for bronchopulmonary dysplasia. J Pediatr 1992;121:420–7.
104. Tyson JE, Wright LL, Oh W, et al. Vitamin A supplementation for extremely-low-birth-weight infants. N Engl J Med 1999;340:1962–8.
105. Gross SJ. Vitamin E. In: Tsang RC, Lucas A, Uauy R, Zlotkin S, editors. Nutritional Needs of the Preterm Infant. Baltimore: Williams & Wilkins; 1993. p. 101–9.
106. Phillips B, Franck LS, Greene HL. Vitamin E levels in premature infants during and after intravenous multivitamin supplementation. Pediatrics 1987;80:680–3.
107. Ehrenkranz RA. Vitamin E and retinopathy of prematurity: Still controversial. J Pediatr 1989;114:801–3.
108. Langenberg P, Bhutani V, Quinn GE. Vitamin E prophylaxis to reduce retinopathy of prematurity: A reappraisal of published trials. J Pediatr 1997;131:844–50.
109. Phelps DL, Rosenbaum AL, Isenberg SJ, et al. Tocopherol efficacy and safety for preventing retinopathy of prematurity: A randomized, controlled, double-masked trial. Pediatrics 1987;79:489–500.
110. Puklin JE, Simon RM, Ehrenkranz RA. Influence on retrolental fibroplasia of intramuscular vitamin E administration during respiratory distress syndrome. Ophthalmology 1982;89:96–103.
111. Watts JL, Milner RA, McCormick AO. Failure of vitamin E to prevent RLF. Clin Invest Med 1985;8:A176.
112. Ehrenkranz RA, Ablow RC, Warshaw JB. Effect of vitamin E on the development of oxygen-induced lung injury in neonates. Ann NY Acad Sci 1982;393:452–65.
113. Saldanha RL, Cepeda EE, Poland RL. The effect of vitamin E prophylaxis on the incidence and severity of bronchopulmonary dysplasia. J Pediatr 1982;101:89–93.
114. Watts JL, Milner R, Zipursky A. Failure of supplementation with vitamin E to prevent bronchopulmonary dysplasia in infants <1500 g birthweight. Eur Respir J 1991;4:188–90.
115. Chiswick ML, Johnson M, Woodhall C. Protective effect of vitamin E (DL-alpha-tocopherol) against intraventricular hemorrhage in premature babies. Br Med J 1983;287:81–4.
116. Law MR, Wijewardene K, Wald NJ. Is routine vitamin E administration justified in very low-birthweight infants? Dev Med Child Neurol 1990;32:442–50.
117. Sinha S, Davies J, Toner N, et al. Vitamin E supplementation reduces frequency of periventricular hemorrhage in very preterm babies. Lancet 1987;1:466–70.
118. Moore MC, Greene HL, Phillips B, et al. Evaluation of a pediatrics multiple vitamin preparation for total parenteral nutrition in infants and children. I. Blood levels of water-soluble vitamins. Pediatrics 1986;77:530–8.
119. Greene HL, Smith R, Pollack P, et al. Intravenous vitamins for very-low-birth-weight infants. J Am Coll Nutr 1991;10:281–8.
120. Levy R, Herzberg GR, Andrews WL, et al. Thiamine, riboflavin, folate, and vitamin B_{12} status of low birth weight infants receiving parenteral and enteral nutrition. J Parenter Enteral Nutr 1992;16:241–7.
121. Nutrition & Gastroenterology Clinical Review Committee. Nutrition support. In: Adams JM, Garcia-Prats JA, Schanler RJ, et al, editors. Guidelines for the Acute Care of the Neonate. Houston: Newborn Section, Department of Pediatrics, Baylor College of Medicine; 2002. p. 43–50.
122. Widdowson EM, Colombo VE, Artavanis CA. Changes in the organs of pigs in response to feeding for the first 24 hours after birth. Biol Neonate 1976;28:272–81.
123. Castillo RO, Feng JJ, Stevenson DK, Kwong LK. Altered maturation of small intestinal function in the absence of intraluminal nutrients: Rapid normalization with refeeding. Am J Clin Nutr 1991;53:558–61.
124. Niinikoski H, Stoll B, Kansagra K, et al. Onset of small intestinal atrophy is associated with reduced intestinal blood flow in TPN-fed neonatal piglets. J Nutr 2004;134:1467–74.
125. Lucas A, Bloom R, Aynsley-Green A. Gut hormones and "minimal enteral feeding." Acta Paediatr Scand 1986;75:719–23.
126. Dunn L, Hulman S, Weiner J, Kliegman R. Beneficial effects of early hypocaloric enteral feeding on neonatal gastrointestinal function: Preliminary report of a randomized trial. J Pediatr 1988;112:622–9.
127. Slagle TA, Gross SJ. Effect of early low-volume enteral substrate on subsequent feeding tolerance in very low birth weight infants. J Pediatr 1988;113:526–31.
128. Meetze WH, Valentine C, McGuigan JE, et al. Gastrointestinal priming prior to full enteral nutrition in very low birth weight infants. J Pediatr Gastroenterol Nutr 1992;15:163–70.
129. Berseth CL. Effect of early feeding on maturation of the preterm infant's small intestine. J Pediatr 1992;120:947–53.
130. Schanler RJ, Shulman RJ, Lau C, et al. Feeding strategies for premature infants: Randomized trial of gastrointestinal priming and tube-feeding method. Pediatrics 1999;103:434–9.
131. Shulman RJ, Schanler RJ, Lau C, et al. Early feeding, feeding tolerance, and lactase activity in preterm infants. J Pediatr 1998;133:645–9.
132. Shulman RJ, Schanler RJ, Lau C, et al. Early feeding, antenatal glucocorticoids, and human milk decrease intestinal permeability in preterm infants. Pediatr Res 1998;44:519–23.
133. Weiler HA, Fitzpatrick-Wong SC, Schellenberg JM, et al. Minimal enteral feeding within 3 d of birth in prematurely born infants with birth weight less than or equal to 1200 g improves bone mass by term age. Am J Clin Nutr 2006;83:155–62.
134. Tyson JE, Kennedy KA. Trophic feedings for parenterally fed infants. The Cochrane Database of Systematic Reviews 2005.
135. Davey AM, Wagner CL, Cox C, Kendig JW. Feeding premature infants while low umbilical artery catheters are in place: A prospective, randomized trial. J Pediatr 1994;124:795–9.
136. Berseth CL, Bisquera JA, Paje VU. Prolonging small feeding volumes early in life decreases the incidence of necrotizing enterocolitis in very low birth weight infants. Pediatrics 2003;111:529–34.
137. Atkinson SA, Bryan MH, Anderson GH. Human milk: Difference in nitrogen concentration in milk from mothers of term and premature infants. J Pediatr 1978;93:67–9.
138. Billeaud C, Guillet J, Sandler B. Gastric emptying in infants with or without gastro-oesophageal reflux according to the type of milk. Eur J Clin Nutr 1990;44:577–83.
139. Gaull GE, Rassin DK, Raiha NCR, Heinonen K. Milk protein quantity and quality in low-birthweight infants, III: Effects on sulfur amino acids in plasma and urine. J Pediatr 1977;90:348–55.
140. Rassin DK, Gaull GE, Raiha NCR, Heinonen K. Milk protein quantity and quality in low-birth-weight infants, IV: Effects on tyrosine and phenylalanine in plasma and urine. J Pediatr 1977;90:356–60.
141. Schanler RJ, Goldblum RM, Garza C, Goldman AS. Enhanced fecal excretion of selected immune factors in very low birth weight infants fed fortified human milk. Pediatr Res 1986;20:711–5.
142. Savilahti E, Kuitunen M. Allergenicity of cow milk proteins. J Pediatr 1992;121:S12–20.
143. Neu J, Roig JC, Meetze WH, et al. Enteral glutamine supplementation for very low birth weight infants decreases morbidity. J Pediatr 1997;131:691–9.
144. Vaughn P, Thomas P, Clark R, Neu J. Enteral glutamine supplementation and morbidity in low birth weight infants. J Pediatr 2003;142:662–8.
145. Tubman TR, Thompson SW, McGuire W. Glutamine supplementation to prevent morbidity and mortality in preterm infants. Cochrane Database Syst Rev 2005.
146. Raiha NCR, Heinonen K, Rassin DK, Gaull GE. Milk protein quantity and quality in low-birth-weight infants, I: Metabolic responses and effects on growth. Pediatrics 1976;57:659–74.
147. Moro GE, Fulconis F, Minoli I, et al. Growth and plasma amino acid concentrations in very low birthweight infants fed either human milk protein fortified human milk or whey-predominant formula. Acta Paediatr Scand 1989;78:18–22.
148. Kashyap S, Forsyth M, Zucker C, et al. Effects of varying protein and energy intakes on growth and metabolic response in low birth weight infants. J Pediatr 1986;108:955–63.
149. Kashyap S, Schulze K, Forsyth M, et al. Growth, nutrient retention, and metabolic response in low birth weight infants fed varying intakes of protein and energy. J Pediatr 1988;113:713–21.
150. Groh-Wargo S. Recommended enteral nutrient intakes. In: Groh-Wargo S, Thompson M, Cox J, editors. Nutritional Care for High-Risk Newborns. Chicago: Precept Press; 2000. p. 231–63.
151. Goldman HI, Goldman JS, Kaufman I, Liebman OB. Late effects of early dietary protein intake on low-birth-weight infants. J Pediatr 1974;85:764–9.
152. Kashyap S, Schulze KF, Forsyth M, et al. Growth, nutrient retention, and metabolic response of low-birth-weight infants fed supplemented and unsupplemented preterm human milk. Am J Clin Nutr 1990;52:254–62.
153. Polberger SKT, Axelsson IA, Raiha NCR. Growth of very low birth weight infants on varying amounts of human milk protein. Pediatr Res 1989;25:414–9.
154. Jensen RG, Jensen GL. Specialty lipids for infant nutrition, I: Milks and formulas. J Pediatr Gastroenterol Nutr 1992;15:232–45.
155. Neville MC, Keller RP, Seacat J, et al. Studies on human lactation, I: Within-feed and between-breast variation in selected components of human milk. Am J Clin Nutr 1984;40:635–46.
156. Greer FR, McCormick A, Loker J. Changes in fat concentration of human milk during delivery by intermittent bolus and continuous mechanical pump infusion. J Pediatr 1984;105:745–9.
157. Innis SM. Human milk and formula fatty acids. J Pediatr 1992;120:S56–61.
158. Valentine CJ, Hurst NM, Schanler RJ. Hindmilk improves weight gain in low-birth-weight infants fed human milk. J Pediatr Gastroenterol Nutr 1994;18:474–7.
159. Clandinin MT, Parrott A, Van Aerde JE, et al. Feeding preterm infants a formula containing C_{20} and C_{22} fatty acids simulates plasma phospholipid fatty acid composition of infants fed human milk. Early Hum Dev 1992;31:41–51.
160. Uauy R, Hoffman DR. Essential fatty acid requirements for normal eye and brain development. Semin Perinatol 1991;15:449–55.
161. Carlson SE, Werkman SH, Rhodes PG, Tolley EA. Visual-acuity development in healthy preterm infants: Effect of marine-oil supplementation. Am J Clin Nutr 1993;58:35–42.
162. O'Connor DL, Hall R, Adamkin D, et al. Growth and development in preterm infants fed long-chain polyunsaturated fatty acids: A prospective, randomized controlled trial. Pediatrics 2001;108:359–71.
163. Uauy R, Peirano P, Hoffman D, et al. Role of essential fatty acids in the function of the developing nervous system. Lipids 1996;31:S167–76.
164. Tantibhedhyangkul P, Hashim SA. Medium-chain triglyceride feeding in premature infants: Effects on calcium and magnesium absorption. Pediatrics 1978;61:537–44.
165. Roy CC, Ste-Marie M, Chartrand L, et al. Correction of the malabsorption of the preterm infant with a medium-chain triglyceride formula. J Pediatr 1975;86:446–50.
166. Hamosh M, Bitman J, Liao TH, et al. Gastric lipolysis and fat absorption in preterm infants: Effect of medium-chain triglyceride or long-chain triglyceride-containing formulas. Pediatrics 1989;83:86–97.
167. Whyte RK, Campbell D, Stanhope R, et al. Energy balance in low birth weight infants fed formula of high or low medium-chain triglyceride content. J Pediatr 1986;108:964–71.
168. Huston RK, Reynolds JW, Jensen C, Buist NRM. Nutrient and mineral retention and vitamin D absorption in low-birth-weight infants: Effect of medium-chain triglycerides. Pediatrics 1983;72:44–8.
169. Wu PYK, Edmond J, Auestad N, et al. Medium-chain triglycerides in infant formulas and their relation to plasma ketone body concentrations. Pediatr Res 1986;20:338–41.
170. Rebouche CJ, Panagides DD, Nelson SE. Role of carnitine in utilization of dietary medium-chain triglycerides by term infants. Am J Clin Nutr 1990;52:820–4.
171. Mehta NR, Hamosh M, Bitman J, Wood DL. Adherence of medium-chain fatty acids to feeding tubes during gavage. J Pediatr 1988;112:474–6.
172. MacLean WC, Fink BB. Lactose malabsorption by premature infants: Magnitude and clinical significance. J Pediatr 1980;97:383–8.
173. Ziegler EE, Fomon SJ. Lactose enhances mineral absorption in infancy. J Pediatr Gastroenterol Nutr 1983;2:288–94.
174. Atkinson SA, Bryan MH, Anderson GH. Human milk feeding in premature infants: Protein, fat and carbohydrate balances in the first two weeks of life. J Pediatr 1981;99:617–24.
175. Butte NF, Garza C, Johnson CA, et al. Longitudinal changes in milk composition of mothers delivering preterm and term infants. Early Hum Dev 1984;9:153–62.
176. Schanler RJ. Calcium and phosphorus absorption and retention in preterm infants. Exp Med 1991;2:24–36.
177. Koo WWK, Sherman R, Succop P, et al. Sequential bone mineral content in small preterm infants with and without fractures and rickets. J Bone Miner Res 1988;3:193–7.
178. Atkinson SA, Radde IC, Anderson GH. Macromineral balances in premature infants fed their own mothers' milk or formula. J Pediatr 1983;102:99–106.
179. Aiken CGA, Sherwood RA, Lenney W. Role of plasma phosphate measurements in detecting rickets of prematurity and in monitoring treatment. Ann Clin Biochem 1993;30:469–75.

180. Lucas A, Brooke OG, Baker BA, et al. High alkaline phosphatase activity and growth in preterm neonates. Arch Dis Child 1989;64:902–9.
181. Fewtrell MS, Cole TJ, Bishop NJ, Lucas A. Neonatal factors predicting childhood height in preterm infants: Evidence for a persisting effect of early metabolic bone disease? J Pediatr 2000;137:668–73.
182. Salle B, Senterre J, Putet G, Rigo J. Effects of calcium and phosphorus supplementation on calcium retention and fat absorption in preterm infants fed pooled human milk. J Pediatr Gastroenterol Nutr 1986;5:638–42.
183. Horsman A, Ryan SW, Congdon PJ, et al. Bone mineral accretion rate and calcium intake in preterm infants. Arch Dis Child 1989;64:910–8.
184. Schanler RJ, Garza C. Improved mineral balance in very low birth weight infants fed fortified human milk. J Pediatr 1987;112:452–6.
185. Schanler RJ, Rifka M. Calcium, phosphorus, and magnesium needs for low birth weight infants. Acta Paediatr 1994;83:111–6.
186. Bronner F, Salle BL, Putet G, et al. Net calcum absorption in premature infants: Results of 103 metabolic balance studies. Am J Clin Nutr 1992;56:1037–44.
187. Schanler RJ, Abrams SA. Postnatal attainment of intrauterine macromineral accretion rates in low birth weight infants fed fortified human milk. J Pediatr 1995;126:441–7.
188. Dauncey MJ, Shaw JCL, Urman J. The absorption and retention of magnesium, zinc, and copper by low birth weight infants fed pasteurized human breast milk. Pediatr Res 1977;11:1033–9.
189. Tyrala EE. Zinc and copper balances in preterm infants. Pediatrics 1986;77:513–7.
190. Ehrenkranz RA, Gettner PA, Nelli CM, et al. Zinc and copper nutritional studies in very low birth weight infants: Comparison of stable isotope extrinsic tag and chemical balance methods. Pediatr Res 1989;26:298–307.
191. Schanler RJ, Shulman RJ, Lau C. Feeding strategies for premature infants: Beneficial outcomes of feeding fortified human milk *vs* preterm formula. Pediatrics 1999;103:1150–7.
192. Obladen M, Loui A, Kampmann W, Renz H. Zinc deficiency in rapidly growing preterm infants. Acta Paediatr 1998;87:685–91.
193. Bilinski DL, Ehrenkranz RA, Cooley-Jacobs J, McGuire J. Symptomatic zinc deficiency in a breast-fed, premature infant. Arch Dermatol 1987;123:1221–4.
194. Siimes MA, Vuori E, Kuitunen P. Breast milk iron a declining concentration during the course of lactation. Acta Paediatr Scand 1979;68:29–31.
195. Dauncey MJ, Davies CG, Shaw JCL, Urman J. The effect of iron supplements and blood transfusion on iron absorption by low birth weight infants fed pasteurized human breast milk. Pediatr Res 1978;12:899–904.
196. Moody GJ, Schanler RJ, Abrams SA. Utilization of supplemental iron by premature infants fed fortified human milk. Acta Paediatr 1999;88:763–7.
197. Lundström U, Siimes MA, Dallman PR. At what age does iron supplementation become necessary in low birthweight infants? J Pediatr 1977;91:878–83.
198. Ehrenkranz RA, Sherwonit EA, Nelli CM, Janghorbani M. Recombinant human erythropoietin stimulates incorporation of absorbed iron into RBCs in VLBW infants. Pediatr Res 1994;35:311A.
199. Roy RN, Chance GW, Radde IC, et al. Late hyponatremia in very low birthweight infants. Pediatr Res 1976;10:526–31.
200. Heinonen K, Mononen I, Mononen T, et al. Plasma vitamin C levels are low in premature infants fed human milk. Am J Clin Nutr 1986;43:923–4.
201. American Academy of Pediatrics, Committee on Nutrition. Vitamin and mineral supplement needs in normal children in the United States. Pediatrics 1980;66:1015–21.
202. Narayanan I, Prakash K, Bala S, et al. Partial supplementation with expressed breast-milk for prevention of infection in low-birth-weight infants. Lancet 1980;2:561–3.
203. Contreras-Lemus J, Flores-Huerta S, Cisneros-Silva I, et al. Disminucion de la morbilidad en neonatos pretermino alimentados con leche de su propia madre. Biol Med Hosp Infant Mex 1992;49:671–7.
204. Hylander MA, Strobino DM, Dhanireddy R. Human milk feedings and infection among very low birth weight infants. Pediatrics 1998;102:e38.
205. El-Mohandes AE, Picard MB, Simmens SJ, Keiser JF. Use of human milk in the intensive care nursery decreases the incidence of nosocomial sepsis. J Perinatol 1998;17:130–4.
206. Lucas A, Cole TJ. Breast milk and neonatal necrotizing enterocolitis. Lancet 1990;336:1519–23.
207. Furman L, Taylor G, Minich N, Hack M. The effect of maternal milk on neonatal morbidity of very low-birth-weight infants. Arch Pediatr Adolesc Med 2003;157:66–71.
208. Lucas A, Morley R, Cole TJ, et al. Breast milk and subsequent intelligence quotient in children born preterm. Lancet 1992;339:261–4.
209. Horwood LJ, Fergusson DM. Breastfeeding and later cognitive and academic outcomes. Pediatrics 1998;101:E91–7.
210. Horwood LJ, Mogridge N, Darlow BA. Cognitive, educational, and behavioral outcomes at 7 to 8 years in a national very low birthweight cohort. Arch Dis Child Fetal Neonatal 1998;79:F12–20.
211. Horwood LJ, Darlow BA, Mogridge N. Breast milk feeding and cognitive ability at 7-8 years. Arch Dis Child Fetal Neonatal 2001;84:F23–7.
212. Vohr BR, Poindexter BB, Dusick AM, et al. Beneficial effects of breast milk in the neonatal intensive care unit on the developmental outcome of extremely low birth weight infants at 18 months of age. Pediatrics 2006;118:e115–23.
213. Hack M, Flannery DJ, Schluchter M, et al. Outcomes in young adulthood for very-low-birth-weight infants. N Engl J Med 2002;346:149–57.
214. Schanler RJ, Oh W. Composition of breast milk obtained from mothers of premature infants as compared to breast milk obtained from donors. J Pediatr 1980;96:679–81.
215. Cooper PA, Rothberg AD, Pettifor JM, et al. Growth and biochemical response of premature infants fed pooled preterm milk or special formula. J Pediatr Gastroenterol Nutr 1984;3:749–54.
216. Gross SJ. Growth and biochemical response of preterm infants fed human milk or modified infant formula. N Engl J Med 1983;308:237–41.
217. Schanler RJ, Garza C, Smith EO. Fortified mothers' milk for very low birth weight infants: Results of macromineral balance studies. J Pediatr 1985;107:767–74.
218. Greer FR, McCormick A. Improved bone mineralization and growth in premature infants fed fortified own mother's milk. J Pediatr 1988;112:961–9.
219. Abrams SA, Schanler RJ, Tsang RC, Garza C. Bone mineralization in former very low birth weight infants fed either human milk or commercial formula: One year follow-up observation. J Pediatr 1989;114:1041–4.
220. Kumar SP, Sacks LM. Hyponatremia in very low-birth-weight infants and human milk feedings. J Pediatr 1978;93:1026–7.
221. Lucas A, Fewtrell MS, Morley R, et al. Randomized outcome trial of human milk fortification and developmental outcome in preterm infants. Am J Clin Nutr 1996;64:142–51.
222. Schanler RJ, Garza C, Nichols BL. Fortified mothers' milk for very low birth weight infants: Results of growth and nutrient balance studies. J Pediatr 1985;107:437–45.
223. Barrett-Reis B, Hall RT, Schanler RJ, et al. Enhanced growth of preterm infants fed a new powdered human milk fortifier: A randomized controlled trial. Pediatrics 2000;106:581–8.
224. Berseth CL, Van Aerde JE, Gross S, et al. Growth, efficacy, and safety of feeding an iron-fortified human milk fortifier. Pediatrics 2004;114:e699–706.
225. Moody GJ, Schanler RJ, Lau C, Shulman RJ. Feeding tolerance in premature infants fed fortified human milk. J Pediatr Gastroenterol Nutr 2000;30:408–12.
226. Jocson MAL, Mason EO, Schanler RJ. The effects of nutrient fortification and varying storage conditions on host defense properties of human milk. Pediatrics 1997;100:240–3.
227. Schanler RJ. Human milk fortification for premature infants. Am J Clin Nutr 1996;64:249–50.
228. Schanler RJ, Lau C, Hurst NM, Smith EO. Randomized trial of donor human milk versus preterm formula as substitutes for mothers' own milk in the feeding of extremely premature infants. Pediatrics 2005;116:400–6.
229. Schanler RJ, Abrams SA, Garza C. Bioavailability of calcium and phosphorus in human milk fortifiers and formula for very low birth weight infants. J Pediatr 1988;113:95–100.
230. Jadcherla SR, Kleigman RM. Studies of feeding intolerance in very low birth weight infants: Definition and significance. Pediatrics 2002;109:516–7.
231. Mihatsch WA, von Schoenaich P, Fahnenstich H, et al. The significance of gastric residuals in the early enteral feeding advancement of extremely low birth weight infants. Pediatrics 2002;109:457–9.
232. Aynsley-Green A, Adrian TE, Bloom SR. Feeding and the development of enteroinsular hormone secretion in the preterm infant: Effects of continuous gastric infusion of human milk compared with intermittent boluses. Acta Paediatr Scand 1982;71:379–83.
233. Premji S, Chessell L. Continuous nasogastric milk feeding versus intermittent bolus milk feeding for premature infants less than 1500 grams. Cochrane Database Syst Rev 2003.
234. DeVille KT, Shulman RJ, Berseth CL. Slow infusion feeding enhances gastric emptying in preterm infants compared to bolus feeding. Clin Res 1993;41:787A.
235. Parker P, Stroop S, Greene H. A controlled comparison of continuous versus intermittent feeding in the treatment of infants with intestinal disease. J Pediatr 1981;99:360–4.
236. McGuire W, McEwan P. Transpyloric versus gastric tube feeding for preterm infants. The Cochrane Database of Systematic Reviews 2002.
237. Koenig WJ, Amarnath RP, Hench V, Berseth CL. Manometrics for preterm and term infants: A new tool for old questions. Pediatrics 1995;95:203–6.
238. Berseth CL, Nordyke CK, Valdes MG, et al. Responses of gastrointestinal peptides and motor activity to milk and water feedings in preterm and term infants. Pediatr Res 1992;31:587–90.
239. McKeown RE, Marsh D, Amarnath U, et al. Role of delayed feeding and of feeding increments in necrotizing enterocolitis. J Pediatr 1992;121:764–70.
240. Rayyis SF, Ambalavanan N, Wright L, Carlo WA. Randomized trial of "slow" versus "fast" feed advancements on the incidence of necrotizing enterocolitis in very low birth weight infants. J Pediatr 1999;134:293–7.
241. Patole SK, de Klerk NH. Impact of standarised feeding regimens on incidence of neonatal necrotising enterocolitis: A systematic review and meta-analysis of observational studies. Arch Dis Child Fetal Neonatal Ed 2005;90:147–51.
242. Olsen IE, Richardson DK, Schmid CH, et al. Dietitian involvement in the neonatal intensive care unit: More is better. J Am Diet Assoc 2005;105:1224–30.
243. Usher R, McLean F. Intrauterine growth of live-born Caucasian infants at sea level: Standards obtained from measurements in 7 dimensions of infants born between 25 and 44 weeks of gestation. Pediatrics 1969;74:901–10.
244. Wilson DC, Cairns P, Halliday HL, et al. Randomised controlled trial of an aggressive nutritional regimen in sick very low birthweight infants. Arch Dis Child Fetal Neonatal 1997;77:F4–F11.
245. Nutrition of the Preterm Infant: Scientific Basis and Practical Guidelines. Cincinnati, OH: Digital Educational Publishing Inc; 2005 .
246. Kleinman RE. Pediatric Nutrition Handbook. Elk Grove Village, IL: American Academy of Pediatrics; 2004 .
247. Nordenstrom J, Thorne A. Comparative studies on a new concentrated fat emulsion: Intralipid 30% vs. 20%. Clin Nutr 1993;12:160–7.
248. Schanler RJ. The low birth weight infant: Perinatal nutrition. In: Walker WA, Watkins JB, editors. Nutrition in Pediatrics: Basic Science and Clinical Applications. Hamilton, Ontario, Canada: B.C. Decker Inc; 1996. p. 387–407.
249. Gross SJ, David RJ, Bauman L, Tomarelli RM. Nutritional composition of milk produced by mothers delivering preterm. J Pediatr 1980;96:641–4.
250. Specker BL, Greer F, Tsang RC. Vitamin D. In: Tsang RC, Nichols BL, editors. Nutrition During Infancy. Philadelphia, PA: Hanley & Belfus Inc; 1988. p. 264–76.
251. Schanler RJ. Water-soluble vitamins for premature infants. In: Tsang RC, Uauy R, Koletzko B, Zlotkin S, editors. Nutrition of the Preterm Infant. Scientific Basis and Practical Guidelines. Cincinnati: Digital Educational Publishing, Inc; 2005. p. 173–99.
252. Schanler RJ, Atkinson SA. Human milk. In: Tsang RC, Uauy R, Koletzko B, Zlotkin S, editors. Nutrition of the Preterm Infant. Scientific Basis and Practical Guidelines. Cincinnati, OH: Digital Educational Publishing Inc; 2005. p. 333–56.

Nutritional Management of Preterm Infants Postdischarge

William C. Heird, MD

The usual recommendation for feeding prematurely born infants is to provide sufficient nutrients to support rates of growth and nutrient accretion equal to intrauterine rates.[1] The protein and energy intakes required to achieve this goal, provided the intakes of all other necessary nutrients are adequate, ~2.8 g/kg/d and 462 to 504 kJ (110 to 120 kcal)/kg/d, respectively.[2] However, many infants do not tolerate the enteral intake necessary to provide these requirements until 2 to 3 weeks of age and do not regain birthweight until approximately the same age. By this time, their weight, even if appropriate for gestational age (AGA) at birth, is usually less than the tenth percentile of the gestational, or postmenstrual, age reference. As a consequence, unless rates of growth higher than the intrauterine rates are achieved after birthweight is regained, these infants will remain small at discharge relative to the fetus of the same postmenstrual age.[3]

The prevalence of postnatal growth restriction is illustrated by the growth characteristics of infants weighing between 501 and 1,500 g at birth who were admitted to one of the National Institutes of Child Health and Development (NICHD) Neonatal Research Network Centers between August 1994 and August 1995.[4] Infants born after 24 to 25 weeks gestation had a mean birthweight somewhat above the fiftieth percentile for gestational age (weight, ~725 g). However, they did not reach the usual discharge weight of 2,000 g until ~12.5 weeks after birth, approximately 5.5 weeks later than the normally growing fetus of the same postmenstrual age. Moreover, weight at this time was considerably less than the tenth percentile of the intrauterine reference. Those born with a birthweight at the fiftieth percentile after 26 to 27 weeks gestation (weight, ~900 g) did not reach 2,000 g until about 10.5 weeks after birth, at which time they were about 5 weeks behind the fetus of the same postmenstrual age and also weighed considerably less than the tenth percentile of the intrauterine reference. Infants born after 28 to 29 weeks gestation with a birthweight at the fiftieth percentile (weight, ~1,150 g) fared somewhat better. They reached 2,000 g in about 7 weeks, almost 4 weeks later than the fetus of the same postmenstrual age.

Infants who were small for gestational age (SGA) at birth fared somewhat better. They regained birthweight sooner and grew somewhat more rapidly after birthweight was regained than infants whose weight at birth was AGA. However, their rate of growth was not sufficiently more rapid to result in a major advantage relative to the intrauterine growth reference. Infants with conditions such as chronic lung disease, intraventricular hemorrhage and necrotizing enterocolitis were even older when they reached discharge weight. Those who weighed between 1,100 and 1,300 g at birth and experienced such conditions did not reach 2,000 g until almost a week later than infants without morbidities and those with morbidities who weighed between 500 and 700 g at birth did not reach 2,000 g until almost 2 weeks later than those without.

These data reflect the in-hospital growth of infants born prematurely in 1994–1995. The situation appears to have improved somewhat, but not dramatically. Only 89% of 401 to 1,000 g infants who were born at the participating NICHD Neonatal Network centers in 2000 to 2001, versus 99% of infants born in 1994 to 1995, weighed less than the tenth percentile of the intrauterine reference at 36 weeks corrected age, or discharge.[5]

From 1994–1995 to 2000–2001, the mean age at initiation of parenteral nutrition decreased by almost a day, from 2.5 ± 3.0 to 1.7 ± 2.5 days, the mean age of beginning enteral nutrition decreased by about 2 days, from 6.8 ± 6.5 to 4.7 ± 6.0 days, the age at which full enteral feedings were achieved decreased by about a week, from 25.3 ± 15.6 to 19.3 ± 15.1 days, and the day birthweight was regained decreased almost 4 days, from 16.2 ± 7.6 to 12.5 ± 6.6 days. It is likely that early nutritional management of LBW infants can be further improved without increasing morbidity (see below) but, until this happens, most infants will continue to be discharged weighing considerably less than a fetus of the same postmenstrual age. This illustrates the importance of continued attention to nutritional management of these infants after discharge, which is the focus of this chapter.

Since postdischarge nutrition primarily concerns catch-up growth, the chapter begins with a discussion of the consequences of inadequate early nutrition or inadequate catch-up growth. Next, recognizing that predischarge and postdischarge nutrition are a continuum, several aspects of predischarge nutrition are discussed. For example, if the duration of inadequate early growth can be reduced or if more catch-up growth can be achieved before discharge, postdischarge nutrition assumes less importance. Thus, strategies for reducing early nutritional deficits as well as enhancing growth prior to discharge are discussed. Finally, data from studies of different strategies of postdischarge nutritional management are discussed followed by an attempt to arrive at an evidence-based approach to postdischarge nutritional management.

CONSEQUENCES OF INADEQUATE EARLY NUTRITION

From the previous discussion, it is clear that many—in fact, most—prematurely born infants, even if AGA at birth, become SGA soon after birth and remain SGA at discharge. The consequences of the infant's weighing less than a fetus of comparable postmenstrual age from shortly after birth until hospital discharge or longer are not known with certainty, in large part because it is difficult to separate the effects of a growth deficit or a less-than-optimal rate of growth from the many other problems of prematurity. Moreover, some of the weight loss during the first few days after birth is excess extracellular fluid rather than endogenous nutrient stores. Since loss of extracellular fluid reflects adaptation to extrauterine life, it probably is of little or no consequence nutritionally. However, the proportion of postnatal weight loss attributable to loss of excess extracellular fluid versus loss of endogenous nutrient stores is not known with certainty. The best estimates are that each contribute ~50% to the total loss of at least 10% and up to 20% of body weight over the first week of life.[6] Thus, correcting for this loss of extracellular fluid versus endogenous nutrient stores will not change the fact that many small infants who are AGA at birth become SGA shortly after birth and remain SGA at hospital discharge. Those who are SGA at birth may become "less SGA" but the majority of these infants also remain SGA at hospital discharge.

Data from a number of studies (see Table 1) show that the LBW infant who receives no protein or amino acid intake during early life experiences urinary nitrogen losses during this time ranging from 90 to 180 mg/kg/d.[7–15] This is equivalent to a daily loss of body protein stores of from 0.6 to 1.2 g/kg. Continued mobilization of endogenous protein at these rates clearly will

Table 1 Nitrogen Balance of LBW Infants While Receiving Glucose Alone versus Glucose and Amino Acids During the First Week of Life

Study	Birthweight (g)	Energy Intake (kcal/kg/d)	Amino Acid Intake (g/kg/d)	Nitrogen Balance (mg/kg/d)
Anderson et al.[7]	1,600	60	0	–132
		60	2.5	178
Saini et al.[8]	1,087	36	0	–133
		45	1.8	120
Mitton et al.[9]	1,470	34	0	–91
	1,480	35	0	–125
Mitton and Garlick[10]	1,280	31	0	–139
		83	2.6	259
	1,330	30	0	–137
		88	2.6	283
van Lingen et al.[11]	1,400	47	0	–96
	1,510	48	2.3	224
Rivera et al.[12]	1,090	35	0	–135
	1,050	54	1.6	88
van Goudoever et al.[13]	1,439	26	0	–110
	1,356	29	1.2	10
Kashyap and Heird[14]	996	30	0	–183
	996	50	2.0	114
Thureen et al.[15]	945	42	0.85	–40
	947	49	2.65	176

result eventually in muscle weakness or failure, which could be particularly hazardous for infants with already compromised pulmonary function. In addition, the inhibitory effect of inadequate nutrition on immune function is likely to enhance susceptibility to infection. These possibilities are supported by data showing that AGA and SGA preterm infants as well as SGA term infants have much higher rates of neonatal morbidity and mortality than term or near-term AGA infants.[16]

On average, SGA infants who weigh <2,500 g at birth weigh ~5 kg less and are ~5 cm shorter as adolescents and young adults than AGA infants.[17] Of even greater concern is the fact that the mean IQ of former LBW infants, both SGA and AGA, is lower at school age and beyond than that of a normal birthweight population.[18]

The consequences of inadequate early nutrition with respect to growth and development of the central nervous system is of particular concern. This stems, in part, from data demonstrating that malnutrition during a "critical" period of central nervous system development, unless corrected during the "critical" period, results in irrecoupable deficits.[19] The "critical" period for growth and development of the entire central nervous system of the human infant is thought to span the first 18 to 24 months of life.[20] Thus, in theory, correction of early malnutrition within this period should circumvent deficits secondary to inadequate nutrition. However, specific developmental events occur in various regions of the central nervous system during more finite periods and little is known about the finite "critical period" for any specific developmental event or the effect of inadequate nutrition during this period. The high prevalence of subtle developmental problems observed in LBW infants during childhood and early adolescence (eg, behavioral problems, poor attention, and specific learning problems) may reflect inadequate nutrition during the finite "critical period" of a specific neurodevelopmental event.[21]

The neurodevelopmental consequences of early nutrition have been studied by Lucas et al. These investigators randomly assigned prematurely born infants to receive either a term formula or a preterm formula with a higher content of protein (and other nutrients) from the time birthweight was regained until discharge (~4 weeks). Those who received the preterm formula had higher neurodevelopmental indices at both 18 months and 7.5 to 8 years of age.[22,23]

PREVENTION OF EARLY GROWTH DEFICITS

Accepting the premise that the postnatal growth deficit of most prematurely born infants relative to the fetus of comparable postmenstrual age is not desirable raises the important question of whether the growth deficit can be prevented. The answer to this question is not clear. Although further reduction of morbidities associated with prematurity obviously will help, improved nutritional management also is likely to be necessary. A number of strategies can be envisioned to accomplish this and, hence, reduce early growth deficits. One obvious strategy is to further decrease the time required to regain birthweight. Another is to enhance growth once birthweight is regained. If either or a combination of these strategies is not successful, catch-up growth must continue postdischarge.

Modern preterm formulas which contain more protein and energy as well as more of some vitamins and minerals than standard term formulas were designed to enhance growth during hospitalization and they achieve this goal, particularly in the larger, more mature infant for whom they were designed. However, these formulas were introduced ~25 years ago and many of today's preterm infants are both smaller and more immature than those for whom the formulas were intended. Hence, the nutritional management of today's infants is more difficult. In addition, their nutritional requirements may be different.

According to the recent data from the NICHD Neonatal Research Network Centers discussed above, much of the delay in reaching 2,000 g is related to the time required to regain birthweight—about 3 weeks for infants born after 24 to 25 weeks gestation, about 2.5 weeks for those born after 26 to 27 weeks gestation and about 2 weeks for those born after 28 to 29 weeks.[4] Thus, had the infants regained birthweight sooner, they would have reached 2,000 g sooner, although not necessarily within the same period as the fetus whose growth rate was sufficient to maintain weight at the fiftieth percentile of the intrauterine reference.

The data summarized in Table 1, in addition to illustrating the magnitude of nitrogen losses in the absence of amino acid intake, show that an amino acid intake of only about 1.0 g/kg/d maintains nitrogen equilibrium and, more important, that higher intakes result in positive nitrogen balance. Equally important, an early parenteral amino acid intake of as much as 2.0 to 2.5 g/kg/d, even with a very modest concomitant energy intake, does not result in disturbing metabolic consequences.[14,15]

Theoretically, abolishing a negative nitrogen balance of about 160 mg/kg/d, equivalent to 1 g/kg/d of protein, will decrease the magnitude of early weight loss by approximately 5 g/kg/d (ie, 1 g of endogenous protein plus an accompanying 4 g of intracellular fluid). Likewise, achievement of a positive balance of 160 mg/kg/d should result in lean body mass deposition of about 5 g/kg/d (again, 1 g/kg/d of protein plus accompanying intracellular fluid). An even higher parenteral amino acid intake, particularly if positive energy balance is achieved, will result in an even higher rate of lean body mass deposition. The protein and energy intakes needed to support the intrauterine rate of protein deposition (without catch-up) is thought to be about 3 g/kg/d and 420 to 504 kJ (100 to 120 kcal)/kg/d.[24] Although the data summarized in Table 1 illustrate that positive nitrogen balance can be achieved with an energy intake as low as 126 to 147 kJ (30 to 35 kcal)/kg/d, tolerance of an amino acid intake greater than 2.5 to 3.0 g/kg/d has not been evaluated in infants with poor tolerance of parenteral glucose and lipid and, hence, limited energy intake. Nonetheless, while an energy intake in the range of 294 to 336 kJ (70 to 80 kcal)/kg/d clearly will improve utilization of the administered amino acids and help promote anabolism, it is unlikely that an amino acid intake of 3 g/kg/d will result in disturbing metabolic derangements, even if not optimally utilized.

Based on the data summarized above, infants who receive no amino acids or protein can be expected to experience a protein deficit of about 3 g/kg/d from loss of endogenous protein stores

(1.1 g/kg/d) plus failure to deposit protein at the intrauterine rate (1.9 g/kg/d). If this continues for the first week of life, the cumulative protein deficit at the end of this time will be 21 g. Since only about 72% of enteral protein intake is retained under optimal circumstances, a minimum protein intake of 29 g/kg will be required to replace this deficit once enteral intake is tolerated. On average, 1 kg infants usually do not tolerate full enteral feeding until at least 14 days of age. Thus, those who receive a parenteral amino acid intake of less than 3 g/kg/d or do not receive a combined parenteral and enteral intake of at least this amount will experience additional protein deficits during the second and, perhaps, third week of life. An additional 10.5 g deficit during the second week of life is not unusual. Assuming no further deficits after the second week of life, this theoretical infant will begin adequate enteral feeding with a cumulative protein deficit of 31.5 g. The additional protein intake required to restore this deficit after birthweight is regained is ~44 g.

According to the reference intrauterine growth data of Alexander et al, a 1,000 g fetus reaches 2,000 g, a reasonable discharge weight, in about 5 weeks (35 days).[3] The protein required to replace the assumed protein deficit of 44 g within this period is about 1.25 g/d (about 0.85 g/kg/d). This will increase the total protein requirement during this period to at least 3.65 g/kg/d (2.8 g/kg/d to support the intrauterine rate of weight gain plus 0.85 g/kg/d to replace the early protein deficit). This is not an impressively high protein intake but it is somewhat higher than provided by usual intakes (150 mL/kg/d) of most currently available preterm infant formulas and considerably higher than provided by usual intakes of term formulas or unfortified human milk. Moreover, in this example, the infant weighed the same as at birth but was 2 weeks old. This means that the protein deficit must be replaced in 21, not 35, days if the infant is to weigh the same at discharge as a fetus of the same postconceptional age. This increases the protein requirement for total catch-up to 4.9 g/kg/d (2.8 g/kg/d to support the intrauterine rate of growth plus 2.1 g/kg/d to replace the deficit incurred during the first 2 weeks of life).

The protein intake calculated to restore the early protein deficit within 35 days can be achieved by increasing the usual volume of preterm formula by ~30 mL/kg/d. The higher volume also will increase energy intake (from 504 kJ (120 kcal)/kg/d at 150 mL/kg/d to 144 kcal/kg/d at 180 mL/kg/d). The higher energy intake, in turn, will result in a rate of fat deposition in excess of the intrauterine rate but, since the theoretical infant probably also experienced a deficit in energy intake prior to achieving full enteral feedings, the higher energy intake may be desirable.

Embleton et al recently documented an energy deficit (from the assumed requirement of 504 kJ (120 kcal)/kg/d) of 1705 ± 386 kJ (406 ± 92 kcal)/d over the first week of life and a deficit of 3415 ± 2276 kJ (813 ± 542 kcal) over the first 5 weeks of life in infants born prior to 30 weeks gestation.[25] Smaller deficits were documented in infants born after 31 weeks gestation, almost all during the first 1 to 2 weeks of life. Interestingly, the additional 101 kJ (24 kcal)/kg/d incident to 180 mL/kg/d versus 150 mL/kg/d of preterm formula (3,528 kJ (840 kcal) over a 35 day period) is only slightly more than the energy deficit documented by Embleton et al over this period.

The protein deficits (from 3 g/kg/d) documented by Embleton et al in infants born prior to 30 weeks gestation were 14 ± 3 g over the first week of life and 23 ± 12 g over the first 5 weeks of life.[25] This is less than the deficit calculated above for the hypothetical infant who received no amino acid or protein intake during the first week of life, largely because the infants surveyed by Embleton et al received about 1 g/kg/d of amino acids during the first week of life.

These examples illustrate the potential impact of more optimal protein and/or amino acid intake during the first few weeks of life and, hence, the subsequent requirements to restore the usual growth deficit.

ENHANCING GROWTH AFTER BIRTHWEIGHT IS REGAINED

Another approach to reducing the growth deficits of LBW infants is to provide the nutrient requirements to support both the intrauterine rate of growth and catch-up growth (ie, that required to correct the deficit incurred prior to regaining birthweight) after the infant is more stable, usually after birthweight is regained. This approach differs minimally from the most common current approach to nutritional management but the current approach places little direct emphasis on the nutrient requirements for catch-up growth.

According to Forbes, catch-up occurs when the magnitude of growth above the normal growth curve equals the magnitude of growth below the normal curve as the growth deficit was incurred.[26] In other words, the requirements for catch-up growth are a function of the amount of catch-up to be achieved and the duration over which it is achieved. For example, the daily requirements to produce catch-up of 500 g over 50 days are those necessary to produce an additional 10 g of weight gain daily (which, of course, will vary depending upon the composition of the weight gain). The daily requirements to achieve this catch-up growth within 25 days, obviously, will be greater and those for achieving it in 100 days will be less. In all cases, of course, the requirements for catch-up are additional to those for normal growth.

Kashyap et al using data from a series of studies of growth and nutrient retention of infants weighing between 750 and 1,750 g at birth and fed varying intakes of protein (2.25 to 3.9 g/kg/d) and energy 483 to 630 kJ (115 to 150 kcal)/kg/d, derived multiple regression equations relating rates of postnatal weight gain, protein accretion and fat accretion to dietary intakes of protein and energy.[27] These equations were then used to predict the relationship between dietary protein and energy intakes of prematurely born infants and the rate as well as the composition of weight gain. A key feature of these predictions was to maintain the same relationship between postnatal rates of protein and fat accretion as observed during the last trimester of gestation, ie, a ratio of protein accretion (not lean body mass accretion) to fat accretion of 1.055.[28] However, any ratio could have been chosen.

These data indicated that protein accretion and fat accretion, respectively, were functions of protein and energy intake.[27] Thus, the ratio of reported postnatal rates of protein and fat accretion expressed as functions of protein and energy intakes was set equal to the intrauterine ratio (ie, protein accretion/fat accretion = 1.055) and this equation was solved for protein (or energy) intake which, in turn, was substituted in a multiple regression equation expressing rate of weight gain as a function of protein and energy intakes. This allowed calculation of the gross protein and energy intakes needed, in theory, to produce desired rates of weight gain with the same composition as that of the fetus during the same period of development. Finally, the predicted protein and energy intakes were fed to another group of infants and shown to result, on average, in the expected growth outcomes.[27]

The principles used by Kashyap et al can be used to estimate the total protein and energy needs of infants of any birthweight who regain birthweight at various ages. For an infant who weighs 1,000 g at birth (27 weeks gestation) and regains birthweight at 2 weeks of age to achieve complete catch-up (ie, to weigh the same and have the same body composition as a fetus of the same postmenstrual age by the time of discharge at a weight of 2,200 g), weight must increase from 1,000 to 2,000 g in 21 rather than 35 days, as would have occurred had the infant remained in utero. The rate of weight gain necessary to achieve this goal is 57 g/d (~36 g/kg/d). The protein and energy intakes required to support this rate of weight gain with the same composition as that which would have occurred in utero are 6.5 g/kg/d and 609 kJ (145 kcal)/kg/d. This predicted protein intake is higher than has been studied in recent years and, further, is not likely to be utilized completely, even at an energy intake of 609 kJ (145 kcal)/kg/d. Moreover, based on studies reported several decades ago, a protein intake of this magnitude may result in undesirable metabolic consequences (eg, metabolic acidosis, hyperaminoacidemia).[29,30]

Although complete catch-up in 21 days seems impossible, it might be possible to recoup at least some of the weight deficit incurred during the 2-week period prior to regaining birthweight. In theory, a protein intake of 4.8 g/kg/d and an energy intake of 508 kJ (121 kcal)/kg/d will support a rate of weight gain of sufficient magnitude (25.8 g/kg/d) to result in the infant's being only a week behind the fetus of the same postconceptional age at discharge. This protein intake also is unlikely to be utilized completely at the predicted energy intake, but the energy intake could be increased, although the higher energy intake will result in a higher rate of fat deposition than occurs in utero.

To achieve catch-up later—by 35 rather than by 32 weeks postmenstrual age, the infant must increase in weight from 1,000 to 2,800 g in 6 weeks rather than 8 weeks. According to the model developed above, this will require a protein intake of 4.1 g/kg/d with a concomitant energy intake of 462 kJ (110 kcal)/kg/d from the time birthweight is regained until weight reaches 2,800 g. This combination of protein and energy intakes is unlikely to result in disturbing metabolic abnormalities. A greater energy intake will improve utilization of this protein intake and also result in a somewhat greater rate of weight gain (in theory, about 1 g/kg/d for each 42 kJ (10 kcal)/kg/d increase in energy intake). However, as indicated previously, this additional weight gain will be predominantly fat.

More modest protein and energy intakes after discharge, but more than provided by "term" formulas which many LBW infants currently are fed after discharge, may also enhance catch-up growth (see below). Whether catch-up over a shorter period (ie, by discharge, by a postmenstrual age of 35 weeks or by term) is preferable remains to be established. In fact, recent studies suggest that rapid catch-up growth, while beneficial for brain development, may be detrimental with respect to subsequent cardiovascular health.[31–34]

ENHANCING GROWTH AFTER HOSPITAL DISCHARGE

It is clear that catch-up can occur throughout childhood, and, particularly during adolescence. However, the extent to which LBW infants catch-up is not clear. Moreover, this appears to depend upon how catch-up is defined. If defined as reaching a weight and/or length above the third percentile of the intrauterine reference, most infants eventually catch-up. For example, Hack et al reported that 54% of 249 infants (BW <1,500 g) born in 1977 to 1979 weighed more than 2 SD below the reference weight and 60% had lengths more than 2 SD below the reference length at 40 weeks postmenstrual age.[35] By 8 months of age (corrected for gestation), only 33 and 22% had weights and lengths more than 2 SD below the weight and length references, respectively, and by 20 months of age (corrected), only 17.5 and 15.5% still had weights and lengths, respectively, more than 2 SD below the references. By 8 years of age, the number with subnormal weights and heights had decreased further with only 8% being more than 2 SD below the reference for both weight and height.

Further catch-up has been shown to occur between 8 years of age and adolescence. Peralta-Carcelen et al found that fewer than 6% of ELBW infants born between 1978 and 1984 had weights more than 2 SD below the reference at ~15 years of age.[36] However, 26.5% had weights more than 1 SD below the reference mean and 34% weighed less than the twenty-fifth percentile. Corresponding percents with lengths more than 2 SD and more than 1 SD below the reference mean and less than the twenty-fifth percentile, respectively, were 5.7, 21, and 36%. The subgroup of ELBW infants who were SGA at birth had lower weight and height Z-scores at ~15 years of age than those who were AGA at birth.

Thus, although VLBW infants as a group catch-up, some remain small compared to infants of normal birthweight. Moreover, it is not clear that the available data concerning weight and height of LBW infants at adolescence, which were obtained in adolescents born 15 to 25 years earlier, are applicable to today's LBW infants, especially today's ELBW infants. Survival of ELBW infants has improved considerably over the past 10 to 15 years making it likely that today's survivors are sicker during the immediate postnatal period and, hence, have greater deficits at term and perhaps from term to adolescence than survivors 15 to 25 years ago.

The deficits in weight and height of former LBW infants are not the major concerns. Rather, it appears that the deficits in nutrient intake which result in the subsequent size deficits may have other consequences. One such consequence is the lower head circumference of former LBW versus normal birthweight infants, children and adolescents, and the likelihood that this may contribute to the lower standardized intelligence test scores of former LBW infants as well as their greater prevalence of behavioral and learning problems. This, as well as other concerns, has resulted in attempts to further reduce the early growth deficits sustained by most surviving LBW infants, particularly those who weigh less than 1,000 g at birth.

Although earlier and more aggressive parenteral and enteral nutrition practices during hospitalization are possible and likely to be beneficial, postdischarge interventions are also possible and, in reality, both in-hospital and postdischarge interventions will probably be necessary to achieve complete or even near-complete catch-up of VLBW infants. Thus, formulas providing more protein as well as other nutrients (eg, calcium, phosphorus, trace minerals, and many vitamins) and somewhat more energy than term formulas but less nutrient-dense than preterm formulas (see Table 2) have been developed and these formulas, called postdischarge formulas, have been evaluated by several investigators.

In the earliest such evaluation, Lucas et al found that infants (BW <1,850 g) fed a postdischarge (n = 16) versus a standard term formula (n = 16) from hospital discharge at a postmenstrual age of ~36 week (weight, ~2,400 g) through a postnatal age of 9 months weighed more and were longer at 9 months of age.[37] The mean weight of both groups at entry was between the third and tenth percentiles of a standard growth reference. At 9 months of age, the mean weight of the term formula group was still between the third and tenth percentiles for age whereas that of the postdischarge formula group was near the twenty-fifth percentile. The mean length of both groups at entry was near the twenty-fifth percentile. That of infants assigned to the term formula remained in this range through 9 months of age, but that of infants assigned to the postdischarge formula was near the fiftieth percentile by 4 months of age and remained at this level through 9 months of age.

Chan, in contrast, found no statistically significant difference in weight gain among infants (BW ~1,200 g) who were randomized to be fed a standard term formula, a preterm formula or a postdischarge formula for 8 weeks postdischarge followed by a standard term formula until 16 weeks postdischarge.[38] At 2 weeks postdischarge, infants fed the preterm formula were heavier than the reference group of breast-fed infants and all formula-fed groups were heavier than the breast-fed group at 8 and 16 weeks postdischarge. The rate of increase in length over the entire study period was greater in the preterm formula and postdischarge formula groups than in the breast-fed group. At 8 weeks postdischarge, bone mineral content of the group assigned to the preterm formula was higher than that of the other formula groups as well as the breast-fed group. At 16 weeks, bone mineral content of all formula groups was higher than that of the breast-fed group but there was no difference in bone mineral content among the formula groups.

Table 2 Approximate Content of Selected Nutrients (Amount/L) in Human Milk, Term Formulas, Preterm Formulas, and Postdischarge Formulas

Nutrient	Human Milk	Term Formula	Preterm Formula	Postdischarge Formula
Energy (kcal)	670	670	810	730
Protein (g)	10	14	24	21
Fat (g)	35	36	43	40
Carbohydrate (g)	70	73	87	76
Calcium (mg)	280	530	1,400	835
Phosphorus (mg)	147	320	740	475
Sodium (mmol)	8	8	18	11
Iron (mg)	0.4	12.2	14.6	13.3
Zinc (mg)	1.2	6	12.2	9
Vitamin A (mg)	0.7	0.6	3.0	1.0
Vitamin D (μg)	0.5	10	40	14

Carver et al studied growth of infants (BW <1,800 g) who were assigned randomly at hospital discharge (weight, ~2,100 g) to receive either a postdischarge or a standard term formula for the first 12 months of life.[39] Mean birthweights of the two groups, respectively, were 1,292 and 1,249 g. Differences at various ages in mean weight, length, and head circumference of infants assigned to the postdischarge formula versus the term formula are shown in Table 4. Differences in weight, length, and/or head circumference between the two groups were observed at all times but some of these differences were not statistically significant. Moreover, differences were more marked in smaller infants and in male infants. Of note is the fact that differences were apparent shortly after discharge and persisted throughout the period of observation but did not increase appreciably or consistently thereafter, suggesting that any benefit of the postdischarge formula with respect to catch-up occurred quite early. However, this early period differs somewhat for catch-up in weight, length and head circumference. The growth benefits achieved during this early period appear to have persisted through 12 months corrected age.

In a similar study, Lucas et al randomly assigned infants (mean gestational age, 31 weeks) to receive a postdischarge (n = 113) or a term formula (n = 116) from discharge (mean postmenstrual age, 36.5 weeks) through 9 months postdischarge.[40] Growth was monitored through 18 months postdischarge and development was assessed at both 9 months and 18 months. A reference group (n = 65) was breast-fed for at least 6 weeks postterm. As shown in Table 3, those fed the postdischarge formula versus the term formula were heavier and longer after 6 weeks and remained heavier and longer through 18 months of age although, as also observed by Carver et al,[39] the differences were not statistically significant at all ages. At 6 weeks postterm, the exclusively breast-fed group was 490 g lighter and 1.5 cm shorter than those fed the postdischarge formula and they remained lighter and shorter at 9 months postterm. In general, the breastfed infants also were lighter and shorter than those fed the term formula. The postdischarge formula group had a somewhat higher Bayley psychomotor developmental index at 18 months (91.7 ± 12.7 vs 89.0 ± 14.8) but this difference was not statistically significant. As observed by Carver et al,[39] differences between infants fed the postdischarge versus the term formula were apparent early and persisted but did not increase (Table 4).

Table 3 Differences in Mean Weight, Length, and Head Circumference (OFC) Between Preterm Infants Assigned to a Postdischarge Formula (PDF) and Those Assigned to a Standard Term Formula (TF) From Discharge to 1 Year of Age[39]

Age	ΔWeight (g)	ΔLength (cm)	ΔOFC (cm)
Enrollment	−15	−0.14	−0.3
Term	186*	0.7	0.3‡
1 mo	265†	0.7	0.4
2 mo	244†	0.7	−0.1
3 mo	268	1.1	0.2
6 mo	458‡	1.6†	0.5‡
9 mo	298	1.0	0.6
12 mo	510§	1.1	0.3‡

*p < .05, male infants BW <1,250 g; †p < .05; ‡p < .05, BW <1,250 g; §p < .05, male infants BW <1,250 g.

Table 4 Differences in Mean Weight, Length and Head Circumference (OFC) Between Preterm Infants Assigned to a Postdischarge Formula and Those Assigned to a Standard Term Formula from Discharge to 9 Months of Age[40]

Age	ΔWeight (g)	ΔLength (cm)	ΔOFC (cm)
Randomization	−10	0.1	−0.20
6 wk	223*	1.06†	0.10
12 wk	160	0.65	−0.18
26 wk	180	0.72*	−0.10
9 mo	370*	1.10‡	0
18 mo	94	0.82	−0.38

*$p \leq .05$; †$p < .001$; ‡$p < .01$.

Fewtrell et al randomly assigned term SGA infants (gestation > 37 weeks; birthweight < tenth percentile) to receive the same postdischarge (n = 152) and term (n = 147) formulas studied by Lucas et al The formulas were fed for the first 9 months of life and weight, length, and head circumference were monitored through 18 months of age.[41] A reference group of 175 breast-fed term SGA infants also was included. As shown in Table 5, SGA infants assigned to the postdischarge versus the term formula group were longer at 9 and 18 months of age and occipitofrontal head circumference was greater at 18 months of age. However, there was no statistically significant difference in weight of the two groups at any time although, as shown in Table 5, the postdischarge formula group was 130 to 150 g heavier than the term formula group from 12 weeks to 18 months of age. In this study, interestingly, breast-fed infants weighed more (400 g), were longer (1.6 cm) and had a greater head circumference (0.5 cm) than the term formula group at 18 months of age but, after controlling for age, parental size and birth order, these differences were no longer statistically significant. Of note is the fact that females fed the enriched formula had a significant developmental disadvantage at 9 months but not 18 months postterm.[42] This led the investigators to conclude that use of the enriched formula for term SGA children should not be promoted until after further long-term follow-up.

Table 5 Differences in Mean Weight, Length, and Head Circumference (OFC) of SGA Term Infants Assigned to a Postdischarge versus a Standard Term Formula from Discharge to 9 Months of Age[41]

Age	ΔWeight (g)	ΔLength (cm)	ΔOFC (cm)
Enrollment	−70	−0.3	−0.3
6 wk	10	0.1	0
12 wk	130	0.1	0.1
26 wk	140	1.0*	0.1
9 mo	140	1.0*	0.1
18 mo	150	0.8*	0.38

*$p \leq .05$

Wheeler and Hall also studied postdischarge growth of preterm infants fed a postdischarge versus a standard formula.[43] These investigators assigned infants (BW < 1,800 g) randomly at discharge to receive a postdischarge versus a standard term formula from shortly before discharge to 8 weeks postdischarge and monitored growth through 12 weeks postdischarge. Length of the group assigned to the postdischarge formula was greater than that of the group assigned to the standard formula from 4 through 12 weeks postdischarge and the head circumference of this group was greater from 2 through 12 weeks postdischarge. However, there was no statistically significant difference in weight of the two groups at any time. This study also included parental reports of the volume of formula intake, which was higher in the term formula group; thus, differences in protein and energy intakes between the two groups were minimal. On the other hand, calcium and phosphorus intakes of the enriched formula group were considerably higher than intakes of the term formula group.

The latest study comparing growth of preterm infants fed term versus postdischarge formula after hospital discharge showed no advantage of the postdischarge formula; in fact, it showed an apparent advantage of the term formula.[44] In this study, infants with a median birthweight and gestational age of 1,250 g (range 630 to 1,620 g) and 29 weeks (range 24 to 34 weeks), respectively, were assigned randomly at discharge to receive one of the two formulas for a year after discharge. During this time, those assigned to the term formula weighed from 352 g (at 2 mo of age) to 864 g (at 9 mo of age) more than those assigned to the postdischarge formula, were from 1.0 cm (at 2 mo of age) to 2.7 cm (at 9 mo of age) longer and had a 0.8 cm (at 2 mo of age) to 1.1 cm (at 4 and 9 mo of age) greater head circumference. Unfortunately, no intake data were obtained.

This study also included serial measurements of body composition by dual-energy X-ray absorptiometry, which showed that the term formula group had slightly higher bone mineral content, fat mass, and lean mass than the postdischarge formula group. However, after controlling for birthweight, the term formula group had a slightly higher fat mass percent and a somewhat lower lean mass percent.

Only one study has evaluated continuation of preterm formula postdischarge. In this study, Cooke et al assigned formula-fed infants (BW <1,750 g) at discharge to one of three postdischarge feeding regimens: A preterm formula from discharge through 6 months corrected age; A term formula for the same period; A preterm formula from discharge to term followed by a term formula through 6 months corrected age.[45,46] Growth was monitored frequently through

6 months corrected age and, then, at 12 and 18 months of age. Differences in weight between male infants assigned to the preterm versus the term formula are shown in Table 6. Although the study formulas were terminated at 6 months of age, the group that received the preterm formula during this time was heavier than the group that received the term formula at all ages studied from term through 18 months corrected age. Moreover, the advantages of the preterm formula over the term formula were much more marked than those observed by Carver et al and Lucas et al in preterm infants assigned to a postdischarge versus a term formula.[39,40] This most likely reflects the greater protein content of the preterm versus postdischarge formulas and the difference in protein intake between the two groups (close to 1 g/kg/d in the study of Cooke et al versus <0.5 g/kg/d in the study of Carver et al). Also of note is that the early advantages of the preterm formula, which were noted as early as term, persisted for up to a year after the assigned formula was terminated. At 18 months of age, male infants assigned to the preterm formula through 6 months of age were 1,000 g heavier, 2 cm longer, and had a 1 cm greater head circumference than those assigned to the term formula for the same period. Interestingly, Cooke et al observed no difference in growth of female infants assigned the preterm versus the term formula. They also observed no statistically significant differences in Bayley MDI or PDI scores between the preterm and term formula groups at 18 months of age.

Considering the fact that the advantages of the nutrient-enriched formula observed by Cooke et al, Carver et al, and Lucas et al were apparent by term or shortly thereafter with no apparent subsequent advantage, it is surprising that Cooke et al did not observe a difference in growth between infants assigned to the preterm formula from discharge to term followed by the term formula until 6 months of age versus those assigned to the term formula for the entire period. This may reflect the fact that intake of the combined group was lower from term until 8 weeks corrected age.

Table 6 Differences in Mean Weight Between Preterm Male Infants Assigned to a Preterm Formula versus a Standard Term Formula from Discharge to 6 Months of Age.[45,46]

Age	ΔWeight (g)*
Birth	−9
Enrollment	118
Term	700
4 weeks	900
8 wk	800
12 wk	800
4 mo	700
5 mo	700
6 mo	1,000
12 mo	960
18 mo	1,000

*All differences from term through 18 months of age are statistically significant ($p < .05$).

In conclusion, the studies described above demonstrate that most LBW infants, regardless of how they are fed postdischarge, eventually catch-up, although not completely. The majority of the studies also suggest that feeding nutrient-enriched formulas postdischarge confers some advantage with respect to growth not only during the time they are fed, but also up to 12 months after the formula is stopped. Interestingly, none of the studies that included neurodevelopmental assessment showed a developmental advantage of the postdischarge formula[40,42,46] and one such study in term SGA infants showed a developmental disadvantage for females at 9, but not 18 months postterm.

In most studies, the growth advantage of the postdischarge formula is apparent quite early and, despite continuation of the formula, does not increase. This suggests that there is a finite period during which catch-up in response to higher nutrient intakes is most likely. This period appears to include the time from discharge through term and, perhaps, the first 1 to 2 months postterm. If so, it is likely that feeding even higher protein and energy intakes than provided by currently available preterm formulas and fortified human milk during hospitalization and at least through 40 to 48 weeks postmenstrual age (PMA) will be the most effective strategy. However, the failure of Cooke et al to observe a growth advantage of feeding the postdischarge formula from discharge to term suggests otherwise.

The concept that there may be a finite period during which response to higher nutrient intakes is optimal, is consistent with findings that muscle protein synthesis of both rats and pigs is more responsive to protein intake shortly after birth than at weaning.[47,48] Further, at a constant protein intake, muscle protein synthesis of piglets also is more responsive to exogenous insulin during the newborn period than at weaning.[49]

APPROACH TO POSTDISCHARGE NUTRITION

It is clear from the foregoing section that there is no universally acceptable approach to postdischarge nutritional management of preterm infants. The majority of studies addressing this issue indicate that postdischarge growth of infants fed a nutrient-enriched formula is somewhat greater than that of infants fed a formula intended for term infants or unsupplemented human milk. However, there are a few exceptions—eg, the study of Koo et al[44] comparing a postdischarge versus a term formula and the study of Fewtrell et al,[41] in term SGA infants that showed an advantage for length and head circumference but not weight. Further, a Cochrane review of the same studies discussed above showed that the only statistically significant difference in growth was a <1 cm greater length in those who received a postdischarge versus a term formula but many of the studies discussed above did not meet the criteria for inclusion in the meta-analysis.[50] Moreover, most studies indicate that growth advantages of the postdischarge formula either are greater in male infants or are limited to male infants; female infants experience either no advantage or a very limited advantage.

Despite the lack of a clear advantage of the nutrient-enriched postdischarge formulas for all preterm infants, most discussions of postdischarge nutrition recommend that preterm infants be discharged on a postdischarge formula.[5,51–53] However, there is less agreement concerning how long the postdischarge formula should be continued. Some recommend 6 months, some 9 months, and some as long as a year but data supporting any of these periods are limited. A priori, it seems reasonable to continue the nutrient-enriched formula until the infant's weight is near the fiftieth percentile for postmenstrual age. Those advocating a longer duration of feeding such formulas cite the need to provide sufficient nutrients to allow the infant to reach his or her growth potential which, for some infants, is obviously greater than the fiftieth percentile for postmenstrual age. However, the growth potential of others is obviously less than the fiftieth percentile for postmenstrual age.

A review of the studies cited above indicates that the growth advantage of a preterm versus a term formula is greater than that of a postdischarge versus a term formula. However, preterm formulas are intended for use during hospitalization and are both expensive and difficult to obtain for postdischarge use. Moreover, use of these formulas postdischarge constitutes an "off-label" use. Since preterm formulas contain more of some vitamins and minerals than postdischarge formulas, there is concern that the intakes of these nutrients may be excessive. However, Cooke et al[45,46] observed no problems in infants fed a preterm formula during hospitalization and until 6 months postterm.

An increasing number of preterm infants are fed human milk during hospitalization and the parents of many of these wish to breast-feed the infant after discharge. The postdischarge nutritional management of these infants is particularly problematic. While there are clear developmental and other advantages of breastfeeding, growth of breast-fed infants is inferior to that of infants fed a preterm, a postdischarge or, even, a term formula. Moreover, the common in-hospital practice of fortifying human milk with a breast milk fortifier is less likely to be successful postdischarge and, further, is likely to interfere with the natural lactation/breastfeeding process. Since most breast-fed infants receive some formula the most common recommendation is to continue breastfeeding, but provide at least one bottle of nutrient-enriched formula daily. There are few, if any, data available concerning the efficacy of this approach but it is clear that a single bottle of nutrient-enriched formula per day will not provide the same nutrient intakes provided by exclusive feeding of a nutrient-enriched formula. The number of feedings of nutrient-enriched formula provided, of course, can be increased but more than about two such feedings per day is likely to interfere with breast milk production and/or diminish the beneficial effects of breastfeeding.

An alternative approach is to start complementary feedings earlier than usually recommended (ie, when the infant weighs 5 kg, has lost the extrusion reflex and is able to eat from a spoon).[54] This approach has some appeal but, in term infants, developmental readiness for complementary feedings (eg, able to sit unassisted) is considered a better indicator for starting complementary foods than a specific weight or age.[55] Further, it is likely that some infants will be ready for complementary foods before they weigh 5 kg whereas others may not be ready at 5 kg. Finally, complementary feedings should be started early enough to help the infant develop tastes for several foods and become accustomed to different textures but not earlier than developmentally ready. Unfortunately, very little is known about any aspect of complementary feeding of term infants and even less is known bout this issue in preterm infants.

There are a few "official" guidelines or recommendations for postdischarge nutritional management of preterm infants. The American Academy of Pediatrics (AAP) appears to endorse use of postdischarge formulas, but provides no specific recommendations.[56] The European society of Pediatric Gastroenterology, Hepatology and Nutrition (ESPGHAN) Committee on Nutrition is somewhat more specific.[57] This Committee recommends that infants whose weight are appropriate for postmenstrual age at discharge (likely to be a very small number depending upon how "appropriate for postmenstrual age" is defined) be breast-fed when possible or fed a standard term formula. It further recommends that infants with a subnormal weight for postmenstrual age at discharge, if breast-fed, should be supplemented to provide an adequate intake of all nutrients (eg, with a breast milk fortifier). If formula-fed, the Committee recommends a postdischarge formula at least until a postconceptional age of 40 weeks and possibly longer. The Committee states that further research is required to determine the specific nutrient needs of infants with both prenatal and postnatal growth restriction and to evaluate the effects of nutritional interventions on long-term growth as well as neurodevelopmental and other health outcomes.

In summary, a number of studies have addressed the possibility of improving growth of preterm infants postdischarge. The majority of these have compared growth of infants assigned at discharge to receive a conventional term formula or a postdischarge formula for varying periods, usually 9 to 12 months but at least one study has compared growth of infants assigned at discharge to continue the preterm formula or be switched to a conventional term formula. Most of these studies have shown some growth advantage of the nutrient-enriched formula, up to 1,000 g for the preterm versus the term formula and up to 300 to 500 g for the postdischarge versus the term formula. These advantages were apparent after a few weeks and did not increase further despite continuation of the enriched formula but the growth advantage persisted for up to a year after the enriched formula was stopped. Some studies have included a reference group of breast-fed infants whose growth, in most studies, was less than that of infants fed the term formula but whose neurodevelopmental status at 18 months of age was superior to that of either formula group. These studies do not indicate clearly that any postdischarge feeding strategy is more efficacious than another. However, most authors recommend that the postdischarge formulas be used routinely or that breast-fed infants receive a nutrient supplement, which of course is problematical and may interfere with normal lactation and breastfeeding. Clearly, as concluded by the ESPGHAN Committee on Nutrition, more studies are needed in order to support any single recommendation for feeding preterm infants postdischarge.

REFERENCES

1. American Academy of Pediatrics, Committee on Nutrition. Nutritional needs of low birth weight infants. Pediatrics 1985;75:976–86.
2. Kashyap S, Schulze KF, Forsyth M, et al. Growth, nutrient retention, and metabolic response in low birth weight infants fed varying intakes of protein and energy. J Pediatr 1988;113:713–21.
3. Alexander GR, Himes JH, Kaufman RB, et al. A United States national reference for fetal growth. Am J Obstet Gynecol 1996;87:163–8.
4. Ehrenkranz RA, Younes N, Lemons JA, et al. Longitudinal growth of hospitalized very low birth weight infants. Pediatrics 1999;104:280–9.
5. Dusick AM, Poindexter BB, Ehrenkranz RA, Lemons JA. Growth failure in the preterm infant: Can we catch up? Semin Perinatol 2003;27:302–10.
6. Van Der Wagen A, Okken A, Zweens J, Zulstra WG. Composition of postnatal weight loss and subsequent weight gain in small for dates newborn infants. Acta Paediatr Scand 1985;74:57–61.
7. Anderson TL, Muttart C, Bieber MA, et al. A controlled trial of glucose vs. glucose amino acids in premature infants. J Pediatr 1979;94:947–51.
8. Saini J, MacMahon P, Morgan JB, Kovar IZ. Early parenteral feeding of amino acids. Arch Dis Child 1989;64:1362–6.
9. Mitton SG, Calder AG, Garlick PJ. Protein turnover rates in sick, premature neonates during the first few days of life. Pediatr Res 1991;30:418–22.
10. Mitton SG, Garlick PJ. Changes in protein turnover after the introduction of parenteral nutrition in premature infants: Comparison of breast milk and egg protein-based amino acid solutions. Pediatr Res 1992;32:447–54.
11. van Lingen RA, van Goudoever JB, Luijendijk IHT, et al. Effects of early amino acid administration during total parenteral nutrition on protein metabolism in pre-term infants. Clin Sci 1992;82:199–203.
12. Rivera A, Bell EF, Bier DM. Effect of intravenous amino acids on protein metabolism of preterm infants during the first three days of life. Pediatr Res 1993;33:106–11.
13. van Goudoever JB, Colen T, Wattimena JLD, et al. Immediate commencement of amino acid supplementation in preterm infants: Effect on serum amino acid concentrations and protein kinetics on the first day of life. J Pediatr 1995;127:458–65.
14. Kashyap S, Heird WC. Protein requirements of low birthweight, very low birthweight, and small for gestational age infants. In: Räihä NCR, editor. Protein Metabolism During Infancy. New York: Raven Press; 1994. p. 133–46.
15. Thureen P, Melara D, Fennessey PV, Hay WW, Jr. Effect of low versus high intravenous amino acid intake on very low birth weight infants in the early neonatal period. Pediatr Res 2003;53:24–32.
16. Ashworth A. Effects of intrauterine growth retardation on mortality and morbidity in infants and young children. Eur J Clin Nutr 1998;52:S34–42.
17. Martorell R, Ramakrishnan U, Schroeder DG, et al. Intrauterine growth retardation, body size, body composition and physical performance in adolescence. Eur J Clin Nutr 1998;52:S43–53.
18. Martorell R. Undernutrition during pregnancy and early childhood and its consequences for cognitive and behavioral development. In: Young ME, editor. Investing in Our Children's Future. Amsterdam: Elsevier; 1997. p. 39–83.
19. Dobbing J. Nutritional growth restriction and the nervous system. In: Davison AN, Thompson RHS, editors. The Molecular Bases of Neuropathology. London: Edward Arnold; 1981. p. 221–33.
20. Dobbing J, Sands J. Comparative aspects of the brain growth spurt. Early Hum Dev 1970;3:79–83.
21. Hack M, Breslau N, Weissman B, et al. Effect of very low birthweight and subnormal head size on cognitive abilities at school age. NEJM 1991;325:231–37.
22. Lucas A, Morley R, Cole TJ, et al. Early diet in preterm babies and developmental status at 18 months. Lancet 1990;335:1477–81.
23. Lucas A, Morley R, Cole TJ. Randomised trial of early diet in preterm babies and later intelligence quotient. Br Med J 1998;317:1481–7.
24. Zlotkin SH, Bryan MH, Anderson GH. Intravenous nitrogen intakes and energy intakes required to duplicate in utero nitrogen accretion in prematurely born human infants. J Pediatr 1981;99:115–20.
25. Embleton NE, Pang N, Cooke RJ. Postnatal malnutrition and growth retardation: An inevitable consequence of current recommendations in preterm infants? Pediatrics 2001;107:270–3.
26. Forbes GB. A note on the mathematics of catch-up growth. Pediatr Res 1974;8:929–31.
27. Kashyap S, Schulze KF, Ramakrishnan R, et al. Evaluation of a mathematical model for predicting the relationship between protein and energy intakes of low-birth-weight infants and the rate and composition of weight gain. Pediatr Res 1994;35:704–12.
28. Ziegler EE, O'Donnell AM, Nelson SE, Fomon SJ. Body composition of the reference fetus. Growth 1976;40:329.
29. Goldman HI, Freudenthal R, Holland B, Karelitz S. Clinical effects of two different levels of protein intake on low birth weight infants. J Pediatr 1969;74:881–9.
30. Goldman HI, Liebman OB, Freudenthal R, Reuben R. Effects of early dietary protein intake on low-birth-weight infants: Evaluation at 3 years of age. J Pediatr 1971;78:126–9.
31. Singhal A, Cole TJ, Lucas A. Early nutrition in preterm infants and later blood pressure: two cohorts after randomised trials. Lancet 2001;357:413–9.
32. Singhal A, Fewtrell M, Cole TJ, Lucas A. Low nutrient intake and early growth for later insulin resistance in adolescents born preterm. Lancet 2003;361:1089–97.
33. Singhal A, Sadaf Farooqi I, O'Rahilly S, et al. Early nutrition and leptin concentrations in later life. Am J Clin Nutr 2002;75:993–9.
34. Singhal A, Cole TJ, Fewtrell M, et al. Is slower early growth beneficial for long-term cardiovascular health. Circulation 2004;109:1108–13.
35. Hack M, Weissman B, Borawski-Clark E. Catch-up growth during childhood among very low-birth-weight children. Arch Pediatr Adoles Med 1996;150:1122–29.
36. Peralta-Carcelen M, Jackson DS, Goran MI, et al. Growth of adolescents who were born at extremely low birth weight without major disability. J Pediatr 2000;136:633–40.
37. Lucas A, Bishop NJ, Cole TJ. Randomized trial of nutrition for preterm infants after discharge. Arch Dis Child 1992;67:324–7.
38. Chan GM. Growth and bone mineral status of discharged very low birth weight infants fed different formulas or human milk. J Pediatr 1993;123:439–43.
39. Carver JD, Wu PYK, Hall RT, et al. Growth of preterm infants fed nutrient-enriched or term formula after hospital discharge. Pediatrics 2001;107:683–9.
40. Lucas A, Fewtrell MS, Morley R, et al. Randomized trial of nutrient-enriched formula versus standard formula for postdischarge preterm infants. Pediatrics 2001;108: 703–11.
41. Fewtrell MS, Morley R, Abbott RA, et al. Catch-up growth in small-for-gestational-age term infants: A randomized trial. Am J Clin Nutr 2001;74:516–23.
42. Morley R, Fewtrell MS, Abbott RA, et al. Neurodevelopment in children born small for gestational age: A randomized trial of nutrient-enriched versus standard formula and comparison with a reference breastfed group. Pediatrics 2004;113:515–21.
43. Wheeler RE, Hall RT. Feeding of premature infant formula after hospital discharge of infants weighing less than 1800 grams at birth. J Perinatol 1996;16:111–6.
44. Koo WWK, Hockman EM. Posthospital discharge feeding for preterm infants: Effects of standard compared with enriched milk formula on growth, bone mass, and body composition. Am J Clin Nutr 2006;84:1357–64.

45. Cooke RJ, Griffin IJ, McCormick K, et al. Feeding preterm infants after hospital discharge: Effect of dietary manipulation on nutrient intake and growth. Pediatr Res 1998;43:355–60.
46. Cooke RJ, Embleton ND, Griffin IJ, et al. Feeding preterm infants after hospital discharge: Growth and development at 18 months of age. Pediatr Res 2001;49:719–22.
47. Davis TA, Fiorotto ML, Nguyen HV, et al. Response of muscle protein synthesis to fasting in suckling and weaned rats. Am J Physiol 1991;261:R1373–80.
48. Davis TA, Burrin DG, Fiorotto ML, Nguyen HV. Protein synthesis in skeletal muscle and jejunum is more responsive to feeding in 7- than in 26-day-old pigs. Am J Physiol 1996;270:E802–9.
49. Wray-Cahen D, Beckett PR, Nguyen HV, Davis TA. Insulin-stimulated amino acid utilization during glucose and amino acid clamps decreases with development. Am J Physiol 1997;273:E305–14.
50. Henderson G, Fahey T, McGuire W. Calorie and protein-enriched formula versus standard term formula for improving growth and development in preterm or low birth weight infants following hospital discharge. Cochrane Database Syst Rev2005; Issue 2, Art. No.: CD004696.
51. Schanler RJ. Post-discharge nutrition for the preterm infant. Acta Paediatr 2005;94:68–73.
52. Fewtrell MS. Growth and nutrition after discharge. Semin Neonatol 2003;8:169–76.
53. Greer FR. Feeding the preterm infant after hospital discharge. Pediatr Ann 2001;30:658–65.
54. Department of Health. Weaning and the Weaning Diet. Report on Health and Subjects No. 45. London: HMSO; 1994.
55. Butte N, Cobb K, Dwyer J, Graney L, Heird W, Rickard K. The start healthy feeding guidelines for infants and toddlers. J Am Diet Assoc 2004;104:442–54.
56. The Committee on Nutrition, American Academy of Pediatrics. Nutritional needs of preterm infants. In: Pediatric Nutrition Handbook, 5th edition. IL, USA: American Academy of Pediatrics; 2004. p. 72–3.
57. Aggett PJ, Agostoni C, Axelsson I, et al. for the ESPGHAN Committee on Nutrition. Feeding preterm infants after hospital discharge: A commentary by the ESPGHAN Committee on Nutrition. J Pediatr Gastroenterol Nutr 2006;42:596–603.

The Term Infant

Ekhard E. Ziegler, MD
Samuel J. Fomon, MD
Susan J. Carlson, MMSc, RD

THE GOALS OF INFANT FEEDING

The goals of infant feeding are to meet all nutritional needs, to aid mother–infant bonding, to aid the infant in making the transition from the predominantly liquid diet of the infant to the predominantly solid food diet of the child and adult, and to aid in establishing habits of eating in moderation. The goals can best be met by breast feeding. However, in industrialized countries, feeding of commercially available infant formulas, although not ideal, is an acceptable substitute. Breast feeding, besides meeting all nutritional needs, offers protection against infectious illnesses, may foster optimal neurocognitive development, and may offer some protection against conditions in adulthood such as obesity and atherosclerosis. Whether feeding practices during infancy can aid in establishing the goal of eating in moderation is unknown. Nevertheless, in various animal models habits established during infancy have been difficult to extinguish later in life, and it therefore seems plausible that habits of eating in moderation should be established during infancy because they may facilitate eating in moderation later in life.

TRENDS IN INFANT FEEDING

Historically, in situations where breast feeding was not possible, survival of the infant was in jeopardy. The feeding of preparations based on various mammalian milks was associated with high morbidity and mortality. Success at formula feeding gradually improved from the end of the nineteenth century through the first half of the nineteenth century. The objective was to make available safe and effective feedings for situations where breast milk was not available. In the 1920s the use of evaporated milk for formula preparation together with a number of improvements in formula preparation and storage contributed to successful formula feeding. By the 1950s, formulas reached a point where they provided adequate nutrition and appeared to be reasonably safe. In the absence of convincing evidence of the inferiority of formula feeding, many parents and physicians adopted formula feeding, presumably because of the supposed greater convenience. The prevalence of formula feeding increased and the prevalence of breast feeding decreased.

The decrease in the prevalence of breast feeding was associated with earlier introduction into the infant's diet of complementary foods and cow's milk. By the end of the 1950s, feeding of complementary foods was common during the first month of life and most infants were fed complementary foods before the end of the second month of life. Whole or reduced-fat cow's milk commonly replaced formula by 4 to 6 months of age.[1]

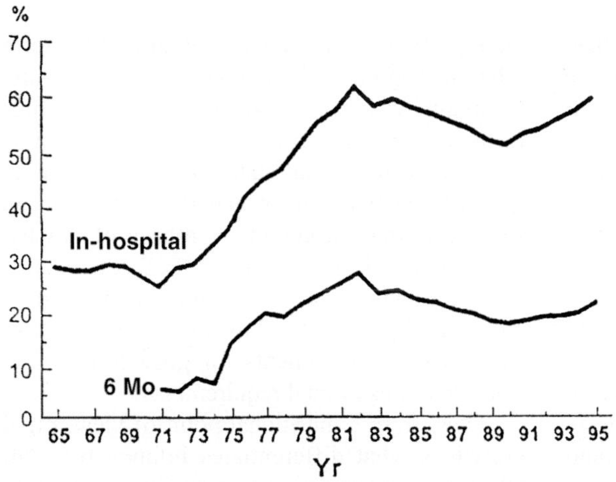

Figure 1 Prevalence of breast-feeding in the United States 1965 through 1995. (With permission from Ryan.[2])

A resurgence of breast feeding began about 1971 (Figure 1). The reason(s) for the initial increase in breast feeding prevalence are poorly understood. But enthusiasm for breast feeding was sustained, at least in part, by the ever-increasing number of reports on the demonstrated or assumed advantages of breast feeding. As Figure 2 indicates, in 2001 about 70% of infants were breast-fed for at least some time. The relatively quick decrease in breast feeding prevalence with age is at least partially explained by mothers' returning to work. Despite the pressures of work, the number of women who breast-feed for 6 months and longer has continued to increase.

In association with the increase in breast feeding, infants were increasingly fed formula after cessation of breast feeding (Figure 3). Thus, formula feeding largely displaced feeding of cow's milk in older infants (Figure 4). Also, complementary foods were less commonly fed during the early months of life and it is now very uncommon to see complementary foods fed before 4 months of age.

Trends in Formula Composition

The formulas fed in the United States in the late 1920s were generally prepared in the home with evaporated milk or fresh cow's milk and sugar.

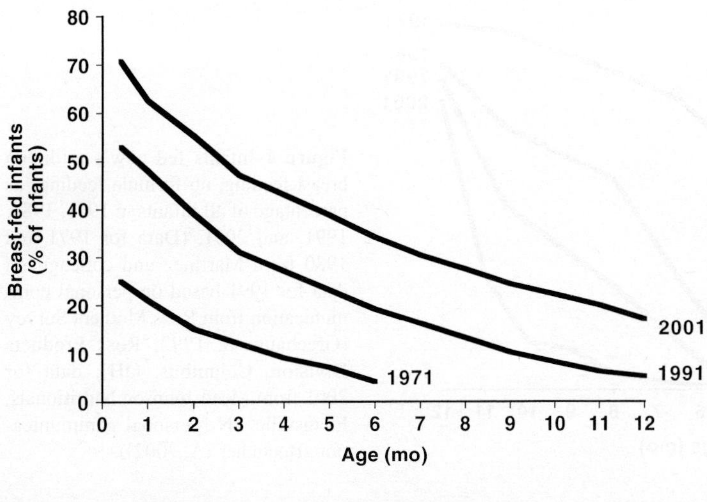

Figure 2 Exclusively and partially breast-fed infants as a percentage of all infants in 1971, 1991, and 2001. (Data for 1971 from Martinez and Nalezienski[3] and for 1991 based on personal communication from Ross Mothers Survey [Greenbaum S, 1992, Ross Products Division, Columbus, OH]; data for 2001 from Mead Johnson Nutritionals, Evansville, IN [personal communication, Boettcher JA, 2002]).

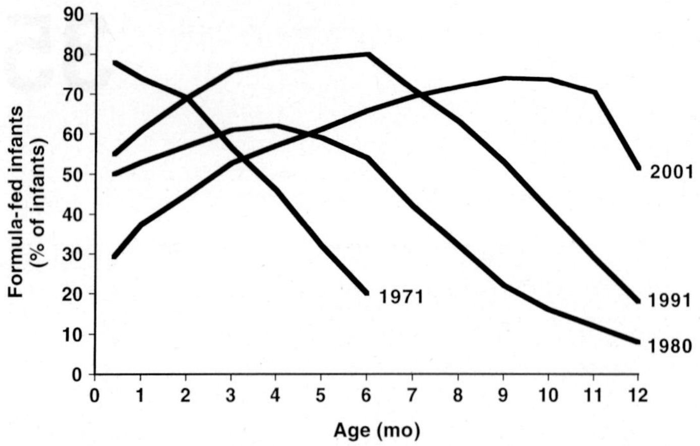

Figure 3 Formula-fed infants (including infants also breast-fed) as percentage of all infants in 1971, 1980, 1991, and 2001. (Data for 1971 and 1980 from Martinez and colleagues[4]; data for 1991 based on personal communication from Ross Mothers Survey [Greenbaum S, 1992, Ross Products Division, Columbus, OH]; data for 2001 from Mead Johnson Nutritionals, Evansville, IN [personal communication, Boettcher JA, 2002]).

The protein content was considerably greater than that of current formulas, the fat was butterfat, the added carbohydrate was corn syrup or sucrose, and neither vitamins nor minerals were added. Prepared powdered formulas (to be diluted with water before use) were available but their use was quite limited until the 1950s. With the introduction of concentrated liquid formulas (requiring only the addition of an equal volume of water before use), commercially prepared formulas gradually replaced home-prepared formulas. Over the years, formulas underwent a number of changes: the protein content was decreased and whey proteins were included to result in a whey protein–casein ratio more like that of human milk; vegetable oils replaced butterfat; the added carbohydrate was lactose rather than corn syrup, and vitamins and minerals were included. See below for detailed composition of currently available formulas.

NUTRIENT REQUIREMENTS

The approach to estimating nutrient requirements of the infant differs considerably from that for adults. The normal adult requires regular intake of energy and specific nutrients to maintain the size and composition of the body (ie, requirements for "maintenance"), whereas infants and young children need, in addition, energy and nutrients for growth. The ratio of need for growth to need for maintenance is greatest for the fetus, the rapidly growing preterm infant and the term infant during the early months of life. Therefore, to obtain reasonable estimates of the requirements for energy and nutrients of the infant, it is desirable to have quantitative data on the increments in energy storage and the increments in specific nutrients needed for synthesis of new tissue. Defining the requirements of energy or nutrients for growth is much less important for children more than 2 years old and for adolescents because by then the requirements for growth are quite small fractions of total requirements.

Thus, from a nutritional point of view, rapid growth is what differentiates infancy from all other ages. Nutrient requirements are exceedingly high primarily because of nutrients needed to support rapid growth. But growth is not only very rapid, it also changes dramatically in velocity as well as in composition. These dynamic changes are illustrated in Figure 5, which depicts rate as well as composition of growth of a "reference infant." The rapid decline in the rate of growth during the first year of life is readily appreciated. It is also evident that during the first 4 months of life, infants deposit large amounts of body fat. During that period fat accounts for as much as 40% of weight gain, and the energy necessary for deposition of this fat accounts for about 20% of energy requirements. Toward the end of the first year of life, fat deposition slows down markedly, and so does the proportion of energy requirement explained by fat deposition. Although accretion of protein as a percentage of weight gain increases with age, absolute protein accretion is highest during the first 2 months of life.

Nutrient requirements of infants are obtained chiefly by two methods: the observational method and the factorial method. Each approach has its difficulties and limitations. The *observational method* relies on the model of the breast-fed infant. The main difficulty with this approach is the determination of representative concentrations of nutrients in breast milk. Concentrations of many nutrients change markedly with the duration of lactation and are in many cases influenced by maternal dietary intakes. Also, the breast-fed infant is not a reliable model in the case of certain nutrients, for example, iron, that are not provided in breast milk in amounts that meet the infant's needs. The *factorial method* yields good estimates for certain nutrients, such as protein, for which estimates of rates of accretion by the infant are available. Nutrient requirements, largely because of the dynamic changes of the needs for growth, are strongly age-dependent. Stating nutrient requirements in relation to energy requirements diminishes the age dependency of nutrient requirements somewhat, but does not eliminate it completely.

Energy Requirement

Because the infant possesses the ability to self-regulate energy intake, it may be assumed that energy intakes observed in infants receiving feedings with normal energy density represent energy requirements. Table 1 presents energy intakes observed in breast-fed and formula-fed infants. The data illustrate the markedly higher energy intakes during the early months of life compared to later infancy, a reflection of the deposition of large amounts of fat as energy stores. The data also show that formula-fed infants consume somewhat more energy than breast-fed infants, especially during the first 3 months of life. Therein may lie (part of) the reason for the somewhat more rapid growth of formula-fed infants. Gender-related differences in energy intake, although quite small, are nevertheless consistently present.

Protein Requirement

Table 2 presents estimates of requirements for protein by the factorial method as well as protein intakes observed in breast-fed infants. The close agreement between the factorial estimate and observed intake is striking. During the first month of life, growth accounts for over 50% of protein requirement. But by the end of the first year of life, the proportion needed for growth is less than 20%.

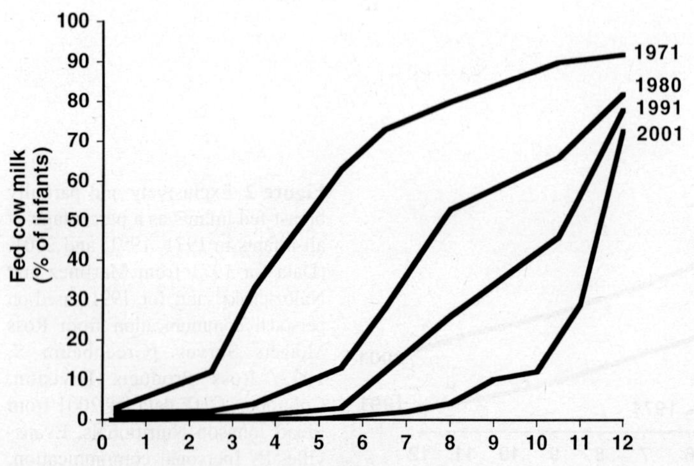

Figure 4 Infants fed cow's milk (no breast feeding, no formula feeding) as percentage of all infants in 1971, 1980, 1991, and 2001. (Data for 1971 and 1980 from Martinez and colleagues[4]; data for 1991 based on personal communication from Ross Mothers Survey [Greebaum S, 1992, Ross Products Division, Columbus, OH]; data for 2001 from Mead Johnson Nutritionals, Evansville, IN [personal communication, Boettcher JA, 2002]).

THE BREAST-FED INFANT

Energy and Protein Intakes

The breast-fed infant receives water, energy, and specific nutrients in amounts that meet the needs of the infant at all times, notwithstanding the fact that the needs change with age of the infant. A prime example is protein. Through a combination of a sharp decrease in protein concentration and an increase in milk volume, a close match between intake of protein and protein requirement is achieved (Table 2). In the case of energy, whose content in breast milk does not change with the duration of lactation, the match between intake and need (Table 1) is achieved solely through a decrease in volume of milk consumed per kilogram of body weight. Most other nutrients fall somewhere between protein and energy, that is, a match between intake and need is brought about through a combination of concentration changes and volume increase. Formulas, on the other hand, must be designed to meet the highest possible needs, that is, those of the youngest infants in the target age group. Consequently, as the infant grows, nutrient intakes from formulas exceed needs by an increasing margin.

Although it is well established that infants generally do not obtain all the milk that is synthesized by the mammary gland,[8] the cause of the failure to consume all the available milk is not known. One possible reason is infant fatigue, since the process of obtaining milk from the breast requires considerable effort on the part of the infant. Whatever the mechanism, failure to consume all available milk may be one of the reasons breast-fed infants consistently consume less energy than formula-fed infants, as shown in Table 1. It has been surmised that because the milk remaining in the breast is not visible to the mother, contrary to formula remaining in the bottle, she may be more prone to stop feeding at the earliest sign of satiety on the part of the infant than if the infant is fed by bottle.

Growth

Formula-fed infants grow more rapidly than breast-fed infants.[9,10] Differences in energy consumption may explain the difference in growth. However, inconsistent with this explanation is the fact that growth is similar during the first 6 weeks of life and only begins to differ significantly thereafter,[9] whereas the difference in energy consumption seems to be largest during the first 2 months of life. Therefore, there may be other explanations. When the average intake is close to the average requirement for a nutrient, there is the likelihood that for some individuals intake falls short of requirement. That is the case for protein (Table 2) and also for zinc,[11] a nutrient whose deficient intake can limit growth. Thus, it is possible that inadequate intakes of protein or zinc, or both, occur among breast-fed infants and explain the slower growth. But it must be stressed that the reason for the growth differential is not actually known. By the same token, it is not known whether there are any long-term consequences, beneficial or detrimental, due to the slower growth of breast-fed infants, or due to the lower nutrient intake that is causing it.

Flavor

Breast milk contains a variety of flavoring substances derived from the maternal diet and there is clear evidence that the infant recognizes flavors and responds to them.[12] Thus, contrary to the formula-fed infant, the breast-fed infant is exposed to a variety of tastes from the earliest age. The nutritional significance of early exposure to flavor variety, perhaps even in the long term, is that it leads to greater acceptance and apparent enjoyment of novel flavors later on.[13,14]

Oligosaccharides

Breast milk contains substantial amounts (5–8 g/L) of oligosaccharides, a complex group of substances derived from lactose.[15,16] These oligosaccharides share similarities with epithelial cell surface carbohydrates and adhesion molecules. They exert a number of important functions, from blocking the adhesion of bacteria to intestinal cell surfaces[17] to being responsible for the predominance of the bifidus flora in the breast-fed infant. Consonant with these important functions is the fact that oligosaccharides are only minimally digested in the upper gastrointestinal tract and undergo fermentation in the colon, thereby

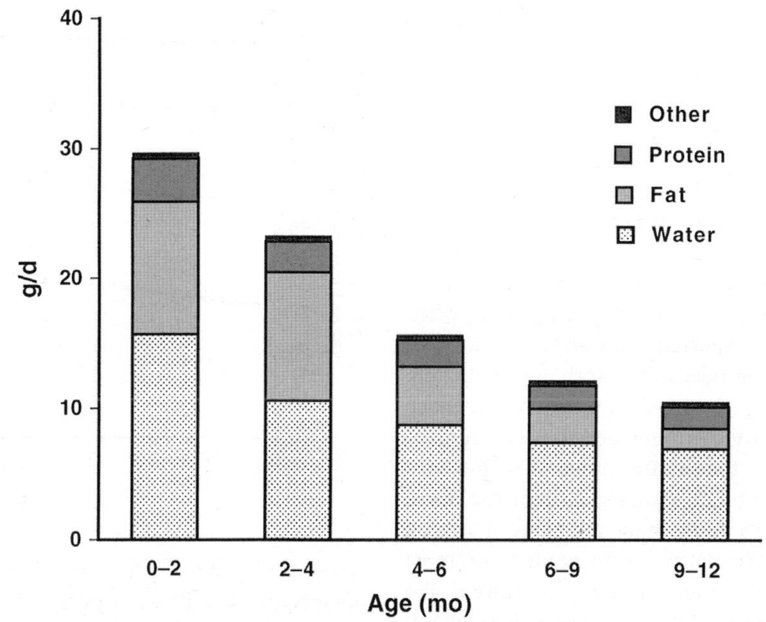

Figure 5 Gain in weight and in major body components of a "reference infant" (an infant with weight and length and body composition at the 50th centile for age). (Based on Fomon and Nelson.[5])

Table 1 Energy Intakes (kcal/kg/d) of Infants

	Breast-Fed		Formaula-Fed			
	Males (mean)	Females (mean)	Males		Females	
Age Interval (mo)			50th	10th–90th	50th	10th–90th
0 to 1	115	111	118	99–137	116	96–136
1 to 2	104	101	113	99–131	111	94–130
2 to 3	95	93	100	88–116	100	87–114
3 to 4	91	91	95	83–106	95	83–107
4 to 5	89	89	94	78–112	97	81–113
5 to 6	86	85	95	64–113	94	78–113
6 to 9	81	81				
9 to 12	92	92				

Modified from reference 6.

Table 2 Protein Requirements of Infants

Age Interval (mo)	Growth (g/kg/d)	Intake of Losses (g/kg/d)	Growth Requirement (g/kg/d)	Breast-fed infant (g/kg/d)	Requirement (g/100 kcal)	Requirement (%)
0 to 1	1.03	0.95	1.98	2.09	1.7	52
1 to 2	0.78	0.93	1.71	1.59	1.5	46
2 to 3	0.56	0.90	1.46	1.18	1.5	38
3 to 4	0.38	0.89	1.27	1.06	1.4	30
4 to 5	0.30	0.88	1.18	1.00	1.3	25
5 to 6	0.29	0.89	1.18	0.95	1.3	24
6 to 9	0.26	0.91	1.17		1.3	22
9 to 12	0.20	0.94	1.14		1.2	18

From reference 7.

accounting for much of the hydrogen gas that is exhaled by breast-fed infants.

Iron

Most infants are born with generous iron stores that render him or her independent of an exogenous supply of iron for the first 5 to 6 months of life. Breast milk provides a small amount of highly bioavailable iron that allows the infant to absorb about 0.15 mg each day. Beginning when iron stores are exhausted at around 5 to 6 months of age, the infant needs to absorb approximately 0.75 mg each day to avoid iron deficiency. Since breast milk provides only about 0.15 mg/d of absorbed iron, the infant must absorb about 0.6 mg/d from other sources. Except for meat, which provides a highly bioavailable form of iron (heme iron), the natural iron content of most complementary foods is low. Therefore, the breast-fed infant can obtain an adequate intake of iron, besides meat, only from iron-fortified foods such as infant cereals. Other options for securing an adequate iron intake include medicinal iron and iron-fortified formula. Although none of these options has ever been demonstrated to be effective in preventing iron deficiency during prolonged breast feeding, prudence nevertheless dictates that attention be paid to ensuring an adequate intake of iron for breast-fed infants. Concerns that exogenous iron might exert adverse effects on the infant are theoretical in nature.

Some infants are born with diminished iron stores[18] and these infants may become dependent on an exogenous iron supply sooner than infants born with more generous iron stores. Because these infants may be prone to developing iron deficiency at a young age and thus be particularly vulnerable to the adverse effects of iron deficiency, it is advisable to start ensuring an adequate iron intake for all infants beginning at 4 months of age.

FORMULAS

Formulas provide macronutrients and micronutrients in amounts and proportions that permit infants to grow normally. Like breast milk, formulas provide energy in roughly equal amounts from carbohydrate and fat. Contrary to breast milk, the protein level is fixed and set at a level that meets the needs of the fastest-growing infants within the target age group. Formulas provide water in amounts that allow the infant to dispose of waste products with a satisfactory margin of safety. Owing to the higher potential renal solute load of formulas,[19] that margin is somewhat narrower than in the breast-fed infant, a difference that is not known to be of clinical consequence.

An enumeration of the myriad substances that are provided by breast milk but are absent from formulas is beyond the scope of this chapter. A number of substances, including macrominerals, trace minerals, and vitamins, are provided in formulas in greater concentration than in breast milk. Some substances that are believed to be biologically important for the infant are added to formulas in amounts similar to breast milk. Some formulas, notably the soy protein-based formulas, provide substances that are not provided by breast milk. Of considerable nutritional importance is the presence of *phytate* because of its potential to inhibit the absorption of macrominerals and, especially, trace minerals. A group of substances collectively referred to as *phytoestrogens* is provided by soy formulas.[20] These substances are not nutritionally important but are biologically active, exerting estrogenic as well as antiestrogenic activities. Phytoestrogens are readily absorbed by the infant[20] but produce no clinically or otherwise recognizable effects. When followed into young adulthood, women who had been exposed to soy formulas as infants had somewhat greater menstrual flow and experienced more discomfort with menstruation.[21] Although these effects are not clinically important, they are biologically significant because they demonstrate that relatively brief exposure during a susceptible period can have effects that last for decades.

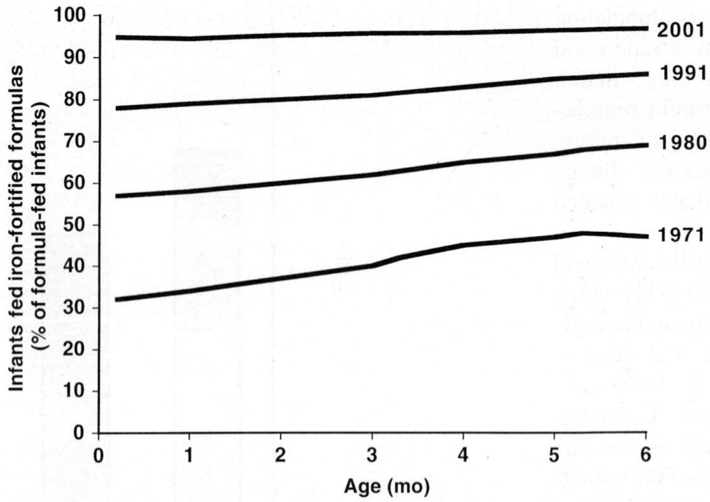

Figure 6 Infants fed iron-fortified formulas as percentage of formula-fed infants in 1971, 1980, 1991, and 2001. (Data for 1971 and 1980 from Martinez and colleagues[4]; data for 1991 based on personal communication from Ross Mothers Survey [Greebaum S, 1992, Ross Products Division, Columbus, OH]; data for 2001 from Mead Johnson Nutritionals, Evansville, IN [personal communication, Boettcher JA, 2002]).

Carbohydrates. Milk-based formulas currently contain lactose as the sole carbohydrate and lack the oligosaccharides that make up a substantial proportion of the carbohydrate of breast milk. Formulas may, however, in the future contain a limited number of oligosaccharides. Oligosaccharides are responsible in large part for the differences in colonic flora between breast-fed and formula-fed infants. Although they are essentially unabsorbable in the upper gastrointestinal tract, the colonic microflora is quite effective in fermenting the oligosaccharides. The fermentation products, acetate and butyrate, are absorbed from the colon.

The *fat* of formulas is made up of various combinations of plant oils, selected to provide major fatty acids in approximately the proportions found in breast milk. The absorbability of the fat of formulas is similar to that of breast milk fat. Many formulas contain added polyunsaturated fatty acids (arachidonic acid and docosahexaenoic acid) from single-cell organisms.

Protein. Although formulas provide bulk casein and whey proteins in approximately the same proportions as breast milk, the individual whey proteins show little resemblance to those provided in breast milk. Manufacturers are able to selectively decrease and/or increase individual whey proteins and thereby alter the biologic quality and amino acid composition of the protein mix. The protein concentration of formulas is set to meet the highest needs, that is, those of the youngest infants in the target age group. Consequently, older infants in the formulas' target group, who have lower protein needs than the younger infants, receive protein intakes that exceed their needs by some margin. In contrast, breast-fed infants receive protein intakes that approximately match their needs at all times.

Iron. Formulas fortified with quite large amounts of iron (1.8 mg/100 kcal) were introduced in 1959 and were shown to be effective in preventing iron deficiency. Although non–iron-fortified formulas continued to be used, the use of formulas providing iron at 1.8 mg/100 kcal gradually increased, as illustrated in Figure 6. In 1971 iron-fortified formulas accounted for less than 50% of formula sales in the United States, and in the year 2001 they accounted for about 95% of formula sales. At present, all formulas contain added iron. Some of the routine formulas are available with an iron level of about 0.6 mg/100 kcal. These formulas are not labeled as iron fortified. All other formulas provide iron at 1.8 mg/100 kcal. Iron fortification is not associated with adverse effects on gastrointestinal function.[22]

Formula Composition

The formulas for *routine use* are rather uniform in composition, as is evident from Table 3. Some formulas provide partially hydrolyzed whey proteins. The latter type of formula is sometimes referred to as "hypoallergenic." Formulas whose iron content is listed as 1.8 mg/100 kcal bear the designation "with iron." They are also available without that designation, in which case the level of fortification iron is 0.6 mg/100 kcal.

The composition of *lactose-free formulas* is listed in Table 4. While those based on soy protein isolate (with methionine supplementation) have been available for many years, those based on cow's milk have been introduced more recently. Although the scientific basis for the widespread use of these formulas is uncertain, it is fairly certain that these formulas provide all essential nutrients and support normal growth. The carbohydrates

Table 3 Formulas for Routine Infant Feeding

Formula	Manu-facturer	Protein: Source	Protein: g/100 kcal (g/dL)	CHO: Source	CHO: g/100 kcal (g/dL)	Fat: Source	Fat: g/100 kcal (g/dL)	Sodium: mEq/100 kcal (mEq/dL)	Potassium: mEq/100 kcal (mEq/dL)	Calcium: mg/100 kcal (mg/dL)	Phosphorus: mg/100 kcal (mg/dL)	Iron: mg/100 kcal (mg/dL)	Osmolality mOsm/kg
Enfamil +/− Lipil	Mead Johnson	Reduced minerals whey and nonfat milk	2.1 (1.4)	Lactose	10.9 (7.5)	Palm olein, soy, coconut, high-oleic sunflower, +/− DHA, ARA	5.3 (3.5)	1.2 (0.8)	2.8 (1.9)	78 (53)	43 (29)	1.8 (1.2)	300
Enfamil Gentlease Lipil	Mead Johnson	Partially hydrolyzed nonfat milk and whey protein	2.3 (1.5)	Lactose and corn syrup solids	10.8 (7.2)	Palm olein soy, coconut, high-oleic sunflower, DHA, ARA	5.3 (3.5)	1.4 (0.9)	2.8 (1.9)	82 (55)	46 (31)	1.8 (1.2)	220
Similac +/− Advance	Ross	Nonfat milk and whey protein concentrate	2.1 (1.4)	Lactose	10.8 (7.3)	High-oleic safflower, soy, coconut, +/− DHA, ARA	5.4 (3.6)	1.0 (0.7)	2.7 (1.8)	78 (53)	42 (28)	1.8 (1.2)	300
Good Start Essentials	Nestlé	Demineralized whey fraction and skim milk	2.2 (1.4)	Lactose, maltodextrin	11.2 (7.4)	Palm olein, soy, coconut, high-oleic safflower	5.1 (3.4)	1.2 (0.8)	2.8 (1.9	64 (43)	36 (24)	1.5 (1)	265
Good Start Supreme +/− DHA and ARA '+/− Natural cultures	Nestlé	Partially hydrolyzed whey	2.2 (1.5)	Lactose, maltodextrin	11.2 (7.4)	Palm olein, soy, coconut, high-oleic safflower, +/− DHA, ARA	5.1 (3.4)	1.2 (0.8)	2.8 (1.9)	64 (43)	36 (24)	1.5 (1)	265
Store brand generic +/− organic	PBM Products	Nonfat milk and whey protein concentrate	2.2 (1.5)	Lactose	10.6 (7.2)	Palm, coconut, oleic, soy, +/− DHA , ARA	5.3 (3.5)	0.9 (0.6)	2.1 (1.4)	63 (43)	42 (28)	1.8 (1.2)	280

Table 4 Lactose-Free Formulas

Formula	Manu-facturer	Protein: Source	Protein: g/100 kcal (g/dL)	Carbohydrate: Source	Carbohydrate: g/100 kcal (g/dL)	Fat: Source	Fat: g/100 kcal (g/dL)	Sodium: mEq/100 kcal (mEq/dL)	Potassium: mEq/100 kcal (mEq/dL)	Calcium: mg/100 kcal (mg/dL)	Phosphorus: mg/100 kcal (mg/dL)	Iron: mg/100 kcal (mg/dL)	Osmolality mOsm/kg
Cow milk based													
Lactofree Lipil	Mead Johnson	Milk protein isolate	2.1 (1.5)	Corn syrup solids	10.9 (7.3)	Palm olein, soy, coconut, high-oleic sunflower, DHA, ARA	5.3 (3.6)	1.3 (0.9)	2.8 (1.9)	82 (55)	46 (31)	1.8 (1.2)	200
Similac Lactose Free Advance	Ross	Milk protein Isolate	2.1 (1.5)	Corn syrup solids, sucrose	10.7 (7.2)	Soy, high-oleic safflower, coconut, DHA, ARA	5.4 (3.6)	1.3 (0.9)	2.7 (1.8)	84 (57)	56 (38)	1.8 (1.2)	200
Soy protein based													
Good Start Supreme Soy DHA, ARA	Nestlé	Hydrolyzed soy protein isolate	2.5 (1.7)	Maltodextrin, sucrose	11.1 (7.4)	Palm olein, soy, coconut, high-oleic safflower, DHA, ARA	5.1 (3.4)	1.7 (1.1)	3.0 (2.0)	105 (70)	63 (43)	1.8 (1.2)	200
Isomil	Ross	Soy protein isolate	2.4 (1.6)	Corn syrup solids, sucrose	10.3 (7.0)	High-oleic safflower, soy, coconut	5.5 (3.7)	1.9 (1.3)	2.8 (1.9)	105 (71)	75 (51)	1.8 (1.2)	200
ProSobee +/− Lipil	Mead Johnson	Soy protein isolate	2.5 (1.7)	Corn syrup solids	10.6 (7.2)	Palm olein, soy, coconut, high-oleic sunflower, +/- DHA, ARA	5.3 (3.6)	1.6 (1.0)	3.1 (2.1)	105 (71)	69 (46)	1.8 (1.2)	200
Store brand generic	PBM Products	Soy protein isolate	2.7 (1.8)	Corn syrup solids, sucrose	10.4 (6.9)	Palm, coconut, oleic, soy	5.3 (3.6)	1.3 (0.9)	2.7 (1.8)	90 (61)	63 (43)	1.8 (1.2)	200

Table 5 Extensively Hydrolyzed Protein and Elemental Formulas

Formula	Manufacturer	Protein Source	Protein g/100 kcal (g/dL)	Carbohydrate Source	Carbohydrate g/100 kcal (g/dL)	Fat Source	Fat g/100 kcal (g/dL)	Sodium mEq/100 kcal (mEq/dL)	Potassium mEq/100 kcal (mEq/dL)	Calcium mg/100 kcal (mg/dL)	Phosphorus mg/100 kcal (mg/dL)	Iron mg/100 kcal (mg/dL)	Osmolality mOsm/kg
Protein hydrolysate													
Nutramigen Lipil	Mead Johnson	Extensively hydrolyzed casein	2.8 (1.9)	Corn syrup solids, modified corn starch	10.3 (6.9)	Palm olein, soy, coconut, high-oleic sunflower, DHA, ARA	5.3 (3.5)	2.0 (1.4)	2.8 (1.9)	94 (64)	52 (35)	1.8 (1.2)	320
Protein hydrolysate, modified fat													
Alimentum Advance	Ross	Extensively hydrolyzed casein	2.7 (1.9)	Sucrose, modified tapioca starch	10.2 (6.8)	Safflower, MCT (33%), soy, DHA, ARA	5.5 (3.7)	1.9 (1.3)	3.0 (2.0)	105 (71)	75 (51)	1.8 (1.2)	370
Pregestimil +/− Lipil	Mead Johnson	Extensively hydrolyzed casein	2.8 (1.9)	Corn syrup solids, dextrose, modified corn starch	10.2 (6.8)	MCT (55%) soy, corn, high-oleic safflower, +/- DHA, ARA	5.6 (3.7)	2.0 (1.1)	2.8 (1.9)	115 (78)	75 (51)	1.8 (1.2)	280
Elemental													
EleCare	Ross	L-Amino acids	3.0 (2.0)	Corn syrup solids	10.7 (7.2)	High-oleic safflower, MCT (33%), soy	4.8 (3.2)	2.0 (1.3)	3.9 (2.6)	108 (73)	81 (55)	1.8 (1.2)	335
Neocate Infant +/− DHA, ARA	SHS	L-Amino acids	3.1* (2.1)*	Corn syrup solids	11.7 (7.8)	Soy, coconut, high-oleic sunflower, +/- DHA, ARA	4.5 (3.0)	1.6 (1.1)	4.0 (2.7)	124 (83)	93 (62)	1.8 (1.2)	342

that are provided in lieu of lactose include sucrose and fractions of corn syrup. The protein concentration of soy-based formulas is generally higher than that of milk-based formulas, reflecting the (presumed) somewhat lesser quality (per unit of weight) of methionine-supplemented isolated soy protein. All lactose-free formulas contain iron at 1.8 mg/100 kcal. In the case of soy-based formulas, this includes a substantial amount of iron provided by the soy protein isolate. Little is known about the bioavailability of this iron.

Table 5 lists the *extensively hydrolyzed formulas* (also referred to as predigested) and *elemental formulas*. These formulas are characterized by the absence of intact protein as well as lactose. The source of nitrogen is hydrolyzed casein or, in the case of elemental formulas, free amino acids. Three of the formulas provide a sizable proportion of their fat in the form of medium-chain triglycerides.

Table 6 lists the composition of formulas designed for *specific medical indications*. Enfamil AR is of thicker than usual consistency and is intended for use in infants with severe gastroesophageal reflux. Isomil DF is intended for infants recovering from diarrhea. Similac PM 60/40 is low in sodium and phosphorus and is used in infants with renal failure.

Formulas for older infants and toddlers. Although the concept of age-specific formulas is not widely embraced in the United States, the feeding of unmodified cow's milk to older infants was practiced for many years. A number of formulas are now available for the older infant and toddler (Table 7). The scientific rationale for the higher protein content compared to routine formulas is not clear since the protein requirement of the older infant is lower rather than higher than that of the young infant. It appears possible that the higher protein content is designed to ensure an adequate protein intake for those infants who consume a sizable amount of complementary foods, which tend to be low in protein content.

Substances Added to Formulas

Of the many bioactive substances that are present in human milk but are contained in cow's milk in lower concentration or are completely absent from cow's milk, some are added to formulas. Evidence that the addition ameliorates an otherwise existing deficiency is not always very convincing. However, it appears reasonable to add a

Table 6 Formulas for Medical Indications

Formula Description	Manufacturer	Protein Source	Protein g/100 kcal (g/dL)	Carbohydrate Source	Carbohydrate g/100 kcal (g/dL)	Fat Source	Fat g/100 kcal (g/dL)	Sodium mEq/100 kcal (mEq/dL)	Potassium mEq/100 kcal (mEq/dL)	Calcium mg/100 kcal (mg/dL)	Phosphorus mg/100 kcal (mg/dL)	Iron mg/100 kcal (mg/dL)	Osmolality mOsm/kg
Enfamil AR Lipil Milk based with rice starch Thickener	Mead Johnson	Nonfat milk	2.5 (1.7)	Lactose, rice starch, maltodextrin	11.0 (7.4)	Palm olein, soy, coconut, high-oleic sunflower, DHA, ARA	5.1 (3.5)	1.7 (1.2)	2.8 (1.9)	78 (53)	53 (36)	1.8 (1.2)	240
Isomil DF Soy based with soy fiber	Ross	Soy protein isolate	2.7 (1.8)	Corn syrup, sucrose	10.1 (6.8)	Soy, coconut	5.5 (3.7)	1.9 (1.3)	2.8 (1.9)	105 (71)	75 (51)	1.8 (1.2	240
Similac PM 60/40 Milk based with reduced minerals	Ross	Whey protein concentrate, sodium caseinate	2.2 (1.5)	Lactose	10.2 (6.9)	Corn, coconut, soy	5.6 (3.8)	1.0 (0.7)	2.2 (1.5)	56 (38)	28 (19)	0.7 (0.5)	280

Table 7 Formulas for Older Infants and Toddlers

Formula (Indicated Age for Use)	Manufacturer	Protein Source	Protein g/100 kcal (g/dL)	Carbohydrate Source	Carbohydrate g/100 kcal (g/dL)	Fat Source	Fat g/100 kcal (g/dL)	Sodium mEq/100 kcal (mEq/dL)	Potassium mEq/100 kcal (mEq/dL)	Calcium mg/100 kcal (mg/dL)	Phosphorus mg/100 kcal (mg/dL)	Iron mg/100 kcal (mg/dL)	Osmolality mOsm/kg
Cow milk based													Good
Start 2 Essentials (4 to 12 mo)	Nestlé	Nonfat milk	2.6 (1.7)	Corn syrup solids, lactose, maltodextrin	13.2 (8.8)	Palm olein, soy, coconut, high-oleic safflower	4.1 (2.7)	1.7 (1.1)	3.5 (2.3)	120 (80)	80 (54)	1.8 (1.2)	326
Next Step (>6 mo)	Mead Johnson	Nonfat milk	2.6 (1.8)	Corn syrup solids, lactose	11.1 (7.5)	Palm olein, soy, coconut, high-oleic sunflower	5.0 (3.4)	1.8 (1.2)	3.3 (2.2)	120 (82)	84 (57)	1.8 (1.2)	270
Similac 2 (6 to 18 mo)	Ross	Nonfat milk, whey protein concentrate	2.1 (1.6)	Lactose	10.6 (7.2)	High-oleic safflower, coconut, soy	5.5 (3.7)	1.0 (0.7)	2.7 (1.8)	118 (80)	64 (43)	1.8 (1.2)	300
Store brand generic (4 to 12 mo)	Wyeth	Whey, casein	2.6 (1.7)	Lactose	10.1 (6.8)	Oleo, coconut, soy, oleic	5.4 (3.7)	1.4 (0.9)	3.2 (2.2)	120 (82)	84 (57)	1.8 (1.2)	280
Soy protein based													
Good Start 2 Soy Essentials (4 to 12 mo)	Nestlé	Soy protein isolate	3.1 (2.1)	Maltodextrin, sucrose	13.2 (8.8)	Palm olein, soy, coconut, high-oleic safflower	4.4 (2.9)	1.8 (1.2)	3.0 (2.0)	135 (90)	90 (60)	1.8 (1.2)	200
Isomil 2 (6 to 18 mo)	Ross	Soy protein isolate	2.4 (1.7)	Corn syrup solids, sucrose	10.3 (7.0)	High-oleic safflower, coconut, soy	5.5 (3.7)	1.9 (1.3)	2.8 (1.9)	135 (91)	90 (61)	1.8 (1.2)	200
Next Step Soy (>6 mo)	Mead Johnson	Soy protein isolate	3.3 (2.2)	Corn syrup solids, sucrose	11.8 (8.0)	Palm olein, soy, coconut, high-oleic sunflower	4.4 (3.0)	2.1 (1.4)	3.8 (2.6)	115 (78)	90 (61)	1.8 (1.2)	260

substance when its presence in breast milk seems "intentional" and when its absence from the infant's diet is associated with deficits in serum or tissue concentrations relative to the breast-fed infant. A prerequisite for the addition of any substance is, of course, the availability of the technology necessary for making the addition feasible. The list of substances added to formulas now includes taurine, carnitine, nucleotides, and long-chain polyunsaturated fatty acids (LC-PUFAs).

Taurine. Taurine is an amino sulfonic acid found in high concentration in certain parts of the developing brain and in the retina. In infants taurine also plays a role in the conjugation of bile acids and it has osmoregulatory functions. Taurine is synthesized from cysteine and the term infant (but perhaps not the preterm infant) appears to possess ample capacity to carry out the conversion. Breast milk contains appreciable quantities of taurine, whereas the taurine content of cow's milk and hence of cow's milk-based formulas is only a fraction of that of breast milk. However, except for low plasma taurine concentrations, adverse effects due to low taurine intakes have not been demonstrated convincingly. Nevertheless, all formulas contain added taurine.

Carnitine. Carnitine plays an essential role in the entry of fatty acids into the mitochondria and is hence necessary for fatty acid oxidation. Carnitine is derived from endogenous synthesis as well as the diet. Breast milk, cow's milk and hence milk-based formulas, and meat provide ample amounts of carnitine. When carnitine is absent from the diet, plasma concentrations of infants are low and certain biochemical abnormalities are observed, whose clinical significance is uncertain. Carnitine is added to all non-milk formulas.

Nucleotides. Breast milk contains free RNA nucleosides (adenine, cytosine, guanine and uridine) as well as their respective nucleotides (ie, nucleosides with one sugar moiety and one or more phosphate groups attached), and some polymeric RNA.[23,24] For purposes of quantification, they are collectively referred to as "total potentially available nucleosides."[23] The amount of available nucleosides in breast milk is considerably higher than in cow's milk. It is thought that during times of high demand, that is, during rapid growth, dietary nucleosides are useful and may be conditionally essential. Animal studies have shown nucleosides to enhance T-cell function and gastrointestinal maturation. Fortification of infant formula with the four main nucleotides found in human milk led to enhanced antibody responses to *H. influenzae* type b and diphtheria.[25]

Long-chain Polyunsaturated Fatty Acids (LC-PUFAs). These fatty acids have received enormous attention in recent years. Although the consequences, especially those in the long term, of a lack of these fatty acids in the infant's diet remain controversial, formula manufacturers are now offering many formulas with and without added LC-PUFAs. Formulas with added LC-PUFAs are specially designated. The fatty acids in question are docosahexaenoic acid (DHA) and arachidonic acid (ARA). DHA is a C22 n-3 fatty acid with six double bonds. It is derived from dietary α-linolenic acid by a series of chain elongation and desaturation steps. ARA is a C20 n-6 fatty acid with four double bonds. It is derived from dietary linoleic acid. Breast milk contains preformed DHA (about 0.2% of fatty acids) and ARA (about 0.5% of fatty acids). The plant oils used in manufacturing formulas do not contain DHA and ARA and formulas are devoid of DHA and ARA unless these fatty acids are specifically added from other sources.

Infants, including premature infants, have the ability to synthesize DHA and ARA from their respective precursors, but the synthetic capacity appears to be insufficient to keep up with the high demands for growth, especially for DHA. DHA is needed for incorporation into cortical gray matter and the retina. In infants who are fed formulas devoid of DHA, concentrations in gray matter and retina are substantially lower than in breast-fed infants[26,27] The same is true for concentrations in plasma and erythrocyte membrane lipids.[28] Infants fed DHA-free formulas show evidence of impaired retinal function during the early months of life.[29] However, this effect seems to be transient and is no longer demonstrable in older infants. The presence of DHA and ARA in formulas is considered desirable because these fatty acids are present in breast milk and because their absence from the infant's diet produces abnormal concentrations in brain, retina, erythrocytes, and plasma.

WEANING AND BEIKOST (COMPLEMENTARY FOODS)

Weaning is the withdrawal or displacement of breast feeding. The weaning period begins with the first introduction of a food other than breast milk (water and vitamin–mineral supplements are not considered to be food) and extends until the complete discontinuation of breast feeding. We do not apply the term *weaning* to the withdrawal and displacement of formula. Beikost denotes foods other than milk or formula fed to infants.[30] These foods are also referred to as complementary foods or weaning foods.

Age of Introduction of Beikost

Evidence that infants can tolerate beikost before the currently recommended age of its introduction into the diet was provided by the experience in the 1950s and 1960s, when various beikost items were fed to many infants even during the early weeks of life.[1] However, there is at least a theoretic objection to feeding beikost during the early months of life because at this time there is greater permeability of the gastrointestinal tract to macromolecules than later. But the major reason for deferring introduction of beikost until 4 to 6 months of age relates to establishment of eating habits.[31,32] By about 4 months of age most infants can sit with support and have adequate neuromuscular control of trunk and neck.[33] At this developmental stage, the caretaker can interact with the infant to permit the infant to discontinue eating at the earliest sign of willingness to do so. Weaning should generally begin within a month or 6 weeks after the infant is developmentally ready. In industrialized countries there is no compelling argument for delaying introduction of beikost beyond 6 months of age.

Choices of Beikost

There is no evidence that the sequence of introduction of various beikost items is a matter of great importance. It is convenient to begin with cereal because a small amount of the dry powder can be mixed with human milk for the breast-fed infant or formula for the formula-fed infant at quite low expense. Initially, only a small amount, less than a teaspoonful, should be given at one time. Whether pureed fruits or vegetables are then introduced seems of little consequence. However, single foods rather than combinations should be offered. It is generally recommended that one food be fed for several days before introducing another. It is desirable to work toward acceptance of variations in tastes and textures.

The exclusively breast-fed infant consumes an adequate intake of protein but, once beikost begins to comprise a substantial portion of the total energy intake, it is important to include some high-protein foods. Deficiency of iron and zinc in breast-fed infants is not rare. Meats, especially red meats, are a good source of protein, zinc, and a highly bioavailable form of iron. We recommend for the breast-fed infant that soft-cooked meats be introduced within a month or two of beikost feeding (by 5 or 6 months of age). We consider the risk of iron and zinc deficiency to be greater than the risk of sensitization to meat proteins.

With the exception of providing sources of iron and zinc of high bioavailability for the breast-fed infant, the goal of feeding beikost is to begin the transition from the infant's primarily liquid diet to the predominantly solid food diet of the child. Therefore, as infancy progresses, the variety of flavors and textures offered to the infant should gradually be increased.

Fruit juices should be fed sparingly and only by cup. Fruit juices are associated with adverse reactions[34] and do not provide nutrients that are lacking in the diet of the breast-fed or formula-fed infant.

COW'S MILK

Feeding of cow's milk during the first year of life is undesirable because such feeding is associated with the development of iron deficiency. It is unclear which of the several mechanisms is mainly accountable for the iron deficiency. It has long been recognized that ingestion of large quantities of cow's milk may result in low intakes of other foods that contain more generous amounts of iron. In addition, there is considerable evidence that ingestion of cow's milk causes occult gastrointestinal blood loss.[35–37] Finally, the high intake provided by cow's milk of casein and calcium, potent inhibitors of iron absorption, may contribute to the development of iron deficiency.[38]

The potential renal solute load provided by cow's milk is undesirably high.[19] Feeding of whole cow's milk does not interfere with maintenance of water balance in normal infants under most circumstances. But in a hot environment or during febrile illness, especially if associated with decreased fluid intake, the infant is at greater risk of dehydration if fed cow's milk than if breast fed or formula fed. The margin of safety is greater with breast feeding or feeding of infant formulas than with feeding of cow's milk.[19]

REFERENCES

1. Fomon SJ. Infant feeding in the 20th century: Formula and beikost. J Nutr 2001;131:409S–20S.
2. Ryan AS. The resurgence of breastfeeding in the United States. Pediatrics 1997;99:e12.
3. Martinez GA, Nalezienski JP. The recent trend in breast-feeding. Pediatrics 1979;64:686–92.
4. Martinez GA, Dodd DA, Samartgedes JA. Milk feeding patterns in the United States during the first 12 months of life. Pediatrics 1981;68:863–58.
5. Fomon SJ, Nelson SE. Body composition of the male and female reference infants. Annu Rev Nutr 2002;22:1–17.
6. Fomon SJ, Bell EF. Energy. In: Fomon SJ, editor. Nutrition of Normal Infants. St. Louis, MO: Mosby; 1993. p. 103–20.
7. Fomon SJ. Requirements and recommended dietary intakes of protein during infancy. Pediatr Res 1991;30:391–5.
8. Daly SEJ, Owens RA, Hartmann PE. The short-term synthesis and infant-regulated removal of milk in lactating women. Exp Physiol 1993;78:209–20.
9. Nelson SE, Rogers RR, Ziegler EE, et al. Gain in weight and length during early infancy. Early Hum Devel 1989;19: 223–39.
10. Dewey KG, Heinig MJ, Nommsen LA, et al. Growth of breast-fed and formula-fed infants from 0 to 18 months: The DARLING study. Pediatrics 1992;89:1035–41.
11. Krebs NF, Hambidge KM. Zinc requirements and zinc intakes of breast-fed infants. Am J Clin Nutr 1986;43:288–92.
12. Menella JA, Beauchamp GK. Maternal diet alters the sensory qualities of human milk and the nursling's behavior. Pediatrics 1991;88:737–44.
13. Menella JA, Jagnow CP, Beauchamp GK. Prenatal and postnatal flavor learning by human infants. Pediatrics 2001;107:e88.
14. Gerrish CJ, Mennella JA. Flavor variety enhances food acceptance in formula-fed infants. Am J Clin Nutr 2001;73:1080–5.
15. Kunz C, Rudloff S, Baier W, et al. Oligosaccharides in human milk: Structural, functional and metabolic aspects. Annu Rev Nutr 2000;20:699–722.
16. Miller JB, Bull S, Miller J, et al. The oligosaccharide composition of human milk: Temporal and individual variations in monosaccharide components. J Pediatr Gastroenterol Nutr 1994;19:371–6.
17. Newburgh DS. Do the binding properties of oligosaccharides in milk protect human infants from gastrointestinal bacteria. J Nutr 1997;127:980S–4S.
18. Georgieff MK, Landon MB, Mills MM, et al. Abnormal iron distribution in infants of diabetic mothers: Spectrum and maternal antecedents. J Pediatr 1990;117:455–61.
19. Fomon SJ, Ziegler EE. Renal solute load and potential renal solute load in infancy. J Pediatr 1999;134:11–14.
20. Setchell KDR, Zimmer-Nechemias L, Cai J, et al. Exposure of infants to phytoestrogens from soy-based infant formula. Lancet 1997;350:23–27.
21. Strom BL, Schinnar R, Ziegler EE, et al. Exposure to soy-based formula in infancy and endocrinological and reproductive outcomes in young adulthood. JAMA 2001;286:807–14.
22. Nelson SE, Ziegler EE, Copeland AM, et al. Lack of adverse reaction to iron-fortified formula. Pediatrics 1988;81:360–4.
23. Leach JL, Baxter JH, Molitor BE, et al. Total potentially available nucleosides of human milk by stage of lactation. Am J Clin Nutr 1995;61:1224–30.
24. Thorell L, Sjöberg L-B, Hernell O. Nucleotides in human milk: Sources and metabolism by the newborn infant. Pediatr Res 1996;40:845–52.
25. Pickering LK, Granoff DM, Erickson JR, et al. Modulation of the immune system by human milk and infant formula containing nucleotides. Pediatrcis 1998;101:242–9.
26. Makrides M, Neumann MA, Byard RW, et al. Fatty acid composition of brain, retina, and erythrocytes in breast- and formula-fed infants. Am J Clin Nutr 1994;60:189–94.
27. Farquharson J, Jamieson EC, Abbasi KA, et al. Effect of diet on the fatty acid composition of the major phospholipids of infant cerebral cortex. Arch Dis Child 1995;72:198–203.
28. Hoffman DR, Birch EE, Birch DG, et al. Impact of early dietary intake and blood lipid composition of long-chain polyunsaturated fatty acids on later visual development. J Pediatr Gast Nutr 2000;31:540–53.
29. SanGiovanni JP, Berkey CS, Dwyer JT, et al. Dietary essential fatty acids, long-chain polyunsaturated fatty acids, and visual resolution acuity in healthy full term infants: a systematic review. Early Hum Dev 2000;57:165-88.
30. Fomon SJ. Infant Nutrition. 2nd edition. Philadelphia, PA: Saunders;1974. p. 408.
31. Fomon SJ. Recommendations for feeding normal infants. In: Fomon SJ, editor. Nutrition of Normal Infants. St. Louis, MO: Mosby; 1993. p. 455–8.
32. Fomon SJ. Feeding normal infants: Rationale for recommendations. J Am Dietet Assoc 2001;101:1002–6.
33. Harris G, Thomas A, Booth DA. Development of salt taste in infancy. Dev Psychol 1990;26:534–8.
34. Bock SA. Prospective appraisal of complaints of adverse reactions to foods during the first 3 years of life. Pediatrics 1983;79:683–8.
35. Fomon SJ, Ziegler EE, Nelson SE, et al. Cow milk feeding in infancy: Gastrointestinal blood loss and iron nutritional status. J Pediatr 1981;98:540–5.
36. Ziegler EE, Fomon SJ, Nelson SE, et al. Cow milk feeding in infancy: Further observations on blood loss from the gastrointestinal tract. J Pediatr 1990;116:11–18.
37. Ziegler EE, Jiang T, Romero E, et al. Cow's milk and intestinal blood loss in late infancy. J Pediatr 1999;135:720–6.
38. Fomon SJ. Iron. In: Fomon SJ, editor. Nutrition of Normal Infants. St. Louis, MO: Mosby; 1993. p. 239–60.

Complementary Feeding

Kenneth H. Brown, MD

INTRODUCTION

The World Health Organization defines *complementary feeding* as the feeding practice whereby other foods and/or energy-containing liquids are provided to the young child along with breast milk.[1] Thus, complementary foods can be considered as the non–breast-milk components of the mixed diets that are consumed by young children while they are still breast-feeding. In societies where breast-feeding is not universally initiated or is discontinued prematurely—and in clinical situations where breast-feeding is contraindicated because of pathological conditions of the mother or infant—other specially designed dietary regimens and child feeding practices are necessary.[2] This chapter will focus only on the former conditions, that is, when mothers and infants are able to initiate and maintain breast-feeding.

Ideally, the period of complementary feeding lasts from approximately 6 months of age, when these foods are first introduced, until at least 2 years. This stage of life represents an especially challenging period for children's nutrition because their elevated metabolic rates per unit body weight and rapid rates of growth impose relatively high nutrient requirements. Moreover, the continuing development of young children's gastrointestinal tract, neuromuscular coordination, and immunological function during this period limits the types of foods that they are able to consume and elevates their susceptibility to food-borne infections and food allergies. For these reasons, recommendations on optimal child feeding must take into consideration not only the children's age-specific physiological requirements for essential nutrients, but also the appropriate food (or other) sources of these nutrients and the proper methods of preparing and feeding these foods.

For the present review, the definitions of infant feeding practices proposed by the World Health Organization will be adopted.[3] In particular, *exclusive breast-feeding* is defined as the consumption of no other food or liquids except breast milk and possibly small amounts of medicines or vitamin–mineral supplements. The term *predominant breast-feeding* is applied when the infant's major source of nourishment is breast milk, but water and water-based drinks, such as flavored water, teas, and herbal infusions, or fruit juices are also consumed. As indicated above, complementary feeding refers to the consumption of both breast milk and other foods, usually during the period from 6 to ~24 months of age, or until the child ceases to nurse at the breast and begins to consume the same foods as the rest of the family.

Several documents focusing on child feeding in lower income settings have been published by the World Health Organization[1,4]; other authorities have issued guidelines targeted to children in industrialized countries.[5–7] The physiological requirements of children in these respective environments do not differ, so general feeding recommendations are similar in each setting. Nevertheless, proper feeding of young children is generally more difficult to achieve in resource-poor settings because of the families' limited access to high-quality, nutrient-rich foods, a lack of clean sources of water and proper facilities for food preparation and storage, and inadequate environmental sanitation. The severe nutritional challenges faced by children in lower income countries during this stage of life is evidenced by the frequent occurrence of growth faltering relative to international reference patterns, which typically coincides with the period of complementary feeding.[8] Thus, recommendations for appropriate breast-feeding and food-handling practices assume even greater importance for children raised in these circumstances. Although the appearance of HIV infection in some of these same countries has complicated infant feeding recommendations,[9] standard feeding guidelines still apply for the vast majority of children worldwide, so these general recommendations will be the focus of the present chapter. In particular, information will be presented on (1) the optimal duration of exclusive breast-feeding, (2) the amounts of energy and nutrients required from complementary foods, and (3) appropriate food sources and available strategies for satisfying the energy and nutrient needs of young children during the particularly vulnerable period of complementary feeding.

APPROPRIATE DURATION OF BREAST-FEEDING

According to the results of observational studies conducted in lower income countries, such as Peru and the Philippines, exclusive breast-feeding during the first months of life is associated with dramatically reduced rates of diarrhea and respiratory infections.[10,11] Furthermore, in a large intervention trial conducted in Belarus, in which families of more than 17,000 newborns were randomly assigned by clinic to receive counseling designed to promote appropriate breast-feeding practices, infants in the intervention group were more likely to be breast-fed exclusively at 3 months of age (43.3% vs 6.4%) and they had a significantly lower occurrence of one or more episodes of diarrhea (9.1% vs 13.2%) and atopic eczema (3.3% vs 6.3%).[12] Thus, it appears that infants who adhere to a regimen of exclusive breast-feeding have lower rates of selected illnesses, particularly enteric infections and respiratory illnesses, regardless of the environment in which they are reared. Indeed, several observational studies in the United States also discovered that children who were fully breast-fed for longer periods of time had lower rates of diarrhea, otitis media, and pneumonia.[13,14]

Current recommendations for the optimal duration of exclusive breast-feeding are based on a systematic review of intervention trials and observational studies carried out in both lower income and more affluent countries, in which the growth velocity and/or rates of infections were assessed among infants who were breast-fed exclusively for 6 months versus those who were partially breast-fed or non–breast-fed.[15] Two of the three available controlled intervention trials were conducted by a research group in Honduras.[16,17] In the first of these studies, infants were randomly assigned to one of three feeding regimens: (1) exclusive breast-feeding until 6 months of age, (2) exclusive breast-feeding until 4 months of age at which time high-quality, packaged complementary foods were started and breast-feeding was continued ad libitum, or (3) exclusive breast-feeding until 4 months at which time complementary feeding was initiated as above along with explicit encouragement to maintain the same breast-feeding frequency as practiced before the intervention.[16] There were no significant differences in the children's total energy intakes at 4 to 6 months of age, despite the additional energy provided by complementary foods, and there were no differences in the children's growth velocities during this interval. In other words, provision of complementary foods prior to 6 months of age simply displaced breast milk intakes. The authors concluded that there was no advantage of introducing complementary foods before 6 months, whereas there may be considerable risks of inadequate nutrient intakes and food-borne infections, as described above, if the nutritional and hygienic quality of the foods cannot be ensured. The second Honduras study yielded similar results, even though all infants enrolled weighed less than 2,500 g at birth.[17] Thus, the same conclusions pertain to low-birth-weight infants.

Based on these intervention trials in Honduras, the aforementioned study in Belarus, and other published observational studies, a review commissioned by the World Health Organization concluded that "the available evidence demonstrates no apparent risk in recommending, as public health policy, exclusive breast-feeding in both developing and developed country settings,"[15] and the major international health agencies now recommend that exclusive breast-feeding should be maintained until about 6 months postpartum based on this body of evidence.

Breast-feeding not only reduces the incidence of selected infections, as described above, but a multicenter study coordinated by the World Health Organization in Brazil, Pakistan, and the Philippines found that exclusive and predominant breast-feeding both were associated with reduced infant mortality.[18] In these latter studies, the protective effect of breast-feeding was greatest during the early months of life, although benefits were still detectable in late infancy. In particular, the pooled odds ratios of mortality associated with non–breast-feeding declined progressively with increasing infant age, ranging from 5.8 [95% CI 3.4, 9.8] during the first 2 months of life and 4.1 [2.7, 6.4] for 2- to 3-month-olds to 1.4 [0.8, 2.6] for 9- to 11-month-olds. Thus, continued breast-feeding beyond the first 6 months of life still confers some protection against infection, even after other foods are introduced. Moreover, breast milk remains an important source of nutrients well into the second year of life, as described below.

ENERGY REQUIREMENTS FROM COMPLEMENTARY FOODS

Despite these remarkable benefits of exclusive breast-feeding during the early months of life, additional foods are required by about 6 months because breast milk is no longer sufficient as a sole source of energy and most micronutrients beyond that age. The amounts of energy and nutrients required from complementary foods can be estimated as the difference between the total age-specific requirements of these nutrients and the mean amounts provided by breast milk for children of different ages.[1] The estimates of energy requirements from complementary foods were revised recently,[19] using new information on young children's total daily energy requirements, which were based on direct measurements of energy expenditure and physical growth, including body composition.[20] According to these updated estimates of total energy requirements and previously summarized information on the amount of breast milk energy consumed by children of different ages,[1] the new estimates of the average amounts of energy required from complementary foods are approximately 200, 300, and 550 kcal/d for young children 6 to 8, 9 to 11, and 12 to 23 months of age, respectively (Table 1).

Table 1 Estimated Average Total Energy Requirements, Breast Milk Energy Transferred from Mother to Infant, and Energy Required from Complementary Foods, by Age Group*

Energy Requirements and Energy Sources	Age Group (mo) 6–8	9–11	12–23
Average total energy requirement (kcal/d)†	615	686	894
Average amount of energy transferred from mother to infant in breast milk (kcal/d)‡	403	379	346
Average amount of energy required from complementary foods (kcal/d)	212	307	548

*Adapted from Dewey and Brown.[19]
†Data from Butte et al.[20]
‡Data from Brown et al.[1]

Several caveats must be noted regarding these estimates of average energy requirements from complementary foods. First, the estimates of children's total energy requirements represent the averages of measurements among multiple children in the specified age ranges, and there is considerable interindividual variation in these figures. Second, the composition of human milk and the amounts of energy transferred from mother to child by breast milk vary among different women. Thus, the stated average amounts of energy required from complementary food at different ages should be considered as just a first approximation of the true energy needs of an individual child. This total amount of energy can be offered to the child and then adjusted accordingly in response to the child's actual consumption and subsequent pattern of growth.

ENERGY DENSITY AND FREQUENCY OF FEEDING COMPLEMENTARY FOODS

The total daily amount of energy that a child consumes from complementary foods is a product of the frequency of feeding (number of servings per day) and the energy density of the foods (kcal/g food).[21,22] Specifically, total daily energy intakes from complementary foods increase with greater meal frequency, and, at any particular level of feeding frequency, total energy consumption rises with greater energy density of the diet,[21] as illustrated in Figure 1. Thus, when more meals are provided each day, the complementary foods can be prepared with lower energy density and still provide adequate total energy intakes, and vice versa. Using empirical data derived from several studies,[21,23] the energy density that is minimally adequate to meet energy requirements has been estimated for children of several age groups, considering different levels of feeding frequency (Table 2).[19] It should be noted, however, that most of the available information on young children's food intakes that was used for these estimates was collected from non–breast-fed children, so additional data are still needed from those who are continuing to nurse at the breast.

There is some evidence that higher energy densities of complementary foods and greater feeding frequencies may have a negative impact on total breast milk consumption, at least in the short term.[22] For example, several recent studies have found that increasing the energy density of complementary foods reduced breast milk intakes slightly, although the effects on total daily energy intakes were inconsistent.[22,24] In one study, total energy intake was increased when the density of complementary foods was raised from 0.5 to 1.5 kcal/g,[22] despite small reductions in breast milk intake. However, no such effect on total

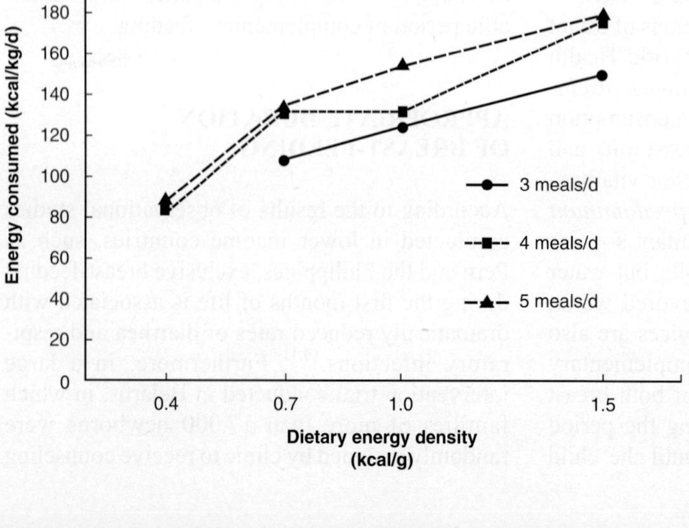

Figure 1 Effects of dietary energy density and frequency of feeding on total daily energy intakes by young children recovering from severe malnutrition. (Reproduced from reference 21 with permission by the American Journal of Clinical Nutrition. © Am J Clin Nutr. American Society for Nutrition.)

Table 2 Minimum Dietary Energy Density Needed to Permit Energy Intakes Consistent with Energy Requirements from Complementary Food at Different Ages*

Number of Meals/d	Energy Density (kcal/g Food), by Age Group (mo)		
	6–8	9–11	12–23
2	0.71	0.84	1.12
3	0.48	0.56	0.75
4	0.36	0.42	0.56
5	0.29	0.34	0.45

*Adapted from Dewey and Brown.[19] Analysis based on average level of breast milk intake and assumed gastric capacity of 30 g/kg reference body weight in each age group.

energy intake was noted in another study when energy density was boosted from 0.20 to 0.55 kcal/g by adding oil to a cereal–legume mixture.[24] The different outcomes of these two studies may be due to the distinct ranges of energy density of the foods that were served or the fact that the latter study provided each diet for 1 day only, so the children may not yet have reached a constant level of intake. Additional longer term studies with a greater number of permutations of energy density and feeding frequency are needed to address these issues. Studies are also needed to assess the effects of the complementary feeding regimen on longer term breast milk intakes and continuation of breast-feeding. Of concern, one study in India found that providing infants with a supplemental milk-containing infant cereal decreased the proportion who continued to breast-feed at 1 year.[25]

Another possible preoccupation regarding the energy content of complementary foods is that continuous exposure to high-energy-density diets could contribute to excessive energy intakes and thereby predispose children to subsequent obesity. However, little information is available on this issue, so it is not yet possible to establish upper levels of desirable energy density for populations at risk for obesity. Of related concern, there is some evidence to suggest that substitution of energy-containing (sweetened) beverages in place of water may promote excessive energy intakes,[26] so consumption of these drinks should be discouraged.

NUTRIENT REQUIREMENTS FROM COMPLEMENTARY FOODS

Estimates of the amounts of specific nutrients required from complementary foods can be calculated using the same conceptual framework as described above for energy. However, these calculations regarding micronutrients are complicated by the fact that there are notable inconsistencies in the different sets of estimates of young children's total nutrient requirements, such as those estimates prepared by the Institute of Medicine[27] and the World Health Organization.[28] In many cases these estimated requirements are simply extrapolated from older age groups or are expressed as "adequate intakes" (AIs), which are based on the observed intakes by apparently healthy children rather than derived from direct measurements of physiological requirements. For estimates based on AIs, which is the case for most of the recommendations published by the Institute of Medicine, many children in the population from which the estimates were derived were likely to be consuming substantially more than their true physiological needs. Thus, the dietary recommendations obtained from these observations may be considerably greater than necessary. The dilemmas imposed by relying on the different sets of existing estimated nutrient requirements have been described elsewhere in more detail, along with their implications for estimating the requirements from complementary foods.[19] Focused research on the nutrient requirements of young children and harmonization of estimates prepared by different expert groups remain pressing needs.

Notwithstanding these difficulties, the amounts of nutrients required from complementary foods have been estimated using the aforementioned sets of recommendations of young children's total nutrient requirements. Examples of these estimates, expressed as desirable nutrient densities in relation to the average amounts of energy required from these foods (ie, the amount of each nutrient per 100 kcal of complementary foods), are presented in Table 3. As indicated in the table, the estimated desired nutrient densities based on the DRI and WHO recommendations are reasonably consistent for protein, iron, riboflavin, thiamine, niacin, folate, and pyridoxine. However, there are sizable discrepancies for vitamins A and C, calcium, and zinc for most age groups, mainly due to the different approaches that were used to estimate the requirements.

The optimal fat content of complementary foods remains somewhat controversial. Whereas a minimum amount of dietary fat is necessary to provide essential long-chain fatty acids and is useful to help achieve adequate energy density and palatability of the diet,[29] some authors have emphasized the desirability of encouraging low-fat intakes beginning early in childhood to establish appropriate dietary habits among older children and adults.[30] Because of the high fat content of human milk (~3.5 g/100 mL or nearly 50% of milk energy content), fully breast-fed infants less than 1 year of age require very little additional fat from complementary foods to achieve fat intakes that are 30% of total energy intakes.[19] A noteworthy study designed to encourage young children to consume <35% of energy as fat and a 1:1:1 ratio of polyunsaturated–mononunsaturated–saturated fats beginning at 6 months of age found slightly lower total fat intakes (~30% of energy vs ~33% of energy at 2 to 3 yr) and lower serum total cholesterol concentrations among the intervention children (although no difference in ratios of HDL cholesterol/total cholesterol), and no difference in their physical growth, compared with control children.[30] These results suggest that total fat intakes less than or equal to 30% of energy are safe and desirable, even in early childhood.

PROBLEM MICRONUTRIENTS AND STRATEGIES TO PROVIDE ADEQUATE MICRONUTRIENTS

As indicated above, the nutrient requirements from complementary foods can be estimated as the difference between the total theoretical nutrient

Table 3 Recommended Nutrient Densities (Amount per 100 kcal) of Complementary Foods for Children 6 to 8 and 9 to 11 Months, Based on the Institute of Medicine Dietary Reference Intakes and World Health Organization Recommendations

Nutrient	Age 6–8 mo		Age 9–11 mo		Age 12–23 mo	
	DRIs*	WHO†	DRIs*	WHO†	DRIs*	WHO†
Protein (g/100 kcal)	1.0	1.0	1.0	1.0	0.9	0.9
Calcium (mg/100 kcal)	40	105	32	74	63	63
Iron (mg/100 kcal)‡	5.3	4.5	3.5	3.0	1.2	1.0
Zinc (mg/100 kcal)	1.1	1.6	0.7	1.1	0.4	0.6
Vitamin A (μg RAE/100 kcal)	81	31	63	30	5	23
Riboflavin (mg/100 kcal)	0.08	0.08	0.06	0.06	0.06	0.06
Thiamine (mg/100 kcal)	0.08	0.08	0.06	0.06	0.07	0.07
Niacin (mg/100 kcal)	1.5	1.5	1.0	1.0	0.9	0.9
Folate (μg/100 kcal)	11	11	9	9	19	21
Vitamin B_6 (mg/100 kcal)	0.12	0.12	0.08	0.08	0.08	0.08
Vitamin C (mg/100 kcal)	11	1.5	8	1.7	0	1.5

*Dietary Reference Intakes, Institute of Medicine.[27]
†World Health Organization, 2002.[28]
‡Assumes medium bioavailability of iron.

requirements and the amounts of these nutrients transferred to the child in breast milk. Figure 2 provides examples of the estimated percentages of different nutrients that must be provided by complementary foods for children of different ages. As indicated, human milk is a good source of protein, vitamin A, folate, vitamin B_{12}, vitamin C, iodine, and copper in most age groups and a fair source of riboflavin, thiamine, calcium, and zinc. However, breast milk transfer of most vitamins depends on adequate maternal status, and in all cases breast milk is a relatively poor source of some nutrients, like niacin, pyridoxine, vitamin D, vitamin K, and iron. Thus, complementary foods must be the primary source of these latter nutrients to allow young children to meet their required intakes, and adequate maternal nutrition must be ensured for the former nutrients.

Despite the difficulties in establishing clear guidelines on adequate micronutrient densities of complementary foods, as described above, several groups of investigators have attempted to identify specific "problem nutrients" by comparing the observed nutrient intakes from complementary foods in different low-income settings with the range of currently estimated requirements.[19,31,32] *Problem nutrients* can be defined as those for which there is the greatest discrepancy between their content in traditional complementary foods and the estimated requirements, regardless of the particular set of estimated requirements that are applied. Analyses of dietary intake data indicate that iron, zinc, calcium, selected B vitamins, and occasionally vitamin A may be present in limited amounts in home-available complementary foods relative to the estimated requirements for these nutrients from complementary foods.

Available strategies to supply these problem nutrients include promotion of greater consumption of animal-source foods or other generous food sources of these nutrients; provision of fortified, centrally processed complementary foods; or delivery of additional nutrients through home-based fortification or micronutrient supplementation. The remaining sections of this chapter will focus on different nutrient-rich foods that might be incorporated in the complementary feeding regimen and other possible exogenous (nondietary) sources of these problem nutrients. An analytic approach, based on linear programming, has been described for identifying local foods that can be used to supply nutrient shortfalls, using dietary intake data and local food prices to model potential nutrient intakes from different combinations of foods at more affordable costs.[33]

Animal-Source Foods

Incorporating animal-source foods, such as animal flesh and organs, dairy products, eggs, and fish, is often the only way to supply the aforementioned problem nutrients through natural foods. Animal-flesh foods are excellent sources of highly bioavailable heme iron and zinc, along with a number of B vitamins, so inclusion of these foods in young children's diets should be encouraged. These foods are also rich in high-quality protein, although traditional complementary feeding regimens generally contain adequate amounts of protein, unless they are composed mainly of low-protein tubers, like cassava or sweet potato, or refined starches. Availability of animal-source foods may be very restricted in the poorest countries,[33] and their relatively high cost frequently limits the amounts consumed in poorer households. Moreover, religious proscriptions or cultural taboos may prevent their use in some societies. Nevertheless, if these foods are adequately cooked and finely minced, experience shows that they can be consumed without difficulty by young children. A recent study in the United States, for example, demonstrated the feasibility of including meat in the feeding regimens of young infants.[34] Another study carried out in slum communities in Peru found that, following an intensive educational campaign, even poor households were able to increase children's consumption of animal source foods, and the linear growth of children in the intervention communities was significantly greater than in the control areas, reducing rates of stunting by two-thirds at 12 months.[35] Thus, it may be possible to increase children's consumption of these foods in some settings, by using appropriately targeted educational interventions.

Nonhuman animal milks and related dairy products, like yogurt and some cheeses, are alternative sources of high-quality protein. These foods are also rich in calcium and selected B vitamins, but low in iron. Moreover, if they are not properly heat treated, these milks can cause gastrointestinal bleeding in infants, producing a further threat to their iron status.[36] Furthermore, because of the relatively high total fat and saturated fatty acid contents of these products, some authorities recommend using partially skimmed milk.[30] However, there is little evidence of any long-term adverse effects of milk fat intake in early childhood on the subsequent risk of cardiovascular disease, so some child-feeding guidelines suggest that reduced fat milks should not be introduced before 2 to 3 years of age to limit the possibility of inadequate energy intakes.[5]

Cereal Products

Cereal products are commonly used as a major component of complementary feeding regimens. Such foods provide energy, mostly as carbohydrate, and they contribute some protein. However, cereal protein is limited in certain amino acids (eg, lysine in wheat and rice and lysine and tryptophan in maize), compared with reference protein

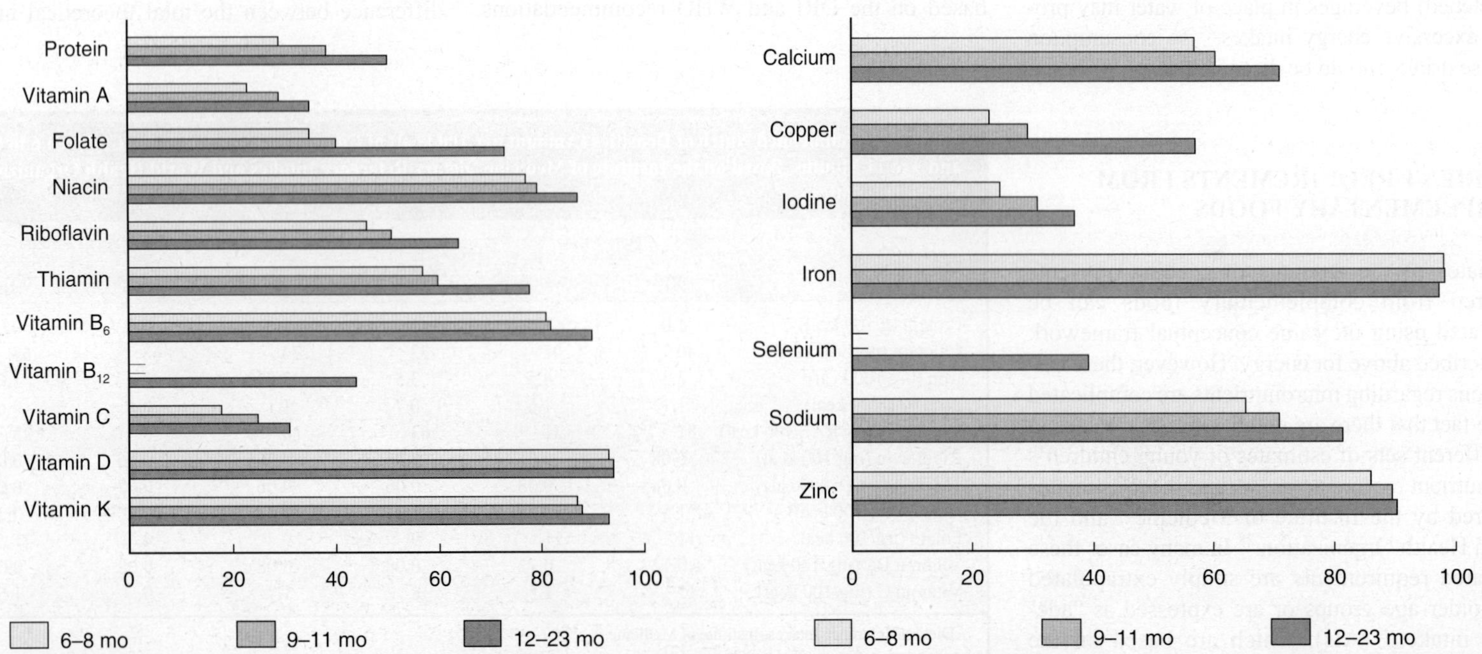

Figure 2 Estimated percentage of total nutrient requirements that must be provided from complementary foods, by age group. (Adapted from reference 19. Assumes adequate maternal nutritional status with regard to those nutrients whose transfer in breast milk depends on maternal status.)

(egg albumin or milk protein) and the digestibility of cereal proteins is generally less than that of proteins derived from animal source foods, so total protein intakes from cereals must be adjusted for their equivalent amount of reference protein. Nevertheless, as indicated above, protein intake is usually sufficient from most complementary feeding regimens that have been examined. Although cereals provide essential minerals, especially when consumed as whole grain products, concerns have been raised about mineral bioavailability from these foods because their high phytate content can inhibit mineral absorption. However, a recent study of Swedish infants who were randomly assigned to receive cereal-based diets with and without phytate reduction from 6 to 12 months of age found no long-term differences in their iron or zinc status.[37]

Processed Complementary Foods

Distribution of processed, fortified complementary foods, either through public sector programs or through commercial channels, offers an alternative food-based approach to supply problem nutrients.[38] Although such foods can successfully cover current nutrient shortfalls of the home diet, the rapid changes in young children's nutrient requirements during the period of complementary feeding make it difficult to design a single product that meets the nutrient needs of all children in this age range without imposing the risk of excessive intakes by some children.[39] Moreover, the impact of these foods on children's growth has been inconsistent, possibly related to the timing, amount, and composition of these foods, as well as the underlying nutritional status of the study populations.[40–42] Despite the inconsistent growth responses observed in these earlier studies, several recent studies have found positive effects on iron status and/or developmental milestones among children who received these products.[43–45]

Micronutrient Supplements

Addition of micronutrients to current feeding regimens, either through home-based food fortification or direct child supplementation, offers a lower cost strategy than providing a processed, nutritionally complete complementary food. Home-based fortification involves the addition of a prepackaged micronutrient supplement to the child's food once daily at the time of serving. One such formulation, "Sprinkles," which contains iron as microencapsulated ferrous fumarate (to avoid adverse organoleptic effects of iron on the food), and vitamins A and D, folic acid, ascorbic acid, and zinc, has been shown to reduce rates of anemia among consumers, although evidence of its positive impact on other indicators of micronutrient status and growth are still lacking.[46]

Micronutrient supplements may be supplied as liquid formulations; chewable, crushable, or dispersable tablets[47]; or fat-based food pastes.[48] A complete review of these products and related issues is beyond the scope of the present publication. Nevertheless, each of these formulations has been found to yield positive impacts on selected indicators of micronutrient status, depending on the specific formulation, the preexisting nutritional status of the target population, and the presence of conditions that may interfere with nutrient absorption or utilization; but there is only limited evidence of any positive effects of these products on child growth. A recent study compared the effects of Sprinkles, Nutritabs (crushable multiple-micronutrient tablets), and Nutributter (a micronutrient-enriched peanut butter mixture) in Ghanaian children.[49] Each type of the supplements was well accepted, and there were no differences in adherence to treatment by intervention group. After 6 months of study, children in the three supplementation groups had greater concentrations of serum ferritin and lower concentrations of transferrin receptors than those in a nonintervention comparison group. Children who received Nutributter had greater final weight-for-age and length-for-age Z scores compared with the other two intervention groups and the nonintervention comparison group. Thus, all three products enhanced iron status, but only Nutributter increased the infants' growth. Additional research is still required to define optimal dosing regimens of multiple-micronutrient formulations added to complementary foods, interactions among nutrients in the various preparations, and any possible adverse effects on child growth and other health outcomes in particular settings.

SUMMARY

Important advances in knowledge have been achieved in recent years with regard to the multiple advantages of exclusive breast-feeding during the early months of life, the optimal timing of introduction of complementary foods, and the appropriate energy density, feeding frequency, and micronutrient composition of these foods. However, adequate understanding of the effects of different complementary feeding regimens on breast milk intakes and the ultimate duration of breast-feeding is still lacking. Likewise, more information is needed on the ideal micronutrient composition of fortified complementary foods and the impact of alternative micronutrient delivery systems on young children's nutritional status, physical growth, and neurobehavioral development.

REFERENCES

1. World Health Organization. Complementary Feeding of Young Children in Developing Countries: A Review of Current Scientific Knowledge. Brown KH, Dewey KG, Allen LH, editors. Geneva, Switzerland: World Health Organization (WHO/NUT/98.1); 1998.
2. World Health Organization. Feeding the Non-breastfed Child 6–24 Months of Age. Geneva, Switzerland: World Health Organization (WHO/FCH/CAH/04.13); 2004.
3. World Health Organization. Indicators for Assessing Breast Feeding Practices. Geneva, Switzerland: World Health Organization, 1991.
4. World Health Organization. Complementary Feeding. Family Foods for Breastfed Children. Geneva, Switzerland: World Health Organization (WHO/NHD/00.1); 2000.
5. Committee on Medical Aspects of Food Policy. Weaning and the Weaning Diet. Report of the Working Group on the Weaning Diet. London: HMSO; 1994.
6. Canadian Pediatric Society, Dieticians of Canada and Health Canada. Nutrition for Healthy Term Infants. Ottawa, Canada: Minister of Public Works and Government Services; 1998.
7. Michaelsen KF, Weaver L, Branca F, Robertson A. Feeding and nutrition of infants and young children in the WHO European Region with emphasis on former soviet countries. Copenhagen, Denmark: WHO/UNICEF. WHO Regional Publications European Series, no. 87, 2000.
8. Shrimpton R, Victora CG, de Onis M, et al. Worldwide timing of growth faltering: Implications for nutritional interventions. Pediatrics 2001;107:E75.
9. World Health Organization. Executive Summary of a Scientific Review. Consultation on Nutrition and HIV/AIDS in Africa: Evidence, Lessons and Recommendations for Action. Geneva: World Health Organization; 2005.
10. Brown KH, Black RE, Lopez de Romana G, Creed de Kanashiro H. Infant-feeding practices and their relationship with diarrheal and other diseases in Huascar (Lima), Peru. Pediatrics 1989;83:31–40.
11. Popkin BM, Adair L, Akin JS, et al. Breast-feeding and diarrheal morbidity. Pediatrics 1990;86:874–82.
12. Kramer MS, Chalmers B, Hodnett ED, et al. Promotion of Breastfeeding Intervention Trial (PROBIT): A randomized trial in the Republic of Belarus. JAMA 2001;285:413–20.
13. Scariati PD, Grummer-Strawn LM, Fein SB. A longitudinal analysis of infant morbidity and the extent of breastfeeding in the United States. Pediatrics 1997;99:E5.
14. Chantry CJ, Howard CR, Auinger P. Full breastfeeding duration and associated decrease in respiratory tract infection in US children. Pediatrics 2006;117:425–32.
15. Kramer MS, Kakuma R. The Optimal Duration of Exclusive Breast Feeding: A Systematic Review. Geneva, Switzerland: World Health Organization; 2002.
16. Cohen RJ, Brown KH, Canahuati J, et al. Effects of age of introduction of complementary foods on infant breast milk intake, total energy intake, and growth: A randomised intervention study in Honduras. Lancet 1994;344:288–93.
17. Dewey KG, Cohen RJ, Brown KH, Rivera LL. Age of introduction of complementary foods and growth of term, low-birth-weight, breast-fed infants: A randomized intervention study in Honduras. Am J Clin Nutr 1999;69:679–86.
18. WHO Collaborative Study Team on the Role of Breastfeeding on the Prevention of Infant Mortality. Effect of breastfeeding on infant and child mortality due to infectious diseases in less developed countries: A pooled analysis. Lancet 2000;355:451–5.
19. Dewey KG, Brown KH. Update on technical issues concerning complementary feeding of young children in developing countries and implications for intervention programs. Food Nutr Bull 2003;24:5–28.
20. Butte NF, Wong WW, Hopkinson JM, et al. Energy requirements derived from total energy expenditure and energy deposition during the first 2 yr of life. Am J Clin Nutr 2000;72:1558–69.
21. Brown KH, Sanchez-Griñan M, Perez F, et al. Effects of dietary energy density and feeding frequency on total daily energy intakes of recovering malnourished children. Am J Clin Nutr 1995;62:13–8.
22. Islam MM, Peerson JM, Ahmed T, et al. Effects of varied energy density of complementary foods on breast-milk intakes and total energy consumption by healthy, breastfed Bangladeshi children. Am J Clin Nutr 2006;83:851–8.
23. Stephenson DM, Gardner JM, Walker SP, Ashworth A. Weaning-food viscosity and energy density: Their effects on ad libitum consumption and energy intakes in Jamaican children. Am J Clin Nutr 1994;60:465–9.
24. Bajaj M, Dubey AP, Nagpal J, et al. Short-term effect of oil supplementation of complementary food on total ad libitum consumption in 6- to 10-month-old breastfed Indian infants. J Pediatr Gastroenterol Nutr 2005;41:61–5.
25. Bhandari N, Bahl R, Nayyar B, et al. Food supplementation with encouragement to feed it to infants from 4 to 12 months of age has a small impact on weight gain. J Nutr 2001;131:1946–51.
26. Welsh JA, Cogswell ME, Rogers S, et al. Overweight among low-income preschool children associated with the consumption of sweet drinks: Missouri, 1999–2002. Pediatrics 2005;115:e223–9.
27. Institute of Medicine, Food and Nutrition Board. Dietary Reference Intakes: Recommended Intakes for Individuals. National Academy of Sciences. Available at: http://www.iom.edu/Object.File/Master/21/372/0.pdf. Accessed March 16, 2007.
28. World Health Organization, Food and Agriculture Organization. Vitamin and Mineral Requirements in Human Nutrition.

Report of a Joint FAO/WHO Expert Consultation. Geneva, Switzerland: World Health Organization; 1998.
29. Prentice AM, Paul AA. Fat and energy needs of children in developing countries. Am J Clin Nutr 2000;72:1253S–65S.
30. Simell O, Niinikoski H, Ronnemaa T, et al. Special Turku Coronary Risk Factor Intervention Project for Babies (STRIP). Am J Clin Nutr 2000;72:1316S–31S.
31. Brown KH, Peerson JM, Kimmons JE, Hotz C. Options for achieving adequate intake from home-prepared complementary foods in low income countries. In: Black RE, Fleischer Michaelsen K, editors. Public Health Issues in Infant and Child Nutrition. Philadelphia: Nestec Ltd., Vevey / Lippincott Williams & Wilkins; 2002. p. 239–56.
32. Gibson RS, Ferguson EL, Lehrfeld J. Complementary foods for infant feeding in developing countries: Their nutrient adequacy and improvement. Eur J Clin Nutr 1998;52:764–70.
33. Ferguson EL, Darmon N, Fahmida U, et al. Design of optimal food-based complementary feeding recommendations and identification of key "problem nutrients" using goal programming. J Nutr 2006;136:2399–404.
34. Krebs NF, Westcott JE, Butler N, et al. Meat as a first complementary food for breastfed infants: Feasibility and impact on zinc intake and status. J Pediatr Gastroenterol Nutr 2006;42:207–14.
35. Penny ME, Creed-Kanashiro HM, Robert RC, et al. Effectiveness of an educational intervention delivered through the health services to improve nutrition in young children: A cluster-randomised controlled trial. Lancet 2005;365:1863–72.
36. Fomon SJ, Ziegler EE, Nelson SE, Edwards BB. Cow milk feeding in infancy: Gastrointestinal blood loss and iron nutritional status. J Pediatr 1981;98:540–5.
37. Lind T, Lönnerdal B, Persson LA, et al. Effects of weaning cereals with different phytate contents on hemoglobin, iron stores, and serum zinc: A randomized intervention in infants from 6 to 12 mo of age. Am J Clin Nutr 2003;78:168–75.
38. Brown KH, Lutter CK. Potential role of processed complementary foods in the improvement of early childhood nutrition in Latin America. Food Nutr Bull 2000;21:511.
39. Dewey KG. Nutrient composition of fortified complementary foods: Should age-specific micronutrient content and ration sizes be recommended? J Nutr 2003;133:2950S–2S.
40. Simondon KB, Gartner A, Berger J, et al. Effect of early, short-term supplementation on weight and linear growth of 4–7-month-old infants in developing countries: a four-country randomized trial. Am J Clin Nutr 1996;64:537–45.
41. Caulfield LE, Huffman SL, Piwoz EG. Interventions to improve intake of complementary foods by infants 6 to 12 months of age in developing countries: Impact on growth and on the prevalence of malnutrition and potential contribution to child survival. Food Nutr Bull 1999;20:183–200.
42. Dewey KG. Success of intervention programs to promote complementary feeding. In: Black RE, Fleischer Michaelsen K, editors. Public Health Issues in Infant and Child Nutrition. Philadelphia: Nestec Ltd., Vevey/Lippincott Williams & Wilkins; 2002. p. 199–216.
43. Lartey A, Manu A, Brown KH, et al. A randomized, community-based trial of the effects of improved, centrally processed complementary foods on growth and micronutrient status of Ghanaian infants from 6 to 12 month of age. Am J Clin Nutr 1999;70:391–404.
44. Rivera JA, Sotres-Alvarez D, Habicht JP, et al. Impact of the Mexican program for education, health, and nutrition (Progresa) on rates of growth and anemia in infants and young children: A randomized effectiveness study. JAMA 2004;291:2563–70.
45. Faber M, Kvalsvig JD, Lombard CJ, Benade AJ. Effect of a fortified maize-meal porridge on anemia, micronutrient status, and motor development of infants. Am J Clin Nutr 2005;82:1032–9.
46. Zlotkin SH, Christofides AL, Hyder SM, et al. Controlling iron deficiency anemia through the use of home-fortified complementary foods. Indian J Pediatr 2004;71:1015–9.
47. Smuts CM, Lombard CJ, Benade AJ, et al. Efficacy of a foodlet-based multiple micronutrient supplement for preventing growth faltering, anemia, and micronutrient deficiency of infants: The four country IRIS trial pooled data analysis. J Nutr 2005;135:631S–8S.
48. Lopriore C, Guidoum Y, Briend A, Branca F. Spread fortified with vitamins and minerals induces catch-up growth and eradicates severe anemia in stunted refugee children aged 3–6 yr. Am J Clin Nutr 2004;80:973–81.
49. Adu-Afarwuah S, Lartey A, Brown KH, et al. Randomized comparison of 3 types of micronutrient supplements for home fortification of complementary foods in Ghana: Effects on growth and motor development. Am J Clin Nutr 2007;86:412–20.

37

Energy Metabolism and Requirements in Health and Disease

Jean Louis Bresson, MD

The interpretation of the changes in metabolic rate resulting from either malnutrition or disease finds its roots in the physiologic determinants of daily energy expenditure. The technical aspects of the measurement of energy expenditure and its obligate correlate, body composition, extend beyond the scope of this chapter and have been thoroughly reviewed in the literature.[1,2] Once raw data are available, many factors may confuse cross-sectional and, even more, age-related comparisons. The influence of body components, whether fat-free mass (FFM), fat mass (FM), or organ weight, should be considered first in an attempt to account for the wide differences in metabolic rate among infants, children, and adults. This is also relevant to a better understanding of the responses to underfeeding and malnutrition. Conversely, recent advances in the field of minor contributors to energy expenditure, such as the thermic effect of feeding (TEF) or the thermic response to cold, may help us to understand how physiologic mechanisms may be turned into an energy-losing machinery.

One of the most common findings in the sick child is a reduced food intake, which is widely accepted as the main, if not the only, cause of malnutrition. However, evidence accumulates suggesting that metabolic dysregulations may also participate and, in some instances, be primarily responsible for the nutritional deficit. This may be particularly true for proteins that, unless fat, are not stored but make up functional or structural tissues. Nitrogen balance in the adult or net protein deposition in the growing child results from protein synthesis rates equal to or higher than protein breakdown, respectively. This equilibrium may be disrupted by the overproduction of peptides, otherwise playing a pivotal role in the regulation of the immune system. It results in a protracted increase in protein breakdown over protein synthesis. This mechanism is found in acute as well as in chronic inflammatory syndromes and may lead to severe protein malnutrition, despite apparently normal nutrient intakes. Consequently, underfeeding is clearly not the only factor in malnutrition. Furthermore, these protein losses are not easily controlled by classic dietary treatment and represent a pressing case for developing a specific pharmacologic approach.

PHYSIOLOGIC DETERMINANTS OF ENERGY EXPENDITURE

Basal Metabolic Rate

Comparisons between the rates of energy expended, or heat produced, by individual subjects require that the measurements should be free of the effects of any factor known to increase it. Failure to control for the effects of activity, feeding, and physical environment on metabolic rate would obviously result in spurious interindividual differences. Benedict proposed a set of standard conditions required to perform accurate measurements of the basal metabolic rate (BMR) in adults[3]: the subject should be awake but in complete muscular repose both before and during the measurement, ideally performed in the morning before the patient rises; the subject should be in the postabsorptive state, normally accepted as 12 or more hours after the last meal, and should have received prior to the measurement a maintenance diet ensuring the stability of body weight; the subject should be in emotional repose and familiar with the measurement devices; in women, the measurement should not be made immediately before or during the menses; ambient temperature should be set in the range of the subject's thermal neutrality in order to avoid any thermoregulatory effect on heat production.

Obviously, these requirements may be impractical in infants and young children or in clinical settings. Metabolic rate measurement not performed in the postabsorptive state, but complying with the remaining conditions, and usually termed *resting metabolic rate* (RMR), is about 15% higher than true BMR.[4] It should be pointed out that, even in adults, the conventional period of 12 hours after the last meal may not be a sufficient interval to guarantee that the continuing effects of its metabolism are negligible.[5] Hence, BMR should not be viewed as a measure of the absolute minimal metabolism. Indeed, energy expenditure is about 8 to 12% lower during sleep than under basal conditions,[6] and oxygen consumption rate is then related to the stage of sleep.[7] As it is difficult to quantify the amount of work performed during spontaneous physical activity,[4] measurement of the sleeping metabolic rate (SMR) may be a convenient way to minimize its consequences on energy expenditure in young children. Thus, rather than defining a specific physiologic event, the set of standardized conditions chosen for metabolic rate measurements is primarily aimed at reducing the variance related to uncontrolled factors, in order to increase the power of interindividual or intergroup comparisons. When the rigorous conditions listed by Benedict are fulfilled, repeated measures display a remarkably low level of intraindividual variations. For instance, the coefficient of variation (σ/m) of replicate indirect calorimetry measurements amounts to about 2 to 4%, of which 2% could be accounted for by the variability related to the technique.[4]

The reproducibility of such measurements is high, even over a prolonged investigation.[8] Thus, the range of intraindividual variations in BMR becomes much narrower than the range of interindividual variations that one may observe in cross-sectional studies of normal adult populations. A threefold difference is usually found between the lower and higher BMR individual values, expressed in kcal or kJ/d.[9] Repeated measures confirm that these are true between-subject differences. Furthermore, BMR is about 15% lower in adult females than in adult males.[6] Much of these interindividual differences may be related to body build, as suggested by the significant correlations between BMR and body weight or height, or Quételet index (P/T^2).[10] Multiple regression analysis indicates that FFM accounts for about 65 to 75% of BMR variance between subjects[6,11] and that FM, age, and sex together account for another 5%.[11] It is noteworthy that—exclusive of pregnancy—the contribution of FM to BMR variance is limited,[6,11,12] or even negligible.[4] This may be related to the low metabolic rate of adipose tissue, estimated as 3 to 4.5 kcal/kg fat per day. Thus, large differences in FM would not be expected to contribute greatly to differences in basal energy expenditure. Indeed, BMR becomes comparable in males and females after adjusting for FFM.[6] Thus, FFM, FM, age, and sex account for about 80% of the interindividual variability in BMR, and nearly all the effect of these covariates is attributable to FFM (Figure 1).[13] However, differences between lower and higher individual metabolic rates still amount to about 600 kcal/d even after adjustment for these factors.[11] Further studies showed that family

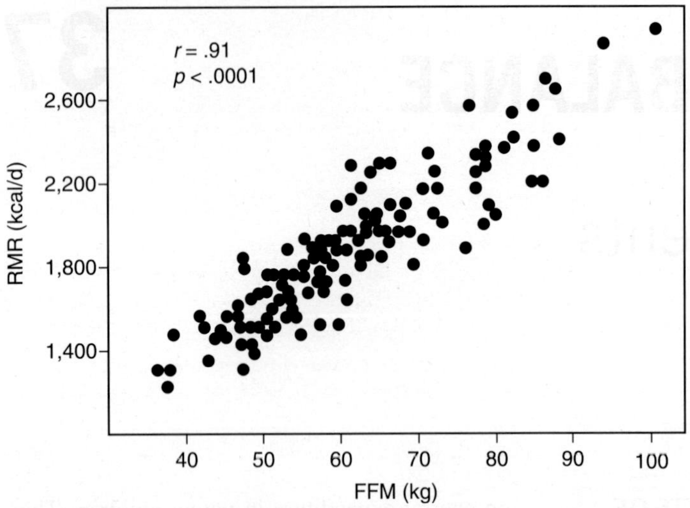

Figure 1 Relationship between resting metabolic rate (RMR) and fat-free mass (FFM) in 130 subjects. (From reference 13, with permission from the New England Journal of Medicine.)

membership is another significant determinant of BMR.[14] In the Pima Indians, metabolic rate among families may vary by nearly 600 kcal/d, whereas the mean variation within families is only about 60 kcal/d.[13] In this population, FFM, age, sex, and family membership account for 94% of the variability in metabolic rate, family membership contributing about 11%. Actually, a metabolic rate lower than that predicted by FFM, age, and sex at the beginning of the study turned out to be a major risk factor for body weight gain during the subsequent follow-up,[11] implying that obesity may just result from an economy in energy expenses. These results emphasize the necessity to express metabolic rate in relation to FFM, its major constituent, rather than in relation to any other parameter such as crude body weight or body area.

However, this mode of expression may still hamper interindividual comparisons in the pediatric population. During growth, RMR expressed either as kcal/kg body weight/d[15] or as kcal/kg FFM/d[16] follows a nonlinear increase, with slopes substantially higher in infants and young children than in adolescents and adults (Figure 2). After a steep increase in the days following birth,[17] RMR falls disproportionately to the rise in body weight[18] or FFM,[16] being about 67 kcal/kg FFM/d at 3 months, 46 kcal/kg FFM/d at 11 years, and 37 kcal/kg FFM/d at 13 years, as compared to adult values of 28 kcal/kg FFM/d (Figure 3). This suggests that the metabolic activity of FFM is changing as a whole[19] or that the relative contribution of tissues with different metabolic rates to the composition of FFM is changing,[20,21] or both.

Holliday pointed out that the brain, heart, liver, and kidney together make up only 5 to 6% of the body weight, but account for 60 to 70% of the BMR in the adult. Conversely, muscle mass, which makes up about 44% of the body weight, accounts for only 15 to 30% of BMR.[15] In contrast, the FFM of infants and young children comprises about 30% muscle and 20% other organs, and that of adolescents averages 42% muscle and 8% other organs.[15] Therefore, the higher metabolic rate of infants and children in relation to FFM could be ascribed to a greater proportion of metabolically active nonmuscle organ mass and to a lesser proportion of less metabolically active muscle mass than in adults (Table 1).[15,16] This is exemplified by experiments carried out on pigs with different nutritional background.[22] A first group was fed to gain steadily 14 kg over 70 days. A second group was fed to gain 19 kg during the first 35 days (high-energy period) and to lose 5 kg during the second 35 days (low-energy period; group HL), and this pattern was reversed (low-energy period first) in a third group (LH). At the end of the 70-day experiment, all animals had achieved the same body weight, but the fasting metabolic rate of the LH group was 25 to 50% higher than that of the HL group and 13 to 40% higher than that of the first one. Furthermore, there was a significant correlation between fasting metabolic rate and organ weights.[22] The consequences of these observations are twofold. First, comparing the BMR/FFM ratio between two groups of subjects may be misleading, when values of FFM are markedly different,[16] mainly because the ratio of the weight of organs (heart, liver, brain, spleen, and kidneys) to total FFM decreases as FFM increases.[23] Second, this raises the possibility that abnormal metabolic rates in disease states may be related to a change in the proportion of metabolically active organs to less active muscles. For instance, a reduction in muscle mass could account for the inverse relationship between RMR per kilogram of body weight and percent ideal body weight observed in patients with Crohn's disease.[24]

Differences in metabolic rate between young and mature animals have also been found in other mammalian species. These weight-related differences further extend to comparisons between mature animals of different species. For instance, mouse metabolic rate is about 5 times greater than man's and about 10 times that of the elephant.[25] Kleiber, and Brody and Proctor proposed a generalization according to which RMR follows a metabolic power function corresponding to weight to the power 0.75 (see references 25 and 26). However, the mass coefficient is not the same in various

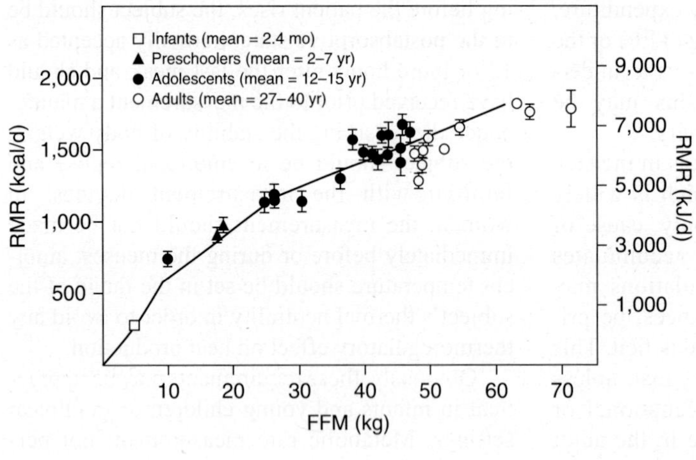

Figure 2 Relationship between resting metabolic rate (RMR) and fat-free mass (FFM) among different age groups. (Adapted from reference 16, with permission from the American Society for Clinical Nutrition.)

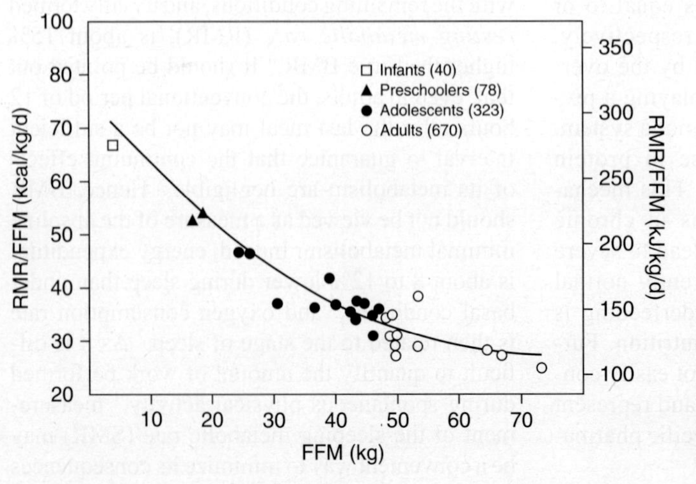

Figure 3 Relationship between resting metabolic rate (RMR) per unit fat-free mass (FFM) (RMR/FFM) to FFM among different age groups. (Adapted from reference 16, with permission from the American Society for Clinical Nutrition.)

Table 1 Relation between Basal Metabolic Rate (BMR) and Muscle and Organ Metabolic Rates with Age

Height (cm)	Weight (kg)	BMR (kcal/d) A	Muscle MR (kcal/d) B	Organ MR (kcal/d) C	B/A
60	5.5	300	21	279	7
80	11.0	590	45	545	7.6
11	19.0	830	117	713	14
14	31.0	1,160	204	956	17.6
160	50.0	1,480	373	1,107	25.2
180	70.0	1,800	500	1,300	27.7

From reference 285.

species, ranging from 0.48 to 0.91, the mean value being 0.67 ± 0.03. As there is no definite value for either the intraspecific or interspecific mass exponents, any attempt to explain the Brody-Kleiber empiric relationship by a general physical principle is most likely to fail.[26] Actually, this statistical relationship may obscure rather than reveal biologically important changes. The relative proportion of metabolically active tissue may contribute to these differences as large mammals have a greater proportion of tissues with low metabolic activity, whereas smaller ones have a greater proportion of tissues with higher metabolic activity. However, Krebs showed that the rates of respiration of homologous tissues are affected by the size of the animal, although there is no strict parallelism between measured tissue oxygen consumption and the BMR of the animals.[27] A comparison between homeo- and poikilotherms might give a hint about a possible cause for this difference. The standard metabolic rate is sevenfold greater in the rat (a typical mammal) than in an ectothermic vertebrate (bearded dragon) of the same body size and at the same body temperature.[28]

This large difference in metabolism is also manifest at the cellular level and may be related to membrane properties.[29] Rat hepatocytes respire fourfold faster than do hepatocytes from the lizard. The inner membrane of isolated rat liver mitochondria has a permeability that is four- to fivefold greater than the proton permeability of the lizard liver mitochondrial membrane.[28] Thus, the greater proton permeability of the mitochondrial inner membrane contributes to the greater metabolic rate of mammals. Actually, this is a major source of heat production (see later), the variations of which might impinge on lifespan.[30] Similarly, plasma membrane permeability to Na^+ and K^+ is higher in mammals than in ectothermic vertebrates, increasing the amount of energy devoted to active Na^+–K^+ exchange.[31] Thus, the activity of the Na^+–K^+-ATPase accounts for about 20% of the total in vitro energy expenditure by mammalian tissues[32] The use of ouabain to inhibit Na^+-K^+-ATPase in vivo leads to a 20 to 30% inhibition of resting oxygen consumption in guinea pigs[33] and to a 20 to 25% inhibition in mice,[34] supporting the idea that active Na^+–K^+ exchange is a significant determinant of resting energy expenditure. In humans, Na^+–K^+-ATPase activity may contribute 20 to 25% to BMR.[35] As in animals, Na^+–K^+-ATPase is subject to chronic control by thyroid hormones, and slight interindividual variations in free T_3 index among healthy adults would account for a between-subject difference in the SMR of 142 kcal/d.[36] Furthermore, the magnitude of Na^+–K^+-ATPase-dependent energy expenditure in tissues appears to be related to the physiologic status, and particularly to age. Muscle preparations from 7- to 21-day-old calves expend 26% more total aerobic energy in support of Na^+–K^+ transport than do the same muscles from 7-month-old calves.[32] Similarly, the Na^+–K^+-ATPase-dependent respiration of skeletal muscle preparations from 4-week-old lambs accounts for a 48% greater amount of energy than similar muscles from adult ewes. Also, energy consumption in support of active Na^+–K^+ exchange by the intercostal muscle from young lambs is 119% greater than for similar preparations taken from adults.[37] Comparable differences exist between hepatocytes obtained from 1- to 8-week-old lambs and from mature sheep.[38] In this latter case, the lower oxygen consumption of hepatocytes isolated from mature sheep is largely attributable (70 to 90%) to the decrease in the Na^+–K^+-ATPase-dependent component of respiration. Thus, membrane-associated processes appear to be significant components of BMR.

It is striking that in quiescent cultured animal cells exposed to mitogens, one of the first events to take place is a rapid, very large increase in the rate of Na+ flow into the cells,[39] which in turn induces increased Na^+–K^+ pumping. Activation of Na^+–K^+-ATPase appears to be an early growth-related event, and it is tempting to speculate that increased energy expended on active Na^+–K^+ transport by young mammals is also related to their higher growth rate.[37] Active ion transport is probably not the sole cause of this difference. Measurement of whole body protein synthesis shows that the smaller mammals display the higher protein synthesis rates in relation to their body weight. Within-species comparisons also indicate that immature animals have higher protein turnover rates than adults. For instance, protein synthesis amounts to 6.7 ± 1.1 g/kg/d in term infants as compared to 3.5 ± 0.6 g/kg/d in adult humans. Simultaneously, basal energy expenditure is 45.1 ± 4.6 and 23.6 ± 3.8 kcal/kg/d in newborns and adults, respectively.[40] Thus, a similar ratio of BMR to whole-body protein synthesis (6.7 to 6.9 kcal/g) applies to both healthy newborn and young adults, suggesting that the turnover of cellular constituents, including proteins, and energy expenditure change in parallel with maturation. Therefore, differences in BMR in relation to body weight or FFM during growth is not merely a matter of proportion between tissues with high or low metabolic rates, but is also related to differences in the amount of work done by the cells to ensure the turnover of their constituents and maintain the membrane electrochemical gradients.[41]

Energy Cost of Growth

An estimate of the energy cost of growth can be obtained in groups of rapidly growing infants from the relationship between growth rate and metabolizable energy intake.[42] The slope of this linear relationship provides an estimate of the total amount of energy stored and expended for synthesis, and its intercept at zero growth indicates the amount of energy required for maintenance. It should be pointed out that maintenance requirement may be higher than BMR by 10% in prematures[43] and 50% in children,[44] as maintenance includes expenses for limited activity and feeding.[45] The energy cost of growth can also be estimated from the independent measurement of stored energy and energy expended for synthesis.[43] An indirect method for calculating the cost of tissue synthesis is to relate weight gain to energy expenditure, assuming that an increase in expenditure is directly related to the increase in cost of synthesis. Unfortunately, the result may be obscured by activity. A direct measurement of the cost of synthesis rests on the assumption that the TEF (ie, the increase in metabolic rate after the meal over the resting value in the postabsorptive state; TEF) is largely accounted for by synthesis. This is supported by the positive correlation observed between weight gain and TEF in rapidly growing individuals.[45] However, the TEF may be grossly underestimated unless the interval between feeds is long enough to allow the metabolic rate to return to postabsorptive levels.

Various estimates of the total cost of growth are in the range of 3 to 6 kcal/g of new tissue. A widely accepted figure in normal infants is 5 kcal/g.[43,44] Metabolic balance and body composition studies indicate that the average composition of weight gain is 28% fat and 16% protein during the first year of life.[46] Assuming crude energy contents of 9.25 kcal/g and 5.65 kcal/g for fat and protein, respectively, it is possible to estimate the amount of energy stored to about 3.5 kcal/g of body weight gain. In contrast, the cost of synthesis is about 1.5 kcal/g of body weight gain. Direct estimates of the amount of energy expended for synthesis usually provide figures in the range of 0.55 to 0.7 kcal/g.[43,47] This discrepancy may be related to an underestimation of the TEF, as it is measured only 2 to 3 hours after the last meal. The so-called fasting metabolic rate used as a baseline is likely to be falsely high owing to the lasting effect of feeding. As the energy stored in weight gain represents about

70% of the total energy cost of growth, one can expect wide differences according to the composition of tissues laid down. For instance, it is possible to calculate that the total amount of energy required to deposit 1 g of protein is about 13.4 kcal/g and is 10.8 kcal/g for fat.[48] Thus, a weight gain comprising 16% protein and no fat would cost about 2.2 kcal/g. Conversely, a weight gain consisting of fat with no protein would cost about 9.7 kcal/g, assuming that adipose tissue may contain up to 90% lipids. These differences may account for the high cost of weight gain found in overfed adults. In these conditions, weight gain consists of about 70% fat and 30% fat-free tissue,[49] the theoretic cost of growth then amounting to approximately 7 kcal/g. Similarly, the average cost of weight gain in patients with anorexia nervosa ranges from 5 to more than 7 kcal/g, suggesting either important changes in the composition of body weight gain during rehabilitation,[50] or an important confounding effect of activity.[51]

The daily energy cost of growth will depend obviously on growth rate as well as on the composition of new tissue. Growth rate is highest during the first 3 months of life, reaching 30 to 35 g/d between birth and 8 weeks of age, or a fractional growth rate of about 1%/d.[46] It decreases rapidly thereafter to 7 to 10 g/d at 1 year of age, or 0.07 to 0.09%/d, and to about 5 g/d (less than 0.03%/d) by 5 years of age. Thus, the cost of growth represents a significant part of daily energy needs (~33%) from birth to 4 months of age. Later on, it decreases to about 7% between the ages of 4 and 12 months, 1.6% between 12 and 24 months, and 1% between 24 and 36 months. Thereafter it is negligible compared to daily energy expenditure. Thus, on the basis of nutrient partition between growth and nongrowth, the 1- to 2-year-old child appears more like the adult than the small, rapidly growing infant.[52]

Thermic Effect of Feeding

It was recognized long ago that fed animals have substantially higher metabolic rates than fasted ones.[53] The effect of specific nutrients was investigated during the nineteenth century showing that the ingestion of proteins induces a greater increase in energy expenditure than carbohydrates or fat. The ingestion of a mixed meal also results in an increased metabolic rate above BMR. Energy expenditure may increase by up to 30% over BMR in response to large energy challenges,[54] a sizable change equivalent to 6 to 10% of the energy intake.[54] Unlike BMR, the TEF appears to be independent of weight, FFM, FM, and Quételet index.[54] In contrast, its duration and magnitude are linearly related to the energy intake,[54] which explains the greater effect of large meals.[55] Duration and magnitude of TEF do not appear to be significantly different when the same meal is ingested or directly delivered into the stomach.[56] However, the magnitude of the thermic effect is significantly greater if the same energy load is delivered in a short time rather than over several hours.[55,57] The route of administration of the nutrients, either intragastric or intravenous, does not seem to affect the magnitude of the response,[58] suggesting that the energy input of luminal digestion, fermentation, mechanical mixing, and nutrient absorption makes only a modest contribution to the TEF in normal subjects. Energy expenditure may still be significantly higher than postabsorptive levels by 5 to 8 hours after a large energy challenge.[54] Furthermore, the effect of the antecedent diet may significantly affect both sleeping and RMRs. For instance, RMR remains elevated by 12% 14 hours after the last meal during short-term overfeeding.[5] In these conditions, the TEF lasts not only for the whole day, but also throughout the night until the following morning, when the effect is still apparent. There is also strong indication that the TEF of one meal merges into the thermic effect of the next meal. Thus, the duration of the TEF should be carefully considered before attempting to determine either BMR or the effect of feeding, particularly in infants.

The composition of the meal bears some importance. In accordance with earlier work, the thermic response to a high-protein meal is greater than that to a high-carbohydrate one.[59] Similarly, the TEF is greater after a high-carbohydrate meal when compared to a high-fat[60] or a mixed diet.[61] Thus, high-fat meals could be a risk factor for obesity in children.[62] However, the ingestion of a mixed meal elicits many simultaneous and complex events, and an experimental account of the thermic response to feeding could only come from a simplified model. The euglycemic–hyperinsulinemic insulin clamp offers several advantages in this regard.[63] It involves a single nutrient and bypasses absorption, allowing one to know precisely the rate of glucose appearance within the body at any time. Combined with indirect calorimetry, it allows one to assess the effect of glucose infusion on glucose oxidation and storage as well as on energy expenditure. When different plasma insulin concentrations are achieved, together with glucose infusion rates appropriate for maintaining euglycemia, it is readily apparent that the increase in energy expenditure secondary to glucose administration is not related to an increase in its oxidation rate. In contrast, the increase in energy expenditure is closely related to the rate of glucose storage.[64] This is supported by studies in insulin-resistant patients showing that their blunted thermic response to glucose infusion is restored when glucose storage rate is matched to controls' by further increasing insulin concentration.[65] Thus, in agreement with Flatt's proposal,[66] the TEF is primarily related to the cost of storage of the nutrients. According to the stoichiometry of these reactions, it is possible to calculate that the synthesis of glycogen costs about 4% of the energy of the glucose stored (0.15 kcal/g), and that this cost increases to 28% (1.05 kcal/g) when glucose is converted to fat. Conversely, the cost of triglyceride synthesis from absorbed fats amounts to about 2% of their energy content. Because of the many ATP-consuming steps involved in the synthesis and breakdown of proteins, the cost of amino acid incorporation into proteins is estimated to about 25%, but might be as high as 55% of their energy content.[66] Indeed, comparing the thermic effect of high-protein and high-carbohydrate diets shows that the former results in a greater thermic response (+45%) than the latter. Simultaneously, the increase in protein turnover is twice as much with the high-protein diet as with the high-carbohydrate diet. The metabolic cost of protein synthesis would thus account for about 68 and 36% of the thermic effect of each diet, respectively, and the combined effect of increased protein synthesis and nitrogen excretion would account for 96% of the thermic effect of the high-protein diet.[59]

The cost of storage may not be the only component of the TEF. Indeed, the increase in energy expenditure related to glucose infusion is substantially higher than predicted from the amount of glucose stored.[64] The fact that overfeeding or the ingestion of a glucose-rich meal elicits an increase in sympathetic nervous system (SNS) outflow,[67] or in plasma noradrenaline concentration and turnover,[68,69] a known thermogenic hormone, suggests that the stimulation of the SNS is involved in the thermic response to feeding. This is supported by the blunting of the glucose-induced increase in energy expenditure by β-adrenergic blockade during insulin clamps. As a result, the residual variation in metabolic rate becomes almost identical to the value predicted from the amount of glucose stored.[70] This implies that the TEF has two components. One is an obligatory component directly related to the intermediary storage of nutrients and accounts for about 60% of the response to feeding. The other is related to the stimulation of the SNS and represents about 30% of the increase in energy expenditure.[71] This partition is confirmed by the use of clonidine, a centrally acting α_2-adrenergic receptor agonist that inhibits SNS outflow. In association with the decreased SNS response to a carbohydrate-rich meal, TEF is blunted by 33%, a value similar to that obtained from peripheral β-adrenergic blockade during insulin clamps.[72] The effect of SNS activity on energy expenditure is not restricted to the hours following meals. Its inhibition by clonidine also decreases RMR. Although the reduction in RMR does not reach significance because of the small number of subjects, the authors aptly point out that a 6% decrease in baseline metabolic rate might account for a greater overall diminution in energy expenditure than the larger 33% blunting of TEF.[72] The contribution of SNS activity to energy expenditure in the postabsorptive state is further confirmed by the 8% reduction in BMR observed in response to a β-adrenergic antagonist that does not affect T_3 production, nadolol.[73] Furthermore, urinary noradrenaline excretion and muscle sympathetic nerve activity are significantly correlated to RMR adjusted for FFM, FM, and age in normal adults, implying that SNS activity is a physiologic determinant of energy expenditure.[74,75] A similar correlation between urinary noradrenaline excretion and oxygen consumption is observed in infants,[76] suggesting that the effects of SNS activity on energy expenditure extend to this age.

Therefore, the TEF involves a short-term meal-related component lasting for several hours, and is accounted for by both nutrient storage (obligatory) and acute stimulation of the SNS (facultative). In rapidly growing infants, this short-term effect also reflects the cost of synthesis of new tissues, as its magnitude is significantly correlated to growth rate.[45] However, the response to feeding also involves a longer-term component, which may affect BMR and SMR.

Thermogenesis

Heat production by living organisms is associated with respiration and concomitant oxidation of nutrients. According to the chemiosmotic hypothesis,[77] the enthalpy of oxidation is transduced by the respiratory chain of the mitochondria into a proton gradient, which powers the ATP synthase. However, the efficiency of the system characterized by the ratio of the amount of energy liberated to that recovered is far from one, even if it is higher than previously estimated from the standard-free energy of ATP, $\Delta G^{0'}$.[1] Attempts to directly evaluate this efficiency in man indicate that about 65% of the energy liberated may be recovered under the form of ATP.[78] Thus, a minimum of 35% is lost as heat, and nutrient oxidation at the level of mitochondrial respiration appears as the primary heat-releasing process. This is consistent with the significant relationship existing between body temperature and BMR or SMR.[79] However, basal heat production may be insufficient to maintain the core temperature within a narrow range of variation, particularly when heat exchange is increased by a low ambient temperature. Extra heat production can be generated by recruiting metabolic processes that do not produce any net work. Isometric muscular contraction, as it may occur during malignant hyperthermia, is a major heat-generating process. Similarly, shivering increases oxygen consumption,[80] and because no external work is performed, the energy appears as heat.

There is some evidence in adult humans that heat production may be increased by other means. For instance, BMR or 24-hour energy expenditure increases significantly (6 to 11%) in response to an ambient temperature drop from 28° to 20–22°C, without any overt sign of shivering or any correlation with activity.[81] Similarly, the metabolic rate of full-term infants increases in response to an ambient temperature lowering from 32° to 23°C. This increase is not correlated with activity and occurs in the absence of shivering. In these conditions, the infants' response is dramatic, amounting to a 100% increase in energy expenditure,[82,83] which suggests that a nonshivering thermogenesis is operative. In the rat, the early stage of cold adaptation is associated with shivering. However, shivering disappears with acclimatization, and a nonshivering heat source eventually takes over all the duties of heat production.[84] It is now well established that cold exposure results in a marked increase in sympathetic activity, largely responsible for the elevated metabolic rate of the rats.[85] The dominant role in nonshivering thermogenesis has been ascribed to brown adipose tissue (BAT), even in adult animals.[86] BAT stimulation is achieved through β-adrenergic receptors, among which is a new type of receptor with pharmacologic properties differing from either β_1 or β_2, thus termed β_3.[87] BAT's prominent characteristic is the synthesis of a specific, 32,000 *M*r protein, known as uncoupling protein–1 (UCP-1; review in reference 88), located in the inner mitochondrial membrane and acting as a proton conductance pathway. UCP-1 dissipates the proton gradient created by respiration, thus bypassing ATP synthase. In turn, the dissipation of the proton gradient causes a dramatic increase in the mitochondrial respiratory rate. Upon β-adrenergic stimulation, BAT substantially increases its respiration. As mitochondrial respiration and phosphorylation are uncoupled, ATP generation accounts for much less than 10% of oxygen consumption,[89] and the enthalpy of oxidation of the nutrients is essentially dissipated as heat, making BAT a tissue specialized in thermogenesis. Acute cold exposure leads to a rapid and pronounced elevation of the level of the mRNA coding for UCP-1, and UCP-1 synthesis is evident within 15 minutes.[90] In contrast, hypothyroid rats are unable to maintain a normal body temperature when placed at 4°C, despite increased noradrenaline turnover rates.[91] The response of UCP mRNA to adrenergic stimulation in hypothyroid brown adipocytes is readily restored by T_4 through mechanisms requiring its intracellular conversion to T_3.[92] For a full UCP-1 response to cold, near-saturation of the nuclear T_3 receptor is required.[92] BAT contains a type II 5'deiodinase (5'D-II), which locally generates T_3 and allows it to reach a very high level of receptor occupancy despite the low physiologic plasma T_3 levels.[93] Indeed, T_4 appears to be a much more efficient source of T_3 for BAT than plasma T_3 when the 5'D-II is activated. Conversely, iopanoic acid, an inhibitor of 5'D-II, abolishes the T_4-induced restoration of both UCP-1 response and normothermia in hypothyroid rats.[92] In turn, 5'D-II activity is stimulated by SNS,[94] and nuclear T_3 receptors are nearly saturated within 4 hours of cold exposure.[93] Thus, SNS, through cAMP generation, and thyroid hormones act synergistically on BAT. T_3 affects the *UCP-1* gene expression at a transcriptional[95] and posttranscriptional level.[96] However, this effect of T_3 is not sufficient to elevate UCP-1 mRNA cellular content in the absence of significant levels of transcription, explaining why T_3 cannot increase UCP-1 mRNA in vivo in the absence of adrenergic stimulation.[97] Thus, T_3 amplifies the effects of the adrenergic stimulation on UCP-1 gene expression, allowing BAT to reach its full thermogenic capacity. Conversely, pretreatment of rats with corticosterone abolishes the UCP-1 mRNA response to noradrenaline and cold by inhibiting UCP-1 gene expression.[98] Interestingly, this effect is antagonized by the action of the corticotropin-releasing hormone (under feedback control by glucocorticoid) on the central nervous system, stimulating SNS outflow[99] and leading to an increased expression of UCP-1.[100] The simultaneous expression of several proteins (uncoupling protein, 5'D-II, and β_3-adrenoreceptors) appears to characterize functionally active BAT, although only UCP-1 is tissue specific.

The first attempts to settle the controversy about the presence or absence of BAT in humans involved the characterization of UCP-1. This protein was first reported in human fat depots from patients with pheochromocytoma.[101] It was subsequently isolated from newborn brown fat.[102] Later on, UCP-1 was found in humans at all ages, but its content was highest in children.[103] Since then, human *UCP-1* gene has been cloned. Its sequence is 80% homologous to rat UCP-1, both at the nucleotidic and amino acid levels.[104] Both UCP-1 and UCP-1 mRNA are present in infants and in an unexpected number of adult patients, UCP-1 mRNA being detected in the periadrenal adipose tissue of all the subjects studied.[105] UCP-1 transcripts are abundant in an infant's perirenal fat, but are low in quantity in subcutaneous depots.[106] Full-term newborn interscapular UCP-1 content is equal to, or even higher than, the level found in 3-week-old mice acclimatized at 20°C. In contrast, ATPase content is low in infant BAT, similar to that found in animal BAT mitochondria, compared with heart and liver mitochondria[107] The specific content of UCP-1 in infant BAT increases twofold between 25 and 32 weeks of gestation and remains nearly constant thereafter.[107] Infant BAT also expresses a 5'D-II. Strikingly, 5'D-II content follows the same pattern as UCP-1 and achieves levels comparable to 5'D-II activities found in animals stimulated during the neonatal period by exposure to cold or increased cAMP levels.[107] Moreover, β_3-adrenoreceptor mRNA content in children and adults parallels that of UCP-1 mRNA.[106] This coexpression of UCP-1, 5'D-II, and β_3-adrenoreceptor strongly suggests that functional BAT exists in humans from birth to old age. Measurements performed in vitro on isolated cell preparations as well as in vivo suggest that the heat-dissipating capacity of BAT is in the range of 300 W/kg of tissue.[108] Thus, 16 g of BAT would be sufficient to account for the 25 to 30 W/m^2 increase in energy expenditure observed in newborns exposed at 23°C.[83] This would represent about 3% of the adipose tissue mass of newborns, or a figure similar to the amount of BAT found in adult rats acclimated to cold.[86]

Adrenaline-mediated thermogenesis also occurs in human muscle,[109] even if its mechanism is still uncertain. Adrenaline infusion causes a 25% increase in whole body energy expenditure and stimulates forearm muscle oxygen consumption by as much as 90%. Assuming that forearm muscle is representative of total body musculature, skeletal muscle would then account for up to 40% of the adrenaline-infusion–induced thermogenesis in humans.[110] More recently, it was shown that T_3 administration to normal adults results in a significant increase in the activity of muscle tricarboxylic acid (TCA) cycle, without any change in the rate of ATP synthesis.[111] The disproportionate increase in TCA cycle flux compared with ATP synthesis suggests that T_3 induces an increase in muscle thermogenesis by promoting mitochondrial energy uncoupling. This might be achieved through an increase in UCP-3 protein expression, which is specific to skeletal muscle and upregulated by thyroid hormones. In this regard, it is noteworthy that intraindividual variations in BMR are tightly correlated to small, spontaneous changes in thyroid hormone concentrations in healthy adults,[36,112] a mechanism that could contribute to cold adaptation.

Besides mitochondrial uncoupling, the thermogenic potential for Ca^{2+} cycling is exemplified by the pathological syndrome of malignant hyperthermia, a dominant pharmacogenetic myopathy that occurs in humans and several other mammalian species. Ca^{2+}-cycling mediated thermogenesis in skeletal muscle cells is a well-characterized mechanism for nonshivering thermogenesis in fish and recently in birds. It could prove to be an important source of heat in mammals lacking large amounts of BAT. In any cases, the biochemical properties of muscle (ie, fast-twitch vs slow oxidative fibers) do contribute to the interindividual variability in SMR and 24-hour energy expenditure in the adult.[113,114] However, the respective contributions of BAT and muscle to the overall thermogenic response remain difficult to ascertain. Some studies in adults suggest that a ~700 g BAT would contribute 25% to adrenaline-induced thermogenesis, whereas the ~34-kg muscle mass would account for 50% of the thermic response.[115] Despite the uncertainties about its effectors, the reality of a β-sympathetically mediated thermogenesis is now well recognized in humans.[75,116]

Twenty-Four-Hour Energy Expenditure

The measurement of 24-hour energy expenditure (24hEE) in free-living conditions over relatively long time intervals can be assessed by determining the turnover rates of isotopes of hydrogen (^2H) and oxygen (^{18}O) in total body water.[117] Despite its cost and its methodological limits, the doubly labelled water technique is quite suited for studies in infants and children. Actually, it led to recognize that recommended dietary allowances overestimated energy requirements by a significant extent in these age groups.[118]

BMR represents a major determinant of 24hEE. For instance, it amounts to about 60% of 24hEE in sedentary adults.[119] The difference between BMR and 24hEE comprises thermogenesis, the TEF and the amount of energy expended on physical activity, be it exercise or nonexercise activity. Obviously, this is the most variable component of total energy expenditure.

In 1985, the FAO/WHO/UNU expert committee on energy requirements expressed the energy needs as multiple of BMR. The 24hEE-to-BMR ratio was subsequently referred to as physical activity level (PAL). Although not entirely satisfactory, PAL offers a convenient means of assessing and comparing physical activity, which is its main source of variance. Extreme PALs range from about 1.2 in the completely chair- or bed-bound subjects to about 4.7 in Tour de France cyclists.[120] PALs >4 represent levels of expenditure which are not sustainable on a permanent way of life. On the contrary, a PAL range of 1.2 to 2.5 corresponds to sustainable lifestyles, where 2.5 represents a very physically active one. Actually, a PAL of 1.35 is now considered as the lowest value compatible with long-term maintenance in normal adults and a PAL range of 1.55 to 1.65 represents the average of the so-called sedentary lifestyle. Data suggest that activities do not have to be obviously strenuous for relatively high PAL values to be achieved. In adults, the time spent at activities with low and moderate intensity determines the activity level, while high-intensity activities do not have much impact.[121] In other words, the cumulative impact of low- to moderate-intensity activities of prolonged duration is of greater energetic significance than short bursts of high-intensity activities. In children, PALs show an inverse relation with the time spent on low-intensity activities[122] and, as in adults, engagement in vigorous-intensity activities does not significantly influence 24hEE.[123] It is noteworthy that the fraction of time spent on low-intensity activities appears lower in 8-year-old children than in young adults and elderly persons.[122] PAL values vary from about 1.4 to 1.5 in boys and from 1.7 to 1.9 in girls between 1 year of age and adolescence.[124] Indirect estimates suggest that the energy cost of spontaneous activity represents only 5 to 10% of 24hEE in premature infants,[47] but amounts to 20 to 26% of 24hEE between 1 and 4 months of age[125] and up to 50% in 8- to 12-year-old children. A mean PAL of 1.5 was reported in 10 to 13 years old boys and girls. In this latter case, the variability of the 24hEE-to-BMR ratio is quite large, reflecting important individual differences in the amount of energy expended for activity (range 1.20 to 1.87).[126]

Of note, PAL is negatively associated with body fat in 5 to 10.5 years[127] or 6 to 8 years old children.[128] This suggests that the amount of energy expended on physical activity may significantly affect energy balance, a potential asset in the prevention and treatment of obesity. Although most cross-sectional studies support a relationship between body fat and activity in children,[129] the results of interventions aimed at preventing childhood obesity through the implementation of physical activity programs remain inconclusive.[130] This is intriguing, as obesity may develop from a remarkably small daily net imbalance between energy intake and expenditure (median of estimated energy accumulation: 15 kcal/d),[131] a difference well within the range of moderate-intensity physical activity expenses.

On the contrary, it is not quite unexpected that most studies in obese adults demonstrate that participating in routine endurance exercise activities for up to a year does not induce a significant weight loss in the absence of an energy-restricted diet. Obesity represents the storage of a large energy surplus (over 100 Mcal in adults) and any attempt to reduce this imbalance, even by a small amount, would require a very significant increase in energy expenditure. Indeed, diminishing such reserves by 1% would imply a net negative balance of ≥1,000 kcal. For a 100 kg-overweight individual, this would translate into more than 2 hours of brisk walking (4 mph) or light jogging every day in order to expend about 700 kcal/d.[132] Thus, a negative outcome with exercise alone may be related to a failure to achieve an adequate level of physical activity.

Nonexercise, spontaneous physical activity, also known as nonexercise activity thermogenesis (NEAT), encompasses the daily expenditure of living activities (mainly ambulation) and the energy cost of all nonvolitional muscle activity, such as muscle tone, posture maintenance, and fidgeting. NEAT may play a significant role in the maintenance of energy balance. Spontaneous physical activity measured within the confines of a respiratory chamber accounts for an average 348 kcal/d, with individual extremes of 100 to 800 kcal/d.[4] NEAT appears to be a familial trait, amounting to as much as 13% of 24hEE.[119] Thus, NEAT may be—independently of volitional exercise—an important mediator of resistance to fat gain. Changes in NEAT account for differences in fat storage between individuals, and failure to activate NEAT in the face of excess energy may lead to weight gain.[133] The comparison of mildly obese and control adults suggests that obese individuals may save up to 352 kcal/d (269 to 477 kcal/d) by staying seated 164 minutes longer per day than their lean counterparts, an economy not matched by a similar reduction in energy intake.[134] The contribution of NEAT to 24hEE in childhood is unknown, but might be quite significant. The regulation of NEAT is also unknown. However, familial resemblance in twin pairs' physical activity is predominantly explained by shared environmental factors rather than by genetic variability.[135]

Thus, components other than BMR and the energy cost of activity contribute modestly to the 24hEE of normal infants and children. However, an increase in the energy expended by these minor components (SNS activity and thermogenesis) may significantly alter energy balance in disease states.

EFFECTS OF UNDERFEEDING AND MALNUTRITION

Effects on Energy Expenditure

Underfeeding healthy or obese adults results in a consistent 20 to 30% reduction in BMR and 24hEE expressed either in absolute terms or related to body weight, body surface area, body weight to the 0.73 power[136] or FFM.[137] It should be pointed out that this effect has important implications for the clinical management of obesity, as this compensatory change opposes the maintenance of a body weight that is different from the usual weight.[137] The decrease in BMR is rapid during the first weeks, then proceeds at a slower rate.[136,138] Thus, the initial, rapid decrease in BMR is not entirely accounted for by a corresponding loss of metabolically active tissue.[136,139] An analysis of fasting and semistarvation studies suggests that about 25 to 30% of the short-term decrease in BMR may be independent of the loss in lean body mass, indicating either a change in the composition of FFM or an alteration of cellular metabolism.[138] The dramatic effect of refeeding on BMR, which returns to normal within a few days without a parallel increase in body weight,[136] further supports the hypothesis that the decrease in metabolic rate during acute dietary restriction is of larger magnitude than that of tissue losses. A downregulation of BMR might be related to the decrease in noradrenaline appearance rate,[69,140] and in thyroid hormones,[69,141,142] in response to fasting or semistarvation. This possibility is supported by the prevention or the reversal of the metabolic response to acute energy restriction by replacement with either levodopa or T_3.[141,142] The enhancement of the thermic response to adrenaline infusion by prior starvation is consistent with a reduction in SNS activity.[143] A decrease in SNS outflow might also explain the significant reduction in the energy cost of glucose storage observed after underfeeding normal adults for 7 days.[144] Similarly, it might account for the absence of any increase in the metabolic rate of undernourished patients exposed to mild cold. As their thermic response to adrenaline is conserved, the defect in cold-induced thermogenesis following weight loss cannot be ascribed to a decrease in tissue responsiveness. In these patients, the thermic response to mild cold is fully restored after weight gain.[145] Similar functional defects are apparent in children. Malnourished infants switched from 28° to 24°C respond with a progressive fall in central temperature. When recovered, these infants increase their BMR by 20% in response to temperature lowering, and are able to maintain their body temperature within the normal range without shivering.[146] A decrease in skeletal muscle respiration proportional to the change in BMR in malnourished infants further supports a decrease in cellular metabolism.[147] However, metabolic rate measurements in chronically undernourished children may provide results that apparently conflict with those observed during acute energy restriction in adults.

Surprisingly, BMR may be approximately normal relative to body weight, and may even appear higher in those infants who are the most wasted.[148] Similar results are obtained in chronically undernourished adults. BMR related to body weight appears higher in the undernourished than in the controls, although in absolute terms it is significantly lower.[149] Body cell mass (BCM) is reduced even in moderate deficiency, but muscle mass seems to decrease linearly with the increasing severity of undernutrition, while visceral cell mass shows limited changes. For instance, body fat and BCM are reduced by 29% while muscle mass is decreased by 41% in severe undernutrition.[150] This is in general agreement with animal experiments, although a larger range in the weight change of some organs in response to nutritional manipulations may be observed.[151] Thus, taking into account the respective metabolic rate of tissues,[14] it is not surprising that BMR related to BCM or FFM may appear falsely high in some cases of severe malnutrition. This increase in metabolic rate related to FFM or body weight does not preclude an overall depression of tissue metabolism.[148,152] In infants, protein turnover, synthesis, and breakdown rates are significantly lower (~40%) before than after recovery from malnutrition.[153] Diminished substrate cycling is observed in adults during short-term underfeeding, and the resulting decrease in both protein turnover and glucose cycling may account for about 35% of the reduction in 24hEE.[154] Conversely, the malnourished infants' increase in energy expenditure in response to dietary treatment is an early event,[148] concurrent with a dramatic increase in growth rate[45] and in protein turnover,[155] suggesting that it may not be entirely accounted for by the change in body composition. Fasting metabolic rate (related to body weight) during rapid growth is equal to, or even higher than,[148,152] the recovered values, a fact that further strengthens this possibility. Another way to look at the reality of metabolic rate downregulation would be to measure the cost of growth, which might be decreased by a higher metabolic efficiency. Although an overall increase in food efficiency may exist during the early period of catch-up growth,[45] the cost of growth during recovery from malnutrition generally appears similar to that of the normal infant.[155] However, longitudinal studies may easily overlook any enhancement in metabolic efficiency if it is short-lived.[156]

Effects on Substrate Use

The classic studies of starvation showed that endogenous glucose production amounts to about 180 g/d after a few days' fast, of which 80% is oxidized by the brain.[157] The bulk of gluconeogenic precursor is provided by body proteins.[157] After 5 or 6 weeks of starvation, ketone bodies have replaced glucose as the predominant fuel for brain metabolism,[158] and glucose production has decreased to about 86 g/d, of which about 50% comes from recycled lactate and pyruvate.[159] Thus, fasting endogenous glucose production relies on gluconeogenesis much earlier than previously expected[160] and both decrease as peripheral glucose uptake diminishes. The reduced demand in gluconeogenic precursors is paralleled by a significant reduction in protein breakdown, which favors sparing of tissue proteins.[161] In parallel, there is a state of insulin resistance at both the hepatic and peripheral levels, which is restored after refeeding.[162] From the beginning, fat is the predominant fuel, the respiratory quotient falling to 0.70 by the fourth day of fasting.[157] Observations made in malnourished children are consistent with these results. Protein contributes little to total energy expenses.[163] The average daily amount of glucose oxidized is also lower, and glucose oxidation decreases more rapidly in response to fasting before recovery than after recovery,[163] which does not demonstrate, but is suggestive of, a reduction in glucose production.[157] It is striking that the reduction in urinary nitrogen output, which occurs in lean, starving adults, is proportionate to the simultaneous decrease in metabolic rate, suggesting that protein sparing might result from the general reduction in fuel use rather than from a specific fat-related mechanism.[164] However, the protein-conserving effect of growth hormone (GH) under fasting conditions has been ascribed to the stimulation of lipolysis,[165] thus demonstrating that free fatty acids are important protein-sparing agents.

Therefore, underfeeding results in a significant decrease in metabolic rate related to tissue loss and, to a lesser extent, to a reduction in the activity of the remaining tissues. This reduction in metabolic rate can be viewed as an attempt to save energy in the face of reduced intakes. However, such an economy goes far beyond the physiologic range of adaptation, as it is obtained at the expense of growth and body composition. Furthermore, its only flexibility depends on the use of remaining functional tissues as a source of substrates. Thus, any interfering increase in energy demand may entirely jeopardize this precarious balance.

EFFECTS OF DISEASE STATES

The compromise achieved by malnourished infants may be imperiled in two obvious ways. The first one would be to increase energy expenditure, for example, through fever. The other one would be to disrupt the adaptation of protein metabolism by a selective increase in protein breakdown, leading to a rapid net loss of nitrogen.

Effects on Protein Metabolism

It has been known for a long time that urinary nitrogen output is dramatically increased during infection and trauma, in sharp contrast with what is observed during malnutrition. In vivo studies reveal that this is accounted for by a disproportionate increase in protein breakdown over synthesis.[166,167] However, infusion of counterregulatory hormones to healthy adults falls short of reproducing the massive 20 to 40 g/d nitrogen losses observed after trauma or thermal injury, although it does induce plasma hormone elevations typical of severe stress.[168] In contrast, peptides isolated from the plasma of patients with sepsis or trauma are able to specifically induce a dramatic increase in protein breakdown, without affecting synthesis.[169,170] This specific effect on protein breakdown is reproduced in vitro by incubating muscle biopsies with the culture medium of activated macrophages, suggesting that cytokines are involved.[171] Cytokines are a large family of cellular regulators that include interleukins (ILs), tumor necrosis factors (TNFs), interferons (IFNs), and others. They play a pivotal role in the immune system, but their effects extend far beyond the immune cells. Each cytokine may interact with different cell types, thus exhibiting pleiotropic functions in different target cells.[172] Conversely, many different cytokines may exert the same biological actions—a property known as redundancy. Administration of recombinant tumor necrosis factor (rTNF) or recombinant interleukin-1α (rIL-1α) to animals results in accelerated muscle proteolysis.[173,174] Chronic administration of either rTNF or rIL-1α induces muscle wasting.[173,175] Furthermore, there is a synergistic effect between TNF and IL-1 on the stimulation of proteolysis.[173] In contrast with earlier expectations, the effect of cytokines on protein breakdown is only partially abolished by inhibitors of prostaglandin (PG) E_2 synthesis.[176] Moreover, proteolysis in response to rIL-1α is not mediated by glucocorticoids.[174] In humans, administration of rTNF also results in a dose-dependent rise in the amino acid efflux from muscle,[177] confirming the central role of cytokines in the protein losses associated with various acute and chronic diseases. In muscle, the underlying mechanism involves the induction of E3 ubiquitin ligase gene (Atrogin-1 and muscle-specific ring finger protein 1 or MuRF1) leading to muscle atrophy through the selective action of the ubiquitin-dependent proteasome on muscle cell gene products. The induction of these ubiquitin ligases does not depend upon glucocorticoids and can be downregulated by insulin-like growth factor I (IGF-I).[178] As in adults, the rates of protein synthesis and breakdown increase markedly in response to infection in children. However, breakdown increases more than synthesis, leading to a net loss of nitrogen.[179] Although malnutrition blunts the response to infection, infected malnourished children have protein turnover rates twice as high as uninfected ones, the relative increase in protein breakdown resulting in a negative protein balance.[179] Increased protein breakdown was first noted in sepsis or trauma patients, but a significant change may also be observed in response to much less severe conditions, such as vaccinations,[180,181] suggesting that even mild infections are likely to offset the fragile equilibrium of undernourished children.

It should be pointed out that protein metabolism imbalance per se (ie, protein breakdown rates greater than synthesis) results in a net protein loss and thus may lead to protein deficiency. Growth failure in Crohn's disease might be accounted for by such a mechanism. Growth failure is often associated with Crohn's disease[182] and may even precede symptoms. These patients have a short stature, but in most cases their body weight is close to the expected weight for height.[183] Obviously, their FFM is significantly lower than in age-matched controls.[184] As GH secretion is normal,[185] a search for nutritional deficiencies was undertaken. A reduction in energy intakes is noted in some reports[186] but not all,[187,188] whereas protein intakes appear consistently within the ranges of recommended dietary allowances.[186,187] Furthermore, energy losses in the feces are not different from those of normal children,[183,187] and intestinal protein losses are only slightly increased over control values.[183,187] When measured, energy expenditure related to FFM is comparable to results in matched controls[184,189] and the preserved FM argues against a significant energy deficit.[190] Despite the lack of evidence in favor of nutritional deficiencies, energy supplements do result in a significant increase in growth rate,[187,188] suggesting that a nutritional deficiency is indeed responsible for growth failure in Crohn's disease. That such a deficiency could not be ascribed to an overt imbalance between intakes and needs suggests that it might result from an abnormal utilization of available substrates. Indeed, abnormal protein turnover rates are consistently found in these patients.[191,192] Moreover, alterations in protein metabolism are correlated with the intensity of the inflammatory syndrome[191,192] and are consistent with an increased production of TNFα and IL-1.[193] Besides the dramatic effect of energy supplements, another line of evidence points toward a nutritional deficiency in Crohn's disease. The plasma concentration of IGF-I is significantly depressed in these patients and further correlates with growth rates.[194] Reduced plasma IGF-I concentrations, despite normal or increased circulating GH levels, is a trait of malnutrition and measurements of IGF-I levels have been proposed as a highly efficient way of monitoring nutritional rehabilitation.[195] Of particular interest is the fact that plasma IGF-I concentration is closely correlated with protein balance in both animal and man.[195,196] In the rat, IGF-I level is also correlated with protein intake.[197] Furthermore, low fasting IGF-I concentrations cannot be restored to normal levels by refeeding protein-free diets.[196] This is related to the direct modulation of IGF-I expression by essential amino acid availability, independently of insulin and glucocorticoid contributions.[198] Likewise, IGF-I levels in infected-malnourished children are sensitive to dietary protein alterations.[199] High-protein diets result in higher IGF-I levels and in improved growth rates,[199] despite the possible direct effect of some cytokines on IGF-1 expression.[200] Therefore, the decrease in IGF-I levels in Crohn's disease pinpoints the critical importance of protein metabolism in growth failure. Indeed, nutritional supplementation results in elevated IGF-I concentrations and increased growth rates.[194] Food supplements induce a significant increase in protein synthesis, which results in an increase in protein balance.[184] In contrast, nutritional support does not seem to affect the elevated breakdown rates.[191] The favorable effect of the nutritional supplements could then be accounted for by the specific induction of protein synthesis by amino acids.[201] Therefore, growth failure in Crohn's disease may be primarily related to an abnormal utilization of substrates, due to an imbalance between protein synthesis and breakdown rates, the latter being specifically increased by the associated inflammatory syndrome. Reduction in food intake would only exaggerate the protein debt by further reducing the synthesis-to-breakdown ratio, whereas nutritional support compensates for the increased breakdown rates by promoting protein synthesis.

Findings in rheumatoid arthritis (RA) are also consistent with a dominant effect of inflammatory syndromes on protein metabolism. RA is associated with a chronic inflammatory syndrome involving local cytokine production.[202] The immunologic response occurs in affected joints and can also be observed and monitored in peripheral blood. The circulating level of some cytokines (IL-6) is significantly correlated with the commonly used markers of inflammatory syndromes, indicating that it is related to disease activity.[203] The measurement of ^{40}K and total body water in RA patients shows that their BCM is decreased, as compared to controls. In addition, there is a strong dose response between RA severity and the amount of BCM adjusted for stature: the more severe the RA, the lower the BCM.[204] BCM is also inversely associated with TNF-α production.[205] This decrease in BCM is important in two regards: it amounts to about one-third of what is thought to be a survivable loss and it occurs in patients with energy and protein intakes comparable to those of controls. Surprisingly, the FM measured by dual-energy X-ray absorptiometry is not very different in RA adult patients and in controls.[204,206] This last observation suggests that the covert nutritional deficiency responsible for the decrease in BCM in adults is not primarily related to energy imbalance. Alternatively, the increase in protein breakdown rates observed in these situations might account for the preferential loss in FFM,[207] particularly in muscle.[208]

A comparable increase in protein breakdown may be induced by ammonium chloride infusion to healthy volunteers,[209] an effect also found in chronic renal failure (CRF). For instance, proteolysis may be increased in children with CRF by up to threefold in relation to metabolic acidosis.[210] In contrast with cytokine-mediated protein breakdown, net proteolysis is related to changes in plasma cortisol levels, suggesting that it plays an important role in protein metabolism during metabolic acidosis.[211] It should be pointed out that the acidosis-induced increase in net proteolysis may be quite deleterious to infants and children with inherited diseases of amino acid metabolism.

Therefore, the disruption of protein metabolism regulation in the favor of breakdown, by cytokines overproduction during chronic inflammatory syndromes or by some glucocorticoid-mediated mechanisms during CRF, might well constitute an entry into severe malnutrition, independent of decreased food consumption.

Effects on Energy Expenditure and Energy Substrate Utilization

Obviously, fever is a common event in children. It is also an efficient way to increase energy expenditure. DuBois emphasized the striking similarity between fevers of greatly different origins by showing that metabolic rate has a much closer relationship with body temperature than with the nature of diseases. This relationship indicates that metabolic rate increases by an average 13% for each 1°C above normal temperature.[80] A comparable relationship is found in children, resting energy expenditure increasing by about 12% for each 1°C above normal temperature.[212] For instance, during acute malaria the mean increment in RMR is about 30%.[212,213] This would amount to a 1,200 kcal/d expenditure in a 5-year-old child, or to a 250 to 300 g/d weight loss, should the child not eat.[212] It is noteworthy that the increase in RMR for each degree of increase in temperature is positively correlated to the expected weight for height, suggesting that undernutrition blunts the RMR response to fever.[212] Although the rise in metabolic rate was first related to shivering,[80] there is some evidence that other mechanisms are operative. An endotoxin bolus delivered to healthy volunteers induces a significant pyrogenic response (+2°C in body temperature) within 90 minutes, maximal at 180 minutes, and sustained for more than 6 hours. Total body oxygen consumption is increased by 28% at 2 hours, when body temperature is about half-maximal, and remains elevated at 6 hours. Coordinately, splanchnic oxygen consumption is increased by 64% at 2 hours and is still increased by 47% at 4 hours.[214] The increase in splanchnic oxygen extraction represents approximately 80% of the increase in whole-body oxygen consumption at 2 hours, suggesting that shivering is not the major source of heat production at this time, although body temperature is still rising. This interpretation is consistent with the absence of increase in leg oxygen extraction at 2 hours.[214]

Both the traditional pharmacological approach and the recent gene knockout technology stress the importance of cytokines in the development of this thermic response. However, some discrepancies persist, which may be related to cytokine redundancy and to the models used. For instance, IL-1β and IL-1 type 1 receptor (IL-1r1) knockout mice challenged with low or high doses of lipopolysaccharide (LPS) display a thermic response similar to wild-type mice, whereas the fever, anorexia, and weight loss resulting from turpentine injection are completely abolished.[215] Similarly, the significant increase in plasma IL-6 levels observed in wild-type mice injected with turpentine is virtually absent in the IL-1β knockout mice.[216] Injection of turpentine into IL-6 knockout mice also fails to induce fever, anorexia, and weight loss.[217] All these data support the direct implication of IL-1β and IL-6, but also TNFα, in the induction of fever and sickness behaviors. The thermic response to LPS is dependent upon PG synthesis, as it is blocked by indometacin, as well as by cyclooxygenase 2 or PG receptor gene disruption.[218,219] PG receptor (subtype EP3) knockout mice fail to mount a febrile response to LPS, IL-1β, and PGE2. The pyrogenic effect of IL-1β may also be inhibited by pretreatment with either a receptor antagonist or a monoclonal antibody to corticotropin-releasing hormone.

In parallel to their effects on energy expenditure, cytokines affect food intake in both animals[220] and humans.[221] Chronic administration of IL-1 to rats causes persistent inhibition of feeding.[220] Strikingly, this effect is not obtained in fish oil–fed rats.[222] Anorexia induced by IL-1 is mediated by CRF,[222] melanocortin-3/4 receptors[223] and, to a lesser extent, by PGs.[227] Other cytokines, including IL-2, IL-6, and interferon-α also stimulate hypothalamic CRF expression and/or release.[225] Thus, CRF seems to modulate both aspects of energy balance regulation in the rat, that is, food intake and energy expenditure. CRF effect on energy expenditure is mediated by a stimulation of SNS outflow, as reflected by a dramatic increase in the secretion of both adrenaline and noradrenaline,[99,226] explaining that the increase in body temperature and oxygen consumption induced by experimental inflammatory syndromes may be significantly reduced by β-adrenoreceptor blockade.[227,228] Urocortin, a member of the CRF family, also increases leptin and affects mitochondrial uncoupling proteins.[229] The chronic administration of IL-1β thus induces a sustained rise in body temperature and a reduction in food intake. The simultaneous increase in energy expenditure and decrease in energy intake result in a significant reduction in body weight gain of the experimental rats compared to controls, indicating that low levels of IL-1β release, maintained over periods of several days, could be responsible for changes in energy balance during chronic infection or inflammation.[230]

Chronic cytokine overproduction also affects energy expenditure in humans. In RA, for instance, RMR adjusted for BCM is about 12% higher than in adult controls. Furthermore, there is a positive correlation between cytokine production and the increase in RMR, cytokine production and BCM accounting for about 20 and 50% of RMR variability, respectively.[204] RMR adjusted for FFM is increased by about 20% in children with systemic juvenile rheumatoid arthritis as compared to controls. As a result, they are stunted and their FFM is reduced. Oligo and polyarticular juvenile rheumatoid arthritis children still display an 8% increase in RMR over controls.[231] Similarly, RMR is increased in stable cystic fibrosis (CF) patients by 10 to 25% above control values,[232,233] a change that is not accounted for by the increase in the oxygen cost of breathing.[232] There is a positive relationship between RMR and TNFα levels,[234] and adrenaline levels, TNFα accounting for about 27% of RMR variability. Contrary to RA patients who have a significant reduction in FFM but a relatively conserved FM, in CF patients FFM and FM are both significantly reduced.[235] Thus, besides the dramatic thermic response to infectious disease or injury, cytokines may also mediate lower-magnitude increases in metabolic rate, which might lead to a progressive depletion of energy stores if sustained for weeks or month.

Infection also induces important changes in the production or utilization of energy substrates. Infected patients present glucose intolerance, irrespective of the severity of the infection and of the infective agent.[236] There is a significant increase in endogenous glucose production, which is not suppressible by glucose infusion[237] and partially accounts for the increase in plasma glucose concentration. The stimulation of hepatic glucose production is principally mediated by increased levels of catecholamines and an increased glucagon-to-insulin ratio.[238] Although whole-body glucose turnover is increased, the ability of insulin to stimulate glucose uptake is reduced. Indeed, peripheral glucose utilization is impaired when compared to controls.[239,240] It is noteworthy that marked insulin resistance is present in previously healthy individuals with uncomplicated viral infections.[241] Insulin resistance is readily apparent 4 hours after the administration of LPS to healthy volunteers.[242] The increase in glucose turnover and the peripheral insulin resistance may be partially accounted for by a sustained β2 stimulation[243] and by the increase in free fatty acid appearance rate in infected humans and animals,[238,239] an increase related to adrenergic stimulation.[238] Cytokines, particularly TNFα, also contribute to insulin resistance by a direct effect on the insulin signaling cascade[244] and by increasing free fatty acid appearance rate by a stimulation of adipose tissue lipolysis.[245] Similarly, IL-6 is a potent modulator of fat metabolism in humans, increasing lipolysis and fatty acid oxidation.[246] This might be related to the suppression of adipocyte glyceroneogenesis, through the inhibition of cytosolic phosphoenolpyruvate carboxykinase (PEPCK-C) gene expression, which results in a dramatic increase in free fatty acid release by adipose tissue.[247]

When compared to healthy controls, fat oxidation is increased in septic patients and falls by a much lesser percentage in response to glucose and insulin.[239] Indeed, at the end of an insulin clamp, fat oxidation still contributes about 58% to metabolic rate in the septic patients, whereas it amounts to only 23% in controls.[239] Moreover, fat oxidation rate appears to be positively related to the severity of sepsis. Despite an increase in glucose turnover, fat thus appears as a preferred calorie source during sepsis.[248] Endotoxin administration to humans induces an increase in adrenaline and cortisol levels, while glucagon and insulin do not change.[214] Simultaneously, there is a significant rise in free fatty acid levels. Splanchnic glucose output is also increased and a progressive hyperglycemia ensues. The reduction in glucose utilization, like that observed in sepsis, is related to impaired nonoxidative glucose disposal and not to abnormal glucose oxidation.[242] Increases in plasma glucose, free fatty acid turnover (126%), and fat oxidation (60%), and similar variations in hormone concentrations follow the injection of rTNF to human volunteers, further supporting the role of cytokines in the development of the metabolic response to acute infection or injury.[249] It is interesting that an increase in both free fatty acid and glycerol concentrations is also observed in CF patients despite a reduction in FM, suggesting that chronic inflammatory syndromes may result in changes in the pattern of substrate utilization qualitatively comparable to those observed during acute infection.

ENERGY REQUIREMENTS IN DISEASE

Energy

The Food and Agricultural Organization of the World Health Organization (FAO/WHO) has published detailed estimates for energy requirements in infants and children of various ages.[250] In the adult, baseline energy needs, that is, energy needed to cover the metabolic response to food and the energy cost of minor activities, are assumed to be equal to 1.35 × BMR, and the time spent sleeping equal to BMR. This is considered as a survival requirement and is of practical value only for estimating the short-term needs of inactive and dependent individuals. Otherwise, estimates should include the energy cost of various occupational activities. However, it is not possible to specify with any confidence the allowance that should be made for a desirable level of physical activity in infants and children. Thus, energy requirements from birth to 10 years have been derived from the observed intakes of healthy children growing normally. Beyond 10 years, calculations are based on published BMR measurements, incremented for the cost of growth and for a cost of activity assumed to be about 1.6 × BMR. Free-living measurements of 24hEE corrected for the energy deposited during growth show that estimated energy requirements are substantially higher than total energy expenditure.[251] Furthermore, calculated energy expenditure also exceeds the energy intakes of 10- to 17-year-old children and adolescents.[251] Clearly, the difficulties encountered in achieving an accurate prediction of the energy needs in healthy infants and children would make unrealistic any such attempt in sick children, as the issue is further confused by the contradictory effects of underfeeding and disease on energy expenditure. Then the only option left is to try to identify some agreement about the range of variations in metabolic rate induced by diseases.

Studies in children with acute measles-associated underfeeding suggest that negative energy balance is related to a dramatic reduction in gross energy intake concomitant with a sustained level of energy expenditure. Metabolic rate after recovery is not significantly different from the values obtained during acute infection, although an average 20% increase would have been expected from the presence of fever.[252] The surprising stability of metabolic rate during acute infection might be accounted for by the balanced effects of underfeeding and infection. In any case, maintenance energy requirement determined at zero energy balance is 64 kcal/kg/d,[252] a figure similar to the maintenance energy requirement of thriving immature infants.[42] In these infants, the safe level of energy intake is estimated to be between 91 and 100 kcal/kg/d, or about 1.5 × RMR,[252] as compared to the 81 to 87 kcal/kg/d free-living 24hEE of normal infants,[251] or the average 103 kcal/kg/d estimated energy requirements for the same age group. It is further possible to evaluate the consequences of sepsis and trauma on energy expenditure. Earlier measurements in adults indicated 20 to 50% increases in metabolic rate in response to severe infection or multiple trauma. Studies performed in critically ill patients without malnutrition indicate that the mean increase in fasting metabolic rate ranges between 5%[253] and 14 to 18% over predicted values.[254] This is consistent with reports comparing septic patients to matched controls and showing a 15 to 19% increase in fasting metabolic rate over normal values.[255] Comparable estimates are obtained in traumatized children. RMR peaks at 3 days after injury, representing an 8% increase over predicted values or a 14% increase over replicate measurements obtained after discharge.[256] After surgery, the mean increase in RMR over baseline reaches about 15%. In these conditions, RMR peaks at 4 hours postoperatively and returns to baseline levels by 12 hours, thus resulting in a modest overall change in metabolic rate. Furthermore, the increase in RMR is related to the nature of the surgical procedure, the maximal rise being about 5% for minor surgery and 19% for major operations.[229] A similar trend toward decreasing estimates is observed regarding the energy expenses following burn injury. RMR in burned infants is independent of burn size and of the time elapsed between burn injury and measurements. Indeed, these two factors only account for 24 and 21% of the variation in RMR above predicted values, which is primarily dependent on body size.[258] Furthermore, ß-adrenergic blockade induces a substantial decrease in RMR in severely burned children.[228] As a result, the amount of energy required to achieve energy balance may be much lower than previously estimated. Actually, caloric delivery in excess of 1.2 × RMR might only result in increased FM without changes in lean body mass.[259] A comparable reevaluation of the change in metabolic rate resulting from severe head injury suggests that patients who are properly taken care of have a lower than expected increase in RMR.[260] Therefore it is likely that an energy intake equivalent to 1.5 × BMR would meet the requirements of most septic, traumatized, or burned infants and children. That increases in RMR after trauma, sepsis, and burn injuries are somewhat comparable is consistent with the existence of common mediators. Although the increase in energy expenditure resulting from disease appears to be substantially lower than previously estimated, applying equations that were originally developed for healthy, nonhospitalized individuals to predict the energy requirements of critically ill children could result in significant errors and may lead to provision of inappropriate nutritional support.[261]

Energy Substrates and Amino Acids

Energy intake should provide glucose and fat in amounts adapted to insulin resistance and to the preferential oxidation of lipids.[262,263] Physiologic considerations also suggest that the amount of glucose infused to malnourished, uninfected patients be limited. In adults, glucose oxidation levels off at about 4 mg/kg/min in response to increasing glucose infusion rates.[264] A similar limitation exists in 6-month-old infants, with a maximal oxidative glucose disposal rate of 12 mg/kg/min.[18] Furthermore, this maximal oxidative disposal decreases in parallel to energy expenditure with age, amounting to about 9 mg/kg/min at 6 years and about 6 mg/kg/min at 10 years.[18] In the uninfected infant, glucose infusion in excess of the maximal oxidative glucose disposal rate only results in inhibiting fat oxidation whether of endogenous or exogenous origin,[18] and may adversely affect protein metabolism and net protein deposition.[265] Thus, expecting some benefit from high glucose intakes in infected infants seems hazardous. On the contrary, glucose intakes should be lower because of the glucose intolerance. Indeed, the insulin-resistance—related decrease in peripheral glucose uptake is accounted for by impaired nonoxidative glucose disposal and not by abnormal glucose oxidation.[242] Glucose intakes in the range of the physiologic endogenous glucose production of the corresponding age range[266] are sufficient to meet the needs of glucose-requiring tissues. In these conditions, the clearance of intravenous emulsions as well as their oxidation are enhanced in septic patients.[262] The other goal is to equilibrate the increased proteolysis by promoting protein synthesis. In the healthy adult, protein synthesis is primarily regulated by amino acid inflow.[201] Similarly, amino acid infusion decreases net nitrogen losses in septic patients; the higher the amino acid intake, the more rapid the effect.[267] In burned infants and toddlers, amino acid intakes in the range of 2.5 to 3 g/kg/d efficiently support recovery.[268]

The Inflammatory Syndrome: A Case for a Pharmacologic Approach

Providing nutrients may not be enough in many of these situations. Nutritional support should be aimed at avoiding unnecessary increases in metabolic rate or, better, at controlling the disease-induced increase in energy expenditure. Obviously, attention should be given to ambient temperature and humidity, particularly in infants and burn patients. Furthermore, the use of inhibitors of either cytokine expression or cyclooxygenase, as well as of blockers of SNS peripheral effects, should be considered. As glucocorticoids suppress the production and the action of several cytokines as well as the production of PGs, it appeared warranted to test their effects in vivo in septic patients. The results are disappointing and do not support their use in sepsis, probably because corticoids could be administered only after cytokine release.[269] The use of molecules (antibodies or receptor analogs) directed against cytokines[270] or modulating inflammation[271] seems to offer interesting possibilities. Another way to curb the inflammatory response is to interfere with signal transduction in target cells through inhibitors of the cyclooxygenase. Indeed, pretreatment with ibuprofen results in the complete suppression of fever, tachycardia, and increase in stress hormones after endotoxin injection, as compared to the subjects who were not pretreated, despite an identical rise in TNF in both groups.[272] Similarly, the use of β-adrenergic receptor antagonists may substantially diminish energy expenditure.[228] If these dispositions may reduce metabolic rate, in many cases they will have little effect on the accelerated protein breakdown.

A pharmacologic intervention would be even more pressing when nutrition support fails to prevent protein losses, as it is the case in sepsis or during cancer cachexia. Animal models confirm that protein wasting is not accounted for by the effects of underfeeding in these situations,[176] thus requiring an approach other than dietary therapy. Besides their effect of boosting proteolysis, glucocorticoids have an inhibitory effect on protein synthesis,[273] which could further exaggerate cytokine-induced protein losses. Unfortunately, cyclooxygenase inhibitors seem to have only a partial and transient effect.[176] One remaining possibility is to directly inhibit cytokine production by new agents. Pretreatment with pentoxifylline inhibits TNF secretion and partially suppresses anorexia, weight loss, and muscle protein wasting in septic rats,[274] although fever, myalgia, and increased cortisol levels are unaffected in pretreated, endotoxin-injected humans.[275] However, these molecules are effective when administered prior to endotoxin or TNF injection, but little is known about their efficacy as therapeutic agents.

The other possibility is to antagonize the effects of cytokines on protein metabolism. Recombinant growth hormone (rGH) administered to postoperative patients induces a dramatic change in nitrogen balance, despite low energy intakes.[276] Furthermore, rGH treatment is able to reverse net whole-body and skeletal muscle protein catabolism in cancer patients.[277] This positive effect has been confirmed in severe sepsis and in patients with HIV-related wasting. Similarly, rIGF-I infusion to rTNF-treated animals preserves its anabolic action and induces a significant reduction in net protein losses in the face of high TNF levels.[278] It is noteworthy that decreased IGF-I levels, a common finding in acutely ill patients, may enhance protein catabolism. The protein anabolic effects of both rGH and rIGF-I may be substantially increased by using both agents simultaneously,[279] a synergy that might prevent acquired GH resistance. Although recombinant hormones are not the only agents favoring net protein synthesis, available evidence suggests that they are the best candidates to date for improving the nutritional therapy of protein-wasting inflammatory syndromes through direct pharmacologic intervention. Indeed, data suggest that rGH treatment improves growth and clinical conditions of CF patients,[280] in children with CRF[281] or juvenile arthritis,[282] increases linear growth and lean body mass in patients with Crohn's disease[283] and, by and large, has substantial anabolic effects on whole-body protein and bone metabolisms in children on chronic steroid therapy.[284]

REFERENCES

1. McLean JA, Tobin G. Animal and Human Calorimetry. Cambridge: Cambridge University Press; 1987.
2. Lukaski HC. Methods for the assessment of human body composition: Traditional and new. Am J Clin Nutr 1987;46:537–56.
3. Benedict FG. Vital Energetics. A Study in Comparative Basal Metabolism, Publication No. 503. Washington, DC: Carnegie Institute; 1938.
4. Ravussin E, Lillioja S, Anderson TE, et al. Determinants of 24-hour energy expenditure in man. Methods and results using a respiratory chamber. J Clin Invest 1986;78:1568–78.
5. Dauncey MJ. Metabolic effects of altering the 24h energy intake in man, using indirect and direct calorimetry. Br J Nutr 1980;43:257–69.
6. Ferraro R, Lillioja S, Fontvieille AM, et al. Lower sedentary metabolic rate in women compared with men. J Clin Invest 1992;90:780–4.
7. Brebbia DR, Altshuler KZ. Oxygen consumption rate and electroencephalographic stage of sleep. Science 1985;150:1621–3.
8. Henry CJK, Hayter J, Rees DG. The constancy of basal metabolic rate in free-living male subjects. Eur J Clin Nutr 1989;43:727–31.
9. Ravussin E, Swinburn BA. Energy metabolism. In: Stunkard AJ, Wadden TA, editors. Obesity: Theory and Therapy. New York: Raven Press; 1993. p. 97–123.
10. Schofield WN. Predicting basal metabolic rate, new standards and review of previous work. Hum Nutr Clin Nutr 1985;39:5–41.
11. Ravussin E, Lillioja S, Knowler WC, et al. Reduced rate of energy expenditure as a risk factor for body weight gain. N Engl J Med 1988;318:467–72.
12. Garby L, Garrow JS, Jørgensen B, et al. Relation between energy expenditure and body composition in man: Specific energy expenditure in vivo of fat and fat-free tissue. Eur J Clin Nutr 1988;42:301–5.
13. Bogardus C, Lillioja S, Ravussin E, et al. Familial dependence of the resting metabolic rate. N Engl J Med 1986;315:96–100.
14. Toubro S, Sorensen TI, Ronn B, et al. Twenty-four-hour energy expenditure: The role of body composition, thyroid status, sympathetic activity, and family membership. J Clin Endocrinol Metab 1996;81:2670–4.
15. Holliday MA. Metabolic rate and organ size during growth from infancy to maturity and during late gestation and early infancy. Pediatrics 1971;47:169–79.
16. Weinsier RL, Schutz Y, Bracco D. Reexamination of the relationship of resting metabolic rate to fat-free mass and to metabolically active components of fat-free mass in humans. Am J Clin Nutr 1992;55:790–4.
17. Chessex P, Reichman BL, Verellen G, et al. Influence of postnatal age, energy intake, and weight gain on energy metabolism in the very-low-birth-weight infant. J Pediatr 1981;99:761–6.
18. Bresson JL, Narcy P, Putet G, et al. Energy substrate utilization in infants receiving total parenteral nutrition with different glucose to fat ratios. Pediatr Res 1989;25:645–8.
19. Sparti A, DeLany JP, de la Bretonne JA, et al. Relationship between resting metabolic rate and the composition of the fat-free mass. Metabolism 1997;46:1225–30.
20. Illner K, Brinkmann G, Heller M, et al. Metabolically active components of fat free mass and resting energy expenditure in nonobese adults. Am J Physiol 2000;278:E308–15.
21. Heymsfield SB, Gallagher D, Kotler DP, et al. Body-size dependence of resting energy expenditure can be attributed to nonenergetic homogeneity of fat-free mass. Am J Physiol 2002;282:E132–8.
22. Koong LJ, Nienaber JA, Mersmann HJ. Effects of plane of nutrition on organ size and fasting heat production in genetically obese and lean pigs. J Nutr 1983;113:1626–31.
23. Garby L, Lammert O. An explanation for the non-linearity of the relation between energy expenditure and fat-free mass. Eur J Clin Nutr 1992;46:235–6.
24. Chan ATH, Fleming CR, O'Fallon WM, et al. Estimated versus measured basal energy requirements in patients with Crohn's disease. Gastroenterology 1986;91:75–8.
25. Blaxter K. Energy Metabolism in Animals and Man. Cambridge: Cambridge University Press; 1989.
26. Heusner AA. What does the power function reveal about structure and function in animals of different body size? Annu Rev Physiol 1987;49:121–133.
27. Krebs HA. Body size and tissue respiration. Biochim Biophys Acta 1950;4:249–269.
28. Brand MD, Couture P, Else PL, et al. Evolution of energy metabolism. Proton permeability of the inner membrane of liver mitochondria is greater in a mammal than in a reptile. Biochem J 1991;275:81–6.
29. Hulbert AJ, Else PL. Membranes and the setting of energy demand. J Exp Biol 2005;208:1593–9.
30. Speakman JR. Body size, energy metabolism and lifespan. J Exp Biol 2005;208:1717–30.
31. Else PL, Hulbert AJ. Evolution of mammalian endothermic metabolism: "leaky" membranes as a source of heat. Am J Physiol 1987;253:R1–7.
32. Gregg VA, Milligan JP. In vitro energy cost of Na^+,K^+-ATPase activity and protein synthesis in muscle from calves differing in age and breed. Br J Nutr 1982;48:65–71.
33. Swaminathan R, Chan ELP, Sin LY, et al. The effect of ouabain on metabolic rate in guinea-pigs: Estimation of energy cost of sodium pump activity. Br J Nutr 1989;61:467–73.
34. Lin MH, Romsos DR, Akera T, et al. Functional correlates of Na^+,K^+-ATPase in lean and obese (ob/ob) mice. Metabolism 1981;30:431–8.
35. Poehlman ET, Toth MJ, Webb GD. Sodium-potassium pump activity contributes to the age-related decline in resting metabolic rate. J Clin Endocrinol Metab 1993;76:1054–7.
36. Astrup A, Buemann B, Christensen JN, et al. The contribution of body composition, substrates, and hormones to the variability in energy expenditure and substrate utilization in premenopausal women. J Clin Endocrinol Metab 1992;74:279–86.
37. Milligan LP, McBride BW. Shifts in animal energy requirements across physiological and alimentational states. Energy costs of ion pumping by animal tissues. J Nutr 1985;115:1374–82.
38. McBride BW, Milligan LP. Magnitude of ouabain-sensitive respiration in the liver of growing, lactating and starved sheep. Br J Nutr 1985;54:293–303.
39. Rosengurt E. Stimulation of Na influx, Na-K pump activity and DNA synthesis in quiescent cultured cells. Adv Enzyme Regul 1981;19:61–85.
40. Denne SC, Kalhan SC. Leucine metabolism in human newborn. Am J Physiol 1987;253:E608–5.
41. Gill M, France J, Summers M, et al. Simulation of the energy costs associated with protein turnover and the Na^+,K^+-transport in growing lambs. J Nutr 1989;119:1287–99.
42. Brooke OG, Alvear J, Arnold M. Energy retention, energy expenditure, and growth in healthy immature infants. Pediatr Res 1979;13:215–20.
43. Reichman BL, Chessex P, Putet G, et al. Partition of energy metabolism and energy cost of growth in the very low-birth-weight infant. Pediatrics 1982;69:446–51.
44. Payne PR, Waterlow JC. Relative energy requirement for maintenance, growth, and physical activity. Lancet 1971;2:210–1.
45. Ashworth A. Metabolic rates during recovery from protein-calorie malnutrition: The specific need for a new concept of specific dynamic action. Nature 1969;223:407–9.
46. Fomon SJ, Haschke F, Ziegler EE, et al. Body composition of reference children from birth to age 10 years. Am J Clin Nutr 1982;35:1169–75.
47. Heim T, Verellen G, Chessex P, et al. Partition of energy metabolism in the very-low-birth-weight infant. In Stern L, Bard H, Friis-Hansen B, editors. Intensive Care of the Newborn. New York: Masson Publishing Inc; 1983. p. 169–81.
48. Roberts SB, Young VR. Energy costs of fat and protein deposition in the human infant. Am J Clin Nutr 1988;48:951–5.
49. Forbes GB, Brown MR, Welle SL, et al. Deliberate overfeeding in women and men: Energy cost and composition of the weight gain. Br J Nutr 1986;56:1–9.
50. Walker J, Roberts SL, Halmi KA, et al. Caloric requirements for weight gain in anorexia nervosa. Am J Clin Nutr 1979;32:1396–400.
51. Kaye WH, Gwirtsman HE, Obarzanek E, et al. Relative importance of calorie intake needed to gain weight and level of physical activity in anorexia nervosa. Am J Clin Nutr 1988;47:989–94.
52. Fomon SJ. Infant Nutrition. Philadelphia: WB Saunders Company; 1974.
53. Séguin A, de Lavoisier AL. Premier mémoire sur la respiration des animaux. Mémoires de l'Académie des Sciences; 1789.
54. D'Alessio DA, Kavie EC, Mozzoli MA, et al. Thermic effect of food in lean and obese men. J Clin Invest 1988;81:1781–9.
55. Tai MM, Castillo P, Pi-Sunyer FX. Meal size and frequency: Effect on the thermic effect of food. Am J Clin Nutr 1991;54:783–7.
56. Hill JO, DiGirolamo M, Heymsfield SB. Thermic effect of food after ingested versus tube-delivered meals. Am J Physiol 1985;248:E370–4.
57. Nacht CA, Schutz Y, Vernet O, et al. Continuous versus single bolus enteral nutrition: Comparison of energy metabolism in humans. Am J Physiol 1986;251:E524–9.
58. Vernet O, Christin L, Schutz Y, et al. Enteral versus parenteral nutrition: Comparison of energy metabolism in lean and moderately obese women. Am J Clin Nutr 1986;43:194–209.

59. Robinson SM, Jaccard C, Persaud C, et al. Protein turnover and thermogenesis in response to high-protein and high-carbohydrate feeding in men. Am J Clin Nutr 1990;52:72–80.
60. Schwartz RS, Ravussin E, Massari M, et al. The thermic effect of carbohydrate versus fat feeding in man. Metabolism 1985;34:285–93.
61. Hurni M, Burnand B, Pittet P, et al. Metabolic effects of a mixed and a high-carbohydrate low-fat diet in man, measured over 24 h in a respiration chamber. Br J Nutr 1982;47:33–42.
62. Maffeis C, Schutz Y, Grezzani A, et al. Meal-induced thermogenesis and obesity: Is a fat meal a risk factor for fat gain in children? J Clin Endocrinol Metab 2001;86:214–9.
63. DeFronzo RA, Tobin JD, Andres R. Glucose clamp technique: A method for quantifying insulin secretion and resistance. Am J Physiol 1979;237:E214–23.
64. Thiebaud D, Schutz Y, Acheson K, et al. Energy cost of glucose storage in human subjects during glucose-insulin infusions. Am J Physiol 1983;244:E216–21.
65. Ravussin E, Acheson KJ, Vernet O, et al. Evidence that insulin resistance is responsible for the decreased thermic effect of glucose in human obesity. J Clin Invest 1985;76:1268–73.
66. Flatt JP. The biochemistry of energy expenditure. In Bray G, editor. Recent Advances in Obesity Research. II. London: Newman Publishing Ltd;1978. p. 211–28.
67. Berne C, Fagius J, Niklasson F. Sympathetic response to oral carbohydrate administration. Evidence from microelectrode nerve recording. J Clin Invest 1989;84:1403–1409.
68. Welle S, Lilavivat U, Campbell RG. Thermic effect of feeding in man: Increased plasma norepinephrine levels following glucose but not protein or fat consumption. Metabolism 1981;30:953–8.
69. O'Dea K, Esler M, Leonard P, et al. Noradrenaline turnover during under- and overeating in normal weight subjects. Metabolism 1982;31:896–9.
70. Acheson K, Jéquier E, Wahren J. Influence of β-adrenergic blockade on glucose-induced thermogenesis in man. J Clin Invest 1983;72:981–6.
71. Acheson KJ, Ravussin E, Wahren J, et al. Thermic effect of glucose in man. Obligatory and facultative thermogenesis. J Clin Invest 1984;74:1572–80.
72. Schwartz RS, Jaeger LF, Veith RC. Effect of clonidine on the thermic effect of feeding in humans. Am J Physiol 1988;254:R90–4.
73. Welle S, Schwartz RG, Statt M. Reduced metabolic rate during β-adrenergic blockade in humans. Metabolism 1991;40:619–22.
74. Spraul M, Ravussin E, Fontvieille AM, et al. Reduced sympathetic nervous activity. A potential mechanism predisposing to body weight. J Clin Invest 1993;92:1730–5.
75. Monroe MB, Seals DR, Shapiro LF, et al. Direct evidence for tonic sympathetic support of resting metabolic rate in healthy adult humans. Am J Physiol 2001;280:E740–4.
76. Weinstein MR, Bell EF, Oh W. Energy intake, norepinephrine excretion, and oxygen consumption in low birthweight infants. J Pediatr Gastroenterol Nutr 1985;4:774–7.
77. Mitchell P. Vectorial chemistry and the molecular mechanics of chemiosmotic coupling: Power transmission by proticity. Biochem Soc Trans 1976;4:399–430.
78. Flatt JP, Pahud P, Ravussin E, et al. An estimate of the P:O ratio in man. Trends Biochem Sci 1984;9:466–8.
79. Rising R, Keys A, Ravussin E, et al. Concomitant interindividual variation in body temperature and metabolic rate. Am J Physiol 1992;263:E730–4.
80. DuBois EF. The basal metabolic rate in fever. JAMA 1921;77:352–55.
81. Warwick PM, Busby R. Influence of mild cold on 24h energy expenditure in "normally" clothed adults. Br J Nutr 1990;63:481–8.
82. Brück K. Temperature regulation in the newborn infant. Biol Neonat 1961;3:65–119.
83. Hey E. Thermal neutrality. Br Med Bull 1975;31:69–74.
84. Davis TRA, Johnston DR, Cremer FCB, et al. Regulation of shivering and nonshivering heat production during acclimation of rats. Am J Physiol 1960;198:471–5.
85. Himms-Hagen J. Cellular thermogenesis. Annu Rev Physiol 1976;38:315–51.
86. Foster DO, Frydman ML. Nonshivering thermogenesis in the rat, II: Measurements of blood flow with microspheres point to brown adipose tissue as the dominant site for the calorigenesis induced by noradrenaline. Can J Physiol Pharmacol 1978;56:110–22.
87. Arch JRS, Ainsworth AT, Cawthorne MA, et al. Atypical β-adrenoreceptor on brown adipocytes as target for anti-obesity drugs. Nature 1984;309:163–5.
88. Pecqueur C, Couplan E, Bouillaud F, et al. Genetic and physiological analysis of the role of uncoupling proteins in human energy homeostasis. J Mol Med 2001;79:48–56.
89. Nicholls DG, Locke RM. Thermogenic mechanisms in brown fat. Physiol Rev 1984;64:1–64.
90. Ricquier D, Bouillaud F, Toumelin P, et al. Expression of uncoupling protein mRNA in thermogenic or weakly thermogenic brown adipose tissue. Evidence for a rapid β-adrenoreceptor-mediated and transcriptionally regulated step during activation of thermogenesis. J Biol Chem 1986;261:13905–10.
91. Bianco AC, Silva JE. Intracellular conversion of thyroxine to triiodothyronine is required for the optimal thermogenic function of brown adipose tissue. J Clin Invest 1987;79:295–300.
92. Bianco AC, Silva JE. Optimal response of key enzymes and uncoupling protein to cold in BAT depends on local T_3 generation. Am J Physiol 1987;253:E255–63.
93. Bianco AC, Silva JE. Cold exposure rapidly induces virtual saturation of brown adipose tissue nuclear T_3 receptors. Am J Physiol 1988;255:E496–503.
94. Silva JE, Larsen PR. Adrenergic activation of triiodothyronine production in brown adipose tissue. Nature 1983;305:712–3.
95. Bianco AC, Kieffer JD, Silva JE. Adenosine 3',5' -monophosphate and thyroid hormone control of uncoupling protein messenger ribonucleic acid in freshly dispersed brown adipocytes. Endocrinology 1992;130:2625–33.
96. Rehnmark S, Bianco AC, Kieffer JD, et al. Transcriptional and posttranscriptional mechanisms in uncoupling protein mRNA response to cold. Am J Physiol 1992;262:E58–67.
97. Silva JE. Full expression of uncoupling protein gene requires the concurrence of norepinephrine and triiodothyronine. Mol Endocrinol 1988;2:706–13.
98. Moriscot A, Rabello R, Bianco AC. Corticosterone inhibits uncoupling protein gene expression in brown adipose tissue. Am J Physiol 1993;265:E81–7.
99. Brown MR, Fisher LA, Spiess J, et al. Corticotrophin-releasing factor: Actions on the sympathetic nervous system and metabolism. Endocrinology 1982;111:928–31.
100. Arase K, York DA, Shimizu H, et al. Effects of corticotropin-releasing factor on food intake and brown adipose tissue thermogenesis in rats. Am J Physiol 1988;255:E255–9.
101. Ricquier D, Nechad M, Mory G. Ultrastructural and biochemical characterization of human brown adipose tissue in pheochromocytoma. J Clin Endocrinol Metab 1982;54:803–7.
102. Lean MEJ, James WPT. Uncoupling protein in human brown adipose tissue mitochondria: Isolation and detection by specific antiserum. FEBS Lett 1983;163:235–240.
103. Lean MEJ, James WPT, Jennings G, et al. Brown adipose tissue uncoupling protein content in human infants, children and adults. Clin Sci 1986;71:291–7.
104. Cassard AM, Bouillaud F, Mattei MG, et al. Human uncoupling protein gene: Structure, comparison with rat gene, and assignment to the long arm of chromosome 4. J Cell Biochem 1990;43:255–64.
105. Garutti G, Ricquier D. Analysis of uncoupling protein and its mRNA in adipose tissue deposits of adult humans. Int J Obes 1992;16:383–90.
106. Krief S, Lönnqvist F, Raimbault S, et al. Tissue distribution of β_3-adrenergic receptor mRNA in man. J Clin Invest 1993;91:344–9.
107. Houstek J, Vizek K, Pavelka S, et al. Type II iodothyronine 5'-deiodase and uncoupling protein in brown adipose tissue of human newborns. J Clin Endocrinol Metab 1993;77:382–7.
108. Girardier LB. Fat: An energy dissipating tissue. In Girardier L, Stock MJ, editors. Mammalian Thermogenesis. London: Chapman and Hall; 1983. p. 50–98.
109. Astrup A, Bülow J, Christensen NJ, et al. Facultative thermogenesis induced by carbohydrate: A skeletal muscle component mediated by epinephrine. Am J Physiol 1986;250: E226–9.
110. Simonsen L, Bulow J, Madsen J, et al. Thermogenic response to epinephrin in the forearm and abdominal subcutaneous adipose tissue. Am J Physiol 1992;263:E850–5.
111. Lebon V, Dufour S, Falk Petersen K, et al. Effect of triiodothyronine on mitochondrial energy coupling in human skeletal muscle. J Clin Invest 2001;108:733–7.
112. Boivin M, Camirand A, Carli F, et al. Uncoupling protein-2 and -3 messenger ribonucleic acids in adipose tissue and skeletal muscle of healthy males: Variability, factors affecting expression, and relation to measures of metabolic rate. J Clin Endocrinol Metab 2000;85:1975–83.
113. Zurlo F, Larson K, Bogardus C, et al. Skeletal muscle metabolism is a major determinant of resting energy expenditure. J Clin Invest 1990;86:1423–7.
114. Schrauwen P, Xia J, Bogardus C, et al. Skeletal muscle uncoupling protein 3 expression is a determinant of energy expenditure in Pima Indians. Diabetes 1999;48:146–9.
115. Astrup A, Bülow J, Madsen J, et al. Contribution of BAT and skeletal muscle to thermogenesis induced by ephedrine in man. Am J Physiol 1985;248:E507–15.
116. Blaak EE, Van Baak MA, Kempen KPG, et al. Role of α- and β-adrenoreceptors in sympathetically mediated thermogenesis. Am J Physiol 1993;264:E11–7.
117. Lifson N, McClintock R. Theory of use of the turnover rates of body water for measuring energy and material balance. J Theoret Biol 1966;12:46–74.
118. Prentice AM, Lucas A, Vasquez-Velasquez L, et al. Are current dietary guidelines for young children a prescription for overfeeding? Lancet 1988;2:1066–9.
119. Zurlo F, Ferraro RT, Fontvieille AM, et al. Spontaneous physical activity and obesity: Cross-sectional and longitudinal studies in Pima Indians. Am J Physiol 1992; 263:E296–300.
120. Black AE, Coward WA, Prentice AM. Human energy expenditure in affluent societies: An analysis of 574 doubly-labelled water measurements. Eur J Clin Nutr 1996;50:72–92.
121. Westerterp KR. Pattern and intensity of physical activity. Nature 2001;410:539.
122. Hoos MB, Kuipers H, Gerver WJ, et al. Physical activity pattern of children assessed by triaxial accelerometry. Eur J Clin Nutr 2004;58:1425–8.
123. Montgomery C, Reilly JJ, Jackson DM, et al. Relation between physical activity and energy expenditure in a representative sample of young children. Am J Clin Nutr 2004;80:591–6.
124. Torun B, Davies PSW, Livingstone MBE, et al. Energy requirements and dietary energy recommandations for children and adolescents 1 to 18 years old. Eur J Clin Nutr 1996;50:S37–81.
125. Butte NF, Wong WW, Ferlic L, et al. Energy expenditure and deposition of breast-fed and formula-fed infants during early infancy. Pediatr Res 1990;28:631–40.
126. Henry CJ, Webster-Gandy JD, Elia M. Physical activity levels in a sample of Oxford school children aged 10–13 years. Eur J Clin Nutr 1999;53:840–3.
127. Abbott RA, Davies PS. Habitual physical activity and physical activity intensity: Their relation to body composition in 5.0–10.5-y-old children. Eur J Clin Nutr 2004;58:285–91.
128. Rennie KL, Livingstone MBE, Wells JCK, et al. Association of physical activity with body-composition indexes in children aged 6–8 y at varied risk of obesity. Am J Clin Nutr 2005;82:13–20.
129. Rowlands AV, Ingledew DK, Eston RG. The effect of type of physical activity measure on the relationship between fatness and habitual physical activity in children: A meta-analysis. Ann Hum Biol 2000;27:479–97.
130. Summerbell CD, Waters E, Edmunds LD, et al. Interventions for preventing obesity in children. Cochrane Database Syst Rev 2005, CD001871.
131. Hill JO, Wyatt HR, Read GW, et al. Obesity and the environment: Where do we go from here. Science 2003; 299:853–5.
132. Ross R, Dagnonne D, Jones P, et al. Reduction in obesity and related comorbid conditions after diet-induced weight loss or exercise-induced weight loss in men: A randomized, controlled trial. Ann Intern Med 2000;133:92–103.
133. Levine JA, Eberhardt NL, Jensen MD. Role of nonexercise activity thermogenesis in resistance to fat gain in humans. Science 1999;283:212–4.
134. Levine JA, Lanningham-Foster LM, McCrady S, et al. Interindividual variation in posture allocation: Possible role in human obesity. Science 2005;307:584–6.
135. Franks PW, Ravussin E, Hanson RL, et al. Habitual physical activity in children: The roles of genes and the environment. Am J Clin Nutr 2005;82:901–8.
136. Grande F, Anderson JT, Keys A. Changes in basal metabolic rate in man in semistarvation and refeeding. J Appl Physiol 1958;12:230–8.
137. Leibel RL, Rosenbaum M, Hirsch J. Changes in energy expenditure resulting from altered body weight. N Engl J Med 1995;332:621–8.
138. Luke A, Schoeller DA. Basal metabolic rate, fat-free mass, and body cell mass during energy restriction. Metabolism 1992;41:450–6.
139. Heilbronn LK, de Jonge L, Frisard MI, et al. Effect of 6-moth calorie restriction on biomarkers of longevity, metabolic adaptation, and oxidative stress in overweight individuals. JAMA 2006;295:1539–48.
140. Landsberg L, Young JB. Fasting, feeding and the regulation of the sympathetic nervous system. N Engl J Med 1978;298:1295–301.
141. Shetty PS, Jung RT, James WPT. Effect of catecholamine replacement with levodopa on the metabolic response to semistarvation. Lancet 1979;1:77–9.
142. Welle SL, Campbell RG. Decrease in resting metabolic rate during rapid weight loss is reversed by low doses of thyroid hormones. Metabolism 1986;35:289–91.
143. Mansell PI, Fellows IW, MacDonald IA. Enhanced thermogenic response to epinephrine after 48-h starvation. Am J Physiol 1990;258:R87–R93.
144. Gallen IW, MacDonald IA. The effects of underfeeding for 7 d on the thermogenic and physiological response to

glucose and insulin infusion (hyperinsulinaemic euglycaemic clamp). Br J Nutr 1990;64:427–37.
145. Mansell PI, Fellows IW, MacDonald IA, et al. Defect in thermoregulation in malnutrition reversed by weight gain. Physiological mechanisms and clinical importance. Q J Med 1990;76:817–29.
146. Brooke OG, Harris M, Salvosa CB. The response of malnourished babies to cold. J Physiol (Lond) 1973;233:75–91.
147. Nichols BL, Barnes DJ, Ashworth A, et al. Relationship between total body and muscle respiratory rates in infants with malnutrition. Nature 1968;217:475–6.
148. Montgomery RD. Changes in the basal metabolic rate of the malnourished infant and their relation to body composition. J Clin Invest 1962;41:1653–63.
149. Soares MJ, Shetty PS. Basal metabolic rates and metabolic economy in chronic undernutrition. Eur J Clin Nutr 1991;45:363–73.
150. Barac-Nieto M, Spurr GB, Lotero H, et al. Body composition in chronic undernutrition. Am J Clin Nutr 1978; 31:23–40.
151. Koong LJ, Ferrell CL. Effects of short term nutritional manipulation on organ size and fasting heat production. Eur J Clin Nutr 1990;44:73–7.
152. Brooke OG, Cocks T. Resting metabolic rate in malnourished babies in relation to total body potassium. Acta Paediatr Scand 1974;63:817–25.
153. Golden MHN, Waterlow JC, Picou D. Protein turnover, synthesis and breakdown before and after recovery from protein-energy malnutrition. Clin Sci Mol Med 1977;53:473–7.
154. Stein TP, Rumpler WV, Leskiw MJ, et al. Effect of reduced dietary intake on energy expenditure, protein turnover, and glucose cycling in man. Metabolism 1991;40:478–83.
155. Spady DW, Payne PR, Picou D, et al. Energy balance during recovery from malnutrition. Am J Clin Nutr 1976; 29:1073–8.
156. Dulloo AG, Girardier L. Adaptive role of energy expenditure in modulating body fat and protein deposition during catch-up growth after early undernutrition. Am J Clin Nutr 1993;58:614–21.
157. Cahill GF, Herrera MG, Morgan AP, et al. Hormone-fuel interrelationships during fasting. J Clin Invest 1966;45:1751–69.
158. Owen OE, Morgan AP, Kemp HG, et al. Brain metabolism during fasting. J Clin Invest 1967;46:1589–95.
159. Owen OE, Felig P, Morgan AP, et al. Liver and kidney metabolism during prolonged starvation. J Clin Invest 1969;48:574–83.
160. Rothman DL, Magnusson I, Katz LD, et al. Quantitation of hepatic glycogenolysis and gluconeogenesis in fasting humans with ^{13}C NMR. Science 1991;254:573–6.
161. Felig P, Owen OE, Wahren J, et al. Amino acid metabolism during prolonged starvation. J Clin Invest 1969;48: 584–94.
162. Pénicaud L, Kandé J, Le Magnen J, et al. Insulin action during fasting and refeeding in rat determined by euglycemic clamp. Am J Physiol 1985;249:E514–8.
163. Kerr DS, Stevens MCG, Robinson HM. Fasting metabolism in infants, I: Effect of severe undernutrition on energy and protein utilization. Metabolism 1978;27:411–35.
164. Henry CJK, Rivers JPW, Payne PR. Protein and energy metabolism in starvation reconsidered. Eur J Clin Nutr 1988;42:543–9.
165. Nørrelund H, Nair KS, Nielsen S, et al. The decisive role of free fatty acids for protein conservation during fasting in humans with and without growth hormone. J Clin Endocrinol Metab 2003;88:4371–8.
166. Rennie MJ, Harrison R. Effects of injury, disease, and malnutrition on protein metabolism in man. Lancet 1984;1:323–5.
167. Bloesch D, Keller U, Spinas GA, et al. Effects of endotoxin on leucine and glucose kinetics in man: Contribution of prostaglandin E_2 assessed by a cyclooxygenase inhibitor. J Clin Endocrinol Metab 1993;77:1156–63.
168. Gelfand RA, Matthews DE, Bier DM, et al. Role of counterregulatory hormones in the catabolic response to stress. J Clin Invest 1984;74:2238–48.
169. Clowes GHA, Jr, George BC, Villee CA, Jr, et al. Muscle proteolysis induced by a circulating peptide in patients with sepsis or trauma. N Engl J Med 1983;308:545–52.
170. Baracos V, Rodeman HP, Dinarello CA, et al. Stimulation of muscle protein degradation and prostaglandin E_2 release by leukocytic pyrogen (interleukin-1). N Engl J Med 1983;308:553–8.
171. Moldawer LL, Svaninger G, Gelin J, et al. Interleukin-1 and tumor necrosis factor do not regulate protein balance in skeletal muscle. Am J Physiol 1987;253:C766–73.
172. Kitamura T, Ogorochi T, Miyajima A. Multimeric cytokine receptors. Trends Endocrinol Metab 1994;5:8–14.
173. Fong Y, Moldawer LL, Marano M, et al. Cachectin/TNF or IL-1(α induces cachexia with redistribution of body proteins. Am J Physiol 1989;256:R659–65.
174. Zamir O, Hasselgren PO, Von Allmen D, et al. In vivo administration of interleukin-1α induces muscle proteolysis in normal and adrenalectomized rats. Metabolism 1993;42:204–8.
175. Hoshino E, Pichard C, Greenwood CE, et al. Body composition and metabolic rate in rat during a continuous infusion of cachectin. Am J Physiol 1991;260:E27–36.
176. Tessitore L, Costelli P, Baccino FM. Pharmacological interference with tissue hypercatabolism in tumor-bearing rats. Biochem J 1994;299:71–8.
177. Starnes HF, Jr, Warren RS, Jeevanadam M, et al. Tumor necrosis factor and the acute metabolic response to tissue injury in man. J Clin Invest 1988;82:1321–5.
178. Lang CH, Huber D, Frost RA. Burn-induced increase in atrogin-1 and MuRF-1 in skeletal muscle is glucocorticoid-independent but down regulated by IGF-I. Am J Physiol 2006 [Epub ahead of print].
179. Tomkins AM, Garlick PJ, Schofield WN, et al. The combined effects of infection and malnutrition on protein metabolism in children. Clin Sci 1983;65:313–24.
180. Garlick PJ, McNurlan MA, Fern E, et al. Stimulation of protein synthesis and breakdown by vaccination. Br Med J 1980;190:263–5.
181. Cayol M, Tauveron I, Rambourdin F, et al. Whole-body protein turnover and hepatic protein synthesis are increased by vaccination in man. Clin Sci 1995;89:389–96.
182. Motil KJ, Grand RJ, Davis-Kraft L, et al. Growth failure in children with inflammatory bowel disease: A prospective study. Gastroenterology 1993;105:681–91.
183. Kelts DG, Grand RJ, Shen G, et al. Nutritional basis of growth failure in children and adolescents with Crohn's disease. Gastroenterology 1979;76:720–7.
184. Motil KJ, Grand RJ, Matthews DE, et al. Whole body leucine metabolism in adolescents with Crohn's disease and growth failure during nutritional supplementation. Gastroenterology 1982;82:1359–68.
185. Gotlin RW, Dubois RS. Nyctohemeral growth hormone levels in children with growth retardation and inflammatory bowel disease. Gut 1973;14:191–5.
186. Hodges P, Gee M, Grace M, et al. Protein-energy intake and malnutrition in Crohn's disease. J Am Diet Assoc 1984;84:1460–4.
187. Kirschner BS, Klich JR, Kalman SS, et al. Reversal of growth retardation in Crohn's disease with therapy emphasizing oral nutritional restitution. Gastroenterology 1981;80:10–5.
188. Belli DC, Seidman E, Bouthillier L, et al. Chronic intermittent elemental diet improves growth failure in children with Crohn's disease. Gastroenterology 1988;94:603–10.
189. Kushner RF, Schoeller DA. Resting and total energy expenditure in patients with inflammatory bowel disease. Am J Clin Nutr 1991;53:161–5.
190. Burnham JM, Schults J, Semeao E, et al. Body-composition alterations consistent with cachexia in children and young adults with Crohn's disease. Am J Clin Nutr 2005;82:413–20.
191. Powell-Tuck J, Garlick PJ, Lennard-Jones JE, et al. Rates of whole body protein synthesis and breakdown increase with the severity of inflammatory bowel disease. Gut 1984;25:469–74.
192. Thomas AG, Miller V, Taylor F, et al. Whole body protein turnover in childhood Crohn's disease. Gut 1992;33:675–7.
193. Murch SH, Lamkin VA, Savage MO, et al. Serum concentrations of tumor necrosis factor α in childhood chronic inflammatory bowel disease. Gut 1991;32:913–7.
194. Kirschner BS, Sutton MM. Somatomedin-C levels in growth-impaired children and adolescents with chronic inflammatory bowel disease. Gastroenterology 1986;91:166–76.
195. Donahue SP, Phillips LS. Response of IGF-I to nutritional support in malnourished hospital patients: A possible indicator of short-term changes in nutritional status. Am J Clin Nutr 1989;50:962–9.
196. Phillips LS, Orawski AT, Belosky DC. Somatomedin and nutrition, IV: Regulation of somatomedin activity and growth cartilage activity by quantity and composition of diet in rats. Endocrinology 1978;103:121–7.
197. Dardevet D, Manin M, Balage M, et al. Influence of low- and high-protein diets on insulin and insulin-like growth factor-1 binding to skeletal muscle and liver in the growing rat. Br J Nutr 1991;65:47–60.
198. Harp JB, Goldstein S, Phillips LS. Nutrition and somatomedin, XXIII: Molecular regulation of IGF-I by amino acid availability in cultured hepatocytes. Diabetes 1991;40:95–101.
199. Pucilowska JB, Davenport ML, Kabir I, et al. The effect of dietary protein supplementation on insulin-like growth factors (IGFs) and IGF-binding proteins in children with shigellosis. J Endocrinol Metab 1993;77:1516–21.
200. Thissen JP, Verniers J. Inhibition by interleukin-1β and tumor necrosis factor-alpha on the insulin-like growth factor 1 messenger ribonucleic acid in response to growth hormone in rat hepatocyte primary culture. Endocrinology 1997;138:1078–84.
201. Castellino P, Luzi L, Simonson DC, et al. Effect of insulin and plasma amino acid concentration on leucine metabolism in man. J Clin Invest 1987;80:1784–93.
202. Guerne PA, Zuraw BL, Vaughan JH, et al. Synovium as a source of interleukin 6 in vitro. Contribution to local and systemic manifestations of arthritis. J Clin Invest 1989;83:585–92.
203. Houssiau FA, Devogelaer JP, Van Damme J, et al. Interleukin-6 in synovial fluid and serum of patients with rheumatoid arthritis and other inflammatory arthritis. Arthritis Rheum 1988;31:784–8.
204. Roubenoff R, Roubenoff RA, Cannon JG, et al. Rheumatoid cachexia: Cytokine-driven hypermetabolism accompanying reduced body cell mass in chronic inflammation. J Clin Invest 1994;93:2379–86.
205. Walsmith J, Abad L, Kehavias J, et al. Tumor necrosis factor-alpha production is associated with less body cell mass in women with rheumatoid arthritis. J Rheumatol 2004;31:23–9.
206. Roubenoff R. Sarcopenic obesity: Does muscle loss cause fat gain? Ann NY Acad Sci 2000;904:553–7.
207. Rall LC, Rosen CJ, Dolnikowski G, et al. Protein metabolism in rheumatoid arthritis and aging. Effects of muscle strength and tumor necrosis factor alpha. Arthritis Rheum 1996;39:1115–24.
208. Gibson JNA, Poyser NL, Morrison WL, et al. Muscle protein synthesis in patients with rheumatoid arthritis: Effect of chronic corticosteroid therapy on prostaglandin F_{2a} availability. Eur J Clin Invest 1991;21:406–12.
209. Reaich D, Channon SM, Scrimgeour CM, et al. Ammonium chloride-induced acidosis increases protein breakdown and amino acid oxidation in humans. Am J Physiol 1992;263:E735–9.
210. Boirie Y, Broyer M, Gaganadoux MF, et al. Alterations in protein metabolism by metabolic acidosis in children with chronic renal failure. Kidney Int 2000;58:236–41.
211. Garibotto G, Russo R, Sofia A, et al. Skeletal muscle protein synthesis and degradation in patients with chronic renal failure. Kidney Int 1994;45:1432–9.
212. Stettler N, Schutz Y, Whitehead R, et al. Effect of malaria and fever on energy metabolism in Gambian children. Pediatr Res 1992;31:102–6.
213. Berclaz PY, Benedek C, Jéquier E, et al. Changes in protein turnover and resting energy expenditure after treatment of malaria in Gambian children. Pediatr Res 1996;39:401–9.
214. Fong Y, Marano MA, Moldawer LL, et al. The acute splanchnic and peripheral tissue metabolic response to endotoxin in humans. J Clin Invest 1990;85:1896–904.
215. Leon LR. Cytokine regulation of fever: Studies using gene knockout mice. J Appl Physiol 2002;92:2648–55.
216. Zheng H, Fletcher D, Kozak W, et al. Resistance to fever induction and impaired acute-phase response in interleikin-1β deficient mice. Immunity 1995;3:9–19.
217. Kozak W, Kluger MJ, Soszynski D, et al. IL6 and IL-1β in fever. Studies using cytokine-deficient (knockout) mice. Ann NY Acad Sci 1998;856:33–47.
218. Li S, Matsumura K, Ballou LR, et al. Cyclooxygenase-2 mediates the febrile response of mice to interleukin-1β. Brain Res 2001;910:163–73.
219. Ushikubi F, Segi E, Sugimoto Y, et al. Impaired febrile response in mice lacking the prostaglandin E receptor subtype EP3. Nature 1998;395:281–4.
220. Hellerstein MK, Meydani SN, Meydani M, et al. Interleukin-1-induced anorexia in the rat. Influence of prostaglandins. J Clin Invest 1989;84:228–35.
221. Reichenberg A, Kraus T, Haack M, et al. Endotoxin-induced changes in food consumption in healthy volunteers are associated with TNF-α and IL-6 secretion. Psychoneuroendocrinol 2002;27:945–56.
222. Uehara A, Sekika C, Takasugi Y, et al. Anorexia induced by interleukin-1: Involvement of corticotropin-releasing factor. Am J Physiol 1989;257:R613–7.
223. Lawrence CB, Rothwell NJ. Anorexic but not pyrogenic actions of inteleukin-1 are modulated by central melanocortin-3/4 receptors in the rat. J Neuroendocrinol 2001;13:490–5.
224. Johnson PM, Vogt SK, Burney MW, et al. COX-2 inhibition attenuates anorexia during systemic inflammation without impairing cytokine production. Am J Physiol 2002;282: E650–6.
225. Plata-Salaman CR. Central nervous system mechanisms contributing to the cachexia-anorexia syndrome. Nutrition 2000;16:1009–12.
226. De Fanti BA, Martinez JA. Central urocortin activation of sympathetic-regulated energy metabolism in Wistar rats. Brain Res 2002;930:37–41.
227. Cooper AL, Rothwell NJ. Mechanisms of early and late hypermetabolism and fever after localized tissue injury in rats. Am J Physiol 1991;261:E698–705.

228. Herndon DN, Hart DW, Wolf SE, et al. Reversal of catabolism by beta-blockade after severe burns. N Engl J Med 2001;345:1223–9.
229. Kotz CM, Wang C, Levine AS, et al. Urocortin in the hypothalamic PVN increases leptin and affects uncoupling proteins-1 and -3 in rats. Am J Physiol 2002;282:R546–51.
230. Busbridge NJ, Dascombe MJ, Rothwell NJ. Chronic effects of interleukin-1β on fever, oxygen consumption and food intake in the rat. Horm Metab Res 1993;25:222–7.
231. Knops N, Wulfraat N, Lodder S, et al. Resting energy expenditure and nutritional status in children with juvenile rheumatoid arthrtis. J Rheumatol 1999;26:2039–43.
232. Bell SC, Saunders MJ, Elborn JS, et al. Resting energy expenditure and oxygen cost of breathing in patients with cystic fibrosis. Thorax 1996;51:126–31.
233. McCloskey M, Redmond AO, Pyper S, et al. Total energy expenditure in stable patients with cystic fibrosis. Clin Nutr 2001;20:235–41.
234. Burdet L, Hugli O, Aubert JD, et al. Effect of elective antibiotic therapy on resting energy expenditure and inflammation in cystic fibrosis. Eur J Pediatr 1999;158:711–6.
235. Stettler N, Kawchak DA, Boyle LL, et al. Prospective evaluation of growth, nutritional status, and body composition in children with cystic fibrosis. Am J Clin Nutr 2000;72:407–13.
236. Sammalkorpi K. Glucose intolerance in acute infections. J Intern Med 1989;225:15–19.
237. Long CL, Kinney JM, Geiger JW. Nonsuppressability of gluconeogenesis by glucose in septic patients. Metabolism 1976;25:193–202.
238. Wolfe RR, Shaw JHF. Glucose and FFA kinetics during sepsis: Role of glucagon and sympathetic nervous system activity. Am J Physiol 1985;248:E236–43.
239. White RH, Frayn KN, Little RA, et al. Hormonal and metabolic responses to glucose infusion in sepsis studied by the hyperglycemic glucose clamp technique. J Parent Ent Nutr 1987;11:345–53.
240. Henderson AA, Frayn KN, Galasko CSB, et al. Dose-response relationships for the effects of insulin on glucose and fat metabolism in injured patients and control subjects. Clin Sci 1991;80:25–32.
241. Yki-Järvinen H, Sammalkorpi K, Koivisto VA, et al. Severity, duration, and mechanisms of insulin resistance during acute infections. J Clin Endocrinol Metab 1989;69:317–23.
242. Agwunobi AO, Reid C, Maycock P, et al. Insulin resistance and substrate utilization in human endotoxemia. J Clin Endocrinol Metab 2000;85:3770–8.
243. Lang CH. Sepsis-induced insulin resistance in rats is mediated by a β-adrenergic mechanism. Am J Physiol 1992;263:E703–11.
244. Rosenzweig T, Braiman L, Bak A, et al. Differential effects of tumor necrosis factor-alpha on protein kinase C isoforms alpha and delta mediates inhibition of insulin receptor signaling. Diabetes 2002;51:1921–30.
245. Gasic S, Tian B, Green A. Tumor necrosis factor alpha stimulates lipolysis in adipocytes by decreasing Gi protein concentrations. J Biol Chem 1999;274:6770–5.
246. Van Hall G, Steenberg A, Saccheti M, et al. Interleukin-6 stimulates limolysis and fat oxidation in humans. J Clin Endocrinol Metab 2003;88:3005–10.
247. Hanson RW, Reshef L. Glyceroneogenesis revisited. Biochimie 2003;85:1199–205.
248. Levinson MR, Groeger JS, Jeevanandam M, et al. Free fatty acid turnover and lipolysis in septic mechanically ventilated cancer-bearing patients. Metabolism 1989;37:618–25.
249. Van der Poll T, Romijn JA, Endert E, et al. Tumor necrosis factor mimics the metabolic response to acute infection in healthy humans. Am J Physiol 1991;261:E457–65.
250. World Health Organizations. Energy and Protein Requirements. Geneva: WHO Technical Report Series 724;1985.
251. Butte NF, Henry CJK, Torun B. Report of the working group on energy requirements of infants, children and adolescents. Eur J Clin Nutr 1996;50:S188–9.
252. Duggan MB, Milner RDG. The maintenance energy requirement for children: An estimate based on a study of children with infection associated underfeeding. Am J Clin Nutr 1986;43:870–8.
253. Baker JP, Detski AS, Stewart S, et al. Randomized trial of total parenteral nutrition in critically ill patients: Metabolic effects of varying glucose-lipid ratios as the energy source. Gastroenterology 1984;87:53–59.
254. Roulet M, Detsky AS, Marliss EB, et al. A controlled trial of the effect of parenteral nutritional support on patients with respiratory failure and sepsis. Clin Nutr 1983;2:97–105.
255. Arnold J, Leinhardt D, Carlson G, et al. Thermogenic and hormonal responses to amino acid infusion in septic humans. Am J Physiol 1992;263:E129–35.
256. Wintrop AL, Wesson DE, Pencharz PB, et al. Injury severity, whole body protein turnover and energy expenditure in pediatric trauma. J Pediatr Surg 1987;22:534–7.
257. Jones MO, Pierro A, Hammond P, et al. The metabolic response to operative stress in infants. J Pediatr Surg 1993;28:1258–63.
258. Goran MI, Broemeling L, Herndon DH, et al. Estimating energy requirements in burned children: A new approach derived from measurements of energy expenditure. Am J Clin Nutr 1991;54:35–40.
259. Hart DW, Wolf SE, Herndon DN, et al. Energy expenditure and caloric balance after burn: Increased feeding leads to fat rather than lean mass accretion. Ann Surg 2002;235:152–61.
260. Matthews DS, Bullock RE, Matthews JN, et al. Temperature response to severe head injury and the effect on body energy expenditure and cerebral oxygen consumption. Arch Dis Child 1995;72:507–15.
261. Fung EB. Estimating energy expenditure in critically ill adults and children. AACN Clin Issues 2000;11:480–97.
262. Nordenstrom J, Carpentier YA, Askanazi J, et al. Metabolic utilization of intravenous fat emulsion during total parenteral nutrition. Ann Surg 1982;196:221–31.
263. Coss-Bu JA, Klish WJ, Walding D, et al. Energy metabolism, nitrogen balance, and substrate utilization in critically ill children. Am J Clin Nutr 2001;74:664–9.
264. Wolfe RR, O'Donnell TF, Jr, Stone MD, et al. Investigation of factors determining the optimal glucose infusion rate in total parenteral nutrition. Metabolism 1980;29:892–900.
265. Bresson JL, Bader B, Rocchiccioli F, et al. Protein-metabolism kinetics and energy-substrate utilization in infants fed parenteral solutions with different glucose-fat ratios. Am J Clin Nutr 1991;54:370–6.
266. Bier DM, Leake RD, Haymond MW, et al. Measurement of "true" glucose production rates in infancy and childhood with 6,6-dideuteroglucose. Diabetes 1977;26:1016–23.
267. Greig PD, Elwyn DH, Askanazi J, et al. Parenteral nutrition in septic patients: Effect of increasing nitrogen intake. Am J Clin Nutr 1987;46:1040–7.
268. Cunningham JJ, Lydon MK, Russell WE. Calorie and protein provision for recovery from severe burns in infants and young children. Am J Clin Nutr 1990;51:553–7.
269. Bone RC, Fisher CJ, Clemmer TP, et al. A controlled clinical trial of high-dose methylprednisolone in the treatment of severe sepsis and septic shock. N Engl J Med 1987;317:653–8.
270. Cooney R, Kimball SR, Eckman R, et al. TNF-binding protein ameliorates inhibition of skeletal muscle protein synthesis during sepsis. Am J Physiol 1999;276:E611–9.
271. Bernard GR, Vincent JL, Laterre PF, et al. Efficacy and safety of recombinant activated protein C for severe sepsis. N Engl J Med 2001;344:699–709.
272. Michie HR, Manogue KR, Spriggs DR, et al. Detection of circulating tumor necrosis factor after endotoxin administration. N Engl J Med 1988;318:1481–6.
273. Rannels SR, Rannels DE, Pegg AE, et al. Glucocorticoid effects on peptide-chain initiation in skeletal muscle and heart. Am J Physiol 1978;235:E134–9.
274. Breuille D, Farge MC, Rose F, et al. Pentoxifylline decreases body weight loss and muscle protein wasting characteristics of sepsis. Am J Physiol 1993;265:E660–6.
275. Zabel P, Wolter DT, Schönharting MM, et al. Oxpentifylline in endotoxemia. Lancet 1989;2:1474–7.
276. Ponting GA, Halliday D, Teale JD, et al. Postoperative positive nitrogen balance with intravenous hyponutrition and growth hormone. Lancet 1988;1:438–40.
277. Wolf RF, Pearlstone DB, Newman E, et al. Growth hormone and insulin reverse net whole body and skeletal muscle protein catabolism in cancer patients. Ann Surg 1992;216: 280–90.
278. Douglas RG, Gluckman PD, Breier BH, et al. Effects of recombinant IGF-I on protein and glucose metabolism in rTNF-infused lambs. Am J Physiol 1991;261:E606–12.
279. Kupfer SR, Underwood LE, Baxter RC, et al. Enhancement of the anabolic effects of growth hormone and insulin-like growth factor I by use of both agents simultaneously. J Clin Invest 1993;91:391–6.
280. Hardin DS, Adams-huet B, Brown D, et al. Growth hormone treatment improves growth and clinical status in prepubertal children with cystic fibrosis—results of a multicenter randomized controlled trial. J Clin Endocrinol Metab 2006 [Epub ahead of print].
281. Haffner D, Schaefer F, Nissel R, et al. Effect of growth hormone treatment on the adult height of children with chronic renal failure. N Engl J Med 2000;343:923–30.
282. Bechtold S, Ripperger P, Bonfig W, et al. Growth hormone changes bone geometry and body composition in patients with juvenile idiopathic arthritis requiring glucocorticoïd treatment: A controlled study using peripheral quantitative computed tomography. J Clin Endocrinol Metab 2005;90:3168–73.
283. Slonim AE, Bulone L, Damore MB, et al. A preliminary study of growth hormone in Crohn's disease. N Engl J Med 2000;342:1633–7.
284. Mauras N. Growth hormone therapy in the glucocorticosteroid-dependent child: Metabolic and linear growth effects. Horm Res 2001;56:13–8.
285. Blaxter K. Energy Metabolism in Animals and Man. Cambridge, UK: Cambridge University Press; 1989.

Energy and Substrate Regulation in Obesity

Susan B. Roberts, PhD
Daniel J. Hoffman, PhD

Overweight and obesity are widely considered to be the major public health problem in affluent countries[1,2] and are becoming increasingly common in some economically disadvantaged societies as well.[3,4] Previously considered a problem mainly occurring in adults, overweight and obesity are now prevalent in children, with an estimated 17% of children aged 2 to 19 years thought to be affected.[5]

DEFINITION OF OBESITY

The definition of obesity is deceptively simple: it is a state of excessive accumulation of body fat. However, the translation of this simple definition into working standards for excess body fat and body weight has been complicated for several reasons. First, because body fatness is a continuum, the cutoff point for the definition of obesity is necessarily arbitrary.[1] In addition, the harmful effects of obesity result primarily from the excessive accumulation of fat, but there is no simple method for the direct measurement of this body compartment in individuals of any age. These concerns notwithstanding, the Centers for Disease Control and Prevention (CDC) have published new body mass index (BMI; kg/m^2) percentiles for children aged up to 20 years (see Appendix I), together with usable definitions for "risk of overweight" and "overweight."[6] These definitions recognize that BMI is a better indicator of relative weight than weight for height, even if it is not precisely aligned with body fatness in all population groups.[7]

The CDC charts provide an improved set of reference growth data that have been updated and smoothed using statistical techniques. However, as reviewed elsewhere,[8] it should be noted that the latest national survey data for children aged 6 years and over were not included in the data set used to calculate the BMI percentiles because of the marked increase in weight of children 6 and older in the latest survey (Third National Health and Nutrition Examination Survey [NHANES III]) compared with previous surveys. The inclusion of the latest survey data would have shifted the percentiles up and resulted in a relative underclassification of the prevalence of overweight. Because the 85th percentile of BMI is used to classify risk of overweight and the 95th percentile is used to classify overweight,[7] the data used effectively define overweight as a fixed percentage relative to population surveys prior to NHANES III. Thus, the BMI charts can be considered more as recommendations for the healthy range of BMI rather than as current population values because they are designed primarily to provide a reference for the diagnosis of overweight. They can also potentially be used to diagnose underweight (eg, at the 10th or 5th percentiles), but accepted definitions for underweight are needed.

One concern with using BMI to identify overweight children is the potential for misclassification.[8] The relationship between weight and height and body fat content can be weak,[9] and, especially in children younger than 5 years when the high BMI percentiles are very close together, factors such as enhanced muscular development, large head size, and a high torso-to-leg ratio could all falsely elevate the BMI of a child with a healthy amount of body fat into an overweight range. For example, differences in head circumference between a 3-year-old child on the 10th head circumference percentile and one on the 90th percentile translate into a body weight difference of approximately 0.75 kg (assuming that the head weighs 1.7 g/cm^3 and is a sphere). A 3-year-old child's BMI would therefore vary by approximately 0.85 units depending on whether head circumference was on the 10th or 90th percentile. This could mean the difference between the 75th and 85th to 90th percentile for BMI—in other words, the difference between no weight concern and a diagnosis of risk of overweight. The effect of the relative length of torso and legs can also be predicted using theoretical calculations. Assuming that the proportion of standing height attributed to torso varies from 0.35 to 0.38 and that for a given contribution to height, torso weight is twice that of legs or neck, 10 BMI would vary by approximately 0.4 units. These calculations highlight the potential for misclassification of individuals, especially those between the 85th and 95th percentiles. Until improved methods for determining body fatness are routinely available, some individual judgment is needed in applying standard BMI definitions for overweight in individual children.

At the same time that the 2000 CDC percentiles were published, Cole and colleagues reported internationally derived, age-specific BMI values for children equivalent to BMI definitions of overweight (BMI = 25 or more) and obesity (BMI = 30 or more) in adults.[11] The adult cutoff values of 25 and 30 were originally developed based on increased health risks[12]; the theoretical advantage of creating equivalent values for children is that they would provide absolute standards for fatness rather than standards relative to population fatness at any given period of survey.[13,14] It should be noted that it is not currently known whether equivalent percentiles in childhood confer similar risk to those found in adults, but because BMI tends to track from childhood through adult life, the approach seems a reasonable one.

As reviewed elsewhere,[8] Cole and colleagues obtained national survey data from six countries (Brazil, the United Kingdom, Hong Kong, the Netherlands, Singapore, and the United States).[11] For each country, the percentiles equivalent to BMI values of 25 and 30 at age 18 years were determined and then BMI values at different childhood ages were obtained for the same percentiles. There was substantial agreement in childhood BMI values among the six countries; thus, mean values for different ages were computed to give age-specific BMI cutoffs equivalent to adult BMIs of 25 and 30 kg/m^2. Figure 1 shows a comparison of the CDC 85th and 90th percentiles with the overweight and obesity cutoff points for BMI provided by Cole and colleagues. For both boys and girls, the 2000 CDC definition of overweight (95th percentile) is markedly higher than the Cole and colleagues'[11] definition of overweight,[11] except for the period between age 4 and 5 years. In other words, by the current US definition, many fewer children in the United States and worldwide are overweight. In fact, the 2000 CDC definition of risk of overweight (85th percentile) most closely approximates the Cole and colleagues definition of overweight, with the Cole and colleagues values tending to be slightly higher for ages 2 to 10 years and slightly lower for 17 years and older.[11] In addition, the CDC BMI definition of overweight is not similar to the Cole and colleagues definition of either overweight or obesity, but the CDC 97th BMI percentile is similar to the Cole and colleagues definition of obesity for the period between 7 and 14 years.[11]

These comparisons raise the important issue that greater agreement is needed among national and international agencies with regard to definitions

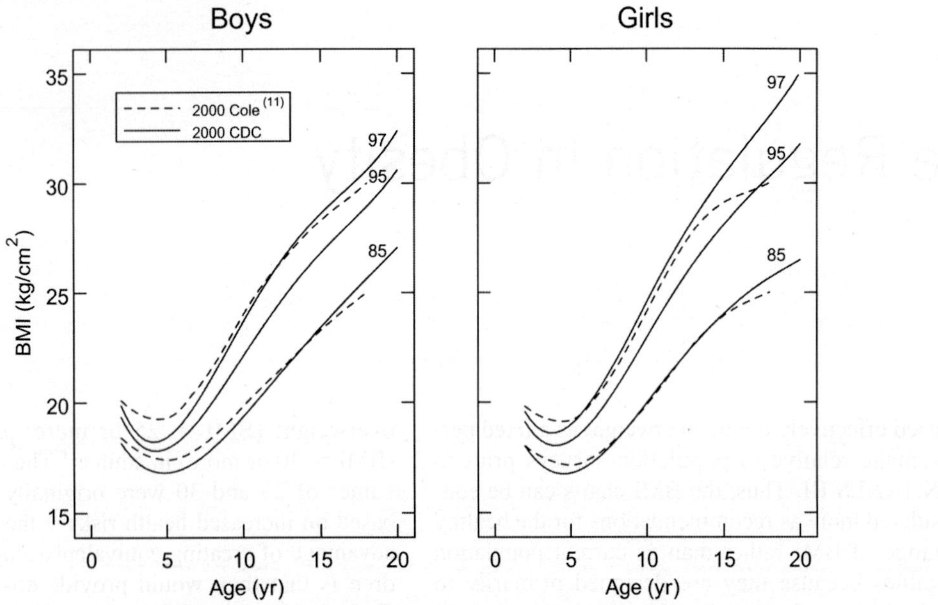

Figure 1 Comparison of Cole and colleagues'[11] BMI definitions of overweight and obesity during childhood (*broken line*) with 2000 CDC 85th and 95th percentiles (defined as risk of overweight and overweight, respectively) and the CDC 97th percentile (*solid line*). (Reproduced from reference 8.)

of what age-specific BMI values appropriately define overweight and obesity. In the meantime, the 2000 CDC percentiles for BMI might be most appropriate for assessing different degrees of overweight in US children, and the BMI cutoffs of Cole and colleagues could be used for international comparisons of obesity prevalence.[11]

RISKS OF OBESITY

The short-term risks of overweight in children and adolescents extend to reduced scholastic performance, psychological problems, and a number of significant health risks, including hyperlipidemia.[15] In addition, obese children are at increased risk of becoming overweight or obese adults compared with children of normal weight[16] and therefore are at long-term risk of the substantially increased morbidity and mortality, psychological problems, reduced economic achievement, and discrimination that are seen in obese adults.[17] In a summary of [17] studies investigating the long-term risks of childhood overweight for the development of adult obesity, Serdula and colleagues observed that 26 to 41% of overweight preschool children go on to become obese adults, with the risk of adult obesity increased to 2.0 to 2.6 times that of nonoverweight children.[18]

The risk of adult obesity in overweight children increases progressively with age. Data from Braddon and colleagues[19] on changes in the risk of adult obesity according to the age of childhood manifestation are shown in Figure 2. In that study, which was conducted in a cohort of English children, the percentage of obese adults who were overweight at age 7 years was only 2.6% for men and 7.5% for women, whereas values increased to 13.9% for men and 25.5% for women who were overweight at age 14 years. In addition, these figures might substantially underestimate the true relationship between early fatness and later obesity because 28.6% of obese men and 36.5% of obese women were already obese or overweight by age 7, a substantially increased percentage relative to the group of children who were categorized as overweight, and again there was an increase in the number of obese adults who were overweight in childhood as age increased (Figure 2).

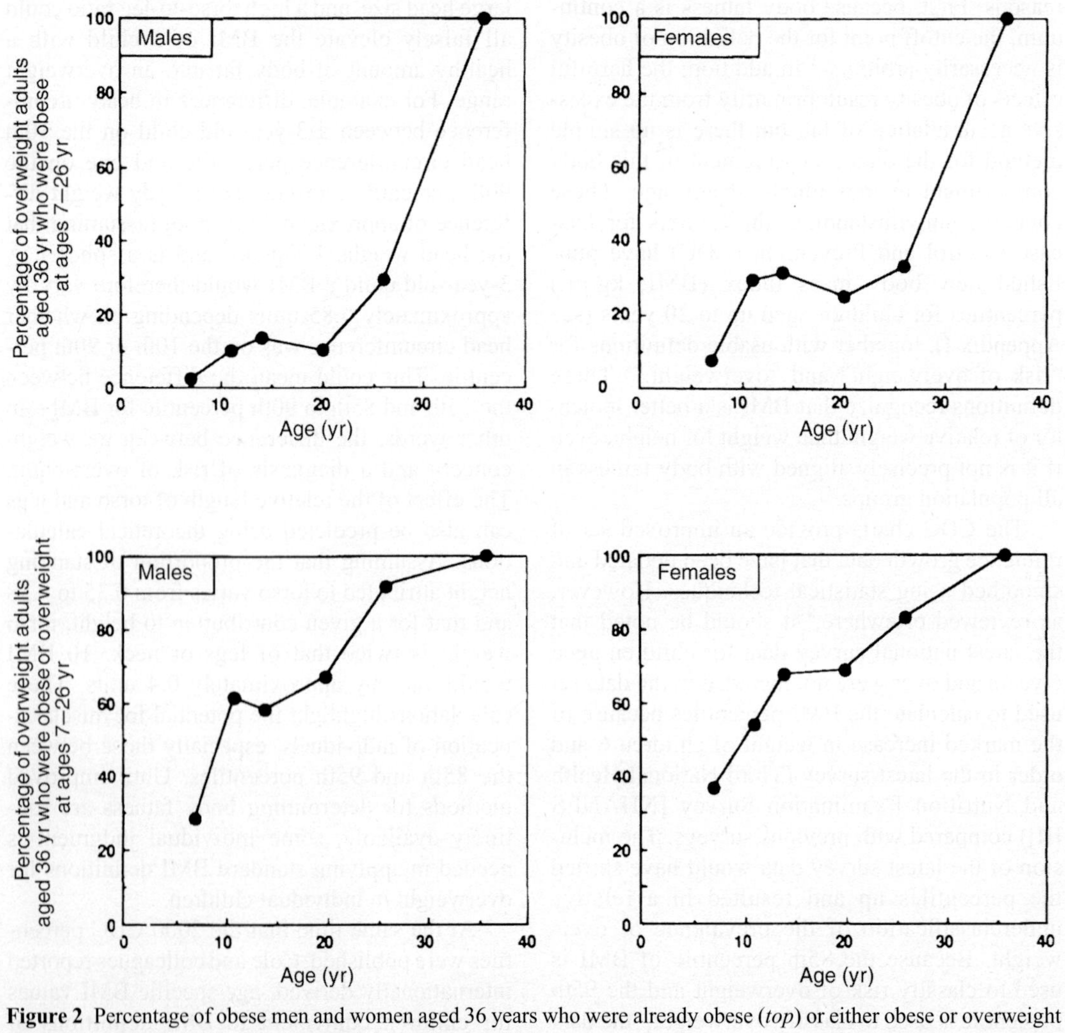

Figure 2 Percentage of obese men and women aged 36 years who were already obese (*top*) or either obese or overweight (*bottom*) by ages 7 to 26 years. (Adapted from reference 19.)

A further issue relevant to the risks of childhood overweight is that there is evidence to suggest that *severe* overweight developing early in life is particularly likely to lead to adult obesity. Whitaker and colleagues showed that childhood overweight was increasingly likely to predict adult obesity from age 3 years and older.[16] Similarly, Abraham and Nordsieck reported that 72.2% of severely overweight children (weighing more than 120% of the average for the population) became obese adults[20]; a similar result was found by others.[21] Although these data illustrate the substantial risk of childhood overweight leading to adult obesity, it is also important to note that many overweight children do not become obese adults. Data from Poskitt indicate that only one in nine overweight infants remain obese as adults in England,[22] whereas other studies similarly indicate that a minority of overweight children remain overweight.[19]

Recent studies have also raised the issue of whether, in addition to increasing the risk of adult obesity, obesity in childhood could also exert an independent influence on adult morbidity and mortality. In an analysis of longitudinal anthropometric data from the Third Harvard Growth Study (1922–1935), Must and colleagues observed that over a 55-year period, men who were overweight in adolescence had significantly increased all-cause mortality (relative risk 1.8) compared with men who were lean during adolescence.[23] This effect of adolescent weight, confirming a similar result found previously by Mossberg,[24] persisted even when weight at age 53 years was controlled. The implication of this finding is that the effects of adolescent weight on morbidity and mortality resulted from the adolescent obesity directly rather than from the effects of adolescent obesity on adult weight.[24] There was no association between adolescent weight and adult mortality in females in the study of Must and colleagues,[23] and gender was not distinguished in the study by Mossberg.[24]

The mechanisms by which adolescent weight might exert an influence on adult morbidity independent of adult fatness in men and possibly in women are not known. However, reports of increased plaque deposition in the arterial walls of overweight children suggest that there could be long-term effects of early body weight on morphology or metabolism that are not easily reversible. Consistent with this suggestion is the fact that overweight girls have been shown to have a reduced age of menarche, a risk factor for developing breast cancer.[25–27] This effect appears to be primarily related to increased body size rather than to differences in dietary intake in the obese.[28–30] A study by Meyer and colleagues suggested that the lowered age of menarche in overweight girls might be associated with increased weight rather than with increased fat mass.[31]

It is important to note that not all studies of the relationship between childhood weight and adult morbidity have reported positive associations. The study of Barker and colleagues reported an opposite trend, with a negative association between weight at 1 year of age and vascular disease in adult life.[32] Further studies are needed to clarify this issue and in particular to determine whether the long-term effects of early obesity could be important at some ages during childhood but not at other ages.

GENETIC VERSUS ENVIRONMENTAL FACTORS IN THE DEVELOPMENT OF OBESITY

Studies in Animals

In animals, there is substantial evidence that obesity can be transmitted genetically.[33] Several genetically obese animal strains exist, such as the Zucker rat and the ob/ob mouse, which have substantially more adipose tissue than lean counterpart animals. The fat gain in genetically obese animals is caused by a variety of mechanisms, including hyperphagia and an increased efficiency of energy use. The increased energy efficiency can be attributed primarily to a reduced thermogenesis for body temperature regulation. It is likely that some degree of imbalance in the autonomic nervous system contributes to the defective thermogenesis, as indicated by reduced sympathetic nervous drive in response to mildly cold ambient temperatures and in response to overeating.[34] In addition, parabiotic studies, in which the circulatory systems of lean and genetically obese animals are joined, have indicated that unidentified circulating factors (or the ability to respond to them correctly) are also important in the development of obesity.[35]

Animal studies also demonstrate that obesity can result from environmental factors, most particularly the availability of high-fat or high-variety diets. Some—but not all—strains of laboratory rodents gain substantial weight and fat when offered cafeteria diets containing a variety of snack foods such as cookies, cheese, cakes, processed meats, nuts, and so forth. Similar results have also been produced by offering synthetic high-fat diets, as well as by providing sucrose solutions in addition to standard rat chow. It could be noteworthy that physical activity does not have as much of an influence on body fat content as does diet in these rodent species. The fact that only some strains of animals, and only some animals within a strain, are susceptible to this diet-induced obesity[36,37] strongly indicates that "environmentally induced" obesity occurs only in genetically susceptible individuals and should therefore really be viewed as a genotype–environment effect. In relation to this observation, it is important to note that the willingness to overconsume food is not entirely a result of absolute standards of taste in animals. Instead, in studies that have separated the process of eating from the process of digestion by the use of esophageal cannulas, it has been shown that unidentified postingestion factors play a dominant role in determining food preferences.[36]

Studies in Humans

Studies on the importance of genetic inheritance versus environmental factors in the development of overweight and obesity have been harder to conduct in humans. It is widely accepted that body fat mass and fat distribution are subject to significant familial transmission[38–43]; in other words, the body compositions of children to a large extent reflect those of their parents. There remains a great deal of uncertainty, however, over the relative importance of genetic inheritance and environmental transmission (transmission between generations through the sharing of common environmental circumstances) in determining body fat content. Reported values for genetic heritability range from negligible to 0.8, implying that genetic inheritance accounts for between 0 and 80% of the variability in body fat mass in the community, and rates of environmental transmission range almost as much.[39,41,43–55]

This uncertainty over the relative importance of genetic and environmental transmission probably relates in large part to the methods that have been used to measure body composition and to the populations that have been studied. Most previous studies have used simple anthropometric indicators of body fat mass (such as weight corrected for height or one or more skinfold thicknesses).[39,43–48,50–55] However, the relationship between anthropometric parameters and fat mass can be very weak.[9] In addition, muscle mass, bone size, and height appear to be strongly inherited.[43] This could help explain the genetic inheritance of indicators of apparent fatness based on weight and could indicate that weight measurements will tend to result in an overestimation of the genetic inheritance of fat mass.

Probably the best data available on the inheritance of body composition come from Bouchard and colleagues, who have been the only group to use hydrostatic weighing (a gold standard method) for assessment of body composition.[49,56] Data from these investigations indicate that there are significant genetic and environmental components to the transmission of body density, with genetic inheritance accounting for 25% and environmental transmission for 30%. Thus, it appears that the family environment is at least as important as genetic inheritance in determining body fat mass.

Other lines of evidence from studies that effectively separate genetic inheritance from environmental factors confirm the importance of environmental factors in human overweight and obesity. For example, the body fat content of unrelated married couples becomes more similar over time.[40] In addition, the prevalence of obesity varies by the season of the year (it is highest in the fall and winter) and location within a country.[57] As further evidence, surveys show that the prevalence of childhood obesity has increased in the United States during the past two decades despite a relatively stable population pool.

METABOLIC PROGRAMMING IN THE DEVELOPMENT OF OBESITY

There is increasing awareness of the possibility that there might be critical periods during the life span when diet and other environmental factors exert a long-term influence on body fat content and the risk of adult obesity in humans,[58–61] a potential event that has been termed "metabolic programming." As emphasized by Lucas, the fact that this tremendously important issue has not yet been resolved reflects the relative lack of randomized dietary intervention trials with long-term follow-up in infants and children.[58,59] More studies of this type are needed despite the complex ethical issues involved.

Evidence consistent with the view that metabolic programming of adult body fatness might exist at different ages comes from several different sources, in particular indicating that either long-term energy insufficiency or long-term energy excess in childhood can lead to excess body fat content in adult life. In 1976, Ravelli and colleagues published the first study suggesting that nutrition of the mother during the intrauterine period might have a long-term influence on the risk of obesity.[62] Specifically, the investigators followed the incidence of obesity among men whose mothers lived in Holland during the Dutch "Hunger Winter," a time when the food supply was reduced in specific areas of the country at the end of the Second World War. A significant *increase* in the incidence of obesity at age 19 years was noted among the male offspring of mothers whose energy intake was reduced to famine levels (estimated at approximately 600 kcal/d) specifically during the first trimester of pregnancy, whereas a significant *decrease* in the risk of obesity was observed in women who had undergone energy deprivation during the third trimester. Although "metabolic programming" of intrauterine malnutrition can explain this result, it is also possible that other factors were important. For example, the mothers who were deprived of food might have been particularly concerned about feeding their infants substantial amounts of food after giving birth. In addition, the food provided by the Allied Forces after the famine was extremely high in fat, and the possibility cannot yet be ruled out that this might have had an important long-term effect.

Nevertheless, recent studies in animal models have also reported that malnutrition during the early part of pregnancy can be associated with increased body fat in adult life,[63,64] supporting the belief that long-term metabolic changes can be induced through diet. Although the mechanism for this effect is not known, Anguita and colleagues suggest that morphologic changes in the hypothalamus might be important.[64]

Similar to in utero energy insufficiency, childhood stunting (which is widely considered an indicator of chronic energy insufficiency during early childhood and typically occurs before age 5) has also been correlated with high BMI in several transitional countries, such as Brazil, China, and South Africa.[4,65–68] The risk for obesity and overweight for adults who were stunted as children and adolescents varies among countries but is consistently positive. The relative risk for obesity for an adult who was stunted in childhood is 1.7 in Brazil, 2.6 in South Africa, and 7.8 in Russia.[65] Mechanisms to explain these associations remain unclear; however, recent studies have offered possible metabolic as well as behavioral evidence that might explain part of this association.

In perhaps the first piece of evidence that early nutrition has long-term effects on metabolism that predispose a child to subsequent obesity, Hoffman and colleagues reported that nutritionally stunted children have a higher respiratory quotient and lower fat oxidation compared with healthy children from the same environment (Figure 3).[69] In the same series of experiments, stunted children also appeared to have impaired regulation of food intake compared with control children from the same environment,[70] resulting in greater energy consumption per kilogram of body weight when the stunted children were exposed to an abundant, ad libitum diet (Table 1). The results of this study need to be replicated but are consistent with the hypothesis that exposure to food insecurity early in life can disrupt normal perceptions of hunger and satiety. Taken together, these studies provide multiple lines of evidence consistent with the suggestion that undernutrition during early life can have long-term metabolic effects that can promote obesity later in life.

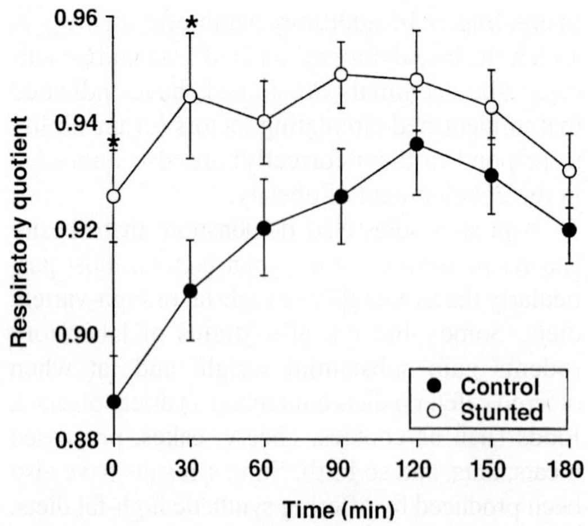

Figure 3 Fasting and postprandial respiratory quotient (RQ) in stunted and control children.[69] Values are means ±SEM. The stunted children had a significantly higher fasting RQ compared with control children ($t = 0$) and postprandially at $t = 30$ minutes ($p < .05$). The average postprandial RQ was not significantly different between the two groups ($p = .10$). (Reproduced with permission from reference 69.)

The first months after birth have received considerable attention as another potential time when metabolic programming, through the choice of diet (breast milk or formula) and the time of weaning, could have a long-term influence on body fatness. In particular, although several studies have suggested no effect of formula feeding on body fatness, the more recent studies have consistently indicated that breast-fed infants tend to become leaner adults.[71–79] The finding of a tendency for formula feeding to promote later body fatness in full-term babies is consistent with preliminary findings from randomized studies in preterm infants[80] and also with the well-known effect of early overfeeding in rodent models (resulting in a permanent increase in body weight and fat content).[81] Additionally, similar results have been demonstrated in nonhuman primates.[82]

Further studies are needed to determine whether metabolic or behavioral influences of formula versus breast-feeding are responsible for the differences observed. However, of potential relevance to this issue is the fact that Singhal and colleagues conducted a prospective study of preterm infants who were fed either a standard infant formula, banked breast milk, or an enriched preterm formula (5 g protein/L and 9 g fat/L greater than the standard formula) to examine long-term effects on circulating leptin.[80] Between the ages of 13 and 16 years, the children were measured for body fatness and leptin concentrations. It was found that the children who had received the preterm formula had a 30% higher ratio of leptin to fat mass compared with both of the other groups,[80] suggesting that the excess energy intake or altered nutrient composition of the preterm formula might have programmed higher circulating leptin during adolescence.

ENERGY AND SUBSTRATE REGULATION IN OBESITY

Energy Regulation

Average nonoverweight children consume more than 2 million kilojoules a year, but their body fat stores increase only modestly if growth is normal and energy expenditure approximates energy intake. A change of only 10%, either in intake or output, can lead to a 15 lb change in body fat in a single year, in addition to that deposited as a normal consequence of growth. The majority of children, who are of normal weight, do not exhibit such undesirable changes in body weight and fat, implying that normal energy regulation must be remarkably sensitive.

Until recently, our understanding of the underlying cause of this sensitive energy regulation was dominated by the guiding principle of energy balance:

$$\text{Energy stored} = \text{Energy intake} - \text{Energy expenditure}$$

Thus, it has been recognized that high levels of body fat (ie, energy) could not have been accumulated without energy intake being unusually high or energy expenditure being unusually low, or a combination of these two options. Similar calculations to those given above can illustrate that the dysregulation of energy in obesity needs to be only very small for excess adipose tissue to accumulate. For example, a child who becomes 100 lb overweight by the age of 15 years needs to have eaten less than an extra 100 MJ/d between the ages of 5 and 15 years. There has been considerable interest in defining whether energy intake or energy expenditure is the

Table 1 Energy Intake and Ratio of Energy Intake to Resting Energy Expenditure

	Girls		Boys	
Variable	Control ($n = 15$)	Stunted ($n = 13$)	Control ($n = 14$)	Stunted ($n = 14$)
Energy (kJ/kg) body weight*	60 ± 15	74 ± 14	67 ± 18	81 ± 9
Energy intake (kcal/d)/resting energy expenditure*	1.67 ± 0.4	1.89 ± 0.3	1.69 ± 0.4	1.93 ± 0.2

Adapted from reference 70.
*$p < .05$ between groups.

primary factor determining this energy dysregulation in obese individuals, as well as seeking to identify metabolic mechanisms that determine the separate regulation of these parameters. As described below, most of the investigations conducted in children have been cross-sectional in nature, that is, comparing measurements of energy intake and expenditure between lean and obese individuals or examining the relationship between these parameters in groups of individuals differing widely in body composition. It is also important to recognize that there may have been changes in the relative importance of excess energy intake and low-energy expenditure over time, reflecting shifting food behavior patterns and physical activity norms.

Energy Intake

The energy intake of an individual is usually understood to be that energy available to the body after obligatory losses of energy in urine and stools. Although complex metabolic balance studies are needed to precisely determine this "metabolizable energy," it can also be predicted from the dietary intakes of protein, fat, carbohydrate, and alcohol using the standard conversion factors of 4.0, 9.0, 4.0, and 7.0 kcal/g, respectively, which take into account the obligatory losses.

The regulation of food intake clearly plays an important part in the sensitive energy regulation in children of normal weight. More than 70 years ago, Davis demonstrated that very young children of normal body weight are capable of choosing a balanced diet and maintaining normal growth without dietary intervention from adult caregivers.[83] This remained true over periods of several days or longer, although food choices at individual meals were frequently extremely erratic. More recently, Birch and colleagues[84] and Shea and colleagues[85] provided additional strong evidence in support of an important role for the regulation of food intake in the energy regulation of young children of normal body weight. These investigators showed that although there might be substantial meal-to-meal fluctuations in energy and nutrient intakes, prompt and appropriate compensation occurs spontaneously so that the 24-hour energy intake remains relatively stable. A further report by Birch and colleagues also demonstrated that young children are able to compensate for the inclusion of low-calorie fat substitutes in a meal to maintain a constant energy intake.[86]

These studies clearly demonstrate that in children of normal body weight, energy regulation through the regulation of food intake occurs and plays an important role in the maintenance of a stable pattern of body composition change throughout childhood. However, a caveat to these studies is that the observed capacity for normal energy regulation may occur only when relatively healthy foods are offered, and the ability of young children to accurately regulate energy intake when offered many highly energy-dense foods of low nutritional value has not been systematically explored.

Individual studies of differences in reported energy intake between overweight and nonoverweight children have been conflicting, but taking all of the data together, reported energy intakes of overweight children are not significantly greater than those of nonoverweight children of the same age and are significantly less when expressed in relation to body weight.[29,85,87–105] However, it is known that overweight individuals, including adolescents,[106] underreport their energy intake to a greater degree than do individuals of normal weight, which indicates that the finding of normal food intake in overweight children might be owing to methodologic error.

In contrast to the studies of reported energy intake, studies from psychological investigations of eating behavior in overweight children suggest that already overweight children consume more total energy than do nonoverweight subjects. Studies by several groups have suggested that overweight children and adolescents are faster eaters, chew less, prefer high-fat foods, and do not exhibit the normal pattern of decelerating eating toward the end of a meal, as seen in children of normal weight.[107–110] Furthermore, obese parents have been reported to give more encouragement to their children to eat than do parents of nonobese children and serve them larger portions of food.[111] These findings are also consistent with results from studies in adults.[112] In addition, overweight children may have an abnormal pattern of energy consumption within the day, with a reduced percentage of calories being consumed at breakfast, which is a meal widely recognized to be associated with prevention of weight gain in adults.[113] As described below, studies of total energy expenditure (TEE) might be more reliable for estimating the energy intake of overweight children than studies of reported energy intake and confirm that already overweight children consume more total energy than children of normal weight. A recent summary of TEE data in children concluded that high-energy intake rather than low TEE could explain secular increases in body weight during the period 1985 to 1995, a suggestion that is consistent with increases in per capita food supply during this time.[114]

Energy Expenditure

The TEE of an individual, which is equal to the metabolizable energy intake when body energy stores remain constant, can be divided into compartments that relate to the different types of energy expenditure measurements that are made. Typically, three major compartments are defined. The resting energy expenditure is the energy expended at rest after an overnight fast and is the major compartment, comprising at least half of the TEE in a typical individual. The thermic effect of feeding is the increase in energy expenditure above baseline resulting from the consumption and processing of food and comprises 7 to 15% of TEE on average. This thermic effect of feeding has been further subdivided into facultative and obligatory components, where obligatory energy expenditure is the expenditure for necessary aspects of digestion and assimilation, whereas the facultative component has been proposed as a form of energy wasting that can perhaps serve to burn off surplus dietary energy. The final component of TEE is the energy expended for physical activity and arousal, which is generally the second largest component of TEE and the most variable because to a large extent it is under voluntary control.

The role of energy expenditure in the regulation of energy balance has been controversial in the past but is perhaps less so currently. Studies in both adults[115–118] and adolescents[119] have suggested that humans have a relatively limited capacity for dissipating surplus dietary energy by thermogenesis. In these studies, subjects have been overfed, and changes in energy expenditure and energy storage have been measured to assess the fate of the excess dietary energy. In all carefully controlled studies, the ability to dissipate excess energy, seen as an increase in TEE or components of energy expenditure, has represented a relatively minor component of the excess dietary intake.[115–118] Thus, the majority of the surplus energy was stored, primarily in the form of additional body fat. Studies of this kind highlight the importance of the regulation of food intake, rather than thermogenesis, in the short-term regulation of energy balance.

It is possible, however, that energy expenditure plays other critical roles in energy regulation that these studies do not address. In particular, it has been speculated that low-energy expenditure in one or more of the components of expenditure could have an association with increased body fatness over the long term. This could be a result of the low-energy expenditure promoting increased fatness or of an underlying mechanism promoting fat gain that precipitates low-energy expenditure to provide the surplus energy needed for the weight gain. Studies of differences in components of energy expenditure between obese and nonobese children are discussed below. These cross-sectional studies do not define the causal role of energy expenditure in obesity but do serve to define the energy expenditure of children who are already obese in relation to normal values. Prospective studies that have investigated the role of energy expenditure in the weight gain in obesity are discussed below under "Roles of Energy Intake and Expenditure in the Development of Obesity."

Concerning resting energy expenditure, a summary of studies in otherwise healthy overweight and nonoverweight children reveals that the overweight individuals do not have reduced resting energy expenditure. In relation to age, the resting energy expenditure of overweight children appears to be within the normal range at 8 to 10 years and increases subsequently compared

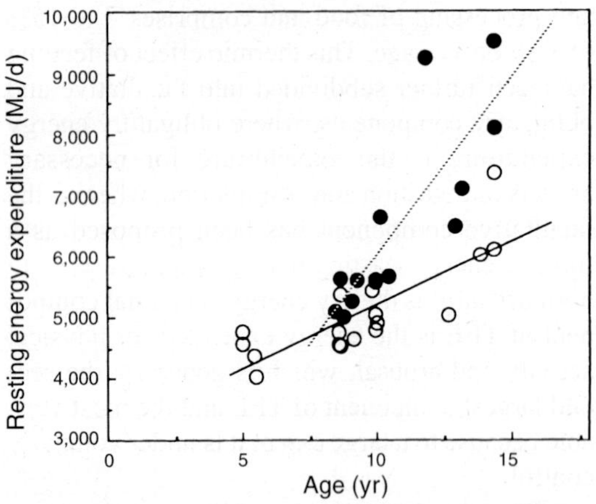

Figure 4 Relationship between resting energy expenditure (in kJ/d, where 1 kJ = 0.239 kcal) and age in nonoverweight (*solid line*) and overweight (*broken line*) boys and girls aged 5 to 15 years.[171] Data points are group means reported between 1989 and 1994.[92,103,122,132,137,141,144,172–178] There was a significant effect of obesity status on the relationship between resting energy expenditure and age ($p <$ .001), and the relationship between resting energy expenditure and age was significant in both nonoverweight (r^2 = .630, $p <$ .000) and overweight children (r^2 = .682, $p <$ .000).

with values of normal children (Figure 4). Values for energy expenditure per unit of fat-free mass (the metabolically active component of the body because fat mass is relatively metabolically inactive) are somewhat lower in overweight compared with nonoverweight children. However, this is an inappropriate method of expressing resting energy expenditure in individuals of different sizes because there is a wide variability in the energy expenditure of different tissues that comprise the lean mass. Tissues such as brain and heart have a very high energy expenditure and tissues such as muscle have a low-energy expenditure. It appears that overweight and nonoverweight individuals have more similar amounts of tissues with high-energy expenditure than they have tissues with low-energy expenditure. Thus, it is more appropriate to examine the relationship between fat-free mass and resting energy expenditure than to compare resting energy expenditure per unit of fat-free mass between different groups.

As seen in Figure 5, neither the intercept nor the slope of the relationship differs between obese and nonobese individuals, demonstrating that there is no difference in the resting energy expenditure of overweight and nonoverweight children when the data are appropriately normalized for metabolically active tissue. This result, obtained by combining data from studies in which data from at least two groups of subjects were available, is compatible with results from regression analyses in a group of children with a wide range of body compositions,[120] as well as with results of numerous studies in adults.[121]

Several studies on the thermic effect of feeding demonstrate a normal energy expenditure in overweight compared with nonoverweight children and adolescents,[119,122,123] a result that contrasts with the numerous studies that indicate a reduced thermic effect of feeding in obese adults.[124,125] There is one report of a reduced thermic effect of feeding in obese children,[126] and the duration of obesity has been implicated as a possible explanation for differences in results among different studies.[122] This explanation could also help explain the fact that the thermic effect of feeding is reduced in obese adults.

Concerning physical activity, several studies have reported no difference in physical activity between lean and overweight children,[71,87,127,128] whereas other studies have reported low[114,129,130–132] or even high[133] levels of physical activity in overweight children relative to nonoverweight controls. Television viewing has also been investigated separately as a marker for low physical activity and for its relationship to body composition in children.[134] Although the mechanism by which television viewing might influence body fat mass is not known, a reduction in physical activity is strongly implicated as part of the mechanism because television viewing is a sedentary activity that might replace more strenuous ones, together with the possibility that dietary intake could be increased as well.[135,136] Studies in this area have not produced consistent results, with some studies reporting a negative association between the time spent watching television and body fatness[135] and other studies failing to substantiate this result.[128,137]

This controversy might reflect the fact that inactivity during television viewing can potentially be compensated for by strenuous activity at other times; more research is needed to elucidate the relationship between body fat mass and physical activity in children as well as in adults. A further

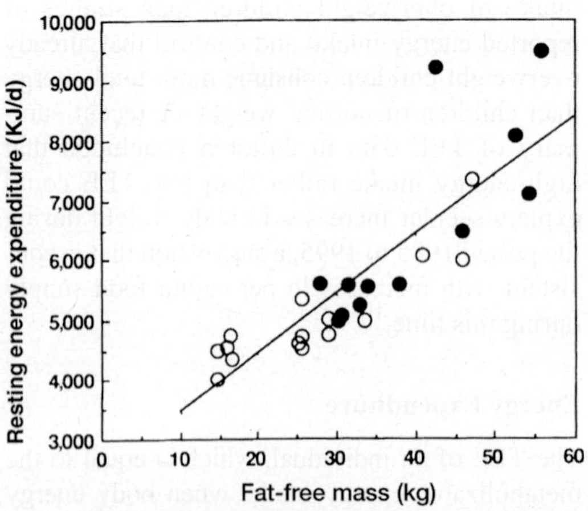

Figure 5 Relationship between resting energy expenditure and fat-free mass in nonoverweight and overweight boys and girls aged 5 to 15 years.[171] Data points are group means (in kJ/d, where 1 kJ = 0.239 kcal) reported between 1989 and 1993.[103,122,132,141,144,172–178] There was no significant effect of overweight status on resting energy expenditure in multiple regression analyses, including fat-free mass as an independent variable. The relationship between resting energy expenditure and fat-free mass is significant (r^2 = .712, $p <$ .000).

unresolved aspect of the literature on television viewing is that there are reports of both a decreased[127] and normal[138] resting energy expenditure during television viewing in obese children compared with nonobese controls. On the basis of the studies described above, it cannot be concluded that the obese child is necessarily inactive, or that inactivity is an important cause of obesity. However, this conclusion does not exclude an important role for physical activity in obese children, and further studies are needed to clarify this important issue.

Studies on TEE as determined using the doubly labeled water technique[139,140] have been conducted as a way to examine the combined effects of different components of energy expenditure in normal-weight and overweight children and also as a more accurate way to assess energy expenditure for physical activity (when combined with measurements of resting energy expenditure). Using this method, several studies in children and adults have indicated an inverse association between energy expenditure for physical activity and body fat mass when values for physical activity are normalized for body size by the use of the ratio of total to resting energy expenditure as a physical activity index,[106,141,142] and one recent study reported no difference between lean and overweight children despite differences in sedentary behavior and sports participation.[143] The mechanism of this association is not known but is likely to include the fact that inactivity promotes insulin resistance and could enhance fat oxidation.[144] Although this ratio of total to resting energy expenditure is reduced with increasing body fat content, the TEE for physical activity is typically high. This is because resting energy expenditure and the energy costs of most activities increase with body size. These consistent findings contrast with the substantial controversy over the effects of obesity on physical activity when studies using reported estimates of physical activity are considered.

Doubly labeled water measurements of TEE have also been used to examine differences in energy intake and energy requirements between normal-weight and overweight children. The recent Dietary Reference Intakes for macronutrients[145] summarized all available data on TEE in childhood to report that there is no substantial difference between normal-weight and overweight children in the relationship between TEE and body weight, height, and age, with equations suitable for all children based on summaries of all available doubly labeled water data:

$$\text{TEE (kcal/d)} = 89 \times \text{weight (kg)} - 100 \text{ (boys and girls 0 to 2 yr)}$$

$$\text{TEE} = 88.5 - 61.9 \times \text{age (yr)} + \text{PA} \times 26.7 \times \text{weight (kg)} + 903 \times \text{height (mm)} \text{ (boys 3 to 18 yr)}$$

$$\text{TEE} = 135.3 - 30.8 \times \text{age (yr)} + \text{PA} \times 10.0 \times \text{weight (kg)} + 934 \times \text{height (mm)} \text{ (girls 3 to 18 yr)}$$

where PA is a physical activity coefficient used for children 3 years and older:

PA = 1.00 if physical activity level is sedentary
PA = 1.13 if physical activity level is low
PA = 1.27 if physical activity level is active
PA = 1.45 if physical activity level is very active

TEE does not equal energy intake in children, because there is additional consumed energy used for growth that is deposited in the form of lean tissue and fat. However, except during the early months of life and during the peak of pubertal development, energy used for energy deposition is only 20 to 25 kcal/d[145]; thus, TEE closely reflects energy intake. The equations given above indicate that children who are overweight do indeed need more energy to maintain current body weight than do normal-weight children. For example, a child more than 3 years of age who is already overweight by 10 kg compared with normal-weight children will have increased TEE and hence energy intake of 100 to 267 kcal/d. Table 2 summarizes estimated energy requirements for children of reference weights, based on the above equations with an increment added for the energy deposition in normal growth.

A final issue to consider when comparing differences in energy expenditure between lean and overweight individuals is the energy expenditure response to overfeeding. As detailed above, an ability to burn off surplus dietary energy has been suggested as potentially important in the regulation of energy balance. However, in a study of overweight and nonoverweight adolescents, Bandini and colleagues found no difference between groups in the ability to dissipate excess energy intake.[146] This finding is consistent with the view, outlined above, that diet-induced thermogenesis plays only a small role in the regulation of energy balance.

SUBSTRATE BALANCE

As an extension of the energy balance principles detailed above, it has been suggested that body carbohydrate balance could play a critical role in overall energy regulation.[147] The basic principle behind this theory of energy regulation, which is in keeping with the earlier glucostatic theory of energy regulation, is that balance of the primary energy substrates, fat and carbohydrate, have to be considered separately.[147] Thus,

Fat stored = Fat intake − Fat oxidation

Carbohydrate stored = Carbohydrate intake − Carbohydrate oxidation

Because the energy in carbohydrate stores is very small in relation to that in fat stores, the carbohydrate stores have a high turnover rate and are liable to be depleted quickly and frequently. The essential requirement of key tissues for glucose suggests that signals should exist to efficiently monitor and correct body carbohydrate balance. An extension of this theory of nutrient regulation is that dietary macronutrient composition plays an important role in determining body fat content.[147] This is because the higher the dietary fat content, the more total food (and energy) needs to be consumed to maintain carbohydrate intake and therefore carbohydrate stores, and the fatter the individual will be because of increased energy intake.

Flatt has also suggested that the increase in body fat induced by a high-fat diet could be self-limiting because reduced insulin sensitivity and increased circulating free fatty acids tend to occur with increased body fat content, promoting increased fat oxidation and preservation of carbohydrate stores, resulting in a stabilization of hunger and satiety signals from body carbohydrate stores and stability of food intake and body fat stores.[147] This model provides a potential explanation for body fat regulation that does not rely on the concept of a novel "signal" from fat stores that detects and corrects a body set point.

Support for the importance of nutrient balance in the overall regulation of energy balance can be derived from several sources, although there is currently little information available on infants and children. Flatt has demonstrated in mice the critically important idea that energy balance is indeed adjusted on a day-to-day basis to maintain stable body carbohydrate balance, through adaptive fluctuations in food intake.[147] Studies in humans have indicated that carbohydrate balance is more closely regulated than is fat balance.[148,149] Concerning the effect of dietary composition on energy intake and body composition, animal studies have repeatedly demonstrated that hyperphagia and obesity can be induced in many strains of normal-weight rodents by feeding a high-fat diet as described above.[36]

In humans, results from some,[150–153] although not all,[154–156] short-term intervention studies in adults indicate that energy intake increases with consumption of a high-fat diet. The fact that not all human studies have found an increase in energy intake with consumption of a high-fat diet does not invalidate the nutrient balance theory of energy regulation because a high-fat diet could induce positive energy balance by decreasing energy expenditure, rather than increasing energy intake as suggested by both animal and adult human studies.[157,158] Also consistent with the nutrient balance model are the data from cross-sectional

Table 2 Estimated Energy Requirements*

Age	Reference Weight (kg)	Activity Level (kcal/d)			
		Sedentary	Low Active	Active	Very Active
Boys					
1 mo	4.4	472	(No activity level specified before 3 yr)		
6 mo	7.9	645			
12 mo	10.3	844			
18 mo	11.7	961			
24 mo	12.7	1,050			
3 yr	14.3	1,162	1,134	1,485	1,683
6 yr	20.7	1,328	1,535	1,742	1,997
9 yr	28.6	1,530	1,787	2,043	2,359
12 yr	40.5	1,798	2,113	2,428	2,817
15 yr	56.3	2,223	2,618	3,013	3,499
18 yr	67.2	2,383	2,823	3,263	3,804
Girls					
1 mo	4.2	438	(No activity level specified before 3 yr)		
6 mo	7.2	593			
12 mo	9.5	768			
18 mo	11.0	899			
24 mo	12.1	997			
3 yr	13.9	1,080	1,243	1,395	1,649
6 yr	20.2	1,247	1,451	1,642	1,961
9 yr	29.0	1,415	1,660	1,890	2,273
12 yr	41.6	1,617	1,909	2,183	2,640
15 yr	52.0	1,731	2,057	2,363	2,870
18 yr	56.2	1,690	2,024	2,336	2,858

*Values are estimated average requirements from reference 145.

studies that indicate that consumption of a high-fat diet is frequently associated with high–body-fat mass in adults.[159–163] Thus, as predicted by the nutrient balance model above, obese and overweight adults tend to consume a higher fat diet than do nonobese subjects and, at least in the short term, might be hyperphagic.

Some,[132,133] but not all,[87] studies in children and adolescents support the view that high–dietary-fat intake is associated with obesity. It is possible that this controversy could be owing to the fact that the fiber content of the diet and its energy density might have significant effects on food intake. Although high-fat diets tend to be low in fiber and have a high energy density, this is not always so, and differences in these aspects of the diet (unreported in the studies described above) might have been important. However, an impairment in total fat oxidation is unlikely to explain an association between dietary fat intake and the development of obesity in review of the several recent reports in children[164–166] that rates of total fat oxidation are equivalently responsive to change in dietary intake in both lean and overweight children. There is also some suggestion that endogenous fuels are less readily oxidized in overweight to lean individuals[167] which requires further study. An additional important consideration in relation to dietary intake is that on theoretical grounds, saturated fat can be expected to have more adverse effects on body fat mass than other fats do because of its influence on insulin sensitivity,[144] and indeed several recent studies have reported lower oxidation of saturated fats than mono- or polyunsaturated fats.[168,169]

ROLES OF ENERGY INTAKE AND EXPENDITURE IN THE DEVELOPMENT OF OBESITY

As described above, the majority of published investigations into the causes of early overweight have been cross-sectional in nature; that is, they have related measurements of body fat mass to energy expenditure or other parameters measured at the same time. This approach provides important information on energy intake, energy expenditure, and substrate oxidation in individuals who are already obese but does not address the question of what happens during the development of the obese state. A finding, for example, of high-energy intake in overweight children does not preclude the possibility that energy intake was normal or even low during the period of excess weight gain. Recent prospective studies have addressed the issue of causality in overweight by investigating whether energy expenditure is low in individuals with increased susceptibility to overweight (because of parental obesity). Although the results have been conflicting, with reports of both low-energy expenditure[170–174] and normal-energy expenditure[175–177] in the pre-overweight state, the current weight of evidence indicates that low-energy expenditure is a contributing factor in some circumstances.[178]

SUMMARY AND IMPLICATIONS FOR THE TREATMENT OF OBESITY

The excess fat mass that characterizes obesity is attributable to both genetic susceptibility and environmental factors and results from energy intake exceeding energy expenditure plus the energy requirement for normal growth over a prolonged period of time. However, this increment in energy intake over energy expenditure can be as little as 400 MJ/d or less if it persists over a period of years. The studies summarized in this chapter do not provide definitive evidence as to whether this differential between energy intake and energy expenditure is caused primarily by decreased energy expenditure or by increased energy intake. However, the weight of evidence currently indicates that both overeating and underexpending can be primary causes of overweight in childhood, and that once a child is overweight, energy intake is higher than that of normal-weight children. In addition, dietary fat, in particular saturated fat, can promote fat deposition through its influence on energy intake.

Further studies are needed in this area, in particular to delineate the usual roles of high-energy intake and low-energy expenditure as causal factors in excessive weight gain leading to overweight in childhood. Current prescriptions for the treatment of childhood overweight, taking into account the degree of caution that is appropriate for a disorder in which the treatment can itself have detrimental consequences, should be based on individualizing for each child a decrease in energy intake relative to energy expenditure by a combination of moderate dietary therapy and promotion of energy expenditure from physical activity (see Chapter 54, "Evaluation and Management of Obesity").

REFERENCES

1. Committee on Diet and Health, Food and Nutrition Board, Commission on Life, National Research Council. Diet and Health: Implications for Reducing Chronic Disease. Washington, DC: National Academy Press; 1989.
2. Livingstone MBE. Childhood obesity in Europe: A growing concern. Public Health Nutr 2001;4:109–16.
3. Popkin BM. The nutrition transition in low-income countries: An emerging crisis. Nutr Rev 1994;52:285–98.
4. Sawaya AL, Dallal G, Solymos G, et al. Obesity and malnutrition in a shantytown population in the city of Sao Paulo, Brazil. Obes Res 1995;3:107S–15S.
5. Department of Health and Human Services, Centers for Disease Control and Prevention. Available at: http://www.cdc.gov/index.htm.
6. Kuczmarski RJ, Ogden CL, Grummer-Strawn LM, et al. Advance Data from Vital and Health Statistics. No. 314, Volume. 314. Hyattsville, MD: National Center for Health Statistics; 2000.
7. Himes JH, Dietz WH. Guidelines for overweight in adolescent preventive services: Recommendations from an expert committee. Am J Clin Nutr 1994;59:307–16.
8. Roberts SB, Dallal GE. The new childhood growth charts. Nutr Rev 2001;59:31–6.
9. Garn SM, Leonard WR, Hawthorne VM. Three limitations of the body-mass index. Am J Clin Nutr 1986;44:996.
10. Trowbridge FL, Marks JS, de Romana GL, et al. Body composition of Peruvian children with short stature and high weight-for-height. II. Implications for the interpretation for weight-for-height as an indicator of nutritional status. Am J Clin Nutr 1987;46:411–8.
11. Cole TJ, Bellizzi MC, Flegal KM, Dietz WH. Establishing a standard definition for child overweight and obesity worldwide: International survey. BMJ 2000;320:1240–3.
12. World Health Organization. Obesity: Preventing and managing the global epidemic. Report of a WHO Consultation; 3–5 June 1995; Geneva, Switzerland Geneva: World Health Organization; 1998.
13. Dietz WH, Robinson TN. Use of the body mass index (BMI) as a measure of overweight in children and adolescents. J Pediatr 1988;132:191–3.
14. Bellizzi MC, Dietz WH. Workshop on childhood obesity: Summary of the discussion. Am J Clin Nutr 1999;70: 173S–5S.
15. Dietz WH. Prevention of childhood obesity. Pediatr Clin North Am 1986;33:823–33.
16. Whitaker RC, Wright JA, Pepe MS, et al. Predicting obesity in young adulthood from childhood and parental obesity. N Engl J Med 1997;337:869–73.
17. Wadden TA, Stunkard AJ. Psychosocial consequences of obesity and dieting. In: Stunkard AJ, Wadden TA, editors. Obesity: Theory and Therapy. New York: Raven Press; 1993. p. 163–77.
18. Serdula MK, Ivery D, Coates RJ, et al. Do obese children become obese adults? A review of the literature. Prev Med 1993;22:167–77.
19. Braddon FEM, Rodgers B, Wadsworth MEJ, Davies JMC. Onset of obesity in a 36 year birth cohort study. BMJ 1986; 293:299–303.
20. Abraham S, Nordsieck M. Relationship of excess weight in children and adults. Public Health Rep 1960;75:263–73.
21. Rimm IJ, Rimm AA. Association between juvenile onset obesity and severe adult obesity in 73,532 women. Am J Public Health 1976;66:479–81.
22. Poskitt EME. Do fat babies stay fat? BMJ 1977;6052:7–9.
23. Must A, Jaques PF, Dallal GE, et al. Long-term morbidity and mortality of overweight adolescents. A follow-up of the Harvard Growth Study of 1922 to 1935. N Engl J Med 1992; 327:1350–5.
24. Mossberg H-O. 40-year follow-up of overweight children. Lancet 1989;ii:491–3.
25. Staszewski J. Age at menarche and breast cancer. J Natl Cancer Inst 1971;47:935–40.
26. Kelsey JL. A review of the epidemiology of human breast cancer. Epidemiol Rev 1979;1:74–109.
27. MacMahon B, Trichopoulos D, Brown J. Age at menarche, urine estrogens, and breast cancer risk. Int J Cancer 1982;30:427–31.
28. Moisan J, Meyer F, Gingras S. A nested case-control study of the correlates of early menarche. Am J Epidemiol 1990;132:953–61.
29. Maclure M, Travis LB, Willet W, MacMahon B. A prospective cohort study of nutrient intake and age of menarche. Am J Clin Nutr 1991;54:649–56.
30. Post GB, Kemper HCG. Nutrient intake and biological maturation during adolescence. The Amsterdam growth and health longitudinal study. Eur J Clin Nutr 1993;47: 400–8.
31. Meyer F, Moisan J, Marcoux D, Bouchard C. Dietary and physical determinants of menarche. Epidemiology 1990;1:377–81.
32. Barker DJP, Osmond C, Winter PD, et al. Weight in infancy and death from ischaemic heart disease. Lancet 1989;ii: 577–80.
33. Bray GA, York DA. Hypothalamic and genetic obesity in experimental animals: An autonomic and endocrine hypothesis. Physiol Rev 1979;59:719–809.
34. York DA. Genetic models of animal obesity. In: Bjorntorp P, Brodoff BN, editors. Obesity. Philadelphia, PA: JB Lippincott; 1992. p. 233–40.
35. Harris RB, Hervey E, Hervey GR. Body composition of lean and obese Zucker rats in parabiosis. Int J Obes 1987;11: 274–80.
36. Sclafani A. Dietary-induced overeating. Ann N Y Acad Sci 1989;575:281–91.
37. West DB, Boozer CN, Moody DL, Atkinson RL. Dietary obesity in nine inbred mouse strains. Am J Physiol 1992;262: R1025–32.
38. Biron P, Mongeau JG, Bertrand D. Familial resemblance of body weight and height in 374 homes with adopted children. Pediatrics 1977;91:555–8.
39. Garn SM, Bailey SM, Cole PE. Similarities between parents and their adopted children. Am J Phys Anthropol 1979;45:539–44.
40. Garn SM, Cole PE, Bailey SM. Living together as a factor in family-line resemblances. Hum Biol 1979;51:565–87.
41. Savard R, Bouchard C, Leblanc C, Tremblay A. Familial resemblance in fatness indicators. Ann Hum Biol 1983;10:111–8.
42. Heller R, Garrison RJ, Havlik RJ, et al. Family resemblances in height and relative weight in the Framingham Heart Study. Int J Obes 1984;8:399–405.

43. Devor EJ, McGue M, Crawford MH, Lin PM. Transmissible and nontransmissible components of anthropometric variation in the Alexanderwohl Mennonites: Resolution by path analysis. Am J Phys Anthropol 1986;69:83–92.
44. Borjeson M. The aetiology of obesity in children. Acta Paediatr Scand 1976;65:279–87.
45. Hartz A, Giefer E, Rimm AA. Relative importance of the effect of family environment and heredity on obesity. Ann Hum Genet (Lond) 1977;41:185–93.
46. Bray GA. The inheritance of corpulence. In: Cioffi LA, editor. The Body Weight Regulatory System: Normal and Disturbed Mechanisms. New York: Raven Press; 1981. p. 185–95.
47. Annest JL, Sing CF, Biron P, Mongeau JG. Familial aggregation of blood pressure and weight in adoptive families. Am J Epidemiol 1983;117:492–506.
48. Byard PJ, Sharma K, Russell JM, Rao DC. A family study of anthropometric traits in a Punjabi community: An investigation of familial transmission. Am J Phys Anthropol 1984;64:97–104.
49. Bouchard C, Savard R, Despres JP, et al. Body composition in adopted and biological siblings. Hum Biol 1985;57: 61–75.
50. Stunkard AJ, Sorensen TIA, Hanis C, et al. An adoption study of human obesity. N Engl J Med 1986;314:193–8.
51. Price RA, Cadoret RJ, Stunkard AJ, Troughton E. Genetic contributions to human fatness: An adoption study. Am J Psychiatry1987;144:1003–8.
52. Newman B, Selby JV, Quesenberry CP, et al. Nongenetic influences of obesity on other cardiovascular disease risk factors: An analysis of identical twins. Am J Public Health 1990;80:675–8.
53. Stunkard AJ, Harris JR, Pedersen NL, McClearn GE. The bodymass index of twins who have been reared apart. N Engl J Med 1990;322:1483–7.
54. Fabsitz RR, Carmelli D, Hewitt JK. Evidence for independent genetic influences on obesity in middle age. Int J Obes 1992;16:657–66.
55. Sorensen T, Holst C, Stunkard A. Correlations of body mass index of adult adoptees and their biological and adoptive relatives. Int J Obes 1992;16:227–36.
56. Bouchard C, Perusse L. Heredity and body fat. Annu Rev Nutr 1988;8:259–77.
57. Dietz WHJ, Gortmaker SL. Factors within the physical environment associated with childhood obesity. Am J Clin Nutr 1984;39:619–24.
58. Lucas A. Does early diet program future outcome? Acta Paediatr Scand Suppl 1990;365:58–67.
59. Lucas A. Programming by early nutrition in man. In: Bock GR, Whelan J, editors. The Childhood Environment and Adult Disease. London: John Wiley & Sons; 1991. p. 38–55.
60. Dietz WH. Critical periods in childhood for the development of obesity. Am J Clin Nutr 1994;59:955–9.
61. Martorell R, Stein AD, Schroeder DG. Early nutrition and later adiposity. J Nutr 2001;131:874S–80S.
62. Ravelli GP, Stein ZA, Susser MW. Obesity in young men after famine exposure in utero and early infancy. N Engl J Med 1976;295:349–53.
63. Jones AP, Simson EL, Friedman MI. Gestational undernutrition and the development of obesity in rats. J Nutr 1984;114:1482–4.
64. Anguita RM, Sigulem DM, Sawaya AL. Intrauterine food restriction is associated with obesity in young rats. J Nutr1993;123:1421–8.
65. Popkin BM, Richards MK, Monteiro CA. Stunting is associated with overweight in children of four nations that are undergoing the nutrition transition. J Nutr 1996;126:3009–16.
66. Sawaya AL, Grillo LP, Verreschi I, et al. Mild stunting is associated with higher susceptibility to the effects of high-fat diets: Studies in a shantytown population in Sao Paulo, Brazil. J Nutr 1998;128:415S–20S.
67. Schroeder DG, Martorell R, Flores R. Infant and child growth and fatness and fat distribution in Guatemalan adults. Am J Epidemiol 1999;149:177–85.
68. Florencio TM, Ferreira HS, de Franca AP, et al. Obesity and undernutrition in a verylow-income population in the city of Maceio, northeastern Brazil. Br J Nutr 2001;86:277–84.
69. Hoffman DJ, Sawaya AL, Verreschi I, et al. Why are nutritionally stunted children at increased risk of obesity? Studies of metabolic rate and fat oxidation in shantytown children from Sao Paulo, Brazil. Am J Clin Nutr 2000;72:702–7.
70. Hoffman DJ, Roberts SB, Verreschi I, et al. Regulation of energy intake may be impaired in nutritionally stunted children from the shantytowns of Sao Paulo, Brazil. J Nutr 2000;130:2265–70.
71. Wilkinson PW, Pearlson J, Parkin JM, et al. Obesity in childhood: A community study in Newcastle upon Tyne. Lancet 1977;i:350–2.
72. Dine MS, Gartside PS, Glueck CJ, et al. Where do the heaviest children come from? A prospective study of white children from birth to 5 years of age. Pediatrics 1979;63:1–7.
73. Vobecky JS, Vobecky J, Shapcott D, Demers P-P. Nutrient intake patterns and nutritional status with regard to relative weight in early infancy. Am J Clin Nutr 1983;38:730–8.
74. Kramer MS, Barr RG, Leduc DG, et al. Infant determinants of childhood weight and adiposity. J Pediatr 1985;107:104–7.
75. Warrington S, Storey DM. Comparative studies on Asian and Caucasian children. 2. Nutrition, feeding, practices and health. Eur J Clin Nutr 1988;42:68–80.
76. Agras WS, Kraemer HC, Berkowitz RI, Hammer LD. Influence of early feeding style on adiposity at 6 years of age. J Pediatr 1990;116:805–9.
77. Strubak V, Skultetyova M, Hromadova M, et al. Late effects of breast-feeding and early weaning: Seven-year prospective study in children. Endocrine Regul 1991;25:53–7.
78. Elliot KG, Kjohede CL, Gournis E, Rasmussen KM. Duration of breastfeeding associated with obesity during adolescence. Obes Res 1997;5:538–41.
79. von Kries R, Koletzko B, Sauerwald T, et al. Breast feeding and obesity: Cross sectional study. BMJ 1999;319:147–50.
80. Singhal A, Farooqi IS, O'Rahilly S, et al. Early nutrition and leptin concentrations in later life. Am J Clin Nutr 2002;75:993–9.
81. Hahn P. Effect of litter size on plasma cholesterol and insulin and some liver and adipose tissue enzymes in adult rodents. J Nutr 1984;114:1231–4.
82. Lewis DS, Bertrand HA, McMahan CA, et al. Influence of preweaning food intake on body composition of young adult baboons. Am J Physiol 1989;275:R1128–35.
83. Davis CM. Self selection of diet by newly weaned infants: An experimental study. Am J Dis Child 1928;36:651–79.
84. Birch LL, Johson SL, Andresen G, et al. The variability of young children's energy intake. N Engl J Med 1991;324:232–5.
85. Shea S, Stein AD, Basch CE, et al. Variability and self-regulation of energy intake in young children in their everyday environment. Pediatrics 1992;90:542–6.
86. Birch LL, Johnson SL, Jones MB, Peters JC. Effects of a nonenergy fat substitute on children's energy and macronutrient intake. Am J Clin Nutr 1993;58:326–33.
87. Stefanik PA, Heald FP, Mayer J. Caloric intake in relation to energy output of obese and non-obese adolescent boys. Am J Clin Nutr 1959;7:55–62.
88. Durnin JVGA, Lonergan ME, Good J, Ewan A. A cross-sectional nutritional and anthropometric study, with an interval of 7 years, on 611 young adolescent schoolchildren. BMJ 1974;32:169–78.
89. Morgan KJ, Zabik ME, Leveille GA. The role of breakfast in nutrient intake of 12-year-old children. Am J Clin Nutr 1981;34:1418–27.
90. Persson LA, Carlgren G. Measuring children's diets: Evaluation of dietary assessment techniques in infancy and childhood. Int J Epidemiol 1984;13:506–17.
91. Griffiths M, Rivers JPW, Payne PR. Energy intake in children at high and low risk of obesity. Hum Nutr Clin Nutr 1987;41C:425–30.
92. Epstein LH, Wing RR, Cluss P, et al. Resting metabolic rate in lean and obese children: Relationship to child and parent weight and percent-overweight change. Am J Clin Nutr 1989;49:331–6.
93. Bandini LG, Schoeller DA, Cyr HN, Dietz WH. Validity of reported energy intake in obese and nonobese adolescents. Am J Clin Nutr 1990;54:421–5.
94. Butte NF, Wong WW, Garza C, et al. Energy requirements of breast-fed infants. J Am Coll Nutr 1991;10:190–5.
95. Drake MA. Anthropometry, biochemical iron indexes, and energy and nutrient intake of preschool children: Comparison of intake at day care center and at home. J Am Diet Assoc 1991;91:1587–8.
96. Miller WC. Diet composition, energy intake, and nutritional status in relation to obesity in men and women. Med Sci Sports Exerc 1991;23:280–4.
97. Nicklas TA, Webber LS, Berenson GS. Studies of consistency of dietary intake during the first four years of life in a prospective analysis: Bogalusa Heart Study. J Am Coll Nutr 1991;10:234–41.
98. Pelto GH, Urgello J, Allen LH, et al. Household size, food intake and anthropometric status of school-age children in a highland Mexican area. Soc Sci Med 1991;33:1135–40.
99. Stein AD, Shea S, Basch CE, et al. Variability and tracking of nutrient intakes of preschool children based on multiple administrations of the 24-hour dietary recall. Am J Epidemiol 1991;134:1427–37.
100. Albertson AM, Tobalmann RC, Engstrom A, Asp EH. Nutrient intake of 2- to 10-year-old American children: 10-year trends. J Am Diet Assoc 1992;92:1492–5.
101. Livingstone MBE, Prentice AM, Coward WA, et al. Validation of estimates of energy intake by weighed dietary record and diet history in children and adolescents. Am J Clin Nutr 1992;56:29–35.
102. Rasanen L, Ylonen K. Food consumption and nutrient intake of one- to two-year-old Finnish children. Acta Paediatr Scand 1992;81:7–11.
103. Maffeis C, Schutz Y, Zoccante L, et al. Meal-induced thermogenesis in lean and obese prepubertal children. Am J Clin Nutr 1993;57:481–5.
104. Nicklas TA, Bao W, Webber LS, Berenson GS. Breakfast consumption affects adequacy of total daily intake in children. J Am Diet Assoc 1993;93:886–91.
105. Nicklas TA, Webber LS, Srinivasan R, Berenson GS. Secular trends in dietary intakes and cardiovascular risk factors of 10-year-old children: The Bogalusa Heart Study (1973–1988). Am J Clin Nutr 1993;57:930–7.
106. Schoeller DA, Fjeld CF. What have we learned from the doubly labeled water method? Annu Rev Nutr 1991;11:355–75.
107. Marston AR, London P, Cooper LM. A note on the eating behaviour of children varying in weight. J Child Psychol Psychiatry 1976;17:221–4.
108. Drabman RS, Cordua GD, Hammer D, et al. Development trends in eating rates of normal and overweight preschool children. J Child Dev 1979;50:211–6.
109. Barkeling B, Ekman S, Rossner S. Eating behaviour in obese and normal weight 11-year-old children. Int J Obes 1992;16:355–60.
110. Fisher JO, Birch LL. Fat preferences and fat consumption of 3- to 5-year-old children are related to parental adiposity. J Am Diet Assoc 1995;95:759–64.
111. Ray JW, Klesges RC. Influences on the eating behavior of children. In: Williams CL, Kimm SYS, editors. Childhood Obesity, Volume. 699. New York: New York Academy of Sciences; 1993. p. 57–69.
112. Spitzer L, Rodin J. Human eating behavior: A critical review of studies in normal weight and overweight individuals. Appetite 1981;2:293–329.
113. Bellisle F, Rolland-Cachera M-F, Deheeger M, Guilloud-Bataille M. Obesity and food intake in children: Evidence for a role of metabolic and/or behavioral daily rhythms. Appetite 1998;11:111–8.
114. Swinburn BA, Jolley D, Kremer PJ, et al. Estimating the effects of Energy imbalance on changes in body weight in children. Am J Clin Nutr 2006;83:859–63.
115. Dauncy MJ. Metabolic effects of altering the 24 h energy intake in man, using direct and indirect calorimetry. Br J Nutr 1980;43:257–69.
116. Ravussin E, Schutz Y, Acheson KJ, et al. Short-term, mixed-diet overfeeding in man: No evidence for "luxuskonsumption." Am J Physiol Endocrinol Metab 1985;249: E470–7.
117. Forbes GF, Brown MR, Welle SL, Lipinski BA. Deliberate overfeeding in women and men: Energy cost and composition of the weight gain. Br J Nutr 1986;56:1–9.
118. Roberts SB, Young VR, Fuss P, et al. Energy expenditure and subsequent nutrient intakes in overfed young men. Am J Physiol 1990;259:R461–9.
119. Bandini LG, Schoeller DA, Edwards J, et al. Energy expenditure during carbohydrate overfeeding in obese and nonobese adolescents. Am J Physiol 1989;256:E357–67.
120. Goran MI, Kaskoun M, Johnson R. Determinants of resting energy expenditure in young children. J Pediatr 1995;126:679–80.
121. Ravussin E, Bogardus C. Relationship of genetics, age, and physical fitness to daily energy expenditure and fuel utilization. Am J Clin Nutr 1989;49:968–75.
122. Molnar D, Varga P, Rubecz I, et al. Food-induced thermogenesis in obese children. Eur J Pediatr 1985;144:27–31.
123. Maffeis C, Schutz Y, Pinelli L. Postprandial thermogenesis in obese children before and after weight reduction. Eur J Clin Nutr 1992;46:577–83.
124. Segal KR, Lacayanga I, Dunaif A, et al. Impact of body fat mass and percent fat on metabolic rate and thermogenesis in men. Am J Physiol 1989;256:E573–9.
125. Segal KR, Edano A, Tomas MB. Thermic effect of a meal over 3 and 6 hours in lean and obese men. Metabolism 1990; 39:985–92.
126. Katch VL, Moorehead CP, Becque MD, Rocchini AP. Reduced short-term thermic effect of a meal in obese adolescent girls. Eur J Appl Physiol Occup Physiol 1992;65: 535–40.
127. Klesges RC, Shelton ML, Klesges LM. Effects of television on metabolic rate: Potential implications for childhood obesity. Pediatrics 1993;91:281–6.
128. Wolf AM, Gortmaker SL, Cheung L, et al. Activity, inactivity, and obesity: Racial, ethnic, and age differences among schoolgirls. Am J Public Health 1993;83:1625–7.

129. Waxman M, Stunkard AJ. Caloric intake and expenditure of obese boys. J Pediatr 1980;96:187–93.
130. Berkowitz RI, Agras WS, Korner AF, et al. Physical activity and adiposity: A longitudinal study from birth to childhood. J Pediatr 1985;106:734–8.
131. Sunnegardh J, Bratteby L-E, Hagman U, Samuelson G. Physical activity in relation to energy intake and body fat in 8- and 13-year-old children in Sweden. Acta Paediatr Scand 1986;75:955–63.
132. Eck LH, Klesges RC, Hanson CL, Slawson D. Children at familial risk for obesity: An examination of dietary intake, physical activity and weight status. Int J Obes 1992;16:71–8.
133. Gazzaniga JM, Burns TL. Relationship between diet composition and body fatness, with adjustment for resting energy expenditure and physical activity, in preadolescent children. Am J Clin Nutr 1993;58:21–8.
134. Robinson TN. Television viewing and childhood obesity. Pediatr Clin North Am 2001;48:1–8.
135. Dietz WH, Jr, Gortmaker SL. Do we fatten our children at the television set? Obesity and television viewing in children and adolescents. Pediatrics 1985;75:807–12.
136. Coon KA, Goldberg J, Rogers BL, Tucker KL. Relationships between use of television during meals and children's food consumption. Pediatrics 2001;107:E7.
137. Robinson TN, Hammer LD, Killen JD, et al. Does television viewing increase obesity and reduce physical activity? Cross-sectional and longitudinal analyses among adolescent girls. Pediatrics 1993;91:273–80.
138. Dietz WH, Bandini LG, Morelli JA, et al. Effect of sedentary activities on resting metabolic rate. Am J Clin Nutr 1994;59:556–9.
139. Schoeller DA. Measurement of energy expenditure in freeliving humans by using doubly labeled water. J Nutr 1988;118:1278–89.
140. Roberts SB. Use of the doubly labeled water method for measurement of energy expenditure, total body water, water intake, and metabolizable energy intake in humans and small animals. Can J Physiol Pharmacol 1989;67:1190–8.
141. Roberts SB, Heyman MB, Evans WJ, et al. Dietary energy requirements of young adult men, determined by using the doubly labeled water method. Am J Clin Nutr 1991;54: 499–505.
142. Goran MI, Carpenter WH, Poehlman ET. Total energy expenditure in 4- to 6-year-old children. Am J Physiol 1993;264:E706–11.
143. Salbe AD, Weyer C, Lindsay RS, et al. Assessing Risk factors for obesity between childhood and adolescence: I. Birth weight, Childhood adiposity, parental obesity, insulin, and leptin. Pediatrics 2002;110:299–306.
144. Parker DR, Weiss ST, Troisi R, et al. Relationship of dietary saturated fatty acids and body habitus to serum insulin concentrations: The Normative Aging Study. Am J Clin Nutr 1993;58:129–36.
145. National Academy of Sciences. Dietary Reference Intakes for Macronutrients. Washington, DC: National Academy of Sciences; 2002.
146. Bandini LG, Schoeller DA, Dietz WH. Energy expenditure in obese and nonobese adolescents. Pediatr Res 1990;27:198–203.
147. Flatt JP. Importance of nutrient balance in body weight regulation. Diabetes Metab Res Rev 1988;4:571–81.
148. Flatt JP, Ravussin E, Acheson KJ, Jequier E. Effects of dietary fat on postprandial substrate oxidation and on carbohydrate and fat balances. J Clin Invest 1985;76:1019–24.
149. Abbott WGH, Howard BV, Christin L, et al. Short-term energy balance: Relationship with protein, carbohydrate, and fat balances. Am J Physiol 1988;255:E332–7.
150. Lissner L, Levitsky DA, Strupp BJ, et al. Dietary fat and the regulation of energy intake in human subjects. Am J Clin Nutr 1987;46:886–92.
151. Tremblay A, Plourde G, Despres JP, Bouchard C. Impact of dietary fat content and fat oxidation on energy intake in humans. Am J Clin Nutr 1989;49:799–805.
152. Kendall A, Levitsky DA, Strupp BJ, Lissner L. Weight loss on a low-fat diet: Consequences of the imprecision of the control of food intake in humans. Am J Clin Nutr 1991;53:1124–9.
153. Sheppard L, Kristal AR, Kushi LH. Weight loss in women participating in a randomized trial of low-fat diets. Am J Clin Nutr 1991;54:821–8.
154. Foltin RW, Fischman MW, Moran TH, et al. Caloric compensation for lunches varying in fat and carbohydrate content by humans in a residential laboratory. Am J Clin Nutr 1990;52:969–80.
155. DeGraaf C, Hulshof T, Weststrate J, Jas P. Short-term effects of different amounts of protein, fat and carbohydrate on satiety. Am J Clin Nutr 1992;55:33–8.
156. Foltin RW, Rolls BJ, Moran TH, et al. Caloric, but not macronutrient, compensation by humans for required-eating occasions with meals and snacks varying in fat and carbohydrate. Am J Clin Nutr 1992;55:331–42.
157. Storlien LH, James DE, Burleigh KM, et al. Fat feeding causes widespread in vivo insulin resistance, decreased energy expenditure, and obesity in rats. Am J Physiol 1986;251:E576–83.
158. Prewitt TE, Schmeisser D, Bowen PE, et al. Changes in body weight, body composition, and energy intake in women fed high and low fat diets. Am J Clin Nutr 1991;54:304–10.
159. Castro DE. Macronutrient relationships with meal patterns and mood in the spontaneous feeding behavior of humans. Physiol Behav 1987;39:561–9.
160. Dreon ME, Frey-Hewitt B, Ellsworth N, et al. Dietary fat: Carbohydrate ratio and obesity in middle aged men. Am J Clin Nutr 1988;47:995–1000.
161. Romieu I, Willet WC, Stampfer MJ. Energy intake and other determinants of relative weight. Am J Clin Nutr 1988;47:406–12.
162. Miller WC, Lindeman AK, Wallace J, Niederpruem M. Diet composition, energy intake and exercise in relation to body fat in men and women. Am J Clin Nutr 1990;52:426–30.
163. Tucker LA, Kano MJ. Dietary fat and body fat: A multivariate study of 205 adult females. Am J Clin Nutr 1992;56: 616–22.
164. Sunehag AL, Toffolo G, Treuth MS, et al. Effects of dietary macronutrient content on glucose metabolism in children. J Clin Endocrinol Metab 2002;87:5168–78.
165. Treuth MS, Sunehag AL, Trautwein LM, et al. Metabolic adaptation to high-fat and high-carbohydrate diets in children and adolescents. Am J Clin Nutr 2003;77:479–89.
166. Maffeis C, Schutz Y, Grezzani A, et al. Meal-induced thermogenesis and obesity: Is a fat meal a risk factor for fat gain in children? J Clin Endocrinol Metab 2001;86:214–9.
167. Sun M, Schutz Y, Maffeis C. Substrate metabolism, nutrient balance and obesity development in children and adolescents: A target for intervention? Obes Rev 2004;5:183–8.
168. Piers LS, Walker KZ, Stoney RM, et al. The influence of the type of dietary fat on postprandial fat oxidation rates: Monosaturated (olive oil) vs saturated fat (cream). Int J Obes Relat Metab Disord 2002;26:814–21.
169. DeLany JP, Windhauser MM, Champagne CM, Bray GA. Differential oxidation of individual dietary fatty acids in humans. Am J Clin Nutr 2000;72:905–11.
170. DeLany JP, Bray GA, Harsha DW, Volaufova J. Energy expenditure in African American and white boys and girls in a 2-year follow-up of the Baton Rouge Children's Study. Am J Clin Nutr 2004;79:268–73.
171. Treuth MS, Butte NF, Sorkin JD. Predictors of body fat gain in nonobese girls with a familial predisposition to obesity. Am J Clin Nutr 2003;78:1212–8.
172. Griffiths M, Payne PR. Energy expenditure in small children of obese and non-obese parents. Nature 1976;260:698–700.
173. Roberts SB, Savage J, Coward WA, et al. Energy expenditure and energy intake in infants born to lean and overweight mothers. N Engl J Med 1988;318:461–6.
174. Goran MI, Carpenter WH, McGloin A, et al. Energy expenditure in children of lean and obese parents. Am J Physiol 1995;268:E917–24.
175. Goran MI, Kaskoun M, Johnson R. Determinants of resting energy expenditure in young children. Pediatrics 1994;125:362–7.
176. Davies PS, Wells JC, Fieldhouse C, et al. Parental body composition and infant energy expenditure. Am J Clin Nutr 1995;61:1026–9.
177. Treuth MS, Butte NF, Wong W. Effects of familial predisposition to obesity on energy expenditure in multiethnic prepubertal girls. Am J Clin Nutr 2000;71:893–900.
178. DeLany JP. Role of energy expenditure in the development of pediatric obesity. Am J Clin Nutr 1998;68:950S–5S.

Evaluation and Management of Obesity

Alison G. Hoppin, MD

INTRODUCTION

At the beginning of the twenty-first century, poverty and under-nutrition have worsened in some countries, while over-nutrition and obesity have reached epidemic levels in many others.[1,2] Currently, obesity is the most important nutritional problem globally, and the associated medical problems account for substantial morbidity, mortality, and healthcare costs in developed countries. In developing countries undergoing rapid changes in economic and technological development, the population is exposed to rapid changes in diet and energy balance; this "nutrition transition" presents unique health challenges.[3,4] Understanding the mechanisms causing obesity and associated medical problems will be essential to reverse the global trend toward obesity and its threats to public health.

DEFINITION

Any definition of obesity is useful only if it predicts medical disability or complications. Since most medical complications of obesity are associated with excess body fat and not muscle mass, measures of obesity represent an attempt to estimate the adipose compartment. At present, there is no precise clinically practical method to measure body fat, so most metrics rely on measurements of body weight as a surrogate for adiposity. Such approaches are imperfect, as they may misclassify a patient with an unusual proportion of fat to lean body mass, but they are inexpensive and practical for use in the clinical setting and in epidemiological studies.

Current definitions of overweight and obesity rely on calculations of the body mass index (BMI), defined as the weight in kilograms divided by the height in meters squared (kg/m^2). Although BMI does not directly measure body fat, it has been established as a useful predictor of adiposity in adults, adolescents, and children. Like other estimates of adiposity, BMI also predicts risks for present or future medical complications of obesity.[5] BMI in children is not only correlated with other predictors of body fat but also with blood pressure,[6,7] lipid levels[8,9] and insulin levels.[10]

In adults, standard ranges of BMI can be used to define risk categories for obesity. However, during childhood and adolescence, BMI varies with age and gender. Therefore, BMI percentiles are used to define risk categories for children and adolescents, and BMI growth charts or standard deviation scores are used to track an individual against established standards for clinical purposes.

In 2000, the Center for Disease Control (CDC) established new growth charts using data from five large surveys representing the U.S. population.[11] These growth charts do not include data from the previous decade because of the sharp rise in BMI during that period. These growth charts are similar but not identical to those developed by the International Obesity Task Force (IOTF).[12] For the IOTF charts, data were drawn from six different countries, and the curves were smoothed to meet the adult cutoff points for overweight and obesity at 18 years of age. Both reference standards are strong predictors of obesity and coronary heart disease risk factors in adulthood.[13] In April 2006, the World Health Organization released new growth curves for exclusively breastfed infants and young children. The WHO BMI curves cover a wider age range (from infancy through age 5 years), and provide different norms for children than the 2000 CDC standards.[14] See Chapter 2, "Clinical Assessment of Nutritional Status," for further discussion of the derivation and applicability of these WHO standards.

The nomenclature applied to BMI risk categories also varies. The CDC and American Academy of Pediatrics use the term "at risk for overweight" for BMI above the 85th percentile but below the 95th percentile, and "overweight" for BMI above the 95th percentile. In contrast, the Institute of Medicine and the IOTF use the term "overweight" for BMI between the 85th and 95th percentiles, and "obesity" for BMI above the 95th percentile. The latter categories correspond more closely to the terms used BMI categories in adults (see Table 1). For the following discussion, the term "obesity" is used to refer to BMI above the 95th percentile.

BMI also depends on pubertal stage, reflecting disproportionate gains in fat-free as compared to fat mass.[15] In addition, there is some evidence that BMI varies with ethnicity.[16] Therefore, research studies that aim for the most precise estimates of obesity risk using BMI should consider not only age and gender, but also pubertal stage and ethnicity. However, for clinical purposes, the CDC or IOTF reference standards are adequate for determining obesity-related risk groups.

EPIDEMIOLOGY

Relevance and Significance

Presently 16% of children and adolescents in the United States are overweight, and 17% of children and adolescents in the United States have obesity (above the 85th and 95th percentiles for age and gender, respectively).[17] Since the 1960s, the prevalence of obesity in US children and adolescents has tripled. Similar but more gradual trends are seen worldwide. Determining the specific causes of this rapid increase in rates of obesity is clearly essential, yet remarkably complex. Both genetic and environmental factors have been shown to contribute significantly to this problem. In general, genetic factors explain a large part of the variation of body weight within a given population in a common

Table 1 Nomenclature for BMI Ranges

Term	Adults	Children and Adolescents (CDC and AAP)	Children and Adolescents (IOM and IOTF)
Underweight	<18.5	<5th percentile	<5th percentile
Healthy weight	18.5–24.9	5th to 85th percentile	5th to 85th percentile
At risk for overweight		85th to 95th percentile	
Overweight	25–29.9	≥95th percentile	85th to 95th percentile
Obesity	≥30		≥95th percentile
Class I obesity	30–34.9		
Class II obesity	35–39.9		
Class III obesity	≥40		

AAP = American Academy of Pediatrics; CDC = Centers for Disease Control; IOM = Institute of Medicine; IOTF = International Obesity Task Force.

environment, while environmental factors tend to explain changes in obesity over time in that population.

The study of Pima Indians provides an important example of the interaction between environmental and genetic factors.[18] The Pima Indians who live in the southwestern United States are strongly predisposed to obesity and diabetes, and these traits assort in patterns indicating genetic inheritance. The genetically similar Pima living as subsistence farmers in Mexico have substantially lower rates of obesity and diabetes. Genetic factors clearly explain a large part of the obesity among Pima Indians in this country, while environmental factors likely explain the dramatic difference in rates of obesity between the two Pima populations.

Epidemiologists have used cohort studies and case-control designs to determine which environmental factors may contribute to obesity. Such studies have pointed to dietary trends, sedentary lifestyle, decreases in structured physical activity, psychosocial stressors, and cultural trends as likely contributors to the obesity epidemic.[3] A number of dietary factors have been proposed to play important roles. These include the easy availability, high caloric content and effective marketing techniques of the fast food industry, and general trends toward consumption of foods that are highly processed, contain high carbohydrates and/or total calories (including sugary beverages), with decreased consumption of fiber and low–density foods. Other factors include decreases in structured physical activity, particularly for children, as well as decreasing lifestyle activity (occupations and transportation require less movement than in the past), and increasing sedentary activities (particularly television viewing and computer use). However, it is important to note that to date *no single factor* among these has been shown to play a pivotal role in the increasing prevalence of obesity.

Tracking

"Tracking" describes the risk for a disease state persisting over time. In the case of obesity, there is a moderate risk of childhood obesity persisting into adulthood, and that risk increases if the child remains overweight as he or she grows older (Figure 1). As an example, in one population with a high frequency of obesity, there was substantial tracking within weight categories from late childhood (age 9 to 11) to young adulthood (19 to 35 years).[19] Tracking varied by gender and ethnicity: 73% of European–American women tracked within their weight category, while 49% of European–American men tracked. Among African–American participants, 60% of both men and women remained in the same weight category between childhood and adulthood.

A child's risk for having obesity in adulthood also depends on the weight status of his parents. A toddler without obese parents has an 8% risk of developing obesity by adulthood; a 10- to 14-year-old child with at least one obese parent has a 79% risk

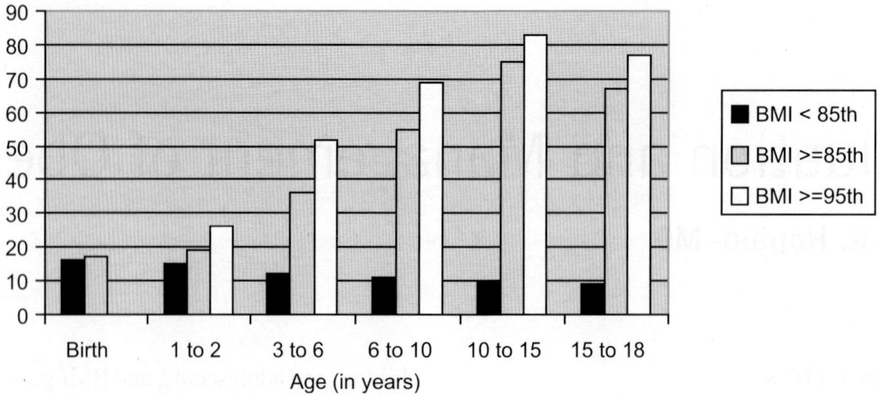

Figure 1 Proportion of children (%) who will become obese adults, as predicted by childhood weight status. (Adapted from reference 20.)

of developing obesity by adulthood.[20] Before three years of age, the primary predictor of obesity in adulthood was the parents' obesity status, and the child's obesity status was not an important indicator of the risk of adult obesity. By contrast, after seven years of age, the child's own obesity status became the more important predictor of his risk for obesity in adulthood.

Obesity in childhood thus confers a higher risk of obesity in adulthood. Moreover, adults who were obese in childhood have a greater risk of morbidity and mortality, independent of their BMI in adulthood, family history of cardiovascular diseases or cancer, and smoking.[21–23] In the Harvard Growth study, overweight adolescents were shown to have an increased risk for developing obesity-related medical problems in adulthood, including cardiovascular disease and diabetes, as compared to adults with more recent onset of obesity.[21] Likewise, Sinaiko and colleagues showed that weight gain during childhood and adolescence predicts cardiovascular risk in young adults.[24]

Heritable Factors

Studies of twins and adoptees provide useful estimates of the role of heritable factors in determining an individual's body weight.[25] Adoption studies tend to generate the lowest heritability estimates (30%), whereas twin studies provide highest heritability estimates (70%). The variability in these estimates of heritability depends in part on definitions of obesity: more severe obesity tends to have a greater heritability factor than lesser variations in BMI.[26]

Observations of a genetic contribution to obesity gave rise to the "thrifty genotype hypothesis,"[27] which posits that genes predisposing to energy conservation were preserved as a survival characteristic in former times of famine, but become a liability in environments with plentiful food and low required physical activity. Possible mechanisms through which genetic polymorphisms can translate to differences in body weight regulation are discussed below.

Fetal Programming

Several decades ago, David Barker and colleagues showed that poor fetal growth, resulting in low birthweight, is associated with an increased risk for type 2 diabetes and other elements of the metabolic syndrome. They proposed that poor nutrition during gestation imprints permanent changes in glucose and insulin metabolism.[28] Interestingly, many more recent studies have also shown clear associations between *high* birthweight and several components of the metabolic syndrome,[29,30] suggesting that newborns at both ends of the weight spectrum are at risk for obesity–associated disease. This concept of "fetal programming" has now been supported by numerous studies in other human populations and in animals.[31]

The fetal programming hypothesis has been extended to include the possibility that postgestational influences can participate to create a lifelong metabolic phenotype.[32] For example, a study of adults in Finland showed that the development of type 2 diabetes mellitus was associated with the combination of low birthweight followed by accelerated gain in height and weight during childhood and with high maternal BMI.[33] Similarly, a study of adults in England showed that accelerated weight gain in early childhood added to the effect of low birthweight on risk of high blood pressure in adulthood.[34] Indeed, populations in transition from conditions of low- to high-nutrition may be at the greatest risk for such obesity-related complications because of the combination of fetal undernutrition and childhood overnutrition.[35]

A few studies strongly support the idea that the intrauterine environment affects obesity risk independently from genetic factors, thus distinguishing the concept of a "thrifty *phenotype*" from that of the "thrifty *genotype*." In a study of the effects of wartime famine in the Netherlands, infants exposed to famine in utero had higher rates of obesity and diabetes in adulthood as compared to a genetically similar cohort not exposed to famine, and this effect was largely independent of birthweight.[36] Furthermore, the timing of the famine exposure during gestation appeared to have important effects, as fetuses exposed to famine during the first trimester of gestation were more severely affected than those exposed later in gestation. These observations are supported by animal studies, which also demonstrate lasting effects of intrauterine and postpartum nutrition.[37] A recent study showed that children of mothers who had undergone gastric bypass surgery prior to pregnancy have reduced risk of obesity as compared to the offspring of mothers who had not undergone the surgery.[38] The mechanism underlying the observed associations, including the contributions of maternal hyperglycemia, insulinemia, and postnatal growth to the development of later complications, is an important subject for future studies. See Chapter 27, "Fetal, Infant and Childhood Growth, and Disease in Later Life," for further discussion of the influence of the prenatal environment on obesity and other nutritional diseases.

BIOLOGY

Regulation of Body Weight

Mature animals and adult humans have a strong tendency to maintain a stable body weight over time, due to a close but sometimes imperfect matching of energy intake with energy expenditure. Animal studies in which energy intake is manipulated reveal powerful homeostatic mechanisms defending body weight. Similarly, the poor long-term results of weight reduction therapies in humans (about 95% of adults regain all weight after dieting), suggest there are mechanisms that defend a highly individualized "set point" for body weight. When an individual has a heritable or acquired susceptibility to positive energy balance, superimposed on these native homeostatic mechanisms, he or she has a tendency to become obese.

Animal models of obesity have been invaluable in establishing an understanding of the complex mechanisms regulating body weight. Our growing understanding of these pathways is likely to lead to better-targeted interventions, both pharmacologic and behavioral. This is an area of vigorous ongoing research; the major elements of the pathways as we currently understand them are outlined below.

Afferent Pathways. Circulating *insulin*, which reflects recent nutrient intake and metabolic demands, is an important regulator of nutrient partitioning in peripheral tissues and also communicates to centers regulating appetite in the brain. Peptides (such as *cholecystokinin*, *peptide YY*, and *glucagon-like peptide 1*) secreted by the gastrointestinal tract in response to intraluminal nutrients, and plasma concentrations of the macronutrients themselves also provide independent signals to the central nervous system affecting short–term appetite and satiety.[39]

Ghrelin is a peptide secreted by the stomach that is an important short–term mediator of appetite. Its name is derived from its ability to stimulate growth hormone release from the pituitary, but it also stimulates appetite through specific receptors in the ventromedial hypothalamus.[40] Ghrelin is released from the stomach during periods of fasting, and is suppressed by nutrient administration.[41] The specific stimulants of ghrelin release are not clear, but volumetric stretching of the stomach wall has no effect. Several reports show that ghrelin is suppressed in humans who lose weight after gastric bypass surgery, but not in the setting of weight loss through caloric restriction.[41,42] These findings suggest that ghrelin may be the mechanism for the appetite–suppressing effect and high success rates of gastric weight loss surgery.

Leptin is an important regulator of body fat, first identified in 1994 through studies of the leptin-deficient obese mouse.[43] It is produced primarily in adipose tissue, and provides feedback to specific receptors in the ventromedial hypothalamus, an important center for regulation of appetite and energy expenditure. The leptin signal decreases appetite, increases both voluntary and resting energy expenditure, permits fertility,[44] and even activates central "reward" pathways that may in turn affect appetitive behavior.[45] The leptin-deficient animal or human therefore has hyperphagia, and decreased thermo-genesis and physical activity, all of which are reversible by leptin administration.

The central mechanisms through which leptin exerts these diverse effects have been partly elucidated through studies in other animal models. Animals with defects in the leptin receptor (the *diabetes* mouse and Zucker rat) predictably have phenotypes indistinguishable from leptin deficiency itself.

Central Nervous System. The leptin signal activates a network of regulatory neuropeptides in the central nervous system, and particularly in the arcuate nucleus of the hypothalamus. The anatomy of this network is the subject of ongoing research, but many important elements have been described. Some of the pathways are orexigenic (favoring energy intake), others anorexigenic (inhibiting energy intake). In general, leptin-generated signals tend to inhibit the orexigenic pathways, and to stimulate the anorexigenic pathways, thus decreasing appetite. The network also participates in leptin's effects on the reproductive system and energy expenditure (Figure 2).

The **melanocortin** pathway is among the most important links downstream of leptin. Leptin appears to directly increase expression of proopiomelanocortin (POMC), which is cleaved by prohormone convertase (PC) to alpha-melanocyte stimulating hormone (α-MSH),[46] as well as β-endorphin. Alpha-MSH in turn stimulates the melanocortin-4 receptor (MC4-R),[47] a potent inhibitory influence on the lateral hypothalamus. Meanwhile, leptin also directly inhibits the expression agouti-related protein (AgRP), which opposes α-MSH action at the melanocortin receptors.[47] The melanocortin pathway appears to be a particularly important regulator of body weight homeostasis because it exhibits less redundancy than other leptin-related pathways; an interruption in the melanocortin pathway can produce severe obesity, as seen in the Agouti mouse.

Leptin also decreases appetite through melanocortin-independent pathways. It inhibits the expression of the orexigenic agent neuropeptide Y (NPY) while increasing expression of cocaine and amphetamine-related transcript (CART). In addition to decreasing appetite, CART has actions on the paraventricular nucleus (PVN) of the hypothalamus and spinal sympathetic preganglionic neurons, where it affects energy expenditure via the autonomic nervous system[46] (Figure 2).

Efferent Pathways. This leptin-responsive network of neuropeptides in the hypothalamus acts on effector pathways in the cerebral cortex, pituitary–adrenal axis, and autonomic nervous system. Most signals regulating appetite and

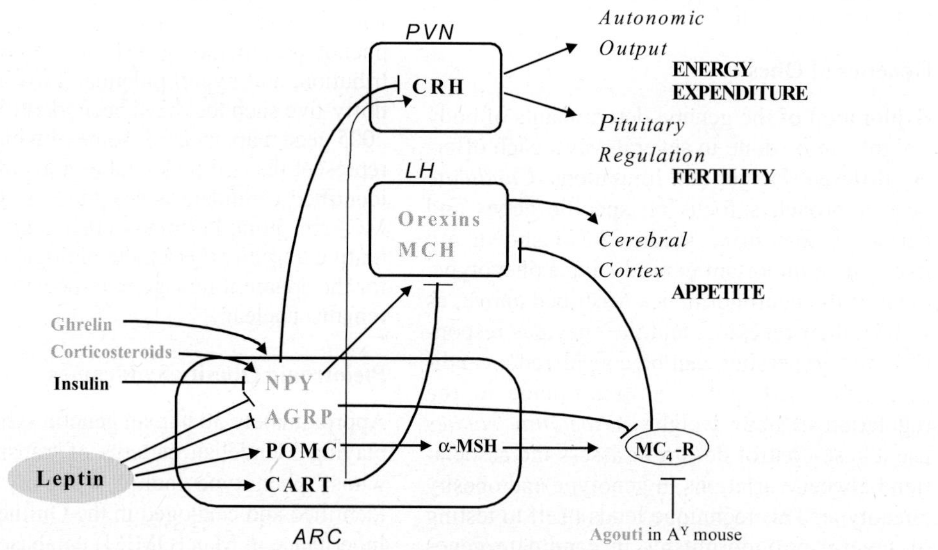

Figure 2 Central nervous system pathways regulating appetite and energy metabolism. Leptin positively regulates proopiomelanocortin (POMC) while negatively regulating agouti-related protein (AGRP)-releasing neurons in the arcuate nucleus (ARC) of the hypothalamus. POMC is a precursor of α-melanocyte-stimulating hormone (α-MSH) which is an antagonist at the MC_4 receptor (MC_4-R). AGRP and agouti protein are antagonists at MC_4-R. The MC_4-R pathway negatively regulates appetite, perhaps acting through appetite-stimulating neuropeptides in the lateral hypothalamus (LH), including melanin-concentrating hormone (MCH) and the orexins. Meanwhile, leptin has some actions that are independent of the POMC pathway, including negatively regulating neuropeptide Y (NPY), itself a potent appetite stimulant. Ghrelin also appears to act to stimulate appetite through the NPY pathway. NPY also influences autonomic and pituitary output through the paraventricular nuclues (PVN), acting in part through corticotropin-releasing hormone (CRH).

satiety meet in the nucleus tractus solitarius in the medulla, where they are further modulated by afferent signals from the autonomic nervous system. The pituitary–adrenal axis mediates leptin's effects on fertility, and likely also affects energy expenditure. Indeed, adrenalectomy prevents the development of obesity in most animal models.[48]

Efferent signals to regulate energy expenditure are integrated in the locus ceruleus, from which the sympathetic nervous system stimulates lipolysis in white adipose tissue, and mediates processes that facilitate voluntary energy expenditure and heat generation. Genetically engineered animal models have clarified some elements of these effector pathways. Animals in which uncoupling protein-1 (UCP-1) in brown adipose tissue is knocked out have increased body fat, decreased cold tolerance, and decreased thermogenic response to food,[49] but the related peptides UCP-2 and -3 which are more widely expressed are more likely to be relevant to human adiposity.[50] A knockout of the β-3 adrenergic receptor has a similar phenotype, suggesting that elements of the sympathetic nervous system are involved in increasing energy expenditure to match energy intake.[51] Parasympathetic efferent signals through the vagus nerve increase insulin secretion in the pancreatic β-cells, and may be a mechanism for the hyperinsulinemia in some groups of obese people.[52]

In addition to these autonomic processes, energy expenditure has a "voluntary" component (5 to 50% of total energy expenditure, depending on the level of exercise),[53] and a component of "fidgeting," or nonexercise activity thermogenesis (NEAT). NEAT has been proposed as a genetically determined system of protection from obesity, and may also be mediated by the sympathetic nervous system.[54]

Genetics of Obesity

Exploration of the genetic determinants of body weight can be done in several ways, each offering different insight and limitations. *Candidate gene* approaches focus on specific genes and pathways that prior studies have shown are likely to be important in producing a phenotype. Each of the neurohormones described above, as well as their receptors and the enzymes responsible for processing, can be considered a candidate gene with potential importance in the regulation of body weight. *Association studies* use a case-control design to assess the association between variations in genotype and obesity phenotype. This technique lends itself to testing of several polymorphisms in candidate genes within a population, however it is also prone to substantial false-positive and false-negative results, depending on sample size. The results of such studies therefore are most compelling if similar gene associations can be demonstrated in several different populations. *Linkage studies* rely on genome-wide scans of large populations to assess the strength of the association between variations in a genomic locus and the phenotype. This technique does not rely on a priori assumptions about the biologic significance of a particular gene, and is therefore important in identifying new areas for inquiry. However, it also has relatively low sensitivity and can easily overlook linkages that are common contributors to less extreme phenotypes (eg, common genes predisposing to moderate degrees of obesity). A complete list of published linkages to obesity phenotypes is summarized yearly.[55]

Candidate Genes. Any of the genes encoding a component of the mechanism for regulating body weight homeostasis, including those mentioned above, could be considered a "candidate gene" for a predisposition or resistance to obesity. Specific mutations in a few of these genes have been shown to cause obesity in rare kindreds. Mutations with strong effects were found in the genes encoding leptin, the leptin receptor, POMC, Proprotein Convertase (PCSK1), SIM-1, melanocortin 3 receptor (MC3R) and melanocortin 4 receptor (MC4R). The latter is the most common gene in which specific mutations cause obesity, accounting for up to 6% of severe early-onset obesity, but it is still very rare, approximately 1 in 2,000 humans overall.[63]

Association Studies. Association studies have analyzed many other candidate genes from the afferent and efferent pathways mentioned above in genetically similar populations (siblings, twins, or kindreds). By 2005, polymorphisms linked to 127 candidate genes had been shown to have some association with obesity phenotypes,[55] including ghrelin,[64] peroxisome proliferation-activated receptor gamma,[65] uncoupling proteins,[66] and the β-3 adrenoreceptor genes.[67]

Linkage Studies. Linkage studies in large populations have identified many chromosomal loci with associations to a variety of obesity-related phenotypes, including BMI, leptin levels, fat distribution, and hyperlipidemia. Two hundred and thirty-five such loci have been identified as of the 2005 gene map update,[55] some of which appear to represent the chromosomal regions of previously identified candidate genes such as the leptin or MC_4 receptors. For many other regions or quantitative trait loci (QTL), the biologic mechanisms for the apparent linkage with obesity phenotypes remains unclear.

Pleiotropic Obesity Syndromes

Approximately 30 human genetic syndromes displaying Mendelian patterns of transmission and whose phenotype includes obesity have been identified and cataloged in the Online Mendelian Inheritance in Man (OMIM) database.[68] Many of these syndromes have been mapped to one or more chromosomal locations.

The most common syndrome with severe obesity is *Prader–Willi* syndrome (infantile hypotonia, hyperphagia, hypogonadotropic hypogonadism, cognitive deficits), mapped to 15q 11–13, a region containing several candidate genes for which a mechanistic explanation for the Prader–Willi phenotype is being sought.[55,63] The syndrome occurs in approximately 1 in 25,000 live births. Because the defect almost always arises sporadically, recurrence within a family is extremely rare. Interestingly, individuals with Prader–Willi syndrome also have elevated levels of ghrelin, providing a potential mechanism for their marked hyperphagia.

The *Bardet–Biedl* syndrome requires a mutation at one of eight loci[63,69] and includes polydactyly and retinopathy. It is rare, occurring in fewer than 1 in 100,000 live births. Molecular studies suggest that the syndrome may be caused by loss of function of ciliated hypothalamic neurons. *Alstrom* syndrome (obesity, hyperinsulinemia, retinopathy and deafness, with or without cognitive defects),[70] and *Cohen* syndrome (hypotonia, retinopathy, and cognitive deficits)[71] have been mapped to one location each, and candidate genes have been identified but the mechanism through which mutations in these genes causes obesity is still unknown.[63] Each of these syndromes have characteristic findings as outlined in Table 2 and in the OMIM database,[68] and can usually be distinguished from common obesity by a thorough medical history and physical examination (Table 2).

EVALUATION

Medical Assessment

The initial step for the assessment of the overweight child is to exclude potential associated syndromes or endocrinopathies, and to diagnose possible associated complications. Several syndromes associated with obesity should be considered, including the Mendelian syndromes mentioned above. Obesity may also accompany the more common, easily recognizable syndromes of Trisomy 21, Fragile X, and Turner. In most cases these syndromes can be distinguished on the basis of their unique features (listed in Table 2 and detailed in some excellent reviews)[63,72–74] and specific laboratory testing is valuable for confirmation, but not for screening. For Prader–Willi syndrome, a cognitive deficit and history of hypotonia are particularly strong predictors of the syndrome. The presence of these characteristics is useful indication for performing genetic testing, which is highly sensitive and specific for the syndrome.[75]

The pathophysiology of medical conditions related to overweight (Table 3) is discussed in Chapter 40, "Complications of Obesity: Metabolic Syndrome," but the laboratory assessment of these conditions is discussed below.[76] The value of screening for obesity-related medical problems has been debated,[77] but can be useful to establish whether there is dyslipidemia, steatohepatitis, or evidence of glucose intolerance, particularly as specific treatments for some of these disorders are increasingly considered.[78,79] Blood testing should be done in a fasting state if practical. Thyroid stimulating hormone, total cholesterol, very low-density lipoprotein, low-density lipoprotein, high-density lipoprotein,

Table 2 Characteristics of the Major Syndromes Associated with Obesity

Syndrome	Cognitive Deficit	Obesity	Features
Albright[74]	Mild	Variable (general) Early onset	Neuroendocrine anomalies Normal or short Skin hyperpigmentation/vitiligo Polydactily Bone fibrous dysplasia Precocious puberty
Alstrom[70]	None	Moderate (central) Onset age 2–5 yr	Retinitis pigmentosa Deafness Neuroendocrine anomalies Normal or short stature Normal or hypogonadism
Bardet-Biedl[63]	Moderate	Moderate (central) Onset age 1–2 yr	Normal or short stature Hypotonia Compulsive behavior Retinitis Heart anomalies Polydactyly Renal dysfunction Hypogonadism
Carpenter[188]	Mild	Central	Acrocephaly Polydactyly Syndactyly Short stature Flat nasal bridge High arched palate Heart anomalies Hypogonadism
Cohen[71,72]	Mild	Variable (central) Mid childhood	Short or tall stature Hypotonia Microcephaly Retinochoroidal dystrophy Short philtrum Low hairline Heart anomalies Normal or hypogonadism
POMC mutation[58] (autosomal dominant)	None	Early onset	Red hair ACTH deficiency hyperphagia
Prader-Willi[75]	Mild to moderate	Moderate to severe (generalized) Onset 1–3 yr	Hypotonia Almond-shaped eyes V-shaped mouth Neuroendocrine anomalies Short stature Compulsive behavior High arched palate Hypogonadism

aspartate aminotransferase and alanine aminotransferase have been recommended to screen for possible hypothyroidism, dyslipidemia, and steatohepatitis, respectively.

Fasting or random glucose levels are used to screen for diabetes mellitus or impaired fasting glucose (Table 4).[80] However, these tests lack both sensitivity and specificity for diagnosing type 2 diabetes or impaired glucose tolerance in children, so oral glucose tolerance testing should be used when possible in high-risk individuals.[81,82] Insulin levels will provide information on carbohydrate metabolism and insulin resistance and may predict a risk for diabetes. Specific guidelines to screen for type 2 diabetes in overweight children have been developed (Table 5), but are also controversial, because of the large number of adolescents fitting the screening criteria (currently about 2.5 million in the United States) and the relatively low yield of the suggested screening tests.[83]

Table 4 Definitions for Impaired Fasting Glucose, Impaired Glucose Tolerance, and Diabetes Mellitus

	Impaired Fasting Glucose	Impaired Glucose Tolerance	Diabetes Mellitus
Fasting glucose	100–125 mg/dL (5.6–6.9 mmol/L)		≥126 mg/dL (7.0 mmol/L)
Blood glucose 2 h after load	<140 mg/dL	140–199 mg/dL (7.8–11.0 mmol/L)	≥200 mg/dl (11.1 mmol/L)
Random glucose			≥ 200 mg/dl (11.1 mmol/L) and symptoms

Adapted from reference 80.

Table 3 Diseases Associated with Obesity in Children

Endocrine
- Type 2 Diabetes
- Impaired glucose tolerance
- Polycystic Ovaries

Gastrointestinal
- Gallstones
- Fatty liver disease (nonalcoholic steatohepatitis)
- Gastroesophageal reflux disease
- Constipation and encopresis

Orthopedic
- Slipped capital femoral epiphysis
- Blount's disease

Respiratory
- Sleep apnea
- Asthma

Further laboratory testing may be useful in selected cases but can be expensive and some tests are not readily available. Sleep studies can and should be performed if there are clinical symptoms of sleep apnea, including consistent snoring. Radiographic evaluation is necessary when slipped capital femoral epiphysis or Blount disease is suspected. Indirect calorimetry can be used to predict the energy deficit necessary for weight loss.[84] This might be useful when poor compliance or abnormally low energy requirements are suspected and at times may be useful to provide concrete caloric goals to support dietary changes. Bone age may be helpful in supporting the diagnosis of an endocrinopathy. Consultations with specialists in sleep disorders, neurology, otorhinolaryngology, pulmonology/allergy, endocrinology, genetics, ophthalmology, and surgery may be necessary to manage specific complications.

The medical history should include assessment of concomitant medical diseases for their potential to contribute to weight gain (such as a history of significant head trauma or hypothalamic dysfunction) and to identify barriers to treatment (factors limiting mobility or ability to be physically active). A variety of drugs used for the treatment of psychiatric disease, epilepsy, diabetes, and migraines are associated with weight gain. The atypical antipsychotic drugs[85,86] and mood stabilizers[87–89] are particularly likely to promote weight gain. However, the weight-promoting effects of other commonly used classes of drugs, including tricyclic antidepressants,[88,90] selective serotonin reuptake inhibitors,[91] anticonvulsants,[92] and antidiabetic agents[93,94] are less widely recognized. Identifying these as a likely trigger of weight gain may prompt consideration

Table 5 ADA Guidelines for the Assessment of Type 2 Diabetes in Children with Overweight or Obesity

Children and adolescents should undergo specific testing for diabetes if they are:

Overweight, as defined by:

1. BMI >85th percentile for age and sex, or
2. Weight for height >85th percentile, or
3. Weight >120% of ideal (50th percentile for height), and

And have at least two of the following risk factors:

1. Have a family history of type 2 diabetes in first- and second-degree relatives
2. Belong to one of the following specific race/ethnic groups
   –American Indians
   –African-Americans
   –Hispanic Americans
   –Asians/South Pacific Islanders
3. Have one or more of the following signs of insulin resistance or conditions associated with insulin resistance
   –Acanthosis nigricans
   –Hypertension
   –Dyslipidemia
   –Polycystic ovary syndrome (PCOS)

Testing should consist of either:

1. fasting plasma glucose (8th fast), or
2. Oral glucose tolerance test (blood glucose level 2 h post challenge)

Further study is called for to determine the predictive value of HgbA1C and fasting insulin levels in determining risks for type 2 diabetes in children.

Adapted from reference 189.

of alternate drugs (Table 6). There is limited empiric information about the weight-related effects of many psychoactive drugs, and the long-term effects are particularly unclear. Most of these drugs should be considered potential contributors to weight gain even if they are said to be "relatively" weight neutral.

Nutritional Assessment

Nutritional evaluation should include, at a minimum, anthropometric measurements, and a history of the onset of obesity, as well as of weight loss attempts. Periods of adiposity rebound and potential triggers for excess weight gain should be identified. Family history of obesity and related medical problems should be evaluated to help establish the genetic factors underlying the weight disorder, and the potential future medical risks.

Assessing dietary intake by recalled food frequency helps to identify diet composition, but in most cases does not provide a good estimate of energy intake, as underreporting of food intake by obese subjects is well described.[95] Estimating the proportion of each macronutrient and fiber in the diet may help identify targets for dietary change, if the diet is particularly skewed toward fat or energy-dense foods. In addition, the diet recall may be useful to assess the diet for deficiencies in micronutrients, particularly calcium and vitamins A, D and E, beta carotene, folic acid, and other B vitamins; excessive energy intake does not always mean adequate intake of micronutrients.

To identify possible areas for intervention, the amount and type of dairy products, fruits, vegetables, and legumes should be assessed, with particular attention to the consumption of sugary beverages including juices and soda. Excessive consumption of sugary beverages has been associated with excess weight gain and increased rate of obesity,[96] and is an important early target for dietary change. Similarly, the frequency of use of fast-food restaurants and of other restaurant meals should be examined, as these meals often contain excessive caloric content and set appropriate portion standards. The diet history should also explore usual meal patterns, with attention to whether there is regular skipping of meals, binge pattern of eating, and the social context of meals, particularly if there are routine family dinners. Each of these factors may become a target for intervention to establish regular meal-based eating patterns.

Finally, the potential role of exercise and sedentary behaviors should be evaluated, with particular attention to determining the frequency of television and computer use. Several studies have suggested specific causal effects of television viewing on obesity,[97] and the American Academy of Pediatrics recommends limiting television viewing to one to two hours per day.[98] Assessment and encouragement of lifestyle exercise, in the form of outdoor play or regular walking (eg, walking to school) is as important as assessing structured exercise (eg, participation in sports programs).

Behavioral Assessment

The psychosocial complications of obesity are often subjective and difficult to measure in a standard fashion, but undoubtedly represent one of the greatest burdens of obesity in children and adolescents. In many cases, psychosocial issues are best understood as consequences of the disease, brought on by feelings of discouragement and criticism by family, peers, or self. In other instances the psychological issues precede or exacerbate the obesity.[99] Regardless of the causality, it is important to acknowledge and assess these behavioral and psychological issues in each individual to best target treatment.

Depressive symptoms,[100,101] anxiety,[102,103] binge-eating disorder,[104,105] decreased self-esteem,[106] and problems with social interactions[107,108] have generally been found more frequently in obese children and adolescents than in their lean peers. Negative psychosocial associations also persist into early adulthood, when obesity is associated with lower educational attainment and household income and lower rates of marriage, independent of baseline education and aptitude.[109,110] Many of these problems can be attributed to the widespread and culturally entrenched bias against obese individuals in our society.[110,111]

Optimal assessment of the psychosocial issues contributing to and stemming from obesity in a particular patient has not been established, and varies greatly between centers and providers. Whether or not standardized instruments are used, some effort should be made to assess mood,

Table 6 Selected Drugs Associated with Weight Gain

Drugs with Weight Gain Potential	Alternatives with Less Potential for Weight Gain
Atypical antipsychotics[85, 86]	
• Clozapine ++++ (gain 4–12 kg)	• Quetiapine
• Olanzapine ++++	• Ziprasidone
• Risperidone ++	
Mood Stablizers[87–89]	
• Divalproex sodium +++	• Lamotrigine (weight neutral)
• Lithium +++ (10 kg over 6–10 yr)	• Adjunctive topiramate (6% of weight lost at 1 yr)
Tricyclic Antidepressants[88]	
• Amitriptyline ++	• Desipramine
• Impramine ++	• Nortriptylene
MAO inhibitors[190]	
• Phenelzine > isocarboxazide	• Tranylcypromine
SSRIs[91]	
• Paroxetine ++ (3.6% gain at 6 mos; 25% of patients gained more than 7% of body weight)	• Fluoxetine
• Sertraline +	
Atypical antidepressants[191]	
	• Buproprion (weight loss)
Anticonvulsants[92]	
• Valproate +++ (10–60% of patients gain weight average gain 8–20 kg)[192]	• Zonisamide
• Carbamazepine ++ (15 kg/3 mos)	• Topiramate (weight loss)
• Gabapentin ++ (23% gained >10% of weight)	
Antidiabetic agents	
• Insulin +++ (avg 4 kg over 10 yr)[93]	• Metformin (2–3 kg weight loss over 6 mo)[94]
• Thiazolidinediones ++ (2–5 kg gain)[94]	

Table 7 Stages of Change

1. Precontemplation
   - Unaware of, denies, or minimizes the problem
   - Needs: encouragement to reevaluate current behavior; encouragement of self-exploration, NOT action. Provide information, personalizing the risks
2. Contemplation
   - Aware of the problem, ambivalent about change
   - Needs: gentle confrontation, information and rationale for change, clarification of any misinformation
3. Preparation
   - Has decided to make change, plans to do so within the next month, or is gathering information
   - Needs: assistance in identifying and overcoming obstacles; assistance to identify social supports, encouragement to take small initial steps
4. Action
   - Plan is in progress, attitudinal and behavioral changes have begun
   - Needs: tools and techniques to implement goals, positive reinforcement; support to deal with obstacles and losses, focusing on long-term benefits
5. Maintenance/relapse
   - Action maintained over six months (maintenance) or return to old habits (relapse)
   - Needs: self-monitoring tools for successful maintenance, feedback and encouragement; stress management, use of support systems

Adapted from reference 194.

motivation, school and social performance, self-image, and eating attitudes and behaviors. It is also important to assess these issues in parents or close caretakers of the patient, as factors such as motivation, mood disorders, and eating disorders in a parent will have substantial impact on the child's attitudes, behaviors, and ability to respond to treatment.[108] The family's financial resources and level of cognitive stimulation in the household also predict the development of obesity,[112] and may also affect the family's ability to respond to treatment. A "stages of change" model may be helpful in establishing the readiness of the patient and family for making lifestyle changes (Table 7). If the patient or family is in an early stage of change (precontemplation or contemplation), efforts should be focused on helping them forward into the next stage, perhaps using motivational interviewing techniques.

TREATMENT

Nutritional Therapy

Long-term studies of nutrition and exercise interventions for *prevention* of pediatric obesity are sparse and generally inconclusive. However, studies with short and moderate lengths of follow-up have shown benefits from a variety of "lifestyle" interventions, including nutritional education (in 3- to 9-year-old school children),[113,114] exercise, and measures to decrease sedentary activity.[115,116] All of these interventions have some effects in specific settings, although similar interventions in different settings failed to show an effect.[117–120] These studies are the subject of several recent reviews.[121–123] Most such studies target a school-based population and do not include the family in the intervention. The interpretation of such studies is hampered by high attrition rates, lack of standardization in definitions of obesity and treatment techniques, and limited generalizability. Long-term observational studies aiming to identify specific risk factors for the development of obesity are planned.[124] Such studies will be valuable to identify the most important targets for intervention.

There is better information available about *treatment* interventions for preadolescents and adolescents with established obesity, but the majority of studies still do not provide long-term data, and many issues such as optimal macronutrient composition of diets and strategies to change food preference have not been adequately studied. A few studies have suggested that structured exercise increases weight loss as compared to diet alone,[125,126] and treatments focusing on increasing lifestyle exercise and reducing sedentary behaviors have also shown beneficial effects.[127,128] In general, regimens that combine hypocaloric diets with exercise and behavior modification have been particularly effective.[126,129] One study showed a medically significant long-term effect after an 8-month family-based behavioral intervention for families with children 6 to 11 years old. The improvement persisted 10 years after the intervention was completed.[130] The design of this study supports the conclusion that the behavioral intervention was a critical component of the success.

Typically, dietary recommendations for adults and children with obesity have consisted of reduction in dietary fat and energy intake as a balanced, hypocaloric diet. Recommendations have been developed by the American Academy of Nutrition as summarized in the *Pediatric Nutrition* handbook[131] and are similar to those supported by other governmental agencies, as described in a recent review.[132] The goal of the intervention is to reach a healthy weight without affecting linear growth. Specific recommendations include limiting beverages and foods with high caloric density and low nutritional value, including sugary beverages, full-fat or low-fat baked goods and candies, and encouraging whole grains, fruits and vegetables. Simple behavioral measures such as meal planning and label reading during grocery shopping are also generally encouraged to support the implementations of these nutritional guidelines.

The "traffic-light diet" provides a structured, balanced, hypocaloric diet in a simple format, and has been used effectively for preadolescent[126,130] and preschool children.[133] It uses a simple color-coding scheme to categorize foods into categories for free consumption (low-density foods; "green"), moderate consumption (moderate-density and protein-containing foods; "yellow") and very limited consumption (foods with high caloric density, and/or with high sugar or fat content; "red"). The prescribed caloric content of the diet is generally between 900 and 1,300 kcal/d.

The Protein-Sparing Modified Fast diet (PSMF) provides high-quality lean protein while strictly limiting total calories. It has been used to treat severe obesity in a variety of settings including hospitalized patients and school-based interventions. This diet has been effectively used in settings where short-term weight loss is medically necessary, but there is no data to suggest that it reliably improves obesity in the long term. The principles of this diet are described in Table 8 and have been reviewed elsewhere, with sample menus.[134,135] Typically patients start with a hypocaloric diet for two weeks before the PSMF diet is started (1,200 kcal/d); the PSMF diet continues for about 12 weeks (600 to 800 kcal/d) and is followed by a maintenance diet (balanced, 1,200 kcal/d). Of note, one report documented an 11.2 kg weight loss after 10 weeks of a PSMF diet, substantially more than that achieved by less restrictive measures, but by 15 months follow-up the weight loss achieved by the two groups was similar.[136] Potential complications of the diet include protein losses, hypokalemia, inadequate calcium intake, cholelithiasis, and intravascular volume depletion with orthostatic hypotension.

While the caloric content of a diet has been shown to relate to treatment success at one year,[137] to date there is little evidence to suggest that alterations in *specific macronutrients* yield long-term weight reduction. A variety of popular diets have arisen around alterations of specific macronutrients, with or without limitations on total caloric intake. Many of these show good short-term weight loss, but whether these diets achieve long-term effects on obesity is unclear as no adequate long-term studies (with five or more years of follow-up) of these diets in representative adult or pediatric populations have been published. These popular diets are reviewed in Chapter 41, "Popular Diets for Obesity." Several dietary approaches have focused on limiting carbohydrates, and in general this approach has modest efficacy, which is similar to that achieved with low-fat diets at one year.[138] The most

Table 8 A Protein-Sparing Modified Fast Diet

1. High-protein, hypocaloric diet for 12 wk
   - 600–800 kcal
   - Protein 2 g/kg/d (max 100 g/d; approximately 50% of calories)13–20 oz/d lean meat or substitute
   - Fat approximately 30–40% of calories
   - Carbohydrate 10–20% calories
     As low-starch vegetables, may include one fruit
   - Ad libitum: tea, bouillion, pickles, spices, mustard
   - 2 L of water per day
   - Supplements:
     multivitamin with minerals
     elemental calcium supplement to meet RDI
     monitor serum potassium and supplement as needed
2. Maintenance diet (36 wk)
   - Balanced macronutrients
   - 1200 kcal/day

Adapted from reference 134.

rigorously studied such diet emphasizes foods with a low glycemic index to reduce insulin release and excursions of blood sugar. A few studies have shown short-term decreases in weight, appetite, and some cardiovascular disease risk factors during a hypocaloric low-glycemic-index diet as compared with a hypocaloric low-fat diet in young adults.[139,140] However, other studies have not shown beneficial effects of targeting low-glycemic-index foods,[141,142] and none have examined long-term outcomes of this type of diet. One intriguing study examined the effects of reducing the glycemic index during pregnancy; there was no difference in maternal weight gain during pregnancy, but infants born to the mothers on the low-glycemic-index diet were less likely to be large for gestational age.[143] Because high birthweight has some association with later risk for obesity, this study raises the theoretical possibility that intervention with a low-glycemic diet during pregnancy could have beneficial effects on the obesity risk of the offspring.

The results of studies that focus on adult populations should be interpreted with caution, since there is compelling evidence that at least some "lifestyle" approaches to obesity are more effective in children than they are in adults.[144] Some dietary approaches might prove to have long-term results in children even if none can be demonstrated for adults.

As rates of obesity rise, obese children represent an increasing proportion of hospital inpatients.[145] Whether or not the child is hospitalized for an obesity-related condition such as gallstones, diabetes, sleep apnea, or orthopedic problems, their nutritional needs must be considered. It is particularly important to recognize that the obesity is a chronic problem, and will not resolve by attempting weight loss acutely during the inpatient stay. Moreover, acute severe caloric restriction is inappropriate and can lead to metabolic problems including refeeding syndrome, even in children with adequate or excessive energy stores. Guidelines for nutritional care of the obese adult inpatients have been developed,[146] but this issue has not been well examined in children. It may be appropriate to prescribe a modest reduction in caloric intake, guided by indirect calorimetry or by calculations based on adjusted body weights, and using a stress factor that is appropriate to the child's condition. The inpatient stay may also present a valuable opportunity for nutritional education, and for engaging the patient and family in a therapeutic plan to address the obesity beyond the hospital stay.

Behavior Therapy

As discussed above, some interventions in childhood have demonstrated long-term improvement of obesity with 5[147] or 10 years[130] follow-up, thus children appear to have a more consistent and durable response to therapy than adults in the same family,[144] or adult populations in general. The importance of including behavior therapy in the treatment of obesity in children has been demonstrated, at least in a family-based setting.[148] Although many interventions use combinations of dietary, exercise, and behavioral interventions, it is notable that the few studies with long-term results have had a rigorous and structured behavioral component.[129]

Commonly used techniques include self-monitoring of food intake and weight, modeling, positive reinforcement (praise), contingency management (certain behaviors are paired with predictable, reinforcing responses), and stimulus control (learning to avoid situations that are cues to overeat). Some studies have tested specific elements of these behavioral techniques. These have shown superiority of family-based over patient-focused treatment,[130] of positive reinforcement over restrictive or critical approaches,[128] and of frequent (daily) over less frequent (weekly) positive reinforcement.[149] The value of problem-solving techniques has not consistently been shown.[150,151] Thus, there is ample evidence to support the use of behavioral modification techniques in the treatment and possibly the prevention of obesity in children. Behavior therapy should be thought of as a tool to achieve long-term changes in diet and exercise. By contrast, there is little data to support the use of behavior "micromanaging" techniques such as rate of eating and bite size.

Weight Loss Drugs

Many of the drugs used for the treatment of obesity in adults in the past are characterized by unproven claims, highly variable efficacy, or dangerous side effects. Nonetheless, the incomplete but growing understanding of the mechanisms underlying the homeostatic control of body weight and the increased rigor applied to clinical drug trials hold promise for the development and use of pharmacologic agents to treat this chronic disease. In the short term, drugs can be important for a patient whose medical condition requires acute weight loss. Drugs may also have a role in treating the chronic component of obesity. Modification of the environmental and societal pressures contributing to obesity should be thought of as an important ultimate goal, but the use of drugs to promote weight loss may keep an individual patient engaged in the "lifestyle" component of treatment, and might even change some of the consumer pressures that contribute to our obesity-promoting environment. Thus, pharmacotherapy for obesity is not at odds with lifestyle-changing approaches. As increasingly specific drugs are developed, efficacy and safety improve, and pharmacotherapy may ultimately be an essential tool to treat an otherwise refractory and devastating disease. Whether pharmacologic treatment is cost-effective depends in large part on whether it prevents the medical complications of obesity and associated costs of medical care.

Current options for the pharmacologic treatment of obesity are limited but may have some clinical utility. In general the drugs demonstrate only modest efficacy, but minimal side effects. Sibutramine (Meridia®) and orlistat (Xenical®) are the two drugs approved by the US Food and Drug Administration (FDA) for treating obesity in adults for periods of up to one year. Both demonstrate only modest efficacy, but also have few side effects. Weight regain typically occurs upon discontinuation of the medication. Concurrent efforts to reduce energy intake and increase exercise are important. Long-term studies (up to five years) of these drugs in adults are in progress. Based on current literature, the modest weight loss achieved by the use of current available drugs in conjunction with reduced calorie diets is not adequate to treat individuals with severe life-threatening complications of obesity, but the drugs may be considered to boost weight loss, assist weight loss maintenance, and to reinforce lifestyle change. Whether phenotypic or genotypic analysis can be used to select for patients who respond relatively well to these agents is an important subject for future study.

Sibutramine is an appetite suppressant that has been the subject of extensive clinical trials, and was approved by the FDA for use in adults with obesity in conjunction with a dietary regimen. It is an inhibitor of both norepinephrine and serotonin, and also weakly inhibits dopamine reuptake. At doses of 10 or 15 mg/d, combined with a reduced calorie diet, modest weight loss is achieved in most patients (loss of 5 to 8% of baseline weight as compared to 1 to 4% of weight on placebo)[152–154] but the range of weight loss varies greatly. Weight loss is sustained for most patients as long as the drug is continued (up to three years observation periods reported),[155] but generally is regained after the drug is discontinued. Side effects include modest increases in blood pressure (2 mm Hg on average) and heart rate, dry mouth, constipation, and insomnia. Most side effects are transient and lead to discontinuation of the drug in about 5% of patients. Importantly, no evidence of valvular heart disease such as that associated with fenfluramine treatment has been found in rigorous studies. Metabolic abnormalities associated with obesity, including hyperlipidemia and insulin resistance, tend to improve commensurate with weight loss.

The safety and effectiveness of sibutramine in adolescents and children have not been established. However, a large multicenter randomized placebo-controlled trial of sibutramine in adolescents with concurrent behavioral therapy demonstrated significantly more weight loss than placebo (8.4 kg more than placebo), as well as reductions in triglyceride levels and insulin levels, and improvements in insulin sensitivity. Adverse effects were similar to those seen in adults and included modest increases in tachycardia (2.5 bpm more than placebo).[156]

Orlistat acts by inhibiting gastrointestinal lipases, reducing fat digestion and absorption by about 30%. Predictably, its side effects are related to fat malabsorption, consisting of steatorrhea when high-fat meals are taken, and decreases in serum levels of fat-soluble vitamins, primarily vitamin D.[157] Daily administration of a multivitamin is therefore recommended. Modest weight loss (3.2% more than placebo)[157] is generally achieved, and sustained use partially prevents weight regain during a second year of treatment.[158]

Metformin improves insulin sensitivity and also promotes modest weight loss in adults.[159] By contrast to other antihyperglycemic agents, metformin does not increase insulin secretion, but decreases hepatic glucose production and improves insulin sensitivity in both diabetic and nondiabetic adults.[160] Small open-label trials of metformin have suggested that it may be useful in ameliorating psychotropic drug-induced weight gain in children.[161,162] Two small randomized trials of metformin in adolescents with hyperinsulinemia showed improved glucose tolerance, and a modest decrease in BMI.[163,164] Larger trials of metformin in adolescents are in progress. Careful review of these results will be necessary before pharmacotherapy outside of clinical trials can be recommended in adolescents or children.

Phentermine, diethylproprion, phendimetrazine, and benzphetamine are noradrenergic agents with appetite-suppressant effects but are studied and approved for short-term use only in adults (generally 12 weeks or less)[152] The latter two drugs are considered to have some potential for abuse and are listed on schedule III of the Drug Enforcement Agency. The use of any agent with only short-term goals for weight loss in children and adolescents, and particularly one with any potential for abuse, is highly questionable.

Dietary "supplements" or herbal medicines are popular, and consumers spend more than 1 billion dollars on these products annually in the United States.[165] However they are unregulated and relatively untested. The commonly used herbal supplements are listed in Table 9. Supplements that could be used with caution in adults include conjugated linoleic acid,[166] ginseng, chromium,[167,168] hydroxycitric acid, DHEA, hydroxymethylbutyrate, chitosan,[169] and St. John's Wort, but there is little or evidence for effectiveness for these drugs.[170] Substances that have questionable safety and should be discouraged include Ephedra (or Ma Huang), horsetail, herbal laxatives, and some forms of some forms of caffeine and fiber.[171,172] All products containing ephedra were banned from the US market in 2004 because of evidence of significant adverse health outcomes, including heart attack and stroke.[173] To the best of our knowledge, there are no well-designed studies of dietary supplements and weight loss in children, and no supplements for weight loss can be recommended or even considered with caution. These supplements are subject to minimal regulation in the United States. Individuals desiring acute weight loss, including adolescents and athletes, often use these supplements, and are also at risk for unhealthy dieting techniques. In contrast to gradual weight loss, acute weight loss is almost always unhealthy and should only be targeted when medically necessary and closely supervised by a physician and dietitian.

Weight Loss Surgery

During the past 15 years, surgically induced weight loss has emerged as an important option for adults with severe obesity. In contrast to poor long–term success rates for nonsurgical treatments of obesity, surgical approaches generally produce durable and substantial weight loss. Over 80% of patients lose at least half of their excess body weight during the first year. Weight generally stabilizes 12 to 24 months after surgery, and 10 to 20% of patients regain a significant portion of the lost weight. If a patient maintains weight loss for five years, there is an excellent likelihood that the weight loss will persist for at least 14 years.[174] Studies have shown improvement or resolution of many of the medical complications of obesity, including diabetes mellitus, hypercholesterolemia, and obstructive sleep apnea.[175]

The jejunoileal bypass was an early surgical procedure for weight loss and caused global malabsorption, and is no longer performed. It caused frequent and unacceptable side effects including intractable diarrhea, nutrient deficiencies, kidney stones, and hepatic failure. The two most common operations performed today are the Roux-en-Y gastric bypass (RYGB) and vertical banded gastroplasty (VBG) (Figure 3), both of which reduce gastric capacity in order to restrict caloric intake. In contrast to the jejunoileal bypass, these operations do not cause significant malabsorption, and their safety profile is substantially better. The mechanism through which these operations cause weight loss is not fully understood, although recent studies suggest that it may suppress gastric production of ghrelin, thereby reducing appetite.[176] About 10% of patients have important complications of these procedures, which include anastomotic strictures, incisional hernias, and gallstone formation requiring cholecystectomy. Anastomotic leaks, staple-line disruptions, and dumping syndrome can occur but have been reduced to 1 to 2% each by modifications in surgical technique.[177,178] While protein–calorie malabsorption is rare, malabsorption of selected micronutrients, particularly iron and vitamin B_{12}, are common and require postoperative monitoring and treatment.[179] One report suggested that individuals undergoing weight loss surgery may develop thiamine deficiency and symptomatic beriberi,[180] and adolescents may be particularly at risk for this complication.[181]

Table 9 Dietary Supplements for Weight Loss

Dietary supplement	Other names	Mechanism	Effectiveness	Safety
Ephedra alkaloids	Ma Huang Norepinephrine	Thermogenic	Yes, only in combination with caffeine	Unsafe (hypertension, palpitation, tachycardia, stroke, seizures, death)
Caffeine	Guarana (*Paullinia cupana*) Yerba Maté (*Ilex paraguayansis*)	Thermogenic	No, when used alone	High doses or combina tions may be unsafe (hypertenstion, tachycardia, nausea, dizziness)
Chromium	Chromium picolinate	↑ insulin sensitivity	Uncertain	Uncertain
Ginseng	Korean ginseng (*Panax ginseng*) American ginseng (*Panax quinquefolux*) Siberian ginseng (*Eleutherococcus senticosus*)	↑ insulin sensitivity Thermogenic ↑ lipolysis	Uncertain	Uncertain May interfere with anticoagulant effect of warfarin
Fiber	Guar gum Psyllium Flaxseed Glucomannan	Malabsorption ↑ insulin sensitivity	Unlikely	Generally safe, but some forms may have risk of GI obstruction
Hydroxycitric Acid	Malabar tamarind (*Garcinia cambogia*)	↓ denovo fatty acid synthesis	Unlikely	Uncertain
Dehydro-epiandrosterone (DHEA)	Adrenal steroid hormone	↓ fat synthesis	Uncertain	Uncertain Metabolites may stimulate breast and prostate tissue
Chitosan	Chitin (crustacean shells)	Blocks dietary fat absorption	Uncertain	Uncertain
Horsetail	*Equisetum* sp.	Diuretic	Uncertain	Unsafe (may be K+-wasting)
Senna Cascara	*Cassia* sp. *Rhamnus pushiana*	Laxatives	Uncertain	Unsafe for treatment of obesity
St. John's Wort	"Herbal phen-fen" *Hypericum perforatum*	Antidepressant	Unlikely	Uncertain Phototoxicity; drug interactions with many psychoactive drugs

Adapted from references 165 and 170 to 172.

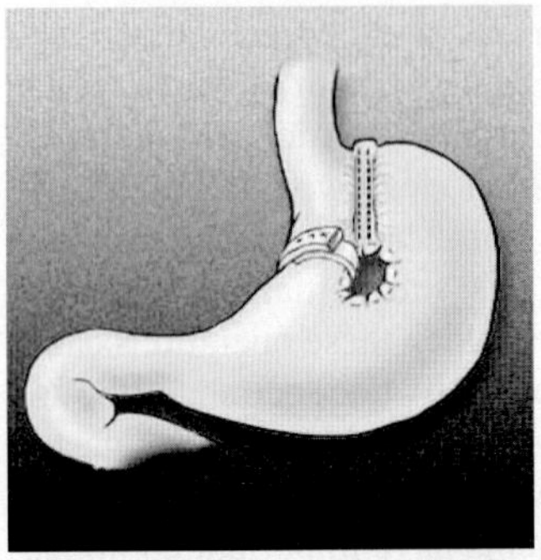

Vertical Banded Gastroplasty (VBG)

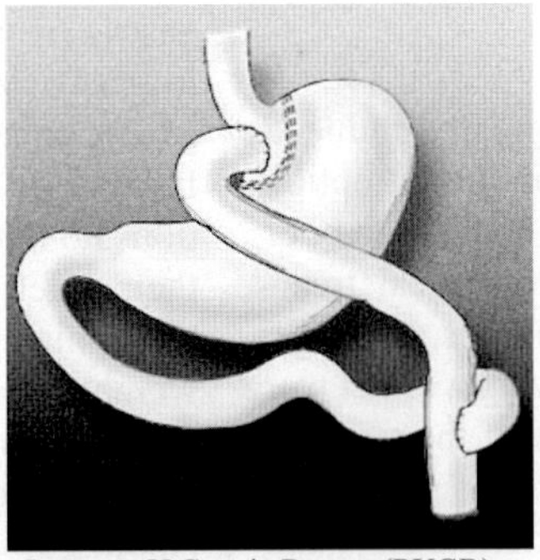

Roux-en-Y Gastric Bypass (RYGB)

Figure 3 Gastric restrictive surgery for weight loss.

Adjustable laparascopic gastric banding is a surgical weight loss procedure in which a restrictive band is placed around the fundus of the stomach to restrict nutrient flow. The band is adjusted periodically to optimize weight loss while minimizing side effects, which include vomiting and dysphagia. As compared to the gastric bypass, adjustable gastric banding may be somewhat less effective and may be more dependent on patient compliance with diet and follow-up. Data on complication rates are also limited, but short-term complication rates may be somewhat less than those of the gastric bypass procedure. Because the stomach and proximal small intestine are not bypassed, micronutrient deficiencies are probably less common than in gastric bypass. A few reports present optimistic short-term outcomes with efficacy approaching that of gastric bypass and low complication rates.[182] However, other groups report substantially higher complication rates,[183] and overall there is still very limited data on long-term outcomes, including potential complications and performance in younger age groups.

Gastric restrictive procedures for weight loss are thus an appropriate treatment option for adults with medically significant obesity, but there is still significant uncertainty regarding optimal patient selection. To date, no psychological or physiological factors have been defined that will determine which patients are most likely to suffer weight regain after surgery (approximately 20% of patients regain most or all of their lost weight), or to suffer medical or psychological complications of surgery. Similarly, there is limited data on the outcomes of weight loss surgery in adolescent patients, but a few series have been published,[178,184–186] and these suggest that short- and long-term outcomes and complications in adolescents are probably similar to those seen in adults.

Weight loss surgery may therefore be appropriate in selected severely obese adolescents. Given the limited data available on outcomes in this age group, these procedures should be limited to patients who have exhausted other management approaches, and have significant medical complications of their obesity. To optimize long-term outcomes, any concomitant psychiatric disorders should be carefully assessed and under good control before surgery, and measures should be taken to ensure long-term follow-up for medical, surgical, and nutritional issues, ideally in the setting of a multidisciplinary obesity treatment center with substantial experience in surgical treatment of obesity. Guidelines for patient selection, choice of surgical technique, and pre- and postoperative management have been developed,[187] but these recommendations will evolve rapidly as more data become available. The indications for weight loss surgery in adolescents as outlined in these guidelines are more conservative than those in adults (Table 10). In addition, there are many more subjective judgments that contribute to responsible decision making, including whether the patient has legitimately exhausted less invasive approaches to weight loss, and their history of and likelihood of reliably returning for medical follow-up postoperatively.

Future Directions

With the exception of surgery, current treatments for established obesity have disappointing long-term outcomes. However, research is likely to lead to advances in several important arenas. Perhaps most importantly, public recognition of the obesity problem should lead to public education and public programs designed to *prevent* obesity during childhood. Such population-wide approaches are more likely to be effective than treatment approaches targeting individual patients with resource-intensive and weakly effective therapies. However, the identification of which preventative strategies will be most effective is important before they can be implemented widely. Second, improved understanding of the genetic determinants and neural pathways underling the homeostatic control of body weight is likely to lead to pharmacologic interventions that are more specific, and therefore safer and more effective. Third, rigorously scientific and detailed analysis of specific environmental factors contributing to obesity, including issues of diet composition and meal patterns, may lead to more focused dietary and behavioral interventions to *treat* obesity. Finally, education of the public and healthcare community to recognize and reverse the commonly held bias against obese individuals should help to minimize the stigma and therefore much of the psychological burden associated with the disease.

Table 10 Indications for Weight Loss Surgery in Adolescents

- BMI > 40 with substantial comorbidities (eg, sleep apnea or diabetes)
- BMI > 50 with more minor comorbidities
- Failed more than six months of "organized" weight loss attempts
- Skeletal maturity

Adapted from reference 187.

USEFUL WEB SITES

Nutrition and Exercise

Body and Mind, an informational and motivational Web site designed by the Centers for Disease Control for children 9 to 13 years old: http://www.bam.gov/

Healthy eating and physical activity across the lifespan: helping your child. (In English and Spanish): http://win.niddk.nih.gov/publications/child.htm

Anthropometric Measurements

New growth charts (2000): www.cdc.gov/growthcharts

Nutritional Supplements and Alternative Therapies

NIH: http://nccam.nih.gov/
USDA: http://www.nal.usda.gov/fnic/pubs/bibs/gen/dietsupp.html
Peer-reviewed journal that analyzes the claims of alternative medicine:http://www.quackwatch.com/04ConsumerEducation/sram.html

Genetics

The Human Obesity Gene Map: http://obesity-gene.pbrc.edu/
Online Mendelian Inheritance in Man (OMIM): http://www.ncbi.nlm.nih.gov/entrez/query.fcgi?db=OMIM

REFERENCES

1. Strauss RS, Pollack HA. Epidemic increase in childhood overweight, 1986–1998. JAMA 2001;286:2845–8.
2. Wang Y, Monteiro C, Popkin BM. Trends of obesity and underweight in older children and adolescents in the United States, Brazil, China, and Russia. Am J Clin Nutr 2002;75:971–7.
3. McLellan F. Obesity rising to alarming levels around the world. Lancet 2002;359:1412.
4. Popkin BM. The nutrition transition in low–income countries: An emerging crisis. Nutr Rev 1994;52:285–98.
5. Dietz WH, Robinson TN. Use of the body mass index (BMI) as a measure of overweight in children and adolescents. J Pediatr 1998;132:191–3.
6. Lauer RM, Clarke WR, Mahoney LT, Witt J. Childhood predictors for high adult blood pressure. The Muscatine Study. Pediatr Clin North Am 1993;40:23–40.
7. Gutin B, Basch C, Shea S, et al. Blood pressure, fitness, and fatness in 5- and 6-year-old children. JAMA 1990;264:1123–7.
8. Laskarzewski P, Morrison JA, Mellies MJ, et al. Relationships of measurements of body mass to plasma lipoproteins in schoolchildren and adults. Am J Epidemiol 1980;111:395–406.
9. Zwiauer K, Widhalm K, Kerbl B. Relationship between body fat distribution and blood lipids in obese adolescents. Int J Obes 1990;14:271–7.

10. Ronnemaa T, Knip M, Lautala P, et al. Serum insulin and other cardiovascular risk indicators in children, adolescents and young adults. Ann Med 1991;23:67–72.
11. Kuczmarski RJ, Ogden CL, Guo SS, et al. 2000 CDC Growth Charts for the United States: Methods and development. Vital Health Stat 2002;11:1–190.
12. Cole TJ, Bellizzi MC, Flegal KM, Dietz WH. Establishing a standard definition for child overweight and obesity worldwide: International survey. BMJ 2000;320:1240–3.
13. Janssen I, Katzmarzyk PT, Srinivasan SR, et al. Utility of childhood BMI in the prediction of adulthood disease: Comparison of national and international references. Obes Res 2005;13:1106–15.
14. de Onis M, Garza C, Onyango AW, Borghi E. Comparison of the WHO child growth standards and the CDC 2000 growth charts. J Nutr 2007;137:144–8.
15. Horlick M. Body mass index in childhood—measuring a moving target. J Clin Endocrinol Metab 2001;86:4059–60.
16. Rosner B, Prineas R, Loggie J, Daniels SR. Percentiles for body mass index in U.S. children 5 to 17 years of age. J Pediatr 1998;132:211–22.
17. Ogden CL, Carroll MD, Curtin LR, et al. Prevalence of overweight and obesity in the United States, 1999–2004. JAMA 2006;295:1549–55.
18. Ravussin E, Valencia ME, Esparza J, et al. Effects of a traditional lifestyle on obesity in Pima Indians. Diabetes Care 1994;17:1067–74.
19. Deshmukh-Taskar P, Nicklas TA, Morales M, et al. Tracking of overweight status from childhood to young adulthood: The Bogalusa Heart Study. Eur J Clin Nutr 2006;60:48–57.
20. Whitaker RC, Wright JA, Pepe MS, et al. Predicting obesity in young adulthood from childhood and parental obesity. N Engl J Med 1997;337:869–73.
21. Must A, Jacques PF, Dallal GE, et al. Long–term morbidity and mortality of overweight adolescents. A follow–up of the Harvard Growth Study of 1922 to 1935. N Engl J Med 1992;327:1350–5.
22. Vanhala M, Vanhala P, Kumpusalo E, et al. Relation between obesity from childhood to adulthood and the metabolic syndrome: Population based study. BMJ 1998;317:319.
23. van Dam RM, Willett WC, Manson JE, Hu FB. The relationship between overweight in adolescence and premature death in women. Ann Intern Med 2006;145:91–7.
24. Sinaiko AR, Donahue RP, Jacobs DR, Jr, Prineas RJ. Relation of weight and rate of increase in weight during childhood and adolescence to body size, blood pressure, fasting insulin, and lipids in young adults. The Minneapolis Children's Blood Pressure Study. Circulation 1999;99:1471–6.
25. Loos RJ, Bouchard C. Obesity—is it a genetic disorder? J Intern Med 2003;254:401–25.
26. Katzmarzyk PT, Perusse L, Rao DC, Bouchard C. Familial risk of obesity and central adipose tissue distribution in the general Canadian population. Am J Epidemiol 1999;149:933–42.
27. Neel JV. Diabetes mellitus: A "thrifty" genotype rendered detrimental by "progress"? Am J Hum Genet 1962;14:353–62.
28. Hales CN, Barker DJ. Type 2 (non-insulin-dependent) diabetes mellitus: the thrifty phenotype hypothesis. Diabetologia 1992;35:595–601.
29. Huang RC, Burke V, Newnham JP, et al. Perinatal and childhood origins of cardiovascular disease. Int J Obes (Lond) 2007;31:236–44.
30. Parsons TJ, Power C, Manor O. Fetal and early life growth and body mass index from birth to early adulthood in 1958 British cohort: Longitudinal study. BMJ 2001;323:1331–5.
31. Oken E, Gillman MW. Fetal origins of obesity. Obes Res 2003;11:496–506.
32. Hales CN, Barker DJ. The thrifty phenotype hypothesis. Br Med Bull 2001;60:5–20.
33. Eriksson JG, Forsen T, Tuomilehto J, et al. Effects of size at birth and childhood growth on the insulin resistance syndrome in elderly individuals. Diabetologia 2002;45:342–8.
34. Law CM, Shiell AW, Newsome CA, et al. Fetal, infant, and childhood growth and adult blood pressure: A longitudinal study from birth to 22 years of age. Circulation 2002;105:1088–92.
35. Dowse GK, Zimmet PZ, Finch CF, Collins VR. Decline in incidence of epidemic glucose intolerance in Nauruans: Implications for the "thrifty genotype." Am J Epidemiol 1991;133:1093–104.
36. Ravelli AC, van der Meulen JH, Michels RP, et al. Glucose tolerance in adults after prenatal exposure to famine. Lancet 1998;351:173–7.
37. Waterland RA, Garza C. Potential mechanisms of metabolic imprinting that lead to chronic disease. Am J Clin Nutr 1999;69:179–97.
38. Kral JG, Biron S, Simard S, et al. Large maternal weight loss from obesity surgery prevents transmission of obesity to children who were followed for 2 to 18 years. Pediatrics 2006;118:e1644–9.
39. Bray GA. Afferent signals regulating food intake. Proc Nutr Soc 2000;59:373–84.
40. Wang L, Saint–Pierre DH, Tache Y. Peripheral ghrelin selectively increases Fos expression in neuropeptide Y-synthesizing neurons in mouse hypothalamic arcuate nucleus. Neurosci Lett 2002;325:47–51.
41. Cummings DE, Purnell JQ, Frayo RS, et al. A preprandial rise in plasma ghrelin levels suggests a role in meal initiation in humans. Diabetes 2001;50:1714–9.
42. Korner J, Inabnet W, Conwell IM, et al. Differential effects of gastric bypass and banding on circulating gut hormone and leptin levels. Obesity (Silver Spring) 2006;14:1553–61.
43. Zhang Y, Proenca R, Maffei M, et al. Positional cloning of the mouse obese gene and its human homologue. Nature 1994;372:425–32.
44. Ahima RS, Dushay J, Flier SN, et al. Leptin accelerates the onset of puberty in normal female mice. J Clin Invest 1997;99:391–5.
45. Fulton S, Woodside B, Shizgal P. Modulation of brain reward circuitry by leptin. Science 2000;287:125–8.
46. Thornton JE, Cheung CC, Clifton DK, Steiner RA. Regulation of hypothalamic proopiomelanocortin mRNA by leptin in ob/ob mice. Endocrinology 1997;138:5063–6.
47. Wardlaw SL. Clinical review 127: Obesity as a neuroendocrine disease: Lessons to be learned from proopiomelanocortin and melanocortin receptor mutations in mice and men. J Clin Endocrinol Metab 2001;86:1442–6.
48. Bray GA, York DA. Clinical review 90: Leptin and clinical medicine: A new piece in the puzzle of obesity. J Clin Endocrinol Metab 1997;82:2771–6.
49. Hagen T, Vidal-Puig A. Mitochondrial uncoupling proteins in human physiology and disease. Minerva Med 2002;93:41–57.
50. Otabe S, Clement K, Dubois S, et al. Mutation screening and association studies of the human uncoupling protein 3 gene in normoglycemic and diabetic morbidly obese patients. Diabetes 1999;48:206–8.
51. Jimenez M, Leger B, Canola K, et al. Beta(1)/beta(2)/beta(3)–adrenoceptor knockout mice are obese and cold-sensitive but have normal lipolytic responses to fasting. FEBS Lett 2002;530:37–40.
52. DeFronzo RA, Ferrannini E. Insulin resistance. A multifaceted syndrome responsible for NIDDM, obesity, hypertension, dyslipidemia, and atherosclerotic cardiovascular disease. Diabetes Care 1991;14:173–94.
53. DeLany JP, Lovejoy JC. Energy expenditure. Endocrinol Metab Clin North Am 1996;25:831–46.
54. Levine JA, Eberhardt NL, Jensen MD. Role of nonexercise activity thermogenesis in resistance to fat gain in humans. Science 1999;283:212–4.
55. Rankinen T, Zuberi A, Chagnon YC, et al. The human obesity gene map: The 2005 update. Obesity (Silver Spring) 2006;14:529–644.
56. Montague CT, Farooqi IS, Whitehead JP, et al. Congenital leptin deficiency is associated with severe early-onset obesity in humans. Nature 1997;387:903–8.
57. Clement K, Vaisse C, Lahlou N, et al. A mutation in the human leptin receptor gene causes obesity and pituitary dysfunction. Nature 1998;392:398–401.
58. Krude H, Biebermann H, Luck W, et al. Severe early–onset obesity, adrenal insufficiency and red hair pigmentation caused by POMC mutations in humans. Nat Genet 1998;19:155–7.
59. Jackson RS, Creemers JW, Ohagi S, et al. Obesity and impaired prohormone processing associated with mutations in the human prohormone convertase 1 gene. Nat Genet 1997;16:303–6.
60. Faivre L, Cormier-Daire V, Lapierre JM, et al. Deletion of the SIM1 gene (6q16.2) in a patient with a Prader–Willi–like phenotype. J Med Genet 2002;39:594–6.
61. Lee YS, Poh LK, Loke KY. A novel melanocortin 3 receptor gene (MC3R) mutation associated with severe obesity. J Clin Endocrinol Metab 2002;87:1423–6.
62. Yeo GS, Farooqi IS, Aminian S, et al. A frameshift mutation in MC4R associated with dominantly inherited human obesity. Nat Genet 1998;20:111–2.
63. Farooqi IS, O'Rahilly S. Monogenic obesity in humans. Annu Rev Med 2005;56:443–58.
64. Ukkola O, Ravussin E, Jacobson P, et al. Mutations in the preproghrelin/ghrelin gene associated with obesity in humans. J Clin Endocrinol Metab 2001;86:3996–9.
65. Hasstedt SJ, Ren QF, Teng K, Elbein SC. Effect of the peroxisome proliferator–activated receptor–gamma 2 pro(12)ala variant on obesity, glucose homeostasis, and blood pressure in members of familial type 2 diabetic kindreds. J Clin Endocrinol Metab 2001;86:536–41.
66. Esterbauer H, Schneitler C, Oberkofler H, et al. A common polymorphism in the promoter of UCP2 is associated with decreased risk of obesity in middle–aged humans. Nat Genet 2001;28:178–83.
67. Oizumi T, Daimon M, Saitoh T, et al. Genotype Arg/Arg, but not Trp/Arg, of the Trp64Arg polymorphism of the beta(3)–adrenergic receptor is associated with type 2 diabetes and obesity in a large Japanese sample. Diabetes Care 2001;24:1579–83.
68. OMIM. On-line Mendelian Inheritance in Man. http://www3.ncbi.nlm.nih.gov/omim. Accessed 10/14/06 2006.
69. Katsanis N, Ansley SJ, Badano JL, et al. Triallelic inheritance in Bardet–Biedl syndrome, a Mendelian recessive disorder. Science 2001;293:2256–9.
70. Alstrom CH, Hallgren B, Nilsson LB, Asander H. Retinal degeneration combined with obesity, diabetes mellitus and neurogenous deafness: A specific syndrome (not hitherto described) distinct from the Laurence–Moon–Bardet–Biedl syndrome: A clinical, endocrinological and genetic examination based on a large pedigree. Acta Psychiatr Neurol Scand Suppl 1959;129:1–35.
71. Cohen MM, Jr, Hall BD, Smith DW, et al. A new syndrome with hypotonia, obesity, mental deficiency, and facial, oral, ocular, and limb anomalies. J Pediatr 1973;83:280–4.
72. Kivitie-Kallio S, Norio R. Cohen syndrome: Essential features, natural history, and heterogeneity. Am J Med Genet 2001;102:125–35.
73. Beales PL, Elcioglu N, Woolf AS, et al. New criteria for improved diagnosis of Bardet–Biedl syndrome: Results of a population survey. J Med Genet 1999;36:437–46.
74. Shapira H, Friedman E, Mouallem M, Farfel Z. Familial Albright's hereditary osteodystrophy with hypoparathyroidism: Normal structural Gs alpha gene. J Clin Endocrinol Metab 1996;81:1660–2.
75. Gunay-Aygun M, Schwartz S, Heeger S, et al. The changing purpose of Prader–Willi syndrome clinical diagnostic criteria and proposed revised criteria. Pediatrics 2001;108:E92.
76. Barlow SE, Dietz WH. Obesity evaluation and treatment: Expert Committee recommendations. The Maternal and Child Health Bureau, Health Resources and Services Administration and the Department of Health and Human Services. Pediatrics 1998;102:E29.
77. Strauss RS. Childhood obesity. Pediatr Clin North Am 2002;49:175–201.
78. Dufour JF, Oneta CM, Gonvers JJ, et al. Randomized placebo–controlled trial of ursodeoxycholic Acid with vitamin e in nonalcoholic steatohepatitis. Clin Gastroenterol Hepatol 2006;4:1537–43.
79. Ueno T, Sugawara H, Sujaku K, et al. Therapeutic effects of restricted diet and exercise in obese patients with fatty liver. J Hepatol 1997;27:103–7.
80. Genuth S, Alberti KG, Bennett P, et al. Follow-up report on the diagnosis of diabetes mellitus. Diabetes Care 2003;26:3160–7.
81. Gomez-Diaz R, Aguilar-Salinas CA, Moran-Villota S, et al. Lack of agreement between the revised criteria of impaired fasting glucose and impaired glucose tolerance in children with excess body weight. Diabetes Care 2004;27:2229–33.
82. Conwell LS, Batch JA. Oral glucose tolerance test in children and adolescents: Positives and pitfalls. J Paediatr Child Health 2004;40:620–6.
83. Fagot-Campagna A, Saaddine JB, Engelgau MM. Is testing children for type 2 diabetes a lost battle? Diabetes Care 2000;23:1442–3.
84. Foster GD, McGuckin BG. Estimating resting energy expenditure in obesity. Obes Res 2001;9:367S–72S; discussion 373S–4S.
85. Guille C, Sachs GS, Ghaemi SN. A naturalistic comparison of clozapine, risperidone, and olanzapine in the treatment of bipolar disorder. J Clin Psychiatry 2000;61:638–42.
86. Sussman N. Review of atypical antipsychotics and weight gain. J Clin Psychiatry 2001;62:5–12.
87. Garland EJ, Remick RA, Zis AP. Weight gain with antidepressants and lithium. J Clin Psychopharmacol 1988;8:323–30.
88. Ness-Abramof R, Apovian CM. Drug-induced weight gain. Timely Top Med Cardiovasc Dis 2005;9:E31.
89. Guille C, Sachs G. Clinical outcome of adjunctive topiramate treatment in a sample of refractory bipolar patients with comorbid conditions. Prog Neuropsychopharmacol Biol Psychiatry 2002;26:1035–9.
90. Sussman N, Ginsberg DL, Bikoff J. Effects of nefazodone on body weight: A pooled analysis of selective serotonin reuptake inhibitor- and imipramine-controlled trials. J Clin Psychiatry 2001;62:256–60.
91. Fava M, Judge R, Hoog SL, et al. Fluoxetine versus sertraline and paroxetine in major depressive disorder: Changes in weight with long-term treatment. J Clin Psychiatry 2000;61:863–7.
92. Pijl H, Meinders AE. Bodyweight change as an adverse effect of drug treatment. Mechanisms and management. Drug Saf 1996;14:329–42.

93. Rendell MS, Kirchain WR. Pharmacotherapy of type 2 diabetes mellitus. Ann Pharmacother 2000;34:878–95.
94. DeFronzo RA. Pharmacologic therapy for type 2 diabetes mellitus. Ann Intern Med 2000;133:73–4.
95. Bandini LG, Schoeller DA, Cyr HN, Dietz WH. Validity of reported energy intake in obese and nonobese adolescents. Am J Clin Nutr 1990;52:421–5.
96. Ludwig DS, Peterson KE, Gortmaker SL. Relation between consumption of sugar-sweetened drinks and childhood obesity: A prospective, observational analysis. Lancet 2001;357:505–8.
97. Robinson TN. Reducing children's television viewing to prevent obesity: A randomized controlled trial. JAMA 1999;282:1561–7.
98. American Academy of Pediatrics: Children, adolescents, and television. Pediatrics 2001;107:423–6.
99. Goodman E, Whitaker RC. A prospective study of the role of depression in the development and persistence of adolescent obesity. Pediatrics 2002;110:497–504.
100. Pine DS, Goldstein RB, Wolk S, Weissman MM. The association between childhood depression and adulthood body mass index. Pediatrics 2001;107:1049–56.
101. Anderson SE, Cohen P, Naumova EN, Must A. Association of depression and anxiety disorders with weight change in a prospective community-based study of children followed up into adulthood. Arch Pediatr Adolesc Med 2006;160:285–91.
102. Becker ES, Margraf J, Turke V, et al. Obesity and mental illness in a representative sample of young women. Int J Obes Relat Metab Disord 2001; 25:S5–9.
103. Morgan CM, Yanovski SZ, Nguyen TT, et al. Loss of control over eating, adiposity, and psychopathology in overweight children. Int J Eat Disord 2002;31:430–41.
104. Berkowitz R, Stunkard AJ, Stallings VA. Binge–eating disorder in obese adolescent girls. Ann N Y Acad Sci 1993;699:200–6.
105. Maloney MJ, McGuire J, Daniels SR, Specker B. Dieting behavior and eating attitudes in children. Pediatrics 1989;84:482–9.
106. French SA, Story M, Perry CL. Self–esteem and obesity in children and adolescents: A literature review. Obes Res 1995;3:479–90.
107. Epstein LH, Wisniewski L, Weng R. Child and parent psychological problems influence child weight control. Obes Res 1994;2:509–15.
108. Epstein LH, Myers MD, Anderson K. The association of maternal psychopathology and family socioeconomic status with psychological problems in obese children. Obes Res 1996;4:65–74.
109. Sargent JD, Blanchflower DG. Obesity and stature in adolescence and earnings in young adulthood. Analysis of a British birth cohort. Arch Pediatr Adolesc Med 1994;148:681–7.
110. Gortmaker SL, Must A, Perrin JM, et al. Social and economic consequences of overweight in adolescence and young adulthood. N Engl J Med 1993;329:1008–12.
111. Canning H, Mayer J. Obesity – its possible effect on college acceptance. N Engl J Med 1966;275:1172–1174.
112. Strauss RS, Knight J. Influence of the home environment on the development of obesity in children. Pediatrics 1999;103:e85.
113. Simonetti D'Arca A, Tarsitani G, Cairella M, et al. Prevention of obesity in elementary and nursery school children. Public Health 1986;100:166–73.
114. Fitzgibbon ML, Stolley MR, Schiffer L, et al. Two-year follow-up results for Hip-Hop to Health Jr.: A randomized controlled trial for overweight prevention in preschool minority children. J Pediatr 2005;146:618–25.
115. Gortmaker SL, Peterson K, Wiecha J, et al. Reducing obesity via a school-based interdisciplinary intervention among youth: Planet Health. Arch Pediatr Adolesc Med 1999;153:409–18.
116. Yin Z, Gutin B, Johnson MH, et al. An environmental approach to obesity prevention in children: Medical College of Georgia FitKid Project year 1 results. Obes Res 2005;13:2153–61.
117. Donnelly JE, Jacobsen DJ, Whatley JE, et al. Nutrition and physical activity program to attenuate obesity and promote physical and metabolic fitness in elementary school children. Obes Res 1996;4:229–43.
118. Mo-suwan L, Pongprapai S, Junjana C, Puetpaiboon A. Effects of a controlled trial of a school-based exercise program on the obesity indexes of preschool children. Am J Clin Nutr 1998;68:1006–11.
119. Sahota P, Rudolf MC, Dixey R, et al. Randomised controlled trial of primary school based intervention to reduce risk factors for obesity. BMJ 2001;323:1029–32.
120. Reilly JJ, Kelly L, Montgomery C, et al. Physical activity to prevent obesity in young children: Cluster randomised controlled trial. BMJ 2006;333:1041.
121. Goran MI, Treuth MS. Energy expenditure, physical activity, and obesity in children. Pediatr Clin North Am 2001;48:931–53.
122. Summerell CD, Waters E, Edmunds LD, et al. Interventions for preventing obesity in children. Cochrane Database Syst Rev 2005;3:CD001871.
123. Reilly JJ, Wilson ML, Summerbell CD, Wilson DC. Obesity: Diagnosis, prevention, and treatment; evidence based answers to common questions. Arch Dis Child 2002;86:392–4.
124. Landrigan PJ, Trasande L, Thorpe LE, et al. The National Children's Study: A 21-year prospective study of 100,000 American children. Pediatrics 2006;118:2173–86.
125. Becque MD, Katch VL, Rocchini AP, et al. Coronary risk incidence of obese adolescents: Reduction by exercise plus diet intervention. Pediatrics 1988;81:605–12.
126. Epstein LH, Wing RR, Penner BC, Kress MJ. Effect of diet and controlled exercise on weight loss in obese children. J Pediatr 1985;107:358–61.
127. Epstein LH, Valoski AM, Vara LS, et al. Effects of decreas ing sedentary behavior and increasing activity on weight change in obese children. Health Psychol 1995;14:109–15.
128. Epstein LH, Saelens BE, Myers MD, Vito D. Effects of decreasing sedentary behaviors on activity choice in obese children. Health Psychol 1997;16:107–13.
129. Epstein LH, Paluch RA, Gordy CC, Dorn J. Decreasing sedentary behaviors in treating pediatric obesity. Arch Pediatr Adolesc Med 2000;154:220–6.
130. Epstein LH, Valoski A, Wing RR, McCurley J. Ten-year follow-up of behavioral, family-based treatment for obese children. JAMA 1990;264:2519–23.
131. Committee on Nutrition AAoP. Obesity in children. Oak Grove, IL: American Academy of Pediatrics, 1998.
132. Ikeda JP, Mitchell RA. Dietary approaches to the treatment of the overweight pediatric patient. Pediatr Clin North Am 2001;48:955–68, ix.
133. Epstein LH, Valoski A, Koeske R, Wing RR. Family–based behavioral weight control in obese young children. J Am Diet Assoc 1986;86:481–4.
134. Suskind RM, Blecker U, Udall JN, Jr, et al. Recent advances in the treatment of childhood obesity. Pediatr Diabetes 2000;1:23–33.
135. Yanovski JA. Intensive therapies for pediatric obesity. Pediatr Clin North Am 2001;48:1041–53.
136. Figueroa–Colon R, von Almen TK, Franklin FA, et al. Comparison of two hypocaloric diets in obese children. Am J Dis Child 1993;147:160–6.
137. Amador M, Ramos LT, Morono M, Hermelo MP. Growth rate reduction during energy restriction in obese adolescents. Exp Clin Endocrinol 1990;96:73–82.
138. Nordmann AJ, Nordmann A, Briel M, et al. Effects of low-carbohydrate vs low-fat diets on weight loss and cardiovascular risk factors: A meta-analysis of randomized controlled trials. Arch Intern Med 2006;166:285–93.
139. Ebbeling CB, Leidig MM, Sinclair KB, et al. Effects of an ad libitum low–glycemic load diet on cardiovascular disease risk factors in obese young adults. Am J Clin Nutr 2005;81:976–82.
140. Pereira MA, Swain J, Goldfine AB, et al. Effects of a low–glycemic load diet on resting energy expenditure and heart disease risk factors during weight loss. JAMA 2004;292:2482–90.
141. Raatz SK, Torkelson CJ, Redmon JB, et al. Reduced glycemic index and glycemic load diets do not increase the effects of energy restriction on weight loss and insulin sensitivity in obese men and women. J Nutr 2005;135:2387–91.
142. Thompson WG, Rostad Holdman N, Janzow DJ, et al. Effect of energy–reduced diets high in dairy products and fiber on weight loss in obese adults. Obes Res 2005;13:1344–53.
143. Moses RG, Luebcke M, Davis WS, et al. Effect of a low–glycemic–index diet during pregnancy on obstetric outcomes. Am J Clin Nutr 2006;84:807–12.
144. Epstein LH, Valoski AM, Kalarchian MA, McCurley J. Do children lose and maintain weight easier than adults: A comparison of child and parent weight changes from six months to ten years. Obes Res 1995;3:411–7.
145. Wang G, Dietz WH. Economic burden of obesity in youths aged 6 to 17 years: 1979–1999. Pediatrics 2002;109:E81–1.
146. Choban PS, Flancbaum L. Nourishing the obese patient. Clin Nutr 2000;19:305–11.
147. Knip M, Nuutinen O. Long-term effects of weight reduction on serum lipids and plasma insulin in obese children. Am J Clin Nutr 1993;57:490–3.
148. Epstein LH, Wing RR, Steranchak L, et al. Comparison of family-based behavior modification and nutrition education for childhood obesity. J Pediatr Psychol 1980;5:25–36.
149. Coates TJ, Jeffery RW, Slinkard LA. Frequency of contact and monetary reward in weight loss, lipid change, and blood pressure reduction with adolescents. Behav Ther 1982;1:175–85.
150. Graves T, Meyers AW, Clark L. An evaluation of parental problem–solving training in the behavioral treatment of childhood obesity. J Consult Clin Psychol 1988;56:246–50.
151. Duffy G, Spence SH. The effectiveness of cognitive self–management as an adjunct to a behavioural intervention for childhood obesity: A research note. J Child Psychol Psychiatry 1993;34:1043–50.
152. Yanovski SZ, Yanovski JA. Obesity. N Engl J Med 2002;346:591–602.
153. Fanghanel G, Cortinas L, Sanchez-Reyes L, Berber A. A clinical trial of the use of sibutramine for the treatment of patients suffering essential obesity. Int J Obes Relat Metab Disord 2000;24:144–50.
154. Ryan DH. Use of sibutramine and other noradrenergic and serotonergic drugs in the management of obesity. Endocrine 2000;13:193–9.
155. James WP, Astrup A, Finer N, et al. Effect of sibutramine on weight maintenance after weight loss: A randomised trial. STORM Study Group. Sibutramine Trial of Obesity Reduction and Maintenance. Lancet 2000; 356:2119–25.
156. Berkowitz RI, Fujioka K, Daniels SR, et al. Effects of sibutramine treatment in obese adolescents: A randomized trial. Ann Intern Med 2006;145:81–90.
157. Heck AM, Yanovski JA, Calis KA. Orlistat, a new lipase inhibitor for the management of obesity. Pharmacotherapy 2000;20:270–9.
158. Davidson MH, Hauptman J, DiGirolamo M, et al. Weight control and risk factor reduction in obese subjects treated for 2 years with orlistat: A randomized controlled trial. JAMA 1999;281:235–42.
159. Lee A, Morley JE. Metformin decreases food consumption and induces weight loss in subjects with obesity with type II non-insulin-dependent diabetes. Obes Res 1998;6:47–53.
160. Kirpichnikov D, McFarlane SI, Sowers JR. Metformin: An update. Ann Intern Med 2002;137:25–33.
161. Morrison JA, Cottingham EM, Barton BA. Metformin for weight loss in pediatric patients taking psychotropic drugs. Am J Psychiatry 2002;159:655–7.
162. Klein DJ, Cottingham EM, Sorter M, et al. A Randomized, Double-Blind, Placebo-Controlled Trial of Metformin Treatment of Weight Gain Associated With Initiation of Atypical Antipsychotic Therapy in Children and Adolescents. Am J Psychiatry 2006;163:2072–2079.
163. Freemark M, Bursey D. The effects of metformin on body mass index and glucose tolerance in obese adolescents with fasting hyperinsulinemia and a family history of type 2 diabetes. Pediatrics 2001;107:E55.
164. Srinivasan S, Ambler GR, Baur LA, et al. Randomized, controlled trial of metformin for obesity and insulin resistance in children and adolescents: Improvement in body composition and fasting insulin. J Clin Endocrinol Metab 2006;91:2074–80.
165. Eisenberg DM, Davis RB, Ettner SL, et al. Trends in alternative medicine use in the United States, 1990–1997: Results of a follow–up national survey. JAMA 1998;280:1569–75.
166. Gaullier JM, Halse J, Hoye K, et al. Supplementation with conjugated linoleic acid for 24 months is well tolerated by and reduces body fat mass in healthy, overweight humans. J Nutr 2005;135:778–84.
167. Kleefstra N, Houweling ST, Jansman FG, et al. Chromium treatment has no effect in patients with poorly controlled, insulin–treated type 2 diabetes in an obese Western population: A randomized, double-blind, placebo-controlled trial. Diabetes Care 2006;29:521–5.
168. Pittler MH, Stevinson C, Ernst E. Chromium picolinate for reducing body weight: Meta-analysis of randomized trials. Int J Obes Relat Metab Disord 2003;27:522–9.
169. Mhurchu CN, Dunshea-Mooij C, Bennett D, Rodgers A. Effect of chitosan on weight loss in overweight and obese individuals: A systematic review of randomized controlled trials. Obes Rev 2005;6:35–42.
170. Pittler MH, Ernst E. Dietary supplements for body–weight reduction: A systematic review. Am J Clin Nutr 2004;79:529–36.
171. Cohen MH, Eisenberg DM. Potential physician malpractice liability associated with complementary and integrative medical therapies. Ann Intern Med 2002;136:596–603.
172. Allison DB, Fontaine KR, Heshka S, et al. Alternative treatments for weight loss: A critical review. Crit Rev Food Sci Nutr 2001;41:1–28; discussion 39–40.
173. FDA issues regulation to prohibit sale of dietary supplements containing ephedrine alkaloid; http://www.fda.gov/bbs/topics/NEWS/2004/NEW01021.html. Accessed February 6, 2007.
174. Pories WJ, Swanson MS, MacDonald KG, et al. Who would have thought it? An operation proves to be the most effective therapy for adult-onset diabetes mellitus. Ann Surg 1995;222:339–50; discussion 350–2.
175. Schauer PR, Ikramuddin S, Gourash W, et al. Outcomes after laparoscopic Roux-en-Y gastric bypass for morbid obesity. Ann Surg 2000;232:515–29.

176. Cummings DE, Weigle DS, Frayo RS, et al. Plasma ghrelin levels after diet–induced weight loss or gastric bypass surgery. N Engl J Med 2002;346:1623–30.
177. Kellum JM, DeMaria EJ, Sugerman HJ. The surgical treatment of morbid obesity. Curr Probl Surg 1998;35:791–858.
178. Strauss RS, Bradley LJ, Brolin RE. Gastric bypass surgery in adolescents with morbid obesity. J Pediatr 2001;138:499–504.
179. Malinowski SS. Nutritional and metabolic complications of bariatric surgery. Am J Med Sci 2006;331:219–25.
180. Al–Fahad T, Ismael A, Soliman MO, Khoursheed M. Very early onset of Wernicke's encephalopathy after gastric bypass. Obes Surg 2006;16:671–2.
181. Towbin A, Inge TH, Garcia VF, et al. Beriberi after gastric bypass surgery in adolescence. J Pediatr 2004;145:263–7.
182. Nadler EP, Youn HA, Ginsburg HB, et al. Short–term results in 53 US obese pediatric patients treated with laparoscopic adjustable gastric banding. J Pediatr Surg 2007;42:137–41; discussion 141–2.
183. Angrisani L, Favretti F, Furbetta F, et al. Obese teenagers treated by Lap–Band System: The Italian experience. Surgery 2005;138:877–81.
184. Anderson AE, Soper RT, Scott DH. Gastric bypass for morbid obesity in children and adolescents. J Pediatr Surg 1980;15:876–81.
185. Sugerman HJ, Sugerman EL, DeMaria EJ, et al. Bariatric surgery for severely obese adolescents. J Gastrointest Surg 2003;7:102–7; discussion 107–8.
186. Inge TH. Bariatric surgery for morbidly obese adolescents: Is there a rationale for early intervention? Growth Horm IGF Res 2006;16:S15–9.
187. Apovian CM, Baker C, Ludwig DS, et al. Best practice guidelines in pediatric/adolescent weight loss surgery. Obes Res 2005;13:274–82.
188. Cohen DM, Green JG, Miller J, et al. Acrocephalopolysyndactyly type II—Carpenter syndrome: Clinical spectrum and an attempt at unification with Goodman and Summit syndromes. Am J Med Genet 1987;28:311–24.
189. Type 2 diabetes in children and adolescents. American Diabetes Association. Diabetes Care 2000;23:381–9.
190. Cantu TG, Korek JS. Monoamine oxidase inhibitors and weight gain. Drug Intell Clin Pharm 1988;22:755–9.
191. Gadde KM, Parker CB, Maner LG, et al. Bupropion for weight loss: An investigation of efficacy and tolerability in overweight and obese women. Obes Res 2001;9:544–51.
192. Sachs GS, Guille C. Weight gain associated with use of psychotropic medications. J Clin Psychiatry 1999;60: 16–9.
193. Levisohn PM. Safety and tolerability of topiramate in children. J Child Neurol 2000;15:S22–6.
194. Prochaska JO, DiClemente CC, Norcross JC. In search of how people change. Applications to addictive behaviors. Am Psychol 1992;47:1102–14.

Complications of Obesity: Metabolic Syndrome

Stavroula K. Osganian, MD, ScD
Sarah de Ferranti, MD, MPH

INTRODUCTION

The rising rates of obesity in children and adults have been accompanied by an increase in the cooccurrence of obesity-associated metabolic abnormalities known as the metabolic syndrome. The metabolic syndrome is described as a constellation of metabolic abnormalities including obesity, dyslipidemia, impaired glucose metabolism, and elevated blood pressure that represent major risk factors for cardiovascular disease (CVD).[1,2] Adults with the syndrome have a significantly increased risk for developing type 2 diabetes and morbidity and mortality from CVD.[3,4] The clustering of major components of the syndrome, including obesity, dyslipidemia, hypertension, and insulin resistance, has been demonstrated in youth,[5–7] and clustering of these risk factors has also been shown to track into adulthood.[8] Obesity is thought to play a significant role in the development of metabolic syndrome in children and adults.[5,6,9] Obese children have a significantly higher prevalence of metabolic syndrome than nonobese children,[10–12] and greater body weight and central adiposity predisposes children to each of the metabolic complications of high blood pressure, dyslipidemia, impaired glucose tolerance, and hyperinsulinemia.[13] The Executive Committee of the Third Report of the National Cholesterol Education Program (NCEP) Expert Panel on Detection, Evaluation and Treatment of High Blood Cholesterol in Adults (Adult Treatment Panel III) has recognized metabolic syndrome as a condition that warrants clinical intervention.[14] The ATP III report identifies metabolic syndrome as an independent risk factor for CVD and considers it an indication for intensive lifestyle intervention. Although comparable guidelines for the treatment of metabolic syndrome in children have not been developed, the available data suggest that obese youth are a high-risk population to target for screening, prevention, and intervention. [5–7] As with adults, treatment should emphasize lifestyle modification and target reduction of levels of the individual metabolic risk factors.

DEFINITION OF METABOLIC SYNDROME

The metabolic syndrome was first identified by Reaven as syndrome X and described as the coexistence of multiple metabolic derangements that included hyperinsulinemia, glucose intolerance, hypertension, decreased high-density lipoprotein (HDL) cholesterol, and elevated triglycerides.[15] The clustering of a set of specific metabolic risk factors remains the defining element of the syndrome; however, the terminology has shifted away from syndrome X and insulin-resistance syndrome to metabolic syndrome in order to avoid the emphasis on insulin resistance as a requisite factor or as the underlying etiologic mechanism.[1,16,17] At this time, there is no universal or consensus definition for metabolic syndrome in children or adults. Among adults, three national expert committees, the World Health Organization (WHO),[18,19] National Cholesterol Education Program—Third Adult Treatment Panel (NCEP ATP III),[2,16,17] and the International Diabetes Federation (IDF),[20] have developed clinical definitions of the metabolic syndrome (Table 1). In general, all definitions include a measure of obesity, insulin resistance, elevated blood pressure, and atherogenic dyslipidemia among the components that define the cluster, yet, the threshold values for the risk factors and the number and combinations of components used to define the syndrome vary considerably.

The WHO and NCEP ATP III are the most commonly used criteria among adult studies and

Table 1 Definitions of Metabolic Syndrome in Adults

World Health Organization[18,19]	International Diabetes Federation[20]	National Cholesterol Education Panel Adult Treatment Panel III[2]
One of the following: • Type 2 diabetes (fasting plasma glucose ≥126 mg/dL or 2 h postglucose load ≥200 mg/dL) • Impaired fasting glucose (fasting glucose from 110–125 mg/dL) • Impaired glucose tolerance (2 h postglucose load from 140–199 mg/dL) • Insulin resistance (glucose uptake below the lowest quartile for the background population under investigation under hyperinsulinemic, euglycemic conditions) *And any two of the following*: • SBP ≥140 mm Hg or DBP ≥ 90 mm Hg and/or antihypertensive medication • Fasting triglycerides ≥150 mg/dL and/or HDL cholesterol <35 mg/dL in men or HDL cholesterol <39 mg/dL in women • BMI >30 kg/m^2 and/or waist:hip ratio >0.9 in men or >0.85 in women • Urinary albumin excretion rate ≥20 µg/min or albumin:creatinine ratio ≥30 mg/g	*Central obesity*: • Waist circumference >94 cm in Europoid men or >80 cm in Eurupoid women with ethnicity-specific values for other groups *And any two of the following*: • Fasting glucose ≥100 mg/dL or previously diagnosed type 2 diabetes • SBP ≥130 or DBP ≥85 mm Hg or treatment of previously diagnosed hypertension • Fasting triglycerides ≥150 mg/dL or specific treatment for this abnormality • HDL cholesterol <40 mg/dL in men or <50 mg/dL in women or specific treatment for this abnormality	***Any three of the following:*** • Fasting glucose ≥100 mg/dL or drug treatment for elevated glucose • SBP ≥130 or DBP ≥ 85 mm Hg and/or drug treatment for hypertension • Fasting triglycerides ≥150 mg/dL or treatment with medication for this abnormality • HDL cholesterol <40 mg/dL in men or <50 mg/dL in women or drug treatment for this abnormality • Waist circumference ≥102 cm in men or ≥88 cm in women with lower thresholds for individual or ethnic groups prone to insulin resistance

BMI = Body mass index; DBP=diastolic blood pressure; HDL= high-density lipoprotein; SBP= systolic blood pressure.

modifications of these criteria have been used in several pediatric studies (Table 2). The WHO definition emphasizes insulin resistance as a primary component for diagnosis and requires the presence of type 2 diabetes, impaired fasting glucose, impaired glucose tolerance, or if fasting glucose is normal, then an abnormality on hyperinsulinemic, euglycemic clamp testing is a necessary criterion for diagnosis. In addition, any two of the following criteria may be present: elevated blood pressure (systolic ≥140 mm Hg or diastolic ≥90 mm Hg) or on medications for high blood pressure, triglycerides ≥150 mg/dL and/or HDL cholesterol <35 mg/dL in men or <39 mg/dL in women, body mass index (BMI) >30 kg/m^2 or waist-to-hip ratio >0.9 in men and >0.85 in women, and urinary albumin excretion rate ≥20 μg/min or albumin-to-creatinine ratio ≥30 mg/g. A major limitation of this definition has been the requirement for hyperinsulinemic, euglycemic clamp testing, which is not feasible in clinical practice or in large-scale, population-based research studies. The NCEP ATP III definition overcomes this limitation by using measures that are readily available or feasible in clinical practice. It also differs from WHO in that its primary goal is to define a syndrome that characterizes individuals who are at increased risk for CVD.[1,16,21] Thus, it uses criteria shown to be strongly predictive of CVD in adults. Furthermore, there is not an emphasis on any single component as necessary to define the syndrome. The most recent and revised NCEP ATP III definition requires the presence of any three out of the following five criteria to define metabolic syndrome: abdominal obesity with waist circumference ≥102 cm in men and ≥88 cm women, triglycerides ≥150 mg/dL or drug treatment for elevated triglycerides, HDL cholesterol <40 mg/dL in men or <50 mg/dL in women or drug treatment for reduced HDL cholesterol, elevated blood pressure (systolic ≥130 mm Hg or diastolic ≥85 mm Hg) or treatment for hypertension, or fasting glucose ≥100 mg/dL or drug treatment for elevated glucose. The criteria allow for adjustment of waist circumference to lower thresholds among groups prone to insulin resistance, specifically Asian-Americans (waist circumference ≥90 cm in men and ≥80 cm in women).[2,16] The IDF criteria closely resemble those from NCEP ATP III but place a greater emphasis on central obesity, defined by increased waist circumference, as a necessary component of the syndrome and use additional ethnic specific waist circumference criteria to define central obesity with greater sensitivity. The rationale was based on data showing that waist circumference is highly correlated with abdominal obesity and insulin resistance and more feasible to measure in clinical practice.[20] Specifically, the IDF criteria require central obesity defined as waist circumference ≥94 cm for Europoid men and ≥80 cm for Eupoid women with ethnic and gender-specific values for South Asians, Chinese, and Japanese men and women as well as any two of the following: triglycerides ≥150 mg/dL or treatment for elevated triglycerides, HDL cholesterol <40 mg/dL in men or <50 mg/dL in women or treatment for low HDL cholesterol, elevated blood pressure (systolic ≥130 mm Hg or diastolic ≥85 mm Hg) or treatment for hypertension, or fasting glucose ≥100 mg/dL or previously diagnosed type 2 diabetes. If fasting glucose is elevated, an oral glucose tolerance test is recommended but not required to meet the criteria.

The most commonly used definitions of metabolic syndrome in children have been adaptations of the WHO and NCEP ATP III definitions for adults.[5,6] The major difference has been in the use of age- and gender-specific percentiles from national reference data or study-specific distributions to define the thresholds for abnormalities of the individual components of the syndrome. Cruz[6] and others[10,12] have proposed that a definition in children be comparable to adults, using the same set of risk factors as those proposed for adults. However, agreement has not been reached on the threshold values or cutoffs for the individual risk factors during childhood that will be most sensitive to predicting future risk of CVD. These cutoffs may need to be less stringent than the cutoffs that are presently used to define abnormally high levels of each individual risk factor in childhood or adolescence.

EPIDEMIOLOGY OF METABOLIC SYNDROME

Prevalence

Several epidemiologic studies have described the prevalence of metabolic syndrome and risk factor clustering in children and adolescents (Table 2). Studies in youth suggest that the syndrome does develop during childhood and adolescence and the prevalence is higher in overweight youth.[5,6] Based on nationally representative samples of US adolescents and adults,[10,22,23] the prevalence in adolescents is substantially lower than the prevalence in adults, and the higher prevalence among those who are overweight or obese has been demonstrated for all ages. Among US adults,[22,23] approximately 22% have metabolic syndrome, and the prevalence is similar between men and women. It is significantly more prevalent among obese (60%) and overweight (22%) adults as compared to normal-weight adults (5%). Racial and ethnic differences have also been observed; metabolic syndrome was more prevalent in Mexican Americans (32%) compared to Whites (24%) and African-American Americans (22%). In a nationally representative sample of 2,430 US adolescents,[10] the overall prevalence of the syndrome was 4.2%, and males (6.1%) were more likely to be affected than females (2.1%). The syndrome was more common in Mexican American (5.6%) and White (4.8%) youth when compared to Black youth (2.0%). The majority of youth with metabolic syndrome were overweight, with the prevalence of the syndrome among those who were at or above the 95th percentile for BMI being 28.7% compared to 6.8% among those who were at risk of overweight (BMI at the 85th to less than the 95th percentile) and only 0.1% among those with a BMI below the 85th percentile. Among overweight youth, abdominal obesity (increased waist circumference) was the most prevalent component (74.5%), followed by dyslipidemia (51%), elevated blood pressure (11.2%), and impaired fasting plasma glucose (2.6%). Analysis of data on 991 adolescents from the 1999 to 2000 follow-up NHANES survey showed a significant increase in the overall prevalence to 6.4%.[11] Gender and race subgroup differences were similar to the earlier survey. The syndrome was again more prevalent among overweight adolescents (32.1% among adolescents with a BMI at or above the 95th percentile for age and sex) than among those at risk of overweight (7.1% among those with BMI at the 85th to below the 95th percentile for age and sex) or normal-weight adolescents (0.1% among those with a BMI below the 85th percentile for age and sex).[11] de Ferranti and colleagues[12] conducted an analysis of both the 1988 to 1994 and 1999 to 2000 surveys using less stringent cutoffs for waist circumference and triglycerides and found a somewhat higher prevalence of the syndrome, overall and for all subgroups.

Although variability exists between studies (Table 2), the overall prevalence of metabolic syndrome or risk factor clustering is also generally low among community- or school-based samples of both young children and adolescents.[13,24–31] The higher prevalence (18.6%) of metabolic syndrome in a community-based sample of Oji-Cree children is thought to be consistent with an excess burden of cardiovascular risk factors in native Canadian children.[32] Among youth, the prevalence has not differed significantly between the age groups studied. Younger children have a similar prevalence of metabolic syndrome or risk factor clustering when compared to older adolescents.[24,25,31] The strikingly higher prevalence of metabolic syndrome and clustering of cardiovascular risk factors among overweight adolescents from national data has been found in other community-based and clinic-based samples of both children and adolescents.[33–36] The prevalence is highest in the more severely obese. Weiss and colleagues[34] studied a clinic-based sample of very obese youth (BMI above the 97th percentile for age and sex) and found a high prevalence of metabolic syndrome that was associated with severity of obesity. The prevalence of metabolic syndrome was 38.7% among the moderately obese (BMI Z score 2.0 to 2.5) and nearly 50% among the severely obese youth (BMI Z score >2.5). Invitti and colleagues[36] also found that among obese youth the prevalence of the syndrome increased significantly with increasing tertiles of BMI Z scores, 16, 23, and 31%, respectively. Unlike findings for overweight or obese youth, significant differences in prevalence between race or gender subgroups have not been consistently observed across studies in youth.[10,11,24–26,28,31,32,36–38]

Table 2 Summary of Epidemiologic Studies of Metabolic Syndrome or Risk Factor Clustering in Youth

Author	Study Population	Risk Factor Cutoffs	Definition	Prevalence
		I. Population-based samples of children and adolescents		
de Ferranti et al., 2006[12] NHANES (1988–1994) NHANES (1999–2000)	Nationally representative sample of 12–19-yr-old US adolescents 1,960 participants	• ≥75th percentile WC for age and sex of study cohort • ≥90th percentile SBP or DBP for age, sex, and height[128] • ≥100 mg/dL TG • ≤45 mg/dL HDL in boys 15–19 yr and < 50 mg/dL HDL for all others • ≥110 mg/dL fasting glucose	Three or more criteria	NHANES 1988–1994 Overall: 9.2% Males: 9.5% Females: 8.9% Non-Hispanic White: 10.9% Non-Hispanic Black: 2.5% Mexican American: 12.9% At Risk/Overweight: 31.2% NHANES 1999–2000 Overall: 12.7% Males: 13.8%% Females: 11.6% Non-Hispanic White: 12.5% Non-Hispanic Black: 10.2% Mexican American: 16.9 At Risk/Overweight: 38.6%
Duncan et al., 2004[11] NHANES (1999–2000)	Nationally representative sample of 12–19-yr-old US adolescents 991 participants	• ≥90th percentile WC for age and sex of study cohort • ≥90th percentile SBP or DBP for age, sex, and height[128] • ≥110 mg/dL TG • ≥40 mg/dL HDL • ≥110 mg/dL fasting glucose	Three or more criteria	Overall: 6.4% Males: 9.1% Females: 3.7% Non-Hispanic White: 7.2% Non-Hispanic Black: 5.1% Mexican American: 8.5% Overweight: 32.1%
Cook et al., 2003[10] NHANES III (1988–1994)	Nationally representative sample of 12–19-yr-old US adolescents 2,430 participants	• ≥90th percentile WC for age and sex of study cohort • ≥90th percentile SBP or DBP for age, sex, and height[128] • ≥110 mg/dL TG • ≥40 mg/dL HDL • ≥110 mg/dL fasting glucose	Three or more criteria	Overall: 4.2% Males: 6.1% Females: 2.1% Non-Hispanic White: 4.8% Non-Hispanic Black: 2.0% Mexican American: 5.6% Overweight: 28.7%
Raitakari et al., 1994[25] Cardiovascular Risk in Young Finns Study	Population-based cohort of 3–18-yr-old Finnish children and adolescents 3,457 participants	Study cohort percentiles for age and sex • ≥75th percentile of sum of biceps, subscapular, and triceps skinfolds • ≥75th percentile SBP • ≥75th percentile of LDL	All three criteria	Overall: 3.1% Males: 3.56% Females: 2.64% Ages 3–6 Males: 2.69% Females: 2.21% Ages 9–12 Males: 3.48% Females: 2.80% Ages 15–18 Males: 4.49% Females: 2.92%
		II. Community- or clinic-based samples of children and adolescents		
Retnakaran et al., 2006[32]	Community-based sample of Oji-Cree Canadian children ages 10–19 yr 236 participants	• ≥90th percentile WC for age and sex[129] • ≥90th percentile SBP or DBP for age, sex, and height[122] • ≥1.1 mmol/L TG • HDL < 1.2 mmol/L in boys 15–19 yr and HDL < 1.3 mmol/L < in all others • ≥110 mg/dL fasting glucose	Three or more criteria	Overall: 18.6% Males: 14.3% Females: 21.4%
Morrison et al., 2005[26] National Heart, Lung, and Blood Institute Growth and Health Study	School-based cohort of US Black and White girls ages 9 and 10 yr fol lowed-up for 10 years 2,270 participants	• >88 cm WC • >130 mm Hg SBP or >85 mm Hg DBP • >150 mg/dL TG • <50 mg/dL HDL cholesterol • ≥110 mg/dL fasting glucose	Three or more criteria	Ages 9–10 yr Black girls:0.2% White girls:0.2% Ages: 18–19 yr Black girls: 3.5% White girls: 2.3%
Braunschweig et al., 2005[30]	School-based US sample of urban African-American children in grades 3–6 90 participants	• ≥90th percentile WC for age and sex[129] • ≥90th percentile DBP or SBP for age, sex, and height[128] • ≤40 mg/dL HDL • ≥110 mg/dL TG • ≥110 mg/dL fasting glucose	Three or more criteria	Overall: 5.6% Males: 5.0% Females: 4.0% Overweight: 13.8%
Rodriguez-Moran et al., 2004[27]	Community-based sample of 10–18-yr-old Mexican children and adolescents 965 participants	Study cohort percentiles for age and sex • ≥90th percentile BMI • ≥90th percentile TG • ≥90th percentile SBP or DBP • ≥110 mg/dL fasting glucose	Three or more criteria	Overall: 6.5%

Continued

Table 2 Summary of Epidemiologic Studies of Metabolic Syndrome or Risk Factor Clustering in Youth (*continued*)

Author	Study Population	Risk Factor Cutoffs	Definition	Prevalence
Goodman et al., 2004[28]	School-based sample of White, Black and Hispanic US adolescents ages 12–19 yr 1,513 participants	• ≥102 cm WC in males and ≥88 cm WC in females or ≥95th percentile BMI for age and sex (WHO) • ≥85 mm Hg DBP or ≥130 mm Hg SBP • ≤40 mg/dL HDL in males or ≤50 mg/dL HDL in females (NCEP) • ≤35 mg/dL HDL in males or ≤39 mg/dL HDL in females (WHO) • ≥150 mg/dL TG • ≥110 mg/dL fasting glucose • ≥75th percentile fasting insulin of study cohort (WHO)	NCEP definition used any three or more criteria WHO definition required impaired fasting glucose, type 2 diabetes, or hyperinsulinemia plus any two of the other criteria	Overall NCEP: 4.2% WHO: 8.4% Males NCEP: 3.8% WHO: 7.5% Females NCEP: 4.7% WHO: 9.5% Obese NCEP: 19.5% WHO: 38.9%
Lambert et al., 2004[24] The Quebec Child and Adolescent Health and Social Survey	School-based sample of Canadian youth ages 9, 13, and 16 yr 1,369 participants	Study cohort percentiles for age and sex (and height for BP) • ≥85th percentile BMI • ≥75th percentile SBP or DBP • ≥75th percentile TG • ≥25th percentile HDL • ≥75th percentile fasting insulin • ≥110 mg/dL fasting glucose	Definition 1 Hyperinsulinemia plus two or more risk factors. Definition 2 Any three or more risk factors.	Definition 1 Overall: 11.5% Males Age 9 yr: 10.7% Age 13 yr: 11.9% Age 16 years: 12.2% Females Age 9 yr: 12.0% Age 13 yr: 11.8% Age 16 yr: 10.8% Definition 2 Overall: 14.0% Males Age 9 yr: 13.1% Age 13 yr: 14.3% Age 16 yr: 15.2% Females Age 9 yr: 14.4% Age 13 yr: 14.7% Age 16 yr: 12.4%
Katzmarzyk et al., 2004[37] Boglausa Heart Study	School-based US cohort of 5–18-yr-old children and adolescents 2,597 participants	Study cohort percentiles for age • ≥80th percentile SBP or DBP • ≥80th percentile LDL • ≥80th percentile TG • ≤20th percentile HDL • ≥80th percentile fasting insulin • ≥80th percentile fasting glucose	Three or more criteria	Males White: 18.2% Black: 17.3% Females White: 16.5% Black: 16.6%
Srinivasan et al., 2002[13] Bogalusa Heart Study	School-based US cohort of 8–17-yr-old Black and White children, 745 participants	Study cohort percentiles for age, sex, race, and study year • ≥75th percentile BMI • ≥75th percentile SBP or MAP • ≥75th percentile cholesterol-to-HDL ratio or TG-to-HDL ratio • ≥75th percentile fasting insulin	All four criteria	Overall: 3.6% No race or sex differences
Chen et al., 1999[31] Bogalusa Heart Study	School-based cohort of 5–17-yr-old US Black and White children and adolescents 2,515 participants	Study cohort percentiles for age, race, and sex • ≥75th percentile ponderal index (weight/height^3) • ≥75th percentile SBP or DBP • ≥75th percentile TG and/or HDL • ≥75th percentile fasting insulin	All four criteria	Ages 5–11 yr White: 4.8 % Black: 3.7% Ages 12–17 yr White: 3.0% Black: 2.7%
Freedman et al., 1999[38] Bogalusa Heart Study	School-based US cohort of 5–17-yr-old Black and White children and adolescents 9,167 participants	Study cohort percentiles for age, race, and sex • ≥95th percentile SBP or DBP • ≥130 mg/dL TG • ≥130 mg/dL LDL • <35 mg/dL HDL • ≥95th percentile fasting insulin	Three or more criteria	Ages 5–10 yr Overall: 2% Overweight: 11% Ages 11–17 yr Overall: 2% Overweight: 10% No race differences
Chu et al., 1998[29] Tapei Children's Heart Study	School-based sample of 12–16-yr-old Chinese adolescents from 1,366 participants	Study cohort percentiles for age and sex • ≥90th percentile of SBP or DBP • ≥90th percentile TG or TC • ≥90th percentile of fasting glucose	All three criteria	Nonobese Males: 0.5% Females: 0.3% Obese Males: 2.0% Females: 4.0%

Continued

Table 2 Summary of Epidemiologic Studies of Metabolic Syndrome or Risk Factor Clustering in Youth (*continued*)

Author	Study Population	Risk Factor Cutoffs	Definition	Prevalence
		III. School- or clinic-based samples of overweight or obese children and adolescents		
Viner et al., 2006[33]	Clinic-based sample of 2–18-yr-old youth undergoing obesity evaluation in the United Kingdom 103 participants	• ≥95th percentile BMI for age and sex[130] • Abnormal glucose homeostasis (fasting hyperinsulinemia prepubertal ≥15 mg/L, midpuberty ≥30 mg/L, postpubertal ≥20 mU/L; impaired fasting glucose ≤110 mg/dL; impaired glucose tolerance min ≥140 mg/dL) • ≥95th percentile SBP or DBP for age and sex[131] • dyslipidemia (elevated triglycerides ≥1.75 mM/L, low HDL ≤ 0.9 mM/L, high TC ≥ 95th percentile)[132]	Three or more criteria	Obese: 33% Males: 34% Females: 33% 12–18 yr: 36% 2–11 yr: 30% White: 37% Black: 13% Asian: 22%
Invitti et al., 2006[36]	Clinic-based sample of 6–16-yr-old obese Italian youth undergoing an evaluation in Italy 588 participants	• Glucose intolerance (fasting glucose ≥100 mg/dL and/or 2 h postload glucose ≥140 mg/dL) and/or insulin resistance defined by being ≥ the median of the Tanner stage (I–V) specific HOMA-IR values (2.4, 2.8, 3.0, 4.1, or 3.0) • BMI or waist circumference ≥97th percentile of a control population • HDL cholesterol ≤5th percentile of a control population • Triglycerides ≥95th percentile of a control population • Blood pressure ≥95th percentile of a control population	Glucose intolerance/ Insulin resistance plus two or more of the other factors	Obese: 23.3% BMI tertiles I Z =2.0–3.5: 16% II Z = 3.6–4.1: 23% II Z = 4.2–6.2: 31% No sex differences
Yoshinaga et al., 2005[133]	School-based sample of 6–11-yr-old Japanese overweight or obese youth 471 participants	• ≥90th percentile WC for age and sex of study cohort • ≥120 SBP or ≥70 mm Hg DBP for grades 1–3 or ≥130 SBP or ≥80 mm Hg DBP for grades 4–6 • <40 mg/dL HDL • >120 mg/dL TG • >100 mg/dL fasting glucose	Three or more criteria	Obese: 17.7% Overweight: 8.7%
Sherry et al., 2005[134]	Clinic-based sample of obese 2–10-yr-old US children of Dominican ancestry 193 participants	• Z score >2.0 for BMI in study cohort • <40 mg/dL HDL • >150 mg/dL TG • ≥90th percentile SBP or DBP for age, sex, and height[122] • ≥100 mg/dL fasting insulin	BMI plus any two of the other risk factors	Obese: 14.3%
Cruz et al., 2004[35]	Clinic-based US sample of obese 8–13-yr-old Hispanic youth with a family history of type 2 diabetes 126 participants	• ≥90th percentile WC for age, gender, and ethnicity[129] • ≥90th percentile SBP or DBP for age, sex, and height[128] • ≥90th percentile TG for age and sex[132] • ≤10th percentile HDL for age and sex[132] • OGTT 2 h glucose 140–199 mg/dL	Three or more criteria	Obese: 30% No sex differences
Weiss et al., 2004[34]	Clinic-based US sample of obese 4–20 yr-old children and adolescents 439 participants	• >97th percentile BMI or Z score ≥2.0 in study cohort • >95th percentile TG for age, sex, and race (NGHS)[26] • <5th percentile HDL for age, sex, and race (NGHS)[26] • OGTT 2 h glucose 140–199 mg/dL • >95th percentile SBP or DBP for age, sex, and height[128]	Three or more criteria	Moderately obese: 38.7% Severely obese: 49.7%
Csabi et al., 2000[40]	Hospital-based sample of 8–18-yr-old Hungarian children and adolescents 180 obese children	110 mg/dL TG • >200 mg/dL TC • <35 mg/dL HDL • OGTT 2 h glucose 140–200 mg/dL • >18.7 µU/mL fasting insulin	Four or more criteria	Obese: 8.9%

DBP = diastolic blood pressure; HDL = high-density lipoprotein; LDL = low-density lipoprotein; MAP = mean arterial pressure; NCEP = National Cholesterol Education Program; OGTT = oral glucose tolerance test; SBP = systolic blood pressure; TC = total cholesterol; TG = triglycerides; WC = waist circumference; WHO = World Health Organization.

CDC growth charts were used to define percentiles of BMI for age and sex unless otherwise noted.[135]

The variability in the magnitude of estimates of prevalence across studies is at least in part due to differences in the definitions or criteria used to define the syndrome. Goodman[28] used NCEP criteria and WHO criteria to compare the presence of metabolic syndrome in the same school-based sample of adolescents and found large differences in prevalence. The prevalence was approximately two times higher when using the WHO versus the NCEP definition, overall and for subgroups defined by gender and BMI, although missing data on blood pressure for half the sample may also have affected the differences in the prevalence estimates. Chi and colleagues[39] examined the prevalence of metabolic syndrome in two cohorts of preadolescent girls from California, a community-based study of 261 Black preadolescent females (Girls Health Enrichment MultiSite studies, GEMS) and a school-based, cross-sectional study of 240 ethnically diverse preadolescent females [Girls Activity, Movement and Environmental Strategy (GAMES)] using several different definitions published in the literature on children. In general, agreement among the various pediatric definitions of metabolic syndrome was poor. The prevalence of metabolic syndrome and cardiovascular risk factor clustering ranged from 0.4 to 23.0% for the GEMS cohort and 2.0 to 24.6% for the GAMES cohort when using definitions adapted from the NCEP ATP III, and 0 to 15.3% for the GEMS cohort and 0.4 to 15.8% for the GAMES cohort when using modified criteria from the WHO. The prevalence of the syndrome was also shown to be much higher when internal study cohort percentiles were used to define cut points of risk factors rather than national pediatric reference data. The Bogalusa Heart Study has similarly reported large differences in the prevalence of risk factor clustering within the same cohort of youth, depending on the type and number of criteria used to define clustering.[13,31,37,38] In addition, studies that have not included a measure of total of central adiposity in the definition[29,40] or have required more than three criteria[13,31,40] have reported a lower prevalence.

Obesity

Obesity is an accepted major risk factor for metabolic syndrome in both children and adults.[7,41–44] Greater overall body weight and central adiposity predispose children to having the metabolic syndrome and the individual metabolic complications of hypertension, dyslipidemia, impaired glucose tolerance, and hyperinsulinemia.[38,45–48] In the Bogalusa Heart Study cohort, Freedman and colleagues[38] found that overweight children, defined as having a BMI at or above the 85th percentile, were more likely to have elevated total cholesterol (OR = 2.4; 95% CI 2.0 to 3.0), diastolic blood pressure (OR = 2.4; 95% CI 1.8 to 3.0), systolic blood pressure (OR = 4.5; 95% CI 3.6 to 5.8), LDL cholesterol (OR = 3.0; 95% CI 2.4 to 3.6), triglycerides (OR = 7.1; 95% CI 5.8 to 8.6), insulin (OR = 12.6; 95% CI 10 to 16), and low HDL (OR = 3.4; 95% CI 2.8 to 4.2). Overweight children were also much more likely to have clustering of risk factors with the odds ratio for having four or more risk factors being 43.5 and 29.8 in 5- to 10-year-old and 11- to 17-year-old children, respectively when compared to children who were not overweight. In this cohort, central or abdominal distribution of body fat was related to adverse concentrations of risk factors, and waist circumference showed the most consistent and strongest positive association with insulin levels and adverse concentrations of lipids.[47,48] Compared with subjects in the 10th percentile of waist circumference, a child in the 90th percentile had on average higher concentrations of LDL cholesterol (+0.17 mmol/L) and triacylglycerols (+0.11 mmol/L) and lower concentrations of HDL cholesterol (−0.07 mmol/L). Maffeis and colleagues[46] found similar associations with adiposity in a sample of children ages 3 to 11 years. ApoA1/ApoB, HDL cholesterol, total cholesterol/HDL cholesterol, and systolic as well as diastolic BP were significantly associated with waist circumference and triceps and subscapular skinfolds, independently of BMI. Children with a waist circumference greater than the 90th percentile were more likely to have multiple risk factors (low HDL, high LDL, and high blood pressure) than children with a waist circumference less at or below the 90th percentile. The relationship between waist circumference and risk factor clustering has been attributed to the effects of excess visceral fat. Intra-abdominal fat has been shown to be highly and positively correlated with basal insulin levels (r = .55) and triacylglycerols (r = .53) and negatively correlated with HDL cholesterol (r = −.54) in obese adolescent girls.[49] Similar associations have been observed between visceral adipose tissue and cardiovascular risk factors in obese adolescent boys and girls (r = .27 for triglycerides; r = .30 for systolic blood pressure; r = .27 for LDL cholesterol; and r = –.26 for HDL cholesterol).[50]

In longitudinal analyses, childhood obesity and central obesity have also been shown to be highly predictive of developing the metabolic syndrome in young adulthood. In the Bogalusa Heart Study, childhood obesity was the strongest predictor of developing metabolic syndrome in adult life. Those youth in the highest versus lowest quartile of BMI were 11.7 times (95% CI 3.4 to 39.7) more likely to develop risk factor clustering as adults.[13] Vanhala and colleagues[51] found that childhood obesity increased the risk for developing metabolic syndrome as an adult nearly threefold (OR = 2.9; 95% CI 1.1 to 7.6). In a follow-up evaluation of the National Heart Lung and Blood Institute (NHLBI) Girls Growth and Health (NGHS) cohort of 2,379 Black and White girls ages 9 and 10 years at baseline, waist circumference at 10- to 11-years-old was an independent predictor of the development of metabolic syndrome at ages 18 to 19 years (OR = 1.16; 95% CI 1.07 to 1.27), and baseline BMI was not significant after adjusting for waist circumference.[26] The tracking coefficient for waist circumference was strong with 72% of girls maintaining increased central adiposity during the follow-up period. These data highlight the importance of obesity prevention and treatment in childhood and adolescence to prevent development of the metabolic syndrome in adulthood. In addition, waist circumference, as well as BMI, may be an important measure that can be used to identify high-risk youth in clinical practice.

Insulin Resistance

Insulin resistance has been shown to be associated with clustering of cardiovascular risk factors in both cross-sectional and longitudinal studies.[34,35,52–54] The degree to which this association is a result of obesity and the temporal relationship between obesity and insulin resistance is still uncertain.[9] It is not clear whether the influence of obesity is entirely or only in part accounted for by insulin resistance.[9] Among a cohort of Finnish children and young adults, serum insulin correlated positively with BMI, serum triglycerides, and blood pressure and inversely with HDL cholesterol.[53] High levels of these risk factors clustered among subjects in the highest quartile of insulin levels. The proportion of subjects having at least two risk factors was approximately 24% in the highest quartile of insulin compared to 9% in the lowest quartile of insulin. Weiss and colleagues[34] found that insulin resistance according to the homeostatic-model assessment was significantly associated with presence of the metabolic syndrome in obese youth who exceeded the 97th percentile for BMI (OR = 1.12 for each unit increase in insulin resistance; 95% CI 1.07 to 1.18), independently of degree of obesity. Among Hispanic children, insulin sensitivity as measured by the modified frequently sampled IV glucose tolerance test decreased significantly as the number of features of the metabolic syndrome increased and was associated with all the individual components of the metabolic syndrome whereas total fat mass as measured by DEXA was not.[35] Insulin sensitivity but not fat mass was independently and negatively related to triglycerides and blood pressure, and positively related to HDL. Insulin sensitivity, adjusted for fat mass, was 62% lower in overweight youth with metabolic syndrome as compared to youth without the metabolic syndrome. Similar associations have been observed prospectively in the Bogalusa Heart Study and Cardiovascular Risk in Young Finns Study. Among subjects from the Bogalusa Study cohort ages 5- to 23-years-old at baseline, those with insulin levels consistently in the highest quartile compared to those in the lowest quartile showed higher BMI (+9 kg/m^2), triglycerides (+58 mg/dL), LDL cholesterol (+11 mg/dL), systolic blood pressure (+7 mm Hg) and diastolic blood pressure (+3 mm Hg), and lower levels of HDL cholesterol (−4 mg/dL) as adults.[54] As adults, those with consistently elevated insulin compared to those with persistently low insulin had an increased prevalence of obesity (71.6% vs 1.9%), dyslipidemia (35.1% vs 13.6%), and hypertension (14.5% vs 6.3%). In the Cardiovascular

Risk in Young Finns cohort who were ages 6 to 24 years at baseline, fasting insulin at baseline was positively related to the development of clustering of high triglycerides, low HDL cholesterol, and high systolic blood pressure after 6 years of follow-up, even after adjusting for baseline obesity and changes in obesity status over time.[52]

In contrast, other studies have found that adiposity has a stronger contribution to clustering of risk factors than insulin resistance, and the effect of insulin resistance is accounted for by obesity. In a school-based sample of youth, both insulin and BMI were strongly associated with clustering individually; however, the independent contribution of adiposity defined by BMI (OR = 2.8; 95% CI 1.9 to 3.2) was stronger than fasting insulin (OR = 1.4; 95% CI 1.0 to 2.0) when these measures were modeled simultaneously.[24] The Bogalusa Heart Study found that the increased risk for developing clustering as an adult was independently associated with childhood BMI but not fasting insulin.[13] These findings suggest that more than one pathophysiologic process may be accounting for the development of risk factor clustering or the metabolic syndrome in youth.

BIOLOGY

The pathophysiologic mechanisms underlying the development of the metabolic syndrome are multifactorial and incompletely understood[9,17,41,42,55,56;] however, obesity has a fundamental role. The effect of obesity is thought to be mediated, at least in part by the role of the adipocyte in controlling circulating free fatty acids and the development of insulin resistance.[9,56] Obesity is accompanied by high levels of nonesterified fatty acids released from adipose tissue that cause insulin resistance in skeletal muscle and overload the liver with lipid, producing fatty liver and atherogenic dylipidemia.[57,58] If free fatty acids are elevated over an extended period, inadequate insulin may be released for the degree of insulin resistance, resulting in hyperglycemia and type 2 diabetes.[59,60] Functional defects among the obese with type 2 diabetes have included decreased insulin-stimulated glucose transport and metabolism in adipocytes and skeletal muscle and impaired suppression of hepatic glucose release.[59] The increased free fatty acids associated with obesity are metabolized to triglycerides, which accounts in part for the associated hypertriglyceridemia.[41,61] This is also associated with a reduction in lipoprotein lipase action in peripheral tissues and the liver and leads to decreased clearance of VLDL and hypertriglyceridemia.[62] The mechanism for the decreased HDL cholesterol is less well understood but is thought to be secondary to the delayed metabolism of triglyceride-rich lipoproteins.[61] The increased triglyceride-rich LDL is rapidly lipolyzed by hepatic lipase to small, dense LDL, and increases in small, dense LDL particles are observed.[61] Nearly 50% of hypertensive adults are insulin resistant, and several mechanisms have been proposed for the link between insulin resistance and hypertension.[63] Insulin increases sodium retention and is associated with increased sympathetic nervous system activity and stimulation of vascular smooth muscle cell growth.[64] Central or intra-abdominal adiposity is more strongly linked to insulin resistance than peripheral distribution and this may be in part attributed to the more lipolytically active intra-abdominal adipocytes and their capacity to release free fatty acids into the liver via the portal circulation, although exact mechanisms are still uncertain.[61] Animal models support the major role of visceral fat. Rats whose visceral fat is removed do not develop insulin resistance.[65]

Adipocytes have been shown to have endocrine functions and release factors that may also help explain the major role of obesity and clustering of metabolic risk factors.[57] Adipose tissue secretes a variety of proteins known as adipocytokines including tumor necrosis factor-alpha (TNF-α), adiponectin, and interleukin-6 (IL-6), which suggest a role for inflammation in the pathway for development of metabolic syndrome. Elevations of inflammatory markers are associated with the development of metabolic risk factors and the metabolic syndrome[66–69] and accelerated atherosclerosis.[70] Treatments with anti-inflammatory mechanisms of action further support a causal role of inflammation. It is known that lipid-lowering therapies (statins) have anti-inflammatory properties and they may also lower risk of type 2 diabetes.[71] Insulin-sensitizing agents such as thiazolinediones[72] and exercise[73] also appear to be anti-inflammatory. Therefore, although the pathophysiology for developing risk factor clustering appears to be largely attributable to insulin resistance, a proinflammatory state likely contributes to the development of the syndrome and its adverse cardiovascular health outcomes.

ADVERSE HEALTH OUTCOMES

The adverse cardiovascular health outcomes associated with the metabolic syndrome have been well described in adults. Adults with the syndrome are at increased risk for morbidity and mortality from CVD.[3,4] Several large prospective cohort studies have shown that metabolic syndrome confers an approximate two-fold increase in the relative risk for atherosclerotic cardiovascular disease events.[4,74–78] Gami and colleagues[79] recently conducted a meta-analysis of longitudinal studies that examined cardiovascular health outcomes in subjects with metabolic syndrome. Among 37 eligible studies that included 43 cohorts established from 1971 to 1997 and 172,573 individuals, those with metabolic syndrome had a 1.78 times (95% CI 1.58 to 2.00) increased risk of cardiovascular events and death when compared to those without the syndrome. The association was stronger in women than men (RR= 2.63 vs 1.98, p = .09) and in studies using the WHO definition versus the NCEP definition (RR= 2.06 vs 1.67, p = .005). The association was attenuated but remained significant after adjusting for traditional cardiovascular risk factors (RR = 1.54, 95% CI 1.32 to 1.79). The value of the diagnosis of metabolic syndrome in clinical practice has been questioned[21,80] and some have suggested that the diagnosis does not provide unique clinical information beyond the risks associated with the individual metabolic risk factors.[21] However, these data suggest that the metabolic syndrome is a clinical entity that increases risk of CVD independent of the risk associated with its individual components, and thus individuals with the syndrome warrant evaluation and targeted intervention in clinical practice.

The longer term health implications of metabolic syndrome for youth, and in particular overweight youth, are still unknown. The available data suggest that the clustering of risk factors in youth can have significant health consequences with the potential for the earlier presentation of type 2 diabetes and cardiovascular disease. This is supported by the concomitant rising rates of obesity[81,82] and type 2 diabetes in youth[83,84] and the presence of early lesions of atherosclerosis.[85] Childhood obesity is a significant and growing public health problem. National data from 1999 to 2002 show that 16% of children and adolescents aged 6 to 19 years are overweight, indicating a 45% increase from 1994 to 1998 surveys and more than a doubling from 1980.[81,82] Along with the increasing prevalence of obesity, there has been an increase in the prevalence of youth with type 2 diabetes, largely and almost exclusively among obese youth. Type 2 diabetes had previously been estimated to account for less than 5% of all childhood diabetes[83]; however, recent national data have suggested a significant increase to 29% of all childhood diabetes.[86] Furthermore, autopsy studies of youth have shown an association between early lesions of atherosclerosis and obesity or the presence of metabolic risk factors.[85,87] In the Pathobiological Determinants of Atherosclerosis in Youth (PDAY) study, obesity was shown to accelerate the progression of coronary atherosclerosis in adolescent and young men based on measurement of fatty streaks and raised atherosclerotic lesions of the coronary arteries found at autopsy.[85] Berenson and colleagues[87] evaluated the presence of aortic and coronary atherosclerosis in young individuals who died of accidental causes and found a striking increase in the extent of lesions with obesity and an increasing number of metabolic syndrome risk factors. Among the cardiovascular risk factors, BMI, systolic and diastolic blood pressure, and serum concentrations of total cholesterol, triglycerides, LDL cholesterol, and HDL cholesterol, the cluster was strongly associated with the extent of lesions in the aorta and coronary arteries (r = .70; p < .001). Youth with none, 1, 2, and 3 or 4 risk factors had 19.1, 30.3, 37.9, and 35% of the intimal surface of the aorta covered with fatty streaks (p for trend = .01), respectively. This trend was similar for fatty streaks and collagenous fibrous plaques of the coronary arteries. As the number of cardiovascular risk factors increased, so did the severity of asymptomatic coronary and aortic atherosclerosis in young people.

The association of cardiovascular risk factor levels and the metabolic syndrome with carotid artery intima thickness, a subclinical marker of atherosclerotic heart disease and predictor of adult clinical coronary artery disease, implies that having high levels of these risk factors in childhood can lead to premature onset of disease and an increased risk of CVD in adulthood. Iannuzzi and colleagues[88] studied 100 obese children aged 6 to 14 years and found that common carotid stiffness was significantly higher in the group of obese children with metabolic syndrome compared to those without metabolic syndrome (1.29 ± 0.06 mm vs 1.12 ± 0.04 mm, respectively; $p < .03$). In the Bogalusa Heart Study, the levels of cardiovascular risk factors in childhood were associated with carotid intima-media thickness (IMT) in young adulthood.[89] Specifically, increasing LDL cholesterol and BMI were significantly and positively associated with carotid IMT. The odds ratio associated with being in the highest quartile of carotid IMT compared to the lower three quartiles was 1.45 (95% CI 1.14 to 1.78) for every unit increase in LDL cholesterol and 1.25 (95% CI 1.01 to 1.54) for every unit increase in BMI. The cumulative effect of HDL cholesterol levels measured from childhood to adulthood was protective. Increasing HDL cholesterol was inversely associated with carotid IMT (OR = 0.75, 95% CI 0.58 to 0.97). The Cardiovascular Risk in Young Finns study similarly found that cardiovascular risk factor levels assessed in 12- to 18-year-old adolescents, including elevated BMI, LDL cholesterol, and systolic blood pressure, were significantly associated with increased carotid IMT in young adulthood.[90] Likewise, having low levels of metabolic syndrome variables in childhood can be beneficial in adulthood. In the Bogalusa Heart Study, mean carotid IMT values in adulthood decreased significantly as the number of risk variables at the lowest quartiles in childhood increased (p for trend = .013).[91]

The occurrence of risk factor clustering in childhood is also more likely to be maintained into adulthood. Limited prospective data have also shown that clustering of metabolic risk factors in childhood track into adulthood and predict the development of metabolic syndrome in adulthood. In the Bogalusa Heart Study, a multiple risk index, calculated as sum of the race-, sex-, and age-specific rankings of systolic blood pressure, insulin level, and total to HDL cholesterol ratio, was shown to significantly track over an 8-year follow-up period in all race–sex groups (correlations ranged from 0.54 to 0.67). The magnitude of the overall multiple risk index tracking correlation ($r = .64$) was significantly stronger than the individual risk factor correlations ($r = .34$ to .57). Among subjects who were initially in the highest quintile of the multiple risk index at baseline, 61% remained there 8 years later.[8] Furthermore, after an average follow-up period of 15.8 years, there was a significant positive relationship between childhood and adulthood clustering of cardiovascular risk factor variables. Children with clustering of three or more versus less than three risk factor variables that included BMI, SBP, HOMA-IR, and total cholesterol to HDL cholesterol ratio had a nearly three-fold higher prevalence of metabolic syndrome in adulthood (12.9% vs 4.6%, respectively; $p = .005$).[91]

More immediate comorbidities for children and adolescents as well as adults with metabolic syndrome are polycystic ovary syndrome (PCOS) and nonalcoholic fatty liver disease (NAFLD). The cooccurrence of both conditions with metabolic syndrome may be accounted for in part by obesity and insulin resistance. Studies have shown that between 35 and 75% of women with PCOS are obese,[92] and NAFLD has been estimated to affect 22.5 to 52.8% of obese children.[93] Azziz[94] compared the prevalence of metabolic syndrome among 129 women, aged 18 to 49 years, with PCOS to normal controls and found that the metabolic syndrome was diagnosed in 34.9% of women with PCOS compared to 6.8% of the controls. Adolescent girls with PCOS have a similarly higher prevalence of metabolic syndrome. In a sample of 49 adolescent girls with PCOS and 165 adolescents from the Third National Health and Nutrition Examination Survey (NHANES III) of similar age and ethnicity, 37% of adolescent girls with PCOS had metabolic syndrome compared with 5% of NHANES III girls ($p < .0001$).[95] None of the girls of normal BMI with PCOS had metabolic syndrome, whereas 11% of overweight and 63% of obese girls with PCOS also had metabolic syndrome. After adjusting for BMI, the increased prevalence of metabolic syndrome among those with PCOS was substantially attenuated but significant (OR = 4.5; 95% CI 1.1 to 17.7; $p = .03$). Gluek and colleagues[96] compared 37 adolescent girls with PCOS to two samples of normal controls and found that girls with PCOS had higher levels of several metabolic risk factor variables including BMI, waist circumference, insulin, LDL-C, triglycerides, systolic blood pressure and diastolic blood pressure, and lower levels of HDL-C. After matching on BMI and age, only waist circumference and free testosterone remained higher. In this sample, central obesity appeared to be a common causal link between having PCOS and metabolic risk factors.

Data also support an association between NAFLD and the metabolic syndrome.[97] Among adults, the metabolic syndrome is a strong predictor for the development of nonalcoholic fatty liver disease. Hamaguchi and colleagues[98] examined the role of the metabolic syndrome in the development of NAFLD among 4,401 Japanese men and women. Men and women who met the criteria for the metabolic syndrome at baseline were four times more likely to develop NAFLD during follow-up (95% CI 2.63 to 6.08), and nonalcoholic fatty liver disease was less likely to regress in those participants with the metabolic syndrome at baseline. Metabolic syndrome has also been shown to be an independent risk factor for severity of fatty liver. Kang and colleagues[99] found that metabolic syndrome was a significant risk factor for global NASH severity (OR =3.48; 95% CI 1.22 to 9.85). Patients with metabolic syndrome had higher scores for steatosis, NASH activity, and global NASH score compared with those without metabolic syndrome. Data in children are limited to use of liver transaminases as a surrogate marker of liver steatosis but suggest a similar association. Among Korean adolescents, the metabolic syndrome was strongly associated with elevated ALT concentrations, and this association existed in a graded fashion across the number of metabolic components.[100] The odds ratio for having an elevated ALT among those with metabolic syndrome versus those not having the syndrome was 6.2 (95% CI 2.3 to 16.8). The risk was graded and increased with the number of components of the syndrome; the odds ratios for elevated ALT were 1.5 (95% CI 0.7 to 3.1), 2.6 (95% CI 1.1 to 6.2), and 6.2 (95% CI 2.3 to 16.8) in the adolescents with 1, 2, and 3 or more risk factors, respectively.

SCREENING, PREVENTION, AND TREATMENT

At this time, general screening of all children for metabolic syndrome is not recommended. Given the strong association with obesity, overweight or obese children should be carefully evaluated for components of the metabolic syndrome. Evaluation of overweight or obese children should include screening for metabolic risk factors including blood pressure, fasting glucose and insulin, HbA1C, fasting lipids, as well as the complications of obesity, which include a history of irregular menstrual periods, acne, and hirsutism for PCOS in adolescent girls and liver enzymes for NAFLD in males and females.[101]

National guidelines for the treatment of metabolic syndrome in youth are lacking. In the absence of national guidelines, recommendations for adults can be extended to children. The ATP III panel[17] and IDF[20] recommend lifestyle intervention as the primary approach to multiple risk factor prevention and reduction. The major lifestyle interventions include weight loss in overweight or obese subjects, increased physical activity, and improved dietary quality. These changes are expected to produce a reduction in all of the metabolic risk factors simultaneously.[2] Weight reduction of 10 to 15% has been shown to improve insulin sensitivity and prevent type 2 diabetes and metabolic syndrome in adults with glucose intolerance and may be as effective in obese children. Toumilehto and colleagues[102] demonstrated that a lifestyle intervention can significantly decrease the proportion of persons with impaired glucose tolerance who progress to type 2 diabetes. The Diabetes Prevention Study lifestyle intervention consisted of advice on how to decrease weight by 5% or more, decrease intake of total and saturated fat, and increase fiber, and individual guidance on increasing physical activity to 30 min/d, including counseling on ways to improve cardiorespiratory fitness as well as muscle strength. The trial found an overall 58% lower incidence of type 2 diabetes in the intervention compared to control group (RR = 0.4; 95% CI 0.3 to 0.7). A benefit was observed even among those who did not achieve the weight loss goal but achieved the physical activity goal of 4 h/wk in the first year (RR = 0.2; 95% CI 0.3 to 1.1). The Diabetes Prevention Program Research Group also demonstrated that a lifestyle intervention consisting of a low-fat, low-calorie diet and moderate physical activity for 150 min/wk significantly reduced the incidence of diabetes by 58% (95% CI 48 to 66%) among nondiabetic adults with elevated fasting or postload glucose compared to placebo.[103] This reduction was greater than the 31% (95% CI 17 to 43%) reduction achieved by metformin (850 mg twice daily) alone. The incidence of developing metabolic syndrome was reduced by 41% in the lifestyle group ($p < .001$) and by 17% in the metformin group ($p = .03$) compared with placebo.[104]

Large randomized trials of lifestyle interventions in youth are lacking; however, small, short-term lifestyle interventions have shown beneficial effects on the metabolic syndrome and its individual components. Overweight youth aged 8 to 16 years participated in a nonrandomized 12-week family lifestyle-centered intervention that included weekly moderate to vigorous exercise sessions and healthy eating education to reduce or limit intake of total and saturated fat, cholesterol, and carbohydrates.[105] At baseline, 49.5% had metabolic syndrome and 10% impaired glucose metabolism. Although weight did not decrease, BMI, lipids, and 2 h post-OGTT glucose all improved significantly, and improvements in metabolic factors were independent of changes in BMI. Chen and colleagues[106] placed 16 children on a high-fiber, low-fat diet in a 2-week residential program where food was provided ad libitum, and daily aerobic exercise was performed. Before the intervention, 7 of the 16 children were classified as having metabolic syndrome and none had the syndrome after the intervention. BMI showed a significant decrease from 33.2 to 31.8 ($p < .01$). All the components of the syndrome decreased significantly except HDL, which showed no significant change. The study demonstrates that a short-term rigorous diet and exercise program can reverse the metabolic syndrome. In a randomized crossover trial, 4 months of a 40 min exercise program significantly improved measures of total body fat, plasma triglycerides, and fasting insulin levels in obese children ages 7- to 11-years-old.[107] In addition to favorable changes in cardiovascular risk factors, Wunsch and colleagues[108] have shown that in obese children who participated in an intensive 1-year outpatient lifestyle intervention, those with substantial reductions in BMI (mean 2.2 unit decrease in BMI) had significant decreases in carotid IMT as well as lipids, blood pressure, and insulin. Lifestyle interventions in children can improve metabolic risk factors and potentially reverse early atherosclerotic changes and future risk of adult onset CVD.

In both adults and children, there is no specific drug recommended or approved for the treatment of metabolic syndrome independent of those agents that are most appropriate for specific risk factors. Recommendations for drug therapy are based on current clinical guidelines established for each specific risk factor. For each risk factor, lifestyle intervention is generally the first-line therapy. The American Heart Association recommends the following dietary and physical activity goals to promote a healthy lifestyle in youth and reduce cardiovascular risk.[109] The diet should include a variety of fruits and vegetables, whole grains, dairy products, fish, legumes, poultry, and lean meat. After age 2 years, saturated fat should be limited to less than 10% of total calories per day, cholesterol should be limited to less than 300 mg/d, and intake of foods high in trans fatty acids should be minimal. Salt intake should also be limited to less than 6 g/d for order children and adolescents and intake of sugar should be limited. They also advise youth to participate in at least 60 min of moderate to vigorous physical activity every day. Adolescents may combine 10 to 15 min of resistance training in the overall activity program. Sedentary time should be limited, and TV time should be no more than 2 h/d. For patients whose risk factors are not improved with lifestyle changes or weight loss, pharmacologic interventions to reduce triglycerides, blood pressure, or control blood glucose may be indicated. Finally, although bariatric surgery is not a specific indication for patients with metabolic syndrome, it has been shown to have a dramatic effect on the metabolic syndrome in morbidly obese adults due to its profound effect on weight loss. Among 645 consecutive morbidly obese adult patients, aged 18 to 63 years with mean BMI 43 kg/m^2 who presented for bariatric surgery, 52.2% met ATP III criteria for metabolic syndrome.[110] Laparoscopic vertical banding was performed in 528 patients and gastric bypass in 117 patients, and mean weight loss after 1 year was 38.4 g and 35.1 kg, respectively. Substantial and significant improvements were observed in blood pressure, weight, glucose triglycerides, and total cholesterol. Among those with metabolic syndrome, mean weight decreased to 38.2 kg, and average reductions of individual risk factors were 11.0 mm Hg for systolic blood pressure, 11.4 mm Hg for diastolic blood pressure, 46.1 mg/dL for glucose, 196.6 mg/dL for triglycerides, and 33.7 mg/dL for total cholesterol. These risk factor reductions resulted in a 95.6% resolution of metabolic syndrome that did not differ between procedures after 1 year. Table 3 summarizes the clinical guidelines and recommendations for the treatment of the individual risk factors for the metabolic syndrome in children and adolescents.

Overweight or Obesity

The current lifestyle strategies for the treatment of overweight in children are similar to those in adults and focus on dietary modification and physical activity to achieve treatment goals.[101] Treatment goals for youth depend on age, severity of obesity, and presence of comorbid conditions. For children, goals may include a slowed rate of weight gain, weight maintenance to improve BMI with increasing height, or gradual weight loss.[101] Children who are at or above the 95th percentile for BMI with comorbid conditions as well as adolescents who are at or above the 95th percentile for BMI without comorbid conditions should seek to achieve a gradual weight loss of 1 to 2 kg/mo and the need for additional treatment of any associated conditions should be evaluated. In addition to lifestyle intervention for weight loss, the only pharmacologic agent approved for use in adolescents (12 yr and older) as an adjunct to diet therapy is Orlistat.[111] However, weight loss has been modest and gastrointestinal side effects can be significant.[112] Bariatric surgery may be considered for the very obese adolescents with serious comorbidities who have failed organized weight loss efforts.[113]

Dyslipidemia

Mild elevations of triglycerides (150 to 400 mg/dL) can be treated with lifestyle intervention that focuses on diet and exercise.[114] Dietary modifications include limiting intake of simple sugars and refined carbohydrates, reducing saturated fat intake, and increasing intake of dietary fish rich in DHA and EPA. Fish oil supplementation with marine-derived n-3 fatty acids, DHA, and EPA are known to dramatically decrease triglyceride levels in adults and may serve as an important adjunct to lifestyle strategies.[115–118] Approximately 3 to 4 g/d of combined EPA and DHA in the form of supplements lowers triglycerides 25 to 30%.[117–118] One study has examined supplementation of omega-3 fatty acids in children[119] but at lower than therapeutic doses of only DHA (1.2 g/d). There was a small (11%) nonsignificant decrease in fasting triglycerides from 133 mg/dL to 119 mg/dL (SD = 71) in the treated group. Lifestyle intervention is also advised for levels between 400 and 1,000 mg/dL; however, if levels are not responsive to dietary intervention, pharmacotherapy is advised.[109] Triglyceride levels above 1,000 mg/dL are associated with significant risk of pancreatitis[120] and pharmacotherapy in combination with lifestyle is recommended. If uncontrolled diabetes is not the root cause, and this should be evaluated, fibrates should be considered to lower triglycerides. Gemfibrozil in the dose of 600 mg/d, or fenofibrate, has been used in adults with preexisting cardiovascular disease, and has been shown to lower rates of further events by 22%.[121] It acts by increasing the production of lipoprotein lipase, which helps clear triglycerides and VLDL, and via hepatic peroxisome proliferator activated receptor (PPAR)-α to increase fatty acid oxidation. Fenofibrate is supplied in micronized and nonmicronized forms; the dose depends on the form. A generic formulation is available. Gemfibrozil may increase LDL and is not appropriate as monotherapy for those with combination disorders in which the LDL is elevated. These medications carry with them a risk of mypopathy,

Table 3 Metabolic Syndrome Risk Factor Reduction Guidelines

At Risk of Overweight or Overweight/Obese	Reduction Guidelines
• At Risk: BMI from 85th to below 95th percentile for age and sex • Overweight/Obese: BMI ⩾95th percentile for age and sex	• For children who are at risk of overweight (85th to below the 95th percentile for age and sex) or overweight/obese (>95th percentile) for age and sex, a weight management program should be initiated with lifestyle changes to support appropriate energy balance achieved through changes in diet and physical activity • Match energy needs for normal growth and development • Maintain weight or slow rate of weight gain for younger children to achieve healthy BMI with growth in height • Gradual weight loss (1–2 kg/mo) in overweight adolescents or in very overweight younger children or in those with comorbid conditions such as hypertension or insulin resistance
Dyslipidemia	
• Fasting triglycerides >150 mg/dL	• Lifestyle intervention to promote achievement of appropriate weight (BMI < 85th percentile for age and sex) with appropriate energy intake and energy expenditure • Decrease intake of simple sugars • Evaluate for secondary causes such as diabetes, thyroid disease, renal disease, and alcohol abuse • Pharmacologic interventions are not recommended in children for isolated elevation of fasting TG unless this is very marked elevation. Treatment with gemfibrozil or fenofibrate may be initiated at TG >400 mg/dL to protect against postprandial TG of 1,000 mg/dL or greater, which may be associated with an increased risk of pancreatitis
• HDL cholesterol <35 mg/dL	• Lifestyle intervention to promote achievement of appropriate weight (BMI <85th percentile for age and sex) with appropriate energy intake and energy expenditure • Promote increased physical activity to at least 60 min of moderate to vigorous physical activity daily • Pharmacologic intervention is not currently recommended for treatment of isolated low HDL
Elevated blood pressure	
• Prehypertension: Systolic and/or diastolic blood pressure from the 90th to <95th percentile for age, sex, and height, or if blood pressure exceeds 120/80 mm Hg in an adolescent • Stage 1: Systolic and/or diastolic blood pressure from the 95th to the 99th percentile for age, sex, and height plus 5 mm Hg • Stage 2: Systolic and/ or diastolic blood pressure >99th percentile for age, sex, and height plus 5 mm Hg	• Lifestyle intervention to promote achievement of appropriate weight (BMI <85th percentile for age and sex) with appropriate energy intake and energy expenditure • Reduce sodium in the diet. Emphasize increased consumption of fruits and vegetables • Evaluate for secondary causes (eg, renal disease, coarctation of the aorta) • Consider pharmacologic therapy for individuals above the 95th percentile if lifestyle modification brings no improvement and there is evidence of target organ changes (left ventricular hypertrophy, microalbuminuria, retinal vascular abnormalities). Angiotensin converting enzyme inhibitor or angiotensin receptor blocker are appropriate first-line treatments in patients with metabolic syndrome
Insulin resistance	
• Fasting plasma glucose 100–125 mg/dL and /or • OGTT 2 h glucose 140–199 mg/dL	• Lifestyle intervention to promote achievement of appropriate weight (BMI <85th percentile for age and sex) with appropriate energy intake and energy expenditure and decreased intake of simple sugars • Consider pharmacologic therapy in patients who are not responsive to lifestyle intervention or who have additional cardiovascular risk factors, a significant family history of type 2 diabetes, or liver steatosis, or for females, those who also have polycystic ovary syndrome. Insulin-sensitizing agents such as metformin may be considered

BMI = body mass index; HDL = high-density lipoprotein; OGTT = oral glucose tolerance test; TG = triglycerides.
Adapted from reference 109.

particularly when combined with a statin, and the two are rarely combined in children. Other side effects include hepatotoxicity (increases in liver function tests), and increase in fibrinolysis, as well as gastrointestinal upset. There is no FDA indication for either medication in pediatrics and their use is generally confined to extreme cases and older adolescents.

Low HDL levels, although associated with increased atherosclerotic burden and increased cardiovascular risk in adults, are not at this time the target of pharmacotherapy in pediatric patients. They are, however, modifying risk factors for those with elevated LDL and most practitioners consider low levels when contemplating recommending LDL-lowering agents. HDL levels are increased by statins, niacin, exercise, and monounsaturated fats. At present, isolated low HDL has not generally been treated by pharmacotherapy in pediatrics.

Hypertension

Blood pressure elevations should be assessed using established recommendations described in the *Fourth Report on the Diagnosis, Evaluation and Treatment of High Blood Pressure in Children and Adolescents.*[122] Lifestyle modification, which includes aerobic exercise, weight reduction, and salt restriction, should be part of the approach to treatment of all patients with hypertension.[123] If hypertension is either severe (step 2 hypertension, blood pressure at or above the 99th percentile for age, sex, and height) or accompanied by end-organ effects (left ventricular hypertrophy, renal scarring, ophthalmologic changes), pharmacotherapy should also be initiated. As children or adolescents with metabolic syndrome necessarily have other cardiovascular risk factors, earlier rather than later use of pharmacotherapy should be considered. Although many medications are appropriate as first-line therapy in unselected groups of children, those with metabolic syndrome are likely best served by starting with an angiotensin converting enzyme inhibitor or angiotensin receptor blocker, as it may serve to protect renal function by minimizing albuminuria, an element of the metabolic syndrome. Beta-blockers cause slight increases in serum glucose levels and are likely not the best choice for this group of patients. Thiazides can increase triglyceride levels and glucose levels, and are also not ideal first-line therapy for this patient population.

Insulin Resistance

The main modality for treating insulin resistance in children and adolescents is again lifestyle modification. In general, studies in adults have shown that lifestyle interventions appear to be equally as effective as pharmacologic interventions with oral diabetic agents in preventing type 2 diabetes among patients with impaired glucose tolerance.[124] However, some practitioners are initiating metformin in older adolescents in an effort to prevent progression to type 2 diabetes mellitus in patients with clear metabolic syndrome who have borderline elevated fasting glucose levels (100 to 125 mg/dL) or impaired 2 h oral glucose tolerance tests (140 to 199 mg/dL). Metformin has been shown to be an effective treatment of type 2 diabetes in children[125] and to increase insulin sensitivity in hyperinsulinemic, obese adolescents,[126,127] but data on its effectiveness in the prevention of type 2 diabetes in youth are lacking. Metformin may also be a valuable adjunct to treatment of obese patients with PCOS or liver steatosis.[111] Generally, starting at 500 mg twice a day induces a small amount of weight loss or at least weight stabilization, along with some improvement in lipid levels. Monitoring of renal function (BUN and creatinine) is recommended and the effect can be assessed by measuring HgbA1C levels. There is no FDA approval for this indication in children, and studies are ongoing.

FUTURE DIRECTIONS

The high prevalence of metabolic syndrome in obese youth, the tendency for risk factors in childhood to track into adulthood, and the increased association of metabolic risk factors with subclinical markers of atherosclerotic disease underscore the importance of defining and better understanding the health implications of metabolic syndrome in children and adolescents. A clinically useful consensus definition and national guidelines are needed for proper screening, evaluation, and treatment of overweight children.[5–7] Additional research is also needed to understand the pathophysiology of the syndrome and identify and evaluate new treatment strategies in children. An improved understanding of the pathophysiology may provide insights into a single therapy that can target a common etiologic factor and affect multiple risk factors simultaneously.[9]

REFERENCES

1. Grundy SM. Metabolic syndrome: Connecting and reconciling cardiovascular and diabetes worlds. J Am Coll Cardiol 2006;47:1093–100.
2. Grundy SM, Cleeman JI, Daniels SR, et al. Diagnosis and management of the metabolic syndrome: An American Heart Association/National Heart, Lung, and Blood Institute scientific statement. Curr Opin Cardiol 2006;21:1–6.
3. Ferrannini E, Stern MP, Galvan AQ, et al. Impact of associated conditions on glycemic control of NIDDM patients. Diabetes Care 1992;15:508–14.
4. Isomaa B, Almgren P, Tuomi T, et al. Cardiovascular morbidity and mortality associated with the metabolic syndrome. Diabetes Care 2001;24:683–9.
5. Bitsori M, Kafatos A. Dysmetabolic syndrome in childhood and adolescence. Acta Paediatr 2005;94:995–1005.
6. Cruz ML, Goran MI. The metabolic syndrome in children and adolescents. Curr Diab Rep 2004;4:53–62.
7. Steinberger J. Diagnosis of the metabolic syndrome in children. Curr Opin Lipidol 2003;14:555–9.
8. Bao W, Srinivasan SR, Wattigney WA, Berenson GS. Persistence of multiple cardiovascular risk clustering related to syndrome X from childhood to young adulthood. The Bogalusa Heart Study. Arch Intern Med 1994;154:1842–7.
9. Miranda PJ, DeFronzo RA, Califf RM, Guyton JR. Metabolic syndrome: Definition, pathophysiology, and mechanisms. Am Heart J 2005;149:33–45.
10. Cook S, Weitzman M, Auinger P, et al. Prevalence of a metabolic syndrome phenotype in adolescents: Findings from the third National Health and Nutrition Examination Survey, 1988–1994. Arch Pediatr Adolesc Med 2003;157:821–7.
11. Duncan GE, Li SM, Zhou XH. Prevalence and trends of a metabolic syndrome phenotype among U.S. Adolescents, 1999–2000. Diabetes Care 2004;27:2438–43.
12. de Ferranti SD, Gauvreau K, Ludwig DS, et al. Inflammation and changes in metabolic syndrome abnormalities in US adolescents: Findings from the 1988–1994 and 1999–2000 National Health and Nutrition Examination Surveys. Clin Chem 2006;52:1325–30.
13. Srinivasan SR, Myers L, Berenson GS. Predictability of childhood adiposity and insulin for developing insulin resistance syndrome (syndrome X) in young adulthood: The Bogalusa Heart Study. Diabetes 2002;51:204–9.
14. Executive Summary of the Third Report of the National Cholesterol Education Program (NCEP) Expert Panel on Detection, Evaluation, and Treatment of High Blood Cholesterol in Adults (Adult Treatment Panel III). JAMA 2001;285:2486–97.
15. Reaven GM. Banting lecture 1988. Role of insulin resistance in human disease. Diabetes 1988;37:1595–607.
16. Grundy SM, Brewer HB, Jr, Cleeman JI, et al. Definition of metabolic syndrome: Report of the National Heart, Lung, and Blood Institute/American Heart Association conference on scientific issues related to definition. Circulation 2004;109:433–8.
17. Grundy SM, Hansen B, Smith SC, Jr, et al. Clinical management of metabolic syndrome: Report of the American Heart Association/National Heart, Lung, and Blood Institute/American Diabetes Association conference on scientific issues related to management. Circulation 2004;109:551–6.
18. Alberti KG, Zimmet PZ. Definition, diagnosis and classification of diabetes mellitus and its complications. Part 1: Diagnosis and classification of diabetes mellitus provisional report of a WHO consultation. Diabet Med 1998; 15:539–53.
19. Definition, diagnosis and classification of diabetes mellitus and its complications. Report of a WHO consultation. Part 1. Diagnosis and classification of diabetes mellitus. Geneva, World Health Organization, 1999 (document WHO/NCD/NCS/99.2).
20. The IDF consensus worldwide definition of the metabolic syndrome. Part 1. Worldwide definition for use in clinical practice. Available at: www.idf.org. Accessed December 1, 2006.
21. Reaven GM. The metabolic syndrome: Is this diagnosis necessary? Am J Clin Nutr 2006;83:1237–47.
22. Park YW, Zhu S, Palaniappan L, et al. The metabolic syndrome: Prevalence and associated risk factor findings in the US population from the Third National Health and Nutrition Examination Survey, 1988–1994. Arch Intern Med 2003;163:427–36.
23. Ford ES, Giles WH, Dietz WH. Prevalence of the metabolic syndrome among US adults: Findings from the third National Health and Nutrition Examination Survey. JAMA 2002;287:356–9.
24. Lambert M, Paradis G, O'Loughlin J, et al. Insulin resistance syndrome in a representative sample of children and adolescents from Quebec, Canada. Int J Obes Relat Metab Disord 2004;28:833–41.
25. Raitakari OT, Porkka KV, Viikari JS, et al. Clustering of risk factors for coronary heart disease in children and adolescents. The Cardiovascular Risk in Young Finns Study. Acta Paediatr 1994;83:935–40.
26. Morrison JA, Friedman LA, Harlan WR, et al. Development of the metabolic syndrome in black and white adolescent girls: A longitudinal assessment. Pediatrics 2005;116: 1178–82.
27. Rodriguez-Moran M, Salazar-Vazquez B, Violante R, Guerrero-Romero F. Metabolic syndrome among children and adolescents aged 10–18 years. Diabetes Care 2004;27:2516–7.
28. Goodman E, Daniels SR, Morrison JA, et al. Contrasting prevalence of and demographic disparities in the World Health Organization and National Cholesterol Education Program Adult Treatment Panel III definitions of metabolic syndrome among adolescents. J Pediatr 2004;145:445–51.
29. Chu NF, Rimm EB, Wang DJ, et al. Clustering of cardiovascular disease risk factors among obese schoolchildren: The Taipei Children Heart Study. Am J Clin Nutr 1998;67:1141–6.
30. Braunschweig CL, Gomez S, Liang H, et al. Obesity and risk factors for the metabolic syndrome among low-income, urban, African American schoolchildren: The rule rather than the exception? Am J Clin Nutr 2005;81:970–5.
31. Chen W, Srinivasan SR, Elkasabany A, Berenson GS. Cardiovascular risk factors clustering features of insulin resistance syndrome (Syndrome X) in a biracial (Black-White) population of children, adolescents, and young adults: The Bogalusa Heart Study. Am J Epidemiol 1999;150:667–74.
32. Retnakaran R, Zinman B, Connelly PW, et al. Nontraditional cardiovascular risk factors in pediatric metabolic syndrome. J Pediatr 2006;148:176–82.
33. Viner RM, Segal TY, Lichtarowicz-Krynska E, Hindmarsh P. Prevalence of the insulin resistance syndrome in obesity. Arch Dis Child 2005;90:10–4.
34. Weiss R, Dziura J, Burgert TS, et al. Obesity and the metabolic syndrome in children and adolescents. N Engl J Med 2004;350:2362–74.
35. Cruz ML, Weigensberg MJ, Huang TT, et al. The metabolic syndrome in overweight Hispanic youth and the role of insulin sensitivity. J Clin Endocrinol Metab 2004;89:108–13.
36. Invitti C, Maffeis C, Gilardini L, et al. Metabolic syndrome in obese Caucasian children: Prevalence using WHO-derived criteria and association with nontraditional cardiovascular risk factors. Int J Obes (Lond) 2006;30:627–33.
37. Katzmarzyk PT, Srinivasan SR, Chen W, et al. Body mass index, waist circumference, and clustering of cardiovascular disease risk factors in a biracial sample of children and adolescents. Pediatrics 2004;114:e198–205.
38. Freedman DS, Dietz WH, Srinivasan SR, Berenson GS. The relation of overweight to cardiovascular risk factors among children and adolescents: The Bogalusa Heart Study. Pediatrics 1999;103:1175–82.
39. Chi CH, Wang Y, Wilson DM, Robinson TN. Definition of metabolic syndrome in preadolescent girls. J Pediatr 2006;148:788–92.
40. Csabi G, Torok K, Jeges S, Molnar D. Presence of metabolic cardiovascular syndrome in obese children. Eur J Pediatr 2000;159:91–4.
41. DeFronzo RA, Ferrannini E. Insulin resistance. A multifaceted syndrome responsible for NIDDM, obesity, hypertension, dyslipidemia, and atherosclerotic cardiovascular disease. Diabetes Care 1991;14:173–94.
42. Liese AD, Mayer-Davis EJ, Haffner SM. Development of the multiple metabolic syndrome: An epidemiologic perspective. Epidemiol Rev 1998;20:157–72.
43. Palaniappan L, Carnethon MR, Wang Y, et al. Predictors of the incident metabolic syndrome in adults: The Insulin Resistance Atherosclerosis Study. Diabetes Care 2004;27:788–93.
44. Edwards KL, Burchfiel CM, Sharp DS, et al. Factors of the insulin resistance syndrome in nondiabetic and diabetic elderly Japanese-American men. Am J Epidemiol 1998;147:441–7.
45. Esmaillzadeh A, Mirmiran P, Azizi F. Clustering of metabolic abnormalities in adolescents with the hypertriglyceridemic waist phenotype. Am J Clin Nutr 2006;83:36–46; quiz 183–4.
46. Maffeis C, Pietrobelli A, Grezzani A, et al. Waist circumference and cardiovascular risk factors in prepubertal children. Obes Res 2001;9:179–87.
47. Freedman DS, Serdula MK, Srinivasan SR, Berenson GS. Relation of circumferences and skinfold thicknesses to lipid and insulin concentrations in children and adolescents: The Bogalusa Heart Study. Am J Clin Nutr 1999;69: 308–17.
48. Freedman DS, Srinivasan SR, Burke GL, et al. Relation of body fat distribution to hyperinsulinemia in children and adolescents: The Bogalusa Heart Study. Am J Clin Nutr 1987;46:403–10.
49. Caprio S, Hyman LD, McCarthy S, et al. Fat distribution and cardiovascular risk factors in obese adolescent girls: Importance of the intraabdominal fat depot. Am J Clin Nutr 1996;64:12–7.
50. Owens S, Gutin B, Barbeau P, et al. Visceral adipose tissue and markers of the insulin resistance syndrome in obese black and white teenagers. Obes Res 2000;8:287–93.
51. Vanhala M, Vanhala P, Kumpusalo E, et al. Relation between obesity from childhood to adulthood and the metabolic syndrome: Population-based study. BMJ 1998;317:319–320.
52. Raitakari OT, Porkka KV, Ronnemaa T, et al. The role of insulin in clustering of serum lipids and blood pressure in children and adolescents. The Cardiovascular Risk in Young Finns Study. Diabetologia 1995;38:1042–50.
53. Ronnemaa T, Knip M, Lautala P, et al. Serum insulin and other cardiovascular risk indicators in children, adolescents and young adults. Ann Med 1991;23:67–72.
54. Bao W, Srinivasan SR, Berenson GS. Persistent elevation of plasma insulin levels is associated with increased cardiovascular risk in children and young adults. The Bogalusa Heart Study. Circulation 1996;93:54–9.
55. Grundy SM, Brewer HB, Jr, Cleeman JI, et al. Definition of metabolic syndrome: Report of the National Heart, Lung, and Blood Institute/American Heart Association conference on scientific issues related to definition. Arterioscler Thromb Vasc Biol 2004;24:e13–8.
56. Bergman RN, Kim SP, Catalano KJ, et al. Why visceral fat is bad: Mechanisms of the metabolic syndrome. Obesity (Silver Spring) 2006;14:16S–19S.
57. McPherson R, Jones PH. Editorial Review: The metabolic syndrome and type 2 diabetes: role of the adipocyte. Curr Opin Lipidol 2003;14:549–53.
58. Wyne KL. Free fatty acids and type 2 diabetes mellitus. Am J Med 2003;115:29S–36S.
59. Kahn BB, Flier JS. Obesity and insulin resistance. J Clin Invest 2000;106:473–81.
60. Scheen AJ. From obesity to diabetes: Why, when and who? Acta Clin Belg 2000;55:9–15.
61. Ruotolo G, Howard BV. Dyslipidemia of the metabolic syndrome. Curr Cardiol Rep 2002;4:494–500.
62. Avramoglu RK, Qiu W, Adeli K. Mechanisms of metabolic dyslipidemia in insulin resistant states: Deregulation

of hepatic and intestinal lipoprotein secretion. Front Biosci 2003;8:d464–76.
63. Zavaroni I, Mazza S, Dall'Aglio E, et al. Prevalence of hyperinsulinaemia in patients with high blood pressure. J Intern Med 1992;231:235–40.
64. Reaven GM. Insulin resistance/compensatory hyperinsulinemia, essential hypertension, and cardiovascular disease. J Clin Endocrinol Metab 2003;88:2399–403.
65. Gabriely I, Ma XH, Yang XM, et al. Removal of visceral fat prevents insulin resistance and glucose intolerance of aging: An adipokine-mediated process? Diabetes 2002;51:2951–8.
66. Ford ES, Ajani UA, Mokdad AH. The metabolic syndrome and concentrations of C-reactive protein among U.S. youth. Diabetes Care 2005;28:878–81.
67. Rutter MK, Meigs JB, Sullivan LM, et al. C-reactive protein, the metabolic syndrome, and prediction of cardiovascular events in the Framingham Offspring Study. Circulation 2004;110:380–5.
68. Frohlich M, Imhof A, Berg G, et al. Association between C-reactive protein and features of the metabolic syndrome: A population-based study. Diabetes Care 2000;23:1835–9.
69. Festa A, D'Agostino R, Jr, Howard G, et al. Chronic subclinical inflammation as part of the insulin resistance syndrome: The Insulin Resistance Atherosclerosis Study (IRAS). Circulation 2000;102:42–7.
70. Grundy SM. Inflammation, hypertension, and the metabolic syndrome. JAMA 2003;290:3000–2.
71. Palinski W. New evidence for beneficial effects of statins unrelated to lipid lowering. Arterioscler Thromb Vasc Biol 2001;21:3–5.
72. Thiemermann C. Ligands of the peroxisome proliferator-activated receptor-gamma and heart failure. Br J Pharmacol 2004;141:1–3.
73. Smith JK, Dykes R, Douglas JE, et al. Long-term exercise and atherogenic activity of blood mononuclear cells in persons at risk of developing ischemic heart disease. JAMA 1999;281:1722–7.
74. Lakka HM, Laaksonen DE, Lakka TA, et al. The metabolic syndrome and total and cardiovascular disease mortality in middle-aged men. JAMA 2002;288:2709–16.
75. Wilson PW, D'Agostino RB, Parise H, et al. Metabolic syndrome as a precursor of cardiovascular disease and type 2 diabetes mellitus. Circulation 2005;112:3066–72.
76. McNeill AM, Rosamond WD, Girman CJ, et al. The metabolic syndrome and 11-year risk of incident cardiovascular disease in the atherosclerosis risk in communities study. Diabetes Care 2005;28:385–90.
77. Malik S, Wong ND, Franklin SS, et al. Impact of the metabolic syndrome on mortality from coronary heart disease, cardiovascular disease, and all causes in United States adults. Circulation 2004;110:1245–50.
78. Hunt KJ, Resendez RG, Williams K, et al. National Cholesterol Education Program versus World Health Organization metabolic syndrome in relation to all-cause and cardiovascular mortality in the San Antonio Heart Study. Circulation 2004;110:1251–7.
79. Gami AS, Witt BJ, Howard DE, et al. Metabolic syndrome and risk of incident cardiovascular events and death: A systematic review and meta-analysis of longitudinal studies. J Am Coll Cardiol 2007;49:403–14.
80. Grundy SM. Does a diagnosis of metabolic syndrome have value in clinical practice? Am J Clin Nutr 2006;83:1248–51.
81. Hedley AA, Ogden CL, Johnson CL, et al. Prevalence of overweight and obesity among US children, adolescents, and adults, 1999-2002. JAMA 2004;291:2847–50.
82. Ogden CL, Flegal KM, Carroll MD, Johnson CL. Prevalence and trends in overweight among US children and adolescents, 1999-2000. JAMA 2002;288:1728–32.
83. Fagot-Campagna A, Pettitt DJ, Engelgau MM, et al. Type 2 diabetes among North American children and adolescents: An epidemiologic review and a public health perspective. J Pediatr 2000;136:664–72.
84. Rosenbloom AL, Joe JR, Young RS, Winter WE. Emerging epidemic of type 2 diabetes in youth. Diabetes Care 1999;22:345–54.
85. McGill HC, Jr, McMahan CA, Herderick EE, et al. Obesity accelerates the progression of coronary atherosclerosis in young men. Circulation 2002;105:2712–8.
86. Duncan GE. Prevalence of diabetes and impaired fasting glucose levels among US adolescents: National Health and Nutrition Examination Survey, 1999–2002. Arch Pediatr Adolesc Med 2006;160:523–8.
87. Berenson GS, Srinivasan SR, Bao W, et al. Association between multiple cardiovascular risk factors and atherosclerosis in children and young adults. The Bogalusa Heart Study. N Engl J Med 1998;338:1650–6.
88. Iannuzzi A, Licenziati MR, Acampora C, et al. Carotid artery stiffness in obese children with the metabolic syndrome. Am J Cardiol 2006;97:528–31.
89. Li S, Chen W, Srinivasan SR, et al. Childhood cardiovascular risk factors and carotid vascular changes in adulthood: The Bogalusa Heart Study. JAMA 2003;290:2271–6.
90. Raitakari OT, Juonala M, Kahonen M, et al. Cardiovascular risk factors in childhood and carotid artery intima-media thickness in adulthood: The Cardiovascular Risk in Young Finns Study. JAMA 2003;290:2277–83.
91. Chen W, Srinivasan SR, Li S, et al. Metabolic syndrome variables at low levels in childhood are beneficially associated with adulthood cardiovascular risk: The Bogalusa Heart Study. Diabetes Care 2005;28:126–31.
92. Ehrmann DA. Polycystic ovary syndrome. N Engl J Med 2005;352:1223–36.
93. Angulo P. Nonalcoholic fatty liver disease. N Engl J Med 2002;346:1221–31.
94. Azziz R. How prevalent is metabolic syndrome in women with polycystic ovary syndrome? Nat Clin Pract Endocrinol Metab 2006;2:132–3.
95. Coviello AD, Legro RS, Dunaif A. Adolescent girls with polycystic ovary syndrome have an increased risk of the metabolic syndrome associated with increasing androgen levels independent of obesity and insulin resistance. J Clin Endocrinol Metab 2006;91:492–7.
96. Glueck CJ, Morrison JA, Friedman LA, et al. Obesity, free testosterone, and cardiovascular risk factors in adolescents with polycystic ovary syndrome and regularly cycling adolescents. Metabolism 2006;55:508–14.
97. Collantes RS, Ong JP, Younossi ZM. The metabolic syndrome and nonalcoholic fatty liver disease. Panminerva Med 2006;48:41–8.
98. Hamaguchi M, Kojima T, Takeda N, et al. The metabolic syndrome as a predictor of nonalcoholic fatty liver disease. Ann Intern Med 2005;143:722–8.
99. Kang H, Greenson JK, Omo JT, et al. Metabolic syndrome is associated with greater histologic severity, higher carbohydrate, and lower fat diet in patients with NAFLD. Am J Gastroenterol 2006;101:2247–53.
100. Park HS, Han JH, Choi KM, Kim SM. Relation between elevated serum alanine aminotransferase and metabolic syndrome in Korean adolescents. Am J Clin Nutr 2005;82:1046–51.
101. Daniels SR, Arnett DK, Eckel RH, et al. Overweight in children and adolescents: Pathophysiology, consequences, prevention, and treatment. Circulation 2005;111:1999–2012.
102. Tuomilehto J, Lindstrom J, Eriksson JG, et al. Prevention of type 2 diabetes mellitus by changes in lifestyle among subjects with impaired glucose tolerance. N Engl J Med 2001;344:1343–50.
103. Knowler WC, Barrett-Connor E, Fowler SE, et al. Reduction in the incidence of type 2 diabetes with lifestyle intervention or metformin. N Engl J Med 2002;346:393–403.
104. Orchard TJ, Temprosa M, Goldberg R, et al. The effect of metformin and intensive lifestyle intervention on the metabolic syndrome: The Diabetes Prevention Program randomized trial. Ann Intern Med 2005;142:611–9.
105. Monzavi R, Dreimane D, Geffner ME, et al. Improvement in risk factors for metabolic syndrome and insulin resistance in overweight youth who are treated with lifestyle intervention. Pediatrics 2006;117:e1111–8.
106. Chen AK, Roberts CK, Barnard RJ. Effect of a short-term diet and exercise intervention on metabolic syndrome in overweight children. Metabolism 2006;55:871–8.
107. Ferguson MA, Gutin B, Le NA, et al. Effects of exercise training and its cessation on components of the insulin resistance syndrome in obese children. Int J Obes Relat Metab Disord 1999;23:889–95.
108. Wunsch R, de Sousa G, Toschke AM, Reinehr T. Intima-media thickness in obese children before and after weight loss. Pediatrics 2006;118:2334–40.
109. Kavey RE, Daniels SR, Lauer RM, et al. American Heart Association guidelines for primary prevention of atherosclerotic cardiovascular disease beginning in childhood. Circulation 2003;107:1562–6.
110. Lee WJ, Huang MT, Wang W, et al. Effects of obesity surgery on the metabolic syndrome. Arch Surg 2004;139:1088–92.
111. Freemark M. Pharmacotherapy of Childhood Obesity: An evidence-based, conceptual approach. Diabetes Care 2007;30:395–402.
112. Chanoine JP, Hampl S, Jensen C, et al. Effect of orlistat on weight and body composition in obese adolescents: A randomized controlled trial. JAMA 2005;293:2873–83.
113. Inge TH, Krebs NF, Garcia VF, et al. Bariatric surgery for severely overweight adolescents: concerns and recommendations. Pediatrics 2004;114:217–23.
114. Coughlan BJ, Sorrentino MJ. Does hypertriglyceridemia increase risk for CAD? Growing evidence suggests it plays a role. Postgrad Med 2000;108:77–84.
115. Carpentier YA, Portois L, Malaisse WJ. N-3 fatty acids and the metabolic syndrome. Am J Clin Nutr 2006;83: 1499S–504S.
116. Bucher HC, Hengstler P, Schindler C, Meier G. N-3 polyunsaturated fatty acids in coronary heart disease: A meta-analysis of randomized controlled trials. Am J Med 2002;112:298–304.
117. Harris WS. N-3 fatty acids and serum lipoproteins: Human studies. Am J Clin Nutr 1997;65:1645S–54S.
118. Harris WS, Ginsberg HN, Arunakul N, et al. Safety and efficacy of Omacor in severe hypertriglyceridemia. J Cardiovasc Risk 1997;4:385–91.
119. Engler MM, Engler MB, Malloy MJ, et al. Effect of docosahexaenoic acid on lipoprotein subclasses in hyperlipidemic children (the EARLY study). Am J Cardiol 2005;95:869–71.
120. Toskes PP. Hyperlipidemic pancreatitis. Gastroenterol Clin North Am 1990;19:783–91.
121. Staels B, Dallongeville J, Auwerx J, et al. Mechanism of action of fibrates on lipid and lipoprotein metabolism. Circulation 1998;98:2088–93.
122. National High Blood Pressure Education Program Working Group on Hypertension Control in Children and Adolescents: The fourth Report on the diagnosis, evaluation, and treatment of high blood pressure in children and adolescents. Pediatrics 2004;114:555–76.
123. Pappadis SL, Somers MJ. Hypertension in adolescents: A review of diagnosis and management. Curr Opin Pediatr 2003;15:370–8.
124. Gillies CL, Abrams KR, Lambert PC, et al. Pharmacological and lifestyle interventions to prevent or delay type 2 diabetes in people with impaired glucose tolerance: Systematic review and meta-analysis. BMJ 2007;334:299.
125. Urakami T. How should we treat type 2 diabetes in youth? Pediatr Endocrinol Rev 2005;3:33–9.
126. Kay JP, Alemzadeh R, Langley G, et al. Beneficial effects of metformin in normoglycemic morbidly obese adolescents. Metabolism 2001;50:1457–61.
127. Freemark M, Bursey D. The effects of metformin on body mass index and glucose tolerance in obese adolescents with fasting hyperinsulinemia and a family history of type 2 diabetes. Pediatrics 2001;107:E55.
128. National High Blood Pressure Education Program Working Group on Hypertension Control in Children and Adolescents: Update on the 1987 Task Force Report on High Blood Pressure in Children and Adolescents: A working group report from the National High Blood Pressure Education Program. National High Blood Pressure Education Working Group on Hypertension Control in Children and Adolescents. Pediatrics 1996;98:649–58.
129. Fernandez JR, Redden DT, Pietrobelli A, Allison DB. Waist circumference percentiles in nationally representative samples of African-American, European-American, and Mexican-American children and adolescents. J Pediatr 2004;145:439–44.
130. Cole TJ, Freeman JV, Preece MA. Boy Mass Index Reference Curves for the UK 1990. Arch Dis Child 1995;73:25–9.
131. Task Force on Blood Pressure Control in Children. Report of the Second Task Force on Blood Pressure Control in Children-1987. Pediatrics 1987;79:1–25.
132. Hickman TB, Briefel RR, Carroll MD, et al. Distributions and trends of serum lipid levels among United States children and adolescents ages 4–19 years. Data from the Third National Health and Nutrition Examination Survey. Prev Med 1998;27:879–80.
133. Yoshinaga M, Tanaka S, Shimago A, et al. Metabolic syndrome in overweight and obese Japanese children. Obes Res 2005;13:1135–40.
134. Sherry N, Hassoun A, Oberfield SE, et al. Clinical and metabolic characteristics of an obese, Dominican, pediatric population. J Pediatr Endocrinol Metab 2005;18:1063–71.
135. Kuczmarski RJ, Ogden CL, Grummer-Strawn LM, et al CDC Growth Charts: United States. Adv Data 2000;314:1–27.

41

Popular Diets for Obesity

Kendrin Sonneville, MS, RD, LDN

INTRODUCTION

As the prevalence of overweight in children and adolescents increases, so does the demand for effective treatment strategies. Without active intervention, resolution of the pediatric overweight epidemic and its associated comorbidities is unlikely.[1] Commercial weight-loss programs and diet books are often used by adults who desire to lose weight, although the popularity and success of these diets far outweigh the evidence to support their use.[2] Application of popular commercial diets to pediatric populations comes with an additional degree of complexity because treatment goals vary based on age and degree of overweight.[3] Further, treatment of overweight in children must take into account age-specific demands for growth to prevent a disruption in linear growth and loss of lean body mass.[4] Consequences other than physical risks must also be considered since popular diets may encourage unhealthy behaviors such as the thought that there is only one potential solution to weight loss.[5]

DESCRIPTION OF DIETS

Weight-reduction strategies vary substantially between popular diet plans. Principles emphasized in popular diets include portion control and caloric restriction (Weight Watchers), limiting carbohydrate intake without reduction in dietary fat intake (Atkins), eating moderate amounts of low–glycemic-index carbohydrates combined with lean proteins and heart-healthy fats (South Beach), macronutrient balance (Zone), and fat restriction (Pritkin and Ornish).[6] In addition to the dietary advice offered by each popular diet, lifestyle recommendations including physical activity and meditation are often also made.

To date, popular diets have not been studied for safety or efficacy in trials with children and adolescents. Two randomized trials have compared the dietary recommendations made by these diets in adults. In a trial by Dansinger and colleagues, adherence rates and effectiveness of the dietary recommendations of four popular diets (Atkins, Zone, Weight Watchers, and Ornish) were compared and a modest reduction in weight was observed in each of the four groups.[6] The amount of weight loss after 1 year did not differ between diet types, although increased adherence was associated with greater weight loss. Although there is no consensus regarding the effect of macronutrient composition on energy expenditure, weight loss, and weight control,[7] this finding suggests that offering a variety of diet options which can be matched to an individual's food preferences and may help to improve the effectiveness of popular diets in adults.[6] In the *A TO Z Weight Loss Study*, Gardner and colleagues compared the effectiveness of four weight loss diet plans in overweight and obese nondiabetic, premenopausal women.[8] Participants were randomly assigned to follow diets outlined by one of four popular diet books: *Dr Atkins' New Diet Revolution, Enter the Zone*[9] by Barrry Sears, *The LEARN Manual for Weight Management*[10] by Kelly Brownell, or *Eat More, Weigh Less*[11] by Dean Ornish. The primary outcome, weight loss at 12 months, was greatest for women following the Atkins diet. Mean weight loss at 12 months for the Atkins diet was −4.7 kg, compared to −1.6 kg for the Zone diet, −2.6 kg for LEARN, and −2.2 kg for the Ornish plan.

Despite this limited evidence, commercial diets remain popular among adult consumers, further underscoring the need for more trials to demonstrate their effectiveness and safety,[12] particularly among children and adolescents who may adopt dieting behaviors used by their parents. In the absence of data on popular diets per se, data from the existing, albeit heterogeneous, trials of weight-loss diets can be used to identify elements of popular diets which may be efficacious in treating childhood overweight. The American Dietetic Association's (ADA) Evidence Analysis Library[13] examined the evidence from two overarching categories of diets: balanced macronutrient diets and altered macronutrient diets.[13] A brief review of this analysis will be summarized here.

SUMMARY OF EVIDENCE

Balanced Macronutrient Diets

The ADA's Evidence Analysis concluded that trials of reduced calorie diets (>1,200 kcal/d) in 6- to 12-year-olds have shown inconsistent results[13–24]; however, low-calorie diets (900 to 1,200 kcal/d) show consistent reduction in short-term and long-term adiposity measures.[13,25–30] All of the studies of reduced calorie diets (>1,200 kcal/d) utilize the Traffic Light Diet (sometimes called the Stop Light Diet) developed by Leonard H. Epstein and colleagues[31] for use in their family based childhood overweight research.[13] The goal of the diet is to encourage foods that maximize nutrient intake while keeping caloric intake to a minimum (see Table 1 for a description of the Traffic Light Diet). Although the outcomes were not completely consistent, the research does show that in both the short term and long term, reduced calorie diets (>1,200 kcal/d) may be an effective part of a multicomponent weight-management (weight-loss or weight-stabilization) program in children aged 6 to 12 years.[13] It is unclear, however, what proportion of this effect may be attributed exclusively to the dietary component of this multicomponent approach.[13] The use of low-calorie diets in adolescents has been less well studied and findings are much more variable.[13,32–37]

Altered Macronutrient Diets: Altered Carbohydrate

Two types of altered carbohydrate diets are commonly used: an ad libitum low-glycemic diet and an ad libitum low-carbohydrate diet.[13]

Low Glycemic. Studies using the low-glycemic approach have found a reduction in caloric intake and therefore weight loss on these diets which may be at least partly due to an inadvertent reduction in caloric intake.[13] Three studies have examined the use of a low–glycemic-load diet in the treatment of childhood overweight and all reported a significant decrease in at least one measure of adiposity.[13,32,38,39] The use of an ad libitum low-glycemic diet may be effective for modest, short-term weight loss in children (age 6 to 12 years), and may be effective for longer term weight loss in adolescents.[13]

Low Carbohydrate. The definition of a low-carbohydrate diet varies substantially throughout the literature. In the ADA's Evidence Analysis Library, a diet was considered "low carbohydrate" only if the dietary prescription for percent of daily energy intake for carbohydrates was lower than Dietary Reference Intake (DRI) recommendations (45 to 65%).[13] The single low-carbohydrate diet study analyzed indicated that adolescents on ad libitum, low-carbohydrate diets lose weight and improve BMI in the short term; however, there is too little research to be able to determine whether calorie-unrestricted low-carbohydrate diets would be effective in long term (>1 year).[13,33] Until more data from clinical trials are available on the safety and efficacy of low-carbohydrate diets in children and adolescents, this approach should not be recommended for general pediatric use.[40]

Table 1 Traffic Light Diet[13]

At a minimum, Epstein's Traffic Light Diet has the following characteristics:

- Foods are divided into five categories:
  1. Fruits and vegetables
  2. Grains
  3. Milk and dairy
  4. Protein
  5. Other
- Foods in each category are color coded according to caloric density per average serving:
  1. *Green foods:* foods containing < 20 cal per average serving
  2. *Yellow foods:* staples of the diet that provide most of the nutrition
  3. *Red foods:* foods high in fat and simple carbohydrates (eg, sweets and sugared drinks)
- Daily calorie intake is determined for program participants with a minimum of 900 cal and a maximum of 1,200 cal (a range of 1,200–1,500 cal in some later studies)
- Families are provided with a food reference guide listing foods according to their color code and group
- Families are given two goals:
  1. Stay within the prescribed calorie range
  2. Eat no more than four red foods a week
- Families are also strongly encouraged to remove all red foods from their homes
- When participants reach the obesity criterion, they are provided instructions in developing a maintenance calorie level, which involves gradually increasing energy intake in 100 kcal/d increments each week until weight gain occurs

In addition to the basic diet, participants in Epstein's family based research program may also be provided with a number of other supports to help them adhere to the diet. These include:

- *Self-monitoring training and support:* Families are taught how to use a food diary, how to chart their weight, and if appropriate, how to record their physical activity. Parents are encouraged to review their children's records for accuracy and completeness
- *Praise and modeling:* Parents and children are taught the importance of serving as models for other family members as well as the importance of praise for family members who make their goals
- *Therapist contact:* Each family may also receive therapist contact, (The amount and type of contact may vary by research study.) Family members may have weekly to monthly contact with the therapist for help with self-monitoring, feedback, to answer questions, and new materials. In some cases, parents may even engage in activity with the therapist
- *Contracting:* Families are provided a financial incentive to complete the program. For instance, money paid up front for participation in the program may be refunded in increments, as the family completes different stages of the program

Altered Macronutrient Diets: Altered Protein

High-protein, low-carbohydrate, very low calorie diets, often called "protein sparing modified fast" diets, are discussed in Chapter 39, "Evaluation and Management of Obesity." Some experts suggest that there are a number of theoretical benefits to this approach, including increased thermogenesis and satiety associated with higher protein diets.[13] The ADA's Evidence Analysis Library concluded that there is insufficient evidence to suggest that high-protein, low-carbohydrate, very low calorie diets result in greater long-term weight loss in children compared to balanced macronutrient diets at the same calorie intake level.[13,41–47] Because all studies on the use of a protein sparing modified fast diet were from the same pediatric weight-loss program,[42–47] it is difficult to quantify the contribution of the dietary recommendations of the multicomponent program on the effectiveness of the program.

CONCLUSIONS AND RECOMMENDATIONS

Current research has begun to examine the use of caloric and macronutrient manipulation in the treatment of pediatric overweight; however, insufficient evidence exists to recommend a standardized approach for weight loss. Until conclusive evidence is available, clinicians must rely on the best available, rather than best possible, evidence. Individualized approaches that encourage behavior modification that involve changes in energy intake and/or energy expenditure with the ultimate goal of achieving negative energy balance should be adopted. In a recent review of treatment options for pediatric obesity, Kirk and colleagues recommend the following strategies for improving diet quality and reducing caloric intake:

- establish a regular meal and snack pattern;
- eat smaller portions at meals and snacks;
- limit second helpings to fresh fruit or nonstarchy vegetables;
- drink more water and other sugar-free drinks to replace sweetened beverages;
- select lower fat dairy products;
- eat more foods that are baked, broiled, grilled, or boiled, instead of fried;
- select healthful snacks that include a low-fat protein source along with fresh fruit, vegetables, or whole-grain bread or cereals; and
- when eating out, select more healthful options or split larger servings to share with other family members or peers.[48]

In conjunction with these dietary strategies, an increase in physical activity and a reduction in sedentary activities, particularly television viewing, should be encouraged. Kirk and colleagues also recommend adopting effective strategies used in adult weight management, such as using motivational interviewing to increase readiness for health behavior changes, modifying the carbohydrate content of the diet, using culturally appropriate messages and materials, and improving cultural competency of health care providers.[48]

Family based changes are likely to be more sustainable and less stigmatizing than behavior change recommendations directed at an individual child and are encouraged for families with overweight children. Changes that will benefit all members of the family such as removing sugary drinks and juices, keeping fast food consumption to a minimum, and limiting the television viewing should be promoted. Practical family based changes, recommended by W. Allan Walker in his book *Eat, Play, and Be Healthy*, include eating meals together as a family as often as possible, planning meals that include fiber-rich foods like fruits, vegetables, whole grains, and legumes, and scheduling time for daily physical activity as a family.[49]

FUTURE DIRECTIONS

Treatment recommendations for childhood overweight will be revised and improved as new literature in the field emerges. As such, reliance on Web-based resources for up-to-date information is essential. Some popular sites that may be consulted include:

http://www.cdc.gov/nccdphp/dnpa/obesity/childhood/index.htm
The Centers for Disease Control and Prevention's Childhood Overweight Web site provides up-to-date information on trends, contributing factors, and consequences of childhood overweight.

http://www.cdc.gov/HealthyYouth/overweight/index.htm
The Centers for Disease Control and Prevention's Healthy Youth Web site provides data and statistics, science-based strategies, and policy guidance for clinicians and school personnel.

http://www.aap.org/obesity/
The American Academy of Pediatrics' Overweight and Obesity Web site offers downloadable publications, chapters, and policy statements, as well as links to endorsed campaigns and initiatives.

http://www.nichq.org/NICHQ/Programs/ConferencesAndTraining/ChildhoodObesityActionNetwork.htm
The National Initiative for Children's Healthcare Quality (NICHQ) Childhood Obesity Action Network, a Web-based national network aimed at rapidly sharing knowledge and successful practices, offers tools, resources, and technical assistance for health care providers.

http://www.nhlbi.nih.gov/health/public/heart/obesity/wecan/index.htm
The National Heart, Lung, and Blood Institute's *We Can!* (Ways to Enhance Children's Activity & Nutrition) Web site offers resources and materials for patients and families.

REFERENCES

1. Steinbeck K. Childhood obesity. Treatment options. Best Pract Res Clin Endocrinol Metab 2005;19:455–69.
2. Astrup A. Atkins and other low-carbohydrate diets: Hoax or an effective tool for weight loss? Lancet 2004;364:897–9.
3. Dietz WH, Robinson TN. Clinical practice. Overweight children and adolescents. N Engl J Med 2005;352:2100–9.
4. Epstein LH, Myers MD, Raynor HA, et al. Treatment of pediatric obesity. Pediatrics 1998;101:554–70.
5. Moyad MA. Fad diets and obesity—Part IV: Low-carbohydrate vs. low-fat diets. Urol Nurs 2005;25:67–70.
6. Dansinger ML, Gleason JA, Griffith JL, et al. Comparison of the Atkins, Ornish, Weight Watchers, and Zone diets for weight loss and heart disease risk reduction: A randomized trial. JAMA 2005;293:43–53.
7. Schoeller D, Buchholz A. Energetics of obesity and weight control: Does diet composition matter? J Am Diet Assoc 2005;105:24–8.
8. Gardner CD, Kiazand A, Alhassan S, et al. Comparison of the Atkins, Zone, Ornish, and LEARN Diets for change in weight and related risk factors among overweight premenopausal women: The A to Z weight loss study: A randomized trial. JAMA 2007;297:969–77.
9. Sears B, Lawren W. Enter the Zone. New York: Harper Collins; 1995.
10. Brownell K. The LEARN Manual for Weight Management. Dallas, TX: American Health Publishing; 2000.
11. Ornish D. Eat More, Weigh Less. New York: Harper Collins; 2001.
12. Lara-Castro C, Garvey WT. Diet, insulin resistance, and obesity: Zoning in on data for Atkins dieters living in South Beach. J Clin Endocrinol Metab 2004;89:4197–205.
13. American Dietetic Association. Evidence-Based Nutrition Practice Guideline on Pediatric Weight Managment; 2007. http://www.adaevidencelibrary.com. Accessed on September 13, 2007
14. Goldfield GS, Epstein LH, Kilanowski CK, et al. Cost-effectiveness of group and mixed family-based treatment for childhood obesity. Int J Obes Relat Metab Disord 2001;25:1843–9.
15. Epstein LH, Wing RR, Penner BC, et al. Effect of diet and controlled exercise on weight loss in obese children. J Pediatr 1985;107:358–61.
16. Epstein LH, Wing RR, Koeske R, et al. A comparison of lifestyle exercise, aerobic exercise, and calisthenics on weight loss in obese children. Behav Ther 1985;16:345–56.
17. Epstein LH, Wing RR, Koeske R, et al. Effects of diet plus exercise on weight change in parents and children. J Consult Clin Psychol 1984;52:429–37.
18. Epstein LH, Wing RR, Koeske R, et al. Effect of parent weight on weight loss in obese children. J Consult Clin Psychol 1986;54:400–1.
19. Epstein LH, Valoski AM, Vara LS, et al. Effects of decreasing sedentary behavior and increasing activity on weight change in obese children. Health Psychol 1995;14:109–15.
20. Epstein LH, Valoski A, Wing RR, et al. Ten-year follow-up of behavioral, family-based treatment for obese children. JAMA 1990;264:2519–23.
21. Epstein LH, Valoski A, Wing RR, et al. Ten-year outcomes of behavioral family-based treatment for childhood obesity. Health Psychol 1994;13:373–83.
22. Epstein LH, Paluch RA, Gordy CC, et al. Decreasing sedentary behaviors in treating pediatric obesity. Arch Pediatr Adolesc Med 2000;154:220–6.
23. Epstein LH, Paluch RA, Gordy CC, et al. Problem solving in the treatment of childhood obesity. J Consult Clin Psychol 2000;68:717–21.
24. Epstein LH, Paluch RA, Raynor HA. Sex differences in obese children and siblings in family-based obesity treatment. Obes Res 2001;9:746–53.
25. Flodmark CE, Ohlsson T, Ryden O, et al. Prevention of progression to severe obesity in a group of obese schoolchildren treated with family therapy. Pediatrics 1993;91:880–4.
26. Golan M, Weizman A, Apter A, et al. Parents as the exclusive agents of change in the treatment of childhood obesity. Am J Clin Nutr 1998;67:1130–5.
27. Levine M, Ringham R, Kalarchian M, et al. Is family-based behavioral weight control appropriate for severe pediatric obesity? Int J Eat Disord 2001;30:318–28.
28. Nuutinen O. Long-term effects of dietary counseling on nutrient intake and weight loss in obese children. Eur J Clin Nutr 1991;45:287–97.
29. Eliakim A, Kaven G, Berger I, et al. The effect of a combined intervention on body mass index and fitness in obese children and adolescents—a clinical experience. Eur J Pediatr 2002;161:449–54.
30. Chen W, Chen SC, Hsu HS, et al. Counseling clinic for pediatric weight reduction: Program formulation and follow-up. J Formos Med Assoc 1997;96:59–62.
31. Epstein LH, Squires S. The Stoplight Diet for Children. Toronto, Canada: Little, Brown & Company; 1988.
32. Ebbeling CB, Leidig MM, Sinclair KB, et al. A reduced-glycemic load diet in the treatment of adolescent obesity. Arch Pediatr Adolesc Med 2003;157:773–9.
33. Sondike SB, Copperman N, Jacobson MS. Effects of a low-carbohydrate diet on weight loss and cardiovascular risk factor in overweight adolescents. J Pediatr 2003;142:253–8.
34. Wadden T, Stunkard A, Rich L, et al. Obesity in black adolescent girls: A controlled clinical trial of treatment by diet, behavior modification, and parental support. Pediatrics 1990;85:345–52.
35. Saelens B, Sallis J, Wilfley D, et al. Behavioral weight control for overweight adolescents initiated in primary care. Obes Res 2002;10:22–32.
36. Rolland-Cachera MF, Thibault H, Souberbielle JC, et al. Massive obesity in adolescents: Dietary interventions and behaviours associated with weight regain at 2 y follow-up. Int J Obes Relat Metab Disord 2004;28:514–9.
37. Maffiuletti NA, De Col A, Agosti F, et al. Effect of a 3-week body mass reduction program on body composition, muscle function and motor performance in pubertal obese boys and girls. J Endocrinol Invest 2004;27:813–20.
38. Spieth LE, Harnish JD, Lenders CM, et al. A low-glycemic index diet in the treatment of pediatric obesity. Arch Pediatr Adolesc Med 2000;154:947–51.
39. Young P, West S, Ortiz K, et al. A pilot study to determine the feasibility of the low glycemic diet as a treatment for overweight children in primary care practice. Ambul Pediatr 2004;4:28–33.
40. Kirk S, Scott B, Daniels S. Pediatric obesity epidemic: Treatment options. J Am Diet Assoc 2005;105:44–51.
41. Figueroa-Colon R, von Almen TK, Franklin FA, et al. Comparison of two hypocaloric diets in obese children. Am J Dis Child 1993;147:160–6.
42. Brown R, Sothern M, Suskind R, et al. Racial differences in the lipid profiles of obese children and adolescents before and after significant weight loss. Clin Pediatr 2000;39:427–31.
43. Sothern M, Schumacher H, von Almen T, et al. Committed to kids: An integrated, four level team approach to weight management in adolescents. J Am Diet Assoc 2002;102:S81–5.
44. Sothern M, Udall J, Suskind R, et al. Weight loss and growth velocity in obese children after very low calorie diet, exercise and behavior modification. Acta Paediatr 2000;89:1036–43.
45. Sothern M, Despinasse B, Brown R, et al. Lipid profiles of obese children and adolescents before and after significant weight loss: Differences according to sex. South Med J 2000;93:278–82.
46. Sothern M, Hunter S, Suskind R, et al. Motivating the obese child to move: The role of structured exercise in pediatric weight management. South Med J 1999;92:577–84.
47. Sothern M, Loftin M, Udall J, et al. Safety, feasibility and efficacy of a resistance training program in preadolescent obese children. Am J Med Sci 2000;319:370–5.
48. Kirk S, Scott BJ, Daniels SR. Pediatric obesity epidemic: Treatment options. J Am Diet Assoc 2005;105:44–51.
49. Walker WA. Eat, Play, and Be Healthy. New York: McGraw-Hill; 2005.

V NUTRITIONAL ASPECTS OF SPECIFIC DISEASE STATES

Feeding Difficulties

Thomas M. Foy, MD
Danita I. Czyzewski, PhD

Although primary nutrient deficiencies are now rare in developed countries, and despite substantial improvements in the health and feeding of infants in the modern era, feeding difficulties continue to challenge those who care for infants and children. It is estimated that up to 54% of infants and toddlers have problematic feeding behavior and that in 25% of children, feeding problems prompt parents to seek professional advice.[1,2] Feeding difficulties may persist and in 1 to 2% of infants will lead to retarded growth.[3,4] A survey of children with cerebral palsy found that in the first 12 months of life, 38% had problems with swallowing, 57% had problems with sucking, and more than 90% had significant oral-motor dysfunction.[5]

For infants with feeding difficulties, the goal of therapy is to achieve normal nutritional status by securing adequate intake with developmentally appropriate feedings. This chapter examines the basis of feeding disorders in infants and young children and current approaches to their evaluation and treatment.

Table 1 Normal Feeding Development

Age	Reflexes	Oral-Motor Skills	Self-Feeding
15–18-wk gestation		Sucking movement	
34–35-wk gestation		Adequate suck–swallow coordination	
Term	Phasic bite Rooting Gag	Jaw and tongue move up and down Air swallowing common	
3–4 mo	Phasic bite disappearing	Tongue protrudes in anticipation of feeding	Visual recognition of bottle/nipple
5–6 mo	Rooting diminishes	Munching begins, smacks lips together, strained foods introduced	Puts hands on breast/bottle, begins finger feeding
7 mo	Mature gag	Tongue begins lateral shift	Plays with spoon
9 mo		Lip closure, lateral tongue movement to transfer food	Holds bottle
12 mo		Rotary chewing, controlled, sustained bite	Finger feeds independently, brings spoon to mouth
18 mo		Swallows without food loss, tongue elevates intermittently or consistently	Cup drinking with two hands, spoon feeds messily
24 mo		Lips contain food/saliva within mouth, tongue transfers food one side to other side	Fills spoon with finger, spoon to mouth without inversion

Adapted from references 6 and 7.

NORMAL DEVELOPMENT AND MECHANICS

Feeding problems represent a deviation from normal feeding skill development and mechanics.[6–8] Maturation of deglutition, which begins in utero and is completed by 3 years of age, depends on integration of oral-motor, fine-motor, gross-motor, sensory, and behavioral skills. An outline of feeding development in normal infants is seen in Table 1. Whereas sucking movements can be seen at 15 to 18 weeks' gestation, adequate coordination of suck, swallow, and breathing to permit significant nutrient intake is not present until 34 to 35 weeks[2] gestation. Reflex behaviors present at term may disappear later in infancy (rooting, phasic bite) or may persist (gag, swallow).[9]

For the infant, successful feeding depends on coordination of suck, swallow, and breathing. This is facilitated by the oral anatomy of the infant, where a relatively large tongue and buccal fat pads enhance suckling, and the high position of the larynx helps to separate the digestive and respiratory tracts. As the infant grows, the larger oral cavity permits more complex oral tasks, and the deepening pharynx enlarges the common channel for swallowing and breathing. This permits advancement of the diet and requires more complex oral-motor skills.[8–10]

Sucking itself has a developmental progression, with the earliest tongue movements described as "suckling" and characterized by an in–out horizontal movement. "Sucking" appears later in infancy, indicates an up–down tongue movement with firm lip approximation, and is used in a general sense in this discussion. Swallowing, or deglutition, occurs in at least three phases, as shown in Figure 1.[9,10] The oral phase includes bolus formation of solid food or liquid by the tongue, with the soft palate lowering to prevent food from entering the pharynx and initiating a swallow. The pharyngeal phase is both voluntary and involuntary and begins as a swallow is initiated. As food enters the pharynx, the soft palate elevates to protect the nasopharynx and the larynx elevates and closes to

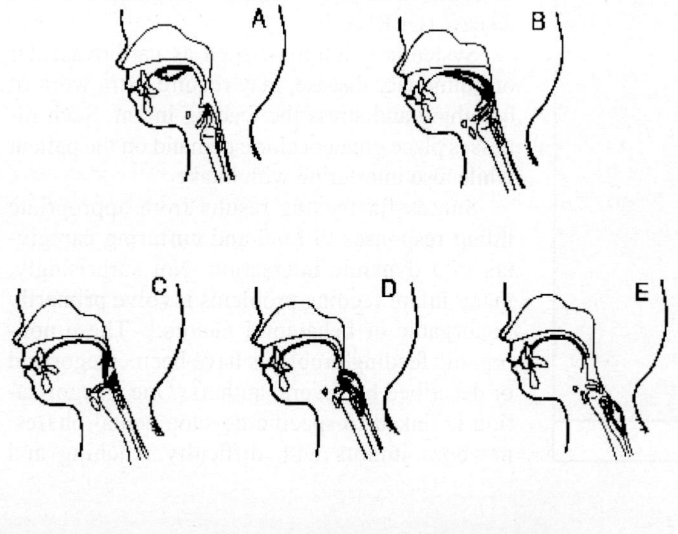

Figure 1 Schematic drawing to show oral, pharyngeal, and esophageal phases of normal swallow in a young child. (A) Oral phase showing formed bolus moving posteriorly through the oral cavity; (B) beginning of pharyngeal phase; (C) bolus moving through the pharynx with adequate airway protection; (D) end of pharyngeal phase as cricopharyngeus opens; (E) esophageal phase with bolus in the cervical esophagus. (From reference 9. Reprinted with permission of Delmar Learning, a division of Thomson Learning: www.thomsonrights.com.)

protect the airway. The final or esophageal phase begins with relaxation of the upper esophageal sphincter (cricopharyngeus muscle) and carries the bolus to the stomach under involuntary control. The return of the upper esophageal sphincter to its tonically contracted state prevents laryngeal penetration or aspiration of esophageal contents or reflux of the bolus back into the pharynx.

ETIOLOGY

Infants with feeding problems are usually referred for evaluation when inadequate intake has led to growth faltering or eventually failure to thrive, or perhaps less frequently when a caregiver perceives significant difficulty in feeding the infant even if weight has not declined.[11] The feeding problem may be the primary cause of poor growth, secondary to other disease processes, or both.

Table 2 Causes of Feeding Difficulties

Altered appetite
- Abnormal feeding patterns
- Supplemental feedings
- Metabolic disorders
- Inflammatory bowel disease

Diet
- Food allergy
- Inappropriate foods

Dysphagia
- Anatomic
  - Macroglossia
  - Cleft lip and palate
  - Submucous cleft palate
  - Pierre Robin sequence
  - Laryngeal cleft
  - Tracheoesophageal fistula
  - Vascular ring
  - Foreign body
- Neuromuscular
  - Prematurity
  - Cerebral palsy
  - Isolated neonatal swallowing dysfunction
  - Bulbar palsy
  - Infant botulism
  - Muscular dystrophy
  - Pseudo-obstruction
  - Connective tissue disease
  - Repaired tracheoesophageal fistula
- Inflammatory
  - Viral stomatitis
  - Candida stomatitis, pharyngitis
  - Peptic esophagitis
  - Mucositis (graft vs host disease)
- Systemic
  - Cardiac disease
  - Pulmonary disease

Behavioral
- Poor parent–infant interaction
- Autonomy struggles
- Picky eater
- Failure to imbibe
- Delayed introduction of solids
- Oral aversion
- Conditioned dysphagia
- Posttraumatic eating disorder
- Vulnerable child
- Parental responses

Adapted from references 8, 14, and 20.

Understanding which patients are at risk for feeding disorders will promote early intervention.[12,13]

Table 2 presents selected etiologies for feeding difficulties. Appetite will be altered if the timing or volume of feedings is inappropriate, an example being the "grazing" behavior of toddlers.[14] A common iatrogenic alteration of appetite occurs with the use of supplemental tube feedings. Although these may be necessary for adequate weight gain, they eventually interfere with normal hunger-satiety cycles. Anorexia may complicate disorders of organic acid or urea cycle metabolism.[15] Decrease of appetite combined with early satiety contributes to the poor nutrient intake responsible for growth failure in Crohn's disease.[16]

The diet of an infant may lead to difficult feedings, as cow's milk allergy was shown to be an unsuspected cause of vomiting or irritability with feeds in up to 41% of infants with gastroesophageal reflux.[17] Age-appropriate foods are essential for acquiring normal feeding behaviors.

Dysphagia specifically refers to difficulty with swallowing and implies an organic basis.[18,19] Illingworth distinguished between anatomic, neuromuscular, and inflammatory factors for dysphagia.[20] Anatomic lesions range from the cleft lip and palate that present at birth to the more subtle anomalies such as submucous cleft palate or vascular ring. The neurologic immaturity of the premature infant results in predictable feeding concerns based on the gestational age and general medical conditions.[21] Other neuromuscular disorders may affect coordination of suck and swallow or esophageal peristalsis (isolated neonatal swallowing dysfunction, muscular dystrophy, repaired tracheoesophageal fistula).[22,23]

Although not specifically related to difficulty in producing a swallow, as with neuromuscular and anatomic causes, the term dysphagia is also applied when the act of eating or swallowing produces pain or other discomfort. Acute inflammatory disorders are usually infectious, and chronic conditions are likely acid related (peptic esophagitis) or allergic (eosinophilic esophagitis). A review of 600 infants with gastroesophageal reflux found that 4% had severe feeding resistance sufficient to warrant tube feedings, and this feeding resistance was often the initial or only symptom.[24] Dysphagia may be the first complaint in older children with gastroesophageal reflux disease (GERD).[25]

Systemic conditions, such as cardiovascular or pulmonary disease, may require extra work of breathing and stress the feeding infant. Such illnesses place greater caloric demand on the patient while also interfering with intake.[26,27]

Successful feeding results from appropriate infant responses to food and nurturing caregivers in a dynamic interaction. Not surprisingly, many infant feeding problems involve primarily nonorganic or behavioral factors.[13] These nonorganic feeding problems have been categorized or described by several authors. One categorization is linked to specific developmental phases: newborn infants with difficulty reaching and maintaining a state of calm alertness for feeding, young infants (2 to 8 mo) with poor or dyssynchronous parent–infant interaction, the toddler (12 to 36 mo) with autonomy struggles, and the less affected "picky eater" who is not yet malnourished.[28] Others describe a popu-lation of nonorganic failure to thrive as "failure to imbibe" in young infants with poor intake but no apparent problems with mother–infant interactions.[29,30]

When the introduction of feedings is delayed beyond a sensitive or critical period, acquisition of feeding skills may be difficult.[31] Medical or surgical disorders early in life may necessitate the use of nasogastric or gastrostomy feedings or parenteral nutrition to maintain adequate nutrition. If supplemental feeding is required on a short-term basis, growth is maintained, and generally the infant quickly resumes normal feeding behavior. However, if long-term tube feeding or intravenous alimentation is required, especially if the infant has had little previous positive experience with normal feeding, the child is at risk for the development of an aversion to oral feedings. Intrusive oral procedures such as nasogastric tube placement, endotracheal intubation, and oropharyngeal suctioning have been associated with aversion to oral feedings. The long-term pairing of eating and pain, as occurs in GERD, may establish a negative feeding experience and a "conditioned dysphagia."[25,32–34]

Even in the case in which medical conditions impact nutrition, the parental reaction to feeding can play a pivotal role. Parents may be faced with innumerable negative feeding interactions because of the need to push the child's nutrient intake. These experiences can change feeding from a satisfying parent–child interaction to a grim, anxiety-producing chore. Further, infants with early medical problems may be perceived as "vulnerable" by their parents, who consequently may have difficulty setting age-appropriate limits, in this case around eating.[2,35] Therefore, even after an organic disorder is resolved, the feeding interaction remains stressed.

Research supports the idea that multiple etiologies, organic and nonorganic, are often present in the child being evaluated for poor feeding. In 50 infants with feeding disorders, Budd and colleagues found that 64% had problems with both organic and nonorganic symptoms, contributing to their insufficient food intake.[36] Burklow and colleagues reviewed 103 children with complex feeding problems, identifying 80% with a significant behavioral component and 85% with multiple conditions leading to the feeding disorder.[37] Of 700 infants referred for severe feeding difficulty over a 5.5-year period in Belgium, almost 50% had coexisting medical and oral-related conditions, and behavioral feeding problems occurred in 18%.[38] Careful study of infants with a diagnosis of nonorganic failure to thrive has revealed that subtle oral-motor dysfunction may be responsible for inadequate feeding skills, contributing to their poor weight gain.[39,40] In children with multiple risk factors, these problems may coexist or evolve separately in time, with the nonorganic component remaining after the organic problem is resolved.

EVALUATION

The presence of feeding difficulties may be first noted by the infant's caregiver, primary care physician, early intervention specialist, or other healthcare personnel. The type and severity of the feeding problem will usually lead to the involvement of several allied professionals (Figure 2). Often an interdisciplinary team approach facilitates an efficient evaluation.[14,41]

The first step in evaluating feeding difficulties is a complete history and physical examination. The prenatal history, gestational age, birth weight, and neonatal course may suggest particular risk factors. The answers to questions regarding general psychomotor developmental progress will inform an understanding of feeding progress and why it might be delayed. The review of systems can identify those infants with chronic lung disease, cardiac malformations, or neurologic conditions that are likely to affect feeding (see Table 2). Symptoms of GERD should be sought because feeding resistance may be one of the early manifestations.[24]

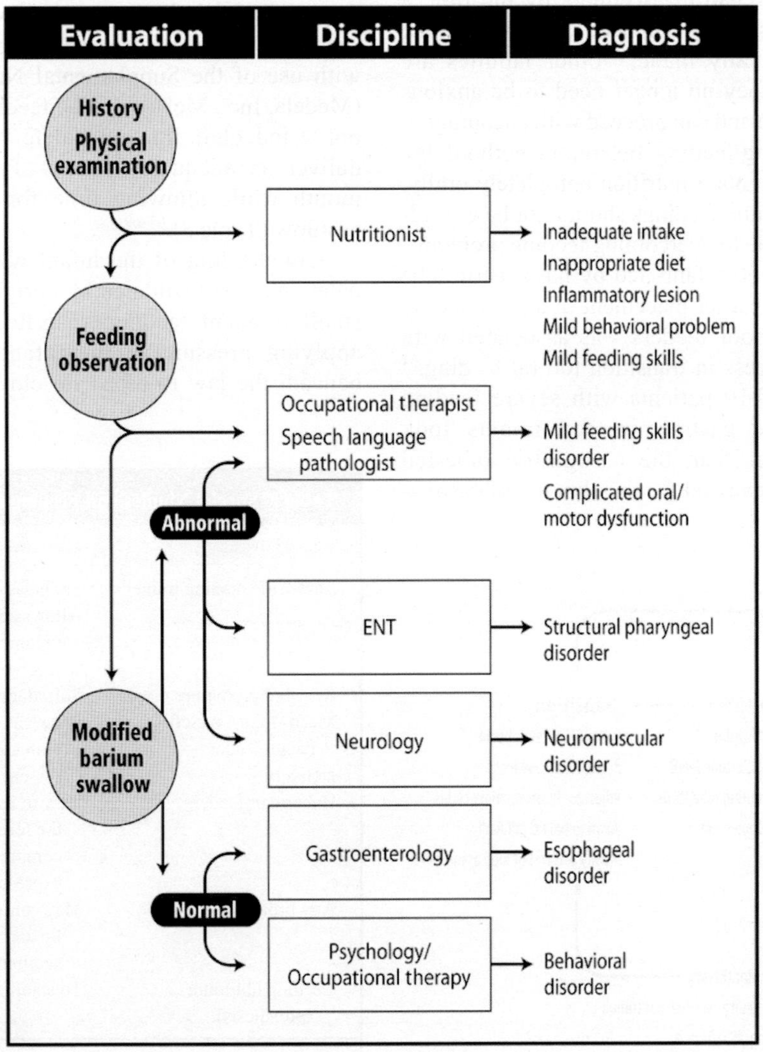

Figure 2 Steps in the evaluation of feeding difficulties.

The nutritionist has a major role in obtaining the diet history, which will include the type, amount, and nutritional value of what is offered to the infant or child, as well as what is actually ingested. A 24 h diet recall or a more formal 3-day diet record assists in calculating fluid, calorie, mineral, and vitamin intake. This information, together with a review of feeding methods, will often suggest inadequate calorie intake or developmentally inappropriate food choices indicative of a feeding skill disorder.

Physical examination begins with careful anthropometric measurement, which can be plotted on the appropriate growth charts. Progressive movement away from previous growth percentiles may indicate inadequate intake and the need for further investigation. Weight-for-length ratio is a sensitive measure of acute malnutrition. Oral examination should evaluate lip closure, tongue position and movement, and palatal movement. Nonnutritive sucking can be evaluated by allowing the infant to suck on the examiner's gloved finger. Infants with oral-motor problems may have poor coordination of suck, swallow, and breathing; poor mouth closure; decreased tongue movement; decreased jaw stability; or sustained or prolonged jaw closure. Oral hypersensitivity with increased gag reflex is common after mechanical ventilation or tube feeding.[42] Further neurologic examination may reveal cranial nerve deficits associated with dysphagia, as well as problems with posture, head and neck control, muscle tone, and persistence of primitive reflexes.[43]

A thorough feeding evaluation is not typically done in the medical encounter alone. An observation of feeding including the parent–child feeding interaction is central to the evaluation of a feeding disorder. An occupational therapist or speech-language pathologist can assist in assessing nutritive sucking and feeding by the primary caregiver, which may detect subtle disorders of feeding skills.[9,39] A prospective study of neonates found that those with disorganized or dysfunctional sucking patterns were more likely to have feeding problems at 6 and 12 months of age.[44] A psychologist on the treatment team can be crucial to understanding the development of the problem and the best way to approach the family.[45] Behavioral assessment includes a thorough feeding history, including details of both the infant's feeding and the parental responses, intake history over several days to demonstrate the pattern of feedings, and feeding observation live or on videotape.[46] A psychologist will observe parent–child interactions around feeding, to assess factors such as how the food is presented, which foods an infant prefers, and the parental responses to good and inappropriate feeding behaviors.

Several imaging methods are available to evaluate more complex oral-motor dysfunction. The primary technique is the modified barium swallow, also referred to as a videofluoroscopic swallow study.[47] It requires involvement of a feeding specialist (occupational therapist or speech-language pathologist) and radiologist. Unlike standard upper gastrointestinal barium contrast radiographs, in this study, the infant is placed in a standard feeding position and presented with a variety of textures. This study is the best method of evaluating the pharyngeal phase of swallowing. Clinically unapparent difficulties with suck and swallow, nasopharyngeal reflux, ineffective pharyngeal closure, and aspiration can be seen and taped for later review. Aspiration is often subclinical, for both liquids and solids.[48] Knowledge of aspiration risk and the ability to handle food of different consistencies will assist in developing a safe feeding program.[49]

Ultrasonography is ideal for evaluating the oral preparatory phase of swallow.[50] The infant and feeder can be studied in a more physiologic state, with repeated observations of swallow possible. No contrast material is needed, and there is no radiation exposure. Ultrasound study of the pharyngeal phase is difficult owing to air-filled spaces, and aspiration will not be detected.

Flexible endoscopic evaluation of swallowing is another technique that allows for evaluation of swallowing, particularly the pharyngeal phase.[51] After topical anesthesia of nasal tissues, a nasopharyngoscope is passed transnasally for observation of the anatomy and function of the palate, pharynx, and larynx. Next, swallowing function is evaluated with administration of food. The ability to handle liquids and risk of aspiration can be directly assessed. The study can be repeated as often as necessary because there is no preparation needed and no radiation exposure.[52]

Manometry is used to assess the esophageal phase of swallowing. It will detect abnormalities of upper esophageal sphincter relaxation or esophageal peristalsis but may be impractical during early infancy or childhood.

Magnetic resonance imaging should be considered in infants with cranial nerve involvement suggesting brain stem or spinal cord disorders, and has been useful in evaluating patients with dysphagia and aspiration due to Arnold–Chiari malformation.[8,19] Upper gastrointestinal endoscopy may detect the presence of inflammatory conditions while ruling out anatomic lesions of the esophagus.

TREATMENT

Treatment of feeding problems, which are often complex, should emanate from the interdisciplinary assessment. Generally, not all aspects of the plan are begun simultaneously. Medical conditions causing pain or discomfort during eating should be resolved. Initial attention should be directed to providing sufficient intake for maintenance and catch-up growth. The dietician will assist in the design of a feeding plan appropriate for the age and abilities of the infant. As nutritional status improves, the occupational therapist, speech therapist, and psychologist can help develop a program to establish normal feeding skills and parent–child interactions.

Whenever possible, oral feeding should be maintained even if alternative feeding is also used. This preserves the sensory function of taste and smell and the neuromotor skills of suck and swallow. Oral feeding promotes speech development and provides what should be a pleasurable social experience for the infant. If the patient is malnourished, nonoral supplementation should be a priority. Figure 3 provides an algorithm for steps in nutritional rehabilitation. No advantage is achieved in delaying nutritional therapy in children with feeding problems because malnutrition is the primary cause of growth retardation and altered body composition in chronic illness.[53] Details of enteral and parenteral feeding are described later in this text.

Nutrient administration is based on patient needs and limitations. Nasogastric or orogastric tubes are easy to place, with feedings given on an intermittent (bolus) or continuous basis. Bolus feeds are more physiologic in preserving hunger-satiety cycles and allow greater mobility for the patient and family. Continuous feedings may be preferable when there is delayed gastric emptying or decreased gut absorptive capacity.[54] Although gastric feeding is preferable, transpyloric tube placement is indicated when there is an increased risk of aspiration.[55]

For most clinical situations, a flexible polyurethane or silicone elastic tube is appropriate for the patient. These tubes produce minimal sensation when the child swallows, do not interfere with feeding, and can remain in place for up to several weeks.[56] Less frequent tube changes decrease noxious oral–facial stimuli for the child, which may help reduce the likelihood of future negative feeding behaviors. Nocturnal feedings have been shown to provide excellent nutritional support while not interfering with daytime activities.[57,58]

Percutaneous endoscopic gastrostomy and use of low-profile gastrostomy buttons facilitate the care of patients on long-term enteral support.[59,60] While some families have had significant distress regarding feedings by the time a gastrostomy is placed and need support when the decision is finally made,[61] other families are relieved that they no longer need to be anxious about nutrition and can proceed with encouraging adaptive eating/feeding behaviors without the pressure to maintain nutrition completely orally. Gastrostomy tube feedings should not be considered an obstacle to overcoming feeding problems. A review of 100 infants fed by nasogastric tube indicated that earlier placement of a gastrostomy tube for the poor feeders was associated with improved success in transition to oral feeding.[62] In a study of 19 patients with severe feeding refusal, those gastrostomy-fed infants took slightly longer than the nasogastric tube-fed infants to achieve oral feeding, but use of gastrostomy feedings did not adversely affect eventual transition to oral feeds.[63]

Various approaches to advancing feedings are available.[64] Tolerance can be assessed by gastric residuals and the absence of vomiting, diarrhea, or abdominal pain. Infants with chronic diarrhea and malnutrition can be successfully managed with enteral therapy, but the volume of the infusion should be increased gradually.[65] Attention to adequate water intake will prevent problems of dehydration owing to formulas with a high renal solute load.[66] Careful attention to appropriate techniques for the provision of proper diets can be of great benefit to children with major feeding difficulties. Two examples of such clinical problems are discussed below.

ORAL–FACIAL ANOMALIES

The newborn with cleft lip or palate has an immediate feeding problem. With a minor cleft lip or palate, the feeding problem is usually related to the inability to generate adequate negative pressure for suction. Apart from its nutritional advantages, breast-feeding may best facilitate intake because the soft tissue of the breast can help seal the cleft during feedings. When there is cleft lip and palate, the breast-fed infant may be unable to generate sufficient negative pressure to hold the nipple and areola in place for compression, and the bottle-fed infant may not develop efficient suction on a nipple. Breast-feeding may be assisted with use of the Supplemental Nursing System (Medela, Inc., McHenry, IL); feeding devices for bottle-fed cleft lip and palate infants should deliver an adequate volume of milk into the mouth while allowing time for the infant to swallow (Table 3).[67–69]

Oral feeding of the infant with cleft lip or palate may be facilitated by upright positioning, small frequent feedings, careful burping, and applying pressure to the infant's cheek and beneath the jaw to assist lip closure and suck-

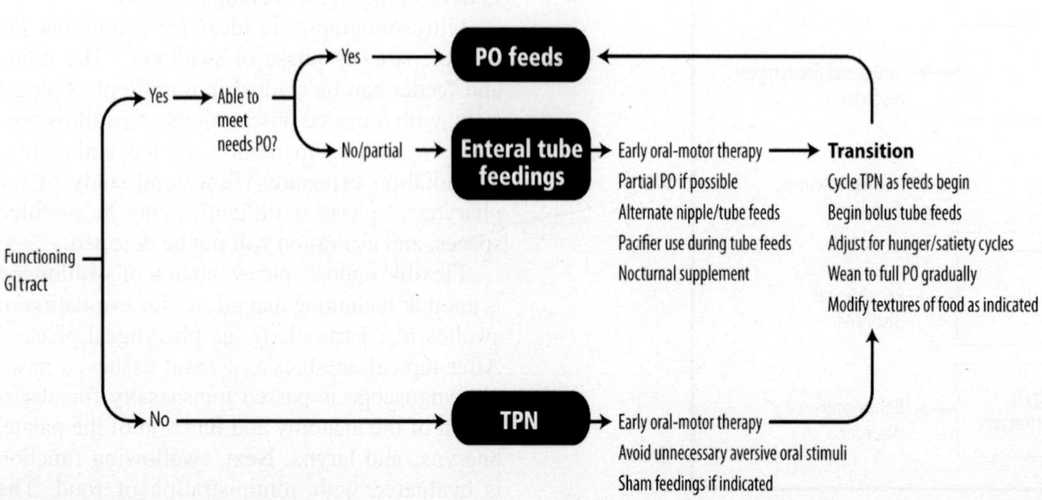

Figure 3 Treatment of feeding difficulties.

Table 3 Special Nipples and Feeding Devices

Nipple/Device	Characteristics
Lact-Aide nursing trainer	For breast-feeding infants Allows control of volume of milk from reservoir
Ross red premature nipple	Soft, durable
Mead–Johnson cleft palate feeder	Squeeze bottle helps with control of milk
Delivery	Cross-cut nipple
Haberman feeder	Easy to use, with nipple the feeder can compress to help express milk
Any broad-based nipple	May conform to a cleft lip and help attain suction
Feeding obturator (prosthesis)	To stabilize wide cleft

Adapted from reference 76.

ing.[70] Nonoral feedings become necessary if significant risk of aspiration is present or if the infant fails to thrive because of either inadequate volume intake or prolonged feeding sessions. When micrognathia and glossoptosis occur with cleft palate (the Robin sequence), respiratory distress may preclude oral feeding. These infants have feeding difficulties caused by inadequate suction, swallowing difficulties, and compromised breathing owing to airway obstruction by the tongue.[21] Some infants will require surgical tongue–lip adhesion, use of a nasopharyngeal airway, or even tracheostomy.[71] These operative procedures are reserved for patients with the inability to maintain a stable airway using conservative measures. The incidence of failure to thrive was reduced when the families of infants with Robin sequence received assistance from a feeding-support nurse and supervised airway management.[72]

CEREBRAL PALSY

Cerebral palsy is the most common form of chronic motor disability that begins in childhood, with a prevalence of 2 of 1,000 infants. Children with cerebral palsy represent a spectrum of developmental disabilities, including mental retardation, epilepsy, and abnormalities of vision, hearing, speech, cognition, and behavior.[73] As a disorder of movement and posture, most patients demonstrate spasticity of the extremities. Swallowing difficulties result from supranuclear bulbar palsies. In a large survey of families with children with neurologic impairment, prolonged feeding times of 3 or more hours per day were common.[74] Early on, affected infants may have decreased sucking reflex and weak or uncoordinated sucking behavior; later, one may observe tonic bite, tongue thrust or lip retraction, and lip pursing.[75,76]

Before oral feeds are begun, nonnutritive sucking can be encouraged at the breast (emptied by pumping) or with a pacifier. Nonnutritive sucking during gavage feeds has been shown to help the maturation of the sucking reflex in premature infants and may improve integration of oral and pharyngeal reflexes in the infant with an immature nervous system.[77]

Treatment techniques are available to enhance oral feeding at the breast and with bottle feeding.[68,76,78] For the older infant, the texture of foods can be adjusted, and with thicker liquids passing more slowly from mouth to throat, they will often be better tolerated. The use of a spoon requires that the infant opens the mouth wide enough so that lateral tongue movements are adequate to remove the food and that jaw control is adequate. Spoons are designed with narrow, shallow bowls, and are made of durable, plastic material; they may have specialized handles to help with the grasp. Cups are available with cutout rims (to allow easier lifting), covers to decrease spillage, and wide bases to prevent tipping. The feeder can use techniques to provide external jaw and cheek support and to stabilize head position. Adaptive equipment is available to improve postural alignment during feedings. The feeder may hold an infant in the lap or use a foam-filled Tumble-Forms (Sammons Preston Rolyan, Bolingbrook, IL) seat. The older infant or toddler with fair sitting stability can use the Rifton chair (Rifton Equipment, Chester, NY) or other adaptive seating device for upright positioning with foot rests, arm supports, and pelvic strapping.[76]

Oral sensorimotor therapy may be effective in promoting oral-motor function, but may not improve oral feeding efficiency, calorie intake, or weight gain. Consequently, some children with an inability to meet nutritional needs orally will require a feeding gastrostomy.[79] The safety of oral feedings and risk of aspiration can be evaluated with videofluoroscopy of swallowing. Early attention to treatment of feeding disorders in these patients can result in significantly improved nutritional status.[80]

BEHAVIORAL APPROACHES TO FEEDING

Principles of learning are used to understand the development of feeding disorders and to design treatment programs for children with feeding problems. Conceptualizing feeding problems in this way is especially important when there is no apparent organic disease or when correction of an organic disorder or oral-motor deficit does not result in normal feeding.[14,81–83] Both classical and operant conditioning models play a role in the understanding and treatment of feeding disorders. Respondent learning or classic conditioning posits that the occurrence of some behaviors is increased or decreased based on their association with normal physiologic reactions, in this case hunger or pain. A common example is that eating has been associated with pain and therefore eating behavior is decreased even after the pain-producing condition is resolved. In the experience of children with feeding disorders, the positive association between hunger, eating, and satiety is inconsistent, disrupted by tube feeding or nonperiodic oral-feeding schedules that are not paired with hunger.

Interventions for feeding disorders often manipulate hunger to prompt eating behaviors. The rationale is that children (all animals) are more likely to emit eating behaviors (show interest in food, accept food put into their mouth, put food into the mouth, swallow food) when they are hungry. Hunger may be manipulated in several ways.[81] For the child fed by the mouth, the timing of meals should be regulated, and between-meal eating and drinking should be minimized or eliminated so that the child is hungry at mealtime. The length of meals is limited to 20 to 30 min, regardless of the amount of food ingested. After 20 to 30 min, it is assumed that rising blood sugar from the food that has been consumed leads to diminished sensation of hunger. From the respondent learning perspective, keeping meals short continues to reinforce the association of hunger–eating–satiety.

For children who are tube fed, the timing and amount of the feeding should be regulated to maximize hunger. Bolus, rather than continuous feeding, and daytime rather than nighttime feeding, will more closely mimic meals and thus move the child toward normal eating patterns. Tube feeding after, rather than before, an oral feeding session is generally recommended. Modestly decreasing the calories received by tube will, in many patients, increase appetite and better motivate the child to eat by mouth.

One caveat is necessary with respect to the manipulation of hunger. Although a modest amount of calorie restriction ($\approx$25%) is typically helpful to encouraging eating behavior, severe calorie restriction is not. Naive interveners, both lay and professional, have found that the statement "He'll eat when he gets hungry enough" is not true for those with feeding disorders seen in a tertiary care center.

Operant learning principles posit that behaviors are increased or decreased based on the responses to the behaviors. Parental behaviors during meals are a common factor in the development and maintenance of feeding disorders. Specifically, parental attention through cajoling, offering preferred foods after nonpreferred are refused, and ending meals because of protest are all ways in which noneating behaviors are reinforced and therefore likely to reoccur. In behavioral feeding therapies, operant techniques are used to increase desired behaviors (acceptance of food) and decrease undesirable behaviors.[82] In the treatment of mild-to-moderate feeding problems, a commonly used and effective operant treatment technique is differential attention.[83] During the meal, the child receives positive reinforcement or attention for specific behaviors related to feeding and no attention for inappropriate or off-task behaviors. Positive attention is often social interaction and praise from the caregiver, but depending on the child, it can be music or access to a preferred food. Inappropriate and off-task behaviors include tantrums, not approaching the food, and playing with the food. These behaviors are ignored, ie, receive no positive reinforcement while the child is required to stay at the table or in the high chair. The target behaviors (behaviors to be increased) are changed as the treatment progresses. For example, the child may initially be reinforced for allowing nonpreferred food on this plate, then for food to be put in his mouth, then for self-feeding, and, finally, for self-feeding a sufficient quantity in a specified time. Depending on the child's feeding problem, physical guidance of appropriate feeding behaviors may be used along with differential attention.[84] The physical guidance is decreased and then stopped as the child progresses through the program.

Extinction is the operant principle that suggests that a behavior will eventually cease if it is never reinforced. Extinction-based techniques have been used in the treatment of severe feeding refusal. Most typically, these are children who, for medical reasons and from a very early age, have not been fed successfully by mouth. When faced with oral feeding these children produce strong rejecting behaviors such as screaming, spitting food, and physically resisting placement of food in the mouth. When the caregiver stops the feeding in response to these rejecting behaviors, the child's behaviors have been reinforced (by escaping the negative situation). Extinction techniques dictate that feeding should not stop in response to rejecting behaviors. Thus, spoonfuls of food (sometimes very little food) are put into the child's mouth repeatedly despite the child's protest. Eventually, when the child's protest behavior does not stop the feeding (ie, the protest behavior is not reinforced), the protest behavior stops. These extinction techniques are successful in cases of severe feeding refusal,[63,85,86] but they must be carefully planned and executed in an inpatient or intensive outpatient setting.

The role of parents in carrying out behavioral treatment programs for feeding must be fully appreciated and supported.[14] As discussed earlier in this chapter, parental anxiety about nutrition is an important factor in the development and maintenance of many feeding problems, because unhelpful parent feeding behavior is typically motivated by their own anxiety. To begin to change these behaviors parental concerns and anxiety must by addressed specifically. The entire treatment team should know and agree on the treatment plan for the child's nutritional and behavioral feeding problem, and this consensus plan should be presented to the family. Most parents need help to understand that the multiple components of their child's feeding problem cannot all be addressed at once. They need to understand that the team has a plan to resolve all of the concerns in time and that the child's nutritional status will not be in danger during this process. Parental lack of understanding of this process can severely impede the progress of treatment. For example, parents will not follow guidelines to stop meals after 30 min and may give in to inappropriate feeding rituals if they fear that the child's nutritional status will be harmed by shortened meals.

For the child with mild-to-moderate feeding problems, most parents can and should be taught behavioral treatment techniques to be carried out at home. Some combination of written and verbal explanation, modeling, and rehearsal can provide motivated parents with the requisite feeding skills.[87] The behavioral feeding plan needs to be carried out consistently, that is, at every meal, to change the child's negative feeding behaviors. Thus, training the parent to carry out the treatment at each meal is far superior to an "expert feeder" who treats the child weekly or even several times per week. Parents will need to understand the behavioral principles and the importance of consistency in applying these techniques. For children with very severe feeding refusal, especially if extinction procedures are used, inpatient treatment or intensive outpatient treatment with alternative feeders will likely be necessary. In these cases, parents must initially understand and support the treatment and then must be taught to carry out the procedures themselves as feeding is transferred to the more normal parent–child interaction and home environment.

TRANSITION TO ORAL FEEDS

When medical or surgical disorders necessitate nonoral feedings or parenteral nutrition, planning for transition to oral feedings should begin early. Oral-motor intervention can begin with the assessment of feeding skills and swallowing ability. Oral feedings, even in small amounts, should continue if at all possible to maintain oral-motor skills.

Manipulation of the appetite by adjustment of enteral and parenteral feedings is essential.[45] Even with the young infant the cycling of parenteral nutrition can begin while advancing enteral feedings.[88] Continuous tube feedings should be converted to bolus feedings to simulate a meal schedule. Eventually tube feeding volume must be reduced to allow the child to experience hunger prior to oral feedings.[76] The premature infant will benefit from nonnutritive sucking during tube feedings, with the use of nipple feeds during the daytime and tube feedings at night.[89] A semidemand feeding protocol for preterm infants shortened the transition to oral feedings by several days.[90] Attention to eating-related behaviors, the feeding environment, and hunger-satiety cycles will help normalize feedings.[91] Ongoing communication with and support for the family will enhance the transition to normal feeding behavior.

REFERENCES

1. Reau N, Senturia Y, Lebailly S, Christoffel K. Infant and toddler feeding patterns and problems: Normative data and a new direction. J Dev Behav Pediatr 1996;17:149–53.
2. Singer L. When a child won't or can't eat. Contemp Pediatr 1990;7:60–76.
3. Dahl M, Sundelin C. Early feeding problems in an affluent society. I. Categories and clinical signs. Acta Paediatr Scand 1986;75:370–9.
4. Babbitt RL, Hoch T, Coe D, et al. Behavioral assessment and treatment of pediatric feeding disorders. J Dev Behav Pediatr 1994;15:278–91.
5. Reilly S, Skuse D, Poblete X. Prevalence of feeding problems and oral motor dysfunction in children with cerebral palsy: A community survey. J Pediatr 1996;129:877–82.
6. Glass RP, Wolf LS. Feeding and oral-motor skills. In: Case-Smith J, editor. Pediatric Occupational Therapy and Early Intervention. Boston: Andover Medical Publishers; 1993. p. 225.
7. Cloud H, Ekvall SW, Hicks L. Feeding problems of the child with special health-care needs. In: Ekvall SW, Ekvall VK, editors. Pediatric Nutrition in Chronic Diseases and Developmental Disorders, 2nd edition. Oxford: Oxford University Press; 2005. p. 172–82.
8. Rudolph CD, Link DT. Feeding disorders in infants and children. Pediatr Clin North Am 2002;49:97–112.
9. Arvedson J, Brodsky L. Pediatric Swallowing and Feeding: Assessment and Management, 2nd edition. San Diego: Singular Publishing Group; 2002.
10. Logan WJ, Bosma JF. Oral and pharyngeal dysphagia in infancy. Pediatr Clin North Am 1967;14:47–61.
11. Gahagan S. Failure to thrive: A consequence of undernutrition. Pediatr Rev 2006;27:e1–11.
12. Lindberg L, Osterberg M, Isacson IM, Dannaeus M. Feeding disorders related to nutrition. Acta Pediatr 2006;95:425–9.
13. Blackman J. Children who refuse food. Contemp Pediatr 1998;15:198–216.
14. Kedesdy JH, Budd KS. Childhood Feeding Disorders: Biobehavioral Assessment and Intervention. Baltimore: Paul H. Brookes Publishing; 1998.
15. Hyman SL, Porter C, Page T, et al. Behavior management of feeding disturbances in urea cycle and organic acid disorders. J Pediatr 1987;111:558–62.
16. Seidman E. Nutritional treatment of growth failure and disease activity in children with inflammatory bowel disease. In: Suskind RM, Lewinter-Suskind L, editors. Textbook of Pediatric Nutrition, 2nd edition. New York: Raven Press; 1993. p. 341–52.
17. Iacono G, Carroccio A, Montalto G, et al. Gastroesophageal reflux and cow's milk allergy in infants: A prospective study. J Allergy Clin Immunol 1996;97:822–7.
18. Green M. Pediatric Diagnosis: Interpretation of Symptoms and Signs in Infants, Children, and Adolescents, 5th edition. Philadelphia: WB Saunders; 1992.
19. Dusick A. Investigation and management of dysphagia. Semin Pediatr Neurol 2003;10:255–64.
20. Illingworth RS. Sucking and swallowing difficulties in infancy: Diagnostic problem of dysphagia. Arch Dis Child 1969; 44:655–65.
21. Wolf LS, Glass RP. Feeding and Swallowing Disorders in Infancy: Assessment and Management. Tucson, AZ: Therapy Skill Builders; 1992.
22. Tilton A, Miller M, Khoshoo V. Nutrition and swallowing in pediatric neuromuscular patients. Semin Pediatr Neurol 1998;5:106–15.
23. Heuschkel RB, Fletcher K, Hill A, et al. Isolated neonatal swallowing dysfunction. Dig Dis Sci 2003;48:30–5.
24. Dellert S, Hyams J, Treem W, Geertsma MA. Feeding resistance and gastroesophageal reflux in infancy. J Pediatr Gastroenterol Nutr 1993;17:66–71.
25. Catto-Smith AG, Machida H, Butzner J, et al. The role of gastroesophageal reflux in pediatric dysphagia. J Pediatr Gastroenterol Nutr 1991;12:159–65.
26. Ford CF, Pietsch JB. Home enteral tube feeding in children after chemotherapy or bone marrow transplantation. Nutr Clin Pract 1999;14:19–22.
27. Morris B, Miller-Loncar C, Landry S, et al. Feeding, medical factors, and developmental outcome in premature infants. Clin Pediatr 1999;38:451–7.
28. Chatoor I. Feeding disorders in infants and toddlers: Diagnosis and treatment. Child Adolesc Psychiatric Clin Am 2002;11:163–83.
29. Tolia V. Very early onset nonorganic failure to thrive in infants. J Pediatr Gastroenterol Nutr 1995;20:73–80.
30. Lichtman S, Maynor A, Rhoads J. Failure to imbibe in otherwise normal infants. J Pediatr Gastroenterol Nutr 2000;30:467–71.
31. Illingworth RS, Lister J. The critical or sensitive period, with special reference to certain feeding problems in infants and children. J Pediatr 1964;65:839–48.
32. DiScipio WJ, Kaslon K, Ruben RJ. Traumatically acquired conditioned dysphagia in children. Ann Otol 1978;87: 509–14.
33. Manikam R, Perman J. Pediatric feeding disorders. J Clin Gastroenterol 2000;30:34–46.
34. Benoit D, Coolbear J. Post-traumatic feeding disorders in infancy: Behaviors predicting treatment outcome. Inf Ment Health J 1998;19:409–21.
35. Green M, Solnit A. Reactions to the threatened loss of a child: A vulnerable child syndrome. Pediatrics 1964;65:538–66.
36. Budd KS, McGraw T, Farbisz R, et al. Psychosocial concomitants of children's feeding disorders. J Pediatr Psychol 1992;17:81–94.
37. Burklow K, Phelps A, Schultz J, et al. Classifying pediatric feeding disorders. J Pediatr Gastroenterol Nutr 1998;27: 143–7.
38. Rommel N, De Meyer AM, Feenstra L, Veereman-Wauters G. The complexity of feeding problems in 700 infants and young children presenting to a tertiary care institution. J Pediatr Gastroenterol Nutr 2003;37: 75–84.
39. Ramsay M, Gisel E, Boutry M. Non-organic failure to thrive: Growth failure secondary to feeding-skills disorder. Dev Med Child Neurol 1993;35:285–97.
40. Reilly S, Skuse D, Wolke D, Stevenson J. Oral-motor dysfunction in children who fail to thrive: Organic or non-organic? Dev Med Child Neurol 1999;41:115–22.
41. Bithoney W, McJunkin J, Michalek J, et al. Prospective evaluation of weight gain in both nonorganic and organic

failure-to-thrive children: An outpatient trial of a multidisciplinary team intervention strategy. J Dev Behav Pediatr 1989;10:27–31.
42. Baker S, Boullard-Backunas K, Davis A. Common oral motor and gastrointestinal-nutritional problems in children referred to early intervention programs. Semin Pediatr Gastroenterol Nutr 1993;4:3–8.
43. Hill A, Volpe J. Disorders of sucking and swallowing in the newborn infant: Clinicopathological correlations. Prog Perinatal Neurol 1981;33:157–81.
44. Hawdon J, Beauregard N, Slattery J, Kennedy G. Identificationof neonates at risk of developing feeding problems in infancy. Dev Med Child Neurol 2000;42:235–9.
45. Linscheid TR. Behavioral treatments for pediatric feeding disorders. Behav Modifi 2006;30:6–23.
46. Czyzewski D. Feeding and eating disorders in young children. In: Roberts M, Walker C, editors. Casebook of Child and Pediatric Psychology. New York: Guilford Press; 1989. p. 255–80.
47. Benson J, Lefton-Greif M. Videofluoroscopy of swallowing in pediatric patients: A component of the total feeding evaluation. In: Tuchman D, Walter R, editors. Disorders of Feeding and Swallowing in Infants and Children. San Diego: Singular Publishing Group; 1994. p. 187–200.
48. DeMatteo C, Matovich D, Hjartarson A. Comparison of clinical and videofluoroscopic evaluation of children with feeding and swallowing difficulties. Dev Med Child Neurol 2005;47:149–57.
49. Newman LA, Keckley C, Peterson MC, Hamner A. Swallowing function and medical diagnoses in infants suspected of dysphagia. Pediatrics 2001;108:e106.
50. Bu'Lock R, Woolridge M, Baum J. Development of coordination of sucking, swallowing and breathing: Ultrasound study of term and preterm infants. Dev Med Child Neurol 1990;32:669–78.
51. Willging J, Miller C, Hogan M, Rudolph C. Fiberoptic evaluation of swallowing in children: A preliminary report of 100 procedures. Dysphagia 1996;11:162.
52. Bastian R. The videoendoscopic swallowing study: An alternative and partner to the videofluoroscopic swallowing study. Dysphagia 1993;8:359–67.
53. Motil K. Aggressive nutritional therapy in growth retardation. Clin Nutr 1985;4:75–84.
54. Ghishan F. Nutritional management of pediatric gastrointestinal disorders. Pediatr Ann 1999;28:123–8.
55. Panadero E, Lopez-Herce J, Caro L, et al. Transpyloric enteral feeding in critically ill children. J Pediatr Gastroenterol Nutr 1998;26:43–8.
56. Fuchs G. Enteral support of the hospitalized child. In: Suskind R, Lewinter-Suskind L, editors. Textbook of Pediatric Nutrition. New York: Raven Press; 1993. p. 239–46.
57. Motil K, Altchuler S, Grand R. Mineral balance during nutritional supplementation in adolescents with Crohn disease and growth failure. J Pediatr 1985;107:473–9.
58. Claris-Appiani A, Ardissino G, Dacco V, et al. Catch-up growth in children with chronic renal failure treated with long-term enteral nutrition. J Parenter Enteral Nutr 1995;19:175–8.
59. Brant C, Stanich P, Ferrari A. Improvement of children's nutritional status after enteral feeding by PEG: An interim report. Gastrointest Endosc 1999;50:183–8.
60. van der Merwe WG, Brown RA, Ireland JD, Goddard E. Percutaneous endoscopic gastrostomy in children-a 5 year experience. S Afr Med J 2003;93:781–5.
61. Spalding K, McKeever P. Mothers' experiences caring for children with disabilities who require a gastrostomy tube. J Pediatr Nurs 1998;13:234–43.
62. Bazyk S. Factors associated with the transition to oral feeding in infants fed by nasogastric tubes. Am J Occup Ther 1990; 44:1070–8.
63. Foy T, Czyzewski D, Phillips S, et al. Treatment of severe feeding refusal in infants and toddlers. Inf Young Child 1997;9:26–35.
64. Nevin-Folino N, Miller M. Enteral nutrition. In: Samour PQ, King K, editors. Handbook of Pediatric Nutrition, 3rd edition. Sudbury: Jones and Bartlett Publishers; 2005. p. 499–524.
65. Maclean W, Lopez de Romana G, Massa E, Graham G. Nutritional management of chronic diarrhea and malnutrition: Primary reliance on oral feeding. J Pediatr 1980;97:316–23.
66. Pardoe E. Tube feeding syndrome revisited. Nutr Clin Pract 2001;16:144–6.
67. Clarren SK, Anderson B, Wolf LS. Feeding infants with cleft lip, cleft palate, or cleft lip and palate. Cleft Palate J 1987;24:244–9.
68. Lawrence RA, Lawrence RM. Breastfeeding: A Guide for the Medical Profession, 6th edition. Philadelphia: Elsevier-Mosby; 2005. p. 515–57.
69. Glenny AM, Hooper L, Shaw WC, et al. Feeding interventions for growth and development ininfants with cleft lip, cleft palate or cleft lip and palate. Cochrane Database Syst Rev 2004;(3):CD003315.
70. Balluf M. Nutritional needs of an infant or child with a cleft lip or palate. Ear Nose Throat J 1986;65:44–9.
71. Lewis MB, Pashayan HM. Management of infants with Robin anomaly. Clin Pediatr 1980;19:519–28.
72. Pandya A, Boorman J. Failure to thrive in babies with cleft lip and palate. Br J Plast Surg 2001;54:471–5.
73. Johnston MV. Encephalopathies. In: Behrman RE, Kliegman RM, Jenson HB, editors. Nelson Textbook of Pediatrics, 17th edition. Philadelphia: WB Saunders; 2004. p. 2023–5.
74. Sullivan PB, Lambert B, Rose M, et al. Prevalence and severity of feeding and nutritional problems in children with neurological impairment: Oxford feeding study. Dev Med Child Neurol 2000;42:674–80.
75. McBride MC, Danner SC. Sucking disorders in neurologically impaired infants: Assessment and facilitation of breastfeeding. Clin Perinatol 1987;14:109–30.
76. Case-Smith J, Humphry R. Feeding intervention. In: Case-Smith J, editor. Occupational Therapy for Children, 4th edition. St. Louis: Mosby; 2001. p. 453–88.
77. Bernbaum JC, Pereira GR, Watkins JB, Peckham GJ. Non-nutritive sucking during gavage feeding enhances growth and maturation in premature infants. Pediatrics 1983;71:41–5.
78. Camp KM, Kalscheur MC. Nutritional approach to diagnosis and management of pediatric feeding and swallowing disorders. In: Tuchman DN, Walter RS, editors. Disorders of Feeding and Swallowing in Infants and Children. San Diego: Singular Publishing; 1994. p. 153–86.
79. Rogers B. Feeding method and health outcomes of children with cerebral palsy. J Pediatr 2004;145:S28–32.
80. Schwarz S, Corredor J, Fisher-Medina J, et al. Diagnosis and treatment of feeding disorders in children with development disabilities. Pediatrics 2001;108:671–6.
81. Linscheid TR, Budd KS, Rasnake LK. Pediatric feeding problems. In: Roberts MC, editor. Handbook of Pediatric Psychology, 3rd edition. New York: Guilford Press; 2003. p. 481–98.
82. Kerwin MLE. Empirically supported treatments in pediatric psychology: Severe feeding problems. J Pediatr Psychol 1999; 24:193–214.
83. Stark LJ, Powers SW, Jelalian E, et al. Modifying problematic mealtime interactions of children with cystic fibrosis and their parents via behavioral parent training. J Pediatr Psychol 1994;19:751–68.
84. Ahearn WH, Kerwin MLE, Eicher PS, et al. An alternating treatments comparison of two intensive interventions for food refusal. J Appl Behav Anal 1996;29:321–32.
85. Blackman JA, Nelson C. Rapid introduction of oral feedings to tube-fed patients. J Dev Behav Pediatr 1987;8:63–7.
86. Benoit D, Wang E, Zlotkin S. Discontinuation of enterostomy tube feeding by behavioral treatment in early childhood: A randomized controlled trial. J Pediatr 2000;137:498–503.
87. Mueller MM, Piazza CC, Moore JW, et al. Training parents to implement pediatric feeding protocols. J Appl Behav Anal 2003;36:545–62.
88. Collier S, Crough J, Hendricks K, Caballero B. Use of cyclic parenteral nutrition in infants less than 6 months of age. Nutr Clin Pract 1994;9:65–8.
89. Field T, Ignatoff E, Stringer S, et al. Nonnutritive sucking during tube feedings: Effects on preterm neonates in an intensive care unit. Pediatrics 1982;70:381–4.
90. McCain GC, Gartside PS, Greenberg JM, Lott JW. A feeding protocol for healthy preterm infants that shortens time to oral feeding. J Pediatr 2001;139:374–9.
91. Schauster H, Dwyer J. Transition from tube feedings to feedings by mouth in children: Preventing eating dysfunction. J Am Diet Assoc 1996;96:277–81.

Failure to Thrive: Malnutrition in the Pediatric Outpatient Setting

Robert Markowitz, MD
John B. Watkins, MD
Christopher Duggan, MD, MPH

HISTORY, BACKGROUND, AND DEFINITION OF TERMS

Pediatricians have described malnourished children with the words "failure to thrive" (FTT) since at least the nineteenth century.[1] There continues to be a notable lack of progress regarding a valid and reliable definition of the term.[2] One review of general pediatric and pediatric nutrition text-books failed to find a consensus definition, with various anthropometric and nonquantitative descriptive terms being employed.[3] Olsen reviewed the pediatric literature and general text books and found many failed to provide specific criteria defining FTT. It was found, however, one or another anthropometrical indicator, with weight gain predominating, was used.[4] Vinton and Dietz have rightly suggested that the term is a mere euphemism for undernutrition,[5] though growth failure may result from medical conditions which involve other factors.[6]

The child termed "failed to thrive" in the office of a pediatrician in industrialized countries would more likely (and more accurately) be described in developing countries as malnourished or suffering from protein-energy malnutrition.[7] The continued use of vague terminology such as failure to thrive limits the ability to scientifically study the nutritional status of a population as well attempts to determine the etiologies of poor growth and weight gain.

Nonetheless, if only owing to the strength of historical precedent, the term failure to thrive will continue to be used to describe infants and young children with malnutrition. It is recommended that quantitative criteria be employed. Commonly used criteria include: (1) a child whose weight (or weight for height) is more than 2 SD below the mean for sex and age and/or (2) a child whose weight curve has crossed downward more than 2 major percentile lines (defined as 5th, 10th, 25th, 50th, 75th, 90th, and 95th percentiles)[8] on the Centers for Disease Control and Prevention (CDC) growth charts after having achieved a previously stable pattern.

Alternative wordings of the first criterion include "less than the 3rd percentile" or "a weight-for-age (or weight for height) z-score (or standard deviation score) less than −2.0." z-scores are calculated by the following formula:

$$\text{Z score} = \frac{\text{actual weight} - \text{median weight}}{\text{standard deviation}}$$

where standard deviation is the age- and sex-specific standard deviation of weight and median weight is the median value for age and sex. Expressing anthropometric measures in terms of z-scores is recommended by the World Health Organization (WHO), especially when describing groups of subjects.[9] Z-scores allow more precision in describing anthropometric status than does the customary placement "near" or "below" a certain percentile curve. For example, the phrase "below the 3rd percentile" does not distinguish between a child just below this point (whose z-score may be −2.1) from one with severe growth faltering (whose z-score may be −3.5 or lower) (Figure 1). Similarly, 3% of normal children will weigh less than the 3rd percentile, but a z-score significantly lower than −2.0 clearly indicates a growth problem. There are CDC computer programs that calculate anthropometric data such as weight for height for age and weight for height; these are expressed as percentiles, z-scores, and percentage of the median without making recourse to plotting points by hand.[10] Software for palm-based computers is also available.

The second criterion is a more functional definition of growth failure that takes into account that weight loss or even lack of normal growth during infancy and childhood is abnormal and patients should not have attained low anthropometric scores before appropriate evaluation and treatment are instituted. What constitutes a "stable pattern" can be difficult to define. Edwards and colleagues addressed this issue by defining the true percentile as the maximum achieved between 4 and 8 weeks of age because weight at this point was found to correlate more strongly with weight at age 12 months than did birthweight.[11] They proposed a functional definition of failure to thrive as "a child whose weight deviates downwards across two or more major centiles from the maximum centile achieved at 4 to 8 weeks for a period of a month or more."

Anthropometric assessment of nutritional status can also be categorized to help determine chronicity of nutritional deprivation. The simple use of a weight-for-age cut-off to define malnutrition is obviously nonspecific because patients included can be either well proportioned and just constitutionally small or truly of low weight. A classic distinction between acute malnutrition ("wasting" or low weight for height) and chronic malnutrition ("stunting" or low height for age) was proposed by Waterlow and has been widely adopted.[12] Table 1 recounts this classification scheme, in which percentage of the median is calculated by the following formula:

$$\%\ \text{median} = \frac{\text{actual weight} \times 100}{\text{median}}\ \text{weight}$$

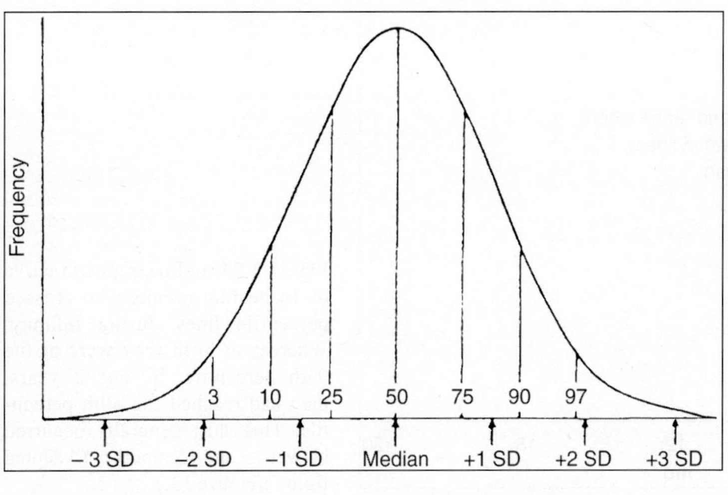

Figure 1 Comparison of percentiles vs. standard deviation or z-scores. Two SDs below (or above) the mean corresponds to the 3rd (or 97th) percentile. (Adapted from reference 17.)

Table 1 Waterlow Criteria for Categorizing Type and Chronicity of Malnutrition

Type of Malnutrition	Acute (Weight for Height) (% of Median)	Chronic (Height for Age) (% of Median)
Normal	>90	>95
Mild	80–90	90–95
Moderate	70–80	85–90
Severe	<70	<85

Abnormalities of weight for height are termed "wasting" and those of height for age are called "stunting."
Adapted from reference 12.

where median weight is the median value for age and sex.

Caution should be exercised when a subject's height faltering is used to call attention to nutritional status. Genetic and constitutional causes of short stature need to be ruled out before implicating chronic malnutrition as the cause of poor height growth. Knowledge of the family growth history (parents and siblings) with interpretation of growth parameters in light of midparental height and familial growth patterns can be helpful in this regard. In addition, an individual may not track consistently along a percentile for any given index. Smith and colleagues have pointed out that the National Center for Health Statistics (NCHS) standard curves were mathematical averages based on large numbers of children (ie, cross-sectional curves) and not growth lines along which individual children should be expected to grow (ie, longitudinal).[13] This is also true for the currently recommended CDC growth curves. They demonstrated that infants manifest a growth rate at birth that is predominantly determined by maternal factors, with a shift to one that then is increasingly determined by genetic background. Thirty percent of healthy, full-term, white infants crossed one percentile line and 23% crossed two lines as they moved from birth to age 2 years. Children whose birth lengths were near the 10th percentile but whose subsequent lengths were closer to the 50th percentile tended to catch up at an average of 11.5 months; those born near the 90th percentile and moving down to the 50th percentile did so at an average age of 13 months (Figure 2). Karlberg and colleagues analyzed the length curves of healthy children in the first 3 years of life.[14] Children were found to have nonlinear decelerations in their growth rates starting during infancy. During the second year of life, the variation in the growth rate was found to increase, with greater gains in linear growth during the spring/summer than fall/winter. During the third year, the growth pattern stabilized. Thus, fluctuations in length percentiles are a normal phenomenon in infant growth and, especially in the face of normal weight gain, should not prompt evaluation for nutritional disease. Horner and colleagues have demonstrated that a more significant decline in the linear growth rate occurs in children with constitutional short stature.[15] This fall in the growth rate generally first became apparent in the first 6 to 9 months of life and was greatest during the first 2 years. These children fell more than 2 SD below the mean for height by 3 years of age. Subsequently, their growth rate was the same as that of normal children but below and parallel to the 3rd percentile. Mei et al.[8] studied the growth trends of over 10,000 children in the first 60 months of life using data from the California Child Health and Development Study. Though the data was collected between 1959 and 1967, and does not include Latinos, it does include children from a wide range of socioeconomic backgrounds. The frequency of crossing 2 major percentiles for the indices of height for age, weight for age, and weight for height was determined. Sex differences were not found. For children 0 to 6 months of age, 32% did so for height for age, 39% for weight for age, and 62% for weight for height. For children 6 to 24 months of age 13 to 15% did so for height for age, 6 to 15% for weight for age, 20 to 27% for weight for height. From the ages of 24 to 60 months, 2 to 10% did so for height for age, 1 to 5% for weight for age, and 6 to 15% for weight for height. Whether a child displayed catch-up or catch-down growth depended on initial measurements, with a tendency to regress towards the mean.

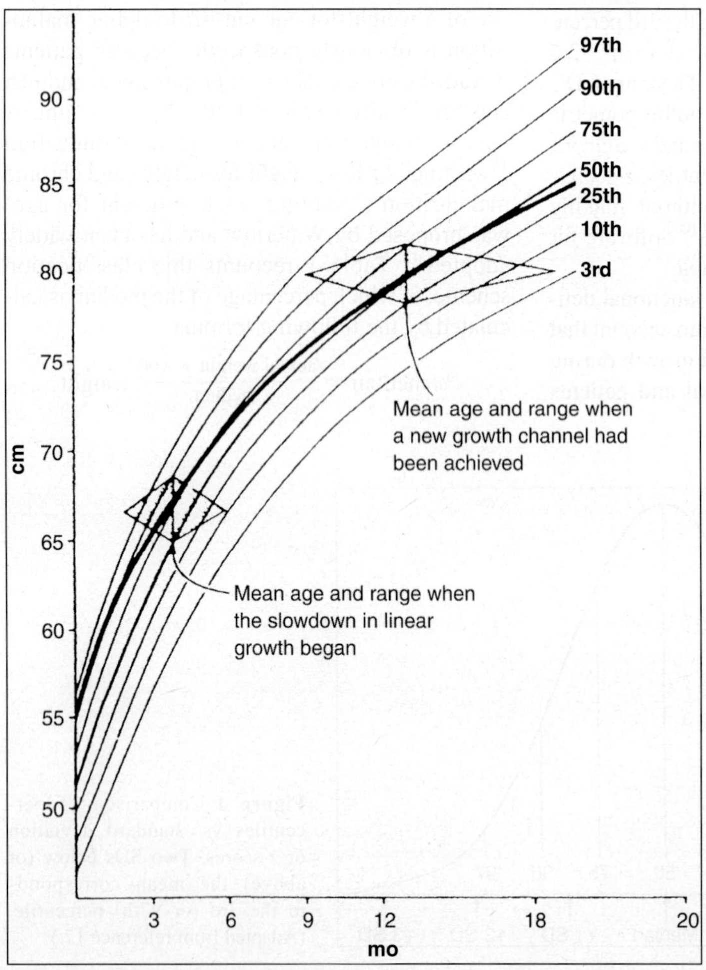

Figure 2 Mean linear growth curve of 16 healthy infants who crossed percentile lines during infancy. Whereas at birth they were at the 90th percentile, by age 2 years, they had reached the 40th percentile. This shift generally occurred between 3 and 13 months. (Adapted from reference 13.)

Alternative or supplemental anthropometric criteria for FTT have been proposed, including decreased weight velocity, low triceps skinfold (TSF) values, and midarm circumference (MAC). For example, data have been published on incremental gains in the length and weight of the infants enrolled in the Iowa and Fels studies.[16] Measurement and interpretation of skinfold thickness and growth velocity have the disadvantage of requiring special equipment and/or graphically represented standards and may not add specificity or sensitivity to the screening criteria noted above. Depleted fat stores and slowed growth velocity are often concomitant findings in the patient with malnutrition, and their presence or absence can be noted on detailed clinical evaluation. However, for standard screening purposes in most US settings, the anthropometric measurements of weight, height, and age are usually sufficient.

Any diagnosis of malnutrition requires accurate measurements of weight, length, head circumference, and age. An infant's length should be measured supine on a length board until age 2 years, after which time they should be measured upright. Infants and children should be weighed with minimal clothing on scales accurate to at least 100 g. If possible, one person in the office should be designated as solely responsible for weighing and measuring patients. Detailed summaries of anthropometric techniques have been published elsewhere.[17]

Measurements should be plotted on appropriate graphs (see Appendix I). When plotting infants with a history of premature birth, their chronologic age should be corrected by gestational age until 24 months for weight, 40 months for length, and 18 months for head circumference.[18]

In 2000, the CDC developed new growth curves for infants from birth to 36 months and for children from 2 to 20 years of age.[19] These curves are now recommended for use in the United States. The new growth charts were developed to rectify deficiencies of the 1977 NCHS curves.[19] The CDC curves are more representative of a cross-section of the ethnicity of the children living in the United States. Data from breastfed infants are also included so that the mix of formula-fed and breastfed infants is more accurately represented. The distribution of birthweights now more closely matches the national distribution. Statistical methods have been employed to smooth the disjunction between length and height. Finally, curves for body mass index (BMI) are available for children from ages 2 to 20 years. On the NCHS charts, weight-for-stature charts were available but stopped at age 10 years for girls and 11 years for boys.

A somewhat misleading distinction in the medical literature is still written of concerning organic versus nonorganic failure to thrive (eg, Rosenn and colleagues[20]). The former is malnutrition attributable to an underlying medical condition that has presumably limited the intake, absorption, or use of adequate calories. Nonorganic failure to thrive, in contrast, implies a primary social dysfunction of the family, mother–child dyad, or societal unit, the net result of which is inadequate nutrional intake. Berwick and colleagues reviewed the records of 122 children between the ages 1 and 25 months who were hospitalized for FTT.[21] Thirty-three percent had no specific diagnosis, 32% were felt to have a social or environmental explanation, and 31% were given a specific medical diagnosis. Gahagan[6] emphasizes that FTT is not a disease, but a symptom representing the final common pathway of medical, psychosocial, and environmental processes. Furthermore, rather than being classified as organic or nonorganic, it should be viewed as undernutrition resulting from an interaction of biological and environmental factors. The most common situation will be multifactorial or "mixed" FTT where both medical and nonmedical factors are identified resulting in a "layering of risk" which interact resulting in growth failure.[6,22,23] This is not surprising and reflects the difficulty in any attempt to dichotomize between physiologic and social influences on health in general and nutrition specifically.

EPIDEMIOLOGY

Significant pediatric undernutrition in the United States is often cited to occur in 10% of low-income children.[24] The prevalence of underweight children can range from 1 to 10%, depending on the clinical setting.[25] Unfortunately, the definitions of undernutrition or FTT used to support such claims do not always employ well-established anthropometric criteria. Factors that can interfere with an accurate survey of FTT infants have been reviewed.[26]

National surveys have been undertaken that provide information on the prevalence of inadequate growth.[25] The National Health and Nutrition Surveys [NHANES I (1971 to 1974), II (1976 to 1980), and III (1988 to 1991)] studied the prevalence of low height for age and weight for height among 2- to 5-year-olds. In the 1988 to 1991 survey, the prevalence was found to be 5.2% and 2.7%, respectively. The Pediatric Nutrition Surveillance System (PedNSS) measured the prevalence of inadequate growth in predominantly less than 5-year-old low-income children who participated in publicly funded nutrition and public health programs. In 1996, the prevalence for low height for age was 5.8% and low weight for height was 2.6% in 2- to 5-year-olds. Furthermore, the PedNSS reported in 1996 that infants from birth to 2 months experienced the highest prevalence for both indicators. In this group, 12% had low height for age and 4.1% low weight for height. Finally, blacks had the highest rates for both of these indicators. The prevalence of low weight for age amongst children 2 to 6 years has dropped over the past three decades from 5.5 to 4.1%, with the prevalence of low weight for height remaining relatively stable at 2.5%.[6]

In recent years, pediatric health care providers have encountered growing numbers of international adoptees and the children of new immigrants. Every year, 3 million children ages 0 to 19 years of age immigrate to the United States mainly from Asia, Western Europe, and North Africa.[27] Immigrant children have been found to be deficient for height for age and weight for age.[28] They may also have developmental delays, infectious diseases, a variety of health problems, and psychosocial stressors.[27,28,30] Fifteen thousand foreign-born children are adopted by American citizens each year.[27] Since 1990, the majority were adopted from China and the countries of the former Soviet Union.[27] Nason and Narad report that poor growth is the most common and consistent problem observed upon arrival in this and other western nations of adoptees from foreign orphanages.[29] Among the children adopted from China, z-scores were <-2 SD in 39% for height, 18% for weight, and 24% for head circumference.[30] Developmental delays, both global and in specific areas, were common, as were parasite infestations, infections, and chronic medical conditions.[30] The degree of growth failure is proportional to the length of time spent in an orphanage.[29] Psychosocial growth failure has been postulated as a possible contributing factor.[29]

MEDICAL RISK FACTORS FOR MALNUTRITION

There are many well-known medical and psychosocial risk factors for the development of FTT (Table 2), which can generally be viewed as relating to the infant or to the family. Almost all chronic medical conditions in a child can lead to poor weight gain by a variety of factors.[31] These include decreased caloric intake (anorexia, food withholding, altered mental status), increased caloric requirements (fever, infections), and/or inefficient use of ingested calories (maldigestion, malasorption, and metabolic disorders). Nutritional recommendations for specific disease states are found elsewhere in this textbook.

Table 2 Risk Factors for the Development of Failure to Thrive

Infant characteristics
Any chronic medical condition resulting in
- Inadequate intake (eg, swallowing dysfunction, central nervous system depression, or any condition resulting in anorexia)
- Increased metabolic rate (eg, bronchopulmonary dysplasia, congenital heart disease, fevers)
- Maldigestion or malabsorption (eg, AIDS, cystic fibrosis, short gut, inflammatory bowel disease, celiac disease)
- Premature birth (especially intrauterine growth retardation)
- Developmental delay
- Congenital anomalies
- Intrauterine toxin exposure (eg, alcohol)
- Plumbism and/or anemia

Family characteristics
- Poverty
- Unusual health and nutrition beliefs
- Social isolation
- Disordered feeding techniques
- Substance abuse or other psychopathology (including Munchausen syndrome by proxy)
- Violence or abuse

An important medical risk factor for undernutrition in childhood is premature birth. Growth data are available for low birthweight preterm infants (see Appendix I).[32–35] Growth curves for the use with hospitalized very-low birthweight growth curves have been developed.[36] Standard growth curves should be used once the infant has achieved a gestational age of 40 weeks. As noted above, correction for prematurity should be done when plotting an infant's anthropometric measurements on the CDC growth curves to correctly assess growth. Even with correction for gestational age, however, Casey and colleagues have shown that patients who were both low birthweight and premature have smaller mean lengths, weights, and head circumferences than their term counterparts in the first 3 years of life.[33,34] The lower the birthweight, the greater the depression of the mean.

The infant who is small for gestational age is a special case because prenatal factors may have already exerted a deleterious effect on somatic growth. The reasons for in utero growth failure may include genetic abnormalities (chromosomal aberrations, syndromes), environmental influences (maternal smoking, malnutrition, exposure to drugs or other toxins), and infection. Infants with symmetric growth retardation (where weight, height, and head circumference are equivalently depressed) are less likely to respond to nutritional supplementation with catch-up growth. Conversely, asymmetrically growth-retarded infants where weight is disproportionately low have more truly suffered in utero malnutrition and can therefore be expected to achieve better growth after birth.[37] Strauss and Dietz have observed that infants who are labeled intrauterine growth retarded (IUGR) often have mothers and non-IUGR siblings who are smaller and lighter and come from families in which there is an increased prevalence of IUGR infants.[38] They concluded that some of these infants may be genetically small, which may limit their catch-up growth.

A prospective case-control study of premature infants has identified some risk factors for poor weight gain after hospital discharge.[39] Among 914 infants with birth weights ≤2,500 g, 19.7% were diagnosed with FTT at some point in the first 3 years of life. Multivariate analysis revealed that among infants with growth failure, significantly more had birthweights less than 1,500 g, were small for gestational age, had an abnormal neurological examination at 40 weeks gestational age, or had a mother whose height was less than 159 cm. This study found that infants born to mothers who were college graduates or who were living with the infant's father were at higher risk of FTT. Family income, prenatal care, and maternal race were not found to be significant factors. Dusick et al.[40] report that amongst very low birthweight (VLBW) infants, the presence and degree of intrauterine growth restriction predicts a higher incidence of growth failure (as defined as < 10th %) both early on and at 18 to 22 months for length, height, and head circumference. They also found that other significant predictive factors for increased risk of growth delay in these children are white race and Grade III/VI intracranial hemorrhage/periventricular leukomalacia. Furthermore, they determined that significant postdischarge risk factors for poor growth at 18 months include abnormal swallow and abnormal neurological examination. They did not find, however, that the mother's educational level was associated with poor growth.

The child with neurological disease, especially cerebral palsy, is at risk for abnormalities of growth and nutritional status.[41–44] Many children with developmental delay are short for their age, and although stunting owing to chronic malnutrition is a possible cause, genetic programming caused by an underlying condition or altered neuroendocrine axis may also be an etiology. In addition, children with developmental delay may suffer from swallowing dysfunction, gastroesophageal reflux, constipation, and other gastrointestinal diseases that, in addition to their underlying neurological dysfunction, may alter their caloric intake. Children with hypertonia and movement disorders can have excessive energy expenditure, which may be an additional factor contributing to poor growth. Conversely, children with cerebral palsy often have limited physical activity and therefore lower energy requirements than similarly aged children, thereby placing them at risk for obesity.

Anthropometric evaluation of children with spastic cerebral palsy can be difficult because of contractures or scoliosis. Furthermore, interpretation of growth needs to be done in light of the growth potential of any known underlying medical condition or syndrome. Due to the difficulty of correctly measuring and interpreting the linear growth of these children, emphasis should instead be placed on obtaining alternative measures of growth and nutritional status. Weight for height can be used, but in cerebral palsy patients may underestimate their degree of malnutrition.[41] Stallings and Spender and their colleagues have found that linear growth in children with quadriplegic, hemiplegic, and diplegic cerebral palsy can be assessed by measurement of upper arm and lower leg lengths.[42,45] Growth curves are available for these parameters.[45] In children with quadriplegic cerebral palsy, upper arm length and lower leg length were found to correlate with TSF and MAC.[42] Samson-Fang and Stevenson have recommended the use of TSF for the nutritional screening of children with cerebral palsy.[41] A TSF less than the 10th percentile indicates the need to more fully assess a child's nutritional status, growth, and overall health.

Table 3[46] lists suggested energy requirements in developmentally delayed children based on calorie per centimeter of height. Experience has shown that estimating needs by Recommended Dietary Allowance (RDA) and weight for these children often leads to excessive energy intake.

Children born with congenital anomalies are also at nutritional risk. For example, infants born with cleft lip and/or palate may have significant oral-motor dysfunction requiring special nipples and feeding instructions. Some of these infants may require feedings by nasogastric tube or gastrostomy. Montagnoli et al.[47] determined the incidence of growth impairment as defined by height or weight less than the 10% in 881 Brazilian children with cleft lip and/or palate. They report that in the first 2 years of life, amongst children with isolated cleft lip, about 20% demonstrated impairment for weight and height. For children with cleft lip and palate or isolated cleft palate, the incidence of growth impairment was similar, occurring in roughly one-third for both weight and height. It is important to remember that the presence of cleft lip and/or palate or other congenital anomalies may be a manifestation of an underlying syndrome or association of which intrauterine growth retardation, poor growth, or short stature is a component. If available, syndrome-specific growth curves should be used. Weight for height, BMI, or TSF and MAC may also be helpful in these children as well.

Table 3 Estimated Energy Needs for Developmentally Delayed Children

	Daily Caloric Condition Recommendation
Ambulatory, ages 5–12 yr	13.9 kcal/cm height
Nonambulatory, ages 5–12 yr	11.1 kcal/cm height
Cerebral palsy with decreased levels of activity	10 kcal/cm height
Cerebral palsy with increased levels of activity	15 kcal/cm height
Athetoid cerebral palsy, adolescence	Up to 6,000 kcal
Down syndrome, boys ages 5–12 yr	16.1 kcal/cm height
Down syndrome, girls ages 5–12 yr	14.3 kcal/cm height
Myelomeningocele	Approximately RDA for age may need as little as 7 cal/cm height

Adapted from reference 46.
RDA = recommended dietary allowance.

Lead intoxication is a medical risk for poor growth.[48] High blood lead levels probably correlate with poor nutrition based on the fact that a high-fat, low-iron diet promotes lead absorption from the intestine. What is less clear is to what extent the anorexia and other behavioral problems seen with iron deficiency and/or lead poisoning are contributing factors to malnutrition.

PSYCHOSOCIAL RISK FACTORS

Factors that predispose to poor growth in the United States may be social or behavioral in origin. Poverty is a significant and has been stated to be the greatest single risk factor for FTT.[49,50] Frank and Zeisel report that 13% of their patients are homeless and noted that inadequate medical care can exacerbate the tendency of acute illnesses to lead to poor growth.[24] The degree to which Federal food aid to poor families in the United States helps improve the nutritional status of this population is controversial,[51] though it is reported that food stamps have been shown to increase the intake of nutrients in children of impoverished families.[52] Food insecurity has been cited as a factor as well.[6] Families experience food insecurity when the availability of food is limited or uncertain, often associated with intermittent hunger.[6] In 1999, 10.9% of families reported food insecurity.[52] For those living below the poverty line, food insecurity was reported by 46%.[52] Casey et al.[52] report that welfare reform has lead to the reduction in food stamp benefits, increased food insecurity, as well as an association with positive maternal depression screens. Depression can also have deleterious effects on child growth as described below.

Feeding-related behavioral disorders are not uncommon in children with poor growth.[53–58] and may extend beyond mealtimes.[57] These children are perceived as having more difficult temperamental characteristics and are rated by their parents as being more negative, irregular, dependent, and unstoppable.[55] There may be a temperamental mismatch between the child and mother.[54] Chatoor and colleagues developed diagnostic criteria for infantile anorexia.[55,56] The diagnostic criteria of this disorder include: (1) refusal to consume adequate amounts of food for at least 1 month, (2) onset of food refusal before 3 years of age, most often during the transition from spoon to self-feeding between 9 to 12 months of age, (3) child does not effectively communicate hunger signals, lacks interest in food but shows interest in exploration and/or interaction with caregiver, (4) demonstrates significant growth deficiency, (5) food refusal did not follow a traumatic event, and (6) food refusal is not due to an underlying medical condition or illness. Some behaviors may have a medical basis or have had roots in prior medical problems experienced by the child leading to food aversion[53,54,59] or the perception that the child is vulnerable or fragile.[57]

Maternal developmental delay, learning disorders, anxiety, psychiatric disease, substance abuse, and difficulties with maternal attachment all may impact the feeding and nurturing of a child aswell.[54,55,58] Indeed, an extensive literature has arisen around the transactional model of FTT,[18] which emphasizes the interrelationships between medical, behavioral, and developmental characteristics of the infant on the one hand and the familial, psychosocial, and economic environment of the child's caretakers on the other. Such a multifactorial approach to the problem of poor growth has direct implications for treatment modalities, as discussed below.

Depression is common in women of all ages, especially young women who are mothers of young children.[52] Puerperal mood disorders are common as well.[61] Postpartum blues, characterized by mood swings, tearfulness, generalized anxiety, and irritability affects 85% of women in the first 5 to 7 postpartum days.[61] If resolved by 10 days postpartum, treatment or referral is not indicated.[62] Postnatal depression affects 5 to 25% of women of childbearing age.[61] Maternal depression is known to affect the mother–child interaction in many ways.[52,62] It has been associated with an increased probability of behavioral problems and a significant negative impact on development.[52] There is a growing body of literature describing the association of maternal depression and poor growth. O'Brien et al.[62] identified children less than 2 years of age with faltering growth and screened their mothers for depression with a standardized tool. On this basis, they found that the mothers of children with faltering growth were at increased risk of postnatal depression and anxiety.

Table 4 Recognition of FTT Secondary to Neglect or Abuse

The risk factors that should alert the pediatrician to the possibility of neglect as the cause of FTT include:

- Parental depression, stress, marital strife, divorce
- Parental history of abuse as a child
- Mental retardation and psychological abnormalities in the parent(s)
- Young and single mothers without social supports
- Domestic violence
- Alcohol or other substance abuse
- Previous child abuse in the family
- Social isolation and/or poverty
- Parents with inadequate adaptive and social skills
- Parents who are overly focused on career and/or activities away from home
- Failure to adhere to medical regimens
- Lack of knowledge of normal growth and development
- Infant with low birth or prolonged hospitalization

Moreover, concerns of abuse or neglect should be raised during the course of intervention and monitored if the following become evident:

- Intentional withholding of food
- Strong beliefs in health and/or nutrition regimens that jeopardize a child's well- being; and or
- Family that is resistant to recommended interventions despite multidisciplinary team approach

Adapted from reference 50.

Other psychosocial risk factors for FTT include the health and nutrition beliefs and concerns of the family, including a fear of obesity or cardiovascular disease.[63] Such concerns can lead to suboptimal caloric intake or a diet low in fat, resulting in poor growth. Also in this category are infants who are exclusively breastfed for longer than is recommended. Breast milk as the sole source of nutrition is inadequate for optimal growth after 6 to 8 months.[64] It should be noted that although growth failure in the neonatal period owing to breast milk insufficiency can be serious, FTT in the older breastfed infant is more likely attributable to underlying medical problems.[65,66] There have also been reports of severe malnutrition caused by the inappropriate use of health food beverages. Carvalho and colleagues reported two cases of children who developed severe nutritional deficiencies caused by the consumption of health food beverages.[67] One received a soy-based beverage and was placed on a strict vegan diet in accordance with the dietary practices of the parents. Another was reported who received a rice beverage because of perceived milk intolerance. Concern about food allergies is widespread, with one quarter of American households altering their dietary intake based on the perception that one or more household members suffer from food allergies.[68,69] These concerns can lead to the unnecessary restriction of a child's diet.[69]

Parenting skills (especially feeding skills), life stresses, and social isolation are also factors that can contribute to growth failure. Most studies examining the role of stress and other social factors in pediatric malnutrition have been retrospective and therefore unable to say whether stress preceded or was caused by the infant's nutritional status. Altemeier and colleagues performed a prospective, case-control study among mothers at risk for having children with poor growth by performing prenatal interviews and monitoring subsequent growth.[70] They found that a combined measure of life stress of the parents correlated significantly with subsequent FTT, as did maternal characteristics such as frequent separations, arguments, and reconciliations with the child's father. Self-reported drug and alcohol use, self-image, and attitude toward pregnancy were not correlated with infant growth. Of note, mothers whose children grew poorly reported unhappy childhoods and being subjected to physical abuse more often than did mothers whose children grew normally. In one series, 66% of mothers of infants with growth failure reported having been abused as children themselves compared with 26% of controls from a similar socioeconomic group.[71]

The children of immigrants and international adoptees may experience unique stressors, including those related to relocating to a new country, language barriers, having spent extended periods in orphanages, or having witnessed war and other atrocities.[27,28,30]

Unfortunately, the theme of abuse and violence runs throughout much of the lives of children who grow poorly. Frank childhood neglect (or the maternal deprivation syndrome) was first hypothesized to be the etiology of many cases of growth failure, as implied by past uses of the term failure to thrive.[72] Food withholding has also been reported to occur in some cases of growth failure.[73] A case series of children diagnosed with Munchausen syndrome by proxy indicated that 29% had been diagnosed with FTT, and 17% of their siblings had had either nonaccidental injury, neglect, inappropriate medication administration, or FTT.[74] Kellogg and Lukefahr reviewed 12 cases of criminal starvation of infants and children.[75] The median age of the children was 2.7 years, with a range of about 2 months to 13.5 years. Though rare, the consequences to the children were dire, with most suffering from severe wasting and stunting, half with past or present evidence of physical or sexual abuse, and half dying shortly after presentation to medical care or law enforcement. These reports all underscore the fact that infants and children with growth failure may represent a flag for serious social and psychological problems in the family. Block et al. list the risk factors which should alert care providers of the possibility that FTT is the result of neglect[50]

APPROACH TO THE PATIENT WITH FTT

Evaluation of a child with growth failure should begin (and often end) with a thorough history and physical examination because the diagnostic benefits of additional laboratory tests are minimal.[21,76] The identification of psychosocial issues that may be confronting the family or care givers should be done concurrently. Because many children with poor growth suffer from behavioral and developmental problems as well as social and economic disadvantages, a multidisciplinary approach has been advocated as an effective method of diagnosis and therapy.[77–79] The use of home visits in conjunction with a multidisciplinary growth and nutrition clinic may provide further benefit.[80] Evaluation by a social worker, behavioral specialist, and/or psychologist supplement the medical and nutritional evaluation. Translators are often necessary to permit adequate communication with immigrant or non–English-speaking families.

Table 5 Historical Evaluation of Infants and Children with Growth Failuree

Prenatal
- General obstetric history
- Recurrent miscarriages
- Was the pregnancy planned?
- Use of medications, drugs, or cigarettes

Labor, delivery, and neonatal events
- Neonatal asphyxia or Apgar scores
- Prematurity
- Small for gestational age
- Birthweight and length
- Congenital malformations or infections
- Maternal bonding at birth
- Length of hospitalization
- Breastfeeding support
- Feeding difficulties as neonate

Medical history of child
- Regular physician
- Immunizations
- Development
- Medical or surgical illnesses
- Frequent infections

Growth history
- Plot previous growth points

Nutrition history
- Feeding behavior and environment
- Perceived sensitivities or allergies to foods
- Quantitative assessment of intake (3-d diet record, 24-h food recall)

Family history
- Maternal and paternal height and weight
- Growth of other siblings
- Gastrointestinal and other systemic diseases

Social history
- Age and occupation of parents
- Who feeds the child?
- Life stresses (loss of job, divorce, death in family)
- Social and economic supports (WIC, AFDC)
- Perception of growth failure as a problem
- History of violence or abuse by or of caretaker

Review of systems/clues to organic disease
- Anorexia
- Change in mental status
- Dysphagia
- Stooling pattern and consistency
- Vomiting or gastroesophageal reflux
- Recurrent fevers
- Dysuria, urinary frequency
- Activity level, ability to keep up with peers

AFDC = aid to families and dependent children; WIC = special supplemental nutrition program for women, infants and children.

In the medical assessment, important historical points to consider (Table 5) include maternal history (especially use of drugs, possible congenital infections, maternal nutrition, and health during pregnancy), labor, delivery, and neonatal events. Altemeier and colleagues showed that although postpartum complications of the mother did not predict subsequent FTT, unresolved health questions at nursery discharge (eg, bilirubin levels) and difficulty feeding in the neonatal period were associated with later growth problems.[70]

A thorough history and review of systems is crucial, as almost any medical condition may present with poor growth. This should include intercurrent illnesses, medication use, and immunization history. Acute infections can embarrass nutritional status by the increased metabolic demands of fever and stress response, as well as by reducing caloric intake through anorexia. At the same time, a history of recurrent or unusual infections should increase the clinician's suspicion for the presence of an immunodeficiency, including acquired immune deficiency syndrome (AIDS). A developmental history should be obtained. Any suggestion of oromotor or feeding difficulties should also be sought. Assessment by an interdisciplinary feeding team may be helpful and effective.[59]

The growth history should be reviewed by careful plotting of past growth points on the CDC or syndrome-specific curves. The growth pattern over time can either provide important clues to an underlying medical condition, or in fact lead to a diagnosis of health. The growth curve should be interpreted in the context of the family's growth history and pattern. Specific growth curves are available for a number of syndromes. These should be used once the diagnosis has been established (see Appendix I).[81–83] The quality of data for ethnic-specific growth curves may be suspect and their use is probably not advisable.

Dietary history should include an assessment of the foods taken, quantities, schedule of feedings and fluid intake, setting of meals, who provides the meals, if self-feeding is permitted when appropriate, force feeding, meal duration, indication of oromotor difficulties (eg., choking, gagging, pouching), oral-aversive behaviors, adverse reactions to foods, overnight feedings, formula preparation, frequency of breastfeeding, adequacy of breast milk supply, dietary restrictions, juice and soda intake, feeding history, and the organization of the household at mealtimes. Culturally-based food preferences and feeding practices should also be ascertained. Intake can be determined based upon a 24-hour food recall. A more accurate assessment is a diary of food consumed over 3 to 5 days, though some families may find this challenging to do.[84] Calculation of intake with respect to the US RDAs for age can then be performed and the need for dietary supplementation of micro- and/or macronutrients determined.

Excessive fruit juice consumption, especially in toddlers, can lead to poor nutrition. Besides the role some juices can play in the etiology of chronic diarrhea, they may displace more calorically dense and nutritionally balanced foods from the diet.[85,86] Reduction of juice intake has been shown to be associated with improved weight gain in a series of eight children who were referred for evaluation of growth failure.[87]

Family history should include the growth parameters and patterns of siblings and parents. The average of maternal and paternal heights can be calculated to derive a midparental height using the following formula:

$$\frac{\text{maternal + paternal heights}}{2} \begin{array}{l} +\ 5\text{ cm if a boy} \\ -\ 5\text{ cm if a girl} \end{array}$$

Comparison with published values can then be done to predict adult stature.[88] The family history should be complete, searching for any family history suggestive of genetic or constitutional short stature, endocrinopathy, syndromes, or any disorder of a major organ system, psychiatric disorders, and eating disorders.

A social history that documents the caretaker's economic status is crucial to help guide diagnostic and therapeutic efforts. Elicitation of the social risk factors outlined above should be performed, as well as the parent's perception of the child's nutritional status. The family's ability to afford, store, and prepare food should also be determined.

A home visit performed by an appropriately trained professional may be helpful. The child and family can be evaluated in a more natural setting, aiding the assessment of the child's environment and mealtimes and allowing for the modeling of behaviors. These visits can even be extended to the child's other significant caregivers (eg, other family members, day care, or preschool). Another method that may be helpful is to ask the child's primary caretaker to videotape the child eating a meal. This tape can then be reviewed with the family, with specific advice and praise offered based upon the observed child and caretaker feeding behaviors recorded.

Screening for organic disease should also include a thorough review of systems. Questions regarding gastrointestinal function (dysphagia, vomiting, abdominal pain, bloating, diarrhea, etc.) are especially important. The presence of fevers or other metabolic stresses should be assessed.

The physical examination of a child with poor growth must be comprehensive, as any physical findings may implicate organic and/or socioeconomic causes of growth failure, as well as potentially providing reassurance regarding the child's growth and health status. The importance of accurate anthropometric measurements has already been stressed. The pattern of growth failure itself is often indicative of whether medical, genetic, or environmental factors are to blame. Genetically small children often maintain normal weight for height, have proportionately low weights, lengths, and head circumferences, and can grow parallel to but lower than the 5th percentile curve. Alternatively, children with caloric deprivation or malabsorption fall off their weight curves first, followed by length, then by head circumference. They will therefore acutely show a deficit of weight for length and then more chronically a deficit of height for age. Figure 3[89] illustrates characteristic linear growth curves for children with intrinsic shortness, constitutional growth delay, and attenuated growth (as might be seen with caloric deprivation or gastrointestinal disease).

A critical aspect of the physical examination is an assessment of caregiver-child interaction, such as physical proximity, verbalization toward each other, and eye contact. The affect of the care provider should also be assessed. Evidence of child neglect should be sought by paying attention to

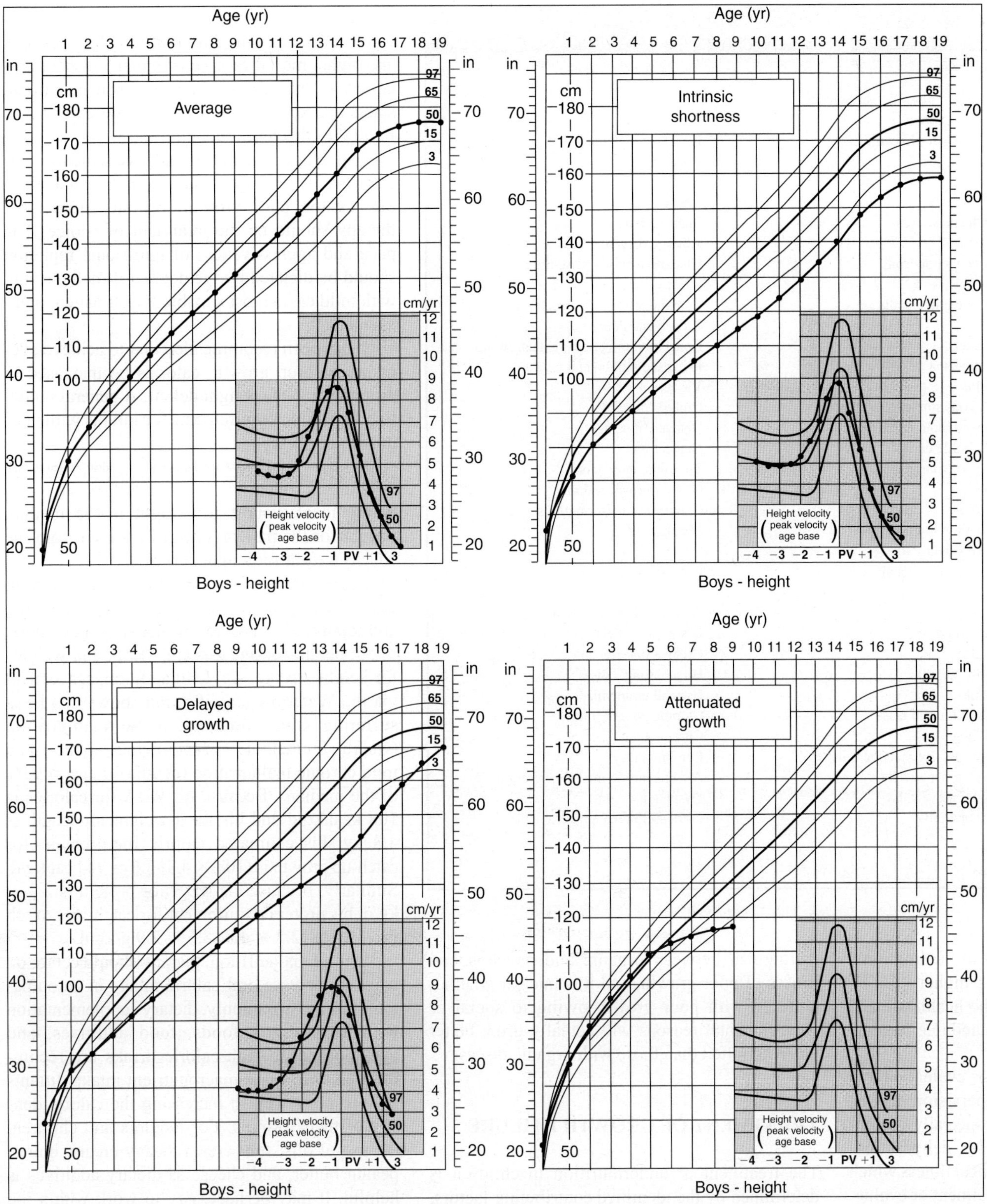

Figure 3 Linear growth curves (and height velocity curves, *insets*) of four different patterns of growth: average, intrinsic shortness, delayed growth, and attenuated growth. The last pattern is more characteristic of malnutrition. (Adapted from reference 89.)

general hygiene, oral health, and evidence of physical abuse. The possibility of organic disease can be evaluated by examination of all major organ systems. Table 6[90] gives a summary of possible findings on physical examination in children with growth failure, which should prompt further evaluation for underlying medical problems.

Unfortunately, the extensive differential diagnosis that can be engendered by the consideration of a child with poor growth (which Tunnessen compared to the index of any pediatric textbook[91]) can lead to excessive diagnostic testing. Sills' landmark study in 1978 succinctly showed the lack of utility of many laboratory tests in children with poor growth.[76] In 185 children less than 3-years-old admitted for evaluation of FTT, only 36 of 2,607 laboratory tests performed (1.4%) were helpful in making a diagnosis, and all of these 36 positive results were suspected on clinical grounds. Berwick and colleagues also demonstrated the importance of a thorough history and examination over extensive testing.[21] Therefore, a thorough history, family history, social history, review of the growth pattern as revealed by the curves, and physical examination are the most effective screening tools for the presence of organic disease.

Laboratory testing should be minimized. Some basic screening tests may include complete blood count, blood urea nitrogen, albumin, erythrocyte sedimentation rate, lead concentration, and urinalysis. Screening for celiac disease should also be considered. An increased incidence of this disorder has been noted,[92,93] with a significant number not presenting with the classic triad of chronic diarrhea, abdominal distension, and FTT, but suboptimal growth. The diagnostic yield of screening

Table 6 Physical Examination of Infants and Children with Growth Failure

	Abnormality	Considerations
Vital signs	Adrenal or thyroid insufficiency	
	Hypertension	Renal disease
	Tachypnea/tachycardia	Increased metabolic demands
Skin	Pallor	Anemia
	Poor hygiene	Neglect
	Eccyhmoses	Abuse
	Candidiasis	Immunodeficiency
	Eczema	Allergic disease
	Erythema nodusom	Ulcerative colitis, vasculitis
HEENT	Hair loss	Stress
	Chronic otitis media	Immunodeficiency, structural orofacial defect
	Cataracts	Congenital infections, galactosemia
	Papilledema	Increased intracranial pressure
	Uveitis	Vasculitis
	Aphthous stomatitis	Crohn's disease
	Delayed tooth eruption	Delayed bone age
	Milk bottle caries	Neglect
	Thyroid enlargement	Thyroid enlargement
Chest	Wheezes	Cystic fibrosis, asthma
Cardiovascular	Murmur	Congenital malformations
Abdomen	Distention, hyperactive bowel sounds	Malabsorption
	Hepatosplenomegaly	Liver disease, glycogen storage, tumor
Genitourinary	Anomalies	Associated endocrinopathies
	Diaper rashes	Diarrhea, neglect
Rectum	Fistulae	Crohn's disease
	Empty ampulla	Hirschprung's disease
Extremities	Edema	Hypoalbuminemia
	Loss of muscle mass	Chronic malnutrition
	Clubbing	Chronic lung disease
Nervous system	Abnormal deep tendon reflexes	Cerebral palsy
	Developmental delay	Altered caloric intake or requirements
	Cranial nerve palsy	Dysphagia
Behavior	Uncooperative	Difficult to feed temperament

Adapted from reference 90.
HEENT = head, eyes, ears, nose, and throat.

tests of immigrant children and international adoptees with undernutrition is higher.[27–30,94,95] Current recommendations for the healthcare and screening of immigrant children and international adoptees are covered elsewhere.[27,28]

Admission to the hospital for evaluation and observation of growth under supervision may be indicated.[96] Admission should especially be considered for those children with dehydration, severe malnutrition, serious medical illness which would benefit from inpatient treatment or evaluation, significant impairment of the care provider (mental illness, drug use), or if there is concern about abuse or the safety of the child's environment. It is hoped that the combination of the provision of adequate calories and extraction from an unfavorable environment may lead to a rapid weight gain in patients with FTT and children with medical reasons for their poor nutritional status will be correctly identified. Unfortunately, once a child is hospitalized, the tendency to perform diagnostic tests often increases, which may, in turn, interfere with feeding the child (multiple consultants, tests requiring nil by mouth status, etc.). Berwick and colleagues pointed out that weight gain or loss in the hospital did not distinguish between organic and psychosocial causes of poor growth, and it is unclear whether children with poor growth owing to social or environmental reasons will actually grow better when admitted than those with organic disease.[21]

TREATMENT OF GROWTH FAILURE

The treatment of undernutrition in children is determined by the identified contributing factors, be they biologic, psychiatric, or socioeconomic. Rarely, simple dietary advice regarding correct formula preparation may be all that is needed to ensure adequate caloric intake. Much more likely is the need for a long-term treatment and a follow-up plan, involving nutritional advice, behavioral modification, and social work intervention. As noted above, the multidisciplinary team approach to management has advantages and may even result in better nutritional outcomes for patients.[76,78–80]

If a heretofore unsuspected medical illness is diagnosed, treatment of the underlying problem should proceed. However, nutritional aspects of the medical illness should not be ignored, given the well-recognized propensity of poorly nourished individuals to suffer more complications and higher mortality rates with many disease processes.[97] The relationships between nutritional status and specific disease states are explored in Part IV of this text.

If medical and nutritional assessments indicate that inadequacy of caloric intake is the etiology of the poor growth, primary nutritional therapy should be the treatment of choice. The pace and aggressiveness of nutritional repletion should be dictated by the degree of malnutrition, with mild cases most suitable for outpatient management.[98]

It has been recommended that to achieve adequate catch-up growth, calories be increased in proportion to the weight deficit. A general guideline for caloric requirements for infants with poor growth is

$$\text{kcal per kg required} = \frac{\text{RDA for age (kcal/kg)} \times \text{ideal weight for age}}{\text{actual weight}}$$

where ideal weight for height is the median weight for the patient's height (as read from the NCHS weight for height curves).

For example, a 3-month-old boy with a weight of 3.6 kg and length of 57 cm has the following anthropometric measures: weight-for-age z-score, -2.50; height-for-age z-score, -1.55; and weight-for-height z-score, -2.11. In addition, assessment via the Waterlow classification shows that he is suffering from moderate acute malnutrition (weight for height = 74% of the median) and mild chronic malnutrition (height for age = 93% of the median). Because his RDA for calories is 108 kcal/kg/d and his ideal weight for length is 4.8 kg, his estimated caloric requirement for catch-up growth is $(108 \times 4.8)/3.6 = 144$ cal/kg/d. Similarly, because his RDA for protein is 2.2 g/kg/d, his protein requirement for catch-up growth is closer to $(2.2 \times 4.8)/3.6 = 2.9$ g/kg/d.

In mild malnutrition, therapy should center on ways to increase oral caloric intake in an outpatient setting. Commonly, dietary supplementation with high-calorie foods, food additives, and age-appropriate high-calorie drinks are recommended to increase macronutrient intake. Infants may respond well to increasing the caloric density of their formula. For toddlers and children, the use of oils, sour cream, heavy cream, butter, peanut butter, and cheese as dietary additives is helpful. It may be necessary to work within the framework of the traditional food preferences and feeding practices of immigrant families and adoptees. For micronutrients, routine supplementation with a zinc- and iron-containing multivitamin is probably prudent, with the need for further iron therapy determined by laboratory evidence of deficiency.

Commenting upon children with LBW and the growth faltering of infants after weaning in developing nations, Weaver raises the issue of the "catch-up growth dilemma".[99] Referring to both animal and human studies, the author points out that accelerated growth early in life does appear to provide the benefits of improved survival, nutritional status, and infection resistance.

Table 7 Classification of Feeding Disorders in Infants and Children with Growth Failure

Disorder Type	Age of Onset	Associated Medical Conditions	Features of Infants	Features of Caretakers	Treatment
Homeostasis	0–2 mo	Limited experience with oral feeds (eg, respiratory occupational therapy distress) and swallow	Excitable; irritable; passive	Anxious; depressed; over- or under-feeds; stimulates infants resuck	Pacifier during nastogastric
Attachment	2–6 mo	Sad; hypervigilant; or separation from mother; developmental delay	Detached; depressed; arches or resists when picked up	Emotional nurtur-ance; holds infant loosely	Developmental stimulation; education of caretaker regarding needs of infant
Individua-tion or sepa-ration	6 mo–3 yr	(eg, diabetes, celiac)	Refuses food; defiant; plays with food	Frustrated does not allow infant to self-feed	Regularly scheduled sepa-rate mealtimes from playtimes; encourage self-feeding

Adapted from reference 101.

However, there may also be a high price to be paid later in life with obesity, insulin resistance, bone demineralization, and cardiovascular disease. It is urged that this dilemma be considered when approaching feeding recommendations.

Possible indications for hospitalization for evaluation and treatment are as above. A common error among hospitalized patients with growth failure is to underestimate their caloric requirements for growth because these can be quite high. Children recovering from severe malnutrition may gain weight safely on caloric intakes as high as 170 kcal/kg/d and protein intakes of 4 to 5 g/kg/d.[100] It should be noted that such extremes in caloric requirements are unusual in the average patient admitted for growth failure in the United States. It is also important to note that any calculations used to judge caloric requirements are merely estimates and that the sufficiency of any diet is proven by the occurrence of subsequent weight and, eventually, height gain. These parameters should be measured and charted graphically to allow assessment of the dietary intervention.

In addition to nutritional therapy, evaluation of family dynamics and economic situation (eg, eligibility for state and federal assistance) should be performed. As mentioned above, visits to the home or other settings where the child receives care by a nurse or other appropriate personnel can also be enlightening in this regard. Regular outpatient and/or home visits should occur to document adequate weight gain and compliance with dietary management and to address any ongoing behavioral issues.

Behavioral modification should center on improving feeding techniques, removing conflict or struggles from mealtimes, reducing between-meal snacking or "grazing," and eliminating television and other distractions during mealtimes. Caregivers are encouraged to establish an eating routine with specific times, as well as a consistent setting and place for meals. It is also recommended that the duration of meals be limited to 30 minutes. Table 7[101] recounts a helpful schema in which three developmental stages of feeding disorders are described, with typical features of effected infants and caretakers. As noted, the approach to therapy will largely be determined by the type of feeding disorder and age of the patient.

PROGNOSIS

The ultimate growth potential of a child with growth failure is determined by a variety of factors, including genetic potential, the timing of malnutrition (intrauterine vs neonatal vs later infancy), and the severity of malnutrition (weight alone affected vs weight, height, and head circumference). The presence of underlying medical problems and their ability to be successfully managed are also important variables. Some premature infants fail to catch up normally. For instance, Kitchen and colleagues showed that in a cohort of children whose birthweights had been less than 1,500 g and who had weights or heights less than the 10th percentile at age 2 years, half were still less than the 10th percentile at age 8 years.[102] Casey and colleagues have reported that low-birthweight premature infants demonstrated little catch-up growth in the first 3 years of life.[33,34] Subsequent studies have demonstrated that these children may demonstrate catch-up growth through childhood and even into adolescence, ultimately achieving predicted genetic height.[103,104] One study compared adolescents born with an extremely low birthweight (ELBW, < 1,000 g) without significant neurodevelopmental disability with a matched group who had a normal birthweight.[105] It was found that those who were ELBW attained growth parameters within 2 SD of the mean, although they had smaller heights, weights, and head circumferences than their normal birthweight peers. The effect was most marked for those who were ELBW and small for gestational age. There were no significant differences in sexual maturation.

Long-term data on the growth of full-term children with a history of growth failure have been limited. In one cohort of 40 children who had been admitted for malnutrition, 17 (42.5%) had weights or heights below the 3rd percentile on follow-up after a mean of 3.4 years.[106] In another series of 30 children diagnosed before age 2 years, mean weights were 15% lower and mean heights were 5% lower than a control group in years 3 through 6 of life.[107] The interpretation of these types of studies is made difficult by biases introduced by patient selection and follow-up rate because patients requiring admission obviously represent a more severely affected spectrum of disease. Thus, not all children referred for growth failure are expected to suffer long-term growth problems.

International adoptees from orphanages often demonstrate significant postadoption catch-up growth.[29] Age and height at the time of adoption are negative predictors of growth, BMI is a positive predictor.[29] It is recommended that adoptive parents should be counseled to allow 3 to 6 months for evidence of improved growth velocity before further intervention is undertaken in the absence of a potential medical issue.[29]

The long-term growth pattern of international adoptees is still unknown.[29] However, there are an increasing number of reports of precocious puberty, especially in girls, in those who have experienced rapid catch-up growth with the depression of ultimate adult height.[29] The "catch-up growth dilemma" and the later consequences of rapid catch-up growth have been previously discussed.

A major concern remains the impact of poor growth and nutrition upon cognitive, behavioral, and social development. As alluded to above and as further developed elsewhere in this textbook, the human neurologic system continues to develop and grow postnatally, making nutritional and environmental influences early in life crucial in any effort to achieve genetic potential. The effects of early iron-deficiency anemia upon development are well known.[6] It would be reasonable to assume that deficiencies of nutrients, micronutrients, and calories could be deleterious to the growing and developing brain as well. There are reports of a significant association between the severity of growth deficiency and IQ, with some maintaining that up to 55% of infants with FTT demonstrated developmental delay, and that those with a history of FTT may continue to demonstrate learning difficulties and developmental delay 5 years after initial presentation .[108]

To help clarify the role of malnutrition per se in the genesis of developmental and intellectual delay, a classic study assessed the intellectual, motor, and social functioning of 41 patients who had suffered malnutrition in infancy.[109] Many of these patients had a history of cystic fibrosis, none had socioeconomic deprivation. Although controls scored higher than their previously malnourished siblings on intelligence testing at 2 to 5 years, this difference was not seen at later ages. Tests of motor development and social maturity were also similar between the two groups. Subsequent studies have supported the concept that appropriate psychosocial stimulation is important for cognitive development both early and later in the child's life.[110,111] How the generally milder degree of malnutrition seen in US children with growth failure impacts on subsequent cognitive, behavior, and emotional development is less clear. Corbett and Drewett[112] reviewed studies of the cognitive development of children with FTT and noted a decline in IQ of 4.2 points. They were unable to attribute this difference purely to poor nutrition versus other confounding factors such as environment or birthweight, nor were they able to demonstrate that the typical interventions were effective in reversing or preventing the difference in IQ. Chatoor et al.[108] studied 88 toddlers up to 33-month-old who were classified as healthy eaters, picky eaters, or having infantile anorexia. It was found that the last two groups had lower developmental scores than the healthy eater group, though still within the normal range. The correlation with body weight and developmental scores for the infantile anorexia group approached statistical significance. It was also found that more problematic and conflictive mother–toddler feeding and play interactions were associated with lower developmental scores as well.

PREVENTION

Because, in the United States, most causes of poor growth stem from or are complicated by social and economic adversity, amelioration of these conditions is the ultimate path to improved nutritional status of children. In the meantime, clinicians caring for these children should have an increased awareness of the medical and psychosocial factors that may predispose to growth failure, should classify such patients along the anthropometric guidelines mentioned above, and should recognize the benefits of multidisciplinary approach to difficult management situations.

REFERENCES

1. Holt LE. The Diseases of Infancy and Childhood. New York: Appleton and Company; 1899.
2. Stickler GB. Failure to thrive or failure to define. Pediatrics 1984;74:57–61.
3. Wilcox WD, Nieburg P, Miller DS. Failure to thrive: A continuing problem of definition. Clin Pediatr 1989;28:391–4.
4. Olsen EM. Failure to thrive: Still a problem of definition. Clin Pediatr 2006;45:1–6.
5. Vinton NE, Dietz WH. Undernutrition. In: Gellis SS, Kagan BM, editors. Current Pediatric Therapy, Vol 13. Philadelphia: WB Saunders; 1990. p. 1–3.
6. Gahagan S. Failure to thrive: A consequence of undernutrition. Pediatr Rev 2006; 27:e1–11.
7. Black M, Dubowitz H. Failure to thrive: Lessons from animal models and developing countries. J Dev Behav Pediatr 1991; 12:259–67.
8. Mei Z, Grummer-Strawn LM, Thompson D, et al. Shifts in percentiles of growth during early childhood: Analysis of longitudinal data from the California child health and development study. Pediatrics 2004;113:e617–27.
9. Waterlow JC, Buzina R, Keller W, et al. The presentation and use of height and weight data for comparing the nutritional status of groups of children under the age of 10 years. Bull World Health Organ 1977;55:489–98.
10. Dean AD, Dean JA, Burton AH, et al. Epi Info, Version 5: A Word Processing Database, and Statistics Program for Epidemiology on Micro-computers. Stone Mountain (GA): USD, Incorporated; 1990. A newer version of this software should be cited
11. Edwards A, Halse P, Parkin M, et al. Recognising failure to thrive in early childhood. Arch Dis Child 1990;65:1263–5.
12. Waterlow JC. Classification and definition of protein-calorie malnutrition. BMJ 1972;3:566–9.
13. Smith DA, Truog W, Rogers, et al. Shifting linear growth during infancy: Illustration of genetic factors in growth from fetal life through infancy. J Pediatr 1976;89:225–30.
14. Karlberg J, Engstrom I, Karlberg P, et al. Analysis of linear growth using a mathematical model. (Pt I) From birth to three years. Acta Paediatr Scand 1987;76:478–88.
15. Horner JM, Thorsson AV, Hintz RL. Growth deceleration patterns in children with constitutional short stature: An aid to diagnosis. Pediatrics 1978;62:529–34.
16. Guo S, Roche AF, Fomon SJ, et al. Reference data on gains in weight and length during the first two years of life. J Pediatr 1991;119:355–62.
17. Jeliffe DB, Jelliffe EFP, Zerfas A, et al. Community Nutritional Assessment. New York: Oxford University Press; 1989.
18. Bithoney WG, Dubowitz H, Egan H. Failure to thrive/growth deficiency. Pediatr Rev 1992;13:453–9.
19. Ogden CL, Kuczmarski RJ, Flegal KM, et al. Centers for Disease Control and Prevention 2000 growth charts for the United States: Improvements to the 1977 National Center for Health Statistics version. Pediatrics 2002;109:45–60.
20. Rosenn DW, Loeb LS, Jura MB. Differentiation of organic from non-organic failure to thrive syndrome in infancy. Pediatrics 1980;66:698–704.
21. Berwick DM, Levy JC, Kleinerman R. Failure to thrive: Diagnostic yield of hospitalization. Arch Dis Child 1982;57:347–51.
22. Homer C, Ludwig S. Categorization of etiology of failure to thrive. Am J Dis Child 1981;135:848–51.
23. Schwartz ID. Failure to thrive: An old nemesis in the new millennium. Pediatr Rev 2000;21:257–64.
24. Frank DA, Zeisel SH. Failure to thrive. Pediatr Clin North Am 1988;35:1187–206.
25. Sherry B. Epidemiology of inadequate growth. In: Kessler DB, Dawson P, editors. Failure to Thrive and Pediatric Undernutrition: A transdisciplinary approach. Baltimore: Paul H. Brookes; 1999. p. 19–36.
26. Drotar D. Sampling issues in research with nonorganic failure to thrive children. J Pediatr Psychol 1990;15:255–72.
27. Jenista JA. The immigrant, refugee, or internationally adopted child. Pediatr Rev 2001;22:419–29.
28. American Academy of Pediatrics. Health care for children of immigrant families. Pediatrics 1997;100:153–6.
29. Mason P, Narad C. Long-term growth and puberty concerns in international adoptees. Pediatr Clin N Am 2005;52:1351–68.
30. Miller LC, Hendrie NW. Health of children adopted from China. Pediatrics [Serial online] 2000;105:1–6. http://www.pediatrics.org/cgi/content/full/105/6/e76 (accessed June 22, 2002). Update date of citation
31. Blecker U, Mehta DI, Davis R, et al. Nutritional problems in patients who have chronic disease. Pediatr Rev 2000;21:29–32.
32. Guo SS, Wholihan K, Roche AF, et al. Weight-for-length reference data for preterm, low-birth-weight infants. Arch Pediatr Adolesc Med 1996;150:964–70.
33. Casey PH, Kraemer HC, Bernbaum J, et al. Growth patterns of low birth weight preterm infants: A longitudinal analysis of a large, varied sample. J Pediatr 1990;117:298–307.
34. Casey PH, Kraemer HC, Bernbaum J, et al. Growth status and growth rates of a varied sample of low birth weight, preterm infants: A longitudinal cohort from birth to three years of age. J Pediatr 1991;119:599–605.
35. Guo SS, Roche AF, Chumlea WC, et al. Growth in weight, recumbent length, and head circumference for preterm low birthweight infants during the first three years of life using gestation-adjusted ages. Early Hum Dev 1997;47:305–25.
36. Ehrenkranz RA, Younes N, Lemons JA, et al. Longitudinal growth of hospitalized very low birth weight infants. Pediatrics 1999;104:280–9.
37. Villar J, Smeriglio V, Martorell R, et al. Heterogeneous growth and mental development of intrauterine growth-retarded infants during the first 3 years of life. Pediatrics 1984; 74:783–91.
38. Strauss RS, Dietz WH. Growth and development of term children born with low birth weight: Effects of genetic and environmental factors. J Pediatr 1998;133:67–72.
39. Kelleher KJ, Casey PH, Bradley RH, et al. Risk factors and out-comes for failure to thrive in low birth weight preterm infants. Pediatrics 1993;91:941–8.
40. Dusick AM, Poindexter BB, Ehrenkranz RA, et al. Growth failure in the pretern infant: Can we catch up? Semin Perinat 2003:27;302–10.
41. Samson-Fang LJ, Stevenson RD. Identification of malnutrition in children with cerebral palsy: Poor performance of weight for-height centiles. Dev Med Child Neurol 2000;42:162–8.
42. Stallings VA, Charney EB, Davies JC, et al. Nutrition-related growth failure of children with quadriplegic cerebral palsy. Dev Med Child Neurol 1993;35:126–38.
43. Stallings VA, Charney EB, Davies JC, et al. Nutritional status and growth of children with diplegic or hemiplegic cerebral palsy. Dev Med Child Neurol 1993;35:997–1006.
44. Stallings VA, Cronk CE, Zemel BS, et al. Body composition of children with spastic quadriplegic cerebral palsy. J Pediatr 1995;126:833–9.
45. Spender QW, Cronk CE, Charney EB, et al. Assessment of linear growth of children with cerebral palsy: Use of alternative measures to height or length [published erratum appears in Dev Med Child Neurol 1990;32:1032]. Dev Med Child Neurol 1989;31:206–14.
46. Pemberton CM, Moxness KE, German MJ, Nelson JK, Gastineau CF, editors. Mayo Clinic Diet Manual. Philadelphia: BC Decker Inc; 1988.
47. Montagnoli LC, Barbieri MA, Bettiol H, et al. Growth impairment of children with different types of lip and palate clefts in the first two years of life: A cross-sectional study. J Pediatr (Rio J) 2005;81:461–5.
48. Bithoney WG. Elevated lead levels in children with nonorganic failure to thrive. Pediatrics 1986;78:891–5.
49. Listernick R, Christoffel K, Chiaramonte J. Severe primary malnutrition in US children. Am J Dis Child 1985; 139;1157–60.
50. Block RW, Krebs NF, the Committees on Child Abuse and Neglect and on Nutrition. Failure to thrive as a manifestation of Child Neglect. Pediatrics 2005;116:1234–7.
51. Graham GG. Poverty, hunger, malnutrition, prematurity, and infant mortality in the United States. Pediatrics 1985;75:117–25.
52. Casey P, Goolsby S, Berkowitz C, et al. Maternal depression, changing public assistance, food security, and child health status. Pediatrics 2004;113:298–304.
53. Blackman JA. Children who refuse food. Contemp Pediatr 1998;15:198–216.
54. Robb AS. Eating disorders in children: Diagnosis and age-specific treatment. Psychiatr Clin North Am 2001;24:259–70.
55. Chatoor I, Ganiban J, Hirsch R, et al. Maternal characteristics and toddler temperament in infantile anorexia. J Am Acad Child Adolesc Psychiatr 2000;39:743–51.
56. Chatoor I, Ganiban J, Surles J, et al. Physiological regulation and infantile anorexia: A pilot study. J Am Acad Child Adolesc Psychiatry. 2004;43:1019–25.
57. Stein MT, Robinson J. Feeding problems, sleep disturbances, and negative behaviors in a toddler. Pediatrics 2001;107:888–92.
58. Black MM, Cureton PL, Berenson-Howard J. Behavior problems in feeding: Individual, family, and cultural influences. In: Kessler DB, Dawson P, editors. Failure to Thrive and Pediatric Undernutrition: A transdisciplinary approach. Baltimore: Paul H. Brookes; 1999. p. 151–69.
59. Rudolph CD, Link DT. Feeding disorders in infants and children. Pediatr Clin North Am 2002;49:97–112.
60. Graham GG. Poverty, hunger, malnutrition, prematurity, and infant mortality in the United States. Pediatrics 1985;75:117–25.
61. Currie ML, Radermacher R. The pediatrician's role in recognizing and intervening in postpartum depression. Pediatr Clin N Am 2004;51:785–801.
62. O'Brien LM, Heycock EG, Hanna M, et al. Postnatal depression and faltering growth: A community study. Pediatrics 2004;113:1242–7.
63. Pugliese MT, Weyman-Daum M, Moses N, et al. Parental health beliefs as a cause of non-organic failure to thrive. Pediatrics 1987;80:175–82.
64. Weston JA, Stage JA, Hathaway P, et al. Prolonged breastfeeding and nonorganic failure to thrive. Am J Dis Child 1987;141:242–3.
65. Roddey OF, Jr, Martin ES, Swetenburg RL. Critical weight loss and malnutrition in breast-fed infants. Am J Dis Child 1981;135:597–9.

66. Lukefahr JL. Underlying illness associated with failure to thrive in breastfed infants. Clin Pediatr 1990;29:468–70.
67. Carvalho NF, Kenney RD, Carrington PH, et al. Severe nutritional deficiencies in toddlers resulting from health food milk alternatives. Pediatrics [Serial online]2001;107:1–7. http://www.pediatrics.org/cgi/content/ full/107/4/e46 (accessed June 22, 2002).
68. Sampson HA. Food allergy: Immunopathogenesis and clinical disorders. J Allergy Clin Imm 1999;103:717–28.
69. Burks AW. The spectrum of food hypersensitivity: Where does it end? J Pediatr 1998;133:175–6.
70. Altemeier WA, O'Connor SM, Sherrod KB, et al. Prospective study of antecedents for non-organic failure to thrive. J Pediatr 1985;106:360–5.
71. Weston JA, Colloton M, Halsey S, et al. A legacy of violence in nonorganic failure to thrive. Child Abuse Neglect 1993;17:709–14.
72. Powell GF, Brasel JA, Blizzard RM. Emotional deprivation and growth retardation simulating idiopathic hypopituitarism. N Engl J Med 1967;267:1272.
73. Krieger I. Food restriction as a form of child abuse in ten cases of psychological deprivation dwarfism. Clin Pediatr 1974;13:127–33.
74. Bools CN, Neale BA, Meadow SR. Co-morbidity associated with fabricated illness (Munchausen syndrome by proxy). Arch Dis Child 1992;67:77–9.
75. Kellogg ND, Lukefahr JL. Criminally prosecuted cases of child starvation. Pediatrics 2005;116:1309–16.
76. Sills RH. Failure to thrive: The role of clinical and laboratory evaluation. Am J Dis Child 1978;132:967–9.
77. Peterson KE, Washington J, Rathbun JM. Team management of failure to thrive. J Am Diet Assoc 1984;84:810–5.
78. Bithoney WG, McJunkin J, Michake J, et al. The effect of a multidisciplinary team approach on weight gain in nonorganicfailure to thrive in children. J Dev Behav Pediatr 1991;12:254–8.
79. Sampson P. Interdisciplinary teamwork. In: Kessler DB, Dawson P, editors. Failure to Thrive and Pediatric Undernutrition: A transdisciplinary approach. Baltimore: Paul H. Brookes; 1999. p. 303–5.
80. Black MM, Dubowitz H, Berenson-Howard J, et al. A randomized clinical trial of home intervention for children with failure to thrive. Pediatrics 1995;95:807–14.
81. American Academy of Pediatrics. Health supervision for children with achondroplasia. Pediatrics 1995;95:443–51.
82. American Academy of Pediatrics. Health supervision for children with Turner syndrome. Pediatrics 1995;96:1166–73.
83. American Academy of Pediatrics. Health supervision for children with Williams syndrome. Pediatrics 2001;107:1192 204.
84. Witschi JC. Short-term dietary recall and recording methods. In: Willet W, editor. Nutritional Epidemiology. New York: Oxford University Press; 1990. p. 52–68.
85. Hyams JS, Leichtner AM. Apple juice: An underappreciated cause of chronic diarrhea. Am J Dis Child 1985;139:503–5.
86. Lifshitz F, Ament ME, Kleinman RE, et al. Role of juice carbohydrate malabsorption in chronic nonspecific diarrhea in children. J Pediatr 1992;120:825–9.
87. Smith MM, Lifshitz F. Excess fruit juice consumption as a contributing factor in nonorganic failure to thrive. Pediatrics 1994;93:438–43.
88. Garn SM, Rohman CC. Interaction of nutrition and genetics in timing of growth. Pediatr Clin North Am 1966;13:353.
89. Schaff-Blass E, Burstein S, Rosenfield RL. Advances in diagnosis and treatment of short stature, with special reference to the role of growth hormone. J Pediatr 1984;104:801–13.
90. Collins J, Mezey AP. Failure to thrive. In: Shelov SP, Mezey AP, Edelman CM, Barnett HL, editors. Primary Care Pediatrics. Norwalk (CT): Appleton-Century-Crofts; 1984. p. 327–9.
91. Tunnessen WW. Signs and Symptoms in Pediatrics. Philadelphia: JB Lippincott Co.; 1983.92.Steens RF, Csizmadia CGDS, George EK, et al. A national prospective study on childhood celiac disease in the Netherlands 1993–2000: An increasing recognition and a changing clinical picture. J Pediatr 2005;147:239–43.
93. Hoffenberg EJ, Emery LM, Barriga KJ, et al. Clinical features of children with screening-identified evidence of celiac disease. Pediatrics 2004;113:1254–9.
94. Saiman L, Aronson J, Zhou J, et al. Prevalence of infectious diseases among internationally adopted children. Pediatrics 2001;108:608–12.
95. Hostetter MK, Iverson S, Thomas W, et al. Medical evaluation of internationally adopted children. N Engl J Med 1991; 325:479–85.
96. Ellerstein NS, Ostrov BE. Growth patterns in children hospitalized because of caloric-deprivation failure to thrive. Am J Dis Child 1985;139:164.
97. Chen LC, Chowdhury AKMA, Huffman SL. Anthropometric assessment of energy-protein malnutrition and subsequent risk of mortality among preschool aged children. Am J Clin Nutr 1980;33:1836–45.
98. Schmitt BD, Mauro RD. Nonorganic failure to thrive: An outpatient approach. Child Abuse Neglect 1989;13:235–48.
99. Weaver LT. Rapid growth in infancy: Balancing the interests of the child. JPGN 2006;43:428–32.
100. Fjeld CR, Schoeller DA, Brown KH. Body composition of children recovering from severe protein-energy malnutrition at two rates of catch-up growth. Am J Clin Nutr 1989;50:1266–75.
101. Chatoor I, Dickson L, Schaefer S, et al. A developmental classification of feeding disorders associated with failure to thrive: Diagnosis and treatment. In: Drotar D, editor. New Directions in Failure to Thrive: Implications for Research and Practice. New York: Plenum Press; 1985. p. 235–58.
102. Kitchen WH, Doyle LW, Ford GW, et al. Very low birth weight and growth to age 8 years. I. Weight and height. Am J Dis Child 1992;146:40–5.
103. Hack M, Weissman B, Borawski-Clark E. Catch-up growth during childhood among very-low-birth-weight children. Arch Pediatr Adolesc Med 1996;150:1122–9.
104. Hirata T, Bosque E. When they grow up: The growth of extremely low birth weight (≤1000 gm) infants at adolescence. J Pediatr 1998;132:1033–5.
105. Peralta-Carcelen M, Jackson DS, Goran MI, et al. Growth of adolescents who were born at extremely low birth weight without major disability. J Pediatr 2000;136:633–40.
106. Glaser HH, Heagarty MC, Bullard DM, et al. Physical and psychological development of children with early failure to thrive. J Pediatr 1968;73:690–8.
107. Mitchell WG, Gorrell RW, Greenberg RA. Failure to thrive: Study in the primary care setting-epidemiology and follow-up. Pediatrics 1980;65:971–7.
108. Chatoor I, Surles J, Ganiban J, et al. Failure to thrive and cognitive development in toddlers with infantile anorexia. Pediatrics 2004;113:e440–7.
109. Lloyd-Still JD, Hurwitz I, Wolff PH, et al. Intellectual development after severe malnutrition in infancy. Pediatrics 1974;54:306–11.
110. Grantham-McGregor S, Schofield W, Harris L. Effect of psychosocial stimulation on mental development of severely malnourished children: An interim report. Pediatrics 1983; 72:239–43.
111. Grantham-McGregor S, Schofield W, Powell C. Development of severely malnourished children who received psychosocial stimulation: Six-year follow-up. Pediatrics 1987;79:247–54.
112. Corbett SS, Drewett RF. To what extent is failure to thrive in infancy associated with poorer cognitive development? A review and meta-analysis. J Child Psychol Psychiatr 2004;45:641–54.

Nutritional Assessment of the Hospitalized Patient

Stephanie H. Abrams, MD
Robert J. Shulman, MD

Evaluating the nutritional status of the hospitalized child presents a unique challenge to the practitioner. While assessment of dietary status upon hospital admission intuitively seems to be similar to assessment of a patient in the clinic setting, the severity of the illness can obscure the current nutritional condition. The metabolic needs of a hospitalized child will depend largely on their pre-hospitalization nutritional status, as well as the current disease state. Acute factors such as fever, stress, or pain may affect caloric requirements. The presence of a chronic disease with a superimposed acute medical condition, such as infection, may further cloud a practitioner's ability to assess the patient's current metabolic needs.

Chronically malnourished children are at risk for infectious diseases, especially in developing countries, a phenomenon likely related to decreased humoral and cellular immunity.[1,2] Poor nutritional status is associated with higher rates of complications, longer lengths of stay in the hospital, and higher mortality rates.[3] For the malnourished hospitalized child, improvement in nutritional status has been associated with decreased mortality.[4] Likewise, the practitioner should be cognizant of the nutritional status during the hospitalization of previously well-nourished children, as the hospitalized child is at risk for developing acute malnutrition. Because many illnesses are associated with anorexia, the current disease process may limit the method by which nutrition may be provided. Additionally, diagnostic tests or treatment may necessitate periods of restricted oral intake. Alternatively, the practitioner should be mindful of the potential for excessive weight gain. For example, in the critically ill patient who is muscle relaxed and sedated, the metabolic needs may be overestimated.

EPIDEMIOLOGY

According to the CDC, 4.7% of all US children less than 5 years of age are underweight, with non-Hispanic blacks and Asian/Pacific Islanders being most affected (up to 6% malnourished).[5] While severe protein energy malnutrition occurs more frequently in developing countries, the United States is not spared completely. Risk factors for malnutrition during childhood include low birth weight (<2500 g), low socioeconomic status, large family size, low parental education level, and chronic infections.[6–9] Most of the studies performed regarding undernutrition in the hospitalized child are from the 1970s. These studies have shown a prevalence of malnutrition in hospitalized patients in developed countries between 20 and 40% by Waterlow's criteria.[10–12] In 1995, Hendricks et al[13] reported the prevalence of acute protein energy malnutrition in hospitalized children to be 24.7%.

Conversely, 14.2% of all children less than 5 years of age are obese.[5] According to the National Health and Nutrition Examination Survey (NHANES, 2004), 36.2% of children between 6 and 19 years of age are obese. Using the definition of obesity as greater than 120% of weight for height, Hendricks et al[13] reported that 25% of hospitalized children were obese. In Istanbul, one study (using weight for height) reported that 15.9% of hospitalized children from 1 month to 23 years were overweight or obese.[14]

NUTRITION SCREENING

Nutrition screening of all pediatric patients has been implemented by most hospitals in order to provide quality health care and to comply with the recommendations by the Joint Commission on Accreditation of Healthcare Organizations Board of Directors.[15] Additionally, the American Society for Parenteral and Enteral Nutrition (A.S.P.E.N.) has recommended standards for nutrition screening and support in hospitalized pediatric patients. These recommendations include screening of all patients within 24 hours of admission to the hospital, nutritional assessment for those at risk, development of a nutrition care plan, implementation of the plan, patient monitoring, reassessment of the care plan, reevaluation of the care setting, and finally either reformulation of the care plan or termination of therapy.[16]

The admitting nurse or a dietitian usually performs the initial nutrition screening. At a minimum, screening should include chronological age, gestational age (when appropriate), gender, anthropometric measurements, and percentile for age and gender by growth chart.[16] Screening may also include other risk factors such as altered diets/special formulas, recent change in body weight or dietary intake, ability to eat and retain food, medical condition, symptoms interfering with feeding, or history of growth failure.[2,17] Table 1 summarizes many of the conditions associated with specific nutritional requirements or problems that may impact the ability of a patient to thrive while being hospitalized. Identification of at risk children should prompt consultation of a dietitian for further nutritional assessment.

NUTRITIONAL ASSESSMENT

The rationale for nutritional assessment of hospitalized patients is supported by data that confirm a strong relationship between underlying nutritional status and complications during hospitalization.[18] Guidelines by A.S.P.E.N. delineate the purposes of the nutritional assessment to document baseline nutritional parameters, identify nutritional risk factors, and determine if specific nutritional deficits exist. Additionally, it establishes the patient's nutritional needs, while developing the dietary management plan. Psychosocial, medical, and socioeconomic factors that may influence the administration of dietary assistance should be identified.[17] These may include behavioral issues revolving around food or mealtime, chronic disease increasing the child's caloric demand, or insufficient funds to buy nutritious food.

Table 1 Medical Conditions That Should Prompt a Full Nutritional Assessment

Prematurity
Ill newborn
Critically ill patient
Eating disorders (anorexia nervosa, bulimia, obesity)
Patient receiving home health nutritional support
Necrotizing enterocolitis
Short bowel syndrome
Inflammatory bowel disease
Gastrointestinal pseudoobstruction
Chronic diarrhea
Liver disease
Organ or bone marrow transplantation
Diabetes mellitus
Bronchopulmonary dysplasia
Cystic fibrosis
Cancer
Central nervous system disorders
Inborn errors of metabolism
Chronic renal failure

Clinical, subjective, and objective data are all important pieces of the nutritional assessment. Clinical data gathered for the nutritional assessment should include admitting diagnosis, allergies, medications, and any coexisting medical problems that may affect nutritional status. Subjective assessment includes the caregiver's perception of the previous growth history. Objective assessment includes physical examination findings, anthropometric evaluation, dietary history, and laboratory evaluations.

History

Thorough medical and dietary histories are crucial pieces of the evaluation of a child's nutritional status. The history may reveal medical conditions, unusual eating behaviors, religious factors, or cultural factors that may influence nutrient intake. A developmental history regarding milestones and the child's ability to chew/swallow can give insight into current dietary issues. The practitioner should query about acute and chronic disease states or medications that may alter the child's appetite, metabolism, or ability to absorb nutrients appropriately. A detailed family history also is imperative as it may reveal short stature or heritable diseases associated with growth issues.

Diet records, food frequency questionnaires, and diet histories are all instruments that can provide some insight into the historical intake of the patient. While 24-hour dietary recall may be performed quickly to get an idea of intake, its validity is limited by recall bias.[19] Underreporting occurs in up to 85% of dietary recalls; likewise, overreporting occurs up to 39% of the time.[1,20] While portion size estimation and retrieval of dietary information from memory may prove to be problematic, a 3- or 7-day diet diary may improve the quality of dietary information.[20–22] Families or nurses are instructed to record everything the child eats or drinks, as well as the volume or portion size. A history of at least 72 hours of intake decreases the subjectiveness of diet recall and accounts for normal variability in the diet. A dietitian is an important member of the medical team who is best equipped to interpret food diaries. Various computer programs exist to aid the dietitian in analyzing food diaries. Additionally, the United States Department of Agriculture (USDA) maintains web sites that provide a wealth of information regarding the nutrient content of dietary foodstuffs.[23] Chapter 16, Nutritional Epidemiology, also reviews dietary intake methodology.

Among hospitalized children, diet records are the most commonly used way to gather intake data. Advantages of this technique include that the patient is often under the watchful eyes of nursing and medical staff, thus allowing accurate data to be collected. However, inaccuracies and incomplete collections can still occur, especially if surgical, radiologic, or other procedures result in the interruption of enteral nutrition intake, or if frequent rotation of hospital staff lead to inaccurate data collection. Butterworth[24] reviewed the several ways in which hospitalized patients are prone to develop undernutrition, such as failure to provide food in a timely fashion.

Physical Exam

A comprehensive physical examination is an integral part of a nutritional assessment. The examiner may appreciate stigmata of nutrient deficiencies. Additionally, the exam may reveal dysmorphic or syndromic features that can provide clues to the expected genetic potential for growth of the child (eg, Down syndrome). Careful examination of the oropharynx may reveal an anatomic explanation for inadequate dietary intake. Abdominal examination may reveal organomegaly or tenderness, which may be related to inadequate intake or increased caloric needs. Among hospitalized patients, examination for peripheral edema (as occurs with hypoalbuminemia), temporal wasting, thin extremities, or other signs of malnutrition is imperative.

The Subjective Global Nutritional Assessment (SGNA) combines elements of the history and physical exam.[25] This nutritional assessment is performed by a dietician who assesses (1) recent and historical changes in growth parameters; (2) parental growth; (3) dietary intake; (4) frequency and duration of gastrointestinal symptoms; (5) current functional capacity; (6) exam findings of fat storage, muscle wasting, or edema; and (7) the presence or absence of historical features, metabolic demands of a disease process, and physical signs of malnutrition to assign a global assessment of the patient as well-nourished, moderately malnourished, or severely malnourished patients. This assessment has been validated in pediatric surgical patients and may be predictive of hospital course. Although only English-speaking patients were included in this study, Secker et al[25] found that malnourished surgical patients had significantly higher rates of infectious complications. Additionally, the malnourished patients had longer postoperative stays than well-nourished children. While this global assessment tool has been validated across different practitioners and has some predictive value in surgical patients, anthropometry provides the advantage of qualitative, objective measure of nutritional status.

Anthropometrics

Basic anthropometric data are helpful upon admission and should be reassessed at various intervals throughout the hospitalization. Numerous measures are used in a nutritional assessment because no single measurement can characterize the nutritional status completely. Anthropometric assessment requires precision equipment that should be checked regularly for accuracy. Anthropometrists should be well trained regarding the application of measurement techniques and the use of various instruments to ensure exact and reproducible measurements. Disease-specific growth charts exist (Table 2) for conditions such as achondroplasia, cerebral palsy, and Down's syndrome, which may help with understanding the limitations of the treatment regimen.[26] (See growth charts for several specific conditions in the Appendix I. Also, Chapter 2, Clinical Assessment of Nutritional Status, reviews the acquisition and interpretation of pediatric anthropometric data.) Monitoring changes in weight on a daily basis (for infants) or thrice weekly for older children gives a more accurate measure of the nutritional status over time. Weight also is the most accurate measure of fluid status.[27] Repeat measurements during the hospitalization should be carried out using the same scale to reduce variability. Further evaluation of the patient's nutritional status/needs by a qualified dietitian should be considered for any patient with a weight <5th or >95th percentile for age and gender. Given that infants and children normally are in a constant state of weight gain, consultation also may be considered for any child who has had demonstrable weight loss (>5% over a month in a child and over 2 weeks in an infant).

Measurement of height or length is also an important way to assess nutritional status, but is often not performed among inpatients, especially those who are critically ill. Fredriks et al[28] investigated various measures of height, which may be applied to critically ill children, including sitting height, leg length, and a sitting height/height ratio. Infants are another population that may present difficulties in measuring length. To simplify the technical difficulty of measuring infants, many infant lengths are measured by a tape measure. However, Corkins et al[29] have found that the length board is more accurate, with an average of 2.2 cm difference between length board and tape measure. In fact, a change in length with measurement by length board resulted in a change in the weight for height percentile range in over 50% of patients measured.

Weight for height, based on age and sex, can be used as an indicator of wasting and acute malnutrition (Table 3, Waterlow Criteria).[30] A weight for height graph also is used to define the ideal body weight (IBW) for an individual. IBW is the weight at the 50th percentile on the weight for height/length curve. Alternatively, body mass index (BMI) may be used to calculate IBW. IBW

Table 2 Conditions with Disease-Specific Growth Charts Available[19,23]
Achondroplasia
Cerebral palsy
Down syndrome
Duchenne muscular dystrophy
Fragile X syndrome
Low birth weight
Marfan syndrome
Noonan syndrome
Prader-Willi syndrome
Silver-Russell syndrome
Turner syndrome
Williams syndrome

is the BMI at the 50th percentile for age and sex multiplied by the height in meters squared. BMI should be calculated for all children greater than 2 years of age and is the best indicator of adiposity. BMI is the weight in kilograms divided by the square of the height in meters (kg/m^2). It also can be calculated by dividing the weight in pounds by the height in inches squared, multiplied by 703 (lbs/in^2 × 703). BMI may be a useful tool in monitoring changes in body weight and determining nutritional risk (Table 4).

Skin-fold thickness may be used to monitor changes in body fat in the hospitalized child. While soft tissue mass is generally more difficult to reproducibly and reliably measure, triceps skin-fold thickness correlates well with total body fat stores.[26] Another advantage of the triceps skin-fold thickness is that excellent reference data from childhood to adulthood are available.[31] One examiner should perform serial measurements in triplicate using calipers to measure to the nearest millimeter. The maximum allowable range across the three measurements should be 20%. Measures should be repeated in triplicate if this range is exceeded.[32]

Among hospitalized patients, the interpretation of standard anthropometric data can be challenging. Changes in body weight, as noted above, often are related to acute changes in body water, which are common in patients with intercurrent illnesses or who are receiving intravenous fluids. Acute weight loss is the gold standard for the diagnosis of dehydration, a finding that may inhibit accurate assessment of malnutrition.[33] Conversely, in patients with inflammatory or infectious illnesses, an acute phase response has been associated with increased capillary permeability, and expansion of extracellular fluid. In the acute phase reaction, patients have decreased albumin synthesis and retention of body salt and water.[34] This may falsely elevate weight and clinically manifest as edema, complicating the practitioner's assessment of the patient's subcutaneous tissue and true "dry weight."

Laboratory Assessment

Interpretation of laboratory data in hospitalized patients may be complicated due to concomitant changes in the synthesis of acute phase proteins. Human and animal data show important changes in circulating blood concentrations of a variety of minerals, vitamins, and electrolytes. As mentioned above, an acute phase reaction may begin within hours of the onset of infection and fever. Practitioners must consider the possibility of alterations in acute phase proteins when interpreting the laboratory data that is typically collected to monitor a child's nutritional status. Decreases in serum zinc and iron have been described in the acute phase response, making these levels difficult to interpret.[35] Similarly, as noted above, assessing serum proteins such as albumin, prealbumin, or transferrin are difficult in the acute phase. Interpretation becomes particularly problematic when an acute phase response is overlaid on malnutrition and/or chronic infections.[36] In these situations, it is particularly important to combine the results of the history, physical examination, and laboratory evaluation to reach an accurate assessment of the patient's nutritional status.

Hematologic and protein analyses should be performed on all at-risk patients as determined by nutritional screen. Complete blood count (CBC) is an inexpensive test commonly performed during the nutritional assessment. CBC may reveal anemia secondary to vitamin B_{12}, folate, or iron deficiencies. Anemia is a late manifestation of these insufficiencies; therefore, assays for these nutrients may prove helpful in identifying subclinical deficiencies.[37] CBC may also demonstrate lymphopenia, a feature of severe protein-energy malnutrition. In general, humoral immunity is preserved until severe malnutrition occurs but cell-mediated immunity is affected early in reduced nutritional states.[2] Delayed-type hypersensitivity testing is a commonly used measure of cellular immunity. However, cutaneous anergy is associated with many nonspecific factors including malnutrition, infections, critical illness, steroids, and immunosuppression. Malnutrition severe enough to cause anergy is associated with an increased risk of surgical complications.[38]

Serum protein concentrations often are used as an indicator of visceral protein status. However, serum proteins may be affected by sepsis, inflammation, hydration status, burns, surgical drains, liver disease, and renal disease.[2] Albumin frequently is monitored but does not reflect acute nutritional changes since it has a half-life of 18 to 20 days. Transferrin, the major iron transport protein may be a better estimate of acute nutritional status given that it has a shorter half-life of 8 to 9 days. In patients with hepatic dysfunction albumin and transferrin are not reliable indices of nutrition since they are synthesized in the liver. Prealbumin (transthyretin) helps in the transport of vitamin A and thyroxine and has a very short half-life (24 to 48 hours). However, like albumin and transferrin, prealbumin is influenced by vascular integrity and hepatic dysfunction and may be decreased by inflammation. Some have suggested that an elevated C-reactive protein infers that serum proteins are low as part of an inflammatory response.[39] In the presence of normal renal function and hydration the blood urea nitrogen (BUN) can be used as an estimate of inadequate or excessive protein intake. A BUN ≤ 5 mg/dL suggests an inadequate protein intake whereas a BUN ≥ 18 mg/dL suggests an excessive protein intake.

Severe micronutrient and vitamin deficiencies may co-exist in patients with certain diseases, such as protein-energy malnutrition. These deficiencies may be obvious clinically and may affect the patient's ability to respond to an infectious process. Anemia due to iron deficiency is widespread among all age groups, especially in developing countries.[40] Assessment of iron status may be useful in anemic children since iron deficiency is known to alter cell-mediated immune functions in children and impact the ability of the patient to respond to infection.[40] Zinc levels may be useful in the patient who is at risk for deficiency, such as patients with inflammatory bowel disease or with severe protein-energy malnutrition. Because zinc excretion is primarily through the gut lumen, patients with ongoing GI losses (eg, nasogastric suction, ostomy, chronic diarrhea) are at particular risk for zinc deficiency. Zinc is essential for DNA synthesis, and low plasma zinc levels are associated with growth failure, diarrhea, poor wound healing, and respiratory infections.[41] Patients with liver disease or other conditions that contribute to fat malabsorption are at risk for subclinical fat-soluble vitamin deficiencies. In these patients vitamin A, D, E, and K status should be assessed and followed on a regular basis as clinically indicated.[2]

Table 4 Body Mass Index (BMI) and Nutritional Risk

BMI Percentile for Age and Gender	Nutritional Risk
<5th percentile	Underweight
5th–85th percentile	Normal weight
85th–95th percentile	At risk for overweight
>95th percentile	Overweight
>97th percentile	Morbidly obese

Table 3 Waterlow Criteria for Acute and Chronic Malnutrition[18]

$$\text{Acute Malnutrition (Wasting)} = \frac{\text{Actual weight (kg)}}{\text{Expected wt (kg) for ht (cm) at 50th percentile}} \times 100$$

Grade 0	Normal	>90%
Grade I	Mild	81–90%
Grade II	Moderate	70–80%
Grade III	Severe	<70%

$$\text{Chronic Malnutrition (Stunting)} = \frac{\text{Actual weight (kg)}}{\text{Expected ht (cm) for age at 50th percentile}} \times 100$$

Grade 0	Normal	>95%
Grade I	Mild	90–95%
Grade II	Moderate	85–89%
Grade III	Severe	<85%

Nutrient Requirements

For most children, 60 to 70% of total daily energy expenditure is determined by resting energy expenditure (REE).[41] While various disease states may alter a child's requirements, determination of REE may provide valuable information when formulating the dietary plan of the hospitalized child. In fact, the World Health Organization (WHO) Expert Consultation on Energy and Protein Requirements recommends that energy requirements be based on measurement of expenditure whenever possible.[42] Indirect calorimetry is a method of measuring oxygen and carbon dioxide exchange in vivo to estimate REE. However, indirect calorimetry may be impractical for clinical application secondary to cost, availability of equipment, and the necessity of a period of fasting. Equations commonly are used to predict the REE of children (Table 5); unfortunately, no one equation may be applied to all patient populations. For example, the Harris-Benedict formulas were created based on subjects, who were 15 to 74 years old.[43] The WHO formulas were validated down to neonates; however, the Schofield height/weight based (HW) equations have been reported to be most accurate in predicting REE in a mixed population of obese and nonobese children and adolescents.[42,44] This equation also was found to be least likely to underestimate the REE in infants and toddlers (birth to 3 years) with failure to thrive.[45]

The Institute of Medicine has delineated dietary reference intakes for children. They recommend that for healthy children above 3 years of age, about 10 to 30% of caloric intake should be from protein, 45 to 65% from carbohydrate, and 25 to 35% from fat (Table 6).[46] Dietary guidelines also specify that most fats should be from sources of polyunsaturated and monounsaturated fatty acids such as vegetable oils, nuts, or fish.[47] Specific guidelines regarding grams per day of protein, carbohydrate, and fat per age also are available; however, these values may not be applicable to hospitalized patients whose disease processes and activity levels can alter dietary needs. As noted above, approximately 30% of daily energy expenditure may be accounted for by activity. In a patient who is confined to bed or may even be mechanically ventilated, caloric repletion based on requirements for healthy children likely will lead to overfeeding.[48,49] Overfeeding may lead to metabolic complications such as hyperglycemia, respiratory compromise secondary to excessive carbon dioxide production, and/or hypertriglyceridemia.[50]

Table 6 Dietary Reference Intakes (DRI) for Macronutrients[38]

Macronutrient	Children 1–3 yr old (% of energy intake)	Children 4–18 yr old (% of energy intake)
Fat*	30–40	25–35
Carbohydrate	45–65	45–65
Protein	5–20	10–30

*Approximately 10% of total fat from long chain *n*-3 or *n*-6 fatty acids.

Critically Ill Patient

The critically ill patient presents a challenge when it comes to nutritional assessment. Acute trauma, sepsis, or illness leads to an intense whole body protein catabolic response as evidenced by increased urinary nitrogen, which may lead to severe protein-energy malnutrition.[2] It is recommended that the health care team provide adequate dietary protein to promote positive nitrogen balance while recognizing that carbohydrate is poorly utilized and fat is used preferentially for oxidation.[51] Protein anabolism can occur in these patients with early administration of protein, followed by carbohydrate and finally lipids.[52] Fat should be started at 1 g/kg/d and advanced to a goal of 3 g/kg/d, accounting for a maximum of 30 to 50% of total caloric intake.[53]

After the acute response, energy expenditure by calorimetry in critically ill children is significantly lower than predicted energy expenditure or recommended dietary intakes; it is even lower in the presence of multiple organ system failure.[54] As noted above overfeeding can be associated with clinically significant complications and underfeeding may result in delayed wound healing, muscle wasting, and increased susceptibility to infection.[55] Both underfeeding and overfeeding may increase morbidity and mortality and may prolong the hospitalization.[56] To avoid errors in estimating energy requirements over the long term (ie, 2 to 3 weeks or more) indirect calorimetry should be considered and can be performed on the ventilated patient. While predictive equations have been used to assess energy expenditure in critically ill children, Coss-Bu et al[57] found that neither the Harris-Benedict nor the Talbot methods predict REE with acceptable precision for clinical use (Table 5). In the absence of indirect calorimetry, particularly close attention must be paid to the calculation of energy and protein requirements as well as observation of changes in weight, fluid status, and serum chemistries (eg, albumin, BUN) even with their limitations.

Nutritional assessment/management of the obese, critically ill patient can be particularly challenging especially if issues of glycemic control arise. Acutely injured obese individuals have a catabolic response to injury that is similar to that of normal weight patients. Therefore, even with excess body fat stores, they are at risk for protein-energy malnutrition.[58] The debate over whether to use actual body weight or IBW when using equations to predict energy expenditure continues. Ireton-Jones et al[59] reported that in adults, actual body weight correlated more accurately with basic metabolic needs than IBW. In healthy obese children the WHO equations (Table 5) were found to be predictive of measured REE.[60] However, their predictive value in critically ill obese children remains largely unknown. As with the normal weight critically ill patient, indirect calorimetry remains the gold standard for evaluation of energy expenditure.

Table 5 Equations Used to Predict Resting Energy Expenditure (REE)[34,36,37]

Authors	Equation for REE	
Harris-Benedict	Female:	655.10 + 9.56W + 1.85H − 4.68A
	Male:	66.47 + 13.75W + 5.0H − 6.76A
FAO/WHO/UNU	Female 0–3 yr:	61W − 51
	Male 0–3 yr:	60W − 54
	Female 3–10 yr:	22.5W + 499
	Male 3–10 yr:	22.7W + 495
	Female 10–18 yr:	17.5W + 651
	Male 10–18 yr:	12.2W + 746
Schofield-HW	Female 0–3 yr:	16.252W + 1023.2H − 413.5
	Male 0–3 yr:	0.167W + 11517.4H − 617.6
	Female 3–10 yr:	16.97W + 1.618H + 371.2
	Male 3–10 yr:	19.6W + 1.033H + 414.9
	Female 10–18 yr:	8.365W + 4.65H + 200
	Male 10–18 yr:	16.25W + 1.372H + 515.5

REE: kcal/24 h; W: weight (kg); H: height (cm); A: age (years).

The Need for an Individualized and Multidisciplinary Approach

An individualized approach to each child is recommended. Each child will cope with his or her hospitalization differently. Anxiety about hospitalization or pain may play an important role in the child's dietary compliance. Disruption of a child's usual feeding schedule may be a necessary part of the hospitalization; however, it may impede dietary management.

A multidisciplinary approach is recommended for each patient with involvement of a dietitian, child life specialist, nurse, physician, and pharmacist.[16] A qualified dietitian is an invaluable part of the team approach to managing the hospitalized child by providing detailed evaluation and calculation of the patient's intake. Similarly, they may aid in determining the nutrient needs of the child as well as providing expertise on defined diets (ie, prepackaged commercially available, nutritionally complete feedings) that may be useful. Consulting a child life specialist when issues arise related to anxiety about hospitalization or dealing with the 24-hour schedule of the hospital setting may help a child cope and allow the child to achieve dietary goals in an expeditious manner. Nurses can provide objective data regarding parental feeding techniques as well as information related to the child's desire and tolerance for feedings. A pharmacist can help prevent adverse dietary and medication interactions.

The team approach also may include consultation with other medical services such as otolaryngology or speech therapy in patients who have anatomic abnormalities of the oropharynx or an abnormal swallow function test. Similarly, consultation with occupational, physical, and/or speech therapists may be helpful for a child who has impaired feeding abilities such as deconditioning caused by a prolonged period without oral intake. Physical rehabilitation may improve a child's strength, providing the motivation and the energy for them to comply with dietary recommendations.

CONCLUSION

Provision of appropriate dietary intake to the hospitalized child presents unique challenges to the health care team. Nutritional status upon admission can provide diagnostic and prognostic information regarding a child's recovery from the acute disease state. Acute processes may be superimposed on chronic illnesses, making assessment of caloric requirements challenging. Thorough history, physical, anthropomorphic, and laboratory analyses are imperative to appropriate evaluation of the nutritional status. While equations may prove to be helpful in predicting energy requirements, indirect calorimetry remains the gold standard for the evaluation of REE. An individualized approach to the dietary assessment and treatment of each child using a multidisciplinary approach is recommended. It gives the practitioner a more complete representation of the child's nutritional status and provides for optimal treatment of the patient.

REFERENCES

1. Man WD, Weber M, Palmer A, et al. Nutritional status of children admitted to hospital with different diseases and its relationship to outcome in the Gambia, West Africa. Trop Med Int Health 1998;3:678–86.
2. Taylor RM, Dhawan A. Assessing nutritional status in children with chronic liver disease. J Gastroenteral Hepatol 2005;20:1817–24.
3. Correia MI, Waitzberg DL. The impact of malnutrition on morbidity, mortality, length of hospital stay and costs evaluated through a multivariate model analysis. Clin Nutr 2003;22:235–9.
4. Bahwere P, De Mol P, Donnen P, et al. Improvements in nutritional management as a determinant of reduced mortality from community-acquired lower respiratory tract infection in hospitalized children from rural Central Africa. Pediatr Infect Dis J. 2004;23:739–47.
5. Pediatric and Pregnancy Nutrition Surveillance System. Growth Indicators by Race/Ethnicity and Age. http://www.cdc.gov/pednss/pednss_tables/pdf/national_table16.pdf
6. From the Centers for Disease Control and Prevention. Severe malnutrition among young children-Georgia, January 1997–June 1999. JAMA 2001;285:2573–4.
7. Lima Mde C, Motta ME, Santos EC, et al. Determinants of impaired growth among hospitalized children: A case-control study. Sao Paolo Med J 2004;122:117–23.
8. Ayaya SO, Esamai FO, Rotich J, et al. Socioeconomic factors predisposing under five-year-old children to severe protein energy malnutrition at the Moi Teaching and Referral Hospital, Eldoret, Kenya. East Afr Med J 2004;81:415–21.
9. Lima MC, Motta ME, Santos EC, et al. Determinants of impaired growth among hospitalized children—A case-control study. Sao Paulo Med J 2004;122:117–23.
10. Waterlow JC. Some aspects of childhood malnutrition as a public health problem. BMJ 1974;4:88–9.
11. Waterlow JC. Classification and definition of protein calorie malnutrition. BMJ 1972;2:566–9.
12. Merritt RJ, Suskind R. Nutritional survey of hospitalized pediatric patients. Am J Clin Nutr 1979;32:1320–5.
13. Hendricks KM, Duggan C, Gallagher L, et al. Malnutrition in hospitalized pediatric patients: Current prevalence. Arch Pediatr Adolesc Med 1995;149:1118–22.
14. Dogan Y, Erkan T, Yalvac S, et al. Nutritional status of patients hospitalized in pediatric clinic. Turk J Gastroenterol 2005;16:212–16.
15. Joint Commission on Accreditation of Healthcare Organizations Board of Directors. 2003 Comprehensive Accreditation Manual for Hospitals: The Official Handbook. Oakbrook Terrace, IL: Joint Commission Resources; 2003.
16. A.S.P.E.N. Board of Directors Task Force on Standards for Specialized Nutrition Support for Hospitalized Pediatric Patients. Standards for Specialized Nutrition Support: Hospitalized Pediatric Patients. Nutr Clin Pract 2005;20:103–16.
17. Sermet-Gaudelus I, Poisson-Salomon AS, Colomb V, et al. Simple pediatric nutritional risk score to identify children at risk of malnutrition. Am J Clin Nutr 2000;72:64–70.
18. Naber THJ, Schermer T, de Bree A, et al. Prevalence of malnutrition in nonsurgical hospitalized patients and its association with disease complications. Am J Clin Nutr 1997;66:1232–9.
19. Westerterp KR, Goris AHC. Validity of the assessment of dietary intake: Problems of misreporting. Curr Opin Clin Nutr Metab Care 2002;5:489–93.
20. Novotny JA, Rumpler WV, Riddick H, et al. Personality characteristics as predictors of underreporting of energy intake on 24-hour dietary recall interviews. J Am Diet Assoc 2003;103:1146–51.
21. Livinston MBE, Robson PJ. Measurement of dietary intake in children. Proc Nutr Soc 2000;59:279–93.
22. Maurer J, Taren DL, Teixeira PJ, et al. The psychosocial and behavioral characteristics related to energy misreporting. Nutr Rev 2006;64:53–66.
23. http://www.nal.usda.gov/fnic/foodcomp/search/
24. Butterworth CE. The skeleton in the hospital closet. Nutr Today 1974;9:4–8.
25. Secker DJ, Jeejeebhoy KN. Subjective global nutritional assessment for children. Am J Clin Nutr 2007;85:1083–9.
26. Ranke MB. Disease-specific standards in congenital syndromes. Horm Res 1996;45:35–41.
27. Centers for Disease Control and Prevention. The management of acute diarrhea in children: Oral rehydration, maintenance, and nutritional therapy. Morb Mortal Wkly Rep 1992;41:13.
28. Fredriks AM, van Buuren S, van Heel WJM, et al. Nationwide age references for sitting height, leg length, and sitting height/height ratio, and their diagnostic value for disproportionate growth disorders. Arch Dis Child 2005;90:807–12.
29. Corkins MR, Lewis P, Cruse W, et al. Accuracy of infant admission lengths. Pediatrics 2002;109:1108–11.
30. Waterlow J. Classification and definition of protein-calorie malnutrition. BMJ 1972;3:566–9.
31. Frisancho AR. New norms of upper limb fat and muscle areas for assessment of nutritional status. Am J Clin Nutr 1981;34:2540–5.
32. Lohman TG, Ring K, Schmitz KH, et al. Associations of body size and composition with physical activity in adolescent girls. Med Sci Sports Exerc 2006;38:1175–81.
33. Gorelick MH, Shaw KN, Murphy KO. Validity and reliability of clinical signs in the diagnosis of dehydration in children. Pediatrics 1997;99:e6.
34. Gruys E, Toussaint MJM, Niewold TA, et al. Acute phase reaction and acute phase proteins. J Zhejiang Univ Sci 2005;6B:1045–56.
35. Ingenbleek M, Young V. Transthyretin (prealbumin) in health and disease: Nutritional implications. Ann Rev Nutr 1994;14:495–533.
36. Morlese JF, Forrester T, Jahoor F. Acute-phase protein response to infection in severe malnutrition. Am J Physiol Endocrinol Metabol 1998;38:E112–17.
37. Viteri FE, Gonzalez H. Adverse outcomes of poor micronutrient status in childhood and adolescence. Nutr Rev 2002;60:S77–83.
38. Moesgaard E, Lykkegaard-Nielsen M. Preoperative cell-mediated immunity and duration of antibiotic prophylaxis in relation to postoperative infectious complications. Acta Chir Scand 1989;155:281–6.
39. Feitelson-Winkler M, Gerrior SA, Pomp A, et al. Use of retinal-binding protein and prealbumin as indicators of response to nutrition therapy. J Am Diet Assoc 1989;89:684–7.
40. Bhaskaram P. Micronutrient malnutrition, infection, and immunity: An overview. Nutr Rev 2002;60:S40–5.
41. Bahl R, Bhandari N, Hambidge KM, et al. Plasma zinc as a predictor of diarrhea and respiratory morbidity in an urban slum setting. Am J Clin Nutr 1998;68:414S–417S.
42. World Health Organization. Energy and protein requirements. Report of a joint FAO/WHO/UNU Expert Consultation. (WHO Technical Report Series No. 724). Geneva: World Health Organization; 1985.
43. Harris JA, Benedict FG. A biometric study of basal metabolism in man. Publication no. 279. Washington, DC: Carnegie Institute of Washington; 1919.
44. Rodriguez G, Moreno LA, Sarria A, et al. Resting energy expenditure in children and adolescents: Agreement between calorimetry and prediction equations. Clin Nutr 2000;21:255–60.
45. Sentongo TA, Tershakovec AM, Mascarenhas MR, et al. Resting energy expenditure and prediction equations in young children with failure to thrive. J Pediatr 2000;136:345–50.
46. United States Department of Agriculture. Dietary guidelines for Americans, 2005. http://www.health.gov/dietaryguidelines/dga2005/document/pdf/dga2005.pdf
47. Food and Nutrition Board, Institute of Medicine, National Academies. Dietary Reference Intakes (DRIs). 2006. http://www.iom.edu/Object.File/Master/21/372/0.pdf
48. Schwals WJ. Metabolism and nutritional frontiers in pediatric surgical patients. Surg Clin North Am 1992;72:1237–66.
49. Schwals WJ, Fernandez M, Charles BC. Adjustment of nutritional repletion using bedside indirect calorimetry in infants recovering from surgical stress. Crit Care Med 1992;20:11–19.
50. Falcao MC, Tannuri U. Nutrition for the pediatric surgical patient: Approach in the peri-operative period. Rev Hosp Clin Fac Med S Paulo 2002;57:299–308.
51. Coss-Bu J, Klish WJ, Walding D, et al. Energy metabolism, nitrogen balance, and substrate utilization in critically ill children. Am J Clin Nutr 2001;74:664–9.
52. Elamin EM. Nutritional care of the obese intensive care unit patient. Curr Opin Crit Care 2005;11:300–3.
53. Irving SY, Simone SD, Hicks FW, et al. Nutrition for the critically ill child: Enteral and parenteral support. AACN Clin Issues Adv Pract Acute Crit Care 2000;11:541–58.
54. Briassoulis G, Venkataraman S, Thompson AE. Energy expenditure in critically ill children. Crit Care Med 2000;28:1166–72.
55. Albina JE. Nutrition and wound healing. JPEN 1994;18:367–76.
56. McClave SA, Snider HL. Use of indirect calorimetry in clinical nutrition. Nutr Clin Pract 1992;7:207–21.
57. Coss-Bu JA, Jefferson LS, Walding D, et al. Resting energy expenditure in children in a pediatric intensive care unit: Comparison of Harris-Benedict and Talbot predictions with indirect calorimetry values. Am J Clin Nutr 1998;67:74–80.
58. Shikora SA, Muskat PC. Protein-sparing modified fast total parenteral nutrition formulation for critically ill morbidly obese patient. Nutrition 1994;10:155–8.
59. Ireton-Jones C, Turner WW. Actual or ideal body weight: Which should be used to predict energy expenditure? J Am Diet Assoc 1991;91:193–5.
60. Derumeaux-Burel H, Meyer M, Morin L, et al. Prediction of resting energy expenditure in a large population of obese children. Am J Clin Nutr 2004;80:1544–50.

45

Developmental Disabilities

Babette Zemel, PhD
Virginia A. Stallings, MD

Children with moderate-to-severe disabilities have a markedly increased risk for malnutrition. Neurologic abnormalities—resulting in altered physical activity (voluntary and involuntary), fine motor patterns, and oral-motor patterns—will often significantly affect food intake and nutrient requirements. Chronic undernutrition, characterized by growth failure and reductions in fat stores and lean body mass, is the most common form of malnutrition, but overweight and obesity also occur. Despite these clinical observations, only limited research-based information on the nutrient needs and nutritional status of children with severe disabilities is available. Consequently, recommended nutrient intakes and growth pattern expectations for this group of patients are poorly defined and must be approached on an individual basis.

Nutritional status assessment is essential for identifying the undernourished or overnourished child, estimating the optimum energy intake to promote growth and well-being, and monitoring treatment. In children with moderate-to-severe disabilities, nutritional assessment is complicated by the interaction of the primary disease process (eg, muscle atrophy, contractures, central nervous system pathology, or movement disorders) and both chronic and acute malnutrition. Cerebral palsy (CP), a common disability with significant risk for malnutrition, will be used as a model to describe the nutritional needs and nutritional status of children with severe disabilities.

The scope of problems relating to feeding difficulties and malnutrition is now being described through community or registry surveys. Studies have revealed that close to 90% of children with neurologic impairment require at least some assistance with feeding based upon oral-motor dysfunction.[1,2] A large, multicenter, community-based study in North America reported that 30 to 40% of children with CP had severe feeding difficulties.[3] A recent population-based cohort study in the United Kingdom demonstrated that feeding difficulty at 4 weeks and 6 months of age was associated with subsequent impairment and poor weight gain and developmental outcomes later in childhood.[4] The association of feeding difficulties and nutritional status has been demonstrated in every population studied.[1–7] Feeding difficulties and nutritional status are also associated with increased healthcare utilization and decreased societal participation by the child and parents.[8,9] A pattern of inadequate food intake, growth failure, and disease-specific nutritional concerns is still evident.

Several important nutritional issues were recognized in these studies. Assistance with feeding, prolonged feeding times, and choking significantly affect food intake.[1,2] In addition, gastrointestinal problems, such as reflux, vomiting, and constipation, and some medications, such as those used to treat seizures, contribute to alterations in both nutritional intake and requirements.[2,10] Food intake low in energy density is of particular concern because of the marked linear growth failure,[5,6,9] delayed skeletal[11–14] and sexual maturation,[15] poor weight gain, and reduced energy reserves seen in patients with CP.[16] Abnormal body composition, with reductions in muscle and fat stores, and a high prevalence of undernutrition (failure to thrive and marasmus) and less frequently overnutrition (overweight and obesity) have also been noted.[16–18] Some specific nutrients are at risk, particularly vitamins C, A, and D, iron, and calcium. Low bone density,[17,19–21] associated with degree of immobilization, hypovitaminosis D, feeding difficulties, and lower triceps skinfold measurements in children with CP, also has been reported. Recently, risk of fracture in children with moderate-to-severe CP was associated with greater body fat, feeding by gastrostomy tube, and prior history of fracture.[22]

For children with CP, the drug–nutrient interactions of anticonvulsant medications and vitamin D were demonstrated by several investigators in the 1970s. Vitamin D deficiency and insufficiency continues to be a concern in the nutritional care of these children.[23–25] Some classes of anticonvulsants, through the action of the hepatic microsomal enzymes, cause increased vitamin D catabolism. In a survey of 125 noninstitutionalized children with heterogeneous types of CP in the United States, nearly 20% had low-serum 25-hydroxyvitamin D levels. However, low vitamin D status was not associated with severity of CP, growth failure, or use of anticonvulsants.[25] Another study of institutionalized children in South Africa found that anticonvulsant therapy was associated with long-bone fracture, and that 3 months of vitamin D and calcium supplementation resulted in marked improvement in serum calcium and phosphorus, and reduced alkaline phosphatase and fracture rate.[26] Another vitamin D and calcium supplementation study demonstrated improved bone mineral density (BMD) in children with CP.[25] Weight-bearing physical activity also has a beneficial effect on bone density.[27] Thus, in addition to anticonvulsants, low dietary intake of vitamin D and calcium, limited physical activity, and low sunlight exposure also contribute to rickets, osteopenia, and pathologic fractures in children with CP.[28–31]

Nutritional assessment of children with severe disabilities has several components, including evaluation of dietary intake, growth status, body composition, energy expenditure, bone density, and laboratory data in the context of the nutritional risk factors related to the medical history, physical examination, diagnosis, and current therapy. The need for interdisciplinary evaluation and treatment of nutrition and feeding abnormalities for children and adults with CP has been addressed by numerous investigators and position papers.[32–36] Inadequate caloric intake is a primary concern. Children with CP have abnormal growth and body composition. Therefore, conventional methods for estimating energy requirements based on age and gender group, or prediction equations that use body weight or surface area, may be inappropriate for nonambulatory children with CP.[37,38] The new Dietary Reference Intake (DRI) recommendations for energy from the US Food and Nutrition Board[39] base the estimated energy requirement (EER) on age group, gender, physical activity level, height, weight, and weight status (healthy weight vs overweight), so these recommendations may prove to be more appropriate for children with CP who have impaired growth and reduced physical activity than the previous recommended daily allowance (RDA) approach.[40] The importance of determining energy requirements and meeting those requirements in children with CP is underscored by several nutrition intervention trials in which caloric supplementation by gastrostomy or nasogastric feeding tube resulted in improvements in various components of nutritional status.[41–45]

Another approach to determining energy needs in children with severe CP has been to determine the extent of growth failure and poor nutritional status and their relationship to nutritional and disease-related factors and energy expenditure. A recent multicenter study of growth and health outcomes in North America documented the association of growth failure with indicators of overall health and social participation across the spectrum of CP, showing that children with the best growth status had lower healthcare utilization and fewer days of social participation missed.[9] In a large single-center study ($N = 142$), children aged 2 to 18 years with spastic quadriplegic cerebral palsy (SQCP) participated in a survey of growth and nutritional status.[5,6] Linear growth, assessed by upper-arm and lower-leg lengths, was significantly reduced (z-scores, –1.57 to –2.38) relative to healthy children.[46] Weight and triceps skinfold thickness were, on average, about 65% of age- and sex-specific medians for children in the United States; subscapular skinfold thickness was 81% of the median. Poor nutritional status was evident in children as young as 2 to 4 years of age. Linear growth retardation in upper-arm and lower-leg length was significantly associated with poor nutritional status (arm muscle area and percent body fat), after adjusting for disease severity (diagnosis, cognitive ability, oral-motor function, ambulatory status, gastrostomy feeding, and dyskinetic component) and nondisease variables (age, gender, race, pubertal status, and midparental height). This analysis demonstrated that the large effect of poor nutritional status on linear growth was independent of, and additive to, the effects of the severity of the CP and nondisease factors.

Energy expenditure and dietary intake were measured in a subsample of these children with SQCP. Resting energy expenditure (REE), expressed as the percentage of the predicted value from World Health Organization (WHO)[47] prediction equations, was considerably lower than in normal children (91% predicted in CP vs 105% in controls). REE was lowest (88% predicted) among the majority group of poorly nourished children with CP.[10] Total energy expenditure, measured by the doubly labeled water method, was also lower than in control children, in keeping with reduced physical activity in children with severe SQCP. The physical activity factor, or ratio of total to REE, was 1.23 for children with CP as opposed to 1.57 for controls. This is similar to the patterns of resting and total energy expenditure observed in adults[48] with CP. Thus, in children with SQCP, energy requirements are lower than in normal children. However, determination of energy intake proved to be far more difficult. The ratio of total caloric intake, measured by a 3-day weighed food intake diary, to total energy expenditure indicated a large—about 50%—overestimation of food intake by the caregivers of these children with poor oral-motor function.

These findings illustrate the complexity of assessing energy requirements in disabled children. Although total energy requirements are lower in children with severe CP, dietary intake is likely to be grossly overestimated in the clinical setting. The prevalence of chronic undernutrition and growth failure in many children with SQCP indicates that energy needs are not being met. The next sections outline an approach to determining energy requirements in children with CP or other severe disabilities. The first step is the assessment of growth and nutritional status to identify those children whose energy needs are not being met and the degree of past or current undernutrition. Methods for estimating energy requirements based on nutritional status and related factors are reviewed.

NUTRITION STATUS ASSESSMENT

Inadequate energy intake appears to be a major cause of nutrition-related growth failure in children with CP. Thus, two clinical management needs arise: (1) methods to assess nutritional and growth status to identify patients who are undernourished or overnourished and (2) methods to determine the caloric requirement of the individual patient. The elements of complete nutritional assessment are based on the standard pediatric medical evaluation and are presented in more detail in Chapters 2 and 3.

The medical history includes assessment of acute and chronic medical problems and medications. In addition, a nutritional history, including review of a "typical" day's food intake; dietary history; use of caloric, vitamin, mineral, herbal, or other nutritional supplements; and unusual food practices by the child or family are obtained. The past growth patterns, including pubertal history and growth charts, are reviewed. The history includes a review of systems, with emphasis on dental and oral-motor function and on the gastrointestinal tract (emesis, gastroesophageal reflux, diarrhea, and constipation).

The physical examination includes current pubertal status[49]; weight; height, length, or alternative linear growth measures; head circumference; midarm circumference; and skinfold measurements. Details of the recommended methods, equipment, and reference standards for the anthropometric measurements are in the following section. (For an overview of some of the physical findings associated with nutritional deficiencies, see Appendix, Table I-9.)

The laboratory evaluation is focused by recognizing the risk factors identified from the history and physical examination for each individual patient. The primary nutritional problem is usually inadequate caloric intake, and laboratory assessment of this pattern of malnutrition is of limited use. Both serum albumin and prealbumin can be indicators of the adequacy of calorie and protein intake, with albumin reflecting the past month (half-life, approximately 18 to 20 days) and prealbumin reflecting the past week (half-life, approximately 2 to 3 days) of nutrient intake. However, these are often in the normal range with the chronic undernutrition associated with CP. Iron-deficiency anemia is seen in groups of patients who have limited caloric intake or who have monotonous food intake with few iron-rich foods. Iron status evaluation includes a complete blood count (hemoglobin, hematocrit, and red cell indices) as a screen, followed by other iron studies (serum iron, total iron-binding capacity, transferrin, and ferritin) as indicated. Response to iron therapy is monitored by changes in the components of the complete blood count and a reticulocyte count.

Laboratory tests are selected depending on the patient's history and physical examination and could include serum values for vitamin D, calcium, phosphorus, and alkaline phosphatase, and radiologic examination of long bones to diagnose rickets. Clinically significant osteopenia often occurs without rachitic changes and can be diagnosed by determining bone mineral content or bone density [dual-energy X-ray absorptiometry (DXA)]. Bone density of the distal femur has been proposed as a measure for children with CP and contractures who are difficult to position for standard measurement sites.[50–52] Skeletal age determination[53,54] is useful for diagnosing nutritional dwarfism in children with a delay of 2 or more years in bone age and for determining the potential for catch-up growth. Blood values for selected vitamins and minerals are available when indicated.

ANTHROPOMETRY

Anthropometric evaluation of growth and nutritional status is an essential component of nutritional care. It is a rapid, inexpensive, noninvasive means of determining both short- and long-term nutritional status. A well-trained anthropometrist is required in order to ensure accurate, reproducible measurements. Numerous anthropometric measures are used in the assessment of nutritional status. Each measure offers different information, and no single measure is sufficient for characterization of nutritional status. Proper equipment must be used, and calibrated regularly to ensure accurate measurements. When accurate measurements are obtained and compared to appropriate reference standards, the clinician obtains a current classification of nutritional status and an opportunity to see changes in status over time. Guidelines for anthropometric measurement techniques are available[55] and are summarized below with consideration of the child with developmental disabilities.

MEASUREMENT OF GROWTH

Weight, stature or length, and head circumference should be measured at routine office visits and every hospital admission. Current status and increments in growth between visits are very informative, especially for tracking progress in the individual patient. For children with severe disabilities, alternative measures of linear growth—upper-arm length and lower-leg length—are described below for assessment when a length or stature measurement is not possible.

WEIGHT

Because growth retardation is common in children with severe disabilities, it is of extra importance that both weight and linear growth are measured at the same time. Because excess weight can be attributable to excess fat, excess water caused by edema, or organomegaly, other anthropometric measures, such as arm circumference and skinfold thicknesses, are important complements to interpreting a weight measurement.

Equipment, Measurement Technique, and Reference Standards

Weight should be measured on a digital electronic or beam balance scale. The scale should be checked weekly with known calibration weights. The measurement should be taken to the nearest 0.1 kg in older children and to the nearest 0.01 kg in infants.

The scale should be reset to zero prior to placing a child on it. Children should be weighed wearing little or no outer clothing and without shoes. Infants should be measured without diapers. Wheelchair-accessible scales are available for older children who cannot stand unattended on a scale. The measured weight of the wheelchair alone is deducted from the weight of the child (with little or no clothing) in the wheelchair.

For reference standards for weight, see the Centers for Disease Control and Prevention (CDC) 2000 growth charts.[56] Reference values for infant weight gain are also available.[57]

LENGTH OR STATURE

Linear growth is a measure of a child's nutritional history and genetic potential and helps to distinguish between short- and long-term nutritional problems. Length or stature measurements are appropriate for children who can be properly positioned, as described below. For children less than 2 years of age or children older than 2 who are not able to stand erect unsupported, a supine length measurement is taken. Standing height, or stature, is measured at age 2 and older. In older children with developmental disabilities, a length measurement is often required past 2 years of age. When comparing a supine length measurement to a growth chart for stature, the length should be decreased by approximately 2 cm[58] to adjust for the known difference between length and stature measurements.

Equipment, Measurement Technique, and Reference Standards

To measure supine length, an infantometer or an inflexible length board with a fixed headboard and a movable footboard should be used. Length is measured to the nearest 0.1 cm. Infantometers and stadiometers with digital counters should be calibrated daily with a calibration bar of fixed length.

Measurement of supine length requires two people to position and hold the child. The head should be placed at the top of the board, with the Frankfurt plane perpendicular to the floor.[59] The Frankfurt plane extends from the lower margin of the orbit to the upper margin of the auditory meatus (Figure 1). An assistant is needed to hold the head firmly in this position. The knees should be flattened to fully extend the legs. The feet should be together and flexed to a 90° angle by the footboard with the infant fully stretched.

To measure stature, the child should stand with the heels, buttocks, and back of the head against the stadiometer. The arms should be down and relaxed and the heels together. The position of the head should be adjusted so that the Frankfurt plane is parallel to the floor. Stature should be measured using a stadiometer with a head paddle that glides smoothly but is firmly perpendicular to the back of the stadiometer. Alternatively, a tape measure permanently fixed to a wall

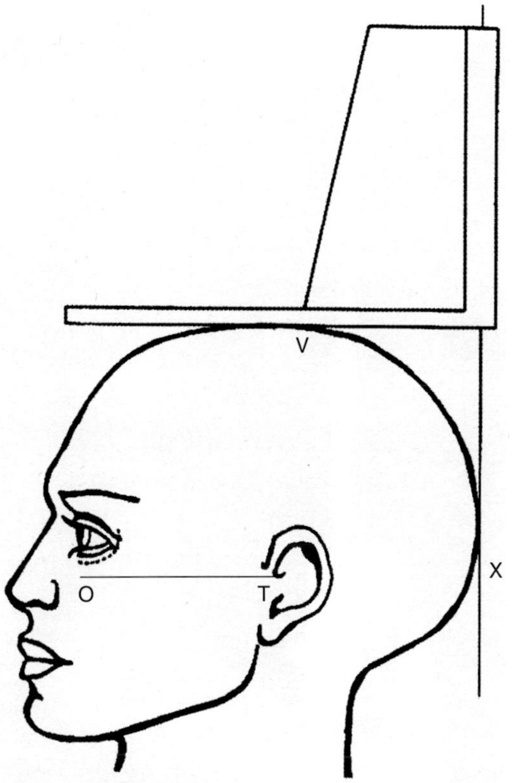

Figure 1 The Frankfurt plane extends from the auditory meatus to the lower border of the orbit. This plane should be parallel to the paddle or headboard when measuring stature or length. (Reproduced from Ross et al.[59])

or doorframe can be used, provided that a head paddle is available that will fit at a 90° angle to the wall. Both length and stature measurements should be accurate to 0.1 cm.

Length and stature measures are inappropriate for children with spinal curvature, contractures, or other conditions that prevent proper positioning for the measurement. Upper-arm length and lower-leg length are alternatives under these conditions (see below).

For both length and stature, measurements should be taken in triplicate, with the measurements in agreement within 0.5 cm, and the mean recorded. Whenever possible, the statures of both biological parents should be obtained and midparental stature computed (the average stature of the mother and father). Adjustment of stature or length measurements using midparental stature charts is a technique that recognizes and corrects for differences in the genetic potential for linear growth.[60]

For reference standards for length and stature, see the CDC 2000 growth charts.[56] Related information is found in several other publications.[57,60–63]

WEIGHT-FOR-HEIGHT INDICES

Weight-for-length and weight-for-height indices are important in the assessment of nutritional status to ensure energy reserves adequate for maintaining growth and overall health. In infants and young children, weight-for-height charts are available[56] to assess nutritional status. For children more than 2 years of age, the body mass index (BMI) can be used. BMI is calculated as weight in kilograms divided by height in meters squared (wt/ht^2). BMI percentile charts are available for children from age 2 to 20 years.[56] Use of these charts is essential for interpretation of BMI in the pediatric range.

HEAD CIRCUMFERENCE

Brain growth is most rapid in the first 3 years of life. Head circumference is a good indicator of brain growth and therefore should be included in the assessment of growth and nutritional status. Because of the high risk of growth failure in children with developmental disabilities, it is important to measure head circumference until age 3, or longer in some children, to determine whether growth of the brain and head is also compromised. However, head circumference is of limited use in nutritional status assessment of patients with central nervous system damage and micro- or megalocephaly of nonnutritional etiology.

Equipment, Measurement Technique, and Reference Standards

A flexible metal or nonstretch plastic-coated measuring tape scaled to 0.1 cm should be used. The tape is placed over the supraorbital ridge and around the occiput so that a maximum circumference is obtained. Care should be taken that the tape is evenly placed on all sides and is flat against the skull. Three measurements should be obtained and the mean recorded.

For reference standards for head circumference, see the CDC 2000 growth charts for children up to 3 years of age,[56] and for older children see Roche and colleagues.[64]

UPPER-ARM AND LOWER-LEG LENGTH

Upper-arm length and lower-leg length are alternative measures of linear growth when length or stature measurements are not possible. This commonly occurs in children with developmental disabilities. Both upper-arm and lower-leg length should be measured because they provide measures of upper- and lower-body long-bone growth. Frequently, lower-leg length is more compromised than upper-arm length in children who are nonambulatory.

Equipment, Measurement Technique, and Reference Standards

For young infants, sliding calipers (0 to 200 mm) are used. For older infants and children, an anthropometer (50 to 570 mm) is used. All measurements should be taken in triplicate to the nearest 0.1 cm and repeated every 3 months. For infants and young children up to 24 months of age, upper-arm length is measured as shoulder-to-elbow length. With the arm flexed at a 90° angle, the upper arm is measured from the superior lateral surface of the acromion to the inferior surface of the elbow. In children 2 to 18 years of age, upper-arm length is measured from the

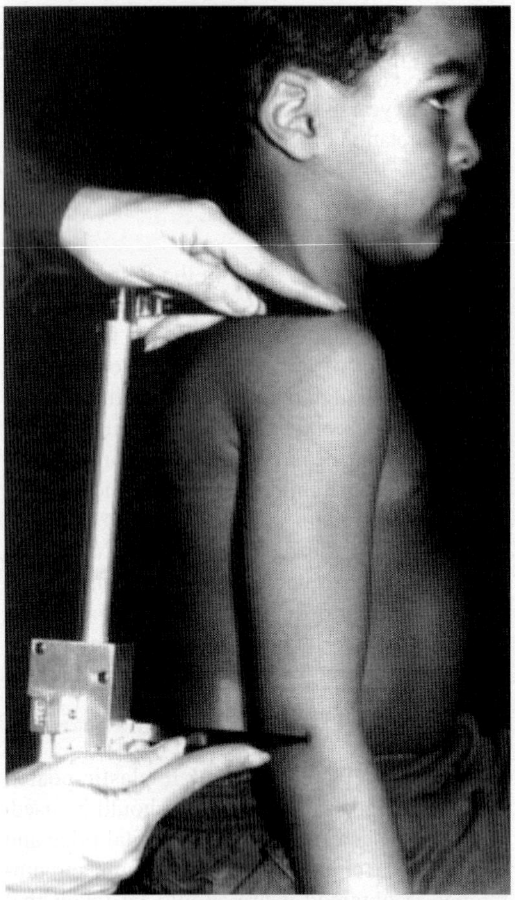

Figure 2 Upper-arm length measurement technique.

superior lateral surface of the acromion to the radiale (head of the radius) with the arm relaxed, as shown in Figure 2.

For infants and young children, lower-leg length is measured as a knee-to-heel length. With the infant lying supine—with the leg flexed to 90° at the hip, the knee, and the ankle—the lower-leg length is measured from the heel to the superior surface of the knee. For children 2 to 18 years of age, the lower-leg length measure is taken from the lower border of the medial malleolus (sphyrion) to the medial tip of the tibia while the patient is sitting in a relaxed position, as shown in Figure 3. The right side should be measured unless there is unilateral involvement affecting the right side. The least affected side should be measured and thus noted on the growth chart so that repeat measures are always taken on the same limb. Reference percentiles for upper-arm length and lower-leg length for infants are given in Figures 4 and 5 and for older children (3 to 18 yr) in Figures 6 through 9.

For reference standards for upper-arm length and lower-leg length, see Spender and colleagues[46] and Snyder and colleagues.[65]

NUTRITIONAL STATUS

Anthropometric indicators of nutritional status consist of measurements of lean and fat tissues at sites known to be sensitive indicators of nutrition and health. Upper-arm anthropometry, the measurement of arm circumference and skinfold

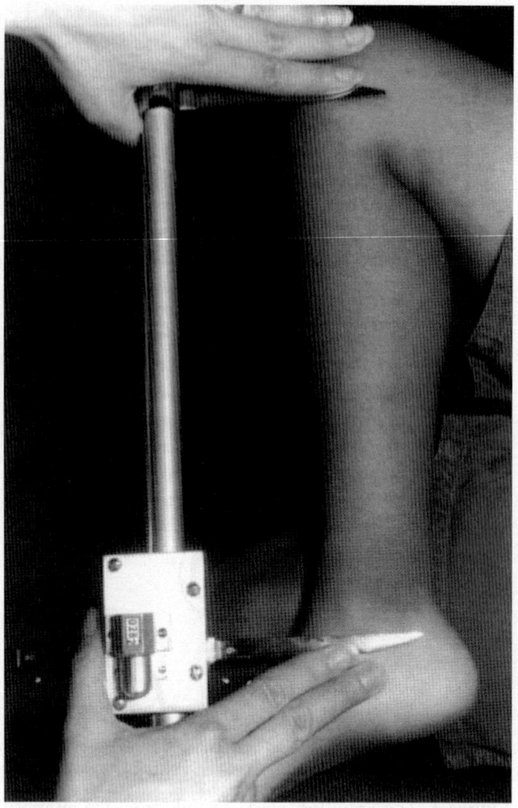

Figure 3 Lower-leg length measurement technique.

thickness, is particularly useful because excellent reference data are available for clinical interpretation. An additional measure of subcutaneous fat on the trunk, the subscapular skinfold thickness measure, is helpful for further assessing total body fat stores, especially when fat distribution is abnormal.

MID-UPPER-ARM CIRCUMFERENCE

Mid-upper-arm circumference is a composite measure of muscle, fat, and bone in the arm. It is sensitive to current nutritional status and can be used in combination with the triceps skinfold thickness measure to estimate upper-arm muscle area and upper-arm fat area.

Equipment, Measurement Technique, and Reference Standards

A nonstretch flexible tape measure is used. All measurements should be taken in triplicate to the nearest 0.1 cm. The midpoint of the upper arm is located by measuring the length of the upper arm (from the tip of the acromion to the olecranon with the arm flexed at 90° and the palm facing upward) and marking the midpoint with a washable ink pen. The midarm circumference is taken with the arm down and in a fully relaxed position. Gently shaking the arm usually ensures that it is relaxed. The tape is placed over the midpoint perpendicular to the long axis of the arm. Care should be taken so that there is no pinching or gaping of the tape as it encircles the arm. This process improves the accuracy and reproducibility of the measure.

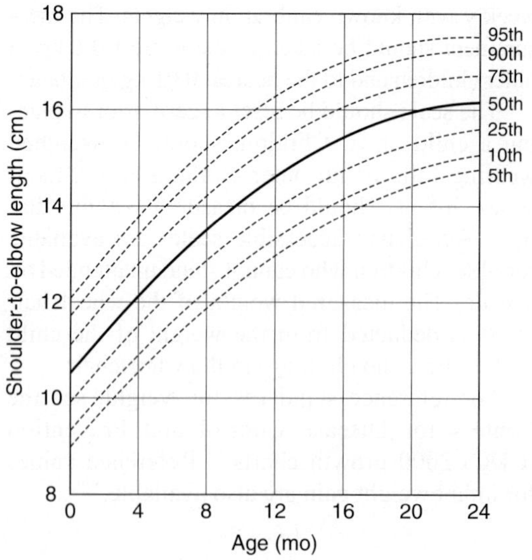

Figure 4 Shoulder-to-elbow lengths for boys and girls from birth to age 2 years. (Reproduced from Stallings VA and Zemel.[75])

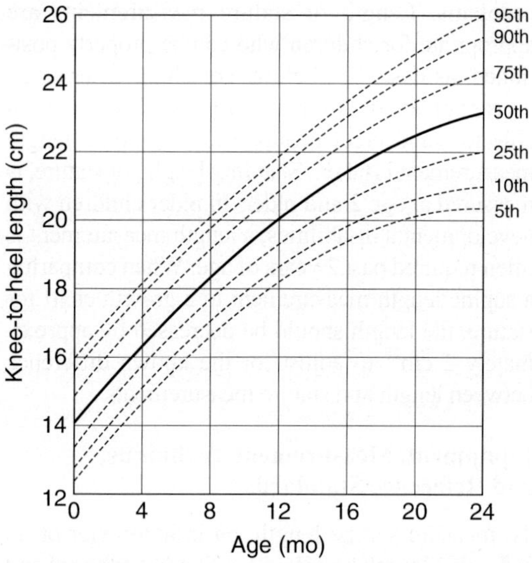

Figure 5 Knee-to-heel lengths for boys and girls from birth to age 2 years. (Reproduced from Stallings and Zemel.[75])

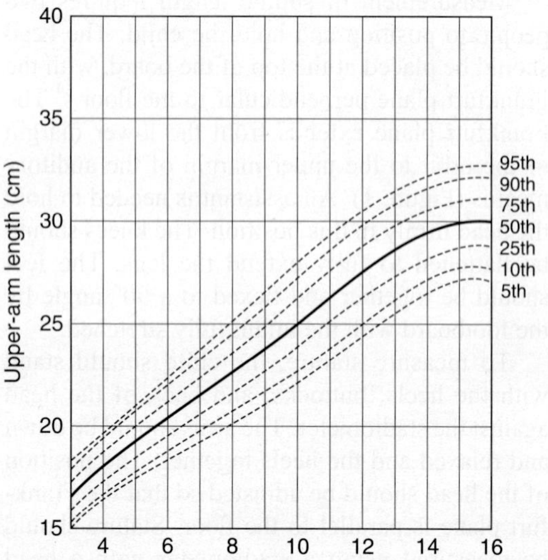

Figure 6 Upper-arm lengths for girls 3 to 16 years of age. (Reproduced from Stallings and Zemel.[75])

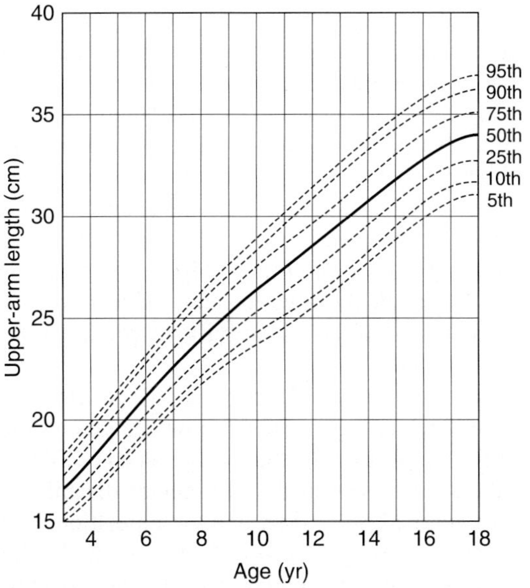

Figure 7 Upper-arm lengths for boys 3 to 18 years of age. (Reproduced from Stallings and Zemel.[75])

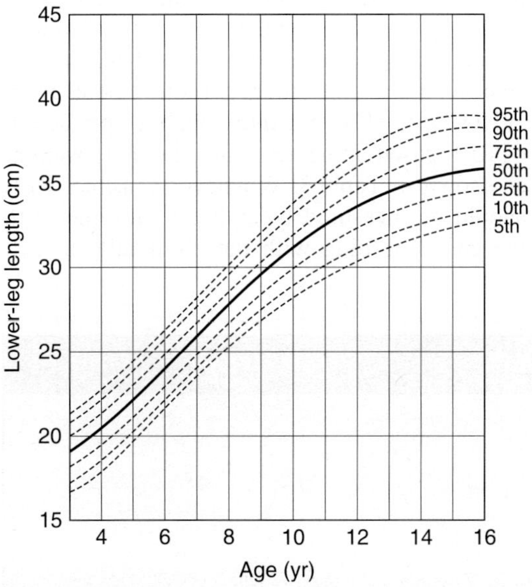

Figure 8 Lower leg length for girls 3 to 16 years of age. Reproduced from Stallings VA, Zemel BA. Nutritional assessment of the disabled child. In: Sullivan PR, Rosenbloom L, editors. Clinics in developmental medicine: feeding the disabled child. London: Cambridge Univ. Press; 1996. p. 62–76.

For reference standards for mid-upper-arm circumference, see Frisancho.[66]

SKINFOLD THICKNESS

Skinfold thickness measures assess subcutaneous fat at specified sites. The triceps and subscapular skinfold measures are indicators of total body fat stores and are sensitive to changes in nutrient intake and nutritional status. Depletion of fat stores at the triceps site is common in children with CP and in other chronically undernourished groups, whereas fatness at the subscapular site is not affected as severely.[5,6,67] Reference data for the sum of these two skinfold measures are available[68] and are used in the research setting as a characterization of total body fat.

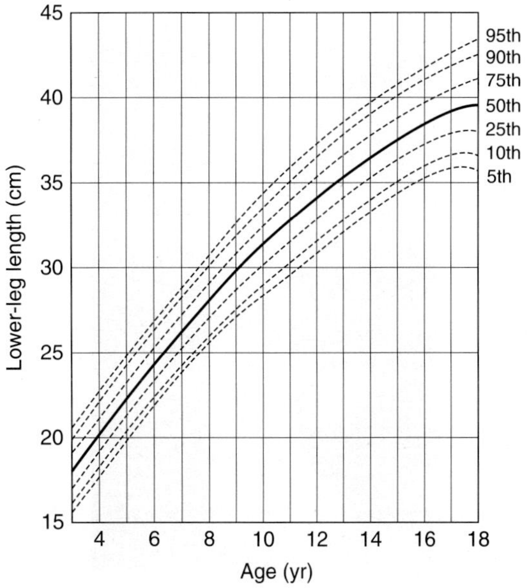

Figure 9 Lower leg length for boys 3 to 18 years of age. Reproduced from Stallings VA, Zemel BA. Nutritional assessment of the disabled child. In: Sullivan PR, Rosenbloom L, editors. Clinics in developmental medicine: feeding the disabled child. London: Cambridge Univ. Press;1996. p. 62–76.

Equipment, Measurement Technique, and Reference Standards

Holtain skinfold calipers are preferred because they are scaled to 0.2 mm. Lange calipers can be used, but with some loss of accuracy as they are scaled to the nearest 0.5 mm. Calipers that are not spring loaded and therefore do not provide a constant tension are not recommended.

The triceps skinfold thickness is measured over the triceps muscle, along the back of the arm. The measurement is taken at the same level at which the mid-upper-arm circumference is measured. The patient should be upright with the arm down and fully relaxed for the measurement. The fold of fat and skin is lifted away from the underlying muscle and held throughout the measurement. The calipers are placed on the skin next to the fingers lifting up the skinfold; the skinfold is held in position while the thickness is measured with calipers, and the reading should be taken 3 to 4 seconds after releasing the caliper's handles.

For the subscapular skinfold, the patient should be upright with the arm and shoulder down and fully relaxed. The skinfold is lifted 1 cm below the tip of the scapula at a 45° angle following the natural contour of the body. The fold is held in place, and the calipers are placed next to the fingers holding the fold. The reading should be taken 3 to 4 seconds after releasing the caliper's handles.

For reference standards for skinfold thickness, see Frisancho,[68] Cronk and Roche,[69] and Johnson and colleagues.[70]

BODY COMPOSITION

Body composition assessment, the measurement of fat and lean body mass stores, is an essential component of nutritional assessment of the disabled child. Whereas linear growth reflects the longer term nutritional history and genetic potential and is often compromised in children with disabilities, fat and lean body mass stores reflect short-term nutritional adequacy. Body composition can be estimated using the prediction equations of Slaughter and colleagues[71] in children aged 8 to 18 years. These equations use the triceps and subscapular skinfold thickness measures shown in Table 1. Specific equations are given based on race, gender, and pubertal status groups.

Body composition values estimated from these anthropometric prediction equations have been compared with measures determined from total body water[16] in children with severe SQCP. Fat mass measured by these two methods is significantly correlated (r = .69), indicating that the anthropometric prediction equations can be used as a clinical, noninvasive method to estimate total body fat in children with CP. Other methods, such as bioelectrical impedance analysis (BIA) and DXA, are possible. However, motion artifact and inability to properly position the patient could increase the measurement error and give inconsistent results in children with moderate-to-severe disabilities. In addition, BIA requires a height measurement. For children whose height can be estimated only from long-bone measures, the measurement error is greatly increased so that these methods become less effective measures of body composition.

BONE DENSITY ASSESSMENT

Children with moderate-to-severe CP are at increased risk of osteopenia and fracture,[21,22] so assessment of bone density is often warranted. Bone density is measured by DXA, a rapid, noninvasive technique that involves very low levels of ionizing radiation. The current recommendation of the International Society for Clinical Densitometry[72] for assessment of bone density in children is to measure the BMD of the

Table 1 Anthropometric Equations for Prediction of Percent Fat (Ages 8–18 yr)

White males	
Prepubescent:	1.21 (triceps + subscapular) − 0.008 (triceps + subscapular)^2 − 1.7
Pubescent:	1.21 (triceps + subscapular) − 0.008 (triceps + subscapular)^2 − 3.4
Postpubescent:	1.21 (triceps + subscapular) − 0.008 (triceps + subscapular)^2 − 5.5
Black males	
Prepubescent:	1.21 (triceps + subscapular) − 0.008 (triceps + subscapular)^2 − 3.2
Pubescent:	1.21 (triceps + subscapular) − 0.008 (triceps + subscapular)^2 − 5.2
Postpubescent:	1.21 (triceps + subscapular) − 0.008 (triceps + subscapular)^2 − 6.8
All females	1.33 (triceps + subscapular) − 0.013 (triceps + subscapular)^2 − 2.5
If (triceps + subscapular) greater than 35 mm:	
Males	0.783 (triceps + subscapular) + 1.6
Females	0.546 (triceps + subscapular) + 9.7

Adapted from reference 71.

lumbar spine and whole body, and compare the results to age- and gender-specific reference data to determine the z (standard deviation) score. A z-score between −1 and −2 may be considered "low normal" and a z-score less than −2 may be considered "low" or "abnormal" BMD.[73]

For many children with developmental disabilities, particularly for those with CP, a whole body and spine measurement may not be feasible due to altered posture, spasticity, voluntary and involuntary movements, and metal spine implants.[52] In addition, the BMD measure is influenced by height and weight, so for children with developmental disabilities and growth failure, a low BMD may be related to poor growth rather than bone strength.[73] An alternative scan technique with accompanying reference data for the distal femur has been developed.[50–52] This has proven to be a more feasible approach for assessing BMD in children with CP. An example of a distal femur image is given in Figure 10. Peripheral quantitative computed tomography (pQCT) has also been used in the research setting to assess bone strength in children with CP.[20] This is not a clinically available assessment technique at this time.

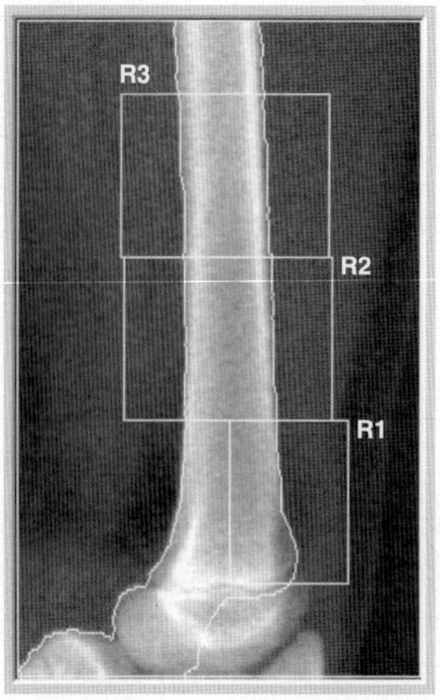

Figure 10 DXA scan of a lateral distal femur for assessment of bone mineral density in children. The bone mineral density of regions R1, R2, and R3 are determined separately.

ENERGY INTAKE RECOMMENDATIONS

Assessment of energy intake compared to requirement is an essential component of the nutritional care of children with significant disabilities. Undernutrition and overnutrition are the common nutritional pathologies and are the result of energy imbalance. True energy intake is difficult to determine accurately in children with poor oral-motor function and other gastrointestinal problems. Food loss during feeding and regurgitation contribute to the inaccurate estimation of energy intake, even when weighed food diaries recorded over several days are obtained.[10] Daily energy expenditure and its components can be measured in individuals in a research setting (doubly labeled water, 24 h indirect room calorimetry, REE, thermic effect of food, physical activity). Only REE by indirect calorimetry, a measurement of basal metabolic needs, is available as a clinical evaluation and can be used with estimates of physical activity to predict total caloric needs.

The accuracy of the revised DRI recommendations for energy intake,[39] now designated the EER, for estimating the energy needs of individual patients with developmental disabilities with atypical body size, body composition, and physical activity has not been evaluated. The EER is based on gender, age, height, weight, and level of physical activity and may be more accurate in estimating the energy needs of children with developmental disabilities than the previous RDA recommendations which were based on age and gender only. The formulas for determining the EER are given in Table 2. The formulas for energy requirement from WHO[47] also allow for individualized prediction of REE based on gender, age, and body weight, as shown in Table 3. Whenever possible, REE should be measured by indirect calorimetry in the early morning with the child fully at rest

Table 2 Prediction Equations for Estimated Energy Requirements (kcal/day) for Healthy Children[39]

Infants	Prediction Equations				
0 to 3 mo	89*weight (kg) − 100 + 175				
3 to 6 mo	89*weight (kg) − 100 + 56				
6 to 12 mo	89*weight (kg) − 100 + 22				
12 to 24 mo	89*weight (kg) − 100 + 20				
Males	**General Prediction Equation***	**Sedentary PA Coefficient**	**Low Active PA Coefficient**	**Active PA Coefficient**	**Very Active PA Coefficient**
3 through 8 yr	88.5 − 61.9*age + PAL*((26.7* weight) + 903* (height)) + 20	1.00	1.13	1.26	1.42
9 through 18 yr	88.5 − 61.9*age + PAL*((26.7* weight) + 903* (height)) + 25	1.00	1.13	1.26	1.42
>18 yr	662 − 9.53*age + PAL*((15.91* weight) + 539.6* (height))	1.00	1.11	1.25	1.48
Overweight 3 through 18 yr	114 − 50.9*age + PAL*((19.5* weight) + 1,161.4* (height))	1.00	1.12	1.24	1.45
Females	**General Prediction Equation***	**Sedentary PA Coefficient**	**Low Active PA Coefficient**	**Active PA Coefficient**	**Very Active PA Coefficient**
3 through 8 yr	135.3 − 30.8*age + PAL*[(10* weight) + 934* (height)] + 20	1.00	1.16	1.31	1.56
9 through 18 yr	135.3 − 30.8*age + PAL*[(10* weight) + 934* (height)] + 25	1.00	1.16	1.31	1.56
>18 yr	354 − 6.91*age + PAL*[(9.36* weight) + 726* (height)]	1.00	1.12	1.27	1.45
Overweight 3 through 18 yr	389 − 41.2*age + PAL*[(15* weight) + 701.6* (height)]	1.00	1.18	1.35	1.60

*Each prediction equation uses weight (kg) and height (cm), and requires that a physical activity coefficient (PA) be included in the calculation of the estimated energy requirement. The PA categories, based on the physical activity level (PAL, calculated as the ratio of total energy expenditure to resting energy expenditure), are as follows: sedentary: PAL is estimated to be ≥1.0 and <1.4; low active: PAL is estimated to be ≥1.4 and <1.6; active: PAL is estimated to be ≥1.6 and <1.9; very active: PAL is estimated to be ≥1.9 and <2.5.

Table 3 Equations for Predicting Resting Energy Expenditure (kcal/d) from Body Weight (w)

Age (yr)	Male	Female
0–3	60.9 W − 54	61.0 W − 51
3–10	22.7 W + 495	22.5 W + 499
10–18	17.5 W + 651	12.2 W + 746
18–30	15.3 W + 679	14.7 W + 496
30–60	11.6 W + 879	8.7 W + 829
>60	13.5 W + 487	10.5 W + 596

Adapted from reference 47.

and in a fasting state. Under these conditions, measurements obtained over 30 to 60 minutes of inactivity can provide an excellent estimate of resting energy needs. The value for REE, whether from indirect calorimetry or a prediction equation, is adjusted by an activity factor to determine total energy expenditure and daily energy requirements. In normally active healthy children and in adults with light or moderate activity, the activity factors range between 1.50 and 1.89 times the REE. Research suggests that the physical activity factor for well-nourished children with spastic quadriplegia is much lower, about 1.3 times the REE, and about 1.5 in malnourished children with CP.[10]

Two other methods for estimating caloric requirements have been published. Culley and Middleton developed a method for disabled children that takes level of motor function into account.[74] The caloric consumption based on motor function status was 14.7 kcal/cm of height and 77 kcal/kg for children without motor dysfunction, 13.9 kcal/cm and 75 kcal/kg for ambulatory children with some motor dysfunction, and 11.1 kcal/cm and 64 kcal/kg for nonambulatory children with motor dysfunction. In addition, Krick and colleagues reported a factorial method approach to determining caloric needs in children with CP.[38] This method accounts for caloric intake based on estimated REE needs, muscle-tone alterations, normal growth needs, and catch-up growth or nutritional repletion in malnourished children. The formula is summarized as

$$\text{kcal/d} = \text{resting energy needs} \times \text{tone factor} + \text{growth factor(s)}$$

SUMMARY

Monitoring nutrition and growth status in children and adults with CP and other severe types of developmental disabilities is an essential component of care. This chapter summarizes the previous work in the area and outlines clinical approaches to determining nutritional status and estimating caloric needs. Although data are not available to provide precise definitions of the levels of severity of malnutrition and growth failure and their effect on long-term outcome, it is clear that many patients with moderate-to-severe CP or other disabilities have malnutrition and growth failure as the result of inadequate caloric intake. Nutritional status assessment every 3 to 6 months will enable the clinical care team to identify malnutrition and growth failure and will provide an objective means of following the response to nutritional intervention.

REFERENCES

1. Reilly S, Skuse D, Poblete X. Prevalence of feeding problems and oral motor dysfunction in children with cerebral palsy: A community survey. J Pediatr 1996;129:877–82.
2. Sullivan PB, Lambert B, Rose M, et al. Prevalence and severity of feeding and nutritional problems in children with neurological impairment: Oxford Feeding Study. Dev Med Child Neurol 2000;42:674–80.
3. Fung EB, Samson-Fang L, Stallings VA, et al. Feeding dysfunction is associated with poor growth and health status in children with cerebral palsy. J Am Diet Assoc 2002;102:361–73.
4. Motion S, Northstone K, Emond A, et al. Early feeding problems in children with cerebral palsy: Weight and neurodevelopmental outcomes. Dev Med Child Neurol 2002;44:40–3.
5. Stallings VA, Charney EB, Davies JC, Cronk CE. Nutritional status and growth of children with diplegic or hemiplegic cerebral palsy. Dev Med Child Neurol 1993;35:997–1006.
6. Stallings VA, Charney EB, Davies JC, Cronk CE. Nutrition-related growth failure of children with quadriplegic cerebral palsy. Dev Med Child Neurol 1993;35:126–38.
7. Troughton KE, Hill AE. Relation between objectively measured feeding competence and nutrition in children with cerebral palsy. Dev Med Child Neurol 2001;43:187–90.
8. Samson-Fang L, Fung E, Stallings VA, et al. Relationship of nutritional status to health and societal participation in children with cerebral palsy. J Pediatr 2002;141:637–43.
9. Stevenson RD, Conaway M, Chumlea WC, et al. Growth and health in children with moderate-to-severe cerebral palsy. Pediatrics 2006;118:1010–8.
10. Stallings VA, Zemel BS, Davies JC, et al. Energy expenditure of children and adolescents with severe disabilities: A cerebral palsy model. Am J Clin Nutr 1996;64:627–34.
11. Gilbert SR, Gilbert AC, Henderson RC. Skeletal maturation in children with quadriplegic cerebral palsy. J Pediatr Orthop 2004;24:292–7.
12. Henderson RC, Gilbert SR, Clement ME, et al. Altered skeletal maturation in moderate to severe cerebral palsy. Dev Med Child Neurol 2005;47:229–36.
13. Kong CK, Tse PW, Lee WY. Bone age and linear skeletal growth of children with cerebral palsy. Dev Med Child Neurol 1999;41:758–65.
14. Roberts CD, Vogtle L, Stevenson RD. Effect of hemiplegia on skeletal maturation. J Pediatr 1994;125:824–8.
15. Worley G, Houlihan CM, Herman-Giddens ME, et al. Secondary sexual characteristics in children with cerebral palsy and moderate to severe motor impairment: A cross-sectional survey. Pediatrics 2002;110:897–902.
16. Stallings VA, Cronk CE, Zemel BS, Charney EB. Body composition in children with spastic quadriplegic cerebral palsy. J Pediatr 1995;126:833–9.
17. Chad KE, McKay HA, Zello GA, et al. Body composition in nutritionally adequate ambulatory and non-ambulatory children with cerebral palsy and a healthy reference group. Dev Med Child Neurol 2000;42:334–9.
18. Suresh-Babu MV, Thomas AG. Nutrition in children with cerebral palsy. J Pediatr Gastroenterol Nutr 1998;26:484–5.
19. Henderson RC, Lark RK, Gurka MJ, et al. Bone density and metabolism in children and adolescents with moderate to severe cerebral palsy. Pediatrics 2002;110:e5.
20. Binkley T, Johnson J, Vogel L, et al. Bone measurements by peripheral quantitative computed tomography (pQCT) in children with cerebral palsy. J Pediatr 2005;147:791–6.
21. Henderson RC, Lin PP, Greene WB. Bone-mineral density in children and adolescents who have spastic cerebral palsy. J Bone Joint Surg Am 1995;77:1671–81.
22. Stevenson RD, Conaway M, Barrington JW, et al. Fracture rate in children with cerebral palsy. Pediatr Rehabil 2006;9:396–403.
23. Bergqvist AG, Schall JI, Stallings VA. Vitamin D status in children with intractable epilepsy, and impact of the ketogenic diet. Epilepsia 2007;48:66–71.
24. Henderson RC. Vitamin D levels in noninstitutionalized children with cerebral palsy. J Child Neurol 1997;12:443–7.
25. Jekovec-Vrhovsek M, Kocijancic A, Prezelj J. Effect of vitamin D and calcium on bone mineral density in children with CP and epilepsy in full-time care. Dev Med Child Neurol 2000;42:403–5.
26. Bischof F, Basu D, Pettifor JM. Pathological long-bone fractures in residents with cerebral palsy in a long-term care facility in South Africa. Dev Med Child Neurol 2002;44:119–22.
27. Chad KE, Bailey DA, McKay HA, et al. The effect of a weight-bearing physical activity program on bone mineral content and estimated volumetric density in children with spastic cerebral palsy. J Pediatr 1999;135:115–7.
28. Crosley CJ, Chee C, Berman PH. Rickets associated with long-term anticonvulsant therapy in a pediatric outpatient population. Pediatrics 1975;56:52–7.
29. Lifshitz F, Maclaren NK. Vitamin D-dependent rickets in institutionalized, mentally retarded children receiving long-term anticonvulsant therapy. I. A survey of 288 patients. J Pediatr 1973;83:612–20.
30. Mimaki T, Walson PD, Haussler MR. Anticonvulsant therapy and vitamin D metabolism: Evidence for different mechanisms for phenytoin and phenobarbital. Pediatr Pharmacol (New York) 1980;1:105–12.
31. Tolman KG, Jubiz W, Sannella JJ, et al. Osteomalacia associated with anticonvulsant drug therapy in mentally retarded children. Pediatrics 1975;56:45–50.
32. Position of the American Dietetic Association: Nutrition in comprehensive program planning for persons with developmental disabilities. J Am Diet Assoc 1992;92:613–5.
33. Position of the American Dietetic Association: Nutrition in comprehensive program planning for persons with developmental disabilities. J Am Diet Assoc 1997;97:189–93.
34. Boyle J. Nutritional management of the developmentally disabled child. Pediatr Surg Int 1991;6:76–81.
35. Johnson RK, Maeda M. Establishing outpatient nutrition services for children with cerebral palsy. J Am Diet Assoc 1989;89:1504–6.
36. Wodarski LA. An interdisciplinary nutrition assessment and intervention protocol for children with disabilities. J Am Diet Assoc 1990;90:1563–8.
37. Eddy TP, Nicholson AL, Wheeler EF. Energy expenditures and dietary intakes in cerebral palsy. Dev Med Child Neurol 1965;7:377–86.
38. Krick J, Murphy PE, Markham JF, Shapiro BK. A proposed formula for calculating energy needs of children with cerebral palsy. Dev Med Child Neurol 1992;34:481–7.
39. Food and Nutrition Board. Institute of Medicine. Dietary Reference Intakes for Energy, Carbohydrate, Fiber, Fat, Fatty Acids, Cholesterol, Protein, and Amino Acids (Macronutrients). Washington, DC: National Academies Press; 2002.
40. National Research Council. Recommended Dietary Allowances. Washington, DC: National Academy Press; 1989.
41. Fried MD, Pencharz PB. Energy and nutrient intakes of children with spastic quadriplegia. J Pediatr 1991;119: 947–9.
42. Patrick J, Boland M, Stoski D, Murray GE. Rapid correction of wasting in children with cerebral palsy. Dev Med Child Neurol 1986;28:734–9.
43. Rempel GR, Colwell SO, Nelson RP. Growth in children with cerebral palsy fed via gastrostomy. Pediatrics 1988;82:857–62.
44. Sanders KD, Cox K, Cannon R, et al. Growth response to enteral feeding by children with cerebral palsy. JPEN J Parenter Enteral Nutr 1990;14:23–6.
45. Shapiro BK, Green P, Krick J, et al. Growth of severely impaired children: neurological versus nutritional factors. Dev Med Child Neurol 1986;28:729–33.
46. Spender QW, Cronk CE, Charney EB, Stallings VA. Assessment of linear growth of children with cerebral palsy: Use of alternative measures to height or length. Dev Med Child Neurol 1989;31:206–14.
47. World Health Organization. Energy and Protein Requirements. Geneva: World Health Organization Technical Report Series No. 724; 1985.
48. Johnson RK, Hildreth HG, Contompasis SH, Goran MI. Total energy expenditure in adults with cerebral palsy as assessed by doubly labeled water. J Am Diet Assoc 1997;97:966–70.
49. Tanner JM. Growth at Adolescence. Oxford: Blackwell Scientific Publication; 1962.
50. Harcke HT, Taylor A, Bachrach S, et al. Lateral femoral scan: An alternative method for assessing bone mineral density in children with cerebral palsy. Pediatr Radiol 1998;28:241–6.
51. Henderson RC, Lark RK, Newman JE, et al. Pediatric reference data for dual X-ray absorptiometric measures of normal bone density in the distal femur. AJR Am J Roentgenol 2002;178:439–43.
52. Moyer-Mileur LJ, Mughal Z, Fung EB. Children with Special Considerations. In: Sawyer AJ, Bachrach LK, Fung EB, editors. Bone Densitometry in Growing Patients. Totowa, NJ: Humana Press; 2006. p. 137–58.

53. Greulich W, Pyle S. Radiographic Atlas of Skeletal Development of the Hand and Wrist. Stanford University Press; 1950.
54. Tanner J, Healy M, Goldstein H, Cameron N. Assessment of Skeletal Maturity and Prediction of Adult Height (TW3) Method. London, WB: Saunders; 2001.
55. Lohman TG, Roche AR, Martorell R. Anthropometric Standardization Reference Manual. Champaign, IL: Human Kinetics; 1988.
56. Ogden CL, Kuczmarski RJ, Flegal KM, et al. Centers for Disease Control and Prevention 2000 growth charts for the United States: Improvements to the 1977 National Center for Health Statistics version. Pediatrics 2002;109:45–60.
57. Guo SM, Roche AF, Fomon SJ, et al. Reference data on gains in weight and length during the first two years of life. J Pediatr 1991;119:355–62.
58. Roche AF, Davila GH. Differences between recumbent length and stature within individuals. Growth 1974;38:313–20.
59. Ross W, Carr RV, Carter JL. Anthropometry Illustrated. The Human Animal Series, Volume 1. Surrey, BC: Turnpike Electronic Publications; 1999.
60. Himes JH, Roche AF, Thissen D, Moore WM. Parent-specific adjustments for evaluation of recumbent length and stature of children. Pediatrics 1985;75:304–13.
61. Roche AF, Himes JH. Incremental growth charts. Am J Clin Nutr 1980;33:2041–52.
62. Berkey CS, Dockery DW, Wang X, et al. Longitudinal height velocity standards for U.S. adolescents. Stat Med 1993;12:403–14.
63. Tanner JM, Davies PS. Clinical longitudinal standards for height and height velocity for North American children. J Pediatr 1985;107:317–29.
64. Roche AF, Mukherjee D, Guo SM, Moore WM. Head circumference reference data: Birth to 18 years. Pediatrics 1987;79:706–12.
65. Snyder RG, Schneider L, Owings S. Anthropometry of infants, children and youths of age 18 for project safety design. Bethesda: Consumer Product Safety Commission Report No. UM-HSR1-77-17; 1977.
66. Frisancho AR. New norms of upper limb fat and muscle areas for assessment of nutritional status. Am J Clin Nutr 1981;34:2540–5.
67. Spender QW, Cronk CE, Stallings VA, Hediger ML. Fat distribution in children with cerebral palsy. Ann Hum Biol 1988;15:191–6.
68. Frisancho AR. Anthropometric Standards for the Assessment of Growth and Nutritional Status. Ann Arbor, MI: University of Michigan Press; 1990.
69. Cronk CE, Roche AF. Race- and sex-specific reference data for triceps and subscapular skinfolds and weight/stature. Am J Clin Nutr 1982;35:347–54.
70. Johnson CL, Fulwood R, Abraham S, Bryner JD. Basic data on anthropometric measurements and angular measurements of the hip and knee joints for selected age groups 1–74 years of age. Vital Health Stat 1981;11:1–68.
71. Slaughter MH, Lohman TG, Boileau RA, et al. Skinfold equations for estimation of body fatness in children and youth. Hum Biol 1988;60:709–23.
72. Leib ES, Lewiecki EM, Binkley N, Hamdy RC. Official positions of the International Society for Clinical Densitometry. J Clin Densitom 2004;7:1–6.
73. Zemel BS, Petit M. Evaluation. In: Sawyer AJ, Bachrach LK, Fung EB, editors. Bone Densitometry in Growing Patients. Totowa, NJ: Humana Press; 2006. p. 115–25.
74. Culley WJ, Middleton TO. Caloric requirements of mentally retarded children with and without motor dysfunction. J Pediatr 1969;75:380–4.
75. Stallings VA and Zemel BS. Nutritional assessment of the disabled child. In: Sullivan PR, Rosnebloom L, editors. Clinics in Developmental Medicine: Feeding the Disabled Child. Cambridge University Press; 1996. p. 62–76.

46

46.1 Inborn Errors of Fasting Adaptation: Glycogen Storage Disease

Angelina I. Valladares, MD
Lisa C. Kemlage, MS, RD
David A. Weinstein, MD, MMSc

Glycogen storage disease (GSD) is caused by a defect in any of multiple enzymes involved in the synthesis or utilization of glycogen.[1,2] Glycogen is stored predominantly in the liver and muscles, and the symptoms of the disorder depend on the location of the defect. Hypoglycemia is the cardinal manifestation of the hepatic glycogenoses due to the inability to utilize glycogen as a source of glucose in a fasting state. Weakness, muscle cramps, and myopathy are the main features of the muscle forms of GSD. Since the disease processes are very different, this chapter is focused on the hepatic glycogenoses which are more dependent upon nutritional therapies.

NORMAL PHYSIOLOGY OF GLUCOSE METABOLISM

Following consumption of a meal, carbohydrates absorbed into the blood stream provide fuel for the brain, muscle, red blood cells, and kidneys. The liver is freely permeable to glucose. After being taken up by the liver, glucose is phosphorylated by glucokinase to form glucose-6-phosphate (G6Pase). Glucose-6-phosphate (G6P) is subsequently converted to glucose-1-phosphate, and glycogen synthase creates chains of glucose molecules by catalyzing the formation of α-1,4-linkages. A branching enzyme forms α-1,6-linkages approximately every 10 glucose units along the chain. During periods of fasting, debranching enzyme hydrolyzes the α-1,6-linkages at branch points and leads to the formation of free glucose. In addition, a cascade of enzymatic reactions activates hepatic glycogen phosphorylase, the rate-limiting enzyme in glycogenolysis, which hydrolyzes the α-1,4-linkages from the outer branches of glycogen to form G6P. G6P catalyzes the terminal reaction of glycogenolysis and gluconeogenesis, the hydrolysis of G6P to glucose and inorganic phosphate in hepatocytes and renal epithelial cells, allowing glucose to be released into the systemic circulation.[3]

Glucose is stored predominantly in muscle, liver, and kidneys as glycogen for use during fasting. Although muscle stores at least twice as much glycogen as the liver, muscle lacks G6Pase. Thus, muscle is unable to release glucose for systemic use, and the muscle forms of GSD are not associated with hypoglycemia. There are five major types of hepatic GSD that affect glucose homeostasis. The location of each of the enzymatic defects is shown in Figure 1.

The clinical severity of the GSDs varies widely depending upon multiple factors including the degree of impairment of glycogenolysis, whether endogenous glucose can be produced by gluconeogenesis, and the availability of alternative fuels (lactate, ketones) during periods of hypoglycemia. Patients with severely limited endogenous glucose production (GSD I) present with seizures, failure to thrive, or developmental delay. In contrast, patients with normal gluconeogenesis and abundant alternative fuels have a milder phenotype (GSD 0 or GSD IX), and they can be asymptomatic until an illness impairs normal dietary carbohydrate intake.

HEPATIC GLYCOGEN SYNTHASE DEFICIENCY (GSD TYPE 0)

Type 0 GSD (GSD 0) is caused by a deficiency in hepatic glycogen synthase, which leads to a marked decrease in liver glycogen content.[4] GSD 0 is due to mutations in the GYS2 gene located on chromosome 12p12.2 and is inherited in an autosomal recessive manner. To date, 15 different mutations have been reported with no identified dominant mutation. Although no high-risk population has been identified, a common mutation, R246X, has been found in people of Italian ancestry.[5]

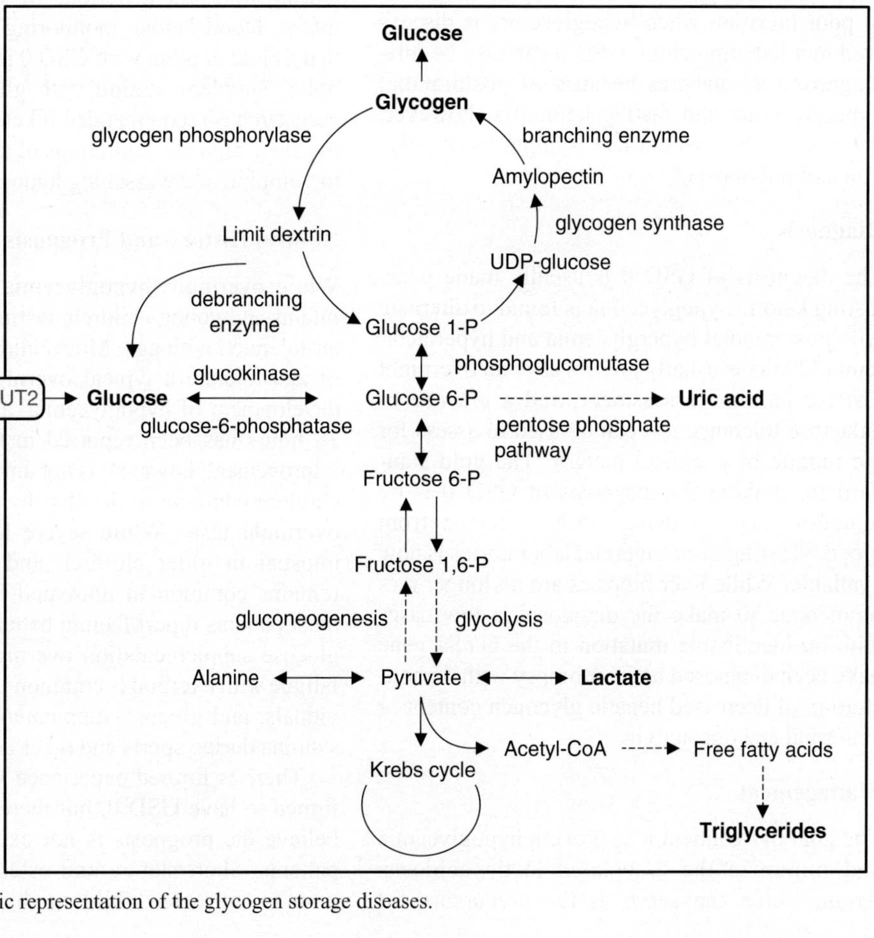

Figure 1 Schematic representation of the glycogen storage diseases.

Pathophysiology

After consumption of carbohydrate, the inability to store glucose as glycogen in the liver results in postprandial hyperglycemia. Glucose taken up by the liver gets shunted down the glycolytic pathway leading to postprandial hyperlactatemia. During fasting, fatty acid oxidation is robust leading to formation of high concentrations of ketones which can be used as an alterative fuel during period of hypoglycemia. Amino acids and lactate can also undergo gluconeogenesis, and these alternative fuels can serve as substrate for endogenous glucose production.

Presentation

The typical presentation of GSD 0 is recurrent ketotic hypoglycemia associated with intercurrent illness.[6] The physical examination is usually normal, and the liver is not enlarged unlike the other hepatic glycogenoses. During infancy, fasting ketotic hypoglycemia develops upon cessation of nighttime feeding. Weaning from overnight feeds proves to be difficult with hypoglycemia and symptoms of agitation and fussiness are often misconstrued as colic. Significant ketonemia develops with fasting and serves as an alternative energy source for the brain.[7] The protection from the prominent ketonemia may explain why developmental delay has only been described in 22% of children with GSD 0.[8] Other manifestations are often subtle including short stature, failure to thrive, hyperlipidemia, or elevation of hepatic transaminase concentrations.[5]

Most children with GSD 0 are identified incidentally during a gastrointestinal illness or period of poor nutrition when hypoglycemia is discovered in a lethargic child. GSD 0 can also be misdiagnosed as diabetes because of postprandial hyperglycemia and fasting ketonuria; however, this presentation would lack symptoms of polyuria and polydipsia.[8]

Diagnosis

The diagnosis of GSD 0 is usually made when fasting ketotic hypoglycemia is found to alternate with postprandial hyperglycemia and hyperlactatemia.[8] Patients usually present after an overnight fast for baseline assessment, and a glucose or galactose tolerance test can be used to assess for the unique biochemical pattern. The gold standard for making the diagnosis of GSD 0 is by mutation analysis using DNA extracted from blood.[4] Testing in commercial laboratories is now available. While liver biopsies are no longer recommended to make the diagnosis, a few cases with no identifiable mutation in the GYS2 gene have been diagnosed by liver biopsy with demonstration of decreased hepatic glycogen content or abnormal enzyme activity.

Management

The goal of treatment is to prevent hypoglycemia and minimize the associated lactic acidosis. Amino acids can serve as the precursors for gluconeogenesis, and thus a high-protein diet is preferred (2 to 3 g/kg). Since hyperlactatemia and hyperlipidemia occur after ingestion of carbohydrates, a low carbohydrate diet is preferred. Low glycemic index complex carbohydrates are preferred over simple sugars.

Infants with GSD 0 are usually asymptomatic due to frequent feeds. As children grow, however, it may be difficult to wean the infant from overnight frequent feeds without additional support. In children, uncooked cornstarch (UCS) with 1 to 1.5 g/kg administered at bedtime is used to prevent hypoglycemia in conjunction with a high-protein, low-carbohydrate diet as previously discussed. In addition to the bedtime cornstarch dose, some children require frequent snacks every 2 to 4 hours during the day to prevent hypoglycemia.[5] Daytime cornstarch is occasionally used (0.5 g/kg) for children and adults who have higher energy needs secondary to an active lifestyle.

In addition to assessing the patient's intake to monitor compliance with the above guidelines, it is critical to ensure that patients receive adequate calories and that no vitamin or mineral deficiencies are present. Unlike other forms of GSD that have a more restricted diet, vitamin and mineral deficiencies are rare in GSD 0. Osteoporosis, however, is common in GSD 0 due to abnormal bone mineralization in the setting of acidosis, and it is important to ensure that appropriate calcium and vitamin D intake is occurring.

Monitoring of blood glucose and blood ketone concentrations is recommended on a routine basis. Cornstarch therapy overnight is titrated to keep blood ketone concentrations under 0.5 mmol/L. During illness and periods of suboptimal food intake, blood ketone monitoring is the first clue that a child or adult with GSD 0 is becoming catabolic. Supplementation with glucose and extra cornstarch is recommended if ketones are increasing since high concentrations of ketones may lead to vomiting and worsening hypoglycemia.

Natural History and Prognosis

While overnight hypoglycemia is common in infants and young children, fasting is usually better tolerated with age. Most children over 7 years of age tolerate a typical overnight fast without development of hypoglycemia, and fasting up to 18 hours has been reported in teenagers.[9] This improvement, however, is not universal, and some children continue to develop hypoglycemia with overnight fasts. While severe hypoglycemia is unusual in older children and adults, ketosis remains common in untreated individuals, and most patients report feeling better with continued glucose supplementation overnight. In addition, fatigue with exertion is common in untreated individuals, and glucose supplementation improves stamina during sports and other active periods.

There is limited experience with adults confirmed to have GSD 0, but there is no reason to believe the prognosis is not excellent for these patients. Short stature and osteopenia are common in untreated children, but improve with prevention of hypoglycemia, lactic acidosis, and ketosis. The long-term complications commonly seen in the other forms of GSD, such as hepatic adenomas, cirrhosis, kidney dysfunction, and muscular abnormalities, have not been reported in teenagers and adults with GSD 0. There are no formal guidelines for screening in this condition.

G6PASE DEFICIENCY (TYPE I GSD; VON GIERKE DISEASE)

G6Pase converts G6P to glucose in the final step of both glycogenolysis and gluconeogenesis.[10] The enzyme is present in the liver, kidneys, and intestines, but it is not present in muscle. At the cellular level, G6Pase is a complex enzyme system located in the endoplasmic reticulum (ER) membrane and consists of a catalytic unit that faces into the ER lumen, a calcium-binding protein, and three transport proteins that facilitate transport of G6Pase (T1), phosphate (T2), and glucose (T3).[11] Abnormalities of any of these components can cause abnormal enzyme function and the clinical phenotype of GSD I. There are three major subtypes of GSD I. More than 85% of patients have mutations that impair the catalytic function of the enzyme (GSD type Ia). Defects in the T1 G6Pase transporter account for most other cases (GSD type Ib). Abnormality of the phosphate transporter (GSD type Ic) is rare.

GSD TYPE IA (VON GIERKE DISEASE)

GSD Ia is caused by mutations in the *G6PC* gene on chromosome 17q21 which encodes for G6Pase.[12] The disease is inherited in an autosomal recessive manner, and the incidence is estimated to be 1 in 100,000 live births. GSD Ia is particularly common in people of Ashkenazi Jewish heritage, and 1 in 68 individuals in this population have been reported to be carriers of the disease.[13] While GSD Ia occurs in all ethnic groups, common mutations have also been reported in people of Chinese, Japanese, and Mexican heritage.

Pathophysiology

The inability to convert G6P to glucose results in hypoglycemia whenever exogenous glucose administration is not occurring. Increased concentrations of G6P develop in hepatocytes and shunting into alternative pathways results in the following:

- Lactic acidosis (as a result of increased glycolysis)[14];
- Hyperuricemia (as a consequence of shunting into the pentose phosphate shunt leading to increased synthesis of uric acid; decreased renal excretion also occurs since lactate and uric acid share the same transporter in the kidney);
- Hypertriglyceridemia (as a result of increased synthesis of acetyl CoA).[15]

With prevention of hypoglycemia and glycogenolysis, all metabolic abnormalities abate.

Presentation

Most children do not present with symptoms until 3 to 6 months of age although hypoglycemia may occur soon after birth. During infancy, as the time period between feeds increases or as an acute illness disrupts normal feeding, symptomatic hypoglycemia develops. The symptoms of agitation and fussiness associated with hypoglycemia may go unrecognized until the child presents with failure to thrive, tachypnea (from lactic acidosis), seizures, lethargy, and developmental delay. If hypoglycemia in infancy is missed, GSD I occasionally is diagnosed when hepatomegaly and a protuberant abdomen are discovered during a routine physical exam.

Diagnosis

The simplest and most rapid means of determining the defect in a child with hypoglycemia suspected to have GSD is to obtain serial blood measurements of glucose, lactate, and ketones during a fasting study. Hypoglycemia and lactic acidosis will manifest in a child with GSD type Ia after a brief fast of 3 to 4 hours. During the study, children should have secure intravenous access to allow for rapid correction since hypoglycemia can develop precipitously. Glucagon must be administered with extreme caution since it will not rescue the child from hypoglycemia, and it can exacerbate lacticacidemia. Typically, glucose concentrations are monitored every 15 to 30 minutes after the initial 2 hours. After the plasma glucose has fallen below 50 mg/dL, a sample for blood glucose and lactate determination should be obtained. Since many of the portable meters are inaccurate in the setting of lactic acidosis, close clinical observation is needed during the test. As soon as the test is completed, intravenous glucose is administered to bring down lactate concentrations and maintain euglycemia.

Mutation analysis on DNA extracted from leukocytes is the recommended test for confirming the diagnosis in a child suspected of having GSD Ia. A total of 82 different mutations have been reported. Since many of the genetic tests for GSD Ia are designed to pick up only the common mutations, complete gene sequencing is recommended for anyone not in a high-risk population.[16] Mutation analysis allows for noninvasive diagnosis, and the technique can be utilized for preimplantation screening and prenatal diagnosis. Liver biopsy is no longer recommended for diagnosing a patient with suspected GSD I, and it should be reserved for those patients in whom GSD Ia is suspected but the mutation analysis is nondiagnostic.

Nutritional Management of the Infant with Type I

Treatment consists of providing a continuous dietary source of glucose to prevent blood glucose from falling below the threshold for glucose counter-regulation, approximately 70 mg/dL (4 mmol/L).[17] A continuous source of glucose can be provided by nocturnal intragastric infusion (via nasogastric tube or gastrostomy) or by using UCS. An estimate of the minimum amount of glucose required can be obtained by using the following formula to calculate the basal glucose production rate:

$$y = 0.0014x^3 - 0.214x^2 + 10.411x - 9.084$$

where y = milligram glucose per minute, and x = body weight in kilogram. In order to avoid excessive caloric intake, the optimum feeding schedule and amounts of cornstarch are determined by metabolic monitoring to ensure that the biochemical goals of therapy are achieved. Cornstarch doses should be weighed on a gram scale to avoid overtreatment which commonly occurs when doses are estimated.

Since nonglucose sugars cannot be converted back to glucose, patients with GSD I must restrict intake of fructose, sucrose, and galactose. Mothers of infants with type I GSD are often encouraged not to breastfeed since the main source of carbohydrate in breast milk is lactose. The formulas most commonly used to treat GSD type I are outlined in Table 1.[18]

The formula chosen must not contain the nonutilizable sugars. Prosobee is the most commonly used formula as it is a nonspecialized, standard infant formula that is easy to obtain and less expensive than the other specialized formulas. The specialized formulas may be indicated, however, if there is a medical necessity, such as malabsorption or intolerance. Tolerex is commonly used for sick-day management since a smaller volume is required to meet the carbohydrate needs of the child. It is well tolerated in infants even though it is an adult formula, but it should not be used as the primary source of nutrition due to the relatively low concentration of protein.

Hypoglycemia is prevented in the infant with GSD I through formula feeds provided every 1.5 to 3 hours. As a result of the need to frequently eat, feeding aversions commonly develop. When solids are introduced, complex carbohydrates such as pastas, legumes, and oatmeal are encouraged. UCS is typically not tolerated in infants younger than 6 months of age due to lack of pancreatic and intestinal amylase which is required to digest cornstarch. The ability to digest UCS, however, differs for each infant, and many infants cannot absorb cornstarch adequately until around 12 months of age.[17] Pancreatic enzyme replacement therapy has been attempted in some infants who develop severe diarrhea with cornstarch. Variable response to this intervention has occurred, and some patients have worsened due to possible over-digestion of cornstarch.

While it is commonly theorized that UCS therapy can lead to obesity in GSD I patients, it must be noted that this is a misconception. In comparing an infant receiving overnight cornstarch supplementation with overnight continuous formula feeds, the infant receiving the cornstarch actually receives fewer calories and a more optimal feeding schedule is promoted. For example, a typical 12-month-old patient with GSD I requires approximately 4 g/h of glucose. To meet the glucose needs, 60 mL/h of Prosobee is required providing ~480 kcal over the 12-hour period. In contrast, when treated with 15 g cornstarch in 2 ounces Prosobee every 4 hours, only 284 calories are administered during the same 12-hour period. Not only is there the 41% reduction in calories, but the cornstarch therapy is associated with lower insulin concentrations and more stability in the morning.

In addition to saving calories, cornstarch therapy is associated with fewer neurologic

Table 1 Commonly Used Formulas in GSD Type I

Formula	Carbohydrate Source	Grams Carbohydrate per 100 mL	Calories/ Ounce	General Comments
Enfamil Prosobee Lipil (Mead Johnson)	Corn syrup solids	7.2	20	• Most commonly used formula
Nutramigen Lipil (Mead Johnson)	Corn syrup solids and modified cornstarch	7	20	• Used with protein allergies and malabsorption issues
Pregestimil (Mead Johnson)	Corn syrup solids, dextrose, modified cornstarch	6.9	20	• High content of MCT as fat (55% of fat calories)
Neocate (SHS)	Corn syrup solids	7.9	20	• Commonly used with food allergies
Elecare (Ross)	Corn syrup solids	7.2	20	• Commonly used with food allergies, malabsorption
Tolerex (Novartis)	Maltodextrin, modified corn starch	23	30	• Commonly used in sick-day management
Vivonex RTF (Novartis)	Maltodextrin, modified corn starch	17.5	30	• Can also be used in sick-day management
Osmolite (Ross)	Maltodextrin	15.1	30	• Isotonic • Kosher

Information obtained from reference 18.

complications when compared with continuous feeds. If a continuous feed is interrupted due to a mechanical problem or leakage of formula, severe hypoglycemia rapidly develops due to the high insulin state. In contrast, the low insulin state associated with cornstarch administration minimizes plasma glucose fluctuations, and blood lactate concentrations increase sufficiently to provide the brain with an alternative fuel. This decreases the risk of hypoglycemia-induced seizures.

Nutritional Management of Children and Adolescents with Type I

Children and adolescents with GSD I are usually treated with UCS therapy bolused around the clock. Dietary fat should be restricted to about 20% of the total energy intake and cholesterol is restricted to <300 mg/d. Carbohydrates, mostly in the form of starches, typically provide about 60 to 65% of the daily calories, of which cornstarch accounts for 30 to 45%. Dietary galactose and fructose continue to be restricted along with restriction of sucrose.

Due to dependence on starch and the restriction of fruit and dairy products, patients often have dietary intakes that are deficient in vitamins and essential minerals. Calcium supplementation is extremely important in combination with a daily multivitamin. Adult multivitamins can be used in children as long as the patient is monitored to avoid vitamin A toxicity. It is also important for iron concentrations to be monitored as iron absorption is typically abnormal in GSD I due to effects of cornstarch and abnormal hepcidin regulation.

Natural History and Prognosis

Prior to the 1970s, many children with GSD I died in infancy or early childhood. Recurrent severe hypoglycemia can cause brain damage, but the prognosis has improved dramatically with early diagnosis and long-term maintenance of optimal metabolic control.[19]

Both acute and long-term complications are common in GSD Ia (Figure 2). Lactate is generated as a consequence of counter-regulation associated with hypoglycemia or secretion of stress hormones (cortisol, epinephrine, glucagon, growth hormone). During illness, lactic acidosis alters gastric motility and causes vomiting. Anesthesia and the stress of surgery cause increased secretion of counter-regulatory hormones, and severe lactic acidosis can develop despite maintenance of normal blood glucose concentrations.

Hepatic adenomas are detected in approximately 50% of patients by the end of puberty.[20] The mean age at diagnosis is approximately 15 years, but adenomas occasionally develop during childhood.[21] There is no gender predisposition, and no difference has been found in the rate of adenoma formation in patients treated with cornstarch compared with those treated with continuous overnight intragastric drip-feeding. Most adenomas remain stable over time, but they may be associated with hemorrhage or degenerate into hepatocellular carcinoma.[22] High alkaline phosphatase concentrations and elevation in the erythrocyte sedimentation rate (ESR) may be seen in patients with adenomas. Ultrasonography is the preferred screening method. When malignant transformation is a concern, magnetic resonance imaging using ferumoxide contrast provides greater definition and may be the best at differentiating benign adenomas from hepatocellular carcinoma.[23] Imaging is recommended at least annually after 5 years of age, and every 6 months if adenomas appear to be enlarging. Both α-fetoprotein and carcinoembryonic antigen have proven unreliable markers for determining malignant transformation.[22]

Treated children usually show no significant impairment of renal function except glomerular hyperfiltration. Some patients have a distal renal tubular acidification defect associated with hypercalciuria.[24] Urinary citrate excretion normally increases with age, whereas in GSD Ia, there is an inverse relationship between age and citrate excretion.[25] The combination of low citrate excretion and hypercalciuria appears to be important in the pathogenesis of nephrocalcinosis and nephrolithiasis. Citrate supplementation may prevent or ameliorate nephrocalcinosis and the development of urinary calculi. Increased albuminuria may be observed in adolescents. More severe renal injury with proteinuria, hypertension, and decreased creatinine clearance due to focal segmental glomerulosclerosis and interstitial fibrosis, which ultimately progresses to renal failure, may be seen in young adults.[26] Patients with persistently elevated concentrations of blood lactate, lipids, and uric acid appear to be at increased risk of nephropathy.[27] Normalization of metabolic parameters decreases proteinuria, and optimal therapy from an early age may delay or prevent renal disease.[19,27]

Anemia is common in patients with GSD Ia and is associated with suboptimal metabolic control.[19] Whereas anemia is usually mild, an unusual, unremitting iron-resistant anemia occurs in a subset of patients.[28] The anemia can be profound with hemoglobin concentrations as low as 4 g/dL and is characterized by microcytosis (mean corpuscular volume 50 to 70 fL), widening of the red-cell distribution width, and iron studies consistent with iron deficiency. Neither erythropoietin nor treatment with oral and intravenous iron significantly improves the anemia. This form of iron-resistant anemia has been associated with large hepatic adenomas (>7 cm in diameter) which inappropriately express hepcidin, a peptide that inhibits intestinal absorption of iron and macrophage recycling of iron. Resection of the hepatic adenomas has been associated with rapid correction of the anemia.[28]

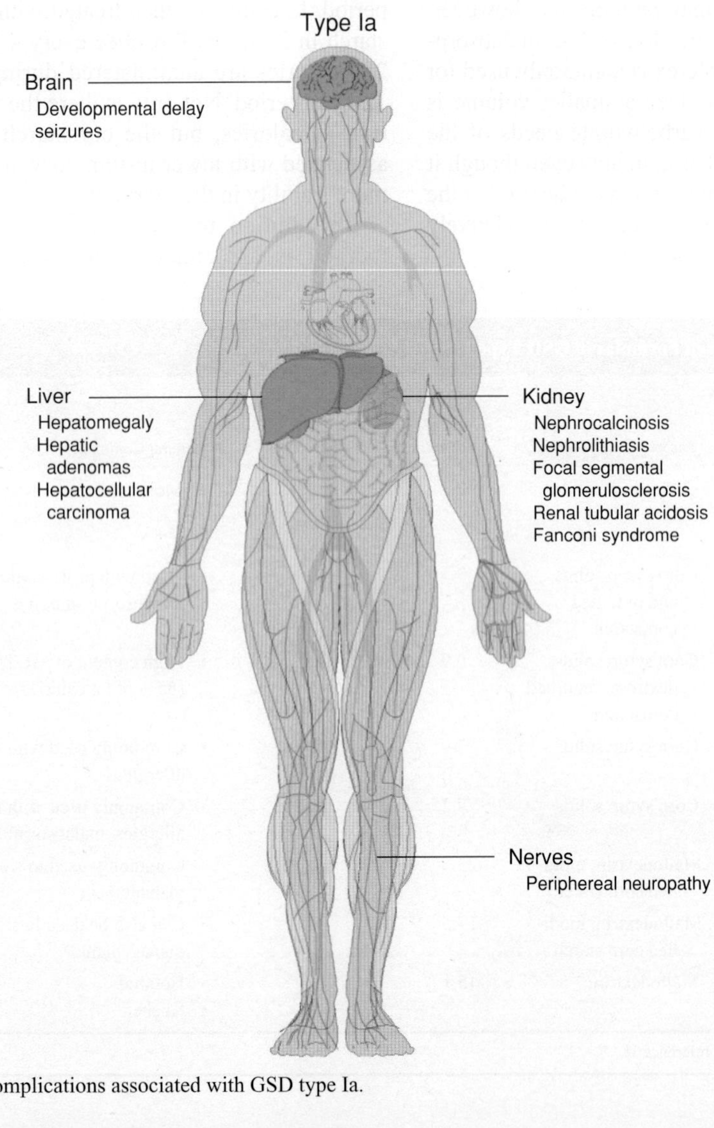

Figure 2 Complications associated with GSD type Ia.

With patients surviving into adulthood, osteoporosis is likely to be a common cause of morbidity. Osteoporosis develops without abnormalities in calcium, phosphate, parathyroid hormone, or vitamin D metabolism.[29] Poor metabolic control has been associated with decreased bone mineral content. The etiology is likely multifactorial, including systemic acidosis, elevated cortisol concentrations, delayed pubertal development, inadequate dietary calcium, and lack of physical activity.[30]

Other complications, seen rarely in type Ia GSD, include pancreatitis, polycystic ovaries, and a bleeding diathesis.[31] Pancreatitis is related to hyperlipidemia, and treatment with Gemfibrozil (600 mg administered twice daily) or Niacin is recommended when hypertriglyceridemia persists despite attempts to improve metabolic control. Pancreatitis has been associated with use of growth hormone and glucocorticoids due to stimulation of glycogenolysis and worsening hypertriglyceridemia. Polycystic ovaries is common in poorly controlled GSD, but it does not appear to be inherent to the disease. Fertility appears to be unaffected and more than 50 children have been born to mothers with GSD Ia. Platelet dysfunction associated with hyperlipidemia and acidosis is also a consequence of poorly controlled GSD. Bleeding is usually not a problem in patients in good metabolic control.

GSD TYPE IB

Type Ib GSD is caused by defects in the G6Pase transporter T1 which is responsible for transport of G6P into the lumen of the ER. The transporter is encoded by *G6PT1* gene on chromosome 11q23 and is inherited in an autosomal recessive manner.[32] The incidence is estimated to be 1 in 1,000,000 live births with no high-risk ethnic group identified.

Pathophysiology

The inability of G6P to interact with the G6Pase enzyme prevents endogenous glucose production. Similar to GSD Ia, hepatomegaly and hypoglycemia develop shortly after birth. In contrast, however, patients with GSD Ib also manifest neutropenia and inflammatory bowel disease (IBD).[33] Immune dysfunction develops as a consequence of both disturbed myeloid maturation and functional defects of circulating neutrophils and monocytes. IBD is also attributed to neutropenia and impaired neutrophil function but persists despite granulocyte colony stimulating factor (G-CSF) therapy.[34]

Presentation

Symptomatic hypoglycemia may occur soon after birth, but most children present around 3 to 6 months of age. Neutropenia is occasionally the first abnormality noted during an evaluation for a serious bacterial infection usually from *Staphylococcus aureus, Streptococcus pneumoniae, and Escherichia coli.* IBD typically develops in the second decade, but it can rarely present within the first few years of life.

Diagnosis

Full gene sequencing is commercially available. To date, approximately 69 mutations in the *G6PT* gene have been described.[35] Diagnosis by liver biopsy is not recommended; if performed, differentiation between the types requires an analysis of G6Pase activity in intact and fully disrupted microsomes as enzyme activity normalizes in type Ib when freezing disrupts the integrity of the ER. Typically the diagnosis is made clinically when a patient with biochemical features of GSD I develops neutropenia and/or IBD.

Nutritional Management

The nutritional management of GSD Ib is the same as GSD Ia. While GSD Ib is easier to manage metabolically, restriction of nonutilizable sugars is also critical in this condition.

Natural History and Prognosis

Long-term complications appear to be less frequent than in GSD Ia (Figure 3). IBD is the major cause of morbidity, and a Crohn's-like IBD almost universally develops by the end of puberty.[33,36] While the IBD responds to therapy with G-CSF, this comorbidity continues to occur even when neutropenia is treated.[37] Periodic screening of inflammatory markers is recommended. Colonoscopy should be performed when IBD is suspected based upon clinical features and laboratory studies. The IBD in GSD Ib may be isolated to the small intestine; consequently, a capsule endoscopy may reveal disease in patients in whom a colonoscopy reveals no evidence of bowel inflammation.

Neutropenia is documented before the age of 1 year in two-thirds of patients, but neutropenia is first noted between the ages of 6 and 9 years in 18% of patients.[33] Most patients have intermittent neutropenia without any clear cyclical course. Children with GSD Ib are prone to oral complications, including recurrent mucosal ulceration, gingivitis, and rapidly progressive periodontal disease. Therapy with recombinant human G-CSF improves infection-related morbidity by increasing numbers of circulating neutrophils and improving in vitro neutrophil function.[34]

DEBRANCHING ENZYME DEFICIENCY (TYPE III GSD; CORI DISEASE; FORBES DISEASE)

Type III GSD is caused by a deficiency of the glycogen debranching enzyme. The incidence of GSD III is estimated to be 1 in 100,000 live births.

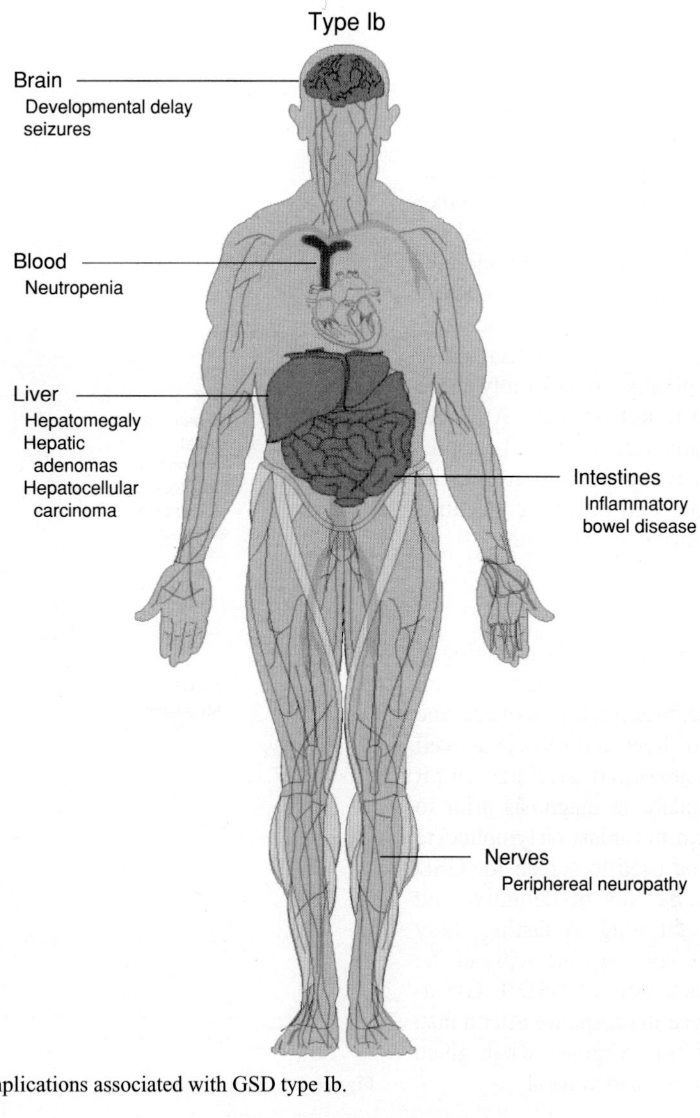

Figure 3 Complications associated with GSD type Ib.

It is particularly frequent in Jews of North African descent living in Israel with a carrier frequency of 1:35.[38] GSD III is inherited in an autosomal recessive manner with the gene for the debranching enzyme located on chromosome 1p21.[39] There are four distinct isoforms with differentially expressed clinical phenotypes associated with specific mutations.[40] Type IIIa affects both liver and muscle and accounts for 80 to 85% of patients with GSD III in the United States; type IIIb affects only the liver and accounts for approximately 15% of patients.[2]

Pathophysiology

Release of glucose from glycogen requires sequential action of both glycogen phosphorylase and glycogen debranching enzyme. After glycogen phosphorylase has acted on the outer branches of glycogen leaving four glucose residues, the debranching enzyme utilizes two distinct catalytic activities to remove them. The first is a transferase activity which transfers three of the four glucosyl residues distal to the glycogen branch point to the outer end of an adjacent chain. Secondly, the amylo-1,6-glucosidase activity of the same enzyme also hydrolyzes the branch point glucose residue. Without the function of the debranching enzyme, the breakdown of glycogen is interrupted with an abnormal form (limit dextrin) left to accumulate in affected tissues.[3]

Presentation

Type III GSD exhibits wide clinical and genetic variability. In infancy and early childhood, fasting hypoglycemia and hepatomegaly may be indistinguishable from GSD I; however, unlike GSD I, blood levels of lactate and uric acid are normal. Biochemical abnormalities include elevated aspartate transaminase (AST), alanine transaminase (ALT), creatine kinase concentrations, and hyperlipidemia.[41] Serum transaminase concentrations are typically considerably more elevated than in GSD I, and often the AST and ALT concentrations are over 1,000 U/L at presentation. Creatine kinase concentrations may be normal at presentation, and normal concentrations do not exclude muscle involvement.

Diagnosis

Mutation analysis from full gene sequencing is commercially available for the diagnosis of both type IIIa and IIIb GSD. Measurements of enzyme activity from biopsy of liver and muscle as well as demonstration of abnormal glycogen (limit dextrin) were the standard in diagnosis prior to mutation analysis. Skin fibroblast or lymphocyte enzyme activity can be used to screen for GSD III, but these studies may not be definitive and cannot be used for subtyping. A fasting study demonstrates ketotic hypoglycemia without the hyperlactatemia characteristic of GSD I. Glucagon fails to elicit a glycemia response after a fast, but does elicit a glycemic response when given 2 hours after a carbohydrate-rich meal.

Nutritional Management

In this type of GSD, gluconeogenesis can occur and protein can therefore be utilized as a substrate for endogenous glucose production. In infancy, hypoglycemia can be problematic, and patients are treated with a high-protein diet (3 g/kg) along with intermittent cornstarch therapy. Without cornstarch, hypoglycemia and ketosis invariably occur, but treatment with 1 to 1.75 g/kg at 6-hour intervals during both day and night maintains normoglycemia, increases growth velocity, and decreases serum transaminase concentrations.[42] As patients get older, hypoglycemia is less common, and the minimum amount of cornstarch is used to maintain normoglycemia. Continuous nocturnal feeding of a nutrient mixture consisting of glucose or glucose oligosaccharides, and protein or amino acids, combined with intermittent high-protein feedings during the day, may be especially beneficial for patients who have significant growth retardation and myopathy.[43] In GSD III, galactose and fructose can be converted into glucose, and restriction of these sugars is not necessary. Concentrated sweets, however, are avoided to prevent excessive glycogen storage.

Natural History and Prognosis

Patients with type III GSD typically do well throughout childhood and as young adults, but complications can occur as patients get older (Figure 4). Hepatic adenomas occur in approximately 25% of adults with GSD III and cases of hepatocellular carcinoma have been reported.[21] Hepatic fibrosis is common in children with both GSD IIIa and IIIb, but cirrhosis and portal hypertension rarely develop.

With GSD IIIa, complications related to the muscle disease become increasingly common with aging. In the third to fourth decades of life, myopathy becomes prominent with slowly progressive muscle weakness.[44] Exercise is restricted because it causes elevations in serum creatine kinase and aldolase concentrations. Cardiac complications may also develop in the muscle forms. Usually by the time a child has finished puberty, concentric left ventricular hypertrophy is detectable by echocardiography. Ventricular function is usually normal, but severe cardiac dysfunction and arrhythmias can occur.[45] Rare cases of severe cardiomyopathy in infants and children have been reported, so annual echocardiograms are recommended for all children with GSD IIIa.

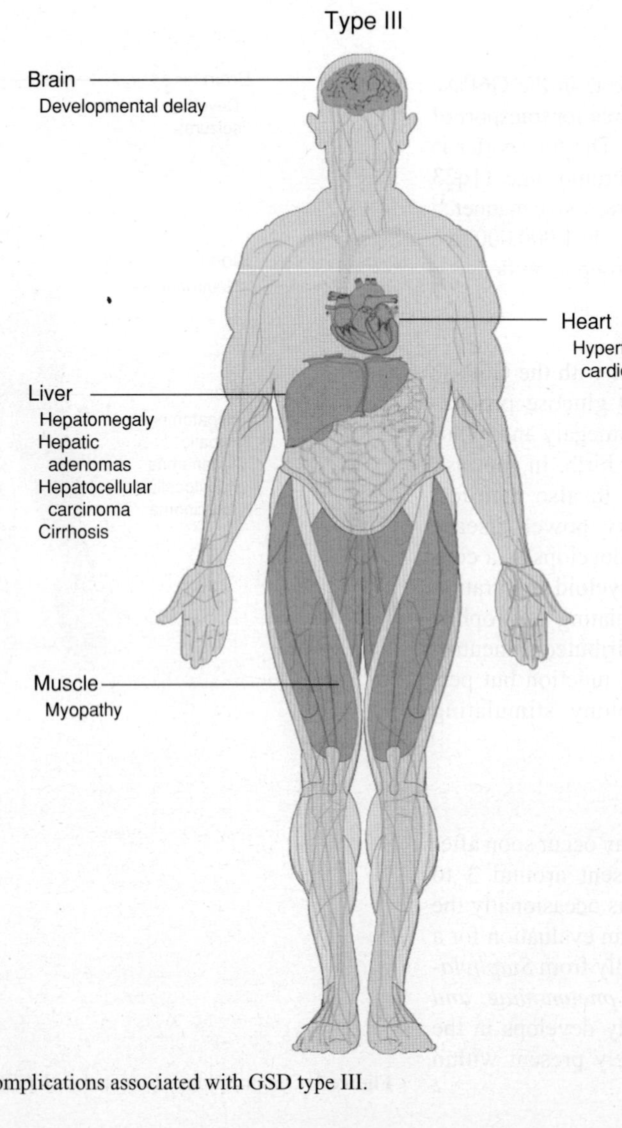

Figure 4 Complications associated with GSD type III.

The limited experience of transplantation in children with GSD III does not allow for adequate assessment of myopathy following liver transplantation. There is no evidence, however, that transplantation will decrease the morbidity associated with the muscle involvement. In fact, several of the immunomodulators, including cyclosporine, may exacerbate the myopathy leading to earlier clinical deterioration. Since liver pathology is not the major source of morbidity in GSD IIIa, liver transplantation should only be performed when there is high risk for hepatocellular carcinoma or evidence of substantial cirrhosis or liver dysfunction.

GLYCOGEN PHOSPHORYLASE DEFICIENCY (TYPE VI GSD; HERS DISEASE) AND GLYCOGEN PHOSPHORYLASE KINASE (PHK) DEFICIENCY (TYPE IX GSD)

Both types VI and IX GSD result from impaired glycogenolysis. Type VI GSD is due to hepatic phosphorylase deficiency while type IX GSD results from abnormal PHK activity, the enzyme that activates hepatic phosphorylase. Phenotypically, these diseases are the same, and they are therefore discussed as one entity in this section. Their estimated prevalence is approximately 1 in 100,000, but this is thought to be an underestimation. Together, they account for approximately 25 to 30% of all cases of GSD.[46] Type IX GSD is more common in people of Scandinavian heritage, and 1 in 1,000 people of Mennonite heritage have type VI GSD.[47]

The hepatic glycogen phosphorylase gene *(PYGL)* is located on chromosome 14q21-22 and is inherited in an autosomal recessive manner.[2] PHK present in liver and muscle is a complex enzyme consisting of four subunits: α, β, δ, and γ. The α-subunit is encoded by the PHKA2 gene located on Xp22.2-p22.1 and is inherited as an X-linked disease. The β-subunit is encoded by PHKB2 gene on chromosome 16q12-q13, and mutations are inherited as an autosomal recessive variant of GSD IX. The γ-subunit, encoded by the PHKG2 gene on chromosome 16p11-p12, contains the catalytic site of the PHK enzyme and is inherited autosomal recessively.[2]

Pathophysiology

Glycogen phosphorylase is the rate-limiting step in glycogenolysis stimulating the hydrolysis of the outer branches of glycogen. Glycogen PHK deficiency results in failure to activate glycogen phosphorylase. Fortunately, these disorders are typically mild and can be confused with "ketotic hypoglycemia." Mild hyperlipidemia and elevation in liver enzyme concentration are common in untreated children while lactic acid and uric acid concentrations are typically normal.

Presentation

Fasting ketotic hypoglycemia is the cardinal manifestation although typically milder than GSD I and III. Children are usually discovered when hepatomegaly is detected on a routine physical examination or when hypoglycemia occurs as a consequence of prolonged fasting during an intercurrent illness.[48]

Diagnosis

It is possible to diagnose glycogen PHK deficiency by assaying the activity of the enzyme in leukocytes and erythrocytes. The blood assay, however, lacks sensitivity as there are liver, muscle, heart, and brain isoforms of this enzyme. Mutation analysis is commercially available for the X-linked variant of GSD IX, but full gene sequencing is still not routinely performed. Definitive diagnosis requires demonstration of abnormal enzyme activity in biopsies of affected tissues, but this is not routinely performed due to the mild clinical phenotype. Mutation analysis likely will become the standard for diagnosis of GSD VI, but this is still only performed in research laboratories at present.

Nutritional Management

The goal of treatment is to prevent hypoglycemia, normalize plasma glucose concentrations, and minimize systemic acidosis. Frequent small meals are supplemented with UCS (1.5 to 2 g/kg given 1 to 2 times/d). Even when more prolonged fasting can be tolerated without development of hypoglycemia, most children and adults report improved energy and well-being with bedtime cornstarch administration because ketosis is prevented.[49] A high-protein, complex carbohydrate diet is recommended; no dietary restriction is necessary.

Natural History and Prognosis

The prognosis of patients with GSD VI and IX is excellent.Treatment, however, improves growth and stamina in patients with these milder forms of GSD. While most patients do very well, a more severe variant associated with significant hepatic transaminase elevation, hepatic fibrosis, and cirrhosis has been described in patients with mutations in the *PHKG2* gene.[50] Muscle symptoms occur occasionally, and these disorders are rarely associated with a proximal renal tubular acidosis and neurologic abnormalities.[51] A severe cardiac-specific PHK variant that can lead to cardiac failure has been reported.[52] Hyperlipidemia is common in untreated children and adults, and untreated adults may be at higher risk for cardiovascular disease.

REFERENCES

1. Wolfsdorf JI, Weinstein DA. Glycogen storage disease. Rev Endocr Metab Disord 2003;4:95–102.
2. Elpeleg ON. The molecular background of glycogen metabolism disorders. J Ped Endocr Metab 1999;12:363–79.
3. Roach PJ. Glycogen and its metabolism. Curr Mol Med 2002;2:101–20.
4. Orho M, Bosshard N, Buist NR, et al. Mutations in the liver glycogen synthase gene in children with hypoglycemia due to glycogen storage disease type 0. J Clin Invest 1998;102:507–15.
5. Weinstein DA, Correia CE, Saunders AC, et al. Hepatic glycogen synthase deficiency: An in frequently recognized cause of ketotic hypoglycemia. Mol Genet Metab 2005;87:284–8.
6. Aynsley-Green A, Williamson DH, Gitzelmann R. Hepatic glycogen synthetase deficiency. Definition of syndrome from metabolic and enzyme studies on a 9-year-old girl. Arch Dis Child 1977;52:573–9.
7. Hasselbalch SG, Knudsen GM, Jakobsen J, et al. Blood-brain barrier permeability of glucose and ketone bodies during short-term starvation in humans. Am J Physiol 1995;268:E1161–6.
8. Bachrach BE, Weinstein DA, Orho-Melander M, et al. Glycogen synthase deficiency (glycogen storage disease type 0) presenting with hyperglycemia and glucosuria: Report of three new mutations. J Pediatr 2002;140:781–3.
9. Dykes JR, Spencer-Peet J. Hepatic glycogen synthetase deficiency. Further studies on a family. Arch Dis Child 1972;47:558–63.
10. Nordlie RC, Foster JD, Lange AJ. Regulation of glucose production by the liver. Annu Rev Nutr 1999;19:379–406.
11. Burchell A. The molecular basis of the type 1 glycogen storage diseases. Bioessays 1992;14:395–400.
12. Lei KJ, Shelly LL, Pan CJ, et al. Mutations in the glucose-6-phosphatase gene that cause glycogen storage disease type 1a. Science 1993;262:580–3.
13. Ekstein J, Rubin BY, Anderson SL, et al. Mutation frequencies for glycogen storage disease Ia in the Ashkenazi Jewish population. Am J Med Genet A 2004;129:162–4.
14. Fernandes J, Berger R, Smit GP. Lactate as a cerebral metabolic fuel for glucose-6-phosphatase deficiency. Pediatr Res 1984;18:335–9.
15. Alaupovic P, Fernandes J. The serum apolipoprotein profile of patients with glucose-6-phosphatase deficiency. Pediatr Res 1985;19:380–4.
16. Rake JP, Berge AM, Visser G, et al. Glycogen storage disease type Ia: Recent experience with mutation analysis, a summary of mutations reported in the literature and a newly developed diagnostic flow chart. Eur J Pediatr 2000;159:322–30.
17. Wolfsdorf JI, Keller RJ, Landy H, Crigler JR. Glucose therapy for glycogenosis type 1 in infants: Comparison of intermittent uncooked cornstarch and continuous overnight glucose feedings. J Pediatr 1990;117:384–91.
18. Texas Children's Hospital. Pediatric Nutrition Reference Guide, 7th edition, Houston, TX, 2005.
19. Weinstein DA, Wolfsdorf JI. Effect of continuous glucose therapy with uncooked cornstarch on the long-term clinical course of type 1a glycogen storage disease. Eur J Pediatr 2002;161:S35–9.
20. Bianchi L. Glycogen storage disease I and hepatocellular tumours. Eur J Pediatr 1993;152:S63–70.
21. Labrune P, Trioche P, Duvaltier I, et al. Hepatocellular adenomas in glycogen storage disease type I and III: A series of 43 patients and review of the literature. J Pediatr Gastroenterol Nutr 1997;24:276–9.
22. Franco LM, Krishnamurthy V, Bali D, et al. Hepatocellular carcinoma in glycogen storage disease type Ia: A case series. J Inherit Metab Dis 2005;28:153–62.
23. Pauleit D, Textor J, Bachmann R, et al. Hepatocellular carcinoma: Detection with gadolinium and ferumoxides-enhanced MR imaging of the liver. Radiology 2002;222:73–80.
24. Restaino I, Kaplan BS, Stanley C, Baker L. Nephrolithiasis, hypocitraturia, and a distal renal tubular acidification defect in type 1 glycogen storage disease. J Pediatr 1993;122:392–6.
25. Weinstein DA, Somers MJ, Wolfdorf JI. Decreased urinary citrate excretion in type 1a glycogen storage disease. J Pediatr 2001;138:378–82.
26. Chen Y-T, Coleman RA, Scheinman JI, et al. Renal disease in type I glycogen storage disease. N Engl J Med 1988;318:7–11.
27. Wolfsdorf JI, Laffel LMB, Crigler JF. Metabolic control and renal dysfunction in type I glycogen storage disease. J Inher Metab Dis 1997;20:559–68.
28. Weinstein DA, Roy CN, Fleming MD, et al. Inappropriate expression of hepcidin is associated with iron refractory anemia: Implications for the anemia of chronic disease. Blood 2002;100:3776–81.
29. Lee PJ, Patel JS, Fewtrell M, et al. Bone mineralization in type I glycogen storage disease. Eur J Pediatr 1995;154:483–7.
30. Wolfsdorf JI. Bones benefit from better biochemical control in type I glycogen storage disease. J Pediatr 2002;141:308–10.
31. Lee PJ, Leonard JV. The hepatic glycogen storage diseases – problems beyond childhood. J Inher Metab Dis 1995;18:462–72.
32. Annabi B, Hiraiwa H, Mansfield BC, et al. The gene for glycogen-storage disease type 1b maps to chromosome 11q23. Am J Hum Genet 1998;62:400–5.
33. Visser G, Rake JP, Fernandes J, et al. Neutropenia, neutrophil dysfunction, and inflammatory bowel disease in glycogen storage disease type Ib: Results of the European Study on Glycogen Storage Disease Type I. J Pediatr 2000;137:187–91.

34. Visser G, Rake JP, Labrune P, et al. Granulocyte colony-stimulating factor in glycogen storage disease type Ib. Results of the European Study on Glycogen Storage Disease Type I. Eur J Pediatr 2002;161:S83–7.
35. Chen LY, Pan CJ, Shieh JJ, Chou JY. Structure-function analysis of the glucose-6-phosphate transporter deficient in glycogen storage disease type Ib. Hum Mol Genet 2002;11:3199–207.
36. Roe TF, Thomas DW, Gilsanz V, et al. Inflammatory bowel disease in glycogen storage disease type Ib. J Pediatr 1986;109:55–9.
37. Roe TF, Coates TD, Thomas DW, et al. Treatment of chronic inflammatory bowel disease in glycogen storage disease type Ib with colony-stimulating factors. N Engl J Med 1992;326:1666–9.
38. Parvari R, Moses S, Shen J, et al. A single-base deletion in the 3'-coding region of glycogen debranching enzyme is prevalent in glycogen storage disease type IIIA in a population of North African Jewish patients. Eur J Hum Genet 1997;5:266–70.
39. Bao Y, Dawson TL, Chen YT. Human glycogen debranching enzyme gene (AGL): Complete structural organization and characterization of the 5' flanking region. Genomics 1996;38:155–65.
40. Shen J, Bao Y, Liu HM, et al. Mutations in exon 3 of the glycogen debranching enzyme gene are associated with glycogen storage disease type III that is differentially expressed in liver and muscle. J Clin Invest 1996;98:352–7.
41. Coleman RA, Winter HS, Wolf B, Chen YT. Glycogen debranching enzyme deficiency: Long-term study of serum enzyme activities and clinical features. J Inherit Metab Dis 1992;15:869–81.
42. Borowitz SM, Greene HL. Cornstarch therapy in a patient with type III glycogen storage disease. J Ped Gastroeneterol Nutr 1987;6:631–4.
43. Slonim A, Weisberg C, Benke P, et al. Reversal of debrancher deficiency myopathy by the use of high-protein nutrition. Ann Neurol 1982;11:420–2.
44. Moses S, Gadoth N, Bashan N, et al. Neuromuscular involvement in glycogen storage disease type III. Acta Paediatr Scand 1986;75:289–96.
45. Lee PJ, Deanfield JE, Burch M, et al. Comparison of the functional significance of left ventricular hypertrophy in hypertrophic cardiomyopathy and glycogenosis type III. Am J Card 1997;79:834–8.
46. Kiliman MW. Glycogen storage disease due to phosphorylase kinase deficiency. In: Swallow DM, Edwards YH, editors. Protein Dysfunction in Human Genetic Disease. Oxford: BIOS Scientific; 1997. p. 57–75.
47. Chang S, Rosenberg MJ, Morton H, et al. Identification of a mutation in liver glycogen phosphorylase in glycogen storage disease type VI. Hum Mol Genet 1998;7:865–70.
48. Willems PJ, Gerver WJ, Berger R, Fernandes J. The natural history of liver glycogenosis due to phosphorylase kinase deficiency: A longitudinal study of 41 patients. Eur J Pediatr 1990;149:268–71.
49. Nakai A, Shigematsu Y, Takano T, et al. Uncooked cornstarch treatment for hepatic phosphorylase kinase deficiency. Eur J Pediatr 1994;153:581–3.
50. Burwinkel B, Rootwelt T, Kvittingen EA, et al. Severe phenotype of phosphorylase kinase-deficient liver glycogenosis with mutations in the PHKG2 gene. Pediatr Res 2003;54:834–9.
51. Nagai T, Matsua N, Tsuchiya Y, et al. Proximal renal tubular acidosis associated with glycogen storage disease, type 9. Acta Paediatr Scand 1988;77:460–3.
52. Servidei S, Metlay LA, Chodosh J, DiMauro S. Fatal infantile cardiopathy caused by phosphorylase b kinase deficiency. J Pediatr 1988;113:82–5.

46.2 Inborn Errors of Metabolism and the Liver

Charles P. Venditti, MD, PhD
Gerard T. Berry, MD

INTRODUCTION

The liver is a nutritional clearing house, metabolizing, partitioning, and distributing dietary nutrients and their metabolites both within the liver and among the different organs in the body. Inborn errors of metabolism involve small molecules, as well as large complex molecules and organelles.[1] It is not surprising that the liver with its varied array of anabolic and catabolic pathways features prominently in hereditary enzyme deficiencies, solute transport defects, and perturbations in organelle biogenesis.

Furthermore, the liver plays a central role in whole body metabolism. Hepatocytes, functionally heterogeneous in their spatial distribution along the tracts from the periportal to the centrilobular zones, are the prime movers in a complex process that involves (1) transport of water and solutes across membrane bilayers; (2) biosynthesis of small and complex molecules, the latter of which are largely destined for export; (3) interconversion of metabolites assimilated from ingested food such as amino acids; (4) catabolism of decaying macromolecules; (5) oxidation of fuels such as the free fatty acids, oleic, stearic, and palmitic acids, the most important energy source for hepatocytes; and (6) synthesis and export of glucose, as well as the hormonal regulation of its storage form, glycogen, the first line of defense in fasting adaptation.

The experiments of nature that result in the heritable defects in glycogenolysis, gluconeogenesis, mitochondrial fatty acid oxidation, carnitine metabolism, ketogenesis, and glucose transport underscore the essential role of the liver in fasting adaptation. The endocrine system and especially circulating insulin governs the interorgan flux of metabolites that are converted to glucose in the liver or to the ketone bodies, acetoacetate, and 3-hydroxybutyrate, that spare glucose. The liver is the site of ketogenesis but oxidation of ketone bodies only occurs in extrahepatic tissues as the hepatocytes are devoid of succinyl-CoA:3-oxyacid-CoA transferase activity (SCOT), the enzyme needed to utilize ketone bodies. Hepatic ketogenesis hinges on the carnitine-dependent translocation of long-chain fatty acids across the inner mitochondrial membrane. The temporal regulation of glycogen phosphorolysis, glucose-6-phosphate hydrolysis, gluconeogenic enzyme activities, carnitine palmitoyltransferase activity and, hence, fatty acid oxidation and ketogenesis depends on changing concentrations of hormones such as insulin and glucagon. Fasting produces a decrease in the ratio of insulin to glucagon, and the magnitude of this alteration depends on the duration of fasting. Inborn errors of hepatic glucose release and export, glycogenolysis, gluconeogenesis, and fatty acid oxidation/ketogenesis characteristically surface at different postprandial times following the last meal. Specifically, hypoglycemia may occur within just a few postprandial hours in a patient with glucose-6-phosphatase deficiency, whereas, of all the inborn errors, a defect in fatty acid oxidation requires the longest period of fasting to result in hypoglycemia.

INBORN ERRORS OF METABOLISM

Many inborn errors of metabolism affect the liver. In some of these biochemical genetic disorders, such as phenylketonuria (PKU), the enzyme function in the hepatocyte is defective, but the complications related to accumulation of phenylalanine metabolites are extrahepatic. Other disease types globally affect the hepatocyte or damage one or more organelles. In addition to hepatocytes, the liver contains other cell populations, such as the Kupffer cells, which can also be affected; this may lead to alterations in hepatic function or size. Mechanisms of hepatic injury, including discrete involvement of organelles (as evidenced by biochemical or pathologic findings) are discussed for selected disorders of amino acid, ammonia, organic acid, carbohydrate, glycogen, fatty acid, complex lipid, cholesterol, bile salt, glycosaminoglycan, glycoprotein, and metal metabolism.

TIMING OF THE PRESENTATION OF INBORN ERRORS OF METABOLISM

Inborn errors of metabolism, especially as envisioned by Garrod in 1908, are most commonly thought of as being the so-called small molecule diseases, in which the pathophysiology is usually a result of the excess of a potentially toxic intermediate. The absence of a necessary substrate more often concerns the symptoms in small molecular diseases. Nutritional treatment approaches typically focus on minimizing pathometabolite production, usually by dietary precursor restriction, while trying to balance demands for substrate utilization and interconversion with obligatory metabolism. Anaplerotic strategies, aimed at relieving product deficiency past the site of a block in a pathway, also have a place in the treatment of inborn errors of metabolism. Yet, the large molecule or complex macromolecule disorders, and, in particular, the storage diseases are now the subject of intense scrutiny as enzyme replacement therapy has transformed molecular history. This division is artificial in that all of the biochemical genetic diseases arise as a result of abnormalities in protein structure and function. In turn, these abnormalities are caused by alterations in nuclear or mitochondrial genes and their expression.

Most disorders of intermediary metabolism may not show signs in the fetus. The placenta and maternal circulation provide a constant supply of calories, which reduces the metabolic stress on the affected pathway of the fetus. Maternal hepatic function is also a means of elimination of many of the toxic metabolites that would otherwise cause symptoms. The free exchange of metabolites from the affected fetus to the maternal circulation has been demonstrated in a number of disorders. However, a metabolic toxicity syndrome featuring maternal liver disease can be seen when the fetus is affected with one of several disorders. The best-described syndrome is when the fetus is affected with long-chain hydroxylacyl-CoA dehydrogenase (LCHAD) deficiency.[2] Other inborn errors in which this can be seen include carnitine palmitoyl transferase type I (CPT I) deficiency[3] and short-chain acyl-CoA dehydrogenase (SCAD) deficiency.[4] A history of maternal illness during pregnancy should always be sought when evaluating patients for metabolic disease.

Prenatal effects can be seen in several different classes of inborn errors. Lesions of the electron transport chain can feature multiple antenatal effects such as intrauterine growth retardation.[5] Other disorders of energy metabolism such as deficiencies of pyruvate carboxylase, pyruvate dehydrogenase, and fumarase deficiency can feature central nervous system (CNS) dysgenesis.[6] Renal cystic changes are seen in multiple acyl-CoA dehydrogenase deficiency,[7] the neonatal variant of carnitine palmitoyl transferase II (CPT II) deficiency,[8] and in the congenital disorders of glycosylation (CDG).[9] Peroxisomal disorders may have a combination of dysmorphic features and hepatocellular involvement by birth.[10] A number of sterol synthetic defects—including Smith-Lemli-Opitz syndrome, lathosterolosis, desmosterolosis, and Conradi-Hunerman syndrome—can feature multiple malformations.[11] These patients can develop cholestatic liver disease and may secrete inadequate quantities of normal bile acids. More specifically, hepatobiliary malformations and developmental defects have been noted to also occur in the setting of hereditary metabolic disease such as ductal plate malformations, which is seen in phosphomannose isomerase deficiency,[12] a CDG; and biliary atresia, which has been documented in one set of siblings with Niemann-Pick type C disease[13] and one patient with deficiency of the mitochondrial trifunctional protein.[14]

A few storage disorders may appear with prenatal or peripartum pathology caused by the accumulation of normal cellular materials as the result of a block at one or more steps of their degradation. Examples in which the disease may be evident at birth include several lysosomal storage disorders, glycogen storage disease (GSD) type IV, CDG type Ik, and Niemann-Pick type C.[15] The recognition of accumulated material in the liver and in other tissues, or the secondary alteration of the somatic structure as a result of the perturbations in metabolism, may take months to occur. Early nutritional manipulations have not been studied in the settings described above.

Each inborn error of metabolism can arise as the result of more than one DNA mutation within the gene. Each mutation can have different effects on the phenotype because of varying levels of residual function of the affected protein. In the case of multimeric proteins, the net activity of the complex may be different based on the structure of the altered subunits. The residual activity, the net metabolic stress on the body (in the case of catabolic errors in intermediary metabolism), and the amount of substrate combine to determine the timing of the recognition of the altered phenotype. Epigenetic or nongenic factors also can influence the phenotype seen in recessive enzymopathies in a less predictable fashion, best evidenced in the intrafamilial variability seen in cystic fibrosis.

CATEGORIES OF INBORN ERRORS OF METABOLISM INVOLVING THE LIVER AND GASTROINTESTINAL TRACT

Table 1 outlines many of the disorders that have a known disturbance in the structure or function of the liver and GI tract as a result of inborn errors of metabolism in the pediatric population. Selected examples of these disorders are discussed briefly in the subsection on mechanisms of pathogenesis and comments on the nutritional approaches to management are highlighted in the text and listed in Table 1.

A few examples of metabolic diseases in which the liver serves the primary role in maintaining normal extrahepatic concentrations of metabolites and in which the signs are exclusively extrahepatic should be mentioned. A prime example of the importance of hepatic metabolism as it relates to CNS effects is PKU due to defects in phenylalanine hydroxylase. The enzymatic blockage prevents the conversion of phenylalanine to tyrosine. Consequences of the increased phenylalanine and lowered tyrosine concentrations include alterations in the transport of neutral aromatic amino acids into the brain and the production of neurotransmitters. As a result, mental retardation and seizures can occur. By lowering the blood phenylalanine concentration, many of the effects on cognition can be prevented or reversed. Hepatic size, synthetic functions, and laboratory tests are normal. A low phenylalanine diet provides the mainstay of therapy for these patients.

Nonketotic hyperglycinemia (NKH) is due to defects in the glycine cleavage system. Although the system is found in the brain and kidney, the vast majority of the activity is expressed in the liver. Except in the atypical form, the failure of the cleavage system results in the accumulation of glycine in all tissues; however, the pathophysiology is due to elevated glycine levels in the CNS. Unlike PKU, in which no symptoms are seen in the early neonatal period, infants with NKH may present with intractable seizures within hours of birth. Glycine levels are massively elevated in the cerebrospinal fluid in the neonatal period, implying that intrauterine elevations are a feature of this disorder. The liver in these patients is unremarkable.

Another example of an inborn error of metabolism where the liver is responsible for whole body metabolism is hyperoxalosis type I, a disorder of glyoxyalate metabolism. It is caused by a deficiency of alanine-glyoxylate aminotransferase, which is due to either a mutant protein or a mistargeting event whereby the enzyme localizes to the mitochondria in lieu of the peroxisomes, where it normally participates in glyoxyalate metabolism. Patients with this disorder progressively deposit calcium oxalate crystals throughout the body because of increased production of oxalate by the liver. The liver is spared, but many other organs—including the kidneys, heart, skin, retina, peripheral nerves, arteries, and skeleton—are not. Nephrocalcinosis eventually leads to end-stage renal failure and ultimately death. Liver or combined liver–kidney transplantation is needed to treat this disorder, depending on the duration and magnitude of the blood oxalate elevation. A liver is transplanted to stop the production of oxalate and provide a reserve for the defective enzyme, and in patients with coexisting renal failure, kidney transplantation is also required to provide essential functions and ensure adequate oxalate clearance.

The last group of metabolic disorders includes those in which the signs and symptoms can be hepatic and extrahepatic. Included are a large number of conditions, such as the urea cycle, fatty acid oxidation, and organic acid disorders, as well as others that affect storage and transport. Liver transplantation has been employed as a treatment modality in some of these diseases with variable success.[16]

Hepatic Injury

The metabolic processes within the hepatocyte, as in any cell, are closely regulated and interactive; they are responsive to external as well as internal stimuli. Central to the well-being of any cell are adequate stores of energy or the means to produce energy from readily available substrates as needed. With this energy, the cell maintains its homeostasis, grows, synthesizes material for export, exports, transports, and recycles unneeded or decaying materials. All of these processes are affected by one or more biochemical genetic disorders.

Compartmentalization of cellular functions is a necessary part of the synthetic and degradative pathways, as well as being essential for the production and maintenance of electrochemical gradients in energy production. Hepatic metabolism is quantitatively and even qualitatively different in the periportal inflow zone compared to the perivenous outflow area. Periportal cells are responsible for the majority of gluconeogenesis, glycogen synthesis by the indirect pathway, urea synthesis, and fatty acid oxidation. This regionalization may allow for discontinuous histopathologic findings during acute and less than massive metabolic insult. As the degree of hepatic injury becomes more severe, or as the duration of repeat injury increases and fibrosis occurs, the distinctions become less obvious.

Pathophysiology

For many of the biochemical genetic disorders, common histologic appearance and laboratory perturbations exist, precluding exact diagnosis without the use of extraordinary testing. The common pathways of hepatic pathophysiology include inflammation, necrosis, and cholestasis as the result of alterations in homeostasis; steatosis as the result of the accumulation of intermediates and the response to metabolic stress; and the accumulation of relatively nontoxic macromolecules, which usually alter cellular function on the basis of mass effects rather than chemical composition. It is also clear that the pathophysiology in some instances is different with many metabolic diseases if the patient is a newborn infant rather than a child or an adult. A factor that can confound diagnosis of a metabolic disorder is the nonspecific mal-handling of metabolites by a diseased liver, particularly methionine and tyrosine.

Cholestasis and Hepatobiliary Disease

Cholestasis can result from multiple groups of metabolic disorders. Defects in bile acid metabolism, absence of peroxisomes, and disorders of amino acid, lipid, carbohydrate, or complex molecule degradation, metal metabolism, and transport can lead to the recognition of cholestasis.

Table 1 Metabolic Disorders That Feature Liver Disease/Gastrointestinal Dysfunction

Class of Disorder	Enzyme Defect	Treatment and Comments
Carbohydrate metabolism		
Galactosemia	Galactose-1-phosphate uridyltransferase	Remove lactose and galactose from diet
Hereditary fructose intolerance	Fructose 1-phosphate aldolase	Remove sucrose, fructose and sorbitol from diet
Fructose 1,6-bisphosphatase deficiency	Fructose 1,6-bisphosphatase	Avoidance of fasting; remove sucrose, fructose and sorbitol from diet
Glycogen synthase defect	Glycogen synthase	Avoidance of fasting
Glycogen storage disease (GSD), type I	Glucose-6-phosphatase	Continuous calories, nocturnal cornstarch feedings Liver transplantation?
GSD, type III	Amylo-1,6-glucosidase (debrancher enzyme)	High carbohydrate diet, frequent feedings may be needed
GSD, type IV	Amylo 1,4 -> 1,6 transglucosidase (brancher enzyme)	Pts may need liver transplantation
GSD, type VI	Liver phosphorylase	Therapy depends on symptoms
Phosphorylase kinase deficiency	Phosphorylase kinase	Therapy depends on symptoms
Fanconi Bickel syndrome	GLUT2	Patients always have a renal Fanconi syndrome
Transaldolase deficiency	Transaldolase	One patient had cirrhosis and rock-hard hepatomegaly[35]
Amino and organic acid disorders		
Tyrosinemia, type I	Fumarylacetoacetate hydrolase	NTBC, dietary tyrosine restriction Eventual need for liver transplantation
Maple syrup urine disease	Branch chain oxoacid dehydrogenase	Leucine restriction; isoleucine and valine supplementation usually needed thiamine in responders Liver transplantation?
Propionic acidemia	Propionyl-coenzyme A carboxylase A	Branched chain amino acid restriction, carnitine supplementation Liver transplantation?
Methylmalonic acidemia	L-Methylmalonyl coenzyme A mutase (*mut* class) MMAA (*cblA* class) MMAB (*cblB* class)	Branched chain amino acid restriction, carnitine supplementation, hydroxylcobalamin IM (not all patients respond) Liver transplantation?
Urea cycle and related disorders		
Carbamyl phosphate synthase deficiency	Carbamyl phosphate synthetase	Stringent dietary protein restriction Sodium benzoate and/or Sodium phenylbutyrate L-Citrulline Liver transplantation?
Ornithine transcarbamylase (OTC) deficiency	Ornithine transcarbamylase	Stringent dietary protein restriction Sodium benzoate and/or sodium phenylbutyrate L-Citrulline Liver transplantation?
Citrullinemia	Argininosuccinate synthase	Stringent dietary protein restriction Sodium benzoate and/or Sodium phenylbutyrate L-Arginine Liver transplantation?
Argininosuccinic acidemia	Argininosuccinate lyase	Stringent dietary protein restriction Sodium benzoate and/or Sodium phenylbutyrate L-Arginine Liver transplantation?
N-Acetyl glutamate synthase deficiency	*N*-Acetyl glutamate synthetase	Stringent dietary protein restriction Sodium benzoate and/or Sodium phenylbutyrate L-Citrulline *N*-Carbamyl glutamate Liver transplantation?
Hyperornithinemia-hyperammonemia-homocitrullinuria (HHH) syndrome	ORNT1 mitochondrial ornithine transporter	Stringent dietary protein restriction Sodium benzoate and/or sodium phenylbutyrate L-Citrulline
Lysinuric protein intolerance	SLC7A7	Stringent dietary protein restriction L-Citrulline, HSM
Fatty acid oxidation defects		
Carnitine palmitoyltransferase-I (CPT-I) deficiency	Carnitine palmitoyltransferase-I	Avoidance of fasting Carnitine may be useful Can be associated with maternal HELLP syndrome
Carnitine palmitoyltransferase-II (CPT-II) deficiency	Carnitine palmitoyltransferase-II	Avoidance of fasting Carnitine may be useful Can be associated with dysplastic kidneys and brain malformations
Carnitine-acylcarnitine translocase deficiency	Carnitine-acylcarnitine translocase	Neonatal lethality in most cases
Very long chain acyl-CoA dehydrogenase (VLCAD) deficiency	Very long chain acyl-CoA dehydrogenase	Avoidance of fasting Carnitine may be useful

(Continued)

Table 1 Metabolic Disorders That Feature Liver Disease/Gastrointestinal Dysfunction *(Continued)*

Class of Disorder	Enzyme Defect	Treatment and Comments
Long-chain 3-hydroxyl acyl-CoA dehydrogenase (LCHAD) deficiency	Long-chain 3-hydroxy acyl-CoA dehydrogenase	Avoidance of fasting Carnitine therapy may promote dysrhythmias Can be associated with maternal HELLP syndrome
Medium-chain acyl-CoA dehydrogenase deficiency	Medium-chain acyl-CoA dehydrogenase	Avoidance of fasting Carnitine may be useful
Short-chain acyl-CoA (SCAD) dehydrogenase deficiency	Short-chain acyl-CoA dehydrogenase	Can be associated with maternal HELLP syndrome
HMG-CoA lyase deficiency	3-Hydroxy-3-methylglutaryl-CoA lyase	Avoidance of fasting
Multiple acyl-CoA dehydrogenase deficiency	ETFA, ETFB, ETFDH	Can be associated with congenital anomalies
Mitochondrial energy production/Primary lactic acidosis syndromes		
Electron transport chain (ETC) deficiencies	Complexes I, II, III, IV (Cytochrome c oxidase), V (ATPase) of the ETC	Clinically heterogeneous, Can have prenatal manifestations
GRACILE syndrome	BCS1L gene defect	Neonatal lethality
Pyruvate carboxylase deficiency	Pyruvate carboxylase	Features neurodegeneration
PEPCK deficiency	Phosphoenolpyruvate carboxykinase	Extremely rare, may be associated with cirrhosis
DNA depletion syndromes	Deoxyguanosine kinase (DGOUK)	Hepatic Failure
	Polymerase-gamma (POLG)	Hepatic Failure
	MPV 17	Hepatic Failure
	Succinyl-CoA synthase (SUCLG1)	Hepatomegaly, Leigh disease
	Thymidine phosphorylase (MNGIE)	Intestinal pseudo-obstruction
Storage disorders		
Gaucher, type II	β-Glucosidase	Can feature nonimmune hydrops fetalis
Niemann Pick, type A	Acid sphingomyelinase	
Niemann Pick, type C	NPC1, NPC2	Can feature nonimmune hydrops fetalis
Sialidosis, type II	Neuraminidase	Can feature nonimmune hydrops fetalis
Galactosialidosis	Protective protein deficiency	Can feature nonimmune hydrops fetalis
Sialic acid transport disorder (infantile free sialic acid storage disease)	SLC17A5	Can feature nonimmune hydrops fetalis
I-cell disease	*N*-Acetylglucosaminyl-1-phosphotransferase	Can feature nonimmune hydrops fetalis
GM1 gangliosidosis	Beta-galactosidase	Can feature nonimmune hydrops fetalis
Multiple sulfatase deficiency	SUMF1 (sulfatase-modifying factor-1 gene)	
Wolman disease	Acid lipase	Can feature nonimmune hydrops fetalis
Farber Disease type I	Ceramidase	Can feature nonimmune hydrops fetalis
Mucopolysaccharidosis, type VII	β-Glucuronidase	Can feature nonimmune hydrops fetalis
Congenital disorders of glycosylation	Multiple enzymopathies; phosphomannomutase (type I), *N*-acetylglucosaminyl-transferase II (type II), GDP-Man:GlcNAc2-PP-dolicholmannosyltransferase	Can feature hyperinsulinism, protein-losing enteropathy, nonimmune hydrops fetalis Oral mannose for phosphomannomutase deficiency
Sterol synthesis defects		
Smith-Lemli-Opitz syndrome	7-Dehydrocholesterol reductase	Malformation syndrome
Lathosterolosis	3B-Hydroxy steroid-Δ5 desaturase	Malformation syndrome
Desmosterolosis	24-Dehydrocholesterol reductase	Malformation syndrome
Conradi-Hunermann syndrome	3B-Hydroxysteroid-8,7-isomerase, others	Malformation syndrome
Mevalonic acidemia	Mevalonate kinase	Dysmorphic features, HSM
Peroxisomal biosynthesis and function		
Zellweger disease	Peroxisomal biogenesis defects	Dysmorphic features, malformations
Infantile Refsum disease	Peroxisomal biogenesis defects	Dysmorphic features
Bile salt metabolic defects	Δ(4)-3-Oxosteroid 5β reductase, 3β-Hydroxy-Δ5 steroid dehydrogenase-isomerase, Oxysterol 7α-hydroxylase	Cholestatic liver disease Treat first two with chenodeoxycholic acid +/− Cholic acid
Metal metabolism		
Neonatal iron storage disease/perinatal hemochromatosis	Defect(s) uncertain	Prenatal and neonatal lethality
Juvenile hemochromatosis	Hemojuvelin; hepcidin antimicrobial peptide	Liver transplantation?
Hemochromatosis, other	HFE 3 (transferrin receptor-2)	
	HFE4 (ferroportin)	Autosomal dominant inheritance
	Atransferrinemia	
	Aceruloplasminemia	Neurological syndrome
Wilson disease	ATP7B	Penicillamine
Indian childhood cirrhosis	Defect(s) uncertain	
Idiopathic copper toxicosis	Defect(s) uncertain	

Table 1 Metabolic Disorders That Feature Liver Disease/Gastrointestinal Dysfunction *(Continued)*

Class of Disorder	Enzyme Defect	Treatment and Comments
Other disorders		
Glycine-*N*-methyltransferase	Glycine-*N*-methyltransferase	A cause of hypermethionemia
Progressive Familial Intrahepatic Cholestasis Syndromes (PFIC1–4), including Byler disease (PFIC1)	ATP8B1, ABCB11, ABCB4; 3-β-Hydroxy-Δ5-C27-steroid oxidoreductase	PFIC1–3 may encode transporter proteins
Vitamin malabsorption disorders and chronic diarrhea		
Congenital folate malabsorption	Unknown etiology	IM folinic acid
Imerslund-Grasbeck disease	CUBN (cubilin)	IM OH cobalamin
Intestinal biotin transporter defect	Unknown etiology	One patient reported to date
Chronic diarrhea	Congenital chloride diarrhea	High chloride diet, electrolyte replacement
	Congenital secretory diarrhea due to defective sodium/hydrogen exchange	Electrolyte replacement, acid base balance
	Glucose–galactose malabsorption	Remove glucose and galactose from diet, provide fructose
	Lactase deficiency	Avoid lactose
	Sucrase–isomaltase deficiency	Avoid sucrose, symptomatic relief with oral yeast and yeast–enzyme extracts

Cystic fibrosis, an extremely common autosomal recessive disease, is due to defects in the cystic fibrosis transmembrane conductance regulator (CFTR), whose gene is located on chromosome 7q31.2. Although respiratory disease, pancreatic exocrine insufficiency, and failure to thrive are easily recognized as components of the clinical spectrum, hepatobiliary disease may be seen in very early infancy with impaired intrahepatic and extrahepatic biliary drainage. CFTR is localized to the intrahepatic biliary epithelium and is a regulator of cholangiocellular bile production. Cholestasis is felt to be secondary to defective chloride transport across this epithelium. Focal biliary cirrhosis can occur early with later evidence of steatosis and fibrosis. In a minority of patients, prolonged neonatal jaundice with cirrhotic change is seen. In rare instances, liver transplantation may be required (see Chapter 52, "Exocrine Pancreatic Disease including Cystic Fibrosis").

Other transport system defects can also cause a cholestatic change in the liver. A series of disorders—the progressive familial intrahepatic cholestasis syndromes—feature mutations in a variety of proteins likely involved in cannilicular transport. Four distinct genetic loci exist, and mutations have been demonstrated in patients from diverse backgrounds, including the Old Order Amish[17] and an Eskimo isolate from Greenland.[18] Three of the genes appear to encode transport-related proteins while the fourth encodes a steroid oxidoreductase.[19–21]

Bile acid synthetic defects can present with cholestatic liver disease and progress to cirrhosis.[23] A number of these rare enzymopathies are known to exist and it is likely that others remain to be discovered. Cheondeoxycholic acid and cholic acid can be used to treat patients with these disorders, in some instances, with great efficacy.

The genetic basis of other cholestatic syndromes, such as North American Indian childhood cirrhosis,[22] appears to involve novel proteins and illustrate that the current understanding of the mechanisms of cholestasis are far from complete[23] (see Chapter 53, "Acute and Chronic Liver Disease").

Hepatocellular Necrosis

Hepatocellular necrosis manifesting with jaundice, edema, ascites, hepatic synthetic failure, or hepatic encephalopathy is a major common pathology due to catabolic errors. The laboratory studies show variable degrees of elevation of serum transaminases, hypoglycemia, hyperammonemia, hypofibrinogenemia, and hypoprothrombinemia. The clinical picture is similar to that of sepsis, and the laboratory findings can be indistinguishable from those of a severe viral hepatitis (see Chapter 59, "The Critically Ill Child").

Galactosemia is a typical example of a disorder in this group. Classic galactosemia is due to a severe deficiency of hepatic galactose-1-phosphate uridyl transferase (GALT) activity. As a result of significant impairment of the function of the enzyme, a syndrome of neonatal-onset toxicity occurs when the at-risk infant is exposed to significant amounts of dietary lactose or galactose. The toxic metabolites are galactose-1-phosphate (a substrate of the enzyme) and galactitol (the result of aldose reductase activity on the sugar). Because there is trapping of cellular phosphate as galactose-1-phosphate, hepatic intracellular ATP/ADP ratios may be altered. Interference with other enzymatic systems has been postulated. Both mechanisms can lead to severe acute hepatocellular damage, which is reversible if treated immediately. The acute manifestations of the disease in the extended neonatal period often are noted within a few days of the onset of milk feedings. Vomiting and diarrhea are common. Most patients present with jaundice caused by an unconjugated hyperbilirubinemia. Severe hemolysis occurs in some patients so that the clinical presentation resembles erythroblastosis fetalis. Ascites has been a prominent early finding. With the progression of hepatic disease, bile stasis, pseudoacinar formation, and portal fibrosis are seen. An end-stage cirrhotic liver can result whose histology is indistinguishable from that of other metabolic etiologies. Laboratory findings include derangements of hepatic function, albuminuria, hyperaminoaciduria, hyperchloremic metabolic acidosis, hypergalactosuria, and elevated blood galactose concentrations. There is increased production and elimination of galactitol and the presence of increased concentrations of tissue galactose-1-phosphate. In the untreated state, alterations in carbohydrate composition of glycoproteins, such as transferrin, can be seen paralleling the CDG.

The other affected organ systems in the neonate include the lens of the eye, the CNS, the immune system, and the renal tubules. Increased synthesis of galactitol in the lens is associated with cataract formation. CNS findings in the infant include alterations in the level of consciousness and hypotonia. Cerebral edema and increased intracranial pressure can occur. A high frequency of *Escherichia coli* sepsis has been noted with fulminant courses. With prompt supportive therapy and the elimination of lactose and galactose from the diet, the acute toxicity syndrome resolves. Chronic, or long-term, effects of GALT deficiency occur in the CNS and ovary. Dietary therapy attempts to minimize offensive carbohydrates precursors from the diet but may never eliminate aberrant metabolites derived from endogenous production.

Hereditary fructose intolerance (HFI) usually presents with vomiting, diarrhea, and sometimes hypoglycemia. Symptoms are related to the ingestion of fructose or sucrose. The pathophysiology includes phosphate trapping, with resultant similar intrahepatic pathologic progression in the face of additional carbohydrate, and, as in galactosemia, there is renal tubular dysfunction. Beneficial effects from the withdrawal of the offending carbohydrates are seen in 2 to 3 days. Older patients characteristically avoid sucrose and have an unusual history of not having any dental caries. Two common mutations are known in the Caucasian population and molecular diagnosis is possible in some cases. Dietary therapy to eliminate fructose is completely effective at preventing the complications of this disorder.

Neonatal iron storage disease, or perinatal hemochromatosis, is a disorder resulting from severe prenatal hepatic disease. There is no single etiology for the disease; nor is there a clear genetic link to any single enzymatic defect, although a recessive pattern of inheritance seems likely. The liver shows diffuse fibrosis with hepatocellular nodular regeneration and ductal transformation. Siderosis in the apical cytoplasm of the tubular hepatocytes is typical. Some patients have had Down syndrome. A newer entity, GRACILE, reported in Finish infants, presents with growth retardation, lactic acidemia, anemia, and hemochromatosis.[24] The defect is in the BCS1L gene, involved in the assembly of complex III of the respiratory chain, and has been mapped to a locus on 2q33.37 and cloned. Other conditions may features neonatal hemochromatosis, such as the tricho-hepato-enteric syndrome.[25] The neonatal onset cases, regardless of distinct etiology, all seem to be severe entities with a difficult clinical course. Although liver transplantation can be curative, some patients may benefit from antioxidant treatment without surgical intervention.

Juvenile hemochromatosis, another form of primary hemochromatosis, can be caused by mutations in hemojuvelin[26] or the gene encoding hepcidin antimicrobial peptide.[27] This condition, like the more commonly seen adult variant caused by mutations in the HFE gene, can feature severe iron overload with hepatocytic iron deposition, liver fibrosis, hypogonadotrophic hypogonadism, and cardiac involvement. Two other genetic forms of primary hemochromatosis are also known. HFE3 is caused by mutations in the gene encoding transferrin receptor-2 and is intermediate in severity.[28] HFE4, the only documented autosomal dominant form of the disease, is caused by a mutant ferroportin gene.[29] Dietary restriction of iron is usually not effective in patients with hemochromatosis and many adults require prophylactic phlebotomy to reduce body iron stores.

Other inborn errors of metabolisms can feature hepatocytic iron deposition by unclear mechanisms. Atransferrinemia, caused by mutation in the structural gene for transferrin, produces a syndrome of microcytic anemia and iron overload and is treated by plasma infusions to provide functional transferrin. Aceruloplasminemia produces a syndrome of hepatic and CNS iron deposition. The basal ganglia seem to be most affected and the syndrome is dominated by a neurological signs. Ceruloplasmin is low, as is serum iron, but excessive iron deposition is seen in the liver, brain, and pancreas (see Chapter 9, "Iron").

Disorders of copper metabolism are another group of important metal metabolic diseases. The prototype is Wilson disease, an autosomal recessive disorder characterized by intracellular

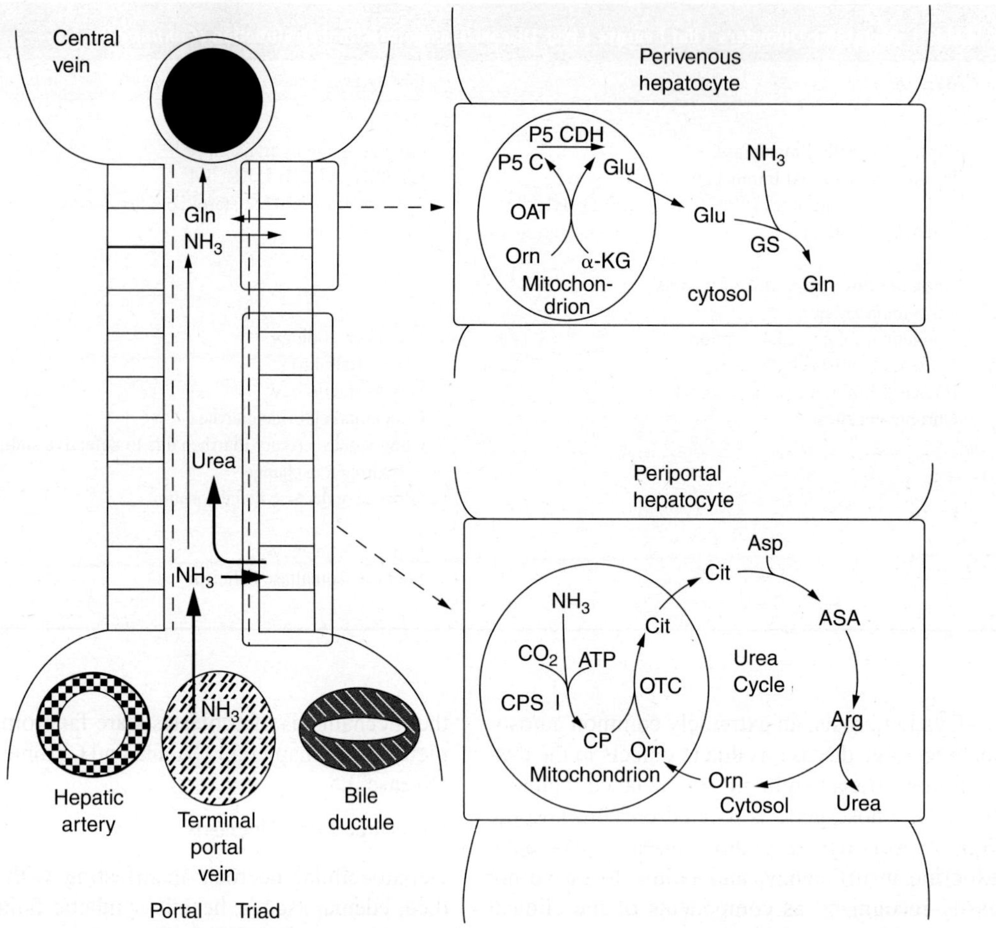

Figure 1 Nonhomogeneous distribution of enzymes in the hepatocytes of an acinar sinusoid as they are linearly distributed from the protal triad to the region of the central vein or terminal hepatic venule. The specific enzymatic reactions shown are for an individual periportal and perivenous hepatocyte. The glutamine synthetase (GS) and ornithine aminotransferase (OAT) enzyme activities are expressed exclusively in the first three cell layers that surround the central vein (i.e., the region of zone 3 of the liver lobule), whereas the urea cycle enzymes are concentrated within the periportal hepatocytes. However, the urea cycle enzyme activities are higher in zone 1 (immediately surrounding the portal triad) than in zone 2. Squares represent hepatocytes, circles represent hepatic mitochondria, and the interrupted line on either side of the linear array of hepatocytes represents the lining of the space of Disse. α-KG = α-ketoglutarate; Arg = arginine; ASA = argininosuccinate; Asp = aspartate; ATP = adenosine triphosphate; Cit = citrulline; CO_2 = carbon dioxide or bicarbonate; CP = carbamoyl phosphate; CPS I = carbamoyl phosphate synthetase I; Gln = glutamine; Glu = glutamate; NH_3 = ammonia; Orn = ornithine; P5C = delta[1] -pyrroline 5-carboxylate; P5CDH = 1-pyrroline-5-carboxylate dehydrogenase. (Adapted from reference 30.)

hepatic copper accumulation, cirrhosis, and, in a sizable number of patients, neurologic abnormalities. The primary defect resides in the ATP7B gene, which encodes a polypeptide that acts as a membrane copper-transport protein. The protein likely plays a role in intracellular copper delivery as well as release of copper into the bile. Like galactosemia and hereditary fructose intolerance, patients with Wilson disease can have a renal tubulopathy featuring aminaciduria and phosphaturia. Neurological and psychiatric presentations are well described. Chelation therapy can be used to enhance copper excretion. Some patients with hepatic failure will need liver transplantation. Another group of less well-characterized disorders of copper overload exist; these include Indian childhood cirrhosis and idiopathic copper toxicosis. The exact basis of these disorders is not known at present.

Urea cycle enzyme disorders may appear as early as 1 to 3 days of age. Figure 1 shows a functional overview of the urea cycle and highlights the compartmentalization of metabolism within the cellular zones of the liver.[30] Infants show combinations of vomiting, lethargy, increased respiratory drive, and CNS dysfunction that may progress to seizure activity. Their glucose concentrations are normal, with normal or slightly alkalotic blood pHs. Markedly elevated plasma ammonium concentrations are a common feature. Blood urea nitrogen concentrations may be low. The common pathogenesis is an inability to detoxify ammonia, which is produced as the result of the catabolism of amino acids. Thus, either protein ingestion or catabolic stress can trigger hyperammonemia. The presentation of the individual disorders is nonspecific, and specialized laboratory testing such as quantitative plasma amino acid analysis and measurement of urinary orotic acid concentration is used to separate the diseases. The enzymes of ureagenesis are present in intestinal, renal, and hepatic compartments, but only in the liver is the full complement of activities of the urea cycle present to enable the conversion of NH_3 to urea. In the liver, only the proximal enzymes *N*-acetyl glutamate synthase, carbamoylphosphate synthetase, and ornithine transcarbamylase are localized within the mitochondrial matrix. In biopsied material examined by electron microscopy, pleomorphic mitochondria with swollen cristae and electron-dense matrices are seen. Other hepatocellular changes include alterations in the appearance of the endoplasmic reticulum. Chronic injury, as the result of either prolonged hyperammonemia or repeated episodes of metabolic crisis, may cause portal fibrosis. Synthetic function of the liver is normal, although elevations in serum transaminases can occur. Such elevations may be present between episodes of hyperammonemia and despite the use of ammonia-trapping agents and enhancers of alternative nitrogen metabolic pathways. In the acute hyperammonemic crisis, detoxification by hemodialysis or hemofiltration may be essential.

In alpha1-antitrypsin deficiency due to the PI ZZ phenotype, the protein has a lysine residue instead of a glutamic acid at position 342. The altered protein is not secreted, because the reactive loop center of one molecule is inserted into the beta-pleated sheet structure of a second molecule. This protein is retained within the endoplasmic reticulum, as is reflected by the accumulation of periodic acid–Schiff (PAS)–positive diastase-resistant material. In some susceptible individuals, the accumulation of the abnormal protein damages the endoplasmic reticulum or Golgi membranes, leading to hepatocellular damage and cirrhosis. Liver transplantation is required in some instances.

Tyrosinemia type I can present in early infancy with varying degrees of hepatomegaly and a mild elevation of serum transaminases. The biochemical lesion is a defect in fumarylacetoacetate hydrolase. Common features also include abnormalities of coagulation, with clotting factors often markedly reduced. Vitamin K does not correct the disorder. Renal dysfunction is usually evident. A porphyuric presentation with neuropathy due to increased succinylacetone can be seen in the acute setting. Specialized testing (ie, quantitive analysis of plasma amino acids by anion exchange chromatography) usually reveals hypertyrosinemia, an increased urinary excretion of succinylacetone, and an elevated serum alpha-fetoprotein concentration. The hepatic disease is progressive and advances from microscopic cirrhosis, which can be seen in the first weeks of life, to macronodular cirrhosis with regenerating nodules. Hepatocellular carcinomas are frequent. In this disorder, biochemical abnormalities may be seen prenatally. The molecular mechanism of the hepatic and renal damage is not known, although the intracellular compartmentalization of toxic metabolites has been proposed to induce local damage. The inhibition of 4-hydroxyphenylpyruvate dioxygenase by fumarylacetoacetate is a major factor in the recognized biochemical abnormalities, and treatment with 2-(nitro-4-trifluoromethylbenzoyl)-1,3-cyclohexanedione

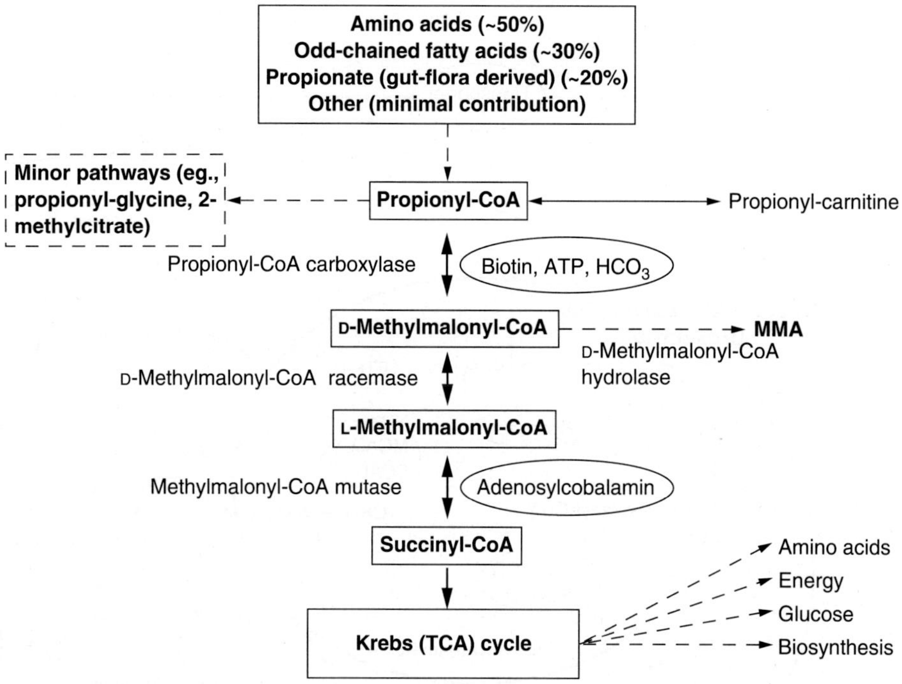

Figure 2 Major pathway of the conversion of propionyl-CoA, a major 3-carbon metabolite, into succinyl-CoA. The precursors are indicated with their approximated contribution to whole body propionate metabolism. The biotin-dependent enzyme, propionyl-CoA carboxylase converts propionyl-CoA into D-methylmalonyl-CoA that is then racemized into L-methylmalonyl-CoA and isomerized into succinyl-CoA, a Krebs cycle intermediate. The L-methylmalonyl-CoA mutase reaction requires adenosylcobalamin, an activated form of vitamin B_{12}. The formation of adenosylcobalamin requires intracellular metabolism of cobalamin. (Adapted from reference 31.)

(NTBC) corrects these but does not always prevent the progression to hepatocellular carcinoma. Dietary therapy consists of limiting tyrosine intake in conjunction with NTBC administration. Serum alpha-fetoprotein, a marker of hepatocellular carcinoma, and routine liver imaging studies are longitudinally followed to help decide which patients need to undergo liver transplantation.

Steatosis

Steatosis can be associated at some point in the natural history of a number of the organic acidopathies that result from enzymatic defects in the metabolism of branched-chain amino acids or odd-chain fatty acids. Propionic acidemia and methylmalonic acidemia, due to defects in either subunit of the heterodimeric propionyl coenzyme A carboxylase or the activity of the enzyme methylmalonyl-CoA mutase, are the prototypes for these disorders. Figure 2 displays the location of the blocks in the pathway of propionyl-CoA metabolism.[31] Affected infants present with severe metabolic acidosis, refusal to feed, vomiting, and alterations in CNS function. Hepatomegaly is found in a fraction of the patients. The livers at autopsy have shown fatty infiltration and necrosis, and the reticuloendothelial cells may have increased iron deposits. The exact mechanism of the fat deposition is unknown but may relate to an imbalance between the rate of fat synthesis and the rate of export of lipoproteins. Laboratory findings of a metabolic ketoacidosis with hyperammonemia and hyperglycinemia are characteristic during the initial presentation and subsequent metabolic crises.

Almost all the disorders of beta-oxidation of fatty acids from defects in carnitine palmitoyltransferase I, carnitine/acylcarnitine translocase, and carnitine palmitoyltransferase II through to the utilization of hydroxy-, medium-chain or short-chain fatty acids have been associated with some degree of hepatic dysfunction and fat accumulation. An overview of these disorders is depicted in Figure 3.[32] In the majority of cases when histology has been performed, the accumulation occurs as macrovesicular lipid storage. Hypothetical mechanisms of fat accumulation in these disorders include effects of a constant supply of fatty acids with a block in their utilization, increased availability of glycerol, and net intracellular accumulation. Dietary management of this group of disorders varies with the nature of the block but generally includes avoidance of fasting, restriction of dietary amino acid (for organic acidurias) and fat intake and careful monitoring for nutritional status. Anaplerotic therapy remains investigational.

Hepatic Pathology Resulting from Peroxisomal Disease

The absence of hepatocyte organelles and their functions can result in recognized hepatic disease in late fetal or early infant life. The best characterized group of these disorders includes those due to the peroxisomal diseases, which comprise a group of disorders with effects on multiple viscera, skeletal development, and the CNS. Zellweger disease, the paradigm for peroxisomal disorders, is caused by biosynthetic defects in the formation of the peroxisome. As a

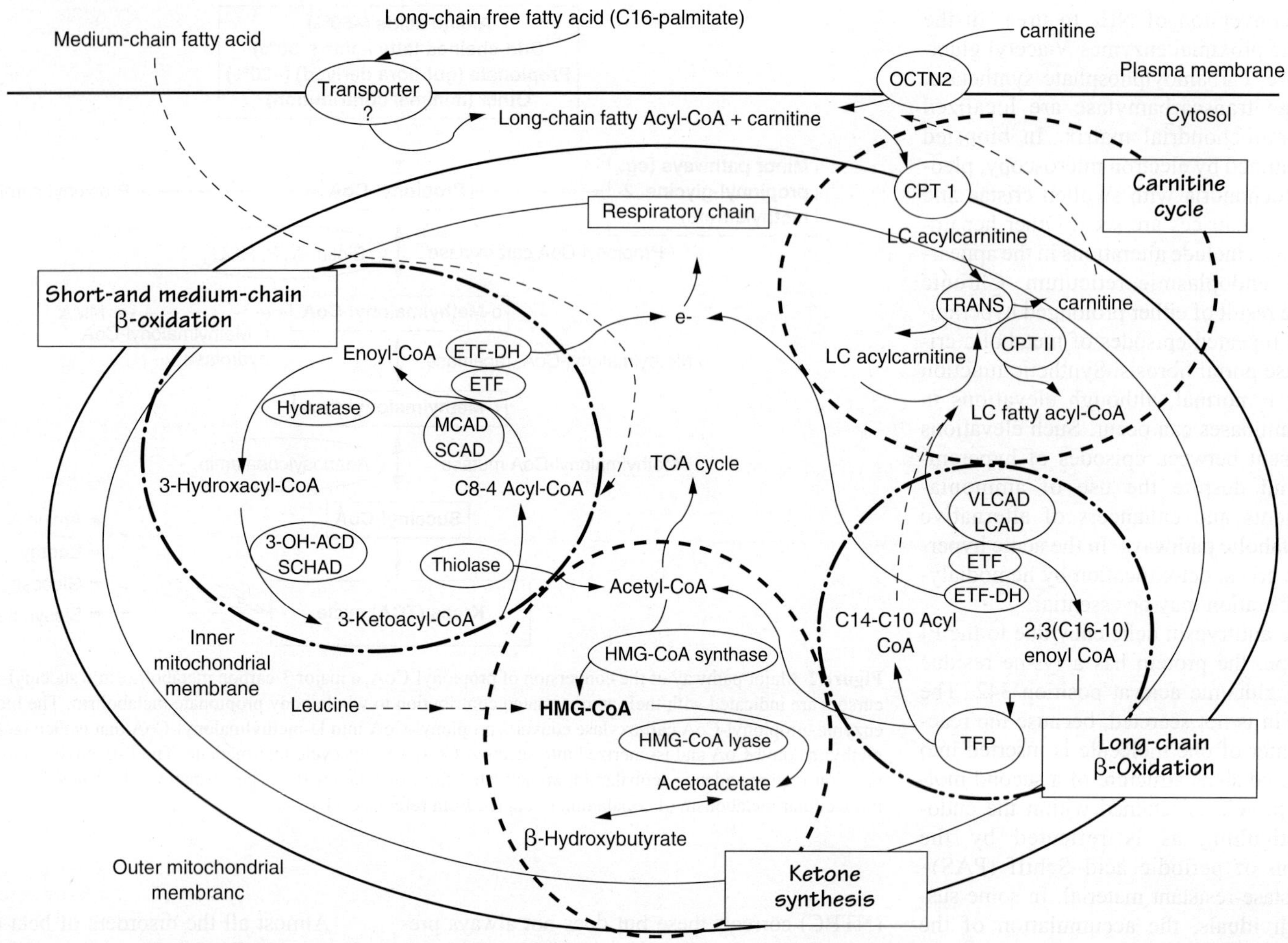

Figure 3 An overview of Mitochondrial fatty acid oxidation. Carnitine enters the cell through the action of the organic cation/carnitine transporter (OCTN2). Palmitate, a typical 16-carbon long-chain fatty acid, is transported across the plasma membrane and can be activated to form a long-chain (LC) fatty acyl-CoA. It then enters into the carnitine cycle, where it is transesterified by carnitine palmitoyltransferase-I (CPT-I), translocated across the inner mitochondrial membrane by carnitine/acylcarnitine translocase (TRANS), and then reconverted into a long-chain fatty acyl CoA by carnitine palmitoyltransferase-II (CPT-II) to undergo β-oxidation. Very long chain acyl-CoA dehydrogenase (VLCAD/LCAD) leads to the production of (C16-10) 2,3 enoyl-CoA. Trifunctional protein (TFP) contains the activities of enoyl-CoA hydratase (hydratase), 3-OH-hydroxyacyl CoA dehydrogenase (3-OH-ACD), and β-ketothiolase (thiolase). Acetyl CoA, FADH, and NADH are produced. Medium- and short-chain fatty acids (C8-4) can enter the mitochondrial matrix independent of the carnitine cycle. Medium-chain acyl-CoA dehydrogenase (MCAD), short-chain acyl-CoA dehydrogenase (SCAD), and short-chain hydroxy acyl-CoA dehydrogenase (SCHAD) are required. Acetyl-CoA can then enter the Krebs (TCA) cycle. Electrons are transported from FADH to the respiratory chain via the electron-transfer flavoprotein (ETF) and the electron-transfer flavoprotein dehydrogenase (ETF-DH). NADH enters the electron transport chain through complex I. Acetyl-CoA can be converted into hydroxymethylglutaryl-CoA (HMG-CoA) by β-hydroxy-β-methylglutaryl-CoA synthase (HMG-CoA synthase) and then the ketone body acetoacetate by the action of β-hydroxy-β-methylglutaryl-CoA lyase (HMG-CoA lyase). (Adapted from reference 32.)

result, more than 50 enzymes involved in multiple pathways can be perturbed. The peroxisomes are responsible for the oxidation of amino acids, alcohols, dicarboxylic acids, pipecolic acid, and phytanic acid, as well as very long chain fatty acids. They are also essential for the synthesis of bile acids, ether phospholipids such as the plasmalogens, and cholesterol, and they are a major reservoir of the hydrogen peroxide–degrading enzyme, catalase. Zellweger disease was also called cerebrohepatorenal disease because of the organ systems involved in the neonate. The infants have distinct dysmorphic features, an enlarged fontanelle, profound hypotonia, hepatomegaly, and neurodegeneration. Neuronal migratory defects are often seen. The liver has micronodular cirrhosis and fibrosis on examination. The laboratory abnormalities are explained by the missing multiple enzyme functions. Diagnosis can be strongly suspected by the constellation of physical findings and is confirmed by the abnormalities in very long chain fatty acid metabolism. The dysmorphia varies with the severity of the defect. For example, infantile Refsum disease, considered to be a milder phenotype of the peroxisomal biogenesis disorders, generally presents with failure to thrive and milder degrees of hepatocellular dysfunction in older infants or toddlers with dysmorphic facial features.

Hepatic Disease Due to Glycosylation Defect

Disorders of glycosylation result from various defects in the formation or processing of the carbohydrate residues attached by N- or O-linkages of peptides. These disorders can be considered "prelysosomal" storage disorders, as improperly glycosylated proteins initially accumulate in the endoplasmic reticulum. This may, in turn, lead to cellular dysfunction via the unfolded peptide response. The most common hepatic pathology is steatosis, but hydrops and severe hepatocellular dysfunction have been reported. Common clinical manifestations include failure to thrive, GI dysfunction or dysmotility, hypotonia, cognitive delays, and alterations in fat distribution. Mannose supplementation has been used as a treatment for mannose phosphate isomerase deficiency (CDG 1b).

Hepatic Disease Due to Mitochondrial Dysfunction

Multiple reports have described infants with severe or fatal hepatic disease of early onset due to a mitochondrial depletion syndrome. In some cases, increased fat has been seen histologically; however, ultrastructural examination of other patients' tissues has shown increased numbers of mitochondria with morphologic abnormalities, and even glycogen storage within the mitochondria. Focal biliary necrosis has been reported, but fibrosis is a later finding. Lactic acidosis, hypoglycemia, and synthetic defects have also been reported. In all cases, activities of the electron transport chain complexes with subunits encoded by mitochondrial DNA have been reduced. The amount of mitochondrial DNA has been reduced to less than 10% of normal. Mutations in the nuclear genes encoding deoxyguanosine kinase (DGOUK), thymidine phosphorylase (MNGIE), MPV17 (causing Navajo hepatoencephalopathy), polymerase-gamma (POLG), and succinyl-CoA synthase (SUCLG1) genes have been identified in some patients. The gastrointestinal phenotypes are variable and can feature hepatic failure, seen in patients with mutations in DGUOK, POLG, and MP17[33]; hepatomegaly with encephalopathy, seen in the one patient with succinyl-CoA synthase deficiency and intestinal pseudo-obstruction, a prominent feature of thymidine phosphorylase (MNGIE) deficiency.[34]

Hepatic Disease Due to Storage Disorders

Material either synthesized within the cell or accumulated through endocytic processes as part of the body's recycling of macromolecules is the sine qua non of the heterogeneous storage disorders. In the GSDs type I, III, or IV presenting in early infancy, there is accumulation of glycogen as well as fat. GSD type I should also be thought of as a steatosis disorder. In Niemann-Pick type A, sphingomyelin accumulates in hepatocytes, as well as in the reticuloendothelial elements, but in Niemann-Pick type C, the accumulated material includes both sphingomyelin and cholesterol. In the latter disorder, hepatocellular necrosis and a progression to fibrosis can also occur, blurring the distinctions made here about disorders primarily associated with hepatocytic dysfunction or storage with minimally altered hepatocytes. The accumulation and storage of glucocerebroside in Kupffer cells in Gaucher disease and of glycolipids and complex lipids in other disorders leads to liver enlargement but relatively little hepatocellular functional abnormality. In many cases, the histopathology and histochemical staining patterns can identify the disorder.

Hepatic Disease Due to Porphyrias

The heme biosynthetic pathway begins in the mitochondria with a condensation reaction of glycine and succinyl-CoA and ends with the production of heme, which is then used for hemoglobin formation in the bone marrow and, of equal importance, for cytochrome formation. Defects in any of the steps in this pathway represent a group of eight disorders that can feature cutaneous, psychiatric, neurologic, and hepatic symptoms. One disorder of this group, protoporphyria, can be associated with severe liver disease that can require liver transplantation.

Other Disorders with Primary Gastrointestinal Disturbances

Chronic diarrhea can be a manifestation of a number of inborn errors of metabolism, including lactase and sucrase–isomaltase deficiencies, glucose–galactose malabsorption, congenital chloride diarrhea, and congenital secretory diarrhea due to defective sodium/hydrogen exchange. Diarrhea, malabsorption, and protein-losing enteropathy can also be features of other disorders discussed in this chapter, such as cystic fibrosis, lysinergic protein intolerance, and phosphomannose isomerase deficiency. Selective vitamin malabsorption disorders, such as congenital folate malabsorption, the intestinal biotin transporter defect,[36] and Imerslund-Grasbeck disease[37] might also be included as metabolic disorders where the primary defect lies in the GI tract.

CONCLUSION

A wide variety of catabolic, anabolic, and transport defects affecting the GI tract can be recognized. The age of presentation ranges from mid-gestation to adulthood and encompasses a wide range of symptoms and signs, some of which are nonspecific. For some disorders, the pathophysiology has been delineated and molecular determinants characterized, but in the majority only the broader features are currently comprehended. The vast array of biochemical genetic diseases, these unfortunate experiments of nature, continue to provide great insight into the secrets of normal hepatic metabolism in man.

REFERENCES

1. Scriver CR, Beaudet AL, Sly WS, et al, editors. The Metabolic and Molecular Bases of Inherited Disease. McGraw-Hill, 2001. p. 2165–2192.
2. Ibdah JA, Bennett MJ, Rinaldo P, et al. A fetal fatty-acid oxidation disorder as a cause of liver disease in pregnant women. N Engl J Med 1999;340:1723–31.
3. Innes AM, Seargeant LE, Balachandra K, et al. Hepatic carnitine palmitoyltransferase I deficiency presenting as maternal illness in pregnancy. Pediatr Res 2000;47:43–5.
4. Matern D, Hart P, Murtha AP, et al. Acute fatty liver of pregnancy associated with short-chain acyl-coenzyme A dehydrogenase deficiency. J Pediatr 2001;138:585–8
5. von Kleist-Retzow JC, Cormier-Daire V, Viot G, et al. Antenatal manifestations of mitochondrial respiratory chain deficiency. J Pediatr 2003;143:208–12.
6. Kerrigan JF, Aleck KA, Tarby TJ, et al. Fumaric aciduria: Clinical and imaging features. Ann Neurol 2000;47:583–8.
7. Chisholm CA, Vavelidis F, Lovell MA, et al. Prenatal diagnosis of multiple acyl-CoA dehydrogenase deficiency: Association with elevated alpha-fetoprotein and cystic renal changes. Prenat Diagn 2001;21:856–9.
8. Strom EH, Stromme P, Westvik J, et al. Renal cysts in the carbohydrate-deficient glycoprotein syndrome. Pediatr Nephrol 1993;7:253–5.
9. Wanders RJ. Metabolic and molecular basis of peroxisomal disorders: A review. Am J Med Genet A 2004;126:355–75.
10. Elpeleg ON, Hammerman C, Saada A, et al. Antenatal presentation of carnitine palmitoyltransferase II deficiency. Am J Med Genet 2001;102:183–7.
11. Kelley RI, Herman GE. Inborn errors of sterol biosynthesis. Annu Rev Genomics Hum Genet 2001;2:299–341.
12. de Koning TJ, Nikkels PG, Dorland L, et al. Congenital hepatic fibrosis in 3 siblings with phosphomannose isomerase deficiency. Virchows Arch 2000;437:101–5.
13. Adam G, Brereton RJ, Agrawal M, et al. Biliary atresia and meconium ileus associated with Niemann-Pick disease. J Pediatr Gastroenterol Nutr 1988;7:128–31.
14. Matthews RP, Russo P, Berry GT, et al. Biliary atresia associated with a fatty acid oxidation defect. J Pediatr Gastroenterol Nutr 2002;35:624–8.
15. Stone DL, Sidransky E. Hydrops fetalis: Lysosomal storage disorders in extremis. Adv Pediatr 1999;46:409–40.
16. Leonard JV, Walter JH, McKiernan PJ. The management of organic acidaemias: The role of transplantation. J Inherit Metab Dis 2001;24:309–11.
17. Bull LN, van Eijk MJ, Pawlikowska L, et al. A gene encoding a P-type ATPase mutated in two forms of hereditary cholestasis. Nature Genet 1998;18:219–24.
18. Klomp LW, Bull LN, Knisely AS, et al. A missense mutation in FIC1 is associated with Greenland familial cholestasis. Hepatology 2000;32:1337–41.
19. Schwarz M, Wright AC, Davis DL, et al. The bile acid synthetic gene 3-beta-hydroxy-delta-5-C27-steroid oxidoreductase is mutated in progressive intrahepatic cholestasis. J. Clin. Invest 2000;106:1175–84.
20. Strautnieks SS, Bull LN, Knisely AS, et al. A gene encoding a liver-specific ABC transporter is mutated in progressive familial intrahepatic cholestasis. Nat Genet 1998; 20:233–8.
21. de Vree JM, Jacquemin E, Sturm E, et al. Mutations in the MDR3 gene cause progressive familial intrahepatic cholestasis. Proc Natl Acad Sci U S A 1998;95:282–7.
22. Chagnon P, Michaud J, Mitchell G, et al. A missense mutation (R565W) in cirhin (FLJ14728) in North American Indian childhood cirrhosis. Am J Hum Genet 2002;71:1443–9.
23. Bove KE, Heubi JE, Balistreri WF, et al. Bile acid synthetic defects and liver disease: A comprehensive review. Pediatr Dev Pathol 2004;7:315–34.
24. Visapaa I, Fellman V, Vesa J, et al. GRACILE syndrome, a lethal metabolic disorder with iron overload, is caused by a point mutation in BCS1L. Am J Hum Genet 2002;71: 863–76.
25. Verloes A, Lombet J, Lambert Y, et al. Tricho-hepato-enteric syndrome: Further delineation of a distinct syndrome with neonatal hemochromatosis phenotype, intractable diarrhea, and hair anomalies. Am J Med Genet 1997;68:391–5.
26. Papanikolaou G, Samuels ME, Ludwig EH, et al. Mutations in HFE2 cause iron overload in chromosome 1q-linked juvenile hemochromatosis. Nat Genet 2004;36:77–82.
27. Roetto A, Papanikolaou G, Politou M, et al. Mutant antimicrobial peptide hepcidin is associated with severe juvenile hemochromatosis. Nat Genet 2003;33:21–2.
28. Camaschella C, Roetto A, Cali A, et al. The gene TFR2 is mutated in a new type of haemochromatosis mapping to 7q22. Nature Genet 2000;25:14–5.
29. Njajou OT, Vaessen N, Joosse M, et al. A mutation in SLC11A3 is associated with autosomal dominant hemochromatosis. Nat Genet 2001;28:213–4.
30. Tuchman M, Lichenstein GR, Rajagopal BS, et al. Hepatic glutamine synthetase deficiency in fatal hyperammonemia after lung transplantation. Ann Intern Med 1997;127:447.
31. Chandler RJ, Venditti CP. Genetic and Genomic Systems to Study Methylmalonic Acidemia. Mol Genet Metab 2005;86:34–43.
32. Venditti CP, Stanley CA. Disorders of Mitochondrial Fatty Acid Oxidation. In Behrman RE, Kliegman RM, Jenson HB, editors. Nelson Textbook of Pediatrics, 17th edition. Philadelphia, PA: WB Saunders; 2003.
33. Alberio S, Mineri R, Tiranti V, et al. Depletion of mtDNA: Syndromes and genes. Mitochondrion 2007;7:6–12.
34. Nishino I, Spinazzola A, Hirano M. Thymidine phosphorylase gene mutations in MNGIE, a human mitochondrial disorder. Science 1999;283:689–92.
35. Verhoeven NM, Huck JH, Roos B, et al. Transaldolase deficiency: Liver cirrhosis associated with a new inborn error in the pentose phosphate pathway. Am J Hum Genet 2001;68:1086–92.
36. Mardach R, Zempleni J, Wolf B, et al. Biotin dependency due to a defect in biotin transport. J Clin Invest 2002;109:1617–23.
37. Aminoff M, Carter JE, Chadwick RB, et al. Mutations in CUBN, encoding the intrinsic factor-vitamin B_{12} receptor, cubilin, cause hereditary megaloblastic anaemia 1. Nat Genet 1999;21:309–13.

47

Persistent Renal Disease

Nancy M. Rodig, MD
Nancy Spinozzi, RD, LDN
William Harmon, MD

This chapter will outline principles for the nutritional management of children with both acute and chronic disturbances of renal function. A decline in glomerular filtration rate (GFR) is common to both disorders, which results in altered renal physiologic functions. The impairment of nitrogenous waste-product excretion and altered regulation of water, electrolyte, and acid-base homeostasis may challenge the provision of optimal nutrition. The discussion will begin with the nutritional management of acute renal failure (ARF), which is defined by a rapid decline in GFR. Given the extreme physiologic abnormalities that may accompany severe ARF, the nutritional care of the critically ill child will be emphasized. The discussion will then focus on the care of children with chronic kidney disease (CKD), who are at increased risk for malnutrition and growth impairment. Noting the shared issues faced by children with chronic renal insufficiency (CRI) and those on maintenance dialysis, the nutritional management of these children will be discussed together. The nutritional care of children who have received renal transplantations will then be reviewed. As the range of clinical manifestations of both acute and chronic renal failure is broad, the need for individualized nutritional management is emphasized throughout.

ESTIMATION OF GFR

GFR is equal to the sum of the filtration rates of all functioning nephrons and reflects functioning renal mass. Estimation of GFR allows clinicians to determine the severity and course of both acute and chronic disturbances of renal function and permits anticipation of necessary changes in therapy, including adjustments of nutritional support. The "gold standard" for measurement of GFR is an inulin clearance. Despite being accurate, performance of an inulin clearance is cumbersome and rarely employed in routine clinical practice. Alternatively, creatinine clearance based on a timed urine collection is readily available. However, the collection itself is inconvenient, prone to error, and impractical in children who are not toilet trained.

Estimation of GFR based on serum creatinine is both convenient and easy to perform. The accuracy of this estimation in pediatric patients can be improved by using predictive equations that take into account the patient's height, age, and gender. Recent guidelines provided by the National Kidney Foundation (NKF) recommend estimation of GFR from predictive equations,[1] and the Schwartz formula has gained widespread clinical use in North America (Table 1).[2,3,4] Given the tubular secretion of creatinine, the Schwartz formula tends to overestimate GFR, and this overestimation increases with decreasing GFR.[5,6] If an exact measurement of GFR is necessary, this can be determined by an inulin clearance or the clearance of other filtration markers such as radioactive and nonradioactive iothalamate, iohexol, ^{51}Cr-ethylenediaminetetra-acetic acid (EDTA), and Tc 99m-diethylenetriaminepentaacetic acid (DTPA). However, using predictive formulas such as the Schwartz calculation is usually sufficient in general practice.

Table 1 Estimation of GFR by the Schwartz Formula

$$C_{cr} = k \times L/S_{cr}$$

C_{cr} = creatinine clearance in mL/min/1.73 m^2
K = proportionality constant
L = length (cm)
S_{cr} = serum creatinine (mg/dL)
k values:
– Full-term babies during first year of life = 0.45
– Children greater than 1 yr and adolescent girls = 0.55
– Adolescent boys = 0.7

Adapted from references 2–4.

ACUTE RENAL FAILURE

ARF is defined by a rapid deterioration in GFR resulting in impairment of nitrogenous waste-product excretion. Depending on the severity of the insult, disturbances in waste excretion may be accompanied by impairment of acid–base homeostasis and loss of water and electrolyte regulation. In mild cases, nonoliguric ARF may be asymptomatic and only be detected when serum laboratory studies are performed. When severe, oliguric ARF may result in significant derangements of electrolyte and volume balance and necessitate the initiation of renal replacement therapy.

The etiology of ARF appears to be changing with advancement of medical and surgical practice, and this trend is most apparent in tertiary care centers. In referral centers, ARF due to primary renal disease is now less frequent than failure secondary to ischemia, drug toxicity, or sepsis in children. This was illustrated in a retrospective study from a large pediatric tertiary center, which reviewed the course of 254 episodes of ARF in 248 children during the period of January 1998 and June 2001.[7] Approximately two-thirds of these children had underlying comorbid conditions. Only 7% of cases of ARF were due to primary renal disease, and the most common causes of ARF were renal ischemia (21%), nephrotoxic agents (16%), and sepsis (11%). As in adults, the reported mortality for children with ARF is high, reaching 30 to 40% and is greatest for those who require dialysis.[8–11] Preexisting or hospital-acquired malnutrition has been identified as a contributing factor to the poor outcome of severe ARF,[12] and therefore providing adequate nutrition should be viewed as a crucial element in the therapeutic effort.

To provide nutritional support necessitates the provision of volume, either in the form of enteral feeds, intravenous nutrition, or a combination of both. If ARF is accompanied by anuria or oligoanuria (urine flow $<$0.5 to 1 mL/kg/h), nutrition will be limited or volume status will be aggravated unless renal replacement therapy is initiated. The modality of renal replacement therapy is chosen based on the clinical status of the patient and the expertise of the center. Options for renal replacement therapy include peritoneal dialysis (PD) and hemodialysis, and hemodialysis may be performed on an intermittent or continuous basis. For hemodynamically stable patients with ARF, intermittent hemodialysis is typically performed daily for 2 to 4 hours, depending on the size of the patient. During the several-hour treatment, ultrafiltration of the daily fluid requirement in addition to any other desired fluid removal is attempted as hemodynamically tolerated. If the patient is hemodynamically unstable, continuous renal replacement therapy (CRRT) allows for gradual ultrafiltration of fluid and is the modality of choice in such patients. Two commonly used modalities of CRRT are continuous venovenous hemodiafiltration (CVVHD) and continuous venovenous hemofiltration (CVVH). CVVHD uses primarily diffusive with added convective clearance, whereas CVVH uses solely convective clearance.

ARF: Energy Metabolism and Requirements

Careful assessment of energy requirements in children with ARF is essential. Inadequate caloric provision will result in poor protein retention, and excessive nutrition increases the risk for metabolic derangement and fluid excess. Total energy requirements include resting energy expenditure, energy needed for physical activity, and diet-induced thermogenesis. In patients with uncomplicated ARF, energy expenditure has been shown to be comparable to healthy subjects as measured by indirect calorimetry.[13] ARF associated with sepsis or multiorgan dysfunction results in increased energy expenditure, and the increase in expenditure is believed to be proportionate to the underlying process leading to the critical illness.[14] One study of critically ill adult patients compared the energy expenditure of patients who required dialysis for severe ARF to those who had normal or only moderately impaired renal function. All of the patients demonstrated increased energy expenditure due to their critical illness, though there was significant individual variation. The measured energy expenditure was greater for those who required only supportive measures when compared to those who required dialysis with average hypermetabolism measured at 42% and 28%, respectively. It was proposed that ARF reduced energy demand secondary to diminished renal metabolic activity.[15]

Given the significant clinical variability, predicting the energy requirements of critically ill patients remains a great challenge. The use of indirect calorimetry allows nutrition to be tailored to the needs of the individual patient and is the preferred method when available. When assessment by indirect calorimetry is not possible, energy expenditure can be estimated by one of the calculations for predicting energy requirements. The reader is referred to Chapter 11 for further reading regarding the use and limitations of these calculations.

The general recommendation for adult patients with ARF is that energy provided be tailored to the individual patient and not exceed 130% of the patient's resting energy expenditure.[13,16–18] Pediatric data and guidelines for energy requirements in ARF are lacking, and assessment should address individual needs. Pediatric patients who are relatively well and not oliguric are unlikely to have increased energy requirements, and those who are critically ill will have increased expenditures. A group of critically ill pediatric patients on CRRT were provided calories 20 to 30% above their resting energy expenditures based on indirect calorimetry.[14] Despite providing this nutritional care, positive nitrogen balance was often not met. For practical purposes, it is reasonable to start at the recommended dietary caloric intake for an aged-matched healthy child and adjust as clinically indicated based on predictive equations or indirect calorimetry. Nutrition regimens should be modified to account for obligatory caloric delivery when dextrose containing intravenous fluids and dextrose containing dialysate solutions are used.

Hyperglycemia is not uncommon in critically ill patients with ARF. The potential for altered carbohydrate metabolism must be considered given that standard nutrition provides the majority of calories from dextrose, and patients on dialysis are delivered additional dextrose from dialysate. Hyperglycemia is a consequence of both accelerated hepatic gluconeogenesis and insulin resistance. Increased hepatic gluconeogenesis results from conversion of amino acids released during protein catabolism.[19] Additionally, the kidney plays a direct role in glucose homeostasis, which is regulated by insulin.[20] Critically ill patients with ARF may demonstrate insulin resistance as evidenced by higher blood glucose and insulin concentrations.[21,22] During acute renal injury, insulin resistance may be more likely given the loss of the kidney as a major target organ for insulin action. The consequences of insulin resistance and hyperglycemia have been shown to be significant. Both were associated with increased mortality in critically ill adults with ARF.[22] In addition, reports indicate that critically ill infants and children who demonstrated sustained hyperglycemia suffered a 3-fold increase in mortality over those with well-controlled glycemia.[23] By employing a strategy of strict glycemic control with intensive insulin therapy to maintain blood glucose level between 80 and 110 mg/dL, the morbidity and mortality among adult patients in a surgical intensive care unit were significantly reduced.[24] Given the association of hyperglycemia with increased complications and worse prognosis, efforts to maintain normoglycemia should be made.

ARF: Protein Metabolism and Requirements

ARF is a state of increased catabolism, which parallels the severity of the underlying illness. During metabolic stress, counterregulatory hormones and cytokines are produced with subsequent release of large amounts of glucose, fatty acids, and amino acids from the body's stores. The catabolism of skeletal muscle allows for the generation of glucose, which is the preferred substrate for the brain, red blood cells, and renal medulla. This stress response is an effective short-term adaptation, though a prolonged response is maladaptive and can result in reduction of lean body mass.

Studies evaluating critically ill adults with ARF have reported high protein catabolic rates of 1.4 to 1.8 g/kg/d.[18,25,26] Virtually all nitrogen arising from amino acids liberated during protein degradation is converted to urea, and the extent of protein catabolism may be assessed by calculating urea nitrogen appearance (UNA). In dialysis patients, UNA equals the sum of the urea in the dialysis ultrafiltrate, urine, and the change in the body nitrogen pool. The UNA was studied in a group of critically ill children with anuric ARF maintained CRRT and measured to be >180 mg/kg/d.[27] This compares to a mean UNA of 103 mg/kg/d in well children on stable PD.[28] Increased protein catabolic rate was confirmed in a subsequent report of critically ill pediatric patients on CVVH and CVVHD with a mean UNA of 291 and 245 mg/kg/d, respectively. Nitrogen balance, defined as the difference between nitrogen intake and UNA, was often negative in these patients despite the provision of 1.5 g/kg/d of protein.[14]

If the care of a patient with ARF requires dialysis, the modality of dialysis must be considered when determining protein requirements. Hemodialysis leads to nitrogen loss, as amino acids and small peptides are filtered across the dialysis membrane.[29,30] During continuous dialysis, there will be continuous nitrogen loss. A study to compare amino acid losses between CVVHD and CVVH in children was undertaken by Maxvold and colleagues.[14] CVVH provides clearance solely by convection, as compared to clearance by CVVHD, which is primarily diffusive. With the exception of glutamic acid, individual free amino acid clearances were greater on CVVH than on CVVHD, though over the 48-hour period of the study, there was no significant difference in daily loss of amino acid when comparing the two modalities. Amino acid losses by dialysis clearance represented 12% and 11% of daily protein intake on CVVH and CVVHD, respectively. PD can result in significant protein losses through the dialysis effluent, and the degree of protein loss varies inversely with the body surface area of the child. Peritoneal protein loss when assessed in children on chronic PD was highest in infants (277 ± 22 mg/kg/d) and lowest in children who were above 50 kg (91 ± 15 mg/kg/d).[31]

Currently, a few studies have attempted to define protein or amino acid requirements for adult patients with ARF, and no studies exist for pediatric patients. Protein requirements in children are dependent on age and severity of illness. A child with uncomplicated ARF (not critically ill) should be provided protein in the amount recommended for age with adjustment to provide ongoing needs. While protein intake is increased, electrolytes, acid-base balance, and uremia should be assessed daily. Protein requirements in children who are critically ill will be increased, though data specific to ARF are lacking. Protein should be provided based on recommendations for critically ill children and adjusted for individual needs. The American Society for Parental and Enteral Nutrition (ASPEN) has put forth recommendations for protein intake and estimated protein losses for children with ARF supported with dialysis (Table 2).[32] Adjustment of protein intake should be made to maintain blood urea nitrogen (BUN) >40 mg/dL and <80 mg/dL, if clinically appropriate. Few studies are available that allow estimation of optimal protein to energy ratio in critically ill children, though provision of 10 to 20% of total energy as protein is often reasonable.

Table 2 Recommended Protein Intake and Estimated Protein Losses During Dialysis Therapy for Acute Renal Failure

Age (weight range)	RDI	Estimated PD Losses	Estimated HD Losses	Estimated CRRT Losses	Daily Protein Intake Goal
Infant age					
< 2 yr (≤ 10 kg)	1.6–2.2	2.0–4.0	0.5–1.0	2.0–3.0	2.0–6.0
Small child age					
1–6 yr (> 10 ≤ 25 kg)	1.0–1.2	2.0–3.0	0.5–1.0	2.0–3.0	1.0–3.0
Older child					
age 7–14 yr					
(> 25 ≤ 40 kg)	0.8–1.2	1.0–2.0	0.5–1.0	2.0–3.0	1.0–2.0
Adolescent					
age 15–21 yr 0.8–1.0					
(> 40)	0.8–1.2	1.0–2.0	0.5–1.0	2.0–3.0	1.0–2.0

Adapted from reference 32.
Values are expressed as grams of protein/kg/d.
CRRT = continuous renal replacement therapy; HD = hemodialysis; PD = peritoneal dialysis; RDI = recommended dietary intake for normal children.

ARF: Micronutrient Requirements

Trace-element requirements in ARF are not clearly defined. Most recommendations for requirements in ARF are extrapolated from data in patients with chronic renal failure. In addition, many of the findings regarding trace element metabolism in ARF may represent the effect of the acute phase response and not necessarily reflect specific effects induced by ARF. As trace elements have small molecular weights and critical illness results in altered protein binding, hemodialysis may alter trace element homeostasis. In vitro data have shown that trace elements are cleared during CVVH, including selenium, chromium, copper, and zinc.[33] The ultrafiltration rate, or rate of convective fluid removal, was a significant factor affecting clearance. However, the assessments of losses in patients on CRRT have been variable.[34,35] Variations likely stem from differences in patient population, CRRT method, and assays employed. One study confirmed removal of copper, selenium, and zinc.[36] As selenium is cofactor for the antioxidant glutathione peroxidase enzymes, impaired defense against antioxidant stress is of concern. Further studies are needed to determine trace-element requirements in renal failure. For patients on parenteral nutrition (PN), standard supplements of trace elements should be provided.

Recommendations for vitamin supplementation during ARF are provided by the ASPEN guidelines.[32] Additional water-soluble vitamins should be administered if the patient is on hemodialysis to replace expected losses. Supplementation with folate, B_{12}, pyridoxine, thiamine, and riboflavin is recommended. Vitamin C is metabolized to oxalate, which can accumulate in patients with CKD. Oxalate accumulation has not been adequately studied in ARF. Supplementation of vitamin C should not exceed the dietary reference intake (DRI) (see Appendix II, Table II-1). Fat-soluble vitamins may accumulate in CKD, as they are not removed with dialysis. Little data regarding fat-soluble vitamins in ARF are available, though deficiencies, with the exception of vitamin K, have been reported.[37] ASPEN guidelines recommend supplementation of fat-soluble vitamins if the duration of ARF is limited (ie, <2 weeks).[32]

ARF: Electrolyte Considerations

ARF predisposes the patient to electrolyte and acid-base disorders, including hyperkalemia, hyperphosphatemia, hypocalcemia, and acidosis. Full discussion of electrolyte physiology in the setting of normal and altered renal function is beyond the scope of this chapter. A limited discussion is provided to serve as a basis for nutritional planning.

Given the potential for life-threatening arrhythmias, hyperkalemia is a dreaded consequence of ARF. Potassium is the most abundant intracellular cation, with less than 2% of total body potassium present in the extracellular fluid. As potassium is primarily renally excreted, decreased GFR and renal tubular damage may result in significant hyperkalemia. In addition to decreased excretion, hyperkalemia may result from transcellular shift induced by acidosis and increased extracellular load secondary to enhanced cell turnover, hemolysis, and transfusion of red blood cells. Therefore, potassium should be withheld during evolving ARF until acceptable potassium homeostasis is assured. If significant hyperkalemia results (≥6.0 mEq/L), treatment with a potassium exchange resin (ie, sodium polystrene sulfonate) should be considered. If dialysis is initiated, potassium clearance should be anticipated if the dialysate contains no or little potassium. While on CRRT, potassium will be cleared continuously. If clinically appropriate, potassium salts may be added to the dialysate (typically up to 3 mEq/L) to mitigate the tendency for hypokalemia.

Similar to hyperkalemia, hyperphosphatemia is a common complication of oliguric and anuric renal failure. Phosphorus is the major intracellular anion with less than 1% present in the extracellular space. Serum phosphorus occurs in two forms, organic and inorganic. The inorganic fraction is the principal circulating form and routinely assayed for clinical use. When GFR is within the normal range and renal tubular function is intact, approximately 80 to 90% of serum inorganic phosphorus is filtered, and typically more than 80% of filtered phosphorus is reabsorbed. In ARF, hyperphosphatemia may cause hypocalcemia as a result of calcium-phosphate precipitation, which typically begins when the calcium × phosphorus product is greater than 70. Treatment of hyperphosphatemia includes restricting phosphorus intake and administering oral phosphate binders with enteral feeds. If needed, nutritionally complete formulas designed for acute and chronic renal failure are available and have lower phosphorus content. These formulas include Similac PM 60/40 (Ross Products) for infants and Suplena (Abbott) for children and adults (see Appendix III, Table III-1). Calcium carbonate and calcium acetate are commonly used phosphorus binders and will provide supplemental calcium, which will be beneficial if hypocalcemia is present.

ARF: Routes of Nutrition

After estimating the nutritional needs of a child with ARF, the next challenge is to determine the appropriate route of nutrition. If allowable, enteral nutrition is the preferred method of support. Proposed benefits of enteral nutrition include intestinal trophism, reducing bacterial translocation, stimulation of the immune system, and cost effectiveness.[38–41] Early initiation of enteral nutrition was shown to reduce septic complications in adult surgical patients when compared to PN[42] and was well tolerated in critically ill pediatric patients.[43] A specific benefit of enteral feeds is the potential for providing concentrated nutrition, which minimizes fluid intake.

Though enteral feeds are preferred, they may not be tolerated in critically ill patients. The underlying illness and need for vasoactive medications may compromise gastrointestinal perfusion. An additional concern in the setting of ARF is the detrimental effect of uremia on gastrointestinal motility. However, nasogastric feeds were well tolerated when applied carefully to a population of adult patients with ARF without significant increase in major gastrointestinal complications.[44] To decrease the risk of aspiration and improve tolerance of feeds when gastric emptying is delayed, transpyloric feeds should be considered. When critically ill children with and without ARF were compared, continuous transpyloric feeds were associated with increased gastrointestinal complications, including abdominal distension and excessive gastric residue. However, transplyloric feeds were overall effective and well tolerated.[45,46]

If enteral feeds are initiated, both standard formulas and formulas appropriate for decreased renal function are available. Feeds should be initiated with hypo- or normocaloric formula at low rates of 0.5 to 1 mL/kg/h with gradual increase to normal caloric delivery for age over 36 to 48 hours as tolerated. Gastric residuals and abdominal exams should be monitored closely with advancement.[46] If the patient is volume restricted, the rate should be increased to the target volume and then gradually fortified using modular components to meet nutritional needs (Table 3). To optimize digestibility, similar proportions of fat, protein, and carbohydrate as in the base formula should be used. In patients on CRRT, amino acid and small peptide losses may challenge the ability to supply adequate protein enterally. If indicated, administration of 10% amino acids can be provided to achieve desired goals.[44]

In critically ill patients with ARF, enteral feeds often cannot meet nutritional needs. PN combined with enteral support or total parental nutrition may be necessary. A balanced PN regimen usually provides 10 to 20% of total calories by amino acids, 50 to 60% of calories by dextrose, and 20 to 30% by lipid emulsion. Modification of PN should be performed based on amino acid losses and dextrose absorption from dialysis therapies. Electrolyte composition should be guided by regular assessment of the patient's laboratory studies.

CHRONIC KIDNEY DISEASE

CKD is defined as kidney damage based on persistent structural or functional abnormalities, which may be associated with reduced or normal GFR. In children, CKD arises more commonly from congenital than acquired renal disease. When reviewing registry data of children with CRI, the most common primary diseases were obstructive uropathy (21.6%), renal aplasia, hypoplasia, and dysplasia (17.6%), and reflux nephropathy (8.4%). Focal segmental glomerulosclerosis, an acquired glomerulopathy, accounted for 8.7% of cases.[47]

When kidney damage is significant, there is a progressive loss of functioning nephron mass leading to end-stage renal disease (ESRD). To avoid or delay this outcome, providing supportive measures to retard progression should be provided. Critical measures to be taken include treating hypertension and reducing proteinuria when proteinuria is significant. In 2002, the Kidney Disease Outcomes Quality Initiative (K/DOQI) of the NKF put forth definition criteria and a classification scheme defining the stages of CKD (Table 4). Given the importance of early detection and intervention, guidelines to facilitate the detection of kidney disease in children and adults were provided and have been summarized.[1,48] When compared to adult onset CKD, persistent kidney disease during childhood poses unique challenges, including growth impairment. Despite advances in medical management, growth in children with CKD remains suboptimal.

Data regarding growth of children with CKD are provided by the North American Pediatric Renal Trials and Collaborative Studies (NAPRTCS). NAPRTCS is a research effort, which studies the clinical course and natural history of children with CRI (GFR <75 mL/min/1.73 m^2), on maintenance dialysis, and after renal transplantation with the ultimate goal of improving care. Review of the registry reveals little change in the mean height standard deviation score (HtSDS) of children enrolled between 1994 and 2001. Analysis of data in 1996, 1998, and 2001, revealed a relatively static mean HtSDS of −1.5 (1,725 patients),[49] −1.4 (3,863 patients),[50] and −1.4 (4,666 patients),[51] respectively. A recent analysis of the NAPRTCS registry reviewed the stature of children with CKD and included data submitted through January of 2004. Defining severe growth delay as HtSDS of less than −1.88, 36.9% of children were found to have severe growth impairment at entry. There was a strong correlation with worsening renal function and short stature at entry. The mean HtSDSs for children with creatinine clearance of 10 to 25 mL/min/1.73 m^2 and greater than 50 mL/min/1.73 m^2 were −1.92 and −0.89, respectively.[52]

Table 4 Stages of Chronic Kidney Disease

Stage	Description	GFR (mL/min/1.73 m^2)
1	Kidney damage with normal or increased GFR	≥ 90
2	Kidney damage with mildly decreased GFR	60–89
3	Moderately decreased GFR	30–59
4	Severely decreased GFR	15–29
5	Kidney failure	< 15 (or dialysis)

Adapted from reference 1.
Chronic kidney disease is defined as either kidney damage or GFR < 60 mL/min/1.73 m^2 persisting for 3 months or more.
Kidney damage is defined as pathologic abnormalities or makers of damage, including abnormalities in blood or urine tests or imaging studies.

The youngest children with CKD comprise the most vulnerable population at risk for severe growth deficiency. In the healthy state, growth rate is rapid during the first 2 years of life. It is during this critical time that the most significant loss of height potential can occur. The European Study Group for nutritional treatment of chronic renal failure in childhood identified that infants with early onset chronic renal failure had already lost approximately 1 SD of height during fetal life and another standard deviation lost by the third postnatal month.[53] This finding was consistent with reported average birth length of –0.74 SDS in 12 infants with chronic renal failure.[54] Multivariate analysis of the NAPRTCS registry revealed that infants with congenital renal disease who entered with a low estimated GFR had the most severe growth attenuation.[52]

Though the etiology of growth failure is multifactorial, inadequate nutrition will adversely affect growth outcome.[55,56] In addition to impacting somatic growth, malnutrition is clearly associated with increased morbidity and mortality in children with CKD. Serum albumin has been identified as a surrogate marker for nutritional status, though levels may reflect factors such as inflammation, hemodilution, and glomerular loss. Due to nutritional concerns, the K/DOQI Nutritional Guidelines recommend including serum albumin as part of the routine nutritional assessment of maintenance dialysis patients.[57] In the adult population, hypoalbuminemia at dialysis initiation and during the maintenance of chronic dialysis has been shown to be predictive of future mortality.[58,59,60] The same association of hypoalbuminemia with increased risk for mortality has been found in pediatric patients.[61] When serum albumin was

Table 3 Nutrient Content of Selected Modular Products*

Modular Product (Manufacturer)	Energy (kcal)	Protein (g)	Fat (g)	Carb (g)	Na (mg)	K (mg)	P (mg)
Carbohydrate (per 100 g)							
–Moducal (Mead Johnson)	375	0	0	95	70	5	Trace
–Polycose (Ross Products)	380	0	0	95	110	10	12
Fat (per 100 mL)							
–Canola oil	813	0	92	0	0	0	0
–Microlipid (Mead Johnson)	449	0	51	0	0	0	0
Carbohydrte and fat (per 100 g)							
–Duocal (SHS International)	492	0	73	22	≤ 20	≤ 5	≤ 5
Protein (per 100 g)							
–Beneprotein (ReSource)	357	86	0	0	214	500	286

Adapted from reference 11.
Carb = carbohydrate; K = potassium; Na = sodium; P = phosphorus.
*For the most current nutrient content, see product labels.

analyzed in over 1,700 pediatric patients at initiation of dialysis, each –1 g/dL difference in albumin was associated with a 54% higher risk of death. This finding was independent of the causes of CKD and other potentially confounding variables. This study also found that HtSDS was inversely associated with mortality risk and consistent with previous findings of growth failure and mortality.[62,63]

CKD: Spontaneous Nutritional Intake

Several studies have demonstrated altered spontaneous nutritional intake in children with CKD, underscoring the importance of nutritional counseling in the management of these children. An Italian study reviewed 4-day weighed dietary records from 50 children with creatinine clearance of 15 to 65 mL/min/1.73 m^2 and 93 healthy controls.[64] The mean energy intake was 76 to 88% of the recommended dietary allowance (RDA) in children with CKD compared with 90 to 93% in healthy subjects. Protein intake was also 33% lower in children with CKD with intake of 1.6 to 2.7 g/kg/d compared with 2.1 to 3.1 g/kg/d in healthy controls. Other studies have confirmed decreased caloric intake in children with CKD, though protein intake has been high. The energy intake of 15 children with moderate renal insufficiency in Spain was evaluated and expressed as percentages of international recommendations. Mean energy and protein intakes were 87% and 223%, respectively.[65] Foreman and colleagues assessed nutrient intake in children with CRI and found that the mean caloric and protein intake were 80% and 153% of the RDA, respectively.[66] The caloric intake decreased with increasing age, though the caloric intake was normal when factored by body weight. There was no relationship found between the degree of renal insufficiency and caloric or protein intake.[66] However, other studies have demonstrated decreased energy intake with increasing severity of renal insufficiency.[65,67]

The etiology of decreased spontaneous energy intake is in children with CKD is unclear, though altered cytokine levels are likely significant. The effect of inflammation and cytokines on appetite and cachexia in CKD has recently been reviewed.[68,69] It has been suggested that the term malnutrition is misapplied in CKD, and cachexia more accurately describes the process.[70] Cachexia is typified by loss of body weight in which muscle mass is replaced by fatty tissue and is associated with declining serum proteins. Anorexia combined with increased metabolism of fat and lean mass leads to cachexia. Leptin is produced by adipocytes and exerts sustained inhibitory effect on food intake while increasing energy expenditure. Leptin is cleared from the circulation by glomerular filtration and then undergoes degradation in the renal tubules.[71] Circulating concentrations of cytokines such as leptin, tumor necrosis factor-α, and interleukins 1 and 6 are elevated in CKD and correlate with the degree of cachexia.[72,73] Further studies are needed to elucidate the underlying mechanisms of inflammation-associated cachexia in CKD.

CKD: Supplemental Feedings

The difficulties associated with feeding infants and young children with CKD are well recognized and may result from refusal of feeds, gastroesophageal reflux (GER), and vomiting.[74] As nutritional intake may be suboptimal in children with CKD, the use of supplemental enteral feedings has been studied and recently reviewed.[70] Given that growth velocity is maximal in infancy and predominantly dependent on nutrition, most studies have focused on the younger child. An early study by Brewer noted improved growth in a group of infants and small children (<10 kg) on PD who received nasogastric feeds. The weight SDS (WtSDS) and HtSDS improved in 11 and 10 of 14 patients, respectively.[75] At Great Ormond Street Hospital for Children, nasogastric and gastric feeds were initiated in 35 children up to age 5 years with GFR < 26 mL/min/1.73 m^2. The aim of supplemental feedings was to provide at least 100% of estimated average requirement for energy and 100% of the reference nutrient intake for protein for height age. The benefit was most apparent in the 0 to 2-year age group (n = 26) with improved mean WtSDS from −3.1 at the initiation of feeds to −1.4 at 2 years. Improvement in HtSDS was also significant with mean Ht SDS −2.9 at initiation and −2.1 at two years.[76] A subsequent report from the same unit studied the growth outcome of 81 children who presented with chronic renal failure (GFR < 20 mL/min/1.73 m^2) in the first 6 months of life. Supplemental enteral feeds were commenced in 81% of patients when growth became subnormal. The mean HtSDS was within the normal range at 1 year of age and continued to improve thereafter.[77] Other studies have supported improvement in growth with supplemental feeds.[78,79,80]

In addition to ensuring sufficient energy and protein intake, the effect of providing supplemental sodium and water to young children with polyuric, salt-wasting forms of chronic renal failure was studied. It was proposed that these children experience growth delay due to chronic intravascular depletion and negative sodium balance, and that the provision of low-caloric density, high-volume, sodium-supplemented feeds would promote normal growth. The treatment group consisted of 24 children diagnosed with polyuric renal insufficiency (<65 mL/min/1.73 m^2) in the first year of life and were compared to a historical population control and a literature control. The nutritional therapy prescribed consisted of formula diluted with water to a caloric density of 0.3 to 0.5 kcal/mL and supplemented with 2 to 4 mEq of sodium per 100 mL of formula. The average energy intake for the treatment group was 104 kcal/kg/d (102% RDA), and the average protein intake was 2.45 g/kg/d (153% RDA). None of the children received growth hormone (GH). The treatment group maintained their height SDS at 1 and 2 years, with a net gain of height SDS of 0.15 during the 2 years. The change in height SDS by regressional analysis was significantly greater in the treatment group than in the control groups.[81]

Though supplemental feeds resulted in improved growth in some studies, others have not demonstrated the same benefit. Several studies have shown stabilization of linear growth without significant catch-up growth.[82,83] Abitbol and colleagues studied 12 infants with congenital renal insufficiency and provided controlled feeding regimens starting at 3 months of age. Six of these infants received supplemental nasogastric or gastric tube feedings. The average energy intake was 95% RDA with average protein intake of 141% RDA. The study revealed that the major height deficit was incurred during the first 6 months of life, as the length SDS fell from −0.7 at birth to approximately −1.9 at 6 months. There was no catch-up growth noted as indicated by the length SDS of −2.0 at 24 months.[54] The only multicenter experience comes from the NAPRTCS survey, which reviewed the impact of supplemental feedings on growth and mortality in children < 6 years of age at dialysis initiation. Questionnaires were completed on 137 patients, 70% of whom received supplemental feedings and outcome was compared to those who did not receive supplements. Significantly more children prior to 2 years of age were given supplemental feedings when compared to children initiating dialysis from 2 to 5 years (~ 80% vs 41%). Despite supplemental feedings, there was no difference in height and weight, and height and weight SDS did not improve over time with supplementation. In addition, mortality was unaffected.[84]

Though inadequate nutrition will negatively impact growth in children with CKD, the variable response to nutritional support highlights the complexity of growth impairment in these patients. Alterations in the GH/insulin-like growth factor-1 (IGF-1) axis independently affect growth in the uremic milieu. Although serum GH and IGF-1 levels are usually normal or high in growth-retarded children with CKD, uremic serum has high IGF-1-binding capacity which results in low IGF-1 bioactivity.[85] In conjunction with optimal medical and nutritional management, recombinant human growth hormone (rhGH) therapy significantly improves linear growth.[86–88] Despite evidence of efficacy and safety, only 22.2% of growth-impaired children which entered into the NAPRTCS CRI registry were receiving rhGH at their 12-month visit.[47] Recommendations for evaluation and treatment of growth failure in children with CRI have been published and include recommendations for rhGH therapy.[89] Secondary hyperparathyroidism and chronic metabolic acidosis are additional factors that impair growth. To optimize the utilization of nutrition for growth and response to GH, appropriate correction of secondary hyperparathyroidism and metabolic acidosis is critical.

Supplemental feedings are an accepted standard of practice in the care of children with CKD who do not meet the RDA for energy and protein. Studies thus far identify younger children as the group most likely to need this support, and the choice of nasogastric versus gastric feedings depends on the needs and comorbidities of the individual patient. Complications associated with nasogastric and gastrosomy feedings include emesis, exit-site infection, and leakage. Additional risks for patients on PD include peritonitis. It is prudent to provide supplementation in children who demonstrate inadequate intake or decline in growth, though prospective studies defining the optimal approach to nutritional supplementation are needed.

CKD: Assessment of Nutritional Status

The importance of nutritional status has been emphasized in numerous clinical practice guidelines for care of patients with CKD.[57,90] Nutritional status is a complex concept, and no single measurement is comprehensive. Therefore a multistaged evaluation of body composition is necessary. Measurements of nutritional parameters are complicated in CKD given the potential for fluid overload and possible abnormalities in the distribution of fat and lean tissue. Children with chronic renal failure and after renal transplantation have been found to have discordant body composition with relatively high fat mass and low lean mass.[91] Additionally, assessment methods recommended for children with CKD were developed in healthy children, and the validity may be limited in CKD. A comprehensive review has been published summarizing the methods recommended for nutritional assessment of children with CKD and details the advantages and disadvantages of these methods.[92]

The most recently published *K/DOQI Clinical Practice Guideline for Nutrition in Chronic Renal Failure* addresses the protein-energy nutritional status for children receiving maintenance dialysis. The recommended measures include an assessment of dietary intake, serum albumin, and anthropometric measurements. In addition, K/DOQI guidelines recommend measurement of the protein equivalent of nitrogen appearance (PNA) for children maintained on PD, which allows estimation of protein intake.[57] The measures and suggested frequency are summarized in Table 5. Reflecting growth challenges faced by the younger child, the frequency of measurement is increased in children <2 years. These guidelines outline the minimum frequency of assessment, and more frequent assessment may be appropriate and should be tailored to the individual patient. In particular, infants and children with comorbid conditions in addition to ESRD may need more frequent monitoring.

Though there is strong evidence that children with mild to moderate CRI are at risk of growth impairment,[65,67,93,94] there are no formal guidelines available for pediatric patients with CRI prior to the onset of ESRD. In the absence of guidelines, it has been recommended that the same assessment for children with ESRD be undertaken in children with CRI, though the frequency of assessment is guided by the degree of insufficiency and should be individualized.[92] Infants in particular are at high risk of malnutrition and may benefit monthly evaluation regardless of the degree of insufficiency.

Nutritional Management of CKD

The following will detail nutritional management and guidelines for children with CRI, on maintenance dialysis, and after renal transplantation. To avoid repetition, the dietary management of children with CRI and on maintenance dialysis will be discussed together. A separate discussion of the nutritional management of patients after renal transplantation will follow. Tables 6 and 7 outline nutrient recommendations for children with CRI and on maintenance dialysis, respectively. Modifications should be made based on individual response or clinical need, such as suboptimal growth or catabolic stress due to acute illness. In general, the use of chronological age is recommended for determining requirements. However, when chronological and height age are significantly different (ie, height <2%), basing requirements for energy and protein on height age may be more appropriate to promote improved growth and "catch-up" growth.

To increase energy intake and improve compliance, dietary modifications for children are typically less restrictive than those prescribed to adults. Dietary guidelines for adults often recommend specific amounts of a restricted nutrient, such as a "2 g sodium diet." In pediatrics, restrictions are imposed only when clinically indicated and usually take the form of a "low-nutrient X diet" with education on which foods are high or low in that nutrient. Clinical indications for restriction include hypertension and edema, which would warrant the recommendation for a low sodium diet. Guidance is provided to substitute or avoid that food. The specified amount of nutrients provided in Tables 6 and 7 can be used as a general references. Depending on the response to the diet, the restriction can be liberalized or tightened.

If available, the support of a renal dietician is indispensable in optimizing the dietary management of children with CKD. The modification of food and fluid intake proves to be a great challenge for many. Every child with CKD and appropriate family member or caretaker should receive nutrition counseling based on individual needs. In addition to addressing the specifics of the renal disease process, the education level and social influences of the family must be considered when counseling is provided. The dietary care plan requires ongoing modification based on the changes in the child's age, nutritional status, renal function, treatment modality, and medication regimen. Depending on the disease time course, a renal dietician may support an individual through the various stages of renal insufficiency, maintenance dialysis, and renal transplantation. Families need continual guidance and support to establish and consistently enforce prescribed dietary guidelines. Nutritional specialists can ease the burden of restrictions and increase the likelihood of success by providing practical suggestions for modifying or replacing favorite foods or fluids.

Table 5 Suggested Nutritional Parameters and Minimum Schedule of Measurements for Children on Dialysis

Parameter	Minimal Interval: Age < 2 yr	Minimal Interval: Age ≥ 2 yr
Length	Monthly	Not applicable
Standing height	Not applicable	3–4 mo
Head circumference	Monthly	3–4 mo until age 36 mo
Estimated dry weight	Monthly	3–4 mo
Weight/height index	Monthly	3–4 mo
Height SD score	3–4 mo	Monthly
Serum albumin	Monthly	Monthly
Skinfold thickness	No agreement	3–4 mo
Midarm anthropometric measures	3–4 mo	3–4 mo
Dietary interview	Monthly	3–4 mo
Urea kinetic modeling	3–4 mo	3–4 mo

Adapted from reference 57.
mo = months; SDS = standard deviation score.

NUTRITIONAL MANAGEMENT OF CRI AND MAINTENANCE DIALYSIS

CRI and Maintenance Dialysis: Energy Requirements

Energy requirements for children with CRI and on maintenance dialysis have been based on requirements for healthy children, as there is lack of evidence to suggest that these children have increased needs. Therefore, the initial prescribed energy intake for infants, children, and adolescents with CKD should be the DRI for chronologic age (see Appendix II, Table II-5). Adequate energy intake is not only critical to allow optimal growth but prevents the utilization of protein stores as an energy source. Energy-malnourished children may require additional energy to restore normal growth and allow "catch-up" growth if possible.

Table 6 Daily Nutrient Recommendations for Children with Chronic Renal Insufficiency

	Infant		Toddler	Child	Adolescent	
Nutrient	0–6 mo	7–12 mo	1–2 yr	3–8 yr	9–13 yr	14–18 yr
Energy (kcal/kg/d)						
Boys	95	80–85	85–90	85–90	60–65	50–55
Girls	85– 90	75	80–85	80–85	60	45
Protein (g/kg/d)	1.5	1.1–1.5	0.9–1.1	0.8–0.95	0.8–0.95	Boys: 0.75–0.85 Girls: 0.7–0.85
Sodium:	If clinically appropriate, no restriction necessary. If edema or HTN: no salt shaker and avoid salty foods (restrict to ~1–3 mEq/kg/d)					
Potassium	If hyperkalemia develops, avoid foods with high potassium content (restrict to ~1–3 mEq/kg/d)					
Calcium	100% of the DRI Monitor total calcium load, including calcium derived from phosphate binders					
Phosphorus	Consider low phosphorus formula if serum levels are elevated despite use of phosphate binders		≤400–600 mg/d when serum levels are elevated		≤600–800 mg/d when serum levels are elevated	
Vitamins	If needed, supplement to 100% of DRI. Supplement with Vitamin D metabolite if needed to prevent hyperparathyroidism and renal osteodystrophy.					
Minerals	If needed, supplement to 100% of DRI. Iron supplementation will be needed if receiving erythropoietin therapy.					

Adapted from reference 110.

Table 7 Daily Nutrient Recommendations for Children on Maintenance Dialysis

	Infant		Toddler	Child		Adolescent	
Nutrient	0–6 mo	7–12 mo	1–3 yr	4–6 yr	7–10 yr	11–14 yr	15–18 yr
Energy (kcal/kg/d)	110	100	105	90	70	Boys: 55 Girls: 50	Boys: 45 Girls: 40
Protein (g/kg/d) HD Patients	2.6	2.0	1.6	1.6	1.4	Boys: 1.4 Girls: 1.4	Boys: 1.3 Girls: 1.2
PD patients	2.9–3.0	2.3–2.4	1.9–2.0	1.9–2.0	1.7–1.8	Boys: 1.7–1.8 Girls: 1.7–1.8	Boys: 1.4–1.5 Girls: 1.4–1.5
Sodium	In general, no salt shaker and avoid salty foods. For infants and small children, sodium supplementation may be needed due to losses from dialysis.						
Potassium	Avoid foods with high potassium content (restrict to ~1–3 mEq/kg/d).						
Calcium	100% of the DRI.						
Phosphorus	Consider low phosphorus formula if serum levels are elevated despite use of phosphate binders.			≤400–600 mg/d		≤600–800 mg/d	
Vitamins	If needed, supplement to 100% DRI for thiamin, riboflavin, pyridoxine, folic acid, and vitamin B_{12}, and 100% RDA for vitamins A, C, E, and K. Supplement with vitamin D metabolites to prevent secondary hyperparathyroidism and renal osteodystrophy.						
Minerals	If needed, supplement to 100% of the DRI for copper and zinc. Iron supplements will be needed while on erythropoietin therapy.						

Adapted from reference 110.
DRI = daily recommended intake; RDA = recommended daily allowance.

Achieving energy goals for infants and toddlers can be challenging due to anorexia and GER, and supplemental feedings may be necessary to achieve intended goals. Oral supplementation is preferred, though tube feedings may be necessary. Tube feeds can be provided via nasogastric, gastrostomy, or gastrojejeunostomy tubes and be infused by intermittent bolus or continuous infusion.[95,96] To encourage daytime oral intake and provide oral stimulation, continuous overnight feeds are generally preferred. Infants and toddlers who have been supported with tube feedings may experience oral feeding dysfunction and need the counseling of a multidisciplinary feeding team.[97,98]

Management of CRI and maintenance dialysis may require volume restriction if urine output is low. Volume restriction is most problematic if intake of solid nutrition is low due to age or oral aversion. If volume restriction is indicated, fortification of feeds to increase caloric density will be necessary. Caloric density may be increased gradually by 2 to 4 kcal/oz increments up to 60 kcal/oz as needed,[99] and the tempo of fortification will depend on individual tolerance. Both breast milk and commercial formulas may be fortified. It is not advisable to increase the energy density of formula by concentration alone due to the increased sodium, potassium, phosphorus, and overall renal solute load. Carbohydrate and fat modular products, or a combination of both, can be added to achieve the desired caloric density. See Table 3 for the nutrient content of selected modular products. Readily available oils such as canola, corn, or safflower may be used for fat supplementation. The benefit of fat modular products is the process of emulsification, which prevents the fat from separating out of the formula during continuous feeds. When making a formula with increased energy density, an attempt should be made to preserve the proportionate distribution of energy from carbohydrate, protein, and fat as in the base formula.

For older children, minimizing the number of restrictions as allowable by metabolic balance will increase the likelihood of achieving energy goals. Individuals with poor appetites may respond to small, frequent meals and snacks. Energy can be added to foods by adding heart-healthy oils or margarines, creams, syrups, or carbohydrate modules. Low-calorie or calorie-free drinks should be restricted. If the child does not meet energy requirements, supplemental nutrition should be provided. As for infants, oral supplementation is preferred, though tube feedings may be required. Nonrenal pediatric feedings designed for children older than 1 year have relatively high phosphorus and potassium content, which may result in electrolyte disturbance. Nutritionally complete renal formulas designed to be energy dense, high or low in protein, and low in electrolytes including phosphorus may be given to children older than 1 year. Suplena (Ross Products) is designed for the predialyzed patient and Nepro (Abbott) is intended for patients on maintenance dialysis (see Appendix III, Table III-2). Serum magnesium should be monitored if used in younger children, as the magnesium content is higher in adult renal products than in infant or pediatric formulas.

Energy intake and requirement issues specific to PD include early satiety or anorexia due to the pressure exerted by the indwelling dialysate volume and the effect of glucose absorption.[100,101] When calculating energy intake, intraperitoneal dialysate glucose absorption should also be considered. Approximately 7 to 10 kcal/kg/d are absorbed by children on CAPD.[102] If the need for tube feeds is anticipated, placement of gastrostomy or gastrojejeunostomy tubes should be performed well before initiating PD. Allowing sufficient time to heal will reduce technical challenges, such as leakage of dialysate at the site of tube placement.

Protein Requirements

Care for patients with CRI emphasizes supportive measures for the benefit of retarding disease progression. There has been concern that higher protein intake would induce intraglomerular hypertension and hyperfiltration injury and hasten progression of kidney disease. Given the finding that a low-protein diet was able to slow the deterioration of renal function in rodent studies,[103,104] prospective clinical studies prescribing low-protein diets were conducted in both adults[105–108] and children.[109] The results of prospective clinical studies in adults were contradictory. Overall the progression rate was not significantly influenced by protein restriction over a period of 2 to 3 years, though a low-protein diet postponed the development of uremic symptoms and start of dialysis for patients with advanced renal failure. In the pediatric study, a low-protein diet of 0.8 to 1.1 g/kg/d was provided for 2 to 3 years. This diet did not affect the rate of decline in creatinine clearance or adversely affect growth.

Given the current lack of evidence that a low-protein diet provides renal protection, children with CRI should be prescribed protein intake according to the DRI (see Appendix II, Table II-4). Requirements are increased by significant proteinuria, catabolism due to intercurrent illness, and use of glucocorticoids. Inadequate protein intake will impact body composition with reduction of lean mass and limit growth. Even if protein intake exceeds recommended levels, protein malnutrition may occur if overall energy intake is low. Protein intake may exceed recommended levels if serum urea and phosphate remain acceptable. Goals in CRI should focus on avoiding excessive protein intake, which may exacerbate uremia or hyperphosphatemia. It has been advocated that approximately 60 to 70% of protein should be of high biological value,[110] which will minimize urea production by reusing circulating nonessential amino acids for protein maintenance. Regardless, emphasis should be placed on palatability of the protein form to optimize intake. Modular protein products are available if needed (Table 3).

For children undergoing maintenance PD, protein intake must provide at least 100% DRI plus an allowance for replacement of transperitoneal losses of protein and amino acids. Transperitoneal protein losses demonstrate significant variability, and an inverse correlation between body surface area and peritoneal protein loss has been demonstrated. Infants were shown to have nearly 2-fold greater peritoneal protein losses per meter square body surface area than older children weighing more than 50 kg.[31] In addition, transperitoneal protein losses were twice as great in patients requiring maintenance PD due to steroid-resistant nephrotic syndrome when compared to children without nephrotic syndrome.[111] Given the significant variability in losses, regular assessment of growth, serum albumin, and urea levels is essential to determine if adjustment in protein intake is necessary.

For children undergoing chronic hemodialysis, the K/DOQI recommends the RDA for age and an additional increment of 0.4 g/kg/d for dialysis protein losses to achieve positive nitrogen balance.[57] Future revisions to the K/DOQI nutrition guidelines will need to consider the newer DRI for protein intake (DRI). Regular assessment of predialysis urea levels may allow assessment of protein intake, though other clinical factors affecting BUN must be considered. A predialysis BUN greater than 70 to 80 mmol/L may indicate excessive protein intake. However inadequate dialysis, recirculation of blood, and increased catabolism will also increase the predialysis BUN. Alternatively, persistently low predialysis BUN of <20 mmol/L may indicate inadequate protein intake.

Vitamin and Micronutrient Requirement

Little is known about specific vitamin requirements in children with CKD, underscoring the need for further study. It has been recommended that intake be the same as for normal children.[70] When intake is considerably less than recommended, vitamin supplementation is indicated. Children on dialysis have additional risk for vitamin deficiency due to losses of water-soluble vitamins through dialysis. The K/DOQI guidelines recommend that dietary intake should achieve 100% of the DRI for thiamin (B_1), riboflavin (B_2), pyridoxine (B_6), vitamin B_{12}, and folic acid. An intake of 100% RDA for vitamins A, C, E, and K, copper, and zinc is also recommended (see Appendix II, Tables II-1 and II-2).[57] When studied, the dietary intake of vitamins in children on PD was lower than the RDA, and supplementation resulted in intakes that exceeded recommended amounts.[112–114] Routine assessment of dietary intake should be performed before providing supplements. If supplements are indicated, infants and small children may be given liquid or chewable multivitamin preparations and additional folic acid dosed for age. Older children and adults may be provided B complex vitamins containing folic acid, such as Nephrocaps (Fleming & Company) and NephroVite (R&D Laboratories, Inc.). Excessive amounts of vitamin A and vitamin C should be avoided. Excessive vitamin A can lead to hypercalcemia,[115] anemia, and hyperlipidemia. Vitamin C is metabolized into oxalate, which is renally excreted. Excessive vitamin C may result in elevated oxalate levels and complications of retention.[116]

In CKD, the need for vitamin D supplementation should be assessed regularly. The most active form of vitamin D is 1,25-dihydroxycholecalciferol ($1,25[OH]_2D_3$), and the enzymatic step of 1α- hydroxylation occurs in the kidney. With progressive renal insufficiency, secondary hyperparathyroidism and defective bone mineralization may ensue due to inadequate $1,25(OH)_2D_3$ levels. Secondary hyperparathyroidism can begin as early as stage 2 CKD. An early study of renal osteodystrophy in 29 children with moderate to severe CRI found that PTH levels were elevated in all children with GFR < 45 mL/min/1.73 m^2. "Early" renal osteodystrophy characterized by elevated PTH but normal serum chemistries detected in one quarter of the patients.[117]

Recent guidelines recommend assessment of 25-cholecalciferol ($25[OH]D_3$) in CKD stages 2 to 4 and supplementation with vitamin D_2 (ergocalciferol) if the level is <30 ng/mL. In stage 5 CKD, supplementation with ergocalciferol will not be effective, as this cannot be converted to the active form. If indicated based on serum levels of PTH and vitamin D metabolites, supplementation with activated vitamin D should be provided. Calcitriol is commonly used, with recommended initiation doses in CKD stages 2 to 4 of 0.05 μg every other day for infants <10 kg, 0.1 to 0.15 μg/d for children 10 to 20 kg, and 0.25 μg/d for children <20 kg. For children with CKD stage 5, recommended initial calcitriol dosing ranges from 0.0075 to 0.025 μg/d given three times per week, depending on serum PTH level.[118] If the child is on maintenance hemodialysis, intravenous calcitriol may be provided at dialysis sessions. Due to potent effect on intestinal calcium absorption, calcitriol treatment can induce hypercalcemia and preclude its use at therapeutic doses. Newer vitamin D analogues have been developed which minimize intestinal calcium and phosphorus absorption while suppressing PTH levels as effectively as calcitriol.[119,120] Currently available active vitamin D sterols with less hypercalcemic effect include paracalcitol and doxercalciferol, though only paracalcitol has been studied in children.[121,122]

Adjustment of active vitamin D sterol dosing should be made to achieve target PTH levels for CKD stage. In CKD stage 5 (GFR <15 mL/min/1.73 m^2), recommendations are to adjust supplementation to keep PTH levels 200 to 300 pmol/L.[118] A potential risk of active vitamin D sterol therapy is subnormal bone formation. Excessive doses of calcitriol may suppress osteoblastic activity, and care should be taken to avoid excessive reduction in PTH levels, as this may be associated with adynamic bone disease.[123]

Children with CKD are at risk for anemia secondary to erythropoietin deficiency and iron deficiency. The introduction of recombinant erythropoietin (rHuEPO) therapy in 1988 provided a highly effective treatment in correcting anemia associated with CKD.[124] Iron deficiency is the most common factor that limits the response to rHuEPO, and children on rHuEPO usually require large amounts of supplemental iron. For children on maintenance hemodialysis, it is strongly recommended that iron be given intravenously. For children who are predialysis or on maintenance PD, iron may be provided either orally or intravenously. Dosing of iron supplementation is guided by serum ferritin and transferrin saturation.[125]

Hyperhomocysteinemia is associated with folate deficiency and has been identified as an independent risk factor for cardiovascular disease in adults with chronic renal disease.[126,127] Hyperhomocysteinemia has also been found in children with CKD, though a clear relation to vascular disease remains to be seen.[128] When children with and without CKD were studied, plasma homocysteine levels where found to increase with deterioration of renal function. Hyperhomocysteinemia was found in 5.2% of controls, 35.7% of nondialyzed CKD, and 86.6% of children with ESRD on dialysis. Folate levels were also lower in patients than controls.[129] When children on PD and hemodialysis were provided folic acid supplementation of 2.5 mg daily, plasma homocysteine concentrations were significantly reduced.[130] Currently there is no standard for monitoring homocysteine levels in children with CKD. Guidelines recommend that dietary intake for folic acid should achieve 100% the RDI. If dietary intake of folic acid is inadequate, supplementation should be considered.

Electrolyte Disturbances

Electrolyte disturbances commonly seen in CKD include hyperphosphatemia, hypocalcemia, and hyperkalemia. Though serum levels of sodium are typically within normal range, the inability to maintain sodium homeostasis will have significant clinical effect. Kidney disease associated with sodium retention may result in hypertension and edema. Alternatively, sodium losses from urine wasting in polyuric kidney disease or losses from dialysis effluent may require sodium supplementation to ensure normal serum concentration and adequate growth. Dietary restrictions of electrolytes may pose significant challenges to the child and family and contribute to inadequate energy intake overall. Restrictions should be applied only when indicated.

Hyperphosphatemia in CKD can lead to significant morbidity due to metastatic calcification, secondary hyperparathyroidism, and renal osteodystrophy. More commonly seen when GFR falls <50 mL/min/1.73 m^2, hyperphosphatemia contributes to secondary hyperparathyroidism by lowering the serum ionized calcium, inhibiting the production of $1{,}25(OH)_2D_3$, and directly stimulating PTH secretion. Therefore normal levels of serum phosphorus should be maintained to prevent renal osteodystrophy and poor growth. Guidelines recommend that dietary phosphorus intake be restricted to the DRI (see Appendix II, Table II-2) for age when the serum PTH is above the target range for the stage of CKD and the serum phosphorus is within the normal range for age. Phosphorus intake should be restricted further if both the serum PTH and phosphorus levels are elevated.[118] In children who require phosphorus restriction, intake of milk, milk products, eggs, nuts, dried beans, peanut butter, whole grains, chocolate, and other high-phosphorus containing foods should be limited. Restriction of dietary phosphorus can challenge efforts to achieve adequate protein intake, as protein and phosphorus are often found in the same foods. Animal proteins have relatively favorable phosphorus to protein ratios when compared to the ratios in eggs, dairy products, legumes, and lentils. If supplementation with formula is indicated, children and adults may be provided Nepro (Ross Products) and Suplena (Ross Products), which are formulated for patients who are predialysis and on maintenance dialysis, respectively (see Appendix II, Table II-5).

In addition to limiting dietary phosphorus, intestinal absorption of phosphorus can be decreased with the use of phosphate binders. Options for phosphate binders include both calcium-based (calcium acetate, calcium carbonate) and noncalcium-, nonmetal-containing binders (sevelamer hydrochloride, lanthanum carbonate). Aluminum-containing binders are available, but long-term use has resulted in retention and toxicity.[131–133] First-line therapy for hyperphosphatemia in children is often a calcium-based binder, and calcium acetate results in less calcium absorption than calcium carbonate. However, children who receive calcium-based binders may experience hypercalciemia with associated risks of joint, vessel, and soft tissue metastatic calcification.[134] Sevelamer hydrochloride has been shown to be effective and safe when studied in pediatric populations and is associated with less hypercalcemia.[135–137] Lanthanum carbonate has not been studied in children. The only phosphate binder readily available in a liquid or powdered form is calcium carbonate, limiting the options for small children and infants. Recently, methods to prepare sevelamer hydrochloride oral suspension have been published.[138]

In formula-fed infants with CRI or on maintenance dialysis, it is our center's practice to attempt feeds with standard formulas and use phosphate binders when indicated. Good Start Supreme (Nestle Clinical Nutrition) has a lower phosphorus content compared to other standard cow's milk-based formula. Should hyperphosphatemia develop and persist despite prescription of phosphate binders, a low-phosphorus formula such as Similac PM 60/40 (Ross Products) may be provided. The calcium content of Similac PM 60/40 is lower than that of standard infant formulas (see Appendix III, Table III-1). Therefore ensuring adequate calcium intake is critical to promote normal bone mineralization. When indicated, calcium supplementation should be provided. Recommended tolerable upper limit of calcium intake for children less than 1 year has not been determined. In children older than 1 year and adults, dietary and supplemental calcium intake should not exceed 2.5 g/d. The calcium content of phosphate binders should be included in the daily calcium intake.

As with the development of hyperphosphatemia, progressive decline in kidney function predisposes to hyperkalemia. However, hyperkalemia does not typically occur in early stages of CKD due to adaptive changes of individual nephrons as GFR declines. When hyperkalemia develops and persists, high potassium-containing foods should be limited. Unfortunately many high-postassium foods are favored by children and include potato products, tomato products, bananas, oranges, and chocolate. If necessary, potassium exchange resins, such as sodium polystyrene sulfonate can be prescribed. Formula-fed infants with significant CKD may require scheduled doses of sodium polystyrene sulfonate daily, though this may be met with increased spitting, aversion, sorbitol-induced diarrhea, and enteral tube obstruction. Methods to lower the potassium content of formula by pretreatment of the formula with sodium polystyrene sulfonate have been published. This resulted in 62 ± 2 .6% reduction of potassium content, though the sodium content of the formula was disproportionately increased (234 ± 37%). The disproportionate effect was due, in part, to exchange for calcium and magnesium.[139] Increased sodium content was seen in a subsequent report of formula pretreatment with sodium polystyrene sulfonate.[140] Should similar methods be employed, the potential complications of increase sodium intake and electrolyte abnormalities should be monitored for.

Sodium balance is directly linked to volume status. Kidney disease characterized by oliguria or anuria typically requires sodium and fluid restrictions to avoid clinical signs of volume excess, such as hypertension and edema. Children at risk for sodium retention are directed to limit dietary intake, including salty snacks, processed luncheon meats, canned soups, and packaged entrees. Food from fast food restaurants should also be limited.

Prior to the initiation of maintenance dialysis, diuretics may be used to improve sodium balance. After the initiation of maintenance dialysis, children continue to limit sodium intake, especially if hypertension is present. Infants on PD may require sodium supplementation due to sodium losses during dialysis coupled with the relatively low sodium concentration found in formula. To avoid hyponatremia and ensure adequate extracellular volume, sodium supplements may be needed (ie, 3 to 5 mEq/kg/d) with close monitoring of electrolytes, volume balance, and growth.[141]

NUTRITIONAL MANAGEMENT AFTER RENAL TRANPLANATION

Renal transplantation is recognized as the preferred treatment for children with Stage 5 CKD, as restoration of normal renal physiologic function can greatly improve the child's quality of life. If the renal allograft functions well, normalization of fluid and dietary intake is allowed. Children often have improvement in appetite after transplantation, though immunosuppressive drugs may cause nausea, vomiting, constipation, diarrhea, or anorexia. These symptoms are typically treated symptomatically. The following section will discuss growth and metabolic disorders after renal transplantaion. General guidelines for nutritional management will follow. If the renal allograft has decreased function, principles of nutritional care for children with chronic renal insufficiency should be applied.

Growth after Kidney Transplantation

Though growth typically improves after transplantation, many children demonstrate suboptimal growth overall.[142–144] During the first years following successful renal transplantation, infants and younger children may display "catch-up" growth; however accelerated growth is often not maintained thereafter. In older children catch-up growth is generally not observed and targeted final adult height is not achieved. Impairment of growth is multifactorial and includes corticosteroid use and decreased renal function. With each 1 mg/dL increase in serum creatinine, a 0.17 decrease in height SDS was observed.[142] To date, strong effort is being made to introduce steroid-sparing regimens utilizing early dose reduction, withdrawal, or avoidance of steroids.[145,146] If growth is poor, initiation of GH should be considered, weighing the potential benefits of improved linear growth with stimulatory effects upon leukocyte function.[147,148] Analysis of the NAPRTCS database comparing growth and allograft function in transplant recipients would suggest that this therapy is effective and safe.[149] In addition to poor linear growth, children may demonstrate discordant body composition with relatively low lean mass, high fat mass, and increased central adiposity after renal transplantation.[91] Given the association of truncal obesity with increased cardiovascular morbidity in adults, this may suggest additional lifetime risks in these pediatric patients.

Hyperlipidemia after Renal Transplantation

Hyperlipidemia is a common and significant disorder after renal transplantation and occurs in up to 70% of adult recipients.[150,151] A known cause of cardiovascular disease, hyperlipidemia leads to increased morbidity and mortality in adult transplant recipients, a population which is already burdened with numerous cardiovascular risks.[152] Children also have a high incidence of lipid abnormalities after renal transplantation, reported in as many as 50% of children.[153] Though well documented in adults, the cardiovascular effects of hyperlipidemia in children are not currently known.[154,155] In addition to potential cardiovascular risks, there is growing concern that hyperlipidemia may promote allograft injury with increased risk of chronic transplant nephropathy and graft failure.[156,157]

Known risk factors for hyperlipidemia in adult renal transplant recipients include renal dysfunction, hypoalbuminemia, pretransplant hyperlipidemia, family history of hyperlipidemia, obesity, and specific diseases resulting in ESRD.[158] When risk factors for hypercholesterolemia or hypertriglyceridemia were studied in pediatric recipients, only pretransplant hyperlipidemia, increased years since transplantation, and reduced GFR correlated.[153] A subsequent study confirmed pretransplant hyperlipidemia to be a significant risk factor for the development of lipid abnormalities after transplantation.[159] Immunosuppressive medications have also been associated with dislipidemias, in particular steroids,[150,160] calcinuerin inhibitors,[161,162] and sirolimus.[163,164] When comparing calcinuerin inhibitors, the incidence of hyperlipidemia appears to be higher in patients receiving cyclosporine (CsA) than those receiving tacrolimus.[151,165,166] A longitudinal study of pediatric renal transplant recipients demonstrated that the prevalence hyperlipidemia declined from 1 to 10 years posttransplant, and this was thought to be due to the reduction of immunosuppressive therapy. Elevated total cholesterol and total triglycerides declined from 70 to 35% and 46 to 15%, respectively.[167]

Children who receive renal transplants are at increased risk for hyperlipidemia, and this risk will be lifelong given the current therapeutic options of dialysis or transplantation for treatment of ESRD. It is standard practice to monitor serum lipids after renal transplantation. Should hyperlipidemia develop, dietary modifications to reduce the intake of saturated fats should be employed. Delucci and colleagues offered the Step II American Heart Association diet (no more than 30% of total calories from fat, no more that 7% of calories from saturated fatty acids) to pediatric renal transplant patients with hyperlipidemia. Of 22 eligible patients, only 12 children were willing to participate. After 12 weeks of the diet, total cholesterol and LDL cholesterol declined modestly by 11% and 14%, respectively.[168] When the practical benefit of lifestyle change is limited, pharmacologic treatment should be considered. Lipid-lowering agents such as HMGCoA-reductase inhibitors, or "statins" have been used in pediatric renal transplant recipients with success.[159,169–171] However, these studies were small and larger controlled studies are needed to more clearly define efficacy and risk.

Diabetes Mellitus after Renal Transplantation

Hyperglycemia and posttransplant diabetes mellitus (PTDM) are well-known complications of solid-organ transplantation. The reported incidence of PTDM in pediatric renal transplant recipients ranges from 2 to 10%,[172–174] and the risk for development of PTDM is associated with the immunosuppression regimen prescribed. Both corticosteroids and calcineurin inhibitors are known to affect carbohydrate metabolism. Corticosteroids alter carbohydrate metabolism by impairing peripheral utilization of glucose, elevating plasma glucagon concentration, and increasing gluconeogenesis.[175] CsA and tacrolimus have been shown to inhibit insulin secretion from beta cells.[176,177] When tacrolimus became widely prescribed in adult renal transplantation, the rate of acute rejection decreased and renal allograft outcomes improved. However, there was an increased incidence of side effects, particularly of diabetes mellitus.[165,178]

Initial pediatric studies and reports also demonstrated that tacrolimus-based immunosuppression regimens increased the risk for PTDM when compared with CsA-based regimens.[179] The odds ratio for PTDM was 9.1 (95% CI 1.1 to 76.0, $p = .04$) for tacrolimus use at PTDM diagnosis compared to CsA.[173] However, as the use of tacrolimus has become more widespread, optimal dosing has targeted lower trough levels, and the incidence of PTDM has decreased. More recently, a large European multicenter study comparing the efficacy and safety of tacrolimus with microemulsion CsA found no difference in the incidence of PTDM (3% in tacrolimus and 2.2% in CsA).[172,180] Other reported risk factors for PTDM in pediatric renal transplantation include family history of type 2 DM, hyperglycemia in the 2 weeks after transplantation, and African-American race.[173,179] Increased weight or body mass index was not identified as a risk factor.

In 2001, NAPRTCS published a report of 36 children who developed PTDM after renal transplantation.[179] The majority of patients (63.6%) presented within the first 6 months of transplantation. The diagnosis was most frequently made by the detection of hyperglycemia on routine laboratory follow-up (64%). Three patients (9%) presented with diabetic ketoacidosis. The development of PTDM was a transient disorder in the majority, as less than one-third of patients remained on insulin therapy at follow-up. Another analysis of 16 children who developed PTDM noted that for patients who presented early after transplantation (mean 0.3 years), the disorder was more likely to be transient. Those who presented later (mean 2.7 years) were more likely to have persistent PTDM. The authors proposed that the transient course reflects insulin resistance due to acute stress on beta-cell function and initial exposure to high doses of corticosteroids, and the persistent course reflects permanent beta-cell injury. They questioned as to whether permanent injury in some resulted from long-term exposure to tacrolimus or CsA.[173]

Nutritional Management after Renal Transplantation

For children who have well-functioning renal allografts, macronutrient intake should be guided by recommendations for healthy children. Energy requirements and intake should generally match that for the normal population. However, if the immunosuppressive regimen includes corticosteroids, this may increase appetite and result in excessive energy intake. Up to 12% of transplanted children become obese,[181] and efforts to control total energy intake may be necessary. In addition, if hyperglycemia or PTDM develops, intake of simple carbohydrates should be adjusted. When considering protein requirements, some have recommended providing 1 to 1.5 times the DRI for the first 3 months after transplantation.[110] This is due to the catabolic effect of surgery and glucocorticoid therapy, if steroids are provided. Should the posttransplant course be relatively unremarkable, reducing protein intake to the DRI after approximately 3 months is appropriate. With respect to fat intake, if hyperlipidemia develops, dietary modification of fat intake remains the first line of therapy. If patients have an insufficient result from dietary modification, pharmacologic intervention should be considered.

Recommendations for micronutrient intake after renal transplantation are also based on the recommended intake for healthy children, though there are some specific considerations. Multivitamin supplementation is generally not necessary after successful renal transplantation. When corticosteroids are used for immunosuppression, calcium intake should meet 100% of the DRI (see Appendix II, Table II-2). Supplementation may be necessary for those who are unable to achieve adequate dietary intake. Sodium restriction should be applied to patients who develop hypertension after transplantation. Hypertension after transplantation may result from corticosteroid and calcineurin inhibitor use and often improves or resolves as immunosuppressant doses are decreased to maintenance levels.

The most recent NAPRTCS data report that the 5-year graft survival for living donor and deceased donor renal transplantation are 85.1% and 76.9%, respectively.[47] Renal allograft function decreases over time due to many factors including acute rejection episodes, chronic rejection, and effects of nephrotoxic agents. If a child has a renal transplant with decreased function, nutritional therapy should be based on guidelines for nutrition in the setting of CRI.

SUMMARY

Acute and chronic disturbances of kidney function require a well-developed nutritional plan. Providing adequate and appropriate nutrition should be viewed as a critical element in the care of these children, as inadequate nutrition may negatively impact outcome, growth, and development. Alterations in renal function and clinical status during the disease course require repeated evaluations and adjustments of the nutritional care plan. If available, the assessment and counseling provided by a renal dietician is an indispensable resource for the child, caregivers, and clinicians.

REFERENCES

1. K/DOQI clinical practice guidelines for chronic kidney disease: Evaluation, classification, and stratification. Am J Kidney Dis 2002;39:S1–266.
2. Schwartz GJ, Haycock GB, Edelmann CM, Jr, Spitzer A. A simple estimate of glomerular filtration rate in children derived from body length and plasma creatinine. Pediatrics 1976;58:259–63.
3. Schwartz GJ, Feld LG, Langford DJ. A simple estimate of glomerular filtration rate in full-term infants during the first year of life. J Pediatr 1984;104:849–54.
4. Schwartz GJ, Gauthier B. A simple estimate of glomerular filtration rate in adolescent boys. J Pediatr 1985;106:522–6.
5. Springate JE, Christensen SL, Feld LG. Serum creatinine level and renal function in children. Am J Dis Child 1992;146:1232–5.
6. Seikaly MG, Browne R, Bajaj G, Arant BS, Jr. Limitations to body length/serum creatinine ratio as an estimate of glomerular filtration in children. Pediatr Nephrol 1996;10:709–11.
7. Hui-Stickle S, Brewer ED, Goldstein SL. Pediatric ARF epidemiology at a tertiary care center from 1999 to 2001. Am J Kidney Dis 2005;45:96–101.
8. Vachvanichsanong P, Dissaneewate P, Lim A, McNeil E. Childhood acute renal failure: 22-year experience in a university hospital in southern Thailand. Pediatrics 2006;118: e786–91.
9. Plotz FB, Hulst HE, Twisk JW, et al. Effect of acute renal failure on outcome in children with severe septic shock. Pediatr Nephrol 2005;20:1177–81.
10. Maxvold NJ, Smoyer WE, Gardner JJ, Bunchman TE. Management of acute renal failure in the pediatric patient: Hemofiltration versus hemodialysis. Am J Kidney Dis 1997;30:S84–8.
11. Zobel G, Ring E, Zobel V. Continuous arteriovenous renal replacement systems for critically ill children. Pediatr Nephrol 1989;3:140–3.
12. Fiaccadori E, Lombardi M, Leonardi S, et al. Prevalence and clinical outcome associated with preexisting malnutrition in acute renal failure: A prospective cohort study. J Am Soc Nephrol 1999;10:581–93.
13. Schneeweiss B, Graninger W, Stockenhuber F, et al. Energy metabolism in acute and chronic renal failure. Am J Clin Nutr 1990;52:596–601.
14. Maxvold NJ, Smoyer WE, Custer JR, Bunchman TE. Amino acid loss and nitrogen balance in critically ill children with acute renal failure: A prospective comparison between classic hemofiltration and hemofiltration with dialysis. Crit Care Med 2000;28:1161–5.
15. Soop M, Forsberg E, Thorne A, Alvestrand A. Energy expenditure in postoperative multiple organ failure with acute renal failure. Clin Nephrol 1989;31:139–45.
16. Marin A, Hardy G. Practical implications of nutritional support during continuous renal replacement therapy. Curr Opin Clin Nutr Metab Care 2001;4:219–25.
17. Druml W. Nutritional management of acute renal failure. J Ren Nutr 2005;15:63–70.
18. Druml W. Nutritional management of acute renal failure. Am J Kidney Dis 2001;37:S89–94.
19. Cianciaruso B, Bellizzi V, Napoli R, et al. Hepatic uptake and release of glucose, lactate, and amino acids in acutely uremic dogs. Metabolism 1991;40:261–9.
20. Stumvoll M, Chintalapudi U, Perriello G, et al. Uptake and release of glucose by the human kidney. Postabsorptive rates and responses to epinephrine. J Clin Invest 1995;96:2528–33.
21. May RC, Clark AS, Goheer MA, Mitch WE. Specific defects in insulin-mediated muscle metabolism in acute uremia. Kidney Int 1985;28:490–7.
22. Basi S, Pupim LB, Simmons EM, et al. Insulin resistance in critically ill patients with acute renal failure. Am J Physiol Renal Physiol 2005;289:F259–64.
23. Srinivasan V, Spinella PC, Drott HR, et al. Association of timing, duration, and intensity of hyperglycemia with intensive care unit mortality in critically ill children. Pediatr Crit Care Med 2004;5:329–36.
24. van den Berghe G, Wouters P, Weekers F, et al. Intensive insulin therapy in the critically ill patients. N Engl J Med 2001;345:1359–67.
25. Chima CS, Meyer L, Hummell AC, et al. Protein catabolic rate in patients with acute renal failure on continuous arteriovenous hemofiltration and total parenteral nutrition. J Am Soc Nephrol 1993;3:1516–21.
26. Macias WL, Alaka KJ, Murphy MH, et al. Impact of the nutritional regimen on protein catabolism and nitrogen balance in patients with acute renal failure. JPEN J Parenter Enteral Nutr 1996;20:56–62.
27. Kuttnig M, Zobel G, Ring E, et al. Nitrogen and amino acid balance during total parenteral nutrition and continuous arteriovenous hemofiltration in critically ill anuric children. Child Nephrol Urol 1991;11:74–8.
28. Mendley SR, Majkowski NL. Urea and nitrogen excretion in pediatric peritoneal dialysis patients. Kidney Int 2000;58:2564–70.
29. Ikizler TA, Flakoll PJ, Parker RA, Hakim RM. Amino acid and albumin losses during hemodialysis. Kidney Int 1994;46:830–7.
30. Hynote ED, McCamish MA, Depner TA, Davis PA. Amino acid losses during hemodialysis: Effects of high-solute flux and parenteral nutrition in acute renal failure. JPEN J Parenter Enteral Nutr 1995;19:15–21.
31. Quan A, Baum M. Protein losses in children on continuous cycler peritoneal dialysis. Pediatr Nephrol 1996;10:728–31.
32. Abitbol CL, Rossique M, Rios M, editors. Nutritional support of the pediatric patient with acute renal failure. In: American Society of Parenteral and Enteral Nutrition. The A.S.P.E.N. Nutrition Support Practice Manual. Silver Spring, MD: American Society of Parenteral and Enteral Nutrition; 2005. p. 287–95.
33. Nakamura AT, Btaiche IF, Pasko DA, et al. In vitro clearance of trace elements via continuous renal replacement therapy. J Ren Nutr 2004;14:214–9.
34. Wooley JA, Btaiche IF, Good KL. Metabolic and nutritional aspects of acute renal failure in critically ill patients requiring continuous renal replacement therapy. Nutr Clin Pract 2005;20:176–91.
35. Story DA, Ronco C, Bellomo R. Trace element and vitamin concentrations and losses in critically ill patients treated with continuous venovenous hemofiltration. Crit Care Med 1999;27:220–3.
36. Berger MM, Shenkin A, Revelly JP, et al. Copper, selenium, zinc, and thiamine balances during continuous venovenous hemodiafiltration in critically ill patients. Am J Clin Nutr 2004;80:410–6.
37. Druml W, Schwarzenhofer M, Apsner R, Horl WH. Fat-soluble vitamins in patients with acute renal failure. Miner Electrolyte Metab 1998;24:220–6.
38. de Lucas C, Moreno M, Lopez-Herce J, et al. Transpyloric enteral nutrition reduces the complication rate and cost in the critically ill child. J Pediatr Gastroenterol Nutr 2000;30:175–80.
39. Major K, Lefor AT, Wilson M. Route of nutrition support. Nutrition 2002;18:445–6.
40. Jolliet P, Pichard C, Biolo G, et al. Enteral nutrition in intensive care patients: A practical approach. Working Group on Nutrition and Metabolism, ESICM. European Society of Intensive Care Medicine. Intensive Care Med 1998;24:848–59.
41. Guidelines for the use of parenteral and enteral nutrition in adult and pediatric patients. JPEN J Parenter Enteral Nutr 2002;26:1SA–138SA.
42. Moore FA, Feliciano DV, Andrassy RJ, et al. Early enteral feeding, compared with parenteral, reduces postoperative septic complications. The results of a meta-analysis. Ann Surg 1992;216:172–83.
43. Chellis MJ, Sanders SV, Webster H, et al. Early enteral feeding in the pediatric intensive care unit. JPEN J Parenter Enteral Nutr 1996;20:71–3.
44. Fiaccadori E, Maggiore U, Giacosa R, et al. Enteral nutrition in patients with acute renal failure. Kidney Int 2004;65:999–1008.
45. Lopez-Herce J, Sanchez C, Carrillo A, et al. Transpyloric enteral nutrition in the critically ill child with renal failure. Intensive Care Med 2006;32:1599–605.
46. Sanchez C, Lopez-Herce J, Carrillo A, et al. Early transpyloric enteral nutrition in critically ill children. Nutrition 2007;23:16–22.

47. North American Pediatric Renal Trials and Collaborative Studies. NAPRTCS 2006 Annual Report. North American Pediatric Renal Trials and Collaborative Studies, 2006.
48. Hogg RJ, Furth S, Lemley KV, et al. National Kidney Foundation's Kidney Disease Outcomes Quality Initiative clinical practice guidelines for chronic kidney disease in children and adolescents: Evaluation, classification, and stratification. Pediatrics 2003;111:1416–21.
49. Fivush BA, Jabs K, Neu AM, et al. Chronic renal insufficiency in children and adolescents: The 1996 annual report of NAPRTCS. North American Pediatric Renal Transplant Cooperative Study. Pediatr Nephrol 1998;12:328–37.
50. Lewy JE. Treatment of children in the U.S. with end-stage renal disease (ESRD). Med Arh 2001;55:201–2.
51. Seikaly MG, Ho PL, Emmett L, et al. Chronic renal insufficiency in children: The 2001 Annual Report of the NAPRTCS. Pediatr Nephrol 2003;18:796–804.
52. Seikaly MG, Salhab N, Gipson D, et al. Stature in children with chronic kidney disease: Analysis of NAPRTCS database. Pediatr Nephrol 2006;21:793–9.
53. Karlberg J, Schaefer F, Hennicke M, et al. Early age-dependent growth impairment in chronic renal failure. European Study Group for Nutritional Treatment of Chronic Renal Failure in Childhood. Pediatr Nephrol 1996;10:283–7.
54. Abitbol CL, Zilleruelo G, Montane B, Strauss J. Growth of uremic infants on forced feeding regimens. Pediatr Nephrol 1993;7:173–7.
55. Simmons JM, Wilson CJ, Potter DE, Holliday MA. Relation of calorie deficiency to growth failure in children on hemodialysis and the growth response to calorie supplementation. N Engl J Med 1971;285:653–6.
56. Holliday MA. Calorie deficiency in children with uremia: Effect upon growth. Pediatrics 1972;50:590–7.
57. Clinical practice guidelines for nutrition in chronic renal failure. K/DOQI, National Kidney Foundation. Am J Kidney Dis 2000;35:S1–140.
58. Avram MM, Mittman N, Bonomini L, et al. Markers for survival in dialysis: A seven-year prospective study. Am J Kidney Dis 1995;26:209–19.
59. Iseki K, Uehara H, Nishime K, et al. Impact of the initial levels of laboratory variables on survival in chronic dialysis patients. Am J Kidney Dis 1996;28:541–8.
60. Owen WF, Jr, Lew NL, Liu Y, et al. The urea reduction ratio and serum albumin concentration as predictors of mortality in patients undergoing hemodialysis. N Engl J Med 1993;329:1001–6.
61. Wong CS, Hingorani S, Gillen DL, et al. Hypoalbuminemia and risk of death in pediatric patients with end-stage renal disease. Kidney Int 2002;61:630–7.
62. Wong CS, Gipson DS, Gillen DL, et al. Anthropometric measures and risk of death in children with end-stage renal disease. Am J Kidney Dis 2000;36:811–9.
63. Furth SL, Hwang W, Yang C, et al. Growth failure, risk of hospitalization and death for children with end-stage renal disease. Pediatr Nephrol 2002;17:450–5.
64. Ratsch IM, Catassi C, Verrina E, et al. Energy and nutrient intake of patients with mild-to-moderate chronic renal failure compared with healthy children: An Italian multicentre study. Eur J Pediatr 1992;151:701–5.
65. Orejas G, Santos F, Malaga S, et al. Nutritional status of children with moderate chronic renal failure. Pediatr Nephrol 1995;9:52–6.
66. Foreman JW, Abitbol CL, Trachtman H, et al. Nutritional intake in children with renal insufficiency: A report of the growth failure in children with renal diseases study. J Am Coll Nutr 1996;15:579–85.
67. Norman LJ, Coleman JE, Macdonald IA, et al. Nutrition and growth in relation to severity of renal disease in children. Pediatr Nephrol 2000;15:259–65.
68. Mak RH, Cheung W, Cone RD, Marks DL. Orexigenic and anorexigenic mechanisms in the control of nutrition in chronic kidney disease. Pediatr Nephrol 2005;20: 427–31.
69. Mak RH, Cheung W, Cone RD, Marks DL. Leptin and inflammation-associated cachexia in chronic kidney disease. Kidney Int 2006;69:794–7.
70. Rees L, Shaw V. Nutrition in children with CRF and on dialysis. Pediatr Nephrol 2007.
71. Cumin F, Baum HP, de Gasparo M, Levens N. Removal of endogenous leptin from the circulation by the kidney. Int J Obes Relat Metab Disord 1997;21:495–504.
72. Stenvinkel P, Pecoits-Filho R, Lindholm B. Leptin, ghrelin, and proinflammatory cytokines: Compounds with nutritional impact in chronic kidney disease? Adv Ren Replace Ther 2003;10:332–45.
73. Herbelin A, Nguyen AT, Zingraff J, et al. Influence of uremia and hemodialysis on circulating interleukin-1 and tumor necrosis factor alpha. Kidney Int 1990;37:116–25.
74. Ruley EJ, Bock GH, Kerzner B, et al. Feeding disorders and gastroesophageal reflux in infants with chronic renal failure. Pediatr Nephrol 1989;3:424–9.
75. Brewer ED. Growth of small children managed with chronic peritoneal dialysis and nasogastric tube feedings: 203-month experience in 14 patients. Adv Perit Dial 1990;6:269–72.
76. Ledermann SE, Shaw V, Trompeter RS. Long-term enteral nutrition in infants and young children with chronic renal failure. Pediatr Nephrol 1999;13:870–5.
77. Kari JA, Gonzalez C, Ledermann SE, et al. Outcome and growth of infants with severe chronic renal failure. Kidney Int 2000;57:1681–7.
78. Ledermann SE, Scanes ME, Fernando ON, et al. Long-term outcome of peritoneal dialysis in infants. J Pediatr 2000;136:24–9.
79. Claris-Appiani A, Ardissino GL, Dacco V, et al. Catch-up growth in children with chronic renal failure treated with long-term enteral nutrition. JPEN J Parenter Enteral Nutr 1995;19:175–8.
80. Strife CF, Quinlan M, Mears K, et al. Improved growth of three uremic children by nocturnal nasogastric feedings. Am J Dis Child 1986;140:438–43.
81. Parekh RS, Flynn JT, Smoyer WE, et al. Improved growth in young children with severe chronic renal insufficiency who use specified nutritional therapy. J Am Soc Nephrol 2001;12:2418–26.
82. Reed EE, Roy LP, Gaskin KJ, Knight JF. Nutritional intervention and growth in children with chronic renal failure. J Ren Nutr 1998;8:122–6.
83. Ramage IJ, Geary DF, Harvey E, et al. Efficacy of gastrostomy feeding in infants and older children receiving chronic peritoneal dialysis. Perit Dial Int 1999;19:231–6.
84. Ellis EN, Yiu V, Harley F, et al. The impact of supplemental feeding in young children on dialysis: A report of the North American Pediatric Renal Transplant Cooperative Study. Pediatr Nephrol 2001;16:404–8.
85. Roelfsema V, Clark RG. The growth hormone and insulin-like growth factor axis: Its manipulation for the benefit of growth disorders in renal failure. J Am Soc Nephrol 2001;12:1297–306.
86. Fine RN, Attie KM, Kuntze J, et al. Recombinant human growth hormone in infants and young children with chronic renal insufficiency. Genentech Collaborative Study Group. Pediatr Nephrol 1995;9:451–7.
87. Hokken-Koelega A, Mulder P, De Jong R, et al. Long-term effects of growth hormone treatment on growth and puberty in patients with chronic renal insufficiency. Pediatr Nephrol 2000;14:701–6.
88. Haffner D, Schaefer F, Nissel R, et al. Effect of growth hormone treatment on the adult height of children with chronic renal failure. German Study Group for Growth Hormone Treatment in Chronic Renal Failure. N Engl J Med 2000;343:923–30.
89. Mahan JD, Warady BA. Assessment and treatment of short stature in pediatric patients with chronic kidney disease: A consensus statement. Pediatr Nephrol 2006;21:917–30.
90. Locatelli F, Fouque D, Heimburger O, et al. Nutritional status in dialysis patients: A European consensus. Nephrol Dial Transplant 2002;17:563–72.
91. Rashid R, Neill E, Smith W, et al. Body composition and nutritional intake in children with chronic kidney disease. Pediatr Nephrol 2006;21:1730–8.
92. Foster BJ, Leonard MB. Measuring nutritional status in children with chronic kidney disease. Am J Clin Nutr 2004;80:801–14.
93. Abitbol CL, Warady BA, Massie MD, et al. Linear growth and anthropometric and nutritional measurements in children with mild to moderate renal insufficiency: A report of the Growth Failure in Children with Renal Diseases Study. J Pediatr 1990;116:S46–54.
94. Betts PR, Magrath G. Growth pattern and dietary intake of children with chronic renal insufficiency. Br Med J 1974;2:189–93.
95. Watson AR, Coleman JE, Warady BA. When and how to use nasogastric and gastrostomy feedings for nutritional support in infants and children on CAPD/CCPD. In: Fine RN, Alexander SR, Warady BA, editors. CAPD/CCPD in Children. Boston, MA: Kluwer Academic Publishers; 1998. p. 281–300.
96. Coleman JE. Supplemental tube feedings. In: Warady BA, Alexander SR, Fine RN, editors. Pediatric Dialysis. Boston, MA: Kluwer Academic Publishers; 2004.
97. Dello Strologo L, Principato F, Sinibaldi D, et al. Feeding dysfunction in infants with severe chronic renal failure after long-term nasogastric tube feeding. Pediatr Nephrol 1997;11:84–6.
98. Schauster H, Dwyer J. Transition from tube feedings to feedings by mouth in children: Preventing eating dysfunction. J Am Diet Assoc 1996;96:277–81.
99. Yiu V, Harmon WE, Spinozzi N, et al. High-calorie nutrition for infants with chronic renal disease. J Ren Nutr 1996;6:203–6.
100. Ikizler TA, Hakim RM. Nutrition in end-stage renal disease. Kidney Int 1996;50:343–57.
101. Wolfson M. Nutritional management of the continuous ambulatory peritoneal dialysis patient. Am J Kidney Dis 1996;27:744–9.
102. Salusky IB, Fine RN, Nelson P, et al. Nutritional status of children undergoing continuous ambulatory peritoneal dialysis. Am J Clin Nutr 1983;38:599–611.
103. Motomura K, Okuda S, Sanai T, et al. Importance of early initiation of dietary protein restriction for the prevention of experimental progressive renal disease. Nephron 1988;49:144–9.
104. Baudoin P, Provoost AP. Effects of age at the time of unilateral nephrectomy and dietary protein on long-term renal function in rats. Pediatr Nephrol 1993;7:536–42.
105. Klahr S, Levey AS, Beck GJ, et al. The effects of dietary protein restriction and blood-pressure control on the progression of chronic renal disease. Modification of Diet in Renal Disease Study Group. N Engl J Med 1994;330: 877–84.
106. D'Amico G, Gentile MG, Fellin G, et al. Effect of dietary protein restriction on the progression of renal failure: A prospective randomized trial. Nephrol Dial Transplant 1994;9:1590–4.
107. Rosman JB, Langer K, Brandl M, et al. Protein-restricted diets in chronic renal failure: A four year follow-up shows limited indications. Kidney Int Suppl 1989;27:S96–102.
108. Rosman JB, Ter Wee PM, Meijer S, et al. Prospective randomised trial of early dietary protein restriction in chronic renal failure. Lancet 1984;2:1291–6.
109. Wingen AM, Fabian-Bach C, Schaefer F, Mehls O. Randomised multicentre study of a low-protein diet on the progression of chronic renal failure in children. European Study Group of Nutritional Treatment of Chronic Renal Failure in Childhood. Lancet 1997;349:1117–23.
110. Rock J, Secker DJ. Nutrition management of chronic kidney disease in the pediatric patient. In: Byham-Gray L, Wiesen K, editors. A Clinical Guide to Nutrition Care in Kidney Disease. Chicago, IL: American Dietetic Association; 2004. p. 127–49.
111. Kopanati S, Baum M, Quan A. Peritoneal protein losses in children with steroid-resistant nephrotic syndrome on continuous-cycler peritoneal dialysis. Pediatr Nephrol 2006;21:1013–9.
112. Kriley M, Warady BA. Vitamin status of pediatric patients receiving long-term peritoneal dialysis. Am J Clin Nutr 1991;53:1476–9.
113. Warady BA, Kriley M, Alon U, Hellerstein S. Vitamin status of infants receiving long-term peritoneal dialysis. Pediatr Nephrol 1994;8:354–6.
114. Pereira AM, Hamani N, Nogueira PC, Carvalhaes JT. Oral vitamin intake in children receiving long-term dialysis. J Ren Nutr 2000;10:24–9.
115. Doireau V, Macher MA, Brun P, et al. Vitamin A poisoning revealed by hypercalcemia in a child with kidney failure. Arch Pediatr 1996;3:888–90.
116. Pru C, Eaton J, Kjellstrand C. Vitamin C intoxication and hyperoxalemia in chronic hemodialysis patients. Nephron 1985;39:112–6.
117. Norman ME, Mazur AT, Borden St, et al. Early diagnosis of juvenile renal osteodystrophy. J Pediatr 1980;97:226–32.
118. National Kidney Foundation. K/DOQI Clinical practice guidelines for bone metabolism and disease in children with chronic kidney disease. Available at: http://www.kidney.org/professionals/KDOQI/guidelines_pedbone/index.htm (Accessed July 12, 2007).
119. Salusky IB. Are new vitamin D analogues in renal bone disease superior to calcitriol? Pediatr Nephrol 2005;20:393–8.
120. Slatopolsky E, Dusso A, Brown A. New analogs of vitamin D_3. Kidney Int Suppl 1999;73:S46–51.
121. Greenbaum LA, Benador N, Goldstein SL, et al. Intravenous paricalcitol for treatment of secondary hyperparathyroidism in children on hemodialysis. Am J Kidney Dis 2007;49:814–23.
122. Seeherunvong W, Nwobi O, Abitbol CL, et al. Paricalcitol versus calcitriol treatment for hyperparathyroidism in pediatric hemodialysis patients. Pediatr Nephrol 2006;21:1434–9.
123. Goodman WG, Ramirez JA, Belin TR, et al. Development of adynamic bone in patients with secondary hyperparathyroidism after intermittent calcitriol therapy. Kidney Int 1994;46:1160–6.
124. Erslev AJ. Erythropoietin. N Engl J Med 1991;324:1339–44.
125. KDOQI; National Kidney Foundation, III. Clinical practice recommendations for anemia in chronic kidney disease in children. Am J Kidney Dis 2006;47:S86–108.

126. Chauveau P, Chadefaux B, Coude M, et al. Hyperhomocysteinemia, a risk factor for atherosclerosis in chronic uremic patients. Kidney Int Suppl 1993;41:S72–7.
127. Robinson K, Gupta A, Dennis V, et al. Hyperhomocysteinemia confers an independent increased risk of atherosclerosis in end-stage renal disease and is closely linked to plasma folate and pyridoxine concentrations. Circulation 1996;94:2743–8.
128. Poyrazoglu HM, Dusunsel R, Yikilmaz A, et al. Carotid artery thickness in children and young adults with end stage renal disease. Pediatr Nephrol 2007;22:109–16.
129. Merouani A, Lambert M, Delvin EE, et al. Plasma homocysteine concentration in children with chronic renal failure. Pediatr Nephrol 2001;16:805–11.
130. Schroder CH, de Boer AW, Giesen AM, et al. Treatment of hyperhomocysteinemia in children on dialysis by folic acid. Pediatr Nephrol 1999;13:583–5.
131. Salusky IB, Foley J, Nelson P, Goodman WG. Aluminum accumulation during treatment with aluminum hydroxide and dialysis in children and young adults with chronic renal disease. N Engl J Med 1991;324:527–31.
132. Sedman AB, Miller NL, Warady BA, et al. Aluminum loading in children with chronic renal failure. Kidney Int 1984;26:201–4.
133. Sedman AB, Wilkening GN, Warady BA, et al. Encephalopathy in childhood secondary to aluminum toxicity. J Pediatr 1984;105:836–8.
134. Goodman WG, Goldin J, Kuizon BD, et al. Coronary-artery calcification in young adults with end-stage renal disease who are undergoing dialysis. N Engl J Med 2000;342:1478–83.
135. Pieper AK, Haffner D, Hoppe B, et al. A randomized cross-over trial comparing sevelamer with calcium acetate in children with CKD. Am J Kidney Dis 2006;47:625–35.
136. Salusky IB, Goodman WG, Sahney S, et al. Sevelamer controls parathyroid hormone-induced bone disease as efficiently as calcium carbonate without increasing serum calcium levels during therapy with active vitamin D sterols. J Am Soc Nephrol 2005;16:2501–8.
137. Mahdavi H, Kuizon BD, Gales B, et al. Sevelamer hydrochloride: An effective phosphate binder in dialyzed children. Pediatr Nephrol 2003;18:1260–4.
138. McElhiney LF. Sevelamer suspension in children with end stage renal disease. Int J Pharm Compound 2007;11:20–4.
139. Bunchman TE, Wood EG, Schenck MH, et al. Pretreatment of formula with sodium polystyrene sulfonate to reduce dietary potassium intake. Pediatr Nephrol 1991;5:29–32.
140. Rivard AL, Raup SM, Beilman GJ. Sodium polystyrene sulfonate used to reduce the potassium content of a high-protein enteral formula: A quantitative analysis. JPEN J Parenter Enteral Nutr 2004;28:76–8.
141. Bunchman TE. Chronic dialysis in the infant less than 1 year of age. Pediatr Nephrol 1995;9:S18–22.
142. Tejani A, Fine R, Alexander S, et al. Factors predictive of sustained growth in children after renal transplantation. The North American Pediatric Renal Transplant Cooperative Study. J Pediatr 1993;122:397–402.
143. Fine RN, Ho M, Tejani A. The contribution of renal transplantation to final adult height: A report of the North American Pediatric Renal Transplant Cooperative Study (NAPRTCS). Pediatr Nephrol 2001;16:951–6.
144. Harmon WE, Jabs K. Factors affecting growth after renal transplantation. J Am Soc Nephrol 1992;2:S295–303.
145. Vidhun JR, Sarwal MM. Corticosteroid avoidance in pediatric renal transplantation. Pediatr Nephrol 2005;20:418–26.
146. Sarwal MM, Vidhun JR, Alexander SR, et al. Continued superior outcomes with modification and lengthened follow-up of a steroid-avoidance pilot with extended daclizumab induction in pediatric renal transplantation. Transplantation 2003;76:1331–9.
147. Jabs K, Van Dop C, Harmon WE. Growth hormone treatment of growth failure among children with renal transplants. Kidney Int Suppl 1993;43:S71–5.
148. Ulinski T, Cochat P. Longitudinal growth in children following kidney transplantation: From conservative to pharmacological strategies. Pediatr Nephrol 2006;21:903–9.
149. Fine RN, Stablein D. Long-term use of recombinant human growth hormone in pediatric allograft recipients: A report of the NAPRTCS Transplant Registry. Pediatr Nephrol 2005;20:404–8.
150. Ong CS, Pollock CA, Caterson RJ, et al. Hyperlipidemia in renal transplant recipients: Natural history and response to treatment. Medicine (Baltimore) 1994;73:215–23.
151. Satterthwaite R, Aswad S, Sunga V, et al. Incidence of new-onset hypercholesterolemia in renal transplant patients treated with FK506 or cyclosporine. Transplantation 1998;65:446–9.
152. Kasiske BL. Risk factors for accelerated atherosclerosis in renal transplant recipients. Am J Med 1988;84:985–92.
153. Silverstein DM, Palmer J, Polinsky MS, et al. Risk factors for hyperlipidemia in long-term pediatric renal transplant recipients. Pediatr Nephrol 2000;14:105–10.
154. Silverstein DM. Risk factors for cardiovascular disease in pediatric renal transplant recipients. Pediatr Transplant 2004;8:386–93.
155. Parekh RS, Carroll CE, Wolfe RA, Port FK. Cardiovascular mortality in children and young adults with end-stage kidney disease. J Pediatr 2002;141:191–7.
156. Roodnat JI, Mulder PG, Zietse R, et al. Cholesterol as an independent predictor of outcome after renal transplantation. Transplantation 2000;69:1704–10.
157. Massy ZA, Guijarro C, Wiederkehr MR, et al. Chronic renal allograft rejection: Immunologic and nonimmunologic risk factors. Kidney Int 1996;49:518–24.
158. Lowry RP, Soltys G, Mangel R, et al. Type II hyperlipoproteinemia, hyperapobetalipoproteinemia, and hyperalphalipoproteinemia following renal transplantation: Prevalence and precipitating factors. Transplant Proc 1987;19:2229–32.
159. Butani L. Prospective monitoring of lipid profiles in children receiving pravastatin preemptively after renal transplantation. Pediatr Transplant 2005;9:746–53.
160. Vathsala A, Weinberg RB, Schoenberg L, et al. Lipid abnormalities in cyclosporine-prednisone-treated renal transplant recipients. Transplantation 1989;48:37–43.
161. Kuster GM, Drexel H, Bleisch JA, et al. Relation of cyclosporine blood levels to adverse effects on lipoproteins. Transplantation 1994;57:1479–83.
162. Markell MS, Armenti V, Danovitch G, Sumrani N. Hyperlipidemia and glucose intolerance in the post-renal transplant patient. J Am Soc Nephrol 1994;4:S37–47.
163. Ponticelli C, MacDonald AS, Rajagopalan P, et al. Phase III trial of Rapamune versus placebo in primary renal allograft recipients. Transplant Proc 2001;33:2271–2.
164. Hocker B, Feneberg R, Kopf S, et al. SRL-based immunosuppression vs CNI minimization in pediatric renal transplant recipients with chronic CNI nephrotoxicity. Pediatr Transplant 2006;10:593–601.
165. Pirsch JD, Miller J, Deierhoi MH, et al. A comparison of tacrolimus (FK506) and cyclosporine for immunosuppression after cadaveric renal transplantation. FK506 Kidney Transplant Study Group. Transplantation 1997;63:977–83.
166. Ferraris JR, Ghezzi L, Waisman G, Krmar RT. Potential cardiovascular risk factors in paediatric renal transplant recipients. Pediatr Nephrol 2006;21:119–25.
167. Milliner DS, Morgenstern BZ, Murphy M, et al. Lipid levels following renal transplantation in pediatric recipients. Transplant Proc 1994;26:112–4.
168. Delucchi A, Marin V, Trabucco G, et al. Dyslipidemia and dietary modification in Chilean renal pediatric transplantation. Transplant Proc 2001;33:1297–301.
169. Butani L, Pai MV, Makker SP. Pilot study describing the use of pravastatin in pediatric renal transplant recipients. Pediatr Transplant 2003;7:179–84.
170. Krmar RT, Ferraris JR, Ramirez JA, et al. Use of atorvastatin in hyperlipidemic hypertensive renal transplant recipients. Pediatr Nephrol 2002;17:540–3.
171. Argent E, Kainer G, Aitken M, et al. Atorvastatin treatment for hyperlipidemia in pediatric renal transplant recipients. Pediatr Transplant 2003;7:38–42.
172. Trompeter R, Filler G, Webb NJ, et al. Randomized trial of tacrolimus versus cyclosporin microemulsion in renal transplantation. Pediatr Nephrol 2002;17:141–9.
173. Greenspan LC, Gitelman SE, Leung MA, et al. Increased incidence in post-transplant diabetes mellitus in children: A case-control analysis. Pediatr Nephrol 2002;17:1–5.
174. El-Husseini AA, Foda MA, Osman YM, Sobh MA. Characteristics of long-term live-donor pediatric renal transplant survivors: A single-center experience. Pediatr Transplant 2006;10:288–93.
175. Ruiz JO, Simmons RL, Callender CO, et al. Steroid diabetes in renal transplant recipients: Pathogenetic factors and prognosis. Surgery 1973;73:759–65.
176. Nielsen JH, Mandrup-Poulsen T, Nerup J. Direct effects of cyclosporin A on human pancreatic beta-cells. Diabetes 1986;35:1049–52.
177. Carroll PB, Boschero AC, Li MY, et al. Effect of the immunosuppressant FK506 on glucose-induced insulin secretion from adult rat islets of Langerhans. Transplantation 1991;51:275–8.
178. Mayer AD, Dmitrewski J, Squifflet JP, et al. Multicenter randomized trial comparing tacrolimus (FK506) and cyclosporine in the prevention of renal allograft rejection: A report of the European Tacrolimus Multicenter Renal Study Group. Transplantation 1997;64:436–43.
179. Al-Uzri A, Stablein DM, A Cohn R. Posttransplant diabetes mellitus in pediatric renal transplant recipients: A report of the North American Pediatric Renal Transplant Cooperative Study (NAPRTCS). Transplantation 2001;72:1020–4.
180. Filler G, Webb NJ, Milford DV, et al. Four-year data after pediatric renal transplantation: A randomized trial of tacrolimus vs. cyclosporin microemulsion. Pediatr Transplant 2005;9:498–503.
181. Hanevold CD, Ho PL, Talley L, Mitsnefes MM. Obesity and renal transplant outcome: A report of the North American Pediatric Renal Transplant Cooperative Study. Pediatrics 2005;115:352–6.

48

Inflammatory Bowel Disease

Robert Heuschkel, MB, BS, MRCPCH

INTRODUCTION

From the earliest clinical descriptions of children with Crohn's disease (CD), it was clear that significant undernutrition is a major feature of the disease. Furthermore, growth retardation, which may have a nutritional component, is a common clinical manifestation. While on occasion undernutrition and short stature may be a feature of chronic ulcerative colitis (UC) in children, these manifestations are less prominent in this disease.

Early reports of nutritional therapy in children with inflammatory bowel disease (IBD) were thus aimed at the restoration of normal nutrition. More recently a body of evidence has shown that in children with CD nutritional therapy has a specific anti-inflammatory action in addition to its ability to restore their nutritional status to normal. Unfortunately there is no such firm evidence in children with UC, yet here also the provision of adequate nutrition still remains important.

The value of nutritional therapy in CD chiefly centers upon the use of exclusive enteral nutrition (EEN) in the treatment of active disease. Enteral nutrition may be defined as the provision of a liquid formula diet by mouth or by tube into the gastrointestinal tract.[1] Bottle feeding of normal infants is excluded from this definition. While it is now clear that oral feeding may be highly effective, research began with liquid formulas administered by intragastric tubes. The technique of tube feeding goes back at least as far as 1872, with a report by Clouston in the Lancet on "Forcible Feeding,"[2] while the work of Elsie Widowson (1947) drew attention to the adverse effect of malnutrition upon human disease in general.[3] The advent of effective parenteral nutrition then made clinicians aware how dramatic the benefits of nutritional rehabilitation from malnutrition could be. The development of a range of complete formula diets of varying compositions, designed for a range of situations, has now made enteral nutrition a highly desirable and practical alternative to parenteral nutrition.

It was Giorgini and colleagues in 1973 who first suggested that treatment of malnutrition could lead to resolution of inflammation in a child with CD.[4] They described resolution of terminal ileal inflammation on barium follow-through after a period of elemental diet. In adults with CD, Logan and colleagues produced evidence that protein and lymphocyte loss from the gut decreased during feeding with an elemental diet.[5] Then in Quebec, Moran and colleagues described four children with CD whose growth failure responded to an elemental diet[6] and this was confirmed in larger studies.[7,8] In France, an elemental diet was given to children with CD by continuous nasogastric infusion. This was called constant rate enteral alimentation (CREN), but was a cumbersome technique not popular with the children. They used a complex regimen using oligopeptides, whereas others reported the use of a high-osmolality amino acid-based elemental formula. At St. Bartholomew's Hospital in London a semielemental diet using extensively hydrolyzed milk protein given intragastrically was shown in a small study to be as effective as conventional steroids in the induction of a clinical remission.[9] Most importantly though this study showed there was no short-term growth while on steroid therapy, whereas enteral nutrition lead to short-term growth acceleration. In subsequent follow-up studies it was shown that this could on occasion be sustained for sometime if the child remained in remission even when back on a normal diet after the period of nutritional therapy.[10] Central to this approach to therapy was the concept of a period of 6 to 8 weeks of enteral nutrition followed by a graded return to a normal diet.

ROLE OF DIET IN ETIOLOGY OF IBD

The etiology of IBD remains one of the greatest challenges in gastroenterology today. The presence of unexplained gut inflammation has inevitably led researchers to try and identify factors in our diet that may trigger, or even cause, IBD. While it appears highly likely that there are several environmental factors involved in the etiopathogenesis of IBD,[11,12] the evidence that some of these may be dietary remains tempting.

It was initially suggested that the adoption of an urban lifestyle may lead to an increase in the incidence of IBD, with increases occurring much more rapidly than could be explained by genetic factors alone.[13,14]

Patients with a recent diagnosis of CD have been shown to consume greater quantities of sucrose than control groups,[15] although this was not confirmed in patients with UC.[16] Whether or not a diet low in fiber leads to an increased risk of CD remains disputed.[17] Many of these studies have had methodological problems and as a result make it difficult to confirm that dietary differences antedated the development of disease. Reif and colleagues,[18] however, again showed that a high level of sucrose intake (>92 g/d) occurred before symptom onset in patients with both UC and CD (OR: 5.3 and 2.8, respectively), in contrast, fructose and fiber consumption were both negatively associated with a risk for IBD. This carefully controlled study also reported an increase in fat consumption prior to a diagnosis of IBD. These findings were mirrored by Geerling and colleagues[19] who reported an increased risk of developing UC in those with a high consumption of monounsaturated and polyunsaturated (mainly n-6 PUFA) fats as well as Vitamin B6. Overall, these findings suggest no more than that a low residue; highly refined diet is associated with the development of IBD, while a high-fiber diet, rich in fruit and vegetables, may be more protective. Large, prospective epidemiological studies will be necessary to adequately control for the many confounding variables that could affect this type of data.

Conflicting evidence is also available on the role of butyrate in the pathogenesis of UC. Data suggest that butyrate levels decrease in the distal colon,[20] with the ability of colonic mucosa to utilize butyrate being reduced even in macroscopically "normal" mucosa of patients with quiescent UC.[21] However, the response of distal UC and so-called diversion colitis to butyrate enemas has not been striking.[22,23] Dietary sulfates have been implicated in reducing the ability of colonocytes to utilize butyrate by their conversion to toxic sulfides like H_2S,[24] although luminal levels of sulfides do not appear to be significantly higher in patients with UC than in normal controls.[25] However, along with a putative role of oxidant injury in the pathogenesis of UC, all these mechanisms appear more likely to be involved as mediators of the injury in UC, rather than primary etiological factors.

It is also of note that researchers have been accumulating evidence over a number of years implicating the food borne pathogen *Mycobacterium avium* subsp. *paratuberculosis* in the pathogenesis of CD. while a detailed discussion of this is beyond the scope of this chapter, the presence of this organism in the food chain and its persistence in milk despite pasteurization, along with the characteristic Th1 immune response it evokes, continue to hold interest.[26] However, well-controlled clinical trials have failed to show any benefit of anti-tuberculous therapy.[27] Larger, population-based cohort studies are still needed to better define the importance of this and other specific dietary risk factors.

NUTRITIONAL COMPLICATIONS OF IBD

The chronic and relapsing nature of intestinal inflammation inevitably impacts on a patient's nutritional status. However, their nutritional state is not only determined by the dietary intake, but also by the patient's age, type of disease, disease distribution as well as their disease activity. These factors all contribute to the wide range of nutritional complications seen; from almost none in a child with mild distal UC, to the most severe nutritional consequences of chronically active disease in a child with pan-enteric CD. Nutritional complications are rarer in children with UC, although a severe pancolitis may present with acute weight loss and significant iron-deficiency anemia.

Caloric Deficiency and Growth Failure

The mechanisms surrounding the anorexia and undernutrition seen in IBD are complex and still poorly understood. As well as food avoidance as a result of abdominal pain or diarrhea, the reduction in caloric intake is due to the consequences of the systemic inflammatory response.[28] Protein-energy malnutrition may occur as a result of unchecked disease activity, with the associated anorexia being largely mediated by the proinflammatory cytokines IL-1 and TNF. Activity of these cytokines leads to lean tissue loss,[29] reduced voluntary motor activity,[30] and protein synthesis, with a concomitant increase in protein catabolism.[31] This state of increased need may not be met during active inflammation, and thus leads to chronic undernutrition. Winter and colleagues elegantly demonstrated the recovery of impaired pancreatic and gastric secretory activity with increasing body mass index (BMI) in severely malnourished (BMI ~ 14) adults with CD.[32] Protein intakes up to 1.5 g/kg body weight may be required per day to achieve adequate nutrition, with excessive supplementation perhaps even being counterproductive during the acute inflammatory state.[33] Increased protein oxidation and worsening of the nitrogen balance may result if overfeeding occurs during inflammation.[34] Calorie intake in children with CD cannot be accurately determined by using estimates of average requirements (EARs), as four in five children will consume about 120% of EAR (range 100 to 149%) while taking EEN as primary therapy at diagnosis.[35] Only the initial BMI was a predictor of subsequent weight gain on EEN, with a median of 11% being achieved over an 8-week course of treatment. Other authors have reported the intake in active disease to be 43 to 82% of recommended values, yet with adequate calorie supplementation, improvements in linear growth can be achieved.[36–38] However, simple nutritional restitution may be insufficient to achieve adequate growth, suggesting that other factors are also important in mediating growth retardation.[39] An elegant study by Azcue and colleagues[40] demonstrated an inappropriately maintained resting energy expenditure (REE) in children with moderately active CD when compared to children with anorexia nervosa and similar degrees of malnutrition. This relative increase in energy expenditure, together with the voluntary reduction in intake, further compromises nutritional status and hence optimal growth. Careful animal experiments, which did not look at body composition, suggest that it is the reduced caloric intake that is largely responsible for the weight loss seen in active colitis. However, in this animal study, while able to restore calorie intake and body weight to normal, nutritional supplementation was unable to restore linear growth. At least in this animal model, 30 to 40% of growth impairment is likely to be a direct result of the inflammatory process.[41]

Particularly in children with CD, active disease can have a profound and lasting effect on long-term growth,[42] and this is covered in greater detail later in the chapter. Although it is well documented that up to 90% of children with CD may present with impaired height velocity,[43] Hildebrand and colleagues also reported a subnormal growth velocity (< -2 SD) in 24% of prepubertal children with UC, compared to 40% in those with CD.[44]

Osteoporosis

Owing to the fact that this complication is largely a problem of adult life, it is easy to forget that the accumulation of peak bone mass occurs during adolescence and early adult life. The implications of a substantial interruption in this process are only now becoming clearer as better long-term bone density data are becoming available.

Much attention has focused on trying to tease out the relative importance of the factors that lead to reduction in bone mineral density (BMD) in patients with IBD. As the most important determinants of peak bone mass appear to be age and genetic potential, these confound almost all studies in IBD trying to identify possible predictors such as nutritional status, disease duration, activity and distribution, and steroid therapy. However, despite these shortcomings, it appears that up to 40% of adults with established IBD have osteopenia ($T \leq -1.0$; -1 to -2.5 SD from the mean), while around 10% have osteoporosis ($T \leq -2.5$; > 2.5 SD from the mean) when compared to age- and sex-matched controls.[45] The relative importance of disease activity, nutritional status, and cumulative steroid consumption remains debated. A large adult study did identify chronic steroid exposure as the only significant risk factor for the staggering 40% increased risk in osteoporotic fractures in adults with CD.[46,47] Furthermore, it appears that BMD is no different to healthy age-matched adult controls within the first 6 months following symptom onset.[48] Interpretation of BMD in the pediatric IBD population remains a problem in the face of significant pubertal and bone age delay.[49] However up to 30% of children are still likely to have a significantly reduced BMD,[49,50] with children with CD tending to be more affected. Overall, therefore, both unchecked inflammation and chronic steroid exposure lead to loss of bone mass.[51]

The impact of nutritional status is unclear, as the correlation with BMD may well be confounded by disease activity. Ahmed and colleagues suggest that the growth failure seen in children with CD leads to a reduction in the size/length of their bones, thereby leading to falsely low values of BMD. If adjustments for bone size are made, bone mass in children with active CD appears to be better than previously reported. If bone area is not considered, up to 65% of children with CD would be labeled with moderate to severe osteopenia, while this falls to 22% if appropriate corrections are made.[52] While aggressive nutritional restitution is likely to minimize the chance of nutritionally dependent bone loss, whether or not supplementation with vitamin D and/or calcium provides added benefits remains to be determined by placebo-controlled studies. Identification of children at greatest risk is important as urinary calcium excretion, plasma 25-OH vitamin D levels, and a baseline bone density scan allow monitoring and subsequent supplementation of documented deficiencies. There is great potential for bone remodeling if children are in good clinical remission. Following presentation with osteoporotic vertebral fractures and in a good nutritional state, a 16-year-old with CD displayed a dramatic recovery of vertebral height within 3 years of largely steroid-free therapy that controlled his disease activity.[53]

The fact that the consequences of osteoporosis occur so long after the diagnosis of IBD in childhood makes it imperative for pediatricians to be aware of the BMD data now accumulating on adults with IBD. Several larger series are now reporting the clear association with lifetime steroid dose and the increased risk of osteoporotic fractures.[46] An ideal combination may be enteral nutrition and azathioprine/6-MP in the treatment of children with more severe CD. It is now clear that treatment regimens minimizing steroid therapy, and relying on nutritional therapy or other steroid-sparing agents, do not lead to the reduction in BMD seen in patients receiving corticosteroids. Although the mechanism is still unclear, infliximab has now been shown as increase markers of bone formation.[54,55] Patients with a lifetime steroid exposure of 12.9 g have a significantly lower BMD than normal controls, while those with <2 g lifetime exposure are comparable to age-matched healthy controls.[56] However, it is also clear that osteopenia does occur in steroid-naïve patients.[57] Unchecked inflammatory activity may lead to calcium and vitamin D malabsorption, which in turn increases parathyroid hormone secretion and further bone resorption.[58] Patients with small-bowel disease and/or resections are therefore also at risk of long-term osteoporosis.

Micronutrient Deficiencies

Identifying and treating macro- and micronutrient deficiencies are problematic for two main reasons. There is the initial difficulty of finding an accurate and reliable measure for each specific nutrient deficiency, followed by the inherent variability of a disease characterized by a remitting/relapsing course. There is also the impact of medical therapies and surgical interventions on nutrient status, eg, sulfasalazine inhibiting folate absorption and corticosteroids limiting calcium absorption. Clinically relevant micronutrient deficiencies in patients with IBD are unusual, and most are likely to occur when receiving long-term TPN.[59] Nonetheless, significant subclinical deficiencies in vitamins (B1, B6, C) and certain trace elements (magnesium, copper, and zinc) have been reported.[60]

Vitamin B12 deficiency occurs most often in patients with active terminal ileal CD, or following a resection of this part of the intestine. In addition to the usual consequences of these deficiencies, low serum B12 and folate levels may result in an elevation of homocysteine and hence contribute to a hypercoagulable state,[61] with folate supplementation leading to a reduction in homocysteine levels.[62] Patients with IBD are also at risk of developing fat-soluble vitamin deficiency. A significant deficiency of both vitamin A and E has been documented in 16% of children with IBD, with moderate to severe disease activity leading to a deficiency in over 40% of children.[63] Whether or not this was a consequence of a poor dietary intake or disease activity was not made clear. The range of vitamin deficiencies in patients with long-standing IBD is wide. Two comprehensive studies documented deficiencies in biotin, folate, β-carotene, thiamine, and vitamins A, E, and C in 40 to 90% of adults, despite inactive disease and adequate dietary intakes.[64,65]

Iron-deficiency anemia is difficult to diagnose in children with CD. Both the anemia of chronic disease and the variability in serum ferritin as part of the acute phase response make clear guidelines impossible. Low values of serum ferritin (<15 μg/dL) certainly confirm iron deficiency, but this may also be present at much higher values. Combining the more stable serum transferrin receptor (sTfR) with serum ferritin has been of benefit in adults,[66] while a small pediatric study suggested basic red cell ferritin was a more reliable measure in the presence of inflammation.[67] Variable absorption and the common gastrointestinal adverse effects of oral iron also make the response to treatment difficult to interpret.[68] This, together with the potential exacerbation of colitis by the oxidative stress of oral iron supplementation, has led to successful trials of parenteral iron and erythropoietin use.[69,70]

Trace elements are reduced in up to 50% of patients with active IBD,[65] with zinc deficiency being the most common.[71] The latter has been implicated in the maintenance of intestinal barrier function by regulating tight-junction permeability, with supplementation leading to a reduction in gut permeability in both animal models of colitis and adults with active CD.[72] Authors have shown significantly reduced fractional zinc absorption in adolescents with stable CD compared to normal controls. This appears to be due to unusually high fecal zinc losses.[73]

Many micronutrients are also antioxidants (Vitamin A, E, C, and selenium), and thus adequate supplementation may help counteract some of the oxidative stress that contributes to ongoing gut inflammation. Both serum selenium and erythrocyte glutathione peroxidase activity have been inversely correlated to plasma TNF-α levels in patients with active CD.[74]

OTHER NUTRITIONAL CONSEQUENCES OF IBD

Patients with long-standing IBD may of course also suffer the nutritional consequences of their therapies. Sulfasalazine is most notable for its impact on folate metabolism by competitively inhibiting dihydropteroate reductase, but folate rarely requires supplementation. Patients with severe ileitis or a significant ileal resection may develop steatorrhea, which in turn binds available free calcium, thus preventing calcium from binding to oxalate. High concentrations of luminal oxalates may lead to hyperoxaluria and renal calculi. A significant decrease in essential fatty acids has been correlated with a BMI <50th centile and active CD,[75] irrespective of dietary intake.

INDICATIONS FOR NUTRITIONAL TREATMENT

The indications for nutritional intervention differ among the different types of IBD. However, adequate nutritional support is an essential part of the long-term management of any chronic inflammatory disorder. In most cases this involves the provision of nutritional supplements to complement an otherwise inadequate intake and may involve anything from overnight nasogastric feeds to long-term support on home parenteral nutrition. For UC, no exclusively nutritional therapy has been shown to be therapeutically effective. In contrast, over many years patients with active CD have responded well to EEN. There have only been anecdotal reports of patients with indeterminate colitis responding to EEN, although the responders are likely to be those with a more Crohn's-like phenotype.

UC

There have been no studies showing that any form of nutritional intervention, used as sole therapy, can induce a remission in patients with active UC. Two randomized, prospective studies[76,77] clearly showed there was no role for exclusive total parenteral nutrition and bowel rest in the management of acute UC. Although there were some nutritional advantages in the group on TPN, these were outweighed by the complications reported at the time.

Table 1 Contraindications to Enteral Feeding

- Massive hemorrhage
- Intestinal obstruction
- Bowel perforation
- Toxic dilatation

Although often not as severe as in patients with CD, malnutrition does occur in children with UC.[78] However, while exclusively nutritional therapies are of no benefit in treating acute UC, nutritional support plays a vital role in minimizing further morbidity. Up to 10% of children with UC present with weight/height z-scores ≤ -2,[79] and inevitably nutrition is compromised in acute disease, both by a reduced oral intake and by increased losses of both protein and blood from the gut mucosa.[80] Although the concept of continuing enteral feeds during an episode of acute colitis may raise concerns in some, the evidence clearly suggests that equal nutritional improvement occurs with TPN and total enteral nutrition (TEN) in active colitis.[81] Not only does the latter lead to fewer complications, it is less costly, more physiological, and much simpler to provide. However, there continue to be absolute contraindications to enteral nutrition (Table 1).

Although dietary supplementation plays a role in acute UC, there is no evidence that specific dietary exclusions are of benefit in the long-term. Well-balanced, healthy diets that include normal amounts of dietary fiber are to be encouraged. Short-term studies suggest improved gastrointestinal symptoms on isphaghula husk,[82] although initial data that suggested diets low in fiber were linked to an increased risk of colon cancer have now been refuted in large epidemiological surveys in women.[83]

CD

In children with CD there are several reasons for nutritional intervention (Table 2).

Exclusive Enteral Nutrition. EEN is indicated as a first-line therapy in any child with acute CD, provided there are no absolute contraindications to enteral nutrition per se. The issue of whether or not enteral nutrition is as effective as steroid therapy at inducing a remission has been hotly

Table 2 Indications for Nutritional Therapy in Crohn's Disease

- Exclusive enteral nutrition for active disease
- Perioperative parenteral nutrition and bowel rest
- Supplemental enteral nutrition for maintenance of disease remission
- Nutritional support to maintain adequate weight gain
- Dietary supplementation of specific vitamins/minerals

debated for some time. However, what is clear from the pediatric literature over the past 20 years is that an exclusively nutritional therapy can be highly effective at inducing a remission from active disease.[84–86] The best results appear to be in those children with newly diagnosed disease,[87] although the pediatric evidence does remain limited in terms of the number of children reported. Large adult studies,[88,89] as well as some of the smaller pediatric studies,[86] suggest disease distribution does not affect the efficacy of the treatment. Colonic disease appears to respond as well as terminal ileal disease, with a similar reduction in inflammatory markers, disease activity, and improved mucosal histology.[85] More recent retrospective data however suggest that clinical remission with isolated colonic disease may only be about 50%, compared to about 75 to 80% in the presence of any macroscopic ileal involvement.[90] Although there is only anecdotal evidence on the response of oral and perianal CD to EEN,[91] the authors have made use of EEN as an adjunct in treating severe perianal CD.

Adverse effects to using EEN in CD are very rare. However, we reported a case of refeeding syndrome in a child following her presentation with severe Crohn's colitis. A rapid loss of weight over the preceding 4 weeks, followed by treatment with exclusive polymeric nutrition, led to a dramatic fall in serum phosphate and signs of hypervolemia in the first few days of treatment.[92] It is important to remain aware of this complication when refeeding previously malnourished children with CD, as adequate supplementation in the first few days can prevent serious complications.

Perioperative Nutritional Support. Preoperative undernutrition has long been known to adversely affect surgical outcome. Although surgical outcome is related to the nutritional state of the patient,[93] short-term preoperative use of TPN is insufficient to dramatically improve the nutritional status. Even 7 to 10 days of preoperative parenteral nutrition in malnourished "cancer" patients achieved only a 10% reduction in postoperative complications.[94] Parenteral nutrition may replace acute nutritional deficits in the immediate perioperative period and may also reduce length of small-bowel resection in adults with CD.[95,96] Uncontrolled studies in adults with IBD also suggest there is a reduction in postoperative complications following preoperative parenteral nutrition,[97] yet it appears most effective in patients with severe malnutrition and highly active disease.[98]

Improvements in the medical management of children with IBD are likely to continue reducing the need for surgery, yet recent studies still suggest that almost 60% of adults with CD will require an operation.[99] Older pediatric data showed that up to 80% of children with CD were needing surgery in the 15 years following diagnosis.[100] Emergency surgery may be unavoidable in a small number of children who present with fulminant colitis; however the majority will require surgery for treatment-resistant disease.

While a child with acute, severe UC will require close monitoring of fluid and electrolytes in the perioperative period, they are less likely to have had a long period of active disease leading to chronic malnutrition.

Despite persistently active, treatment-resistant disease, surgery can often be planned some weeks in advance. In these circumstances, optimizing nutrition over a period of 4 to 6 weeks is likely to result in a much better postoperative course. Provided inflammatory activity and symptoms allow, several weeks of EEN in children with severe CD can lead to nutritional restitution prior to surgery. In isolated cases, the use of TPN for a several weeks may also be justified in preparation for if enteral access is impossible. However, clinicians can be forced to compromise in the face of severe treatment-resistant disease, where disease activity does not allow time for any improvement in nutritional state and surgery should then not be delayed.

Postoperative support for all children, irrespective of the type of abdominal/perianal surgery, should involve institution of enteral feeds as soon as possible. Adult evidence demonstrates no increase in complications when patients are fed enterally within 48 hours of colectomy.[101] Very early use of enteral supplements reduces early postoperative complications even in undernourished adults, and leads to a better weight gain, as well as an improvement in physical and mental quality of life.[102] Routine use of postoperative TPN in well-nourished patients should be discouraged as it increases complication rates.[103] However provision for TPN should still be made if enteral feeding is likely to be delayed for more than 1 to 3 days in any undernourished child who is likely to suffer a long convalescence without achieving full enteral feeds.

NUTRITIONAL TREATMENT OF ACTIVE CD

In severe malnutrition there is clear evidence of a secondary immune dysregulation.[104] Both T-cell numbers and secretory IgA levels are consistently reduced, and there are also defects in bacterial phagocytosis, lysozyme, and interferon production. While today's children with CD are not often severely malnourished, they are certainly well below their expected centile for weight.[105] It is therefore quite clear that this degree of malnutrition does little to attenuate tissue damaging immune responses.

Parenteral Nutrition

The advent of parenteral nutrition in the early 1970s proved useful in managing intractable cases of CD[106] and its use became more widespread as an alternative primary therapy for severe disease.[107] As would later be clearly demonstrated for enteral nutrition,[42] it was parenteral nutrition that was first shown to reverse growth failure in children and adolescents with active CD.[37,108] However, as awareness of the septic and thrombotic complications associated with an indwelling line increased, the use of parenteral nutrition in CD declined. While it still appears to be as effective as elemental nutrition in the short-term treatment of acute disease,[109] its complications, practical difficulties, and expense, limit its use. Furthermore, total parenteral nutrition induces mucosal atrophy and increases bacterial translocation,[110] something that is entirely preventable by luminal nutrition.

The combination of intravenous nutritional support and complete bowel rest has not been shown to be more effective in treating active disease than either EEN or TPN with oral feeding.[111] In a controlled study, 58 to 71% of all groups achieved a clinical remission, indicating that bowel rest per se has no added effect on the disease, but that improved nutrition in any form has clinical benefit. However, there have also been a number of case series suggesting that exclusive parenteral nutrition may be of significant benefit in severe Crohn's colitis,[95] with at least one study documenting endoscopic healing of mucosal ulcers on exclusive PN.[112] Despite this, the preference for nutritional support in most cases remains an enteral feed.

There has been limited success (35%) in achieving fistula closure on exclusive TPN,[113] with any improvement not being sustained once back on a normal diet. In view of other therapies, such as octreotide and anti-TNFα antibody, TPN now has only a very limited role in the management these fistulae.

Children only rarely have bowel resections large enough to require long-term home parenteral nutrition support. However, in adults less than 100 cm of jejunum, or less than 50 cm of small bowel with an intact colon remain, long-term parenteral nutrition is often necessary.[114] Yet over 70% of these patients will be on a full oral diet within 12 months of starting home parenteral nutrition.[115]

Enteral Nutrition

Elemental Diet. An elemental feed is a chemically defined diet whose protein source is amino acids or short-chain peptides, with short-chain carbohydrates and added fat, minerals, and vitamins. The National Aeronautics and Space Administration (NASA) had initially designed elemental diets for astronauts.[116] This was with the intention of providing a nutritionally complete diet of which as much as possible would be absorbed. However, while absorption was limited mainly to the upper small bowel, the diet did not prevent the production of stool as had been hoped.

Nutrition was initially used in IBD as an adjunct in malnourished patients with growth failure. Elemental diets were developed and first used as sole therapy for IBD in adults in the 1970s.[117] It was then shown that nutrition had a beneficial effect on disease by reducing the increased gut permeability characteristic of CD.[5] Logan and colleagues studied seven adults with extensive jejunoileal CD. They showed a reduction in both gut protein and gut lymphocyte loss during a period of elemental feeding. This was the first report that an elemental diet could directly improve gut function, probably by reducing bowel inflammation.

In 1973 Giorgini and colleagues[4] reported the first successful use of enteral nutrition in treating a child with acute CD. It was then shown that enteral nutrition was effective in treating a series of children with CD. Successful use in combination with drug therapy led on to a further study by the same group, which first showed exclusive CREN to be as effective as steroid therapy at inducing a remission.[118] While both these studies had a few patients, they gave the first insights into the possible benefits of nutritional therapy as treatment for childhood CD. In addition to achieving disease remission, nutritional therapy was also found to have beneficial effects on inflammatory masses and fistulae.[6,118] Simultaneously, both Morin and colleagues[6] and O'Morain and colleagues,[119] documented that an elemental diet improved linear growth in several children with active CD.

A variety of devices, formulas, and regimens were then used to feed patients intragastrically. Continuous feeding[7,8] and then overnight feeds predominated[9] for the induction of remission. Supplementation of an elemental diet with glutamine, a gut-specific metabolic fuel, did not further improve efficacy, although the small numbers in this study make conclusions difficult.[120]

Semielemental Diet. Once elemental diets had achieved their first successes, short-chain peptide-containing diets were suggested as a better nitrogen source than amino acids.[121] Silk and colleagues refuted previous evidence that free amino acids were better absorbed than di- and tripeptides. By using an intestinal perfusion technique in adults, he was able to demonstrate better absorption of amino acids from both casein and lactalbumin hydrolysates, than from an equimolar feed of free amino acids. Not only was there a more uniform absorption of amino acids, but the hydrolysates had a beneficial effect on jejunal absorption of water and electrolytes. There followed the first small randomized study of 7 to 8 children in each group, in which overnight nasogastric feeding of a semielemental diet was compared to prednisolone treatment in children with predominant small bowel CD.[9] A 4–5-chain amino acid-based diet was as effective as steroids at achieving a remission in active CD. It again confirmed the North American finding that there was a clear acceleration in growth in the group not taking steroids.

Polymeric Diet. It therefore appeared that steroids may have a similar efficacy to semielemental feeds in the induction of remission. Several adult studies reported the efficacy of whole-protein diet compared to both that of elemental diets and to steroids. Raouf and colleagues[122] and others all found polymeric diets to be as effective as an elemental diet at inducing remission.

Polymeric diets were also shown to be as effective as conventional steroid treatment. Gonzalez-Huix and colleagues [123] confirmed this in adults, and Ruuska and colleagues [86] and Beattie and colleagues [84] in children. Ruuska and colleagues,[86] in a well-planned but small study ($n = 19$), showed a polymeric diet to be as effective as steroids in inducing a remission in children with acute CD. A further great advantage in using a polymeric diet then became clear. While almost all children previously required feeding by intragastric tube, whole protein formulas such as AL110 (Nestlé-Clintec), used by Beattie and colleagues[84] and Nutrison Standard (Nutricia), used by Ruuska and colleagues,[86] were palatable enough for daily oral consumption. Children rarely required a nasogastric tube to complete their entire nutritional needs. This provided a considerable improvement in the quality of life for children on several weeks of nutritional therapy.

The most recent, and most definitive cohort study to date, by Fell and colleagues,[85] shows that a whole casein, polymeric diet CT 3211 (now known as Modulen IBD, Nestlé Clinical Nutrition), rich in transforming growth factor β, is well tolerated and achieves a clinical and histologic remission. Twenty-nine consecutive patients were treated with the exclusive enteral diet for an 8-week period. Although over half had mild disease, 12 had moderate to severe disease with a pediatric Crohn's disease activity index (PCDAI) >30.[124] A nasogastric tube was only required in one patient for the first 2 weeks of treatment. Only 2 of 29 patients failed to show any clinical response, one with severe colonic disease, the other with an inflammatory mass requiring surgery. Twenty-three of 29 patients achieved a complete remission on PCDAI scoring. The PCDAI fell dramatically within 2 weeks of starting the diet, but continued to fall until 8 weeks of treatment. There was significant macroscopic and histologic improvement after treatment, with mucosal healing occurring in the terminal ileum and colon of 8 and 2 patients, respectively. Serum TNFα and mucosal mRNA for IL-1β and IL-8 were significantly reduced in both the terminal ileum and the colon after treatment. IFN-γ was significantly reduced and transforming facton beta (TGF-β) was elevated in the terminal ileum alone. There is no direct evidence that the TGF-β in the enteral formula is responsible for the upregulation of mucosal TGF-β. Nonetheless, this study strengthens the findings by Breese and colleagues [125] that polymeric enteral nutrition alone can achieve an improvement in histology and a complete normalization of some of the mucosal messenger RNA of proinflammatory cytokines involved in tissue damage. Bannerjee and colleagues documented the most rapid reduction in proinflammatory cytokines to date, in children receiving EEN for active CD.[126] Within 3 days of starting an exclusive polymeric diet, there was a significant reduction in IL-6 and ESR. This, together with improvements in CRP, IGF-1, and PCDAI by Day 7, predated any measures of nutritional restitution (mid-upper arm circumference/triceps skinfold thickness). Further evidence that nutritional therapy in this situation is providing more than an optimal calorie intake.

The lipid composition of some polymeric diets has been held responsible for some of the variability in their efficacy.[127] High LCT concentrations have been associated with a poorer response in treating active CD, with suggestions that the high linoleic acid concentration may be responsible,[128] although high concentrations of MCT in the feed does not effect its short-term efficacy.[129] However, the only two randomized studies have been unable to show a difference in efficacy between formulas containing either low or high amounts of long-chain triglyceride.[130] Only one randomized study appeared to show a significant difference in remission rates depending on the fatty acid composition of the polymeric feeds. Gassull and colleagues report a significantly better clinical remission rate in adults after 4 weeks of an exclusive enteral feed rich in n-6 fatty acids, compared to one high in monounsaturated fats (52% vs 20%, respectively).[127] Why this conflicts with previous evidence[123] remains unclear, although the high percentage of synthetic oleate (79% of total fat) in this study may mask beneficial effects previously seen with formulae containing different fatty acid profiles.

There is limited evidence of milk intolerance in adults with active CD. True lactase deficiency is an unusual cause of symptoms in adults with active CD[131]; however up to 46% complained of gastrointestinal symptoms related to milk intake. In contrast, exclusive enteral feeding with lactose-free, whole-casein diets has not been associated with intolerance in children with active disease.

Steroids Versus Enteral Nutrition. Contrary to these striking pediatric findings, large adult trials[81,88,132] as well as meta-analyses of the adult data, have found steroids to be more effective than enteral nutrition at inducing remission in active CD.[133] The meta-analysis by Griffiths and colleagues,[133] while including both children and adults, excluded most of the smaller pediatric studies. This large review ($n = 413$) reported that steroids were significantly more effective at achieving a remission than enteral diets (OR: 0.35; 95% CI 0.32 to 0.58). Like other analyses, this study also relies on clinical disease activity indices to document clinical remission rates, but these tend to favor steroid therapy by their reliance on a patient's general feeling of well-being. As a result, conclusions from these studies are frequently and inappropriately applied to children, despite there being clear differences between adult and pediatric patients. Most children have had much shorter disease duration and tend to be much more compliant with therapy. Furthermore, no comment is made on the differing adverse effects and abilities of the two treatments to heal gut mucosa, with steroids having been well-documented to have limited effects on gut inflammation.[134] As yet no analysis has detected a significant difference in efficacy between elemental or polymeric diets.[135]

Despite the several small pediatric studies that suggest a useful role for enteral nutrition in active CD, the view has thus prevailed that enteral nutrition is less effective than steroid therapy. A meta-analysis of pediatric data was performed to maximize the available pediatric data.[136] Despite limited numbers of truly randomized children, sensitivity analyses allowed the authors to arrive at valid and important conclusions. The summary data clearly showed enteral nutrition to be as effective as steroids in the treatment of children with active CD. Furthermore, to overturn this finding and demonstrate that steroids were significantly more effective than enteral nutrition would be close to impossible given the outcomes of the pediatric studies reported to date. All these studies principally address efficacy as their primary outcome measure, largely ignoring the very different side effect profiles of each therapy. Corticosteroids have many significant adverse effects, while oral enteral nutrition has almost none. Prospective observational studies have also highlighted that even in the pediatric age group about 30% of children with CD, treated with corticosteroids within 30 days of diagnosis, are corticosteroid dependent at 1 year.[137]

Enteral Nutrition and Crohn's Colitis. There remains the further question of whether enteral nutrition is less effective at treating Crohn's colitis than Crohn's ileitis. Early use of enteral feed was limited to children with predominantly small bowel disease,[138] with a suggestion that colonic disease was unresponsive to nutritional management.[139] More recent evidence from Thomas and colleagues,[140] Ruuska and colleagues,[86] and Fell and colleagues,[85] however, supports the value of nutritional therapy in large bowel and small bowel disease. The improvement in colonic mucosal cytokine profiles after enteral nutrition[85] provides hard evidence that there is an effect on colonic disease. Larger studies in adults also confirm that disease location does not appear to influence the response to treatment.[88,132,133]

However, a more recent retrospective analysis of 60 children treated with EEN suggested disease distribution may be relevant in the response to nutritional therapy. Children with any macroscopic ileal inflammation were significantly more likely to achieve a clinical remission than those children with colonic involvement alone (75% vs 50%).[141] Despite this, many individuals with Crohn's colitis continue to respond extremely well, still making EEN the first choice for any child with CD, irrespective of their disease distribution.

Food Reintroduction

There has long been uncertainty as to the best way of reintroducing adults and children onto their "normal" diet after a period of EEN. The evidence for any of these different practices is very limited, with most approaches having been selected by experienced clinicians on the basis of theories prevalent at the time.

The best-described reintroduction program is based on the stepwise introduction foods, starting with the least allergenic.[142] One new food is introduced every 48 hours and if not tolerated, reintroduced at the end of the program. This systematic, but quite laborious program not only allows individual foods to be identified if causing immediate symptoms, but also gives the patients several more weeks on reasonable quantities of enteral nutrition while their normal diet is re-established. The most frequently implicated foods causing discomfort in adults are cereals, dairy products, and yeast,[142] although in children only a very small minority require exclusion of specific items from their diet. In a 2-year follow-up study of about 100 adults, the relapse rate was only just significantly lower in the group excluding dietary products that caused symptoms compared to those maintaining a normal diet ($p = .048$). However, in a randomized controlled trial of an exclusion diet following a remission induced with an elemental diet, subsequent rechallenge and double-blinded challenges in adults with CD proved that specific dietary exclusions did not persist.[143] There is thus insufficient evidence to routinely suggest exclusion of specific food items in children with CD.

Other units use less evidence-based, but more practical, reintroduction programs which range from the immediate introduction of a full diet, to a graded introduction over 3 weeks with the "ad libitum" diet increasing by 25% each week, along with the simultaneous reduction in enteral nutrition.

ENTERAL NUTRITION AS MAINTENANCE THERAPY IN CD

There has been much interest in whether dietary modification may prolong a remission in CD.

Initial studies suggested intermittent use of EEN for 1 month in every four could not only reduce steroid requirement and reduce disease activity, but also increase long-term growth rate in children with CD.[144] While this intermittent use of EEN may have had a role in managing patients with otherwise intractable disease and a previous good response to enteral nutrition, repeated and prolonged use of exclusive enteral diets in most adolescents is difficult and mostly unnecessary. Given the availability of other, currently more effective maintenance agents, compliance with supplements of enteral nutrition is likely to be much greater if these can be shown to be effective.

Low-residue diets are not indicated in the maintenance of remission in CD. Unless required as a dietary modification in the presence of fibrosing/stricturing disease, they have not been shown to prevent disease relapse.[145]

A retrospective study in which a normal "ad libitum" diet of children with CD was supplemented with an additional 30% of the recommended daily calorie intake as polymeric feed led to the halving of relapse rates within the first 12 months.[146] Small controlled studies also suggest an advantage to simple long-term calorie supplementation per se,[147] although larger, more definitive studies are still awaited. However, it is highly likely that a long-term nutritional supplement, in combination with a well-tolerated immunosuppressant, will provide the optimal maintenance therapy for most children with moderate to severe CD.

Attempts at supplementing diets with specific antiinflammatory agents continue, with fish oils receiving particular attention. Their effects on reducing mucosal eicosanoids (particularly leukotriene B4 and thromboxane A2)[148] have been widely reported. The n-3 fatty acids present in fish oils may also inhibit interleukin-1β and TNF production.[149] In addition, they also decrease platelet responsiveness,[150] and thus may act to reduce the multifocal gastrointestinal infarctions that have been reported as early pathogenic steps of CD.[151] Several large placebo-controlled, randomized studies have been performed on adults with both CD and UC,[152,153] but unfortunately much of the data remain conflicting. Although different methodology makes generalizations difficult, several important issues are raised. While low-dose regimens cause no appreciable adverse effects,[154] compliance with high-dose fish oils in adults is poor, making long-term maintenance therapy in children even less attractive. Belluzzi and colleagues[152] found that supplementation with 2.7 g of n-3 fatty acids reduced the relapse rate in adults with CD, while another large study failed to confirm any benefit over placebo in using either >5 g/d of n-3 fatty acids, or maintaining a diet low in carbohydrate (84 g/d).[153] However, despite no clear-cut clinical benefits, significant changes are reported on a mucosal level. Colonic inflammatory cell infiltrates are reduced and the synthesis of LTB4 and TXA2 downregulated after supplementation with n-3 fatty acids.[153] It may therefore be that further refining of the composition, formulation, and dose is required before fish-oil supplements become an accepted part of maintenance therapy. A small prospective study in children with CD ($n = 38$) suggests that adjunctive therapy with enteric-coated omega-3 fatty acids and mesalazine (50 mg/kg/d) reduces relapse rates at 12 months compared to mesalazine alone.[155]

Other, more specific dietary interventions have been reported to prolong remission in CD. Although none of these has been assessed in larger, placebo-controlled studies, they offer interesting clues to the role dietary modification may play in maintaining disease remission. A small study randomizing patients to a diet low in microparticles[156] suggested significant benefits in disease activity and remission rates after 4 months when compared to 10 patients on a normal diet. Diets low in refined sugars have been not been found to prevent relapse rates in adults with CD.[157] Similarly, the presence of yeast in the diet of patients with CD may potentiate disease relapse, but larger studies are necessary before firm conclusions may be drawn.[158]

As the importance of gut microflora in the etiology of IBD is increasingly recognized, so the prospect of modulating it by means of "functional foods" has gained much support. Although discussion is beyond the scope of this chapter, the mechanisms of action and potential implications of this exciting new field are great for patients with chronic intestinal disease driven by enteric flora. It is quite clear that over the next few years we are likely to see larger, placebo-controlled trials of both pro- and prebiotics. Prebiotics are the complex sugars, such as fructo-oligosaccharides and inulin, which pass into the colon undigested where they may be selectively fermented by certain probiotic species.[159] Attempts to maintain remission in both UC and pouchitis with combined probiotic combinations has proved quite successful,[160] while *Lactobacillus GG* alone may have a role in improving gut barrier function and clinical status in children with CD.[161]

If long-term nutritional support is required, most children will tolerate a more palatable polymeric formula by mouth. However, some children will require supplementation by tube. While short-term support can be given via a nasogastric tube, longer term needs should be met via a more permanent device. Where nutritional support is needed for several months, placement of a percutaneous endoscopic gastrostomy (PEG) is ideal. Despite initial reservations about possible complications from fistulous tracts formation, PEG placement has now been documented to be uncomplicated in selected adults and children with IBD.[162] In patients receiving corticosteroids adhesion of the gastric to the abdominal wall may be delayed, and thus early "pulling" of the PEG could lead to tract disruption.

THE ROLE OF ENTERAL NUTRITION ON GROWTH AND DEVELOPMENT

Epidemiology of Growth Failure

After the onset of symptoms, but before a diagnosis of CD is made, up to 46% of children will have a reduced height velocity, with only 12% having a normal height velocity up to the time of diagnosis.[43] In contrast, only 3 to 10% of children with UC may present with reduced height velocities at diagnosis.[44] Although much of this data are now over 10 years old, and an accurate diagnosis may now be made more quickly, it is clear that untreated CD has profound implications on a child's growth potential. Motil and colleagues reported in a cross-sectional study of their pediatric IBD patients that 23% had a z-score <-1.64, with 50% of these having a bone age delayed by >1 year over their chronological age. Physicians caring for children with IBD, particularly CD, therefore, have the unique opportunity to try and modify the impact that both disease and therapy has on the growth rate of their patients. Sawzcenko and colleagues recently reported that children with the IL6-174 promoter polymorphism are more growth-retarded at diagnosis than those without.[163] Although levels of CRP were highest in children with this polymorphism, they appeared to be at no increased risk of developing CD than the other polymorphisms compared to 351 healthy controls. The authors speculate that IL-6 mediates growth failure in these children, and that genotyping at an early stage would allow the use of specific growth sparing/focused biological therapies.

A delay in presentation is associated with a significantly greater degree of growth impairment at diagnosis.[79] The length of this delay appears to correlate with a lower height z-score at diagnosis, and hence with a lower final adult height.[164] A delay in diagnosing the more subtle presenting symptoms of jejunal CD may at least in part explain the more significant reduction in adult height seen in this particular group of children. Despite management within tertiary centers, 49 to 65% of children with CD have a reduced height velocity in early puberty, with growth velocity remaining less than 4 cm/yr during the first 1 to 2 years of therapy.[44,165] Hildebrand and colleagues report a mean z-score for height of -0.6, 2 years after diagnosis in 46 consecutive children with CD. Griffiths and colleagues reported that of 67 consecutively diagnosed children with CD followed to maturity, about two-third maintained or increased their z-scores for height.

The outcome of many of these studies reflects management where the mainstay of therapy was often corticosteroids, and so does not include the more recent move to the earlier use of steroid-sparing agents. However, although the most recent follow-up data show that the majority of children diagnosed with CD are closer to their expected adult height, almost 20% will be at least 8 cm below the height expected by mid-parental centile (Sawczenko, 2006 3070/id). Earlier diagnosis and identification of those children at risk of growth failure remain a significant problem for clinicians wanting to optimize growth outcomes.

Etiology of Growth Failure

The growth failure seen in children with IBD is multi-factorial, with inflammation, undernutrition, and steroid therapy being its principal determinants.

Initial evidence suggested that chronic under nutrition was the main factor in the growth failure seen in children with IBD,[37] with studies confirming that simple nutritional restitution improved the linear growth of children with CD.[36,38] Children with active CD have a relative insufficiency of dietary intake when compared with children of the same age,[140] although they may compensate with an increased intake between disease relapses.[165] However, simply increasing the calorie intake, as seen in patients on steroids, does not confer the same benefit on growth as a lower calorie-intake received on EEN.[140] The presence of low levels of insulin-like growth factor-1 (IGF-1) in children with active CD strengthens this association, as the relationship between IGF-1 and malnutrition is now clear.[167] Both IGF-1 and its carrier protein IGF-binding protein-3 are increased significantly by treatment with EEN.[168,169] Further evidence that inflammation, and not only nutritional factors, plays a role in determining growth can be seen in studies of children undergoing surgery for active IBD. While postoperative catch-up growth is not documented by all authors, several authors show a clear growth-spurt occurring after the removal of an inflamed segment of bowel.[170] Although this is most striking in prepubertal children, the benefit is still substantial if surgery is carried out before the final stages of puberty.[171] This response may of course in part be the result of improved postoperative nutrition. However, Varille and colleagues neatly documented that even children undergoing localized resections for stricturing disease had a significant reduction in REE and increase in nitrogen utilization 4 weeks after surgery, despite maintaining preoperative nutritional and steroid regimens.[172]

There now seems little doubt that ongoing inflammatory activity plays a key role in the inhibition of growth.[173] Downregulation of proinflammatory cytokines by enteral nutrition may partly improve growth by reducing IL-6, a potent inhibitor of IGF-1.[174] There is a dramatic reduction in CRP, with concomitant increase in IGF-1 and IGFBP-3, within 14 days of commencing EEN.[84,85] This clearly indicates that enteral nutrition also has a more rapid, direct antiinflammatory action in addition to its longer term nutritional benefits. As has been confirmed in children with rheumatoid arthritis,[175] systemic inflammation, as well as malnutrition, reduces IGF-1. Direct inhibitory effects of proinflammatory cytokines such as TNFα on developing growth plates[176] and a downregulation of IGF-1 by IL-6 are both likely to contribute to growth retardation.[177] The additional suppression of appetite by TNFα,[178] the failure to downregulate the REE during malnutrition in CD,[40] and the exacerbation of bowel symptoms by food intake, all add to the final reduction in height velocity.

Enteric losses during active disease can also contribute to the decline in nutritional state. Children with small bowel CD have varying degrees of malabsorption, with some of the hypoalbuminemia occurring as a result of enteric losses.[179] The most important determinant of hypoalbuminemia is the systemic inflammatory response. Although protein loss through an inflamed mucosa does occur, it is usually modest, nonspecific, and occurs in association with loss of globulins. The hypoalbuminemia seen in CD is more frequently associated with the hypergammaglobulinemia occurring as a result of the acute-phase protein synthesis. The latter is principally mediated by IL-6.[180] Furthermore, a sustained protein intake of less than 0.4 g/kg/d[181] is necessary to achieve any reduction in serum albumin.

Bile acid malabsorption may not only occur in children with active terminal ileitis, as systemic effects of ileal inflammation may lead to malabsorption in the proximal small bowel.[182] As a result fat malabsorption may occur in some children with CD. In addition, low concentrations of vitamins A, E, and zinc have been shown to correlate more with disease activity than nutritional state,[63,183] suggesting depletion occurs during the acute inflammation rather than as a result of chronic malabsorption.

Ongoing growth failure in the first years after diagnosis may be due to several factors. Growth velocity can be delayed well beyond nutritional restitution and normalization of inflammatory indices. This, together with the frequent use of high-dose steroids to achieve the initial remission, up to 85% of children in some studies,[166,184] may arrest normal growth for many months after diagnosis. However, the most recent data suggest that it is neither the disease distribution nor pubertal stage at diagnosis that determines final adult height,[185] but rather the use of corticosteroids during puberty. Children who were diagnosed with CD during puberty and were treated with corticosteroids were significantly shorter as adults when compared to those who did not receive corticosteroids. In this study, this was the only independent predictor of final adult height.

Nutritional Treatment of Growth Failure

Over 20 years ago several small studies confirmed the central role of nutrition in the long-term management of growth failure in children with IBD. Motil and colleagues[186,187] concluded that neither low-grade chronic inflammation nor low-dose corticosteroid uses reduced whole-body protein synthesis, and that it was adequate dietary supplementation that led to a significant increase in growth velocity of children with growth failure. This, confirmed by others as nutritional therapies, became more practical for the treatment of acute CD.[6,36] Sanderson and colleagues were the first to establish the benefit of enteral nutrition over steroid therapy on short-term growth in children with newly diagnosed CD.[9]

MECHANISM OF ENTERAL NUTRITION

Despite the wealth of information that exists about the benefits of enteral nutrition, the mechanisms of action remain largely unclear (Table 3)

The most frequently advanced theory is that the bacterial flora within the gut lumen is modified by enteral nutrition. The clinical evidence of any difference in flora between patients with CD and normal controls remains slim. It was shown in the late 1970s that there are higher bacterial counts within the terminal ileum of patients with active disease.[188] Studies at that time also suggested a reduction in fecal flora after enteral nutrition.[189] It is now clear that increasing severity of systemic disease is associated with an increase in the adherence of fecal bacteria to the enterocytes,[190] and this does not appear to be related to the degree of local mucosal inflammation. The response of acute CD to antibiotic therapy further implicates the bacterial flora in the disease pathogenesis,[191] although antibiotics such as the quinolones and metronidazole have other immunomodulatory effects in addition to their antimicrobial actions.[192] The organisms that appear increased in the lumen of patients with CD include Bacteroides, Eubacteria, and Peptostreptococcus.[193] Elegant work on mice that develop spontaneous colitis (TCRα-/-) has confirmed that feeding with an elemental diet prevents bowel inflammation.[194] Unlike the mice fed elemental diet, the mice fed regular chow and then develop colitis are colonized by *Bacteroides vulgatus* in >80% of cases. Furthermore, instilling this strain into the rectum of the elementally fed mice led to development of a typical Th-2 type, T-cell induced colitis. Further animal work has shown that elemental diet may reduce progression of granulomatous enteritis by modulating the activation of T cells, the production of NO, and the generation of oxygen free radicals.[194–196]

Table 3 Exclusive Enteral Nutrition

- Alteration in bacterial flora
- Reduction in antigenic load
- Whole body nutritional restitution
- Provision of enterocyte nutrition
- Direct immunoregulatory effect
- Increased concentrations of Transforming Factor βeta
- Low lipid and fiber content

The reduction in antigenic load that accompanies EEN may also contribute, at least in part, to bowel rest. However, a whole-protein diet, and even an ad libitum diet together with some parenteral nutrition, appears to be as effective as an exclusive elemental diet at inducing a remission.[85,86,111,197] The efficacy of polymeric diets and recent evidence that dietary supplementation with enteral nutrition may prolong a remission,[146] both suggest that reducing luminal antigens may only play a modest role in the efficacy of this therapy.

Whether enteral nutrition per se has either a direct and/or indirect immuno-regulatory effect remains speculative. Degrees of moderate protein malnutrition have been associated with poor immune function. In rodents, protein deprivation leads to impairment of the mucosal immune response, as well as depleting a population of T cells that control oral tolerance.[198,199] This would suggest that poor nutrition inhibits T cells that downregulate the gut's response to foreign antigens. Enteral feeding may therefore have an indirect effect of on the immune response by restoring an adequate nutritional status.

More recently, the direct influence of luminal content on immune function has been studied. Sanderson and colleagues provided evidence that luminal content can influence epithelial cell gene expression within the gut.[200] Short-chain fatty acids, such as butyrate, are bacterial metabolites from unabsorbed carbohydrates. Butyrate induces secretion of insulin growth factor-binding proteins (IGFBPs) by a complex process involving histone deacetylation.[201] Butyrate has also been shown to potentiate the secretion of IL-8 by intestinal epithelial cells (Caco-2) if these are stimulated with either lipopolysaccharide (LPS) or IL-1β. LPS was only able to induce IL-8 secretion if these cells were preincubated with butyrate, implying direct effects of the latter on gene regulation.[202] Epithelial cell-gene regulation by luminal products thus appears to be able to influence intestinal inflammation through release of suc inflammatory cytokines. Upregulation of the chemokine macrophage-inflammatory-protein-2 (MIP-2) increases local neutrophil recruitment.[203]

It has also been suggested that the presence, or absence, of individual components of enteral feeds is important in immune regulation. The putative advantage of high TGF-β levels in both AL110 and CT3211 (~24 p.p.m.) is based on the large body of experimental evidence that this cytokine has the ability to downregulate other proinflammatory cytokines.[204] Fell and colleagues[85] demonstrated mucosal upregulation of TGF-β within the terminal ileum after an 8-week course of TGF-β-rich CT3211. It is still unclear whether this is related to the increased luminal presence of TGF-β or is simply an epi-phenomenon of tissue repair.

It may also be that enteral nutrition plays a direct role in promoting the mechanisms involved in epithelial healing. There are numerous peptides involved in the restoration of a disrupted epithelial barrier. The ulcer-associated cell lineage (UACL)[205] secretes cytoprotective peptides that promote epithelial healing. Among them are epidermal growth factor (EGF), TGF-α, human spasmolytic peptide (hSP), and the family of trefoil peptides.[205] The trefoil peptides in particular have been shown to be vital in protecting against mucosal damage.[206] Enteral nutrition may contribute toward the maintenance of mucosal integrity by boosting the proliferation of the UACL.[207]

While the theory of "bowel rest" has its supporters, others continue to feel it is adequate nutrition alone that could induce remission and growth in these patients.[208] Kirschner and colleagues[36] demonstrated improved growth in children simply fed an extra 1,000 kcal/d. The same group later confirmed that improved nutrition not only increased linear growth, but also returned previously low levels of IGF-1 to normal in children with active CD.[209] Thomas and colleagues[168] confirmed this finding with an elemental feed, which was as effective at increasing IGF-1 as prednisolone, yet better promoted linear growth.

There are likely to be many mechanisms responsible for the clinical efficacy of enteral nutrition. It is clear, however, that the luminal environment is crucial to the expression of mucosal disease. Our ability to regulate specific aspects of this environment by nutritional or other means remains a great challenge. The multitude of variables that may be important in achieving a disease remission makes identification of single factors extremely difficult. Current attention is focused on modifying enteral formulas in line with the recent evidence on dietary fats, while continuing to ensure their clinical efficacy and tolerability.

Mucosal Healing

Attention has focused on the ability of treatments to achieve mucosal healing.[210] Breese and colleagues[125] gave an initial indication that enteral nutrition was able to downregulate intestinal mucosal inflammation. Enteral nutrition was as effective as cyclosporin and steroids in reducing the percentage of IL-2 secreting cells in the terminal ileum after treatment, while it appeared more effective than steroids at reducing the percentage of IFN-γ secreting cells. Furthermore, it was only the enterally fed group that showed significant histologic improvement.

Despite being only a small study, Breese and colleagues raised two important issues. First, that

Table 4 Data Showing mRNA Transcripts (10^3)/μg Total RNA from Biopsies Taken before and after Treatment with CT3211 and Normal Controls

	Terminal Ileum			Colon		
	Control	Pre-treatment	Post-treatment	Control	Pre-treatment	Post-treatment
IL-1β	15**	350	16*	0.54**	130	18*
IFN-γ	1**	8.6	1.1*	1.1**	3.5	1.2
IL-8	50	660	150	4.8**	1500	130*
IL-10	1.5	1.7	1.3	3.7**	1.9	1.2
TGF-β	16	4.2	34*	11	15	15

Adapted from reference 85.

*Significant change ($p < .05$) with treatment assessed by *t*-test.

**Significant difference between pre-treatment (diseased) and control values assessed by Mann–Whitney U-test.

enteral nutrition may be able to heal mucosa, second, that mucosal cytokine analysis following treatment did not necessarily correlate with either clinical or histologic indices of remission.

The mucosal cytokine responses of a much larger cohort of children were reported by Fell and colleagues.[85] While clear clinical and histologic remission was achieved in over 70% of children, cytokine profiles also dramatically improved with a polymeric diet alone. The dramatic downregulation of the potent proinflammatory cytokines IL-1β, IFN-γ, and IL-8 is the most concrete evidence to date that enteral nutrition acts at the mucosal level (Table 4).

The issue of whether clinical, endoscopic, histologic, or immunologic remission should be the gold standard remains a matter of personal practice.[210] If we are to believe that the presence of chronic inflammation predisposes to long-term complications and malignancy,[211] it may be a state of immunologic remission at the mucosal level that should be achieved in children with a lifetime of CD ahead of them.

BODY COMPOSITION, ENERGY EXPENDITURE, AND PROTEIN METABOLISM

It has become clear that both in adults and children, active gut inflammation is associated with alterations in body composition. While substrate metabolism during active CD resembles that during starvation, it is more a consequence of malnutrition and may be easily reversed by treatment with EEN.[40,212] BMI, lean body mass (LBM), and fat mass are all decreased in children with IBD, and this may be related to poor calorie intake.[186,213] A higher BMI and LBMs were both positively correlated with increased BMD, factors that again stress the importance of adequate nutrition in maximizing long-term BMD.

EEN provides a simple but effective treatment for children with CD. Not only does it appear to influence disease activity directly, it also appears to have clear benefits on growth and nutrition.

Early evidence suggested that REE was increased in patients with inactive CD.[214] It now appears, however, that if the REE is calculated per unit of LBM, it is the same in active CD as it is in normal controls.[40] The REE/LBM was found to be significantly lower in children with anorexia nervosa than in normal controls. When comparing these malnourished noninflammatory disease-controls with children with active CD, the authors showed that the appropriate physiological response to starvation is lost during active inflammation. Thus this inappropriately elevated REE further contributes to weight loss. On treatment with elemental feed, their absolute REE did increase to above normal levels, but per unit of LBM only remained within the normal range. This study also showed that an elemental diet was significantly better than steroids at accruing lean body tissue and was again better at achieving linear growth.

Despite the documented increase in energy intake by children on steroids compared to those on an elemental diet,[168] the latter group have a significantly greater rise in their median height velocity standard deviation score (SDS) after 4 weeks on an elemental diet. Adequate calorie intake alone in the presence of steroid therapy (124% of RDA) is thus unable to achieve optimal growth. The short-term growth suppressant effects of prednisolone[215] probably override any advantage conferred by the improved calorie intake. IGF-1 levels appeared greater after steroid treatment than after enteral nutrition, yet a significant increase in IGF-1 was only associated with greater height velocity after an elemental diet.[168]

The rate of protein turnover in seven children with chronically active CD receiving steroids was considered to be similar to that of normal adolescent controls,[186] although their nitrogen balance was found to increase 4-fold during nutritional supplementation. Another small study compared the effect of steroids ($n = 6$) and elemental feed ($n = 6$) after the first 7 days of treatment in acute CD.[216] Labeled L-leucine studies showed an equal increase in protein turnover after 7 days of treatment, whereas in the steroid treated group this was at the expense of total body protein stores. Clinical improvement was similar in each group. In a more recent study by Thomas and colleagues,[217] rates of protein turnover were also elevated in active CD. Labeled L-leucine studies and mass spectrometry analysis showed an equal reduction in protein turnover to normal levels, both by steroids ($n = 4$) and by elemental feed ($n = 6$). This study only assessed protein turnover after several weeks of treatment, and only after effective recovery and nutritional restitution were almost complete.

Royall and colleagues[218] published evidence in 30 adults with active CD that proportionate increases in body fat, protein, and water occurred after 21 days of elemental nutrition. In this study, a sustained remission was only achieved in patients who showed a gain in total body nitrogen.

Further evidence that optimizing nutrition may contribute to a clinical remission arises from the study by Slonim and colleagues.[219] The combination of a protein-rich diet (> 2 g/d) and subcutaneous growth hormone (GH) led to a significant reduction in CDAI within 4 months, in a small group of adults with moderate to severe CD. Increased uptake of amino acids[220] and improved intestinal and muscle protein synthesis are mechanisms that are likely to be important in mediating this effect.[221] Direct effects of GH on IGF-1 are not felt to be as significant, as no correlation was found between IGF-1 levels and clinical response.

FUTURE DIRECTIONS

From the above discussion it is abundantly clear that nutrition still has a major role to play in the management of children with IBD, and in particular those with CD. While EEN is clearly effective in many children with active CD, it remains difficult for some children and their families to complete prolonged courses. Work is continuing to assess whether long-term supplementation of a normal diet prolongs remission.

Palatable whole-protein formulae are being modified to include higher percentages of n-3 fatty acids, while the addition of probiotics to feeds is also already underway.

Work also continues on isolating the specific factors within formulas that may directly act on mucosal inflammation. Upregulation of mucosal TGF-β may be a direct result of higher levels of TGF-β within a formula (Modulen IBD, Nestle), while further characterization of the gut microflora in children with IBD may allow specific supplementation with specific prebiotics, substrates that selectively stimulate the growth of certain favorable probiotic species.

CONCLUSIONS

Despite the ever-increasing choice of therapies available to children with IBD, the role of nutrition remains central to their optimal management. The impact of bowel inflammation on growth and development cannot be underestimated. As final adult height is determined during the pubertal growth spurt, it is crucial to minimize the impact that both the disease and its therapies may have on a child's growth potential.

Advances in identifying children at particular risk of growth failure may, in the future, allow specific interventions to maximize growth.

We strongly suggest that EEN remains the best primary therapy for the treatment of all children presenting with a new diagnosis of CD, apart from those with severe perianal disease. Thereafter the challenge is to maintain a lasting remission, particularly during puberty. This is likely to be best achieved with early use of immunosuppressants such as azathioprine/6-mercaptopurine, hoping to minimize steroid use. Continued vigilance of undernutrition and appropriate use of dietary supplementation remain essential to an optimal outcome.

The consequences of developing a chronic inflammatory disease during childhood will be felt long after a child is handed over to our adult physician colleagues. Increased risks of osteoporotic fractures, high rates of surgery, and a reduced final height are only some of the areas where nutritional therapy is vitally important. The ability of therapies to achieve healing of the gut mucosa is of utmost importance in children who have a lifetime ahead of them. Although dietary therapies do not yet play a significant therapeutic role in maintenance therapy for IBD, it is likely that evidence about potential disease-modifying dietary supplements will continue to appear. It is important that as more potent immunologic agents become available to treat these diseases, we do not forget the therapeutic role of nutrition in CD its absence of adverse effects, and its proven impact on growth and gut mucosa.

While newer therapies may require less commitment from families and medical teams, their unknown long-term safety profile still makes enteral nutrition an excellent choice for children with CD for many years to come.

REFERENCES

1. Guidelines for use of home total parenteral nutrition. A.S.P.E.N. Board of Directors. American Society for Parenteral and Enteral Nutrition. JPEN J Parenter Enteral Nutr 1987;11:342–4.
2. Clouston TS. Forcible feeding. Lancet 1872;i:797–8.
3. Widdowson E.M. A Study of Individual Children's Diets. MRC Special Report 1947;257.
4. Giorgini GL, Stephens RV, Thayer WRJ. The use of "medical by-pass" in the therapy of Crohn's disease: Report of a case. Am J Dig Dis 1973;18:153–7.
5. Logan RF, Gillon J, Ferrington C, Ferguson A. Reduction of gastrointestinal protein loss by elemental diet in Crohn's disease of the small bowel. Gut 1981;22:383–7.
6. Morin CL, Roulet M, Roy CC, Weber A. Continuous elemental enteral alimentation in children with Crohn's disease and growth failure. Gastroenterology 1980;79:1205–10.
7. Morin CL, Roulet M, Roy CC, et al. Continuous elemental enteral alimentation in the treatment of children and adolescents with Crohn's disease. JPEN J Parenter Enteral Nutr 1982;6:194–9.
8. O'Morain C, Segal AW, Levi AJ. Elemental diet as primary treatment of acute Crohn's disease: A controlled trial. Br Med J (Clin Res Ed) 1984;288:1859–62.
9. Sanderson IR, Udeen S, Davies PS, et al. Remission induced by an elemental diet in small bowel Crohn's disease. Arch Dis Child 1987;62:123–7.
10. Savage MO, Beattie RM, Camacho-Hubner C, et al. Growth in Crohn's disease. Acta Paediatr Suppl 1999;88:89–92.
11. Dalwadi H, Bo W, Braun J. Defining new pathogens and nonculturable infectious agents associated with inflammatory bowel disease. Curr Opin Gastroenterol 2000;16:56–9.
12. Feeney MA, Murphy F, Clegg AJ, et al. A case-control study of childhood environmental risk factors for the development of inflammatory bowel disease. Eur J Gastroenterol Hepatol 2002;14:529–34.
13. Gilat T, Hacohen D, Lilos P, Langman MJ. Childhood factors in ulcerative colitis and Crohn's disease. An international cooperative study. Scand J Gastroenterol 1987;22:1009–24.
14. Mahmud N, Weir DG. The urban diet and Crohn's disease: Is there a relationship? Eur J Gastroenterol Hepatol 2001;13:93–5.
15. Russel MG, Engels LG, Muris JW, et al. Modern life' in the epidemiology of inflammatory bowel disease: A case-control study with special emphasis on nutritional factors. Eur J Gastroenterol Hepatol 1998;10:243–9.
16. Thornton JR, Emmett PM, Heaton KW. Diet and ulcerative colitis. Br Med J 1980;280:293–4.
17. Persson PG, Ahlbom A, Hellers G. Diet and inflammatory bowel disease: A case-control study. Epidemiology 1992;3:47–52.
18. Reif S, Klein I, Lubin F, et al. Pre-illness dietary factors in inflammatory bowel disease. Gut 1997;40:754–60.
19. Geerling BJ, Dagnelie PC, Badart-Smook A, et al. Diet as a risk factor for the development of ulcerative colitis. Am J Gastroenterol 2000;95:1008–13.
20. Roediger WE. The colonic epithelium in ulcerative colitis: An energy-deficiency disease? Lancet 1980;2:712–5.
21. Chapman MA, Grahn MF, Boyle MA, et al. Butyrate oxidation is impaired in the colonic mucosa of sufferers of quiescent ulcerative colitis. Gut 1994;35:73–6.
22. Scheppach W, Christl SU, Bartram HP, et al. Effects of short-chain fatty acids on the inflamed colonic mucosa. Scand J Gastroenterol Suppl 1997;222:53–7.
23. Steinhart AH, Hiruki T, Brzezinski A, Baker JP. Treatment of left-sided ulcerative colitis with butyrate enemas: A controlled trial. Aliment Pharmacol Ther 1996;10:729–36.
24. Roediger WE, Duncan A, Kapaniris O, Millard S. Sulphide impairment of substrate oxidation in rat colonocytes: A biochemical basis for ulcerative colitis? Clin Sci (Lond) 1993;85:623–7.
25. Pitcher MC, Beatty ER, Cummings JH. The contribution of sulphate reducing bacteria and 5-aminosalicylic acid to faecal sulphide in patients with ulcerative colitis. Gut 2000;46:64–72.
26. Harris JE, Lammerding AM. Crohn's disease and Mycobacterium avium subsp. paratuberculosis: Current issues. J Food Prot 2001;64:2103–10.
27. Thomas GA, Swift GL, Green JT, et al. Controlled trial of antituberculous chemotherapy in Crohn's disease: A five year follow up study. Gut 1998;42:497–500.
28. McCartney S, Ballinger A. Growth failure in inflammatory bowel disease. Nutrition 1999;15:169–171.
29. Ling PR, Schwartz JH, Bistrian BR. Mechanisms of host wasting induced by administration of cytokines in rats. Am J Physiol 1997;272:E333–9.
30. Smith BK, Conn CA, Kluger MJ. Experimental cachexia: Effects of MCA sarcoma in the Fischer rat. Am J Physiol 1993;265:R376–84.
31. Flores EA, Bistrian BR, Pomposelli JJ, et al. Infusion of tumor necrosis factor/cachectin promotes muscle catabolism in the rat. A synergistic effect with interleukin 1. J Clin Invest 1989;83:1614–1622.
32. Winter TA, O'Keefe SJ, Callanan M, Marks T. Impaired gastric acid and pancreatic enzyme secretion in patients with Crohn's disease may be a consequenece of a poor nutritional state. Inflamm Bowel Dis 2004;10:618–625.
33. Chikenji T, Elwyn DH, Gil KM, et al. Effects of increasing glucose intake on nitrogen balance and energy expenditure in malnourished adult patients receiving parenteral nutrition. Clin Sci (Lond) 1987;72:489–501.
34. Macias WL, Alaka KJ, Murphy MH, et al. Impact of the nutritional regimen on protein catabolism and nitrogen balance in patients with acute renal failure. JPEN J Parenter Enteral Nutr 1996;20:56–62.
35. Gavin J, Anderson CE, Bremner AR, Beattie RM. Energy intakes of children with Crohn's disease treated with enteral nutrition as primary therapy. J Hum Nutr Diet 2005;18:337–42.
36. Kirschner BS, Klich JR, Kalman SS, et al. Reversal of growth retardation in Crohn's disease with therapy emphasizing oral nutritional restitution. Gastroenterology 1981;80:10–15.
37. Kelts DG, Grand RJ, Shen G, et al. Nutritional basis of growth failure in children and adolescents with Crohn's disease. Gastroenterology 1979;76:720–7.
38. Aiges H, Markowitz J, Rosa J, Daum F. Home nocturnal supplemental nasogastric feedings in growth-retarded adolescents with Crohn's disease. Gastroenterology 1989;97:905–10.
39. Markowitz J, Grancher K, Rosa J, et al. Growth failure in pediatric inflammatory bowel disease. J Pediatr Gastroenterol Nutr 1993;16:373–80.
40. Azcue M, Rashid M, Griffiths A, Pencharz PB. Energy expenditure and body composition in children with Crohn's disease: Effect of enteral nutrition and treatment with prednisolone. Gut 1997;41:203–8.
41. Ballinger AB, Camacho-Hubner C, Croft NM. Growth failure and intestinal inflammation. QJM 2001;94:121–5.
42. Walker-Smith JA. Management of growth failure in Crohn's disease. Arch Dis Child 1996;75:351–4.
43. Kanof ME, Lake AM, Bayless TM. Decreased height velocity in children and adolescents before the diagnosis of Crohn's disease. Gastroenterology 1988;95:1523–7.
44. Hildebrand H, Karlberg J, Kristiansson B. Longitudinal growth in children and adolescents with inflammatory bowel disease. J Pediatr Gastroenterol Nutr 1994;18:165–73.
45. Compston JE. Review article: Osteoporosis, corticosteroids and inflammatory bowel disease. Aliment Pharmacol Ther 1995;9:237–50.
46. Bernstein CN, Blanchard JF, Leslie W, et al. The incidence of fracture among patients with inflammatory bowel disease. A population-based cohort study. Ann Intern Med 2000;133:795–9.
47. Arden NK, Cooper C. Osteoporosis in patients with inflammatory bowel disease. Gut 2002;50:9–10.
48. Schoon EJ, Blok BM, Geerling BJ, et al. Bone mineral density in patients with recently diagnosed inflammatory bowel disease. Gastroenterology 2000;119:1203–8.
49. Herzog D, Bishop N, Glorieux F, Seidman EG. Interpretation of bone mineral density values in pediatric Crohn's disease. Inflamm Bowel Dis 1998;4:261–7.
50. Gokhale R, Favus MJ, Karrison T, et al. Bone mineral density assessment in children with inflammatory bowel disease. Gastroenterology 1998;114:902–11.
51. Picado C, Luengo M. Corticosteroid-induced bone loss. Prevention and management. Drug Saf 1996;15:347–59.
52. Ahmed SF, Horrocks IA, Patterson T, et al. Bone mineral assessment by dual energy X-ray absorptiometry in children with inflammatory bowel disease: Evaluation by age or bone area. J Pediatr Gastroenterol Nutr 2004;38:276–80.
53. Thearle M, Horlick M, Bilezikian JP, et al. Osteoporosis: An unusual presentation of childhood Crohn's disease. J Clin Endocrinol Metab 2000;85:2122–6.
54. Abreu MT, Geller JL, Vasiliauskas EA, et al. Treatment with infliximab is associated with increased markers of bone formation in patients with Crohn's disease. J Clin Gastroenterol 2006;40:55–63.
55. Pazianas M, Rhim AD, Weinberg AM, et al. The effect of anti-TNF-alpha therapy on spinal bone mineral density in patients with Crohn's disease. Ann N Y Acad Sci 2006;1068:543–56.
56. Dear KL, Compston JE, Hunter JO. Treatments for Crohn's disease that minimise steroid doses are associated with a reduced risk of osteoporosis. Clin Nutr 2001;20:541–6.
57. Habtezion A, Silverberg MS, Parkes R, et al. Risk factors for low bone density in Crohn's disease. Inflamm Bowel Dis 2002;8:87–92.
58. Jahnsen J, Falch JA, Mowinckel P, Aadland E. Vitamin D status, parathyroid hormone and bone mineral density in patients with inflammatory bowel disease. Scand J Gastroenterol 2002;37:192–9.
59. Quercia RA, Korn S, O'Neill D, et al. Selenium deficiency and fatal cardiomyopathy in a patient receiving long-term home parenteral nutrition. Clin Pharm 1984;3:531–5.
60. Filippi J, Al Jaouni R, Wiroth JB, et al. Nutritional deficiencies in patients with Crohn's disease in remission. Inflamm Bowel Dis 2006;12:185–191.
61. Chowers Y, Sela BA, Holland R, et al. Increased levels of homocysteine in patients with Crohn's disease are related to folate levels. Am J Gastroenterol 2000;95:3498–502.
62. Mahmud N, Molloy A, McPartlin J, et al. Increased prevalence of methylenetetrahydrofolate reductase C677T variant in patients with inflammatory bowel disease, and its clinical implications. Gut 1999;45:389–94.
63. Bousvaros A, Zurakowski D, Duggan C, et al. Vitamins A and E serum levels in children and young adults with inflammatory bowel disease: Effect of disease activity. J Pediatr Gastroenterol Nutr 1998;26:129–35.
64. Geerling BJ, Badart-Smook A, Stockbrugger RW, Brummer RJ. Comprehensive nutritional status in recently diagnosed patients with inflammatory bowel disease compared with population controls [In Process Citation]. Eur J Clin Nutr 2000;54:514.
65. Fernandez-Banares F, Mingorance MD, Esteve M, et al. Serum zinc, copper, and selenium levels in inflammatory bowel disease: Effect of total enteral nutrition on trace element status. Am J Gastroenterol 1990;85:1584–9.
66. Thomas C, Thomas L. Biochemical markers and hematologic indices in the diagnosis of functional iron deficiency. Clin Chem 2002;48:1066–76.
67. Maherzi A, Galan P, Cezard JP, et al. Assessment of iron status in children and adolescents with Crohn's disease: Value of basic red cell ferritin. Ann Nutr Metab 1996;40:331–5.
68. Oldenburg B, Koningsberger JC, Berge Henegouwen GP, et al. Iron and inflammatory bowel disease. Aliment Pharmacol Ther 2001;15:429–38.

69. Gasche C, Dejaco C, Waldhoer T, et al. Intravenous iron and erythropoietin for anemia associated with Crohn disease. A randomized, controlled trial. Ann Intern Med 1997;126:782–7.
70. Schreiber S, Howaldt S, Schnoor M, et al. Recombinant erythropoietin for the treatment of anemia in inflammatory bowel disease [see comments]. N Engl J Med 1996;334:619–23.
71. Geerling BJ, Badart-Smook A, Stockbrugger RW, Brummer RJ. Comprehensive nutritional status in patients with long-standing Crohn disease currently in remission [see comments]. Am J Clin Nutr 1998;67:919–26.
72. Sturniolo GC, Di LV, Ferronato A, et al. Zinc supplementation tightens "leaky gut" in Crohn's disease. Inflamm Bowel Dis 2001;7:94–98.
73. Griffin IJ, Kim SC, Hicks PD, et al. Zinc metabolism in adolescents with Crohn's disease. Pediatr Res 2004;56:235–9.
74. Reimund JM, Hirth C, Koehl C, et al. Antioxidant and immune status in active Crohn's disease. A possible relationship. Clin Nutr 2000;19:43–8.
75. Trebble TM, Wootton SA, May A, et al. Essential fatty acid status in paediatric Crohn's disease: Relationship with disease activity and nutritional status. Aliment Pharmacol Ther 2003;18:433–42.
76. Dickinson RJ, Ashton MG, Axon AT, et al. Controlled trial of intravenous hyperalimentation and total bowel rest as an adjunct to the routine therapy of acute colitis. Gastroenterology 1980;79:1199–204.
77. McIntyre PB, Powell-Tuck J, Wood SR, et al. Controlled trial of bowel rest in the treatment of severe acute colitis. Gut 1986;27:481–5.
78. Seidman EG. Nutritional management of inflammatory bowel disease. Gastroenterol Clin North Am 1989;18:129–55.
79. Spray C, Debelle GD, Murphy MS. Current diagnosis, management and morbidity in paediatric inflammatory bowel disease. Acta Paediatr 2001;90:400–5.
80. Powell-Tuck J. Protein metabolism in inflammatory bowel disease. Gut 1986;27:67–71.
81. Gonzalez-Huix F, Fernandez-Banares F, Esteve-Comas M, et al. Enteral versus parenteral nutrition as adjunct therapy in acute ulcerative colitis. Am J Gastroenterol 1993;88:227–32.
82. Hallert C, Kaldma M, Petersson BG. Ispaghula husk may relieve gastrointestinal symptoms in ulcerative colitis in remission. Scand J Gastroenterol 1991;26:747–50.
83. Fuchs CS, Giovannucci EL, Colditz GA, et al. Dietary fiber and the risk of colorectal cancer and adenoma in women. N Engl J Med 1999;340:169–76.
84. Beattie RM, Schiffrin EJ, Donnet-Hughes A, et al. Polymeric nutrition as the primary therapy in children with small bowel Crohn's disease. Aliment Pharmacol Ther 1994;8:609–15.
85. Fell JM, Paintin M, Arnaud-Battandier F, et al. Mucosal healing and a fall in mucosal pro-inflammatory cytokine mRNA induced by a specific oral polymeric diet in paediatric Crohn's disease. Aliment Pharmacol Ther 2000;14:281–9.
86. Ruuska T, Savilahti E, Maki M, et al. Exclusive whole protein enteral diet versus prednisolone in the treatment of acute Crohn's disease in children. J Pediatr Gastroenterol Nutr 1994;19:175–80.
87. Seidman E, Griffiths A, Jones A, Issenman R. Semi-elemental diet vs prednisolone in pediatric Crohn's disease. Gastroenterology 1993;104:778.
88. Lochs H, Steinhardt HJ, Klaus-Wentz B, et al. Comparison of enteral nutrition and drug treatment in active Crohn's disease. Results of the European Cooperative Crohn's Disease Study. IV [see comments]. Gastroenterology 1991;101:881–8.
89. Malchow H, Ewe K, Brandes JW, et al. European Cooperative Crohn's Disease Study (ECCDS): Results of drug treatment. Gastroenterology 1984;86:249–66.
90. Afzal NA, Davies S, Paintin M, et al. Colonic Crohn's disease in children does not respond well to treatment with enteral nutrition if the ileum is not involved. Dig Dis Sci 2005;50:1471–5.
91. Lim S, Dohil R, Meadows N, et al. Treatment of orofacial and ileo-colonic Crohn's disease with total enteral nutrition. J R Soc Med 1998;91:489–90.
92. Afzal NA, Addai S, Fagbemi A, et al. Refeeding syndrome with enteral nutrition in children: A case report, literature review and clinical guidelines. Clin Nutr 2002;21:515–20.
93. Dempsey DT, Mullen JL, Buzby GP. The link between nutritional status and clinical outcome: Can nutritional intervention modify it? Am J Clin Nutr 1988;47:352–6.
94. Klein S, Simes J, Blackburn GL. Total parenteral nutrition and cancer clinical trials. Cancer 1986;58:1378–86.
95. Shiloni E, Coronado E, Freund HR. Role of total parenteral nutrition in the treatment of Crohn's disease. Am J Surg 1989;157:180–5.
96. Lashner BA, Evans AA, Hanauer SB. Preoperative total parenteral nutrition for bowel resection in Crohn's disease. Dig Dis Sci 1989;34:741–6.
97. Rombeau JL, Barot LR, Williamson CE, Mullen JL. Preoperative total parenteral nutrition and surgical outcome in patients with inflammatory bowel disease. Am J Surg 1982;143:139–43.
98. Jacobson S, Kallner A. Effect of total parenteral nutrition on serum concentrations of eight proteins in Crohn's disease. Am J Gastroenterol 1984;79:501–5.
99. Loftus EV, Jr, Schoenfeld P, Sandborn WJ. The epidemiology and natural history of Crohn's disease in population-based patient cohorts from North America: A systematic review. Aliment Pharmacol Ther 2002;16:51–60.
100. Puntis J, McNeish AS, Allan RN. Long term prognosis of Crohn's disease with onset in childhood and adolescence. Gut 1984;25:329–36.
101. Beier-Holgersen R, Boesby S. Influence of postoperative enteral nutrition on postsurgical infections. Gut 1996;39:833–5.
102. Beattie AH, Prach AT, Baxter JP, Pennington CR. A randomised controlled trial evaluating the use of enteral nutritional supplements postoperatively in malnourished surgical patients. Gut 2000;46:813–8.
103. Perioperative total parenteral nutrition in surgical patients. The Veterans Affairs Total Parenteral Nutrition Cooperative Study Group. N Engl J Med 1991;325:525–32.
104. Chandra RK. Interactions of nutrition, infection and immune response. Immunocompetence in nutritional deficiency, methodological considerations and intervention strategies. Acta Paediatr Scand 1979;68:137–44.
105. Seidman E, LeLeiko N, Ament M, et al. Nutritional issues in pediatric inflammatory bowel disease. J Pediatr Gastroenterol Nutr 1991;12:424–38.
106. Anderson DL, Boyce HWJ. Use of parenteral nutrition in treatment of advanced regional enteritis. Am J Dig Dis 1973;18:633–40.
107. Fischer JE, Foster GS, Abel RM, et al. Hyperalimentation as primary therapy for inflammatory bowel disease. Am J Surg 1973;125:165–75.
108. Layden T, Rosenberg F, Nemchausky G, et al. Reversal of growth arrest in adolescents with Crohn's disease after parenteral alimentation. Gastroenterology 1976;70:1017–21.
109. Wright RA, Adler EC. Peripheral parenteral nutrition is no better than enteral nutrition in acute exacerbation of Crohn's disease: A prospective trial. J Clin Gastroenterol 1990;12:396–9.
110. Deitch EA, Xu D, Naruhn MB, et al. Elemental diet and IV-TPN-induced bacterial translocation is associated with loss of intestinal mucosal barrier function against bacteria [see comments]. Ann Surg 1995;221:299–307.
111. Greenberg GR, Fleming CR, Jeejeebhoy KN, et al. Controlled trial of bowel rest and nutritional support in the management of Crohn's disease. Gut 1988;29:1309–15.
112. Fuchigami T, Ohgushi H, Imamura K, et al. Effects of total parenteral nutrition on colonic lesions in Crohn's disease: Radiographic and endoscopic study. Gastroenterol Jpn 1982;17:521–529.
113. Himal HS, Allard JR, Nadeau JE, et al. The importance of adequate nutrition in closure of small intestinal fistulas. Br J Surg 1974;61:724–6.
114. Spiliotis J, Briand D, Gouttebel MC, et al. Treatment of fistulas of the gastrointestinal tract with total parenteral nutrition and octreotide in patients with carcinoma. Surg Gynecol Obstet 1993;176:575–80.
115. Howard L, Heaphey L, Fleming CR, et al. Four years of North American registry home parenteral nutrition outcome data and their implications for patient management. JPEN J Parenter Enteral Nutr 1991;15:384–93.
116. Greenstein JP, Birnbaum SM, Winitz M, Otey M. Quantitative nutritional studies with water soluble chemically defined diets. 1. Growth, reproduction and lactation in rats. Arch Biochem Biophys 1957;72:396–416.
117. Voitk AJ, Echave V, Feller JH, et al. Experience with elemental diet in the treatment of inflammatory bowel disease. Is this primary therapy? Arch Surg 1973;107:329–33.
118. Navarro J, Vargas J, Cezard JP, et al. Prolonged constant rate elemental enteral nutrition in Crohn's disease. J Pediatr Gastroenterol Nutr 1982;1:541–6.
119. O'Morain C. Crohn's disease treated by elemental diet. J R Soc Med 1982;75:135–6.
120. Akobeng AK, Miller V, Stanton J, et al. Double-blind randomized controlled trial of glutamine-enriched polymeric diet in the treatment of active Crohn's disease. J Pediatr Gastroenterol Nutr 2000;30:78–84.
121. Silk DB, Fairclough PD, Clark ML, et al. Use of a peptide rather than free amino acid nitrogen source in chemically defined "elemental" diets. JPEN J Parenter Enteral Nutr 1980;4:548–53.
122. Raouf AH, Hildrey V, Daniel J, et al. Enteral feeding as sole treatment for Crohn's disease: Controlled trial of whole protein v amino acid based feed and a case study of dietary challenge. Gut 1991;32:702–7.
123. Gonzalez-Huix F, de Leon R, Fernandez-Banares F, et al. Polymeric enteral diets as primary treatment of active Crohn's disease: A prospective steroid controlled trial. Gut 1993;34:778–82.
124. Hyams JS, Ferry GD, Mandel FS, et al. Development and validation of a pediatric Crohn's disease activity index. J Pediatr Gastroenterol Nutr 1991;12:439–47.
125. Breese EJ, Michie CA, Nicholls SW, et al. The effect of treatment on lymphokine-secreting cells in the intestinal mucosa of children with Crohn's disease. Aliment Pharmacol Ther 1995;9:547–52.
126. Bannerjee K, Camacho-Hubner C, Babinska K, et al. Anti-inflammatory and growth-stimulating effects precede nutritional restitution during enteral feeding in Crohn disease. J Pediatr Gastroenterol Nutr 2004;38:270–5.
127. Gassull MA, Fernandez-Banares F, Cabre E, et al. Fat composition may be a clue to explain the primary therapeutic effect of enteral nutrition in Crohn's disease: Results of a double blind randomised multicentre European trial. Gut 2002;51:164–8.
128. Miura S, Tsuzuki Y, Hokari R, Ishii H. Modulation of intestinal immune system by dietary fat intake: Relevance to Crohn's disease. J Gastroenterol Hepatol 1998;13:1183–90.
129. Sakurai T, Matsui T, Yao T, et al. Short-term efficacy of enteral nutrition in the treatment of active Crohn's disease: A randomized, controlled trial comparing nutrient formulas. JPEN J Parenter Enteral Nutr 2002;26:98–103.
130. Leiper K, Woolner J, Mullan MM, et al. A randomised controlled trial of high versus low long chain triglyceride whole protein feed in active Crohn's disease. Gut 2001;49:790–4.
131. von Tirpitz C, Kohn C, Steinkamp M, et al. Lactose intolerance in active Crohn's disease: Clinical value of duodenal lactase analysis. J Clin Gastroenterol 2002;34:49–53.
132. Malchow H, Steinhardt HJ, Lorenz-Meyer H, et al. Feasibility and effectiveness of a defined-formula diet regimen in treating active Crohn's disease. European Cooperative Crohn's Disease Study III. Scand J Gastroenterol 1990;25:235–44.
133. Griffiths AM, Ohlsson A, Sherman PM, Sutherland LR. Meta-analysis of enteral nutrition as a primary treatment of active Crohn's disease. Gastroenterology 1995;108:1056–67.
134. Modigliani R, Mary JY, Simon JF, et al. Clinical, biological, and endoscopic picture of attacks of Crohn's disease. Evolution on prednisolone. Groupe d'Etude Therapeutique des Affections Inflammatoires Digestives. Gastroenterology 1990;98:811–8.
135. Zachos M, Tondeur M, Griffiths AM. Enteral nutritional therapy for inducing remission of Crohn's disease. Cochrane Database Syst Rev 2001;CD000542.
136. Heuschkel RB, Menache CC, Megerian JT, Baird AE. Enteral nutrition and corticosteroids in the treatment of acute Crohn's disease in children. J Pediatr Gastroenterol Nutr 2000;31:8–15.
137. Markowitz J, Hyams J, Mack D, et al. Corticosteroid therapy in the age of infliximab: Acute and 1-year outcomes in newly diagnosed children with Crohn's disease. Clin Gastroenterol Hepatol 2006;4:1124–9.
138. Murch SH, Walker-Smith JA. Nutrition in inflammatory bowel disease. Baillieres Clin Gastroenterol 1998;12.
139. Rigaud D, Cosnes J, Le Quintrec Y, et al. Controlled trial comparing two types of enteral nutrition in treatment of active Crohn's disease: Elemental versus polymeric diet. Gut 1991;32:1492–7.
140. Thomas AG, Taylor F, Miller V. Dietary intake and nutritional treatment in childhood Crohn's disease. J Pediatr Gastroenterol Nutr 1993;17:75–81.
141. Afzal NA, Davies S, Paintin M, et al. Colonic Crohn's disease in children does not respond well to treatment with enteral nutrition if the ileum is not involved. Dig Dis Sci 2005;50:1471–5.
142. Riordan AM, Hunter JO, Cowan RE, et al. Treatment of active Crohn's disease by exclusion diet: East Anglian multicentre controlled trial [see comments]. Lancet 1993;342:1131–4.
143. Pearson M, Teahon K, Levi AJ, Bjarnason I. Food intolerance and Crohn's disease. Gut 1993;34:783–7.
144. Polk DB, Hattner JA, Kerner JAJ. Improved growth and disease activity after intermittent administration of a defined formula diet in children with Crohn's disease. JPEN J Parenter Enteral Nutr 1992;16:499–504.
145. Levenstein S, Prantera C, Luzi C, D'Ubaldi A. Low residue or normal diet in Crohn's disease: A prospective controlled study in Italian patients. Gut 1985;26:989–93.
146. Wilschanski M, Sherman P, Pencharz P, et al. Supplementary enteral nutrition maintains remission in paediatric Crohn's disease. Gut 1996;38:543–8.

147. Verma S, Kirkwood B, Brown S, Giaffer MH. Oral nutritional supplementation is effective in the maintenance of remission in Crohn's disease. Dig Liver Dis 2000;32:769–74.
148. Rampton DS, Collins CE. Review article: Thromboxanes in inflammatory bowel disease–pathogenic and therapeutic implications. Aliment Pharmacol Ther 1993;7:357–67.
149. Endres S, Ghorbani R, Kelley VE, et al. The effect of dietary supplementation with n-3 polyunsaturated fatty acids on the synthesis of interleukin-1 and tumor necrosis factor by mononuclear cells. N Engl J Med 1989;320:265–71.
150. Jaschonek K, Clemens MR, Scheurlen M. Decreased responsiveness of platelets to a stable prostacyclin analogue in patients with Crohn's disease. Reversal by n-3 polyunsaturated fatty acids. Thromb Res 1991;63:667–72.
151. Wakefield AJ, Sawyerr AM, Dhillon AP, et al. Pathogenesis of Crohn's disease: Multifocal gastrointestinal infarction [see comments]. Lancet 1989;2:1057–62.
152. Belluzzi A, Brignola C, Campieri M, et al. Effect of an enteric-coated fish-oil preparation on relapses in Crohn's disease [see comments]. N Engl J Med 1996;334:1557–60.
153. Lorenz-Meyer H, Bauer P, Nicolay C, et al. Omega-3 fatty acids and low carbohydrate diet for maintenance of remission in Crohn's disease. A randomized controlled multicenter trial. Study Group Members (German Crohn's Disease Study Group). Scand J Gastroenterol 1996;31:778–85.
154. Middleton SJ, Naylor S, Woolner J, Hunter JO. A double-blind, randomized, placebo-controlled trial of essential fatty acid supplementation in the maintenance of remission of ulcerative colitis. Aliment Pharmacol Ther 2002;16:1131–5.
155. Romano C, Cucchiara S, Barabino A, et al. Usefulness of omega-3 fatty acid supplementation in addition to mesalazine in maintaining remission in pediatric Crohns disease: A double-blind, randomized, placebo-controlled study. World J Gastroenterol 2005;11:7118–21.
156. Lomer MC, Harvey RS, Evans SM, et al. Efficacy and tolerability of a low microparticle diet in a double blind, randomized, pilot study in Crohn's disease. Eur J Gastroenterol Hepatol 2001;13:101–6.
157. Ritchie JK, Wadsworth J, Lennard-Jones JE, Rogers E. Controlled multicentre therapeutic trial of an unrefined carbohydrate, fibre rich diet in Crohn's disease. Br Med J (Clin Res Ed) 1987;295:517–20.
158. Barclay GR, McKenzie H, Pennington J, et al. The effect of dietary yeast on the activity of stable chronic Crohn's disease. Scand J Gastroenterol 1992;27:196–200.
159. Gibson GR. Dietary modulation of the human gut microflora using the prebiotics oligofructose and inulin. J Nutr 1999;129:1438S–41S.
160. Gionchetti P, Rizzello F, Venturi A, et al. Oral bacteriotherapy as maintenance treatment in patients with chronic pouchitis: A double-blind, placebo-controlled trial. Gastroenterology 2000;119:305–9.
161. Gupta P, Andrew H, Kirschner BS, Guandalini S. Is lactobacillus GG helpful in children with Crohn's disease? Results of a preliminary, open-label study. J Pediatr Gastroenterol Nutr 2000;31:453–7.
162. Israel DM, Hassall E. Prolonged use of gastrostomy for enteral hyperalimentation in children with Crohn's disease. Am J Gastroenterol 1995;90:1084–8.
163. Sawczenko A, Azooz O, Paraszczuk J, et al. Intestinal inflammation-induced growth retardation acts through IL-6 in rats and depends on the -174 IL-6 G/C polymorphism in children. Proc Natl Acad Sci U S A 2005;102:13260–5.
164. Sawczenko A, Ballinger AB, Savage MO, Sanderson IR. Clinical features affecting final adult height in patients with pediatric-onset Crohn's disease. Pediatrics 2006;118:124–9.
165. Motil KJ, Grand RJ, Davis-Kraft L, et al. Growth failure in children with inflammatory bowel disease: A prospective study. Gastroenterology 1993;105:681–91.
166. Griffiths AM, Nguyen P, Smith C, et al. Growth and clinical course of children with Crohn's disease. Gut 1993;34:939–43.
167. Thissen JP, Underwood LE, Ketelslegers JM. Regulation of insulin-like growth factor-I in starvation and injury. Nutr Rev 1999;57:167–76.
168. Thomas AG, Holly JM, Taylor F, Miller V. Insulin like growth factor-I, insulin like growth factor binding protein-1, and insulin in childhood Crohn's disease. Gut 1993;34:944–7.
169. Beattie RM, Camacho-Hubner C, Wacharasindhu S, et al. Responsiveness of IGF-I and IGFBP-3 to therapeutic intervention in children and adolescents with Crohn's disease. Clin Endocrinol (Oxf) 1998;49:483–9.
170. Davies G, Evans CM, Shand WS, Walker-Smith JA. Surgery for Crohn's disease in childhood: Influence of site of disease and operative procedure on outcome. Br J Surg 1990;77:891–4.
171. Evans CM, Kirk JM, Savage MO, Walker-Smith JA. Growth after gut resection for Crohn's disease. Arch Dis Child 1991;66:370.
172. Varille V, Cezard JP, de Lagausie P, et al. Resting energy expenditure before and after surgical resection of gut lesions in pediatric Crohn's disease. J Pediatr Gastroenterol Nutr 1996;23:13–9.
173. Murch SH, Lamkin VA, Savage MO, et al. Serum concentrations of tumour necrosis factor alpha in childhood chronic inflammatory bowel disease. Gut 1991;32:913–7.
174. Mingrone G, Greco AV, Benedetti G, et al. Increased resting lipid oxidation in Crohn's disease. Dig Dis Sci 1996;41:72–6.
175. Davies UM, Jones J, Reeve J, et al. Juvenile rheumatoid arthritis. Effects of disease activity and recombinant human growth hormone on insulin-like growth factor 1, insulin-like growth factor binding proteins 1 and 3, and osteocalcin. Arthritis Rheum 1997;40:332–40.
176. Koniaris SG, Fisher SE, Rubin CT, Chawla A. Experimental colitis impairs linear bone growth independent of nutritional factors. J Pediatr Gastroenterol Nutr 1997;25:137–41.
177. De Benedetti F, Alonzi T, Moretta A, et al. Interleukin 6 causes growth impairment in transgenic mice through a decrease in insulin-like growth factor-I. A model for stunted growth in children with chronic inflammation. J Clin Invest 1997;99:643–50.
178. Braegger CP, Nicholls S, Murch SH, et al. Tumour necrosis factor alpha in stool as a marker of intestinal inflammation [see comments]. Lancet 1992;339:89–91.
179. Beeken WL, Busch HJ, Sylwester DL. Intestinal protein loss in Crohn's disease. Gastroenterology 1972;62:207–15.
180. Moshage H. Cytokines and the hepatic acute phase response. J Pathol 1997;181:257–66.
181. Gersovitz M, Munro HN, Udall J, Young VR. Albumin synthesis in young and elderly subjects using a new stable isotope methodology: Response to level of protein intake. Metabolism 1980;29:1075–86.
182. Stelzner M, Somasundaram S, Khakberdiev T. Systemic effects of acute terminal ileitis on uninflamed gut aggravate bile acid malabsorption. J Surg Res 2001;99:359–64.
183. Schoelmerich J, Becher MS, Hoppe-Seyler P, et al. Zinc and vitamin A deficiency in patients with Crohn's disease is correlated with activity but not with localization or extent of the disease. Hepatogastroenterology 1985;32:34–8.
184. Markowitz J, Daum F. Growth impairment in pediatric inflammatory bowel disease. Am J Gastroenterol 1994;89:319–26.
185. Alemzadeh N, Rekers-Mombarg LT, et al. Adult height in patients with early onset of Crohn's disease. Gut 2002;51:26–9.
186. Motil KJ, Grand RJ, Maletskos CJ, Young VR. The effect of disease, drug, and diet on whole body protein metabolism in adolescents with Crohn disease and growth failure. J Pediatr 1982;101:345–51.
187. Motil KJ, Altchuler SI, Grand RJ. Mineral balance during nutritional supplementation in adolescents with Crohn disease and growth failure. J Pediatr 1985;107:473–79.
188. Peach S, Lock MR, Katz D, et al. Mucosal-associated bacterial flora of the intestine in patients with Crohn's disease and in a control group. Gut 1978;19:1034–42.
189. Axelsson CK, Justesen T. Studies of the duodenal and fecal flora in gastrointestinal disorders during treatment with an elemental diet. Gastroenterology 1977;72:397–401.
190. Swidsinski A, Ladhoff A, Pernthaler A, et al. Mucosal flora in inflammatory bowel disease. Gastroenterology 2002;122:44–54.
191. Rutgeerts P, Hiele M, Geboes K, et al. Controlled trial of metronidazole treatment for prevention of Crohn's recurrence after ileal resection [see comments]. Gastroenterology 1995;108:1617–21.
192. Pourtaghi N, Radvar M, Mooney J, Kinane DF. The effect of subgingival antimicrobial therapy on the levels of stromelysin and tissue inhibitor of metalloproteinases in gingival crevicular fluid. J Periodontol 1996;67:866–70.
193. Linskens RK, Huijsdens XW, Savelkoul PH, et al. The bacterial flora in inflammatory bowel disease: Current insights in pathogenesis and the influence of antibiotics and probiotics. Scand J Gastroenterol Suppl 2001;234:29–40.
194. Kishi D, Takahashi I, Kai Y, et al. Alteration of V beta usage and cytokine production of CD4+ TCR beta beta homodimer T cells by elimination of Bacteroides vulgatus prevents colitis in TCR alpha-chain-deficient mice. J Immunol 2000;165:5891–9.
195. Tanaka S, Miura S, Kimura H, et al. Amelioration of chronic inflammation by ingestion of elemental diet in a rat model of granulomatous enteritis. Dig Dis Sci 1997;42:408–19.
196. Tanaka S, Miura S, Kimura H, et al. Amelioration of chronic inflammation by ingestion of elemental diet in a rat model of granulomatous enteritis. Dig Dis Sci 1997;42:408–19.
197. Beattie RM, Walker-Smith JA. Treatment of active Crohn's disease by exclusion diet. J Pediatr Gastroenterol Nutr 1994;19:135–6.
198. Koster F, Pierce NF. Effect of protein deprivation on immunoregulatory cells in the rat mucosal immune response. Clin Exp Immunol 1985;60:217–24.
199. Lamont AG, Gordon M, Ferguson A. Oral tolerance in protein-deprived mice. II. Evidence of normal 'gut processing' of ovalbumin, but suppressor cell deficiency, in deprived mice. Immunology 1987;61:339–43.
200. Sanderson IR. Dietary regulation of genes expressed in the developing intestinal epithelium [In Process Citation]. Am J Clin Nutr 1998;68:999–1005.
201. Nishimura A, Fujimoto M, Oguchi S, et al. Short-chain fatty acids regulate IGF-binding protein secretion by intestinal epithelial cells. Am J Physiol 1998;275:E55–63.
202. Fusunyan RD, Quinn JJ, Ohno Y, et al. Butyrate enhances interleukin (IL)-8 secretion by intestinal epithelial cells in response to IL-1beta and lipopolysaccharide. Pediatr Res 1998;43:84–90.
203. Ohtsuka Y, Lee J, Stamm DS, Sanderson IR. MIP-2 secreted by epithelial cells increases neutrophil and lymphocyte recruitment in the mouse intestine. Gut 2001;49:526–33.
204. Kulkarni AB, Huh CG, Becker D, et al. Transforming growth factor beta 1 null mutation in mice causes excessive inflammatory response and early death. Proc Natl Acad Sci U S A 1993;90:770–4.
205. Wright NA, Poulsom R, Stamp G, et al. Trefoil peptide gene expression in gastrointestinal epithelial cells in inflammatory bowel disease. Gastroenterology 1993;104:12–20.
206. Babyatsky MW, deBeaumont M, Thim L, Podolsky DK. Oral trefoil peptides protect against ethanol- and indomethacin-induced gastric injury in rats [see comments]. Gastroenterology 1996;110:489–97.
207. Beattie RM, Bentsen BS, MacDonald TT. Childhood Crohn's disease and the efficacy of enteral diets. Nutrition 1998;14:345–50.
208. Kirschner BS. Nutritional consequences of inflammatory bowel disease on growth. J Am Coll Nutr 1988;7:301–8.
209. Kirschner BS, Sutton MM. Somatomedin-C levels in growth-impaired children and adolescents with chronic inflammatory bowel disease. Gastroenterology 1986;91:830–6.
210. Walker-Smith JA. Mucosal healing in Crohn's disease [letter; comment]. Gastroenterology 1998;114:419–20.
211. Munkholm P, Langholz E, Davidsen M, Binder V. Intestinal cancer risk and mortality in patients with Crohn's disease. Gastroenterology 1993;105:1716–23.
212. Schneeweiss B, Lochs H, Zauner C, et al. Energy and substrate metabolism in patients with active Crohn's disease. J Nutr 1999;129:844–8.
213. Boot AM, Bouquet J, Krenning EP, de Muinck Keizer-Schrama SM. Bone mineral density and nutritional status in children with chronic inflammatory bowel disease. Gut 1998;42:188–94.
214. Zoli G, Katelaris PH, Garrow J, et al. Increased energy expenditure in growing adolescents with Crohn's disease. Dig Dis Sci 1996;41:1754–9.
215. Friedman M, Strang LB. Effect of long-term corticosteroids and corticotrophin on the growth of children. Lancet 1966;2:569–72.
216. O'Keefe SJ, Ogden J, Rund J, Potter P. Steroids and bowel rest versus elemental diet in the treatment of patients with Crohn's disease: The effects on protein metabolism and immune function. JPEN J Parenter Enteral Nutr 1989;13:455–60.
217. Thomas AG, Miller V, Taylor F, et al. Whole body protein turnover in childhood Crohn's disease. Gut 1992;33:675–7.
218. Royall D, Greenberg GR, Allard JP, et al. Total enteral nutrition support improves body composition of patients with active Crohn's disease [see comments]. JPEN J Parenter Enteral Nutr 1995;19:95–9.
219. Slonim AE, Bulone L, Damore MB, et al. A preliminary study of growth hormone therapy for Crohn's disease. N Engl J Med 2000;342:1633–7.
220. Inoue Y, Copeland EM, Souba WW. Growth hormone enhances amino acid uptake by the human small intestine. Ann Surg 1994;219:715–22.
221. Lo HC, Ney DM. GH and IGF-I differentially increase protein synthesis in skeletal muscle and jejunum of parenterally fed rats. Am J Physiol 1996;271:E872–8.

49

Pediatric HIV Infection

Colleen Hadigan, MD, MPH

There are many nutritional challenges clinicians face in the care of human immunodeficiency virus (HIV)-infected children. Important interactions between the immune system and nutritional status, which will be discussed in this and other chapters, has led to the recognition that treatment of nutritional problems plays a critical role in the health and well-being of HIV-infected children. Careful attention to the nutritional needs of children with HIV can help optimize growth, and more importantly may improve clinical outcomes, such as reduced hospitalization rates and increased survival. This chapter will provide current background information on pediatric HIV infection and the associations between nutrition and HIV. Focus will also be given to the emerging problem of the metabolic disturbances associated with HIV-infection and its therapies. Furthermore, the growth patterns of HIV-infected children, pathogenesis of nutritional disorders, and current diagnostic and therapeutic interventions will be presented. It is hoped that this chapter will provide both practical advice to clinicians caring for HIV-infected children, as well as serve as a basis to stimulate much needed scientific research in this area.

THE PEDIATRIC AIDS EPIDEMIC

Despite the dramatic progress that has been made over the past decade regarding the prevention, detection, diagnosis, and treatment of HIV infection, HIV continues to be a global epidemic. In some regions of the world, such as the United States, HIV has evolved into a chronic disease which carries significant morbidity and mortality. The World Health Organization (WHO) and the UN AIDS report on the global AIDS Epidemic estimated that 38.6 million people worldwide were living with HIV/AIDS in 2005.[1] There is increasing disparity between the United States and developing nations with regard to pediatric HIV/AIDS. While there were 48 documented new cases of perinatally acquired HIV in the United States in 2004, nearly one-third of women presenting to prenatal clinics in regions in sub-Saharan Africa are HIV-infected; there are an estimated 2 million children under age 15 years living with HIV/AIDS in this region, and there were some 12 million orphans living in sub-Saharan Africa in 2005. In addition, more than 70% of deaths in infants under 5 years of age are attributable to AIDS in this part of the world. Finally, children in developing countries who have HIV infection are especially vulnerable to the endemic problems of protracted diarrhea and severe malnutrition.

HIV AND TREATMENT

HIV, an RNA virus that belongs to the lentivirus family, was first isolated in 1983. The virus has a particular tropism for the CD4 surface antigen of cells, and the binding of HIV to the CD4 receptor initiates the viral life cycle, which is mediated by the HIV-1 envelope glycoprotein gp120. The binding of gp120 to CD4 leads to events that cause fusion of the virus into the host membrane, with subsequent steps leading to replication of the virus within the host cell. The proviral DNA within the host cell may also remain latent for varying amounts of time until cellular activation occurs. Human T lymphocytes and monocyte or macrophages are the primary cells that are infected with HIV, although numerous other cell lines have been reported to be infected as well. The net biological effect on the immune system of children with HIV infection is the progressive decline in CD4-positive T lymphocytes, leaving children susceptible to opportunistic and recurrent bacterial infections. Treatment of HIV with antiretroviral medications suppresses HIV viral replication and permits reconstitution of the immune system with a compensatory rise in the CD4-positive T cells. Despite significant clinical and immune benefits of therapy, it is important to note that, even among patients with undetectable HIV viral RNA in the blood while on treatment, virtually all patients will develop detectable virus after withdrawal of therapy.

NUTRITION AND IMMUNITY

Nutritional status and immunity have long been linked, and malnutrition is the most common cause of immunodeficiency worldwide. Long before HIV was described, opportunistic infections such as *Pneumocystis carinii* pneumonia were described in otherwise healthy, but malnourished individuals in developing nations.[2] This association led investigators to conclude that nutrition alone can impact on the immunologic response of an individual. In malnourished children, there is a profound involution of lymphoid tissues, including thymic atrophy and diminished paracortical regions of lymph nodes.[3] In young infants and children, protein calorie malnutrition increases the risk of death by several fold by increasing the susceptibility to infection.[4] In many countries, mortality rates increase from 0.5% in children whose weight-for-height percent of standard is greater than 80%, to a mortality rate of 18% in children whose weight-for-height percent of standard is less than 60%.[5] Biochemically, protein-calorie malnutrition leads to changes in several aspects of the immune system that are similar to the immunologic changes in HIV infection. Cell-mediated immunity, antimicrobial function of phagocytes, complement systems, secretory antibodies, and antibody affinity, are consistently impaired in patients with significant malnutrition. Additionally, deficiencies of micronutrients, especially zinc and vitamin A, as well as many others, may also have deleterious effects on the immune system. Other aspects of immunity that are altered by protein-calorie malnutrition include impaired chemotaxis of neutrophils, decreased lysozyme levels in serum and secretions, and decreased interferon production in antibody response to T-cell dependent antigens. A child with protein-calorie malnutrition may also have impaired mucosal immunity with lowered concentrations of secretory IgA in saliva, nasopharynx, and tears compared to well-nourished control children. Table 1 illustrates the significant and close interaction between nutrition and immunity. This topic is discussed in greater detail in Chapter 22, "Immunophysiology and Nutrition of the Gut," and Chapter 23, "Malnutrition and Host Defenses."

Because many of the immunologic changes in malnutrition are similar to those found in

Table 1 Immunologic Abnormalities Associated with Malnutrition and Human Immunodeficiency Virus (HIV) Infection

	Protein Energy Malnutrition	HIV Infection
CD4 T-lymphocyte number	↓	↓
CD8 T-lymphocyte number	↓	↓
CD4/CD8 ratio	↓	↓
Proliferative response to mitogens	↓	↓
Serum immunoglobulins	↑	↑
Circulating immune complexes	Normal or ↑	↑
Serologic response after immunization	↓	↓
Chemotaxis	↓	↓
Bacterial killing	↓	↓
Natural killer activity	?	↓
Serum complement	↓	Normal

children infected with HIV, malnutrition has been proposed to act as a cofactor of immune dysfunction by influencing both susceptibility to HIV infection and progression of the disease. It is logical to expect that augmenting the nutritional status of an HIV-infected child may improve the function of an already compromised immune system. Preliminary evidence to support this notion is presented later in this chapter.

GROWTH AND BODY COMPOSITION OF HIV-INFECTED CHILDREN

Growth

Impaired growth and malnutrition are common among infants and children with HIV infection and are closely associated with morbidity and mortality in this population. In 1998, HIV-wasting or failure to thrive became the second most common AIDS defining illness in children in the United States.[6] Most, if not all children with HIV infection, will experience nutritional abnormalities during the course of their illness that may impact growth and development. Even in the era of antiretroviral therapy, failure to thrive defined as weight for age Z-score ≤ -2.0 SD is common in HIV-infected children in the United States and was found in 37% of perinatally infected children at 1 year of age.[7] In this study, failure to thrive was also associated with a significantly increased mortality rate by 36 months of age (36.3% vs 14.3% among HIV-infected children without failure to thrive). Further, in one of the early studies of antiretroviral therapy in pediatric HIV ($n = 434$), low height-for-age Z-score, a sensitive marker of stunting and chronic nutritional deprivation, was associated with increased mortality, independent of age or HIV viral load.[8] These findings indicate the ongoing importance of assessing nutritional status and growth in the management of HIV-infected children.

Weight loss and gastrointestinal symptoms are one of the most common presenting symptoms of HIV disease in developing countries. In Tanzania, 200 children with severe malnutrition and nonmalnourished controls who were matched for age, sex, and area of residence, were screened for evidence of HIV infection.[9] Twenty-five percent of the malnourished group was HIV-positive compared with 1.5% of the control group. These authors recommend routine screening for HIV infection in malnourished children in developing nations, since there is a high likelihood that they will be HIV-positive.

Among HIV-infected infants in developing nations, mortality remains high and strongly linked with nutritional status. For example, of 62 HIV-infected infants studied in the first 2 years of life in Nairobi, Kenya, 52% died with a median survival of 6.2 months.[10] Importantly, low birthweight, weight, length, and head circumference $\leq$ 5th percentile at 1 month of age and formula feeding were all strong predictors of infant mortality. Similar observations were made in Kampala, Uganda, where HIV-infected infants experienced a 54% mortality by 2 years of age and growth failure (defined as weight-for-age Z- score < -1.5) was associated with mortality.[11] A study in New Delhi, India identified 109 HIV-infected children and noted that 81.3% presented with failure to thrive, 50.5% with diarrhea, and virtually all of the children had poor nutritional status.[12] Therefore, early recognition of growth failure and provision of appropriate nutritional support may significantly improve the health and survival of HIV-infected children.

Growth abnormalities may not be present at birth in perinatally infected infants. In the United States, children with HIV infection have similar birthweights and are at no higher risk of prematurity than children who are not HIV-infected, but who are born to HIV-infected women.[13] In a prospective study of infants born to HIV-infected women in the United States, as early as 6 months of age and up through age 5 years, HIV-infected children had significantly lower weight-for-age, height-for-age Z-scores,[7] and weight-for-height[13] than there HIV-exposed, but uninfected counterparts. Thus, growth abnormalities may begin postnatally and may develop even in asymptomatic children.

The natural history of somatic growth in pediatric HIV infection was reported in 1996 in the United States [Women and Infants Transmission Study (WITS)]. An analysis of 282 infants born to HIV-infected women revealed that at birth, HIV-infected infants were 0.28 kg lighter and 1.64 cm shorter than uninfected infants, and these differences persisted after controlling for the effects of maternal drug and alcohol use.[14] HIV-infected children had a progressive decrement in weight, length, and BMI extending to 18 months of age. There were also early and sustained decrements in head circumference. Preliminary data from 10 years of follow-up in this same study demonstrate considerable progressive growth decrements with as much as an 8.9 kg weight and 8.0 cm height deficits among HIV-infected children at 9 years of age.[15] Additional studies in children with hemophilia who were HIV-infected documented poor growth as a prognostic indicator to progression to AIDS. HIV-positive children with hemophilia who downwardly crossed 15 percentile points in height- or weight-for-age on two repeated measurements were found to have a greater likelihood to progress to AIDS.[16]

In developing nations, other confounding factors may exist which can explain different outcomes relating to growth. In one study of 822 HIV-infected pregnant women from Tanzania, low birthweight was associated with maternal advanced stage HIV; however malaria, helminthic infections, and intestinal parasites were also strong predictors of low birthweight.[17] Infant HIV infection was not associated with low birthweight, but was predictive of being small for gestational age. In a study from Malawi, 362 children born to HIV-infected women (92 infants HIV-infected) and 686 infants born to noninfected women were evaluated at birth and followed for 2 years.[18] HIV-infected infants had significantly lower weight-for-age at birth and lower length-for-age by 5 months of age. Infants born to HIV-infected mothers who were not perinatally infected initially weighed less and were shorter than infants born to HIV-seronegative mothers, but this difference disappeared by 24 months. A prospective cohort study from Rwanda[19] of 318 HIV-infected and 309 seronegative women was conducted to determine growth parameters in their offspring. Birthweight was significantly lower among infants born to HIV-infected mothers compared to those born to seronegative mothers. These data demonstrate the importance of maternal health in fetal growth and birthweight.

Body Weight and Composition

Accurate assessment of weight, linear growth, and evaluation of body composition are key components in determining nutritional status in all children. Weight loss, or a decrease in growth velocity is a simple marker used to diagnose the wasting syndrome in children with HIV infection. However, using weight as the only marker of nutritional status can be misleading, since weight can be confounded by symptoms such as vomiting and diarrhea. In addition, hydration status and edema can influence weight measurements and obscure the true nutritional condition. Mid-upper arm circumference, or MUAC, is a useful and simple tool used globally to determine nutritional status in adults and children. When available, a more accurate measure of nutritional status is body-cell-mass which refers to the nonadipose cellular mass and is equivalent roughly to the intracellular water volume and can be determined using bioelectrical impedance.

Anthropometry and body composition studies can provide insight into the potential etiology of a nutritional disorder. The body's first (and normal) response to starvation (inadequate food intake) is the preferential loss of body fat which can be reflected in diminished triceps skinfold thickness measurements or other measurements of body fat. When fat stores are depleted, wasting of lean body mass occurs. In contrast, cachexia or wasting refers to the preferential and inappropriate loss of lean body mass over fat mass, with or without concomitant weight loss. Cachexia has been described previously in patients with cancer, but more recently has been found in patients with HIV infection, including children. Cachexia may be mediated by chemical intermediates such as cytokines and will be discussed in the section on pathogenesis.

Earlier studies utilizing various methods to assess body composition have been performed in HIV-infected children. Body composition measurements of 89 children born to HIV-infected women, (52 children were HIV-infected) found lean body mass measured by arm muscle circumference was significantly less in the HIV-infected group by 2 years of age. There were no differences in fat mass between the two groups of children.[13] In a cross-sectional study of HIV-infected children treated with nucleoside reverse transcriptase inhibitors, Fontana and colleagues compared bioelectrical impedance measurements of fat-free mass (FFM) in 86 HIV-infected children (mean age 6.9 years) and 113 healthy controls (mean age 7.7 years).[20] These investigators found FFM was lower in HIV-infected children compared to controls; however, when FFM was evaluated as a percentage of total body weight, there was no difference between groups. Weight for age and FFM *Z*-scores <–2.0 were associated with increased risk of death (RR 11.4 and 5.1, respectively), with weight-for-age serving as a stronger prognostic indicator than FFM. Arpadi and colleagues used dual energy X-ray absorptiometry (DXA) and also found reduced FFM but normal fat stores among HIV-infected children compared to uninfected controls, regardless of whether or not growth failure was also present.[21] These findings indicate that poor growth and decreased FFM are a considerable problem for children living with HIV infection and that these parameters have a significant deleterious effect on survival.

The introduction of highly active or combination antiretroviral therapy (HAART) has revolutionized the management of HIV infection in adults and children. Much recent attention has focused on the potential impact of HAART on growth and body composition as well as immune function and survival. One of the first reports came as part of the Pediatric AIDS Clinical Trials Group 219 Study evaluating the effects of the introduction of protease inhibitor (PI) therapy in 906 HIV-infected children between 3 months and 18 years of age.[22] Initiation of PI treatment was associated with small but statistically significant increases in height and weight *Z*-scores. More recently, Nachman and colleagues[23] reported that, in addition to a significant relationship between HIV viral RNA levels and indices of poor height and weight, the introduction of HAART was associated with improved weight gain. Importantly, height growth achieved essentially normal levels after 2 years of therapy.

There is further evidence that abnormalities in growth parameters may be linked to virologic and immune response to antiretroviral therapy. Verweel and colleagues found that both weight and height improved after initiation of HAART, but only in a subset of children who demonstrated virologic response defined as 1.5 or greater log reduction in HIV RNA.[24] Furthermore, a Swiss study assessing a cohort of 44 prepubertal HIV-infected children found that children with stunting prior to initiation of PI-based therapy experienced statistically significant increases in height for age *Z*-scores after 72 weeks of treatment.[25] In this study, there was a significant positive correlation between change in CD4 T-cell count and change in height *Z*-score. Combined, these data represent mounting evidence that effective viral suppression and immune reconstitution with HAART can substantially ameliorate the growth deficits in HIV-infected children. As will be covered in the next section of this chapter, in addition to improvements in overall growth, unanticipated effects of HAART have been identified including metabolic alterations and abnormal patterns of body fat distribution or lipodystrophy. Further longitudinal information is needed to determine the potential long-term benefits of antiretroviral therapy and it effects on growth and body composition.

HIV-ASSOCIATED LIPODYSTROPHY

Shortly after the widespread introduction of highly active antiretroviral therapy (HAART), a constellation of metabolic abnormalities and changes in body fat distribution were recognized among many HIV-infected patients (Table 2). The loss of subcutaneous fat as well as increased adiposity of the abdomen and hypertrophy of the dorsocervical fat pad were reminiscent of congenital and acquired forms of lipodystrophy and this term has been used in the HIV population. There is increasing evidence that both protease inhibitors and nucleoside reverse transcriptase inhibitors contribute directly to lipodystrophy and other identified metabolic complications.[26–28]

In addition to significant and often disturbing changes in fat distribution, patients may develop hyperlipidemia, insulin resistance, and diabetes.[29,30] The long-term effects of insulin resistance, hyperlipidemia, and fat redistribution have not yet been fully realized, but there is growing evidence of increased cardiovascular disease in HIV-infected patients. The Data Collection on Adverse Events of anti-HIV Drugs (DAD) study evaluated 23,468 HIV-infected adults and found that hypertriglyceridemia and total cholesterol increased with exposure to antiretroviral medications. The study also established increased rates of myocardial infarction with increasing years of exposure to antiretroviral therapy.[31]

Several studies have been conducted to evaluate whether pediatric patients with HIV-infection receiving HAART are also experiencing changes in body fat distribution and metabolic abnormalities. For example, Arpadi and colleagues[32] assessed body fat distribution in 28 prepubertal HIV-infected children with DEXA scans and 29% had evidence of lipodystrophy (defined as fat atrophy and trunk fat accumulation). The presence of lipodystrophy was positively associated with protease inhibitor use (OR 7.0) and stavudine use (OR 9.0) in this population. A multicenter 2-year prospective evaluation of 130 HIV-infected children on antiretroviral therapy was completed in Paris, France.[33] Nearly one quarter of the participants had evidence of lipodystrophy. Other metabolic disturbances were frequently identified in this cohort including low HDL cholesterol, increased total cholesterol, and triglycerides. Insulin resistance, defined as a fasting insulin >95th percentile for normoglycemic children matched for pubertal status, doubled in frequency over the 2-year study period from 13.2 to 25.6%. Important predictors of hyperinsulinemia and dyslipidemia were development of puberty, exposure to protease inhibitors, and pretreatment severity of HIV disease. More research is needed to determine the effects of HAART on fat redistribution, lipids, and glucose homeostasis in children, particularly given the potential lifelong exposure to HAART which may be required for HIV viral suppression. In addition to the potential increased risk of diabetes and cardiovascular disease, children may also experience as yet unappreciated abnormalities in pubertal development and bone health in relation to metabolic complications of HIV and lipodystrophy.

Table 2 Clinical and Biochemical Abnormalities Associated with the Lipodystrophy Syndrome in Children

Clinical Features	Laboratory Features
Increased abdominal (visceral) fat	Hyperlipidemia
–Increased waist-to-hip ratio	–Increased triglycerides
(not reliable in growing children)	–Increased total cholesterol
Buffalo hump	–Increased LDL
Fat atrophy	–Decreased HDL
–Loss of fat in extremities	Insulin resistance
–Loss or thinning of facial fat, prominence of nasolabial fold	–Normal to increased serum glucose
–Loss of fat of buttocks	–Increased insulin
	–Increased C peptide
No change to increased weight	–Decreased glucose tolerance/insulin resistance
Fatigue and weakness	Elevated lactate levels

WASTING IN HIV-INFECTED CHILDREN: PATHOGENESIS

Globally, severe weight loss, growth failure, and wasting remain a central component of HIV infection in adults and children. The pathogenesis of malnutrition, or the wasting syndrome, in pediatric HIV disease is most likely multifactorial. A limited number of studies have determined the risk factors for malnutrition in HIV-infected patients, and even fewer have been performed in children. Identified risk factors include fever, diarrhea, acute and opportunistic infections, anorexia as well as social factors such as ill parents and availability of food and clean water. Four potential mechanisms for weight loss include inadequate oral intake, impaired gastrointestinal absorption, abnormal or increased energy utilization, and psychosocial

Table 3 Causes of Malnutrition in HIV-Infected Children

Etiology	Mechanism
Decreased nutrient intake	
Peptic disease	Pain
Opportunistic infections of upper gastrointestinal tract (Candida, CMV, HSV)	Pain, dysphagia
Pancreatic/hepatobiliary disease	Pain
Encephalopathy	Discoordinated swallow
Aphthous ulcers	Pain
Primary anorexia	Nausea, CNS, cytokines
Gastrointestinal malabsorption	
Mucosal disease	
Infectious	Bacterial, parasitic, viral
Inflammatory	HIV enteropathy
Disaccharidase deficiency	Infectious, inflammatory
Protein-losing enteropathy	Infectious, inflammatory
Fat malabsorption	Infectious, inflammatory
Hepatobiliary	
Sclerosing cholangitis	Infectious
Chronic pancreatitis	Infectious, drug-induced
Cirrhosis	HBV, HCV
Increased nutritional requirements or tissue catabolism	
Protein wasting	Fever, infections, sepsis
Hypermetabolism	Neoplasms (Kaposi's sarcoma, lymphoma)
Futile metabolic cycling	Medications
	Release of catabolic factors (cytokines, tumor necrosis factor)
Psychosocial factors	
Poverty	
Illness in biological family members	
Limited access to health care	
Substance abuse	

CMV = cytomegalovirus; CNS = central nervous system; HBV= hepatitis B virus; HCV = hepatitis C virus; HSV = herpes simplex virus.

influences. In many cases several factors may be operating simultaneously.

Energy Intake

A variety of potential factors may lead to abnormal intake as outlined in Table 3. For example, inflammation and ulcers of the upper gastrointestinal tract can lead to anorexia owing to odynophagia, dysphagia, or abdominal pain that is associated with eating. In one series, 70% of upper gastrointestinal endoscopies in HIV-infected children revealed abnormal histologic findings.[34] These lesions may be due to acid-related injury or infectious agents such as *Candida albicans*, cytomegalovirus, or herpes simplex virus, all of which may cause inflammation and pain with swallowing or after eating.

Pancreatic and biliary tract disease can also cause vomiting and abdominal pain in HIV-infected children leading to poor oral intake. Pancreatic disease has been linked to medications (eg, NRTIs, PIs, sulfonamides) and opportunistic infections (eg, cytomegalovirus and mycobacterial disease). Biliary tract disease with sclerosing cholangitis and papillary stenosis has been associated with *Cryptosporidium*, cytomegalovirus, and *Microsporidia* infection. It is postulated that increased cytokine production [eg, tumor necrosis factor (TNF), interleukins 1 and 6] may be associated with anorexia. In animal models, administration of exogenous TNF has produced anorexia and cachexia. In a small cohort of 36 HIV-infected adults evaluated in 1997, TNFα plasma levels were significantly increased in those with AIDS wasting compared to asymptomatic HIV-infected subjects or healthy controls.[35] However, there were no associations between TNFα levels and parameters of malnutrition. There are currently more than 20 agents approved by the Food and Drug Administration for the treatment of HIV and many of these as well as other medications frequently used in HIV-infected children may result in gastric irritation, vomiting, and nausea (See Table 4).

There are increasing data suggesting decreased energy intake among HIV-infected children who have more symptomatic infection and/or growth failure. For example, Arpadi and colleagues[36,37] found, in the absence of active secondary infections or other illnesses, HIV-infected children with growth failure had significantly lower mean energy intake (77% of the RDA) compared with HIV-infected children without growth failure (103% of the RDA). In this study, when energy balance was assessed as the difference between energy intake and total energy expenditure (TEE), HIV-infected children with growth failure had a 674-kJ/d deficit whereas those without growth failure had a surplus intake of 1,448 kJ/d. Therefore, energy intake below the RDA during stable periods of disease, as well as inadequate energy intake occurring during symptomatic periods of disease, may contribute to growth failure in HIV-infected children.

Gastrointestinal Absorption

Adequate nutrient absorption is essential to maintain growth and nutrition in infants and children. HIV-infected patients are at risk for developing malabsorptive disorders which can potentially impact on their growth and nutritional status. Possible reasons for gastrointestinal malabsorption in HIV-infected children include infections of the gastrointestinal tract and/or direct and indirect effects of HIV on the intestinal epithelial cell. Infections that are known to affect the small bowel and that may promote malabsorption of nutrients include *Cryptosporidium, Isospora belli, Microsporidia, Mycobacterium*

Table 4 Common Gastrointestinal Side Effects Associated with Medications Used in HIV Care

Side Effect	Medications
Nausea	• NRTI: abacavir, didanosine (ddI), emtricitabine, lamivudine, stavudine, zidovudine • NNRTI: efavarenz, nevirapine • PI: atazanavir, darunavir, indinavir, nelfinavir, ritonavir, saquinavir, tipranavir • Antiviral: acyclovir, ganciclovir • Antibacterial: macrolides, sulfonamides, rifampin • Antiparasitic: pentamadine
Abdominal Pain	• NRTI: abacavir, didanosine (ddI), emtricitabine, lamivudine, stavudine, tenofovir, zidovudine • NNRTI: nevirapine • PI: amprenavir, atazanavir, darunavir, indinavir, nelfinavir, ritonavir, saquanivir • Antibacterial: macrolides, sulfonamides, ciprofloxacin, rifampin • Antiparasitic: pentamadine
Vomiting	• NRTI: abacavir, didanosine (ddI), emtricitabine, lamivudine, stavudine, zidovudine • NNRTI: efavarenz • PI: amprenavir, atazanavir, indinavir, nelfinavir, ritonavir • Antiviral: ganciclovir • Antibacterial: macrolides, sulfonamides, ciprofloxacin, rifampin • Antiparasitic: pentamadine
Pancreatitis	• NRTI: abacavir, didanosine (ddI), lamivudine, stavudine, tenofovir • PI: lopinavir/ritonavir, ritonavir, saquanivir, tipranavir • Antibacterial: sulfonamides, ciprofloxacin • Antiparasitic: pentamadine

NRTI = nucleoside analogue reverse transcriptase inhibitor; NNRTI = nonnucleoside analogue reverse transcriptase inhibitor; PI = protease inhibitor.

avium intracellulare complex (MAC), *Giardia lamblia*, and *rotavirus*. These pathogens can injure the intestinal epithelial cell where critical digestive enzymes are present to digest essential nutrients. Enteric infections may also decrease bowel transit time, thus shortening nutrient contact with the epithelial cell and causing malabsorption. Malnutrition alone can cause villous blunting and secondary malabsorption of nutrients which would further impact on nutritional status. Malabsorption has also been linked to an "HIV enteropathy" where the villi are blunted with a hypercellular lamina propria and absence of a detectable enteric pathogen.[38] Investigation into the pathogenesis of diarrhea related to mucosal HIV infection in the absence of identifiable enteric infection is ongoing. While HIV appears to penetrate the mucosal epithelium via CCR5 binding in a receptor-mediated fashion, the lymphocytes in the lamina propria are recognized as the primary target of viral infection in the intestine. There is evidence for enterocyte cell death or apoptosis which occurs in both infected and uninfected cells.[39] In addition, in vitro studies of enterocytes show that HIV exposure and/or exposure to gp120 may have evoked disruption of microtubules, and tight junctions as well as impaired ion flux, suggesting a pathophysiologic mechanism for HIV enteropathy and malabsorption.[39,40]

In the pre-HAART era, a few studies provided evidence of malabsorption in HIV-infected children.[41–44] For example, of 28 HIV-infected children evaluated for gastrointestinal malabsorption in the United States, over 60% were found to have some degree of carbohydrate malabsorption by D-xylose testing or lactose hydrogen breath testing.[41] Carbohydrate malabsorption, however, was not associated with nutritional status or gastrointestinal symptoms. Abnormal D-xylose absorption was associated with an active enteric infection. Yolken and colleagues[42] documented clinically significant lactose malabsorption and weight loss in a cohort of HIV-infected children. In an Italian study,[43] intestinal function of 47 symptomatically infected children was compared with 50 noninfected children with diarrhea and 48 healthy children. Intestinal absorption was measured using the steatocrit method to determine fat absorption, fecal concentration of α-1-antitrypsin as a measure of protein absorption, and D-xylose absorption. Fecal fat loss was detected in 30%, carbohydrate malabsorption in 32%, and protein loss in 17% of HIV-infected children. Investigators found intestinal dysfunction was not associated with diarrhea, poor growth, enteric agents, or degree of immune dysfunction, but was significantly different than healthy control children. In a similar series, Sentongo and colleagues[44] identified fat malabsorption in 39% of 44 HIV-infected children, but no patient had exocrine pancreatic insufficiency and there was no relationship between steatorrhea, growth, HIV viral load, or CD4 count. Thus, although malabsorption is fairly common, it cannot completely account for the gastrointestinal symptoms or malnutrition in HIV-infected children.

Metabolism

Increased energy metabolism of HIV-infected children can contribute to malnutrition by increasing the child's caloric demands to maintain weight and sustain growth. Total daily energy expenditure is the sum of energy needed to maintain a child at rest, the energy needed for activities of daily living, the thermic effect of feeding, energy needs for growth, and obligatory energy losses. Measurements of resting energy expenditure (REE) through indirect calorimetry and total daily energy expenditure through techniques such as doubly labeled water studies and whole room calorimetry enables investigators to determine metabolic rates of HIV-infected patients.

There are several studies in the pediatric HIV population which delineate resting or total daily energy expenditure, although more studies have been performed in the adult HIV population. The literature in children with HIV infection generally shows no differences in REE[45–47] or TEE[47,48] between children with growth failure and those with normal rates of growth. However, these studies have been performed in clinically stable children; metabolism in sicker children is likely to be much higher. One study determined whole body protein turnover in children with HIV and found increased protein turnover is associated with low weight and height.[49] Interestingly, Hardin and colleagues[50] showed the use of a protease inhibitor in the treatment of HIV resulted in decreased protein catabolism and was associated with improvement in lean tissue mass in HIV-infected children tested pre- and posttherapy.

In adults, there have been a number of different studies evaluating REE; Batterham recently reported on the results of a meta-analysis summarizing data from over 50 studies with 32 studies comparing HIV-infected patients to HIV-negative control groups.[51] This investigation found a mean increase in REE according to FFM of approximately 630 to 661 kJ/d in HIV compared to control subjects. In a subset analysis, subjects with symptomatic HIV/AIDS had the highest REE, but the size and number of the studies limited more detailed comparisons. Interestingly, this study made a similar observation to that of Shevitz and colleagues[52] that patients receiving HAART tended to have higher REE compared to HIV-infected subjects who were not using HAART. Further investigation is needed to more fully understand the role of alterations in REE in weight regulation, particularly as it pertains to use of HAART and lipodystrophy.

Cytokines

Elevated cytokine expression may contribute to altered metabolic rates and weight regulation abnormalities in HIV and this hypothesis is supported by experimental and animal studies. The cachectin hypothesis was first described by Beutler and cerami[53] who noticed that patients with chronic infections have significant weight loss that is associated with hypertriglyceridemia and reduced clearance of triglycerides by lipoproteins. They postulated that a decrease in triglyceride clearance could lead to a decrease in fat storage and wasting of lean body mass as a result of the inability to utilize fats as a reserve source for energy. In animal studies, supernatants from activated macrophages induced weight loss when given daily to rodents.[54] This factor in the supernatant was subsequently isolated and named cachetin; later discovered to be the cytokine, TNF. Other cytokines, such as interleukin-1 (IL-1) and the interferons, have similar effects.

Cytokines are known to alter metabolic processes in non-HIV populations. In patients with HIV, cytokines can cause ineffective use of energy substrates. Hellerstein[55] studied hepatic lipogenesis in HIV-infected adult patients and correlated it with peripheral cytokine levels. Both symptomatic HIV-infected patients with normal CD4 counts and HIV-infected patients with weight loss had elevated hepatic lipogenesis, compared to noninfected controls. Hepatic lipogenesis correlated with interferon-alpha levels in the fasted state in the patients with HIV infection and weight loss. Other cytokines were not correlated with increased hepatic lipogenesis. In addition to increasing the hepatic synthesis of fatty acids, TNF also mobilizes free fatty acids by stimulating peripheral lipolysis. The net result, "futile cycling," the process by which fatty acids are shuttled from adipose tissue to liver and back to adipose tissue, utilizes energy inefficiently. The process results in increased metabolic rates, with greater caloric needs to maintain nutrition.

The net effect of cytokines for patients infected with HIV is nonproductive use of energy substrates. Approximately 28% of calories are lost if lipogenesis from carbohydrate precedes its oxidation. Roubenoff and colleagues[56] found that loss of lean body mass was driven by catabolic cytokines and not by inadequate dietary intake or hypogonadism. Other investigators have found similar associations, independent of viral load.[57] Limited studies in children showed increased IL-6 activity, as well as low IGF-1 and increased viral load to be associated with growth impairment.[48] The net effect of elevated cytokine levels may contribute to the relative hypermetabolism seen in HIV-infected patients. Since depression of immune function secondary to malnutrition is potentially reversible, nutritional rehabilitation in HIV-infected children may significantly lower serum cytokine levels by positively improving immunologic function, decreasing opportunistic infection, and diminishing HIV replication. This, in turn, would decrease cytokine production. With lower TNF and IL-1 production, promotion of HIV replication would be decreased and the systemic effects of these cytokines such as the wasting and malabsorptive symptoms would be reduced.

Psychosocial Factors

Psychosocial factors are also important contributors to suboptimal nutrition of HIV-infected children. An unstable home environment and inadequate emotional and social support have been shown to be a factor for growth problems in both HIV-1-infected[58] and non-HIV-infected children by many mechanisms, including growth hormone (GH) deficiencies.[59,60] Children with HIV infection are at risk for living with parents who are ill, who have limited access to social services and support, and who may have ongoing problems with drug and substance abuse.[61] Investigators have found maternal crack and cocaine use during pregnancy to be a predictor of growth and nutritional problems for the child.[7,14] This finding is not unique for HIV, as it has been reported in other non-HIV cohorts.[62] Children born to drug-using women are often small, suggesting that drugs have a prenatal effect, but the postnatal home environment is likely to influence growth as well. Current studies have also found that home care providers can both positively or negatively influence functional status of HIV-infected children.[58]

MICRONUTRIENTS

Several micronutrients have been linked to immunomodulation, both in vivo and in vitro. For example, deficiencies of pyridoxine, folic acid, vitamin A, vitamin C, and vitamin E result in impaired cell-mediated immunity and reduced antibody responses. Vitamin B_6 deficiency results in decreased lymphocyte response to mitogens, yet a moderate increase in beta-carotene intake may enhance immune responses. With zinc deficiency, there is lymphoid atrophy and decreased delayed cutaneous hypersensitivity responses. Likewise, zinc deficiency in animals can reduce the number of antibody-forming cells in the spleen and impair natural killer activity. Clinically, wound healing is impaired in zinc deficiency, whereas, excessive zinc can depress neutrophil function and lymphocyte responses. Iron is important for bacterial growth as well as neutrophil and lymphocytes function. Deficiencies of iron may reduce bacterial multiplication, but may also impair lymphocyte proliferation response to mitogens and antigens. In patients with iron deficiency, lymphocyte response to tetanus toxoid and herpes simplex antigen is low. Overall, in animal models it is clear that selected vitamin and micronutrient deficiencies impact on immune function in many ways. See Chapter 8, "Trace Elements," Chapter 9, "Iron," and Chapter 10, "Vitamins" for full discussions of trace elements, iron, and vitamins.

Because of the close link between immunologic function and micronutrients, it is logical to expect that low micronutrient levels can affect susceptibility to infection. For HIV-infected children, whose immunologic function is already compromised, further alterations of immunologic function, through micronutrient deficiencies or excesses, may synergistically decrease resistance to infections. Available studies of micronutrients and HIV infection, particularly among children, will be outlined in the following sections.

General Studies

There is increasing data available on the micronutrient status of children with HIV infection. Eley and colleagues[63] evaluated 60 HIV-infected children in Cape Town, South Africa and, using blood nutrient concentrations, vitamin deficiencies were frequently identified: vitamin A (80%), retinol-binding protein (85%), vitamin B_6 (37%), vitamin E (37%), zinc (20%), and copper (25%). Sixty-two percent of children had two or more deficiencies and deficiencies were more common and more severe in children older than 24 months. Only 5% of patients were found to have low vitamin B_{12} levels. In a large series of symptomatic HIV-infected children (n = 71) in Italy, 48% were iron deficient and 66% had anemia and this was positively associated with markers of malabsorption.[64]

In a large cohort of HIV-infected children and adolescents in the United States (n = 264), there were no differences in intake of vitamins A, C, iron or zinc, compared to uninfected controls (n = 127).[65] Approximately one-third of the children studied reported use of a daily vitamin/mineral supplement. The investigators noted intake below the estimated average requirement of the dietary reference intakes (DRI) in 40% of children for vitamin E, 19% for vitamin A, and 10% for zinc. However, there were no identified differences in the prevalence of micronutrient inadequacy when evaluated according to HIV status or CD4 T-cell strata. Therefore, there appears to be important regional variation in the prevalence of micronutrient deficiencies in children.

Vitamin A

Vitamin A is arguably one of the most frequently studied vitamins in relationship to immune function and HIV. In adults, Tang and colleagues[66] showed a relationship between total vitamin A intake and progression to AIDS, but the relationship was U-shaped, the lowest and highest quartiles of intake did less well than the two middle quartiles in terms of progression to AIDS. In a multinutrient model, low vitamin A and niacin were significantly associated with progression to AIDS while vitamin C was only marginally significant. In earlier work, Semba and colleagues[67] studied the association between plasma vitamin A, immunologic status, and clinical outcome during HIV infection. In a cohort of 179 subjects with intravenous drug use, 15% of HIV-positive patients had low plasma vitamin A levels. Vitamin A deficiency was associated with increased mortality in HIV-infected patients, with a relative risk of 6.3, (95% CI, 2.1 to 18.6). Data available from HIV-infected children in North America,[68] however, found vitamin A deficiency to be relatively uncommon and vitamin A concentrations did not appear to be related to mortality in this population.

Vitamin A deficiency and supplementation, however, may have a significant role in HIV disease transmission and progression in areas of the world where vitamin A deficiency is more prevalent.[69–74] In a trial of vitamin A supplementation in Tanzania, HIV-infected children experienced a 63% reduction in all-cause mortality with vitamin A supplementation compared to placebo.[71] In a longitudinal observational study of 194 HIV-infected children in Uganda, low plasma β-carotene levels, but not vitamin A levels, were predictive of increased mortality. This and other studies, however, show a relationship between low vitamin A levels and poor growth in HIV-infected children.[71,72] For example, in a placebo-controlled trial of vitamin A supplementation in Tanzania, including 50 HIV-infected children, vitamin A-treated children under 18 months of age experienced a 2.8 cm greater height increase compared to placebo.[73] One potential mechanism for this beneficial effect on growth may be improved gut permeability (ie, reduced permeability with vitamin A) which was shown with perinatal vitamin A supplementation in HIV-infected infants.[74]

Observational data that linked low maternal vitamin A concentrations with a higher risk of vertical transmission[69,70] prompted a number of placebo-controlled clinical trials of vitamin A in HIV-infected pregnant women. Results from Malawi and South Africa showed no reduction in vertical transmission with vitamin A supplementation, whereas a trial from Tanzania showed that vitamin A alone increased the risk of HIV transmission (RR 1.38; 95% CI 1.09 to 1.76). More recent data of postpartum vitamin A supplementation to HIV-infected mothers and their neonates have shown conflicting evidence of its efficacy in reducing morbidity and mortality.[75]

B Vitamins and Folate

Baum and colleagues[76] studied vitamin B_6 status in HIV-infected adults. In this study, vitamin B_6 deficiency was associated with decreased lymphocyte responsiveness to mitogens and suggested as a cofactor in reduced natural killer cell cytotoxicity. However, vitamin B_6 was not related to CD4 T-cell number. Dowling and colleagues[77] studied vitamin B_{12} and folate in 35 HIV-infected men, of whom 16 were asymptomatic. Serum B_{12} was normal, or above normal in all patients, coincident with high B_{12} intake. Lower RBC folate was found in only 3 patients, but levels were lower overall in the more symptomatic group. Folate intake was low in nearly half of patients. Folic acid absorption was studied[78] in 25 HIV-infected patients after an oral folic acid dose, with blood samples taken sequentially over 3 hours. Absorption of folic acid was significantly impaired in patients, regardless of the stage of the disease. Thus, intestinal absorption of folate and other nutrients may be responsible for abnormal blood levels.

Supplementation with B vitamins, vitamin C, and vitamin E was evaluated in a large clinical trial of pregnant HIV-infected women in Tanzania. In addition to improved birth outcomes (lower risk of both preterm delivery and low birthweight), maternal supplementation was associated with lowered infant morbidity and higher CD4 counts[79] as well as a reduced rate of mortality and AIDS progression in mothers.[80]

Antioxidants

Oxygen-free radicals are generated during normal metabolism, yet production may increase during infection, malnutrition, stress, or drug therapy. Endogenous antioxidant activity such as catalase production and exogenous antioxidants (eg, vitamin E and selenium) may be important in HIV. Selenium is a potent antioxidant and is also an important cofactor for immune function in humans. In vivo studies have shown the importance of this element in protecting cells from HIV activation and the effects of TNF, through increasing glutathione peroxidase activity.[81] In one cross-sectional study, HIV-infected children had low glutathione levels which correlated with CD4 cell count.[82] Low plasma selenium levels were associated with increased risk of mortality of children born to HIV-infected mothers in Tanzania,[83] supporting a potential relationship with nutritional antioxidant and immunity.

Trace Metals

Zinc's role in metabolic function has been well studied. It is important in the stabilization and function of metabolic enzymes including those involved in protein synthesis, catabolism, energy metabolism, and RNA and DNA synthesis. Regeneration of gut epithelium, stabilization of brush border enzymes, and improved immune function are all proposed mechanisms for zinc's beneficial effects in acute diarrhea.[84] A study by Graham and colleagues[85] showed that serum copper levels were higher and zinc levels lower in HIV-infected adult patients who progressed to AIDS than in seropositive patients who did not progress. In a logistic regression model, they found that higher serum copper levels (OR 2.23; 95% CI 1.02, 4.87) and lower serum zinc levels (OR 0.3; 95%CI 0.14, 0.66) predicted progression to AIDS independently of baseline CD4 lymphocyte levels, age, and calorie-adjusted dietary intake of both of these nutrients. In an open treatment study of HIV-infected children with a CD4 count < 500/mm^3, supplemental zinc was administered for 1 month. Although 69% of the children had low zinc levels at baseline, supplementation did not have an effect on p24 antigen or CD4 count. The prevalence of zinc deficiency among HIV-infected children, which was estimated at 20% in one South African study[63] and the observed reduction in episodes of watery diarrhea in HIV-infected children who received zinc supplementation compared to a placebo,[87] points to a potential benefit for zinc supplementation in children with HIV.

DIAGNOSTIC EVALUATION

Malnutrition and wasting are common in HIV-infected children, and therefore routine nutritional assessment should be performed at regular intervals, particularly under 24 months of age, in every child who is at risk for acquiring HIV infection. Careful consideration of the pattern of growth will lead to an investigation of nutritional versus endocrine dysfunction. Subtle changes in growth and altered nutrient intake can be detected. The nutritional assessment should include measures of weight, height, head circumference, triceps skinfold thickness (to measure fat mass), and mid-upper arm circumference or MUAC (to assess muscle mass). A detailed dietary history and recall should be ascertained regardless of the child's nutritional condition. Dietary advice or encouragement should be reinforced at each visit. Figure 1 outlines a clinical algorithm of diagnosis and management of HIV-infected children with nutritional abnormalities.

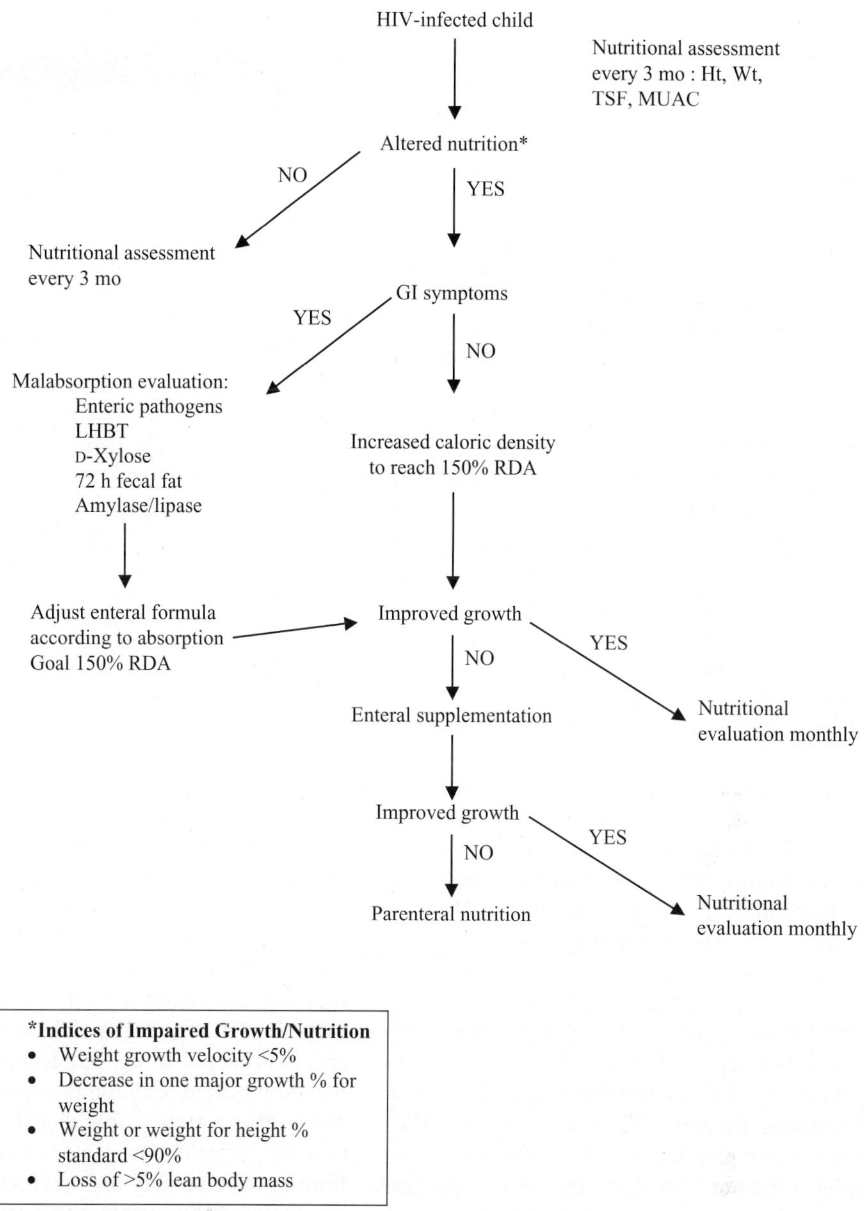

Figure 1 Algorithm for monitoring, diagnosing, and treating malnutrition associated with human immunodeficiency (HIV) disease in infants and children. GI = gastrointestinal; Ht = height; LHBT = lactose hydrogen breath test; MUAC = mid upper arm circumference; RDA = recommended dietary allowance; TSF = tricep skin fold; Wt = weight.

If a child shows evidence of malnutrition (Table 5), nutrient losses should be evaluated in addition to nutrient intake. Clinical symptoms should be determined with the focus on gastrointestinal problems, such as vomiting, abdominal pain, and diarrhea. A complete physical examination will provide clues. The child should be evaluated for oral thrush, abdominal pain, and gross or occult blood in the stool. Laboratory studies should include a complete blood count, liver function studies, pancreatic enzyme levels, and a complete evaluation for enteric pathogens. Studies such as an upper gastrointestinal contrast series, upper gastrointestinal endoscopy, and an abdominal ultrasound may provide a definitive diagnosis. If clinical symptoms warrant, a gastrointestinal absorption evaluation should be performed; including a lactose hydrogen breath test, D-xylose absorption study, and/or 72-hour fecal fat collection.

Serum micronutrients should be assessed in malnourished or wasted HIV-infected children. Vitamins A, E, and D should be measured,

Table 5 Clinical Indicators of Malnutrition in HIV-Infected Children

Clinical Features
Weight growth velocity <5% for more than 2 mo
Decrease in 1 major growth percentile for weight
Weight or weight-for-height percent standard <90%
Weight-for-height <5th%
Loss of >5% of lean body mass
Serum albumin <3 g/dL

especially if there is liver, biliary tract, or pancreatic disease. Serum zinc and selenium should be measured and may be low; if so, they should be replaced to optimize immune function. As other micronutrients such as B_6, B_{12}, and iron may be depressed, they should also be measured in malnourished children.

It may also be useful, where able, to evaluate a child's energy needs. Although the use of doubly labeled water as a measure of TEE remains a research test, clinical centers are increasingly able to perform indirect calorimetry as a bedside test of REE in children. In a practical sense, the best estimation of energy needs for an HIV-infected child is the child's response to a diet enriched in calories, with accurate documentation of caloric intake and type of food.

Among HIV-infected children receiving chronic antiretroviral therapy, it is also important to monitor for potential changes in body fat distribution and abnormalities in metabolic parameters that have been linked to the use of HAART. For example, skin fold thickness measurements obtained using standardized calipers by trained bionutritionist can be effective in identifying and monitoring peripheral lipoatrophy.[88] This combined with annual anthropometric assessment of waist and hip circumference with calculation of a waist-to-hip ratio may be very useful in detecting alterations in body fat distribution that develop over time with exposure to HAART.

It is currently recommended that HIV infected adults have fasting serum glucose and lipids checked prior to initiation of antiretroviral therapy and then repeated biannually after initiation of therapy as well as following any changes in antiretroviral therapy. While there are no HIV-specific recommendations for performing more detailed screening for diabetes such as on oral glucose tolerance testing, this may be beneficial in cases where there is concern for insulin resistance or documented impaired fasting glucose (fasting glucose $>$100 mg/dL).

NUTRITIONAL INTERVENTIONS

Oral Supplementation

Nutritional interventions should be instituted when the child fails to meet growth standards as defined in Table 5. In general, a proactive approach to nutritional guidance is preferred when early nutritional interventions are more effective, than during the later stages of HIV disease. Nutritional therapies should be instituted in parallel with treatment for other ongoing systemic or gastrointestinal diseases. Oral nutritional therapies, in most patients, should be tried initially. Formula caloric density should be increased by concentration or adding fat or carbohydrate. If the child is eating solids, adding a high-fat supplement, such as butter or margarine may be helpful. Efforts should be made to increase formula volume as much as tolerated. Since a precise estimation of caloric needs is usually not available, the caloric goal, in general, should be targeted at 50% above the RDA for age and sex for a child with growth failure. Other nutritional requirements are shown in Table 6, although these requirements are considered minimal, and more may be required if the child has clinical and biochemical evidence of nutritional deficiencies. Formula composition should be prescribed according to the extent of nutrient malabsorption. If a child has clinical symptoms indicating malabsorption of lactose (eg, diarrhea, bloating, flatulence), a lactose-free diet is indicated. Caution is advised, however, in prescribing a lactose-free diet if the child has no clinical symptoms of lactose malabsorption, as limiting lactose may also restrict the foods that are the most enjoyable and richest in calories. In addition, an oral lactase supplement may be added in some cases of lactose intolerance. A protein hydrolysate formula should be considered if the child has evidence of gastrointestinal mucosal dysfunction with malabsorption of fats and proteins.

Table 6 Nutritional Requirements for HIV-Infected Children

Nutrient	Requirements/d*
Total calories	100–150% RDA for age and sex
Protein	100–150% RDA for age and sex
Vitamin A	400–1,000 μg retinol
Vitamin D	400 IU
Vitamin E	3–10 mg d-alpha tocopherol
Vitamin K	5–80 μg
Vitamin C	30–60 mg
Thiamin	0.3–1.1 mg
Riboflavin	0.4–1.3 mg
Niacin	5–15 mg
Vitamin B_6	0.3–1.6 mg
Folate	25–180 μg
Vitamin B_{12}	0.3–2.0 μg
Iron	6–15 mg
Zinc	5–12 mg
Selenium	10–55 μg

Ranges reflect variations in needs based on age and sex.
*Requirements reflect the clinical nutritional status of the child; more or less may be needed depending on evidence of deficiency.

Breast milk is generally considered the best nutrition for infants worldwide, since it contains factors that protect the infant against pathogens. Breast-feeding also fosters the maternal–infant bond. Unfortunately, women with HIV infection can transmit the virus to their infant through breast milk and therefore breast-feeding in this circumstance is strongly discouraged in countries where other safe feeding options exist. WHO recommendations issued in 2001 stated that only "when replacement feeding is acceptable, feasible, affordable, sustainable and safe, avoidance of breast-feeding by HIV-infected mothers is recommended. Otherwise, exclusive breast-feeding is recommended during the first months of life." This position was further supported by the observations of Iliff and colleagues that exclusive breast-feeding among HIV-infected women in Zimbabwe was associated with a decreased risk of postnatal HIV transmission compared to early mixed feeding or supplemented feeding.[89]

Enteral Supplementation

If oral interventions fail, because the child cannot consume adequate calories to sustain growth, enteral supplementation should be considered. Nasogastric tube feedings should be instituted first, to document the child's ability to gain weight with supplemental enteral feedings. Nighttime feedings are most practical, since they allow the child to eat normally throughout the day. Complications relating to nasogastric tube feedings include sinusitis and the technical inability of the caretaker to administer the feedings or place the tube. If delivery of feedings through a nasogastric tube improves growth than placement of a more permanent device, such as a gastrostomy tube should be considered. A gastrostomy tube provides easy access to the stomach with less physical and emotional trauma to the child. In addition, studies show that gastrostomy tube placement results in significant improvements in medication compliance and reductions in medication administration time in children with HIV infection.[90,91]

In a study of 23 HIV-infected children,[92] weight and weight-for-height *Z*-scores increased with gastrostomy tube feedings. This increase in weight and weight-for-height was coincident with an increase in caloric intake. Fat stores, as measured by triceps skinfold thicknesses, increased in parallel with weight and weight-for-height, with no appreciable effect on lean body mass. Additionally, children who gained weight with gastrostomy-tube feedings were hospitalized less in the 6 months after gastrostomy tube placement and had a 2.8-fold reduction in risk of dying. Guarino and colleagues[93] evaluated the effects of enteral (n = 16) and parenteral (n = 46) nutritional therapy for HIV infected children with malnutrition and evidence of diarrhea or malabsorption. More than 80% of patients receiving enteral therapy gained $>$5% of their baseline weight and enteral therapy was associated with significant increases in CD4 cell count. In addition, enteral therapy improved gut absorption with 75% of patients experiencing normalization in the xylose absorption test. Combined, these findings suggest that early nutritional intervention is indicated in children with HIV infection and may improve morbidity and survival.

Parenteral Nutrition

Parental Nutrition (PN) should be reserved for HIV-infected children who continue to lose weight on an aggressive enteral program, who have severe recurrent or chronic pancreatic or biliary tract disease, or have intractable diarrhea with weight loss. The placement of a central venous catheter can provide venous access that is often difficult to obtain in terminal stages. Central venous catheters present an additional risk for sepsis, and studies in adults and children with HIV infection present conflicting results regarding the risk of infection.

Limited data are available on the benefits of PN in children with HIV infection. In the series reported by Guarino and colleagues,[93] 46 HIV-infected children with malnutrition and malabsorption received a median of 157 days of PN. While CD4 cell count, weight, and xylose absorption all improved significantly in the patients receiving enteral therapy (n = 16), these measures improved on PN, but not significantly. One possible explanation for the difference in findings between PN and enteral nutritional support is that this was an observational study and patients on PN had more advanced disease as indicated by a lower baseline CD4 count (154 cells/mm^3 for enteral patients vs 55 cells/mm^3 for PN patients). In addition, 58.7% of PN patients versus 18.8% of enteral patients died during the follow-up period which may be related to increased risk of infection with central lines and PN, but may also reflect the practice of reserving PN for late and end-stage patients. In resource-poor settings with more advanced HIV disease, the availability of PN is usually limited as well.

Other Nutritional Therapies/Appetite Stimulants

Megestrol acetate, a synthetic orally active progesterone, widely used to treat breast cancer, has shown promising results as an appetite stimulant in adults with HIV infection. The mechanism of weight gain with megestrol acetate is under investigation, but research suggests that it has an effect both on behavior (ie, food intake) and metabolism, by the induction of lipogenic enzymes and fat synthesis. There are few reports on the use of megestrol acetate in children with HIV infection. Clarick and colleagues[94] evaluated the effects of megestrol acetate in 19 HIV-infected children for a median of 7 months at doses between 4.0 to 8.5 mg/kg/d and found increased weight Z-scores with continued therapy, but no improvement in linear growth. The authors also reported that poor weight gain and/or weight loss occurred after megestrol acetate was withdrawn. Adrenal suppression was also noted in 7 of 10 HIV-infected children treated with megestrol acetate compared to 0 of 10 HIV-infected children not on megestrol acetate.[95] Therefore, use of megestrol acetate may be beneficial for weight gain and improved appetite in HIV-infected children, but caution is warranted particularly when discontinuing or withdrawing therapy.

Dronabinol (delta-9-tetrahydrocannabinol) is another appetite stimulant that has been used in adult HIV-infected patients. It was approved for use in the United States in 1986 for treatment of chemotherapy-induced nausea and vomiting, although it was found to stimulate appetite as well. A randomized, placebo-controlled study of dronabinol[96] was performed on 139 patients. Appetite stimulation, measured by visual analog scale, was maintained or increased in patients receiving dronabinol. After at least 2 months of treatment with dronabinol, 38% of patients gained greater than or equal to 2 kg of weight. Altered mental status was the primary adverse effect for this medication. Currently there are no dosing recommendations for children.

Growth Hormone

Growth hormone (GH) can be used as a therapeutic agent to improve lean body mass and weight in HIV-infected patients. This application is based on observations of GH disturbances in HIV infected populations. Heijligenberg and colleagues examined 24-hour GH and IGF-1 levels, in eight asymptomatic HIV-infected men, eight clinically stable AIDS patients, and eight healthy controls.[97] No differences were demonstrated in 24-hour GH profiles or IGF-I levels between the three groups, suggesting that HIV disease per se does not affect the GH-IGF-I axis. In contrast, abnormalities in the GH axis have been demonstrated among patients with AIDS wasting[98] and in the setting of HIV associated lipodystrophy.[99,100]

A study examining IGF-1 secretion of HIV-infected children showed IGF-1 secretion was diminished in both asymptomatic (45% of children) and symptomatic (86% of children) HIV-infected children and was associated with growth failure. Less clear association with thyroid function was found.[101] GH is anabolic, improves nitrogen balance and serum protein levels, and promotes lipid mobilization and protein synthesis in some clinical setting. In a small trial of HIV-infected children with growth failure (n = 6), Hardin and colleagues found that administration of recombinant human GH was associated with reduced protein catabolism and improvements in height and weight, including increased lean tissue mass.[102] These data are similar to results seen in larger trials of GH in HIV-infected adults with wasting,[103] but more research is needed to determine the safety and long-term efficacy of this approach in children.

Numerous other therapies have been employed to initiate weight gain in patients with HIV infection. These include essential fatty acid supplementation (n-3 fatty acids), specific vitamin and antioxidant replacements, pancreatic enzymes, testosterone replacement, and cytokine inhibitors such as pentoxifylline and thalidomide. As well, studies are underway evaluating the effects of exercise and aerobic training in patients with HIV infection. Unfortunately, there are no therapies discovered to date that universally prevent or reverse nutritional derangements in HIV-infected patients. However, the improved nutritional status observed with the use of antiretroviral therapy supports the importance of suppression of viral replication and avoidance of opportunistic infections in the maintenance of nutritional health.

CONCLUSION

Great strides have been made over the past two decades regarding the detection, prevention, and virologic treatment of HIV in childhood, with the basic understanding of the interaction between nutritional status and HIV becoming better understood. The cause of nutritional problems in patients with HIV infection is complex and likely multifactorial. It is clear, however, that malnutrition of HIV-infected children is among the most serious, chronic, and difficult to treat problems confronting clinicians caring for HIV-infected children, especially in developing countries. Clinicians should be aware of nutritional problems, and close surveillance of nutrition should be conducted on all children who are at risk for HIV infection. Early, aggressive nutritional interventions are indicated. As a treatment strategy, improving nutritional status of HIV-infected children, may improve clinical outcome.

While the incidence of malnutrition in developed countries has decreased with HAART therapy, other metabolic problems can arise. The long-term risks of HAART on HIV-infected children are unknown. Close surveillance for the emergence of insulin resistance, dyslipidemias, and premature cardiovascular disease will be important as children with perinatally acquired HIV age into adulthood. Further investigations on the short- and long-term nutritional and metabolic effects of HAART therapy are needed. Investigators should continue to study the effects of oral hypoglycemic agents, lipid-lowering medications, and life style changes on cardiovascular risk factors for HIV-infected children with lipodystrophy.

REFERENCES

1. World Health Organization/UNAIDS. AIDS Epidemic Update, August 2006.
2. Hughes WT, Price RA, Sisko F, et al. Protein-calorie malnutrition: A host determinant for *Pneumocystis carinii* infection. Am J Dis Child 1974;128:44–52.
3. Chandra RK. Immunocompetance of Nutritional Disorders. London: Arnold; 1980.
4. Chandra RK, Newbuerne PM. Nutrition, Immunity and Infection: Mechanisms of Interactions. New York: Plenum; 1977.
5. Scrimshaw NS, Taylor CE, Gordon JE. Interactions of Nutrition and Infection. WHO Monograph Series 57, 1968.
6. Lindegren ML, Steinberg S, Byers RH. Epidemiology of HIV/AIDS in children. Ped Clin N Amer 2000;47:1–20.
7. Miller TL, Easley KA, Zhang W, et al. Maternal and infant factors associated with failure to thrive in children with vertically transmitted human immunodeficiency virus-1 infection: The prospective P2C2 human immunodeficiency virus multicenter study. Pediatrics 2001;108:1287–96.
8. Chantry CJ, Byrd RS, Englund JA, et al. Growth, survival and viral load in symptomatic childhood human immunodeficiency virus infection. Pediatr Infect Dis J 2003;22:1033–8.
9. Mgone CS, Mhalu FS, Shao JF, et al. Prevalence of HIV-1 infection and symptomatology of AIDS in severely malnourished children in Dar Es Salaam, Tanzania. J Acquir Immune Defic Syndr 1991;4:910–3.
10. Obimbo EM, Mbori-Ngacha DA, Ochieng JO, et al. Predictors of early mortality in a cohort of human immunodeficiency virus type-1-infected African children. Pediatr Infect Dis J 2004;23:536–43.
11. Berhane R, Bagenda D, Marum L, et al. Growth failure as a prognostic indicator of mortality in pediatric HIV infection. Pediatrics 1997;100: E7.
12. Lodha R, Upadhyay A, Kapoor V, et al. Clinical profile and natural history of children with HIV infection. Indian J Pediatr 2006;73:201–4.
13. Miller TL, Evans S, Orav EJ, et al. Growth and body composition in children with human immunodeficiency virus-1 infection. Am J Clin Nutr 1993;57:588–92.

14. Moye J, Rich KC, Kalish LA, et al. Natural history of somatic growth in infants born to women infected by human immunodeficiency virus. Women and Infants Transmission Study Group. J Pediatr 1996;128:58–69.
15. Moye J, Frederick M, Chantry C, et al. 10-year follow-up of somatic growth in children born to women infected by human immunodeficiency virus. 8th Conference on Retroviruses and Opportunistic Infections; Feb 2001, Chicago, Abs 514.
16 Brettler DB, Forsberg A, Bolivar E, et al. Growth failure as a prognostic indicator for progression to acquired immunodeficiency syndrome in children with hempohilia. J Pediatr 1990;117:584–8.
17 Dreyfuss ML, Msamanga GI, Speigelman D, et al. Determinants of low birth weight among HIV infected pregnant women in Tanzania. Am J Clin Nutr 2001;74:814–26
18. Henderson RA, Miotti PG, Saavedra JM, et al. Longitudinal growth during the first 2 years of life in children born to HIV-infected mothers in Malawi, Africa. Pediatr AIDS HIV Infect 1996;7:91–7.
19. Bulterys M, Chao A, Munyemana S, et al. Maternal human immunodeficiency virus 1 infection and intrauterine growth: A prospective cohort study in Butare, Rwanda. Pediatr Infect Dis J 1994;13:94–100.
20. Fontana M, Zuin G, Plebani A, et al. Body composition in HIV-infected children: Relations with disease progression and survival. Am J Clin Nutr 1999;69:1282–6.
21. Arpadi SM, Horlick MN, Wang J, et al. Body composition in prepubertal children with human immunodeficiency virus type 1 infection. Arch Pediatr Adolesc Med 1998;152:688–93.
22. Buchacz K, Cervia JS, Lindsey JC, et al. Impact of protease inhibitor-containing combination antiretroviral therapies on height and weight growth in HIV-infected children. Pediatrics 2001;108:E72
23. Nachman SA, Lindsey JC, Moye J, et al. Growth of human immunodeficiency virus-infected children receiving highly active antiretroviral therapy. Pediatr Inf Dis J 2005;24:352–7.
24. Verweel G, van Rossum AMC, Hartwig NG, et al. Treatment with highly active antiretroviral therapy in human immunodeficiency virus type-1-infected children is associated with a sustained effect on growth. Pediatrics 2002;109:E275.
25. Steiner F, Kind C, Aebi C, et al. Growth in human immunodeficiency virus type 1-infected children treated with a protease inhibitor. Eur J Pediatr 2001;160:611–6.
26. Mallal SA, John M, Moore CB, et al. Contribution of nucleoside analogue reverse transcriptase inhibitors to subcutaneous fat wasting in patients with HIV infection. AIDS 2000;14:1309–16.
27. Purnell JQ, Zambon A, Knopp RH, et al. Effect of ritonavir on lipids and post-heparin lipase activities in normal subjects. AIDS 2000;14:51–7.
28. Noor M, Lo J, Mulligan K, et al. Metabolic effects of indinavir in healthy HIV-seronegative men. AIDS 2001;15:F11–8.
29. Grinspoon S, Carr A. Cardiovascular risk and body-fat abnormalities in HIV-infected adults. N Engl J Med. 2005;352:48–62.
30. Brown TT, Cole SR, Li X, et al. Antiretroviral therapy and the prevalence and incidence of diabetes mellitus in the multicenter AIDS cohort study. Arch Intern Med 2005;165:1179–84.
31. Friis-Moller N, Sabin CA, Weber R, et al. Data collection on adverse events of anti-HIV drugs (DAD) study group. Combination antiretroviral therapy and the risk of myocardial infarction. N Engl J Med 2003;349:1993–2003.
32. Arpadi SM, Cuff PA, Horlick M, et al. Lipodystrophy in HIV infected children is associated with high viral load and low CD4+ lymphocyte count and CD4+ lymphocyte percentage at baseline and use of protease inhibitors and stavudine. J Acquir Immune Def Syndr 2001;27:30–4.
33. Beregszaszi M, Dollfus C, Levine M, et al. Longitudinal evaluation and risk factors of lipodystrophy and associated metabolic changes in HIV-infected children. J Acquir Immune Defic Syndr 2005;40:161–8.
34. Miller TL, Martin SR, Cooper ER, et al. Gastrointestinal inflammation and carbohydrate intolerance in HIV-infected children. Pediatr Res 1990;27:650.
35. Arnalich F, Martinez P, Hernanz A, et al. Altered concentrations of appetite regulators may contribute to the development and maintenance of HIV-associated wasting. AIDS 1997;11:1129–34.
36. Arpadi SM, Cuff PA, Kotler DP, et al. Growth velocity, fat-free mass and energy intake are inversely related to viral load in HIV-infected children. J Nutr 2000;130:2498–502.
37. Zuin G, Comi D, Fontana M, et al. Energy and nutrient intakes in HIV-infected children. Pediatr AIDS HIV Infect: Fetus Adolesc 1994;5:159–61.
38. Ullrich R, Zeitz M, Heise W, et al. Small intestinal structure and function in patients infected with human immunodeficiency virus (HIV): Evidence for HIV-induced enteropathy. Ann Intern Med 1989;111:15–21
39. Kotler DP. HIV infection and the gastrointestinal tract. AIDS 2005;19:107–17.
40. Delezay O, Yahi N, Tamalt C, et al. Direct effect of type-1 human immunodeficiency virus (HIV-1) on intestinal epithelial cell differentiation: Relationship to HIV-1 enteropathy. Virology 1997;238:231–42.
41. Miller TL, Orav EJ, Martin SR, et al. Malnutrition and carbohydrate malabsorption in children with vertically transmitted human immunodeficiency virus 1 infection. Gastroenterology 1991;100:1296–302.
42. Yolken RH, Hart W, Oung I, et al. Gastrointestinal-dysfunction and diasaccharide intolerance in children infected with human immunodeficiency virus. J Pediatr 1991;118:359–63.
43. The Italian Paediatric Intestinal/HIV Study Group. Intestinal malabsorption of HIV-infected children: Relationship to diarrhoea, failure to thrive, enteric micro-organisms and immune impairment. AIDS 1993;7:1435–40.
44. Sentongo TA, Rutstein RM, Stettler N, et al. Association between steatorrhea, growth, and immunologic status in children with perinatally acquired HIV infection. Arch Pediatr Adol Med 2001;155:149–52.
45. Alfaro MP, Siegel RM, Baker RC, et al. Resting energy expenditure and body composition in pediatric HIV infection. Pediatr AIDS HIV Infect 1995;6:276–80.
46. Henderson RA, Talusan K, Hutton N, et al. Resting energy expenditure and body composition in children with HIV-1 infection. J Acquir Immne Defic Syndr Hum Retrovirol 1998;19:150–7.
47. Arpadi SM, Cuff PA, Kotler DP, et al. Growth velocity, fat-free mass and energy intake are inversely related to viral load in HIV-infected children. J Nutr 2000;130:2498–502.
48. Johann-Liang R, O'Neill L, Cervia J, et al. Energy balance, viral burden, insulin-like growth factor-1, interleukin-6 and growth impairment in children infected with human immunodeficiency virus. AIDS 2000;14:683–90.
49. Henderson RA, Talusan K, Hutton N, et al. Whole body protein turnover in children with human immunodeficiency virus (HIV) infection. Nutrition 1999;15:189–94.
50. Hardin DS, Ellis KJ, Rice J, et al. Protease inhibitor therapy improves protein catabolism in prepubertal children with HIV infection. J Pediatr Endocrinol Metab 2004;17:321–5.
51. Batterham M. Investigating heterogeneity in studies of resting energy expenditure in persons with HIV/AIDS: A meta-analysis. Am J Clin Nutr 2005;81:702–13.
52. Shevitz AH, Knox TA, Spiegelman D, et al. Elevated resting energy expenditure among HIV-seropositive persons receiving highly active antiretroviral therapy. AIDS 1999;13:1351–7.
53. Beutler B, Cerami A. Cachectin: More than a tumor necrosis factor. N Engl J Med 1987;316:379–85.
54. Beutler B. Cytokines and cancer cachexia. Hosp Pract 1993;28:45–52.
55. Hellerstein MK, Grunfeld C, Wu K, et al. Increased de novo hepatic lipogenesis in human immunodeficiency virus infection. J Clin Endocrinol Metabol 1993;76:559–65.
56. Roubenoff R, Grinspoon S, Skolnick PR, et al. Role of cytokines and testosterone in regulating lean body mass and resting energy expenditure in HIV-infected men. Am J Physiol Endocrinol Metab 2002;283:E138–45.
57. Galhardo MC, de Carvalho MG, Georg I, et al. Nutritional status impairments in HIV-infected patients are associated with increased TNF-alpha and IL-6 serum levels, but not with viral load. Infection 2001;29:257–61.
58. Missmer S, Speigelman D, Gorbach SL et al. Predictors of change in the functional status of children with human immunodeficiency virus infection. Pediatrics 2000;106:E24.
59. Money J. The syndrome of abuse dwarfism (psychosocial dwarfism or reversible hyposomatotropism). Am J Dis Childhood 1977;131:508–13.
60. Boulton TJ, Smith R, Single T. Psychosocial growth failure: A positive response to growth hormone and placebo. Acta Paediatr 1992;81:322–5.
61. Anonymous. Children whose mothers are infected with HIV. Communicable Disease Report. CDR Weekly 1995;5:111.
62. Lifschitz MH, Wilson GS, Smith EO, et al. Fetal and postnatal growth of children born to narcotic-dependent women. Pediatrics 1983;102:686–90.
63. Eley BS, Sive AA, Abelse L, et al. Growth and micronutrient disturbances in stable, HIV-infected children in Cape Town. Ann Trop Paediatr 2002;22:19–23.
64. Castaldo A, Tarallo L, Palombo E, et al. Iron deficiency and intestinal malabsorption in HIV disease. J Pediatr Gastroenterol Nutr 1996;22:359–63.
65. Kruzich LA, Marquis GS, Carriquiry AL, et al. US youths in the early stages of HIV disease have low intakes of some micronutrients important for optimal immune function. J Am Diet Assoc 2004;104:1095–101.
66. Tang AM, Graham NM, Kirby AJ, et al. Dietary micronutrient intake and risk of progression to acquired immunodeficiency syndrome (AIDS) in human immunodeficiency virus type 1 (HIV-1)-infected homosexual men. Am Journal Epidemiol 1993;138:937–51.
67. Semba RD, Graham MH, Caiaffa WT, et al. Increased mortality associated with vitamin A deficiency during human immunodeficiency virus type 1 infection. Arch Intern Med 1993;153:2149–54.
68. Read JS, Bethel J, Harris DR, et al. Serum vitamin A concentrations in a North American cohort of human immunodeficiency virus type-1-infected children. National Institute of Child Health and Human Development Intravenous Immunoglobulin Clinical Trial Study Group. Pediatric Infect Dis J 1999;18:134–42.
69. Semba RD, Miotti PG, Chiphangwi JD, et al. Maternal vitamin A deficiency and mother-to child transmission of HIV-1. Lancet 1994;343:1593–7.
70. Greenberg BL, Semba RD, Vink PE, et al. Vitamin A deficiency and maternal-infant transmission of HIV in two metropolitan areas in the United States. AIDS 1997;11:325–32.
71. Fawzi WW, Mbise RL, Hertzmark E, et al. A randomized trial of vitamin A supplements in relation to mortality among human immunodeficiency virus-infected and uninfected children in Tanzania. Pediatric Infect Dis J 1999;18:127–33.
72. Melikian G, Mmiro F, Ndugwa C, et al. Relation of vitamin A and carotenoid status to growth failure and mortality among Ugandan infants with human immunodeficiency virus. Nutrition 2001;17:567–72.
73. Villamor E, Mbise R, Speigelman D, et al. Vitamin A supplements ameliorate the adverse effect of HIV-1, malaria, and diarrheal infections on child growth. Pediatrics 2002;109:E6.
74. Filteau SM, Rollins NC, Coutsoudis A, et al. The effect of antenatal vitamin A and beta-carotene supplementation on gut integrity of infants of HIV-infected South African women. J Pediatr Gastroenterol Nutr 2001;32:464–70.
75. Humphrey JH, Iliff PJ, Marinda ET, et al. ZVITAMBO Study Group. Effects of a single large dose of vitamin A, given during the postpartum period to HIV-positive women and their infants, on child HIV infection, HIV-free survival, and mortality. J Infect Dis 2006;193:860–71.
76. Baum MK, Mantero-Atienza E, Shor-Posner G, et al. Association of Vitamin B6 status with parameters of immune function in early HIV-1 infection. J Acquir Immune Defic Syndr 1991;4:1122–32.
77. Dowling S, Lambe J, Mulcahy F. Vitamin B_{12} and folate status in human immunodeficiency virus infection. Eur J Clin Nutr 1993;47:803–7.
78. Rubell P, O'Doherty J, Tang A, et al. Folic acid absorption in patients infected with the human immunodeficiency virus. J Intern Med 1991;230:227–31.
79. Fawzi WW, Msamanga GI, Wei R, et al. Effect of providing vitamin supplements to human immunodeficiency virus-infected, lactating mothers on the child's morbidity and CD4+ cell counts. Clin Inf Dis 2003;36:1053–62.
80. Fawzi WW, Msamanga GI, Spiegelman D, et al. A randomized trial of multivitamin supplements and HIV disease progression and mortality. N Engl J Med 2004;351:23–32.
81. Sappey C, Legrand-Poels S, Best-Belpomme M, et al. Stimulation of glutathione peroxidase activity decreases HIV type 1 activation after oxidative stress. AIDS Res Hum Retrovir 1994;10:1451–61.
82. Rodriguez JF, Cordero J, Chantry C, et al. Plasma glutathione concentrations in children infected with human immunodeficiency virus. Pediatr Infect Dis J 1998;17:236–41.
83. Kupka R, Msamanga GI, Spiegelman D, et al. Selenium levels in relation to morbidity and mortality among children born to HIV-infected mothers. Eur J Clin Nutr. 2005;59:1250–8.
84. Sazawal S, Black RE, Bhan MK, et al. Zinc supplementation in young children with acute diarrhea in India. N Eng J Med 1995;333:839–44.
85. Graham NMH, Sorenson D, Odaka N, et al. Relationship of serum copper and zinc levels to HIV-1 seropositivity and progression to AIDS. J Acquir Immune Defic Syndr 1991;4:976–80.
86. Reich EN, Church JA. Oral zinc supplementation in the treatment of HIV-infected children. Pediatr AIDS HIV Infect 1994;5:357–60.
87. Bobat R, Coovadia H, Stephen C, et al. Safety and efficacy of zinc supplementation for children with HIV-1 infection in South Africa: A randomized double-blind placebo-controlled trial. Lancet 2005;366:1862–67.
88. Saint Marc T, Partisini M, Poizot-Martin I, et al. Fat distribution evaluated by computed tomography and metabolic abnormalities in patients undergoing antiretroviral therapy: Preliminary results of the LIPCO study. AIDS 2000;14: 37–49.

89. Iliff PJ, Piwoz EG, Tavengwa NV, et al. ZVITAMBO study group. Early exclusive breastfeeding reduces the risk of postnatal HIV-1 transmission and increases HIV-free survival. AIDS 2005;19:699–708.
90. Shingadia D, Viani RM, Yogev R, et al. Gastrostomy tube insertion for improvement of adherence to highly active antiretroviral therapy in pediatric patients with human immunodeficiency virus. Pediatrics 2000;105:E80.
91. Temple ME, Koranyi KI, Nahata MC. Gastrostomy tube placement in nonadherent HIV-infected children. Ann Pharmacother 2001;35:414–8.
92. Miller TL, Awnetwant EL, Evans S, et al. Gastrostomy tube supplementation for HIV-infected children. Pediatrics 1995;96:696–702.
93. Guarino A, Spagnuolo MI, Canani RB, et al. Effects of nutritional rehabilitation on intestinal function and CD4 cell number in children with HIV. J Pediatr Gastroenter Nutr 2002;34:366–71.
94. Clarick RH, Hanekom MB, Yogev R, et al. Megestrol acetate treatment of growth failure in children with human immunodeficiency virus. Pediatrics 1997;99:354–57.
95. Stockheim JA, Daabul JJ, Yogev R, et al. Adrenal suppression in children with the human immunodeficiency virus treated with megestrol acetate. J Pediatr 1999;134:368–70.
96. Beal JE, Olson R, Laubenstein L, et al. Dronabinol as a treatment for anorexia associated with weight loss in patients with AIDS. J Pain Symptom Manage 1995;10:89–97.
97. Heijligenberg R, Sauerwein HP, Brabant G, et al. Circadian growth hormone secretion in asymptomatic human immune deficiency virus infection and acquired immunodeficiency syndrome. J Clin Endocrinol Metab 1996;81:4028–32.
98. Grinspoon S, Corcoran C, Lee K, et al. Loss of lean body and muscle mass correlates with androgen levels in hypogonadal men with acquired immunodeficiency syndrome and wasting. J Clin Endocrinol Metab 1996;81:4051–8.
99. Rietschel P, Hadigan C, Corcoran C, et al. Assessment of growth hormone dynamics in human immunodeficiency virus-related lipodystrophy. J Clin Endocrinol Metab 2001;86:504–10.
100. Vigano A, Mora S, Brambilla P, et al. Impaired growth hormone secretion correlates with visceral adiposity in highly active antiretroviral treated HIV-infected adolescents. AIDS 2003;17:1435–41.
101. Matarazzo P, Palomba E, Ciuti E, et al. Growth impairment, IGF-1 hyposecretion and thyroid dysfunction in children with perinatal HIV-1 infection. Acta Paediatr 1994;83:1029–34.
102. Hardin DS, Rice J, Doyle ME, et al. Growth hormone improves protein catabolism and growth in prepubertal children with HIV infection. Clin Endocrinol (Oxf) 2005;63:259–62.
103. Schambelan M, Mulligan K, Grunfeld C, et al. Recombinant human growth hormone in patients with HIV-associated wasting. A randomized, placebo-controlled trial. Serostim Study Group. Ann Intern Med 1996;125:873–82.

Celiac Disease

Dascha C. Weir, MD
Ciaran Kelly, MD

Celiac disease (CD) is an immune-mediated enteropathy secondary to permanent sensitivity to wheat gluten and related proteins in rye and barley. It results in characteristic histologic changes consisting of inflammation, crypt hyperplasia, and villous atrophy of the small intestine in genetically susceptible individuals. Significant variability in the clinical presentation of CD in the pediatric population complicates recognition of the disease in many patients. Treatment for CD consists of a lifelong strict gluten-free diet (GFD). Adherence to this diet is associated with resolution of most related signs and symptoms and a decreased risk of related complications. With an explosion of new knowledge over the span of two decades, our understanding of CD has changed dramatically. CD has gone from a rare condition causing gastrointestinal symptoms in children of European origin to a common disorder causing symptoms that affect multiple organ systems in all ages virtually worldwide.[1]

The overall prevalence of CD is similar in Europe and North America affecting up to 1% of the population.[2,3] A large multicenter study in the United States, using serologic screening with biopsy confirmation to identify cases of CD, showed a prevalence of CD of 1:133 in individuals with no evident risk factors. Prevalence of CD in symptomatic patients was 1:56. The prevalence of diagnosed CD is much lower, especially in the United States. This reflects underrecognition and underdiagnosis related to the wide clinical spectrum of disease and the presence of silent disease.[4] In the United States, the prevalence of CD in people of non-European descent is not known. Limited studies suggest that, in the United States, Hispanic and African-American populations have a lower prevalence of CD than non-Hispanic Caucasians. For example, a study in Colorado showed that the incidence of positive serology in Hispanic children was three times lower than in non-Hispanic Whites.[5] African-Americans also represent a small number of patients currently diagnosed with CD. A large center in New York City reported that African-Americans comprised 1.3% of their patients with biopsy-proven CD.[6] This is likely partially because of genetic differences in these populations. However, given the increasing recognition of CD in non-Caucasian populations internationally, serious consideration should be given to the possibility of underdiagnosis in minority populations in the United States.

CD is being increasingly diagnosed in other parts of the world, involving populations that were not traditionally thought to be affected by the disease. Reports from Mexico, South America, North India, the Middle East, Turkey, and North Africa have changed previous assumptions that CD is a European affliction.[7–15] CD is rare in people of Japanese, Chinese, and purely African-Caribbean descent.[16]

CD is associated with several autoimmune conditions and genetic disorders and often presents atypically or silently in these populations. In children, it is associated with autoimmune thyroid disease and with type I diabetes mellitus with a 7.8 and 4.5% prevalence of CD in affected children.[17,18] Up to 7% of patients with a selective IgA deficiency also have CD.[19] Patients with Trisomy 21, Turner syndrome, and Williams syndrome have also been found to be at higher risk of CD than the general population.[19–22]

PATHOGENESIS

Environmental, immunologic, and genetic factors are all important contributors to the pathogenesis of CD. Clearly, enteric exposure to specific proteins in wheat, rye, and barley are essential to disease activation in a genetically susceptible person. Wheat, rye, and barley have common ancestry and are all derived from the Triticeae tribe of the grass family. Broadly termed "gluten," the specific proline- and glutamine-rich proteins that activate disease are gliadins in wheat, secalins in rye, and hordeins in barley. Gluten, the second major protein fraction of wheat gluten, is likely involved to a lesser degree. Multiple toxic antigenic epitopes have been described (Figure 1).

These peptides activate immune cells causing a chain of events that result in tissue damage. The mechanisms for this activation are incompletely understood and are likely a combination of adaptive and innate immunity. Partially because of their high proline content, these large cereal peptides are resistant to digestion by intestinal proteases and pass through the epithelium and into the lamina propria in an intact state. The mechanisms of this passage through the intestinal barrier are not well understood. Tissue transglutaminase deamidates these peptides in the lamina propria causing them to become negatively charged as the glutamine residues are converted to glutamic acid. Deamidated peptides bind with far greater affinity to specific positively charged residues on the peptide-binding groove of HLA-DQ2 or HLA-DQ8 major histocompatibility complex (MHC) Class II molecules. These peptides are then presented by HLA-DQ2 or HLA-DQ8 to activate gliadin-specific CD4+ T cells thereby activating an intestinal inflammatory response leading to the characteristic histopathologic changes of CD. Intraepithelial lymphocytes, T cells that are markedly increased in the intestinal biopsies of patients with active CD, are also likely involved. It is now evident that gluten can

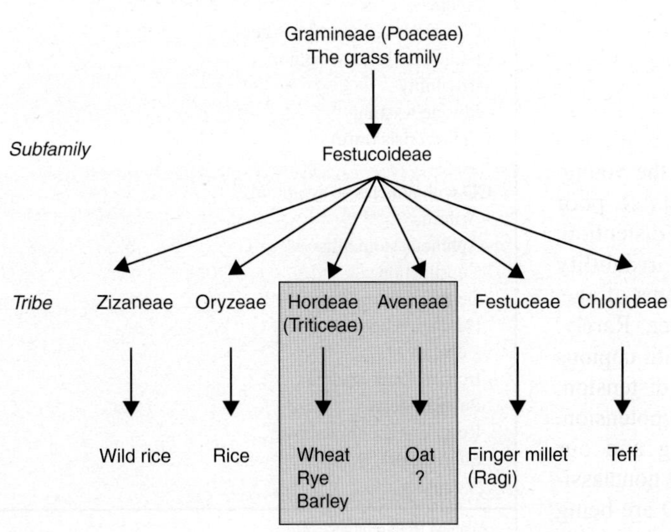

Figure 1 The grass family: Grains in the tribe *Triticeae* mediate celiac disease. Species of interest in the *Festucoideae* subfamily of the grass family are depicted. It seems likely that, for most patients with celiac disease, only grains in the tribe *Triticeae* mediate celiac disease. (Adapted from reference 23.)

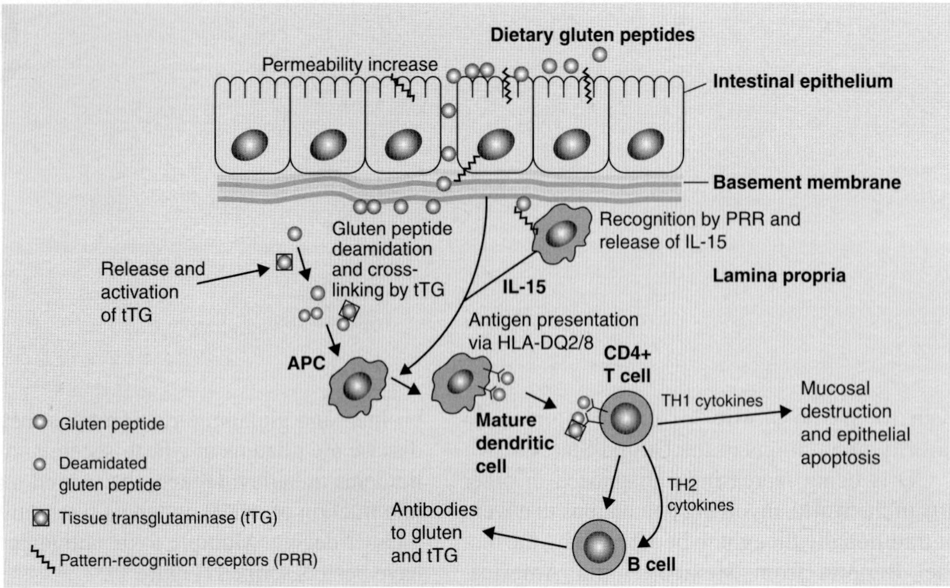

Figure 2 Adaptive and innate immune system responses in celiac disease. Cross-linking of gluten by tTG potentiates presentation of peptides by antigen-presenting cells (APC); deamidation of gluten improves binding to HLA-DQ2 or HLA-DQ8, triggering adaptive T-cell responses (inflammation and tissue remodeling (Th1) or antibody production (Th2)). Cells of the innate system recognize gluten peptides directly via pattern recognition receptors, and release cytokines (IL-15) that drive adaptive responses. Dendritic and T cells circulate to mesenteric lymph nodes (where they encounter T cells) and back to lamina propria. (Adapted from reference 26.)

stimulate interleukin-15 production, leading to the transformation of some T cells into natural killer cells and ultimately to enterocyte destruction (Figure 2).[1,24,25]

Genetics are clearly a factor in the development of CD. Among monozygous twins, there is a 70 to 75% CD concordance rate and first-degree relatives have a 10% risk of disease.[27,28] CD is strongly associated with HLA class II genes that map to the DQ locus. The HLA-DQ2 heterodimer is expressed in up to 95% of celiac patients with most of the remaining 5% expressing HLA-DQ8 heterodimer. These HLA types are present in 30% of the general population. Additionally, CD is concordant in only 30 to 40% of HLA-matched siblings. Clearly, these HLA types are necessary but not sufficient for CD to develop and other genes are likely to be involved. Candidate susceptibility genes include MY09B (myosin IXB) and regions of chromosome 5, 6, 11, and 19.[1,29] Investigation in this area is ongoing.

CLINICAL PRESENTATION

Traditionally, CD was thought to present primarily with gastrointestinal symptoms in the young. This "classical" presentation consists of poor growth, chronic diarrhea, abdominal distention, muscle wasting, poor appetite, and irritability typically seen in patients 6 to 24 months of age. Edema, pallor, and emesis are also seen. Rarely, children can present in celiac crisis with copious watery diarrhea, marked abdominal distension, dehydration, electrolyte imbalances, hypotension, and lethargy.[30] As serologic testing and our understanding of CD have improved, "nonclassical" or "atypical" presentations of CD are being increasingly recognized. In pediatric patients, this form of presentation is characterized by delayed onset with gastrointestinal complaints, such as nausea, bloating, recurrent abdominal pain, or constipation.[19] Many patients have no gastrointestinal complaints but have extraintestinal manifestations such as short stature, osteopenia, joint pains, pubertal delay, iron-deficiency anemia, dental enamel defects, neurologic disorders, or elevated transaminases. Some patients, with classic histologic changes on intestinal biopsy, are entirely asymptomatic and are described as having "silent" CD.[16,30]

CD is being increasingly diagnosed in adults. In fact, the mean age of diagnosis is now in midadult life (circa 45 years of age).[1] Many of these patients have likely had CD since childhood. Adults can present with gastrointestinal symptoms such as diarrhea, flatulence, abdominal bloating, and discomfort but often present with extraintestinal manifestations such as iron-deficiency anemia, macrocytic anemia, osteopenia, malaise, infertility, obstetrical complications, and neurologic conditions. Dermatitis herpetiformis, a pruritic blistering skin disorder, is also seen with CD but rarely occurs in pediatric patients (Table 1 and Figure 3).[16,30]

DIAGNOSIS

While the pathogenesis of CD and the genetic factors involved are being still elucidated, the resulting inflammation and tissue damage causes characteristic and well-recognized histopathologic changes. Small intestinal biopsy histology remains the gold standard in the diagnosis of CD. The spectrum of histopathologic changes in CD have been classified by Marsh with additional more recent modifications.[31] Marsh I lesions, an early but often nonspecific finding, are characterized by increased intraepithelial lymphocytes (>30 IEL per 100 enterocytes) and normal villous architecture. Marsh II lesions consist of crypt hyperplasia in the setting of increased numbers of intraepithelial lymphocytes (>30 per 100 epithelial cells). Marsh III lesions, type a–c, are characterized by partial to total villous atrophy in addition to crypt hyperplasia and increased numbers of intraepithelial lymphocytes. To avoid misinterpretation, biopsies are best reviewed by an experienced gastrointestinal pathologist. Because of patchy distribution of these histopathologic changes, multiple biopsies taken from the duodenal mucosa are indicated (Figure 4).[32]

Table 1 Clinical Manifestation of Celiac Disease in Children

Manifestations Secondary to Untreated CD	Associated Diseases (or Diseases Secondary to Untreated CD)
CD with classic symptoms	Autoimmune diseases
–Abdominal distension	–Type 1 diabetes
–Anorexia	–Thyroiditis
–Chronic or recurrent diarrhea	–Sjogren's syndrome
–Failure to thrive/weight loss	
–Irritability	Neurologic and psychologic disturbances
–Muscle wasting	–Ataxia
–Celiac crisis (rare)	–Depression
	–Epilepsy with intracranial calcifications
CD with nonclassic symptoms	
–Arthritis	Other disorders
–Aphthous stomatitis	–IgA nephropathy
–Constipation	–Osteopenia/osteoporosis
–Dental enamel defects	
–Dermatitis herpetiformis	Genetic disorders
–Hepatitis	–Down syndrome
–Iron-deficient anemia	–Turner syndrome
–Pubertal delay	–Williams syndrome
–Recurrent abdominal pain	–IgA deficiency
–Short stature	
–Vomiting	

Adapted from reference 30.

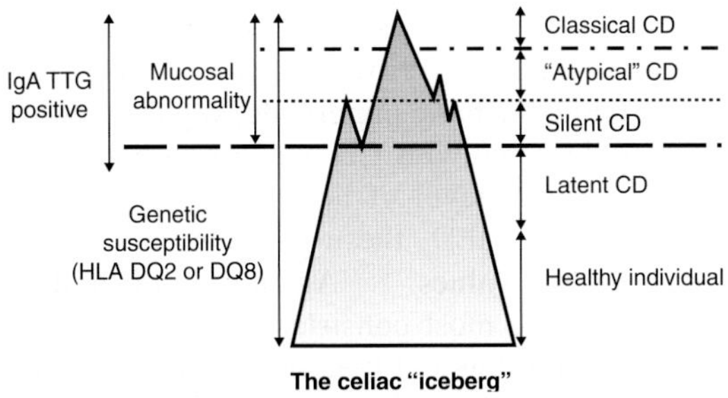

Figure 3 Clinical manifestations of celiac disease—the celiac iceberg. Celiac disease (CD) presents with a wide range of symptoms. Classical CD with prominent diarrhea and malabsorption is now less common than atypical CD presenting with iron-deficiency anemia or other disease manifestations with mild or absent gastrointestinal symptoms. Many individuals have silent CD with no symptoms or disease manifestations despite positive tTG serology and abnormal small bowel histology. Only a subset of individuals with CD has been diagnosed. This subgroup is often referred to as the "tip of the celiac iceberg." Most individuals with genetic susceptibility (HLA DQ2 or DQ8 positive) do not develop CD.

The development of accurate serologic markers has markedly improved our ability to identify patients with untreated CD and to monitor them after diagnosis. Serologic testing, coupled with clinical assessment and histopathologic confirmation, has become a cornerstone of diagnosis. IgA endomysial antibodies (EMA IgA) can be detected by indirect immunofluorescence using human umbilical cord or monkey esophagus. In pediatric patients, the sensitivity ranges from 89 to 94% and the specificity ranges from 99 to 100%.[33,34] However, this test is expensive and heavily operator dependent. IgA tissue transglutaminase (TTG IgA) is a less expensive, less operator-dependent assay. Its sensitivity ranges from 84.6 to 100% and specificity ranges from 76 to 97.4% in the pediatric population.[33,35,36] These tests perform less well in pediatric patients compared to adults, especially in patients under the age of 2 years. False negatives can also occur in the setting of mild enteropathy and in patients with IgA deficiency. TTG IgA and EMA IgA have largely replaced the older IgA and IgG antigliadin antibody tests. Antigliadin antibodies have poorer test performance, with low specificity in all but the youngest patients. However, in patients under 2 years of age, they may still be useful. Serologic markers also have a role in monitoring disease control once a GFD has been initiated. TTG IgA gradually normalizes within 3 to 12 months on a GFD depending upon the initial antibody concentration. TTG IgA has greater sensitivity than EMA IgA in monitoring for continued gluten intake but may not be sensitive enough to detect occasional or minor dietary errors.[33,37]

Positive TTG or EMA serology and/or resolution of symptoms on a GFD are not sufficient to make a definitive diagnosis of CD and do not replace the need for duodenal biopsies to make the initial diagnosis. However, repeat biopsies are no longer routinely recommended. Historically, repeat intestinal biopsies were used to confirm diagnosis and to monitor disease control. However, the availability of more accurate serologic markers has greatly reduced the use of repeat biopsies in patients with CD. A second biopsy is now limited to patients with poor clinical response to a strict GFD. Gluten rechallenge, once a mainstay of diagnosis, has also largely fallen by the wayside, especially in the pediatric population. Rechallenge is now indicated only in patients on a GFD in whom the diagnosis remains in doubt (Figure 5).[16]

First-degree relatives of people with CD have a 10% risk of disease. In family members, symptoms may be subtle or differ significantly from those in the affected child. It is controversial whether or not to perform serologic screening of all symptomless family members. However, case finding by a careful review of symptoms or signs of possible CD in first-degree relatives should be sought routinely when a child or adolescent is diagnosed with CD.

EFFECT OF CD ON GROWTH AND BODY COMPOSITION

Short stature is a common presenting sign of CD, especially in the pediatric population. It may be the only manifestation.[39–43] The pathophysiology of CD growth retardation is not fully defined but is traditionally thought to be secondary to associated malnutrition. With the initiation of a GFD and nutritional rehabilitation, children with CD undergo significant growth acceleration. This catch-up growth appears to be most evident during the first year on a GFD.[44] There is some evidence that, even when diagnosed early, monitored closely, and kept on a strict GFD, many children do not catch up completely and remain slightly below average height for age and skeletal age into adolescence.[45,46] New evidence suggests overlap of CD with growth hormone deficiency.[47,48] When catch-up growth on a GFD is not observed, further evaluation and possible growth hormone replacement is warranted.

In addition to linear growth, body composition is also significantly affected by CD. Longitudinal study of children and adolescents with newly diagnosed CD has shown significantly decreased weight, fat mass, and muscle mass compared to controls.[49] Decreased fat mass has also been described in children presenting with asymptomatic disease.[50] Similar findings have also been described in the adult population.[51] After 1 year on a GFD, affected children have been found to have complete restoration of body composition with no significant differences in weight, fat mass, or lean mass of the limbs compared to healthy controls. This restoration appears to occur faster and more completely when the GFD is initiated in childhood or adolescence compared to adulthood. It also appears to be a lasting effect, as body composition in young adults who had initiated a GFD in childhood or adolescence was entirely normal.[49] Even without strict adherence, long-term

(A)
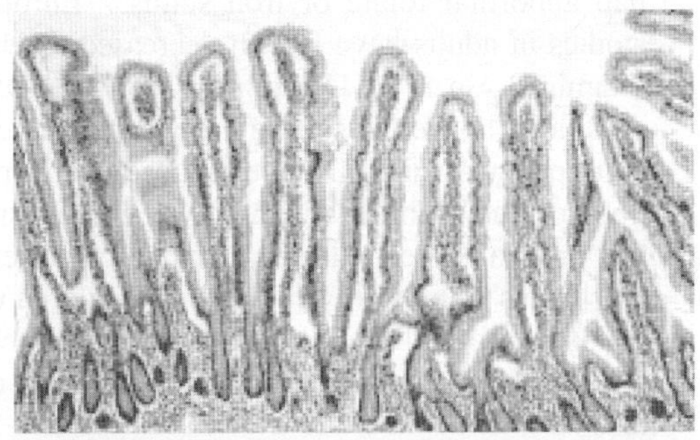
(B)
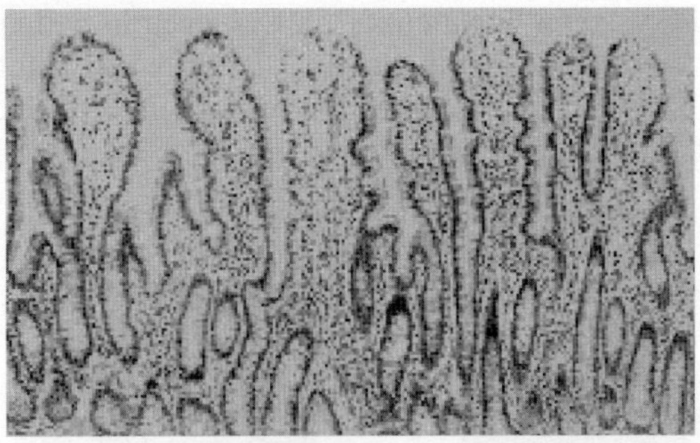
(C)
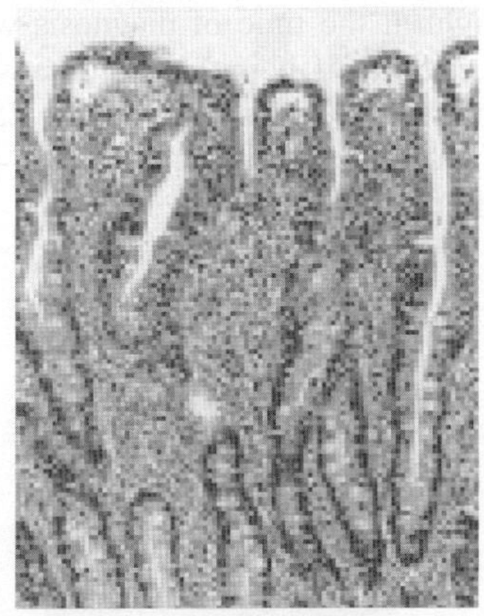
(D)
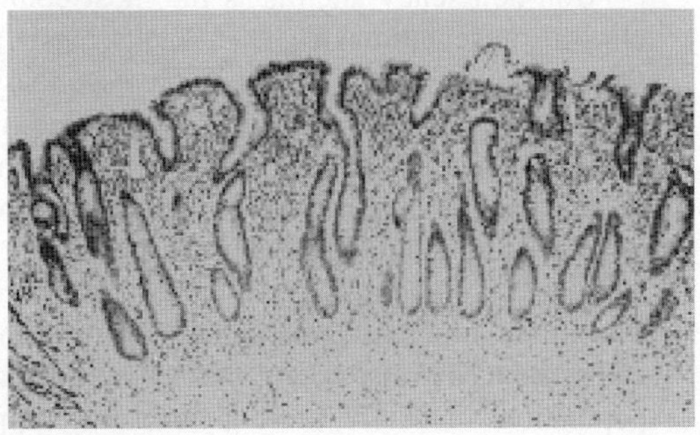
(E)
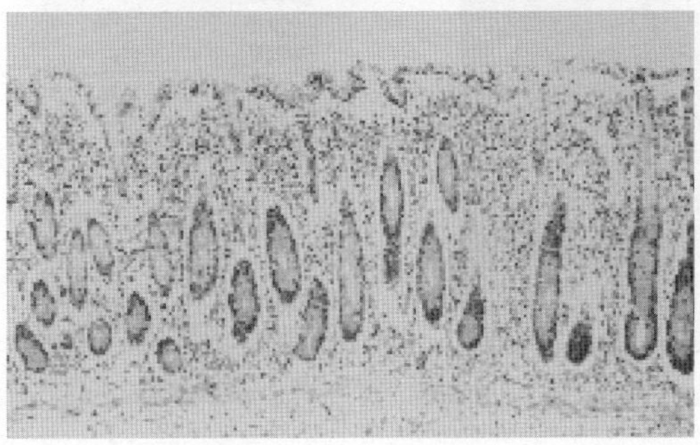

Figure 4 The spectrum of intestinal damage in celiac disease, Marsh classification. **(A)** Marsh I: Increased intraepithelial lymphocytes. **(B)** Marsh II: Increased intraepithelial lymphocytes and crypt hyperplasia. **(C)** Marsh IIIA: Partial villious atrophy. **(D)** Marsh IIIB: Subtotal villious atrophy. **(E)** Marsh IIIC: Total villous atrophy. (Adapted from reference 119.)

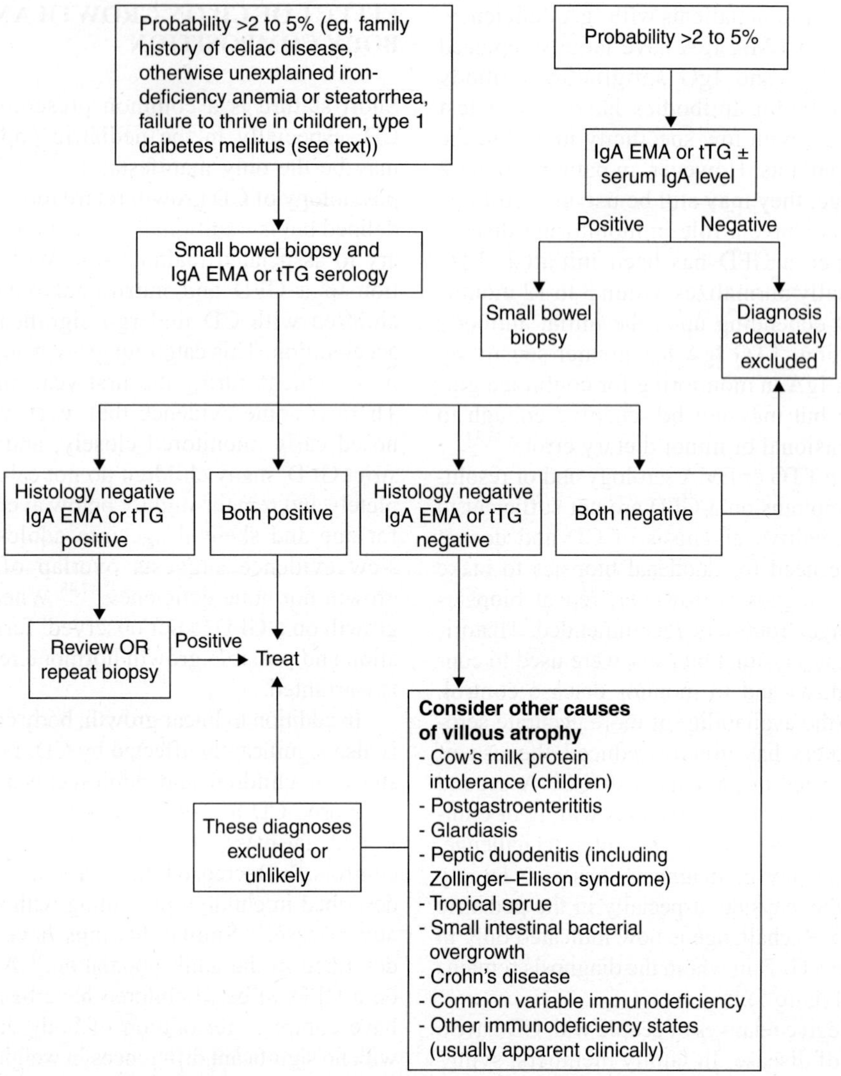

Figure 5 Making the diagnosis of celiac disease. (Adapted from reference 38.)

maintenance of the diet through adolescence was associated with improvements in body composition.[52] As nonclassical forms of CD are being increasingly recognized, these characteristic changes in body composition may not be found consistently. A recent analysis of adults with CD in the United States showed that only 18% were underweight at the time of diagnosis with 21% meeting criteria of being either overweight or obese (specifically defined as a BMI > 25).[53] This has not yet been demonstrated in the pediatric population (Figures 6 and 7).

Osteoporosis, rickets, and osteomalacia are all seen with CD. The specific mechanism of bone disease associated with CD is unclear but is likely related to malabsorption of calcium and vitamin D, and a possible effect of increased interleukins and other inflammatory mediators. Decreased bone mineral density is frequently seen in patients with CD, even in patients with clinically silent CD.[54] In untreated adult celiac patients, the reported prevalence of decreased bone mineral content is 22 to 80%. In children and adolescents with CD, bone mineral density is often decreased at the time of diagnosis (3 to 39% prevalence).[55] However, after 1 year on a strict GFD, the bone mineral density of children and adolescents with CD appears to normalize and reach the level of healthy controls. After 4 years of a GFD, these patients continue to have normal values.[54,56] Again, this restoration appears to be most consistent in the setting of early recognition and treatment.[57] Interestingly, patients who are poorly compliant did not appear to achieve peak bone mineralization.[56] The effect of the GFD on bone mineral density in adult studies has shown conflicting results. Some studies report improvement of bone mineral density on the diet and others show no such effect.[51,58–60] The age at diagnosis and initiation of the GFD seems to be a determining factor in bone restoration perhaps because of the increased activity of bone metabolism in childhood and adolescence.[61] There are conflicting data, however, on whether fracture risk is increased in adult patients with CD so the clinical significance of this osteoporosis is not clear.[62,63]

Another characteristic change associated with celiac disease involves dentition. Dental enamel defects of permanent teeth involving symmetric and chronologic distribution are well recognized in CD affecting up to 96% of children with CD and 83% of adults.[64]

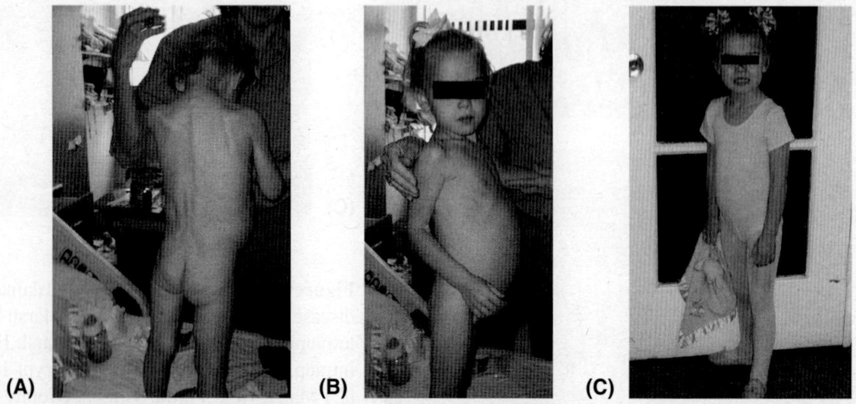

Figure 6 A toddler with "classic" presentation of celiac disease: **(A)** at the time of diagnosis (1); **(B)** at the time of diagnosis (2); **(C)** 1 year on a gluten-free diet.

NUTRITIONAL DEFICIENCIES

Nutritional deficiencies associated with CD are well recognized and should be an important consideration at the time of diagnosis and in continued management. Abnormal folate, iron, and vitamin B_{12} levels are found in children, adolescents, and adults with newly diagnosed or untreated CD. This appears to be true in patients with clinically silent disease as well as those with more "classic" manifestations. A study of screening-detected adolescent cases of CD in Finland (30% asymptomatic) found that 1 of 3 had abnormal folate or iron status.[65] European studies in adults have shown decreased levels of vitamin B_{12} in 11 to 41% of patients with CD.[66,67] Additionally, there is some evidence that untreated adult patients with CD have reduced endogenous pools of zinc.[68] Children with active gastrointestinal CD have also been shown to have lower serum zinc levels than healthy controls and children with celiac on the GFD.[69] Fat-soluble vitamins such as vitamin E, vitamin D, and vitamin K levels may also be low.

Iron-deficiency anemia is the most common clinical presentation of CD in adults but is also seen in children.[70,71] This is likely secondary to decreased absorption of iron in the proximal small bowel but may also be related to inadequate dietary intake as a result of CD-associated anorexia or chronic inflammation. Megoblastic anemia due to folate or vitamin B12 deficiency is also seen. Thrombocytopenia, leukopenia, and prolonged coagulation have also been reported in the pediatric population.[72] Notably, these abnormalities appear

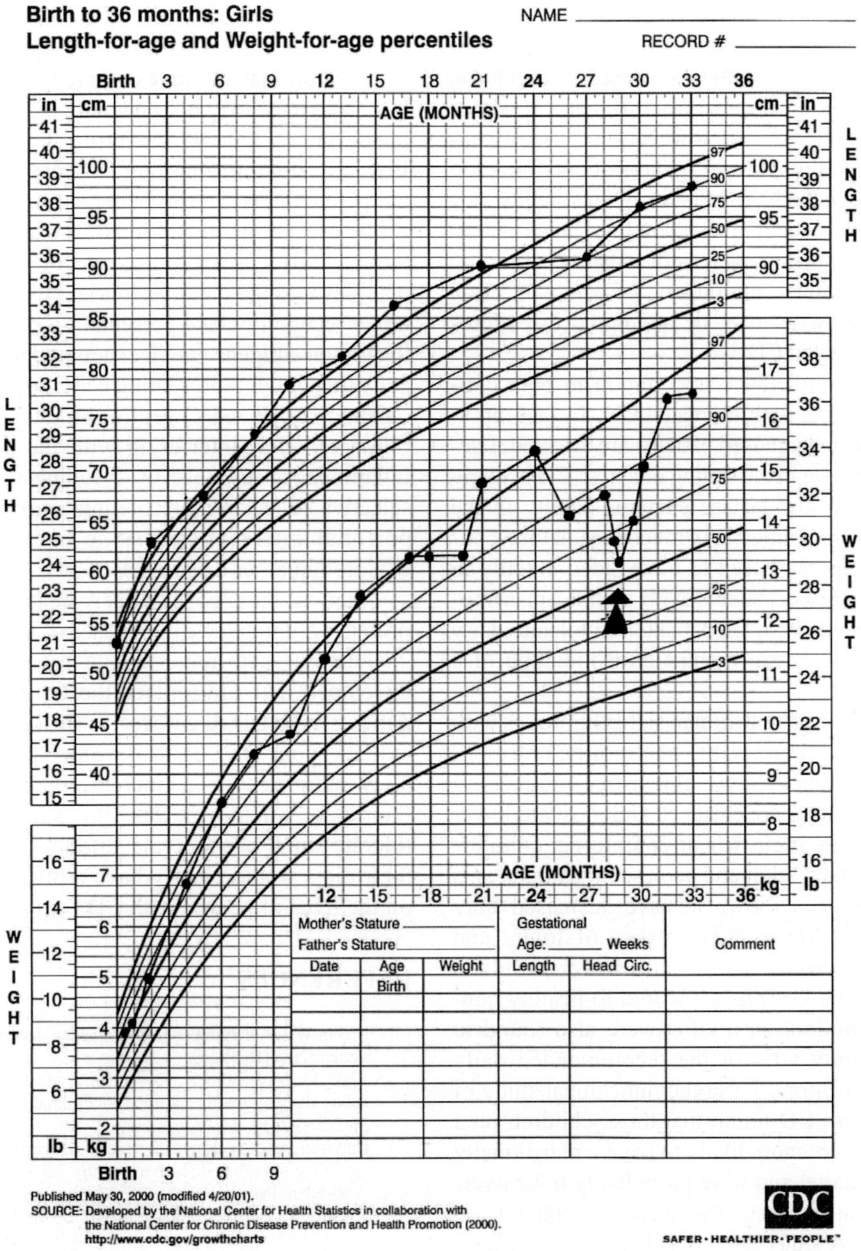

Figure 7 Growth chart of a classically presenting toddler with celiac disease. The arrow indicates time of diagnosis and initiation of a gluten-free diet.

to resolve with treatment. For example, up to 95% of patients have correction of their anemia after 1 year on the GFD.[73]

OTHER EXTRAINTESTINAL MANIFESTATIONS

Hepatic involvement is seen in adult and pediatric patients with CD. In a European study of 114 consecutive pediatric patients with CD, mild hypertransaminasemia was observed in 32% of patients at the time of diagnosis. In 5 patients (4.3%), it was the only manifestation of CD. In these children, aminotransferases normalized within 1 year of initiating a GFD either before or at the same time as serologic marker normalization. Hypertransaminasemia does not seem to be related to malnutrition in these patients and the mechanism of hepatic injury is not clear.[74] Similar findings have been reported in the adult celiac population.[75] Severe liver disease that resolved with a GFD has also been reported in adults with CD.[76]

Pubertal delay can occur in both boys and girls with CD. Hypogonadism, infertility, and sexual dysfunction have all been described in the literature. Boys have been found to have an abnormal pattern of androgen resistance. Girls with untreated CD have been shown to have delayed menarche compared to their mothers and to girls with CD who are on a GFD.[77,78] Increased risk for recurrent miscarriage, premature delivery, and lower birth weight babies have each been reported in women with untreated CD.[79–81]

Neurologic complications are a rare but recognized manifestation of CD. In fact, there are a growing number of reports linking neurologic symptoms with CD, sometimes as the presenting manifestation. Cerebellar ataxia, peripheral neuropathy, and epilepsy have been described primarily in the adult celiac population. Depression and anxiety have also been described to affect up to a third of patients with CD.[82–84] The syndrome of bilateral occipital cerebral calcifications and seizures, also known as CD, epilepsy, and cerebral calcifications (CEC syndrome), has been well described in association with CD. It presents primarily in childhood.[85]

There are limited studies on other neurologic complications of CD in pediatrics. Headache appears to be the most common neurologic complaint in children affecting almost a third of patients. Neurologic disorders such as hypotonia, developmental delay, learning disabilities, attention deficit hyperactivity disorder, headache, and ataxia have been described in up to 52% of patients with CD diagnosed in childhood which was significantly higher than a healthy control group. Epilepsy unrelated to CEC syndrome was not strongly associated with CD in children. There is no increase in the incidence of tics in patients with CD.[86] Despite previous reports to the contrary an association between CD and autism has not been confirmed.[30,84,87]

The spectrum of neurologic complications responds variably to a GFD. Up to half of children experiencing headaches improved on the diet. High rates of response in transient infantile hypotonia associated with classical early onset CD have also been reported, perhaps because of resolution of nutritional deficiencies.[86] In cases of epilepsy, improved seizure control has been reported but not seizure resolution. Depressive symptoms and anxiety may improve with a GFD in some patients but depression remains common in the treated celiac population. A few reports describe improvement of neuropathy and ataxia on a GFD but for most patients these neurologic problems persist or progress despite gluten avoidance.[84]

NATURAL HISTORY

Overall mortality in patients with CD has been described as two times that of the general population. The risk of increased mortality appears higher in patients with malabsorptive symptoms with no increased risk in patients with minor or no symptoms. Increased mortality has also been observed in association with delayed diagnosis and with poor adherence to the GFD.[88,89]

Specifically, an increased risk of malignancy has been associated with CD since the 1960s. Patients with CD appear to be at increased risk for non-Hodgkin lymphoma, especially small-intestinal T-cell lymphoma, small-intestinal adenocarcinoma, squamous cell carcinomas of the esophagus, mouth, and pharynx, and other gastrointestinal tract tumors. However, the absolute risk for malignancy remains small and recent data suggest that the risk while present is less than previously estimated and is low in patients with clinically silent CD.[89,90–93] The mechanism for this increased risk of cancer is not well understood but is perhaps related to chronic inflammation, increased exposure to environmental carcinogens secondary to intestinal permeability, immune surveillance abnormalities, or nutritional deficits.

Increased mortality and malignancy appear to be issues that primarily effect adult patients with CD. Few cases of cancer in children and adolescents with CD have been reported and increased risk of malignancy in this population has not been shown clearly.[91,93–95] Nonetheless, prompt identification of CD and appropriate treatment likely has long-term effects into adulthood. Adult patients with CD who were diagnosed in childhood appear to have a normal mortality rate presumably a benefit of long-term adherence to a GFD.[89] Additionally, patients who adhere to a GFD appear to have decreased malignancy risk that approaches that of the general population.[93,94]

The prevalence of autoimmune disorders is higher in adolescents and adults with CD and in their relatives as compared to the general population.[97–99] This association is likely related to the common genetic background including HLA type. It has been suggested that the risk of autoimmunity is related to the duration of gluten exposure and the age of diagnosis.[97] However, other studies have disputed this theory.[100,101]

TREATMENT

Gluten and related proteins in rye and barley are clearly implicated in the pathogenesis of CD and eliminating these proteins from the diet is currently the mainstay of treatment. Adherence to a strict GFD leads to histopathologic remission, serologic normalization, resolution of most of the related symptoms, and likely prevention of long-term complications.

However, the GFD is often challenging and sometimes overwhelming to people with CD. Wheat-based foods are a major staple of the American diet and finding palatable gluten-free alternatives can be difficult and expensive. Additionally, gluten is a hidden ingredient in many foods and medications and labeling can be confusing. The initiation of a strict GFD can have significant implications on quality of life. In fact, both adults and children with CD report negative feelings toward the diet and report difficulties with adherence especially related to eating out of the home, traveling, and social events.[102,103] Thus it is not surprising that adherence to the GFD is a major issue in CD management. This is true across all ages but especially in adolescents and young adults. Strict adherence to a GFD in this age group has been reported to be between 45 to 65%.[104,105] A very young age of diagnosis is associated with higher rates of adherence.[106] Screening detected disease, with either atypical or silent features, is associated with poorer compliance.[107] Patient and family education and support help the transition to a GFD and increase adherence. Intensive support is best given via a team approach with involvement of both a physician and a dietitian experienced in CD. Involvement in support groups is also helpful.[102,103]

The role of oats in the GFD has been somewhat controversial. In Europe, they are often included as part of a GFD. Various studies show that the inclusion of oats is safe for the majority of children and adults with CD. In some individuals, the avenin proteins in oats can trigger a response similar to gluten.[108–110] However, because of concerns about high levels of cross-contamination with wheat in the North American oats supply, it is not yet widely recommended in the United States. As uncontaminated sources of oats become more available, gradual introduction of oats with close clinical follow-up may be attempted in patients with well-treated CD.

Lactose intolerance is common in both children and adults with untreated CD. In fact, up to half of newly diagnosed patients are affected. Lactose intolerance in the setting of active CD is likely secondary to low lactase enzyme activity in the damaged small intestinal mucosa. Lactose-containing foods may need to be avoided initially in newly diagnosed patients with significant symptoms. Fortunately, most patients can tolerate dairy intake within 3 to 6 months after initiation of a GFD.[111,112]

While general nutritional status improves with treatment, a lifelong GFD may not be nutritionally well balanced. Few gluten-free products in the United States are enriched and most are lower in fiber than their wheat-containing counterparts.[108] In fact, adult and adolescent patients on a GFD have been shown to have decreased fiber intake.[113,114] Mean daily intakes of folate and vitamin B_{12} were significantly lower in adults with CD on a GFD as compared to healthy controls.[115] Children on a GFD were also found to consume only 60% of the recommended daily allowance of iron.[116] Another nutritional study of children with CD found that those children on a strict diet were more likely to have a nutritionally unbalanced diet and were more likely to be overweight than children who were not adherent to the diet.[117] A study in adult celiac patients after 8 to 12 years of GFD with biopsy-proven remission showed that 56% showed signs of poor vitamin status, specifically with lower plasma levels of folate, vitamin B_6, and elevated levels of homocysteine (a metabolic marker of folate, vitamin B_6, and vitamin B_{12} deficiency).[115] Thus the use of a daily gluten-free multivitamin supplement is often recommended.[108]

Please refer to Chapter 71, "Special Diets," for additional information about a gluten-restricted diet and celiac resources and support groups.

BEYOND THE GFD

While highly effective, a GFD is not an ideal therapeutic option for many individuals with CD because of the challenges associated with diet adherence and the negative impact on quality of life. Developing grains, through selective breeding and transgenic technology, that have low or nontoxic peptide sequences and acceptable baking qualities is technically challenging. Fortunately, as our understanding of the pathophysiology of CD has grown, several potential targets for new treatments have been identified. Alternatives to the GFD are currently being investigated.

Intraluminal therapies, such as endoproteolytic enzymes, may help degrade gluten peptides in the lumen thereby rendering them nontoxic. Blocking zonulin, a protein that regulates intestinal permeability, is also being explored and may act by preventing disruption of the intestinal epithelial barrier and the passage of toxic gluten peptides into the lamina propria. Other strategies target recognition and presentation of the offending gluten antigens via blockade of dendritic cells and other antigen-presenting cells, specific antagonization of HLA-DQ peptide binding or by inhibition of TTG. Interfering with the subsequent inflammatory response by cytokine therapy and selective adhesion molecule inhibition is another potential intervention that is currently being explored in other disease processes.[118]

Many of these potential new treatments, while promising, are in the early phases of investigation.

Ideally, a safe and effective treatment will be developed that can replace the GFD and allow patients with CD to eat freely. However, a more realistic goal may be to develop therapies that allow patients with CD increased flexibility with their diet. A treatment that allows individuals to tolerate small or moderate amounts of gluten in their diets would clearly have a positive impact on the lives of people with CD.

REFERENCES

1. Treem WR. Emerging concepts in celiac disease. Curr Opin Pediatr 2004;16:552–9.
2. Maki M, Mustalahti K, Kokkonen J, et al. Prevalence of celiac disease among children in Finland. N Engl J Med 2003;348:2517–24.
3. Carlsson AK, Axelsson IE, Borulf SK, et al. Serological screening for celiac disease in healthy 2.5-year-old children in Sweden. Pediatrics 2001;107:42–5.
4. Fasano A, Berti I, Gerarduzzi T, et al. Prevalence of celiac disease in at-risk and not-at-risk groups in the United States: A large multicenter study. Arch Intern Med 2003;163:286–92.
5. Hoffenberg EJ, MacKenzie T, Barriga KJ, et al. A prospective study of the incidence of childhood celiac disease. J Pediatr 2003;143:308–14.
6. Brar P, Lee AR, Lewis SK, et al. Celiac disease in African-Americans. Dig Dis Sci 2006;51:1012–5.
7. Remes-Troche JM, Ramirez-Iglesias MT, Rubio-Tapia A, et al. Celiac disease could be a frequent disease in Mexico: Prevalence of tissue transglutaminase antibody in healthy blood donors. J Clin Gastroenterol 2006;40:697–700.
8. Melo SB, Fernandes MI, Peres LC, et al. Prevalence and demographic characteristics of celiac disease among blood donors in Ribeirao Preto, State of Sao Paulo, Brazil. Dig Dis Sci 2006;51:1020–5.
9. Sood A, Midha V, Sood N, et al. Prevalence of celiac disease among school children in Punjab, North India. J Gastroenterol Hepatol 2006;21:1622–5.
10. Rawashdeh MO, Khalil B, Raweily E. Celiac disease in Arabs. J Pediatr Gastroenterol Nutr 1996;23:415–8.
11. Masjedizadeh R, Hajiani E, Hashemi J, et al. Celiac disease in South-West of Iran. World J Gastroenterol 2006;12:4416–9.
12. Ertekin V, Selimoglu MA, Kardas F, Aktas E. Prevalence of celiac disease in Turkish children. J Clin Gastroenterol 2005;39:689–91.
13. Catassi C, Ratsch IM, Gandolfi L, et al. Why is coeliac disease endemic in the people of the Sahara? Lancet 1999;354:647–8.
14. Bdioui F, Sakly N, Hassine M, Saffar H. Prevalence of celiac disease in Tunisian blood donors. Gastroenterol Clin Biol 2006;30:33–6.
15. al-Tawaty AI, Elbargathy SM Coeliac disease in north-eastern Libya. Ann Trop Paediatr 1998;18:27–30.

16. Farrell RJ, Kelly CP. Celiac sprue. N Engl J Med 2002;346:180–8.
17. Larizza D, Calcaterra V, De Giacomo C, et al. Celiac disease in children with autoimmune thyroid disease. J Pediatr 2001;139:738–40.
18. Holmes GK. Screening for coeliac disease in type 1 diabetes. Arch Dis Child 2002;87:495–8.
19. Hill ID, Dirks MH, Liptak GS, et al. Guideline for the diagnosis and treatment of celiac disease in children: Recommendations of the North American Society for Pediatric Gastroenterology, Hepatology and Nutrition. J Pediatr Gastroenterol Nutr 2005;40:1–19.
20. Bonamico M, Pasquino AM, Mariani P, et al. Prevalence and clinical picture of celiac disease in Turner syndrome. J Clin Endocrinol Metab 2002;87:5495–8.
21. Ivarsson SA, Carlsson A, Bredberg A, et al. Prevalence of coeliac disease in Turner syndrome. Acta Paediatr 1999;88:933–6.
22. Giannotti A, Tiberio G, Castro M, et al. Coeliac disease in Williams syndrome. J Med Genet 2001;38:767–8.
23. Jabri B, Kasarda DD, Green PH. Innate and adaptive immunity: The yin and yang of celiac disease. Immunol Rev 2005;206:219–31.
24. Kagnoff MF. Overview and pathogenesis of celiac disease. Gastroenterology 2005;128:S10–8.
25. Hourigan CS. The molecular basis of coeliac disease. Clin Exp Med 2006;6:53–9.
26. Schuppan D, Esslinger B, Dieterich W. Innate immunity and coeliac disease. Lancet 2003;362:3–4.
27. Greco L, Romino R, Coto I, et al. The first large population based twin study of coeliac disease. Gut 2002;50:624–8.
28. van Heel DA, Hunt K, Greco L, Wijmenga C Genetics in coeliac disease. Best Pract Res Clin Gastroenterol 2005;19:323–39.
29. Stepniak D, Koning F. Celiac disease–sandwiched between innate and adaptive immunity. Hum Immunol 2006;67:460–8.
30. Fasano A. Clinical presentation of celiac disease in the pediatric population. Gastroenterology 2005;128:S68–73.
31. Marsh MN. Gluten, major histocompatibility complex, and the small intestine. A molecular and immunobiologic approach to the spectrum of gluten sensitivity ('celiac sprue'). Gastroenterology 1992;102:330–54.
32. Bonamico M, Mariani P, Thanasi E, et al. Patchy villous atrophy of the duodenum in childhood celiac disease. J Pediatr Gastroenterol Nutr 2004;38:204–7.
33. Baudon JJ, Johanet C, Absalon YB, et al. Diagnosing celiac disease: A comparison of human tissue transglutaminase antibodies with antigliadin and antiendomysium antibodies. Arch Pediatr Adolesc Med 2004;158:584–8.
34. Tonutti E, Visentini D, Bizzaro N, et al. The role of antitissue transglutaminase assay for the diagnosis and monitoring of coeliac disease: A French-Italian multicentre study. J Clin Pathol 2003;56:389–93.
35. Barker CC, Mitton C, Jevon G, Mock T. Can tissue transglutaminase antibody titers replace small-bowel biopsy to diagnose celiac disease in select pediatric populations? Pediatrics 2005;115:1341–6.
36. Hansson T, Dahlbom I, Rogberg S, et al. Recombinant human tissue transglutaminase for diagnosis and follow-up of childhood coeliac disease. Pediatr Res 2002;51:700–5.
37. Bazzigaluppi E, Roggero P, Parma B, et al. Antibodies to recombinant human tissue-transglutaminase in coeliac disease: Diagnostic effectiveness and decline pattern after gluten-free diet. Dig Liver Dis 2006;38:98–102.
38. Kelly C. Diagnosis of celiac disease. In: Rose BD, editor. Waltham, MA: Up To Date, Inc; 2006.
39. Bonamico M, Scire G, Mariani P, et al. Short stature as the primary manifestation of monosymptomatic celiac disease. J Pediatr Gastroenterol Nutr 1992;14:12–6.
40. Rosenbach Y, Dinari G, Zahavi I, Nitzan M. Short stature as the major manifestation of celiac disease in older children. Clin Pediatr (Phila) 1986;25:13–6.
41. Knudtzon J, Fluge G, Aksnes L. Routine measurements of gluten antibodies in children of short stature. J Pediatr Gastroenterol Nutr 1991;12:190–4.
42. Groll A, Candy DC, Preece MA, et al. Short stature as the primary manifestation of coeliac disease. Lancet 1980;2:1097–9.
43. Cacciari E, Salardi S, Lazzari R, et al. Short stature and celiac disease: A relationship to consider even in patients with no gastrointestinal tract symptoms. J Pediatr 1983;103:708–11.
44. Bosio L, Barera G, Mistura L, et al. Growth acceleration and final height after treatment for delayed diagnosis of celiac disease. J Pediatr Gastroenterol Nutr 1990;11:324–9.
45. Gemme G, Vignolo M, Naselli A, Garzia P. Linear growth and skeletal maturation in subjects with treated celiac disease. J Pediatr Gastroenterol Nutr 1999;29:339–42.
46. Patwari AK, Kapur G, Satyanarayana L, et al. Catch-up growth in children with late-diagnosed coeliac disease. Br J Nutr 2005;94:437–42.
47. Giovenale D, Meazza C, Cardinale GM, et al. The prevalence of growth hormone deficiency and celiac disease in short children. Clin Med Res 2006;4:180–3.
48. Salardi S, Cacciari E, Volta U, et al. Growth and adult height in atypical coeliac patients, with or without growth hormone deficiency. J Pediatr Endocrinol Metab 2005;18:769–75.
49. Barera G, Mora S, Brambilla P, et al. Body composition in children with celiac disease and the effects of a gluten-free diet: A prospective case-control study. Am J Clin Nutr 2000;72:71–5.
50. Mazure RM, Vazquez H, Gonzalez D, et al. Early changes of body composition in asymptomatic celiac disease patients. Am J Gastroenterol 1996;91:726–30.
51. Bode S, Hassager C, Gudmand-Hoyer E, Christiansen C. Body composition and calcium metabolism in adult treated coeliac disease. Gut 1991;32:1342–5.
52. Carbone MC, Pitzalis G, Ferri M, et al. Body composition in coeliac disease adolescents on a gluten-free diet: A longitudinal study. Acta Diabetol 2003;40:S171–3.
53. Brar P, Egbuna I, Ramakrishnan S, et al. BMI in the celiac disease patients of United States—Abstract. XII International Celiac Disease Symposium; 2006. p. D-325.
54. Kavak US, Yuce A, Kocak N, et al. Bone mineral density in children with untreated and treated celiac disease. J Pediatr Gastroenterol Nutr 2003;37:434–6.
55. Bernstein CN, Leslie WD, Leboff MS. AGA technical review on osteoporosis in gastrointestinal diseases. Gastroenterology 2003;124:795–841.
56. Mora S, Barera G, Beccio S, et al. A prospective, longitudinal study of the long-term effect of treatment on bone density in children with celiac disease. J Pediatr 2001;139:516–21.
57. Scotta MS, Salvatore S, Salvatoni A, et al. Bone mineralization and body composition in young patients with celiac disease. Am J Gastroenterol 1997;92:1331–4.
58. Caraceni MP, Molteni N, Bardella MT, et al. Bone and mineral metabolism in adult celiac disease. Am J Gastroenterol 1988;83:274–7.
59. Molteni N, Caraceni MP, Bardella MT, et al. Bone mineral density in adult celiac patients and the effect of gluten-free diet from childhood. Am J Gastroenterol 1990;85:51–3.
60. McFarlane XA, Bhalla AK, Robertson DA. Effect of a gluten free diet on osteopenia in adults with newly diagnosed coeliac disease. Gut 1996;39:180–4.
61. Ciacci C, Maurelli L, Klain M, et al. Effects of dietary treatment on bone mineral density in adults with celiac disease: Factors predicting response. Am J Gastroenterol 1997;92:992–6.
62. Moreno ML, Vazquez H, Mazure R, et al. Stratification of bone fracture risk in patients with celiac disease. Clin Gastroenterol Hepatol 2004;2:127–34.
63. Thomason K, West J, Logan RF, et al. Fracture experience of patients with coeliac disease: A population based survey. Gut 2003;52:518–22.
64. Aine L, Maki M, Collin P, Keyrilainen O. Dental enamel defects in celiac disease. J Oral Pathol Med 1990;19:241–5.
65. Haapalahti M, Kulmala P, Karttunen TJ, et al. Nutritional status in adolescents and young adults with screen-detected celiac disease. J Pediatr Gastroenterol Nutr 2005;40:566–70.
66. Dickey W. Low serum vitamin B12 is common in coeliac disease and is not due to autoimmune gastritis. Eur J Gastroenterol Hepatol 2002;14:425–7.
67. Dahele A, Ghosh S. Vitamin B12 deficiency in untreated celiac disease. Am J Gastroenterol 2001;96:745–50.
68. Crofton RW, Aggett PJ, Gvozdanovic S, et al. Zinc metabolism in celiac disease. Am J Clin Nutr 1990;52:379–82.
69. Naveh Y, Lightman A, Zinder O. A prospective study of serum zinc concentration in children with celiac disease. J Pediatr 1983;102:734–6.
70. Bonamico M, Vania A, Monti S, et al. Iron deficiency in children with celiac disease. J Pediatr Gastroenterol Nutr 1987;6:702–6.
71. Kalayci AG, Kanber Y, Birinci A, et al. The prevalence of coeliac disease as detected by screening in children with iron deficiency anaemia. Acta Paediatr 2005;94:678–81.
72. Fisgin T, Yarali N, Duru F, et al. Hematologic manifestation of childhood celiac disease. Acta Haematol 2004;111:211–4.
73. Green PHR, Stavropoulos SN, Panagi SG, et al. Characteristics of adult celiac disease in the USA: Results of a national survey. Am J Gastroenterol 2001;96:126–31.
74. Farre C, Esteve M, Curcoy A, et al. Hypertransaminasemia in pediatric celiac disease patients and its prevalence as a diagnostic clue. Am J Gastroenterol 2002;97:3176–81.
75. Bardella MT, Fraquelli M, Quatrini M, et al. Prevalence of hypertransaminasemia in adult celiac patients and effect of gluten-free diet. Hepatology 1995;22:833–6.
76. Kaukinen K, Halme L, Collin P, et al. Celiac disease in patients with severe liver disease: Gluten-free diet may reverse hepatic failure. Gastroenterology 2002;122:881–8.
77. Rujner J. Age at menarche in girls with celiac disease. Ginekol Pol 1999;70:359–62.
78. Bona G, Marinello D, Oderda G. Mechanisms of abnormal puberty in coeliac disease. Horm Res 2002;57:63–5.
79. Sher KS, Mayberry JF. Female fertility, obstetric and gynaecological history in coeliac disease: A case control study. Acta Paediatr Suppl 1996;412:76–7.
80. Smecuol E, Maurino E, Vazquez H, et al. Gynaecological and obstetric disorders in coeliac disease: Frequent clinical onset during pregnancy or the puerperium. Eur J Gastroenterol Hepatol 1996;8:63–89.
81. Ludvigsson JF, Montgomery SM, Ekbom A. Celiac disease and risk of adverse fetal outcome: A population-based cohort study. Gastroenterology 2005;129:454–63.
82. Hadjivassiliou M, Grunewald RA, Kandler RH, et al. Neuropathy associated with gluten sensitivity. J Neurol Neurosurg Psychiatry 2006;77:1262–6.
83. Muller AF, Donnelly MT, Smith CM, et al. Neurological complications of celiac disease: A rare but continuing problem. Am J Gastroenterol 1996;91:1430–5.
84. Bushara KO. Neurologic presentation of celiac disease. Gastroenterology 2005;128:S92–7.
85. Gobbi G, Bouquet F, Greco L, et al. Coeliac disease, epilepsy, and cerebral calcifications. The Italian Working Group on Coeliac Disease and Epilepsy. Lancet 1992;340: 439–43.
86. Zelnik N, Pacht A, Obeid R, Lerner A. Range of neurologic disorders in patients with celiac disease. Pediatrics 2004;113:1672–6.
87. Pavone L, Fiumara A, Bottaro G, et al. Autism and celiac disease: Failure to validate the hypothesis that a link might exist. Biol Psychiatry 1997;42:72–5.
88. Corrao G, Corazza GR, Bagnardi V, et al. Mortality in patients with coeliac disease and their relatives: A cohort study. Lancet 2001;358:356–61.
89. Logan RF, Rifkind EA, Turner ID, Ferguson A. Mortality in celiac disease. Gastroenterology 1989;97:265–71.
90. Swinson CM, Slavin G, Coles EC, Booth CC. Coeliac disease and malignancy. Lancet 1983;1:111–5.
91. Askling J, Linet M, Gridley G, et al. Cancer incidence in a population-based cohort of individuals hospitalized with celiac disease or dermatitis herpetiformis. Gastroenterology 2002;123:1428–35.
92. Mearin ML, Catassi C, Brousse N, et al. European multi-centre study on coeliac disease and non-Hodgkin lymphoma. Eur J Gastroenterol Hepatol 2006;18:187–94.
93. Catassi C, Bearzi I, Holmes GK. Association of celiac disease and intestinal lymphomas and other cancers. Gastroenterology 2005;128:S79–86.
94. Cereda S, Cefalo G, Spreafico F, et al. Celiac disease and childhood cancer. J Pediatr Hematol Oncol 2006;28:346–9.
95. Schweizer JJ, Oren A, Mearin ML. Cancer in children with celiac disease: A survey of the European Society of Paediatric Gastroenterology, Hepatology and Nutrition. J Pediatr Gastroenterol Nutr 2001;33:97–100.
96. Holmes GK, Prior P, Lane MR, et al. Malignancy in coeliac disease—effect of a gluten free diet. Gut 1989;30:333–8.
97. Ventura A, Magazzu G, Greco L. Duration of exposure to gluten and risk for autoimmune disorders in patients with celiac disease. SIGEP Study Group for Autoimmune Disorders in Celiac Disease. Gastroenterology 1999;117:297–303.
98. Petaros P, Martelossi S, Tommasini A, et al. Prevalence of autoimmune disorders in relatives of patients with celiac disease. Dig Dis Sci 2002;47:1427–31.
99. Cataldo F, Marino V. Increased prevalence of autoimmune diseases in first-degree relatives of patients with celiac disease. J Pediatr Gastroenterol Nutr 2003;36:470–3.
100. Segatna Guidetti C, Solerio E, Scaglione N, et al. Duration of gluten exposure in adult coeliac disease does not correlate with the risk for autoimmune disorders. Gut 2001;49:502–5.
101. Viljamaa M, Kaukinen K, Huhtala H, et al. Coeliac disease, autoimmune diseases and gluten exposure. Scand J Gastroenterol 2005;40:437–43.
102. Case S. The gluten-free diet: How to provide effective education and resources. Gastroenterology 2005;128: S128–34.
103. Pietzak MM. Follow-up of patients with celiac disease: Achieving compliance with treatment. Gastroenterology 2005;128:S135–41.
104. Mayer M, Greco L, Troncone R, et al. Compliance of adolescents with coeliac disease with a gluten free diet. Gut 1991;32:881–5.
105. Bardella MT, Molteni N, Prampolini L, et al. Need for follow up in coeliac disease. Arch Dis Child 1994;70:211–3.
106. Hogberg L, Grodzinsky E, Stenhammar L. Better dietary compliance in patients with coeliac disease diagnosed in early childhood. Scand J Gastroenterol 2003;38:751–4.

107. Fabiani E, Catassi C, Villari A, et al. Dietary compliance in screening-detected coeliac disease adolescents. Acta Paediatr Suppl 1996;412:65–7.
108. Kupper C. Dietary guidelines and implementation for celiac disease. Gastroenterology 2005;128:S121–7.
109. Janatuinen EK, Kemppainen TA, Julkunen RJ, et al. No harm from five year ingestion of oats in coeliac disease. Gut 2002;50:332–5.
110. Janatuinen EK, Pikkarainen PH, Kemppainen TA, et al. A comparison of diets with and without oats in adults with celiac disease. N Engl J Med 1995;333:1033–7.
111. Bode S, Gudmand-Hoyer E. Incidence and clinical significance of lactose malabsorption in adult coeliac disease. Scand J Gastroenterol 1988;23:484–8.
112. Roggero P, Ceccatelli MP, Volpe C, et al. Extent of lactose absorption in children with active celiac disease. J Pediatr Gastroenterol Nutr 1989;9:290–4.
113. Kemppainen T, Uusitupa M, Janatuinen E, et al. Intakes of nutrients and nutritional status in coeliac patients. Scand J Gastroenterol 1995;30:575–9.
114. Hopman EG, le Cessie S, von Blomberg BM, Meari n ML Nutritional management of the gluten-free diet in young people with celiac disease in The Netherlands. J Pediatr Gastroenterol Nutr 2006;43:102–8.
115. Hallert C, Grant C, Grehn S, et al. Evidence of poor vitamin status in coeliac patients on a gluten-free diet for 10 years. Aliment Pharmacol Ther 2002;16:1333–9.
116. Hjelt K, Krasilnikoff PA. The impact of gluten on haematological status, dietary intakes of haemopoietic nutrients and vitamin B12 and folic acid absorption in children with coeliac disease. Acta Paediatr Scand 1990;79:911–9.
117. Mariani P, Viti MG, Montuori M, et al. The gluten-free diet: A nutritional risk factor for adolescents with celiac disease? J Pediatr Gastroenterol Nutr 1998;27:519–23.
118. Sollid LM, Khosla C. Future therapeutic options for celiac disease. Nat Clin Pract Gastroenterol Hepatol 2005;2:140–7.
119. Green PH, Rostami K, Marsh MN. Diagnosis of coeliac disease. Best Pract Res Clin Gastroenterol 2005;19:389–400.

Food Allergies

Hugh Sampson, MD
Jennifer Maloney, MD

DEFINITION

The term "allergy" is subject to a wide range of interpretations. Many conditions are labeled as allergic disorders; however, a clear immunologic basis for disease is not present. As a result, a clear definition is necessary before delving into the subject of food allergy.

Adverse reactions to food include food allergic and nonallergic reactions (see Figure 1). Immunologic interactions, through either IgE or non–IgE-mediated mechanisms, result in the development of food allergy. Nonallergic adverse food reactions include intolerances which result from host factors,[1] such as enzyme deficiencies, for example, lactase deficiency, which results in the bloating, abdominal pain, and occasionally diarrhea of lactose intolerance. Toxic food reactions represent a separate category, which result from inherent toxicities or properties of the food, for example, histamine-mediated symptoms due to scromboid fish poisoning.[1]

PREVALENCE

Food allergy affects approximately 6 to 8% of children under age 3 years, although the public's perception of food allergy prevalence is greater.[2] Investigators sought to determine the prevalence of food allergy in an unselected population of children and adults within families ($n = 1834$) and found that self-reported food allergy occurred in 16.6% of participants.[3] A pivotal prevalence study, which followed a cohort of 480 children from birth, determined the prevalence of food reactions in their population. Twenty-eight percent of the cohort displayed adverse symptoms, which either a physician or a family member attributed to food ingestion. Food challenges confirmed food reactions in 8% of the study cohort.[2] A more recent prevalence study of food allergy in adolescent patients revealed that two cohorts (11-year-old and 15-year-old children) reported adverse reaction to foods with frequencies of 11.6 and 12.4%, respectively. Prick skin testing to food allergens revealed sensitization rates of 5.1 and 4.9% for the 11- and 15-year-old cohorts. When supported by oral food challenges, the authors concluded that the prevalence of food hypersensitivity in both cohorts was 2.3%.[4] This result is similar to the estimated 3.5 to 4% prevalence of food allergy in the general population.[5]

Cow's milk allergy affects approximately 2.5 to 2.8% of infants in their first year of life.[2,6,7] IgE-mediated processes account for approximately 60% of cases. Hypersensitivity to egg affects approximately 1.3% of children[8] and peanut affects approximately 0.8% of children.[9] Interestingly, over a 5-year period, the rate of peanut allergy in the United States appears to have doubled in young children.[9,10] Similarly, a cohort of children from the Isle of Wight was compared with a previous cohort in terms of peanut clinical reactivity and sensitization, and a twofold increase in clinical reactivity and a threefold increase in peanut sensitization was reported.[11]

The persistence of symptomatic food allergy varies depending upon the food. The majority of children outgrow milk and egg hypersensitivities, 85% by age 8.6 years for milk and 66% by age 5 for egg.[12,13] Approximately, 20% of children become tolerant to peanut,[14,15] and it has been recently shown that at least 9% of young children outgrow tree nut allergy.[16]

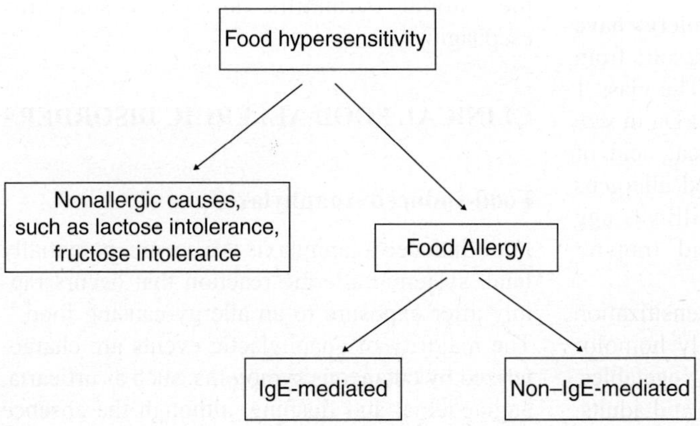

Figure 1 Classification of food hypersensitivities.

Pollen-food allergy syndrome (also known as oral allergy syndrome) is a common symptom complex, which usually provokes isolated oral symptoms following exposure to heat-labile proteins in uncooked fruits and vegetables. Pollen allergic individuals are at risk due to the homology between specific pollen proteins and proteins in certain foods. Of patients with allergic rhinitis, it has been estimated that 23 to 76% of patients experience oral symptoms to at least one food.[17] The cooked version of the foods is typically tolerated due to disruption of the protein conformation or tertiary structure.

Food allergy commonly presents in patients with or who will develop other atopic diseases. Approximately, one-third of children and adolescents with moderate–severe atopic dermatitis have IgE-mediated food allergy,[18] and some investigators have reported a correlation between the rise in the rate of food allergy with increasing severity of atopic dermatitis.[19] The presence of food allergy increases the probability of developing allergic airway disease[20,21] and has been shown to be an independent predictor of a persistent wheezing phenotype.[22] Despite the concomitant existence of food allergy and asthma, asthma is rarely an isolated finding in a food allergic reaction. Positive food challenges in food allergic, asthmatic patients are rarely characterized by only asthmatic symptoms.[23]

PATHOPHYSIOLOGY

Food allergy results from an atypical response of the mucosal immune system to orally consumed antigens. The gastrointestinal mucosa is an extensive structure responsible for digestion and absorption of nutrients as well as protection from pathogenic organisms. A nonspecific physical barrier works with immune and nonimmune cells and cytokines to maintain immunologic homeostasis.

The physical constituents of the gastrointestinal (GI) mucosa are composed of epithelial cells, the mucin glycoprotein lining, trefoil factors, proteolytic enzymes, and bile salts. The epithelial cells are attached by intercellular tight junctions. The mucin lining traps large particles due to its viscous nature and functions as a reservoir for secretory IgA, which entraps bacteria and viruses. Trefoil peptides maintain barrier function by restoring its integrity if defects occur. Proteolytic enzymes, bile salts, and exposures to wide ranges of pH gradients work to eliminate pathogenic organisms and modify the immunogenicity of proteins due to proteolysis and emulsification.[24]

Furthermore, the mucosal immune system provides an active line of defense through both the innate and adaptive arms. Peyer's patches (organized lymphoid structures of the small intestine and rectum), sIgA, dendritic cells, antigen-presenting macrophages, major histocompatibility complex (MHC) class I and II bearing T lymphocytes, intestinal epithelia cells, as well as other cytokine-producing cells allow for immunologic responsiveness.[25] Despite the complex interplay of the mucosal system, approximately 2% of intact food proteins are absorbed through the mature GI tract and reach the lymphatic and portal circulation.[26,27] The intestinal permeability is increased during infancy, and young children's vulnerability is further augmented by the nature of their immature mucosal barrier, which has decreased gastric acid production and reduced pancreatic and intestinal enzymatic activity.[28] Consequently, there is increased absorption of intact food proteins which may cause stimulation of the immune system and generation of IgE antibody.[28]

Oral tolerance allows individuals to encounter immense quantities of dietary protein and commensal bacteria without inciting a dynamic immune response. Antigenic factors and host factors are involved in the generation of oral tolerance (see Table 1). Antigenic factors, which influence oral tolerance, include the form and the dose of the antigen. Soluble antigens are more tolerogenic than particulate antigens.[29] Antigenic dose is also a key component to tolerance development. Experiments in mice have shown that oral tolerance can be induced by the administration of a single high dose of allergen or repeated low doses.[30] High-dose oral tolerance may occur through Fas-mediated apoptosis[31] or through the generation of anergy. Anergy occurs when T cells encounter antigens in the absence of co-stimulatory signaling.[32] Low-dose tolerance develops as a result of regulatory T-cell activation. The best categorized regulatory T cells are CD4+ cells (Th3 via TGF-β, TR1 via IL-10, CD4+CD25+ cells possibly via surface-bound TGF-β), CD8+ suppressor cells, and NK1.1+T cells.[25,33]

Table 1 Factors Influencing the Development of Oral Tolerance

Antigenic factors
- Form—Soluble antigens are more tolerogenic than particulate antigens
- Dose—Tolerance is induced by single high dose or repeated low doses

Host factors
- Age—Ability to generate oral tolerance increases with age
- Genetics—Genetic composition influences oral tolerance
- Gut flora—Contributes to the development of oral tolerance

Host factors involved in the generation of oral tolerance include age, genetics, and GI flora. The ability to become tolerant to food antigens appears to become more effective with age. Neonates develop a stronger immunologic response to dietary proteins in their first few months of life, as demonstrated by rapid increases in circulating antibodies when fed milk or soy formulas.[34] Host genetic composition influences the development of oral tolerance or food hypersensitivity, as demonstrated in murine models and human disease. Induction of oral tolerance in mice differs depending upon the strain of mouse.[35,36] In humans, a higher frequency of three HLA class II genotypes has been found in peanut allergic patients.[37] Additionally, monozygotic twins have been shown to have a high concordance rate of peanut allergy,[38] supporting the interplay of genetic influence on oral tolerance and food hypersensitivity.

Commensal gut flora takes residence in the GI tract within 24 hours after birth at a concentration that has been estimated to be between 10^{12} and 10^{14} bacteria per gram of colon tissue.[24] The impact of gut flora on oral tolerance is supported by the finding that mice raised in germ-free environments following birth are unable to develop tolerance to orally administered ovalbumin (OVA).[39] Furthermore, both mice with tall-like receptor 4 (TLR) 4 deficiency plus normal GI flora and mice with intact TLR 4 signaling but are raised in germ-free conditions are susceptible to the induction of allergy,[40] suggesting that cooperation between the innate immune system and the gut flora is essential for oral tolerance induction. The effects of administering probiotics (supplemental microbes) on the downregulation of allergic disease have generated great interest. Recent publications suggest that the ingestion of probiotics by lactating mothers and their infants may be beneficial in the prevention of atopic disease, specifically atopic dermatitis.[41,42]

FOOD ALLERGENS

Despite the wide range of foods that humans consume, surprisingly few foods account for the vast majority of food allergies. Milk, egg, peanut, wheat, and soy are responsible for most food-induced reactions in American children, while peanut, tree nuts, fish, and shellfish cause most reactions in adults.[1]

Two forms of IgE-mediated food allergy have been proposed. Class 1 food allergy results from sensitization through the GI tract.[43] The class 1 food allergens are generally 10 to 70 kDa in size and highly stable when subjected to heat, acid, or proteases.[28] Examples of class 1 food allergens include milk (caseins), peanut (vicillins), egg (ovomucoid), and nonspecific lipid transfer proteins.[44]

Class 2 food allergy results from sensitization to inhalant allergens that are partially homologous to proteins in certain fruits and vegetables, and principally occurs in adolescents and adults. Class 2 allergens are heat labile and susceptible to digestive processes.[43] Consequently, symptoms occur when the food is ingested in the raw form, but not when cooked. For example, Bet v 1, a major allergen of birch pollen, shares homology with class 2 allergens in various fruits and vegetables (eg, apple, Mal d 1; carrot, Dau c 1). A similarity in the three-dimensional structures (rather than the overall sequence identity) between birch pollen epitopes and the epitopes of specific foods has been demonstrated.[45] IgE antibody recognition of structurally related epitopes among pollens and foods likely results in the fruit–vegetable–pollen cross-reactive allergy syndromes (also known as oral allergy syndrome).

REACTION MECHANISMS

IgE-Mediated Reactions

Food allergic reactions involving IgE antibodies occur when IgE binds to and cross-links the high-affinity IgE receptor (FcεRI) on mast cells and basophils. Following mast cell and basophil activation, preformed and newly synthesized mediators are released. The mediators include histamine, leukotrienes, numerous cytokines, chemokines, and proteases.[46]

Perivascular mast cells are present in significant concentrations in areas that border the external environment, such as skin, and the respiratory and GI tracts. When activated, mediator release produces vasodilation, bronchoconstriction, and mucus production, which lead to the symptoms of an immediate hypersensitivity reaction. Six to 24 hours after the initial allergen encounter, a late-phase reaction may occur which is characterized by edema and an inflammatory cell influx.[46]

IgE-mediated reactions usually occur within minutes to 1 hour following ingestion of the causal food. Multiple organ systems may be involved including the skin, respiratory tract, GI tract, and cardiovascular system.

Non–IgE-Mediated Reactions

Several food hypersensitivity disorders exist that are not solely IgE mediated. Cell-mediated hypersensitivity reactions, orchestrated by antigen-sensitized T cells, may be responsible for the manifestations of certain conditions. A few diseases are thought to result from cooperation between cell-mediated and IgE-mediated mechanisms, for example, atopic dermatitis, allergic eosinophilic esophagitis.

CLINICAL FOOD ALLERGIC DISORDERS

Food-Induced Anaphylaxis

Food-induced anaphylaxis is a severe, potentially fatal, systemic allergic reaction that occurs rapidly after exposure to an allergy-causing food.[47] The majority of anaphylactic events are characterized by cutaneous symptoms, such as urticaria, angioedema, and flushing, although the absence of skin involvement does not exclude the diagnosis. For example, cardiovascular collapse with resultant shock may occur without cutaneous symptoms due to decreased blood supply to the skin.[48] In fact, in a report of six food-induced, fatal and seven near-fatal anaphylactic reactions, 38% ($n = 13$) of reactions were not accompanied by cutaneous symptoms.[49]

As with any IgE-mediated reaction, there may be a late-phase response associated with anaphylaxis. The incidence of such reactions is described to occur in up to 20% of food-induced events.[47] The only published series of anaphylactic episodes in a pediatric population reports the incidence of biphasic reactions to be 6%.[50] With biphasic reactions, a period of recovery after the initial reaction is followed by a recurrence of symptoms. Late-phase reactions are variable, may be severe, and severity cannot be predicted based on earlier symptoms.

Food-associated exercise-induced anaphylaxis usually occurs when exercise follows the ingestion of a specific food (such as wheat, shellfish, and celery) by approximately 2 to 4 hours. A less common form of food-associated exercise-induced anaphylaxis occurs with the ingestion of any food prior to exercise. The pathogenesis of food-dependent exercise-induced anaphylaxis is unclear.[51,52]

Cutaneous Food Hypersensitivity Reactions (Table 2)

Acute urticaria and angioedema are the most common manifestations of food-induced allergic reactions.[1] The onset of symptoms may occur minutes after ingestion. Urticaria also frequently develops as a result of direct skin contact with food allergens. Contact reactions are typically localized to areas of direct exposure and are unlikely to provoke systemic reactions, unless inadvertent ingestion occurs.[53] Chronic urticaria and angioedema are defined as the presence of symptoms for more than 6 weeks and are infrequently due to food allergy.[54]

Atopic dermatitis is a mixed IgE-mediated and cellular disorder. It is a chronic skin condition which often starts in childhood and is characterized by a relapsing and remitting course. Acute lesions are intensely pruritic and appear as erythematous macular and papulovesicular lesions. Scratching results in excoriation with crusting and exudation. The rash may progress to a subacute form with erythematous, scaling papules, and further advances with the chronic changes of skin thickening or lichenification.[55]

Table 2 Cutaneous Food Hypersensitivity Disorders

IgE mediated
- Urticaria and angioedema, skin erythema, morbilliform rash

Mixed IgE and cell mediated
- Atopic dermatitis

Cell mediated
- Contact dermatitis, dermatitis herpetiformis

The cutaneous lesions of atopic dermatitis usually occur on the face, scalp, and extensor surfaces in young infants. The distribution tends to shift as children get older, affecting the flexural surfaces of the extremities.[55] Atopic dermatitis skin lesions are characterized by a Th2 cytokine profile (acute lesions IL-4, IL-5, IL-13; chronic lesions IL-5, IL-13). These cytokines result in an inflammatory state with upregulation of adhesion molecules on vascular endothelial cells, upregulation of the high-affinity IgE receptor on Langerhan cells and other antigen-presenting cells, recruitment of inflammatory cells to the skin, and local production of IgE.

Approximately, one-third of children and adolescents with moderate–severe atopic dermatitis have IgE-mediated food hypersensitivity.[18] When patients with food allergy–related atopic dermatitis undergo food challenges, positive challenges are usually hallmarked by cutaneous symptoms such as pruritic, morbilliform, or macular eruptions with a tendency to occur in skin areas affected by atopic dermatitis. In addition to affecting the skin, the majority of positive food challenges trigger other organ system involvement (gastrointestinal or respiratory). Egg, milk, wheat, peanut, tree nuts, and soy are the most frequent foods to which patients are clinically reactive,[56] with egg affecting approximately two-thirds of patients with food allergy and atopic dermatitis.[57] If the history reveals food-related symptoms and tests for specific IgE to the food are positive, elimination is the best initial approach. However, caution is needed because although removal of a causal food may improve the skin disease, the patient develops an increased probability of an acute allergic reaction, even anaphylaxis, with reintroduction of the food.[58]

Dermatitis herpetiformis is a polymorphous, pruritic rash characterized by erythematous, urticarial plaques, papules, and vesicles. It develops as a result of gluten sensitivity, usually in association with gluten-sensitive enteropathy (celiac disease). Patients with dermatitis herpetiformis have serum IgA autoantibodies to epidermal transglutaminase.[59]

Contact dermatitis is a cell-mediated skin condition which may be provoked by food exposures. In a study investigating the causes of occupational skin diseases, food handlers were at risk for developing food-induced contact dermatitis.[60]

Respiratory Food Hypersensitivity Reactions (Table 3)

Food-induced respiratory symptoms usually occur in conjunction with other organ system reactions.[61] Respiratory symptoms consist of rhinoconjunctivitis, laryngeal edema, cough, and bronchospasm. Food-induced respiratory symptoms, specifically asthmatic reactions, are a risk factor for fatal and near-fatal anaphylactic events.[62] Not only is asthma a risk factor for more severe food allergic reactions, but also having a food allergy has been shown to be associated with life-threatening asthma. In a case-control study, it was demonstrated that children requiring intubation at the time of asthma exacerbation were 5.9 times more likely to have a food allergy compared with matched children who had milder asthma exacerbations.[63]

Table 3 Respiratory Food Hypersensitivity Disorders

IgE mediated
- Bronchospasm, cough, rhinitis, congestion, rhinorrhea, sneeze

Mixed IgE and cell mediated
- Asthma

Cell mediated
- Heiner's syndrome

Rhinitis and nasal symptoms are commonly seen in patients who have reactions during food challenges. Just as it is uncommon to have isolated food-induced asthmatic symptoms, it is very unusual to have nasal symptoms as the only manifestation of an acute allergic reaction.[64]

Allergic reactions can develop as a result of inhalation of airborne proteins. This modality of exposure is more significant when vapors or steams (from foods like fish or eggs) are being emitted during the cooking process.[65] Inhalation reactions secondary to peanuts, such as particulate matter from peanut dust when shells are opened, have also been reported.[66] In contrast, exposure of peanut allergic patients to the smell of peanut butter, a material that is unlikely to result in release of airborne allergens, has not been shown to result in systemic or respiratory symptoms.[53]

Food-induced pulmonary hemosiderosis (Heiner's syndrome) is a non–IgE-mediated hypersensitivity reaction primarily to milk, which results in the development of recurrent pneumonia, hemosiderosis, GI blood loss, iron-deficiency anemia, and failure to thrive. Removal of milk from the diet results in symptom resolution.[61]

GI Food Hypersensitivity Disorders (Table 4)

Food-induced reactions affecting the GI tract may be IgE mediated, cell mediated, or due to an interplay of IgE and cell mediated reactivity. Gastrointestinal anaphylaxis is an IgE-mediated reaction that includes symptoms of acute nausea, abdominal pain, colic, vomiting, and/or diarrhea. More indolent symptoms may occur in infants with atopic dermatitis and food allergy who are chronically ingesting the allergen. In these patients, intermittent vomiting and failure to thrive may be part of the symptom constellation.[28]

Pollen-food allergy syndrome (also known as oral allergy syndrome) is also an IgE-mediated reaction that occurs in pollen-allergic individuals due to homologous proteins shared between foods and specific airborne pollens.[67] Patients with birch allergy may develop symptoms with raw apple, carrot, potato, celery, pear, kiwi, stone

Table 4 Gastrointestinal Food Hypersensitivity Disorders

IgE mediated
- Nausea, abdominal pain, colic, vomiting, diarrhea
- Pollen food allergy syndrome–usually only oropharygeal symptoms

Mixed IgE and cell mediated
- Allergic eosinophilic esophagitis, eosinophilic gastroenteritis

Cell mediated
- Food protein-induced enterocolitis, proctocolitis, celiac disease

fruits, hazelnut, almond, and peanut; patients with ragweed allergy may be sensitive to various melons and banana; patients with grass allergy might become symptomatic with tomato, melons, and kiwi; and patients with mugwort allergy may develop symptoms with celery, carrots, and spices.[68] Symptoms of pollen-food allergy syndrome are usually confined to the oropharygeal cavity, and the foods are usually tolerated in the cooked form because the allergens do not retain their structure with high temperatures.

Eosinophilic esophagitis and gastroenteritis are disorders mediated by IgE-dependent and/or cell-mediated mechanisms. Eosinophils infiltrate the walls of the esophagus, stomach, and small intestine. Peripheral eosinophilia is found in approximately half of the patients.[69] When evaluating these patients, other known causes of eosinophilia must be excluded, such as drug reactions, parasitic infections, and malignancy.[70] Patients with GI eosinophilic disorders have a high incidence of concomitant atopy, with many having sensitizations to foods and environmental allergens.[71]

In a disease-free state, eosinophils are usually not present in the esophagus. Eosinophilic esophagitis may occur at any age from infancy through adolescence and into adulthood. Symptoms include abdominal pain, spitting-up or vomiting, food refusal, and gastroesophageal reflux symptoms in younger patients, and dysphagia and food impaction in adolescents and adults, with a poor response to antireflux medications in both age groups. This symptom complex in association with esophageal biopsies revealing greater than 24 eosinophils per high-powered field is diagnostic. Eosinophils may be located in the proximal and distal esophagus. Esophageal tissue may have thickened mucosa, papillary elongation, and basal zone hyperplasia. On gross appearance, the esophagus may have furrowing (vertical, linear creases), mucosal rings, strictures, ulcerations, and whitish papules.[69,70,72]

Allergic eosinophilic gastroenteritis may occur at any age. Most notably, patients frequently present with weight loss and failure to thrive. Additional symptoms include abdominal pain, emesis, nausea, and diarrhea.[69,71] Especially in young infants, presentation may consist of gastric outlet obstruction or symptoms resembling pyloric stenosis.[70] Diagnosis is made through biopsies, which reveal significant eosinophilic infiltration of the gastric and/or duodenal mucosa, with no other identifiable medical cause (ie, infection, inflammatory bowel disease, drug reaction).[73] A subgroup of patients develop anemia and hypoalbuminemia, likely secondary to fecal loss of blood and protein resulting in protein-losing enteropathy.[29]

Allergic proctocolitis is a non–IgE-mediated, eosinophilic disorder that typically presents in the first few weeks to months of life. Infants appear in good health; however, they have blood and mucus in the stool, which increases in frequency unless the causal allergen is removed from the diet.[74] Growth delay and poor weight gain are not usual presenting features. Case series reveal that patients with proctocolitis may have peripheral eosinophilia, elevated serum IgE, and a family history of atopic disease.[75–77]

Proctocolitis commonly occurs in breast-fed infants (as many as 60% of cases),[76,78,79] with milk and soy formulas being the causative foods in the majority of the remaining cases.[75,77,80] For infants who develop proctocolitis while breast-feeding, it is believed that cow's milk proteins consumed by the mother are the triggering agents in breast milk, and it has been demonstrated that β-lactoglobulin (one of the major allergens in milk) is detectable in the majority of breast milk samples following maternal cow's milk consumption.[81] Elimination of cow's milk from the mother's diet will usually bring about gradual resolution of symptoms[76,78,79]; however, if cessation of bleeding does not occur with maternal dietary manipulation, a casein hydrolysate formula or in rare instances, an amino acid–based formula[82] eliminates gross symptoms, typically within 48 to 72 hours. For formula-fed infants drinking cow's milk formula, a large percentage who have milk-induced proctocolitis will also become symptomatic to other foods if introduced in the first 6 months of life, for example, soy ingestion.[75,83] A casein hydrolysate or amino acid formula is the recommended treatment.

Food protein-induced enterocolitis syndrome (FPIES) is a non–IgE-mediated food allergy, which usually occurs in formula-fed infants, although it has been reported to a variety of foods (especially cereal grains) in older infants, and is characterized by irritability, excessive, vigorous vomiting, and diarrhea. Diarrhea may have occult blood and stool smears may reveal leukocytes and eosinophils. The stool may also be positive for reducing substances. Depending on the severity of symptoms, patients may develop dehydration with accompanying hypotension and lethargy. Metabolic derangements such as acidosis and hyponatremia can occur as does leukocytosis and a "left shift."[84–86] In severe cases, children may even present with methemoglobinemia.[87]

Symptoms may follow a more indolent course for children who are fed the causal food from birth or shortly thereafter. Failure to thrive and hypoalbuminemia in conjunction with chronic emesis and diarrhea may be presenting features. When the causal food is removed and later reintroduced, extreme vomiting within 2 to 3 hours and late-onset diarrhea occur.[88,89] Milk and soy are most frequently the causative foods in FPIES; however, solid foods (such as oat, barley, rice, chicken, and turkey) may be responsible.[88,89] Approximately 50% of patients reactive to milk also develop reactivity to soy,[85,88] necessitating treatment with a casein hydrolysate formula or, in rare instances, an amino acid–based formula.[90] FPIES due to a grain, for example, oat, increases the risk of reactivity to other grains, milk, soy, meats, and legumes, necessitating cautious food introduction, especially in the first 6 to 8 months of life.

Celiac disease is a chronic inflammatory disorder of the small intestine (see Chapter 50, Celiac Disease for more details). An interplay between genetic risk factors and dietary triggers are thought to result in the manifestations of this disease, which include intestinal villus atrophy, malabsorption, and chronic inflammation of the small intestinal mucosa. The major associated haplotypes are HLA-DQ2 and HLA-DQ8, with approximately 95% of patients having HLA-DQ2. Celiac disease is strongly associated with dermatitis herpetiformis, and patients with celiac disease are at increased risk for other autoimmune conditions, such as type 1A diabetes mellitus and autoimmune thyroiditis.[91]

As a result of the immunologic imbalance, patients with celiac disease react to peptide sequences of gluten proteins. Responsible gluten proteins are present in wheat, rye, and barley. Unlike IgE-mediated allergy to wheat, barley, or rye, the T-cell cytokine profile from patients with celiac disease has a Th1 bias. Removal of gluten from the diet leads to symptom resolution. Patients with untreated disease are at increased risk for T-cell non–Hodgkin's lymphoma.[91]

The diagnostic gold standard for celiac disease is the intestinal biopsy, which demonstrates a loss of villi, lymphocytic and plasma cell infiltration of the lamina propria and intraepithelial compartments, and crypt lengthening. Enzyme-linked immunosorbent assays for IgA anti-recombinant human tissue transglutaminase can be utilized as a screening tool. Antigliadin antibodies alone should not be used for screening due to high rates of false-positive results.[91] Importantly, testing for celiac disease, either by biopsy or through serologic studies, must be performed while the patient has a diet that includes gluten; otherwise, false-negative results may occur.

DIAGNOSIS

The diagnosis of food allergies (Table 5) requires a comprehensive history, specifically focusing on adverse reactions to particular foods, the time frame of such reactions, whether other contributing factors were present (ie, exercise), the extent of organ system involvement, and required treatment. Attention to accompanying atopic conditions in the patient and family history of allergy are important. Diet diaries may be helpful in recognizing patterns of reactivity, in identifying commonly consumed allergens, and in identifying foods that may have "hidden allergens" which have provoked the reaction.

Table 5 Methods of Diagnosing Food Allergy

History ± diet diary
Oral food challenge
IgE-mediated and mixed disease
• Prick skin testing
• Serum-specific IgE testing
Cell-mediated and mixed disease
• One patch testing

The history may be more helpful in situations when food ingestions are causally linked to a reaction, such as the development of urticaria and cough immediately after cashew consumption. For chronic disorders, such as atopic dermatitis, asthma, and GI disorders, the history has a poor predictive value. This point is highlighted by a study in which double-blind placebo-controlled food challenges (DBPCFCs) were conducted in 38 children with severe persistent asthma, where the asthma symptoms were attributed to food allergy. Only 20% of the food challenges (70 challenges conducted) resulted in symptoms. Furthermore, the challenges elicited symptoms predominantly affecting the GI tract despite the chronic respiratory complaints.[92]

Diagnostic Modalities for IgE-Mediated Disorders

Prick skin testing is a rapid screening method for IgE-mediated food hypersensitivity. A small amount of food allergen extract is placed on the skin and then subjected to a prick or puncture, which breaks the skin integrity. A negative control (saline) and a positive control (histamine) are also placed on the skin. Wheals which are 3 mm larger than the negative control are considered positive.

Unfortunately, the positive predictive value of a positive prick skin test is less than 50% when compared to results of DBPCFCs.[93] Therefore, the medical history becomes important because tests must be interpreted in light of the clinical situation. Positive skin tests may be helpful especially when a clear-cut history of food reactivity is present. Additionally, when hypersensitivity is suspected to milk, egg, or peanut, "diagnostic prick skin test (SPT) mean wheal diameters" have been defined (cow's milk ⩾8 mm, egg ⩾7, peanut ⩾8; for children ⩽2 years of age, cow's milk ⩾6 mm, egg ⩾5 mm, peanut ⩾4 mm).[94] However, test results are highly dependent on reagents used (which are not standardized), application technique, and interpretation by the physician. Negative skin tests essentially exclude IgE-mediated allergy.

Intradermal skin testing has no place in the diagnosis of food allergy. In addition to having poor specificity and positive predictive value, fatalities have been reported with the use of this diagnostic modality.[95]

Detection of food-specific IgE antibodies (ie, UniCAP System FEIA, Phadia, Inc.; Uppsala, Sweden) has been shown to be predictive in symptomatic IgE-mediated food allergy.[96,97] The Phadia UniCAP system contrasts with qualitative RAST assays because standardized allergens are used, the dose-response curve is calibrated against the World Health Organization IgE standard and the matrix binds more antigen, which provides a steep dose-response curve.[96] Diagnostic "decision points" have been generated for common food allergens, namely, milk, egg, peanut, and fish (see Figure 2). The decision points indicate reaction likelihood (a greater than 95% probability of reaction), but do not predict reaction severity.[96] As serum-specific IgE levels decrease to undetectable, the likelihood of reaction decreases. However, reactions may still occur for a subset of patients when serum-specific IgE levels are undetectable. One study notes that 32 of 120 patients (especially young infants), who reacted to milk,

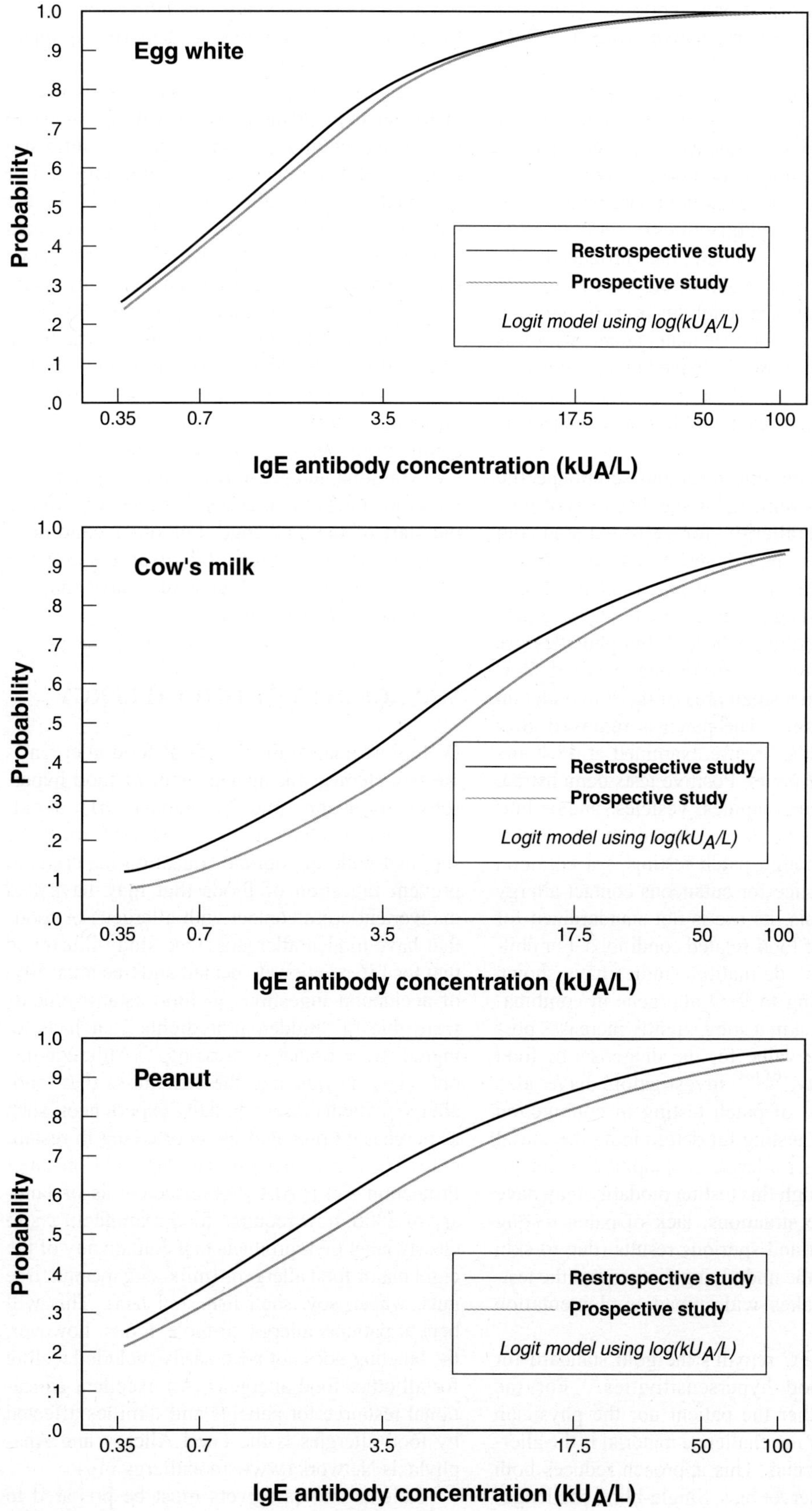

Figure 2 Diagnostic decision points for specific foods.

egg, or peanut challenges, had negative serum-specific IgE levels to the food.[98]

With newer technologies, it has been possible to map sequential allergenic epitopes of many major food allergens. So far it has been shown that detection of IgE antibodies against specific epitopes can be used as a marker for persistent allergy,[99] and some patients who produce IgE antibodies to sequential epitopes have more persistent allergy compared with patients who produce antibodies to conformational epitopes (epitopes dependent upon tertiary, native structure).[100,101] Recent enthusiasm has been generated by the microarray immunoassay, which allows for the determination of IgE binding to thousands of overlapping peptide sequences. This technique is an attractive epitope recognition assay because it has the potential for screening a large number of patients with minimal quantities of sera to a wide variety of antigens. To date, data produced with this methodology have shown that peanut-allergic patients with severe reaction histories recognize a greater number of epitopes than patients with less severe reaction histories.[102] In the future, microarray may become a useful clinic-based diagnostic modality for determination of transient versus persistent allergy.

Whereas prick skin tests and serum-specific IgE tests are instrumental in the diagnosis of IgE-mediated food allergy, for cell-mediated and mixed disorders, their diagnostic utility has little or no value. Patch testing is a modality being considered for diagnosing delayed-contact hypersensitivity reactions, where T lymphocytes are the major effector cell. For testing, the food allergen is placed on a small area of the skin under an occlusive dressing. The patch is removed after 48 hours, and the area is examined at 48 hours and again at 72 hours. Positive tests demonstrate erythema, edema, papules, vesicles, and/or bullae, and are graded 0 to 3 based on severity of reactivity. Although patch testing is a common diagnostic practice for cutaneous contact allergy due to chemicals, its use is not standardized for the diagnosis of food-related conditions. For children with atopic dermatitis, studies have shown that patch testing to food allergens in combination with prick skin testing slightly increases positive predictive value for the diagnosis of food hypersensitivity.[103,104] Investigators have also studied the use of patch testing in conjunction with prick skin testing for determining the causal foods that trigger allergic eosinophilic esophagitis.[105,106] Although this testing modality may have utility in some situations, lack of patch testing standardization and spurious results (due to skin irritation from the underlying disease and the testing media) makes widespread implementation complex.

The DBPCFC remains the gold standard for diagnosing food hypersensitivities.[93] For the DBPCFC, neither the patient nor the physician knows whether the challenge material is the allergen or the placebo. This approach reduces both patient and observer bias. Single-blind challenges and open challenges are other options best utilized for foods that are unlikely to produce a reaction. For single-blind challenges, the physician knows the content of the challenge material and the patient is blinded, and for open challenges, all participants know the challenge content. The decision to pursue a food challenge should be based on the clinical history in conjunction with prick skin test and serum-specific IgE results. Food challenges are not benign procedures. Positive challenges may produce mild, moderate, or severe symptoms, and often require treatment[107,108]; therefore, a properly equipped environment is essential.

Prior to food challenges, patients should be instructed to avoid medications that may interfere with interpretation of results, such as antihistamines and β-adrenergic bronchodilators. For IgE-mediated food allergies, the aim is for the patient to eat approximately 8 g of dry food mixed within a vehicle.[107] A negative-blinded challenge must be followed by an open challenge to assure that the patient can ingest the food safely in natural, meal-sized portions. For non–IgE-mediated FPIES, 0.3 to 0.6 g of protein per kilogram of body weight is given in one or two doses.[84] A reaction typically occurs 1 to 3 hours later, but when symptoms occur, they may be severe with excessive vomiting and possibly result in hypotension; therefore, intravenous access is necessary prior to the start of the challenge. For other conditions such as the eosinophilic GI disorders, several feedings of the food over a few days may be necessary to induce symptoms.[1]

MANAGEMENT OF FOOD ALLERGY

Dietary avoidance of the causal food allergen is the key element for management of food hypersensitivity at this time. To practice strict avoidance, patients and their caregivers must be supplied with appropriate education materials to prevent ingestion of foods that may have had inadvertent cross contact with allergens or foods that have hidden allergens. One study illustrated that for 156 reactions to peanut and tree nuts, 50% of accidental ingestions in food establishments were due to "hidden ingredients," such as an ingredient in a sauce or dressing.[109] Although just one study, it illustrates the difficulties that food-allergic patients face with daily experiences, such as purchasing prepared foods or eating in restaurants. The Food Allergen Labeling and Consumer Protection Act (FALCPA), effective as of January of 2006, now requires food manufacturers to clearly label their products that contain any of the eight major food allergens (milk, egg, peanut, tree nuts, wheat, soy, shell fish, and fish). This will benefit patients allergic to those foods; however, the labeling does not necessarily include labeling for all other food allergens. An excellent educational resource for patients and families affected by food allergies is the Food Allergy and Anaphylaxis Network (www.foodallergy.org).

Patients and caregivers must be prepared to respond in case of an accidental ingestion. Written anaphylaxis action plans should explicitly state the symptoms of anaphylaxis and when epinephrine should be administered (Table 6). Antihistamines are useful in treating mild symptoms, particularly cutaneous and oral symptoms, but will not reverse systemic reactions. Epinephrine is the treatment of choice for acute anaphylaxis (1:1000 dilution, 0.2 to 0.5 mL; 0.01 mg/kg in children with a maximum of 0.3 mg). Fatalities from anaphylactic events often appear to result from the late administration of epinephrine and subsequent irreversible cardiopulmonary complications.[48]

Table 6 Treatment Approach to Food Allergy

Food avoidance
- Anaphylaxis action plan
  - Epinephrine, antihistamines, six corticosteroids
- FPIES action plan
  - Intravenous fluids six corticosteroids
- Possible future therapies
  - Monoclonal anti-IgE
  - Recombinant protein immunotherapy
  - Sublingual immunotherapy
  - Traditional Chinese herbal medicine

The treatment of eosinophilic disorders requires allergen avoidance. Frequently, multiple foods must be eliminated from the diet. Corticosteroids result in clinical and histopathologic improvement[72,110]; however, the side effects which accompany prolonged corticosteroid therapy are unacceptable, and the disease typically returns with discontinuation of the medication. Many patients with eosinophilic GI disorders have evidence of sensitization to foods (by prick skin tests and/or serum-specific IgE assays); however, immediate reactions to foods are infrequently reported. Dietary elimination based on prick skin test and serum-specific IgE results alone is frequently insufficient to promote disease resolution of eosinophilic disorders. Multiple foods may be causative in the same patient, with the most common ones including milk, soy, egg, and wheat.[111] A common approach is to place the patient on an elemental (L-amino acid) formula and slowly add foods back into the diet when symptoms have resolved. Several weeks on an elemental formula is usually required for diminution of symptoms and for regression of the GI eosinophilic infiltrate.[112] Open challenges with the causative foods, following elimination, have been shown to frequently provoke symptoms indistinguishable to those experienced before the elimination diet.[111] Recently a six-food elimination diet has been proposed for the initial evaluation of food-induced symptoms; resolution of symptoms reportedly occurs in about two-thirds of patients.[113]

For proctocolitis, progression to a normal diet, including the eliminated allergen, is usually possible by 1 to 2 yeas of age.[69,78] If the prick skin tests and serum-specific IgE levels are negative, gradual introduction typically takes place at home. For FPIES, action plans must be in place in the event of accidental ingestions. First-line treatment is fluid resuscitation rather than epinephrine and antihistamines (although these medications should be administered if there is concomitant IgE-mediated disease). Corticosteroids should be considered, especially when past history reveals serious reactions. Corticosteroids likely suppress a presumed T-cell immune response. When food reintroduction is considered, challenges in a properly equipped environment are necessary, and challenges are not recommended until the patient has had at least 18 months with no reactions to the causal food. The high risk of developing FPIES to multiple foods, for example, milk and soy, multiple cereal grains, often necessitates multiple food challenges. Up to 50% of patients reactive to milk may react to soy; up to 65% of patients reactive to grains may react to milk or soy; up to 50% of patients reactive to one grain may react to another grain.[114] More than half of the patients with FPIES due to milk become tolerant by age 3 years. Resolution of FPIES varies by age and is influenced by the primary causative food and the presence of concomitant IgE-mediated disease.[114]

Much recent attention has focused on means of altering the immune system to either eliminate food allergy or increase tolerance to allergenic food. Allergen immunotherapy with peanut extract administered subcutaneously has been attempted to increase oral tolerance to peanut. Although increased tolerance was achieved in four of six patients studied, the adverse reactions from such treatment were not tolerable.[115] Sublingual immunotherapy with standardized hazelnut extract was compared to placebo in a group of hazelnut allergic individuals, and subjects receiving the active treatment developed increased tolerance to hazelnut while remaining on therapy.[116] The implementation of recombinant proteins with an altered IgE-binding epitope may be a form of immunotherapy that holds future promise. The altered IgE-binding epitopes prevent binding of the patient's IgE to the engineered protein within the vaccine. In a murine model of peanut anaphylaxis, recombinant proteins coadministered with heat-killed *Listeria monocytogenes* or *Escherichia coli* markedly decreased symptoms when mice were challenged to peanut.[117,118]

Allergen nonspecific forms of treatment include anti-IgE therapy and Traditional Chinese medicine. Humanized IgG1 monoclonal antibody against IgE (TNX-901) was tested in peanut-allergic subjects and was shown to enable subjects to tolerate increased quantities of peanut following therapy. Although, not a cure for food allergy, the medication offered protection in the event of inadvertent ingestion.[119] Recent enthusiasm has been generated by the potential value of Traditional Chinese medicine, which has been used in Asia for centuries, as an effective form of treatment for allergic disease. Experiments administering a Chinese herbal medicine formula have been able to block anaphylaxis in a murine model of peanut allergy.[120]

SUMMARY

Food allergy is a general term that includes a wide range of conditions. The pathogenesis involves IgE-mediated and/or cell-mediated processes with varying manifestations depending on the mechanisms of disease. Diagnosis requires a skillful history, physical examination, and targeted diagnostic testing. Treatment requires avoidance of the causal allergen(s). Hopefully, in the future, diagnostic modalities will be more fine tuned and additional treatment options will be available.

REFERENCES

1. Sampson HA. Update on food allergy. J Allergy Clin Immunol 2004;113:805,19; quiz 820.
2. Bock SA. Prospective appraisal of complaints of adverse reactions to foods in children during the first 3 years of life. Pediatrics 1987;79:683–8.
3. Osterballe M, Hansen TK, Mortz CG, et al. The prevalence of food hypersensitivity in an unselected population of children and adults. Pediatr Allergy Immunol 2005; 16:567–73.
4. Pereira B, Venter C, Grundy J, et al. Prevalence of sensitization to food allergens, reported adverse reaction to foods, food avoidance, and food hypersensitivity among teenagers. J Allergy Clin Immunol 2005;116:884–92.
5. Sicherer SH, Munoz-Furlong A, Sampson HA. Prevalence of seafood allergy in the United States determined by a random telephone survey. J Allergy Clin Immunol 2004;114:159–65.
6. Schrander JJ, van den Bogart JP, Forget PP, et al. Cow's milk protein intolerance in infants under 1 year of age: A prospective epidemiological study. Eur J Pediatr 1993;152:640–4.
7. Hide DW, Guyer BM. Cows milk intolerance in Isle of Wight infants. Br J Clin Pract 1983;37:285–7.
8. Nickel R, Kulig M, Forster J, et al. Sensitization to hen's egg at the age of twelve months is predictive for allergic sensitization to common indoor and outdoor allergens at the age of three years. J Allergy Clin Immunol 1997;99:613–7.
9. Sicherer SH, Munoz-Furlong A, Sampson HA. Prevalence of peanut and tree nut allergy in the United States determined by means of a random digit dial telephone survey: A 5-year follow-up study. J Allergy Clin Immunol 2003;112:1203–7.
10. Sicherer SH, Munoz-Furlong A, Burks AW, Sampson HA. Prevalence of peanut and tree nut allergy in the US determined by a random digit dial telephone survey. J Allergy Clin Immunol 1999;103:559–62.
11. Grundy J, Matthews S, Bateman B, et al. Rising prevalence of allergy to peanut in children: Data from 2 sequential cohorts. J Allergy Clin Immunol 2002;110:784–9.
12. Saarinen KM, Pelkonen AS, Makela MJ, Savilahti E. Clinical course and prognosis of cow's milk allergy are dependent on milk-specific IgE status. J Allergy Clin Immunol 2005;116:869–75.
13. Boyano-Martinez T, Garcia-Ara C, Diaz-Pena JM, Martin-Esteban M. Prediction of tolerance on the basis of quantification of egg white-specific IgE antibodies in children with egg allergy. J Allergy Clin Immunol 2002;110:304–9.
14. Hourihane JO, Roberts SA, Warner JO. Resolution of peanut allergy: Case-control study. BMJ 1998;316:1271–5.
15. Skolnick HS, Conover-Walker MK, Koerner CB, et al. The natural history of peanut allergy. J Allergy Clin Immunol 2001;107:367–74.
16. Fleischer DM, Conover-Walker MK, Matsui EC, Wood RA. The natural history of tree nut allergy. J Allergy Clin Immunol 2005;116:1087–93.
17. Sicherer SH. Clinical implications of cross-reactive food allergens. J Allergy Clin Immunol 2001;108:881–90.
18. Eigenmann PA, Sicherer SH, Borkowski TA, et al. Prevalence of IgE-mediated food allergy among children with atopic dermatitis. Pediatrics 1998;101:E8.
19. Guillet G, Guillet MH. Natural history of sensitizations in atopic dermatitis. A 3-year follow-up in 250 children: Food allergy and high risk of respiratory symptoms. Arch Dermatol 1992;128:187–92.
20. Tariq SM, Matthews SM, Hakim EA, Arshad SH. Egg allergy in infancy predicts respiratory allergic disease by 4 years of age. Pediatr Allergy Immunol 2000;11:162–7.
21. Zeiger RS, Heller S. The development and prediction of atopy in high-risk children: Follow-up at age seven years in a prospective randomized study of combined maternal and infant food allergen avoidance. J Allergy Clin Immunol 1995;95:1179–90.
22. Csonka P, Kaila M, Laippala P, et al. Wheezing in early life and asthma at school age: Predictors of symptom persistence. Pediatr Allergy Immunol 2000;11:225–9.
23. Novembre E, de Martino M, Vierucci A. Foods and respiratory allergy. J Allergy Clin Immunol 1988;81:1059–65.
24. Mayer L. Mucosal immunity. Pediatrics 2003;111:1595–600.
25. Chehade M, Mayer L. Oral tolerance and its relation to food hypersensitivities. J Allergy Clin Immunol 2005;115:3,12; quiz 13.
26. Husby S, Foged N, Host A, Svehag SE. Passage of dietary antigens into the blood of children with coeliac disease. Quantification and size distribution of absorbed antigens. Gut 1987;28:1062–72.
27. Warshaw AL, Walker WA, Isselbacher KJ. Protein uptake by the intestine: Evidence for absorption of intact macromolecules. Gastroenterology 1974;66:987–92.
28. Sampson HA. Food allergy. Part 1: Immunopathogenesis and clinical disorders. J Allergy Clin Immunol 1999;103:717–28.
29. Chehade M, Magid MS, Mofidi S, et al. Allergic eosinophilic gastroenteritis with protein-losing enteropathy: Intestinal pathology, clinical course, and long-term follow-up. J Pediatr Gastroenterol Nutr 2006;42:516–21.
30. Friedman A, Weiner HL. Induction of anergy or active suppression following oral tolerance is determined by antigen dosage. Proc Natl Acad Sci U S A 1994;91:6688–92.
31. Chen Y, Inobe J, Marks R, et al. Peripheral deletion of antigen-reactive T cells in oral tolerance. Nature 1995;376:177–80.
32. Appleman LJ, Boussiotis VA. T cell anergy and costimulation. Immunol Rev 2003;192:161–80.
33. Ko J, Mayer L. Oral tolerance: Lessons on treatment of food allergy. Eur J Gastroenterol Hepatol 2005;17:1299–303.
34. Eastham EJ, Lichauco T, Grady MI, Walker WA. Antigenicity of infant formulas: Role of immature intestine on protein permeability. J Pediatr 1978;93:561–4.
35. Lamont AG, Mowat AM, Browning MJ, Parrott DM. Genetic control of oral tolerance to ovalbumin in mice. Immunology 1988;63:737–9.
36. Morafo V, Srivastava K, Huang CK, et al. Genetic susceptibility to food allergy is linked to differential TH2-TH1 responses in C3H/HeJ and BALB/c mice. J Allergy Clin Immunol 2003;111:1122–8.
37. Howell WM, Turner SJ, Hourihane JO, et al. HLA class II DRB1, DQB1 and DPB1 genotypic associations with peanut allergy: Evidence from a family-based and case-control study. Clin Exp Allergy 1998;28:156–62.
38. Sicherer SH, Furlong TJ, Maes HH, et al. Genetics of peanut allergy: A twin study. J Allergy Clin Immunol 2000;106:53–6.
39. Sudo N, Sawamura S, Tanaka K, et al. The requirement of intestinal bacterial flora for the development of an IgE production system fully susceptible to oral tolerance induction. J Immunol 1997;159:1739–45.
40. Bashir ME, Louie S, Shi HN, Nagler-Anderson C. Toll-like receptor 4 signaling by intestinal microbes influences susceptibility to food allergy. J Immunol 2004;172:6978–87.
41. Kalliomaki M, Salminen S, Poussa T, et al. Probiotics and prevention of atopic disease: 4-year follow-up of a randomised placebo-controlled trial. Lancet 2003;361:1869–71.
42. Rautava S, Kalliomaki M, Isolauri E. Probiotics during pregnancy and breast-feeding might confer immunomodulatory protection against atopic disease in the infant. J Allergy Clin Immunol 2002;109:119–21.
43. Breiteneder H, Ebner C. Molecular and biochemical classification of plant-derived food allergens. J Allergy Clin Immunol 2000;106:27–36.
44. Sicherer SH, Sampson HA. Food allergy. J Allergy Clin Immunol 2006;117:S470–5.
45. Jenkins JA, Griffiths-Jones S, Shewry PR, et al. Structural relatedness of plant food allergens with specific reference to cross-reactive allergens: An in silico analysis. J Allergy Clin Immunol 2005;115:163–70.
46. Prussin C, Metcalfe DD. IgE, mast cells, basophils, and eosinophils. J Allergy Clin Immunol 2003;111:S486–94.
47. Sampson HA, Munoz-Furlong A, Campbell RL, et al. Second symposium on the definition and management of anaphylaxis: Summary report–Second National Institute of Allergy and Infectious Disease/Food Allergy and Anaphylaxis Network symposium. J Allergy Clin Immunol 2006;117:391–7.
48. Joint Task Force on Practice Parameters. American Academy of Allergy, Asthma and Immunology, American College of Allergy, Asthma and Immunology, Joint Council of Allergy, Asthma and Immunology. The diagnosis and management of anaphylaxis: An updated practice parameter. J Allergy Clin Immunol 2005;115:S483–523.
49. Sampson HA, Mendelson L, Rosen JP. Fatal and near-fatal anaphylactic reactions to food in children and adolescents. N Engl J Med 1992;327:380–4.

50. Lee JM, Greenes DS. Biphasic anaphylactic reactions in pediatrics. Pediatrics 2000;106:762–6.
51. Johansson SG, Hourihane JO, Bousquet J, et al. A revised nomenclature for allergy. An EAACI position statement from the EAACI nomenclature task force. Allergy 2001;56:813–24.
52. Sampson HA. Food anaphylaxis. Br Med Bull 2000; 56:925–35.
53. Simonte SJ, Ma S, Mofidi S, Sicherer SH. Relevance of casual contact with peanut butter in children with peanut allergy. J Allergy Clin Immunol 2003;112:180–2.
54. Greaves M. Chronic urticaria. J Allergy Clin Immunol 2000;105:664–72.
55. Blauvelt A, Hwang ST, Udey MC. Allergic and immunologic diseases of the skin. J Allergy Clin Immunol 2003;111: S560–70.
56. Burks W. Skin manifestations of food allergy. Pediatrics 2003;111:1617–24.
57. Sampson HA. Food sensitivity and the pathogenesis of atopic dermatitis. J R Soc Med 1997;90:2–8.
58. Flinterman AE, Knulst AC, Meijer Y, et al. Acute allergic reactions in children with AEDS after prolonged cow's milk elimination diets. Allergy 2006;61:370–4.
59. Karpati S. Dermatitis herpetiformis: Close to unravelling a disease. J Dermatol Sci 2004;34:83–90.
60. Judd L. A descriptive study of occupational skin disease. N Z Med J 1994;107:147–9.
61. James JM. Respiratory manifestations of food allergy. Pediatrics 2003;111:1625–30.
62. Bock SA, Munoz-Furlong A, Sampson HA. Fatalities due to anaphylactic reactions to foods. J Allergy Clin Immunol 2001107:191–3.
63. Roberts G, Patel N, Levi-Schaffer F, et al. Food allergy as a risk factor for life-threatening asthma in childhood: A case-controlled study. J Allergy Clin Immunol 2003;112:168–74.
64. James JM, Bernhisel-Broadbent J, Sampson HA. Respiratory reactions provoked by double-blind food challenges in children. Am J Respir Crit Care Med 1994;149:59–64.
65. Roberts G, Golder N, Lack G. Bronchial challenges with aerosolized food in asthmatic, food-allergic children. Allergy 2002;57:713–7.
66. Sicherer SH, Furlong TJ, DeSimone J, Sampson HA. Self-reported allergic reactions to peanut on commercial airliners. J Allergy Clin Immunol 1999;104:186–9.
67. Valenta R, Kraft D. Type 1 allergic reactions to plant-derived food: A consequence of primary sensitization to pollen allergens. J Allergy Clin Immunol 1996;97:893–5.
68. Nowak-Wegrzyn A, Sampson HA. Adverse reactions to foods. Med Clin North Am 2006;90:97–127.
69. Sampson HA, Anderson JA. Summary and recommendations: Classification of gastrointestinal manifestations due to immunologic reactions to foods in infants and young children. J Pediatr Gastroenterol Nutr 2000;30:S87–94.
70. Rothenberg ME. Eosinophilic gastrointestinal disorders (EGID). J Allergy Clin Immunol 2004;113:11,28; quiz 29.
71. Guajardo JR, Plotnick LM, Fende JM, et al. Eosinophil-associated gastrointestinal disorders: A world-wide-web based registry. J Pediatr 2002;141:576–81.
72. Markowitz JE, Liacouras CA. Ten years of eosinophilic oesophagitis: Small steps or giant leaps? Dig Liver Dis 2006;38:251–3.
73. Sampson HA, Sicherer SH, Birnbaum AH. AGA technical review on the evaluation of food allergy in gastrointestinal disorders. American Gastroenterological Association. Gastroenterology 2001;120:1026–40.
74. Lake AM. Food-induced eosinophilic proctocolitis. J Pediatr Gastroenterol Nutr 2000;30:S58–60.
75. Jenkins HR, Pincott JR, Soothill JF, et al. Food allergy: The major cause of infantile colitis. Arch Dis Child 198459:326–9.
76. Pumberger W, Pomberger G, Geissler W. Proctocolitis in breast fed infants: A contribution to differential diagnosis of haematochezia in early childhood. Postgrad Med J 2001;77:252–4.
77. Goldman H, Proujansky R. Allergic proctitis and gastroenteritis in children. Clinical and mucosal biopsy features in 53 cases. Am J Surg Pathol 1986;10:75–86.
78. Lake AM, Whitington PF, Hamilton SR. Dietary protein-induced colitis in breast-fed infants. J Pediatr 1982;101:906–10.
79. Machida HM, Catto Smith AG, Gall DG, et al. Allergic colitis in infancy: Clinical and pathologic aspects. J Pediatr Gastroenterol Nutr 1994;19:22–6.
80. Odze RD, Bines J, Leichtner AM, et al. Allergic proctocolitis in infants: A prospective clinicopathologic biopsy study. Hum Pathol 1993;24:668–74.
81. Kilshaw PJ, Cant AJ. The passage of maternal dietary proteins into human breast milk. Int Arch Allergy Appl Immunol 1984;75:8–15.
82. Vanderhoof JA, Murray ND, Kaufman SS, et al. Intolerance to protein hydrolysate infant formulas: An underrecognized cause of gastrointestinal symptoms in infants. J Pediatr 1997;131:741–4.
83. Odze RD, Wershil BK, Leichtner AM, Antonioli DA. Allergic colitis in infants. J Pediatr 1995;126:163–70.
84. Powell GK. Food protein-induced enterocolitis of infancy: Differential diagnosis and management. Compr Ther 1986;12:28–37.
85. Powell GK. Milk- and soy-induced enterocolitis of infancy. Clinical features and standardization of challenge. J Pediatr 1978;93:553–60.
86. Powell GK. Enterocolitis in low-birth-weight infants associated with milk and soy protein intolerance. J Pediatr 1976;88:840–4.
87. Murray KF, Christie DL. Dietary protein intolerance in infants with transient methemoglobinemia and diarrhea. J Pediatr 1993;122:90–2.
88. Sicherer SH, Eigenmann PA, Sampson HA. Clinical features of food protein-induced enterocolitis syndrome. J Pediatr 1998;133:214–9.
89. Nowak-Wegrzyn A, Sampson HA, Wood RA, Sicherer SH. Food protein-induced enterocolitis syndrome caused by solid food proteins. Pediatrics 2003;111:829–35.
90. Kelso JM, Sampson HA. Food protein-induced enterocolitis to casein hydrolysate formulas. J Allergy Clin Immunol 1993;92:909–10.
91. James SP. Immunologic, gastroenterologic, and hepatobiliary disorders. J Allergy Clin Immunol 2003;111:S645–58.
92. May CD. Objective clinical and laboratory studies of immediate hypersensitivity reactions to foods in asthmatic children. J Allergy Clin Immunol 1976;58:500–15.
93. Sampson HA. Food allergy. Part 2: Diagnosis and management. J Allergy Clin Immunol 1999;103:981–9.
94. Sporik R, Hill DJ, Hosking CS. Specificity of allergen skin testing in predicting positive open food challenges to milk, egg and peanut in children. Clin Exp Allergy 2000;30:1540–6.
95. Lockey RF. Adverse reactions associated with skin testing and immunotherapy. Allergy Proc 1995;16:293–6.
96. Sampson HA. Utility of food-specific IgE concentrations in predicting symptomatic food allergy. J Allergy Clin Immunol 2001;107:891–6.
97. Sampson HA, Ho DG. Relationship between food-specific IgE concentrations and the risk of positive food challenges in children and adolescents. J Allergy Clin Immunol 1997;100:444–51.
98. Perry TT, Matsui EC, Kay Conover-Walker M, Wood RA. The relationship of allergen-specific IgE levels and oral food challenge outcome. J Allergy Clin Immunol 2004;114:144–9.
99. Jarvinen KM, Beyer K, Vila L, et al. B-cell epitopes as a screening instrument for persistent cow's milk allergy. J Allergy Clin Immunol 2002;110:293–7.
100. Cooke SK, Sampson HA. Allergenic properties of ovomucoid in man. J Immunol 1997;159:2026–32.
101. Vila L, Beyer K, Jarvinen KM, et al. Role of conformational and linear epitopes in the achievement of tolerance in cow's milk allergy. Clin Exp Allergy 2001;31:1599–606.
102. Shreffler WG, Beyer K, Chu TH, et al. Microarray immunoassay: Association of clinical history, in vitro IgE function, and heterogeneity of allergenic peanut epitopes. J Allergy Clin Immunol 2004;113:776–82.
103. Roehr CC, Reibel S, Ziegert M, et al. Atopy patch tests, together with determination of specific IgE levels, reduce the need for oral food challenges in children with atopic dermatitis. J Allergy Clin Immunol 2001;107:548–53.
104. Isolauri E, Turjanmaa K. Combined skin prick and patch testing enhances identification of food allergy in infants with atopic dermatitis. J Allergy Clin Immunol 1996;97:9–15.
105. Spergel JM, Beausoleil JL, Mascarenhas M, Liacouras CA. The use of skin prick tests and patch tests to identify causative foods in eosinophilic esophagitis. J Allergy Clin Immunol 2002;109:363–8.
106. Spergel JM, Andrews T, Brown-Whitehorn TF, et al. Treatment of eosinophilic esophagitis with specific food elimination diet directed by a combination of skin prick and patch tests. Ann Allergy Asthma Immunol 2005;95:336–43.
107. Sicherer SH, Morrow EH, Sampson HA. Dose-response in double-blind, placebo-controlled oral food challenges in children with atopic dermatitis. J Allergy Clin Immunol 2000;105:582–6.
108. Perry TT, Matsui EC, Conover-Walker MK, Wood RA. Risk of oral food challenges. J Allergy Clin Immunol 2004;114:1164–8.
109. Furlong TJ, DeSimone J, Sicherer SH. Peanut and tree nut allergic reactions in restaurants and other food establishments. J Allergy Clin Immunol 2001;108:867–70.
110. Liacouras CA, Wenner WJ, Brown K, Ruchelli E. Primary eosinophilic esophagitis in children: Successful treatment with oral corticosteroids. J Pediatr Gastroenterol Nutr 1998;26:380–5.
111. Kelly KJ, Lazenby AJ, Rowe PC, et al. Eosinophilic esophagitis attributed to gastroesophageal reflux: Improvement with an amino acid-based formula. Gastroenterology 1995;109:1503–12.
112. Markowitz JE, Spergel JM, Ruchelli E, Liacouras CA. Elemental diet is an effective treatment for eosinophilic esophagitis in children and adolescents. Am J Gastroenterol 2003;98:777–82.
113. Kagalwalla AF, Sentongo TA, Ritz S, et al. Effect of six-food elimination diet on clinical and histologic outcomes in eosinophilic esophagitis. Clin Gastroenterol Hepatol 2006;4:1097–102.
114. Sicherer SH. Food protein-induced enterocolitis syndrome: Case presentations and management lessons. J Allergy Clin Immunol 2005;115:149–56.
115. Nelson HS, Lahr J, Rule R, et al. Treatment of anaphylactic sensitivity to peanuts by immunotherapy with injections of aqueous peanut extract. J Allergy Clin Immunol 1997;99:744–51.
116. Enrique E, Pineda F, Malek T, et al. Sublingual immunotherapy for hazelnut food allergy: A randomized, double-blind, placebo-controlled study with a standardized hazelnut extract. J Allergy Clin Immunol 2005;116:1073–9.
117. Li XM, Srivastava K, Huleatt JW, et al. Engineered recombinant peanut protein and heat-killed Listeria monocytogenes coadministration protects against peanut-induced anaphylaxis in a murine model. J Immunol 2003;170:3289–95.
118. Li XM, Srivastava K, Grishin A, et al. Persistent protective effect of heat-killed Escherichia coli producing "engineered," recombinant peanut proteins in a murine model of peanut allergy. J Allergy Clin Immunol 2003;112:159–67.
119. Leung DY, Sampson HA, Yunginger JW, et al. Effect of anti-IgE therapy in patients with peanut allergy. N Engl J Med 2003;348:986–93.
120. Srivastava KD, Kattan JD, Zou ZM, et al. The Chinese herbal medicine formula FAHF-2 completely blocks anaphylactic reactions in a murine model of peanut allergy. J Allergy Clin Immunol 2005;115:171–8.

Exocrine Pancreatic Disease Including Cystic Fibrosis

Kevin Gaskin, MD, FRACP
Jane Allen, PhD

Exocrine pancreatic diseases (EPDs) associated with maldigestion are characterized clinically by excessive losses of undigested fat and protein with resultant oily stools and severe hypoproteinemia with edema. Descriptions of "bacon fat, melted butter, or cheese" stools are commonplace, and stress the excessive fat and energy losses resulting in often severe undernutrition in patients with EPDs.[1] This chapter will highlight the variety of disorders associated with EPD in childhood and their consequences, investigation, and management from a nutritional perspective.

EXOCRINE PANCREATIC DISEASES IN CHILDHOOD

Subsequent to the original reports describing the pathology of cystic fibrosis (CF) of the pancreas,[2,3] a variety of inherited and acquired EPDs of childhood have been recognized, as per Table 1. CF is the commonest inherited disorder, occurring in 1 in 2,500 to 1 in 4,000 live births,[4] with Shwachman–Diamond syndrome (SDS)[5,6] estimated to be of the order of 1 in 10,000 to 1 in 100,000.[7] The other inherited disorders are rare with only isolated anecdotal reports.[8–11] Worldwide one would suspect that protein-energy malnutrition and tropical calcific pancreatitis are the commonest causes of EPD in children, but the exact proportions of such patients with pancreatic dysfunction or pancreatic insufficiency with malabsorption are essentially unknown.

Although the inherited disorders are uncommon, their discovery and the elucidation of their pathophysiology have helped considerably in our understanding of normal pancreatic physiology and the mechanism of normal fat and protein digestion in the small intestine. SDS patients, for instance, have severe pancreatic lipomatosis with acinar hypoplasia and markedly impaired pancreatic enzyme secretion.[12] Their pancreatic ductal function is, however, well preserved.[12] As such the SDS pancreas is a "ductal" model of pancreatic function and the fluid and electrolyte secretion data from SDS patients have been instrumental in helping to understand the pancreatic fluid and electrolyte secretion deficits in CF.[12,13] If one considers the inherited defects of lipase and colipase, it is not too surprising that pancreatic lipase deficiency is associated with severe steatorrhea.[14] However, what occurs if there is a deficiency of colipase? In vitro, pure pancreatic lipase is inhibited by supramicellar concentration of bile acids normally found in duodenal fluid.[15–18] The lipase cofactor, colipase, relieves this inhibition and thus in in vivo colipase deficiency one could predict is also associated with severe steatorrhea. The latter has been demonstrated both in cases with inherited colipase deficiency[19] and in some CF and SDS patients who have a relative colipase deficiency.[20]

Table 1 Exocrine Pancreatic Disorders in Childhood

Inherited
• Cystic fibrosis
• Shwachman–Diamond syndrome
• Pearson's pancreas/marrow syndrome
• Johanson–Blizzard syndrome
• Pancreatic agenesis
• Hereditary pancreatitis
• Isolated enzyme deficiencies
–Trypsinogen
–Lipase/colipase
–Enterokinase*
Acquired
• Malnutrition
• Tropical calcific pancreatitis
• Chronic pancreatitis

*Small intestinal brush border enzyme which initiates proteolytic cascade.

Further, in terms of protein digestion pancreatic proteases are secreted into the duodenum in an inactive zymogen form. Trypsinogen is cleaved by the small intestinal enzyme, enterokinase, to active trypsin which sets into motion the proteolytic cascade with trypsin cleaving further molecules of trypsinogen and other zymogens. Lack of enterokinase thus leads to significant maldigestion and malabsorption of protein and subsequent severe diarrhea and hypoproteinemia from birth.[21]

PANCREATIC PHENOTYPE

As alluded to in the introduction, most patients with inherited pancreatic disease on presentation have a history of oily bowel movements and have steatorrhea. However, only a few centers have quantitated fat malabsorption in their patients with formal 5-day fat balance studies (ie, assessment of oral fat intake from food records over 5 days and measurement of fecal fat output over the final 3 days).[1,20,22] Of importance, these clinics have consistently found that either CF or SDS patients who have normal fat absorption do not require oral enzyme replacement therapy (OERT).[6,22]

Currently patients with fat malabsorption (fecal fat >7% of oral fat intake on 5-day balance studies in older children or >10% in bottle-fed infants and >2 g/d in breast-fed infants <6 months of age[22]) are referred to as pancreatic insufficient (PI) and those with normal fat absorption as pancreatic sufficient (PS). This terminology is based on a study assessing pancreatic colipase/lipase secretion in patients with CF, SDS, and controls undergoing quantitative pancreatic stimulation tests and fecal fat measurements.[20] The results demonstrated in terms of colipase secretion that all patients with fat malabsorption had colipase secretion rates <1% of the average controls value. In contrast, those with normal fat absorption had colipase secretion rates >1% and up to within the normal range. Consequently, those PI patients had insufficient endogenous enzyme secretion to produce normal absorption and conversely those PS patients had sufficient enzyme output to produce normal absorption. This terminology will be used throughout the remainder of this chapter.

MOLECULAR BASIS/ PATHOPHYSIOLOGY OF EPDS

The molecular genetics for most of the inherited diseases, CF, SDS, Pearson's marrow-pancreas syndrome (PMPS), pancreatic agenesis, and inherited pancreatitis, have been found over the last decade. The following is a summary of these developments, with an account of the pathophysiology of the individual disorders.

CYSTIC FIBROSIS (CF)

The CF transmembrane conductance regulator (*CFTR*) gene was located on the long arm of chromosome 7 in 1989.[23,24] The gene product, the CFTR protein, was subsequently demonstrated to be a c-AMP-dependent chloride channel on the apical membrane of the epithelial cells.[25] There are now well over 1,200 *CFTR* mutations recognized, with most being rare, personal mutations. The most common, ΔF508, is found in patients of mid- and northern European origin, with 50 to 55% being ΔF508 homozygotes, 35 to 40% ΔF508 compound heterozygotes, and 5 to 10% non-ΔF508 compound heterozygotes.[26] In southern European and other Mediterranean populations ΔF508 is less common, occurring on 50% of CF chromosomes in White southern Europeans[27] and only 30% of chromosomes of Ashkenazi Jewish patients.[28]

Table 2 Classification of CFTR Mutations Reflecting Biosynthetic Defects and Function

Class I	• Defective protein production • Frameshift and nonsense mutations • Unstable messenger ribonucleic acid
Class II	• Defective *CFTR* processing (includes ΔF508 as most common mutation)
Class III	• Defective regulation of *CFTR* • Mutations can dramatically impair channel function, G551D
Class IV	• Defective channel conduction, eg R117H
Class V	• Abnormal splicing of *CFTR* • Reduction in normally functioning channels

Adapted from reference 29.

As per Table 2, *CFTR* mutations have been categorized into five classes according to defects in the biosynthesis and function of the mutated CFTR protein.[29] In Class I and II the mutated CFTR protein fails to localize in the cell membrane and in Class III, although locating in the cell membrane, channel function is very impaired. In Class IV and V the CFTR protein locates appropriately in the cell membrane. However, in Class IV conductance of Cl^- is reduced, and in Class V although Cl^- conductance is normal, the splice mutations result in a reduction of the amount of CFTR protein produced thus effectively reducing net Cl^- transport.

These groups of mutations have been correlated with disease severity particularly pancreatic phenotype. In any large CF population 80 to 90% of patients are PI with malabsorption and 10 to 20% PS with normal absorption.[30] Not surprisingly, Class I, II, and III mutations with very low to absent CFTR function are associated with the PI phenotype and Class IV and V mutations with residual channel function with the PS phenotype.[31] Patients with PI have two Class I to III mutations with few exceptions and PS patients at least one Class IV or V "mild" mutation, for example, R117H, noting that even if combined with a severe I to III mutation, the "mild" mutation is dominant and confers the PS status.[32,33]

From a pathology perspective the CF pancreatic disease appears to result from extensive duct obstruction. This occurs from early infancy and may account for the elevation of serum trypsinogen and other pancreatic enzymes at this age, noting that this phenomenon is the basis for newborn screening.[4] Duct obstruction is accompanied by destruction of acinar tissue and acinar atrophy, dense fibrosis and cyst formation, and eventually extensive fatty replacement of the pancreas.[34,35] The first clue as to the underlying pathophysiology of EPD came from the discovery that CF patients had impaired fluid and HCO_3^- secretion in comparison to non-CF controls.[36] Although a seminal finding, it remained uncertain as to whether this was a primary abnormality directly linked to the gene defect or related to the extensive fibrosis and fatty replacement reflecting pancreatic destruction. In subsequent studies[12,13] this issue was resolved in that as acinar function declined fluid and electrolyte secretion declined in both CF patients and non-CF controls (reflecting pancreatic tissue destruction). However, of importance at any level of acinar function CF patients had significantly lower electrolyte and fluid secretion, indicating that the deficit was not only related to pancreatic destruction but also related to the primary disease process; that is, the defect was present irrespective of the degree of pancreatic destruction.

Following the description of the *CFTR* gene and the recognition that it encoded for the cAMP-dependent chloride channels, in vitro studies of cultured pancreatic ductal cells have been undertaken to explain the secretion anomalies in CF. One model suggested that *CFTR* mutations impaired cAMP-stimulated acinar-ductal Cl^- secretion and luminal Cl^- concentration was low.[37] Low luminal Cl^- in turn did not drive the Cl^-/HCO_3^- exchanger, and thus ductal HCO_3^- secretion was also impaired. However, in normal duct cell models, secretin-driven HCO_3^- secretion occurs in the absence of luminal Cl^-[38] and possibly occurs by a conductive pathway. Moreover, others have shown that HCO_3^- accumulates in normal ductal cells via a basolateral cell membrane Na^+–$nHCO_3^-$ cotransporter which is dependent on the electrogenic gradient due to membrane depolarization caused by CFTR cAMP-dependent Cl^- secretion on the luminal apical cell membrane.[39] *CFTR* mutations interfere with Cl^- secretion, membrane depolarization, and thus HCO_3^- entry and secretion from the cell.

While the investigation of the mechanisms of impaired Cl^- and HCO_3^- ductal secretion continue, there is little debate regarding the inadequate alkalinization of pancreatic duct contents in CF patients. In a CF mouse model this defect in alkalinization has been shown to interfere with the normal endocytosis of zymogen granule membranes and the solubilization of zymogen granule–associated proteins including glycoprotein-2 (GP-2).[40] Consequent dilatation of the lumen and accumulation and aggregation of GP-2 is consistent with the known early pancreatic pathology in CF humans, that is, duct protein accumulation and obstruction.

NON-CF DISORDERS

The molecular genetics of SDS, PMPS, pancreatic agenesis, and hereditary pancreatitis have now been determined. In SDS, the Shwachman–Bodian–Diamond syndrome (*SBDS*) gene has been located at 7q11 as a 1.6 kb transcript with 5 exons and encodes a protein with 250 amino acids.[41–43] The function of *SBDS* is unknown but may be important in RNA metabolism. Three common recurring mutations resulting from conversion of exon 2 segments and leading to premature protein truncation were noted in the original 15 families. In the unrelated SDS patients, 60% carried conversion mutations in both alleles and 89% on one allele. Mitochondrial DNA base pair deletions have been demonstrated in PMPS[44] and in a case of pancreatic agenesis a single nucleotide deletion within codon 63 of the insulin promoter factor gene at 13q22.1.[45] Furthermore, mutations in the cationic trypsinogen gene at 7q35 have been associated with autosomal-dominant hereditary pancreatitis.[46]

SDS, PMPS, Johanson–Blizzard syndrome (JBS), and pancreatic agenesis can all be associated with PI in early life. SDS and JBS have severe lipomatosis of the pancreas and PMPS-extensive pancreatic fibrosis.

CLINICAL MANIFESTATIONS

The majority of the patients with inherited EPDs are PI and they are thus at risk from both macro- and micronutrient deficiencies. Of significance, most of these disorders are multisystem diseases and the nonpancreatic involvement may also contribute to the nutritional problems experienced. It is thus worth discussing the clinical manifestations of these disorders and the nutritional implications for the patients involved.

CF

The clinical manifestations of CF are summarized in Table 3. Pulmonary disease accounts for over 90% of the mortality and remains the major cause of morbidity and hospitalization.

Pulmonary Disease. CF lung disease results from thick tenacious secretions obstructing the bronchial tree, and with recurrent infections patients develop bronchiectasis, extensive lung fibrosis, cyst formation/emphysema, and, terminally, respiratory failure. The presentation and course of the pulmonary disease vary considerably, with some patients developing severe disease during childhood and others with relatively mild disease persisting into adulthood.[47] Many factors contribute to this variability, including early diagnosis and treatment, nutritional status, pseudomonas lung colonization, the emergence of antibiotic-resistant infections, the cross contamination of patients with infections, and the genetic variability of the disease. PS patients maintain an average near-normal lung function to age 30,[30] and have a median survival into the mid-50s, although this is not an invariable phenomenon. On the other hand, the majority of PI patients experience deterioration of lung function during their early adult years and median survival at best is to 40 years. The longer survival of PS patients is likely genetic in origin and although the more severe disease in the PI group is at least partly genetic, the large variation in lung disease and progression at any one age suggests that other gene modifiers or environmental effects contribute to this variation.[48]

The effect of lung disease on nutritional status is multifactorial. Recurrent infections, antibiotic

Table 3 Clinical Manifestations of Cystic Fibrosis

- Pulmonary disease
  - Recurrent infections
    - –*Staphylococcus*
    - –*Pseudomonas*
    - –*Burkholderia*
    - –Fungal
  - Bronchiectasis
  - Lung fibrosis
  - Pneumothorax
  - Emphysema
  - Respiratory failure
- Pancreatic disease
  - Pancreatic insufficiency
  - Pancreatic sufficiency ± pancreatitis
- Gut disease
  - Gastroesophageal reflux
  - Esophagitis
  - Giardiasis
  - Celiac disease
  - Neonatal meconium ileus
  - Distal intestinal obstruction syndrome
  - Intussusception
  - Appendicitis
  - Appendiceal mucocele ± abscess
  - Fibrosing colonopathy
  - Crohn's disease
  - Fecal retention, megacolon
  - Rectal prolapse
- Biliary tract/liver disease
  - Microgallbladder
  - Nonfunctioning gallbladder
  - Obstructed cystic duct
  - Cholelithiasis
  - Common bile duct stenosis
  - Common bile duct stones
  - Hepatosteatosis
  - Focal biliary fibrosis
  - Multilobular biliary cirrhosis
    - ± portal hypertension
    - ± liver failure
- Dermatological
  - Salt wasting
  - Hyponatremic dehydration

therapy, and severe pulmonary dysfunction are anorexigenic. Severe disease with recurrent coughing and the effect of physiotherapy can also exacerbate gastroesophageal reflux with esophagitis and further impair appetite. These interdependent effects are critical and may even reduce the energy intake below that recommended for normal subjects.[49] In addition, in lung disease and infections, inflammatory mediators and drugs, for example, β agonists, can substantially increase energy expenditure in excess of 20% above normal energy expenditure in some patients interfering with the maintenance of normal nutritional status.[50–52]

Gut and Liver Disease. CF patients experience a wide variety of gut and liver complications as summarized in Table 3. Gastroesophageal reflux disease (GERD) with esophagitis affects near 10% of the population.[53] Many patients accept reflux symptoms as part of the disease and admit to symptoms of waterbrash and heartburn only on direct questioning. Some will have anorexia and weight loss as the only presentation of their esophagitis. The presence of the typical symptoms or unexplained anorexia and weight loss should alert the physician to the possibility of GERD. For those with typical GERD symptoms, for example, heartburn and waterbrash, an empirical trial of a proton pump inhibitor (PPI) should be considered. Depending on the severity of lung disease those with anorexia should be considered for esophageal pH monitoring and endoscopy and esophageal biopsy prior to institution of PPI therapy.

Patients with distal intentinal obstruction syndrome (DIOS), gallstones, or biliary tract disease present with recurrent abdominal pain postprandially and they may limit food intake to alleviate their pain. DIOS should be apparent clinically with a mass palpable usually in the right iliac fossa. An abdominal ultrasound can confirm the diagnosis and also exclude the possibility of appendiceal masses. Simple DIOS without obstruction can be treated with laxatives. More resistant cases will need lavage therapy with the colonoscopy preparation solutions, for example, Golytely, to wash out the impacted fecal masses. Failure of this therapy should initiate further investigation, including contrast radiography and/or colonoscopy to exclude other diseases including fibrosing colonopathy (FC), Crohn's disease, and in the adult patient colonic/ileal malignancy. Patients with biliary tract disease and biliary colic will require an abdominal ultrasound to exclude cholelithiasis and biliary tract dilatation and hepatobiliary scintigraphy to screen for bile duct stenosis.[54,55] Persistent pain with associated weight loss and deterioration of liver function tests may necessitate further imaging with contrast cholangiography[54] or MRI cholangiography prior to possible surgical intervention.

Giardiasis and celiac disease (CD) can contribute to the nutritional problems of CF patients as both induce anorexia and exacerbate problems with diarrhea and malabsorption. In one study using a fecal antigen test, 30 of 107 (28%) of CF patients tested positive for giardia.[56] The positivity increased with age with 44% of those over 20 years testing positive for the antigen in contrast to the controls where 11% aged <5 years and none over 10 years were antigen positive. Giardiasis commonly causes a watery diarrhea in non-CF patients but it can be associated with steatorrhea and also severe protein malabsorption and hypoproteinemia. These data and the suggested increased susceptibility of CF patients to acquire giardiasis, as in the above study, indicate that those with diarrheal symptoms outside of their normal bowel movement pattern should be investigated further and treated appropriately with metronidazole.

CD is an alternative diagnosis for patients with anorexia, persistent steatorrhea, or deterioration of bowel movement pattern despite compliance to adequate enzyme therapy. It has been documented in CF adults with a prevalence of 1 in 1,258 in the US CF survey,[57] and it may be even higher in European communities where screening of non-CF populations suggest prevalence rates of >1 in 100.[58] As yet there are no studies confirming the reliability of antiendomysial or transglutaminase antibody testing in CF populations and small bowel biopsy remains the gold standard test for this disorder. Given the similarity of symptoms of CD with giardiasis, small bowel biopsy would be the ideal test to prove or exclude these complications in the absence of reliable noninvasive tests.

Since the early 1990s a new entity, FC, has been described in CF patients.[59] Pathologically, there are extensive areas of noninflammatory fibrosis affecting the lamina propria causing bowel wall thickening and long fusiform strictures in the ascending, transverse, and/or descending colon. Clinically, patients can present with intestinal obstruction, abdominal pain, anorexia, weight loss, diarrhea, and/or chylous ascites and may require surgical intervention to alleviate the obstruction.[60] Two case-control studies have attributed FC to the use of high-dose lipase pancreatic enzyme replacement therapy at a dose in excess of 20,000 U of lipase/kg/d or in excess of 6,000 U of lipase/kg/meal.[61,62] Current recommendations encourage patients to restrict their total daily dose to <10,000 U of lipase/kg of body weight.

Pancreatic Disease. As indicated previously, there are two pancreatic phenotypes in CF, PI and PS, based on the presence or absence of fat malabsorption, respectively. In older childhood/adult populations, 80 to 90% are PI and 10 to 20% are PS.[30] However, in newborn screened populations, in the first 2 months of life 60 to 70% are PI and 30 to 40% PS.[22] These data reflect the higher preservation of acinar function in early life, but later a deterioration of function so that approximately 50% of the PS patients become PI.[22,23] This deterioration mainly occurs in the first 5 years and almost invariably in those with two Class I, II, or III mutations. In contrast, those with persistent PS have at least one "mild" Class IV or V mutation, similar to older PS patients.[33,64] The latter group are at risk from recurrent pancreatitis in later life[65,66] and potentially they could become PI but this has been an infrequent occurrence to date.[33,66]

Untreated PI patients have an average fecal fat loss of 40% of fat intake, but it may exceed 50% and extend up to 80%.[1,67] There is a wide range of fat malabsorption (from >7 to 80%) in PI patients which is largely unaccounted for. Fecal fat increasing from 10 to 25% of fat intake may be attributed to the minimal decline in residual enzyme/cofactor secretion, that is, from <1 to <0.5% of average normal values.[20] However, the increase of fecal fat above the 25% level is enigmatic. The variable output of nonpancreatic pregastric lipases, duodenal bile salt concentrations,[68] or the interference of nonhydrolyzed phospholipids on triglyceride digestion may contribute to the varying fecal fat levels.[69] Irrespective of the cause, the nutritional consequences of these high losses are evident in patients from nonscreened populations at presentation and include wasting, stunting, hypoproteinemia, essential fatty acid deficiency, and associated fat-soluble vitamin deficiencies.

As alluded to above (pancreatic phenotype section) PS patients have sufficient endogenous enzyme secretion for normal absorption. It is imperative therefore to determine the pancreatic phenotype and thus the necessity or otherwise for OERT. The conventional gold standard test is a 3- to 5-day fat balance study with expression of fecal fat as a percentage of fat intake. It provides reliable and accurate data, as evident by comparison with pancreatic stimulation test data and follow-up data of individual patients in assessing response to OERT.[20] However, many laboratories and clinics refuse to undertake fat balance studies as handling fecal material is unaesthetic, undesirable, and potentially hazardous.

Consequently there has been a proliferation of tests, including serum measurements of pancreatic enzymes, for example, trypsinogen and the PABA (para-aminobenzoic acid) test, and ^{13}C triglyceride-labeled breath tests.[70] Others have used spot fecal samples for measurements of pancreatic enzymes, including chymotrypsin and fecal elastase (FE-1).[71–75] Sensitivity and specificity of ^{13}C-labeled breath tests for assessing PI and PS are high at over 90%, but are noninformative regarding the degree of steatorrhea in PI patients or the degree of residual pancreatic function in PS patients. FE-1 has been touted as a simple test with ease of collection and performance on spot fecal samples.[71] However, until recently the vast majority of the patients studied were PI-CF patients or normal subjects and little was known regarding other childhood pancreatic or intestinal disease.[72,73] Nevertheless in non-CF adults with chronic pancreatitis FE-1 was more sensitive and specific and had higher practicability and lower cost than the ^{13}C mixed triglyceride breath test for assessing pancreatic function.[70] One study evaluated FE-1 in PI and PS of CF and non-CF origin and in patients with intestinal diseases alone, in comparison with controls.[74] The test had a sensitivity of 98% and specificity of 93.6% to identify patients with steatorrhea due to PI with a positive predictive value of 89.9% and a negative predictive value of 99%. Sensitivity and specificity in CF patients in predicting PI were both 100%, but noteworthy among the PS non-CF group 30% had low FE-1 (<100 μg/g stool). This finding was similar to one of the large original adult studies in non-CF patients with chronic pancreatitis wherein a group classified as having moderate pancreatic disease (approximately less than 25% of normal enzyme secretion on pancreatic stimulation tests and with normal fat absorption) over 50% had a low FE-1 (<50 μg/g stool) and would have been misclassified as PI on the basis of the FE-1 alone.[75] The results in the CF population are encouraging but less so in the non-CF group with pancreatic disease. One should be aware that FE-1 has not provided information to date on the degree of residual function in PS patients and cannot be used as a specific guide as to the efficacy of enzyme therapy.

Current therapy for patients with proven PI consists of microspheric enzyme preparations. Prior to their development in the 1980s, OERT was given as either a porcine pancreatic powder or with the powder contained in a gelatine capsule. Administration of either of these preparations exposed the pancreatic enzymes to gastric acid pepsin inactivation and not surprisingly efficacy in most patients was poor, with average fecal fat decreasing from 40 to 25 to 30% of fat intake. The microspheric preparations were designed so that the enzyme extract is contained in microspheres which in turn are contained in a gelatine capsule. The latter readily undergoes acid dissolution in the stomach releasing the microspheres. The microspheres, however, remain intact in the stomach as they have an acid-resistant coating which dissolves and releases the enzyme only in the more alkaline environment of the duodenum and upper small intestine. There are now multiple microspheric preparations available and the reader is referred to the section on nutritional management for further information on the use of microspheric therapy.

Other Pancreatic Diseases

The above discussion of pancreatic dysfunction is also relevant to the non-CF pancreatic diseases. Specific features of these diseases are described in Table 4. In addition to maldigestion and malabsorption of nutrients, other factors including recurrent infections and antibiotic therapy in SDS, severe sideroblastic anemia and transfusion therapy in PMPS, diabetes in pancreatic agenesis, and developmental delay in PMPS and JBS may contribute to poor intake and exacerbate undernutrition in these patients. Long-term outcome in the non-CF disorders in the main is unknown given most are rare and have been recognized only in the last two to three decades. There is a known propensity for SDS patients to develop bone marrow malignancies, such as acute myeloid leukemia, and currently research activity is underway to determine factors or markers which may predict this occurrence, including myelodysplasia and the presence of monosomy 7 and isochromosome-7q.[6] An interesting feature of SDS is that while most are PI at diagnosis in the first year of life, up to 50% will become PS at a later age.[76] Reasons for this improvement in pancreatic function are unknown, but it will be important to determine if it is mutation related and whether such patients have less of a risk for developing bone marrow malignancy.

Table 4 Noncystic Fibrosis Pancreatic Diseases

Shwachman–Diamond syndrome (SDS)
- Pancreatic acinar cell hypoplasia with lipomatosis
- Bone marrow dysfunction
  - –Neutropenia
  - –Thrombocytopenia
  - –Red cell hypoplasia
  - –Myelodysplastic syndrome
  - –Acute myeloid leukemia
- Bone disease
  - –Metaphyseal dysplasia
  - –Shortened splayed ribs
  - –Short stature
- Miscellaneous
  - –Developmental delay
  - –Eczematous skin lesions
  - –Hepatosteatosis
  - –Renal tubular dysfunction

Pearson's marrow-pancreas syndrome (PMPS)
- Pancreatic fibrosis with pancreatic insufficiency
- Severe macrocytic anemia
- Vacuolated cells and ringed sideroblasts in bone marrow aspirates
- Developmental delay

Johanson–Blizzard syndrome (JBS)
- Pancreatic lipomatosis with PI
- Aplasia or hypoplasia of alae nasi
- Congenital deafness
- Hypothyroidism
- Short stature ± growth hormone deficiency
- Imperforate anus
- Absence of permanent teeth

Pancreatic agenesis
- Pancreatic insufficiency
- Diabetes mellitus

NUTRITION IN EPDS

The foregoing description of EPDs emphasizes they are multisystem disorders and as such not only the pancreatic disease but other organ involvement contribute to the nutritional status of the individual patient. To date, most of the clinical nutritional research has been directed at CF but there are large gaps in our knowledge about the nutritional outcomes of the non-CF disorders, mostly related to their rare occurrence. The remainder of this chapter is thus mostly concerned with the nutritional status of CF patients.

Background

The first reports on growth and nutritional status in CF demonstrated wasting and stunting,[77,78] and growth failure was considered inherent to the underlying disease. However, in a large cross-sectional study the Toronto clinic demonstrated, as per Table 5,[49] that over 40% of their patients had achieved the 50th percentile for height and only 10% were at or below the 3rd percentile.[79] Males had achieved similar percentiles for weight, but females appeared disadvantaged with 16% being below the 3rd percentile over age 8 years. These data contrasted with other clinics, including our own clinic at Sydney, where 13% of males and 21% of females were stunted (<3rd percentile for height) over age 8 years and 33 and 42% of males and females, respectively, were wasted.[49] The Toronto findings indicated that CF patients could achieve near-normal linear growth and suggested that growth failure was not related to the underlying disease process. Other investigators observed[80] that the growth advantage achieved in the Toronto clinic was directly related to dietary policy; that is, their patients had adhered to a high-quantity normal-quality diet with at least 40% of the energy intake as long-chain triglyceride[81] in contrast to the more universal policy of using a low-fat diet in order to control malabsorption. Energy intakes on low-fat diets averaged 80% of the recommended dietary intake (RDI) for energy, compared to the 113% achieved on the higher fat diet in Toronto.[49,81,82] Subsequently, others demonstrated improvement in growth

Table 5 Comparison of Height and Weight Data between RAHC (1984) and the Toronto Clinic in 1980, and RAHC Data from 1994*

	Gender	RAHC <8 yr	RAHC ≥8 yr	Toronto <8 yr	Toronto ≥8 yr
RAHC 1984 vs Toronto in 1980					
Height					
≤3rd percentile	Male	9	13	16	6
	Female	6	21	8.5	12.5
≥50th percentile	Male	29	41	48	37
	Female	25	29	40	40
Weight					
≤3rd percentile	Male	21	33	5	8
	Female	29	42	5	16
≥50th percentile	Male	20	22	40	41
	Female	15	18	34	26
RAHC Height and Weight Data in 1994					
Height					
≤3rd percentile	Male	0	13		
	Female	7	5		
≥50th percentile	Male	33	37		
	Female	43	41		
Weight					
≤3rd percentile	Male	0	9		
	Female	4	2		
≥50th percentile	Male	29	30		
	Female	32	36		

Adapted from reference 49.
*Presented as a percentage of male and female patients in each age group.
RAHC = Royal Alexandra Hospital for Children.

Table 6 Origin of Nutritional Problems in Cystic Fibrosis

Inadequate intake
- Inappropriate therapy
  - Low fat diets
- Anorexia
  - Lung infections
  - Lung disease
  - Malnutrition
  - Antibiotics
  - Esophagitis
  - Gut and biliary tract disease
  - Psychosocial factors
  - Salt depletion
  - Micronutrient deficiency, eg, zinc

Malabsorption
- Hypoproteinemia and edema
- Increased fecal bile acid losses and cholelithiasis
- Essential fatty acid deficiency
- Fat-soluble vitamin deficiency resulting from pancreatic insufficiency

Excessive energy expenditure
Related to:
- Underlying gene defect
- Female gender
- Lung disease
- Infections and inflammatory mediators

Bone disease
- Vitamin D deficiency due to pancreatic insufficiency and climate
- Osteoporosis
  - Dietary
  - Corticosteroid use
  - Cytokines

parameters over the short term with reversal of the low-fat diet policy.[83] We have also observed a marked improvement in both linear growth and weight, particularly in the female population as seen in Table 5 following an increase in dietary fat intake. These data provided further evidence supporting the concept that growth failure in CF was nutritionally related and could be reversed and improved with the consumption of a normal to high-fat-quantity diet.

Significantly, in 1980, the Toronto clinic also reported median survival of their population to the early 30s, and at least 10 years better than other Canadian and US clinics.[79] Although retrospective, these data suggested that the Toronto nutritional policy had contributed to the difference in survival. Subsequently, a direct comparison between the Toronto clinic with a "high"-fat diet policy and the Boston clinic with a "low"-fat diet policy demonstrated a near-10-year survival advantage to the Toronto patients, although average spirometric lung function parameters at 20 years were virtually identical.[84] Most clinics have now reversed their dietary policy to emulate the Toronto clinic and have not only shown improvement in growth but also shown an improvement in median survival to at least the late 30s. These findings emphasize that maintenance of normal nutritional status and growth contributes to longevity in CF and thus the importance of determining the basis of the nutritional complications to enable development of appropriate treatment strategies. In this regard, early diagnosis through neonatal screening has enabled early introduction of enzyme therapy and nutritional care with subsequent significant improvements in growth,[22,85,86] micronutrient status,[87,88] and cognitive function.[88] These improvements may well account for improved pulmonary function and survival as reported by others.[89,90]

Longitudinal growth studies for most non-CF diseases are not available, except for SDS. The latter appear to maintain a normal linear growth velocity, but usually at or below the 3rd percentile throughout childhood.[91] The linear growth percentile is similar in both PI- and PS-SDS patients and does not increase with the institution of OERT in PI patients. These data suggest that short stature in SDS is unrelated to the pancreatic disease but inherent to the disorder and probably related to the underlying bone dysplasia. Radiologically, the dysplasia is often mild and apparently resolves during puberty. This may account for the improvement in linear growth during puberty with some patients achieving final heights within the normal range.

Nutritional Problems in CF

The major nutritional problems in CF include linear growth failure and wasting, consequences of maldigestion and malabsorption, namely hypoproteinemia and fat-soluble vitamin, and essential fatty acid deficiency and bone disease. The origins of these problems are summarized in Table 6 and in general relate to nutrient balance; that is, the nutrient intake must be adequate for maintenance of normal function and growth and to compensate for excessive nutrient losses or excessive utilization.

Macronutrients. Macronutrient intakes have been documented in several studies of CF patients using recall methods, food frequency charts, and weighed diets.[49,80–83] Protein intakes are usually well in excess of RDI reaching in one study an average 200% RDI in a group of well-nourished patients on normal- to high-fat diets and 170% in a malnourished group on relatively low-fat diets.[49] Protein intake can, however, be compromised in patients with severe anorexia occurring with lung and liver disease and in those with imposed dietary restriction/fasting postabdominal surgery. In addition, prediagnosis breast-fed infants in regions without neonatal screening are at risk of hypoproteinemia due to the combined effects of the lower protein content of breast milk and pancreatic insufficiency. Energy intakes on the "higher" fat diet regimen recommended by the Toronto clinic averaged 113% of the recommended in one of the original studies. However, the low-fat diet regimens are clearly inadequate with energy intakes reaching only 80 to 90% of the normal RDI without even compensating for losses due to malabsorption or excessive expenditure. Not surprisingly, these patients develop malnutrition with wasting and in the longer term stunting.

Recovery from this downhill nutritional spiral is difficult as energy intakes may have to reach over 150% RDI to compensate for losses, excessive expenditure, and to ensure catch-up growth. In the presence of anorexia, which a high proportion experience, this task is virtually impossible. These individuals require assessment reanorexigenic components of their disease, as outlined in Table 6. Although the severity of lung disease is usually self-evident, it is worthwhile intensifying antibiotic therapy at regular even 3-monthly intervals to determine if appetite and growth improve over a 6- to 12-month interval.

During this time dietary counseling and support can also be intensified and other problems, particularly esophagitis or micronutrient deficiencies, excluded or treated. Many patients also have concurrent psychosocial problems, which will require investigation and management,[92,93] including behavioral therapy.[94]

Macronutrient Losses. Macronutrient losses associated with maldigestion and malabsorption are cardinal features of PI patients, with nitrogen malabsorption averaging 30% and varying up to 50% of nitrogen intake, and fat malabsorption averaging near 40% and varying up to 80% of fat intake on 5-day fat balance studies. It is thus imperative as indicated previously that PI is recognized and documented at diagnosis and OERT commenced in order to avoid the nutritional complications that would ensue without therapy. Optimal microspheric OERT in the large majority of patients will improve fat malabsorption to less than 20% of fat intake, with an average excretion of 10 to 15%.[95–97]

Historically in CF there was a vogue to use medium-chain triglyceride (MCT)-containing formulas for infants and as a dietary supplement in older children. This practice was based on data that demonstrated that fat absorption was much improved in infants who received MCT formula alone and avoided the need for OERT.[98,99] In both studies, however, fecal fat was measured by the Van de Kamer method which measures LCT but not MCT and thus the fecal fats were underestimated. Infants on MCT-based formulas still require OERT.[100]

Increased Energy Expenditure. Increased energy expenditure also contributes to the negative energy balance in patients with CF. Feigel and Shapiro first demonstrated a doubling of oxygen consumption in cultured fibroblasts from CF patients compared with controls,[101] a finding confirmed by others when studying CF nasal epithelium.[102] Several studies subsequently reported varying elevation of resting energy expenditure (REE) in CF subjects[50–52] and suggested that the elevation was directly related to the combination of malnutrition and lung disease. However, Shepherd and colleagues contended that the increase was intrinsic to the underlying disease, as total energy expenditure (TEE) in CF infants seemingly with minimal lung disease was increased when compared to controls.[103] Two later studies disputed these findings.[104,105] Fried and colleagues in a group of male CF adolescents/young adults with normal lung function were unable to demonstrate significant differences in REE between two groups (ΔF508 homozygotes and ΔF508 compound heterozygotes) with PI and another with PS, and average values were only minimally above (104%) World Health Organization (WHO) normal predicted values.[104] Furthermore, in a retrospective analysis they showed a curvilinear relationship between REE and FEV_1 so that as FEV_1 decreased below 75% predicted, REE increased exponentially.[104] These findings were also supported by a study of newly diagnosed CF infants where there was no difference in energy expenditure between controls and various genotypic groups of CF infants.[105] However, in the study of Fried and colleagues there were only nine patients in both the ΔF508 compound heterozygote PI and PS groups. Moreover, there was a near 20% reduction in REE in the PS group when REE was expressed per kilogram fat-free mass despite having lower average lung function than the PI group. The results of this study thus remain in question considering the inadequacy of the sample size and also because of the lack of an actual control group. When considering the second study of CF infants the standard deviation among the groups of CF infants varied from 30 to 70% of the average values compared to only 21% in the controls. Values for the PS infants were not provided and thus it was difficult to determine whether the CF results were unduly influenced by lower results in this PS group.

Other larger studies in terms of participants support the original in vitro studies and the Shepherd and colleagues' contention that the elevated EE is intrinsic to the disease. O'Rawe and colleagues demonstrated in three genotypic groups (ΔF508/ΔF508, ΔF508/other, and non-ΔF508/non-ΔF508) average REE of 121, 109, and 104%, respectively,[106] and regression analysis did not show a relationship with pulmonary dysfunction. However, average FEV_1 percent predicted was low in the ΔF508/ΔF508 group (56%) and the ΔF508/other group (63%), and thus these data did not exclude an effect of lung dysfunction on REE. In a more recent study[107] of 104 CF patients with near-normal lung function (average FEV_1 percent predicted 87 and 83% for males and females, respectively), and 131 age-matched controls, average REE predicted from controls was highly significantly elevated in CF females (111% of predicted), but less elevated in males (104% of predicted), confirming the preliminary findings in a smaller study from other investigators.[108] Importantly also, average REE in PI patients adjusted for fat-free mass was 110% of the PS value despite the similarity of pulmonary function, in the two pancreatic phenotype groups. If pancreatic phenotype is a surrogate marker of genotype, that is, PI patients have the more "severe" Class I to III mutations and PS the "milder" Class IV or V mutations, then one can conclude that the elevated REE in PI patients is intrinsic to the more severe genotype, particularly in the presence of minimal or no lung disease. The finding that REE is more elevated in the CF females remains enigmatic. In a further study of the effect of puberty and the menstrual cycle on females REE, neither appears to influence these already elevated values.[109] Clearly, further work is required to explore this relationship as it is already recognized that CF female patients are disadvantaged in terms of survival. Two of the above studies,[106,107] although suggesting that elevated REE is related to the intrinsic disease, could not exclude an effect of lung dysfunction or disease as shown retrospectively by Fried and colleagues[104] as the O'Rawe study had small numbers and our own study[109] did not include patients with significant lung disease. In addition, although we conducted our study on patients without apparent acute exacerbation of their lung infections, we could not exclude the effect of chronic Pseudomonas infection and inflammatory disease. Others, for instance, have demonstrated an average 4% decrease in REE during an uncontrolled study assessing the effect of intravenous antibiotics on EE, but no effect on TEE.[110]

Essential Fatty Acid Metabolism

EFA deficiency (EFAD) associated with malabsorption is well documented in PI patients. [111,112] Clinical deficiency manifests as seborrhoeic dermatitis, poor wound healing, thrombocytopenia, anemia, and an increased propensity for infections and may be present in PI infants prior to treatment of PI, but is far less evident in older PI patients receiving a normal diet and appropriate OERT.[113] Older PI patients, however, have subclinical/biochemical deficiencies of blood and tissue EFA levels, particularly showing decreases of linoleic acid and increased palmitoleic, oleic, and eicosatrienoic acids. Although some have suggested that EFAD is a primary abnormality and unrelated to malabsorption,[114] others have demonstrated that EFAD is evident only in patients with <5% of normal exocrine pancreatic function and the EFAD can be improved by optimizing OERT and dietary intake.[115]

There has been considerable recent interest in EFA metabolism in a CF-knockout mouse model,[40] without functional *CFTR*. These animals demonstrate an elevated arachidonic acid (AA)-to-docosahexanoic acid (DHA) ratio in tissues which normally express CFTR, for example, lungs, pancreas, and small intestine, compared with wild-type controls. Of interest, the early dilatation of pancreatic ductules in the CF mouse can be normalized with supplemental DHA and normalization of tissue AA-to-DHA. In CF humans the average AA-to-DHA in nasal epithelium and monocytes from PI patients is two to three times that observed in controls. The same phenomenon was observed in six PS patients, although four of these had values in the control range. Given the small numbers involved, these data are difficult to interpret and require clarification.[116] In addition, as the mouse model has no functional *CFTR,* one is left to assume that the effect of DHA on improving the pancreatic pathology is by upregulating non-CFTR chloride and fluid secretion, but this also needs confirmation. Until these studies are completed one would have to caution against routine DHA supplementation of human CF patients.

Micronutrients

Micronutrient deficiencies present in EPD include fat-soluble vitamin deficiencies, vitamin B_{12} deficiency, trace metal deficiencies, and salt depletion.

Fat-Soluble Vitamins. Fat-soluble vitamin deficiencies A, D, E, and K are well documented in CF PI patients.[117–126] Most descriptions of deficiencies have occurred in patients prior to diagnosis and commencement of OERT and in an era particularly when therapy was suboptimal, that is, prior to microspheric therapy. Clinical evidence of deficiency is unusual in patients on optimal diets and OERT but has been described in noncompliant patients and those with evidence of liver disease. Policies regarding vitamin supplementation vary, though it would appear unnecessary in PS patients and in PI patients who normalize their fat absorption on OERT and maintain normal serum vitamin levels and coagulation profiles. A recent report of elevated serum retinol concentrations in CF patients receiving a vitamin A intake similar to the NHANES study suggests that some CF patients may be at risk from long-term vitamin A toxicity,[127] and cautions against excessive use of vitamin A supplementation. Further work is required to determine the minimal A intake to maintain normal retinal function. Omitting fat-soluble vitamin supplementation in PS patients is also important as, in fact, declining serum levels in this group is a useful monitoring strategy of pancreatic function alerting the physician to the development of PI.

Vitamin A. Infants with vitamin A deficiency may present with a bulging fontanelle due to benign intracranial hypertension.[117] Older patients present with night blindness, and if the deficiency persists, xerophthalmia, corneal xerosis, and ulceration with Bitôt spots.[118] Although night blindness is usually associated with very low serum A levels (<0.5 μmol/L), subtle impairment of dark adaptation tests have occurred with serum levels between 0.2 to 1.4 μmol/L.

Vitamin D. Clinical rickets or osteomalacia are unusual phenomena in CF populations.[119] However, subclinical/biochemical rickets with low-serum 25-hydroxy-cholecalciferol levels does occur in patients from countries in the northern hemisphere with prolonged winters and little exposure to sunlight.[120,121] In contrast, in hotter countries with milder winters and year-round sunlight exposure low 25-hydroxyvitamin-D levels are unusual.

Vitamin E. Vitamin E deficiency has been described in CF patients,[122–124] but probably occurs more often in non-CF patients with either persistent cholestasis or in the rare disorders, abeta- or hypobetalipoproteinemia. Early signs include loss of deep tendon reflexes and impaired position and vibration sensations. Untreated prolonged deficiency may be associated with the development of ataxia, tremors, dysarthria, proximal muscle weakness, and external ophthalmoplegia. Of importance, these more severe symptoms may be less responsive to vitamin E repletion therapy and thus it is imperative to diagnose the deficiency and institute therapy prior to the onset of these symptoms. In regions without neonatal screening, infants with CF have presented with a vitamin E–deficient hemolytic anemia in the presence of severe malabsorption and hypoproteinemia.[128] In those diagnosed by neonatal screening at the time of diagnosis up to 40% will have low-serum α-tocopherol levels, and in some 10%, low levels may persist despite seemingly optimal oral replacement.[129] In older CF children and adolescents clinical symptomatology and low-serum vitamin E levels are unusual. Vitamin E deficiency has not been described in patients with persistent PS, but does occur in PS patients who develop PI. As such, regular monitoring of serum vitamin E levels should be undertaken in both PI and PS patients with supplementation to maintain levels >7 μg/mL would appear appropriate. If low-serum vitamin E levels occur in a PS patient, this could indicate that the patient has become PI and further investigation for malabsorption is mandatory.

Vitamin K. Vitamin K deficiency is associated with a coagulopathy and hemorrhagic manifestations. It has been described in CF infants prior to diagnosis and in patients with persistent cholestasis.[125,126] Monitoring and maintenance of normal coagulation profiles, particularly in patients with persistent steatorrhea, is appropriate.

Water-Soluble Vitamins. Water-soluble vitamins are well absorbed by CF patients. The exception is vitamin B_{12}. Normally, the vitamin B_{12} intrinsic factor complex is bound to R proteins and prior to binding to the specific terminal ileal receptors the R proteins need to be separated from the vitamin B_{12} intrinsic factor complex. This process requires pancreatic proteases and thus there is a theoretical possibility that untreated PI CF patients can develop B_{12} deficiency. This is unlikely to occur in patients receiving optimal OERT with the exception of patients who have undergone ileal resection.

Trace Metals. Trace metal deficiencies, of zinc and selenium, have been described in CF patients usually in association with protein-energy malnutrition. Clinical zinc deficiency with acrodermatitis has not been described, but mildly low serum zinc levels are common in hypoproteinemia. Clinical selenium deficiency associated with a cardiomyopathy in Cheshen's disease reported in non-CF populations is possibly related to a soil deficiency of selenium, a geographic phenomenon. The fact that it was not evident in a US CF study,[130] but present in a Scottish study[131] suggests that a geographic problem and patients from known selenium-deficient areas should be monitored and treated appropriately if deficient.

Salt Depletion. Salt depletion due to excessive sweat salt losses occurs in patients from or visiting warm to hot climates. Depending on activity and ambient temperature salt losses in older patients can exceed 10 g/d. The subsequent salt craving and an access to ingestion of salt usually prevent severe depletion. However younger patients, particularly infants without similar access to salt, are at risk from salt depletion. Symptoms are nonspecific and include lethargy, anorexia, nausea, and vomiting, but they may rapidly escalate and produce frank signs of dehydration, poor perfusion, and collapse. Classically, on measuring serum electrolytes patients are hyponatremic and hypochloremic, and have secondary hyperaldosteronism with hypokalemia and a metabolic alkalosis. Gut symptoms with nausea, vomiting, and abdominal distension may predominate as a result of hypokalemia and the ensuing gut dysmotility with paralytic ileus. Patients presenting in this manner may be misdiagnosed as having mechanical intestinal obstruction, and not receive appropriate salt replacement until circulatory collapse ensues. Intravenous salt replacement is usually required to treat these severely symptomatic patients. Those with evidence of poor perfusion and dehydration require intravenous therapy with a bolus dose of normal saline 10 to 20 mL/kg immediately and replacement therapy continued with normal saline depending on the patient's response. Potassium can be replaced following establishment of urine flow and monitored by measurement of serum electrolytes. Patients less severely compromised may respond to oral electrolyte solutions or simple oral salt replacement, but if nausea and vomiting prevail, intravenous replacement will be required.

Nutritional Assessment

Nutritional assessment is mandatory. At diagnosis, all patients require examination with height and weight, head circumference measurements, assessment of muscle and subcutaneous fat wasting, and examination for macro- and micro nutrient deficiencies including edema. Baseline biochemical parameters should include fat-soluble vitamin levels, coagulation profile, hemogram, serum albumin, and if available, serum essential fatty acid levels. Pancreatic status should be assessed preferably with a 3- to 5-day fat balance study, but if unavailable, one of the other tests as indicated previously. Beyond infancy a fecal fat in excess of 7% indicates PI and conversely $\leq 7\%$ PS and the necessity or not respectively for OERT. In infants <6 months of age a fecal fat $>10\%$ of fat intake or if breast-fed >2 g/d indicates PI and the necessity to start OERT.

In follow-up, accurate growth measurements are the simplest and most important clinical data to obtain to assess patient well-being from a nutritional point of view. Maintenance of previously obtained normal percentiles for both height and weight usually indicates the adequacy of nutrient assimilation. Although the US CF Foundation recommends using the percentage of ideal body weight (%IBW) for assessing malnutrition, a recent study[132] suggests that the body mass index percentile (BMIp) is more appropriate. BMI and %IBW are, for instance, very comparable when assessing children of average stature (height-for-age percentiles between 25th and 75th), but %IBW underestimates the severity of malnutrition in short patients (height for age <25th percentile) and overestimates malnutrition in tall patients (height for age >75th percentile). Patients should be questioned in regard to their appetite, the occurrence of heartburn, waterbrash, abdominal pain and constipation, and exacerbation of chest symptoms. Abdominal examination should be undertaken to look for hepatomegaly and splenomegaly and the presence of fecal masses in the right lower quadrant. Older patients can be asked about night blindness to assess for vitamin A deficiency. Deep tendon reflexes should be elicited to determine early onset vitamin E deficiency and the ribs and long bones examined for evidence of rickets. Biochemically, patients should have at least on an annual basis, a hemogram, coagulation profile, serum electrolytes, albumin, liver function tests, fat-soluble vitamin levels, and a blood glucose performed. A limited nutritional assessment of dietary intake by recall is used by our clinic at the annual review, but a more detailed weighed food record is required in those with anorexia and persistent weight loss.

More elaborate nutritional studies, including indirect calorimetry and body composition studies, are performed at some clinics, but usually in the context of a clinical research project. The possible exception is the routine measurement of bone mineral density (BMD) with DXA because of the reported high incidence of osteoporosis, osteopenia in older children, and adolescence with CF.[123]

Repeat assessments of pancreatic function are required in PS patients who have developed symptomatology suggestive of steatorrhea or in PI patients who are not responding to their OERT. The latter can be reliably tested only with formal fat balance studies and if fat malabsorption is in excess of 20% of fat intake on a standard OERT regimen, the patient may require adjunctive gastric acid suppression with histamine (H_2) receptor antagonists or PPIs.[133]

Nutritional Management

Nutritional guidelines for the management of EPD are outlined in Table 7. The aim of these nutritional guidelines is to ensure that PI patients achieve normal linear growth and weight gain. Diets for children in Western countries ensure a high-protein intake well in excess of the recommended. Energy requirements, however, will vary from patient to patient depending on physical activity, the degree of residual malabsorption in response to OERT, and the variable increase of energy expenditure.

Standard management of malabsorption focuses on OERT. Prior to microspheric OERT powdered extracts of porcine pancreas were used either directly or as a powder or in an encapsulated form. Fecal fat excretion as a percent of intake improved from an average near 40% off OERT to 25 to 30% on doses of up to 50 capsules daily with a lipase content of near 5,000 IU per capsule. A sizable proportion had minimal or no improvement in their fecal fat excretions. With the advent of microspheric therapy there was a significant improvement in fat malabsorption in most patients.[96,97] Most of the studies were performed in older children and adolescents over at least 25 kg in weight. A regime of using one capsule (5,000 IU) of lipase/kg of body weight/d to a maximum of 30 capsules/d improved fecal fat excretion to between 10 and 15% of fat intake with 80 to 90% of patients having fat excretions <20% of intake and up to 40% with near-normal excretion, that is, <10% of fat intake. Considering the higher fat intake of infants of up to 4 g/kg/d with declining rate to near 1 to 2 g/kg/d in adolescents and adults, we have used a regimen of a standard capsule containing 5,000 lipase IU/kg/d to a maximum of 30 capsules/d. On this regimen, growth has been near normal,[22] as also indicated in the 1994 data from our Clinic in Table 5. In a variable 10 to 15% of patients this regimen appears suboptimal with patients maintaining fat excretion in excess of 10% of intake. One early study of microspheric therapy indicated that however, the latter could be improved with the use of adjunctive gastric acid suppressant therapy.[96] The latter was proposed to elevate upper small intestinal pH ensuring dissolution of the acid-resistant enteric-coated microspheres. In general, most patients with ongoing malabsorption will improve their fat excretion with PPIs, but if not, they will need further investigation to exclude intestinal disease (celiac disease and giardiasis) and biliary tract complications. Inclusion of bicarbonate in microspheric OERT to provide a more optimal pH for enzyme activity has not improved fat excretion in this subgroup,[134] but preliminary results using acid-resistant lipases are encouraging although not impressive.[135]

To improve compliance to OERT, manufacturers produced higher dose lipase capsules in increments of 2,000 to 5,000 IU of lipase from a standard 5,000 IU capsule up to those containing 25,000 IU of lipase during the early 1990s. Many clinics permitted self-modulation of capsule dose which resulted in an incremental "dose-creeping effect" with many consuming in excess of 20,000 IU/kg/d, and in some up to at least 50,000 IU/kg/d. Less than 5 years after marketing of these high-dose preparations a new disease complication appeared, namely FC.[59] In two subsequent epidemiological studies FC was linked to the introduction of high-dose enzyme ingestion[61,62] and it is now recommended that enzyme dose be restricted to less than 10,000 IU of lipase/kg/d and preferably less than 5,000 IU/kg/d.[63]

Energy intake should also be modified depending on the variability of energy expenditure. CF patients, for instance, with chronic lung disease, or those experiencing acute exacerbations of their lung disease, can demonstrate REE in excess of 150% of predicted. Failure to meet these requirements leads to weight loss and if persistent to growth failure. Thus, while recommendations for average energy intake of 115 to 120% of RDI are not unreasonable in between exacerbations of pulmonary disease and residual malabsorption, a degree of flexibility is required in terms of dietary advice. Female PI patients, for instance, may require an extra 10 to 20% for excessive energy expenditure and a further 10 to 20% to compensate for malabsorption. If growth failure does occur in individual patients, a fat balance study should be undertaken to determine whether there is excessive malabsorption (>20% of fat intake) despite compliance to diet and optimal OERT (≈5,000 IU of lipase/kg/d). If there is, adjunctive gastric acid suppressant therapy should be trialled, but if no improvement occurs the malabsorption should be investigated further as above. In the absence of excessive malabsorption growth failure is either related to suboptimal intake and/or excessive energy utilization. Both the latter can be related to exacerbation of lung disease and deterioration of lung function and intensification of lung therapy including 3- to 6-monthly admission for intravenous antibiotics

Table 7 Nutrient Requirements in Pancreatic Insufficiency Including Cystic Fibrosis

Nutrient	Requirement	
Protein	>120% of RDI	
Energy	Variable, depending on disease status, patient should average near 120% RDI with 40% as LCT and 3 to 5% as EFA	
Vitamins		
A	5,000 IU/d*	1 to 3 yr of age
	10,000 IU/d*	>3 yr of age
D	400 to 800 IU/d†	
E	200 to 400 IU/d*	
K	5 mg twice weekly*	
Salt intake‡		
Age		
0 to 6 mo	0.5 g/d	
6 to 12 mo	1 g/d	
1 to 5 yr	2 g/d	
>5 yr	3 to 5 g/d	

*If serum levels and coagulation profile are normal, patients may not need supplement.
†Not required if exposed to sunlight throughout the year.
‡Double salt dose in hot weather or during strenuous exercise.
Can use vitamins A, D, E, and K (Scandipharm) or vitamins A, B, D, E, and K (Technipro): 4–10 yr, 1 cap daily; >10 yr, 2 caps daily; 0–1 yr, 1 mL daily; 1–3 yr, 2 mL daily; or Micelle A & E, 1–2 mL daily or Aquasol E (Rover Pharmaceutical, PA), 1 mL daily
EFA = essential fatty acid; LCT = long-chain triglyceride; PI = pancreatic insufficiency; RDI = recommended dietary intake.

and/or prolonged inhalational antibiotic therapy should be trialled. Failure to improve growth over 6 to 12 months usually indicates that the patients are failing to meet the excessive requirements to compensate for their losses and excessive utilization and intensive dietary therapy possibly with invasive nutrition will be required.

The recommendations for micronutrient supplements also have to be considered in regard to the presence and degree of malabsorption. PS patients usually maintain normal serum vitamin levels and coagulation profiles without supplementation. Similarly, a large proportion of PI patients on optimal OERT have normal fat absorption and do not demonstrate vitamin deficiencies based on serum vitamin levels. Vitamin supplementation is of questionable value in this group. We would recommend at least annual monitoring rather than encumber the patients with yet another medication. The recommendation for salt supplementation applies specifically to those children residing in warm to hot climates or those in more temperate climates who undertake strenuous exercise.

Special Circumstances

Infant Nutrition. From the foregoing, in the premicrospheric OERT era, enzyme therapy for infants was delivered in a powdered form, usually mixed with food, but many developed mouth ulcers. CF infants in this era also presented at diagnosis with hypoproteinemia and edema and steatorrhea, and thus semielemental hydrolyzed protein/amino acid and MCT-containing formulas were developed to aid protein and fat absorption without using OERT. However, as indicated above (Macronutrient Losses section) the premise regarding MCT not requiring digestion before absorption was incorrect and thus infants on semielemental diets still require OERT.

Until recently, breast-feeding had not been recommended for CF infants because of its lower protein content and the frequent occurrence of hypoproteinemia at presentation in PI patients in unscreened populations. In the early 1980s, several centers commenced neonatal screening for CF and as a result PI patients were diagnosed and commenced on OERT at an early age. A reevaluation of breast-feeding in this population demonstrated that breast-fed PI infants could maintain normal average growth to age 2 years. It was at least comparable to those given humanized cow's milk formulas,[136] and clearly better than those on predigested formulas who had suboptimal standardized weight scores.[137] Breast-feeding is thus entirely appropriate in the context of neonatal screening where there is early recognition and treatment of PI, but has yet to be evaluated in a nonscreened population where older PI infants may be severely malnourished and hypoproteinemic at diagnosis.

Invasive Nutrition. Most patients with CF adhering to a high-quantity energy intake with normal quality diets in terms of fat content achieve normal growth rates throughout childhood and adolescence.[79] Nevertheless, as per Table 5, a substantial proportion of patients are both underweight and stunted even in the modern era. An anecdotal study demonstrated that parenteral nutrition in this group of patients can improve weight gain and linear growth and with restoration to previous normal growth channels.[138] There was not only an improvement in growth but also an improvement in spirometric lung function and a decline in pulmonary infections. However, this and other studies were uncontrolled with small numbers and thus the beneficial effects on lung disease could not be determined.

Subsequently, three large studies over at least 12 months were conducted at three different centers.[139–141] They demonstrated improvement in growth and while one demonstrated a mild improvement in FEV_1 percent predicted in the treatment group, the other two suggested that the expected decline in lung function was prevented in the treatment group. However, the number of patients in each study was small, that is, 10 to 20 per treatment or control cell, and thus the effect of improving growth on pulmonary function in malnourished subjects remains contentious. Recommendations regarding the type of formula used (elemental, polymeric), the feeding technique (nasogastric, gastrostomy, jejunostomy), duration of use, etc, vary from clinic to clinic. We have used a nocturnal feeding regimen with a polymeric formula, Ensure Powder (Abbott), which on reconstitution has a fat content of 35.5 g/L. We have advised patients to use an enzyme dose providing approximately 1,000 lipase U/g of fat, so if receiving a liter of the formula, they would take 7 × 5,000 IU capsules, with half the dose given prior to sleep and the other half on awakening.

Nocturnal feeding regimens are demanding on the patients and their families and the psychological/emotional impact of this therapy is not well documented. Some cope extraordinarily well, but for others the burden of the therapy is overwhelming and unsuccessful. Given that improvement of lung function with these regimens is questionable and without information on whether they improve survival one has to be cautious about recommending this type of therapy. Families need to have education and thorough discussions regarding the commitments needed to ensure success of the therapy and a psychological evaluation to assess their ability to cope with this extra treatment burden. It may well be that this type of therapy in the future will be restricted to compliant patients and potential lung or liver transplant recipients. As indicated recently, the education process could be enhanced by discussions with patients with successful gastrostomies and the development of a video to emphasize the positive benefits of such therapy.[142]

In view of the difficulties frequently encountered with "invasive" nutrition regimens there has been considerable interest generated by three studies on the use of megestrol acetate as an appetite stimulant in CF patients.[143–147] The drug acts directly via the hypothalamus to stimulate appetite and has been used in other anorexigenic/cachetic illness.[147] The most recent study,[145] a double-blind placebo-controlled study, demonstrated a substantial improvement in average weight gain in the treatment versus control group (5.3 kg vs 1.5 kg, respectively) over 6 months. This is an encouraging result, but the study numbers were small (10 vs 7, respectively), and there is still some uncertainty about long-term adverse events, including adrenal suppression and the occurrence of diabetes mellitus, although they did not occur in this study. BMD was also said to be stable over the 6 months, but only seven patients had dual-energy X-ray absorptiometry (DXA) evaluation of their BMD. While one can be cautiously optimistic about these reports, clearly further long-term studies are required to evaluate the potential for adverse events and to determine which patients are likely to benefit from such therapy. One would hope that it could be avoided in the 90 to 95% of patients who in general maintain normal growth, but it may well have application in the 5 to 10% of patients who do not respond to routine regimens.

CF-Related Bone Disease

A variable 40 to 70% of CF adult patients have osteopenia and/or osteoporosis and in those with severe lung disease virtually all have decreased BMD.[148,149] This is particularly important in those awaiting lung transplantation[150] where an estimate of a 100-fold increased risk of vertebral fractures and a 10-fold increased risk of rib fractures has been documented in this group.[151] Significantly, loss of BMD occurs in early adolescence with often failure to reach peak bone density.

The problem is multifactorial with contributing factors including inflammatory mediators/cytokines released during pulmonary exacerbations, malnutrition, vitamin D and K deficiencies, decreased gonadal sterol levels, corticosteroid use, and decreased weight-bearing exercise.[148] Others have found an increase in osteoclast precursors and stimulation of osteoclast activity leading to bone loss during respiratory exacerbations.[152] Interestingly, there is a reduction in bone formation and increased bone resorption in the *CFTR*-null mouse.[153] Current recommendations for screening include a baseline BMD in all 18-year-old patients.[154] The Consensus Committee also recommended a BMD at age 8 if the following risk factors were present:

1. Ideal body weight <90%
2. FEV1 percent predicted <50%
3. On corticosteroids ≥5 mg for >90 d/yr
4. Delayed puberty
5. History of fracture.

The standard lumbar spine and hip DXA should be performed. Patients with t- or z-scores of −1.0 or better should have monitoring with repeat DXA scans not more than 5-yearly; those with BMD −1.0 to −2.0, 2- to 4-yearly; and those below −2.0, annually. Current recommendations

Table 8 Prevention and Treatment of Bone Disease in Cystic Fibrosis*

Prevention
Maintain normal serum 25-OH vitamin D levels >30 to 40 ng/mL
Vitamin K supplements 0.3 to 0.5 mg/d
Daily calcium intake up to 1,500 mg/d
BMI >25th percentile
Outdoor weight-bearing exercise
Intensive treatment of lung exacerbations
Decrease use of corticosteroids
Treat diabetes
Endocrine referral for treatment of delayed puberty with sex hormones
For t-/z-scores −1.0 to −2.0
–Oral bisphosphonates to be considered
For t-/z-scores below −2.0
–Oral bisphosphonates, but if not tolerated, IV bisphosphonates
If not responding, consider teriparatide

*Adapted from references 148 and 154.

for prevention and treatment of bone disease are outlined in Table 8.

CONCLUSION

Many of the EPDs, including CF, are multisystem disorders and require a team approach for delivery of optimal care. Personnel with nutritional expertise are required for monitoring the patient's nutritional status and growth, and for educating the patients and their families regarding dietary intake and OERT. Patients consuming high-energy intakes by avoiding low-fat diets can achieve normal growth and with appropriate vitamin intake can avoid most micronutrient deficiencies. In addition, it is essential to monitor growth and micronutritional status, and to ensure appropriate but not excessive OERT ingestion to avoid iatrogenic disease such as FC. Some patients, despite optimal advice and care, experience growth and nutritional problems and may be candidates for invasive nutrition if they clearly fail to demonstrate a response to specific oral supplementation regimens.

REFERENCES

1. Forstner GG, Gall G, Corey M, et al. Digestion and absorption of nutrients in cystic fibrosis. In: Sturgess JM, editor. Proceedings of the 8th International Congress on CF. Mississauga (ON): Imperial Press Ltd; 1980. p. 137–48.
2. Fanconi G, Uehlinger E, Knauer C. Das coelioksyndrom bei angeborener zystisher pankreas fibromatose and bronchicktasis. Wein Med Wochensch 1936;86:753–6.
3. Anderson D. Cystic fibrosis of the pancreas and its relation to celiac disease. Am J Dis Child 1938;56:344–99.
4. Wilcken B, Brown AR, Urwin R, Brown DA. Cystic fibrosis screening by dried blood spot trypsin assay: Results in 75,000 newborn infants. J Pediatr 1983;102:383–7.
5. Shwachman H, Diamond LK, Oski FA, Khaw KT. The syndrome of pancreatic insufficiency and bone marrow dysfunction. J Pediatr 1964;65:645–63.
6. Mack DR, Forstner GG, Wilschanski M, et al. Shwachman syndrome: Exocrine pancreatic dysfunction and variable phenotypic expression. Gastroenterology 1996;1593–602.
7. Woods WG, Roloff JS, Lukens JN, Krivit W. The occurrence of leukemia in patients with the Shwachman syndrome. J Pediatr 1981;99:425–8.
8. Pearson HA, Lobel JS, Kocoshis SA, et al. A new syndrome of refractory anemia with vacuolization of marrow precursors and exocrine pancreatic dysfunction. J Pediatr 1979;95:976–84.
9. Johanson A, Blizzard R. A syndrome of congenital aplasia of the alae nasi, deafness, hypothyroidism, dwarfism, absent permanent teeth, and malabsorption. J Pediatr 1971;79:982–7.
10. Howard CP, Go VLW, Infante AJ, et al. Long-term survival in a case of functional pancreatic agenesis. J Pediatr 1980;97:786–9.
11. Wilschanski M. Other hereditary and acquired pancreatic disorders. In: Walker WA, Durie PR, Hamilton JR, editors. Pediatric Gastrointestinal Disease, 3rd edition. Hamilton: BC Decker Inc; 2000. p.1378–81.
12. Gaskin KJ, Durie PR, Corey M, et al. Evidence for a primary defect in pancreatic HCO32 secretion in cystic fibrosis. Pediatr Res 1982;16:554–7.
13. Kopelman H, Corey M, Gaskin KJ, et al. Impaired chloride secretion, as well as bicarbonate secretion, underlies the fluid secretory defect in the cystic fibrosis pancreas. Gastroenterol 1988;95:349–55.
14. Sheldon W. Congenital pancreatic lipase deficiency. Arch Dis Child 1964;39:268–71.
15. Morgan R, Barrowman J, Borgstrom B. The effect of sodium taurodeoxycholate and pH on the gel filtration behaviour of rat pancreatic protein and lipases. Biochim Biophys Acta 1969;175:65–75.
16. Maylie MF, Charles M, Gache C, Desnuelle P. Isolation and partial identification of pancreatic colipase. Biochim Biophys Acta 1971;229:286–9.
17. Morgan R, Hoffman N. The interaction of lipase, lipase cofactor and bile salts in triglyceride hydrolysis. Biochim Biophys Acta 1971;248:143–8.
18. Gaskin KJ, Durie PR, Hill RE, et al. Colipase and maximally activated pancreatic lipase in normal subjects and patients with steatorrhoea. J Clin Invest 1982;69:427–34.
19. Ghishan FK, Moran JR, Durie PR, et al. Isolated congenital lipase-colipase deficiency. Gastroenterol 1984;86:1580–2.
20. Gaskin KJ, Durie PR, Hill RE, et al. Colipase and lipase secretion in childhood onset pancreatic insufficiency: Delineation of patients with steatorrhoea secondary to relative colipase deficiency. Gastroenterol 1984;86:1–7.
21. Ghishan FK, Lee PC, Lebenthal E, et al. Isolated congenital enterokinase deficiency: Recent findings and review of the literature. Gastroenterology 1983;85:727–31.
22. Waters DL, Dorney SFA, Gaskin KJ, et al. Pancreatic function in infants identified as having cystic fibrosis in a neonatal screening program. N Engl J Med 1990;322:303–8.
23. Riordan JR, Rommens JM, Kerem BS, et al. Identification of the cystic fibrosis gene: Cloning and characterization of complementary DNA. Science 1989;245:1066–72.
24. Rommens JM, Iannuzzi MC, Kerem B, et al. Identification of the cystic fibrosis gene: Chromosome walking and jumping. Science 1989; 245:1059–65.
25. Bear CE, Li C, Kartner N, et al. Purification and functional reconstitution of the cystic fibrosis transmembrane conductance regulator (CFTR). Cell 1992;68:809–18.
26. Kerem E, Corey M, Kerem B, et al. The relation between genotype and phenotype in cystic fibrosis-analysis of the most common mutation (DF508). N Engl J Med 1990;323:1517–22.
27. Novelli G, Sangiuolo F, Maceratesi P, et al. The up-to-date molecular genetics of cystic fibrosis. Biomed Pharmacother 1994;48:455–63.
28. Kerem E, Kalman YM, Yahav Y, et al. Highly variable incidence of cystic fibrosis and different mutation distribution among different Jewish ethnic groups in Israel. Hum Genet 1995;96:193–7.
29. Wilschanski M, Zielenski J, Markiewicz D, et al. Correlation of sweat chloride concentration with classes of the cystic fibrosis transmembrane conductance regulator gene mutations. J Pediatr 1995;127:705–10.
30. Gaskin KJ, Gurwitz D, Durie PR, et al. Improved respiratory prognosis in CF patients with normal fat absorption. J Pediatr 1982;100:857–62.
31. Kristidis P, Bozon D, Corey M, et al. Genetic determination of exocrine pancreatic function in cystic fibrosis. Am J Hum Genet 1992;50:1178–84.
32. Hamosh A, Corey M. Correlation between genotype and phenotype in patients with cystic fibrosis: The Cystic Fibrosis Genotype-Phenotype Consortium. N Engl J Med 1993;329:1308–13.
33. Ahmed M, Corey M, Forstner G, et al. Molecular consequences of cystic fibrosis transmembrane regulator (CFTR) gene mutations in the exocrine pancreas. Gut 2003;52:1159–64.
34. Daneman A, Gaskin K, Martin DJ, et al. Pancreatic changes in cystic fibrosis: CT and sonographic appearances. Am J Radiol 1983;141:653–5.
35. Vawter GF, Shwachman H. Cystic fibrosis in adults. An autopsy study. Pathol Ann 1979;14:357–82.
36. Hadorn B, Johansen PG, Anderson CM. Pancreozymin secretin test of exocrine pancreatic function in cystic fibrosis and the significance of the result for the pathogenesis of the disease. Can Med J 1968;98:377–84.
37. Case RM, Argent BE. Pancreatic duct cell secretion. Control and mechanisms of secretion. In: Go LW, editor. The Pancreas: Biology, Pathobiology and Disease. New York: Raven Press; 1993. p. 301–50.
38. Ishiguro H, Steward C, Wilson RW, Case RM. Bicarbonate secretion in interlobular ducts from guinea pig pancreas. J Physiol 1996;495:179–91.
39. Shumaker H, Amlal H, Frizzell R, et al. CFTR drives Na+ 2nHCO32 cotransport in pancreatic duct cells: A basis for defective HCO3-secretion in CF. Am J Physiol 1999;276: C16–25.
40. Freedman SD, Katz MH, Parker EM, et al. A membrane lipid imbalance plays a role in the phenotypic expression of cystic fibrosis in cftr(2/2) mice. Proc Natl Acad Sci U S A 1999; 96:13995–14000.
41. Goobie S, Popovic M, Morrison J, et al. Shwachman-Diamond syndrome with exocrine pancreatic dysfunction and bone marrow failure maps to the centromeric region of chromosome 7. Am J Hum Genet 2001;68:1048–54.
42. Popovic M, Goobie S, Morrison J, et al. Fine mapping of the locus for Shwachman–Diamond syndrome at 7q11, identification of shared disease haplotypes, and exclusion of SBDS TPST1 as a candidate gene. Eur J Hum Genet 2002;10: 250–8.
43. Boocock GR, Morrison JA, Popovic M, et al. Mutations in SBDS are associated with Shwachman–Diamond syndrome. Nat Genet 2003;33:97–101.
44. Sano T, Ban K, Ichiki T, et al. Molecular and genetic analyses of two patients with Pearson's marrow-pancreas syndrome. Pediatr Res 1993;34:105–10.
45. Stoffers DA, Zinkin NT, Stanojevic V, et al. Pancreatic agenesis attributable to a single nucleotide in the human IPF1 gene coding sequence. Nat Genet 1997;15:106–10.
46. Gorry MC, Gabbaizedeh D, Furey W, et al. Mutations in the cationic trypsinogen gene are associated with recurrent acute and chronic pancreatitis. Gastroenterol 1997;113:1063–8.
47. Gurwitz D, Corey M, Francis PWI, et al. Perspectives in cystic fibrosis. Pediatr Clin North Am 1979;26:603–15.
48. Santis G, Osborne L, Knight RA, Hodson ME. Independent genetic determinants of pancreatic and pulmonary status in cystic fibrosis. Lancet 1990;336:1081–4.
49. Soutter VL, Kristidis P, Gruca MA, Gaskin KJ. Chronic undernutrition, growth retardation in cystic fibrosis. Clin Gastroenterol 1986;15:137–55.
50. Pencharz P, Hill R, Archibald E, et al. Energy needs and nutritional rehabilitation in undernourished adolescents and adults with cystic fibrosis. J Pediatr Gastroenterol Nutr 1984;3:147–53.
51. Vaisman N, Pencharz PB, Corey M, et al. Energy expenditure of patients with cystic fibrosis. J Pediatr 1987;111:496–500.
52. Buchdahl RM, Cox M, Fulleylove C, et al. Increased resting energy expenditure in cystic fibrosis. J Appl Physiol 1988;64:1810–6.
53. Scott RB, O'Loughlin EV, Gall DG. Gastroesophageal reflux in patients with cystic fibrosis. J Pediatr 1985;106:223–7.
54. Gaskin KJ, Waters DLM, Howman-Giles R, et al. Liver disease and common-bile-duct stenosis in cystic fibrosis. N Engl J Med 1988;318:340–6.
55. Gaskin KJ. The liver and biliary tract in cystic fibrosis. In: Suchy FJ, editor. Liver Disease in Children, 2nd edition. Philadelphia: Lippincott Williams and Wilkins; 2000. p. 549–63.
56. Roberts DM, Craft JC, Mather FJ, et al. Prevalence of giardiasis in patients with cystic fibrosis. J Pediatr 1988;112:555–59.
57. Lloyd-Still JD. Crohn's accounts for increased prevalence of inflammatory bowel disease (IBD) in CF [abstract]. Pediatr Pulmonol 1992:307–8.
58. Collin P, Reunala T, Mäki M. New diagnostic strategy for coeliac disease. In: Mäki M, Collin P, Visakorpi JK, editors. Coeliac Disease. Vammala: Vammalan Kirjapaino Oy; 1997. p. 47–51.
59. Smyth RL, van Velzen D, Smyth AR, et al. Strictures of ascending colon in cystic fibrosis and high-strength pancreatic enzymes. Lancet 1994;343:85–6.
60. Gaskin KJ. Intestines. In: Yankaskas JR, Knowles MR, editors. Cystic Fibrosis in Adults. Philadelphia: Lippincott-Raven Publishers; 1999. p. 325–42.
61. FitzSimmons SC, Burkhart GA, Borowitz D, et al. High-dose pancreatic-enzyme supplements and fibrosing colonopathy in children with cystic fibrosis. N Engl J Med 1997;336: 1283–9.
62. Smyth RL, Ashby D, O'Hea U, et al. Fibrosing colonopathy in cystic fibrosis: Results of a case-control study. Lancet 1985;346:1247–51.

63. Borowitz DS, Grand RJ, Durie PR, et al. Use of pancreatic enzyme supplements for patients with cystic fibrosis in the context of fibrosing colonopathy. J Pediatr 1995;127:681–4.
64. Cipolli M, Gaskin. Pancreatic phenotype in infants with CF identified by two mutational screening programs. J Cystic Fibrosis 2005;4 (abstract).
65. Noone PG, Zhou Z, Silverman LM, et al. Cystic fibrosis gene mutations and pancreatitis risk: Relation to epithelial ion transport and trypsin inhibitor gene mutations. Gastroenterology 2001;121:1310–9.
66. Durno C, Corey M, Zielenski J, et al. Genotype and phenotype correlations in patients with cystic fibrosis and pancreatitis. Gastroenterology 2002;123:1857–64.
67. Lapey A, Kirkpatrick J, di Sant'Agnese P, Laster L. Steatorrhoea and azotorrhoea and their relation to growth and nutrition in adolescents and young adults with cystic fibrosis. J Pediatr 1974;84:328–34.
68. Roy CC, Weber AM, Lepage G, et al. Digestive and absorptive phase anomalies associated with the exocrine pancreatic insufficiency of cystic fibrosis. J Pediatr Gastroenterol Nutr 1988;7:51–7.
69. Borgstrom B. Importance of phospholipids, pancreatic phospholipase A2 and fatty acids for the digestion of dietary fat: In vitro experiments with the porcine enzymes. Gastroenterology 1980;78:954–62.
70. Löser CHR, Brauer C, Aygen S, et al. Comparative clinical evaluation of the ^{13}C-mixed triglyceride breath test as an indirect pancreatic function test. Scand J Gastroenterol 1998;33:327–34.
71. Soldan W, Henker J, Sprössig C. Sensitivity and specificity of quantitative determination of pancreatic elastase 1 in feces of children. J Pediatr Gastroenterol Nutr 1997;24:53–5.
72. Wallis C, Leung TH, Cubitt D, Reynolds A. Stool elastase as a diagnostic test for pancreatic function in children with cystic fibrosis. Lancet 1997;350:1001.
73. Walkowiak J, Cichy WK, Herzig KH. Comparison of fecal elastase-1 determination with the secretin-cholecystokinin test in patients with cystic fibrosis. Scand J Gastroenterol 1999;34:202–7.
74. Bebarry S, Ellis L, Corey M, et al. How useful is fecal pancreatic elastase 1 as a marker of exocrine pancreatic disease? J Pediatr 2002;141:84–90.
75. Löser CHR, Möllgaard A, Fölsch UR. Faecal elastase 1; A novel, highly sensitive, and specific tubeless pancreatic function test. Gut 1996;39:580–6.
76. Hill RE, Durie PR, Gaskin KJ, et al. Steatorrhoea and pancreatic insufficiency in Shwachman's syndrome. Gastroenterol 1982;83:22–7.
77. Sproul A, Huang H. Growth patterns in children with cystic fibrosis. J Pediatr 1964;65:664–76.
78. Berry HK, Kellog FW, Hunt MM, et al. Dietary supplement and nutrition in children with cystic fibrosis. Am J Dis Child 1975;129:165–71.
79. Corey ML. Longitudinal studies in cystic fibrosis. In: Sturgess JM, editor. Perspectives in Cystic Fibrosis. Toronto: The Imperial Press Ltd; 1980. p. 246–55.
80. Roy CC, Darling P, Weber AM. A rational approach to meeting macro- and micronutrient needs in cystic fibrosis. J Pediatr Gastroenterol Nutr 1983;3:154–62.
81. Bell L, Durie P, Forstner GG. What do children with cystic fibrosis eat? J Pediatr Gastroenterol Nutr 1984;3: 137–46.
82. Chase HP, Long MA, Lavin MH. Cystic fibrosis and malnutrition. J Pediatr 1979;95:337–47.
83. Parsons HG, Beaudry P, Dumas A, Pencharz PB. Energy needs and growth in children with cystic fibrosis. J Pediatr Gastroenterol Nutr 1983;2:44–9.
84. Corey M, McLaughlin FJ, Williams M, Levison H. A comparison of survival, growth and pulmonary function in patients with cystic fibrosis in Boston and Toronto. J Clin Epidemiol 1988;41:588–91.
85. Farrell PM, Kosorok MR, Laxova A, et al. Nutritional benefits of neonatal screening for cystic fibrosis. N Engl J Med 1997;337:963–9.
86. Farrell PM, Kosorok MR, Rock MJ, et al. Early diagnosis of cystic fibrosis through neonatal screening prevents severe malnutrition and improves long term growth. Pediatrics 2001;107:1–13.
87. Huang SH, Schall JI, Zemel BS, Stallings VA. Vitamin E status in children with cystic fibrosis and pancreatic insufficiency. J Pediatr 2006;148:556–9.
88. Koscik RL, Lai HJ, Laxova A, et al. Preventing early, prolonged vitamin E deficiency: An opportunity for better cognitive outcomes via early diagnosis through neonatal screening. J Pediatr 2005;147:S51–6.
89. Peterson ML, Jacobs DR, Jr, Milla CE. Longitudinal changes in growth parameters are correlated with changes in pulmonary function in children with cystic fibrosis. Pediatrics 2003;112:588–92.
90. Lai HJ, Cheng Y, Farrell PM. The survival advantage of patients with cystic fibrosis diagnosed through neonatal screening: Evidence from the United States Cystic Fibrosis Foundation registry data. J Pediatr 2005;147:S57–63.
91. Ginzberg H, Shin J, Ellis L, et al. Shwachman syndrome: Phenotypic manifestations of sibling sets and isolated cases in a large patient cohort are similar. J Pediatr 1999;135:81–8.
92. Willis E, Miller R, Wyn J. Gendered embodiment and survival for young people with cystic fibrosis. Soc Sci Med 2001;53:1163–74.
93. Stark LJ, Mulvihill MM, Jelalian E, et al. Descriptive analysis of eating behaviour in school-age children with cystic fibrosis and healthy control children. Pediatrics 1997;99:665–71.
94. Powers SW, Mitchell MJ, Patton SR, et al. Mealtime behaviours in families of infants and toddlers with cystic fibrosis. J Cyst Fibros 2005;4:175–82.
95. Mitchell EA, Quested C, Marks RD, et al. Comparative trial of viokase, pancreatin and Pancrease(r) pancrelipase (enteric-coated beads) in the treatment of malabsorption in cystic fibrosis. Aust Paediatr J 1982;18:114–7.
96. Gow R, Bradbear R, Francis P, Shepherd RW. Comparative study of varying regimens to improve steatorrhoea and creatorrhoea in cystic fibrosis. Lancet 1981;i:1071–4.
97. Gaskin KJ. Impact of nutrition in cystic fibrosis. A review. J Ped Gastroenterol Nutr 1988;7:12–7.
98. Duhamel DJ, Lenoir G, Brouard J, et al. Prise en charge nutritionelle des nouveau-nés et nourrissons atteints de fibrose kystique du pancréas et dépistés à la naissance. Proceedings of the International Conference on Neonatal Screening for Cystic Fibrosis. Caen, France: University of Caen; 1988. p. 183–99.
99. Kuo PT, Huang NN. The effect of medium-chain triglycerides upon fat absorption and plasma lipids and deposition of fat of children with cystic fibrosis of the pancreas. J Clin Invest 1965;44:1924–9.
100. Durie PR, Newth CJ, Forstner GG, Gall DG. Malabsorption of medium-chain trigylcerides in infants with cystic fibrosis: Correction with pancreatic enzyme supplements. J Pediatr 1980;96:862–4.
101. Feigel RJ, Shapiro BL. Mitochondrial calcium uptake and oxygen consumption in cystic fibrosis. Nature 1979;178:276–7.
102. Stutts MJ, Knowles MR, Gatzy JT, Boucher RC. Oxygen consumption and ouabain binding-sites in cystic fibrosis nasal epithelium. Pediatr Res 1986;20:1316–20.
103. Shepherd RW, Holt TL, Vasques-Velasquez L, et al. Increased energy expenditure in children with cystic fibrosis. Lancet 1988;i:1300–3.
104. Fried MD, Durie PR, Tsui L-C, et al. The cystic fibrosis gene and resting energy expenditure. J Pediatr 1991;119:913–6.
105. Bines JE, Truby HD, Armstrong DS, et al. Energy metabolism in infants with cystic fibrosis. J Pediatr 2002;140:527–33.
106. O'Rawe A, McIntosh I, Dodge JA, et al. Increased energy expenditure in cystic fibrosis is associated with specific mutations. Clin Sci 1992;82:71–6.
107. Allen JR, McCauley J, Selby A, et al. Differences in resting energy expenditure between male and female children with cystic fibrosis. J Pediatr 2003;142:15–9 (editorial p. 4–6).
108. Zemel BS, Kawchak DA, Cnaan A, et al. Prospective evaluation of resting energy expenditure, nutritional status, pulmonary function, and genotype in children with cystic fibrosis. Pediatr Res 1996;40:578–86.
109. Barclay A, Allen JR, Byler E, et al. Resting energy expenditure in females with cystic fibrosis—is it affected by puberty? Eur J Clin Nutr 2007 1–6. doi: 10.1038/sj.ejcn.1602637.
110. Beghin L, Gottrand F, Michaud L, et al. Impact of intravenous antibiotic therapy on total daily energy expenditure and physical activity in cystic fibrosis children with pseudomonas aeruginosa pulmonary exacerbation. Pediatr Res 2003;54:756–61.
111. Farrell PM, Mischler EH, Engle MJ, et al. Fatty acid abnormalities in cystic fibrosis. Pediatr Res 1985;19:104–9.
112. Hubbard VS, Dunn GD. Fatty acid composition of erythrocyte phospholipids from patients with cystic fibrosis. Clin Chim Acta 1980;102:115–8.
113. Parsons HG, O'Loughlin EV, Forbes D, et al. Supplemental calories improve essential fatty acid deficiency in cystic fibrosis patients. Pediatr Res 1988;24:353–6.
114. Rogiers V, Dab I, Crokaert R, et al. Long chain non-esterified fatty acid pattern in plasma of cystic fibrosis patients and their parents. Pediatr Res 1980;14:1088–91.
115. Forstner G, Durie P, Corey M. Cystic fibrosis, progress in gastroenterology and nutrition. Proceedings of the 10th International Cystic Fibrosis Congress; 1988 (Sydney). Hong Kong: Excerpta Medica, Asia Ltd. Asia Pacific Congress Series. 1988;74:154–60.
116. Freedman SD, O'Sullivan BP, Martinez-Clark P, et al. An abnormality in AA/DHA metabolism is present in CFTR-regulated tissues from CF patients. Pediatr Pulmonol 2000:158–59.
117. Abernathy RS. Bulging fontanelle as presenting sign in cystic fibrosis. Am J Dis Child 1976;130:1360–2.
118. Rayner RJ, Tyrell JC, Hiller EJ, et al. Night blindness and conjunctival xerosis due to vitamin A deficiency in cystic fibrosis. Arch Dis Child 1989;64:1151–6.
119. Scott J, Elias E, Moult PJA, et al. Rickets in adult cystic fibrosis with myopathy, pancreatic insufficiency and proximal renal tubular dysfunction. Am J Med 1977;63:488–92.
120. Hubbard VS, Farrell PM, di Sant'Agnese PA. 25-Hydroxycholecalciferol levels in patients with cystic fibrosis. J Pediatr 1979;94:84–6.
121. Reiter EO, Brugman SM, Pike JW, et al. Vitamin D metabolites in adolescents and young adults with cystic fibrosis: Effects of sun and season. J Pediatr 1985;106:21–5.
122. Farrell PM, Bieri JG, Fratantoni JF, et al. The occurrence and effects of human vitamin E deficiency. A study in patients with cystic fibrosis. J Clin Invest 1977;60:233–41.
123. Elias E, Muller DPR, Scott J, et al. Association of spinocerebellar disorders with cystic fibrosis or chronic childhood cholestasis and low serum vitamin E. Lancet 1981;ii:1319–21.
124. Sitrin MD, Lieberman F, Jensen WE, et al. Vitamin E deficiency and neurologic disease in adults with cystic fibrosis. Ann Intern Med 1987;107:51–4.
125. Walters TR, Koch HF. Hemorrhagic diathesis and cystic fibrosis in infancy. Am J Dis Child 1972;124:641–7.
126. Komp DM, Selden RF. Coagulation abnormalities in cystic fibrosis. Chest 1970;58:501–8.
127. Graham-Maar RC, Schall JI, Stettler N, et al. Elevated vitamin A intake and serum retinol in preadolescent children with cystic fibrosis. Am J Clin Nutr 2006;84:174–82.
128. Bines JE, Israel EJ. Hypoproteinemia, anaemia and failure to thrive in an infant. Gastroenterol 1991;101:848–56.
129. Sokol RJ, Reardon MC, Accurso FJ, et al. Fat-soluble vitamin status during the first year of life in infants with cystic fibrosis identified by screening of newborns. Am J Clin Nutr 1989;50:1064–71.
130. Castillo R, Landon C, Eckhardt K, et al. Selenium and vitamin E status in cystic fibrosis. J Pediatr 1981;99:583–5.
131. Ward KP, Arthur JR, Russell G, Aggett PJ. Blood selenium content and glutathione peroxidase activity in children with cystic fibrosis, coeliac disease, asthma, and epilepsy. Eur J Pediatr 1984;142:21–4.
132. Zhang Z, Lai HJ. Comparison of the use of body mass index percentiles and percentage of ideal body weight to screen for malnutrition in children with cystic fibrosis. Am J Clin Nutr 2004;80:982–91.
133. Tran TMD, Van den Neucker A, Hendriks JJE, et al. Effects of a proton-pump inhibitor in cystic fibrosis. Acta Pediatr 1998;87:553–8.
134. Kalnins D, Ellis L, Corey M, et al. Enteric-coated pancreatic enzyme with bicarbonate is equal to stand enteric-coated enzyme in treating with malabsorption in cystic fibrosis. J Pediatr Gastroenterol Nutr 2006;42:256–61.
135. Borowitz D, Goss CH, Limauro S, et al. Study of a novel pancreatic enzyme replacement therapy in pancreatic insufficient subjects with cystic fibrosis. Pancreas 2006;32:258–63.
136. Holliday KE, Allen JR, Waters DL, et al. Growth of human milk-fed and formula-fed infants with cystic fibrosis. J Pediatr 1991;118:77–9.
137. Marcus MS, Sondel SA, Farrell PM, et al. Nutritional status of infants with cystic fibrosis associated with early diagnosis and intervention. Am J Clin Nutr 1991;54:578–85.
138. Shepherd R, Cooksley EGE, Donvill Cooke WD. Improved growth and clinical, nutritional and respiratory changes in response to nutritional therapy in cystic fibrosis. J Pediatr 1980;97:351–7.
139. Levy LD, Durie PR, Pencharz PB, Corey ML. Effects of long-term nutritional rehabilitation on body composition and clinical status in malnourished children and adolescents with cystic fibrosis. J Pediatr 1985;107:225–30.
140. Boland MP, Stocki DS, Macdonald NE, et al. Chronic jejunostomy feeding with a non-elemental formula in undernourished patients with cystic fibrosis. Lancet 1986;i:232–4.
141. Shepherd RW, Holt TL, Thomas BJ, et al. Nutritional rehabilitation in cystic fibrosis: Controlled studies of the effects on nutritional growth retardation, body protein turnover and cause of pulmonary disease. J Pediatr 1986;109:788–94.
142. Gunnell S, Christensen NK, McDonald C, Jackson D. Attitudes towards percutaneous endoscopic gastrostomy placement in cystic fibrosis patients. J Pediatr Gastroenterol Nutr 2005;40:334–8.
143. Nasr SZ, Hurwitz ME, Brown RW, et al. Treatment of anorexia and weight loss with megestrol acetate in patients with cystic fibrosis. Pediatr Pulmonol 1999;28:380–2.
144. Marchand V, Baker SS, Start TJ, Baker RD. Randomized, double-blind, placebo-controlled pilot trial of megestrol acetate in malnourished children with cystic fibrosis. J Pediatr Gastroenterol Nutr 2000;31:264–9.

145. Eubanks V, Koppersmith N, Wooldridge N, et al. Effects of megestrol acetate on weight gain, body composition, and pulmonary function in patients with cystic fibrosis. J Pediatr 2002;140:439–44.
146. Feliu J, Gonzalez-Baron M, Berrocal A, et al. Usefulness of megestrol acetate in cancer cachexia and anorexia. Am J Clin Oncol 1992;15:432–40.
147. Oster MH, Enders SR, Samuels SJ, et al. Megesterol acetate in patients with AIDS and cachexia. Ann Intern Med 1994;121:400–8.
148. Boyle MP. Update on maintaining bone health in cystic fibrosis. Curr Opin Pulm Med 2006;12:453–8.
149. Haworth CS, Selby PL, Webb AK, et al. Low bone mineral density in adults with cystic fibrosis. Thorax 1999;54:961–7.
150. Aris RM, Neuringer IP, Weiner MA, et al. Severe osteoporosis before and after lung transplantation. Chest 1996;109:1176–83.
151. Aris RM, Renner JB, Winders AD, et al. Increased rate of fractures and severe kyphosis: Sequelae of living into adulthood with cystic fibrosis. Ann Intern Med 1998;128:186–93.
152. Shead EF, Haworth CS, Gunn E, et al. Osteoclastogenesis during infective exacerbations in patients with cystic fibrosis. Am J Respir Crit Care Med 2006;174:306–11.
153. Dif F, Marty C, Baudoin C, et al. Severe osteopenia in CFTR-null mice. Bone 2004;35:595–603.
154. Aris RM, Merkel PA, Bachrach LK, et al. Guide to bone health and disease in cystic fibrosis. J Clin Endocrinol Metab 2005;90:1888–96.

Acute and Chronic Liver Disease

Deirdre Kelly, MD, FRCP, FRCPI, FRCPCH

The liver has a central role in energy metabolism, nutritional homeostasis, and absorption of nutrients. Severe liver disease, whether acute or chronic, leads to multiorgan failure, which can have significant effects on growth and development in the long term. The pathophysiology of malnutrition in liver disease is complex and multifactorial and has extensive implications (Table 1). It is most severe in infants with chronic cholestatic liver disease, who are particularly vulnerable to the effects of malnutrition because of their high-energy and growth requirements.[1] This chapter reviews the pathophysiology of malnutrition in pediatric liver disease and current treatment strategies, including liver transplantation.

PATHOPHYSIOLOGY OF MALNUTRITION IN LIVER DISEASE

Prevalence of Malnutrition

Malnutrition is common in children with chronic liver disease. Estimates vary from 50 to 80% in studies from North America and Europe.[2–5] In general; children who present with acute liver disease such as viral hepatitis or fulminant hepatitis are not malnourished at presentation but can become so as a result of their illness.[6]

Reduced Energy Intake

Anorexia is a common symptom in children with either acute or chronic liver disease. They often take in less than the recommended requirements or less than is appropriate for their energy requirements because of increased energy expenditure.[7] The consequent reduction in enteral intake can lead to considerable loss of body stores or lean body mass, which alters body composition.

In children with chronic liver disease, the complications of portal hypertension, such as ascites and hepatosplenomegaly, can lead to malabsorption of nutrients. The treatment of ascites, which includes fluid restriction, the prescription of unpalatable feeds, or both, can exacerbate anorexia and reduce energy intake further.[3]

Table 1 Pathophysiology of Malnutrition in Liver Disease

Reduced calorie intake anorexia
• Fat malabsorption
• Use of bile salt resins
• Portal hypertension
• Unpalatable feeds
Inappropriate substrate use
• Abnormal nitrogen metabolism
• Reduction in glycogen stores
• Negative protein balance
Increased metabolic needs
• Energy expenditure
• Calorie requirements
Hormonal dysregulation
• Growth hormone/IGF-I insulin resistance

IGF = Insulin-like factor.

Carbohydrate Metabolism

Under normal circumstances, the liver receives portal vein blood rich in absorbed glucose, which can be stored in the liver as glycogen or circulated to extrahepatic tissues, especially muscle, where lactate, pyruvate, and alanine are generated by glycolysis.[8,9] In children with liver disease, this substrate supply and use can be abnormal. The loss of glycogen stores in chronic liver disease leads to fasting hypoglycemia and an inability to meet energy demands. In addition, any significant hepatocyte loss, especially in acute liver failure,[10] has an immediate effect on glucose metabolism, leading to hypoglycemia.

In cirrhotic adults, the pancreas secretes increased amounts of insulin, which is not metabolized, either because of portosystemic shunting around the liver or because of reduced degradation owing to hepatic dysfunction[11] or reduced glucose uptake by hepatocytes.[12] Although there is increased circulation of insulin, glucose uptake in the peripheral tissues, especially muscles, is reduced as a result of insulin resistance. Adult studies suggest that this could be attributable to impaired glycogen synthesis in the muscle, either because of abnormal insulin receptor numbers or affinity.[13,14] These data have not been confirmed in children, but it is possible that similar mechanisms occur, although few children (apart from those with cystic fibrosis) develop overt diabetes mellitus, unlike adults.[13]

Protein Metabolism

Amino acids are absorbed by the intestine directly into the portal vein and transferred to the liver, where they are synthesized into protein or used for energy. The liver is responsible for approximately 10% of plasma protein synthesis; thus, amino acids are constantly recycled.[9,15] Nonessential amino acids are oxidized in both liver and muscle. The seven aromatic essential amino acids (AAAs; arginine, histidine, lysine, methionine, phenylalanine, tryptophan, and threonine) are metabolized in the liver, whereas the three branched-chain essential amino acids (BCAAs; leucine, isoleucine, and valine) are metabolized predominantly in muscle and pass unaltered through the liver to the periphery, where their uptake is regulated by insulin.[16] The liver is also responsible for detoxification of nitrogenous wastes via the urea cycle, leading to the production of ammonia-hence the rise of plasma ammonia in both acute and chronic liver failure.[17]

Reduced hepatic and muscle glycogen stores lead to early recruitment of fat and increased dependence on amino acids as an alternative fuel.[18] Abnormal protein use by the liver leads to a rise in AAAs and a reduction in the BCAAs, which are metabolized in muscle in both children and adults.[19–21] An abnormal ratio of BCAAs to AAAs correlates with histologic damage and encephalopathy in adults[22] and children.[20]

Studies in adults demonstrating abnormalities in BCAA metabolism using studies of BCAA fluxes and protein turnover have given conflicting results. It is possible that the hyperinsulinemia detected in cirrhosis could cause the decreased BCAA levels by increasing BCAA uptake in muscle or adipose tissue. Alternatively, it is possible that there is an increase in liver transamination of BCAAs in addition to abnormal protein turnover.[23] Three adult studies demonstrated that protein synthesis can be increased or decreased depending on clinical condition and that muscle wasting is attributable to a relative increase in protein breakdown.[24–26] Those patients who had more efficient protein retention were less malnourished.

A study of protein metabolism in infants with liver disease, which used a whole-body leucine turnover model, demonstrated that muscle protein degradation and protein oxidation were increased, possibly as a result of a reduction in carbohydrate metabolism and the use of protein as an energy supply.[27] In contrast to normal children, muscle protein degradation continued in these children even when they were fed, suggesting that this could be a factor in the muscle loss common in infants with chronic liver disease. A recent study in cholestatic children also documented increased leucine oxidation in the postabsorptive state, but not in the fed state, but these children had less severe liver disease than the above study.[28]

In addition to protein synthesis and degradation, the liver is the site of synthesis of all of the coagulation factors except factor VIII, von Willebrand's factor, which is synthesized by vascular endothelial cells.[29,30] Thus, coagulopathy is an early sign of significant acute or chronic liver failure.

In chronic liver disease, these metabolic changes result in muscle wasting, hyperammonemia, hypoalbuminemia, hypoglycemia, hypolipidemia, and reduced circulating triglyceride levels secondary to the increased fat oxidation. Hypoalbuminemia is associated with a reduction in plasma oncotic pressure, exacerbating the development of ascites and peripheral edema. In acute liver failure, the main effects of deranged protein metabolism are hyperammonemia and abnormal coagulation.

Fat Metabolism

Most dietary fat is in the form of long-chain triglycerides (LCT) and is an excellent energy source.[31] The first step in fat digestion is emulsification in the stomach, followed by hydrolysis of triglycerides by pancreatic lipase in the intestinal lumen and then micellar solubilization of di- and monoglycerides by bile acids, which are then transported into the enterocytes. Once in the enterocytes, fatty acids are reesterified and chylomicrons are formed and removed via the lymphatics through the portal system to the liver and other tissues.[31]

In contrast, medium-chain triglycerides (MCTs) do not depend on micellar solubilization for absorption and can be transferred directly from the enterocytes to the portal circulation without reesterification.[31,32] In the liver, free fatty acids are metabolized into triglycerides or oxidized for energy. The very-low-density lipoproteins (VLDL) and high-density lipoproteins (HDL) are synthesized in the liver, as is cholesterol, which is the precursor for many hormones, vitamins, and bile acids.

In all forms of chronic liver disease, there is reduction in the synthesis and secretion of bile salts, although this is more severe in cholestatic diseases such as biliary atresia. Up to 50% of LCTs, fat-soluble vitamins, and essential polyunsaturated fatty acids (PUFAs) might not be absorbed because of reduced biliary secretion and reduction in intraluminal bile concentration.[33–35] In contrast, 95% of water-soluble lipids, such as MCTs, which do not depend on bile solubility, are absorbed even in cholestatic infants[36] and form the basis for nutritional replacement.[37]

Fat malabsorption can also be affected by portal hypertension, which leads to congested gastric and intestinal mucosa, and by small bowel overgrowth in the Roux-en-Y blind loop created by a Kasai portoenterostomy. In addition, therapy such as cholestyramine to reduce pruritus can exacerbate steatorrhea because it binds bile salts, decreasing micellar solubilization.

Pancreatic function is usually normal except in children with Alagille syndrome, in which pancreatic lipase can be reduced.[36,38]

Long-Chain Polyunsaturated Fatty Acids

Long-chain polyunsaturated fatty acids (LCPs) such as arachidonic acid and docosahexaenoic acid (DHA) are essential nutrients in infancy. LCPs, in particular DHA, play a major role in the development of visual acuity and mental development in the first year of life, particularly in preterm infants.39–42 The main source of LCPs is maternal, in the last trimester of pregnancy and through breast-feeding, because breast milk is a rich source of LCPs, containing both arachidonic acid and DHA in a combination of phospholipid and triglyceride forms.

Studies in adults have demonstrated that LCP deficiency can develop either from malabsorption of long-chain fat and essential fatty acids or from reduced synthesis or function of the A-6-desaturase enzyme required for the de novo synthesis of very-long-chain (20 to 22) carbon PUFAs from their essential fatty acid 18-carbon dietary precursors.[43,44]

A recent study which compared plasma and liver levels of very long chain PUFAs in adults undergoing liver transplantation with controls undergoing hepatic resection demonstrated low plasma but normal liver levels in cirrhotic adults suggesting that tissue stores were not affected.[45] It is unclear how this would compare with infants who are growing rapidly and certainly deficiencies have been described in pretransplant infants.[46]

Children with cholestatic liver disease have normal LCP and DHA levels at birth but can become deficient within 8 to 12 weeks,[47] either from malabsorption of LCTs, from prescription of formula feeds rich in MCTs, or as a result of inadequate liver desaturase enzyme activity.[43,48,49]

Fat-Soluble Vitamin Deficiency

Chronic liver disease affects vitamin absorption, metabolism, and storage. Reduction in bile salt secretion leads to malabsorption of the fat-soluble vitamins A, D, E, and K. Fat-soluble vitamin deficiency can develop within 6 to 12 weeks of birth, depending on body stores and availability of vitamin supplementation. Vitamin A deficiency can also develop secondary to reduction in protein synthesis or depletion of hepatic stores. Vitamin D deficiency can occur either from fat malabsorption or from reduction in hepatic 25-hydroxylation. Vitamin K deficiency arises partly from fat malabsorption and partly from a reduction in intake, particularly in breast-fed infants and may be prevalent even with supplementation in severely cholestatic children.[50]

Because the liver has a central role in lipoprotein metabolism and cholesterol synthesis, hypercholesterolemia and hypertriglyceridemia are common in chronic liver disease. There can be increased synthesis of cholesterol esters as a result of loss of hepatic lecithin cholesterol acyltransferase, which can alter lipoprotein fractions. In cholestatic liver disease such as Alagille syndrome, unusual lipoproteins, such as lipoprotein X, are produced with cutaneous xanthomata and hemolysis from alterations in red cell and platelet membranes.[51]

In terminal liver disease, however, the reduction in cholesterol synthesis leads to hypocholesterolemia, which is a poor prognostic sign.[52]

Growth Hormone/Insulin-Like Growth Factor Axis

Growth failure in chronic liver disease can be exacerbated by an impaired growth hormone/insulin-like growth factor (IGF-I) axis,[53,54] because IGF-I and its major circulating binding protein, IGF-BP3, are synthesized in the liver. It seems that IGF-I is nutritionally regulated[55] because there is animal evidence that nutrients influence synthesis and action of IGF-I and its binding proteins at many levels, including defects in pre- and posttranslational expression. Thus, protein malnutrition not only decreases the IGF-I production rate but can also increase serum clearance and degradation. Evaluation of growth hormone, growth hormone-binding proteins, and IGF-I in children with protein-energy malnutrition, before and after nutritional rehabilitation, has confirmed the role of malnutrition in these hormones.[56]

Children with chronic liver disease have low plasma levels of IGF-I despite elevated levels of growth hormone, which could be a result of diminished hepatic synthesis or malnutrition or related to end-organ insensitivity to IGF-I.[57,58]

Increased Energy Expenditure

Adult studies have produced conflicting data on energy expenditure, but the situation is different in a growing child. A number of studies have indicated an increase in energy requirements of up to 140% in children with chronic liver disease.[59,60] Mechanisms implicated include portosystemic shunting and ascites, abnormal intermediate metabolism, and the energy demands of specific complications, such as sepsis and variceal hemorrhage. A recent study has confirmed that children with end-stage liver disease have a hypermetabolic state with increased metabolic activity in the body cell mass with excess lipid oxidation during fasting and at rest, once again confirming the necessity for appropriate nutrition and the avoidance of prolonged fasting in these children.[61] In contrast, children with stable liver disease such as Alagille's syndrome did not have increased energy expenditure, suggesting that abnormal energy expenditure is related to severity of liver disease.[62] Children with acute liver failure also have excess energy expenditure and requirements because of multiorgan failure, but this has not been specifically studied.

Trace Elements and Metals

Biochemical deficiencies of water-soluble vitamins such as thiamin and pyridoxine can occur and lead to nutritional cardiomyopathy and peripheral neuropathy.[63] Trace metal deficiencies include iron deficiency secondary to gastrointestinal bleeding or diminished intake and zinc and selenium deficiencies caused by reduced enteral intake, malabsorption, or increased losses.

Consequences of Malnutrition

Many different nutrient deficiencies occur in children with chronic liver disease (Table 2), and malnutrition per se can increase liver dysfunction because of the energy required for synthesis, storage, and detoxification. Children with progressive cholestasis, such as those with biliary atresia or Alagille syndrome, develop significant fat malabsorption, which leads to steatorrhea, fat-soluble vitamin deficiency, essential fatty acid deficiency, loss of fat stores, and a reduction in growth (Tables 2 and 3). Essential fatty acid deficiency can present with a skin rash, whereas DHA deficiency is associated with abnormalities in visual function, as demonstrated by electroretinograms in cholestatic infants.[47]

Fat-soluble vitamin deficiency is more common and can be detected biochemically before clinical symptoms, which are obvious only when severe deficiencies, appear. Clinical signs and symptoms of vitamin A deficiency are rare but include night blindness, xerophthalmia, and keratomalacia.[64] Vitamin D deficiency leads to hypocalcemia, hypophosphatemia, rickets, and pathologic fractures, particularly in infants who are rarely exposed to sunlight or who have inherited metabolic liver disease and a renal tubular disorder. Deficiency of vitamin E leads to hemolysis, peripheral neuropathy, and occasionally visual loss.[65,66] Vitamin K deficiency can present as hemorrhagic disease of the newborn, particularly in breast-fed babies who are given insufficient vitamin K at birth.[67] It leads to coagulopathy, which is exacerbated by decreased synthesis of liver-dependent clotting factors. In vitamin K deficiency secondary to fat malabsorption, parenteral vitamin K will improve the coagulation profile, whereas it will be ineffective in parenchymal liver disease.[68]

Table 2 Clinical Manifestations of Malnutrition in Liver Disease

Nutritional Deficit	Clinical Manifestation
Protein-energy malnutrition	Stunting, muscle wasting, motor developmental delay
Fat malabsorption	Steatorrhea, loss of fat stores
Essential fatty acid deficiency	Peeling skin rash
Vitamin A deficiency	Conjunctival and corneal drying, night blindness
Vitamin E deficiency	Peripheral neuropathy, ophthalmoplegia, ataxia, hemolysis
Vitamin D deficiency	Osteopenia, rickets, fractures, reduced bone density
Vitamin K deficiency	Bruising, epistaxis, coagulopathy
Zinc deficiency	Acrodermatitis, anorexia, poor growth
Hypercholesterolemia	Xanthomata
Immunosuppression secondary to reduced cell-mediated immunity	Systemic infections

Table 3 Anthropometric Definitions in Children with Liver Disease

Acute malnutrition	Decreased weight-for-heigh Decreased triceps skinfold or midarm muscle area
Chronic malnutrition	Decreased weight-for-height
Severe malnutrition	<2 SDS below the mean <3rd percentile

SDS = Standard deviation scores (*Z*-scores), 0 = 50th percentile.

Metabolic bone disease with reduced bone density is usually observed in end-stage liver disease[69] and has been related to fat absorption rather than dietary intake.[70] Although malabsorption of vitamin D is a factor, the etiology is more complex as normal levels of vitamin D do not prevent bone demineralization.[69] Children with liver disease have a higher incidence of dental caries and enamel hypoplastic defects, which could be related to nutritional deficiency or to bone disease. They also have discolored teeth as a result of hyperbilirubinemia.[71]

Trace element and mineral deficiencies include iron deficiency with anemia and zinc deficiency, which leads to acrodermatitis, immunodeficiency, and altered protein metabolism; both zinc and selenium deficiency can exacerbate growth failure and poor protein synthesis.[2]

In the course of chronic liver failure, fat malnutrition develops first, as demonstrated by loss of fat stores. Protein malnutrition is a late development and is associated with a reduction in muscle bulk, stunting, and significant motor developmental delay. In time, children with significant malnutrition will have impaired growth and psychosocial development[72,73]; thus, malnutrition is not only an important indication for liver transplantation Severe malnutrition has a significant effect on mortality and morbidity and correlates with a prolonged hospital stay[74] and is one of the most important prognostic factors for survival post–liver transplantation.[72–75]

NUTRITIONAL ASSESSMENT

Accurate nutritional assessment is essential to the management of children with acute or chronic liver disease. It is important to start with a comprehensive clinical history, feeding history, and careful physical examination. Serial anthropometric examination is critical and can identify early malnutrition. Standard weight and height ratios are of little value in children with liver disease because of misinterpretation caused by fluid overload, ascites, and visceromegaly. Many researchers, using sophisticated methods such as whole-body potassium and dual-energy X-ray absorptiometry (DXA) scanning, have demonstrated that body weight underestimated the incidence of malnutrition by 50% in both adults and children,[3,13] and for this reason, simple methods of measuring body composition, such as body impedance analysis, are not reliable in children with liver disease.[76,77]

Thus, the assessment of malnutrition should be performed using a number of parameters, such as triceps or subscapular skinfolds, midarm circumference, and arm muscle measurements (midarm muscle area).[1,78] Triceps skinfold and midarm circumference are useful indicators of body fat and protein and serial recordings demonstrate early loss of fat stores before weight and height changes become obvious.[1,78] Although linear growth is a sensitive parameter, it is a late sign of growth failure in infancy; stunting (or negative height velocity) might not be apparent until 1 year of age (Table 3).[79]

Growth data are best expressed as standard deviation scores (or *Z*-scores) related to the median value for the child's age and sex in which the *Z*-score of 0 = 50th percentile. This is particularly useful for comparisons between centers and for evaluation of new feeds.

Biochemical evaluation of vitamin deficiency is a useful adjunct to nutritional assessment. Plasma vitamin A levels can be measured but might not reflect hepatic stores.[80] Plasma betacarotene, or the ratio of plasma retinol to retinol-binding protein, can be helpful.[80] Vitamin E deficiency is monitored by serum vitamin E levels or the ratio of vitamin E to total lipids. Vitamin D deficiency is evaluated by measuring serum levels of calcium, phosphate, and alkaline phosphatase, whereas the diagnosis of rickets is confirmed by radiographic examination of the wrist or knee. In some centers, it is possible to measure 25-hydroxyvitamin D levels. Vitamin K deficiency is usually identified by measuring coagulation times and monitoring the response to parenteral vitamin K, but a more accurate assessment can be obtained by measuring the plasma PIVKA-II (protein induced in Vitamin K absence).[50]

Acute malnutrition is evidenced by loss of weight compared to height and loss of fat stores, whereas chronic malnutrition is documented by stunting and reduction in the height-for-age index (Table 3).

INDICATIONS FOR NUTRITIONAL THERAPY

The aim of nutritional therapy is to prevent or treat malnutrition by providing adequate calories for energy and sufficient nitrogen for protein synthesis, to restore plasma amino acid imbalance, to prevent vitamin and trace element deficiency, and to achieve normal growth and activity. The need for nutritional support is often underestimated, particularly in infants with liver disease, who might have an increased appetite in the first few months of life.

Children who are at particular risk for developing malnutrition include the following:

- Children under 2 years of age who have severe cholestasis [serum bilirubin >70 mmol/L (4 mg/dL)]
- Those with progressive liver disease such as biliary atresia or severe familial intrahepatic cholestasis

- Those with end-stage liver failure awaiting liver transplantation
- Children with recurrent hepatic complications such as ascites and bleeding varices

STRATEGIES FOR NUTRITIONAL SUPPORT

Increased Energy Intake

Because the resting energy requirements of infants and children with liver disease are increased,[59] it is important to increase the energy intake to 140 to 200% of estimated average requirements. In cholestatic infants, this can be achieved by using concentrated formulas (the formula is concentrated by 13 to 15%, which increases the number of kilocalories from 67 to 80 per 100 mL) or by supplementing milk feedings with extra carbohydrate and fat to produce a feed with an energy density of 4.18 kJ/mL (1 kcal/mL or more). As such a feed can have a high osmolality (500 to 800 mmol/L), it should be introduced gradually to establish intestinal tolerance (Table 4). Caloric supplementation added to drinks can be effective for older children. If there is no response to an increase in energy intake alone, nocturnal enteral feeding by nasogastric tube might be required (Figure 1).

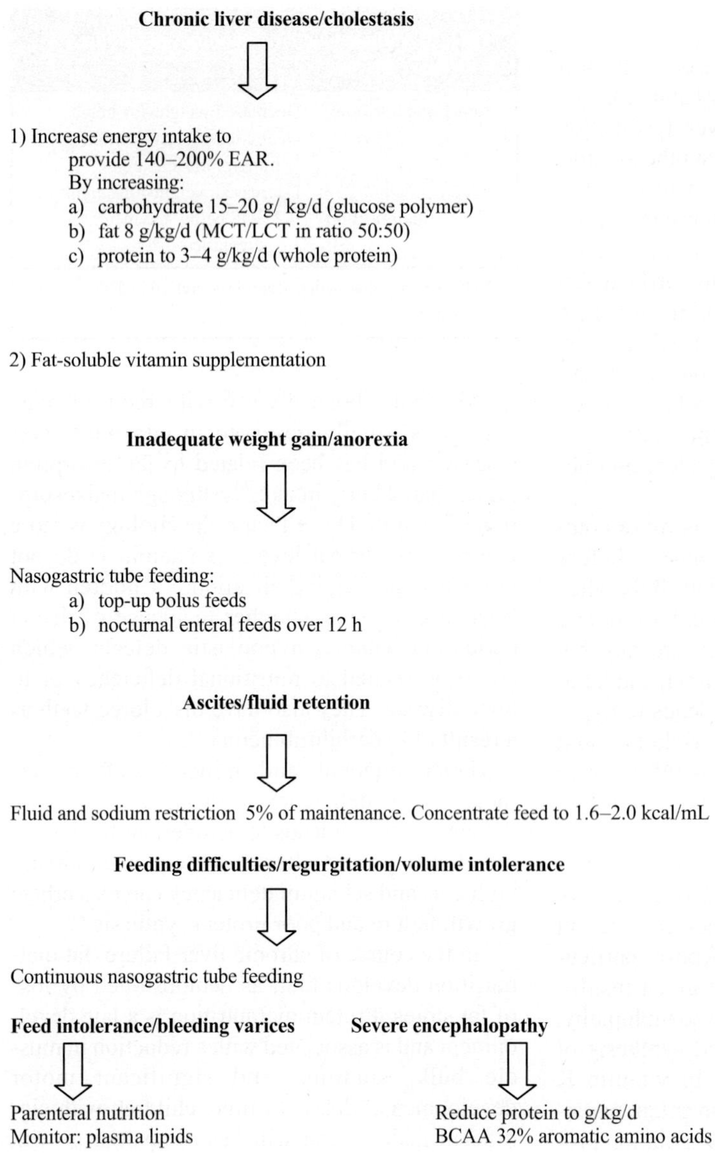

Figure 1 Nutritional support for chronic liver disease. BCAA = branched-chain amino acid; EAR = estimated average requirement; LCT = long-chain triglyceride; MCT = medium-chain triglyceride.

Medium-Chain Triglycerides

Because fat is an important calorie source, with an energy value of 8 to 9 kcal/g, it is a major source of energy for infants. Because absorption is deranged in liver disease, the fat content of the diet needs careful consideration. Low-fat diets are no longer considered appropriate, but an increase in the MCT content will reduce steatorrhea.[34,37,48] Hydrolyzed-protein infant formulas, such as Pregestimil (Mead Johnson), which contain 50% MCTs, will maximize fat absorption and improve steatorrhea,[48,81] but formulas with more than 80% MCTs can lead to essential fatty acid deficiency.[48] Although MCTs are a useful energy source, there is no evidence that growth improves with formulas with a high MTC content,[82,83] so it is necessary to increase the total fat intake with both LCTs and MCTs. This will increase the overall amount of fat absorbed and improve growth despite increasing steatorrhea.[37] In practice, this means supplementing feeds with approximately 50% MCTs with essential fatty acids. In older children, MCT oil can be added to meals and should be balanced by fats with high LCP content.

Table 4 Formulas for Children with Liver Disease*

Formula	Kcal/kJ	Protein (g)	Fat (% MCT)	Sodium (mmol)	Essential Fatty Acids (omega-6: omega-3)
Pregestimil†	68/285	1.9	55	1.26	10:1
Peptijunior‡	67/280	1.8	50	0.9	7:1
Caprilon§	66/276	1.5	75	0.8	7.5:1
Generaid Plus§	102/428	2.4	32%	0.7	4:1
MCT Pepdite§	68/285	2	75	1.5	6.9:1
MCT PEPDITE 1+	90	2.8		1.8	
Modular feed§	Flexible	Flexible	0–100	Flexible	None

*Per 100 mL.
†Mead Johnson.
‡Cow and Gate.
§Scientific Hospital supplies.
MCT = medium-chain triglyceride.

Low-Chain Polyunsaturated Fatty Acids

The malabsorption of long-chain fats in chronic liver disease means that it is important to ensure adequate intake of LCPs. The minimal intake of linoleic acid recommended for infants is 1 to 2% of energy in a ratio of linoleic to linolenic acid of 5:15.1.[41]

The LCPs, or PUFAs, can be supplemented by the addition of soybean or rapeseed oil, whereas LCP supplementation is provided in dietary products such as egg yolk (which is rich in arachidonic acid) or fish oil (which is rich in DHA). Alternatively, infants can be given conventional LCP-supplemented formulas, which are commercially available.[84]

Structured Lipids

Recently, chemically defined structured lipids have been developed to increase absorption of both medium- and long-chain and essential fatty acids.[85] These lipids combine pure MCTs with LCTs, resulting in a triglyceride that contains combinations of short-, medium-, and long-chain fatty acids on a single glycerol backbone, which should be absorbed like MCTs. To date, clinical studies in adults have evaluated structured lipids in postoperative patients receiving parenteral nutrition and demonstrated that they were safe and effective when compared to LCP emulsion.[86,87] Although clinical studies of these modified lipids in children are currently in the preliminary stages,[88] studies in rats have demonstrated improved fat absorption and reversal of essential fatty acid deficiency in vitro in caco-2 cells.[89,90] If successful, there might be considerable benefit for cholestatic infants.

Carbohydrate

Carbohydrate is a major source of energy and is particularly useful for increasing calorie intake. It can be given as a monomer, short-chain polymer, or starch, but complex carbohydrates such as maltodextrin or glucose polymer restrict the osmolality of the feed while maintaining a high-energy density of more than 1 kcal/mL. This allows fluid restriction if necessary while providing up to 20 g/k/d of carbohydrate. In infants, glucose polymers are best added to milk feeds, whereas in older children, they can be provided as supplemental drinks.

Protein

Historical advice, which restricted protein in advanced end-stage liver disease, is now considered inappropriate in both children and adults.[91,92] Children with end-stage liver disease require minimal protein intake of approximately 2 to 3 g/kg/d but will tolerate up to 4 g/kg/d without developing encephalopathy or a significant increase in plasma amino abnormalities.[93] Severe protein restriction (less than 2 g/kg/d) might be required for acute, severe encephalopathy but should be avoided in the long term as it can lead to endogenous muscle protein consumption.[59] There is no necessity to use semielemental diets or protein hydrolysates because there is no evidence of protein malabsorption.

In view of the abnormal aromatic acid-to-BCAA ratio, there has been considerable interest in the use of a modified amino acid formulation designed to improve this imbalance. Numerous studies in adults have not demonstrated a clear benefit for BCAA nutritional supplementation, despite the evidence that BCAAs did improve nitrogen retention and protein synthesis; their effect on patient outcome was not proven.[94]

The necessity for BCAA supplementation may persist posttransplant as demonstrated in a recent study in five clinically stable children, although the requirement was less than pretransplant.[95]

There is both animal and clinical evidence that suggests that BCAA-enriched formulas could have significant nutritional benefit in children. BCAAs increased weight gain, protein and muscle mass, body composition, and bone mineral density in an animal model of biliary obstruction.[86] A study that compared a feed containing 32% BCAAs with a standard feed demonstrated improved lean body mass in children awaiting liver transplantation but no improvement in amino acid levels.[97] In another study in infants with liver disease, the effect of a modified amino acid feed containing 50% BCAAs was compared with an isonitrogenous formula containing 22% BCAAs by measuring whole-body protein turnover.[60] The BCAA-supplemented feed improved protein retention when compared with the standard formula by suppressing endogenous protein catabolism and normalizing the plasma amino acid profile. Formulas rich in BCAAs, complete with MCTs and vitamin and mineral supplements, have been developed for use in infants, and oral supplements rich in BCAAs are available for older children, but both are particularly unpalatable.

Attempts to use BCAA supplementation to treat hepatic encephalopathy in adults could be of value in those patients with advanced encephalopathy,[98] but similar studies have not been performed in children.

Vitamin and Mineral Supplementation

Both water- and fat-soluble vitamins should be supplemented in children with chronic liver disease. Supplementation should be based on plasma levels of selenium, zinc, calcium, and magnesium. Iron supplementation might be required in children with chronic blood loss.

Fat-soluble vitamins are required in all children with prolonged or cholestatic liver disease (Table 5). Most children will be maintained adequately on oral fat-soluble vitamin administration, but monthly intramuscular administration is occasionally required for children with severe cholestasis.

Mode of Delivery

Nutritional supplementation should be provided enterally for as long as possible because it has a number of advantages over parenteral feeding. Not only is it cheaper and more physiologic, but it maintains gastrointestinal tract immunity, reduces bacterial overgrowth, and maintains the integrity of the gut barrier to microorganisms.[99,100] It is also essential to maintain normal feeding behavior. Few children with end-stage liver disease will be able to tolerate the increased calorie intake necessary to prevent or reverse malnutrition orally; thus, nasogastric tube feeding is indicated for children who have no nutritional response to an increase in calorie intake or who become anorexic.

Despite anxiety about using nasogastric feeding in children with esophageal varices, there is no evidence that the use of modern soft silastic nasogastric tubes is harmful. Nocturnal feeding is the method of choice because it allows calorie supplementation while maintaining normal oral feeding during the day. For infants with severe liver disease, nocturnal feeding can be beneficial because it will prevent fasting hypoglycemia and reduce protein catabolism. Continuous enteral infusion might be required in children with severe malabsorption or feed intolerance. Intensive enteral nasogastric feeding has effectively reversed malnutrition in infants and children with liver disease and can transform the child's affect and increase voluntary intake.[37,93,101] Under normal circumstances, it should be possible to provide nocturnal or continuous nasogastric feeding at home with appropriate support from a nutritional care team including a dietitian, a liaison nurse, and clinicians.

Gastrostomy tube placements might be preferable in older children but should be avoided in children with severe portal hypertension because of the development of stomal varices. In children with stable compensated liver disease (eg, cystic

Table 5 Assessment and Management of Nutritional Deficiency in Pediatric Liver Disease

Deficit	Investigation	Investigation
Energy	Calorie intake, energy expenditure (body cell mass [TBK], DXA)	Increase calorie intake, achieve 130–150% EAR, nocturnal enteral nutrition, continuous enteral nutrition
Protein	Plasma proteins (albumin), BCAA/AAA ratio, protein stores (muscle mass, TBN)	Provide adequate protein, (3–4 g/kg/d), BCAA-enriched protein (32%), albumin infusion (if serum albumin < 25 g/L)
Fat	Triceps skinfolds, body composition, EFA deficiency, plasma lipid profile	Improve fat absorption (MCT/LCT, 50:50), provide saturated fats high in EFA, supplement DHA
Fat-soluble vitamins	Plasma 25-OH-D (skeletal X-rays, DXA), prothrombin time [(< 138 c) INR = 1], plasma vitamin E and A	Light exposure, vitamin D-1-a (50 ng/kg), vitamin K (2.5–5 mg/d), vitamin E (50–400 IU/day as TPGS), vitamin A (5,000–10,000 IU/d)
Water-soluble count vitamins	Specific levels, blood	Supplement as requested
Minerals	Specific levels, cardiac evaluation	Supplement as requested

AAA = aromatic amino acids; BCAA = branched chain amino acids; DHA = docosahexaenoic acid; DXA = dual-energy X-ray absorptiometry; EAR = estimated average requirement; EFA = essential fatty acids; INR = international normalized ratio; LCT = long-chain fatty acids; MCT = medium-chain fatty acids; TBK = total body potassium; TBN = total body nitrogen; TPGS = tocopherol polyethylene glycol-1000 succinate.

fibrosis), percutaneous endoscopic gastrostomy might be beneficial.

Growth Hormone Therapy

In view of the disruption of the growth hormone/IGF-I axis, it is tempting to prescribe growth hormone therapy for children with significant growth failure, but this has not proven beneficial in two studies of its use in children with end-stage liver disease.[102,103]

Parenteral Nutrition

In view of the well-recognized hepatobiliary complications that occur in premature infants with short-gut syndrome or intestinal failure, parenteral nutrition has been used cautiously in children with liver disease. Particular concern has focused on whether the potentially toxic components of parenteral nutrition could be exacerbated in children with established chronic liver disease or cholestasis. There is no evidence that amino acids, carbohydrates, or lipid emulsions are any more toxic in children with established liver disease, although amino acid levels and plasma lipids need careful monitoring.

Although aluminum toxicity is well recognized in parenteral nutrition and can lead to bone disease, there is no evidence that it is implicated in parenteral nutrition liver disease or that it exacerbates the metabolic bone disease associated with chronic liver disease.[104,105] In contrast, chromium toxicity has been reported in animals on parenteral nutrition. Although both serum and urine chromium levels are higher in children on long-term parenteral nutrition, there is no correlation with liver disease.[106]

Manganese toxicity in children on long-term parenteral nutrition has recently been reported, however.[107–109] Although 79% of children on long-term parenteral nutrition had whole-blood manganese concentrations above the reference range, children with impaired liver function had the highest manganese levels. There was a significant correlation between whole-blood manganese levels, aspartate amino transferase ($r = .63, p = < .001$), and total plasma bilirubin ($r = .64, p = < .001$). Eleven children had both high manganese levels and cholestasis; four of these died. In the seven survivors, whole-blood manganese declined when the supplements were reduced or withdrawn. Although manganese is toxic to both brain and liver, it is not clear whether the high manganese levels led to cholestasis or were secondary to it because manganese is excreted in the bile. Nevertheless, it is likely that manganese toxicity exacerbates cholestasis in children with established liver disease; thus, monitoring of manganese levels is particularly important in this group.[110]

In general, the use of parenteral nutrition in children with established liver disease is for short-term purposes only; thus, they are unlikely to develop biliary sludge and gallstones from the prescription of parenteral nutrition alone,[111,112] although prescription of ursodeoxycholic acid (15 to 20 mg/kg) might be of value.[113]

Parenteral nutrition should be considered in children with chronic liver disease only if they cannot be enterally fed because of feed intolerance or secondary to complications such as recurrent variceal bleeding or abdominal sepsis. As stated above, there is no evidence that short-term parenteral nutrition is associated with hepatobiliary dysfunction or an increase in cholestasis; it can improve nutritional status in the short term. Standard amino acid and lipid solutions are well tolerated in stable patients, and lipids can be particularly beneficial in achieving adequate calorie intake. If encephalopathy develops, the amino acid content of the feed can be reduced to 1 to 2 g/kg/d; lipid administration requires careful monitoring in children with severe liver dysfunction, hepatic encephalopathy, or sepsis.

Although MCT emulsions have been suggested for adults with advanced liver failure, intravenous MCTs should be used with caution in children because incomplete oxidation can occur, producing metabolic acidosis.[114] Parenteral structural lipid emulsions have not yet been evaluated in children.

The use of parenteral nutrition is particularly important for children with acute fulminant hepatitis who are awaiting liver transplantation because they are hypercatabolic. Standard formulas should be used, although the volume needs to be restricted to 75% of maintenance and the concentration should be increased to maintain glucose levels (>4 mmol/L). There is no need to reduce protein content, particularly if the patient is electively ventilated. As indicated above, intravenous use of BCAAs for the treatment of hepatic encephalopathy or coma has not been evaluated in children, although they can be of value in adults.

Behavioral Feeding Problems

Behavioral feeding problems are common in this group of children, particularly in infants who have had long-term nasogastric feeding. Feeding problems are compounded by the use of unpalatable feeds, medications, and excess parental anxiety about feeding and growth.

Strategies to prevent behavior problems include daytime feeding to provide oral stimulation and encouraging children to experiment with flavors and textures appropriate to their age. The success of these techniques is dependent on a multidisciplinary approach involving a clinician, nurse specialist, dietitian, clinical psychologist, speech therapist, and play therapist.[37]

SPECIFIC DISEASE STATES

Acute Liver Disease

Most children with acute viral or autoimmune hepatitis require no nutritional supplementation. Fulminant hepatic failure requires careful management of protein to prevent hepatic encephalopathy and to reduce excess protein catabolism. Protein should be restricted only for short periods of time to treat severe encephalopathy (see above). Fluid volume can be reduced to prevent or treat cerebral edema; it is critical to maintain adequate glucose levels by infusing 6 to 8 mg/kg/min of glucose to prevent hypoglycemia. Enteral nutrition should be continued as long as the child is conscious and in the early stages of elective ventilation. Once the requirement for liver transplantation becomes obvious, parenteral nutrition should be started to provide sufficient calories to prevent additional protein catabolism (see above).

Chronic Liver Disease

The majority of children with chronic liver disease will have cholestasis, either from biliary atresia, Alagille syndrome, or familial intrahepatic cholestasis and should be managed as indicated above. Children who are not jaundiced require similar support, although their requirement for fat-soluble vitamin supplementation will be less.

Problems can arise with children who have ascites and fluid retention; fluid restriction might be required. In these circumstances, modular feeds, which allow individual prescription of protein, sodium, and water and to which complex carbohydrate polymers, fats, vitamins, and mineral are added to produce a highly energy-dense feed, can be of value.

Inborn Errors of Metabolism

A number of inborn errors of metabolism rely on dietary modification as part of therapy. These include galactosemia, hereditary fructose intolerance, and tyrosinemia type I.

Galactosemia is an autosomal recessive disorder in which there is a reduction in the enzyme activity of galactose-1-phosphate uridyl transferase, which prevents the conversion of galactose to glucose. Dietary treatment includes removing all products containing galactose (ie, milk and milk products).[115]

Hereditary fructose intolerance is an autosomal recessive disorder caused by a deficiency or absence of the enzyme aldolase B, which leads to cirrhosis and renal tubular disorders. Dietary management consists of elimination of fructose, sucrose, and sorbitol from the diet; this must be maintained for life. This means that all fruit and fruit juices are eliminated from the diet and only certain vegetables are permitted. Commercial products such as breads and cereals can also contain small amounts of sucrose, as can medications and toothpaste.[116]

Tyrosinemia type I is an autosomal recessive disorder caused by a defect in the enzyme fumarylacetoacetase, which leads to hypertrophic cardiomyopathy, cirrhosis, and renal tubular acidosis. For many years, dietary treatment was the only method of therapy and included restriction of phenylalanine, tyrosine, and methionine. Although restriction of these amino acids was effective in normalizing plasma amino acids, it did not prevent the progression of liver failure or the development of metabolic crises. The development of NTBC (2-[2-nitro-4-trifluoromethylbenzoyl]-1,3-cyclohexenedione) in association with dietary treatment has altered the natural history and outcome of the disease.[117]

Glycogen Storage Disease

The hepatic glycogen storage disorders are a group of autosomal recessive inherited disorders that lead to defects in the metabolism of glycogen. Liver and skeletal muscle are usually affected but heart, kidney, bones, and brain can also be involved. The presentation and biochemical features depend on the precise enzyme deficiency. Nevertheless, the treatment is dietary: to provide a continuous supply of exogenous glucose, either intravenously or enterally, to maintain normal glucose, and to suppress counterregulatory responses. In infants this is best achieved by frequent daytime feedings or continuous nocturnal enteral glucose feeding. In older children, the oral feeding of uncooked cornstarch (1 to 2 g/kg every 4 hours), which is hydrolyzed in the gut to release glucose slowly, can reduce the need for frequent daytime feedings or continuous nocturnal feeding.[116] Glycogen storage disease type III requires similar treatment but with a higher protein intake (3 g/kg). In most instances, dietary management is successful and can prevent the long-term complications of these diseases.

PREPARATION FOR LIVER TRANSPLANTATION

Liver transplantation is indicated for both acute and chronic liver failure. Nutritional support is of particular importance for children with chronic liver failure because malnutrition is a significant risk factor for mortality and morbidity related to liver transplantation.[72,75,76]

Chin and colleagues prospectively studied 26 children pre- and posttransplantation. They identified a significant difference in the 2-year actual survival for children with standard deviation scores (SDS) for weight of greater than –1 (57%) compared with those with scores less than –1 (95%) at the time of transplantation.[76] Similar data were obtained from Moukarzel and colleagues using height SDS. Children who were less stunted (height SDS <-1) had less morbidity and mortality (91% 1-year survival) compared with those who were more stunted (height SDS >-1), who had a 1-year survival rate of 75%[72] These data have recently been confirmed in a study that evaluated a number of risk factors, including malnutrition, in infants undergoing liver transplantation.[75] and in a separate study which correlated morbidity and prolonged hospital stay with malnutrition.[74]

Children awaiting liver transplantation require intensive nutritional support, depending on the etiology of their liver failure, as documented above, but the main principle is to provide a sufficient energy intake (Table 6).

Table 6 Nutritional Support in Children Before and After Liver Transplantation

Requirement	Preoperative	Postoperative
Carbohydrate	Glucose polymer 15–20	Glucose polymer 6–8 (g/kg/d)
Protein (g/kg/d)	Low-salt protein 3–4	Whole protein 2.5–3
Fat (g/kg/d)	50–70% medium-chain triglyceride 8	Long-chain triglyceride 5–6
Energy intake (estimated average requirement)	130–150%	120%

EFFECT OF LIVER TRANSPLANTATION ON NUTRITIONAL STATUS

Many recent studies have documented the nutritional rehabilitation achieved by successful liver transplantation.[5,76,79,118]

Following liver transplantation, surviving children experience a rapid return to normal midarm muscle area and midarm fat within 3 to 6 months.[79,118] Initial weight gain can be rapid because of the effects of corticosteroids on appetite and salt and water retention, but most children return to a normal weight once corticosteroids are reduced or discontinued. Linear growth is often delayed by 6 to 24 months, depending on the rate of hepatic complications and the withdrawal or reduction of corticosteroids.[119–121]

Preoperative nutritional status has a strong influence on posttransplantation growth. Children who were less stunted at transplantation grew slowly initially but finally achieved normal growth velocity, whereas older children who were more stunted (height SDS >-2) grew more quickly initially posttransplantation but did not achieve normal height.[122,123] There are no differences in catch-up growth between the sexes or with pretransplantation disease, apart from Alagille syndrome, which is associated with growth failure before and after transplantation in 50% of patients.[124,125]

Although successful liver transplantation reverses most aspects of malnutrition, it can be some months or years before bone density returns to normal. Persistent osteoporosis and bone fractures have been described at 3 to 6 months following transplantation[126] and were exacerbated by the effects of corticosteroid therapy. Clinical studies to evaluate the use of bisphosphonates in the treatment of metabolic bone disease before and after transplantation are under evaluation.

Likewise, it may take some time before long-chain PUFA and BCAA metabolism return to normal[46,95] and these factors should be taken into consideration when planning posttransplant nutrition.

EFFECT OF GROWTH HORMONE AND INSULIN-LIKE GROWTH FACTOR

As indicated earlier, both growth hormone and IGF-I are necessary for normal growth, and it has been shown that plasma IGF-I levels are low in children with chronic liver disease, despite elevated serum growth hormone. Although posttransplantation IGF-I and IGF-BP3 rise significantly and IGF levels return to normal, abnormalities in the IGF-binding proteins BP1, BP2, and BP3 remain for some months.[54]

PREVENTION OF GROWTH FAILURE AFTER TRANSPLANTATION

The nutritional strategy for the prevention of growth failure before and after liver transplantation begins with intensive nutritional support preoperatively. Children who are malnourished before transplantation should be maintained with parenteral nutrition perioperatively until normal nutrition is resumed, whereas children with normal nutritional status should start enteral feeding with a rapid buildup of calorie intake 3 to 5 days following transplantation.

It is important to ensure sufficient energy intake (at least 120% of estimated average requirement) following the operation. This can be provided as a modular feed or supplemental nocturnal enteral nasogastric formula feedings in infants who refuse oral feeding and as diet in older children with calorie supplements. The energy intake should include 2.5 to 3 g protein/d and glucose polymer (6 to 8 g/kg/d), but fat can now be provided entirely as long-chain fat (5 to 6 g/kg/d) unless cholestasis secondary to chronic rejection is a complication (Table 6).[127]

Glucocorticoids, used to prevent organ rejection, interfere with growth hormone excretion. As growth hormone, IGF-I, IGF-BP1, IGF-BP2, and IGF-BP3 remain abnormal following transplantation, it is rational to consider whether growth hormone therapy might be helpful. Recombinant human growth hormone has been evaluated in eight growth-retarded children following liver transplantation.[128] The median growth rate increased from 3.2 to 7.1 cm/yr (p = .025) and height SDSs increased from –2.9 to –3.1 (p = .036) during the first year of growth hormone treatment. Both IGF-I and insulin IGF-BP3 levels increased significantly during treatment. There was no effect on graft function, and no child developed rejection or any other complication, but growth velocity was not maintained beyond the first year.

CONCLUSION

The essential role of the liver in energy and growth has particular relevance for infants and children with end-stage liver failure. Considerable progress has been made in understanding the pathophysiology of malnutrition in liver disease, and this has improved our ability to support these children. Nutritional rehabilitation has been achieved by intensive nutritional support, and mortality following liver transplantation has been reduced. Its success depends on a multidisciplinary approach based on early intervention and prevention of malnutrition.

REFERENCES

1. Sokal RJ, Stall C. Anthropometric evaluation of children with chronic liver disease. Am J Clin Nutr 1990;52:203–8.
2. Chin SE, Shepherd RW, Thomas BJ, et al. The nature of malnutrition in children with end stage liver disease. Am J Clin Nutr 1992;56:164–8.
3. Trocki O, Wotton MJ, Cleghorn GJ, et al. Value of total body potassium in assessing the nutritional status of children with end-stage liver disease. Ann N Y Acad Sci 2000;904:400–5.
4. Kaufman SS, Murray ND, Wood RP, et al. Nutritional support for the infant with extrahepatic biliary atresia. J Pediatr 1987;110:679–86.
5. Beath S, Pearmain G, Kelly D, et al. Liver transplantation in babies and children with extra hepatic biliary atresia: Preoperative condition, complications, survival and outcome. J Pediatr Surg 1993;28:1044–7.
6. Novy MA, Schwarz KB. Nutritional considerations and management of the child with liver disease. Nutrition 1997;13:177–84.
7. Roggero P, Cataliotti E, Ulla L, et al. Factors influencing malnutrition in children waiting for liver transplants. Am J Clin Nutr 1997;65:1852–7.
8. Romijn JA, Endert E, Sauerwein HP. Glucose and fat metabolism during short term starvation in cirrhosis. Gastroenterology 1991;100:731–7.
9. Hellerstein MK, Munro HN. Interaction of liver, muscle and adipose tissue in the regulation of metabolism in response to nutritional and other factors. In: Arias IM, editor. The Liver: Biology and Pathobiology, 3rd edition. New York: Raven Press; 1994. p. 1169–91.
10. Felig P, Brown V, Levine RA, et al. Glucose homeostasis in viral hepatitis. N Engl J Med 1970;283:1436–40.
11. Petrides AS, Defronzo RA. Glucose and insulin metabolism in cirrhosis. J Hepatol 1989;8:107–14.
12. Nielson MF, Caumo A, Aagaard NK, et al. Contribution of defects in glucose uptake to carbohydrate intolerance in liver cirrhosis: Assessment during physiological glucose and insulin concentration. Am J Gastrointest Liver Physiol 2005;288:G1135–43.
13. Cabre E, Gassull MA. Nutritional issues in cirrhosis and liver transplantation. Curr Opin Clin Nutr Metab Care 1999;2:373–80.
14. Petrides AS, Strohmeyer G, DeFronzo RA. Insulin resistance in liver disease and portal hypertension. Prog Liver Dis 1992;10:311–28.
15. Yudkoff M, Nissin I, McNellis W, et al. Albumin synthesis in premature infants: Determination of turnover with (15N) glycine. Pediatr Res 1987;21:49–53.
16. Miller LL. The role of the liver and the non-hepatic tissues in the regulation of free amino acid levels in the blood. In: Holden JI, editor. Amino Acid Pools. Amsterdam: Elsevier; 1962. p. 708–9.
17. Powers Lee SG, Meister L. Urea synthesis and ammonia metabolism. In: Arias M, Jakoby WB, Popper H, et al., editors. The Liver: Biology and Pathobiology. New York: Raven Press; 1988. p. 317–30.
18. McCullough AJ, Mullen KD, Smanik EJ, et al. Nutritional therapy and liver disease. Gastroenterol Clin North Am 1989; 18:619–43.
19. Weisdorf SA, Freese DK, Fath JJ, et al. Amino acid abnormalities in infants with extrahepatic biliary atresia and cirrhosis. J Pediatr Gastroenterol Nutr 1987;6:860–4.
20. Protheroe S, Jones R, Kelly DA. Evaluation of the role of branched chain amino acids in the treatment of protein malnutrition in infants with liver disease [abstract]. Gut 1995; 37:A30.
21. Weisdorf SA. Nutrition in liver disease. In: Lebenthal E, editor. Textbook of Gastroenterology and Nutrition in Infancy, 2nd edition. New York: Raven Press; 1993. p. 665–76.
22. Casccino A, Cangiano C, Calcaterra V, et al. Plasma amino acid imbalance in patients with liver disease. Am J Dig Dis 1978;23:591–8.
23. Blonde-Cynober F, Aussel C, Cynober L. Abnormalities in branched-chain amino acid metabolism in cirrhosis: Influence of hormonal and nutritional factors and directions for future research. Clin Nutr 1999;18:5–13.
24. Tessari P, Barazzoni R, Biolo G, et al. Response of phenylalanine and leucine kinetics to branched chain-enriched amino acids and insulin in patients with cirrhosis. Gastroenterology 1996;111:252–5.
25. Dichi I, Dichi JB, Papini-Berto SJ, et al. Protein-energy status and 15N-glycine kinetic study of a child, a cirrhotic patient fed low to high protein energy diets. Nutrition 1996;12:519–23.
26. Kondrup J, Nielsen K, Juul A. Effect of long-term refeeding on protein metabolism in patients with cirrhosis of the liver. Br J Nutr 1997;77:197–212.
27. Protheroe S, McNurlan M, Garlick P, et al. Failure to suppress protein breakdown contributes towards malnutrition in infants with liver disease [abstract]. Hepatology 1996;24:141A.
28. Mager DR, Wykes LJ, Roberts EA, et al. Mild to moderate chronic cholestatic liver disease increases leucin oxidation in children. J Nutr 2006;136:965–70.
29. Kelly DA, Summerfield JA. Hemostasis in liver disease. Semin Liver Dis 1987;7:182–91.
30. Wion KL, Kelly DA, Summerfield JA, et al. Distribution of factor VIII mRNA and antigen in human liver and other tissues. Nature 1985;317:726–9.
31. Van Dyke RW. Mechanisms of digestion and absorption of food. In: Sleisenger MH, Fordtran JS, editors. Gastrointestinal Disease, Pathophysiology, Diagnosis, Management, 4th edition. Philadelphia: WB Saunders Co; 1989. p. 1062–88.
32. Carey M, Small DM, Bliss CM. Lipid digestion and absorption. Annu Rev Physiol 1983;45:651–77.
33. Greenberger NJ, Skillman TG. Medium chain triglycerides. N Engl J Med 1969;280:1045–58.
34. Glasgow JFT, Hamilton JR, Sass-Kortsak A. Fat absorption in congenital obstructive liver disease. Arch Dis Child 1973;48:601–7.
35. Phan CT, Tso CS. Intestinal lipid absorption and transport. Front Biosci 2001;6:D299–319.
36. Beath S, Hooley I, Willis K, et al. Long chain triacyglycerol malabsorption and pancreatic function in children with protein energy malnutrition complicating severe liver disease [abstract]. Proc Nutr Soc 1993;52:252A.
37. Beath SV, Kelly DA, Booth IW. Nutritional support in liver disease. Arch Dis Child 1993;69:545–9.
38. Chong SKF, Lindridge J, Moniz C, et al. Exocrine pancreatic insufficiency in syndromic paucity of interlobular bile ducts. J Pediatr Gastroenterol Nutr 1989;9:445–9.
39. Makrides M, Neuman M, Simmer K, et al. Are long-chain polyunsaturated fatty acids essential nutrients in infancy? Lancet 1995;345:1463–8.
40. Koletzko B, Thiel I, Springer S. Lipids in human milk: A model for infant formulae? Eur J Clin Nutr 1992;46:S45–55.
41. Koletzko B, Agostoni C, Carlson SE, et al. Long chain polyunsaturated fatty acids (LC-PUFA) and postnatal development. Acta Paediatr 2001;90:460–4.
42. Hoffman DR, Birch EE, Birch DG, et al. Effects of supplementation with omega 3 long-chain polyunsaturated fatty acids on retinal and cortical development in premature infants. Am J Clin Nutr 1993;57:807S–12S.
43. Burke PA, Ling PR, Forse RA, et al. Conditionally essential fatty acid deficiencies in end-stage liver disease. Nutrition 1999;15:302–4.
44. Cabre E, Gassull MA. Polyunsaturated fatty acid deficiency in liver diseases: Pathophysiological and clinical significance. Nutrition 1996;12:542–8.
45. Burke PA, Ling PR, Forse RA, et al. Sites of conditional essential fatty acid deficiency in end stage liver disease. J Parenter Enteral Nutr 2001;25:188–93.
46. Lapillonne A, Hakme C, Mamoux V, et al. Effects of liver transplantation on long-chain polyunsaturated fatty acid status in infants with biliary atresia. J Pediatr Gastroenterol Nutr 2000;30:528–32.
47. Spray CH, Beath SV, Willis KD, et al. Docosahexaenoic acid (DHA) and visual function in infants with fat malabsorption secondary to liver disease [abstract]. Proc Nutr Soc 1995; 54:108A.
48. Kaufman SS, Scrivener DJ, Murray ND, et al. Influence of Portagen and Pregestimil on essential fatty acid status in infantile liver disease. Pediatrics 1992;89:151–4.
49. Larque E, Zamora S, Gil A. Dietary trans fatty acids in early life: A review. Early Hum Dev 2001;65:S31–41.
50. Mager DR, McGee PL, Furuya KN, et al. Prevalence of vitamin K deficiency in children with mild to moderate chronic liver disease. J Pediatr Gastroenterol Nutr 2006;42:71–6.
51. Powell EE, Kroon PA. Liver lipoproteins and disease. II. Clinical relevance of disordered cholesterol metabolism in liver disease. J Gastroenterol Hepatol 1992;7:225–31.
52. Malatack JJ, Schald DJ, Urbach AH, et al. Choosing a paediatric recipient of orthotopic liver transplantation. J Pediatr 1987;112:479–89.
53. Quirk P, Owens P, Moyse K, et al. Insulin-like growth factors I and II are reduced in plasma from growth retarded children with chronic liver disease. Growth Regul 1994;4:35–8.
54. Holt RI, Jones JS, Stone NM, et al. Sequential changes in insulin-like growth factor (IGF-1) and IGF-binding proteins in children with end-stage liver disease before and after successful orthotopic liver transplantation. J Clin Endocrinol Metab 1996;81:160–8.
55. Ketelslegers JM, Maiter D, Maes M, et al. Nutritional regulation of insulin-like growth factor-I. Metabolism 1995;44:50–7.
56. Zamboni G, Dufillot D, Antoniazzi F, et al. Growth hormone-binding proteins and insulin-like growth factor-binding proteins in protein energy malnutrition, before and after nutritional rehabilitation. Pediatr Res 1996;39:410–4.
57. Bucuvalas JC, Horn JA, Slusher J, et al. Growth hormone insensitivity in children with biliary atresia. J Pediatr Gastroenterol Nutr 1996;23:135–40.
58. Holt RI, Miell JP, Jones JS, et al. Nasogastric feeding enhances nutritional status in paediatric liver disease but does not alter circulating levels of IGF-1 and IGF binding proteins. Clin Endocrinol 2000;52:217–24.
59. Pierro A, Koletzko B, Carnielli V, et al. Resting energy expenditure is increased in infants with extra hepatic biliary atresia and cirrhosis. J Pediatr Surg 1989;24:534–8.
60. Protheroe SM, McKiernan PJ, Kelly DA. Can measurement of dietary-induced thermogenesis (DIT) predict response to nutritional intervention in infants with liver disease? Clin Nutr 1996;15:39.
61. Greer R, Lehnert M, Lewindon P, et al. Body composition and components of energy expenditure in children with end-stage liver disease. J Pediatr Gastroenterol Nutr 2003;36:358–63.
62. Rovner AJ, Stallings VA, Piccoli DA, et al. Resting energy expenditure is not increased in prepubertal children with Alagille syndrome. J Pediatr 2006;148:680–2.
63. Rossouw JE, Labadarous D, Davis M, et al. Water soluble vitamins in severe liver disease. S Afr Med J 1978;54:183–90.
64. Mourey MS, Siegenthaler G, Amed EE, et al. Regulation of metabolism of retinal binding protein by vitamin A in children with biliary atresia. Am J Clin Nutr 1990;51:638–43.
65. Guggenheim MA, Ringel SP, Silverman A, et al. Progressive neuromuscular disease in children with chronic cholestasis and vitamin E deficiency. J Pediatr 1982;100:51–7.
66. Sokol RJ, Heubi JE, Iannacone ST, et al. Mechanism causing vitamin E deficiency during chronic childhood cholestasis. Gastroenterology 1983;85:1172–82.
67. Hope PL, Hall MA, Millward-Sadler GH. a1-antitrypsin deficiency presenting as a bleeding diathesis in the newborn. Arch Dis Child 1982;57:69–79.
68. Yanofskyi RA, Jackson VG, Lilly JR, et al. The multiple coagulopathies of biliary atresia. Am J Hematol 1984;16:171–80.
69. Argao EA, Balistreri WF, Hollis BW, et al. Effect of orthotopic liver transplantation on bone mineral content and serum vitamin D metabolites in infants and children with chronic cholestasis. Hepatology 1994;20:598–603.
70. Olsen IE, Ittenbach RF, Rovner AJ, et al. Deficits in size-adjusted bone mass in children with Alagille syndrome. J Pediatr Gastroenterol Nutr 2005;4076–82
71. Hosey MT. Dental care of children with liver disease. In: Kelly DA, editor. Diseases of the Liver and Biliary System in Children. Oxford: Blackwell Science; 1999. p. 241–52.
72. Moukarzel AA, Najm I, Vargas J, et al. Effect of nutritional status on outcome of orthotopic liver transplantation in pediatric patients. Transplant Proc 1990;22:1560–3.
73. Wayman KL, Cox KL, Esquivel CO. Neurodevelopmental out-come of young children with extrahepatic biliary atresia after liver transplantation. J Pediatr 1997;131:894–7.
74. Barshes NR, Chang IF, Karpen SJ, et al. Impact of pretransplant growth retardation in pediatric liver transplantation. J Pediatr Gastroenterol Nutr 2006;43:89–94.
75. Rodeck B, Melter M, Kardorff R, et al. Liver transplantation in children with chronic end stage liver disease; factors influencing survival after transplantation. Transplantation 1996;62:1071–6.
76. Chin SE, Shepherd RW, Cleghorn GJ, et al. Survival, growth and quality of life in children after orthotopic liver transplantation: A 5 year experience. J Pediatr Child Health 1991;27:380–5.
77. Holt TL, Cui CT, Thomas BJ, et al. Clinical applicability of bioelectric impedance as a measure of body composition in health and disease. Nutrition 1994;10:21–4.
78. Shepherd RW, Chin SE, Cleghorn GJ, et al. Malnutrition in children with chronic liver disease accepted for liver transplantation: Clinical profile and effect on outcome. J Pediatr Child Health 1991;27:295–9.

79. Van Mourik IDM. Long term nutrition and neurodevelopmental outcome of liver transplantation in infants aged less than 12 months. J Pediatr Gastroenterol Nutr 2000;30:269–76.
80. Amedee-Manesme O, Furr HC, Alvarez F, et al. Biochemical indicators of vitamin A depletion in children with cholestasis. Hepatology 1985;5:1143–8.
81. Hochman J, Balistreri WF. In: Balistreri WF, Ohi R, Todani T, Tsuchida Y, editors. Neonatal Cholestasis: Differential Diagnosis, Evaluation and Management in Hepatobiliary, Pancreatic and Splenic Disease in Children. Amsterdam: Elsevier Science; 1997. p. 157–93.
82. Beath SV, Johnson S, Willis KD, et al. Growth and luminal fat solubilisation in cholestatic infants on medium chain triglyceride (MCT) [abstract]. J Pediatr Gastroenterol Nutr 1996;22:443.
83. Pettei MJ, Daftary S, Levine JJ. Essential fatty acid deficiency associated with the use of a medium-chain-triglyceride infant formula in paediatric hepatobiliary disease. Am J Clin Nutr 1991;53:1217–21.
84. Socha P, Koletzko B, Jankowska I, et al. LCP-supplementation in infants with cholestasis. J Pediatr Gastroenterol Nutr 2000;30:528–32.
85. Stein J. Chemically defined structured lipids: Current status and future directions in gastrointestinal diseases. Int J Colorectal Dis 1999;14:79–85.
86. Bellantone R, Bossola M, Carriero C, et al. Structured versus long-chain triglycerides: A safety, tolerance, and efficacy randomised study in colorectal surgical patients. JPEN J Parenter Enteral Nutr 1999;23:123–7.
87. Sandstrom R, Hyltander A, Korner U, et al. Structured triglycerides were well tolerated and induced increased whole body fat oxidation compared with long-chain triglycerides in postoperative patients. JPEN J Parenter Enteral Nutr 1995;19:381–6.
88. Carnielli VP, Luijendijk IHT, Van Goudoever JB, et al. Structural position and amount of palmitic acid in infant formulas: Effects on fat, fatty acid and mineral balance. J Pediatr Gastroenterol Nutr 1996;23:553–60.
89. Spalinger JH, Seidman EG, Lepage G, et al. Uptake and metabolism of structured triglyceride by caco-2 cells: Reversal of essential fatty acid deficiency. Am J Physiol 1998;275:G652–9.
90. Straarup EM, Hoy CE. Structured lipids improve fat absorption in normal and malabsorbing rats. J Nutr 2000;130:2802–8.
91. Lochs H, Plauth M. Liver cirrhosis: Rationale and modalities for nutritional support—the European Socicty of Parenteral and Enteral Nutrition consensus and beyond. Curr Opin Clin Nutr Metab Care 1999;2:345–9.
92. Protheroe SM. Feeding the child with chronic liver disease. Nutrition 1998;4:796–800.
93. Charlton CPJ, Buchanan E, Holden C, et al. The use of enteral feeding in the dietary management of children with chronic liver disease. Arch Dis Child 1992;67:603–7.
94. Platell C, Kong SE, McCauley R, et al. Branched-chain amino acids. J Gastroenterol Hepatol 2000;15:706–17.
95. Mager DR, Wykes LJ, Roberts EA, et al. Effect of orthotopic liver transplantation (OLT) on branded-chain amino acid requirement. Pediatr Res 2006;59:829–34.
96. Sokal EM, Baudoux MC, Collette E, et al. Branched chain amino acids improve body composition and nitrogen balance in a rat model of extra-hepatic biliary atresia. Pediatr Res 1996;40:66–71.
97. Chin SE, Shepherd RW, Thomas BJ, et al. Nutritional support in children with end-stage liver disease: A randomised crossover trial of a branched-chain amino acid supplement. Am J Clin Nutr 1992;56:158–63.
98. Mizock BA. Nutritional support in hepatic encephalopathy. Nutrition 1999;15:220–8.
99. Parker P, Stroop S, Greene H. A controlled comparison of continuous versus intermittent feeding in the treatment of infants with intestinal disease. J Pediatr 1981;99:360–3.
100. Stringer MD, Puntis JWL. Short bowel syndrome. Arch Dis Child 1995;73:170–3.
101. M oreno LA, Gottrand F, Hoden S, et al. Improvement of nutritional status in cholestatic children with supplemental nocturnal enteral nutrition. J Pediatr Gastroenterol Nutr 1991;12:213–6.
102. Bucuvalas JC, Cutfield W, Horn J, et al. Resistance to the growth promoting in metabolic effect of GH in children with chronic liver disease. J Pediatr 1990;117:397–402.
103. Bucuvalas JC, Horn JA, Chernausek SD. Resistance to growth hormone in children with chronic liver disease. Pediatr Transplant 1997;1:73–9.
104. Moreno A, Guez C, Ballibriga A. Aluminium in the neonate related to parenteral nutrition. Acta Paediatr 1994;83:25–7.
105. Rabinow BE, Ericson S, Shellgren T. Aluminium in parenteral products: Analysis, reduction and implications for paediatric TPN. J Parenter Sci Technol 1989;43:132–6.
106. Bougle D, Beaureax F, Deschrepel G, et al. Chromium and parenteral nutrition in children. J Pediatr Gastroenterol Nutr 1993;17:72–5.
107. Reynolds AP, Kiely E, Meadows N. Manganese in long term paediatric parenteral nutrition. Arch Dis Child 1994;71:527–9.
108. Fell JME, Reynolds AP, Meadows N, et al. Manganese toxicity in children receiving long-term parenteral nutrition. Lancet 1996;347:1218–20.
109. Huang C, Chu N, Lu C. Chronic manganese intoxication. Arch Neurol 1989;46:1014–8.
110. Plaa GL, Delamirande E, Lewittes M, et al. Liver cell plasma lipids in manganese-bilirubin induced intrahepatic cholestasis. Biochem Pharmacol 1982;31:3698–703.
111. Messing B, Bories C, Kunstlinger F, et al. Does total parenteral nutrition induce gallbladder sludge formation and lithiasis? Gastroenterology 1983;84:1012–5.
112. Lirosa F, Vaja S, Murphy GM, et al. Cholestasis of total parenteral nutrition: Bile acid and bile lipid metabolism in parenterally nourished rats. Gastroenterology 1989;96:493–6.
113. Linco PD, Burnes J. Ursodeoxycholic acid for the treatment of home parenteral nutrition-associated cholestasis. A case report. Gastroenterology 1991;101:250–4.
114. Glynn MJ, Powell-Tuck J, Reaveley DA, et al. High lipid parenteral nutrition improves port-systemic encephalopathy. JPEN J Parenter Enteral Nutr 1988;12:457–61.
115. Wenz E. Galactosemia. In: Ekvall SW, editor. Pediatric Nutrition in Chronic Diseases and Developmental Disorders. New York: Oxford Univ. Press; 1993. p. 363–79.
116. Green A, Kelly DA. Metabolic liver disease in older children. In: Kelly DA, editor. Diseases of the Liver and Biliary System in Children. Oxford: Blackwell Science; 1999. p. 157–66.
117. Lindstedt S, Holme E, Lock EA, et al. Treatment of hereditary tyrosinaemia type I by inhibition of 4-hydroxyphenylpyruvate dioxygenase. Lancet 1992;340:813–7.
118. Holt RI, Broide E, Buchanan CR, et al. Orthotopic liver transplantation reverses the adverse nutritional changes of end-stage liver disease in children. Am J Clin Nutr 1997;65:534–42.
119. Codoner-Franch P, Bernard O, Alvarez F. Long-term follow-up growth in height after successful liver transplantation. J Pediatr 1994;124:368–73.
120. Rodeck B, Melter M, Hoyer PF, et al. Growth in long-term survivors after orthotopic liver transplantation in childhood. Transplant Proc 1994;26:165–6.
121. McKiernan PJ, Pearmin GD, Johnson T, et al. Catch up growth in children following orthotopic liver transplantation. Hepatology 1992;16:567.
122. Sarna S, Sipila I, Jalanko H, et al. Factors affecting growth after pediatric liver transplantation. Transplant Proc 1994;26:161–4.
123. Bartosh SM, Thomas SE, Sutton MM, et al. Linear growth after pediatric liver transplantation. J Pediatr 1999;135:624–31.
124. Cardona J, Houssin D, Gauthier F, et al. Liver transplantation in children with Alagille syndrome—a study of twelve cases. Transplantation 1995;60:339–42.
125. Quiros-Tejeira RE, Ament ME, Heyman MB, et al. Does liver transplantation affect growth pattern in Alagille syndrome? Liver Transpl 2000;6:582–7.
126. Hill SA, Kelly DA, John PR. Bone fractures in children under-going orthotopic liver transplantation. Pediatr Radiol 1995;25:s112–7.
127. Kelly DA. Posttransplant growth failure in children. Liver Transpl Surg 1997;3:S32–9.
128. Sarna S, Sipila I, Ronnholm K, et al. Recombinant human growth hormone improves growth in children receiving glucocorticoid treatment after liver transplantation. J Clin Endocrinol Metab 1996;81:1476–82.

Cancer Prevention

Erika K. Nakamoto, MS
A. Lindsay Frazier, MD, ScM

INTRODUCTION

Cancer is undeniably a disease with an established genetic basis, but the field of epidemiology has shown that the development of cancer is the result of an interaction between genes and the environment. A simple example are migrant studies that show an increase in cancer risk in the second generation after migration but not in the first generation, theoretically after sufficient exposure to the environment of the new country has taken place. These studies strongly suggest that it is environment that modifies underlying genetic risk. Diet has long been postulated to one of the most important environmental factors in the etiology of cancer.[1]

Pinpointing exactly which elements of diet are implicated in the pathogenesis of cancer is complicated; diet itself is inherently complex and can simultaneously contain both cancer-promoting and cancer-preventing substances. Moreover, diet does not occur in a vacuum but takes place in the context of other human behaviors, and these other risk factors must be collectively taken into account. Precise measurement of diet is challenging due to the day-to-day variability in consumption; measurement is also dependent on the accurate recall and estimation by the individual (see Chapter 16, "Nutritional Epidemiology," for details). Finally, the critical time of the exposure may vary by type of cancer. For instance, in the case of breast cancer, the theory has advanced to the following: There is a critical period for carcinogenic exposures between onset of menarche and age of first birth due to hormone-induced proliferation that occurs with each menstrual cycle prior to the differentiation of the breast (which occurs at the time of pregnancy and lactation). Diet during this adolescent period may have different implications for breast cancer than diet in later life. Despite this substantial list of caveats, the evidence has accumulated that diet throughout the life course, beginning with in utero exposures and extending through adult life, has an impact on the risk of malignancy, both in childhood and in adulthood.

The evidence for the relationship between nutritional intake and cancer comes in several forms. The simplest line of evidence is the relationship between growth and risk of malignancy. Although studies showing a relationship between birth weight, height, or growth velocity do not help to identify a causative agent, these studies do confirm that what one eats, and therefore what fuels growth, is related to cancer. The second line of evidence attempts to identify the causative agent through the use of dietary records, either in the setting of a case-control study or in a prospective cohort study. Animal studies in which diet can be more tightly controlled can either suggest or support observations in humans.

In this chapter, we will review the evidence that childhood nutrition can impact the risk of subsequent malignancy. Using a wide lens, we will examine several different aspects of nutrition. The first principle will be to examine the impact of diet over the entire span of childhood, beginning with in utero exposures through adolescence. Secondly, we will consider the impact of childhood diet on the incidence of both childhood and adult malignancies. To do so, we will review the evidence linking childhood growth and cancer, making the argument that growth is a proxy for nutrition. In addition, using case-control studies, we will review the specific associations between childhood diet and cancer. Last, we will review the evidence that for breast cancer at least, the period of childhood and adolescence may be the critical period for exposures that ultimately determines risk of disease as an adult (see Figure 1).

THE CONNECTION BETWEEN GROWTH AND CANCER

Cancer, simply put, is uncontrolled growth. Where does the uncoupling occur between controlled and uncontrolled growth? In pediatrics, there are a set of clinical syndromes notable for "overgrowth," or excessive growth in the pre- and postnatal periods that occur at a frequency of approximately 1 of 10,000 children. Over 20 pediatric overgrowth syndromes have been described, each with the shared feature of excessive growth, but also with unique abnormalities due to the specific underlying genetic cause. Most of these syndromes are also associated with an increased risk of cancer, principally embryonal tumors. These syndromes are provocative paradigms of the malignant hazards of excessive growth.

The most widely recognized of pre- and postnatal growth syndromes is Beckwith–Wiedemann syndrome (BWS). BWS is often associated with advanced bone age, macroglossia, hemihypertrophy, neonatal hypoglycemia, and umbilical hernia or omphalocele. These children are at a moderately increased risk for Wilms' tumor and hepatoblastoma. Genetic abnormalities have been located primarily to the short arm of chromosome 11. This region is heavily imprinted; the paternal gene for insulin-like growth factor II (IGF-II) is normally constitutively activated. The presence of not just one but two active copies of the IGF-II gene, due to paternal uniparental disomy, which is demonstrable in 10 to 20% of BWS patients, is hypothesized to be one of the molecular causes of the syndrome.

Simpson–Golabi–Behmel syndrome (SGBS) is an X-linked disorder that has many of the same clinical features as BWS: pre- and postnatal overgrowth, macroglossia, cleft plate, advanced bone age, and umbilical hernia. SGBS patients

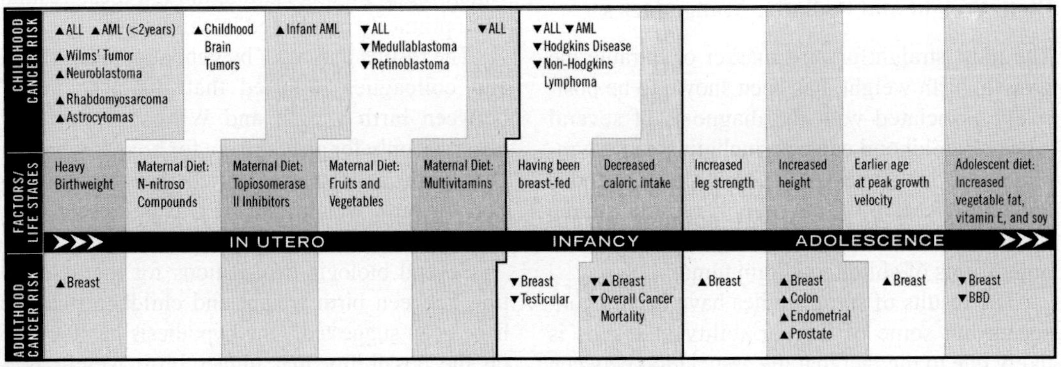

Figure 1 Nutritional factors in childhood and lifetime prevention of cancer.

often have other features including coarse facies, downslanting palpebrae, polydactyly, syndactyly, intracardiac defects, and cardiac conduction defects. SGBS is caused by a deletion in the glypican 3 gene on the X chromosome. Glypican 3 is a heparan sulfate proteoglycan that is attached to the cell surface via a glycosylphosphatidylinositol anchor. Its role in the cell is to regulate the growth and differentiation of predominately mesodermal cells through modulating the interaction of growth factors, particularly IGF-II, with their receptors. Glypican 3 is usually expressed in embryonic tissues and downregulated in adult tissues. Glypican 3 is found to be overexpressed in Wilms' tumor, hepatocellular carcinoma, and neuroblastoma. It is interesting that the IGF-II gene is implicated in two of the most common pediatric overgrowth syndromes: BWS and SGBS. Understanding the molecular basis for these overgrowth syndromes will likely highlight genes critical for the proper balance of growth during childhood and may help us to understand the link between the genetics of growth and the genetics of cancer and the environmental influences, such as diet, which can tip the balance in favor of malignant growth.

IN UTERO EXPOSURES AND INFANT LEUKEMIAS AND OTHER CHILDHOOD CANCERS

When does cancer begin? The genetic evidence is now quite compelling that infant leukemias are initiated in utero. Infant leukemias have certain pathognomic translocations such as t(12;21), t(4,11), or t(8:21). Among infants who developed leukemia in the first 2 years of life, scientists used neonatal blood spots collected to neonatal screening purposes at birth to get a picture of the chromosomal makeup of the child at birth. They have been able to identify the leukemia-causing translocation clone present at birth, even though the leukemia itself did not become manifest for several months or years.[2,3] Epidemiologic evidence supports the notion that in utero exposures are etiologic in cancer causation. For instance, there is strong association between birth weight and childhood cancer, especially leukemia. Other environmental factors, particularly maternal—or in utero—diet, have also been shown to influence the risk of certain childhood cancers, particularly leukemia and central nervous system tumors in children.

Birth Weight and Pediatric Malignancies

The most straightforward marker of intrauterine growth, birth weight, has been shown to be positively associated with the diagnosis of several types of childhood cancers, including acute lymphoblastic leukemia (ALL), acute myelogenous leukemia (AML), Wilms' tumor, neuroblastoma, rhabdomyosarcma, and astrocytomas (but not other forms of childhood brain tumors).[4–8]

The results of some studies have been inconsistent but some of the variability in results is likely due to the fact that the association between birth weight and cancer may operate for only one gender and not the other, or only for certain histologic subtypes, or only for earlier age at diagnosis, depending on the underlying mechanism responsible for the association. Reviewing the adequacy of stratified analyses is imperative in interpreting the findings.

The data linking higher birth weight and childhood malignancy are most consistent for childhood leukemias. A meta-analysis of 18 studies of birth weight and childhood leukemia[9] estimated that for each one kilogram (kg) increase in birth weight, risk of ALL increased by 14% (95% CI 1.08 to 1.20) and risk of AML increased by 29% (95% CI 0.73 to 2.20).[9] There was evidence of a dose–response relationship for both types of leukemia, although it was stronger for ALL (likely because ALL is more prevalent than AML and hence there is more power to detect an association). The association is strongest in children under the age of 2 years; in fact, for AML, the association appears to be limited to children diagnosed before age 2.[10] Indeed, for children under age 2, risk of leukemia may increase by as much as 100% for children who weigh >4,000 g (>8.8 lbs) at birth.[11] Interestingly, both the prevalence of children who are large for gestational age (birth weight >90th percentile) and the incidence of childhood leukemia and brain tumors have been increasing in parallel in the United States over the past several decades.[4]

Several studies report no relationship between birth weight and soft-tissue sarcoma, but soft-tissue sarcoma encompasses a very wide range of histologies and subgroup analysis is important. For instance, in a recent report from the United Kingdom, there was no association between birth weight and embryonal rhabomyosarcoma, but there was an association observed between alveolar rhabdomyosarcoma and heavier birth weight.[12] Of note, alveolar rhabodmyosarcoma is the subtype associated with BWS, a syndrome of fetal and pediatric overgrowth.

A case-control study of the risk of osteosarcoma was conducted in orthopedic surgery departments in 10 US medical centers between 1994 and 2000. Controls (n = 151) were from the same departments as cases (n = 158) and the study included both children and adults. The study found that a higher birth weight was associated with an increased risk of osteosarcoma and the odds were greater for females.[107] However, these results were inconsistent with two prior studies which found no association, though these results were primarily conducted in children.[108–109]

The results may vary by gender as well. Birch and colleagues reported that the association between birth weight and Wilms' tumor was observed only for girls and not for boys,[12] whereas Dorak and colleagues reported that the association for birth weight and ALL was present only for boys and not for girls.[13]

Several biologic explanations for the association between birth weight and childhood cancer have been suggested. One hypothesis has focused on the possibility that higher birth weight is a simple proxy for a greater number of cells proliferating at any one time and therefore, greater absolute number of cells that are at potential risk for malignant transformation. Another possible mechanism may be a surfeit of IGF-I, which is known to be associated with higher birth weight. Others have suggested that excess of iron, which has also been linked to both increased birth weight and enhanced cancer cell growth, may explain the relationship between birth weight and childhood cancer. The major hemochromatosis allele, HFE C282Y, which is associated with increased serum iron levels in 15 to 25% of heterozygotes, is also present in higher frequency among boys diagnosed with childhood ALL than controls.[14]

It should be noted that a variety of studies have also reported an association between birth weight and cardiovascular disease, but in the opposite direction as that observed for cancer. Low birth weight has been associated with an increased risk of ischemic heart disease, as well as many of the intermediate markers of cardiovascular disease, such as blood pressure, body mass index, waist/hip ratio, serum lipids, plasma clotting factors, and impaired glucose tolerance.[15] Adverse conditions in utero, whether it is a surfeit of growth (linked to cancer) or a paucity of growth (linked to cardiovascular disease), appear to have long-lasting implications on the human for risk of subsequent disease (see Chapter 27, "Human Growth and Disease in Later Life," for details).

In Utero Diet (Maternal Diet) and Childhood Cancer

Topoisomerase II Inhibitors and Infant Leukemias. Infant leukemias, although rare, clearly represent a unique subset of childhood leukemia because of their high resistance to standard chemotherapy (20% survival), in contrast to leukemias that occur later in childhood (80% survival). The majority of infant leukemias display a gene rearrangement at 11q23 in the *MLL* gene. This gene has been shown to play a major role in normal hematopoesis.

The same gene, *MLL*, is implicated in secondary leukemias that result from treatment with a class of drugs, epipodophyllotoxins, that inhibit the function of DNA topoisomerase II (DNAt2). DNAt2 first relaxes the supercoiled DNA double helix by cleaving the bonds between the strands and then religates the two strands. Epipodophyllotoxins act by inhibiting religation by the enzyme thereby triggering apoptosis. Topoisomerase inhibitors have wide activity against a number of different types of malignancies, but a small percent of treated patients will develop secondary leukemia, usually AML, with a characteristic cytogenetic marker of an 11q23 abnormality.

The de novo presence of the *MLL* abnormalities in infant leukemias led Ross and colleagues to propose in 1994 that there might be a link between in utero exposure to DNAt2 inhibitors and infant leukemias.[16] The principal source of DNAt2 inhibitors in the environment is diet, primarily flavinoids, genistein, and catechins. Flavinoids, such as quercetin, are found in citrus fruits, apples, onions, parsley, tea, red wine, and dark berries, such as blueberries and blackberries; genistein is found in soy products and catechins are found in green and black tea, cocoa and, red wine. In the largest case-control study to date ($n = 240$), an increase in the odds of infant AML but not infant ALL was observed.[17] The effect was limited to in infants who were MLL+. Mothers in the top quartile of consumption of DNAt2-containing foods during pregnancy had 3.2 times (95% CI 0.9 to 11.9) the odds of having an infant with AML (MLL+); however, the p-value for the test for trend was 0.10 likely due to the fact that the study was based only on 29 patients in this subgroup.

***N*-nitroso Compounds and Brain Tumor.** Animal experiments have definitively shown that feeding pregnant animals nitrosamides causes nervous system tumors in the offspring. In the human diet, cured meats are the major source of nitrites and vegetables a major source of nitrates. Cured meats are treated with nitrites to prevent spoilage and unappealing changes in the color of the meat. The most common types of cured meats consumed include hotdogs, bacon, sausage, cured ham, and packaged lunchmeats. In the acid environment of the stomach, nitrates and nitrites are converted to *N*-nitroso compounds, which can cause the formation of DNA adducts. Vitamins C and E block the nitrosation reactions in the intestines and have been shown in animals to protect against the carcinogenic effect of *N*-nitroso compounds.

Numerous case-control studies have examined the relationship between maternal consumption of nitrate- and nitrite-containing foods and childhood brain tumors; a consistent relationship has been seen for cured meats but not for vegetables.[18,19] In a meta-analysis of maternal cured meat consumption during pregnancy and the risk of childhood brain tumors that included seven observational studies, the pooled RR was 1.68.[20] As part of the US West Coast Childhood Brain Tumor Study, Preston-Martin and colleagues examined the mitigating effects of vitamin supplementation on risk of childhood brain tumors among women who consumed cured meat.[21] Risk of diagnosis of a brain tumor in her offspring was greater among women who did not take supplemental prenatal vitamins than among women who did take vitamins (OR 2.4 vs 1.3). In the group overall, daily use of prenatal vitamins decreased risk of childhood brain tumors by nearly 50% (OR 0.54).

Multivitamins Supplementation during Pregnancy and Childhood Cancer. Three studies have examined how the use of multivitamins periconceptually and during pregnancy affect cancer risk in offspring. Two studies have shown a decreased risk of childhood ALL, but not AML, among the offspring of women who took vitamins at time of pregnancy. In a case-control study of children with Down syndrome, chosen as the study population because of their 20-fold increase in risk of leukemia, vitamin use by the mother in the periconceptual period was associated with a reduced risk of ALL (OR 0.63, 95% CI 0.39 to 1.00), whereas vitamin use later in pregnancy was associated with an increase in risk.[22] Two other case-control studies have shown that the protective effect was stronger for folate in particular than for multivitamins.[22,23] A third study showed a reduced risk of neuroblastoma among the offspring of women with daily vitamin use before and during pregnancy; the lower odds of cancer were slightly stronger for vitamin use in last two trimesters of pregnancy.[24]

Fruit and Vegetable Intake during Pregnancy and Childhood Cancers. Two studies have examined the relationship between fruit and vegetable consumption of the mother during pregnancy and risk of childhood ALL and both have shown an inverse association.[25,26] One of these studies also showed an increase in the risk of ALL in the offspring among mothers who had higher sugar/sweets consumption and higher consumption of meat and meat products.[26] Another study has shown a moderate association between maternal consumption of fruits and vitamin C and a decreased risk of medulloblastoma/PNET in the offspring.[27] An additional case-control study from Mexico City has shown that incidence of sporadic retinoblastoma in the offspring is associated with lower maternal intake of fruits and vegetables, in particular folate and lutein/zeaxanthin.[28]

Birth Weight and Adult Malignancies

The association between birth weight and breast cancer is the most studied; evidence for other adult malignancies is limited. The hypothesis that the roots of breast cancer could originate in utero was proposed by Trichopoulos in 1990.[29] He suggested that higher levels of maternal estrogens and other intrauterine growth factors could produce higher birth weight[30] and simultaneously affect the developing fetal breast tissue,[31,32] both of which might contribute to a higher risk of breast cancer.

There is a strong relationship between high birth weight and increased risk of premenopausal breast cancer. Evidence is remarkably consistent across study types (ie, case-control vs cohort), exposure ascertainment (birth records vs self-reported birth weight), and even countries including populations in Scandinavia, United Kingdom, and the United States.[31] To date, 12 of the 15 studies provide supportive evidence of a relation between premenopausal breast cancer and high birth weight.[31] In meta-analyses of birth weight and premenopausal breast cancer, cohort studies showed a 20% (95% CI 1.07 to 1.35) increase whereas case-control studies showed a 36% (95% CI 1.15 to 1.61) increase in risk with each 1,000 g (2.2 lbs) increase in birth weight.[31] In an analysis that combined data from the Nurses' Health Study and Nurses' Health Study II ($n = 152{,}608$ women), women with low birth weights [<2.2 kg (<5.5 lbs)] had a 34% reduction in risk of premenopausal breast cancer incidence (95% CI 0.47 to 0.93) compared to high birth weight [≥3.9 kg (≥8.5 lbs)].[33] The association of birth weight was stronger in ER+ (estrogen-receptor–positive) and PR+ (progesterone-receptor–positive) tumors, indicating that steroid hormones are a possible mediator between birth weight and breast cancer.[33] Finally, the association of birth weight and future risk of premenopausal breast cancer was independent of other factors later in life (ie, age of menarche, family history of breast cancer), with the exception of adult height,[33] another risk factor for breast cancer that is established during childhood (see Figure 2).

In contrast, all but one study to date report no association between birth weight and postmenopausal breast cancer.[31] The pooled analysis of birth

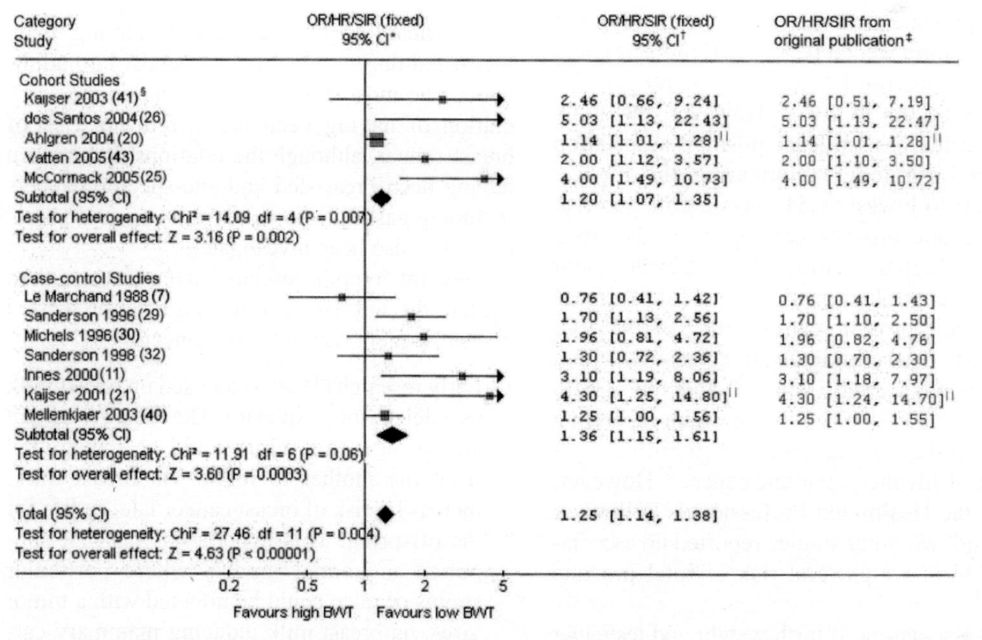

Figure 2 Studies on birthweight and the risk of breast cancer among premenopausal women.* OR = odds ratio; HR = hazard ratio; SIR = standardized incidence ratio; CI = confidence interval. The square indicates the odds ratio, hazard ratio, or standardized incidence ratio; the size of the square indicates the statistical weight each study contributes to the overall estimate; the line indicates the 95% confidence interval.† Odds ratios, hazard ratios, standardized incidence rate ratios, and 95% confidence intervals generated by Revman through the generic inverse variance method used in the analysis.‡ Odds ratios, hazard ratios, standardized incidence rate ratios, and 95% confidence intervals from original publication.§ The number following the last name of the first author indicates the year of publication; the number in parentheses indicates the reference number of publication. ||Effect estimate associated with each 1,000 g (2.2 lbs) increase in birth weight. (From reference 31.)

weight and postmenopausal breast cancer reported a relative risk of 1.04 (95% CI 0.91 to 1.19) in cohort studies and an RR of 1.04 in (95% CI 0.66 to 1.64) case-control studies.[31] The data from the combined Nurses Health Study (NHS) cohorts also support this meta-analysis, reporting an RR of 0.97 (CI 0.08 to 1.16) of postmenopausal breast cancer comparing women with a birth weight >3.9 kg (>8.5 lbs) compared to those ≤2.5 kg (≤5.5 lbs)[33]

Overall, there is a strong association of birth weight and risk of total breast cancer, although these results should be interpreted through the findings of pre- and postmenopausal breast cancer. Specifically, in a meta-analysis of cohort and case-control studies, there was a 24% (95% CI 1.10 to 1.40) and 21% (95% CI 1.06 to 1.38) increase in total breast cancer risk, respectively, in women with high birth weight compared to those women with low birth weights[31]; Ahlgren and colleagues reported a similar significant increase in risk, in one of the largest cohort studies to date.[34] In this study, school health records were collected in Copenhagen, Denmark, from 1930 to 1974 in a cohort of 91,601 women with a total of 2,074 incidence total breast cancer cases. There was a 17% increase in risk of total breast cancer in women in the highest [>8.8 lbs (>4,000 g)] compared to the lowest [<5.5 lbs (<2,500 g)] birth weight categories. Overall, 17 of the 27 individual studies support an association of high birth weight and increased risk of total breast cancer.[31]

The relationship between birth weight and other cancers have been investigated, although the data are sparse. Several studies have investigated the relationship between prostate cancer and birth weight but results are inconclusive. In a large Norweigian cohort (n = 19,681), a weak positive association was found between birth weight and risk of prostate cancer comparing the highest quartile of birth weight [≥8.6 lbs (≥3,925 g)] and the lowest quartile [<7.2 lbs (<3,260 g)] (RR 1.3, 95% CI 0.8 to 2.0).[35] However, the study also reported a significant positive association between birth length comparing the highest (≥53 cm) to lowest (<51 cm) quartile and risk for metastatic prostate cancer (n = 33). Also, men in the highest quartiles for both birth weight and birth length had nearly a four-fold increase in metastatic prostate cancer (RR: 3.8, 95% CI 1.2 to 2.0). These findings are consistent with a small Swedish cohort study[36] and the Health Professionals Follow-up Study which reported a weak positive association between birth weight and risk of advanced prostate cancer.[37] However, to date, the Health and Professionals Follow-up Study and two other studies reported no association of birth weight and risk of total prostate cancer.[37–39]

The association of birth weight and testicular cancer is also unclear. A large cohort study of Swedish men (n = 337,249) found no association between birth weight and total testicular cancer (n = 144) nor in a subset of nonseminomatous testicular cancer (n = 120),[40] although three previous case-control studies had reported a positive association.[41–43]

Two case-control studies have been conducted regarding birth weight and colorectal cancer.[44,45] Of note, in one case-control study, lower birth weight was associated with increased risk, though the trend across categories was not consistent.[44] Another prior study reported a J-shaped relationship between birth weight and colorectal cancer; the study was based on only a few cases and included both men and women in analyses.[45]

Breast-feeding and Childhood Malignancy

Breast-feeding already has many proven benefits for the mother and child, including potentially decreasing the mothers' own risk for ovarian and breast cancer.[46,47] Breast-feeding likely also reduces risk of hematologic malignancy in the offspring.[48,49] Children who have been breast-fed for at least 6 months have approximately a 30% lower likelihood of developing ALL and AML.[50] The effect appears restricted to pre-B-cell ALL and M_0, M_1, and M_2 subtypes of AML. Other studies have suggested a reduction in risk for non-Hodgkin's lymphoma, although not all studies have reached statistical significance due to small number of cases.[48,51,52] The risk of Hodgkin's Disease also appears reduced in two studies,[51,53] but inference is limited in other studies due to small sample size.[50,52] The mechanism by which breast-feeding protects against hematologic malignancies in children is thought to be immunomodulatory, protecting against an inappropriate lymphoproliferative response to an infection or other antigen challenge, rather than due to the nutritive components of breast milk.

Having Been Breast-fed and Adult Malignancies

The anticarcinogenic effects of having been breast-fed during infancy may persist into adulthood. The most studied relationship is the association of having been breast-fed and risk of breast cancer, although the relationship between having been breast-fed and site-specific cancers including gastric, colorectal, prostate, and testicular have also been investigated.[54]

Several hypotheses have been advanced to explain the link between having been breast-fed and subsequent risk of breast cancer.

- Early research (1930's) focused on breast milk as a deleterious exposure. The theory was that an "oncogenetic" virus could be transmitted from the mother to infant via breast milk, increasing risk of breast cancer later in life for the offspring. This hypothesis was first supported in animal models where particular strains of mice could be infected with a tumor virus via breast milk inducing mammary carcinogenesis.[55] Additionally, there is evidence of viral DNA, RNA, and antigen in human breast tissue and milk, and thus there has been continued interest in the possible viral etiology of breast cancer.[56–59]
- Organochlorines, such as PCBs (polychlorinated biphenyls) and DDT (dichloro-diphenyl-trichloroethane), are carcinogenetic substances that are preferentially secreted into breast milk.[60] It has been postulated that breast-feeding is a method used by the body to reduce the mother's burden of these chemicals, and women with higher levels of these chemicals are associated with increased lactation,[61] thereby possibly reducing breast cancer risk for the mother.[62] However, the infant is exposed to these carcinogenetic substances which are implicated in increasing risk of cancer (including breast) in adulthood. This physiologic situation raises the question as to the optimal duration of breast-feeding, balancing the positive attributes of breast milk against possible extended exposure to carcinogens secreted into the breast milk.[63] At present, the World Health Organization recommends exclusive breast-feeding for the first 6 months of life because of well-documented benefits to both the mother and the child.[64]
- Breast milk contains many bioactive components not present in formula such as prostaglandins, hormones, and cytokines, present at especially high levels in colostrum[65] that may affect the offspring's normal breast development but in addition reduce overall child morbidity.[64] Breast-fed children may have altered patterns of growth which may impact subsequent risk of breast cancer risk later in life, as reviewed later in this chapter.[57]
- A protein fraction of breast milk, multimeric alpha-lactalbumin (MAL), is a potent agent inducing apoptosis in tumor and immature cells, while sparing mature cells. This unique property of MAL has been proposed as possibly guiding the breast epithelieum of the infant toward healthy maturation and away from neoplasm.[66]

The Boyd Orr cohort is one of the few cohort studies with prospective data (rather than recalled data) on breast-feeding and subsequent risk of cancer. The Boyd Orr cohort comprised 4,999 children who were ages 0 to 19 when enrolled as part of Carnegie Survey of Family Diet and Health in Pre-War Britain (1937 to 1939). In 1988, the children who had been part of the study were recontacted by a team of researchers who were then able to link their childhood exposures with adult disease outcomes. Using data from the National Health Services Central Registry, cancer outcomes from 1948 to 2003 were available on 88% of the original cohort. Martin and colleagues reported the association of having been breast-fed with risk of total cancer, smoking-related, and nonrelated cancers, as well as site-specific cancers including breast, prostate, testicular, colorectal, and gastric cancers. For each cancer site, Martin and colleagues also conducted a meta-analysis of data on breast-feeding and cancer using data available from other cohort and case-control studies.[54]

Analysis of cases from the Boyd Orr cohort itself showed no association between total cancer incidence nor any of the individual cancers (prostate, breast, colorectal, gastric). In the meta-analyses using data pooled from other studies, there was an 18% reduction in risk for testicular cancer and having been breast-fed, though the association failed to reach statistical significance (95% CI 0.62 to 1.10).[54] This result was consistent with an individual case-control study included in the meta-analysis, which found that men who had been breast-fed >6 months compared to those never breast-fed had a reduction in risk of 55% of borderline statistical significance in a dose-responsive manner (95% CI 0.41 to 1.04, $p = .05$).[67]

Having been breast-fed is associated with a lower risk of premenopausal breast cancer. The Boyd Orr meta-analysis of breast-feeding and premenopausal breast cancer which included nine studies and a total of 3,346 premenopausal breast cancer incident cases showed a 12% reduction in risk for premenopausal breast cancer (95% CI 0.79 to 0.98).[54] This is consistent with the majority of case-control studies, although the prospective NHS and NHS II cohorts reported a nonsignificant reduction in risk of having been breast-fed and premenopausal breast cancer.[54,57,68] In contrast, the Boyd Orr meta-analysis that focused solely on postmenopausal breast cancer reported no association (RR 1.0, 95% CI 0.86 to 1.16) ($n = 5{,}069$)[54] and is consistent with individual studies.

There are several limitations to the research of having been breast-fed and later risk of cancer in adulthood. First, in the meta-analyses described above, subjects were born in 1874 to 1972 when alternatives to breast-feeding were primarily unmodified cows' milk. Preparations of infant formula have changed dramatically over time. Rates of breast-feeding have decreased as depicted in NHS cohort, in which 82% of women were breast-fed as infants as compared to the younger cohort of women in NHS II, among whom only 31% report having been breast-fed as an infant; there was also a decrease in exclusive breast-feeding, likely resulting in mixed feeding.[57] This raises a concern of generalizability of past research to modern day populations worldwide. Second, ascertainment of breast-feeding exposure was generally a simple yes/no question, a rather crude estimate and breast-feeding duration was ascertained in only three studies.[30] Third, timing of breast-feeding initiation is a possible important question since colostrum is dense with immulogical factors, a possible mechanism of protection in childhood cancers with possible implications for disease in adulthood. Lastly, residual confounding is possible since infant feeding practices are associated with social, educational, and economical factors.

ADOLESCENCE AND BREAST CANCER: CRITICAL TIME PERIOD FOR BREAST CARCINOGENESIS

Data from both animal and human studies suggest strongly that the breast is particularly sensitive to carcinogenic exposures that occur after menarche and prior to first pregnancy. In the rat, Russo and Russo have elegantly studied the underlying biology of mammary gland development that explains the phenomenon of this time-sensitive window for exposure.[69,70] The mammary gland, a specialized accessory organ of the skin, is unusual in that, unlike most other organs in the body, it develops entirely postnatally. It is the terminal end of the duct, farthest from the nipple, or terminal end bud (TEB) that undergoes growth and differentiation at the time of puberty. With the advent of menarche and the monthly surges in progesterone and estrogen, the TEB undergoes further cleavage into alveolar buds (AB). At the time of pregnancy, these AB differentiate into lobules that are capable of lactation. Pregnancy permanently alters the architecture of the mammary gland; the multiparous rat's mammary gland has virtually no TEBs and the number of lobules is four times that seen in an age-matched virgin rat.[69,70]

This change in structure is important in terms of carcinogenesis because of the concomitant change that has occurred within the epithelial cells that line these three developmentally distinct structures. The epithelial cells that line the TEB likely represent a pluripotent stem cell that can differentiate into either a myoepithelial cell or a ductal cell. Cell kinetics of TEB are quite different than their more differentiated counterparts. Compared to cells that line the AB, cells in the TEB have much higher DNA labeling index, as measured by incorporation of ^{3}H thymidine, and fewer cells in the G_0 portion of the cell cycle.[69,70] Higher rates of cell proliferation and less time in the G_0 phase of the cell cycle allow less time for DNA repair, which may be one reason that TEB are more susceptible to carcinogenic exposures than the more differentiated structure of the AB or lobule.

In animals, one of the most reproducible ways to decrease cancer incidence is to restrict calories. The effect of caloric restriction is most pronounced for hormone-sensitive cancers. The effect of reducing calories during different age periods of the rat has been tested and restricting the peripubertal diet of the rat, as compared to the adult diet, is the most potent inhibitor of future cancer risk.[69,70] If the caloric intake of the rats is restricted early in life, the architecture of the mammary gland is permanently altered, with more TEBs and lower rates of proliferation in the gland overall.[71] These structural changes remain evident into the adulthood of the rat, and persist even after pregnancy-induced differentiation. Some insight into the mechanism by which a reduction in calories also reduces risk of cancer is evident from experiments in the worm *Caenorhabditis elegans*. In *C. elegans*, reduced food induces a decrease in an IGF-I-like compound, *daf*, that results in the induction of "diapause," a hibernation-like state of the larva between the juvenile state and adulthood. The breast may also be undergoing a similar developmental arrest.[72]

Few human studies exist on the effect childhood caloric intake and risk of cancer as it is rare to have a study that has data on both childhood diet and adult cancer risk. Analysis of the data from the Boyd–Orr cohort did show that for each one megajoule (Mj) increase in total calories during childhood, there was a 20% increase in nonsmoking-related cancers observed as an adult.[73]

Sadly, the Second World War has provided another mechanism to study the effect of war-induced famine on human health. The residents of Norway experienced a chronic reduction in calories due to rationing over the entire time period of the war. Females who were adolescents during the war subsequently had a 13% reduction in risk of breast cancer.[74] A famine in the Netherlands at the end of the war, known as "the Hunger Winter," was more abrupt and severe.[75] The Dutch government in exile ordered a railroad strike to try to cripple the German army; the Nazis retaliated with a transport embargo that severely limited the transport of all food and fuel. Average caloric intake dropped to 600 kcal/d. Women exposed to the famine as children had, as expected, a later age at menarche, reduced height and earlier age at menopause, three factors shown to reduce risk of breast cancer. The effects were strongest for prepubertal children who were 2 to 9 years old during the Hunger Winter. However, Dutch scientists found that paradoxically the risk of breast cancer was increased, not decreased, among childhood survivors of the famine. Consistent with this increased risk of breast cancer, scientists showed that hormone levels of estrone sulfate were higher in the women exposed to the famine as children, measured 60 years postexposure. Likewise, IGF-I was also higher among the women who had been exposed to the famine. The authors propose that the immediate effects of the famine were as predicted, but that the effect of severe deprivation followed by refeeding reset hypothalamic setpoints, resulting in lifelong elevations in IGF-I and steroid hormones. This resetting overrode the short-term results of famine that should have reduced risk of breast cancer and resulted in higher observed rates of breast cancer among the famine exposed. These two experiences of famine indicate the complexity of the human organism's response to environmental exposures and how the response can be modulated by dose (severity of the famine) and by susceptibility of the organism (age at exposure).

Other animal experiments, and human experiences, have highlighted how the age at which exposure occurs can influence the risk of subsequent breast cancer. For instance, chemical induction of tumors in the rat is most potent when the carcinogen is administered *after* week 30 and *before* week 60, the time period analogous to the window between menarche and first pregnancy.[76] In humans, women who survived the atomic bombs in Japan have an elevated risk of breast cancer, but increase in risk is inversely proportional to age at the time of the bombing. Interestingly, no increase in risk at all was observed among women 35 years and older at the time of the bombing. Effects of the treatment for Hodgkin's disease is another example of the importance of age of exposure to radiation in determining subsequent risk of breast cancer. When the mediastinal lymph nodes are involved with lymphoma, Hodgkin's disease patients receive what is known as "mantle irradiation," a radiation field that includes the breast. Women who survive Hodgkin's disease have a markedly increased risk of developing breast cancer, but again, risk is dependent on age at exposure to the ionizing radiation.[77] Similar to the experience of women who were exposed in Japan to the radiation fall out of the atomic bomb, no increase in risk of breast cancer is observed among women who were over age 30 at the time of treatment; however, risk rises exponentially to the younger the woman who was at the time of her mantle irradiation for Hodgkin's disease.

Migrant studies are another indicator of the importance of age at exposure. Migrant studies examine how risk of disease changes when an individual migrates from a country with a low incidence of disease to a country with a high incidence of disease. In the case of breast cancer, studies of Japanese immigrants (low incidence) to Hawaii (higher incidence), rates of breast cancer did not approximate with those of US citizens for the immigrants themselves but only for their children and grandchildren.[78] The interpretation of this data is that the immigrant must grow up in the adopted country to "inherit" the cancer risk of the country, pinpointing again the importance of early life and adolescent exposures in breast cancer risk induction.

Childhood and Adolescent Growth, Adult Height, and Breast Cancer

Adult height has been correlated with several adult-onset cancers, including colon, prostate, and endometrial cancer, but tall stature has been most consistently observed in terms of risk of breast cancer, primarily postmenopausal breast cancer. A review of 24 prospective studies[79] found a positive relationship in all but one and since the publication of that review, several more studies have confirmed the relationship.[34,80] On average, risk of breast cancer increases by 11% for each 5 cm increase in height.[34,81]

Height is the composite of leg length plus trunk length. Interestingly, leg length and trunk length, though both strongly correlated with total height, are poorly correlated with one another ($r = 0.1$ to 0.2)[80,82] and appear to be determined by different factors during childhood and at different times during childhood growth.[83] Growth immediately after birth is due in larger part to leg length than trunk growth. This is demonstrated by the changing ratio of trunk length: height over time. At birth, the ratio is around 0.66 but by puberty, this ratio has declined to 0.50.[83] After puberty, linear growth occurs proportionately in the trunk and the leg. It has been suggested therefore that separate analysis of these two components of height may help elucidate the biologic connections between growth and breast cancer.

Insight on the determinants of leg and trunk height has been gleaned from the 1946 national birth cohort.[82] The 1946 national birth cohort study ($n = 5{,}362$) is a social-class–stratified sample of all legitimate births in England, Scotland, and Wales from March 3 to 9, 1946, who have been followed up on 21 separate occasions between birth and age 53. Adult leg and trunk height were measured by a research nurse at home visit when the subjects were 43 years old. The most important predictor of leg length was early childhood nutrition: having been breast-fed (reported at age 2) and total energy intake (reported at age 4).[82] Lack of overcrowding, a proxy for socioeconomic conditions, was also associated with longer leg length. The determinants of trunk length are less clear than those of leg length. Prolonged childhood illness (greater than 3 months or requiring hospital admission) was associated with shorter trunk length as was parental separation, whereas childhood nutrition was not associated with trunk length.

In one analysis, both leg length and trunk length were found to be associated with increased risk of breast cancer; the magnitude of the associations for the two components of height was similar. In contrast, using data from the Boyd–Orr cohort, Gunnell and colleagues argue that the effect of stature on cancer risk is more strongly correlated with leg length; in fact, the authors report that no association was observed between trunk length and risk.[84] Overall, Gunnell reports an 80% increase in risk of nonsmoking-related cancers with each one z-score increase (approximately 3 to 4 mm) in leg length; this effect was even more pronounced in sex hormone–dependent cancers, like breast cancer. Further elucidation of the separate contributions of trunk length and leg length to the overall association of height and breast cancer may provide insight into the key developmental periods for initiation of breast cancer risk.

Earlier age at onset of peak growth velocity and more total growth during puberty have also been associated with increased risk of breast cancer, independent of total stature.[34] A study from Denmark linked school health records in Copenhagen from 1930 to 1975 to the Danish Cancer Registry, resulting in a cohort of 117,415 women, among whom 3,340 cases of breast cancer had been diagnosed. Age at peak growth was divided into quintiles. Girls whose peak growth occurred in the oldest quintile (median age 13.5 years) had a decreased risk of breast cancer (RR 0.84) compared to those whose peak growth occurred in the youngest quintile (median age: 10.4 years). Earlier age at peak growth velocity is associated with earlier onset of menarche and therefore more prolonged exposure of the never pregnant and thus undifferentiated breast to the higher levels of estrogens postpuberty. In the Danish study, age at menarche was a significant predictor of subsequent risk of breast cancer in univariate analysis but not when age at peak growth velocity was also included in the model, indicating that both are likely a measure of onset of puberty. Larger increases in height during puberty (between ages 8 and 14) conferred an increased risk of breast cancer, whereas total height accrued prior to age 8 was not significantly associated with risk of breast cancer.

Adolescent Diet and Breast Cancer

The totality of the data on the critical importance of adolescence for the induction of breast cancer has lead investigators to also study adolescent diet and breast cancer. The study of adolescent diet and breast cancer is challenging in that it is based on recall of diet from the past, which undermines its accuracy due to measurement error.[85] In addition, in the situation where the recall of adolescent diet is collected after the diagnosis of breast cancer, there is the potential for recall bias.

In the NHS and the NHS II, the reproducibility of the recall of adolescent diet has been assessed and effort made to estimate validity of diet recalled from 15 to 30 years previously.[86,87] In NHS, a short 24-item food frequency questionnaire (FFQ) was added to the main questionnaire in 1986. In NHS II, participants were asked on the main questionnaire if they would be willing to fill out a supplemental questionnaire on adolescent diet. The 124-item supplemental adolescent diet FFQ was completed by 45,947 NHS II participants in 1998. In both cohorts, a subset of the nurse participants who had completed the initial FFQ on adolescent diet were asked to complete a second survey 4 to 8 years later. In both cohorts, the reproducibility of recall of both foods and nutrients was reasonable [$r = 0.5$ to 0.6 (NHS) and $r = 0.6$ to 0.7 (NHS II)]. The mothers of the participants from the NHS II were also asked to recall their daughters' diets as adolescents. The correlation between the report of the mother versus the daughter was moderate ($r = 0.4$) but implies some modicum of validity especially when one acknowledges that the mother of an adolescent no longer has the control over diet that a mother has at an earlier age and therefore may have been unaware of what the daughter was eating outside the home. As an additional approach to assessing the validity of the report, the basal metabolic rate of the NHS II participant as an adolescent was calculated on the basis of her reported weight at age 18. This predicted basal metabolic rate was then used to calculate expected total energy intake. The expected energy intake was compared to the reported energy intake. Participants were categorized as under-, over-, or acceptable reporters. Correlation between the two reports of adolescent diet did not differ by reporter status. In addition, in both cohorts, current diet was minimally correlated ($r = 0.2$) with report of adolescent diet which implies minimal confounding by the content of the current diet. Finally, foods and nutrients were ranked into quintiles. Eighty percent of the reports on the two surveys of adolescent diet were within one quintile of each other. These data in sum show that recall of adolescent diet using a FFQ provides a reasonable estimate, given the many limitations of the method.

In the NHS II, vegetable fat was also observed to be protective (RR 0.58, 95% CI 0.38 to 0.86) as was vitamin E (RR 0.61, 95% CI 0.42 to 0.89).[86] Vitamin E is a fat-soluble vitamin, and vegetable fat (principally peanut butter) is the major source of vitamin E in the adolescent diet of the NHS II participant. In addition, in the analysis of the adolescent diet of the NHS II participant, foods with a higher glycemic index, which are foods that invoke a steeper rise in blood sugar and therefore a compensatory rise in insulin and IGFs, were associated with an increase in the risk of breast cancer (RR 1.47, 95% CI 1.04 to 2.08). In the NHS, a significant protective effect was also observed for higher dietary intake of vegetable fat (RR 0.85) and risk of breast cancer.[88]

Other retrospective case-control studies have examined the issue of adolescent diet and breast cancer. In a case-control study using cases identified through the Surveillance Epidemiology and End Results (SEER) registry in three sites, Potischman and colleagues found a borderline effect for high-fat meats.[89] In another case-control study that used a limited version of the Bloch FFQ to assess only foods high in fat and fiber, Pryor and colleagues reported that higher intake of fat from dairy sources was associated with decreased risk of breast cancer for both pre- and postmenopausal women.[90] In the same study, higher intake of fiber decreased risk among premenopausal women, whereas higher intake of fiber was associated with an increased risk of breast cancer among postmenopausal women. Hislop and colleagues conducted a case-control study in British Columbia among 846 incident cases of breast cancer between 1980 and 1982.[91] Women were asked to recall dietary intake of 31 foods during early childhood (up to age 13). Among premenopausal women, consumption of meat with visible fat during childhood was associated with increased risk of breast cancer (RR for "three or more times per week" compared to "less than once per month" = 2.69; 95% CI 1.26 to 5.80) Consumption of vegetable oils was associated with reduced risk among premenopausal women (RR = 0.48, 95% CI 0.25 to 0.89), analogous to the findings from the NHS and NHS II.

Adolescent Soy Intake and Breast Cancer

Several recent studies have focused on adolescent soy intake and breast cancer. Phytoestrogens have been shown in animal models to promote differentiation of the mammary gland by enhancing the transition from TEBs to ABs or lobules.[92] All three case-control studies to date have shown a protective effect for adolescent soy intake,[93–95] which was especially pronounced in one study that measured both adolescent and adult intake. Those individuals who indicated high intake in both time periods had 50% reduction in risk of breast cancer.[94]

Adolescent Diet and Benign Breast Disease

Benign breast disease (BBD) is catch-all phrase that includes several different types of pathologic lesions, some with no relation to breast cancer and some that dramatically heighten risk. Nonproliferative BBD has no bearing on subsequent risk of breast cancer, whereas women with proliferative lesions without atypia have 1.5- to 2-fold greater risk; women who have proliferative lesions with atypia have a 3.5- to 5-fold greater risk of breast cancer.[96] A mathematical model of breast cancer has also shown that BBD confers an increased risk of breast cancer, even when adult risk factors are included in the model, suggesting that it is early life events that determine risk. Therefore, proliferative BBD is considered an intermediate marker of risk for breast cancer that reflects adolescent exposures in particular.

In an analysis from the NHS, a retrospective analysis of diet during adolescence and subsequent risk of proliferative BBD showed that higher intakes of vegetable fat, vitamin E, and fiber during adolescence were inversely related to risk. In addition, it was shown that whereas recent alcohol did not affect risk of BBD, remote consumption of alcohol between ages 18 to 22 increased risk for both proliferative and nonproliferative BBD.[97]

Childhood Diet and Age at Menarche

Earlier age at menarche is a strong risk factor for breast cancer. In fact, it has been estimated that risk of breast cancer increases by 4% for each yearly decrease in age at menarche.[98] Earlier age at menarche is also a risk factor for endometrial cancer. Examination of the dietary predictors of age at menarche has been sparse. Most dietary hypotheses have had null results.[99–101] A study in Germany showed that energy-adjusted fat intake was associated with accelerated menarche,[102] but this finding was not replicated in a study in Canada.[102] In fact, the Canadian study reported that higher intake of monounsaturated fat was associated with a delay in menarche. Several studies have shown an association between higher intakes of dietary fiber and later age at menarche.[103–106]

SUMMARY

Data from a variety of sources support the notion that diet during childhood, beginning in utero and extending through adolescence, has an impact on the incidence of childhood as well as adult malignancies. Some of the evidence is based on the relationship between childhood growth and cancer, both abnormal growth patterns as in the BWS, and "normal" growth, for instance, the relationship between birth weight and childhood ALL or height and breast cancer. Other studies have been able to pinpoint foods or nutrients that may impact risk of cancer, such as nitrate-containing meats and pediatric brain tumors, or topoisomerase II inhibitors and infant AML. Timing of the exposure is a key variable; for instance, topoisomerase II inhibitors are not implicated in the genesis of AML that develops later in childhood and vegetable oil has not been found to have an effect when consumed in the adult diet, only in the adolescent diet. The availability of validated tools such as the FFQ that allow diet to be measured efficiently and accurately in prospective large-scale, population-based studies will allow for the ascertainment of further relationships between diet and cancer, avoiding the inherent recall bias of case-control studies. Finally, the interaction between nutrition, genes, and cancer will become more interesting as the interrelationships are elucidated and we understand more about how diet interacts with genetic susceptibility.

REFERENCES

1. Doll R, Peto R. The Causes of Cancer. New York: Oxford University Press; 1981.
2. Wiemels JL, Cazzaniga G, Daniotti M, et al. Prenatal origin of acute lymphoblastic leukaemia in children. Lancet 1999;354:1499–503.
3. Gale KB, Ford AM, Repp R, et al. Backtracking leukemia to birth: Identification of clonotypic gene fusion sequences in neonatal blood spots. Proc Natl Acad Sci U S A 1997;94:13950–4.
4. Ross JA. High birth weight and cancer: Evidence and implications. Cancer Epidemiol Biomarkers Prev 2006;15:1–2.
5. Heuch JM, Heuch I, Akslen LA, et al. Risk of primary childhood brain tumors related to birth characteristics: A Norwegian prospective study. Int J Cancer 1998;77:498–503.
6. Emerson JC, Malone KE, Daling JR, et al. Childhood brain tumor risk in relation to birth characteristics. J Clin Epidemiol 1991;44:1159–66.
7. Von Behren J, Reynolds P. Birth characteristics and brain cancers in young children. Int J Epidemiol 2003;32:248–56.
8. Mogren I, Malmer B, Tavelin B, et al. Reproductive factors have low impact on the risk of different primary brain tumours in offspring. Neuroepidemiology 2003; 22:249–54.
9. Hjalgrim LL, Westergaard T, Rostgaard K, et al. Birth weight as a risk factor for childhood leukemia: A meta-analysis of 18 epidemiologic studies. Am J Epidemiol 2003;158:724–35.
10. Yeazel MW, Ross JA, Buckley JD, et al. High birth weight and risk of specific childhood cancers: A report from the Children's Cancer Group. J Pediatr 1997;131:671–7.
11. Hjalgrim LL, Rostgaard K, Hjalgrim H, et al. Birth weight and risk for childhood leukemia in Denmark, Sweden, Norway, and Iceland. J Natl Cancer Inst 2004;96:1549–56.
12. Birch J. "Fetal growth, birth weight and childhood cancers" Abstract S7.03; International Society of Pediatric Oncology, SIOP XXXVIII Congress Meeting: Contents and Abstracts. Pediatr Blood Cancer 2006;47:355–532.
13. Dorak MT, Pearce MS, Hammal DM, et al. Examination of gender effect in birth weight and miscarriage associations with childhood cancer (United Kingdom). Cancer Causes Control 2007;18:219–28.
14. Dorak MT, Burnett AK, Worwood M, et al. The C282Y mutation of HFE is another male–specific risk factor for childhood acute lymphoblastic leukemia. Blood 1999;94:3957.
15. Barker DJ. Growth in utero and coronary heart disease. Nutr Rev 1996;54:S1–7.
16. Ross JA, Potter JD, Robison LL. Infant leukemia, topoisomerase II inhibitors, and the MLL gene. J Natl Cancer Inst 1994;86:1678–80.
17. Spector LG, Xie Y, Robison LL, et al. Maternal diet and infant leukemia: The DNA topoisomerase II inhibitor hypothesis: A report from the children's oncology group. Cancer Epidemiol Biomarkers Prev 2005;14:651–5.
18. Preston-Martin S, Yu MC, Benton B, et al. N-Nitroso compounds and childhood brain tumors: A case-control study. Cancer Res 1982;42:5240–5.
19. Kuijten RR, Bunin GR, Nass CC, et al. Gestational and familial risk factors for childhood astrocytoma: Results of a case-control study. Cancer Res 1990;50:2608–12.
20. Huncharek M, Kupelnick B. A meta-analysis of maternal cured meat consumption during pregnancy and the risk of childhood brain tumors. Neuroepidemiology 2004;23:78–84.
21. Preston-Martin S, Pogoda JM, Mueller BA, et al. Maternal consumption of cured meats and vitamins in relation to pediatric brain tumors. Cancer Epidemiol Biomarkers Prev 1996;5:599–605.
22. Ross JA, Blair CK, Olshan AF, et al. Periconceptional vitamin useand leukemia risk in children with Down syndrome: A Children's Oncology Group study. Cancer 2005;104:405–10.
23. Thompson JR, Gerald PF, Willoughby ML, et al. Maternal folate supplementation in pregnancy and protection against acute lymphoblastic leukaemia in childhood: A case-control study. Lancet 2001;358:1935–40.

24. Olshan AF, Smith JC, Bondy ML, et al. Maternal vitamin use and reduced risk of neuroblastoma. Epidemiology 2002;13:575–80.
25. Jensen CD, Block G, Buffler P, et al. Maternal dietary risk factors in childhood acute lymphoblastic leukemia (United States). Cancer Causes Control 2004;15:559–70.
26. Petridou E, Ntouvelis E, Dessypris N, et al. Maternal diet and acute lymphoblastic leukemia in young children. Cancer Epidemiol Biomarkers Prev 2005;14:1935–9.
27. Bunin GR, Kushi LH, Gallagher PR, et al. Maternal diet during pregnancy and its association with medulloblastoma in children: A children's oncology group study (United States). Cancer Causes Control 2005;16:877–91.
28. Orjuela MA, Titievsky L, Liu X, et al. Fruit and vegetable intake during pregnancy and risk for development of sporadic retinoblastoma. Cancer Epidemiol Biomarkers Prev 2005;14:1433–40.
29. Trichopoulos D. Hypothesis: Does breast cancer originate in utero? Lancet 1990;335:939–40.
30. Potischman N, Troisi R. In utero and early life exposures in relation to risk of breast cancer. Cancer Causes Control 1999;10:561–73.
31. Michels KB, Xue F. Role of birth weight in the etiology of breast cancer. Int J Cancer 2006;119:2007–25.
32. de Assis S, Khan G, Hilakivi-Clarke L. High birth weight increases mammary tumorigenesis in rats. Int J Cancer 2006;119:1537–46.
33. Michels KB, Xue F, Terry KL, et al. Longitudinal study of birth weight and the incidence of breast cancer in adulthood. Carcinogenesis 2006;27:2464–8.
34. Ahlgren M, Melbye M, Wohlfahrt J, et al. Growth patterns and the risk of breast cancer in women. N Engl J Med 2004;351:1619–26.
35. Nilsen TI, Romundstad PR, Troisi R, et al. Birth size and subsequent risk for prostate cancer: A prospective population-based study in Norway. Int J Cancer 2005;113:1002–4.
36. Tibblin G, Eriksson M, Cnattingius S, et al. High birth weight as a predictor of prostate cancer risk. Epidemiology 1995;6:423–4.
37. Platz EA, Giovannucci E, Rimm EB, et al. Retrospective analysis of birth weight and prostate cancer in the Health Professionals Follow-up Study. Am J Epidemiol 1998;147:1140–4.
38. Ekbom A, Hsieh CC, Lipworth L, et al. Perinatal characteristics in relation to incidence of and mortality from prostate cancer. BMJ 1996;313:337–41.
39. Ekbom A, Wuu J, Adami HO, et al. Duration of gestation and prostate cancer risk in offspring. Cancer Epidemiol Biomarkers Prev 2000;9:221–3.
40. Rasmussen F, Gunnell D, Ekbom A, et al. Birth weight, adult height, and testicular cancer: Cohort study of 337,249 Swedish young men. Cancer Causes Control 2003;14:595–8.
41. Moller H, Skakkebaek NE. Testicular cancer and cryptorchidism in relation to prenatal factors: Case-control studies in Denmark. Cancer Causes Control 1997;8:904–12.
42. Akre O, Ekbom A, Hsieh CC, et al. Testicular nonseminoma and seminoma in relation to perinatal characteristics. J Natl Cancer Inst 1996;88:883–9.
43. Brown LM, Pottern LM, Hoover RN. Prenatal and perinatal risk factors for testicular cancer. Cancer Res 1986;46:4812–6.
44. Nilsen TI, Romundstad PR, Troisi R, et al. Birth size and colorectal cancer risk: A prospective population based study. Gut 2005;54:1728–32.
45. Sandhu MS, Luben R, Day NE, et al. Self-reported birth weight and subsequent risk of colorectal cancer. Cancer Epidemiol Biomarkers Prev 2002;11:935–8.
46. Siskind V, Green A, Bain C, et al. Breastfeeding, menopause, and epithelial ovarian cancer. Epidemiology 1997;8:188–91.
47. Lipworth L, Bailey LR, Trichopoulos D. History of breast-feeding in relation to breast cancer risk: A review of the epidemiologic literature. J Natl Cancer Inst 2000;92:302–12.
48. Davis MK. Review of the evidence for an association between infant feeding and childhood cancer. Int J Cancer 1998;78:29–33.
49. Parker L. Breast-feeding and cancer prevention. Eur J Cancer 2001;37:155–8.
50. Shu XO, Linet MS, Steinbuch M, et al. Breast-feeding and risk of childhood acute leukemia. J Natl Cancer Inst 1999;91:1765–72.
51. Davis MK, Savitz DA, Graubard BI. Infant feeding and childhood cancer. Lancet 1988;2:365–8.
52. Bener A, Denic S, Galadari S. Longer breast-feeding and protection against childhood leukaemia and lymphomas. Eur J Cancer 2001;37:234–8.
53. Schwartzbaum JA, George SL, Pratt CB, et al. An exploratory study of environmental and medical factors potentially related to childhood cancer. Med Pediatr Oncol 1991;19:115–21.
54. Martin RM, Middleton N, Gunnell D, et al. Breast-feeding and cancer: The Boyd Orr cohort and a systematic review with meta-analysis. J Natl Cancer Inst 2005;97:1446–57.
55. Bittner J. Some possible effects of nursing on the mammary gland tumor incidence in mice. Science 1936;84:162.
56. Titus-Ernstoff L, Egan KM, Newcomb PA, et al. Exposure to breast milk in infancy and adult breast cancer risk. J Natl Cancer Inst 1998;90:921–4.
57. Michels KB, Trichopoulos D, Rosner BA, et al. Being breastfed in infancy and breast cancer incidence in adult life: Results from the two nurses' health studies. Am J Epidemiol 2001;153:275–83.
58. Wang Y, Holland JF, Bleiweiss IJ, et al. Detection of mammary tumor virus env gene-like sequences in human breast cancer. Cancer Res 1995;55:5173–9.
59. Levine PH, Mesa-Tejada R, Keydar I, et al. Increased incidence of mouse mammary tumor virus-related antigen in Tunisian patients with breast cancer. Int J Cancer 1984;33:305–8.
60. Jensen A, Slorach SA, editors. Chemical Contaminants in Human Milk. Boca Roton, FL: CRC Press; 1991.
61. Nickerson K. Environmental contaminants in breast milk. J Midwifery Womens Health 2006;51:26–34.
62. Dewailly E, Yotte PA, Brisson J. Protective effect of breast feeding on breast cancer and body burden. J Natl Cancer Inst 1994;86:603.
63. Rogan W, Ragan N. Chemical contaminants, pharmacokinetics, and lactating mother. Environ Health Perspect 1994;102:89–95.
64. Chantry CJ, Howard CR, Auinger P. Full breastfeeding duration and associated decrease in respiratory tract infection in US children. Pediatrics 2006;117:425–32.
65. Freudenheim JL, Marshall JR, Graham S, et al. Exposure to breastmilk in infancy and the risk of breast cancer. Epidemiology 1994;5:324–31.
66. Hakansson A, Zhivotovsky B, Orrenius S, et al. Apoptosis induced by a human milk protein. Proc Natl Acad Sci U S A 1995;92:8064–8.
67. Coupland CA, Forman D, Chilvers CE, et al. Maternal risk factors for testicular cancer: A population-based case-control study (UK). Cancer Causes Control 2004;15:277–83.
68. Barba M, McCann SE, Nie J, et al. Perinatal exposures and breast cancer risk in the Western New York Exposures and Breast Cancer (WEB) Study. Cancer Causes Control 2006;17:395–401.
69. Russo IH, Russo J. Mammary gland neoplasia in long-term rodent studies. Environ Health Perspect 1996;104:938–67.
70. Russo J, Russo IH. Toward a physiological approach to breast cancer prevention. Cancer Epidemiol Biomarkers Prev 1994;3:353–64.
71. Engelman RW, Day NK, Good RA. Calorie intake during mammary development influences cancer risk: Lasting inhibition of C3H/HeOu mammary tumorigenesis by peripubertal calorie restriction. Cancer Res 1994;54:5724–30.
72. Dillin A, Crawford DK, Kenyon C. Timing requirements for insulin/IGF-I signaling in C. elegans. Science 2002;298:830–4.
73. Frankel S, Gunnell DJ, Peters TJ, et al. Childhood energy intake and adult mortality from cancer: The Boyd Orr Cohort Study. BMJ 1998;316:499–504.
74. Tretli S, Gaard M. Lifestyle changes during adolescence and risk of breast cancer: An ecologic study of the effect of World War II in Norway. Cancer Causes Control 1996;7:507–12.
75. van Noord PAH. Breast cancer and the brain: A neurodevelopmental hypothesis to explain the opposing effects of caloric deprivation during the Dutch famine of 1944–1945 on breast cancer and its risk factors. J Nutr 2004;134:3399S–406S.
76. Ariazi JL, Haag JD, Lindstrom MJ, et al. Mammary glands of sexually immature rats are more susceptible than those of mature rats to the carcinogenic, lethal, and mutagenic effects of *N*-nitroso-*N*-methylurea. Mol Carcinog 2005;43:155–64.
77. Hancock SL, Tucker MA, Hoppe RT. Breast cancer after treatment of Hodgkin's disease. J Natl Cancer Inst 1993;85:25–31.
78. Ziegler RG, Hoover RN, Pike MC, et al. Migration patterns and breast cancer risk in Asian-American women. J Natl Cancer Inst 1993;85:1819–27.
79. Gunnell D, Okasha M, Smith GD, et al. Height, leg length, and cancer risk: A systematic review. Epidemiol Rev 2001;23:313–42.
80. Lawlor DA, Okasha M, Gunnell D, et al. Associations of adult measures of childhood growth with breast cancer: Findings from the British Women's Heart and Health Study. Br J Cancer 2003;89:81–7.
81. Tretli S. Height and weight in relation to breast cancer morbidity and mortality. A prospective study of 570,000 women in Norway. Int J Cancer 1989;44:23–30.
82. Wadsworth ME, Hardy RJ, Paul AA, et al. Leg and trunk length at 43 years in relation to childhood health, diet and family circumstances; Evidence from the 1946 national birth cohort. Int J Epidemiol 2002;31:383–90.
83. Gunnell D. Can adult anthropometry be used as a "biomarker" for prenatal and childhood exposures? Int J Epidemiol 2002;31:390–4.
84. Gunnell DJ, Smith GD, Holly JM, et al. Leg length and risk of cancer in the Boyd Orr cohort. BMJ 1998;317:1350–1.
85. Friedenreich CM, Orenstein MR. Physical activity and cancer prevention: Etiologic evidence and biological mechanisms. J Nutr 2002;132:3456S–64S.
86. Frazier AL, Willett WC, Colditz GA. Reproducibility of recall of adolescent diet: Nurses' Health Study (United States). Cancer Causes Control 1995;6:499–506.
87. Maruti SS, Feskanich D, Colditz GA, et al. Adult recall of adolescent diet: Reproducibility and comparison with maternal reporting. Am J Epidemiol 2005;161:89–97.
88. Frazier AL, Ryan CT, Rockett H, et al. Adolescent diet and risk of breast cancer. Breast Cancer Res 2003;5:R59–64.
89. Potischman N, Weiss HA, Swanson CA, et al. Diet during adolescence and risk of breast cancer among young women. J Natl Cancer Inst 1998;90:226–33.
90. Pryor M, Slattery ML, Robison LM, et al. Adolescent diet and breast cancer in Utah. Cancer Res 1989;49:2161–7.
91. Hislop TG, Coldman AJ, Elwood JM, et al. Childhood and recent eating patterns and risk of breast cancer. Cancer Detect Prev 1986;9:47–58.
92. Hilakivi-Clarke L, Onojafe I, Raygada M, et al. Prepubertal exposure to zearalenone or genistein reduces mammary tumorigenesis. Br J Cancer 1999;80:1682–8.
93. Shu XO, Jin F, Dai Q, et al. Soyfood intake during adolescence and subsequent risk of breast cancer among Chinese women. Cancer Epidemiol Biomarkers Prev 2001;10:483–8.
94. Wu AH, Wan P, Hankin J, et al. Adolescent and adult soy intake and risk of breast cancer in Asian-Americans. Carcinogenesis 2002;23:1491–6.
95. Thanos J, Cotterchio M, Boucher BA, et al. Adolescent dietary phytoestrogen intake and breast cancer risk (Canada). Cancer Causes Control 2006;17:1253–61.
96. Schnitt SJ, Connolly JL. Pathology of benign breast disorders. In: Harris JR, Lippmann ME, Osborne CK, editors. Diseases of the Breast, 2nd edition. Philadelphia, PA: Lippincott Williams & Wilkins; 2000.
97. Baer HJ, Schnitt SJ, Connolly JL, et al. Early life factors and incidence of proliferative benign breast disease. Cancer Epidemiol Biomarkers Prev 2005;14:2889–97.
98. Kvale G, Heuch I. Menstrual factors and breast cancer risk. Cancer 1988;62:1625–31.
99. Maclure M, Travis LB, Willett W, et al. A prospective cohort study of nutrient intake and age at menarche. Am J Clin Nutr 1991;54:649–56.
100. Koprowski C, Ross RK, Mack WJ, et al. Diet, body size and menarche in a multiethnic cohort. Br J Cancer 1999;79:1907–11.
101. Meyer F, Moisan J, Marcoux D, et al. Dietary and physical determinants of menarche. Epidemiology 1990;1:377–81.
102. Merzenich H, Boeing H, Wahrendorf J. Dietary fat and sports activity as determinants for age at menarche. Am J Epidemiol 1993;138:217–24.
103. Koo MM, Rohan TE, Jain M, et al. A cohort study of dietary fibre intake and menarche. Public Health Nutr 2002;5:353–60.
104. Soriguer FJ, Gonzalez-Romero S, Esteva I, et al. Does the intake of nuts and seeds alter the appearance of menarche? Acta Obstet Gynecol Scand 1995;74:455–61.
105. Hughes RE, Jones E. Intake of dietary fibre and the age of menarche. Ann Hum Biol 1985;12:325–32.
106. de Ridder CM, Thijssen JH, Van 't Veer P, et al. Dietary habits, sexual maturation, and plasma hormones in pubertal girls: A longitudinal study. Am J Clin Nutr 1991;54:805–13.
107. Troisi R, Masters MN, Joshipura K, et al. Perinatal factors, growth and development, and osteosarcoma risk. Br J Cancer 2006;1603–7.
108. Gelberg KH, Fitzgerald EF, Hwang S-A, et al. Growth and development and other risk factors for osteosarcoma in children and young adults. Int J Epidemiol 1997;26:272–78.
109. Operskalski EA, Preston-Martin S, Henderson BE, et al. A case: Control study of osteosarcoma in young persons. Am J Epidemial 1987;126:118–26.

55

Cancer Treatment

Lori J. Bechard, MEd, RD, LDN
Christopher Duggan, MD, MPH

INTRODUCTION

The nutritional implications of childhood cancer have evolved from a chronicle of extensive malnutrition to a complex scenario of nutritional diagnoses resulting from disease and treatment. Nutritional assessment of the child with cancer is important for identifying and treating malnutrition, and also in ensuring the appropriate provision of nutrients to promote recovery and long-term health. Being overweight or underweight has been associated with greater treatment-related mortality.[1] Changes in nutrient metabolism[2] and body composition[3] in pediatric cancer patients occur as a result of disease and subsequent treatment. These changes can obscure nutritional deficits for growing children. Increased survival rates and improvements in supportive care therapies have shed light on several late effects of cancer treatment, including obesity, hyperlipidemia, and variations of the so-called "metabolic syndrome,[4–6] which have emerged as important entities in the ever-growing population of childhood cancer survivors. Chronic health conditions, many of which have a relationship with nutritional intake, are common among survivors of pediatric cancer.[7,8] Families of children with cancer place a strong emphasis on weight[9] and nutritional therapy, both for the important psychosocial aspects of eating[10] and for the potential for synergistic intervention with medical therapies.[11] We review the metabolic effects of pediatric cancers and their treatment, highlighting the nutritional conditions and interventions encountered by children from diagnosis to long-term survival.

PREVALENCE OF MALNUTRITION IN PEDIATRIC CANCER

The incidence of childhood cancer in the United States during 2000 to 2003 was 16.4 cases per 100,000 children under age 18 years; the most common pediatric malignancy was acute lymphocytic leukemia (ALL), followed by brain and other central nervous system (CNS) tumors.[12] Malnutrition among cancer patients is determined by host susceptibility, tumor type and location, and treatment regimen. Relapsed malignant disease, hematopoietic stem cell transplantation (HSCT), tumors of the abdomen, head, or neck, and other advanced-stage solid tumors are clinically associated with poorer nutritional status than lower risk diseases. In general, children with solid tumors have a greater incidence of malnutrition.[13,14] Most patients with low-risk ALL, those with nonmetastatic solid tumors, and patients in remission are generally able to maintain a normal weight. Some children become obese during or following treatment.[15,16] A variety of pediatric cancer diagnoses can be grouped according to their nutritional risk (Table 1).

Weight loss may be considered the final step in a long process of nutritional perturbation in patients with cancer, and as such may not be a useful indicator of malnutrition. Even the use of body mass index (BMI) for a marker of nutritional status may be inaccurate due to its inability to access changes in lean body mass. At presentation for HSCT, most children appear well nourished by BMI criteria; however, reduced body cell mass is common and does not correlate well with BMI.[17] Overt signs of malnutrition do not typically present at diagnosis with leukemia, although elevations in cytokine antagonists and reductions in plasma proteins, compared to controls, have been observed, suggestive of an early malnourished state.[18] A study of prepubertal children with low-risk ALL followed body weight and lean body mass over time (as measured by sum of four skinfold measurements and bioelectrical impedance). Although body weight in the cancer patients was no different than age- and sex-matched controls, lean body mass declined substantially with the use of chemotherapy.[3] Similarly, when comparing arm anthropometry to weight for height in children newly diagnosed with solid tumors, 27% were malnourished by arm anthropometry, while weight for height did not reveal this observation.[19] Consequently, dependence on body weight alone to inform nutritional status may lead to an underestimate of the incidence of malnutrition.

Table 1 Nutritional Risk Groupings of Pediatric Malignancies and Associated Conditions

High risk
Relapsed disease
High-risk acute lymphocytic leukemia
Acute myelogenous leukemia
Advanced-stage solid tumors
Neuroblastoma
Wilm's tumor
Lymphoma (Hodgkin's and non-Hodgkin's)
Hepatoblastoma
Medulloblastoma
Tumors involving the head, neck, or abdomen
Hemophagocytic lymphohistiocytosis (HLH)
Hematopoietic stem cell transplantation
Low risk
Standard-risk leukemia
Early stage solid tumors
Obesity risk
Acute lymphocytic leukemia
Brain tumors with hypothalamic damage

Definition of Cancer Cachexia

Cachexia has been classically defined as a severe state of malnutrition characterized by anorexia, weight loss, muscle wasting, and anemia.[20,21] In its broader sense, cancer cachexia has also been used to describe a variety of metabolic events including hypoalbuminemia, hypoglycemia, lactic acidosis, hyperlipidemia, impaired hepatic function, glucose intolerance with insulin resistance, elevated gluconeogenesis, skeletal muscle atrophy, visceral organ atrophy, and anergy.[22]

Wasting is defined as involuntary weight loss, and is found in many patients with chronic disease, including cancer, kidney disease, cardiac disease, and advanced HIV infection. Overall loss of body weight, including fat and fat-free mass, occurs as a result of the energy imbalance caused by disease. Cachexia, in contrast with wasting,[23] is defined as involuntary loss of lean body mass in the setting of minimal or no overall weight loss. In this scenario, patients of normal weight can still be malnourished due to diminished lean body mass. This loss of muscle is known to negatively influence recovery and reduce survival in patients with cardiac disease and cancer.[24] Since this decline in lean body mass has important functional and prognostic significance, even in the setting of stable or increasing weight, this type of malnutrition is important to identify.

Differential loss of body fat versus fat-free mass implies a different etiology and prognosis of malnutrition; therefore, the pattern of weight loss and changes in body composition in patients with illness is of considerable significance. For example, prolonged fasting in the absence of metabolic perturbation (as can be seen in adolescents with anorexia nervosa) leads to a predictable decrement first in body fat and then in body protein stores.[25] In this case, energy repletion is usually successful with the careful provision of adequate energy, protein, and micronutrients.

In contrast, weight loss in the setting of cancer, infection, or other metabolic stress is composed of both fat and fat-free mass.[26] Since the energy density of fat-free mass is lower than that of fat, body's use of lean body mass as an energy and amino acid source can lead to weight loss that can be quite profound and rapid. It is this loss of fat-free mass that is of significance, since loss of lean body mass is associated with important functional changes, including loss of strength, decreased immune function, decreased pulmonary function, increased disability, and death.[27–31]

The provision of nutritional support to these patients may not be adequate to reverse the catabolic effects of their underlying condition. In the early days of parenteral nutrition use, it was hypothesized that aggressive parenteral nutrition could overcome the catabolism of cancer and other critical illnesses[32]; however, this has not proven to be the case. In a meta-analysis of parenteral nutrition (PN), the authors concluded that the benefits of PN in cancer and HSCT were unclear due to conflicting data.[33] Methodologies and nutritional prescriptions for children with cancer are explored in subsequent sections.

METABOLIC EFFECTS OF CANCER

The presence of malignancy results in several important changes in macronutrient (carbohydrates, fats, and protein) metabolism and these metabolic alterations can in turn affect energy balance. Metabolic effects of cancer are variable, and depend in part on tumor types and sizes, chemotherapy treatment protocols, as well as a number of host factors, including nutritional status at baseline. A general understanding of these aberrations is, however, useful in anticipating potential metabolic complications as well as planning nutritional therapy.

Carbohydrate

Multiple metabolic shifts in glucose homeostasis tend to increase blood concentrations of glucose in cancer. These include increased gluconeogenesis (the conversion of amino acid carbon skeletons to glucose),[34] and increased Cori cycling (the hepatic conversion of lactate to glucose).[35] Increased conversion of lactate to glucose may be due in part to increased lactate production by selected tumors. Combined with insulin resistance,[36–38] the enhanced production of glucose provides the tumor with ample substrate that is readily metabolized under both aerobic and anaerobic conditions.

Lipid

Multiple changes in lipid metabolism in cancer include increased free fatty acid turnover, increased free fatty acid oxidation, increased glycerol turnover, greater lipolysis, and lower rates of lipogenesis. A lipid-mobilizing factor has been isolated from the urine of cachectic cancer patients and shows bioactivity with isolated murine adipocytes.[39] In addition, there can be a marked loss of body fat that can occur early in the evolution of the malignancy.[40] Hypertriglyceridemia can be observed among children with ALL, those with widespread solid tumors, and those treated with L-asparaginase.[41] The provision of glucose does not seem to resolve the high rates of fatty acid and glycerol turnover evident in weight-losing cancer patients.[42] Treatment with chemotherapy is associated with decreased fat utilization in children newly diagnosed with ALL.[2]

Protein

Cancer is often associated with an acute-phase-response blood profile, with low synthesis rates of albumin, prealbumin, and transferrin, and increased rates of synthesis of C-reactive protein, fibrinogen, and ferritin.[43] Some tumors such as hepatocellular cancer exhibit very high rates of protein turnover and increased protein degradation.[44] An increase in muscle protein breakdown mobilizes amino acids that may assist tumor growth as well as fuel gluconeogenesis. This increased protein breakdown in pediatric cancer patients may be related to falling levels of insulin-like growth factor (IGF-1), and insulin-like growth factor binding proteins.[45] In other patients, decreased skeletal muscle protein synthesis seems to be of primary importance.[46] Although the mechanism remains uncertain, a net loss of skeletal muscle protein is a common finding with malignancy and is particularly problematic in the growing child.

Cytokines

Proinflammatory cytokines commonly associated with cancer cachexia include tumor necrosis factor-alpha (TNF-α), interleukin-6 (IL-6), interleukin-1 (IL-1), and interferon-gamma (INF-γ). These cytokines are secreted by macrophages and lymphocytes and may represent the host response to cancer. Administering TNF-α to humans produces effects associated with cancer cachexia, including increased fatty acid turnover, elevated glycerol turnover, and increased whole-body protein turnover.[47] Not all patients with cancer cachexia have detectable levels of TNF-α; hence, a paracrine or autocrine mechanism of action may be responsible. Other factors also seem to be involved with the catabolic response to cancer. Circulating IL-6 levels are generally elevated in cancer patients and animal models support its role in causing cachexia.[48] As with TNF-α, the precise mechanism of action of IL-6 is unknown. The metabolic roles of IL-1 and interferon-γ are less well characterized in tumor models; however, like TNF-α and IL-6, they appear to inhibit lipoprotein lipase and hence facilitate lipolysis. Drugs with cytokine inhibitory properties such as pentoxyfylline, thalidomide, anti-COX-2, and megesterol acetate are being evaluated as possible therapies for cancer cachexia.[49]

Energy Balance

While early studies suggested that the energy needs of rapidly dividing cells of the tumor increased basal metabolic demands of the host from 20 to 90% over predicted needs, more recent studies provide conflicting data. Energy expenditure measurements of children with cancer have been observed in a variety of clinical scenarios with mixed outcomes. Stallings et al measured resting energy expenditure (REE) in nine patients with ALL and found that patients with a higher tumor burden (elevated WBC count, and organomegaly) had an increased REE.[2] On the contrary, study of 26 patients with ALL or solid tumors in remission showed no elevations in resting energy expenditure, when compared to age- and sex-matched healthy controls.[50] Reilly et al[51] studied 20 preadolescent children with ALL with doubly labeled water. Compared to healthy controls matched for age, sex, and body composition, children with ALL had significantly lower TEE than controls by an average of 282 kcal/d. Most of this reduction was due to reduced physical activity. Any deviation in energy expenditure can result in energy imbalance and potentially undesirable weight loss or gain; thus, a careful look at changes in expenditure is worthwhile.

Lean body mass is the primary predictor of energy expenditure, so it follows that cancer treatment, which is known to alter lean body mass, could affect energy expenditure. Patients with head and neck cancer experienced changes in REE, as measured by indirect calorimetry, when prospectively evaluated prior to treatment, at weeks 2, 4, and 6 during treatment, at the end of treatment, and 2 weeks following completion of treatment. While REE was higher than that predicted by standardized equations in this small group of adults, REE declined significantly over time and followed a U-shaped curve from pretreatment to posttreatment.[52] Ringwald-Smith et al compared weekly measured REE in 34 children undergoing autologous or allogeneic SCT to standardized equations and found that REE was significantly lesser than predicted except at 14 days posttransplant.[53] Furthermore, a prospective study of 37 children undergoing allogeneic transplantation described a significant decline in REE from baseline to week 3 after HSCT, as well as a significant reduction in midarm muscle area.[54] These three studies suggest that treatment-related changes in REE occur, which may be related to reductions in lean body mass. Further explorations of REE as it relates to changes in body composition in children with cancer are needed.

METABOLIC EFFECTS OF TREATMENT

Treatments used in pediatric cancer cause systemic side effects that exacerbate the symptoms of the tumor itself. A combination of agents, including radiotherapy, chemotherapeutic drugs, and surgery, is commonly used to treat pediatric cancers, particularly high-risk diseases. Radiation therapy, widely used in the treatment of leukemias and brain tumors, is known to cause localized end-organ damage. Diarrhea and malabsorption with fluid and electrolyte losses may result when the abdomen or pelvis is radiated.[55] Radiation to the head and neck areas may similarly cause damage to taste, chewing, and swallowing functions. Nutritional status may be affected with surgical interventions depending on the site of the tumor and the extent of the resection.[55] The efficient digestion, ingestion, absorption, and utilization of food is a complex process. Surgical disruption with impaired swallowing, decreased gastric reserve, or reduction in intestinal length can result in decreased oral intake as well as absorption of nutrients.[56]

Chemotherapeutic agents are known to cause anorexia, with or without nausea and vomiting, enteritis with malabsorption and diarrhea, mucositis, and constipation. Taste perception is also altered in cancer patients receiving chemotherapy; this phenomenon contributes further to anorexia and reduced food intake. Mucosal damage is generally dose related, with increased risk of mucosal toxicity with high-dose induction therapy, escalating dosage patterns, continuous infusion (vs bolus doses), and combination chemotherapy treatments. Oral and gastrointestinal mucositis represents a major nonhematologic complication of cytotoxic chemotherapy and radiotherapy which is associated with significant morbidity, pain, and odynophagia.[57] Mucositis often leads to a decreased intake of liquids and solids as well as nausea and vomiting. Examples of commonly used chemotherapies and applicable nutrition-related toxicities are presented in Table 2.

Myeloablative HSCT is typically reserved for those cases without other reasonable options, since it is known to be a high-risk, highly toxic intervention (Table 3). High-dose chemotherapy and total body irradiation as conditioning for HSCT frequently cause prolonged oral and gastrointestinal mucositis that can diminish nutritional intake for days to weeks. Another adverse effect of HSCT is hepatic veno-occlusive disease (VOD), a syndrome of hepatomegaly, jaundice, and fluid retention, which in its severe form may cause renal and respiratory failure. Hepatic VOD has nutritional implications in that its cholestasis and fluid management will almost certainly impact nutrient and fluid provision. Graft-versus-host disease (GVHD), a condition involving the attack of newly engrafted cells on the host recipient, can occur following allogeneic HSCT. Acute gastrointestinal GVHD can cause symptoms ranging from mild nausea and anorexia to profuse, bloody diarrhea. Acute skin GVHD can similarly manifest as a mild rash, or progress to severe epithelial sloughing, akin to a burn injury. Other organ systems may also be affected. Most children with acute GVHD will require intensive, individualized nutrition support, while high-dose immunosuppression is used to treat the disease process.

Chronic GVHD typically occurs more than 100 days following transplant, and while its

Table 2 Nutrition-Related Side Effects of Commonly Used Chemotherapies in Childhood Cancer

Chemotherapies	Diseases Targeted	Toxicities
Alkylating Agents		
Mechlorethamine (nitrogen mustard)	Hodgkin's disease	N&V, phlebitis, mucositis
Cyclosphosphamide	Lymphomas, leukemias, sarcomas, neuroblastoma	N&V, cystitis, water retention, cardiac (HD)
Ifosfamide	Sarcomas, germ cell	N&V, cystitis, renal, cardiac (HD)
Melphalan	Rhabdomyosarcoma, sarcomas, neuroblastoma, leukemias (HD)	N&V, mucositis, diarrhea (HD)
Lomustine, carmustine (CCNU, BCNU)	Brain tumors, lymphoma, Hodgkin's disease	N&V, renal, pulmonary
Busulfan	CML, leukemias (HSCT)	Pulmonary, N&V, mucositis, hepatic (HD)
Cisplatin	Testicular, other germ cell, brain tumors, osteosarcoma, neuroblastoma	N&V, renal
Carboplatin	Brain tumors, germ cell, neuroblastoma, sarcomas	N&V, hepatic
Dacarbazine	Neuroblastoma, sarcomas, Hodgkin's disease	N&V, flulike syndrome, hepatic
Temozolomide	N&V	Brain tumors
Procarbazine	Hodgkin's disease, brain tumors	N&V, rash, mucositis
Antimetabolites		
Methotrexate	Leukemia, lymphoma, osteosarcoma	Mucositis, rash, hepatic, renal
Mercaptopurine (6MP)	Leukemia (ALL, CML)	Hepatic, mucositis
Thioguanine	Leukemia (ALL, AML)	N&V, mucositis, hepatic (VOD)
Cytarabine (Ara-C)	Leukemia, lymphoma	N&V, mucositis, GI, flulike syndrome, ocular, skin (HD)
Fluorouracil (5FU)	Carcinomas, hepatic tumors	Mucositis, N&V, diarrhea, skin, ocular, cardiac
Antitumor antibiotics		
Doxorubicin (adriamycin), daunomycin, idarubicin	Leukemia (ALL, ANLL), lymphomas, solid tumors	Mucositis, N&V, diarrhea, cardiac
Mitoxantrone	Leukemia (ALL, ANLL), lymphomas	Mucositis, N&V, bluish color to urine, veins, sclerae, nails
Bleomycin	Lymphoma, testicular, other germ cell	Lung, skin, fever, mucositis, Raynaud's, N&V
Dactinomycin (actinomycin-D)	Wilm's sarcomas	N&V, mucositis, hepatic (VOD)
Plant products		
Vincristine	Leukemia (ALL), lymphomas, solid tumors	SIADH, hypotension, constipation
Vinblastine	Histiocytosis, Hodgkin's disease, testicular	Mucositis
Etoposide	Leukemias (ALL, ANLL), lymphomas, neuroblastoma, sarcomas, brain tumors	N&V, mucositis, hypotension, secondary leukemia, diarrhea (PO dosing)
Teniposide	Leukemia (ALL)	N&V, mucositis, hypotension
Topotecan	Neuroblastoma, rhabdomyosarcoma	Diarrhea, mucositis, N&V, rash, hepatic
Irinotecan	Rhabdomyosarcoma	Diarrhea, N&V, hepatic, dehydration, ileus
Other agents		
Corticosteroids (prednisone, methylprednisolone, dexamethasone, decadron)	Leukemia, lymphomas, brain tumors	Increased appetite, centripedal obesity, myopathy, osteoporosis, pancreatitis, hypertension, diabetes, growth failure, impaired wound healing
Asparaginase	Leukemia (ALL), lymphoma	Pancreatitis, hepatic
All-*trans*-Retinoic acid (ATRA, tretinoin)	Acute promyelocytic leukemia	Retinoic acid syndrome (weight gain, respiratory distress, cardiac & renal failure), cheilitis, dry skin, ↑triglycerides
13-*cis*-Retinoic acid (isotretinoin, accutane)	Minimal residual disease neuroblastoma	Cheilitis, dry mouth, bone & joint pain, ↑triglycerides, ↑Ca^{2+}
Imatinib mesylate (gleevec)	Ph chromosome+ CML	N&V, fatigue, GI, hepatic

Adapted from reference 58.

ALL = acute lymphoblastic leukemia; AML = acute myelogenous leukemia; ANLL = acute nonlymphoblastic leukemia; CLL = chronic lymphocytic leukemia; CML = chronic myelocytic leukemia; GI = gastrointestinal; HD = high dose; HSCT = hematopoietic stem cell transplantation; N&V = nausea and vomiting; SIADH = syndrome of inappropriate antidiuretic drug hormone secretion; VOD = veno-occlusive disease; ↑, increased.

Table 3 Diseases Commonly Treated with Hematopoietic Stem Cell Transplantation

Autologous Transplantation	Allogeneic Transplantation	
Non-Hodgkin's lymphoma	*Cancers*	*Other diseases*
Hodgkin's disease	Acute myeloid leukemia	Aplastic anemia
Acute myeloid leukemia	Acute lymphoblastic leukemia	Fanconi's anemia
Neuroblastoma	Chronic myeloid leukemia	Blackfan–Diamond anemia
Germ cell tumors	Myelodysplastic syndrome	Thalassemia major
	Non-Hodgkin's lymphoma	Sickle cell anemia
	Hodgkin's disease	Severe combined immunodeficiencies
	Juvenile chronic myeloid leukemia	Wiskott–Aldrich syndrome

Adapted from reference 59.

presentation tends to be less severe than acute GVHD, it is associated with significant long-term morbidity and mortality.[60–62] Skin, liver, mouth, and eyes are the most commonly affected sites.[63] Single-organ disease incurs less weight loss than multiorgan disease, and requires significantly shorter length of therapy. Multiorgan disease often affects the skin and oral cavity, as well as the lung and liver, while single-organ disease is more frequently found in the liver or skin.[64] The incidence of chronic GVHD is lower in children than adults; however, its manifestations are uniquely problematic to children. Malnutrition and accompanying growth failure is common, but poorly understood.[64] Other complications include bone loss, steroid induced weight gain, dysphagia, and depression. Treatment of chronic GVHD typically employs therapy beyond first-line immunosuppression with steroids and calcineurin inhibitors.

ETIOLOGY OF ANOREXIA IN CANCER TREATMENT

As indicated in the above sections, malignancies and their treatment can have a considerable effect on a child's nutritional status. Frequently occurring nutritional problems with cancer treatment are depicted in Figure 1. Anorexia can be a side effect of any disease. Food aversion and anorexia may be linked with nausea and vomiting. While the pathophysiology of cancer undoubtedly causes nutritional risk in children with cancer, eating problems are multifactorial in nature. Psychological factors are also important to consider in evaluating the reasons behind inadequate dietary intake. Depression-related anorexia is probably underappreciated as a cause.

The ability of children to eat at their appropriate developmental level may affect the nutritional adequacy of their diet. Anorexia, mucositis, and other effects of cancer treatment may interrupt the normal progression of feeding skills in infants and young children. Once arrested, the development of these skills may be difficult to restore. The resumption of eating can be a lengthy and difficult process and may extend the time frame of cancer recovery. Poor swallowing and chewing abilities will lengthen the time required to complete a meal and thus may lead to inadequate consumption of many required nutrients. Children may refuse to eat their preferred foods due to adverse associations or other impairments and thus may self-restrict their intake.

The impact of a cancer diagnosis on family dynamics and related behaviors should not be overlooked. Relationships between patients and caregivers influence nutritional intake, both positively and negatively. Appetite and feeding behaviors are inherently complicated activities of all children, and this behavior can obviously be affected by the onset of illness, its treatment, as well as the psychosocial impact that cancer has on the child and family. The nature of cancer medical care is such that parents often feel that they are relinquishing much of their usual caregiving behavior to the medical and nursing staff. Some parents understandably cling to the provision of food and nutrients as a critical part of parenting. Occasionally, such strong feelings concerning food and dietary intake can cause conflict between parent and child, and be counterproductive to the goal of optimal nutrition. Discord among family members can lead to further negative consequences to the feeding relationship.

NUTRITIONAL ASSESSMENT OF THE CHILD WITH CANCER

The assessment of a child with cancer includes standard elements of a nutritional evaluation: history of past and present illness, review of dietary intake, physical examination, and anthropometric measurements. Attention should also be directed to the significance of body composition changes as well as a review of pertinent laboratory measures.

History

A detailed medical history is essential to the nutritional evaluation of a patient. Important oncologic history includes the type and stage of the tumor, the intensity of the antitumor therapy, and the presence or absence of remission. Nutritional history entails (1) current symptoms of cancer and its therapy and their effect on nutrient intake, absorption, and retention; (2) past history, including growth data, and previous antitumor therapy and its effects on nutritional status; (3) developmental status, with special attention to milestones of feeding skills and swallowing function; (4) known or perceived food allergies or intolerances; (5) medications, with special attention to those with gastrointestinal and metabolic side effects; (6) family history, parental heights, and sibling growth patterns; (7) social history, food preferences/beliefs, and food availability; and (8) a thorough diet history obtained from the patient and/or caregivers.

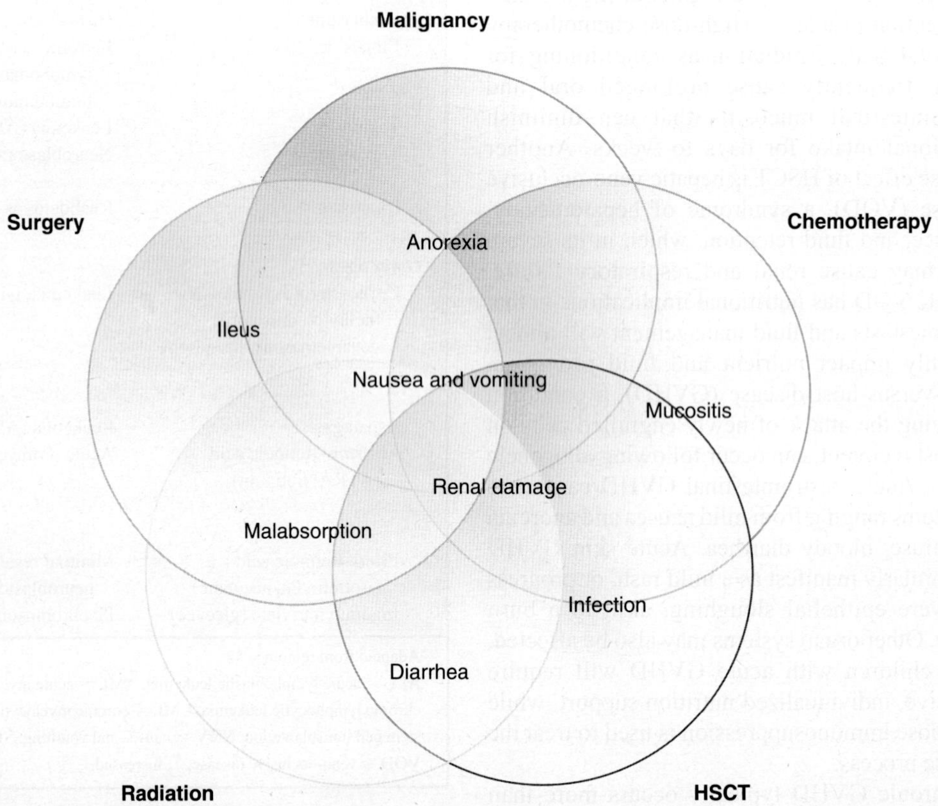

Figure 1 Nutrition-related problems in pediatric cancer treatment.

Physical Examination

The physical characteristics of a child with cancer may suggest the presence of nutritional problems. Indeed, the predisposition of chemotherapy to affect tissues of rapid turnover (eg, hair and gastrointestinal mucosa) parallels the symptoms of deficiency of several nutrients (eg, stomatitis with some B vitamins, alopecia with biotin deficiency). Careful inspection and palpation of subcutaneous fat and muscle stores are particularly important in the physical examination, since deficits of these two components of body stores are common in malnutrition.

The general physical examination may show edema as a result of low concentrations of circulating albumin. This can be a subtle finding with only mild hypoalbuminemia. Edema may actually mask progressive muscle wasting and loss of lean body mass. Hypoalbuminemia may be due to poor liver function related to tumor or treatment, inadequate protein intake, or nutrient losses in excess of intake.[65] Painful mouth or esophageal sores caused by mucositis can negatively impact a child's oral intake and thus be an impetus to consider nutritional support.[66] Children who have limited mobility due to impairment by disease or treatment side effects may experience changes in appetite or satiety. Recognition of these aspects of the physical examination is a valuable component of the overall nutritional assessment of the child with cancer.

Anthropometrics

Weight and height measured over time are the foundation of nutritional monitoring and evaluation.[67] These objective measures of nutritional status provide the most information for the least inconvenience and cost. Weight should be measured daily in the hospital setting and at each office visit for outpatients. Height/length measurements should be recorded monthly. Accurate technique is critical to the validity of the measures; detailed methodologies are reviewed in Chapter 2, "Clinical Assessment of Nutritional Status."

The incidence of weight and height deficits in children with cancer has been reported to be quite high, depending on the severity and type of cancer and its treatment.[68,69] However, with the increased incidence of obesity in children,[70] and the predisposition of some pediatric cancer patients to become obese, it is also important to screen for overweight. For children under the age of 3 years, this can be done by calculating the weight-for-height percent standard using the National Center for Health Statistics (NCHS) growth curves. For older children, BMI[71] is a more suitable measure of body fatness. Children with BMIs greater than the 85th percentile for age and sex are termed at risk for overweight, and those with BMIs greater than the 95th percentile are overweight. Reference values for BMIs are available[72] and are also included with the NCHS growth curves (see Appendix I, "Nutritional Assessment").

Arm Anthropometrics

Arm anthropometrics are an inexpensive, noninvasive, and widely accepted technique for estimating body composition against established normal values (see Chapter 2, "Clinical Assessment of Nutritional Status"). Triceps skinfold, mid-upper arm circumference and computed values of midarm muscle area, and midarm fat area correlate well with more accurate and sensitive measures of body composition.[73] Percentiles and standards for comparisons for triceps skinfolds and midarm muscle area are available[74] and may indicate the presence of malnutrition when weight or height is unavailable or unreliable, as in the case of a growing tumor mass.

A study of 16 boys with newly diagnosed cancer revealed no significant deviation from normal with respect to weight, height, and weight for height. However, when comparing the midarm circumference, triceps skinfold, and subscapular skinfold to normal values, significant reductions were found in the patients with cancer.[75] Another study compared weight-for-height values to MUAC and TSF of children with solid tumors and controls. While all children presented with normal weights and heights compared to national standards, children with solid tumors, particularly those with intra-abdominal tumors, had significantly lower values of MUAC and TSF.[19] These studies suggest that arm anthropometrics may be more sensitive indicators of undernutrition in the child with malignancy than are weight and height.

Other Measures of Body Composition

Anthropometric measurements may be confounded by technique, inaccuracy of equipment, lack of patient cooperation, and poor interindividual reliability. Since lean body mass is the metabolically active component of the body, it would be ideal, therefore, to characterize weight by an accurate and dependable measure of lean body mass in order to assess the need for and/or response to nutritional intervention.[75] Patients with solid tumors prior to reduction or excision are particularly susceptible to inaccurate weight measurements. In a study of 19 children with malignant solid tumors, regional ultrasonography of the femoral quadriceps muscle was more sensitive than anthropometrics and measurements of visceral proteins in detecting reduced muscle protein reserves compared to age- and sex-matched controls,[76] suggesting the need for further analysis of body composition in assessing nutritional status.

Dual-energy X-ray absorptiometry (DXA) is becoming increasingly available for clinical use. A whole-body DXA assessment measures total body bone mineral content, nonbone lean tissue, and fat, as well as bone mineral density, thereby providing body composition information using a three-compartment model. Elevations in body fat mass measured by DXA without a concomitant rise in body mass index (BMI, kg/m^2) have been reported in several studies of cancer survivors.[77–79] Others have shown similar trends in body fat mass measurements. Warner et al found that a group of children treated for ALL with chemotherapy and cranial radiation had significantly greater percent body fat, as measured by DXA, than age-matched groups with other malignancies or healthy controls.[80] When combining the DXA measurements of fat-free mass with measures of total body water and total body potassium, children with ALL in this cohort had a significantly lower hydration and potassium state of their fat-free mass than those with other malignancies and controls. Conversely, a cross-sectional study of children in remission from ALL showed a significantly higher hydration fraction of fat-free mass compared to healthy, age- and sex-matched controls, using DXA and a four-component model of body composition assessment.[81] Another study of 25 children who had undergone allogeneic HSCT at least 4 years previously showed that their mean BMI was 0.45 Z scores lower ($p < .05$) but that percent body fat as measured by DXA was 1.1 Z scores higher than controls ($p < .001$).[82] These studies confirm the utility of assessing body composition in children with cancer to reveal clinically important changes relevant to nutrient provision. While the ultimate applicability of DXA scanning to nutritional assessment is still evolving,[83] it is now widely used as a reasonable method of body composition[84] in both the clinical and research setting.

Laboratory Evaluation

Although laboratory evaluation of the pediatric cancer patient is commonly performed to assess the hematologic and metabolic response to cancer and its treatment, nutritional status should also be monitored with select biochemical parameters. Serum electrolytes and mineral concentrations are commonly deranged during treatment of cancer, especially when nephrotoxic agents are employed. A specific metabolic emergency termed "tumor lysis syndrome" occurs in the early stages of tumor diagnosis and treatment as a result of tumor cell breakdown. The massive cell lysis can lead to life-threatening electrolyte abnormalities, including hyperphosphatemia, hyperkalemia, hyperuricemia, and resultant renal failure.

Visceral proteins synthesized by the liver are often used to assess nutritional status, since decreased levels presumably reflect a reduced supply of amino acid precursors and/or decreased hepatic and other visceral protein mass. Blood concentrations of these proteins, however, are dependent on their rates of synthesis, degradation, and escape from the circulatory system. Serum proteins are also affected by infectious or catabolic processes. The concentrations of positive acute-phase proteins (eg, C-reactive protein, ferritin, and ceruloplasmin) are increased in infectious or other catabolic illnesses, whereas negative acute-phase proteins (eg, albumin, prealbumin, transferrin, and retinol-binding protein) are decreased in these circumstances.

Albumin is the most abundant serum protein, the least expensive, and easiest protein to measure, and therefore is commonly used to assess protein status. It is, however, a relatively insensitive marker of nutritional status owing to its long half-life of 20 days and its ability to be mobilized from extravascular stores even in the presence of prolonged energy and protein deficiency. Hypoalbuminemia can occur in situations of decreased synthesis (eg, liver disease, age over 70 years, and malignancy), increased losses (eg, nephrosis, protein-losing enteropathy, and burn injuries), or increased losses to extravascular spaces (eg, acute catabolic stress with capillary leak syndrome), and is not necessarily related to the presence of malnutrition. Fluid overload, a condition common to acutely ill cancer patients, can also dilute albumin concentrations.

Prealbumin is a more sensitive measure of visceral protein status than albumin because of its short half-life (2 days) and high ratio of essential to nonessential amino acids. Studies have shown prealbumin to correlate well with nitrogen balance.[85,86] A small study of children with solid tumors correlated disease status and treatment intensity with changes in prealbumin levels, suggesting that it is likely the best available serum marker of nutritional status.[87] Like albumin, its concentrations fall with an acute-phase protein response or liver disease. Levels increase with renal failure.

In a study of 170 children with an assortment of cancers, albumin and prealbumin levels were significantly lower on presentation in patients than in controls, while the acute-phase indicator C-reactive protein was elevated. After 6 months of chemotherapy, however, the C-reactive protein levels were comparable in the groups but the visceral protein levels were still lower in those with cancer.[88] This suggests that even though the acute-phase response is responsible for some alterations in visceral protein levels, cancer patients still have poorer visceral protein nutrition than controls.

Assessment of vitamin and mineral nutriture, particularly in the patient on total enteral or parenteral nutritional support, may also be helpful. At the time of diagnosis, the effect of tumor burden on metabolic processes may be profound, as demonstrated by laboratory analysis. In a study of 40 children with ALL >70% of children had low plasma 1,25-dihydroxy vitamin D levels, 73% had low osteocalcin levels, and 64% had hypercalciuria at the time of diagnosis. This is an indication of the effect of leukemia on vitamin D metabolism and bone turnover. The use of steroids and nephrotoxic agents may worsen hypercalciuria, putting patients at a greater risk for osteopenia and fractures. Excessive renal losses of magnesium during treatment with these medications were also demonstrated, with only 50% of patients able to maintain normal serum magnesium levels despite parenteral supplementation.[89]

Antioxidant nutrients, including vitamins A and E, beta-carotene, zinc, and selenium, have also been studied. Children newly diagnosed with a variety of cancers had lower concentrations of retinol, beta-carotene, vitamin E, and zinc prior to treatment compared to healthy controls in a multicenter French study. After 6 months of treatment, most of these parameters were largely unchanged; however, zinc concentrations in patients with CNS tumors and malignant bone tumors showed significant decline, suggesting the possibility of losses related to therapy, or a reduction in intake.[88] Zinc deficiency was also found to be common in children following SCT. Nineteen of 28 children developed biochemical zinc deficiency at a median of 7 days posttransplant. Zinc blood levels were positively correlated with serum concentrations of alkaline phosphatase, a zinc-dependent enzyme.[90] An observational study of 120 adults examined concentrations of retinol and vitamin E in the first month following SCT. Plasma retinol levels declined significantly from baseline to day 7 posttransplant, and were associated with severity of mucositis.[91] Another study of 103 children with ALL examined plasma antioxidant levels and chemotherapy side effects at diagnosis, 3 months, and 6 months after diagnosis. After adjustment for multiple comparisons, there was a significant relationship between shorter length of hospital stay and higher total carotenoid to total cholesterol ratio at diagnosis. Additionally, subjects were more likely to experience a treatment-related toxicity if they had a low plasma total carotenoid level.[92] More research is needed to further elucidate the relationship of these nutrient levels with clinical outcomes in cancer.

NUTRITION INTERVENTION

Food Safety

Since cancer and its treatment inherently cause immunosuppression to varying degrees, low microbial diets have historically been used in an effort to minimize risk of illness from foodborne pathogens.[93] Although there is little evidence to support efficacy of these regimens in preventing clinical infections, it is intuitive to rule out possible causes when little potential harm is involved. Versions of the neutropenic or low microbial diet are widely used throughout pediatric cancer treatment centers, though the impact of diet adherence and quality of life must be considered when comparing to food safety guidelines.[94] Chapter 17, "Food Safety," reviews these practices applicable to all children; Table 4 summarizes the prudent principles recommended for HSCT recipients.

Indications for Feeding Modalities

The method of nutrition support selected for the child with cancer is determined by a timely clinical assessment and estimation of the child's nutrient requirements.[96] Some children may thrive well on volitional oral intake, while others may require specialized enteral or parenteral support. Available evidence suggests that enteral support is a less expensive, safer, and effective way of nourishing the child with cancer than parenteral nutrition.[97–99] However, there is no standardized approach to nutrition intervention in pediatric oncology.[100] It is axiomatic that enteral feeding should be considered prior to the initiation of parenteral nutrition, and that oral supplements should be offered before considering tube feeding. The choice of diet for the child with cancer is often complicated by many medical and psychosocial issues; the most appropriate feeding method must provide nutrient requirements with least risk.[101] Patients and their family members should of course be included in the discussion of nutrition options, with mention of the risks and benefits of appropriate methods for the patient's current situation.

In the case of malnutrition, it is imperative to consider the manifestations of refeeding the body in a starved state. A profound hypophosphatemia, in particular, can characterize the rapid cellular influx of nutrients during the anabolic phase following starvation. The risk of this complication is especially present with parenteral nutrition. Severe metabolic complications may be avoided by the slow advancement of macronutrients over a period of days to weeks as well as close laboratory monitoring of electrolytes, glucose, and minerals.

Oral Diet

Since painful oral mucositis is a common side effect of chemotherapy with few effective treatments, a soft diet is often better tolerated. A diet high in magnesium or potassium may be useful for the child with excessive urinary losses of minerals due to chemotherapies or antibiotics. Other diet alterations may be indicated for a variety of comorbidities, for example, a reduced sodium diet for hypertension, a bland, low residue diet for gastrointestinal GVHD.[102] Most commonly, however,

Table 4 Food Safety Recommendations for HSCT Recipients

In addition to careful attention to food safety guidelines recommended for all children, those who have undergone HSCT should adhere to the following recommendations for 3 months, or until immunosuppresive medications have been discontinued:

- Avoid raw or undercooked meat, including beef, poultry, pork, lamb, venison, sweetbreads, and other game meat
- Avoid any foods containing undercooked meat, including sausages and casseroles
- Avoid raw or undercooked eggs or foods that contain them, such as hollandaise sauce, homemade eggnog, homemade mayonnaise, or salad dressing
- Avoid raw or undercooked seafood, such as clams, oysters, and sushi
- Avoid raw fruits and vegetables from developing countries
- Drink only tap water that has been treated and tested, or bottled water
- Avoid unpasteurized milk or other dairy products
- Avoid unpasteurized fruit juices
- Avoid food and drinks from street vendors

Adapted from reference 95.

calorie enhancement is the primary manipulation in an effort to promote weight gain or weight maintenance during treatment-associated anorexia. This can be accomplished with usual foods, or in combination with commercial supplemental drinks, bars, or calorie additives (see Chapter 71, "Special Diets," for further specifications of the high-calorie diet). Some children, including those with standard risk ALL and long-term survivors of cancer with activity limitations, may be aided by calorie moderation when excessive weight gain is a concern.

Enteral Feeding

If children are unable to meet their nutrient needs orally, tube feedings should be considered to preserve or achieve optimal nutritional status. Nasogastric tubes have been used with success in many pediatric oncology patients. In 21 children newly diagnosed with cancer, nasogastric tube feedings were given in addition to volitional oral intake. After 16 weeks of feedings, weights increased significantly.[103] Several studies have reported the use of nasogastric feedings in children after SCT with varying results. One group demonstrated improved weight gain in 21 patients, compared to eight children receiving dietary counseling alone. There was a positive correlation between increases in weight and midarm circumference and the duration of enteral feedings. However, 8 of the 21 patients stopped feedings after 10 days due to vomiting or diarrhea. Six of these patients were then switched to parenteral nutrition support.[104] Langdana et al retrospectively analyzed their intensive enteral feeding protocol for children undergoing HSCT, which included routine insertion of nasogastric tubes during conditioning or when oral intake had decreased. Of their 49 evaluable patients, 86% (42) were maintained on enteral nutrition alone, including 8% who took adequate oral intake.[105] Another study compared tube feeding to parenteral nutrition in a group of children undergoing allogeneic HSCT, with just 3 of 34 patients supported exclusively by tube feeding; the remainder required partial or total parenteral nutrition. Cholestasis occurred significantly less often in children who received at least some tube feeding compared to children who were exclusively parenterally fed; nutritional costs were also less in children receiving tube feeding.[106]

These studies suggest the feasibility of nasogastric feeding as a method of nutrition support for pediatric cancer and HSCT patients, although clearly some patients will be unable to tolerate the adequate volumes to support their nutritional needs. Gastrostomy tube feedings are generally considered to be more cosmetically acceptable and comfortable than nasogastric feedings while still providing the same advantages over parenteral nutrition. In a number of studies, significant weight gain in pediatric cancer patients has been demonstrated with the use of surgically placed or percutaneous endoscopic gastrostomy (PEG) feedings.[97,107–109] Although some patients may ultimately require parenteral support due to gastrointestinal intolerance, the use of enteral nutrition substantially reduces the amount and duration of parenteral nutrition required, thus reducing the risks and costs with which it is associated.[97,98,106–108]

Nutritionally complete formulas for oral supplementation or tube feeding are available for a variety of ages and conditions (see Appendix III, "Enteral Products"). Most pediatric cancer patients will tolerate intact protein, one kilocalorie per milliliter formulas either orally or via tube feeding. On rare occasions, a specialized formula for tube feeding may be indicated. Formulas with elemental (free amino acids) or semielemental (small peptides) protein are available, primarily for the purpose of allergy or intolerance. Medium-chain triglycerides are also used in many formulas intended for patients with fat malabsorption. An abundance of defined formula diets are available for varying conditions and ages.

Parenteral Feeding

When the gastrointestinal tract is nonfunctional or unavailable, nutrients may be infused via central venous catheters. Peripheral venous lines may also be used temporarily to provide a nutrient solution with <900 mOsm/L, usually 10% dextrose and 1.5 to 2% amino acids. PN has been widely used in the oncology population due to the cytotoxic effects of many treatment regimens. Most chemotherapies commonly cause some degree of nausea and vomiting. Radiation therapy, when directed to gastrointestinal organs, also causes cell damage that may impair digestive or absorptive function. High-dose chemotherapeutic regimens and total body irradiation, used in preparation for SCT, may cause a severe mucositis and enteritis, making significant oral or enteral intake difficult for many patients to achieve for several weeks. Gastrointestinal GVHD, a complication of allogeneic SCT, typically causes impaired absorption of nutrients, either due to anorexia and diminished oral intake in its mildest cases, or as profuse, bloody diarrhea in its more severe cases.

The value of parenteral nutrition in cancer patients has been questioned; in fact, its routine use in cancer treatment has been discouraged due to the risks of infectious complications.[110] A small study of pediatric cancer patients with severe, chemotherapy-induced mucositis failed to demonstrate a significant benefit of parenteral nutrition over standard intravenous fluid. This prospective, randomized trial compared body composition measurements (bioelectrical impedance analysis), laboratory parameters, and other clinical outcomes after 10 days of therapy. Only total weight gain was greater in the parenteral nutrition group, with similar measures of fat-free mass, thus implying exclusive accumulation of body fat in the PN group.[111] HSCT, however, is one of the few clinical situations where PN has historically demonstrated benefit. In a study of 22 patients receiving prophylactic PN compared to age- and diagnosis-matched historical controls, engraftment occurred significantly sooner in patients receiving prophylactic PN; there was no significant difference in overall clinical outcome.[112] In a subsequent prospective trial, patients were randomized to receive either PN or a 5% dextrose solution with additives for 1 week prior to and 4 weeks following transplantation. Although engraftment was not different among the two groups, overall survival, time to relapse, and disease-free survival were significantly better in the group receiving PN.[113] This study was instrumental in making PN an integral part of supportive care to HSCT patients.

Since the publication of these studies in the mid-1980s, however, there have been relatively few well-designed trials to further advance the science of nutrition support in children with cancer. For instance, one group evaluated the effect of PN on visceral protein levels in children undergoing HSCT and reported that concentrations of albumin and prealbumin rose significantly from day 0 until the end of PN administration. However, all subjects received the same PN regimen and no control data were presented.[114] Another study of 20 children receiving PN during HSCT attempted to clarify a relationship between changes in parenteral energy intake and clinical outcomes. A greater difference between expected and actual parenteral energy intake was associated with longer time to engraftment in this retrospective analysis. Actual energy expenditure and oral intake were not reported.[115]

The use of lipids in parenteral nutrition has been questioned with regard to infectious risk and immunosuppressive effects. Clinical and metabolic effects of a lipid-based PN (67% total energy from fat) versus a glucose-based PN (lipid-free, isocaloric, isonitrogenous) were analyzed and suggested a lower incidence of lethal acute GVHD and hyperglycemia in the lipid-based PN group. No significant differences in survival, time to engraftment, incidence of infections, or rate of relapse were seen.[116] This implies that intravenous lipids, due to their possible immunosuppressive effects, may have an effect on the severity of GVHD. More research, particularly in children, is warranted.

When clearly indicated, parenteral nutrition should be initiated according to standard recommendations (see Chapter 69, "Parenteral Nutrition"). Goals for parenteral nutrition infusions will be based upon estimated nutrient requirements, fluid requirements, and available venous access. Electrolytes are added to promote metabolic homeostasis; pediatric multivitamin and trace element preparations are generally used as well. Attention should also be directed to concomitant and expected medication use, particularly those with known nutritional interactions.

The risks of PN can be significant, and include infections, hepatotoxicity, suppression of oral intake, and metabolic abnormalities. Most children undergoing aggressive cancer treatment will require indwelling central venous catheters for chemotherapy, but the use of PN has been associated with a 2.4-fold increase in the risk of infection in children receiving chemotherapy who have central access devices in place.[117] The specific role of intravenous fats in increasing infectious complications was evaluated in a randomized trial of more than 500 children and adults undergoing BMT. There was no increased risk of bacteremia or fungal infections in those receiving standard amounts intravenous lipids (25 to 30% of energy) versus those receiving only 6 to 8% of energy as fat.[118]

Many of the medicines used in oncologic treatment can cause liver injury. The use of PN, singly or in combination with these medicines, may cause biliary dysfunction or steatosis.[119] Another potential risk of PN administration is the generation of peroxide compounds, which may have harmful effects in neonates and others with immune dysfunction and/or reduced antioxidant defenses.[120] Covering PN bags and intravenous tubing with opaque plastic coloring may reduce this effect.[121]

Parenteral nutrition may also cause early satiety and decreased oral intake. In a randomized controlled trial of children and young adults following marrow transplantation, outpatient PN delayed resumption of oral intake by 6 days as compared to 5% dextrose hydration. The clinical outcome of both groups was not significantly different.[122] Metabolic derangements are also associated with PN. Over- or underhydration, electrolyte imbalance, hyperglycemia, and hypoglycemia are among the most common concerns.[123] While there remains a role for PN in selected pediatric cancer patients, close monitoring of laboratory values, clinical condition, and ability to enterally or orally feed are important to maintain.

The significant metabolic and nutritional ramifications of cancer and its therapy have lead investigators to evaluate whether the addition of various nutrients may improve clinical outcomes. Glutamine, an important amino acid for rapidly turning over cells, has a documented role in ameliorating the mucosal atrophy seen in prolonged states of parenteral nutrition[124,125] in the healing of gastrointestinal mucosa after damage from radio- or chemotherapy,[126,127] and in reducing episodes of clinical sepsis.[128,129] Evidence supporting its use in cancer treatment has been conflicting, however, and pediatric data are minimal. Omega-3 fatty acids, derived from the essential fatty acid α-linolenic acid, have also been under consideration, owing to the antiangiogenic and antitumoral properties observed in animal models, and the anticachectic effect seen in a small number of clinical studies.[130] Controlled study of these nutrients has not been performed in children. Further research is needed to advance this science as it pertains to the nutritional therapy of pediatric cancer.

NUTRITIONAL CONCERNS OF CHILDHOOD CANCER SURVIVORS

Many nutritional issues during childhood cancer treatment are associated with weight loss or poor growth, but more recently, the risk of obesity and excess body fat accumulation has been elucidated. The Childhood Cancer Survivor Study, a multicenter, retrospective cohort study of adults who survived pediatric cancer >5 years, described a greater prevalence of overweight and obesity in cancer survivors who experienced high-dose cranial radiation (≥20 Gy) compared to their healthy siblings. The effect was present only when cancer was diagnosed at a young age (<15 yr), and the association was strongest in females.[131] Mayer et al also found an increase in obesity rates among survivors of ALL treated with cranial radiation, which correlated with significant reductions in REE and physical activity.[132] Another study, using a combination of indirect calorimetry and ambulatory heart rate monitoring to measure basal metabolic rate and TEE, also concluded that ALL survivors have lower levels of energy expenditure for activity.[133] As many as half of childhood leukemia survivors in one study became obese young adults.[15] Another study of ALL survivors compared BMI values and whole-body percent fat as measured by DXA to controls. ALL survivors had significantly higher percent body fat, while their BMI remained similar to controls,[77] suggesting the need for body composition measurements to elucidate changes in body fat. While this phenomenon may be primarily or exclusively present in the ALL population,[16,134] its impact is substantial since ALL is the most common and most curable pediatric cancer.

The impact of cancer treatment on linear growth has also been examined. A cohort of HSCT survivors, engrafted before or at the onset of puberty, had a significant decrease in final height, compared to pretransplant height standard deviation scores. However, most of the patients achieved a height considered to be normal.[135] Similarly, another study of HSCT survivors, who were treated with total body irradiation, found a reduction in peak height velocity following transplant.[136] Again, radiation therapy seems to be the common element. Growth failure has also been described in children with brain tumors.[137] Nutritional intervention may play a key role in limiting the extent of growth faltering, though the primary cause is likely a deficiency of growth hormone caused by radiation damage. While the clinical significance of this growth stunting is as yet unclear, the relationship of height to nutrient intake, body weight, and body composition is certainly notable.

Conflicting reports of a greater prevalence of osteopenia in childhood cancer survivors have been published,[138–141] perhaps related to differences in treatment, time of follow-up, or variability in measurements. Bone loss has been described in adult HSCT survivors,[142] likely related to steroid treatment posttransplant. Declines in bone mineral density Z scores have also been observed in children following HSCT. One study demonstrated an increasing incidence of osteopenia (defined as Z score between 1 and 2 SD below the mean) and osteoporosis (defined as Z score more than 2 SD below the mean) in a prospective look at bone mineral density at time of HSCT, 100 days, 6 months, and 1 year after HSCT.[143] These changes in bone mass have yet to be correlated with clinical findings, such as fractures; however, their relationship to the overall health of the growing group of childhood cancer survivors may be substantial.

A significant incidence of insulin resistance and dyslipidemia among survivors of HSCT has been reported.[4,144] Likewise, features of the metabolic syndrome have been found in ALL survivors[6]; however, the findings appear to be most pronounced in those receiving HSCT.[145] Unquestionably, complications of oncologic treatment, including obesity and insulin resistance, need further evaluation and attention. Children should be taught healthy diet principles and acceptable activity options for weight maintenance.

CONCLUSION

From the time of diagnosis to many years after treatment, nutrition is an important aspect of the care and recovery of the pediatric cancer patient. The effects of cancer and its treatment have lifelong implications. Children must maintain acceptable growth and development during extended treatment courses as well as following the completion of therapy. Serial nutritional assessments should be performed regularly with appropriate interventions taken. Malnutrition should not be accepted as an inevitable consequence of cancer and/or its treatment. Similarly, effort should be made to prevent obesity and other nutrition-related chronic diseases in long-term cancer survivors. Effective supportive care of the pediatric cancer patient involves nutritional intervention and counseling with a multidisciplinary approach, emphasizing the quality of life of each child.

REFERENCES

1. Lange BJ, Gerbing RB, Feusner J, et al. Mortality in overweight and underweight children with acute myeloid leukemia. JAMA 2005;293:203–11.
2. Stallings VA, Vaisman N, Chan HS, et al. Energy metabolism in children with newly diagnosed acute lymphoblastic leukemia. Pediatr Res 1989;26:154–7.
3. Delbecque-Boussard L, Gottrand F, Ategbo S, et al. Nutritional status of children with acute lymphoblastic leukemia: A longitudinal study. Am J Clin Nutr 1997;65:95–100.
4. Shalitin S, Phillip M, Stein J, et al. Endocrine dysfunction and parameters of the metabolic syndrome after bone marrow transplantation during childhood and adolescence. Bone Marrow Transplant 2006;37:1109–17.
5. Gurney JG, Kadan-Lottick NS, Packer RJ, et al. Endocrine and cardiovascular late effects among adult survivors of childhood brain tumors: Childhood Cancer Survivor Study. Cancer 2003;97:663–73.
6. Gurney JG, Ness KK, Sibley SD, et al. Metabolic syndrome and growth hormone deficiency in adult survivors of childhood acute lymphoblastic leukemia. Cancer 2006;107:1303–12.
7. Oeffinger KC, Mertens AC, Sklar CA, et al. Chronic health conditions in adult survivors of childhood cancer. N Engl J Med 2006;355:1572–82.
8. Dickerman JD. The late effects of childhood cancer therapy. Pediatrics 2007;119:554–68.
9. Gerhardt CA, Baughcum AE, Johnston A, et al. Parent perceptions of nutritional issues during their child's treatment for cancer. J Pediatr Hematol Oncol 2006;28:454–60.
10. Wolfe J, Grier HE, Klar N, et al. Symptoms and suffering at the end of life in children with cancer. N Engl J Med 2000;342:326–33.

11. Kemper KJ, Wornham WL. Consultations for holistic pediatric services for inpatients and outpatient oncology patients at a children's hospital. Arch Pediatr Adolesc Med 2001;155:449–54.
12. Ries LHD, Krapcho M, Mariotto A, et al. SEER Cancer Statistics Review, 1975–2003. http://seer.cancer.gov/csr/1975_2003/National Cancer Institute. Bethesda, MD, 2006. Accessed February 11, 2007.
13. Brennan BM, Gill M, Pennells L, et al. Insulin-like growth factor I, IGF binding protein 3, and IGFBP protease activity: Relation to anthropometric indices in solid tumours or leukaemia. Arch Dis Child 1999;80:226–30.
14. Garofolo A, Lopez FA, Petrilli AS. High prevalence of malnutrition among patients with solid non-hematological tumors as found by using skinfold and circumference measurements. Sao Paulo Med J 2005;123:277–81.
15. Didi M, Didcock E, Davies HA, et al. High incidence of obesity in young adults after treatment of acute lymphoblastic leukemia in childhood. J Pediatr 1995;127:63–7.
16. Nathan PC, Jovcevska V, Ness KK, et al. The prevalence of overweight and obesity in pediatric survivors of cancer. J Pediatr 2006;149:518–25.
17. White M, Murphy AJ, Hastings Y, et al. Nutritional status and energy expenditure in children pre-bone-marrow-transplant. Bone Marrow Transplant 2005;35:775–9.
18. Schmid I, Schmitt M, Streiter M, et al. Effects of soluble TNF receptor II (sTNF-RII), IL-1 receptor antagonist (IL-1ra), tumor load and hypermetabolism on malnutrition in children with acute leukemia. Eur J Med Res 2005;10:457–61.
19. Oguz A, Karadeniz C, Pelit M, Hasanoglu A. Arm anthropometry in evaluation of malnutrition in children with cancer. Pediatr Hematol Oncol 1999;16:35–41.
20. Tisdale MJ. Cancer cachexia: Metabolic alterations and clinical manifestations. Nutrition 1997;13:1–7.
21. Kern K, Norton J. Cancer cachexia. JPEN J Parenter Enteral Nutr 1988;12:286–98.
22. Picton SV. Aspects of altered metabolism in children with cancer. Int J Cancer Suppl 1998;11:62–4.
23. Roubenoff R, Heymsfield SB, Kehayias JJ, et al. Standardization of nomenclature of body composition in weight loss. Am J Clin Nutr 1997;66:192–6.
24. Wolfe RR. The underappreciated role of muscle in health and disease. Am J Clin Nutr 2006;84:475–82.
25. Moley JF, Aamodt R, Rumble W, et al. Body cell mass in cancer-bearing and anorexic patients. JPEN J Parenter Enteral Nutr 1987;11:219–22.
26. Tisdale M. Wasting in cancer. J Nutr 1999;129:243S–6S.
27. Cunningham JJ. Body composition and nutrition support in pediatrics: What to defend and how soon to begin. Nutr Clin Pract 1995;10:177–82.
28. Castaneda C, Charnley JM, Evans WJ, Crim MC. Elderly women accommodate to a low-protein diet with losses of body cell mass, muscle function, and immune response. Am J Clin Nutr 1995;62:30–9.
29. Arora NS, Rochester DF. Respiratory muscle strength and maximal voluntary ventilation in undernourished patients. Am Rev Respir Dis 1982;126:5–8.
30. Briend A, Garenne M, Maire B, et al. Nutritional status, age, and survival: The muscle mass hypothesis. Eur J Clin Nutr 1989;43:715–26.
31. Kotler DP, Tierney AR, Wang J, Pierson RN, Jr. Magnitude of body-cell-mass depletion and the timing of death from wasting in AIDS. Am J Clin Nutr 1989;50:444–7.
32. Brennan MF. Total parenteral nutrition in the cancer patient. N Engl J Med 1981;305:375–82.
33. Koretz RL, Lipman TO, Klein S. AGA technical review on parenteral nutrition. Gastroenterology 2001;121:970–1001.
34. Lundholm K, Holm G, Schersten T. Insulin resistance in patients with cancer. Cancer Res 1978;38:4665–70.
35. Holroyde CP, Gabuzda TG, Putnam RC, et al. Altered glucose metabolism in metastatic carcinoma. Cancer Res 1975;35:3710–4.
36. Bennegard K, Lundgren F, Lundholm K. Mechanisms of insulin resistance in cancer associated malnutrition. Clin Physiol 1986;6:539–47.
37. Copeland GP, Leinster SJ, Davis JC, Hipkin LJ. Insulin resistance in patients with colorectal cancer. Br J Surg 1987;74:1031–5.
38. Yoshikawa T, Noguchi Y, Doi C, et al. Insulin resistance was connected with the alterations of substrate utilization in patients with cancer. Cancer Lett 1999;141:93–8.
39. Todorov PT, McDevitt TM, Meyer DJ, et al. Purification and characterization of a tumor lipid-mobilizing factor. Cancer Res 1998;58:2353–8.
40. Kralovic RC, Zepp FA, Cenedella RJ. Studies of the mechanism of carcass fat depletion in experimental cancer. Eur J Cancer 1977;13:1071–9.
41. Halton JM, Nazir DJ, McQueen MJ, Barr RD. Blood lipid profiles in children with acute lymphoblastic leukemia. Cancer 1998;83:379–84.
42. Shaw JH, Wolfe RR. Fatty acid and glycerol kinetics in septic patients and in patients with gastrointestinal cancer. The response to glucose infusion and parenteral feeding. Ann Surg 1987;205:368–76.
43. Fearon KC, McMillan DC, Preston T, et al. Elevated circulating interleukin-6 is associated with an acute-phase response but reduced fixed hepatic protein synthesis in patients with cancer. Ann Surg 1991;213:26–31.
44. O'Keefe SJ, Ogden J, Ramjee G, Rund J. Contribution of elevated protein turnover and anorexia to cachexia in patients with hepatocellular carcinoma. Cancer Res 1990;50:1226–30.
45. Attard-Montalto SP, Camacho-Hubner C, Cotterill AM, et al. Changes in protein turnover, IGF-I and IGF binding proteins in children with cancer. Acta Paediatr 1998;87:54–60.
46. Dworzak F, Ferrari P, Gavazzi C, et al. Effects of cachexia due to cancer on whole body and skeletal muscle protein turnover. Cancer 1998;82:42–8.
47. Starnes HF, Jr, Warren RS, Jeevanandam M, et al. Tumor necrosis factor and the acute metabolic response to tissue injury in man. J Clin Invest 1988;82:1321–5.
48. Black K, Garrett IR, Mundy GR. Chinese hamster ovarian cells transfected with the murine interleukin-6 gene cause hypercalcemia as well as cachexia, leukocytosis and thrombocytosis in tumor-bearing nude mice. Endocrinology 1991;128:2657–9.
49. Muscaritoli M, Bossola M, Aversa Z, et al. Prevention and treatment of cancer cachexia: New insights into an old problem. Eur J Cancer 2006;42:31–41.
50. Bond SA, Han AM, Wootton SA, Kohler JA. Energy intake and basal metabolic rate during maintenance chemotherapy. Arch Dis Child 1992;67:229–32.
51. Reilly JJ, Ventham JC, Ralston JM, et al. Reduced energy expenditure in preobese children treated for acute lymphoblastic leukemia. Pediatr Res 1998;44:557–62.
52. Garcia-Peris P, Lozano MA, Velasco C, et al. Prospective study of resting energy expenditure changes in head and neck cancer patients treated with chemoradiotherapy measured by indirect calorimetry. Nutrition 2005;21:1107–12.
53. Ringwald-Smith KA, Heslop HE, Krance RA, et al. Energy expenditure in children undergoing hematopoietic stem cell transplantation. Bone Marrow Transplant 2002;30:125–30.
54. Duggan C, Bechard L, Donovan K, et al. Changes in resting energy expenditure among children undergoing allogeneic stem cell transplantation. Am J Clin Nutr 2003;78:104–9.
55. Donaldson SS. Effects of therapy on nutritional status of the pediatric cancer patient. Cancer Res 1982;42:729S–36S.
56. Sheard N, Clark N. Nutritional management of pediatric oncology patients. In: Baker S, Baker R, Davis A, editors. Pediatric Enteral Nutrition. New York: Chapman & Hall, 1994. p. 387–98.
57. Kostler WJ, Hejna M, Wenzel C, Zielinski CC. Oral mucositis complicating chemotherapy and/or radiotherapy: Options for prevention and treatment. CA Cancer J Clin 2001;51:290–315.
58. Adamson PC, Balis FM, Berg S, Blaney SM. General principles of chemotherapy. In Pizzo PA, Poplack DG, editors. Principles and Practice of Pediatric Oncology. Philadelphia: Lippincott, Williams, & Wilkins; 2006. p. 290–365.
59. Copelan EA. Hematopoietic stem-cell transplantation. N Engl J Med 2006;354:1813–26.
60. Wingard JR, Piantadosi S, Vogelsang GB, et al. Predictors of death from chronic graft-versus-host disease after bone marrow transplantation. Blood 1989;74:1428–35.
61. Stern JM, Chesnut CH, III, Bruemmer B, et al. Bone density loss during treatment of chronic GVHD. Bone Marrow Transplant 1996;17:395–400.
62. Jacobsohn DA, Margolis J, Doherty J, et al. Weight loss and malnutrition in patients with chronic graft-versus-host disease. Bone Marrow Transplant 2002;29:231–6.
63. Bhushan V, Collins RH, Jr. Chronic graft-vs-host disease. JAMA 2003;290:2599–603.
64. Browning B, Thormann K, Seshadri R, et al. Weight loss and reduced body mass index: A critical issue in children with multiorgan chronic graft-versus-host disease. Bone Marrow Transplant 2006;37:527–33.
65. Papadopoulou A, Nathavitharana K, Williams M, et al. Diarrhea and weight loss after bone marrow transplantation in children. Pediatr Hematol Oncol 1994;11:601–11.
66. Tyc V, Vallelunga L, Mahoney S, et al. Nutritional and treatment-related characteristics of pediatric oncology patients referred or not referred for nutritional support. Med Pediatr Oncol 1995;25:379–88.
67. Motil KJ. Sensitive measures of nutritional status in children in hospital and in the field. Int J Cancer Suppl 1998;11:2–9.
68. Mauer AM, Burgess JB, Donaldson SS, et al. Special nutritional needs of children with malignancies: A review. JPEN J Parenter Enteral Nutr 1990;14:315–24.
69. Bakish J, Hargrave D, Tariq N, et al. Evaluation of dietetic intervention in children with medulloblastoma or supratentorial primitive neuroectodermal tumors. Cancer 2003;98:1014–20.
70. Freedman D, Srinivasan S, Valdez R, et al. Secular increases in relative weight and adiposity among children over two decades: The Bogalusa Heart Study. Pediatrics 1997;99:420–26.
71. Dietz WH, Bellizzi MC. Introduction: The use of body mass index to assess obesity in children. Am J Clin Nutr 1999;70:123S–5S.
72. Must A, Dallal GE, Dietz WH. Reference data for obesity: 85th and 95th percentiles of body mass index (wt/ht2) and triceps skinfold thickness. Am J Clin Nutr 1991;53:839–46.
73. Chomtho S, Fewtrell MS, Jaffe A, et al. Evaluation of arm anthropometry for assessing pediatric body composition: Evidence from healthy and sick children. Pediatr Res 2006;59:860–5.
74. Frisancho AR. New norms of upper limb fat and muscle areas for assessment of nutritional status. Am J Clin Nutr 1981;34:2540–5.
75. Brennan BM. Sensitive measures of the nutritional status of children with cancer in hospital and in the field. Int J Cancer Suppl 1998;11:10–13.
76. Taskinen M, Saarinen-Pihkala UM. Evaluation of muscle protein mass in children with solid tumors by muscle thickness measurement with ultrasonography, as compared with anthropometric methods and visceral protein concentrations. Eur J Clin Nutr 1998;52:402–6.
77. Nysom K, Holm K, Michaelsen KF, et al. Degree of fatness after treatment for acute lymphoblastic leukemia in childhood. [erratum appears in J Clin Endocrinol Metab 2001;86:1758]. J Clin Endocrinol Metab 1999;84:4591–6.
78. Jarfelt M, Lannering B, Bosaeus I, et al. Body composition in young adult survivors of childhood acute lymphoblastic leukaemia. Eur J Endocrinol 2005;153:81–9.
79. Kyle UG, Chalandon Y, Miralbell R, et al. Longitudinal follow-up of body composition in hematopoietic stem cell transplant patients. Bone Marrow Transplant 2005;35:1171–7.
80. Warner JT, Evans WD, Webb DK, Gregory JW. Pitfalls in the assessment of body composition in survivors of acute lymphoblastic leukaemia. Arch Dis Child 2004;89:64–8.
81. Murphy AJ, Wells JC, Williams JE, et al. Body composition in children in remission from acute lymphoblastic leukemia. Am J Clin Nutr 2006;83:70–4.
82. Nysom K, Holm K, Michaelsen KF, et al. Degree of fatness after allogeneic BMT for childhood leukaemia or lymphoma. Bone Marrow Transplant 2001;27:817–20.
83. Roubenoff R, Kehayias J, Dawson-Hughes B, Heymsfield S. Use of dual-energy X-ray absorptiometry in body-composition studies: Not yet a "gold standard." Am J Clin Nutr 1993;58:589–91.
84. Warner JT, Evans WD, Webb DK, Gregory JW. Body composition of long-term survivors of acute lymphoblastic leukaemia. Med Pediatr Oncol 2002;38:165–72.
85. Fletcher JP, Little JM, Guest PK. A comparison of serum transferrin and serum prealbumin as nutritional parameters. JPEN J Parenter Enteral Nutr 1987;11:144–7.
86. Hawker FH, Stewart PM, Baxter RC, et al. Relationship of somatomedin-C/insulin-like growth factor I levels to conventional nutritional indices in critically ill patients. Crit Care Med 1987;15:732–6.
87. Elhasid R, Laor A, Lischinsky S, et al. Nutritional status of children with solid tumors. Cancer 1999;86:119–25.
88. Malvy DJM, Arnaud J, Burtschy B, et al. Antioxidant micronutrients and childhood malignancy during oncological treatment. Med Pediatr Oncol 1997;29:213–7.
89. Atkinson SA, Halton JM, Bradley C, et al. Bone and mineral abnormalities in childhood acute lymphoblastic leukemia: Influence of disease, drugs and nutrition. Int J Cancer Suppl 1998;11:35–9.
90. Papadopoulou A, Nathavitharana K, Williams MD, et al. Diagnosis and clinical associations of zinc depletion following bone marrow transplantation. Arch Dis Child 1996;74:328–31.
91. High KP, Legault C, Sinclair JA, et al. Low plasma concentrations of retinol and alpha-tocopherol in hematopoietic stem cell transplant recipients: The effect of mucositis and the risk of infection. Am J Clin Nutr 2002;76:1358–66.

92. Kennedy DD, Ladas EJ, Rheingold SR, et al. Antioxidant status decreases in children with acute lymphoblastic leukemia during the first six months of chemotherapy treatment. Pediatr Blood Cancer 2005;44:378–85.
93. Moody K, Charlson ME, Finlay J. The neutropenic diet: What's the evidence? J Pediatr Hematol Oncol 2002; 24:717–21.
94. Moody K, Finlay J, Mancuso C, Charlson M. Feasibility and safety of a pilot randomized trial of infection rate: Neutropenic diet versus standard food safety guidelines. J Pediatr Hematol Oncol 2006;28:126–33.
95. Centers for Disease Control and Prevention. Guidelines for preventing opportunistic infections among hematopoietic stem cell transplant recipients: Recommendations of CDC, the Infectious Disease Society of America, and the American Society of Blood and Marrow Transplantation. MMWR 2000;49:50–2.
96. Bowman LC, Williams R, Sanders M, et al. Algorithm for nutritional support: Experience of the Metabolic and Infusion Support Service of St. Jude Children's Research Hospital. Int J Cancer Suppl 1998;11:76–80.
97. Aquino VM, Smyrl CB, Hagg R, et al. Enteral nutritional support by gastrostomy tube in children with cancer. J Pediatr 1995;127:58–62.
98. Pietsch JB, Ford C, Whitlock JA. Nasogastric tube feedings in children with high-risk cancer: A pilot study. J Pediatr Hematol Oncol 1999;21:111–4.
99. Deswarte-Wallace J, Firouzbakhsh S, Finklestein JZ. Using research to change practice: Enteral feedings for pediatric oncology patients. J Pediatr Oncol Nurs 2001;18:217–23.
100. Ladas EJ, Sacks N, Brophy P, Rogers PC. Standards of nutritional care in pediatric oncology: Results from a nationwide survey on the standards of practice in pediatric oncology. A Children's Oncology Group study. Pediatr Blood Cancer 2006;46:339–44.
101. Ladas EJ, Sacks N, Meacham L, et al. A multidisciplinary review of nutrition considerations in the pediatric oncology population: A perspective from children's oncology group. Nutr Clin Pract 2005;20:377–93.
102. Imataki O, Nakatani S, Hasegawa T, et al. Nutritional support for patients suffering from intestinal graft-versus-host disease after allogeneic hematopoietic stem cell transplantation. Am J Hematol 2006;81:747–52.
103. den Broeder E, Lippens RJ, van't Hof MA, et al. Effects of naso-gastric tube feeding on the nutritional status of children with cancer. Eur J Clin Nutr 1998;52:494–500.
104. Papadopoulou A, MacDonald A, Williams MD, et al. Enteral nutrition after bone marrow transplantation. Arch Dis Child 1997;77:131–6.
105. Langdana A, Tully N, Molloy E, et al. Intensive enteral nutrition support in paediatric bone marrow transplantation. Bone Marrow Transplant 2001;27:741–6.
106. Hopman GD, Pena EG, Le Cessie S, et al. Tube feeding and bone marrow transplantation. Med Pediatr Oncol 2003;40:375–9.
107. Mathew P, Bowman L, Williams R, et al. Complications and effectiveness of gastrostomy feedings in pediatric cancer patients. J Pediatr Hematol Oncol 1996;18:81–85.
108. Pedersen AM, Kok K, Petersen G, et al. Percutaneous endoscopic gastrostomy in children with cancer. Acta Paediatr 1999;88:849–52.
109. Skolin I, Hernell O, Larsson MV, et al. Percutaneous endoscopic gastrostomy in children with malignant disease. J Pediatr Oncol Nurs 2002;19:154–63.
110. American College of Physicians. Parenteral nutrition in patients receiving cancer chemotherapy. Ann Intern Med 1989;110:734–6.
111. Schmid I, Schmitt M, Streiter M, et al. Parenteral nutrition is not superior to replacement fluid therapy for the supportive treatment of chemotherapy induced oral mucositis in children. Eur J Cancer 2006;42:205–11.
112. Weisdorf S, Hofland C, Sharp H, et al. Total parenteral nutrition in bone marrow transplantation: A clinical evaluation. J Pediatr Gastroenterol Nutr 1984;3:95–100.
113. Weisdorf S, Lysne J, Wind D, et al. Positive effect of prophylactic total parenteral nutrition on long-term outcome of bone marrow transplantation. Transplantation 1987;43:833–38.
114. Uderzo C, Rovelli A, Bonomi M, et al. Total parenteral nutrition and nutritional assessment and leukaemic children undergoing bone marrow transplantation. Eur J Cancer 1991;27:758–62.
115. Forchielli ML, Azzi N, Cadranel S, Paolucci G. Total parenteral nutrition in bone marrow transplant: What is the appropriate energy level? Oncology 2003;64:7–13.
116. Muscaritoli M, Conversano L, Torelli G, et al. Clinical and metabolic effects of different parenteral nutrition regimens in patients undergoing allogeneic bone marrow transplantation. Transplantation 1998;66:610–16.
117. Christensen ML, Hancock ML, Gattuso J, et al. Parenteral nutrition associated with increased infection rate in children with cancer. Cancer 1993;72:2732–8.
118. Lenssen P, Bruemmer BA, Bowden RA, et al. Intravenous lipid dose and incidence of bacteremia and fungemia in patients undergoing bone marrow transplantation. Am J Clin Nutr 1998;67:927–33.
119. Copeman MC. Use of total parenteral nutrition in children with cancer: A review and some recommendations. Pediatr Hematol Oncol 1994;11:463–70.
120. Laborie S, Lavoie JC, Chessex P. Paradoxical role of ascorbic acid and riboflavin in solutions of total parenteral nutrition: Implication in photoinduced peroxide generation. Pediatr Res 1998;43:601–6.
121. Laborie S, Lavoie JC, Pineault M, Chessex P. Protecting solutions of parenteral nutrition from peroxidation. JPEN J Parenter Enteral Nutr 1999;23:104–8.
122. Charuhas PM, Fosberg KL, Bruemmer B, et al. A double-blind randomized trial comparing outpatient parenteral nutrition with intravenous hydration: Effect on resumption of oral intake after marrow transplantation. JPEN J Parenter Enteral Nutr 1997;21:157–61.
123. Davis AM. Initiation, Monitoring, and Complications of Pediatric parenteral nutrition. In: Baker RD, Jr, Baker SS, Davis AM, editors. Pediatric Parenteral Nutrition. New York: Chapman & Hall, 1997. p 212–37.
124. Tamada H, Nezu R, Imamura I, et al. The dipeptide alanyl-glutamine prevents intestinal mucosal atrophy in parenterally fed rats. JPEN J Parenter Enteral Nutr 1992;16:110–16.
125. Van der Hulst R, van Kreel B, von Meyenfeldt M, et al. Glutamine and the preservation of gut integrity. Lancet 1993;334:1363–65.
126. Klimberg V, Souba W, Dolson D, et al. Prophylactic glutamine protects the intestinal mucosa from radiation injury. Cancer 1990;66:62–68.
127. Fox A, Kripke S, DePaula J, et al. Effect of glutamine-supplemented enteral diet on methotrexate-induced enterocolitis. JPEN J Parenter Enteral Nutr 1988;12:325–31.
128. Ziegler TR, Young LS, Benfell K, et al. Clinical and metabolic efficacy of glutamine-supplemented parenteral nutrition after bone marrow transplantation. A randomized, double-blind, controlled study. Ann Intern Med 1992;116:821–8.
129. Neu J, Roig J, Meetze W, et al. Enteral glutamine supplementation for very low birth weight infants decreases morbidity. J Pediatr 1997;131:691–9.
130. Hardman WE. (n - 3) fatty acids and cancer therapy. J Nutr 2004;134:3427S–30S.
131. Oeffinger KC, Mertens AC, Sklar CA, et al. Obesity in adult survivors of childhood acute lymphoblastic leukemia: A report from the Childhood Cancer Survivor Study. J Clin Oncol 2003;21:1359–65.
132. Mayer EI, Reuter M, Dopfer RE, Ranke MB. Energy expenditure, energy intake and prevalence of obesity after therapy for acute lymphoblastic leukemia during childhood. Horm Res 2000;53:193–9.
133. Warner JT, Bell W, Webb DK, Gregory JW. Daily energy expenditure and physical activity in survivors of childhood malignancy. Pediatr Res 1998;43:607–13.
134. Meacham LR, Gurney JG, Mertens AC, et al. Body mass index in long-term adult survivors of childhood cancer: A report of the Childhood Cancer Survivor Study. Cancer 2005;103:1730–9.
135. Cohen A, Rovelli A, Van-Lint M, et al. Final height of patients who underwent bone marrow transplantation during childhood. Arch Dis Child 1996;74:437–40.
136. Bakker B, Oostdijk W, Geskus RB, et al. Patterns of growth and body proportions after total-body irradiation and hematopoietic stem cell transplantation during childhood. Pediatr Res 2006;59:259–64.
137. Meacham LR, Mason PW, Sullivan KM. Auxologic and biochemical characterization of the three phases of growth failure in pediatric patients with brain tumors. J Pediatr Endocrinol Metab 2004;17:711–7.
138. Kadan-Lottick N, Marshall JA, Baron AE, et al. Normal bone mineral density after treatment for childhood acute lymphoblastic leukemia diagnosed between 1991 and 1998. J Pediatr 2001;138:898–904.
139. Arikoski P, Komulainen J, Riikonen P, et al. Reduced bone density at completion of chemotherapy for a malignancy. Arch Dis Child 1999;80:143–8.
140. Marinovic D, Dorgeret S, Lescoeur B, et al. Improvement in bone mineral density and body composition in survivors of childhood acute lymphoblastic leukemia: A 1-year prospective study. Pediatrics 2005;116:e102–8.
141. Ruza E, Sierrasesumaga L, Azcona C, Patino-Garcia A. Bone mineral density and bone metabolism in children treated for bone sarcomas. Pediatr Res 2006;59:866–71.
142. Schulte CM, Beelen DW. Bone loss following hematopoietic stem cell transplantation: A long-term follow-up. Blood 2004;103:3635–43.
143. Petryk A, Bergemann TL, Polga KM, et al. Prospective study of changes in bone mineral density and turnover in children after hematopoietic cell transplantation. J Clin Endocrinol Metab 2006;91:899–905.
144. Taskinen M, Saarinen-Pihkala U, Hovi L, Lipsanen-Nyman M. Impaired glucose tolerance and dyslipidemia as late effects after bone marrow transplantation in childhood. Lancet 2000;356:993–97.
145. Neville KA, Cohn RJ, Steinbeck KS, et al. Hyperinsulinemia, Impaired glucose tolerance, and diabetes mellitus in survivors of childhood cancer: Prevalence and risk factors. J Clin Endocrinol Metab 2006;91:4401–7.

Diabetes Mellitus

Joseph Wolfsdorf, MB, BCh
Maryanne Quinn, MD
Karen Warman, MS, RD, LDN

Meal planning is a cornerstone of diabetes management, and nutrition education is an essential component of a comprehensive program of diabetes education for patients and their families.[1,2] Recommendations for medical nutrition therapy (MNT) of diabetes mellitus have changed repeatedly since the advent of insulin therapy in 1922. In this chapter, we briefly review the history of MNT, the scientific basis upon which the general principles are founded, and recent investigations that implicate dietary factors in the etiology of immune-mediated or type 1a diabetes mellitus. Finally, we discuss the goals of treatment, principles of meal planning, and formulation of an individualized meal plan based on current evidence as recommended by the Food and Nutrition Committee of the American Diabetes Association (ADA).[3]

PREVALENCE, DEFINITION, CLINICAL DESCRIPTION OF DIABETES MELLITUS

Diabetes mellitus is not a single entity but a group of metabolic diseases characterized by hyperglycemia that is caused by defects in insulin secretion, insulin action, or both.[4,5] Most cases of diabetes fall into two broad etiologic categories: Type 1 diabetes, caused by an absolute deficiency of insulin secretion, is the most common form in children and adolescents,[6] whereas type 2 diabetes is the most common form of diabetes worldwide, comprising 80 to 90% of the overall diabetic population, and is caused by a combination of resistance to insulin action and impaired insulin secretion.[7,8] Type 2 diabetes usually has its onset in middle life and is often associated with abdominal (visceral) obesity and hypertension. Until relatively recently, immune-mediated or type 1a diabetes was the only type of diabetes prevalent among children in the United States, and 1 to 2% of children had type 2 or other rare forms of diabetes. Throughout the developed world, however, the prevalence of type 2 diabetes in youth has increased at an alarming rate[9–13] and recent reports indicate that 8 to 45% of children with newly diagnosed diabetes have nonimmune-mediated diabetes.[14] The variation in incidence appears to depend on race/ethnicity and sampling strategy. Most of these children have type 2 diabetes, but other types, especially maturity-onset diabetes of youth (MODY) or monogenic diabetes, are being increasingly identified in adolescents and young adults.[15]

Changes in energy intake and expenditure have resulted in an epidemic of obesity in children and adolescents in the United States,[16] which has been temporally associated with an alarming increase in the prevalence of type 2 diabetes in children and adolescents, especially in minority populations, in the past decade. Almost 95% of patients are either overweight or frankly obese.[14]

Simple obesity, even in the absence of glucose intolerance, is associated with impaired insulin action on target tissues.[17–19] In children, body composition is also a major determinant of insulin sensitivity. Adiposity accounts for 55% of the variance in insulin sensitivity in white children.[20] An inverse relationship between increasing adiposity and insulin sensitivity also has been demonstrated in black children. As body mass index (BMI) and percent adiposity increase, insulin sensitivity decreases and serum insulin levels increase.[21]

The incidence of type 1 diabetes varies widely among geographic regions, from 0.1 per 100,000 per year in China and Venezuela to 54 per 100,000 per year in Finland.[22,23] In 2001, there were approximately 155,000 youth with diagnosed diabetes in the United States.[6] The estimated crude prevalence rate was 1.82 cases per 1,000 youth, being lower for children 0 to 9 years of age (0.79 cases per 1,000 youth) than for those 10 to 19 years of age (2.80 cases per 1,000 youth). Among younger children, type 1 diabetes accounted for at least 80% of diabetes, whereas among older youth the proportion of type 2 diabetes ranged from 6% for non-Hispanic white youth to 76% for American Indian youth.[6]

Type 1a diabetes occurs in genetically predisposed individuals as a consequence of immune-mediated destruction of the insulin secreting β cells of the pancreatic islet.[24] The onset of clinically overt diabetes represents a late stage in the process of chronic progressive immune-mediated β-cell destruction and occurs when the majority of β-cells have been destroyed.[25] The disease typically presents with the rapid onset of polyuria, polydipsia, and weight loss. The cardinal features are attributable to an absolute deficiency of insulin, which leads to hyperglycemia (the result of decreased uptake and utilization of glucose by liver, muscle, and adipose tissue and uncontrolled hepatic gluconeogenesis), unregulated release of free fatty acids from adipose tissue, and increased ketogenesis.

Patients with type 1 diabetes depend on exogenous insulin to survive. Insulin normally is secreted in an oscillatory fashion at a low basal rate upon which are superimposed periodic increases in secretion in response to ingestion of food. In contrast, when insulin is injected subcutaneously, it is absorbed from the injection site in a somewhat predictable fashion depending on the specific type and combination of insulins used. Each type of insulin has a characteristic time of onset of action and maximum effect, duration of peak effect, and total duration of action (Table 1). When short- or intermediate-acting insulins are used, meals and snacks have to be timed to match the pharmacodynamics of insulin. Rapid-acting insulin analogs, delivered by injection or via continuous subcutaneous insulin infusion (CSII, insulin pump therapy), significantly reduce the variation in absorption

Table 1 Insulin Preparations Classified According to their Pharmacodynamic Profiles

	Onset of Action (h)	Peak Action (h)	Duration of Action (h)
Rapid-acting*			
Insulin lispro (Humalog®)†	0.25–0.5	0.5–2.5	≤ 5
Insulin aspart (Novolog®)†	<0.25	1–3	3–5
Insulin glulisine (Apidra®)†	<0.25	0.5–1.5	3–4
Short-acting*			
Regular (soluble)	0.5–1	2–4	5–8
Intermediate-acting*			
NPH (isophane)	1–2	2–8	14–24
Long-acting*			
Insulin glargine (Lantus ®)†	2–4	Peakless	20–24
Insulin detemir (Levemir ®)†	2–4	6–8	6–23

*Premixed combinations of intermediate-acting and either rapid- or short-acting insulins are available whose pharmacodynamic profiles have a bimodal pattern reflecting the two insulin components.
†Insulin analog developed by modifying the amino acid sequence of the human insulin molecule.

of insulin and permits greater flexibility in matching insulin delivery to glucose absorption after meals and snacks.

Children with idiopathic or nonimmune-mediated type 1 diabetes may be difficult to distinguish from those with immune-mediated diabetes. In the United States, most patients with idiopathic type 1 diabetes are African-American and have so called atypical diabetes mellitus or Flatbush diabetes.[26,27] They typically have a positive family history of early-onset diabetes in several relatives and in multiple generations. Although insulin may not be required for survival after the episode of acute metabolic deterioration has resolved, blood glucose control usually is poor without insulin therapy and ketoacidosis may recur.

MODY is a form of diabetes caused by monogenic defects in β-cell function inherited in an autosomal dominant pattern.[15] The clinical spectrum of MODY is broad ranging from asymptomatic hyperglycemia to a severe acute presentation. MODY occurs in all racial and ethnic groups, and molecular diagnostic testing is required for specific classification.[15]

Individuals with nonimmune-mediated diabetes may have clinical presentations indistinguishable from those of patients with immune-mediated type 1 diabetes. This is especially relevant because as the number of children with type 2 diabetes increases, it is important to classify correctly the cause of the child's diabetes to be able to institute appropriate therapy.

Acute, life-threatening consequences of diabetes are hyperglycemia with ketoacidosis or the hyperosmolar nonketotic syndrome.[28] Long-term complications of chronic hyperglycemia include: retinopathy with potential loss of vision, nephropathy leading to hypertension and renal failure, and peripheral and autonomic neuropathy with associated risk of foot ulcers and limb amputation, gastrointestinal, genitourinary, and cardiovascular symptoms.[29] Glycation of tissue proteins and other macromolecules and excess production of polyol compounds from glucose are among the mechanisms thought to produce tissue damage from chronic hyperglycemia.[30]

The initial classification usually is based on the clinical picture at presentation. Children with immune-mediated type 1 diabetes are typically not overweight, have a short duration of symptoms, frequently have ketosis, and approximately 15 to 70% of new onset patients in North America and Europe present with ketoacidosis.[31] As the childhood population in the United States has become increasingly overweight, the percentage of children with immune-mediated type 1 diabetes who are coincidentally overweight, if not obese, has increased.[32] After metabolic stabilization, they may have an initial period of diminished insulin requirement (the honeymoon period) after which they require daily insulin replacement for survival and are always at risk for ketoacidosis. In contrast, approximately 95% of children with type 2 diabetes are either overweight or obese at the time of diagnosis and typically present with glucosuria, absent or mild polyuria and polydipsia, and a little or no weight loss. Up to 33% have ketonuria at diagnosis, and 5 to 25% of patients classified as having type 2 diabetes present with ketoacidosis. Children with type 2 diabetes usually are more than 10 years old and are in middle to late puberty, 45 to 80% have at least one parent with diabetes and 74 to 100% have a first- or second-degree relative with type 2 diabetes. Children and adolescents of African-American, Hispanic, Asian, American Indian, and Pacific Islander descent are disproportionately represented.[6,33]

HISTORY OF MNT FOR TYPE 1 DIABETES MELLITUS

Until the advent of insulin therapy in 1922, the only available treatment was diet and exercise. Meal plans severely restricted the total intake of energy and were low in carbohydrate and high in fat.[34] Nutrition recommendations were often based on dogma and a limited understanding of the metabolic derangements. After the introduction of insulin, nutrition recommendations changed, but generally involved restriction of carbohydrate to a maximum of 40% of total energy because this was thought to reduce the severity of hyperglycemia.[35,36] By early in the twentieth century, several studies had shown that a high-carbohydrate meal plan, provided it was restricted in total energy, had beneficial metabolic effects.[37–39] Change was slow and despite evidence to the contrary, patients continued to be indoctrinated to use a low-carbohydrate, high-fat meal plan until 1971 when the Committee on Food and Nutrition of the ADA formally recommended liberalizing the consumption of carbohydrate.[40] Sucrose had not been permitted in the meal plans of people with diabetes mellitus; however, considerable scientific evidence has shown that sucrose as part of the meal plan does not impair blood glucose control in people with either type 1 or type 2 diabetes (vide infra).

In 1950, the ADA, the American Dietetic Association, and the United States Public Health Service introduced the exchange system for meal planning to assist patients to choose foods consistent with current nutrition recommendations.[41] The exchange system established portion sizes and grouped foods with similar macronutrient contents. The goal of the system was to enable individuals with diabetes to exchange foods within a group and still receive comparable amounts of macro- and micronutrients. The exchange system was an important advance because it antedated the widespread availability of standardized food composition analysis. Legislation mandating food labeling was not introduced in the United States until 1974. The exchange system has undergone four revisions. The 1976 revision improved the accuracy of the calorie content of foods within the lists and stratified foods by their fat content. The 1986 revision developed a database for nutrient composition and increased the carbohydrate content of fruits from 10 to 15 g, which is closer to their actual carbohydrate content. The 1995 revision grouped carbohydrate-containing foods into a single category, which allowed for greater flexibility in meal planning. This revision also added many new food items (eg, fat-modified, vegetarian, and fast foods) to reflect the US population's changing dietary habits and food choices. The most recent revision, in 2003, liberalized the use of sugar in the diet by establishing a food list titled "Sweets, Desserts and Other Carbohydrates that could be exchanged for Grains, Fruits and Dairy." Another new category, "Combination foods," was added in response to the increased availability of processed foods.

Modifications to the exchange system reflect societal changes in dietary habits, including the increased marketing and consumption of prepared foods, frequency of eating outside the home, and the modification of natural foods to lower their fat and carbohydrate content. The 2003 revision of the exchange system also includes the nutrient profiles of food items reflecting their increasing use by the general public. It is important, however, to recognize that the portion size on food labels may differ from the portion size and carbohydrate content listed in the exchange system. Although some food manufacturers list diabetes exchanges on their products, most do not. Since the introduction of mandatory food labeling, the general public is becoming more accustomed to reading nutrition facts provided on food labels. It is no longer essential, therefore, for people with diabetes to rely on the exchange system as the sole source of information regarding macronutrients for dietary planning.[42]

Increasingly widespread use of intensive insulin therapy (either multiple daily injections, referred to as basal–bolus or flexible insulin therapy, or CSII using an insulin pump) in combination with carbohydrate counting (utilizing item-specific nutrient content from food labels, readily available reference books and software) allows patients with type 1 diabetes to have considerably more dietary choices and to live more normal lifestyles without compromising glycemic control. Carbohydrate counting is discussed in more detail later in this chapter.

DIETARY FACTORS IN THE PATHOGENESIS OF TYPE 1a DIABETES MELLITUS

The nature of the interaction among genetic, environmental, and immunologic factors in the etiology of type 1a diabetes remains poorly understood. The genetic predisposition to diabetes is associated with specific DQ and DR alleles in the HLA region of chromosome 6, but the observation of less than 50% concordance for type 1 diabetes in identical twins indicates that environmental factors are also involved. The role of diet, particularly cow's milk protein, in the pathogenesis of human type 1a diabetes is controversial.[43] Changes in food, particularly its protein content, influence the onset of diabetes in rodent models of autoimmune diabetes. These observations have been invoked as evidence that complex natural ingredients in standard human and rodent diets may be involved in the autoimmune-mediated destruction of ß cells. It has been suggested that a dietary antigen may play a role as the factor driving the disease process toward clinical type 1 diabetes, and bovine insulin is thought to be an attractive candidate because an immune response, initially induced by bovine insulin, cross-reacts with and may target human insulin in the β-cell.[43]

Antibodies reactive against a peptide sequence contained within bovine serum albumin (BSA) occur in humans, BB rats, and NOD mice, which cross-react with an islet antigen designated p69. Together with suggestive epidemiological data, these observations have given rise to the controversial theory that dietary cow's milk may contribute to the pathogenesis of type 1a diabetes in susceptible individuals.[44] Removal of bovine proteins from the diet prevents diabetes in NOD mice.[45] Some investigators have shown that diets containing cow's milk are diabetogenic in the BB rat; however, this has not been confirmed by others.[46] Diet clearly has a major diabetogenic effect in BB rats[47,48] and NOD mice,[48] but the exact chemical identity of the food diabetogen(s) is still not clear.

Insulin is a crucial autoantigen in type 1 diabetes and is the only β-cell-specific autoantigen in postnatal life.[49] Insulin autoantigens (IAAs) are the first or among the first autoantibodies to appear when the disease process leading to type 1 diabetes is initiated in young children.[50,51] Because cow's milk formulas are generally the first and most common dietary source of foreign complex proteins to which infants are exposed in developed countries, the question has been asked whether early exposure to cow's milk formula results in an immune response to bovine insulin (which differs from human insulin in 3 amino acids) present in formulas. Infants who were exclusively breastfed, at least up to the age of 3 months, had substantially lower IgG class antibodies to bovine insulin than those who were exposed to formula before 3 months of age.[52] Follow-up demonstrated that the IgG class insulin antibodies started to decrease slowly after the age of 3 months as a sign of the development of oral tolerance in those infants who were given formula before the age of 3 months, whereas in those exclusively breastfed, at least to the age of 3 months, the antibody levels increased up to the age of 12 months before titers leveled off. It has been suggested that young children who present with early signs of β-cell autoimmunity lack the capacity to develop oral tolerance to bovine insulin.[43] Accordingly, the initial immune response to bovine insulin may be diverted into a response targeting human insulin in such individuals.

Data from three population-based case-control studies on cow's milk intake before the diagnosis of type 1 diabetes have yielded conflicting results. In New South Wales, Australia, cow's milk intake was higher in prediabetic children than in control children,[53] and in Finland, a high consumption of cow's milk in childhood was associated with a more frequent appearance of diabetes-associated autoantibodies and type 1 diabetes in a prospective cohort of initially unaffected siblings of children with type 1 diabetes.[54] In contrast, a Swedish retrospective survey indicated that the frequency of milk consumption had been lower among children who presented with type 1 diabetes than among unaffected children.[55]

Gluten or other cereal-derived proteins have also been implicated as potential driving antigens in type 1 diabetes. In small intervention studies performed in family members positive for diabetes-associated pancreatic autoantibodies, elimination of gluten from the diet did not significantly affect autoantibody titers, nor did titers change when gluten was reintroduced into the diet.[56,57] These trials indicated that a gluten-free diet has no effect on the signs of ß-cell autoimmunity in first-degree relatives of affected patients.

Early exposure to cereals may increase the risk of seroconversion to positivity for diabetes-associated autoantibodies.[58,59] Both early (before the age of 4 months) and late (at the age of ≥7 months) exposures to cereals (either gluten- or nongluten-containing) were associated with increased risk of β-cell autoimmunity,[58] whereas another study implied that an increased risk was related to exposure to cereals before the age of 3 months.[59] It has been speculated that dietary gliadin may trigger intestinal inflammation in subjects with type 1 diabetes (because of the HLA DQ2/DQ8 genotype capable of binding gliadin-derived peptides).[60] Wheat gliadin could thus affect the immune activation stage of the gut immune system in individuals at genetic risk for type 1 diabetes and modify the autoimmune process involved in β-cell destruction.[43]

There is seasonal variation in the appearance of the first pancreatic autoantibodies in young children with increased HLA-conferred susceptibility to type 1 diabetes.[51] In addition to seasonal variation in viral infections, there is a marked seasonal variation in the amount of daylight and sunshine hours, especially in Northern Europe, which has the highest incidence of type 1 diabetes in the world.[22] Without oral supplementation, sunlight-dependent synthesis of vitamin D in the skin is the most important source of this immunologically active prohormone. The lack of oral vitamin D supplementation in infancy may increase the subsequent risk of type 1 diabetes[61] and vitamin D supplementation during infancy confers partial protection against type 1 diabetes. There is countervailing evidence, however, arguing against the role of vitamin D deficiency as a trigger of β-cell autoimmunity.

A pilot intervention study conducted mainly in Finland has sought to determine whether weaning to hydrolyzed formula over the first 6 to 8 months of life decreases the cumulative incidence of diabetes-associated autoantibodies. Preliminary evidence indicates that such a dietary intervention results in a decreased frequency of positivity for islet cell antibodies and at least one diabetes-associated autoantibody by the age of 6 years[62] On the basis of these pilot data, in 2002 a randomized double-blind trial (Trial to Reduce IDDM in the Genetically at Risk, TRIGR) was initiated to determine whether it is possible to reduce the frequency of diabetes-associated autoantibodies and/or clinical type 1 diabetes by the age of 6 years and the cumulative incidence of type 1 diabetes by the age of 10 years by weaning to a highly hydrolyzed formula over the first 6 to 8 months of life.

Increased weight gain in infancy is a risk factor for type 1 diabetes later in childhood.[63] Children with type 1 diabetes are both heavier and taller in infancy[64] and increased height and weight later in childhood are also a risk factor for type 1 diabetes.[65] Accelerated linear growth and weight gain result in an enhanced β-cell load and increasing insulin resistance. Rapid growth and weight gain may induce β-cell stress; and active β-cells, as compared to resting β-cells, are more prone to cytokine-induced damage.

At present, no definitive nutrition recommendations can be made for preventing type 1 diabetes; however, increasing BMI is associated with a younger age at diagnosis of type 1 diabetes among those US youth with reduced β-cell function.[66] Avoiding excessive weight gain during childhood is clearly a desirable goal for many reasons.

GOALS OF MEDICAL NUTRITION THERAPY (MNT)

MNT is the process by which the nutrition prescription is individually tailored for the patient with diabetes based on medical, lifestyle, and personal factors and is an integral component of diabetes management and diabetes self-management education.[3] The goals of MNT for children and adolescents are shown in Table 2.

The Diabetes Control and Complications Trial (DCCT) and the succeeding observational follow-up of the DCCT cohort in the Epidemiology of Diabetes Interventions and Complications (EDIC) study confirmed that long-term maintenance of blood glucose levels near to normal delays or prevents the microvascular complications of type 1 diabetes,[67] and the benefits of intensive treatment extend well beyond the period of its most vigorous implementation.[68] The DCCT also demonstrated that intensive management of type 1 diabetes is associated with an increased risk of severe hypoglycemia[69] and a tendency to gain weight.[70] Obesity (greater than 120% of ideal body weight or BMI >95th percentile) was more common in intensively treated patients.[70] Weight gain in intensively treated patients with type 1 diabetes has been primarily attributed to the elimination of glucosuria (70% of the weight gain) and a 5% reduction in daily energy expenditure (30% of the weight gain).[71] Recurrent symptomatic hypoglycemia requiring oral carbohydrate to restore euglycemia also contributes to the tendency to gain weight in some intensively treated patients.

Our ability to help patients achieve these objectives is still limited by the imperfection of insulin

Table 2 Goals of Medical Nutrition Therapy for Diabetes Mellitus

Goals that apply to all persons with diabetes	1. Attain and maintain optimal metabolic outcomes including a. Blood glucose levels in the normal range or as close to normal as is safely possible. b. A lipid and lipoprotein profile that reduces the risk for vascular disease c. Blood pressure levels in the normal range or as close to normal as is safely possible 2. To prevent, or at least slow, the rate of development of the chronic complications of diabetes by modifying nutrient intake and lifestyle. 3. To address individual nutrition needs, taking into account personal and cultural preferences and willingness to change 4. To maintain the pleasure of eating by only limiting food choices when indicated by scientific evidence
Goals specific to type 1 diabetes	To provide adequate energy to ensure normal growth and development, integrate insulin regimens into usual eating and physical activity habits
Goals specific to type 2 diabetes	To facilitate changes in eating and physical activity habits that reduce insulin resistance and improve metabolic control
Goals specific to patients on insulin or insulin secretagogs	To provide self-management education for treatment and prevention of hypoglycemia, acute illnesses, and exercise-related blood glucose problems

Adapted from reference 3.

Table 3 American Diabetes Association Recommended Glycemic Targets[2]

	Blood Glucose Goal Range (mg/dL)		
	Preprandial	Bedtime	HbA1c %
Toddlers and preschool age children (<6 yr)	100–180	110–200	<8.5
School age children (6–12 yr)	90–180	100–180	<8%
Adolescents and young adults	90–130	90–150	<7.5%*

*Ideal is <7% if this can be achieved safely without frequent or severe hypoglycemia.

replacement, which does not precisely mimic normal physiology, the lack of methods to continuously monitor blood glucose concentrations, and the risk of severe hypoglycemia when glucose levels are near to normal but insulin delivery is not regulated by a closed-loop feedback system.[72] Target blood glucose and hemoglobin A1c goals vary by age, primarily because young children are frequently unable to recognize hypoglycemia and are at greater risk for severe hypoglycemia (Table 3).[2]

The child with diabetes and his or her family must assume primary responsibility for daily management, whereas the role of the healthcare professional is that of educator, advisor, and motivator. Even modest objectives are not achievable in all patients because educational, psychosocial, and economic factors make it impossible for some children and their families to perform daily *all* the tasks that comprise a comprehensive treatment program.[73,74] The goals of therapy can, however, be accomplished in most patients most of the time by the use of flexible insulin regimens and dosage algorithms, frequent self-monitoring of blood glucose, individualized meal planning, and by educating older children and adolescents leading to patient empowerment and independent decision-making.

GENERAL PRINCIPLES OF NUTRITION MANAGEMENT

There is a little or no research on the nutrient requirements of children and adolescents with either type 1 or type 2 diabetes nor is there evidence that their nutritional needs differ from those of healthy children. Therefore, nutrient recommendations are based on the requirements of healthy children and adolescents.[75–79] Meal plans for children with diabetes should begin with the key recommendations outlined in The Dietary Guidelines for Healthy Americans 2005.[80] This important document provides guidelines that should serve as the foundation for nutrition management within each of the following areas: adequate nutrients within calorie needs, weight management, physical activity, food groups that should be encouraged, fats, carbohydrates, sodium and potassium, alcoholic beverages, and food safety. The guidelines address issues specific to children and may require further definition as they relate to diabetes management. For example, the guidelines suggest that carbohydrate choices should include fiber-rich fruits, vegetables and whole grains, and added sugar should be minimized.[80] People with diabetes treated with insulin or insulin secretagogues must be aware of the total amount of carbohydrate eaten at a meal.

Energy

Clinical dietitians frequently use equations such as the Schofield, WHO, Harris–Benedict, or RDA for age to calculate energy requirements (see Appendix II, "Nutritional Requirements". The following simpler equation can be used to provide a crude approximation for children up to 12 years of age:

Basal daily needs for all children = 1,000 kcal;
for boys add to the basal needs
125 kcal × age in years,
and for girls add 100 kcal × age in years.

Add up to 20% more kilocalories for very active children.

It is important to assess a child's usual dietary intake before the onset of symptomatic hyperglycemia to assist with the formulation of the initial meal plan. Because energy requirements change with age, physical activity, and growth rate, an assessment of height, weight, and energy intake is recommended every 3 to 6 months.[81] Good metabolic control is essential for normal growth and development.[82]

Growth is an excellent indicator of the adequacy of energy intake, which should be evaluated by regularly plotting weight and stature on the Centers for Disease Control and Prevention (CDC) pediatric growth charts (http://www.cdc.gov/growthcharts). If growth is not optimal, the diet should be reviewed and, in patients with type 1 diabetes, screening for symptoms and signs of inadequate insulin delivery,[83] hypo- or hyperthyroidism, celiac disease, and adrenal insufficiency is warranted.

For overweight and obese children and adolescents with either type 1 or type 2 diabetes, energy is reduced to arrest weight gain while supporting normal linear growth and physical development.

Distribution of Macronutrients

Many studies have attempted to determine the optimal mix of macronutrients that should comprise total energy intake. The general consensus is that a single prescription does not exist.[3] The Dietary Reference Intake (DRI) is cited as a guideline that should be used to formulate the initial prescription. The DRI reports suggest a mix of 45 to 65% of calories from carbohydrate, 20 to 35% from fat, and 10 to 35% from protein. Once the nutrition prescription has been determined, the proportion of macronutrients can be modified, as necessary, according to blood glucose and plasma lipid goals and requirements for growth and development.

Carbohydrate

Control of blood glucose in an effort to achieve normal or near-normal levels is the primary goal of diabetes management. Because dietary carbohydrate is the major determinant of postprandial glucose levels, food and nutrition interventions that reduce postprandial blood glucose excursions are important.[84] Blood glucose concentrations after a meal are primarily determined by the rate of appearance of glucose in the blood (digestion and absorption) and its disappearance from the circulation. The normal insulin secretory response maintains blood glucose in a narrow range; however, in patients with diabetes, defects in insulin secretion, insulin action, or both impair regulation of postprandial blood glucose concentrations in response to dietary carbohydrate. The amount, type, and source of carbohydrates in foods, as well as the dose and time interval between administration of rapid- or short-acting insulin and consumption of the meal influence postprandial glucose levels.

The diet should include carbohydrates from fruits, vegetables, whole grains, legumes, and low-fat dairy products.[3] Dietary dogma in diabetes had been to avoid simple sugars and replace them with complex carbohydrates. This belief was based on the assumption that simple sugars are more rapidly digested and absorbed than starches and would lead to more pronounced hyperglycemia. During the past two decades, the blood glucose responses to various carbohydrate-containing foods have been extensively investigated and there is little scientific evidence to support this notion. Although insulin and glucose-lowering medications for type 2 diabetes can adequately control the glycemic impact of added sucrose and other sugars, their impact on total caloric intake suggests that moderation in the use of added sugars is still warranted.

Numerous factors influence the glycemic response to food, including the amount of carbohydrate,[85] the type of sugar (glucose, fructose, sucrose, lactose),[86] the nature of the starch (amylose, amylopectin, resistant starch),[87] cooking and food processing (degree of starch gelatinization, particle size, cellular form),[88] and food structure,[89] as well as other food components (fat and natural substances that slow digestion—lectins, phytates, tannins, fiber, and starch-protein and starch-lipid combinations).[90,91] Furthermore, the glycemic response to a particular carbohydrate food is dependent on whether it is eaten alone or as part of a mixed meal.[92] Fasting and preprandial blood glucose concentrations,[93–96] the severity of glucose intolerance,[97] and the second meal effect[98] are other factors that can affect the glycemic response to foods.

The glycemic index (GI), proposed in 1981 as an alternative system for classifying carbohydrate-containing food, measures the glycemic response after ingestion of carbohydrate. Carbohydrates were previously classified only on the basis of their chemical structure: sugars, starches, or fiber. GI is defined as the incremental area under the plasma glucose response curve over 2 hours after consumption of a standard amount (usually a 50 g portion) of carbohydrate from a test food relative to that of a control food, either white bread or glucose.[99] The glycemic and hormonal responses to a large number of ingested carbohydrates have been systematically examined and their GIs defined.[99–105] As a result of these studies, the validity of the dogma that ingestion of simple sugars causes a rapid and pronounced rise in blood glucose, whereas complex carbohydrates produce only modest increments in blood glucose concentration began to be disputed.[106] It is now clear that there is a wide spectrum of biologic responses to different complex and simple carbohydrates, with so much overlap that they cannot be simply classified into two distinct groups. Even a single food produces a substantially different glycemic response when it is prepared in different ways. For example, a pureed apple causes a greater increment in blood glucose than does an apple eaten whole.[107] Similarly, ground rice or rice flour causes a greater glycemic and insulinemic response than does whole cooked rice,[103] and cooking increases the glycemic response to starch.[108] Blood glucose levels after ingesting wheat flour in the form of pasta are lower than after an equal amount of wheat flour in bread.[109] Thus, the form of a carbohydrate-containing food, in addition to its chemical composition, influences its glycemic effect. The effect of food form alters the rate of digestion and absorption and, therefore, affects postprandial glycemia. Fruits (eg, apples GI 40, Sunkist oranges GI 48, peaches GI 42, pears GI 38 vs. watermelon GI 72) and milk (eg, whole milk GI 27, skim milk GI 32)[110–112] cause a lower glycemic response than most starches, and sucrose causes a glycemic response similar to that of bread, rice, and potatoes. In general, most refined starchy foods eaten in the United States have a high GI, whereas nonstarchy vegetables, fruits, and legumes tend to have a low GI (Table 4).

Use of the GI of a food alone ignores the glycemic response if the portion is other than 50 g. The concept of glycemic load was introduced to describe more accurately the postprandial glycemic response to a food when eaten in a realistic portion size. The glycemic load is determined by multiplying the GI of a food by the amount (grams) of carbohydrate in the portion size actually consumed. For example, 12 medium carrots contain 50 g of carbohydrate. Whereas carrots have a high GI, a usual portion would not significantly increase the glycemic load of the meal. The glycemic load of a meal reflects the sum of the contributions of each food that is eaten.

Table 4 Glycemic Indexes of Common Foods

Low GI (<55)	Moderate GI (55–70)	High GI (>70)
Apples, apple juice, bananas, grapefruit, kiwi, mango, oranges, peaches, pears, plums, grapes, strawberries	Pineapple, raisins, cantaloupe, cranberry juice cocktail	Watermelon
Whole-grain pumpernickel	Hamburger bun, whole wheat pita bread, stoned wheat thins, oatmeal cookies, plain	Bagel, white bread
Sourdough wheat bread, sourdough rye bread, 100% stone-ground wheat bread		Saltines, rice cakes
Sweet potato or yam		Mashed potato, baked potato
Corn		
Oatmeal, from steel-cut oats, milk, yogurt		Rice Krispies, Cheerios

The practical usefulness of low-GI diets in type 1 diabetes is controversial and there are limited data available in children. A meta-analysis of randomized controlled trials (virtually all adult studies) shows that choosing low-GI foods in preference to conventional or high-GI foods has a small (0.4% decrement in HbA1c) but clinically beneficial effect on medium-term glycemic control in patients with diabetes.[113]

Using a low-GI diet as the only approach to nutrition management is not recommended, but substituting lower-GI foods of approximately equal carbohydrate and nutritional value is a useful approach to improve glycemic control, especially in patients with pronounced postprandial hyperglycemia. When making recommendations regarding GI and glycemic load, it is important to focus on encouraging low- and moderate-GI foods from the food groups recommended in the Dietary Guidelines for Americans 2005 report: grains, fruits, vegetables, and low-fat dairy products.[80] For example, a chocolate bar (moderate GI) would not be a suitable substitute for French fries (high GI); whereas oven "fried" sweet potato (low GI) would be an appropriate substitute. A food with a low GI and glycemic load that is high in fat and low in vitamins and minerals is not a healthy substitute unless it is replacing an item of equally poor nutritional value.

Concerns about the acceptance of lower-GI foods have been expressed as a reason not to introduce a low-GI diet. At a diabetes summer camp for 7- to 16-year-old children, satisfaction ratings were equal when dinner and snacks containing lower-GI foods replaced standard food choices; however, they were lower (although within the acceptable range) at breakfast and lunch.[114] Children 8 to 13 years old who received low-GI dietary advice did not report more limited food choices or compromise their macronutrient intake as compared to children who continued to use a traditional carbohydrate-exchange diet.[115]

Once patients have mastered the concept of matching carbohydrate intake to insulin, or distributing carbohydrate throughout the day to optimize glycemic control, we recommend providing additional guidance on how to lower the GI of the diet.

Fiber

Fiber refers to the portion of a plant that is not digestible in the human small intestine. It was thought to have no nutritive value and in the past century, the quantity of fiber in the American diet has declined. During the last two decades, however, considerable attention has been focused on the various plant fibers because of their influence on gastrointestinal physiology. It is now known that fiber markedly influences the digestion, absorption, and metabolism of many nutrients.[116–119] Cellulose, lignins, and certain hemicelluloses, the fibers present in vegetables and grains are usually insoluble in water. Many fruits and certain legumes are rich in water-soluble fibers such as pectins, guar, and storage polysaccharides. When carbohydrate is ingested together with soluble fiber, the resulting increase in blood glucose concentration is less than when carbohydrate is ingested alone.[120] A large test meal containing carbohydrate, protein, and fat normally causes significantly less postprandial glycemia when the meal is supplemented with guar.[121] The attenuated increment in blood glucose concentration that occurs when guar is added to ingested carbohydrate is due to delayed rather than incomplete absorption of carbohydrate.[122]

Short-term studies using large amounts of fiber (>30 g/d) in small numbers of suboptimally controlled type 1 diabetic subjects suggested a positive effect of fiber on glycemia.[123–126] However, in subjects using intensive insulin therapy, 56 g of fiber had no beneficial effect on glycemic control.[127] Subjects receiving ≥ 2 injections per day and with baseline HbA1c levels of 7 to 10% were randomized to either a high-fiber (50 g/d) low-GI diet, or a low-fiber (15 g/d) high-GI diet for 24 weeks. The high-fiber diet significantly decreased mean daily blood glucose concentrations, number of hypoglycemic events, and, in the subgroup of patients compliant with diet, HbA1c levels, but had no beneficial effect on cholesterol, HDL cholesterol, or triglyceride concentrations.[128] Conversely, a cross-sectional analysis of dietary fiber in type 1 diabetes patients enrolled in EURODIAB IDDM showed that a higher intake of fiber was independently associated with higher levels of HDL cholesterol in both men and women, and lower LDL cholesterol levels in men but not in women.[129] No substantial differences were observed between soluble- and insoluble-fiber intakes.

These observations suggest that inclusion of plant fiber in the diet may benefit patients with diabetes by diminishing postprandial hyperglycemia. Furthermore, certain soluble plant fibers significantly reduce serum cholesterol concentrations and decrease fasting serum triglyceride levels in diabetics with hypertriglyceridemia.[118] The mechanism responsible for the effects on cholesterol and triglycerides is not known.

People with diabetes are encouraged to choose a variety of fiber-containing foods such as legumes, fiber-rich cereals (≥5 g fiber per serving), fruits, vegetables, and whole grain products because they provide vitamins, minerals, and other substances important for good health.[3] Patients should be encouraged to achieve the fiber intake goals set for the general population of 14 g per 1,000 kcal.[75] Dietary fiber recommendations for children with diabetes are the same as for nondiabetic children. Children older than 2 years should have an amount of dietary fiber equal to or greater than their age plus 5 g/d.[130]

Protein

Protein requirements are not increased when diabetes is well controlled; therefore, children with diabetes should follow the RDA guidelines suggested for children without diabetes. The physiologic requirement, determined by the amount of protein necessary to sustain normal growth, is based on ideal weight-for-height and varies with age, being highest in infancy and early childhood. The protein requirement (per kilogram body weight) of infants, children, and adolescents is higher than that of adults. It is recommended that for individuals with diabetes and normal renal function, the protein content of the diet should be the same as for nondiabetic children and adolescents. The 2005 DRIs for children 1 to 3 years old is 5 to 20% and for children 4 to 18 years of age 10 to 30%, respectively, of total energy intake. The recommendation for adults with diabetes is to maintain protein intake at less than 20% of energy needs. Any ingested protein that exceeds the body's requirement for new protein synthesis enters the carbon pool and is converted into either glucose or fat.

Dietary protein should be derived from both animal and vegetable sources; however, the source of protein is not especially important provided that all the essential amino acids are available in adequate amounts. Good quality protein sources include meat, poultry, fish, eggs, milk, cheese, and soy. To lower the consumption of saturated fat, less protein should be derived from red meat, whole milk, and high-fat dairy foods than is customary in the United States. With the onset of nephropathy, lower intakes of protein should be considered. A protein intake similar to the adult RDA (0.8 g/kg body weight per day), ~10% of daily energy, is sufficiently restrictive and is recommended for individuals with evidence of nephropathy. With protein intake of 0.6 g per kg per day, evidence of protein under-nutrition has been reported.[131]

Fat

Cardiovascular disease (CVD) is more prevalent among patients with type 1 and type 2 diabetes than among those without diabetes.[132,133] Type 1 diabetes is associated with at least a 10-fold increase in CVD as compared with an age-matched nondiabetic population.[133,134] Its major clinical consequences are atherosclerosis of the coronary, cerebral, and lower extremity large arteries. In Westernized populations, atherosclerotic vascular disease is the major cause of mortality and morbidity in patients with diabetes. About 75% of patients with diabetes in Europe and North America die of coronary heart disease. This terrible toll is not inevitable. In other parts of the world, patients with diabetes who escape atherosclerosis have low serum cholesterol levels and live on diets that are usually high in starch and have a low content of saturated fat. Cognizance of these facts compels us to focus attention on the amount and type of fat consumed by persons with diabetes. The recent DCCT/EDIC report on the effect of intensive diabetes therapy on CVD in type 1 diabetes showed that higher total and LDL cholesterol levels at baseline were significantly associated with the occurrence of CVD independent of treatment assignment.[135]

To reduce the risk for CVD, the goal is to limit the consumption of saturated fatty acids, *trans* fatty acids, and cholesterol, and to increase intake of omega-3 fatty acids and unsaturated fat. These recommendations are consistent with those of the Dietary Guidelines for Americans 2005, the American Academy of Pediatrics, and the American Heart Association.[136] Saturated and *trans* fatty acids are the principal dietary determinants of plasma LDL cholesterol. In nondiabetic individuals, reducing the consumption of saturated and *trans* fatty acids, and cholesterol decreases plasma total and LDL cholesterol levels. Reducing saturated fatty acids may also reduce HDL cholesterol and, importantly, the ratio of LDL cholesterol to HDL cholesterol is not adversely affected (Table 5).

Table 5 Practical Guidelines for Implementing the American Heart Association Dietary Guidelines

- Reduce added sugars, including sugar-sweetened drinks and juices
- Use canola, soybean, corn, safflower oil, or other unsaturated oil in place of solid fats during food preparation
- Use fresh, frozen, and canned vegetables and fruits and serve at every meal; be careful with added sauces and sugar
- Introduce and regularly serve fish as an entrée
- Remove the skin from poultry before eating
- Use only lean cuts of meat and reduced-fat meat products
- Limit high-calorie sauces such as Alfredo, cream sauces, cheese sauces, and hollandaise
- Eat whole-grain breads and cereals rather than refined products, read labels and ensure that "whole grain" is the first ingredient on the food label of these products
- Eat more legumes (beans) and tofu in place of meat for some entrees
- Breads, breakfast cereals, and prepared foods, including soups, may be high in salt and sodium and/or sugar; read food labels for content and choose high-fiber, low-salt/low-sugar alternatives

Children and adolescents with well-controlled type 1 diabetes are not at high risk for developing lipid abnormalities, but should be screened and monitored according to guidelines issued by the National Cholesterol Education Program (NCEP) and by the American Academy of Pediatrics.[137] For children and adolescents who are growing and developing normally and have normal plasma lipid levels, it is recommended that less than 10% of energy comes from saturated fat, the daily intake of cholesterol should be less than 300 mg per day, and consumption of *trans* fatty acids should be minimal. Total fat should be reduced in the obese child to reduce total energy consumption. The consumption of saturated fat can be reduced by drinking less whole milk and more low-fat milk and eating less red meat and high-fat dairy foods, and by eating more poultry, fish, and vegetable proteins.

The NCEP Step II diet guidelines should be implemented in the patient with elevated LDL cholesterol (>100 mg/dL).[138] The guidelines recommend that total fat represent no more than 30%

of total calories, less than 7% of calories are from saturated fat, and dietary cholesterol is 200 mg/d.

Recent survey data of a representative sample of US youth with diabetes (89% with type 1) show that percent consumption of energy from total fat is 37 to 38% across subgroups of age (10 to 14 years, >15 years). Only 6.5% of the cohort met ADA recommendations of <10% of energy from saturated fat and less than 50% met recommendations for total fat, vitamin E, fiber, fruits, vegetables, and grains. It is evident that there is a critical need for improvement in dietary intake in youth with diabetes.[139]

Sodium

The average consumption of salt in populations correlates well with the prevalence of hypertension[140] and a high intake of sodium causes high blood pressure in susceptible individuals. Most processed foods contain considerably more sodium than similar foods prepared from raw ingredients. Sodium is present in the form of sodium chloride; it may also be present as sodium glutamate, added to enhance flavor, or as sodium nitrite included as a preservative. The leaders in sodium content are take-out or "fast foods," which account for an ever-increasing proportion of the US diet. It has been estimated that 70% of the sodium in the US diet is derived from prepared foods.

Sodium consumption in persons with diabetes should be the same as for the general population, between 2,400 mg[141] and 3,000 mg daily.[142] A reduction in salt intake lowers blood pressure in both normotensive and hypertensive individuals. In nondiabetic adults, a reduction in salt consumption lowers systolic blood pressure by 4 to 5 mm Hg[143,144]; therefore, for diabetic patients with hypertension (in children and adolescents defined as the average of three separate systolic and/or diastolic blood pressures >95th percentile for age, sex, and height), a reduction in salt intake to 2,400 mg daily is recommended. Note, however, that sodium restriction has not been tested in the diabetic population in controlled clinical trials.[145] To achieve these goals, patients should be taught to reduce their use of table salt and decrease their consumption of convenience foods.

MEDICAL NUTRITIONAL THERAPY

A registered dietitian skilled in MNT is the diabetes team member who plays the leading role in providing nutrition care; however, it is important that all members of the diabetes team, including physicians and diabetes nurse educators, be knowledgeable about MNT and help to support its implementation.[3]

MNT begins with a nutrition history and assessment, taking heed of the ethnic, religious, and economic factors that pertain to the individual patient and his or her family. Family eating patterns, meal preparation methods, and nutrition beliefs must be identified. The initial evaluation of eating styles and nutrition beliefs within the family assist the dietitian to determine how best to begin educating the patient and family to achieve nutrition guidelines for optimal management of the disease. The first priority is to teach families how diet and insulin (or other medications) affect blood glucose levels. Thereafter, it is important to teach dietary habits that will help patients reduce their risk of CVD.

The way meals are planned should be understandable to the patient and family. A great deal of lay literature about diet is available to the general public; some accurately describes evidence-based research, but much does not. Families that have received and applied advice consistent with the recommendations of the American Heart Association, American Academy of Pediatrics, and Dietary guidelines for Americans 2005 will benefit by an approach that builds on their current practices.

Changing how we think about our food and beverage selections on a day-to-day basis is, perhaps, the most difficult aspect of diabetes management. Before discovering that a member of the family has diabetes, families may give significant thought to their food purchases, but planning when and the precise amount to be eaten at a meal are not common in the general population.

Patients with both type 1 and type 2 diabetes have the same goals; namely, to achieve and maintain target blood glucose and glycated hemoglobin levels (Table 2). The initial focus of MNT, however, differs between the two major types of diabetes.[14] Children with type 2 diabetes typically are obese at presentation and there is great emphasis on weight loss, limiting caloric intake, and distributing meals evenly throughout the day. Even modest weight reduction alone increases sensitivity to insulin and improves fasting and postprandial plasma glucose levels.[18] Similarly, moderate calorie reduction decreases plasma glucose levels in type 2 diabetes.[146,147] Studies in adults provide evidence that structured, intensive lifestyle programs involving participant education, individualized counseling, reduced energy and fat intake (~30% of total energy), regular physical activity, and frequent participant contact are necessary to produce long-term weight loss of 5 to 7% of starting weight.[148] Accordingly, lifestyle changes that lead to weight loss are the cornerstone of therapy in patients with type 2 diabetes. In contrast, in the child with type 1 diabetes, the primary goal is to match insulin delivery and carbohydrate consumption to achieve blood glucose levels in the age-specific target range.

Considerations When Formulating a Meal Plan for Type 1 Diabetes

Newly diagnosed children usually present with weight loss and are hungry for the first few days to weeks after starting insulin therapy. Therefore, the child's initial dietary allowance is determined by appetite. The meal plan should be formulated to restore and then maintain an appropriate body weight and allow for normal growth and development. Energy requirements vary with age, height, weight, and gender, as well as with physical activity, season of the year, and stage of puberty. If the child's usual food intake cannot be adequately determined, the nutrition prescription can be based on a formula for estimating energy and protein allowances (see above under Energy).

The daily eating patterns of young children generally include three meals and two or three snacks, depending on the length of time between meals, the age of the child, and level of physical activity. Although their daily energy intake is relatively constant over time, young children adjust their energy intake at successive meals.[149,150]

Dietary strategies principally are determined by the patient's insulin replacement regimen (Table 6). Rapid-acting insulin combined with

Table 6 General Approaches to Meal Management

Type 1 diabetes Split-mixed insulin regimen	• Three meals and 2 or 3 snacks daily • Meals and snacks spaced 2–3 hours apart • Consistent carbohydrate intake • Snack before bed to decrease risk of overnight hypoglycemia • Meal times consistent from day-to-day • Continued education and assessment of readiness to change lifestyle to achieve Heart Healthy diet
Basal–bolus or insulin pump therapy	• Carbohydrate content can vary • Must accurately count carbohydrate and match insulin dose to predetermined insulin:carbohydrate ratio • Should eat at least 3 meals daily • Snack before bed to decrease risk of overnight hypoglycemia • Should not eat less than a predetermined amount of carbohydrate per day • Continued education and assessment of readiness to change lifestyle to achieve Heart Healthy diet
Type 2 diabetes	• Meal plan to assist with evenly spaced carbohydrate intake and increased emphasis on reducing calories to promote weight loss

Age related issues: Children's activities often differ on weekdays compared to weekends and holidays, and appropriate allowance must be made for these differences.
The meal plan must take into account the child's school schedule, early or late lunches, gym classes, and after-school physical activity.

intermediate-acting (neutal protamine Hagedorn, NPH) insulin is often used at the outset because glycemia can be controlled with two or three daily injections: typically at breakfast, dinner, and/or bedtime. Rapid-acting insulin and intermediate-acting insulin are released from the subcutaneous injection site into the circulation reaching peak effects 1 to 2 hours and 4 to 10 hours after injection, respectively. A meal plan is formulated to provide a consistent carbohydrate intake because the breakfast dose of NPH will have its peak effect between lunch and dinner and the dose is based on the glycemic load provided by lunch and a mid-afternoon snack. Therefore, over- or undereating carbohydrate will result in hyper- or hypoglycemia, respectively. The use of fixed doses of rapid- or short-acting together with intermediate-acting insulin is not ideal for families whose lifestyles do not allow for consistent meal times. Similarly, very young children whose appetites are highly variable present significant challenges when rigid meal timing and constant carbohydrate intake are required to match a fixed dose of insulin. Using are insulin regimen that includes administering rapid-acting insulin after the meal provides a practical solution to this problem.[151]

Because the energy needs of children continuously change, food intake should be re-evaluated at 3- to 6-month intervals depending on the age of the child.[152,153] Whenever the quantity of carbohydrate in the meal plan is changed, the insulin dose must be reviewed. If a pattern of premeal hyperglycemia is identified, it should be treated by adjusting the insulin dose and not by withholding food. Trends in hunger and satiety should be tracked. Additional servings of protein- and fat-rich foods should not be routinely offered to satisfy hunger, and force-feeding carbohydrate to achieve meal plan goals is discouraged. Instead, the meal plan should be adjusted when an abnormal trend in growth is observed, when the child frequently complains of being too full to eat the prescribed meal, or frequently complains of being hungry after meals. Occasional hunger between meals need not lead to a major dietary change.

In general, more physiologic and flexible insulin-replacement strategies are preferred. These employ CSII using an insulin pump or multiple daily doses of rapid-acting insulin in conjunction with a long-acting (basal) insulin. Meal plans need not be rigid with respect to the time meals are eaten or the amount of carbohydrate that has to be consumed at each meal. Patients adjust the premeal insulin dose of rapid-acting insulin to match ("cover") the carbohydrate content of the meal. There is a strong relationship between the premeal insulin dose and the postprandial response[154]; therefore, patients who use these regimens are encouraged to perform pre- and postprandial blood glucose monitoring to optimize prandial insulin doses. Variation in the carbohydrate content of meals does not modify the patient's basal insulin requirement. The patient's blood glucose level prior to the meal and the carbohydrate content of the meal are used to determine the mealtime insulin dose. In contrast to patients receiving intermediate-acting insulin, patients who use basal–bolus insulin therapy or an insulin pump should not have excessive insulin action between meals and, therefore, are not obliged to eat snacks, unless they engage in strenuous or prolonged physical activity. They must, however, inject rapid-acting insulin or give a bolus of insulin via the pump each time they consume carbohydrate.

The concept of total carbohydrate intake determining the premeal insulin dosage is supported by data from the DCCT. Individuals who adjusted their premeal insulin dosages based on the carbohydrate content of their meals had a 0.5% lower HbA1c level than those who did not adjust premeal insulin doses.[155] It should, also, be noted that day-to-day consistency in the amount and source of carbohydrate is associated with lower HbA1c levels in individuals who receive fixed doses of short-acting (or rapid-acting) and intermediate-acting insulin.[156]

Formulation of a Meal Plan for Type 2 Diabetes

Treatment aims for type 2 diabetes are to normalize fasting and postprandial blood glucose and hemoglobin A1c values, to identify and treat associated comorbidities such as hypertension and hyperlipidemia,[1] and to minimize the risk of acute and chronic complications associated with diabetes. Early onset of type 2 diabetes is associated with a high incidence of diabetic nephropathy[157] and vascular disease may already be present at diagnosis.[158,159] The early age of onset of type 2 diabetes in children can be expected to increase the risk of microvascular complications, which are directly related to the duration of diabetes and hyperglycemia.

MNT for patients with type 2 diabetes emphasizes healthy eating to support optimal growth and weight management. A careful history of an individual's usual eating and physical exercise habits can assist in determining the best approach to formulating a meal plan. Patients and their family members should be encouraged to adopt healthy eating habits. Guidance should be offered on behavior-modification strategies to change their lifestyle, decrease their consumption of high-energy, high-fat foods,[160] and incorporation of daily aerobic physical activity in their lives. In order to increase children's physical activity, the amount of time devoted to sedentary activities such as viewing television, playing video games, and sitting in front of a computer, must be strictly limited.[161,162] Recommendations outlined by the American Heart Association (Table 5) that include but are not limited to simple suggestions such as eliminating sugar-containing sodas and juices, and decreasing consumption of calorie-dense "fast foods" and high-fat snacks, can improve blood glucose levels and achieve weight loss. Patients who have no regularly scheduled meals and eat large amounts of food toward the end of the day can also see improvements in glycemic control when carbohydrate intake is more evenly distributed throughout the day. If weight loss is not achieved by targeting identified eating habits and food selections, a more structured approach such as a low-glycemic load diet or a diet with defined portions and calories is warranted. These diets are based on energy requirements calculated from resting energy expenditure equations and modified based on weight change. Younger children can achieve weight loss and better glycemic control when weight is maintained or the rate of weight gain is slowed so that over time with linear growth their weight-for-height gradually returns toward normal. A child whose BMI exceeds the 95th percentile, however, should be encouraged to lose weight. When the diet is implemented linear growth should be monitored to assure that the decrease in calories does not adversely affect linear growth velocity.

Individuals with type 2 diabetes who do not achieve satisfactory glycemic control with a combination of weight loss, portion control, and optimal meal spacing require drug therapy. The meal plan then needs to be formulated based on the prescribed medical regimen.

Teaching Individual Nutrition and Meal Plans

The dietitian has the important task of evaluating the patient's and family's understanding of basic principles of nutrition and then providing sufficient knowledge to help clients implement their individualized meal plan. The aim is to lay a foundation for lifelong, healthy eating habits for the child and family. Even the most intensive regimens of insulin administration are not successful without careful attention to meal planning.[155] Nutrition education, like all aspects of diabetes education, has to be an ongoing process, with periodic review and revision of the meal plan. The child's and parents' levels of comprehension, ability to solve problems, and adherence to the nutrition goals should be regularly reassessed. Teaching should be followed by systematic assessment of the patients' ability to perform in an environment that approximates as closely as possible the behaviors expected in the natural environment.[163]

Healthcare professionals need to communicate recommendations in practical terms and teach clients how to minimize the daily burden of food calculations, maintain the pleasure of eating, and enjoy a wide variety of food choices whose use is supported by scientific evidence. A successful nutrition plan is effective only when it enables patients to achieve their healthcare goals. When implementing a nutrition plan, the use of commonly used educational materials and approaches will help a client's other healthcare providers assist in evaluating their patient's understanding of and adherence to the plan. Appreciation of a patient's or family's learning style, math and reading skills, and attention to detail is important when devising and implementing the plan.

Several commonly employed meal planning approaches are available. These include: exchange or carbohydrate choices, carbohydrate counting, experience-based estimation,[164] low-GI diet,[115] and a method based on the food guide pyramid. Although it is well accepted that diet is integral to successful diabetes care, methods of dietary education remain controversial and poorly evaluated and there is little evidence to support the superiority of one method over another.[164,165]

Exchange System and Carbohydrate Choices

The exchange system approach for meal planning has been most widely used. It was originally developed in 1950 by a joint committee of the ADA, the American Dietetic Association, and the Diabetes–Arthritis Program of the US Public Health Service, and was last updated in 2003.[166] The system was based on six exchange lists: milk, fruit, vegetable, starch, meat, and fat. Each list indicates the appropriate size or volume of each food exchange. Each portion of food within a group was exchangeable because it contained approximately the same nutritional value in terms of calories, carbohydrate, protein, and fat. The food groups have been more recently categorized into three groups to simplify the teaching of carbohydrate consistency concepts (Table 7). Thus, by prescribing the meal plan in terms of a number of exchanges for each meal, consistency of total calories and the proportions of nutrients can be maintained, while allowing the patient to choose among numerous foods (Table 8). Accurate measurement of portion sizes has to be learned, and weighing and measuring foods help to achieve familiarity with the sizes of food portions specified in the exchange list. Weighing food is an educational exercise to train the eye and need not be continued indefinitely. If blood glucose control appears inexplicably to deteriorate, however, it is useful to resume weighing and measuring food portions to ensure that amounts are not excessive. The exchange system should not be used in isolation; rather, it should be one component of a nutritional program directed by a trained dietitian.

An example of how this system is applied to an individual patient is illustrated below. An 11-year-old girl's height is 144 cm (50th percentile on the CDC growth chart) and weight is 37.4 kg (50th percentile). Her daily energy requirement based on the RDA to support growth in the 50th percentile is 1,756 kcal. An appropriate distribution of macronutrients could be 50% of the total calories from carbohydrate, 20% as protein, and 30% as fat.

	kcal	g
50% carbohydrate	878	219
20% protein	351	88
30% fat	527	59
Total	1,756	

Table 7 shows how this patient's daily food allowance is distributed among the six food groups.

Recognizing that added sugar in the diet is not deleterious to glycemic control, the food exchanges have been modified to include foods that contain simple sugars. Exchanges that provide 15 g of carbohydrate per serving have been combined and are currently referred to as Carbohydrate Choices (Table 7). This allows for more flexibility in the patient's food choices while maintaining a constant carbohydrate intake. For example, a patient who wishes to substitute a serving of milk for a cookie cannot do so, because while the carbohydrate content will remain constant, other nutrients will be affected (eg, calcium intake will decrease) (Table 7).

Dietitians face new challenges when instructing patients how to use the exchange system. Food selections have become more numerous, patients are eating more meals outside the home, and manufacturers are altering the usual composition of food items in response to the public's interest in low-fat and low-carbohydrate diets. Foods previously assumed to have a uniform composition now can markedly vary in their carbohydrate content. For example, according to the exchange system a 1 ounce slice of bread provides 15 g (1 exchange) of carbohydrate; however, a 1 ounce slice of "low carb bread" provides only 8 to 10 g of carbohydrate. Therefore, it would be incorrect to count a slice of "low carb bread" as 1 exchange. To avoid errors in calculating exchanges, patients should be instructed to use the nutrition facts on a product's food label. Taking the example above, two slices of "low carb bread" could be considered 1 exchange. Patients may find it easier to count grams of carbohydrate rather than exchanges, by looking at food labels and pocket reference books, since this allows for a wider selection of foods. Most food labels do not provide diabetic exchange values, but all provide carbohydrate values.

Carbohydrate Counting

Carbohydrate counting is a meal planning method based on determining the amount (grams) of carbohydrate eaten during a meal (Tables 9 and 10). When educating patients and their families about this approach, the process begins by describing the primary sources of carbohydrate in the diet. It is also important to describe foods that provide little carbohydrate. An introduction to carbohydrate counting utilizes the "carbohydrate choice" defined as 15 g of carbohydrate. The food exchanges groups, milk, starch, fruit, and starchy vegetables have been merged and are referred to as Carbohydrate Choices (Table 7). In addition to the basic exchange groups, desserts and sweets have been added. A typical breakfast of 2 starch

Table 7 Calorie and Macronutrient Content of Exchange Lists

Groups/Lists	Carbohydrate (g)	Protein (g)	Fat (g)	Calories
Carbohydrate choices				
Starch	15	3	0–1	80
Fruit	15	0	0	60
Milk				90–150
Fat-free, low fat	12	8	0–3	90
Reduced Fat	12	8	5	120
Whole	12	8	8	150
Other carbohydrates	15	Varies	Varies	Varies
Nonstarchy vegetable (when using carbohydrate choices, a single serving is "free"; 3 servings = 1 carbohydrate choice)	5	2	0	25
Meat and meat substitutes				
Very lean	0	7	0–1	35
Lean	0	7	3	55
Medium fat	0	7	5	75
High fat	0	7	8	100
Fats	0	0	5	45

Table 8 Distribution of Daily Food Allowance among Six Food Groups for the Child Described in Text

Group	Exchanges	Carbohydrate	Protein	Fat
Starch	8	120	16	
Fruit	4	60		
Milk	3 low-fat (1%)	36	24	9
Vegetables	1	5	2	
Meat	6 medium-fat		42	30
Fat	4			20
Grams		221	84	59
Calories (%)		884 (50.5)	336 (19.2)	531 (30.3)

Table 9 Sample Menu Based on the Daily Food Allowance*

Foods	Exchanges	Carbohydrate Choices	Carbohydrate (g)
Breakfast			
$\frac{3}{4}$ cup cornflakes + 1 slice toast	2 starches	$3\frac{1}{2}$	32
$\frac{1}{2}$ cup 1% fat milk	$\frac{1}{2}$ low-fat milk		6
1 small banana (6 inch)	1 fruit		23
1 tsp margarine	1 fat		
Snack			
1 oz. Granola bar	1 starch	1	20
Lunch			
2 slices bread	2 starches	4	30
1 cup 1% fat milk	1 low-fat milk		12
1 small apple ($2\frac{1}{2}$ inches diameter)	1 fruit		15
Lettuce + tomato	"free vegetable"		
Mustard	"free food"		
1 slice turkey, 1 slice cheese	2 meat		
Snack			
17 grapes	1 fruit	2	15
3 cups low-fat popcorn	1 starch		12
Supper			
$\frac{1}{2}$ cup mashed potatoes	1 starch	4	15
1 cup 1% low-fat milk	1 low-fat milk		12
1 small orange ($2\frac{3}{8}$ inch diameter)	1 fruit		11
$1\frac{1}{2}$ cup % broccoloi	3 vegetable		15
3 oz chicken	3 meat		
1 teaspoon margarine	1 fat		
Snack			
3 graham cracker squares	1 starch	$1\frac{1}{2}$	15
$\frac{1}{2}$ cup 1% fat milk	$\frac{1}{2}$ cup low-fat milk		6
2 Tbsp. peanut butter	1 meat + 2 fats		6

*For child described in text.

exchanges, 1 fruit exchange, and 1 milk exchange is equal to 4 carbohydrate choices or 60 g of carbohydrate (Table 9). Patients are taught to evaluate food labels. The "Nutrition Facts" on food labels show the portion size and the total amount of carbohydrate measured in grams per serving. Foods not included in the exchange lists may be more easily incorporated into a meal plan. Table 9 shows a sample menu that includes exchange servings, carbohydrate choices, and grams of carbohydrate for the child described in the text.

Although food labels are available to determine the carbohydrate content of foods, it is important that sample food labels be reviewed and that patients demonstrate proficiency in utilizing the Nutrition Facts to determine portions per container and the amount of carbohydrate in the portion that they actually consume. Among 200 adult participants recruited from a primary care setting, 89% reported regularly using nutrition facts, but only 37% accurately calculated the carbohydrate content of a 20-fluid ounce soda when 2.5 servings was indicated as the number of servings per container. Ninth grade or greater reading skills were identified in 77% of the participants and ninth grade math skill or greater in 37%.[167]

Advanced Carbohydrate Counting

Advanced carbohydrate counting is encouraged for patients on basal–bolus insulin regimens or those utilizing insulin pump therapy (Table 10). This approach attempts to more precisely count carbohydrates, and insulin doses are titrated to match anticipated or consumed carbohydrate intake. Portion sizes should first be determined by weighing or measuring foods to help to develop excellent visual estimation skills. The Nutrition Facts on food labels and nutrition composition reference guides are then used to determine the carbohydrate content of the portion eaten. The total carbohydrate should be adjusted for fiber and sugar alcohol content to account for their decreased impact on glycemic response. General guidelines are to subtract fiber if it accounts for more than 5 g of the total carbohydrate in the meal, and half that from sugar alcohols. For practical purposes, it may be easier and provide a clearer message to subtract the entire amount of fiber, especially if a patient usually maintains a high-fiber diet. Currently, insulin doses are not adjusted for GI or glycemic load. Although fat intake does not contribute to glycemic load, a high-fat diet prolongs hyperglycemia due to delayed digestion and absorption of the meal.

Patients should be encouraged to keep records of food, medication, physical activity, and blood sugar levels to facilitate recognition of glycemic patterns. In individuals using intensive insulin therapy, if the premeal insulin is correctly adjusted to the carbohydrate content of the meal, the glycemic response 2 to 4 hours after the meal should be within 40 to 80 mg/dL of the premeal blood glucose value. Advanced features available on insulin pumps (eg, dual wave and extended bolus) should be exploited to optimize postprandial blood glucose control when macronutrient distribution is skewed. Diets with limited food choices are inconvenient and difficult to maintain. The broader the understanding of the relationship between food and exercise-related glycemic responses and cardiovascular health, the greater the likelihood that preferred foods can be included in the diet. By measuring pre- and postprandial glucose levels, many individuals use experience to evaluate and achieve postprandial glucose goals with a variety of foods. Reviewing these data with the clinical

Table 10 Constant Carbohydrate Plan and Basal–Bolus Insulin Plan

(A) Constant Carbohydrate Plan

	Day 1	Grams	Choices	Day 2	Grams	Choices
Breakfast						
Time: 7:30 am	1 cup 1% milk	12	1	1 cup 1% milk	12	1
Carbohydrate	$\frac{1}{2}$ cup oatmeal	12	1	1 slice wheat bread	15	1
Grams 45 or	1 (6 inch) banana	23	1	1 egg	0	0
Choices 3		47	3	$1\frac{1}{4}$ cup strawberries	15	1
					42	3

(B) Basal–Bolus Insulin Plan

	Day 1	Grams	Choices	Day 2	Grams	Choices
Insulin:carbohydrate ratio is 1:10	1 cup 1% milk	12	1	$\frac{1}{2}$ cup 1% milk	6	0.5
	$\frac{1}{2}$ cup oatmeal	12	1	1 slice wheat bread	15	1
	1 (6 inch) banana	23	1	1 egg	0	0
		47	3		21	1.5
	The patient would take 5 units of rapid-acting insulin			The patient would take 2 units of rapid-acting insulin		

A. Foods are selected in amounts that provide approximately equal amounts of carbohydrate from day-to-day.
B. An insulin:carbohydrate ratio is individually determined for each patient and evaluated by measurement of premeal and 2–3 hour postprandial blood glucose levels.

dietitian experienced in MNT of diabetes can assist patients to optimize glycemic control and consume preferred foods.

Nutrition education is an ongoing process with periodic review of the meal plan and assessment of accuracy of carbohydrate counting. The patient with newly diagnosed diabetes and his or her parents should meet a dietitian several times during the first several weeks after diagnosis. Within a few weeks of the child resuming his or her usual schedule, the patient and family should review the meal plan with a dietitian who should also be available to patients and their families for telephone consultation. Because children's energy needs change with growth and variations in physical activity, food intake should be re-assessed every 3 to 6 months in young children.[153]

Once the family is able to accurately apply the principles of nutrition management directed toward glycemic control, focus should turn to identifying food choices and cooking methods that will be consistent with guidelines aimed at lowering the risk of CVD. If the patient's glycemic control is poor, growth is failing, weight gain is excessive, or the insulin regimen is changed, the dietitian should be reconsulted to review the meal plan and to make any necessary dietary recommendations.

The use of individually applied imaginative teaching methods and materials will engage the attention and co-operation of children and parents more effectively than abstract concepts of nutritional principles and detailed diet sheets that list the composition of individual foodstuffs. Incorporating visual demonstrations with exercises such as sorting pictures, first for their carbohydrate content and then according to healthier carbohydrate choices, will keep the patient and family engaged. This approach also provides the dietitian with an opportunity to assess the patient's understanding of the topic.

Exercise

Regular exercise improves blood glucose control, reduces cardiovascular risk factors, and helps to reach and maintain a healthy weight.[168] School age children should participate daily in at least 60 minutes of moderate to vigorous physical activity that is developmentally appropriate, enjoyable, and involves a variety of activities.[169]

Patients with type 1 diabetes should measure their blood glucose levels before exercise to determine whether additional carbohydrate is needed to prevent exercise-induced hypoglycemia. The amount of supplemental carbohydrate depends on the intensity and duration of exercise. If blood glucose is <100 mg/dL before exercise, added carbohydrate is required. If exercise is planned and the individual is familiar with his glycemic response to exercise, the insulin dose at the meal preceding exercise can be decreased in preference to increasing carbohydrate intake. This approach is especially appropriate for overweight patients, attempting to lose weight, who do not want added calories to offset the energy expenditure from exercise.

Adherence

Adherence to a meal plan is one of the behaviors patients must maintain for optimal management of type 1 diabetes and strongly correlates with blood glucose control in children less than 16 years old and in adults.[155] For many patients this is the most difficult aspect of diabetes management.[170–173] Patients frequently do not adhere to their prescribed meal plan[73,74,174,175] and parents often have difficulty helping their young child to follow a meal plan.[173] Furthermore, many children (and their parents) do not possess the knowledge and skill required for good dietary adherence regardless of motivation.[163,176] Approximately 60% of Finnish adolescents reported at least a satisfactory level of adherence to their meal plans.[177] In the Unites States, a self-report survey of 144 adolescents who attended a tertiary care diabetes program showed that 15% took extra insulin to cover inappropriate food intake, 73% ate inappropriate foods, and 50% missed meals and snacks.[178] A recent survey of usual dietary intake among a large ethnically diverse cohort of youth with diabetes aged 10 years or older (89% type 1) showed that only 6.5% of the cohort met ADA recommendations of <10% of energy from saturated fat and 40% of youth with diabetes had a BMI of ≥85th percentile. Less than 50% met recommendations for total fat, vitamin E, fiber, fruits, vegetables, and grains.[139] There clearly is a critical need for improvement in dietary intake in youth with diabetes in the United States. In contrast, in Northern Italy, where the national diet is already low in total fat, high in monounsaturated fat, and the intake of fruits and vegetables is consistent with recommended allowances, dietary recommendations and good glycemic control can be achieved.[179]

Management of diabetes is difficult for children and adolescents and, as children progress through adolescence and into young adulthood, satisfactory adherence to therapy and optimal glycemic control become increasingly difficult to achieve and maintain.[180] To achieve better diabetes outcomes, families must remain actively involved in their youngster's diabetes management, regardless of the child's age, even as the primary responsibility for diabetes care shifts from parent to adolescent.[181–183]

Eating disorders are a significant health problem among adolescents. Although there has been variation in the reported magnitude of the problem in type 1 diabetes, the combination of an eating disorder and type 1 diabetes has major adverse health consequences.[184] Adolescent girls and young women with type 1 diabetes frequently decrease or omit insulin doses to maintain or lose weight.[185,186] Family meals are an important defense against disordered eating in adolescents with diabetes.[187]

An important role of healthcare professionals involved in the care of children with diabetes is to motivate their patients to overcome the barriers to adherence so that they will be able to enjoy the benefits of good diabetes control.[67,188] Empirical research shows that adherence to the meal plan can be improved by psychosocial factors such as promoting a positive attitude toward the illness and its treatment, and fostering supportive relationships with family, peers, and the healthcare team.[177] Frequent follow-up and ongoing education aims to individualize the meal plan and set attainable goals are necessary to teach the patient and his or her family how to match insulin to exercise and food.[189,190] Self-monitoring of blood glucose and carbohydrate counting provides patients with a greater degree of dietary flexibility and enables adolescents to take a more active and informed role in their diabetes nutritional management.[183,191,192]

SUMMARY

Nutrition recommendations for treatment of diabetes have repeatedly changed since the preinsulin era, in which a starvation diet with negligible carbohydrate and 70% of calories from fat was the recommended treatment. Today, there is no one "diabetic diet." The recommended diet can only be defined as a meal plan based on a nutrition assessment and mutually accepted treatment goals and desired outcomes. Nutrition therapy should be individualized and consideration given to usual eating habits and other lifestyle factors. Monitoring clinical and metabolic parameters including blood glucose, glycated hemoglobin, lipids, blood pressure, and body weight, as well as quality of life, is crucial to ensure successful outcomes. Modern diabetes management, combining frequent self-monitoring of blood glucose with multiple-dose insulin regimens, or insulin pump therapy, and mastery of carbohydrate counting, has made it possible for children and adolescents with diabetes to have considerable dietary flexibility while maintaining near normal glycemic control.[193]

Although, the introduction of insulin analogs, flexible insulin regimens, and insulin pump therapy has permitted greater flexibility in carbohydrate intake, timing of meals, variety of food choices, and overall quality of life, these therapeutic innovations may also have encouraged unhealthy food choices. Education must continue to emphasize dietary recommendations that maintain normal body weight and improve cardiovascular risk factors, including reduction of total fat, and especially saturated and *trans* fats, and promote consumption of cardioprotective foods such as those containing monounsaturated fats and antioxidants.[164]

REFERENCES

1. American Diabetes Association. Standards of medical care in diabetes—2006. Diabetes Care 2006;29:S4–42.
2. Silverstein J, Klingensmith G, Copeland K, et al. Care of children and adolescents with type 1 diabetes: A statement of the American Diabetes Association. Diabetes Care 2005;28:186–212.
3. Bantle JP, Wylie-Rosett J, Albright AL, et al. Nutrition recommendations and interventions for diabetes—2006: A position statement of the American Diabetes Association. Diabetes Care 2006;29:2140–57.
4. Report of the expert committee on the diagnosis and classification of diabetes mellitus. Diabetes Care 2003;26:S5–20.
5. Craig ME, Hattersley A, Donaghue K. ISPAD Clinical Practice Consensus Guidelines 2006–2007 Definition, epidemiology and classification. Pediatr Diabetes 2006;7:343–351.

6. Liese AD, D'Agostino RB Jr, Hamman RF, et al. The burden of diabetes mellitus among US youth: Prevalence estimates from the SEARCH for Diabetes in Youth Study. Pediatrics 2006;118:1510–8.
7. DeFronzo RA. Lilly lecture 1987. The triumvirate: Beta-cell, muscle, liver. A collusion responsible for NIDDM. Diabetes1988;37:667–87.
8. Boden G. Pathogenesis of type 2 diabetes. Insulin resistance. Endocrinol Metab Clin North Am 2001;30:801–15.
9. Pinhas-Hamiel O, Dolan LM, Daniels SR, et al. Increased incidence of non-insulin-dependent diabetes mellitus among adolescents. J Pediatr 1996;128:608–15.
10. Dabelea D, Hanson RL, Bennett PH, et al. Increasing prevalence of Type II diabetes in American Indian children. Diabetologia 1998;41:904–10.
11. Kitagawa T, Owada M, Urakami T, Yamauchi K. Increased incidence of non-insulin dependent diabetes mellitus among Japanese schoolchildren correlates with an increased intake of animal protein and fat. Clin Pediatr (Phila) 1998;37:111–5.
12. Fagot-Campagna A, Pettitt DJ, Engelgau MM, et al. Type 2 diabetes among North American children and adolescents: An epidemiologic review and a public health perspective. J Pediatr 2000;136:664–72.
13. Bloomgarden ZT. Type 2 diabetes in the young: The evolving epidemic. Diabetes Care 2004;27:998–1010.
14. American Diabetes Association. Type 2 diabetes in children and adolescents (Consensus statement). Diabetes Care 2000;23:381–9.
15. Hattersley A, Bruining J, Shield J, et al. ISPAD Clinical Practice Consensus Guidelines 2006–2007: The diagnosis and management of monogenic diabetes in children. Pediatr Diabetes 2006;7:352–60.
16. Ogden CL, Carroll MD, Curtin LR, et al. Prevalence of overweight and obesity in the United States, 1999–2004. JAMA 2006;295:1549–55.
17. Archer JA, Gorden P, Roth J. Defect in insulin binding to receptors in obese man. Amelioration with calorie restriction. J Clin Invest 1975;55:166–74.
18. DeFronzo RA, Soman V, Sherwin RS, et al. Insulin binding to monocytes and insulin action in human obesity. J Clin Invest 1978;62:204–13.
19. Kolterman OG, Insel J, Saekow M, Olefsky JM. Mechanisms of insulin resistance in human obesity. Evidence for receptor and postreceptor defects. J Clin Invest 1980;65:1273–84.
20. Arslanian S, Suprasongsin C. Insulin sensitivity, lipids, and body composition in childhood: Is "syndrome X" present? J Clin Endocrinol Metab 1996;81:1058–62.
21. Arslanian S, Danadian K. Insulin secretion, insulin sensitivity and diabetes in black children. Trends Endocrinol Metab 1998;9:194–9.
22. Karvonen M, Viik-Kajander M, Moltchanova E, et al. Incidence of childhood type 1 diabetes worldwide. Diabetes Mondiale (DiaMond) Project Group. Diabetes Care 2000;23:1516–26.
23. Tuomilehto J, Karvonen M, Pitkaniemi J, et al. Record-high incidence of Type I (insulin-dependent) diabetes mellitus in Finnish children. The Finnish Childhood Type I Diabetes Registry Group. Diabetologia 1999;42:655–60.
24. Atkinson MA, Eisenbarth GS. Type 1 diabetes: New perspectives on disease pathogenesis and treatment. Lancet 2001;358:221–29.
25. Gianani R, Eisenbarth GS. The stages of type 1A diabetes: 2005. Immunol Rev 2005;204:232–49.
26. Winter WE, Maclaren NK, Riley WJ, et al. Maturity-onset diabetes of youth in black Americans. N Engl J Med 1987;316:285–91.
27. Banerji M. Impaired beta-cell and alpha-cell function in African-American children with type 2 diabetes mellitus— "Flatbush diabetes." J Pediatr Endocrinol Metab 2002 15:493–501.
28. Wolfsdorf J, Glaser N, Sperling MA. Diabetic ketoacidosis in infants, children, and adolescents: A consensus statement from the American Diabetes Association. Diabetes Care 2006;29:1150–9.
29. Daneman D. Early diabetes-related complications in adolescents: Risk factors and screening. Horm Res 2005;63:75–85.
30. Brownlee M. The pathobiology of diabetic complications: A unifying mechanism. Diabetes 2005;54:1615–25.
31. Dunger DB, Sperling MA, Acerini CL, et al. ESPE/LWPES consensus statement on diabetic ketoacidosis in children and adolescents. Arch Dis Child 2004;89:188–94.
32. Libman IM, Pietropaolo M, Arslanian SA, et al. Changing prevalence of overweight children and adolescents at onset of insulin-treated diabetes. Diabetes Care 2003;26:2871–5.
33. Gahagan S, Silverstein J. Prevention and treatment of type 2 diabetes mellitus in children, with special emphasis on American Indian and Alaska Native children. American Academy of Pediatrics Committee on Native American Child Health. Pediatrics 2003;112:e328.
34. Allen FM, Stillman E, Fitz R. Total dietary regulation in the treatment of diabetes, Volume 11. New York: Monographs of the Rockefeller Institute for Medical Research; 1919.
35. Mayer J. Dietary control of diabetes: I. Trial and error. II. Present nutritional basis. Postgrad Med 1971;50:43–5,55–7.
36. Pollack H. Fat content of the diabetic diet. Diabetes 1960;9:145–6.
37. Richardson R. High carbohydrate diets in diabetes mellitus. Am J Med Sci 1929;177:426–30.
38. Sansum WD, Blatherwick NR, Bowden R. The use of high carbohydrate diets in the treatment of diabetes mellitus. JAMA 1926;86:178–81.
39. Rabinowitch IM. Effects of the high carbohydrate-low calorie diet upon carbohydrate tolerance in diabetes mellitus. Can Med Assoc J 1935;33:136–44.
40. Bierman EL, Albrink MJ, Arky RA, et al. Special report: Principles of nutrition and dietary recommendations for patients with diabetes mellitus. Diabetes 1971;20:633–4.
41. Caso EK. Calculation of diabetic diets. J Am Diet Assoc 1950;26:575–83.
42. Wheeler ML. Nutrient database for the 2003 exchange lists for meal planning. J Am Diet Assoc 2003;103: 894–920.
43. Knip M, Veijola R, Virtanen SM, et al. Environmental triggers and determinants of type 1 diabetes. Diabetes 2005;54: S125–36.
44. Schrezenmeir J, Jagla A. Milk and diabetes. J Am Coll Nutr 2000;19:176S–90S.
45. Martin JM, Trink B, Daneman D, et al. Milk proteins in the etiology of insulin-dependent diabetes mellitus (IDDM). Ann Med 1991;23:447–52.
46. Malkani S, Nompleggi D, Hansen JW, et al. Dietary cow's milk protein does not alter the frequency of diabetes in the BB rat. Diabetes 1997;46:1133–40.
47. Scott FW, Trick KD. Dietary modification of spontaneous diabetes in the BB Wistar rat. Proc Calif Fed Biol Soc 1983;26:222.
48. Scott FW, Marliss EB. Conference summary: Diet as an environmental factor in development of IDDM. Can J Physiol Pharmacol 1991;69:311–9.
49. Nakayama M, Abiru N, Moriyama H, et al. Prime role for an insulin epitope in the development of type 1 diabetes in NOD mice. Nature 2005;435:220–3.
50. Ziegler AG, Hummel M, Schenker M, Bonifacio E. Autoantibody appearance and risk for development of childhood diabetes in offspring of parents with type 1 diabetes: The 2-year analysis of the German BABYDIAB Study. Diabetes 1999;48:460–8.
51. Kimpimaki T, Kupila A, Hamalainen AM, et al. The first signs of beta-cell autoimmunity appear in infancy in genetically susceptible children from the general population: The Finnish Type 1 Diabetes Prediction and Prevention Study. J Clin Endocrinol Metab 2001;86:4782–8.
52. Vaarala O, Knip M, Paronen J, et al. Cow's milk formula feeding induces primary immunization to insulin in infants at genetic risk for type 1 diabetes. Diabetes 1999;48:1389–94.
53. Verge CF, Howard NJ, Irwig L, et al. Environmental factors in childhood IDDM. A population-based, case-control study. Diabetes Care 1994;17:1381–9.
54. Virtanen SM, Laara E, Hypponen E, et al. Cow's milk consumption, HLA-DQB1 genotype, and type 1 diabetes: A nested case-control study of siblings of children with diabetes. Childhood diabetes in Finland study group. Diabetes 2000;49:912–7.
55. Dahlquist GG, Blom LG, Persson L-A, et al. Dietary factors in the risk of developing insulin-dependent diabetes in childhood. Br Med J 1990;300:302–6.
56. Hummel M, Bonifacio E, Naserke HE, Ziegler AG. Elimination of dietary gluten does not reduce titers of type 1 diabetes-associated autoantibodies in high-risk subjects. Diabetes Care 2002;25:1111–6.
57. Pastore MR, Bazzigaluppi E, Belloni C. Six months of gluten-free diet do not influence autoantibody titers, but improve insulin secretion in subjects at high risk for type 1 diabetes. J Clin Endocrinol Metab 2003;88:162–5.
58. Norris JM, Barriga K, Klingensmith G, et al. Timing of initial cereal exposure in infancy and risk of islet autoimmunity. JAMA 2003;290:1713–20.
59. Ziegler AG, Schmid S, Huber D, et al. Early infant feeding and risk of developing type 1 diabetes-associated autoantibodies. JAMA 2003;290:1721–8.
60. Auricchio R, Paparo F, Maglio M, et al. In vitro-deranged intestinal immune response to gliadin in type 1 diabetes. Diabetes 2004;53:1680–3.
61. Hypponen E, Laara E, Reunanen A, et al. Intake of vitamin D and risk of type 1 diabetes: A birth-cohort study. Lancet 2001;358:1500–3.
62. Akerblom HK, Virtanen SM, Ilonen J, et al. Dietary manipulation of beta cell autoimmunity in infants at increased risk of type 1 diabetes: A pilot study. Diabetologia 2005;48:829–37.
63. Akerblom HK, Vaarala O, Hyoty H, et al. Environmental factors in the etiology of type 1 diabetes. Am J Med Genet 2002;115:18–29.
64. Hypponen E, Kenward MG, Virtanen SM, et al. Infant feeding, early weight gain, and risk of type 1 diabetes. Childhood Diabetes in Finland (DiMe) Study Group. Diabetes Care 1999;22:1961–5.
65. Hypponen E, Virtanen SM, Kenward MG, et al. Obesity, increased linear growth, and risk of type 1 diabetes in children. Diabetes Care 2000;23:1755–60.
66. Dabelea D, D'Agostino RB Jr, Mayer-Davis EJ, et al. Testing the accelerator hypothesis: Body size, beta-cell function, and age at onset of type 1 (autoimmune) diabetes. Diabetes Care 2006;29:290–4.
67. The Diabetes Control and Complications Trial Research Group. The effect of intensive treatment of diabetes on the development and progression of long-term complications in insulin-dependent diabetes mellitus. N Engl J Med 1993;329:977–86.
68. The Diabetes Control and Complications Trial/Epidemiology of Diabetes Interventions and Complications Research Group. Effect of intensive therapy on the microvascular complications of type 1 diabetes mellitus. JAMA 2002;287:2563–9.
69. The Diabetes Control and Complications Trial Research Group. Hypoglycemia in the Diabetes Control and Complications Trial. The Diabetes Control and Complications Trial Research Group. Diabetes 1997;46:271–86.
70. The DCCT Research Group. Weight gain associated with intensive therapy in the Diabetes Control and Complications Trial. Diabetes Care 1988;11:567–73.
71. Carlson MG, Campbell PJ. Intensive insulin therapy and weight gain in IDDM. Diabetes 1993;42:1700–7.
72. Cryer PE, Davis SN, Shamoon H. Hypoglycemia in diabetes. Diabetes Care 2003;26:1902–12.
73. Jacobson AM, Hauser ST, Lavori P, et al. Adherence among children and adolescents with insulin-dependent diabetes mellitus over a four-year longitudinal follow-up: I. The influence of patient coping and adjustment. J Pediatr Psychol 1990;15:511–26.
74. Hauser ST, Jacobson AM, Lavori P, et al. Adherence among children and adolescents with insulin-dependent diabetes mellitus over a four-year longitudinal follow-up: II. Immediate and long-term linkages with the family milieu. J Pediatr Psychol 1990;15:527–42.
75. Institute of Medicine. Dietary Reference Intakes: Energy, Carbohydrate, Fiber, Fat, Fatty Acids, Cholesterol, Protein, and Amino Acids. Washington, DC: National Academies Press; 2002.
76. Institute of Medicine Food and Nutrition Board. Dietary Reference Intakes for Thiamine, Riboflavin, Niacin, Vitamin B6, Folate, Vitamin B12, Pantothenic Acid, Biotin, and Choline. Washington, DC: National Academies Press; 1998.
77. Institute of Medicine Food and Nutrition Board. Dietary Reference Intakes for Vitamin C, Vitamin E, Selenium and Carotenoids. Washington, DC: National Academies Press; 2000.
78. Institute of Medicine Food and Nutrition Board. Dietary Reference Intakes for Vitamin A, Vitamin K, Arsenic, Boron, Chromium, Copper, Iodine, Iron, Manganese, Molybdenum, Nickel, Silicon, Vanadium, and Zinc. Washington, DC: National Academies Press; 2001.
79. Institute of Medicine Food and Nutrition Board. Dietary Reference Intakes for Calcium, Phosphorus, Magnesium, Vitamin D, and Fluoride. Washington, DC: National Academies Press; 2001.
80. Dietary Guidelines for Americans 2005. http://www.health.gov/DietaryGuidelines/.
81. Kulkarni K, Castle G, Gregory R, et al. Nutrition practice guidelines for type 1 diabetes mellitus positively affect dietitian practices and patient outcomes. The Diabetes Care and Education Dietetic Practice Group. J Am Diet Assoc 1998;98:62–70.
82. Wise JE, Kolb EL, Sauder SE. Effect of glycemic control on growth velocity in children with IDDM. Diabetes Care 1992;15:826–30.
83. Quinn M, Ficociello LH, Rosner B. Change in glycemic control predicts change in weight in adolescent boys with type 1 diabetes. Pediatr Diabetes 2003;4:162–7.
84. Sheard NF, Clark NG, Brand-Miller JC, et al. Dietary carbohydrate (amount and type) in the prevention and management of diabetes: A statement by the American Diabetes Association. Diabetes Care 2004;27:2266–71.
85. Gannon MC, Nuttall FQ, Westphal SA, et al. Acute metabolic response to high-carbohydrate, high-starch meals compared with moderate-carbohydrate, low-starch meals in subjects with type 2 diabetes. Diabetes Care 1998;21:1619–26.

86. Wolever TM, Nguyen PM, Chiasson JL, et al. Determinants of diet glycemic index calculated retrospectively from diet records of 342 individuals with non-insulin-dependent diabetes mellitus. Am J Clin Nutr 1994;59:1265–9.
87. O'Dea K, Snow P, Nestel P. Rate of starch hydrolysis in vitro as a predictor of metabolic responses to complex carbohydrate in vivo. Am J Clin Nutr 1981;34:1991–3.
88. Snow P, O'Dea K. Factors affecting the rate of hydrolysis of starch in food. Am J Clin Nutr 1981;34:2721–7.
89. Jarvi AE, Karlstrom BE, Granfeldt YE, et al. The influence of food structure on postprandial metabolism in patients with non-insulin-dependent diabetes mellitus. Am J Clin Nutr 1995;61:837–42.
90. Hughes TA, Atchison J, Hazelrig JB, Boshell BR. Glycemic responses in insulin-dependent diabetic patients: Effect of food composition. Am J Clin Nutr 1989;49:658–66.
91. Bornet FR, Costagliola D, Rizkalla SW, et al. Insulinemic and glycemic indexes of six starch-rich foods taken alone and in a mixed meal by type 2 diabetics. Am J Clin Nutr 1987;45:588–95.
92. Jenkins DJA, Taylor RH, Wolever TMS. The diabetic diet, dietary carbohydrate, and differences in digestibility. Diabetologia 1982;23:477–84.
93. Nielsen H, Nielsen GL. Preprandial blood glucose values: Influence on glycemic response studies. Am J Clin Nutr 1989;49:1243–46.
94. Rasmussen O, Hermansen K. Preprandial blood glucose values and glycemic responses in insulin-dependent diabetes mellitus at constant insulinemia. Am J Clin Nutr 1991;53:520–3.
95. Fraser RJ, Horowitz M, Maddox AF, et al. Hyperglycaemia slows gastric emptying in type 1 (insulin-dependent) diabetes mellitus. Diabetologia 1990;33:675–80.
96. Schvarcz E, Palmer M, Aman J, et al. Hypoglycaemia increases the gastric emptying rate in patients with type 1 diabetes mellitus. Diabet Med 1993;10:660–3.
97. Parillo M, Giacco R, Ciardullo AV, et al. Does a high-carbohydrate diet have different effects in NIDDM patients treated with diet alone or hypoglycemic drugs? Diabetes Care 1996;19:498–500.
98. Jenkins DJ, Wolever TM, Taylor RH, et al. Slow release dietary carbohydrate improves second meal tolerance. Am J Clin Nutr 1982;35:1339–46.
99. Jenkins DJA, Wolever TMS, Taylor RH, et al. Glycemic index of foods: A physiological basis for carbohydrate exchange. Am J Clin Nutr 1981;34:362–6.
100. Crapo PA, Reaven GM, Olefsky JM. Postprandial plasma glucose and insulin responses to different complex carbohydrates. Diabetes 1977;26:1178–83.
101. Crapo PA, Kolterman OG, Waldeck N, et al. Post-prandial hormonal responses to different types of complex carbohydrate in individuals with impaired glucose tolerance. Am J Clin Nutr 1980;33:1723–8.
102. Jenkins DJA, Wolever TMS, Taylor RH, et al. Rate of digestion of foods and post-prandial glycemia in normal and diabetic subjects. Br Med J 1980;2:14–17.
103. O'Dea K, Nestel PJ, Antonoff L. Physical factors influencing post-prandial glucose and insulin responses to starch. Am J Clin Nutr 1980;33:760–5.
104. Jenkins DJA, Ghafari H, Wolever TMS, et al. Relationship between the rate of digestion of foods and post-prandial glycemia. Diabetologia 1982;22:450–5.
105. Bantle JP, Laine DC, Castle GW, et al. Post-prandial glucose and insulin responses to meals containing different carbohydrates in normal and diabetic subjects. N Engl J Med 1983;309:7–12.
106. Crapo PA, Olefsky JM. Food fallacies and blood sugar. N Engl J Med 1983;309:44–5.
107. Haber GB, Herton KW, Murphy D, Burroughs LF. Depletion and disruption of dietary fiber: Effects on satiety, plasma glucose and serum insulin. Lancet 1977;2:679–82.
108. Collings P, Williams C, MacDonald I. Effect of cooking on serum glucose and insulin responses to starch. Br Med J 1981;282:1032.
109. Jenkins DJA. Lente carbohydrate: A newer approach to the dietary management of diabetes. Diabetes Care 1982;5:634–41.
110. Foster-Powell K, Brand-Miller J, Colagiuir S, Wolever T. The Glucose Revolution Pocket Guide to Diabetes. New York: Marlowe and Company; 2000.
111. Brand-Miller J, Foster-Powell K, Gilbertson H. The Glucose Revolution Pocket Guide to Childhood Diabetes. New York: Marlowe and Company; 2004.
112. Foster-Powell K, Holt SH, Brand-Miller JC. International table of glycemic index and glycemic load values: 2002. Am J Clin Nutr 2002;76:5–56.
113. Brand-Miller J, Hayne S, Petocz P, Colagiuri S. Low-glycemic index diets in the management of diabetes: A meta-analysis of randomized controlled trials. Diabetes Care 2003;26:2261–7.
114. Nansel TR, Gellar L, Zeitoff L. Acceptability of lower glycemic index foods in the diabetes camp setting. J Nutr Educ Behav 2006;38:143–50.
115. Gilbertson HR, Thorburn AW, Brand-Miller JC, et al. Effect of low-glycemic-index dietary advice on dietary quality and food choice in children with type 1 diabetes. Am J Clin Nutr 2003;77:83–90.
116. Kritchevsky D. Dietary fiber: What it is and what it does? Ann N.Y. Acad Sci 1977;300:283–9.
117. Kelsay JL. A review of research on the effects of fiber intake on man. Am J Clin Nutr 1978;31:142–59.
118. Anderson JW, Chen WJL. Plant fiber: Carbohydrate and lipid metabolism. Am J Clin Nutr 1979;32:346–63.
119. Eastwood MA, Kay RM. An hypothesis for the action of dietary fiber along the gastrointestinal tract. Am J Clin Nutr 1979;1979:364–7.
120. Jenkins DJA, Leeds AR, Gassull MA, et al. Decrease in postprandial insulin and glucose concentrations by guar and pectin. Ann Intern Med 1977;86:20–23.
121. Goulder TJ, Alberti KGMM, Jenkins DJA. The effect of added fiber on the glucose and metabolic response to a mixed meal in normal and diabetic subjects. Diabetes Care 1978;1:351–5.
122. Jenkins DJA, Wolever TMS, Leeds AR, et al. Dietary fibers, fiber analogues, and glucose intolerance: Importance of viscosity. Br Med J 1978;1:1392–4.
123. Vaaler S, Hanssen KF, Aagenaes O. Effect of different kinds of fibre on postprandial blood glucose in insulin-dependent diabetics. Acta Med Scand 1980;208:389–91.
124. Chenon D, Phaka M, Monnier LH, et al. Effects of dietary fiber on postprandial glycemic profiles in diabetic patients submitted to continuous programmed insulin infusion. Am J Clin Nutr 1984;40:58–65.
125. Riccardi G, Rivellese A, Pacioni D, et al. Separate influence of dietary carbohydrate and fibre on the metabolic control in diabetes. Diabetologia 1984;26:116–21.
126. Nygren C, Hallmans G, Lithner F. Effects of high-bran bread on blood glucose control in insulin-dependent diabetic patients. Diabete Metab 1984;10:39–43.
127. Lafrance L, Rabasa-Lhoret R, Poisson D, et al. Effects of different glycaemic index foods and dietary fibre intake on glycaemic control in type 1 diabetic patients on intensive insulin therapy. Diabet Med 1998;15:972–8.
128. Giacco R, Parillo M, Rivellese AA, et al. Long-term dietary treatment with increased amounts of fiber-rich low-glycemic index natural foods improves blood glucose control and reduces the number of hypoglycemic events in type 1 diabetic patients. Diabetes Care 2000;23:1461–6.
129. Toeller M, Buyken AE, Heitkamp G, et al. Fiber intake, serum cholesterol levels, and cardiovascular disease in European individuals with type 1 diabetes. EURODIAB IDDM Complications Study Group. Diabetes Care 1999;22:B21–8.
130. Williams CL, Bollella M, Wynder EL. A new recommendation for dietary fiber in childhood. Pediatrics 1995;96:985–8.
131. Brodsky IG, Robbins DC, Hiser E, et al. Effects of low-protein diets on protein metabolism in insulin-dependent diabetes mellitus patients with early nephropathy. J Clin Endocrinol Metab 1992;75:351–7.
132. Krolewski AS, Kosinski EJ, Warram JH, et al. Magnitude and determinants of coronary artery disease in juvenile-onset, insulin-dependent diabetes mellitus. Am J Cardiol 1987;59:750–5.
133. Laing SP, Swerdlow AJ, Slater SD, et al. Mortality from heart disease in a cohort of 23,000 patients with insulin-treated diabetes. Diabetologia 2003;46:760–5.
134. Dorman JS, Laporte RE, Kuller LH, et al. The Pittsburgh Insulin-Dependent Diabetes Mellitus (IDDM) Morbidity and Mortality Study. Mortality results. Diabetes 1984;33:271–6.
135. Nathan DM, Cleary PA, Backlund JY, et al. Intensive diabetes treatment and cardiovascular disease in patients with type 1 diabetes. N Engl J Med 2005;353:2643–53.
136. Gidding SS, Dennison BA, Birch LL, et al. Dietary recommendations for children and adolescents: A guide for practitioners. Pediatrics 2006;117:544–59.
137. American Academy of Pediatrics. Committee on Nutrition. Cholesterol in childhood. Pediatrics 1998;101:141–7.
138. National Cholesterol Education Program. Report of the Expert Panel on Blood Cholesterol Levels in Children and Adolescents. Pediatrics 1992;89:525–84.
139. Mayer-Davis EJ, Nichols M, Liese AD, et al. Dietary intake among youth with diabetes: The SEARCH for Diabetes in Youth Study. J Am Diet Assoc 2006;106:689–97.
140. Altschul AM, Grommet JK. Sodium intake and sodium sensitivity. Nutr Rev 1980;38:393–402.
141. National High Blood Pressure Education Program. Working Group Report on Primary Prevention of Hypertension. Bethesda, MD: U. S. Department of Health and Human Services, National Institutes of Health; 1993.
142. American Heart Association Nutrition Committee. Treatment of hypertension in diabetes (consensus statement). Circulation 1993;88:3009–29.
143. Cutler JA, Follmann D, Allender PS. Randomized trials of sodium reduction: An overview. Am J Clin Nutr 1997;65:643S–51S.
144. Midgley JP, Matthew AG, Greenwood CM, Logan AG. Effect of reduced dietary sodium on blood pressure: A meta-analysis of randomized controlled trials. JAMA 1996;275:1590–7.
145. Arauz-Pacheco C, Parrott MA, Raskin P. The treatment of hypertension in adult patients with diabetes. Diabetes Care 2002;25:134–47.
146. Henry RR, Wallace P, Olefsky JM. Effects of weight loss on mechanisms of hyperglycemia in obese non-insulin-dependent diabetes mellitus. Diabetes 1986;35:990–8.
147. Campbell PJ, Gerich JE. Impact of obesity on insulin action in volunteers with normal glucose tolerance: Demonstration of a threshold for the adverse effects of obesity. J Clin Endocrinol Metab 1990;70:1114–8.
148. Klein S, Sheard NF, Pi-Sunyer X, et al. Weight management through lifestyle modification for the prevention and management of type 2 diabetes: Rationale and strategies: A statement of the American Diabetes Association, the North American Association for the Study of Obesity, and the American Society for Clinical Nutrition. Diabetes Care 2004;27:2067–73.
149. Birch LL, Johnson SL, Andresen G, et al. The variability of young children's energy intake. N Engl J Med 1991;324:232–5.
150. Forbes GB. Children and food—order amid chaos. N Engl J Med 1991;324:262–3.
151. Rutledge KS, Chase HP, Klingensmith GJ, et al. Effectiveness of postprandial Humalog in toddlers with diabetes. Pediatrics 1997;100:968–72.
152. National Diabetes Advisory Board. National standards and review criteria for diabetes patient education programs. Diabetes Educ 1986;12:286–91.
153. Connell JE, Thomas-Dobersen D. Nutritional management of children and adolescents with insulin- dependent diabetes mellitus: A review by the diabetes care and education dietetic practice group. J Am Diet Assoc 1991;91:1556–64.
154. Rabasa-Lhoret R, Garon J, Langelier H, et al. Effects of meal carbohydrate content on insulin requirements in type 1 diabetic patients treated intensively with the basal–bolus (ultralente-regular) insulin regimen. Diabetes Care 1999;22:667–73.
155. Delahanty LM, Halford BN. The role of diet behaviors in achieving improved glycemic control in intensively treated patients in the Diabetes Control and Complications Trial. Diabetes Care 1993;16:1453–8.
156. Wolever TM, Hamad S, Chiasson JL, et al. Day-to-day consistency in amount and source of carbohydrate associated with improved blood glucose control in type 1 diabetes. J Am Coll Nutr 1999;18:242–7.
157. Eppens MC, Craig ME, Cusumano J, et al. Prevalence of diabetes complications in adolescents with type 2 compared with type 1 diabetes. Diabetes Care 2006;29:1300–6.
158. Bao W, Srinivasan SR, Berenson GS. Persistent elevation of plasma insulin levels is associated with increased cardiovascular risk in children and young adults. The Bogalusa Heart Study. Circulation 1996;93:54–9.
159. Raitakari OT, Juonala M, Kahonen M, et al. Cardiovascular risk factors in childhood and carotid artery intima-media thickness in adulthood: The Cardiovascular Risk in Young Finns Study. JAMA 2003;290:2277–83.
160. Willett WC, Dietz WH, Colditz GA. Guidelines for healthy weight. N Engl J Med 1999;341:427–34.
161. Gortmaker SL, Must A, Sobol AM, et al. Television viewing as a cause of increasing obesity among children in the United States, 1986–1990. Arch Pediatr Adolesc Med 1996;150:356–362.
162. Epstein LH, Paluch RA, Gordy CC, Dorn J. Decreasing sedentary behaviors in treating pediatric obesity. Arch Pediatr Adolesc Med 2000;154:220–6.
163. Lorenz RA, Christensen NK, Pichert JW. Diet-related knowledge, skill, and adherence among children with insulin-dependent diabetes mellitus. Pediatrics 1985; 75:872–6.
164. Waldron S. Dietary education and outcomes for young people with type 1 diabetes. Can J Diabetes 2005;29:133–41.
165. Pastors JG, Warshaw H, Daly A, et al. The evidence for the effectiveness of medical nutrition therapy in diabetes management. Diabetes Care 2002;25:608–13.
166. Diabetes Care and Education Dietetic Practice Group of the American Dietetic Association. Meal Planning Approaches for Diabetes Management, 2nd edition. Chicago, IL: American Dietetic Association; 1994.
167. Rothman RL, Housam R, Weiss H, et al. Patient understanding of food labels: The role of literacy and numeracy. Am J Prev Med 2006;31:391–8.

168. Riddell MC, Iscoe KE. Physical activity, sport, and pediatric diabetes. Pediatr Diabetes 2006;7:60–70.
169. Strong WB, Malina RM, Blimkie CJ, et al. Evidence based physical activity for school-age youth. J Pediatr 2005;146:732–7.
170. Anderson BJ, Miller JP, Auslander WF, Santiago JV. Family characteristics of diabetic adolescents: Relationship to metabolic control. Diabetes Care 1981;4:586–94.
171. Lockwood D, Frey ML, Gladish NA, Hiss RG. The biggest problem in diabetes. Diabetes Educator 1986;12:30–3.
172. Brink SJ. Pediatric, adolescent, and young-adult nutrition issues in IDDM. Diabetes Care 1988;11:192–200.
173. Powers SW, Byars KC, Mitchell MJ, et al. Parent report of mealtime behavior and parenting stress in young children with type 1 diabetes and in healthy control subjects. Diabetes Care 2002;25:313–8.
174. Christensen NK, Terry RD, Wyatt S, et al. Quantitative assessment of dietary adherence in patients with insulin-dependent diabetes mellitus. Diabetes Care 1983;6:245–50.
175. Schmidt LE, Klover RV, Arfken CL, et al. Compliance with dietary prescriptions in children and adolescents with insulin-dependent diabetes mellitus. J Am Diet Assoc 1992;92:567–70.
176. Delameter AM, Smith JA, Kurtz SM, White NH. Dietary skills and adherence in children with type 1 diabetes mellitus. Diabetes Educ 1988;14:33–36.
177. Kyngas H. Compliance of adolescents with diabetes. J Pediatr Nurs 2000;15:260–7.
178. Weissberg-Benchell J, Glasgow AM, Tynan WD, et al. Adolescent diabetes management and mismanagement. Diabetes Care 1995;18:77–82.
179. Pinelli L, Mormile R, Gonfiantini E, et al. Recommended dietary allowances (RDA) in the dietary management of children and adolescents with IDDM: An unfeasible target or an achievable cornerstone? J Pediatr Endocrinol Metab 1998;11:335–46.
180. Bryden KS, Peveler RC, Stein A, et al. Clinical and psychological course of diabetes from adolescence to young adulthood: A longitudinal cohort study. Diabetes Care 2001;24:1536–40.
181. La Greca AM, Auslander WF, Greco P, et al. I get by with a little help from my family and friends: Adolescents' support for diabetes care. J Pediatr Psychol 1995;20:449–76.
182. Wysocki T, Taylor A, Hough BS, et al. Deviation from developmentally appropriate self-care autonomy. Association with diabetes outcomes. Diabetes Care 1996;19:119–25.
183. Anderson B, Ho J, Brackett J, et al. Parental involvement in diabetes management tasks: Relationships to blood glucose monitoring adherence and metabolic control in young adolescents with insulin-dependent diabetes mellitus. J Pediatr 1997;130:257–65.
184. Peveler RC, Bryden KS, Neil HA, et al. The relationship of disordered eating habits and attitudes to clinical outcomes in young adult females with type 1 diabetes. Diabetes Care 2005;28:84–8.
185. Polonsky WH, Anderson BJ, Lohrer PA, et al. Insulin omission in women with IDDM. Diabetes Care 1994;17:1178–85.
186. Kelly SD, Howe CJ, Hendler JP, Lipman TH. Disordered eating behaviors in youth with type 1 diabetes. Diabetes Educ 2005;31:572–83.
187. Mellin AE, Neumark-Sztainer D, Patterson J, Sockalosky J. Unhealthy weight management behavior among adolescent girls with type 1 diabetes mellitus: The role of familial eating patterns and weight-related concerns. J Adolesc Health 2004;35:278–89.
188. The Diabetes Control and Complications Trial Research Group. Effect of intensive diabetes treatment on the development and progression of long-term complications in adolescents with insulin- dependent diabetes mellitus: Diabetes Control and Complications Trial. J Pediatr 1994;125:177–88.
189. Travis T. Patient perceptions of factors that affect adherence to dietary regimens for diabetes mellitus. Diabetes Educ 1997;23:152–6.
190. Williamson AR, Hunt AE, Pope JF, Tolman NM. Recommendations of dietitians for overcoming barriers to dietary adherence in individuals with diabetes. Diabetes Educ 2000;26:272–9.
191. Daneman D, Siminerio L, Transue D, et al. The role of self-monitoring of blood glucose in the routine management of children with insulin-dependent diabetes mellitus. Diabetes Care 1985;8:1–4.
192. Templeton CL, Burkhart MT, Anderson BJ, Bacon GE. A group approach to nutritional problem solving using self-monitoring of blood glucose with diabetic adolescents. Diabetes Educ 1988;14:189–91.
193. Wolfsdorf J. Improving diabetes control in adolescents with type 1 diabetes. In: Anderson BJ, Rubin RR, editors. Practical Psychology for Diabetes Clinicians. Alexandria, VA: American Diabetes Association; 1996. p. 23–33.

Diarrheal Diseases

Tyler Burpee, MD
Christopher Duggan, MD, MPH

Diarrheal diseases are a major cause of pediatric morbidity and mortality worldwide, with a median incidence of 3.2 episodes per child-year and 2.5 million deaths of children under 5 years of age estimated to occur annually.[1] If these statistics appear daunting, they should be compared with data from 1992, when 3.3 million annual deaths were estimated,[2] and 1982, when 4.6 million deaths were estimated.[3] The story underlying these statistics is the remarkable success of worldwide campaigns to treat acute diarrhea with oral rehydration therapy (ORT). The development of ORT is among the most successful collaborations ever between basic and applied biomedical research and one of the most significant applications of nutritional therapy to the management of acute disease. Interestingly, it is also a case of reverse technology transfer,[4] in which work originally carried out for benefit of those in countries with less developed economies has changed the standard of practice, even in industrialized settings.

It is, however, clear that the full benefits of the fluid, electrolyte, and nutritional therapy of acute diarrhea have not been realized. Shortcomings in treatment are significant, as they result in added morbidity and costs in both developing and industrialized societies. In the United States alone, acute gastroenteritis accounts for greater than 1.5 million outpatient visits, 200,000 hospitalizations, and roughly 300 deaths per year.[5] It has been reported that 13% of all childhood hospitalizations in the United States are associated with diarrhea, with a median hospital charge of nearly $3,000.[6] It may be argued that the full implementation of ORT for treatment of acute diarrhea in countries with developed market economies has lagged behind its use in less developed countries, perhaps because of the ingrained use of intravenous therapy or the reduced appeal of a technologically simple solution.[7] In addition, it has been difficult to establish continued feeding during diarrheal episodes as normative therapy, in spite of a wealth of in vitro and in vivo data supporting the role of continued nutrition in improving measurements of gastrointestinal function, as well as anthropometric, biochemical, and clinical outcomes.[8,9] This chapter reviews the historical background and scientific basis of ORT and provides a framework for assessing and treating the dehydrated patient or the patient at risk for dehydration. The discussion focuses on common clinical scenarios and traditional practices, especially with regard to feeding. The limitations of ORT are discussed, as well as areas of ongoing research.

HISTORICAL BACKGROUND

Early attempts at treating dehydration resulting from diarrhea were first described in the medical literature in the 1830s, during epidemics of *Vibrio cholerae* infections.[10,11] It was not until 100 years later that the use of intravenous fluids became widespread. Accurate chemical analysis of diarrheal stools eventually permitted the formulation of physiologically appropriate replacement solutions, leading to the successful treatment of cholera with intravenous fluids by the 1940s.[12] Further research into intestinal electrolyte transport led to the development of oral solutions for rehydration.[13,14] In 1971, these were put to the test in the field with the large-scale treatment of refugees from the Bangladesh war of independence.[15] The remarkable success of oral solutions hastened the development of the World Health Organization (WHO) guidelines for ORT and production of standard packets of oral rehydration salts. It may be argued that the initial application of ORT to cholera epidemics in the developing world hindered the acceptance of this therapy's relevance in the United States and Europe. With time, however, ORT has become accepted as the standard of care for clinically efficacious and cost-effective management of acute diarrhea,[5,16] although it remains underused in settings in which parenteral rehydration has been the established practice.[17–20]

PHYSIOLOGIC BASIS FOR THE USE OF ORAL REHYDRATION SOLUTIONS

Fluid must be absorbed and reabsorbed for survival. Under the best of circumstances, the adult intestinal epithelium must handle 6,500 mL fluid per day, the combination of oral intake, salivary, gastric, pancreatic, biliary, and upper intestinal secretions. This is typically reduced to 1,500 mL by the distal ileum and is further reduced in the colon to stool output less than 250 mL/d.[21] Were it not for this ability for net absorption, there would be no balance of fluid to replace insensible losses and that necessary for renal filtration. During disease, the volume of intestinal fluid output is remarkably increased, overwhelming reabsorptive capacity, leading to diarrhea.

Applied clinical research, first carried out among cholera patients, showed that diarrhea in cholera is not the result of a failure of intestinal reabsorption but a state of extreme output in which reabsorptive mechanisms remain intact.[22] Not only *V. cholerae* but many strains of *Escherichia coli*, *Shigella*, *Salmonella*, and other pathogenic bacteria have been shown to produce toxins that bind to enterocyte receptors, causing chloride-mediated secretion stimulated by second messengers, such as cyclic adenosine monophosphate, cyclic guanosine monophosphate, and calcium.[23,24] Even those infectious agents typically classified as causing osmotic diarrhea may, in some cases, also increase enterocyte secretion. *Rotavirus*, for instance, damages the villous brush border, causing osmotic diarrhea, but also produces an enterotoxin that causes a Ca^{2+}-mediated secretory diarrhea.[25,26]

Basic scientific studies of intestinal solute transport mechanisms were also crucial in outlining the processes by which solute absorption is maintained. Water passively follows the osmotic gradient generated by the transcellular transport of electrolytes and nutrients. Although three principal mechanisms of sodium absorption have been described,[21] that essential to the efficacy of oral rehydration solutions (ORSs) was shown to result from the stoichiometric cotransport of sodium and glucose molecules at the intestinal brush border.[27] Figure 1 provides a schematic of the cotransport process. Cotransport across the luminal membrane is facilitated by the protein SGLT1.[28] Once in the enterocyte, the transport of glucose into the blood is facilitated by GLUT 2 in the basolateral membrane. The Na^+–K^+ adenosine triphosphatase provides the gradient that drives the process. Clinical studies have demonstrated that this mechanism remains intact even in patients with severe diarrhea.[22]

In 1975, the WHO and the United Nations Children's Fund (UNICEF) agreed to promote a single solution (WHO-ORS) containing (in mmol/L) sodium 90, potassium 20, chloride 80, base 30, and glucose 111 (2%). This composition was selected to allow a single solution to be used among diverse populations in different countries. Although this solution performed well over 25 years, subsequent clinical research, documented

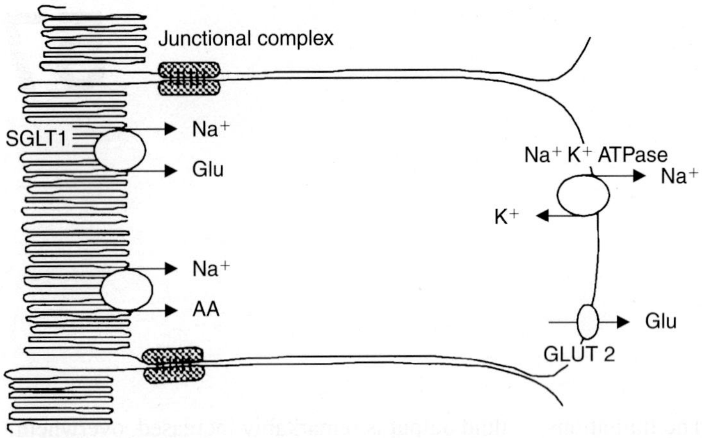

Figure 1 Solute-coupled sodium absorption. AA = amino acid; ATPase = adenosine triphosphatase; Glu = glucose; SGLT1 = sodium glucose transporter-1. (Adapted from reference 5.)

in numerous controlled trials and summarized in a recent meta-analysis,[29] has favored the adoption of a lower osmolarity standard solution. Based on these findings, UNICEF and WHO organized an expert consultation on oral rehydration that recommended a reduced osmolarity solution.[30] In May 2002, WHO announced a new ORS formulation consistent with these recommendations, with sodium concentration 75 mEq/L, glucose 75 mmol/L, and total osmolarity 245 mmol/L[31] (see Table 1 for a comparison of the two solutions).

HOME MANAGEMENT OF ACUTE DIARRHEA

The simplicity of treatment based on ORSs makes possible the management of uncomplicated cases of diarrhea at home. As long as caretakers are properly instructed with regard to the need for clinical assessment when children appear significantly ill or appear to be failing treatment, then it is appropriate to begin therapy at home. Early intervention may reduce complications such as dehydration and poor nutrition. In developed, as in developing settings, early administration of ORS may lead to fewer office or emergency room visits,[32] hospitalizations, or deaths.

In fact, it has always been the case that mothers and other caretakers begin treatment of diarrhea at home.[33] The advent of ORT allows a therapy that is more effective and less harmful than many traditional home therapies. All families should be encouraged to have a supply of ORS in the home at all times, much in the same way that acetaminophen and adhesive bandages are viewed as staples of the medicine chest. As soon as diarrhea begins, one of the commercially available products can be started at home. Although it is possible to produce a homemade solution with appropriate concentrations of glucose and sodium, possibilities for serious error abound, so that standard commercial oral rehydration preparations should be recommended where they are readily available and not prohibitively expensive. Regardless of the fluid used, an age-appropriate diet should be given as well.[8] The most crucial aspect underlying home management of diarrhea is the need to give increased volumes of fluid as well as to maintain adequate caloric intake. Infants should be offered more frequent feeds at the breast or bottle, and children should also be given more fluids.

Caretakers should be educated to recognize signs of illness or treatment failure that necessitate medical intervention. Infants with acute diarrhea are more prone to become dehydrated than are older children because they have a higher body surface-to-volume ratio, a higher metabolic rate, and relatively smaller fluid reserves and depend on others for fluid. For this reason, parents should seek medical care promptly for infants with diarrhea, even before the first signs of dehydration are evident. Indications for prompt medical evaluation are summarized in Table 2. No guidelines have established a specific age under which evaluation is mandated, but, in general, infants should be evaluated by a health professional when there is risk of dehydration; in general, the smaller the child, the lower the threshold for hands-on evaluation. When fever is present, infants and children should be evaluated according to current guidelines. Naturally, underlying conditions, including history of prematurity, metabolic disorders, immune compromise, and recent recovery from surgical interventions, may prompt early evaluation, as may concurrent illness, even a concurrent respiratory infection. Children with dysentery (visible blood or mucus in stool) should be brought in for medical evaluation.

Naturally, parents or other caretakers cannot be assumed to have skills of assessment comparable to a clinician, but their report of any of the easily recognized signs of dehydration may indicate the need for immediate evaluation. Reports of changing mental status are particularly concerning. When the child's condition is in doubt, there should be a low threshold for recommending office or acute care evaluation. The hands-on visit provides an opportunity for physical assessment, including vital signs, more detailed history, and better family instruction.

Table 1 Composition of Commercial Oral Rehydration Solutions as well as Commonly Consumed Beverages

Solution	CHO (g/L)	Glucose (mmol/L)	Na (mmol/L)	Na:Glu	K (mmol/L)	Cl (mmol/L)	Base[*] (mmol/L)	Osmolarity
WHO-ORS (2002)	13.5	75	75	1.1	20	65	10	245
WHO-ORS (1975)	20	111	90	0.8:1	20	80	10	311
ESPGHAN ORS	16	89	60	0.7:1	20	60	10	240
ReSoMal	22.5	125	45	0.4:1	40	70	21	300
Enfalyte[#]	30	167	50	0.3:1	25	45	34	200
Pedialyte[†]	25	139	45	0.3:1	20	35	30	250
Rehydralyte[†]	25	139	75	0.5:1	20	65	30	305
Apple Juice[‡]	120	—	0.4	—	44	45	—	730
Coca Cola[§]	112	—	1.6	—	—	—	13.4	650
Gatorade[‖]	58	—	23	—	3	17	3	330
Chicken Broth[‡]	8	—	260	—	0.5	260	—	450
Brewed Tea[‡]	4	—	—	—	6	—	—	6

Adapted from reference 5.
[*]Actual or potential bicarbonate (eg, lactate, citrate, or acetate).
[†]Ross Laboratories, Columbus, OH. (Data for flavored and freezer pop pedialyte are identical.)
[‡]US Department of Agriculture.
[§]Coca-Cola Corporation, Atlanta, GA. (Figures do not include electrolytes, which may be present in local water used for bottling; base = phosphate.)
[‖]The Gatorade Company, Chicago, IL.
[#]Mead-Johnson Laboratories, Princeton, NJ.
CHO = carbohydrate; ESPGHAN = European Society of Pediatric Gastroenterology, Hepatology and Nutrition; Glu = glucose; ORS = oral rehydration solution; WHO = World Health Organization.

Table 2 Indications for Medical Evaluation

- Young age, with low threshold for evaluating all children under 10 kg and lowest threshold for those under 6 months
- History of prematurity, underlying chronic medical conditions, or concurrent illness
- Fever ≥38°C for infants under 3 months, ≥39°C ages 3 to 36 months
- Visible blood in the stools
- High output, including large-volume diarrhea and persistent vomiting
- Caretaker's report of signs consistent with dehydration, including sunken eyes, decreased tears, and dry mucous membranes
- Poor apparent response to ORT already given or inability to administer ORT

Adapted from reference 5.
ORT = oral rehydration therapy.

CLINICAL ASSESSMENT

Diarrhea may be characterized by the passage of three or more loose, watery stools per day. The volume of fluid lost through the stools can vary from 5 mL/kg/d (near normal) to 200 mL/kg/d or more.[34] Dehydration (loss of body water) and electrolyte losses follow untreated diarrhea and cause the primary morbidity of acute gastroenteritis. Loose stools may be among the presenting signs of nongastrointestinal illnesses, including meningitis, bacterial sepsis, pneumonia, otitis media, and urinary tract infection. Vomiting alone can be the first symptom of metabolic disorders, congestive heart failure, toxic ingestions, or trauma. To rule out other serious illnesses, a detailed history and physical examination should not be neglected in the diagnosis of acute gastroenteritis.

History taking should include questions about the onset, frequency, quantity, and character (including the presence of bile, blood, mucous) of vomiting and diarrhea. Recent oral intake, including food, fluids, and breast-feeding, as well as urine output, should be carefully noted and previous weight recorded, if known. Associated symptoms, including fever or changes in mental status, should be noted. Past medical history should include questions regarding underlying significant medical problems, history of other recent infections, and human immunodeficiency virus (HIV) status, if known. Relevant social history may include the number and nature of caretakers and their ability to return for reevaluation, which may affect instructions regarding follow-up care.

As part of the complete physical examination, an accurate body weight must be obtained, along with temperature, heart rate, respiratory rate, and blood pressure. When premorbid weight is not known but a previous growth curve is available, an estimate of fluid loss may be obtained by subtracting current weight from expected weight based on previous weight-for-age percentile.[35] The quality of this estimate will vary, depending on the number and variability of prior data points. The general condition of the patient should be assessed, with special concern given to infants and children who appear listless, apathetic, or less reactive. The appearance of the eyes should be noted, including the degree to which they are sunken and the presence or absence of tears. The condition of the lips, mouth, and tongue may yield important clues as to the degree of dehydration, even if the patient has recently taken fluid. Deep respirations may be suggestive of metabolic acidosis. Faint or absent bowel sounds may suggest ileus. Extremities should not be neglected, as general perfusion, capillary refill, and skin turgor can help the assessment of dehydration. Visual examination of the stool can confirm abnormal consistency and determine the presence of blood or mucus.

The clinical signs and symptoms of dehydration are outlined in Table 3. A recently published comprehensive literature review found that the three most useful individual signs for predicting 5% dehydration in pediatric patients are abnormal capillary refill time, abnormal skin turgor, and an abnormal respiratory pattern.[36] The assessment of the anterior fontanel, though helpful in select instances, can be unreliable or misleading.[37,38] In infants and children, a fall in blood pressure is a late sign that signifies the development of uncompensated shock and may correspond to fluid deficits greater than 10%. Increases in heart rate and slowed peripheral perfusion may be more sensitive indicators of moderate dehydration, although both may be difficult to interpret as both can vary with the degree of fever. Decreased urine output is a sensitive but nonspecific sign.[35] Urine output may be difficult to measure in infants with diarrhea, although increased urine-specific gravity may indicate dehydration when urinalysis is indicated.

Previous guidelines, including the CDC's 2003 recommendations[5] and the American Academy of Pediatrics (AAP) 2004 guidelines,[16] divide patients into subgroups for mild (3 to 5% fluid deficit), moderate (6 to 9% fluid deficit), or severe dehydration (>10% shock or near shock). Other classification schemes, including 2005 WHO[39] and 2001 European Society of Pediatric Gastroenterology, Hepatology and Nutrition (ESPGHAN) guidelines,[40] divide patients into those showing no signs of dehydration (<5%), some signs of dehydration (5 to 10%), and severe dehydration (>10%). Studies that have looked carefully at the correlation of clinical signs of dehydration with posttreatment weight gain suggest that the first signs of dehydration may not be evident until 3 to 4% dehydration, with more numerous clinical signs evident at 5% dehydration and those signs indicating severe dehydration not evident until fluid loss of 9 to 10%.[35,37] Because of this threshold effect, it may be difficult to distinguish between mild and moderate dehydration based on clinical signs alone. For this reason, Table 3 groups together patients with mild-to-moderate dehydration and notes that these signs may be seen over a relatively wide range of fluid loss, from 3 to 9%. The magnitude of ongoing losses and the patient's oral intake will determine the success of ORT as much as current status. The goal of assessment is not to determine the patient's hydration status once and for all but to provide a starting point for treatment and conservatively determine which patients may be safely sent

Table 3 Signs of Dehydration

	Minimal or No Dehydration	Mild-to-Moderate Dehydration	Severe Dehydration
Mental status	Well, alert	Normal, fatigued or restless, irritable	Apathetic, lethargic, unconscious, floppy
Thirst	Drinks normally, may refuse	Thirsty, eager to drink	Drinks poorly, unable to drink
Heart rate	Normal	Normal to increased	Tachycardia, with bradycardia in most severe cases
Quality of pulses	Normal	Normal to decreased	Weak, thready, or impalpable
Breathing	Normal	Normal, fast	Deep
Eyes	Normal	Slightly sunken	Deeply sunken
Tears	Present	Decreased	Absent
Mouth and tongue	Moist	Dry	Parched
Skinfold	Instant recoil	<2 s	>2 s
Capillary refill	Normal	Prolonged	Prolonged, minimal
Extremities	Warm	Cool	Cold, mottled, cyanotic
Urine output	Normal to decreased	Decreased	Minimal
Loss of body weight	<3%	3–9%	>9%

Adapted from reference 5.

Table 4 Treatment of Acute Gastroenteritis—the "Seven Pillars of Good Treatment"

I.	Use of ORS for rehydration
II.	Fast oral rehydration, over 3–4 h
III.	Rapid realimentation with age-appropriate unrestricted diet
IV.	Formula continuity: use of diluted formula is unjustified; special formula is usually not necessary
V.	Continuation of breast-feeding at all times
VI.	Additional ORS for ongoing losses
VII.	No unnecessary laboratory tests or medications

Adapted from reference 40.
ORS = oral rehydration solution.

home for therapy, which should remain for observation during therapy, and which should receive more intensive therapy immediately.

Supplementary laboratory studies in the assessment of the patient with acute diarrhea are usually unnecessary, including serum electrolytes.[39] Stool cultures are indicated in the case of dysentery but are generally not indicated in acute, watery diarrhea in the immunocompetent patient. Laboratory studies should not, however, be neglected where they may give important clues as to underlying or alternative causes of illness. For instance, urine cultures should not be neglected where there is reason to be concerned for urinary tract infection, and blood cultures and white blood cell count with differential are indicated where the clinical presentation suggests possible sepsis.

THERAPY OF ACUTE GASTROENTERITIS BASED ON DEGREE OF DEHYDRATION

Table 4 outlines the "Seven Pillars of Good Treatment of Acute Gastroenteritis," adapted from ESPGHAN guidelines,[40] and Table 5 provides a summary of specific treatment recommendations synthesized from CDC, WHO, AAP, and ESPGHAN guidelines.[5,39,16,40] Although the first pillar, the use of ORS, should seem self-evident, one recent national survey of physicians in emergency care facilities in the United States showed that many would treat mild dehydration with intravenous therapy, and half would always or almost always use intravenous therapy for a moderately (5 to 10%) dehydrated child under age 2.[20] Treatment should include two phases: rehydration and maintenance. In the rehydration phase, the fluid deficit is replaced quickly, over 3 to 4 hours, and clinical hydration is attained. In the maintenance phase, maintenance calories and fluids are given. Rapid realimentation should follow rapid rehydration, with a goal of rapid return to an age-appropriate unrestricted diet, including solids. Gut rest is not indicated. If anything, diet should be increased as soon as tolerated to make up for lost caloric intake during the acute illness. Lactose restriction is generally not necessary, nor are changes in formula usually indicated. Full-strength formula is generally tolerated and allows more rapid return to full caloric intake. Breast-feeding should be continued at all times, even during the initial rehydration phases. In both phases, fluid losses from vomiting and diarrhea are replaced in an ongoing manner. No unnecessary medications should be used, and laboratory studies should be limited to those necessary to guide management.

Minimal Dehydration

For those patients with minimal or no dehydration, treatment is aimed at replacing ongoing losses. Children with diarrhea must have increased fluid intake to make up for losses and to cover maintenance needs. In principle, 1 mL of fluid should be given for each gram output. In hospital settings, soiled diapers can be weighed (without urine) and the estimated dry weight of the diaper can be subtracted. When losses are not easily measured, a reasonable rule of thumb is that one may give 10 mL/kg additional fluid allotted for each watery stool or 2 mL/kg for each episode of emesis. Nutrition should not be restricted. Instructions regarding dietary therapy are summarized in Table 5.

Mild-to-Moderate Dehydration

Children who are found on assessment to have mild-to-moderate dehydration should have their estimated fluid deficit rapidly replaced, with additional fluid given for ongoing losses. Current guidelines recommend giving 50 to 100 mL ORS per kilogram over 2 to 4 hours to replace estimated fluid deficit, with additional ORS given to replace ongoing losses. WHO guidelines recommend a maximum rate of 20 mL/kg/h,[39] but the rate may be individualized. Using a teaspoon, syringe, or medicine dropper, small volumes of fluid (eg, one teaspoon) should be offered at first, with the amount gradually increased as tolerated. If a child appears to want more than the estimated amount of ORS solution, more can be offered. Although it is safe to give ORS very rapidly, vomiting may be increased with larger boluses. Frequent, small bolus feedings will generally be tolerated. Nasogastric (NG) feeding allows continuous administration of ORS at a slow, steady rate. Clinical experience supports the use of NG feedings even in vomiting patients. Rehydration via NG tube may be particularly useful in an emergency department setting where rapid correction of hydration may prevent unnecessary hospitalization. Although rapid intravenous hydration may also prevent unnecessary hospital admissions, one recent study showed that rapid NG rehydration was well tolerated, more cost-effective, and associated with fewer complications.[41]

Outpatient Observation

Because a certain percentage of children with mild-to-moderate dehydration will fail to improve with ORT, it is prudent to observe dehydrated children until signs of dehydration subside. Similarly, children who do not show clinical signs of dehydration but who demonstrate unusually high

Table 5 Summary of Treatment Plans

Degree of Dehydration	Rehydration Therapy	Replacement of Losses	Nutrition
Minimal or no dehydration	N/A	1 mL ORS for each gram lost to vomiting or diarrhea or 10 mL/kg for each diarrheal stool, 2 mL/kg for each episode of emesis	Continue breast-feeding; resume age-appropriate normal diet after initial hydration, including adequate caloric intake for maintenance*
Mild-to-moderate dehydration	ORS 50–100 mL/kg over 3 to 4 h	Same as above	Same as above
Severe dehydration	LR or NS in 20 mL/kg IV boluses until perfusion and mental status improve. Then give 100 mL/kg ORS over 4 h or 100 mL/kg D5 ½ NS IV over 8 h	Same as above; if unable to drink, give via NG tube or give IV D5 ¼ NS with 20 mmol KC1/L	Begin oral or enteral feedings after initial hydration, acidosis corrected

Adapted from reference 5.
*Overly restricted diets should be avoided during acute diarrhea. Breast-fed infants should continue to nurse ad libitum even during acute rehydration. Infants too weak to eat may be given breast milk or formula via NG tube. Full-lactose formulas are generally well tolerated. If lactose malabsorption appears clinically significant, lactose-free formulas may be used. Complex carbohydrates, fresh fruits, lean meats, yogurt, and vegetables are all recommended.
IV = intravenous; LR = lactated Ringer's; N/A = not applicable; NS = normal saline; ORS = oral rehydration solution.

output may be held for observation. Hydration status should be reassessed on a regular basis, with more frequent monitoring given to those patients whose status is more tenuous. This may be carried out in an emergency room, office, or other outpatient setting. Once dehydration is corrected, if ORT appears to be going well and if the child's caretakers demonstrate comprehension of home rehydration techniques, understand indications for returning for further evaluation, and have the means to do so, then further management may be carried out at home. Even among those whose illness appears uncomplicated on initial assessment, a small percentage may fail ORT, so that some plan for reassessment must be in place. Caretakers should be encouraged to return to medical attention should they have any concerns, if they are not sure that rehydration is proceeding well, or, naturally, should new or worsening symptoms develop.

Management in the Hospital

Indications for management of the child in the hospital include (1) inability of caretakers to manage ORT at home; (2) significant difficulties administering ORT, including vomiting, ORS refusal, or inadequate intake; (3) concern for possible comorbidity, complicating course; (4) failure of treatment, including worsening diarrhea or dehydration in spite of ORT; (5) severe (>9%) dehydration; (6) social or logistical issues that may prevent return evaluation if necessary; (7) or any factors, for example, very young age, unusual irritability or drowsiness, progressive course of symptoms, or uncertainty of diagnosis, which may indicate close observation.

Severe Dehydration

Severe dehydration constitutes a medical emergency. Intravenous rehydration should begin immediately. Twenty milliliters per kilogram boluses of lactated Ringer's (LR) solution, normal saline, or a similar isotonic solution should be given until pulse, perfusion, and mental status return to normal. This may require two intravenous lines or even alternative access sites (eg, intraosseous infusion, venous cutdown). The patient should be closely observed during this period and vital signs monitored on a regular basis. Where available, serum electrolytes, bicarbonate, blood urea nitrogen, creatinine, and serum glucose should be obtained, although it is safe to commence rehydration therapy without these results, as normal saline or LR infusion is the appropriate first step in either hyponatremic or hypernatremic dehydration. Hypotonic solutions should not be used for acute parenteral rehydration.[42]

The severely dehydrated patient may require several boluses, which may be carried out in short succession. Practically speaking, overly rapid rehydration is unlikely to occur as long as weight-based boluses are given with close observation. Errors occur most commonly in settings in which adult dosing is given to infants. (for example, "500 cm^3 normal saline intravenous bolus × ii" would provide 200 mL/kg for the average 2-to 3-month-old.) Edema of the eyelids and extremities may indicate overhydration. Diuretics should not be given. Once the edema has subsided, the patient may be reassessed for continued therapy. With very frail or malnourished infants, it may be prudent to proceed with 10 mL/kg boluses because of their poorer ability to increase cardiac output and because it may be especially difficult to distinguish dehydration from sepsis in these patients. The smaller boluses will also facilitate closer evaluation (please see Chapter 13, "Protein-Energy Malnutrition: Pathophysiology, Clinical Consequences, and Treatment," for details). In general, frequent reassessment of hydration status should be performed to follow the adequacy of replacement therapy. Failure to respond to fluid bolus should raise the suspicion of alternative or concurrent diagnoses, including, as mentioned, septic shock, as well as metabolic, cardiac, or neurologic disorders.

As soon as the patient's level of consciousness returns to normal, therapy can often be changed to the oral route, with the patient taking by mouth the remaining estimated deficit. An NG tube may be helpful for patients too weak to drink adequately but with normal mental status. Although no studies have specifically documented increased aspiration risk with NG tube use in obtunded patients, intravenous therapy is ordinarily favored in these patients. If further intravenous therapy is necessary after initial resuscitation, ESPGHAN guidelines call for the use of 5% dextrose, 0.45% saline over 8 hours to replace calculated deficit, followed by 5% dextrose, 0.18% saline solution (with 20 mmol/L potassium once urine output is documented) for ongoing losses and maintenance.[40] Although it is reasonable to leave intravenous access in place in these patients should it be needed, early reintroduction of ORS is safer. The use of intravenous catheters is associated with frequent minor complications, including extravasation of intravenous fluid, and rare significant complications, including the inadvertent administration of inappropriate fluid, such as those containing excessive potassium. In addition, early ORS will likely encourage earlier resumption of feeding, and some recent data suggest that resolution of acidosis may be more rapid with ORS compared with intravenous fluid.[41]

Dietary Therapy

Recommendations for maintenance dietary therapy depend on the age and diet history of the patient. Breast-fed infants should continue nursing on demand. Those on formula should continue their usual formula immediately upon rehydration in amounts sufficient to satisfy energy and nutrient requirements. Lactose-free or lactose-reduced formulas are usually not necessary. A meta-analysis of clinical trials shows no advantage of lactose-free formulas over lactose-containing formulas for most infants, although some infants with malnutrition or severe dehydration recover more quickly when given lactose-free formula.[43] Patients with true lactose intolerance will have exacerbation of diarrhea when a lactose-containing formula is introduced. The presence of low pH (<6.0) or reducing substances (>0.5%) in the stool in the absence of clinical symptoms is not diagnostic of lactose intolerance. Although medical practice has often favored beginning feeds with diluted (eg, half or quarter strength) formula, there is insufficient evidence to justify this practice; in general, full caloric intake should be restored as soon as possible.

Soy formulas containing soy fiber, specifically Isomil® DF, have been widely marketed to physicians and consumers in the United States. Brown and colleagues showed that added soy fiber reduced liquid stools without changing overall stool output.[44] This "cosmetic" effect might have some benefits with regard to diminishing diaper rash and encouraging early resumption of normal diet but is probably not sufficient to merit its use as standard of care. A more recent trial by Burks and colleagues showed a reduction in the duration of antibiotic-associated diarrhea in older infants and toddlers fed soy formula with added soy fiber.[45]

Children receiving semisolid or solid foods should continue to receive their usual diet during diarrhea. Foods high in simple sugars should be avoided, as the osmotic load may worsen diarrhea. For this reason, large amounts of juice, gelatin desserts, and other highly sugared liquids should be avoided. Some guidelines have recommended avoiding fatty foods, but it is difficult to maintain adequate calories without some fat. Additionally, fat may in fact reduce intestinal motility. The practice of withholding food for 24 hours is inappropriate. Early feeding may decrease changes in intestinal permeability brought about by infection,[46] reduce illness duration, and improve nutritional outcomes.[8,9] Highly specific diets, such as the BRAT (bananas, rice, applesauce, and toast) diet, have been commonly recommended. Although one recent study has shown some benefit from green bananas and pectin in persistent diarrhea (PD),[47] the BRAT diet is unnecessarily restrictive and, like juice-centered diets, may provide suboptimal nutrition for the patient's nourishment and recovering gut.

Many children in poor countries have multiple episodes of diarrhea in a single season, so that diarrhea may contribute to poor nutrition, which may, in turn, worsen the course of subsequent episodes.[48] For this reason, ESPGHAN guidelines call for increased nutrition in the 2 weeks following an episode of diarrhea.[40] WHO guidelines recommend caloric supplements following episodes of diarrhea, such as added cereal in milk, oil in cereal, and foods with high nutrient density.[39] In general, current guidelines call for age-appropriate unrestricted diets, including complex carbohydrates, meats, yogurt, fruits, and vegetables. Children should maintain caloric intake during acute episodes as best possible and should subsequently receive additional nutrition to make up for any shortfalls arising during the illness.

Limitations of ORT

Although ORT is recommended for all age groups and for diarrhea of any etiology, some restrictions to its use do exist. In children presenting in shock, the administration of oral solutions may be contraindicated, as airway-protective reflexes may be impaired. Likewise, patients with abdominal ileus should not be given oral fluids until bowel sounds are audible. It should be remembered that intestinal intussusception may present with diarrhea, including bloody diarrhea. Radiographic and surgical evaluations are warranted when the diagnosis is in question.

Stool output in excess of 10 mL/kg/h has been associated with a lower rate of success of oral rehydration.[49] No patient, however, should be denied ORT simply because of a high purging rate because most patients will respond well if given adequate replacement fluid.

A small proportion of infants with acute diarrhea experience carbohydrate malabsorption, with a dramatic increase in stool output following the administration of ORS. The presence of stool-reducing substances alone is not sufficient to make the diagnosis because this is a common finding in patients with diarrhea and does not in itself predict failure of oral therapy. Patients with true glucose malabsorption will also show an immediate reduction in stool output when ORS is replaced with intravenous therapy. The incidence of clinically significant glucose malabsorption during acute diarrhea is probably less than 1%, although rates as high as 8% have been reported in selected populations.[50]

Many patients with acute diarrhea have concomitant vomiting. Most, however, can be successfully rehydrated with oral fluids if small volumes of ORS (5 mL) are given every 5 minutes, with a gradual increase in the amount consumed. Administration via a spoon or syringe with close supervision helps guarantee a gradual progression in the amount taken. Often, correction of acidosis and dehydration lessens the frequency of vomiting. Continuous slow NG infusion of ORS via a feeding tube may be helpful. Even if some emesis occurs after NG administration of fluid, treatment may not be adversely affected.[41] The physician may characteristically meet some resistance in implementing NG rehydration in the vomiting child. Education of the hospital staff may be helpful, as the NG tube may not only help the initial rehydration but may also speed tolerance of refeeding, leading to improved patient disposition and quicker discharge.

Hypernatremic Dehydration

Patients with hypernatremic dehydration respond well to ORT. Those with severe dehydration should first receive intravenous hydration, as outlined above. Subsequent hydration may be achieved with ORS.[51] As with normonatremic dehydration, ORS should be given both to replace the calculated deficit and for ongoing losses. ORS is safer than intravenous therapy because it is less likely to lead to a precipitous decline in serum sodium, which may increase intracranial pressure.[40] ESPGHAN guidelines recommend slow intravenous rehydration only should ORT fail, replacing the calculated deficit with 5% dextrose/0.45% saline over 8 hours, followed by repeat plasma sodium. If the patient is still hypernatremic, then this may be repeated, followed by maintenance with 5% dextrose/0.18% saline.

PHARMACOLOGIC THERAPY

Antibiotics

Because viral agents are the predominant cause of acute diarrhea (eg, rotavirus, astrovirus, enteric adenovirus, norovirus, and sapovirus), the routine use of antimicrobial agents for the treatment of diarrhea wastes resources and may lead to increased microbial resistance. Especially in the hospital setting, bacterial causes of diarrhea are unusual. A survey of stool cultures submitted over several years to the microbiology laboratory at Children's Hospital in Boston, Massachusetts, revealed such infrequent occurrence of bacterial infections that the practice of sending stool cultures in patients who develop diarrhea while hospitalized has been abandoned.[52] Hospitalized patients and patients with a history of recent antibiotic use are, however, at risk for infections with *Clostridium difficile*. Infections with *C. difficile* documented by toxin assay should be treated with metronidazole 30 mg/kg divided three times daily given orally. Oral vancomycin is also effective but should be reserved as a second-line agent, given its expense and concern over the possible emergence of vancomycin-resistant *Enterococcus*.

Even when a bacterial cause is suspected, antibiotic therapy is generally not indicated because the majority of cases of acute diarrhea are self-limited and not shortened by antibiotics. In addition, antibiotics may cause harm. There is evidence that antibiotic use may increase the risk of hemolytic uremic syndrome from *E. coli* infections.[53] There remains some concern that treatment of *Salmonella enteritis* may increase the risk of the carrier state, although patients under 3 months old or with bacteremia should be treated.[54] Patients with underlying disorders, including immunodeficiency, provide exceptions to these rules. Detailed information regarding the appropriate use of antimicrobial therapy for infectious causes of acute diarrhea is beyond the scope of this chapter and is available in a variety of other resources.[55–58]

Nonantibiotic Drug Therapies

The use of nonspecific antidiarrheal agents such as adsorbents (eg, kaolin-pectin), antimotility agents (eg, loperamide), antisecretory drugs, or toxin binders (eg, cholestyramine) is a common practice. Few data are available to support their efficacy. The side effects of these drugs are well known, in particular among the antimotility agents, including opiate-induced ileus, drowsiness, and nausea owing to atropine effects and binding of nutrients and other drugs. One report from Pakistan detailed 18 cases of severe abdominal distention in association with use of loperamide, including at least 6 deaths.[59] Bismuth subsalicylate has shown some efficacy in traveler's diarrhea and other causes of acute gastroenteritis in children,[60] and although the side effects are less than antimotility agents, some theoretic concerns over the potential toxicity of salicylate remain. In any event, reliance on antidiarrheal agents shifts the therapeutic focus away from appropriate fluid, electrolyte, and nutritional therapy and adds unnecessarily to the economic cost of the illness.

It should be noted that none of the drugs mentioned above specifically address the underlying causes of diarrhea, specifically increased secretion by intestinal crypt cells. Racecadotril, an enkephalinase inhibitor, preserves the antisecretory activity of enkephalins, first discovered in 1975. It does not slow intestinal transit or promote bacterial overgrowth.[61] Its use has shown promise in two controlled clinical trials in children, significantly reducing acute watery diarrhea compared to placebo.[62,63] As long as its cost is reasonable and its use does not distract from ORT and education regarding home management of diarrhea, racecadotril may prove to be a useful adjunct to the treatment of watery diarrhea.

Similarly, the use of antiemetics may be warranted in some cases. Phenothiazines can interfere with oral rehydration by causing sleepiness. There are, however, two recent randomized, double-blind, placebo-controlled pediatric trials that have shown ondansetron, a 5HT3 receptor antagonist, to be effective in decreasing vomiting and limiting hospital admission when administered either by oral[64] or by intravenous[65] route. A third trial showed that a single oral dose of ondansetron, given to pediatric emergency department patients with gastroenteritis and dehydration, significantly decreased the likelihood and frequency of vomiting. There was no significant decrease in the rate of hospitalization, however, the ondansetron group was significantly less likely to require intravenous hydration, had increased oral intake, and had a shorter mean length of stay in the emergency department.[66] The cost is not trivial, and nausea is frequently self-limited, but where admission or even the need for outpatient intravenous therapy is avoided, this intervention may be cost-effective.

Functional Foods

Functional foods may be defined as those that have an effect on physiologic processes separate from their established nutritional function.[67] Probiotics, live microorganisms found in fermented foods and intended to promote intestinal health, are the classic functional food. The modern interest in probiotics may date from Metchnikoff's hypothesis that fermented milk products were responsible for the longevity of Bulgarian peasants.[68] Although a number of recent reviews[69]and journal supplements[70] have more broadly evaluated their use, numerous recent studies have looked specifically at their use in reducing the severity or duration of diarrheal illnesses in children, especially those caused by *Rotavirus*[71] or associated with antibiotic use.[72] Generally, these have included various species of lactobacilli or bifidobacteria, or the nonpathogenic yeast *Saccharomyces boulardii*. The mechanism of action may include competition with pathogenic bacteria, either for receptor sites or for intraluminal nutrients, production of antibiotic substances, and enhancement of host immune defenses.[73,74]

One recently published meta-analysis concludes that *Lactobacillus* spp are both safe and effective as treatment for children with infectious diarrhea, reducing diarrhea duration by 0.7 days and diarrhea frequency by 1.6 stools per day.[75] A recent comprehensive review concluded that there is evidence for the efficacy of a wide variety of probiotics in acute gastroenteritis, especially *Rotavirus*.[76] A positive recommendation also emerges from a recent meta-analysis of probiotic use in antibiotic-associated diarrhea.[77] Probiotics may be effective in terms of prevention as well. A recent meta-analysis of studies predominately executed in developed countries concluded that probiotics reduced the risk of acute diarrhea among children by 57% and that of antibiotic-associated diarrhea by 52%.[78] In this analysis, the protective effect did not vary significantly among the variety of probiotic strains examined.

These reviews included some trials with limited sample size and are susceptible to potential publication bias, as it must be noted that trials with negative results may not have been published. Furthermore, as these products are generally not regulated, there is potential for great variability among products. As such, it may be difficult for the prescribing physician to make an informed recommendation. That being said, the safety and relatively low cost of probiotics may make recommendation of specific products worthwhile, especially where doing so may improve compliance with ORT.

Prebiotics differ from probiotics in that they are nutrients, rather than organisms, used to preferentially stimulate the growth of health-promoting intestinal flora.[79] Presumably, their use could be synergistic with probiotics. The oligosaccharides found in breast milk have been called the prototypic prebiotic in that they foster the growth of lactobacilli and bifidobacteria in the colon of breast-fed neonates.[80] The prebiotic effects of inulin and fructose oligosaccharides have been studied primarily in vitro and in animal model studies.[81] Two randomized, blinded trials on prebiotic-supplemented infant cereal in an urban, economically depressed area did not demonstrate a reduced incidence of diarrheal disease.[82] Specific recommendations regarding the use of prebiotics should await further well-controlled human trials. In the meantime, it should be noted that dietary fiber may serve both as a prebiotic and as a modifying agent of intestinal motility. Current guidelines recommend fiber-containing fruits and vegetables as part of the diet of children recovering from acute gastroenteritis.

Supplemental Zinc Administration

Many reports have linked diarrhea and abnormal zinc status,[83] including increased stool zinc loss,[84] negative zinc balance,[85] and reduced tissue levels of zinc.[86] It has long been observed that diarrhea may occur with severe zinc deficiency, as in acrodermatitis enteropathica, but the broader clinical question is whether more incremental deficiencies of zinc may play a role in childhood diarrhea and whether supplementation may be of benefit, either for improved outcomes in acute or chronic diarrhea or as prophylaxis against diarrheal disease.

A large number of studies have addressed these questions. One early study showed reduced duration of acute diarrhea in patients with low rectal zinc levels.[86] In Bangladesh, zinc supplements also improved markers of intestinal permeability in children with diarrhea.[87] In India, zinc supplementation was associated with a decrease in both the mean number of watery stools per day and the number of days with watery diarrhea.[88] More recently, prophylactic zinc supplementation in India was associated with substantially reduced incidence of severe and prolonged diarrhea, two of the most important determinants of malnutrition and diarrhea-related mortality.[89] In Nepal, this effect was shown to be independent of concomitant vitamin A administration, with very few side effects noted in a substantial number of patients, apart from a slight increase in emesis.[90] In Peru, zinc administration was also associated with a reduction in duration of PD when given during the illness[91] and a decreased incidence of diarrhea, dysentery, and other morbidity when given prophylactically.[92] In the latter study, zinc supplementation alone, compared to zinc supplementation and a multivitamin, had a greater decrease in morbidity. In two different pooled analyses of randomized, controlled trials in developing countries, the Zinc Investigators' Collaborative Group reviewed evidence that zinc supplementation is beneficial for the treatment of acute and Persistent diarrhea[93] and as a prophylactic supplement for decreasing the incidence of diarrheal disease and pneumonia. Among infants and young children who received supplemental zinc for 5 or 7 days per week for 12 to 54 weeks, the pooled odds ratio for diarrhea incidence was 0.82 [95% confidence interval (CI) 0.72 to 0.93] and that for pneumonia incidence was 0.59 (95% CI 0.41 to 0.83).[94]

WHO and UNICEF now recommend that all children with acute diarrhea receive zinc supplementation for a total of 10 to 14 days during and after diarrhea (10 mg/d for infants under 6 months of age and 20 mg/d for children greater than 6 months of age).[39,95] Zinc supplementation in more developed settings may not be as efficacious. A recent randomized, double-blind, placebo-controlled trial of zinc supplementation in breast-fed infants in the United States did not show a significant difference in the frequency of diarrhea between the treatment and control groups.[96] Further research is needed to identify the mechanism of action and to determine optimal schemes for delivery of zinc to the neediest populations.

OTHER CLINICAL SCENARIOS

Acute Bloody Diarrhea (Dysentery)

Dysentery is defined as acute bloody diarrhea caused by invasive microbial infection. This does not include occult blood (detected by guaiac card only), streaks of blood on the surface of formed stool, or melena. The reader is referred to WHO guidelines, which discuss the evaluation and management of dysentery at length.[34,39,97] AAP,[16] CDC,[5] and ESPGHAN guidelines[40] do not specifically address dysentery.

The treatment of dehydration in dysentery follows the same principles as the treatment of acute watery diarrhea. The child with bloody diarrhea is at higher risk for complications, including sepsis and other systemic disease, so that the threshold for admission to the hospital for close observation is lower. Stool cultures are indicated in the setting of acute bloody diarrhea and are helpful for guiding therapy. Food should not be withheld in dysentery any more than in other cases of diarrhea. Because patients with dysentery may have significant anorexia, they should be coaxed to eat.[34] More frequent, smaller meals may be better tolerated. Children convalescing from dysentery should be given extra food to help them regain nutrition lost during the acute illness.

Cholera

Cholera differs from other causes of acute diarrhea in that (1) it may occur in large epidemics involving adults and children; (2) it produces voluminous diarrhea, which may lead to shock and death by dehydration in a very short period; and (3) certain antibiotics may shorten the course.[39] Management of cholera may be carried out using the methods for assessment of dehydration and treatment plans outlined above and summarized in Tables 3, 4, and 5. The health worker must be prepared to deliver prodigious quantities of fluid, either by ORS or intravenously, to overcome ongoing losses. These losses should be quantified so that treatment may be updated and modified under continuous close observation. Unlike diarrhea from other causes, where cereal-based ORSs are equivalent to standard ORSs, there may be some advantages in using rice-based ORS in treating cholera.[98] Traditional wisdom held that sodium concentrations of ORS used in treating cholera should be higher than those for other causes of diarrhea (based on measured stool sodium losses), but a CHOICE study group trial showed no clinical difference between those treated with the lower osmolarity solution compared with a standard solution, apart from some increased incidence of asymptomatic hyponatremia.[99] In Bangladesh, a recently published study of over 50,000 monitored patients with uncomplicated watery diarrhea found no evidence for an increase in symptomatic hyponatremia in those treated with reduced osmolarity ORS. In fact, the incidence rate of developing symptomatic hyponatremia was significantly lower in those treated the newer, reduced osmolarity formulation.[100]

Persistent Diarrhea

Persistent diarrhea may be defined as diarrhea of acute onset that lasts more than 14 days in a child who either fails to gain or loses weight. Globally, PD accounts for a substantial proportion of diarrhea-related morbidity and between 36 and 54% of all diarrhea-related deaths.[101] A recent community-based study suggested that PD is experienced by roughly one in five young children per year in the United States, though with far less morbidity and mortality.[102]

In developing countries, the most important epidemiological risk factor for acquiring PD is malnutrition, further emphasizing the importance of aggressive nutritional therapy in the treatment of acute diarrhea. Other risk factors include immune status (including HIV), zinc deficiency, lack of breast-feeding, male sex, and infection with enteropathogenic or enteroaggregative *E. coli* or *Cryptosporidium*.[103] Malnutrition can also significantly increase mortality from PD, with a study of diarrheal deaths in Bangladesh demonstrating a 17-fold higher relative risk of death from PD in malnourished children compared to those with lesser degrees of malnutrition.[104]

The approach to the patient with PD should include assessing and treating diarrhea, as in the acute presentations. Worldwide, the most important predisposing factor is an acute diarrheal episode triggered by an enteric infection.[103] Particularly in the developing world, bacterial and parasitic infections are common and warrant aggressive diagnosis and therapy. In areas where HIV infection is endemic, chronic gastrointestinal infections with organisms such as *Cryptosporidium parvum* are even more likely.

When infection has been carefully excluded, other specific etiologies must be considered. These include food allergy and dietary protein intolerances, celiac disease, disaccharide (ie, lactose) intolerance, cystic fibrosis and other causes of pancreatic insufficiency, and inflammatory bowel disease. For further details on the diagnosis and nutritional management of these disorders, please refer to Chapters 48 ("Inflammatory Bowel Disease"), 50 ("Celiac Disease"), 51 ("Food Allergies"), 52 ("Exocrine Pancreatic Disease Including Cystic Fibrosis"), and 61 ("Carbohydrate Absorption and Malabsorption").

In the developed world, chronic nonspecific diarrhea of childhood (or "toddler's diarrhea") is a common, nonpathologic phenomenon seen in children between the ages of 6 and 36 months. It is characterized by the passage of two or more loose, voluminous stools per day for over 4 weeks, in the absence of abdominal pain or growth inhibition. Its pathophysiology remains unknown, but it will often respond to dietary alterations.[105] Diets either low in fat (which modulates intestinal motility), low in fiber (which may promote balanced intestinal flora) and/or high in high-osmolarity carbohydrate drinks, particularly sorbitol-containing fruit juice, may all contribute to PD in the developed world. In such cases, dietary modification should be attempted before undertaking an extensive diagnostic evaluation.

Attention to nutrition is critical in the treatment of PD, with restoration of a nutritious diet, including adequate calories, being a key element of therapy. As with acute diarrhea, recommended foods include age-appropriate unrestricted diets, including complex carbohydrates, meats, yogurt, fruits, and vegetables.[5] As previously discussed, zinc supplementation has been shown to be effective in reducing the duration and severity of PD and should be continued for prophylaxis against additional episodes after appropriate therapy is complete.[94] In cases of infectious etiologies, education regarding sanitation and hygiene may reduce rates of reinfection.

For details of PD in the setting of protein-energy malnutrition, please refer to Chapter 13, "Protein-Energy Malnutrition: Pathophysiology, Clinical Consequences, and Treatment."

Table 6 ORS for the Severely Malnourished Child

Simple ORS for the Severely Malnourished Child	More Effective ORS for the Severely Malnourished Child
Dilute 1 L WHO-ORS to make 2 L	Dilute 1 L WHO-ORS to make 2 L
Add 45 mL KCl solution from stock solution containing 100 g KCl/L	Add the following salts:
Add and dissolve 50 g sucrose	3.6 g KCl
	1.3 g K citrate
Children given this solution should also receive:	1.2 g MgCl
2 mL 50% $MgSO_4$ solution (4 mEq Mg/mL) IM once	130 mg Zn acetate
Zinc chloride solution (10 g/L) 1 mL/kg/d until diarrhea stops	22 mg $CuSO_4$
	0.44 mg $NaSeO_4$
	0.20 mg KI
	Add and dissolve 50 g sucrose

Adapted from reference 39.
IM = intramuscularly; ORS = oral rehydration solution.

Diarrhea with Severe Malnutrition

Assessment of the malnourished child is difficult because many of the signs outlined in Table 3 may be unreliable. Skin turgor may appear poor owing to the absence of subcutaneous fat. Eyes may be sunken from loss of periorbital fat. Irritability or apathy from malnutrition may complicate the assessment of mental status. When possible, malnourished children with diarrhea should be referred to a hospital. A severely malnourished child with signs of dehydration without a history of increased stool output should be treated for septic shock.[39] Because of the increased risk of bacteremia in severely malnourished children, and, in fact, in a broad range of children with diarrhea in a less developed setting,[106] the use of empiric antibiotics is not unreasonable where blood cultures cannot be obtained, although the literature regarding choice of antibiotics, doses, and duration is sparse.

Because intravenous therapy may cause overhydration and heart failure in the severely malnourished child, except for treatment of shock, slow oral rehydration is the treatment of choice. An NG tube may be used for children who drink poorly. Rehydration should begin with 10 mL/kg over 2 hours. This rate may be adjusted based on the child's thirst or ongoing stool losses. Increasing edema may be evidence of overhydration.

Full-strength WHO-ORS contains too much sodium and inadequate potassium for the severely malnourished child. WHO guidelines recommend modified solutions such as ReSoMal, as outlined in Tables 1 and 6. Feeding should begin as soon as possible once hydration has been achieved and should continue every 2 to 3 hours day and night. Malnourished children often exhibit anorexia and require coaxing to eat. For greater details, the reader is again referred to Chapter 13. "Protein-Energy Malnutrition: Pathophysiology, clinical consequences, and Treatment".

CHOICE OF ORS

Table 1 outlines the composition of several commonly available ORSs, as well as other beverages frequently used for inappropriate rehydration. The vast discrepancy between the composition of the WHO-ORS and beverages inappropriately recommended for rehydration should be noted. In July 2002, WHO and UNICEF recommended a significant change in ORS composition, including a reduction in sodium and glucose to maintain a 1:1 molar ratio and to decrease total osmolarity to 245 mOsm/L. The change was prompted by clinical trials showing that this solution resulted in less use of supplemental intravenous fluid therapy as well as lower stool output and less vomiting compared with the previous WHO standard ORS.[29,107] Although the differences in measured stool output resulting from different ORS formulations may be modest, reduction in intravenous fluid use is a substantial economic and health benefit of the new solution. The composition of the new solution is also more in line with solutions more commonly used in industrialized countries.

New Solutions

Numerous improved ORSs have been attempted. These have generally included additional substrates for sodium cotransport (such as the amino acids glycine, alanine, and glutamine)[108,109] or, as reviewed by Fontaine and colleagues,[98] substituting complex carbohydrates for the glucose (rice and other cereal-based ORSs) to reduce osmolarity while preserving glucose–sodium cotransport. Given trials to date, the amino acid preparations do not appear to be more effective than traditional ORSs and are more costly. Rice-based ORS may be recommended where training is adequate and home preparation is preferable and appears to be particularly effective in treating diarrhea from cholera.[98,110] Nevertheless, given the simplicity and safety of ORS packets in developing countries and commercially available ORSs in developed countries, these remain the first choice for most clinicians.

A recent publication investigated the addition of recombinant human lactoferrin and lysozyme, two breast milk proteins with antimicrobial activity, to a cereal-based ORS. This novel ORS resulted in a decreased duration of acute diarrhea in Peruvian children compared to a mixed control of standard cereal- and rice-based ORS.[111]

Other potential additives to ORS include substances capable of liberating short-chain fatty acids. These include amylase-resistant starch derived from corn[112] and partially hydrolyzed guar gum.[113] The presumed mechanism of action is the enlistment of increased colonic sodium uptake coupled to short-chain fatty acid transport. Recently, a controlled trial of children with acute diarrhea demonstrated significantly decreased diarrhea duration in those given amylase-resistant starch-fortified ORS compared to those receiving the standard WHO-ORS formulation.[114]

Future possible ORS composition changes include the addition of probiotics, prebiotics, and zinc. Until further data are accumulated regarding all these additional substrates, no definitive recommendations can be made for their use.

Barriers to ORT

Barriers to the use of ORS and continued nutrition during diarrheal disease include, among patients, cultural practices[33] and lack of information[115] and, among physicians, preference for intravenous hydration, even where evidence suggests improved results from oral rehydration.[18,20,116] At the other extreme from the development of the ultimate ORS, it remains distressingly common for patients, even at times under physician supervision, to attempt rehydration with solutions bearing no resemblance to physiologically based ORS. Table 1 includes a number of fluids commonly used in treating diarrhea which do not contain physiologically sound concentrations of carbohydrates and electrolytes. An informal survey of numerous hospital Web sites reveals outdated recommendations for the treatment of diarrhea that include nonstandard fluids. A recent case report of one child whose care was compromised by following advice obtained from a prominent hospital's Internet site highlights the continued gap between knowledge and practice and the ongoing need to disseminate accurate information regarding oral rehydration.[117]

CONCLUSION

The treatment of acute diarrhea has for many years been shown to rely on the simple but overwhelmingly effective therapy of oral rehydration. More recently, the important coprinciple of early refeeding of children immediately upon rehydration has also gained wider acceptance. The combination of oral rehydration and early nutritional support promises to safely and effectively guide a patient through a bout of diarrhea. If the principles of therapy outlined above are accepted by all levels of the medical community, and if education of parents includes beginning ORT at home, then numerous deaths and unnecessary hospitalizations can be avoided. Meanwhile, we await further technological breakthroughs (eg, improved vaccines, superior rehydration solutions) to better combat one of the most important public health problems today.

REFERENCES

1. Kosek M, Bern C, Guerrant RL. The global burden of diarrhoeal disease, as estimated from studies published between 1992 and 2000. Bull World Health Organ 2003;81:197–204.
2. Bern C, Martines J, de Zoysa I, Glass R. The magnitude of the global problem of diarrhoeal disease: A ten year update. Bull World Health Organ 1992;70:705–14.
3. Snyder JD, Merson MH. The magnitude of the global problem of acute diarrhoeal disease: A review of active surveillance data. Bull World Health Organ 1982;60:605–13.
4. Santosham M, Keenan EM, Tulloch J, et al. Oral rehydration therapy for diarrhea: An example of reverse transfer of technology. Pediatrics 1997;100:E10.
5. King CK, Glass R, Bresee JS, Duggan C. Centers for Disease Control and Prevention. Managing acute gastroenteritis among children: Oral rehydration, maintenance, and nutritional therapy. MMWR Morb Mortal Wkly Rep 2003;52:1–16.
6. Malek MA, Curns AT, Holman RC, et al. Diarrhea- and rotavirus-associated hospitalizations among children less than 5 years of age: United States, 1997 and 2000. Pediatrics 2006;117:1887–92.
7. Hoekstra JH. Acute gastroenteritis in industrialized countries: Compliance with guidelines for treatment. J Pediatr Gastroenterol Nutr 2001;33:S31–5.
8. Duggan C, Nurko S. "Feeding the gut": The scientific basis for continued enteral nutrition during acute diarrhea. J Pediatr 1997;131:801–8.
9. Sandhu BK. Rationale for early feeding in childhood gastroenteritis. J Pediatr Gastroenterol Nutr 2001;33:S13–6.
10. O'Shaughnessy W. Experiments on blood in cholera. Lancet 1831;1:490.
11. Latta T. Malignant cholera: Documents communicated by the Central Board of Health London, relative to the treatment of cholera by copious injection of aqueous and saline fluids into the veins. Lancet 1832;2:274.
12. Phillips RA. Twenty years of cholera research. JAMA 1967;202:610–4.
13. Nalin D, Cash R, Islam R, et al. Oral maintenance therapy for cholera in adults. Lancet 1968;ii:370–2.
14. Hirschhorn N, Kinzie J, Sachar D, et al. Decrease in net stool output in cholera during intestinal perfusion with glucose-containing solutions. N Engl J 1968;279:176–81.
15. Hirschhorn N, Greenough WB. Progress in oral rehydration therapy. Sci Am 1991;264:50–6.
16. Centers for Disease Control and Prevention. Managing Acute Gastroenteritis Among Children: Oral rehydration, maintenance, and nutritional therapy. Pediatrics 2004;114:507.
17. Snyder J. Use and misuse of oral therapy for diarrhea: Comparison of US practices with American Academy of Pediatrics recommendations. Pediatrics 1991;87:28–33.
18. Merrick N, Davidson B, Fox S. Treatment of acute gastroenteritis: Too much and too little care. Clin Pediatr (Phila) 1996;35:429–35.
19. Perlstein PH, Lichtenstein P, Cohen MB, et al. Implementing an evidence-based acute gastroenteritis guideline at a children's hospital. Jt Comm J Qual Improv 2002;28:20–30.
20. Ozuah PO, Avner JR, Stein RE. Oral rehydration, emergency physicians, and practice parameters: A national survey. Pediatrics 2002;109:259–61.
21. Acra SA, Ghishan GK. Electrolyte fluxes in the gut and oral rehydration solutions. Pediatr Clin North Am 1996;43:433–49.
22. Pierce N, Banwell J, Mitra R, et al. Effect of intragastric glucose-electrolyte infusion upon water and electrolyte balance in Asiatic cholera. Gastroenterology 1968;55:333–42.
23. Acheson DW. Enterotoxins in acute infective diarrhoea. J Infect 1992;24:225–45.
24. Field M, Rao MC, Chang EB. Intestinal electrolyte transport and diarrheal disease (1). N Engl J Med 1989;321:800–6.
25. Huang H, Schroeder F, Zeng C, et al. Membrane interactions of a novel viral enterotoxin: Rotavirus nonstructural glycoprotein NSP4. Biochemistry 2001;40:4169–80.
26. Morris AP, Scott JK, Ball JM, et al. NSP4 elicits age-dependent diarrhea and Ca(2+)mediated I(−) influx into intestinal crypts of CF mice. Am J Physiol 1999;277:G431–44.
27. Curran P. NaCl and water transport by rat ileum in vitro. J Gen Physiol 1960;43:1137–48.
28. King JC. The risk of maternal nutritional depletion and poor outcomes increases in early or closely spaced pregnancies. J Nutr 2003;133:1732S–6S.
29. Hahn S, Kim Y, Garner P. Reduced osmolarity oral rehydration solution for treating dehydration due to diarrhoea in children: Systematic review. BMJ 2001;323:81–5.
30. World Health Organization. Reduced Osmolarity Oral Rehydration Salts (ORS) Formulation. New York: UNICEF House; 2001.
31. World Health Organization. Oral rehydration salts (ORS): A new reduced osmolarity formulation. Geneva: WHO; 2002.
32. Duggan C, Lasche J, McCarty M, et al. Oral rehydration solution for acute diarrhea prevents subsequent unscheduled follow-up visits. Pediatrics 1999;104:e29.
33. Mull JD, Mull DS. Mothers' concepts of childhood diarrhea in rural Pakistan: What ORT program planners should know. Soc Sci Med 1988;27:53–67.
34. World Health Organization. The Treatment of Diarrhoea: A Manual for Physicians and Other Senior Health Workers. Geneva: WHO; 1995.
35. Gorelick M, Shaw K, Murphy K. Validity and reliability of clinical signs in the diagnosis of dehydration in children. Pediatrics 1997;99:E6. http://www.pediatrics.org/cgi/content/full/99/5/e6.
36. Steiner MJ, DeWalt DA, Byerley JS. Is this child dehydrated? JAMA 2004;291:2746–54.
37. Duggan C, Refat M, Hashem M, et al. How valid are clinical signs of dehydration in infants? J Pediatr Gastroenterol Nutr 1996;22:56–61.
38. MacKenzie A, Barnes G, Shann F. Clinical signs of dehydration in children. Lancet 1989;2:605–7.
39. World Health Organization. Department of Child and Adolescent Health and Development. The Treatment of Diarrhoea: A Manual for Physicians and Other Senior Health Workers, 4th revised edition. Geneva: World Health Organization; 2005.
40. Sandhu BK. Practical guidelines for the management of gastroenteritis in children. J Pediatr Gastroenterol Nutr 2001;32:S36–9.
41. Nager AL, Wang VJ. Comparison of nasogastric and intravenous methods of rehydration in pediatric patients with acute dehydration. Pediatrics 2002;109:566–72.
42. Jackson J, Bolte RG. Risks of intravenous administration of hypotonic fluids for pediatric patients in ED and prehospital settings: Let's remove the handle from the pump. Am J Emerg Med 2000;18:269–70.
43. Brown K, Peerson J, Fontaine O. Use of nonhuman milks in the dietary management of young children with acute diarrhea: A meta-analysis of clinical trials. Pediatrics 1994;93:17–27.
44. Brown K, Perez F, Peerson J, et al. Effect of dietary fiber (soy polysaccharide) on the severity, duration and nutritional outcome of acute, watery diarrhea in children. Pediatrics 1993;92:241–7.

45. Burks AW, Vanderhoof JA, Mehra S, et al. Randomized clinical trial of soy formula with and without added fiber in antibiotic-induced diarrhea. J Pediatr 2001;139:578–82.
46. Isolauri E, Juntunen M, Wiren S, et al. Intestinal permeability changes in acute gastroenteritis: Effects of clinical factors and nutritional management. J Pediatr Gastroenterol Nutr 1989;8:466–73.
47. Rabbani GH, Teka T, Zaman B, et al. Clinical studies in persistent diarrhea: Dietary management with green banana or pectin in Bangladeshi children. Gastroenterology 2001;121:554–60.
48. Checkley W, Gilman R, Black R, et al. Effects of nutritional status on diarrhea in Peruvian children. J Pediatr 2002;140:210–8.
49. Sack DA, Islam S, Brown KH, et al. Oral therapy in children with cholera: A comparison of sucrose and glucose electrolyte solutions. J Pediatr 1980;96:20–5.
50. Salazar-Lindo E, Sack RB, Chea-Woo E, et al. Bicarbonate versus citrate in oral rehydration therapy in infants with watery diarrhea: A controlled clinical trial. J Pediatr 1986;108:55–60.
51. Santosham M, Daum RS, Dillman L, et al. Oral rehydration therapy of infantile diarrhea: A controlled study of well-nourished children hospitalized in the United States and Panama. N Engl J Med 1982;306:1070–6.
52. Zaidi AK, Macone A, Goldmann AD. Impact of simple screening criteria on utilization of low-yield bacterial stool cultures in a Children's Hospital. Pediatrics 1999;103:1189–92.
53. Wong CS, Jelacic S, Habeeb RL, et al. The risk of the hemolytic-uremic syndrome after antibiotic treatment of *Escherichia coli* O157:H7 infections. N Engl J Med 2000;342:1930–6.
54. American Academy of Pediatrics. Salmonella. In: Pickering L, editor. Red Book: Report of the Committee on Infectious Diseases, 25th edition. Elk Grove Village, IL: American Academy of Pediatrics; 2000. p. 501–6.
55. Guerrant RL, Van Gilder T, Steiner TS, et al. Practice guidelines for the management of infectious diarrhea. Clin Infect Dis 2001;32:331–51.
56. Pickering LK, Cleary TG. Therapy for diarrheal illness in children. In: Blaser M, Smith P, Ravdin J, et al, editors. Infections of the Gastrointestinal Tract, 2nd edition. New York: Raven Press; 2002. p. 1223–40.
57. American Academy of Pediatrics. Drugs for parasitic infections. In: Pickering LK, editor. Red Book: 2003 Report of the Committee on Infectious Diseases, 26th edition. Elk Grove, IL: AAP; 2003. p. 744–70.
58. Centers for Disease Control and Prevention. Diagnosis and management of foodborne illnesses: A primer for physicians. MMWR 2001;50:1–69.
59. Bhutta TI, Tahir KI. Loperamide poisoning in children. Lancet 1990;335:363.
60. Gorbach SL. Bismuth therapy in gastrointestinal diseases. Gastroenterology 1990;99:863–75.
61. Schwartz JC. Racecadotril: A new approach to the treatment of diarrhoea. Int J Antimicrob Agents 2000;14:75–9.
62. Salazar-Lindo E, Santisteban-Ponce J, Chea-Woo E, Gutierrez M. Racecadotril in the treatment of acute watery diarrhea in children. N Engl J Med 2000;343:463–7.
63. Cezard JP, Duhamel JF, Meyer M, et al. Efficacy and tolerability of racecadotril in acute diarrhea in children. Gastroenterology 2001;120:799–805.
64. Ramsook C, Sahagun-Carreon I, Kozinetz CA, Moro-Sutherland D. A randomized clinical trial comparing oral ondansetron with placebo in children with vomiting from acute gastroenteritis. Ann Emerg Med 2002;39:397–403.
65. Reeves JJ, Shannon MW, Fleisher GR. Ondansetron decreases vomiting associated with acute gastroenteritis: A randomized, controlled trial. Pediatrics 2002;109:e62.
66. Freedman SB, Adler M, Seshadri R, Powell EC. Oral ondansetron for gastroenteritis in a pediatric emergency department. N Engl J Med 2006;354:1698–705.
67. Duggan C, Gannon J, Walker WA. Protective nutrients and functional foods for the gastrointestinal tract. Am J Clin Nutr 2002;75:789–808.
68. Metchnikoff E. The Prolongation of Life. New York: Putnam and Sons; 1908.
69. Vanderhoof JA, Young RJ. Use of probiotics in childhood gastrointestinal disorders. J Pediatr Gastroenterol Nutr 1998;27:323–32.
70. Wu S, Cai W. Bacterial colonization of the gut and the use of prebiotics and probiotics: Proceedings of a symposium. J Pediatr Gastroenterol Nutr 2000;30:S1–39.
71. Guandalini S, Pensabene L, Zikri MA, et al. Lactobacillus GG administered in oral rehydration solution to children with acute diarrhea: A multicenter European trial. J Pediatr Gastroenterol Nutr 2000;30:54–60.
72. Vanderhoof JA, Whitney DB, Antonson DL, et al. Lactobacillus GG in the prevention of antibiotic-associated diarrhea in children. J Pediatr 1999;135:564–8.
73. Lu L, Walker WA. Pathologic and physiologic interactions of bacteria with the gastrointestinal epithelium. Am J Clin Nutr 2001;73:1124S–30S.
74. Walker WA. Role of nutrients and bacterial colonization in the development of intestinal host defense. J Pediatr Gastroenterol Nutr 2000;30:S2–7.
75. Van Niel CW, Feudtner C, Garrison MM, Christakis DA. Lactobacillus therapy for acute infectious diarrhea in children: A meta-analysis. Pediatrics 2002;109:678–84.
76. Szajewska H, Mrukowicz JZ. Probiotics in the treatment and prevention of acute infectious diarrhea in infants and children: A systematic review of published randomized, double-blind, placebo-controlled trials. J Pediatr Gastroenterol Nutr 2001;33:S17–25.
77. D'Souza AL, Rajkumar C, Cooke J, Bulpitt CJ. Probiotics in prevention of antibiotic associated diarrhoea: Meta-analysis. BMJ 2002;324:1361–6.
78. Sazawal S, Hiremath G, Dhingra U, et al. Efficacy of probiotics in prevention of acute diarrhoea: A meta-analysis of masked, randomised, placebo-controlled trials. Lancet Infect Dis 2006;6:374–82.
79. Roberfroid MB. Prebiotics: Preferential substrates for specific germs? Am J Clin Nutr 2001;73:406S–9S.
80. Dai D, Walker WA. Protective nutrients and bacterial colonization in the immature human gut. Adv Pediatr 1999;46:353–82.
81. Roberfroid MB, Delzenne NM. Dietary fructans. Annu Rev Nutr 1998;18:117–43.
82. Duggan C, Penny ME, Hibberd P, et al. Oligofructose-supplemented infant cereal: 2 randomized, blinded, community-based trials in Peruvian infants. Am J Clin Nutr 2003;77:937–42.
83. Hambidge K. Zinc and diarrhea. Acta Pediatr 1992;2:82–86.
84. Castillo-Duran C, Vial P, Uauy R. Trace mineral balance during acute diarrhea in infants. J Pediatr 1988;113:452–7.
85. Castillo-Duran C, Vial P, Uauy R. Oral copper supplementation: Effect on copper and zinc balance during acute gastroenteritis in infants. Am J Clin Nutr 1990;51:1088–92.
86. Sachdev HP, Mittal NK, Mittal SK, Yadav HS. A controlled trial on utility of oral zinc supplementation in acute dehydrating diarrhea in infants. J Pediatr Gastroenterol Nutr 1988;7:877–81.
87. Roy S, Behrens R, Haider R, et al. Impact of zinc supplementation on intestinal permeability in Bangladeshi children with acute diarrhoea and persistent diarrhoea syndrome. J Pediatr Gastroenterol 1992;15:289–96.
88. Sazawal S, Black RE, Bhan MK, et al. Zinc supplementation in young children with acute diarrhea in India. N Engl J Med 1995;333:839–44.
89. Bhandari N, Bahl R, Taneja S, et al. Substantial reduction in severe diarrheal morbidity by daily zinc supplementation in young North Indian children. Pediatrics 2002;109:e86.
90. Strand TA, Chandyo RK, Bahl R, et al. Effectiveness and efficacy of zinc for the treatment of acute diarrhea in young children. Pediatrics 2002;109:898–903.
91. Penny ME, Peerson JM, Marin RM, et al. Randomized, community-based trial of the effect of zinc supplementation, with and without other micronutrients, on the duration of persistent childhood diarrhea in Lima, Peru. J Pediatr 1999;135:208–17.
92. Penny ME, Marin RM, Duran A, et al. Randomized controlled trial of the effect of daily supplementation with zinc or multiple micronutrients on the morbidity, growth, and micronutrient status of young Peruvian children. Am J Clin Nutr 2004;79:457–65.
93. Zinc Investigators Collaborative Group. Therapeutic effects of oral zinc in acute and persistent diarrhea in children in developing countries: Pooled analysis of randomized controlled trials. Am J Clin Nutr 2000;72:1516–22.
94. Zinc Investigators' Collaborative Group, Bhutta ZA, Black RE, et al. Prevention of diarrhea and pneumonia by zinc supplementation in children in developing countries: Pooled analysis of randomized controlled trials. J Pediatr 1999;135:689–97.
95. WHO/UNICEF. WHO/UNICEF joint statement: Clinical management of acute diarrhoea. New York, NY, and Geneva, Switzerland: World Health Organization/The United Nations Childrens Fund; 2005. p. 1–8.
96. Heinig MJ, Brown KH, Lonnerdal B, Dewey KG. Zinc supplementation does not affect growth, morbidity, or motor development of US term breastfed infants at 4–10 mo of age. Am J Clin Nutr 2006;84:594–601.
97. World Health Organization. The management of bloody diarrhoea in young chldren. Geneva: WHO; 1994.
98. Fontaine O, Gore SM, Pierce NF. Rice-based oral rehydration solution for treating diarrhoea. Cochrane Database Syst Rev 2000:CD001264.
99. Alam NH, Majumder RN, Fuchs GJ, CHOICE Study group. Efficacy and safety of oral rehydration solution with reduced osmolarity in adults with cholera: A randomised double-blind clinical trial. Lancet 1999;354:296–9.
100. Alam NH, Yunus M, Faruque ASG, et al. Symptomatic hyponatremia during treatment of dehydrating diarrheal disease with reduced osmolarity oral rehydration solution. JAMA 2006;296:567–73.
101. Anonymous. Evaluation of an algorithm for the treatment of persistent diarrhoea: A multicentre study. International Working Group on Persistent Diarrhoea. Bull World Health Organ 1996;74:479–89.
102. Vernacchio L, Vezina RM, Mitchell AA, et al. Characteristics of persistent diarrhea in a community-based cohort of young US children. J Pediatr Gastroenterol Nutr 2006;43:52–8.
103. Bhutta ZA, Ghishan F, Lindley K, et al. Persistent and chronic diarrhea and malabsorption: Working Group report of the second World Congress of Pediatric Gastroenterology, Hepatology, and Nutrition. J Pediatr Gastroenterol Nutr 2004;39:S711–6.
104. Fauveau V, Henry FJ, Briend A. Persistent diarrhea as a cause of childhood mortality in rural Bangladesh. Acta Paediatr Suppl 1992;381:12–4.
105. Kneepkens CM, Hoekstra JH. Chronic nonspecific diarrhea of childhood: Pathophysiology and management. Pediatr Clin North Am 1996;43:375–90.
106. Mitra AK, Albert MJ, Alam AN. Bacteraemia and meningitis among hospital patients with diarrhoea. Trans R Soc Trop Med Hyg 1993;87:560–3.
107. CHOICE Study Group. Multicenter, randomized, double-blind clinical trial to evaluate the efficacy and safety of a reduced osmolarity oral rehydration salts solution in children with acute watery diarrhea. Pediatrics 2001;107:613–8.
108. Silva AC, Santos-Neto MS, Soares AM, et al. Efficacy of a glutamine-based oral rehydration solution on the electrolyte and water absorption in a rabbit model of secretory diarrhea induced by cholera toxin. J Pediatr Gastroenterol Nutr 1998;26:513–9.
109. Duggan C. Glutamine-based oral rehydration solutions: The magic bullet revisited? J Pediatr Gastroenterol Nutr 1998;26:533–5.
110. Bhan MK, Mahalanabis D, Fontaine O, Pierce NF. Clinical trials of improved oral rehydration salt formulations: A review. Bull World Health Organ 1994;72:945–55.
111. Zavaleta N, Figueroa D, Rivera J, et al. Efficacy of a rice-based ORS containing recombinant human lactoferrin and lysozyme in Peruvian children with acute diarrhea. J Pediatr Gastroenterol Nutr 2007;44:258–64.
112. Ramakrishna BS, Venkataraman S, Srinivasan P, et al. Amylase-resistant starch plus oral rehydration solution for cholera. N Engl J Med 2000;342:308–13.
113. Alam NH, Meier R, Schneider H, et al. Partially hydrolyzed guar gum-supplemented oral rehydration solution in the treatment of acute diarrhea in children. J Pediatr Gastroenterol Nutr 2000;31:503–7.
114. Raghupathy P, Ramakrishna BS, Oommen SP, et al. Amylase-resistant starch as adjunct to oral rehydration therapy in children with diarrhea. J Pediatr Gastroenterol Nutr 2006;42:362–8.
115. Anidi I, Bazargan M, James FW. Knowledge and management of diarrhea among underserved minority parents/caregivers. Ambul Pediatr 2002;2:201–6.
116. Szajewska H, Hoekstra JH, Sandhu B. Management of acute gastroenteritis in Europe and the impact of the new recommendations: A multicenter study. The Working Group on acute Diarrhoea of the European Society for Paediatric Gastroenterology, Hepatology, and Nutrition. J Pediatr Gastroenterol Nutr 2000;30:522–7.
117. Crocco AG, Villasis-Keever M, Jadad AR. Two wrongs don't make a right: Harm aggravated by inaccurate information on the Internet. Pediatrics 2002;109:522–3.

58

Intestinal Failure, Short Bowel Syndrome, and Intestinal Transplantation

Daniel Kamin, MD
Olivier Goulet, MD, PhD

Care for infants and children with intestinal failure (IF) challenges nutritional medicine fundamentally: it attempts to provide nutrition that supports normal growth and development, even though the very organ fulfilling this role has failed. Before the advent of intravenous (IV) nutrition, patients with IF often succumbed to malnutrition and dehydration. Many patients are now able to grow and develop normally on long-term parenteral nutrition (PN) for many patients, and methods exist to transition patients from parenteral to enteral nutrition (EN). For those suffering severe complications, novel medical and surgical therapies increase hope for successful transition to enteral feeding. Outcomes after intestinal transplantation have improved substantially since its inception, so that motivation for choosing this therapy is no longer a "last ditch" effort to rescue very ill children. With these points in mind, we will review the etiology, complications, and medical management of pediatric IF including intestinal transplantation, the nutritional physiologic principles motivating this management, and highlight nutritional outcomes of various management strategies.

DEFINITIONS AND DISEASES

Definitions

The term "intestinal failure" is now often used to describe a state wherein gastrointestinal function is insufficient to support normal growth in children and physiologic balance in both adults and children. "Gastrointestinal function" refers to the ability to absorb enteral nutrients and fluid. While this definition is broadest, its consistent application relies on uniformity in defining "normal growth" or "physiologic balance." Some have suggested that IF be defined by the extent of energy loss in stool rather than the inability to provide enteral energy. Another practical approach is to define IF according to the amount of PN required to maintain normal growth in children and physiologic balance in adults. For patients with short bowel syndrome (SBS), length or percentage of small bowel remaining might also figure into a definition.

Laboratory assessment has promise for helping to define IF. For instance, serum citrulline level has recently been proposed as a marker for functional small intestinal mass. It is a nonstructural amino acid net-produced only in presumably functionally capable enterocytes.[1] Clinical studies in enteropathy[2] and SBS[3,4] support its use as a valid marker of functional enterocyte mass and absorptive function. Rhoads and colleagues[5] studied 24 children of age 3 weeks to 4 years with SBS and found that a serum citrulline level of >19 µmol/L had a 94% sensitivity and 67% specificity for predicting weaning off PN over a 24 month period. Citrulline has not enjoyed uniform success[6] as a proxy for intestinal adaptation or function.

A recent consensus report settled on the following: "IF results from obstruction, dysmotility, surgical resection, congenital defect, or disease-associated loss of absorption and is characterized by the inability to maintain protein-energy, fluid, electrolyte, and micronutrient balance (without IV support)." For children, an additional criterion would be the inability to preserve normal growth.[7]

Underlying Diseases

Most cases of IF (Table 1) are caused by surgical resection of the small intestine. The most common conditions are necrotizing enterocolitis, gastroschisis, and congenital intestinal atresias. Resections may be classified according to the amount of residual small intestine, as measured distal to the ligament of Treitz along the antimesenteric border. Multiple studies have linked prognosis of IF patients with residual small bowel length.

Congenital diarrheal diseases lead to IF because of the severe relentless electrolyte and nutrient losses, which prevent successful EN. These diseases result from defects in enterocyte structure and/or function, and often there is villus atrophy. Microvillus inclusion disease (MVID) is characterized by microvillus "inclusions" in enteroytes and colonocytes when viewed with an electron microscope. Severe watery diarrhea usually begins in the newborn period, and IV support may be required from the outset. The disease is clearly inherited, as multiple siblings may be affected and ethnic clustering exists among individuals of Navajo decent. The prognosis is generally unfavorable without transplantation, but individual case reports describe patients with more moderate symptoms and improvement over time.[9]

Tufting enteropathy (or intestinal epithelial dysplasia) presents in infancy with watery diarrhea and impaired growth. Many patients have unusual facial features. Focal epithelial "tufts" of closely packed enterocytes with rounded apical plasma membranes constitute the distinguishing features of this condition. As with MVID, the cause is unknown, but ethnic clustering and families with multiple affected individuals support a genetic cause. Prognosis is felt to be less dire than MVID[10]; a case report describes an adult woman off PN for many years who was able to give birth to a healthy infant.[11]

Table 1 Causes of Intestinal Failure in Children

Category	Disorder	
Short bowel syndrome	Infant Gastroschisis Necrotizing enterocolitis Small intestinal atresia Malrotation with volvulus	Older child Crohn's disease Mesenteric infarction Radiation enteritis Tumors Trauma
Motility	Hirschsprung's disease Pseudo-obstruction Neuronal intestinal dysplasia	
Mucosa	Primary epithelial Microvillus inclusion disease Tufting enteropathy	Immune-mediated Autoimmune enteropathy Immunodeficiency syndromes
Miscellaneous	Enteroendocrine cell hypoplasia	

Reproduced with permission from Kamin D and Duggan C.[8]

Severe motility disorders include long-segment Hirschprung disease and chronic idiopathic intestinal pseudo-obstruction (CIPO). Long-segment Hirschprung disease refers to the characteristic aganglionosis usually isolated to the colon extending for various lengths into the small bowel. This condition causes functional SBS because the involved "paralysed" intestine will not support aboral flow of intestinal contents. Additionally, the colon will always be affected and cannot be used for electrolyte and water recovery. Significant difficulty weaning PN may be expected with residual functional small bowel lengths less than 50 cm.[12]

CIPO is a heterogeneous mix of conditions sharing a common clinical presentation of apparent intestinal obstruction without surgical findings. CIPO is often further classified according to histologic and manometric criteria.[13] Myopathic CIPO refers to the primary defect localized in the smooth muscle; often these patients have dysfunction of other smooth muscle, most commonly in the genitourinary tract (eg, megacystis-microcolon-intestinal hypoperistalsis syndrome). This form of CIPO is generally thought to be more severe, resulting in more debilitating symptoms because dysmotility is more extensive or more complete. Neuropathic CIPO indicates that the enteric nervous system is disordered, resulting in motor responses that poorly propel intestinal contents forward. In both conditions, presentation is usually in the first 5 years of life, patients often undergo multiple laparotomies before diagnosis, and attempts are made to establish intestinal function by avoiding diseased intestine, which usually results in gastrostomies, jejunostomies, and diverting ileostomies. Nevertheless, the most severely affected individuals will still not be able to tolerate sufficient EN to support growth, and long-term PN is required.

Epidemiology

IF is a relatively rare condition. Unlike rare cancers, bona fide prospective registries do not yet exist in North America to track patient number and outcomes. A standard proxy is the use of home PN. Using Medicare and Oley Foundation information, Howard and colleagues estimated that 40,000 people were using home PN in 1992.[14] Extrapolation based on the 1994 Oley Foundation report demonstrates that roughly 40% of patients used home PN because of a primary gastrointestinal cause of IF. Children of 14 years and younger accounted for approximately 25% of this group. Based on the 40,000 estimate noted above, approximately 4,000 US children of 14 years and younger were on home PN because of primary gastrointestinal IF in 1992.[14] A more recent multicenter European study estimated the prevalence of pediatric home PN use at 2 to 6.8 children/million population.[15] Finally, a 2005 Italian survey that recorded all patients receiving artificial home nutrition reported 1.2 children/million inhabitants as using home PN.[16]

It is difficult to estimate the prevalence of individual causes of IF. Very limited published data exits for pediatrics. Certainly SBS constitutes the majority diagnosis, and all are relatively rare. Table 2 displays the causes and proportions of neonatal SBS from larger published series.

Table 2 Distribution of Causes of Neonatal SBS

Study	Andorsky et al, 2001[17] (% of total)	Goulet et al, 2005[109] (% of total)	Wales et al, 2005[18] (% of total)
Total	30	87	40
Necrotizing enterocolitis	13 (43)	13 (15)	NA (35)
Intestinal atresia	9 (30)	34 (39)	NA (10)
Gastroschisis	5 (17)	13 (15)	NA (12)
Malrotation/volvulus	3 (10)	21 (24)	NA (10)
Other*	NA	6 (7)	(32)

Adapted with permission from Goulet O and Sauvat F.[19]
NA = not available; SBS = short bowel syndrome.
*Includes diagnoses such as long segment Hirshsprung's disease, complicated meconium ileus, spontaneous perforations.

PHYSIOLOGY AND PATHOPHYSIOLOGY

Normal Intestinal Growth

In utero intestinal growth is most marked during the last trimester, nearly doubling over this period of time.[20] This has obvious implications for prognosis, as acquisition of IF in early infancy or after premature birth (eg, necrotizing enterocolitis) may lead to improved outcomes because of the growth potential of residual small intestine. An average small intestinal length for full-term infants measured from the ligament of Treitz to ileocecal valve (ICV) was 250 to 300 cm,[20,21] with maximal increase in length occuring in the first year of life.[21] Normal adult small intestinal lengths range from 275 to 850 cm,[22] a generous span owing to the variable contexts (eg, radiologic, intra-operative, postmortem) and/or methods used. Bowel length directly correlates with body length/height (Figure 1).[21,23] Note that in Figure 1, the curve levels off at approximately 100 cm, the average height of a 3- to 4-year-old child.

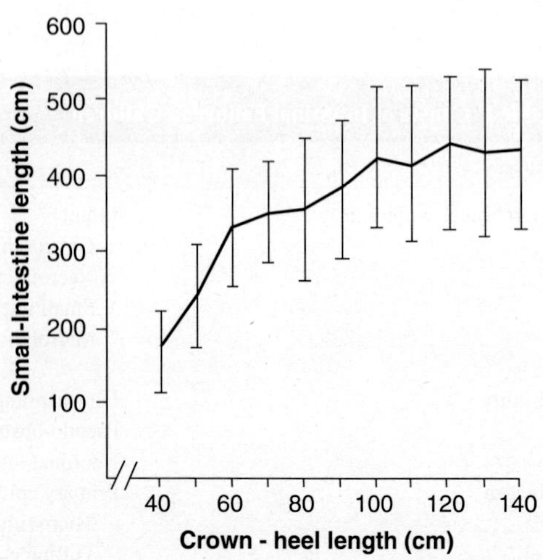

Figure 1 Small-intestine length versus crown-heel length, showing means and standard deviations. (Reproduced with permission from Siebert JR.[21])

Adaptation

Intestinal adaptation refers to the gross anatomic, histologic, and functional changes that occur in the intestine, maximizing digestive and absorptive capacity in the context of loss of intestinal function from either resection or disease. The phenomenon has been recognized for over a century.[24] Experimental work in dogs and clinical experience led Flint[25] to conclude in 1912 that as much as 50% of the small intestine might be removed without culminating in inexorable weight loss and death, and that neither colon nor stomach could compensate for the loss. Today, while this estimate can be pushed further, the principles and observations derived from experiments years ago are still apt.[22]

Adaptive changes in humans may begin 12 to 24 hours after massive intestinal resection and will continue for a year or longer after resection.[26] It is generally thought that maximal adaptation occurs after 1 to 3 years in children[27] and 1 to 4 years in adults.[28] However, these data are based on retrospective review of patients on long-term PN with variable diagnoses, treatment strategies, and time periods. Medical, surgical, and nutritional innovations may extend these ranges.

Structural Adaptation

Animal data. Rodent data indicate that structural adaptation can be marked. Gross morphologic changes occur after extensive small intestinal resections (>70%) such as thickening, increase in length, and dilation.[29] Adult female Sprague-Dawley rats were examined 1 week after 80% small bowel resections (distal ileum and colon intact). The wet weight of the small intestine increased fivefold, up to 70% of the preresection weight. However, there were no further increases in intestinal mass when assessed 5 and 10 weeks postresection, and there was no recovery of the pre-resection intestinal length (Figure 2). In the juvenile domestic pig 16 weeks after surgery, bowel diameter and length increased proportionally more in those that received 75% mid-small intestinal resections as compared to animals who received transactions.[30] Discrepancies between studies showing recovery of intestinal length may depend on species and timing. It is not clear whether intestinal length can be recovered only within species-specific "window periods."

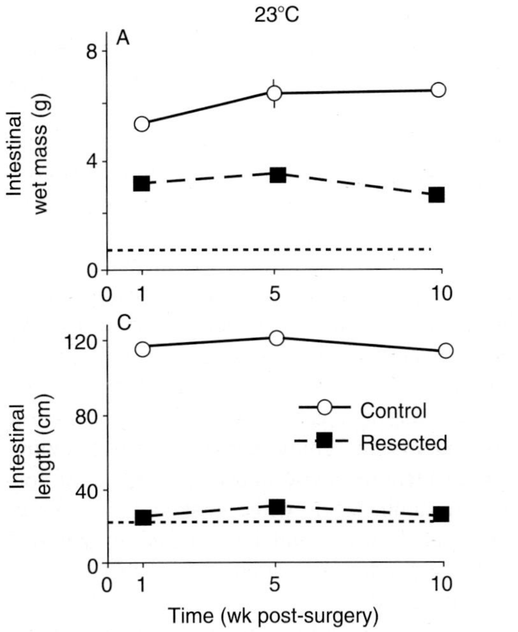

Figure 2 Effect of resection on wet mass (upper graph) and intestinal length (lower graph) in female Sprague-Dawley rats. Dotted line represents estimated wet mass or length immediately after resection. Eighty percent small intestinal resections were performed (dark square) while control animals (open circles) had sham operations. (Reproduced with permission from O'Connor TP et al.[31])

Adapted rodent intestinal mucosa is characterized by elongated crypts and wider, taller villi.[32] There is increased cellularity, which is manifested by increased DNA and protein content in adapted intestine.[33] These processes are more marked when resection is more extensive,[34] and when the residual intestine is ileum.[35,36] Moreover, enterocyte turnover is altered in adapted rat mucosa. As compared to ileal mucosa from mice that received sham operations (intestinal transections), mucosa from rodents receiving 50% proximal small intestinal resections displayed heightened cellular proliferation and apoptosis at 24 hours and 7 days postresection.[37] More specifically, hyperplasia characterized the adaptive response in C57BL/6J mouse jejunum after resection, while ileum displayed enterocyte hypertrophy.[38]

The rodent has obvious significant limitations as a model for human disease. Mucosal responses to adaptation likely differ between species. For instance, resection often causes crypt-villus elongation in rodents, while similar structural changes have not been routinely noted in humans.[39] The neonatal piglet model has recently been offered as an alternative,[40,41] and has been used to show efficacy of surgical[42] and medical[43] therapies for IF.

Human data. There is adequate documentation that human intestine can adapt by improving nutrient absorption following injury or resection.[25,44,45] The macroscopic changes of intestinal hypertrophy and lengthening have been observed in many case series,[39] but the crypt-villus architectural modifications observed in rodents have not been recapitulated.[44,46] For example, duodenal mucosa from an adult patient with significant SBS demonstrated hyperplasia of crypts and villi as compared to specimens from normal adult humans, but cell proliferation, crypt depth, and villus height were equivalent.[47] However, a small case series of patients who received segmental small intestinal transplants found that villus length did increase by 50% over baseline at 6 months, suggesting that intestinal adaptation in the human may include morphologic changes in the villus that maximize surface area.[48]

Functional Adaptation

Animal data. Functional adaptation is characterized by an increase in the absorption of carbohydrate, protein, water, or electrolytes per unit length of intestine. Within 6 hours of intestinal resection, upregulation of the sodium-glucose cotransporter occurs in enterocytes, leading to enhanced electrolyte and water absorption.[49] Physiologic mechanisms underlying these changes may be upregulation of total available transporters, a larger number of functional enterocytes, or upregulation of efficiency of individual nutrient transporters.[50] Work using a rabbit model of SBS, which examined nutrient transport across jejunal sections isolated from animals with and without significant distal small bowel resections indicates that changes in the lipid content of the brush border membrane may account for enhanced passive absorption of free fatty acids in small intestine.[51–53] Dowling and Booth[35] in their classic paper on rat SBS found that per unit length of remaining intestine that glucose absorption was increased 2 weeks later, and that this affect was more pronounced in ileum than jejunum.

It is worth noting that structural changes do not entirely correlate with functional adaptations. For instance, total mucosal glucose absorption reached 33% of the preresection value after 80% small bowel resection in the Sprague-Dawley rat, while mucosal weight increased to an average two-thirds that of the preresection weight.[54]

Delayed transit through the GI tract, affording luminal nutrients more contact time with the intestinal absorptive surface, may be considered an adaptive mechanism after small intestinal resection. Few studies have documented this well[55]; others have found transit time normal or shortened.[56,57] Moreover, the lack of correlation between small intestinal transit time and residual bowel length complicates generation of simple theories.[56] Transit time may even be delayed because of bowel dilation and stasis, both concerns that could contribute to maladaptive physiology.

Human data. Segmental intestinal transplant from living human donors provides some insight on the adaptive process. When 200 cm of ileum was transplanted into an HLA-matched sibling who suffered traumatic loss of his entire jejunum, ileum, and right colon, *d*-xylose and fat balance studies were markedly abnormal 1 month after transplant, but were considered normal at 6 months.[58] Ziegler and colleagues[59] compared small intestinal biopsies from 13 adult SBS patients on long-term PN to those obtained from 33 adult control subjects undergoing endoscopy without histories of intestinal resection, inflammation, or infection. All 13 SBS patients were also consuming oral nutrition. Small intestinal villus height, width, and crypt depth were no different between the groups, suggesting that intestinal adaptation in humans does not depend on sheer size of the crypt-villus structure. Interestingly, Ziegler did identify upregulated expression of the peptide transporter PepT1 in colonic mucosa of SBS patients, a finding that could indicate that colon may salvage not just carbohydrates (see below) in patients with small intestinal malabsorption.

Mineral absorption may adapt over an extended period of time. Gouttebel and colleagues investigated calcium absorption in 30 adults with SBS, comparing those whose resections were <2 years ago to those >2 years. While *d*-xylose absorption was equivalent, calcium absorption continued to increase in the later group, suggesting that adaptation may be a prolonged, slowly evolving process.[60]

Little information exists that characterizes intestinal adaptation with respect to motility in the human. Moreover, much of the phenotype of intestinal adaptation in humans has not been fully described (eg, bowel flora and immunologic function), and molecular mechanism is just beginning to be understood.

Molecular Adaptation. Adaptation can be characterized on the molecular level.[61–63] For instance, cDNA isolated from residual ileum 48 hours after 70% resection in rats suggested significant upregulation (as compared to sham-operated rats) of genes encoding proteins responsible for nutrient trafficking, cell cycle control, and protein processing.[63] Further, Stern and colleagues[62] used exogenous epidermal growth factor (EGF) in a similar experiment and detected upregulation of a gene product (proline-rich protein 2) not previously thought to play a role in intestinal adaptation. Current and future studies using microarray analysis and other sophisticated molecular techniques will soon offer a much more complete picture of adaptation, and possibility lead to more rational identification of therapies to promote adaptation.

Determinants of Adaptation

By far the most powerful and consistent determinant of adaptation is provision of EN. Directly and/or indirectly, nutrient flow through the intestinal tract promotes structural and functional integrity of the intestine; the amount of EN that is tolerated is a robust predictor of successful adaptation and thus freedom from parenteral therapies.

Earlier Observations. There has been great interest in isolating the component(s) linking provision of EN with enhanced intestinal function. Observations included the effects of direct nutrient contact with the mucosa, pancreatic and hepatobiliary secretions, and circulating hormones. Ileum that is transposed into a proximal position in jejunum will develop larger villi and crypts,[64] suggesting that direct mucosal contact with richer chyme is important for maintaining mucosal structure. When the ampulla of Vater is surgically transposed to distal small intestine, mucosal hyperplasia will occur distally, highlighting the possible importance of hepatobiliary and pancreatic secretions in adaptation.[65] Finally, animal studies support the notion that humoral factors are released secondary to enteral feeding that maintain structure and function of the intestinal mucosa. Feeding an animal with a Thiry-Vella fistula, in which a portion of small intestine is removed completely from the luminal circuit while maintaining physiologic blood supply, will produce mucosal hyperplasia in the fistula when nutrients are administered enterally but not parenterally.[66] Parabiotic animal studies are also revealing. Here, two animals have blood supplies that are surgically cross-circulated, while only one animal has an intestinal resection. Both animals will then develop mucosal hyperplasia of small intestine when the resected animal is fed enterally.[67]

Nutritive Factors

Lipids. The amount, nature, and route of administration of lipids may influence the adaptive process. Studies in rats imply that both saturated and polyunsaturated fatty acids have trophic effects on small intestine.[68,69] Maxton[69] gave female Wistar rats 4 weeks of Vivonex or Vivonex with 50% of calories replaced with either saturated or essential fatty acid-substituted triglycerides, and found that, as compared to the Vivonex, small bowel mucosal weight, protein, and DNA content were each equally higher in the supplemented groups. Alternatively, using a rat model, Vanderhoof and colleagues[70] found that menhaden oil [a marine source of omega-3 polyunsaturated fatty acids (PUFAs)], as compared to safflower oil, stimulated greater small bowel mucosal regeneration during recovery from mucositis induced with subcutaneous methotrexate.

Admittedly, nonresection models may have limited applicability for understanding adaptation after intestinal resection. Manipulation of dietary fat has been explored in rodents with experimental SBS.[71–73] Kollman[73] investigated the effect of various combinations of docosahexaenoic acid (DHA) and arachidonic (AA) acid (major constituents of marine oil) in the diets of small-bowl resected Sprague-Dawley rats. Rats received 80% small bowel resections, leaving distal ileum and ICV intact. Rats were fed varying amounts of DHA and AA (from 5% AA and 3.3% DHA to 45% AA and 30% DHA) while energy from fat was kept constant at 30%. At 14 days, the ileal mucosa removed from rats receiving the highest amount of DHA and AA was significantly heavier (87.38 vs 71.55 expressed as mg/cm) than mucosa removed from animals that received normal diet (10% soy oil and 90% hydrogenated coconut oil). However, sucrase activity did not differ between the groups, nor did the mucosal characteristics from the duodenum.

Changes in nutrient transport have also been explored. A rat model of SBS suggests that a high fat diet, as compared to isocaloric regular chow, enhances fatty acid transport in the remaining small intestine. Three days after 75% small intestinal resection, male Sprague-Dawley rats given a diet with saturated-fat enhanced chow had enhanced fat clearance (based on fat balance studies) than rats that had received usual chow.[74] Earlier, Keelan and colleagues[51] resected the distal half of the small intestine in adult female Sprague-Dawley rats, leaving the ICV intact. Animals were fed regular chow for 3 weeks, and then 2 additional weeks with isocaloric saturated fatty acid (SFA)- or PUFA-enriched chow. Glucose transport was twice as high across mucosa isolated from animals fed the SFA diet as compared to that measured in tissue derived from animals fed the PUFA-enriched diet. The heterogeneity of positive findings, differing models (eg, resection vs chemical injury), and various protocols (eg, age, sex, amount, and type of resection) limit the ability to draw firm conclusions. It is clear that the amount and type of enteral fat [most convincingly saturated long-chain triglycerides (LCTs) or fatty acids] can modify the nature and extent of adaptation.

Carbohydrates. Dietary carbohydrate absorption may be enhanced by altering the amount of administered carbohydrate (the functional "workload" hypothesis). This has been demonstrated carefully in nonresection rat models.[75–77] Diamond and colleagues[76] isolated intestinal sleeves from mice and demonstrated in vitro that dietary carbohydrate significantly increased the V_{max} across the mucosa, suggesting carbohydrate induction of monosaccharide carriers in the intestine. Later, Shu and colleagues[75] found that increasing dietary fructose or sucrose induced in parallel higher expression of GLUT5 mRNA, sucrase activity, and brush border fructose transport. Moreover, enterocytes may acquire transport characteristics only while they are still in the crypt. Using a time-sequenced freeze fraction and transporter staining technique, Ferraris and colleagues[78] found that glucose-dependent regulation of Na^+/D-glucose cotransport (assessed by functional staining technique which quantifies glucose transporter density) was possible only when cells were still in the crypts. Disaccharides may be more trophic on intestinal mucosa than equivalent amounts of monosaccharides, an affect abolished when disaccharide hydrolysis was inhibited.[79]

Other dietary constituents may influence transport of carbohydrates. Using a rat model of ethanol mucosal injury, Thomson and colleagues[80] found that SFA-enriched diet "protected" the in vitro jejunal and ileal transport of glucose, while mucosa derived from rats fed PUFA-enriched diet demonstrated decrements in glucose transport when exposed to ethanol. Alternatively, fish oil seemed to have an opposite influence on Na^+ dependent glucose transport in proximal small intestine membrane vesicles isolated from rats maintained for 4 weeks on Menhaden oil- (unsaturated fat) or butter fat (SFA)-enriched diets.[81] Compared to the SFA diet, V_{max} for glucose was significantly higher in vesicles derived from rats fed the fish oil-enriched diet. Taken together, these data do not clearly support a specific nutrient formulation to enhance carbohydrate absorption; enteral administration of nutrients in general, including a disaccharide or polysaccharide carbohydrate source, positively influences intestinal absorption of carbohydrates.

Protein. Similar to "reflexive" influence of macronutrients on their own absorption, dietary protein influences intestinal amino acid transport. Isocalorically fed mice on high nitrogen diets will increase uptake by 77 to 81% for nonessential amino acids, while increasing uptake only by 32 to 61% for more toxic but essential amino acids.[82] Conversely, nitrogen-deficient diets lead to decrease uptake of nonessential amino acids, while uptake for the essential amino acids was maintained, a finding that suggests independent regulation of individual or groups of amino acids.[83]

The amino acid glutamine has received significant attention as a nutrient that enhances intestinal adaptation.[84] Ziegler and colleagues[85] gave rats receiving 80% intestinal resections either low or glutamine-supplemented diets. Using intestinal DNA content as proxy for intestinal adaptation, Ziegler suggested that feeds supplemented with glutamine for 7 days enhanced intestinal adaptation as compared to rats that received deficient diets. This is not a uniform finding,[86] which is corroborated by the mixed results seen in clinical trials of glutamine supplementation.[87,88] Some amino acids may in fact have detrimental effect on the adaptive response. Parenteral arginine administration led to lower proliferative and higher apoptotic indices in 75% resected rats after 15 days following resection.[89]

Miscellaneous. Pectin and other soluble fibers may facilitate intestinal adaptation. Animal studies document improved caloric and fluid absorption when diets are supplemented with soluble fiber.[90] A rodent SBS study found that the weight, DNA, and protein content of ileum and colonic sections were significantly higher in rats fed diets supplemented with 2% pectin as compared to animals with similar small bowel resections consuming an unsupplemented, isocaloric diet.[91] Proposed mechanisms of action include increased lumen/nutrient contact time, "carbohydrate salvage" via colonic assimilation of short-chain fatty acids (SCFAs) derived by fermentation of the soluble fiber, and direct effects of SCFAs on tissue trophism and nutrient absorption.

"Salvage" occurs when anaerobic bacteria in the colon ferment un- or malabsorbed carbohydrate, producing SCFAs. Study of human subjects with SBS have shown that carbohydrate fermentation does occur.[92] SCFAs are used by the colon as a fuel source,[93] thus increasing the amount of calories assimilated from EN.

SCFAs may also directly enhance intestinal tissue growth and function. SCFAs given intravenously prevented TPN-induced small intestinal mucosal atrophy in rats.[94] Rodent work also suggests that SCFA supplementation augments intestinal assimilation of nutrients and electrolytes. Tappenden and colleagues[95] gave male Sprague-Dawley rats who underwent an 80% jejunoileal resection either isocaloric SCFA-supplemented or unsupplemented PN. Three or seven days later, residual small intestinal mucosal/submucosal weight and DNA content were significantly greater in the supplemented group as compared to the unsupplemented rats. Later, using a similar model, this group found that ileal uptake of D-glucose was substantially higher in the SCFA-supplemented animals, while expression of membrane glucose (GLUT2) and ion transporter (sodium-dependent glucose transporter 1) mRNA were also higher in ileal tissue from rats receiving SCFA-supplemented TPN.[96]

Intestinal trophic factor secretion could be augmented by SCFA supplementation. Tappenden and colleagues[95] found that ileal pro-glucagon mRNA was higher among SBS rats that received SCFA-supplemented versus unsupplemented TPN. More recently, a randomized SBS rodent trial found that, compared to rodents fed fiber-free elemental diets, rats given the same diet supplemented with 2.5% pectin had significantly increased lower intestinal weight and length (ileum, cecum, colon), and serum samples from supplemented rats had significantly increased glucagon-like peptide 2 (GLP-2) concentrations.[97] Taken together, these data suggest that SCFAs enhance bowel adaptation via multiple mechanisms, and further work may help direct how these molecules can be harnessed most usefully in the clinical setting.

Polyamines are dietary constituents that play and important role in cellular growth and differentiation.[98] Polyamines are polycationic compounds present in all prokaryotic and eukaryotic cells, and must be present in sufficient quantities to support cell division and differentiation. Rodent intestinal perfusion studies suggest that polyamines enhance glucose absorption via heightened expression of SGLT1.[99] Moreover, experiments suggest polyamines exert trophic effect on intestinal mucosa and muscle. Enteral diets supplemented with the polyamine precursor ornithine alpha-ketoglutarate lead to mucosal hyperplasia and heighted muscle glutamine repletion in rodents with 80% small intestinal resections.[100] Ornithine decarboxylase, an enzyme responsible for enterocyte polyamine synthesis, is upregulated in hyperplastic ileal mucosa isolated from 80% intestinal resected rodents given SCFA-supplemented TPN.[95] Trophic effects are seen even in nonresected animals fed polyamine-supplemented diets.[101] Taken together, these data indicate that polyamines may mediate some important elements of intestinal adaptation. Well-designed prospective clinical trials can determine the nature of their role in human adaptation, with particular attention to the possibility that polyamines may be "conditionally essential" and thus more or less helpful depending on the age and underlying disease.

Clinical studies. Clinical data suggest that EN maintains and/or promotes intestinal function. In 1975 Greene and colleagues[102] gave 16 infants with protracted diarrhea either PN for 2 to 3 weeks followed by semi-elemental oral formula ($n = 10$), or dilute PN and continuous enteral feeding with elemental formula ($n = 6$). After 2 to 3 weeks of treatment, sucrase and maltase activity in jejunal biopsies improved in both groups, but to the normal range only in the group that received early EN. Additionally, the enteral feeding group stayed in hospital for fewer days (mean 34 vs 46 days; $p < .05$) suggesting that EN brings about recovery more effectively and more quickly than regimens that rely largely on PN. Orenstein[103] later extended these findings by studying 13 infants with intractable diarrhea, malnutrition, and malabsorption. The severe group (defined as D-xylose <10 mg/dL, $n = 8$) was randomized to receive continuous EN using semi-elemental formula or PN for 3 to 4 weeks followed by EN. Diarrhea resolved more quickly for those receiving EN versus PN (2 to 4 weeks vs 7 to 12 weeks; $p = .02$), while malabsorption, assessed by achieving D-xylose >15 mg/dL, also resolved more quickly for those receiving EN (2 to 4 weeks vs 7 to 12 weeks; $p = .02$).

Early introduction of EN influences adaptation. Sondheimer and colleagues[104] identified 44 neonates retrospectively with SBS on PN for at least 3 months. Independent predictors of PN duration included percent of EN at 12 weeks after surgery, suggesting that EN may influence outcomes. These findings were corroborated by Andorsky and colleagues[17] who similarly identified 30 neonates retrospectively who had received at least 3 months of PN because of SBS. The percentage of enteral calories at 6 weeks after surgery of (breast milk or elemental feedings) was associated with shorter duration of PN. While multivariate analysis found that only residual small intestinal length was an independent predictor of PN duration, these data suggest that attention to specific aspects of EN may influence adaptation.

Nonnutritive Factors

Patient and organ-related factors. The age of the patient, amount of residual intestine, type of residual intestine, presence of a proximal ostomy, lack of colon in continuity, absence of ICV, and underlying disease in residual intestine have all been noted as organ and patient-specific characteristics that can influence success of intestinal adaptation. Many of the relationships were identified or suspected first by Wilmore in 1972.[105]

Most studies demonstrate that residual intestinal length robustly predicts the duration of PN, a proxy for the tenor of intestinal adaptation. Based on retrospective studies[104,106–110] and one prospective study,[18] residual small intestinal length less than 15 to 40 cm in an infant, especially with lack of colon in continuity, predicts inability to wean from PN.

The nature of the residual intestine is important.[107,111] Messing and colleagues examined outcomes in 124 consecutive adults referred to their IF center between 1980 to 1992. Depending on the type of resection, adults with IF had a significantly higher chance of remaining PN dependent 2 years post-acquisition of IF when remaining intestine was less than 100 cm for patients with end jejunostomies, while less than 30 cm served as the demarcation for patients with jejunoileocolostomies.[107]

Ileum appears to adapt more readily than jejunum.[35,112] In 1967 Dowling and Booth[35] performed 70% distal or proximal small intestinal resection in rats and then measured efficiency of glucose absorption over time as well as mucosal morophological characteristics in the residual small intestine. Ileal villus height increased on average 53% in rats with residual ileum, while villi from residual jejunum increased only 14%. At the same time, glucose absorption from residual ileum increased 96% compared to baseline, but there was only an 18% increase in sugar absoption from residual jejunum. Human data supports the notion that jejunum has at best modest adaptive capacity. Patients with jejuno-colic anastamosis after extensive resections (>75% small bowel resection) did demonstrate mucosal hyperplasia in residual jejunum,[44,46] while others have reported no hyperplasia or in fact hypoplasia following jejunocolic anastamosis[113] or end jejunostomy.[114]

Debate continues with respect to the importance of the ICV in continuity. Whether the ICV promotes intestinal adaptation or prevents complications that impede adaptation is inescapably confounded by the usual absence of some or all colon when the ICV is removed. Clinical experience and some observational data[28] support the notion that colon in continuity decreases time to PN independence. In any case, most studies report[106,108,109] or suggest[18] that presence of ICV improves likelihood of achieving PN independence. Some of these studies also suggest that colonic resections[108] or lack of continuity[18] predict prolonged PN courses. Corroboration comes from adult series,[107] which clearly indicate that patients lacking colon in continuity or ileum/ICV are at higher risk for requiring long-term PN.

Growth hormone and related factors. Intuition likely resulted in early consideration of growth hormone (GH) as an adaptation-enhancing hormone. Strong animal data supports its role in either promoting mucosal growth/function or preventing mucosal atrophy.[115] Intestinal mucosa atrophies when mice are hypophysectomized, and supplemental GH restores mucosal adaptation in these mice that have had intestinal resections.[116] Insulinlike growth factor-1 (IGF-1) signaling likely accounts for GH effect in small intestine. While not all studies show GH administration causes mucosal growth,[117] the impact may be more on nutrient or ion transport.[118]

Mouse small intestinal resection models have found that GH and glutamine supplemented diet together synergistically increase plasma IGF-1 levels, mucosal DNA content, and villus growth in the residual small intestine.[85,119] Thus many recent clinical trials evaluating GH in SBS have included glutamine supplementation. The physiologic basis for this interaction may be provision of a substrate for ornithine carboxylase, an enzyme responsible for nucleotide production and polyamine synthesis, both important for tissues with rapidly diving cells.[120]

Clinical evaluation of GH has yielded variable results. Adult studies using moderate to high dose GH, glutamine supplementation (enterally or parenterally), and regulated diets have not been promising.[121] Scolapio and colleagues[122] conducted a randomized, blinded, placebo-controlled, crossover trial testing the adaptive impact of GH (0.15 mg/kg/d), oral glutamine (0.63 g/kg/d), and high carbohydrate diet on eight adult SBS patients (average small bowel length, 71 cm; mean duration of TPN, 12.9 years). Treatment with GH transiently increased total body water and electrolyte absorption, but made no difference with regard to multiple measures of nutrient transport or villus morphology. Hyperphagia and normal body composition could be important mediators of optimal adaptation; negative studies may be explained by lack of consideration for these, and other factors.[123,124]

Positive results with GH have been reported.[124–126] A randomized double blind trial in 12 adult SBS patients (duration of PN 7 ± 1 years; small-bowel remnant length, 48 ± 11 cm) on TPN and unrestricted hyperphagic diets were given 3 weeks of low dose (0.05 mg/kg/d) GH or placebo, followed by a period and crossover for additional 3 weeks.[126] Compared to the control group, those receiving GH had improved lean body mass and significantly increased nutrient absorption. Absorption of protein increased by 15% ± 5% ($p < .002$), while enteral caloric absorption improved to 37% ± 16% of total parenteral energy delivery. Later, Byrne and colleagues[124] conducted a randomized placebo-controlled inpatient trial in 41 adult PN-dependent subjects with SBS (average duration PN 4.6 years, average length small bowel 73 cm), comparing glutamine-supplemented diets with and without GH. Compared to those receiving glutamine only, subjects who received GH plus glutamine-supplemented diet were able to wean PN more substantially during the 4-week-treatment trial (mean reduction in PN volume 7.7 L/wk ± 3.2 vs 3.8 L/wk ± 2.4; $p < .001$); these effects were durable 3 months later, but only for the group that received both GH and glutamine diet. It does not appear that any patient was able to completely wean off PN.

There is very limited published experience regarding the GH axis in pediatric IF.[127–131] Retrospective investigations have included few patients and outcomes have primarily focused on somatic growth and not intestinal adaptation. Safety concerns not withstanding, any future prospective investigation will be more meaningful when differences in anatomy, age, dietary compliance, nutritional status, and mucosal disease processes are minimized or accounted for a priori.[132]

An open label clinical trial was performed in infants who received 0.3 IU/kg/day rhGH for a 10-day period of treatment.[133] A significant weight gain during treatment and a tendency to an increase in polyamine concentration in the small bowel mucosa were reported, although no information was given about tolerance to PN weaning. An open-labeled trial involved 8-PN dependent children with neonatal SBS receiving > 50% of their protein-energy requirements from PN.[134] They received 0.6 IU/kg^{-1}/day^{-1} rhGH for 3 months. All were weaned from PN during the treatment period. However, only two children remained free of PN 1 year later.

More recently, PN-dependent children with neonatal SBS received 0.14 mg/kg/day and glutamine for 3 months.[131] Results suggested a beneficial effect of rhGH by the decreasing need for PN, but body composition and gut mucosa changed insignificantly. In addition, there was no apparent benefit from glutamine treatment. Finally, two girls with neonatal SBS received exogenous GH at 0.3 mg/kg per week subcutaneously and concurrent glutamine supplementation, beginning at 6 and 6½ years of age.[127] Treatment duration was 8 and 2.5 years, respectively. Patient weights increased from the fifth to the forty-first percentile and from the seventeenth to the twenty-third percentile, respectively. Height increased from the first to the fifty-seventh percentile in the former patient and increased from less than the first to the seventeenth percentile in the latter. Both patients were weaned from PN, taking enteral nutrition alone. These data show that late exogenous treatment with GH and glutamine supplementation improved growth parameters in pediatric patients with SBS. Earlier use of rhGH in SBS infants or children might be helpful for future management.

IGF-1 physiology may have important role in intestinal adaptation following resection. This has been established in animal studies. Small and large intestinal resections induce IGF-1 mRNA expression in residual colon and ileum.[85,135] As compared to resection alone, exogenous IGF-1 produced heightened IGF-1 mRNA expression in residual ileum[85] and colon,[135] larger increases in small intestinal weight, DNA, and protein content,[85] and enhanced crypt cellular proliferation.[136] Administration of IGF-1 with supplemental glutamine likely has synergistic influences on these processes.[85] Interestingly, IGF-1 signaling from within the smooth muscle layers of the small intestine may exert some control over intestinal adaptation.[137]

Differential physiologic responses have been identified with regard to IGF-1 and intestinal resection. In rat models of SBS, residual colon[138] and ileum[85] underwent adaptive changes in response to intestinal resection, while jejunum had no response to resection alone; changes in colon and ileum correlated with tissue protein expression of IGF-1 binding protein 3. In contrast, exogenous IGF-1 produced adaptive changes in jejunum and ileum, but not colon.[139] This has not been a consistent finding.[135] This complex physiology with respect to IGF-1 provides additional insight on the heterogenous GH findings noted above.

Exogenous administration of IGF-1 may facilitate transition to EN in animal models of SBS. Gillingham and colleagues[140] gave rats who received 60% jejunoileal resection plus cecectomy either IGF-1 or vehicle for 7 days while receiving PN, and then gave 100% EN for an additional 10 days. Rats who received IGF-1 had significantly better preserved lean body mass, and intestinal mucosa demonstrated the expected mucosal hyperplasia while this was not the case for those animals receiving vehicle.

Barksdale and colleagues[128] investigated the relationship between growth failure (defined as weight and length for age <5%) and serum hormone profiles in 40 patients (29 boys; mean age 5.3 years; range 0.5 to 18.6 years) with SBS (73% receiving PN). Thirty-eight percent (11 patients) of the cohort with height measurements ($n = 29$) met criteria for growth failure, and significantly more children with growth failure had low IGF-1 as compared to those without growth failure (64 vs 17%; $p < .05$). GH levels were generally normal in all patients. While patient numbers were small, Barksdale and colleagues speculated that this data serves as indirect evidence that, in a select group of children with poorly adapted intestine, inadequate IGF-1 may have caused growth failure even in context of adequate enteral and/or PN. Larger, prospective studies accounting for confounders such as comorbid illness will be required to validate this potentially important claim.

Epidermal growth factors. EGF is well recognized for its intestinal trophic properties.[141–144] Characterized molecular events which occur with EGF stimulation include redistribution of SGLT1 from microsomal pools to the brush border membrane[145] and intestinal resection-induced movement of EGF receptors from basolateral to the brush border membrane.[146] EGF may prevent enterocyte apoptosis which, although physiologic, could be maladaptive in the project of maximal intestinal adaptation.[147]

In vivo support for EGF's trophic properties mainly comes from animal models of SBS. Mice that receive a sialoadenectomy (the salivary gland is the major source for EGF in mice) and proximal small bowel resection, as compared to mice with small bowel resection with sham sialoadenectomy, have significantly attentuated ileal villus height and tissue weight gain, the differences of which are abolished by exogenous administration of enteral or parenteral EGF.[148] Ileal brush border surface area and glucose transport were enhanced when EGF was administered to rabbits with proximal surgical SBS as compared to those that received saline.[149] Conversely, as compared to mice receiving saline, mice receiving 50% small bowel resections that also received orogastric EGF receptor inhibitor demonstrated poor adaptation (reduced intestinal wet weight, crypt depth, villus height) in residual small intestine.[143] Barrier function and carbohydrate absorption were enhanced in juvenile rats with surgical SBS administered recombinant human EGF as compared to rats with similar operations administered saline.[150] Lastly, one human study[151] is consistent with notion that EGF plays a role in human intestinal mucosal integrity. EGF levels in multiple body fluids from 25 infants with NEC were significantly lower than levels found in 19 gestational age and weight-matched neonates without NEC.

A pilot study has been conducted in five children with severe SBS (defined as <25% small bowel length predicted for age) using exogenous, enterally-administered EGF. As compared to baseline, after 6 weeks of therapy carbohydrate absorption was significantly higher, as was tolerance of enteral feedings. While the trial was successful, soon after it ended three patients developed sepsis.[152] Other human observational studies suggest EGF is important for maintenance of adequate barrier[151] and reparative function. It is important to emphasize the role of oral feeding and subsequent salivary gland EGF release in promoting intestinal adaptation.

Glucagon-like peptide 2. GLP-2 is a pro-glucagon derived peptide produced in distal ileum or proximal colonic L-cells in response to luminal nutrient exposure, providing feedback information to the upper intestine so that fluid and nutrient absorption may be optimal.[153] Animal models of SBS strongly suggest that GLP-2 plays an important role in intestinal adaptation following resection or injury. Rats subjected to 70% jejunal-ileal resections followed by oral feeding sustained persistent elevation in plasma GLP-2 levels as compared to those receiving transection alone, and measures of adaptive growth in the resected animals positively correlated with levels of circulating GLP-2 and pro-glucagon mRNA in residual ileum and colon.[154] Martin and colleagues[155] extended these findings in rats by demonstrating that the magnitude of GLP-2 elevation directly correlated with the extent of intestinal resection, mucosal enterocyte proliferation, and protein and fat malabsorption. This suggested that heightened GLP-2 release may induce intestinal trophism in response to nutrient exposure in distal small and large intestine.

Heightened adaptation occurs when GLP-2 or analogue is administered to animals with induced SBS. Rats given 21 days of GLP-2 analogue in the context of 75% mid-jejunum-ileum resection developed enhanced mucosal adaptation (eg, activity, mucosal weight, villus height, mucosal DNA content) in jejunum, as compared to the adaptive responses to resection alone.[156] GLP-2 treatment for 21 days also restored *d*-xylose absorption to levels in excess of control. A later study using a similar design found that GLP-2 administration, as compared to placebo administration, was capable of accelerating adaptation, decreasing permeability, and increasing SGLT-1 protein abundance after resection even when animals were kept NPO on PN.[157]

GLP-2 has been evaluated in humans. Jeppesen and colleagues[158] gave subcutaneous GLP-2 twice daily to 8 adult patients (4 on home PN) with longstanding SBS and jejunostomies. None of the patients had meal-stimulated GLP-2 responses, but all had supraphysiologic plasma levels after subcutaneous administration. After 35 days, stoma output weight significantly decreased compared to baseline, and energy absorption increased modestly, as reflected by trends toward improved carbohydrate, protein, but not fat absorption. Motility changes were significant in the stomach, while small intestinal transit time was unchanged. Over this small period of time, lean body mass increased significantly by 2.9 ± 1.9 kg. Later, Jeppesen conducted an open-label pilot study[159] investigating the affect of the peptidase-resistant GLP-2 analogue teduglutide on intestinal absorptive capacity in 16 adults with longstanding SBS (12 on parenteral fluids). Ten subjects had end jejunostomies, five had greater than 50% of colon in continuity, and one subject had <50% residual small intestine. Subjects received subcutaneous injections of 0.03 to 0.15 mg/kg/d for 21 days, while nutrient balance and intestinal morphology (via mucosal biopsy) was assessed at baseline, during last 3 days of treatment, and 3 weeks after treatment was discontinued. Treatment decreased average fecal wet weight (−711 +/− 734 g/d; p = .001) and energy losses (−193 +/− 347 kcal/d; p = .04), while for those with jejunostomies villus height, crypt depth, and mitotic index all increased significantly. However, at 21 days, average body weight was not different from baseline, and 3 weeks after the medication was discontinued, all measures had returned to baseline (Figure 3). Further evaluation will be necessary to determine

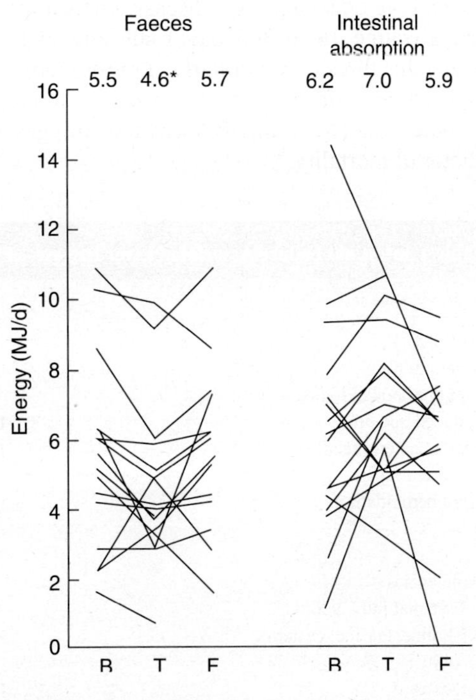

Figure 3 Fecal energy excretion and intestinal absorption in patients with SBS receiving the GLP-2 analogue teduglutide. B baseline; T after 18 to 21 days of treatment; F follow-up. (Reproduced with permission from Jeppsen PB et al.[159])

optimal timing, dose, duration, and safety of teduglutide.[158] Teduglutide has not yet been evaluated in children.

Insulin. Insulin has been shown to influence intestinal structure and absorptive function. The effects of parenteral insulin (INS) on structural intestinal adaptation, cell proliferation, and apoptosis were assessed in rats divided into three experimental groups: sham operated rats underwent bowel transection and reanastomosis, SBS rats underwent a 75% small bowel resection, and SBS-INS rats underwent a 75% small bowel resection and were treated with insulin (1 U/kg, twice daily subcutaneously), from day 3 through day 14.[162] SBS-INS animals demonstrated higher jejunal and ileal bowel and mucosal weights, jejunal and ileal mucosal DNA and protein, and jejunal and ileal crypt depth, as compared with SBS animals. SBS-INS rats also had a greater cell proliferation index in both jejunum and ileum and a trend toward a decrease in enterocyte apoptotic index in jejunum and ileum, as compared with the SBS untreated group. This favorable effect of insulin is relevant and might be considered in patients on PN receiving high intravenous glucose infusion rates that induce insulin release and relative hyperinsulinism.

Other hormones. A variety of other circulating factors have been considered for trophic effect in intestine. See Table 3 for comprehensive list.

Intracellular observations. Differential gene expression certainly underlies the structural and functional changes characterizing intestinal adaptation. Investigations using cDNA microarray technology have recently begun to elucidate these pathways. Erwin and colleagues[61] resected 50% of proximal intestine in male mice and extracted RNA from residual ileum 3 days later. As compared to ileum from mice that received sham operations, resected ileum had upregulation of genes that regulate apoptosis, cell cycle control, stress responses, ion flux, and transcription. The same group extended these findings by giving EGF, with demonstration that a novel gene product, small proline-rich protein 2 (sprr2) was significantly induced above baseline, with further enhancement after EGF administration.[62] Other molecules have been considered, such as peroxisome proliferation-activated receptor α (PPAR α).[123] Molecular techniques will be instrumental for understanding the molecular correlates of adaptation, adaptation failure, and identifying logical pathways amenable to manipulation.[163]

Summary Animal and clinical data indicate that EN, directly or indirectly, enhance intestinal adaptation. Complex macronutrients may enhance adaptation to a larger extent than single amino acid or monosaccharide-containing nutrition (the functional "workload hypothesis"). Specific fatty acids or triglycerides may offer advantages over others, but discrepant findings disallow formulation of an ideal fat composition. Nonnutrient factors such as

Table 3 Peptides and Hormones with Demonstrated Effects (animal or human studies) on Intestinal Adaptation Following Resection

Hormone	Source	Receptor/location	Action/effects
Gastrin	G cells (predominantly antrum and stomach)	CCK-B receptor on ECL cells	Increased gastric acid secretion gastric hyperplasia
Leptin	Fat cells, gastric mucosa	Surface receptors, many kinds/ concentrated in hypothalamus but also diffuse distribution	Enhances carbohydrate absorption in small intestine
Growth hormone	Anterior pituitary	GHR expressed in stomach, small intestine, colon	Increased cellular proliferation, increased absorption of water, sodium, and amino acids
IGF-1	Liver	IGF-IR (ubiquitous)	Increased cellular proliferation, increased weight
Peptide YY	L cell in ileum, colon	Y receptor family/diffusely distributed in intestine and CNS	Decreased gastric emptying, prolonged intestinal transit
GLP-2	L cells in ileum and colon	GLP-2 receptor	Increased cellular proliferation, increased weight
Hepatocyte growth factor	Intestinal fibroblasts	c-Met receptors/intestinal epithelial cells	Increased cellular proliferation, differentiation
Epidermal growth factor	Brunner's glands of duodenum, salivary glands, pancreatic secretions	TGF-α/EGFR receptor found throughout the intestinal epithelium	Increased cellular proliferation
TGF-α	Epthelial cell throughout the GI tract	TGF-α/EGFR receptor found throughout the intestinal epithelium	Increased cellular proliferation
Keritinocyte growth factor	Stromal cells	KGFR/intestinal epithelial cells	Increased cellular proliferation
Interleukin-11	Stromal cells	IL-11R/intestinal epithelial cells	Increased intestinal mass, enhanced absorption
Bombesin	Brain and intestinal tissue	Serveral cell surface receptors/diffuse in GI tract including enteric nerves	Increased enterocyte proliferation, mucosal weight
Retinoic acid	Diet, stored in liver	Nuclear receptors and enterocyte migration	Stimulate crypt cell proliferation
Insulin	Released from enteral feeding		Greater cell proliferation index decrease in enterocyte apoptotic

Adapted with permission from Cisler JJ and Buchman AL.[161]

CCK-B = cholecystokinin B; CNS = central nervous system; ECL = enterochromaffin-like cell; EGFR = epidermal growth factor receptor; GHR = growth hormone receptor; GI = gastrointestinal; GLP = glucagons-like peptide; IGF = insulin-like growth factor; KGF = keratinocyte growth factor receptor; TGF-α = transforming growth factor-α.

peptide hormones may exert important paracrine or endocrine affects, and pharmacologic use may promote adaptation in humans.

Pathophysiology

Intestinal Failure Associated Liver Disease. IF associated liver disease or (IFALD) is a leading cause of mortality in both adults and children with chronic IF, and the primary indication for liver–intestinal transplantation in pediatrics. The prevalence, natural history, and liver histology differ between adults and children. The etiology is still unclear and likely multifactorial (see Table 4).

Cholestasis is primarily a problem in children. Most series have reported 40 to 60% of infants on chronic PN develop cholestasis, whereas 40 to 55% of adults develop steatosis or steatohepatitis.[165] Cavicchi and colleagues[166] conducted a prospective investigation on PN cholestasis in their adult population of 90 home PN patients receiving PN between 1985 and 1996. The group reported that fully 65% of home PN patients developed chronic cholestasis after an average of 6 months on PN (range 3 to 132 months), with complications associated with portal hypertension developing in 41% of patients. Others[167] have reported a lower burden of cholestatic IFALD in adults.

IFALD is a serious complication, leading to increased mortality. Nasr and colleagues[168] recently reviewed all infants in their SBS registry (n = 70) born between 1997 and 2003, and found that those (n = 23) whose direct bilirubin rose above 100 μmol/L (5.8 mg/dL) had a 70% chance of developing end-stage liver disease, on average 60 days (range 10 to 365 days) subsequent to reaching this threshold. Similarly, a retrospective analysis of 90 infants with SBS had also found that cholestasis (>2.5 mg/dL) was the strongest predictor of mortality.[106]

Cholestasis and/or portal hypertension may hamper intestinal adaptation. Weber and Keller[169] stratified a group of 42 infants with SBS/IF by the severity of liver disease, assessed both clinically and with biopsy or measurement of portal venous pressure. As compared to infants with minimal clinical or objective evidence of liver disease, time on PN was markedly longer in those with marked clinical liver disease (80 vs 100 days) or

Table 4 Intestinal Failure Associated Liver Disease—Etiology and Management

Predisposing Factor	Management Response
Prematurity	
Duration of PN	Cycling PN, vigilance in transition to drip enteral nutrition
Length of bowel remnant	
Reduced bile flow	Ursodeoxycholic acid 20–30 mg/kg/d
Lack of enteral feeding	Early introduction of drip feeds
Recurrent sepsis	Daily line care, rigorous education and reinforcement
Lipid peroxidation	Lipid administration not greater than 2.5 g/kg/d, or 1 g/kg/d and less in face of worsening cholestasis and thrombocytopenia
Deficiencies	
Essential fatty acid	Appropriate type and amount of IV lipid
Choline, taurine, cysteine	Pediatric amino acid formulations
Toxicity	
Dextrose	Limit excessive administration; cycling
Phytosterols	Substitute other lipid sources for soy bean
Manganese	Monitor levels
Bacterial overgrowth	Targeted antibiotic therapy, surgical tapering, probiotics

Adapted with permission from Goulet O and Ruemmele F.[164]

PN = parenteral nutrition.

abnormal portal pressures (72 vs 184 days). These data form the basis for the recommendation that select patients with SBS and advanced IFALD be considered for liver intestine transplant (LITx).[170]

Lack of enteral intake. Experimental studies suggest that lack of enteral feeding may indirectly lead to liver toxicity. Intestinal and biliary stasis develop during fasting, likely influenced by a gastrointestinal hormonal milieu dramatically different from the fed state. Intestinal stasis may lead to overgrowth, translocation, and sepsis, while biliary stasis may cause accumulation of hepatotoxic bile acids. Biliary sludge may form in the context of biliary stasis from lack of Cholecystokinin (CCK) stimulation. However, CCK administration to pediatric patients with IF did not influence frequency or severity of cholestasis in this population.[171] Retrospective analysis of clinical data suggests that early introduction of enteral feeding may be protective in this context.[17]

Blood stream infections. Early and repeated blood stream infections likely influence the severity or progession of IFALD. Hermans and colleagues[172] reviewed their experience with IFALD in children on prolonged PN ($n = 30$; mean PN duration 65 months) who had received liver biopsies. Those children with severe fibrosis were more likely to have had more frequent (average 3.2 vs 1.5 events/yr) and earlier (average 1 vs 4 months) sepsis events as compared to those with mild to moderate fibrosis. Earlier retrospective reviews of infants IF have demonstrated strong relationships between cholestasis and early and/or frequency of sepsis events.[173,174]

Gestational age. Gestational age or diagnosis may influence risk for IFALD. Christensen and colleagues[175] reviewed a regional database and extracted data on all neonates receiving PN for >14 days ($n = 1,366$). Groups at highest risk for developing a persistently elevated direct bilirubin of >2 mg/dL (operational definition of IFALD) were those with birth weight <750 g and diagnoses of jejunal atresia or gastroschisis.

Excessive intake or content of lipid emulsions. Clinical evidence suggests that hypertriglyceridemia (>150 mg/dL) may cause or be caused by hepatic dysfunction in neonates receiving >2 weeks of PN.[176] Colomb and colleagues[177] found that for 10 infants on chronic PN, more than half of 23 episodes of cholestasis were preceeded by increases in IV lipid delivery. Improvements were noted with temporary discontinuation or decreasing lipid administration. Among adults, Cavicchi and colleagues[166] found that lipid administration in excess of 1 g/kg/d was an independent predictor of chronic cholestasis in 90 adults with IF followed between 1985 and 1996.

The pathophysiology of IFALD has been explored in vitro and in animals. Mechanisms include lack of enteral processing, direct hepatocyte toxicity, and cytokine-induced injury. As compared to mice fed both PN solution and Intralipid orally, mice given PN solution orally and Intralipid IV developed significantly greater fatty liver and hepatocellular damage after 19 days.[178] In vitro investigations found that Intralipid alters cholesterol metabolism when added directly to hepatocyte cell cultures.[179] Rabbits with PN induced liver injury will show histologic and ultrastructural improvements when supplemented with IV glutathione, an intracellular antioxidant.[180] Phytosterols, which are natural components of the soy oil used to produce IV lipid emulsions, may alter cell membrane properties and decrease bile flow in neonatal pigs.[181] Lastly, rat models of inflammatory injury in the liver[182] show that endotoxemia via the portal vein may upregulate liver macrophages which elaborate injurious cytokines.

Management considerations are listed in Table 4. A critical strategy is the prevention of sepsis. Daily line care, intensive education and reinforcement, and multidisciplinary teams with dedicated staff to manage patients on home PN form the ideal system to prevent infection, monitor nutritional variables carefully, and address dangerous problems quickly.[183] Introduction of small amounts of oral or EN may help promote normal bile flow, although data suggests CCK secretion may not be adequate in SBS/IF in response to enteral stimulus.[184] Recently, Gura and colleagues[185] reported on two infants with IF and severe IFALD who received omega-3 rich, fish oil-derived IV lipid emulsion (Omegaven) instead of the standard Intralipid. Cholestasis improved significantly in both, one patient was removed from the liver transplant list because of resolution of end-stage signs and symptoms, and the other had resolution of cholestasis while continuing to receive full calories parenterally. Well designed clinical trials are urgently needed to corroborate these findings and evaluate the safety of this regimen.

Line Infections and Thrombosis. Any child with a central venous catheter (CVC) is at risk for developing catheter-related bacteremia or fungemia, and patients with IF/SBS may be at particularly high risk[186] because of the abnormal intestinal milieu. Intestinal stasis, bacterial overgrowth, and intestinal inflammation may increase the risk for bacterial translocation from the intestine to blood stream. The organisms can "seed" the venous catheter and not only lead to bacteremia or sepsis but the need for removal of the line. While this scenario has been demonstrated in animal models,[187] definitive evidence in humans does not exist.[188] Suggestive evidence includes isolation of enteric organisms at a much higher frequency from the blood of patients with IF than from patients with CVCs but without IF.[189] Significant concordance has also been found between species isolated from stool or ostomy output and blood culture isolates.[190] Lastly, Weber[191] found that there was a statistically significant increase in enteric organism bacteremia during feeding advancement in 21 infants with IF/SBS as compared to baseline as well as a reference population of infants with CVCs but without IF.

Thrombosis may occur when foreign material is introduced into the vascular space. Scant literature indicates that IF/SBS is a hypercoagulatory state.[192] Whether IF patients compared to other patients with long-term central access have increased incidence of thrombosis has not directly been studied. Moukarzel and colleagues[193] found that for long-term PN dependent pediatric patients, the mean lifespan for a CVC was 22.4 ± 14.7 months (range 1.5 to 178 months); 25% of CVC removals were caused by catheter occlusion. Recurrent vascular occlusion/thrombosis limiting central venous access is particularly worrisome for patients who require central venous nutrition for survival, and this is one of the indications for intestinal transplantation. Nevertheless, true loss of all catheter insertion sites is rare.[26]

Bone disease. Osteopenia and osteomalacia develop frequently in patients with IF. Causative factors include inadequate vitamin D, inability to provide enough calcium and phosphorus parenterally without causing precipitation, magnesium malabsorption, aluminum toxicity, recurrent acidosis, and physical inactivity.[194] In the past, aluminum accumulation may have occurred because of relatively large amounts found in the parenteral protein source.[195] Bone mineral ought to be monitored even after PN has been discontinued, as deficits have been noted in children with a history of PN use.[196] Long-term outcomes have not yet been characterized. Preventive strategies have been attempted in adults using PTH and GH therapy,[197,198] but have not been adequately tested in children.

Bacterial Overgrowth. Small intestinal bacterial overgrowth (SIBO) occurs frequently in patients with IF. The prevalence of SIBO in SBS/IF is widely variable, and primarily depends on the methods chosen to make the diagnosis.[187]

Risk factors for SIBO include abnormal intestinal anatomy, hypomotility, decreased secretion of acid in the stomach and enzymes from the pancreas, and possibly an underlying immune defect. Motility in SBS is abnormal[199]; lack of effective migrating motor complexes during fasting may promote retention of bacteria in the small intestine. The distal ileum, and not the ICV per se, may be responsible for the propulsive function in the distal small intestine[200]; as such, resection of the ICV may be more a marker for SIBO risk than its cause.

SIBO may cause disease because of malabsorption and compromised intestinal epithelial barrier. Bacteria in the upper small intestine may deconjugate bile salts, leading to impaired micelle formation and increased risk for fat maldigestion. Vitamin B_{12} deficiency is thought to occur in SIBO because of sequestration by anaerobic bacteria.

The sequence of SIBO, mucosal inflammation, compromised intestinal epithelial barrier, bacterial translocation, and bacteremia/sepsis has been carefully studied in animals.[187,201] Human experiments have not found clear relationships.

For instance, O'Boyle[202] failed to demonstrate any relationship between humoral measures of permeability, mucosal inflammation or atrophy, and bacterial counts in mesenteric lymph nodes in 43 adults. Nevertheless, SIBO may influence other organs or organ systems. IFALD[203] and sepsis[204] may be influenced not by bacterial translocation directly but instead via cell and humoral immunologic phenomena originating in the intestinal mucosa affected by SIBO.

The diagnosis of SIBO can be challenging, as both invasive and noninvasive determinations have important limitations. Traditionally SIBO has been defined as >100,000 CFU/mL of fluid isolated from the proximal small intestine.[187] Bacteria cultured usually include flora typical of the oropharynx or colon, such as *Streptococci*, members of *Enterobacteriaceae*, and *Staphylococci*. Endoscopic jejunal cultures, while being the "gold standard," are both difficult to obtain and poorly reproducible. Hydrogen breath testing has become the noninvasive test of choice for diagnosing SIBO. Hydrogen is a by-product of carbohydrate fermentation by intestinal bacteria, which can be quantified in the breath. Elevated background levels or early "peaks" after administration of a simple carbohydrate such as lactulose can be considered consistent with SIBO. Multiple reasons for falsely positive and negative tests exist. Moreover, testing will oftentimes be impractical or cumbersome in pediatrics. Thus, empiric antibiotic trials are the norm in the clinical setting.[187]

Management includes selective and periodic use of enteral antibiotics, prokinetic agents, and surgical therapy to relieve partial obstructions or dilated loops of bowel (see below). Antibiotic therapy remains primarily empiric. Single 7 to 10 day courses may be prescribed, but more typical for patients with SBS/IF would be repeated regimens (eg, first week of every month) or a continuous, rotating antibiotic regimen. Pro- and prebiotics likely have a role, but safety and efficacy have not been demonstrated clearly enough in clinical studies to recommend routine use. Further discussion and information regarding antibiotic and probiotic use in SIBO can be found elsewhere.[187]

Renal Calculi. Calcium oxalate nephrolithiasis may occur in patients with SBS because of the hyperabsorption of oxalate.[194] Oxalate is usually complexed with residual calcium, forming nonabsorbable salts. However, in the setting of fatty acid malabsorption with colon in continuity, calcium is instead complexed with fatty acids, leaving the oxalate free to diffuse through the colonic mucosa. Nonabsorbed bile salts may also increase colonic permeability to oxalate.[205] Obligate renal excretion will lead to hyperoxaluria and increased risk for stone formation. Management may include low oxalate diet, calcium supplementation, adequate hydration, resins such as cholestyramine, and medications to alkalinize the urine.

D-Lactic Acidosis. D-Lactic acidosis was first described in 1983[206] and is an uncommon but distinctive complication of SBS. The clinical presentation is highly variable, but usually features altered mental status and anion gap metabolic acidosis. The mental status changes may be subtle, such as apathy or irritability, or dramatic, such as lethargy or even coma. Suspicion for this diagnosis should be raised in any patient with SBS and altered mental status, especially in a patient with known bowel dilation. Confirmation of the diagnosis requires the ability to measure *d*-lactate level in blood or urine. The pathophysiology is presumed to entail the overgrowth of *d*-lactate-producing bacterial organisms in the small bowel. In the setting of a carbohydrate rich feeding, large amounts of *d*-lactate are generated and promptly absorbed. *d*-Lactate is poorly metabolized in humans, such that toxic amounts may accumulate easily.[207] Treatment primarily involves discontinuing enteral feeding, selective bowel decontamination, and sometimes bicarbonate infusions. Prevention may include surgical tapering of dilated bowel loops aimed at reducing stasis and overgrowth.[208] Medical maneuvers using a mixture of antibiotics and long-term probiotics may also be successful.[209] However, antibiotics may occasionally promote the growth of *d*-lactic acid-producing organisms.[210]

MANAGEMENT AND OUTCOMES

Understanding the driving forces behind intestinal adaptation motivates a principled approach to what is primarily a nutritional therapy for children needing intestinal rehabilitation. To be sure, the outcomes are slow to evolve. The results, however, are nothing short of momentous. Success demands patience, persistence, and attention to detail. This can best be achieved through a multidisciplinary approach, providing broad-based medical, nutritional, and surgical support for the patient and longitudinal social support for caregivers.

Medical

What to Feed. Although the general role of EN in intestinal function and structure is well-supported, the specific composition, especially in IF syndromes, has been less well delineated.

Breast milk. Breast milk's special immunologic and anti-infective properties ought to be especially advantageous to infants with IF. Breast milk contains growth factors, nucleotides, long-chain fatty acids, glutamine, and other amino acids that may promote intestinal adaptation. In addition, breastfeeding has been associated with improved immune function, as well as the genesis of a fecal microbiota rich in lactobacilli and bifidobacteria, both of which might improve IF prognosis. On the other hand, breastmilk contains lactose, which is sometimes not well tolerated in patients with reduced intestinal surface area. In a population of 30 infants with SBS (defined as more than 90 days of dependency on PN), the percentage of days that infants received breast milk was strongly correlated with fewer days of PN use ($r = -.821$, $p < .03$).[17] As a result of these theoretical and practical data, best practice may be to use breast milk, if available, for most infants with IF receiving enteral support.

Enteral formulas. For infants with SBS for whom breastmilk is not available, the choice of enteral formulas is controversial. On the one hand, the "functional workload" presented by complex nutrients may promote mucosal cell proliferation,[211] via direct contact with disaccharides[79] or indirectly, whereby distal small intestinal or colonic exposure to luminal nutrients promotes release of trophic factors that stimulate small bowel adaptation.[67,95] On the other hand, the presence of a limited mucosal surface area can lead to lactose, protein, and long-chain fatty acid malabsorption. If this malabsorption is severe, fluid, electrolyte, and metabolic balance can be difficult to achieve.

Carbohydrates may be poorly tolerated by patients with IF, as they are broken down by gastrointestinal bacteria into small, osmotically active organic acids that can present a major osmotic load to the distal small intestine and colon.[212] For this reason, carbohydrate content should generally not exceed 40% of calories, and formulas given to IF patients are usually lactose-free. While lactase activity is significantly lower in the jejunum as compared with sucrase–isomaltase and maltase–glucoamylase activity,[213] unless there is an extensive jejunal resection, most infants and children with SBS will tolerate small to moderate amounts of lactose.[26]

Fiber supplementation may be helpful in the older child with SBS with intact colon. Colonic bacterial fermentation of the unabsorbed fiber produces SCFAs, such as butyrate, which appears to induce trophic changes in animal small intestinal mucosa.[94,214] Moreover, pectin, a fermentable but nondigestable oligosaccharide, increased nitrogen absorption and decreased transit time in a child with SBS,[215] while supplementation improved electrolyte absorption and mucosal permeability for infants with protracted diarrheal illnesses.[216]

Although fat tends to be poorly absorbed in SBS, it is a dense energy source relative to carbohydrate or protein. Considering the relatively greater adverse effect of carbohydrate on osmotic diarrhea, it is usually advantageous for patients with SBS to include at least moderate amounts of fat in their diets.

Medium chain triglycerides (MCTs) may be more reliably absorbed than LCTs. MCTs are efficiently hydrolyzed by gastric and pancreatic lipases, giving rise to relatively water-soluble component fatty acids and monoglycerides which readily diffuse into enterocytes and enter the portal blood directly.[217] This is relevant because infants with dysmotility or SBS often have dilated, poorly motile segments of intestine, conditions which encourage SIBO.[187] Bacteria metabolize and inactivate bile acids, preventing the solubilization necessary for LCT digestion and absorption. On the other hand, excessive provision of MCT oil can cause diarrhea and ketosis, while MCTs do not provides essential fatty acids. Thus, MCT content should not be the sole source of dietary lipid.

Moreover, free fatty acids derived from hydrolyzed LCTs may have strong trophic effects on small intestinal mucosa.[68,69] Specific fatty acids may influence intestinal adaptation, as animal data suggest that Omega-3-, Omega-6-,[70,73] and PUFA-[218] supplemented diets promote mucosal growth and/or function.

An ideal protein source for infants with IF has not yet been determined. Protein itself may have trophic properties. Colostrum protein concentrate improved weight gain and morphometric measures of intestinal adaptation in a piglet model of SBS using polymeric diet plus colostrum versus polymeric diet alone.[43]

Nevertheless, it is not yet clear if the type of protein in infant formulas influences outcomes. Bines and colleagues[219] reported a series of four SBS patients with persistent feeding intolerance. After receiving an elemental amino acid based-formula, all four patients discontinued PN within 15 months. In addition, histologic and physiologic measures of small bowel function improved concurrently. One retrospective review also found better outcomes (shorter duration of PN dependency) with the use of an amino-acid based formula.[17]

Hydrolyzed protein formulas have also been evaluated clinically. Intact protein infant formula was compared to hydrolyzed protein formula in a crossover study of 60 days duration in 10 infants with SBS.[220] No effect of formula type was observed on growth, nitrogen absorption, or mucosal permeability. An earlier study in adult jejunostomy patients produced similar findings.[221]

Concern for the development of IgE[222] and non-IgE mediated sensitization and allergic enteritis has favored the use of protein hydrolysate or amino acid based formulas for children with IF. Noninfectious colitis has been reported in patients with SBS.[223] Allergy may occur in children with IF because of sensitization associated with abnormal mucosal permeability. Increased small intestinal mucosal permeability occurs in the context of intestinal inflammation,[219] oftentimes a complication of SIBO.[224] As noted above, dilated, poorly motile segments of small bowel in close proximity to colon are common in patients with SBS and dysmotility, and the stagnation and contamination that results promotes abnormal growth of bacteria in small intestine.[225]

In summary, animal and some human data support an important role of EN in children with SBS/IF. Modest data support the use of protein hydrolysate or amino acid-based formulas. Most formulas are lactose-free and many include a portion of their fat source as MCTs. Infants with diarrhea and protein losing enteropathies may require formulas with enhanced protein content. Appendix III provides important details on enteral products used in infants and children with IF.

Supplementary fluids, electrolytes, and micronutrients. Excess fluid and electrolyte losses may complicate the management of IF patients, particularly in patients with high output jejunostomies, in pseudo-obstruction patients who incur large gastric/duodenal fluid losses, or in those with persistent secretory diarrhea. Glucose-containing electrolyte solutions (also called oral rehydration solutions) with sodium concentrations of 75 to 90 mEq/L are typically used to replace jejunostomy and diarrheal losses. Replacement fluids, be they enteral or IV, may be adjusted based on electrolyte concentration of the lost fluids. The IV route should be used when there is still net loss of fluid following enteral replacement. Monitoring urine sodium concentration for excessive retention (<10 mEq/L) may indicate the need to provide more sodium, even if serum values are near normal. Excessive magnesium losses can occur with large ostomy volumes, and appropriate magnesium replacement may also improve calcium nutriture.[226]

Zinc[227] and selenium[228] losses increase with watery diarrhea and high ostomy output. Zinc supplements are often used empirically, given that serum values do not reliably reflect body stores. Fat-soluble vitamin supplements should be considered, as fat malabsorption is common when absorptive surface area or micellar function is limited. Vitamin B_{12} monitoring and/or parenteral supplementation is necessary for infants with ileal resection or diversion.

How to Feed. Continuous enteral feeding via a nasogastric or gastrostomy tube is advantageous in the patient with SBS or diarrhea,[103,229] as this permits constant saturation of carrier transport proteins, thus taking full advantage of the available absorptive surface area. A controlled study of intragastric feeds in infants with chronic diarrhea and/or SBS found that continuous feeding was associated with improved nutrient balance and weight gain, as compared to intermittent feeding.[230]

Devices. Most centers recommend percutaneous enteral access for children who will require EN for greater than 3 months. Nevertheless, most infants start with nasogastric or nasoenteric (transpyloric) feedings. Table 5 displays the methods,

Table 5 Devices Used for Enteral Feeding

Devices	Indications	Contraindications	Advantages	Disadvantages
Gastric feeding				
Nasogastric	Nutritional support <3 mo	Serve GE reflux, aspirations slow gastric emptying	Easy to place at home	Frequent dislodgements, nasal symptoms
Percutaneous endoscopic gastrostomy (PEG)	Nutritional support >3 mo	History of abdominal surgery, abnormal abdominal anatomy, portal hypertension with dilated abdominal vessels	Fewer occlusions with large bore, one-step low profile devices available	
Surgical gastrostomy	Nutritional support >3 mo and higher risk for injury to abdominal organs	Coagulopathy, poor candidate for surgery (cardiac or respiratory insufficiency)	Immediate placement of low-profile device, direct visualization of stomach	Open surgery
Transpyloric feeding				
Gastrojejunal (GJ)	Longer-term enteral nutrition for patients with severe GERD, gastric dysmotility or need for gastric decompression	Recent proximal surgical anastamoses	Radiologic placement, transpyloric tube can be passed through existing gastrostomy tube	Requires healing of gastrostomy tract prior to replacement with GJ, intussesception around tube, frequent occlusions of jejunal port
Nasojejunal	Short-term nutritional support for patients with severe GERD, gastric dysmotility, pancreatitis	Recent proximal surgical anastamoses	Radiologic or bedside placement techniques, noninvasive	Frequent dislodgements, intusseception, nasal symptoms
Jejunal	Long-term enteral nutrition for patients with severe GERD, upper intestinal dysmotility	Generalized dysmotility, poor wound healing	Direct access to small intestine	Open surgical procedure, mechanical problems

Reproduced with permission from Kamin D and Duggan C.[8]
GE = gastroesophageal; GERD = gastroesophageal reflux disease.

contraindications, and important features of enteral feeding strategies.

Methods for advancement. A protocol for enteral advancement in SBS, or in IF in general, is outlined in Table 6. Strict adherence to an ostomy/stool output maximum is unwise, and enteral advancement can occur so long as fluid and electrolyte balance is maintained. Small quantities of oral feedings should be introduced in infants two- or three-times a day to stimulate sucking and swallowing and to minimize the chances of feeding aversion in the future. Frequent setbacks are not unusual. Enteral feedings may eventually be transitioned to oral/bolus feedings, or oral/bolus and nocturnal feedings, to allow more freedom from the feeding pump.

Surgical

Surgery plays a crucial role in the lives of children with IF/SBS. Half of children with SBS will have more than one laparotomy.[231] The underlying gastrointestinal disease may demand urgent or emergent operative repair. Subsequent surgical management of IF/SBS alters the bowel physically to effect improvement in bowel function or to address complications. Reestablishment of intestinal continuity, relief of strictures (stricturoplasty), resections employing serosal patches, and bowel tapering for reestablishment of normal intestinal caliber (tapering enteroplasty) are essential surgical tools designed to repair common intestinal complications while preserving intestinal length. These techniques are considered standard of care.[232]

Surgery may also assuage intestinal pathophysiology by altering normal intestine. Patients with SBS may have malabsorption of nutrients and electrolytes because of insufficient contact time with intestinal mucosa. Intestinal valves using sutures or synthetic material, denervation of intestinal segments, and intussusception of intestinal loops have been attempted in animals, but there is minimal published clinical data to support their use in increasing transit time.[12] Segments of intestine may be reversed, which create antiperistaltic "valves" that slow transit enough to improve absorption.[233,235] Colon segments have been transposed into small intestine for similar reasons, in either iso- or antiperistaltic fashion.[234,236] These techniques have not gained wide acceptance because short and dilated intestine would not be well-suited for this approach, reversal segment length choice is unclear, and disrupting normal bowel continuity is counterintuitive.

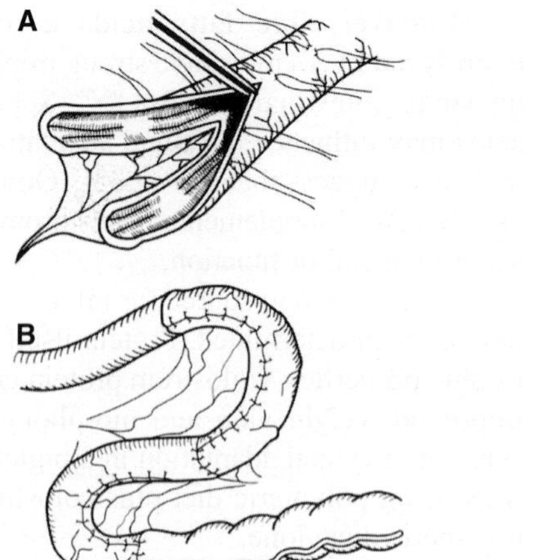

Figure 4 Longitudinal intestinal lengthening and tailoring. (A) Depiction of the separation of two leaflets of mesentery each attached to longitudinally split piece of small intestine. (B) Final results after each piece of intestine sewed together longitudinally, and then end-to-end anastamosis made in series. (Reproduced with permission from Bianchi A.[244])

Longitudinal intestinal lengthening and tailoring (LILT) (Figure 4) and serial transverse enteroplasty (STEP) (Figure 5) represent advanced techniques that at once taper dilated segments of bowel and increase intestinal length. Digestive function may improve not only because aboral flow is facilitated by the normal caliber lumen, but also because subsequent adaptation may lead to increased intestinal surface area.

LILT was first described in 1980 by Bianchi[237] and has since been used at many centers.[12] The technique involves separating the leaflets of mesentery, preserving the segmental blood supply to each side of the intestine. The intestine is then split longitudinally, maintaining the blood supply to each half. Two lumens are formed by closing the halves along the longitudinal axis, finally forming an end-to-end anastamosis in isoperistaltic fashion. The resultant bowel is half diameter and up to twice as long. Data regarding efficacy come from retrospective and prospective observation case series. A recent review of 19 pediatric IF patients (mean age at procedure 1.62 years ± 1.62; mean follow-up period 7.74 years ± 4.75) receiving LILT between 1984 to 2004 found that 79% were living, 60% were sent for intestinal transplantation, and 44% were able to completely wean from TPN after LILT. Nearly half of the patients completely weaned from TPN require supplemental IV fluids, and bowel dilation in the LILT segment was common.[238] Earlier Weber[239] described his experience with 16 children (age range 3 months to 14 years) who received LILT in an 8-year-period of time. By 12 months post-procedure, 14 of 16 (88%) were receiving all nutrition enterally. High[240,241] and modest[242,243] success rates with LILT have been the norm. Standardized indications, contraindications, and surgical guidelines have not been developed, which may explain inconsistent

Table 6 Enteral Advancement Methodology

A. Feeding initiation
Audible bowel sounds?
Functioning ostomy (if applicable)?
No contraindications?*
No, then continue IVF/PN/NPO
Yes, then start feeds (NG/NJ/G-tube/J-tube)
Day 1: breastmilk (full strength) or formula (20 cal/oz) @ 10–20 ml/kg/d continuously† ×24 h

B. Feeding advancement
Principle 1: quantify feeding intolerance primarily by stool or ostomy output and secondarily by reducing substances. Reducing substances should be measured twice daily. Persistent vomiting may also be indication of intolerance
Principle 2: tolerance assessed no more than twice per 24 h. No more than one advance per 24 h period
Principle 3: ultimate goals: 150–200 mL/kg/d, 100–140 kcal/kg/d
Principle 4: if ostomy/stool output precludes advancement at 20 cal/oz for 7 d, then increasing caloric density of the formula can be performed.
Principle 5: isocaloric reductions in PN support should be undertaken simultaneous with feeding advancement.

1. Stool output	
If $<$ 10 g/kg/d or $<$10 stools/d	advance rate by 10–20 mL/kg/d
If 10–20 g/kg/d or 10–12 stools/d	no change
If $>$20 g/kg/d or $>$12 stools/d	reduce rate or hold feeds‡
2. Ileostomy output	
If $<$2 g/kg/h	advance rate by 10–20 mL/kg/d
If 2–3 g/kg/h	no change
If $>$3 g/kg/h	reduce rate or hold feeds‡
3. Stool reducing substances	
If $<$1%	advance feeds per stool or ostomy output
If $=$1%	no change
If $>$1%	reduce rate or hold feeds‡

Reproduced with permission from Kamin D and Duggan C.[8]
PN = parenteral nutrition.
*Contraindications to enteral feeding: (1) paralytic or drug-induced ileus; (2) grossly bloody stools or ostomy output and/or radiological changes of intestinal ischemia; (3) shock/poor perfusion due to cardiac or respiratory insufficiency; (4) bilious and/or persistent vomiting (defined as more than three episodes of emesis in 12 hour); (5) clinical suspicion of obstruction or ileus (severe abdominal distension, decreased ostomy or stool output, and/or radiologic changes of obstruction or ileus); (6) electrolyte instability; (7) ostomy or stool volumes $>$3 mL/kg/h.
†Oral feeds may only be offered as follows: (1) infant is developmentally able to feed by mouth (po); (2) *one hour's* worth of continuous feeds may be offered PO QD-TID after 5 days of continuous feeds. During this time, tube feeds should be held; (3) *more than 1 hour's* worth of continuous feeds may be offered PO once the infant has reached full volume of feeds by continuous route *or* at least 7 days have passed on the feeding advancement protocol.
‡Feeds should generally be held for 8 hour, then restarted at three-fourth of the previous rate.

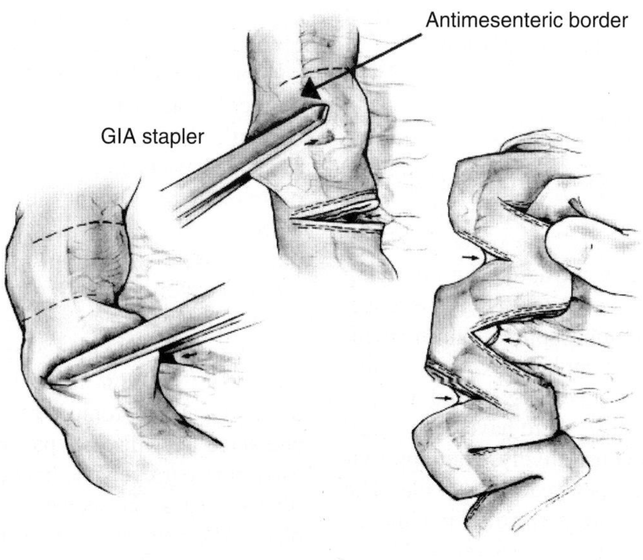

Figure 5 Depiction of surgical technique used to perform serial transverse enteroplasty (STEP). (Reproduced with permission from Javid PJ et al.[307])

results reported in literature.[244] Complications such as anastamotic leaking, obstruction, and dilatation are not rare, and lead to significant ongoing morbidity or mortality.[241] Criteria for LILT vary but generally require greater than 20 cm of symetrically dilated intestine in the context of residual intestine >40 cm.[12]

STEP involves the application of a staple gun incompletely across the intestine, on opposite sides in serial fashion, creating a "zig-zag" pattern that results in a lumen both narrower and longer. Since its description by Kim and colleagues[245] in 2003, it has become an excepted technique at many IF centers. Potential advantages over LILT include no enterotomies, the ability to modulate lumen diameter based on the density of staple firings, and the feasibility even if intestinal dilation is in unusual locations or dilation is not of uniform caliber.[42] A STEP registry recently prospectively characterized the pooled experience with the procedure from 19 centers in 3 different countries between September 2004 and April 2006.[246] Thirty-eight patients (mean age 1.3 years) underwent STEP (29 primary indication SBS) with median follow-up of 12.6 months. Survival was 92%. Ten of the 29 (34%) SBS patients have been completely weaned off of TPN, and the average percentage of total calories supplied enterally increased from 31 to 67%. Complications were noted in 5 patients, none of which led to long-term sequelae. Three deaths were from sepsis in the context of progressive liver failure. Nine patients included in the Registry underwent STEP for bacterial overgrowth ($n = 6$) and neonatal bowel repair ($n = 3$), and results were generally encouraging, consistent with recent published case reports.[247,248] "Re-STEP" also appears feasible.[249] Longer term follow-up will be critical.

The nature of and mechanisms for specific physiologic adaptations have not been well characterized in SBS. Intestine subjected to lengthening procedures has only rarely been studied in this manner.[239] A recent study investigated mechanisms in young pigs ($n = 10$) who received 90% intestinal resections, half of whom had STEP to remaining bowel.[42] After 6 weeks on oral diet, STEP animals showed improved *D*-xylose absorption, higher serum citrulline levels (a biomarker for intestinal mass), and no gram-negative bacterial overgrowth. The impact of nontransplant surgery on intestinal motility, mucosal immune/barrier function, and gastroendocrine function is not known.

Long-term Outcomes

Quality of life (QOL), mortality, and morbidity have all been characterized in patients with IF, but, generally speaking, the retrospective nature of ascertainment and single center experiences have limited the ability to apply findings confidently to individual patients.

QOL has been assessed mostly in adults. Not surprisingly, scoring on QOL tests are usually lowest during the first year on chronic PN, especially if before acquisition of IF the patient had been healthy, for example, mesenteric infarction. QOL slowly improves over the next year, leveling off at 60 to 70 (100 is "best quality of life") after 5 years of PN.[250] Factors associated with more favorable QOL include strong self-esteem in the patient and good family support.[251] Moreover, participation in strong peer support networks is associated with reduced incidence of sepsis and depression.[252] Personal stories demonstrating the possibility for meaningful life on chronic PN[253] imbue these statistics with meaning.

Pironi and colleagues[254] recently compared health-related QOL (using the SF-36 questionnaire) between adult patients on stable chronic PN ($n = 18$) and those with intestinal transplants ($n = 12$). The results were nearly equivalent, with the exception of subjective physical health, which was significantly higher in the transplant group because of less body pain. If long-term outcomes after intestinal transplantation continue to improve (see below), larger QOL studies that can confirm these findings may broaden the indications for intestinal transplantation beyond life-threatening complications associated with failing PN. Gottrand and colleagues conducted a cross-sectional, national, multicenter QOL survey of children and adolescents on home parenteral nutrition because of digestive disease.[255] Of the 104 eligible patients, 72 (70%) agreed to participate. QOL was high at all ages and comparable to scores from a healthy pediatric reference population. QOL was significantly impaired in parents, especially mothers, and in adolescents with ileostomies. This study suggests that children with IF on home PN cope reasonably well, whereas parents perceive their own lives as significantly limited because of their children's illnesses.

The growth pattern in children on chronic PN for gastrointestinal disorders can be favorable, but may be difficult to consistently achieve. Colomb and colleagues[256] examined school-age girls and boys ($n = 16$) on home PN for an average of 10 years. Only four subjects had consistently normal weight and height, velocities, while the others had fluctuating periods of regular (velocity >50%) and slow (velocity <25%) growth, not necessarily associated with illness. Analysis did suggest that inadequate nitrogen provision was closely associated with these periods of slower growth. Consistent with earlier reports[257] normal growth can be achieved on PN, but careful and repeated evaluation and biochemical monitoring is essential.

It is critical to confirm that normal growth can be maintained once PN and/or artificial nutrition is weaned. Goulet and colleagues[109] reviewed all cases ($n = 87$) of neonatal SBS at their institution born between 1975 and 1991, who had been followed for an average of 15 years. The subgroup that had weaned from artificial nutrition (parenteral and enteral) grew up with normal puberty and achievement of expected height based on the parents. Gonzalez and colleagues[258] evaluated 10 children in cross-sectional fashion with history of SBS (mean age 7.4 years; range 3 to 12 years) who had been off PN for at least 2 years. Eight children had normal weight for height, although height-for-age was low in 5 children who had SBS in early life. The values were not adjusted for parental height. Body fat mass calculated from anthropometric measures was low in 5 subjects. These data are motivation enough for all patients with a history of IF to be followed prospectively; publications based on prospectively obtained data will be instrumental for assessing nutritional outcomes in this population.

Cognitive development and outcomes have been sporadically studied in infants and children on long-term PN. It is difficult to separate the affect of the artificial nutrition from that of the underlying illness. Ralston and colleagues[259] examined a group of nine infants who were receiving home PN through to age 3 years. While somatic growth was normal by 2 years of age, neurocognitive development in two patients worsened inexplicably to "mildly retarded" at 3 years of age, while for the others development appeared normal. More recently, Beers and colleagues[260] performed detailed neuropsychiatric testing in eight school-age patients with SBS, comparing results to eight patients with cystic fibrosis. Specific deficits were noted in visual-spatial performance, including left but not right-sided upper extremity deficits in dexterity and psychomotor speed. The authors suggest that right-hemispheric central nervous system impairments may be present in patients with SBS. Earlier work also suggested the same pattern of deficits.[261] Studied confirming and/or extending these findings have not been published.

Mortality for patients with IF on home PN is of particular interest, because decisions with respect to referring for intestinal transplant depend heavily on comparative mortality. Most data are derived from retrospective chart reviews of patients treated over a span of many years. Adult studies suggest that deaths are typically unrelated directly to PN, such as line sepsis or decompensated cirrhosis. Messing and colleagues[107] studied 124 adults with SBS diagnosed between 1980 and 1992 and found that end enterostomy and residual bowel length <50 cm were independent predictors of mortality, not PN dependence. Mortality was 86 and 49% after 2 and 5 years of PN dependence, respectively. More recently, Lloyd and colleagues[262] shared there experience with IF spanning 1979 to 2003 in 188 patients, reporting mortality rates of 96, 77, 73, and 71% after 1, 3, 5, and 10 years on PN respectively. Importantly, most deaths were due to complications from primary disease; only 9% could be attributed to complications from PN. These data suggest that unless the primary disease itself carries a grave prognosis, home PN has superior outcomes as compared to intestinal transplantation (see below).

In contrast, it appears that mortality in infants and children with IF may be more attributable to complications from PN. Colomb and colleagues[263] reviewed their experience in Paris with 302 children on home PN between 1980 and 1999. Survival was 97, 89, 81, and 72% after 2, 5, 10, and 15 years on home PN. For children on home PN because of gastrointestinal disorders, half of deaths were attributable to PN complications such as liver disease or line sepsis, although only 9% (21 patients) of children with gastrointestinal diagnoses died during the study period. Earlier, Quiros-Tejeira and colleagues[108] found that early cholestasis was a strong predictor of mortality (cumulative survival 73%) in a retrospective review of 78 children diagnosed between 1975 and 2000 with SBS on chronic PN.

Wales and colleagues[18] conducted an unusually rigorous prospectives cohort study of 40 infants diagnosed between 1997 to 1998 with SBS on PN, comparing outcomes to a well-chosen group of infants with non-SBS surgical disorders. His findings were sobering, as fully 37% of SBS patients on PN died, usually of liver failure or sepsis, while only 13% of infants with non-SBS diagnoses died. These data indicate that a large minority of infants and children may do very poorly on chronic PN; predicting which children are at particular risk may lead to early referral for intestinal transplantation. Outcomes after intestinal transplant may thus be superior for select groups of infants and children (see below).

TRANSPLANTATION

Intestinal transplantation was introduced into clinical practice in 1989 with the advent of modern immunosuppressive agents. The purpose was to save the lives of children and adults with IF dying from complications related to PN. Experience, surgical technique, immunosuppression, and medical/nutritional management have evolved significantly since then, as have organ and patient survival. As of May 2007, there have been 1,720 intestinal transplants cumulatively, with approximately 150 performed per year worldwide. The majority of transplants are performed in children 28% <2 years, 31%> 2 and <18 years. [264] The cost of an intestinal transplant has been estimated to be $200,000 to $300,000[265] per patient, which is beyond the reach of most families. Medicare began covering intestinal transplantation in 2001[266] and most major instance companies have followed suit.

Indications

Because intestinal transplantation still has formidable immediate and long-term risks, strict criteria have been proposed[26,267] or even required by insurance companies.[268] Current consensus regards intestinal transplant as appropriate therapy for permanent IF when one or more of the following complications related to PN have occurred: (1) Serious liver disease, with evidence of portal hypertension and/or coagulopathy; (2) Thrombosis of major venous access points (>2 thrombosis in jugular, subclavian, or femoral veins); (3) Recurrent catheter-related sepsis events; and (4) Frequent hospitalizations caused by severe water and electrolyte abnormalities or surgical emergencies.[26] Common underlying conditions for patients receiving transplants are displayed in Table 7.

The definition of "permanent" is sometimes obvious. For instance, conditions such as severe congenital diarrhea from MVID, SBS with duodenocolic anastamosis, and extensive Hirshsprung's disease with minimal functional small intestine have been unequivocally associated with permanent IF. On the other hand, CIPOS and SBS that is less extensive may have rehabilitation potential that is more or less obvious depending on local experience and over time, as surgical and medical innovations evolve.

It would be best to evolve towards an objective score that uses clinical and biological data to predict survival on chronic PN.[270,271] Akin to model for end-stage liver disease, patients could be referred early before irreversible liver disease ensues and/or illness ensues that jeopardizes survival posttransplant. Alternatively, a valid scoring system would prevent premature or inappropriate referrals. Achieving this degree of sophistication is problematic, because intestinal transplantation is rare and the patient population is so heterogeneous.

Particular details and adherence to fulfilling transplant criteria may vary depending on organ availability and local experience. For instance, it may be appropriate to consider intestinal transplantation for a patient with CIPOS on chronic PN who, while not meeting any of the above criteria, has persistent medical and psychological problems that severely limits QOL and productivity. Alternatively, one could find motivation to list a patient with ultrashort SBS for isolated intestinal transplant who may not yet fulfill any of the criteria but for whom complications from PN are likely to develop in the future.[272]

Recently Pironi[273] surveyed all IF and intestinal transplant programs in Europe with the goal of identifying the number and nature of patients referred for transplant, as well as the reasons for doing so. Between January and March 2004, European IF centers were caring for 688 adult (>18 years) and 166 pediatric patients on PN for

Table 7 Indications for Intestinal Transplantation in Children and Adults, 1985–2007*

	Worldwide Cases, *N* (1,720 Patients)	
Underlying Diagnosis	Children, % of Worldwide Cases	Adults, % of Worldwide Cases
Short bowel syndrome	63	30
Gastroschisis	20	
Volvulus	17	7
Necrotizing enterocolitis	13	
Intestinal atresias	8	
Crohn's disease		12
Other	5	11
Motility	15	10
Agangionosis/Hirschsprung	7	
Pseudo-obstruction	8	
Microvillus inclusion disease	6	
Other causes	2	
Retransplant	8	7
Tumor	1	13
Trauma		9
Ischemia/thrombosis		24

*Adapted from Ruiz P, Kato T, and Tzakis A[269] and Intestinal Transplant Registry.[264]

nononcologic causes of chronic IF (SBS, chronic motility disorders, intestinal fistulas, and extensive mucosal diseases). Centers reported that 16% of adults and 34% of children were candidates for intestinal transplant. For adults, primary indication was failure of TPN (62%) while for pediatrics, underlying disease (eg, intractable diarrhea or ultrashort-segment SBS) accounted for the majority (60%). Very few patients were judged as needing "immediate" transplant (roughly 15% of adult and pediatric patients). While relatively few patients were being considered for transplant because of liver failure (22 adults and 7 children), less than half in each group were considered "immediate." While this study has flaws,[271] the findings suggest that "preemptive transplantation" is the predominant reason for referral in children, and that IF centers often consider transplant as a therapeutic option but uncommonly as an immediate therapy, even for those with significant liver disease. In the future, a robust model based on outcomes will hopefully make timing and reasons for referral equitable and consistent.

Graft Considerations

The intestine may be transplanted alone or in combination with other abdominal organs. Isolated intestinal transplantation (ITx) is performed when significant liver disease is not present. These grafts (usually entire jejunum and ileum) may include ileo-cecal valve and some amount of colon, but majority of transplants include only the small intestine. Living donor ITx can be performed,[274] in which a segment (approximately 200 cm) would be used.

Most pediatric intestinal transplants include the liver.[264] Modern techniques have evolved so that en bloc methods are used to implant the graft without having to do complex biliary and vascular anastamoses. Thus, when there is serious liver disease but normal function of stomach and duodenum, an en bloc organ unit composed of graft duodenum, pancreas, small intestine, and liver can be implanted after removal of native small LITx. The graft duodenum exists in addition to the native duodenum but serves only as a conduit for biliary secretions.

Multivisceral transplantation (MVTx) consists of removal and replacement of the entire foregut and midgut. The graft consists of stomach, duodenum, pancreas, jejunoileum, sometimes spleen, and most often the liver. This graft type would be reserved for patients with abdominal catastrophes so extensive that other graft types would be impossible or too difficult to implant. However, this graft-type has recently been used in younger patients who might only have needed LITx.[275] Advantages include more available space for placement of organs, and improved hemostasis. Coagulopathy and portal hypertension can cause major hemorrhage during native organ explantation. Bleeding can be effectively controlled by ligating the celiac and superior mesenteric arteries during surgery when hemorrhage is severe.[276] This necessitates full foregut removal as the blood supply has been severed; thus a MVTx is indicated to replace vital organs.

Children with SBS and significant liver disease have received isolated liver transplants. As mentioned above, significant liver disease may hamper intestinal adaptation, so that isolated liver transplant may allow for more complete adaptation and avoid the need to intestinal transplantation. Botha and colleagues[277] reported on their results in 23 children with SBS and end-stage liver disease who received isolated liver transplants between 1995 and 2004. Children were only evaluated if they had achieved at least 50% of calories enterally, were less than 2 years of age, and had no underlying intestinal disease. After a median follow-up of 54 months, 17 children were alive, 14 of whom had achieved full enteral autonomy at a median of 3 months post-transplantation. These results indicate that isolated liver transplant is feasible in this population, and given the lower immunosuppression required after isolated liver transplant, careful patient selection can lead to highly satisfactory outcomes.

Post-transplantation Management and Care

Care for pediatric intestinal transplant recipients is comprised of immunosuppression and allograft rejection monitoring, prevention or early detection and treatment of immune and nonimmune complications related to immunosuppression, infection prevention, prophylaxsis, and treatment and nutrition support. Aside from nutrition support, the other aspects of care are in principle identical to care for children with other solid organ transplants, and have been reviewed elsewhere.[278] There are no studies demonstrating superiority of any method of nutritional management postintestinal transplantation. What follows is an amalgam of personal experience and expert opinion deduced from informal communication at conferences and review of consensus statements.

PN is resumed usually in the first 1 to 2 days post-transplantation. Most transplant programs will introduce enteral fluids within 7 days of transplant, and usually sooner if recovery from surgery is demonstrable with good ileostomy output and bowel sounds.[278] Many centers will secure access into the upper graft with a gastro-jejunal tube, such that the tip of the feeding catheter lies well beyond the anastamosis and sits in the graft jejunum. Gastroparesis is expected after intestinal or MVTx, and recovery may take weeks. The jejunal access enables increasing EN in this context, so that full volume and calorie provision may be achieved enterally while the stomach and upper native intestine recover function. If gastric secretions are significantly bile tinged and pH is 5 or greater, some or all of the lost fluids can be "refed" into the jejunal port along with the EN. Without Surgical or medical complications, PN can typically be discontinued between 3 and 4 weeks after transplantation.

Hypoallergenic, MCT-oil supplemented formulas are considered standard for intestinal transplant recipients. These recommendations flow from suppositions that anticipated abnormal barrier function[279] and lack of physiologic lymphatic drainage may increase the chance of allergic sensitization and fat malabsorption, respectively. Maternal breast milk is rarely available by the time young children receive transplants, but administration of banked BM has not been well documented. Full strength feeds are usually commenced after 1 to 2 days of clear fluid administration. Advancement is homologous to standards set forth for children with SBS.

Transition to gastric or oral feeds is based on individual patient tolerance and clinical context. The nature and timing of the recommended foods varies considerably between transplant centers. For infants/young children, it may by prudent to avoid highly allergenic foods,[280] as symptoms of GI allergy may be confused with allograft rejection. Nevertheless, food avoidance may have no influence on whether patients ultimately develop allergy or not. Food allergies have developed after intestinal transplantation.[281,282] However, in addition to risk from abnormal mucosal barrier function, immunosuppression may also increase the potential for allergic responses to environmental stimuli.[283]

Some centers prefer that patients consume low-fat diets, as fat absorption is expected to be abnormal with disruption of lymphatic drainage and loss of neural input to exocrine pancreas. Mean coefficient of fat absorption was 86 ± 12% among 22 pediatric intestinal transplant recipients receiving full EN between 43 to 1,000 days post-transplantation.[284] Adequate vitamin E absorption could not be demonstrated until 4 months post-transplant. Individual case reports indicate that fat excretion normalizes by 6 months.[58,285] Finally, pancreatic insufficiency has not commonly developed in patients after MVTx.[286] Fat absorption may equally be a function of frequency and severity of infectious and immune complications. Thus, motivation for strict adherence to low-fat diet is likely less important than careful liberalization and monitoring for individual intolerance.

Similar to patients with SBS, sugar malabsorption can lead to osmotic diarrhea; most centers recommend that patients avoid excessive intake of fruit juices for instance. Sugar absorption has indirectly been evaluated by Kaufman and colleagues.[284] Disaccharidase activities were all within normal ranges from small intestinal mucosal biopsies obtained 15 to 412 days post-transplantation in 22 transplant recipients. Breath testing as a means of obtaining a functional index of carbohydrate tolerance usually will not be helpful, because of lack of colon in continuity and bacterial overgrowth.

As with all immunocompromised patients, good food safety practices should be reviewed carefully and periodically with parents and patients to reduce the risk of food borne illnesses. Excellent resources are available[287] for seeking expert advise on this important subject.

Most intestinal transplant patients receive micronutrient supplements. Patients should receive supplemental fat-soluble vitamins, with attention also to zinc, calcium, magnesium, and iron status. Venick and colleagues[288] found in their cohort of

19 pediatric intestinal transplant recipients who survived greater than 6 months posttransplant that 4 had laboratory evidence of essential fatty acid deficiency, and 17 with zinc deficiency. Iron deficiency was also common. Laboratory monitoring for fat-soluble vitamin, zinc, and iron deficiency should occur two times per year unless clinical context warrants more frequent testing.

Bone density will likely be abnormal in intestinal transplant patients for multiple reasons. One published case report[289] noted low bone density in the femur and femur neck of a pediatric patient who received a living donor graft from an identical twin. Annual bone density scans with appropriate bone-age, size, and sex standards may be prudent, although vigilance with regard to adequate calcium and vitamin D nutriture is appropriate in all cases.

"Functional foods," or nutrients that are beneficial to a bodily structure or function beyond mere caloric value, have not been evaluated clinically. Rodent work suggests that glutamine supplementation enterally[290,291] or parenterally[292] enhances restoration of normal mucosal architecture following intestinal transplantation, which may decrease bacterial translocation as determined by bacterial counts in mesenteric lymph node samples. Preservation injury may also be prevented by administering glutamine to the donor prior to removal of the organ.[293] Omega-3 fatty acids may exert an immunomodulatory affect at the mucosa[294,295] and small vessel[296] level to promote allograft function and prevent allograft vasculopathy. Concern exists with regard to giving probiotics to transplant patients, because immunocompromised patients or premature neonates make up the majority of cases of bacteremia with probiotics in the literature. A mouse study looking at acute graft versus host disease of the bowel found that administration of *Lactobacillus rhamnosus* GG was associated with reduced severity and frequency of graft versus host disease, as well as reduced bacterial translocation assessed in the mesenteric lymph nodes.[297] Well-designed multi-institutional studies could investigate whether these "nutrients" are beneficial in human intestinal transplant recipients.

Because intestinal rejection causes significant organ dysfunction and increases the likelihood for bacterial translocation and sepsis, resumption of PN is not uncommon especially during moderate or severe episodes of rejection. Severe acute cellular rejection may result in loss of the intestinal graft, which would necessitate resuming lifelong PN unless another transplant is attempted. Chronic intestinal rejection results in the slow but progressive and irreversible loss of graft function, and ultimately leads to requirement for long-term PN as well. Venous access may be challenging,[298] and invasive measures may be required to maintain access because of stenosis and collateralization of the usual large venous structures.

Outcomes

In the 1990s, graft and patient survival after intestinal transplantation were poor, with patient survival rates less than 50 and 40% at 1 and 3 years posttransplantation, respectively.[299] However, beginning in 2002 to 2003, overlapping with the usage of lymphocyte depleting agents for induction, survival rates improved markedly. In experienced hands, some centers are reporting 1 and 3 year patient survivals of greater than 85%.[300] Patient survival between 2002 and 2007, based on survey data collected by the intestinal transplant registry, is depicted graphically in Figure 6. Univariate positive predictors of graft and patient survival included home location at time of organ offer, and first transplant.[264, 301] Important nonsignificant predictors were recipient age, gender, underlying diagnosis, and graft type. Nutritional status was not considered. Unfortunately, 5-year and longer patient and graft survival rates remain low (see Figure 7),[264] Opportunistic infections, sepsis, malignancy, and chronic rejection account for the majority of graft and life loss, similar to recipients of other solid organs.

QOL after intestinal transplantation in children appears favorable, although small sample size and/or nonideal study design render conclusions preliminary. International transplant registry results found that for 334 pediatric recipients surviving >6 months, modified Karnofsky scores were 90 to 100% in approximately 80% of recipients, comparing favorably with results from the adult sample.[264] Sudan and colleagues[302] administered the validated child health questionnaire to 29 pediatric intestinal transplant recipients (at least 1 year post-transplantation) and their parents. Comparison was made to published norms for healthy children. Intestinal recipients (average 5 years post-transplant; mean 11 years of age) rated QOL the same as healthy children in all domains. Prospective analysis of QOL in 46 consecutive adult intestinal transplant recipients[303] has demonstrated significant and durable improvement in multiple QOL measures 6 months, 1, and 2 years post-transplantation as compared to results pretransplantation, and all recipients were eventually free of parenteral and enteral support (average 22 and 83 days respectively). In summary, it appears QOL

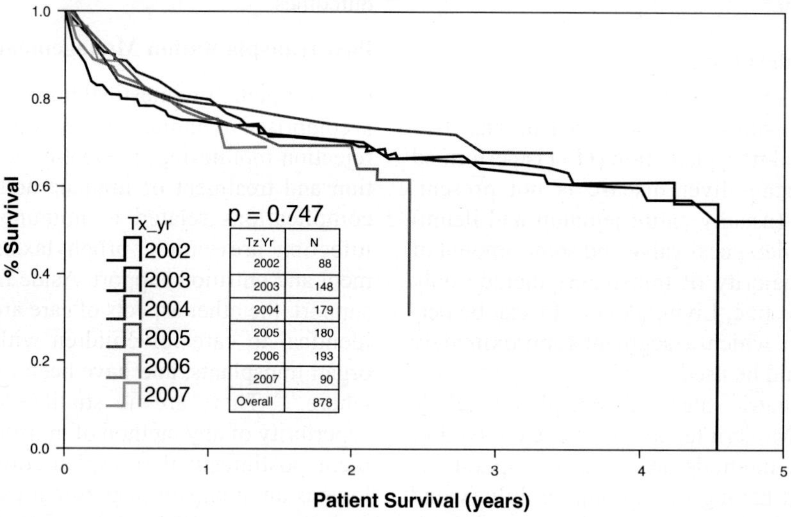

Figure 6 Patient survival after intestinal transplantation by year of transplant 2002–2007. (Adapted with permission from the Intestinal Transplant Registry.[264])

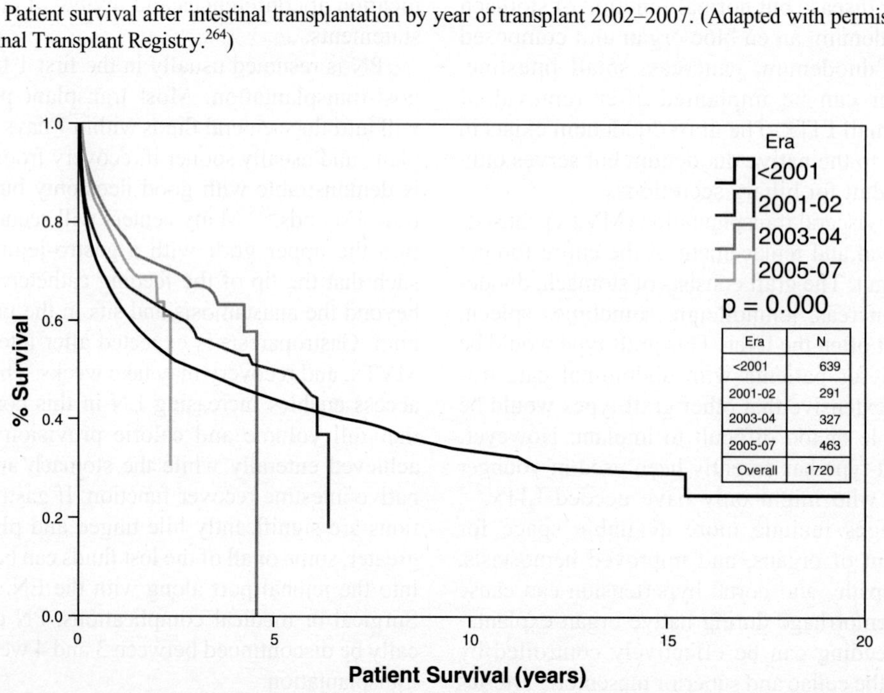

Figure 7 Long-term patient survival after intestinal transplantation. (Adapted with permission from the Intestinal Transplant Registry.[264])

Table 8 Growth Parameters in Children After Intestinal Transplantation

	Nucci et al[282]	Venick et al[288]	Rivas et al[304]	Iyer et al[305]	Lacaille et al[306]
N (at time of transplant)	24	19	23	46	31
Median age, years (range)	3.2 (0.7–17.4)	2.9	1.1	3.7 (0.4–16.6)	5.0 (0.4–13)
Mean height *Z*-score					
Transplant	−1.9	−2.8	−3.8	−1.9	−1.2
One-year posttransplant	−2.4*	−2.2	NA	−1.9	−1.3
Two-year posttransplant	−1.8	−2.0*	−2.2	−2.0	−1.2
Mean weight *Z*-score					
Transplant	−0.7	−1.0	−2.3	−0.8	−0.2
One-year posttransplant	−1.0	−0.2	NA	−0.8	+0.1
Two-year posttransplant	−1.0	−0.3	−1.0	−0.8	+0.3

NA = not available.
*Significantly different from transplant, $p \leq .04$.

is well-preserved in patients that are doing well posttransplantation. Should these results be confirmed, with respect to permanent IF, intestinal transplantation may soon be considered an alternative to chronic PN, provided that long-term transplant morbidity and mortality also show improvement.[272]

Nutritional outcomes following intestinal transplantation and predictors thereof have not yet been well-characterized. Until recently, survival limited interest and ability to identify relationships and trends. Five centers have published growth outcomes after intestinal transplantation, as displayed in Table 8. It is expected that at transplant many patients would be stunted and underweight. Posttransplantation, improvements in Z-scores can be appreciated but it is not yet clear whether and how much length/height "catch-up" growth can be achieved. Rigorous prospective assessment controlling for bone-age and parental height will be essential. Predictors of growth might be expected to be the number and severity of infections and rejection, as well as exposure to steroids. However, at least one publication was unable to show this, although power was limited by the sample size.

CONCLUDING REMARKS

IF is a debilitating, life-threatening condition that predisposes children to develop significant medical, nutritional, and psychological disorders. Repair and rehabilitation require intimate knowledge of the process of intestinal adaptation, the nutritional principles guiding management of IV support for children of all ages (Chapter 69, "Parenteral Nutrition"), and vigilance for medical and nutritional complications associated with IF. Medical and surgical innovations have changed the therapeutic landscape for children with IF, while early and persistent EN remains a cornerstone of therapy. Intestinal transplantation has become a viable treatment option when PN fails, and may become an alternative to chronic PN for patients with IF. Patients with intestinal transplants have different but nevertheless significant nutritional needs posttransplantation, demanding ongoing monitoring and repair of abnormal growth and micronutrient deficiencies. In the future, "immunonutrition" will combine the goals of graft tolerance and nutrition support, with the prospect for withdrawal of traditional medications that negatively affect growth, glucose homeostasis, and cardiovascular health.

REFERENCES

1. Wu G. Synthesis of citrulline and arginine from proline in enterocytes of postnatal pigs. Am J Physiol 1997;272:G1382–90.
2. Crenn P, Vahedi K, Lavergne-Slove A, et al. Plasma citrulline: A marker of enterocyte mass in villous atrophy-associated small bowel disease. Gastroenterology 2003;124:1210–9.
3. Crenn P, Coudray-Lucas C, Thuillier F, et al. Postabsorptive plasma citrulline concentration is a marker of absorptive enterocyte mass and intestinal failure in humans. Gastroenterology 2000;119:1496–505.
4. Jianfeng G, Weiming Z, Ning L, et al. Serum citrulline is a simple quantitative marker for small intestinal enterocytes mass and absorption function in short bowel patients. J Surg Res 2005;127:177–82.
5. Rhoads JM, Plunkett E, Galanko J, et al. Serum citrulline levels correlate with enteral tolerance and bowel length in infants with short bowel syndrome. J Pediatr 2005;146:542–7.
6. Luo M, Fernandez-Estivariz C, Manatunga AK, et al. Are plasma citrulline and glutamine biomarkers of intestinal absorptive function in patients with short bowel syndrome? JPEN J Parenter Enteral Nutr 2007;31:1–7.
7. O'Keefe SJ, Buchman AL, Fishbein TM, et al. Short bowel syndrome and intestinal failure: Consensus definitions and overview. Clin Gastroenterol Hepatol 2006;4:6–10.
8. Kamin D, Duggan C. Enteral support for children with intestinal failure. In: Langnas A, Goulet O, Quigley E, Tappenden K, editors. Intestinal Failure: Diagnosis, Management and Transplantation. Malden: Blackwell Publishing; 2007.
9. Ruemmele FM, Schmitz J, Goulet O. Microvillous inclusion disease (microvillous atrophy). Orphanet J Rare Dis 2006;1:22.
10. Goulet O, Salomon J, Ruemmele F, et al. Intestinal epithelial dysplasia (tufting enteropathy). Orphanet J Rare Dis 2007;2:20.
11. Cameron DJ, Barnes GL. Successful pregnancy outcome in tufting enteropathy. J Pediatr Gastroenterol Nutr 2003;36:158.
12. Goulet O, Ruemmele F, Lacaille F, et al. Irreversible intestinal failure. J Pediatr Gastroenterol Nutr 2004;38:250–69.
13. Stanghellini V, Cogliandro RF, de Giorgio R, et al. Chronic Intestinal pseudobstruction: Manifestations, natural history and management. Neurogastroenterol Motil 2007;19:440–52.
14. Howard L, Ament M, Fleming CR, et al. Current use and clinical outcome of home parenteral and enteral nutrition therapies in the United States. Gastroenterology 1995;109:355–65.
15. Van Gossum A, Vahedi K, Abdel M, et al. Clinical, social and rehabilitation status of long-term home parenteral nutrition patients: Results of a European multicentre survey. Clin Nutr 2001;20:205–10.
16. Pironi L, Candusso M, Biondo A, et al. Prevalence of home artificial nutrition in Italy in 2005: A survey by the Italian Society for Parenteral and Enteral Nutrition (SINPE). Clin Nutr 2006;26:123–132.
17. Andorsky DJ, Lund DP, Lillehei CW, et al. Nutritional and other postoperative management of neonates with short bowel syndrome correlates with clinical outcomes. J Pediatr 2001;139:27–33.
18. Wales PW, de Silva N, Kim JH, et al. Neonatal short bowel syndrome: A cohort study. J Pediatr Surg 2005;40:755–62.
19. Goulet O, Sauvat F Short bowel syndrome and intestinal transplantation in children. Curr Opin Clin Nutr Metab Care 2006;9:304–13.
20. Touloukian RJ, Smith GJ. Normal intestinal length in preterm infants. J Pediatr Surg 1983;18:720–3.
21. Siebert JR. Small-intestine length in infants and children. Am J Dis Child 1980;134:593–5.
22. Nightingale J, Woodward JM. Guidelines for management of patients with a short bowel. Gut 2006;55:iv1–12.
23. Reiquam CW, Allen RP, Akers DR. Normal and abnormal small bowel lengths: An analysis of 389 autopsy cases in infants and children. Am J Dis Child 1965;109:447–51.
24. Senn N. An experimental contribution to intestinal surgery with special reference to the treatment of intestinal obstruction. Ann Surg 1888;7:99–115.
25. Flint J. The effect of extensive resections of the small intestine. Bull Johns Hopkins Hosp 1912;23:127–44.
26. American Gastroenterological Association. Medical position statement: Short bowel syndrome and intestinal transplantation. Gastroenterology 2003;124:1105–10.
27. Vanderhoof JA, Langnas AN. Short-bowel syndrome in children and adults. Gastroenterology 1997;113:1767–78.
28. Nightingale JM, Lennard-Jones JE, Gertner DJ, et al. Colonic preservation reduces need for parenteral therapy, increases incidence of renal stones, but does not change high prevalence of gall stones in patients with a short bowel. Gut 1992;33:1493–7.
29. Nygaard K. Resection of the small intestine in rats. 3. Morphological changes in the intestinal tract. Acta Chir Scand 1967;133:233–48.
30. Sigalet DL, Lees GM, Aherne F, et al. The physiology of adaptation to small bowel resection in the pig: An integrated study of morphological and functional changes. J Pediatr Surg 1990;25:650–7.
31. O'Connor TP, Lam MM, Diamond J. Magnitude of functional adaptation after intestinal resection. Am J Physiol 1999;276:R1265–75.
32. Haxhija EQ, Yang H, Spencer AU, et al. Influence of the site of small bowel resection on intestinal epithelial cell apoptosis. Pediatr Surg Int 2006;22:37–42.
33. Weale AR, Edwards AG, Bailey M, et al. Intestinal adaptation after massive intestinal resection. Postgrad Med J 2005;81:178–84.
34. Hanson WR, Osborne JW, Sharp JG. Compensation by the residual intestine after intestinal resection in the rat. I. Influence of amount of tissue removed. Gastroenterology 1977;72:692–700.
35. Dowling RH, Booth CC. Structural and functional changes following small intestinal resection in the rat. Clin Sci 1967;32:139–49.
36. Booth CC, Evans KT, Menzies T, et al. Intestinal hypertrophy following partial resection of the small bowel in the rat. Br J Surg 1959;46:403–10.
37. Helmrath MA, Erwin CR, Shin CE, et al. Enterocyte apoptosis is increased following small bowel resection. J Gastrointest Surg 1998;2:44–9.
38. Haxhija EQ, Yang H, Spencer AU, et al. Intestinal epithelial cell proliferation is dependent on the site of massive small bowel resection. Pediatr Surg Int 2007;23:379–90.
39. Tavakkolizadeh A, Whang EE. Understanding and augmenting human intestinal adaptation: A call for more clinical research. JPEN J Parenter Enteral Nutr 2002;26:251–5.
40. Lauronen J, Pakarinen MP, Kuusanmaki P, et al. Intestinal adaptation after massive proximal small-bowel resection in the pig. Scand J Gastroenterol 1998;33:152–8.
41. Heemskerk VH, van Heurn LW, Farla P, et al. A successful short-bowel syndrome model in neonatal piglets. J Pediatr Gastroenterol Nutr 1999;29:457–61.
42. Chang RW, Javid PJ, Oh JT, et al. Serial transverse enteroplasty enhances intestinal function in a model of short bowel syndrome. Ann Surg 2006;243:223–8.
43. Nagy ES, Paris MC, Taylor RG, et al. Colostrum protein concentrate enhances intestinal adaptation after massive small bowel resection in juvenile pigs. J Pediatr Gastroenterol Nutr 2004;39:487–92.
44. Weinstein LD, Shoemaker CP, Hersh T, et al. Enhanced intestinal absorption after small bowel resection in man. Arch Surg 1969;99:560–2.
45. Pullan JM. Massive intestinal resection. Proc R Soc Med 1959;52:31–7.
46. Porus RL. Epithelial hyperplasia following massive small bowel resection in man. Gastroenterology 1965;48:753–7.
47. Pironi L, Paganelli GM, Miglioli M, et al. Morphologic and cytoproliferative patterns of duodenal mucosa in two patients after long-term total parenteral nutrition: Changes with oral refeeding and relation to intestinal resection. JPEN J Parenter Enteral Nutr 1994;18:351–4.
48. Jao W, Sileri P, Holaysan J, et al. Morphologic adaptation following segmental living related intestinal transplantation. Transplant Proc 2002;34:924.
49. Hines OJ, Bilchik AJ, Zinner MJ, et al. Adaptation of the Na^+/glucose cotransporter following intestinal resection. J Surg Res 1994;57:22–7.
50. Helliwell PA, Richardson M, Affleck J, et al. Regulation of GLUT5, GLUT2 and intestinal brush-border fructose

absorption by the extracellular signal-regulated kinase, p38 mitogen-activated kinase and phosphatidylinositol 3-kinase intracellular signalling pathways: Implications for adaptation to diabetes. Biochem J 2000;350:163–9.
51. Keelan M, Walker K, Thomson AB. Resection of rabbit ileum: Effect on brush border membrane enzyme markers and lipids. Can J Physiol Pharmacol 1985;63:1528–32.
52. Thomson AB. Resection of rabbit ileum: Effect on jejunal structure and carrier-mediated and passive uptake. Q J Exp Physiol 1986;71:29–46.
53. Thomson AB, McIntyre Y, MacLeod J, et al. Dietary fat content influences uptake of hexoses and lipids into rabbit jejunum following ileal resection. Digestion 1986;35:78–88.
54. O'Connor TP, Lam MM, Diamond J. Magnitude of functional adaptation after intestinal resection. Am J Physiol 1999;276:R1265–75.
55. Althausen TL, Doig RK, Uyeyama K, et al. Digestion and absorption after massive resection of the small intestine. II. Recovery of the absorptive function as shown by intestinal absorption tests in two patients and a consideration of compensatory mechanisms. Gastroenterology 1950;16:126–39.
56. Fallingborg J, Pedersen P, Jacobsen BA. Small intestinal transit time and intraluminal pH in ileocecal resected patients with Crohn's disease. Dig Dis Sci 1998;43:702–5.
57. Neal DE, Williams NS, Barker MC, et al. The effect of resection of the distal ileum on gastric emptying, small bowel transit and absorption after proctocolectomy. Br J Surg 1984;71:666–70.
58. Benedetti E, Baum C, Cicalese L, et al. Progressive functional adaptation of segmental bowel graft from living related donor. Transplantation 2001;71:569–71.
59. Ziegler TR, Fernandez-Estivariz C, Gu LH, et al. Distribution of the H+/peptide transporter PepT1 in human intestine: Up-regulated expression in the colonic mucosa of patients with short-bowel syndrome. Am J Clin Nutr 2002;75:922–30.
60. Gouttebel MC, Saint Aubert B, Colette C, et al. Intestinal adaptation in patients with short bowel syndrome. Measurement by calcium absorption. Dig Dis Sci 1989;34:709–15.
61. Erwin CR, Falcone RA, Jr, Stern LE, et al. Analysis of intestinal adaptation gene expression by cDNA expression arrays. JPEN J Parenter Enteral Nutr 2000;24:311–6.
62. Stern LE, Erwin CR, Falcone RA, et al. cDNA microarray analysis of adapting bowel after intestinal resection. J Pediatr Surg 2001;36:190–5.
63. Dodson BD, Wang JL, Swietlicki EA, et al. Analysis of cloned cDNAs differentially expressed in adapting remnant small intestine after partial resection. Am J Physiol 1996;271:G347–56.
64. Menge H, Robinson JW. Functional and structural characteristics of the rat intestinal mucosa following ileo-jejunal transposition. Acta Hepatogastroenterol (Stuttg) 1978;25:150–4.
65. Altmann GG. Influence of bile and pancreatic secretions on the size of the intestinal villi in the rat. Am J Anat 1971;132:167–77.
66. Dworkin LD, Levine GM, Farber NJ, et al. Small intestinal mass of the rat is partially determined by indirect effects of intraluminal nutrition. Gastroenterology 1976;71:626–30.
67. Williamson RC, Buchholtz TW, Malt RA. Humoral stimulation of cell proliferation in small bowel after transection and resection in rats. Gastroenterology 1978;75:249–54.
68. Jenkins AP, Thompson RP. Trophic effect of Efamol on the rat small-intestinal mucosa. Clin Sci (Lond) 1989;77:555–9.
69. Maxton DG, Cynk EU, Jenkins AP, Thompson RP. Effect of dietary fat on the small intestinal mucosa. Gut 1989;30:1252–5.
70. Vanderhoof JA, Blackwood DJ, Mohammadpour H, et al. Effect of dietary menhaden oil on normal growth and development and on ameliorating mucosal injury in rats. Am J Clin Nutr 1991;54:346–50.
71. Hart MH, Grandjean CJ, Park JH, et al. Essential fatty acid deficiency and postresection mucosal adaptation in the rat. Gastroenterology 1988;94:682–7.
72. Grey VL, Garofalo C, Greenberg GR, et al. The adaptation of the small intestine after resection in response to free fatty acids. Am J Clin Nutr 1984;40:1235–42.
73. Kollman KA, Lien EL, Vanderhoof JA. Dietary lipids influence intestinal adaptation after massive bowel resection. J Pediatr Gastroenterol Nutr 1999;28:41–5.
74. Sukhotnik I, Gork AS, Chen M, et al. Effect of a high fat diet on lipid absorption and fatty acid transport in a rat model of short bowel syndrome. Pediatr Surg Int 2003;19:385–90.
75. Shu R, David ES, Ferraris RP. Dietary fructose enhances intestinal fructose transport and GLUT5 expression in weaning rats. Am J Physiol 1997;272:G446–53.
76. Diamond JM, Karasov WH, Cary C, et al. Effect of dietary carbohydrate on monosaccharide uptake by mouse small intestine in vitro. J Physiol 1984;349:419–40.
77. Cheeseman CI, Harley B. Adaptation of glucose transport across rat enterocyte basolateral membrane in response to altered dietary carbohydrate intake. J Physiol 1991;437:563–75.
78. Ferraris RP, Diamond JM. Crypt/villus site of substrate-dependent regulation of mouse intestinal glucose transporters. Proc Natl Acad Sci U S A 1993;90:5868–72.
79. Weser E, Babbitt J, Hoban M, et al. Intestinal adaptation. Different growth responses to disaccharides compared with monosaccharides in rat small bowel. Gastroenterology 1986;91:1521–7.
80. Thomson AB, Keelan M, Clandinin MT. Feeding rats a diet enriched with saturated fatty acids prevents the inhibitory effects of acute and chronic ethanol exposure on the in vitro uptake of hexoses and lipids. Biochim Biophys Acta 1991;1084:122–8.
81. Brasitus TA, Dudeja PK, Bolt MJ, et al. Dietary triacylglycerol modulates sodium-dependent D-glucose transport, fluidity and fatty acid composition of rat small intestinal brush-border membrane. Biochim Biophys Acta 1989;979:177–86.
82. Karasov WH, Solberg DH, Diamond JM. Dependence of intestinal amino acid uptake on dietary protein or amino acid levels. Am J Physiol 1987;252:G614–25.
83. Vanderhoof JA, Grandjean CJ, Burkley KT, et al. Effect of casein versus casein hydrolysate on mucosal adaptation following massive bowel resection in infant rats. J Pediatr Gastroenterol Nutr 1984;3:262–7.
84. Duggan C, Gannon J, Walker WA. Protective nutrients and functional foods for the gastrointestinal tract. Am J Clin Nutr 2002;75:789–808.
85. Ziegler TR, Mantell MP, Chow JC, et al. Gut adaptation and the insulin-like growth factor system: Regulation by glutamine and IGF-I administration. Am J Physiol 1996;271:G866–75.
86. Wiren ME, Permert J, Skullman SP, et al. No differences in mucosal adaptive growth one week after intestinal resection in rats given enteral glutamine supplementation or deprived of glutamine. Eur J Surg 1996;162:489–98.
87. Duggan C, Stark AR, Auestad N, et al. Glutamine supplementation in infants with gastrointestinal disease: A randomized, placebo-controlled pilot trial. Nutrition 2004;20:752–6.
88. Albers MJ, Steyerberg EW, Hazebroek FW, et al. Glutamine supplementation of parenteral nutrition does not improve intestinal permeability, nitrogen balance, or outcome in newborns and infants undergoing digestive-tract surgery: Results from a double-blind, randomized, controlled trial. Ann Surg 2005;241:599–606.
89. Sukhotnik I, Mogilner JG, Lerner A, et al. Parenteral arginine impairs intestinal adaptation following massive small bowel resection in a rat model. Pediatr Surg Int 2005;21:460–5.
90. Roth JA, Frankel WL, Zhang W, et al. Pectin improves colonic function in rat short bowel syndrome. J Surg Res 1995;58:240–6.
91. Koruda MJ, Rolandelli RH, Settle RG, et al. The effect of a pectin-supplemented elemental diet on intestinal adaptation to massive small bowel resection. JPEN J Parenter Enteral Nutr 1986;10:343–50.
92. Royall D, Wolever TM, Jeejeebhoy KN. Evidence for colonic conservation of malabsorbed carbohydrate in short bowel syndrome. Am J Gastroenterol 1992;87:751–6.
93. Marsman KE, McBurney MI. Dietary fiber increases oxidative metabolism in colonocytes but not in distal small intestinal enterocytes isolated from rats. J Nutr 1995;125:273–82.
94. Koruda MJ, Rolandelli RH, Bliss DZ, et al. Parenteral nutrition supplemented with short-chain fatty acids: Effect on the small-bowel mucosa in normal rats. Am J Clin Nutr 1990;51:685–9.
95. Tappenden KA, Thomson AB, Wild GE, et al. Short-chain fatty acids increase proglucagon and ornithine decarboxylase messenger RNAs after intestinal resection in rats. JPEN J Parenter Enteral Nutr 1996;20:357–62.
96. Tappenden KA, Thomson AB, Wild GE, et al. Short-chain fatty acid-supplemented total parenteral nutrition enhances functional adaptation to intestinal resection in rats. Gastroenterology 1997;112:792–802.
97. Fukunaga T, Sasaki M, Araki Y, et al. Effects of the soluble fibre pectin on intestinal cell proliferation, fecal short chain fatty acid production and microbial population. Digestion 2003;67:42–9.
98. Tabor CW, Tabor H. 1,4-Diaminobutane (putrescine), spermidine, and spermine. Annu Rev Biochem 1976;45:285–306.
99. Uda K, Tsujikawa T, Ihara T, et al. Luminal polyamines upregulate transmural glucose transport in the rat small intestine. J Gastroenterol 2002;37:434–41.
100. Dumas F, De Bandt JP, Colomb V, et al. Enteral ornithine alpha-ketoglutarate enhances intestinal adaptation to massive resection in rats. Metabolism 1998;47:1366–71.
101. Raul F, Gosse F, Galluser M, et al. Functional and metabolic changes in intestinal mucosa of rats after enteral administration of ornithine alpha-ketoglutarate salt. JPEN J Parenter Enteral Nutr 1995;19:145–50.
102. Greene HL, McCabe DR, Merenstein GB. Protracted diarrhea and malnutrition in infancy: Changes in intestinal morphology and disaccharidase activities during treatment with total intravenous nutrition or oral elemental diets. J Pediatr 1975;87:695–704.
103. Orenstein SR. Enteral versus parenteral therapy for intractable diarrhea of infancy: A prospective, randomized trial. J Pediatr 1986;109:277–86.
104. Sondheimer JM, Cadnapaphornchai M, Sontag M, et al. Predicting the duration of dependence on parenteral nutrition after neonatal intestinal resection. J Pediatr 1998;132:80–4.
105. Wilmore DW. Factors correlating with a successful outcome following extensive intestinal resection in newborn infants. J Pediatr 1972;80:88–95.
106. Spencer AU, Neaga A, West B, et al. Pediatric short bowel syndrome: Redefining predictors of success. Ann Surg 2005;242:403–9; discussion 09–12.
107. Messing B, Crenn P, Beau P, et al. Long-term survival and parenteral nutrition dependence in adult patients with the short bowel syndrome. Gastroenterology 1999;117:1043–50.
108. Quiros-Tejeira RE, Ament ME, Reyen L, et al. Long-term parenteral nutritional support and intestinal adaptation in children with short bowel syndrome: A 25-year experience. J Pediatr 2004;145:157–63.
109. Goulet O, Baglin-Gobet S, Talbotec C, et al. Outcome and long-term growth after extensive small bowel resection in the neonatal period: A survey of 87 children. Eur J Pediatr Surg 2005;15:95–101.
110. Kurkchubasche AG, Rowe MI, Smith SD. Adaptation in short-bowel syndrome: Reassessing old limits. J Pediatr Surg 1993;28:1069–71.
111. Carbonnel F, Cosnes J, Chevret S, et al. The role of anatomic factors in nutritional autonomy after extensive small bowel resection. JPEN J Parenter Enteral Nutr 1996;20:275–80.
112. Thompson JS, Ferguson DC. Effect of the distal remnant on ileal adaptation. J Gastrointest Surg 2000;4:430–4.
113. De Francesco A, Malfi G, Delsedime L, et al. Histological findings regarding jejunal mucosa in short bowel syndrome. Transplant Proc 1994;26:1455–6.
114. Cisler JJ, Buchman AL. Intestinal adaptation in short bowel syndrome. J Investig Med 2005;53:402–13.
115. Lund PK. Molecular basis of intestinal adaptation: The role of the insulin-like growth factor system. Ann N Y Acad Sci 1998;859:18–36.
116. Taylor B, Murphy GM, Dowling RH. Pituitary hormones and the small bowel: Effect of hypophysectomy on intestinal adaptation to small bowel resection in the rat. Eur J Clin Invest 1979;9:115–27.
117. Ljungmann K, Grofte T, Kissmeyer-Nielsen P, et al. GH decreases hepatic amino acid degradation after small bowel resection in rats without enhancing bowel adaptation. Am J Physiol Gastrointest Liver Physiol 2000;279:G700–6.
118. Berni Canani R, Cirillo P, Mallardo G, et al. Growth hormone regulates intestinal ion transport through a modulation of the constitutive nitric oxide synthase-nitric oxide-cAMP pathway. World J Gastroenterol 2006;12:4710–5.
119. Gu Y, Wu ZH, Xie JX, et al. Effects of growth hormone (rhGH) and glutamine supplemented parenteral nutrition on intestinal adaptation in short bowel rats. Clin Nutr 2001;20:159–66.
120. Dowling RH. Cellular and molecular basis of intestinal and pancreatic adaptation. Scand J Gastroenterol Suppl 1992;193:64–7.
121. Jeppesen PB, Szkudlarek J, Hoy CE, et al. Effect of high-dose growth hormone and glutamine on body composition, urine creatinine excretion, fatty acid absorption, and essential fatty acids status in short bowel patients: A randomized, double-blind, crossover, placebo-controlled study. Scand J Gastroenterol 2001;36:48–54.
122. Scolapio JS, Camilleri M, Fleming CR, et al. Effect of growth hormone, glutamine, and diet on adaptation in short-bowel syndrome: A randomized, controlled study. Gastroenterology 1997;113:1074–81.
123. Drozdowski L, Thomson AB. Intestinal mucosal adaptation. World J Gastroenterol 2006;12:4614–27.
124. Byrne TA, Wilmore DW, Iyer K, et al. Growth hormone, glutamine, and an optimal diet reduces parenteral nutrition in patients with short bowel syndrome: A prospective, randomized, placebo-controlled, double-blind clinical trial. Ann Surg 2005;242:655–61.
125. Byrne TA, Persinger RL, Young LS, et al. A new treatment for patients with short-bowel syndrome. Growth hormone, glutamine, and a modified diet. Ann Surg 1995;222:243–54; discussion 54–5.
126. Seguy D, Vahedi K, Kapel N, et al. Low-dose growth hormone in adult home parenteral nutrition-dependent short bowel syndrome patients: A positive study. Gastroenterology 2003;124:293–302.

127. Ladd AP, Grosfeld JL, Pescovitz OH, et al. The effect of growth hormone supplementation on late nutritional independence in pediatric patients with short bowel syndrome. J Pediatr Surg 2005;40:442–5.
128. Barksdale EM, Jr, Koehler AN, Yaworski JA, et al. Insulin-like growth factor 1 and insulinlike growth factor 3: Indices of intestinal failure in children. J Pediatr Surg 1999;34:655–61; discussion 61–2.
129. Nucci AM, Finegold DN, Yaworski JA, et al. Results of growth trophic therapy in children with short bowel syndrome. J Pediatr Surg 2004;39:335–9; discussion 35–9.
130. Velasco B, Lassaletta L, Gracia R, et al. Intestinal lengthening and growth hormone in extreme short bowel syndrome: A case report. J Pediatr Surg 1999;34:1423–4.
131. Lifschitz C, Duggan C, Langston C, et al. Growth hormone therapy in children with short bowel syndrome: A randomized, placebo controlled trial. Gastroenterology 2003;124:A–64.
132. Matarese LE, Seidner DL, Steiger E. Growth hormone, glutamine, and modified diet for intestinal adaptation. J Am Diet Assoc 2004;104:1265–72.
133. Socha J, Ksiazyk J, Fogel WA, et al. Is growth hormone a feasible adjuvant in the treatment of children after small bowel resection. Clin Nutr 1996;15:185–88.
134. Dabbas-Tyan M, Colomb V, Rosilio M, et al. Evaluation of the effect of recombinant human growth hormone (rhGH) treatment of children with short bowel syndrome. J Pediatr Gastroenterol Nutr 2000;31:5165–66.
135. Mantell MP, Ziegler TR, Adamson WT, et al. Resection-induced colonic adaptation is augmented by IGF-I and associated with upregulation of colonic IGF-I mRNA. Am J Physiol 1995;269:G974–80.
136. Dahly EM, Guo Z, Ney DM. IGF-I augments resection-induced mucosal hyperplasia by altering enterocyte kinetics. Am J Physiol Regul Integr Comp Physiol 2003;285: R800–8.
137. Knott AW, Juno RJ, Jarboe MD, et al. Smooth muscle overexpression of IGF-I induces a novel adaptive response to small bowel resection. Am J Physiol Gastrointest Liver Physiol 2004;287:G562–70.
138. Gillingham MB, Kritsch KR, Murali SG, et al. Resection upregulates the IGF-I system of parenterally fed rats with jejunocolic anastomosis. Am J Physiol Gastrointest Liver Physiol 2001;281:G1158–68.
139. Gillingham MB, Dahly EM, Carey HV, et al. Differential jejunal and colonic adaptation due to resection and IGF-I in parenterally fed rats. Am J Physiol Gastrointest Liver Physiol 2000;278:G700–9.
140. Gillingham MB, Dahly EM, Murali SG, et al. IGF-I treatment facilitates transition from parenteral to enteral nutrition in rats with short bowel syndrome. Am J Physiol Regul Integr Comp Physiol 2003;284:R363–71.
141. Yang H, Teitelbaum DH. Novel agents in the treatment of intestinal failure: Humoral factors. Gastroenterology 2006;130:S117–21.
142. Opleta-Madsen K, Hardin J, Gall DG. Epidermal growth factor upregulates intestinal electrolyte and nutrient transport. Am J Physiol 1991;260:G807–14.
143. O'Brien DP, Nelson LA, Williams JL, et al. Selective inhibition of the epidermal growth factor receptor impairs intestinal adaptation after small bowel resection. J Surg Res 2002;105:25–30.
144. Erwin CR, Helmrath MA, Shin CE, et al. Intestinal overexpression of EGF in transgenic mice enhances adaptation after small bowel resection. Am J Physiol 1999;277: G533–40.
145. Chung BM, Wallace LE, Winkfein RK, et al. The effect of massive small bowel resection and oral epidermal growth factor therapy on SGLT-1 distribution in rabbit distal remnant. Pediatr Res 2004;55:19–26.
146. Avissar NE, Wang HT, Miller JH, et al. Epidermal growth factor receptor is increased in rabbit intestinal brush border membrane after small bowel resection. Dig Dis Sci 2000;45:1145–52.
147. Helmrath MA, Shin CE, Erwin CR, et al. The EGF/EGF-receptor axis modulates enterocyte apoptosis during intestinal adaptation. J Surg Res 1998;77:17–22.
148. Helmrath MA, Shin CE, Fox JW, et al. Adaptation after small bowel resection is attenuated by sialoadenectomy: The role for endogenous epidermal growth factor. Surgery 1998;124:848–54.
149. Hardin JA, Chung B, O'Loughlin EV, et al. The effect of epidermal growth factor on brush border surface area and function in the distal remnant following resection in the rabbit. Gut 1999;44:26–32.
150. Sham J, Martin G, Meddings JB, et al. Epidermal growth factor improves nutritional outcome in a rat model of short bowel syndrome. J Pediatr Surg 2002;37:765–9.
151. Shin CE, Falcone RA, Jr, Stuart L, et al. Diminished epidermal growth factor levels in infants with necrotizing enterocolitis. J Pediatr Surg 2000;35:173–6; discussion 77.
152. Sigalet DL, Martin GR, Butzner JD, et al. A pilot study of the use of epidermal growth factor in pediatric short bowel syndrome. J Pediatr Surg 2005;40:763–8.
153. Wallis K, Walters JR, Forbes A. Review article: Glucagon-like peptide 2—current applications and future directions. Aliment Pharmacol Ther 2007;25:365–72.
154. Dahly EM, Gillingham MB, Guo Z, et al. Role of luminal nutrients and endogenous GLP-2 in intestinal adaptation to mid-small bowel resection. Am J Physiol Gastrointest Liver Physiol 2003;284:G670–82.
155. Martin GR, Wallace LE, Hartmann B, et al. Nutrient-stimulated GLP-2 release and crypt cell proliferation in experimental short bowel syndrome. Am J Physiol Gastrointest Liver Physiol 2005;288:G431–8.
156. Scott RB, Kirk D, MacNaughton WK, et al. GLP-2 augments the adaptive response to massive intestinal resection in rat. Am J Physiol 1998;275:G911–21.
157. Martin GR, Wallace LE, Sigalet DL. Glucagon-like peptide-2 induces intestinal adaptation in parenterally fed rats with short bowel syndrome. Am J Physiol Gastrointest Liver Physiol 2004;286:G964–72.
158. Jeppesen PB, Hartmann B, Thulesen J, et al. Glucagon-like peptide 2 improves nutrient absorption and nutritional status in short-bowel patients with no colon. Gastroenterology 2001;120:806–15.
159. Jeppesen PB, Sanguinetti EL, Buchman A, et al. Teduglutide (ALX-0600), a dipeptidyl peptidase IV resistant glucagon-like peptide 2 analogue, improves intestinal function in short bowel syndrome patients. Gut 2005;54:1224–31.
160. Jeppesen PB. Glucagon-like peptide-2: Update of the recent clinical trials. Gastroenterology 2006;130:S127–31.
161. Cisler JJ, Buchman AL. Intestinal adaptation in short bowel syndrome. J Investig Med 2005;53:402–13.
162. Sukhotnik I, Mogilner J, Shamir R, et al. Effect of subcutaneous insulin on intestinal adaptation in a rat model of short bowel syndrome. Pediatr Surg Int 2005;21:132–7.
163. Sanderson IR, Naik S. Dietary regulation of intestinal gene expression. Annu Rev Nutr 2000;20:311–38.
164. Goulet O, Ruemmele F. Causes and management of intestinal failure in children. Gastroenterology 2006;130:S16–28.
165. Kelly DA. Intestinal failure-associated liver disease: What do we know today? Gastroenterology 2006;130:S70–7.
166. Cavicchi M, Beau P, Crenn P, et al. Prevalence of liver disease and contributing factors in patients receiving home parenteral nutrition for permanent intestinal failure. Ann Intern Med 2000;132:525–32.
167. Chan S, McCowen KC, Bistrian BR, et al. Incidence, prognosis, and etiology of end-stage liver disease in patients receiving home total parenteral nutrition. Surgery 1999;126:28–34.
168. Nasr A, Avitzur Y, Ng VL, et al. The use of conjugated hyperbilirubinemia greater than 100 micromol/L as an indicator of irreversible liver disease in infants with short bowel syndrome. J Pediatr Surg 2007;42:359–62.
169. Weber TR, Keller MS. Adverse effects of liver dysfunction and portal hypertension on intestinal adaptation in short bowel syndrome in children. Am J Surg 2002;184:582–6; discussion 86.
170. Horslen SP, Sudan DL, Iyer KR, et al. Isolated liver transplantation in infants with end-stage liver disease associated with short bowel syndrome. Ann Surg 2002;235:435–9.
171. Teitelbaum DH, Tracy TF, Jr, Aouthmany MM, et al. Use of cholecystokinin-octapeptide for the prevention of parenteral nutrition-associated cholestasis. Pediatrics 2005;115:1332–40.
172. Hermans D, Talbotec C, Lacaille F, et al. Early central catheter infections may contribute to hepatic fibrosis in children receiving long-term parenteral nutrition. J Pediatr Gastroenterol Nutr 2007;44:459–63.
173. Sondheimer JM, Asturias E, Cadnapaphornchai M. Infection and cholestasis in neonates with intestinal resection and long-term parenteral nutrition. J Pediatr Gastroenterol Nutr 1998;27:131–7.
174. Beath SV, Davies P, Papadopoulou A, et al. Parenteral nutrition-related cholestasis in postsurgical neonates: Multivariate analysis of risk factors. J Pediatr Surg 1996;31:604–6.
175. Christensen RD, Henry E, Wiedmeier SE, et al. Identifying patients, on the first day of life, at high-risk of developing parenteral nutrition-associated liver disease. J Perinatol 2007;27:284–290.
176. Toce SS, Keenan WJ. Lipid intolerance in newborns is associated with hepatic dysfunction but not infection. Arch Pediatr Adolesc Med 1995;149:1249–53.
177. Colomb V, Jobert-Giraud A, Lacaille F, et al. Role of lipid emulsions in cholestasis associated with long-term parenteral nutrition in children. JPEN J Parenter Enteral Nutr 2000;24:345–50.
178. Javid PJ, Greene AK, Garza J, et al. The route of lipid administration affects parenteral nutrition-induced hepatic steatosis in a mouse model. J Pediatr Surg 2005;40:1446–53.
179. Whitfield PD, Clayton PT, Muller DP. Effect of intravenous lipid emulsions on hepatic cholesterol metabolism. J Pediatr Gastroenterol Nutr 2000;30:538–46.
180. Hong L, Wu J, Cai W. Glutathione decreased parenteral nutrition-induced hepatocyte injury in infant rabbits. JPEN J Parenter Enteral Nutr 2007;31:199–204.
181. Clayton PT, Whitfield P, Iyer K. The role of phytosterols in the pathogenesis of liver complications of pediatric parenteral nutrition. Nutrition 1998;14:158–64.
182. Doi F, Goya T, Torisu M. Potential role of hepatic macrophages in neutrophil-mediated liver injury in rats with sepsis. Hepatology 1993;17:1086–94.
183. Beath SV, Booth IW, Murphy MS, et al. Nutritional care and candidates for small bowel transplantation. Arch Dis Child 1995;73:348–50.
184. Ling PR, Sheikh M, Boyce P, et al. Cholecystokinin (CCK) secretion in patients with severe short bowel syndrome (SSBS). Dig Dis Sci 2001;46:859–64.
185. Gura KM, Duggan CP, Collier SB, et al. Reversal of parenteral nutrition-associated liver disease in two infants with short bowel syndrome using parenteral fish oil: Implications for future management. Pediatrics 2006;118:e197–201.
186. Diamanti A, Basso MS, Castro M, et al. Prevalence of life-threatening complications in pediatric patients affected by intestinal failure. Transplant Proc 2007;39:1632–3.
187. Quigley EM, Quera R. Small intestinal bacterial overgrowth: Roles of antibiotics, prebiotics, and probiotics. Gastroenterology 2006;130:S78–90.
188. Lichtman SN. Translocation of bacteria from gut lumen to mesenteric lymph nodes—and beyond? J Pediatr Gastroenterol Nutr 1991;13:433–4.
189. Piedra PA, Dryja DM, LaScolea LJ, Jr. Incidence of catheter-associated gram-negative bacteremia in children with short bowel syndrome. J Clin Microbiol 1989;27:1317–9.
190. Kurkchubasche AG, Smith SD, Rowe MI. Catheter sepsis in short-bowel syndrome. Arch Surg 1992;127:21–4; discussion 24–5.
191. Weber TR. Enteral feeding increases sepsis in infants with short bowel syndrome. J Pediatr Surg 1995;30:1086–8; discussion 88–9.
192. Inaki I, Paloma P, Iske G, et al. Long-term parenteral nutrition outcome and incidence of pulmonary emboli. IXth International Small Bowel Transplantation Symposium, Brussels, 2005.
193. Moukarzel AA, Haddad I, Ament ME, et al. 230 patient years of experience with home long-term parenteral nutrition in childhood: Natural history and life of central venous catheters. J Pediatr Surg 1994;29:1323–7.
194. Nightingale JM. Hepatobiliary, renal and bone complications of intestinal failure. Best Pract Res Clin Gastroenterol 2003;17:907–29.
195. Vargas JH, Klein GL, Ament ME, et al. Metabolic bone disease of total parenteral nutrition: Course after changing from casein to amino acids in parenteral solutions with reduced aluminum content. Am J Clin Nutr 1988;48:1070–8.
196. Dellert SF, Farrell MK, Specker BL, et al. Bone mineral content in children with short bowel syndrome after discontinuation of parental nutrition. J Pediatr 1998;132:516–9.
197. Pazianas M, Compher C, Schiavone-Gatto P, et al. Intestinal failure-associated metabolic bone diseases and response to teriparatide. Nutr Clin Pract 2006;21:605–9.
198. Tangpricha V, Luo M, Fernandez-Estivariz C, et al. Growth hormone favorably affects bone turnover and bone mineral density in patients with short bowel syndrome undergoing intestinal rehabilitation. JPEN J Parenter Enteral Nutr 2006;30:480–6.
199. Quigley EM, Thompson JS. The motor response to intestinal resection: Motor activity in the canine small intestine following distal resection. Gastroenterology 1993;105:791–8.
200. Quigley EM, Phillips SF, Dent J. Distinctive patterns of interdigestive motility at the canine ileocolonic junction. Gastroenterology 1984;87:836–44.
201. Zhang SC, Wang W, Ren WY, et al. Effect of cisapride on intestinal bacterial and endotoxin translocation in cirrhosis. World J Gastroenterol 2003;9:534–8.
202. O'Boyle CJ, MacFie J, Dave K, et al. Alterations in intestinal barrier function do not predispose to translocation of enteric bacteria in gastroenterologic patients. Nutrition 1998;14:358–62.
203. Solga SF, Diehl AM. Non-alcoholic fatty liver disease: Lumen-liver interactions and possible role for probiotics. J Hepatol 2003;38:681–7.
204. Alverdy J, Holbrook C, Rocha F, et al. Gut-derived sepsis occurs when the right pathogen with the right virulence genes meets the right host: Evidence for in vivo virulence expression in Pseudomonas aeruginosa. Ann Surg 2000;232:480–9.
205. Kathpalia SC, Favus MJ, Coe FL. Evidence for size and charge permselectivity of rat ascending colon. Effects of ricinoleate and bile salts on oxalic acid and neutral sugar transport. J Clin Invest 1984;74:805–11.
206. Perlmutter DH, Boyle JT, Campos JM, et al. D-Lactic acidosis in children: An unusual metabolic complication of small bowel resection. J Pediatr 1983;102:234–8.

207. Halperin ML, Kamel KS. D-lactic acidosis: Turning sugar into acids in the gastrointestinal tract. Kidney Int 1996;49:1–8.
208. Modi BP, Langer M, Duggan C, et al. Serial transverse enteroplasty for management of refractory D-lactic acidosis in short-bowel syndrome. J Pediatr Gastroenterol Nutr 2006;43:395–7.
209. Uchida H, Yamamoto H, Kisaki Y, et al. D-lactic acidosis in short-bowel syndrome managed with antibiotics and probiotics. J Pediatr Surg 2004;39:634–6.
210. Coronado BE, Opal SM, Yoburn DC. Antibiotic-induced D-lactic acidosis. Ann Intern Med 1995;122:839–42.
211. Bines JE, Taylor RG, Justice F, et al. Influence of diet complexity on intestinal adaptation following massive small bowel resection in a preclinical model. J Gastroenterol Hepatol 2002;17:1170–9.
212. Jirapinyo P, Young C, Srimaruta N, et al. High-fat semielemental diet in the treatment of protracted diarrhea of infancy. Pediatrics 1990;86:902–8.
213. Gray G, Santiago N. Disaccharide absorption in normal and diseased human intestine. Gastroenterology 1966;51:489.
214. Pirman T, Ribeyre MC, Mosoni L, et al. Dietary pectin stimulates protein metabolism in the digestive tract. Nutrition 2007;23:69–75.
215. Finkel Y, Brown G, Smith HL, et al. The effects of a pectin-supplemented elemental diet in a boy with short gut syndrome. Acta Paediatr Scand 1990;79:983–6.
216. Rabbani GH, Teka T, Saha SK, et al. Green banana and pectin improve small intestinal permeability and reduce fluid loss in Bangladeshi children with persistent diarrhea. Dig Dis Sci 2004;49:475–84.
217. Jeppesen PB, Mortensen PB. Colonic digestion and absorption of energy from carbohydrates and medium-chain fat in small bowel failure. JPEN J Parenter Enteral Nutr 1999;23:S101–5.
218. Sagher FA, Dodge JA, Moore R, et al. Modulation of fluid absorption and the secretory response of rat jejunum to cholera toxin by dietary fat. Gut 1990;31:1256–61.
219. Bines J, Francis D, Hill D. Reducing parenteral requirement in children with short bowel syndrome: Impact of an amino acid-based complete infant formula. J Pediatr Gastroenterol Nutr 1998;26:123–8.
220. Ksiazyk J, Piena M, Kierkus J, et al. Hydrolyzed versus nonhydrolyzed protein diet in short bowel syndrome in children. J Pediatr Gastroenterol Nutr 2002;35:615–8.
221. McIntyre PB, Fitchew M, Lennard-Jones JE. Patients with a high jejunostomy do not need a special diet. Gastroenterology 1986;91:25–33.
222. Mazon A, Solera E, Alentado N, et al. Frequent IgE sensitization to latex, cow's milk, and egg in children with short bowel syndrome. Pediatr Allergy Immunol 2007.
223. Taylor SF, Sondheimer JM, Sokol RJ, et al. Noninfectious colitis associated with short gut syndrome in infants. J Pediatr 1991;119:24–8.
224. Vanderhoof JA, Young RJ. Hydrolyzed versus nonhydrolyzed protein diet in short bowel syndrome in children. J Pediatr Gastroenterol Nutr 2004;38:107.
225. O'Keefe SJ. Bacterial overgrowth and liver complications in short bowel intestinal failure patients. Gastroenterology 2006;130:S67–9.
226. Buchman AL. Etiology and initial management of short bowel syndrome. Gastroenterology 2006;130:S5–S15.
227. Hambidge KM. Zinc and diarrhea. Acta Paediatr Suppl 1992;381:82–6.
228. Rannem T, Hylander E, Ladefoged K, et al. The metabolism of [^{75}Se]selenite in patients with short bowel syndrome. JPEN J Parenter Enteral Nutr 1996;20:412–6.
229. Weizman Z, Schmueli A, Deckelbaum RJ. Continuous nasogastric drip elemental feeding. Alternative for prolonged parenteral nutrition in severe prolonged diarrhea. Am J Dis Child 1983;137:253–5.
230. Parker P, Stroop S, Greene H. A controlled comparison of continuous versus intermittent feeding in the treatment of infants with intestinal disease. J Pediatr 1981;99:360–4.
231. Thompson JS. Reoperation in patients with the short bowel syndrome. Am J Surg 1992;164:453–6; discussion 56–7.
232. Wales PW. Surgical therapy for short bowel syndrome. Pediatr Surg Int 2004;20:647–57.
233. Hakami M, Moslehy A, Mosavy SH. Reversed jejunal segment used to treat the short bowel syndrome. Am Surg 1975;41:432–5.
234. Glick PL, de Lorimier AA, Adzick NS, et al. Colon interposition: An adjuvant operation for short-gut syndrome. J Pediatr Surg 1984;19:719–25.
235. Panis Y, Messing B, Rivet P, et al. Segmental reversal of the small bowel as an alternative to intestinal transplantation in patients with short bowel syndrome. Ann Surg 1997;225:401–7.
236. Trinkle JK, Bryant LR. Reversed colon segment in an infant with massive small bowel resection: A case report [passim]. J Ky Med Assoc 1967;65:1090–1.
237. Bianchi A. Intestinal loop lengthening-a technique for increasing small intestinal length. J Pediatr Surg 1980;15:145–51.
238. Walker SR, Nucci A, Yaworski JA, et al. The Bianchi procedure: A 20-year single institution experience. J Pediatr Surg 2006;41:113–9; discussion 13–9.
239. Weber TR. Isoperistaltic bowel lengthening for short bowel syndrome in children. Am J Surg 1999;178:600–4.
240. Sudan D, DiBaise J, Torres C, et al. A multidisciplinary approach to the treatment of intestinal failure. J Gastrointest Surg 2005;9:165–76; discussion 76–7.
241. Waag KL, Hosie S, Wessel L. What do children look like after longitudinal intestinal lengthening. Eur J Pediatr Surg 1999;9:260–2.
242. Hosie S, Loff S, Wirth H, et al. Experience of 49 longitudinal intestinal lengthening procedures for short bowel syndrome. Eur J Pediatr Surg 2006;16:171–5.
243. Bianchi A. Longitudinal intestinal lengthening and tailoring: Results in 20 children. J R Soc Med 1997;90:429–32.
244. Bianchi A. From the cradle to enteral autonomy: The role of autologous gastrointestinal reconstruction. Gastroenterology 2006;130:S138–46.
245. Kim HB, Fauza D, Garza J, et al. Serial transverse enteroplasty (STEP): A novel bowel lengthening procedure. J Pediatr Surg 2003;38:425–9.
246. Modi BP, Javid PJ, Jaksic T, et al. First report of the international serial transverse enteroplasty data registry: Indications, efficacy, and complications. J Am Coll Surg 2007;204:365–71.
247. Ismail A, Alkadhi A, Alnagaar O, et al. Serial transverse enteroplasty in intestinal atresia management. J Pediatr Surg 2005;40:E5–6.
248. Wales PW, Dutta S. Serial transverse enteroplasty as primary therapy for neonates with proximal jejunal atresia. J Pediatr Surg 2005;40:E31–4.
249. Ehrlich PF, Mychaliska GB, Teitelbaum DH. The 2 STEP: An approach to repeating a serial transverse enteroplasty. J Pediatr Surg 2007;42:819–22.
250. Howard L. Home parenteral nutrition: Survival, cost, and quality of life. Gastroenterology 2006;130:S52–9.
251. Smith CE. Quality of life in long-term total parenteral nutrition patients and their family caregivers. JPEN J Parenter Enteral Nutr 1993;17:501–6.
252. Smith CE, Curtas S, Werkowitch M, et al. Home parenteral nutrition: Does affiliation with a national support and educational organization improve patient outcomes? JPEN J Parenter Enteral Nutr 2002;26:159–63.
253. Fairman J, Compher C, Morris J, et al. Living long with short bowel syndrome: A historical case of twenty-nine years of living with home parenteral nutrition. JPEN J Parenter Enteral Nutr 2007;31:127–34.
254. Pironi L, Paganelli F, Lauro A, et al. Quality of life on home parenteral nutrition or after intestinal transplantation. Transplant Proc 2006;38:1673–5.
255. Gottrand F, Staszewski P, Colomb V, et al. Satisfaction in different life domains in children receiving home parenteral nutrition and their families. J Pediatr 2005;146:793–7.
256. Colomb V, Dabbas M, Goulet O, et al. Prepubertal growth in children with long-term parenteral nutrition. Horm Res 2002;58:2–6.
257. Amarnath RP, Fleming CR, Perrault J. Home parenteral nutrition in chronic intestinal diseases: Its effect on growth and development. J Pediatr Gastroenterol Nutr 1987;6:89–95.
258. Gonzalez HF, Perez NB, Malpeli A, et al. Nutrition and immunological status in long-term follow up of children with short bowel syndrome. JPEN J Parenter Enteral Nutr 2005;29:186–91.
259. Ralston CW, O'Connor MJ, Ament M, et al. Somatic growth and developmental functioning in children receiving prolonged home total parenteral nutrition. J Pediatr 1984;105:842–6.
260. Beers SR, Yaworski JA, Stilley C, et al. Cognitive deficits in school-age children with severe short bowel syndrome. J Pediatr Surg 2000;35:860–5.
261. O'Connor MJ, Ralston CW, Ament ME. Intellectual and perceptual-motor performance of children receiving prolonged home total parenteral nutrition. Pediatrics 1988;81:231–6.
262. Lloyd DA, Vega R, Bassett P, et al. Survival and dependence on home parenteral nutrition: Experience over a 25-year period in a UK referral centre. Aliment Pharmacol Ther 2006;24:1231–40.
263. Colomb V, Dabbas-Tyan M, Taupin P, et al. Long-term outcome of children receiving home parenteral nutrition: A 20-year single-center experience in 302 patients. J Pediatr Gastroenterol Nutr 2007;44:347–53.
264. Intestinal Transplant Registry Data. Available at: http://www.intestinaltransplant.org/. Accessed July 15, 2007.
265. Kocoshis SA, Beath SV, Booth IW, et al. Intestinal failure and small bowel transplantation, including clinical nutrition: Working Group report of the second World Congress of Pediatric Gastroenterology, Hepatology, and Nutrition. J Pediatr Gastroenterol Nutr 2004;39:S655–61.
266. Abu-Elmagd K, Bond G, Reyes J, et al. Intestinal transplantation: A coming of age. Adv Surg 2002;36:65–101.
267. Kaufman SS, Atkinson JB, Bianchi A, et al. Indications for pediatric intestinal transplantation: A position paper of the American Society of Transplantation. Pediatr Transplant 2001;5:80–7.
268. Cigna Healthcare Coverage Position—Intestinal and Multivisceral Transplant. Available at: http://www.cigna.com/customer_care/healthcare_professional/index.html. Accessed July 5.
269. Ruiz P, Kato T, Tzakis A. Current status of transplantation of the small intestine. Transplantation 2007;83:1–6.
270. Fishbein TM, Matsumoto CS. Intestinal replacement therapy: Timing and indications for referral of patients to an intestinal rehabilitation and transplant program. Gastroenterology 2006;130:S147–51.
271. O'Keefe SJ. Candidacy for intestinal transplantation. Am J Gastroenterol 2006;101:1644–6.
272. Abu-Elmagd KM. Intestinal transplantation for short bowel syndrome and gastrointestinal failure: Current consensus, rewarding outcomes, and practical guidelines. Gastroenterology 2006;130:S132–7.
273. Pironi L, Hebuterne X, Van Gossum A, et al. Candidates for intestinal transplantation: A multicenter survey in Europe. Am J Gastroenterol 2006;101:1633–43; quiz 79.
274. Benedetti E, Holterman M, Asolati M, et al. Living related segmental bowel transplantation: From experimental to standardized procedure. Ann Surg 2006;244:694–9.
275. Kato T, Tzakis AG, Selvaggi G, et al. Intestinal and multivisceral transplantation in children. Ann Surg 2006;243:756–64; discussion 64–6.
276. Ruiz P, Kato T, Tzakis A. Current status of transplantation of the small intestine. Transplantation 2007;83:1–6.
277. Botha JF, Grant WJ, Torres C, et al. Isolated liver transplantation in infants with end-stage liver disease due to short bowel syndrome. Liver Transpl 2006;12:1062–6.
278. Horslen SP. Optimal management of the post-intestinal transplant patient. Gastroenterology 2006;130:S163–9.
279. Gabe SM, Bjarnason I, Tolou-Ghamari Z, et al. The effect of tacrolimus (FK506) on intestinal barrier function and cellular energy production in humans. Gastroenterology 1998;115:67–74.
280. Nucci AM, Barksdale EM, Jr, Yaworski JA, et al. Enteral formula use in children after small bowel transplant. Nutr Clin Pract 2002;17:113–7.
281. Chehade M, Nowak-Wegrzyn A, Kaufman SS, et al. De novo food allergy after intestinal transplantation: A report of three cases. J Pediatr Gastroenterol Nutr 2004;38:545–7.
282. Nucci AM, Barksdale EM, Jr, Beserock N, et al. Long-term nutritional outcome after pediatric intestinal transplantation. J Pediatr Surg 2002;37:460–3.
283. Nowak-Wegrzyn AH, Sicherer SH, Conover-Walker MK, et al. Food allergy after pediatric organ transplantation with tacrolimus immunosuppression. J Allergy Clin Immunol 2001;108:146–7.
284. Kaufman SS, Lyden ER, Brown CR, et al. Disaccharidase activities and fat assimilation in pediatric patients after intestinal transplantation. Transplantation 2000;69:362–5.
285. Berney T, Genton L, Buhler LH, et al. Five-year follow-up after pediatric living related small bowel transplantation between two monozygotic twins. Transplant Proc 2004;36:316–8.
286. Loinaz C, Mittal N, Kato T, et al. Multivisceral transplantation for pediatric intestinal pseudo-obstruction: Single center's experience of 16 cases. Transplant Proc 2004;36:312–3.
287. Diagnosis and management of foodborne illnesses—a primer for physicians and other health care professionals. In: Agriculture USDo, Volume 53. 2004. p. 1–33.
288. Venick RS, Farmer DG, Saikali D, et al. Nutritional outcomes following pediatric intestinal transplantation. Transplant Proc 2006;38:1718–9.
289. Genton L, Raguso CA, Berney T, et al. Four year nutritional follow up after living related small bowel transplantation between monozygotic twins. Gut 2003;52:659–62.
290. Yagi M, Sakamoto K, Hasebe K, et al. Effect of a glutamine-enriched diet on small bowel allograft during immunosuppressive therapy. Nutrition 1997;13:778–82.
291. Zhang W, Frankel WL, Bain A, et al. Glutamine reduces bacterial translocation after small bowel transplantation in cyclosporine-treated rats. J Surg Res 1995;58:159–64.
292. Zhang W, Frankel WL, Singh A, et al. Improvement of structure and function in orthotopic small bowel transplantation in the rat by glutamine. Transplantation 1993;56:512–7.
293. Lew JI, Zhang W, Koide S, et al. Glutamine improves cold-preserved small bowel graft structure and function following ischemia and reperfusion. Transplant Proc 1996;28:2605–6.
294. Wu XT, Li JS, Zhao XF, et al. Effects of n-3 fatty acid, fructose-1,6-diphosphate and glutamine on mucosal cell

proliferation and apoptosis of small bowel graft after transplantation in rats. World J Gastroenterol 2003;9:1323–6.
295. Ogita K, Suita S, Taguchi T, et al. Effects of omega-3 fatty acids in rat allogenic small intestinal transplantation. Pediatr Surg Int 2003;19:157–61.
296. Ma H, Wang J, Wang J, et al. Fish oil ameliorates the allograft arteriosclerosis of intestine on rats. Pediatr Transplant 2007;11:173–9.
297. Gerbitz A, Schultz M, Wilke A, et al. Probiotic effects on experimental graft-versus-host disease: Let them eat yogurt. Blood 2004;103:4365–7.
298. Rodrigues AF, van Mourik ID, Sharif K, et al. Management of end-stage central venous access in children referred for possible small bowel transplantation. J Pediatr Gastroenterol Nutr 2006;42:427–33.
299. Grant D, Abu-Elmagd K, Reyes J, et al. 2003 report of the intestine transplant registry: A new era has dawned. Ann Surg 2005;241:607–13.
300 Scientific Registry of Transplant Recipients. Available at: http://www.ustransplant.org/. Accessed August 21.
301. Goulet O, Sauvat F, Ruemmele F, et al. Results of the Paris program: Ten years of pediatric intestinal transplantation. Transplant Proc 2005;37:1667–70.
302. Sudan D, Horslen S, Botha J, et al. Quality of life after pediatric intestinal transplantation: The perception of pediatric recipients and their parents. Am J Transplant 2004;4:407–13.
303. O'Keefe SJ, Emerling M, Koritsky D, et al. Nutrition and quality of life following small intestinal transplantation. Am J Gastroenterol 2007;102:1093–100.
304. Rivas K, Kato T, Ueno T, et al. Growth after intestinal transplantation in children. IXth International Small Bowel Transplantation Symposium. Brussels, 2005.
305. Iyer K, Horslen S, Iverson A, et al. Nutritional outcome and growth of children after intestinal transplantation. J Pediatr Surg 2002;37:464–6.
306. Lacaille F, Vass N, Sauvat F, et al. Long-term outcome, growth and digestive function in children 2 to 18 years after intestinal transplantation. Gut 2008, in press.
307. Javid PJ Kim HB, Duggan CP, et al. Serial transverse enteroplasty is associated with successful short-term outcomes in infants with short bowel syndrome. J Pediatr Surg 2005;40:1019–23.

59

The Critically Ill Child

Nilesh M. Mehta, MD, DCH, MRCPCH
Tom Jaksic, MD, PhD

The prevalence of malnutrition among critically ill patients, especially those with a protracted clinical course, has remained largely unchanged over the last two decades.[1,2] The profound and stereotypic metabolic response to critical illness and failure to provide optimal nutritional support during the intensive care unit (ICU) stay are the principal factors contributing to malnutrition in this cohort. The nutritional status of children is expected to affect physiological responses and influence outcome during critical illness. Malnutrition is associated with increased physiological instability and longer ICU stay with increased utilization of resources.[3] Accurate individual assessment of energy requirements and provision of optimal nutritional support through the appropriate route is an important goal of pediatric critical care.

Over a half century ago, Sir David Cuthbertson described the fundamental aspects of the metabolic response to injury in the adult.[4] An acute catabolic phase precedes the metabolic process of recovery and repair. This metabolic response to trauma can be conceptually divided into two phases. The initial *ebb phase* is characterized by decreased enzymatic activity and oxygen consumption, low cardiac output with core temperature that may be subnormal. This is followed by the hypermetabolic *flow phase* characterized by increased cardiac output, oxygen consumption, and glucose production. During this phase, fat and protein mobilization is associated with increased urinary nitrogen excretion and weight loss. The catabolic response may in part be mediated by a surge in cytokines and the characteristic endocrine response to trauma or surgery that results in availability for food substrates essential for healing. Research regarding the pediatric stress response has shown that although neonates and children share similar qualitative metabolic sequelae to illness with adults, significant quantitative differences exist. An understanding of the metabolic events that accompany critical illness and surgery of the child is the first step in implementing adequate nutritional support. The goal of nutritional supportive therapy in this setting is to augment the short-term benefits of the pediatric stress response while minimizing the long-term harmful consequences. Ultimately, an individualized determination of nutrient requirements must be made to provide appropriate amounts of both macro- and micronutrients.

The metabolic response to critical illness differs from the response during prolonged nutrient deprivation or starvation. Increased ketone bodies produced during prolonged starvation replace glucose as the major energy substrate especially for the brain. If starvation is not reversed, protein catabolism persists and involves all protein compartments, including heart, lungs, and intestine, resulting in significant organ dysfunction and increasing morbidity and mortality. However, nitrogen loss associated with starvation can be suppressed by administration of glucose, which reduces gluconeogenesis and conserves nitrogen in proportion to the amount of glucose supplied.[5] Therefore, starvation is a reversible process if energy intake is provided. This is fundamentally different from the metabolic response during critical illness.

METABOLIC RESPONSE TO CRITICAL ILLNESS: AN OVERVIEW OF THE HYPERMETABOLIC OR STRESS RESPONSE

Children, similar to adults, rely on the metabolic breakdown and transfer of protein, carbohydrates, and lipid to meet the catabolic demands of critical illness. Figure 1 illustrates the basic pathways involved in the pediatric metabolic response. In general, the metabolic stress response is characterized by an increase in net muscle protein degradation and enhanced movement of the free amino acid products through the circulation. These amino acids serve as the building blocks for rapid synthesis of proteins that act as inflammatory mediators for tissue repair and the inflammatory response. Remaining amino acids not used in this way are channeled through the liver, where their carbon skeletons are used to create glucose through gluconeogenesis. Although the catabolism of muscle protein is an effective short-term adaptation for the child, it is of limited duration and potentially damaging owing to relative reduction in lean body mass. Carbohydrate and lipid turnover is also increased severalfold during the pediatric metabolic response. Although these metabolic alterations would be expected to increase overall energy requirements, recent data show that any increase is variable and far less than originally proposed. Overall, the energy needs of the critically ill child are governed by the severity and persistence of the underlying illness. Accurate assessment of energy requirement in individual patients will allow optimal caloric supplementation and avoid the deleterious effects of both under- and overfeeding. Moreover, recent reports have convincingly linked hyperglycemia with increased mortality and established the

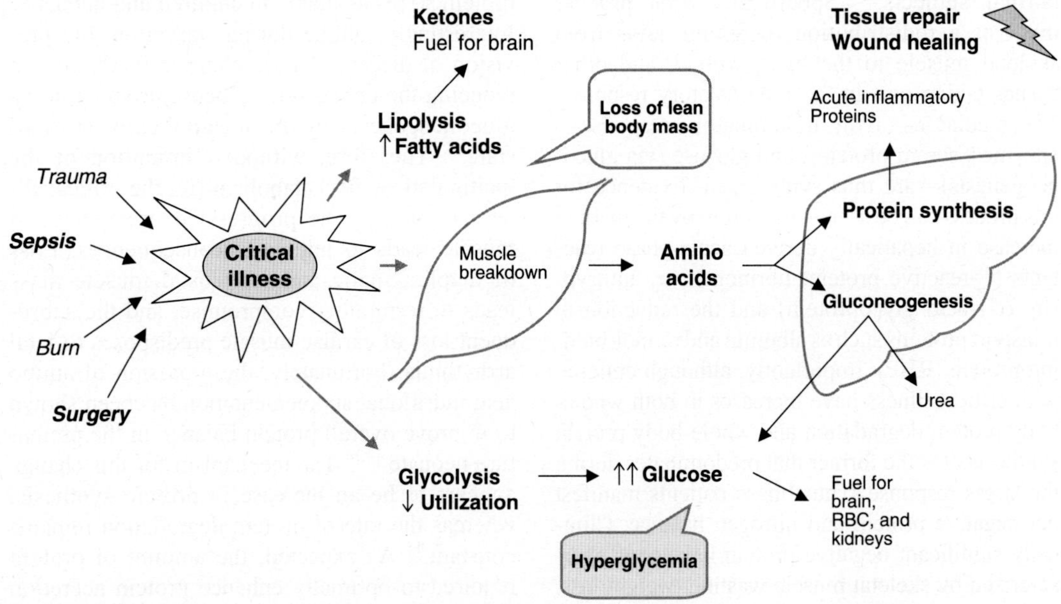

Figure 1 Basic pathways of the metabolic stress response.

role of insulin-assisted tight glycemic control in improving outcomes in the critically ill adults.[6] Finally, a unique hormonal and cytokine profile is found in the child with critical illness. Such patients demonstrate an elevation in serum levels of insulin, the catabolic hormones (glucagons, cortisol, catecholamines), and specific cytokines known to interact with the inflammatory process.[89] Current research in this field is focused on ways to manipulate these hormonal and cytokine alterations to minimize the deleterious consequences induced by the stress response itself. The individual nutrient metabolism during the stress response during critical illness is further elaborated in subsequent parts of this chapter.

NUTRIENT METABOLISM AND THE METABOLIC CONSEQUENCES OF THE STRESS RESPONSE

Protein Metabolism

Amino acids are the key building blocks required for growth and tissue repair. The vast majority (98%) is found in existing proteins, with the remainder residing in the free amino acid pool. Proteins themselves are not static as they are continually degraded and synthesized in the process of protein turnover. The reuse of amino acids released by protein breakdown is extensive; protein turnover contributes more than two times the amino acids derived from protein intake. As a reference, healthy newborns have a protein turnover of approximately 6.7 g/kg/d, and adults have a protein turnover of approximately 3.5 g/kg/d.[7] An advantage of high protein turnover is that a continuous flow of amino acids is available for synthesis of new proteins. In this way, maximal physiologic adaptability is present at times of injury or illness. In the metabolically stressed patient, such as adults with severe burn injury or children with significant cardiorespiratory failure requiring extracorporeal membrane oxygenation (ECMO), protein turnover is double that of normal subjects.[8,9] Specifically, this process involves a redistribution of amino acids from skeletal muscle to the liver, wound, and other tissues taking part in the inflammatory response. The mediators of the inflammatory response—enzymes, serum proteins, and glucose (via gluconeogenesis)—are thus synthesized. Evidence for this process can be seen in the serum by the marked increase in hepatically derived acute-phase reactants (C-reactive protein, fibrinogen, α_1-antitrypsin, α-1-acid glycoprotein) and the reduction in transport proteins such as albumin and retinol-binding protein (RBP). Importantly, although children with critical illness have increases in both whole-body protein degradation and whole-body protein synthesis, it is the former that predominates during the stress response. Thus, these patients manifest net negative protein and nitrogen balance. Clinically significant negative protein balance is characterized by skeletal muscle wasting, weight loss, and immune dysfunction. Apart from the need for acute-phase protein production in the inflammatory response, another driving force for increased protein catabolism is the obligate production of glucose from amino acids through the process of gluconeogenesis. This process is essential as glucose is the preferred substrate for the brain, erythrocyte, and renal medulla and is a versatile energy source for tissues involved in the inflammatory response. In this process, free alanine and glutamine are first produced by muscle protein degradation. These amino acids are then transported to the liver for glucose production. Alanine, through deamination to pyruvate, contributes a three-carbon unit toward gluconeogenesis, in the glucose-alanine cycle.[10] Glutamine is first converted to alanine in the intestinal mucosa and then transported through the portal vein to the liver, to be used in glucose production.[108] Whereas in fasting subjects, alanine and glutamine account for over 60% of total amino acids released from muscle, this ratio is further accentuated in critical illness. From neonates to adults, increased gluconeogenesis is known to occur during illness and injury. On a per kilogram basis, this process is particularly prominent in patients with low body weight, presumably because of an elevated brain-to-body weight ratio and hence an increased requirement for glucose as an energy source.[11] Because hepatic gluconeogenesis incorporates deamination of these amino acids to cleave the carbon skeleton, the ammonia moiety by-product is detoxified by the liver through the urea cycle. Urea is thus generated as a soluble and relatively nontoxic metabolite that can be safely excreted in the urine. In addition, glycolysis is often initiated for energy production given the anaerobic environment of injured tissue. Although this process is exceedingly inefficient compared to the aerobic oxidation of glucose, its end product, lactate, can eventually be reduced to pyruvate and shunted back into gluconeogenesis via the Cori cycle.

Although the catabolism of muscle protein to generate glucose and inflammatory response proteins is an excellent short-term adaptation, it is ultimately limited because of the reduced protein stores available in children and neonates. Interestingly, unlike during starvation, the provision of dietary glucose alone is ineffective in reducing the endogenous glucose production via gluconeogenesis in the metabolically stressed state.[12] Therefore, without elimination of the inciting stress for catabolism (ie, the critical illness or injury) the progressive breakdown of muscle leads to untoward consequences. Loss of diaphragmatic and intercostal muscle mass leads to respiratory compromise, and the subsequent loss of cardiac muscle predisposes to fatal arrhythmia. Fortunately, the provision of amino acid nutritional supplementation has been shown to improve overall protein balance in the premature neonate.[13,14] The mechanism for this change appears to be an increase in protein synthesis, whereas the rate of protein degradation remains constant.[15] As expected, the amount of protein required to optimally enhance protein accretion is higher in critically ill than in healthy children. Infants demonstrate 25% higher protein degradation after surgery, a 100% increase in urinary nitrogen excretion with bacterial sepsis, and a 100% increase in net protein breakdown while on ECMO.[8,15] Children under treatment for cancer have also been shown to have increased net protein breakdown.[16] The provision of dietary protein sufficient to optimize protein synthesis, facilitate wound healing and the inflammatory response, and preserve skeletal muscle protein mass is the single most important nutritional intervention in critically ill children. The quantities of protein recommended for critically ill neonates and children are outlined in Table 1.[8] Certain severely stressed states, such as significant burn injury or patients requiring ECMO, may require additional protein supplementation to meet metabolic demands. Hence, growth rates and other indices for protein accretion (ie, prealbumin levels) must be monitored closely in chronically ill patients. Excessive protein administration should be avoided as toxicity has been documented, particularly in children with marginal renal and hepatic function. Studies using high protein allotments of 4 to 6 g/kg/d have been associated with adverse effects such as azotemia, metabolic acidosis, and neurodevelopmental abnormalities.[17] A similar evaluation of the effects of high protein administration using newer formulas is desirable.

Although the precise amino acid composition to best increase whole-body protein balance has yet to be fully determined, stable isotope techniques now exist to study this issue.[18–20] Neonates, in particular, have immature biosynthetic pathways that may alter their ability to synthesize specific amino acids. For example, histidine is a conditionally essential amino acid until 6 months of age, and data suggest that biosynthetic pathways for cysteine, taurine, and proline may be of limited capacity in the premature neonate.[18–22] These immature amino acid pathways may have clinical relevance. Given that cysteine is essential for the production of the antioxidant glutathione, our laboratory has demonstrated that, in very low birth weight neonates, glutathione concentrations in erythrocytes are only 30 to 40% of that in normal infants (T. Jaksic, personal communication). In addition, proline demand has been shown to increase significantly in patients with severe burns.[9] Therefore, it is likely that specific disease states may accentuate specific amino acid requirements, and further research is needed to determine optimal dietary protein supplementation for such conditions.

In summary, during critical illness and recovery from trauma or surgery, there is increased

Table 1 Estimated Protein Requirements for Injured Children of Various Age Groups

Age (yr)	Estimated Protein Requirement (g/kg/d)
0–2	2.0–3.0
2–13	1.5–2.0
13–18	1.5

protein catabolism. The short-term adaptive benefit of this response is, in time, outweighed by the loss of protein in critical organs and the consequent morbidity seen after the exhaustion of limited protein reserves. This sustained protein breakdown cannot be stopped by optimal caloric provision alone (as in starvation), but protein balance may be restored by optimal (probably individual and disease-specific) quantities of protein intake during this state. Future studies may also elucidate if specific amino acid mixtures may be of benefit to select subpopulations.

ENERGY METABOLISM (ASSESSMENT OF ENERGY EXPENDITURE)

During critical illness, increases in the metabolic turnover of protein, carbohydrate, and lipid result in an increased basal energy requirement for the pediatric patient. However, the question of whether total energy expenditure (TEE) is actually increased in this cohort has drawn much interest. The question is important as the caloric provision for the critically ill child has significant consequences. For example, in adults, protein retention can be optimized by an adequate caloric allotment, and this is particularly true when protein intake is marginal.[23] Conversely, the dietary provision of excess calories from glucose results in an increased production of carbon dioxide (CO_2), with no change in loss of lean body mass.[24,25] Recent data in neonates on ECMO therapy have also shown a possible paradoxical increase in net protein degradation from excess carbohydrate intake.[26] Administration of high-caloric (glucose load) diets in the early phase of critical illness may exacerbate hyperglycemia, increase carbon dioxide generation with increased load on the respiratory system, promote hyperlipidemia resulting from increased lipogenesis, and result in a hyperosmolar state. On the other hand, hypocaloric diet may have a protein-sparing effect and demonstrable benefits in the adult critically ill obese patients. Some investigators have recently proposed hypocaloric diets during critical illness in adult patients.[27,28] Although, overfeeding critically ill children is also associated with net lipogenesis, hepatic steatosis, and liver dysfunction, as well as increased CO_2 production and difficulty in ventilator weaning,[29] it is uncertain if administration of lower caloric intakes are appropriate for this group. The risks and benefits of a hypocaloric regimen will need to be carefully examined in children before its implementation in practice. Thus, a careful appraisal of energy requirements in the critically ill pediatric patient is mandatory.

The components of TEE for a sedentary individual are (1) resting energy expenditure (REE)—70%, (2) diet-induced thermogenesis (DIT)—10%, and (3) energy expended during physical activity (PA)—20%. The sum of these components determines the energy requirement for an individual. Previous recommendations for energy requirements were based on estimates of basal metabolic rate (BMR) or REE derived either by indirect calorimetry or by standard equations.[30] REE can be measured using direct or indirect methods. The direct calorimetric method measures the heat released by a subject at rest and is based on the principle that all energy is eventually converted to heat. In practice, the patient is placed in a thermally isolated chamber, and the heat dissipated is measured for a given period of time.[31] This method is the true gold standard for measured energy expenditure. Although precise, direct calorimetry is not practical for most hospitalized critically ill patients. On the other hand, REE estimates using standardized World Health Organization (WHO) predictive equations are unreliable, particularly in the underweight subjects.[32–34] Newer equations have attempted to improve the prediction of REE in children by accounting for weight-based groups or including pubertal staging, with variable success.

The challenges of accurate REE estimation are further compounded in critically ill children. Their energy requirements show individual variation and are dependent on severity of injury. For instance, an infant with respiratory distress on pressure support is likely to have high energy requirement due to increased work of breathing. The same patient when placed on mechanical ventilatory support, with muscle relaxants, is unlikely to have sustained high-energy requirements. Infants with congenital diaphragmatic hernia on ECMO support have been shown to have energy expenditures of approximately 90 kcal/kg/d. Following extubation, the same patients may have energy requirements as high as 140 kcal/kg/d. Although stress factors ranging from 1.0 to 2.7 have been applied to correct for these variations,[35,36] calculated standardized energy expenditure equations have not been satisfactorily validated in critically ill children.[36–39]

The indirect methods estimate energy production based on quantities of O_2 consumption or CO_2 production by the whole body during a specific time interval. The classic indirect method, *indirect calorimetry*, measures VO_2 (the volume of oxygen consumed) and VCO_2 (the volume of CO_2 produced) and uses a correlation factor based on urinary nitrogen excretion to calculate the overall rate of energy production.[40] Historically, indirect calorimetry has been regarded as the standard bedside method for energy expenditure estimation. This method uses the *metabolic cart*, a leak-free system with a computer-controlled gas exchange measurement device as well as 24-hour urine collection. Indirect calorimetry provides a measurement of the overall respiratory quotient (RQ), defined as the ratio of CO_2 produced to O_2 consumed, for a given patient. However, this method is not accurate in the setting of air leaks around the endotracheal tube, ventilator circuit or through a chest tube, or in subjects supported on ECMO support. High, inspired oxygen fraction ($FiO_2 > 0.6$) will also affect indirect calorimetry results.

Another method of determination of energy expenditure is based on the use of doubly labeled water (DLW). Stable isotope technique has been available for many years and was first applied for energy expenditure measurement in humans in 1982.[41] Isotope studies using DLW have since been validated and have been followed with intense and skeptical scrutiny.[42–44] Orally administered stable isotopes of water (^2H_2O and $H_2{}^{18}O$) mix with the body water and the ^{18}O is lost from the body as both water and CO_2, while the ^2H is lost from the body only as water. The difference in the rates of loss of the isotopes ^{18}O and ^2H from the body reflects the rate of CO_2 production, which can be used to calculate the TEE. This method is noninvasive and isotope dilution is measured over two half-lives of the isotope, giving an average estimate of TEE over a period of few days. However, the DLW method has its limitations and is not widely used.[42] The critically ill child with active capillary leak, decreased urine output, fluid overload, and diuretic use would pose major challenges to the assumptions made in the use of this technique. Moreover, this technique is not widely available and due to the technical challenges is not often used outside dedicated laboratories.

Despite the limitations of available methods, studies have tried to address the issue of estimating energy expenditure in the heterogeneous population in the pediatric ICU. Using ^{13}C-labeled bicarbonate and DLW ($^2H_2{}^{18}O$), studies in pediatric surgical patients have accurately measured TEE.[8,44] These techniques have been shown to correlate well with indirect calorimetry and have been used to measure energy expenditure of critically ill neonates in a variety of settings.[45] A common theme in these studies is the observation that the severity and duration of the critical illness govern the energy needs of the ill child. In general, any increase in energy expenditure during illness or after surgery is variable, and recent studies suggest that the increase is far less than originally hypothesized. In children with severe burns, the initial REE during the flow phase of injury is increased by 50% but then returns to normal during convalescence.[46] In neonates with bronchopulmonary dysplasia, in which the illness increases the patient's work of breathing, a 25% elevation in energy requirement is evident.[47] Newborns undergoing major surgery have only a transient 20% increase in energy expenditure that returns to baseline values within 12 hours postoperatively provided that no major complications develop.[48,49] Stable, extubated neonates, 5 days following surgery, have been shown to have REEs comparable to normal infants.[50] Effective anesthetic and analgesic management may play a significant role in muting the stress response of the neonate. Studies have demonstrated no discernable increase in REE in neonates undergoing patent ductus arteriosus ligation who receive intraoperative fentanyl anesthesia and postoperative intravenous analgesic regimens.[49] Finally, by using stable isotopic methods, we have found that the mean energy expenditures of critically ill neonates on ECMO are nearly identical to age- and diet-matched nonstressed controls.[51] These studies suggest that critically ill neonates have only a small and perhaps negligible increase in energy expenditure. Although critically ill children have increased energy requirements from increased metabolic turnover, their growth is often halted or slowed during physiologic stress.[52] In critically ill mechanically ventilated children, use of sedation and muscle paralysis decreases the component of energy requirement related to PA,[53] and caloric needs in the critically ill child may be lower than previously considered. Thus, energy requirement estimates in some select groups of patients remain variable and possibly overestimated. Many studies reporting the energetic needs of critically ill children have been conducted on heterogeneous populations under various conditions. Thus, for practical purposes, the recommended dietary caloric intake for healthy children represents a reasonable starting point for the upper limit of caloric allotment in the critically ill child.[54]

In summary, due to the high individual variability in energy expenditure in critically ill patients, actual measurement of REE (ie, by indirect calorimetry) is recommended. Since predictive equations, used with stress factors to account for the degrees of illness, have proven inaccurate in determining individual energy expenditures, the preferred method to measure energy expenditure remains indirect calorimetry, when available.[33] Once protein needs have been met, safe caloric provisions using carbohydrate and lipid energy sources have similar beneficial effects on net protein synthesis and overall protein balance in critically ill patients. The rational partitioning of these substrates requires knowledge of carbohydrate and lipid handling in critical illness.

CARBOHYDRATE METABOLISM

Glucose production and availability are a priority of the metabolic response in critically ill children. Glucose is the primary energy used by the brain, erythrocyte, and renal medulla and is useful in the repair of injured tissue. Glycogen stores are limited and quickly depleted in illness or injury, resulting in the need for gluconeogenesis. In injured and septic adults, a three-fold increase in glucose turnover and oxidation has been demonstrated as well as an elevation in gluconeogenesis.[55,56] As mentioned earlier, a significant feature of the metabolic stress response is that the provision of dietary glucose does not halt gluconeogenesis. Consequently, the catabolism of muscle protein to produce glucose continues unabated.[12] However, it is clear that a combination of dietary glucose and amino acids effectively improves net protein balance in critical illness. This occurs primarily through the augmentation of protein synthesis and has little, if any, effect on protein breakdown.[15,57] In early nutritional support regimens for critically ill patients, excessive glucose allotments were used to attempt to overcome the need for gluconeogenesis and, in effect, protein degradation. As expected, the excess glucose was converted to fat, resulting in the net generation of CO_2. The synthesis of fat from glucose has an RQ of approximately 8.7. Clinically, this high RQ is not attained, as glucose is never purely used for fatty acid synthesis. Nonetheless, the provision of excess glucose results in an elevated RQ and thus increases the ventilatory burden on the child. The mean RQ in postsurgical neonates fed a high-glucose diet is approximately 1.0, whereas comparable neonates fed with reduced quantities of glucose in combination with a standard concentration of lipid have an RQ of 0.83.[58] Using high-glucose total parenteral nutrition (TPN), hypermetabolic adult patients fed excess caloric allotments have a 30% increase in O_2 consumption, a 57% increase in CO_2 production, and a 71% elevation in minute ventilation.[24] In addition, aforementioned studies have found that excess glucose provisions may worsen negative protein balance in neonates requiring ECMO.[26] Thus, avoidance of excess calories from glucose provisions and the use of a mixed-fuel system employing both carbohydrates and lipid are theoretically and practically useful in critically ill children, many of whom already have respiratory challenges from the nature of their illness. This approach also helps to alleviate difficulties with hyperglycemia in the relatively insulin-resistant stressed child.

HYPERGLYCEMIA IN CRITICAL ILLNESS: ROLE OF TIGHT GLYCEMIC CONTROL

Hyperglycemia is prevalent in critically ill children including those in the posttraumatic and postsurgical state.[4] The etiology of hyperglycemia during the stress response is multifactorial with the neuroendocrine response to stress and insulin resistance during critical illness playing a role. A strong correlation between hyperglycemia and mortality has been recently demonstrated.[59,60] Improved outcomes were reported in a cohort, comprising predominantly postcardiac surgery patients in an adult ICU, by implementing strict glycemic control (arterial blood glucose levels below 110 mg/dL) using insulin infusion.[6] A remarkable 43% reduction in mortality was reported in the treatment group with tight glycemic control when compared with patients in the control group (average blood glucose level of 150 to 160 mg/dL) (Figure 2A and B). Secondary benefits observed in the treatment group included reduction in the overall hospital mortality, new-onset renal dysfunction, bacteremia, red cell transfusion requirement, and critical illness neuropathy. Similarly, using a nursing-led insulin protocol for tight glycemic control (blood sugar below 140 mg/dL), in a heterogeneous cohort of adult medical ICU patients, a 29.3% decrease in mortality was observed in the treatment group when compared to historical controls (matched for disease type and severity).[61] Moreover, there was no increase in the frequency of hypoglycemia in the treatment group or resources used for the application of such a protocol. These studies have firmly established the correlation between glycemic control and adult intensive care mortality. The precise mechanism(s) responsible for this beneficial effect of tight glycemic control with insulin protocol remains unanswered. Although the incidence of hyperglycemia in the pediatric intensive care population is high and may be associated with increased mortality and length of stay,[62,63] no data exist currently for similar benefits of tight glycemic control in the pediatric age group. Studies examining the role of tight glycemic control strategy (its benefits and risks) in the pediatric population are currently underway. Although it is prudent to avoid prolonged hyperglycemia in the pediatric ICU patients, in the absence of definitive data, aggressive glycemic control cannot be recommended as yet in the critically ill child.

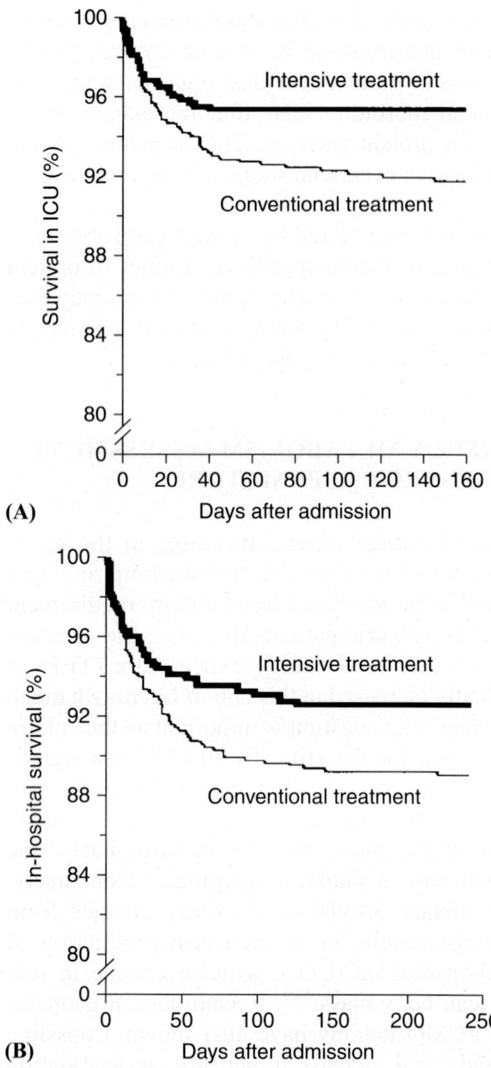

Figure 2 Outcomes data from the Leuven study. (Adapted from reference 6.) Kaplan-Meier curves showing cumulative survival of patients who received intensive insulin treatment (strict glycemic control, blood glucose maintained below 110 mg/dL) or convention treatment in the intensive care unit.

Patients discharged alive from the ICU (A) and from the hospital (B) were considered to have survived. In both cases, differences between the treatment groups were significant.

LIPID METABOLISM

Analogous to protein and carbohydrate metabolism, lipid turnover is generally accelerated by critical illness, surgery, and trauma.[57] Although lipid use is compromised in the initial, brief ebb phase following acute trauma or sepsis, overall lipid turnover increases dramatically during the predominant flow phase. Adult patients demonstrate two- to four-fold increases in lipid turnover compared with healthy controls, and this increase is proportional to the degree of illness.[64] This process involves the recycling of free fatty acids and glycerol into and from triglycerides. Approximately 30 to 40% of the free fatty acid moieties are oxidized for energy, and the RQ values postinjury are approximately 0.8. Infants and children subjected to uncomplicated abdominal surgery have also shown a reduction in RQ along with a decline in plasma triglyceride levels.[65] Recently, it has been shown that critically ill children do, indeed, have a higher rate of fat oxidation.[39] Thus, this suggests that fatty acids are, in fact, the prime source of energy in metabolically stressed children. Glycerol, released along with free fatty acids from the breakdown of triglycerides, may be converted to pyruvate and thereby shunted into the gluconeogenesis pathway. Again similar to protein catabolism, the provision of dietary glucose does not decrease glycerol clearance or overall lipid turnover.

Because of the increased demand for lipid use in critical illness coupled with the limited lipid stores in the pediatric patient, critically ill children are susceptible to the evolution of biochemically detected essential fatty acid deficiency if administered a fat-free diet.[66,67] In infants, linoleic and linolenic acid are considered essential, whereas arachidonic acid and docosahexaenoic acid are thought to be conditionally essential. If the body lacks dietary linoleic acid, the formation of arachidonic acid (a tetraene) by desaturation and chain elongation cannot take place. The same pathway then converts available oleic acid to 5,8,11-eicosatrienoic acid (a triene), resulting in an elevated triene-to-tetraene ratio, which is empirically characteristic of essential fatty acid deficiency.[68] Clinically, this syndrome presents as dermatitis, alopecia, thrombocytopenia, and increased susceptibility to bacterial infection. To avoid essential fatty acid deficiency in critically ill or injured infants, the allotment of linoleic and linolenic acid is recommended at concentrations of 4.5 and 0.5% of total calories, respectively.[69] The provision of commercially available lipid solutions to parenterally fed critically ill children reduces the risk of essential fatty acid deficiency, results in improved protein use, and does not significantly increase CO_2 production or metabolic rate.[70] There are disadvantages, however, with lipid administration, including hypertriglyceridemia, increased rates, of infection, and decreased alveolar oxygen diffusion capacity.[71–73] Most centers, therefore, start lipid supplementation in ill children at 1.0 g/kg/d and advance over a period of days to 2 to 4 g/kg/d, with monitoring of triglyceride levels. Lipid administration is generally restricted to a maximum of 30 to 40% of total calories, although this practice has not been validated by clinical trials. Of note, normal ketone body metabolism is also markedly affected by critical illness. The product of incomplete fatty acid and pryruvate oxidation is acetyl coenzyme A, which forms the ketone bodies acetoacetate and γ-hydroxybutyrate through a condensation reaction within the hepatocyte. In starved healthy subjects, a major adaptation to preserve skeletal muscle mass is the production of these ketone bodies, which can then be used as an energy source for the brain. However, in the 3-day period following trauma, there is a negligible elevation in serum ketone body levels.[74] This observation may be explained in part by the elevated serum insulin concentrations found during the metabolic stress response. Even low concentrations of insulin inhibit ketogenesis, a fact made evident by the absence of ketotic complications in type 2 diabetics. Hence, the elevated insulin concentrations seen in severe illness and injury serve to negate the ketotic adaptation found in starvation.

ELECTROLYTE METABOLISM

Requirements for the basic electrolytes—Na^+, K^+, Cl^-, HCO_3^-, and Ca^{2+}—must be evaluated frequently in the critically ill patient. In addition to routine electrolyte monitoring, careful attention to phosphate and magnesium levels is recommended. Hypophosphatemia may lead to hemolytic anemia and respiratory muscle dysfunction and may also be seen with refeeding syndrome in the ill child. Renal failure can result in the retention of phosphate, and nutritional allotments must be reduced accordingly. Deficiency of magnesium can cause fatal cardiac arrhythmia. Abnormalities of acid–base physiology in the critically ill child can also influence the nutritional regimen. For example, head-injured patients often develop an iatrogenically induced respiratory alkalosis. If a metabolic alkalosis secondary to active diuresis or gastric suction is also present, Cl^- administration should be used to correct the alkalosis. Untreated alkalemia tends to inhibit the respiratory drive, shift potassium intracellularly, and decrease ionized calcium concentrations by increasing the affinity of albumin for calcium. Metabolic acidosis can also be seen in critically ill children, often from associated hypotension or ischemic etiologies. In this case, the provision of acetate instead of Cl^- in the PN regimen should be used so as not to worsen the existing acidemia. The provision of excess acetate at 1 mEq/kg/d is usually a safe adjunct to limit metabolic acidosis.

VITAMIN AND TRACE MINERAL METABOLISM

Vitamin and trace mineral metabolism in critically ill and postoperative patients has not been extensively studied. For the neonate and the child, required vitamins include fat-soluble vitamins (A, D, E, and K) and water-soluble vitamins (ascorbic acid, thiamin, riboflavin, pyridoxine, niacin, pantothenate, biotin, folate, and vitamin B_{12}), and these are routinely administered. Because vitamins are not stoichiometrically consumed in biochemical reactions but rather act as catalysts, the administration of large supplements of vitamins in stressed states is not logical from a nutritional standpoint. The trace minerals required for normal development are zinc, iron, copper, selenium, manganese, iodide, molybdenum, and chromium. Trace minerals are used in the synthesis of active sites of a ubiquitous and extraordinarily important class of enzymes termed metalloenzymes. As with vitamins, the role of metalloenzymes is to act as catalysts. Hence, unless there are excessive losses, such as increased zinc loss with severe diarrhea, large nutritional requirements in critical illness should not be anticipated. The Recommended Dietary Allowances of vitamin and trace mineral needs of healthy children and neonates are reviewed periodically and are well defined in the literature.[54] These recommended levels have been used in critically ill patients, and little evidence exists that they are nutritionally inadequate. In children with severe hepatic failure, copper and manganese accumulation can occur; thus, parenteral trace mineral supplementation should be reduced.

BODY COMPOSITION AND METABOLIC RESERVES

Table 2 outlines the body composition of the neonate, child, and adult patient.[75–77] The most striking difference in body composition between the adult and the child is the quantity of protein in reserve and available at times of illness. Table 3 outlines the relative protein stores in humans at various stages of development.[78] As a percentage of body weight, the protein stores of adults are nearly twice those of the neonate. In contrast, carbohydrate stores remain constant and do not afford significant reserve at any age. Lipid concentrations are low at birth and increase gradually during development; premature infants have even lower proportions of stored lipid at birth. In addition to the reduced macronutrient reserves in the child, both neonates and children have much higher baseline requirements. The REE for neonates is up to three times that for adults when standardized for weight.[79,80] This inverse relationship between energy expenditure and body weight is constant throughout mammalian

Table 2 Body Composition of Neonates, Children, and Nonobese Adults as a Percentage of Total Body Weight

Age	Protein (%)	Fat (%)	Carbohydrate (%)
Neonates	11	14	0.4
Children (age 10 yr)	15	17	0.4
Adults	18	19	0.4

Table 3 Proportion of Skeletal Muscle in the Body of Humans at Various Stages of Development[78]

Stage	Proportion of Skeletal Muscle (%)
Birth	21
Weaning	18
Adolescent	36
Adult	45
Elderly	27

species and is partially related to body surface area. The recommended intakes of macronutrients and water for healthy children and adults can be found in Table 4. The protein requirements of the full-term neonate (per kg body weight) are nearly three times that of the adult. Moreover, premature neonates require a minimum of 2.8 g/kg/d of protein to maintain growth rates similar to *those* in utero, and this is 3.5 times the requirement for protein balance in the adult.[81] Thus, the critically ill child has the potential to be much more susceptible to the harmful effects of protracted catabolic stress, and the prompt implementation of adequate nutritional support must be a priority in the patient's care.

Accurate assessment of body composition is necessary for planning ongoing nutritional intake, monitoring dynamic changes in the body compartments (such as ongoing loss of lean body mass), and assessing the adequacy of nutritional supportive regimens during critical illness. Ongoing loss of lean body mass is an indicator of inadequate dietary supplementation and may have clinical implications in the critically ill child. However, current methods of body composition analysis (such as anthropometry, weight, and biochemical parameters) are either impractical for clinical use or inaccurate in the setting of critical care. One of the principal problems in critically ill children is the presence of capillary leak, manifesting as edema and large fluid shifts. These make anthropometric measurements invalid and other bedside techniques have not been validated. A bedside body composition analysis technique for critically ill children is desirable. Bioelectric impedance monitoring allows accurate prediction of both body compartments and fluid distribution in various compartments in healthy adults. Instruments of potential utility, such as the BIA remain to be evaluated in critically ill children.

ASSESMENT OF NUTRITIONAL STATUS

Nutritional assessment of the critically ill child is challenging and clinicians use a combination of anthropometric and laboratory data to diagnose undernourishment. However, standard methods of nutritional assessment are either difficult to obtain or impossible to interpret in critically ill patients. Carefully elicited past history with details of weight gain, dietary history, recent illness, and medications may allow identification of risk factors for preoperative malnutrition. Weight on admission to the hospital is important and may be the only estimate of the actual dry weight before the capillary leak syndrome lead to edema and weight gain. Regular weight monitoring is a valuable index of nutritional status in these patients. Weight changes during the ICU admission should be interpreted in the context of fluid therapy, other causes of volume overload, and diuresis. Physical examination can be directed toward specific signs of nutritional and metabolic deficiencies. Hair, skin, eyes, mouth, and extremities may reveal stigmata of protein-energy malnutrition or vitamin and mineral deficiencies. The biggest hurdle in applying routine techniques for nutritional assessment in this subgroup is the presence of capillary leak and the consequent alterations in fluid distribution. Commonly used anthropometric methods of body composition (such as the triceps skinfold) may be unreliable in the presence of edema. Objective assessment of fluid shift within the body compartments would allow accurate estimates of true nutritional status. The bioelectric impedance assessment device has been applied in some populations as a noninvasive body composition measurement. Isotope dilution techniques using DLW, deuterium, and sodium bromide allow accurate assessment of the various body compartments and fluid distribution, but remain impractical for routine bedside use.

Laboratory Tests

Serum albumin is frequently used as a tool for nutritional assessment in the ICU. Levels <2.2 g/dL reflect malnutrition. However, the long half-life of albumin (14 to 20 days) makes it less responsive to acute changes in nutritional status. Serum albumin concentrations may be affected by albumin infusion, dehydration, sepsis, trauma, and liver disease, independent of nutritional status. Thus, its reliability as a marker of visceral protein status is questionable.

Prealbumin (also known as transthyretin or thyroxine-binding prealbumin) is a stable circulating glycoprotein synthesized in the liver. It binds with RBP and is involved in the transport of thyroxine as well as retinol. Prealbumin, so named by its proximity to albumin on an electrophoretic strip, has a half-life of 24 to 48 hours and reflects more acute nutritional changes. Prealbumin concentration is diminished in renal and liver disease. Chemistry profile should be monitored on admission and repeated periodically. Other proteins used for nutritional assessment include, RBP, transferrin, fibronectin, and insulin-like growth factor 1 (IGF-1).

Other laboratory tests that help in overall nutritional assessment include serum electrolytes, blood urea nitrogen, glucose, coagulation profile, iron, magnesium, calcium, and phosphate. The adequacy of cellular immunity can be estimated through the measurement of total lymphocyte count (TLC) and by delayed-type hypersensitivity testing with a series of common antigens (eg, Candida, trichophyton, tuberculin). However, critically ill children in the postsurgical state may be anergic for many days, regardless of nutritional status. Anergy is a nonspecific indicator of malnutrition, and may be seen following radiotherapy or immunosuppresion.

ROUTES OF NUTRITIONAL PROVISION

Enteral Nutrition

Following the estimation of energy expenditure and requirement in the critically ill child, the next challenge is to facilitate the provision of this nutritional support. In the critically ill child with a functioning gastrointestinal tract, the enteral route of nutrient administration is preferable to PN. Enteral nutrition is physiologic and has been shown to be more cost-effective

Table 4 Dietary Reference Intakes (DRIs); Recommended Intakes of Macronutrients and Total Water

Age	Total Water (L/day)	Carbohydrate (g/day)	Fat (g/day)	Linoleic Acid (g/day)	alpha-Linoleic Acid (g/day)	Protein (g/day)
0–6 mo	0.7	60	31	4.4	0.5	9.1
7–12 mo	0.8	95	30	4.6	0.5	**11**
1–3 yr	1.3	**130**	ND	7	0.7	**13**
4–8 yr	1.7	**130**	ND	10	0.9	**19**
Males						
9–13 yr	2.4	**130**	ND	12	1.2	**34**
14–18 yr	3.3	**130**	ND	16	1.6	**52**
19–30 yr	3.7	**130**	ND	17	1.6	**56**
31–50 yr	3.7	**130**	ND	17	1.6	**56**
Female						
9–13 yr	2.1	**130**	ND	10	1.0	**34**
14–18 yr	2.3	**130**	ND	11	1.1	**46**
19–30 yr	2.7	**130**	ND	12	1.1	**46**
31–50 yr	2.7	**130**	ND	12	1.1	**46**

Recommended dietary allowances (RDA) are in bold and the rest are adequate intakes (AI). Both RDA and AI may be used as goals for individual intake. ND = not determined. Adapted from: *Dietary Reference Intakes for Energy, Carbohydrate, Fiber, Fat, Fatty Acids, Cholesterol, Protein, and Amino Acids* (2002/2005); *Dietary Reference Intakes for Water, Potassium, Sodium, Chloride, and Sulfate* (2005). These reports may be accessed via http://www.nap.edu.

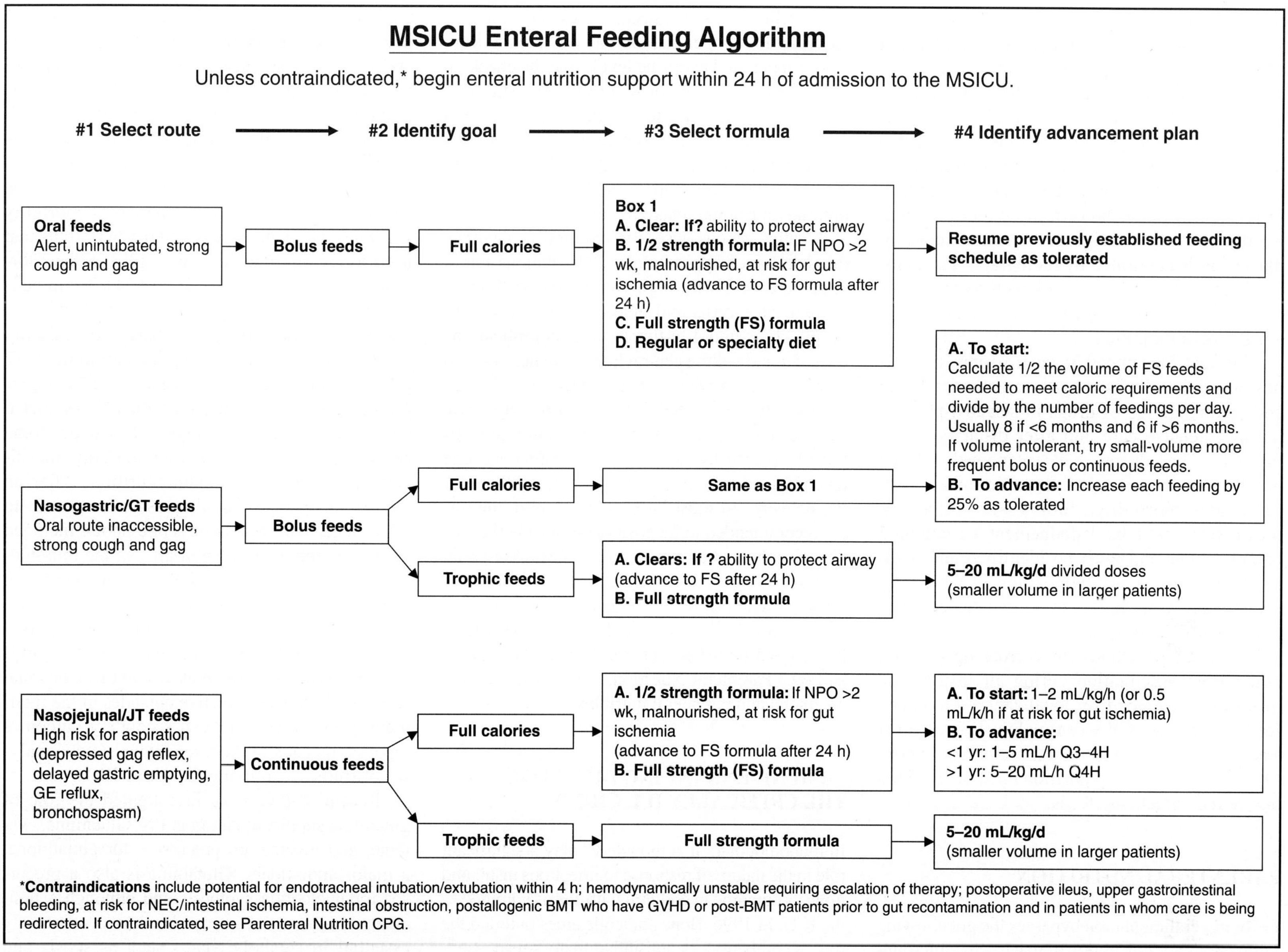

Figure 3 Enteral feeding algorithm at Children's Hospital, Boston.

without the added risk of nosocomial infection inherent in PN.[82,83] The postpyloric feeding tube, placed at the bedside or with fluoroscopic guidance, helps to decrease the risk of aspiration and is a useful tool in the nutritional management of the critically ill child. Continuous feedings using standard formulas can adequately nourish the majority of injured patients. Diarrhea can often be avoided by carefully controlling the infusion rate until tolerance is established. Early enteral nutrition has been shown to decrease infectious episodes and decrease length of hospital stay in critically ill patients.[84] The enteral route has been successfully used for nutritional support of the critically ill child.[85–87] At the time of extubation, tube feeds are held for 6 to 12 hours to lower the corresponding risk of aspiration. It is also recommended not to use enteral feeds with patients who are hypotensive or who have evidence of bowel ischemia so as to limit the risk of small bowel necrosis associated with rapid enteral feeding.[88] Intolerance to enteral feeds may be a limiting factor and supplementation with PN in this group of patients allows optimal nutritional intake. In a subgroup of critically ill patients, TPN may be required for a period before initiation of enteral feeds. However, many studies have shown inability to achieve the set nutritional goal.

In a study examining the endocrine and metabolic response of children with meningococcal sepsis, goal nutrition was achieved in only 25% of the cases.[89,90] Similar observations have been made in a group of 95 children in a pediatric ICU (PICU) where patients received a median of 58.8% (range 0 to 277%) of their estimated energy requirements. In this review, enteral feeding was interrupted on 264 occasions to allow clinical procedures. Consistently underachieved enteral nutrition goals are thought to be perhaps responsible for the absence of beneficial effect in multiple studies and meta-analysis of the efficacy of immunonutrition in preventing infection.[91]

In another review of nutritional intake in 42 patients in a tertiary-level pediatric ICU over 458 ICU days, actual energy intake was compared with estimated energy requirement.[90] Only 50% of patients were reported to have received full estimated energy requirements after a median of 7 days in the ICU. Prolonged fluid resuscitation was a major factor hindering the achievement of estimated energy requirements despite maximizing the energy content of feeds. Other contributing factors included interruption of feeds for procedures, enteral feed intolerance, and cooling. Protocols for feeding use of transpyloric feeding tubes and changing from bolus to continuous feeds during brief periods of intolerance are strategies to achieve estimated energy requirements in this population. In Figure 3 we outline a methodological approach to initiating and advancing enteral nutrition in children on our ICUs.

Enterally administered feeds meet nutritional requirements in critically ill children with functional gastrointestinal system and have the advantages of cost, manageability, safety, and preservation of gastrointestinal function. Early introduction of enteral feeds in critically ill patients helps to achieve positive protein and energy balance and restores nitrogen balance during the acute state of illness. It maintains gut integrity and elicits release of growth factors and hormones that maintain gut integrity and function.[92] Despite its perceived benefits, current practice in ICUs shows a significant proportion of eligible patients deprived of enteral feeds.[93]

Enteral feedings are indicated early on the course of critical illness if peristalsis has been established. Postpyloric feedings are recommended, due to gastric distension and hypomotility. Feeds can be administered into the stomach or jejunum with the aid of feeding tubes inserted nasally or orally. Intragastric or intrajejunal tip placement is confirmed by radiograph. Postpyloric feeding is increasingly adopted to feed children with reflux or delayed gastric emptying who are at risk of aspiration.

Surgical placement of gastrostomy or jejunostomy tube allows long-term enteral feeding and administration of drugs in selected patients during intensive care and after discharge from the ICU. The advent of percutaneously placed gastric and jejunal tubes has minimized cost, time, and morbidity. Stoma site infection, obstruction, and tube dislodgement are common complications and must be identified and managed early. Tube tip malposition is frequently encountered with any of these devices either at placement or during the course of its use. Bedside screening methods for correct tip position range from auscultation during air insufflation to ultrasound-guided tip localization. However, feeds should be held when malposition of tip is suspected and when in doubt, radiographic confirmation of correct tip position must be obtained before recommencing feeds.

PARENTERAL NUTRITION

PN or hyperalimentation bypasses the gut allowing intravenous administration of macro- and micronutrients to meet the nutritional requirements of the body. PN is indicated in children who are unable to tolerate enteral feeds for a prolonged period of time. Intravenous feeding may supplement enteral feeding or replace it entirely as in TPN. Although widespread in its application, PN is associated with mechanical, infectious, and metabolic complications and hence should only be used in carefully selected patients. In the setting of an intact intestinal function, PN is not indicated if enteral feeds alone can maintain nutrition.

Fluid and electrolytes status will guide the initial PN prescription. The patient's hydration, size, age, and underlying disease will dictate the amount of the fluid to be administered. PN should not be used for replacing ongoing losses. PN should be prescribed daily and after reviewing electrolytes and blood sugar in order to allow adjustments in the macro- and micronutrient composition.

Careful biochemical monitoring is mandatory to prevent acute and long-term complications from PN therapy. A PN profile is recommended at initiation of therapy and then weekly. It includes serum levels of sodium, potassium, chloride, glucose, carbon dioxide, blood urea nitrogen, creatinine, albumin, magnesium, phosphate, total and direct bilirubin, and transaminases. For children requiring PN longer than 30 days, selenium, iron, zinc, copper, and carnitine levels may be checked. It is essential to monitor daily vital statistics and routine anthropometry to ensure adequate growth and development. Critical care units benefit from the expertise of a dedicated nutritionist, who should be consulted on a regular basis to guide optimal nutritional intake of patients.

Central venous access is required to facilitate the delivery of hyperosmolar PN solutions into a large-bore vein with high-volume blood flow, to prevent thrombosis and phlebitis. The incidences of infective and life-threatening complications related to indwelling central lines have necessitated extreme caution when using central PN.[94–96] Central line tips are located in the superior vena cava, right atrium, or inferior vena cava. Central line tips must be placed by experienced operators and line tip confirmed on radiographs before using them for PN delivery. At most institutions, central line tips are recommended to be positioned outside the cardiac chambers at all times. At our institution, only central lines are recommended for the delivery of infusates with osmolarity higher than 900 mosm/L (10% dextrose, 2% amino acids with standard additives). (please see Chapters 68, "Enteral Nutrition," and 69, "Parenteral Nutrition," for further reading on enteral and parenteral nutrition.

IMMUNE-ENHANCING DIETS FOR THE CRITICALLY ILL CHILD

Immunomodulation is thought to play a significant role in the nature of response to infectious insult and impacts outcome in children with sepsis admitted to the ICU. In 1996, Bone and colleagues outlined the role of compensatory anti-inflammatory response.[97] The anti-inflammatory response that follows the initial proinflammatory response by the body challenged with an insult or infection is aimed at keeping the proinflammatory response under control. Therapies aimed at modulating or stimulating the immune response have been a focus of many recent studies.

Immune-enhancing diets (IEDs) have been available for many years and their role in the care of critically ill patients remains controversial. Studies examining their role in critically ill patients suffer from heterogeneous clinical populations, methodological flaws, and the heterogeneous nature of the IED formulations used. Thus meta-analyses of these studies have resulted in conflicting conclusions that do not allow for dispelling current doubts regarding the safety and efficacy of these diets. The commercially available diets contain varied compounds in different doses and the role of individual compounds is impossible to interpret. Furthermore, there are no pediatric studies evaluating the role of immunonutrition in critically ill children.

A recent meta-analysis of randomized clinical trials examining the efficacy of enteral immunonutrients in adult patients included 2,419 subjects from 22 studies.[98] There was no difference in mortality between the two groups, although patients who received enteral immunonutrition had a decreased incidence of infective episodes and decreased length of hospital stay, compared to patients who received standard enteral formula. In a subgroup analysis of 13 trials in critically ill patients, the duration of hospital stay was decreased in the experimental arm in this subgroup (ES −0.47; 95% CI −0.93 to −0.01). On further subgroup analysis, increased mortality was reported in the experimental arm of trials that used lower arginine content (6 g/L) in their formula (RR 2.13; 95% CI 1.08 to 4.21). Arginine is a conditionally essential amino acid. It becomes essential in the setting of sepsis. No mortality effect was seen in trials using high arginine (>12 g/L) content. A recent multicenter trial[99] comparing enteral immunonutrition with PN conducted an interim subgroup analysis, based on some reports suggestive of increased mortality in critically ill patients on immunonutrition. After an interim analysis, the study was discontinued. In 39 patients with sepsis or septic shock included in this interim analysis, mortality in the immunonutrition arm (8 of 18, 44.4%) of this subgroup was three times higher than that in the PN arm (3 of 21, 14.3%). The increased mortality reported with certain subgroups and with low-dose arginine is cautionary. Decreased length of hospital stay and decreased infective episodes in the treatment group were beneficial secondary outcomes reported by each of the three reviews/meta-analyses of studies examining the use of IEDs.

Recent studies have investigated the role of glutamine supplementation in PN. Glutamine, cysteine, and glycine are precursors for glutathione, a major antioxidant. Glutamine is also a precursor for nucleotide synthesis and although a nonessential amino acid, it can become conditionally essential in catabolic states such as sepsis and trauma. Its applicability may be widespread and it has been introduced in PN solutions for its presumed benefits, such as restoration of protein and nitrogen balance, attenuation of gastrointestinal mucosal atrophy, reduced bacterial translocation, and reduction in bacteremia after chemotherapy. Pediatric burns patients have been shown to have deficient peripheral glutamine production. Glutamine supplementation was associated with reduced gram-negative bacteremia in severely burned patients in a double-blinded randomized control trial.[100] Glutamine has also been added to enteral feeds as an immunomodulating agent. A recent Spanish study involving 11 ICUs and 84 patients with active inflammation (predominantly septic) compared glutamine-enriched enteral feed with a control matched for nonprotein calories to nitrogen ratio. Although, the ICU mortality and length of stay remained unchanged, there was a decrease in the incidence of nosocomial pneumonia from 33 to 14%. Another study reported improved survival at 6 months and decreased costs per survivor in the treatment arm of a study comparing glutamine-enriched PN to isonitrogenous and isocaloric control nutrition in 84 critically ill adults. Following enteral administration, there is a 50% splanchnic extraction of this amino acid, which attenuates its blood levels attained by this route. A large meta-analysis recently[101] reported a larger benefit from parenteral administration compared with enteral glutamine intake. The National Institute of Child Health and Development (NICHD) neonatal research network did not find significant differences in outcomes; when a multicenter study randomized 1,430 extremely low birth weight neonates to PN containing 20% glutamine or isonitrogenous control. Overall, the studies investigating glutamine in IED have shown no major side effects and this relatively inexpensive additive may be a promising immune nutrient in critically ill patients with anticipated mortality benefits in treatment groups. Arginine, n-3 polyunsaturated fatty acids, and nucleic acids are some of the other compounds found in commercially available IEDs.

In summary, no conclusive data in regard to the beneficial effects of IEDs have been established. The immune-enhancing effect of individual components of these formulations has not been tested.

OMEGA-3 FATTY ACIDS

Substitution of the intralipid component of PN (rich in proinflammatory omega-6 fatty acids) with fish oil has been demonstrated to alleviate some of the toxic effects of long-term PN on the liver. The beneficial effects omega-3 fatty acids have been shown in animal and human models and this is an area of great interest. Omega-3 fatty acids have an anti-inflammatory effect, with decreased cytokine production shown in some models. More recently a commercially available omega-3 fatty acid for parenteral administration has been administered in children with exciting results. In a cohort of PN-dependent children with PN-associated cholestatic liver damage, parenteral fish oil was employed as compassionate use with almost complete recovery of liver function in some cases.[109] A clinical trial to test the benefits of Omegaven in children is currently under way.

MECHANISMS OF THE METABOLIC RESPONSE

Although research continues to elucidate the metabolic changes associated with the pediatric stress response, future studies will aim to uncover the mechanisms behind these metabolic alterations. The goal of this research is ultimately to gain the knowledge necessary to control and modulate the response. In this way, many of the deleterious consequences associated with the metabolic stress response can potentially be circumvented. Two integrated and complex systems are involved: neuroendocrine pathways and inflammatory cytokines. The neuroendocrine response to critical illness is relatively well defined, and its features are common to both children and adults. Beginning soon after the initial insult, a unique hormonal profile takes hold. Catecholamines are released from the adrenal medulla on stimulation by the sympathetic nervous system. The secretion of adrenocorticotropic hormone mediated by the anterior pituitary results in an increase in serum cortisol and aldosterone levels. Growth hormone and antidiuretic hormone are secreted by the anterior and posterior pituitary glands, respectively. In addition, glucagon levels rise with the surge in catecholamines. After a brief, initial decline, a rapid increase in serum insulin concentrations is found.[102–104] Overall, the hormonal changes in neonates and infants have been shown to be of greater magnitude but shorter duration than those found in older children and adults. The alterations in intermediary metabolism inherent in the metabolic response can be attributed, at least in part, to these hormonal changes. The mobilization of amino acids from muscle, the increased rate of gluconeogenesis in the liver, and the increased lipolysis from adipocyte stores can be explained by the elevations in glucagon, cortisol, and the catecholamines. The increase in net protein degradation, however, is not consistent with the persistent elevation of insulin, a known anabolic hormone. In this way, it has been postulated that injury-induced protein degradation is the result of a postreceptor defect in insulin action.[105] This hypothesis is further supported by the finding that burn patients do not demonstrate the same degree of inhibition of protein breakdown compared with normal controls when subjected to hyperinsulinemic euglycemic conditions.[106] The presence of inflammatory cytokines can be found in the circulation within hours of elective surgery or trauma. These peptides are secreted by leukocytes in a variety of settings and help to mediate the inflammatory response. In general, the prototypical cytokine response in neonates does not markedly differ from that of older children or adults. Interleukin (IL)-6 has been found in increased concentrations in the serum of children within hours after surgery, and this increase persists up to 24 to 48 hours postoperatively.[107] IL-6 levels have also been shown to be significantly elevated in critically ill children requiring ECMO.[51] IL-6 levels have been directly correlated with increased protein turnover and catabolism as well as a higher incidence of postoperative complications and mortality.[104,105] Tumor necrosis factor (TNF) has also been shown to increase in neonatal critical illness such as necrotizing enterocolitis and sepsis. It is hypothesized that TNF is involved in the release of prostaglandins, thereby mediating the hypotension associated with the septic state. The release of IL-2, IL-8, IL-11, interferon-γ, and other growth factors is also known to augment the immunologic and hormonal response to injury, although the precise effect of these cytokines on metabolism has not been fully defined.

CONCLUSIONS

The pediatric metabolic response to critical illness and injury is composed of a significant increase in the turnover of protein, carbohydrate, and lipid substrates. This process allows for the production of inflammatory response proteins that participate in the associated inflammation and wound healing. Extreme protein loss, consistent with the severity of the illness or injury, is a hallmark of this metabolic process. Interestingly, recent research has demonstrated that the overall energy expenditure of the child is not necessarily increased during this metabolic response. It is thought that the child shifts energy resources from normal growth and activity to provide fuel for the increased turnover of substrate. Implementing an appropriate nutritional regimen to minimize the protein loss and to meet the energy requirements of the child is of paramount importance in the long-term management of children suffering from critical illness or major injury. Maintaining positive protein balance in the face of protein loss requires substantially increased protein allotments, especially in neonates. Excessive carbohydrate provisions do not blunt the metabolic response and, indeed, have been shown to have deleterious consequences. In addition, because the energy expenditure of these patients does not appear to increase significantly, the recommended caloric intake for healthy children in a similar age group represents a reasonable starting point for the upper limit of caloric allotment in critically ill children. Nutritional therapy in the critically ill child must be provided via the enteral route where possible. PN may be cautiously employed to supplement or replace enteral nutrition in certain cases. Careful monitoring, judicious application, and prompt recourse to enteral feeds, as feasible, will allow safe use of PN in the critically ill child. A dedicated nutritionist and pharmacist are integral to any multidisciplinary critical care team. Finally, exact measurement of energy expenditure using indirect calorimetry should be used in complicated patients and when patients do not respond over time to an appropriate nutritional regimen.

REFERENCES

1. Hulst J, et al. Malnutrition in critically ill children: From admission to 6 months after discharge. Clin Nutr 2004;23:223–32.
2. Pollack MM, et al. Malnutrition in critically ill infants and children. JPEN J Parenter Enteral Nutr 1982;6:20–4.
3. Pollack MM, Ruttimann UE, Wiley JS. Nutritional depletions in critically ill children: Associations with physiologic instability and increased quantity of care. JPEN J Parenter Enteral Nutr 1985;9:309–13.
4. Cuthbertson D. Intensive-care-metabolic response to injury. Br J Surg 1970;57:718–21.
5. O'Connell RC, Morgan AP, Aoki TT, et al. Nitrogen conservation in starvation: Graded responses to intravenous glucose. J Clin Endocrinol Metab 1974;39:555–63.
6. van den Berghe G, Wouters P. Weekers F, et al. Intensive insulin therapy in the critically ill patients. N Engl J Med 2001;345:1359–67.
7. Denne SC, Kalhan SC. Leucine metabolism in human newborns. Am J Physiol 1987;253:E608–15.
8. Keshen TH, et al. Stable isotopic quantitation of protein metabolism and energy expenditure in neonates on- and post-extracorporeal life support. J Pediatr Surg 1997;32:958–62; discussion 962–3.
9. Jaksic T, Wagner DA, Burke JF, et al. Proline metabolism in adult male burned patients and healthy control subjects. Am J Clin Nutr 1991;54:408–13.
10. Felig P. The glucose-alanine cycle. Metabolism 1973;22:179–207.
11. Keshen T, Miller R, Jahoor F, et al. Glucose production and gluconeogenesis are negatively related to body weight in mechanically ventilated, very low birth weight neonates. Pediatr Res 1997;41:132–8.

12. Long CL, Kinney JM, Geiger JW. Nonsuppressability of gluconeogenesis by glucose in septic patients. Metabolism 1976;25:193–201.
13. van Lingen RA, van Goudoever JB, Luijendijk IH, et al. Effects of early amino acid administration during total parenteral nutrition on protein metabolism in pre-term infants. Clin Sci (Lond) 1992;82:199–203.
14. Rivera A, Jr, Bell EF, Bier DM. Effect of intravenous amino acids on protein metabolism of preterm infants during the first three days of life. Pediatr Res 1993;33:106–11.
15. Duffy B, Pencharz P. The effects of surgery on the nitrogen metabolism of parenterally fed human neonates. Pediatr Res 1986;20:32–5.
16. Daley SE, et al. Whole body protein metabolism in children with cancer. Arch Dis Child 1996;75:273–81.
17. Premji S, Fenton T, Sauve R. Does amount of protein in formula matter for low-birthweight infants? A Cochrane systematic review. JPEN J Parenter Enteral Nutr 2006;30:507–14.
18. Miller RG, Jahoor F, Jaksic T. Decreased cysteine and proline synthesis in parenterally fed, premature infants. J Pediatr Surg 1995;30:953–7; discussion 957–8.
19. Miller RG, et al. Compartmentation of endogenously synthesized amino acids in neonates. J Surg Res 1996;63:199–203.
20. Reeds PJ, et al. Integration of amino acid and carbon intermediary metabolism: Studies with uniformly labeled tracers and mass isotopomer analysis. Eur J Pediatr 1997;156: S50–8.
21. Zlotkin SH, Anderson GH. The development of cystathionase activity during the first year of life. Pediatr Res 1982;16:65–8.
22. Shew SB, et al. Assessment of cysteine synthesis in very low-birth weight neonates using a [13C6] glucose tracer. J Pediatr Surg 2005;40:52–6.
23. Calloway DH, Spector H. Nitrogen balance as related to caloric and protein intake in active young men. Am J Clin Nutr 1954;2:405–12.
24. Askanazi J, et al. Respiratory changes induced by the large glucose loads of total parenteral nutrition. JAMA 1980;243:1444–7.
25. Hart DW, et al. Energy expenditure and caloric balance after burn: Increased feeding leads to fat rather than lean mass accretion. Ann Surg 2002;235:152–61.
26. Shew SB, et al. The determinants of protein catabolism in neonates on extracorporeal membrane oxygenation. J Pediatr Surg 1999;34:1086–90.
27. McCowen KC, et al. Hypocaloric total parenteral nutrition: Effectiveness in prevention of hyperglycemia and infectious complications—a randomized clinical trial. Crit Care Med 2000;28:3606–11.
28. Patino JF, et al. Hypocaloric support in the critically ill. World J Surg 1999;23:553–9.
29. MacIntyre NR, Cook DJ, Ely EW, et al. Evidence-based guidelines for weaning and discontinuing ventilatory support: A collective task force facilitated by the American College of Chest Physicians; the American Association for Respiratory Care; and the American College of Critical Care Medicine. Chest 2001;120:375S–95S.
30. Schofield WN. Predicting basal metabolic rate, new standards and review of previous work. Hum Nutr Clin Nutr 1985;39:5–41.
31. Seale JL, Rumpler WV. Comparison of energy expenditure measurements by diet records, energy intake balance, doubly labeled water and room calorimetry. Eur J Clin Nutr 1997;51:856–63.
32. Daly JM, et al. Human energy requirements: Overestimation by widely used prediction equation. Am J Clin Nutr 1985;42:1170–4.
33. Hunter DC, et al. Resting energy expenditure in the critically ill: Estimations versus measurement. Br J Surg 1988;75:875–8.
34. Muller MJ, et al. World Health Organization equations have shortcomings for predicting resting energy expenditure in persons from a modern, affluent population: Generation of a new reference standard from a retrospective analysis of a German database of resting energy expenditure. Am J Clin Nutr 2004;80:1379–90.
35. Elwyn DH, Kinney JM, Askanazi J. Energy expenditure in surgical patients. Surg Clin North Am 1981;61:545–56.
36. Tilden SJ, et al. Measured energy expenditure in pediatric intensive care patients. Am J Dis Child 1989;143:490–2.
37. Phillips R, et al. Nutritional support and measured energy expenditure of the child and adolescent with head injury. J Neurosurg 1987;67:846–51.
38. Chwals WJ, Bistrian BR. Predicted energy expenditure in critically ill children: Problems associated with increased variability. Crit Care Med 2000;28:2655–6.
39. Coss-Bu JA, et al. Energy metabolism, nitrogen balance, and substrate utilization in critically ill children. Am J Clin Nutr 2001;74:664–9.
40. Ferrannini E. The theoretical bases of indirect calorimetry: A review. Metabolism 1988;37:287–301.
41. Schoeller DA, van Santen E. Measurement of energy expenditure in humans by doubly labeled water method. J Appl Physiol 1982;53:955–9.
42. Schoeller DA, Hnilicka JM. Reliability of the doubly labeled water method for the measurement of total daily energy expenditure in free-living subjects. J Nutr 1996;126:348S–54S.
43. Schoeller DA, Kushner RF, Jones PJ. Validation of doubly labeled water for measuring energy expenditure during parenteral nutrition. Am J Clin Nutr 1986;44:291–8.
44. Jones PJ, et al. Validation of doubly labeled water for assessing energy expenditure in infants. Pediatr Res 1987;21:242–6.
45. Shew SB, et al. Validation of a [13C]bicarbonate tracer technique to measure neonatal energy expenditure. Pediatr Res 2000;47:787–91.
46. Jahoor F, et al. Dynamics of the protein metabolic response to burn injury. Metabolism 1988;37:330–7.
47. Weinstein MR, Oh W. Oxygen consumption in infants with bronchopulmonary dysplasia. J Pediatr 1981;99:958–61.
48. Jones MO, et al. The metabolic response to operative stress in infants. J Pediatr Surg 1993;28:1258–62; discussion 1262–3.
49. Shew SB, et al. Ligation of a patent ductus arteriosus under fentanyl anesthesia improves protein metabolism in premature neonates. J Pediatr Surg 2000;35:1277–81.
50. Pierro A, et al. Partition of energy metabolism in the surgical newborn. J Pediatr Surg 1991;26:581–6.
51. Jaksic T, et al. Do critically ill surgical neonates have increased energy expenditure? J Pediatr Surg 2001;36:63–7.
52. Briassoulis G, Venkataraman S, Thompson AE. Energy expenditure in critically ill children. Crit Care Med 2000;28:1166–72.
53. Goran MI, Kaskoun M, Johnson R. Determinants of resting energy expenditure in young children. J Pediatr 1994;125:362–7.
54. National Academy of Sciences. Recommended Dietary Allowances, 10th edition. Washington, DC; National Academy Press; 1989.
55. Long CL, et al. Carbohydrate metabolism in man: Effect of elective operations and major injury. J Appl Physiol 1971;31:110–6.
56. Long CL, et al. Carbohydrate metabolism in normal man and effect of glucose infusion. J Appl Physiol 1971;31:102–9.
57. Jeevanandam M, Young DH, Schiller WR. Nutritional impact on the energy cost of fat fuel mobilization in polytrauma victims. J Trauma 1990;30:147–54.
58. Jones MO, et al. Protein metabolism kinetics in neonates: Effect of intravenous carbohydrate and fat. J Pediatr Surg 1995;30:458–62.
59. Krinsley JS. Association between hyperglycemia and increased hospital mortality in a heterogeneous population of critically ill patients. Mayo Clin Proc 2003;78:1471–8.
60. Laird AM, et al. Relationship of early hyperglycemia to mortality in trauma patients. J Trauma 2004;56:1058–62.
61. Krinsley JS. Effect of an intensive glucose management protocol on the mortality of critically ill adult patients. Mayo Clin Proc 2004;79:992–1000.
62. Faustino EV, Apkon M. Persistent hyperglycemia in critically ill children. J Pediatr 2005;146:30–4.
63. Srinivasan V, et al. Association of timing, duration, and intensity of hyperglycemia with intensive care unit mortality in critically ill children. Pediatr Crit Care Med 2004;5:329–36.
64. Nordenstrom J, et al. Metabolic utilization of intravenous fat emulsion during total parenteral nutrition. Ann Surg 1982;196:221–31.
65. Powis MR, et al. Effect of major abdominal operations on energy and protein metabolism in infants and children. J Pediatr Surg 1998;33:49–53.
66. Paulsrud JR, et al. Essential fatty acid deficiency in infants induced by fat-free intravenous feeding. Am J Clin Nutr 1972;25:897–904.
67. Friedman Z, et al. Rapid onset of essential fatty acid deficiency in the newborn. Pediatrics 1976;58:640–9.
68. Holman RT. The ratio of trienoic: Tetraenoic acids in tissue lipids as a measure of essential fatty acid requirement. J Nutr 1960;70:405–10.
69. Aggett PJ, et al. Comment on the content and composition of lipids in infant formulas. ESPGAN Committee on Nutrition. Acta Paediatr Scand 1991;80:887–96.
70. Van Aerde JE, et al. Metabolic consequences of increasing energy intake by adding lipid to parenteral nutrition in full-term infants. Am J Clin Nutr 1994;59:659–62.
71. Cleary TG, Pickering LK. Mechanisms of intralipid effect on polymorphonuclear leukocytes. J Clin Lab Immunol 1983;11:21–6.
72. Periera GR, et al. Decreased oxygenation and hyperlipemia during intravenous fat infusions in premature infants. Pediatrics 1980;66:26–30.
73. Freeman J, et al. Association of intravenous lipid emulsion and coagulase-negative staphylococcal bacteremia in neonatal intensive care units. N Engl J Med 1990;323: 301–8.
74. Birkhahn RH, et al. A comparison of the effects of skeletal trauma and surgery on the ketosis of starvation in man. J Trauma 1981;21:513–9.
75. Forbes GB, Bruining GJ. Urinary creatinine excretion and lean body mass. Am J Clin Nutr 1976;29:1359–66.
76. Fomon SJ, et al. Body composition of reference children from birth to age 10 years. Am J Clin Nutr 1982;35:1169–75.
77. Munro HN. Nutrition and muscle protein metabolism: Introduction. Fed Proc 1978;37:2281–2.
78. Munro HN. Fifth annual Jonathan E. Rhoads lecture. Metabolic integration of organs in health and disease. JPEN J Parenter Enteral Nutr 1982;6:271–9.
79. Reichman B, et al. Dietary composition and macronutrient storage in preterm infants. Pediatrics 1983;72:322–8.
80. Schulze KF, et al. Energy expenditure, energy balance, and composition of weight gain in low birth weight infants fed diets of different protein and energy content. J Pediatr 1987;110:753–9.
81. Kashyap S, et al. Growth, nutrient retention, and metabolic response in low birth weight infants fed varying intakes of protein and energy. J Pediatr 1988;113:713–21.
82. Kawagoe JY, et al. Risk factors for nosocomial infections in critically ill newborns: A 5-year prospective cohort study. Am J Infect Control 2001;29:109–14.
83. de Lucas C, et al. Transpyloric enteral nutrition reduces the complication rate and cost in the critically ill child. J Pediatr Gastroenterol Nutr 2000;30:175–80.
84. Zaloga GP. Early enteral nutritional support improves outcome: Hypothesis or fact? Crit Care Med 1999;27:259–61.
85. Briassoulis G, Zavras N, Hatzis T. Malnutrition, nutritional indices, and early enteral feeding in critically ill children. Nutrition 2001;17:548–57.
86. Briassoulis GC, Zavras NJ, Hatzis MT. Effectiveness and safety of a protocol for promotion of early intragastric feeding in critically ill children. Pediatr Crit Care Med 2001;2:113–21.
87. Chellis MJ, et al. Early enteral feeding in the pediatric intensive care unit. JPEN J Parenter Enteral Nutr 1996;20:71–3.
88. Munshi IA, Steingrub JS, Wolpert L. Small bowel necrosis associated with early postoperative jejunal tube feeding in a trauma patient. J Trauma 2000;49:163–5.
89. de Groof F, et al. Acute stress response in children with meningococcal sepsis: Important differences in the growth hormone/insulin-like growth factor I axis between nonsurvivors and survivors. J Clin Endocrinol Metab 2002;87:3118–24.
90. Rogers EJ, et al. Barriers to adequate nutrition in critically ill children. Nutrition 2003;19:865–8.
91. Atkinson S, Sieffert E, Bihari D. A prospective, randomized, double-blind, controlled clinical trial of enteral immunonutrition in the critically ill. Guy's Hospital Intensive Care Group. Crit Care Med 1998;26:1164–72.
92. Briassoulis G, et al. Influence of an aggressive early enteral nutrition protocol on nitrogen balance in critically ill children. J Nutr Biochem 2002;13:560.
93. Heyland DK, Cook DJ, Guyatt GH. Enteral nutrition in the critically ill patient: A critical review of the evidence. Intensive Care Med 1993;19:435–42.
94. Agarwal KC, et al. Cardiac perforation from central venous catheters: Survival after cardiac tamponade in an infant. Pediatrics 1984;73:333–8.
95. Collier PE, Ryan JJ, Diamond DL. Cardiac tamponade from central venous catheters. Report of a case and review of the English literature. Angiology 1984;35:595–600.
96. Ziegler M, et al. Route of pediatric parenteral nutrition: Proposed criteria revision. J Pediatr Surg 1980;15:472–6.
97. Bone RC, Grodzin CJ, Balk RA. Sepsis: A new hypothesis for pathogenesis of the disease process. Chest 1997;112:235–43.
98. Heyland DK, et al. Should immunonutrition become routine in critically ill patients? A systematic review of the evidence. JAMA 2001;286:944–53.
99. Bertolini G, et al. Early enteral immunonutrition in patients with severe sepsis: Results of an interim analysis of a randomized multicentre clinical trial. Intensive Care Med 2003;29:834–40.
100. Tubman TR, Thompson SW, McGuire W. Glutamine supplementation to prevent morbidity and mortality in preterm infants. Cochrane Database Syst Rev 2005:CD001457.
101. Novak F, et al. Glutamine supplementation in serious illness: A systematic review of the evidence. Crit Care Med 2002;30:2022–9.
102. Anand KJ, Hickey PR. Pain and its effects in the human neonate and fetus. N Engl J Med 1987;317:1321–9.
103. Anand KJ, et al. Studies on the hormonal regulation of fuel metabolism in the human newborn infant undergoing anaesthesia and surgery. Horm Res 1985;22:115–28.

104. Srinivasan G, et al. Glucose homeostasis during anesthesia and surgery in infants. J Pediatr Surg 1986;21:718–21.
105. Black PR, et al. Mechanisms of insulin resistance following injury. Ann Surg 1982;196:420–35.
106. Jahoor F, et al. Role of insulin and glucose oxidation in mediating the protein catabolism of burns and sepsis. Am J Physiol 1989;257:E323–31.
107. Sweed Y, Puri P, Reen DJ. Early induction of IL-6 in infants undergoing major abdominal surgery. J Pediatr Surg 1992;27:1033–6; discussion 1036–7.
108. Windmueller HG, Spaeth AE. Uptake and metabolism of plasma glutamine by the small intestine. J Biol Chem 1974;249:5070–9.
109. Gura KM, Duggan CP, Collier SB, et al. Reversal of parenteral nutrition-associated liver disease in two infants with short bowel syndrome using parenteral fish oil: Implications for future management. Pediatrics 2006;118:e197–201.

Hyperlipidemia and Cardiovascular Disease Risk

Sarah de Ferranti, MD, MPH, FAAP
Ellis Neufeld, MD, PhD

Atherosclerotic heart disease is a major cause of adult morbidity and mortality in the United States; coronary heart disease (CHD) affected 13.2 million Americans and caused 1 of every 2.7 deaths in 2003. Other atherosclerotic complications, including stroke and peripheral vascular disease, affect millions more.[1] The causes of atherosclerotic cardiovascular disease are multifactorial; however, nutrition is related to many traditional cardiovascular risk factors including hyperlipidemia. Increased total cholesterol is an important risk factor for atherosclerosis and was found in half of the Framingham Heart Study adult cohort who sustained a myocardial infarction.[2] Reducing cholesterol by 8% reduced the risk of CHD by 19%.[3] Other important cardiovascular risk factors, including hypertension and obesity, are significantly affected by diet. Given the recently recognized obesity epidemic with a doubling in rates of overweight and obesity over the past two decades,[4] healthcare providers who deliver care to young persons can be assured that millions of today's youth, and a significant fraction of our clinical practice, will sooner or later fall victim to diabetes and atherosclerotic vascular disease. Pharmacotherapy is not an ideal of treatment modality; nutritional approaches are more advisable ways of treating the cardiovascular risk factors in this young, growing population and will be the focus of this chapter.

Several lines of evidence suggest that atherosclerotic vascular changes begin by adolescence and that early intervention on a population basis and, for severe cases, on an individual basis, is warranted. These lines of evidence, and the arguments for and against various screening and treatment strategies, are laid out in the comprehensive report of the National Cholesterol Education Program (NCEP) Expert Panel on Children and Adolescents.[5] These consensus guidelines were reported in 1992 by the American Academy of Pediatrics.[6] Although they have become somewhat dated in more than a decade since their initial presentation, the guidelines still form the basis for recommendations for pediatric lipid practice from the American Academy of Pediatrics.[7] Whether new guidelines are necessary is debated[8]; they are likely forthcoming.

In this chapter, we present evidence supporting the early onset of atherosclerosis in childhood, including new thinking about pathophysiology and evidence of preclinical disease by noninvasive testing; briefly review lipid biochemistry; and describe different pediatric hyperlipidemias, nutritional and pharmacologic treatments, and practical clinical approaches to children with hyperlipidemia. We make specific note of examples in which our current practice or recommendations diverge from those of the NCEP.

PEDIATRIC ORIGINS OF ADULT ATHEROSCLEROSIS

Atherosclerosis usually takes decades to develop. Symptoms and sequelae from atherosclerotic vascular disease are extremely rare in children and adolescents and are limited to patients with profound genetic dyslipidemias. However, both the disease process itself and the nutritional habits that propagate the disease begin early. Autopsy studies of cohorts as early as the Korean War have shown atherosclerotic coronary artery disease in the second decade of life on gross examination[9] and by microscopy.[10,11] These pathology findings were correlated with hyperlipidemia in US young persons in the landmark study termed Pathological Determinants of Atherosclerosis in Youth (PDAY),[12] among others.[13] In the PDAY study, fatty streak precursor lesions were present by age 15 years in the coronary arteries of children who died of noncardiac causes. Both the prevalence and extent of fatty streaks, and the degree of progression to raised vascular lesions (early atherosclerosis) by young adulthood, were directly related to increased non-high-density lipoprotein (HDL) cholesterol—that is, low-density lipoprotein (LDL) plus very low-density lipoprotein (VLDL)—and decreased HDL cholesterol as measured at the time of death.

EPIDEMIOLOGIC EVIDENCE

Epidemiologic studies have shown that countries with higher rates of CHD have higher pediatric population mean total cholesterol.[14] Cholesterol levels in the pediatric age group are important because they predict adult cholesterol levels to a substantial degree. Cholesterol "tracks" quite well; children with very high cholesterol levels are highly likely to be adults with high cholesterol. This has been demonstrated in a decades-long cohort project in Iowa, the Muscatine Study: nearly half of subjects with high cholesterol as children had high cholesterol levels as adults.[15]

There are data connecting cholesterol levels in young adults with CHD. Starting in the late 1940s, cholesterol levels were available for cohorts of Johns Hopkins University medical students. High total cholesterol values in the students predicted greater risk of CHD, mortality from CHD, and overall mortality later in adult life.[16] This study provides the most compelling link between measured cholesterol levels in young persons and subsequent risk of heart disease 30 or 40 years later. Unfortunately, to date there are no long-term studies demonstrating a link between cholesterol levels in school-aged children and CHD in the fifth and sixth decades of life, or showing that interventions in the pediatric age range prevent future disease; the length of follow-up is daunting. Therefore, the interventions we discuss below are based on inference, adult studies, and short-term interventions in the young.

HIGH-RISK GROUPS

In adult atherosclerosis primary and secondary prevention, guidelines for initiating treatment and goals for therapy are adjusted depending on accompanying cardiovascular risk factors. This concept is more recently being applied to evaluating and treating lipid disorders in children. Recommendations with regard to treatment of and target levels of lipids should be modified in these high-risk groups. These include heart transplant recipients[17,18] and renal transplantation patients,[19,20] in whom the problem is related only in part to chronic transplant rejection. Children with previous Kawasaki Disease, in particular those who had coronary aneurysms in the past, are another high-risk group.[21] Some clinicians believe children with some types of congenital heart disease are at increased risk for atherosclerosis, even if repaired. In particular, coarctation and transposition of the great arteries after the arterial switch operation seem to be at greater risk but patients with Fontan physiology may also be vulnerable.[22–24] Children with diabetes mellitus type 1 and type 2, increasingly more common in adolescence, are also at particular risk for cardiovascular disease in the long run. In assessing risk for individual children, solid-organ transplantation and juvenile-onset diabetes can reasonably each be considered to count as two risk factors in determining whether a child is a candidate for pharmacologic therapy, and should lower the therapeutic goal for treatment. For example, it is our practice to place all children on pravastatin after heart transplantation, regardless of cholesterol levels, due to the risk of coronary artery pathology in this population.

EMERGING CONCEPTS IN ATHEROSCLEROSIS: APPLICATIONS IN CHILDREN AND ADOLESCENTS

The fact that half of adults in the Framingham Heart Study who had myocardial infarctions had normal cholesterol levels,[2] a finding supported by other studies,[25,26] has prompted researchers to search for other contributors to atherosclerosis. Although the prevailing theory of atherosclerotic disease since the 1960s focused on cholesterol, recent thinking places emphasis on vascular and systemic inflammation as instrumental forces in the pathophysiology of atherosclerosis. A simple marker, serum C-reactive protein (CRP), is proving to be a valuable tool for assessing cardiovascular disease risk in adults. CRP is an acute-phase reactant. Transient inflammation, from minor infections for example, can readily raise the CRP level above a population upper limit of normal, 0.5 mg/dL. However, a highly sensitive CRP assay (hsCRP) detects variations in levels of less than 0.1 mg/dL. At these low levels, previously categorized as normal, differences in hsCRP levels in the population predict cardiac risk. Studies examining adults having myocardial infarctions show abnormally elevated hsCRP; higher peak values predict worse outcomes[27] and larger infarcts.[28] Adults who have abnormal hsCRP levels even months or years after an acute coronary event have a significantly greater risk of recurrence.[29,30] Prospective evaluation in large cohort studies reveals that men and women without clinical atherosclerotic disease who have hsCRP values higher than the normal range are at risk for future cardiovascular disease.[31,32] In adults, the relative risk of future cardiovascular disease events is low in those with hsCRP levels <1 mg/L, average in those with hsCRP of 1.0 to 3.0 mg/L, and high in those with hsCRP >3.0 mg/L.[33] The exact physiological relationship between CRP and coronary risk is still unclear. It is likely that ongoing, mild vascular inflammation contributes both to atherosclerosis and to the increased CRP level.

RELATION OF CRP TO PEDIATRIC LIPID DISORDERS AND CARDIAC RISK

Inflammation probably has a role in the increased risk of future cardiovascular disease in pediatric patients. Only a fraction (between 23 and 43%) of the offspring of parents with early myocardial infarction have high LDL cholesterol.[36,37] This suggests that at least part of familial cardiac disease risk is not related to hypercholesterolemia and might be related to a hyperinflammatory state. In fact, one study found that children with first-degree relatives who had myocardial infarctions have abnormally elevated CRP levels.[38] Despite these intriguing results, no data available in 2006 demonstrate a specific role for CRP as a screening tool in pediatric lipid practice. However, the test might be valuable in some individual patients with terrible family history and borderline lipid levels, and will likely have greater use in risk prediction in the future. It is worth bearing in mind that in clinical practice, children with hsCRP levels consistent with increased cardiovascular risk in adults may have either an intercurrent illness (particularly if CRP is >10 mg/L) or excess adipose tissue. Infectious issues can be circumvented with repeat measurement, as is recommended in adults[33]; however the association with adipose tissue is less easily resolved. It is likely that there is a level of hsCRP in children that is ultimately found to be associated with increased cardiovascular risk, even discounting hsCRP elevations related to illness or overweight.

Understanding of the role of inflammation in atherosclerosis has led to new thinking about therapies in adults, including acetylsalicylic acid, vitamins E and C, and betacarotene. However, a recent large adult study on antioxidants found no difference in 5-year mortality, despite increases in serum levels of vitamins E and C and betacarotene.[39] Two small studies have demonstrated improvement in flow-mediated brachial artery dilation with short courses of vitamin E and C supplementation in children with hyperlipidemia.[34,35] The role of antioxidant therapy in children is unclear, however.

HOMOCYSTEINEMIA AND PEDIATRIC EVALUATION FOR CARDIAC RISK

Elevated level of the nonstructural amino acid homocysteine is another coronary artery disease risk factor that has lately become better understood. Three lines of evidence link homocysteine levels to atherosclerotic disease: (1) in large adult cohorts, including the Framingham Heart Study, mild hyperhomocysteinemia is predictive of coronary events[40]; (2) homocysteine itself causes vascular disease in animal models[41]; and (3) young patients with profound hyperhomocysteinemia owing to the rare genetic defect cystathionine-β-synthase deficiency (homocystinuria) have dramatic elevation in thrombosis risk. Dietary deficiencies of vitamin B_{12} (cobalamin), folate, or vitamin B_6 (pyridoxine) can all lead to hyperhomocysteinemia, as can genetic defects in absorption or metabolism of these vitamins.

The most common genetic association is with a heat-labile form of methylenetetrahydrofolate reductase, caused by a 677C-to-T polymorphism and present in more than one-quarter of Caucasians.[42] In the presence of this polymorphism, relative folate deficiency with resultant mild elevation in homocysteine levels is fairly common in adults with poor folate intake. However, just as the significance of relative folate deficiency was becoming clear in the late 1990s, universal folate supplementation of cereals and enriched grain products to prevent neural tube defects was enacted, clouding the data on the relationship between folate supplementation and CHD. In a large cohort of pediatric patients studied for lipid nutritional intervention, the Dietary Intervention Study in Children (DISC), hyperhomocysteinemia was rare among several hundred subjects,[43] and although we measured it regularly for some time, we have rarely identified abnormalities and in general we have not found it to be useful in our clinical practice.

METABOLIC SYNDROME AND PEDIATRIC EVALUATION FOR CARDIAC RISK

Metabolic syndrome, previously called syndrome X, is a collection of cardiovascular risk factors associated with a higher rate of atherosclerotic disease. In adults, metabolic syndrome involves hypertension, elevated fasting glucose levels, central obesity, low HDL, and high triglycerides.[54] Several researchers have described the prevalence of a pediatric metabolic syndrome in adolescents.[55,56] Estimates range between 4 and 12.7% of the population ages 13 to 19 years. Although at the time of writing there was no official definition of metabolic syndrome, it is likely that having a collection of risk factors such as these put an adolescent at increased risk for atherosclerotic disease in adulthood and therefore should alert the clinician to screen for all metabolic risk factors, and to emphasize modification of lifestyle, including diet. Body mass index (BMI) above the 95th percentile for age in childhood is a risk factor for future metabolic syndrome.[57] Metabolic syndrome is discussed more fully elsewhere in this volume.

LIPOPROTEIN (a) AND PEDIATRIC EVALUATION FOR CARDIAC RISK

Lipoprotein (a), or Lp(a), is a variant LDL particle with a covalently bound protein portion, termed apolipoprotein (a). This particle is not measured on standard lipid profiles. High levels are thought to be atherogenic because the particle not only participates in atheromatous plaques (as does LDL) but also impairs fibrinolysis by preventing normal plasminogen activation,[50] and is therefore likely involved in the thrombosis of cardiovascular disease. Lp(a) is genetically determined, and high levels are associated with increased risk of coronary artery disease and stroke. The levels within the population are not normally distributed. The majority of humans have normal levels of less than 74 nmol/L (30 mg/dL), but higher levels are common in pediatric referral lipid clinic settings and the cutoff for increased cardiovascular risk may indeed be closer to 65 mg/dL.[51] Certainly, very high levels (more than 100 mg/dL) deserve particular attention and might serve to modify treatment in patients whose values fall into the "gray zone" for treatment. Pharmacologic doses of niacin lower Lp(a); however most adolescents find it difficult to tolerate this medication, even in the slow or extended release forms (adherence must be as near as possible to 100% to avoid tachyphylaxis). We have rarely used it in children due to frequent side effects, as high as 76% of children in a small series.[52] Lovastatin has produced some mild reduction of Lp(a) in adults,[53] and others with severe CHD or stroke have been treated with plasmapheresis. Attention must be paid to the units among different assays which measure either mass or molarity (mg/dL vs nmol/L).

LIPID BIOCHEMISTRY

Lipids, including cholesterol and other sterols, triglycerides, and free fatty acids, are essential for life. In humans, all but the essential fatty acids can be endogenously synthesized, but diet is a major contributor to total body lipid stores in typical diets in developed countries. Essential fatty acids include the basic precursors of the polyunsaturated fatty acids (eg, linoleic acid or linolenic acid).

Cholesterol is partially absorbed from the diet and partially synthesized by the liver. The only dietary source of absorbed cholesterol is animal products; 30 to 50% of dietary intake is absorbed. Strict vegans synthesize 100% of their cholesterol needs as vegetables contain no cholesterol. After absorption, cholesterol is esterified and carried in the serum on lipoprotein particles, as described below.

Fat, in the form of fatty acids and triglycerides (three fatty acids esterified to glycerol), is derived both from dietary sources and from endogenous synthesis, including excess carbohydrates and even proteins. Fatty acids can be "saturated," with hydrogen at each carbon; "monounsaturated," with one double carbon bond; or "polyunsaturated," with two to six double bonds. Naturally occurring dietary fatty acids are in the *"cis"* configuration at each double bond. Polyunsaturated fats are prone to spoilage by oxygen, light, and heat; therefore, food processing, especially catalytic hydrogenation processing, which is used to avoid rancidity, produces nonnatural fatty acid chemistry, including a *"trans"* bond configuration. Readers will be familiar with "partially hydrogenated" oils from the list of ingredients in many processed foods, especially snack foods. In general, the larger the proportion of partially hydrogenated fats, the larger the proportion of undesirable *trans* conformation fatty acids. *Trans*-fatty acids not only act like saturated fats to increase LDL, but they also decrease HDL and should be minimized in the diet.[44] Dietary cholesterol (usually not much more than 300 mg/d) is re-esterified to fatty acids in plasma. Dietary triglycerides (typically dozens of grams daily) are degraded by lipase in the gut, absorbed, and re-esterified to re-form triglycerides. Dietary fat is distributed to body tissues, primarily the liver, in the form of chylomicrons.

Cholesterol esters and neutral fats such as triglycerides are negligibly soluble in water and therefore are carried in the bloodstream by lipoproteins. Free fatty acids in plasma are carried mainly on albumin and are rapidly taken up by tissues for re-esterification or for combustion as fuel. Lipoproteins are made up of hydrophobic lipids (triglycerides and cholesterol ester) on the inside and apoproteins, phospholipids, and unesterified cholesterol on the outside.

There are several types of lipoproteins, classified by density as determined using plasma ultracentrifugation: chylomicrons, which float as a creamy supernatant, HDL, LDL, and VLDL.

- Chylomicrons are synthesized in the intestine from dietary triglycerides, cholesterol, and apolipoproteins synthesized in the liver. Chylomicrons have the lipoproteins apo A, apo C, and apo C-II. The chylomicron delivers the triglyceride to muscle and adipose tissue, where it is modified by lipoprotein lipase, losing triglycerides, apo A, and apo CE, and gaining apo E. The chylomicron remnants are taken up by the liver via the apo E receptor and degraded.
- HDL is the densest and smallest lipoprotein. The major proteins (apoproteins) in HDL are apo A-I, apo A-II, apo C, and apo E. HDL is the primary lipoprotein responsible for reverse cholesterol transport, returning cholesterol from other tissues back to the liver. HDL also transports cholesterol from other lipoproteins, such as LDL, and cell membranes to VLDL and chylomicrons.
- LDL is the main reservoir of circulating cholesterol esters, supplying cell membranes and tissues. Each LDL particle carries an apolipoprotein B molecule, the protein responsible for LDL clearance by its cognate receptor. Cholesterol synthetic mechanisms are present in nearly all mammalian cell types, but exogenous sources are used prior to endogenous synthesis. Delivery to tissues is regulated by the number of LDL receptors, and a tight negative feedback system prevents cholesterol synthesis and downregulates LDL receptors in normal humans when extracellular LDL is abundant. Recent studies have noted an increased risk of atherosclerotic events in people with small dense LDL particles.[45]
- VLDL is manufactured in the liver, particularly during fasting, as the main source of triglycerides when chylomicrons are absent. VLDL is secreted into the bloodstream and triglycerides are removed in the periphery by lipoprotein lipase. The VLDL remnants are metabolized by the liver and serve as the precursor for LDL production.

HYPERLIPIDEMIA

Cholesterol levels are age dependent; children normally have lower levels than adults do. The NCEP guideline cutoffs for borderline and overt hypercholesterolemia, as well as for normal levels of HDL, triglycerides, and LDL, are shown in Table 1.

ESTABLISHING A DIAGNOSIS

Hypercholesterolemia and hyperlipidemia are both multifactorial and polygenic traits. It is useful to distinguish primary (familial or sporadic) from secondary hyperlipidemia. In pediatrics, most cases of hyperlipidemia are primary; however, secondary causes of hyperlipidemia should be considered, evaluated, and ruled out because several of the secondary causes are treatable. Secondary causes of hyperlipidemia (Table 2) are often readily identified by a medical history and examination, with simple laboratory testing as indicated.

Among those with primary hyperlipidemias, dietary transgressions, lack of exercise, glucose intolerance, and obesity often accompany sporadic high cholesterol levels and complicate familial lipid disorders. Indeed certain individuals have lipid disorders only secondary to these lifestyle issues. With regard to pure primary hypercholesterolemia, several of the familial lipid disorders are dominantly inherited with a gene dosage effect: heterozygous individuals have elevated lipids but are generally asymptomatic until the condition manifests as early stroke, angina, myocardial infarction, or sudden death in the fourth or fifth decade of life. However, homozygotes can manifest xanthomas, arcus cornea, and thickened tendons even before puberty and can have cardiovascular end points in early adulthood or even as teenagers. Although multiple genes affect lipid levels, several monogenic conditions have been distinguished and can be readily recognized if family history and laboratory data are available. A simple guide for diagnosis based on lipid profile and family history is presented in Table 3.

Familial combined hyperlipidemia is the most common type of inherited hyperlipidemia. It is autosomal dominant and is found in 1 in 100 individuals. Of patients with early CHD, 10 to 15% carry this diagnosis. The lipid abnormalities are moderate. About one-third of patients with familial combined hyperlipidemia have increased LDL primarily, one-third have increased triglycerides without altered LDL, and another third have increased triglycerides and increased LDL. The three types frequently coexist within a family.

Familial hypercholesterolemia, though rare, is the genetic lipid disorder best understood at a biochemical level. The cause is genetic defects in the LDL receptor gene. Heterozygotes have a decrease in the number of active receptors and homozygotes have absence or near absence of functional receptors. Heterozygous deficiency has a prevalence of 1 in 500 individuals in the United States (0.2%), but heterozygotes account for 5% of early myocardial infarction survivors. These individuals usually have total cholesterol levels in the range of 200 to 500 mg/dL (5.2 to 13 mmol/L). They have a family history of high cholesterol and

Table 1 NCEP and Population Age-Based Percentiles for Lipid Values in Children

Classification/ Percentile	Total Cholestrol, (mg/dL)*	Low-Density Lipoprotein,† (mg/dL)*	High-Density Lipoprotein, (mg/dL)*	Triglycerides (mg/dL)*
	<170	<110	–	–
Borderline	170–199	110–129	–	–
Elevated	>200	>130	–	–
5th percentile				
Age 5–9 yr				
Boys	125	65	39	31
Girls	130	70	37	33
Age 10–14 yr				
Boys	123	66	38	33
Girls	128	70	38	38
Age 15–19 yr				
Boys	116	64	31	38
Girls	124	61	36	40
50th percentile				
Age 5–9 yr				
Boys	164	93	56	53
Girls	168	101	54	57
Age 10–14 yr				
Boys	160	97	57	61
Girls	163	97	54	72
Age 15–19 yr				
Boys	150	96	47	71
Girls	160	96	53	70
75th percentile				
Age 5–9 yr				
Boys	180	106	65	67
Girls	184	118	63	73
Age 10–14 yr				
Boys	178	112	63	80
Girls	179	113	60	93
Age 15–19 yr				
Boys	170	112	54	94
Girls	177	114	63	90
95th percentile				
Age 5–9 yr				
Boys	209	133	76	104
Girls	211	144	75	108
Age 10–14 yr				
Boys	208	136	76	129
Girls	207	140	72	135
Age 15–19 yr				
Boys	203	134	65	152
Girls	209	141	76	136

Adapted from reference 5.
Acceptable, borderline, and elevated cholesterol values according to the NCEP pediatric guidelines are shown for total cholesterol and low-density lipoprotein (LDL). For comparison, percentile values are shown for these measures and for high-density lipoprotein (HDL) and triglycerides. See reference 5 for full percentile tables.
*Values are reported as serum; to convert to plasma values, divide by 1.03.
†LDL and HDL values for Caucasian subjects.

Table 2 Medical, Physiologic, and Pharmacologic Causes of Secondary Hyperlipidemia

Endocrine and metabolic states
- Diabetes mellitus
  - Type I: With concomitant primary hyperlipidemia, very high vascular risk
  - Type II: Particularly related to high triglycerides insulin resistance states without overt diabetes (check for acanthosis nigricans)
- Pregnancy
- Hypothyroidism
- Hypopituitarism*
- Anorexia nervosa

Hepatic disease
- Hepatitis of any etiology
- Biliary atresia†
- Acute intermittent porphyria
- Glycogen storage disease†
- Genetic and acquired cholestatic disorders

Renal disease
- Nephrotic syndrome†
- Any renal inflammatory state
- Hemolytic uremic syndrome
- Idiopathic hypercalcemia

Lysosomal storage disease
- Cholesterol ester storage disease
- Niemann–Pick disease
- Other conditions, such as Tay–Sachs disease, Gaucher's disease

Recognizable genetic syndromes
- Klinefelter's syndrome
- Progeria (Hutchinson-Gilford disease)

Systemic inflammatory states
- Trivial inflammation (eg, viral illnesses, simple urinary tract infection, sinusitis) can raise triglyceride levels; "healthy day" testing recommended
- Systemic lupus erythematosus: severe vascular risk if combined with primary hyperlipidemia
- Burns

Drugs and other agents
- Corticosteroids (systemic): primarily hypertriglyceridemia
- Thiazides
- Beta-blockers
- Oral contraceptives (third-generation oral contraceptive pills may have beneficial effect on HDL, which can appear as benign elevation in total cholesterol). Should be used in caution in those with severe hyperlipidemia.
- Antiepileptic medications
- Ethanol: low-dose, regular consumption increases salutary HDL; in excess, hypertriglyceridemia

*If hypopituitarism is suspected, thyroid-stimulating hormone alone, as advocated for primary screening, is not sufficient to rule out central hypothyroidism.
†Elevations can be severe with xanthomas.
HDL = high-density lipoprotein.

early coronary disease and require pharmacologic treatment. Premature atherosclerosis is seen in 30% of adults heterozygous for familial hypercholesterolemia.[46]

Some populations with elevated familial hypercholesterolemia prevalence because of founder effects include French Canadians, Dutch Afrikaners in South Africa, and Lebanese Christians. Individuals with homozygous LDL receptor defects are rare, about one in a million individuals, and have very high total cholesterol levels of 500 to 1,000 mg/dL (13 to 25.9 mmol/L). These are children who could have myocardial infarctions and require not pharmacologic treatment, which is usually ineffective, but plasmapheresis or if there is intractable coronary disease, liver transplantation. In the complete absence of LDL receptors (familial hypercholesterolemia patients homozygous for null mutations), statins are utterly ineffective at standard doses. LDL apheresis with devices such as Liposorber columns is very effective, and carries lower risk than does liver transplantation. Gene therapy approaches have been attempted,[47] but long-term benefit remains to be demonstrated.[48]

Familial defective apolipoprotein B is clinically similar to familial hypercholesterolemia, with similar prevalence for heterozygote and homozygote forms. Familial defective apolipoprotein B is attributable to decreased binding of LDL to its receptor because of a mutation in the apolipoprotein B protein itself rather than a receptor mutation. The condition is rare. The biochemical findings in untreated patients are indistinguishable from heterozygous familial hypercholesterolemia. However, response to pharmacologic therapy, including statins and other agents, tends to be poor, because the upregulation of hepatic LDL receptors, a key step in the mechanism of action for statins and for

Table 3 Phenotype and Family History Commonly Found among Pediatric Lipid Clinic Patients

Common Phenotypes	Family History	Likely Diagnosis
Elevated LDL* and total cholesterol only	Xanthomas/early heart disease†	Familial hypercholesterolemia (total cholesterol 500–1,000 mg/dL in homozygotes)
Elevated triglycerides + low HDL, often with obesity	Type 2 diabetes or similar lipid patterns	High risk for metabolic syndrome
Moderately elevated triglycerides and LDL	Elevated triglycerides, LDL, or both	Familial combined hyperlipidemia
Low HDL only	Low HDL, early coronary heart disease	Familial hypoalphalipoproteinemia
High HDL (> 60 mg/dL), normal LDL	Often negative for early heart disease	Normal variant; 20% of children with elevated TC; no intervention

Cholesterol, HDL, and triglyceride values measured in a fasting state.
Combination of phenotype with typical family history suggests diagnosis.
*LDL is calculated from fasting values using the Friedewald formula, in which LDL = TC − (HDL + TG/5).
†Early heart disease is defined as myocardial infarction before age 55 in men and before 65 in women.
HDL = high-density lipoprotein; LDL = low-density lipoprotein; TC = total cholesterol.

bile-binding resins, will not increase clearance of the mutant particles from the blood.

Familial hypertriglyceridemia is characterized by high triglyceride levels, sometimes accompanied by low HDL. This is a very common profile, of polygenic origin, exacerbated by type 2 diabetes and obesity. Rare monogenic disorders cause chylomicronemia and profound hypertriglyceridemia. Homozygous deficiency of lipoprotein lipase or its cofactor, apolipoprotein C-II, causes isolated increase in chylomicrons, presents in children as recurrent pancreatitis, and is autosomal recessive. Affected individuals have xanthomas but increased risk of early myocardial infarction has not been described.

Familial hypoalphalipoproteinemia exists, but in the general population, low HDL is a common trait, and low HDL is especially prevalent among young survivors of myocardial infarction. With notable but rare exceptions, the exact genetic basis of low HDL is obscure. One allele of the apo A-I gene was found in 32% of adults with severe coronary artery disease and in 3 to 4% of those without CHD.[49]

A number of other rare inherited disorders of lipoprotein metabolism have been described. These are beyond the scope of this chapter.

CHOLESTEROL SCREENING

Whom to Screen

The NCEP and the American Academy of Pediatrics have recommended selective screening of children with risk factors for atherosclerosis, including family history of hypercholesterolemia or early coronary artery disease (Figure 1), after age 2 years. Universal screening of all children is not advocated, for these reasons:

- The cost of screening some 60 million young persons is not worth the marginal gain in identifying the small number of patients not identified by family history.
- Based on the NCEP screening algorithm presented in Figure 1, re-screening costs for the 15 million US children above the 75th percentile would be even higher.
- It would be rare to discover children by universal screening who would require medication before adulthood, and all children should follow a prudent (Step One) diet and exercise regularly.
- Labeling children unnecessarily as hypercholesterolemic could cause harm.

Nevertheless, several studies have shown that selective screening misses some children because of its dependence on family history—often the full family history is not available,[58] and very young children might have grandparents too young to have had early heart disease, and family history might be less predictive in black children than in white children.[59,60] Therefore, patients with unknown family histories can be screened at physician discretion. Healthcare providers might also check fasting lipid profiles or total cholesterol in children who have personal risk factors such as obesity, hypertension, or smoking. Children in higher-risk groups, as described above, should be screened; we generally screen these children with a full fasting lipid panel.

What to Test

The 1991 pediatric NCEP guidelines suggest initial screen by nonfasting total cholesterol only for children with a family history of hypercholesterolemia. False-negative and false-positive results are common, based in part on HDL cholesterol variance. By contrast, current NCEP guidelines for adults suggest screening with nonfasting total cholesterol *and* HDL cholesterol rather than total cholesterol alone.[61] Adding HDL to the screen adds to the initial cost but dramatically improves sensitivity and specificity of the screen; we believe it is well worthwhile. We recommend screening nonfasting total cholesterol and HDL cholesterol to primary care colleagues in our practice.

NUTRITION AND CHOLESTEROL IN CHILDREN

Dietary habits among American children have changed over the past several decades. Children, like all Americans, eat out more often, consuming 32% of their calories outside the home between 1994 and 1996 compared with 18% between 1977 and 1978. Food eaten outside the home is usually higher in total and saturated fats and lower in calcium, iron, and fiber than food eaten at home.[63] Indeed, food eaten outside the home is often fast food. Adolescents who eat fast food are more likely to have a poor quality diet, one higher in saturated fat and sugar, and lower in fruits and vegetables.[62] Fruit juice has been recognized as a major source of calories; high intake has been associated both with poor growth and also with obesity, and some studies have

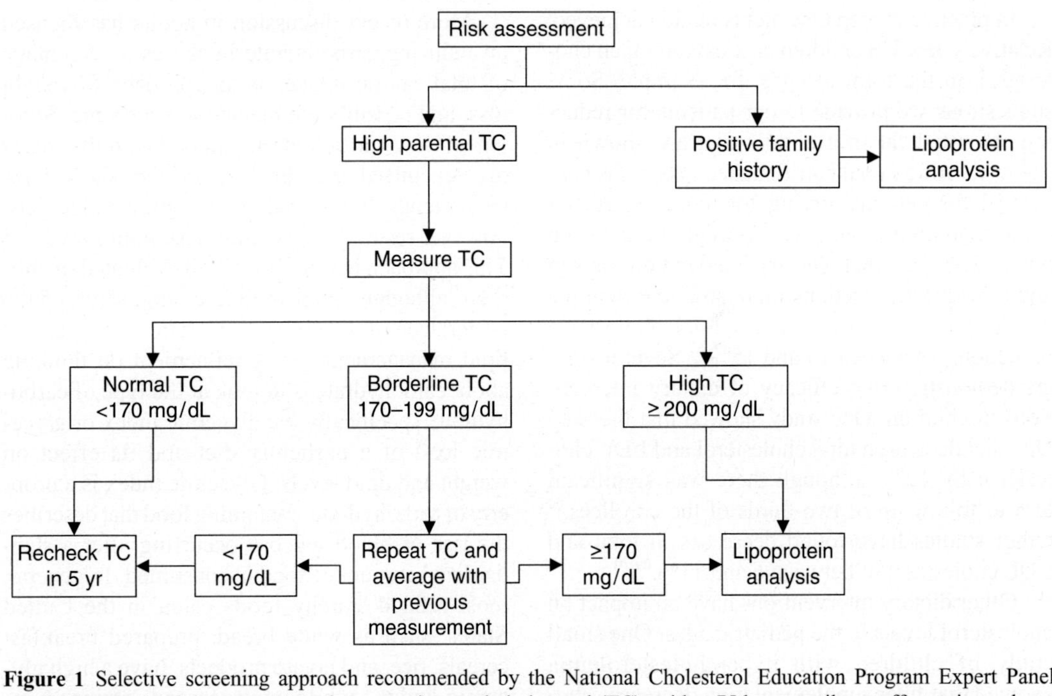

Figure 1 Selective screening approach recommended by the National Cholesterol Education Program Expert Panel on Children and Adolescents. Note that screening total cholesterol (TC), with a 75th percentile cutoff, requires a large volume of retesting because a single value between 170 and 200 mg/dL has limited positive predictive value.[58]

shown higher total cholesterol to HDL ratios and lower absolute HDL with high intake of some types of juice.[64] There have been suggestions in recent years that early exposures in fetal life and infancy can have a significant impact on later cholesterol patterns and cardiovascular risk in adulthood (the so-called Barker or fetal-origins hypothesis).[65] A meta-analysis of 1,532 British children and adults showed that breastfeeding was associated with higher total cholesterol and LDL in childhood, but lower total cholesterol and LDL in adulthood.[66]

Management of obesity is covered elsewhere in this volume (see Chapter 20, "Humoral Regulation of Growth"). From a lipid management point of view, in patients who are prone to hypertriglyceridemia from a genetic basis and for patients with obesity or at family history of type 2 diabetes, trends toward "super-sized" fast-food meals, juice, and sedentary lifestyle are highly detrimental. Lipid disorders of all types are usually worsened by overweight.

TREATMENT FOR DYSLIPIDEMIAS

Dietary treatment is the first line of intervention in all childhood dyslipidemias, as it is in the adult population. Diet modification is emphasized even more in the pediatric age range than for adults because pharmacologic agents have been tested primarily in adults and safety data are somewhat limited in children. The NCEP has recommended a two-level nutritional approach, adopted with variations by the American Heart Association and the American Academy of Pediatrics. Step One reduces total fat intake to less than 30% of total calories, with a goal of saturated fat representing less than 10% of total calories and cholesterol intakes of less than 300 mg/d.[61] The Step Two diet restricts saturated fat intake to less than 7% of daily calories.

In practice, a Step One diet is readily achieved. Relatively few US children now eat too much cholesterol, in the form of eggs, for example. Some suggestions we provide to our patients for reducing saturated fat in a child's diet are shown in Table 4. Professional nutritional counseling is very helpful for patients aiming for more significant changes in lipid values, such as might be achieved with a Step Two diet. Dietary intervention trials in adults with fat reductions more stringent than the NCEP Step One diet show a total cholesterol reduction of between 10 and 15%.[67] Several studies demonstrate the efficacy of dietary interventions in children. One study showed that the Step One diet decreased total cholesterol and LDL cholesterol by 12%, although there was significant loss to follow-up of two-thirds of the enrollees.[68] Other studies have found decreases in total and LDL cholesterol of between 6 and 11%.[69,70]

Other dietary interventions have an impact on cholesterol levels in the pediatric ages. One small study of children with hypercholesterolemia showed that fiber supplementation decreases cholesterol while preserving HDL, and is more effective than simply following the Step One diet alone.[71] Fiber seems to have an independent effect of reducing cholesterol in children.[72] Recently, counseling has focused not on eliminating fat from the diet so much as exchanging saturated fat for monounsaturated fat. Unfortunately, fat elimination can lead to substitution with refined sugars and carbohydrates that increase triglyceride levels, whereas increased intake of monounsaturated fats can raise HDL levels and improve the cardiovascular risk profile. The Mediterranean diet, one focusing on mono- and polyunsaturated fats, has been associated with a reduced risk of cardiac mortality and morbidity in adults after their first myocardial infarction.[73] It has not been systematically evaluated in children, although many practitioners recommend it to their patients and families.

Table 4 Simple Substitutions for the Step One Diet

For	Substitute
Fatty meats	Fish, skinless chicken, lean beef, and pork
Saturated fat (eg, butter)	Monounsaturated fat
Partially hydrogenated oils (*trans*-fatty acids) in regular margarines	Canola or olive oil, monounsaturated margarines (eg, Smart Balance)
Regular peanut butter (partially hydrogenated)	"Natural" peanut butter
Ice cream	Frozen yogurt
Whole milk	Skim or 1% milk
Regular cheese	Low-fat cheese
Lunch meats	Low-fat equivalents
Chocolate (saturated oils)	Cocoa flavoring
Less healthful school lunch purchased	Lunch packed at home

More recent discussion in adults has focused on reducing carbohydrate intake as a percentage of total caloric intake, as an approach to weight loss, and possibly the metabolic syndrome. Studies of low carbohydrate diets in adults show greater initial weight loss in the short term (~ 6 months) compared to low-saturated fat diets, however results at 1 year are less impressive.[74,75] This approach has not been well evaluated in children, although small trials are supportive of the importance of dietary carbohydrate in weight and lipid management.[76,77] A refinement on thinking about carbohydrate is to look at the type of carbohydrate, specifically the glycemic index or glycemic load of a particular diet and its effect on weight and lipid levels. Glycemic index is a property of carbohydrate-containing food that describes the rise of blood glucose occurring after a standardized amount of food is consumed. In general, most refined starchy foods eaten in the United States, such as white bread, prepared breakfast cereals, rice, and potato products, have a high glycemic index, while unprocessed grains, nonstarchy vegetables, fruits, and legumes tend to have a low glycemic index. Several studies in children have demonstrated greater weight loss in children on low glycemic index diets.[78,79] Although some studies in adults suggest low glycemic index diets have a favorable effect on lipid profiles,[80] the data in children are lacking. However, weight loss in children has been shown to effectively decrease total cholesterol and triglycerides and to increase HDL,[81] and is a goal of many nutritional interventions if the child is overweight.

Some pediatric practitioners have raised concerns that these diets will hamper pediatric growth and development; however, the DISC demonstrated that children on a Step One diet had the same growth and development, with somewhat lower cholesterol levels, than did children on a diet close to the usual American intake.[82] The Special Turku Coronary Risk Factor Intervention Project (STRIP) showed that dietary consumption of fat, saturated fat, and total cholesterol did not affect neurodevelopment, although higher protein intake was associated with better neurodevelopmental outcome in boys, demonstrating that some degree of fat restriction is safe even in children less than 5 years old.[83]

Other interventions that have been explored, but not well exploited, are community-based programs. For example, school-based interventional strategies show some promise. In one study, after 5 years of group nutritional teaching, 2 hours per week, average total cholesterol was lower in children at the intervention schools than in the comparison groups.[84] Another similar study in Greece showed smaller increases in BMI and fat, saturated fat intake, and larger decreases in total cholesterol in the intervention schools than in the control schools.[85] The DISC is the largest published experience with school-based interventions. The investigators found that even in the control schools, with modest education rather than formal interventions, cholesterol values improved. The American Heart Association Web site (<http://www.americanheart.org>) is an excellent resource for community-based interventions. One such program, jumpstart, offers a curriculum for third to fifth graders (<http: //www.nhlbi.nih.gov/health/prof/heart/other/jumpstrt.htm>).

SPECIAL NUTRITIONAL INTERVENTIONS: STANOL-CONTAINING MARGARINES AND OMEGA-3 FATTY ACIDS

Several specific nutritional tools modify lipid profiles. Certain sterols, similar in structure to cholesterol but not absorbed by the small intestines, lower cholesterol by inhibiting absorption of cholesterol, both dietary and in the form of bile acids. As part of a low-fat diet in adults, stanols decrease total cholesterol by 8 to 10%, in addition to the 7% reduction from the low-fat diet alone.[86] A few studies have been performed in children; one trial of stanol ester margarine in 24 children found a decrease from pretreatment levels in total and LDL cholesterol by 14 and 18%, respectively, after 12 weeks, although betacarotene and tocopherol levels also decreased.[87] In adults, n-3 polyunsaturated fatty acids (omega-3 fatty acids) have been shown to reduce the risk of cardiovascular mortality after a myocardial infarction,[88] but, of course, no such data are available for children. Fish are a rich source of omega-3 fatty acids and should be recommended. Flax oil and ground flaxseed are reasonable substitutes for fish for children who will not eat fish. For children with high triglycerides, particularly those who do not consume many omega-3 fatty acids, supplements can be recommended; care should be taken in regard to DHA and EPA content as this varies substantially in over-the-counter preparations and is not standardized. Several name brands were tested for content, including mercury contaminant and were found to have minimal amounts of mercury and contain amounts of DHA and EPA as labeled.[89] We have used a dose of 1,000 mg per day. Side effects (unpleasant fishy taste) are minimized by keeping the supplements in the freezer, and taking them at night. A prescription form of purified omega-3 fatty acids is available (Omacor, Reliant Pharmaceuticals); however the pills are expensive and to date have not been reimbursed for children by health insurance. At the time of writing, there is no FDA indication for the prescription form of this medication in children.[90]

PHARMACOLOGIC INTERVENTION

Adult studies demonstrate significant reduction in cardiovascular morbidity and mortality with cholesterol-lowering medications, not just in severely affected patients or those who have existing heart disease, but also as primary prevention in patients with only moderate hypercholesterolemia.[91] As in adults, lipid-lowering drugs can be very effective in children. However, not enough data are available to weigh the potential long-term benefit against very low short-term risk of heart disease in young patients, together with the expense and potential risk of the medications.

In addressing this difficulty, national guidelines take a compromise approach: after approximately a year of nutritional and lifestyle changes, children aged 10 years or older with severe hyperlipidemia, defined as LDL cholesterol of >190 mg/dL or >160 mg/dL with two additional risk factors for cardiovascular disease, are eligible for consideration for pharmacologic treatment. In practice, we follow this guideline approximately, with the following modifications: we are less likely to consider medication in prepubertal patients if the beneficial HDL levels are high (consistent with the current adult guidelines, which take HDL cholesterol of more than 60 mg/dL as a negative risk factor). Conversely, we occasionally consider and treat children less than 10 years of age with medication for very abnormal profiles with severe family history. Furthermore, we are more inclined to treat children who are in a high-risk group such as a diabetic child, or a child with a history of Kawasaki Disease, as discussed above. Usual dosages are shown in Table 5.

The few pediatric trials show efficacy rates for decreasing cholesterol levels that are similar to those of adults. Cholestyramine and colestipol are resins that bind to bile acids in the gut, which prevents their reabsorption and prompts the body to convert more cholesterol to bile acids, thereby lowering cholesterol by 10 to 15%.[92,93] These medications may also decrease dietary cholesterol absorption from the gut, and have been demonstrated to increase LDL receptor expression and HMGCoA reductase activity.[94] The bile acid-binding medications are not absorbed into the blood stream, so there are no systemic effects; however, they have a gritty texture in powdered form and can cause constipation, so many children cannot tolerate them. Tablet forms of colestipol and cholestyramine are presently off the market. Colesevelam tablets are available and can be used in patients who do not tolerate the powdered forms but are old enough to swallow the large pills. Because they bind to lipophilic and acidic drugs, bile-binding agents are challenging to use in patients on multiple crucial medications such as posttransplantation immunosuppressive agents. In these special patients, it would be reasonable to consider statin use earlier in a patient's course. Compliance with bile acid-binding medications can be a problem that limits their usefulness, particularly in the younger child who might not understand the point of a preventive medication. Teenagers might have compliance issues as well, particularly with medications that require multiple doses per day.

Other lipid-lowering medications are systemically absorbed and are used with even more caution in children. Niacin can be an effective adjunct to lipid therapy in some adult settings, but flushing, abdominal discomfort, and risk of hepatotoxicity limit its use in children.[95] 3-hydroxy-3-methylglutaryl CoA reductase inhibitors, or statins, are the clear first-line agents for adults with elevated LDL cholesterol levels and have been used in selected, high-risk pediatric and adolescent patients for many years, but there are relatively few formal pediatric studies of safety and efficacy. Pravastatin was tested in 8- to 16-year-old boys and found to decrease total cholesterol by 25% and LDL cholesterol by 33%,

Table 5 Dosages of Medications Commonly Used in Hyperlipidemia

Lipid-Lowering Medications	Dosage Forms	Typical Dosage Range	Comments
Bile acid binding resins			
Cholestyramine powder (Questran, Lo-Cholest)	Generic powder is unflavorcd; Questran Light and Lo-Cholest are flavored	Weight <40 kg: start with 2 g bid, increase to 4 g bid if well tolerated; weight >40 kg: start as above, to 6 g bid; max. adult dose, 24 g/d	Not systemically absorbed; side effects of bloating, constipation fairly common
Colesevelam (Welchol)	625 mg tablets	Adult dose: 1,875 mg bid; pediatric dose: approx. 30 mg/kg bid, with liquids	Tablets are large; can be difficult for children to swallow
Colestipol (Colestid)	Powder or tablet (2 gm)	5–30 gm of powder div bid (supplied as 5 gm packets or scoops) 2–16 gm tablet form, div bid	As above
Absorption inhibitor†			
Ezetimibe (Zetia)	10 mg tablets	10 mg po qd	Inadequate LDL control on statins, sitosterolemia
Statins††			
Lovastatin (Mevacor, generic)	10, 20, 40 mg tablets	Pediatric dose:* 10–20 mg qd or divided bid; adult dose: 20–80 mg qd or divided bid	Generic form available, inexpensive; works best with bid dosing; is the drug with longest experience and most pediatric safety data available
Pravastatin (Pravachol, generic)	10, 20, 40, 80 mg tablets	Adult dose: 10–40 mg qhs	
Simvastatin (Zocor, generic)	5, 10, 20, 40, 80 mg tablets	5–80 mg qhs	
Atorvastatin (Lipitor)	10, 20, 40, 80 mg tablets		

Dosages are provided as a guide only and should be reviewed independently prior to prescribing.

*Children heavier than 40 kg are considered nearly adult sized and are dosed as adults.

†Side effects are minimal in adults and include gastrointestinal upset. No long-term studies in children.

††Statin therapy is contraindicated in pregnancy. Liver function tests (LFTs) should be monitored at baseline, after 4 weeks therapy, and then intermittently if normal. Caution patients about rare rhabdomyolysis; creatine phosphokinase should be checked if patient has myalgias. Sleep disturbances and abdominal discomfort are infrequent side effects.

without side effects, after 12 weeks of follow-up[96]; other short-term studies have supported these findings.[97,98] A longer trial of a statin, a 48-week follow-up trial in boys, showed significant efficacy, with a reduction of LDL cholesterol by 25% and no long-term endocrinologic or other sequelae.[99] Additional trials of similar length are consistent with these findings, with good efficacy and no serious side effects[100–102]; regardless, trials are too small and too short to definitively rule out long-term sequelae or the major but very rare adverse effect of rhabdomyolysis, or the theoretical modification of sex-steroid production. Gemfibrozil and fenofibrate are indicated for hypertriglyceridemia in adults but are used only for teenagers at risk for pancreatitis (triglycerides >1,000 mg/dL), and almost never in younger patients. There are no official pediatric targets for triglycerides; we generally think of triglycerides >150 mg/dL as abnormally high. An interesting new medication approved for use in adults by the US Food and Drug Administration in late 2002 is ezetimibe, a selective inhibitor of cholesterol absorption that reduces LDL by approximately 20% in 12 weeks, with minimal side effects.[106] It is now used in adults with relative frequency in addition to a statin, permitting a lower dose of statin to be used with a lower side-effect profile. This trial included seven participants aged 12 to 17 years, with no particular mention of ill effects in these children; however, the medication has not yet been systematically studied in pediatric patients. We have used it in pediatric and aged patients to keep statin doses low; a pediatric trial is ongoing. It is the primary medication recommended for sitosterolemia, a rare genetic cause of early atherosclerotic disease associated with xanthomata and only moderately elevated LDL levels. We have used it in pediatric-aged patients to keep statin doses low; pediatric trials are ongoing.

OTHER APPROACHES FOR SEVERE HYPERCHOLESTEROLEMIA

For patients with severe hypercholesterolemia unresponsive to diet or pharmacologic intervention, plasmapheresis or LDL apheresis with a Liposorber column has been successfully used in adults, lowering total cholesterol, LDL, triglycerides, and Lp(a), and perhaps a slowing of the progression of atherosclerosis.[104] The technique has also been used in selected pediatric patients with success,[105] although the issue of vascular access is a difficult one. Drugs that raise HDL have been studied in adults without, as yet, good results for the general population; they have not been used in children. There are no pediatric treatment recommendations for HDL at present.

MULTIDISCIPLINARY CLINIC APPROACH

Because atherosclerosis has a complex and multifactorial pathophysiology, pediatric lipid treatment programs that employ a multidisciplinary approach are more likely to be successful. In our center, the approach is combined nutritional and aerobic activity counseling, along with risk assessment and lipid monitoring. Our impression is that lifestyle habits can be more malleable in children, and changes put into place in younger children might be more likely to have an impact for years to come. This is the prime rationale for seeing children at young ages, along with their families, even if they will not require medication before adulthood. Contrary to the trend in adult lipid practice, we, along with most groups who see many children with hyperlipidemias, strive to avoid pharmacotherapy and reserve medication for use in the most severely affected patients. Figure 2 describes one such approach to patient management.

Clinic sessions should include group and individual nutritional education, laboratory work (or a review of previously obtained laboratory results), and a session with a clinician. A 3-day food recall provides a basis for individual nutritional counseling at the initial visit and in follow-up. Patient and family group education can include the basics of "good" and "bad" cholesterol, saturated and *trans*-fatty acids, protein, sugars, and fiber, and so on. Parents can be taught to read labels and to read between the lines on labels, and children can learn the concept of budgeting their fat and sugar intake so that birthday cake, for example, is not completely off limits but requires a lean period in compensation. It is useful to show children the actual amount of sugar in a can of soda or a serving of juice, or the appearance of fat clogging a tube that represents an artery. Methods of "dieting" for children can include using the plate method (Figure 3). We stress that "diet" does not mean weight loss for slender patients with genetic hyperlipidemia, but weight loss is paramount in patients with moderate to severe obesity, even when genetic hyperlipidemia is present. In general, emphasizing substitution of foods, as opposed to restricting or eliminating food, is more positive and seems more effective. Table 4 presents some simple suggestions for dietary modifications in hyperlipidemia.

The physician or nurse practitioner portion of the visit should involve a review of family history, general medical history, level of physical activity (or lack thereof), and an evaluation of lipid values. Twelve-hour fasting lipid values are the most valuable for children referred to a specialist clinic as it is important to have accurate triglyceride and LDL levels, at least on one or two occasions. At the Children's Hospital, Boston clinic, a healthful breakfast is provided to children after their laboratory samples are drawn, allowing modeling of good eating habits. Because severely affected children in a pediatric lipid setting usually have severely affected parents, we have found that often the most pressing issue affecting the child's well-being is having his or her parents tested for hyperlipidemia. It is important to ask about cigarette smoke exposure, to encourage children not to smoke, and to encourage parents not to smoke around their children because children exposed to cigarette smoking have lower HDL levels.[107,108] We stress the need to find physical activities that the child will enjoy.

We try to emphasize that for most children, these issues are not an emergency but rather are long-term modifications that are important not for present health but for cardiovascular and endocrine risk 30 to 40 years in the future (a nearly unimaginable length of time for most children). This helps parents and children to view this as a long-term project and removes the pressures of enforcing an immediate turnaround. Having only appropriate food in the home is helpful in making

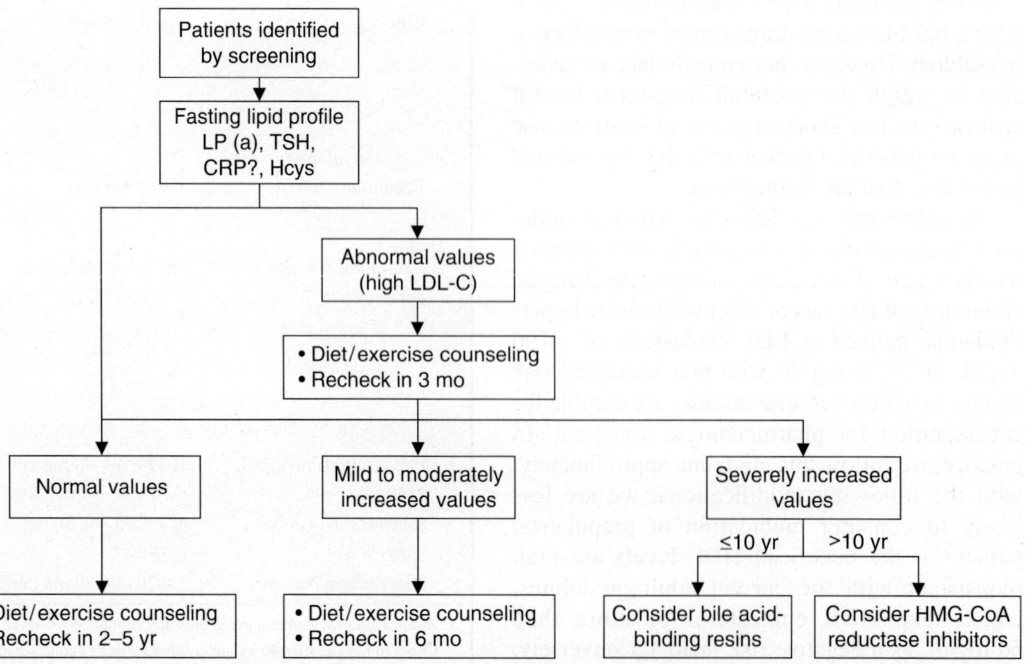

Figure 2 Proposed approach to young patients ascertained to have high cholesterol on screening. Thyroid-stimulating hormone (TSH) serves as an inexpensive screen for primary hypothyroidism. Lipoprotein (a) [Lp(a)] is an independent risk factor for premature atherosclerosis. The role of highly sensitive C-reactive protein (hsCRP) or homocysteine (Hcys) screening is not defined in pediatrics. HMG CoA = 3-hydroxy-3-methylglutaryl coenzyme A.

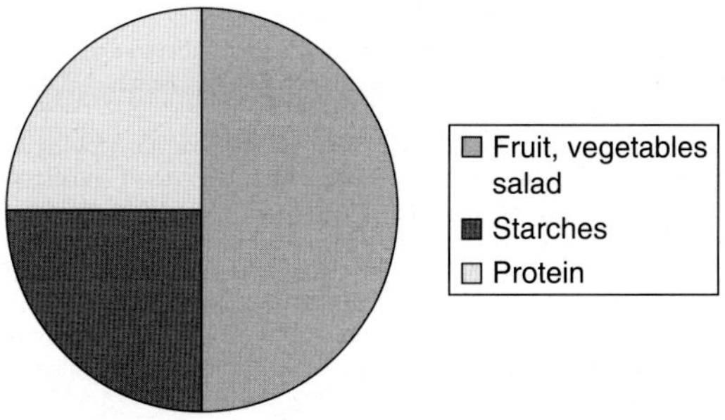

Figure 3 The "plate method" is a simple means for balancing the diet and reducing carbohydrate consumption without counting calories or grams of fat. Half the plate should contain fruits and vegetables, while one quarter should contain starch and the final quarter protein. Some practitioners use 1/3, 1/3, 1/3. The method is highly effective for hypertriglyceridemia and for obesity, if given with a few suggestions: (1) the entire family, not just the patient, should try the method for 4 to 6 weeks and then recheck lipids and weight; (2) the patient must finish the entire plate before having second helpings; and (3) "seconds" cannot be just starches but must again be balanced.

choices easier. Lifestyle changes seem to be more effectively made if the entire family joins in the effort. Often, suggested changes are indicated for multiple family members, even if only one child in the family was referred. Follow-up is crucial for monitoring progress, medication compliance, and somatic growth.

SUMMARY

Pediatric lipid disorders contribute to future cardiovascular risk and as such should be addressed aggressively. Yet at the same time, in the majority of cases, pediatric hyperlipidemias might be most safely, and perhaps most effectively, treated with a multidisciplinary approach that includes aerobic activity, nutritional counseling, and individualized interventions. Care should be exercised to prevent the establishment of negative behavioral patterns because the health implications of dyslipidemias are, for the most part, far in the future. Future research should focus on longer term evaluation of antihyperlipidemic medications in young patients, on the utility of markers of preclinical either blood or vascular testing, that can be used to evaluate the efficacy of interventions for atherosclerosis prevention.

REFERENCES

1. Thom T, Haase N, Rosamond W, et al. Heart disease and stroke statistics—2006 update: A report from the American Heart Association Statistics Subcommittee. Circulation 2006;113;85–151.
2. Kannel WB. Range of serum cholesterol values in the population developing coronary artery disease. Am J Cardiol 1995;76:69C–77C.
3. Lipid Research Clinics Program. The Lipid Research Clinics Coronary Primary Prevention Trial results II: The relationship of reduction in incidence of coronary heart disease to cholesterol lowering. JAMA 1984;251:365–74.
4. Committee on Nutrition. Policy Statement: Prevention of pediatric overweight and obesity. Pediatrics 2003;112:424–30.
5. National Cholesterol Education Program. Report of the expert panel on blood cholesterol levels in children and adolescents. Department of Health and Human Services (US); 1991 Sept. NIG Publication No. 91–2732.
6. Committee on Nutrition, American Academy of Pediatrics. Statement on cholesterol. Pediatrics 1992;90:469–73.
7. Committee on Nutrition, American Academy of Pediatrics. Cholesterol in childhood. Pediatrics 1998;101:141–7.
8. Gidding SS. New cholesterol guidelines for children? Circulation 2006;114:989–91.
9. Holman RL, Anderson JL, Cannon RO, III, et al. The natural history of atherosclerosis. Am J Pathol 1958;34:209–35.
10. Stary HC. Evolution and progression of atherosclerotic lesions in coronary arteries of children and young adults. Arteriosclerosis 1989;9:I19–32.
11. Prevalence and extent of atherosclerosis in adolescents and young adults: Implications for prevention from the Pathobiological Determinants of Atherosclerosis in Youth Study. JAMA 1999;24:727–35.
12. McGill HC, Jr, McMahan CA. Determinants of atherosclerosis in the young. Pathobiological Determinants of Atherosclerosis in Youth (PDAY) Research Group. Am J Cardiol 1998;82:30T–6T.
13. Solberg LA, Strong JP. Risk factors and atherosclerotic lesions: A review of autopsy studies. Arteriosclerosis 1983;3:187–98.
14. Knuiman JT, West CE, Katan MB, Hautvast JG. Total cholesterol and high density lipoprotein cholesterol levels in populations differing in fat and carbohydrate intake. Arteriosclerosis 1987;7:612–9.
15. Lauer RM, Lee J, Clarke WR. Factors affecting the relationship between childhood and adult cholesterol levels: The Muscatine Study. Pediatrics 1988;82:309–18.
16. Klag MJ, Ford DE, Mead LA, et al. Serum cholesterol in young men and subsequent cardiovascular disease. N Engl J Med 1993;328:313–8.
17. Tuzcu EM, Kapadia SR, Tutar E, et al. High prevalence of coronary atherosclerosis in asymptomatic teenagers and young adults: Evidence from intravascular ultrasound. Circulation 2001;103:2705–10.
18. Mulla NF, Johnston JK, Vander Dussen L, et al. Late rejection is a predictor of transplant coronary artery disease in children. J Am Coll Cardiol 2001;37:243–50.
19. Pennisi AJ, Heuser ET, Mickey MR, et al. Hyperlipidemia in pediatric hemodialysis and renal transplant patients. Associated with coronary artery disease. Am J Dis Child 1976;130:957–61.
20. Sharma AK, Myers TA, Hunninghake DB, et al. Hyperlipidemia in long-term survivors of pediatric renal transplantation. Clin Transplant 1994;8:252–7.
21. Newburger JW, Takahashi M, Gerber MA, et al. Diagnosis, treatment, and long-term management of Kawasaki Disease: A statement for health professionals from the Committee on Threumatic Fever, Endocarditis, and Kawasaki Disease, Council on Cardiovascular Disease in the Young, American Heart Association. Circulation 2004;110:2747–71.
22. Hauser M, Bengel FM, Kuhn A, et al. Myocardial perfusion and coronary flow reserve assessed by positron emission tomography in patients after Fontan-like operations. Pediatr Cardiol 2003;24:386–92.
23. Bengel FM, Hauser M, Duvernoy CS, et al. Myocardial blood flow and coronary flow reserve late after anatomical correction of transposition of the great arteries. J Am Coll Cardiol 1998;32:1955–61.
24. Hauser M, Bengel FM, Kuhn A, et al. Myocardial blood flow and flow reserve after coronary reimplantation in patients after arterial switch and ross operation. Circulation 2001;103:1875–80.
25. Rubins HB, Robins SJ, Collins D, et al. Distribution of lipids in 8,500 men with coronary artery disease. Am J Cardiol 1995;75:1196–201.
26. EUROASPIRE Study Group. A European Society of Cardiology survey of secondary prevention of coronary heart disease: Principal results. Eur Heart J 1997;18:1569–82.
27. de Beer FC, Hind CRK, Fox KM, et al. Measurement of serum C-reactive protein concentration in myocardial ischaemia and infarction. Br Heart J 1982;47:239–43.
28. Kushner I, Broder ML, Karp D. Control of the acute phase response: Serum C-reactive protein kinetics after acute myocardial infarction. J Clin Invest 1978;61:235–42.
29. Thompson SB, Kienast J, Pyke SD, et al. Hemostatic factors and the risk of myocardial infarction or sudden death in patients with angina. N Engl J Med 1995;332:635–41.
30. Ridker PM, Rifai N, Pfeffer MA, et al. Inflammation, pravastatin, and the risk of coronary events after myocardial infarction in patients with average cholesterol levels. Circulation 1998;98:839–44.
31. Ridker PM, Cushman M, Stampfer MJ, et al. Inflammation, aspirin, and risks of cardiovascular disease in apparently healthy men. N Engl J Med 1997;336:973–9.
32. Ridker PM, Hennekens CH, Buring JE, Rifai N. C-reactive protein and other markers of inflammation in the prediction of cardiovascular disease in women. N Engl J Med 2000;342:836–43.
33. Pearson TA, Mensah GA, Alexander RW, et al. Markers of inflammation and cardiovascular disease: Application to clinical and public health practice: A statement for healthcare professionals from the Centers for Disease Control and Prevention and the American Heart Association. Circulation. 2003;107:499–511.
34. Mietus-Snyder ML, Malloy MJ. Endothelial dysfunction occurs in children with three genetic hyperlipidemias: Improvement with antioxidant therapy. J Pediatr 1998;133:35–40.
35. Engler MM, Engler MB, Malloy MJ, et al. Antioxidant vitamins C and E improve endothelial function in children with hyperlipidemia: Endothelial Assessment of Risk from Lipids in Youth (EARLY) trial. Circulation. 2003;108:1059–63.
36. Lee J, Lauer RM, Clarke WR. Lipoproteins in the progeny of young men with coronary disease: Children with increased risk. Pediatrics 1986;78:330–7.
37. Bistritzer T, Rosenzweig L, Barr J, et al. Lipid profile with paternal history of coronary heart disease before age 40. Arch Dis Child 1995;73:62–5.
38. Margaglione M, Cappucci G, Colaizzo D, et al. C-reactive protein in offspring is associated with the occurrence of myocardial infarction in first-degree relatives. Arterioscler Thromb Vasc Biol 2000;20:198–203.
39. Collins R, Armitage J, Parish S, et al. for the Heart Protection Study Collaborative Group. MRC/BHF Heart Protection Study of antioxidant vitamin supplementation in 20,536 high-risk individuals: A randomized placebo-controlled trial. Lancet 2002;360:23–33.
40. Bostom AG, Silbershatz H, Rosenberg IH, et al. Nonfasting plasma total homocysteine levels and all-cause and cardiovascular disease mortality in elderly Framingham men and women. Arch Intern Med 1999;159:1077–80.
41. Welch GN, Loscalzo J. Homocysteine and atherothrombosis. N Engl J Med 1998;338:1042–50.
42. Online Mendelian Inheritance in Man #236250. Available at: http://www.ncbi.nlm.nih.gov/entrez/query.fcgi?db=OMIM.
43. Obarzanek E, Kimm SY, Barton BA, et al. and the DISC Collaborative Research Group. Long-term safety and efficacy of a cholesterol-lowering diet in children with elevated low-density lipoprotein cholesterol: Seven-year results of the Dietary Intervention Study in Children (DISC). Pediatrics 2001;107:256–64.
44. Mensink RP, Katan MB. Effect of dietary trans fatty acids on high-density and low-density lipoprotein cholesterol levels in healthy subjects. N Engl J Med. 1990;323:439–45.
45. Packard CJ. Small dense low-density lipoprotein and its role as an independent predictor of cardiovascular disease. Curr Opin Lipidol 2006;17:412–7.
46. Vuorio AF, Turtola H, Piilahti KM, et al. Familial hypercholesterolemia in the Finnish North Karelia: A molecular, clinical and genealogical study. Arterioscler Thromb Vasc Biol 1997;17:3127–38.
47. Grossman M, Rader DJ, Muller DW, et al. A pilot study of ex vivo gene therapy for homozygous familial hypercholesterolemia. Nat Med 1995;1:1148–54.
48. Brown MS, Goldstein JL, Havel RJ, Steinberg D. Gene therapy for cholesterol. Nat Genet 1994;7:349–50.
49. Online Mendelian Inheritance in Man #107680. Available at: http://www.ncbi.nlm.nih.gov/entrez/query.fcgi?db=OMIM.
50. Angles-Cano E, de la Pena Diaz A, Loyau S. Inhibition of fibrinolysis by lipoprotein(a). Ann N Y Acad Sci 2001;936:261–75.
51. Suk Danik J, Rifai N, Buring JE, Ridker PM. Lipoprotein(a), measured with an assay independent of apolipoprotein(a) isoform size, and risk of future cardiovascular events among initially healthy women. JAMA. 2006;296:1363–70.
52. Colletti RB, Neufeld EJ, Roff NK, et al. Niacin treatment of hypercholesterolemia in children. Pediatrics 1993;78–82.
53. Leren TP, Hjermann I, Foss OP, et al. Long-term effect of lovastatin alone and in combination with cholestyramine on lipoprotein (a) in familial hypercholesterolemic subjects. Clin Investig 1992;70:711–8.
54. Ford ES, Giles WH, Dietz WH. Prevalence of the metabolic syndrome among US adults: Findings from the third National Health and Nutrition Examination Survey. JAMA 2002;287:356–9.
55. de Ferranti SD, Gauvreau K, Ludwig DS, et al. Prevalence of the metabolic syndrome in american adolescents: Findings from the Third National Health and Nutrition Examination Survey. Circulation. 2004;110:2494–7.
56. Cook S, Weitzman M, Auinger P, et al. Prevalence of a metabolic syndrome phenotype in adolescents: Findings from the third National Health and Nutrition Examination Survey, 1988-1994. Arch Pediatr Adolesc Med 2003;157:821–7.
57. Vanhala MJ, Vanhala PT, Keinanen-Kiukaanniemi SM, et al. Relative weight gain and obesity as a child predict

metabolic syndrome as an adult. Int J Obes Relat Metab Disord 1999;23:656–9.

58. Dennison BA, Jenkins PL, Pearson TA. Challenges to implementing the current pediatric cholesterol screening guide-lines into practice. Pediatrics 1994;94:296–302.
59. Dennison BA, Kikuchi DA, Srinivasan SR, et al. Parental history of cardiovascular disease as an indication for screening for lipoprotein abnormalities in children. J Pediatr 1989;115:186–94.
60. Rifai N, Neufeld E, Ahlstrom P, et al. Failure of current guide-lines for cholesterol screening in urban African-American adolescents. Pediatrics 1996;98:383–8.
61. National Cholesterol Education Program. Expert Panel on Detection, Evaluation and Treatment of High Cholesterol in Adults (Adult Treatment Panel III), executive summary, third report. National Cholesterol Education Program, National Heart, Lung and Blood Institute, National Institutes of Health; 2001 May. Publication No. 01–3670.
62. Bowman SA, Gortmaker SL, Ebbeling CB, et al. Pediatrics. Effects of fast-food consumption on energy intake and diet quality among children in a national household survey. 2004;113:112–8.
63. Guthri JF, Lin BH, Frazao E. Role of food prepared away from home in the American diet, 1977–78 versus 1994–96: Changes and consequences. J Nutr Educ Behav 2002;34:140–50.
64. Dennison BA, Rockwell HL, Nichols MJ, Jenkins P. Children's growth parameters vary by type of fruit juice consumed. J Am Coll Nutr 1999;18:346–52.
65. Mone SM, Gillman MW, Miller TL, et al. Effects of environmental exposures on the cardiovascular system: Prenatal period through adolescence. Pediatrics. 2004;113:1058–69.
66. Owen CG, Whincup PH, Odoki K, et al. Infant feeding and blood cholesterol: A study in adolescents and a systematic review. Pediatrics 2002;110:597–608.
67. Nguyen TT. Cholesterol-lowering trials and coronary heart disease in the United States. In: Postgraduate Medicine Special Report: New Developments in the Dietary Management of High Cholesterol. New York: McGraw-Hill; 1998. p. 15–26.
68. Polansky SM, Bellet PS, Sprecher DL. Primary hyperlipidemia in a pediatric population: Classification and effect of dietary treatment. Pediatrics 1993:91:92–6.
69. Glueck CJ, Fallat RW, Mellies M, Tsang RC. Pediatric familial type II hyperlipoproteinemia: Therapy with diet and colestipol resin. Pediatrics 1976;57:68–74.
70. Kwiterovitch PO, Jr, Bachorik PS, Franklin FA, Jr, et al. Effect of dietary treatment on the plasma levels of lipids, lipoprotein, cholesterol and LDL B protein in children with type II hyperlipoproteinemia. Prog Clin Biol Res 1985;188:123–37.
71. Glassman M, Spark A, Berezin S, et al. Treatment of type IIa hyperlipidemia in childhood by a simplified American Heart Association diet and fiber supplementation. Am J Dis Child 1990;144:973–6.
72. Zavoral JH, Hannan P, Fields DJ, et al. The hypolipidemic effect of locust bean gum products in familial hypercholesterolemic adults and children. Am J Clin Nutr 1983;38: 285–94.
73. de Lorgeril M, Salen P, Martin JL, et al. Mediterranean diet, traditional risk factors, and the rate of cardiovascular complications after myocardial infarction: Final report of the Lyon Diet Heart Study. Circulation 1999;99:779–85.
74. Yancy WS, Jr, Olsen MK, Guyton JR, et al. A low-carbohydrate, ketogenic diet versus a low-fat diet to treat obesity and hyperlipidemia: A randomized, controlled trial. Ann Intern Med 2004;769–77.
75. Samaha FF, Iqbal N, Seshadri P, et al. A low-carbohydrate as compared with a low-fat diet in severe obesity. N Engl J Med 2003;2074–81.
76. Sondike SB, Copperman N, Jacobson MS. Effects of a low-carbohydrate diet on weight loss and cardiovascular risk factor in overweight adolescents. J Pediatr 2003;253–8.
77. Lindquist CH, Gower BA, Goran MI. Role of dietary factors in ethnic differences in early risk of cardiovascular disease and type 2 diabetes. Am J Clin Nutr 2000;725–32.
78. Young PC, West SA, Ortiz K, Carlson J. A pilot study to determine the feasibility of the low glycemic index diet as a treatment for overweight children in primary care practice. Ambul Pediatr 2004;28–33.
79. Spieth LE, Harnish JD, Lenders CM, et al. A low-glycemic index diet in the treatment of pediatric obesity. Arch Pediatr Adolesc Med 2000;947–51.
80. Pereira MA, Swain J, Goldfine AB, et al. Effects of a low-glycemic load diet on resting energy expenditure and heart disease risk factors during weight loss. JAMA 2004;2482–90.
81. Epstein LH, Kuller LH, Wing RR, et al. The effect of weight control on lipid changes in obese children. Am J Dis Child 1989;143:454–7.
82. Writing Group, DISC Collaborative Research Group. Efficacy and safety of lowering dietary intake of fat and cholesterol in children with elevated LDL lipoprotein cholesterol: The Dietary Intervention Study in Children (DISC). JAMA 1995;273:1429–35.
83. Rask-Nissila L, Jokinen E, Terho P, et al. Effects of diet on the neurologic development of children at 5 years of age: The STRIP project. J Pediatr 2002;140:328–33.
84. Walter HJ, Hofman A, Vaughan RD, Wynder EL. Modification of risk factors for coronary heart disease. Five-year results of a school-based intervention trial. N Engl J Med 1988;318:1093–100.
85. Manios Y, Moschandreas J, Hatzis C, Kafatos A. Health and nutrition education in primary schools of Crete: Changes in chronic disease risk factors following a 6-year intervention programme. Br J Nutr 2002;88:315–24.
86. Hallikainen MA, Uusitupa MI. Effects of 2 low-fat stanol ester-containing margarines on serum cholesterol concentrations as part of a low fat diet in hypercholesterolemic subjects. Am J Clin Nutr 1999;69:403–10.
87. Vuorio AF, Gylling H, Turtola H, et al. Stanol ester margarine alone and with simvastatin lowers serum cholesterol in families with familial hypercholesterolemia caused by the FHNorth Karelia mutation. Arterioscler Thromb Vasc Biol 2000;20:500–6.
88. Marchioli R, Barzi F, Bomba E, et al. Early protection against sudden death by n-3 polyunsaturated fatty acids after myocardial infarction: Time-course analysis of the results of the Gruppo Italiano per lo Studio della Sopravvivenza nell'Infarto Miocardico (GISSI)-Prevenzione. Circulation 2002;105:1897–903.
89. Omega-3 oil: Fish or pills? Available at: http:/www.consumerreports.org/cro/health-fitness/drugs-supplements/fishoil-pills-703. Accessed 11/27/06.
90. The medical letter on drugs and therapeutics. Fish oil supplements 2006;1239:59–60.
91. Downs JR, Clearfield M, Weis S, et al. Primary prevention of acute coronary events with lovastatin in men and women with average cholesterol levels: Results of AFCAPS/TexCAPS. Air Force/Texas Coronary Atherosclerosis Prevention Study. JAMA 1998;279:1615–22.
92. Tonstad S, Knudtzon J, Siversten M, et al. Efficacy and safety of cholestyramine therapy in peripubertal and prepubertal children with familial hypercholesterolemia. J Pediatr 1996;129:42–9.
93. McCrindle BW, O'Neill MB, Cullen-Dean G, Helden E. Accept-ability and compliance with two forms of cholestyramine in the treatment of hypercholesterolemia in children: A randomized cross-over trial. J Pediatr 1997;130:266–73.
94. Reihnir E, Angelin B, Rudling M, et al. Regulation of hepatic cholesterol metabolism in humans: Stimulatory effects of cholestyramine on HMG-CoA reductase activity and low density lipoprotein receptor expression in gallstone patients. J Lipid Res 1990;31:2220–6.
95. Stein EA. Treatment of familial hypercholesterolemia with drugs in children. Arteriosclerosis 1989;9:1451–511.
96. Knipscheer HC, Boelen CC, Kastelein JJ, et al. Short-term efficacy and safety of pravastatin in 72 children with familial hypercholesterolemia. Pediatr Res 1996;39:867–71.
97. Lambert M, Lupien PJ, Gagne C, et al. Treatment of familial hypercholesterolemia in children and adolescents: Effect of lovastatin. Canadian lovastatin in children's study group. Pediatrics 1996;97:619–28.
98. Duplaga BA. Treatment of childhood hypercholesterolemia with HMG-CoA reductase inhibitors. Ann Pharmacother 1999;33:1224–7.
99. Stein EA, Illingworth DR, Kwiterovich PO, et al. Efficacy and safety of lovastatin in adolescent males with heterozygous familial hypercholesterolemia: A randomized controlled trial. JAMA 1999;281:137–44.
100. Ducobu J, Brasseur D, Chaudron JM, et al. Simvastatin use in children. Lancet 1992;339:1488.
101. de Jongh S, Ose L, Szamosi T, et al. Efficacy and safety of statin therapy in children with familial hypercholesterolemia: A randomized, double-blind, placebo-controlled trial with simvastatin. Circulation 2002;2231–7.
102. Wiegman A, Hutten BA, de Groot E, et al. Efficacy and safety of statin therapy in children with familial hypercholesterolemia: A randomized controlled trial. JAMA 2004;331–7.
103. McCrindle BW, Helden E, Cullen-Dean G, Conner WT. A randomized crossover trial of combination pharmacologic therapy in children with familial hyperlipidemia. Pediatr Res 2002;715–21.
104. Schiel R, Bambauer R, Muller U. Low-density lipoprotein apheresis versus lipid lowering drugs in the treatment of severe hypercholesterolemia: Four years' experience. Artif Organs 1996;20:318–23.
105. Zwiener RJ, Uauy R, Petruska ML, Huet BA. Low-density lipoprotein apheresis as long-term treatment for children with homozygous familial hypercholesterolemia. J Pediatr 1995;126:728–35.
106. Gagne C, Gaudet D, Bruckert E for the Ezetimibe Study Group. Efficacy and safety of ezetimibe coadministered with atorvastatin or simvastatin in patients with homozygous familial hypercholesterolemia. Circulation 2002;105: 2469–75.
107. Moskowitz WB, Schwartz PF, Schieken RM. Childhood passive smoking, race, and coronary artery disease risk: The MCV Twin Study. Arch Pediatr Adolesc Med 1999;153:446–53.
108. Neufeld EJ, Mietus-Snyder M, Beiser AS, et al. Passive cigarette smoking and reduced HDL cholesterol levels in children with high-risk lipid profiles. Circulation 1997;96:1403–7.

Carbohydrate Absorption and Malabsorption

Doron D. Kahana, MD
Martin H. Ulshen, MD
Martín G. Martin, MD, MPP

INTRODUCTION

Carbohydrates account for about half of our total caloric intake after early infancy, with an average dietary intake of 200 to 300 g/d in adults.[1] Carbohydrates (CHO) include starch derived from cereals and plants (eg, amylose, amylopectin), sugars derived from fruits and vegetables (glucose, fructose, sucrose), milk (lactose), refined processed foods (eg, sucrose, fructose, oligo- and polysaccharides), and fiber derived from plant wall polysaccharides (eg, cellulose, pectin, gum, and lignin). The disaccharide lactose (glucose linked with galactose) is the principal CHO ingested by most suckling infants, whether fed human milk or commercial formula. Other CHOs are introduced progressively into the diet as solids and juices, and by early childhood, starch becomes the major dietary CHO.

Starch consists of long chains of glucose molecules joined together by α-1,4 (linear) linkages (ie, amyloses) and both α-1,4 and α-1,6 branched linkages (ie, amylopectins; see Figures 1 and 2). Dietary fiber is ingested mostly in the form of cellulose that consists of glucose molecules joined together by β-1,4 linear and branched linkages which are resistant to hydrolysis by α-amylase (see Figures 1 and 3). Lactase-phlorizin hydrolase (LPH), sucrase-isomaltase (SI), and glucoamylase are the primary hydrolyzing enzymes that process the majority of dietary saccharides. Polysaccharides and disaccharides cannot pass the brush border membrane and must be broken down into the monosaccharides glucose, galactose, and fructose in order to be absorbed.

The process of digestion and absorption is termed *nutrient assimilation*, which is a dynamic process that can adapt to changes in environmental conditions and metabolic homeostasis. CHO assimilation is unique from protein and fat assimilation in that undigested saccharides undergo colonic fermentation by the microbiota that colonizes the distal bowel and colon. The intestine is inhabited by more than 500 unique species of microorganisms that form a symbiotic relationship with the mucosa and depend on a continuous supply of luminal nutrients.[2]

The process of nutrient assimilation may be best modeled into nutritive *loads* and luminal digestive and absorptive *capacities*. Similar to most engineered machines (eg, elevators, cranes, bridges), physiologic processes are designed with certain safety factors (capacity × load^{-1} = safety factor) that ensure that capacities exceed loads.[3,4] However, studies in quantitative evolutionary design, the study of the relation between biological capacities and natural loads, have demonstrated that nutritive processing has a limited safety factor. That is, our ability to assimilate nutrients is designed in the short-term to match the average nutritive load rather than to dramatically exceed it.[5] Furthermore, long-term consumption of an excessive (either generalized or specific nutrients) dietary load results in gut adaptation and improved capacity to assimilate nutrients.[5–7] However, the adaptive process is not limitless, as upper limits have been well established in rodent models and are frequently encountered in the management of patients with short bowel syndrome.[5] Nevertheless, a homeostatic balance between metabolic needs that varies dramatically with age and dietary intake must be achieved in order to maintain health; a disturbance in this balance can result in either obesity or malnourishment. Homeostasis is achieved through complex molecular interactions between metabolic, genetic, and physiologic systems, including endocrine, paracrine, autocrine, and nervous, some of which will be discussed in this chapter.[8]

One of the benefits of a limited safety factor in nutritive processing is the provision of nutritive resources for the gut flora. The symbiotic relationship between the microflora and its host depends on the ingestion of certain nutritive resources. When nutrient load breeches

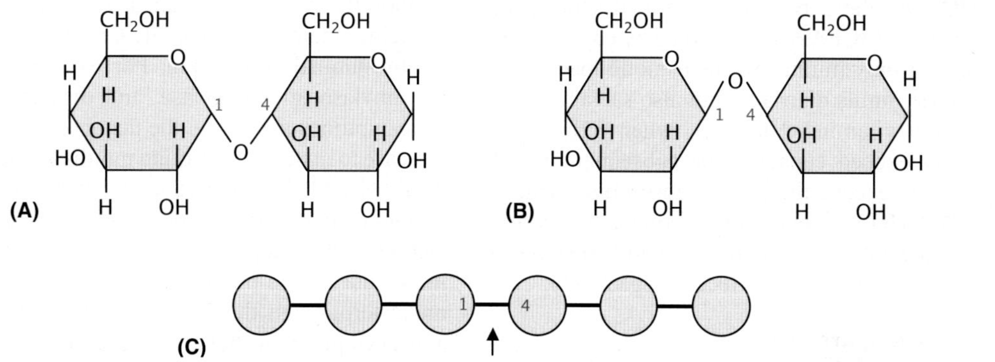

Figure 1 (**A**) D-glucose molecules linked by an α-1,4 bond. (**B**) D-glucose molecules linked by β-1,4 bonds, as seen in plant cellulose. (**C**) Amylose (starch) is a polymer consisting exclusively of α-1,4 linkage of D-glucose; α-amylase cleaves α-1,4 bonds (*arrow*), forming maltose and maltotriose. Cellulose digestion requires the activity of β-amylase which humans do not make.

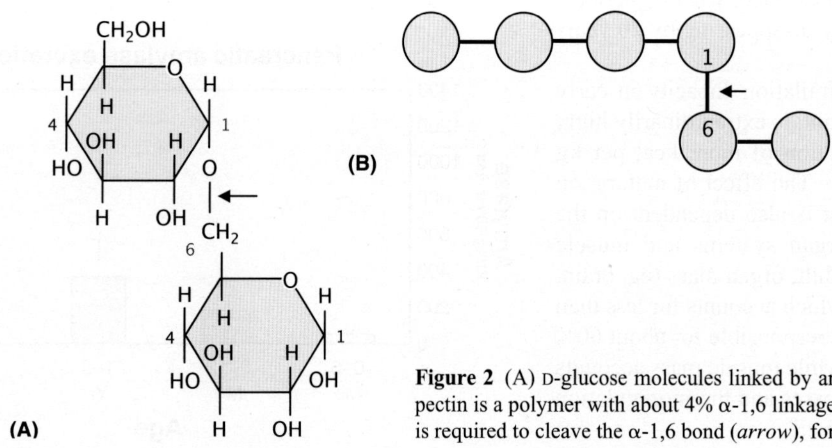

Figure 2 (A) D-glucose molecules linked by an α-1,6 bond. (B) Amylopectin is a polymer with about 4% α-1,6 linkage of D-glucose; isoamylase is required to cleave the α-1,6 bond (*arrow*), forming α-limit dextrins.

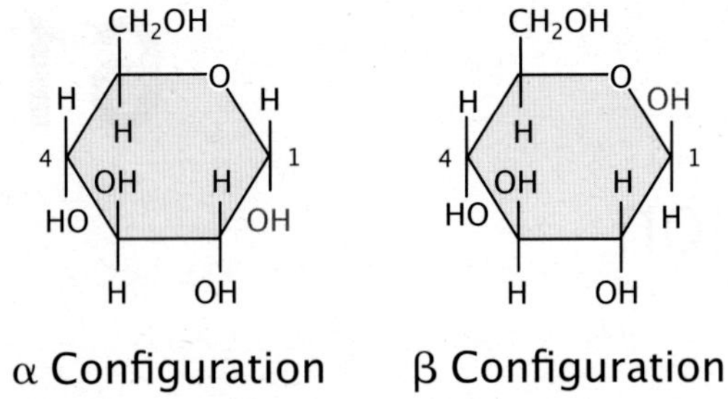

Figure 3 α and β isomers of D-glucose.

capacity, resident microflora process some of the undigested and unabsorbed nutrients, especially CHO, and the subsequently formed short-chain fatty acids (SCFAs) are absorbed by colonocytes. This not only minimizes the osmotic load of the stool (ie, limits diarrhea), but also salvages calories and vitamins. However, when CHO loads greatly exceed capacity, the subsequent SCFA load may exceed the colonic absorptive capacity or the CHO may exceed the fermentative capacity of the gut flora, resulting in acidified stools or frank CHO spillage into feces, respectively.

Energy Requirements

Energy balance is tightly regulated. Most infants and children grow in regular fashion and many adults maintain a stable body weight for long periods. In infants and young children, growth rate is a very good bioassay for adequate energy intake, with studies showing a good linear relationship between total energy expenditure (TEE) and body weight.[9] TEE includes basal metabolism, the metabolic response to food, thermoregulation, physical activity, and growth. Energy that is consumed but unused may be stored as fat and protein, or excreted. During the first 3 months of life, when weight gain is about 30 g/d, the energy cost of growth is about 6 kcal/g of new tissue, or about 30 to 40% of TEE. By 6 months of age, weight gain falls to about 18 g/d and only 2.8 kcal/g of new tissue, or about 10 to 20% of calories, are expanded for growth, with more energy expanded in physical activity.[10] By 1 year of age, the energy needs for growth represent less than 10% of the total energy intake but still require between 8 to 12 kcal/g of new tissue.[11] Energy requirement for growth falls to less than 2% of TEE in the second year of life and remains there through mid-adolescence, when it periodically jumps, eventually disappearing by 20 years of age.[12,13]

Thus, nutrient assimilation capacity in early infancy, per body weight, is extraordinarily high, allowing the consumption of more kcal per kg than at any other time. The effect of maturation on energy requirement is also dependent on the needs of different organ systems and muscle mass. In an average adult, organ mass (eg, brain, liver, heart, kidney), which accounts for less than 6% of body weight, is responsible for about 60% of metabolic energy, while muscle mass accounts for only 20 to 25%. Losses and thermoregulation make up most of the rest.[14]

Infant Nutrient Assimilation

Human milk has a very high lactose content compared to the milks of other mammals; human milk and cow's milk contain about 37 and 42% of their calories, respectively, in the form of lactose.[15] Oligosaccharides represent about 10% of total milk CHO in human milk and less than 1% in cow's milk. Use of soy-based formulas has increased over the past 30 years, and as many as 25% of infants in the United States now receive these formulas.[16] Soy-based formulas contain CHOs in the form of sucrose, cornstarch, cornstarch hydrolysate, or tapioca starch rather than lactose.

The gut's capacity to assimilate CHOs is temporally regulated, with several enzymatic capacities maturing during late gestation and others by luminal stimulation. For example, luminal amylase, glucoamylase, and disaccharidase concentrations are low in the neonatal period but increase to mature levels quite rapidly in the postnatal period.[17–19] About 25% of 1-week-old term infants exhibit some lactose malabsorption, and lactase activity appears to be induced by lactose intake during the premature period.[20–22] Lactose malabsorption in the neonate is generally mild and asymptomatic but may be associated with feeding intolerance in premature infants. Unabsorbed lactose is largely salvaged in the colon with bacterial fermentation and production of SCFAs.[23] Along with other nondigestible CHOs (ie, galacto- and fructooligosaccharides) in breast milk, the malabsorbed lactose may actually help select for particular microbiota species that colonize the colon (eg, *Lactobacillus, Bifidobacteria*).[24]

Starch digestion is limited in newborn infants, and pancreatic secretion of α-amylase may remain insufficient for several months. Thus, CHO needs in infancy are met largely via the digestion of lactose into its components, glucose and galactose, and the need for α-amylase digestion is minimal until weaning. Weaning is also the point at which time all studied nonhuman mammals, and most humans, begin to experience a decline in lactase levels.

By 12 months of age, table foods should account for most of the calories in an infant's diet, and milk consumption is usually limited to 24 oz/d. An average diet for an older child or adult consists of about 50% of the CHOs in the form of starch, while lactose accounts for a decreased proportion of the total CHO calories, becoming only a minor fraction for many adults.

CARBOHYDRATE ASSIMILATION

Starch

Most dietary starch consists of amylose, straight chains of glucose linked by α-1,4 bonds, and amylopectin, straight chains with about 5% interspersed α-1,6 branches (Figures 1 and 2). Amylopectin is the major form of starch in the human diet. The primary enzyme of starch digestion, α- amylase, acts only on the interior α-1,4 linkages of starch, releasing oligo- and disaccharides such as maltose (two glucose units), maltotriose (three glucose units), and the α-limit dextrins (oligosaccharides consisting of up to six glucose units with or without α-1,6 links). The amount of glucose released during amylose and amylopectin digestion is negligible, and therefore the products of starch hydrolysis require further digestion prior to absorption.

Carbohydrate digestion really begins in the mouth, with oral exposure to salivary α-amylase, and in breast-fed infants, α-amylase produced by mammary glands.[25,26] Human milk amylase levels do not seem to vary between preterm and term milk, throughout a feeding, or between feedings.[27] As a whole, these amylases, like salivary α-amylase, may partially compensate for the low level of pancreatic α-amylase secretion in the duodenum of newborns.[27] Although the enzyme in vitro becomes largely inactivated at gastric pH, its activity is protected by food.[28,29] In fact, infants less than 6 months of age typically have low concentration of pancreatic-derived α-amylase activity and a concomitant inability to completely hydrolyze amylopectin following a test meal containing this starch (Figure 4).[30–32] Infants can digest various cooked starches in limited quantities: up to 10 g/d at 1 month of age and 23 g/d at 3 months of age. By the end of the first year of life, infants have adequate concentrations of α-amylase activity in their duodenal fluid, and their capacity for digestion of a test meal of starch is comparable to that of adults. In adults, the pancreas secretes α-amylase in excess of the normal requirements for hydrolysis (ie, capacity exceeds load), and by the time intestinal contents reach the distal

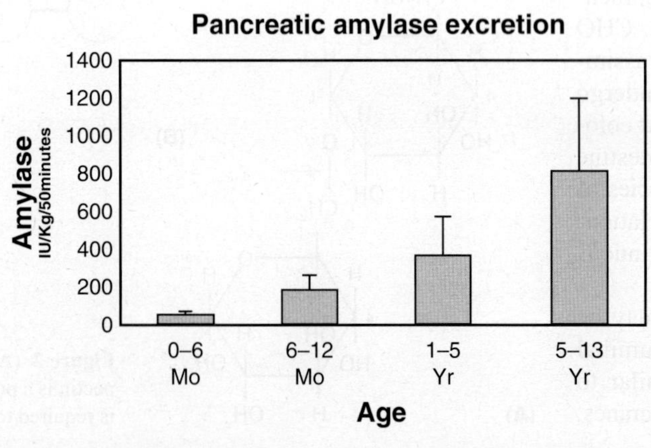

Figure 4 Pancreozymin-secretin test in 30 children without pancreatic disease. Output of pancreatic amylase in different age groups is expressed in international units (IU) per kilogram per 50 minutes. Note the age-dependent increase in pancreatic excretory output. (Adapted from reference 31.)

duodenum, hydrolysis is essentially complete.[33] Even patients with pancreatic insufficiency and secondary steatorrhea are usually able to digest starch adequately despite decreased levels of pancreatic α-amylase.

The form of starch consumed greatly influences the degree to which it is digested. As much as 10 to 20% of the CHOs in bread composed of whole-wheat flour may pass unabsorbed in the small intestine, whereas the starch from low-gluten wheat or rice bread appears to be completely digested and absorbed.[34,35] Whole-wheat flour consists of granules of starch surrounded by a protein shell, or husk, and this layering effect may interfere with digestion.

Table 1 Principal Enzymes of Carbohydrate Digestion in Humans and Their Common Substrates

Enzyme	Substrate
α-Amylase	Starch (interior α-1, 4 links)
Oligosaccharidases Sucrase-isomaltase	Sucrose Maltose Maltotriose α-Limit dextrins
Maltase-glucoamylase	Short glucose polymers with α-1, 4 links; activity greatest for linear polymers. Starch (interior α-1, 4 links)
Lactase	Lactose

Oligosaccharides

Oligosaccharides are generally composed of 3 to 20 monosaccharides and are normally the products of starch and glycogen digestion, since they are not commonly found naturally. Hydrolysis of the oligosaccharides occurs at the luminal surface of the small bowel and is catalyzed by a group of oligosaccharidases (ie, disaccharidases) which reside on the exterior surface of the brush border (containing the microvillus membrane) of the surface epithelium. These glycoproteins are composed of a hydrophobic region which serves as an anchor in the lipid-rich brush border membrane and a hydrophilic region which extends into the small bowel lumen and contains the active site.[36]

The oligosaccharidases are classified into α -glucosidases (ie, sucrase-isomaltase and maltase-glucoamylase) and a β-galactosidase (ie, lactase), depending on the type of linkage that they split (Figure 3). As shown in Table 1, a number of the oligosaccharidases have the ability to cleave more than one substrate. The α-limit dextrins that result from amylose and amylopectin hydrolysis are digested by α-glucosidases.[37] Glucose monomers are removed in sequence from the nonreducing end of the oligosaccharide by cleavage of the α-1,4 links. Isomaltase appears to be most active when four or more glucose residues remain; sucrase is most active for three or less glucose residues (ie, maltotriose and maltose). Only isomaltase is capable of splitting the α-1,6 branches. Glucoamylase is especially active with straight-chain glucose polymers with about six glucose units.[38]

Oligosaccharidase synthesis occurs along the crypt-villus axis. The surface of the small bowel is covered by a continuous sheet of epithelium consisting of different cell types that are derived from a common intestinal progenitor cell.[39] The epithelium proliferates in the crypts and migrates up the villus to the tip over a period of 3 to 5 days. During this migration, enterocytes mature both morphologically and functionally and synthesize digestive enzymes and signaling proteins. Immature enterocytes within the crypt do not express digestive enzymes and a gradual increase in oligosaccharidase activity along the villus-crypt axis is observed, with maximal activity in the mid-villus. Activity also varies along the length of the small intestine, with maximal levels in the proximal jejunum and minimal levels in the proximal duodenum and terminal ileum.[40] Data from mRNA studies in rats document the developmental changes along the crypt-villus axis for both sucrase and lactase activities.[41–43] In both rodents and humans, sucrase-isomaltase and lactase mRNAs appear to be minimal in crypt epithelial cells and most prominent in the lower to mid-villus enterocytes.[44–46]

The half life of the oligosaccharidases in vivo is in the range of 4 to 16 hours. Since migration of the enterocyte up to the villus tip occurs over several days, there must be continued synthesis and degradation of these enzymes. Pancreatic proteases and bile acids play a role in the degradation of these enzymes.[47–48] In laboratory animals, removal of pancreatic enzymes or bile from the intestinal lumen resulted in increased level of activity of the oligosaccharidases, accompanied by a decreased enzyme turnover.[47–49] Moreover, treatment of pancreatic insufficiency with enzyme replacement returns oligosaccharidase activity to normal.[50]

Disaccharides

Lactase-Phlorizin Hydrolase. The disaccharide lactose is composed of glucose and galactose monosaccharides and is hydrolyzed by lactase-phlorizin hydrolase (LPH; E.C. 3.2.1.108) at the β-1,4-glycosidic linkage. LPH is a large 1972-amino acid protein whose short hydrophobic carboxyl-terminus spans the brush border membrane once, and the majority of the protein, including the catalytic domain, is situated luminally (Figure 5). Details of the synthesis and processing of the polypeptide as it proceeds from the endoplasmic reticulum to its final destination as an active hydrolase on the apical membrane have been thoroughly studied.[51] The precursor molecule is *N*- and *O*-glycosylated and eventually proteolytically cleaved at two locations, yielding a mature 145 kDa LPH enzyme protein with two distinct enzymatic sites for lactase and phlorizin hydrolysis.[52]

The oligosaccharidases, with the exception of lactase, have the capacity to hydrolyze faster than the rate at which the resultant monosaccharide products can be absorbed.[53,54] Therefore, monosaccharide absorption, rather than oligosaccharide digestion, is the rate-limiting step for assimilation of these sugars. Lactase is unique in that it splits lactose at a lower rate than that of the mucosal uptake of the glucose and galactose products, thus lactase activity is the rate-limiting step of lactose assimilation rather than absorption.[53]

LPH is produced almost exclusively in the small intestine, where it has a distinct pattern

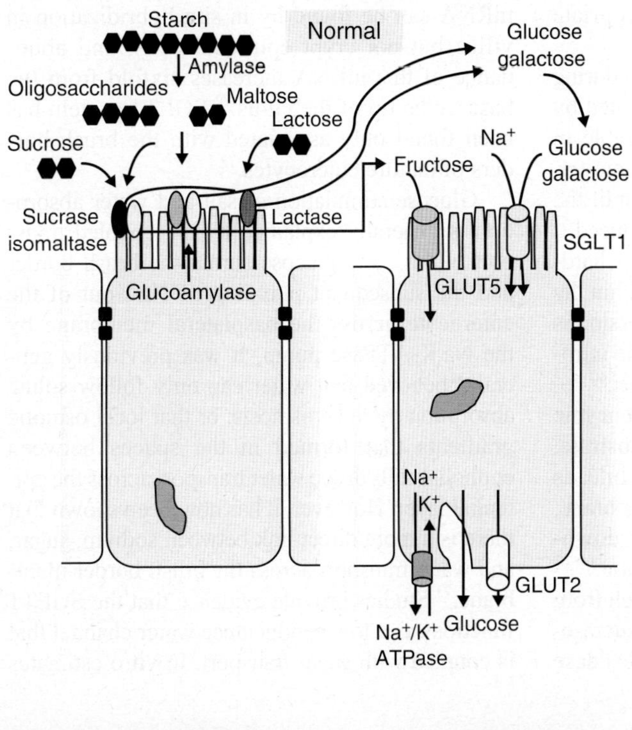

Figure 5 Normal assimilation of carbohydrates in the intestine.

of expression along the proximo-distal axis of the intestine. Mature protein is localized to enterocytes, and is most abundant in the distal duodenum and jejunum.[55] The spatial and developmental pattern of LPH expression is regulated predominately at the level of transcription and appears to be orchestrated largely by a series of transcription factors that bind specific and well-defined elements located in the immediate promoter region of the human and rodent LPH. The factors include caudal-related homeodomain proteins (Cdx-2), hepatocyte nuclear factor 1 (HNF-1), and GATA-4/5/6 function collectively to direct expression along the gut.[56,57]

Sucrase-Isomaltase Hydrolase. Sucrase-isomaltase (SI; EC 3.2.1.48/10) is a type II integral membrane glycoprotein that forms a noncovalent homodimer complex. The human isoform is an 1827-amino acid polypeptide that undergoes posttranslational glycosylation prior to sorting to the apical membrane where it is further processed by luminal proteases to sucrase and isomaltase (Figure 5). These functional subunits remain associated by hydrostatic interactions, with the isomaltase site hydrolyzing the α-1,4-glycosidic linkage of maltose and the α-1,6-glucose bonds of α-limit dextrins and isomaltose. In contrast, the sucrase site cleaves the α-1,4-glucose bonds of maltotriose and maltose and the identical linkage of sucrose into glucose and fructose. Redundant hydrolysis of the α-1,4-glucose linkage is provided by maltase-glucoamylase; however, 80% of the intestinal maltase activity is provided by the sucrase-isomaltase.

Wide-ranging studies done primarily in rodents have defined the transcriptional basis of SI's spatial, developmental, and dietary regulation.[58] The 5′-flanking region of the *SI* gene contains many functional *cis*-acting DNA elements that are sufficient to drive SI expression in the appropriate tissue and developmental-specific manner. The transcriptional factors that bind to the immediate promoter region of the SI gene include HNF-1, Cdx2, and GATA-4 which work in a combinatory manner to drive appropriate expression.[59]

Sucrase-isomaltase expression changes during development and, unlike lactase, is modulated by diet. In humans, SI expression is measurable in the small bowel by the end of the first trimester, while it remains undetectable in rodents until the time of weaning when it is dramatically induced.[58] This developmental pattern of expression is hard-wired and is controlled by *cis*-elements within the 5′-flanking region of the *SI* gene. SI expression is also induced by both corticosteroids and the introduction of either sucrose or starch to the diet.[60]

Many factors are known to influence enzyme activity, including the presence of substrate, hydrolytic products, pancreatic enzymes, bile, as well as damage to the brush border membrane. The α-glucosidases are able to up- or down-regulate in response to luminal stimulation.[61–63] In fact, the elimination of sucrose and starch from the diet is accompanied by conversion of sucrase-isomaltase to its inactive form.[64] β-Galactosidase (ie, lactase) is unable to up-regulate after weaning and in fact shows down-regulation despite maintenance of lactose in the diet, the cause of widespread lactose intolerance for most individuals (more below).

Monosaccharides

Most of the monosaccharides that are present in the intestinal lumen result from hydrolysis of dietary starch and oligosaccharides. Monosaccharides released at the brush border by the oligosaccharidases can either be absorbed directly or can diffuse back into the lumen of the intestine to be absorbed at another site. Because of the size and hydrophilic nature of the monosaccharides, they are not able to move across the brush border membrane by diffusion. Glucose and galactose are absorbed by the same carrier-mediated active process, whereas fructose moves across the brush border membrane by facilitated transport in association with a different carrier[65–67] (Figure 5).

Na^+/glucose cotransporter (SGLT1). Evidence from in vitro studies has clearly demonstrated that Na^+-coupled active transport is the primary mechanism for absorption of glucose and galactose[65,66] In the human intestine, about 95% of the dietary glucose ingested by an adult is absorbed by carrier-mediated transport.[68] Transport of each sugar is saturable, and competitive inhibition suggests that both sugars are transported by the same membrane carrier.

The Na^+/glucose cotransporter (SGLT1), a transmembrane protein, is responsible for active transport across the brush border membrane.[69,70] Glucose absorption by enterocytes occurs in two steps. First, glucose binds to the extracellular domain of SGLT1 in the presence of Na^+; this interaction causes a conformational change in this transmembrane protein, moving glucose into the cell.[70] Second, glucose moves out of the enterocyte by facilitated diffusion across the basolateral membrane in association with the transporter GLUT2.[71] In studies in rabbit intestine, SGLT1 mRNA can be found by in situ hybridization in villus but not crypt epithelial cells, and abundance of this mRNA increases sixfold from the base to the tip of the villus.[72] SGLT1 protein has been found only associated with the brush borders of mature enterocytes.[72]

Glucose stimulation of salt and water absorption is generally explained by the coupled transport of Na^+ and glucose across the brush border and the subsequent pumping of Na^+ out of the enterocyte across the basolateral membrane by the Na,K-ATPase pump. It was previously generally believed that water can only follow solute absorption by local osmosis; or that local osmotic gradients that formed in the spaces between epithelial cells drove water transport across the epithelial layer. However, it has now been shown that there is a more direct link between sodium, sugar, and water transport across the brush border membrane.[73] Studies provide evidence that the SGLT1 functions as a low conductance water channel that is coupled with sugar transport. In vitro estimates of water transport suggest that one-third of the transport occurred via Na^+-glucose cotransport, while the remaining occurred by local osmosis. This link between salt, sugar, and water absorption provides the rationale for the use of oral rehydration therapy in patients with various forms of acute diarrhea including those of infectious origin.[74] See Chapter 57, "Diarrheal Diseases," for more details on oral rehydration solutions.

Although glucose is absorbed down a concentration gradient during meals, absorption continues as intraluminal glucose concentrations drop below tissue levels. Sodium concentration gradients appear to be the driving force for this transport system. The basolateral membrane transporter GLUT2 maintains a low intracellular concentration. Therefore, while glucose movement is against a concentration gradient, it is coupled to Na^+ movement down an electrochemical gradient. In studies in which Na^+ had been removed from a solution bathing the intestine, in vivo or in vitro, glucose transport was reduced or eliminated.[75,76]

Facilitated Fructose Transporter (GLUT5). Fructose absorption occurs by facilitated diffusion (ie, carrier-mediated but not active transport). Fructose assimilation occurs at the brush border in association with a high affinity transporter GLUT5.[77] Fructose then crosses the basolateral membrane associated with the carrier GLUT2 (Figure 5). Expression of both transporters is increased by the presence of fructose. Recent studies have identified GLUT7 as a high affinity glucose and fructose carrier on the brush border membrane of enterocytes located in the distal intestine.[78] New studies are also emerging in rats implying that brush border GLUT2 plays a major role in the absorption of fructose.[79] The capacity of the small intestine to absorb fructose in humans is limited and can be surpassed in some individuals during ingestion of a diet rich in fructose.[80] Excess fructose in the diet of infants, in addition to sorbitol, can be a factor in the development of toddler's diarrhea.[81]

Current data suggest that fructose absorption in the small intestine occurs via GLUT5, since it has a much higher K_m (and thereby higher capacity) for fructose than GLUT7.[82,83] Fructose absorption is independent of glucose absorption and remains intact in patients with glucose-galactose malabsorption (GGM), for example. Studies performed primarily in rodents have confirmed that GLUT5 expression is regulated in a tissue- and development-specific manner and is induced by dietary fructose.[84] Specifically, GLUT5 mRNA and protein levels are found at very low levels prior to weaning and increase dramatically in the proximal small intestine in weaned animals. An analysis of the age dependence of GLUT5 levels in human intestine has not been performed; however, fructose malabsorption as determined by the breath hydrogen test is certainly more common during early infancy when compared to adults.[85] Likewise, whether or not the fructose malabsorption that is so common in toddler's diarrhea is secondary to insufficient GLUT5 expression has yet to be formally established.

CONSEQUENCES OF CARBOHYDRATE MALABSORPTION

The physiologic consequences of CHO malabsorption are similar for all CHOs, and the range of symptoms and the nutritional effects of CHO malabsorption have been well characterized. The complete symptom complex of CHO malabsorption can include nausea, crampy abdominal pain, intestinal gas, bloating, abdominal distention, and watery diarrhea. However, not all of these symptoms need occur in every individual with CHO intolerance. Patients may have abdominal pain with little or no diarrhea. Likewise, diarrhea may be present without other symptoms. Because a delay in the onset of symptoms after CHO ingestion can occur, the association may not be obvious.

The net capacity of the small bowel for CHO absorption is influenced by several variables: (1) the functional capacity of the bowel mucosa for each of the steps (hydrolysis and absorption) of CHO assimilation, (2) the amount of small bowel surface area available (influenced by bowel resection or mucosal damage), and (3) the rate of transit of luminal contents through the intestine. In the past, the small intestine was thought to be the only region of the gastrointestinal tract in which CHOs could be absorbed. However, more recent data indicate that the colon is not only capable of conserving malabsorbed CHOs but is also dependent on it for its own nourishment.[86–88]

Chronic diarrhea is the most common clinical symptom of disorders that are secondary to abnormalities of nutrient assimilation.[89] Categorizing the type of diarrhea into either malabsorptive or secretory is a useful initial step in the evaluation of any patient with chronic diarrhea. Classifying the type of diarrhea may be done with either a trial of fasting or by analysis of stool electrolytes while on a complete diet. To compute the stool osmotic gap, either cations such as Na^+ and K^+ or anions such as Cl^- and HCO_3^- may be measured in liquid fecal samples.[90,91] If the sum of twice the value of cations (or anions) is lower (< 50 mOsm) than the obligatory fecal osmolality of 290 mOsm, an osmotic gap provided by the ingested osmotically active nutrient or a nonmeasured ion (eg, Mg^{+2}) likely accounts for the gap. SCFA, osmotic anions that are products of fermented CHO formed by the intestinal microflora, may contribute to the final osmotic load if insufficiently absorbed by colonocytes. In contrast, a low osmotic gap (<50 mOsm) is seen in secretory diarrheas, which are generally large volume (2 to 3 L) and fail to subside with fasting.

The surface of the gastrointestinal tract provides a hydrophobic barrier to the passive diffusion of CHOs. Therefore, if any step in the assimilation of CHO is blocked, CHO remain in the luminal contents and pass distally. The stomach and proximal small bowel are permeable to water and electrolytes; therefore, nonabsorbed CHO in the lumen of the gastrointestinal tract is diluted with water and electrolytes that have moved across the mucosa to maintain isotonicity. It has been shown that normal subjects absorbed 92 to 100% of a 12.5 g lactose load in the small bowel while subjects with lactase deficiency absorbed only 22 to 60% of the load. This estimate was derived by collecting ileal contents after ingestion of a mixture of ^{14}C-labeled lactose and a nonabsorbable marker.[76]

When normal individuals were challenged with a mixture of lactose and a nonabsorbable marker, polyethylene glycol (PEG), dilution of PEG occurs in the duodenum, and progressive concentration of PEG is found in aspirates from the distal small bowel.[92] The increased concentration of PEG represents a decrease in intraluminal volumes resulting from net fluid absorption, since PEG does not cross the small bowel surface. For lactose-intolerant individuals, dilution of the lactose solution occurs in the duodenum as well; however, the concentration of PEG remains low throughout the distal small bowel, suggesting a lack of subsequent reabsorption of intraluminal water. Although net absorption of fluid does occur in the colon in these subjects, it is at a decreased rate. Furthermore, increased transit through the small bowel has been found to occur when CHO is incompletely absorbed.[93] The net secretion of fluid and electrolyte in the small bowel, decreased reabsorption in the colon, and possibly the rapid transit through the small bowel all contribute to the production of a watery diarrhea rich in electrolyte. This has been called an osmotic diarrhea since the diarrhea results from the presence of a poorly absorbed osmotically active solute in the intestinal lumen.[90] These diarrheas are characterized by (1) the fact that they stop when the solute is removed from the diet, and (2) a stool osmolality that is at least 50 mOsm greater than twice the sum of stool sodium and potassium concentrations (ie, there is another osmotically active solute present in addition to electrolyte).[90–93]

Unabsorbed CHO reaching the colon is fermented by bacteria, which produce SCFAs, CO_2, hydrogen, and methane. This process increases the osmolality of the colonic contents and stool by splitting CHO into smaller units. Gas production and the increased fluid volumes in the intestine probably cause abdominal cramps by distention and altered motility. It is estimated that 1 g of malabsorbed CHO (including the resultant short-chain fatty acids) results in an increase in stool weight of about 30 to 35 g.[94,95]

Much of the CHO malabsorbed in the small bowel may be conserved in the colon. In patients with lactose intolerance, a greater amount of ^{14}C from radiolabeled lactose is recovered in ileal aspirates than in the stool.[76] Germ-free animal studies have demonstrated that CHOs are not absorbed intact in the colon; however, SCFAs (including acetic, propionic, and butyric acids) are rapidly absorbed by colonocytes.[77,96] Absorption of ^{14}C-labeled sucrose has been compared in healthy subjects and patients with jejunoileal bypass.[75] The bypass patients were unable to absorb up to 84% of a 50 g dose of ^{14}C sucrose. For most of these patients, more than 60% of the ^{14}C that passed through the ileum unabsorbed was fermented and absorbed in the colon. Normal individuals absorbed 95 to 98% of the sucrose load in the small bowel, and less than 1% of the ^{14}C was recovered in the stool. These studies suggest that in clinical situations in which there is malabsorption of CHO, a large proportion of the CHO can be salvaged by colonic fermentation and conversion to SCFA which are then absorbed. Of the ^{14}C that remained in the feces, a major portion was nondialyzable (either incorporated into macromolecules or bound to nondialyzable components of the feces) and was, therefore, neither available for absorption nor osmotically active. It has been calculated that up to 540 kcal/d in the form of SCFA may be absorbed in the colon of an adult.[96] In the normal subjects, the amount of sucrose reaching the terminal ileum was only a small part of the total dose, but was great enough to cause an osmotic diarrhea if not removed in the colon. Variability of the factors influencing this mechanism of colonic conservation of CHO (ie, changes in colonic flora) may explain, in part, the wide range of symptoms that can occur with similar degrees of CHO malabsorption. Variability of other gastrointestinal disorders, such as irritable bowel, chronic constipation, and antibiotic-related diarrhea, may have a similar basis.

The influence of lactose malabsorption on the absorption of other nutrients has been controversial. Studies are inconclusive as to whether lactose intolerance does or does not lead to malabsorption of protein and fat; however, lactose malabsorption is associated with increased recovery of calcium, magnesium, and phosphate from the ileum.

TESTS OF CARBOHYDRATE INTOLERANCE

Carbohydrates unabsorbed in the small intestine can either be metabolized by colonic bacteria into SCFAs and gas, or be excreted as feces. When the CHO load dramatically exceeds the capacity of assimilation, the microbiota serve as a salvaging unit with a limited capacity to metabolize CHO. At limited quantities, fermentation results in SCFAs that are absorbed by colonocytes that use them as unique energy source, thereby limiting the osmotic load of the feces and subsequent diarrhea. At excessive quantities, CHOs exit unfermented; excessive production of SCFAs may also exceed absorptive capacity of colonocytes and provide additional osmoles and acidify the stools. As discussed earlier, unabsorbed CHOs and organic acids can lead to an osmotic diarrhea by increasing the solute load in the colon, with water following passively. Fecal excretion of CHOs and monosaccharides in normal subjects under control conditions is only about 3 g/d or about 1% of all ingested CHOs. Depending on the consumption of dietary fiber, about 10% of CHO intake may initially reach the colon under normal physiologic conditions. Thus, the human colon and its bacterial flora are very efficient in salvaging unabsorbed CHOs. Even under conditions of an osmotic diarrhea (eg, intake of polyethylene glycol or sodium sulfate), fecal excretion of CHOs rises only slightly despite a marked increase in fecal water output. In fact, up to 45 g of undigested CHOs can reach the colon daily before fecal excretion of CHOs or organic acids will exceed the normal 3 g/d.

Tests of CHO intolerance have not achieved overwhelming innovation in the past few years. Moreover, none of the current tests available correlates perfectly with clinical symptoms. Most of the tests evaluate bowel function by confirming CHO absorption or recording malabsorption; disaccharidase assays measure mucosal enzyme activity directly but do not measure absorption. Clinical suspicion of CHO intolerance should arise if the introduction of a particular CHO into the diet results in diarrhea, bloating, and/or abdominal pain. A typical example would be diarrhea that starts when sucrose-containing solids (eg, fruits) are introduced into the diet of an infant with congenital sucrase-isomaltase deficiency. Likewise, the resolution of diarrhea with the removal of a CHO from the diet should be a clue to the diagnosis. For example, diarrhea following viral gastroenteritis may be due to transient lactase deficiency which will resolve when lactose is removed from the diet. Routine lactose restriction is unnecessary, however, during most episodes of acute diarrhea.

Screening Tests

Screening tests for CHO malabsorption include evaluation of stool-reducing substances and pH, as well as measurement of stool osmolality and electrolyte concentration.[97]

Examination of stool for reducing sugars is a simple bedside test that is semiquantitative. The test is done using Clinitest tablets (Benedict's reagent), and the method is similar to that for measuring glucose in the urine. Clinitest was originally introduced by Bayer in 1941, under the name Miles Laboratories. The reagent is copper sulfate ($CuSO_4$) which reacts with reducing substances (containing an aldehyde group) to convert to cuprous oxide (Cu_2O). An aldehyde group (CHO) is oxidized to carboxylic acid (COOH) and Cu^{2+} is reduced to Cu^{+}. The result is a color change, from blue to green to yellow to orange-red, depending on the amount of reaction present (ie, the amount of reducing substances). All of the hexose monosaccharides (ie, fructose, glucose, galactose), certain pentoses (eg, xylose), and disaccharides (eg, lactose) contain an aldehyde group when in noncyclic form and are therefore reducing substances. Sucrose (a disaccharide), starch, and cellulose do not contain an aldehyde group and are, therefore, not reducing and will result in a false-negative Clinitest. Nonreducing substances can be converted to reducing sugars via boiling in calcium chloride and hydrochloric acid.

Neonates normally maldigest to some degree and will have some detectable lactose in the stool; therefore, a weakly positive Clinitest reaction in this group is not abnormal. False-positive tests can result from consuming large quantities of ascorbic acid, nalidixic acid (quinolone antibiotics), and cephalosporins. A purple Clinitest reaction has been reported in an infant with phenolphthalein-induced factitious diarrhea.[98] If the quantity of CHO that reaches the colon is completely metabolized by fermentation, then the diarrhea is likely to be mainly secondary to the osmotic effect of organic acids, and associated cations and the Clinitest may be falsely negative. But as the amount of malabsorbed CHO increases, unmetabolized substrates make a larger contribution to the diarrhea and the Clinitest will be positive.[99]

Stool pH is also a good sign of CHO malabsorption. The fermentation products of organic acids (ie, short-chain fatty acids) lower the stool pH, and a fecal pH <5.3 has been shown to be a reliable indicator of CHO malabsorption.[90–100] A low pH may be noted at times despite a negative Clinitest, indicating the presence of organic acids but no reducing substances.

Comparing the predicted (stool is always isoosmolar) or measured fecal osmolality with the contribution of the main ions (ie, twice the concentrations of sodium and potassium) distinguishes between an osmotic diarrhea versus a secretory one. Stool osmolality greater than twice the sum of the sodium and potassium concentration in the stool (accounting for the respective anions) implies an osmotic diarrhea. Malabsorbed CHOs and osmotic cathartics are the most common reasons for an osmotic diarrhea.

Starch maldigestion and excretion rarely a clinical problem, usually seen only in the setting of severe pancreatic insufficiency. No routine clinical studies specifically identify this disorder, but Lugol solution (iodine potassium-iodide, IKI) can be used as an indicator for the presence of starches. The solution reacts by turning dark blue/black, a result of the interaction of IKI with the coil structure of the polysaccharide; IKI solution does not detect simple sugars. Starch maldigestion can also be assessed by measuring duodenal amylase activity using the secretin-pancreozymin test, which involves collection and analysis of duodenal fluid after an intravenous injection of secretin and pancreozymin.[31–32] However, this test has been correlated with exocrine pancreatic function including amylase secretion, but not CHO malabsorption.

Carbohydrate Tolerance Tests

Carbohydrate tolerance tests are readily available and easy to perform; in the past, they were widely done as a simple test for CHO absorption. Following the ingestion of a CHO, the patient is evaluated for a rise in blood sugar which, when present, suggests that absorption has occurred. Symptoms that develop during the test can also be correlated with the results. The advantages of such a test include its simplicity, lack of sophisticated equipment, relatively noninvasive character, and potential correlation with symptoms. The disadvantages include a high rate of both false-positive and false-negative studies, and the necessity to draw repeated blood specimens. Factors other than an individual's capacity for CHO assimilation may alter the blood sugar level, including the rate of gastric emptying, hormonal influence on blood glucose, and the rate of peripheral metabolism of glucose. Delayed gastric emptying has been a common cause of false-positive results in children. This problem can be circumvented by administering the CHO directly into the duodenum using a nasoduodenal tube; however, this method increases the complexity and reliability of the test.

Tolerance tests have been used most commonly to study the absorption of glucose, xylose, lactose, and sucrose; however, none of these tests has been standardized. The quantity of sugar administered can vary from 0.5 to 2 g/kg (maximum 25 to 50 g), usually given in a 10% aqueous solution. The timing for collection of blood samples varies from 0, 15, 30, 45, 60, 90, and 120 minutes to a single sample 45 to 60 minutes after ingestion. Generally, a rise above baseline in blood sugar of 20 mg/dL is interpreted to represent significant absorption.

D-xylose, a pentose that is not metabolized, has been used to assess the glucose-galactose carrier system (ie, SGLT1). However, in humans D-xylose is poorly absorbed (Km ~100 mM), compared to that of D-glucose (0.5 mM). Xylose is given as 0.5 g/kg, and fasting and 1 hour blood samples are collected for measurement of blood xylose concentration levels. A 5-hour urine sample can be collected and analyzed to determine the percentage of the xylose that is excreted. There are studies that both support and question the usefulness of xylose absorption as a screening test for mucosal damage.[101–104]

Disaccharide tolerance tests have been useful in screening for lactase and sucrase deficiencies. However, the breath hydrogen test, which is described below, is simpler and more accurate and has largely replaced the use of tolerance tests. Since glucose is released on hydrolysis of both lactose and sucrose, absorption should lead to an elevation of blood glucose. In one study of the standard lactose tolerance test performed in adults with normal lactase activity (demonstrated by small bowel biopsy), 28% of the subjects had a maximal rise of blood glucose of less than 20 mg/dL.[105] When the administration of 50 or 100 g of lactose was compared, there was no difference in the percentage of individuals with normal curves. In 50% of the individuals, the blood glucose value had peaked at 15 minutes.

Some investigators have felt that the reliability of tolerance tests can be increased by the use of capillary samples rather than venous blood.[106] In another test, the ingestion of ethanol with lactose inhibits the conversion of galactose to glucose, and the blood galactose level is measured. This test is rarely performed now.

Disaccharidase Assay

Quantitation of oligosaccharidase activity in the mucosa of the small intestine has been the standard against which other tests of disaccharide intolerance have been measured.[107] Tissue from the distal duodenum or proximal jejunum is obtained for study by endoscopic biopsy. If the tissue is immediately frozen, these enzymes will remain stable for months. Assays are done by homogenizing the tissue in buffer, incubating the homogenate with the appropriate substrate (usually a disaccharide) at 37°C, and measuring the quantity of glucose released during a given period of time.[108] Although disaccharidase assays are generally performed in this manner, there are minor variations among laboratories, including the type of buffer used and the pH at which the incubation is done. Therefore, mean values and ranges may vary somewhat from one laboratory to another for any specific substrate studied. The enzyme activities most commonly assayed are sucrase, lactase, and maltase, each incubated with the respective substrate. Measurement of isomaltase activity uses the substrate palatinose since highly purified isomaltose is not readily available. Activity is usually expressed as milligram of mucosal protein per gram of mucosal wet weight (ie, specific activity). Inappropriate handling or storage of tissue samples either by delayed freezing, or freeze thawing, will result in false-negative enzyme activity. Suspicion of the quality of the results should be raised by a broad decline (ie, multiple enzymes) in activity in the presence of normal histological tissue.

Disaccharidase activity can be easily quantified in this manner; however, activity levels do not always correlate well with symptoms.[109] Moreover, the small bowel biopsy is only a small sample and may not be representative of the total oligosaccharidase activity in the bowel. This problem may occur with a disorder that causes patchy damage to the bowel (eg, Crohn's disease) or with small bowel rejection following intestinal transplantation.

Breath Testing

The breath hydrogen test remains the most widely used method of analysis of CHO intolerance.[110] CHOs malabsorbed in the small bowel are fermented by bacteria in the colon, releasing hydrogen, carbon dioxide, and methane gasses. A large proportion of these gasses are absorbed and subsequently expired in the breath (about 15 to 20% of the hydrogen).[109,111] Although the original technique for measuring expired hydrogen involved a continuous, closed, rebreathing system for collection, sampling is now usually done at 30-minute intervals over 2 to 4 hours. A rise in breath hydrogen content of more than 10 to 20 parts per million (ppm) over the fasting value (measured by gas chromatography) is considered consistent with CHO malabsorption; a threshold of 10 ppm (over two consecutive periods) is associated with greater sensitivity but lower specificity as compared to 20 ppm. For infants and children, identification of either lactose or sucrose intolerance is done by collecting three samples at 30-minute intervals after ingestion of 1 to 2 g/kg (up to 25 g) of the sugar of interest.[110,112,113]

The measurement of breath hydrogen content has gained validity as an indirect, semiquantitative test of CHO malabsorption. It offers the advantages of being simple, noninvasive, and sensitive. The method for collection of breath samples has been adapted for infants and children, and samples may be collected in the field and stored for later analysis.[112]

Breath methane concentrations can be used to enhance the reliability of the test, although methane production is low before 3 years of age, and individuals who produce methane and not hydrogen gas are rare. Additionally, for lactose malabsorption, the sensitivity and specificity of breath methane testing have been shown to be lower than for breath hydrogen testing.[114]

Bond and Levitt demonstrated excellent correlation of breath hydrogen content with lactose malabsorption by studying lactose-tolerant and intolerant adults who had ingested 12.5 g of radiolabeled lactose.[87] Lactose malabsorption was determined by measuring radiolabeled lactose concentration in aspirates from a per-oral tube placed in the distal ileum and compared to breath samples collected simultaneously and analyzed for hydrogen content. For each subject, breath hydrogen was also analyzed after the ingestion of the unabsorbable CHO, lactulose. By comparing the two tests, it was shown to be possible to quantify the amount of CHO malabsorbed by an individual through measurement of the hydrogen excreted in the breath.

Breath hydrogen testing can be used to identify isolated lactose or sucrose intolerance, small bowel mucosal damage, decreased surface area, and bacterial overgrowth. However, potential problems in interpretation of the test do exist. As with all of the other tests for CHO intolerance, a positive study does not always correlate well with symptoms. Since breath hydrogen analysis is a more sensitive measure of CHO intolerance than many of the previously available tests, it is likely that identification of subclinical CHO malabsorption will occur more frequently. Conversely, about 10% of the population lack the bacterial flora necessary to produce hydrogen gas in the colon and can therefore have a negative test despite CHO malabsorption.[110] The use of antibiotics shortly before the test may alter the intestinal flora and influence colonic fermentation, reducing the amount of hydrogen produced. If the ability of an individual to produce hydrogen gas is in question, lactulose ingestion can be used as a control, as it normally leads to detectable hydrogen production. Diarrhea or abnormally rapid transit may affect results as well. Interestingly, breath hydrogen concentrations may rise during certain activities, such as sleep and cigarette smoking, and a lower rate of hydrogen production has been demonstrated when lactose was given in whole milk rather than in an aqueous solution.[110] Finally, breath testing of patients with an ileostomy has not been standardized and may be of limited value.

PRIMARY DISORDERS OF CARBOHYDRATE ASSIMILATION

Disturbances of CHO assimilation may be secondary to defective enzymatic processing of complex sugars and disaccharides or failure to transport monosaccharides across the apical membrane (Figure 6). As outlined earlier, CHO intolerance is characterized by diarrhea that subsides shortly after CHOs are reduced or eliminated from the diet. Therefore, abnormal CHO assimilation results in the presence of major osmotic forces in colonic luminal fluid derived from oligosaccharides, lactose, sucrose, or glucose. As reviewed earlier, unabsorbed CHOs are fermented by the resident colonic microflora to gas and volatile SCFA. A proportion of these

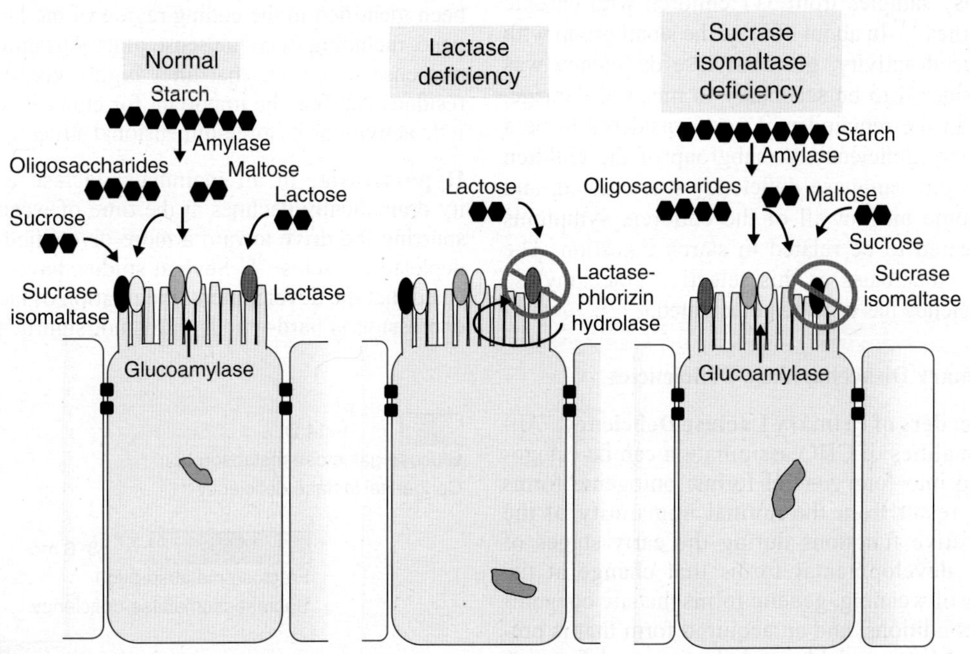

Figure 6 Disorders of disaccharidase deficiency.

SCFAs are absorbed across the colonic epithelium by poorly defined diffusion and transporter-mediated mechanisms.[115] The absorbed SCFAs are metabolized preferentially by colonic epithelia, where they are an important energy source and also facilitate the absorption of NaCl. Therefore, SCFA absorption leads to a reduction of luminal osmolality and thereby facilitates the colonic absorption of water. Nevertheless, diarrhea may result when the ileal effluent exceeds the salvaging capacity of the colon. Specifically, the passage of unabsorbed and unfermented CHOs and SCFA into the distal colon provides an additional osmotic load that results in the retention of water in the gut and subsequent diarrhea.

Starch Intolerance

Clinically apparent starch malabsorption is uncommon. Infants less than 6 months of age normally have very low levels of α-amylase activity in the duodenum and therefore do have the potential for starch malabsorption.[110] Although starch malabsorption is uncommon, there have been several descriptions of patients with chronic diarrhea that appears to have been secondary to starch intolerance.[116,117] Selective deficiency of α-amylase is likely an autosomal recessive disorder, and mutations in the amylase gene have yet to be identified. In a 1-month-old infant, starch provided 7% of the infant's dietary calories, and this proportion had increased to 16% by age 4 months. However, no α-amylase activity was found in a duodenal aspirate. Treatment by removal of starches from the diet resulted in improved stools, accelerated growth, and a drop in the intake from 300 to 120 kcal/kg/d. When the infant reached 1 year of age, the duodenal fluid contained low levels of α-amylase activity. At that time starches were reintroduced into the diet without incident.

Reduced glucoamylase activity has been identified in 3% of assays performed in small bowel biopsy samples from 511 children with chronic diarrhea.[107] In about 40% of the small group with reduced activity, glucoamylase deficiency was considered to be secondary to mucosal damage, and in the remainder, it was considered to be a primary deficiency. A subgroup of the children with glucoamylase deficiency was studied, and in some but not all of the children, symptoms appeared to be related to starch ingestion. The molecular basis of this selective glucoamylase deficiency has not been elucidated.

Primary Disaccharidase Deficiencies

Disorders of Primary Lactase Deficiency. Abnormalities of CHO assimilation can be categorized into four general forms: ontogenic forms that result from the normal immaturity of the digestive functions during the early stages of life, developmental forms that change at the time of weaning, genetic forms that are congenital conditions, and an acquired form that is preceded by a variable period of normal function (Figure 7).

Developmental or Neonatal Lactase Deficiency. Lactase, unlike the other commonly measured disaccharidases, develops to the level of activity seen in full-term newborns late in the third trimester of gestation[21]. Lactase deficiency and lactose intolerance have been described in premature infants less than 34 weeks of gestation, as lactase is the final disaccharidase to develop in premature infants. Therefore, it is thought that premature infants commonly have low levels of lactase activity proportionate to their degree of immaturity. MacLean and Fink evaluated a group of 22 healthy infants, ranging from 29 to 38 weeks of gestational age, who received a commercial infant formula containing lactose[118]. Serial measurements of breath hydrogen excretion were made, and hydrogen excretion increased during the first 3 weeks of life consistent with the diagnosis of lactose intolerance. This study suggests that most premature infants probably do malabsorb lactose.

While it is generally believed that the lactose intolerance seen in premature infants is rarely symptomatic, the addition of lactase to formula in this population was shown in a prospective randomized study to result in improved weight gain.[119] Similarly, a low lactose-containing diet has been shown to improve feeding tolerance including weight gain and caloric intake in premature infants.[120]

Congenital Lactase Deficiency. The rarest form of lactose intolerance is the autosomal recessive congenital form (MIM #223000) that presents during the immediate postnatal period as severe watery diarrhea while on a lactose-containing diet[121,122] (Figure 7). This form can be distinguished clinically as a selective lactase deficiency as symptoms subside on a non–lactose-containing diet. The diagnosis of the congenital form requires severely reduced or absent small bowel lactase activity in the newborn period in association with normal mucosal histology and normal levels of the other disaccharidases (Figure 6). Recently, five distinct mutations have been identified in the coding region of the lactase gene, including three nonsense mutations and two missense mutations that alter highly conserved residues that may be important for either its catalytic activity or its three-dimensional structure.[123]

Hypolactasia. In all mammals, lactase activity dramatically declines at the time of weaning, spurring the drive toward a more diversified diet depleted of lactose.[124] Several studies have indicated that the developmental regulation of lactase expression is hard-wired, and is not significantly modified by exposure to lactose-containing dietary load.[125] Hypolactasia (MIM #223100), or lactase nonpersistence, results from this hard-wired developmental decline of LPH activity that occurs in the majority of humans at a prevalence that varies based on race and ethnicity[121–122] (Figure 7).

Clinical Background. The decline in lactase levels seen in hypolactasia is nearly 90% as early as 3 years of age in children from Thailand and Bangladesh, and by 10 years of age for others of Asian, African, and Latin descent.[126] Lactose intolerance is common among adult Semitics, Asians, Africans, Eskimos, and American Indians, occurring in up to 80 to 90% of unmixed populations.[127,128] However, it is rare in Northern Europeans as well as in several tribes from Africa and India, occurring in only 10 to 20% of unmixed populations. In the United States, up to 70% of African descent but less than 20% of Caucasian have been found to be lactose intolerant.[127] Many of these studies suggest that lactose intolerance is inherited as an autosomal recessive manner.[129]

Despite the name "late-onset hypolactasia," the age of onset of this entity is quite variable among ethnic backgrounds, and it often occurs in early childhood. In Thailand, nearly all native adults have been lactose intolerant, and 85% of Thai children were found to be lactose intolerance by 2 years of age.[130] In an American Indian population where two-thirds of individuals were lactose intolerant, lactase deficiency was already present by 5 years of age.[128]

Hypolactasia, identified by the standard lactose tolerance test, has been found to develop in African-Americans between the age of 6 and the teenage years.[131] Other studies have suggested that the reduced lactase levels of late-onset lactose intolerance may develop by as early as 3 years of age in this population.[132] In contrast, abnormal lactase levels are not seen before 5 years of age in the Caucasian population.[132–133] As in African-Americans, the incidence of symptomatic late-onset lactose intolerance probably increases gradually into the teenage years. These findings have led to the observation that if evidence of lactose intolerance (by breath hydrogen) is found in African-Americans under 3 years of age or a Caucasian under 5 years of age, one should always consider the possibility that there has been damage to the intestinal mucosa.[134]

The identification of lactose intolerance by screening tests does not necessarily correlate

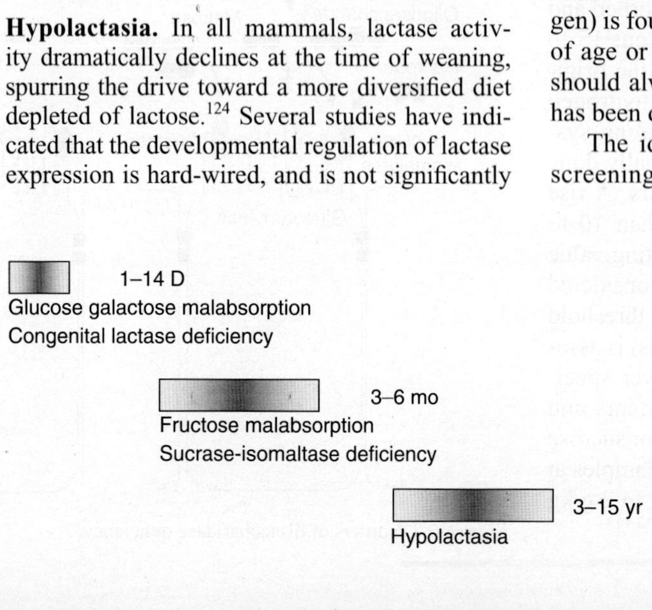

Figure 7 Carbohydrate assimilation: age at onset.

with the presence of symptoms and has resulted in confusion in the interpretation of these tests. Although the quantity of lactose that an individual ingests influences the degree of symptoms of lactose intolerance, the threshold for development of these symptoms varies among individuals. This observation may result from variation in the levels of residual lactase activity along the length of the bowel but is more likely to be related to factors that influence the colonic conservation of CHO. Among individuals with hypolactasia, symptomatic tolerance for lactose may range from the quantity present in one-half glass up to one quart or more of milk. An evaluation of the threshold for symptoms of lactose malabsorption among 20 adults with lactose intolerance (6 of whom were asymptomatic), found that 75% developed symptoms; including abdominal fullness, bloating, flatulence, or diarrhea, within 4 hours after ingesting 12 g or less of lactose.[135] This amount is equivalent to the quantity of lactose in one glass of milk. However, only about two-thirds of the subjects who developed these complaints had a previous history of symptomatic intolerance in association with the ingestion of one glass of milk. When lactose consumption exceeded the lactase capacity for an individual, symptoms became more severe with greater loads. Interestingly, the capacity, or threshold did not appear to correlate well with the jejunal lactase level. However, more recently, individuals who considered themselves to have severe lactose intolerance were able to tolerate as much lactose as in 8 ounce glass of milk daily without symptoms.[136] Lactose malabsorbed in those subjects that were lactose tolerant was up to 8% of a 12.5 g lactose load; whereas intolerant individuals malabsorbed 42 to 75% of the load in the small bowel.[87] Individuals who do become symptomatic with the ingestion of lactose should tolerate an equivalent amount of a glucose and galactose mixture without any problem.[127]

Studies of school children and hospitalized adults suggest that lactose-intolerant individuals as a group do tend to drink less milk than individuals who are lactose tolerant.[127] In fact, among individuals with lactase deficiency, symptomatic lactose intolerance is more common in adults than in children.[128] Likewise, when subjects were given 50 g of lactose (or 2 g/kg if this were lower), children were less likely to develop symptoms than adults at an equivalent quantity of lactose per kilogram of body weight. In a double-blind study of the symptoms associated with lactose intolerance among healthy teenagers, no statistical difference was found for the occurrence of symptoms noted by either group after drinking 8 ounces of either a lactose-containing or placebo drink.[137] After ingesting 16 ounces of the lactose drink, however, 16% of the intolerant subjects did have symptoms that seemed to be related to the lactose.

The extent to which late-onset lactose intolerance contributes to the etiology of recurrent abdominal pain of childhood (RAP) has been an area of great interest. RAP is probably the most common chronic symptom of childhood, occurring in more than 10% of school-age children.[138] In one study, nearly 40% of a group of 80 children with RAP studied prospectively were lactose malabsorbers, as defined by the breath hydrogen test.[113] However, among these lactose-intolerant children, it was not possible by history to associate symptoms with lactose ingestion. Although there was a trend toward more frequent symptoms following a lactose load among the lactose-intolerant individuals, two-thirds of the tolerant individuals complained of symptoms that could have been associated with lactose malabsorption as well. Of the malabsorbers who participated in diet trials with and without lactose, 71% reported more frequent symptoms on the lactose-containing diet. Although this study suggests that lactose intolerance might have an important etiologic role in RAP, the diet trial was neither blinded nor controlled. Considering all of these studies, it seems that lactose intolerance is undoubtedly the cause of RAP in a small proportion of patients.

Perhaps of greater importance is the possibility that lactose intolerance might exacerbate the symptoms of other gastrointestinal disorders, for example, inflammatory bowel disease (IBD). Since hypolactasia is common, it is inevitable that among individuals with another disorder, a subgroup will have lactose intolerance as well. Despite the clinical impression that lactose intolerance can at times contribute to symptoms in IBD, lactose intolerance has been observed to be no more common in a group of children with IBD than in a group with RAP.[139] Although a comparison with normal subjects was not made, the prevalence of lactose intolerance is probably no greater in patients with IBD than in a healthy population of similar ethnic background. As mentioned previously, normal individuals commonly malabsorb small amounts of ingested lactose in the small bowel.[87] Patients with other gastrointestinal diseases, such as IBD, may be unable at times to compensate for even the small quantity of lactose that normally reaches the colon, and this factor may contribute to their symptoms.

Molecular Basis. In individuals without adult-onset hypolactasia (ie, those who have persistently high small bowel lactase activity as adults), lactase mRNA is found uniformly in all villus enterocytes, and lactase protein as well as lactase activity is present uniformly at the brush border.[140] Individuals with adult-onset hypolactasia may have different patterns of development of lactase deficiency as a result of alterations primarily at the transcriptional level.[141–143] Even on a single villus from an individual with adult-onset hypolactasia, some enterocytes may have (1) no detectable lactase mRNA, (2) lactase mRNA but no detectable brush border lactase protein, (3) lactase protein but no activity, or (4) lactase protein and lactase activity.[140,144] Some enterocytes contain as much lactase mRNA as seen in the enterocytes of individuals without hypolactasia. Thus, enterocytes with different phenotypes are present on the same villus. Enterocytes with different patterns of lactase expression occur in a patchy distribution, indicating that they are not arising in a clonal pattern. The mechanism of this variable expression remains to be fully elucidated; however, it is generally believed that this mosaic pattern of lactase expression is attributable to differential expression in enterocytes originating for distinct stem cell populations.

The long sought out breakthrough in the molecular basis of lactase nonpersistence was recently made with linkage disequilibrium analysis of nine well-characterized Finnish families.[122] Sequence analysis revealed two distinct areas of sequence variability that precisely associated with low levels of lactase activity. Specifically, $C/T_{-13,910}$, a DNA variant located 13,910 base pairs upstream from the *LCT* gene, and a $G/A_{-22,018}$ polymorphism located 8 kb further upstream, showed complete cosegregation with the nonpersistence trait. The $C/T_{-13,910}$ variant was also associated with hypolactasia in a large cohort of non-Finnish subjects in four different populations.

The $T_{-13,910}$ polymorphism was associated with lactase persistence in the European population but not in African descendants, while the C variant was limited to the nonpersistence population.[124] These polymorphisms are located in a potent enhancer whose transcriptional activity is augmented by the T variant which binds Oct-1 at higher avidity than the C variant.[145,146] Binding sites for other transcription factors, including HNF-4, GATA, and were identified in the vicinity of the −13,910 polymorphism. It is currently thought that in the presence of the T variant, this transcriptional enhancer is of sufficient potency to sustain LPH activity despite the natural age-dependent decline that is driven by elements residing in the genes immediate to promoter region.

Diagnostic Criteria. The diagnosis of lactose intolerance is suggested by the resolution of clinical symptoms when subjects are placed on a strict lactose elimination diet for 2 weeks and recurs once lactose is reintroduced. However, it should be recognized that dietary history is frequently unreliable to establish the diagnosis of lactose intolerance.[136] The inconsistency of dietary history has been attributable to several factors including the patient's age, dose of lactose, and confounding clinical conditions as described earlier. Genetic tests have been developed to assess for the homozygote CC (-13910) genotype that is associated with hypolactasia. Several studies have confirmed that genotyping is as reliable as breath hydrogen testing in adults and older children.[120]

Treatment. As with all other disorders of CHO assimilation, symptoms resulting from lactose intolerance may be minimized by the avoidance of milk and dairy products. Commercially available milk products that are either lactose-free or contain a reduced lactose content including rice and soy-based products may be used as substitutes. Since the malabsorptive symptoms are dose-dependent, the consumption of small quantities (4 to 8 ounces) may be encouraged, either alone or with the use of oral lactase replacement. Since milk and other dairy products are a rich dietary source of calcium and vitamin D, alternative sources should be recommended to patients with lactose intolerance that severely limits their intake of dairy products in order to reduce the long-term risk of abnormal bone density and fractures. Live culture yogurt is often tolerated by individuals with lactose intolerance (see section "Treatment of Carbohydrate Intolerance").

Congenital Sucrase-Isomaltase Deficiency

Clinical Background. In humans, a congenital deficiency of small intestinal sucrase is always associated with a deficiency of isomaltase and is known as congenital sucrase-isomaltase deficiency (CSID) (MIM #222900)[147–149] (Figure 6). CSID is a rare autosomal recessive disorder that leads to malabsorptive diarrhea with the ingestion of sucrose and oligosaccharides.[150] This deficiency is much less common than hypolactasia, but more common than congenital lactase deficiency. It is found in about 0.2% of North Americans and in up to 10% of Greenland Eskimos.[151] The association of these two enzyme deficiencies is, in fact, no surprise since these enzymes are synthesized together, inserted into the brush border membrane as one large protein, and subsequently cleaved into two units which continue to remain closely associated.[152]

Characteristically, CSID first presents at the time of introduction of sucrose into the diet (Figure 7). This sugar may be introduced in a sucrose-containing formula (usually soy-based) or in solid foods (especially fruits). The symptoms are typical of all the syndromes of CHO malabsorption: diarrhea, bloating, flatulence, and cramps. Failure to thrive may be a prominent component in young infants.[147] A rarer presentation has been protracted diarrhea in infants fed glucose polymer formula.[149] Older children with CSID can develop an aversion to sucrose-containing foods, which limit their intake of this sugar.

Molecular Basis. Multiple germ-line mutations have been identified in patients with CSID that result in a decline in sucrase and/or isomaltase activity. Specifically, mutations have been characterized that result in either a selective decline in enzymatic activity, or abnormalities in the processing and sorting of the SI protein.[153] The majority of the mutations of the sucrase isomaltase gene results in improper targeting to the brush border membrane; glucoamylase depletion also occurs, but is not clinically significant because of the redundancy provided by α-amylase.[154–156]

Diagnostic Criteria. The resolution of chronic diarrheal symptoms in a patient on a strict sucrose and glucose polymer-free diet is suggestive of the diagnosis of CSID. Diarrhea induced by large complex CHOs is usually an indication of abnormal exocrine pancreatic function, such as seen with cystic fibrosis, but may also be attributed to a deficiency of glucoamylase synthesis or CSID.[107,157] Distinguishing between these various disorders can be accomplished by analyzing small bowel disaccharidase activity and with CHO-specific breath hydrogen testing.[110] A selective deficiency of mucosal sucrase activity would be consistent with the congenital form of this disorder, while a general decline in multiple disaccharidases would suggest a secondary form of sucrase-isomaltase deficiency. Breath hydrogen test can also be performed with sucrose; however, evidence of malabsorption should be followed by testing with each monosaccharide (glucose and fructose) in order to confirm the specific disaccharidase deficiency.

Treatment. Sacrosidase, an invertase (β-fructofuranosidase) preparation with sucrase activity isolated from *Saccharomyces cerevisiae*, has been studied in the treatment of congenital sucrase-isomaltase deficiency.[158] This treatment has been shown to decrease symptoms of gas, abdominal cramps, bloating, and diarrhea.

Congenital Trehalase Deficiency. Trehalase deficiency is a common disaccharidase deficiency in Greenland, occurring in about 8% of the population.[159] However, this deficiency does not appear to have nutritional importance.

Primary Monosaccharide Intolerance

Glucose-Galactose Malabsorption. Glucose-galactose malabsorption (GGM) is a rare disorder that causes severe life-threatening diarrhea and dehydration during the neonatal period (MIM #182380). GGM was first established when investigators demonstrated evidence of an inherited disorder of active glucose and galactose transport.[160] Conformation was provided by in vitro studies on GGM duodenal biopsies which demonstrated that enterocytes were unable to accumulate galactose owing to a reduction in the number of transporters in the brush border membrane[161–163] (Figure 8). Expression studies confirmed that glucose and galactose are transported by the sodium-dependent transporter, SGLT1, which is defective in patients with GGM.[69]

Clinical Background. The majority of patients with GGM present clinically with severe life-threatening diarrhea during the neonatal period; however, on several occasions the diagnosis was not established until adulthood[164] (Figure 7). Diarrhea is most frequently detected during the first week of life, and will result in a severe metabolic acidosis and hyperosmolar dehydration. If not properly diagnosed in a timely manner and if dietary management is not implemented, GGM is frequently fatal. Isolated and profuse CHO malabsorption is distinctly unusual during the first several days of life, and its presence should initiate the workup for both GGM and primary lactase deficiency.

Lactose, the principal CHO of human milk, consists of glucose and galactose subunits, and therefore infants with this disorder will not be spared symptoms by nursing. Furthermore, infants with congenital glucose–galactose malabsorption will not tolerate sucrose (glucose–fructose), sugar (glucose + fructose), or glucose polymers. In fact, this diagnosis should be considered when a neonate has diarrhea in association with CHO malabsorption and is found to tolerate fructose alone.[165]

Molecular Basis. In vitro studies with radiolabeled glucose and galactose have demonstrated that the small bowel mucosa from patients with GGM cannot concentrate these sugars, in contrast to the mucosa from normal subjects.[161–162] Small bowel perfusion studies have also demonstrated decreased absorption of these sugars in vivo.[165] The mucosal histologic appearance and the capacity for absorption of fructose have both been shown to be normal.[166]

The primary CHO present in breast milk is lactose that is hydrolyzed by lactase on the external surface of the intestinal brush border. The liberated glucose and galactose are then transported across the brush border membrane by SGLT1 and accumulated within the enterocyte.

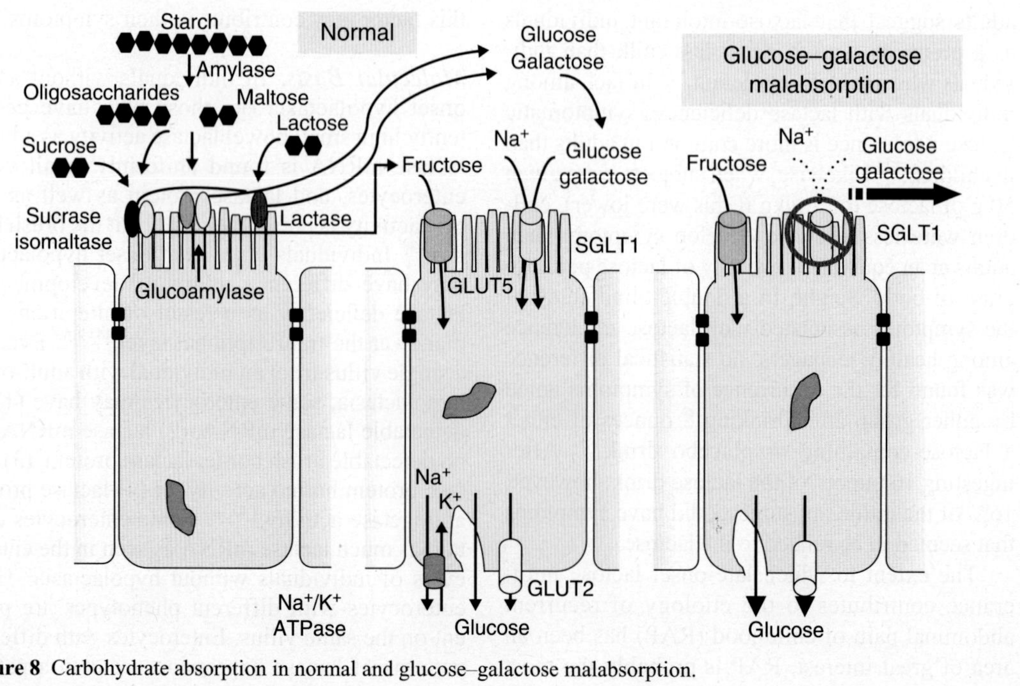

Figure 8 Carbohydrate absorption in normal and glucose–galactose malabsorption.

Complex CHOs provide the major source of glucose in older children and adults. Until recently, the facilitated carrier GLUT2 was believed to be responsible for transport of glucose and galactose across the basolateral membrane; however, this is now doubtful in light of studies on humans and mice with mutations of GLUT2 and no evidence of osmotic diarrhea.[167,168]

SGLT1 is responsible for the tight coupling of two Na^+ ions and one sugar molecule across the membrane during one catalytic turnover. The basolateral Na,K-ATPase pump maintains the low intracellular sodium concentration by pumping sodium out of the cell, and this results in the net absorption of sodium (chloride and bicarbonate), sugar, and water across the epithelium.[169] Because the osmolality of stool in both secretory and malabsorptive diarrhea is always isomolar with serum, the addition of undigested solutes (glucose and galactose) and SCFA that reach the colon of patients with GGM will result in an excessive amount of water loss to maintain the obligatory fecal osmolality.

The relative abundance of GGM in consanguineous unions and the absence of vertical transmission suggest an autosomal recessive pattern of inheritance. Genetic testing performed on 82 patients in 74 unrelated families and identified 46 mutations in the SGLT1 gene of patients with GGM.[170–173] The majority of the mutations are missense; however, six nonsense and seven frame-shift mutations, producing truncated, nonfunctional proteins, have been identified. All missense mutations that caused a defect in sugar transport were in amino acids that were conserved within the 18 closely related genes, including eight *SGLT1*s from different species (Figure 9).

Diagnostic Criteria. Three key features are necessary to establish the diagnosis of GGM: elimination of glucose and galactose (and lactose) from the diet results in the complete resolution of diarrheal symptoms, a normal intestinal biopsy, and an abnormal glucose breathe hydrogen test. When considering the diagnosis of GGM, several tests should be performed. Patients should have standard stool analysis, including pH, occult blood, and leukocyte analysis and evaluation for the presence of reducing and non-reducing sugars. Patients with GGM have been identified using the breath hydrogen test with a relatively small glucose challenge (0.1 g per kg) in the absence of any associated symptoms.[165] With greater quantities of glucose or galactose (0.5 or 1.0 g per kg, respectively), loose, acidic stool developed and contained reducing substance; however, fructose (2.0 g per kg) was well tolerated.

Treatment. With GGM, as with other disorders of CHO malabsorption, symptoms resolve on an elimination diet free of glucose and galactose. Several formulas are available for managing GGM patients during early infancy, for example, Ross Carbohydrate Free Formula (Ross Products, Columbus, OH), Galactomin 19 (Nutricia, Holland). Care should be exercised with formulas containing fructose as fructose absorptive capacity is rather limited in young children. The dietary management becomes particularly challenging as children enter into late infancy and begin to exert more independence. Guidance from a well-trained dietitian is frequently invaluable. Highly motivated parents will generally benefit from dietary manuals that list the sugar content of selected foods. While the obligatory lifelong glucose- and galactose-free diet may have significant long-term renal and cardiovascular consequences; none has been reported in several adult patients.

Fructose Malabsorption. Fructose malabsorption has been implicated in both toddler's diarrhea and in a rare and poorly defined autosomal recessive disorder named isolated fructose malabsorption (IFM). Distinguishing between the more common toddler's diarrhea and IFM is particularly difficult, and it is unclear if they represent distinct disorders. The clinical and genetic features of IFM are not as well defined as its counterpart CHO transport disorder, GGM. Although the ability of GLUT5 to transport fructose has been demonstrated, there remains insufficient information confirming that GLUT5 represents the main fructose facilitative carrier in the intestine.[174] Recent studies have identified GLUT7 as a high affinity glucose and fructose carrier on the brush border membrane of enterocytes located in the distal intestine.[78] New studies are also emerging in rats implying that brush border GLUT2 plays a major role in the absorption of fructose.[79]

Clinical Background. Fructose is the primary monosaccharide found in fruits and fruit juices. Fruit juices that contain a high proportion of fructose to glucose or an excessive amount of the non-absorbable CHO sorbitol have been associated with infant diarrhea and abdominal pain[175–176] (Figure 7). Malabsorption of fruit juices is dose-dependent, with diarrheal symptoms associated with the daily consumption of juice that exceeds 15 mL/kg. Whether children with toddler's diarrhea have a reduced capacity to absorb fructose than other similarly aged children has yet to be defined. Intolerance to dietary fructose has also been identified in infants with colic and adults with irritable bowel syndrome.[177,178]

Molecular Basis. Eight patients with clinical evidence suggestive of IFM were previously evaluated for mutations in the *GLUT5* gene.[179] Analysis of both the coding region and intron and exon boundaries of the *GLUT5* gene failed to identify a deleterious mutation that could account for defective transport.

Clinical Manifestations. Fructose malabsorption can be assessed by either placing the patient on a fructose elimination diet or performing a fructose breath hydrogen test. Fructose given at 1 g/kg body weight or a maximum of 25 g can be used to perform these studies.[110] Concomitant administration of glucose can attenuate the malabsorption of fructose as assessed by breath testing presumably by improving solvent drag.[180] To determine whether the malabsorption is fructose-specific, intestinal biopsies should reveal normal intestinal histology, and malabsorption should be limited to fructose and not other monosaccharides.

Diagnostic Criteria and Treatment. Patients experiencing significant fructose-induced diarrhea should either reduce or eliminate their dietary fructose load to resolve symptoms. It has been established in rodent models that GLUT5 levels are dependent on the chronic load of dietary fructose; therefore, it is conceivable that fructose malabsorption may resolve by initiating a feeding regimen of incrementally increasing amounts of fructose. Because fructose malabsorption is generally limited to early infancy, attempts to reintroduce fructose should be considered as patients enter into the school-age years.

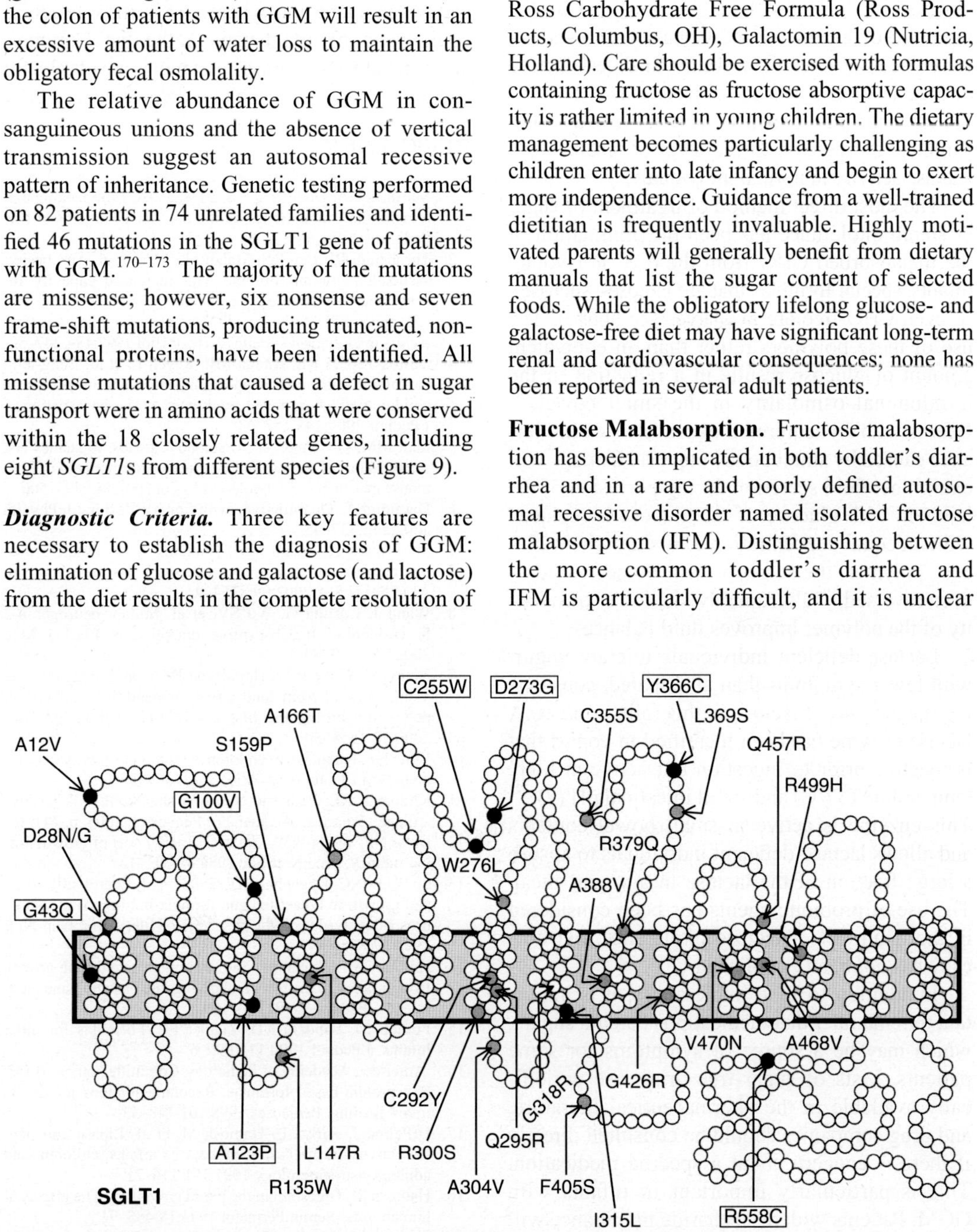

Figure 9 Location of missense mutations in sodium-coupled glucose transporter (SGLT1) in patients with glucose-galactose malabsorption.

SECONDARY DISORDERS OF CARBOHYDRATE ABSORPTION

Many forms of injury to the mucosa of the small bowel may lead to transient CHO intolerance. Often, histologic abnormalities will be noted to be concomitant with the CHO intolerance; however, the mucosa can appear relatively normal by light microscopy, especially with a transient disaccharide intolerance. Infants seem to be more prone to secondary disorders than older individuals, and CHO intolerance commonly occurs in association with infantile gastroenteritis. Intolerance for disaccharides alone or in combination with monosaccharides may occur, but the former is more common. Acquired monosaccharide intolerance usually suggests severe small bowel mucosal damage, manifested as moderate to severe villous atrophy on light microscopy and damaged microvilli on electron microscopy.[181]

During acute infantile diarrhea, malabsorption of both monosaccharides and disaccharides has been demonstrated by small bowel intubation studies.[182] Occasionally, transient lactose intolerance can persist for a period of months. The likelihood that this will occur seems to correlate with the severity of the diarrheal illness and the degree of malnutrition.[183] A substantial proportion of childhood infectious diarrhea is caused by viruses (primarily rotavirus); the pathogenesis of this diarrhea involves acute damage to mature villus epithelial cells with replacement by rapidly migrating but immature crypt epithelial cells.[184] These immature epithelial cells exhibit decreased disaccharidase activity as well as decreased capacity for glucose absorption. When a group of patients with rotavirus gastroenteritis were evaluated with a lactose breath hydrogen test during the acute illness, an abnormal study was noted in most of these children; but 1 week later, the test was normal in all.[185]

A deficiency of sucrase-isomaltase may result from either a selective congenital deficiency or as a global decline in disaccharidase activity that occurs with infection and inflammation. Secondary SI deficiency may result from the general decline in small bowel surface area associated with villus blunting, or because of transcriptional repression that can be induced by cytokines such as IL-6 and interferon-γ.[186]

Bacterial overgrowth in the small intestine may be associated with both mono- and disaccharide intolerance.[187] An animal model for bacterial overgrowth, which has been extensively studied, has been surgically prepared blind loops of bowel in the rat.[188–191] A reduction of disaccharidase activity in these blind loops appears to be secondary to an increase in brush border glycoprotein degradation rather than decreased synthesis.[189] Although increased amounts of deconjugated bile salts have been thought to be a mediator of the disaccharidase deficiency in bacterial overgrowth, this may not be the case.[191] Bacterial extracts prepared from anaerobic organisms isolated from blind loops have been shown to have the ability to remove disaccharidases from isolated brush borders, most likely as a result of an elastase-like protease activity.[190]

Some species of *Bacteroides* have been shown to have what appears to be a unique ability to secrete proteases, which release maltase and sucrase when incubated with human brush borders.[192] Similar protease activity has been found in fluid aspirated from the small intestine of patients with bacterial overgrowth. Other clinical disorders that have been associated with secondary CHO intolerance include giardiasis, gluten-sensitive enteropathy, cow's milk protein intolerance, and protracted diarrhea of infancy.

TREATMENT OF CARBOHYDRATE INTOLERANCE

Attempts to induce enzyme activity as a treatment for patients with oligosaccharidase (disaccharidase) deficiencies have not been successful. Chronic ingestion of lactose by individuals with hypolactasia does not alter their ability to digest lactose or their level of small bowel lactase activity.[130,193] Although the ingestion of a diet rich in fructose will stimulate an increase in the level of small bowel sucrase activity in normal individuals,[194]

The most direct method of treatment of sugar or starch intolerance has been the elimination of the malabsorbed CHO from the diet. For young infants, special formulas that are lactose-, sucrose-, or even CHO-free are available (see above). The use of these polymers rather than an equivalent amount of glucose results in a reduction in the intraluminal osmolality in the small bowel.[195] Infants with an acquired monosaccharide intolerance caused by small bowel mucosal damage will exhibit net fluid secretion during perfusion of the jejunum with glucose. If the glucose is replaced with an equal concentration of a short-chain glucose polymer, the secretion will be decreased or even reversed.[196] Presumably, the lower osmolality of the polymer improves fluid balance.

Lactase-deficient individuals tolerate yogurt with fewer symptoms than anticipated, considering the amount of lactose in this milk product. A lactase enzyme has been identified in yogurt that is inactive prior to ingestion but active at body temperature (37°C) and small intestinal pH (7).[197] This enzyme is active in small bowel contents and allows lactase-deficient individuals to absorb a large fraction of the lactose in a yogurt meal. The use of probiotic agents has been considered in the treatment of lactose intolerance, but efficacy has not been established.[198]

In addition to food intolerances, it is important to remember that medications contain sugars, which may be a source of symptoms for some patients. Lists of sugar-free drugs are periodically available in the pharmaceutical literature, and drug companies should be consulted directly if there is concern about a specific medication. This is particularly important in infants with GGM. Patients with disaccharide intolerance will usually tolerate sugar substitutes, although it is important to keep in mind that the use of these products does restrict the caloric intake. Sorbitol, a poorly absorbed polyalcohol sugar used in many sugar-free products, may produce an osmotic diarrhea as well as gas, bloating, and cramps.[199] For patients on low-sugar diets, it is important to consider sorbitol as a potential cause of chronic symptoms suggestive of sugar intolerance.

Commercially produced lactase enzyme products are available to add to foods or take with meals containing lactose in order to reduce symptoms.[200] This enzyme is prepared by extraction of bacterial or yeast β-galactosidases. If added to cow's milk at room or refrigerator temperature and when allowed to sit for a specified period of time, it will hydrolyze up to 95% of the lactose. Taste acceptance of the milk prepared in this manner is good. This kind of product allows for bulk production of low-lactose dairy products. This technical advance may have excellent possibilities in areas of the world where the majority of individuals are lactase-deficient and where cow's milk products could be an important staple in the diet. Commercially produced sucrase enzyme is available for congenital sucrase-isomaltase deficiency as well.

REFERENCES

1. Martinez GA, Dodd DA, Samartgedes JA. Milk feeding patterns in the United States during the first 12 months of life. Pediatrics 1981;68:863–8.
2. Turnbaugh PJ, Ley RE, Mahowald MA, et al. An obesity-associated gut microbiome with increased capacity for energy harvest. Nature 2006;444:1027–31.
3. Alexander RM. A theory of mixed chains applied to safety factors in biological systems. J Theor Biol 1997;184:247–52.
4. Quiros-Tejeira RE, Ament ME, Reyen L, et al. Long-term parenteral nutritional support and intestinal adaptation in children with short bowel syndrome: A 25-year experience. J Pediatr 2004;145:157–63.
5. Lam MM, O'Connor TP, Diamond J. Loads, capacities and safety factors of maltase and the glucose transporter SGLT1 in mouse intestinal brush border. J Physiol 2002;542:493–500.
6. Diamond J. Quantitative evolutionary design. J Physiol 2002;542:337–45.
7. Steyermark AC, Lam MM, Diamond J. Quantitative evolutionary design of nutrient processing: Glucose. Proc Natl Acad Sci U S A 2002;99:8754–9.
8. Wang J, Cortina G, Wu SV, et al. Mutant neurogenin-3 in congenital malabsorptive diarrhea. N Engl J Med 2006;355:270–80.
9. Butte NF, Wong WW, Hopkinson JM, et al. Energy requirements derived from total energy expenditure and energy deposition during the first 2 y of life. Am J Clin Nutr 2000;72:1558–69.
10. Butte NF. Fat intake of children in relation to energy requirements. Am J Clin Nutr 2000;72:1246S–52S.
11. Kleinman RE. Pediatric Nutrition Handbook. Elk Groove Village: American Academy of Pediatrics; 2004. p. 241–6.
12. Butte NF, Wong WW, Garza C. Energy cost of growth during infancy. Proc Nutr Soc 1989;48:303–12.
13. de Bruin NC, Degenhart HJ, Gal S, et al. Energy utilization and growth in breast-fed and formula-fed infants measured prospectively during the first year of life. Am J Clin Nutr 1998;67:885–96.
14. Holliday MA. Metabolic rate and organ size during growth from infancy to maturity and during late gastation and early infancy. Pediatrics 1971;47:169.
15. Fomon SJ, Sanders KD, Ziegler EE. Formulas for older infants. J Pediatr 1990;116:690–6.
16. American Academy of Pediatrics. Committee on Nutrition. Soy protein-based formulas: Recommendations for use in infant feeding. Pediatrics 1998;101:148–53.
17. DiPalma J, Kirk CL, Hamosh M, et al. Lipase and pepsin activity in the gastric mucosa of infants, children, and adults. Gastroenterology 1991;101:116–21.
18. Hamosh M. Digestion in the premature infant: The effects of human milk. Semin Perinatol 1994;18:485–94.
19. Hamosh M, Scanlon JW, Ganot D, et al. Fat digestion in the newborn. Characterization of lipase in gastric aspirates of premature and term infants. J Clin Invest 1981;67:838–46.

20. Shulman RJ, Schanler RJ, Lau C, et al. Early feeding, feeding tolerance, and lactase activity in preterm infants. J Pediatr 1998;133:645–9.
21. Antonowicz I, Chang SK, Grand RJ. Development and distribution of lysosomal enzymes and disaccharidases in human fetal intestine. Gastroenterology 1974;67:51–8.
22. Raul F, Lacroix B, Aprahamian M. Longitudinal distribution of brush border hydrolases and morphological maturation in the intestine of the preterm infant. Early Hum Dev 1986;13:225–34.
23. Kien CL, Liechty EA, Myerberg DZ, Mullett MD. Dietary carbohydrate assimilation in the premature infant: Evidence for a nutritionally significant bacterial ecosystem in the colon. Am J Clin Nutr 1987;46:456–60.
24. Topping DL, Clifton PM. Short-chain fatty acids and human colonic function: Roles of resistant starch and nonstarch polysaccharides. Physiol Rev 2001;81:1031–64.
25. Jones JB, Mehta NR, Hamosh M. alpha-Amylase in preterm human milk. J Pediatr Gastroenterol Nutr 1982;1:43–8.
26. Lindberg T, Skude G. Amylase in human milk. Pediatrics 1982;70:235–8.
27. Hegardt P, Lindberg T, Borjesson J, Skude G. Amylase in human milk from mothers of preterm and term infants. J Pediatr Gastroenterol Nutr 1984; 3:563–6.
28. Murray RD, Kerzner B, Sloan HR, McClung HJ, Gilbert M, Ailabouni A. The contribution of salivary amylase to glucose polymer hydrolysis in premature infants. Pediatr Res 1986; 20:186–91.
29. Rosenblum JL, Irwin CL, Alpers DH. Starch and glucose oligosaccharides protect salivary-type amylase activity at acid pH. Am J Physiol 1988;254:G775–80.
30. Auricchio S, Della PD, Vegnente A. Studies on intestinal digestion of starch in man. II. Intestinal hydrolysis of amylopectin in infants and children. Pediatrics 1967;39:853–62.
31. Hadorn B, Zoppi G, Shmerling DH, et al. Quantitative assessment of exocrine pancreatic function in infants and children. J Pediatr 1968;73:39–50.
32. Zoppi G, Andreotti G, Pajno-Ferrara F, et al. Exocrine pancreas function in premature and full term neonates. Pediatr Res 1972;6:880–6.
33. Fogel MR, Gray GM. Starch hydrolysis in man: An intraluminal process not requiring membrane digestion. J Appl Physiol 1973;35:263–7.
34. Anderson IH, Levine AS, Levitt MD. Incomplete absorption of the carbohydrate in all-purpose wheat flour. N Engl J Med 1981;304:891–2.
35. Stephen AM, Haddad AC, Phillips SF. Passage of carbohydrate into the colon. Direct measurements in humans. Gastroenterology 1983;85:589–95.
36. Maroux S, Louvard D. On the hydrophobic part of aminopeptidase and maltases which bind the enzyme to the intestinal brush border membrane. Biochim Biophys Acta 1976;419:189–95.
37. Gray GM, Lally BC, Conklin KA. Action of intestinal sucrase-isomaltase and its free monomers on an alpha-limit dextrin. J Biol Chem 1979;254:6038–43.
38. Kelly JJ, Alpers DH. Properties of human intestinal glucoamylase. Biochim Biophys Acta 1973;315:113–22.
39. Bjerknes M, Cheng H. Gastrointestinal stem cells. II. Intestinal stem cells. Am J Physiol Gastrointest Liver Physiol 2005;289:G381–7.
40. Newcomer AD, McGill DB. Distribution of disaccharidase activity in the small bowel of normal and lactase-deficient subjects. Gastroenterology 1966;51:481–8.
41. Leeper LL, Henning SJ. Development and tissue distribution of sucrase-isomaltase mRNA in rats. Am J Physiol 1990;258:G52–8.
42. Buller HA, Kothe MJ, Goldman DA, et al. Coordinate expression of lactase-phlorizin hydrolase mRNA and enzyme levels in rat intestine during development. J Biol Chem 1990;265:6978–83.
43. Krasinski SD, Estrada G, Yeh K-Y, et al. Transcriptional regulation of intestinal hydrolase biosynthesis during postnatal development in rats. Am J Physiol Gastrointest Liver Physiol 1994;267:G584–94.
44. Traber PG, Yu L, Wu GD, Judge TA. Sucrase-isomaltase gene expression along crypt-villus axis of human small intestine is regulated at level of mRNA abundance. Am J Physiol 1992;262:G123–30.
45. Rings EH, de Boer PA, Moorman AF, et al. Lactase gene expression during early development of rat small intestine. Gastroenterology 1992;103:1154–61.
46. Maiuri L, Rossi M, Raia V, et al. Mosaic regulation of lactase in human adult-type hypolactasia. Gastroenterology 1994;107:54–60.
47. Alpers DH, Tedesco FJ. The possible role of pancreatic proteases in the turnover of intestinal brush border proteins. Biochim Biophys Acta 1975;401:28–40.
48. Cook RM, Powell PM, Moog F. Influence of biliary stasis on the activity and distribution of maltase, sucrase, alkaline phosphatase, and leucylnaphthylamidase in the small intestine of the mouse. Gastroenterology 1973;64:411–20.
49. Ulshen MH, Herbst CA. Effect of removal of pancreaticobiliary secretions on adaptation to short bowel in orally nourished rats. Am J Clin Nutr 1984;39:762–70.
50. Arvanitakis C, Olsen WA. Intestinal mucosal disaccharidases in chronic pancreatitis. Am J Dig Dis 1974;19: 417–21.
51. Naim HY, Jacob R, Naim H, et al. The pro region of human intestinal lactase-phlorizin hydrolase. J Biol Chem 1994;269:26933–43.
52. Jacob R, Weiner JR, Stadge S, Naim HY. Additional N-glycosylation and its impact on the folding of intestinal lactase-phlorizin hydrolase. J Biol Chem 2000;275:10630–7.
53. Gray GM, Santiago NA. Disaccharide absorption in normal and diseased human intestine. Gastroenterology 1966;51:489–98.
54. McMichael HB, Webb J, Dawson AM. The absorption of maltose and lactose in man. Clin Sci 1967;33:135–45.
55. Lorenzsonn V, Lloyd M, Olsen WA. Immunocytochemical heterogeneity of lactase-phlorizin hydrolase in adult lactase deficiency. Gastroenterology 1993;105:51–9.
56. Fang R, Olds LC, Sibley E. Spatio-temporal patterns of intestine-specific transcription factor expression during postnatal mouse gut development. Gene Expr Patterns 2006;6:426–32.
57. Bosse T, Piaseckyj CM, Burghard E, et al. Gata4 is essential for the maintenance of jejunal-ileal identities in the adult mouse small intestine. Mol Cell Biol 2006;26:9060–70.
58. Traber PG, Silberg DG. Intestine-specific gene transcription. Annu Rev Physiol 1996;58:275–97.
59. Boudreau F, Rings EH, Van Wering HM, et al. Hepatocyte nuclear factor-1 alpha, GATA-4, and caudal related homeodomain protein Cdx2 interact functionally to modulate intestinal gene transcription. Implication for the developmental regulation of the sucrase-isomaltase gene. J Biol Chem 2002;277:31909–17.
60. Emvo EN, Raul F, Koch B, Neuville P, Foltzer-Jourdainne C. Sucrase-isomaltase gene expression in suckling rat intestine: Hormonal, dietary, and growth factor control. J Pediatr Gastroenterol Nutr. 1996;23:262–9.
61. Deren JJ, Broitman SA, Zamcheck N. Effect of diet upon intestinal disaccharidases and disaccharide absorption. J Clin Invest 1967;46:186–95.
62. Rosensweig NS, Stifel FB, Zakim D, Herman RH. Time response of human jejunal glycolytic enzymes to a high sucrose diet. Gastroenterology 1969;57:143–6.
63. Ulshen MH, Grand RJ. Site of substrate stimulation of jejunal sucrase in the rat. J Clin Invest 1979;64:1097–102.
64. Quan R, Gray GM. Sucrase-alpha-dextrinase in the rat. Postinsertional conversion to inactive molecular species by a carbohydrate-free diet. J Clin Invest 1993;91:2785–90.
65. Crane RK. Na+-dependent transport in the intestine and other animal tissues. Fed Proc 1965;24:1000–6.
66. Crane RK. Hypothesis for mechanism of intestinal active transport of sugars. Fed Proc 1962;21:891–5.
67. Guy MJ, Deren JJ. Selective permeability of the small intestine for fructose. Am J Physiol 1971;221:1051–6.
68. Fine KD, Santa Ana CA, Porter JL, Fordtran JS. Effect of D-glucose on intestinal permeability and its passive absorption in human small intestine in vivo. Gastroenterology 1993;105:1117–25.
69. Hediger MA, Coady MJ, Ikeda TS, Wright EM. Expression cloning and cDNA sequencing of the Na+/glucose co-transporter. Nature 1987;330:379–81.
70. Wright EM, Turk E, Zabel B, et al. Molecular genetics of intestinal glucose transport. J Clin Invest 1991;88:1435–40.
71. Thorens B, Cheng Z-Q, Brown D, Lodish HF. Liver glucose transporter: A basolateral protein in hepatocytes and intestine and kidney cells. Am J Physiol Cell Physiol 1990;259: C279–85.
72. Hwang ES, Hirayama BA, Wright EM. Distribution of the SGLT1 Na+/glucose cotransporter and mRNA along the crypt-villus axis of rabbit small intestine. Biochem Biophys Res Commun 1991;181:1208–17.
73. Loo DD, Wright EM, Zeuthen T. Water pumps. J Physiol 2002;542:53–60.
74. Wright EM, Hirayama BA, Loo DF. Active sugar transport in health and disease. J Intern Med 2007;261:32–43.
75. Bieberdorf FA, Morawski S, Fordtran JS. Effect of sodium, mannitol, and magnesium on glucose, galactose, 3-O-methylglucose, and fructose absorption in the human ileum. Gastroenterology 1975;68:58–66.
76. Schultz SG, Frizzell RA. An overview of intestinal absorptive and secretory processes. Gastroenterology 1972;63:161–70.
77. Burant CF, Takeda J, Brot-Laroche E, et al. Fructose transporter in human spermatozoa and small intestine is GLUT5. J Biol Chem 1992;267:14523–6.
78. Li Q, Manolescu A, Ritzel M, et al. Cloning and functional characterization of the human GLUT7 isoform SLC2A7 from the small intestine. Am J Physiol Gastrointest Liver Physiol 2004;287:G236–42.
79. Kellett GL, Brot-Laroche E. Apical GLUT2: A major pathway of intestinal sugar absorption. Diabetes 2005;54: 3056–62.
80. Ravich WJ, Bayless TM, Thomas M. Fructose: Incomplete intestinal absorption in humans. Gastroenterology 1983;84:26–9.
81. Lifshitz F, Ament ME, Kleinman RE, et al. Role of juice carbohydrate malabsorption in chronic nonspecific diarrhea in children. J Pediatr 1992;120:825–9.
82. Beaudet AL, Tsui L-C. A Suggested nomenclature for designating mutations. Hum Mutat 1993;2:245–8.
83. Ferraris RP. Dietary and developmental regulation of intestinal sugar transport. Biochem J 2001;360:265–76.
84. Cui XL, Soteropoulos P, Tolias P, Ferraris RP. Fructose-responsive genes in the small intestine of neonatal rats. Physiol Genomics 2004;18:206–17.
85. Barnes G, McKellar W, Lawrance S. Detection of fructose malabsorption by breath hydrogen test in a child with diarrhea. J Pediatr 1983;103:575–7.
86. Bond JH, Currier BE, Buchwald H, Levitt MD. Colonic conservation of malabsorbed carbohydrate. Gastroenterology 1980;78:444–7.
87. Bond JH, Levitt MD. Quantitative measurement of lactose absorption. Gastroenterology 1976;70:1058–62.
88. Bond JH, Jr, Levitt MD. Fate of soluble carbohydrate in the colon of rats and man. J Clin Invest 1976;57:1158–64.
89. Fine KD, Schiller LR. AGA technical review on the evaluation and management of chronic diarrhea. Gastroenterology 1999;116:1464–86.
90. Eherer AJ, Fordtran JS. Fecal osmotic gap and pH in experimental diarrhea of various causes. Gastroenterology 1992;103:545–51.
91. Duncan A, Robertson C, Russell RI. The fecal osmotic gap: Technical aspects regarding its calculation. J Lab Clin Med 1992;119:359–63.
92. Christopher NL, Bayless TM. Role of the small bowel and colon in lactose-induced diarrhea. Gastroenterology 1971;60:845–52.
93. Debongnie JC, Newcomer AD, McGill DB, Phillips SF. Absorption of nutrients in lactase deficiency. Dig Dis Sci 1979;24:225–31.
94. Ameen VZ, Powell GK, Jones LA. Quantitation of fecal carbohydrate excretion in patients with short bowel syndrome. Gastroenterology 1987;92:493–500.
95. Hammer HF, Fine KD, Santa Ana CA, et al. Carbohydrate malabsorption. Its measurement and its contribution to diarrhea. J Clin Invest 1990;86:1936–44.
96. Ruppin H, Bar-Meir S, Soergel KH, et al. Absorption of short-chain fatty acids by the colon. Gastroenterology 1980;78:1500–7.
97. Perman JA, Modler S, Olson AC. Role of pH in production of hydrogen from carbohydrates by colonic bacterial flora. Studies in vivo and in vitro. J Clin Invest 1981;67:643–50.
98. Devore CD, Ulshen MH, Cross RE. Phenolphthalein Laxatives and Factitious Diarrhea. Clin Pediatr 1982;21:573–4.
99. Hammer HF, Santa Ana CA, Schiller LR, Fordtran JS. Studies of osmotic diarrhea induced in normal subjects by ingestion of polyethylene glycol and lactulose. J Clin Invest 1989;84:1056–62.
100. Soeparto P, Stobo EA, Walker-Smith JA. Role of chemical examination of the stool in diagnosis of sugar malabsorption in children. Arch Dis Child 1972;47:56–61.
101. Buts JP, Morin CL, Roy CC, et al. One-hour blood xylose test: A reliable index of small bowel function. J Pediatr 1978;92:729–33.
102. Christie DL. Use of the one-hour blood xylose test as an indicator of small bowel mucosal disease. J Pediatr 1978;92:725–8.
103. Lamabadusuriya SP, Packer S, Harries JT. Limitations of xylose tolerance test as a screening procedure in childhood coeliac disease. Arch Dis Child 1975;50:34–9.
104. Schaad U, Gaze H, Hadorn B. Value of 1-hour blood-xylose test in diagnosis of childhood coeliac disease. Arch Dis Child 1978;53:420–2.
105. Newcomer AD, McGill DB. Lactose tolerance tests in adults with normal lactase activity. Gastroenterology 1966;50:340–6.
106. McGill DB, Newcomer AD. Comparison of venous and capillary blood samples in lactose tolerance testing. Gastroenterology 1967;53:371–4.
107. Lebenthal E, Khin-Maung-U, Zheng B-Y, et al. Small intestinal glucoamylase deficiency and starch malabsorption: A newly recognized alpha-glucosidase deficiency in children. J Pediatr 1994;124:541–6.

108. Dahlqvist A. Assay of intestinal disaccharidases. Anal Biochem 1968;22:99–107.
109. Gupta SK, Chong SK, Fitzgerald JF. Disaccharidase activities in children: Normal values and comparison based on symptoms and histologic changes. J Pediatr Gastroenterol Nutr 1999;28:246–51.
110. Romagnuolo J, Schiller D, Bailey RJ. Using breath tests wisely in a gastroenterology practice: An evidence-based review of indications and pitfalls in interpretation. Am J Gastroenterol 2002;97:1113–26.
111. Levitt MD. Production and Excretion of Hydrogen Gas in Man. N Engl J Med 1969;281:122–7.
112. Perman JA, Barr RG, Watkins JB. Sucrose malabsorption in children: Noninvasive diagnosis by interval breath hydrogen determination. J Pediatr 1978;93:17–22.
113. Barr RG, Levine MD, Watkins JB. Recurrent abdominal pain of childhood due to lactose intolerance. N Engl J Med 1979;300:1449–52.
114. Myo K, Bolin TD, Khin MO, et al. Ineffectiveness of breath methane excretion as a diagnostic test for lactose malabsorption. J Pediatr Gastroenterol Nutr 1999;28:474–9.
115. Kunzelmann K, Mall M. Electrolyte transport in the mammalian colon: Mechanisms and implications for disease. Physiol Rev 2002;82:245–89.
116. Lilibridge CB, Townes PL. Physiologic deficiency of pancreatic amylase in infancy: A factor in iatrogenic diarrhea. J Pediatr 1973;82:279–82.
117. Sjolund K, Haggmark A, Ihse I, et al. Selective deficiency of pancreatic amylase. Gut 1991;32:546–8.
118. MacLean WC, Jr, Fink BB. Lactose malabsorption by premature infants: Magnitude and clinical significance. J Pediatr 1980;97:383–8.
119. Griffin MP, Hansen JW. Can the elimination of lactose from formula improve feeding tolerance in premature infants? J Pediatr 1999;135:587–92.
120. Rasinpera H, Savilahti E, Enattah NS, et al. A genetic test which can be used to diagnose adult-type hypolactasia in children. Gut 2004;53:1571–6.
121. Savilahti E, Launiala K, Kuitunen P. Congenital lactase deficiency. A clinical study on 16 patients. Arch Dis Child 1983;58:246–52.
122. Enattah NS, Sahi T, Savilahti E, et al. Identification of a variant associated with adult-type hypolactasia. Nat Genet 2002;30:233–7.
123. Kuokkanen M, Kokkonen J, Enattah NS, et al. Mutations in the translated region of the lactase gene (lct) underlie congenital lactase deficiency. Am J Hum Genet 2006;78:339–44.
124. Swallow DM. Genetics of lactase persistence and lactose intolerance. Annu Rev Genet 2003;37:197–219.
125. Diamond JM. Hard-wired local triggering of intestinal enzyme expression. Nature 1986;324:408.
126. Heyman MB. Lactose intolerance in infants, children, and adolescents. Pediatrics 2006;118:1279–86.
127. Bayless TM, Rothfeld B, Massa C, et al. Lactose and milk intolerance: Clinical implications. N Engl J Med 1975;292:1156–9.
128. Newcomer AD, Thomas PJ, McGill DB, Hofmann AF. Lactase deficiency: A common genetic trait of the American Indian. Gastroenterology 1977;72:234–7.
129. Sahi T, Isokoski M, Jussila J, et al. Recessive inheritance of adult-type lactose malabsorption. Lancet 1973;2:823–6.
130. Keusch GT, Troncale FJ, Miller LH, et al. Acquired lactose malabsorption in Thai children. Pediatrics 1969;43:540–5.
131. Huang SS, Bayless TM. Lactose intolerance in healthy children. N Engl J Med 1967;276:1283–7.
132. Welsh JD, Poley JR, Bhatia M, Stevenson DE. Intestinal disaccharidase activities in relation to age, race, and mucosal damage. Gastroenterology 1978;75:847–55.
133. Lebenthal E, Antonowicz I, Shwachman H. Correlation of lactase activity, lactose tolerance and milk consumption in different age groups. Am J Clin Nutr 1975;28:595–600.
134. Hyams JS, Stafford RJ, Grand RJ, Watkins JB. Correlation of lactose breath hydrogen test, intestinal morphology, and lactase activity in young children. J Pediatr 1980;97:609–12.
135. Bedine MS, Bayless TM. Intolerance of small amounts of lactose by individuals with low lactase levels. Gastroenterology 1973;65:735–43.
136. Suarez FL, Savaiano DA, Levitt MD. A comparison of symptoms after the consumption of milk or lactose-hydrolyzed milk by people with self-reported severe lactose intolerance [see comments]. N Engl J Med 1995;333:1–4.
137. Kwon PH, Jr, Rorick MH, Scrimshaw NS. Comparative tolerance of adolescents of differing ethnic backgrounds to lactose-containing and lactose-free dairy drinks. II. Improvement of a double-blind test. Am J Clin Nutr 1980;33:22–6.
138. Walker LS, Lipani TA, Greene JW, et al. Recurrent abdominal pain: Symptom subtypes based on the Rome II Criteria for pediatric functional gastrointestinal disorders. J Pediatr Gastroenterol Nutr 2004;38:187–91.
139. Kirschner BS, DeFavaro MV, Jensen W. Lactose malabsorption in children and adolescents with inflammatory bowel disease. Gastroenterology 1981;81:829–32.
140. Maiuri L, Rossi M, Raia V, et al. Mosaic regulation of lactase in human adult-type hypolactasia. Gastroenterology 1994;107:54–60.
141. Witte J, Lloyd M, Lorenzsonn V, et al. The biosynthetic basis of adult lactase deficiency. J Clin Invest 1990;86:1338–42.
142. Sterchi EE, Mills PR, Fransen JA, et al. Biogenesis of intestinal lactase-phlorizin hydrolase in adults with lactose intolerance. Evidence for reduced biosynthesis and slowed-down maturation in enterocytes. J Clin Invest 1990;86:1329–37.
143. Lloyd M, Mevissen G, Fischer M, et al. Regulation of intestinal lactase in adult hypolactasia. J Clin Invest 1992;89:524–9.
144. Rossi M, Maiuri L, Fusco MI, et al. Lactase persistence versus decline in human adults: Multifactorial events are involved in down-regulation after weaning. Gastroenterology 1997;112:1506–14.
145. Lewinsky RH, Jensen TG, Moller J, et al. T-13910 DNA variant associated with lactase persistence interacts with Oct-1 and stimulates lactase promoter activity in vitro. Hum Mol Genet 2005;14:3945–53.
146. Olds LC, Sibley E. Lactase persistence DNA variant enhances lactase promoter activity in vitro: Functional role as a cis regulatory element. Hum Mol Genet 2003;12:2333–40.
147. Ament ME, Perera DR, Esther LJ. Sucrase-isomaltase deficiency-a frequently misdiagnosed disease. J Pediatr 1973;83:721–7.
148. Antonowicz I, Lloyd-Still JD, Khaw KT, Shwachman H. Congenital sucrase-isomaltase deficiency. Observations over a period of 6 years. Pediatrics 1972;49:847–53.
149. Newton T, Murphy MS, Booth IW. Glucose polymer as a cause of protracted diarrhea in infants with unsuspected congenital sucrase-isomaltase deficiency. J Pediatr 1996;128:753–6.
150. Treem WR. Congenital sucrase-isomaltase deficiency. J Pediatr Gastroenterol Nutr 1995;21:1–14.
151. Gray GM, Conklin KA, Townley RR. Sucrase-isomaltase deficiency. Absence of an inactive enzyme variant. N Engl J Med 1976;294:750–3.
152. Cezard JP, Conklin KA, Das BC, Gray GM. Incomplete intracellular forms of intestinal surface membrane sucrase-isomaltase. J Biol Chem 1979; 254:8969–75.
153. Keiser M, Alfalah M, Propsting MJ, et al. Altered folding, turnover, and polarized sorting act in concert to define a novel pathomechanism of congenital sucrase-isomaltase deficiency. J Biol Chem 2006;281:14393–9.
154. Ouwendijk J, Moolenaar CE, Peters WJ, et al. Congenital sucrase-isomaltase deficiency. Identification of a glutamine to proline substitution that leads to a transport block of sucrase-isomaltase in a pre-Golgi compartment. J Clin Invest 1996;97:633–41.
155. Jacob R, Zimmer KP, Schmitz J, Naim HY. Congenital sucrase-isomaltase deficiency arising from cleavage and secretion of a mutant form of the enzyme. J Clin Invest 2000;106:281–7.
156. Spodsberg N, Jacob R, Alfalah M, et al. Molecular basis of aberrant apical protein transport in an intestinal enzyme disorder. J Biol Chem 2001;276:23506–10.
157. Etemad B, Whitcomb DC. Chronic pancreatitis: Diagnosis, classification, and new genetic developments. Gastroenterology 2001;120:682–707.
158. Treem WR, McAdams L, Stanford L, et al. Sacrosidase therapy for congenital sucrase-isomaltase deficiency. J Pediatr Gastroenterol Nutr 1999;28:137–42.
159. Gudmand-Hoyer E, Fenger HJ, Skovbjerg H, et al. Trehalase deficiency in Greenland. Scand J Gastroenterol 1988;23:775–8.
160. Lindquist B, Meeuwisse GW. Chronic diarrhoea caused by monosaccharide malabsorption. Acta Paediatr 1962;51:674–85.
161. Schneider AJ, Kinter WB, Stirling CE. Glucose-galactose malabsorption. Report of a case with autoradiographic studies of a mucosal biopsy. N Engl J Med 1966;274:305–12.
162. Meeuwisse GW, Dahlqvist A. Glucose-galactose malabsorption. A study with biopsy of the small intestinal mucosa. Acta Paediatr Scand 1968;57:273–80.
163. Stirling CE, Schneider AJ, Wong M-D, Kinter WB. Quantitative radioautography of sugar transport in intestinal biopsies from normal humans and a patient with glucose-galactose malabsorption. J Clin Invest 1972;51:438–51.
164. Hughes WS, Senior JR. The glucose-galactose malabsorption syndrome in a 23-year-old woman. Gastroenterology 1975;68:142–5.
165. Douwes AC, van Caillie M, Fernandes J, et al. Interval breath hydrogen test in glucose-galactose malabsorption. Eur J Pediatr 1981;137:273–6.
166. Elsas LJ, Lambe DW, Jr. Familial glucose-galactose malabsorption: Remission of glucose intolerance. J Pediatr 1973;83:226–31.
167. Stumpel F, Burcelin R, Jungermann K, Thorens B. Normal kinetics of intestinal glucose absorption in the absence of GLUT2: Evidence for a transport pathway requiring glucose phosphorylation and transfer into the endoplasmic reticulum. Proc Natl Acad Sci U S A 2001;98:11330–5.
168. Santer R, Groth S, Kinner M, et al. The mutation spectrum of the facilitative glucose transporter gene SLC2A2 (GLUT2) in patients with Fanconi-Bickel syndrome. Hum Genet 2002;110:21–9.
169. Loo DDF, Zeuthen T, Chandy G, Wright EM. Cotransport of water by the Na^+/ glucose cotransporter. Proc Natl Acad Sci U S A 1996;93:13367–70.
170. Martin MG, Turk E, Lostao MP, et al. Defects in Na^+ glucose cotransporter (SGLT1) trafficking and function cause glucose-galactose malabsorption. Nature Genet 1996;12:216–20.
171. Martin MG, Lostao MP, Turk E, et al. Compound missense mutations in the sodium/D-glucose cotransporter result in trafficking defects. Gastroenterology 1997;112:1206–12.
172. Lam JT, Martin MG, Turk E, et al. Missense mutations in SGLT1 cause glucose-galactose malabsorption by trafficking defects. Biochimt Biophys Acta-Molecular Basis of Disease 1999;1453:297–303.
173. Turk E, Zabel B, Mundlos S, et al. Glucose/galactose malabsorption caused by a defect in the Na+/glucose cotransporter. Nature 1991;350:354–6.
174. Rand EB, Depaoli AM, Davidson NO, et al. Sequence, tissue distribution, and functional characterization of the rat fructose transporter GLUT5. Am J Physiol Gastrointest Liver Physiol 1993;264:G1169–76.
175. Nobigrot T, Chasalow FI, Lifshitz F. Carbohydrate absorption from one serving of fruit juice in young children: Age and carbohydrate composition effects. J Am CollNutr 1997;16:152–8.
176. Hoekstra JH. Fructose breath hydrogen tests in infants with chronic non-specific diarrhoea. Eur J Pediatr 1995;154:362–4.
177. Fernandez-Banares F, Esteve-Pardo M, De Leon R, et al. Sugar malabsorption in functional bowel disease: Clinical implications. Am J Gastroenterol 1993;88:2044–50.
178. Duro D, Rising R, Cedillo M, Lifshitz F. Association between infantile colic and carbohydrate malabsorption from fruit juices in infancy. Pediatrics 2002;109:797–805.
179. Wasserman D, Hoekstra JH, Tolia V, et al. Molecular analysis of the fructose transporter gene (*GLUT5*) in isolated fructose malabsorption. J Clin Invest 1996;98:2398–402.
180. Kellett GL. The facilitated component of intestinal glucose absorption. J Physiol 2001;531:585–95.
181. Klish WJ, Udall JN, Rodriguez JT, et al. Intestinal surface area in infants with acquired monosaccharide intolerance. J Pediatr 1978;92:566–71.
182. Rodriguez-de-Curet H, Lugo-de-Rivera C, Torres-Pinedo R. Studies on infant diarrhea. IV. Sugar transit and absorption in small intestine after a feeding. Gastroenterology 1970;59:396–403.
183. Lifshitz F, Coello-Ramirez P, Gutierrez-Topete G, Cornado-Cornet MC. Carbohydrate intolerance in infants with diarrhea. J Pediatr 1971;79:760–7.
184. Davidson GP, Gall DG, Petric M, et al. Human rotavirus enteritis induced in conventional piglets. Intestinal structure and transport. J Clin Invest 1977;60:1402–9.
185. Hyams JS, Krause PJ, Gleason PA. Lactose-malabsorption following rotavirus infection in young-children. J Pediatr 1981;99:916–8.
186. Ziambaras T, Rubin DC, Perlmutter DH. Regulation of sucrase-isomaltase gene expression in human intestinal epithelial cells by cytokines. J Biol Chem 1996;271:1237–42.
187. King CE, Toskes PP. Small-intestine bacterial overgrowth. Gastroenterology 1979;76:1035–55.
188. Giannell RA, Rout WR, Toskes PP. Jejunal brush-border injury and impaired sugar and amino-acid uptake in blind loop syndrome. Gastroenterology 1974;67:965–74.
189. Jonas A, Flanagan PR, Forstner GG. Pathogenesis of mucosal injury in blind loop syndrome—brush-border enzyme-activity and glycoprotein degradation. J Clin Invest 1977;60:1321–30.
190. Jonas A, Krishnan C, Forstner G. pathogenesis of mucosal injury in blind loop syndrome-release of disaccharidases from brush-border membranes by extracts of bacteria obtained from intestinal blind loops in rats. Gastroenterology 1978;75:791–5.
191. Jonas A, Forstner G. Effect of biliary diversion on mucosal enzyme-activity and brush-border glycoprotein degradation in rats with self-filling blind loops. Eur J Clin Invest 1979;9:167–73.

192. Riepe SP, Goldstein J, Alpers DH. Effect of secreted bacteroides proteases on human intestinal brush-border hydrolases. J Clin Invest 1980;66:314–22.
193. Gilat T, Gelmanma E, Russo S, Aldor TAM. Lactase in man—nonadaptable enzyme. Gastroenterology 1972;62:1125–7.
194. Rosensweig NS, Herman RH. Control of jejunal sucrase and maltase activity by dietary sucrose or fructose in man. A model for the study of enzyme regulation in man. J Clin Invest 1968;47:2253–62.
195. Daum F, Cohen MI, Mcnamara H, Finberg L. Intestinal osmolality and carbohydrate-absorption in rats treated with polymerized glucose. Pediatr Res 1978;12:24–6.
196. Klish WJ, Udall JN, Calvin RT, Nichols BL. The effect of intestinal solute load on water secretion in infants with acquired monosaccharide intolerance. Pediatr Res 1980;14:1343–6.
197. Kolars JC, Levitt MD, Aouji M, Savaiano DA. Yogurt—An autodigesting source of lactose. N Engl J Med 1984;310:1–3.
198. Saltzman JR, Russell RM, Golner B, et al. A randomized trial of *Lactobacillus acidophilus* BG2FO4 to treat lactose intolerance. Am J Clin Nutr 1999;69:140–6.
199. Hyams JS. Sorbitol intolerance—an unappreciated cause of functional gastrointestinal complaints. Gastroenterology 1983;84:30–3.
200. Biller JA, King S, Rosenthal A, Grand RJ. Efficacy of lactase-treated milk for lactose-intolerant pediatric-patients. J Pediatr 1987;111:91–4.

62

Nutritional Anemias

Ellen Butensky, PhD, PNP
Paul Harmatz, MD
Bertram Lubin, MD

INTRODUCTION

Anemia is defined as a circulating red blood cell mass inadequate to prevent tissue hypoxia. Anemia can be related to blood loss, decreased red cell production, increased red cell destruction, or a combination of these events. When anemia occurs as a consequence of a nutritional deficiency, any of these pathologic processes may be involved, either singly or in combination. Vitamin deficiencies that have been implicated as causes of anemia in humans include vitamin A, members of the vitamin B group [pyridoxine (B_6), riboflavin (B_2), folate (B_9), and cyanocobalamin (B_{12})], vitamin C, and vitamin E. Among minerals, iron and copper are recognized as essential for optimal erythropoiesis. Complex nutritional disturbances, such as those observed in starvation and protein/calorie deficiency states, can also result in anemia.

Hemoglobin, hematocrit, and red cell indices (mean cell volume, MCV, mean corpuscular hemoglobin, MCH, and mean corpuscular hemoglobin concentration, MCHC) are the initial laboratory assessments used to diagnose and classify an anemia. It is important to recognize and adjust for the age-related changes in these parameters when assessing anemia in the pediatric age group (Table 1).[1,2] These parameters can help classify the anemia (Figure 1)[3] as one due to decreased red cell production versus increased red cell destruction, acute blood loss, or impaired hemoglobin production. If the anemia is secondary to inhibited hemoglobin synthesis, the anemia will be characterized from these laboratory parameters as microcytic and hypochromic (decreased red cell indices). Conversely, if the anemia results as a consequence of a disturbance in cell maturation, the anemia may be described as macrocytic (increased red cell indices). If the deformability of the red cell membrane is altered, the anemia will have a hemolytic component, an elevated reticulocyte count, and normocytic or macrocytic red cell indices. Nutritional deficiency states often result in combinations of decreased hemoglobin synthesis, abnormal red cell maturation, increased red cell destruction, or decreased RBC production, making straightforward classification as shown in Figure 1 difficult.

The most common nutritional deficiency responsible for anemia is iron deficiency. Nutritional deficiencies of folic acid or vitamin B_{12} are also occasionally encountered in clinical practice and patients with chronic illness may have other vitamin, mineral, and protein deficiencies contributing to anemia. In this chapter, we will review relationships between nutritional deficiencies and anemia and discuss responsible mechanisms. The etiology of the vitamin and mineral deficiencies will not be discussed in detail as this information is provided elsewhere in this book.

MEGALOBLASTIC ANEMIAS: FOLATE AND VITAMIN B_{12} DEFICIENCIES

Nutrient deficiency of either folate or vitamin B_{12} results in a megaloblastic anemia. The fundamental biochemical defect related to vitamin B_{12} or folate deficiencies is decreased synthesis of deoxyribonucleoprotein (DNA). This appears to be the result of the inadequate conversion of deoxyuridylate to thymidylate related to inadequate quantities of 5,10-methylene tetrahydrofolate for the single carbon transfer reaction.[4] Vitamin B_{12} is required for the release of folate from its methyl form so that it can return to the tetrahydrofolate pool for conversion to 5,10-methylene tetrahydrofolate. In vitamin B_{12} deficiency, folate is trapped as methylfolate which is metabolically inactive. This abnormality of folate metabolism is known as the "folate trap" hypothesis.[5–7]

The morphologic representation of this decreased DNA synthesis is the megaloblast. Megaloblasts are nucleated red blood cells that display lacy nuclear chromatin and prominent parachromatin pattern, and an apparent dyssynchrony of maturation between the nucleus and the cytoplasm. This dyssynchrony is produced by the slow DNA synthesis in the nucleus in relation to the near-normal synthesis of RNA in the cytoplasm. Although these morphologic abnormalities in the maturing erythroid precursors are regarded as the hallmark of folic acid or vitamin B_{12} deficiency, these same abnormalities are also evident in the myeloid and megakaryocytic cell lines.

In an established case of megaloblastic anemia, the circulating red cells are macrocytic, with an MCV increased to a range of 105 to 160 femtoliters (fl). The presence of simultaneous iron deficiency may obscure the macrocytosis resulting in a normocytic anemia. Polychromia and fine

Table 1 Red Blood Cell Values at Various Ages: Mean and Lower Limit of Normal (–2 SD)

	Hemoglobin (g/dL)		Hematocrit (%)		MCV (fl)	
	Mean	Lower Limit	Mean	Lower Limit	Mean	Lower Limit
Age						
Birth (cord blood)	16.5	13.5	51	42	108	98
1–3 d (capillary)	18.5	14.5	56	45	108	95
1 wk	17.5	13.5	54	42	107	88
2 wk	16.5	12.5	51	39	105	86
1 mo	14.0	10.0	43	31	104	85
3–6 mo	11.5	9.0	35	28	96	77
0.5–1.9 yr	11.5	9.5	35	29	91	74
2–4 yr	12.0	11.0	37	33	77	70
5–7 yr	12.5	11.0	38	34	79	73
8–11 yr	13.0	11.5	39	35	81	75
12–14 yr	13.5	12.0	40	36	83	76
Female	13.5	12.0	41	36	85	78
Male						
15–17 yr	14.0	12.5	43	37	84	77
Female	14.0	12.0	41	36	87	79
Male						
19–49 yr	15.0	13.0	46	38	86	78
Female	14.0	12.0	42	37	90	80
Male	16.0	14.0	47	40	90	80

Adapted from references 1 and 2.
MCV = mean corpuscular volume.

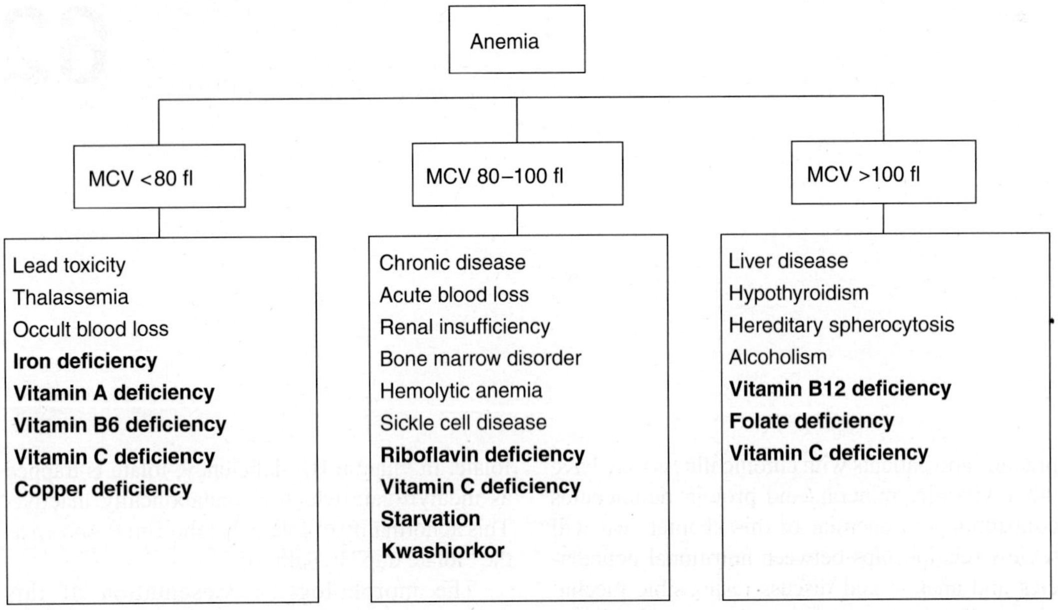

Figure 1 Initial laboratory evaluation of anemia. (Adapted from reference 3.)

basophilic stippling of the erythrocytes are observed and Howell–Jolly bodies, nuclear remnants normally extruded from the erythrocyte during cell maturation, may be present. The concentration of serum iron and nontransferrin bound iron is increased due to impaired erythrocytosis.[8] The red cell life span is modestly reduced, perhaps due to an abnormality in membrane properties related to the dyserythropoietic state. A significant degree of ineffective erythropoiesis is present,[9] which may be reflected by increases in serum bilirubin, serum LDH,[10] and nontransferrin bound iron.[8]

The earliest morphologic change in the megaloblastic anemias is alteration in the circulating granulocytes, which become hypersegmented. In the normal child, the average number of nuclear segments is 2.6. In megaloblastic anemias, the average number of segments generally exceeds a mean value of 3.0 and is often six or greater.[10] In severe forms of deficiency, both neutropenia and thrombocytopenia may be present.

Deficiencies of either folate or B_{12}, from any mechanism, are uncommon in the pediatric population in the United States. However, when they do occur, it may be as a result of inadequate ingestion, absorption, or utilization due to congenital or acquired defects. Not all megaloblastic anemias are due to a lack of these vitamins. Megaloblastosis can also be seen in thiamine deficiency, Lesch–Nyhan syndrome, congenital dyserythropoietic anemias, or as a side effect of chemotherapeutic agents (methotrexate and cytosine arabinoside), antimalarials, and antibacterials (trimethoprim). These antifolates have an affinity for dehydrofolate reductase (DHFR). When intracellular folate concentrations are low, they may inhibit DHFR activity and cause folate deficiency.

FOLIC ACID DEFICIENCY

The clinical manifestations of folate deficiency include megaloblastic changes (not necessarily anemia or pancytopenia), gastrointestinal symptoms such as glossitis, anorexia, gastrointestinal discomfort or occasional diarrhea, humoral and cellular immune defects, and neurologic abnormalities including depression, poor judgment, and some affective disorders.[11]

Folate is present in a wide variety of foods. Cow's milk, human milk, and proprietary infant formulas normally provide approximately 50 μg/L. In contrast, goat's milk contains only 2 to 11 μg/L, and the feeding of goat's milk to infants as the sole source of nutrition will result in the appearance of a megaloblastic anemia.[13] Although dietary folic acid deficiency appears to be unusual in the United States, it is a common cause of megaloblastic anemia in developing countries. Folate deficiency may accompany kwashiorkor, and its incidence has been found to range from 10 to 70%. This variation presumably reflects regional dietary practices such as overcooking of foods or boiling of milk can reduce the folate content by approximately 50%.[14] Both malabsorption and chronic infection may also contribute to this folic acid deficiency.

Table 2 Etiologic and Pathophsiologic Classification of Folate Deficiency

I. Nutritional causes
  A. Decreased dietary intake
    1. Poverty and famine (associated with kwashiorkor, marasmus)
    2. Institutionalized individuals (psychiatric and nursing homes)
    3. Chronic debilitating disease
    4. Goat's milk, special diets (phenylketonuria, maple syrup urine disease, slimming)
    5. Cultural/ethnic cooking techniques (food folate destroyed) or habits (folate-rich foods not consumed)
  B. Decreased diet and increased requirements
    1. Physiologic
      (a) Pregnancy
      (b) Lactation
      (c) Prematurity, infancy
    2. Pathologic
      (a) Intrinsic hematologic disease [autoimmune hemolytic anemia, drugs; malaria, hemoglobinopathy (ie, sickle cell disease, thalassemia); membrane defects; hereditary spherocytosis, paroxysmal nocturnal hemoglobinuria]
      (b) Abnormal hematopoiesis (leukemia, lymphoma, myelodysplastic syndrome, agnogenic myeloid metaplasia with myelofibrosis)
      (c) Infiltration with malignant disease
      (d) Dermatologic (psoriasis, methotrexate dermatopathies)

II. Folate malabsorption
  A. With normal intestinal mucosa
    1. Some drugs (controversial)
    2. Congenital folate malabsorption
  B. With mucosal abnormalities
    1. Tropical sprue
    2. Nontropical sprue
    3. Regional enteritis

III. Defective cellular folate uptake
  A. Familial aplastic anemia

IV. Inadequate cellular utilization
  A. Folate antagonists (methotrexate)
  B. Hereditary enzyme deficiencies involving folate

V. Drugs (multiple effects on folate metabolism)
  A. Alcohol
  B. Sulfasalazine
  C. Triamterene
  D. Pyrimethamine
  E. Trimethopirm-sulfamethoxazole
  F. Anticonvulsants (diphenylhydantoin, barbiturates)

VI. Acute folate deficiency

Adapted from reference 12.

Developmental changes in folate balance are seen during infancy. Serum and red cell folate concentrations are higher in both preterm and term infants than in normal adults.[15] After birth, serum values decline rapidly, but the decline is most severe in infants weighing less than 1,700 g at birth. Approximately two-thirds of low-birth-weight infants may display subnormal serum folate concentrations between 1 and 3 months of age, but they rarely have a megaloblastic anemia. Administration of supplemental folic acid, in the absence of megaloblastic anemia, has not been demonstrated to produce any increase in the hemoglobin concentration. The normal preterm infant absorbs folic acid without difficulty and the dietary provision of 20 to 50 μg/d appears adequate to prevent the development of a deficiency. The presence of chronic infection or diarrhea may impair absorption or increase needs in these small infants.

Folate requirements appear greater in the preterm infant, in pregnant women, in whom folate is shunted to the developing fetus and urinary folate loss is increased, and in lactating women, who secrete 50 μg or more into each liter of milk.[16] Other groups of patients with higher than normal folate requirements include those with celiac disease and other diseases of the small intestine, those taking antiepileptic medication or birth control pills, and persons with hemolytic anemia, including those with sickle cell anemia and thalassemia.[11]

Laboratory Diagnosis of Folate Deficiency

In addition to the characteristic laboratory findings of megaloblastic anemia, such as macrocytosis, multilobulated polymorphonuclear cells, increased LDH and bilirubin, bone marrow showing megaloblastic changes, increased plasma iron and transferrin saturation, and decreased serum cholesterol and lipids, specific measurements provide direct evidence of deficiency of folate. These include decreased serum folate, decreased erythrocyte folate, homocysteinemia, and sometimes homocystinuria.[11] RBC folate is considered a better indicator of folate status than serum folate. RBC levels are significantly higher than normal serum levels and thus less subject to processing artifacts. Red cell folate also has been reported to parallel tissue stores and is, therefore, more useful than serum folate for documenting the presence of a long-standing deficiency.[17] The normal range of serum folate is 3 to 15 ng/mL. Serum folate values in the 1.5 to 3.0 range are regarded as "indeterminate." The red cell folate normally ranges from 150 to 600 ng/mL, and values of less than 150 ng/mL are diagnostic of deficiency.

VITAMIN B_{12} DEFICIENCY

Vitamin B_{12}, or cobalamin, is an organometallic complex consisting of two major moieties: a corrin nucleus containing a covalently bound cobalt atom, and a nucleotide base lying at right angles to the corrin nucleus. Hydroxycobalamin is the predominant dietary form of the vitamin. Vitamin B_{12} is synthesized by bacteria, is present in animal foods, and is not present in plants; therefore it does not occur in vegetables or fruit.

Only two metabolic functions for the vitamin B_{12} coenzymes, 5-adenosylcobalamin and methylcobalamin, have been identified in humans. The first of these is the conversion of L-methylmalonyl-CoA to succinyl-CoA, a reaction catalyzed by methylmalonyl-CoA mutase and requiring 5-adenosylcobalamin. Defects in the conversion of L-methylmalonyl-CoA to succinyl-CoA result in methylmalonic acidemia (MMA) and methylmalonic aciduria. The second reaction in which vitamin B_{12} is a cofactor is the homocysteine 5-methyl-tetrahydrofolate methyltransferase reaction. This reaction generates methionine from homocysteine using methionine synthase and produces tetrahydrofolic acid from 5-methyl-tetrahydrofolic acid.[18]

Dietary vitamin B_{12}, primarily in the form of hydroxycobalamin, is absorbed in the terminal ileum and requires the presence of intrinsic factor that has been secreted in the parietal cells of the stomach. Nutritional deficiency of vitamin B_{12} is extremely rare in infants and children.

It is estimated that the older child and adult require 1.0 μg of vitamin B_{12}/d, and the infant 0.1 μg/d, to maintain normal erythropoiesis. The normal diet usually contains far more B_{12} than this minimal requirement. Western diets usually contain 5 to 10 μg daily. The highest concentrations are found in liver, kidney, meat muscle, fowl, shellfish, and dairy products. There is probably no vitamin B_{12} in fruits, vegetables, nuts, or cereal unless they are contaminated with vitamin B_{12}-producing bacteria. Vitamin B_{12} is usually not destroyed by cooking. Under alkaline conditions and the presence of ascorbic acid, some vitamin B_{12} may be lost when milk is boiled or when meat is overcooked.

The average daily vitamin B_{12} output in breast milk is approximately 0.3 μg and closely parallels the serum vitamin B_{12} concentration of the mother.[19] The term infant receives approximately 30 μg of vitamin B_{12} from the mother during the course of gestation. Liver stores are about 26 μg in term infants but only 10 μg in premature infants.[20] Serum vitamin B_{12} values in the newborn are normally much higher than those of the mother. Because of this adequate endowment, vitamin B_{12} deficiency due to inadequate ingestion in the first year or two of life is seen only when an infant is born to a severely vitamin B_{12}-deficient mother and is exclusively breastfed by her or placed on a strict vegetarian diet. Megaloblastic anemia in the infants of strict vegetarian mothers has been reported from India.[21] Megaloblastic anemia in breastfed infants of mothers who either have untreated pernicious anemia[22] or are on vegetarian diets has also been observed in 5- to 6-month-old infants in the United States.[23] In many of these cases, the infant presents with evidence of neurologic involvement as well as a macrocytic anemia. Both resolve following treatment with vitamin B_{12}.

The juvenile form of pernicious anemia resembles that seen in adults. These children have gastric atrophy, gastric achlorhydria, absent intrinsic factor, and a high incidence of antibody against intrinsic factor. Some children with pernicious anemia, like adults, have associated endocrinopathies such as hypoparathyroidism, hypothyroidism, and Addison's disease. An association of selective IgA deficiency with juvenile pernicious anemia has also been observed.

The biochemical changes associated with vitamin B_{12} deficiency include MMA and aciduria. The secondary effects of MMA accumulation including acidosis, hyperglycinemia, and possibly inhibition of other enzymes and of bone marrow stem cells by accumulated MMA,[24–27] homocystinemia, and homocystinuria, can be found. Inadequate levels of THF in cells, producing defective rates of polyglutamyl folate synthesis and deficiency of folates required for some intracellular reactions, are observed. Defective thymidylate synthesis, defective synthesis of endogenous purines, defective detoxification of formate, and accumulation of formiminoglutamate, 5(4)-amidoimidazole-4(5) carboxyribonucleotide and other intermediates of folate-dependent reactions are present. Biochemical central nervous system (CNS) changes, which might relate to defective methylation of myelin basic protein, have been reported.[28–30] Finally, intracellular folate levels are lower than expected for the concentration of folate in plasma.[11]

The onset of symptoms is often insidious and may include pallor, apathy, fatigability, and anorexia. These symptoms are not specific for vitamin B_{12} deficiency. A beefy red and sore tongue with papillary atrophy may be observed. Paresthesias may be reported in the older child. Signs of subacute dorsolateral degeneration are uncommon in children, but loss of vibration and position sense may be seen. When neurologic disease is present, the lower limbs are more severely affected. The neurologic changes may precede the appearance of anemia. A number of gastrointestinal symptoms have been reported. The peripheral blood findings and bone marrow findings in vitamin B_{12} deficiency resemble those observed with folic acid deficiency.

Laboratory Diagnosis of B_{12} Deficiency

The general findings secondary to megaloblastic anemia are similar to those indicated above for deficiency of folic acid. Specific measurements for vitamin B_{12} deficiency include decreased serum cobalamin, excess methylmalonic acid in the urine or serum, homocystinemia and sometimes homocystinuria, and abnormal deoxyuridine suppression test in bone marrow, corrected in vitro by addition of MeCbl or 5-formyl-THF but not by methyl-THF.

The serum vitamin B_{12} level is deficient when it is less than 100 pg/mL (normal 200 to 800 pg/mL). If the dietary history indicates a normal vitamin B_{12} intake, absorption of cobalt-labeled B_{12} should be performed by the Schilling test. For this purpose, a standard dose of the labeled vitamin (0.5 μg) is given orally after an overnight fast, and then a "flushing dose" of 1,000 μg of vitamin B_{12} is given parenterally 2 hours after the oral dose. Less than 7% of the labeled dose will appear in the urine during the 24-hour collection period if there is a lack of intrinsic factor or malabsorption of vitamin B_{12} for any other reason. If absorption is impaired, the Schilling test is repeated with the simultaneous administration of both intrinsic factor and labeled vitamin B_{12}. Improvement in the urinary excretion of the labeled B_{12} confirms the diagnosis of intrinsic factor deficiency. Gastric biopsy, the measurement of gastric acid secretion, and assay of intrinsic factor in gastric juice all help to categorize the nature of the underlying disturbance.

A therapeutic trial may be employed for the diagnosis of vitamin B_{12} deficiency. A dose of 0.5 μg of cyanocobalamin or hydroxycobalamin is given parenterally for 7 to 10 days. A reticulocytosis and increase in hemoglobin concentration should be observed. If the diagnosis has been firmly established, a therapeutic trial may be omitted and the patient may be treated with daily oral doses of 25 to 100 μg. If the patient has any form of B_{12} malabsorption, rather than a primary nutritional deficiency, maintenance therapy should consist of monthly injections of 50 to 1,000 μg, depending on the patient's age and weight. Recently, a nasal gel form of vitamin B_{12} (Questcor Pharmaceuticals, Union City, CA) was approved and has been shown to be safe and effective in treating pernicious anemia.

IRON-DEFICIENCY ANEMIA

Iron deficiency continues to be the most common nutritional cause of anemia worldwide, affecting as many as 4 to 5 billion people.[31] The prevalence of iron deficiency has been declining in industrialized countries over the past few decades, in part, due to an increase in breastfeeding and fortification of infant formulas and cereals.[32] Unfortunately, most of the rest of the world has not experienced such a decline; an estimated 90% of cases occur in developing countries, impacting significantly on morbidity, mortality, and national development.[31]

Iron is a vitally important nutrient that serves multiple functions in the body. It is the functional group in hemoglobin for oxygen transport in the red blood cell and it helps with storage of oxygen in myoglobin in muscle. Iron is also present in peroxidase, catalase, and the cytochromes. Anemia, a treatable condition, is the most common clinical problem associated with iron deficiency. However, the real public health concerns are the cognitive and behavioral impairments seen in infants and children,[33–37] the fatigue and decreased work capability in older children and adults,[33] and the association of severe iron-deficiency anemia in pregnant women with prematurity, perinatal mortality, and low-birth-weight infants.[37–40]

Iron is found in many different food sources; however, the bioavailability is highly variable. Heme iron is more readily absorbed than nonheme iron, as it is absorbed in the intestinal mucosa in the intact protoporphyrin ring. Nonheme iron must be reduced from the ferric state to the ferrous state, which requires a low gastric pH, and its absorption is influenced by many other constituents in the concurrent meal.[41,42] Orange juice facilitates absorption whereas tea hinders it. Other enhancers of iron absorption include fructose, certain amino acids, meat, fish, and poultry. Inhibitors include phosphates, phytates (common in vegetarian diets), tannins, and oxalates.[43,44]

The body, based on its needs, attempts to maintain a balance between iron stores, recycled iron, and dietary iron intake. One-third of an infant's iron needs come from dietary sources; the remainder is recycled from red blood cell breakdown. Over time this changes, so that by adulthood an even greater proportion of iron needs come from recycled iron such that there is less reliance on the diet for iron.[45]

FETAL–MATERNAL RELATIONSHIPS

The iron content of the normal newborn infant is approximately 75 mg/kg as determined by carcass analysis of stillbirths.[46] Studies performed during various stages of pregnancy indicate that the iron content of the fetus and the weight of the fetus increase proportionately with age. Under usual circumstances, 66 to 75% of the infant's iron is present in the red cell mass. Storage iron in the liver and spleen, although subject to great variability, makes up approximately 6% of the total iron while nonhemoglobin iron in the form of cytochromes, myglobin, and other iron-containing enzymes account for approximately 24%.[47]

The bulk of the infant's iron endowment at birth is represented by the red cell mass. As a result, the amount of iron in the body at the time of birth depends on the blood volume and the hemoglobin concentration. Any complications during pregnancy or the perinatal period that result in fetal blood loss will compromise the infant's iron endowment. Unless extreme, the presence of maternal iron deficiency does not appear to compromise the iron endowment of the fetus. The hemoglobin concentration in the cord blood of infants born to anemic iron-deficient mothers does not differ from that of infants born to iron-sufficient mothers until maternal hemoglobin values fall below 6.0 g/dL.[48] With extreme maternal iron-deficiency anemia, the placenta is small and the cord blood hemoglobin concentration is reduced. Some studies have observed that women with low serum iron values tend to have infants with lower than normal serum iron levels[49]; other studies have found no difference in the state of the infant's iron nutrition at 6, 12, and 18 months of age, regardless of whether their mothers had received iron supplementation during pregnancy.[50,51] Employing plasma ferritin concentrations as an index of iron sufficiency, Rios and coworkers were unable to document any correlation between plasma ferritin concentrations in mothers with high and low values and the plasma ferritin concentrations of their infants at birth or at 1.5 months of age.[52] It may be concluded from these studies that, except in the most unusual circumstances, maternal iron deficiency by itself does not result in iron-deficiency anemia in the infant, either at birth or later in the first year of life. Factors such as rate of growth relative to birthweight, initial iron endowment that has been compromised by blood loss, and infant nutrition seem to be far more important in determining the later appearance of anemia.

At birth the newborn has a large number of reticulocytes and a relatively high hemoglobin concentration with a mean of 16.6 g/dL.[53] The hemoglobin increases over the first few days and then, as erythropoiesis slows in the marrow and extramedullary spaces, the hemoglobin falls, reaching a nadir in 6 to 8 weeks. Erythropoiesis is then stimulated and the hemoglobin rises to 12.5 g/dL, which is the mean throughout infancy.[53] Preterm infants have a more dramatic fall in hemoglobin to a mean of about 9 g/dL at the nadir, though the marrow recovery is good, and at 6 months of age these infants have the same mean hemoglobin concentration as a term infant.[54]

Iron Requirements

Iron requirements are age dependent. It is rare for a term infant to become iron deficient before 4 months of age, but a preterm infant can become deficient by 2 to 3 months because of relatively faster growth and smaller iron stores at birth.[53] Children, from birth through adolescence, need iron for growth and increasing blood volume, as well as to replace losses. Although the amounts are small in an infant, averaging 20 μg/kg/d, iron is lost in sweat, urine, bile, desquamation of skin and intestinal cells, and through hair and nail loss.[32] The Committee on Nutrition of the American Academy of Pediatrics made the following recommendation for daily iron requirements for premature infants: (1) breastfed infants, 2 mg/kg/d from 1 month to 12 months of age; (2) formula-fed infants, 1 mg/kg/d through the first year of life.[16] Adequate intake (AI) for infants 0 to 6 months is 0.27 mg/d and the dietary reference intake (DRI) is: 7 to 12 months, 11 mg/d; 1 to 2 years, 7 mg/d; 3 to 8 years, 10 mg/d; 9 to 13 years, 8 mg/d; 14 to 18 years, boys 11 mg/d, girls 15 mg/d; pregnancy 27 mg/d.[55]

Manifestations

With the decline in iron-deficiency anemia in industrialized countries, children with the manifestations of severe longstanding iron-deficiency anemia are rare. Sadly, they are still seen elsewhere. Mild to moderate iron-deficiency anemia is most common. Frequently the first signs and symptoms of iron-deficiency anemia are pallor, fatigue, exercise intolerance, and occasionally palpitations. The pallor is most notable in the nail beds, conjunctiva, and palms, especially if the individual has dark skin. Fatigue and exercise intolerance have been best documented in studies of adults employed at physical labor revealing that even mild anemia can affect exercise tolerance in settings involving strenuous energy expenditure, and that correction of the anemia increased exercise tolerance.[56–58] The phenomenom of pica or compulsive consumption of nonnutritional items such as dirt, clay, cornstarch, laundry detergent, or ice is a characteristic finding of iron-deficiency anemia. Ingestion of these items often exacerbates the underlying iron deficiency by further impairing absorption.[59]

The recognition that iron deficiency produces a broad array of systemic effects has attracted increasing attention.[45,60] A partial list of nonhematologic manifestations of iron deficiency are provided in Table 3.[61] Over time, glossitis, stomatitis, and angular cheilosis may develop. These symptoms may be the result of tissue iron deficiency rather than the anemia itself.[62] Koilonychia, or spooning of the fingernails, is caused by abnormal proliferation of the cells of the nail bed. Other features of severe longstanding iron-deficiency anemia can actually make treatment with oral iron supplementation difficult. The presence of esophageal webs, or Plummer–Vinson syndrome, impairs swallowing, atrophic gastritis, and abnormal duodenal mucosa can each decrease absorption.

There have been numerous studies investigating immune function associated with iron-deficiency anemia.[33,63–72] Paradoxically, iron overload has also been shown to impair normal immune function, decreasing lymphocyte proliferation and the ability of macrophages to kill intracellular pathogens.[73] Similarly, both iron deficiency and iron overload have been associated with increased infection. In one study, anemia was associated with malaria, acute respiratory infection, and diarrhea.[74] and in other studies, individuals with malaria,[75] hepatitis C virus infection[76] and human immunodeficiency virus infection[77] have worse outcomes if they have excess iron. This suggests that there is a level of optimal body iron with deficiency or overload leading to abnormal immune function.

Iron plays an important role in brain development and many studies have indicated that iron deficiency is associated with cognitive impairment, poor motor development, and behavioral problems.[33–36,78–80] This is particularly disturbing as these problems may continue long term, even after correction of the anemia. However, it should be noted that a causal relationship has not been established as important potential confounding variables have not been fully accounted for. It is also not clear that CNS effects can be remedied by iron therapy, as many of the clinical trials have failed to demonstrate benefit from therapy.[81,82]

Iron is essential to the metabolism of certain amine neurotransmitters.[33] Children with iron-deficiency anemia have increased catecholamines in their urine which return to normal levels after iron therapy.[83] There have been animal studies suggesting abnormal dopamine receptor function in association with iron-deficiency anemia.[84] The exact meaning of these findings and how they relate to cognitive and behavioral development remains unclear.

Table 3 Nonhematologic Manifestations of Iron Deficiency

1. Impaired growth
2. Skin and mucous membranes
   (a) Koilonychia
   (b) Angular stomatitis
   (c) Glossitis
3. Gastrointestinal tract
   (a) Anorexia
   (b) Dysphagia with postcricoid webs
   (c) Gastric achlorhydria
   (d) Malabsorption
   (e) Beeturia
   (f) Exudative enteropathy and occult bleeding
4. Central nervous system
   (a) Irritability
   (b) Decreased attention span
   (c) Poor performance in standardized developmental testing
   (d) Breath-holding spells
5. Impaired exercise tolerance
6. Immunologic response
   (a) Impaired lymphocyte mitogen response
   (b) Decreased leukocyte killing

Laboratory Findings

The diagnosis of iron-deficiency anemia is rarely made based on a single laboratory test, but rather on a combination of several tests and the comparison to age-specific norms reflecting the changes that occur as a child grows. Commonly used tests assess the iron storage, erythropoiesis, and severity of the anemia (Table 4). Together these tests can help to rule out other causes of anemia.

Iron deficiency occurs in various stages. First, there is depletion of iron stores in the body. This stage is unlikely to be diagnosed by any routine screening laboratory tests. Next, there is iron deficiency with anemia, initially with a normal MCV. As the deficiency continues, erythropoiesis is significantly impaired, and the diagnosis becomes more evident with obvious hypochromia and microcytosis on peripheral blood smear, in conjunction with some of the nonhematologic manifestations of this condition.

Peripheral Smear. Often microscopic examination of the blood smear can be normal early in iron deficiency, but as the anemia progresses hypochromia, microcytosis, anisocytosis, and occasional target cells and elliptocytes are seen.

Hemoglobin. Anemia starts when this value is greater than 2 standard deviations below the normal mean for age. Thus it is essential to use age-based mean hemoglobin values for accurate interpretation of these results.

Table 4 Laboratory Measurements of Iron Status

1. Storage iron depletion
   (a) Bone marrow iron stain (decreased)
   (b) Serum ferritin (decreased)
   (c) Serum transferrin (increased)
   (d) Transferrin receptor (increased)
   (e) Serum iron (decreased)*
2. Iron deficiency erythropoiesis
   (a) Transferrin saturation (decreased)
   (b) Total iron-binding capacity (increased)
   (c) Free erythrocyte protoporphyrin (increased)
   (d) Zinc protoporphyrin (increased)
   (e) Red cell mean corpuscular volume (decreased)
   (f) Red cell mean corpuscular hemoglobin (decreased)
   (g) Red cell distribution width (increased)
   (h) Reticulocyte heme (decreased)
3. Iron deficiency anemia
   (a) Hemoglobin (decreased)
   (b) Therapeutic trial with increase in hemoglobin concentration

*See text.

Red Cell Distribution Width. This rarely used index may provide early evidence for iron-deficiency anemia.[85] It represents the variation in size of the red blood cells. In thalassemia, infection, and inflammation, it is usually normal, but in iron-deficiency anemia this value is elevated and can be $>20\%$.[45]

MCV. This value represents the average size of the red blood cell and it varies with age. When anemia becomes significant enough to interfere with hemoglobin synthesis microcytosis occurs (low MCV). This is one of the red cell indices readily available in the routine complete blood count (CBC) from an electronic counter in the laboratory.

MCH. As with the MCV, this index is available from an electronic counter. Initially with iron deficiency the MCH is normal, but with advancing anemia the red blood cell becomes more hypochromic and this change is evident by a low MCH.

Serum Ferritin. Ferritin, the primary intracellular iron storage protein, is also found in small amounts in the circulation. Serum ferritin generally correlates with total body iron although, as an acute phase reactant, ferritin may be increased by inflammatory, infectious, and malignant processes, and this correlation becomes less reliable. In contrast, a few conditions, including vitamin C deficiency, reduced serum ferritin, and scurvy, or vitamin C deficiency, should be evaluated as a potential cause of low ferritin. In general, values less than 10 μg/L are indicative of iron deficiency.

Serum Iron. Serum iron has not been a reliable test for iron-deficiency anemia because of its diurnal pattern with a peak in the morning and a trough in the evening. As with serum ferritin it can be elevated by many other conditions. The concentration is usually low in iron-deficiency anemia. However, even a single dose of iron within the 24 hours prior to the test can cause a transient elevation in the serum iron level, thus possibly masking an underlying iron-deficiency anemia.[62]

Total Iron-Binding Capacity (TIBC) and Transferrin Saturation (TS). Most circulating iron is bound to a plasma protein called transferrin. TIBC is a measure of the total transferrin. As the serum iron decreases, the TIBC increases, and the ratio of these variables in iron-deficiency anemia is less than 1:6.[85] TS is the ratio of serum iron to TIBC multiplied by 100 to yield a percentage. It represents the percent of transferrin that is saturated with iron. A low percentage is suggestive of iron deficiency.

Soluble Transferrin Receptor (sTfR). This receptor can be measured in the circulation and is indicative of the concentration of cellular transferrin receptor. Since receptor synthesis increases with iron deficiency but not with anemia of chronic disease, it is a sensitive indicator of iron deficiency.[86] Because sTfR is also elevated in the presence of ineffective erythropoiesis and sideroblastic anemias, this must be taken into account and evaluated appropriately.

Erythrocyte Protoporphyrin (EP). Under normal circumstances iron combines with protoporphryin in the red blood cell to form heme, a reaction catalyzed by the enzyme ferrochelatase. In iron-deficiency anemia there is an elevation in EP, usually >35 μg/dL.[87] Lead poisoning, which often causes a higher level of EP than iron deficiency, does so by inhibiting ferrochelatase. Inflammatory, infectious, and/or malignant processes also can raise the EP level.[62]

Zinc Protoporphyrin (ZPP). In iron deficiency and lead poisoning, ZPP is formed instead of EP because zinc fills the iron pocket in the protoporphyrin molecule. This is a sensitive, inexpensive test that will show an elevation in iron deficiency before anemia is present.[88] When iron stores are sufficient, the ratio of iron to zinc incorporation into protoporphyrin is 30,000 to 1.[89] Iron deficiency produces an increase in the normal ratio of ≤40 umol ZPP/mol heme.[90] This test alone does not differentiate between iron deficiency and lead poisoning, and so further tests must be done. The issue is complicated because iron deficiency increases the absorption of lead so that in many situations the two disturbances exist together. A lead level and a therapeutic trial of oral iron therapy may be necessary to clarify the diagnosis.

Reticulocyte Heme. Reticulocyte hemoglobin content (CHr) measurement by automated flow cytometry assesses the iron status of red blood cells when they are released from the bone marrow as reticulocytes.[91] It can be used to detect early iron deficiency and has been found to be the strongest predictor of iron deficiency when compared to other commonly used laboratory parameters.[92]

Bone Marrow Biopsy. If the usual tests are equivocal or there are confounding factors making the diagnosis of iron deficiency difficult, such as infection or inflammation, the bone marrow iron stores can be assessed. Staining the specimen with Prussian blue and counterstaining with safranin O helps to show the characteristic paucity of ferritin and hemosiderin, the final breakdown product of iron and ferritin.[54] Normally 10 to 20% of red cell precursors in the marrow contain iron granules; however, in iron deficiency few if any will be present.[93]

Therapy

If iron deficiency is diagnosed or suspected based on some or all of the laboratory tests discussed above, treatment with iron should begin immediately. In most circumstances, oral iron supplementation is used since it is inexpensive and easily absorbed. The dose of iron for infants and children is 4 to 6 mg/kg of elemental iron, depending on the severity of the anemia, divided into two to three doses per day. For adolescents the dose is 100 to 300 mg of elemental iron per day.[94] Traditionally, 3-times-daily dosing has been used but recent research has demonstrated that once-daily dosing results in similar treatment of anemia,[94] and once- or twice-weekly dosing results in similar improvement in hemoglobin but not ferritin.[96] Further work in this area is ongoing, in an attempt to reduce side effects, simplify treatment, and improve compliance.

Ferrous iron is more easily absorbed than ferric iron, and thus the usual treatment for infants and children is ferrous sulfate. Premature infants are frequently vitamin E deficient due to decreased intake, decreased stores, and poor absorption of vitamin E. Since iron therapy inhibits absorption of vitamin E, this deficiency must be corrected before iron therapy is started.[97] The absorption of iron on an empty stomach is about twice that of a full stomach; therefore it is recommended that the dose be given about an hour prior to a meal.

The duration of treatment is 2 to 4 months after the hemoglobin has returned to a level normal for age, in order to replenish the iron stores.[45] If these stores are not replenished because iron therapy is discontinued too soon, a rapid recurrence of iron-deficiency anemia may result. Response to treatment is initially evident by a reticulocytosis peaking in 5 to 10 days from the onset of treatment. During the first week of therapy, the hemoglobin rises about 0.25 to 4 g/dL/d and then slows to about 0.1 g/dL/d.[94] It is important to follow up no more than a month later to see if there is improvement, because if there is no change in that period of time on an adequate dose, and compliance is not an issue, further studies must be done to determine the underlying problem.[45] Failure of oral iron therapy can be the result of impaired absorption, incorrect diagnosis, ongoing blood loss greater than hemoglobin generation, inadequate dose, ineffective iron preparation, superimposed malignancy or inflammatory disease, or, most commonly, simple noncompliance. Compliance can be an issue because of the taste of iron, gastrointestinal distress, or concern of parents that the drops will stain the infant's teeth. These problems can be dealt with by giving the iron with a small amount of food or liquid, preferably something that will enhance the absorption, and by giving the drops in the back of the mouth. If noncompliance is suspected but denied, the stool can be examined. In the presence of iron supplements, it should be black. The stool can also be tested specifically for iron if necessary.

Parenteral iron therapy has greater side effects and is therefore reserved for only specific circumstances. These include true intolerance to oral iron (extremely rare), severe gastrointestinal disease that prevents absorption and may be exacerbated by oral iron therapy, chronic bleeding, or repeated noncompliance.[98,99] There are three parenteral preparations available in the United States: iron dextran, iron sucrose, and iron gluconate, and the maximum dose that can be given at once varies among them.[100] The dose is calculated to correct the anemia and replenish the iron stores. The formula is:

$$\text{Normal Hgb} - \text{Initial Hgb} \times \text{blood volume} \times 3.4 \times 1.5 = \text{mg iron } 100$$

The normal hemoglobin should be based on the age. Blood volume is approximately 80 mL/kg of body weight. The value 3.4 converts the grams of hemoglobin to milligrams of iron, and the factor 1.5 provides a little extra iron to supply the iron stores.[98,99]

A small portion of patients have an anaphylactic reaction to dextran-containing iron preparations, and this should be considered when choosing which preparation to use. Whenever iron dextran treatment is used, a test dose must first be given, and if there is no sign of reaction 5 minutes after the test dose, the therapeutic dose may be started. Epinephrine should be kept at the bedside, as well as resuscitation equipment. Less severe side effects are hypotension and flushing (2%), phlebitis (10%), and a delayed rash with or without arthritis (20%).[98,99]

In extreme iron-deficiency anemia with a very low hemoglobin and/or cardiovascular instability, a packed red blood cell transfusion is given first to stabilize the patient. This is usually followed by oral iron therapy. In this situation the transfusion is given slowly, at 5 cc/kg over 4 hours to start. Depending on how much more blood is necessary to increase the hemoglobin to the desired level, the rest of the transfusion can be broken into aliquots and given slowly or at the usual rate for a transfusion.[94]

OTHER VITAMIN AND METAL DEFICIENCY-RELATED ANEMIAS

Vitamin A Deficiency

Chronic vitamin A deficiency results in an anemia with certain characteristics similar to those observed in iron deficiency. Mean red cell volume and MCHC are reduced, anisocytosis and poikilocytosis may be present, and serum iron values are low.[101–104] Unlike iron deficiency, however, liver and marrow iron stores are increased, serum ferritin values are normal, serum transferrin concentration is usually normal or decreased, and the administration of therapeutic doses of iron may not correct the anemia. These findings suggest that this hypochromic, microcytic anemia may be related to a failure of iron transport from storage sites to active metabolic pools.

Several large pediatric studies conducted in developing countries support a relationship between serum concentration of vitamin A and blood hemoglobin concentration.[104–108] This relationship was confirmed in experimental studies showing a correlation between plasma retinol and hemoglobin in adult men with induced vitamin A deficiency.[102] Finally, studies in underdeveloped countries have shown that treating anemia with vitamin A in combination with iron is more effective than iron alone, again supporting a causal relationship.[102,109–112]

Pyridoxine Deficiency

The vitamin B_6 group includes pyridoxal, pyridoxine, and pyridoxamine. These substances are all phosphorylated to pyridoxal-5-phosphate (PLP), which is an essential cofactor in heme biosynthesis mediated by D-aminolevulinic acid synthetase.[113,114] Limited animal and human studies support a relationship between pyridoxine deficiency and anemia. In animals with experimentally induced pyridoxine deficiency, Bottomly and colleagues observed anemia and ringed sideroblasts.[115] Experimental induction of vitamin B_6 deficiency in two infants was associated with a hypochromic, microcytic anemia,[116] and a malnourished patient has been described whose hypochromic anemia failed to respond to iron therapy but subsequently responded to the administration of vitamin B_6.[117]

Nutritional deficiencies of pyridoxine are extremely rare, although patients receiving therapy with antituberculosis drugs such as isoniazid, which interferes with the transport of pyridoxine to cells,[115,118,119] can develop a microcytic anemia. This anemia was corrected with large doses of pyridoxine.[120,121] A small percentage of patients with congenital or acquired sideroblastic anemia improve on treatment with pharmacologic doses of pyridoxine.[122,123] There are also reports of sideroblastic anemia due to vitamin B_6 deficiency occurring in patients on hemodialysis.[113] Administration of pyridoxine with isoniazid or during dialysis may decrease the risk of these complications.

Riboflavin Deficiency

While anemia secondary to riboflavin deficiency has been demonstrated in several animal models, it has been difficult to establish a direct causal role in humans.[124] The best evidence has been provided by experimental studies. Human volunteers with malignancies maintained on a riboflavin-deficient diet and fed the riboflavin antagonist, galactoflavin, developed pure red cell aplasia.[125] Vacuolated erythroid precursors were evident prior to the development of aplasia. Red cell indices were normal and the reticulocyte count was low. This anemia was corrected by the administration of riboflavin. Confirmation of this response to riboflavin supplementation has been seen in both human adult and pediatric populations with anemia.[126,127]

Riboflavin-deficient children given riboflavin demonstrated a decrease in serum iron and TS accompanied by an increase in hemoglobin if the initial hemoglobin was below 13.5 g/mL, supporting a relationship between riboflavin and iron utilization.[127] Abnormal iron utilization as a possible mechanism for riboflavin-induced anemia was explored in rodent studies that have shown that riboflavin deficiency was associated with reduced iron absorption and increased iron loss.[128,129] In addition, ferrokinetic studies in humans receiving the riboflavin-deficient diet and galactoflavin demonstrated distribution of iron primarily to liver and spleen in contrast to bone marrow in normals. Clearly, riboflavin has an important role in erythropoiesis, probably by altering iron metabolism.

Riboflavin deficiency has been shown to produce a decrease in red cell glutathione reductase,[130,131] which is necessary for glutathione peroxidase to effectively regulate cellular redox potential.[132,133] Under normal conditions, the decrease in glutathione reductase activity is not associated with an increased sensitivity of the red cell to oxidant-induced injury.[134] It is theoretically possible that riboflavin deficiency in conjunction with increased oxidant stress leaves the red cell vulnerable to oxidation injury, causing hemolytic anemia; however, this has not been described in humans.

Vitamin C (Ascorbic Acid) Deficiency

It is unclear whether ascorbic acid has a direct role in hematopoiesis or whether the anemia observed in subjects with ascorbic acid deficiency (scurvy) is a result of the interactions of ascorbic acid with folic acid and iron metabolism. Although approximately 80% of individuals with scurvy are anemic,[135] attempts to induce anemia in human volunteers by severe restriction of dietary ascorbic acid have been unsuccessful.[136,137] Confusion arises because the anemia observed in subjects with scurvy may be hypochromic, normocytic, or macrocytic; and the marrow may be hypocellular, normocellular, or hypercellular. In about 10% of patients the marrow is megaloblastic.[135]

Ascorbic acid is required to maintain folic acid reductase in its reduced, or active form. Impaired folic acid reductase activity results in an inability to form tetrahydrofolic acid, the metabolically active form of folic acid. It has been demonstrated that patients with scurvy and megaloblastic anemia excrete 10-formylfolic acid as the major urinary folate metabolite. Following ascorbic acid therapy, 5-methyltetrahydrofolic acid becomes the major urinary folate metabolite in these patients. This observation has led to the suggestion that ascorbic acid prevents the irreversible oxidation of methyltetrahydrofolic acid to formylfolic acid.[138] Failure to synthesize tetrahydrofolic acid or to protect it from oxidation in scurvy ultimately results in the appearance of a megaloblastic anemia. Under these circumstances, ascorbic acid therapy will produce a hematologic response only if sufficient folic acid is present to interact with the ascorbic acid.[139]

Iron deficiency in children often occurs in association with ascorbic acid deficiency. Scurvy may cause iron deficiency as a consequence of external bleeding. Iron balance may be further compromised by ascorbic acid deficiency because this vitamin facilitates intestinal iron absorption.[140] Ascorbic acid increases the bioavailability of iron through two mechanisms. First, it can reduce Fe^{3+} to Fe^{2+}, which is more soluble and less likely to form insoluble hydroxides at low pH than Fe^{3+}. Second, it forms a stable complex with iron, preventing iron from complexing with dietary constituents, such as tannins and phytates, which block transport into gastrointestinal mucosal cells.[141] Patients with scurvy, particularly children, often require both iron and ascorbic acid to correct a hypochromic, microcytic anemia.[142] Rarely, a combination of iron, ascorbic acid, and folate may be required.[143]

Despite the evidence linking ascorbic acid deficiency to alterations in either folic acid or iron metabolism, many patients with scurvy have a normocytic, normochromic anemia accompanied by a persistent reticulocytosis of 5 to 10%. Ascorbic acid has antioxidant properties, and it is possible that a deficiency of this vitamin renders the cell susceptible to oxidant injury. This is of particular interest in regard to the possible reducing effects of ascorbic acid on oxidized vitamin E, much like those described above for folic acid.[144] Administration of ascorbic acid to patients with scurvy who have hemolysis produces an initial increase in reticulocyte count, followed by a rise in hemoglobin concentration and an ultimate correction of hematologic abnormalities.[145]

Vitamin E Deficiency

The human fetus at 5 months gestation has a total body vitamin E content of only 1 mg.[146] A term newborn has a body vitamin E content of 20 mg. The normal adult male averages 50 mg/kg, and the female averages 160 mg/kg. This difference in ratio of body vitamin E to body weight presumably reflects differences in body fat composition. The ratio of vitamin E to fat remains relatively constant throughout gestation and averages 0.27 mg of vitamin E per gram of lipid; ratios of 0.24:1.00 have been described for adult males and 0.46:1.00 for adult females.[147,148]

Plasma vitamin E levels average close to 0.9 mg per 100 mL in the mother at term, with a corresponding value of only 0.2 mg per 100 mL in the infant.[149] Although there is a direct relationship between the plasma level of vitamin E in the infant at birth and that of the mother, infants are not born with values above 0.6 mg per 100 mL, the value regarded as the lower limit of normal for older children and adults. When vitamin E concentrations are expressed as vitamin E-lipid ratios, perhaps a more nutritionally valid means of determining vitamin E deficiency, differences between mothers and their infants disappear. The vitamin E-total lipid ratio of mothers at term has been found to average 1.57:1.00, with a ratio of 2.40:1.00 in cord blood.[150]

Infants, both term and preterm, who are fed colostrum and human milk achieve normal plasma vitamin E concentrations by 1 week of age.[3,151] Most of the simulated human milk formulas presently available will produce vitamin E concentrations within the normal adult range when fed to infants during the first 2 weeks of life. The relationship between iron content and vitamin E in the diet may determine the turnover of vitamin E as iron-mediated reactions stimulate lipid peroxidation and increase the requirements for vitamin E.

Hemolytic Anemia and the Premature Infant

Prior to 1967, despite the fact that it was recognized that most proprietary formulas fed to low-birth-weight infants resulted in a prolonged period of vitamin E deficiency, no hematologic abnormalities could be demonstrated.[152,153] In 1967, the presence of a hemolytic anemia that could be corrected by vitamin E or prevented by maintaining vitamin E sufficiency from early infancy was described.[154]

This syndrome was seen almost exclusively in infants with birth weights of less than 1,500 g and was most pronounced during the period of 6 to 10 weeks of life. The hematologic findings consisted of anemia with hemoglobin of 6 to 8 g/dL, reticulocytosis of 4 to 5% or greater, and thrombocytosis. Red cell morphologic changes included the presence of anisocytosis, poikilocytosis, red cell fragments, and irregularly contracted erythrocytes and spherocytes. The hydrogen peroxide hemolysis test was abnormal, and the red cell life span was reduced.[154,155] These findings were all consistent with alterations in the membrane due to oxidant injury. Treatment with vitamin E, in total doses ranging from 200 to 1,000 mg, produced a prompt rise in hemoglobin, a reduction in the reticulocyte count, and a gradual decline in the platelet count to the normal range. In addition to the hematologic abnormalities, many of the small infants also displayed edema of the lower legs and scrotum, watery nasal discharge, and, on occasion, tachypnea. The mechanisms responsible for these changes are not known.

Melhorn and Gross studied infants of less than 36 weeks gestation receiving a commercial formula and found that, at 6 to 10 weeks of age, infants who had been supplemented with 25 IU of vitamin E per day from Day 8 of life had significantly higher hemoglobin concentrations and lower reticulocyte counts and hydrogen peroxide tests than the unsupplemented infants.[156] It was also found that the daily administration of ferrous sulfate, 10 to 12 mg/kg/d from Day 8, exaggerated the hemolytic anemia in the infants not receiving the vitamin E supplement. Williams and coworkers demonstrated that hemolytic anemia due to vitamin E deficiency occurred in infants receiving iron-fortified formulas only if the formula was unusually rich in polyunsaturated fats.[157]

It has been hypothesized that hemolysis occurs in vitamin E deficiency as a consequence of peroxidation of lipid components of the red cell membrane. The peroxidation is initiated by the generation of a free radical (an unpaired electron) and proceeds autocatalytically in the absence of an antioxidant. Iron, in the reduced state, particularly in the presence of ascorbic acid, is recognized to generate free radicals. The requirements for lipid peroxidation include the presence of a suitable substrate (eg, a long-chain unsaturated fatty acid), a lack of antioxidant (eg, vitamin E), and a source of a free radical generating system (eg, heavy metals, molecular oxygen). Most proprietary formulas have now reduced their polyunsaturated fatty acid (PUFA) content and increased their vitamin E concentration, resulting in vitamin E-PUFA ratios in excess of 0.6:1.00, a value generally regarded as sufficient to prevent the development of vitamin E deficiency.[158] The potential for the development of vitamin E deficiency anemia is present when infants receive intravenous lipid preparations without adequate vitamin E supplementation.

The diagnosis should be suspected in an infant who displays anemia in the presence of persistent reticulocytosis, nonspecific red cell morphologic abnormalities, and thrombocytosis. Confirmation of the diagnosis requires: (1) evidence of a reduced plasma vitamin E concentration (<0.5 mg/dL) or a reduced vitamin E to a total lipid ratio (<0.6); (2) an abnormal hydrogen peroxide hemolysis test (usually >30% hemolysis with a normal laboratory value of <10%); (3) an increase in hemoglobin and a fall in reticulocyte count after vitamin E therapy. Response should be apparent within 10 days, provided correction of criteria 1 and 2 has occurred.

Miscellaneous Conditions

Patients with various forms of malabsorption will become vitamin E deficient. These include patients with exocrine pancreatic insufficiency (cystic fibrosis), congential biliary atresia, abetalipoproteinemia, and extensive small bowel resections. In patients with reduced concentrations of plasma vitamin E, the red cell half-life is usually shortened,[159,160] although anemia is usually not evident or, when present, is usually not correctable by the administration of vitamin E alone. The relative anemia observed in most patients with chronic lung disease with cystic fibrosis will not respond to iron alone but may improve when iron and vitamin E are given concurrently.[161]

Copper Deficiency

Copper is present in a number of metalloproteins. Among the cuproenzymes are cytochrome c oxidase, dopamine-β-hydroxylase, urate oxidase, tyrosine and lysyl oxidase, ascorbic acid oxidase, and superoxide dismutase (erythrocuprein). More than 90% of the copper in the blood is carried bound to ceruloplasmin, an α_2-globulin with ferroxidase activity.

Copper appears to be required for the absorption and utilization of iron. It has been proposed that copper, in the form of ferroxidases, converts and maintains iron in the Fe^{3+} state for its transfer by transferrin.[162] Decreased absorption of iron and anemia have been demonstrated in rats with induced dietary copper deficiency.[107]

Copper deficiency has been described in malnourished children[163] and in both infants[164] and adults[165] receiving parenteral alimentation. Copper deficiency in humans is characterized by (1) a microcytic anemia that is unresponsive to iron therapy, (2) hypoferremia, (3) neutropenia, and usually (4) the presence of vacuolated erythroid precursors in the marrow. In infants and young children with copper deficiency, radiologic abnormalities are generally present. These abnormalities include osteoporosis, flaring of the anterior ribs with spontaneous rib fractures, cupping and flaring of long bone metaphyses with spur formation and submetaphyseal fractures, and epiphyseal separation. These radiologic changes have frequently been misinterpreted as signs of scurvy.

The diagnosis of copper deficiency can be established by the demonstration of a low serum ceruloplasm or serum copper level. Adequate normal values for the first 2 to 3 months have not been well defined and are normally lower than those observed later in life. Despite these limitations, a serum copper level of less than 40 μg/dL or a ceruloplasmin value of less than 15 mg/dL after 1 or 2 months of age can be regarded as evidence of copper deficiency. In later infancy, childhood, and adulthood, serum copper values should normally exceed 70 μg/dL.

Preterm infants are at risk due to their lower hepatic copper stores which largely accumulate in the third trimester.[166] Low serum copper values may be observed in hypoproteinemic states, such as exudative enteropathies and nephrosis, as well as in Wilson's disease. In these circumstances, a diagnosis of copper deficiency cannot be established by serum measurements alone, but instead requires analysis of liver copper content or clinical response after a therapeutic trial of copper supplementation. Dietary zinc decreases copper absorption and may lead to copper deficiency and anemia.[167,168]

The anemia does not respond to iron but is quickly corrected by administration of copper. Therapy in a dose of 0.2 mg/kg of body weight will cause a prompt reticulocytosis and rise in the leukocyte count. This can be given as a 10% solution of copper sulfate ($CuSO_4 \cdot 5H_2O$), which contains about 25 mg of copper per milliliter.

The daily requirement of copper is 0.1 to 1 mg for infants and 1.0 to 5.0 mg for children and adolescents. Copper intake in infants is usually low since breast milk contains only 0.2 to 0.4 mg copper per liter and infant formulas are generally fortified to 0.4 to 0.6 mg/L; however, copper deficiency is rarely seen in healthy term infants. Older infants and children tend to have increased copper intake as cereals and other foods provide more copper than milk.[16]

NUTRITIONAL STATES CAUSING ANEMIAS

Anemia of Starvation

Studies conducted during World War II with conscientious objectors demonstrate that semistarvation for 24 weeks produces a mild to moderate normocytic, normochromic anemia.[169] Marrow cellularity was usually reduced and was accompanied by a decrease in the erythroid-myeloid ratio. Measurements of red cell mass and plasma volume suggested that dilution was a major factor responsible for the reduction in hemoglobin concentration. In persons subjected to complete starvation, either for experimental purposes or to treat severe obesity, anemia was not observed during the first 2 to 9 weeks of fasting.[170] Starvation for 9 to 17 weeks produced a fall in hemoglobin and marrow hypocellularity.[171] Resumption of a normal diet was accompanied by a reticulocytosis and disappearance of anemia. It has been suggested that the anemia of starvation is a response to a hypometabolic state with its attendant decrease in oxygen requirements.

Anemia of Protein Deficiency (Kwashiorkor)

Most cases of Kwashiorkor occur in developing countries as a result of malnutrition and poverty. In the United States, though rare, Kwashiorkor may be observed in individuals consuming restricted diets.[172] The mechanisms for anemia in Kwashiorkor have been examined in several laboratories. Protein deficiency leads to a reduction in oxygen consumption and erythropoietin production, with a subsequent drop in erythropoiesis and reticulocyte count.[173] Red cell maturation is blocked at the erythroblast level and the erythropoietin-sensitive stem cell pool is slightly decreased.[174]

In infants and children with protein-calorie malnutrition, the hemoglobin concentration may fall to 8 g/dL of blood,[175,176] but some children with kwashiorkor are admitted to the hospital with normal hemoglobin levels, probably due to a decreased plasma volume. The anemia is normocytic and normochromic, but there is a considerable variation in size and shape of the red cells on the blood film. The white blood cells and the platelets are usually normal. The marrow is most often normally cellular or slightly hypocellular, with a reduced erythroid-myeloid ratio. Erythroblastopenia, reticulocytopenia, and a marrow containing a few giant pronormoblasts may be found, particularly if these children have an infection. With treatment of the infection, erythroid precursors may appear in the marrow, and the reticulocyte count may rise. When nutrition is improved by feeding high-protein diets (powdered milk or essential amino acids), there is reticulocytosis, a slight fall in hematocrit due to hemodilution, and then a rise in hemoglobin, hematocrit, and red blood cell count. Improvement is slow, however, and during the third or fourth week, when the children are clinically improved and the serum proteins are approaching normal, another episode of erythroid marrow aplasia devoid of giant pronormoblasts may develop. This relapse is not associated with infection, does not respond to antibiotics, and does not remit spontaneously. It does respond to either riboflavin or prednisone, and unless treated with these agents, children who develop this complication may die suddenly. It has been suggested that the erythroblastic aplasia is a manifestation of riboflavin deficiency.[177]

Although the plasma volume is reduced to a variable degree in children with kwashiorkor, the total circulating red cell mass decreases in proportion to the decrease in lean body mass as protein deprivation reduces metabolic demands.[176] During repletion, an increase in plasma volume may occur before an increase in red cell mass, and the anemia may seem to become more severe, despite reticulocytosis. The erythropoietin level increases as the hemoglobin concentration falls[178] and, more important, as oxygen demand increases. The increased oxygen demand may in part account for the reticulocytosis. Also, during the repletion period, occult deficiencies of iron, folic acid, and occasionally of riboflavin, vitamin E, and vitamin B_{12} may become manifest unless these essential nutrients are supplied in adequate amounts.

Anemia and Obesity

The prevalence of obesity has been increasing dramatically in developed countries, particularly over the past two decades.[179] Children who are obese or overweight may not consume more calories than nonobese children,[180,181] and yet they may have inadequate micronutrient intake despite adequate or excessive energy intake.[182] One study of an overweight population found that intake of saturated fat, calcium, fruits, and vegetables was below recommended amounts.[183] Overweight or obese children have been shown to have lower levels of vitamin B_{12},[184] an increased prevalence of iron deficiency,[185] and a greater likelihood of iron-deficiency anemia than children of normal weight.[186] These findings suggest that children who are overweight or obese may be at risk for multiple micronutrient deficiencies that may lead to anemia.

REFERENCES

1. Oski, Brugnara, Nathan. A diagnostic approach to the anemic patient In: Nathan, Orkin, Ginsburg, Look, editors. Nathan and Oski's Hematology of Infancy and Childhood. Philadelphia, PA: Saunders; 2003.
2. Oski Pallor. In: Kay, Oski, Barness, editors. Core Textbook of Pediatrics. Philadelphia, PA: Lippincott; 1989.
3. Karnath BM. Anemia in the adult patient. Hosp Physician. 2004;32–6.
4. Herbert V. Folic acid. In: Shils ME, Olson JA, Shike M, et al., editors. Modern Nutrition in Health and Disease, 9th edition. Philadelphia, PA: Lippincott Williams & Wilkins; 1999.p. 433–46.
5. Herbert V, Zalusky R. Interrelations of vitamin B_{12} and folic acid metabolism: Folic acid clearance studies. J Clin Invest 1962;41:1263.
6. Baumgartner ER, Stokstad ELR, Wick H, et al. Comparison of folic acid coenzyme distribution patterns in patients with mehtylenetetrahydrofolate reductase and methionine synthetase deficiencies. Pediatr Res 1985;19:1288–92.
7. Hoffbrand AV, Jackson BFA. Correction of the DNA synthesis defect in vitamin B_{12} deficiency by tetrahydrofolate: Evidence in favour of the methyl-folate trap hypothesis as the cause of megaloblastic anaemia in vitamin B_{12} deficiency. Br J Haematol 1993;83:642–47.
8. Gafter-Gvili A, Prokocimer M, Breuer W, et al. Non-transferrin-bound serum iron (NTBI) in megaloblastic anemia: Effect of vitamin B_{12} treatment. Hematol J 2004;5:32–34.
9. Finch CA. Erythrokinetics in pernicious anemia. Blood 1956;9:807.
10. Herbert V. Megaloblastic anemia: Mechanism and management. Disease-A-Month. Chicago, IL: Year Book; 1965.
11. Cooper BA, Rosenblatt DS. Disorders of cobalamin and folic acid metabolism. In: Handin RJ, Lux SE, Stossel TP, editors. Blood: Principles and Practice of Hematology. Philadelphia, PA: J.B. Lippincott; 1995.
12. Antony A. Megaloblastic anemias In: Hoffman R, et al., editors. Hematology: Basic Principles and Practice. New York: Churchill Livingstone; 1991.
13. Lanzkowsky P. Megaloblastic anemias and other nutritional anemias. In: Miller DR, et al., editors.Blood Diseases of Infancy and Childhood. St. Louis, MO: Mosby; 1978.
14. Streiff RR. Disorders of folate metabolism. Dis Mon 1972; 1–32.
15. Baker H, Frank O, Thomson AD, et al. Vitamin profile of 174 mothers and newborns at parturition. Am J Clin Nutr 1975;28:59–65.
16. American Academy of Pediatrics. Pediatric Nutrition Handbook, 5th edition. American Academy of Pediatrics, 2004.
17. Hoffbrand AV, Newcomb B, Mollin D. Method of assay of red cell folate activity and the value of the assay as a test for folate deficiency. J Clin Pathol 1966;19:17–28.
18. Rosenblatt DS, Fenton WA. Inherited disorders of folate and cobalamin transport and metabolism. In: Scriver CR, Beaudet AL, Sly WS, et al., editors. The Metabolic and Molecular Bases of Inherited Disease, 8th edition. New York: McGraw-Hill; 2001.
19. Baker SJ, et al. Vitamin B_{12} deficiency in pregnancy and the puerperium. Br Med J 1962;1:1658.
20. Rappazzo ME, Salmi HA, Hall CA. The content of vitamin B_{12} in adult and foetal tissue: A comparative study. Br J Haematol 1970;18:425–33.
21. Jadhav M, et al. Vitamin B_{12} deficiency in Indian infants. Lancet 1962;2:903.
22. Lampkin BC, Shore NA, Chadwick D. Megaloblastic anemia of infancy secondary to maternal pernicious anemia. N Engl J Med 1966;274:1168–71.
23. Higginbottom MC, Sweetman L, Nyhan WL. A syndrome of methylmalonic aciduria, homocystinuria, megaloblastic anemia and neurologic abnormalities in a vitamin B_{12}-deficient breast-fed infant of a strict vegetarian. N Engl J Med 1978;299:317–23.
24. Coulombe JT, Shih VE, Levy HL. Massachusetts metabolic disorders screening program. II. Methylmalonic aciduria. Pediatrics 1981;67:26–31.
25. Halperin ML, Schiller CM, Fritz IB. The inhibition by methylmalonic acid of malate transport by the dicarboxylate carrier in rat liver mitochondria. A possible explantation for hypoglycemia in methylmalonic aciduria. J Clin Invest 1971;50:2276–82.
26. Montgomery JA, Mamer OA, Scriver CR. Metabolism of methylmalonic acid in rats. Is methylmalonyl-coenzyme a racemase deficiency symptomatic in man? J Clin Invest 1983;72:1937–47.
27. Rosenberg LE. The inherited methylmalonic acidemias. Prog Clin Biol Res 1982;103:187–209.
28. Deacon R, Purkiss P, Green R, et al. Vitamin B_{12} neuropathy is not due to failure to methylate myelin basic protein. J Neurol Sci 1986;72:113–17.
29. van Tonder SV, Ruck A, van der WJ, et al. Dissociation of methionine synthetase (EC 2.1.1.13) activity and impairment of DNA synthesis in fruit bats (Rousettus aegyptiacus) with nitrous oxide-induced vitamin B_{12} deficiency. Br J Nutr 1986;55:187–92.
30. Young PR, Waickus CM. Time dependence of the methylation of myelin basic protein from bovine brain; Evidence for protein-methylarginine demethylation. Biochem Biophys Res Commun 1987;142:200–4.
31. World Health Organization. Micronutrient deficiencies: Battling iron deficiency anaemia. http://www.who.int/nut/ida.htm. 3-13-2002.

32. Oski FA. Iron deficiency in infancy and childhood. N Engl J Med 1993;329:190–93.
33. Cook JD, Lynch SR. The liabilities of iron deficiency. Blood 1986;68:803–9.
34. Lozoff B, Brittenham GM, Wolf AW, et al. Iron deficiency anemia and iron therapy effects on infant developmental test performance. Pediatrics 1987;79:981–95.
35. Oski FA, Honig AS. The effects of therapy on the developmental scores of iron-deficient infants. J Pediatr 1978;92: 21–5.
36. Walter T, De AI, Chadud P, et al. Iron deficiency anemia: Adverse effects on infant psychomotor development. Pediatrics 1989;84:7–17.
37. Walter T, Kovalsky J, Stekel A. Effect of mild iron deficiency on infant mental development scores. J Pediatr 1953;102:519.
38. Cook JD, Skikne BS, Baynes RD. Iron deficiency: The global perspective. Adv Exp Med Biol 1994;356:219–28.
39. Lops VR, Hunter LP, Dixon LR. Anemia in pregnancy. Am Fam Physician 1995;51:1189–97.
40. Swain S, Singh S, Bhatia BD, et al. Maternal hemoglobin and serum albumin and fetal growth. Indian Pediatr 1994;31: 777–82.
41. Beard JL, Dawson H, Pinero DJ. Iron metabolism: A comprehensive review. Nutr Rev 1996;54:295–317.
42. Bothwell T. Overview and mechanisms of iron regulation. Nutr Rev 1995;53:237–45.
43. Cook JD, Monsen ER. Food iron absorption in human subjects. III. Comparison of the effect of animal proteins on nonheme iron absorption. Am J Clin Nutr 1976;29:859–67.
44. van Dokkum W. Significance of iron bioavailability for iron recommendations. Biol Trace Elem Res 1992;35:1–11.
45. Dallman PR, Yip R, Oski FA. Iron deficiency and related nutritional anemias. In: Nathan DG, Oski FA, editors. Hematology of Infancy and Childhood. Philadelphia, PA: W.B. Saunders; 1993.
46. Iob V, Swanson WW. Mineral growth of the human fetus. Am J Dis Child 1934;47:302.
47. Dallman PR. Nutritional anemias. In: Rudolph AM, Hoffman JIE, Rudolph CD, editors. Rudolph's Pediatrics, 20th edition. Stamford, CT: Appleton & Lange; 1996.
48. Singla PN, Chand S, Khanna, S et al. Effect of maternal anaemia on the placenta and the newborn infant. Acta Paediatr Scand 1978;67:645–48.
49. Shott RJ, Andrews BF, Thomas PT. Maternal and infant serum iron and total iron binding capacity at birth in a high risk population. Clin Res 1972;20:100.
50. DeLeeuw NKM, Lowenstein L, Hsieh Y-S. Iron deficiency and hydremia in normal pregnancy. Medicine 1966;45:291.
51. Lanzkowsky P. The influence of maternal iron deficiency on the hemoglobin of the infant. Arch Dis Child 1961;36:205.
52. Rios E, Lipschitz DA, Cook JD, et al. Relationship of maternal and infant iron stores as assessed by determination of plasma ferritin. Pediatrics 1975;55:694–99.
53. Brown MS. Physiologic anemia of infancy: Normal red cell values and physiology of neonatal erythropoiesis. In: Stockman JA, Pochedly C, editors. Developmental and Neonatal Hematology. New York: Raven Press; 1988.
54. Bridges KR, Seligman PA. Disorders of iron metabolism. In: Handin RJ, Lux SE, Stossel TP, editors. Blood: Principles and Practice of Hematology. Philadelphia, PA: J.B. Lippincott; 1995.
55. Russell RM. New micronutrient dietary reference intakes from the National Academy of Sciences. Nutr Today 2001;36:163–71.
56. Edgerton VR, Gardner GW, Ohira Y, et al. Iron–deficiency anaemia and its effect on worker productivity and activity patterns. Br Med J 1979;2:1546–49.
57. Gardner GW, Edgerton VR, Senewiratne B, et al. Physical work capacity and metabolic stress in subjects with iron deficiency anemia. Am J Clin Nutr 1977;30:910–17.
58. Viteri RE, Torun B. Anemia and physical work capacity. Clin Hematol 1974;3:609.
59. Moore DF, Jr, Sears DA. Pica, iron deficiency, and the medical history. Am J Med 1994;97:390–93.
60. Oski FA. The nonhematologic manifestations of iron deficiency. Am J Dis Child 1979;133:315–22.
61. Lanzkowsky P. Iron metabolism and iron deficiency anemia. In: Miller DR, et al., editors. Blood Diseases of Infancy and Childhood St. Louis: Mosby, 1978.
62. Fairbanks VF, Beutler E. Iron deficiency. In: Beutler E, editor. Williams Hematology. New York: McGraw–Hill; 1995.
63. Chandra RK, Saraya AK. Impaired immunocompetence associated with iron deficiency. J Pediatr 1975;86:[V20] 899–902.
64. Dallman PR. Iron deficiency and the immune response. Am J Clin Nutr 1987;46:329–34.
65. Feng XB, Yang XQ, Shen J. Influence of iron deficiency on serum IgG subclass and pneumococcal polysaccharides specific IgG subclass antibodies. Chin Med J (Engl) 1994; 107:813–16.
66. Hershko C, Peto TE, Weatherall DJ. Iron and infection. Br Med J (Clin Res Ed) 1988;296:660–4.
67. Joynson DH, Walker DM, Jacobs A, et al. Defect of cell-mediated immunity in patients with iron-deficiency anaemia. Lancet 1972;2:1058–9.
68. Krantman HJ, Young SR, Ank BJ, et al. Immune function in pure iron deficiency. Am J Dis Child 1982;136:840–4.
69. Kulapongs P, Vithayasai V, Suskind R, et al. Cell-mediated immunity and phagocytosis and killing function in children with severe iron-deficiency anaemia. Lancet 1974;2:689–91.
70. Macdougall LG, Anderson R, McNab GM, et al. The immune response in iron-deficient children: Impaired cellular defense mechanisms with altered humoral components. J Pediatr 1975;86:833–43.
71. Srikantia SG, Prasad JS, Bhaskaram C, et al. Anaemia and immune response. Lancet 1976;1:1307–9.
72. Thibault H, Galan P, Selz F, et al. The immune response in iron-deficient young children: Effect of iron supplementation on cell-mediated immunity. Eur J Pediatr 1993;152:120–4.
73. Weiss G. Iron and immunity: A double-edged sword. Eur J Clin Invest 2002;32:70–8.
74. Gebreselassie H. Iron supplementation and malaria infection: Results of a randomized controlled field trial. Montreal, Canada: McGill University;1996.
75. Gordeuk VR, Thuma PE, Mclaren CE, et al. Transferrin saturation and recovery from coma in cerebral malaria. Blood 1995;85:3297–301.
76. Barton AL, Banner BF, Cable EE, et al. Distribution of iron in th eliver predicts the response of chronic hepatitis C infection to interferon therapy. Am J Clin Pathol 1995;103:419–24.
77. de Monye C, Karcher DS, Boelaert JR, et al. Bone marrow macrophage iron grade and survival of HIV-seropositive patients. AIDS 1999;13:375–80.
78. Hurtado EK, Claussen AH, Scott KG. Early childhood anemia and mild or moderate mental retardation. Am J Clin Nutr 1999;69:115–9.
79. Lozoff B, Jiminez E, Hagen J, et al. Poorer behavioral and developmental outcome more than 10 years after treatment for iron deficiency in infancy. Pediatrics 2000;105:E51.
80. Wasserman G, Graziano JH, Factor-Litvak P, et al. Independent effects of lead exposure and iron deficiency anemia on developmental outcome at age 2 years. J Pediatr 1992;121:695–703.
81. Iannotti LL, Tielsch JM, Black MM, et al. Iron supplementation in early childhood: Health benefits and risks. Am J Clin Nutr 2006;84:1261–76.
82. Lozoff B, Georgieff MK. Iron deficiency and brain development. Semin Pediatr Neurol 2006;13:158–65.
83. Voorhess ML, Stuart MJ, Stockman JA, et al. Iron deficiency anemia and increased urinary norepinephrine excretion. J Pediatr 1975;86:542–47.
84. Youdin MBH, Yehuda S, Ben-Shachar D, et al. Behavioral and brain changes in iron-deficient rats: The involvement of iron in dopamine receptor function. In: Politt E, Leibel RL, editors. Iron Deficiency: Brain Biochemistry and Behavior. New York: Raven Press; 1982.
85. Thompson WG, Meola T, Lipkin M, Jr, et al. Red cell distribution width, mean corpuscular volume, and transferrin saturation in the diagnosis of iron deficiency. Arch Intern Med 1988;148:2128–30.
86. Whelby MS, Jones-Garrison S. Clinical use of transferrin receptor assay. Blood 1992;80:278a.
87. Yip R, Schwartz S, Deinard AS. Screening for iron deficiency with the erythrocyte protoporphyrin test. Pediatrics 1983;72:214–9.
88. Siegel RM, LaGrone DH. The use of zinc protoporphyrin in screening young children for iron deficiency. Clin Pediatr (Phila) 1994;33:473–79.
89. Labbe RF, Rettmer RL. Zinc protoporphyrin: A product of iron-deficient erythropoiesis. Semin Hematol 1989;26:40–6.
90. Hastka J, Lasserre J, Schwarzbeck A, et al. Zinc protoporphyrin in anemia of chronic disorders. Blood 1993; 81:1200–4.
91. Brugnara C, Laufer MR, Friedman AJ, et al. Reticulocyte hemoglobin content (CHr): Early indicator of iron deficiency and resonse to therapy. Blood 1994;83:3100–1.
92. Brugnara C, Zurakowski D, DiCanzio J, et al. Reticulocyte hemoglobin content to diagnose iron deficiency in children. J Am Med Assoc 1999;281:2225–30.
93. Ellis LD, Jensen WN, Westerman MP. Marrow iron: An evaluation of depleted stores in a series of 1,322 needle biopsies. Ann Intern Med 1964;61:44.
94. Lanzkowsky P. Iron-deficiency anemia. Manual of Pediatric Hematology and Oncology. New York: Churchill Livingstone; 1995.
95. Zlotkin S, Arthur P, Antwi KT, et al. Randomized, controlled trial of single versus 3-times-daily ferrous sulfate drops for treatment of anemia. Pediatrics 2001;108:613–6.
96. Kianfar H, Kimiagar M, Ghaffarpour M. Effect of daily and intermittent iron supplementation on iron status of high school girls. Int J Vitam Nutr Res 2000;70:172–7.
97. Brown MS. Physiologic anemia of infancy: Nutritional factors and abnormal states. In: Stockman JA, Pochedly C, editors. Developmental and Neonatal Hematology. New York: Raven Press; 1988.
98. Hamstra RD, Block MH, Schocket AL. Intravenous iron dextran in clinical medicine. JAMA 1980;243:1726–31.
99. Wallerstein RO. Intravenous iron-dextran complex. Blood 1968;32:690–5.
100. Macdougall IC. Intravenous administration of iron in epoetin-treated haemodialysis patients-which drugs, which regimen? Nephrol DialTransplant 2000;15:1743–45.
101. Blackfan KD. Vitamin A deficiency in infants, a clinical and pathological study. J Pediatr 1933;3:679.
102. Hodges RE, Sauberlich HE, Canham JE, et al. Hematopoietic studies in vitamin A deficiency. Am J Clin Nutr 1978;31: 876–85.
103. Majia LA, Hodges RE, Arroyave G, et al. Vitamin A deficiency and anemia in Central American children. Am J Clin Nutr 1977;30:1175–84.
104. Mohanram M, Kulkarni KA, Reddy V. Hematological studies in vitamin A deficient children. Int J Vitam Nutr Res 1977;47:389–93.
105. Nutrition Survey of Paraguay, May-August. 1965. Washington, D.C., U.S. Printing Office.
106. Ahmed F, Rahman A, Noor A, et al. Anaemia and vitamin A status among adolescent schoolboys in Dhaka City, Bangladesh. Public Health Nutrit 2006;9:345–50.
107. Hashizume M, Chiba M, Shinohara A, et al. Anaemia, iron deficiency and vitamin A status among school-aged children in rural Kazakhstan. Public Health Nutr 2005;8:564–71.
108. Molla A, Khurshid M, Molla AM, et al. Is anemia an accurate predictor of vitamin A status in Pakistani children? Am J Trop Med Hyg 1993;49:276–9.
109. Ahmed F, Khan MR, Jackson AA. Concomitant supplemental vitamin A enhances the repsonse to weekly supplemental iron and folic acid in anemic teenagers in urban Bangladesh. Am J Clin Nutr 2001;74:108–15.
110. Muslimatun S, Schmidt MK, Schultink W, et al. Weekly supplementation with iron and vitamin A during pregnancy increases hemoglobin concentration but decreases serum ferritin concentration in Indonesian pregnant women. J Nutr 2001;131:85–90.
111. Mwanri L, Worsley A, Ryan P, et al. Supplemental vitamin A improves anemia and growth in anemic school children in Tanzania. J Nutr 2000;130:2691–6.
112. Suharno D, West CE, Muhilal, et al. Supplementation with vitamin A and iron for nutritional anaemia in pregnant women in West Java, Indonesia. Lancet 1993;342:1325–8.
113. Nankivell BJ. Vitamin B_6 deficiency on hemodialysis causing sideroblastic anemia. Nephron 1991;59:674–5.
114. Weissgarten J, Modai D, Oz D, et al. Vitamin B_6 therapy does not improve hematocrit in hemodialysis patients supplemented with iron and erythropoietin. Nephron 2001;87: 328–32.
115. Bottomley SS. Porphyrin and iron metabolism in sideroblastic anemia. Semin Hematol 1977;14:169–85.
116. Snyderman SE, Holt LE, Carretero R, et al. Pyridoxine deficiency in the human infant. J Clin Nutr 1953;1:200.
117. Foy H, Kondi A. Hypochromic anemias of the tropics associated with pyridoxine and nicotine acid deficiencies. Blood 1958;13:1054.
118. Bottomley SS. Sideroblastic anaemia. Clin Haematol 1982;11:389–409.
119. Verwilghen R, Reybrouck G, Callens L, et al. Antituberculous drugsand sideroblastic anemia. Br J Haematol 1965;II:92.
120. Frimpter GW. Pyridoxine (B_6) dependency syndromes. Ann Intern Med 1968;68:1131–2.
121. McCurdy PR, Donohoe RF, Magovern M. Reversible sideroblastic anemia caused by pyrazinoic acid (Pyrazinamide). Ann Intern Med 1966;64:1280–4.
122. Horrigan DL, Harris JW. Pyridoxine-responsive anemia: Analysis of 62 cases. Adv Intern Med 1989;12:103.
123. Raab SO, Haut A, Cartwright GE, et al. Pyridoxine-responsive anemia. Blood 1961;18:285.
124. Alfrey CP, Lane M. The effect of riboflavin deficiency on erythropoiesis. Semin Hematol 1970;7:49–90.
125. Lane J, Alfrey CP. The anemia of human riboflavin deficiency. Blood 1963;22:811.
126. Ajayi OA, Okike OC, Yusuf Y. Haematological response to supplements of riboflavin and ascorbic acid in Nigerian young adults. Eur J Haematol 1990;44:209–12.
127. Buzina R, Jusic M, Milanovic N, et al. The effects of riboflavin administration on iron metabolism parameters in a school-going population. Int J Vitam Nutr Res 1979;49:136–43.
128. Powers HJ, Wright AJ, Fairweather-Tait SJ. The effect of riboflavin deficiency in rats on the absorption and distribution of iron. Br J Nutr 1988;59:381–7.

129. Powers HJ, Weaver LT, Austin S, et al. Riboflavin deficiency in the rat: Effects on iron utilization and loss. Br J Nutr 1991;65:487–96.
130. Beutler E. Effect of flavin compounds on glutathione reductase activity: In vivo and in vitro studies. J Clin Invest 1969;48:1957–66.
131. Beutler E. Glutathione reductase: Stimulation in normal subjects by riboflavin supplementation. Science 1969;165:613–5.
132. Staal FJT, Ela SW, Roederer M, et al. Glutathione deficiency and human immunodeficiency virus infection. Lancet 1992;339:909–12.
133. Delmas-Beauvieux M, Peuchant E, Couchouron A, et al. The enzymatic antioxidant system in blood and glutathione status in human immunodeficiency virus (HIV)-infected patients; effects of supplementation with selenium or B-carotene. Am J Clin Nutr 1996;64:101–7.
134. Beutler E, Srivastava SK. Relationship between glutathione reductase activity and drug induced haemolytic anaemia. Nature 1970;226:759–60.
135. Vilter RW, Woolford RMSTL. Severe scurvy, a clinical and hemaotlogical study. J Lab Clin Med 1946;31:609.
136. Crandon JH, Lund CC, Dill DB. Experimental human scurvy. N Engl J Med 1940;223:353.
137. Hodges RE, Baker EM, Hood J, et al. Experimental scurvy in man. Am J Clin Nutr 1969;22:535–48.
138. Stokes PL, Melikian V, Leeming RL, et al. Folate metabolism in scurvy. Am J Clin Nutr 1975;28:126–9.
138. Cox EV, Meynell MJ, Northan BE, et al. The anemia of scurvy. Am J Med 1966;42:220.
140. Moore CV, Dubach R. Observations on the absorption of iron from foods tagged with radioiron. Trans Assoc Am Physicians 1951;64:245.
141. Fairweather-Tait S, Fox T, Wharf SG, et al. The bioavailability of iron in different weaning foods and the enhancing effect of a fruit drink containing ascorbic acid. Pediatr Res 1995;37:389–94.
142. Zucker W, Hutnoff L, Apt L. Relationship of anemia and scurvy. Am J Dis Child 1949;77:128.
143. Clark N, Sheard NF, Kelleher JF. Treatment of iron-deificiency anemia complicated by scurvy and folic acid deficiency. Nutr Rev 1992;50:134–7.
144. van den Berg JJ, Kuypers FA, Roelofsen B, et al. The cooperative action of vitamins E and C in the protection against peroxidation of parinaric acid in human erythrocyte membranes. Chem Phys Lipid 1990; 53:309–20.
145. Cox EV. The anemia of scurvy. In: Harris RS, Wool IG, Loraine JA, editors. International Symposium on Vitamin-Related Anemias. Vitamins and Hormones. Advances in Research and Applications. New York: Academic; 1968.
146. Dju MV, Mason KE, Filer LJ. Vitamin E in human fetuses and placentae. Etud Neo-Natales 1952;1:49.
147. Durnin JV, Womersley J. Body fat assessed from total body density and its estimation from skinfold thickness: Measurements on 481 men and women aged from 16 to 72 years. Br J Nutr 1974;32:77–97.
148. Quaife ML, Dju MY. Chemical estimation of vitamin E in tissue and the tocopherol content of some normal human tissues. J Biol Chem 1949;180:263.
149. Leonard PJ, Doyle E, Harrington W. Levels of vitamin E in the plasma of newborn infants and of the mothers. Am J Clin Nutr 1972;25:480–4.
150. Martinez FE, Goncalves AL, Jorge SM, et al. Brief clinical and laboratory observations. Vitamin E in placental blood and its interrelationship to maternal and newborn levels of vitamin E. J Pediatr 1981;99:298–300.
151. Wright SW, Filer LJ, Mason RE. Vitamin E blood levels in premature and full term infants. Pediatrics 1951;7:386.
152. Goolbloom RB, Cameron D. Studies of tocopherol requirements in health and disease. Pediatrics 1963;32:36.
153. Hassan H, Hashim SA, Van Itallie TB, et al. Syndrome in premature infants associated with low plasma vitamin E levels and high polyunsaturated fatty acid diet. Am J Clin Nutr 1966;19:147–57.
154. Oski FA, Barness LA. Vitamin E deficiency: A previously unrecognized cause of hemolytic anemia in the premature infant. J Pediatr 1967;70:211–20.
155. Ritchie JH, Fish MB, McMasters V, et al. Edema and hemolytic anemia in premature infants. A vitamin E deficiency syndrome. N Engl J Med 1968;279:1185–90.
156. Melhorn DK, Gross S. Vitamin E-dependent anemia in the premature infant. I. Effects of large doses of medicinal iron. J Pediatr 1971;79:569–80.
157. Williams ML, Shoot RJ, O'Neal PL, et al. Role of dietary iron and fat on vitamin E deficiency anemia of infancy. N Engl J Med 1975;292:887–90.
158. Bell EF, Filer LJ, Jr. The role of vitamin E in the nutrition of premature infants. Am J Clin Nutr 1981;34:414–22.
159. Bieri JG, Corash L, Hubbard VS. Medical uses of vitamin E. N Engl J Med 1983;308:1063–71.
160. Farrell PM, Bieri JG, Fratantoni JF, et al. The occurrence and effects of human vitamin E deficiency. A study in patients with cystic fibrosis. J Clin Invest 1977;60:233–41.
161. Ater JL, Herbst JJ, Landaw SA, et al. Relative anemia and iron deficiency in cystic fibrosis. Pediatrics 1983;71:810–4.
162. Frieden E. The ferrous to ferric cycles in iron metabolism. Nutr Rev 1973;31:41–4.
163. Graham GG, Cordano A. Copper depletion and deficiency in the malnourished infant. Johns Hopkins Med J 1969;124:139–50.
164. Joffe G, Etzioni A, Levy J, et al. A patient with copper deficiency anemia while on prolonged intravenous feeding. Clin Pediatr (Phila) 1981;20:226–8.
165. Dunlap WM, James GW, III, Hume DM. Anemia and neutropenia caused by copper deficiency. Ann Intern Med 1974;80:470–6.
166. Committee on Nutrition AAoP. Pediatric Nutrition Handbook, 4th edition. Elk Grove Village, IL: American Academy of Pediatrics; 1998.
167. Fischer P, Giroux A, L'Abbe M. The effect of dietary zinc on intestinal copper absorption. Am J Clin Nutr 1981;34:1670–5.
168. Forman W, Sheehan D, Cappelli S, et al. Zinc abuse–An unsuspected cause of sideroblastic anemia. West J Med 1990;152:190–2.
169. Keys A, et al. The Biology of Semistarvation Minneapolis: University of Minnesota Press, 1950.
170. Thomson TJ. Treatment of obesity by total fasting for up to 249 days. Lancet 1966;2:992.
171. Drenick EJ, Swendseid ME, Blahd WH, et al. Prolonged starvation as a treatment for severe obesity. J Am Med Assoc 1964;187:100.
172. Fischer P. Commentary. Clin Pediatr 2004;43:306.
173. Delmonte L, Aschenasy A, Eyquen A. Studies on the hemolytic nature of protein deficiency anemia in the rat. Blood 1964;24:49.
174. Naets JP, Wittek M. Effect of starvation on the response to erythropoietin in the rat. Acta Haematol 1974;52:141–50.
175. Adams EB. Observations on the etiology and treatment of anemia in kwashiorkor. Br Med J 1967;3:451.
176. Viteri RE, Alvaredo J, Luthringer DG, et al. Hematological changes in protein-calorie malnutrition. In: Harris RS, Wool IG, Loraine JA, editors. International Symposium on Vitamin-Related Anemias. Vitamins and Hormones. Advances in Research and Applications. New York: Academic; 1968.
177. Foy H, Kondi A. Comparison between erythroid aplasia in marasmus and kwashiorkor and the experimentally induced erythroid aplasia in baboons by riboflavin deficiency. In: Harris RS, Wool IG, Loraine JA, editors. International Symposium on Vitamin-Related Anemias. Vitamins and Hormones. Advances in Research and Applications. New York: Academic; 1968.
178. McKenzie D, Friedman R, Katz S, et al. Erythropoietin levels in anaemia in kwashiorkor. S Afr Med J 1967;41:1044–6.
179. Eisenmann J. Secular trends in variables associated with the metabolic syndrmoe of North American children and adolescents: A review and synthesis. Am J Hum Biol 2003;15:786–94.
180. Rocandio A, Ansotegui L, Arroyo M. Comparison of dietary intake among overwieght and non-overweight schoolchildren. Int J Obes Relat Metab Disord 2001;25:1651–55.
181. Rodriguez G, Moreno L. Is dietary intake able to explain differences in body fatness in children and adolescents? Nutr Metab Cardiovasc Dis 2006;16:294–301.
182. Gillis L, Gillis A. Nutrient inadequacy in obese and non-obese youth. Can J Diet Pract Res 2005;66:237–42.
183. Davy B, Harrell K, Stewart J, et al. Body weight status, dietary habits, and physical activity levels of middle school-aged children in rural Mississippi. South Med J 2004;97:571–7.
184. Pinhas-Hamiel O, Doron-Panush N, Reichman B, et al. Obese children and adolescents: A risk group for low vitamin B12 concentration. Arc Pediatr Adolesc Med 2006;160:933–6.
185. Nead K, Halterman J, Kaczorowski J, et al. Overweight children and adolescents: A risk group for iron deficiency. Pediatrics 2004;114:104–8.
186. Pinhas-Hamiel O, Newfield R, Koren I, et al. Greater prevalence of iron deficiency in overweight and obese children and adolescents. Int J Obes Relat Metab Disord 2003;27:416–18.

63

Function and Nature of the Components in the Oral Cavity

James H. Shaw, DMD, PhD
Linda P. Nelson, DMD, MScD
Catherine Hayes, DMD, DMSc

The position of the oral cavity at the entrance to the gastrointestinal tract requires that it perform functions that need diverse tissues and specialized structures. The foods and other items that children eat and drink vary widely in their particle size and texture, degree of hardness, pH, and other chemical stimuli, as well as wide ranges of temperature. These different characteristics produce stresses on the oral components that must be moderated before swallowing. In the mouth, food items must be subdivided by chewing and simultaneously diluted and buffered with saliva until the bolus is suitable to swallow and pass on to the esophagus and lower areas of the gastrointestinal tract. The amount and composition of saliva secreted on each occasion are in response to the whole experience of eating—from the initial seeing, smelling, and anticipating to the tasting, chewing, and swallowing.[1,2] Especially in young children, many undesirable materials are taken into the mouth, which contribute various kinds of microorganisms and/or other dangerous entities.

The temperature and humidity of the oral cavity, as well as the frequent presence of all required nutrients for cellular growth and multiplication in food and drink, result in the mouth being an ideal incubator for many types of microorganisms from birth onward. An important source of the infant's flora is the primary caregiver.[3] There is evidence of matrilineal transmission of mutans streptococci in very early childhood. Strong correlations between salivary mutans streptococci counts in mothers and their children have been reported. Recent studies indicate that mutans streptococci can colonize the mouth of predentate infants and that horizontal transmission (eg, between family members or children in a day care setting) as well as vertical transmission (between caregiver and child with the major reservoir from mother to infant) occurs.[4] Maternal salivary levels of mutans streptococci infection may influence infection rates of mutans streptococci in their children at ages 6 to 18 months and at 4 to 5 years. Salivary concentrations of 10^5 colony forming units mutans streptococci per milliliter of maternal saliva were associated with a 52% infection rate in their children compared with only a 6% infection rate when the maternal saliva concentration was 10^3 or below.[5,6] The presence of caries in the mother and siblings increases risks for the child, but the most consistent predictor of risk of caries (dental decay) in children is past caries experience.[7] Nutrients and the foods that provide them have numerous relationships to the oral tissues and structures, and these relationships vary depending on the nature of the tissue or structure itself. Some relationships differ from those elsewhere in the body. For example, sugars, when metabolized throughout the body, are wholesome sources of energy for the cells' many and varied functions. However, in contrast to this vital systemic relationship, the sugars have an undesirable local effect in the mouth. On the surfaces of dental enamel, sugars support the metabolism of microorganisms in dental plaque with the production of acid.

In the life history of the soft tissues, a transition occurs at birth as a result of the new, stressful exposure of their outer surfaces to microorganisms and food, meanwhile still being nourished systemically. A much more striking transition occurs for the teeth, especially the enamel surfaces, at the time of their eruption into the oral cavity. Prior to eruption, the external surfaces of enamel are surrounded by the enamel cap, including the enamel-forming cells of ectodermal origin, the ameloblasts; the inner surface of the dentin is covered by the layer of odontoblasts, the dentin-forming cells, which are embryonically of mesodermal origin. Both enamel and dentin throughout their formation and mineralization are related fully to the systemic environment. At eruption, the enamel cap is ruptured, and the outer surfaces of enamel become exposed to the oral milieu of saliva, microorganisms, and food. The odontoblastic layer remains intact in contact with the capillaries of the pulp and continues to metabolize slowly with the centripetal formation of secondary dentin at the expense of the connective tissue in the pulp. The latter process accelerates when toxic metabolites from a deep carious lesion in the dentin trigger a protective response with more rapid production of secondary dentin.

STRUCTURE OF ENAMEL

Enamel and dentin are characteristically different from other tissues in the body. When fully mature, enamel contains only about 1% organic material and 2% water. Its tiny organic component consists of proteins chemically similar to the keratins of skin and is dispersed throughout the inorganic crystals as a network of extremely delicate and intricate fibrils.[8] The rest of enamel is the complex calcium–phosphorus salt hydroxyapatite, which varies somewhat in its composition, depending on the concentrations of anions and cations in the extracellular fluids at the time it crystallizes in the embryonic organic matrix. The hydroxyapatite in enamel has more perfectly formed crystals than those in dentin and bone. After its eruption, enamel contains no cells and is cut off from systemic influences other than through saliva, which bathes it continuously throughout life. Elements in saliva exchange with those on the outer surface of the enamel, especially in the period shortly after eruption.[9] Owing to its acellular nature, enamel has no ability to heal or remodel, with the exception that remineralization of early (precaries) surface lesions with the incorporation of calcium and phosphorus from saliva can occur under suitable conditions.[10,11]

STRUCTURE OF DENTIN

Dentin contains about 20% protein of the collagen family comparable to bone. About 70% of dentin is hydroxyapatite. Although dentin continues to form centripetally at a slow rate, like enamel, it is unable to remodel or repair itself as it does not contain anything comparable to the haversian system of bone. Any developmental errors in the formation of enamel and dentin remain throughout life as chemical or histologic artifacts in the kymographic record.

NUTRITIONAL STUDIES ON THE ORAL TISSUES AND STRUCTURES

Soft Tissues

The soft tissues, mucosa, gingiva, tongue, and taste buds, are especially susceptible to local stresses. Their metabolic activity is high. Oral mucosal cells in rats, for example, are replaced in 3 to 5 days by rapid cell division in the basal layer and sloughing of the surface cells; in contrast, the turnover rate in cheek skin is about 10 days.[12] This high metabolic activity accounts for the rapid healing of injuries to soft tissues within the mouth. However, the high metabolic activity of oral tissues results in a high susceptibility to nutritional deficiencies as adequate nutrients must be available to support the rapid cell multiplication and replacement.

In the early decades of nutrition as a discipline, deficiencies were often recognized first as clinical entities because of manifestations in the oral cavity; scurvy (vitamin C) and pellagra (niacin) are the prime examples.[13] The ease of oral examination for abnormalities with minimal violation of the subject's privacy also contributed to early recognition of nutritional deficiencies that affected oral components.

The increased understanding of nutrition and the attention to preventive nutrition, including legally required fortification of foods, such as niacin for the prevention of pellagra, have led to almost total elimination of such nutritional deficiencies in children of the industrialized nations. However, in the developing nations of the third world, especially in times of famine, such deficiencies still occur.

Mineralized Tissues

In early experimental studies with rats, severe deficiencies of vitamin A caused abnormalities in the ameloblasts, which led to hypoplastic enamel.[14] Severe vitamin C deficiency in guinea pigs, which, unlike rats, require preformed vitamin C in their diets, produced a syndrome in which the odontoblasts produced much less dentin.[15] As a result, the erupting teeth were thin and fragile. Acute deficiencies in rats and dogs of vitamin D or calcium or grossly abnormal calcium-to-phosphorus ratios resulted in inadequate mineralization and hypoplasia of the teeth.[16,17] Little evidence exists to suggest that moderate deficiencies of these nutrients are of clinical significance in children in industrialized countries, although we still see cases of vitamin D-resistant ricketts. In severely malnourished children in developing countries, a linear enamel hypoplasia (natal line) has been described in the anterior teeth of the primary dentition (Figure 1), which is much less frequent or absent in better nourished children in the same communities.[18,19] The poorly mineralized ring around the teeth in this syndrome was being formed about the time the children were born and was highly susceptible to dental caries. All children at birth had low serum vitamin A levels.

Low protein intake during the reproductive cycle of white rat dams resulted in delayed eruption of the molars of their offspring. Their teeth were smaller and more susceptible to tooth decay than those of the offspring of losely related females provided with adequate protein.[20] The increased caries susceptibility in the deprived rats may be attributable to structural abnormalities in the salivary glands produced by the protein deficiency.[21]

Alvarez conducted two cross-sectional and one longitudinal study among Peruvian children in whom malnutrition in early life was prevalent.[22] He studied the influence of malnutrition on the time of tooth eruption and of deciduous tooth exfoliation and the susceptibility of both deciduous and permanent teeth to dental caries. As in the earlier studies with rodents, tooth eruption was delayed significantly among malnourished children. Because rodents have only a single dentition, exfoliation could not be studied in the laboratory. Among the malnourished Peruvian children, their deciduous teeth exfoliated appreciably later than those in better-nourished children in the same communities. When the length of time that the deciduous teeth were exposed to the oral environment was considered, instead of the traditional method of considering only the chronologic age of the children, the deciduous teeth of malnourished children were observed to have a higher incidence of caries than those of the better-nourished children. Even a single episode of moderate malnutrition before 1 year of age also resulted in a higher incidence of dental caries of the permanent incisors and first molars, which were being formed and were starting to mineralize during that interval. The increased incidence of dental caries among these children again paralleled the rodent studies conducted three decades earlier. Alvarez suggested that this observation may result from imperfect formation of dental enamel early in life.

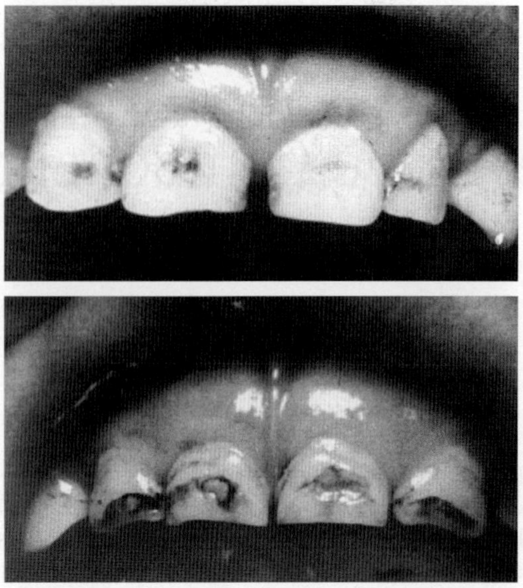

Figure 1 Photographs of linear hypoplasia of the anterior teeth of Guatemalan children. These hypoplastic areas are prone to develop dental caries. (Reproduced with permission from references 18 and 19.)

Several studies, in animals and humans, have evaluated the effect of nutrition and nutrients on the growth and development of oral structures. The conclusion of many studies is that adequate nutrition is essential from the earliest periods of development. Further, a firm diet enhances proper growth and development compared with a soft diet. Specifically, the effect of diet consistency has been shown to affect growth of the mandible and maxilla and proper tooth eruption. Ongoing research on the harmful effects of nutrition on oral growth indicates that excess vitamin A can be a potent teratogen that may contribute to oral defects such as cleft palate. Protective effects of folic acid have been shown in animal studies but not in humans as yet, probably owing to the complexity of other factors also involved.[23]

Adequate amounts of all nutrients should be provided throughout the long periods of tooth formation in children to ensure their normal development, that is, from the last trimester of pregnancy through 16 years of age.

DISEASES OF THE ORAL CAVITY

The two principal diseases of the oral cavity are dental caries (cavities, carious lesions) and periodontal disease (destruction of the tissues that support the teeth in the jaws). Although the latter is the chief cause of tooth loss in adults, juvenile periodontitis occurs infrequently in children, is much more localized than in adults, and may be associated with an immunologic defect in some children. Both diseases are of multifactorial origin, are chronic in nature, and progress slowly and intermittently. Nutrition is not known to have a relationship to juvenile periodontitis except possibly through dietary influences on the dental plaque.

Etiology of Dental Caries

A carious lesion results from an interaction between the carbohydrates in food, especially the sugars, with cariogenic microorganisms in the dental plaque on tooth surfaces and the tooth surface in the presence of saliva; the gross anatomy of the tooth, the composition of the enamel and dentin, and the quantity and quality of saliva all vary in ways that influence the rate of progression of tooth decay. The most serious adverse influence on the ability of the teeth to be maintained in the oral cavity is any reduction in the flow of saliva owing to salivary disease, radiation, or drug use that modifies the ability of the salivary glands to function.[24,25]

Under certain circumstances, the acidic metabolic products of the microorganisms on the tooth surfaces from sugars reduce the pH of plaque sufficiently to demineralize enamel and, later, the dentin progressively until a carious lesion (dental decay) is produced. The epidemiologist commonly speaks of this type of disease production as the relationship of the agent (microorganism[s]), host (the tooth and the person in which it functions), and environment (the components in the milieu around the tooth and the home and community in which the individual lives) (Figure 2).[26] All three parameters must simultaneously be in a caries-producing mode for carious lesions to be initiated and progress to become visually detectable. Periodontal disease also results from the interaction of food, the microorganisms in the crevices between the teeth and the gingiva, and the tissues in the area.

Agent. The microorganisms producing carious lesions are able to colonize the surfaces of the teeth and/or the pits and fissures of the biting

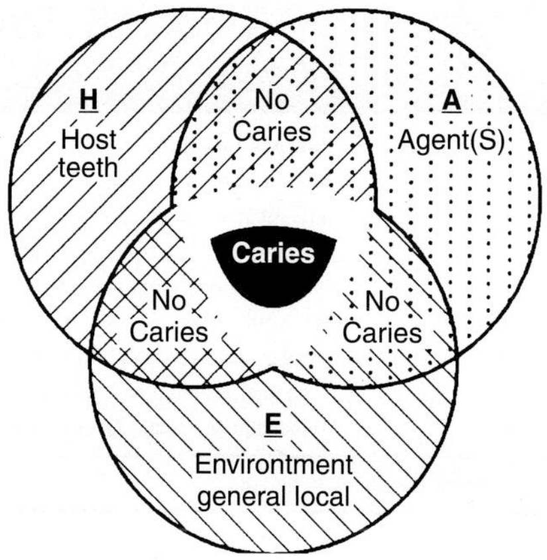

Figure 2 Diagrammatic illustration of the three major parameters simultaneously required for the initiation and progression of carious lesions. (Reproduced with permission from reference 26.)

surfaces.[27] These microbiota are able to produce sufficiently acidic environments (pH around 5) on the tooth surfaces when metabolizing actively to demineralize enamel and later dentin. They must be able to continue to metabolize actively at these low pH values as the lesion progresses deeper into the tooth. The primary sources of energy required by these organisms are the sugars. *Streptococcus mutans* is of special interest because it produces mutans, a polysaccharide of glucose, which enables it to adhere to smooth surfaces and to build up colonies in dental plaque. The nature of plaque is such that the microbial metabolites are produced in close proximity to enamel with restricted access to buffering saliva. In the human mouth, plaque contains numerous species of microorganisms with acid-producing capabilities. The complex nature of the oral milieu makes it virtually impossible to fully apply Koch's principles for identification of a specific causative organism. Probably more than one species is involved in most situations, but especially as lesions progress more deeply into the tooth with the need to metabolize in a strongly acidic environment. The recent recognition that dental plaque is a bacterial biofilm and that it behaves quite differently from its individual constituents has led to research to control plaque formation by preventing bacterial adhesion to the tooth surface. Physical approaches include coating the enamel surface with a polymer, whereas biological approaches to prevent initial colonization include inhibition of plaque matrix formation and inhibition of the bacterial signaling mechanisms.[28]

Host. Evidence of genetic determinants of caries resistance is limited in humans, yet a variety of subtle indications of genetic influences have been reported. Early suggestions that large differences in caries experience between national groups were genetically determined have been largely discredited. The caries prevalence in industrialized nations tended to be routinely higher than in developing countries; however, as the dietary customs of the high-caries industrialized nations were adopted in developing countries with increased sugar consumption and more frequent eating, their low-caries experience has been increasing. Meanwhile, in the last 20 years, dental caries prevalence in the industrialized nations has been decreasing significantly.[29]

Comparison of the dental caries experience of twins indicated that identical twins had more similar caries experiences than fraternal twins.[30] This may not be a truly genetic influence as such environmental experiences as food preferences, frequency of eating, and tooth brushing techniques may be more similar for identical than for fraternal twins. Similarities in dental caries for twins reared separately were considered to be about 50% attributable to genetic influences.[31]

Numerous trials have been conducted to develop animal strains of divergent caries resistance. Superficially, differences attributable to heredity seemed to be produced. However, when so-called resistant strains were heavily challenged early in life with cariogenic microorganisms, carious lesions developed readily, although not always as extensively as in the seemingly more susceptible strains.

Mandel suggested three avenues through which genetic influences may be mediated: (1) salivary components that buffer plaque acids — elevating the pH and influencing the bacterial ecology of plaque, (2) immunologic and nonimmunologic constituents of oral fluids that have the capacity to alter the ability of cariogenic bacteria to attach to enamel, and (3) protein-bound lipids on the surfaces of teeth that may alter the permeability to acids produced in plaque.[32]

Environment. The single most important variable in the oral environment is the frequency of consuming foods containing sugars that adhere to tooth surfaces. The absolute amount of sugars consumed is less important than the frequency of eating. In the 1930s and 1940s, numerous studies were conducted on the relation of frequency of eating to caries experience (Figure 3).[33] Almost invariably, the conclusion was that caries experience increased as frequency of food consumption, especially of between-meal snacks, increased. More recently, this type of trial has been less frequent and the above relationship has not been as readily demonstrable. Since the earlier studies, food habits have changed dramatically. At that time, most food was prepared and eaten at home, and the amount of sugar used was controlled by the home-maker. Between-meal snacks were usually candy and cookies. Today, relatively little food is prepared at home; many items are commercially prepared, with the amount of sugar controlled industrially on the basis of the amount needed for "best" taste. In addition, a much higher percentage of meals is consumed away from the home. Snack consumption is much more frequent, and less dependence is placed on three main meals a day.

The amount of sugar available per capita in a country is a reasonable index of the prevalence of dental caries among its children (Figure 4).[34] The information supporting the pivotal role of sugars in the etiology of dental caries was considered by 1977 to be sufficiently conclusive that Horowitz stated that in human dental experimentation:

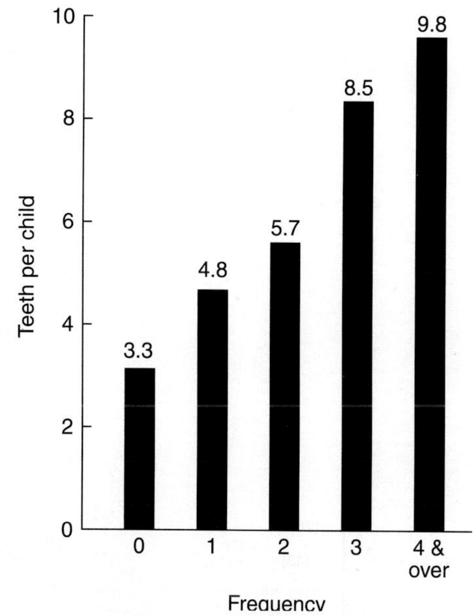

Figure 3 This bar graph compares the number of decayed, missing, and filled deciduous teeth with the frequency of between-meal eating in preschool children in Tennessee. *Includes extracted primary molars. (Reproduced with permission from reference 33.)

> *the control group should not be asked to engage in any practice that may have a harmful effect on the dentition or its surrounding tissues. For example, subjects in a control group should not be given or asked to use chewing gum sweetened with sucrose, nor should they be asked to use sucrose rinses or other agents to produce decalcification of tooth enamel or initiate carious lesions, unless the investigators are certain that they can completely "reverse" the defects.*[35]

Mandel stated that little disagreement exists that differences in amount, form, and frequency of readily fermentable carbohydrates can affect the rate of caries attack, but considerable variation between children exists when intake appears to be generally comparable.[32]

Foods are complex mixtures of many chemicals. As yet, it has not been possible to devise a series of animal trials and evaluations in the human oral cavity that dependably estimate the caries-producing value of a specific food.[36] Some food items that contain relatively little sugar but substantial amounts of starch are more capable of producing caries lesions than expected; others containing high amounts of sugar are less capable of supporting the caries process than expected.

A special case of rampant dental caries limited to the maxillary anterior deciduous teeth and posterior molars has become known as early childhood caries. This problem occurs in young children who are put to bed at night or for rests during the day with a bottle of formula or sweetened juice. When they go to sleep, salivary secretion decreases drastically, and the fermentable carbohydrates in the milk or juice are not diluted or washed away but are readily available to the microorganisms on tooth surfaces.[37] It is believed that the tongue affords protection to the mandibular anterior teeth so that they are pathognomonically

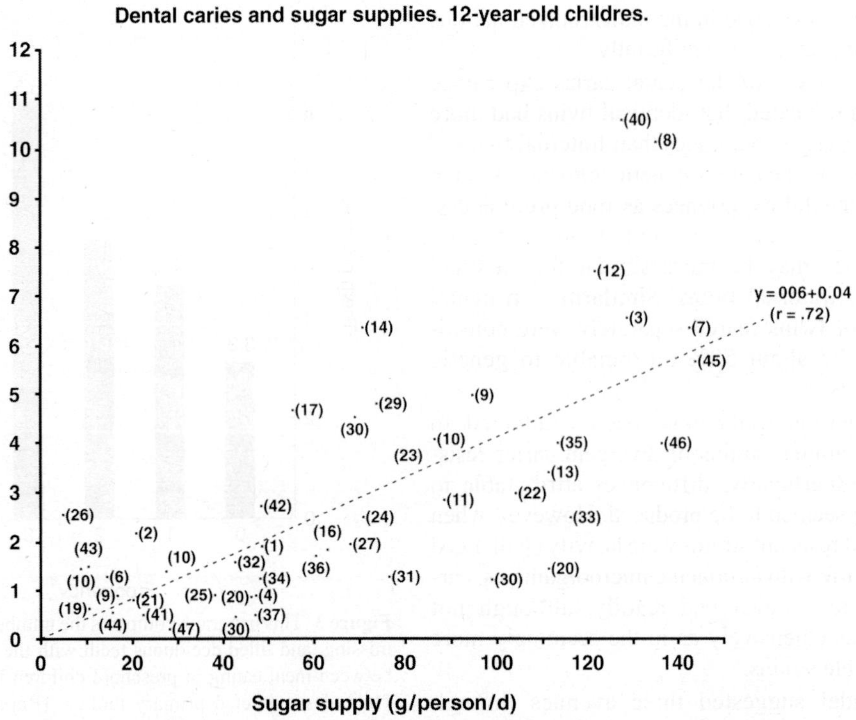

Figure 4 This graph represents a comparison of the number of decayed, missing, and filled permanent teeth with the sugar supply in grams per person per day for 47 countries. (Reproduced with permission from reference 34.)

not affected. Excessive on-demand breast-feeding is also capable of causing the same problem. The sugar, lactose, in human milk is clearly able to support the caries process.

Pediatricians and pediatric dentists on a preventive basis need to urge mothers of young infants to follow feeding practices in which excessive exposure to sweetened fluids and breast milk does not occur. When early childhood caries is already present, appropriate dietary corrections need to be made by less frequent feeding and the use of fewer sweet snacks of all kinds. Appropriate professional dental care is needed, probably including topical fluoride applications, such as a fluoride varnish, coupled with strong oral hygiene procedures at home.[38] The latter will include the parent's brushing of the infant's teeth with fluoridated toothpaste. Care is needed so that excess fluoride is not swallowed.

The importance of maintaining the deciduous teeth is not to be underestimated. They are needed as "space maintainers" as the jaws grow in order that there will be adequate room for eruption of the permanent teeth. Increased likelihood of orthodontic problems accompanies the early loss of deciduous teeth. High levels of untreated caries in the deciduous teeth provide reservoirs of cariogenic microorganisms from which the permanent teeth become quickly infected when they erupt into the oral cavity.

Reduced Ability of Polyols to Support Caries. Measurement of the pH of dental plaque in vivo with tiny, sensitive electrodes has become a convenient means of evaluating how various solutions and foods in the oral cavity affect the metabolism in the dental plaque in proximity to the tooth surface. In 1944, Stephan reported on a sharp depression in the pH of dental plaque after a glucose rinse was swished around the mouth.[37] This depression from the resting value with a pH around 6.6 to 7.0 (the range observed in saliva) to 5.0 or less within minutes after the start of the glucose rinse lasted for a few minutes and then slowly returned to the resting value. Plots of results from this kind of evaluation have become known as Stephen curves (Figure 5).[39,40] The consensus from the Stephen curve concerning the relation of plaque pH to caries production is shown in Table 1.

Both the equipment and the procedures for intraoral tests have been refined and are used widely today. For example, certain varieties of cheese eaten shortly after a sugar rinse or a sweet food prevent the rapid pH drop in dental plaque

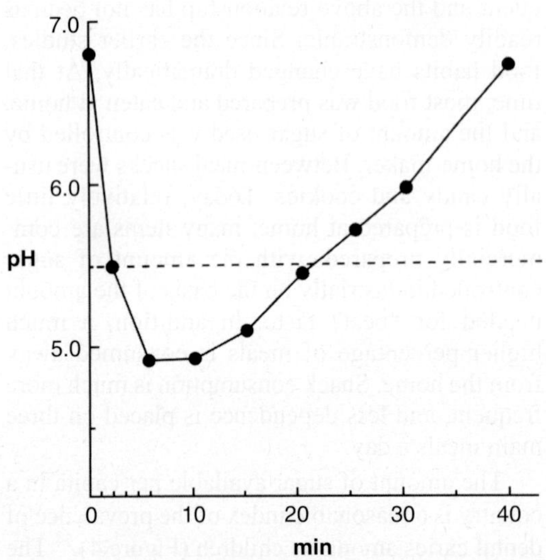

Figure 5 The typical Stephen curve showing the precipitous decrease in pH measured in vivo in dental plaque after a glucose rinse and the slower return to the resting pH. (Adapted from references 39 and 40.)

Table 1 Relation of Plaque pH to Caries Production

Plaque pH	Potential for Caries Initiation and Development
Above 6.0	Safe area; low solubility of enamel; calcium and phosphorous adequate to saturate environment
6.0 to 5.5	Doubtful or very slow progression
Below 5.5	Danger area; high solubility of enamel; calcium and phosphorous inadequate to saturate environment

Adapted from references 39 and 40.

(Figure 6).[40] Likewise, chewing a gum sweetened with a polyol, sorbitol, or xylitol, does not result in a pH decrease, whereas chewing a gum sweetened with sucrose causes the typical caries-producing decrease (Figure 7).

Oral microorganisms have greatly limited abilities to metabolize the polyols, xylitol (5 carbon), sorbitol, and mannitol.[41,42] The effect of sugar substitutes on changes in caries rates has been evaluated in several observational studies as well as clinical trials, with results consistently demonstrating a protective effect of xylitol on caries incidence. Sorbitol was also shown to decrease caries rates compared with controls; however, the reductions in caries rates were greatest when xylitol was the sugar substitute. Some limitations of these studies include a lack of radiographs in caries diagnosis, high loss to follow-up, potential confounding, and bias owing to the nature of long-term community intervention studies. The criteria for causality—consistency, strength association, biologic plausibility, temporal sequence, and dose-response relationship—should be considered. First, these studies are remarkably consistent both in terms of the magnitude of the effect observed as well as the consistent demonstration that xylitol was superior to sorbitol in decreasing the risk of dental caries. Second, the relative risks observed are considered strong (0.19 to 0.4). It is biologically plausible that xylitol can reduce dental caries because the pH of plaque is lowered with xylitol compared with sucrose. Fourth, a dose–response trend was observed in the two studies that evaluated different concentrations of xylitol, with the greatest effect observed in the subjects using the strongest xylitol preparations. The evidence to date suggests a strong caries-protective effect of xylitol.[43]

In vivo pH testing has been used extensively in Switzerland, not only in basic research, but also in the estimation of the potential of a specific product to cause dental caries when used excessively. When a product has been evaluated by approved methods for in vivo testing and is found not to cause an excessive decrease in pH, the Swiss Health Authority grants permission to identify the product as "zahnfreundlich" (friendly or safe for the teeth) and imprint a distinctive logo on the label (Figure 8).[44] This procedure has not been adopted elsewhere because of the inability to find a consensus that this procedure is adequate for the intended purpose.

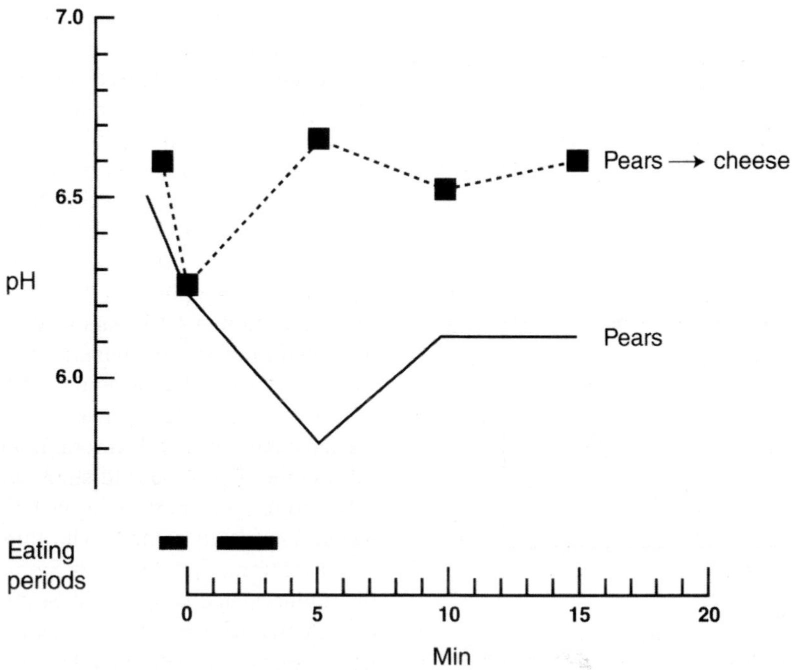

Figure 6 An example of the sharp pH decrease after eating a portion of sweetened pears and the moderating influence of eating cheese immediately after the same portion of pears. (Reproduced with permission from reference 40.)

FLUORIDES AND HUMAN HEALTH

Because fluoride has relationships to dental caries through both the host and the environment, a separate section for fluoride discussion is appropriate. Fluoride ion from any salt of the highly reactive halogen fluorine occurs ubiquitously in water supplies, soils, and foods. Fluoride is also present in all body fluids and tissues, even when the amount of fluoride ingested is low. Probably no nutrient demonstrates more clearly the physiologic spectrum from the influence of an insufficient intake, through normal to toxic levels of ingestion.

TOXICITY OF EXCESS FLUORIDE: MOTTLED ENAMEL

Toxic manifestations of excess fluoride ingestion were observed before recognition of its benefits, unlike other nutrients, for which the effects of deficiencies were described first. In 1901, Eager, a physician in the US Public Health Service stationed in Naples, Italy, described an esthetically disfiguring problem of dental enamel in otherwise healthy adults.[45] Their enamel was variously mottled with brown stains; he attributed the problem to local geologic conditions. In striking contrast, he recognized that the enamel of teeth in

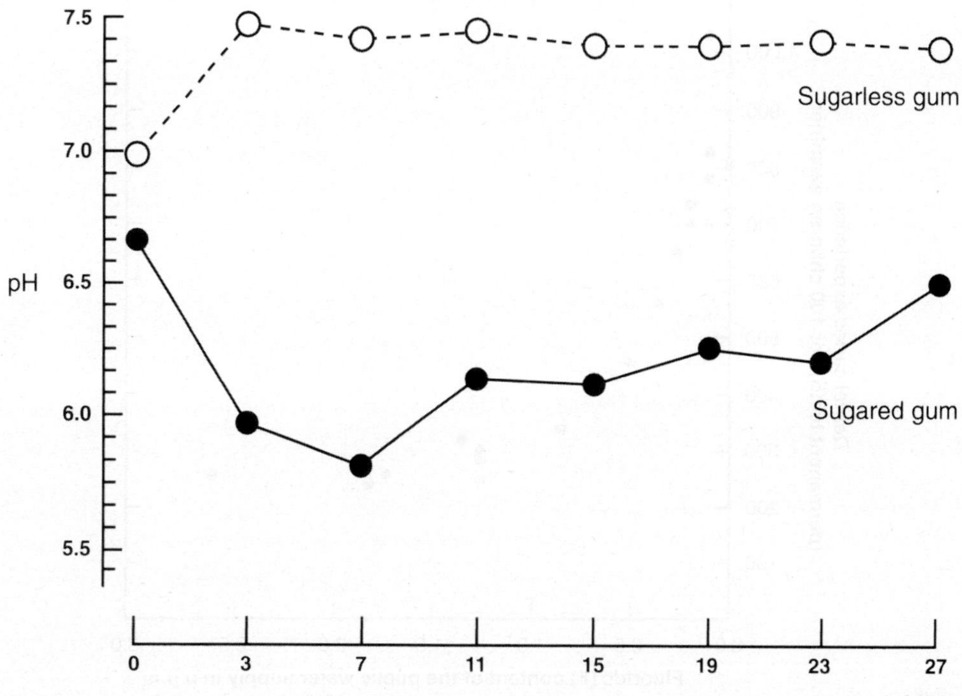

Figure 7 A comparison of the Stephen curve after chewing sucrose-sweetened gum with the pH curve after chewing gum sweetened with a noncariogenic polyol. (Reproduced with permission from reference 40.)

Figure 8 The "safe for teeth" logo approved for use on the label of an approved product in Switzerland. (Reproduced with permission from reference 44.)

young children in the area was normal, which he postulated might be attributable to a recent change known to have occurred in the water supply.

Subsequently, descriptions of mottled enamel were reported from numerous parts of the world in humans as well as in domestic animals.[44] Evidence became increasingly clear in humans that this esthetically disfiguring problem was caused by some agent in community or home water supplies. In animals, the problem sometimes was caused by their water supplies and in other situations was related to rock phosphate supplements added to their feeds as a source of calcium and phosphorus.

By 1931, reports from several widely separated laboratories established that the mottled enamel in humans and experimental animals was attributable to excess ingestion of fluoride from drinking water that contained more than 1.5 ppm fluoride, that is, 1.5 mg/L of water.[47–49] At this point, the popular name, mottled enamel, was superseded by the scientific descriptor, chronic endemic dental fluorosis.

This abnormality was determined to result from some as yet undefined altered relationship(s) in the deposition of crystals of hydroxyapatite in the organic matrix formed by ameloblasts, the enamel-forming cell of ectodermal origin. This developmental interrelationship is apparently the most sensitive process to excess fluoride in the extracellular fluids of any in the body. Higher intake (20 mg) of fluoride per day in industrial exposure causes abnormal calcification in the spine and, after 20 years, serious crippling fluorosis.[50]

CLASSIFICATION SYSTEM FOR MOTTLED ENAMEL

Dean developed a classification system to describe the various visual levels of enamel pathology and a weighting system to provide a community fluorosis index.[51] He used the terms (1) questionable—slight aberrations from the normal glossy translucency of enamel, which the examiner could not be certain was pathologic (weight = 0.5); (2) very mild—small, dull, paper-white areas scattered irregularly over the tooth surface but covering less than 25% of its area (1.0); (3) mild—more extensive white opacities but less than 50% of the area involved (2.0); (4) moderate—all surfaces affected with marked wear on the chewing surface accompanied by brown stains (3.0); and (5) severe—all surfaces affected with marked hypoplasia, discrete or confluent pitting, and widespread brown stains.

The community fluorosis index was calculated by combining the weight for each child with

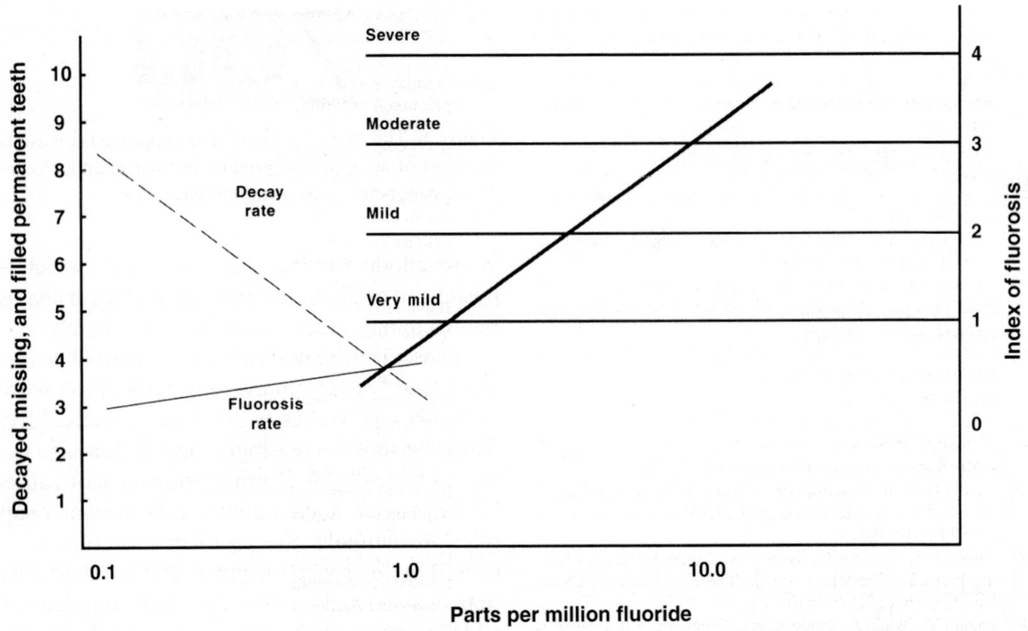

Figure 9 Relation between decayed, missing, and filled per manent teeth (*broken line*), severity of dental fluorosis (*solid line*), and fluoride concentration in the public water supply, with the latter on a logarithmic scale. (Reproduced with permission from reference 52.)

the frequency of occurrence of each grade in the child population. A community fluorosis index over 0.5 was considered undesirable, indicating the need to reduce the water fluoride level.

As shown in Figure 9, mottled enamel does not become a problem until in excess of 1.5 ppm fluoride in drinking water was ingested during tooth development.[50] However, water concentrations beyond this amount caused increasingly severe fluorosis and increasing frequency. As a public health measure, excessively high fluoride amounts must be reduced or a new lower fluoride water supply found. It must be emphasized that mottled enamel cannot result from consuming excessively high amounts of fluoride after the teeth are formed because this abnormality is completely of developmental origin.

DENTAL BENEFITS OF NATURALLY AVAILABLE FLUORIDES

One of the earliest observers of enamel fluorosis in this country, McKay, in Colorado Springs, where the water supply was later shown to contain 2.0 ppm fluoride, reported that teeth with mottled enamel did not seem to have an increased susceptibility to dental caries despite the surface irregularities.[53] In the late 1920s and 1930s, several small studies suggested that fluorosis appeared to be associated with reduced dental caries experience.

A combination of the need to know the permissible upper limit of fluoride in drinking water plus the increasing concern about the generally high incidence of dental caries among American children led to many extensive epidemiologic surveys among children. Numerous increasingly large surveys in the 1930s and 1940s indicated the strong correlation between fluoride ingestion during tooth development and tooth decay. For example, Dean and colleagues reported on data for 7,257 12- to 14-year-old children in 21 cities in four states.[54,55] Figure 10 indicates the convincing relationship between fluorides during development and dental caries experience. They also considered other factors that might be related—composition of diet, hours of sunshine, and hardness of the water—and concluded that none could explain the naturally available fluoride–dental caries relationship.

DENTAL BENEFITS OF WATER FLUORIDATION

By 1945, the dental benefits of fluoride in communal water supplies had been demonstrated to the satisfaction of almost all investigators and many health-related professional organizations. The possibility of pathology elsewhere in the human body or of increased susceptibility to other diseases had been thoroughly studied, with negative results with one exception, the crippling fluorosis described above, which has never been observed at the optimal level for caries reduction.

Hence, in 1945, three clinical trials were initiated to adjust the fluoride concentration of community water supplies to an optimal level, with the expectation that 10 years would be needed for demonstration of the benefits. Grand Rapids, Michigan, was selected as one trial community, with Muskegon, Michigan, to serve as the unfluoridated control city and Aurora, Illinois, as a natural fluoride city. A second study was initiated in Newburgh, New York, with nearby Kingston as the unfluoridated control. The third community was Brantford, Ontario, with Sarnia, Ontario, as the unfluoridated control and Stratford, a nearby community with an optimal fluoride level naturally present. The data soon demonstrated that the results from water fluoridated in the distribution system duplicated those observed where fluoride was naturally present, with caries reductions from 50 to 60% in permanent teeth (Figure 11).[55–59] The benefits in teeth developed during the study began to show up sufficiently rapidly that Muskegon dropped out as the control community for Grand Rapids before the 10-year test period ended and initiated its own water fluoridation program. In addition, some unexpected reductions in caries initiation were observed among the teenage population in teeth formed before fluoridation was begun; this observation suggested that an oral environmental influence was occurring in addition to the expected systemic influence on developing teeth. As in communities with naturally

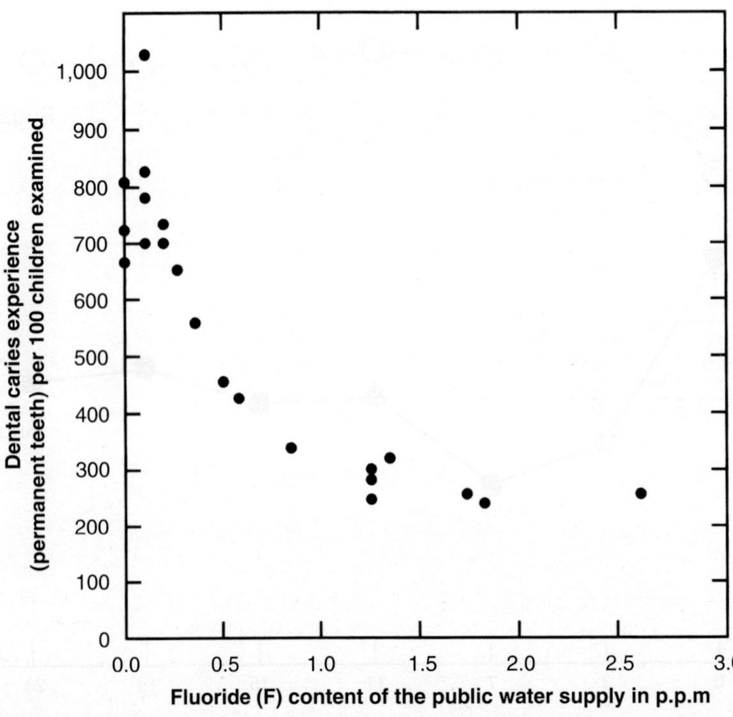

Figure 10 Relationship between the fluoride content naturally available in public water supplies and the number of decayed, missing, and filled permanent teeth per 100 children 12 to 14 years old. (Reproduced with permission from references 54 and 55.)

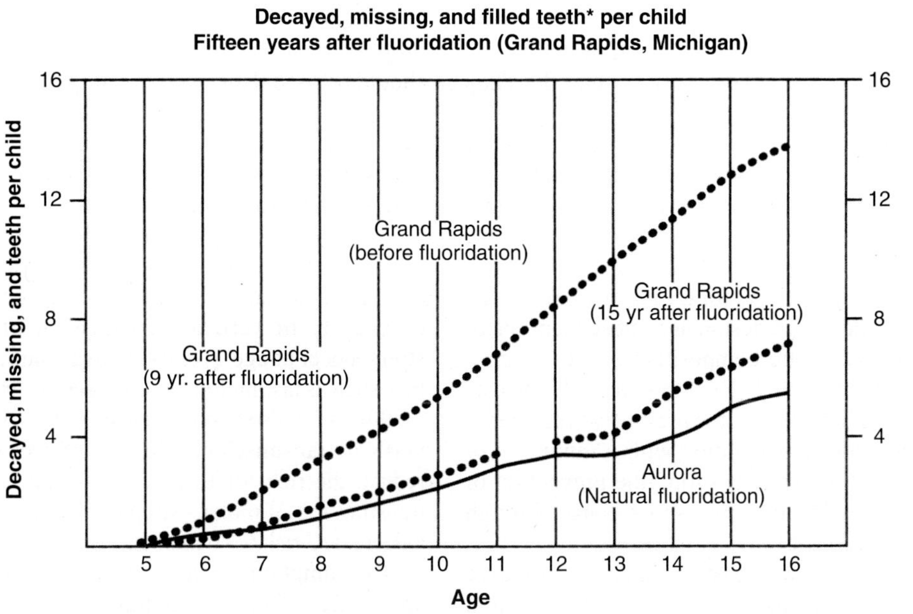

Figure 11 The benefits of fluoridation of the communal water supply in Grand Rapids, Michigan, are shown for the deciduous teeth after 9 years and for the permanent teeth after 15 years. The inclusion of the data for Aurora, Illinois, where the water naturally contains an adequate amount of fluoride, can be used as a basis for comparison of how similar the benefits are between natural fluoride and fluoride introduced at the water treatment facility. (Reproduced with permission from references 56–59.)

available fluoride, the greatest benefit was for the smooth surfaces of the anterior teeth and the least for the carious lesions that develop in the developmental pits and fissures on the grinding surfaces of the posterior teeth. No evidence of esthetically disfiguring mottling was observed in these trials.

Fluoridation of water supplies has been widely adopted in the United States as a valuable and inexpensive public health measure. The Fluoridation Census in 1992 reported that 134.7 million individuals on communal water supplies in 8,572 communities received water fluoridated in the water processing system; in addition, 10.0 million individuals lived in 1,924 communities where the water contained at least 0.7 ppm fluoride naturally.[60] The total percentage of the population benefiting from fluoride in the water in the United States was 62.1.

METABOLISM OF FLUORIDES

The varying evidence of mottled enamel within the child population of any community in both natural fluoride areas and areas where fluoridation is practiced has been the subject of much interest since the first evidence of the fluoride relationships. Some variation undoubtedly occurs in the amount of water consumed by individual children; the amounts of canned fish with bones and the use of tea, the only foods with substantial amounts of fluoride, constitute additional variables.

Fluorides from soluble salts are readily absorbed from the gastrointestinal tract.[61] In the presence of high concentrations of cations that produce much less soluble salts of fluoride, its absorption is reduced. When much less soluble sources of fluoride are ingested, absorption of fluoride is also reduced.

The kidneys are the major route for fluoride removal from the body, which is characterized by variable degrees of tubular resorption. A range in resorption has been reported in humans; in four studies, the average resorption of fluoride after filtration into the tubules varied from 23 to 38%.[62] In general, fluoride clearance tended to increase with increased urinary flow rate. Urinary pH also influenced fluoride excretion. In rats with a urinary pH less than 5.6 induced by administration of ammonium chloride, urinary excretion was less than 5% of the amount filtered; alkaline pH as high as 8.0, induced by administration of sodium bicarbonate, resulted in fluoride excretion approaching 70%. Various factors can chronically alter the acid–base status and affect fluoride relationships. The composition of the diet is normally the major determinant of acid–base balance and urinary pH. In addition, various metabolic and respiratory disorders, level of physical activity, and altitude of residence contribute to acid–base status.

The combination of slightly different levels of fluoride ingestion by children with the above factors, which modify excretion in the urine, is probably adequate to explain the different degrees of mottled enamel in children within the same community.

DENTAL BENEFITS OF FLUORIDE TABLETS, TOOTHPASTES, AND ORAL RINSES

Efforts to extend the systemic benefits of fluoride to populations for whom water-borne fluoride was not available led to the development of fluoride dietary supplements. Three major factors have combined to change the way in which fluoride supplements are used in contemporary practice: (1) a shift in our understanding of fluoride's mode of action from systemic to topical; (2) an increased exposure among children to other sources of fluoride; and (3) concern for the risk of fluorosis in permanent teeth. With those factors in mind it is recommended that prior to prescribing fluoride supplements, assay the child's primary drinking water supply for fluoride content. In addition, practitioners should consider other sources of fluoride exposure for their patients and do a caries risk assessment.[63] The levels recommended by the American Academy of Pediatric Dentistry for different ages and levels of fluoride in the water supply are shown in Table 2.[64] Because young children are prone to swallow toothpaste, use of fluoridated toothpaste (usually containing 1,000 ppm fluoride, ie, 1 mg F per gram) contributes to the level of fluoride ingested. Therefore, it must be used sparingly; the size of a pea on the brush is adequate and must be applied by the child's caregiver. As a safety factor, a maximum of 120 mg of fluoride should be prescribed at one time. This amount would be a certainly lethal dose only for those children weighing less than 8 kg and would be a probably toxic dose for children weighing 24 kg or less.[65]

The overall effectiveness of fluoride supplements has been estimated to provide 20 to 30% reduction in dental disease. The level of evidence for the effectiveness of fluoridated dentifrices in the permanent dentition is high and sufficient to warrant a strong recommendation for their use to reduce the incidence of caries. Unfortunately, there is no evidence regarding their effectiveness in the primary dentition, but logically it should follow that they would be as effective in younger patients.

Fluoridated mouthrinses (0.05NaF) and self-applied gels (stannous fluoride) should be reserved for use with children judged to be at moderate or high risk for dental caries, including children with orthodontic appliances or prosthetic appliances, children with special health care needs, and those with reduced salivary flow. Fluoride mouthrinses should be recommended only for children who have demonstrated mastery of their swallowing reflex.[63]

In children with special health care needs who are especially at risk for dental caries (children with GERD) who cannot control their swallow reflex, it is recommended that the caregiver dip the brush in the mouthrinse before bedtime or use a supplemental gel.

Fluoride varnish recently received FDA approval in 1994 for use as a desensitizig agent and as a cavity liner. It has been used off-label as a

Table 2 Dietary Fluoride Concentration in the Water Supply

	Fluoride Concentration in the Water Supply		
Age of Child	Less Than 0.3 ppm F	0.3–0.6 ppm F	More Than 0.6 ppm F
Birth–6 mo	0	0	0
6 mo–3 yr	0.25 mg	0	0
3–6 yr	0.50 mg	0.25 mg	0
6 yr up to at least 16 yr	1.0 mg	50.50 mg	0

Adapted from Pediatr Dent.[62]

caries preventive agent. Fluoride varnish is easily applied to the teeth, and it sets relatively quickly in contact with moisture. A typical application requires 0.2 to 0.5 mL, resulting in a total fluoride ion application of approximately 5 to 11 mg. The Cochrane Database for Systematic Reviews found a 46% pooled prevented fraction for permanent teeth and 33% for primary teeth. The authors concluded that fluoride varnish provides a substantial caries-inhibiting effect in both dentitions.[66]

The extent to which the various uses of fluorides contribute to the dental health of the United States is demonstrated by a statement by Harold Varmus, Nobel laureate and director of the National Institutes of Health, at a Senate Appropriations Subcommittee Hearing on March 17, 1994.[67] In response to Senator Harkin's question, "Does medical research contribute to long-term cost savings?" Varmus stated that his favorite example of the benefits of research concerned the use of fluorides to prevent dental caries, which alone saves the taxpayer several billion dollars per year.

MECHANISMS OF ACTION OF FLUORIDES

When the dental benefits of fluoride were first observed, systemic mechanisms of action were sought. The degree of crystallinity of hydroxyapatite in enamel increased as its fluoride concentration increased. Acid solubility of hydroxyapatite decreased as its fluoride concentration increased. Enamel surfaces had particularly high fluoride concentrations.[68]

Saliva contains about 0.019 ppm fluoride (1 µmol/L), about one-fiftieth of the concentration in communal water fluoridated at 1 ppm.[69] Even this low concentration appears to be important in the maintenance of the integrity of the tooth surface and in the remineralization of precarious lesions in the enamel. The mechanisms of action of fluoride in caries inhibition include the following: (1) the enhancement of remineralization during the repeated cycles of demineralization/remineralization in the early stages of the caries process, (2) the inhibition of glycolysis by which sugar is metabolized by bacteria to produce acid, and (3).while a preeruptive systemic effect cannot be ruled out, no direct evidence of such an effect has been demonstrated.[70]

TREATMENT OF CARIOUS LESIONS

Because a visually detectable carious lesion is rarely self-limiting, it continues to progress until the pulp is infected, with the probable loss of the tooth, unless specific action is taken to interrupt the progress of the lesion. Decayed enamel and dentin must be removed and replaced with an inert material that is able to resist the forces of mastication and the influences of the oral milieu.

Pit and fissure sealants have been demonstrated to be effective in the primary prevention of caries, and their effectiveness remains strong as long as the sealants are maintained.[6] Sealants are intended to protect caries-susceptible tooth surfaces, which are benefited least by fluoride. They should be placed as soon as possible after the tooth erupts and isolation to prevent moisture contamination during placement can be achieved.

Identification of early carious lesions and treatment with preventive resin restorations have moved dentistry into a new era. This very conservative treatment allows for the removal of just the small pit and fissure lesion and subsequent restoration with esthetic composite resin to which a sealant can be applied. By removing only the carious enamel and dentin, the preventive resin technique provides a restoration with a minimum of tooth reduction while ensuring the prevention of future caries in other pits and fissures through sealant placement.[71]

Amalgam is the least expensive restorative material to purchase and insert. The new high copper amalgams are expected to last over 30 years. Questions have been raised in a few publications about the safety of amalgams because of their gradual release of mercury vapor. The media picked up this concern and exaggerated the problem with regard to both its severity and its frequency. Berglund estimated that 1.7 µg of mercury vapor was inhaled from 12 amalgam fillings in a 24-hour period.[72] He noted that the World Health Organization threshold limit value for mercury vapor in the workplace is 100 times greater than this amount.

Osborne stated that allergies to amalgam has been reported in the literature infrequently but that it is speculative as to which component(s) of amalgam (mercury, silver, tin, or copper) is causative.[73] Owing to their frequent handling of amalgam, dentists and their staffs are exposed to more mercury than any patient. Even though the profession urges great care in amalgam handling and ventilation of dental offices, guidelines that are followed by most dentists, dentists still accumulate a greater body burden of mercury than do nondentists. However, dentists have $2^1/_2$ years longer life expectancies than the population in general, including physicians. Dentists and their staffs do not have elevated levels of spontaneous abortions, and their children do not have a higher incidence of birth defects.[74]

SUMMARY AND RECOMMENDATIONS

Typical of all areas of the body, the mouth and each of its components require a nutritionally well-balanced diet containing adequate amounts of all essential nutrients throughout development and maintenance.

Attention must be drawn to one special requirement for the adequate development and maintenance of the teeth throughout their entire life histories, namely, a source of fluoride. The easiest and least expensive way to provide fluoride is through a communal water supply containing 1.0 ppm fluoride that is present naturally or is added in the local water treatment plant. If, for any reason, water fluoridation is not possible, a proprietary source of fluoride in tablets or drops should be used. However, it is imperative that the diet should not be supplemented if the water already contains 0.7 ppm or more fluoride; an undesirable level of mottling is likely to occur with fluoride from two sources.

Söderling demonstrated that habitual use of xylitol chewing gum by mothers was associated with a statistically significant reduction in the probability of vertical transmission of mutans streptococci at age 2 years. Saliva sharing activities, such as tasting food before feeding and shared toothbrushes also contributes to the horizontal and vertical transmission. Clearly, efforts made to reduce the risk for early vertical and horizontal transmission of mutans streptococci translate into a decreased risk for dental caries in the child.[75]

Consumption of sticky snacks containing sugars should be kept to a minimum and be replaced whenever possible by such noncariogenic snacks as fresh fruits and vegetables, cheese, or nuts. Candy and gum sweetened with a xylitol are good substitutes for products sweetened with sugar.

Good oral hygiene habits need to be followed at least once a day using a small amount of fluoridated toothpaste. Use of a fluoride oral rinse or varnish is appropriate, especially when the child has a high degree of susceptibility and when there is a problem of reduced manual dexterity.

Visits to a dentist regularly are essential to detect and treat early lesions. Usually, every 6 months is sufficient, but when the child is especially susceptible, more frequent visits are important, as suggested by the dentist. Preventive procedures, such as topical fluoride applications to the tooth surfaces and the use of sealants to flow into and fill the susceptible pits and fissures on the occlusal surfaces of the posterior teeth, are to be encouraged.

Children who have special health care needs or have had radiation of the head or neck or chemotherapy may have a reduced salivary flow, which is probably the most serious deleterious influence on caries initiation and progression. Special attention to frequent and careful oral hygiene and frequent use of oral fluoride rinses are imperative.

The most publicized and promising research is an approach developed by Hillman and associates. They have genetically modified a mutans streptococcus bacterium so that it no longer produces acid while competing aggressively for the niche where the wild-type mutans streptococcus is found. In laboratory animals and in limited human trials, once the substitution is introduced, it entirely displaces the disease causing wild-type mutans streptococcus. Not only does this stop the disease process, it also precluded the reemergence of the disease-causing organism and eliminates reinfection.

REFERENCES

1. Baum BJ. Principles of saliva secretion. In: Malamud D, Tabak L, editors. Saliva as a Diagnostic Fluid. Ann N Y Acad Sci 1993;694:17–23.
2. Turner RJ. Mechanisms of fluid secretion by salivary glands. In: Malamud D, Tabak L, editors. Saliva as a Diagnostic Fluid. Ann N Y Acad Sci 1993;694:24–35.

3. Berkowitz RJ, Jordan HV. Similarity of bacteriocins of *Streptococcus mutans* from mother and infant. Arch Oral Biol 1975;20:725–30.
4. Berkowitz RJ, Mutans streptococci: Acquisition and transmission. Pediatr Dent 2006;28:106–9.
5. Berkowitz RJ, Turner J, Green P. Maternal salivary levels of *Streptococcus mutans* and primary oral infection in infants. Arch Oral Biol 1981;26:147–9.
6. Kohler B, Bratthall D. Intrafamilial levels of *Streptococcus mutans* and some aspects of the bacterial transmission. Scand J Dent Res 1978;86:35–42.
7. Diagnosis and management of dental caries throughout life. NIH Consens Statement 2001;18:1–30.
8. Scott DB, Ussing MJ, Sognnaes RF, et al. Electron microscopy of mature dental enamel. J Dent Res 1952;31:74–84.
9. Sognnaes RF, Shaw JH. Salivary and pulpal contributions to the radiophosphorus uptake in enamel and dentin. J Am Dent Assoc 1952;44:489–505.
10. Silverstone LM, Hicks MJ, Featherstone MJ. Dynamic factors affecting lesion initiation and progression in human dental enamel. Part I. The dynamic nature of dental caries. Quintessence Int 1988;19:683–711.
11. Silverstone LM, Hicks MJ, Featherstone MJ. Dynamic factors affecting lesion initiation and progression in human dental enamel. Part II. Surface morphology of sound enamel and caries-like lesions of enamel. Quintessence Int 1988;19:773–85.
12. Cutright DE, Bauer H. Cell renewal in the oral mucosa and skin of the rat. I. Turnover time. Oral Surg 1967;23:249–59.
13. Jolliffe N. The clinical signs. In: Jolliffe N, editor. Clinical Nutrition, 2nd edition. New York: Hoeber Medical Books; 1962. p. 28–87.
14. Wolbach SB, Howe PR. Tissue changes following deprivation of fat-soluble A vitamin. J Exp Med 1925;42:753–7.
15. Wolbach SB, Howe PR. Effect of scorbutic state upon the production of intercellular substances. Proc Soc Exp Biol Med 1925;22:400–2.
16. Mellanby M. An experimental study of the influence of diet on teeth formation. Lancet 1918;ii:767–70.
17. Weinman JP, Schour I. Experimental studies in calcification. I. The effect of a rachitogenic diet on the dental tissues of the white rat. Am J Pathol 1945;21:821–31.
18. Sweeney EA, Guzman M. Oral conditions in children from three highland villages in Guatemala. Arch Oral Biol 1966;11:687–98.
19. Sweeney EA, Cabrera J, Urrutia J, et al. Factors associated with linear hypoplasia of human deciduous incisors. J Dent Res 1969;48:1275–9.
20. Shaw JH, Griffiths D. Dental abnormalities in rats attributable to protein deficiency during reproduction. J Nutr 1963;80:123–41.
21. Menaker L, Navia JM. Effect of undernutrition during the perinatal period on caries development in the rat. III. Effects of undernutrition on biochemical parameters in the developing submandibular salivary gland. J Dent Res 1973;52:688–91.
22. Alvarez JO. Nutrition, tooth development, and dental caries. Am J Clin Nutr 1995;61:410–6.
23. Hayes C. Nutrition and growth and development of oral tissues and structures. In: Palmer C, editor. Diet and Nutrition in Oral Health. Upper Saddle River, NJ: Prentice Hall; 2002.
24. Papas AS, Joshi A, MacDonald SL, et al. Caries prevalence in xerostomic individuals. J Can Dent Assoc 1993;59:171–9.
25. Sreebny LM. Salivary flow and dental caries. In: Guggenheim B, editor. Cariology Today. Basel: S. Karger; 1984. p. 56–69.
26. Keyes PH, Jordan HV. Factors influencing the initiation, trans-mission, and inhibition of dental caries. In: Sognnaes RF, editor. Mechanisms of Hard Tissue Destruction. Washington, DC: American Association for the Advancement of Science; 1963. p. 261–83.
27. Gibbons RJ, van Houte J. Bacteriology of dental caries. In: Shaw JH, et al., editors. Textbook of Oral Biology. Philadelphia, PA: WB Saunders; 1978. p. 975–91.
28. Cummins D. The impact of research and development on the prevention of oral diseases in children and adolescents: An industry perspective. Pediatr Dent 2006;28:118–27.
29. Glass RL, editor. The first international conference on the declining prevalence of dental caries. J Dent Res 1982;61:1301–83.
30. Kent RL, Jr, Moorrees CFA. Associations in interproximal caries prevalence from a longitudinal twin study [abstract]. J Dent Res 1979;58:225.
31. Conroy JP, Messer LB, Boraas JC, et al. Dental caries and treatment characteristics in human twins reared apart. Arch Oral Biol 1993;38:937–43.
32. Mandel ID. Nature versus nurture in dental caries. J Am Dent Assoc 1994;125:1345–51.
33. Weis RL, Trithart AH. Between-meal eating habits and dental caries experience in preschool children. Am J Public Health 1960;50:1097–104.
34. Sreebny LM. Sugar availability, sugar consumption and dental caries. Community Dent Oral Epidemiol 1982;10:1–7.
35. Horowitz HS. Ethical considerations in human experimentation. J Dent Res 1977;56:154–9.
36. Hefferren JJ, editor. Scientific consensus conference on methods for the assessment of the cariogenic potential of foods. J Dent Res 1986;65:1473–543.
37. Dilley GJ, Dilley DH, Machen JB. Prolonged nursing habit: A profile of patients and their families. ASDC J Dent Child 1980;47:102–8.
38. Weinstein P, Domoto P, Koday M, et al. Results of a promising open trial to prevent baby bottle tooth decay: A fluoride varnish study. J Dent Child 1994;61:338–41.
39. Stephan RM. Intra-oral hydrogen-ion concentrations associated with dental caries activity. J Dent Res 1944;23:257–66.
40. Edgar WM. Plaque pH assessments related to food cariogenicity. In: Hefferren JJ, Koehler HM, editors. Foods, Nutrition and Dental Health. Volume 1. Park Forest South, IL: Pathotox; 1981. p. 137–47.
41. Scheinin A, Makinen KK, Tammisalo E, et al. Turku sugar studies. XVIII. Incidence of dental caries in relation to 1-year consumption of xylitol chewing gum. Acta Odontol Scand 1975;33:269–78.
42. Scheinin A, Makinen KK, Ylitalo K. Turku sugar studies. V. Final report on the effect of sucrose, fructose and xylitol diets on the caries incidence in man. Acta Odontol Scand 1975;33:67–104.
43. Hayes C. The effect of non-cariogenic sweeteners on the prevention of dental caries: A review of the evidence. J Dent Educ 2001;65:1112–5.
44. Guggenheim B. Preface. In: Guggenheim B, editor. Cariology Today. Basel, Switzerland: Karger; 1984. p. x-ii.
45. Eager JM. Denti di Chiaie (Chiaie teeth). US Public Health Rep 1901;16:2576–7.
46. McClure FJ. Water Fluoridation. The Search and the Victory. Washington, DC: National Institute of Dental Research, National Institutes of Health, US Department Health, Education and Welfare; 1970.
47. Smith MC, Lantz EM, Smith HV. The Cause of Mottled Enamel, a Defect of Human Teeth. Tempe, AZ: University of Arizona Agricultural Experimentation Station; 1931. Bulletin No.: 32.
48. Churchill HV. Occurrence of fluorides in some waters of the United States. Ind Eng Chem 1931;23:996.
49. Velu H. Le darmous (ou dermes). Fluorose spontanee des zones phosphate. Arch Inst Pasteur Alger 1932;1:41–118.
50. Roholm K. Fluorine intoxication. A Clinical-Hygienic Study with a Review of the Literature and Some Experimental Investigations. London: HK Lewis and Co; 1937.
51. Dean HT. Chronic endemic dental fluorosis (mottled enamel). In: Gordon SM, editor. Dental Science and Dental Art. Philadelphia, PA: Lea & Febiger; 1938. p. 387–414.
52. Hodge HC, Smith FA. Some public health aspects of water fluoridation. In: Shaw JH, editor. Fluoridation as a Public Health Measure. Washington, DC: American Association for the Advancement of Science; 1954. p. 79–109.
53. McKay FS (in collaboration with Black GV). Investigations of mottled teeth: An endemic developmental imperfection of the enamel of the teeth, heretofore unknown in the literature of dentistry. Dent Cosmos 1916;58:627–44, 781–92, 894–904.
54. Dean HT, Jay P, Arnold FA, Jr, et al. Domestic water and dental caries. II. A study of 2,832 children aged 12–14 years of eight suburban Chicago communities, including *L. acidophilus* studies of 1,761 children. US Public Health Rep 1941;56:761–9.
55. Dean HT, Arnold FA, Jr, Elvove E. Domestic water and dental caries. V. Additional studies of relation of fluoride domestic waters to dental caries experience in 4,425 children, aged 12 to 14 years, of 13 cities in 4 states. US Public Health Rep 1942;57:1155–79.
56. Arnold FA, Jr, Dean HT, Jay P, et al. Effect of water fluoridation of public water supplies on dental caries prevalence, tenth year of the Grand Rapids-Muskegon study. US Public Health Rep 1956;71:652–8.
57. Arnold FA, Jr, Likins RC, Russell AL, et al. Fifteenth year of the Grand Rapids fluoridation study. J Am Dent Assoc 1962;65:780–5.
58. Ast DB, Smith DJ, Wachs B, et al. Newburgh-Kingston caries-fluorine study: Combined clinical and roentgenographic dental findings after ten years of fluoride experience. J Am Dent Assoc 1956;52:314–25.
59. Hutton WL, Linscott BW, Williams B. Final report of local studies on water fluoridation in Brantford. Can J Public Health 1956;47:89–92.
60. Fluoridation census, 1992. Atlanta, GA: US Department of Health and Human Services, National Centers for Disease and Prevention, Division of Oral Health; September 1993.
61. Whitford GM. Overview of fluoride metabolism. In: Whitford GM, editor. The Metabolism and Toxicity of Fluoride. Basel, Switzerland: Karger; 1989. p. 1–30.
62. Whitford GM. Renal handling of fluoride. In: Whitford GM, editor. The Metabolism and Toxicity of Fluoride. Basel, Switzerland: Karger; 1989. p. 51–66.
63. Adair S. Evidence-based use of fluoridein comtemporary pediatric dental practice. Pediatr Dent 2006;28:133–141.
64. Clark DC. Appropriate use of fluorides in the 1990s. J Can Dent Assoc 1993;59:272–9.
65. Whitford GM. Fluoride in dental products: Safety considerations. J Dent Res 1987;66:1056–60.
66. Marinho VCC, Higgins JPT, Logan S, et al. Fluoirde varnishes for preventing dental caries in children and adolescents. Cochrane Database Syst Rev 2002, Issue1.
67. Varmus H. 1995 Senate Appropriations Subcommittee Hearing, March 17, 1994.
68. Dawes C. Fluorides: Mechanisms of action and recommendations for use. J Can Dent Assoc 1989;55:721–3.
69. Dawes C, Weatherell JA. Kinetics of fluoride in the oral fluids. J Dent Res 1990;69:638–44.
70. Fejerskov O. Changing paradigms in concepts on dental caries: Consequences for oral health care. Carfies Res 2004;38:182–91.
71. Meiers JC, Jensen ME. Management of the questionable carious fissure: Invasive vs. noninvasive techniques. J Am Dent Assoc 1984;108:64.
72. Berglund A. Estimation by a 24-hour long study of the daily dose of intra-oral mercury vapor inhaled after release from dental amalgam. J Dent Res 1990;69:1646–51.
73. Osborne JW. Dental amalgams and mercury vapor release. In: Effects and Side-Effects of Dental Restorative Materials. An NIH Technology Assessment Conference, National Institute of Dental Research, Bethesda, MD, August 26–28, 1991. Adv Dent Res 1992;6:135–8.
74. Jones DW. The enigma of amalgam in dentistry. J Can Dent Assoc 1993;59:155–66.
75. Söderling E, Isokangas P, Pienihakkinen K, et al. Influence of maternal xylitol consumption on acquisition of mutans streptococci by infants. J Dent Res 2000;79:882–7.

Adolescence: Healthy and Disordered Eating

Ellen S. Rome, MD, MPH
Nancy E. Blazar, RD, LD

Adolescence consists of a period of rapid and often dramatic changes in the teen's physical, cognitive, and emotional states. The pubertal growth spurt, surpassed only by the growth rate in the first 2 years of life,[1] forces each teen to deal with changing body habitus, with resultant shifts in body image. Simultaneously, each teen must deal with the development of primary and secondary sexual characteristics, alterations in mood, and differentiation of cognitive ability.[2,3] Because the onset and speed of these changes can vary considerably, adolescents can be particularly sensitive about their appearance.[4] Many teens attempt to gain control or a sense of mastery over their changing bodies and environment through changes in dietary habits or behaviors.[5–7] Others may engage in exercise for a variety of reasons, ranging from recreation to fitness to use as a means of weight control.[8] Nutrition during this period of rapid growth can be critical for adolescents in ensuring a healthy progression through puberty and achievement of full height, optimal bone density, and, for girls, initiation/continuation of normal menstrual cycles.

Adolescent diets have been shown to contain inadequate amounts of calcium, iron, and other essential nutrients.[9] Teens also may ingest protein, total fats, saturated fats, and cholesterol in higher than recommended doses.[10] Young athletes with higher energy demands may also consume nutrients that are inadequate to ensure growth and development. Moreover, aberrant eating patterns can have their antecedents prior to or early in adolescence, at which point, eating disorders can emerge.[11] A fine line often exists between pursuit of fitness and "healthy" exercising and the more obsessive hyperexercising seen in many teens with eating disorders. This chapter addresses the nutritional concerns of the healthy adolescent as well as the specific dietary concerns for those patients with eating disorders. Topics to be covered include the diagnostic criteria for anorexia nervosa, bulimia nervosa, and eating disorder not otherwise specified and a brief overview of the medical complications associated with these conditions. The role of exercise will also be addressed, including the issues of amenorrhea and osteopenia in the adolescent athlete with and without an eating disorder. Strategies for nutritional intervention in the office setting will be provided with the goal of prevention, early identification, and treatment of adolescents at risk for an eating disorder or experiencing the consequences of nutritional insufficiency.

GUIDELINES FOR THE DIETARY NEEDS OF THE HEALTHY ADOLESCENT

Adolescent dietary needs differ from the needs of younger children in the amount of required calcium, iron, most vitamins and minerals, and calories. The calorie and protein needs of adolescents are influenced by several factors, including gender, age, degree of maturation, and level of activity. The main nutritional goal is for the adolescent to ingest optimal nutrients in a balanced way to promote growth and health. Sometimes this nutritional goal is not achieved owing to adolescent eating practices, lifestyle, behaviors, and, in some cases, inadequate food and income.

Recommended daily caloric and nutrient requirements by age are seen in Appendix II.To look at energy needs in a different way, many dietitians and clinicians use calories and protein per unit height instead of per unit weight as this method takes into account growth better than would a calculation based on weight.[12,13] For instance, if an adolescent girl with anorexia nervosa had her caloric needs estimated by weight, we might underestimate her needs; conversely, an obese adolescent might overestimate caloric needs if using kcal/kg body weight as the basis for determining energy needs. The Recommended Dietary Allowances (RDAs) categorized the calorie and protein needs by chronologic age, without taking into account height. Table 1 shows the comparison between estimated calories based on weight versus height. A concrete example might be the calculation of energy needs for a 15-year-old girl at a weight of 50 kg (110 pounds) and a height of 160 cm. Based on weight, her calorie needs would be 50 kg × 40 kcal/kg = 2,000 kcal. Protein needs based on weight would be 50 kg × 0.08 g/cm = 40 g of protein. Based on height, the calculations change to 160 cm × 13.5 kcal/cm = 2,160 kcal, and for protein, 160 cm × .27 g/cm = 43.2 g protein per day.

The use of the kcal/cm factor provides a quick formula by which to calculate daily needs. For a longer method that takes into account weight, height, and age, basal energy expenditure can be used. The basal metabolic rate (BMR), estimated by the resting energy expenditure (REE), represents the minimum amount of energy needed by the body at rest in the fasting state; measuring REE is usually expensive and inconvenient for the office setting. Estimations of the standard REE for an individual prove more useful for the health care provider and can be calculated from the Harris Benedict equation[14]:

Table 1 Adolescent Nutritional Requirements: Comparison of Recommended Calorie and Protein Needs

		Calories		Protein	
	Age	kcal/kg	kcal/cm	g/kg	g/cm
Males	11–14	55	15.9	1.0	0.29
	15–18	45	17.1	0.9	0.34
	19–24	40	16.4	0.8	0.33
Females	11–14	47	14.0	1.0	0.29
	15–18	40	13.5	0.8	0.27
	19–24	38	13.4	0.8	0.28

Adapted from Subcommittee on the Tenth Edition of the RDAs, Food and Nutrition Board, Commission on Life Sciences, National Research Council.[177]

$$\text{For females, REE} = 665 + (9.6 \times \text{wt in kg}) + (1.7 \times \text{ht in cm}) - (4.7 \times \text{age in years})$$

$$\text{For males, REE} = 66 + (13.7 \times \text{wt in kg}) + (5 \times \text{ht in cm}) - (6.8 \times \text{age in years})$$

Above REE, energy requirements are also determined by activity level and the need for weight gain above basal requirements. Correction factors for activity levels and various disease states are seen in Appendix Table I-12.[15–18] Total energy requirements are estimated by multiplying REE by the activity and stress correction factors. The Mayo Clinic Nomogram can also be used to calculate total energy expenditure from surface area, age, and sex.[19]

Adolescents have high intakes of protein, total and saturated fat, and cholesterol. The intake of fat in a typical adolescent diet is around 33%, which is higher than the amount recommended by the American Heart Association (30% calories from fat). In general, adolescents consume more fat than recommended, and their food intakes are deficient in important vitamins and minerals such as calcium and iron.[20–24] A subset of adolescents are overly concerned about their weight and their appearance.[25] Many are dissatisfied with their weight, especially girls who want to lose weight and boys who are underweight and want to be heavier, with more muscle mass. Many adolescents follow unsafe practices to control their weight and to lose weight. Such practices include the use of diet pills, laxatives, vomiting, diuretics, fasting, and strict diets that can compromise the health and growth of the adolescent.[26] In our health-conscious society, the norm for this subset of teens may be a low-fat diet or a more Atkins-like variant (high protein, low carbs). Teens following a low-fat plan, along with their mothers and/or families, may falsely assume that "low fat" should mean "no fat." Actually, a low-fat diet for a child, teen, or young adult needs to include a minimum of 30 to 50 g of fat per day. Those following an Atkins or South Beach diet may be missing out on other food groups. In terms of calories, the ideal balance for the average teen should be as follows:

Regular diet:	*Low-fat diet:*
50–55% carbohydrate	50–55% carbohydrate
15–20% protein	15–20% protein
30% fat	20–25% fat

So, a teen consuming a 2,100-calorie diet might require 70 g of fat (30% calories), 105 g of protein (20%), and 263 g of carbohydrate (50%). Fluid requirements can be calculated in terms of body weight, using the following formula:

Body weight	*Maintenance fluid needs per day*
1–10 kg	100 mL/kg
11–20 kg	1,000 mL + 50 mL/kg for each kg above 10 kg
Above 20 kg	1,500 mL + 20 mL/kg for each kg above 20 kg

Thus, an adolescent weighing 50 kg (110 pounds) needs around 1,500 mL + (30 kg × 20 mL/kg) = 2,100 mL fluid per day or the equivalent of 8.4 cups (8 oz/cup). The adolescent athlete may require higher calories to meet increased energy demands of their sport, with the difference made up by extra carbohydrates usually to best maximize performance. The nutritionally restricting athlete may run into problems of not meeting basic energy, protein, or dietary fat needs, although sheer percentages may meet an 80 to 15 to 5% distribution. General guidelines for adolescent athletes can be found in Table 2.

Table 2 Guidelines for Adolescent Athletes

General recommendations

- Adolescent athletes need between 6 and 10 g of carbohydrate per kg of body weight per day.
- Food intake should emphasize the consumption of complex carbohydrates and moderate amounts of fat.
- Fat intake should be kept at 30% of calories from fat.
- Protein recommendations for endurance athletes are 1.2 to 1.4 g/kg body weight. For strength-trained athletes, the protein requirements may increase to 1.6 to 1.7 g/kg body weight per day. The increase in protein intake can be easily met through diet without the use of supplements; therefore, protein and amino acid supplements are not recommended.
- Water is the best alternative for fluid. Diluted fruit juices and sport drinks are also acceptable.
- Vitamin and mineral supplements are not recommended unless the adolescent is not consuming adequate amounts of food.
- Vegetarian athletes may be at risk for low calorie, protein, and micronutrient intake.
- There is no scientific evidence to support the notion that supplements improve athletic performance. Liquid supplements should be recommended only to athletes with poor nutrient intake.
- Adolescent athletes and nonathletes are at risk for iron deficiency and low intakes of calcium. Food intake should emphasize the consumption of those two nutrients.
- Adolescent athletes need adequate calories especially at the time of high-intensity training to support growth and to avoid muscle mass losses and menstrual dysfunction.

Before exercise

- Adolescents should eat a light meal about 3 h prior to competition.
- Adolescent athletes should drink between 14 and 22 oz of fluid 2 h before exercise.
- Adolescent athletes should not eat sweet foods or drinks before participation in sports.
- A snack or meal before exercise should be high in carbohydrate, low in fat, moderate in protein, and low in fiber.

During exercise

- The most important goal when the athlete is doing exercise is to replace fluid losses and provide between 30 and 60 g of carbohydrate per hour, especially for endurance events that last over an hour.
- 6 to 12 oz of fluid should be consumed every 15 to 20 min, depending on tolerance.

After exercise

- After exercise, the goal is to provide adequate fluids, energy, and carbohydrates.
- Provide a carbohydrate intake of 1.5 g/kg of body weight during the first 30 min and again every 2 h for 4 to 6 h.
- After exercise, the athlete needs to drink between 16 and 24 oz of fluid for every pound of weight loss during exercise.
- After a strenuous competition, athletes should consume a mixed meal with adequate amounts of carbohydrate, protein, and fats.

Adapted from Nutrition and athletic performance: position of the American Dietetic Association, Dietitians of Canada, and the American College of Sports Medicine. J Am Diet Assoc 2000;100:1543–56.

During the pubertal growth spurt, the adolescent acquires 15% of adult height, 50% of adult weight, and 40% of adult total-body mineral content.[27] Over half of the adult bone calcium is normally deposited during adolescence, with bone calcium content reaching a potential maximum by age 30.[28] During this time, the daily intake of elemental calcium must be above a threshold level to meet the daily demands and add new calcium to bone, in other words, creating a positive calcium balance. Currently, the RDA for calcium in teenagers 12 to 18 years of age is 1,200 mg/day. Some studies have suggested that this amount is insufficient to meet the needs of rapidly growing teens.[29,30] In a calcium balance study, Matkovic and Ilich found that the minimum daily intake of elemental calcium required by adolescents to reach the threshold level is 1,480 mg/day, significantly above the RDA of 1,200 mg/day. The authors recommended a daily intake of 1,600 mg/day to mineralize new bone without depleting current skeletal reserves in growing teens.[31] Without additional calcium supplementation, meeting 1,600 mg calcium daily would require approximately five servings of milk, cheese, or yoghurt a day (for 1,200 mg, that means four of these servings a day). It is noteworthy that most healthy teenagers fail to meet the RDA of 1,200 mg/day,[32] and patients with eating disorders have been shown to ingest insufficient calcium. In teens with anorexia nervosa, intakes have ranged from 300 mg/day to 1,100 mg/day, with most in the range of 500 to 600 mg/day.[33–36]

To create a positive calcium balance, many teens with eating disorders will require calcium supplementation. Several acceptable forms are available, as outlined in Table 3. Calcium supplements vary in their ability to be absorbed. To test the quality of a particular supplement, the tablet can be placed in a glass of vinegar. If the tablet has not dissolved after 10 minutes, it is not readily bioavailable, or an easily absorbed source of calcium.[37] The patient should be reminded not to drink the glass of vinegar, that it is only a test to see if she picked a brand useful for her body. To maximize absorption, clinicians should instruct their patients to take calcium carbonate supplements at mealtime as the presence of food in the stomach increases acid levels, helping with absorption. Although calcium carbonate supplements contain the highest percentage of elemental calcium, they may also cause constipation or flatulence. Calcium citrate supplements have a higher absorption rate (next in line is calcium carbonate, than calcium phosphate). Calcium citrate supplements can be taken at any time, making them easier for patients on a busy schedule. Calcium phosphate can be found in calcium-fortified orange juice, soy milk, and rice milk. Nonchewable supplements should be taken with water to help them dissolve. Absorption is better when a patient ingests no more than 500 mg of calcium at a time. Women's multivitamins with calcium may contain up to 450 mg of calcium, whereas a typical multivitamin may contain significantly less calcium. Other helpful hints include having patients avoid taking calcium with high-fiber meals as fiber reduces the amount of calcium the body can use; avoid preparations with bone meal, dolomite, and oyster shell as they may contain contaminants or toxic ingredients; and avoid taking iron and calcium supplements simultaneously

Table 3 Available Calcium Supplements

Product	Type of Calcium	Manufacturer	Elemental Calcium per Tablet (mg)
Calcet	Calcium lactate, calcium gluconate, calcium carbonate	Mission Pharmacal	153
Calcet Triple Calcium + Vitamin D	Calcium lactate, calcium gluconate, calcium carbonate	Mission Pharmacal	300
Caltrate 600 Plus	Calcium carbonate	Lederle Laboratories	600
Caltrate 600 + Vitamin D	Calcium carbonate	Lederle Laboratories	600
Citracal	Calcium citrate	Mission Pharmacal	200
Citracal + Vitamin D	Calcium citrate	Mission Pharmacal	315
Citracal Liquitabs	Calcium citrate	Mission Pharmacal	500
One a Day for Women multivitamin	Calcium carbonate	Bayer	450
OsCal 500 chewable tablets	Calcium carbonate	Marion Laboratories	500
OsCal 500 + Vitamin D	Calcium carbonate	Marion Laboratories	500
Rolaids	Calcium carbonate	Warner-Lambert	220
Rolaids—extra strength	Calcium carbonate	Warner-Lambert	271
Titralac—extra strength	Calcium carbonate	3M	300
TUMS	Calcium carbonate	Smith Kline Beecham	200
TUMS—extra strength	Calcium carbonate	Smith Kline Beecham	300
TUMS 500	Calcium carbonate	Smith Kline Beecham	500
Viactiv*	Calcium carbonate	McNeil Nutritionals	500
Calcium Soft Chews*	Calcium carbonate	Trader Joe's	500

*Do not use if patient has lactose intolerance.

as they may interfere with each other's absorption. The calcium content of some foods and drinks is seen in Table 4.

EATING DISORDERS: DEFINITIONS

Described as the "relentless pursuit of thinness,"[38] anorexia nervosa is characterized by extreme weight loss, distorted body image, and a morbid fear of obesity.[39,40] Diagnostic criteria have evolved over time, with *DSM-V* currently being formulated. The prior iteration, from the *Diagnostic and Statistical Manual of Mental Disorders, Fourth Edition (DSM-IV)*,[41] is outlined in Table 5. This table includes definitions for anorexia nervosa, bulimia nervosa, and eating disorder not otherwise specified. Of note, in *DSM-IV*,[41] anorexia nervosa can involve either weight loss leading to maintenance of body weight less than 85% of that expected or a failure to gain the expected amount of weight during a period of growth, leading to a body weight of less than 85% of that expected. In other words, a teen with a distorted body image who gains in height but maintains a given weight can cross weight centiles during that period of growth, alerting the astute clinician to a potential problem even before other symptoms have become apparent. The latest revision in *DSM-V* will try to address some of the issues in younger children, with a hope of preventing pathology including failure of growth or brain development. These efforts are supported by such data as that from Swenne and Thurfiell (2003),[42] who found that inadequate weight gain and growth retardation preceded the diagnosis of eating disorders in 45 premenarchal girls. At their maximal weight, girls were 12.5 + 1.7 years old, and found to be significantly lighter, shorter, and leaner than the general population. A year later, these girls had lost 5.8 + 4.3 kg of body weight, were 2.27 standard deviations below expected weight goals, and further stunted in height. What was noteworthy in this study was that two-thirds of the weight deficits and 60% of the height deficit was generated before the onset of weight loss.

Table 4 Comparison of Calcium Content in Various Foods

Food	Serving	Calcium per Serving (mg)
Milk	1 cup	300
American cheese	1 oz	174
Cottage cheese	1/2 cup	77
Tofu	1/2 cup	434
Ice cream	1/2 cup	88
Yogurt	1 cup	345–415
Frozen yogurt	1/2 cup	104
Broccoli (cooked)	1/2 cup	89
Orange juice fortified with calcium	1 cup (8 oz)	300

Typically, the adolescent who is either overweight or dissatisfied with current body image moves from a moderate effort to lose weight to an intense preoccupation with weight loss and eating; eventually, food-related activities interfere with socialization and family activities. School performance is often affected last, if at all. Restrictive anorexic adolescents are often characterized as obsessive-compulsive, perfectionistic, introverted, and emotionally inhibited.[43,44]

Bulimia nervosa, derived from the Greek root meaning "ox hunger,"[45] is characterized by the binge eating behavior, in which one "eats like a bull." Typically, bulimia nervosa begins in a teen who has been trying to control his or her weight with little success; he or she discovers, either spontaneously, from a friend or family member, or from the media, that self-induced vomiting, laxatives, or diet pills can control weight.[40] Binges may develop subsequently and can involve the ingestion of up to 20,000 calories in a 1- to 2-hour period, with resultant abdominal discomfort, distress, or fatigue.[46] For other patients, a "binge" might consist of the same amount a healthy person would consider normal. In the patient with an eating disorder, this volume triggers an inordinate amount of guilt or negative feelings. Binges usually end with compensatory behavior, such as self-induced vomiting, exercise, and abuse of laxatives or diuretics. Other binges end with an exhausted food supply or interruption by family or friends. These patients often display other impulsive behaviors, including stealing, overspending, substance abuse, self-mutilation, and promiscuity.[47] A history of sexual abuse has also been reported in 20 to 50% of patients with bulimia nervosa.[48]

The teen with anorexia nervosa whose actions and thoughts appear to be egosyntonic or consistent with her inner self feels justified in her behaviors and is extremely resistant to therapy. This intrapsychic state depends on a severe level of cognitive denial and disappears when the denial is successfully challenged. In contrast to the adolescent with anorexia nervosa, the bulimic teen's thoughts and actions are egodystonic, causing her to have feelings of guilt, loss of control, and acute distress. Adolescents with bulimia are more likely to seek help, whereas adolescents with anorexia nervosa are often dragged in by concerned family or friends. However, changing the behavior can be just as difficult in a bulimic patient as in a patient with anorexia nervosa.

Challenges of Current Definitions

As mentioned above, the current definitions are limiting in usage, with several factors being particularly problematic. In a retrospective chart review of 588 consecutive admissions to an inpatient treatment program, Watson and Anderson (2003) found that 297 females had some form of anorexia nervosa, with 77.4% meeting *DSM-IV* criteria, while 22.6% with similar core psychopathology and self-starvation met criteria for ED-NOS because of some menstrual function or final weight above 85%.[49] The groups displayed few statistically significant differences in demographics, illness history, psychopathology, bone density, and treatment response. They concluded that neither amenorrhea nor weight below 85% of ideal body weight was a useful diagnostic criterion for the spectrum of anorexia nervosa. In fact, insurance companies may use failure to meet these strict

Table 5 Diagnostic Criteria for Anorexia Nervosa, Bulimia Nervosa, and Eating Disorder not Otherwise Specified

Anorexia nervosa

Intense fear of becoming fat or gaining weight, even when underweight

Refusal to maintain body weight at or above a minimally normal weight for age and height (eg, weight loss leading to maintenance of body weight <85% of that expected or failure to gain weight during a period of growth leading to body weight <85% of weight expected)

Disturbed body image, undue influence of weight or shape on self-evaluation, or denial of the seriousness of the current low body weight

Amenorrhea or absence of at least three consecutive menstrual periods for those postmenarchal (also considered amenorrheic if periods inducible only after estrogen therapy)

Types

Restricting = no regular binges or purges (self-induced vomiting or use of laxatives or diuretics)

Binge eating/purging = regularly binges or purges in patient who also meets the above criteria for anorexia nervosa

Bulimia nervosa

Recurrent episodes of binge eating, characterized by eating a substantially larger amount of food in a discrete period of time (eg, in 2 h) than would be eaten by most people in similar circumstances during that same time period

A sense of lack of control over eating during the binge

Recurrent inappropriate compensatory behavior in order to prevent weight gain, eg, self-induced vomiting, use of laxatives or diuretics, fasting, or hyperexercising

Binges or inappropriate compensatory behaviors occurring, on average, at least twice weekly for at least 3 mo

Self-evaluation unduly influenced by body shape or weight

The disturbance does not occur exclusively during periods of anorexia nervosa

Types

Purging = regularly engages in self-induced vomiting or use of laxatives or diuretics

Nonpurging = uses other inappropriate compensatory behaviors, eg, fasting, hyperexercising, without regular use of vomiting or medicines to purge

***Eating disorder** not otherwise specified (those that do not meet criteria for anorexia nervosa or bulimia nervosa by* DSM-IV)

All criteria for anorexia nervosa except has regular menses

All criteria for anorexia nervosa except weight still in normal range

All criteria for bulimia nervosa except binges less than twice a week or less than 3 mo

A patient with normal body weight who regularly engages in inappropriate compensatory behavior after eating small amounts of food (eg, self-induced vomiting after eating 2 cookies)

A patient who repeatedly chews and spits out large amounts of food without swallowing

Binge eating disorder: recurrent binges without the compensatory behaviors associated with bulimia nervosa

Adapted from the American Psychiatric Association, Diagnostic and Statistical Manual of Mental Disorders, 4th ed. Washington, DC: American Psychiatric Association; 1994.

criteria as a means of withholding needed medical benefits. The Academy for Eating Disorders and other organizations have recently been increasing efforts to advocate for expanded coverage for eating disorder treatment in the United States, with recent deaths of those patients denied care by insurance serving to crystallize the issues.

Younger children with eating disorders may not fit neatly into a specific psychiatric category, compounded by a lack of recognition of eating disorders in younger children by parts of the medical community.[50–53] Another challenge comes from the cognitive differences between children and adults. This issue becomes relevant as more children of younger ages are getting diagnosed with eating disorders. Children tend be less able to voice conscious cognitive processes that underlie behaviors or emotions, which poses a challenge when trying to strictly apply *DSM-IV* criteria. For instance, a child of 8 or 9 years may or may not state that they want to lose weight, but they may refuse food and have all symptomatology otherwise match strict definitions of anorexia nervosa. Our view is that we are looking at the same disorder expressed differently across various cognitive ages and stages, but this view remains to be confirmed. A current working group on challenges of *DSM-V* has commented that it may be better to focus diagnostic criteria on observed behaviors and their consequences rather than mandating verbalized acknowledgment of conscious motivation as reasons for these behaviors.[54]

EPIDEMIOLOGY

Incidence rates for anorexia nervosa have increased steadily from 1975 to 1991 in teens ages 10 to 19 years, although rates in adults have remained relatively constant.[55–57] The prevalence has been most recently estimated to be 0.5 to 3% of adolescent and young adult women, with an increasingly larger number of "healthy" girls expressing worrisome eating attitudes and weight concerns.[39,58–61] The classic image of the overachieving "perfect little girl" from the upper-middle-class family is also being challenged, with more eating disorders seen in males (up to 5 to 10% of all cases) and in teens with a variety of backgrounds, ethnicities, and psychological profiles.[58,61–64] Eating disorders have been found in increasing numbers in Japan, China, and other countries.[65–67] In the United States, eating disorders are on the rise in minority groups such as Hispanics and native Americans.[68]

Bulimia nervosa tends to begin in late adolescence with a teen of normal or high weight. The prevalence of bulimia nervosa has been estimated to be 1 to 19% using DSM-IV criteria.[47,55,58,69,70] Studies of female high school and college students have found symptoms of bulimia in 4.5 and 18%, respectively.[71,72] Higher rates of anxiety (43%), chemical dependency disorders (49%), bipolar disorders (12%), and personality disorders or personality trait disturbances (50–75%) have also been found in patients with bulimia nervosa.[47,73–77] Another series found that 50% of patients with anorexia nervosa and 30% of patients with bulimia nervosa met criteria for major depression.[78]

Anorexia nervosa continues to have two peaks of onset, one in early adolescence (ages 11–14 years) and a second peak in late adolescence (17–19 years),[39,79] although cases have been described in the literature in children as young as 7.[52,80] In our personal experience, we have seen one child meeting full criteria for bulimia nervosa at age 5 years, with symptoms beginning at age $3^1/_2$ years. In a recent study, 959 patients treated between 1997 and 1995 at Stanford's eating disorder program were evaluated to see if differences existed between older adolescents and younger children at initial evaluation.[51] In their study, younger patients (mean age 11.6 years + 1.2 years) were more likely than older adolescents (mean age 15.6 years + 1.4 years) to be male ($p < 0.005$) or diagnosed with EDNOS ($p < 0.05$), and less likely to be diagnosed with bulimia nervosa ($p < 0.001$). No differences in prevalence of anorexia nervosa between the younger and older patients were found. Younger patients were less likely to report purging, binge eating, useing diet pills or laxatives than were older patients. These findings are not surprising, with many younger children with eating disorders anecdotally telling us that they do not have access to use of diet pills or laxatives, or "my mother would kill me," with parental approval carrying more weight for the child than older adolescent. In Dr. Peebles's study, young patients weighed less in percentage ideal body weight, had a shorter duration of disease, and had lost weight more rapidly than had older adolescents. Several other studies have found younger patients with eating disorders more likely to be male.[52,81–84] In school-based studies of 8- to 13-year-olds, 20 to 56% report dieting, 44 to 71% had tried exercising to lose weight, 1.4 to 10% had tried purging or using diet pills or laxatives, and 4 to 6.5% reported binge eating on a regular basis.[84–88]

Many adolescents may show unhealthful eating behaviors even without evidence of a full-blown eating disorder. Adolescents and young adults who are required to reduce their food intake or follow a strict diet owing to a disease state are at high risk for developing an eating disorder.[89] In a study of 4,746 public middle school and high school students in Minnesota, healthful weight control behaviors were used by the majority of teens to control weight (85% adolescent girls, 70% adolescent boys).[90] These behaviors included cutting down on high-fat items and sweets, increasing fruits and vegetables, and exercise. Unhealthful weight control practices included fasting, restricting, using a food substitute (powder or special drink), skipping meals, and smoking more cigarettes; these behaviors were used by 57% of adolescent girls and 33% of adolescent boys. Extreme weight control behaviors, defined as use of diet pills, laxatives, diuretics, or vomiting to control weight, were used by 12% of the girls and 5% of the boys. The authors found that a high percentage of average-weight girls perceived themselves as overweight desired to weigh less, and expressed body dissatisfaction.[90] Their data also found that obese adolescents recognized that they were overweight, with most reporting some steps taken to lose weight. Thus, prevention of both obesity and eating disorders may lie less in recognizing who is overweight and a superficial review of desirable weight control behaviors; rather, interventions may be more effective if more time is spent in building skills in how to engage in healthful weight control behaviors successfully.[90] Further strategies for eating-disorder nutritional management are discussed in more detail later in this chapter.

In the most recent Youth Risk Behavior Surveillance Data from high schools in the United States, 12.3% of students reported fasting for 24 hours to lose weight or to keep from gaining weight, 6.3% had tried diet pills, powders, or liquids to lose weight or keep from gaining, and 4.5% had tried vomiting or use of laxatives to manipulate weight, with more females than males reporting any of these behaviors.[91] The female athlete triad describes the combination of disordered eating, amenorrhea, and osteopenia; in a recent study of the triad among high school athletes, Nichols et al found that 18.2% of girls met the criteria for disordered eating, 23.5% for menstrual irregularity, and 21.8% for low bone mass, with only 5.9% meeting two of the three criteria to earn the definition of the triad and 1.2% meeting criteria for all three components of the triad.[83] This study captures another aspect limiting epidemiologic studies; many represent a snapshot in time, with full aspects of a diagnosable eating disorder only captured over time, rather than at a glance.

In a study in Cleveland, Ohio, 1,268 urban, suburban, and rural high school students were given questionnaires asking about dieting and purging behavior.[5] Laxatives and diuretics were used more frequently by black girls than by white girls (10 vs 3% for laxatives, 5 vs 2% for diuretics). Vomiting was used more commonly by white girls, with 8% vomiting monthly compared with only 1% of black girls. It should be noted that 40% of the boys reported dieting, with similar dieting and purging behaviors between black and white boys. A survey of 36,320 Minnesota public school students in grades 7 through 12 revealed chronic dieting reported by 12.1% of the girls and 2.1% of the boys, with significantly greater numbers of girls dieting as they progressed from junior high through high school. Chronic dieters were more likely to report use of laxatives, ipecac, diuretics, self-induced vomiting, and other maladaptive behaviors.[7] Thus, clinicians should be alerted to the possibility that an adolescent who has reported chronic dieting may be developing an eating disorder.

Some male runners with compulsive exercise patterns have been shown to have bizarre preoccupations with food, concern about weight with strict monitoring of intake, and a high achievement orientation.[92] Such behaviors may indicate the presence of an eating disorder in the male athlete. In a group of 93 elite women runners, 13% had been diagnosed previously with anorexia nervosa, 25% displayed binge eating, 9% binged and purged, and 34% had atypical eating practices.[93] Among college athletes who often engage in highly intense competition, abnormal dietary patterns are prevalent. Self-induced vomiting has been reported in 14%, laxative abuse in 16%, routine use of diet pills in 25%, and at least one unhealthful eating habit in 32% overall.[94] A study of female college gymnasts showed that 62% reported unhealthful eating behaviors, with two-thirds told by their coaches that they were too heavy.[95] Athletes whose coaches had commented on their weights were more likely to engage in unhealthful dietary practices. Athletes should be questioned by their clinicians about body image, weight concerns, menstrual patterns, and eating behaviors.

NUTRITIONAL ASSESSMENT OF THE TEEN WITH AN EATING DISORDER

A careful history and physical examination can reveal much information about the chronicity of the teen's illness, abnormal eating behaviors, and potential strategies for management. The clinician can start the history-taking session by asking the parent and the teen individually why he or she is being seen. This information can be most helpful in revealing hidden agendas or different perceptions of parents and their teenagers. Ideally, the parent and teen each should be given time alone with the provider to promote a sense of individualized caring and listening to each one's needs. Confidentiality should be established immediately, with the explicitly stated caveat that the provider will break confidentiality if the situation is life-threatening or extremely dangerous. The clinician should ask the teen what is the most he or she has ever weighed and when, and at what height. What is the least weight remembered and when, and at what height? What is the current weight and height? For girls, at what age did periods start? When was her last period? Are menses regular, with or without cramps, and how long do they last? Has flow or duration changed? If periods have ceased, at what weight was she when she had her last period? Eating disorders can be associated with both primary and secondary amenorrhea. It is helpful to elicit the age of menarche and regularity of periods of the mother and the teen's female siblings.

The clinician should also ask questions about body image and self-esteem. For instance, does the teen feel underweight, overweight, or just right? At what weight would the teen like to be? How much of his/her day is spent on food, exercise, and body thoughts? Does he or she have any "trouble spots" or areas on the body that cause the teen particular discomfort or concern? With a reticent teen, the clinician might change the phrasing to state that most people have certain parts of their body that they would like to change and then ask the teen if he or she has any "trouble areas." Asking the teen how hard he or she struggles to lose or maintain weight simultaneously gives information on the effort placed in the abnormal eating behaviors and acknowledges the difficulty and stress the teen may feel over weight issues.

The clinician should specifically ask how the teen controls weight. Does the teen vomit to lose weight and, if so, using what methods (finger, toothbrush, or other tool)? A teen who can vomit at will without use of a finger or other item has probably been practicing this behavior frequently or for a long time. Does the teen use diet pills? Diuretics? Laxatives? Ipecac? The latter is most dangerous because it binds irreversibly to cardiac muscle and can lead to fatal arrhythmia if chronically misused; even with the recent ban on ipecac for child ingestions, we still see patients accessing it. If various medicines are used to purge, what kinds, how many per day, and how often? How often does the teen have bowel movements? Are they loose or formed? Any diarrhea or constipation? How much caffeine does he or she consume daily? The amount and kinds of fluids consumed also are important. Use of over-the-counter and illicit drugs, cigarettes, and alcohol should also be assessed.

The provider should determine the amount of time spent in exercise, what kinds of exercise and level of competition, and duration of involvement in a sport (think frequency, intensity, and duration). Exercise can serve as another means of purging behavior. When women with eating disorders exercise, they tend to do so compulsively.[80] Many women pursue abnormally low body weights to participate in ballet, to compete in sports such as track or gymnastics, or to pursue a career in modeling.[97] Menstrual disorders have been associated with eating disorders in gymnasts, runners, ballet dancers, and models.[98] The amount of distress or any physical symptoms caused by missing a workout can be a fairly sensitive way to assess use of exercise as a purging strategy. Asking about level of comfort with taking days off can also get at compulsive exercise. The clinician should also ask the patient and family members whether the teen performs other "anxious" repetitive movements, such as pacing, foot tapping, or excessive trips up and down the stairs.

In obtaining a dietary history, the clinician can ask about the frequency and location of meals and snacks and about the quantity of food consumed. If she states that she eats a bagel for

Table 6 Sample Food Journal

Name						Day and Date						
Time	Place	Description of food and amount		Fluids and amount	Hunger Level*	Fullness Level*	Exercise	Purge	Binge	Pills	Emotions	

*Hunger and fullness scale: 1 =starving/empty; 5 =neutral; 10 = uncomfortably full/stuffed

breakfast, ask how many bites she can manage; in this way, the provider acknowledges his or her awareness of the difficulty in consuming foods. Is he or she able to recognize hunger, and if so, can the teen give himself or herself permission to respond and eat promptly and adequately to that cue? Does the teen usually skip breakfast? Lunch? Dinner? Can the teen comfortably eat food prepared outside the home, for example, at school, restaurants, or friends' houses? Is he or she comfortable eating in front of friends and family? At home, who prepares the food, and are meals eaten alone or with other family members? How many nights a week is there a family dinner? Does he or she ever binge or "pig out?" What constitutes a binge? The provider and the patient may have different concepts about the definition of a binge, so explicit descriptions of the last binge can be helpful. How long does a binge last? Are they planned? What are the rituals around the bingeing?

The clinician should ask if the teen has any "taboo" foods or foods that she simply cannot or will not eat. Certain foods may be deemed "safe," whereas others are "unsafe"; for example, cake and cookies may be assiduously avoided, whereas many patients will eat muffins.[99] Other patients may be sophisticated label readers and eliminate all hidden fats, believing that if less fat is good, then none is better. Foods may be classified as absolutely good or bad, often with episodes of "magical thinking." Extreme examples include avoidance of all fat grams as they will automatically produce body fat, fear of talking about food on the telephone lest the calories move through the telephone and deposit themselves on the patient's body, fear that food consumed by a sibling in the same room may result in calories absorbed by the child/teen, or assumptions that restaurants or companies prepare foods in the most caloric way possible. Some patients may refuse to look in a particular mirror in the house because of the belief that the mirror literally added pounds to the teen's hips and buttocks. Such extreme delusional thinking often resolves with refeeding,[100] but many of the associated eating behaviors can be difficult to change. Families may note unusual use of utensils in eating or ritualistic behaviors, such as cutting food into minuscule pieces or chewing each bite multiple times.

Strict avoidance of fat grams, red meat, or other items can alert the clinician to potential nutritional insufficiencies while simultaneously painting a picture of how rigid the teen's diet currently may be. Many teens begin their eating disorder with a gradual switch to "healthful eating," often heralded by the weight-conscious family as a positive sign. For instance, the teen may cut out red meat, then move to lacto-ovovegetarianism, and then shift to be a "vegan," one who abstains from consumption of meat, fish, fowl, dairy products, and eggs.[101] Although a vegetarian diet can be healthful, the adolescent may use this diet as a means to restrict further, especially in the context of a nonvegetarian family who may be accepting of this seemingly healthful change and not realize the extent of the abnormal eating. Another method for assessing daily intake is by 24-hour recall. Although this technique has achieved some popularity owing to its ease of use, its validity has been questioned.[102,103] Teens with eating disorders may exaggerate or minimize the amounts and types of food consumed, depending on whether they are restricting or bingeing. Having a parent in the room during this part of the interview may serve as a "reality check," with the body language and parents' interruptions "correcting" the teen's potential misrepresentation of amounts. Also, the meals of the teen's previous day may not be "typical," with a change in intake solely in anticipation of "reporting" to the health care provider. The main point of the 24-hour recall lies in distinguishing the types and amounts of foods consumed, including dairy products, fruits and vegetables, sources of fat and protein, and any junk foods. Patients with anorexia nervosa in particular should not be encouraged to count calories or read labels excessively as they may eat even less when attention is given to caloric contents, quantity, and quality of foods ingested. Excessive preoccupation with cooking, food channel viewing, and pro-ana or pro-mia website surfing should be red flags that a child or teen may be developing an unbalanced relationship with food.[104]

For teens with disordered eating, a 3-day food record or a daily food journal can be a useful tool, not only during the dietitian's initial assessment but also to monitor the changes being made during recovery. Specific instructions on how to complete the food record can help improve accuracy of the information. The teen should be given advice on how to quantify food using standard measuring tools (eg, tablespoons or cups rather than "mouthfuls"). Patients with obsessive-compulsive tendencies may benefit from a more generalized approach to journaling and changing behavior patterns, helping them get away from strict calorie or fat gram counting, weighing, and measuring. In contrast, patients with bulimia nervosa can use the information obtained from the food record to identify foods or situations that trigger a binge (see Table 6). Attention can be placed on the emotional state during a binge, timing, or other pertinent aspects. For instance, if a teen always binges on arrival home after school, the clinician can suggest filling the time with more structured activities so that the teen does not automatically enter the kitchen at that time. Such simple interventions can sometimes provide a new behavioral pattern for a teen who is otherwise "stuck." Asking what the teen has tried, if anything, to avoid bingeing can also guide the clinician toward potentially useful interventions. The clinician should determine how the binge/purge pattern functions for the teen (eg, do they need to purge until they feel pain, until they see "all the food," or to compensate for eating too much, or other self-induced criteria). Other questions to assess include how the binge/purge cycle typically ends and whether they engage in compensatory behaviors after a binge. For purgers, the ability to postpone vomiting for even an hour may be a positive first step. Those patients who vomit should be advised to rinse their mouths with water with baking soda or mouthwash in lieu of brushing teeth after vomiting to minimize the impact of acid on the tooth enamel.

The clinician should also ask about more general symptoms. This review of systems should include questions about the level of energy or fatigue, change in mood, depression, and suicidal ideation. Tolerance to cold, headaches, reflux, constipation, and bloating if not already asked, irritability, and changes in skin should also be assessed. Level of school and family functioning should also be determined; patients with anorexia nervosa may slowly isolate themselves from peers and family, and all teens with eating disorders may show an extreme narrowing of interest. Major losses or changes in the family structure can also trigger the onset of an eating disorder.

In the office setting, weights should be obtained in a hospital gown after voiding. Clinicians should be on the alert for weight manipulation during office visits, ranging from simple water loading for weight elevation to hiding of weights or other objects beneath the hospital gown or in various orifices. Many providers weigh patients backwards on the scale, especially if a patient will use a number on the scale to restrict further. A dipstick urinalysis can help assess specific gravity, with a value of 1.005 or less indicating water loading intentionally or perhaps a misguided view on fluid requirements. Urinalysis can also illuminate ketosis, proteinuria, and dehydration. Dehydration may result in an accelerated heart rate, masking a sinus bradycardia. Relevant findings on the physical examination of a patient with an eating disorder are listed in Table 7.

MEDICAL COMPLICATIONS OF EATING DISORDERS

Despite substantial malnourishment, adolescents with eating disorders may have remarkably few physiologic abnormalities at the time of presentation and in follow-up.[40] Medical complications of the eating disorder can be caused directly or indirectly by three processes: (1) caloric restriction, (2) purging behaviors, and (3) binges. Almost every organ system of the body can be affected by these behaviors.[105–108] Pure restrictors can have a different constellation of complications from those found in patients who purge; binges put the patient at risk for a separate set of problems. To clarify the myriad complications, the following sections divide the problems into those caused by caloric restriction, those caused by purging behaviors, and those related to bingeing.

Table 7 Physical Findings in Teens with Eating Disorders

Finding	Cause
Mouth	
Dental caries	Bingeing on sugar-containing foods
Enamel erosions on lingual and occlusal surfaces	Chronic vomiting
Dry mouth	Anxiety, decreased salivary output
Scratches on posterior pharynx or palate	Use of toothbrush, finger, or other object for vomiting
Skin	
Lanugo	Extreme weight loss (primitive response to warm body)
Russell's sign (calluses on the knuckle)	Use of finger for vomiting
Dry, cold, scaly skin	Decreased basal metabolic rate
Orange skin	Hypercarotenemia
Brittle hair and nails	Relative hypothyroidism
Petechiae	Thrombocytopenia from extreme malnutrition, on face from vomiting with Valsalva
Pedal or pretibial edema	Withdrawal from laxatives or diuretics; rapid refeeding
Sallow, loose, or sagging skin	Loss of subcutaneous fat
Callus formation or pressure sores	Pressure from sitting or exercising excessively
Eyes	
Conjunctival hemorrhage	Vomiting with Valsalva
Cheeks	
Parotid enlargement	Chronic vomiting
Cardiac	
Hypotension by pulse or blood pressure, bradycardia	Myocardial wasting, malnutrition
Breasts	
Atrophic tissue	Loss of subcutaneous tissue
Abdomen	
Scaphoid	Loss of subcutaneous tissue
Palpable loops of stool	Slowed gastrointestinal motility; constipation
Genitalia	
Dry, atrophic vagina	Hypoestrogenemia
Extremities	
Cold hands and feet; acrocyanosis	Poor circulation
Muscle wasting	Malnutrition
Other	
Loose-fitting clothes	To hide cachexia

MEDICAL COMPLICATIONS OF CALORIC RESTRICTION

The most serious sequelae of a prolonged starvation state include risk of sudden cardiac death, risk of arrhythmias, and myocardial wasting. In anorexia nervosa, thinning of the left ventricle and decreased cardiac chamber size have been reported,[109,110] along with the associated decreased blood pressure and reduced cardiac output.[39] The teen may complain of cold hands and feet, caused by diminished peripheral circulation owing to increased peripheral vascular tone in the face of decreased cardiac output.[111]

Sinus bradycardia, sinus arrhythmia, and hypotension can be seen as protective mechanisms or adaptations to a state of malnutrition, occurring gradually over time; by themselves, these changes are not thought to be life-threatening.[112] In contrast, direct myocardial impairment can occur more quickly and can be lethal; examples include primary cardiovascular abnormalities such as prolonged corrected QT interval, ventricular dysrhythmias, and reduced myocardial contractility. Thus, the low heart rate of patients with anorexia nervosa is primarily a problem in association with a primary cardiovascular abnormality or electrolyte imbalance predisposing to arrhythmia. However, bradycardia, hypotension, and hypothermia are appropriately used as cues indicating medical compromise and the need for intervention. Varying heart rates (less than 40 to 60 beats per minute) have been used as a criterion for admission in various programs.[45,47,113,114] Gradual refeeding and bed rest under close observation remain the appropriate therapy for profound asymptomatic sinus bradycardia, with the cardiac abnormalities reversible when the teen returns to a more normal weight.[112] Rapid refeeding has been associated with congestive heart failure, probably caused by the large increase in afterload in patients with cardiac wasting.[115] Refeeding can also result in hypophosphatemia, caused by the combination of depletion of total-body phosphorus stores during catabolic starvation and increased cellular influx of phosphorus during anabolic refeeding.[116,117] This extracellular hypophosphatemia is often treated with 500 mg, orally twice a day, of a replacement product such as Nutraphos (250 mg phosphorus, 164 mg sodium phosphate, 278 mg potassium phosphate; Willen), in a dose of two capsules orally twice a day, to provide the RDA of 1,000 mg phosphorus per day during acute refeeding.

For patients presenting with heart rates at 50 or less, an ECG should be performed, looking for prolonged QTc or other arrhythmias, and exercise/caffeine restriction should occur until the heart rate is consistently above 60 and not orthostatic. The teen and parent(s) need to realize that exercise and caffeine, separately or together, can trigger a fatal cardiac event in the face of a diminished cardiac muscle. When reintroducing exercise, strict formulas for adding back 15 minutes, with an additional 250 calories per that time period of exercise, no more than 3 to 4 days a week, of ideally noncompulsive exercise works best. For instance, adding back a solo run may be more provocative of eating disorder thoughts than adding back family bowling; soccer practice and team-oriented sports may be more useful than cross country team, where individual success defines team success.

Many patients develop a pattern consistent with the "euthyroid sick syndrome." Peripheral conversion of thyroxine (T4) to triiodothyronine (T3) is decreased, with a high or high-normal level of reverse T3.[39,118] It is most likely that the decrease in T3 represents another adaptive response to starvation by helping to reduce the metabolic rate in the face of decreased energy stores. Suggestive symptoms include bradycardia, cold intolerance, dry skin, coarse hair, slowed relaxation of reflexes, and hypercarotenemia.[39] Teens with anorexia nervosa should not be given thyroid hormone solely on the basis of a low T4 level.[111]

As with other starved patients, growth hormone and cortisol levels are the only hormones typically above normal in anorexia nervosa.[94] Elevated levels of growth hormone probably reflect the associated decrease in insulin-like growth factor I, which normally inhibits growth hormone secretion at the level of the hypothalamus and the pituitary.[39] With refeeding, growth hormone levels fall to normal within a few days. Hypercortisolemia has been postulated as a cause of the osteopenia associated with eating disorders.[33]

Hematologic changes include pancytopenia, neutropenia without an apparent increased susceptibility to infection, and a normochromic or hypochromic anemia.[40] The bone marrow tends to be hypocellular.[39] Although many patients who have eliminated red meat from their diets may also have iron deficiency anemia, the anemia associated with their malnourished state often resolves with refeeding.

Gastrointestinal manifestations include delayed gastric emptying and slowed motility, with patients often describing feelings of early satiety, bloating, postprandial discomfort, and constipation.[107,108,119] Abnormal liver function tests may reflect fatty infiltration of the liver and usually normalize with weight gain. Teens with anorexia nervosa may also have transient hypercholesterolemia, also reversible with weight gain; in general, checking cholesterol levels in these teens should be avoided as they tend to use an elevated level as an excuse to restrict their daily fat intake further.

An elevated blood urea nitrogen level can also be observed, reflecting dehydration and a decreased glomerular filtration rate.[40] Starvation can also cause total-body sodium and potassium depletion, with 25% of patients with anorexia nervosa found to have peripheral edema with refeeding; it is most likely that this effect is caused by increased renal sensitivity to aldosterone and the action of increased insulin secretion on the renal tubules.[40] A minority of patients may have impaired or erratic release of vasopressin in response to osmotic challenge.[120] These patients may note mild polyuria. Remarkably, almost all patients who lose weight solely by caloric restriction tend to have normal electrolyte levels, even in the face of severe malnutrition.[58] The exception occurs in adolescents who restrict fluid to lower the weight and develop severe dehydration and in adolescents who load water to manipulate the weight prior to a visit to a health care provider and present with significant hyponatremia. Amenorrhea, hypoestrogenism, and osteopenia occur commonly in girls with low weight as well as in patients with bulimia (see Chapter 66, "Adolescence: Bone Disease").

MEDICAL COMPLICATIONS FROM PURGING AND BINGEING

Chronic, self-induced vomiting has been associated with hypokalemic, hypochloremic, metabolic alkalosis.[58,121,122] Loss of hydrogen, chloride, and water from gastric fluid results in chloride and volume depletion, triggering a secondary hyperaldosteronism. Consequently, tubular reabsorption of sodium and excretion of potassium increase. The loss of hydrogen ions, both from tubular excretion and from gastric fluid, further causes an exchange of hydrogen and potassium at the cellular level, with worsening hypokalemia. Sodium levels tend to be low or normal but can also be high. It is unclear why some teens who report vomiting over 20 times per day can have remarkably normal electrolytes, whereas those vomiting only three or four times per week can have values that are markedly abnormal.

Hypokalemia can also cause fatal or life-threatening arrhythmias. In a series of 37 patients with anorexia nervosa, 24% had prolonged corrected QT, with each case except one associated with hypokalemia, hypomagnesemia, or medications.[123] Adults with a protracted course of anorexia nervosa may be at greater risk for fatal arrhythmia.[124] Teens who use ipecac to purge are also at risk for irreversible myocardial damage as well as a diffuse myositis secondary to emetine toxicity.[40] If the myopathy is detected at an early stage, it may be reversible.[125] Diuretic abuse can also result in electrolyte abnormalities through tubular excretion of potassium and hydrogen; it has also been associated with low levels of calcium, magnesium, and zinc in patients with eating disorders.[94,109] Laxative abuse causes loss of fluid and electrolytes in the stool. Those patients who combine vomiting with laxative and diuretic use are most at risk for severe electrolyte imbalances. Significant peripheral edema with accompanying fluid and electrolyte shifts can occur in patients who abruptly stop taking laxatives and diuretics, as might occur on admission to an inpatient unit.[58]

Vomiting can also cause parotid enlargement and a characteristic pattern of dental enamel erosion (perimolysis) on the lingual and occlusal surfaces of the incisors from repeated contact with gastric acid.[90,94] Patients may note thermal hypersensitivity when dental erosion has occurred. Bingeing on foods with high sugar content can also cause an increase in dental caries. Elevated amylase levels have also been found and are probably salivary in origin.[127] Vomiting in a state of decreased consciousness, as would occur in a patient using alcohol or drugs, may result in aspiration pneumonia. Binge eating can cause acute gastric dilatation and even rupture.[128,129] A few patients who binge and vomit have also developed Mallory–Weiss tears and esophageal rupture.[127]

AMENORRHEA AND OSTEOPENIA

Recently, attention has been focused on the "female athlete triad," consisting of amenorrhea, osteopenia, and the presence of an eating disorder.[130] Amenorrhea, one of the cardinal signs of eating disorders, can also be seen in certain athletes, especially those participating in competitive sports that emphasize endurance and/or a slender physique with minimal body fat.[131–137] Binge-purging has also been shown to be a risk factor for secondary amenorrhea, with an odds ratio of 4.17.[138] In eating disorders and in long-distance runners, amenorrhea has been associated with hypothalamic dysfunction, weight loss, decreased body fat, excessive exercise, and stress.[139,140] Typically occurring after a 10 to 15% loss of body weight, amenorrhea can also precede weight loss in 50 to 75% of patients with eating disorders.[131,141,142] The basic mechanism appears to be an alteration in the regulation of gonadotropin-releasing hormone secretion by the hypothalamus, with changes in the dopaminergic and opioid systems found in patients with anorexia nervosa and in athletes.[131] Heavy training (over 18 hours per week) starting before and continuing throughout puberty has been shown to alter growth rate and to reduce growth potential in adolescent gymnasts. The proposed mechanisms include prolonged inhibition of the hypothalamic–pituitary–gonadal axis by exercise combined with the metabolic effects of dieting.[143]

"Athletic amenorrhea" can result in a hypoestrogenic state associated with decreased bone density in adults and delayed or interrupted puberty with decreased bone density in teens.[144,145] The osteopenia occurring with prolonged loss of menses has been associated with increased risk of stress fractures in both athletes and patients with eating disorders.[134,145] The risk factors for osteopenia in athletes and eating disorder patients can be seen as a negative net balance between bone resorption and formation.[145] Increased bone loss through resorption occurs with hypoestrogenism (amenorrhea) and hypercortisolemia (chronic stress). Decreased bone formation occurs with glucocorticoid excess and with inadequate calcium and protein intake. Excess glucocorticoids decrease calcium absorption from the gut and inhibit bone formation through direct, receptor-mediated osteoblast effects.[146,147] Acquisition of bone mineral normally continues through the second decade, with peak bone mass reached only in late adolescence or early adulthood.[148,149] Approximately 40 to 60% of bone mass is acquired during the pubertal growth spurt, occurring in females between the ages of 11 and 13 years; evidence suggests that as much as 5% may be acquired during the third decade.[34] This latter figure gains importance in that an extra 5% can account for a significant decrease in fracture risk.[34] Net gains are positively correlated with physical activity, weight, and calcium and protein intake and negatively associated with age.[34]

Osteopenia has been associated with amenorrhea of even a relatively short duration. Bachrach and colleagues found that 12 of 18 teens with anorexia nervosa had osteopenia, with half of this group having been diagnosed within the previous year.[148] The authors postulate that either osteopenia occurs relatively quickly or each patient had unrecognized illness for a longer period of time. Age at onset and duration of anorexia nervosa correlated significantly with bone density, whereas activity level, duration of amenorrhea, and calcium intake did not show a significant relationship with bone density. In contrast, Rigotti and colleagues found that exercise offered some protection against bone loss in anorexia nervosa.[35] Neither calcium supplementation nor vigorous exercise will protect against osteopenia in teens with severely abnormal eating behaviors.

Therapy for osteopenia and amenorrhea in athletes and patients with eating disorders has not been adequately studied. Estrogen replacement therapy can prove problematic for some teens with eating disorders and for athletes who are concerned about potential weight gain or the development of secondary sexual characteristics. Moreover, in teens who have not achieved final height and show significant pubertal delay, estrogen doses high enough to prevent osteopenia may cause accelerated fusion of the epiphyses, compromising final adult height.[148,150] Although estrogen may have an independent effect on bone mass in adolescents,[151] recent data suggest that hormonal replacement therapy alone is inadequate without weight gain to overcome the detrimental effect of low weight for height on bone density.[152] Stokosch and colleagues recently performed a double-blind placebo-controlled clinical trial of Ethinyl Estradiol/Norgestimate on bone mineral density in females with anorexia nervosa; despite promising findings at 6 months of a significant increase in lumbosacral spine bone density in the treatment group versus the placebo group, the findings were no longer significant at 13 months.[153] Weight gain with associated reestablishment of normal estrogenization appears to be the best means of increasing peak bone mass in teens with eating disorders, with increased bone mineral density seen even before the return of menses.[151,154]

Several noninvasive methods are available and have been used to assess bone density, analyzing either trabecular or cortical bone. Best measured in the vertebral spine, trabecular bone consists of plates traversing the internal cavities of the skeleton. Found in the distal radius and other areas, cortical bone forms the outer layer of the skeleton.[131] Both cortical and trabecular bone mass increase during the pubertal growth spurt. In anorexia nervosa, trabecular bone appears to be most severely affected, with a relative sparing of cortical bone; this discrepancy is probably attributable to the more rapid turnover of trabecular bone, with resultant increased sensitivity to the metabolic changes caused by starvation or stress.[33,145,148] Single-photon absorptiometry, used in Rigotti and colleagues' study,[35] measures only cortical bone, whereas quantitative computed tomography of the spine exclusively measures trabecular bone. This latter method involves 75 times the radiation exposure of absorptiometry and thus has been used primarily in research studies.[155] Dual-photon absorptiometry, or dual-energy X-ray absorptiometry (DXA), measures trabecular bone of the axial skeleton (eg, the lumbar vertebrae or femur). DXA is currently the method of choice in assessing bone density in adolescents because of its precision, accuracy, and minimal dose of radiation.[131]

Several questions remain with respect to the triad of eating disorders, amenorrhea, and osteopenia. First, who should be studied with dual-energy absorptiometry or another methodology? For those with significant osteopenia, who should be treated and with what? Bone density assessments of teens with eating disorders who have had amenorrhea for 6 to 12 months should occur and then followed yearly if symptoms persist or initial loss of bone density has been found. The information can also be used as an impetus for weight gain and/or for improved compliance with calcium supplementation.

The decision for hormonal (estrogen/progestin) replacement should be made on an individual basis, taking into account potential final height and bone age. Those individuals also engaging in sexual activity clearly could benefit from hormonal therapy, with dual purpose, and a reminder that eating disorder patients can still get pregnant! Hope for improvements in bone density should not be focused solely on use of a birth control pill; weight gain remains the essential component in bone recovery. Bachrach and colleagues found that individuals recovered from anorexia nevosa displayed persistent osteopenia, suggesting that deficits in bone density acquired during adolescence may not be completely reversible.[134] The burden, then, should be placed on early detection of eating disorders, initiation of efforts to promote weight gain at the onset, calcium supplementation to ensure intake of 1,200 to 1,600 mg orally per day,[27] and consideration of hormonal replacement or other interventions after 6 to 12 months of hypoestrogenic amenorrhea.

FORMING A NUTRITIONAL PLAN

Treatment of eating disorders should involve a team approach, including a primary care provider to address medical concerns, a therapist, a registered dietitian, and often a family therapist or social worker.[45,108,114] Younger patients in particular can benefit from a family-centered approach with use of the Maudsley method, where the family relearns to take charge of meal planning and are literally coached in strategies to operationalize these methods. For full details on how to implement this method for families, we recommend Daniel LeGrange and James Lock's book *Helping Your Teen Overcome an Eating Disorder.* Nutritional intervention is an essential part of treatment for children, adolescents, and adults. The extreme thought disorder often accompanying severe malnutrition will not change with therapy alone; the initial step must ensure adequate nutrition before any therapy will be effective or even tolerated.[84]

In performing the anthropometric assessment, the clinician needs to determine if the patient weighs less than 85% of the weight expected for her age and height (ideal body weight [IBW]). The body mass index (BMI) is calculated as the weight in kilograms divided by the height in squared centimeters. In adults, a BMI less than 18.5 raises the suspicion of anorexia nervosa. The newer growth charts now help track the BMI and can be found through the Centers for Disease Control and Prevention Web site www.cdc.gov/growthcharts. Adolescents with a BMI less than the 10th percentile are considered to be underweight; a BMI less than the 5% may indicate a higher risk for anorexia nervosa. The clinician should also consider the patient's weight history, body build (muscle versus fat), and stage of development when using the BMI.[62,63,156] The IBW initially can also be determined by using the 10th percentile weight for height (Appendix Tables I-1 and I-2) or the Frisch table at the 10th percentile (Table 8).[157] The latter table establishes a minimum weight for patients with both primary and secondary amenorrhea. The clinician should make clear to the patient that menses will not necessarily resume the moment the teen achieves the target weight; otherwise, the teen may inch herself up to that weight and not budge an ounce above it. The health care provider should emphasize a weight range above which menses are most likely to return, remembering that the weight will probably be at or near that weight at which periods ceased.

Several other methods can be used to determine IBW for patients over 18 years of age. The

Table 8 Minimal Weight for Particular Height Associated with the Onset or Restoration of Menstrual Cycles

Height		Menarche or Primary Amenorrhea (13–15 yr) Minimal Weight (10th Percentile)		Average Weight (50th Percentile)	Secondary Amenorrhea (16–18 yr) Minimal Weight (10th Percentile)		Average Weight (50th Percentile)
in	cm	lb	kg	kg	lb	kg	kg
53.1	135	66.7	30.3	34.9	74.6	33.9	38.9
53.9	137	68.6	31.2	36.0	76.8	34.9	40.1
54.7	139	70.6	32.1	37.0	79.0	35.9	41.2
55.5	141	72.6	33.0	38.0	81.2	36.9	42.4
56.3	143	74.4	33.8	39.0	81.4	37.9	43.5
57.1	145	76.3	34.7	40.1	85.6	38.9	44.7
57.9	147	78.3	35.6	41.1	87.8	39.9	45.8
58.7	149	80.3	36.5	42.1	90.0	40.9	47.0
59.4	151	82.2	37.4	43.1	92.2	41.9	48.1
60.2	152	84.3	38.3	44.2	94.4	42.9	49.3
61.0	155	86.2	39.2	45.2	96.6	43.9	50.4
61.8	157	88.2	40.1	46.2	98.8	44.9	51.5
62.6	159	90.2	41.0	47.2	101.0	45.9	52.7
63.4	161	92.2	41.9	48.3	103.2	46.9	53.8
64.2	163	93.9	42.7	49.3	105.4	47.9	55.0
65.0	165	95.9	43.6	50.3	107.6	48.9	56.1
65.7	167	97.9	44.5	51.4	109.8	49.9	57.3
66.5	169	99.9	45.4	52.4	112.0	50.9	58.4
67.8	171	101.9	46.3	53.4	114.0	51.8	59.6
68.1	173	103.8	47.2	54.4	116.2	52.8	60.7
68.9	175	105.8	48.1	55.5	118.4	53.8	61.8
69.7	177	107.3	49.0	56.5	120.6	54.8	63.0
70.3	179	109.6	49.8	57.5	122.8	55.8	64.1
71.3	181	111.8	50.8	58.5	125.2	56.9	65.3

Adapted from Frisch RE and McArthur JW.[139]

1983 Metropolitan Life Charts provide estimations for weight by age, sex, and appropriate frame size. The Hamwi formula provides a simple means of calculating desirable body weight.[158] For women of medium frame, allow 100 pounds for the first 5 feet and then add 5 pounds for every inch above. For example, a women who is 5 feet and 3 inches would have a Hamwi desired weight of $100 + (3 \times 5) = 115$ pounds (range 112–118 pounds given to the patient). For women of a large frame, add 10%, and for those with a small frame, subtract 10%. In men, the medium frame starting point is 106 pounds, with 6 pounds added per inch.

Overall goals for nutritional management should be spelled out clearly to the teen and family at the start of therapy. The dietitian may be viewed with some fear and mistrust by the adolescent initially[159]; the teen should be reassured that the dietitian hears and understands his or her concerns and will work with the teen to ease the transition back to health.[160] Recognition of the extreme variability between individual patients' diets and identification of the specific diet pattern exhibited by a particular teenager can have practical implications for planning individualized treatment.[161] Proceeding too quickly with nutritional changes may trigger anxiety and cause the patient to become more resistant to therapy.[162] The primary care provider, nutritionist, therapist, and other members of the care team must work together to allay these fears and to stabilize the patient medically and psychologically.

If not following the Maudsley approach, a food plan, developed collaboratively with the teen, will support the gradual transition to a normalized eating pattern. Initially, a daily intake of as little as 1,200 calories may be appropriate to prevent postprandial discomfort after prolonged starvation. Otherwise, a 1,500-calorie diet should be adequate to start, with calories added in 200 to 300 kcal increments every 3 days to produce a rate of weight gain of 0.2 kg per day (⅓ pound) if hospitalized or ½ to 2 pounds per week in the outpatient setting.[107,108,163] Food plans offer an easy way to communicate calorie and nutrient requirements, also offering structure and help eliminating the binge, purge, and restrict patterns common to teens with eating disorders. Food plans allow the teen to eat mechanically until he or she is able reliably to recognize hunger and satiety signals.

Liquid supplements (Ensure, Boost, Resource, or other brands) may be used as needed in patients who initially cannot tolerate the addition of solid foods. Other options include Duocal (SHS) and Benecalorie (Novartis), gel-like tasteless supplements that offer 340 calories in 2 tablespoons that can be mixed into certain foods without a significant change in texture (eg, smoothies, peanut butter, yoghurt). If a teen has a 1,500-calorie-a-day meal plan and can manage only 750 calories as solid food initially, three cans of a liquid supplement (250 calories each) could be substituted.

Nasogastric tube feedings and peripheral alimentation carry increased medical and psychological risks; their use should be limited to those patients unable to consume sufficient calories orally who need urgent or acute stabilization.[163,164] A protocol for inpatient nutritional stabilization is outlined in Table 9.

Metabolic rate or caloric demands may increase quickly in the refeeding anorexia nervosa patient. In one study, during several stages of anorexia nervosa, when weight remained stable, restricting anorexic patients needed to consume a greater number of calories than patients with bulimic anorexia nervosa.[166] Differences in activity did not account for these findings, and bulimic anorexic patients were found to have similar or greater activity than the restricting group. As patients transition from a hypometabolic state to a hypermetabolic state during refeeding, daily caloric intake may need to be increased to as high as 3,500 to 4,000 calories, and sometimes even higher.

The clinician should establish safe ranges for intake of both macronutrients and micronutrients. RDAs for various nutrients are found in Appendix Table I-8. Protein should constitute 20% of total calories, with minimum intake equal to the RDA in g/kg of IBW. Carbohydrates should account for 50 to 55% of total calories, and the clinician can encourage intake of fluids and water-insoluble fiber to treat the constipation that often accompanies refeeding.[99] Many patients with anorexia nervosa eat a relatively large quantity of fruits and vegetables; fiber in other forms, such as whole-wheat breads, cereal, or other grains, should be recommended. The last 20 to 30% of calories should come from ingestion of fat to provide sources of essential fatty acids; in teens ingesting few or no fat grams initially, the nutritionist can use a starting goal of 15% fat intake. This latter dietary change is often the most traumatic for the teen and should occur with a

Table 9 Nutritional Treatment for the Patient with an Eating Disorder During an Inpatient Admissions

I. Initial caloric and protein requirement
   a. Calorie intake at 1,500 kcal per day (females), 1,750 kcal per day (males), until assessed by nutritionist
   b. Maintenance calorie range for weight gain on a long-term basis is determined by adding 500–1,000 kcal to the initial estimated caloric requirement. In some cases, higher calorie levels are necessary.
   c. Minimum protein intake range is per RDA for age based on minimum-weight goal and ideal body weight.
   d. Micronutrient supplementation (daily multivitamin)
   e. Nutraphos, 500 mg orally twice a day for 5 d
   f. Maintenance fluid requirements

II. Nutrition monitoring
   a. Daily weight in a hospital gown after voiding: expect 0.2 kg/d weight gain
   b. Adequate caloric provision, with 30 min bed rest after each meal
   c. Increase calories by 250 calories until steady weight gain is achieved.
   d. Supplements: if <0.2 kg gain after 2 d in hospital, 250-calorie supplements are given, starting with two supplements initially, to be treated as medicine (nonnegotiable). Each day that weight goal is not met, an additional can is added.

III. Patient education

RDA = Recommended Dietary Allowance.

gradual, sequential reintroduction of the patient to "normal" eating. Expanded food selections should be encouraged, but the addition of a multivitamin mineral supplement providing 100% of the RDA for most micronutrients will help ensure an adequate nutrient intake. Iron-containing preparations may aggravate constipation,[83] but the clinician can counter this effect with use of sufficient fiber.

An easy way to communicate the calorie and nutrient requirements is through the use of a food plan. Food plans offer structure and help eliminate the binge, purge, and restrict patterns common to people with eating disorders. Food plans allow the teen to eat mechanically until he or she is able to recognize hunger and satiety signals consistently and reliably.

It is important for the teen to be comfortable eating a wide variety of foods without any fear, guilt, or anxiety. "Forbidden" foods should be gradually reintroduced into the diet. With the help of a parent, creating a list of foods liked and disliked prior to the onset of the eating disorder can help determine whether a food is now avoided out of fear or is one that has always been disliked. It is useful to then develop a hierarchy of identified fear foods and begin reintroducing the least "scariest" foods first.

Vegetarianism is an easy way to justify the elimination of meats, which are often feared because of their fat content. Adherence to a vegetarian diet, if begun with the onset of the eating disorder, should be discouraged during the recovery process to facilitate an adequate nutrient intake and promote comfort with eating a wide variety of foods.

The refeeding process can cause discomfort with bloating, flatulence, constipation, or diarrhea. The dietitian or clinician should remind teens that these symptoms, although bothersome, will gradually resolve as their body adjusts to the changes they are making. Bloating and gas can be reduced by limiting gas-producing foods. Constipation can be corrected by consuming adequate calories and fluids, as well as more soluble fiber found in whole grains.

There are several dietary modifications to consider when refeeding teens with anorexia nervosa. Limiting raw high-fiber foods and consuming only a moderate amount of fat help promote gastric emptying. Eating foods cold or at room temperature helps reduce the feeling of fullness. Choosing to eat smaller, more frequent meals will reduce bloating. Restricting the use of caffeine, gum, sugar substitutes, and diet beverages will improve the teen's ability to recognize hunger and satiety. Calorie and fat gram counting should be discouraged, and access to scales should be limited or prohibited. Social eating should be encouraged, and time limits should be placed on mealtimes to prevent the teen from being at the table all day.

Interventions for teens with bulimia nervosa should focus on creating feelings of satiety and implementing a structured eating behavior pattern. Selecting hot or warm foods with adequate amounts of fat enhances feelings of satiety. Buying foods in single servings whenever possible and avoiding "trigger" foods initially will help control the urge to binge. Eating meals and snacks sitting down and selecting foods that require the use of utensils will slow down the rate of eating and increase satiety. Skipping meals, eating on the run, and eating secretly should be discouraged. Binge purge behaviors should be stabilized before assisting an overweight teen with weight loss. Other helpful hints can be found in Table 10.

Table 10 Guidelines for Adolescents with Eating Disorders

Individualize treatment
Avoid discussing numbers such as weight and calories
Encourage variety of foods
Slowly incorporate unsafe foods
Avoid fat gram and/or calorie counting
Limit meal time to 20–30 min per meal
Encourage small, frequent feedings
Avoid gas-producing foods
Avoid diet beverages, sugar substitutes, gum, and caffeine
If patient is not eating fat, start with 15% calories from fat
Use multivitamin supplement with calcium
Provide concrete ideas to facilitate changes in eating behavior patterns

Attention can be placed on the emotional state during a binge, when and where it occurs, and how hungry the teen is at the time. For instance, if a teen always binges on arrival home after school, the clinician can help identify triggers and explore possible solutions with the teen. If boredom is the trigger, filling the time with more structured activities will be helpful. Effective strategies also include disrupting the automatic behavior chain by entering through a different door and changing the order of activities, for example, checking electronic mail or calling a friend before snacking. Deciding on a snack in advance, encouraging the teen to put leftovers away after assembling the food, sitting down at a predetermined location, and eating without distraction (eg, never in front of a television or computer) will help prevent a binge. If a teen arrives home overly hungry, it makes eating a moderate amount of food nearly impossible. Therefore, encouraging an adequate intake of calories at breakfast and lunch is important in preventing binge eating after school.

For teens with secondary amenorrhea, resumption of menses often occurs as they improve fat intake toward a range of 40 to 60 g per day, although, anecdotally, menses may resume at lower intakes. Hence, if an adolescent girl has regained weight to that weight at which periods had ceased but remains amenorrheic, one intervention could be to increase fat grams to 40 to 60 g of fat per day, a task difficult for many of these patients.

In addition to the above guidelines and concerns, adolescent athletes may also have specific nutritional issues. For instance, much mythology exists about the pre-event meal and the pros and cons of carbohydrate loading. Short-term, high-intensity activities, such as sprinting, diving, or high jump, rely on anaerobic fuel sources. Longer-term activities of lesser intensity, such as long-distance running or crosscountry skiing, require aerobic energy sources.[150] Activities such as tennis, basketball, and soccer use both. A high-carbohydrate diet promotes muscle glycogen storage, which, over time, can enhance endurance. Caloric requirements may be as high as 2,400 to 4,500 calories daily in the high school or college athlete,[8] whereas skilled competitive cyclists riding 19 hours a day may need as many as 9,500 to 14,000 calories per day.[168] The metabolism of additional carbohydrates may also increase requirements of thiamin, riboflavin, and niacin, but a well-balanced diet should supply sufficient amounts of these nutrients. Large doses of vitamins and minerals will not enhance muscle mass or performance.

A strong emphasis on competition can make young athletes vulnerable to nutrition misinformation and unsafe practices thought to enhance performance. During prolonged, strenuous exercise, carbohydrate supplementation has been shown to improve performance.[169] However, carbohydrate ingested prior to competition has not had an effect on performance and, in past years, has even been considered detrimental.[167] One study showed that preexercise candy bar consumption does not cause premature fatigue or decreased endurance.[170] In counseling teens on nutrition to optimize performance, emphasis should be placed on a healthful, balanced diet, with adequate calories and fluids to prevent dehydration and electrolyte imbalances. Carbohydrates should be ingested within 2 hours after prolonged, strenuous exercise and preferably within about 20 minutes because glycogen synthesis rates are 50% higher than at 2 to 4 hours after exercise.[169] Complex carbohydrates are preferred as they facilitate faster gastric emptying when ingested in high concentrations, they are associated with less gastrointestinal stress than found with simple sugars, and they contain fiber, vitamins, and minerals.[171–173]

In sports such as wrestling and lightweight crew, the clinician should use the preparticipation physical as an opportunity to educate and intervene in any unhealthful eating practices detected at that time. Wrestlers have been shown to use profuse sweating, diuretics and laxatives, and spitting into a cup to keep from swallowing saliva as added water weight.[174] Tcheng and Tipton have recommended a desired minimum range of 7 to 10% fat for wrestlers; the athlete should not be allowed to compete below the weight recommended by the physician.[175] The athlete should be asked about desired weight goals, dieting practices, and training activities, with nutritional guidance and appropriate interventions occurring before, during, and after the season as needed.

Teens who engage in weight lifting and similar activities should be discouraged from use of anabolic steroids or protein supplements. Strenuous physical activity does not increase protein requirements[176]; athletes can easily meet their protein needs by following a balanced diet.[167] The RDA for protein is 0.36 kg protein per pound of body weight for the average adult or adolescent athlete[177]; a total of 0.45 g of protein per pound is recommended for marathoners. Diets that provide more than 0.9 g of protein per pound of body weight have not been shown to increase muscle strength.[178,179] Dehydration in combination with use of protein supplements can compromise kidney function with the added load of nitrogen; with nitrogen excretion, further water is lost.[180]

Strenuous physical activity or intense training has been associated with anemia, which can impair performance. Contributing factors include marginal iron intake, increased iron losses, and increased destruction of erythrocytes with extreme exercise.[181] Screening with a yearly hemoglobin or hematocrit level is warranted in teenagers engaging in competitive or strenuous athletics.[182]

CONCLUSION

Adolescents with eating disorders or those who participate in athletics can have specific nutritional needs, most of which can be adequately provided through a healthful, balanced diet. Clinicians and nutritionists can work with patients and families and within the community to target high-risk eating behaviors and to do preventive education. Prevention can target both obesity and eating disorders, without work on the former having to trigger development of the latter. Nutritional education for coaches, parents, and other individuals involved in teens' lives and activities can be provided within the school setting, church, or community. Teens who are deemed to be at high risk can be referred to appropriate centers for further counseling and treatment.

REFERENCES

1. Story M. Nutritional requirements during adolescence. In: McAnarney ER et al, editors. Textbook of Adolescent Medicine. Philadelphia: WB Saunders; 1992. p. 75–84.
2. Simmons RG, Borgeson R, Carlton-Ford S. The impact of cumulative change in early adolescence. Child Dev 1987;58:1220–34.
3. Brooks-Gunn J, Peterson AC, Eichorn D. The study of maturational timing effects in adolescence. J Youth Adolesc 1985;14:149–61.
4. Elkind D. Egocentrism in adolescence. Child Dev 1967;38:1025–34.
5. Emmons L. Dieting and purging behaviors in black and white high school students. J Am Diet Assoc 1992;92:306–12.
6. Mallick MJ, Whipple TW, Huerta E. Behavioral and psychological traits of weight-conscious teenagers: a comparison of eating-disordered patients and high- and low-risk groups. Adolescence 1987;22:157–68.
7. Story M, Rosenwinkel K, Himes JH, et al. Demographic and risk factors associated with chronic dieting in adolescents. Am J Dis Child 1991;145:994–8.
8. McKeag DB. Adolescents and exercise. J Adolesc Health Care 1986;7:121S–9S.
9. Chapman G, Maclean H. "Junk food" and "healthy food": meanings of food in adolescent women's culture. J Nutr Educ 1993;25:108–13.
10. US Department of Agriculture, Agricultural Research Service. Continuing Survey of Food Intakes by Individuals (CSFII) and the Diet and Health Knowledge Survey (DHKS), 1994–1996.
11. Maloney MJ, McGuire J, Daniels SR, et al. Dieting behavior and eating attitudes in children. Pediatrics 1989;84:482–9.
12. Wait B, Blair R, Roberts LJ. Energy intake of well-nourished children and adolescents. Am J Clin Nutr 1969;22:1383.
13. Spear B. Adolescent growth and development. In: Rickert VI, editor. Adolescent Nutrition: Assessment and Management. New York: Chapman & Hall; 1996. p. 3–24.
14. Harris JA, Benedict FG. Standard basal metabolism constants for physiologists and clinicians. In: A Biometric Study of Basal Metabolism in Man, Washington, DC: Carnegie Institute. Philadelphia: Lippincott; 1919. p. 233–50.
15. Wilmore DW. The Metabolic Management of the Critically Ill. New York: New Plenum Press; 1977.
16. Kinney JM. Nutritional Aspects of the Critically Ill. New York: Churchill Livingstone; 1977.
17. Duke HH, Jorgensen SB, Broell JR, et al. Contribution of protein to caloric expenditure following injury. Surgery 1970;68:168.
18. American Academy of Pediatrics, Committee on Nutrition. Pediatric Nutrition Handbook. 2nd ed. Elk Grove Village, IL: American Academy of Pediatrics; 1985.
19. Pike RL, Brown ML. Nutrition: An Integrated Approach. 2nd ed. New York: John Wiley & Sons; 1975.
20. Krebs-Smith SM, Cook A, Subar AF, et al. Fruits and vegetables intakes of children and adolescents in the United States. Arch Pediatr Adolesc Med 1996;150:81–6.
21. Donovan UM, Gibson RS. Dietary intakes of adolescent females consuming vegetarian, semi-vegetarian, and omnivorous diets. J Adolesc Health 1996;18:292–300.
22. Johnson RK, Johnson DG, Wang MQ, et al. Characterizing nutrient intakes of adolescents by sociodemographic factors. J Adolesc Health 1996;15:149–54.
23. Lifshitz F, Tarim O, Smith MN. Nutrition in the adolescent. Endocrinol Metab Clin North Am 1993;22:673–83.
24. Lund EK, Lee-Finglas E, Southon S, et al. Dietary fat intake and plasma lipid levels in adolescents. Eur J Clin Nutr 1992;46:857–64.
25. Moore DC. Body image and eating behavior in adolescents. J Am Coll Nutr 1993;12:505.
26. Story M, French SA, Resnick MD, et al. Ethnic/racial and socioeconomic differences in dieting behaviors and body image perceptions in adolescents. Int J Eat Disord 1995;18:173.
27. Key JD, Key LL. Calcium needs of adolescents. Curr Opin Pediatr 1994;6:379–82.
28. Rolland-Cachera MF. Body composition during adolescence: methods, limitations, and determinants. Horm Res 1993;39:25–40.
29. Schaafsma G. The scientific basis of recommended dietary allowances for calcium. J Intern Med 1992;231:187–94.
30. Spark A. Children's diet and health requirements: preschool age through adolescence. Compr Ther 1992;18:9–20.
31. Matkovic V, Ilich J. Calcium requirements for growth: are current recommendations adequate? Nutr Rev 1993;51:171–80.
32. Post GB, Kemper HCG. Nutrient intake and biological maturation during adolescence. Eur J Clin Nutr 1993;47:297–300.
33. Biller BMK, Saxe V, Herzog DB, et al. Mechanisms of osteoporosis in adult and adolescent women with anorexia nervosa. J Clin Endocrinol Metab 1989;68:548–54.
34. Recker RR, Davies KM, Hinders SM, et al. Bone gain in young adult women. JAMA 1992;92:89–91.
35. Rigotti NA, Nussbaum SR, Herzog DB, et al. Osteoporosis in women with anorexia nervosa. N Engl J Med 1984;311:1601–6.
36. Hay PJ, Hall A, Delahunt JW, et al. Investigation of osteopaenia in anorexia nervosa. Aust N Z J Psychiatry 1989;23:161–268.
37. Zukin J. Dairy free cookbook. Rocklin, CA: Prima Publishing; 1991.
38. Bruch H. Perceptual and conceptual disturbances in anorexia nervosa. Psychosom Med 1962;24:187–94.
39. Herzog DB, Copeland PM. Eating disorders. N Engl J Med 1985;313:295–303.
40. Birnbaum CS, Herzog DB. Eating disorders. Semin Pediatr Gastroenterol Nutr 1992;3:2–8.
41. American Psychiatric Association. Diagnostic and Statistical Manual of Mental Disorders. 4th ed. Washington, DC: American Psychiatric Association; 1994.
42. Swenne I, Thurfjell B. Clinical onset and diagnosis of eating disorders in premenarchal girls is preceded by inadequate weight gain and growth retardation. Acta Pediatrica 2003;92(10):1133–7.
43. Garner DM. Pathogenesis of anorexia nervosa. Lancet 1993;341:1631–4.
44. Garner DM, Garner MV, Rosen LR. Anorexia nervosa "restricters" who purge: implications for subtyping anorexia nervosa. Int J Eat Disord 1993;13:171–85.
45. Harper G. Eating disorders in adolescence. Pediatr Rev 1994;15:72–7.
46. Harris RT. Anorexia nervosa and bulimia nervosa in female adolescents. Nutr Today 1991;26:30–4.
47. American Psychiatric Association. Practice guideline for eating disorders. Am J Psychiatry 2000;157:1–39.
48. Bulik CM, Sullivan PF, Rorty M. Childhood sexual abuse in women with bulimia. J Clin Psychiatry 1989;50:460–4.
49. Watson TL, Andersen AE. A critical examination of the amenorrhea and weight criteria for diagnosing anorexia nervosa. Acta Psychiatr Scand. 2003 Sep;108(3):161–2.
50. Rome ES, Fisher MM, Kaplan DW, et al. Committee on Adolescence, American Academy of Pediatrics.
51. Peebles R, Wilson JL, Lock JD. How do children with eating disorders differ from adolescents with eating disorders at initial evaluation? J Adolesc Health 2006;39:800–5.
52. Nielson GB, Lausch B, Thomsen PH. Three cases of severe early-onset eating disorder: are they cases of anorexia nervosa? Psychopathology 1997;30(1):49–52.
53. Rosen DS. Eating disorders in children and young adolescents: etiology, classification, clinical features, and treatment. Adolesc Med 2003;14(1):49–59.
54. Workgroup for Classification of Eating Disorders in Children and Adolescents. Classification of child and adolescent easting disturbances. Int I Eat Disord 2007;40(SB): S117–5112.
55. Lucas AR, Beard CM, O'Fallon WM, et al. 50-Year trends in the incidence of anorexia nervosa in Rochester, Minnesota: a population-based study. Am J Psychiatry 1991;148:917–22.
56. Lucas AR. The eating disorder "epidemic": more apparent than real? Pediatr Ann 1992;21:746–51.
57. Whitaker AH. An epidemiologic study of anorectic and bulimic symptoms in adolescent girls: implications for pediatricians. Pediatr Ann 1992;21:752–9.
58. Fisher M. Medical complications of anorexia and bulimia nervosa. Adolesc Med 1992;3:487–503.
59. Fisher M, Schneider M, Pegler C, et al. Eating attitudes, health-risk behaviors, self-esteem, and anxiety among adolescent females in a suburban high school. J Adolesc Health 1991;12:377–84.
60. Comerci GD. Eating disorders in adolescents. Pediatr Rev 1988;10:1–11.
61. Committee on Adolescence, American Academy of Pediatrics. Identifying and treating eating disorders. Pediatrics 2003;111:204–11.
62. Fisher M, Golden NH, Datzman KD, et al. Eating disorders in adolescents: a background paper. J Adolesc Health Care 1995;16:420–37.
63. Kreipe RE, Birndorf DO. Eating disorders in adolescents and young adults. Med Clin North Am 2000;84:1027–49.
64. Rogers L, Resnick MD, Mitchell JE, et al. The relationship between socioeconomic status and eating-disordered behaviors in a community sample of adolescent girls. Int J Eating Disord 1997;22:15–23.
65. Pate JE, Pumariega AJ, Hester C, et al. Cross cultural patterns in eating disorders: a review. Am J Child Adolesc Psychiatry 1992.
66. Davis C, Katzman MA. Perfection as acculturation: psychological correlates of eating problems in Chinese male and female students living in the United States. Int J Eat Disord 1999;25:65–70.
67. Davis C, Katzman MA. Chinese men and women in USA and Hong Kong: body and self-esteem ratings as a prelude to dieting and exercise. Int J Eat Disord 1998;23: 99–102.
68. Crago M, Shisslack CM, Estess LS. Eating disturbances among American minority groups: a review. Int J Eat Disord 1996;19:239–48.
69. Chaum E, Herzog DB. New directions in anorexia nervosa and bulimia nervosa. Curr Opin Pediatr 1990;2:641–7.
70. Freund KM, Graham SM, Lesky LG, et al. Detection of bulimia in a primary care setting. J Gen Intern Med 1993;8:236–42.
71. Pyle RL, Mitchell JE, Eckert ED, et al. The incidence of bulimia in freshmen college students. Int J Eat Disord 1983;2:75–85.
72. Halmi KA, Falk JR, Schwartz E. Binge-eating and vomiting: a survey of a college population. Psychol Med 1981;11:697–706.

73. Hudson JI, Pope HG, Jr, Yurgelun-Todd D, et al. A controlled study of lifetime prevalence of affective and other psychiatric disorders in bulimic outpatients. Am J Psychiatry 1987;144:1283–7.
74. Shisslak CM, Perse T, Crago M. Coexistence of bulimia nervosa and mania; a literature review and case report. Compr Psychiatry 1991;32:181–4.
75. Gartner AF, Marcus RN, Halmi K, et al. DSM-II-R personality disorders in patients with eating disorders. Am J Psychiatry 1989;146:1585–91.
76. Yager J, Landsverk J, Edelstein CK, Hyler SE. Screening for axis II personality disorders in women with bulimic eating disorders. Psychosomatics 1989;30:255–62.
77. Zanarini MC, Frankenburg FR, Pope HG Jr, et al. Axis II comorbidity of normal weight bulimia. Compr Psychiatry 1990;31:20–4.
78. Herzog DB. Are anorexic and bulimic patients depressed? Am J Psychiatry 1984;141:1594–7.
79. Halmi KA, Casper RC, Eckert ED, et al. Unique features associated with the age of onset of anorexia nervosa. Psychiatry Res 1979;1:209–15.
80. Bostic JQ, Muriel AC, Hack S, et al. Anorexia nervosa in a 7-year-old girl. J Dev Behav Pediatr 1997;18(5):331–3.
81. Lask B, Bryant-Waugh R. Early-onset anorexia nervosa and related eating disorders. J Child Psychol Psychiatry 1992;33(1):281–300.
82. Bryant-Waugh R, Lask B. Eating disorders in children. J Child Psychol Psychiatry 1995;36(2):191–202.
83. Nicholls D, Chater R, Lask B. Children into DSM don't go: a comparison of classification systems for eating disorders in childhood and adolescence. Int J Eat Disord 2000;28(3):317–24.
84. Austin SB, Field AE, Wiecha J, et al. The impact of a school-based obesity prevention trial on disordered weight-control behaviors in early adolescent girls. Arch Pediatr Adolesc Med 2005;159(3):225–30.
85. Field AE, Ausin SB, Taylor CB, et al. Relation between dieting and weight change among preadolescents and adolescents. Pediatrics 2003;112(4):900–6.
86. Krowchuk DP, Kreiter SR, Woods CR, et al. Problem dieting behaviors among young adolescents. Arch Pediatr Adolesc Med 1998;152(9):884–8.
87. Maloney MJ, McGuire J, Daniels SR, et al. Dieting behavior and eating attitudes in children. Pediatrics 1989;84(3):482–9.
88. McVey G, Tweed S, Blackmore E. Dieting among preadolescent and young adolescent females. Can Med Assoc J 2004;170(10):1559–61.
89. Becker AE, Grinspoon SK, Klibanski A, et al. Eating disorders. N Engl J Med 1999;340:1092–8.
90. Neumark-Sztainer D, Story M, Hanan PJ, et al. Weight-related concerns and behaviors among overweight and nonoverweight adolescents: implication for preventing weight-related disorders. Arch Pediatr Adolesc Med 2002;156:171–8.
91. Centers for Disease Control and Prevention. Youth Risk Behavior Surveillance System. Available at: http://apps.Nccd.cdc.gov/yrbss/CategoryQuestions.as;?Cat=5&desc-Dietary%20Behaviors. Accessed September 25, 2006.
92. Yates A, Leehey K, Shisslak CM. Running-an analog of anorexia? N Engl J Med 1983;308:251–5.
93. Clark N, Nelson M, Evans W. Nutrition education for elite female runners. Physician Sports Med 1988;16:124–36.
94. Rosen LW, McKeag DB, Hough DO. Pathogenic weight-control behavior in female athletes. Physician Sports Med 1986;14:79–86.
95. Rosen LW, Hough DO. Pathogenic weight-control behaviors in female college gymnasts. Physician Sports Med 1988;16:141–4.
96. Yates A, Shisslak C, Allender J, et al. Comparing obligatory and nonobligatory runners. Psychosomatics 1992;33:180–9.
97. McKenna MS. Assessment of the eating disordered patient. Psychiatr Ann 1989;19:467–72.
98. Yates A. Current perspectives on the eating disorders: history, psychological and biological perspectives. J Am Acad Child Adolesc Psychiatry 1989;28:813–28.
99. Schebendach J, Nussbaum MP. Nutrition management in adolescents with eating disorders. Adolesc Med 1992;3:541–58.
100. Beaumont P, Russell J, Touyz S. Treatment of anorexia nervosa. Lancet 1993;341:1635–40.
101. Position of the American Dietetic Association. Vegetarian diets. J Am Diet Assoc 1988;88:351–5.
102. Howat PM, Mohan R, Champagene C, et al. Validity and reliability of reported dietary intake data. J Am Diet Assoc 1994;94:169–73.
103. Eck LH, Klesges RC, Hanson CL. Recall of a child's intake from one meal: Are parents accurate? J Am Diet Assoc 1989;89:784–9.
104. Welson JL, Peebles R, Hardy KK, et al. Surfing for thinness: a pilot study of pro-eating disorder website usage in adolescence with eating disorders. Pediatrics 2006;118(6):el1635–43.
105. Kaplan AS. Biomedical variables in the eating disorders. Can J Psychiatry 1990;35:745–53.
106. Kaplan AS, Woodside DB. Biological aspects of anorexia nervosa and bulimia nervosa. J Consult Clin Psychol 1987;55:645–53.
107. Rome ES, Ammerman S. Medical complications of eating disorders: J Adolesc Health 2003;33:418–26.
108. Rome ES. Eating disorders in adolescents and young adults: what's a primary care clinician to do? Cleve Clin J Med 1996;63:387–95.
109. Gottdiener JS, Gross HA, Henry WL, et al. Effects of self-induced starvation on cardiac size and function in anorexia nervosa. Circulation 1978;58:426–33.
110. Fohlin L. Body composition, cardiovascular and renal function in adolescent patients with anorexia nervosa. Acta Paediatr Scand 1977;268:1–20.
111. Spack NP. Medical complications of anorexia nervosa and bulimia. In: Emmett SW, editor. Eating Disorders. New York: Brunner/Mazel; 1985. p. 5–19.
112. Kreipe JE, Harris JP. Myocardial impairment resulting from eating disorders. Pediatr Ann 1992;21:760–8.
113. Kreipe RE, Uphoff M. Treatment and outcome of adolescents with anorexia nervosa. Adolesc Med 1992;3:519–40.
114. Rome ES, Ammerman S, Rosen DR, et al. Children and adolescents with eating disorders: The state of the art. Pediatrics 2003;e98.
115. Powers PS. Heart failure during treatment of anorexia nervosa. Am J Psychiatry 1982;139:1167–70.
116. Solomon SM, Kirby DF. The refeeding syndrome: a review. J Parenter Enteral Nutr 1990;14:90–7.
117. Sheridan PH, Collins M. Potentially life-threatening hypophosphatemia in anorexia nervosa. J Adolesc Health Care 1983;4:44–6.
118. Moshang T, Jr, Utiger RD. Low triiodothyronine euthyroidism in anorexia nervosa. In: Vigersky RA, editor. Anorexia Nervosa. New York: Raven Press; 1977. p. 263–70.
119. Dubois A, Gross HA, Ebert MH, et al. Altered gastric emptying and secretion in primary anorexia nervosa. Gastroenterology 1979;77:319–23.
120. Gold PW, Kaye W, Robertson GL, et al. Abnormalities in plasma and cerebrospinal-fluid arginine vasopressin in patients with anorexia nervosa. N Engl J Med 1983;308:1117–23.
121. Palla B, Litt IF. Medical complications of eating disorders in adolescents. Pediatrics 1988;81:613–23.
122. Oster JR. The binge-purge syndrome: A common albeit unappreciated cause of acid-base and fluid-electrolyte disturbances. South Med J 1987;80:58–67.
123. Webb JG, Birmingham CL, Macdonald IL. Electrocardiographic abnormalities in anorexia nervosa. Int J Eat Disord 1988;7:785–90.
124. Isner JM, Roberts WC, Heymsfield SB, et al. Anorexia nervosa and sudden death. Ann Intern Med 1985;102:49–52.
125. Palmer EP, Guay AT. Reversible myopathy secondary to abuse of ipecac in patients with major eating disorders. N Engl J Med 1985;313:1457–9.
126. Fonesca V, Havard CWH. Electrolyte disturbances and cardiac failure with hypomagnesemia in anorexia nervosa. Br Med J 1985;291:1680–2.
127. Mitchell JE, Pyle RL, Miner RA. Gastric dilatation as a complication of bulimia. Psychosomatics 1982;23:96–7.
128. Evans DS. Acute dilatation and spontaneous rupture of the stomach. Br J Surg 1968;55:940–2.
129. Mitchell JE, Seim HC, Colon E, et al. Medical complications and medical management of bulimia. Ann Intern Med 1987;107:71–7.
130. Skolnick AA. "Female athlete triad" risk for women. JAMA 1993;270:921–3.
131. Golden NH, Shenker IR. Amenorrhea in anorexia nervosa: etiology and implications. Adolesc Med 1992;3:503–17.
132. Warren MP. Amenorrhea in endurance runners. J Clin Endocrinol Metab 1992;75:1393–7.
133. Brooks-Gunn J, Warren MP, Hamilton LH. The relation of eating problems and amenorrhea in ballet dancers. Med Sci Sports Exerc 1987;19:41–4.
134. Warren MP, Brooks-Gunn J, Hamilton LH, et al. Scoliosis and fractures in young ballet dancers: Relation to delayed menarche and secondary amenorrhea. N Engl J Med 1986;314:1348–53.
135. Highet R. Athletic amenorrhea: An update on aetiology, complications, and management. Sports Med 1989;7:82–108.
136. DeSouza MJ, Metzger DA. Reproductive dysfunction in amenorrheic athletes and anorexic patients: a review. Med Sci Sports Exerc 1991;23:995–1007.
137. Gadpaille WJ, Sanborn CF, Wagner WW. Athletic amenorrhea, major affective disorders, and eating disorders. Am J Psychiatry 1987;144:939–42.
138. Johnson J, Whitaker AH. Adolescent smoking, weight changes, and binge purge behaviors: associations with secondary amenorrhea. Am J Public Health 1992;82:47–54.
139. Schwartz B, Cumming DC, Riordan E, et al. Exercise-associated amenorrhea: A distinct entity. Am J Obstet Gynecol 1981;141:662–70.
140. Kreipe RE, Churchill BH, Strauss J. Long-term outcome of adolescents with anorexia nervosa. Am J Dis Child 1989;143:1322–7.
141. Falk JR, Halmi K. Amenorrhea in anorexia nervosa: Examination of the critical body weight hypothesis. Biol Psychiatry 1982;17:799–806.
142. Theintz GE, Howald H, Weiss U, et al. Evidence for a reduction of growth potential in adolescent female gymnasts. J Pediatr 1993;122:306–13.
143. Mansfield MJ, Emans SJ. Growth in female gymnasts: should training decrease during puberty? J Pediatr 1993;122:237–40.
144. Dhuper S, Warren MP, Brooks-Gunn J, et al. Effects of hormonal status on bone density in adolescent girls. J Clin Endocrinol Metab 1990;71:1083–8.
145. Kreipe RE, Forbes GB. Osteoporosis: A "new morbidity" for dieting adolescents? Pediatrics 1990;86:478–80.
146. Prior JC, Vigna YM, McKay DW. Reproduction for the athletic woman. Sports Med 1992;14:190–9.
147. Chen TL, Aronow L, Feldman DL. Glucocorticoid receptors and inhibition of bone cell growth in primary culture. Endocrinology 1977;100:619–28.
148. Bachrach LK, Guido D, Katzman D, et al. Decreased bone density in adolescent girls with anorexia nervosa. Pediatrics 1990;86:440–7.
149. Gilsanz V, Gibbens DT, Roe TF, et al. Vertebral bone density in children: effect of puberty. Radiology 1988;166:847–50.
150. Ettinger B, Genant HK, Cann CE. Postmenopausal bone loss is prevented by treatment with low-dosage estrogen with calcium. Ann Intern Med 1987;106:40–5.
151. Bachrach LK, Katzman DK, Litt IF, et al. Recovery from osteopenia in adolescent girls with anorexia nervosa. J Clin Endocrinol Metab 1991;72:602–6.
152. Kreipe R, Hicks D, Rosier R, et al. Effects of estrogen/progesterone supplementation on tetracycline-labelled bone histomorphometry in anorexia nervosa. Abstract presented at the Fifth International Conference on Eating Disorders, New York, 1992.
153. Strokosch GR, Friedman AJ, Wu S-C, et al. Effects of an oral contraceptive (Norgestimate/Ethinyl Estradiol) on bone mineral density in adolescent females with anorexia nervosa: a double-blind placebo-controlled study. J Adolesc Health 2006;39:819–27.
154. Charig MJ, Fletcher EWL. Reversible bone loss in anorexia nervosa. Br Med J 1987;295:474–5.
155. Chestnut CH. Noninvasive techniques for measuring bone mass: a comparative review. Clin Obstet Gynecol 1987;30: 812–9.
156. Becker AE, Grinspoon SK, Klibanski A, et al. Eating disorders. N Engl J Med 1999;340:1092–8.
157. Frisch RE, McArthur JW. Menstrual cycles: Fatness as a determinant of minimum weight for height necessary for their maintenance or onset. Science 1974;185:949–51.
158. Davidson JK. Controlling diabetes mellitus with diet therapy. Postgrad Med 1976;59:114–22.
159. Woo LMH. Diet counseling: treatment of anorexia nervosa and bulimia. Top Clin Nutr 1986;1:73.
160. Omizo SA, Oda EA. Anorexia nervosa: Psychological considerations for nutrition counseling. J Am Diet Assoc 1988;88:49–51.
161. Huse DM, Lucas AL. Dietary patterns in anorexia nervosa. Am J Clin Nutr 1984;40:251–4.
162. Garrow JS. Dietary management of obesity and anorexia nervosa. J Hum Nutr 1980;34:137.
163. Luder E, Schebendach J. Nutrition management of eating disorders. Top Clin Nutr 1993;8:48–63.
164. Tolstrup K. The treatment of anorexia nervosa in childhood and adolescence. J Child Psychol Psychiatry 1975;16:75.
165. Garfinkel PE, Garner DM. Anorexia Nervosa: A Multidimensional Perspective. New York: Brunner, Mazel; 1982. p. 214–57.
166. Kaye WH, Gwirtzman HE, Obarzanek E, et al. Caloric intake necessary for weight maintenance in anorexia nervosa: Nonbulimics require greater caloric intakes than bulimics. Am J Clin Nutr 1986;44:435–43.
167. Kris-Etherton PM. Nutrition and athletic performance. Nutr Today 1990;September/October:37.
168. Costill DL. Carbohydrate for exercise: dietary demands for optimal performance. Int J Sports Med 1988;9:1–18.
169. Alberici JC, Farrell PA, Kris-Etherton PM, Shively CA. Effects of preexercise candy bar ingestion on substrate utilization and performance in trained cyclists. Med Sci Sports Exerc 1989;21 Suppl 2:S47.
170. Wheeler KB. Sports nutrition for the primary care physician: the importance of carbohydrate. Physician Sports Med 1989;17:106–17.
171. Mann J. Complex carbohydrates: Replacement energy for fat or useful in their own right? Am J Clin Nutr 1981;45:1202–6.

172. Foster C, Costill DL, Fink NJ. Effects of pre-exercise feeding on endurance. Med Sci Sports Exerc 1979;11:1–5.
173. Hoffman CJ, Coleman E. An eating plan and update on recommended dietary practices for the endurance athlete. J Am Diet Assoc 1991;91:325–30.
174. Yarrows SA. Weight loss through dehydration in amateur wrestlers. J Am Diet Assoc 1988;88:491–3.
175. Tcheng T, Tipton CM. Iowa wrestling study: Anthropometric measurements and the prediction of a "minimal" body weight for high school wrestlers. Med Sci Sports 1973;5(1):1–101.
176. Slavin J. Assessing athletes' nutritional status, making it part of the sports physical. Physician Sports Med 1991;19:79–94.
177. Subcommittee on the Tenth Edition of the RDAs, Food and Nutrition Board, Commission on Life Sciences, National Research Council. Recommended Dietary Allowances. 10th ed. Washington, DC: National Academy Press; 1989.
178. Town GP, Wheeler KB. Nutritional concerns for the endurance athlete. Diet Currents 1987;13:7.
179. American Dietetic Association. Nutrition for physical fitness and athletic performance for adults. J Am Diet Assoc 1987;87:993.
180. Aronson V. Physician Sports Med Issues 1986;14:199–202.
181. Elliot D, Goldberg L. Nutrition and exercise. Med Clin North Am 1985;69:71–83.
182. Raunikar RA, Sabio H. Anemia in the adolescent athlete. Am J Dis Child 1992;146:1201–5.

65

The Adolescent Athlete: Performance-Enhancing Drugs and Dietary Supplements

Ryan P. Calfee, MD
Archna G. Calfee, MD
Paul D. Fadale, MD

INTRODUCTION

The term *ergogenic* is of Greek origin, derived from *ergon*, to work, and *gennan*, to produce. Literally translated to produce work, ergogenic aids are any products utilized to enhance performance. Ergogenic drugs used by athletes are one such aid and include traditional anabolic–androgenic steroids, steroid precursors (prohormones), growth hormone, ephedra alkaloids, and nutritional supplements.

Drug and supplement use is not uncommon today. Two thousand and five hundred metric tons of creatine were consumed in 1999, and it is estimated today that 1 to 3 million US athletes are taking steroids.[1,2] These substances, once confined to professional locker rooms, are now being used by today's youth commonly, without recognizing the risks of such drugs.[3] Children as early as middle school are experimenting with anabolic steroids and supplements to improve physical appearances and performance.

As over 7 million high school students participate in formal athletic teams, the use of both banned and legal "performance-enhancing" substances by amateur athletes today is of significant concern (Figure 1).[4] Adolescent athletes commonly initiate ergogenic drug use with nutritional supplements before illicit substances; former high school athletes using legal sport supplements were over 25 times more likely to have used steroids than those not taking over the countersupplements.[5] The social environment surrounding high school sports during the time of early ergogenic drug use has been associated with continued steroid and supplement use into young adulthood.[5]

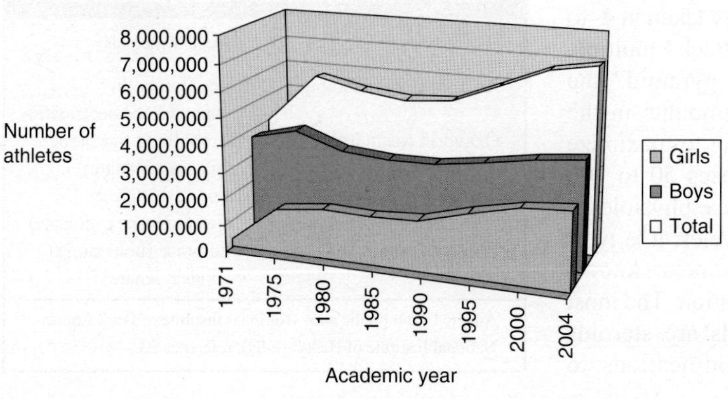

Figure 1 High school sports participation totals in the United States. (Adapted from reference 4.)

Pediatricians, the primary medical contact with the adolescent athlete, must educate themselves as to the true effects of these substances. Young athletes are not expected to volunteer facts about substance use but may respond honestly to direct, nonaccusational questions. Given that school athletic teams require yearly preparticipation physicals, the opportunity for starting such discussions and educating adolescent athletes about these substances is available and should be capitalized on.

This chapter explains the physiologic and performance effects of popular ergogenic substances as well as their prevalence and legal standing. Although the literature regarding these drugs is extensive, it is important for the pediatrician and pediatric nutritionist to note several critical limitations of studies to date. Nearly all investigations into the safety and performance effects of ergogenic drugs have been conducted in the adults. Similar data in growing children and adolescents are generally unavailable. Second, there are no studies to report the health consequences of long-term use of these performance-enhancing substances beginning in the developmental years. Therefore, even those substances appearing benign with short-term use in mature athletes may pose yet unrecognized risk to the adolescent.

HISTORY OF DRUGS IN SPORTS

Although the use of drugs in sports dates back to the Greek Olympians, the landmark discovery for modern ergogenic drugs occurred in 1889. Dr. Brown-Sequard announced at a scientific meeting in Paris that he had found a substance that reversed his 72-year-old body's ailments. He reported injecting himself with the extract of dog and guinea pig testicles under the hypothesis that these organs had "internal secretions that acted as physiologic regulators."[6] This bold statement was confirmed with discovery of hormones in 1905 and the isolation of testosterone in 1935. Soon thereafter in the 1950s, the US Olympic physician teamed with chemists to produce an anabolic steroid for the Americans now known as dianabol.[7] In the decades that followed, steroids and stimulants spread throughout sports, and in 1959, the first reported case of a high school football player abusing steroids surfaced.[8] In the 1960s, the International Olympic Committee (IOC) banned steroids from competition and began formal drug testing in the following decade. During the 1980s, reported positive test results ranged from 2 to 50%, as tests were both scheduled and conducted at random.[9] At the 1988 Seoul Olympics, Canadian sprinter Ben Johnson was the first athlete to have a gold medal in track and field stripped for failing drug tests for an oral anabolic steroid. In 1994, a widely referenced survey was conducted by Goldman who asked aspiring Olympians two simple questions. The first was, "If you were offered a banned performance-enhancing substance that guaranteed that you would win an Olympic medal, and you could not be caught, would you take it?" One hundred and ninety five out of 198 athletes said yes. The second was, "Would you take a banned performance-enhancing drug with a guarantee that you will not be caught, you will win every competition for the next 5 years, but will then die from side effects of the substance?" Still, over 50% of the athletes polled said yes.[10] This survey made it clear that modern athletes often approach their sports with a "win at all costs" mentality. In 2005 information is surfaced to suggest that this mentality is increasingly prevalent, even in high school athletics, with several highly publicized deaths in teenagers who were on steroids, and reports of nine students on one high school football team admitting to steroid abuse.[11]

FACTORS IN SOCIETY TODAY

Several factors unique to our current society may contribute to young people using drugs to succeed in sports. First is the message imparted by professional sport icons. The recent steroid investigations in baseball and books by former players make it clear that steroids and other drugs have played a part in many record-breaking performances. Yet, the fame and respect still garnered by these athletes sends the message that ergogenic drugs are accepted, if not necessary, to reach such success. In a survey conducted following Mark McGwire's highly publicized use of the steroid precursor androstenedione during his record-breaking home-run year in 1998, 24% of United States citizen respondents now wanted to learn more about androstenedione and 22% were interested in taking the prohormone.[12] The deadly consequences of adolescent steroid abuse modeled after their professional heroes have surfaced in the headlines with several suicides by otherwise healthy young athletes while on steroids.[13]

Society today also places a huge emphasis on sports, with collegiate football stadiums seating nearly 100,000 people and countless events featured on national television. From high school basketball all-star games to the Little League World Series, youth today are placed under the national spotlight at exceedingly young ages. With professional scouts now following high school sports and collegiate coaches eyeing even younger talent, the pressure to succeed is now placed on younger, more impressionable shoulders than ever before.

Several economic factors encourage drug use to gain an edge in sports. The money and social stature that accompany athletic success worthy of garnering professional contracts appears to be a motivating factor. One-third of collegiate hockey players surveyed reported anonymously that they would use a banned substance if it would help them earn a National Hockey League contract.[14] Another more subtle but increasingly wide-reaching monetary influence is the rising cost of collegiate education. This has been shown to be a self-reported factor for high school females choosing to use performance-enhancing drugs while competing for prestigious and very valuable athletic scholarships to college.[15,16] As Kurt Gibson, the Illinois High School Association's assistant executive director, said, "You not only get that edge, but you get that notoriety, you get seen and all of a sudden you've got a scholarship on your table. That's a big lure."[17] Whether they turn to ergogenic drugs for the competitive edge or as a means of keeping up with fellow students already using these substances, it is clear that the pressure to do so is significant today.

ANABOLIC–ANDROGENIC STEROIDS

Introduction

Anabolic steroids are the most time-tested group of ergogenic drugs in sports. Properly referred to as anabolic–androgenic steroids, all of these compounds retain male virilizing effects. Adolescent athletes generally turn to steroids in an attempt to increase strength and gain muscle. This is especially desirable in sports such as football and wrestling which place a high premium on power generation. Although not legally attainable for ergogenic purposes, steroids are now cited as the third most common drug offered to children in the United Kingdom, trailing only marijuana and amphetamines.[18]

Physiology

Steroids are hormones derived from cholesterol. Anabolic steroids are synthetic derivatives of the hormone testosterone. The chemical structure has been modified by manufacturers to maximize anabolic effects by delaying metabolism via alkylation of the 17-α position or carboxylation of 19-β hydroxyl group on the sterol D ring.[19] Steroids bind to androgen receptors within the cell cytoplasm. They are then transported into the nucleus before binding DNA and increasing mRNA transcription, which enhances contractile and structural protein synthesis.[7,19]

Steroids have three general effects benefiting the athlete. Binding androgen receptors promotes a positive nitrogen balance in muscle, which produces an anabolic state.[20] However, in the normal physiologic male, endogenous testosterone nearly saturates the available androgen receptors, making this effect of questionable importance. Therefore, it becomes critical that steroids are also anticatabolic. In the overtrained individual, glucocorticoids are increasingly released which promote the breakdown of muscle glycogen for energy.[21] Once available androgen receptors are saturated, exogenous steroids competitively inhibit the binding of catabolic glucocorticoids thereby preserving muscle mass being gained.[22] Finally, anabolic steroids have significant emotional effects. This is often manifest in increased aggression which can push athletes to train more intensely, more often, or for longer duration.[21]

Dosing

Oral, injectable, and newer transdermal steroid preparations are available. Oral forms are short acting and eliminated over days, while injectable steroids have longer lasting effects, but risk positive drug testing up to months after use.[2] Steroids are usually used in the off-season when athletes are strength training and when use is least likely to be detected. Steroids are generally taken in 4- to 12-week cycles. Athletes often "stack" multiple steroids at the same time and "pyramid" the dosing schedule taking highest amounts in the middle of cycles. While attempting to maximize results, athletes may consume doses 50 to 100 times the amount that would replace physiologic steroid levels.[7] Between dosing cycles, it is typical for users to have a period of abstinence known as a "drug holiday" of varying duration. The most recent so-called designer steroids are steroids made with simple chemical modifications to preserve anabolic activity while being undetected during drug testing.[19] Common steroid preparations are presented in Table 1.[23] Athletes have also been found to take additional medications to prevent positive testing (ie, diuretics) or to limit side effects (ie, antiestrogenic medication to prevent gynecomastia) during use.[24]

Effects

Although not every study agrees, the general consensus today is that anabolic steroids do increase athletic measures with objective gains in strength and fat-free mass.[25–27] This fact was conceded in the 1980s by the American College of Sports Medicine.[25] Haupt reviewed the literature in the 1980s and concluded that athletes could not expect aerobic gains, but that strength gains were substantial.[21] Effects were most evident in those with prior weight-training experience and when measuring single repetition maximal efforts. A recent double-blinded study over a 12-week training cycle confirmed significant gains over placebo in ultrasound measured muscle pennation and overall strength on a bench press test.[26] Muscle pennation was measured as the angle that fascicles branched from the aponeurosis, as greater angles are associated with muscles performing higher force contractions. These drugs increase isokinetic and isometric strength, as well as muscle mass via both muscle hypertrophy and the formation of new muscle fibers.[27] Due to ethical concerns, these studies on the effects of anabolic-androgenic steroids as well as those subsequently discussed concerning other ergogenic drugs were performed on adults. However, they offer our best controlled evidence and are presumed to equally represent effects in adolescents.

Side Effects

Nearly 30% of steroid users report experiencing mild subjective side effects.[21] Steroid supplementation has potential adverse effects in multiple organ systems. In the endocrine system, exogenous steroids provide feedback inhibition of luteinizing and follicle stimulating hormones, which causes testicular atrophy and possible infertility. The additional steroids also undergo peripheral aromatization to estrogens, which can lead to irreversible male gynecomastia. It is also common to see premature balding, acne, and precocious

Table 1 Common Anabolic–Androgenic Steroids

Oral Steroids	Injectable Steroids
Anadrol (oxymetholone)	Deca-durabolin (nandrolone decanoate)
Oxandrin (oxandrolone)	Durabolin (nandrolone phenpropionate)
Dianabol (methandrostenolone)	Depo-testosterone (testosterone cypionate)
Winstrol (stanozolol)	Equipoise (boldenone undecylenate)

Adapted from public site—National Institute of Drug Abuse: National Institute of Health (NIH), reference 23.

puberty.[20] Acne results from increased skin lipids as well as increased skin colonization with *Propionibacteria acnes*.[28] Steroids affect the cardiovascular system by adversely altering lipid profiles, raising blood pressure, and producing left ventricular hypertrophy.[29–31] The oral preparations which are 17α-alkylated to inhibit liver inactivation pose the greatest risk to the hepatic system, with common transient disturbances including cholestasis, and nonspecific increases in liver enzymes. These changes are evident in dose-dependent fashion after several months of abuse and are generally reversible with cessation of use.[24] There are also rare cases of peliosis hepatitis with blood-filled liver cysts, and anecdotal reports of hepatocellular carcinoma with proposed links to steroid abuse.[32] The musculoskeletal system, although with grossly increased strength, exhibits dysplastic collagen fibrils which can predispose to muscle strains and ligament sprains.[33] The immature athlete, after initial acceleration of bony growth, may have premature physeal closure, permanently shortening their final adult height.[33] Infections such as HIV, hepatitis B, and hepatitis C remain a concern associated with injectable preparations, as several studies confirm that between 25 and 33% of adolescents on steroids share needles.[34,35] Specific to female users are side effects such as deepened voice, clitoromegaly, and loss of breast tissue, with elements of this virilization being irreversible.[20] Psychologically, steroid users may experience severe mood swings from depression to mania, and aggression that cannot be properly channeled outside of the athletic arena. Using the Diagnostic and Statistical Manual of Mental Disorders (DSM IV), the American Psychiatric Association's standard for defining mental illnesses, it has been reported that nearly 50% of steroid users in a series met criteria for being dependent upon or abusing steroids.[36] Withdrawal symptoms may be seen in up to 88% of steroid abusers.[37]

Apart from medical side effects, several investigators have documented social risks to steroid use. Middleman documented an association with other high-risk activities such as driving under the influence, carrying weapons, and engaging in unsafe sexual practices by young users.[38] Increased use of other illicit substances, including marijuana and alcohol, has also been reported by youths taking steroids.[39]

Legal/Sport Opinion

The Anti-Drug Abuse Act in 1988 first prohibited the distribution of steroids for any purpose other than treatment of a disease. Subsequently, the Anabolic Steroid Control Act of 1990 placed steroids under Schedule III of controlled substances. The illegal possession of anabolic steroids is punishable by 1 year in prison and/or a minimum $1,000 (US) fine, with selling or intent to sell incurring a 5-year prison sentence and/or a $250,000 (US) fine. Steroids are banned from use by all major US sporting leagues, although each governing body has individualized testing and penalization policies. Steroid testing is based on the ratio of testosterone to epitestosterone in urine. A ratio of 6:1 or higher is generally considered a positive test. Physiologically, only 1 in 1,000 men is found to have a ratio as high as 4:1.[19]

Incidence

Current estimates of high school athlete steroid use reach up to 8% in males and up to 6% in females. Buckley and colleagues performed a nationwide survey of over 3,000 males found that 6.6% of male high school seniors had tried steroids, with 67% beginning use by 16 years of age and 40% using multiple cycles.[40] These results were later confirmed in a survey of Indiana high school football players documenting 6% use rate (mean age at first use 14 years),[42] and 2003 nationwide Center for Disease Control (CDC) data finding a 6.4% use of steroids by 12th grade males.[41] Publications have continued to document childhood steroid use with consistent findings of 2 to 3% use of steroids in youths from 9 years old to young teens with numbers reaching 9% among middle school students who identify themselves as gymnasts or weightlifters.[35,43,44] Surveying over 4,000 students in Minnesota, researchers found an annual prevalence of steroid use of 5.7 and 7.6% in middle school girls and boys, respectively.[45] Interestingly, these numbers decreased to 1.4 and 4.4% in high school aged female and male students.[45] The ongoing Monitoring the Future Study, which has the largest nationwide cohort of nearly 50,000 students, reported a 1.1, 1.3, and 1.5% annual prevalence of male steroid users in the 8th, 10th, and 12th grades, respectively, in 2005.[46] Girls in the 12th grade had a 0.4% use rate of steroids in the past year, while the CDC found 3.3% lifetime prevalence of steroid use in 12th grade girls.[41,46] Although the numbers from the Monitoring the Future Survey are more modest than other reports, it is important to remember that these numbers reflect the entire student population, not just athletes. While 57% of 12th graders viewed steroid use as a great risk, the availability of steroids to high school students increases with grade level so that 40% of 12th grade students felt that steroids were either "fairly easy" or "very easy" to obtain.[46]

In the 1980s estimates of steroid use reached 20% for Division I college athletes.[47] Subsequently, the NCAA began surveying its athletes to better define the demographics of substance use in this population. The latest NCAA survey in 2005 polled nearly 20,000 student athletes in all championship sports and all divisions.[48] They reported that 1.2% of these student athletes reported steroid use in the past 12 months. Recent independent studies of college athletes, however, raise the possibility of underreporting to the NCAA as results show up to 9% athletes using steroids on one campus.[49] Furthermore, 76% of users and even 36% of nonusers reported that if desired, they could obtain steroids in less than 2 weeks.[49] Worrisome trends discovered by the NCAA included that nearly 60% of anabolic steroid use began in junior high or high school.[48] This identification of drug use at a young age was consistent for all ergogenic substances.[48] The trend of athletes using steroids to improve performance or appearance as opposed to use for injury recovery has remained constant since 2001. In this population, the most common sources of anabolic steroids were friends/relatives (25%), Web site/mail order (22%), and coach/trainers (17%).

STEROID PRECURSORS (PROHORMONES)

Introduction

Androstenedione and dehydroepiandosterone (DHEA) were catapulted into the public spotlight following report of their use by US professional baseball player Mark McGwire in 1998. These substances were available over the counter at the time and adolescents turned to these prohormones for building muscle mass and strength as an alternative to steroids.

Physiology

Androstenedione and closely related dehydroepiandosterone are two popular steroid precursors, or prohormones. DHEA was identified in 1934 and is a weak androgen produced in the adrenal cortex, while androstenedione, a more potent anabolic–androgenic steroid, is made in the adrenal glands and gonads. DHEA is converted in the body to androstenedione, which can then be transformed into either testosterone or estrone (Figure 2). Athletes use these substances with the belief that they will boost testosterone levels, thereby having ergogenic effects similar to anabolic steroids.

Dosing

DHEA's recommended dosing is in a range of 50 to 100 mg/d for up to 1 year. The number of side effects increases at doses exceeding this amount, although athletes may well take more than recommended amounts. Although now off of the supplement market, androstenedione's upper limit for dosing was 100 to 300 mg/d.

Effects

In 1962, Mahesh reported that androstenedione given to two females resulted in increased testosterone levels.[50] Since that time there has been little support for these precursors having any ergogenic effects, although their popularity soared after Mark McGuire admitted to using androstenedione during his 1998 quest to break Roger Maris's single-season home-run record. Leder in 2000 reported that men given androstenedione had increased blood testosterone concentrations, although this effect was only seen in the first few hours after initial use.[51] Furthermore, the early boost in testosterone levels reached only

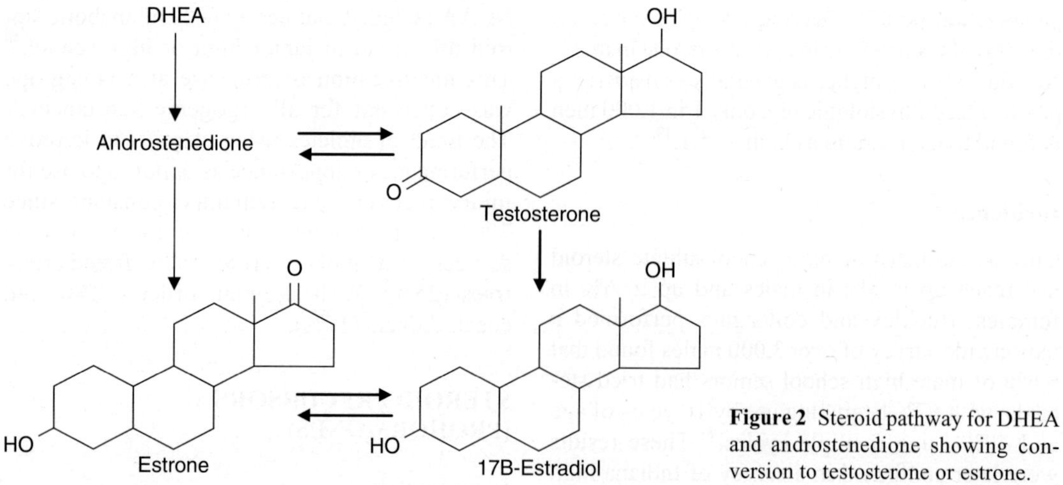

Figure 2 Steroid pathway for DHEA and androstenedione showing conversion to testosterone or estrone.

the upper limit of normal for physiologic males. Later, after several weeks of use, the only hormone level alteration was increased estrogen.[51] Most studies have found no change in testosterone levels, but have confirmed increasing estrogen levels in males.[2] In one investigation, 20 healthy males who underwent 8 weeks of standardized resistance training while being given either androstenedione or placebo in double-blinded fashion. At the conclusion of the testing period, those receiving the drug showed no change in any athletic measure or testosterone levels but were found to have significantly increased estrone and estradiol levels.[52] Thus in the literature to date, there is no convincing evidence that these prohormones have any true benefit for athletes.

Side Effects

Although androstenedione and DHEA are without proven benefit, they are not without risk. As they share a metabolic pathway with anabolic steroids, they share several common side effects. These include adverse changes in lipid profiles as well as potentially irreversible male gynecomastia and female virilization, particularly when taken at higher than recommended doses. Chronic dosing with resultant elevation of sex hormone levels also presents the theoretical risk of associated prostate and uterine cancer.[53] Use of these substances may also downregulate endogenous testosterone over time.[54] Priapism has also been reported and animal studies have found resultant hyperplastic prostatic changes with use.[55,56] Finally, although DHEA is a legal supplement, impurities during production as well as postdigestion metabolites can place athletes at risk for testing positive for a banned substance.

Legal/Sports Opinion

The availability of androstenedione and DHEA has changed over time. Androstenedione was originally sold as a nutritional supplement. In 2004, a new Steroid Control Act was signed which placed androstenedione under Schedule III of controlled substances effective January 2005. Androstenedione is now banned by all major sporting leagues including Olympic and collegiate sports.

Following the initial marketing of DHEA, the compound was removed from distribution by the FDA in 1985 secondary to concerning associations with liver damage.[53] However, the Dietary Supplement Health and Education Act of 1994 reopened the distribution of DHEA as a "nutritional supplement." DHEA was not included in the 2004 Steroid Control Act and remains an over-the-counter nutritional supplement.

Incidence

Sparse literature is available for evaluating the use of androstenedione and DHEA. In 2002, Reeder surveyed 475 high school students and found that 4% of this population of athletes and nonathletes used steroid precursors within the past year.[57] The high number of adolescent users in Reeder's student body cohort suggests that these drugs are being used by adolescents. Importantly, the published data available to estimate adolescent use of steroid precursors predates the reclassification of androstenedione as a controlled substance.

GROWTH HORMONE

Introduction

Fewer adolescents have turned to growth hormone than steroids for ergogenic purposes. Young athletes use growth hormone with little scientific knowledge of its properties beyond the obvious implications of its name, which is exploited in internet advertisements claiming to sell the compound. Young athletes believe it will make them bigger and stronger. In the population of competitive body builders, users aim to decrease subcutaneous fat to allow for a more defined appearance.

Physiology

Growth hormone is a polypeptide secreted by the somatotrope cells in the anterior pituitary. Secretion is pulsatile, and gradually decreases after peaking during early adolescence. Its half-life is approximately 15 to 20 minutes in plasma.[58] After injection, growth hormone's blood concentration peaks within 3 hours before diminishing to levels undetectable by 24 hours.[58] Growth hormone is converted in the liver into insulin-like growth factor 1 (IGF-1), which has several effects throughout the body. Although there is some debate whether IGF-1 is responsible for or merely a marker of growth hormones actions, end results include increased protein synthesis, lipid catabolism, and bone growth.[59]

Dosing

Human growth hormone (hGH) was first used in children who were growth hormone deficient. Typical medicinal doses range from .03 to .05 mg/kg/d. hGH was initially derived from cadavers and its use was associated with the transmission of prion disease. Since 1985, a biosynthetic growth hormone has been available. Growth hormone is manufactured only in injectable form, as orally administered product is completely digested. It may be used several times per month and the cost of 1-month supply can approach $5,000 (US).[60] Athletes taking growth hormone may take supratherapeutic doses in the range of .06 to .11 mg/kg/d and often combine use with anabolic steroids.[3,61]

Effects

Although growth hormone has many benefits for those congenitally deficient, it does not appear to hold similar promise for healthy young athletes. No conclusive evidence exists that growth hormone enhances athletic performance. One double-blinded placebo-controlled trial involving 6 weeks of growth hormone administration to trained athletes failed to show any improvement in strength beyond that gained using identical conditioning with placebo.[62] In fact, acromegaly patients with an excess of endogenous growth hormone may be the most accurate model for the athlete supplementing an already normal hormone level. Acromegaly patients often have weaker muscles due to a growth hormone–induced myopathy and have greater exercise tolerance with reduction of blood growth hormone levels.[63] Even without proven performance benefit, this drug does have several effects that attract athletes. One is that growth hormone causes perceptible fluid shifts within bodily tissues with early use, causing individuals to feel that the drug is "doing something." Second, growth hormone has a repartitioning effect channeling calories into protein synthesis and driving lipolysis, which decreases subcutaneous fat, producing a more toned appearance.[64]

Side Effects

Concern exists that black market growth hormone may still include cadaveric growth hormone, thus posing an infectious disease risk. Injecting the synthetic form still carries with it the well-known risks of hepatitis and HIV transmission with use of nonsterile needles. Due to its interactions with insulin and IGF-1, growth hormone administered at times of inadequate insulin reserves can be catabolic and ketogenic, potentially inciting diabetic ketoacidosis.[58] Even in the normal physiologic state, growth hormone may produce insulin resistance and potentially type 2 diabetes.[64] Fluid retention can produce arthralgias and carpal tunnel syndrome. Additional risks include premature physeal closure, jaw enlargement, hypertension, and slipped capital femoral epiphysis. Rare but severe risks also include reported papilledema with intracranial hypertension.[7]

Legal/Sports Opinion

Growth hormone is banned by all major sporting leagues. However, no reliable blood or urine test to detect use by athletes has yet been developed. Attempts have been made to identify exogenous growth hormone administration based upon circulating isomer composition as well as longer lasting growth hormone–dependent markers, but are yet to be used in competition.[65]

Incidence

Questioning younger athletes, Rickert surveyed 224 males in the 10th grade to assess high school growth hormone use.[3] Nearly 5% reported using growth hormone, over half used growth hormone in conjunction with steroids, and 70% reported use more than once per month. Of concern was the fact that half of the students could not name a single risk associated with taking growth hormone. The most recent NCAA study found that 1.2% of athletes reported using growth hormone in the past 12 months which was lower than the reported 3% in 2001.[48]

NUTRITIONAL SUPPLEMENTS

Nutritional supplements can be legally purchased at any health store. Yearly sales in the US approach $12 to 15 billion (US) with sport supplements being responsible for $1.9 billion (US) in sales during 2004.[66–68] Investigators in one Division I conference found that 88% of athletes used nutritional supplements, and among a high school cohort of 270 athletes, 58% had used some form of supplementation.[69,70] The 1994 Dietary Supplement Health and Education Act permanently changed the landscape for these substances. In this act, dietary supplements were defined as, "A product (other than tobacco), that is intended to supplement the diet. It bears or contains one or more of the following dietary ingredients: a vitamin; a mineral; an herb or other botanical; an amino acid; a dietary substance to supplement the diet by increasing the total daily intake; or a concentrate, a metabolite, constituent, extract, or combination of these ingredients. The product is intended for ingestion in pill, capsule, tablet, or liquid form. The product is not recommended for use as a conventional food or as the sole item of a meal or diet, and it is labeled as a dietary supplement."[71] Besides providing a generously inclusive definition, the act had several other implications. Specifically, there is no FDA approval necessary for a supplement to reach the marketplace. Remarkably, manufacturer claims do not need to be proven before appearing on labels. Claims only require a disclaimer that there is a "lack of proof," while the FDA now has the burden of proof in establishing that claims are actually false. This fact is largely unappreciated by the adolescent athlete, with 48% believing that over-the-counter nutritional supplements have been scientifically tested for efficacy and safety.[72] Proper labeling simply requires that manufacturers list the ingredient(s) and the quantity enclosed, with the product having the strength and identity of the substance is represented to have.[71] Although no specific criteria for this last requirement were made, the US Pharmacopeia adheres to drugs having 90 to 110% of the represented strength for ethical drug production.

The lack of regulation in supplement production can place the consumer at significant risk. Although documented by many investigators, Green, in 2001, illustrated this point quite clearly.[73] Sampling two to four capsules in every bottle of 12 supplement brands, he used liquid and gas chromatography to identify the true ingredients in each package. Stunningly, only one brand met the 1994 labeling requirements detailed above. Eleven out of 12 brands contained less than the stated dose, 1 brand had 177% of the stated dose, and 2 brands contained none of a stated ingredient. While taking an erroneous dose of a supplement can be risky, there was an even larger warning to athletes born out in this study. One brand actually contained 10 mg of testosterone, which as an anabolic steroid, is banned in the sporting arena. With the stringent rules adhered to by today's governing bodies of sports such as the NCAA, this type of contaminated supplement could cost the athlete immediate disqualification. By most leagues today, athletes are held strictly accountable for all substances entering their bodies. A positive drug test is punishable, regardless if the athlete knew they were consuming the drug. Therefore, much caution is warranted when athletes consider using even "legal" nutritional supplements as manufacturing standards are not the same as pharmaceuticals.

These supplements are popular among adolescent athletes looking for ways to boost performance without using illicit substances. Given the lack of quality standards, even adolescents taking supplements as directed may be placing themselves at risk. Multiple studies support the conclusion that up to 20% of high school students are using these supplements. The latest NCAA survey results revealed that 75% of collegiate athletes using nutritional supplements began use either before or during high school.[48] As relatively inexpensive compounds that are readily available at most health food stores, they are often the first ergogenic drugs used by the adolescent athlete. The most common sources for supplement purchase by high school students are presented in Figure 3.[57,74] Friends provide the majority of information on and encouragement for use (Figure 4).[74] As such, the reasons behind use and understanding of actual effects are often rudimentary at best. In a 2001 examination of adolescent supplement users, reasons for use included, "[for an] energy boost… You don't lose energy as fast… To build muscle tissue when working with weights."[75] Approximately 20% of student athletes identify parents as encouraging sport supplement use.[57,74]

CREATINE

Introduction

Creatine is popular among adolescents involved in sports requiring quick bursts of energy. Billed as a safe, legal way to add quick muscle, young athletes appear eager to try creatine supplementation. Most series of young athletes indicate positive subjective enhancement of performance. Generally, the immature athlete fails to perceive any risk in taking creatine and dosing practices vary widely.[74]

Physiology

Creatine (Cr) is formed from glycine, arginine, and methionine and is naturally produced by the liver, kidneys, and pancreas. After production, creatine is transported to muscle, heart, and brain, with 95% of bodily stores remaining in muscle. Type II muscle fibers, which are high powered with fast twitch speeds, have the highest storage

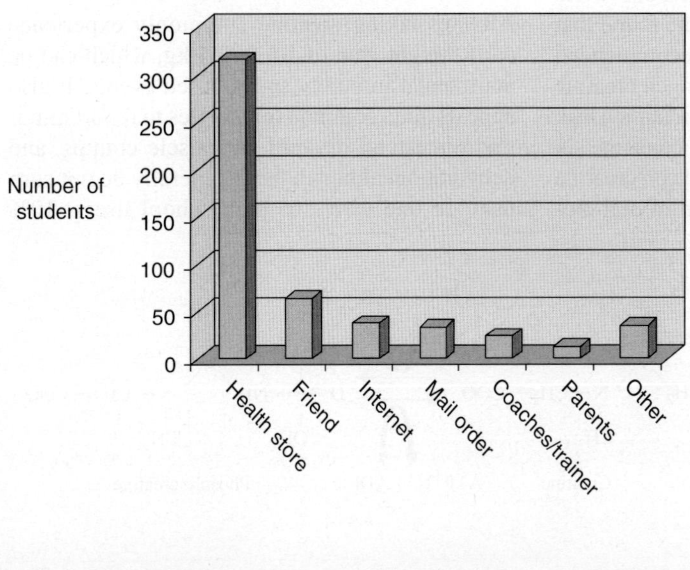

Figure 3 Sources of nutritional supplements for high school students. (Adapted from references 57 and 74.)

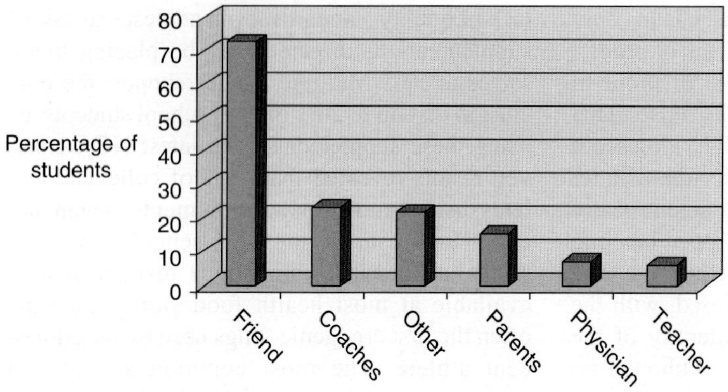

Figure 4 Persons encouraging creatine use in young athletes. (Adapted from reference 74.)

capacity. Creatine is also naturally present in the diet, mainly in meat and fish. The daily metabolic cycling of creatine is 2 g, with one half produced endogenously and the second half supplied from the normal diet. Muscle creatine stores are in a balanced equilibrium with creatine and phosphocreatine (PCr) interconverted via creatine kinase. The dephosphorylation of PCr generates ATP, which provides the source of quick energy for muscular contraction (Figure 5). Aerobic recovery time then allows for the restoration of PCr.[7] PCr availability is considered the limiting factor in short high-intensity activities, as it provides muscle with the major energy source over the first 10 seconds of anaerobic activity after free ATP is consumed in the first 1 second of action (Figure 6).[76]

Investigations into the tissue-level effects of oral creatine appear to show several changes. Supplementation can cause approximately a 20% increase in muscle PCr stores, quicken the replenishment of PCr during recovery, and can buffer lactic acid as hydrogen ions are consumed during the dephosphorylation of PCr, which potentially delays fatigue onset.[77–79]

Dosing

Creatine is most commonly taken as a powder that is dissolved in a drink. It is recommended to be taken first as a loading phase, with athletes consuming 5 g four times per day, for the first 4 to 6 days. The standard dosing is then 2 g daily for the next 3 months. Creatine taken in excess of this amount appears to be excreted via the kidneys.[80] A month of abstinence is standard practice following each use cycle. Notably, one series of high school students taking creatine found that 78% of users either took more than recommended doses or simply did not know how much creatine they were consuming.[81] The Physician's Desk Reference notes that athletes should consume six to eight glasses of water per day while on creatine to prevent dehydration.[82] Absorption of oral creatine does vary with diet. Carbohydrate-rich fluids tend to increase creatine absorption, while caffeine impairs its uptake.[83,84]

Effects

Creatine supplementation does appear to have athletic benefits. However, nearly 30% of athletes do not see benefits with creatine use, thereby falling into a category of "nonresponders" who are theorized to already have maximal PCr stores.[7] Most commonly, performance effects are seen in increasing strength and outcomes in short-duration, anaerobic events. Studies do not show improved endurance performance as expected given that prolonged muscle activity depends on aerobic glycolysis.[85] Ostojic published the only study to date on creatine effects in adolescent athletes. It was a randomized, blinded trial assessing soccer-specific skill enhancement in 20 adolescent players (mean 16.6 years of age).[86] With 7 days of dosing (10 g 3×/d) versus placebo, vertical jump, sprint-power test times, and dribbling test times were all significantly improved on creatine. Endurance abilities were not affected. In another well-controlled setting, Volek performed a double-blinded study examining 12 weeks of creatine use including standard loading and maintenance phases in recreational weightlifters.[87] In those athletes on creatine, significant increases in fat-free body mass, bench press maximal lift, peak power production in sets of repeated jump squats, and in the area of biopsied type I, IIA, and IIAB muscle fibers were demonstrated.

Side Effects

Athletes taking creatine commonly experience early weight gain of 1.6 to 2.4 kg, which can be detrimental in purely speed-based events. It also appears quite common for athletes to report minor gastrointestinal discomfort, muscle cramps, and dehydration, although these generally do not curb use.[2] In one series of high school users, 10% experienced these adverse effects.[74] There have been two case reports of renal function compromise. One was an athlete with diagnosed focal segmental glomerular sclerosis who experienced a transient 50% loss of glomerular filtration rate, while one previously healthy athlete reported transient interstitial nephritis.[88,89] However, at least one study of self-reported use over several years did not show adverse renal effects.[90] While the exact risk that creatine supplementation poses to the kidneys is unknown, it is prudent to be especially concerned about creatine use by athletes with impaired renal function. Three highly publicized deaths have occurred in college wrestlers known to take creatine, although official autopsy results indicated that dehydration and weight loss were at fault, not creatine.[82] Further questions remain, including the effect of increased creatine in the brain, liver, kidney, and lungs as well as potential effects of chronic use, or the effects of creatine use by children.

Legal Sport Aspects

Creatine remains a legal nutritional supplement today. Despite what at least one brand's name suggests, *Teen Advantage*, the American College of Sports Medicine has explicitly recommended that it should not be used by anyone under 18 years of age.[79] Collegiate teams including trainers and coaches are prohibited from supplying creatine or other supplements directly to their student athletes.

Incidence

Reported incidence rates of creatine use range from 5.6% of 10- to 18-year-olds[91] to 8.2% of 14- to 18-year-olds.[81] It was also noted that 12th graders used creatine much like their collegiate counterparts, with that grade reporting 44% use. One of the largest surveys queried over 4,000 Wisconsin high school athletes.[74] Across 37 public schools, 16.7% of the athletes reported creatine use. One quarter of male athletes used creatine, while only 4% of the female population utilized the supplement. In agreement with previous studies, the prevalence peaked in the 12th grade with 25% of the athletes taking creatine. Current estimates of collegiate creatine use vary from 25 to 78% of athletes.[48,92]

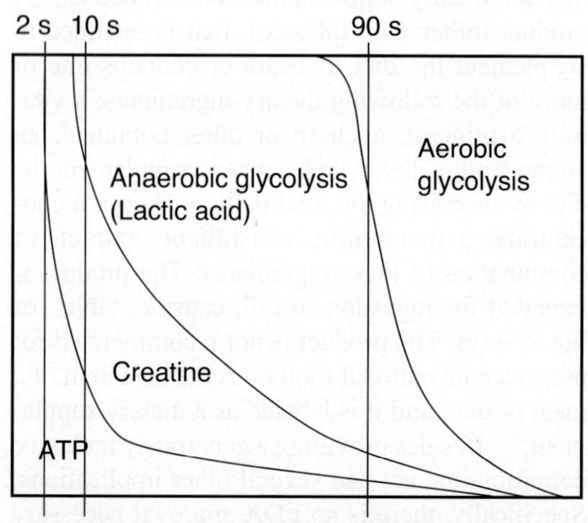

Figure 6 Time-dependent, dominant energy source for muscle activity. (Reprinted with permission from reference 76.)

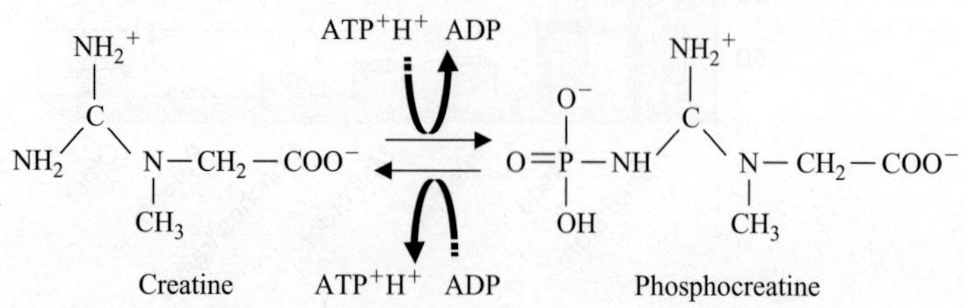

Figure 5 Interconversion of phosphocreatine and creatine producing ATP.

EPHEDRINE

Introduction

Young athletes approach stimulants such as ephedrine and amphetamines similarly. These drugs are abused by adolescents for two purposes. One population uses these drugs to provide quick energy, reduce fatigue, and to enhance speed. Other users are drawn to the stimulant effects on metabolism hoping to lose unwanted weight either as a primary objective or to secondarily improve athletic performance. More recently, athletes have turned to pseudoephedrine due to its availability, hoping for similar effects.

Physiology

Ephedrine is a stimulant with a chemical structure closely related to amphetamine. It is derived from ephedra herbs also known as ma huang. It possesses α- and β-adrenergic agonistic effects, enhances the release of norepinephrine, and stimulates the central nervous system.[93] Pseudoephedrine is a closely related α-adrenergic agonist available without prescription in common decongestants. Physiologic effects include increased blood pressure with heightened peripheral vascular tone, respiratory dilation, relaxation of gastrointestinal muscle, and increased blood flow to skeletal muscle.[94] Ergogenic effects of these compounds are attributed to increasing cardiac output and via its stimulation of the central nervous system. This excitatory effect on the nervous system may decrease fatigue as well as decrease the athlete's perceived effort.[95]

Dosing

Previously available ephedrine compounds included such brands as *Metabolife 356* and *Ripped Fuel*. Prior to being banned in 2004, the FDA recommended that daily ephedra alkaloid intake remain under 25 mg and not be continued longer than 1 week. Pseudoephedrine in cold remedies is taken in maximal amount at 60 mg or as 120 mg in sustained release capsules. Combining ephedrine with caffeine or its herbal form guarana poses significant risk and was prohibited by the FDA in the 1980s.

Effects

Ephedrine has been traditionally used by athletes to provide quick energy and to aid in fat loss, consequently improving speed and appearance. The majority of studies available show no change in athletic performance with ephedrine use. However, investigations have reported improvements in quadriceps strength or stationary cycling, but these have involved high doses of ephedra compounds and were sometimes combined with caffeine, which poses significant risk to the athlete.[94,96] At least one study has reported improved performance in a 1,500 m run following 2.5 mg/kg (average dose 180 mg) dose of pseudophedrine.[95] While supratherapeutic dosing of pseudophedrine may impact athletic performance, further research is needed to definitively answer this question and to identify the health risks associated with such doses.

Side Effects

Bent reported that ephedra accounted for 0.82% of herbal product sales, but was implicated in 64% of adverse herbal reactions in the United States in 2001.[97] Adverse reactions are wide ranging, and include hypertension, arrhythmias, anxiety, tremors, insomnia, seizures, paranoid psychoses, cerebral vascular accident, myocardial infarction, and death.[98] In fact, in athletic performance studies, the most consistent finding is increased heart rate. Haller in 2000 critically evaluated the 140 adverse events reported to the FDA from 1997 to 1999 and concluded that 62% of the adverse events reported were definitely or possibly related to the drug.[98] In that series, 10 users were under 18 years old and there were 10 deaths and 13 cases of permanent disability. These included a 22-year-old male on *Ripped Force* who suffered a cardiac arrest and was left with a permanent neurologic disability, and a 15-year-old female on *Ripped Fuel* who suffered a fatal arrhythmia.

Legal/Sport Aspects

In 2004, ephedrine was the first supplement removed from the market by the FDA since the 1994 Supplement Act. However, in April of 2005 a US District Court judge ruled to overturn the ban stating that the FDA had not proven that a 10 mg dose was dangerous. She ruled that, "[the prior ban] would be directly contrary to the statutory language placing the burden of proof on the government." Although this legal battle is far from over, this ruling may open the door to ephedrine's return to the supplement marketplace. Pseudoephedrine, previously banned by the World Anti Doping Agency, is currently on the monitoring list due to insufficient evidence of its ergogenic effects. The monitoring list includes substances which are not prohibited, but are followed by the World Anti Doping Agency for, "patterns of misuse in sport." The IOC, NCAA, Major League Baseball (MLB), National Basketball Association (NBA), and National Football League (NFL) have all banned the systemic use of ephedrine products.

Incidence

The NCAA has documented that its athletes in 2005 were using ephedra products earlier than in the past with 73% beginning prior to college.[48] Kayton's work in 2002 supported this claim, finding that among 270 high school athletes, 26% of females and 12% of males had tried ephedrine products.[70] The NCAA data reported a 2.5% incidence of ephedrine use, and 4.1% incidence of amphetamine use in the past 12 months for men and women athletes.[48] When examining sport-specific use, marked increases from 2001 were noted with 7.9% of male gymnasts and 11.9% of female hockey players using ephedrine.[48] The NCAA also confirmed that over two-thirds of ergogenic stimulant use was initiated prior to college. A smaller study of collegiate use among five male Division I ice hockey teams noted that 38% of players used ephedrine and 46% used psuedoephedrine in cold remedies hoping to boost performance.[97] Stimulants were common even when examining current use, with over a third of the players using these drugs in the preceeding 30 days.[97] In this survey, the student athletes were well aware of both stimulant side effects and the NCAA ban on the use of such substances. This may represent a change in abuse patterns, which more closely mirror that in professional athletes.

CAFFEINE

Introduction

Present in many of the most popular drinks today, it is easy to overlook caffeine as a potential ergogenic drug. As the most readily available stimulant, adolescents commonly take advantage of caffeinated beverages to give them energy boosts.

Physiology

Caffeine is a dimethylxanthine stimulant and adenosine receptor antagonist.[99] The exact mechanism responsible for potential ergogenic effects has not been identified. The inhibition of adenosine, the enhancement of adrenaline secretion, and the conservation of glucose have been theorized as the basis for performance enhancement.

Dosing

Caffeine dosing for athletic events ranges from 2 to 9 mg/kg, equivalent to 250 to 750 mg per dose. Caffeine is taken in immediate proximity to the performance not more than 1 hour prior to competition. While caffeine tablets contain predetermined amounts, the caffeine content in beverages such as coffee vary greatly with an 8-ounce cup generally containing from 100 to 300 mg.[100]

Effects

In several well-controlled studies, caffeine has shown ergogenic properties, although not every study agrees. Caffeine resulted in improved 1-hour-time trial cycling performance in one double-blind, crossover study.[101] Rowing ability over 2,000 m was also improved after caffeine supplementation in a similarly designed study.[102] Some of the urine testing of athletes in these studies resulted in concentrations that would warrant disqualification by the Olympic Committee.

Side Effects

Caffeine can produce dependency with abstinence causing anxiety and headache. Caffeine is a diuretic, although this property has not produced any documented complications.

Legal/Sports Aspects

Caffeine is available as over-the-counter tablets and in beverages. To our knowledge, high school athletes have not been tested for caffeine abuse. The NCAA and Olympic Committee rely on urinary concentrations of caffeine to detect excessive use. Positive test results are set at 15 µg/mL for collegiate student athletes and at 12 µg/mL for Olympians. It is estimated that 9 mg/kg of caffeine intake is required to produce urinary concentrations of 12 µg/mL, although there is some variability in the results of this urine measurement.[101]

Incidence

Clearly, the number of adolescents with caffeine intake is extremely high. Caffeine is now a prominent ingredient in popular sport and energy drinks. While these beverages are popular, it is difficult to estimate the prevalence of adolescents utilizing caffeine specifically to improve performance. While studies of adolescents and supplements often mention energy drink consumption, no research to date has specifically examined caffeine use in the young athlete.

VITAMINS/MINERAL SUPPLEMENTS

It is clear that athletes of all ages use a variety of sport supplement bars, drinks, and pills. Many vitamin and mineral supplements are available and are marketed as having wide ranging health and performance effects. To date, no vitamin or mineral has been proven to have any ergogenic potential. While they may contribute to overall health, these substances do not improve performance. Examples include chromium and vanadyl which are trace elements marketed to increase muscle mass but lack scientific proof of such effects.[57] β-Hydroxy-β-methylbutyrate also falls into this category. A metabolite of leucine, this product is sold to increase muscle mass and is advertised as being muscle protective. Studies in trained athletes have not demonstrated performance enhancement for this popular compound.[99]

UNIQUE NUTRITIONAL RISKS

The Female Athlete

Although the nutritional aspects of athletics are important for all young athletes, care for the female athlete requires exceptional vigilance. As female athletics have become increasingly competitive, more young women are at risk for disordered eating, menstrual irregularities, and osteoporosis. Termed the "Female Athlete Triad" these entities pose risk to adolescent competitors at a critical time in their development. A study of 170 high school female athletes in 2006 raises concern for the health of these young women. Eighteen percent qualified as having disordered eating, 23% had irregular menses (oligomenorrhea, and amenorrhea), and 22% were found to have low bone mass.[103] Notably, the reduction in bone mass correlated with menstrual irregularity and trended downward for all body sites, reaching statistical significance in the greater trochanter of the hip. Few athletes in this series demonstrated all three variables concurrently but the high prevalence of each individually should raise concern (see Chapter 66, "Adolescence: Bone Disease," for details on adolescent bone health and nutrition).

Wrestlers

Wrestling is unique as a sport that bases the level of individual competition on weight. Athletes strive for strength and agility, yet perceive an advantage to qualifying for competition within the lightest weight class possible. Adolescent wrestlers are infamous for taking extreme measures to achieve rapid weight loss prior to meets. While much anecdotal evidence exists for this unhealthy behavior, the largest series of high school wrestlers involved in a formal study was produced by the University of Michigan.[104] With data on 2,532 wrestlers from all levels of high school competition, the prevalence of dangerous weight loss measures is clear. Beginning at an average of 14 years of age, 66% of the wrestlers attempted to lose weight for competition. Over 60% of the adolescents had lost over 5 lbs in the 5 days leading up to a meet with 16% losing over 10 lbs in the same time period. In fact, 6% of the population used weekly laxatives, diet pills, or diuretics to control their weight during the season. Table 2 summarizes the weight-loss measures employed. This group of young athletes should be monitored carefully as the compounding effects of vigorous exercise, food and drink restriction, and pharmacologic weight-loss drugs can produce potentially deadly dehydration and electrolyte imbalances.

Table 2 Percentage of High School Wrestlers Employing Weight Loss Measures.

	At Least 1×/Week	Monthly	Never
Laxatives	1.9	2	88
Diet pills	2.1	1	90
Diuretics	2.1	2	89
Enemas	1.1	0.2	91
Vomiting	2.1	1	89
Spitting	32	10	52
Plastic suit	11	5	77
Increased exercise	72	5	18
Restricting fluids	35	7	51
Fasting	29	8	57
Restricting food	49	9	35
Gradual dieting	53	8	32

Adapted from reference 104.

ADDRESSING THE PROBLEM

Approaches to combat the use of drugs by young athletes have generally fallen in two categories: changes in rules and testing, and educational initiatives. Collegiate rules now bar any supplement distribution directly from teams, and the NCAA employs rigorous drug testing of student-athletes. Similarly, the National Federation of High Schools position statement reads, "In order to minimize health and safety risks to student athletes, maintain ethical standards and reduce liability risks, school personnel and coaches should never supply, recommend or permit the use of any drug, medication, or food supplement solely for performance enhancing purposes."[74] For high school athletes, the 1995 Supreme Court ruling in the case of Vernonia versus Acton upheld the constitutionality of school drug testing policies, maintaining that testing does not violate participants' Fourth Amendment rights. Only preliminary research examining the efficacy of drug testing in adolescent athletes is available. Initial results of a comparative study of steroid use between two high schools, one with random drug testing (announced before the start of the sports season), are encouraging.[105] Among the students subjected to random in-season drug testing, the incidence of illicit substance use during the previous month decreased fourfold with a threefold decrease in the use of performance-enhancing drugs. In that study, a positive test resulted in parental notification, a counseling referral, and a single game suspension. Students in the school conducting the drug testing had more negative attitudes toward testing, although this may have been a reaction to the newly adopted school policy. Thus it appears likely that testing with immediate consequence may deter ergogenic drug use in the high school population.

Data from the National Federation of State High School Association indicates that only 13% of high schools perform drug testing on athletes.[106] However, only 29% reported testing for anabolic steroids, while the rest tested only for illicit substances such as marijuana, opiates, and alcohol. On June 7, 2006 the New Jersey Interscholastic Athletic Association (NJSIAA) enacted the first state wide random drug-testing program for high school athletes.[68] The testing began during post-season tournament competition and consisted of urine testing for steroids, diuretics, urine manipulators, and HCG (in males). The exact list of banned substances follows those listed by the NCAA and International Olympic Committee. Under the New Jersey plan, any substance use violation results in a 1-year loss of sport eligibility. Five hundered students were tested during the 2006--2007 school year. The results of individual tests are to be kept confidential with only the athlete, their parents, and their school being notified of positive tests. At this time, no cumulative data has been released regarding the rate of positive tests from New Jersey. Other states have considered such testing, but will likely await the results of New Jersey's program before instituting similar programs.

The second approach to combating youth drug use in sports has been educational programs designed to teach students about the facts and myths of these substances. This approach offers potentially wide-reaching and sustainable effects for several reasons. Student athletes have an obvious deficit in ergogenic drug knowledge. Adolescents often see the promise of instant improvement in advertisements and the media without understanding the risk associated with ergogenic drugs. For example, when asked for potential side effects of creatine use, the second most common response at 36% (230/635 athletes) was none.[74] Furthermore, adolescents using supplements receive the majority of encouragement to do so from their peers.[74] This means that educational programs may both help to decrease current use and lessen the motivation for other students to begin use.

The model program for such interventions is the Adolescents Training and Learning to Avoid Steroids (ATLAS) program.[107] This program involved over 3,000 high school football players with the intervention group participating in interactive classroom sessions and exercise training sessions focusing on nutrition, drug effects, and drug-refusal role-playing. The control group received brochures with similar information. The sessions were lead both by student athletes and by educators. At the conclusion of the study, testing showed the intervention group to be more knowledgeable of steroid and other drug effects. They were less likely to believe supplement ads, and were more able to reject drug offers from peers. At the end of the season and 1 year later, supplement use was lower, there were fewer new steroid users, and students remained more knowledgeable about ergogenic drugs in the intervention group. Similar intervention specifically for female athletes also resulted in a significant reduction in use of diet pills, amphetamines, anabolic steroids, supplements, and alcohol as well as safer sexual practices and wearing of seat belts.[108]

ROLE OF THE PHYSICIAN

Caring for the young athletes poses several challenges. This age group is often developing rapidly with physiologic changes that mimic those produced by several of the ergogenic drugs discussed. They are not likely to volunteer information about drug or supplement use to physicians. However, the pediatric community is poised to make a unique impact on this problem. Pediatricians are the primary contact for most young people with the medical community and are in a position to develop long-lasting relationships with their patients. Therefore, it is critical for pediatricians to be aware that drug use in sports is not simply an adult problem. Physicians need to become educated about the drugs being used and the consequences of their use. One must be willing to ask about such ergogenic drug use in the same tone as other routine screening questions during office visits and preparticipation physicals. Physicians should ask about the use of both illicit drugs and nutritional supplements as part of routine visits with adolescent athletes. Questions should be directed to identify which substances are being used, and why the young person is using them. Further history should explore both the sources of the drugs and who has encouraged the behavior. As some parents encourage this substance use, it is important to determine if they are aware of the situation as they too may need to be educated about the risks of such drugs.

When young people do admit to using these substances, having a physician that is able to openly discuss the performance effects, as well as the side effects of ergogenic drugs can be the first step in establishing that physician as a trustworthy source to approach, should the young person consider using other drugs, or begins to experience side effects of these drugs. The physician should present the athlete with alternatives to drug use such as balanced diet and regular strength training. While not every young athlete will abstain from ergogenic drugs, physicians can at least empower the adolescent with accurate information regarding the true effects and risks of their habits. In this way the entire medical community, not just physicians formally caring for athletic teams, can have a significant influence on youth drug use in sports.

REFERENCES

1. Silver MD. Use of ergogenic aids by athletes. J Am Acad Orthop Surg 2001;9:61–70.
2. Cogeni J, Miller S. Supplements and drugs used to enhance athletic performance. Pediatr Clin North Am 2002;49:435–61.
3. Rickert VI, Pawlak-Morello C, Sheppard V, et al. Human growth hormone: A new substance of abuse among adolescents? Clin Pediatr 1992;31:723–36.
4. National Federation of State High School Associations. High Schools Sport Participation Survey 2004–2005. http://www.nfhs.org/scriptcontent (accessed September 14, 2006).
5. Dodge TL, Jaccard JJ. The effect of high school sports participation on the use of performance-enhancing substances in young adulthood. J Adolesc Health 2006;39:367–73.
6. Hoberman JM, Yesalis CE. The history of synthetic testosterone. Sci Am 1995;272:76–81.
7. McDevitt ER. Ergogenic drugs in sports. In: DeLee JC, DrezD, editors. Orthopaedic Sports Medicine: Principles and Practice, Volume 1, 2nd edition. Philadelphia, PA: Saunders; 2003. p. 471–83.
8. Sturmi JE, Diorio DJ. Anabolic agents. Clin Sport Med 1998;17:261–82.
9. Yesalis CE, editor. Anabolic Steroids in Sport and Exercise. Champaign, IL: Kinetic Publishers; 1993. p. 35–47.
10. Bamberger M, Yaeger D. Over the edge :Special report Sports Illustrated 1997;86:64.
11. Scelfo J, Johnson D. Texas, football, and juice. Newsweek 2005:46–7.
12. Brown WJ, Basil MD, Bocarnea MC. The influence of famous athletes on health beliefs and practices: Mark McGwire, child abuse prevention, and androstenedione. J Health Commun 2003;8:41–57.
13. Fainaru-Wada M. Dreams, steroids, death—A ballplayer's downfall. San Francisco Chronicle December 19, 2004.
14. Bents RT, Tokish JM, Goldberg L. Ephedrine, pseudoephedrine, and amphetamine prevalence in college hockey players. Curr Sport Med Rep 2004;3:243–5.
15. Yesalis C, Bahrke M. Doping among adolescent athletes. Clin Endocrin Metab 2000;14:25–35.
16. Gorman C. Girls on steroids: Among young athletes these dangerous drugs are the rage: Is your daughter using them? Time 1998:93.
17. Dennis J. Illinois mulls steroid testing for high schools. Indiana Daily Student; 2006. http//www.idsnews.com (accessed on September 2, 2006).
18. Dawson RT. Drugs in sport—The role of the physician. J Endocrinol 2001;170:55–61.
19. Tokish JM, Kocher MS, Hawkins RJ. Ergogenic Aids: A review of basic science, performance, side effects, and status in sports. Am J Sport Med 2004;32:1543–53.
20. Wilson JD. Androgens. In: Hardman JG, Limbird LE, editors. Goodman and Gilman's the Pharmacological Basis of Therapeutics. New York: McGraw-Hill; 1996. p. 1441–57.
21. Haupt HA, Rovere GD. Anabolic steroids: A review of the literature. Am J Sport Med 1984;12:469–84.
22. Wilson JD. Androgen abuse by athletes. Endocr Rev 1988;9:181–99.
23. National Institute on Drug Abuse. NIDA_Research_Report—Steroid Abuse and Addiction. http://www.drugabuse.gov/ResearchReports/Steroids/AnabolicSteroids.html (accessed on September 14, 2006).
24. Chyka PA. Health risks of selected performance-enhancing drugs. J Pharm Pract 2003;16:37–44.
25. American College of Sports Medicine. Position statement on anabolic–androgenic steroids in sports. Med Sci Sport Exerc 1987;19:534–9.
26. Blazevich AJ, Giorgi A. Effect of testosterone administration and weight training on muscle architecture. Med Sci Sport Exerc 2001;33:1688–93.
27. Kadi F, Eriksson A, Holmner S, Thornell L. Effects of anabolic steroids on the muscle cells of strength trained athletes. Med Sci Sport Exerc 1999;31:1528–34.
28. Scott MJ, Scott AM. Effects of anabolic–androgenic steroids on the pilosebaceous unit. Cutis 1992;50:113–6.
29. Glazer G. Atherogenic effects of anabolic steroids on serum lipid levels: A literature review. Arch Intern Med 1991;151:1925–33.
30. Riebe D, Fernhall B, Thompson PD. The blood pressure response to exercise in anabolic steroid users. Med Sci Sport Exerc 1992;24:633–7.
31. Blue JG, Lombardo JA. Steroids and steroid-like compounds. Clin Sport Med 1999;18:667–89.
32. Haupt HA. Anabolic steroids and growth hormone. Am J Sport Med 1993;21:468–74.
33. Michna H. Tendon injuries induced by exercise and anabolic steroids in experimental mice. Int Orthop 1987;11:157–62.
34. Rich JD, Dickinson BP, Feller A, et al. The infectious complications of anabolic–androgenic steroid injection. Int J Sport Med 1999;20:563–6.
35. Melia P, Pipe A, Greenberg L. The use of anabolic–androgenic steroids by Canadian students. Clin J Sport Med 1996;6:9–14.
36. Copeland J, Peters R, Dillon P. Anabolic–androgenic steroid use disorders among a sample of Australian competitive and recreational users. Drug Alcohol Depend 2000;60:91–6.
37. Evans NA. Gym and tonic: A profile of 100 male steroid users. Br J Sport Med 1997;31:54–8.
38. Middleman AB, Faulkner AH, Woods ER, et al. High risk behaviors among high school students in Massachusetts who use anabolic steroids. Pediatrics 1995;96:268–72.
39. DuRant RH, Escobedo LG, Heath GW. Anabolic-steroid use, strength training, and multiple drug use among adolescents in the United States. Pediatrics 1995;96:23–8.
40. Buckley WE, Yesalis CE, Friedl KE, et al. Estimated prevalence of anabolic steroid use among male high school seniors. JAMA 1988;260:3441–5.
41. Stilger VG, Yesalis CE. Anabolic–androgenic steroid use among high school football players. J community Health 1999;24:131–45.
42. Grunbaum JA, Kann L, Kinchen SA, et al. Youth risk behavior surveillance—United States, 2003. MMWR Surveil Summ 2004;53:1–96.
43. Faigenbaum AD, Zaichowsky LD, Gardner DE, Micheli LJ. Anabolic steroid use by male and female middle school students. Pediatrics 1998;101:e6. http://www.pediatrics.org/cgi/content/full/101/5/e6 (accessed September 15, 2006).
44. Gray M. Youth athletes and anabolic steroid usage. Med Sci Sport Exerc 1990;22:S63.
45. Irving LM, Wall M, Neumark-Sztainer D, Story M. Steroid use among adolescents: Findings from project EAT. J Adolesc Health 2002;30:243–52.
46. US Dep Health Human Services. Monitoring the Future Study, Overview of Key Findings 2005. http://www.monitoringthefuture.org (accessed on September 2, 2006), pp 40–66
47. Dezelsky TL, Toohey JV, Shaw RS. Non-medical drug use behavior at five United States universities: A 15 year study. Bull Narc 1989;37:49–53.
48. NCAA study of substance use habits of college student-athletes 2005. http://www.ncaa.org/library/research.html#substance use habits (accessed September 2, 2006).
49. Berning JM, Adams KJ, Bryant SA, et al. Prevalence and perceived prevalence of anabolic steroid use among college-aged students. Med Sci Sport Exerc 2004:36;S350.
50. Mahesh VB, Greenblatt RB. The in vivo conversion of dehydroepiandosterone and androstenedione to testosterone in the human. Acta Endocrinol 1962;41:400–6.
51. Leder BZ, Longcope C, Catlin DH, et al. Oral androstenedione administration and serum testosterone concentrations in young men. JAMA 2000;283:779–82.
52. King Ds, Sharp RL, Vukovich MD, et al. Effect of oral androstenedione on serum testosterone and adaptations to resistance training in young men: A randomized controlled trial. JAMA 1999;281:2020–8.

53. Armsey TD, Hosey RG. Medical aspects of sports: Epidemiology of injuries, pre-participation physical exam, and drugs in sports. Clin Sport Med 2004;23:255–79.
54. Broeder CE, Quindry J, Brittingham K, et al. The Andro Project: Physiologic and hormonal influences of androstenedione supplementation in men 35 to 65 years old participating in a high-intensity resistance training program. Arch Intern Med 2000;160:3093–104.
55. Kachhi PN, Henderson SO. Priapism after androstenedione intake for athletic performance enhancement. Ann Emerg Med 2000;35:391–3.
56. Habernicht UP, Schwarz K, Neumann F, et al. Induction of estrogen related hyperplastic changes in the prostate of the cynomolgus monkey (Mecaca facicularis) by androstenedione and its antagonization by the aromatase inhibitor 1-methyl-androsta-1,4-diene-3,1 7-dione. Prostate 1987;1:313–26.
57. Reeder BM, Patel DR, Rai A, et al. Nutritional supplement use by high school students: A survey of two high-schools in the United States. Int Ped 2003;18:170–7.
58. Sonksen PH. Hormones and sport: Insulin, growth hormone and sport. J Endocrinol 2001;170:13–25.
59. Rosen CJ. Growth hormone and aging. Endocrine 2000;12:197–201.
60. Rogol AD. Sex steroid and growth hormone supplementation to enhance performance in adolescent athletes. Cur Opin Ped 2000;12:382–7.
61. Dean H. Does exogenous growth hormone improve athletic performance? Clin J Sport Med 2002;12:250–3.
62. Deyssig R, Frisch H, Blum WF, et al. Effect of growth hormone treatment on hormonal parameters, body composition, and strength in athletes. Acta Endocrinol 1993;128:313–8.
63. Colao A, Cuocolo A, Marzullo P, et al. Is the acromegalic cardiomyopathy reversible? Effect of 5 year normalization of growth hormone and insulin like growth factor I levels on cardiac performance. J Clin Endocrin Metab 2001;86:1551–7.
64. Rennie MJ. Claims for the anabolic effects of growth hormone: A case of the emperor's new clothes? Brit J Sport Med 2003;37:100–5.
65. Chung L, Clifford D, Buckley M, Baxter RC. Novel biomarkers of human growth hormone action from serum proteomic profiling using protein chip mass spectrometry. J Clin Endocrinol Metab 2006;91:671–7.
66. Herbal Rx: The promise and pitfalls. Consum Rep 1999:44–8.
67. Zorpette G. The mystery of muscle. Sci Am 1999;10:48–55.
68. Wood G. Supplement use common among school athletes. Bradenton Herald August 12, 2006. http://www.bradenton.com (accessed on September 2, 2006).
69. Burns RD, Schiller MR, Merrick MA, Wolf KN. Intercollegiate student athlete use of nutritional supplements and the role of athletic trainers and dietitians in nutrition counseling. J Am Diet Assoc 2004;104:246–9.
70. Kayton S, Cullen RW, Memken JA, Rutter R. Supplement and ergogenic aid use by competitive male and female high school athletes. Med Sci Sport Exerc 2002;35S:S193.
71. Dietary Supplement Health and Education Act of 1994, Public Law 103–417 (October 25, 1994).
72. Massad SJ, Shier NW, Koceja DM, Ellis NT. High school athletes and nutritional supplements: A study of knowledge and use. Int J Sport Nutr 1995;5:232–45.
73. Green GA, Catlin DH, Starcevic B. Analysis of over the counter dietary supplements. Clin J Sport Med 2001;11:254–9.
74. McGuine TA, Sullivan JC, Bernhard DA. Creatine supplementation in Wisconsin high school athletes. Wis Med J 2002;101:25–30.
75. O'Dea JA. Consumption of nutritional supplements among adolescents: Usage and perceived benefits. Health Educ Res 2003;18:98–107.
76. Jenkins MA. Creatine supplementation in athletes: Review. 1998 Sports Med Web. http://www.rice.edu/~jenky/sports/creatine.html (accessed September 2, 2006).
77. Greenhaff PL, Bodin K, Soderlund K, Hultman E. Effect of oral creatine supplementation on skeletal muscle phosphocreatine resynthesis. Am J Physiol 1994;66:E725–30.
78. Harris RC, Soderlund K, Hultman E. Elevation of creatine in resting and exercised muscle of normal subjects by creatine supplementation. Clin Sci 1992;83:367–74.
79. American College of Sports Medicine Roundtable on the Physiological and Health Effects of Oral Creatine Supplements. Med Sci Sport Exerc 2000;32:706–17.
80. Clark JF. Creatine: A review of its nutritional applications in sport. Nutrition 1998;14:322–4.
81. Smith J, Dahm DL. Creatine use among select population of high school athletes. Mayo Clin Proc 2000;75:1257–63.
82. PDR Health. Creatine. http://www.pdrhealth.com/drug_info/nmdrugprofiles/nutsupdrugs/cre_0086.shtml (accessed December 12, 2005).
83. Green AL, Hultman E, Macdonald IA, et al. Carbohydrate ingestion augments skeletal muscle creatine accumulation during creatine supplementation in humans. Am J Physiol 1997;271:E821–6.
84. Vandenberghe K, Gillis N, Van Leemputte M, et al. Caffeine counteracts the ergogenic action of muscle creatine loading. J Appl Physiol 1996;80:452–7.
85. Engelhardt M, Neuman G, Berbalk A, Reuter I: Creatine supplementation in endurance sports. Med Sci Sport Exerc 1998;30:1123–9.
86. Ostojic SM. Creatine supplementation in young soccer players. Int J Sport Nutr Exerc Metab 2004;14:95–103.
87. Volek JS, Duncan ND, Mazzetti SA, et al. Performance and muscle fiber adaptations to creatine supplementation and heavy resistance training. Med Sci Sport Exerc 1999;31:1147–56.
88. Pritchard NR, Kaira PA. Renal dysfunction accompanying oral creatine supplements. Lancet 1998;351:1252–3.
89. Koshy KM, Griswold E, Schneeberger EE. Interstitial nephritis in a patient taking creatine. N Engl J Med 1999;340:814–5.
90. Poortmans JR, Francaux M. Long-term oral creatine supplementation does not impair renal function in healthy athletes. Med Sci Sport Exerc 1999;31:1108–10.
91. Metzl JD, Levine SR, Gershel JC. Creatine use among young athletes. Pediatrics 2001;108:421–5.
92. Sallis RE, Jones K. Dietary supplement use among college football players. Med Sci Sport Exerc 1999;31S:S118.
93. Hoffman BB, Lefkowitz RJ. Catecholamines, sympathomimetic drugs and adrenergic receptor antagonists. In: Hardman JG, Limbird LE, editors. Goodman and Gilman's the Pharmacological Basis of Therapeutics. New York: McGraw-Hill; 1996. p. 221–4.
94. Gill ND, Shield A, Blazevich AJ, et al. Muscular and cardiorespiratory effects of pseudoephedrine in human athletes. Br J Clin Pharmacol 2000;50:205–13.
95. Hodges K, Hancock S, Currell K, et al. Pseudoephedrine enhances performance in 1500-m runners. Med Sci Sport Exerc 2006;38:329–33.
96. Bell DG, McLellan TM, Sabiston CM. Effect of ingesting caffeine and ephedrine on 10 km run performance. Med Sci Sport Exerc 2002;34:344–9.
97. Bent S, Tiedt TN, Odden MC, Shlipak MG. The relative safety of ephedra compared with other herbal products. Ann Intern Med 2003;138:468–71.
98. Haller CA, Benowitz NL. Adverse cardiovascular and central nervous system events associated with dietary supplements containing ephedra alkaloids. N Engl J Med 2000;343:1833–88.
99. Juhn MS. Popular sports supplements and ergogenic aids. Sport Med 2003;33:921–39.
100. Harland BF. Caffeine and nutrition. Nutrition 2000;16:522–6 .
101. Kovacs EM, Stegen JHCH, Brouns F. Effect of caffeinated drinks on substrate metabolism, caffeine excretion, and performance. J Appl Physiol 1998;85:709–15.
102. Bruce CR, Anderson Me, Fraser SF, et al. Enhancement of 2000 m rowing performance after caffeine ingestion. Med Sci Sport Exerc 2000;32:1958–63.
103. Nichols JF, Rauh MJ, Lawson MJ, et al. Prevalence of the female athlete triad syndrome among high school athletes. Arch Pediatr Adolesc Med 2006;160:137–42.
104. Kiningham RB, Gorenflo DW. Weight loss methods of high school wrestlers. Med Sci Sport Exerc 2001;33:810–3.
105. Goldberg L, Elliot DL, MacKinnon DP, et al. Drug testing athletes to prevent substance abuse: Background and pilot study results of the SATURN (student athlete testing using random notification) study. J Adolesc Health 2003;32:16–25.
106. National Federation of State High School Associations. Sports medicine: High school drug-testing programs: August 2003. http://www.nfhs.org (accessed September 2, 2006).
107. Goldberg L, MacKinnon D, Elliot DL, et al. Preventing drug use and promoting health behaviors among adolescents: Results of the ATLAS program. Arch Pediatr Adolesc Med 2000;154:332–8.
108. Elliot DL, Goldberg L, Moe EL, et al. Preventing substance use and disordered eating: Initial outcomes of the ATHENA (athletes targeting healthy exercise and nutrition alternatives) program. Arch Pediatr Adolesc Med 2004;158:1043–9.

66

Adolescence: Bone Disease

Keith J. Loud, MDCM, MSc
Catherine M. Gordon, MD, MSc

Adolescence is a critical period for lifetime bone health. Evidence has accumulated that an individual's peak bone mass (PBM), which is the strongest predictor of his or her future risk of osteoporosis, is reached by early adulthood. At least half of all adult mineralized calcium is laid down during the adolescent years, with the most rapid bone accretion occurring in late childhood and early adolescence.[1,2] Any condition which impairs this process may create a deficit in bone mass that will have permanent ramifications for future risk of osteoporosis, which afflicted over 10 million Americans and cost more than $18 billion in direct medical expenditures just for fracture care in 2002.[3]

Many disease states, each related to nutritional deficits, can inhibit bone accretion during adolescence, including rickets, eating disorders, the "female athlete triad," inflammatory bowel disease, celiac disease, cystic fibrosis, cancer, and other multisystem or inflammatory disorders. In this chapter, these conditions will be discussed in detail. Adolescent behavior itself may also prevent maximal PBM attainment, as the dietary habits of many teenagers do not optimize calcium and vitamin D intake.

NORMAL BONE PHYSIOLOGY AND DEVELOPMENT

Bones are the fundamental units of the skeletal system, providing an adaptable frame that supports and protects the major organ systems of the body while allowing for locomotion. Due to its role in calcium and phosphate homeostasis, bone can also be considered an organ system. The skeletal system is the reservoir for the calcium used in essential mechanisms ranging from the regulation of cardiac electrical activity, contraction of muscles, and varied inter- and intracellular messaging systems. Each bone, housing lymphoid and myeloid precursor cells within the marrow, is also an organ unto itself. Finally, these organs are composed of a unique tissue substance that is once again called "bone."[4]

Types of Bone

Bone as a tissue takes on two forms in normal health: cortical (dense) and trabecular (cancellous or spongy) bone.[4] Cortical bone, which makes up 80% of the skeletal bone mass, is found in the diaphysis (shaft) of long bones such as the femur, as well as the "walls" of almost all other bones, including the vertebrae. It provides strength against tensile, torsional, and shear forces. The remaining 20% of bone mass consists of trabecular bone, found in the metaphyses (ends) of long bones and the entire bodies of the vertebrae. It is well suited to resist compressive forces. Because of its high surface area-to-volume ratio, trabecular bone occupies greater than 20% of the volume of the skeletal system and has approximately eight times the metabolic activity of cortical bone.[4] Due to its higher metabolic availability, trabecular bone is more significantly affected by disease states.

Histology: The Building Blocks of Bone

Regardless of its structure or ultrastructure, on a microscopic level bone consists of thin layers, or lamellae, of a mineralized protein matrix. This mature lamellar bone is 70% (by dry weight) mineral, predominantly calcium and phosphate in the form of hydroxyapatite crystals [$Ca_{10}(PO_4)_6(OH)_2$] and a less pure, carbonate-rich analogue called bone apatite, which is more soluble and thus more available for metabolic activity.[5] The remaining 30% of the mass is an organic substance called osteoid, primarily protein in the form of type I collagen. Cellular elements, which produce all of the metabolic activity of bone, make up only 2% of the osteoid.

Osteoblasts are bone-forming cells derived from fixed-tissue osteoprogenitor cells.[6] Osteoblasts synthesize osteoid on the surface of already mature lamellar bone, periosteum, or endosteum. They then regulate the process of mineralization of the collagen matrix through the actions of bone-specific alkaline phosphatase (BSAP), which is different than the alkaline phosphatase produced in the liver and can be distinguished from it by specific assays.

Once the osteoid matrix has mineralized, it is considered bone. The osteoblasts, which are synchronized in such a way as to create the parallel lamellae, become trapped inside small caverns called lacunae and mature into osteocytes that communicate via long processes with each other in order to direct mineral homeostasis.

Osteoclasts are multinucleated cells from the marrow monocyte-macrophage cell line.[7] Producing lysosomal enzymes such as acid phosphatase, osteoclasts break down the mineralized bone matrix, mobilizing calcium and phosphorus for participation in homeostasis, in a process called bone resorption.

Growth and Remodeling: The Bone Cycle

Bone is a dynamic tissue. Growth in long bones occurs at the physes (growth plates) and apophyses (secondary centers of ossification) by a process known as endochondral ossification in which osteoblasts lay down bone on a cartilaginous framework that is ultimately resorbed by osteoclasts. Even after skeletal maturity, osteoblasts respond to structural stresses in bone by laying down a new matrix. Osteoclasts concomitantly resorb areas of bone under less stress. Thus, bone is constantly remodeling. At times of growth, bone formation by osteoblasts is greater than resorption by osteoclasts. With disuse, osteoclasts outpace osteoblasts and bone mass decreases. Otherwise, osteoblasts and osteoclasts are tightly "coupled" to keep formation and resorption equally balanced in what is known as "the bone cycle."[4]

Importance of Adolescence

Bones grow at different rates throughout the skeleton. The extremities (appendicular skeleton) have largely completed growth by the time of the pubertal growth spurt (peak height velocity). Increases in estrogen and testosterone during puberty result in growth of the trunk and spine (axial skeleton). These increases in vertebral bone size are accompanied by dramatic increases in bone mineral density (BMD) in cross-sectional studies.[8,9] This trabecular bone reaches its peak BMD by age 20 to 30 years, but steadily declines thereafter.[10] Alarmingly, one animal model showed that calcium restriction in adolescence resulted in a decreased bone volume throughout life, even after restoration to recommended calcium intake in young adulthood.[11]

Adolescence is an essential time for significant bone accretion. Over half of adult bone calcium is laid down during the teenage years.[1] Maximal rates of bone mineral accretion follow peak height velocity (PHV) by 6 to 12 months.[12] As a consequence, at the time of PHV (Tanner pubertal stage II–III in girls, Tanner III–IV in boys), teenagers have reached approximately 90% of their adult height but they have acquired only 60% of their adult total body mineral content, resulting in relatively less mineralized bone.[12] In North America, these pubertal stages are reached by age 11 to 14 in girls and 13 to 17 in boys. Studies by Thientz and colleagues are consistent, showing that girls' BMD may plateau by age 16 (or 2 years post menarche) and boys' by age 20.[2] This is a much earlier window of opportunity than was previously suspected. In fact, 95 to 100% of peak bone mass may be attained by the end of adolescence.[13,14]

Factors Affecting Bone Health (Figure 1)

Genetics. Intrinsic factors dominate the determination of bone density. Males have a higher bone mass than females at nearly all ages.[10] African-American children demonstrate an approximately 10% higher BMD by DXA than do children of other ethnicities,[16] even after correcting for bone size.[14] An interesting finding among African-American and Caucasian girls was that their spinal BMD was similar until puberty, at which point the African-American girls had an increase of 34% while the Caucasian girls an increase of only 11%.[17] Family history of osteoporosis in postmenopausal women predicts lower BMD for their daughters,[18] and both elderly men and women have an increased risk of osteoporosis when other family members have been affected.[19] In all, 60 to 80% of the variance in PBM is attributed to heritable factors.[10] Polymorphisms in the genes encoding receptors for vitamin D, estrogen, type I collagen,[20] insulin-like growth factor I (IGF-I), transforming growth factor beta (TGF-β), and interleukin 6 (IL-6) are under ongoing study,[21] but none have been able, singly or in combination, to account for more than a small percentage of this variance in PBM.

Hormonal Status. A normal hormonal milieu is essential to attain and maintain normal bone formation. Early menarche and regular menses are strong predictors of increased bone mass in women,[22] demonstrating the importance of estrogen.[23] Among adolescent girls, an estimate of estrogen exposure was positively correlated with spinal BMD.[10] Estrogen deficiency may also slow growth in axial bone size[24–26] when it occurs during adolescence, a time when truncal growth typically accelerates.

Androgens exert independent and positive effects on peak bone mass.[27] While men with a history of delayed puberty and documented low serum androgen levels have been shown to have decreased BMD, a meta-analysis of randomized, placebo-controlled clinical trials of testosterone use in males showed only a modest improvement in lumbar spine BMD and inconclusive results at the femoral neck.[28] Nonetheless, androgen replacement therapy to teenage boys may provide skeletal benefits during the formative adolescent years.[29] Patients with androgen insensitivity have a mutation in the androgen receptor, with consequent impaired androgen action, such that there is resistance to even elevated androgen levels. Previous reports have shown that affected individuals have decreased bone mineralization.[30–32] Even after administration of estrogen replacement therapy in these individuals, BMD did not significantly increase, again highlighting the importance of androgens in bone physiology.[30] Women with androgen excess also have been shown to have a higher BMD.[33,34]

Children and adults with childhood-onset growth hormone deficiency have lower BMD than controls.[35,36] While patients on adequate replacement doses of GH have increased BMD compared to GH-deficient patients,[37] those adolescents who discontinued the medication at the completion of linear growth demonstrated decreased spine and hip BMD in long-term follow-up, suggesting that bone mineral accretion continues beyond completion of linear growth.[38] The actions of growth hormone are likely mediated by IGF-I, an anabolic factor that stimulates osteoblast function directly.

Exercise. Patients with impaired activity due to central nervous system or neuromuscular disease develop disuse osteoporosis.[39] It is well established that individuals engaged more intensely in weight-bearing activities have higher measured BMD than less active controls.[40] Even among women with amenorrhea and adolescents with anorexia nervosa, those who are more athletic have higher bone density.[41,42] Unfortunately, swimmers do not consistently reap this benefit, as their activity is largely weightless, highlighting the importance of weight-bearing activities.[43] The increases in BMD are site specific; for example, runners and ballet dancers have higher proximal femur (hip) BMD than controls, while gymnasts have higher measured radial (arm) BMD.[44] These gains in BMD persist years after these athletes have retired from sports.[45] Although not all intervention studies have replicated these findings,[46] most clinical trials of physical activity demonstrate a positive association between exercise and the bone health of children, adolescents, and adults.[47]

Chronic Illness and Systemic Inflammation. Many of the medical conditions associated with impaired bone density are listed in Table 1. Some of those that act by directly causing malnutrition, with concomitant decreases in BMI and absorption of important nutrients, will be described in detail later in this chapter. Many are additionally marked by systemic inflammation, which is increasingly known to result independently in decreased BMD. For example, the magnitude of glucocorticoid use is the single greatest predictor of osteopenia in patients with both ulcerative colitis (UC) and Crohn's disease (CD).[48] Glucocorticoids directly decrease bone formation by inhibiting osteoblast activity. Indirectly, these agents also decrease the secretion of estrogen and testosterone, which are necessary for bone accretion, as well as decrease the absorption of calcium in the gut and reabsorption of calcium in the kidneys.

These adverse effects of glucocorticoids are a concern for other patients with systemic steroid-dependent diseases such as juvenile rheumatoid arthritis (JRA), childhood leukemias, collagen vascular and connective tissue diseases, and solid organ transplant recipients. One study has shown a dose-related loss of BMD at the hip in premenopausal adult women using inhaled glucocorticoids for treatment of their asthma.[49] Although there is a similar concern for children and adolescents, it is largely speculative. Reassuring evidence comes from a study of steroid-responsive nephrotic syndrome in children and adolescents which showed that decreased BMD is not correlated with steroid dosage but with underlying disease severity, for which steroid use is merely a marker. Body mass was also shown to be protective of BMD in that study.[50]

Other autoimmune mediated diseases, allergy, and even chronic infection have been associated with decreased regional and total body bone density, further implicating systemic inflammation as a cause of bone loss.[51] The proinflammatory cytokines IL-1α, IL-1β, IL-6, IL-11, IL-17, tumor necrosis factor (TNF)-α and TNF-β, transforming growth factor (TGF)-α, epidermal growth factor (EGF), and prostaglandin E_2 all activate osteoclastic resorption of bone.[51] TNF-α and IL-1β also decrease osteoblastic bone formation while stimulating the osteoblasts to secrete IL-6, further activating the osteoclasts.[51]

Elegant experiments have begun to elucidate the final common pathways of the signaling cascade that modulates the coupling of the bone remodeling cycle. Of particular interest is the osteoblast surface ligand called the receptor–activator of nuclear factor kappa B ligand, or RANKL. When binding to the osteoclast precursor RANK is predominant, osteoclast differentiation and maturation is favored, leading to increased bone resorption. Osteoprotegerin (OPG) blocks the RANK–RANKL interaction, thus shifting the balance in favor of bone formation.[51] The observation that RANKL also regulates early lymphocyte development and some T-cell

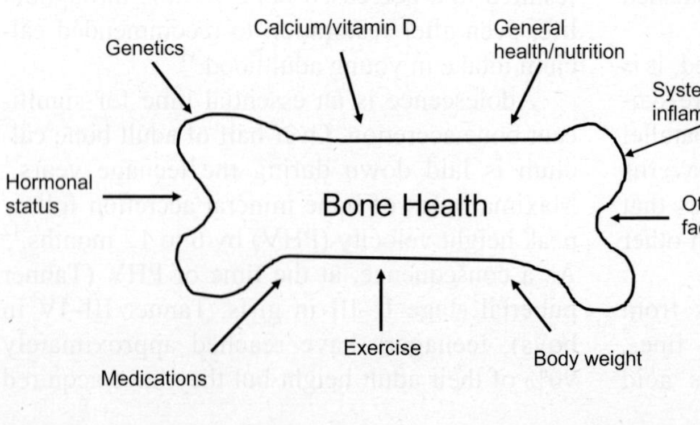

Figure 1 Factors affecting bone health. (Reproduced with permission from reference 15.)

pseudofracture. Serum levels of 25(OH)D are a reliable measure of total vitamin D stores. However, the desirable level for 25(OH)D, including what constitutes the threshold stimulus for rises in PTH, remains a subject of debate.[78,99] Data by Haden and colleagues[115] showed that PTH levels start to increase at a 25(OH)D level of 25 ng/mL, higher than the threshold of 12 to 15 ng/mL previously established for vitamin D deficiency. Treatment consists of ensuring adequate dietary intake of vitamin D, with supplementation as necessary. Commonly prescribed replacement doses for children and adolescents with vitamin D deficiency include ergocalciferol (vitamin D_2), 2,000 international units (IU) by mouth once or twice daily for 6–8 weeks, or 50,000 IU once weekly for the same length of therapy.[64] There are data suggesting an increased efficacy of vitamin D_3 (animal-derived) over vitamin D_2[116,117]; however, only ergocalciferol is available in the United States for providing high-dose therapy. Parenteral dosing of 50,000 to 300,000 IU provided as vitamin D_2 intramuscularly is also used, but must be undertaken cautiously, with assurance of adequate calcium intake and appropriate monitoring of vitamin D and PTH levels.

Osteoporosis

Definitions. In contrast to *osteomalacia,* which refers to a condition in which the bone matrix is poorly mineralized regardless of the actual mass of bone tissue produced, *osteoporosis* is defined as a systemic skeletal disease characterized by low bone mass and microarchitectural deterioration of bone tissue, with a consequent increase in bone fragility and susceptibility to fractures.[118] A related term, *osteopenia,* is used to describe a significant reduction in bone mass for age and sex, but only in postmenopausal women and older adult men.[119] In each of these conditions, the osteoid is mineralized normally to form calcified bone, but there is less of it and its structural arrangement is abnormal.

Diagnosis. Adult osteoporosis is defined by the World Health Organization (WHO) as a BMD below 2.5 standard deviations from the mean peak BMD attained for gender (ie, T-score <-2.5) as measured by dual-energy X-ray absorptiometry (DXA). Osteopenia is the term reserved for BMD with T-score between -1.0 and -2.5.[120] Using these definitions, DXA scanning has become the standard modality for diagnosing osteoporosis in postmenopausal women and older adult men. In adolescents and younger adults, these WHO definitions do not apply; the International Society for Clinical Densitometry (ISCD), in a 2004 position statement, specifies that osteoporosis in these age groups is a clinical diagnosis, requiring evidence of skeletal fragility in addition to decreased BMD.[119]

Dual Energy X-Ray Absorptiometry. DXA utilizes X-rays of two differing photon energies passing through the body to a sensitive detector. The beams are attenuated differentially depending on the tissues through which they pass. A computer then calculates body composition, bone mineral content (BMC), and BMD based on the attenuation. DXA scanners report BMC in grams of mineralized calcium and BMD in grams per area of bone region in squared centimeters (g/cm^2). Advantages of DXA scanning include relatively rapid scanning times (approximately 5 minutes for each scan), low levels of radiation exposure (1/10th of the radiation of a chest X-ray) and precision in the range of 1%. For these reasons, DXA can be used in children, with reliable normative databases consistently available, with some including children as young as 5 years.[96,121]

Limitations of DXA for Adolescents. The major limitation of DXA is that it utilizes a two-dimensional technique to quantify a three-dimensional structure. Density is, by definition, a measure of mass per unit volume. The BMD reported by DXA scanners is areal, or per unit area in g/cm^2. The significance of this calculation is more than academic, as the mechanical properties of bone are dependent on its architecture and geometry, as well as its composition. Good mathematical models have been developed to calculate the approximate volumetric BMD—known as bone mineral apparent density (BMAD) in g/cm^3—although their prognostic value is not well established.[122]

These limitations of DXA are more significant in adolescents. First, not all DXA scanners are equipped with the proper software to evaluate pediatric body composition and, therefore, BMD. Even comparing a single adolescent with him or herself on a single machine with reliable pediatric software is subject to flaws. Presumably, one could measure serial DXA scans over time to assess the effect of a disease state or treatment on BMD. Unfortunately, the growth of the child complicates interpretation. To illustrate, consider quantifying the density of a tree trunk by measuring the shadow cast by the tree in the sun. After 1 year of growth, the tree trunk casts a wider (and perhaps darker) shadow, but the trunk itself may be no denser than it was previously. Using DXA, the "shadow" or areal BMD (aBMD) of this tree would be reported as greater than it was the previous year. The same phenomenon occurs when measuring a growing child's bones. The opposite phenomenon, that of a growing child's measured aBMD remaining constant, should therefore appear ominous to the clinician. Unfortunately, limitations on the actual scores reported for BMD do not allow the clinician to quantify the degree of risk. Fortunately, bone grows stronger as it increases in diameter, even at the same BMD.[123]

As mentioned, interpreting even reliable values for BMD is challenging. The T (or standard deviation) score, which compares an individual adult's BMD to the mean peak BMD (or PBM) attained by young adults of the same gender, provides a valid estimate of the risk of fracture for that adult. The Z-score compares an individual's BMD to the mean BMD (in standard deviation units) for his or her age and gender, which is useful to grade patients with respect to their peers, but has unknown prognostic significance. Reliable pediatric databases report T- and Z-scores, but the T-scores are not informative as most children and adolescents have not reached their peak young adult BMD and therefore may prove confusing to the reader of the report. For this reason, the ISCD has recommended that T-scores do not appear on printouts or reports from DXA scans of children and adolescents younger than 20 years.[119] In the same position statement, ISCD recommends the terms "low bone density for chronologic age" or "below the expected range for age" for Z-scores lower than -2.0 and discourages use of the term osteopenia entirely in this age group.[119]

Furthermore, as bone mineral accretion is strongly influenced by Tanner stage, which does not directly correlate with chronologic age, comparing BMDs based on age alone (as in Z-scores) may be problematic. Finally, most databases include predominantly or exclusively Caucasian populations, which makes the interpretation of BMD data more difficult for patients of different ethnic groups.[121]

Other Imaging Techniques. Quantitative computed tomography (QCT) is a technique of bone densitometry that is rapidly becoming the gold standard in research protocols because it can generate direct measures of bone volume and thus a more accurate volumetric BMD. Pediatric algorithms are available, but the increased time required and significantly increased radiation doses limit its clinical use in this age group. Peripheral QCT (pQCT) is becoming increasingly used as a research tool in pediatric patients as it affords a measure of volumetric BMD in assessment of the appendicular skeleton, and provides insight into bone geometry and strength.[121,124] A final appeal of this methodology is that it involves a minimal radiation dose. Another technology, quantitative ultrasound (QUS), showed promise as it has no associated radiation exposure and demonstrates reasonable precision, but has proven difficult to validate in comparison with DXA and QCT.[125]

Serum Markers. Bone turnover markers are used infrequently in the assessment of metabolic bone disease, primarily for research purposes, to gauge the relative contributions of bone formation versus bone resorption in the bone remodeling cycle.[111] Some endocrinologists also use them to monitor response to medical treatment. Serum alkaline phosphatase levels, particularly bone-specific alkaline phosphatase (BSAP), reflect osteoblast function, as does serum osteocalcin, an osteoblast-specific product. Serum tartrate-resistant acid phosphatase (TRAP) is an osteoclast equivalent for BSAP, while collagen type I cross-linked *N*-telopeptides (NTx) are breakdown products of bone that reflect osteoclast activity and are measured in the urine. Adult studies have shown these markers to be inferior to bone densitometry for diagnosing osteoporosis and monitoring skeletal health, and pediatric reference ranges are limited, as growth, puberty, and diurnal cycling cause wide variation in these values.[96]

NUTRITIONAL DISEASE STATES ASSOCIATED WITH OSTEOPOROSIS

Anorexia Nervosa

Patients with anorexia nervosa (AN) are at risk for profound deficits in BMD that are often irreversible, even with a return to appropriate weight. Patients with chronic AN have a seven-fold increased incidence of fractures and are at increased risk for developing early osteoporosis.[126–129] Because the incidence of anorexia increases during the years of attainment of PBM, the life-long impact on skeletal health in maturity is particularly concerning. The mechanisms of this bone loss are certainly related to decreased dietary intake of calcium, vitamin D, and other macronutrients. Females with AN also develop hypothalamic amenorrhea which results in low circulating levels of estrogen.

It is hypothesized that estrogen helps regulate bone mass by impairing osteoblast-mediated bone resorption. Oral contraceptive (OCP) use by young women with AN was shown in a retrospective cross-sectional study to be associated with a higher BMD.[130] In a small pilot study of women with AN and hypothalamic amenorrhea, estrogen replacement therapy (ERT) resulted in increases in BMD.[131] Unfortunately, ERT alone has not consistently been shown in other controlled studies to be able to reverse the bone loss in patients with AN, with the possible exception of those most profoundly affected (below 70% of ideal body weight).[132] Despite the fact that its effects on bone accretion have been disappointing, ERT remains one of the standard therapies used to help maintain skeletal health in patients with AN,[133] along with psychological support. Ultimately, nutritional rehabilitation and weight restoration are necessary to return menstrual function, circulating estrogen levels, and bone formation to normalcy. Even prior to attainment of menstrual regularity, however, bone density increases with weight gain in adolescent girls with AN.[134]

It has been suggested that bone formation is more profoundly decreased than resorption is increased in patients with AN.[128] This "uncoupling" of the normal bone cycle has led investigators to address both sides of the formation-resorption dyad.[42,135–137] Serum levels of IGF-I have been found to be decreased in patients with AN.[137] Short-term randomized controlled trials of IGF-I administration showed significant increases in bone formation in patients with AN,[138] with greatest improvement in those also given OCPs,[139] arguing for a synergistic effect between ERT and IGF-I. Unfortunately, use of this agent in children and adolescents may be limited due to its availability only as an intravenous or subcutaneous preparation. Longitudinal data are also being collected that document long-term efficacy.

Nutritional Supplements: DHEA. Like IGF-I, levels of the adrenal steroid dehydroepiandrosterone (DHEA)[140] are low in patients with AN. DHEA is positively correlated with BMD in adults[141] and parallels the pattern of bone accretion in that secretion of DHEA peaks during the same adolescent years as bone mass acquisition accelerates.[142,143] DHEA is thought to increase levels of IGF-I, thereby increasing bone formation by stimulating osteoblasts, and also decrease mediators of osteoclast-mediated resorption.

Studies of the administration of oral DHEA, which is currently sold as a nutritional supplement, in adolescent girls with AN have shown that this agent is well-tolerated.[144,145] The adolescents who were given DHEA showed significant decreases in concentrations of NTx, a markers of bone resorption, and increases in osteocalcin and BSAP, markers of formation.[144] In a randomized, double-blind clinical trial, the effect of DHEA on BMD in these patients was the same as that of ERT; both agents resulted in maintenance of BMD, but no significant gains, after controlling for weight gain.[145] However, bone turnover markers again revealed increased bone formation after DHEA, and a more significant suppression of bone resorption after ERT.[145] Since DHEA is unregulated by the FDA, it is potentially unsafe, depending on the purity of the preparation and dosing. For all of these reasons, DHEA cannot yet be recommended as a therapy for patients with bone loss secondary to AN.

The Female Athlete

Athletic participation has become increasingly common among adolescent girls since the enactment of Title IX of the Educational Amendments Act in 1972, which required women's intercollegiate athletic offerings to be proportional to their representation in the student body. As noted previously, an active lifestyle has the potential for improved skeletal health. Unfortunately, some female athletes may develop patterns of unhealthy eating, irregular menstrual cycles, and an ensuing state of low estrogen levels, which can undo the beneficial effects of exercise on bone density.[146] In 1992, 20 years after Title IX, the American College of Sports Medicine coined the term "female athlete triad" to define this interrelatedness of disordered eating, amenorrhea, and osteoporosis in certain female athletes.[147] Owing to its relatively recent definition, the prevalence of the entire female athlete triad has not been well-established. Studies have estimated that 3.4 to 66% of female athletes have experienced amenorrhea,[148,149] compared with only 2 to 5% in the general population, and 15 to 62% of female college athletes demonstrate disordered eating, compared with a 5 to 10% prevalence of eating disorders in the general population.[150,151]

Complete epidemiologic characterization of the female athlete triad may prove elusive, as most athletic women with menstrual irregularities do not meet criteria for osteoporosis nor frank eating disorders. Some of these women even consume adequate calories, leading some clinicians to use the term "athletic amenorrhea," believing it is caused by the stress of exercise. Loucks and colleagues have disputed this concept, showing that low energy availability, defined as a failure to match food intake directly to exercise energy expenditure, not stress of exercise, alters luteinizing hormone (LH) pulse frequency and amplitude.[152] These disturbances in LH pulsatility can cause amenorrhea or more subtle menstrual dysfunction, including irregular, anovulatory, and short luteal phase cycles, all of which can cause a relative estrogen deficiency and increased bone resorption. Work with elite gymnasts and runners has shown that even within-day, hourly energy deficits cause changes in body composition, with greater amplitude and frequency variations in energy balance correlating with increased body fat percentage.[153] The authors suggest that these wide swings also predispose to menstrual dysfunction.[153]

An alternative but complementary hypothesis is that cognitive dietary restraint, defined as the intention to limit food intake to control body weight, regardless of actual food limitation, is associated with higher levels of cortisol, which in turn impairs bone mass accretion by directly decreasing osteoblast activity and indirectly increasing osteoclast activity. In studies by McLean and colleagues, exercising women with high dietary restraint measures by questionnaire had similar BMI and menstrual cycle length compared to those with low restraint, but higher urinary cortisol excretion[154] and lower total body bone mineral content.[155] In either case, it is important to counsel adolescent female athletes to maintain a positive energy balance throughout the day with frequent appropriate pre-, post-, and between-exercise meals.

Celiac Disease

Celiac disease is a disorder of nutrient absorption in the small intestine that affects as many as 1 in 250 people of European descent. In susceptible individuals, an immunologic reaction to gluten (a protein found in wheat, barley, and rye) leads to a chronic enteropathy of the proximal intestine. See Chapter 50, "Celiac Disease" for details.

Low BMD is a common complication of celiac disease, caused by general malnutrition secondary to anorexia (reduced dietary intake) and impaired absorption of nutrients, especially calcium and vitamin D,[156] among other etiologies.

A gluten-free diet (GFD) is the mainstay of treatment for celiac disease, decreasing intestinal manifestations and improving BMD in adults and, in short-term trials, children. A long-term longitudinal study in children and adolescents showed that spinal BMD in patients with celiac disease was significantly lower than in controls at the time of diagnosis. After long-term GFD treatment (4 years), patients had regained bone mineral content and BMD to levels similar to controls, with significant "catch up" gains made in the first year of GFD treatment.[156] Provision of adequate calcium to these patients is critically important for bone mass.[157]

Inflammatory Bowel Disease

Like patients with celiac disease, adolescents with IBD are at risk for low BMD.[158,159] Patients with CD have a higher incidence of osteopenia than those with UC,[160] likely related to the more widespread distribution of intestinal inflammation in the former versus the latter diagnosis. In addition to malabsorption of calcium, phosphate and vitamin D, these patients have generalized malnutrition. They may also have delayed puberty, leading to inadequate levels of estrogen and/or testosterone to promote adequate bone accretion. High concentrations of circulating inflammatory cytokines IL-1β, IL-6, and TNF-α occur in IBD, increasing bone resorption as mentioned previously. Patients with IBD have relatively reduced lean body mass as a percentage of body composition, leading some to describe this deleterious combination of cytokines and malnutrition as "inflammatory cachexia."[161] Finally, extensive mucosal disease or surgical resection of the small bowel, particularly the terminal ileum, seen in CD further impairs calcium and vitamin D absorption.

Cystic Fibrosis

Patients with CF are at increased risk for significant bone disease. A review of the literature from 1988–1998 showed relative BMD decreases for patients with CF, with measured Z-scores ranging from −0.31 to −2.14 in studies with varying age populations and densitometry methods. This decrease in BMD translates into measurable increases in fracture rates and kyphosis (compression of the thoracic vertebrae) in CF patients aged 6 years and older.[162]

As with other chronic diseases, the pathophysiology of bone loss in these patients is felt to be multifactorial, with malabsorption of calcium and vitamin D, general malnutrition, inflammatory cytokines, and systemic corticosteroid use all playing roles. Vitamin D is a fat-soluble vitamin which relies on pancreatic enzymes for optimal absorption and reabsorption via enterohepatic circulation. Patients with CF have been shown to have a high prevalence of vitamin D deficiency, even after exogenous supplementation.[162] CF patients additionally have decreased levels of IGF-I[163] and growth impairment, with height deficits as great as one standard deviation when compared with controls,[162] which impairs maximal bone mineral accretion and may warrant growth hormone replacement. Pubertal delay and hypogonadism ensue, even in adulthood, leading to deficits in the estrogen and testosterone necessary to optimize the bone cycle. Low concentrations of IGF-I have also been directly correlated with decreased bone density.[164] An additional consideration in CF can be a lack of exercise tolerance in patients due to their respiratory disease. Since bones require mechanical loading for remodeling, lack of weight-bearing activity further hinders normal bone mineral acquisition.

EVALUATION AND MANAGEMENT

The conditions described above are only a few of those which predispose children and adolescents to osteoporosis (Table 1). The wide variety of conditions that impair skeletal health necessitates a high index of suspicion and heightened level of concern for bone health on the part of the pediatric health care or nutrition practitioner. The limitations of DXA scanning in pediatric populations detailed earlier have delayed its widespread use. Therefore, there is little evidence on which to make general recommendations as to when and how frequently specific groups of children should have bone density measurements by DXA. The Cystic Fibrosis Foundation (CFF) convened an expert panel in 2002 to develop practice guidelines for the management of bone disease in CF.[165] These guidelines include a screening and treatment protocol calling for a baseline DXA scan at the time of diagnosis on patients age 8 years and older. It may be reasonable to apply this recommendation, and others from the CFF consensus statement, to patients with celiac disease, IBD, JRA, and other chronic diseases. Standard practice in the authors' clinic is to perform DXA scans on girls and young women with AN after 6 months of hypothalamic amenorrhea. Bone density measurement is also recommended for patients with multiple fractures, regardless of etiology, pathologic or atraumatic fractures, and stress fractures. A higher level of suspicion should also be raised in any patient with a strong family history of osteoporosis or with long-term use of systemic corticosteroids. DXA scans should then be repeated over time, but generally not more frequently than annually in clinical practice, as the changes noted over a shorter period are unlikely to be significant.

Patients found to have a subnormal BMD on DXA scanning should have a screening evaluation of calcium and vitamin D homeostasis in addition to any clinically indicated laboratory assessments of their underlying medical conditions. A panel including serum calcium, phosphorus, magnesium, 25(OH)D, PTH, and thyroid stimulating hormone (TSH), as well as a urinary spot calcium-to-creatinine ratio (normal < 0.2) would be sufficient. At the present time, it generally agreed that a teenager with a BMD Z-score less than −2.0 warrants referral to a provider (eg, endocrinologist) experienced in calcium metabolism and skeletal health. Consideration should be given to early referrals for a BMD Z-score less than −1.0 if the adolescent has sustained recurrent fractures or a strong family history of documented osteoporotic fracture.

Management

Management of bone disease in patients with the chronic illnesses described consists primarily of optimizing nutritional status, particularly with respect to calcium and vitamin D, and ensuring a normal hormonal milieu, with exogenous replacement of estrogen, testosterone, and growth hormone, as warranted. Gluten-free diets have already been mentioned for patients with celiac disease. Systemic glucocorticoids should be used judiciously, but should not be withheld if that would jeopardize management of the underlying disease process. As with many decisions in clinical medicine, potential risks and benefits must be balanced for each individual case.

Novel Therapies. The uses of DHEA and IGF-I in patients with AN have already been discussed. The positive effects of each on bone formation may make them attractive candidates for use in other diseases, particularly IGF-I for CF. However, long-term improvements in BMD as well as solutions to the limitations mentioned above (nonstandard preparations for DHEA, parenteral administration for IGF-I) will need to be demonstrated before widespread use can be recommended.

Another class of agents being explored in several clinical trials of patients with AN[166] and some of the other subgroups mentioned above are the bisphosphonates, which are potent and irreversible inhibitors of bone resorption that become incorporated permanently into the mineralized bone matrix. These investigations have been prompted by the successful use of the bisphosphonate pamidronate in children with osteogenesis imperfecta (OI),[167] as well as widespread experience with the bisphosphonate alendronate in postmenopausal women with osteoporosis. The CFF consensus statement includes the bisphosphonate alendronate as a therapeutic option in its screening and treatment protocol.[165] However, concerns still exist around use of bisphosphonates in pediatrics, especially with respect to possible inhibition of primary remodeling of growing bone, increased risk of osteomalacia, long half-life in bone (>10 years), and unknown effects on the growing fetus. Additionally, despite increases in BMD, there is concern that the bone matrix, intercalated with bisphosphonate, may not provide normal mechanical strength. A recent case report of osteopetrosis (excessively dense and brittle bone) induced in an adolescent treated with very high dose bisphosphonates highlights the caution with which these agents should be used.[168] Therefore, although there is great promise to translate the established benefits of bisphosphonates in the elderly and younger patients with specific diagnoses to a wider pediatric population, these agents should currently be used extremely cautiously and/or in the setting of a controlled research study.

Finally, early recognition of the conditions which predispose to low bone density and early identification of patients at risk are essential to the prevention of bone loss in adolescents with chronic illnesses, which may be the most effective way to manage bone disease in these patients.

Prevention

In addition to managing the skeletal complications of chronic illnesses, one of the most important goals of adolescent nutrition is the potential prevention of osteoporosis by maximizing skeletal health in otherwise healthy teenagers. It is essential to ascertain family history of osteoporosis, especially early-onset osteoporosis, or frequent fractures. Dietary sources of calcium and vitamin D should be assessed and inadequacies addressed. Recommended age-appropriate daily calcium, magnesium, and phosphorus intake guidelines have been developed in the United States by the National Institutes of Health and National Academy of Sciences (Table 2)[108] and endorsed by the American Academy of Pediatrics (AAP).[58]

Metabolic studies of calcium retention in adolescent girls[169,170] showed such large variation, however, that it might be necessary to individualize calcium requirements based on postmenarcheal age. Others have argued that gender and physical activity should also modify recommendations for optimal calcium intake.[171]

The recommended age-appropriate intake for vitamin D intake has not yet reached a consensus. The efficiency of conversion of 25(OH)D to active calcitriol in the kidney increases during puberty, suggesting that requirements for vitamin D in adolescents are no higher than in adults[172]; but, as mentioned previously, the prevalence of subclinical vitamin D deficiency in adolescents may be widespread.[100] While this is an area of ongoing research and debate, it is the official recommendation of the AAP that adolescents consume 200 IU of vitamin D daily,[173] but much higher doses are likely needed to attain the 25OHD levels above 30 ng/mL suggested by a recent expert panel to prevent secondary hyperparathyroidism and provide potential benefits to multiple tissues.[174]

The success shown by a single supplementation trial in maintaining increases in BMD several years after discontinuation of concentrated milk protein as the primary calcium source may suggest the superiority of milk over other sources,[93] but further study is necessary to confirm this finding. Adolescent girls may need to be reassured that consuming dairy products instead of calcium supplements will not increase their weight or percent body fat. Indeed, evidence from one large study often cited in the lay press suggests that regular consumption of milk may be protective against weight gain.[175]

The AAP once again reaffirmed the importance of dairy products for bone health in its recent position statement that recommends the increasingly widely available "partially digested" forms of milk, cheese, and yogurt as the primary source of calcium and vitamin D for patients with lactose intolerance due to relative lactase deficiency.[176] Pretreatment with lactase enzyme replacement tablets was also recommended. For those patients with the most severe forms of lactose intolerance or those who will not consume adequate dairy products, there are other dietary sources of calcium (see Table 3), along with calcium supplements as a suitable alternative. Despite concerns to the contrary, chronic consumption of high levels of calcium has not been shown to impair absorption of such essential nutrients as iron,[177] magnesium, and zinc, as long as the intake is held below 2.5 g (2,500 mg) daily.[55]

Table 3 Examples of Dietary Sources of Calcium

Food	Calcium	Serving Size
Milk	300	8 oz
Low-fat yogurt	300–415	8 oz
Calcium-fortified orange juice	300	8 oz
Cheddar cheese	300	1.5 oz
Cooked broccoli	35	$\frac{1}{2}$ cup

Adapted from reference 10.

CONCLUSIONS

The growing body of literature highlighted in this section should alert clinicians in all disciplines to the adverse effects of chronic illnesses and inadequate nutrition on the skeletal health of adolescents. Most clinicians should find the solutions less obscure, however, as the promotion of skeletal health is ultimately no more than the promotion of good general health, including recommending balanced general nutrition, moderate weight-bearing exercise, and avoidance of alcohol and tobacco for all adolescents. The challenge is in helping teenagers modify their behaviors to meet these goals.

REFERENCES

1. Bonjour JP, Thientz G, Buchs B, et al. Critical years and stages of puberty for spinal and femoral bone mass accumulation during adolescence. J Clin Endocrinol Metab 1991;73:555–63.
2. Thientz G, Buchs G, Rizzoli R, et al. Longitudinal monitoring of bone mass accumulation in healthy adolescents: Evidence for a marked reduction after 16 years of age at the levels of lumbar spine and femoral neck in female subjects. J Clin Endocrinol Metab 1992;75:1060–5.
3. National Osteoporosis Foundation. America's Bone Health: The State of Osteoporosis and Low Bone Mass in Our Nation. [Online report] http://www.nof.org/osteoporosis/diseasefacts.htm (accessed October 27, 2006).
4. Dempster DW. Anatomy and functions of the adult skeleton. In: Favus MJ, editor. Primer on the Metabolic Bone Diseases and Disorders of Mineral Metabolism, 6th edition. Durham, NC: American Society for Bone and Mineral Research; 2006. p. 7–11.
5. Robey PG, Boskey AL. Extracellular matrix and biomineralization of bone. In: Favus MJ, editor. Primer on the Metabolic Bone Diseases and Disorders of Mineral Metabolism, 6th edition. Durham, NC: American Society for Bone and Mineral Research; 2006. p. 12–9.
6. Aubin JE, Lian JB, Stein GS. Bone formation: Maturation and functional activities of osteoblast lineage cells. In: Favus MJ, editor. Primer on the Metabolic Bone Diseases and Disorders of Mineral Metabolism, 6th edition. Durham, NC: American Society for Bone and Mineral Research; 2006. p. 20–9.
7. Ross FP. Osteoclast biology and bone resorption. In: Favus MJ, editor. Primer on the Metabolic Bone Diseases and Disorders of Mineral Metabolism, 6th edition. Durham, NC: American Society for Bone and Mineral Research; 2006. p. 30–5.
8. Southard RN, Morris JD, Mahan JD, et al. Bone mass in healthy children: Measurement with quantitative DXA. Radiology 1991;179:735–8.
9. McCormick DP, Ponder SW, Fawcett HD, Palmer JL. Spinal bone mineral density in 335 normal and obese children and adolescents: Evidence for ethnic and sex differences. J Bone Miner Res 1991;6:507–13.
10. Steelman J, Zeitler P. Osteoporosis in pediatrics. Pediatr Rev 2001;22:56–64.
11. Peterson CA, Eurell JAC, Erdman JW. Alterations in calcium intake on peak bone mass in the female rat. J Bone Miner Res 1995;10:81–95.
12. Bailey DA, McKay HA, Mirwald RL, et al. A six-year longitudinal study of the relationship of physical activity to bone mineral accrural in growing children: The University of Saskatchewan Bone Mineral Accrural Study. J Bone Miner Res 1999;14:1672–9.
13. Teegarden D, Proulx WR, Martin BR, et al. Peak bone mass in young women. J Bone Miner Res 1995;10:711–5.
14. Bachrach LK, Hastie T, Marcus R, et al. Bone mineral acquisition in healthy Asian, Hispanic, Black, and Caucasian youth: A longitudinal study. J Clin Endocrinol Metab 1999; 84:4702–12.
15. Loud KJ, Gordon CM. Bone and nutrition in health and disease. Int Semin Pediatr Gastroenterol Nutr 2002;11:1–7.
16. Bell NH, Shary J, Stevens J, Garza M, et al. Demonstration that bone mass is greater in black than in white children. J Bone Miner Res 1991;6:719–23.
17. Gilsanz V, Roe TF, Mora S, et al. Changes in vertebral bone density in black girls and white girls during childhood and puberty. New Engl J Med 1991;325:1597–600.
18. Seeman E, Hopper JL, Bach LA, et al. Reduced bone mass in daughters of women with osteoporosis. N Engl J Med 1989;320:554–8.
19. Pocock NA, Eisman JA, Hopper JL, et al. Genetic determinants of bone mass in adults. J Clin Invest 1987;80:706–10.
20. Brown MA, Haughton MA, Grant SF, et al. Genetic control of bone density and turnover: Role of the collagen 1alpha1, estrogen receptor, and vitamin D receptor genes. J Bone Miner Res 2001;16:758–64.
21. Eisman JA. Genetics of osteoporosis. Endocr Rev 1999;20:788–804.
22. Gerdhem P, Obrant KJ. Bone mineral density in old age: The influence of age at menarche and menopause. J Bone Miner Metab 2004;22:372–5.
23. Riggs BL, Khosla S, Melton LJ. Sex steroids and the construction and conservation of the adult skeleton. Endocr Rev 2002;23:279–302.
24. Bass S, Delmas PD, Pearce G, et al. The differing tempo of growth in bone size, mass and density in girls is region-specific. J Clin Invest 1999;104:795–804.
25. Cameron N, Tanner JM, Whitehouse RH. A longitudinal analysis of the growth of limb segments in adolescence. Ann Hum Biol 1982;9:211–20.
26. Seeman E, Karlsson MK, Duan Y. On exposure to anorexia nervosa, the temporal variation in axial and appendicular skeletal development predisposes to site-specific deficits in bone size and density: A cross-sectional study. J Bone Miner Res 2000;15:2259–65.
27. Buchanan JR, Myers C, Lloyd T, et al. Determinants of peak trabecular density in women: The role of androgens, estrogen and exercise. J Bone Miner Res 1988;3:673–80.
28. Tracz MJ, Sideras K, Bolona ER, et al. Testosterone use in men and its effects on bone health. A systematic review and meta-analysis of randomized placebo-controlled trials. J Clin Endocrinol Metab 2006;91:2011–6.
29. Rogol AD. Pubertal androgen therapy in boys. Pediatr Endocrinol Rev 2005;2:383–90.
30. Munoz-Torres M. Jodar E, Quesada M, Escobar-Jiminez F. Bone mass in androgen-insensitivity syndrome: Response to hormonal replacement therapy. Calcif Tissue Int 1995;57:94–6.
31. Marcus R, Leary D, Schneider DL, et al. The contribution of testosterone to skeletal development and maintenance: Lessons from the androgen insensitivity syndrome. J Clin Endocrinol Metab 2000;85:1032–7.
32. Bertelloni S, Baroncelli GI, Federico G, et al. Altered bone mineral density in patients with complete androgen insensitivity syndrome. Horm Res 1998;50:309–14.
33. Buchanan JR, Hospodar P, Myers C, et al. Effect of excess endogenous androgens on bone density in young women. J Clin Endocrinol Metab 1988;67:937–43.
34. Good C, Tulchinsky M, Mauger D, et al. Bone mineral density and body composition in lean women with polycystic ovary syndrome. Fertil Steril 1999;72:21–5.
35. Shore RM, Chesney RW, Mazess RB, et al. Bone mineral status in growth hormone deficiency. J Pediatr 1980,96.393–6.
36. Boot AM. Body composition and bone mineral density in adolescents with partial growth hormone deficiency. J Clin Endocrinol Metab 2003;88:5099–100.
37. Boot AM, Engels MA, Boerma GJ, et al. Changes in bone mineral density, body composition, and lipid metabolism during growth hormone (GH) treatment in children with GH deficiency. J Clin Endocrinol Metab 1997;82:2423–8.
38. Baroncelli GL, Bertelloni S, Sodini F, Saggese G. Acquisition of bone mass in normal individuals and in patients with growth hormone deficiency. J Pediatr Endocrinol Metab 2003;16:327–35.
39. Ferretti JL. On new opportunities for absorptiometry. J Clin Densitom 1998;1:41–53.
40. Kohrt WM, Bloomfield SA, Little KD, et al. American College of Sports Medicine Position Stand: Physical activity and bone health. Med Sci Sports Exerc 2004;36:1985–96.
41. Marcus R, Cann C, Madvig P, et al. Menstrual function and bone mass in elite women distance runners: Endocrine and metabolic features. Ann Intern Med 1985;102:158–63.
42. Gordon CM, Goodman E, Emans SJ, et al. Physiologic regulators of bone turnover in young women with anorexia nervosa. J Pediatr 2002;141:64–70.
43. Taafe DR, Snow-Harter C, Connolly DA, et al. Differential effects of swimming versus weight-bearing activity on bone mineral status of eumenorrheic athletes. J Bone Miner Res 1995;10:586–93.
44. Duncan CS, Blimkie CJ, Cowell CT, et al. Bone mineral density in adolescent female athletes: Relationship to exercise type and muscle strength. Med Sci Sports Exerc 2002;34:286–94.
45. Bass S, Pearce G, Bradney M, et al. Exercise before puberty may confer residual benefits in bone density in adulthood: Studies in active prepubertal and retired female gymnasts. J Bone Miner Res 1998;13:500–7.
46. Bachrach LK. Acquisition of optimal bone mass in childhood and adolescence. Trends Endocrinol Metab 2001;12:22–8.

47. Strong WB, Malina RM, Blimkie CJR, et al. Evidence based physical activity for school-age youth. J Pediatr 2005;146:732–7.
48. Berstein CN, Seeger LL, Sayre JW, et al. Decreased bone density in inflammatory bowel disease is related to corticosteroid use and not disease diagnosis. J Bone Miner Res 1995;10:250–6.
49. Israel E, Banerjee TR, Fitzmaurice GM, et al. Effects of inhaled glucocorticoids on bone density in premenopausal women. New Engl J Med 2001;345:941–7.
50. Leonard MB, Feldman HI, Shults J. Long-term, high-dose glucocorticoids and bone mineral content in childhood glucocorticoid-sensitive nephrotic syndrome. N Engl J Med 2004;351:868–75.
51. Bernstein CN, Leslie WD. The pathophysiology of bone disease in gastrointestinal disease. Eur J Gastroenterol Hepatol 2003;15:857–64.
52. Blum M, Harris SS, Must A, et al. Weight and body mass index at menarche are associated with premenopausal bone mass. Osteoporos Int 2001;12:588–94.
53. Goulding A, Grant AM, Williams SM. Bone and body composition of children and adolescents with repeated forearm fractures. J Bone Miner Res 2005;20:2090–6.
54. Goulding A, Taylor RW, Jones IE, et al. Overweight and obese children have low bone mass and area for their weight. Int J Obes Relat Metab Disord 2000;24:627–32.
55. Weaver CM, Peacock M, Johnston CC. Adolescent nutrition in the prevention of postmenopausal osteoporosis. J Clin Endorinol Metab 1999;84:1839–43.
56. Cadogan J, Blumsehn A, Barker M, Eastell R. A longitudinal study of bone gain in pubertal girls: Anthropometric and biochemical correlates. J Bone Miner Res 1998;13:1602–12.
57. Need AG, Kemp A, Giles N, et al. Relationships between intestinal calcium absorption, serum vitamin D metabolites and smoking in postmenopausal women. Osteoporos Int 2002;13:83–8.
58. Greer FR, Krebs NF, and the Committee on Nutrition, American Academy of Pediatrics. Optimizing bone health and calcium intakes of infants, children and adolescents. Pediatrics 2006;117:578–85.
59. Heaney RP. Calcium in the prevention and treatment of osteoporosis. J Intern Med 1992;231:169–80.
60. Kalkwarf HJ, Khoury JC, Lamphear BP. Milk intake during childhood and adolescence, adult bone density, and osteoporotic fractures in US women. Am J Clin Nutr 2003;77:257–65.
61. Specker BL. Evidence for an interaction between calcium intake and physical activity on changes in bone mineral density. J Bone Miner Res 1996;11:1539–44.
62. Holick MF, Garabedian M. Vitamin D: Photobiology, metabolism, mechanism of action, and clinical applications. In: Favus MJ, editor. Primer on the Metabolic Bone Diseases and Disorders of Mineral Metabolism, 6th edition. Durham, NC: American Society for Bone and Mineral Research; 2006. p. 106–14.
63. El-Hajj Fuleihan G, Nabulsi M, Choucair M, et al. Hypovitaminosis D in healthy schoolchildren. Pediatrics 2001;107:e53.
64. Hickey L, Gordon CM. Vitamin D deficiency: New perspectives on an old disease. Curr Opin Endocrinol Diab 2004;11:18–25.
65. Parfit AM, Gallagher JC, Heaney RP, et al. Vitamin D and bone health in the elderly. Am J Clin Nutr 1982;32:1014–31.
66. Webb AR, Kline L, Holick MF. Influence of season and latitude on the cutaneous synthesis of vitamin D3: Exposure to winter sunlight in Boston and Edmonton will not promote vitamin D3 synthesis in human skin. J Clin Endocrinol Metab 1988;67:373–8.
67. Krall EA, Sahyoun N, Tannenbaum S, et al. Effect of vitamin D intake on seasonal variation in parathyroid hormones secretion in postmenopausal women. N Engl J Med 1989;321:1777–83.
68. Ala-Houhala M, Parviainen MT, Pyykko K, Visakorpi JC. Serum 25-hydroxyvitamin D levels in Finnish children aged 2–17 years. Acta Pediatr Scand 1984;73:232–6.
69. Juttman JR, Visser TJ, Buurman C, et al. Seasonal fluctuations in serum concentrations of vitamin D metabolites in normal patients. BMJ 1981;282:1349–52.
70. Landin-Wilhelmsen K, Wilhelmsern L, Wilske J, et al. Sunlight increases serum 25-OH vitamin D concentration whereas $25(OH)D_3$ is unaffected: Results from a general population study in Goteborg, Sweden. Eur J Clin Nutr 1995;49:400–7.
71. Poskitt EME, Cole TJ, Lawson DEM. Diet, sunlight, and 25-hydroxyvitamin D in healthy children and adults. BMJ 1979;1:221–3.
72. Vik T, Try K, Srtomme JH. The vitamin D status of man at 70 degrees north. Scan J Clin Lab Invest 1980;80:227–32.
73. Aitken JM, Anderson JB, Horton PW. Seasonal variations in bone mineral content after the menopause. Nature 1973;241:59–60.
74. Krolner B. Seasonal variation of lumbar spine bone mineral content in normal women. Calcif Tissue Int 1983;35:145–7.
75. Vanderschueren D, Gevers G, Dequeucker J, et al. Seasonal variation in bone metabolism in young healthy subjects. Calcif Tissue Int 1991;49:84–9.
76. Dawson-Hughes B, Dallal GE, Krall EA, et al. Effect of vitamin D supplementation on wintertime and overall bone loss in healthy postmenopausal women. Ann Int Med 1991;115:505–12.
77. Overgaard K, Johansen NL, Christiansen C. Lack of seasonal variation in bone mass and biochemical estimates of bone turnover. Bone 1988;9:285–8.
78. Lips P. Vitamin D deficiency and osteoporosis: The role of vitamin D deficiency and treatment with vitamin D analogues in the prevention of osteoporosis-related fractures. Eur J Clin Invest 1996;26:436–42.
79. Krall EA, Dawson-Hughes B. Relation of fractional 47-calcium retention to season and rates of bone loss in healthy postmenopausal women. J Bone Miner Res 1991;6:1323–9.
80. Chapuy MC, Arlot ME, DuBoef F, et al. Vitamin D3 and calcium to prevent hip fractures in elderly women. N Engl J Med 1992;327:1637–42.
81. Dawson-Hughes B, Harris SS, Krall EA, Dallal GE. Effect of calcium and vitamin D supplementation on bone density in men and women 65 years of age and older. N Engl J Med 1997;337:670–6.
82. Baoshe A, Matkovic V. Relation of nutrition, body composition, and physical activity to skeletal development: A cross-sectional study in preadolescent females. J Am Coll Nutr 1998;17:136–47.
83. Ruiz JC, Mandel C, Garabedian M. Influence of spontaneous calcium intake and physical exercise on the vertebral and femoral bone mineral density of children and adolescents. J Bone Miner Res 1995;10:675–82.
84. Boot AM, de Ridder MA, Pols HA, et al. Bone mineral density in children and adolescents: Relation to puberty, calcium intake, and physical activity. J Clin Endocrinol Metab 1997;82:57–62.
85. Gunnes M, Lehmann EH. Physical activity and dietary constituents as predictors of forearm cortical and trabecular bone gain in healthy children and adolescents: A prospective study. Acta Pediatr 1996;85:19–25.
86. Lloyd T, Andon MB, Rollings N, et al. Calcium supplementation and bone mineral density in adolescent girls. JAMA 1993;270:841–4.
87. Chan GM, Hoffman K, McMurry M. Effects of dairy products on bone and body composition in pubertal girls. J Pediatr 1995;126:551–6.
88. Cadogan J, Eastell R, Jones N, Barker ME. Milk intake and bone mineral acquisition in adolescent girls: Randomized, controlled intervention trial. BMJ 1997;315:1255–60.
89. Lee WT, Leung SS, Leung DM, et al. A randomized double-blind controlled calcium supplementation trial, and bone and height acquisition in children. Br J Nutr 1995;74:125–39.
90. Johnston CC, Miller JZ, Slemenda CW, et al. Calcium supplemetation and increases in bone mineral density in children. N Engl J Med 1992;327:82–7.
91. Nowson CA, Green RM, Hopper JL, et al. A co-twin study of the effect of calcium supplementation on bone density during adolescence. Osteoporos Int 1997;7:219–25.
92. Bonjour JP, Carrie AL, Ferrari S, et al. Calcium-enriched foods and bone mass growth in prepubertal girls: A randomized, double-blind, placebo-controlled trial. J Clin Invest 1997;99:1287–94.
93. Bonjour JP, Chevalley T, Ammann P, et al. Gain in bone mineral mass in prepubertal girls 3.5 years after discontinuation of calcium supplmentation: A follow-up study. Lancet 2001;358:1208–12.
94. Lanou AJ, Berkow SE, Barnard ND. Calcium, dairy products and bone health in children and young adults: A reevaluation of the evidence. Pediatrics 2005;115:736–43.
95. Committee on Nutrition, American Academy of Pediatrics. Calcium requirements of infants, children, and adolescents. Pediatrics 1999;104:1152–7.
96. Gordon CM, Bachrach LK, Carpenter TO, et al. Bone health in children and adolescents: A symposium at the annual meeting of the Pediatric Academic Societies/Lawson Wilkins Pediatric Endocrine Society, May 2003. Curr Probl Pediatr Adolesc Health Care 2004;34:226–42.
97. Thomas MK, Lloyd-Jones DM, Thadhani RI, et al. Hypovitminosis D in medical inpatients. N Engl J Med 1998;338:777–83.
98. Guillemant J, Allemandou A, Cabrol S, et al. Vitamin D status in the adolescent: Seasonal variations and effects of winter supplementation with vitamin D_3. Arch Pediatr 1998;5:1211–5.
99. Docio S, Riancho JA, Perez A, et al. Seasonal deficiency of vitamin D in children: A potential target for osteoporosis-preventing strategies? J Bone Miner Res 1998;13:554–8.
100. Gordon CM, DePeter KC, Feldman HA, et al. Prevalence of vitamin D deficiency among healthy adolescents. Arch Pediatr Adolesc Med 2004;158:531–7.
101. Harkness LS, Cromer BA. Vitamin D deficiency in adolescent females. J Adolesc Health 2005;37:75.
102. Sullivan SS, Rosen CJ, Halteman WA. Adolescent girls in Maine are at risk for vitamin D insufficiency. J Am Diet Assoc 2005;105:971–4.
103. Slemenda CW, Peacock M, Hui S, et al. Reduced rates of skeletal remodeling are associated with increased bone mineral density during the development of peak bone mass. J Bone Miner Res 1997;12:676–82.
104. Ferrari SL, Rizzoli R, Slosman DO, Bonjour JP. Do dietary calcium and age explain the controversy surrounding the relationship between bone mineral density and vitamin D receptor gene polymorphisms? J Bone Miner Res 1998;13:363–70.
105. Massey LK, Whiting SJ. Dietary salt, urinary calcium, and bone loss. J Bone Miner Res 1996;11:731–6.
106. Harel Z, Riggs S, Menzies G, et al. Adolescents and calcium: What they do and do not know and how much they consume. J Adolesc Health 1998;22:225–8.
107. Albertson AM, Tobelmann RC, Marquart L. Estimated dietary calcium intake and food sources for adolescent females: 1980–1992. J Adolesc Health 1997;20:20–6.
108. Standing Committee on the Scientific Evaluation of Dietary Reference Intakes, Food and Nutrition Board, Institute of Medicine. DRI: Dietary Reference Intakes for Calcium, Phosphorous, Magnesium, Vitamin D, and Fluoride. Washington, DC: National Academy Press; 1997.
109. Wyshak G, Frisch RE. Carbonated beverages, dietary calcium, the dietary calcium/phosphorous ration, and bone fractures in girls and boys. J Adolesc Health 1994;15:210–5.
110. Wyshak G. Teenaged girls, carbonated beverage consumption, and bone fractures. Arch Pediatr Adolesc Med 2000;154:610–3.
111. Camacho P, Kleerekoper M. Biochemical markers of bone turnover. In: Favus MJ, editor. Primer on the Metabolic Bone Diseases and Disorders of Mineral Metabolism, 6th edition. Durham, NC: American Society for Bone and Mineral Research; 2006. p. 127–33.
112. McGartland C, Robson PJ, Murray L, et al. Carbonated soft drink consumption and bone mineral density in adolescence: The Northern Ireland Young Hearts project. J Bone Miner Res 2003;18:1563–9.
113. Amato D, Araujo F, Paniaqua R. The soda debate fizzes on. J Bone Miner Res 2004;19:521.
114. Putnam JJ, Allhouse JE. Food consumption, prices and expenditures, 1970–1997. Washington, DC: Food and Economics Division, Economic Research Service, US Department of Agriculture: 1999. Statistical Bulletin 965.
115. Haden ST, Fuleihan GEH, Angell JE, et al. Calcidiol and PTH levels in women attending an osteoporosis program. Calcif Tissue Int 1999;64:275–9.
116. Armas LA, Hollis BW, Heaney RP. Vitamin D_2 is much less effective than vitamin D3 in humans. J Clin Endocrinol Metab 2004;89:5387–91.
117. Houghton LA, Vieth R. The case against ergocalciferol (vitamin D2) as a vitamin supplement. Am J Clin Nutr 2006;84:694–7.
118. Consensus Development Conference V, 1993. Diagnosis, prophylaxis, and treatment of osteoporosis. Am J Med 1994;90:646–50.
119. Leib ES and Writing Group for the ISCD Position Development Conference. Diagnosis of osteoporosis in med, premenopausal women, and children. J Clin Densitom 2004;7:17–26.
120. Kanis JA, Melton LJ, III, Christiansen C, et al. The diagnosis of osteoporosis. J Bone Miner Res 1994;9:1137–41.
121. Bachrach LK. Osteoporosis and measurement of bone mass in children and adolescents. Endocrinol Metab Clin North Am 2005;34:521–35.
122. Carter DR, Bouxsein ML, Marcus R. New approaches for interpreting projected bone densitometry data. J Bone Miner Res 1992;7:137–45.
123. Rubin CT, Rubin J. Biomechanics and mechanobiology of bone. In: Favus MJ, editor. Primer on the Metabolic Bone Diseases and Disorders of Mineral Metabolism, 6th edition. Durham, NC: American Society for Bone and Mineral Research; 2006. p. 36–42.
124. Rauch F, Schonau E. Peripheral quantitative computed tomography of the distal radius in young subjects new reference data and interpretation of results. J Musculoskelet Neuronal Interact 2005;5:99–126.
125. Specker BL, Schoenau E. Quantitative bone analysis in children: Current methods and recommendations. J Pediatr 2005;146:726–31.
126. Bachrach LK, Guido D, Katzman D, et al. Decreased bone density in adolescent girls with anorexia nervosa. Pediatrics 1990;86:440–7.

127. Rigotti NA, Neer RM, Skates SJ, et al. The clinical course of osteoporosis in anorexia nervosa. JAMA 1991;265:1133–8.
128. Soyka LA, Grinspoon S, Levitsky L, et al. The effects of anorexia nervosa on bone metabolism in female adolescents. J Clin Endocrinol Metab 1999;84:4489–96.
129. Castro J, Lazaro L, Pons F, et al. Predictors of bone mineral density reduction in adolescents with anorexia nervosa. J Am Acad Child Adolesc Psychiatry 2000;39:1365–70.
130. Seeman E, Szmuckler GI, Formica C, et al. Osteoporosis in anorexia nervosa: The influence of peak bone density, bone loss, oral contraceptive use and exercise. J Bone Miner Res 1992;7:1267–74.
131. Hergenroeder AC, Smith EO, Shypailo R, et al. Bone mineral changes in young women with hypothalamic amenorrhea treated with oral contraceptives, medroxy-progesterone, or placebo over 12 months. Am J Obstet Gynecol 1997;176:1017–25.
132. Klibanski A, Biller BM, Schoenfeld DA, et al. The effects of estrogen administration on trabecular bone loss in young women with anorexia nervosa. J Clin Endocrinol Metab 1995;80:898–904.
133. Robinson E, Bachrach LK, Katzman DK. Use of hormone replacement therapy to reduce the risk of osteopenia in adolescent girls with anorexia nervosa. J Adolesc Health 2000;26:343–8.
134. Bachrach LK, Katzman DK, Litt IF, et al. Recovery from osteopenia in adolescent girls with anorexia nervosa. J Clin Endocrinol Metab 1991;72:602–6.
135. Stefanis N, MacIntosh, Abaha HD, et al. Dissociation of bone turnover in anorexia nervosa. Ann Clin Biochem 1998;35:709–16.
136. Caillot-Augusseau A, Lafage-Prous MH, Margaillan P, et al. Weight gain reverses bone turnover and restores circadian variation of bone resorption in anorexic patients. Clin Endocrinol (Oxf) 2000;52:113–21.
137. Grinspoon S, Miller K, Coyle C, et al. Severity of osteopenia in estrogen-deficient women with anorexia nervosa and hypothalamic amenorrhea. J Clin Endocrinol Metab 1999;84:2049–55.
138. Grinspoon S, Baum H, Lee K, et al. Effects of short-term recombinant insulin-like growth factor administration on bone turnover in osteopenic women with anorexia nervosa. J Clin Endocrinol Metab 1996;81:3864–70.
139. Grinspoon S, Thomas L, Miller K, et al. Effects of recombinant human IGF-I and oral contraceptive administration on bone density in anorexia nervosa. J Clin Endocrinol Metab 2002;87:2883–91.
140. Nicholas V, Prwett A, Bettica P, et al. Age-related decreases in IGF-I and TGF-beta in femoral cortical bone from both men and women: Implications for bone loss with aging. J Clin Endocrinol Metab 1994;78:1011–6.
141. Haden ST, Glowacki J, Hurwitz S, et al. Effects of age and serum dehydroepiandrosterone sulfate, IGF-I and IL-6 levels in women. Calcif Tissue Int 2000;66:414–8.
142. Meikle AW, Daynes RA, Aranco BA. Adrenal androgen secretion and biologic effects. Endocrinol Metab Clin North Am 1991;20:381–400.
143. Labrie F, Diamond R, Cusan L, et al. Marked decline in serum concentrations of adrenal C19 sex steroid precursors and conjugated androgen metabolites during aging. J Clin Endocrinol Metab 1997;82:2396–402.
144. Gordon CM, Grace E, Emans SJ, et al. Changes in bone turnover markers and menstrual function after short-term oral DHEA in young women with anorexia nervosa. J Bone Miner Res 1999;14:136–45.
145. Gordon CM, Grace E, Emans SJ, et al. Effects of oral DHEA on bone density in young women with anorexia nervosa: A randomized trial. J Clin Endocrinol Metab 2002;87:4935–41.
146. Goodman LR, Warren MP. The female athlete and menstrual function. Curr Opin Obstet Gynecol 2005;17:466–70.
147. Otis CL, Drinkwater B, Johnson M, et al. American College of Sports Medicine Position Stand: The Female Athlete Triad. Med Sci Sports Exerc 1997;29:i–ix.
148. Feicht CB, Johnson TS, Martin BJ, et al. Secondary amenorrhea in athletes. Lancet 1978;2:1145–6.
149. Shangold M, Rebar RW, Wentz AC, et al. Evaluation and management of menstrual dysfunction in athletes. JAMA 1990;263:1665–9.
150. Rosen LW, McKeag DB, Hough DO, et al. Pathogenic weight-control behavior in female athletes. Phys Sports Med 1986;14:79–84.
151. Warren BJ, Stanton AL, Blessing DL. Disordered eating patterns in competitive female athletes. Int J Eat Disord 1990;9:565.
152. Loucks AB, Verdun M, Heath EM. Low energy availability, not stress of exercise, alters LH pulsatility in exercising women. J Appl Physiol 1998;84:37–46.
153. Deutz RC, Bernadot D, Martin DE, Cody MM. Relationship between energy deficits and body composition in elite female gymnasts and runners. Med Sci Sports Exerc 2000;32:659–68.
154. McLean JA, Barr SI, Prior JC. Cognitive dietary restraint is associated with higher urinary cortisol excretion in healthy premenopausal women. Am J Clin Nutr 2001;73:7–12.
155. McLean JA, Barr SI, Prior JC. Dietary restraint, exercise, and bone density in young women: Are they related? Med Sci Sports Exerc 2001;33:1292–6.
156. Mora S, Barera G, Beccio S, et al. A prospective, longitudinal study of the long-term effect of treatment on bone density in children with celiac disease. J Pediatr 2001;139:516–21.
157. Pazianas M, Butcher GP, Subhani JM, et al. Calcium absorption and bone mineral density in celiacs after long term treatment with gluten-free diet and adequate calcium intake. Osteoporos Int 2005;16:56–63.
158. Burnham JM, Shults J, Semeao E, et al. Whole body BMC in pediatric Crohn disease: Independent effects of altered growth, maturation, and body composition. J Bone Miner Res 2004;19:1961–8.
159. Sylvester FA. IBD and skeletal health: Children are not small adults. Inflamm Bowel Dis 2005;11:1020–3.
160. Ulivieri FM, Piodi LP, Taioli E, et al. Bone mineral density and body composition in ulcerative colitis: A six-year follow-up. Osteoporos Int 2001;12:343–8.
161. Burnham JM, Shults J, Semeao E, et al. Body-composition alterations consistent with cachexia in children and young adults with Crohn disease. Am J Clin Nutr 2005;82: 413–20.
162. Ott SM, Aitken ML. Osteoporosis in patients with cystic fibrosis. Clin Chest Med 1998;19:555–67.
163. Arumugam R, LeBlanc A, Seilheimer DK, Hardin DS. Serum leptin and IGF-I levels in cystic fibrosis. Endocr Res 1998;24:247–57.
164. Gordon CM, Binello E, LeBoff MS, et al. Relationship between insulin-like growth factor I, dehydroepiandrosterone sulfate and proresorptive cytokines and bone density in cystic fibrosis. Osteoporos Int 2006;17:783–90.
165. Aris RM, Merkel PA, Bachrach LK, et al. Consensus Statement: Guide to bone health and disease in cystic fibrosis. J Clin Endocrinol Metab 2005;90:1888–96.
166. Golden NH, Iglesias IEA Jacobson MS, et al. Alendronate for the treatment of osteopenia in anorexia nervosa: A randomized, double-blind, placebo-controlled trial. J Clin Endocrinol Metab 2005;90:3179–85.
167. Glorieux F, Bishop N, Poltoon H, et al. Cyclic administration of pamidronate in children with severe osteogenesis imperfecta. N Engl J Med 1998;339:947–52.
168. Whyte MP, Wenkert D, Clements KL, et al. Bisphosphonate-induced osteopetrosis. N Engl J Med 2003;349:457–63.
169. Jackman LA, Millane SS, Martin BR, et al. Calcium retention in relation to calcium intake and postmenarcheal age in adolescent females. Am J Clin Nutr 1997;66:327–33.
170. Weaver CM, Peacock M, Martin BR, et al. Calcium retention estimated from indicators of skeletal status in adolescent girls and young women. Am J Clin Nutr 1996;64:67–70.
171. Anderson JJ. Calcium requirements during adolescence to maximize bone health. J Am Coll Nutr 2001;20:186S–91S.
172. Aksnes L, Aarskog D. Plasma concentration of vitamin D metabolites in puberty: effect of sexual maturation and implications for growth. J Clin Endocrinol Metab 1982;55:94–101.
173. Gartner LM, Greer FR. Prevention of rickets and vitamin D deficiency: New guidelines for vitamin D intake. Pediatrics 2003;111:908–10.
174. Bischoff-Ferrari HA, Giovannucci E, Willett WC, et al. Estimation of optimal serum concentrations of 25-hydroxyvitamin D for multiple health outcomes. Am J Clin Nutr 2006;84:18–28.
175. Pereira MA, Jacobs DR, Jr, Van Horn L, et al. Dairy consumption, obesity, and the insulin resistance syndrome in young adults: The CARDIA Study. JAMA 2002;287: 2081–9.
176. Heyman MB for the Committee on Nutrition. Lactose intolerance in infants, children, and adolescents. Pediatrics 2006;118;1279–86.
177. Abrams SA, Griffin IJ, Davila P, Liang L. Calcium fortification of breakfast cereal enhances calcium absorption in children without affecting iron absorption. J Pediatr 2001;139:522–6.

Standard and Specialized Enteral Formulas

Tien-Lan Chang, MD
Ronald E. Kleinman, MD

As research and experience over the past century have advanced our knowledge of the nutrient requirements and digestive functions of infants and children in health and illness, enteral formulas have become more sophisticated and diversified to meet their nutritional and metabolic needs. These liquid meals, together with advances in enteral feeding techniques, have contributed to the increased survival and shorter hospitalizations of pediatric patients with severely compromised intestinal function as well as other children with chronic health conditions. This chapter will provide a brief historical perspective of the development of infant formulas, review the composition of the major groups of available formulas for infants and children, and discuss their use in general. Breast- and formula feeding of infants and the enteral nutrition support of children with specific chronic illnesses are discussed in detail in other chapters. The composition of many formulas available in the United States and other industrialized countries is also listed in detail in Appendix III, grouped by category and by use.

HISTORICAL BACKGROUND

Human milk was the principal source of nutrition for newborns and infants up to the mid-nineteenth century. Wet nurses provided an alternate source of milk when the mother's milk was not adequate or available. Milk from donkeys, horses, and cows was used as a substitute when human milk was not available. The mortality of bottle-fed infants was 4 to 10 times greater than breastfed infants in the early part of twentieth century mainly because of unsanitary methods of preparation and storage of the milks. Innovations toward the end of the nineteenth century and beginning of the twentieth century, such as evaporated cow milk, the rubber nipple, pasteurization, and the introduction of refrigeration into most households in the industrialized world, led to a greater use of formula feeding, and the practice of wet nursing was gradually replaced by cow milk formula.[1,2] In the 1970s infectious diarrhea and malnutrition, two interrelated causes of morbidity and mortality in infants in the developing nations, were linked to the unsanitary and inappropriate preparation of infant formulas. The marketing techniques employed by the infant formula industry were blamed, among other factors, for the decline of breastfeeding in these nations. In 1981 the World Health Organization and UNICEF developed the International Code of Marketing of Breast Milk Substitutes, the purpose of which was to promote breastfeeding. The Code set restrictions on direct marketing of the formulas by manufacturers to the general public, display of formulas in the health care facilities, and distribution of formulas by health workers to mothers of infants.[3] The United States gave endorsement to the Code only in 1994, when it was presented again at the World Health Assembly. Implementation of the Code by member nations has been incomplete, however, and violations of the Code continue.[4]

The modification of cow milk to make it more similar to the nutrient composition of human milk began in a scientific way with the German pediatrician, Philip Biedert, who added cream, whey, and sugar to cow milk to make it suitable for young infants. Meigs' mixture, formulated by the American physician, John Meigs, was similar in composition to Biedert's mixture.[5] In addition to changing the quantity of cow milk constituents, the quality of the protein, fat, and carbohydrate in cow milk was also a subject of research and in some cases changed, as with the acid treatment of casein curds to render them smaller and softer.[6] These early formulas formed the basis for the modern formulas with a defined nutrient composition that are currently fed to human infants.

STANDARD INFANT FORMULAS

In spite of Abraham Jacobi's admonition that "Cow's milk cannot be changed into woman's milk. . . . The efficiency of all alleged improvements in artificial feeding is liable to be overestimated, and not always received with sound criticism,"[7] modern proprietary formulas intended for infants continue to attempt to simulate human milk. In doing this, however, the nutrient composition has also been adjusted to provide what are currently established as the nutrient requirements of growing infants. The levels of nutrients present in all infant formulas in the United States are subjected to regulations established by the FDA (Table 1).[8] For many nutrients, minimal and maximal amounts are specified. Modifications in nutrient and nonnutrient content are generally based on recommendations from the scientific and medical communities. In the United States, the Committee on Nutrition of the American Academy of Pediatrics has had an important role in the development of these recommendations. The Codex Alimentarius Commission, created by the Food and Agriculture Organization of the United Nations (FAO) and the World Health Organization in 1963 to develop global standards for food items, includes a standard for infant formula composition

Table 1 Recommended Nutrient Levels for Infant Formulas (per 100 kcal)

Nutrient	Minimum	Maximum
Protein (g)	1.8	4.5
Fat (g)	3.3	6.0
Calories	30.0	54.0
Essential fatty acids		
Linoleic acid (mg)	300.0	—
Calories	2.7	—
Vitamins		
A (IU)	250.0	750.0
D (IU)	40.0	100.0
K (mcg)	4.0	—
E (IU)	0.7	—
C (ascorbic acid) (mg)	8.0	—
B1 (thiamine) (mcg)	40.0	—
B2 (riboflavin) (mcg)	60.0	—
B6 (pyridoxine) (mcg)	35.0	—
B12 (mcg)	0.15	—
Niacin (mcg)*	250.0	—
Folic acid (mcg)	4.0	—
Pantothenic acid (mcg)	300.0	—
Biotin (mcg)†	1.5	—
Choline (mg)†	7.0	—
Inositol (mg)†	4.0	—
Minerals		
Calcium (mg)	50.0	—
Phosphorus (mg)	25.0	—
Magnesium (mg)	6.0	—
Iron (mg)	0.15	3.0
Iodine (mcg)	5.0	75.0
Zinc (mg)	0.5	—
Copper (mcg)	60.0	—
Manganese (mcg)	5.0	—
Sodium (mg)	20.0	60.0
Potassium (mg)	80.0	200.0
Chloride (mg)	55.0	150.0

From Section 412, Food, Drug and Cosmetic Act.[8]
*Includes niacin (nicotinic acid) and niacinamide (nicotinamide).
†Required only for non–milk-based infant formulas.

that was first adopted in 1981. An update on the global standard was prepared in 2005 by a group of international nutritional experts coordinated by the European Society of Pediatric Gastroenterology, Hepatology and Nutrition at the request of the Codex Committee on Nutrition and Foods for Special Dietary Uses.[9]

The Infant Formula Act of 1980 and the amendments of 1986 mandate the quality control standards under which all infant formulas are manufactured in the United States. These government regulations on good manufacturing practices came about following reported cases of hypochloremia and alkalosis in infants fed with a chloride-deficient soy formula.[10] However, the potential for error in preparation and contamination of infant formulas pre- and postmarketing continues even in the twenty-first century in different parts of the world. Several infants in Israel, which has similar regulatory safeguards as the United States, developed signs of beriberi, including death in two, as a result of a thiamine-deficient soy formula imported from Germany.[11] One infant died of meningitis due to Enterobacter sakazakii in Tennessee, USA,[12] and another infant developed botulism due to Clostridium botulinum type B toxin in the United Kingdom.[13] Bacterial contamination of infant formulas remains an active issue in the formula industry because, unlike liquid formulas, powdered formulas cannot be sterilized during the manufacturing process. Enterobacter sakazaki is the most common organism isolated, though Salmonella species has also been identified in outbreaks.[14] Batches of formulas have also been recalled because of metal pieces found in the formula, or because of an inadequate seal that could lead to oxidation and depletion of vitamin C in the liquid formula.[15,16] These episodes emphasize the continuing need for constant monitoring of infant formula composition and quality as required by statute, including postmarketing surveillance.

The enteral formulas can be categorized either by their protein composition (cow-milk-, soy-, protein hydrolysate-, and amino acid-based), or by the intended consumer groups (eg, premature infants, healthy infants, children with special metabolic needs).

COW-MILK-BASED FORMULAS

Standard cow-milk-based formulas are marketed in ready-to-use, concentrated liquid and powdered forms. All are based on nonfat cow milk, to which lactose and vegetable oils have been added. These formulas are low in cholesterol because the fat is derived from vegetable sources. In addition, emulsifiers (eg, lecithin) and thickeners (eg, carrageenan) have been added. Their mineral and vitamin content have also been adjusted to suit the needs of human infants.

Experience accumulated over the past 50 years has shown that casein-predominant milks support normal growth in both premature and full-term infants.[17] Casein has served as a standard reference protein by which to measure the biologic value of other proteins such as soybean or egg protein. The measure of the biologic value is the grams of weight that reference animal gains for each gram of protein fed. Setting casein as 100%, FDA regulations require protein at a minimum level of 1.8 g/100 kcal of formula. For proteins with a lower biologic value, the formula must contain proportionately more protein. No protein source can be used with a biologic value less than 70% of casein. Cow milk has a relatively greater amount of casein than human milk. Those formulas that are based on casein have an amino acid and mineral composition that more closely resembles that of cow milk than human milk. The osmolality and potential renal solute loads of these standard formulas fall intermediate between human and cow milk, although these values increase, as do those of the other constituent nutrients, if the formulas are prepared to be more concentrated than indicated by the manufacturer.

Renal solute load refers to the sum of solutes filtered by the kidneys. These solutes include amino acids, urea, and electrolytes. The potential renal solute load (PRSL) of an enteral formula refers to the sum total of the solutes present in the preparation, as approximated by the equation[18]

$$\text{PRSL (mOsm)} = \text{N}/28 + \text{Na} + \text{Cl} + \text{K} + \text{P},$$

where N is total nitrogen in mg. Assuming that 1 g of protein contains 0.16 g of nitrogen, the equation can also be written as

$$\text{PRSL (mOsm)} = (\text{Protein(g)} \times 5.714) + \text{Na} + \text{Cl} + \text{K} + \text{P}.$$

As the nutrients are digested, absorbed, and metabolized, and waste products are generated, the actual amount of solutes that reach the kidneys may be quite different. Nevertheless, when the solute load is above the handling capacity of the kidneys, dehydration from osmotic diuresis and metabolic derangement, for example, hypernatremia, metabolic acidosis, and an elevated BUN, may occur.

Infants who are fed a casein-predominant formula have a different profile of amino acids in their serum after feeding than breastfed infants, and some have developed metabolic derangements on casein-predominant formulas.[19] For this reason and others, including attempts by manufacturers to simulate human milk, whey-predominant and whey-only formulas have achieved popularity for both premature and full-term infants. By increasing the amount of whey proteins, mainly alpha-lactalbumin and beta-lactoglobulin, the amino acid composition of the formula is altered so that it resembles human milk more than cow milk. This is particularly so for the sulfated amino acids, cystine, taurine, and methionine. Clinical studies have demonstrated the adequate growth of full-term infants taking these formulas. Serum amino acid profiles of infants fed whey-predominant formulas are different from those fed human or cow milk, with a higher percentage of branched-chain amino acids and threonine in circulation. However, the significance of this finding is unclear.[20,21]

Iron is added to the standard formulas in order to prevent iron deficiency in newborns in the first year of life. Iron supplementation is particularly important for premature or small-for-gestational-age infants, who have reduced iron stores. The amount of iron present in the formulas range from approximately 4.7 to 14.5 mg/L (equivalent to 0.7 mg to 1.8 mg/100 kcal) in the United States and 4 to 7 mg/L in Europe.[22] The proposed global standard is a range of 0.3 mg to 1.3 mg/100 kcal.[9] The designation "low-iron" on infant formulas now refers to an iron content at the lower end of the range.

Nucleotides are now being added to many of the standard cow-milk-based formulas based on the presence of nucleotides in human milk. The addition of nucleotides is supported by the finding of a decreased incidence of diarrheal disease in a few studies of infants fed formulas supplemented with nucleotides.[23,24] Furthermore, nucleotides added to infant formula have also increased plasma lipoproteins and enhanced the growth of small-for-gestational-age infants.[25,26] In a study of term infants, cow-milk-based formula supplemented with nucleotides enhanced antibody responses to Diphtheria and Hemophilus influenzae vaccinations, but antibody responses to polio and tetanus were unaffected.[27] In preterm infants on formula supplemented with nucleotides, serum IgM and IgA levels were higher, while IgG and lymphocyte subsets were unaffected.[28] The full clinical significance of these observations remains to be demonstrated.

The fatty acid composition of infant formulas remains an area of intense investigation. Oils from a variety of plants such as palm, coconut, corn, safflower, and soybean are used instead of the animal fat in cow-milk-based formulas. Formulas that contain palm olein as part of the oil mixture were designed to imitate the palmitic acid profile of human milk. However, several studies have shown that babies fed with formulas with palm olein had lower calcium and fat absorption and lower bone mineralization compared to those on a formula without palm olein.[29,30] The position of the palmitic acid in the triglyceride molecule affects its absorption in the gut. Human milk fat has a greater proportion of triglycerides with palmitic acid in the beta position of the glycerol backbone than palm olein. Infants on a formula with a high portion of triglycerides with palmitic acid in the beta position have better fat and calcium absorption than those on a formula with a low percentage of palmitic acid in the beta position.[31]

Human milk contains relatively more monounsaturated fatty acids than regular infant formulas and also contains long-chain polyunsaturated fatty acids (LCPUFA) such as arachidonic (AA) and docosahexaenoic acids (DHA). Arachidonic acid and DHA are important structural components of cell membranes in the brain and retina. Studies have shown enhanced cognitive development and visual acuity in premature infants fed with formulas supplemented with AA and DHA.[32,33] Another study in preterm infants found increased lean body mass and reduced fat mass by 1 year of age for those fed with AA and DHA supplemented formulas.[34] Studies in term infants, however, have shown mixed results.[35,36] A follow-up study at 39 months of age of these infants who had received AA and DHA supplemented formulas up to 1 year found no difference with respect to their visual and cognitive functions when compared to infants fed either breast milk or unsupplemented formula.[37] LCPUFAs also influence the maturation of the immune system. The expression of CD45RO (mature phenotype) on CD4+ cells and IL-10 production were higher in preterm infants fed human milk and those fed with infant formula supplemented with LCPUFAs compared to those in infants fed with unsupplemented infant formula alone, although it is unclear whether this is a clinically important phenomenon.[38] The supplemented formulas appear to be safe, as all studies have shown no adverse outcomes and no significant difference in the growth parameters for infants on supplemented formulas with appropriate ratios of AA and DHA.[39,40]

Cow-milk-based formulas with lactose are contraindicated for infants with galactosemia, cow milk allergy, or lactose intolerance. However, a lactose-free cow-milk-based formula with corn syrup solids as the carbohydrate is an appropriate choice for infants with lactose intolerance. Another cow-milk-based formula with added rice starch was specifically marketed for infants with uncomplicated gastroesophageal reflux. Rice cereal is frequently added to thicken the formula in the management of uncomplicated gastroesophageal reflux. This practice increases the amount of carbohydrate relative to protein in the feeding and potentially may lead to intake of either excessive calories or inadequate protein by the infant. This formula addresses this concern by replacing part of the lactose with rice starch so that the protein: calorie ratio remains at 2.5 g/100 kcal.

A formula containing oligosaccharides as part of the carbohydrates and the synthetic triglyceride with palmitic acid in the beta position is already commercially available in Europe. Besides lactose, oligosaccharides make up approximately 10% of carbohydrates in human breast milk. The oligosaccharides are a mixture of short chain carbohydrates with sialic acid, fucose, and galactose residues. They are poorly digested like soluble fiber and serve as substrates for intestinal bacterial metabolism. They promote growth of Bifidobacteria and Lactobacillus species in the gut.[41,42] The incidence of moderate to severe diarrheal disease in a group of breastfed infants was found to be inversely related to the concentration of fucosyloligosaccharides in the breast milk.[43] Human infants on a formula with added oligosaccharides had softer and more frequent stools and had a lower risk for atopic dermatitis than those without the oligosaccharide supplement.[44] Future studies will determine whether this type of formula has other long-term advantages over those without the oligosaccharides.

Formulas for Premature Infants

Milk feedings formulated specifically for premature and small-for-gestational-age infants are sold in a liquid ready-to-use form for use in hospitals and postdischarge. These formulas differ from the standard formulas by attempting to meet the nutritional requirements of rapidly growing low-birth-weight infants within the limitations of intestinal and renal functions seen in these infants. These formulas have 20, 22, or 24 kcal/oz. When prepared at 20 kcal/oz, these formulas contain more protein than standard formulas. Fat malabsorption is a common occurrence in the low-birth-weight infant. Therefore, a high percentage of the fat in most of these formulas is in the form of medium-chain triglycerides, which have been shown to reduce steatorrhea, enhance calcium absorption, and improve nitrogen retention in low-birth-weight infants.[45,46] Carbohydrate is provided as a mixture of lactose, maltodextrins, and glucose polymers. Glucose polymers appear to be well tolerated by prematures.[47] Finally, the concentrations of calcium and phosphorus, in a 2:1 ratio, are increased above levels found in standard formulas. These nutrient concentrations are necessary to support a rate of growth similar to that of a full-term infant in utero. Although the breast milk of mothers delivering premature infants has higher protein and vitamin A concentrations than breast milk of mothers of full-term infants, the amounts of these nutrients are still insufficient to provide the daily requirements. A human milk "fortifier" formula can be added to breast milk to provide additional calories, calcium, phosphorus, other minerals, and vitamins.

Soy-Based Formulas

The soy protein formulas were introduced for use in infants who are cow milk intolerant. Although soy formulas are often fed to cow milk-allergic infants, soy protein is also antigenic and concomitant allergic reactions to soy may occur in cow milk allergic infants. Soybean protein is readily available and is a high-quality protein. Soy protein isolate is supplemented with L-methionine and taurine to balance the amino acid composition relative to animal milks and improve its biologic value.[48] Soy formulas are also supplemented with carnitine, which is found only in animal proteins. Nucleotides are not added to the soy formulas, as studies of infants fed nucleotide-supplemented soy formula failed to show any obvious immunological advantages, such as an enhanced response to vaccines or enhanced lymphocyte maturation.[49,50] The carbohydrates in soy formulas consist of sucrose, corn syrup solids, and/or maltodextrin. These formulas are therefore useful in infants with clinically significant lactose intolerance. Infants with acute lactose intolerance fed soy formula may have a shorter duration of diarrhea, although for most infants with acute infectious diarrhea, lactose intolerance is not clinically significant.[51,52]

While earlier studies showed that bone mineralization was reduced in infants fed a soy-based formula compared to infants fed a cow-milk-based formula,[53] studies from the 1990s of soy formula with improved mineral suspension showed no difference in bone mineralization in term infants fed soy- and cow-milk-based formulas.[54,55] The bioavailability of phosphorus, zinc, manganese, copper, and iron is reduced by phytic acid and polysaccharides present in the soy protein isolate.[56] Soy formulas are therefore supplemented with zinc and iron. Iron status appears to be equivalent in infants fed soy and cow milk formulas.[57]

Aluminum has been found in soy formulas at concentrations of 600 to 1,300 ng/mL, compared to concentrations of 4 to 65 ng/mL found in human milk.[58,59] Aluminum is the most abundant metal in the earth's crust and is present in many plants. It is present in the formula as a contaminant of calcium salts and the soy protein isolate. Aluminum-induced encephalopathy has been reported in patients with renal disease and those who were taking aluminum salts as an antacid or as phosphate binders. Aluminum also competes with calcium for absorption and may contribute to the osteopenia seen in infants with compromised renal function. No adverse effects of aluminum have been seen in healthy infants consuming soy formulas.

Soy protein isolate also contains isoflavones with estrogenic activity. Plasma concentrations of the isoflavones in infants fed with soy formulas were two orders of magnitude higher than levels found in infants fed with cow milk formulas or human milk.[60] The high concentrations of isoflavones found in infants fed with soy formulas have raised concern regarding the long-term health effects on infants exposed to soy. While many studies have demonstrated adequate growth for infants fed with soy formulas, up to now only one study has reported on the sexual development of infants fed on soy-based formulas. This retrospective cohort study of young adults who had participated in studies on soy- and cow-milk-based formulas in their infancy found no substantial effects of soy formulas on either growth or sexual maturation of human infants.[61]

Other specific indications for use of the soy formulas, in addition to lactose intolerance, include galactosemia and parents who prefer to avoid feeding their infants animal products, that is, vegetarians, or those whose specific religious dietary laws preclude the use of animal-based milks. The majority of infants with cow milk protein intolerance can tolerate soy formula. However, 15–40% of those with cow milk protein intolerance may have concomitant soy intolerance.[62,63] There is no benefit from the use of soy formulas to treat common problems in infancy such as gastroesophageal reflux, colic, and constipation unless these are symptoms of cow milk intolerance. Weight gain and bone mineralization in preterm infants fed soy formula have been reported to be lower than those fed cow-milk-based formulas.[64,65] Because of this and a concern for aluminum toxicity associated with soy formulas, the American Academy of Pediatrics issued a policy statement that "soy protein-based formulas are not designed or recommended for premature infants who weigh < 1800g."[66] For the same obvious reason, soy formulas should also be avoided in patients with renal disease, and patients with fructose intolerance should avoid soy formulas that contain sucrose.

Other Non–Cow Milk-Based Infant Formulas

Goat milk has been frequently used to feed cow milk-sensitive infants although studies show that it is as antigenic as cow milk. Like almost all mammalian milks (the California sea lion is an exception), lactose is the carbohydrate in goat milk. Goat's milk is high in essential fatty acids and has a higher percentage of medium-chain triglycerides than cow milk. It is low in folate, and because of more useful and effective commercial formula alternatives, its popularity has markedly waned in the United States. Goat milk remains a significant source of nutrition for infants after weaning in other countries. Infants fed with home preparations of goat milk are at risk for nutritional deficiencies and infections if the milk is contaminated. A goat milk formula, commercially produced in New Zealand, has been reported to be equivalent to a cow milk formula in terms of its growth-promoting effect and frequency of adverse events in term infants.[67]

Meat-based formula is yet another lactose-free, cow milk protein-free alternative for infant feeding. Its nutritional adequacy for healthy infants has been demonstrated, and it may be used in the management of children with food-induced atopic dermatitis,[68] but currently there is no commercial preparation of it.

PROTEIN HYDROLYSATE FORMULAS

Protein hydrolysate formulas, sometimes referred to as semielemental formulas (a vague term, implying that the hydrolysis process results in a source of nitrogen close to the free amino acids found in an "elemental" formula), are intended for patients with disorders associated with compromised enteric digestion, such as short bowel syndrome, food protein allergy, autoimmune enteropathy, HIV-associated enteropathy, cystic fibrosis, pancreatic insufficiency, and hepatobiliary disorders such as biliary atresia. The casein or whey in these formulas (Appendix III) is modified by hydrolysis and the addition of free amino acids. The casein hydrolysates are supplemented with L-cystine, L-tyrosine, and L-tryptophan to increase their biologic value to the infant. The major portion of the nitrogen in the formulas is in the form of oligopeptides. While the hydrolyzed protein peptides are less likely to induce an antigenic response than whole protein molecules, they are not nonallergenic.[69–71] One study suggests that peptides consisting of 5, 4, or even 3 amino acids can still activate T cell clones in vitro.[72] There is evidence to support the considerably faster rate of intestinal amino acid uptake from solutions containing dipeptides, tripeptides, or partially hydrolyzed proteins than from solutions composed solely of free amino acids.[73] Formulas with oligopeptides have a lower osmolality than a free amino acid-containing formula, and therefore may have a theoretical advantage over the amino acid-containing formulas for young infants and patients with short bowel syndrome. With immaturity of the intestine or loss of absorptive surface area, either following bowel resection or as a result of inflammation, all of the disaccharidases, but most commonly lactase, may be diminished.[74] The use of sucrose or glucose polymers (partially hydrolyzed corn starch) would therefore be useful in circumventing the absence of lactase or both lactase and sucrase. Monosaccharides are not used exclusively in any of the prepared formulas because of their high osmolality, which may inhibit gastric emptying[75,76] and further impair intestinal function.

Medium-chain triglycerides form a large percentage of the total fat content of these formulas. Medium-chain triglycerides can be absorbed from the intestine with minimal lipolysis to enter the portal circulation. Because of the enhanced solubility of medium-chain fatty acids in aqueous fluids, absorption of this form of fat can also take place in the absence of bile salts in the intestinal lumen and unstirred layer. None of these formulas contains only medium-chain triglycerides since they would then be devoid of the essential fatty acids. Medium-chain triglycerides increase the osmolality of a formula more so than long-chain fatty acids, and the excessive use of this form of fat may also contribute, in some patients, to excessive losses of stool water.

FREE AMINO ACID FORMULAS

The principal difference between these formulas and the peptide-based formulas is in the amino acid composition. The lipid component is a mixture of safflower, coconut (or MCT), and soy oils to provide essential and nonessential fatty acids. The carbohydrate is from corn syrup solids or maltodextrins, which are both derived from corn starch, differing only in the size of glucose polymers. As free amino acids by themselves are nonimmunogenic, these formulas are most useful for infants and children with multiple food allergies that do not tolerate even the peptide-based formulas. Several studies have shown that most infants with cow milk or multiple food allergies are able to grow adequately on amino acid-based formulas.[77,78] However, depending on the manufacturing and purification process, the soy oil may be contaminated by trace amounts of soy protein and may trigger an allergic response in susceptible individuals.[79] Children with severe enteropathy or short bowel syndrome unable to tolerate protein hydrolysates can use the amino acid-based formulas as an alternative or as an adjunct to parenteral nutrition.[80]

FOLLOW-UP FORMULAS

Follow-up formulas are defined by the joint FAO/WHO Codex Alimentarium Commission (1988) as: "A food intended for use as a liquid part of the weaning diet for the infant from the 6th month on and for young children."[81] Currently, several formulas for this use are marketed in the United States. These formulas are either cow milk or soy based, differing from the standard infant formulas only slightly in nutrient concentrations. Even though follow-up formulas are nutritionally adequate, they have no advantage over a combination of solid foods and standard infant formulas and/or human milk and may interfere with the normal weaning process. Ideally, the weaning process should take place over a period of several months, effecting a transition to a solid food diet comprising 30 to 50% of total calories. Solid foods should complement infant formula/breast milk in mineral and vitamin composition.[82]

FORMULAS FOR CHILDREN 1 TO 10 YEARS OF AGE

Although the use of formulas among healthy children decreases significantly after the first year of life, some children may require continued nutritional support with a liquid formula for a variety of reasons, including inadequate nutrient intake, perhaps as a result of chronic infections or single or multiple organ system dysfunction, compromised digestion or absorption, or inherited disorders of metabolism. These formulas can be cow milk-, soy-, peptide-, or amino acid-based. The carbohydrate is usually corn starch-derived glucose polymers and sucrose, and the fat is a blend of vegetable oils, such as safflower, soy, canola, and coconut oil to provide both medium- and long-chain triglycerides. These formulas are different from the infant formulas with a higher caloric density and protein concentration. The mineral and vitamin concentrations are intended to support the daily requirements for this age group.

Children who are unable to chew and swallow adequately due to neurological impairment, but who have intact intestinal motility, digestion, and absorption, exemplify those with a need for such a liquid enteral formula. For these children, the formulas are often administered via a gastrostomy. Children with critical illnesses or conditions who are unable to eat by mouth due to airway issues may use an enteral formula in the short term via a nasogastric or nasojejunal tube. Until recently, both adult and infant formulas have been used for preschool and school-aged children because of a lack of specific formulations for these age groups. If such formulas are "tailored" and their use is monitored to meet individual patient needs, they can be used successfully in this age group. However, vitamin and mineral deficiencies/excesses, osmotic diarrhea, and an excess renal solute load are a few of the concerns with the use of adult products in young children. Current products specifically manufactured for this age group have made it easier provide the nutrients required to optimally support their growth. Some of the formulas have added soy fiber. Studies in adult patients have shown fewer problems with diarrhea (and constipation) when fiber is added to the enteral nutrition.[83,84]

Peptide- and amino acid-based formulas designed for older children are often used for patients with limited digestive and absorptive capacity, such as those with Crohn disease, pancreatitis, and chemotheapy-induced enteropathy, in addition to those disorders mentioned above. In the case of Crohn disease (see also Chapter 48) peptide- and amino acid-based formulas have been used successfully to induce and maintain remission. While a meta-analysis of several randomized, controlled trials indicated that enteral nutrition was less effective than corticosteroids in induction of remission in adults with active Crohn disease,[85] studies in children suggest the opposite.[86] Several studies have also demonstrated that enteral nutrition begun early in the course of acute pancreatitis was superior to parenteral nutrition, with fewer septic complications and lower cost.[87–89] A recent meta-analysis of enteral nutrition in patients with pancreatitis confirms the safety and efficacy of this route of nutrition.[90] Children requiring long-term tube feeding support, without any oral supplementation, should be monitored for the development of macro- and micronutrient deficiencies, for example, vitamin B_{12}, zinc and selenium, especially in those with chronic disease processes and severe diarrhea. Children with severe developmental delay and mental retardation are also at risk for obesity and osteopenia because of a low resting energy expenditure and inactivity. Since vitamins and trace elements in these formulas are present in proportion to the calories, provision of supplemental vitamins and minerals may be necessary if the amount of calories provided is substantially less than the usual recommended dietary allowance for age.

MODULAR FORMULAS

Modular formulas may be complete or intended to supplement the diet, and can be used to satisfy a particular nutrient requirement or to augment an already established feeding regimen (eg, caloric supplementation). For example, a carbohydrate-free product containing protein, fat, vitamins, and minerals can be mixed with another carbohydrate source in the treatment of conditions such as fructose intolerance or galactosemia. Carbohydrate-free formulas are also used in a ketogenic diet for infants and young children with intractable seizure disorders. Protein preparations of casein or whey are available separately without lactose and fat. Human milk fortifiers provide a mixture of protein (cow milk), fat (medium-chain triglycerides), carbohydrate (corn syrup solids), vitamins, and minerals to provide additional nutrients to premature and full-term infants who are fed with breast milk. Problems may arise with their solubility in various commercial formulas, and they may also cause a significant increase in the osmolality of the new mixture.[91] Additionally, when modular formulas are prepared by supplementing a standard liquid diet with extra carbohydrate or fat, changes in the calorie-to-nitrogen ratio occur which may not support optimal growth. In spite of these limitations, when used appropriately, these formulas and additives provide a means of specifically tailoring formulas to meet the nutritional needs of infants and children for whom no standard prepared formula is available. Children with congenital heart disease, renal disease, liver disease, and bronchopulmonary dysplasia are representative of those requiring formulas of increased caloric density because they are often fluid-restricted and have increased calorie requirements.

FORMULAS FOR METABOLIC DISORDERS

Liquid feedings are available to support patients with specific inborn errors of metabolism. These formulas generally use a mixture of amino acids as the protein source, without the specific amino acid(s) that can cause toxicity in patients with that specific metabolic disorder (eg, phenylalanine in phenylketonuria). These formulas are also available for different age groups. Some formulas can be used for more than one metabolic disorder. The formula for patients with Maple Syrup Urine Disease is free of the branched-chain amino acids leucine, isoleucine and valine, and it may also be used for patients with hypervalinemia, methylacetoacetic aciduria, isovaleric acidemia, hyperleucine-isoleucinemia, and leucine-induced hypoglycemia. However, since the omitted amino acid(s) are also essential for growth, a certain minimal amount of additional protein containing the missing amino acid(s) needs to be provided in the diet for these patients. For patients with metabolic disorders of fatty acids, such as long-chain- and very-long-chain acyl CoA dehydrogenase deficiencies, a formula with medium-chain triglycerides as the predominant fat source is used.

The metabolic status of these patients can be easily deranged by an acute viral infection that affects their oral intake. The mainstay of a "sick-day plan" is provision of adequate calories using a glucose polymer to prevent starvation-induced gluconeogenesis and lipolysis and subsequent accumulation of toxic metabolites.[92] Patients must be monitored closely for clinical and laboratory indices of toxicity and deficiency. These formulas include vitamins and minerals age-adjusted to meet the patients' needs. However, one study, based on 3-day diet records, indicated that children with maple syrup urine disease were getting only 21 to 66% of recommended daily allowance for selenium.[93] Until further studies have been completed, the long-term efficacy and safety of some of the metabolic formula products remains to be determined.

FORMULAS INTENDED FOR OLDER CHILDREN WITH CHRONIC ILLNESS

Enteral formulas intended for adults can generally be used for children older than 10 years of age with chronic illness. The osmolality of these formulas varies from 280 to over 600 mosm/L. Sucrose is often one of the carbohydrate ingredients, perhaps to make these formulas more palatable. The sources of protein, carbohydrate, and fat are similar to those used for younger children and infants, but differ in their concentrations. Fiber is added in many of the formulas. In addition to standard formulas for the chronically feeding tube-dependent population, a number of disease-specific formulas are available (see Appendix III). Patients with severe pulmonary compromise may benefit from formulas that provide 40 to 55% of calories from fat, which has a lower respiratory quotient—that is, lower CO_2 production—than carbohydrates.[94] In contrast, formulas with a high-carbohydrate and low-fat content are preferred for patients with burn injury,[95] and patients with renal failure may benefit from formulas with low protein and salt concentrations. Some enteral formulas have increased concentrations of branched-chain amino acids (BCAA) that may be protein-sparing or reduce ammonia production in patients with chronic liver failure. Recently, single photon emission computed tomography (SPECT) in patients with cirrhosis and healthy controls showed that cirrhotic patients had reduced cerebral perfusion in bilateral, central, parietal, angular, and left pericallosal segments as compared to the healthy controls. The cirrhotic patients had improved cerebral perfusion 70 minutes after taking BCAA compared to those given placebo.[96] One randomized, controlled trial in adults with cirrhosis found that those given BCAA supplementation for 1 year had a risk for death or clinical deterioration lower than those given lactalbumin but not lower than those given maltodextrins.[97] A second randomized, controlled trial examined the effect of BCAA supplementation at 12 g/day in comparison to a diet with defined daily protein (1–1.4 g/kg) and caloric (25–35 kcal/kg) intake for 2 years in adults with cirrhosis. The primary end point was a composite of death, liver cancer, rupture of esophageal varices, or progress of hepatic failure, and secondary end points were the serum albumin concentration and quality of life measures. The BCAA group had better outcomes for both primary and secondary endpoints.[98]

FORMULAS FOR CRITICALLY ILL PATIENTS

A number of nutritional substrates may modulate the host response to critical illness including major trauma. Included among these are zinc, glutamine, arginine, and omega-3 fatty acids. Animal, human, and/or epidemiologic data suggest that one or more of these nutrients may be beneficial in the treatment of diseases such as AIDS,[99,100] ulcerative colitis,[101] lupus,[102] rheumatoid arthritis,[103] major burns,[104,105] and coronary heart disease.[106] Possible effects include an improvement in nitrogen balance (arginine), normalization/reduction of platelet aggregation (arginine),[107] substrate availability for energy utilization in rapidly replicating cells such as enterocytes and lymphocytes (glutamine),[108,109] a decrease in the incidence of bacterial translocation (glutamine),[110] and alterations in eicosanoid and cytokine production (omega-3 fatty acids).[111,112]

Some randomized trials have demonstrated decreased infection rates, improved nitrogen balance, a decrease in hospital stay, and decreased cost of care in adult patients on an enteral formula supplemented with glutamine or with added fish oil, arginine and nucleotides.[113–116] These findings were corroborated in a systematic review of 22 randomized, controlled trials involving 2,419 surgical and critically ill patients on either an immune-modulating formula or a standard formula.[117] However, none of the studies has shown any difference in mortality in patients as a result of these supplements, and few studies have been performed in children.

In addition to the "conditional essential nutrients" mentioned above, there is also research interest in the potential therapeutic role of cytokines and growth factors found in the whey fraction of cow milk. Bovine colostrum is currently available as a diet supplement and has been reported to protect against the nonsteroidal antiinflammatory drug-induced increase in intestinal permeability.[118] Studies in vitro have demonstrated that a bovine whey protein concentrate protected against chemotherapy-induced cell injury and suppressed T and B lymphocyte proliferative responses to mitogens.[119,120] Transforming growth factor beta (TGFβ) is present in bovine whey and especially that of colostrum,[121] but it can account for only some of the effects seen with the use of the bovine whey extract or colostrum. An enteral formula with bovine TGFβ administered to 29 children with Crohn disease was effective in causing clinical remission in 79% after 8 weeks, though it was not a randomized or controlled study.[122] Further research will determine whether TGFβ or other factors in bovine whey are useful in the management of patients with severe enteropathies.

In all patients with critical illness on a defined diet, the potential for the development of serious metabolic complications, such as azotemia, hypocalcemia, and hypomagnesemia, is high. Thiamine deficiency has been reported in 10 of 80 critically ill children admitted to the intensive care unit for more than 2 weeks and in 4 of 6 patients on chemotheapy.[123] Thus, in spite of their label as "complete" enteral feedings, chemically defined diets may lack essential nutrients, especially trace nutrients. A regular system for monitoring nutritional adequacy, including anthropometric determinations, must be undertaken. Laboratory tests such as complete blood count, total protein, albumin, ferritin, electrolytes, BUN, creatinine, Ca, Mg, and P require only small volumes of blood, while additional tests such as zinc, copper, folate, B_{12}, vitamin A, vitamin E, and so on may also be indicated, depending on the underlying medical condition.

CONCLUSION

Standard infant formulas have evolved significantly since the turn of the century and now provide some but not all of the advantages seen with breastfeeding. There has also been a significant advance in our ability to provide adequate and appropriate nutrition by the enteral route to infants and children who would otherwise have required extended parenteral nutrition support. In spite of the relative ease of enteral feeding, patients must be carefully observed to ensure that they are growing and developing appropriately and that nutritional deficiencies are not developing. Physicians have the responsibility to inform their patients about the risks of enteral formulas. They must also be informed themselves about the evidence for the purported advantages of various formulas, as research efforts continue to define the role of nutrients and nonnutritive substances in the diet that will promote the health and the normal growth and development of infants and children.

REFERENCES

1. Fomon S. Infant feeding in the 20th century: Formula and beikost. J Nutr 2001; 131:409S–20S.
2. Fomon SJ. Infant feeding. In: Nichols BL, Ballabriga A, Kretchmer N, editors. History of Pediatrics, 1850–1950. Nestle Nutrition Workshop Series, Vol. 22. New York, NY: Raven Press; 1991. p. 77–89.
3. World Health Organization. 1981. International Code of Marketing of Breast Milk Substitutes.
4. Taylor A. Violations of the international code of marketing of breast milk substitutes: Prevalence in 4 countries. BMJ 1998;316:1117–22.
5. Wood AL. The history of artificial feeding in infants. J Am Diet Assoc 1955;31:474.
6. Brennemann J. Artificial feeding of infants. In Abt A, editor. Pediatrics by Various Authors, Vol. 2, Philadelphia: Saunders; 1923.
7. Jacobi A. The gospel of top milk. In Robinson WJ, editor. Colleetana Jacobi, vol. 3. New York: Critic and Guide; 1909.
8. Rules and Regulations. Nutrient requirements for infant formulas (21 CFR 107.100). Fed Reg 1985;50:45106–8.
9. Koletzko B, Baker S, Cleghorn G, et al. Medical Position Paper. Global standard for the composition of infant formula: Recommendations of an ESPGHAN coordinated international expert group. J Pediatr Gastroenterol Nutr 2005;41:584–99
10. Garin EH, Geary D, Richard GA. Soybean formula (NEO-Mull-Soy) metabolic alkalosis in infancy. J Pediatr 1979;95:985–7.
11. Vikhanski L. Fatal flaw in baby formula sparks reform in Israeli ministry. Nat Med 2004;10:7.
12. Center for Disease Control. Enterobacter sakazakii infections associated with the use of powdered infant formula-Tennessee, 2001. MMWR Morb Mortal Wkly Rep 2002;51:297–300.
13. Brett MM, McLauchlin J, Harris A, et al. A case of infant botulism with a possible link to infant formula milk powder: Evidence for the presence of more than one strain of Clostridium botulinum in clinical specimens and food. J Med Microbiol. 2005;54:769–76.
14. FAO/WHO 2004. Enterobacter sakazakii and other microorganisms in powdered infant formulas: Meeting Report (Microbiological Risk Assessment Series No. 6).
15. FDA News. FDA informs public of nationwide infant formula recall. February 22, 2006. http://www.fda.gov/bbs/topics/NEWS/2006/NEW01323.html
16. FDA Recall-Firm Press Release. Abbott voluntarily issues a nationwide recall for one lot of Alimentum, two lots of Similac Advance liquid formula ready-to-feed 32 oz plastic bottles and one lot of hospital discharge kits. September 15, 2006. http://www.fda.gov/oc/po/firmrecalls/abbott09_06.html
17. Fomon SJ. Comparative study of adequacy of protein from human milk and cow's milk in promoting nitrogen retention by normal full term infants. Pediatrics 1960;26:51.
18. Fomon SJ, Ziegler EE. Renal solute load and potential renal solute load in infancy. J. Pediatr 1999;134:11–4.
19. Raiha NCR, Heinonen K, Rassin DK, Gaull GE. Milk protein quantity and quality in low-birth-weight infants. I: Metabolic Responses and Effects on Growth. Pediatrics 1976;57:659–84.
20. Janas LM, Picciano MF, Hatch TF. Indices of protein metabolism in term infants fed human milk, whey-predominant formula, or cow's milk formula. Pediatrics 1985;75:775–84.
21. Jarvenpaa AL, Rassin DK, Raiha NC, Gaull GE. Milk protein quantity and quality in the term infant. II: Effects on acidic and neutral amino acids. Pediatrics 1982;70:221–30.
22. Committee of Nutrition. American Academy of Pediatrics Policy Statement. Iron fortification of infant formulas (RE9865). Pediatrics 1999;104:119–23.
23. Brunser O, Espinoza J, Araya M, et al. Effect of dietary nucleotide supplementation on diarrheal disease in infants. Acta Paediatr 1994;83:188–91.
24. Lama More RA, Gil-Alberdi Gonzalez B. Effect of nucleotides as dietary supplement on diarrhea in healthy infants. An Esp Pediatr 1998;48:371–5.
25. Morillas J, Molto L, Robles R, et al. Lipoprotein changes in small-for-gestational age infants fed nucleotide-supplemented milk formula. Acta Paediatr 1994;83:481–5.
26. Cosgrove M, Davies DP, Jenkins HR. Nucleotide supplementation and the growth of term small for gestational age infants. Arch Dis Child Fetal Neonatal Ed 1996;74:F122–5.
27. Pickering LK, Granoff DM, Erickson JR, et al. Modulation of the immune system by human milk and infant formula containing nucleotides. Pediatrics 1998;101:242–9.
28. Navarro J, Maldonado J, Narbona E, et al. Influence of dietary nucleotides on plasma immunoglobulin levels and lymphocyte subsets of preterm infants. Biofactors 1999;10:67–76.
29. Nelson SE, Frantz JA, Ziegler EE. Absorption of fat and calcium by infants fed a milk-based formula containing palm olein. J Am Coll Nutr 1988;17:327–32.
30. Koo WW, Hammami M, Margeson DP, et al. Reduced bone mineralization in infants fed palm olein-containing formula: A randomized, double-blinded, prospective trial. Pediatrics 2003;111:1017–23.
31. Carnielli VP, Luijendijk IH, Van Goudoever JB, et al. Structural position and amount of palmitic acid in infant formulas: Effects on fat, fatty acid, and mineral balance. J Pediatr Gastroenterol Nutr 1996;23:553–60.
32. O'Connor DL, Hall R, Adamkin D, et al. Ross preterm lipid study. Growth and development in preterm infants fed long-chain polyunsaturated fatty acids: A prospective, randomized controlled trial. Pediatrics 2001;108:359–71.
33. Carlson SE, Salem N, Jr. Essentiality of omega-3 fatty acids in growth and development of infants. In: Simopoulos AP, Kifer RR, Martin RE, Barlow SM, editors. Health Effects of Omega-3 Polyunsaturated Fatty Acids in Seafoods. Basel, Switzerland: Karger; 1991. p. 74.
34. Groh-Wargo S, Jacobs J, Auestad N, et al. Body composition in preterm infants who are fed long-chain polyunsaturated fatty acids: A prospective, randomized, controlled trial. Pediatr Res. 2005;57:712–8.
35. Auestad N, Halter R, Hall RT, et al. Growth and development in term infants fed long-chain polyunsaturated fatty acids: A double-masked, randomized, parallel, prospective, multivariate study. Pediatrics 2001;108:372–81.
36. Hoffman DR, Birch EE, Birch DG, et al. Impact of early dietary intake and blood lipid composition of long-chain polyunsaturated fatty acids on later visual development. J Pediatr Gastroenterol Nutr 2000;31:540–53.
37. Auerstad N, Scott DT, Janowsky JS, et al. Visual, cognitive, and language assessments at 39 months: A follow-up study of children fed formulas containing long-chain polyunsaturated fatty acids to 1 year of age. Pediatrics 2003;112:e177–83.

38. Field CJ, Thomson CA, Van Aerde JE, et al. Lower proportion of CD45RO cells and deficient interleukin-10 production by formula-fed infants, compared with human-fed, is corrected with supplementation of long-chain polyunsaturated fatty acids. J Pediatr Gastroenterol Nutr 2000;31:291–9.
39. Tantibhedyangkul P, Hashim SA. Medium-chain triglyceride feeding in premature infants: Effects on calcium and magnesium absorption. Pediatrics 1978;61:537–45.
40. Tantibhedyangkul P, Hashim SA. Medium-chain triglyceride feeding in premature infants: Effects on fat and nitrogen absorption. Pediatrics 1975;55:359–70.
41. Euler AR, Mitchell DK, Kline R, Pickering LK. Prebiotic effect of fructo-oligosaccharide supplemented term infant formula at two concentrations compared with unsupplemented formula and human milk. J Pediatr Gastroenterol Nutr 2005;40:157–64.
42. Knol J, Scholtens P, Kafka C, et al. Colon microflora in infants fed formula with galacto and fructo-oligosaccharides: More like breast-fed infants. J Pediatr Gastroenterol Nutr 2005;40:36–42.
43. Morrow AL, Ruiz-Palacios GM, Altaye M, et al. Human milk oligosaccharides are associated with protection against diarrhea in breast-fed infants. J Pediatr 2004;145:297–303.
44. Moro G, Arslanoglu S, Stahl B, et al. A mixture of prebiotic oligosaccharides reduces incidence of atopic dermatitis in the first 6 months of life. Arch Dis Child 2006;91:814–9.
45. Tantibhedyangkul P, Hashim SA. Medium-chain triglyceride feeding in premature infants: Effects on calcium and magnesium absorption. Pediatrics 1978;61:537–45.
46. Tantibhedyangkul P, Hashim SA. Medium-chain triglyceride feeding in premature infants: Effects on fat and nitrogen absorption. Pediatrics 1975;55:359–70.
47. Cicco R, Holzman LR, Brown DR, Becker DJ. Glucose polymer tolerance in premature infants. Pediatrics 1981;67:498–501.
48. Fomon SJ, Ziegler EE, Filer LJ, Jr, et al. Methionine fortification of a soy protein formula fed to infants. Am J Clin Nutr 1979;32:2460.
49. Ostrom KM, Cordle CT, Schaller JP, et al. Immune status of infants fed soy-based formulas with or without added nucleotides for 1 year. Part 1: Vaccine responses, and morbidity. J Pediatr Gastroenterol Nutr 2002;34:137–44.
50. Cordle CT, Winship TR, Schaller JP, et al. Immune status of infants fed soy-based formulas with or without added nucleotides for 1 year. Part 2: Immune cell populations. J Pediatr Gastroenterol Nutr 2002;34:145–53.
51. Allen UD, McLeod K, Wang EL. Cow's milk versus soy-based formula in mild and moderate diarrhea: A randomized, controlled trial. Acta Pediatr 1994;83:183–7.
52. Santosham M, Goepp J, Burns B, et al. Role of a soy-based lactose-free formula in the outpatient management of diarrhea. Pediatrics 1991;87:619–22.
53. Steichen JJ, Tsang RC. Bone mineralization and growth in term infants fed soy-based or cow milk-based formula. J Pediatr 1987;110:687–92.
54. Mimouni F, Campaigne B, Neylan M, Tsang RC. Bone mineralization in the first year of life in infants fed human milk, cow milk formula or soy-based formula. J Pediatr 1993;122:348–54.
55. Venkataraman PS, Luhar H, Neylan MJ. Bone mineral metabolism in full term infants fed human milk, cow milk-based and soy-based formulas. Am J Dis Child 1992;146:1302–5.
56. Lonnerdal B. Trace element absorption in infants as a foundation to setting upper limits for trace elements in infant formulas. J Nutr 1989;119:1839–44.
57. Hertrempf E, Cayazzo M, Pizarro F, Stekel A. Bioavailability of iron in soy based formula and its effect on iron nutriture in infancy. Pediatrics 1986;78:640–5.
58. Koo WWK, Kaplan LA, Krug-Wispe SK. Aluminum contamination of infant formulas. JPEN J Parenter Enteral Nutr 1988;12:170–3.
59. Litov R, Sickle VS, Chan GM, et al. Plasma aluminum measurement in term infants fed human milk or a soy-based infant formula. Pediatrics 1989;84:1105–7.
60. Setchell KD, Zimmer-Nechemias L, Cai J, Heubi JE. Exposure of infants to phyto-oestrogens from soy-based infant formula. Lancet 1997;350:23–7.
61. Strom BL, Schinnar R, Ziegler EE, et al. Exposure to soy-based formula in infancy and endocrinological and reproductive outcomes in young adulthood. JAMA 2001;286:807–14.
62. Zeiger RS, Sampson HA, Bock A, et al. Soy allergy in infants and children with IgE-associated cow's milk allergy. J Pediatr 1999;134:614–22.
63. Klemola T, Vanto T, Juntunen-Backman K, et al. Allergy to soy formula and to extensively hydrolyzed whey formula in infants with cow's milk allergy: A prospective, randomized study with a follow-up to the age of 2 years. J Pediatr 2002;140:219–24.
64. Naude SP, Prisloo JG, Haupt CE. Comparison between a humanized cow's milk and a soy product for premature infants. S Afr Med J 1979;55:982–6.
65. Callenbach JC, Sheehan MB, Abramson SJ, Hall RT. Etiologic factors in rickets of very-low-birth-weight infants. J Pediatr 1981;98:800–5.
66. Committee on Nutrition. American Academy of Pediatrics. Soy protein-based formulas: Recommendations for use in infant feeding (RE9806). Pediatrics 1998;101:148–53.
67. Grant C, Rotherham B, Sharpe S, et al. Randomized, double-blind comparison of growth in infants receiving goata milk formula versus cow milk infant formula. J Paediatr Child Health 2005;41:564–8.
68. Martino F, Bruno G, Aprigliano D, et al. Effectiveness of a home-made meat based formula (the Rezza-Cardi diet) as a diagnostic tool in children with food-induced atopic dermatitis. Pediatr Allergy Immunol 1998;9:192–6.
69. Hill DJ, Cameron DJS, Francis DEM, et al. Challenge confirmation of late-onset reactions to extensively hydrolyzed formulas in infants with multiple food protein intolerance. J Allergy Clin Immunol 1995;96:386–94.
70. Saylor JD, Bahn SL. Anaphylaxis to casein hydrolysate formula. J Pediatr 1991;118:71–4.
71. Niggermann B, Nies H, Renz H, et al. Sensitizing capacity and residual allergenicity of hydrolyzed cow's milk formulae: Results from a murine model. Int Arch Allergy Immunol 2001;125:316–21.
72. Hemmer B, Kondo T, Gran B, et al. Minimal peptide length requirements for CD4(+) T cell clones—implications for molecular mimicry and T cell survival. Int Immunol 2000;12:375–83.
73. Mathews DM, Adibi SA. Peptide absorption. Gastroenterology 1976;71:151–61.
74. Phillips AD, Smith MW, Walker-Smith JA. Selective alteration of brush-border hydrolases in intestinal diseases in childhood. Clin Sci 1988;74:193–200.
75. Meeroff JC, Go VL, Phillips SF. Control of gastric emptying by osmolality of duodenal contents in man. Gastroenterology 1975;68:1144–51.
76. Graham GG, Klein GL, Cordano A. Nutritive value of an elemental formula with reduced osmolality. Am J Dis Child 1979;133:795.
77. Sicherer SH, Noone SA, Koerner CB, et al. Hypoallergenicity and efficacy of an amino acid-based formula in children with cow's milk and multiple food hypersensitivities. J Pediatr 2001;138:688–93.
78. Niggermann B, Binder C, Dupont C, et al. Prospective, controlled, multi-center study on the effect of an amino-acid-based formula in infants with cow's milk allergy/intolerance and atopic dermatitis. Pediatr Allergy Immunol 2001; 12:78–82.
79. Awazuhara H, Kawai H, Baba M, Komiyama A. Antigenicity of the proteins in soy lecithin and soy oil in soybean allergy. Clin Exp Allergy 1988;28:1559–64.
80. Andorsky D, Lund D, Lillehei C, et al. Nutritional and other postoperative management of neonates with short-bowel syndrome correlates with clinical outcome. J Pediatr 2001;139:27–33.
81. Fomon SJ. Nutrition of Normal Infants. St. Louis: Mosby-Year Book; 1993.
82. Committee on Nutrition, American Academy of Pediatrics. Follow-up on weaning formulas. Pediatrics 1989;83:1067.
83. Nakao M, Ogura Y, Satake S, et al. Usefulness of soluble dietary fiber for the treatment of diarrhea during enteral nutrition in elderly patients. Nutrition 2002;18:35–9.
84. Homann HH, Kemen M, Fuessenich C, et al. Reduction I diarrhea incidence by soluble fiber in patients receiving total or supplemental enteral nutrition. JPEN J Parenter Enteral Nutr 1994;18:486–90.
85. Griffiths AM, Ohlsson A, Sherman PM, Sutherland LR. Meta-analysis of enteral nutrition as a primary treatment of active Crohn disease. Gastroenterology 1995;108:1056–67.
86. Papadopoulou A, Rawashdeh MO, Brown GA, et al. Remission following an elemental diet or prednisolone in Crohn disease. Acta Paediatr 1995;84:79–83.
87. Olah A, Pardavi G, Belagyi T, et al. Early nasojejunal feeding in acute pancreatitis is associated with a lower complication rate. Nutrition 2002;18:259–62.
88. Windsor AC, Kanwar S, Li AG, et al. Compared with parenteral nutrition, enteral feeding attenuates the acute phase response and improves disease severity in acute pancreatitis. Gut 1998;42:431–5.
89. Kalfarentzos F, Kehagias J, Mead N, et al. Enteral nutrition is superior to parenteral nutrition in severe acute pancreatitis: Results of a randomized prospective trial. Br J Surg 1997;84:1665–9.
90. McClave SA, Chang WK, Dhaliwal R, Heyland DK. Nutritional support in acute pancreatitis: A systematic review. JPEN J Parenter Enteral Nutr 2006;30:143–56.
91. Shike M. Enteral feeding. In: Shils M, et al, editors. Modern Nutrition in Health and Disease, 8th edition. Phildelphia: Lea & Febiger; 1994. p. 1417–29.
92. Dixon MA, Leonard JV. Intercurrent illness in inborn errors of intermediary metabolism. Arch Dis Child 1992;67: 1387–91.
93. Gropper SS, Naglak MC, Nardella M, et al. Nutrient intakes of adolescents with phenylketonuria and infants and children with maple syrup urine disease on semisynthetic diets. J Am Coll Nutr 1993;12:108–14.
94. Ferreira I, Brooks D, Lacasse Y, Goldstein R. Nutritional intervention in COPD: A systemic overview. Chest 2001;119:353–63.
95. Garrel DR, Razi M, Lariviere F, et al. Improved clinical status and length of care with low-fat nutrition support in burn patients. JPEN J Parenter Enteral Nutr 1995;19:482–91.
96. Yamamoto M, Iwasa M, Matsumura K, et al. Improvement of regional cerebral blood flow after oral intake of branched-chain amino acids in patients with cirrhosis. World J Gastroenterol 2005;11:6792–9.
97. Marchesini G, Bianchi G, Merli M, et al (Italian BCAA Study Group). Nutritional supplementation with branched-chain amino acids in advanced cirrhosis: A double blind, randomized trial. Gastroenterology 2003;124:1980–2.
98. Muto Y, Sato S, Watanabe A, et al. Long-Term Survival Study Group. Clin Gastroenterol Hepatol 2005;3(7): 705–13.
99. Bell SJ, Apour CS, Burke PA, Forse RA. Enteral formula: An update. In Torosian M, editor. Nutrition for the Hospitalized Patient: Basic Science and Principles of Practice. New York: Marcel-Dekker; 1995. p. 293–306.
100. Bell SJ, Mascioli EA, Forse RA, Bistrian BR. Nutrition support and the HIV virus. Parasitology 1993;107:S53–67.
101. Hawthorne AB, Daneshmend TK, Hawkey CJ, et al. Treatment of ulcerative colitis with fish oil supplementation: A prospective 12 month randomized controlled trial. Gut 1992;33:922–8.
102. Drevon CA. Marine oils and their effects. Nutr Rev 1992;50:38–45.
103. Kremer JM, Jubiz W, Michalek A, et al. Fish-oil fatty acid supplementation in active rheumatoid arthritis. Ann Intern Med 1987;106:497–503.
104. Trocki O, Heyd TJ, Waymack JP, et al. Effects of fish oil on postburn metabolism and immunity. JPEN J Parenter Enteral Nutr 1987;11:521–8.
105. De-Souza DA, Greene LJ. Pharmacological nutrition after burn injury. J Nutr 1998;128:797–803.
106. Burr ML, Fehily AM, Gilbert JF, et al. Effect of changes in fat, fish, and fibre intakes on death and myocardial infarction: Diet and reinfarction trial (DART). Lancet 1989;2:757–61.
107. Wolf A, Zalpour C, Theilmeier G, et al. Dietary L-arginine supplementation normalizes platelet aggregation in hypercholesterolemic humans. J Am Coll Cardiol 1997;29:479–85.
108. Windmueller HG, Spaeth AE. Respiratory fuels and nitrogen metabolism in vivo in small intestine of fed rats. J Biol Chem 1980;255:107–12.
109. Calder PC. Glutamine and the immune system. Clin Nutr 1994;13:2–8.
110. Gianotti L, Alexander JW, Gennari R, et al. Oral glutamine decreases bacterial translocation and improves survival in experimental gut-origin sepsis. JPEN J Parenter Enteral Nutr 1995;19:69–74.
111. Hwang D. Essential fatty acids and immune responses. FASEB J 1989;3:2052–61.
112. Endres S, Grobani R, Kelley VE, et al. The effect of dietary supplementation with n-3 polyunsaturated fatty acids on the synthesis of interleukin-1 and tumor necrosis factor by mononuclear cells. New Engl J Med 1989;320:265–71.
113. Gottschlich MM, Jenkins M, Warden GD, et al. Differential effects of three enteral dietary regimens on selected outcome variables in burn patients. JPEN J Parenter Enteral Nutr 1990;14:225–36.
114. Daly JM, Lieberman MD, Goldfine J, et al. Enteral nutrition with supplemental arginine, RNA, and omega-3 fatty acids in patients after operation: Immunologic, metabolic, and clinical outcome. Surgery 1992;112:56–67.
115. Bower RH, Cerra FB, Bershadsky B, et al. Early enteral administration of a formula (Impact) supplemented with arginine, nucleotides, and fish oil in intensive care unit patients: Results of a multicenter, prospective, randomized, clinical trial. Crit Care Med 1995;23:436–49.
116. Jones C, Palmer TE, Griffiths RD. Randomized clinical outcome study of critically ill patients given glutamine-supplemented enteral nutrition. Nutrition 1999;15: 108–15.
117. Heyland DK, Novak F, Drover JW, et al. Should immunonutrition become routine in critically ill patients? A systematic review of the evidence. JAMA 2001;286:944.

118. Playford RJ, MacDonald CE, Calnan DP, et al. Co-administration of the health food supplement, bovine colostrum, reduces the acute non-steroidal anti-inflammatory drug-induced increase in intestinal permeability. Clin Sci (Lond) 2001;100:627–33.
119. Cross ML, Gill HS. Modulation of immune function by a modified bovine whey protein concentrate. Immunol Cell Biol 1999;77:345–50.
120. Taylor VL, Goddard C, Read LC. A milk growth factor extract reduces chemotherapeutic drug toxicity in epithelial cells in vitro. In vitro Cell Dev Biol Anim 2001;37: 310–8.
121. Pakkanen R. Determination of transforming growth factor-beta (TGF-beta 2) in bovine colostrum samples. J Immunoassay 1998;19:23–37.
122. Fell JM, Paintin M, Arnaud-Battandier F, et al. Mucosal healing and a fall in mucosal pro-inflammatory cytokine mRNA induced by a specific oral polymeric diet in paediatric Crohn disease. Aliment Pharmacol Ther 2000;14:281–9.
123. Seear M, Lockitch G, Jacobson B, et al. Thiamine, riboflavin, and pyridoxine deficiencies in a population of critically ill children. J Pediatr 1992;121:533–8.

Enteral Nutrition

Maria-Luisa Forchielli, MD, MPH, FACG
Julie Bines, MD, FRACP

The delivery of food via a tube directly into the gastrointestinal tract has been described since pre-Christian times. In ancient Egypt, and later in Greece, feeds were introduced into the rectum, and in the nineteenth century, rudimentary tubes were used to infuse basic foods such as broths, eggs, milk, and even alcohol into the esophagus and stomach.[1] Despite the increasing sophistication in other areas of medical care over the past century, treatment with enteral nutrition had been slow to develop. However, over the past two decades, enteral nutrition therapy has undergone a renaissance.[2–7] Many patients who previously received parenteral nutrition are now successfully managed with enteral nutrition alone or in combination with parenteral nutrition.[2,3,8] This has been made possible by the increasing range of options for gastrointestinal access, improved delivery systems, and advances in enteral nutrition formulas. Home enteral nutrition therapy is now an important adjunct to the management of infants and children with chronic disease or feeding problems.[6]

PRINCIPLES OF ENTERAL NUTRITION

Enteral nutrition therapy has a number of advantages over parenteral nutrition in the management of patients requiring nutritional support. Enteral nutrition aids in the preservation of gastrointestinal function by the provision of enteral nutrients and is easier, safer and less costly to administer. However, despite these relative advantages, the delivery of safe and effective enteral nutrition therapy may still present challenges for families and caregivers in terms of time, technical expertise, and cost.[9]

PRESERVATION OF GASTROINTESTINAL FUNCTION

Enteral nutrition mimics the normal gastrointestinal response following the ingestion of a meal, with the exception of the oral phase. The presence of nutrients within the intestinal lumen provides stimulation of gastrointestinal function and helps to maintain the complex intraluminal environment via a number of key mechanisms.

Intraluminal nutrients stimulate gastrointestinal neuroendocrine function, effecting motility, and digestion through the secretion of digestive enzymes and gastrointestinal hormones. Intestinal functional and structural changes occur through local and systemic interaction of nutrients and neuroendocrine peptides, cytokines, and hormones.[10–12] The list of these mediators is constantly growing and includes gastrin; enteroglucagon; peptide YY; interleukin 3, 11, or 15; epidermal growth factor; growth hormone; insulin-like growth factors I and II; glutathione; fiber; short-chain fatty acids; glutamine; triglycerides; dietary nucleotides; and polyamines.[10–12] Monosaccharides and fatty acids can influence the secretion of enteroglucagon and peptide YY and via these mediators effect mucosal growth and decrease intestinal transit time.[13] Carbohydrate, protein, zinc, magnesium, potassium, or manganese deficiency can modify the effect of growth hormone and insulin-like growth factor II.[14–16]

Intraluminal nutrients assist in the maintenance of gut mucosal mass, including the gut-associated lymphoid tissue (GALT). The GALT consists of the lamina propria, intraepithelial lymphocytes, immunoglobulin A (IgA), Peyer's patches, and mesenteric nodes and is responsible for processing intestinal antigens.[17] During periods of "bowel rest," such as occur with intravenous feeding and starvation, there is a reduction in gut mass and the function of the GALT is suppressed.[17] This has been associated with a reduction in IgA secretion and increased gut permeability resulting in increased bacterial adherence to the intestinal wall, cellular injury, and bacterial penetration with adverse systemic host responses.[17–19] In animal studies, an association between parenteral nutrition and bacterial translocation has been reported; however, these results have not been replicated in humans.[20] Oral or enteral feeding may reduce the potential risk of bacterial translocation, except when disturbances in intestinal permeability are related to an underlying disease process (eg, short-bowel syndrome) or the chemical composition of the enterally provided substance (eg, blue food dye).[17,21–23]

The gastrointestinal tract is a delicate ecosystem with the balance determined and maintained through the interplay between nutrients, bacteria, and the intestinal defense system (luminal, mucosal, and submucosal immune system). Intraluminal nutrients play an important role in the development and function of the gastrointestinal ecosystem through the modulation of the resident bacterial flora. The key contribution of prebiotics to development of normal intestinal flora and the intestinal immune system has been recognized.[24] The interaction between specific bacteria and toll-like receptors located on intestinal enterocytes and lymphoid cell from as early as birth influences the development of physiologic intestinal immune response.[24] The provision of nutrients via the intestine results in improved utilization of digested and absorbed nutrients. Gut and liver work in synchronism utilizing and eliminating nutrients. The actions of digestion and absorption in the gut followed by a first-pass metabolism in the liver contribute to maintenance of physiologic metabolism.

COST

Although enteral nutrition therapy is more costly than standard feeds, compared to parenteral nutrition therapy, enteral nutrition is approximately two- to fourfold cheaper on an inpatient or out-patient basis.[2,3,9,25–27] Based on US Medicare charges, the annual cost of providing enteral nutrition per patient is approximately US$9,605 ± US$9,327 compared with US$55,193 ± US$30,596 for parenteral solutions.[4] In addition, the frequency and cost of hospitalization is higher for patients supported on parenteral nutrition therapy compared with enteral nutrition therapy.[4]

MANAGEABILITY AND SAFETY

Due to advances in technology of enteral feeding tubes and delivery systems, specialization of health professionals, and better education of parents and caregivers, the administration of enteral nutrition has been associated with improved clinical outcome and safety profiles.[28] Enteral nutrition therapy is easier and safer to administer than is parenteral nutrition. Not only are the risks of intravenous access avoided, but there is also a wider margin for error with most metabolic complications. As a result, enteral nutrition therapy is easier to administer in low-intensity hospitals and patient care settings, including the home. However, compared with normal diet, tube feedings require extra time and effort to administer and this additional care need may contribute to increased burden and stress for families and caregivers.[9,29]

INDICATIONS FOR ENTERAL NUTRITION

Enteral nutrition should be considered for any patient with a functional gastrointestinal tract who requires nutritional support. Enteral feeding may be required if adequate oral nutrient intake cannot be provided in children with growth failure, weight faltering, or weight deficit. This may be defined as a child with a weight or weight for height less than 5th percentile below the mean for sex and age and/or crossing of two growth curves on the weight, height, or weight/height percentile charts, no weight gain or weight loss during the last 2–3 months and/or triceps skin fold measurements less than 5th percentile. Children with severe neurological dysfunction may require prolonged periods devoted to oral feeding. Tube feeding can provide welcome respite for families and caregivers who previously may have spent over 6 hours a day assisting with oral feeding. Patients with severe neurological disabilities associated with oropharyngeal dysfunction may be at risk of chronic aspiration. The risk of aspiration may be reduced by tube feeding. Children with cognitive, pyschiatric, and behavioral disorders that interfere with oral feeding may develop nutritional deficiency. Enteral tube feeding may provide a safe and reliable route for the delivery of essential nutrients. Enteral feeding may be an option for children with increased energy needs that are difficult to achieve via the oral route such as may occur in cystic fibrosis or congenital heart disease. Disorders of the gastrointestinal tract that result in excessive gastrointestinal losses, such as short-bowel syndrome, secretory diarrhea, or dysmotility syndromes, may have improved absorption and reduction in losses with small volume continuous enteral feeds of a specialized formula. Due to their composition these formulas are often unpalatable and require tube administration to obtain adequate volumes of administration. Most patients receiving parenteral nutrition will also receive some enteral nutrition. Enteral nutrition usually provides an important transition stage as the patient progresses from parenteral nutrition to oral diet. Although enteral nutrition has mainly a therapeutic intent, it can also be used to prevent the development of malnutrition, such as can occur during cancer chemotherapy.[30] A more recent concept is that of minimal enteral feeding, in which enteral nutrition is provided at a very slow rate and volume with the aim of presenting nutrients to the intestinal mucosa without attempting to contribute significantly to total-body nutrition.[31] Advances in the understanding of the role of nutrients in the modification of inflammation and specific disease processes have led to the development of disease-specific formulas (eg, for Crohn's disease).[32] Enteral nutrition has been advocated as a primary treatment for conditions associated with a metabolic disturbance, such as the use of gastrostomy tube feeding to infuse a ketogenic diet in children with epilepsy.[33]

Indications for enteral nutrition in pediatric patients are listed in Table 1. With developments in options for gastrointestinal access, delivery systems, and enteral formulas, the list of absolute contraindications for enteral nutrition therapy has been reduced significantly. Contraindications include gastrointestinal ischemia, including necrotizing enterocolitis and toxic megacolon, severe intractable vomiting or diarrhea, diffuse peritonitis, and mechanical intestinal obstruction.[7,34] Extreme care should be taken when administering enteral nutrition in patients in whom the gastrointestinal blood flow could be compromised, such as during treatment with hypothermia, low cardiac output, multiorgan failure, chronic occlusion, compression syndromes, or infusions of specific drugs. However, in addition to a reduction of caloric deficits, enteral nutrition has been shown to protect the splanchnic oxygen balance during intraoperative duodenal feedings in severely burned patients.[35]

Table 1 Indications for Pediatric Enteral Nutrition

1. Inability to ingest adequate nutrition orally
   - i. Disorders of sucking and swallowing
     - Prematurity
     - Neurological and neuromuscular disorders (eg, cerebral palsy, dysphagia)
   - ii. Congenital abnormalities of the upper gastrointestinal tract or airways
     - Tracheoesophageal fistula
   - iii. Tumors
     - Oral cancer
     - Head and neck cancer
   - iv. Trauma
   - v. Critical illness
     - Mechanical ventilation
   - vi. Severe gastroesophageal reflux
   - vii. Drug related
     - Chemotherapy
   - vii. Severe food aversion
   - viii. Severe depression
2. Disorders of digestion or absorption
   - i. Cystic fibrosis
   - ii. Short-bowel syndrome
   - iii. Inflammatory bowel disease
   - iv. Congenital abnormalities of the gastrointestinal tract
     - Microvillus inclusion disease
     - Tufting enteropathy
   - v. Enteritis
   - vi. Intractable diarrhea of infancy
   - vii. Auto-immune enteropathy
   - viii. Immunodeficiency
     - AIDS
     - Severe combined immunodeficiency
   - ix. Postgastrointestinal surgery
   - x. Graft-versus-host disease
   - xi. Solid organ transplantation
   - xii. Intestinal fistulae
   - xiii. Chronic liver disease
     - Biliary atresia
     - Alagille's Syndrome
3. Disorders of gastrointestinal motility
   - i. Chronic pseudo-obstruction
   - ii. Ileocolonic Hirschsprung's disease
4. Increased nutritional requirements
   - i. Cystic fibrosis
   - ii. Chronic renal disease
   - iii. Congenital heart disease
   - iv. Chronic pulmonary disease
     - Bronchopulmonary dysplasia
   - v. Burn injury
5. Psychiatric and behavioral disorders that interfere with oral intake
   - i. Anorexia nervosa
   - ii. Severe behavioral disorders
     - Autism
6. Metabolic diseases
   - i. Inborn errors of metabolism
   - ii. Diabetes mellitus
7. Acute or acute/chronic pancreatitis
8. Administration of disease treatment
   - Ketogenic diet in epilepsy
   - Administration of pharmaceutical agents
   - Bowel washouts in severe chronic constipation

ROUTES OF ADMINISTRATION

During enteral nutrition therapy, nutrients are directly delivered via a tube into the stomach, duodenum, or jejunum. The tube is inserted either through the nose or mouth for short-term enteral nutrition (<3 months) or through a surgically or endoscopically created stoma for long-term enteral nutrition (>3 months). The choice of the location and the route of administration will depend on the patient's underlying medical or surgical condition, including gastrointestinal anatomy and function, the indication and duration of enteral nutrition therapy, and psychosocial factors. Additional factors, such as local technical expertise, tube availability, and cost, will also influence the route and type of device selected. As a general principle, tubes that deliver nutrients into the stomach are the preferred choice. Gastric tubes are easier to insert and allow a physiological digestive process with bolus or continuous feeding regimens. However, in the presence of gastric outlet dysfunction, severe gastroesophageal reflux, or gastric paralysis, trans-pyloric access may be indicated.

NONINVASIVE GASTROINTESTINAL ACCESS FOR ENTERAL NUTRITION

Nonsurgical or nonendoscopic placement of a feeding tube through the mouth or nose is the most common method of establishing gastrointestinal access in infants and children due to the ease of placement and cost. The nasal access is usually preferred, except in preterm infants or in patients with nasopharyngeal abnormalities or obstruction as may occur following trauma or with congenital malformations. The tube is generally of small diameter (5 to 12 Fr) and is well suited to nutritional support of short or intermediate duration or intermittent nutritional therapy. However, the small luminal diameter renders these tubes susceptible to blockage particularly when medications or nutrient supplements are infused. To minimize the risk of blockage it is recommended that the tube is flushed after each feed and each infusion of medication.

There is a wide range of enteric feeding tubes available for use in children. Early nasogastric tubes were composed of polyethylene or polyvinyl chloride. Because of their inherent stiffness, they required regular replacement to reduce the risk of skin necrosis, gastric ulceration, and perforation. Current feeding tubes are made from flexible silicone, polyurethane, or elastomer and may require a stylet to assist placement. Despite the increased flexibility, they have a longer life span and may incorporate specialized features. These features may include (1) aids for tube placement and to prevent dislodgment, including water-activated hydrophilic lubricant at the distal end and in the lumen, plastic-coated stylets to minimize the risk of tube perforation, marked reference points on the tubing to allow proper tube selection and positioning, and a rounded, non-weighted bullet-shaped tip to favor insertion; (2) a combination of distal-end and side exit ports to prevent blockage; and (3) a double port at the proximal end to allow for feeding and side injections. Accurate tube positioning is enhanced by radiopaque material within the tube wall. Tube sizes differ in length and port diameter, with the longer tubes suited for jejunal feeding (Table 2). Weighted tips are designed to allow gravity to assist with small-bowel placement and to prevent retrograde displacement. However, with the possible exception of patients requiring mechanical ventilation, the weighted tubes have not been shown to have significant benefit over non-weighted tubes.[36,37]

Nasogastric Tube Placement

With training, nasogastric tubes can be safely inserted by allied health staff, caregivers, family members, and even the patients themselves. Prior to insertion, the desired length of the tube is estimated by measuring the distance from the tip of the nose to the ear and down to the xiphoid. This provides an estimate of the distance between the external nares and the gastroesophageal junction. An additional measurement from the xiphoid to the right or left lateral costal margin provides an estimate of the distance from the gastroesophageal junction to the pylorus. A small amount of lubricant is applied to the nostril and along the length of the tube. The tube is then advanced through the nares past the nasopharynx into the stomach. Voluntary swallowing and head flexion by the patient can aid the passage of the tube. Once the tube is in place, the stylet is removed and the proximal end of the tube is secured close to or behind the ear. The tube location must be verified before commencing the infusion. Fluoroscopy or endoscopy can be used to assist difficult gastric tube placement as well as magnetic assisted devices.

Table 2 A Guide to Pediatric Enteric Tubes

	Tube French size	Tube length (cm)
Premature to neonate	4–5	38–41
Infants to young children	5–8	41–91
Older children to adolescents	8–14	91–114

Nasoduodenal or Nasojejunal Tube Placement

Advances in tube technology and the techniques for placement of nasoenteric tubes in children have provided an opportunity for postpyloric feeding in children in whom gastric feeding is difficult or contraindicated. As a result there has been renewed enthusiasm for the use of postpyloric feeding in the critically ill. Compared to intragastric feeding, postpyloric feeding in the critically ill is associated with a higher caloric intake and avoids complications associated with parenteral nutrition therapy. In a recent study in critically ill children requiring mechanical ventilation the risk of aspiration was similar in patients receiving either postpyloric or intragastric feeding.[38]

Nasoenteric tubes can be placed blindly or under fluoroscopic or endoscopic guidance.[39] The blind tube placement technique relies on the spontaneous passage of an enteric feeding tube from the stomach into the small intestine. This can occur after a period of hours or days and be facilitated by positioning the patient on the right side using the "corkscrew" technique, whereby a wire stylet is twisted when the tube is in the stomach. The use of air insufflation, a pH sensing tube, or the administration of prokinetic drugs, such as metoclopramide, may assist in tube placement.[40,41] The role of erythromycin for postpyloric intubation is controversial, with both positive and negative results observed in children.[42,43] In a randomized controlled trial comparing enteric-tube placement in critically ill children using either the standard technique, the standard technique with gastric insufflation, or the standard technique with erythromycin, a high rate of successful placement was reached at the first attempt (88%) in all groups, with approximately 95% of the tubes placed at the second attempt.[44] The operator's experience rather than the specific technique was correlated with successful placement.

Postpyloric tube placement can also be performed under fluoroscopic guidance.[45] In this method, the passage of the tube is monitored with the aid of the radiopaque markings on the tube. Endoscopic placement of a nasoenteric tube has a number of advantages over the other methods of placement. The tube is placed under direct vision with a guidewire within the tube lumen using a drag and pull technique.[39,46] Endoscopic placement avoids exposure to ionizing radiation and can be performed in high-dependency patient care areas such as the intensive care unit.[39] The application of magnets to guide tubes into small bowel seems promising although pediatric experience using this technique is limited.

INVASIVE ACCESS FOR ENTERAL NUTRITION

Placement of a feeding tube using surgical, radiological, or endoscopic techniques is recommended for long-term enteral nutrition therapy or gastric decompression. There are a number of important advantages of these tubes over nasogastric or nasoenteric tubes in children. The gastrostomy or jejunostomy tube can be maintained in position for a longer period because it is fixed against the anterior abdominal wall. The tube does not interfere with breathing and avoids potential complications of chronic nasal discharge, sinusitis, and developmental abnormalities of the nose. In addition, for some children, repeated insertion of a nasogastric tube is associated with psychological trauma and feeding aversion. Once the decision has been made to place a gastrostomy or jejunostomy tube for long-term home enteral nutrition therapy, education of the patient, parents, and caregivers should be initiated.

Gastrostomy Tube

Gastrostomy tubes are usually large-bore tubes (14–24 Fr) to deliver high feeding volumes and medications with minimal risk of occlusion. The original gastrostomy tubes were made from latex with a balloon retention device, such as the Foley catheter. Today, most gastrostomy tubes are made of a biocompatible material such as silicone or polyurethane, and are anchored in place with either parallel bumpers, or a mushroom or balloon at the gastric site with a retention disk at the skin. This allows the tube to be secured to the stomach wall without sutures. The gastrostomy tube can extend through the stoma with at least two access ports for simultaneous administration of feed and medical medications. A wide range of gastrostomy tubes is available for use in children. These tubes can be summarized into the following types: (i) standard gastrostomy tube with a cupped internal bolster, a sliding external bolster, and a separate cap to be placed at the distal end of the tube with a large feeding infusion port and a small side port for medications; (ii) a balloon gastrostomy replacement tube with a balloon-type internal bolster, a sliding external bolster, and a one-piece external tube ending with three openings for feedings, medications and inflation; (iii) low-profile gastrostomy devices with a balloon-type or a stylet distensible internal bolster and a shaft of a predetermined length to suit the fistula length. The external bolster contains the access infusion port. When in use a connector is used to allow infusion of formula or medications. Most low-profile devices have an antireflux valve to prevent the release of gastric contents when the tube is accessed. This device is easily disguised under clothing and the feeding tube is connected only at the time of infusion; as a result it is particularly popular with older children and adolescents (Figure 1).

The ideal position for gastrostomy tube placement is on the greater curvature of the stomach with the stoma sited on the anterior abdominal wall just below the costal margin with consideration of the axis of bending and clothing. However, if proximity to the small intestine is a priority, such as in the use of the gastric stoma for placement of a jejunostomy tube, placement close

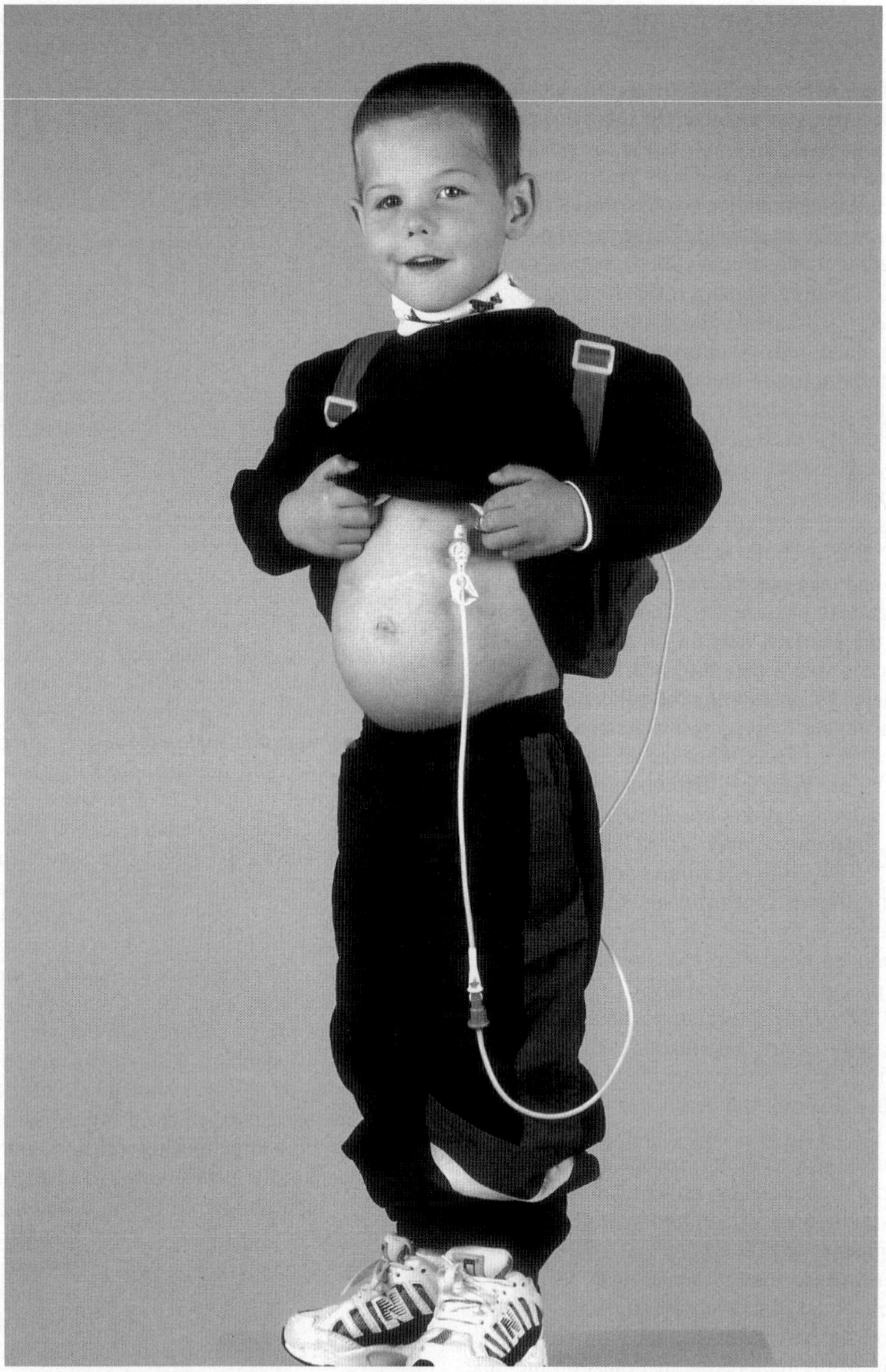

Figure 1 A child with PEG ready for a physical education session.

to the antrum may be preferred. The external bolster should be routinely checked for secure position to avoid tube migration and to prevent injury to the abdominal wall due to compression between the internal and external bolsters. The stomal site requires regular cleaning to avoid chemical injuries from the gastric secretions and infection. Stomal granulomas and skin irritation or infection need prompt attention with referral to a stomal therapist if necessary, to prevent further complications. Eventually gastrostomy tubes will degrade over months to years due to physical or chemical trauma from yeast contamination or medications. The most vulnerable gastrostomy devices are balloon-type skin level devices which have a high rate of inner balloon rupture limiting their longevity to an average of 5 months.[47] However, these devices have been associated with few major complications.

The introduction of the percutaneous endoscopic gastrostomy (PEG) technique has revolutionized the placement of enteric feeding tubes in children.[48] This relatively simple and fast procedure can be performed during esophagogastroduodenoscopy in an endoscopy suite with the use of conscious sedation and local anesthesia or general anesthesia with a success rate of up to 96% even in small infants (<3.5 kg).[49] Although several techniques (Ponsky pull, Sachs-Vine push, Russel introducer) have been developed, all have in common the basic principle that the endoscope locates the site of tube placement from within the stomach while transillumination of the light from the endoscope through the abdominal wall identifies the site of skin incision. Using the Ponsky pull technique, the anterior abdominal wall is indented at the point of maximal transillumination of the endoscope light. This should be seen as a sharp indentation on the gastric wall by the endoscopist. A poorly defined indentation could indicate an overlying viscus (eg, transverse colon) and either an alternative site should be sought or the procedure converted to a surgical gastrostomy. After sterile preparation of the abdominal wall, local anesthetic is instilled and a small incision is made. The endoscopist distends the stomach with air and prepares the snare. A cannula is inserted perpendicular to the abdominal wall through the incision and punctures the gastric wall. The stylet is then removed; a thick suture is introduced along the cannula and is snared by the endoscopist. The endoscope and the suture are retrieved. The gastrostomy tube is tied to the suture and is slowly pulled back, by tension at the abdominal wall, through the mouth, along the esophagus, and into position on the gastric wall under direct vision by the endoscopist. Once the position has been verified by endoscopy, the external bolster can be opposed to the abdominal wall and the tube cut to the desired length. Postinsertion edema at the stoma site is common, and care should be taken not to pull the bolster too tight. To minimize infection at the stoma site, perioperative antibiotic prophylaxis is advocated.[50] The tube can be used within 6 to 24 hours in most patients.

Immediate complications of PEG placement include abdominal wall skin infection, necrosis of the skin or mucosa caused by a tight bolster, perforation of a viscus, hepatogastric-, gastrocolic- or colocutaneous fistula, and pharyngeal or esophageal trauma associated with the passage of the internal fixation device. Pneumoperitoneum is common following PEG placement and does not necessarily indicate a complication of insertion. Long-term complications include gastroesophageal reflux, granulation tissue formation, recurrent stoma-site infection, stoma enlargement, and dislodgment of the tube distally into the small bowel or proximally along the fistula track (ie, buried bumper syndrome).[51] Occlusions are rare events and can be easily treated with warm water instilled by a syringe, pancreatic enzymes and bicarbonate solution, or specific tube cleaning brushes. Contraindications to the PEG technique include gastric varices, severe esophageal stricture, or abnormalities that might restrict the ability to oppose the stomach against the anterior abdominal wall, such as ascites, previous gastrointestinal surgery, or abnormalities in gastrointestinal rotation or position. Extreme care must be taken in patients with musculoskeletal deformities, hyperinflation of the lungs, organomegaly, immunodeficiency disease, cyanotic heart disease, or prior gastrointestinal surgery, including ventriculoperitoneal shunts.

Table 3 Bedside Evaluation Tests for Tube Placement in Children[61–66]

Aspirate	Color and appearance	pH value	Pepsin (μg/mL)	Trypsin (μg/mL)	Bilirubin (mg/dL)
Gastric secretions	Yellow-gray or white-tan; cloudy	< 6	> 100 (> 20)*	< 30 (< 50)*	< 5
Intestinal secretions	Green	> 6	< 100 (< 20)*	> 30 (> 50)*	> 5
Respiratory secretions	Yellow-gray; mucoid	6–8	< 100 (< 20)*	< 30 (< 50)*	< 5

*Trypsin and pepsin ranges specific for children.

Radiological placement of gastrostomy tubes has been shown to be safe and cost-effective in pediatric patients.[52,53] During this procedure, the stomach is distended with air instilled via a nasogastric tube. The stomach is then directly punctured under fluoroscopic control. A guidewire is inserted, followed by an introducer, a dilator, and then finally the feeding tube. The major disadvantage of this procedure is the exposure to ionizing radiation during the procedure.

With the development of the PEG technique surgical placement of a gastrostomy tube has become generally restricted to patients who have a contraindication for PEG placement, had a failed PEG placement, or require another surgical procedure in conjunction with tube placement, such as a fundoplication. Placement of the feeding tube can be performed using an open surgical approach or by laparoscopy. In the classic open gastrostomy technique (Stamm and Witzel techniques), the tube is inserted into the stomach along a serosa-lined tract, whereas in the revised version (Janeway technique), a small portion of the stomach is used to make a mucosa-lined tube attached to the skin as a modified fistula. The procedure for laparoscopic gastrostomy tube placement requires the creation of pneumoperitoneum and insertion of an umbilical catheter. The anterior stomach wall is fastened to the abdominal wall with temporary sutures. An opening (by a needle and a J-wire) is made in the stomach and progressively enlarged using dilators to finally allow the insertion of the feeding tube.[54] In experienced hands, laparoscopic gastrostomy is faster than the open procedure and is associated with reduced length of hospital stay, and patient discomfort.[55] Laparoscopy is also a useful aid during PEG placement by monitoring tube placement by direct vision.[56]

Jejunostomy Tube

The percutaneous endoscopic technique can be used to place an enteric tube using either a direct approach (direct percutaneous endoscopic jejunostomy, DPEJ) or by the creation of a PEG and placement of a specialized double-lumen tube (percutaneous endoscopic gastrostomy jejunostomy, PEJ).[57] The method for the DPEJ is similar to the PEG technique but with the endoscope placed in the jejunum. Transillumination of the bowel through the anterior abdominal wall and a sharp indentation easily seen within the small bowel by the endoscopist is necessary prior to the direct puncture of the duodenum or jejunum.[57] The suture is advanced along the cannula and is grasped by forceps rather than a snare. The PEGJ can be inserted as part of an initial PEG procedure or through an existing gastrostomy stoma. The specialized tube has a gastric lumen and port and another longer lumen and port for the small bowel. This enables gastric decompression during postpyloric feeding. Once the tube is inserted into the stomach, the intestinal lumen of the tube can then be advanced into the duodenum or jejunum under direct endoscopic vision using a guidewire and grasping forceps.

Among the range of surgical techniques described for jejunostomy tube placement, the needle-catheter jejunostomy is the most common. Using this technique, a large-bore needle is tunneled through the seromuscular layers of the jejunum distal to the ligament of Treitz. The jejunum is then anchored to the anterior abdominal wall and the tube is secured to the skin. The tunneling procedure limits reflux of formula and heals quickly upon tube removal. In the presence of intestinal adhesions, severe intestinal disease, or high risk of infection or bleeding, straight insertion of a tube into the jejunum (Stamm technique) or direct jejunal stoma (Maydl technique) might be preferred. Laparoscopic placement of a jejunostomy tube requires two additional cannulae to bring the proximal jejunum into proximity of the abdominal wall and secure it there.[58] Fluoroscopic J-tube positioning is also possible using similar techniques as described above for the insertion of an intragastric tube.

J-tubes are generally smaller in diameter (9–12 Fr) than gastrostomy tubes and tend to have a shorter lifespan (3–6 months). Dislodgement of gastro-jejunal tubes is not uncommon and may be a limiting factor for the use of this type of tube in patients requiring long-term home enteral nutrition.[59]

MONITORING TUBE POSITION AND CONDITION

Before infusing any fluid through a gastric or enteric feeding tube, the position of the tube should be confirmed. Complications owing to incorrect placement or tube dislodgment can potentially be fatal. Plain or contrast radiography is a universally accepted method for assessing tube position. However, repeat radiological studies are impractical and potentially unsafe in patients requiring long-term enteral nutrition therapy. As a result, bedside methods have been developed to screen for correct tube position. These include clinical observation, auscultation, and analysis of tube aspirate. If a nasogastric tube is incorrectly placed in the airways, cough, choking, and pulmonary distress can occur. However, these features can be minimal or absent if the tube is small or if tracheal reflexes are absent (eg, in coma or intubated patients). Although commonly used, auscultation does not reliably distinguish between either gastric and pulmonary placement or gastric and small-bowel placement.[60] Aspirates from either the feeding tube or the lungs can be assessed for color, appearance, pH level, and enzyme measurements (Table 3).[61–66] Aspirate pH value can be measured with a qualitative colorimetric test strip or a quantitative pH meter. Bilirubin can also be measured with spectrophotometer readings, using urine bilirubin test strips, or on the colorimetric visual bilirubin scale. Detection of gastric pepsin in tracheal aspirates relies on a Western blot immunoassay using a rooster polyclonal antibody against human pepsin.[38] Trypsin also can be used to screen for intestinal juice present in the aspirate. Both trypsin and pepsin are secreted at a physiologically lower level in infants and young children compared to adults but continue to be effective tools in the discrimination of tube placement.[64] However, measurement of gastric aspirate may be modified by fasting, intermittent or continuous feeding, and use of gastric acid suppressants. Due to the difficulties in verifying tube position, new approaches are being developed to confirm correct tube position. The measurement of myoelectric slow-wave frequencies has been proposed because these differ in the stomach (3 cycles/min) and the duodenum (11 to 12 cycles/min) and are not influenced by other gastrointestinal contractions.[67] The "bubbling under water" method relies on the exit of bubbles from the external end of the tube when placed under water if the tube has been misplaced in the lungs. However, misplacement of the tube into the bronchioles or pleura will not produce bubbles. Other options under development include electromagnetic navigation devices, self-propelling tubes, fiberoptic tube tips, and ultrasonography-guided tube placement.[68–71]

In the case of PEG or other invasive tube placement it is recommended to routinely examine the stoma tract and the access device to prevent the occurrence of major complications. For instance, incorrect positioning of the external bolster, cracks or ruptures, discoloration or irregular beading of the tube, stoma leaking are examples of initial problems of access devises to be looked for and promptly managed. In patients in whom dislodgment or migration of the gastrostomy or jejunostomy tube is suspected, endoscopy or liquid contrast radiology may assist in defining the tube position.

DELIVERY OF ENTERAL NUTRITION

The method of delivery of enteral nutrition will depend on the route of administration (gastric, duodenal, or jejunal), characteristics of the feeding tube (small- versus large-bore catheter), the desired feeding pattern (bolus, intermittent, cyclic, or continuous), and the cost and availability of equipment (by gravity or syringe, or by infusion pump). Bolus tube infusion usually mimics the normal meal pattern based on age. Intermittent or cyclic feedings are delivered at a specified rate over 1 or more hours, with 4 to 8 hours per day of gut rest allowing freedom from tubes and pumps for a period of the day. Continuous feeding delivers a constant-rate infusion, usually by an infusion pump, over the entire day or a prolonged period. The infusion pump allows accurate nutrient delivery with less intestinal pressure. Some pumps are specifically designed for outdoor activities and may be carried in a small backpack improving mobility for children on long-term enteral nutrition therapy.

Gastric feeding is preferred because it is considered more physiologic, allows bolus feeds through large-bore tubes, and is generally cheaper and easier to administer.[7] Many patients intolerant of bolus feeds can be successfully fed intragastrically using an intermittent or continuous feeding regimen. Jejunal feeding is an option for patients with disorders of gastric or esophageal anatomy or function and in the nutritional management of the critically ill.[2,3,39] Jejunal feedings are usually delivered as an intermittent or continuous infusion because rapid-rate infusion of nutrients is often limited by abdominal discomfort, diarrhea, or dumping syndrome.

There are specific physiologic and metabolic considerations associated with continuous-rate feeding. During continuous intragastric feeding, gastric emptying increases parallel to the rate of infusion if the infusion rate is maintained at less than 3 kcal/minute.[72] However, increased caloric density, fat, and osmolarity of the formula can delay gastric emptying. The protein composition is also an important factor influencing the gastric emptying rate. Whey-based enteral formulas enter the duodenum faster than casein-based enteral formulas.[73] In animals, the absorptive capacity of the proximal small intestine is unchanged during continuous enteral nutrition. However, the protein and DNA content of the distal small intestine and the enzymatic and functional capacity of the distal small intestine and colon are reduced.[72] The relative lack of nutrients reaching the distal gut during jejunal feeding with an elemental or hydrolyzed formula could explain this observation. This might provide an opportunity for the treatment of gastrointestinal inflammatory diseases, such as Crohn's disease, by providing nutrients to the proximal intestine but reducing antigenic stimulation to the distal gut.[74] In addition, energy expenditure owing to the thermic effect of feeding is lower in patients receiving continuous enteral nutrition than in patients receiving the same quantity of nutrients delivered by bolus.[75] The continuous delivery of nutrients into the small intestine affects glycemic control by modifying the typical fluctuating pattern of insulin and glucagon production.[76,77] The reduction in steatosis during continuous enteral nutrition compared with parenteral nutrition with the same carbohydrate intake is also consistent with this observation. Energy intake goals are more successfully achieved in critically ill patients receiving postpyloric feeds compared with those receiving intragastric feeds.[78]

Enteral feedings should be monitored in terms of intestinal tolerance: nausea, vomiting, diarrhea, abdominal distension, and bowel movements. Tube-feeding residuals are an indirect parameter to determine enteral feeding tolerance. Residuals should be checked more frequently during the first days from starting enteral feedings, when changing infusions or during symptoms. Residuals are checked by aspirating through a tube with a syringe gastric or intestinal fluids. Changes in infusions are recommended when residual volume exceeds twice the hourly infusion volume in continuous feedings or 50% of the infusion volume in bolus. Tubes should be irrigated after any infusion (feeding or medication). Irrigation volume to be instilled into tubes after every meal or medication can vary between 3 and 5 mL in infants and between 20 and 30 mL in children and adults.

ENTERAL FORMULAS

In the early days of enteral nutrition, a mixture of blenderized diets and milk products was administered through a large bore feeding tube. This approach was associated with nutritional imbalance, micronutrient deficiencies, feeding intolerance, and tube blockage. Today, there is a wide range of enteral nutrition products suitable for use in infants and children (see Chapter "Enteral Products" in Appendix III). Most formulas are designed to provide complete macro- and micronutrient requirements as the sole nutritional intake. Specific needs of different ages and stages of development are reflected in the composition of preterm infant, full-term infant, and pediatric enteral nutrition formulations. Modular formulas are specialized combinations of nutrients that provide a nutritional supplement or fulfill a specific nutrient requirement. A recent area of development has been the introduction of disease-specific enteral formulas. These formulas aim to modify the metabolic or gastrointestinal response to feeds by limiting some nutrients, supplementing others, or both (eg, branched-chain amino acid formula for hepatic failure and immune-enhancing formula for critical illness).[79–82]

The majority of patients with normal gastrointestinal tracts will tolerate the gastric administration of a polymeric formula. Polymeric formulas are based on intact protein or polypeptides usually derived from cow's milk or soybeans. The nitrogen to nonnitrogen calorie ratio approximates 1 to 150. Carbohydrates are sourced from different starches, including corn and tapioca. Maltodextrin and hydrolyzed cornstarch, glucose-derived saccharides, and corn syrup are commonly used. Formulas can have different lactose contents. Fats are usually present as polyunsaturated fatty acids from corn, safflower, sunflower, or soybean oil or from animal fat. The content of medium-chain tryglicerides is increased in formulas developed for the treatment of patients with malabsorption. Some enteral nutrition formulas contain soluble fiber. The soluble fiber is added primarily to normalize gastrointestinal transit, but after it is converted to short-chain fatty acids it provides an additional source of calories and can exert trophic effects on the colonic mucosa. In all complete enteral formulas, electrolytes, vitamins, and trace elements are added to provide the Dietary Reference Intakes of micronutrients and minerals at the target volume. However, in a study of stable young children receiving long-term enteral feeding and without excessive gastrointestinal losses, the serum vitamin B_{12} and copper levels exceeded the reference range despite receiving a median energy intake of only 75% of their estimated requirement.[83] At standard dilution, the caloric content of infant formula is usually 0.67 kcal/mL, and of standard enteral formula, 1 kcal/mL. Concentrated enteral nutrition formulas are also available (1.5 and 2 kcal/mL). The osmolality of enteral formulas can range widely depending on the nutrient composition and caloric density (~ 200 to 750 mOsm/L).

In patients with underlying gastrointestinal disease or those requiring jejunal feeding, an oligomeric formula might be indicated. The protein in oligomeric formulas has been hydrolyzed to peptides or a combination of peptides and amino acids. The carbohydrate complexity varies among formulas, although many oligomeric formulas are lactose free. A proportion of medium-chain triglycerides is usually provided to improve fat absorption. Elemental formulas contain completely digested macronutrients, such as monosaccharides, medium-chain triglycerides, and amino acids, with an essential to nonessential amino acid ratio reflecting high biologic protein values. Lactose and gluten are absent and residues are low. The unpalatability and high osmotic load of simple sugars and amino acids generally limit the use of elemental formulas to tube feeding when feeding intolerance occurs with other types of formula (eg, severe malabsorption or short-bowel syndrome).

Advances in the understanding of the role of specific nutrients and their effects on metabolism have led to modification of enteral nutrition formulas for treatment of specific diseases. The aim of the disease-specific formulas is to provide therapeutic benefits in addition to the maintenance of general nutritional status. Glutamine-enriched formula has been advocated for the prevention and treatment of intestinal mucosa injury associated with chemotherapy and critical illness.[79,81] Formulas supplemented with arginine, glutamine, ribonucleic acid nucleotides, medium-chain triglycerides, and/or omega-3 fatty acids have been also been advocated as enhancing the immune system of critically ill patients.[79–82] However, whether the benefit of glutamine or immune-enhancing formulas in malnourished and critically ill children outweighs the additional cost of these formulas remains controversial.[84,85] Omega-3 fatty acids have been supplemented in infant formula to enhance neurologic development.[86] Evidence for improved clinical and economic outcomes of many of the disease-specific formulas, compared with

Table 4 Complications Associated with Enteral Tube Feeding

Complication	Possible cause	Prevention and treatment
	Most common tube feeding complications	
Tube occlusion	Failure to flush tube regularly, inappropriate feed or medications placed down tube, inadequately dissolved feed, high-energy feed	Flush tube regularly with water; use prescribed feeds and Medications only
Tube dislodgment	Inadequate securing of tube, inadequate monitoring of tube position	Check tube placement every 8 hours during continuous feeds and before every bolus or intermittent feed
Accidental tube removal	Inadequate securing mechanism, deterioration of tube (balloon rupture)	Review method of securing tube; consider specific dressings or clothing to prevent access to tube; regularly review tube function and integrity; ensure availability of replacement or "emergency" tube to prevent stoma closing prior to reinsertion
Diarrhea	Gastroenteritis, medications (antibiotics, sorbitol-containing drugs), rapid administration or bolus feeds, malabsorption, formula intolerance (lactose, hyperosmolar)	Review for possible causative factors including medications, formula, and gastrointestinal absorptive function; consider changing rate of delivery or formula as indicated (reduced osmolality, fiber enriched, lactose free)
Bloating, abdominal cramps	Gastrointestinal dysmotility, bowel obstruction, intolerance to formula (lactose intolerance), bacterial overgrowth	Reduce or cease feeds according to severity until cause is defined; consider investigations to address possible causes
Constipation	Inadequate fluid intake or large fluid losses, gastrointestinal dysmotility, medications, immobilization, underlying medical condition	Correct fluid losses and provide adequate ongoing fluid requirements; review medications; consider stool softeners or fiber supplementation
Dumping syndrome	Rapid infusion of high-volume or hypertonic feeds into duodenum or jejunum, postgastric surgery or vagotomy, gastrostomy sited in distal gastric antrum	Administer continuous feeds, reduced volume or osmolality of formula; use uncooked cornstarch
Nosocomial infection (bacteremia, pneumonia)	Enteral feed or equipment contamination, aspiration, increased risk with gastric acid suppression in paralyzed or ventilated Patients	Change sets every 24 hours; limit feed hang time; use sterile system and sterile water to reconstitute feeds; culture feeds and equipment if contamination suspected; review for "silent" reflux or aspiration or tube dislodgment
Metabolic complications (increased or decreased glucose, phosphate, potassium or magnesium)	Complication of the primary disease (renal failure) or treatment (amphotericin), refeeding syndrome	Correct any significant electrolyte abnormalities prior to initiating enteral nutrition; undertake regular biochemical monitoring particularly in malnourished patients; gradually increase feed volume and concentration if at risk of refeeding syndrome
Malabsorption	Underlying gastrointestinal disease (cystic fibrosis), inappropriate formula selection or rate of administration	Assess absorptive status and alter formula and rate of delivery as appropriate
Perforation	Tube malposition, wrong type of tube, disorders of mucosal Integrity	Ensure appropriate tube selection and placement technique; regularly check tube position; surgical treatment might be required
	Gastric tube feeding (general)	
Vomiting, nausea	Gastroenteritis, intolerance to formula, rate of infusion too rapid, medications, bacterial contamination of feed, delayed gastric Emptying	Review feeding regime and medications; culture feeds and equipment if contamination is suspected; consider intermittent or continuous infusion, postpyloric administration, or prokinetic agents
Gastroesophageal reflux	Underlying abnormality of esophagus or stomach associated with reflux or medical illness (eg, neurologic, pulmonary diseases), mechanical aspects related to tube	Assess for underlying reflux; consider antireflux therapies or Postpyloric feeding
Large-volume gastric as pirates	Delayed gastric emptying related to underlying medical condition (eg, neurologic disease, critical illness, diabetes, intestinal pseudo-obstruction) or medications	Review medications; consider continuous or postpyloric feeds or prokinetic agents
Pulmonary aspiration	Incorrect tube placement, tube dislodgment, gastroesophageal reflux, gastric stasis, or vomiting (neurologic disorders, coma)	Cease feeds and check tube position; consider postpyloric feeding
Gastrointestinal bleeding	Tube-related irritation, ulceration, or perforation; vitamin K deficiency	Review tube position and gastrointestinal status; assess for alternative tube placement sites; try gastric acid suppression; supplement with vitamin K when indicated
Cellulitis	Postplacement contamination of wound, inadequate cleaning of stoma site, bolster too tight, chronic leakage through stoma	Perioperative antibiotics during tube placement, regular skin care, antibiotic therapy as appropriate; check tube and stoma site for areas of mechanical irritation and poor fit
Stoma leakage	Site infection; incorrect tube size, type, or position; perished tube; gastric stasis (eg, diabetes, pseudo-obstruction); medications	Examine site; assess tube integrity, suitability, and position; check balloon volume; replace with larger or different type of tube if appropriate; treat stoma site infection
	Nasogastric tube feeding	
Nasal airway obstruction	Inappropriate tube size, nasopharynx disorders	Insert smaller-bore tube
Chronic nasal discharge or ulceration	Inappropriate tube size or composition, immunodeficiency, disorder of mucosal or skin integrity	Re-evaluate tube size and type; regularly change tube; assess for alternative sites for tube placement
Epistaxis		
Sinusitis or otitis media		
Feeding aversion	Repeated tube replacement in infants and young children, development implications of tube feeding	Consider alternatives to nasogastric route in infants requiring long-term enteral nutrition; involve speech therapist early
Esophageal perforation	Incorrect tube placement, ulceration related to tube position, underlying disorders of mucosal integrity (eg, epidermolysis bullosa)	Use appropriate tube placement technique; regularly check tube position
Pulmonary intubation	Incorrect tube placement or tube dislodgment	Use appropriate tube placement technique; take particular care in children with neurologic disorders or disturbances of conscious state

(continued)

Table 4 Complications Associated with Enteral Tube Feeding *(continued)*

Complication	Possible cause	Prevention and treatment
	Gastrostomy tube feeding	
Granulation tissue formation	Chronic inflammation at stoma site, leakage, tube moving too freely along tract	Check tube size, type, and position; specialized dressings, corticosteroid cream, or cautery might be required
Site swelling or tenderness	Site infection, migration of tube along tract, tube shaft too short or bolster too tight	Examine site; tube removal and replacement might be required
Fasciitis	Incorrect tube or bolster position	Remove tube; obtain surgical opinion; administer intravenous antibiotics
Buried bumper syndrome	Retaining device and bolster secured too tight	Remove tube; administer antibiotics
Gastritis, gastric ulceration, or perforation	Trauma caused by tube, often of wall opposite insertion site, wrong tube type (composition or design)	Consider change in tube design to minimize trauma and gastric acid suppression
	Duodenal or jejunal tube feeding	
Reflux into stomach	Tube placed in proximal small intestine, dysmotility	Consider more distal placement
Bowel obstruction	Tube too large, tube malposition, disorder of gastrointestinal anatomy	Review tube size and position
Volvulus	Tube providing an abnormal fixation point	Remove tube; obtain surgical review

standard formulas, is still required to justify recommendations of their routine use.[79,81]

COMPLICATIONS OF ENTERAL NUTRITION THERAPY

Despite the potential benefits of enteral nutrition, complications can occur (Table 4).[87–91] Fortunately, life-threatening events are rare. However, problems related to the tube, the method of delivery, or the composition of the formula can seriously interfere with achieving nutritional goals. To minimize complications, prior consideration should be given to the patient's medical and physical condition, including any metabolic or electrolyte abnormalities, previous diet, dietary tolerance, and the time that has elapsed since the last significant oral or enteral nutrition.

GASTROINTESTINAL COMPLICATIONS

Intestinal discomfort, bloating, cramping, diarrhea, nausea, and vomiting can occur during enteral feeding. Whenever symptoms occur, the position and integrity of the tube should be confirmed. In some cases, these symptoms relate to the high osmolality of the formula or the rate of infusion and alterations to the formula composition or infusion rate will be sufficient to improve feeding tolerance. The assessment of a sample of stool from a patient with diarrhea can assist in directing further investigations as required (bacterial culture, guaiac test, absorptive status by pH, microscopy, and reducing substances). The use of concomitant medications should be reviewed for possible drug-nutrient interactions or gastrointestinal side effects. Bacterial contamination of the feed or the tubing can result in diarrhea or vomiting. Therefore the method of formula preparation and storage and the technique of hanging and administering should be reviewed.[87] Samples of the feed, the tubing, and the feeding reservoirs are necessary to confirm this diagnosis.

Patients with a primary gastrointestinal disorder could be at risk of bacterial overgrowth owing to disturbances in gut motility. Bacterial culture of an intestinal biopsy or a lactulose breath hydrogen test will assist in establishing the presence of bacterial overgrowth of the small intestine. Constipation associated with enteral nutrition is uncommon and when it occurs is usually associated with insufficient fluid or fiber intake, intestinal dysmotility or obstruction, or medications. Gastroesophageal reflux can be exacerbated by tube feeding. The nasogastric tube can split open the lower esophageal sphincter, and irritation owing to tube trauma can contribute to lower sphincter incompetence. Placement of a gastrostomy tube plicates the stomach against the anterior abdominal wall, distorting the normal gastric anatomy, with a potential impact on gastric function. Owing to the frequency of this complication in high-risk patients, such as those with cerebral palsy or cystic fibrosis, assessment for gastroesophageal reflux with a 24-hour pH probe and nuclear gastric emptying study may be considered prior to gastrostomy tube placement.

If the gastrostomy or jejunostomy tube is no longer required, the tube can be removed after consideration of the original method of insertion. For tubes inserted using a PEG, DPEJ, or PEGJ technique, the tube can usually be withdrawn and the stoma edges opposed using a dressing or suture. In most cases, this will be sufficient to allow closure of the stoma and tract within days to weeks. This process can be assisted with the use of gastric acid suppression aimed at minimizing gastric secretion. If the gastro- or jejunocutaneous fistula does not close spontaneously, formal surgical closure might be required. Patients in whom the gastrostomy or jejunostomy tube has been inserted using the traditional surgical approach usually require surgical closure of the fistula.

PULMONARY COMPLICATIONS

Aspiration of gastric contents—and pneumonia owing to aspiration—incorrect tube placement, or tube dislodgment into the airway can be fatal. Children at high risk include those with chronic neurologic disease, depressed conscious state, intestinal dysmotility, severe gastroesophageal reflux and patients requiring mechanical ventilation. In addition to checking tube position, tracheal aspirates can be measured for glucose content or fat-laden macrophages. The addition of blue dye to the formula to assess tube position and aspiration patients should be avoided because it has been associated with fatalities.[26]

INFECTIOUS COMPLICATIONS

Irritation due to the mechanical trauma of tube or exposure to gastric or intestinal secretions renders the skin and mucosa susceptible to infection. A well-fitting, well-maintained device specifically designed for enteral nutrition use will limit this complication. Contamination of the formula and the delivery set can occur as a result of preparation or administration of the feed.[87] Bacterial contamination resulted to occur in 35 to 50% of enteral bags at the end of infusions in a pediatric hospital.[92] Feeding devices also harbor biofilm growth of various bacteria and fungi in the outer and inner surfaces with potential risk of local and systemic infections.[93] Longterm nasogastric and nasoenteric tubes are associated with chronic nasal discharge, otitis media, and sinusitis.

MECHANICAL COMPLICATIONS

Mechanical complications related to enteral tube feeding are common. However, these can generally be treated and do not involve the same risks as a central venous catheter in critically ill children.[88–91] Tube occlusion can occur as a result of problems related to the tube (length, caliber, characteristics), the infusion (formula, drugs), pumps and clamps, the method and rate of delivery, and the level of tube care (method, frequency). Infusions that contain a highly viscous formula or crushed or powdered drugs are often associated with tube occlusion. If flushing the tube with warm water is unsuccessful in clearing the blockage, a number of other options are available. The instillation of pancreatic enzyme supplements is sometimes successful in clearing a blockage. The use of meat tenderizer is not recommended because of its high sodium content and the risk of tube breakage during infusion. Cytology brushes, guidewires, neonatal tubes inserted into larger tubes, and specially designed catheters have been developed to treat tube occlusion. A biliary catheter for endoscopic retrograde cholangiopancreatography was described for the treatment of an occlusion in a nasojejunal tube.[94] The key to the prevention of tube occlusion is careful monitoring and repeated flushing of the tube. Mixing of drugs and formula should be avoided.

Irritation can occur anywhere along the interface between the tube and the skin or mucosa, resulting in inflammation, ulceration, or even perforation of any structure present along the tube lining (eg, laceration or bleeding of nasal or oral cavity, perforation of trachea or pulmonary parenchyma, perforation or laceration of the gut). Granulation tissue formation at the stoma site can occur as a result of chronic irritation. The migration of tubes with an internal balloon or retention device distally along the gastrointestinal tract can cause bowel obstruction. Migration of a gastrostomy tube along the fistula tract can cause pain and inflammation around the site or the buried bumper syndrome.[51] Complications such as dislodgment, ampullary obstruction, and jaundice can occur with jejunal tubes.

METABOLIC COMPLICATIONS

Metabolic complications associated with enteral nutrition are uncommon. Patients with chronic malnutrition or cardiac, hepatic, or renal impairment require careful monitoring of fluid and electrolyte status to prevent imbalance.[95] Patients commencing enteral nutrition who have had a period of prolonged fasting, inadequate nutritional intake, or significant weight loss (>10% body weight) should be monitored for the metabolic features of the refeeding syndrome. Daily monitoring of fluid status, serum sodium, potassium, phosphate, and magnesium levels is required until stability has been achieved with feeding advancement. Serum glucose levels, which are usually stable during continuous enteral nutrition therapy, can increase with overfeeding or as part of a stress response during critical illness. Hypoglycemia during intermittent feeding can be prevented with a progressive slowing of the rate of infusion in the period prior to disconnection. Dumping syndrome is reported in patients during enteral feeding in response to the presence of nutrients within the proximal intestine. This is can be associated with a rapid infusion of a formula with a high nutrient density and is treated with modifications to the formula (such as adding uncooked cornstarch) or rate of delivery.

HOME ENTERAL NUTRITION

Over the past two decades, advances in tube design, methods of delivery, and formulas have made enteral nutrition therapy safer, cheaper, and easier to administer for a wide range of disorders in childhood.[5,96,97] With attention to appropriate patient selection, education, and providing adequate technical support, enteral nutrition therapy can be safely and effectively provided in the home.[97] In 1992, data from Medicare and insurance companies estimated that there were about 152,000 patients of all ages receiving home enteral nutrition in the United States.[5] The rapid growth of home enteral nutrition therapy observed in the United States in 1987 had reached a plateau in 1992.[5] In contrast, in Britain, home enteral nutrition therapy has been increasing rapidly—at a rate of up to 20% per year—and is about 10 times more common than home parenteral nutrition therapy.[97] Of patients receiving home enteral nutrition therapy in Britain, 40% are children, compared with 5 to 20% in three US cohorts.[98]

Table 5 List of Common Medications That May Contain Sorbitol

Acetaminophen (Tylenol pediatric elixir, suspension, and maximum strength liquid)
Acyclovir (Zovirax suspension)
Al/MgOH (Maalox suspension and extra strength plus)
Al/MgOH/simethicone (Mylanta cherry cream-, milk cream-, double strength-liquid)
AlOH (Alternagel, Gaviscon liquid) and AlOH gel
Aminocaproic acid (amicar syrup)
Calcium carbonate ($CaCO_3$ oral suspension), calcium glucobionate (neo-calglucon)
Carbamazepine (tegretol susp)
Chloral hydrate (syrup)
Cimetidine (Tagamed liquid)
Clemastine (Tavist syrup)
Dexamethasone (oral solution)
Diazepam (oral solution)
Digoxin (elixir)
Diphenhydramine (Benadryl elixir)
Felbamate (Felbatol susp)
Ferrous sulfate (drops, syrup)
Furosemide (solutions)
Hydroxyzine (Vistaril susp)
Ibuprofen (Pedia-Profen susp)
Lithium citrate
Metaproterenol and metaproterenol sulfate (syrup)
Metoclopramide (syrup, oral solution)
Milk of magnesia
Multivitamins (Iberet 250, 500 liquid)
Naproxen (Naprosyn oral suspension)
Nitrofurantoin (Furadantin suspension)
Oxybutynin (Ditropan syrup)
PE/Tripolidine (Children's actifed liquid)
PE/PPA/chlorpheniramine/phenyltoloxamine (Naldecon Ped drops, syrup)
Potassium chloride (Rum-K)
Prednisolone (Pediapred)
Propanolol (oral solution)
Ranitidine (Zantac syrup)
Sodium polystyrene sulfonate (suspension)
Sucralfate (Carafate suspension)
Tetracyline (sumycin)
Theophylline (oral solution, Slo-phyllin syrup, Theoclear syrup)
Trimethoprim/Sulfamethoxazole (Septra suspension, sulfa/trimethoprim, bactrim susp)
Valproic acid (Depakene syrup)
Vitamin E (Aquasol E drops)

Best-practice guidelines for the administration of safe and effective home enteral nutrition therapy have been developed by national nutrition support organizations.[7,97] These guidelines take into consideration patient selection, assessment, monitoring, and the development of the enteral nutrition plan, including methods of implementation, documentation, and protocols for termination of therapy. Training patients, their families, or caregivers in safe and effective home enteral nutrition therapy is ideally performed by a multidisciplinary team, including the gastroenterologist or surgeon, dietitian, stomal therapist, or nurse specialist.[97] An essential component of a successful home enteral nutrition service is availability of health professionals to provide support to the patient or caregivers at home to address concerns and direct appropriate intervention when necessary. A mechanism should be available to manage after-hours tube malfunction. To facilitate this process, all patients should carry a card with the type and size of tube and the date of last insertion clearly listed. Written documentation of routine tube care, as well as the recommended steps to take in the event of tube malfunction, is invaluable to the patient and caregiver at home.

Regular review by the multidisciplinary home enteral nutrition team is cost-effective and improves quality of care.[99] At regular outpatient appointments, all aspects of the administration of enteral nutrition can be assessed. The tube is examined for size, function, and integrity and can be changed if necessary. The stoma site is examined. The method of delivery is reviewed, along with protocols for formula preparation. The intake of formula is assessed with reference to the nutritional goals. The patient is examined for growth, weight gain, and nutritional status. Laboratory markers of nutritional status can be obtained as indicated.

INTERACTIONS BETWEEN DRUGS AND ENTERAL FEEDING

Administration of medications through an enteral feeding tube, either in combination with formula or alone, is problematic because only a few drugs have been tested and approved for tube delivery. Characteristics of the composition of the tube can influence the binding of drug to the tube wall (eg, carbamazepine reacts with polyvinyl chloride feeding tubes).[7] Interactions between a drug and a nutrient can result in an undesired side effect of the drug or feeding intolerance. Drug-nutrient interactions can result in changes in medication bioavailability, distribution, metabolism, or excretion.[100] Common drug-nutrient interactions are described with substances containing calcium, zinc, and iron, or when acidic and neutral liquid medications are combined with casein or soy protein. Impaired absorption of phenytoin is well documented in the literature and occurs as a result of pharmacokinetic incompatibility.[7] Long-chain fatty acids can enhance the absorption of lipid-soluble drugs but hasten the degradation of other medications (eg, carbamazepine) (Table 5).

Liquid preparations of medications are preferred by children and for enteral administration.

However, liquid drug preparations tend to have a high osmolality (1,000 and 11,000 mOsm/kg) and may cause feeding intolerance when infused into the jejunum. The osmotic properties of these liquids are usually attributable to the presence of sorbitol, propylene glycol, or polyethylene glycol. Although included among the inactive ingredients on drug labels, the amount is not usually quantified. Osmotic diarrhea and delayed gastric emptying can occur if the cumulative dose is more than 20 g (range, 7.5 to 30 g).

CONCLUSION

Advances in tube placement techniques, tube design, delivery systems, and enteral formulas have enabled the safe and effective provision of enteral nutrition therapy for a broad range of disease indications in children. Successful enteral nutrition therapy has limited the use of parenteral nutrition therapy, resulting in important benefits in terms of safety, manageability, and cost. The management of nutritional problems in patients with chronic diseases, such as neurologic disorders, Crohn's and cystic fibrosis, can be enhanced by home enteral nutrition therapy. The development of disease-specific formulas provides new therapeutic options. Further improvements in technology enabling light, simple, feeding pumps and modifications to tube design will continue to assist in the administration of enteral nutrition to children.

REFERENCES

1. Harkness L. The history of enteral nutrition therapy: From raw eggs and nasal tubes to purified amino acids and early post-operative jejunal delivery. J Am Diet Assoc 2002;102:399–404.
2. Braga M, Gianotti L, Gentilini O, et al. Early postoperative enteral nutrition improves gut oxygenation and reduces costs compared with total parenteral nutrition. Crit Care Med 2001;29:242–8.
3. de Lucas C, Moreno M, Lopez-Herce J, et al. Transpyloric enteral nutrition reduces the complication rate and cost in the critically ill child. J Pediatr Gastroenterol Nutr 2000;30:175–80.
4. Reddy P, Malone M. Cost and outcome analysis of home par-enteral and enteral nutrition. JPEN J Parenter Enteral Nutr 1998;22:302–10.
5. North American Home Parenteral and Enteral Nutrition Patient Registry. Annual report with outcome profiles 1985–1992. Albany, NY: Oley Foundation; 1994.
6. Howard L, Ament M, Fleming CR, et al. Current use and clinical outcome of home parenteral and enteral nutrition therapies in the United States. Gastroenterology 1995;109:355–65.
7. Board of Directors and Clinical Guidelines Task Force, American Society for Parenteral and Enteral Nutrition. Guidelines for the use of parenteral and enteral nutrition in adults and pediatric patients. JPEN J Parenter Enteral Nutr 2002;26:18SA–9SA.
8. Braunschweig CL, Levy P, Sheean PM, et al. Enteral compared with parenteral nutrition: A meta-analysis. Am J Clin Nutr 2001;74:534–42.
9. Heyman MB, Harmatz P, Acree M, et al. Economic and psychologic costs for maternal caregivers of gastrostomy-dependent children. J Pediatr 2004;145:511–6.
10. Wong WM, Wright NA. Epidermal growth factor, epidermal growth factor receptors, intestinal growth, and adaptation. JPEN J Parenter Enteral Nutr 1999;23:S83–8.
11. Chen K, Nezu R, Wasa M, et al. Insulin-like growth factor-1 modulation of the intestinal epithelial cell restitution. JPEN J Parenter Enteral Nutr 1999;23:S89–92.
12. Ziegler TR, Estivariz CF, Jonas CR, et al. Interactions between nutrients and peptide growth factors in intestinal growth, repair, and function. JPEN J Parenter Enteral Nutr 1999;23:S174–83.
13. Aponte GW, Fink AS, Meyer JH, et al. Regional distribution and release of peptide YY with fatty acids of different chain lengths. Am J Physiol 1985;249:745–50.
14. Thissen JP, Ketelslegers JM, Underwood LE. Nutritional regulation of the insulin-like growth factors. Endocr Rev 1994;15:80–101.
15. Ninh NX, Thissen JP, Collette L, et al. Zinc supplementation increases growth and circulating insulin-like growth factor I (IGF-1) in growth-retarded Vietnamese children. Am J Clin Nutr 1996;63:514–9.
16. Dorup I. Magnesium and potassium deficiency. Its diagnosis, occurrence and treatment in diuretic therapy and its consequences for growth, protein synthesis and growth factors. Acta Physiol Scand 1994;618:S1–55.
17. Li J, Kudsk KA, Gocinski B, et al. Effects of parenteral and enteral nutrition on gut-associated lymphoid tissue. J Trauma 1995;39:44–51.
18. Alverdy JC, Aoys E, Moss GS. Total parenteral nutrition pro-motes bacterial translocation from the gut. Surgery 1988;104:185–90.
19. Kudsk KA, Li J, Renegar KB. Loss of upper respiratory tract immunity with parenteral feeding. Ann Surg 1996;223:629–38.
20. Sedman PC, MacFie J, Palmer MD, et al. Preoperative total par-enteral nutrition is not associated with mucosal atrophy or bacteria translocation in humans. Br J Surg 1995;82:1663–7.
21. Alverdy JC, Aoys E, Moss GS. Effect of commercially available chemically defined liquid diets on the intestinal microflora and bacterial translocation from the gut. JPEN J Parenter Enteral Nutr 1990;14:1–6.
22. Weber TR. Enteral feeding increases sepsis in infants with short bowel syndrome. J Pediatr Surg 1995;30:1086–9.
23. Maloney JP, Bhargava R, Ryan TA, et al. FD&C Blue No. 1 food dye is a mitochondrial poison that can be absorbed from enteral tube feedings in sepsis: A report of 3 deaths linked to systemic absorption. JPEN J Parenter Enteral Nutr 2001;25:S25.
24. Forchielli ML, Walker WA. The role of gut-associated lymphoid tissues and mucosal defence. Br J Nutrition. 2005;93: S41–8.
25. Adams S, Dellinger P, Wertz MJ, et al. Enteral versus parenteral nutrition support following laparotomy for trauma: A randomized prospective trial. J Trauma 1986;26:882–91.
26. Bower RH, Talamini MA, Sax HC, et al. Postoperative enteral vs parenteral nutrition. Arch Surg 1986;121: 1040–5.
27. Deswarte-Wallace J, Firouzbakhsh S, Finklestein JZ. Using research to change practice: Enteral feedings for pediatric oncology patients. J Pediatr Oncol Nurs 2001;18:217–23.
28. Anonymous. Making health care safer: A critical analysis of patient safety practices. Evid Rep Technol Assess 2001;43:1–668.
29. Enrione EB, Thomlison B, Rubin A. Medical and psychological experiences of family caregivers with children fed enterally at home. JPEN J Parenter Enteral Nutr 2005;29:413–9.
30. Hastings Y, White M, Young J. Enteral nutrition and bone marrow transplantation. J Ped Onc Nurs 2006;23:103–10.
31. Adan D, La Gamma EF, Browne LE. Nutritional management and the multisystem organ failure/systemic inflammatory response syndrome in critically ill preterm neonates. Crit Care Clin 1995;11:751–84.
32. Beattie RM. Enteral nutrition as primary therapy in childhood Crohn's disease: Control of intestinal inflammation and anabolic response. JPEN J Parenter Enteral Nutr 2005;29:S151–9.
33. Hosaid SA, La Vega-Talbott M, Solomon GE. Ketogenic diet in pediatric epilepsy patients with gastrostomy feeling. Pediatr Neurol 2005;32:81–3.
34. Lord L, Harrington M. Enteral nutrition implementation and management. ASPEN Nutrition Support Practice Manual, 2nd edition; 2005. p. 76–89.
35. Andel D, Kamolz LP, Donner A, et al. Impact of intraoperative duodenal feeling on the oxygen bilance of the splanchnic region in severely burned patients. Burns 2005;31:302–5.
36. Zaloga GP. Bedside method for placing small bowel feeding tubes in critically ill patients: A prospective study. Chest 1991;100:1643–6.
37. Lord LM, Weser-Maimone A, Pulhamus M, et al. Comparison of weighted versus unweighted enteral feeding tubes for efficacy of transpyloric intubation. JPEN J Parenter Enteral Nutr 1993;17:271–3.
38. Meert KL, Daphtary KM, Metheny NA. Gastric vs small-bowel feeding in critically ill children receiving mechanical ventilation. Chest 2004;126:872–8.
39. Chellis MJ, Sanders SV, Dean JM, et al. Bedside transpyloric tube placement in the pediatric intensive care unit. JPEN J Parenter Enteral Nutr 1996;20:88–90.
40. da Silva PSL, Paulo CST, de Oliveira, et al. Bedside transpyloric tube placement in the pediatric intensive care unit: A modified insufflation air technique. Intensive Care Med 2002;28:943–6.
41. Kittinger JW, Sandler RS, Heizer WD. Efficacy of metoclopramide as an adjunct to duodenal placement of small-bore feeding tubes: A randomized, placebo-controlled, double-blind study. JPEN J Parenter Enteral Nutr 1987;11:33–7.
42. Di Lorenzo C, Lachman R, Hyman PE. Intravenous erythromycin for post-pyloric intubation. J Pediatr Gastroenterol Nutr 1990;11:45–7.
43. Gharpure V, Meert KL, Sarnaik AP. Efficacy of erythromycin for postpyloric placement of feeding tubes in critically ill children: A randomized, double-blind, placebo controlled study. JPEN J Parenter Enteral Nutr 2001;25:160–5.
44. Phipps LM, Weber MD, Ginder BR, et al. A randomized controlled trial comparing three different techniques of nasojejunal feeding tube placement in critically ill children. J Par Enter Nutr 2005;29:420–4.
45. Guitierrez ED, Balfe DM. Fluoroscopically guided nasoenteric feeding tube placement: Results of a 1-year study. Radiology 1991;178:759–62.
46. Dranoff JA, Angood PJ, Topazian M, et al. Transnasal endoscopy for enteral feeding tube placement in critically ill patients. Am J Gastroenterol 1999;94:2902–4.
47. Michaud L, Guimber D, Blain-Stregloff AS, et al. Longevity of balloon-stabilized skin-level gastrostomy device. J Ped Gastroent Nutr 2004;38:426–9.
48. Gaudener MWL, Ponsky JL, Izant RJ, Jr. Gastrostomy without laparotomy: A percutaneous endoscopic technique. J Pediatr Surg 1980;15:872–5.
49. Wilson L, Oliva-Hemker M. Percutaneous endoscopic gastrostomy in small medically complex infants. Endoscopy 2001;33:433–6.
50. Jonas SK, Neimark S, Panwalker AP. Effect of antibiotic prophylaxis in percutaneous endoscopic gastrostomy. Am J Gastroenterol 1985;80:438–41.
51. Klein S, Heare BR, Soloway RD. The "buried bumper syndrome": A complication of percutaneous endoscopic gastrostomy. Am J Gastroenterol 1990;85:448–51.
52. Chait PG, Weinberg J, Connolly BL, et al. Retrograde percutaneous gastrostomy and gastrojejunostomy in 505 children: A 4 1/2 year experience. Radiology 1996;201:691–5.
53. Barron MA, Duncan DS, Green GJ, et al. Efficacy and safety of radiologically placed gastrostomy tubes in paediatric haematology/oncology patients. Med Pediatr Oncol 2000;34:177–82.
54. Duh QY, Way LW. Laparoscopic gastrostomy using T-fasteners as retractors and anchors. Surg Endosc 1993;7:60–3.
55. Rosser JC, Rodas EB, Blancaflor J, et al. A simplified technique for laparoscopic jejunostomy and gastrostomy tube placement. Am J Surg 1999;177:61–5.
56. Lotan G, Broide E, Efrati Y, et al. Laparoscopicaly monitored percutaneous endoscopic gastrostomy (PEG) in children. Surg Endosc 2004;18:1280–2.
57. Shike M, Latkany L, Gerdes H, et al. Direct percutaneous endoscopic jejunostomies for enteral feeding. Gastrointest Endosc 1996;44:536–40.
58. Duh QY, Way LW. Laparoscopic jejunostomy using T-fasteners as retractors and anchors. Arch Surg 1993; 128:105–8.
59. Fortunato JE, Darbari A, Mitchell SE, et al. The limitations of gastro-jejunal (G-J) feeding tubes in children: A 9-year pediatric hospital database analysis. Am J Gastroenterol 2005;100:186–9.
60. Metheny N, Dettenmeir P, Hampton K, et al. Detection of inadvertent respiratory placement of small-bore feeding tubes: A report of 10 cases. Heart Lung 1990;19:631–8.
61. Westhus N. Methods to test feeding tube placement in children. Am J Mat Child Nurs 2004;29:282–89.
62. Metheny NA, Clouse R, Clark J, et al. pH testing of feeding-tube aspirates to determine placement. Nutr Clin Pract 1994;9:185–90.
63. Metheny NA, Reed L, Berglund B, et al. Visual characteristics of aspirates from feeding tubes as a method of predicting tube location. Nurs Res 1994;43:282–7.
64. Gharpure V, Meert KL, Sarnaik AP, et al. Indicators of postpyloric feeding tube placement in children. Crit Care Med 2000;28:2962–6.
65. Metheny NA, Smith L, Stewart BJ. Development of a reliable and valid bedside test for bilirubin and its utility for improving prediction of feeding tube location. Nurs Res 2000;49:302–9.
66. Ellett MLC, Croffie JMB, Cohen MD, et al. Gastric tube placement in young children. Clin Nurs Res 2005;14:238–52.
67. Cannon RA, Isaac RM, Puryear H. Confirmation of enteral feeding tube placement using duodenal slowwave frequency analysis. Gastroenterology 1989;96:A73.

68. Greenberg M, Bejar R, Asser S. Confirmation of transpyloric feeding tube placement by ultrasonography. J Pediatr 1993;122:413–5.
69. Grathwohl KW, Gibbons RV, Dillard TA, et al. Bedside videoscopic placement of feeding tubes: Development of fiberoptics through the tube. Crit Care Med 1997;25:629–34.
70. Gabriel SA, Ackermann RJ, Castresana MR. A new technique for placement of nasoenteral feeding tubes using external magnetic guidance. Crit Care Med 1997;25:641–5.
71. Ozdemir B, Frost M, Hayes J, et al. Placement of nasoenteral feeding tubes using magnetic guidance: Retesting a new technique. J Am Coll Nutr 2000;19:446–51.
72. Goulet O. Paeditric enteral feeding. Int Semin Paediatr Gastroenterol Nutr 1998;7:1–8.
73. Khoshoo V, Brown S. Gastric emptying of two whey-based formulas of different energy density and its clinical implication in children with volume intolerance. Eur J Clin Nutr 2002;56:656–8.
74. Morin CL, Ling V, Bourass D. Small intestinal colonic changes induced by a chemically defined diet. Dig Dis Sci 1980;25:123–8.
75. Nacht CA, Schutz O, Vernet L, et al. Continuous versus single bolus enteral nutrition: Comparison of energy metabolism. Am J Physiol 1986;251:E524–9.
76. Heymsfield S, Casper K, Grossman GD. Bioenergetic and metabolic response to continuous versus intermittent feeding. Metabolism 1987;36:570–5.
77. Pinchofsky-Devin GD, Kaminsky MV. Visceral protein increase associated with interrupt versus continuous enteral hyperalimentation. JPEN J Parenter Enteral Nutr 1985;9:474–6.
78. Graham TW, Zadrozny DB, Harrington T. The benefits of early jejunal hyperalimentation in the head-injured patient. Neurosurgery 1989;25:729–35.
79. Heyland DK, Novak F, Drover JW, et al. Should immunonutrition become routine in critically ill patients? A systematic review of the evidence. JAMA 2001;286:944–53.
80. Kenler AS, Swails WS, Driscoll DF, et al. Early enteral feeding in postsurgical cancer patients: Fish oil structured lipid-based polymeric formula versus a standard polymeric formula. Ann Surg 1996;223:316–33.
81. Heys S, Walker L, Smith L, et al. Enteral nutritional supplementation with key nutrients in patients with critical illness and cancer. A meta-analysis of randomized controlled clinical trials. Ann Surg 1999;229:467–77.
82. Schloerb P. Immune-enhancing diets: Products, components, and their rationales. JPEN J Parenter Enteral Nutr 2001;25:S3–7.
83. Johnson TE, Janes SJ, MacDonald A, et al. An observational study to evaluate micronutrient status during enteral feeding. Arch Dis Child 2002;86:411–5.
84. Briassoulis G, Filippou O, Hatzi E, et al. Early enteral administration of immunonutrition in critically ill children: Results of a blinded randomized controlled trial. Nutrition 2005;21:799–807.
85. Lima AAM, Brito LFB, Ribeiro HB, et al. Intestinal barrier function and weight gain in malnourished children taking glutamine supplemented enteral formula. J Ped Gastroent Nutr 2005;40:28–35.
86. Uauy-Dagach R, Mena R. Nutritional role of omega-3 fatty acids during the neonatal period. Clin Perinatol 1995;22:157–75.
87. Bott L, Husson MO, Guimber D, et al. Contamination of gastrostomy feeding systems in children in a home-based enteral nutrition program. J Pediatr Gastroenterol Nutr 2001;33:266–70.
88. Ramage IJ, Harvey E, Geary DF, et al. Complications of gastrostomy feeding in children receiving peritoneal dialysis. Pediatr Nephrol 1999;13:249–52.
89. Israel DM, Hassal E. Prolonged use of gastrostomy for enteral hyperalimentation in children with Crohn's disease. Am J Gastroenterol 1995;90:1084–8.
90. Weiss B, Fradkin A, Ben-Akun M, et al. Upper gastrointestinal bleeding due to gastric ulcers in children with gastrostomy tubes. J Clin Gastroenterol 1999;29:48–50.
91. Bastow MD. Complications of enteral nutrition. Gut 1986; 27:51–5.
92. Roy S, Rigal M, Doit C, et al. Bacterial contamination of enteral nutrition in a pediatric hospital. J Hosp Infect 2005;59:311–6.
93. Dautle MP, Wilkinson TR, Gauderer MWL. Isolation and identification of biofilm microorganisms from silicone gastrostomy devices. J Pediatr Surg 2003;38:216–20.
94. Golioto M, Lytle J, Jowell P. Re-establishing patency of a small bore feeding tube with complete occlusion-a novel use for an ERCP catheter. Nutr Clin Pract 2001; 16:284–5.
95. Pardoe EM. Tube feeding syndrome revisited. Nutr Clin Pract 2001;16:144–6.
96. Daveluy W, Guimber D, Mention K, et al. Home enteral nutrition in children: An 11-year experience with 416 patients. Clin Nutr 2005;24:48–54.
97. Elia M, Cottee S, Holden C, et al. Enteral and parenteral nutrition in the community. The British Association for Parenteral and Enteral Nutrition. Berkshire, UK: The Association; 1994.
98. Elia M. Home enteral nutrition: General aspects and a comparison between the United States and Britain. Nutrition 1994;10:115–23.
99. Scott F, Beech R, Smedley F, et al. Prospective, randomized, controlled, single-blind trial of the costs and consequences of systemic nutrition team follow-up over 12 months after percutaneous endoscopic gastrostomy. Nutrition 2005;21:1071–7.
100. Thomson FC, Naysmith MR, Lindsay A. Managing drug therapy in patients receiving enteral and parenteral nutrition. Hosp Pharm 2000;7:155–64.

69

Parenteral Nutrition

John A. Kerner Jr., MD
Melissa Hurwitz, MD

Intravenous nutritional care was introduced more than 65 years ago when protein hydrolysates first became available. In the late 1930s, Shohl and others[1] demonstrated positive nitrogen balance with infusion of glucose plus protein hydrolysates in pediatric patients. In 1944, Helfrick and Abelson[2] infused 50% glucose, 10% casein hydrolysate, and a homogenized emulsion of olive oil and lecithin in an alternating manner into a 5-month-old marasmic infant for 5 days via a peripheral vein. During the next 20 years, parenteral nutrition (PN) in infants and children was unsuccessful, largely because of the inability of peripheral veins to tolerate the hyperosmolar infusates. Significant side effects, including allergic reactions and marked elevations of body temperature, further complicated attempts at PN. Often, there was inadequate provision of calories to allow the nitrogen to be used efficiently. Intravenous fat (IVF) preparations were also used, but they were removed from general use because of toxic side effects, such as thrombosis, embolism, fever, vomiting, rash, eosinophilia, and thrombocytopenia.[3,4]

In the late 1960s, a group of surgeons at the University of Pennsylvania demonstrated, first in beagle puppies and later in an infant, that the continuous intravenous infusion of hypertonic dextrose and amino acids through deep central venous catheters could provide adequate caloric intake safely and allow normal growth and development.[5,6] The development of a safe IVF preparation, Intralipid® (Kabivitrum, Alameda, CA), was another major advance in clinical PN. Fat emulsions offered the dual advantage of high caloric density and isotonicity, thereby meeting caloric requirements with less damage to peripheral veins. In the mid-1970s, protein hydrolysates were replaced by crystalline amino acid solutions. Their composition was more controlled than that of the hydrolysates, reducing the risk of allergic reactions. In the 1980s, crystalline amino acid solutions specifically designed for newborn infants became available. Finally, appreciation of the vitamin and trace element requirements of neonates and older children led to the development of the infusible vitamin and mineral solutions designed to meet these needs.

Indications

PN is indicated for most patients who are unable to tolerate enteral feedings for a significant period of time.[7] Four or five days without adequate oral nutrient intake is an indication for instituting some form of PN. Even 2 to 3 days without adequate nutritional intake for very-low-birth-weight (VLBW) infants or infants with pre-existing nutritional depletion is likely to result in significant depletion of their limited endogenous stores. PN is not indicated in patients with adequate intestinal function, in whom nutrition may be maintained by oral or tube feedings. Relative contraindications to PN include intended use for <5 days, the probability that a patient will die imminently because of underlying disease, and significant hydration or metabolic perturbations that make the provision of PN unsafe or ill advised. Although PN is a potentially life-saving therapy and is now an accepted practice, experience has demonstrated metabolic, mechanical, and infectious complications. Therefore, candidates for PN should be selected carefully. PN is supportive therapy for some illnesses and primary therapy for others (Table 1).

Although PN is used to replenish the malnourished child, it may be started prophylactically in clinical situations in which prolonged starvation is expected. Other indications for PN include a recent loss of more than 10% of body weight, with a concomitant inability to ingest sufficient nutrients to reverse this state, and marginal nutritional reserves in a patient who is unable to ingest sufficient calories to prevent further negative nitrogen balance.

Infants receiving central venous PN retain nitrogen and grow as well as infants fed human milk or standard formulas. PN has been directly credited with improving the survival of infants with intestinal failure by prevention death due to starvation[8] and has also been accepted as a standard part of the medical and nutritional management of premature infants (see Chapter 33, "The Low-Birth-Weight Infant: Inpatient Care").

Parenteral Nutrient Requirements

Calories (Energy). There are many different recommendations and methods to calculate the caloric needs of children. The World Health Organization (WHO) recommendations are based on evaluations of several thousand children and have proven to be relatively accurate for children 1 year of age.[9] The WHO recommendations provide an estimated resting energy expenditure (REE), which may then be multiplied by a factor to adjust for catch-up growth, activity, and medical status, to provide an estimate of total daily caloric needs. In obese patients (>120% ideal body weight), the Schofield height/weight equation more accurately predicts energy needs.[10]

Table 1 Indications for Parenteral Nutrition in Pediatric Patients

Condition	Examples
Surgical gastrointestinal disorders	Gastroschisis, omphalocele, tracheoesophageal fistula, multiple intestinal atresias, meconium ileus and peritonitis, malrotation and volvulus, Hirschsprung's disease with enterocolitis, diaphragmatic hernia
Intractable diarrhea of infancy	
Inflammatory bowel disease	Crohn's disease, ulcerative colitis
Short-bowel syndrome	
Serious acute alimentary diseases	Pancreatitis, pseudomembranous colitis, necrotizing enterocolitis
Severe malabsorption	Idiopathic villous atrophy
Chronic idiopathic intestinal Pseudo-obstruction syndrome	
Gastrointestinal fistulas	Fistulas in Crohn's disease
Hypermetabolic states	Severe burns and trauma
Renal failure	
Low-birth-weight infants	Asphyxiated infants, very low-birth-weight infants, respiratory distress syndrome
Malignancies	Especially those receiving abdominal irradiation (causing radiation enteritis) or chemotherapy, which leads to severe nausea and intestinal dysfunction
Marrow and organ transplantation	
Special circumstances	Anorexia nervosa, cystic fibrosis, cardiac cachexia, hepatic failure, sepsis
Rare disorders	Congenital microvillous inclusion disease, chylothorax and chylous ascites, Cryptosporidium-induced secretory diarrhea

Table 2 Protein and Energy Requirements for Infants

	Preterm	Full Term 0–6 months	Full Term 6–12 months
Energy (kcal/kg/d)	100–120	90–110	80–100
Protein (g/kg/d)	2.5–3.5	2.5–3.0	2.0–2.5

See Tables 2 to 4, for caloric needs for infants and children and for activity and stress adjustment factors. Indirect calorimetry (measurement of oxygen consumption and carbon dioxide production) provides a precise and practical measurement of REE.[11] This measurement should be used when possible, especially for patients with increased needs and for those not responding to nutritional therapy. Indirect calorimetry technology in the nonintubated patient not receiving supplemental oxygen is well standardized, but measurements in the newborn baby and the intubated patient receiving high concentrations of supplemental oxygen (FiO_2 greater than 50%) may be fraught with technical difficulties.

Adequate protein intake must be provided with adequate caloric intake for optimal caloric utilization and growth (Tables 2, 3). In a controlled trial of 114 premature appropriate-for-gestational-age infants, two isocaloric (60 kcal/kg/d) intravenous feeding regimens were compared, one with glucose alone and the other with glucose plus 2.5 g/kg/d of crystalline amino acids.[12] Infants on the glucose-only regimen had a negative mean nitrogen balance, whereas those fed glucose plus amino acids had a positive balance. There was no significant weight gain in either group. Additionally, intravenous intakes of 70 to 90 kcal/kg/d have resulted in weight gain in premature infants, and energy intakes providing more than 70 kcal/kg/d (including intakes of 2.7 to 3.5 g/kg/d of protein) resulted in nitrogen accretion and growth rates similar to in utero values.[13]

"Early aggressive nutritional support" is being practiced in many neonatal ICUs to improve premature infants' nutritional status.[14] In previous practice, preterm infants would start with 0.5 g/kg/d of protein. When given parenteral glucose alone, an infant will lose 1% of body protein stores per day (~1 g/kg/d). Parenteral protein is usually started on day of life 1 to 2 or as soon as serum electrolytes are stable. A number of studies over the past 15 years indicate that most preterm infants will tolerate 1.5 to 2 g/kg/d of parenteral amino acids in the first day of life to reduce catabolism. In one randomized controlled trial, infants of LBW (<1500 g) who received 2.4 g/kg/d of amino acids from birth onward had more positive nitrogen balance and better plasma amino acid profiles than infants who received a graduated increment in protein intake over the first 3 days of life.[15] Several studies have shown that the parenteral intake required to avoid catabolism in extremely low-birth-weight (ELBW) infants may be as low as 1.1 to 1.5 g/kg/d when administered with 30 kcal/kg/d of energy. To achieve intrauterine rates of protein deposition, the upper limits of protein intake is 3 g/kg/d for term infants and up to 4g/kg/d for most preterm infants.[16]

Table 3 Protein Requirements: Children and Adolescents

Age (yr)	Protein (g/kg/d)
1–6	1–2
7–10	1–2
11–14	1–2
15–18 (boys)	0.9–2
15–18 (girls)	0.8–2

Peripheral PN seems best suited for minimally stressed patients undergoing a limited course of PN or for whom PN is not the sole source of energy. Central PN is indicated either for nutritional repletion of a seriously malnourished patient or when PN is the sole nutrient source. Concentrations of glucose up to 30 to 35% may be necessary to provide sufficient carbohydrate calories. The macronutrient composition of PN solutions should be balanced, especially when there is a risk of PN-associated liver disease. Regimens high in carbohydrate increase the respiratory quotient resulting in excessive carbon dioxide retention, which leads to increased difficulty in weaning from the ventilator.

Fluids. Fluid requirements depend on hydration status, size, age, environmental factors, and underlying disease. Daily maintenance fluid requirements for children are outlined in Table 4. Premature infants have unique requirements that are reviewed in Chapter 33, "The Low-Birth-Weight Infant: Inpatient Care." Factors that increase fluid requirements include radiant warmers, conventional single-walled incubators, and phototherapy. Those that decrease fluid requirements include heat shields, thermal blankets, and double-walled incubators. Furthermore, excess fluid intake (>150 mL/kg/d) in LBW infants may be associated with patent ductus arteriosus, bronchopulmonary dysplasia, NEC, and intraventricular hemorrhage.[17]

During PN, it may be necessary to give fluids in excess of maintenance to provide adequate calories, especially if using a peripheral vein, but care must be given to avoid fluid overload. Highly concentrated glucose solutions and 20% fat emulsion are used to decrease total fluid volume. It is important not to use PN for replacing ongoing losses, since the fluid contains not just electrolytes but protein, vitamins, and minerals.

Table 4 Fluid Recommendations for Parenteral Nutrition

Initial volume for patients free of cardiovascular or renal disease
<10 kg = 100 mL/kg/d
10–30 kg = 2,000 mL/m²/d
30–50 kg = 100 mL/h (2.4 L/d)
>50 kg = 124 mL/h (3 L/d)
Volume can be increased by
10 mL/kg/d in infants until the desired caloric intake is achieved (maximum of 200 mL/kg/d, if tolerated)
>10 kg: by 10% of initial volume per day until desired caloric intake is achieved (maximum of 4,000 mL/m²/d, if tolerated)

Carbohydrate. The major source of nonprotein calories in PN is D-glucose, which is provided in the monohydrate form for intravenous use, reducing its caloric yield to 3.4 kcal/g rather than the 4 kcal/g of enteral glucose or other carbohydrates. Glucose provides most of the osmolality in the PN solution; peripheral PN concentrations with more than 10% glucose increase the risk of phlebitis and, thus, decrease the lifespan of peripheral venous lines. The carbohydrate load is initiated in a stepwise fashion to allow an appropriate response of endogenous insulin and thus prevent glucosuria (and subsequent osmotic diuresis). Glucose as the sole calorie source leads to greater water retention than when combined with lipids.[18] A balanced PN solution, including carbohydrate and fat (as nonnitrogen calories) may avoid (1) fatty infiltration of the liver, (2) water retention, and (3) worsening respiratory compromise in acutely ill ventilator-dependent patients. Carbon dioxide production is higher with glucose as the only source of nonprotein calories than when fat emulsion provides some of the total caloric content.[19]

Small, premature infants have poor glucose tolerance in the first days of life, and hyperglycemia (>125 mg/dL of sugar) occurs frequently. Glucose infusions are well tolerated by the newborn infant if the initial rate of administration does not exceed the hepatic rate of glucose production (6 to 8 mg/kg/min). The premature infant or physiologically stressed patient may develop hyperglycemia at even lower rates of infusion. Glucose infusion rates between 5 to 12 mg/kg/min are recommended in neonates and 2 to 5 mg/kg/min in older children and adolescents. Serum glucose measurements should be monitored when PN solutions are abruptly stopped.[20]

The response of premature infants to insulin is highly variable; some develop profound hypoglycemia with minuscule insulin doses, and others have no response. There have been numerous studies in VLBW and ELBW infants (<1,000 g), documenting improved weight gain, increased tolerance to intravenous glucose, normalization of serum glucose concentrations, and increased caloric intake with the use of continuous insulin infusions.[21,22] There are serious concerns about the use of insulin in the neonate because (1) suppression of muscle proteolysis may not be desirable (the glutamine released is an important substrate for intestinal epithelial cells and the immune system); (2) there is a lack of understanding of the composition of the weight gain (especially protein accretion); and (3) it is not known whether increased glucose utilization deprives the brain of this important substrate or whether increased glucose can be efficiently oxidized. In older children and adolescents, insulin may be required to improve caloric intake in the face of hyperglycemia. It is not recommended to add insulin to the PN directly, but rather to deliver the insulin as a separate infusion that can be titrated according to serum glucose, thus avoiding shifts in nutrient delivery rates.

Adult studies have clearly demonstrated the association between hyperglycemia and prolonged hospitalization, prolonged time on the ventilator and increased morbidity and mortality.[23,24] Diya and colleagues found that hyperglycemia in premature infants with sepsis resulted in prolonged mechanical ventilation and longer hospital stays. In addition, infants who did not survive had higher maximum serum glucose levels as compared to infants who did survive.[25] A recent retrospective study examined glycemic control for patients in the pediatric intensive care unit (PICU). A correlation was found between maximal glucose level and prolonged PICU stay and mortality; however, a causal relationship could not be determined.[26]

Protein. The problems of hyperammonemia and poor utilization of nitrogen often seen with parenteral protein hydrolysates have been alleviated by the use of purer, crystalline amino acid formulations. Hyperammonemia, seen with earlier solutions, rarely occurs with the increased amounts of arginine and decreased glycine in the formulations. Hyperchloremic metabolic acidosis, a problem noticed with earlier crystalline amino acid solutions, has been ameliorated by the substitution of acetate for chloride in the salts of lysine and the use of basic salts of histidine. In addition to decreased toxicity, crystalline amino acids promote greater rates of nitrogen retention than do protein hydrolysates. All amino acid formulations currently marketed consist of crystalline amino acids; most were designed according to the requirements of normal, orally fed adult subjects and not for growing infants and children. These solutions produced weight gain and positive nitrogen balance in the stable neonate or infant when adequate nonprotein calories were also provided. However, use of these solutions leads to high plasma concentrations of such amino acids as methionine, glycine, and phenylalanine (a cause for concern regarding safety) and to low plasma concentrations of such amino acids as the branched-chain amino acids (BCAAs), tyrosine, and cysteine.

Heird and Malloy found that free amino acid patterns, total weight, and protein content of brains in beagle puppies that received PN were grossly abnormal, compared with those of suckled puppies.[27] The abnormal free amino acid patterns of the brains of the PN-fed puppies reflected plasma amino acid concentrations. Extensive research led to the production of a parenteral formula, TrophAmine® (B Braun, Irvine, CA), which normalizes plasma amino acid concentrations within the range observed in breastfed infants.[28] TrophAmine® is unique, in that it provides the essential amino acids (including taurine, tyrosine, and histidine) in adequate amounts, as judged by the normalized plasma amino acid profile, plus aspartic acid, glutamic acid, and the dicarboxylic acids at appropriate levels. Studies of this product have been conducted in preterm and term infants and in older children.

Helms and others[29] compared TrophAmine® with a standard amino acid formula (Freamine III®: B Braun, Irvine, CA) in neonates and found that the TrophAmine® group had significantly greater weight gain and nitrogen retention and had plasma amino acid concentrations within the postprandial neonatal target range. Concentrations of methionine, glycine, and phenylalanine were above and tyrosine was below the range when Freamine III® was used. L-Cysteine was supplemented in both groups. Overall imbalance of amino acids or toxicity of one or more amino acids elevated in plasma may also be responsible for hepatic dysfunction and cholestasis.

Of the standard amino acid solutions, Aminosyn® (Abbott Laboratories, North Chicago, IL), with its low pH, allows the addition of greater amounts of calcium and phosphate for growing preterm infants.[30] TrophAmine® has a lower pH than Aminosyn® and allows even larger amounts of calcium and phosphorus to be added to the PN solution without precipitation.[31]

Abbott Laboratories released Aminosyn-PF® in the hope of producing a product comparable with TrophAmine®. TrophAmine® contains 60% essential amino acids and Aminosyn-PF® contains 50%. A large multicenter study comparing TrophAmine ® and Aminosyn-PF in LBW infants described similar nitrogen balance and weight gain in both groups.[32] However, one center reported improved nitrogen balance and better levels of methionine and tyrosine in the TrophAmine® group. Both formulas contain supplemental taurine, as data show potentially deleterious effect of taurine deficiency on the developing brain and retina.[33] Both Aminosyn-PF® and TrophAmine® appear to be better designed to meet the metabolic needs of the preterm infant than do standard amino acid solutions.

Cysteine is considered an indispensable amino acid for infants because hepatic cystathionase activity is absent or low until some time after term birth (cystathionase converts methionine to cysteine). In addition, removal of cysteine from an otherwise adequate diet inhibits the rate of weight gain and nitrogen retention. Enterally fed infants do not have a major problem because both human milk and infant formulas contain cysteine. Because cysteine is unstable and is only sparingly soluble in aqueous solution, parenteral amino acid solutions previously did not contain cysteine. Infants receiving PN have low plasma cysteine concentrations; furthermore, nitrogen retention is usually lower than in infants receiving the same amount of nitrogen enterally. Cysteine hydrochloride (HCl) can be added to PN, but within 24 hours, approximately 50% of it forms a complex with glucose, making D-glucocysteine. Previous studies of this method of cysteine supplementation of PN failed to show improvement in growth or nitrogen retention. This may have been because the regimens used were also deficient in tyrosine. Kashyap and others showed that supplementation of PN with cysteine-HCl (where the amino acid solution contained tyrosine)—by either admixture or piggyback—resulted in cysteine retention, higher plasma cysteine concentrations, possible improved nitrogen retention, and increased acidosis (which required increased acetate to offset).[34]

Glutamine. Glutamine, a primary fuel source for enterocytes, colonocytes, lymphocytes, and macrophages, is a precursor for nucleotide synthesis and for glutathione, an important antioxidant. A nonessential amino acid by definition, cellular uptake of glutamine may exceed synthesis and release from skeletal muscle during catabolic illness, making glutamine essential under these conditions.[35]

Clinical studies of glutamine-supplemental PN were initially positive in a number of patient populations, including bone marrow transplant recipients,[36] short bowel syndrome,[37,41] and in severely burned patients.[38,39] For example, Wilmore and others[41] used supplemental glutamine (0.56 g/kg/d), growth hormone (0.14 mg/kg/d), and a modified enteral diet in adults with short-bowel syndrome and reported improved protein absorption, decreased stool output, and reduction in dependence on PN. Subsequent randomized, blinded, and controlled studies, however, did not confirm this benefit.[42,43]

Preliminary studies in VLBW infants showed benefit of glutamine-supplemented PN. Lacey and colleagues performed a randomized trial in VLBW infants of glutamine-supplemented PN (15 to 20% of administered amino acids as L-glutamine); the infusion was safe, and was associated with improved plasma glutamine concentrations without elevation of ammonia or glutamate.[40] In addition, of the 44 randomized infants, for the group of infants with birthweight <800 grams, the glutamine supplemented group required fewer days on PN (13 vs 21 days), had shorter length of time to reach full feeds (8 vs 14 days), and needed less time on the ventillator (38 vs 47 days).

The NICHD Neonatal Research Network performed a randomized trial of parenteral glutamine supplementation for ELBW infants.[44] Fifteen centers randomized 1,430 infants (birthweight 401 to 1,000 g) to TrophAmine® or an isonitrogenous amino acid solution with 20% glutamine. There were no differences between the two groups for late onset sepsis, NEC, days to full enteral feeds, days to regain birthweight, length of hospital stay, or survival even though glutamine concentrations in plasma significantly increased in the treatment group. Albers studied 80 newborns and infants who underwent digestive tract surgery and compared PN alone to glutamine supplemented PN. This double-blind randomized trial found no significant benefit of glutamine as measured by intestinal permeability, nitrogen balance, or clinical outcomes.[45] In a recent Cochrane review of glutamine supplementation, 2,300 VLBW infants participating in six randomized control trials were reviewed. The authors found no positive effect from parenteral or enteral glutamine for preterm infants in terms of decreasing mortality and sepsis. Overall, they concluded that supplemental glutamine has no statistically significant benefit for preterm infants and does not warrant further investigation.[46]

Guidelines for amino acid requirements in PN are shown in Tables 2 and 3. Preterm neonates given 2.5 to 3.5 g/kg/d of amino acids and approximately 80 kcal/kg/d achieve nitrogen retention at levels that approximate intrauterine nitrogen retention; intakes for older children and adolescents vary from 1.0 to 2.0 g/kg/d. In neonates in our institution, we start at 1.5 to 2.5 g/kg/d of amino acids and increase to the desired goal. In older infants and children, we start at the goal dose except in hepatic or renal insufficiency or disorders of protein metabolism. Solutions high in BCAAs have been used in patients with liver failure and encephalopathy. These solutions are expensive and the data justifying their use is not well substantiated. We often use TrophAmine® (with its higher percentage of BCAAs) in patients age <6 months and those with cholestasis. In an attempt to decrease cholestasis and hepatic dysfunction, consideration should be given to using TrophAmine® for all long-term PN patients.

Calorie-to-Nitrogen Ratio. To promote efficient net protein utilization and not use the protein as an energy source, it is often recommended to provide approximately 150 to 200 nonprotein calories per gram of nitrogen, as follows:

(1) Nitrogen content (g) = protein (g)/6.25; (2) 1 g protein contains 0.16 g nitrogen; (3) therefore, 24 to 32 nonnitrogen calories must be supplied per gram of protein infused to yield a desirable ratio of 150 to 200:1

- Nonnitrogen calories/N (g) = 24/0.16 = 150/1; 32/0.16 = 200/1
- If 2 g/kg/d of protein as amino acids is supplied, then 48 to 64 kcal/kg/d of nonnitrogen calories must be supplied to ensure adequate protein utilization
- If 2.5 g/kg/d of protein is supplied, then 60 to 70 kcal/kg/d of nonnitrogen calories must be supplied

Albumin. Albumin at a concentration of 0.5 to 1.0 g/kg/d may be administered to PN patients who are hypoalbuminemic from nonnutritional causes. Such infusions are for oncotic, not nutritive, benefits. Albumin should be infused separately via a "Y" connector and not placed in the PN solution since (1) albumin is a blood product and should not be hung for more than 8 hours; (2) recent concerns exist about flocculation of albumin in PN solutions; and (3) albumin in PN solutions increases the risk of sepsis.[47]

Fat. IVF is an integral part of the PN regimen. It provides a concentrated isotonic source of calories (20% solution supplies 2.0 kcal/mL) and prevents or reverses essential fatty acid (EFA) deficiency. Patients who cannot tolerate large glucose or fluid loads can receive sufficient calories if IVF is added to the glucose-amino acid regimen.[9] In addition, continuous administration of IVF with the PN regimen prolongs the viability of peripheral intravenous lines in infants who may have limited venous access.[48] The IVF must be infused separately from the PN solution because these solutions may "crack" (disturb) the fat emulsion. It is given using a "Y" connector near the infusion site and beyond the Micropore filter.

The rate of elimination and metabolic fate of IVF particles are the same as those of naturally occurring chylomicrons, so plasma clearance is dependent on the activity of lipoprotein lipase in the capillary endothelial cells, primarily in muscle and adipose tissue. The IVF should be infused over 24 hours, whenever possible. Continuous IVF infusions (24 h/d) are better tolerated than intermittent infusions (8 to 18 h/d)[49,50] with less fluctuation and lower concentrations of plasma lipids especially at higher rates of infusion. Early studies argued against exceeding a rate of 0.15 g/kg/h (3.6 g/kg/d). Slower infusion rates are required for small-for-gestational-age (SGA) infants. Infusion rates of 0.12 g/kg/hr or less resulted in less elevation of plasma lipid concentrations than rates of 0.17 g/kg/hr or more.[50]

The CDC guidelines from 2002 state that lipid emulsions should be hung for 12 hours or less, based on the associated risk with sepsis.[51]

Biochemical evidence of EFA deficiency has been observed in the serum of fasted newborn infants as early as 2 days after initiating fat-free PN.[52] Biochemical evidence precedes clinical signs of deficiency: reduced growth rate, flaky dry skin, poor hair growth, thrombocytopenia, increased susceptibility to infections, and impaired wound healing.[52] An EFA deficiency (EFAD) can be assessed by determination of the ratio of 5,8-11-eicosatrienoic to arachidonic acid (triene-to-tetraene ratio). A ratio >0.4 is generally assumed to be an early indicator of EFA deficiency. Interestingly, 15 mL twice a day of corn oil, sunflower oil, or safflower oil enterally provides as much linoleic acid as 150 mL of 10% IVF at less than 5% of the cost. Many PN patients not on complete bowel rest tolerate such a regimen. An EFA deficiency can be prevented by providing 2 to 4% of total calories as IVF (1 to 2% linoleic acid)—an IVF dose of 0.5 to 1.0 g/kg/d. Linoleic and linolenic acids are EFAs. Too much linolenic acid may inhibit the conversion of linoleic acid to arachidonic acid. These concerns led to the development of Liposyn II® (Abbott Laboratories), a blend of safflower oil (0.1% linolenic acid) and soybean oil (8.0% linolenic acid). Currently used IVF products are shown in Table 5. One study demonstrated that hypertriglyceridemia is more common in preterm infants who receive safflower oil-based as opposed to soybean oil-based IVF.[53] However, studies in newborn babies comparing Liposyn II® and Intralipid® found no difference in the incidence of hypertriglyceridemia between the two products, with comparable plasma fatty acid profiles.

Carnitine is necessary for optimal oxidation of fatty acids. Solutions currently used for intravenous alimentation contain no carnitine, but they do contain all the precursors for its endogenous production. Infants and newborn infants maintained on PN solutions have decreased total plasma and tissue carnitine concentrations. Normalization of serum carnitine levels occurs in infants receiving long-term PN and supplemental oral L-carnitine (50 μmol/kg/d = 8.1 mg/kg/d),[54] or intravenous L-carnitine.[55] The latter study also led to lower peak triglyceride concentrations after delivery of a fat bolus (suggesting an enhanced ability to use fat for energy) and modest increases in growth and nitrogen accretion. The VLBW infants requiring PN developed low carnitine concentrations and impaired ketogenesis that appeared to improve with parenteral carnitine. In VLBW infants on PN supplemented with

Table 5 Currently Available Intravenous Fat Emulsions*

	Oil (%)		Fatty Acid Content (%)				
Product (Distributor)	Safflower	Soybean	Linoleic	Oleic	Palmitic	Linolenic	Stearic
Intralipid† 10% (Fresenius Kabi Clayton)	–	10	50	26	10	9	3.5
Intralipid† 20% (Fresenius Kabi Clayton)	–	20	50	26	10	9	3.5
Intralipid† 30% (Fresenius Kabi Clayton)	–	30	50	26	10	9	3.5
Liposyn II‡ 10% (Abbott)	5	5	65.8	17.7	8.8	4.2	3.4
Liposyn II‡ 20% (Abbott)	10	10	65.8	17.7	8.8	4.2	3.4
Liposyn III‡ 10% (Abbott)	–	10	54.5	22.4	10.5	8.3	4.2
Liposyn III‡ 20% (Abbott)	–	20	54.5	22.4	10.5	8.3	4.2

Product (Distributor)	Egg Yolk Phospholipids (%)	Glycerine (%)	kcal/mL	Osmolarity (mOsm/L)	Phospholipid/ Triglyceride Ratio
Intralipid† 10% (Fresenius Kabi Clayton)	1.2	2.25	1.1	260	0.12
Intralipid† 20% (Fresenius Kabi Clayton)	1.2	2.25	2	260	0.06
Intralipid† 30% (Fresenius Kabi Clayton)	1.2	1.7	3	200	0.04
Liposyn II‡ 10% (Abbott)	1.2	2.5	1.1	276	0.12
Liposyn II‡ 20% (Abbott)	1.2	2.5	2	258	0.06
Liposyn III‡ 10% (Abbott)	1.2	2.5	1.1	284	0.12
Liposyn III‡ 20% (Abbottt)	1.2	2.5	2	292	0.06

*Available in the United States.
†Store at 25°C (77°F) or below; do not freeze.
‡Store at 30°C (86°F) or below; do not freeze.

L-carnitine (50 μmol/kg/d), increased carnitine concentrations and improved tolerance to IVF (only in the infants in the 1,001 to 1,500 g and not 750 to 1,000 g birth-weight range) were noted.

Other studies of carnitine supplementation have failed to demonstrate significant improvement in clinical outcome.[56,57] Some experts recommend 10 mg/kg/d intravenous L-carnitine for VLBW infants. Higher doses of carnitine seem to have pharmacologic effects, leading to increased protein and fat oxidation with associated energy loss. Supplementation with 48 mg L-carnitine/kg/d (about 300 μmol/kg/d) increased the metabolic rate, decreased fat and protein accretion, and prolonged the time to regain birthweight in preterm infants receiving PN with lipids.[58] Our center does not routinely supplement PN solutions with carnitine. Cholestatic infants and children without enteral intake on long-term PN are supplemented when serum carnitine levels are low.

Structured lipids are being considered as an alternative energy source.[59] They contain medium- and long-chain fatty acids esterified to the same glycerol molecule. They are different from physical mixtures of medium-chain triglycerides (MCT) and long-chain triglycerides (LCT). Fat emulsions containing MCTs have been released in Europe; their advantage is that they are not stored in the liver or adipose tissue and they undergo hydrolysis and rapid beta-oxidation independent of the carnitine enzyme system. Although early laboratory and clinical studies demonstrated intravenous MCTs to be a safe, carnitine-independent energy substrate, subsequent studies have shown increased mortality in previously starved animals and central nervous system toxicity in dogs.[60] The potential advantage in pediatric patients would be for cases where endogenous lipoprotein lipase levels are low, as in infants of less than 28 weeks gestation or those with sepsis or trauma. Some reports suggest a benefit of adding MCTs to intravenous preparations, compared with using LCTs alone. Fifty-one newborn infants received Lipofundin® MCT/LCT (50% MCT, 50% LCT) (B. Braun Medical, Germany) or conventional IVF over 20 hours. Triglyceride and fatty acid concentrations were not significantly different in the two groups. After 6 days of IVF, mean plasma cholesterol was 100% higher in the group receiving conventional IVF.[61] A second study of neonates showed elevation of triglycerides and free fatty acids in the MCT/LCT group.[62] Further studies are needed to evaluate the MCT/LCT regimen for pediatric patients. Finally, Canadian investigators were concerned that preterm infants lacked transplacental accretion for eicosapentaenoic acid (EPA) and docosahexaenoic acid (DHA), so they designed a soy emulsion enriched with EPA and DHA and found no toxicity or biochemical abnormalities in piglets. These fatty acids are essential for brain development but are not available in any current IVF products in the United States.

Omegevan® (Fresenius Kabi AG, Bad Homburg, Germany) is a 10% IVF solution enriched in the omega 3 fatty acids EPA and DHA. Its use as an adjunctive IVF has been described in the literature and most recently its use as monotherapy as a IVF source has been reported as a possible therapy for PN-associated liver disease.[63] More trials of this and other IVF are needed to address their role in clinical and nutritional outcomes in children.

Parenteral fat may contribute 30 to 50% of total nonnitrogen calories, but generally, it should not exceed 60% to avoid ketosis. Four grams per kilogram per day of 20% IVF caused less increase of plasma lipids than 2 g/kg/d of 10% IVF. Hyperlipidemia occurs with PN with 10% IVF but not 20% IVF and is caused by an increase in lipoprotein X. The phospholipid/triglyceride ratio is 0.12 in 10% IVF and 0.06 in 20% IVF (see Table 5).[64,65] Phospholipid is believed to inhibit lipoprotein lipase, which is the main enzyme responsible for IVF clearance probably explaining why 20% IVF is cleared more rapidly. Thirty percent IVF has been shown to be safe and has similar metabolic effects to 20% IVF. It is administered as a 3-in-1 solution and cannot be given alone via a peripheral intravenous line.[66] Suggested dosing for IVF is shown in Table 6.

Table 6 Dosing for Intravenous Fat*

Age	Starting Dose	Daily Dose Increase	Maximum Dose
Preterm	0.5–1.0	1.0	3.5
Full term (0–6 month)	1.0–1.5	1.0–1.5	3.5
Older infants (6–12 month)	1.0–1.5	1.0–1.5	3.0
Children (1–10 yr)	1.0	1.0–1.5	3.0
Adolescents (11–18 yr)	1.0	1.0	2.0–3.0

*In grams per kilogram per day.

Electrolytes. The ranges of recommended daily intakes of electrolytes and minerals for PN solutions in pediatrics are shown in Table 7. Calcium and phosphorus requirements change with age and are much greater in preterm infants than in term infants, older children, and adults.[67] During the last 6 to 8 weeks of gestation, calcium and phosphorus are incorporated into the bone matrix. Thus, premature infants are at risk for developing rickets and "handling" fractures. Any radiograph taken should be checked for the early bone changes of rickets. Serum calcium, phosphorus, and alkaline phosphatase should be monitored. Serum calcium concentration will be maintained at the expense of bone (demineralization), so a normal serum calcium does not necessarily mean that adequate amounts of calcium are being delivered. The serum phosphorus concentration does not fluctuate as rapidly and is a better indicator of total body stores. Elevated plasma alkaline phosphatase concentrations should prompt a radiograph to exclude rickets.

Calcium and phosphorus requirements for some patients may exceed the solubility of these two elements in PN solutions, particularly when patients are fluid restricted or have several other intravenous fluid sources. The maximum amounts of calcium and phosphorus that can be admixed in PN solutions are determined primarily by the pH of the solution,[30] which, in turn, is determined primarily by the amino acid product and concentration. Currently, TrophAmine® and Aminosyn-PF® have a low enough pH to allow adequate amounts of calcium and phosphorus for growth. Of the other amino acid solutions designed for use in adults, Aminosyn has the lowest pH and is probably the better choice for use in children with active bone growth. Continuous infusion of calcium in the PN solution is preferable to bolus administration of calcium. With bolus administration, large amounts of calcium are lost in the urine.[69] Also, the potential tissue damage from line infiltration is much greater with concentrated calcium given as a bolus than with dilute calcium as a continuous infusion.

Table 7 Parenteral Provision of Electrolytes and Minerals

Electrolytes and Minerals	Daily Amount
Phosphate	0.5–2.0 mM/kg
Sodium	2.0–4.0 mEq/kg
Potassium	2.0–3.0 mEq/kg
Chloride	2.0–3.0 mEq/kg
Acetate	1.0–4.0 mEq/kg
Magnesium	0.25–0.5 mEq/kg
Calcium gluconate*	50–500 mg/kg

*Gluconate is the recommended calcium salt for use in parenteral nutrition solutions. Calcium chloride dissociates more readily than calcium gluconate solutions and can lead to precipitation problems with phosphate.

Infusions of solutions containing both calcium and phosphorus together result in stable calcium and phosphorus concentrations. Calcium concentrations of 50 mEq/L and phosphate concentrations of 20 mmol/L are compatible in solutions containing 2% TrophAmine, 10% glucose, and 0.08% L-cysteine.[70] Calcium–phosphorus solubility is less in Aminosyn-PF® than in TrophAmine®.[70] A calcium:phosphorus ratio of 1.7:1 by weight (1.3:1 by molar ratio, similar to fetal mineral accretion ratio) allows for a higher absolute retention of both minerals and approaches in utero accretion of calcium and phosphorus.[71,72] This ratio provided 76 mg/kg/d of calcium and 45 mg/kg/d of phosphorus, using Aminosyn-PF® as the amino acid source. There may be an advantage of using calcium glycerophosphate versus conventional calcium gluconate because the former is more soluble.[73,74] Dunham and others [75] have generated calcium and phosphorus precipitation curves for neonatal PN, using TrophAmine®, to guide pharmacists and clinicians to help avoid compounding PN solutions that will precipitate. See Table 8 for recommended amounts of calcium and phosphorus.

Calcium phosphate is more soluble at cooler temperatures than at room or body temperature. Thus, serious concerns have been raised about the recent advocates for 3-in-1 infusates[76] that contain glucose, amino acids, and lipid emulsion in the same bottle or bag with electrolytes, minerals, and vitamins. Because these infusates must be administered without an in-line filter, the presence of lipid in the infusate obscures any visual

Table 8 Recommended Amounts of Calcium and Phosphorus

	Calcium Gluconate	Phosphate
Premature infants	300–500 mg/kg/d	1–1.5 mM/kg/d
Full-term infants	300–400 mg/kg/d	1–1.5 mM/kg/d
Older infants and children	100–200 mg/kg/d	1.0 mM/kg/d
Adolescents	50–100 mg/kg/d	0.5–1.0 mM/kg/d

Table 9 Suggested Intakes of Parenteral Vitamins in Infants and Children

		Preterm Infants (Dose/kg Body Wt Maximum Not to Exceed Full-Term Infant Dose)	
Vitamin	Full-Term Infants and Children (Dose/d)*	Current Suggestions†	Best Estimate for New Formulation‡
Lipid soluble			
A (μg)§	700	280	500
E (mg)§	7	2.8	2.8
K (μg)	200	80	80
D (μg)§	10	4	4
(IU)	400	160	160
Water soluble			
Ascorbic acid (mg)	80	32	25
Thiamin (mg)	1.2	0.48	0.35
Riboflavin (mg)	1.4	0.56	0.15
Pyridoxine	1.0	0.40	0.18
Niacin (mg)	17	6.8	6.8
Pantothenate (mg)	5	2.0	2
Biotin (μg)	20	8.0	6
Folate (μg)	140	56	56
Vitamin B_{12} (μg)	1.0	0.4	0.30

Adapted from Greene HL et al.[80]

*These guidelines for full-term infants and children are identical to those of the American Medical Association (Nutrition Advisory Group) published in 1979.[79] MVI-Pediatric (Armour; currently produced by Astra) meets these guidelines. Recent data indicate that 40 IU/kg/d vitamin D (maximum 400 IU/d) is adequate for full-term and preterm infants. The higher dose of 160 IU/kg/d has not been associated with complications and maintains blood levels within the reference range for fed orally full-term infants. This dosage therefore appears acceptable until further studies using the lower dose formulations indicate their superiority.

†These represent a practical guide (40% of the currently available single-dose vial MVI-Pediatric formulation per kilogram of body weight), which will provide adequate levels of vitamins E, D, and K but low levels of retinal and excess levels of most of the B vitamins. The maximum daily dose is one single-dose vial for any infant.

‡Because of elevated levels of water-soluble vitamins, the current proposal is to reduce intake of water-soluble vitamins and increase retinal as described in the committee's report.[80]

§700 μg retinal equivalents = 2,300 IU; 7 mg α-tocopherol = 7 IU; 10 μg vitamin D = 400 IU.

detection of precipitation that may occur either on removal from refrigeration and warming before administration or during the time of infusion. Their use in LBW infants seems unwise, especially when efforts are being made to maximize calcium and phosphate intakes. One retrospective review of 3-in-1 solutions in infants found their use safe, efficacious, and cost-effective for infants younger than 1 year of age.[77] In the review of Rollins and others,[77] Travenol® was the amino acid solution used: it does not have the lowest pH of the adult standard solutions. Thus, maximal calcium and phosphorus levels cannot be achieved with 3-in-1 solutions and should not be used routinely in the neonate.

In April 1994, a US Food and Drug Administration (FDA) safety alert was issued regarding 3-in-1 solutions, after a report was received from one institution of two deaths and at least two cases of respiratory distress that developed during peripheral infusion of a 3-in-1 (amino acids, carbohydrate, and lipids) PN admixture. Autopsies revealed diffuse microvascular pulmonary emboli containing calcium phosphate. The presence of a lipid emulsion in the PN admixture would have obscured the presence of any precipitate. ASPEN's newest "Safe Practice Guidelines" clearly state that given the limited amount of published stability information available, the use of 2-in-1 formulation with a separate administration of IVF is recommended for neonatal and infant patients.[78]

Vitamins. In 1975, the Nutrition Advisory Group (NAG) of the Department of Food and Nutrition, American Medical Association (AMA) proposed adult and pediatric guidelines for parenteral multivitamins.[79] In the United States, the FDA accepted the AMA adult formulation MVI-12® (Armour Pharmaceutical, Blue Bell, PA). The pediatric formulation MVI-Pediatric® (Armour Pharmaceutical), approved in 1981, has been tested primarily in medically stable infants and children receiving PN. The specific recommendation from a 1988 review is to use one vial of MVI-Pediatric® per day for term infants and children and 2 ml/kg/dup to 5 ml/d for preterm infants.[80] Patients receiving oral multivitamin supplements may need adjustments in parenteral multivitamin dose. For several years, there was a shortage of MVI-Pediatric® resulting in clinical deficiency states, especially thiamine deficiency.[81] See Table 9 for recommended intakes of parenteral vitamins.

Lipid-Soluble Vitamins. Lipid-soluble vitamins must be dispersed in an aqueous solution, if they are to be provided in a single vitamin mixture. To "solubilize" these lipid-soluble molecules for intravenous use, synthetic detergents, such as polysorbate, have been used. There are concerns about the safety of these detergents given intravenously to preterm infants.[82,83] In Europe, Vitalipid® (KabiVitrum, Stockholm) is a preparation containing vitamins A, D, E, and K dissolved in fractionated soybean oil and emulsified with fractionated egg phospholipids in the same manner that Intralipid is prepared. Infants requiring PN receive water-soluble vitamins in the glucose amino acid solution and the lipid-soluble vitamins with IVF (devoid of synthetic emulsifiers).

Intravenous vitamins, including vitamin A, may be lost through adsorption to plastic PN bags and tubing or biodegradation in the presence of light. Using radiolabeled vitamins, researchers found that only 31% of vitamin A, 68% of vitamin D, and 64% of vitamin E were actually delivered to the patient over a period of 24 hours.[84] Retinol depletion during PN is much more severe in VLBW infants because of the higher light intensity in nurseries and lower infusion rates of PN, which result in longer exposure time.[80]

Armour originally recommended that MVI-Pediatric® doses be 5 mL/d for all patients weighing >3 kg and 3.25 mL/d for infants weighing <3 kg. Unfortunately, at the 3.25-mL dose, infants weighing <1 kg displayed elevated vitamin E concentrations (>3.5 mg/dL).[85] Such elevations have been associated with an increased incidence of NEC and sepsis. The manufacturers subsequently modified their recommendations, suggesting that infants weighing <1 kg receive 1.5 mL/d of MVI-Pediatric. At this lower dosage, vitamin E concentrations were <1 mg/dL in 44% of the infants weighing <1 kg,[86] lower than the safe and effective levels (1 to 2 mg/dL) suggested by the American Academy of Pediatrics (AAP).[87] The recommended dose of 40% of a vial (2 mL = 2.8 mg alpha-tocopherol) per kilogram per day results in normal serum vitamin E concentrations within the range of 1.0 to 2.5 mg/dL, even in infants with birth weights between 450 and 1,360 g.[88] However, this dose may be inadequate for some infants weighing 1,000 g or less since 15% of neonates receiving 50% of a vial of MVI-Pediatric® (a larger dose than recommended) had vitamin E concentrations <1 mg/dL. Vitamin D requirements of infants receiving PN are met with the recommended doses of MVI-Pediatric.

Serum concentrations of vitamins A and E should be monitored in high-risk neonates so that adjustments in their PN regimen can be made. The benefits of adding fat-soluble vitamins to IVF solutions (to prevent loss of vitamin A onto the plastic tubing) were further demonstrated by increased plasma retinol levels in premature infants.[88] The authors concluded, however, that 280 μg/kg/d was insufficient to raise the blood levels of all infants into the normal range. Meta-analyses suggest that vitamin A supplementation may reduce chronic lung disease (CLD) and sepsis in ELBW infants. A 14-center randomized trial of vitamin A supplementation was performed in such infants, using a higher dose of vitamin A than that used in most neonatal trials (based on a pilot study)—5,000 IU vitamin A given intramuscularly three times per week for 3 weeks.[90] This regimen reduced biochemical evidence of vitamin A deficiency as well as the incidence of BPD at 36 weeks postconceptional age from 62 to 55% ($p < .03$). The investigators concluded that vitamin A supplementation is safe and reduces the incidence of BPD.

Whereas previous formulations of multivitamins did not include Vitamin K, MVI®-Adult (Mayne Pharmaceuticals, designed for patients >1 years old) now contains 150 μg of vitamin K per 10 ml, so additional Vitamin K no longer needs to be added separately.

MVI®-Pediatric (Mayne Pharmaceuticals) contains 200 μg per vial of phylloquinone (lipid-soluble vitamin K preparation). No deficiency state or toxicity has been reported with this dose.

Water-Soluble Vitamins. Thiamine deficiency was reported in a number of patients who received PN when a national shortage of MVI preparations was experienced.[81,89] As much as one-third of riboflavin in PN solutions is inactivated by light, especially phototherapy lights; riboflavin deficiency causes abnormalities of epithelia (hyperemia and edema of the pharyngeal and oral mucous membranes, cheilosis, stomatitis, glossitis, seborrheic dermatitis) and normocytic anemia.[80] Such deficiency has not been described in children maintained on PN. Findings of riboflavin-induced photohemolysis with excess riboflavin indicate the importance of maintaining normal blood concentrations of this vitamin.

The recommended parenteral dose of pyridoxine in full-term infants (1 mg/d) may be more than necessary, but it has not resulted in toxicity or deficiency. Preterm infants receiving 40% of a unit dose vial of MVI-Pediatric® would receive 0.4 mg/kg/d of pyridoxine. When this dose was given to 8 premature infants, pyridoxine concentrations increased by more than 10-fold over cord-blood and maternal levels[91]; a lower dose of 0.18 mg/kg/d resulted only in two-fold increases and is recommended for future formulations.[80] Pyridoxine is also destroyed by exposure to direct sunlight.

The clinical syndrome resulting from biotin omission from PN is characterized by scaly dermatitis, alopecia, pallor, irritability, and lethargy[92] Biotin is currently included in MVI-Pediatric in doses which are not toxic but adequate to prevent deficiency. Two studies support the continued use of the 1975 AMA NAG guidelines for water-soluble vitamin doses for term infants and children. [93,94]

Table 10 Trace Elements Daily Requirements for Pediatrics*

Trace Element	Preterm Neonates <3 kg (mcg/kg/d)	Term Neonates 3–10 kg (mcg/kg/d)	Children 10–40 kg (mcg/kg/d)	Adolescents >40 kg (per day)
Zinc	400	50-250	50–125	2.0-5.0 mg
Copper	20	20	5–20	200–500 mcg
Manganese	1.0	1.0	1.0	40–100 mcg
Chromium	0.05–0.2	0.2	0.14–0.2	5–15 mcg
Selenium	1.5–2	2.0	1.0–2.0	40–60 mcg

*Assumes normal age-related organ function and normal losses.
†Recommended intakes of trace elements cannot be achieved through the use of a single pediatric multiple trace element product. Only through the use of individualized trace element products can recommended intakes of trace elements be achieved.[80]

Trace Elements. Guidelines for intravenous administration of trace elements to pediatric patients are summarized in Table 10.[78,80,95] Moukarzel and others[96] evaluated the chromium status of children on long-term PN receiving the standard recommendations. Elevated serum chromium levels and lower glomerular filtration rates (GFRs) were noted. The GFRs were significantly inversely correlated with serum chromium concentration. After 1 year of PN without supplemental chromium, the mean serum chromium concentrations had fallen but were still higher than in controls. No change occurred in the GFRs. Unplanned chromium contamination of the PN solutions still provided 0.05 μg/kg of chromium, which is one-fourth of the current recommendation. Routine chromium supplementation seems unnecessary.

Persistent diarrhea or other excessive GI fluid losses from ostomy sites may grossly increase zinc losses. In adult balance studies, the following additional zinc replacement is required: (1) 17.1 mg of zinc per kilogram of stool or ileostomy output and (2) 12.2 mg of zinc per kilogram of small bowel fluid lost via fistula or stoma. Monitoring serum zinc in patients with persistent losses is recommended.

Selenium deficiency causes Keshan disease, an often fatal cardiomyopathy affecting children and young women in a large geographic area of China.[97] Deficiency states associated with long-term PN have been seen in adults and children [98] with intermittent leg muscle pain and tenderness, white fingernails, increases in serum alanine aminotransferase, aspartate aminotransferase, and creatine kinase and cardiomyopathy. Low selenium concentrations were also found in children receiving long-term PN[99] with similar findings and, additionally, profound muscle weakness. Long-term intravenous supplementation with 2 μg/kg/d of selenium resulted in improved clinical and laboratory findings. Suggested selenium requirements are 1.5 μg/kg/d for maintenance and 3.0 μg/kg/d for replacement[100,101] based on extrapolation from selenium intake in breastfed infants, assuming 80% absorption.[80] There is no good evidence that selenium is required for short-term PN.

Molybdenum deficiency symptoms (tachycardia, tachypnea, vomiting, and central scotomas, with rapid progression to coma) have been reported in an adult on long-term PN.[102] The patient had an excellent clinical and biochemical response to 2.5 μg/kg/d of molybdenum. Molybdenum supplementation in PN is not performed routinely.

Iron (Fe). Intravenous iron in PN regimens remains controversial owing to concerns about the risks of adverse effects. Excess Fe is thought to enhance the risk of gram-negative septicemia. Fe has powerful oxidant properties and can enhance the demand for antioxidants, especially vitamin E; particular caution is needed in giving Fe to the preterm infant.[80] Porter and others[103] agree that malnourished patients with low transferrin may be at risk of receiving a substantial infusion of Fe in the free form, which may lead to stimulation of bacterial or fungal growth.

Serum Fe, total iron-binding capacity, percent saturation, and ferritin should be assayed to assess repletion of Fe stores. There is danger of adverse reactions, including death, when Fe dextran is given intramuscularly or as a large infusion.

Pediatric patients have received iron dextran (INFeD®) in their infusates at a daily dose of 0.5 mg to 1 mg of elemental Fe per day. Adults have received 2 mg of elemetnal Fe per day. There have been no published adverse physiochemical or clinical effects. Such use is only with non-IV fat emulsions. INFeD® is not compatible with 3-in-1 PN solutions. Even then, this use of INFeD® requires caution because of compatibility issues. The INFeD® package insert states, "Do not mix INFeD® with other medications or add to PN solutions for intravenous infusion."

We recommend Fe infusions be administered separate from PN. Fe can be provided as sodium ferric gluconate complex in sucrose (Ferrlecit®) or as iron dextran. There are standard equations for Fe supplementation.[104]

Aluminum. Current PN solutions are contaminated with aluminum, which can accumulate in bone after only 3 weeks of PN in infants. Aluminum impairment of bone matrix formation and mineralization may be mediated by its direct effect on bone cells or indirectly by its effect on parathyroid hormone and calcium metabolism. Toxic effects are proportional to tissue aluminum load.[105] Intravenous calcium, phosphorus, and albumin solutions have high aluminum concentrations (>500 μg/L), while crystalline amino acids, sterile water, and dextrose have low (>50 μg/L) levels.[105] Calcium gluconate can contribute up to 80% of the total aluminum load from PN. The FDA has proposed labeling requirements concerning aluminum contents on PN additives, establishing an upper limit permitted in PN additives and has suggested that manufacturers develop validated assay methods.[106] Bishop and others demonstrated developmental delay in premature infants on PN solutions receiving aluminum 45 μg/kg/d.[107] Aluminum intake should be determined in children at high risk for toxicity: preterm infants, infants or children with impaired renal function, and patients on prolonged PN.[80] In July 2004, the FDA mandated labeling requirements for aluminum content in all PN components, and suggested that that not more than 5 μg/kg/d of aluminum be received in PN. We found that even utilizing the lowest current aluminum level PN products, we fell short of the FDA requirement, especially in the neonate.[108,109] Measuring the actual concentration of aluminum in PN solutions may prove to be far more accurate than relying on the manufacturer's label. Manufacturers will also have to improve techniques of reducing aluminum contamination from parenterally infused products.

Heparin. Heparin (1 U/mL) is often added prophylactically to PN solutions to prevent thrombosis. It reduces the formation of a fibrin sheath around the catheter and possibly reduces phlebitis with peripheral PN solutions. No controlled studies have conclusively demonstrated heparin's benefits in PN. One controlled trial has shown that it reduces catheter-related sepsis[110] and that it stimulates lipoprotein lipase release, thereby enhancing clearance of IVF. Heparin decreased total lipid concentrations and turbidity when given as a single injection of 50 to 100 U/kg to SGA infants.[111,112] One unit of heparin per milliliter of PN solution seems safe for full-term infants, children, and adults. In premature babies, no definitive guidelines are available. We routinely give 0.5 mL heparin per milliliter of PN solution to neonates.

Route of Administration

Caloric need is the primary determining factor for selecting the intravenous route for nutritional support. Solutions given in a peripheral vein are less calorically dense than solutions given in a central vein; therefore, centrally alimented patients may receive more calories and gain more weight on a daily basis.

Because peripheral venous PN regimens maintain existing body composition, this route is a reasonable choice for a normally nourished infant or child who is expected to need PN for <2 weeks. Central venous PN is a more reasonable choice for infants and older children, regardless of initial nutritional status, who will be intolerant of enteral feedings for >2 weeks. It is difficult to maintain peripheral venous PN for >2 weeks.

Ziegler and others [113] compared the complication rates of PN using central and peripheral veins. Although infectious complications occurred in approximately 10% of the central-vein group and in none of the peripheral-vein group, morbidity related to the administration of solution (primarily in the form of soft-tissue sloughs) was more prevalent in the peripheral-vein group. Complications, such as pleural effusions and thrombosis, occurred in the central-vein group. The overall complication rate was higher in the central-vein group (20% vs 9% in the peripheral-vein group). However, the complication rates per day between the two groups were not different.

Centrally placed venous catheters not only allow the infusion of hypertonic PN solutions that provide more energy, but they are less prone to noninfectious complications. In a single-center review of percutaneously inserted central catheters (PICC lines), noncentral PICC lines were noted to have a significantly higher incidence of occlusion and leaking problems than central PICCs. Adjusting for patient age, catheter size, gender, and duration of catheter placement, the OR (95% CIs) for complications among the noncentral group was 8.28 (5.11 to 13.43), compared to central group.[114] In a prospective trial among 37 adults randomized to receive a venous catheter placement in a noncentral location (axillary, subclavian or innominate vein) versus a central location (SVC), the incidence of thrombotic complications was significantly higher in the noncentral group.[115] Neither study was large enough to detect differences in infectious complications.

Intradialytic PN (IDPN) given with hemodialysis or peritoneal dialysis can be an additional route of nutrient delivery in patients with chronic renal failure and end-stage renal disease.[116]IDPN is indicated for malnourished patients and can offset the protein losses that occur as part of the dialysis process.

Patients receiving PN while on extracorporeal membrane oxygenation (ECMO) life support may have a glucose–amino acid solution administered through the ECMO circuit.[117] Some centers administer IVF through a peripheral intravenous line because of concerns that the fat may occlude the ECMO filter; however, other centers have not had this experience, and they infuse fat into the ECMO circuit directly.

Central Venous Catheters. To achieve a high caloric intake, a hyperosmolar infusate should be delivered through a central, large-bore vein with high-volume blood flow to minimize the risk of venous thrombosis and phlebitis.

The definition of a Central Venous Catheter (CVC) at Lucile Packard Children's Hospital/Stanford University Medical Center is stated below:

The optimal location for the tip of CVCs is at the junction of the superior vena cava (SVC) and right atrium. Venous catheters will be defined as "central" if the catheter tip is positioned in the distal SVC, SVC/right atrial junction, or in the inferior vena cava (IVC) at or above the level of the diaphragm. Catheter tips positioned other than these locations will be defined as "peripheral catheters". The distal SVC and IVC at or above the level of the diaphragm are the largest veins with the highest flow rate in the venous system. Infusion of cytotoxic, hypertonic, hypotonic, acid, or alkaline solutions or drug admixtures in CVC locations "minimizes" the risk of venous thrombosis, postinsertion malposition, and vessel perforation.

Most institutions recommend that PN solutions infused in a noncentral catheter should be limited in osmolarity to ≤900 mOsm/L (eg, 10% dextrose, 2% amino acids with standard additives). Silastic catheters, which have been used effectively in pediatric central venous PN for many years, are preferred to polyvinyl or polyethylene catheters because of their high degree of flexibility. They do not become rigid when in place for only a short time unlike polyvinyl catheters, which are associated with an increased likelihood of perforation of a vessel.

Two specially designed catheters for long-term PN are the Hickman® and Broviac® catheters (Davol Evermed, Kirkland, WA), which can be placed by either a cut-down incision or a percutaneous method into the SVC. Improved catheter stability and decreased risk of infection are achieved by subcutaneously tunneling the catheter to a distant exit site[118] After the insertion of any type of CVC, chest films are mandatory to confirm proper line placement and to rule out mechanical complications secondary to catheter placement. Infusion of hypertonic PN solutions or fat emulsions should not be initiated until the film has been interpreted and line placement documented. It should be noted that for PICC lines, arm movement can have a substantial impact on the CVC tip location. Standardized methodologies of arm placement during radiographic confirmation is recommended.

Umbilical Artery Catheters

The use of UA catheters for PN is not recommended because this practice is associated with a high incidence of arterial thrombosis.[196]

Initiating Therapy with PN

Before initiating PN, complete nutritional assessment, including anthropometric measurements, should be carried out to determine the potential need for nutritional repletion and to estimate caloric requirements. The PN solutions can be ordered using two formats: customized or standardized. Customized solutions are formulated specifically to meet the daily nutritional requirements of the individual patient and most nutrients are dosed on a gram, mEq, or milligram per kilogram (or per liter) basis. Standardized solutions are designed to provide a formulation that meets most of the nutritional needs of patients with stable biochemical and metabolic parameters. We feel that a customized PN regimen is best suited for pediatric patients' needs.

Preprinted PN order sheets (Figure 1) save time for physicians and pharmacy personnel. In

(addressograph stamp)

A. Please send TPN orders to the pharmacy before 11:00 am DAILY.

B. Order all additives on a 24-hour basis: eg, mEq/kg/day, mM/day, mL/day, mL/kg/day

PERIPHERAL ____________ or CENTRAL ____________ TPN LINE (check one) Today's DATE ____________

DATE DUE ____/____/____ TIME DUE ____________ (am pm)

month day year Today's WEIGHT ____________ kg

TOTAL FLUID INTAKE (mL/kg/day) ____________ Next Bottle # ____________

AMOUNT OF FAT EMULSION (g/kg/day) ____________ Fat Concentration ____ 10% ____ 20% (check one)

How many IV or IA lines exist that will not be used for TPN? ____________

	Line		Line
Enter flow rates (mL/hr):	(1) ________	and % NaCl:	(1) ________
	(2) ________	(e.g., 0.45%)	(2) ________
	(3) ________		(3) ________

If taking enteral feedings, complete the following section (check one):

____ 1. Total fluids administered as parenteral and advancing enteral, ie, "TPN + PO." (Additives are distributed assuming that the total fluids will be given parenterally)

____ 2. Total fluids administered as parenteral and fixed enteral. (Additives are distributed in parenteral fluids only; ignores electrolyte content of enteral fluids.)

Enter Amount: ________ (mis), Frequency: q ____hrs, Calories/mL: ________, Product name: ____________

Enter AMINO ACIDS (g/kg/day)† ________ Enter DEXTROSE CONCENTRATION ________%

TODAY'S ADDITIVES		PROTOCOL RECOMMENDATION
TRACE ELEMENTS AND VITAMINS		
1. PEDIATRIC TRACE ELEMENTS	____mL/kg/day	0.2 mL/kg/day (weight < 20 kg)
2. ADULT TRACE ELEMENTS	____mL/day	5 mL/day (weight > 20 kg)
3. ZINC (additional)	____μg/kg/day	100 μg/kg/day—Preemies only
4. PEDIATRIC M.V.I.	____mL/day	2 mL/kg/day—infants < 2.5 kg
	____mL/day	5 mL/day—infants ≥ 2.5 kg and children up to 11 years of age
5. ADULT MVI–12 (or generic)	____mL/day	10 mL/day—children > 11 years of age
6. VITAMIN K	____mg/day	0.5 mg/day—children > 11 years of age
ELECTROLYTES AND MINERALS		
1. PHOSPHATE*	____mM/kg/day	0.5–2 mM/kg/day
2. SODIUM	____mEq/kg/day	2.4 mEq/kg/day (sodium from other IVs is included)
3. POTASSIUM	____mEq/kg/day	2–3 mEq/kg/day
4. ACETATE*†	____mEq/kg/day	1–4 mEq/kg/day
5. MAGNESIUM	____mEq/kg/day	0.25–0.5 mEq/kg/day
6. CALCIUM GLUCONATE	____mg/kg/day	50–500 mg/kg/day
7. HEPARIN	____Units/mL	0.5–1 Unit/mL
8. INSULIN	____Units/liter	
9. OTHER (specify)	____	
10. OTHER (specify)	____	

*NOTE: Balance of anions will be provided as chloride.

†Each 0.5 g/kg/day of amino acid provides either 0.47 mEq/kg/day of acetate (TrophAmine) or 0.74 mEq/kg/day of acetate (Aminosyn).

RN ____________________ MD ____________________

Figure 1 Example of a physician's order sheet for total parenteral nutrition (TPN)

addition, the order sheet helps to avoid errors of omission, ensuring that all necessary nutrients are ordered. The order sheet provides the necessary input for specific PN computer programs. Protocol recommendations are provided in the right-hand column of the order sheet for reference. For teenage patients, it may be acceptable to use an adult-standard solution. Depending on the patient's electrolyte and nutritional status, calorie, fluid, and electrolyte requirements are determined and the solution ordered appropriately. As mentioned earlier, doses of carbohydrate, fat, and protein are gradually advanced to avoid overtaxing the metabolic capacities of the patient. Our recommended advancing guidelines are shown in Table 11. Clinical pathways have been developed for the administration of PN.[119] To further improve safety and efficiency of the PN process, we employ Windows-based software from Monterey Medical Solutions, Inc (TPN Medsoft v4.0–Salinas, CA). The software drives a Baxa

Table 11 Parenteral Nutrition Advancing Guidelines

	Dextrose	Fat (g/kg/d)	Amino Acids (g/kg/d)
Premature infants			
Initial	4–6 mg/kg/min	0.5	1.5
Advance*	1–2 mg/kg/min	0.5	0.5–1.0
Full-term neonates			
Initial	5%	0.5–1.0	1.5
Advance*	2.5%	0.5	0.5–1.0
Older infants/children			
Initial	10%	1.0	1.5
Advance*	5%	0.5–1.0	1.0
Adolescents and older			
Initial	10%	1.0	1.5
Advance*	5–10%	1.0	1.0

*Rate of advancement might be limited by metabolic tolerance, for example, hyperglycemia, hypertriglyceridemia, or azotemia.

Table 12 Complications of Parenteral Nutrution

Catheter related	
Infection: local (site), tunnel infection, sepsis	
Catheter occlusion	
Air embolus	
Crack, breakage, or aneurysm of catheter	
Noncatheter related	
1. Electrolyte hypo-/hypernatremia	Hypo-/hyperkalemia
2. Mineral hypo-/hypercalcemia	Hypo-/hyperphosphatemia Hypo-/hypermagnesemia
3. Metabolic acidosis	
4. Lipid related hypertriglyceridemia	Hypercholesterolemia Essential fatty acid deficiency Fat overload syndrome
5. Protein related	Hyperammonemia Uremia
6. Carbohydrate related	Hypo-/hyperglycemia
7. Hydration related	Dehydrated/fluid overload
8. Refeeding syndrome	
9. Hepatobiliary disease	
10. Metabolic bone disease	

automated compounder which utilizes bar code technology, eliminates compounding errors, and improves quality control. Daily compounding time has been reduced from 20 to 6 hours at our hospital. We are now piloting computer order entry to further simplify the PN ordering process.[120]

Cyclic PN

The administration of PN over a period of < 24 h/d is termed cyclic PN. It allows for the patient to be more physically active, and allows more flexible PN scheduling.[121] Conditions necessary for instituting cyclic PN include stable metabolic status, electrolyte and fluid requirements, and steady weight gain for at least 2 to 4 days on continuous PN. Patients should be able to handle maintenance fluids over a short period of time and have well-positioned CVCs. Safe administration of cyclic PN has been described in all ages, including infants with weights as low as 5 kg.[122] If the glucose concentration exceeds 10% and/or if the glucose infusion rate is high, some suggest tapering the rate over the last hour by 50%. Almost all home PN patients receive cyclic PN for ease of care. Recent cycling guidelines, with an equation online to do the calculations for users are available at: http://peds.stanford.edu/tpn.html. The cycle calculator can also be downloaded to a handheld computer.

Transition from Parenteral to Enteral Nutrition

There is an approximately 50% decline in enteric mucosal mass in normal animals maintained on intravenous nutrition in positive nitrogen balance without enteric stimulation.[123] Pancreatic atrophy and impairment of function also occur.[124] All segments of the small intestine demonstrate a decrease in the rate of proliferation and migration of the epithelial cells in the parenterally fed versus enterally fed animals. Numerous animal studies have demonstrated the positive impact that luminal nutrients have on maintaining the structural and functional integrity of the GI tract. These trophic effects on the intestinal mucosa may be direct or may be mediated by the GI hormones. Although human data are limited, it seems prudent to maintain a small oral nutritional intake during PN, whenever possible.

In infants with intractable diarrhea, Greene and others have demonstrated more rapid recovery of intestinal disaccharidases with the combination of PN plus elemental enteral feeds than with PN alone.[125] Intestinal development is arrested when animals receive PN with no enteral nutrients, and resumption of intestinal maturation occurs on reintroduction of intraluminal nutrients. Unlike that of the intestine and pancreas, the digestive function of the stomach is not impaired during PN in the very preterm infant. PN without gastric feeds decreases acid and pepsin in human infants, but when these infants are placed on constant-rate enteral infusion, these secretions return to normal.[126]

The transition from parenteral to enteral feeding should be gradual because the sudden cessation of PN may result in severe rebound hypoglycemia (secondary to hyperinsulinemia produced from high glucose intake). Small volumes of oral feedings are begun and then increased to full feeds. The volume of the PN is proportionally decreased. After prolonged PN, many infants and children are reluctant to feed orally for reasons that are not clear.[127] Early involvement of oromotor therapists with these patients (in advance of their starting oral feedings) may prove extremely helpful.

Complications

Patients receiving PN are at risk of technical, infectious, and metabolic complications. These complications can be avoided or minimized only by regular monitoring, strict aseptic technique, and a multidisciplinary nutrition support team (Table 12).

Technical Complications. Possible complications at the time of the catheter insertion include pneumothorax, hemothorax, hydromediastinum, arterial injury, hematoma formation, arterial laceration, arteriovenous fistula and air embolism, catheter embolism, malposition, cardiac perforation, and tamponade. Complications related to ongoing use of the catheter include venous thrombosis, catheter dislodgment, and perforation of the pericardium, pleura, and mediastinum with leakage of the PN solution.

Forty-two newborns who had Broviac catheter placement were followed up prospectively with echocardiograms.[128] Six infants (14%) had thrombus formation after the catheter had been in place for a median of 7 weeks. Those with thrombus formation had significantly lower birth weight and gestational ages than those without thrombus, but there was no correlation of thrombosis with duration of catheter placement. Many nurseries employ percutaneous central venous catheterization. In a study of 481 catheters placed percutaneously in a neonatal intensive care unit over a 3-year period,[129] 50% were placed in infants weighing ≤1 kg. Mean catheter life was 13 days; almost half were removed nonelectively for leaking, clotting, or suspicion of sepsis (6%). Catheter sepsis was confirmed in 1.3%. For catheter-related sepsis, three factors were important: prolonged catheter placement (3 to 5 weeks), infection by Staphylococcus epidermidis, and infant weight ≤1 kg.[129]

Percutaneous central lines result in lower complication rates than those reported with surgically placed venous catheters. Complications with this method are leakage or perforation of the catheter. Placement of the catheter in the atrium can stimulate cardiac arrhythmias or cause the catheter to incorporate itself into the endocardium. Cardiac tamponade can result from atrial perforation by the CVC.[130–132] Regular and meticulous care of the CVC, particularly the catheter exit site, is essential for prolonged, safe complication-free use. Use of the catheter for purposes other than delivery of PN, particularly for blood transfusions and blood sampling, should be avoided.

For long-term venous access, the Broviac catheter continues to demonstrate a lower complication rate than the traditional Silastic catheter.[133] Broviac catheter-associated infections occur more often in VLBW infants (69%), compared with infants weighing >1,500 g (20%).[134] Seventy-eight percent (14 of 18) of these infections were successfully treated with antibiotics without catheter removal. The rate of thrombosis was also higher in VLBW infants.

A prospective study of 8 pediatric patients by Newall demonstrated that warfarin prophylaxis helps decrease the frequency of central vein thrombosis and prolonges the duration of the line.[136] Our center has not adopted this practice for central catheters.

Catheter-Associated Infection. The major catheter-related complication is infection, usually the result of improper care of the catheter. Most of these infections can be treated with the catheter in situ.[137] Staphylococcus epidermidis is the most frequent organism encountered, so vancomycin and gentamicin may be used successfully as initial therapy,[138] pending final culture report and sensitivities. Lack of defervescence of fever and continued positive blood cultures for 2 to 4 days despite antibiotics are indications for catheter removal.[139] Otherwise antibiotics should be continued for 10 to 21 days.[139] The GI tract may be a source of microbial seeding of the bloodstream via the catheter. There is considerable interest in therapies that maintain or improve the integrity of the gut.[140] For example, the role of glutamine in preventing gut atrophy in parenterally fed, enterally fasted patients needs to be further explored[141] because gut atrophy may foster increased intestinal permeability of bacterial pathogens. Guidelines have been published to offer recommendations for preventing catheter-related sepsis in the pediatric setting.[142]

Recently, a prospective study of 300 neonates demonstrated that a closed drug delivery system had no impact on decreasing the incidence of catheter-related sepsis or nosocomial infections.[143] A closed drug delivery system is one in which there are no openings providing a direct pathway between a sterile product and the environment.[144]

Catheter Occlusion. Estimates suggest that 25% of CVCs become occluded, with thrombosis as the most common etiology. Nonthrombotic causes include: deposition of intravenous lipids, calcium–phosphorus precipitates, heparin-induced occlusion, intraluminal drug precipitates, and mechanical occlusion.

Before 1999, the only approved pharmacologic agent for the medical treatment of thrombosed CVCs was urokinase (Abbokinase–Open Cath; Abbott Laboratories, Abbott Park, IL) derived from human neonatal kidney cells. In January 1999, the FDA suspended the distribution of urokinase because of the theoretical concern for the transmission of infectious agents.

Recombinant tissue plasminogen activator (alteplase) has subsequently been shown to be very effective in the restoration of function of CVCs occluded by a thrombus.[145] In September 2001, CathFlo™ Activase® (Alteplase; Genentech Inc., San Francisco, CA) was approved by the FDA for occlusions caused by thrombus. Published pediatric data on alteplase to date had demonstrated both safety and efficacy, but the FDA requested additional safety data in pediatric patients. Therefore, a multicenter phase IV open-label, single-arm study of the safety and efficacy of Cathflo ™ Activase® in in pediatric subjects was conducted; in January 2005 it was concluded that the product was safe for use in patients ages 2 weeks to 17 years.[146]

Should a thrombolytic agent fail to clear an occlusion, alternative causes should be considered. Six pediatric patients with occlusion of CVCs by calcium phosphate crystals were successfully treated by irrigating their catheters with a dilute hydrochloric acid solution.[147] Catheter occlusion caused by lipid material, associated with PN treatment, has been successfully cleared with ethanol after urokinase failed to clear these occlusions.[148,149] A recent review provides specific guidelines for clearance of catheter occlusions.[149]

Metabolic Complications: Use of IVF. The incidence of complications associated with the use of IVF is low. If the IVF infusion exceeds its maximal clearance rate, hyperlipidemia occurs, which may cause impairment of pulmonary function, displacement of albumin-bound bilirubin by plasma free fatty acids (which may lead to kernicterus), and a fat overload syndrome (hypertriglyceridemia, fever, lethargy, liver damage, and coagulopathy). Thus, careful monitoring of the use of IVF emulsions is essential by regularly checking serum triglyceride concentrations. ESPGHAN/ESPEN guidelines state that reduction of lipids should be considered if serum triglyceride levels during infusion exceed 250 mg/dl in infants or 400 mg/dl in older children.[187] ASPEN guidelines recommend that if serum triglyceride levels exceed 200mg/dl, then IVF should be discontinued and then restarted at a rate of 0.5 to 1 g/kg/d.[186] Allergic or hypersensitivity reactions to IVF are extremely rare.[150,151]

After boluses of IVF are infused into newborn infants, several investigators have demonstrated significant drops of arterial oxygen tension (PaO_2) without alteration in other pulmonary function tests.[152] Two hypotheses exist to explain the fall in arterial oxygen saturation: (1) lipid microemboli block pulmonary capillaries and alter perfusion ventilation ratios; and (2) fat metabolism leads to increased production of certain prostaglandins, which leads to pulmonary hypertension. The use of IVF in patients with pulmonary compromise has yielded conflicting results. While fat emboli were found on postmortem examination of pulmonary capillaries in neonates and infants who received Intralipid,[153–156] other reports have found no consistent association.[157] Fat deposition in the pulmonary microcirculation also have been documented in babies who never received IVF.[154]

In rabbits there were no blood gas or prostaglandin changes in lipid-infused normal animals.[158] However, when the rabbits' lungs were damaged with oleic acid and then infused with IVF, significant deterioration in gas exchange occurred. Furthermore, these changes were blocked by indomethacin (implying prostaglandin-mediated effects of IVF). Brans and others [159] found that oxygen diffusion in the lungs of premature infants was not affected by the infusion of up to 4 g/d of Intralipid over 24 hours.

Studies have been performed to evaluate the effect of early infusion of IVF in LBW infants on the development of CLD. Some studies suggested that early administration of IVF was a risk factor for the occurrence of CLD[160,161] A meta-analysis, however, of six randomized controlled trials (n = 522 patients) of early (Day 1 to 5) versus late (Day 5 to 14) introduction of I.V. lipids in preterm, LBW infants, found no significant trend or effect on the incidence of death or CLD (at 28 days or at 36 weeks).[162]

Unsaturated fatty acids are highly susceptible to peroxidation, and the products (hydroperoxides) can interfere with arachidonic acid metabolism or react to form organic free radicals, which can initiate peroxidative injury in tissues. Helbock and others[163] demonstrated significant concentrations of lipid hydroperoxides in Intralipid. These toxic hydroperoxides may represent a significant risk to premature infants, particularly those with preexisting lung disease. Neuzil and others demonstrated oxidation of IVF by ambient and phototherapy lights in a neonatal intensive care unit. [164] Minimizing exposure of lipids to ambient and phototherapy light decreases the hydroperoxide concentrations.

A study by Park and others[165] confirms previous observations that septic infants can develop significant elevations in triglyceride concentrations. A sudden rise in triglycerides not associated with an increase in IVF dose should make caregivers suspicious of sepsis. A study in neonates receiving IVF for 2 weeks or more (n = 162) demonstrated that liver dysfunction and fetal growth retardation were associated with lipid intolerance (elevated triglycerides), perhaps secondary to reduced hepatic lipase activity and, hence, impaired triglyceride clearance. Infection was not independently associated with hypertriglyceridemia.[166]

There is a reluctance to use IVF in patients with low platelet counts, on the basis of reports of varying degrees of thrombocytopenia with earlier IVF preparations and on the basis of one case report with Intralipid. Many anecdotal reports of thrombocytopenia may be secondary to an underlying condition (eg, sepsis) rather than to IVF. Cohen and others[167] could not implicate IVF as a cause of thrombocytopenia in any of the 128 patients studied. In addition, 10 patients with thrombocytopenia secondary to sepsis or chemotherapy had rises in platelet counts, concomitant with the improvement of the septicemia state or with marrow recovery after cessation of chemotherapy. Actually, PN without IVF may lead to EFA deficiency, which, in turn, may cause thrombocytopenia and platelet dysfunction.

Use of Carbohydrate. Hyperglycemia and hypoglycemia can occur with inappropriate dosing of carbohydrate intake. Hyperglycemia can result in glucosuria. If urine glucose by Keto-Diastix® (Ames Company, Elkhart, IN) is 0.25% (250 mg/dL) or greater, it should be monitored with Dextrostix®. If the Dextrostix result is elevated, it should be confirmed with a blood glucose. If glucosuria is present in the absence of hyperglycemia, renal dysfunction may be to blame and PN should not unnecessarily be reduced. If hyperglycemia and glucosuria coexist, better glycemic control should be sought, either with avoidance of high rates of glucose infusion or the addition of insulin. A systematic review of all possible etiologies for glucosuria should consider medications, including steroids, dietary indiscretions, an error in the PN delivery rate, and sepsis.

Use of Protein. Excessive amino acid infusions can result in increased blood urea nitrogen (BUN), increased ammonia production, and metabolic acidosis in at-risk patients with liver or kidney disease and LBW infants who have limited tolerance.[168] Thus, frequent monitoring of serum electrolytes, blood pH, BUN, and even ammonia may be indicated in these patients. In patients with ongoing protein losses and hypoproteinemia despite good protein intake, a 24-hour urine collection for urine urea nitrogen (UUN) may be necessary to determine nitrogen balance. The UUN is measured in milligrams per 100 mL.

N balance = grams of protein (intake) /6.25 − (UUN + 3).

The protein intake should include grams of protein provided by oral or enteral feeds plus those provided by intravenous amino acids. Dividing by 6.25 converts the grams of protein intake into grams of nitrogen. The UUN in this equation is expressed in grams. The constant of 3 in the equation corrects for nonurea nitrogen losses (approximately 2 g/d), fecal losses (approximately 1 g/d), and skin, hair, and nail losses (approximately 0.2 g/d). This constant has been established in adult balance studies; some have used the estimate of 10 mg/kg/d in children.

Osteopenia of Prematurity. Premature infants are subject to a unique condition, "osteopenia" of prematurity or "rickets of prematurity," a common but poorly defined metabolic bone disease causing decreased mineralization. In most cases, decreased bone mineralization is subclinical; this condition is diagnosed only after the development of bone fractures or overt rickets.[169] Experts believe that a deficiency of calcium and phosphorus is more likely than a defect in vitamin D metabolism as the cause of osteopenia in preterm infants.[170]

Hepatobiliary Dysfunction. Hepatic dysfunction, one of the most common and most serious complications of PN, has been reviewed extensively.[171–173] Cholestasis is especially prevalent in very premature infants and in infants on PN for >2 weeks. Other risk factors for PN-associated liver disease (PNALD) include excess energy intake, high parenteral protein or fat intake, earlier age of first bloodstream infection, and longer time with diverting ostomies. Hepatomegaly with mild elevation of serum transaminases in the absence of cholestasis may result from hepatic accumulation of lipid or glycogen secondary to either excess carbohydrate calories or an inappropriate nonnitrogen calorie/nitrogen ratio. Fatty infiltration of the liver as a result of excessive caloric intake is readily reversible in nearly all instances by reduction of total calories administered. Abnormal liver function tests are not uncommon in patients on PN for long periods of time. Those with chronic intestinal conditions complicated by infection and bacterial overgrowth are particularly susceptible to hepatic complications. In most of these patients, elevated liver enzymes improve with the initiation of partial enteral alimentation.

The earliest abnormality (at 2 weeks) noted is an elevated serum GGT or bile acid level. A small percentage of infants and children go on to develop chronic liver disease (CLD) associated with poor growth[174] and even cirrhosis and hepatic failure.[175] A follow-up study of patients on long-term PN documented a wide variety of complications, but all of them (except liver dysfunction) proved to be temporary.[176] In this study, 58% of the children showed liver dysfunction during PN; some showed long-term abnormalities after its cessation. If PNLD is suspected, then excessive caloric and/or protein intake should be avoided, feeds should be advanced as able.[177] PN solution should be cycled, and the percentage of calories from carbohydrates kept between 50 and 55%.

Long-term administration of PN increases the risk of gallstones in patients of all ages[178–180]; children with ileal disease or resection are at particularly high risk.[180] Gallbladder disease appears to be secondary to bile stasis. Clinically, gallbladder disease can be detected by the demonstration of "sludge" or stones in a patient with liver function tests consistent with cholestasis. Messing and others[179] demonstrated sludge in 6% of cases in the first 3 weeks of PN; the incidence increased to 50% between the fourth and sixth weeks and reached 100% after 6 weeks. Roslyn and others[180] recommend periodic ultrasonography in children on prolonged PN, especially if they have an ileal resection or underlying ileal disease. They advised clinicians to suspect cholecystitis in any child on PN who complains of abdominal pain. A review of 246 infants and children receiving PN for more than 4 weeks revealed significant biliary disease.[181]

Refeeding Syndrome. This is the term used to describe the metabolic disturbances that occur when malnourished patients are refed rapidly. Drops in serum phosphorus, potassium, and magnesium, changes in glucose metabolism, vitamin deficiency, and need for fluid resuscitation may occur.[182,183] The most important preventative measure is to identify the at-risk patient and then start caloric intake at 75% of the REE, followed by a cautious increase of caloric intake by 10 to 15% per day, provided the electrolyte, calcium, phosphorus, and magnesium concentrations are within normal limits (see Chapter 13, "Protein-Energy Malnutrition: Pathophysiology, Clinical Consequences, and Treatment," for additional discussion of refeeding syndrome).

Monitoring PN

The suggested schedule for chemical and anthropometric monitoring is shown in Table 13. Such monitoring should allow detection of metabolic complications in sufficient time to permit alteration of the PN infusate, with resultant correction of any abnormality. Detailed guides for monitoring are readily available.[184]

Home PN

For patients who require long-term chronic PN administration and hospitalization solely for the provision of PN, techniques have been developed to provide PN at home. Since the first patients being managed on home parenteral nutrition (HPN) were described by Scribner and others in

Table 13 Monitoring of Parenteral Nutrition

Short-term monitoring
1. Anthropometrics: daily weight check
2. Laboratory studies (baseline): complete blood count, serum electrolytes, triglycerides, cholesterol, calcium, magnesium, phosphorus, alkaline phosphatase, total protein, albumin, BUN, creatinine, ALT, GGTP, bilirubin (total and conjugated), iron studies, prealbumin
3. Daily laboratory studies (initial): serum electrolytes, BUN, creatinine, triglycerides, calcium, phosphorus, magnesium
4. Weekly laboratory studies (the above daily laboratory studies plus): ALT, alkaline, phosphatase, GGTP, bilirubin (total and conjugated), cholesterol, total protein, albumin, prealbumin
Long-term monitoring
1. Anthropometrics: <2 years of age: Weight, length, head circumference, arm anthropometrics (every 2–4 weeks)
>2 years of age: Weight, height, arm anthropometrics (monthly)
2. Every 3 months: Iron studies (serum iron, TIBC, % saturation, ferritin)
3. Every 6 months:
(a) Vitamin A, E, 25-OH vitamin D, PT/PTT
(b) Serum selenium, zinc, copper,* chromium, whole blood manganese
4. Yearly:
(a) Abdominal ultrasonography
(b) Bone mineral density study
(c) Renal clearance

ALT = alanine aminotransferase; BUN = blood urea nitrogen; GGTP = γ-glutamyl transpeptidase; PT = prothrombin time; PTT = partial thromboplastin time; TIBC = total iron-binding capacity.
*Obtain monthly if copper has been removed from total parental nutrition secondary to cholestasis.

1970, the technique has been successfully adapted to children. Over the last two decades, the use of HPN has been greatly expanded, and HPN has come to be accepted as a useful supportive and therapeutic technique for various gastrointestinal diseases and other conditions.[185–190]

Indications. The clinical conditions requiring HPN are the same as those for PN in the hospital, except that the patient no longer requires acute hospital care. Discharge on HPN, although expensive, can save healthcare dollars. The most common indications for HPN[189] are as follows: (1) short-bowel syndrome, with and without the potential for bowel adaptation; (2) motility disorders; (3) intractable diarrhea; (4) acquired immunodeficiency syndrome (AIDS); and (5) cancer-related conditions. Contraindications for HPN include a functional GI tract and lack of vascular access. Patients with anorexia nervosa are generally not candidates for HPN. HPN should also not be used if no parent or family member is dedicated to learning and performing the daily techniques required for a successful program, or when parents and other family members do not have sufficient ability to learn.[185] The Ament group believes that a child should require HPN for a minimum of 30 days to justify the time and expense involved in training family members and establishing the program.[185] However, discharging a patient on HPN may afford overall cost savings to all parties, even if the patient might be able to take adequate oral nutrition in fewer than 30 days after discharge.

Implementation. Preparing a patient for HPN requires a multidisciplinary team approach, including medical specialists, nursing staff, pharmacists, dietitians, social workers, and psychologists or psychiatrists. Social workers need to assess the family's ability to perform HPN and then provide emotional support at home. Before discharge, parents must master the necessary technical skills for providing HPN on a continuous or cyclic basis. Such skills include the following: (1) using aseptic technique, (2) adding medications to the HPN solution, (3) administering HPN through a central venous line, (4) operating the infusion pump, (5) heparin-locking the line, and (6) performing dressing changes. Once the child is home, the family is faced with integrating these procedures into their life, while coping with the child's illness and the demands of normal child development.[191]

General information outlining benefits, risks, and complications are the first aspects of HPN discussed with the family. These discussions with caretakers should also include the expected outcome of PN therapy and the predicted degree of bowel adaptation.[185] Ninety percent of children with short bowel who have at least 25 cm of small intestine and an ileocecal sphincter eventually are able to discontinue PN support.[192] Children who have an intact ileocecal sphincter and 15 to 20 cm of small bowel ultimately may adapt partially or completely.[185,192]

For long-term PN, cuffed silicone elastomer (Silastic) tunneled CVCs, such as the Hickman and Broviac catheters, have been commonly used. Totally implantable venous access systems, for example, Infuse-A-Port® (Intermedics Infusaid Corporation, Norwood, MA) and Port-A-Cath® (Pharmacia Laboratories, Piscataway, NJ), have been used in children for administering blood products, drugs, and PN. The choice of vascular access device should be based on patient needs, capability, lifestyle, preference, and the HPN team's experience and knowledge of the available products. Patients can be freed from multiple intravenous poles, bottles, and tubing with the advent of lightweight portable pumps carried in ambulatory vests or backpacks.

Home nutritional requirements and fluid needs are assessed as stated previously. Generally, patients are stabilized before discharge from hospital. Virtually all patients can receive a cyclic PN schedule. The duration of infusion time may vary from 8 to 18 hours, depending on the age, nutritional requirements, medications, and enteral intake of the patient.

Complications. Complications of HPN are fewer when an experienced team is involved. The three types of complications that can occur are infectious, technical, and metabolic. In the series of De Potter and others,[189] the mean duration of HPN was 615 days (range, 30 to 3,532 days). Twenty-nine patients died, but only 3 deaths were HPN related, 1 because of cirrhosis and 2 because of catheter-related sepsis. Catheter-related complications included sepsis (n = 105), occlusion (n = 10), and dislodgment (n = 9).

The most common HPN-related complication requiring hospital re-admission is catheter sepsis,[185] but these infections are less common in HPN than in hospitalized PN patients.[185] The lower incidence of catheter infection at home reflects the positive impact of one dedicated caregiver, well trained in meticulous catheter care. The incidence of HPN catheter infections is higher in children than in adults.[193] Catheter infections are usually caused by some known or unsuspected break in standard technique for HPN. Fever can occur in children because of catheter infection but also from usual childhood illnesses. With each fever, HPN patients should be seen for a careful physical examination and history. If there is no recognizable source of infection, the most likely possibility is a catheter infection or an intercurrent viral infection. The patient should have central and peripheral venous blood cultures done for aerobes, anaerobes, and fungi, a complete blood cell count, urinalysis, and chest radiography; other tests depend on clinical findings. If infection is found, the patient should be treated with intravenous antibiotics because most HPN patients cannot adequately absorb oral antibiotics. If no source of infection is found, empiric antibiotic coverage may still be considered.

In general, not removing a line is important because of the long-term need for vascular access. Catheter removal is required for the following reasons: (1) fungal infection, (2) septic shock, (3) endocarditis, (4) embolism, (5) persistent fever with positive blood culture growth, or (6) disseminated intravascular coagulation. Tunnel tract infections usually require catheter removal.[193] After a catheter is removed, antimicrobial therapy is continued for 5 to 7 days, and a new catheter is inserted after the patient is afebrile for 72 hours and blood cultures no longer contain the infectious organism.[194] In a large series, 87% of gram-positive and 53% of gram-negative infections were treated successfully without catheter removal. Of exit-site infections, 50% were successfully treated without catheter removal. There was also a longer lifespan with the second catheter as well as a higher incidence of catheter-related complications of HPN in the first 2 years versus later years.[194]

The major technical problem with HPN is catheter occlusion. As stated previously, warfarin has been used to prevent catheter-related thrombosis.[136,195] Of a group of 12 children on HPN,[196] bilateral upper limb venography showed extensive deep vein thrombosis (DVT) in 8. Warfarin treatment lengthened the average lifespan of their catheters, and no catheter-related DVT had occurred on follow-up. The authors advocated venography as the reference test for the diagnosis of central venous line-related DVT. Magnetic resonance imaging (MRI) has been used to diagnose DVT in adults, but there are no comparable studies in children. Lineograms, consisting of injection of contrast media into the central venous line, were found to be insensitive. Sola and others[197] described their 6-year experience with 22 Infusc-A-Ports in 15 cystic fibrosis patients. The overall complication rate was low: 1 in 1,483 catheter days, but the incidence of major thrombotic events in 3 of 22 catheters (14%) led to a policy of administering low-dose aspirin therapy (80 mg/d) in all patients who did not have liver disease or other risks of bleeding.

Metabolic complications of HPN are similar to those previously described. There is a single report in the literature of thrombocytopenia in 7 children on long-term HPN, all of whom were receiving only 1–2 g/kg/d of fat emulsion.[198] Recurrent thrombocytopenia (platelets $<$100,000) occurred in all 7. Platelet lifespan measured with indium-111 was reduced. These data contrast with an 18-year HPN experience at UCLA where no patient receiving long-term daily parenteral fat emulsion has developed significant thrombocytopenia.

Since the guidelines for trace elements and vitamins[80] have been developed, deficiency states previously described rarely occur on long-term HPN. As stated previously, extra zinc supplementation is required in patients who have massive diarrhea and/or malabsorption. If iodide antiseptic solutions are used in central venous line care, this iodide is absorbed through the skin and contributes to normal iodide levels.[188] Now that iodide is not used in central line skin care, some centers are adding 1 μg/kg/d of I.V. iodide in children receiving more than 30 days of PN. Intravenous Fe must be provided in patients who are unable to absorb it enterally. When patients receiving PN develop cholestasis (conjugated bilirubin ⩾2), it is routine to remove or reduce copper and manganese from the PN solution, because both are hepatotoxic and are cleared by the liver (since many centers use a standard solution of 4 trace elements—zinc, copper, manganese, and chromium—the trace element solution is held and zinc is added back separately). Recently, severe copper deficiency has been reported in cholestatic patients associated with symptoms such as pancytopenia, depigmentation of the hair, and pseudoscurvy. In these patients, it is wise to monitor serum copper at least monthly, and replace copper if values come back low.[199]

Manganese (Mn) toxicity has been reported in long-term PN patients. Symptoms have included disturbances in thought processes and gait, hallucinations, and Parkinson's-like symptoms. MRI can detect accumulation of Mn in the brain, and T_1-weighted MRI images have shown high intensity in the basal ganglia, especially in the globus pallidus, in patients receiving PN. Whole blood Mn is the best test to screen for excess levels. In adults, the dose of 1 mcmol Mn/day in PN keeps those blood concentrations normal.[200] Cholestatic patients should have Mn omitted or reduced in their PN.

Carnitine deficiency may be associated with abnormal oxidation of long-chain fatty acids and progressive hepatic dysfunction. In a longitudinal study of 9 children on carnitine-free PN, plasma total and free carnitine were 50% lower than in healthy control subjects, but they did not decrease further during the 3-year prospective follow-up.[201] The mean alanine aminotransferase, aspartate aminotransferase, and alkaline phosphatase were slightly increased at the onset of the study but remained unchanged 3 years later. Low plasma carnitine concentrations appeared to be without clinical consequences after 10 years of carnitine-free HPN.[201]

In the past, patients receiving long-term HPN were seen with bone pain, hypercalciuria with normocalcemia, normal phosphatemia, and normal 1,25-dihydroxyvitamin D, 25-hydroxyvitamin D, and parathyroid hormone concentrations. The pathogenesis of this syndrome was secondary to aluminum toxicity because casein hydrolysates (used as the protein source in PN at some centers) were heavily contaminated with aluminum. This symptomatic bone disease has not been seen since all children have been receiving crystalline amino acid solutions. Osteopenia is a characteristic of patients who receive long-term PN. Such patients have been demonstrated to have a mean loss of 25% of the calcium in their trabecular bone.[202] This osteopenia may be multifactorial. Deficiencies of Mn, fluoride, boron, and silicon have all been suggested as causative factors, as well as reduced amounts of weight-bearing exercise. Additionally, adequate amounts and proportions of calcium and phosphorus are sometimes difficult to achieve in PN solutions. Moukarzel and others[203] found that serum silicon concentrations in children receiving HPN were 50% lower than those in non-HPN controls. Furthermore, a significant correlation between silicon intake and mineralization suggests an involvement of silicon in the pathogenesis of the bone disease.[203]

Buchman and others[204] reported that long-term PN is associated with a marked decrease in both GFR and tubular function. The observed decline could not be entirely explained on the basis of nutritional status, age, duration of PN, the protein load, exposure to nephrotoxic drugs, or the frequency of infectious episodes. A previous study of renal function in children on long-term PN[205] showed that GFR might be reduced in these patients. No nephrocalcinosis or tubular dysfunction was identified in this group of patients.

Long-term effects of PN on the liver and biliary tree have been discussed earlier in this chapter. A comprehensive review[206] concluded that excessive caloric provision, especially in the form of carbohydrate, plays an important role in the pathogenesis of steatosis; and loss of enteric stimulation rather than PN per se may be the critical determinant in the development of cholestasis, biliary sludge, and gallstones.[207]

In recent years, there has been a dramatic reduction in PN-induced liver disease associated with two key differences in management practices: (1) initiation of enteral feedings (even as little as 1 to 5 mL per feed in the preterm neonate), and (2) availability of balanced amino acid solutions (TrophAmine, Aminosyn-PF) specifically designed for infants, reducing the toxicity occurring with adult formulations.

In addition, choline deficiency plays a role in hepatocyte damage. In animal models, choline-deficient diets are associated with fatty infiltration of the liver, a process that is reversible by adding choline to the diet. Buchman and others[208] reported low free-plasma choline in HPN patients. They found that there was a significant correlation ($p < .02$) between low free-plasma choline and elevations in serum aminotransferases. The same group reported the reversal of PN-associated hepatic steatosis in 4 long-term HPN patients using an intravenous choline supplement added to the PN, 1 to 4 g/d for 6 weeks.[209] Fifteen of their HPN patients who had a low free-plasma choline were randomly assigned to receive oral lecithin 40 g/d or placebo for 6 weeks.[210] Lecithin supplementation resulted in increased plasma-free choline and a significant and progressive reduction in hepatic fat as assessed by computed tomography (CT).

A placebo-controlled trial demonstrated proof of a human choline requirement for long-term home PN patients.[211] All 15 study patients had hepatic steatosis confirmed by CT scan. Those randomized to choline received 2 g choline chloride per night, rather than placebo, and experienced resolution of hepatic steatosis along with decreases in serum AST and ALT.

Long-Term Growth and Nutritional Problems. Children receiving only HPN can achieve normal height, weight, midarm circumference, midarm muscle circumference, and triceps skin-fold thickness. The HPN patients receiving 30 to 70% of their total nutrients orally or enterally do gain weight and grow, but not as well as those on exclusive PN.[212] In this latter group, there may be a propensity to underestimate the amount of PN needed by patients who ingest some nutrients.[185] Enteral calories may be malabsorbed to various degrees, depending on the underlying disease of the patients. Periodically, one should assess the amount of nutrients these patients can absorb enterally. Frequently, long-term HPN patients have growth retardation in the face of an apparently adequate caloric support. Causes for such failure of growth might include EFA deficiency, trace element deficiency, various endocrine disorders, or alpha-ketoglutarate deficiency.[213] Six prepubertal children on HPN who were well below their expected 50th percentile for height were studied over two successive 5-month periods. A dose of 15 g of ornithine alpha-ketoglutarate (OKG) was added to the HPN solution in the first 5 months but not in the second 5 months. During this supplementation, height velocity significantly increased, 2 patients started puberty, and insulin-like growth factor I (IGF-I) concentrations increased.[213]

In general, patients on HPN who have been tested by standard developmental tests have had normal or near-normal intelligence and motor function.[214] Parents tend to be overprotective of children on HPN with particular fear of harm to the CVC. Some children have poor muscle development of unknown cause.[185] Most children receiving long-term HPN have deficits in perceptual-motor performance, especially the older children,[214] but their overall ability to sustain normal age-related activity is judged to be partial or complete in more than 95% of cases.[190] In the large series of De Potter and others (156 children on HPN),[189] 86% achieved normal growth, 89% were regularly attending school, 91% took part in physical activities, and 50% were able to go on family vacations.

Visual function may be altered in children receiving long-term HPN.[185] It has been noted that despite normal visual acuity, one-half of the children had at least one and usually two abnormalities on their electroretinograms.[215]

A recent national multicenter study in France[216] concluded that quality of life (QOL) of HPN-dependent children and their siblings is not different from that of healthy children, suggesting that these children actively use effective coping strategies. In contrast, the QOL of parents, especially mothers, of HPN-dependent children is low. Necessary support to families providing this demanding type of care for their children should be offered.

Monitoring. Standards of practice for home nutrition support have been published.[217] As discussed previously, a multidisciplinary team responsible for ongoing nutritional assessments is the optimal way to manage HPN patients. Theoretically, HPN should be feasible and effective for an entire lifespan.

SUMMARY

PN remains a therapy in evolution. New technology to help better assess caloric needs has been designed, and standards for nutritional support in hospitalized pediatric patients and home parenteral patients have been recently updated.[186,187]

REFERENCES

1. Shohl AT, et al. Nitrogen metabolism during the oral and parenteral administration of the amino acids of hydrolyzed casein. J Pediatr 1939;15:469–75.
2. Helfrick FW, Abelson NM. Intravenous feeding of a complete diet in a child. J Pediatr 1939;15:400–3.
3. Forbes AL. Incidence of reactions to an intravenous fat emulsion administered at two different rates. Metabolism 1957;6:645–9.
4. Lehr HL, et al. Clinical experience with intravenous fat emulsions. Metabolism 1957;6:666–72.
5. Dudrick SJ, Wilmore DW, Vars HM. Long-term total parenteral nutrition with growth in puppies and positive nitrogen balance in patients. Surg Forum 1967;18:356–7.
6. Wilmore DW, Dudrick SJ. Growth and development of an infant receiving all nutrients exclusively by vein. JAMA 1968;203:140–4.
7. Levy JS, Winters RW, Heird WC. Total parenteral nutrition in pediatric patients. Pediatr Rev 1980;2:99.
8. Dorsey SF et al., Improved survival in very short small bowel of infancy with use of long-term parenteral nutrition. J Pediatrics 1985;107:521–25
9. WHO: Energy and protein requirements. Tech Rep Ser 1985;724:71.
10. Schoefield WN. Predicting basal metabolic rate, new standards and review of previous work. Hum Nutr Clin Nutr 1985;1:5–41.
11. Pencharz PB, Azcue MP. Measuring resting energy expenditure in clinical practice. J Pediatr 1995;127:269–71.
12. Anderson TL, et al. A controlled trial of glucose versus glucose and amino acids in premature infants. J Pediatr 1979;94:947.
13. Zlotkin SH, Bryan MH, Anderson CH. Intravenous nitrogen and energy intakes required to duplicate in utero nitrogen accretion in prematurely born human infants. J Pediatr 1981;99:115.
14. Thureen PJ. Early aggressive nutrition in the neonate. Pediatr Rev1999;e45–e55. http://pedsinreview.aapjournals.org/cgi/content/full/20/9/e45.
15. te Braake FW, et al. Amino acid administration to premature infants directly after birth. J Pediatr 2005;147:457–61.
16. Porcelli PJ, Jr, Sisk PM. Increased parenteral amino acid administration to extremely low-birth-weight infants during early postnatal life. J Pediatr Gastroenterol Nutr 2002;34:174–79.
17. Kerner JA. Fluid requirements. In: Kerner JA, editor. Manual of Pediatric Parenteral Nutrition. New York: John Wiley and Sons; 1983. p. 69–77.
18. Macfie J, Smith RC, Hill GL. Glucose or fat as a non-protein energy source? A controlled clinical trial in gastroenterological patients requiring intravenous nutrition. Gastroenterology 1981;80:103.
19. Askanazi J, et al. Nutrition for the patient with respiratory failure: Glucose vs fat. Anesthesiology 1981;54:373.
20. Krzywda EA, et al. Glucose response to abrupt initiation and discontinuation of total parenteral nutrition. J Parenter Enter Nutr 1993;17:64–67.
21. Vaucher YE, Walson PD, Morrow G. Continuous insulin infusion in hyperglycemic, very low birth weight infants. J Pediatr Gastroenterol Nutr 1982;1:211.
22. Collins JW, et al. A controlled trial of insulin infusion and parenteral nutrition in extremely-low-birth-weight infants with glucose intolerance. J Pediatr 1991;118:921.
23. Montori VM, Bistrian BR, McMahon MM. Hyperglycemia in acutely ill patients. JAMA 2002;288:2167–9.
24. Van den Berghe G, Wouters P, Weekers F, et al. Intensive insulin therapy in critically ill patients. N Engl J Med 2001;345:1359–67.
25. Alaedeen DI, Walsh MC, Chwals WJ. Total parenteral nutrition-associated hyperglycemia correlates with prolonged mechanical ventilation and hospital stay in septic infants. J Pediatr Surg 2006;41:239–44.
26. Faustino EV, Apkon M. Persistent hyperglycemia in critically ill children. J Pediatr 2005;146:30–4.
27. Heird WC, Malloy MH. Brain composition of beagle puppies receiving total parenteral nutrition. In: Itka V, editor. Nutrition and Metabolism of the Fetus and Infant. The Hague: Nijhoff Publishers; 1979. p. 365.
28. Wu PYK, Edwards NB, Storm MC. Characterization of the plasma amino acid pattern of normal term breast-fed infants. J Pediatr 1986;109:347.
29. Helms RA, et al. Comparison of a pediatric versus standard amino acid formulation in preterm neonates requiring parenteral nutrition. J Pediatr 1987;110:466.
30. Poole RL, Rupp CA, Kerner JA. Calcium and phosphate in neonatal parenteral solutions. J Parenter Enter Nutr 1983;7:358.
31. Fitzgerald KA, MacKay MW. Calcium and phosphate solubility in neonatal parenteral nutrient solutions containing TrophAmine. Am J Hosp Pharm 1986;43:88.
32. Adamkin DH, et al. Comparison of two neonatal intravenous amino acid formulations in preterm infants: A multicenter study. J Perinatol 1991;11:375.
33. Zelikovic I, et al. Taurine depletion in very-low-birth-weight infants receiving prolonged total parenteral nutrition: Role of renal immaturity. J Pediatr 1990;116:301.
34. Kashyap S, Abildskov K, Heird WC. Cysteine supplementation of very-low-birth-weight infants receiving parenteral nutrition. II. Pediatr Res 1992;31:290A.
35. Barton RG. Nutrition support in critical illness. Nutr Clin Prac 1994;9:127.
36. Ziegler TR, et al. Clinical and metabolic efficacy of glutamine-supplemented parenteral nutrition after bone marrow transplantation. Ann Intern Med 1992;116:821.
37. Allen SJ, et al. Glutamine-supplemented parenteral nutrition in a child with short bowel syndrome. J Pediatr Gastroenterol Nutr 1993;17:329.
38. Wischmeyer PE, Lynch J, Liedel J, et al. Glutamine administration reduced gram-negative bacteremia in severely burned patients: A prospective, randomized, double-blind trial versus isonitrogenous control. Crit Care Med 2001;29:2075–80.
39. Gore DC. Deficiency in peripheral glutamine production in pediatric patients with burns. J Burn Care Rehabil 2000;21:171–7.
40. Lacey JM, et al. The effects of glutamine-supplemented parenteral nutrition in premature infants. J Parenter Enter Nutr 1996;20:74–80.
41. Wilmore DW, et al. A new treatment for patients with short-bowel syndrome. Ann Surg 1995;222:243–55.
42. Scolapio JS, Camilleri M, Fleming CR, et al. Effects of growth hormone, glutamine, and diet on adaptation in short bowel syndrome: A randomized, controlled trial. Gastroenterology 1997;113:1074–81.
43. Szkudlarek J, Jeppesen PB, Mortensen PB. Effect of high dose growth hormone with glutamine and no change in diet on intestinal absorption in short bowel patients: A randomized, double blind, crossover, placebo-controlled study. Gut 2000;47:199–205.
44. Poindexter BB, Ehrenkranz RA, Stoll BJ, et al. Parenteral glutamine supplementation does not reduce the risk of mortality or late-onset sepsis in extremely low birth weight infants. Pediatrics 2004;113:1209–1215.
45. Albers MJ, Steyerberg EW, et al. Glutamine supplementation of parenteral nutrition does not improve intestinal permeability, nitrogen balance, or outcome in newborns and infants undergoing digestive-tract surgery: Results from a double-blind, randomized, controlled trial. Ann Surg 2005;241:599–606.
46. Tubman TRJ, Thompson SW, McGuire W. Glutamine supplementation to prevent morbidity and mortality in preterm infants. Cochrane Database of Systemic Reviews 2006; Issue I. Art. No.: CD001457. DOI: 10.1002/14651858.CD001457.pub2.
47. Acra SA, Rollins C. Principles and guidelines for parenteral nutrition in children. Pediatr Ann 1999;28:113–20.
48. Phelps SJ, Cochran EB. Effect of continuous administration of fat emulsion on the infiltration of intravenous lines in infants receiving peripheral parenteral nutrition solutions. J Parenter Enter Nutr 1989;13:628.
49. Kao LC, Cheng MH, Warburton D. Triglycerides, free fatty acids, free fatty acids/albumin molar ratio, and cholesterol levels in serum of neonates receiving long-term lipid infusions: Controlled trial of continuous and intermittent regimens. J Pediatr 1984;104:429.
50. Brans YW, et al. Tolerance of fat emulsions in very-low-birth-weight infants. Am J Dis Child 1988;142:145.
51. O'Grady NP, Alexander M, et al. CDC Guildelines for the prevention of intravascular catheter-related infections. 2002/51(RR10); 1–26.
52. Friedman Z, et al. Rapid onset of essential fatty acid deficiency in the newborn. Pediatrics 1976;58:640.
53. Cooke RJ, Burckhart GJ. Hypertriglyceridemia during the intravenous infusion of a safflower-oil based fat emulsion. J Pediatr 1983;103:959.
54. Helms RA, et al. Enhanced lipid utilization in infants receiving oral L-carnitine during parenteral nutrition (PN) in neonates. J Pediatr 1986;109:984.
55. Helms RA, et al. Intravenous (IV) carnitine during parenteral nutrition (PN) in neonates. J Parenter Enter Nutr 1987;11:9.
56. Stahl GE, Spear ML, Hamosh M. Intravenous administration of lipid emulsions to premature infants. Clin Perinatol 1986;13:133.
57. Innis SM. Fat. In: Tsang RC, Lucas A, Uauy R, Zlotkin S, editors. Nutritional Needs of the Preterm Infant. Baltimore: Williams & Wilkins; 1993. p. 65–86.
58. Sulkers EJ, et al. Effects of high carnitine supplementation on substrate utilization in low-birth-weight infants receiving total parenteral nutrition. Am J Clin Nutr 1990;52:889.
59. Dahn MS. Structured lipids: An alternative energy source [editorial]. Nutr Clin Prac 1995;10:89–90.
60. Hyltander A, Sandstrom R, Lundhold K. Metabolic effects of structured triglycerides in humans. Nutr Clin Prac 1995;10:91–97.
61. Lima LAM, et al. Neonatal parenteral nutrition with a fat emulsion containing medium chain triglycerides. Acta Paediatr Scand 1988;77:332.
62. Bientz J, et al. Medium chain triglycerides in parenteral nutrition in the newborn: A short-term clinical trial. Infusionstherapie 1988;15:96.
63. Gura KM, Duggan CP, et al. Reversal of parenteral nutrition-associated liver disease in two infants with short bowel syndrome using parenteral fish oil: Implications for future management. Pediatrics 2006;118:e197–201.
64. Haumont D, et al. Plasma lipid and plasma lipoprotein concentrations in low birth weight infants given parenteral nutrition with twenty or ten percent lipid emulsion. J Pediatr 1989;115:787.
65. Haumont D, et al. Effect of liposomal content of lipid emulsions on plasma lipid concentrations in low birth weight infants receiving parenteral nutrition. J Pediatr 1992;121:759.
66. Nordenstrom J, Thorne A. Comparative studies on a new concentrated fat emulsion: Intralipid ® 30% vs. 20%. Clin Nutr 1993;12:160–67.
67. Vileisis RA. Effect of phosphorus intake in total parenteral nutrition infusates in premature neonates. J Pediatr 1987;110:586.
68. Kovar I, Mayne P, Barltrop D. Plasma alkaline phosphatase activity: A screening test for rickets in preterm neonates. Lancet 1982;i:308.
69. Goldsmith MA, et al. Gluconate calcium therapy and neonatal hypercalciuria. Am J Dis Child 1981;135:538.
70. Fitzgerald KA, McKay MW. Calcium and phosphate solubility in neonatal parenteral nutrient solutions containing Aminosyn PF. Am J Hosp Pharm 1987;44:1396.
71. Pelegano JF, et al. Simultaneous infusion of calcium and phosphorus in parenteral nutrition for premature infants: Use of physiologic calcium/phosphorus ratio. J Pediatr 1989;114:115.
72. Pelegano JF, et al. Effect of calcium/phosphorus ratio on mineral retention in parenterally fed premature infants. J Pediatr Gastroenterol Nutr 1991;12:351.
73. Hanning RM, Atkinson SA, Whyte RK. Efficacy of calcium glycerophosphate vs conventional mineral salts for total parenteral nutrition in low-birth-weight infants: A randomized clinical trial. Am J Clin Nutr 1991;54:903.
74. Hanning RM, Mitchell MK, Atkinson SA. In vitro solubility of calcium glycerophosphate versus conventional mineral salts in pediatric parenteral nutrition solution. J Pediatr Gastroenterol Nutr 1989;9:67.
75. Dunham B, et al. The solubility of calcium and phosphorus in neonatal total parenteral nutrition solutions. J Parenter Enter Nutr 1991;15:608.
76. Driscoll DF. Total nutrient admixtures: Theory and practice. Nutr Clin Prac 1995;10:114–19.
77. Rollins CJ, et al. Three-in-one parenteral nutrition: A safe and economical method of nutritional support for infants. J Parenter Enter Nutr 1990;14:290.
78. Task force for the revision of safe practices for parenteral nutrition. Safe practices for parenteral nutrition. J Parenter Enter Nutr 2004;28:S39–70.
79. American Medical Association, Department of Foods and Nutrition: Multivitamin preparations for parenteral use: A statement by the Nutrition Advisory Group 1975. J Parenter Enter Nutr 1979;3:258.
80. Greene HL, Hambidge KM, Shanler R, et al. Guidelines for the use of vitamins, trace elements, calcium, magnesium, and phosphorus in infants and children receiving total parenteral nutrition: Report of the Subcommittee on Pediatric Parenteral Nutrient Requirements from the Committee on Clinical Practice Issues of the American Society for Clinical Nutrition. Am J Clin Nutr 1988;48:1324.
81. Hahn JS, et al. Wernicke encephalopathy and beriberi during total parenteral nutrition attributable to multivitamin infusion shortage. Pediatrics 1998;101(100)e10. URL: http://www.pediatrics.org/cgi/content/full/101/1/e10.
82. Alade SL, Brown RE, Paquet A. Polysorbate 80 and E-ferol toxicity. Pediatrics 1986;77:593.

83. MacDonald MG, et al. Propylene glycol: Increase of seizures in low birth weight infants. Pediatrics 1987;79:622.
84. Gillis J, Jones G, Pencharz P. Delivery of vitamins A, D, and E in parenteral nutrition solutions. J Parenter Enter Nutr 1983;7:11–14
85. Kerner JA Jr, et al. High serum vitamin E levels in premature infants receiving MVI-Pediatric. J Pediatr Perinat Nutr 1987;1:75–82
86. Phillips B, Franck LS, Greene HL. Vitamin E levels in premature infants during and after intravenous multivitamin supplementation. Pediatrics 1987;80:680.
87. Poland RL. Vitamin E: What should we do? Pediatrics 1986;77:787.
88. Baeckert PA, et al. Vitamin concentrations in very low birth weight infants given vitamins intravenously in a lipid emulsion: Measurement of vitamins A, D, and E and riboflavin. J Pediatr 1988;113:1057.
89. CDC. Lactic acidosis traced to thiamine deficiency related to nationwide shortage of multivitamins for total parenteral nutrition—United States, 1997. MMWR. 1997;46.
90. Tyson JE, et al. Vitamin A supplementation for extremely-low birth-weight infants. N Engl J Med 1999;340:1962–8.
91. Greene HL, et al. Blood pyridoxine levels in preterm infants receiving TPN. J Parenter Enter Nutr 1989;24:113A.
92. Mock DM, et al. Biotin deficiency: An unusual complication of parenteral alimentation. N Engl J Med 1981;304:820.
93. Moore MC, et al. Evaluation of a pediatric multiple vitamin preparation for total parenteral nutrition in infants and children. I. Blood levels of water-soluble vitamins. Pediatrics 1986;77:530.
94. Marinier E, et al. Blood levels of water soluble vitamins in pediatric patients on total parenteral nutrition using a multivitamin preparation. J Parenter Enter Nutr 1989;13:176.
95. Shils ME, et al. Guidelines for essential trace element preparations for parenteral use. JAMA 1979;241:2051.
96. Moukarzel AA, et al. Excessive chromium intake in children receiving total parenteral nutrition. Lancet 1992;339:385.
97. Keshan Disease Research Group, Chinese Academy of Medical Sciences, Beijing: Observations on effect of sodium selenite in prevention of Keshan disease. Chin Med J 1979;92:471.
98. Kien CL, Ganther HE. Manifestations of chronic selenium deficiency in a child receiving total parenteral nutrition. Am J Clin Nutr 1983;37:319.
99. Vinton NE, et al. Macrocytosis and pseudoalbinism: Manifestations of selenium deficiency. J Pediatr 1987;111:711.
100. Kelly DA, et al. Symptomatic selenium deficiency in a child on home parenteral nutrition. J Pediatr Gastroenterol Nutr 1988;7:783–86.
101. Levander OA, Burk RF. Report on the 1986 ASPEN Research Workshop on Selenium in Clinical Nutrition. J Parenter Enter Nutr 1986;10:595–600.
102. Abumrad NN, et al. Amino acid intolerance during prolonged total parenteral nutrition reversed by molybdate therapy. Am J Clin Nutr 1981;34:2551.
103. Porter KA, Blackburn GL, Bistrian BR. Safety of iron dextran in total parenteral nutrition: A case report. Am J Coll Nutr 1988;7:107.
104. Kumpf VJ. Update on parenteral iron therapy. Nutr Clin Pract 2003;18:318–26.
105. Koo WW, Kaplan LA. Aluminum and bone disorders: With specific reference to contamination of infant nutrients. J Am Coll Nutr 1988;7:1999.
106. Klein GL, Leichtner AM, Heyman MB. Aluminum in large and small volume parenterals used in total parenteral nutrition: Response to the food and drug administration notice of proposed rule by the North American society for pediatric gastroenterology and nutrition. J Pediatr Gastroenterol Nutr 1998;27:457–60.
107. Bishop NJ, et al. Aluminum neurotoxicity in preterm infants receiving intravenous-feeding solutions. N Engl J Med 1997;336:1557–62.
108. Poole RL, Rey LL, Hintz SR, et al. Aluminum exposure from parenteral nutrition: Meeting the new FDA regulation. Clinical Nutrition Week A.S.P.E.N. National Meeting, Dallas, TX, 2006. Program Syllabus, Volume 2, p. 635.
109. Poole RL, Hintz SR, Mackenzie NI, et al. Aluminum exposure in neonates from parenteral nutrition. Pediatric Academic Societies' 2006 Annual Meeting, 2006; Program Syllabus, p. 64.
110. Bailey MJ. Reduction of catheter-associated sepsis in parenteral nutrition using low-dose intravenous heparin. BMJ 1979;1:1671.
111. Gustafson A, et al. Nutrition in low birth weight infants. II. Repeated intravenous injections of fat emulsion. Acta Paediatr Scand 1974;63:177.
112. Berkow SE, et al. Total parenteral nutrition with Intralipid® in premature infants receiving TPN with heparin: Effect on plasma lipolytic enzymes, lipids, and glucose. J Pediatr Gastroenterol Nutr 1987;6:581.
113. Ziegler M, et al. Route of pediatric parenteral nutrition: Proposed criteria revision. J Pediatr Surg 1980;15:472.
114. Racadio JM, Doellman DA, Johnson ND, et al. Pediatric peripherally inserted central catheters: Complication rates related to catheter tip location. Pediatrics 2001;107:e28.
115. Kearns PJ, Coleman S, Wehner JH. Complications of long arm-catheters: A randomized trial of central vs peripheral tip location. J Parenter Enter Nutr 1996;20:20–4.
116. Brewer ED. Pediatric experience with intradialytic parenteral nutrition and supplemental tube feeding. Am J Kidney Dis 1999;33:205–7.
117. Brown RL, Wessel J, Warner BW. Nutrition considerations in the neonatal extracorporeal life support patient. Nutr Clin Prac 1994;9:22–7.
118. Chung DH, Ziegler MM. Central venous catheter access. Nutrition 1998;14:119–23.
119. Fisher AA, et al. Clinical pathway for pediatric parenteral nutrition. Nutr Clin Pract 1997;12:76–80.
120. Kerner JA, Poole R. Patient safety and the neonatal/pediatric TPN process. A.S.P.E.N. Clinical Nutrition Week, Orlando, FL, 2005. Program Syllabus, Volume 1, p. 176–179.
121. Faubion WC, et al. Cycling TPN for hospitalized pediatric patients. Nutr Support Serv 1981;1:24.
122. Collier S, et al. Use of cyclic parenteral nutrition in infants less than 6 months of age. Nutr Clin Pract 1994;9:65–8.
123. Williamson RCN. Intestinal adaptation. N Engl J Med 1978;298:1444.
124. Hughes CA, Prince A, Dowling RH. Speed of change in pancreatic mass and in intestinal bacteriology of parenterally fed rats. Clin Sci 1980;59:329.
125. Greene HL, McCabe DR, Merenstein GB. Protracted diarrhea and malnutrition in infancy: Changes in intestinal morphology and disaccharidase activities during treatment with total intravenous nutrition or oral elemental diets. J Pediatr 1975;87:695.
126. deAngelis GL, et al. Gastric pepsin and acid secretion during total parenteral nutrition and constant-rate enteral nutrition in infancy. J Parenter Enter Nutr 1988;12:505.
127. Geertama MA, et al. Feeding resistance after parenteral hyperalimentation, Am J Dis Child 1985;139:255.
128. Mehta S, et al. Central venous catheters and risk of thrombosis in newborns, J Pediatr Surg 1992;27:18.
129. Chathas MK, Paton JB, Fisher DE. Percutaneous central venous catheterization: 3 years' experience in a neonatal intensive care unit. Am J Dis Child 1990;144:1246.
130. Agarwal KC, et al. Cardiac perforation from central venous catheters: Survival after cardiac tamponade in an infant. Pediatrics 1984;73:333.
131. Collier PE, Ryan JJ, Diamond DL. Cardiac tamponade from central venous catheters: Report of a case and review of the English literature. Angiology 1984;595–600
132. Leibovitz E, et al. Fatal cardiac tamponade complicating total parenteral nutrition via a silastic central vein catheter [letter]. J Pediatr Gastroenterol Nutr 1988;7:306.
133. Yokoyama S, et al. Use of Broviac/Hickman catheter for long-term venous access in pediatric cancer patients. Jpn J Clin Oncol 1988;18:143.
134. Sadig HF. Broviac catheterization in low birth weight infants: Incidence and treatment of associated complications. Crit Care Med 1987;15:47.
135. Weese JL, Trigg ME. Triple lumen venous access for pediatric bone marrow transplantation candidates. J Surg Oncol 1987;36:55.
136. Newall F, Barnes C, et al. Warfarin therapy in children who require long-term parenteral nutrition. Pediatrics 2003;112:e386.
137. Flynn P, et al. In situ management of confirmed central venous catheter-related bacteremia. Pediatr Infect Dis 1987;6:729.
138. Nahata MC, et al. Management of catheter related infections in pediatric patients. J Parenter Enter Nutr 1988;12:58.
139. Wang EEL, et al. The management of central intravenous catheter infections. Pediatr Infect Dis 1984;3:110.
140. Merritt RJ, Mason W. Catheter associated infections in 1988. Nutrition 1988;4:247.
141. Van Der Hulst RRW, et al. Glutamine and the preservation of gut integrity. Lancet 1993;341:1363.
142. O'Grady NP, Alexander M, Dellinger EP, Guidelines for the Prevention of Intravascular Catheter-Related Infections. Pediatrics 2002;110:e51.
143. Reiter PD, Novak K, et al. Effects of a closed drug-delivery system on the incidence of nosocomial and catheter-related bloodstream infections in infants. Epidemiol Infect 2006;134:285–91.
144. United States Pharmacopeia, 2005, Chapter 797, p. 2465.
145. Deitcher SR, Fesen MR, Kiproff PM, et al. Safety and efficacy of alteplase for restoring function in occluded central venous catheters: Results of the cardiovascular thrombolytic to open occluded lines trial. J Clin Oncol 2002;20:317–24.
146. http://www.gene.com/gene/products/information/cardiovascular/cathflo-activase/cvc-fact.jsp
147. Breaux CW Jr, et al. Calcium phosphate crystal occlusion of central venous catheters used for total parenteral nutrition in infants and children: Prevention and treatment. J Pediatr Surg 1987;22:829.
148. Pennington CR, Pithie AD. Ethanol lock in the management of catheter occlusion. J Parenter Enter Nutr 1987;11:507.
149. Kerner JA, Garcia-Careaga MG, et al. Treatment of catheter occlusion in pediatric patients. J Parenter Enter Nutr 2006;30:S73–S81.
150. Market AD, et al. Parenteral nutrition-associated anaphylaxis in a 4-year-old child. J Pediatr Gastroenterol Nutr 1998;26:229–31.
151. Buchman AL, Ament ME. Comparative hypersensitivity in intravenous lipid emulsions. J Parenter Enter Nutr 1991;15:345–6.
152. Pereira GR, et al. Decreased oxygenation and hyperlipemia during intravenous fat infusions in premature infants. Pediatrics 1980;66:26.
153. Barson AJ, Chiswick ML, Doig MC. Fat embolism in infancy after intravenous fat infusions. Arch Dis Child 1978;53:218.
154. Hertel J, Tystrup I, Andersen GE. Intravascular fat accumulation after Intralipid infusion in the very low-birth-weight infant. J Pediatr 1982;100:975.
155. Shulman RJ, Langston C, Schanler RJ. Pulmonary vascular lipid deposition after administration of intravenous fat to infants. Pediatrics 1987;79:99.
156. Puntis JWL, Rushton DI. Pulmonary intravascular lipid in neonatal necropsy specimens. Arch Dis Child 1991;66:26.
157. Shroeder H, Paust H, Schmidt R. Pulmonary fat embolism after Intralipid therapy: A post-mortem artifact? Acta Paediatr Scand 1984;73:461.
158. Hageman J, et al. Intralipid alterations in pulmonary prostaglandin metabolism and gas exchange. Crit Care Med 1983;11:794–8.
159. Brans YW, et al. Fat emulsion tolerance in very low birth weight neonates: Effect on diffusion of oxygen in the lungs and on blood pH. Pediatrics 1986;78:79.
160. Hammerman C, Aramburo MJ. Decreased lipid intake reduces morbidity in sick premature neonates. J Pediatr 1988;113:1083.
161. Alwaidh MH, Bowden L, Shaw B, Ryan SW. Randomized trial of effect of delayed intravenous lipid administration on chronic lung disease in preterm neonates. J Pediatr Gastroenterol Nutr 1996;22:303.
162. Fox GF, Wilson DC, Ohlsson A. Effect of early vs. late introduction of intravenous lipid to preterm infants on death and chronic lung disease (CLD)–results of meta-analyses. Pediatr Res 1998;43:214A.
163. Helbock HJ, Motchnik PA, Ames BN. Toxic hydroperoxides in intravenous lipid emulsions used in preterm infants. Pediatrics 1993;91:83.
164. Neuzil J, et al. Oxidation of parenteral lipid emulsion by ambient and phototherapy lights: Potential toxicity of routine parenteral feeding. J Pediatr 1995;126:785–90.
165. Park W, Paust H, Schroder H. Lipid infusion in premature infants suffering from sepsis. J Parenter Enter Nutr 1984;8:290.
166. Toce SS, Keenan WJ. Lipid intolerance is associated with hepatic dysfunction but not infection. Arch Pediatr Adolesc Med 1995;149:1249–53.
167. Cohen IT, Dahms B, Hays DM. Peripheral total parenteral nutrition employing a lipid emulsion (Intralipid ®): Complications encountered in pediatric patients. J Pediatr Surg 1977;12:7–845.
168. Johnson JD, Albritton WL, Sunshine P. Hyperammonemia accompanying parenteral nutrition in newborn infants. J Pediatr 1972;1:154.
169. Greer FR, Steichen JJ, Tsang RC. Effects of increased calcium, phosphorus, and vitamin D intake on bone mineralization in very-low-birth-weight infants fed formulas with Polycose® and medium-chain triglycerides. J Pediatr 1982;100:951.
170. Tsang RC. The quandary of vitamin D in the newborn infant. Lancet 1983;1:1370.
171. Peden VH, Witzleben DL, Skelton MA. Total parenteral nutrition. J Pediatr 1971;78:180.
172. Sinatra FR. Cholestasis in infancy and childhood. Curr Prob Pediatr 1982;12:6.
173. Sax HC, Bower BH. Hepatic complications of total parenteral nutrition. J Parenter Enter Nutr 1988;12:615.
174. Marino L, Hack M, Dahms B. Two year follow-up: Growth and neonatal PN-associated liver disease. J Parenter Enter Nutr 1981;5:569.
175. Hodes JE, et al. Hepatic failure in infants on total parenteral nutrition (TPN): Clinical and histopathologic observations. J Pediatr Surg 1982;17:463.

176. Suita S, et al. Follow-up studies of the children treated with long-term intravenous nutrition (IVN) during the neonatal period. J Pediatr Surg 1982;17:37.
177. Javid PJ, Collier S, Richardson D, et al. The role of enteral nutrition in the reversal of parenteral nutrition-associated liver dysfunction in infants. J Pediatr Surg 2005;40:1015–8.
178. Benjamin DR, et al. Cholelithiasis in infants: The role of total parenteral nutrition andgastrointestinal dysfunction. J Pediatr Surg 1982;17:386.
179. Messing B, et al. Does total parenteral nutrition induce gallbladder sludge formation and lithiasis? Gastroenterology 1983;84:1012.
180. Roslyn JJ, et al. Increased risk of gallstones in children receiving total parenteral nutrition. Pediatrics 1983;71:784.
181. King DR, et al. Parenteral nutrition with associated cholelithiasis: Another iatrogenic disease of infants and children. J Pediatr Surg 1987;22:593–6.
182. Solomon SM, Kirby DF. The refeeding syndrome: A review. J Parenter Enter Nutr 1990;14:90–7.
183. Havala T, Shronts E. Managing the complications associated with refeeding. Nutr Clin Prac 1990;5:23–9.
184. Kerner JA Jr, Poole RL. Metabolic monitoring and nutritional assessment. In: Yu VYH, MacMahon RA, editors. Intravenous Feeding of the Neonate. London: Edward Arnold; 1992. p. 207–33.
185. Moukarzel AA, Ament ME. Home parenteral nutrition in infants and children. In: Rombeau JL, Caldwell MD, editors. Clinical Nutrition: Parenteral Nutrition, 2nd edition. Philadelphia, PA: WB Saunders; 1993. p. 791–813.
186. ASPEN Board of Directors: Guidelines for the use of parenteral and enteral nutrition in adults and pediatric patients. J Parenter Enter Nutr 2002;26.
187. Koletzko B, Goulet O, et al. Guidelines on Paediatric Parenteral Nutrition of the ESPGHAN and the ESPEN. Supported by the ESPR. JPGN 2005;41:S1–87.
188. Ricour C, et al. Home parenteral nutrition in children: 8 years of experience with 112 patients. Clin Nutr 1990;9:65.
189. De Potter S, et al. Two hundred sixty-three patient-years of home parenteral nutrition in children. Transplant Proc 1992;24:1056.
190. Howard L, et al. Four years of North American registry home parenteral nutrition outcome data and their implications for patient management. J Parenter Enter Nutr 1991;15:384.
191. Berry RK, Jortensen S. Growing with home parenteral nutrition: Adjusting to family life and child development. Pediatr Nurs 1988;14:43.
192. Dorney SF, et al. Improved survival in very short bowel of infancy with use of long-term parenteral nutrition. J Pediatr 1985;107:521.
193. Buchman AL, et al. Catheter-related infections associated with home parenteral nutrition and predictive factors for the need for catheter removal in their treatment. J Parenter Enter Nutr 1994;18:297.
194. Moukarzel AA, Ament ME. Home parenteral nutrition. Home Infusion News 1993;2:3.
195. Andrew M, et al. Oral anticoagulation therapy in pediatric patients: A prospective study. Thromb Haemost 1994;71:265.
196. Andrew M, et al. A cross-sectional study of catheter related thrombosis in children on home total parenteral nutrition. J Pediatr 1995;126:358.
197. Sola JE, et al. Atypical thrombotic and septic complications of totally implantable venous access devices in patients with cystic fibrosis. Pediatr Pulmonol 1992;14:239.
198. Goulet O, et al. Hematologic disorders following prolonged use of intravenous fat emulsion in children. J Parenter Enter Nutr 1986;10:284.
199. Hurwitz M, Garcia MG, Kerner JA. Copper Deficiency During Parenteral Nutrition: A Report of Four Pediatric Cases. Nutr Clin Pract 2004;19:305–8.
200. Takagi Y, Okada A, Sando K, et al. Evaluation of indexes of in vivo manganese status and the optimal intravenous dose for adult patients undergoing home parenteral nutrition. Am J Clin Nutr 2002;75:112–8.
201. Moukarzel AA, et al. Carnitine status of children receiving long-term total parenteral nutrition: A longitudinal prospective study. J Pediatr 1992;120:759.
202. Moukarzel A, et al. Parenteral nutrition bone disease in children. Clin Res 1990;38:190A.
203. Moukarzel A, et al. Is silicon deficiency involved in the pathogenesis of metabolic bone disease of children receiving parenteral nutrition? J Parenter Enter Nutr 1992;16:31S.
204. Buchman AL, et al. Serious renal impairment is associated with long term parenteral nutrition. J Parenter Enter Nutr 1993;17:438.
205. Moukarzel A, Ament M, Buchman A. Renal function of children receiving long term parenteral nutrition. J Pediatr 1991;119:864.
206. Quigley EMM, et al. Hepatobiliary complications of total parenteral nutrition. Gastroenterology 1993;104:286.
207. Quiros-Tejeira RE, Ament ME, Reyen L, et al. Long-term parenteral nutritional support and intestinal adaptation in children with short bowel syndrome: A 25-year experience. J Pediatr 2004;145:157–63.
208. Buchman AL, et al. Low plasma free choline is prevalent in patients receiving long term parenteral nutrition and is associated with hepatic aminotransferase abnormalities. Clin Nutr 1993;12:33.
209. Buchman AL, et al. Choline deficiency causes TPN-associated hepatic steatosis in man and is reversed by choline supplemented TPN. Gastroenterology 1993;104:A881.
210. Buchman AL, et al. Lecithin increases plasma free choline and decreases hepatic steatosis in long-term total parenteral nutrition patients. Gastroenterology 1992;102:1363.
211. Buchman AL, Ament ME, Sohel M, et al. Choline deficiency causes reversible hepatic abnormalities in patients receiving parenteral nutrition: Proof of a human choline requirement: A placebo-controlled trial. J Parenter Enter Nutr 2001;25:260–8.
212. Dahlstrom KA, et al. Nutritional status in children receiving home parenteral nutrition. J Pediatr 1985;107:219.
213. Moukarzel AA, et al. Growth retardation in children receiving long-term total parenteral nutrition: Effects of ornithine alpha-ketoglutarate. J Parenter Enter Nutr 1993;17:24S.
214. O'Connor MJ, Ralston CW, Ament ME. Intellectual and perceptual motor performance of children receiving prolonged home total parenteral nutrition. Pediatrics 1988;81:231.
215. Vinton NE, et al. Visual function in patients undergoing long-term total parenteral nutrition. Am J Clin Nutr 1990;52:895.
216. Gottrand F, et al. Satisfaction in different life domains in children receiving home parenteral nutrition and their families. J Pediatr 2005;146:793–7.
217. ASPEN Board of Directors: Guidelines for use of home total parenteral nutrition. J Parenter Enter Nutr 1987;11:342–4.

Dietary Supplements and Nutraceuticals

Martin Kohlmeier, MD
Steven H. Zeisel, MD, PhD

INTRODUCTION

More Americans than ever use dietary supplements, expecting to enhance their health or improve their physical or mental performance. Supplement use is common across all population segments, including young children and adolescents. It is estimated that approximately 50% of US children receive some form of vitamin and mineral supplements.[1,2] Children whose parents use dietary supplements are more likely to use them.[3] In one birth cohort, nearly a third of the participating 2-year-old children were reported to get nutrient supplements.[4] Many older children and adolescents continue to get vitamins and minerals from dietary supplements.[5] Many children also get dietary supplements with herbal and other nonnutrient ingredients occasionally or regularly. Use of both nutrient and herbal supplements is most common in children with long-term health problems.[6] Supplement use has been studied specifically in children with chronic diseases such as inflammatory bowel diseases,[7] cancer,[8,9] and in some diseases or conditions, such as cystic fibrosis, that limit nutrient absorption from foods or increase requirements, making supplementation a critical component of treatment.[10]

Appropriately dosed dietary supplements are an important source of essential nutrients for some children and adolescents, ensuring adequate intakes (AIs) for optimal growth and development. Dietary supplements that provide higher than adequate amounts of nutrients, or contain nonessential ingredients, on the other hand, often cause concern because of potential health risks and questionable benefits. Interactions of supplement ingredients with prescription or over-the-counter medications must also be considered. The growth of the industry and the lack of product regulation raise serious concerns for the health and safety of children. Because so many children use them, each visit to the pediatrician should include a review of current supplement use (Figure 1). Careful evaluation of individual dietary patterns and specific medical circumstances should then guide the selection of dietary supplements, if any are needed.

Drugs in Our Foods?

It is often difficult to distinguish among nutrients, food additives, and drugs. Independent of the matrix (food or pill) in which it is delivered, a dietary supplement can sometimes be foodlike and other times druglike. Nutrients are defined as having nutritive value (they participate in metabolism or are used to build the structures of our cells) and are presumed to be safe. Food additives enhance the aroma, color, structure, or taste of foods but are not nutritive. Under present conceptualizations, the boundary at which a food ingredient becomes a drug is not well defined; often the health claims made for the substance are used to make the determination.[11] Should a nutrient used as part of a treatment for a defined disease be considered a drug, whereas the same nutrient used to enhance health (reduce the risk of disease) be considered a functional food or dietary supplement? This approach could result in classifying a naturally occurring cholesterol-lowering agent as a drug when it is used to reverse atherosclerosis and as a dietary supplement when it is used to optimize cardiovascular function.

One way to differentiate between foods and drugs is to examine how people are exposed to them.[12] Drugs can sometimes be found naturally in foods, and they can participate in metabolism. However, they are substances that humans are not normally exposed to at the doses at which they exert their beneficial effects. In contrast, a nutrient exerts its effects at doses that correspond to reasonably expected exposures for a given population. Some supplements are druglike when ingested in amounts that could never be achieved in the diet, even though they are essential nutrients when ingested in smaller amounts. At low doses, tryptophan is a necessary amino acid required for metabolism and incorporation into proteins. At high doses it (or the currently used 5-hydroxy-L-tryptophan) increases brain serotonin synthesis and thus acts as a drug that treats insomnia.[13,14] In this case a substance normally part of most foods was administered in doses that exceeded dietary requirements in order to obtain a pharmacologic response and so was druglike in this circumstance. Another case is a substance that is not usually consumed by humans. Some plant constituents (eg, ephedra and digitalis glycosides) are biologically active even at small concentrations and have toxicity relative to this activity at higher concentrations.[15,16] Even small doses of these constituents are beyond common human experience. Foods are presumed to be safe because we can extrapolate from a known history of exposure to them, whereas a drug that has no such widespread exposure history cannot be presumed to be safe. Thus, we must weigh the risk/benefit ratio before large populations of humans are encouraged to ingest drugs or supplements.

What Is a Dietary Supplement?

For a long time, the term dietary supplement lacked a clear legal definition. The Dietary Supplement Health and Education Act (DSHEA) of 1994 defines dietary supplements as products that are intended to complement dietary intake and contain any of the following as their active ingredient: a vitamin, mineral, amino acid, herb, or other botanical, or is a dietary substance used to supplement the diet by increasing the total dietary intake, and is intended for ingestion in the form of a capsule, powder, softgel, or gelcap, and not represented as a conventional food or as a sole item of a meal or the diet (DSHEA, Public Law 103–417, 25 October 1994; Codified at 42 USC 287C-11)]. The act specifically excludes from this definition any tobacco-containing products. The definition of dietary supplements does not include the typical dose intended for use.

DSHEA added dietary supplements as another legal category of commercial products acceptable for oral intake, in addition to foods, food additives, and medical drugs. Extensive laws and regulations govern the production and marketing of foods and medical drugs. Both food additives and medical drugs have to go through tightly regulated evaluation of safety and efficacy before approval is granted. The regulatory burden on dietary supplement products is much lighter. In particular, there is no legal requirement that dietary supplements have to be effective unless such claims are made. Manufacturers and sellers are also not obliged to investigate the safety of their products as long as they observe sanitary practices and use ingredients that were already on the market when DSHEA was passed. It falls to the FDA to demonstrate health risks of such grandfathered ingredients. This high legal threshold of conclusive evidence for harm is very hard to meet.

For new ingredients in dietary supplements, the manufacturers (not the FDA) are responsible for determining that the products they market are safe. The FDA must be notified of a new ingredient in a supplement, and this notice must provide information that supports the manufacturer's conclusion that the ingredient is safe. This is a less rigorous process than is required for review of food additives (used to enhance the aroma, color, structure, or taste of a food) or drugs, for which there is a formal process for evaluation of safety. A manufacturer wishing to use a new food additive or a drug must conduct safety studies in a manner defined by the FDA and must submit the results to the FDA for review and approval before the ingredient or drug can be used in marketed products. This is not the case for dietary supplements in the United States because they are legally in a class by themselves; they can be marketed without the manufacturers satisfying the FDA that they are safe. For more information, see http://www.fda.gov/.

A case study illustrating the high burden of proof that the FDA needs to ban a traditional dietary supplement ingredient is the experience with ephedra (Chinese name Ma Huang), which was a component of many popular weight-loss and performance-enhancing products. The potent ephedrine alkaloids in ephedra induce blood pressure spikes and tachycardia, with potentially fatal consequences. Among several similarly unfortunate cases, the 2003 death of baseball pitcher Steve Bechler after use of an ephedra-containing supplement caught the public's particular attention. The FDA issued a ruling shortly afterward that completely banned ephedrine alkaloids from dietary supplements, but this was immediately challenged in court. Review of 133,000 pages of administrative records eventually convinced a three-judge panel of the Tenth Circuit Court of Appeals to uphold the FDA ruling (United States Court of Appeals Tenth Circuit, Nutraceutical Corporation and Solaray Inc. vs Eschenbach et al, 05-4151). As of this writing, it is still illegal to sell the popular weight-loss and performance-enhancing products with the banned ingredients.

A similar epic battle concerned the determination of the FDA that the red yeast rice ingredient in the dietary supplement cholestin is an unapproved drug, because the product contains pharmacologically active amounts of the cholesterol-lowering medication lovastatin and related metabolites. The ruling was upheld[17] and the manufacturer discontinued marketing of the red yeast rice ingredient in their product.

In another instance, the FDA asked for the voluntary recall of a product containing the herbal ingredient plantain contaminated with *Digitalis lanata* after an individual consuming the product suffered a complete heart block (Federal Register Volume 65, Number 227, November 24, 2000). The FDA also asked for the voluntary recall of supplements containing γ-butyrolactone, because this agent was associated with serious side effects, including coma and death.[18] Due to concerns over severe liver toxicity, the FDA issued a consumer advisory regarding the use of kava (*Piper methysticum*), a product used for relaxation, relief from anxiety, and sleeplessness.[19] The FDA also alerted consumers on several occasions that certain dietary supplement products contain dangerous amounts of aristolochic acid, a constituent of the *Aristolochia, Bragantia,* and *Asarum* plant species, which can cause cancer or kidney failure (http://www.cfsan.fda.gov/%20~dms/addsbot.html, accessed September 1, 2006).

Product Quality

At any dose, there is further reason to regulate the preparation of dietary supplements, nutraceuticals, and functional foods. Some plants contain a wide variety of toxic chemicals that help them to survive in their environmental niche and defend against bacteria, insects, and herbivores. Manufacturers may inadvertently add toxic constituents during the manufacturing process; the recent experience with eosinophilia myalgia syndrome and impurities in tryptophan preparations is an example.[20] Natural ingredients stored improperly can be substrates for molds that make highly dangerous mycotoxins—mold on peanuts forms the potent carcinogen aflatoxin.[21] There is as much reason for oversight of natural supplements as there is for oversight of synthetic drugs and foods.

The dietary supplement industry has adopted a voluntary code of good manufacturing practices (GMPs) (US Pharmacopoeia. www.usp.org., accessed August 10, 2007). The FDA proposed reasonable rules for Current Good Manufacturing Practices for dietary supplement ingredients in 1997,[22] and a public meeting was held in July 1999 but at this time there is no mandatory code established by the FDA. These rules are an essential first step toward a rational oversight of dietary supplements.

In response to growing concerns about the quality of dietary supplements on the market, the US Pharmacopoeia established the Dietary Supplement Verification Program (DVSP) in 2000. Through compliance testing and document review, adherence to good manufacturing principles, and postmarketing surveillance, DSVP is designed to help assure that dietary supplement products contain the declared ingredients in the declared quantities. Participation in the program is voluntary. A supplement that carries the USP DVSP symbol is certified to contain the ingredients stated on the label in the declared amount and strength; meet specified standards for product purity by meeting requirements for known contaminants; and have been manufactured properly by complying with USP and proposed FDA standards for GMPs.

The increased review and regulation of dietary supplements could decrease the access of the public to some beneficial products. For supplements administered at doses that can be found in foods, the adoption of GMPs should not significantly alter availability. For nutraceuticals that expose humans to ingredients at doses they would normally not be exposed to, demonstration of safety should be mandated. This may mean it will take years rather than weeks to introduce a new product, and some products may never be introduced. This seems a reasonable cost to protect the public health. The proposed schema for regulation is also in the interest of supplement manufacturers, in a manner similar to the experience of the pharmaceutical industry after the thalidomide debacle.[23] A dietary supplement harming a large number of individuals, with ensuing publicity, could result in public reaction that would damage the marketplace for all dietary supplements. In addition, with no requirement to show efficacy or safety, corporate investments in research and development of better nutraceuticals are less likely because competitors can jump in without having to amortize the costs of such research. Although DSHEA has fostered a situation that encourages continued market growth, it has not fully protected the public or fostered an atmosphere conducive to continuous quality improvement through an investment in research.

Marketing to Children

As noted earlier, half of children use diet supplements. These children are a critical niche market for dietary supplement manufacturers. The *Nutrition Business Journal*, which tracks the industry, reported 1999 sales of $120 million in herbal and nutritional supplements for children. A study conducted by National Public Radio, the Kaiser Foundation, and the Kennedy School of Government found that 18% of parents were giving their children dietary supplements that were not vitamins or minerals.[24] In Germany, where dietary supplement use in children is lower than in US children, over 100 supplements are marketed directly or indirectly for the use by children with products containing anywhere from 1 to 26 constituents per product.[25] There are myriad reasons for supplement use by children. Parents give dietary supplements to their children to enhance health, as a substitute for good nutrition, to be a good parent, because of personal positive experiences, or at the recommendation of alternative medicine specialists.[26] Teens often use supplements that are touted as appearance, energy, and athletic performance enhancers.

Special Considerations in Pediatrics

Much of the knowledge about important aspects of dietary supplements comes from studies in adults and has been extrapolated to children. Considerable uncertainty exists in regard to estimates about appropriate dosing, effectiveness, and risks for children. With the exception of iron and zinc, guidance for desirable nutrient amounts for the first year of life is estimated only from population-wide typical consumption and listed as AI, because information is just too sparse for the formulation of Recommended Dietary Allowance (RDA). Most RDAs for older children and adolescents are adult values adapted to the smaller body size with an added allowance for growth. The same is true for the upper tolerable levels (UL).

While herbal supplement use is quite common in children, there is even less information about efficacy and risks than for adults. Very young infants, 4 months old or less, have not yet fully developed their hepatic drug metabolizing enzymes and are likely to be more sensitive to herbal phytochemical exposure. Growing tissues, including brain and bones, may continue to be more susceptible to herbal effects than adults, but firm evidence is lacking.

When assessing the safety and efficacy of a dietary supplement for a child, several considerations must be made. Nutrients can compete for absorption and use in the body, making high-dose supplementation with single nutrients potentially dangerous. For example, a high dose of supplemental zinc competes with iron absorption and can lead to iron deficiency.[27] The effect on copper status may be even more insidious, because use of high-dose zinc, possibly to prevent a cold, may significantly deplete copper stores.[28] If anemia were to develop due to copper deficiency, increased iron intake would only worsen the situation due to additional competition with copper absorption.

Essential Nutrients

Good health depends on adequate consumption of water, protein, carbohydrates, essential fatty acids, vitamins, minerals, and trace elements. Additional regular food constituents may provide some benefit in particular situations. Ideally, a varied selection of foods and beverages should provide sufficient amounts of each essential nutrient. A major argument for a prudent food pattern with plentiful consumption of whole-grain staples, fruits, and vegetables is their high content of healthful phytochemicals, including carotenoids and flavonoids. Dietary fiber is another critical component of a well-balanced diet.

While the American Dietetic Association maintains that eating a balanced diet that adheres to the Dietary Guidelines for Americans is the best way to meet nutrient needs, they recommend a daily supplement of 100% of the RDA for selected vitamins and minerals for certain individuals unable to meet needs.[29] The American Academy of Pediatrics sees no evidence for benefits from supplementing the diets of healthy children.[30] However, if dietary intake of nutrients is chronically inadequate, the use of a multivitamin and mineral supplement may be advisable.

It is a fact that many children do not get enough of the nutrients they need. Classical deficiencies continue to make occasional reappearances, and milder forms are even more common. Rickets still occurs in the US, particularly in breast-fed infants of dark-skinned mothers.[31] Children in vegan families are at risk for severe vitamin B_{12} deficiency.[32]

Children with acute or chronic illnesses present their own particular challenges. An example of acute effects on nutrient status is the more than three-fold increase in copper and zinc requirement of children with severe trauma and burns,[33] probably due to increased losses through burn exudate. Conditions that interfere with normal nutrient absorption require careful adjustment of micronutrient intakes to their individual situation. Thus, young patients with cystic fibrosis often have suboptimal status of vitamins D and K, even with relatively high-dosed supplementation; in a recent study of such patients in the UK, more than two-thirds had low vitamin K status.[34] Poor status of either vitamin jeopardizes normal bone growth and mineralization. Celiac disease, which often goes unrecognized in children for a long time, impairs absorption of many micronutrients, including iron and the other divalent trace minerals.[35] These patients also need additional vitamin B_{12} and other vitamins due to chronic malabsorption.[36] Sometimes it is the treatment for a disease that increases diet requirements. Required medication for the treatment of epilepsy can accelerate vitamin D breakdown and threaten bone health.[37] Chronic use of theophylline or aminophylline by patients with asthma can interfere with vitamin B_6 metabolism and increase requirements.[38]

While dosages may be recommended on dietary supplement labels, actual dosages necessary to achieve the desired effects can vary. Bioavailability of the active compound is affected by maturation of the gastrointestinal tract, growth, character of the child's diet, and nutritional status.[39] In addition, the chemical form of the nutrient, the food or supplement matrix in which the nutrient is consumed, and other foods in the diet affect bioavailability.[39] While vitamin and mineral supplements may deliver the dosage listed on the label, numerous reports on herbal supplements have shown that the amount of active substance is not necessarily consistent with what is reported on the label.[40,41] Consequently, a child may take a prescribed dosage and actually get much less or much more of the actual ingredients. Data on the bioavailability and toxicity of micronutrients were used in establishing the Dietary Reference Intake (DRI) values and should be used as guidance for recommendations of acceptable limits for nutrient consumption in children.[42] Supplementation of individual and multiple megadose preparations of vitamins and minerals often provides amounts far in excess of the recommendations. Supplement users assessed in the National Health Interview Survey consumed two times the RDA for vitamin A, seven times the RDA for riboflavin, and 17 times the RDA for vitamin C.[43] The message that excess administration of vitamin/mineral supplements at levels far exceeding the recommendations can result in adverse health effects must be communicated by pediatricians to children and their caregivers.

Probiotics

While widely used in other parts of the world, probiotics are recently achieving popularity in the United States. Often in the form of a functional food such as yogurt, a probiotic is a preparation containing viable, defined microorganisms in sufficient numbers, which alter the microflora (by implantation or colonization) in a compartment of the host and by that exert beneficial health effects on the host.[44] They are marketed in single-bacteria and multiple-bacteria preparations with some of the more common ones being *Lactobacillus casei, Lactobacillus acidophilus,* and *Bifidobacterium bifidum*. While actual colonization by the live bacteria cannot be proven directly, it is inferred by bacterial shedding in the feces after the cessation of supplementation. In children, reports suggest that supplementation with *L. casei* shortens the duration of diarrhea[45] and helps eliminate recurrent *Clostridium difficile* colitis in children where antibiotics had failed.[46] Supplementation with a combination of *B. bifidum* and *Streptococcus thermophilus* shortened the duration of rotavirus shedding in hospitalized children.[47] Also, there is evidence that probiotics improve lactose tolerance when live cultures are present in fermented dairy products. They result in decreased cramping and gas as well as a decrease in the concentrations of exhaled hydrogen.[48] Probiotics have also been reviewed for their roles in immunomodulation, cholesterol levels, cancer prevention, *Helicobacter pylori* infection, allergy, inflammatory bowel disease, and mineral absorption.[49]

Performance Supplements

There is evidence that the use of performance-enhancing supplements is prevalent among young people.[50] In particular, androstenedione, creatine, and ephedra are touted to boost athletic performance, although none of these supplements has been shown to significantly enhance performance and their safety in children is questionable.

Androstenedione is a steroid hormone and a precursor to testosterone that is taken to promote muscle growth and athletic performance. Clinical trials of androstenedione show that it raises estradiol and testosterone levels in healthy men.[51] Long-term use has not been studied but it is thought that effects similar to those seen in chronic steroid use could be seen. Although the use of androstenedione is banned in most sports, both in the United States and in abroad, many young athletes report using it.

Creatine is a nonessential dietary element that is present in meat and fish and is endogenously synthesized in the liver. Skeletal muscle phosphorylates creatine to create phosphocreatine, a high-energy compound. During exercise, if aerobic energy production cannot meet ATP demand, phosphocreatine conversion assists in the production of ATP. There is no evidence that dietary phosphocreatine is necessary for muscle contraction or that creatine stimulates protein synthesis. The American College of Sports Medicine (ACSM) released a consensus statement in 2000 concluding that creatine has potential impact on intense short exercise, such as short-distance sprints that last 6 seconds. They also noted that due to the lack of research in the pediatric population, they do not recommend supplementation for children under 18.[52] One study of 6th to 12th graders in the northeast USA found that 8.8% of surveyed boys and 1.8% of girls used creatine; among 12th grade athletes, usage was at 44%.[53]

Herbal Supplements

Children and adolesscents are increasingly using herbal supplements, often reflecting the use patterns of their parents or other adults in their family. Very little, if any, information is available about age-specific pharmacodynamics, benefits, or risks. All descriptions of herbal product effects are taken from the German Commission E monographs.[54]

Echinacea (*Echinacea purpurea*). Fresh or dried root of *E. purpurea* and its preparations. Contains caffeic acid derivatives, alkamides, polyacetylene derivatives, polysaccharides, glycoproteins, and essential oil. Approved by the Commission E for the treatment of symptoms of upper respiratory infections associated with colds.

Ephedra/Ma huang (*Ephedra sinica*). Dried, young branchlets, harvested in the fall, of *E. sinica* or equivalent *Ephedra* species; the herb contains alkaloids (eg, ephedrine, pseudoephedrine). In the United States, ephedra is regulated under DSHEA in aqueous infusion, alcoholic tincture, and dry extract in capsules or tablets. The alkaloids of ephedra (ephedrine and pseudoephedrine) are approved as over-the-counter ingredients in remedies for the common cold, flu, and allergies by the FDA. Ephedra's use in products for weight loss, athletic performance enhancement, and nervous system stimulation has raised concern with questions about the safety of these products and its use in dietary supplements is now banned. The FDA has received reports of 80 deaths and 1,400 adverse effects associated with ephedra in dietary supplements and ephedra has been linked with heart attack, stroke, seizures, and psychosis.

St. John's Wort (*Hypericum perforatum*). Dried parts above ground, gathered during the flowering season, of the *H. perforatum* and their preparation in effective dosage. The Commission E approved the use of St. John's Wort internally in the treatment of psychovegetative disturbances, depressive moods, anxiety, and nervous unrest. It is thought that the active ingredient for the treatment of depression is hyperforin; however, studies are still being conducted. Oily preparations are approved for external use in the treatment of acute and contused injuries, myalgia, and first-degree burns.

Ginkgo Biloba (*Ginkgo biloba*). Dry extract pharmaceutically prepared to a 35 to 67:1 ratio of dried leaves to final extract containing flavonone glycosides (quercetin and kaempferol), terpene lactones (eg, ginkgolides A, B, and C), and ginkgolic acids. *G. Biloba* has been approved by the Commission E for symptomatic treatment of disturbed performance in organic brain syndrome within a therapeutic regimen; improvement in pain-free walking in peripheral arterial occlusive disease; vertigo and tinnitus.

Garlic (*Allium sativum*). Fresh or dried compound bulbs of *A. sativum* with no less than 0.5% alliin. Active compounds include thiosulfinates (allicin). In clinical trials, garlic has been effective in lowering cholesterol in hyperlipidemia and in treating hypertension. Garlic has antibacterial, antimycotic, lipid-lowering, inhibiting of platelet aggregation, prolonging of bleeding and clotting time, tumor-inhibiting, and fibrinolytic activity enhancing properties. Commission E approved the use of garlic as a support to dietary measures for lowering elevated levels of blood lipids and in age-dependent vascular change prevention. However, limited results in the use of garlic for pediatric patients with hyperlipidemia have been shown.

Chamomile (*Chamomilla recutita*). Fresh or dried flowerheads of *Matricaria recutita* and its preparations in effective dosage. It is a popular ingredient in herbal tea in the United States and is prepared for topical use in rinses, creams, ointments, and vapor baths. In German pediatrics, chamomile is widely used in caring for infants' and children's sensitive skin, particularly for inflammatory skin conditions. The Commission E has approved chamomile for gastrointestinal spasms and inflammatory diseases of the gastrointestinal tract. It is also approved for external use for skin and mucus membrane inflammation, and bacterial skin diseases.

Ginger (*Zingiber officinale*). Peeled, fresh, or dried rhizome of *Z. officinale* and its preparations in effective dosages. Ginger contains oleoresin, volatile oil, carbohydrates, lipids, vitamins niacin and vitamin A, minerals, and amino acids. Ginger is used alone and as a component in digestive, antinausea, and cold and flu dietary supplements in the United States. The Commission E approved ginger for dyspepsia and prevention of motion sickness.

Valerian Root (*Valeriana officinalis*). Fresh underground plant parts or carefully dried parts of *V. officinalis* and its preparations in effective dosages. Valerian roots contain essential oil with monoterpenes and sesquiterpenes. The Commission E approved the product for restlessness and sleeping disorders based on nervous conditions. Clinical data support its action as a mild sedative and sleep-promoting agent. The US Pharmacopoeia does not support the use of valerian due to inadequate clinical studies.

Supplement Interactions and Potential Risks

Another concern is that dietary supplements can interact with pharmaceuticals and either attenuate or dampen treatment effects of drugs and/or cause adverse side effects. For example, St. John's wort activates p450 (CYP3A4) and affects metabolism of antiretroviral protease inhibitors.[55] In 2002, the National Toxicology Program, in partnership with the NIH ODS and FDA, reviewed the safety of a select number of dietary supplements including Aloe Vera Gel, Black Walnut Extract, comfrey, Echinacea purpurea extract, gingko biloba extract, ginseng, goldenseal, grape seed extract, pine bark extract, Kava Kava, milk thistle extract, pulegone, and thujone focusing on characterization of potential adverse health effects (http://ntp.niehs.nih.gov, accessed August 10, 2007). The following are side effects and contraindications for popular herbs excerpted from the Physician's Desk Reference for Herbal Medicines[56] and medical literature.

Echinacea. Because of a conceivable activation of autoimmune and other overreactive immune responses, the drug should not be administered in the presence of multiple sclerosis, leukoses, ollagenoses, AIDS, or tuberculosis.

Ginkgo Biloba. The ginkgolide B component has a potent inhibitory effect on platelet-activiting factor (PAF) by displacing PAF from receptor-binding sites and thus may inhibit platelet activation.

Kava. May potentiate the effectiveness of substances that act on the central nervous system, such as alcohol, barbiturates, and psychopharmacologic agents.

St. John's Wort. The most prominent adverse effect associated with this herb is photosensitivity attributed to its hypericin component. It has also been shown to increase clearance of antiretroviral protease inhibitors.[55]

Ephedra. Contraindications include death, states of anxiety and restlessness, high blood pressure, angle closure glaucoma, cerebral perfusions, prostate adenoma with reisdual urine volume, pheochromocytoma, and thyrotoxicosis.

Eucalyptus. Infants and young children should not have preparations containing the oil applied to their faces as this can lead to glottal spasm or bronchial spasms through asthma-like attacks or even death by asphyxiation.

Physicians Role in Dietary Supplement Use

The FDA maintains the MedWatch Program for reporting adverse events. Physicians should report adverse events experienced by their patients. The program can be accessed online at: https://www.accessdata.fda.gov/scripts/medwatch/. Patients do not always discuss their use of dietary supplements with their physicians. In one survey of patients completing a survey during a routine physical, only 30% of dietary supplement users reported usage.[57] Patients may think that the supplement use is not related to conditions for which care is being sought or may not feel supported by their physician. It is extremely important to obtain a thorough history of supplement use in pediatric patients. Figure 1 provides a reasonable assessment tool for use by physicians. Often, it is helpful to photocopy labels from supplement bottles brought in by patients.

Accessing Information about Dietary Supplements

The National Academies of Science Dietary Reference Intake (DRI) publications provide extensive information on vitamin and mineral needs.[42] Based on exhaustive research, expert analysis, and diverse input, the DRIs are reference values for intake and include three categories: estimated average requirement, RDA, and tolerable upper intake level. The *Estimated Average Requirement* (*EAR*) is the intake value that is estimated to meet the requirement defined by a specified indicator of adequacy in 50% of an age- and gender-specific group. At this level of intake, the remaining 50% of the specified group would not have its needs met.

NAME:
AGE:
DATE:

Supplement	*Brand Name*	*Amount You Take, How Often?*	*Why Are You Taking It?*
Aloe			
Amino acid(s)			
Black cohosh			
Bee pollen			
Calcium			
Cat's claw			
Choline			
Chondroitin			
Chromium			
Coenzyme Q10			
Creatine			
Dong quai			
Echinacea			
Evening primrose oil			
Feverfew			
Fiber			
Fish oil/DHA			
Folic acid			
Garlic			
Ginger			
Ginkgo biloba			
Ginseng			
Goldenseal			
Grapeseed extract			
Iron			
Kava kava			
Licorice			
Lecithin (phosphatidylcholine)			
Milk thistle			
Multiple vitamin			
Peppermint			
Pyruvate			
St. John's wort			
Saw palmetto			
SAM-e			
Valerian			
Vitamin B complex			
Vitamin C			
Vitamin D			
Vitamin E			
Other			

Figure 1 Form for self-reporting commonly used dietary supplement ingredients.

The *RDA* is the dietary intake level that is sufficient to meet the nutrient requirements of nearly all individuals in the group. The *tolerable upper intake level* (UL) is the maximum level of daily nutrient intake that is unlikely to pose risks of adverse health effects to almost all of the individuals in the group for whom it is designed. DRI documents are produced by the Food and Nutrition Board of the Institute of Medicine, National Academies of Science. Full text is available on the Web site at http://www.nap.edu/catalog/dri (accessed on August 10, 2007). (see also Chapter 11, "Dietary Reference Intakes").

There are also several reputable sources for information on other dietary supplements.

Physician's Desk Reference (PDR) for Herbs. Gruenwald J, Brendler T, Jaenicke C, scientific editors. PDR for Herbal Medicines. 1st edition. Montvale, NJ: Medical Economics Co; 1998.

Cochrane Database of Systematic Reviews. It is an evidence-based analysis prepared by the Cochrane Collaboration, an international nonprofit organization, and a part of Britain's National Health Service. It "prepares, maintains, and promotes the accessibility of systematic, up-to-date reviews of health care interventions" (http://www.update-software.com/cochrane/order.htm).

National Center for Complementary and Alternative Medicine (NCCAM). NCCAM is 1 of the 27 institutes and centers that make up the National Institutes of Health (NIH). Its mission is to support rigorous research on complementary and alternative medicine (CAM), to train researchers in CAM, and to disseminate information to the public and professionals on which CAM modalities work, which do not, and why. The Web site offers health, research, training, and clinical trials information (http://nccam.nih.gov/). Another offer is a synopsis of information on dietary supplements (http://nccam.nih.gov/health/bottle).

National Institutes of Health Office of Dietary Supplements (ODS). The ODS plans, organizes, and supports conferences, workshops, and symposia on scientific topics related to dietary supplements. The Web site features dietary supplement fact sheets and the Computer Access to Research on Dietary Supplements (CARDS) Database (http://ods.od.nih.gov/index.asp, accessed August 10, 2007). The ODS produces the International Bibliographic Information on Dietary Supplements (IBIDS), a database of published, international, scientific literature on dietary supplements, including vitamins, minerals, and botanicals. IBIDS assists the public, healthcare providers, educators, and researchers in locating credible, scientific information on dietary supplements (http://ods.od.nih.gov/databases/ibids.html, accessed August 10, 2007).

Finally, the excellent monographs on herbals produced by the American Botanical Council are an excellent resource.[54]

ACKNOWLEDGMENT

This work was supported by a grant from the National Institutes of Health (DK56350) to the University of North Carolina Clinical Nutrition Research Center.

REFERENCES

1. Yu SM, Kogan MD, Gergen P. Vitamin-mineral supplement use among preschool children in the United States. Pediatrics 1997;100:E4.
2. US Department of Agriculture. Agricultural Research Service: Date tables: Results from USDA's 1994–1996 Continuing Survey of Food Intakes by Individuals and 1994–1996 Diet and Health Knowledge Survey. 1997.
3. Lee Y, Mitchell DC, Smiciklas-Wright H, Birch LL. Maternal influences on 5- to 7-year-old girls' intake of multivitamin-mineral supplements. Pediatrics 2002;109:E46.
4. Eichenberger Gilmore JM, Hong L, Broffitt B, Levy SM. Longitudinal patterns of vitamin and mineral supplement use in young white children. J Am Diet Assoc 2005;105:763–72; quiz 773–4.
5. Dwyer JT, Garcea AO, Evans M, et al. Do adolescent vitamin-mineral supplement users have better nutrient intakes than nonusers? Observations from the CATCH tracking study. J Am Diet Assoc 2001;101:1340–6.
6. Ball SD, Kertesz D, Moyer-Mileur LJ. Dietary supplement use is prevalent among children with a chronic illness. J Am Diet Assoc 2005;105:78–84.
7. Heuschkel R, Afzal N, Wuerth A, et al. Complementary medicine use in children and young adults with inflammatory bowel disease. Am J Gastroenterol 2002;97:382–8.
8. Neuhouser ML, Patterson RE, Schwartz SM, et al. Use of alternative medicine by children with cancer in Washington state. Prev Med 2001;33:347–54.
9. Kelly KM, Jacobson JS, Kennedy DD, et al. Use of unconventional therapies by children with cancer at an urban medical center. J Pediatr Hematol Oncol 2000;22:412–6.
10. Hayek KM. Medical nutrition therapy for cystic fibrosis: Beyond pancreatic enzyme replacement therapy. J Am Diet Assoc 2006;106:1186–8.
11. Clydesdale F. A proposal for the establishment of scientific criteria for health claims for functional foods. Nutr Rev 1997;55:413–22.
12. Zeisel SH. Regulation of "nutraceuticals" [see comments]. Science 1999;285:1853–5.
13. Asheychik R, Jackson T, Baker H, et al. The efficacy of L-tryptophan in the reduction of sleep disturbance and depressive state in alcoholic patients. J Stud Alcohol 1989;50:525–32.
14. Schneider-Helmert D, Spinweber CL. Evaluation of L-tryptophan for treatment of insomnia: A review. Psychopharmacology (Berl) 1986;89:1–7.

15. Gurley BJ, Gardner SF, White LM, Wang PL. Ephedrine pharmacokinetics after the ingestion of nutritional supplements containing Ephedra sinica (ma huang). Ther Drug Monit 1998;20:439–45.
16. Goldman P. Herbal medicines today and the roots of modern pharmacology. Ann Intern Med 2001;135:594–600.
17. SoRelle R. Appeals Court says Food and Drug Administration can regulate Cholestin. Circulation 2000;102:E9012–3.
18. From the Centers for Disease Control and Prevention. Adverse events associated with ingestion of gamma-butyrolactone–Minnesota, New Mexico, and Texas, 1998–1999. JAMA 1999;281:979–80.
19. Parkman CA. Another FDA warning: Kava supplements. Case Manager 2002;13:26–8.
20. Williamson BL, Johnson KL, Tomlinson AJ, et al. On-line HPLC-tandem mass spectrometry structural characterization of case-associated contaminants of L-tryptophan implicated with the onset of eosinophilia myalgia syndrome. Toxicol Lett 1998;99:139–50.
21. Hirano S, Shima T, Shimada T. Proportion of aflatoxin B1 contaminated kernels and its concentration in imported peanut samples. Shokuhin Eiseigaku Zasshi 2001; 42:237–42.
22. Current good manufacturing practice in manufacturing, packing, or holding dietary supplements; proposed rule. Fed Regist 1997;62:5699–709.
23. Fraser FC. Thalidomide retrospective: What did we learn? Teratology 1988;38:201–2.
24. Gugliotta G. Diet supplement marketers target kids. Washington Post 2000, July 18.
25. Kersting M, Alexy U. Vitamin and mineral supplements for the use of children on the German market: Products, nutrients, dosages. Ann Nutr Metab 2000;44:125–8.
26. Baker SS. Unregulated dietary supplements: Bitter medicine for children. J Pediatr Gastroenterol Nutr 2001;33:439–41.
27. Donangelo CM, Woodhouse LR, King SM, et al. Supplemental zinc lowers measures of iron status in young women with low iron reserves. J Nutr 2002;132:1860–4.
28. Fiske DN, McCoy HE, III, Kitchens CS. Zinc-induced sideroblastic anemia: Report of a case, review of the literature, and description of the hematologic syndrome. Am J Hematol 1994;46:147–50.
29. Position of the American Dietetic Association: Food fortification and dietary supplements. J Am Diet Assoc 2001;101:115–25.
30. American Academy of Pediatrics. Committee on Nutrition: Pediatric Nutrition Handbook. Elk Grove Village: American Academy of Pediatrics; 1993.
31. Nield LS, Mahajan P, Joshi A, Kamat D. Rickets: Not a disease of the past. Am Fam Physician 2006;74:619–26.
32. Roschitz B, Plecko B, Huemer M, et al. Nutritional infantile vitamin B12 deficiency: Pathobiochemical considerations in seven patients. Arch Dis Child Fetal Neonatal Ed 2005;90: F281–2.
33. Voruganti VS, Klein GL, Lu HX, et al. Impaired zinc and copper status in children with burn injuries: Need to reassess nutritional requirements. Burns 2005;31:711–6.
34. Conway SP, Wolfe SP, Brownlee KG, et al. Vitamin K status among children with cystic fibrosis and its relationship to bone mineral density and bone turnover. Pediatrics 2005;115:1325–31.
35. Lombardo T, Ximenes B, Ferro G. Hypochromic microcytic anemia as a clinical presentation of celiac disease. Clin Lab 2006;52:231–6.
36. Halfdanarson TR, Litzow MR, Murray JA. Hematological manifestations of celiac disease. Blood 2007;109:412–21.
37. Xu Y, Hashizume T, Shuhart MC, et al. Intestinal and hepatic CYP3A4 catalyze hydroxylation of 1alpha, 25-dihydroxyvitamin D(3): Implications for drug-induced osteomalacia. Mol Pharmacol 2006;69:56–65.
38. Delport R, Ubbink JB, Serfontein WJ, et al. Vitamin B6 nutritional status in asthma: The effect of theophylline therapy on plasma pyridoxal-5′-phosphate and pyridoxal levels. Int J Vitam Nutr Res 1988;58:67–72.
39. Krebs NF. Bioavailability of dietary supplements and impact of physiologic state: Infants, children and adolescents. J Nutr 2001;131:1351S–4S.
40. Herbal roulette. Consum Rep 1995:698–705.
41. Koutkia P, Chen TC, Holick MF. Vitamin D intoxication associated with an over-the-counter supplement. N Engl J Med 2001;345:66–7.
42. Institute of Medicine. Dietary Reference Intakes: Applications in Dietary Assessment. A Report of the Subcommittees on Interpretation and Uses of Dietary Reference Intakes and Upper Reference Levels of Nutrients, and the Standing Committee on the Scientific Evaluation of Dietary Reference Intakes, Food and Nutrition Board. Washington, DC: National Academy Press, 2001.
43. Subar AF, Block G. Use of vitamin and mineral supplements: Demographics and amounts of nutrients consumed. The 1987 Health Interview Survey. Am J Epidemiol 1990;132:1091–101.
44. Rastall RA, Maitin V. Prebiotics and synbiotics: Towards the next generation. Curr Opin Biotechnol 2002;13:490–6.
45. Isolauri E, Juntunen M, Rautanen T, et al. A human Lactobacillus strain (*Lactobacillus casei* sp strain GG) promotes recovery from acute diarrhea in children. Pediatrics 1991;88:90–7.
46. Biller JA, Katz AJ, Flores AF, et al. Treatment of recurrent Clostridium difficile colitis with Lactobacillus GG. J Pediatr Gastroenterol Nutr 1995;21:224–6.
47. Saavedra JM, Bauman NA, Oung I, et al. Feeding of Bifidobacterium bifidum and Streptococcus thermophilus to infants in hospital for prevention of diarrhoea and shedding of rotavirus. Lancet 1994;344:1046–9.
48. Lin MY, Savaiano D, Harlander S. Influence of nonfermented dairy products containing bacterial starter cultures on lactose maldigestion in humans. J Dairy Sci 1991;74:87–95.
49. Teitelbaum JE, Walker WA. Nutritional impact of pre- and probiotics as protective gastrointestinal organisms. Annu Rev Nutr 2002;22:107–38.
50. Smith J, Dahm DL. Creatine use among a select population of high school athletes. Mayo Clin Proc 2000;75: 1257–63.
51. Leder BZ, Longcope C, Catlin DH, et al. Oral androstenedione administration and serum testosterone concentrations in young men. JAMA 2000;283:779–82.
52. Terjung RL, Clarkson P, Eichner ER, et al. American College of Sports Medicine roundtable. The physiological and health effects of oral creatine supplementation. Med Sci Sports Exerc 2000;32:706–17.
53. Metzl JD, Small E, Levine SR, Gershel JC. Creatine use among young athletes. Pediatrics 2001;108:421–5.
54. Blumenthal M, Goldberg AJG. The German Commission E Monographs: Therapeutic Monographs on Medicinal Plants for Human Use. Austin, TX: American Botanical Council; 1998.
55. Piscitelli SC, Burstein AH, Chaitt D, et al. Indinavir concentrations and St John's wort. Lancet 2000;355:547–8.
56. The PDR for Herbal Medicines. Montvale NJ: Medical Economics Co.; 1998.
57. Hensrud DD, Engle DD, Scheitel SM. Underreporting the use of dietary supplements and nonprescription medications among patients undergoing a periodic health examination. Mayo Clin Proc 1999;74:443–7.

Special Diets

Melanie V. Connolly, MSc, RD, LDN, CNSD

The role of meeting nutrient requirements in disease, and the importance of providing essential nutrients to prevent disease, have been recognized for centuries. Examples include text from ancient Egyptian writings, the discovery of the dietary etiology of scurvy, and the devotion of Florence Nightingale, the founder of dietetics and modern nursing, to feeding and nursing the sick and wounded during the Crimean War. The concept of diet as an adjunct mechanism to support health and to prevent and treat various disease states has a strong historical foundation.

The term "special diets" refers to diets that are modifications of the normal adequate diet pattern based on the dietary reference intakes suggested by the Food and Nutrition Board of the Institute of Medicine. Modern medical nutrition therapy promotes the use of diet in the prevention and treatment of a variety of diseases.

The majority of healthy children never require special diets. Typically, children thrive on a varied diet with erratic bursts in growth, usually coupled with concomitant changes in appetite. However, many children with chronic diseases require special diets for optimal health, growth, and development. Depending on the condition, the required nutrient adjustments might be acute or chronic. For example, a surgical procedure might necessitate the use of a special diet for a short duration. Other diseases, however, such as insulin dependent diabetes mellitus, phenylketonuria, or celiac disease, require lifelong modifications in nutrient consumption. It is important to recognize that disease is not the only indication for implementation of a special diet. Various situations, including the prevention of unwanted disease, personal religious beliefs, and individual lifestyle preferences, can influence an individual to choose a special diet. In these instances, it is important to evaluate the safety of the special diet for a child.

The rising incidence of obesity in children and the fact that many adults intermittently restrict or alter dietary intake for presumed health effects mean that special or restricted diets may be provided to children more frequently than pediatricians and other clinicians suspect. Therefore, an essential part of the medical history is a review of the diet and eating habits, including timing, consistency, and preparation of meals, as well as the use of dietary supplements.

To implement a medically indicated special diet, adequate education and supervision are key to successful compliance. For children who require permanent alterations of their diet, regular follow-up, ongoing education, reevaluation of the diet, and continual attempts to motivate the family and maintain the child's commitment to the diet are important elements of success. Most special diets can be planned to meet 100% of the dietary reference intakes for nutrients; however, some diets could be deficient in particular nutrients and might require vitamin or mineral supplementation. In particular, chronic use of special diets in the pediatric population necessitates periodic monitoring of macro- and micronutrient status. With the proper use of special diets, optimal growth and development can be achieved.

- This chapter describes commonly used special diets for selected pediatric disorders. Chapter 67, "Standard and Specialized Formula," reviews the rationale and development of types of special formulas, and Appendix III, "Enteral Products," provides a comprehensive list of commercially available enteral formulas. The conditions and diets described here do not comprise a comprehensive list but rather represent the most common diets required in pediatrics. Special diets for clinical conditions such as food allergy, gastrointestinal disease, growth failure, hyperlipidemia, select inborn errors of metabolism, mineral deficiency, and weight control are found in this chapter. Included are descriptions, rationales for implementation, and lists of specific foods allowed and to be avoided. Checking food labels diligently is strongly advised because manufacturers often change product recipes.

FOOD ALLERGY

Food allergies can require major dietary changes, depending on the food antigen in question. Some of the most common allergens in infancy include cow's milk protein, soy protein, fish, eggs, and grains. In older pediatric patients, the list expands to include berries, nuts, peanuts, and chocolate. Cow's milk protein allergy, one of the most common allergies in infancy and early childhood, occurs with a frequency of between 0.5 and 7.0% in the general population. Up to 60% of pediatric patients with immediate hypersensitivity to cow's milk protein are allergic to soy protein as well.[1]

The gold standard for the diagnosis of a potential food allergy is the double-blind placebo-controlled food challenge. Liquid preparations can be used for infants and toddlers, and tablets or capsules can be used for older children. Such studies should be conducted in a hospital or clinic setting to ensure patient safety, especially in cases of suspected immunoglobulin E (IgE) mediation. Although elimination diets remain popular, they are fraught with problems, including the correct identification of the allergen in question, patient compliance, and other potential agents (dietary or otherwise) that could elicit a similar response.[2]

Nutritional management includes complete exclusion of the dietary antigen. Families are instructed to read product labels for terms indicative of the antigen, such as whey and sodium caseinate in the case of cow's milk protein allergy (see "Milk-Free Diet" below for a complete list). For the nonbreastfed infant, a hypoallergenic infant formula is recommended to replace cow's milk-based formula.[3] Fortified soy or rice milk can be substituted for cow's milk in diets for toddlers. When food allergies are severe or multiple, amino acid-based formulas can be used. Children not receiving a complete enteral supplement should be assessed for mineral and vitamin deficiencies. In families with a high risk for the development of one or more food allergies, it would be prudent to initially breast-feed infants, use a hypoallergenic formula, or both, in conjunction with the avoidance of the common food allergens mentioned.

- Periodic patient education updates are necessary. This is especially important with a diagnosis made in infancy because of the introduction of solid foods and the increased possibility of multiple caregivers. Education for family and even extended family should stress the necessity of continued dietary compliance. Support groups, cookbooks, and the like can be beneficial to patients requiring long-term dietary restrictions.

The Food Allergen Labeling and Consumer Protection Act of 2004 went into effect January 1, 2006.[4] This law refers to mandatory guidelines for the labeling of foods containing certain food allergens. It refers to all packaged foods sold in the United States that are regulated under the Federal Food, Drug, & Cosmetic Act. It includes domestically manufactured foods as well as imported foods, and excludes meat and poultry products, egg products, and fruits and vegetables in their natural state. The Food and Drug Administration (FDA) has identified eight major food allergens to which this law applies, which account for 90% of all food allergies: milk, egg, fish, crustacean shellfish, tree nuts, wheat, peanuts, and soybeans. The diets for these major allergens are listed below.

Noteworthy Points

- To comply with the law, labels of food products containing one of the eight major food allergens must either (1) list the ingredient in the ingredient list (eg, "casein (milk)"), or (2) use a "Contains" statement at the end of the ingredient list (eg, "Contains wheat, milk, and soy ingredients").
- Molluscan shellfish (including oysters, clams, mussels, or scallops) are not included in the list of major food allergens.
- The law does not apply to unintentional cross-contamination of a product with a major food allergen, such as on shared manufacturing lines during processing or cross-contact during harvesting or transporting crops. To ensure a desired food product has not come into contact with a major food allergen, consumers are advised to contact the food manufacturer directly.
- Packages on store shelves which were labeled prior to January 1, 2006 are not required to be in compliance with the above law.
- Because either of two methods can be used to communicate the presence of an allergen, consumers are advised to read food labels carefully before each and every purchase, particularly if your child is allergic to a food which is not considered one of the eight major food allergens.

TREE-NUT-FREE DIET

Tree nuts are available in their natural state (with or without shells), as ingredients in dishes, or processed into butters, flours, oils, pastes, milks, or coffees. The following are tree nuts and should be avoided: acorns, almonds, beechnuts, brazil nuts, cashews, chestnuts, hazelnuts (filberts), hickory nuts, macadamia nuts, pecans (mashuga nuts), pine nuts (pignoli), pistachios, shea nut/shea butter, walnuts, and nut oils or nut butters. During processing, tree nuts can contaminate a food which is not intended to contain a tree nut. Although not mandatory under the new food labeling law, many food manufacturers use voluntary labeling (eg, "may contain peanuts or tree nuts" or "processed on equipment which also processes nuts"). It is important to contact the food manufacturer directly to ensure that a processed food has not unintentionally come into contact with a tree nut.

The following foods may contain tree nuts: baked goods, barbeque sauce, candy, cereals, crackers, ice cream, marzipan, mortadella, natural flavoring, nougat, Nutella (or other chocolate/nut spread), pesto.

Noteworthy Points

- Many African, Chinese, Indonesian, Mexican, Thai, and Vietnamese dishes contain tree nuts.
- Avoid natural extracts such as almond extract, which may contain concentrated amounts of tree nut protein.
- Coconut, nutmeg, and water chestnuts are not in the tree nut family.
- Be aware of lotions and sunscreens which may contain shea butter or other nut butter.
- Experts recommend that if a person is allergic to one tree nut, all tree nuts should be avoided due to risk of cross-contamination.
- Artificial nuts (eg, Nu-Nuts) are in fact ground and reshaped tree nuts, and should be avoided.

CORN-FREE DIET

The corn-free diet is for individuals with an allergy to corn and its derivatives. Elimination of the following ingredients is necessary for individuals adhering to a corn-free diet: corn, corn flour, corn meal, cornstarch, corn sweeteners, corn syrup, corn syrup solids, maize, maltodextrin, marshmallow, popcorn, and powdered sugar.

- The following ingredients might contain corn: hydrolyzed plant protein, hydrolyzed vegetable protein, natural flavors, and starch (99% likelihood of cornstarch content).

EGG-FREE DIET

The egg-free diet is for use in people with a suspected or documented allergic reaction to egg-related products. Elimination of the following ingredients is necessary: egg albumin (also called ovalbumin), eggs, egg white, egg yolk, dried egg, egg powder, egg solids, egg substitutes (which contain eggs), eggnog, egg lecithin, globulin, livetin, lysozyme, mayonnaise, meringue, ovoglobulin, ovomucin, ovomucoid, vitellin, Simplesse, and surimi (imitation crabmeat).

Noteworthy Points

- The egg white, or albumin, is the most allergenic part of the egg.
- Many baked products that have a yellow color or shiny glaze are made with eggs or egg whites.
- Egg whites are often used as a clarifying agent in broths or soups. Always check with the chef when eating out.
- Some vaccines are grown on egg embryos and could contain trace amounts of egg protein. Inform your health care provider if your child has an egg allergy.
- Simplesse is used as a fat substitute in ice cream and frozen desserts and is made from either egg or milk protein.
- Even if your child is allergic to egg white or egg yolk only, complete egg elimination is recommended. This includes egg in baked goods.

Tips for Egg-Free Cooking

- Egg substitutes can be used only if they are free of egg whites.
- Two tbsp of pureed vegetables can replace an egg in soups, sauces, and other dishes.
- To bind or thicken fruit desserts, use one tsp dry, unflavored gelatin mixed with two tbsp of liquid to replace one egg.
- Because baked goods without eggs crumble easily, use smaller pans. For example, make cupcakes instead of a cake or muffins instead of bread.
- Xantham gum is excellent for holding baked goods together. Use one tsp for each egg.
- To help leaven baked goods, add an extra half tsp egg-free baking powder for each egg called for in a recipe, along with another egg substitute to bind or thicken.
- For thickening cream dishes and sauces, add extra flour, cornstarch, or xantham gum.
- To enhance the flavor of egg-free cookies or cakes, add extra ingredients such as raisins, nuts, coconut, seeds, or spices.
- Use any of the following as a binder to replace each egg in your egg-free baked goods:
  - Two tbsp tahini (ground sesame seeds)
  - Two tbsp any nut butter
  - Two tbsp oat flour plus one tbsp water
  - One tsp baking powder, one tbsp liquid (water), and one tbsp vinegar
  - One tsp yeast dissolved in one-fourth cup warm water
  - One and a half tbsp water and one and a half tbsp vegetable oil, and one tsp baking powder
  - Two tbsp mashed banana or apricot puree and half tsp baking powder.

MILK-PROTEIN-FREE DIET

The milk-free diet is for use in patients with a documented, or in some cases suspected, allergy to cow's milk protein. It should not be confused with a lactose-free diet. If the patient is taking a fortified milk substitute, then additional supplements might not be necessary. If a fortified milk substitute is not consumed, the diet could be deficient in calcium, phosphorus, and vitamin D, and supplementation may be needed.

- Elimination of the following ingredients is necessary: artificial butter flavor, butter, butter fat, buttermilk, casein, caseinate (ammonium, calcium, magnesium, potassium, sodium), cheese, cottage cheese, cream, crème fraiche, curds, custard, pudding, ghee, half and half cream, hydrolysates (casein, milk protein, protein, whey, and whey protein), Lactaid milk, lactalbumin, lactoglobulin, lactose, milk (derivative, protein, solids, malted, condensed, evaporated, dry, whole, low fat, nonfat, skim), nondairy creamer (check for casein), nougat, organic milk, raw milk, rennet, sour cream, sour cream solids, whey (delactosed, demineralized, protein concentrate), and yogurt. Ingredients that might indicate the presence of milk proteins are brown sugar flavoring, caramel flavoring, chocolate, high-protein flour (protein source could be skim milk powder), lactic acid starter culture, margarine (might contain whey), natural flavoring, nondairy creamer (may contain casein), Simplesse (could be made from eggs or milk protein), and certain brands of soy yoghurt, soy cheese, or soy desserts.

Noteworthy Points

- Products that have KD or $(U)_D$ on their labels indicate the presence of milk in the product. The ingredient list does not always list the milk source. It could be present as the result of cross-contamination from a milk-containing product that is produced in the same facility. Some labels now state "KDE," which indicates that the product is kosher but made on dairy equipment.
- Parve or Pareve on the label indicates that the product may be milk free; check all labels to confirm.
- Certain vitamin and mineral supplements, as well as some prescription and over-the-counter drugs, contain lactose as a filler. Consult a doctor or pharmacist for specific information.
- The brine that surrounds prepackaged deli meats often contains whey or casein. There could also be cross-contamination from other meat or cheese products when meats are sliced in a store's deli area.
- Some brands of canned tuna fish contain casein.
- Goat's milk and sheep's milk are not acceptable cow's milk substitutes.

Suggested Milk-Free Foods

Fats. Kosher margarine, unsalted Mazola margarine, unsalted Fleishmann's stick margarine, lard, vegetable oil, mayonnaise, cocoa butter, Better than Cream Cheese (Tofutti brand), Sour Supreme (Tofutti brand).

Fruits. All types.

Meat, Fish, Poultry, and Eggs. Plain beef, poultry, fish, pork, lamb, bacon, kosher frankfurters, kosher cold cuts (eg, Morrison & Schiff or Hebrew National), tofu, peanut butter, eggs.

Cheese. Soy cheese (without sodium caseinate).

Potatoes, Pasta, and Rice. All except prepackaged (canned or frozen) products, in which casein is added to pasta to maintain shape.

Soups. Clear canned soups and commercial and homemade soups made with allowed ingredients. Be sure to check labels as even some clear soups might contain margarine, which will probably contain milk products.

Beverages. Milk-free infant formulas such as Isomil, ProSobee, and Alsoy; fruit juices; carbonated beverages; Kool-Aid; cocoa without added milk solids; Nut Quick (Ener-G Foods); Westbrae Rice Drink, Amazake Original, Rice Dream; soy milks such as EdenSoy Original, Vitasoy Original, Vitasoy Light Original, and WestSoy Lite Plain.

Bread and Crackers. French, Italian, Vienna, or Syrian bread; bagels are traditionally milk-free but check labels.

Cereals. Most do not contain milk products in the ingredient list but often have the $(U)_D$ symbol, which suggests that the product could contain some milk and should be avoided.

Sweets. Sugar, jams, jellies, syrups, honey, candies such as gum drops, baking chocolate, Marshmallow Fluff.

Desserts. Jello, fruit sorbet, Italian ice (gelato), milk-free Popsicles; baked products made with Crisco, Spry, or allowed margarine; Royal brand instant pudding mix made with appropriate milk substitute; milk-free cake mixes (read labels); Tofutti.

Vegetables. All types.

Miscellaneous. Mustard, relish, ketchup, salt, pepper, spices, soy sauce, cocoa powder, carob powder, potato chips, pretzels (check labels for $(U)_D$), olives, peanut butter without added milk, plain popcorn, corn chips.

PEANUT-FREE DIET

The peanut-free diet is for individuals with a known peanut allergy. The peanut is a legume and not a member of the nut family. Legumes are edible seeds enclosed in pods; others include soybeans, lima beans, carob, and sweet clover. Peanut allergy can be fatal.

- Elimination of the following ingredients is necessary: cold-pressed peanut oil, ground nuts, mixed nuts, peanuts, peanut butter, peanut flour, and nut meats. Foods that could contain peanuts or peanut products include African, Chinese, Indonesian, and Thai dishes; baked goods (eg, pastries, cookies); beer nuts; candy; chili and spaghetti sauce (which might be thickened with peanut butter); chocolate candies; egg rolls (may be sealed with peanut butter); hydrolyzed plant protein; hydrolyzed vegetable protein; ice cream; marzipan (which can be a mixture of nuts); and nougat.

Noteworthy Points

- Peanut allergies are usually not outgrown.
- Skin tests for peanut allergy are positive throughout life.
- Only peanut oil prepared by the hot-solvent extraction processes that are commonly used in the United States is known to be free of protein.[5] However, as not all peanut oils are produced in the same way, caution may warrant complete avoidance of peanut oil.
- Check all candy labels; often they will list peanuts on the label if the product was made in the same facility as another peanut-containing candy. For example, plain M&Ms and Raisinettes both note on the label that they may contain peanuts, but peanuts are not necessarily in the ingredient list.
- Avoid mixed nuts, which often contain peanuts.
- Some kitchens use peanuts in a variety of foods, which makes cross-contamination in restaurants likely.
- Egg rolls are occasionally sealed with peanut butter.
- Avoid crafts which call for peanut butter.

SHELLFISH-FREE DIET

The shellfish-free diet is for individuals with a documented allergy to shellfish. Individuals allergic to one type of shellfish could be allergic to others in the same family. Edible shellfish are usually divided into two categories: mollusks and crustaceans. Mollusks, such as clams and mussels, have two shells, but also include the abalone, which has a shell covering and a soft underpart. The crustaceans, such as the lobster, have segmented bodies that are covered with an armor-like section of thick and thin shells.

Elimination of the following ingredients is necessary: mollusks, such as abalone, calamari, clams, cockle, escargots/snails, mollusk, mussels, octopus, oysters, periwinkle, sea urchin, scallops, and squid, and crustaceans, such as crab, crawfish, crayfish, ecrevisse, lobster, shrimp, prawn, and crevette.

Caution should be exercised at salad bars, where cross-contamination may occur, as well as restaurants with deep fryers shared with shellfish.

SOY-FREE DIET

The soy-free diet is for patients with a documented, or in some cases suspected, soy protein allergy. Patients with a soy protein allergy rarely have difficulty meeting their macro- and micronutrient requirements. However, patients with both cow's milk and soy protein allergies should be monitored for caloric and protein (quality and quantity) intakes, as well as for calcium, phosphorus, and vitamin D intakes. If possible, supplementation with a fortified milk-free, soy-free formula will assist in meeting nutrient requirements for growth.

- Elimination of the following ingredients is necessary: edamame, hydrolyzed soy protein, miso, natto, shoyu sauce, soy beans, soy cheese, soy fiber, soy flour, soy grits, soy milk, soy nut butter, soy nuts, soy protein concentrate, soy protein isolate, soy sauce, soy sprouts, soy yoghurt, soya, tempeh, textured vegetable protein, tofu, and yuba. The following ingredients might indicate the presence of soy protein: flavoring, hydrolyzed vegetable protein, hydrolyzed plant protein, natural flavoring, vegetable broth, vegetable gum, and vegetable starch.

Noteworthy Point

Most people with soy allergies can safely eat soy lecithin and soy oil. Soy lecithin, often used as a stabilizer, emulsifier, or an antioxidant, is a mixture of fatty substances and is a by-product of soybean processing. The processing of most soybean oils removes the protein portion.

Suggested Soy-Free Foods

Beverages. Milk, fruit juices, carbonated beverages, Kool-Aid, cocoa, hot chocolate; infant formulas such as Enfamil, Similac, Nutramigen, Alimentum, and Pregestimil; rice beverages such as Rice Dream and Westbrae Rice Drink.

Bread and Crackers. Syrian and French bread.

Cereals. Oatmeal, cream of rice, cream of wheat; any cold cereals with allowed ingredients; infant cereals without soy (check labels).

Fats. Butter, cream, bacon, soy-free mayonnaise, lard, pure vegetable oil (eg, coconut, corn, cottonseed, olive, peanut, safflower, sunflower).

Meat, Fish, Poultry, Cheese, and Eggs. All types when plain or prepared with allowed ingredients, such as waterpacked tuna; kosher 100% beef hot dogs; eggs; all cheese except soy cheese and imitation cheeses containing soy.

Meat Alternatives. Legumes (eg, baked beans), nuts, and seeds, except soybeans.

Potatoes, Rice, and Pasta. All, including spaghetti, macaroni, and plain noodles.

Vegetables. All except soybeans.

Fruits. All fruit and fruit juices.

Soups. Homemade and canned soups made with allowed ingredients.

Desserts. Fruit, gelatin, homemade puddings (cornstarch, tapioca, rice); ice cream, sherbet, and fruit ices; Popsicles, Fudgsicles; homemade cakes, cookies, and pies made with allowed ingredients; baking chocolate; yogurt.

Sweets. Sugar, jams, jellies, honey, molasses, syrups, marshmallows.

Miscellaneous. Salt, pepper, spices, mustard, relish, ketchup, pickles, olives, coconut; snack foods only if prepared without soy (potato chips, popcorn, dry roasted peanuts).

WHEAT-FREE DIET

The wheat-free diet is for patients with a documented, or in some cases suspected, wheat allergy. The following ingredients should be eliminated from the diet: bread crumbs, bran, bulgur, cereal extract, cous-cous, cracker meal, durum flour, enriched flour, farina, flour, gluten, graham flour, high-gluten flour, high-protein flour, malt vital gluten, matzo, semolina, triticale, wheat bran, wheat grain, wheat gluten, wheat starch, and whole-wheat flour. The following ingredients could have wheat present: gelatinized starch, hot dogs, hydrolyzed vegetable protein, ice cream, imitation crabmeat, modified food starch, natural flavoring, sauces (could be thickened with wheat), soy sauce, starch, vegetable gum, and vegetable starch.

Noteworthy Points

- One and one-eighth cup oat flour, seven-eighth cup rice flour, or one cup yellow/white corn flour can be substituted for one cup wheat flour.
- Spaghetti squash, corn pasta, and rice pasta make great substitutions for regular pasta.
- Fresh, frozen, and canned vegetables are your best choice. Prepackaged vegetables in sauces often contain wheat as fillers.
- Gluten free also means wheat free.
- For thickening, instead of one tbsp wheat flour, use half tbsp cornstarch.
- The white, all-purpose flour which is often used for baking is wheat flour.

Suggested Wheat-Free Foods

Beverages. Milk, fruit juices, carbonated beverages, Kool-Aid, cocoa, hot chocolate.

Breads and Crackers. Only those made with 100% rye, oat, corn, or rice flour with no wheat added; corn tortillas.

Cereals. Any corn, oat, rice, or rye cereal that has no wheat flour added (eg, puffed rice, corn flakes, crispy rice).

Potatoes, Rice, and Pasta. All plain rice and wheat-free pastas.

Fats. Butter, margarine, vegetable oils, lard, bacon, cream, mayonnaise, homemade gravy thickened with cornstarch.

Meat, Fish, Poultry, Eggs, and Cheese. All types when plain or prepared with allowed ingredients; all eggs; all cheeses. Be sure to read the labels of processed cheeses.

Meat Alternatives. Legumes, nuts, seeds (eg, peanut butter, baked beans, tofu).

Vegetables. All types; avoid those prepared with sauces.

Soups. Homemade soups with allowed ingredients.

Desserts. Fruit, gelatin, junket, cornstarch, and tapioca puddings.

Miscellaneous. Salt, pepper, spices, mustard, ketchup, pickles, relish, olives, coconut, baking chocolate, potato chips, corn chips, popcorn.

ALLERGY ORGANIZATIONS, SUPPORT GROUPS, AND RESOURCES

- Food Allergy and Anaphylaxis Network, 11,781 Lee Jackson Highway, Suite 160 Fairfax, VA 22033-3309; telephone: 800-929-4040; fax: 703-691-2713; e-mail: faan@foodallergy.org; www.foodallergy.org. The Food Allergy and Anaphylaxis Network (FAAN) is a national nonprofit organization established to help families living with food allergies and to increase public awareness about food allergies and anaphylaxis. All resources are checked for medical accuracy by FAAN's Medical Advisory Board. There is a subscription fee.
- American Academy of Allergy, Asthma, and Immunology, 800-822-ASMA (2762), www.aaaai.org
- American Academy of Pediatrics, 800-433-9016, www.aap.org
- American College of Allergy, Asthma, and Immunology, 800-842-7777, www.acaai.org
- Asthma and Allergy Foundation of America, 800-7-ASTHMA (727-8462), www.aafa.org
- American Dietetic Association, 800-366-1655, www.eatright.org
- www.peanutallergy.com

GASTROINTESTINAL DISEASES

A number of gastrointestinal diseases require dietary modification, both short- and long-term. Patients can have malabsorption, maldigestion, or both coupled with an inadequate intake, as seen in both celiac disease and Crohn's disease, for example. Patients often require individually tailored diets based on their degree of bowel integrity or function. Enteral formulas, both standard and special, are commonly used with several gastrointestinal disorders (see Appendix III, "Enteral Products"). In addition, Chapter 67, "Standard and Specialized Formula," reviews the rationale and development of many of these formulas. Below, we review the more common diets used in pediatric gastroenterology. Please refer to other chapters for a more detailed discussion of each disorder.

FAT MODIFICATION FOR PANCREATIC DISEASE

A low-fat diet might be indicated in the treatment of chronic pancreatitis, as well as the later stages of acute pancreatitis. Acute pancreatitis usually warrants the discontinuation of oral feedings. As clinical parameters indicate improvement of the disease state, careful reintroduction of food might be allowed, with the eventual return to a normal diet.

Chronic pancreatitis with pancreatic enzyme insufficiency will necessitate enzyme replacement therapy; however, dietary modification is usually not necessary. Children with chronic pancreatitis and pancreatic enzyme sufficiency can consume a diet containing 20 to 30% of calories from fat, unless laboratory and clinical data suggest fat intolerance.

Low-fat diets are based on individual requirements and must be designed by using food tables, reading labels, and following the Food Guide Pyramid; they also must be evaluated for tolerance and acceptance. Caloric consumption should be carefully monitored whenever fat restriction is warranted. Fat restriction to less than 5% of total

Table 1 Dietary Fiber Content of Foods

Food	Little (<0.5 g)	Low (1 g)	Moderate (2 g)	High (3 g)	Very High (>4 g)
Dairy	Milk, yogurt, pudding, ice cream, cheese	–	–	–	–
Protein	Eggs, beef, chicken, pork, turkey, fish	–	2 tbsp peanut butter	1/2 cup garbanzo beans, lima beans	1/2 cup lentils (5 g), northern beans (4 g), navy beans (5 g), pork and beans (6 g), kidney beans (6 g)
Fruit	Fruit juice, watermelon, cherries	1/2 cup canned pears, pineapple, fruit cocktail, peaches, fresh grapes	Fresh: 1 peach, 3 apricots, half a grapefruit; 1/2 cup applesauce, blueberries, strawberries	Fresh: 1 apple, orange, banana, 3 dates; 1/2 cup raspberries; peaches, apricots, apples	Fresh: 1 pear (5 g), half an avocado (4 g), 3 plums (4 g), dried: 1/4 cup raisins, 3 prunes (4 g)
Vegetables	–	1/2 cup tomato, juice lettuce, spinach, celery, cauliflower, cucumber, green beans	1/2 cup tomato, cabbage	1/2 cup sweet potato, broccoli, carrots, peas, potato salad, corn	1 baked potato with skin (4 g)
Breads	1 slice French, Italian, raisin, or white bread; 1 pancake or donut; half a bagel	1 slice cracked wheat, bread; 1 tortilla or whole-wheat pancake	1 slice 100% whole-pumpernickel, or rye	1 slice Branola; wheat bread	1 slice flourless bread (5 g), 1 bran muffin
Cereals	1/2 cup corn flakes, Frosted Flakes, Lucky Charms, Cheerios	1/2 cup oatmeal, Life, Total, Honey Nut Shredded Wheat	1/2 cup shredded wheat, Nutrigrain, Wheaties, n' Raisins, Wheat Chex	1/2 cup Bran Flakes, granola, Crispy Wheats, wheat germ	1/2 cup 100% bran (9 g), Raisin Bran, Grape Nuts, All Bran, (9 g), Fiber 1 (12 g); 1/4 cup unprocessed wheat bran (7 g; 2 g/tbsp)
Pasta and rice	1/2 cup white pasta	1/2 cup egg noodles, white rice	1/2 cup brown rice	–	1/2 cup whole wheat pasta
Crackers	Goldfish, saltines, Ritz	2 graham, 16 Wheat Thins, 1 granola bar	3 Harvest Wheats, 3 Triscuit	1 rye crisp	Metamucil wafers
Desserts	Chocolate chip cookies	Oatmeal cookies	Fig Newtons, Peak Freans, Bran Crunch (3 g)	–	–
Miscellaneous	Beverages, fats, sweets	–	1 cup popcorn	1/4 cup cashews, pecans peanuts, walnuts	1/4 cup almonds, 1/4 cup coconut

Adapted from reference 6.

daily calories places the child at risk for the development of essential fatty acid deficiency.

- For specific foods pertaining to the low-fat diet, see "Low Cholesterol and Low Saturated Fat Diet" below.

HIGH-FIBER DIET

Dietary fiber is a food component that is neither digested nor absorbed by the body. This undigested material can itself absorb water, resulting in the formation of larger, softer stools, which are more easily moved through the intestines and then passed. A high-fiber diet can benefit the whole family. Diets high in fiber have been shown to control constipation, lower the risk of colon cancer, and reduce blood cholesterol levels. Children are more accepting of dietary changes when they are adopted by the entire family.

- A general rule of thumb for recommended daily fiber intake is five plus the age (in years) of the child more than 2 years of age, to a maximum of 35 g/d. For example, a 7 years old should receive 12 g/d (5 + 7 years).

Noteworthy Points

To increase the fiber content in a child's diet, include fruits, vegetables, and whole grains (Table 1). During commercial processing, the fiber content of these sources can be reduced. Therefore:

- Instead of white bread, use 100% whole-grain breads.
- Instead of processed cereals, use whole-grain cereals.
- Instead of canned fruits and juices, use fresh fruits.
- Maintain a well-balanced diet: choose a variety of foods from the Food Guide Pyramid (see Appendix II, "Nutritional Requirements").
- Increase fiber in the diet gradually. A sudden increase in dietary fiber intake can cause gas and bloating.
- If a child refuses high-fiber foods, remember that children often need to be introduced to foods several times before the foods become familiar and acceptable. Slow changes in a child's diet are often better accepted than rapid ones.
- Increase fluid intake with an increase in dietary fiber (Table 2). Inadequate fluid intake can also cause constipation.
- Give children choices as to what they would like to eat but provide appropriate choices.
- Add two to four tbsp of a high-fiber cereal to a favorite hot or cold cereal.
- Add unprocessed wheat bran to yogurt, applesauce, hot or cold cereal, soup, peanut butter, tuna salad, pancake batter, or spaghetti.

GLUTEN-RESTRICTED DIET

The gluten-restricted diet is necessary, for life, for patients diagnosed with celiac disease. The diet is designed to provide adequate nourishment while eliminating foods containing the gliadin fraction of gluten, a protein found in many grains, which causes intestinal injury in susceptible people. Although many cereal grains contain gluten, only wheat, rye, barley, and oats contain the gliadin fraction. Gliadin from these grains is present in many everyday foods, including breads, rolls, crackers, cookies, and breakfast cereals, and might also be present as an incidental ingredient in food additives and derivatives (see the list below). For

Table 2 Recommended Fluid Intake

Child's Weight (lb)	Total Fluid Per 24 h (Cups)
7	2
12	3⅓
21	5
26	6
35	7
44	8
63	9½
99	10½

this reason, food labels must be read carefully. When all sources of gliadin are removed from the diet, the intestine will heal and function normally.

Noteworthy Points

- Despite the restrictions, the gluten-restricted diet should be well balanced based on the Food Guide Pyramid. Table 3 lists foods allowed and restricted while following a gluten-restricted diet. Table 4 provides sample menus for a gluten-restricted diet.
- Read food labels carefully to avoid gluten-containing grains and gluten derivatives such as
  - Flour and cereal products: avoid textured vegetable protein
  - Colorings: avoid hydrolyzed vegetable protein
  - Emulsifiers: avoid hydrolyzed plant protein
  - Flavorings: avoid starch
  - Malt or malt flavoring: avoid modified food starch
  - Preservatives: avoid vegetable gum
  - Vinegar: avoid distilled white or grain vinegar.

Table 3 Gluten-Restricted Diet

Type of Food	Allowed	Avoid
Grains and flours	Arrowroot starch, corn flour, cornstarch, cornmeal; maize and waxy maize; potato flour, potato starch flour; rice bran; rice flours: plain, sweet, brown, and polished rice; soy flour; tapioca starch	Low-gluten flours; all flours containing wheat, rye, barley, and oats; durham wheat, all purpose flour, white enriched flour, wheat germ, whole-wheat flour, wheat starch; wheat bran; oat bran; amaranth; buckwheat, buckwheat groats; bulgar; graham; kasha; matzo; millet; rusks, semolina, sorghum; triticale
Breads	Specially prepared breads using only allowed flours (100% potato, corn, rice, arrowroot, soybean); special commercial gluten-free baking mixes (Ener-G Foods, Dietary Specialties)	All breads, rolls, etc, made with wheat, rye, barley, or oats
Cereals	Hot or cold cereals made from corn meal, rice, hominy*	All containing wheat, rye, barley, oats, farina, bran (except rice bran), graham, wheat germ, kasha, bulgar, buckwheat, millet, triticale. Do not eat cereals that contain malt unless the source is known.
Noodles and pasta	Gluten-free corn pasta; special gluten-free pasta (Aproten and other brands); oriental rice noodles or bean noodles	Regular noodles, spaghetti, macaroni, etc
Crackers and snacks	Pure cornmeal tortillas; rice wafers; rice cakes without added rye or millet;* popcorn; crackers made with allowed flours (100% potato, corn, rice, arrowroot, soybean); some potato chips*	All containing wheat, wheat snack foods, starch, rye, barley, oats, bran (except rice bran), graham, wheat germ, malt, kaska, bulgar, buckwheat, matzo, millet, durham wheat, sorghum, rusks, amaranth, triticale
Milk products	Fresh, dry, evaporated, or condensed milk; cream; sour cream;† whipping cream,† yogurt†	Malted milk; commercially prepared milkshakes; some nondairy cream;* some commercial chocolate drinks*
Meat and alternatives	Fresh meat, fish, poultry, and eggs; fish canned in oil, brine, or water; luncheon meats, frankfurters, and prepared meat products packaged without food starch or gluten derivatives; peanut	Any meat or meat products containing wheat, rye, barley, oats, or gluten derivatives; some canned tuna in vegetable broth,* some sausages,* frankfurters, luncheon meats, and sandwich spreads; canned chili and stews; bread-containing products such as Swiss steak, pot pies, croquettes; selfbasting turkey with hydrolyzed vegetable protein (HPV) injected as part of the basting solution
Cheese	Aged cheese (100% cheddar, Swiss, parmesan, etc); cottage cheese,† cream cheese; processed cheese*	Cheese foods; cheese spreads or dips; imitation cheese products
Fruit and juices	Most fresh, frozen, dried, or canned fruit	Thickened or prepared fruits as in pie fillings*
Vegetables	Most plain, fresh, frozen, or canned vegetables; dried beans, peas, and lentils; tomato puree and paste; white and sweet potatoes; yams; hominy; rice	Vegetables in sauces;* commercially prepared vegetables; canned baked beans; most packaged rice mixes
Fats	Most margarines,* butter, vegetable oil, lard, shortening; nuts; pure mayonnaise made without distilled white vinegar*	Commercial salad dressings and dips,* unless product contents are known
Sweets and desserts	Special commercial gluten-free cakes, cookies, and baking mixes; homemade puddings with cornstarch, rice, or tapioca; some pudding mixes,* gelatin desserts, custards, and ices; sherbet and ice cream if they do not contain gluten stabilizers,* hard candy flavored with sugar, honey, molasses, marshmallow, coconut, or chocolate; most jams and jellies;* most nonbuttered syrups;* some candy*	Most commercially prepared cakes, cookies, and other baked goods; "instant" puddings and bread pudding; ice cream cones; frozen desserts containing gluten stabilizers; check contents of commercial candies
Beverages	Fruit juice; plain tea; brewed coffee; hot chocolate made with pure cocoa powder; carbonated drinks except most root beers; wine and brandy without dyes or preservatives; most rums; vodka distilled from potatoes	"Instant" drinks, such as tea, coffee, cocoa, and fruit punch, which are processed with additives, stabilizers, or emulsifiers;* ground coffee with added grain; some flavored coffees;* some herbal teas;* most root beers;* all beer and ale; all whisky (including corn whisky); bourbon; any liquor made from grain alcohol; vodka distilled from grain
Soups	Homemade broths and soups made with allowed ingredients; special gluten-free commercial soups (Ener-G Foods)	Most canned soups and soup mixes,* bouillon, bouillon cubes or powder
Miscellaneous	Cider, rice, or wine vinegar; salt; black or red pepper; herbs; pure spices; monosodium glutamate (MSG); bicarbonate of soda; pure cocoa; most yeast; baking powder; cream of tartar; flavoring if not made with alcohol (choose imitation)	Distilled white vinegar; most white pepper; some curry powder;* some dry seasoning mixes (such as chili seasoning mix);* some gravy extracts and meat sauces;* yeast flakes;* extracts,* natural flavorings containing alcohol; ketchup,* prepared mustard, and horseradish

Commercially prepared condiments (pickles, ketchup, mustard, mayonnaise, steak sauce) are usually made with distilled white vinegar, which is made with grain.

A very small amount of protein may be carried over into white vinegar during distillation. Moderate use of commercially prepared condiments is allowed by some physicians. However, individuals with newly diagnosed or extreme gluten sensitivity should avoid these condiments.

*Some products may be used if checked with the manufacturer and found to be gluten free.

†Check label for oat gum.

Table 4 Sample Menus for a Gluten-Restricted Diet

Breakfast	Lunch	Dinner	Snack
Orange juice, scrambled egg, gluten-free muffin with margarine, milk	Corn pasta with tomato and meat sauce, fresh fruit, milk	Tossed salad with gluten-free dressing, grilled chicken, rice, ice cream (check label), milk	Potato chips, fruit juice
Grape juice, gluten-free waffles with strawberries or gluten-free syrup, milk	Tacos (pure corn tortilla, beef, cheese, tomato), mixed fruit cup, milk	Oven-fried whitefish (gluten-free beans, cornflake crumbs), french fries, carrot coins, pudding (check label)	Milk, gluten-free pound cake
Apple juice, hot rice cereal, gluten-free toast, milk, margarine, jelly	Grilled cheese on gluten-free bread fresh fruit, gelatin, milk	Baked pork chop, potatoes, corn, applesauce gluten-free cookies	Peanuts and raisins

Table 5 Additives and Ingredients to Avoid on Gluten-Free Diet

Additives*	Modified starch*
Alcohol*	Mono- and diglycerides*
Amaranth	Oat
Barley	Oat groats
Bran*	Oatmeal
Buckwheat	Oat gum
Buckwheat groats	Preservatives*
Bulgur	Rye
Cereal products*	Rusks
Coloring*	Semolina
Distilled white vinegar	Sorghum
Durum wheat	Stabilizers*
Emulsifiers*	Starch*
Farina	Textured vegetable protein (TVP)*
Flavorings*	Triticale
Flour*	Vegetable gum*
Groats	Vegetable protein*
Hydrolyzed plant protein (HPP)*	Wheat
Hydrolyzed vegetable protein (HVP)*	Wheat flour
Kasha	Wheat germ
Malt flavoring	Wheat germ oil
Matzo cake meal	Wheat starch
Matzo farfel	White enriched flour
Matzo meal	Whole-wheat flour
Millet	Wheat stabilizers
Modified food starch*	

*Some products can be used if the manufacturer verifies that they are gluten free.

- Product ingredients can change from one batch to another. To check an ingredient, contact the Celiac Sprue Association/USA, the Gluten Intolerance Group of North America, or the manufacturer of the product. Foods of unknown composition should be omitted. Brand names of gluten-free products are available from the celiac sprue support groups. Table 5 provides a list of additives and ingredients to avoid while following a gluten-free diet; Table 6 lists those that are permitted.
- Many gluten-free foods can be purchased at grocery stores, Asian food markets, and health food stores.
- Eating in restaurants requires planning and a basic knowledge of foods and food preparation. Choose foods prepared simply, such as broiled or roasted meats, plain vegetables, plain salads, and foods without breading, gravies, or sauces.
- A lactose-restricted diet might be necessary in the early treatment of newly diagnosed celiac disease if symptoms of malabsorption are severe. Milk and milk products may be restricted and gradually reintroduced into the diet.
- Ensure prescription and nonprescription medications are gluten-free.
- Use a separate colander and toaster for gluten-free pasta and breads.

Tips For Gluten-Restricted Cooking

Gluten's elasticity is an important element in baked products. Special recipes to compensate for this are required when gluten-free flours are used for baking. Cookbooks specifically for the gluten-restricted diet are available. When gluten-free flour or starch is used as a substitute in baked goods, it is necessary to increase the amount of leavening (baking powder, baking soda, yeast, or eggs) and protein (eggs, milk or powdered milk, soy flour, tofu, or cottage cheese). A mixture of flours gives a better result in gluten-free baking.

The following grains can also be used in the quantities listed as a substitute for one cup of wheat flour:

- Five-eighth cup potato starch flour (half cup plus two tbsp)
- Seven-eighth cup white rice flour (three-fourth cup plus two tbsp)

Table 6 Additives and Ingredients Allowed on Gluten-Free Diet

Adipic acid	Mannitol
Ascorbic acid	Microcrystalline cellulose
BHA	Monosodium glutamate (MSG)
BHT	Niacin
Betacarotene	Polyglycerol
Biotin	Polysorbate 60 and 80
Calcium phosphate	Potassium citrate
Calcium chloride	Potassium iodide
Calcium pantothenate	Propylene glycol monostearate
Carboxymethylcellulose	Propylgallate
Carrageenan	Pyridoxine hydrochloride
Citric acid	Riboflavin
Corn sweetener	Sodium acid pyrophosphate
Corn syrup solids	Sodium ascorbate (ascorbic acid)
Demineralized whey	Sodium benzoate
Dextrimaltose	Sodium caseinate
Dextrose (dextrins)	Sodium citrate
Dioctyl sodium sulfosuccinate	Sodium hexametaphosphate
Folic acid (folacin)	Sodium nitrate
Fructose	Sodium silaco aluminate
Fumaric acid	Sorbitol
Gums: acacia, arabic, carob bean, cellulose, guar, locust bean, tragacanth, xanthan	Sucrose
Invert sugar	Sulfosuccinate
Lactic acid	Tartaric acid
Lactose	Thiamine hydrochloride
Lecithin	Tricalcium phosphate
Magnesium hydroxide	Vanillin
Malic acid	Vitamins and minerals
	Vitamin A (palmitate)

Adapted from reference 7.

- Half cup soy flour plus half cup potato starch flour
- One cup corn flour
- One cup fine cornmeal
- Three-fourth cup coarse cornmeal.

To substitute for one tbsp of wheat flour as a thickener in sauces, gravies, and puddings, use one of the following:

- Half tbsp cornstarch
- Half tbsp potato starch
- Five and half tsp white rice flour
- Five and half tsp arrowroot starch
- Two tsp quick-cooking tapioca.

Celiac Disease Organizations, Support Groups, and Resources

Support groups provide a network for people with celiac disease. Group services provide up-to-date information about celiac disease and the gluten-free diet, and include information and referrals, publications, such as newsletters and gluten free diet instructions, annual conferences, and workshops.

National groups include:

- Celiac Sprue Association/United States of America, Inc. (CSA/USA), PO Box 31700, Omaha, NE 68131-0700; telephone: 877-CSA-4CSA; fax: 402-558-1347; www.csaceliacs.org
- Canadian Celiac Association National Office, 5170 Dixie Rd., Ste. 204, Mississauga, ON L4W IE3; telephone: 800-363-7296; fax: 905-507-4673; www.celiac.ca
- Gluten Intolerance Group of North America (GIG),31,214 124 Avenue SE, Auburn, WA 98092; telephone: 206-246-6652; fax: 206-246-6531; www.gluten.net
- Celiac Disease Foundation, 13251 Ventura Blvd., Ste. 3, Studio City, CA 91604; telephone: 818-990-2354; fax: 818-990-2379; www.celiac.org
- Celiac Support Group; http://www.childrenshospital.org/clinicalservices/Site2166/mainpageS2166P0.html
- Organizations that can be of assistance in following the gluten-free diet include; www.celiac.com
- American Dietetic Association, National Center for Nutrition and Dietetics; telephone: 800-366-1655 (consumer hotline); www.eatright.org
- US FDA, www.fda.gov

LACTOSE-FREE DIET

The lactose-free diet is intended for the individual who must eliminate sources of lactose from the diet, such as patients with galactosemia (an inborn error of metabolism) or those who have difficulty digesting lactose.

Lactose is the primary carbohydrate of dairy products; therefore, foods containing milk or milk products are to be excluded from the diet. People with lactose intolerance might not produce enough intestinal lactase to break down the lactose in their diet. The undigested lactose can cause symptoms such as gas, abdominal pain, diarrhea, and poor weight gain. Table 7 outlines the foods that are permitted and those that should be avoided while following the lactose-free diet.

Table 7 Lactose-Free Diet

Foods Allowed	Foods to Avoid
Milk: none	All milk, milk drinks—including whole, skim, low-fat, dried, evaporated, and condensed milk, breast milk; yogurt (any type, cream or sour)
Soy protein infant formulas	Infant formulas other than those permitted, frappes, ice cream sodas
Fortified soy or rice milk	An enzymatic preparation such as LactAid may be added to milk to convert lactose into digestible sugars; instructions are for conversion of 70 to 95% of the lactose to glucose and galactose; check with your nutritionist or physician before beginning use of LactAid
Eggs: as desired	Eggs prepared with milk—use specific formula; do not prepare with butter
Meats: any except those to be avoided	Creamed or breaded meat, fish, or poultry; prepared meats that contain dried milk solids including bologna and cold cuts, frankfurt, salami, commercially prepared fish sticks, and some sausage; kosher products are milk free
Beverages: powdered, fruit-flavored drinks, ginger ale, tonics	Any made with milk, such as frappes, eggnog, hot chocolate
Cheese: soy or lactose-free cheeses	All types of cheeses and cheese dishes that are not listed as allowed
Breads: breads made without milk, such as French bread, Italian bread, water bagels, or parve breads	Any baked products made with milk; muffins, biscuits, waffles, pancakes, donuts, sweet rolls, commercial mixes
Cereal: any made without milk, cooked or ready to eat. Macaroni, spaghetti, pasta, rice—all prepared without milk	Any prepared cereal that contains dry milk solids
Vegetables and potatoes: all cooked, canned, frozen, or fresh	Any vegetable prepared with milk, butter, milk solids, bread, or bread crumbs; no cheese or cream sauces
Fruit: all	
Desserts: any made without milk or milk products, such as gelatin desserts, fruit crisp, snow puddings, fruit and water sherbets, pie with fruit filling, angel food cake	All commercial cake and cookie mixes, ice cream, custard puddings, junket, ice milk or sherbets that contain milk; frosting made with milk or butter, dessert sauces, cheese cakes
Soup: any prepared without milk or milk products; homemade or canned (eg, chicken rice)	All creamed soups, chowders; no cheese
Fats: milk-free margarine or parve margarine; oils, nuts, peanut butter	Butter, margarine, some commercial salad dressings
Sugar and seasonings: sugar, honey, molasses, maple syrup, corn syrup, jelly and jam, hard candy, gum drops, marshmallow, hard peppermints, fondant; salt, pepper, spices, herbs, condiments, vinegar, ketchup, relish, pickles, olives, tomato sauce, coconut, wheat germ; artificial flavoring or extracts	Any product made from milk, butter, cream, chocolate, toffee, cream mints, caramel candy, candy with cream centers
Miscellaneous	Medications that use lactose as filler or bulk agents; party dips, nonprescription vitamins; spice blends; Easter egg dyes; dietetic foods and foods advertised as high protein sometimes contain lactose or dry milk solids

Adapted from reference 8.

Noteworthy Points

This diet is not intended for those who are sensitive to cow's milk protein. Read labels carefully. Avoid any food containing milk, nonfat milk solids, skim milk, butter, cream, lactose, casein, caseinate, sodium caseinate, or whey.

Calcium Supplements

If a nutritionally complete lactose-free infant formula, enteral product, or nutritional supplement is taken, this diet can be sufficient in all nutrients. If a lactose-free fortified milk substitute is not consumed, the diet could be deficient in calcium, phosphorus, and vitamin D. If a milk-free diet is followed for more than 4 to 6 weeks, calcium and other vitamin or mineral supplementation might be needed. Choose a supplement that is complete, well absorbed, and cost efficient. Calcium supplements are available in several acceptable forms: carbonate, gluconate, lactate, and citrate. Avoid dolomite or bonemeal supplements because they have been linked with lead poisoning.

Low-Lactose Diet Guidelines

These guidelines are intended for individuals who can tolerate small amounts of lactose or those who are reintroducing lactose after following the lactose-free diet. Note that a lactose containing diet is not appropriate for persons with galactosemia.

Some foods that contain lactose might be better tolerated than others owing to natural processing. Examples are naturally aged cheeses and yogurt with live cultures.

After a period of lactose-free intake, the reintroduction of lactose into the diet should be gradual, based on individual tolerance. Better tolerance might be achieved by consuming lactose-containing foods in small amounts. There are products available that are designed to aid in the digestion of lactose. Lactase enzymes are commercially available as chewable tablets and drops. Refer to Table 7 for further information about lactose-containing foods.

GROWTH FAILURE

Growth failure and failure to thrive are terms that describe the condition of infants, children, and young adults whose physical growth deviates significantly from standards or falters from their individual growth pattern. Growth failure can be a result of a variety of factors, including medical, social, and psychological conditions. In most cases, these factors create an environment in which caloric intake is inadequate to meet requirements for normal growth and development (see Chapter 43, "Failure to Thrive: Malnutrition in the Pediatric Outpatient Setting," for more details).

- Nutritional management is the cornerstone of therapy for individuals afflicted with growth failure. Therapy should aim to reverse nutrient deficits, achieve ideal body weight for height, and restore optimal body composition. Diets rich in calories and adequate in protein facilitate reversal of growth failure and failure to thrive. The following section provides guidelines for increasing the caloric content of the diet and outlines sample foods and meal plans designed to promote a high-calorie intake with adequate protein.

HIGH-CALORIE DIET

The high-calorie diet is indicated for promoting weight gain or preventing excessive weight loss during periods of increased nutritional needs (eg, infectious or postoperative states). A well-balanced diet based on the Food Guide Pyramid with an emphasis on foods that are high in protein and calories should be followed.

Suggestions for Increasing Calories and Nutrient Density Milk and Milk Products

- Use high-calorie milk (recipe follows) or half-and-half cream as a beverage and as a substitute for milk or water in cooking whenever possible (pudding, cocoa, milkshakes, cream soup, custard, eggnog).
- Add powdered milk to yogurt, casseroles, bread, muffins, sauces, and gravies.
- Melt cheese on sandwiches, meats, potatoes, vegetables, rice, pasta, and cream sauces; add cheese to salads.
- Have cream cheese or cottage cheese on crackers or added to vegetables or pasta.
- Make Instant Breakfast with whole or high-calorie milk.
- Add whole-milk yogurt to fruit or desserts and use as a topping for cereal, pancakes, and waffles.

Protein Group

- Add small pieces of cooked meat, fish, poultry, or eggs to salads, casseroles, soups, vegetables, omelets, and noodles.
- Use peanut butter (or other nut butter) with all grain products, spread on fruit or vegetables, or blended in milk drinks, ice cream, or yogurt.
- Add nuts to desserts, salads, ice cream, vegetables, or fruits (nuts are not recommended for children under three years of age).
- Add textured vegetable protein or legumes to casseroles or soups.
- Offer simple fried foods such as chicken or fish.
- Serve meat with extra gravy or sauce when appropriate.

Fruits and Vegetables

- Add mashed fruit to milk, yogurt, shakes, ice cream, and pudding.
- Add dried fruits to muffins, cookies, cereal, and grains or combine with vegetables and nuts (children under 3 years of age can be at increased risk for choking with dried fruits and nuts).
- Serve vegetables raw with a dip, cooked cream style, or topped with melted cheese.
- Add butter, sour cream, or mayonnaise to vegetables.

Grains

- Make hot cereals with milk instead of water.
- Use high-protein noodles and grains in casseroles and soups.
- Coat meat with breading or flour before cooking.
- Top muffins, toast, crackers, and pancakes with margarine, cream cheese, syrup, jam, peanut butter, cheese, or honey (honey is not recommended for children under 1 year of age).
- Serve granola over ice cream, frozen yogurt, or fruit or mixed with nuts or dried fruit.

Tips for Increasing Caloric Intake

- Eat small, frequent meals throughout the day.
- Keep snacks handy for nibbling.
- Try eating a snack or drinking a high-calorie beverage before going to bed in addition to other meals.
- Instead of drinking water, select beverages that contain calories, such as high-calorie milk or frappes (see recipes).
- Notice the times of day that appetite is best and eat more at those times.

Sample Meal Plan

The following daily food plan is one example of a high-calorie diet:

Breakfast

Half cup citrus juice

One protein serving (eg, one egg, one-fourth cup cottage cheese, two tbsp peanut butter, 1 oz cheese, or 1 oz meat)

Two servings of whole-grain bread products or enriched cereal margarine, butter, jam, jelly, sugar

One cup high-calorie milk (recipe follows)

Morning Snack

Frappe (recipe follows)

Lunch

Three to four ounces of protein

Half cup vegetable

Two servings whole grain, potato, rice, or other starch

One serving fruit or dessert

Butter, margarine, jelly, sugar

One cup high-calorie milk

Afternoon Snack

Frappe or high-calorie milk

Peanut butter or cheese with crackers or as a sandwich

Dinner

Three to four ounces of protein

Two servings vegetable (one deep-green or yellow vegetable)

Two servings whole grain, potato, rice, or other starch

One serving fruit or dessert

Margarine, butter, jelly, sugar

One cup high-calorie milk

Evening Snack

Frappe or high-calorie milk

Pizza, grilled cheese sandwich, or pudding

Recipes

The following recipes are revised from those developed by clinical nutrition staff at Children's Hospital Boston.

Fortified Milk (180 to 210 cal)

Add two to four tbsp of powdered nonfat dry milk to 8 oz of whole milk

Vanilla Shake/Frappe (400 cal)

Five and half cups ice cream (three to four scoops)

Half cup whole milk

Three tbsp nonfat milk powder (Can also add two tbsp of strawberry, chocolate, or coffee syrup)

Mix in blender

Strawberry Shake/Frappe (530 cal/8 oz)

Two cups whole milk

Two-third cup nonfat dry milk powder or one pkg of Carnation Instant Breakfast

Ten and a half cups strawberry ice cream

Two tbsp heavy cream

Mix in blender

Creamsicle Shake/Frappe (560 cal)

Half cup whole milk

Two tbsp instant nonfat dry milk powder

Half cup orange juice

One cup orange sherbet

One pkg of vanilla Instant Breakfast

Mix in blender

Peanut Butter Shake/Frappe (400 cal)

One cup whole milk

Three tbsp smooth peanut butter

Three tbsp chocolate syrup

Mix in blender

Banana Orange Shake/Frappe (690 to 790 cal)

Half cup milk

Half cup orange juice

One cup vanilla ice cream

Two whole bananas

Mix in blender

Super Pudding (326 cal)

One cup fortified milk

One cup heavy cream

One pkg (20.5 oz) instant pudding

Make into half cup servings.

Super Grilled Cheese

Dip cheese sandwich into egg fortified milk mixture before grilling with lots of butter or margarine. This will be like French toast with cheese in the middle.

CONGENITAL HEART DISEASE AND HYPERLIPIDEMIA

Pediatric patients with congenital heart disease or hyperlipidemia require careful nutritional monitoring to ensure optimal growth and development. Growth failure in congenital heart disease is common and can be attributable to anorexia, hypermetabolism, frequent respiratory infections, decreased peripheral blood flow, malabsorption, or pulmonary hypertension, among other factors.[9,10] Patients requiring dietary fat restriction because of hyperlipidemia are placed at greater risk for caloric deficits, as well as deficits in calcium and iron. Nutrition education with frequent monitoring is necessary to prevent these deficiencies.

- Fluid-restricted and sodium-restricted diets are often used in the management of congenital heart disease.

Table 8 Sodium-Restricted Diet

Type of Food	Allowed	Avoid
Meat, fish, fowl, and cheese	Fresh or frozen beef, lamb, pork, rabbit, veal, chicken, turkey, liver; fresh fish except shellfish, canned salt-free tuna; salt-free cottage cheese; eggs (one per day); salt-free peanut butter	Smoked, processed, or canned meat or fish; frankfurters, ham, sausage, pepperoni, Spam, bacon, luncheon meat, salt-free chipped or corned beef, salted kosher meats, salt pork, smoked tongue, canned tuna or salmon, caviar, salted and dried cod, herring, frozen fish fillets; frozen meat pies, frozen entrees; shellfish: clams, crabs, lobsters, oysters, scallops, shrimp; egg substitutes; cheese (unless low sodium); peanut butter (unless low sodium); anchovies
Breads and cereals	Low-sodium breads, cereals, and cereal products; breads and mixes; rolls made without salt; quick breads made with sodium-free baking powder or potassium bicarbonate and without salt; the following cooked cereals without added salt: pearl barley, cracked wheat, plain farina, Ralston, maltex rolled oats, pettijohns, wheatena, rice; dry cereals: puffed rice, puffed wheat, shredded wheat; macaroni, spaghetti, noodles (cooked without added salt); salt-free melba toast, salt-free venus wafers, low-sodium crackers, plain, unsalted matzo, yeast waffles	Breads and rolls made with salt or commercial mixes; quick breads (pancakes, waffles, cakes, pastries, muffins) made from baking powder, baking soda, salt, monosodium glutamate or commercial mixes; quick cooking and enriched cereals that contain a sodium compound (read label); dry cereals (except those allowed); crackers (except low sodium); "self-rising" flour or cornmeal
Fruits and juices	All fresh; frozen, canned, or dried to which salt, sodium benzoate, or sodium sulfite has not been added; read labels	Regular tomato and vegetable juices, maraschino cherries; any fruit or fruit product that contains salt or sodium benzoates, sodium-preserved dried fruits
Vegetables	Fresh, frozen, or dietetic canned without salt: asparagus, green beans, dried lima beans, dried navy beans, brussels sprouts, cabbage, cauliflower, corn, cowpeas, cucumbers, parsley, parsnips, peas (fresh), peppers, potatoes, sweet potatoes, pumpkin, radishes, rutabaga, soybeans, squash (winter, summer), tomatoes, turnip greens	All regular canned vegetables; beets, beet greens, carrots, celery, dandelion greens, hominy, kale, mustard greens, pickles, sauerkraut, spinach, white turnips, frozen peas or lima beans if processed with salt; commercially seasoned frozen vegetables, frozen mixed vegetables
Desserts	Fruit and fruit juices as allowed above; gelatin (made with plain, unflavored gelatin, sugar, fruit and fruit juices); homemade cornstarch, rice, or tapioca pudding made from part of milk allowance or low-sodium milk; ice cream; candy, cake, cookies, pastry: homemade, salt free, or special low sodium	Commercial candies, cakes, cookies, or homemade unless prepared with allowed ingredients; packaged pudding, Jello or other commercial sweetened gelatin desserts
Fat	Lard, vegetable oil, shortening, salt-free butter or margarine, unsalted nuts	Salted butter or margarine, bacon fat, salt pork, commercial mayonnaise or other salad dressing (except low sodium), salted nuts, olives
Sugar and sweets	Sugar, honey, syrups, jams, marmalades, and jellies that contain no preservatives	Molasses, commercial jams containing sodium benzoate or other sodium preservatives (read labels)
Beverages	Fruit juices, lemonade, milk (regular or low sodium as allowed), coffee, tea, Postum, Hershey's cocoa (made with allowed milk or water)	Fountain beverages, "Dutch process" cocoa, instant cocoa mixes, powdered milk, prepared beverages, mixes including fruit-flavored powders, mineral waters, buttermilk
Seasonings and condiments	All spices, extracts, herbs, except those with sodium as an ingredient; lemon juice, vinegar, salt substitute (with doctor's approval), low-sodium bouillon cube	Salt; celery salt, seeds, and flakes; onion salt, garlic salt, prepared mustard, ketchup, horseradish prepared with salt, barbecue sauce, chili sauce; meat extracts, gravies, and tenderizers; monosodium glutamate (Accent), soy sauce, Worcestershire sauce, saccharin and other sugar substitutes containing salt, regular bouillon cubes, olives, relishes, pickles. Avoid all foods with above seasonings added
Miscellaneous		Canned, dehydrated, or frozen potato; spaghetti, macaroni, or noodle products; preprepared gravies; canned or dehydrated soups, except low sodium; salted popcorn, potato chips, pretzels, and other snack items such as corn chips or Doritos; party spreads and dips; regular baking powder, baking soda (sodium bicarbonate), rennet tablets, laxatives, Chinese/Asian food, Italian food, fast foods, bread stuffing

FLUID-RESTRICTED DIET

The fluid-restricted diet is a modification of the normal diet in which all fluids are limited to a prescribed level. Individuals with renal, liver, or cardiac insufficiency might require it.

Noteworthy Points

- All foods contain water in varying amounts. All foods that are liquid at room temperature are considered to be fluids. These include water, tonic, coffee, tea, fruit and vegetable juices, milk, ice, ice cream, sherbet, Popsicles, fruit ices, gelatins, soups, gravies, sauces, cream, and alcohol.
- Fluid from solid foods is not routinely restricted in a fluid-restricted diet. Solid foods with the highest water content are fruits and vegetables. Excessive consumption of these foods should be avoided.
- Liquid medications and fluids consumed while ingesting medications must be accounted for in the fluid-restricted diet.
- The following measurements are useful in calculating daily fluid allowance:
  - 1 oz = 30 cc = two tbsp
  - 4 oz = 120 cc = half cup
  - 8 oz = 240 cc = one cup
  - 32 oz = 960 cc = four cups = 1 quart
  - 1 L = 1,000 cc = 1 kg

SODIUM-RESTRICTED DIET

The sodium-restricted diet is a modification of the normal diet in which the sodium content is limited to a prescribed level. Many people consume much more than the recommended amount (adequate intake) of sodium. Conditions that might require sodium restriction include hypertension, congestive heart failure, liver disease, renal disease, and corticosteroid therapy. If a strict sodium restriction is necessary, see Table 8 for lists of foods allowed and to avoid. For children, a no added salt diet might be a sufficient restriction.

Suggestions for Limiting Sodium Intake

- Do not use salt in cooking and do not add salt to food at the table. Do not put the saltshaker on the table.
- Read labels carefully on all canned, frozen, and packaged foods. Avoid products with added sodium or salt. Ingredients are listed on the package by weight, from the largest amount to the smallest.
- Use low-sodium or sodium-free canned soups, broth, potato chips, crackers, and nuts.
- Try spices and flavorings such as herbs, onion powder, thyme, or lemon juice to add flavor to foods.
- Limit fast foods and restaurant foods that are high in sodium. Most restaurant meals can be made without added salt or salt-containing ingredients such as monosodium glutamate or soy sauce.
- Evaluate medications for sodium content because some medicines contain sodium. Examples are laxatives (Ex-Lax), antacids (Maalox), and some pain relievers, such as acetaminophen (Tylenol).

Table 9 AHA Diet Recommendations for Lowering Cardiovascular Disease Risk

Nutrient	Recommended Intake
Total fat	25 to 35% of total calories
Saturated fat	<7% of energy
Trans fat	1% of energy
Cholesterol	<300 mg/d
Sodium	<2.3 g/d
Fiber	Minimum 14 g/1,000 kcal

Adapted from references 11 and 12.

LOW-CHOLESTEROL AND LOW-SATURATED FAT DIET

Cardiovascular disease is associated with a variety of risk factors, including hypercholesterolemia. Blood cholesterol levels can be reduced by as much as 10 to 15% by lowering cholesterol and saturated fat consumption. Exercise, in conjunction with dietary modifications, should be encouraged as this can aid in lowering cholesterol, as well as in weight management.

- Low-cholesterol and low-saturated fat diets are used for the management of hypercholesterolemia. The American Heart Association released new dietary guidelines in June 2006 which replaced the Step One and Step Two diets.[11] These new guidelines emphasize the crucial relationship between nutrition and exercise in the prevention and treatment of cardiovascular disease, and encourage a further reduction in saturated and *trans* fatty acid intakes. These dietary recommendations are only for children 2 years of age and older because of the rate of central nervous system development at an earlier age. An earlier report discusses specific recommendations for children less than 2 years of age.[12] Because of the potential risk of insufficient caloric intake, careful monitoring is necessary to ensure normal growth and development in all children on these diets. Table 9 provides target nutrient intake levels to optimize cardiovascular health and promote optimal growth. Table 10 discusses dietary guidelines for hyperlipidemia.

Definition of Dietary Fats

There are four types of fat in the food we eat: saturated fat, polyunsaturated fat, monounsaturated fat, and *trans* fat. Saturated fats are believed to increase blood cholesterol, so the amount of saturated fat in the diet should be limited. Saturated fat is usually solid at room temperature. Examples are butter, shortening, meat fats (suet, lard, salt pork, bacon fat), chicken fat, coconut oil, palm oil, and hydrogenated oils. The fat in whole milk, cheese, yogurt, and cream is also saturated.

- Polyunsaturated fats lower total blood cholesterol, that is, both low-density lipoprotein (LDL) and high-density lipoprotein (HDL) cholesterol. Polyunsaturated fat is liquid at room temperature. Examples are corn, safflower, sunflower, soybean, cottonseed, walnut, and sesame oils, as well as fish, which contains omega-3 polyunsaturated fats. Monounsaturated fat lowers serum LDL while maintaining HDL levels. Examples are olive, canola, and peanut oils, as well as some other nut oils. *Trans* fats are formed when liquid oils are hydrogenated into a solid form. They are found in margarine, cookies, crackers, pastries, baked goods, and many other processed foods and snack foods. Evidence suggests that *trans* fats raise LDL and lower HDL levels. The *trans* fat content of all processed foods is mandatory on US food labels as of January 1, 2006.

Suggestions for Lowering Cholesterol and Saturated Fat Intake

- Limit red meat to a maximum of two or three servings (2 to 3 oz per serving) per week. Use only lean cuts of meat. Cut away any visible fat from meat before cooking.
- Bake, broil, boil, or stir-fry meats, fish, or poultry. Remove skin from poultry.
- Use nonstick fry pans or nonstick spray coatings.
- Eat no more than three or four egg yolks per week. Substitute two egg whites for a whole egg in recipes. Use egg whites to batter meats and vegetables, coat with crumbs moistened with acceptable oil, and then bake. Use low-cholesterol commercial egg substitutes in place of whole eggs.
- Read labels of commercially prepared products and avoid those containing ingredients not allowed.
- Limit all fats and oils to reduce total fat intake.
- Avoid fast foods that could be high in fat (eg, fried chicken, french fries).
- Increase fish intake, especially oily fish, to two servings per week.
- Try some meatless dishes, such as pasta with tomato sauce or vegetarian stir-fry dishes.
- Use high-protein vegetables such as legumes (kidney, red, or pinto beans) and fat-free dairy products to supply protein.
- Limit high-calorie sauces such as cream, cheese, and Alfredo sauce.
- Achieve 60 minutes of moderate to vigorous play or exercise every day.
- Choose whole grains and cereals rather than refined grains.
- Eat skim or low-fat dairy products daily.

To reduce high triglyceride levels, take the following steps to decrease simple carbohydrate intake (if LDL is also high, it will be necessary to also reduce saturated fat intake):

- Avoid sweetened drinks such as soda, fruit juices, and coffee beverages; replace with water, skim or 1% milk, or smoothies made with fat- and sugar-free yogurt and fresh fruit.

Table 10 Diet for Hyperlipidemia

Food Group	Choose	Decrease
Fats and oils	Unsaturated oils—safflower, sunflower, corn, soybean, cotton seed, canola, olive, peanut	Coconut oil, palm kernel oil, palm oil
	Margarine made from unsaturated oils listed above; light or diet margarine	Butter, lard, shortening, bacon fat
	Salad dressings made with unsaturated oils listed above; low fat or oil free	Dressings made with egg yolk, cheese, sour cream, whole milk
	Seeds and nuts—peanut butter, other nut butters	Coconut
	Cocoa powder	Chocolate
Breads and cereals	Breads—whole-grain bread, hamburger and hot dog bun, corn tortilla	Bread in which eggs are a major ingredient, croissants
	Cereals—oat, wheat, corn, multigrain	Granola made with coconut
	Pasta	Egg noodles and pasta containing egg yolk
	Rice	
	Dry beans and peas	
	Crackers—low-fat animal type, graham, saltine type	High-fat crackers
	Homemade baked goods using unsaturated oil, skim or 1% milk, and egg substitute— quick breads, biscuits, cornbread muffins, bran muffins, pancakes, waffles	Commercial baked pastries, muffins, biscuits
Soup	Chicken or beef noodle, minestrone, tomato, vegetarian, potato	Soup containing whole milk, cream, meat fat, poultry skin
Vegetables	Fresh, frozen, or canned	Vegetables prepared with butter, cheese, or cream sauce
Fruits	Fruit—fresh, frozen, canned, or dried	Fried fruit or fruit served with butter or cream sauce
	Fruit juice—fresh, frozen, or canned	
Sweets and modified fat desserts	Beverages—fruit-flavored drinks, lemonade, fruit punch	
	Sweets—sugar, syrup, honey, jam, preserves, candy made without fat (candy corn, gumdrops, hard candy), fruit-flavored gelatin	Candy made with chocolate, coconut oil, palm kernel oil, palm oil
	Frozen desserts—sherbet, sorbet, fruit ice, popsicles	Ice cream and frozen treats made with ice cream
	Cookies, cake, pie, pudding—prepared with egg whites, egg substitute, skim or 1% milk, and unsaturated oil or margarine; gingersnaps; fig bar cookies, angel food cake	Commercial baked pies, cakes, donuts, high-fat cookies, cream pies
Meat, poultry, and fish	Beef, pork, lamb—lean cuts well trimmed before cooking	Beef, pork, lamb—regular ground beef, fatty cuts, spare ribs, organ meats, sausage, regular luncheon meats, wieners, bacon
	Poultry without skin	Poultry with skin, fried chicken
	Fish, shellfish	Fried fish, fried shellfish
	Processed meat—prepared from lean meat (eg, turkey ham, tuna wieners)	Regular luncheon meat (eg, bologna, salami, sausage, wieners)
Eggs	Egg whites (two whites equal one whole egg in recipes), cholesterol-free egg substitute	Egg yolks; includes egg used in cooking
Dairy products	Milk—skim or 1% fat (fluid, powdered, evaporated), buttermilk	Whole milk (fluid, evaporated, condensed), 2% low-fat milk, imitation milk
	Yogurt—nonfat or low-fat yogurt or yogurt beverages	Whole-milk yogurt, whole-milk yogurt beverages
	Cheese—low-fat natural or processed cheese (part-skim mozzarella, ricotta)	Regular cheeses (American, blue, Brie, cheddar, Colby, Edam, Monterey Jack, whole-milk mozzarella, Parmesan, Swiss), cream cheese, Neufchatel cheese
	Cottage cheese-low fat, nonfat, or dry curd (0 to 2% fat)	Cottage cheese (4% fat)
	Frozen dairy dessert—ice milk, frozen yogurt (low fat or nonfat)	Ice cream, cream, half and half, whipping cream, nondairy creamer, whipped topping, sour cream

- Avoid large or frequent servings of sugary foods such as cookies, candy, ice cream, fruit rollups, and regular chewing gum.

To determine how many calories come from fat in a particular product, using the information on the food label, divide the calories coming from fat by the total calories and then multiply by 100. This equals the percentage of calories from fat. If the percentage from fat is less than 30%, the product is appropriate; if it is more than 30%, the product is too high in fat. The goal is to balance any high-fat food with low-fat foods so that at the end of the day, total fat intake is 25 to 35% of calories.

Determining Percentage of Calories From Fat: An Example

Product: Cheez-it

Serving size: 12 crackers (nutrition information is per serving)

Calories: 70; calories from fat: 36

Protein: 2 g

Carbohydrates: 7 g

Fat: 4 g (total fat per serving)

Polyunsaturated fat: less than 1 g

Saturated fat: 1 mg

Cholesterol: less than 2 mg

Sodium: 135 mg

Ingredients: enriched flour, riboflavin, vegetable shortening (contains one or more of the following: partially hydrogenated oils: soybean, cottonseed, canola), skim milk, cheese, salt, paprika, yeast, paprika extractives (vegetable color). (Ingredients are listed in descending order, with the largest amount first.)

- Thirty-six calories from fat divided by 70 cal per serving = 0.51 × 100 = 51; therefore, 51% of calories are from fat. This product is high in fat.

INBORN ERRORS OF METABOLISM

Medical nutritional therapy plays a key role in the management of several metabolic disorders, including those related to carbohydrate, fatty acid, and amino acid metabolism.[13] Dietary alterations are often necessary in reestablishing a balance in metabolic function through provision of deficient products and restriction of toxic substrates. In addition, nutritional management is important in stabilizing altered protein enzymes, replacing cofactors that might be deficient, and supplying products that are deficient owing to an inhibited secondary pathway.

Several formulas currently available for the management of metabolic disorders are age and diagnosis specific (see Appendix III, "Enteral Products"). Frequent monitoring is imperative to ensure optimal growth and neurologic development in these medically complex patients.

Appendix III, "Enteral Products" provides an extensive list of known metabolic disorders and their suggested dietary modifications, including appropriate enteral formulas.

MINERAL-RICH DIETS

A number of acute and chronic pediatric medical conditions might require mineral supplementation, either in the diet or by therapeutic measures during their course. Included in this list is cow's milk protein allergy, lactose intolerance, hypercholesterolemia, renal disease, and celiac disease. Some diets chosen for personal reasons, such as the vegan or lacto-ovo-vegetarian diets, can be inadequate in certain micronutrients.

- Included in this section are lists of food sources high in calcium and iron, the minerals most commonly found to be deficient in the pediatric population. It is recommended that any child on a special diet be assessed for micro- and macronutrient intake periodically to ensure an optimal intake for growth and development.

CALCIUM-RICH DIET

A calcium-rich diet is recommended for all individuals as part of a healthful, well-balanced diet. In particular, growing children have high dietary requirements for calcium. Consuming calcium-rich foods daily will help minimize resorption of calcium from the bones and thus promote dense, strong bones.

Milk and dairy products are the primary source of calcium in the North American diet; the other food groups—breads, meats, fruits, and vegetables (include calcium-fortified juices)—provide the remainder (see Appendix II "Nutritional Requirements," for Dietary Reference Intakes and Table 11 for calcium food sources).

Calcium Information

- Dietary Reference Intakes, National Academy Press: www.nap.edu.
- Pennington JAT. Bowes and Church's Food Values of Portions Commonly Used, 17th edition. Philadelphia: Lippincott-Raven Publishers; 1997.
- National Dairy Council: www.nationaldairycouncil.org.

IRON-RICH DIET

The iron-rich diet might be indicated for individuals with anemia. Anemia can occur as a result of dietary deficiencies, blood loss, or inadequate absorption of iron.

The body more readily absorbs iron from animal sources (heme iron) than from vegetable sources (nonheme iron). Consuming foods high in vitamin C at the same meal can enhance the absorp-

Table 11 Calcium Food Sources

Food Group	Calcium/ Serving (mg)	Food Group	Calcium/ Serving (mg)
Milk and dairy		English muffin	105
Milks, 1 cup	300	Waffles (7")	179
Buttermilk	285	Wonder calcium rich bread (white/whole wheat), 1 slice	290
Chocolate	280	Wonder light calcium enriched bread, 2 slices	290
Malted	347	Vegetables/legumes (1/2 cup cooked)	
Whole	291	Beet greens	82
1% low fat	300	Bokchoy	79
2% low fat	297	Broccoli	89
Skim	302	Butternut squash	42
Soy Plus-West Soy (soy milk)	300	Cabbage	79
Cheeses	77 to 337	Carrots	35
American, pasteurized process, 1 oz	174	Collards	74
Blue, 1 oz	150	Kale	90
Brick, 1 oz	191	Lima beans	35
Caraway, 1 oz	191	Mustard greens	38
Cheddar, 1 oz	191	Okra	50
Cheese food		Pumpkin	31
American, pasteurized process, 1 oz	163	Stewed tomatoes	42
Swiss, pasteurized process, 1 oz	205	Spinach	61
Colby, 1 oz	194	Sweet potatoes	38
Cottage, 2% low fat, 1/2 cup	77	Tomato soup	80
Edam, 1 oz	207	Tomato soup, with milk (1 cup)	159
Monterey, 1 oz	212	Turnip greens	99
Mozzarella, part skim, 1 oz	207	Fruits/juices	
Whole, 1 oz	147	Rhubarb, 1/2 cup	174
Muenster, 1 oz	203	Dried figs, 1/2 cup	144
Ricotta, part skim, 1/2 cup	337	Orange	92
Whole, 1/2 cup	257	Orange juice (calcium fortified) 8 oz	300
Swiss, 1 oz	272	Dates, dried cut, 1/2 cup	53
Frozen desserts, 1/2 cup	88 to 104	Prunes, dried, (4)	49
Ice cream, 1/2 cup	88	Hawaiian Punch (calcium fortified), 8 oz	150
Ice milk, hardened, 1/2 cup	88	Cereal (1 cup)	
Ice milk, soft serve, 1/2 cup	88	Total	282
Sherbet, 1 cup	51	Total raisin bran	200
Frozen yogurt, 1/2 cup nonfat	104	Total corn flakes	200
Yogurt low fat, 1 cup	345 to 415	Basic four	200
Flavored	389	100% Natural	181
Fruit	345	Oatmeal	170
Plain	415	Life	154
Pudding, 1/2 cup	150	Other	
Protein		Molasses blackstrap, 1 tbsp	137
Beans, dried, cooked, 1 cup	90	Carnation breakfast bar, 1 each	500
Clams, 4 oz	100	Combination and fast foods	
Crab, 3 oz	132	Pizza Hut supreme personal pan pizza	520
Cod, 3 oz	136	Lasagna (2½" × 2½")	460
Halibut, 3 oz	191	Macaroni and cheese, homemade (1 cup)	362
Oysters, raw, 1/2 cup	113	Enchilada, cheese (1 enchilada)	324
Perch, 3 oz	117	McDonald's Big Mac (1 sandwich)	256
Salmon, with bones, 3 oz	167	McDonald's Egg McMuffin (1 sandwich)	256
Sardines, with bones, 3 oz	371	Wendy's broccoli and cheese potato (1)	250
Shrimp, canned, 3 oz	98	Chef's salad, without dressing (1½ cups)	235
Tofu, piece, 1/2 cup	434	Quiche (1/8 pie)	224
Trout, 1 serving	210	McDonald's Filet-o-Fish (1 sandwich)	165
Nuts/legumes (1/2 cup)		Cheeseburger, regular (1 sandwich)	182
Almonds	188	Pizza, meat and veg., thin crust (1/4 of 12")	166
Beans, dried, cooked	45	Burger King's Croissan'wich (1 sandwich)	136
Brazil nuts	123	Spaghetti with meat balls (1 cup)	124
Garbanzo beans	150	Submarine sandwich (3 to 4" sub)	95
Hummus	66	Taco Bell's taco (1 taco)	84
Lima beans	35	Dairy Queen's hot dog (1 sandwich)	80
Peanuts	77		
Pistachio	86		
Pork and beans	67		
Refried beans	58		
Soybeans	130		
Walnuts	55		
Grain foods			
Pancakes 1, (2–3")	150		

Table 12 Iron Food Sources

Food	Approximate Measure	Iron (mg)
High-iron sources		
Cream of wheat (quick or instant)*	1/2 cup	7.8
Heart, beef†	2 oz	3.7
Kidney, beef†	2 oz	5.3
Kidney, lamb†	2 oz	6.1
Kidney, pork†	2 oz	5.3
Liver, beef†	2 oz	5.8
Liver, calf†	2 oz	9.0
Liver, chicken†	2 oz	6.0
Liver, lamb†	2 oz	10.9
Liver, pork†	2 oz	15.6
Liverwurst†	2 oz	3.6
Prune juice	1/2 cup	5.1
Moderate-iron sources		
All-bran cereal	1/2 cup	2.9
Almonds, dried unblanched	1/2 cup	3.0
Dried beans and peas		
Baked beans, no pork	1⁄4 cup	1.5
Blackeye peas, cooked	1⁄4 cup	0.8
Broad beans, dry	1⁄4 cup	3.6
Chick peas, dry	1⁄4 cup	3.5
Cow peas, cooked	1⁄4 cup	0.8
Great northern beans, cooked	1⁄4 cup	1.3
Green peas, cooked	1⁄4 cup	1.4
Lentils, dry	1⁄4 cup	3.4
Lima beans, cooked	1⁄4 cup	1.3
Mung beans, dry	1⁄4 cup	3.6
Navy beans, cooked	1⁄4 cup	1.3
Red beans, dry	1⁄4 cup	3.5
Soybeans, cooked	1⁄4 cup	1.4
White beans, dry	1⁄4 cup	3.9
Beef, cooked	2 oz	2 to 3‡
Clams	3 medium	2.1
Ham, cooked	2 oz	1.3
Heart, pork, cooked	2 oz	1.8
Lamb, cooked	2 oz	1.9
Mackerel, canned	1/2 cup	1.0
Malt-o-meal, cooked	1/2 cup	1.4
Oysters	3 to 4 medium	2.8
Peaches, dried	1⁄4 cup	2.4
Peanuts, roasted without skins	3½ oz	3.2
Pork, cooked	2 oz	2 to 3§
Prunes, dried	2 large	1.1
Sardines	8 medium	3.5
Scallops	2 oz	1.6
Turkey, cooked	2 oz	1.7
Veal, cooked	2 oz	2.0
Venison, cooked	2 oz	2.0
Wheat germ	1 oz (3 tbsp)	2.6
Contributing iron sources		
Apricots, dried	4 large halves	1.4
Breads, white enriched	1 slice	.6
Bread, whole wheat	1 slice	.5
Chard	1⁄2 cup	1.5
Chicken	2 oz	1.0
Dandelion greens	1⁄4 cup	0.9
Dates, dried	1⁄4 cup	1.3
Egg, large	1	1.2
Heart, chicken	9 to 10 medium	1.7
Kale	1⁄4 cup	.6
Mustard greens	1⁄4 cup	.9
Macaroni, enriched	1/2 cup	.6
Noodles, enriched	1/2 cup	.7
Peanut butter	2 tbsp	.6
Raisins, dried seedless	1/4 cup	1.25
Rice, long grain or instant	1/2 cup	.6
Salmon, canned	2 oz	.7
Shrimp, raw	2 oz	.9
Spaghetti	1/2 cup	.8
Spinach	1⁄4 cup	1.3
Strawberries, raw cleaned	1 cup	1.5
Tomato juice, canned	1/2 cup	1.05
Tuna, canned	2 oz	1.1
Turnip greens	1⁄4 cup	0.8
Waffle, enriched	5½" diameter	1.3
Approximate iron content of children's favorite foods		
Hamburger, small	1	3.0
Hamburger, large	1	5.2
Big Mac	1	4.3
Quarter pounder	1	5.1
Spaghetti with meatballs	1 cup	3.3
Frankfurters and beans	1 cup	4.8
Pork and beans	1 cup	5.9
Raisins‖	5/8 cup	3.5
Cereals, fortified	1 serving	4.5 to 17.8
Nuts‖	1 cup	5.0 to 7.0
Seeds, sunflower‖	3½ oz	7.1
Chile con carne	1 cup	3.6
Beef burrito	1 medium	4.6
Beef tostado	1 medium	3.4
Cheese pizza	2 slices	3.0
Cheese pizza with beef	2 slices	4.8

*Or other fortified cereals that contain 10 mg of iron per ounce or 100% recommended dietary allowance per serving.

†As organ meats are generally high in cholesterol, these iron-rich foods should be eaten in moderation.

‡Depending on cut. The greatest amounts of iron are generally found in the chuck, flank, and bottom round cuts of beef.

§Depending on cut. The greatest amounts of iron are generally found in the loin, sirloin, tenderloin, and picnic shoulder cuts of pork.

‖Raisins, nuts, and seeds are not generally recommended for children under age 3 because of the risk of choking.

tion of nonheme iron. Vitamin C-rich foods include citrus fruits and juices, cantaloupe, strawberries, tomatoes, and dark-green vegetables (see Appendix II, "Nutritional Requirements," for dietary reference intakes). Table 12 lists iron food sources.

WEIGHT CONTROL

The National Center for Health Statistics reports that the prevalence of overweight in children and adolescents is on the rise and has nearly tripled since the 1970s.[14]

Being overweight is considered to be the result of an imbalance of energy intake and energy expenditure. Many factors can influence the upward trend in the prevalence of overweight in children, such as alterations in nutrient intake, changes in physical activity patterns, television viewing habits, level of nutritional knowledge, genetics, and parental influence (see Chapter 38, "Energy and Substrate Regulation in Obesity," for more information).

- Successful weight reduction and control incorporates a combination of caloric reduction, behavior modification, and exercise. Below are guidelines for healthful eating and weight reduction and control in children.

GOAL 1: PLAN ALL MEALS AND SNACKS

- Preplan menus to avoid impulse food choices.
- Do not skip meals; try to eat at the same times each day. Three meals and two or three snacks are sometimes better than only three large meals. There might be a greater risk of eating fattening snack foods when you are very hungry.
- Keep a box of low-calorie foods ready for between-meal snacks (eg, a variety of raw vegetable strips, rice cakes, popcorn, pretzels, fresh fruit).

- When away from home, take food along or know where appropriate foods can be purchased.
- Help make the shopping list and plan for low-calorie selections.
- Read food labels to limit products that list fats or sugars as main ingredients.
- Avoid fried foods (such as french fries and fried chicken), creamed products, and gravies.
- Avoid empty calories (foods such as chips, cakes, cookies, pies, pastry, regular soda, candy, jellies, and syrups) because these foods have very few nutrients and are high in fat or sugar calories or both.
- Preportion food for meals and snacks. Never eat food directly from the serving container or bag; this makes it too easy to overeat.

GOAL 2: EAT A WELL-BALANCED DIET

Eat a variety of foods from the Food Guide Pyramid to meet nutritional needs. The recommended number of servings and serving sizes for the various food groups are listed below:

- **Milk group:** Skim or 99% fat-free milk; nonfat yogurt (some yogurts contain large amounts of added sugar; compare labels); low-fat cheeses (less than 3 g fat per serving). Recommended number of servings: ages 2 to 8: 2 cups/d. age >8: 3 cups/d.
- **Meat group:** Lean cuts with little fat marbling; trim all fat from meat; remove skin of poultry; choose fish canned in water instead of oil; avoid processed deli meats, bacon, and sausage. Recommended number of servings: 5 oz/d.
- **Breads and cereals group:** Choose whole-grain or enriched products and plain cereals (not presweetened). Recommended number of servings: 6 oz/d.
- **Fruit and vegetables group:** Choose whole fruits that are fresh or canned in water and frozen fruits without added sugar. Choose unsweetened juice and limit to 4 oz (half cup) per day. Choose vegetables that are fresh, canned, or frozen and serve without butter, cheese, or sauces. Recommended number of servings: 4 cups/d.

GOAL 3: PREPARE FOODS THE LOW-CALORIE WAY

- Bake, broil, steam, roast, grill, or stir-fry foods.
- Spray pans with fat-free coating instead of using oil when frying.
- Do not add extra fat (eg, butter, margarine, oil, bacon, gravy) when cooking or for serving. Use herbs and spices to season foods instead of fats. Low-calorie butter substitutes (eg, Butter Buds) can provide the flavor of butter without the fat.
- Trim skin and visible fat off meats.
- Choose fat-free mayonnaise and fat-free salad dressings.
- Skim fat from homemade soups, stews, and gravies (refrigerate or freeze the product until the fat hardens and then spoon it off).
- Use skim milk in place of whole milk or cream when preparing soups, puddings, and home-baked products.

GOAL 4: AVOID EXCESS SUGAR

- Sugar and sugary foods provide many calories and very little nutrition and can cause tooth decay.
- Large amounts of sugar are contained in desserts such as cakes and cookies, as well as in soft drinks and candies.
- Sugar can be "hidden" in foods under such names as corn syrup, honey, fructose, and glucose. Read the label. If a sugar is listed as one of the first three ingredients on a food label, the product is probably very high in sugar.
- Beverages can be a major contributor of sugar and extra calories. Choose sugar-free sodas and sugar-free packaged drink mixes or water. Limit juice intake because even naturally sweetened products contain calories.
- It is not necessary to buy dietetic foods. Products marked "dietetic," "lite," or "light" are not necessarily low in calories. When a treat is desired, choose a lower calorie item such as Popsicles, Italian ice, Fudgsicles, angel food cake, fat-free frozen yogurt, or sugar-free pudding.

GOAL 5: EXERCISE

Activity is an important part of most successful weight control programs. Regular exercise will help burn extra calories all of the time, not just while exercising. Exercise also helps to strengthen the heart and tone muscles. Aim for at least 60 minutes of physical activity (including exercise or active play) most days of the week.[12] A 150-pound person will burn calories as listed in 30 minutes of continuous activity:

- Brisk walking, 93
- Dancing, 126
- Playing baseball, 141
- Cycling, 150 to 360
- Swimming, 180
- Playing basketball, 180 to 270
- Playing soccer, 270
- Running, 300 to 450
- Skipping rope, 300 to 450
- Walking up stairs, 300 to 540

GOAL 6: EAT OUT INTELLIGENTLY

- Limit restaurant and fast-food eating because such foods are generally high in fat and calories.
- Plan food selections to avoid meats and vegetables that have been fried (eg, select baked or broiled chicken in place of fried chicken).
- Choose a baked potato instead of fries.
- Order pizza without sausage, pepperoni, or extra cheese.
- When eating at fast-food restaurants, take advantage of salads, lean hamburgers, and fresh fruit cups.
- When selecting prepared-to-order foods, ask that the food be prepared with as little fat as possible.
- Avoid vegetables, meats, and starches that are topped with cheese, cream sauces, gravy, butter, or margarine.
- Because restaurant portions are often large, plan to take home some of your food.
- Ask for the salad dressing to be served on the side or request a low-calorie topping. If possible, eat salad without any dressing at all.
- Always ask for water with meals. Request low-fat or skim milk or sugar-free beverages.
- Plan ahead for school lunches. Review the menu and take lunch from home when the school lunch is high in fat or sugar.
- Order sandwiches without mayonnaise, special sauce, or extra cheese. Use mustard or fat-free spreads.

GOAL 7: MAKE POSITIVE CHANGES

- Maintain a positive attitude.
- When family members or friends are eating tempting foods, choose a low-calorie food (such as a sugar-free ice cream bar) or noncaloric beverage.
- Slow down the pace of eating to a minimum of 20 minutes per meal. This will allow the feeling of fullness to set in and help you enjoy the flavor of the food. If hunger persists after a meal, wait 20 minutes; if you are still hungry, choose low-calorie items such as plain vegetables or fresh fruit. Try to avoid second helpings of meats, desserts, and other high-calorie foods.
- Eat foods high in fiber, such as fresh fruits, vegetables, and whole grains, because they increase the feeling of fullness.
- Keep a food diary. Record everything eaten in order to become more aware of what and how much is actually eaten.
- Realize that change takes time. Select a few areas to work on and focus just on those until they have been mastered. Then add a few more areas needing change.
- If you eat too much of something, do not give up. Think about the positive changes that have been made and just get back on track.
- Measure weight only every 1 to 2 weeks to monitor progress. Do not get frustrated if sometimes results are not seen. A successful weight control program takes time, and a change in behavior is more important than any one weight measurement.
- Note that if a child has not attained adult height, significant weight loss could interfere with growth. Therefore, a dietitian might advise that weight maintenance rather than weight loss should be the goal while continuing to grow taller. The dietitian and physician

will help to determine weight goals. If a child is on a weight loss program, a 1- to 2-lb weight decrease per week is usually appropriate.

VEGETARIANISM

A vegetarian is typically defined as a person who avoids the consumption of animal flesh, such as meat, poultry, and fish.[15] Dairy products and eggs might be included or avoided. When all dairy and egg sources are avoided, the diet is referred to as a vegan diet. A vegetarian diet can offer health advantages as a result of its high fiber and low saturated fat content. The American Dietetic Association's position statement on vegetarian diets indicates that appropriately planned vegan and lacto-ovovegetarian diets can meet the nutrient needs of infants, children, and adolescents and can promote normal growth.

- Dietary deficiencies, however, are possible with overly restrictive diets. All children following a vegan diet should have a reliable source of vitamin B_{12} and vitamin D (ie, they should receive a vitamin supplement). In addition, emphasis should be placed on the intake of foods rich in calcium, iron, and zinc. Children following a vegetarian diet might need to eat foods higher in fat to meet energy needs for appropriate growth and development.

VEGETARIAN GROUPS AND RESOURCES

Vegetarian Resource Group, PO Box 1463, Baltimore, MD 21203; telephone: 410-366-8343; www.vrg.org

American Dietetic Association. Position statement on vegetarian diets. J Am Diet Assoc 1997;97:1317-21.

Katzen M. The New Enchanted Broccoli Forest. Berkeley, CA: Ten Speed Press; 2000.

Katzen M. New Moosewood Cookbook. Berkeley, CA: Ten Speed Press; 2000.

Lappe FM. Diet for a Small Planet. 20th anniversary edition. New York: Ballantine Books; 1991.

Robertson L, Flinders C, Ruppenthal B. The New Laurel's Kitchen: A Handbook for Vegetarian Cookery and Nutrition. Berkley, CA: Ten Speed Press; 1986.

Vegetarian Times, PO Box 420235, Palm Coast, FL 32142-0235; telephone: 877-717-8923; www.vegetariantimes.com

WEB SITES FOR GENERAL INFORMATION

American Acadamy of Pediatrics: www.aap.org

American Dietetic Association: www.eatright.org

American Heart Association: www.americanheart.org

National Acadamy Press Dietary Reference Intakes: www.nap.edu

United States Department of Agriculture Food and Nutrition Information Center: www.usda.gov

REFERENCES

1. American Academy of Pediatrics. Soy protein-based formulas: Recommendations for use in infant feeding (RE9806). Policy statement of the American Academy of Pediatrics. Pediatrics 1998;101:148–53.
2. Burks AW, Sampson HA. Diagnostic approaches to the patient with suspected food allergies. J Pediatr 1992;121: S64–71.
3. American Academy of Pediatrics. Hypoallergenic infant formulas (RE0005). Policy statement of the American Academy of Pediatrics. Pediatrics 2000;106:346–9.
4. US Food and Drug Administration. Questions and answers regarding food allergens, including the Food Allergen Labeling and Consumer Protection Act of 2004, edition 3; 2006. Available at: http://www.cfsan.fda.gov/~dms/alrguid.html. Accessed September 20, 2006.
5. The Food Allergy and Anaphylaxis Network. Tips for managing a peanut allergy. Available at http://www.foodallergy.org/allergens/peanut.html. Accessed August 16, 2007.
6. DiSanto C, Duggan C. Gastrointestinal diseases. In: Hendricks KM, Duggan C, editors. Manual of Pediatric Nutrition, 4th edition. Hamilton, ON: BC Decker; 2005.
7. Hartsook EI. Gluten-Restricted, Gliadin-Free Diet Instruction. Seattle, WA: Clinical Research Center, University of Washington Hospital; 1987.
8. Stoker TW. Common nutrition problems in pediatrics. In: Hendricks KM, Walker WA, editors. Manual of Pediatric Nutrition, 2nd edition. Toronto: BC Decker Inc; 1990.
9. Cameron JW, Rosenthal A, Olson AD. Malnutrition in hospitalized children with congenital heart disease. Arch Pediatr Adolesc Med 1995;149:1098–20.
10. Salzer HR, Haschke F, Wimmer M, et al. Growth and nutritional intake of infants with congenital heart disease. Pediatr Cardiol 1989;10:17–23.
11. Lichtenstein AH, Appel LJ, Brands M, et al. Diet and lifestyle recommendations revision 2006: A scientific statement from the American Heart Association nutrition committee. Circulation 2006;114:82–96.
12. Gidding SS, Dennison BA, Birch LL, et al. Dietary recommendations for children and adolescents: A guide for practitioners: Consensus statement from the American Heart Association, endorsed by the American Academy of Pediatrics. Circulation 2005;112:2061–75.
13. Acosta PB, Yanicelli S. The Ross Metabolic Formula System Nutrition Support Protocols, 4th edition. Columbus, OH: Abbott Laboratories; 2001.
14. Centers for Disease Control and Prevention, National Center for Health Statistics, US Department of Health and Human Services. 2006. Available at: www.cdc.gov/nchs. Accessed November 26, 2006.
15. American Dietetic Association. Vegetarian diets. Position of the American Dietetic Association. J Am Diet Assoc 1997;97:1317–21.

Appendix I

Nutritional Assessment

Melanie V. Connolly, MSc, RD, LDN, CNSD

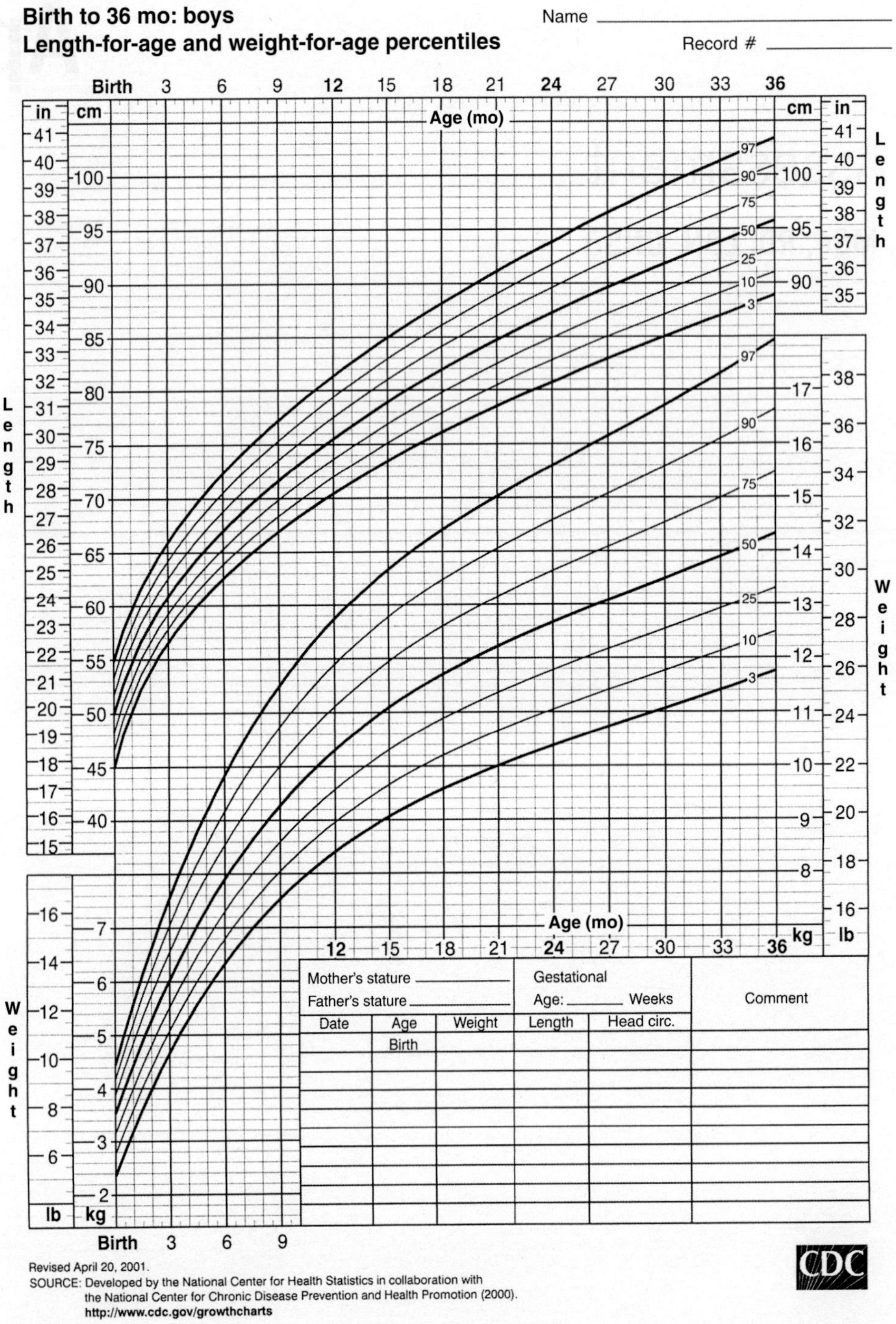

Figure I-1 Birth to 36 months: boys, length-for-age and weight-for-age percentiles. Developed by the National Center for Health Statistics in collaboration with the National Center for Chronic Disease Prevention and Health Promotion (2000). (http://www.cdc.gov/growthcharts)

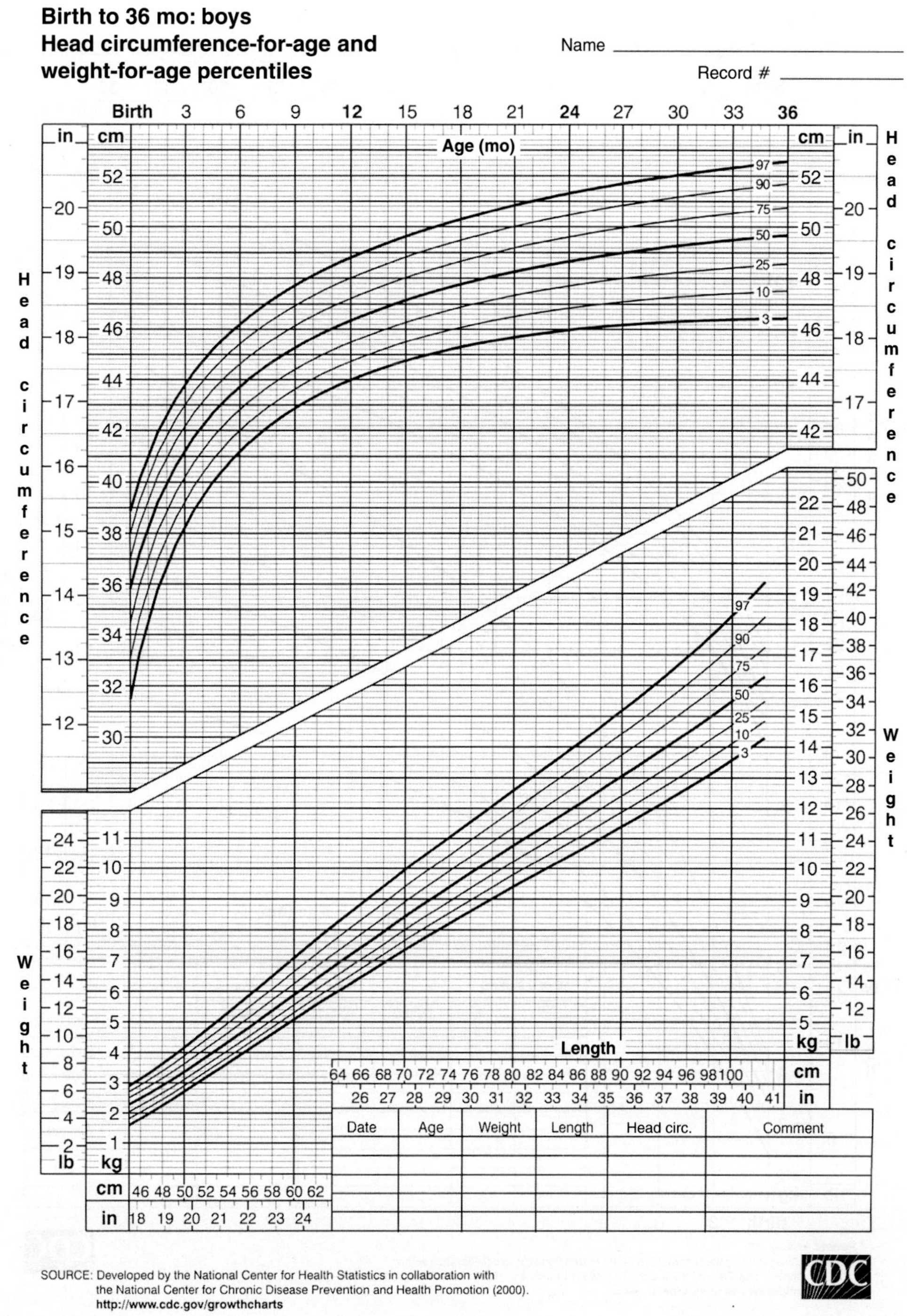

Figure I-2 Birth to 36 months: boys, head circumference-for-age and weight-for-length percentiles. Developed by the National Center for Health Statistics in collaboration with the National Center for Chronic Disease Prevention and Health Promotion (2000). (http://www.cdc.gov/growthcharts)

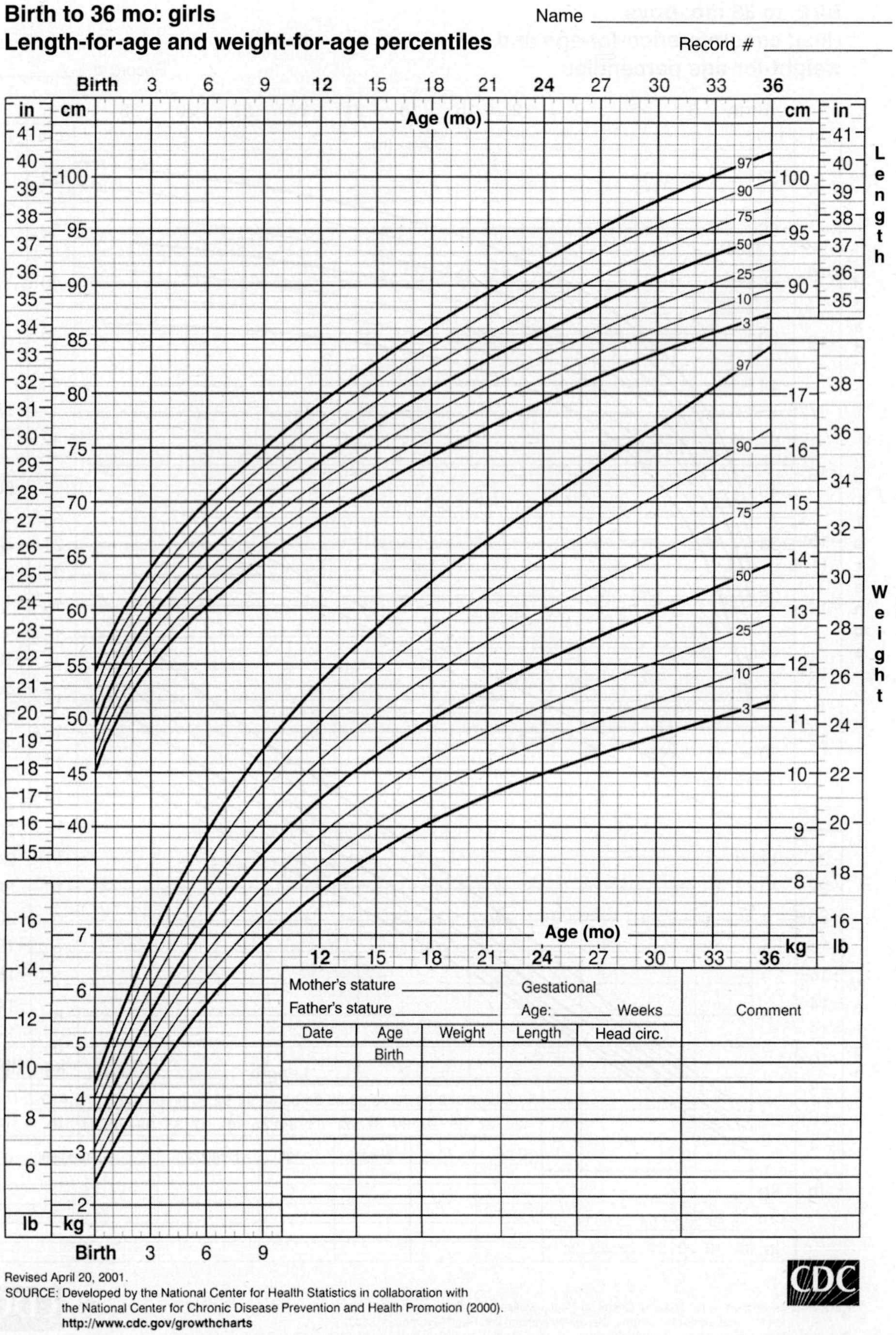

Figure I-3 Birth to 36 months: girls, length-for-age and weight-for-age percentiles. Developed by the National Center for Health Statistics in collaboration with the National Center for Chronic Disease Prevention and Health Promotion (2000). (http://www.cdc.gov/growthcharts)

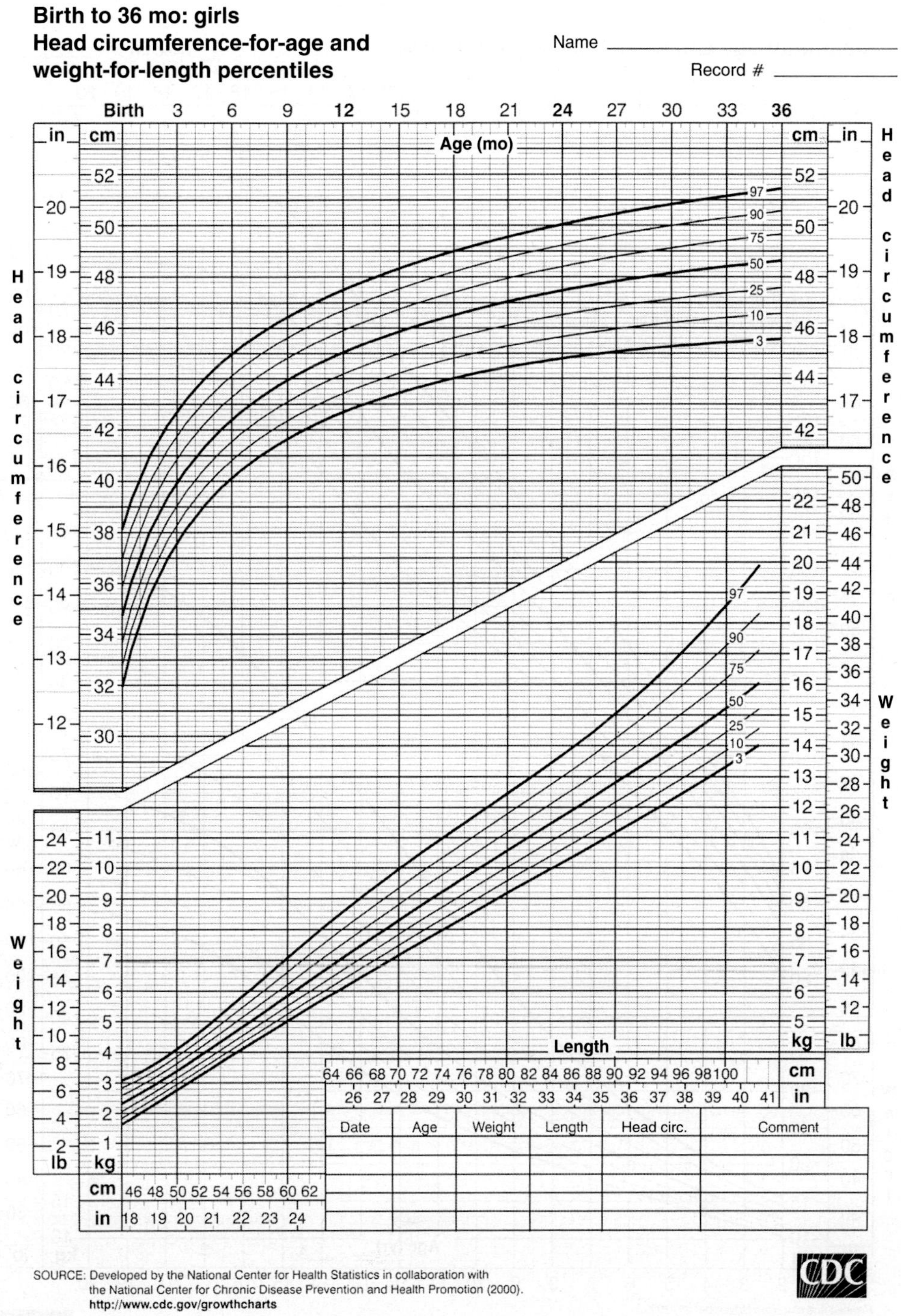

Figure I-4 Birth to 36 months: girls, head circumference-for-age and weight-for-length percentiles. Developed by the National Center for Health Statistics in collaboration with the National Center for Chronic Disease Prevention and Health Promotion (2000). (http://www.cdc.gov/growthcharts)

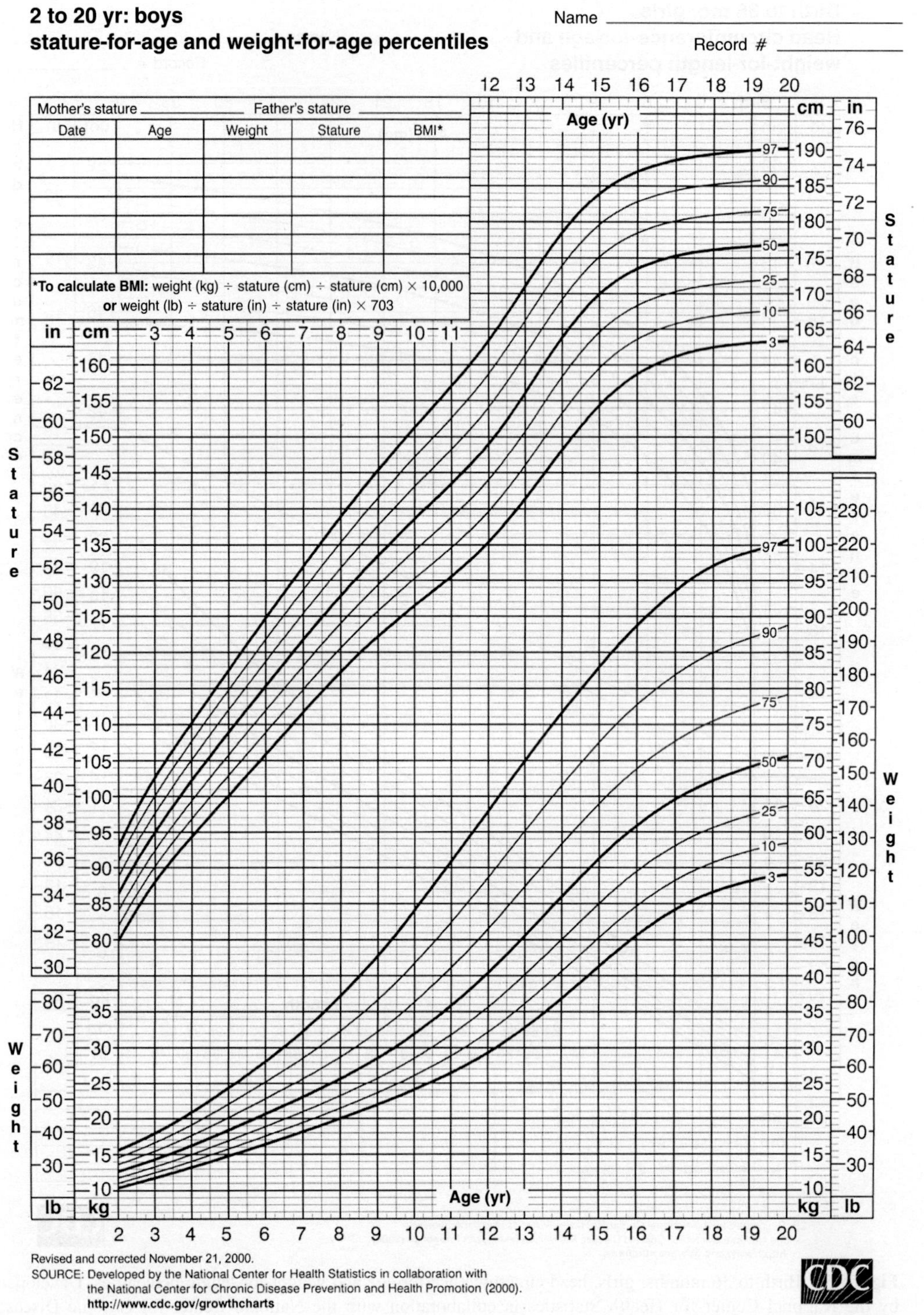

Figure I-5 Two to 20 years: boys, stature-for-age and weight-for-age percentiles. Developed by the National Center for Health Statistics in collaboration with the National Center for Chronic Disease Prevention and Health Promotion (2000).

Name ____________________

Weight-for-stature percentiles: boys

Record # ____________

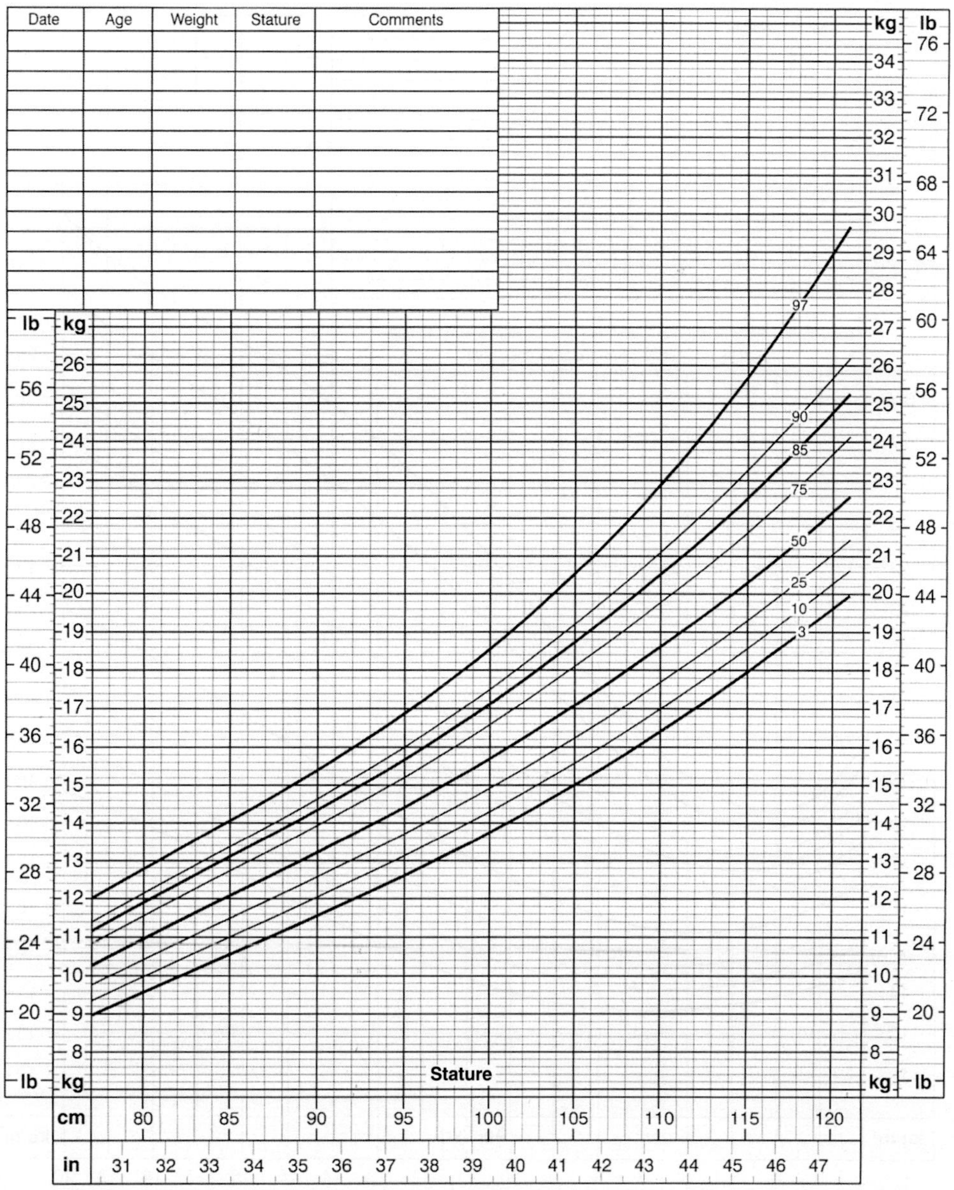

SOURCE: Developed by the National Center for Health Statistics in collaboration with the National Center for Chronic Disease Prevention and Health Promotion (2000).
http://www.cdc.gov/growthcharts

Figure I-6 Boys, weight-for-stature percentiles. Developed by the National Center for Health Statistics in collaboration with the National Center for Chronic Disease Prevention and Health Promotion (2000).

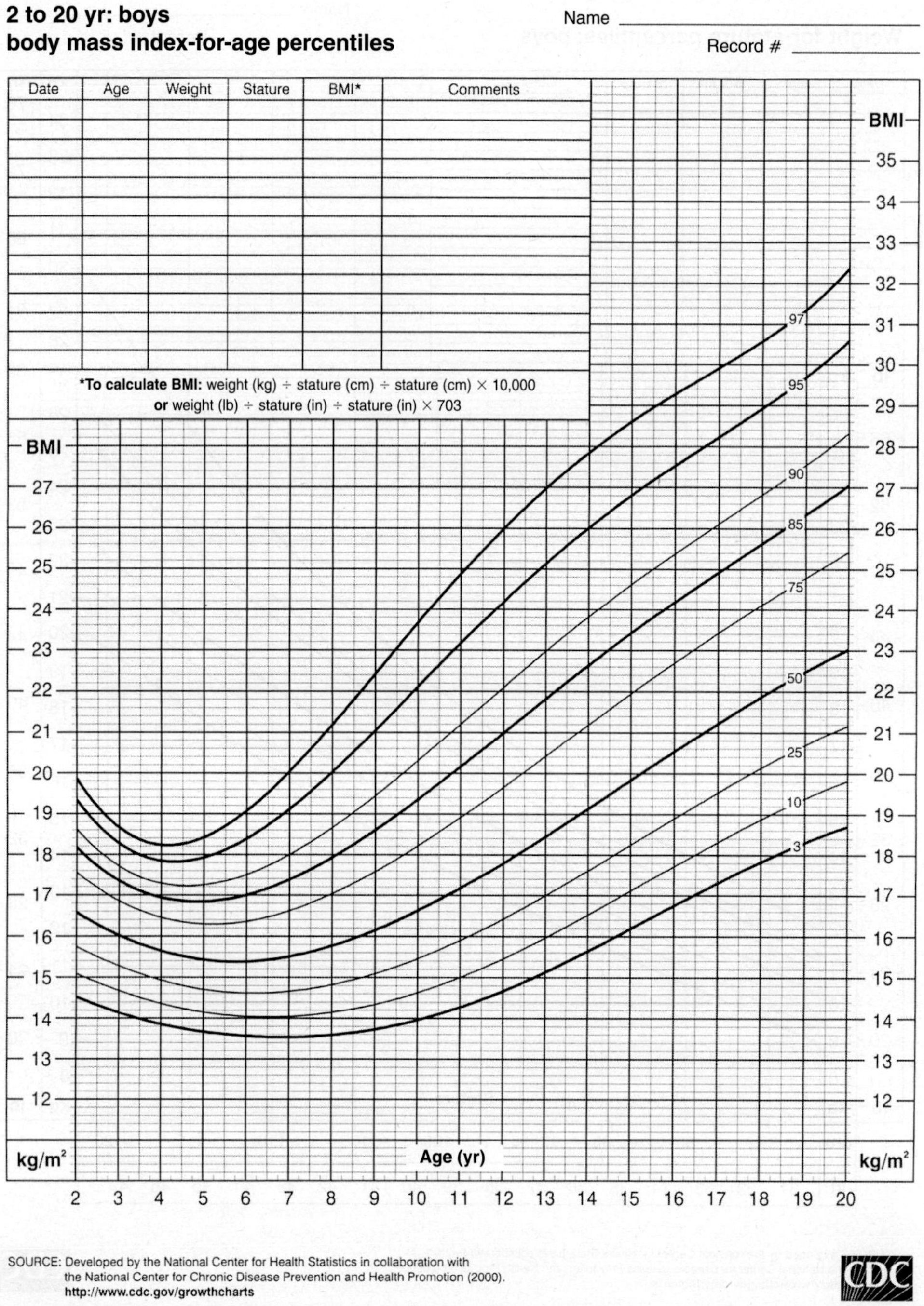

Figure I-7 Two to 20 years: boys, body mass index-for-age percentiles. Developed by the National Center for Health Statistics in collaboration with the National Center for Chronic Disease Prevention and Health Promotion (2000).

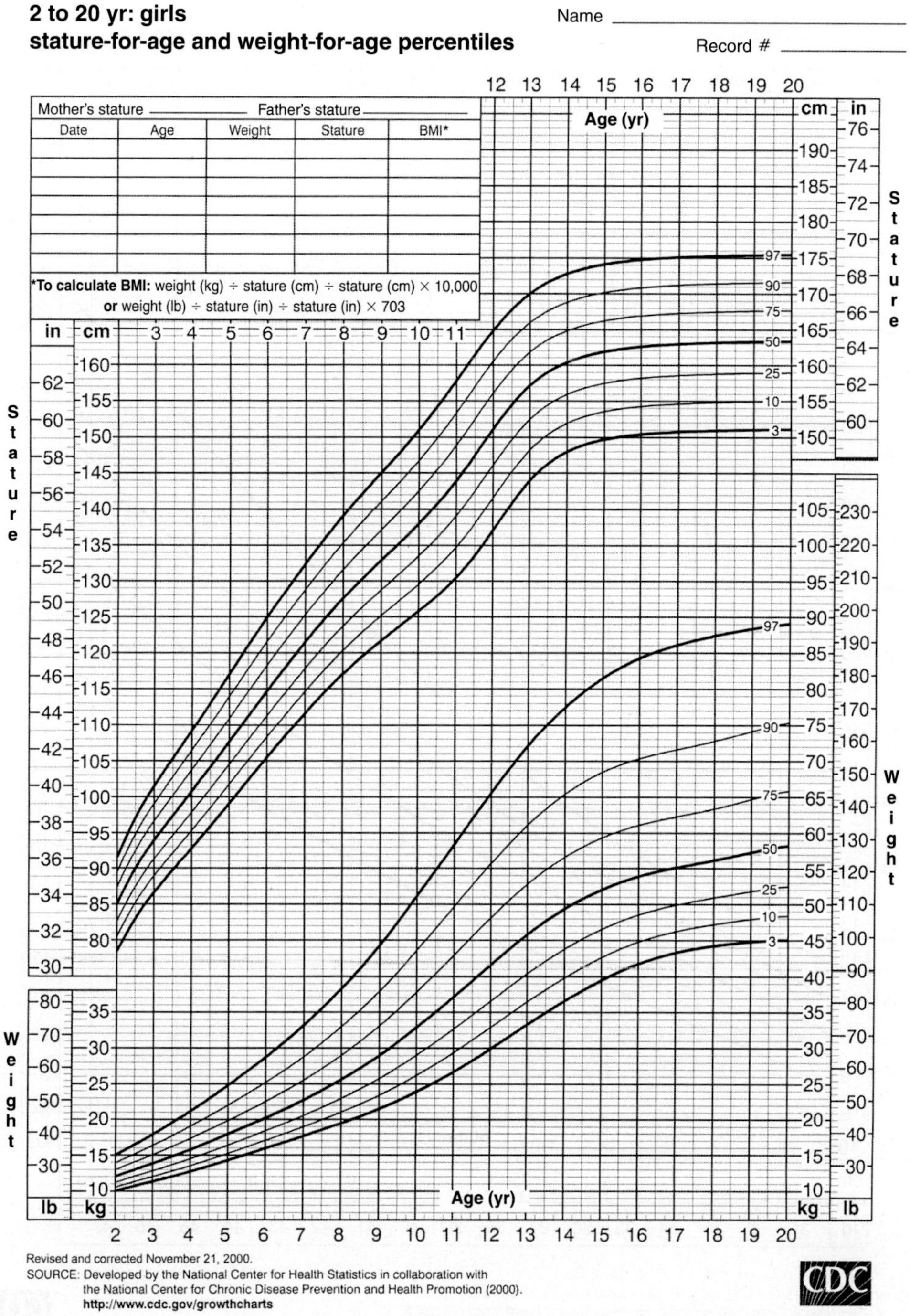

Figure I-8 Two to 20 years: girls, stature-for-age and weight-for-age percentiles. Developed by the National Center for Health Statistics in collaboration with the National Center for Chronic Disease Prevention and Health Promotion (2000).

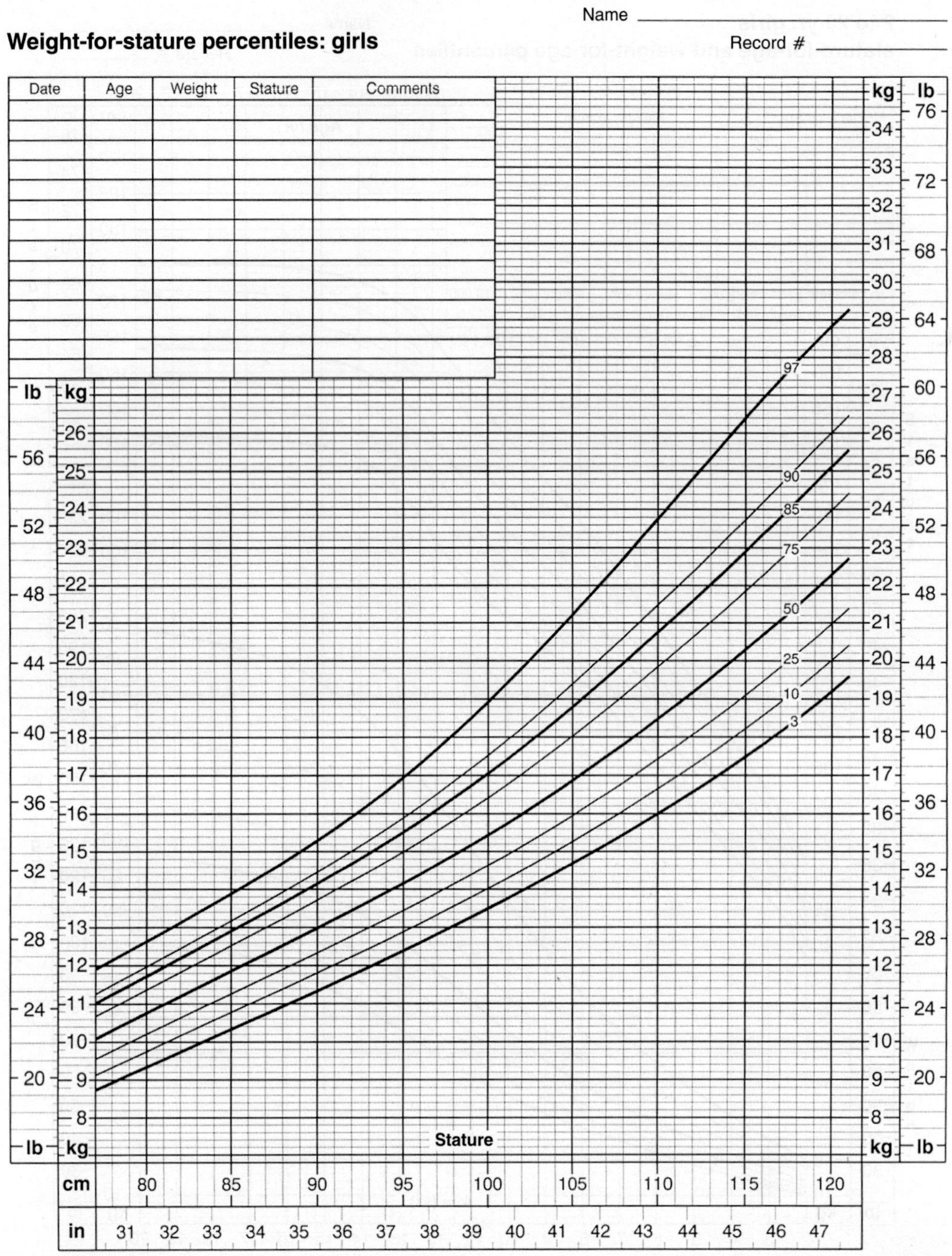

SOURCE: Developed by the National Center for Health Statistics in collaboration with
the National Center for Chronic Disease Prevention and Health Promotion (2000).
http://www.cdc.gov/growthcharts

Figure I-9 Girls: weight-for-stature percentiles. Developed by the National Center for Health Statistics in collaboration with the National Center for Chronic Disease Prevention and Health Promotion (2000).

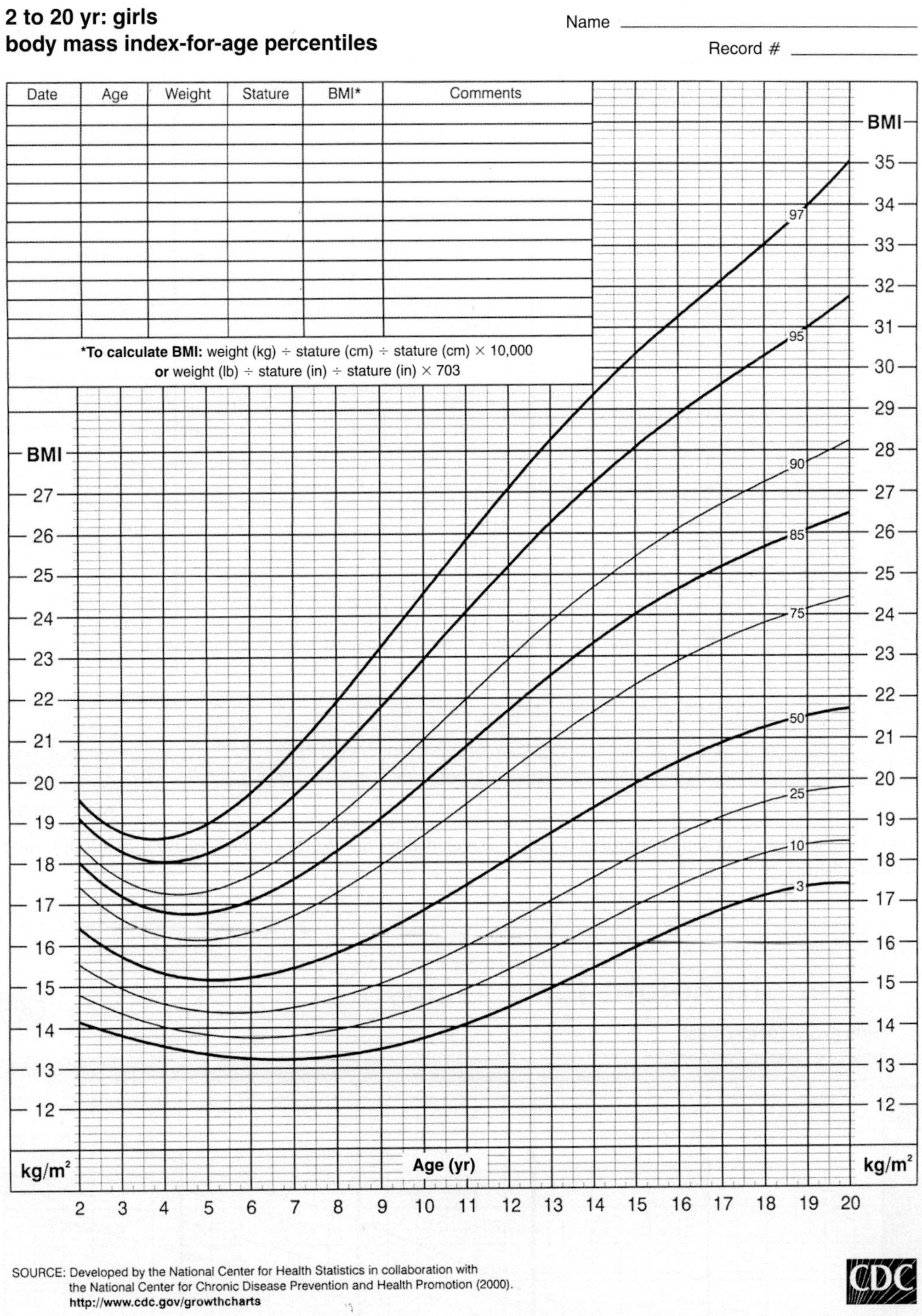

Figure I-10 Two to 20 years: girls, body mass index-for-age percentiles. Developed by the National Center for Health Statistics in collaboration with the National Center for Chronic Disease Prevention and Health Promotion (2000).

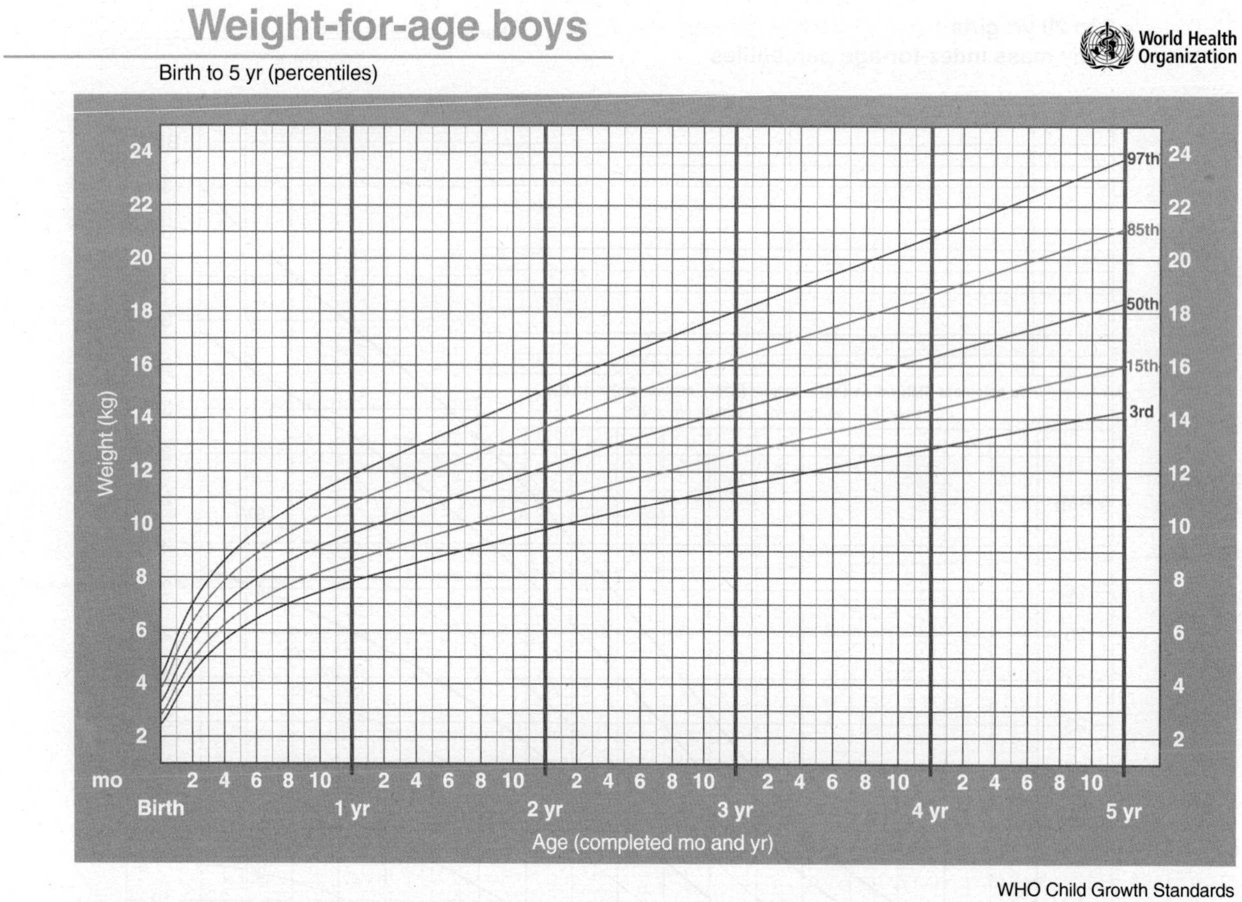

Figure I-11 Boys, weight-for-age percentiles (birth to 5 years). Developed by the World Health Organization (2006). (http://www.who.int/childgrowth/standards/en/)

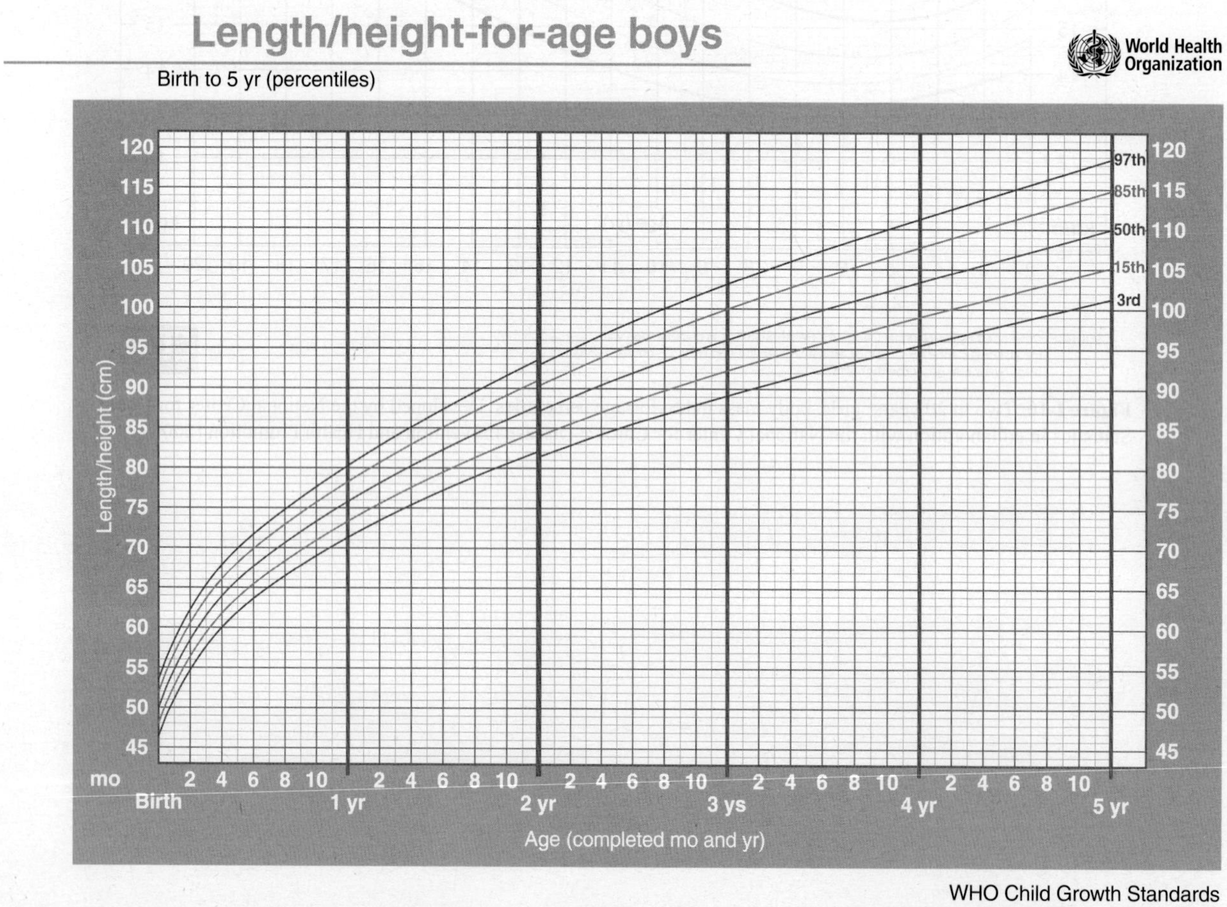

Figure I-12 Boys, length/height-for-age percentiles (birth to 5 years). Developed by the World Health Organization (2006). (http://www.who.int/childgrowth/standards/en/)

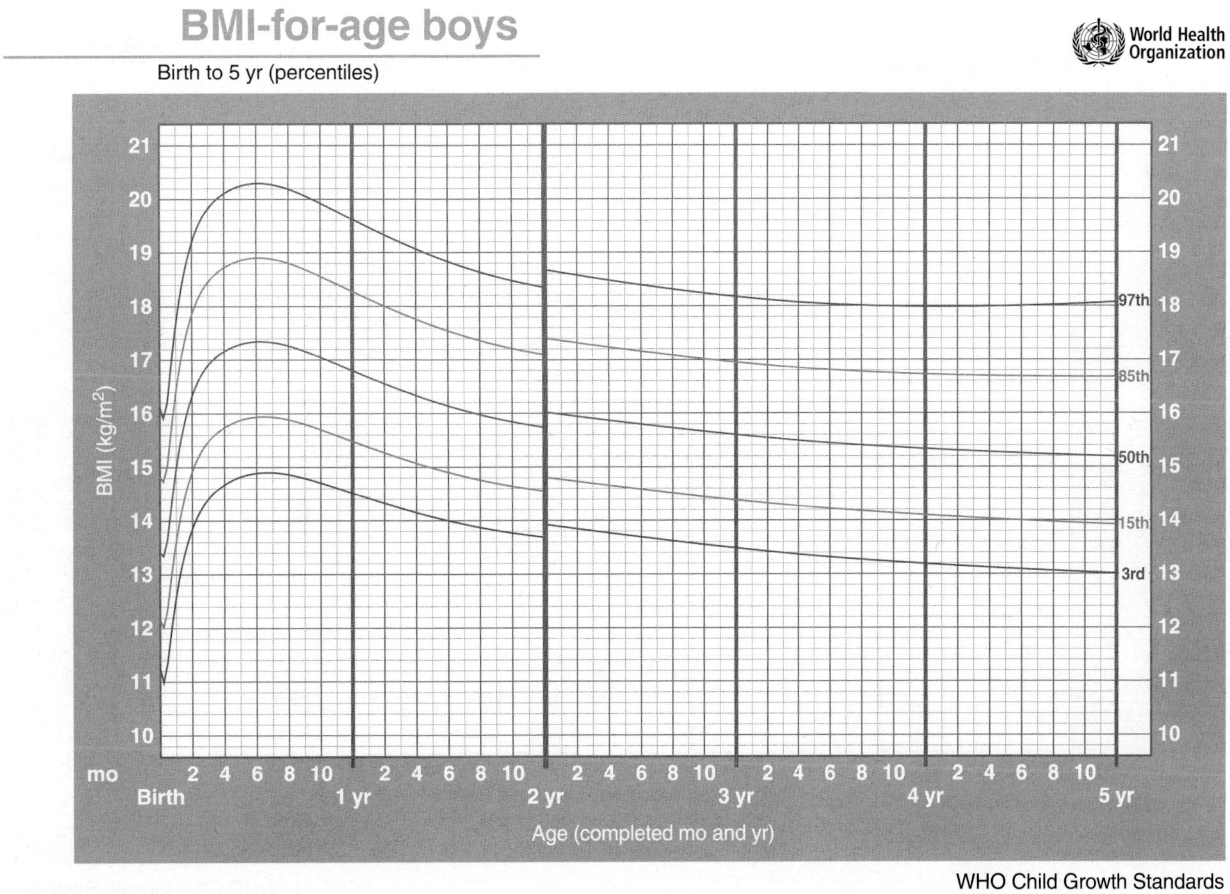

Figure I-13 Boys, BMI-for-age percentiles (birth to 5 years). Developed by the World Health Organization (2006). (http://www.who.int/childgrowth/standards/en/)

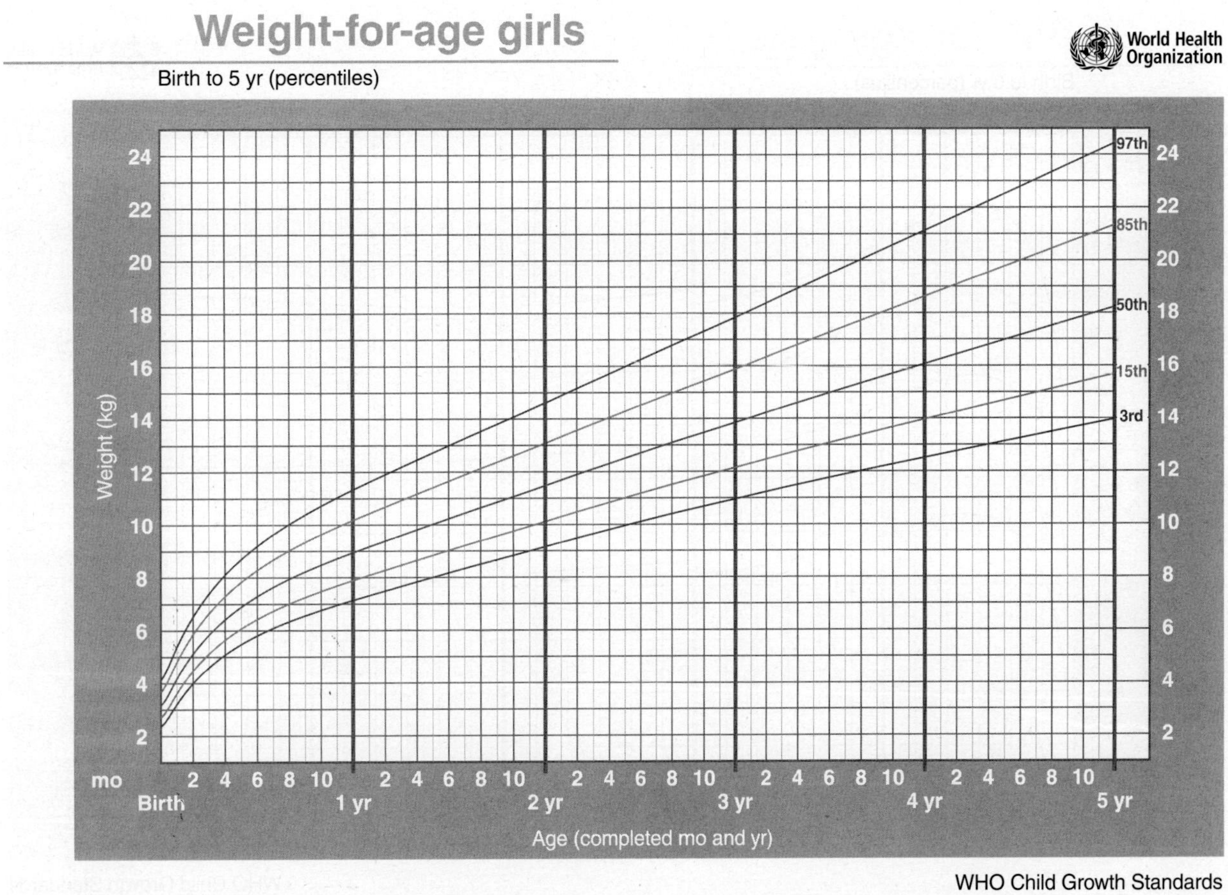

Figure I-14 Girls, weight-for-age percentiles (birth to 5 years). Developed by the World Health Organization (2006). (http://www.who.int/childgrowth/standards/en/)

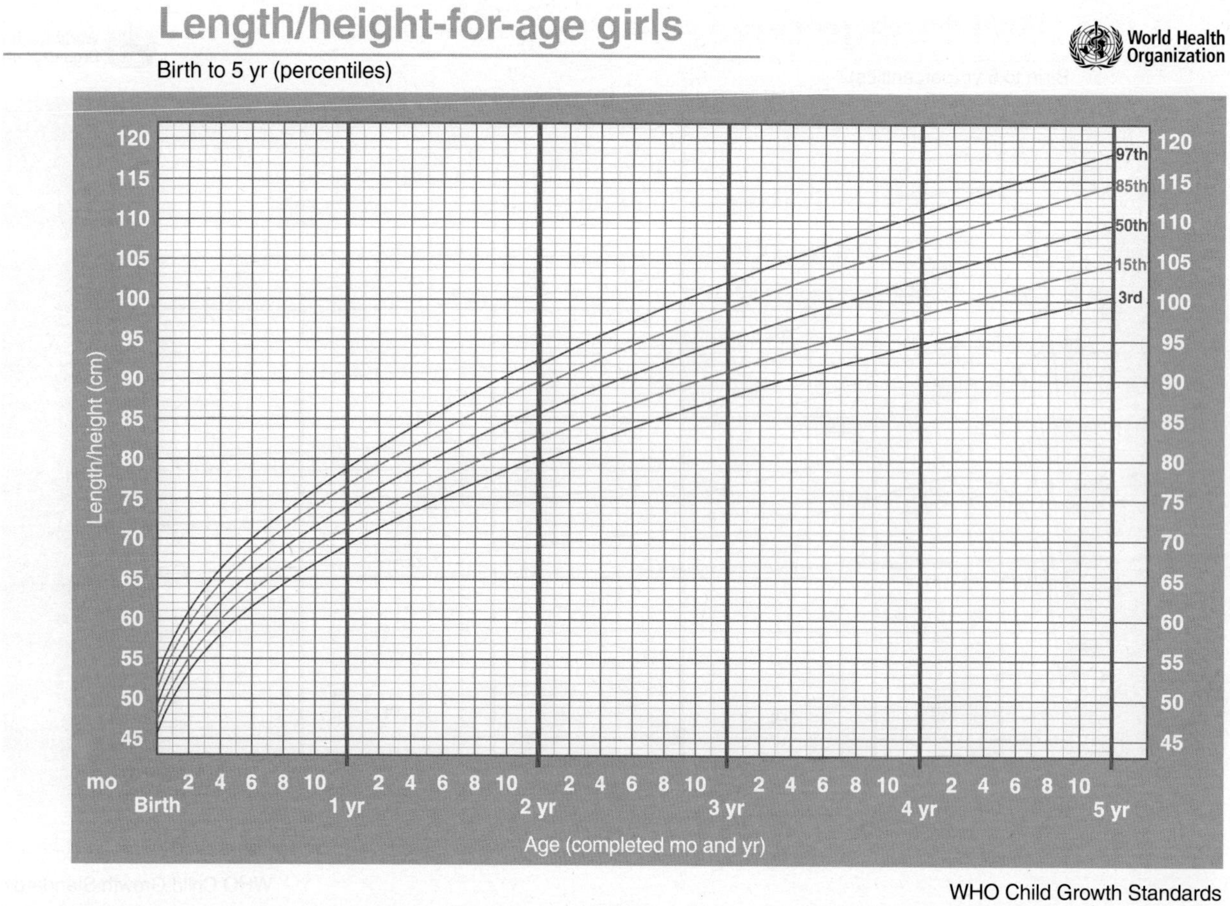

Figure I-15 Girls, length/height-for-age percentiles (birth to 5 years). Developed by the World Health Organization (2006). (http://www.who.int/childgrowth/standards/en/)

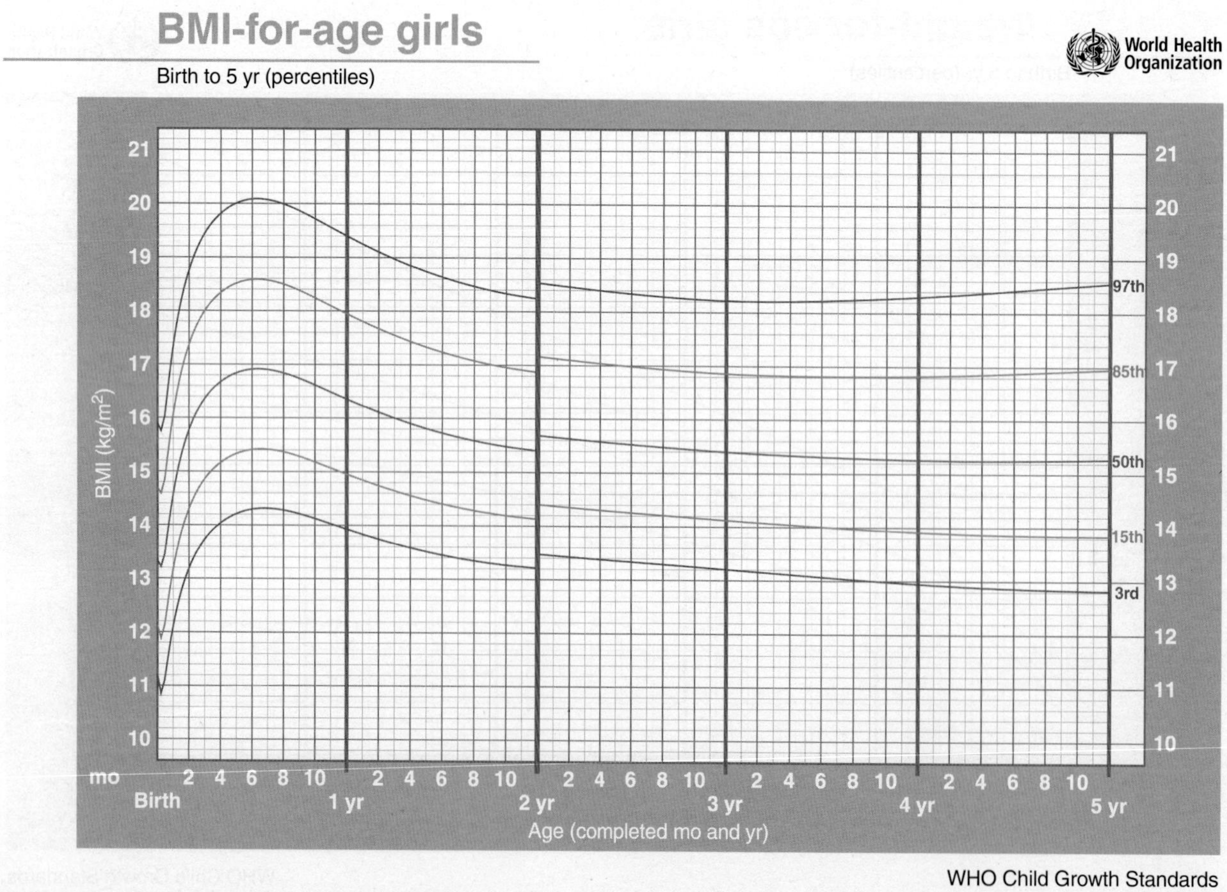

Figure I-16 Girls, BMI-for-age percentiles (birth to 5 years). Developed by the World Health Organization (2006). (http://www.who.int/childgrowth/standards/en/)

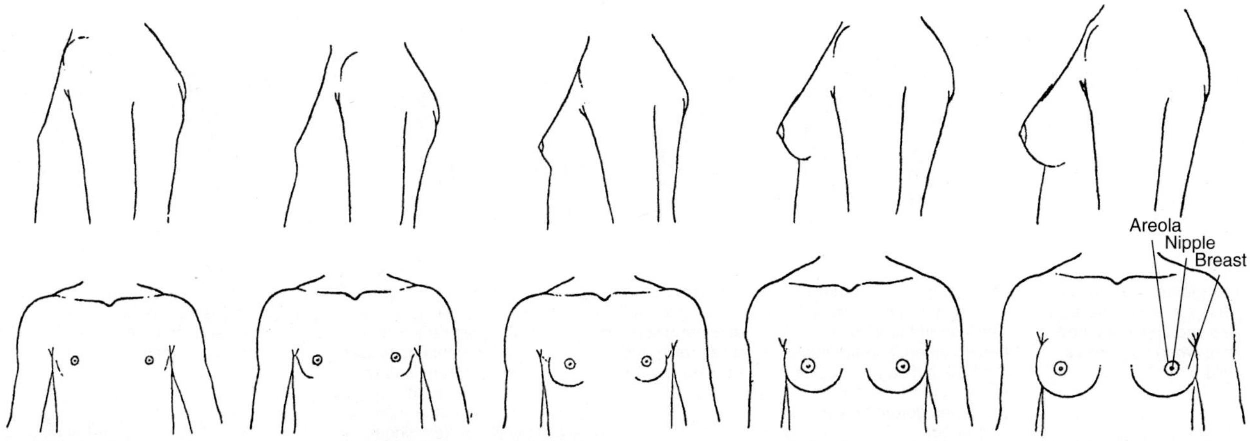

The nipple is raised a little in this stage. The rest of the breast is still flat.

This is the breast bud stage. In this stage the nipple is raised more than in stage 1. The breast is a small mound, the areola is larger than in stage 1.

The areola and the breast are both larger than in satge 2. The areola does not stick out away from the breast.

The areola and the nipple make up a mound that sticks up above the shape of the breast. (Note: This stage may not happen at all for some girls. Some girls develop from stage 3 to stage 5, with no stage 4.)

This is the mature adult stage. The breast are fully developed, only the nipple sticks out in this stage. The areola has moved back to the general shape of the breast.

Figure I-17 Typical progression of female pubertal development. (Reproduced from Morris NM, Udry JR. Validation of a self-administered instrument to assess stage of adolescent development. J Youth Adolesc 1980;9:271–80. With permission from Springer Science and Business Media.)

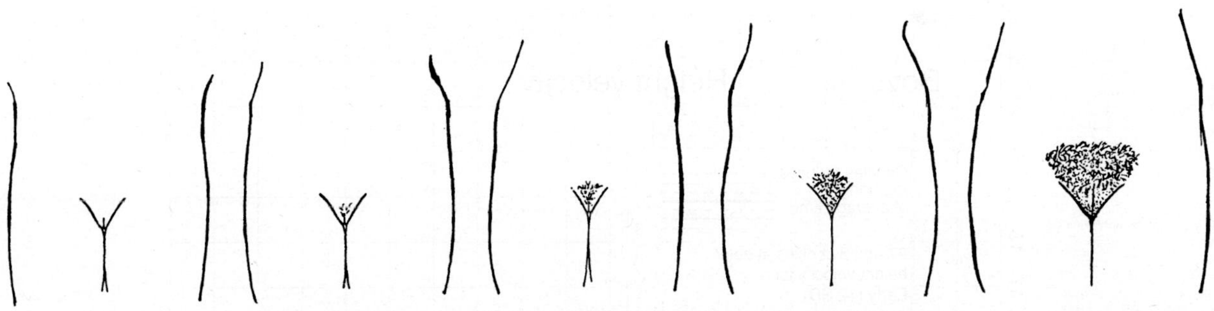

There is no pubic hair.

There is a little long, lightly colored hair. This hair may be straight or a little curly.

The hair is a darker in this stage. It is coarser and more curled. It has spread out and thinly covers a larger area.

The hair is now as dark, curly, and coarse as that of an adult female. However, the area that the hair covers is not as large as that of an adult female. The hair has not spread out to the thighs.

The hair now is like that of an adult female. It also covers the same area as that of the adult female. The hair usually forms a tringular (▽) pattern as it spreads out to the thighs.

Figure I-18 Typical progression of female pubertal development. (Reproduced from Morris NM, Udry JR. Validation of a self-administered instrument to assess stage of adolescent development. J Youth Adolesc 1980;9:271–80. With permission from Springer Science and Business Media.)

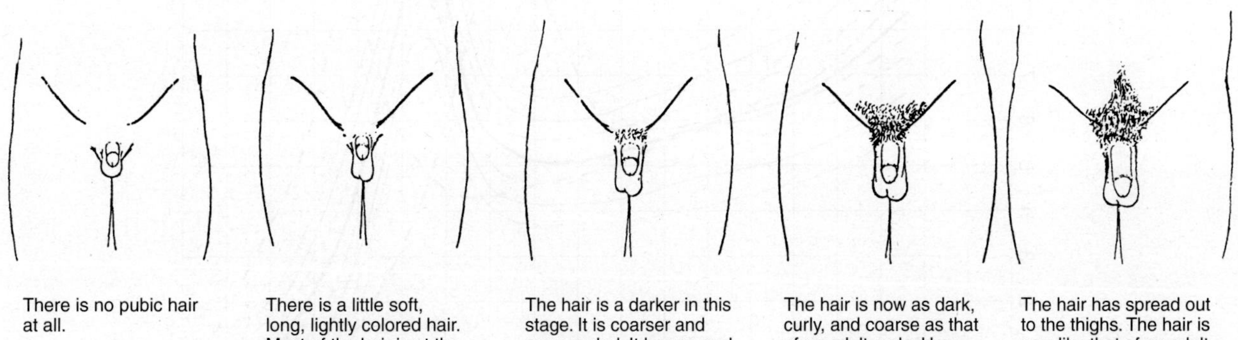

There is no pubic hair at all.

There is a little soft, long, lightly colored hair. Most of the hair is at the base of the penis. This hair may be straight or a little curly.

The hair is a darker in this stage. It is coarser and more curled. It has spread out and thinly covers a somewhat larger area.

The hair is now as dark, curly, and coarse as that of an adult male. However, the area that the hair covers, is not as large as that of an adult male. The hair has not spread out to the thighs.

The hair has spread out to the thighs. The hair is now like that of an adult male. It covers the same area as that of an adult male.

Figure I-19 Typical progression of male pubertal development. (Reproduced from Morris NM, Udry JR. Validation of a self-administered instrument to assess stage of adolescent development. J Youth Adolesc 1980;9:271–80. With permission from Springer Science and Business Media.)

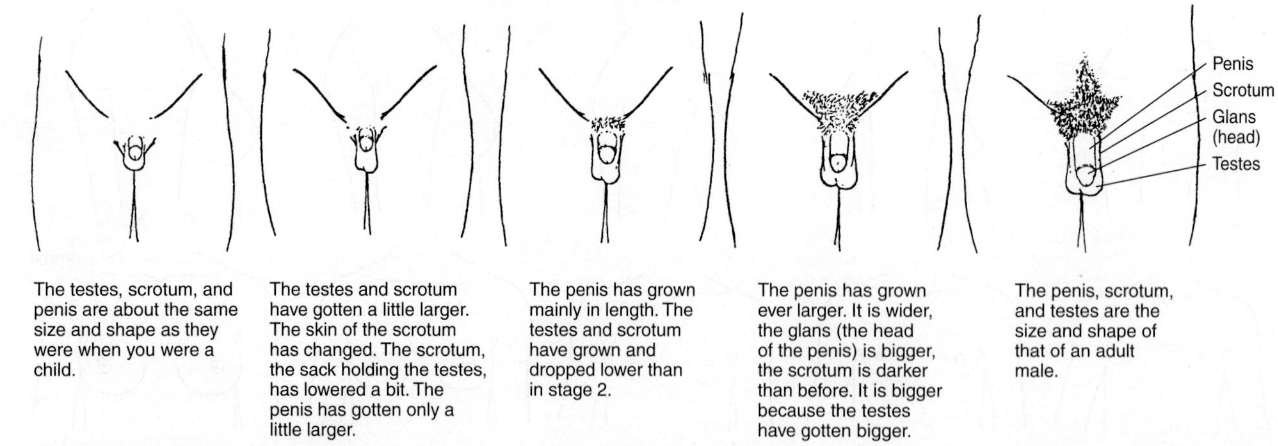

Figure I-20 Typical progression of male pubertal development. (Reproduced from Morris NM, Udry JR. Validation of a self-administered instrument to assess stage of adolescent development. J Youth Adolesc 1980;9:271–80. With permission from Springer Science and Business Media.)

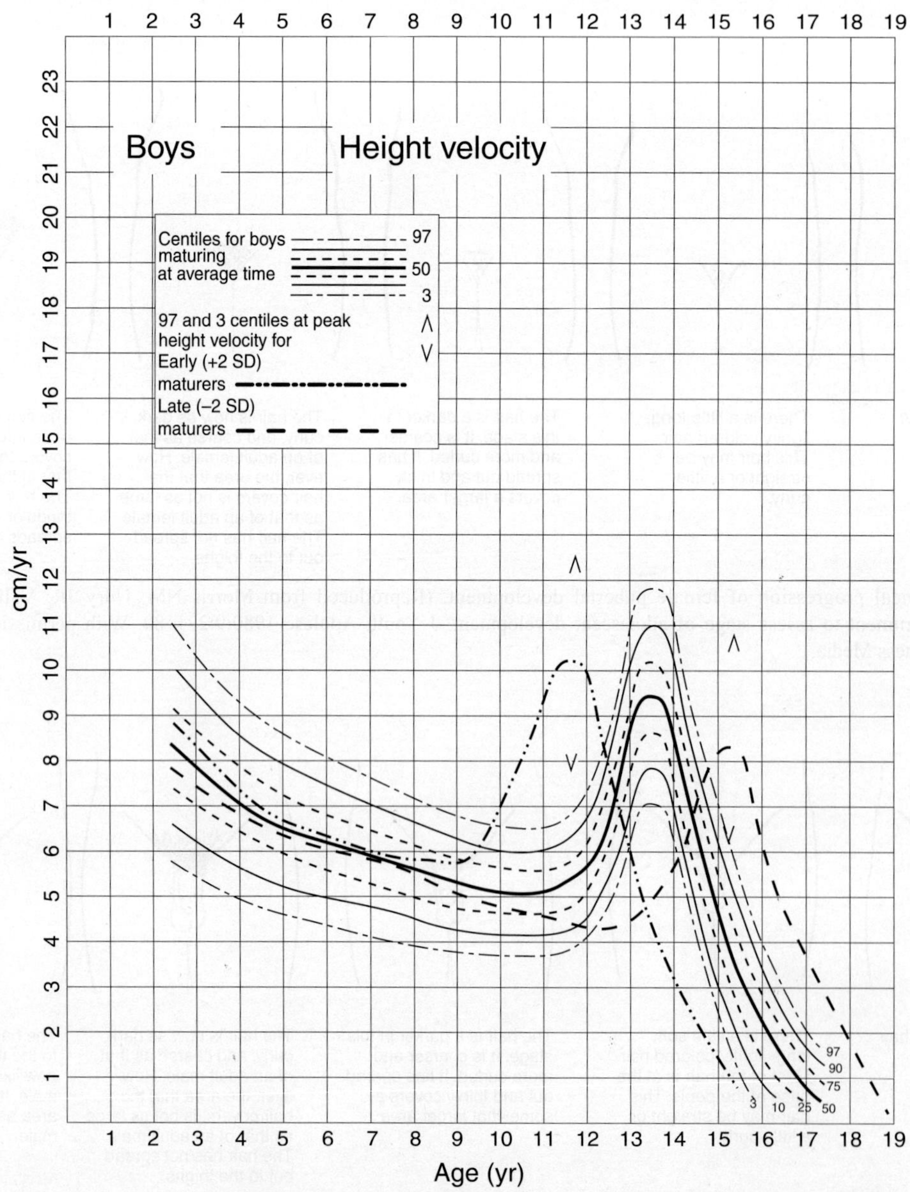

Figure I-21 Height velocity for American boys. (Reproduced from Tanner JM, Davies PSW. Clinical longitudinal standards for height and height velocity for North American children. J Pediatr 1985;107:317–29. With permission from Elsevier.)

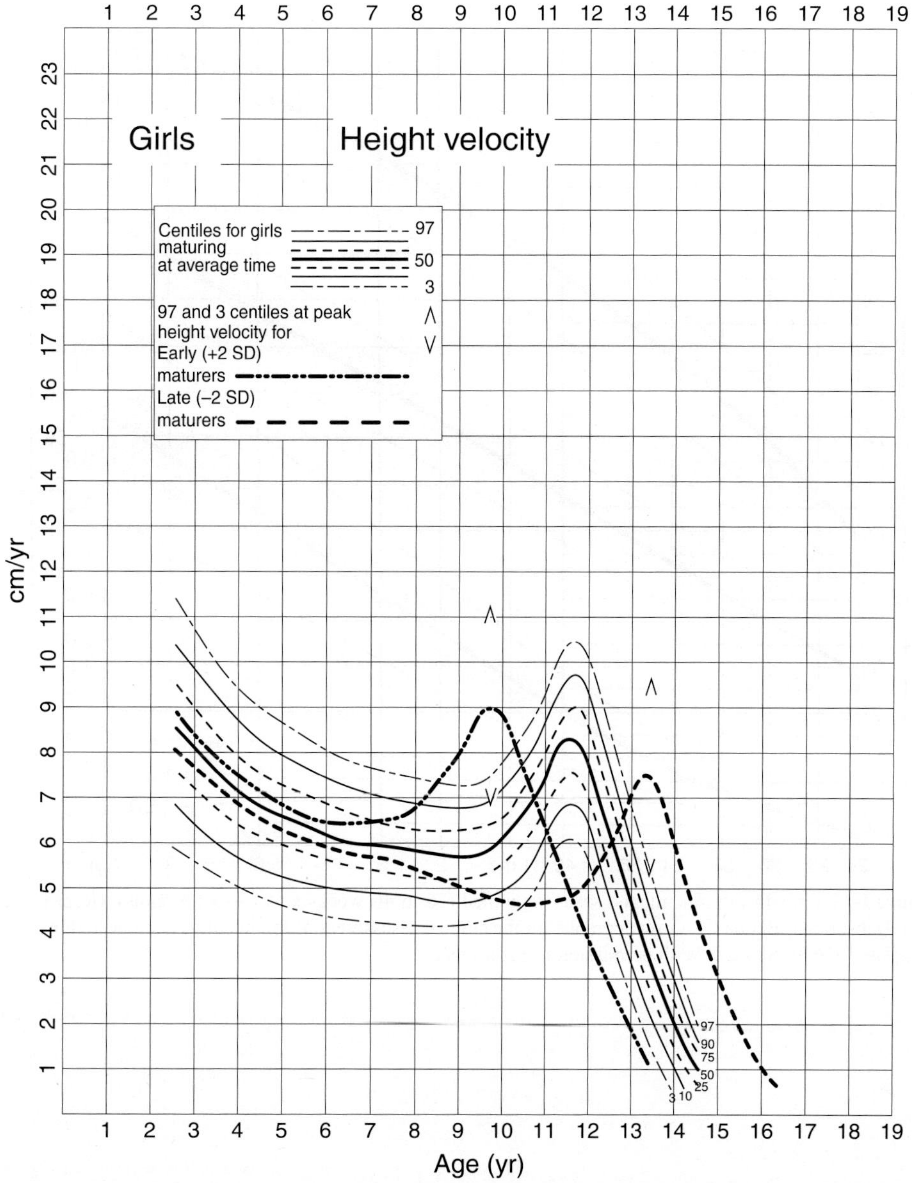

Figure I-22 Height velocity for American girls. (Reproduced from Tanner JM, Davies PSW. Clinical longitudinal standards for height and height velocity for North American children. J Pediatr 1985;107:317–29. With permission from Elsevier.)

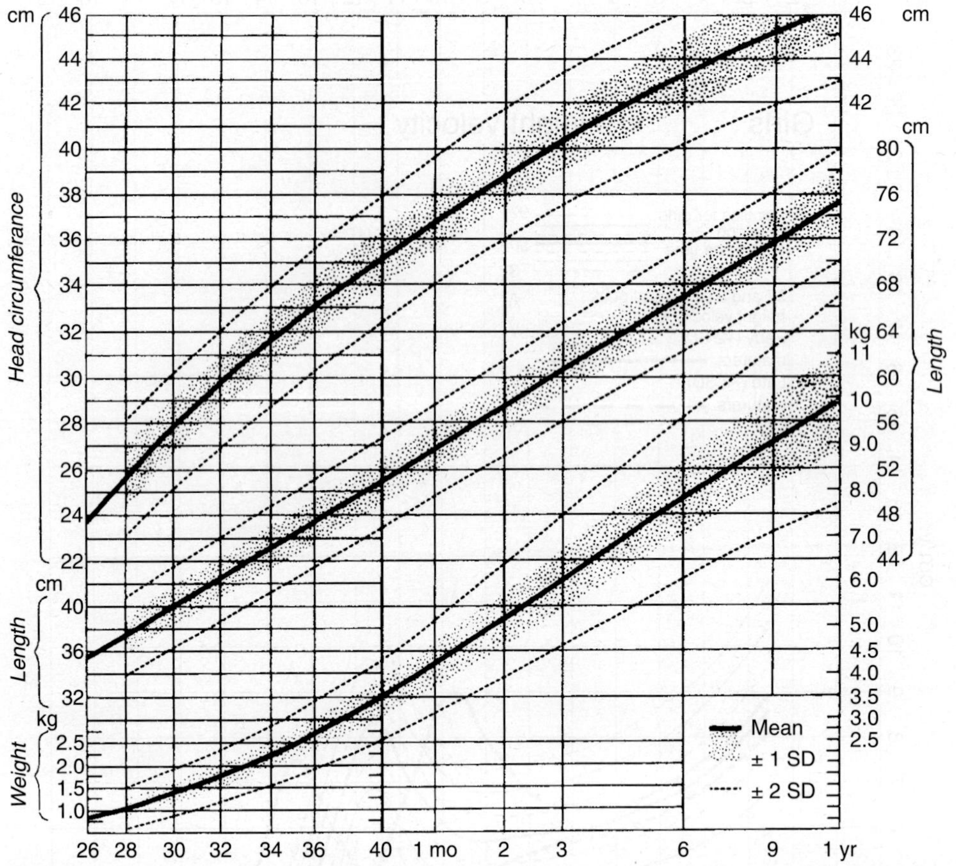

Figure I-23 Growth rate for infants, sexes combined (26 to 40 weeks and 1 to 12 months). (Reproduced from Babson SG, Benda GI. Growth graphs for the clinical assessment of infants of varying gestational age. J Pediatr 1976;89:814–20. With permission from Elsevier.)

Classification of Newborns— Based on Maturity and Intrauterine Growth

Symbols: X - 1st exam O - 2nd exam

Side 2

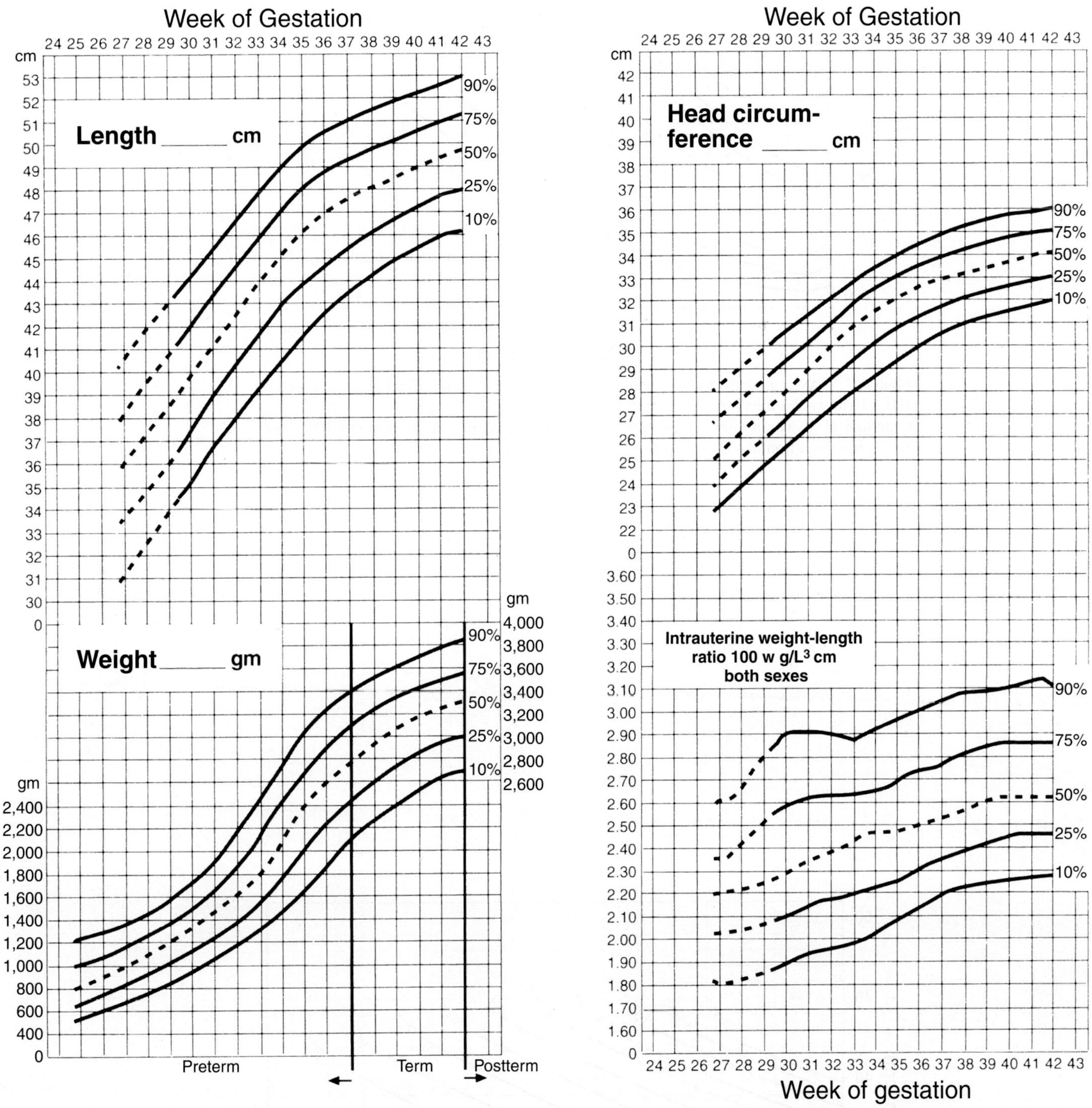

	1st exam (X)	2nd exam (O)
Large for gestational age **(LGA)**		
Appropriate for gestational age **(AGA)**		
Small for gestational age **(SGA)**		
Age at exam	h	h
Signature of examiner	M.D./R.N.	M.D./R.N.

Figure I-24 Classification of newborns, based on maturity and intrauterine growth. (Adapted from Battaglia FC, Lubchenco LO. A practical classification of newborn infants by weight and gestational age. J Pediatr 1967;71:159–63, with permission from Elsevier; and from Lubchenco LO, Hansman C, Boyd E. Intrauterine growth in length and head circumference as estimated from live births at gestational ages from 26 to 42 weeks. Pediatrics 1966;37:403–8. With permission from the American Academy of Pediatrics. ©1988, 1992, 1997, 1999 Mead Johnson & Company, Evansville, Indiana 47721, USA.)

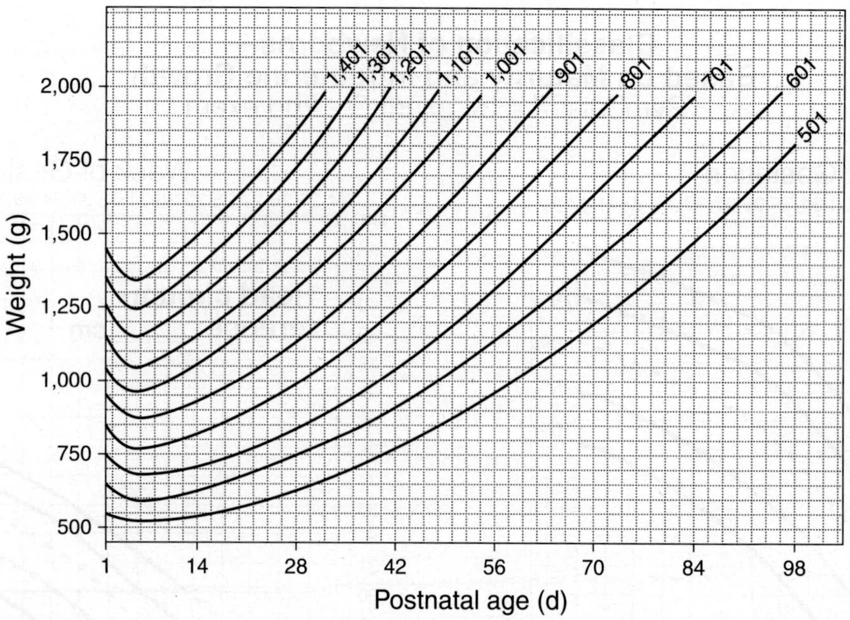

Figure I-25 Average daily body weight versus postnatal age in days for infants stratified by 100 g birth weight intervals. (Reproduced from Ehrenkranz R, Younes N, Lemons JA, et al. Longitudinal growth of hospitalized very low birth weight infants. Pediatrics 1999;104:280–9. With permission from the American Academy of Pediatrics.)

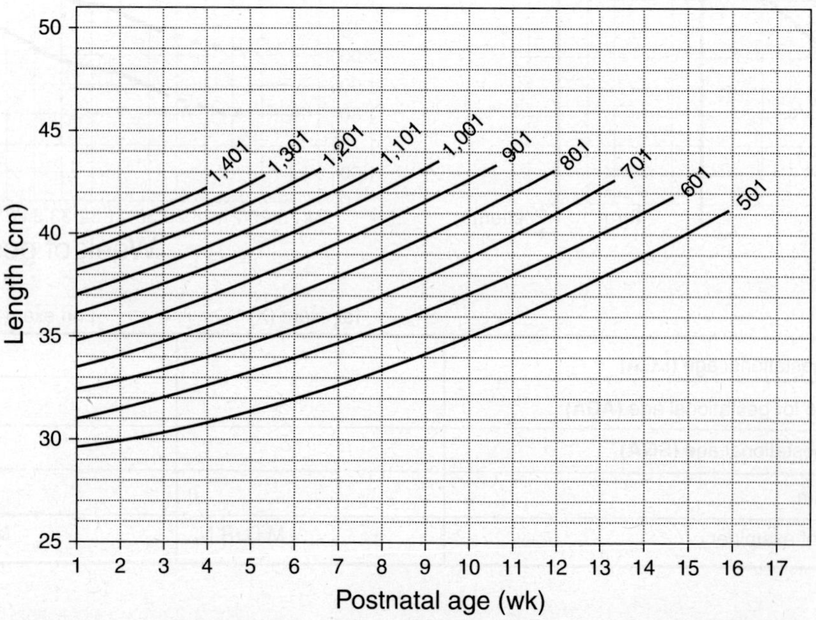

Figure I-26 Average weekly length versus postnatal age in weeks for infants stratified by 100 g birth weight intervals. (Reproduced from Ehrenkranz R, Younes N, Lemons JA, et al. Longitudinal growth of hospitalized very low birth weight infants. Pediatrics 1999;104:280–9. With permission from the American Academy of Pediatrics.)

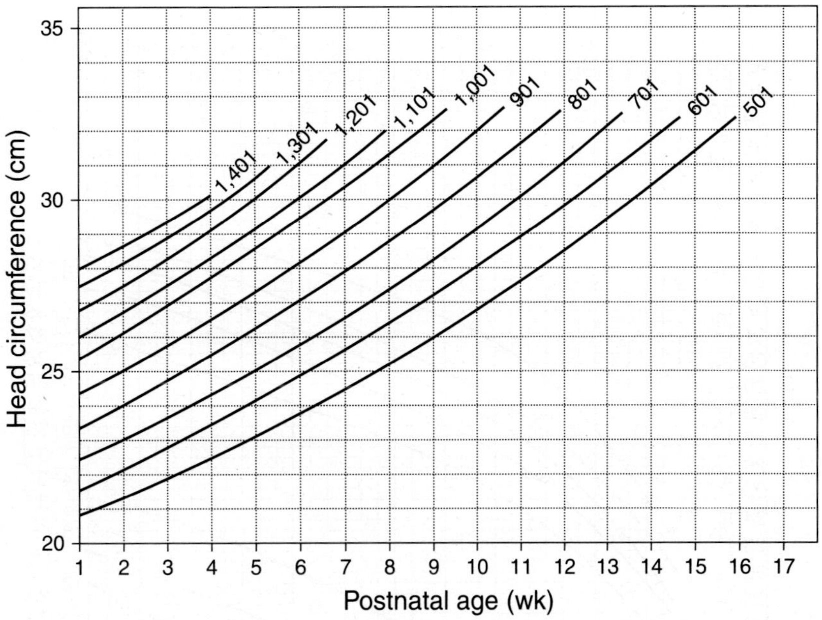

Figure I-27 Average weekly head circumference versus postnatal age in weeks for infants stratified by 100 g birth weight intervals. (Reproduced from Ehrenkranz R, Younes N, Lemons JA, et al. Longitudinal growth of hospitalized very low birth weight infants. Pediatrics 1999;104:280–9. With permission from the American Academy of Pediatrics.)

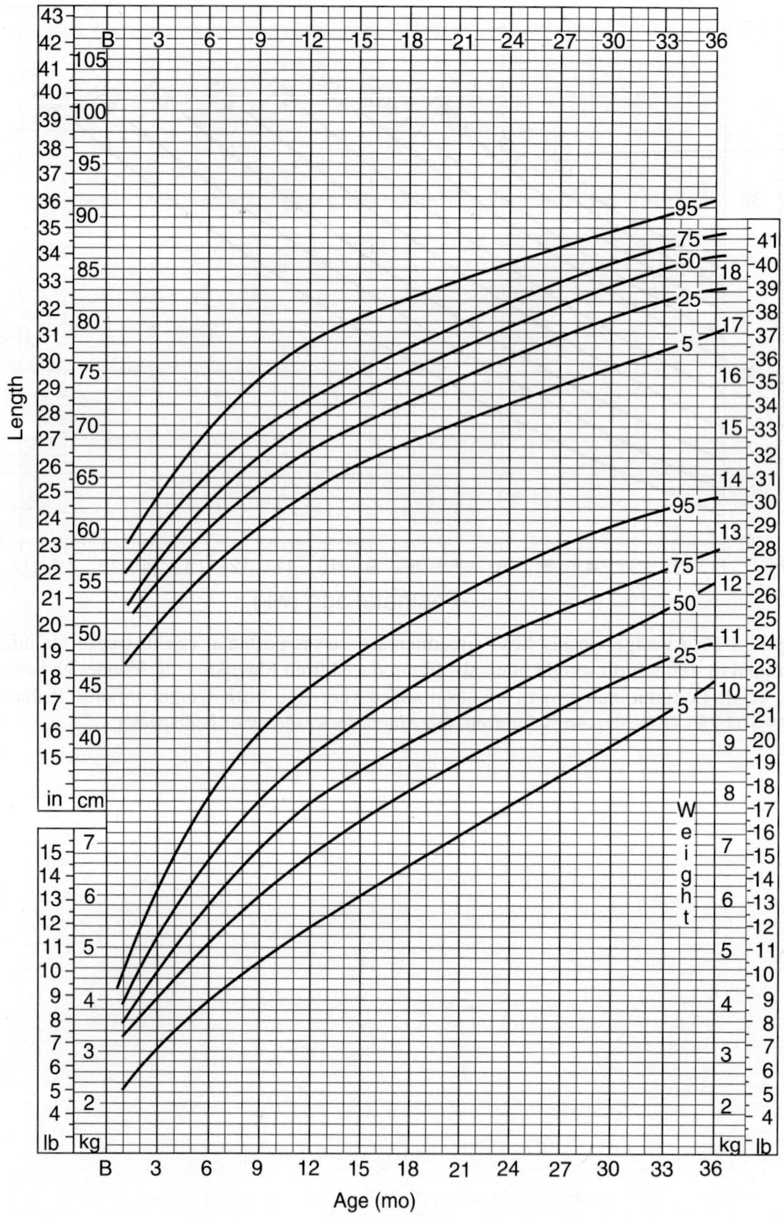

Figure I-28 Physical growth of females with Down syndrome (1 to 36 months). (Reproduced from Cronk C, Crocker AC, Pueschel SM, et al. Growth charts for children with Down syndrome: 1 month to 18 years of age. Pediatrics 1988;81:102–10. With permission from the American Academy of Pediatrics.)

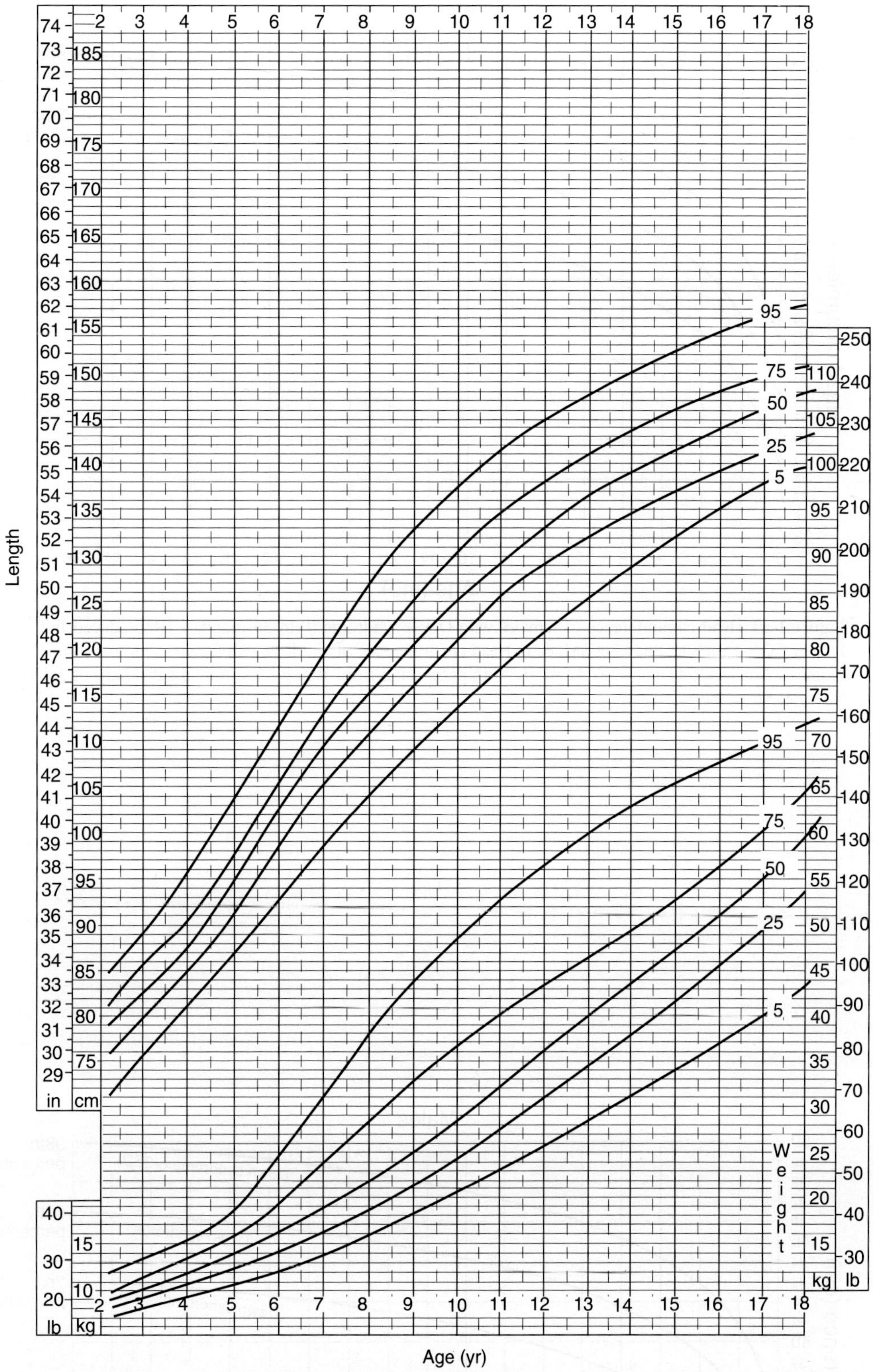

Figure I-29 Physical growth of females with Down syndrome (2 to 18 years). (Reproduced from Cronk C, Crocker AC, Pueschel SM, et al. Growth charts for children with Down syndrome: 1 month to 18 years of age. Pediatrics 1988;81:102–10. With permission from the American Academy of Pediatrics.)

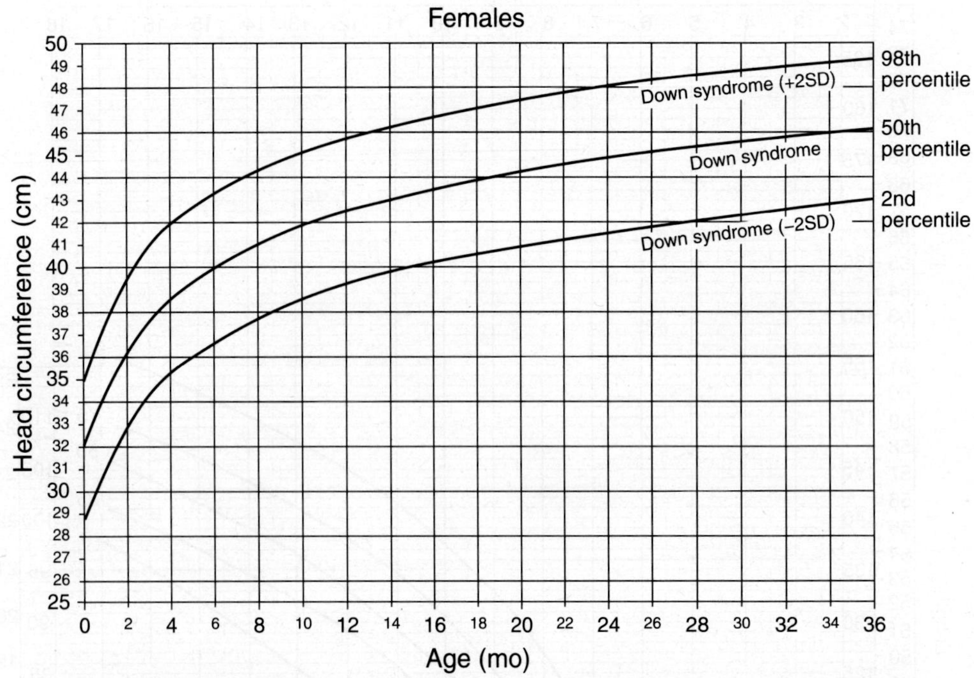

Figure I-30 Head circumference of females with Down syndrome (0 to 36 months). (Reproduced from Palmer CGS, Cronk C, Pueschel SM, et al. Head circumference of children with Down syndrome (0 to 36 months). Am J Med Genet 1992;42:61–7. With permission from Wiley-Liss, Inc., a subsidiary of John Wiley & Sons, Inc.)

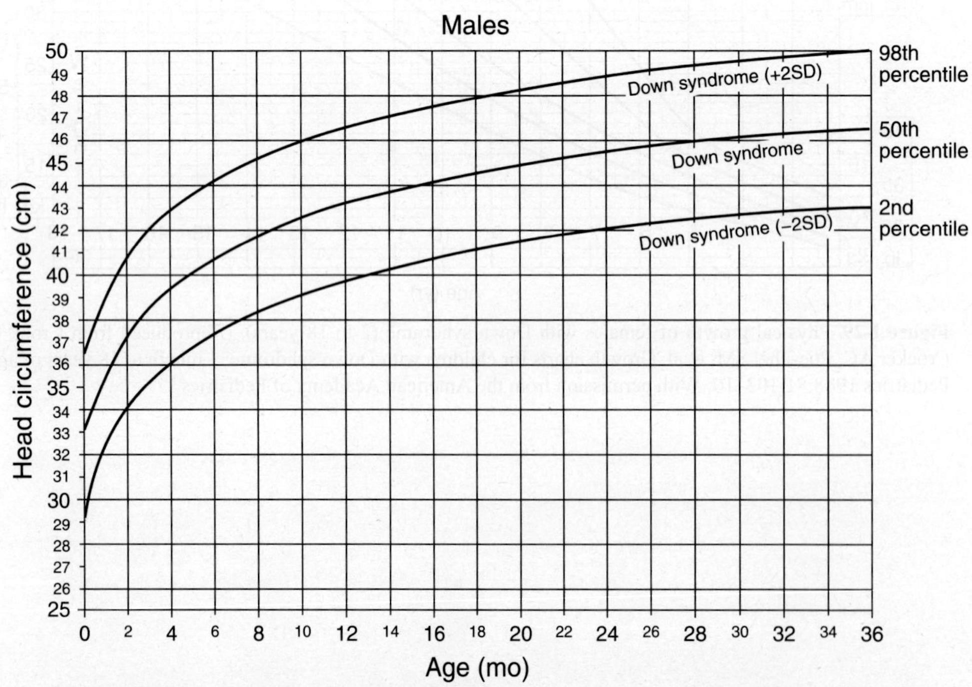

Figure I-31 Head circumference of males with Down syndrome (0 to 36 months). (Reproduced from Palmer CGS, Cronk C, Pueschel SM, et al. Head circumference of children with Down syndrome (0 to 36 months). Am J Med Genet 1992;42:61–7. With permission from Wiley-Liss, Inc., a subsidiary of John Wiley & Sons, Inc.)

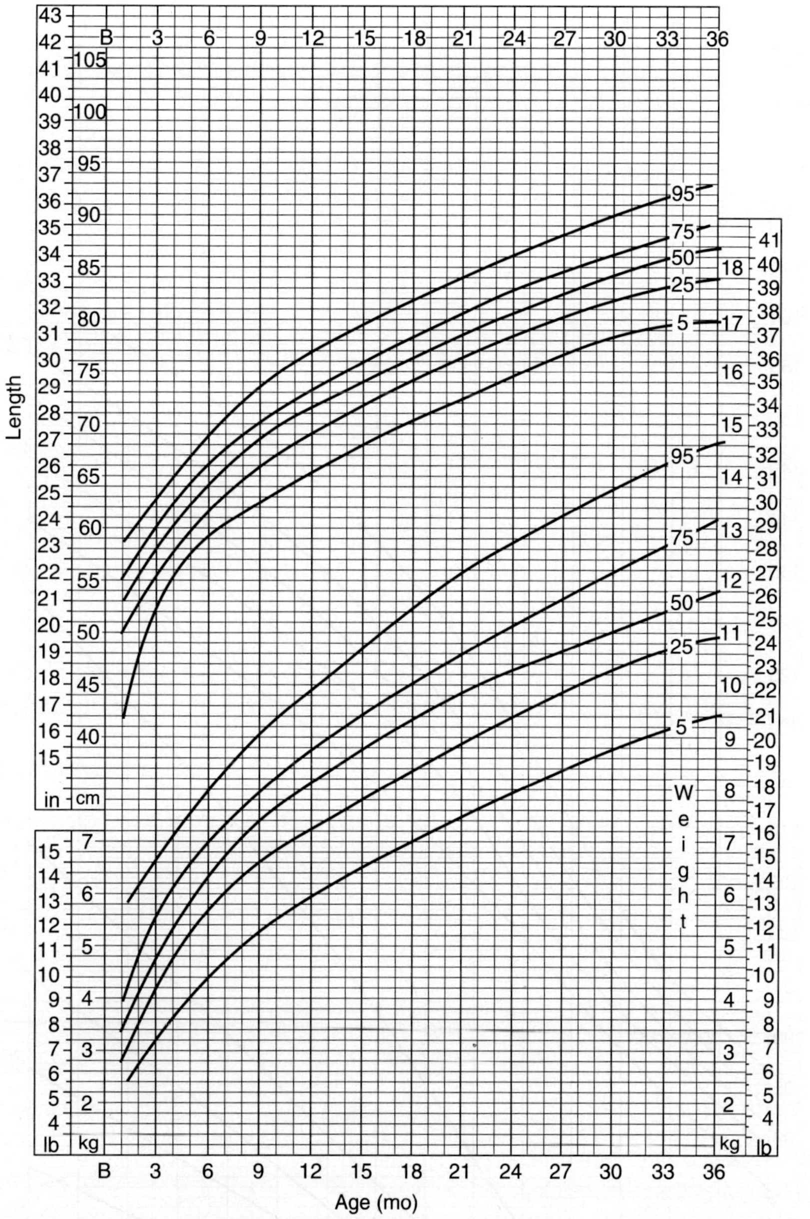

Figure I-32 Physical growth of males with Down syndrome (1 to 36 months). (Reproduced from Cronk C, Crocker AC, Pueschel SM, et al. Growth charts for children with Down syndrome: 1 month to 18 years of age. Pediatrics 1988;81:102–10. With permission from the American Academy of Pediatrics.)

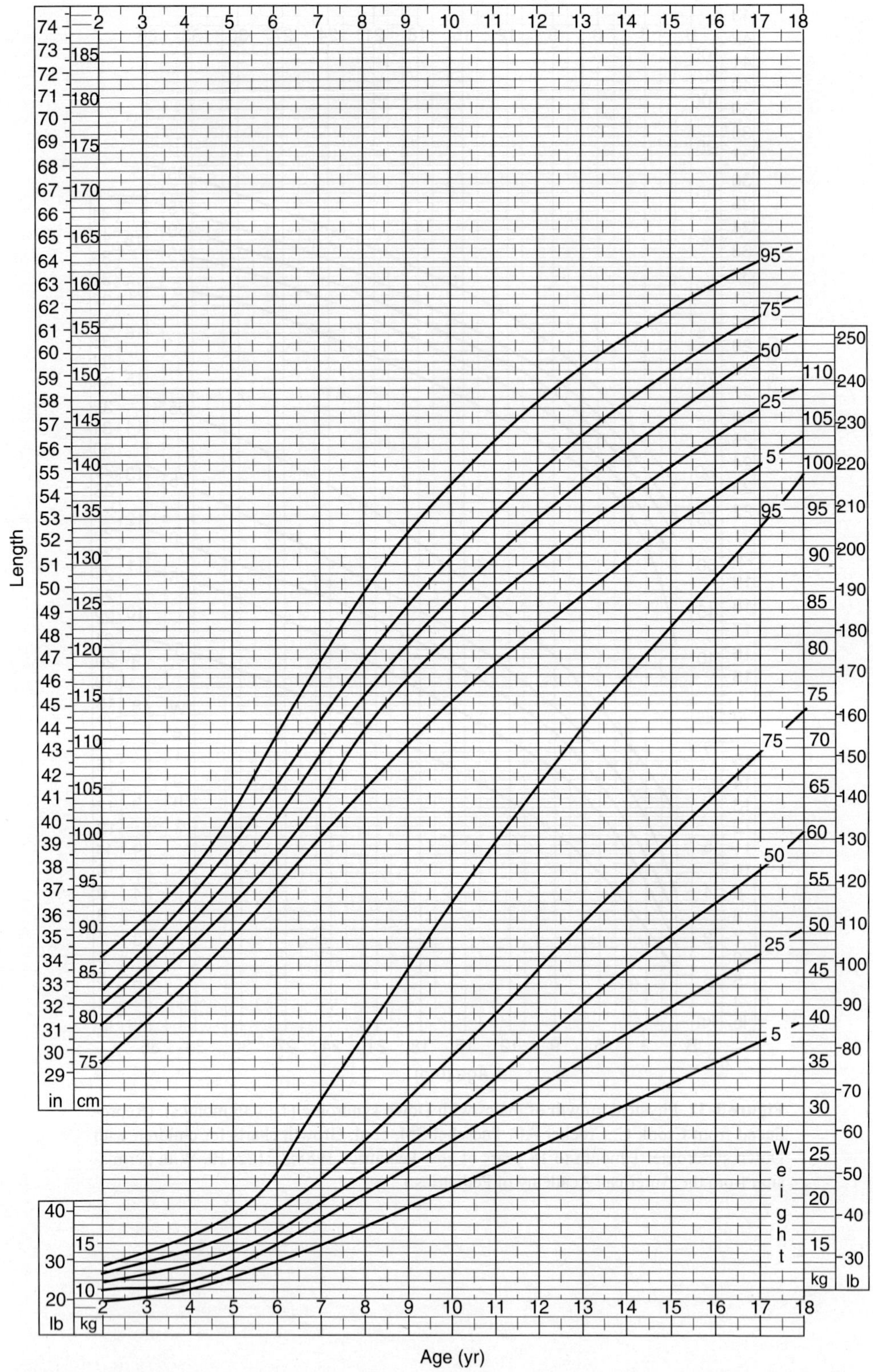

Figure I-33 Physical growth of males with Down syndrome (2 to 18 years). (Reproduced from Cronk C, Crocker AC, Pueschel SM, et al. Growth charts for children with Down syndrome: 1 month to 18 years of age. Pediatrics 1988;81:102–10. With permission from the American Academy of Pediatrics.)

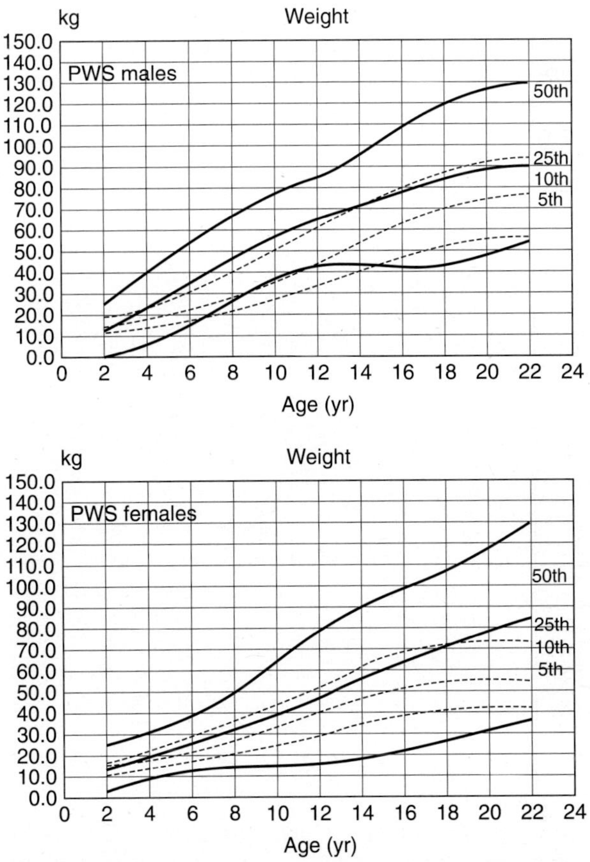

Figure I-34 Weight-for-age percentile curves for males and females with Prader–Willi syndrome (*solid line*) versus healthy individuals (*broken line*). (Reproduced from Butler MG, Meaney FJ. Standards for selected anthropometric measurements in Prader–Willi syndrome. Pediatrics 1991;88:853–60. With permission from the American Academy of Pediatrics.)

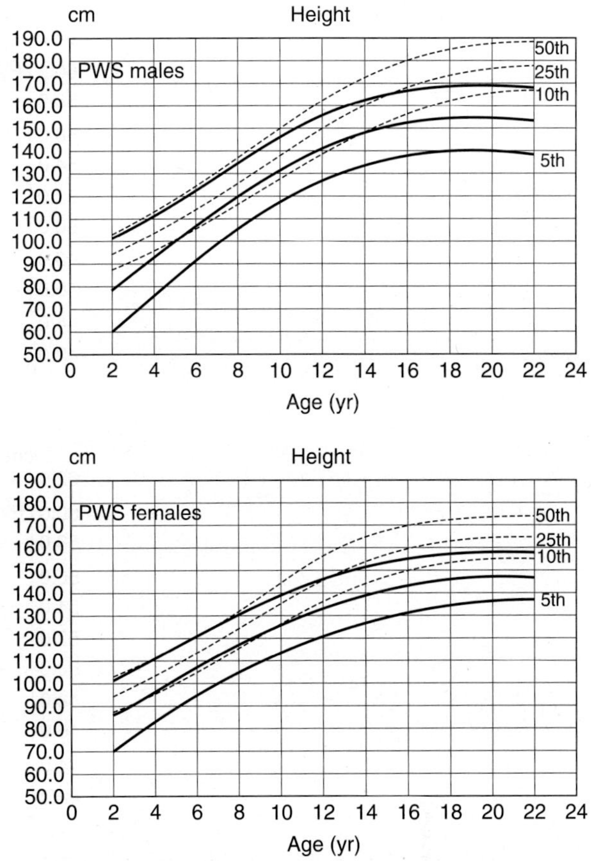

Figure I-35 Height-for-age percentile curves for males and females with Prader–Willi syndrome (*solid line*) versus healthy individuals (*broken line*). (Reproduced from Butler MG, Meaney FJ. Standards for selected anthropometric measurements in Prader–Willi syndrome. Pediatrics 1991;88:853–60. With permission from the American Academy of Pediatrics.)

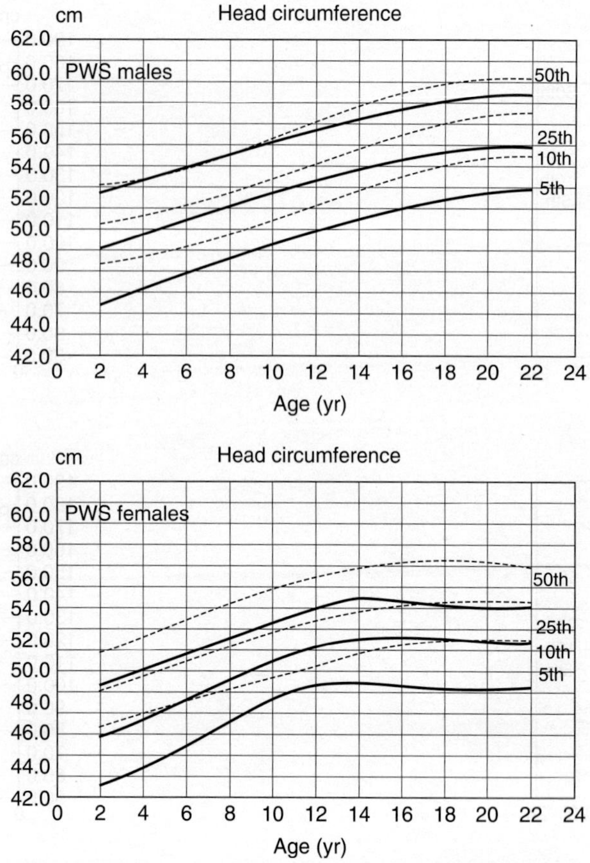

Figure I-36 Head circumference-for-age percentile curves for males and females with Prader–Willi syndrome (*solid line*) versus healthy individuals (*broken line*). (Reproduced from Butler MG, Meaney FJ. Standards for selected anthropometric measurements in Prader–Willi syndrome. Pediatrics 1991;88:853–60. With permission from the American Academy of Pediatrics.)

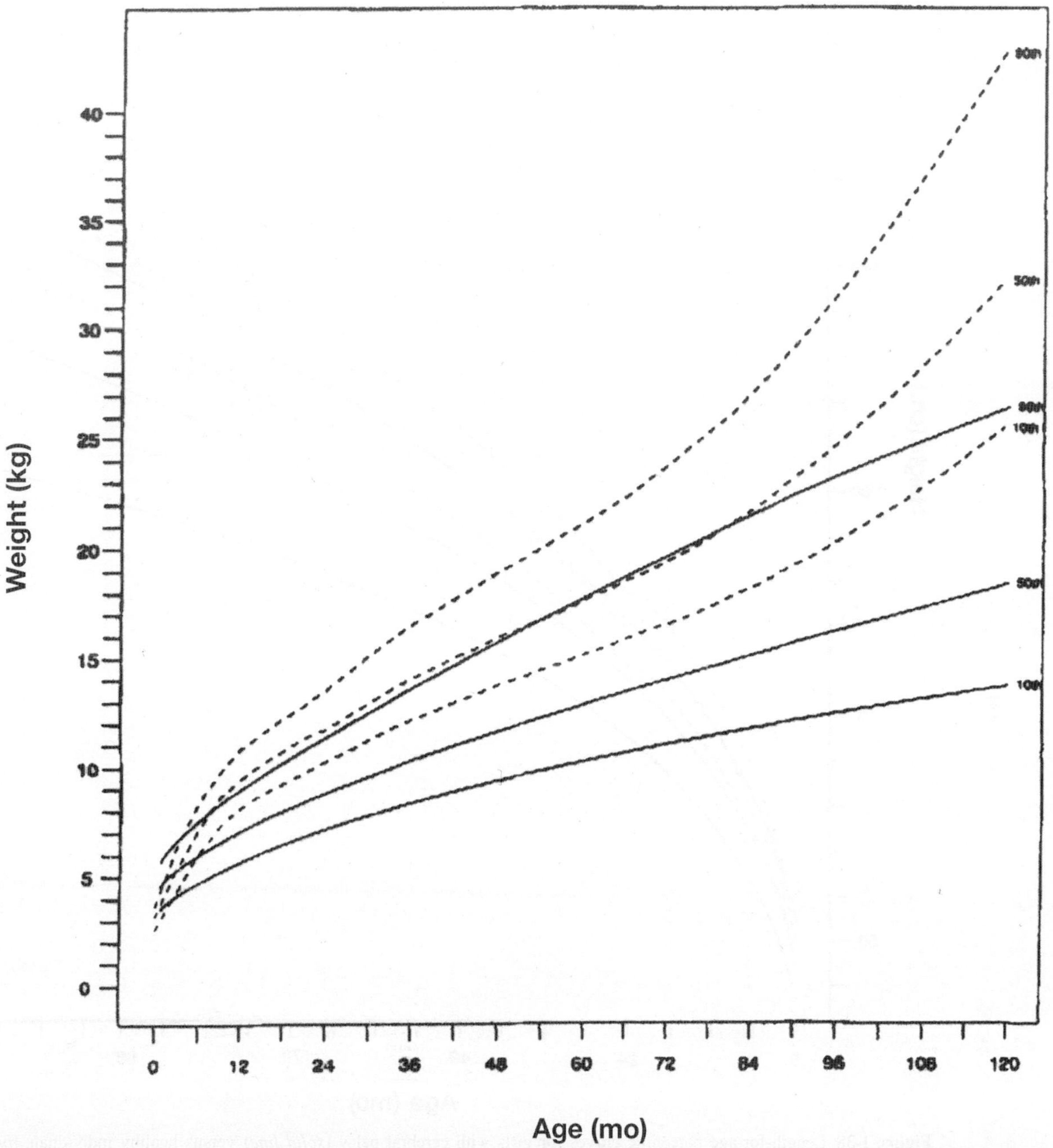

Figure I-37 Weight-for-age percentile curves for girls with cerebral palsy (*solid line*) versus healthy individuals (*broken line*) (0 to 120 months). (Reproduced from Krick J, Murphy-Miller P, Zeger S, et al. Pattern of growth in children with cerebral palsy. J Am Diet Assoc 1996;96:680–85. With permission from Elsevier.)

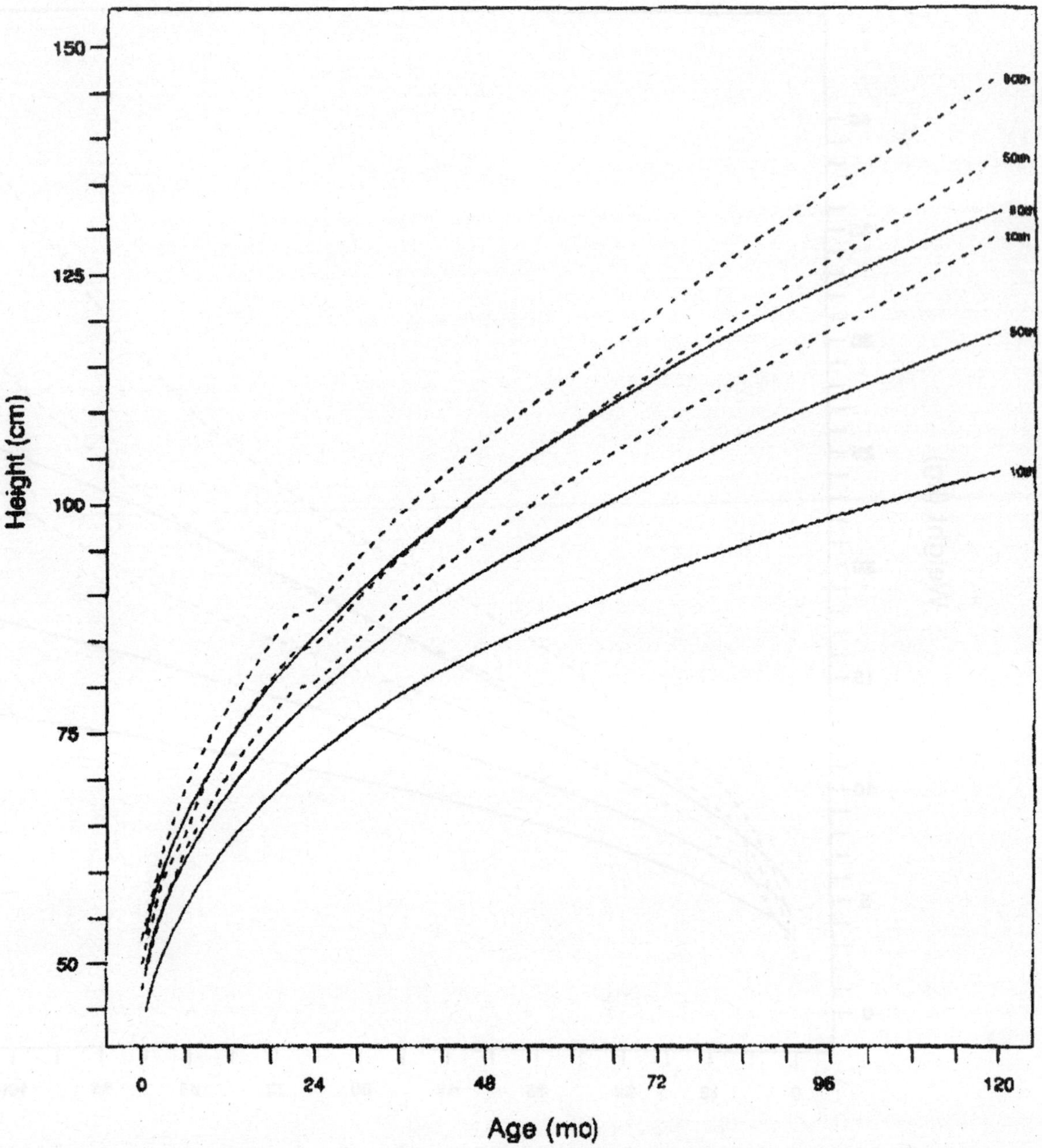

Figure I-38 Length-for-age percentile curves for girls with cerebral palsy (*solid line*) versus healthy individuals (*broken line*) (0 to 120 months). (Reproduced from Krick J, Murphy-Miller P, Zeger S, et al. Pattern of growth in children with cerebral palsy. J Am Diet Assoc 1996;96:680–5. With permission from Elsevier.)

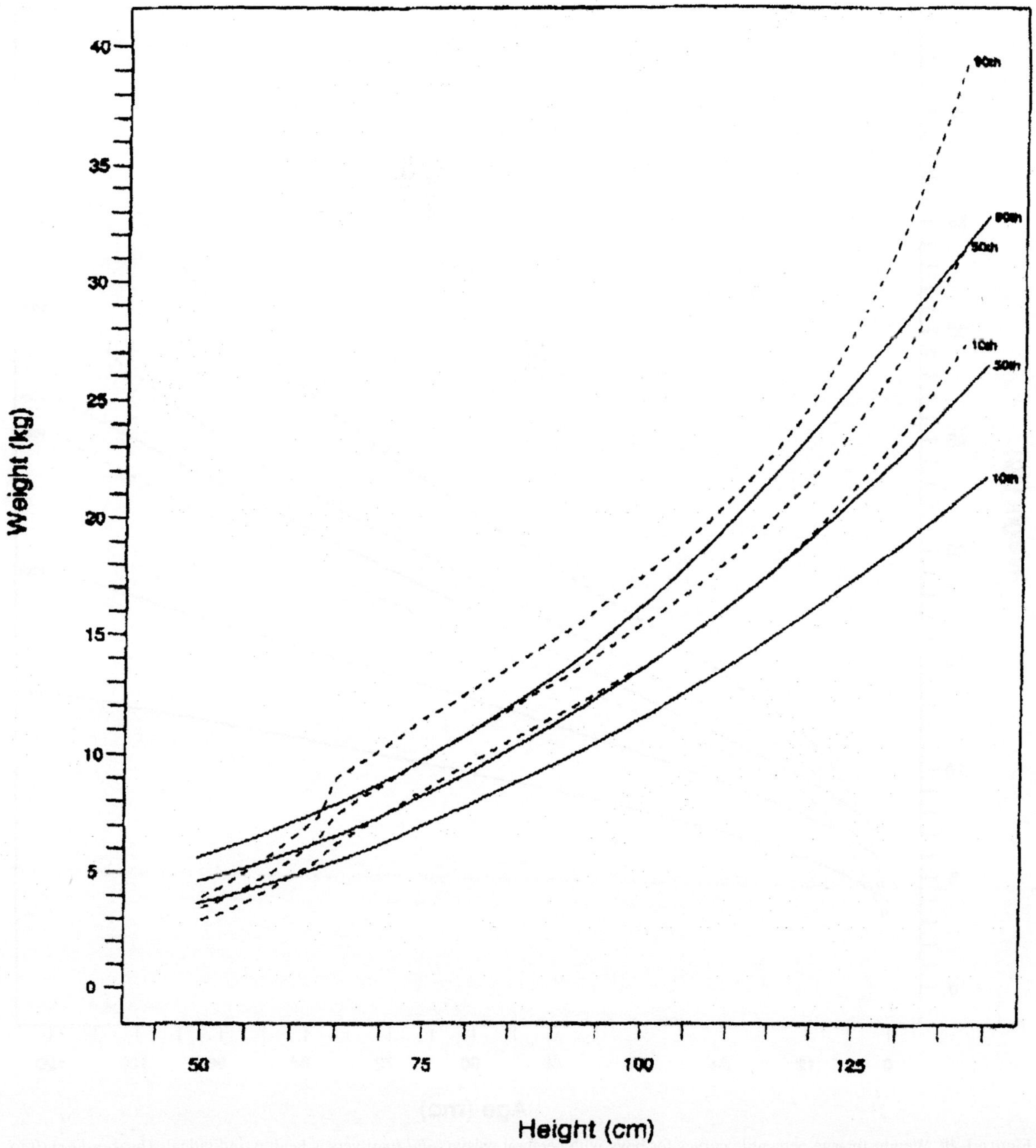

Figure I-39 Weight-for-length percentile curves for girls with cerebral palsy (*solid line*) versus healthy individuals (*broken line*) (0 to 120 months). (Reproduced from Krick J, Murphy-Miller P, Zeger S, et al. Pattern of growth in children with cerebral palsy. J Am Diet Assoc 1996;96:680–5. With permission from Elsevier.)

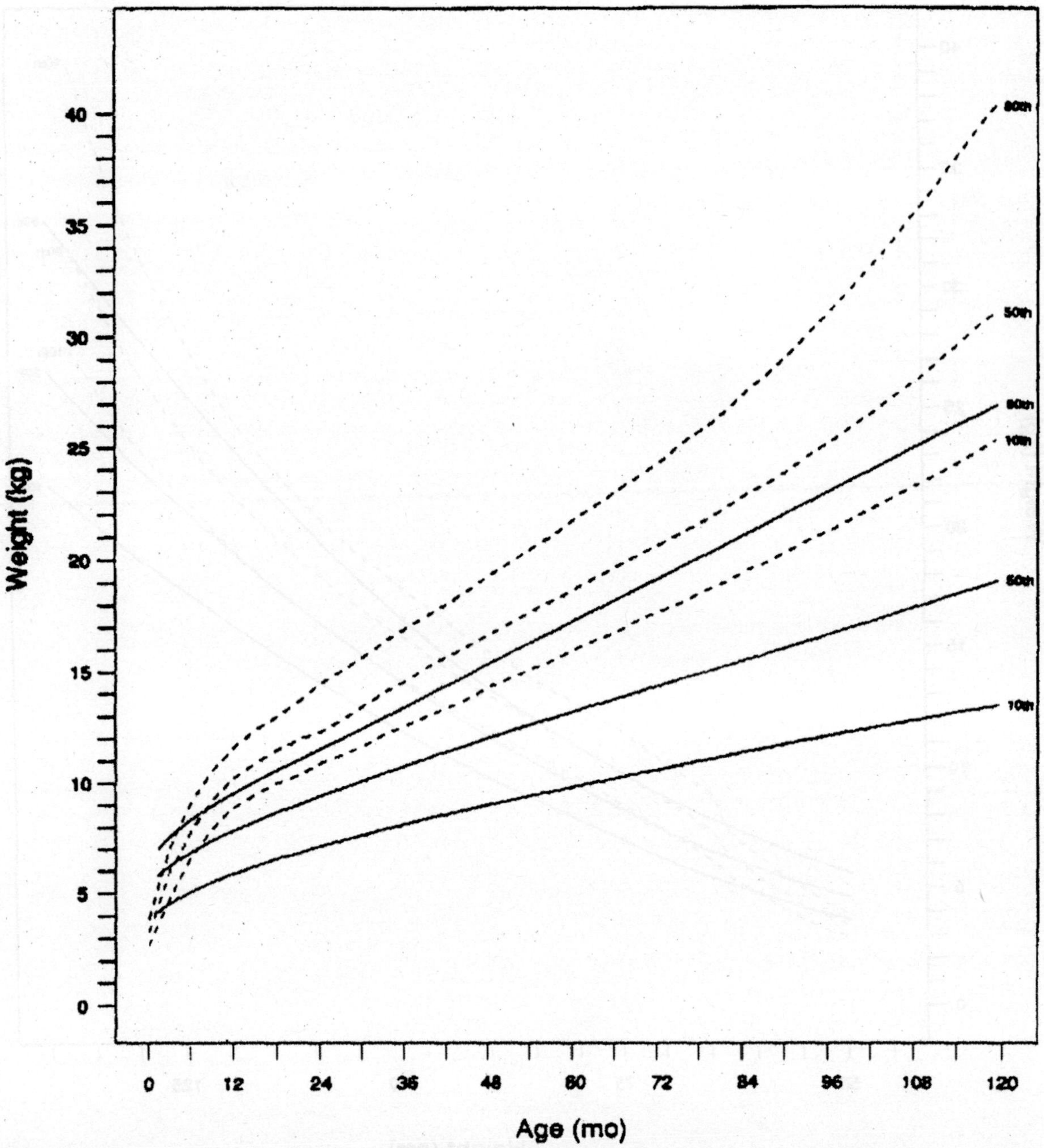

Figure I-40 Weight-for-age percentile curves for boys with cerebral palsy (*solid line*) versus healthy individuals (*broken line*) (0 to 120 months). (Reproduced from Krick J, Murphy-Miller P, Zeger S, et al. Pattern of growth in children with cerebral palsy. J Am Diet Assoc 1996;96:680–5. With permission from Elsevier.)

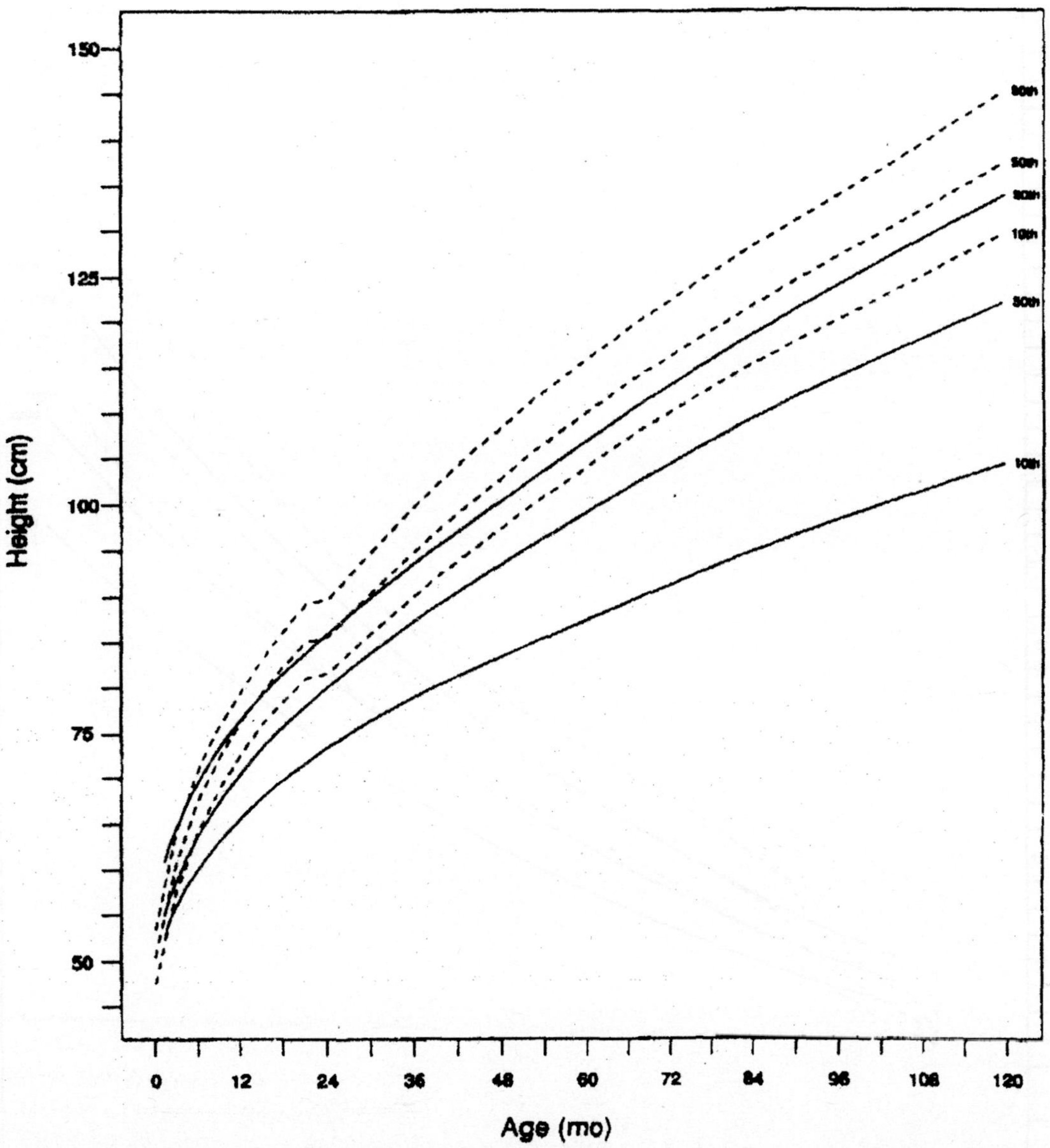

Figure I-41 Length-for-age percentile curves for boys with cerebral palsy (*solid line*) versus healthy individuals (*broken line*) (0 to 120 months). (Reproduced from Krick J, Murphy-Miller P, Zeger S, et al. Pattern of growth in children with cerebral palsy. J Am Diet Assoc 1996;96:680–5. With permission from Elsevier.)

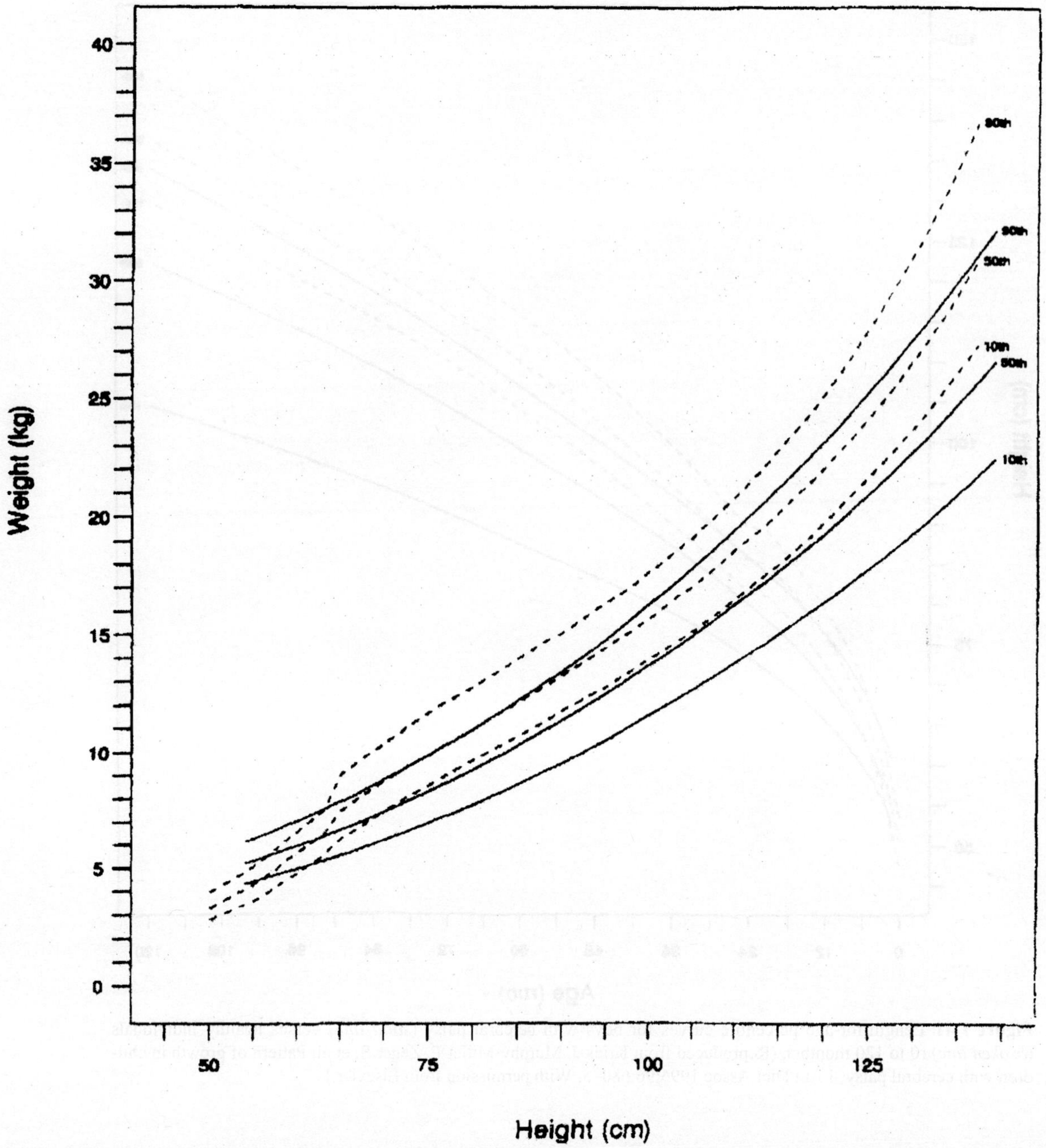

Figure I-42 Weight-for-length percentile curves for boys with cerebral palsy (*solid line*) versus healthy individuals (*broken line*) (0 to 120 months). (Reproduced from Krick J, Murphy-Miller P, Zeger S, et al. Pattern of growth in children with cerebral palsy. J Am Diet Assoc 1996;96:680–5. With permission from Elsevier.)

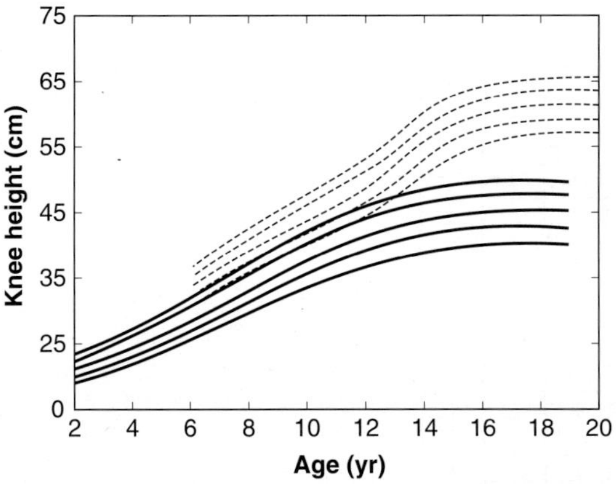

Figure I-43 Knee height percentile curves (10th, 25th, 50th, 75th, 90th) for boys with cerebral palsy (*solid line*) versus healthy individuals (*broken line*) (2 to 20 years). (Reproduced from Stevenson RD, Conaway M, Chumlea WC, et al. Growth and health in children with moderate-to-severe cerebral palsy. Pediatrics 2006;118:1010–8. With permission from the American Academy of Pediatrics.)

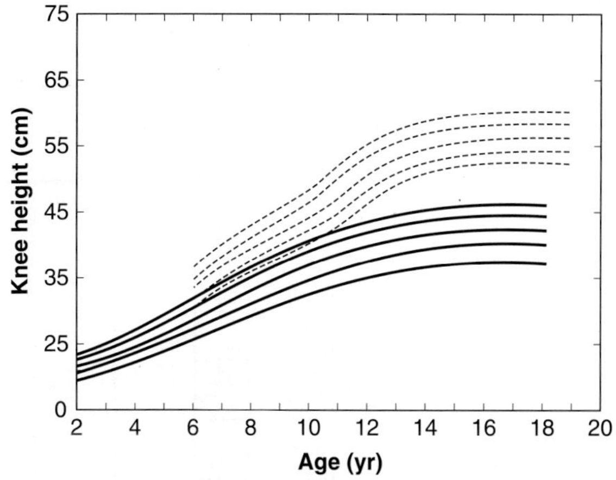

Figure I-44 Knee height percentile curves (10th, 25th, 50th, 75th, 90th) for girls with cerebral palsy (*solid line*) versus healthy individuals (*broken line*) (2 to 20 years). (Reproduced from Stevenson RD, Conaway M, Chumlea WC, et al. Growth and health in children with moderate-to-severe cerebral palsy. Pediatrics 2006;118:1010–18. With permission from the American Academy of Pediatrics.)

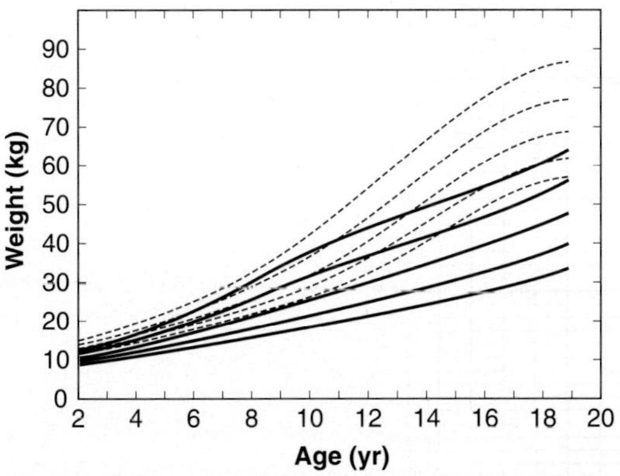

Figure I-45 Weight-for-age percentile curves (10th, 25th, 50th, 75th, 90th) for boys with cerebral palsy (*solid line*) versus healthy individuals (*broken line*) (2 to 20 years). (Reproduced from Stevenson RD, Conaway M, Chumlea WC, et al. Growth and health in children with moderate-to-severe cerebral palsy. Pediatrics 2006;118:1010–18. With permission from the American Academy of Pediatrics.)

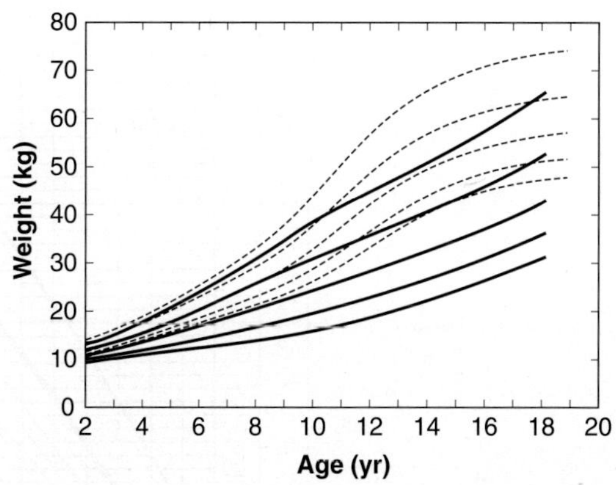

Figure I-46 Weight-for-age percentile curves (10th, 25th, 50th, 75th, 90th) for girls with cerebral palsy (*solid line*) versus healthy individuals (*broken line*) (2 to 20 years). (Reproduced from Stevenson RD, Conaway M, Chumlea WC, et al. Growth and health in children with moderate-to-severe cerebral palsy. Pediatrics 2006;118:1010–18. With permission from the American Academy of Pediatrics.)

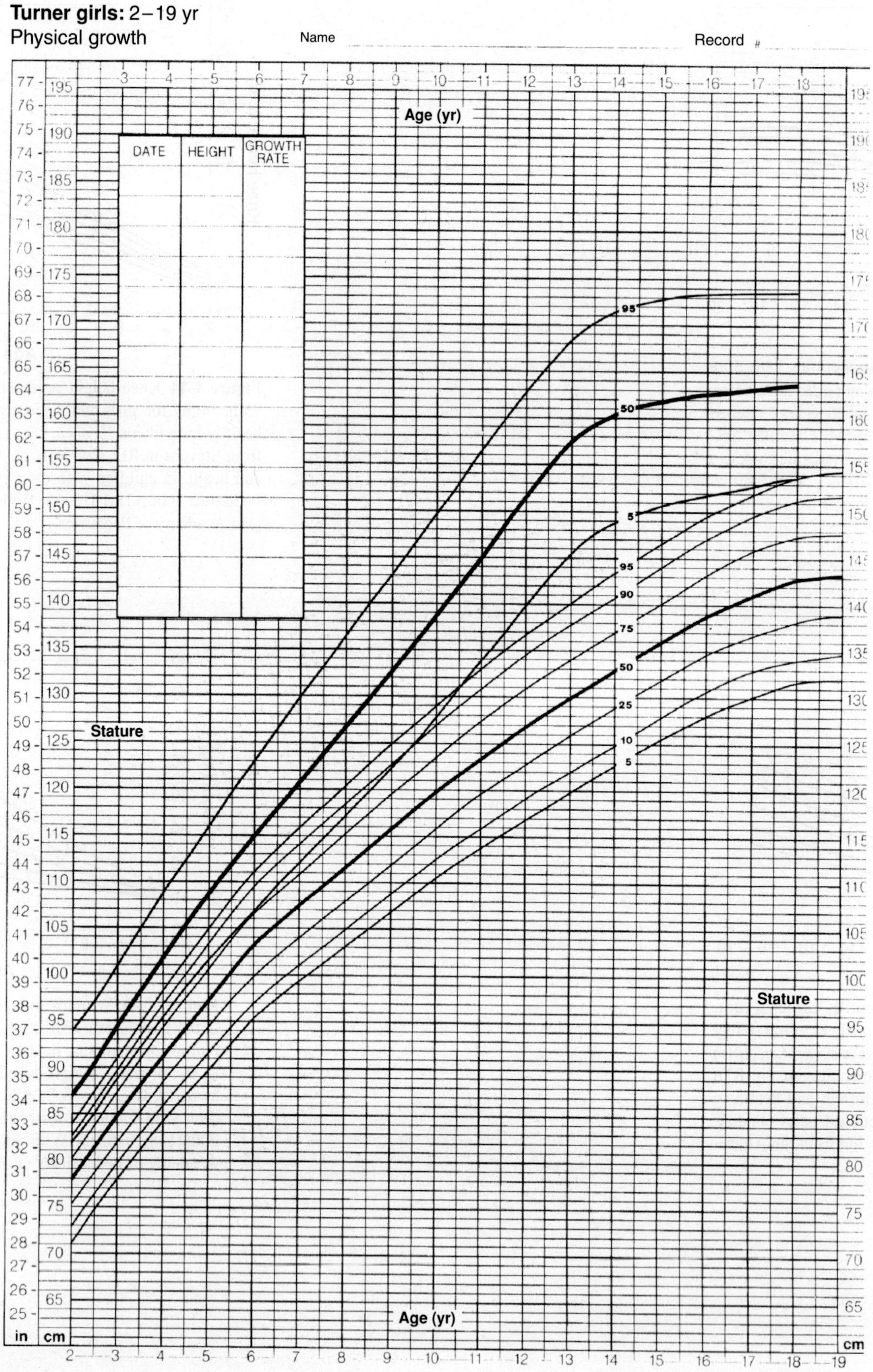

Figure I-47 Physical growth of girls with Turner syndrome (2 to 19 years). (Normal girls' (top three lines) percentiles derived from National Center for Health Statistics. Untreated Turner syndrome growth rates derived from Lyon AJ, Preece MA, Grant DB. Growth curve for girls with Turner syndrome. Arch Dis Child 1985;60:932–5. With permission from the BMJ Publishing Group.)

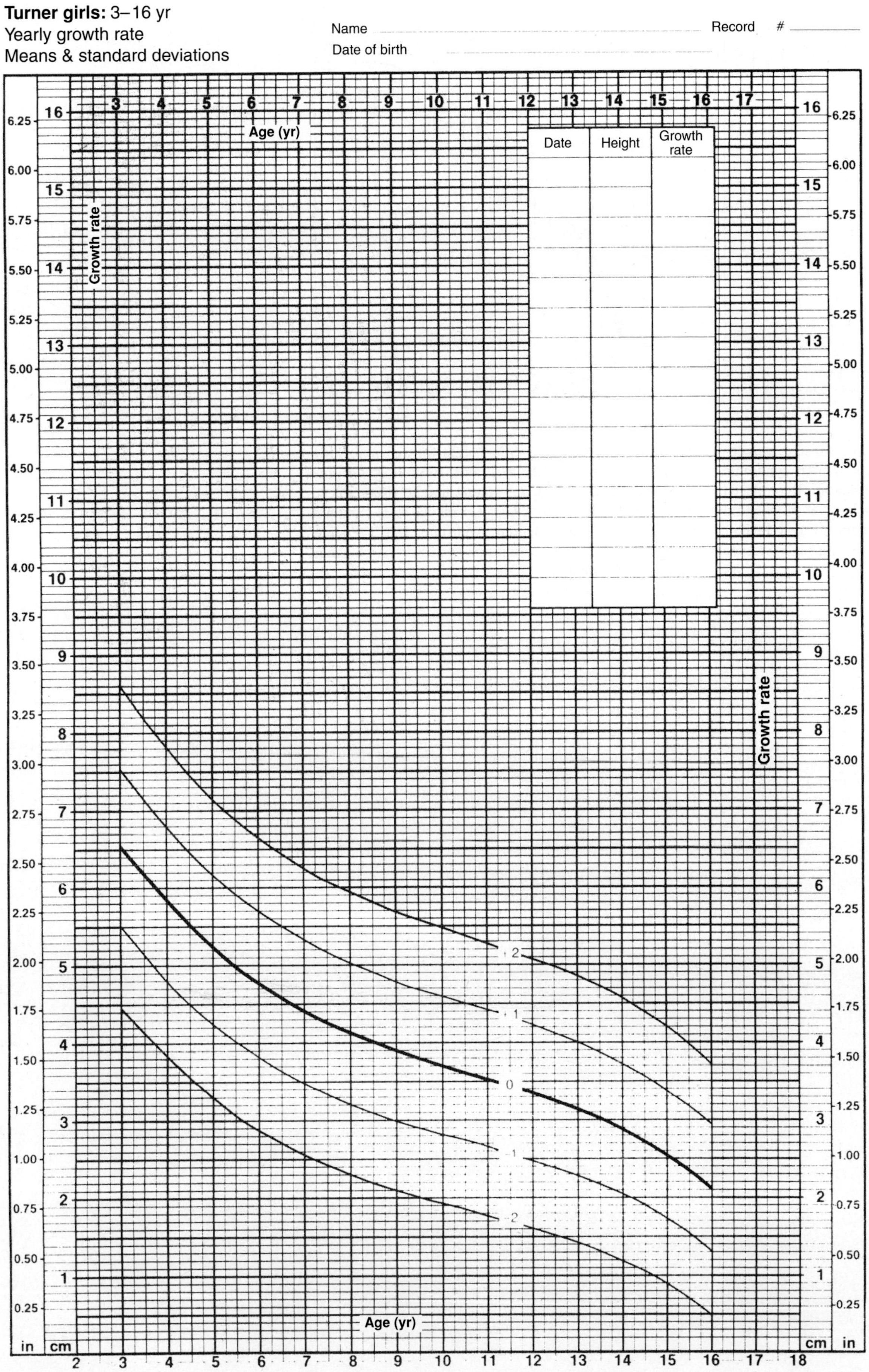

Figure I-48 Yearly growth rate means and standard deviations for girls with Turner syndrome (3 to 16 years). (Turner syndrome growth rates derived from Ranke MB, Pfluger H, Rosendahl W, et al. Turner syndrome: Spontaneous growth in 150 cases and review of the literature. Eur J Pediatr 1983;141:81–8. With permission from Springer Science and Business Media.)

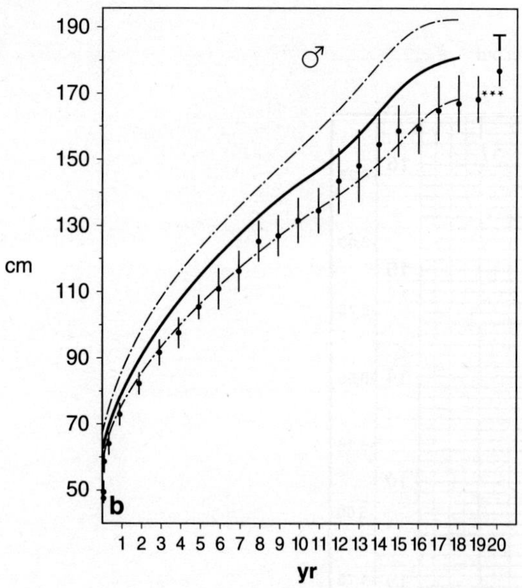

Figure I-49 Mean (±1 SD) height-for-age percentile curves for boys with Williams–Beuren syndrome (6 months to 20 years). *T* = target height. (Reproduced from Pankau R, Partsch C-J, Gosch A, et al. Statural growth in Williams–Beuren syndrome. Eur J Pediatr 1992;151:751–5. With permission from Springer Science and Business Media.)

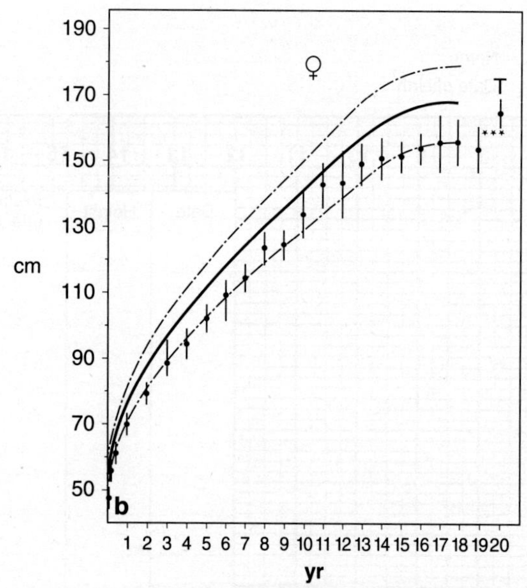

Figure I-50 Mean (±1 SD) height-for-age percentile curves for girls with Williams–Beuren syndrome (6 months to 20 years). *T* = target height. (Reproduced from Pankau R, Partsch C-J, Gosch A, et al. Statural growth in Williams–Beuren syndrome. Eur J Pediatr 1992;151:751–5. With permission from Springer Science and Business Media.)

Table I-1 Thickness of Triceps and Subscapular Skinfolds

		Triceps (mm)		Subscapular (mm)	
Age (mo)	Percentiles	Males	Females	Males	Females
1	<3	2.9	3.5	3.1	3.8
	10	4.0	4.5	4.2	4.9
	25	4.7	5.2	4.8	5.4
	50	5.3	5.8	5.6	6.2
	75	6.2	6.7	6.5	7.0
	90	7.0	7.6	7.5	7.9
	>97	8.1	8.3	8.3	9.0
3	<3	4.5	5.0	3.5	4.7
	10	6.0	6.2	4.9	5.9
	25	6.8	7.2	5.8	6.9
	50	8.1	8.2	6.9	8.0
	75	9.2	9.2	8.1	8.6
	90	10.3	10.5	9.0	9.4
	>97	11.7	11.8	10.7	11.1
6	<3	6.3	6.7	3.8	4.0
	10	7.8	8.2	5.5	5.9
	25	8.6	9.0	6.2	6.9
	50	9.7	10.4	7.1	8.1
	75	11.1	11.3	8.4	8.9
	90	11.8	12.7	10.1	10.3
	>97	13.5	13.9	11.0	12.4
9	<3	6.0	6.7	3.4	4.7
	10	7.5	7.9	5.3	6.0
	25	8.7	8.8	6.0	6.7
	50	9.9	10.1	7.1	7.6
	75	11.2	11.3	8.5	8.8
	90	12.5	12.5	9.7	10.1
	>97	14.0	13.5	11.4	11.1
12	<3	6.2	6.4	3.8	4.5
	10	7.8	7.6	5.3	6.0
	25	8.6	8.7	6.0	6.5
	50	9.8	9.8	7.2	7.5
	75	11.1	11.2	8.6	8.7
	90	12.2	12.2	9.6	9.8
	>97	3.8	13.6	11.0	10.9
18	<3	6.4	6.8	3.9	4.2
	10	7.7	7.9	5.3	5.7
	25	8.6	8.9	6.0	6.2
	50	9.9	10.3	6.8	7.1
	75	11.4	11.3	7.9	8.0
	90	12.2	12.3	9.3	9.0
	>97	13.6	13.6	10.3	10.2
24	<3	5.8	6.5	3.0	3.9
	10	7.4	8.3	4.6	5.3
	25	8.5	8.9	5.4	5.6
	50	9.8	10.1	6.5	6.5
	75	11.6	11.6	7.4	7.3
	90	13.1	12.8	8.3	8.4
	>97	14.2	14.1	10.2	9.5
36	<3	6.6	6.4	2.9	2.6
	10	7.8	8.2	4.5	4.7
	25	9.0	9.4	5.0	5.2
	50	9.8	10.3	5.5	6.1
	75	11.0	11.5	6.4	7.2
	90	12.2	12.5	7.1	8.6
	>97	13.4	14.4	8.9	10.6

Adapted from Karlberg P, Engstrom I, Lichtenstein H, Svennberg I. The development of children in a Swedish urban community: A prospective longitudinal study. III Physical growth during the first three years of life. Acta Paediatr Scand Suppl 1968;187:48–66. With permission from Taylor and Francis Group.

Table I-2 Percentiles of Upper Arm Circumference and Estimated Upper Arm Muscle Circumference

	Arm Circumference (mm)							Arm Muscle Circumference (mm)						
Age Group (yr)	5th	10th	25th	50th	75th	90th	95th	5th	10th	25th	50th	75th	90th	95th
Males														
0.0–0.4	113			134			153							
0.5–1.4	128			152			175							
1–1.9	142	146	150	159	170	176	183	110	113	119	127	135	144	147
2–2.9	141	145	153	162	170	178	185	111	114	122	130	140	146	150
3–3.9	150	153	160	167	175	184	190	117	123	131	137	143	148	153
4–4.9	149	154	162	171	180	186	192	123	126	133	141	148	156	159
5–5.9	153	160	167	175	185	195	204	128	133	140	147	154	162	169
6–6.9	155	159	167	179	188	209	228	131	135	142	151	161	170	177
7–7.9	162	167	177	187	201	223	230	137	139	151	160	168	177	190
8–8.9	162	170	177	190	202	220	245	140	145	154	162	170	182	187
9–9.9	175	178	187	200	217	249	257	151	154	161	170	183	196	202
10–10.9	181	184	196	210	231	262	274	156	160	166	180	191	209	221
11–11.9	186	190	202	223	244	261	280	159	165	173	183	195	205	230
12–12.9	193	200	214	232	254	282	303	167	171	182	195	210	223	241
13–13.9	194	211	228	247	263	286	301	172	179	196	211	226	239	245
14–14.9	220	226	237	253	283	303	322	189	199	212	223	240	260	264
15–15.9	222	229	244	264	284	311	320	199	204	218	237	254	266	272
16–16.9	244	248	262	278	303	324	343	213	225	234	249	269	287	296
17–17.9	246	253	267	285	308	336	347	224	231	245	258	273	294	312
18–18.9	245	260	276	297	321	353	379	226	237	252	264	283	298	324
19–24.9	262	272	288	308	331	355	372	238	245	257	273	289	309	321
25–34.9	271	282	300	319	342	362	375	243	250	264	279	298	314	326
35–44.9	278	287	305	326	345	363	374	247	255	269	286	302	318	327
45–54.9	267	281	301	322	342	362	376	239	249	265	281	300	315	326
55–64.9	258	273	296	317	336	355	369	236	245	260	278	295	310	320
65–74.9	248	263	285	307	325	344	355	223	235	251	268	284	298	306
Females														
0.0–0.4	107			127			150							
0.5–1.4	125			146			170							
1–1.9	138	142	148	156	164	172	177	105	111	117	124	132	139	143
2–2.9	142	145	152	160	167	176	184	111	114	119	126	133	142	147
3–3.9	143	150	158	167	175	183	189	113	119	124	132	140	146	152
4–4.9	149	154	160	169	177	184	191	115	121	128	136	144	152	157
5–5.9	153	157	165	175	185	203	211	125	128	134	142	151	159	165
6–6.9	156	162	170	176	187	204	211	130	133	138	145	154	166	171
7–7.9	164	167	174	183	199	216	231	129	135	142	151	160	171	176
8–8.9	168	172	183	195	214	247	261	138	140	151	160	171	183	194
9–9.9	178	182	194	211	224	251	260	147	150	158	167	180	194	198
10–10.9	174	182	193	210	228	251	265	148	150	159	170	180	190	197
11–11.9	185	194	208	224	248	276	303	150	158	171	181	196	217	223
12–12.9	194	203	216	237	256	282	294	162	166	180	191	201	214	220
13–13.9	202	211	223	243	271	301	338	169	175	183	198	211	226	240
14–14.9	214	223	237	252	272	304	322	174	179	190	201	216	232	247
15–15.9	208	221	239	254	279	300	322	175	178	189	202	215	228	244
16–16.9	218	224	241	258	283	318	334	170	180	190	202	216	234	249
17–17.9	220	227	241	264	295	324	350	175	183	194	205	221	239	257
18–18.9	222	227	241	258	281	312	325	174	179	191	202	215	237	245
19–24.9	221	230	247	265	290	319	345	179	185	195	207	221	236	249
25–34.9	233	240	256	277	304	342	368	183	188	199	212	228	246	264
35–44.9	241	251	267	290	317	356	378	186	192	205	218	236	257	272
45–54.9	242	256	274	299	328	362	384	187	193	206	220	238	260	274
55–64.9	243	257	280	303	335	367	385	187	196	209	225	244	266	280
65–74.9	240	252	274	299	326	356	373	185	195	208	225	244	264	279

Data collected from whites in the United States Health and Nutrition Examination Survey 1 (1971–1974).

Adapted from Frisancho AR. Triceps skin fold and upper arm muscle size norms for assessment of nutritional status. Am J Clin Nutr 1974;27:1052–58 and Frisancho AR. New norms of upper limb fat and muscle areas for assessment of nutritional status. Am J Clin Nutr 1981;34:2540–5. With permission from the American Society for Nutrition.

Table I-3 Percentiles of Triceps Skinfolds

Age Group (yr)	5th	10th	25th	50th	75th	90th	95th
Males							
1–1.9	6	7	8	10	12	14	16
2–2.9	6	7	8	10	12	14	15
3–3.9	6	7	8	10	11	14	15
4–4.9	6	6	8	9	11	12	14
5–5.9	6	6	8	9	11	14	15
6–6.9	5	6	7	8	10	13	16
7–7.9	5	6	7	9	12	15	17
8–8.9	5	6	7	8	10	13	16
9–9.9	6	6	7	10	13	17	18
10–10.9	6	6	8	10	14	18	21
11–11.9	6	6	8	11	16	20	24
12–12.9	6	6	8	11	14	22	28
13–13.9	5	5	7	10	14	22	26
14–14.9	4	5	7	9	14	21	24
15–15.9	4	5	6	8	11	18	24
16–16.9	4	5	6	8	12	16	22
17–17.9	5	5	6	8	12	16	19
18–18.9	4	5	6	9	13	20	24
19–24.9	4	5	7	10	15	20	22
25–34.9	5	6	8	12	16	20	24
35–44.9	5	6	8	12	16	20	23
45–54.9	6	6	8	12	15	20	25
55–64.9	5	6	8	11	14	19	22
65–74.9	4	6	8	11	15	19	22
Females							
1–1.9	6	7	8	10	12	14	16
2–2.9	6	8	9	10	12	15	16
3–3.9	7	8	9	11	12	14	15
4–4.9	7	8	8	10	12	14	16
5–5.9	6	7	8	10	12	15	18
6–6.9	6	6	8	10	12	14	16
7–7.9	6	7	9	11	13	16	18
8–8.9	6	8	9	12	15	18	24
9–9.9	8	8	10	13	16	20	22
10–10.9	7	8	10	12	17	23	27
11–11.9	7	8	10	13	18	24	28
12–12.9	8	9	11	14	18	23	27
13–13.9	8	8	12	15	21	26	30
14–14.9	9	10	13	16	21	26	28
15–15.9	8	10	12	17	21	25	32
16–16.9	10	12	15	18	22	26	31
17–17.9	10	12	13	19	24	30	37
18–18.9	10	12	15	18	22	26	30
19–24.9	10	11	14	18	24	30	34
25–34.9	10	12	16	21	27	34	37
35–44.9	12	14	18	23	29	35	38
45–54.9	12	16	20	25	30	36	40
55 64.9	12	16	20	25	31	36	38
65–74.9	12	14	18	24	29	34	36

Adapted from Frisancho AR. New norms of upper limb fat and muscle areas for assessment of nutritional status. Am J Clin Nutr 1981;34:2540–5. With permission from the American Society for Nutrition.

Table I-4 Percentiles for Estimates of Upper Arm Muscle Area and Upper Arm Fat Area

	Arm Muscle Area (mm)							Arm Fat Area (mm)						
Age Group (yr)	5	10	25	50	75	90	95	5	10	25	50	75	90	95
Males														
1–1.9	956	1,014	1,133	1,278	1,447	1,644	1,720	452	486	590	741	895	1,036	1,176
2–2.9	973	1,040	1,190	1,345	1,557	1,690	1,787	434	504	578	737	871	1,044	1,148
3–3.9	1,095	1,201	1,357	1,484	1,618	1,750	1,853	464	519	590	736	868	1,071	1,151
4–4.9	1,207	1,264	1,408	1,579	1,747	1,926	2,008	428	494	598	722	859	989	1,085
5–5.9	1,298	1,411	1,550	1,720	1,884	2,089	2,285	446	488	582	713	914	1,176	1,299
6–6.9	1,360	1,447	1,605	1,815	2,056	2,297	2,493	371	446	539	678	896	1,115	1,519
7–7.9	1,497	1,548	1,808	2,027	2,246	2,494	2,886	423	473	574	758	1,011	1,393	1,511
8–8.9	1,550	1,664	1,895	2,089	2,296	2,628	2,788	410	460	588	725	1,003	1,248	1,558
9–9.9	1,811	1,884	2,067	2,288	2,657	3,053	3,257	485	527	635	859	1,252	1,864	2,081
10–10.9	1,930	2,027	2,182	2,575	2,903	3,486	3,882	523	543	738	982	1,376	1,906	2,609
11–11.9	2,016	2,156	2,382	2,670	3,022	3,359	4,226	536	595	754	1,148	1,710	2,348	2,574
12–12.9	2,216	2,339	2,649	3,022	3,496	3,968	4,640	554	650	874	1,172	1,558	2,536	3,580
13–13.9	2,363	2,546	3,044	3,553	4,081	4,502	4,794	475	570	812	1,096	1,702	2,744	3,322
14–14.9	2,830	3,147	3,586	3,963	4,575	5,368	5,530	453	563	786	1,082	1,608	2,746	3,508
15–15.9	3,138	3,317	3,788	4,481	5,134	5,631	5,900	521	595	690	931	1,423	2,434	3,100
16–16.9	3,625	4,044	4,352	4,951	5,753	6,576	6,980	542	593	844	1,078	1,746	2,280	3,041
17–17.9	3,998	4,252	4,777	5,286	5,950	6,886	7,726	598	698	827	1,096	1,636	2,407	2,888
18–18.9	4,070	4,481	5,066	5,552	6,374	7,067	8,355	560	665	860	1,264	1,947	3,302	3,928
19–24.9	4,508	4,777	5,274	5,913	6,660	7,606	8,200	594	743	963	1,406	2,231	3,098	3,652
25–34.9	4,694	4,963	5,541	6,214	7,067	7,847	8,436	675	831	1,174	1,752	2,459	3,246	3,786
35–44.9	4,844	5,181	5,740	6,490	7,265	8,034	8,488	703	851	1,310	1,792	2,463	3,098	3,624
45–54.9	4,546	4,946	5,589	6,297	7,142	7,918	8,458	749	922	1,254	1,741	2,359	3,245	3,928
55–64.9	4,422	4,783	5,381	6,144	6,919	7,670	8,149	658	839	1,166	1,645	2,236	2,976	3,466
65–74.9	3,973	4,411	5,031	5,716	6,432	7,074	7,453	573	753	1,122	1,621	2,199	2,876	3,327
Females														
1–1.9	885	973	1,084	1,221	1,378	1,535	1,621	401	466	578	706	847	1,022	1,140
2–2.9	973	1,029	1,119	1,269	1,405	1,595	1,727	469	526	642	747	894	1,061	1,173
3–3.9	1,014	1,133	1,227	1,396	1,563	1,690	1,846	473	529	656	822	967	1,106	1,158
4–4.9	1,058	1,171	1,313	1,475	1,644	1,832	1,958	490	541	654	766	907	1,109	1,236
5–5.9	1,238	1,301	1,423	1,598	1,825	2,012	2,159	470	529	647	812	991	1,330	1,536
6–6.9	1,354	1,414	1,513	1,683	1,877	2,182	2,323	464	508	638	827	1,009	1,263	1,436
7–7.9	1,330	1,441	1,602	1,815	2,045	2,332	2,469	491	560	706	920	1,135	1,407	1,644
8–8.9	1,513	1,566	1,808	2,034	2,327	2,657	2,996	527	634	769	1,042	1,383	1,872	2,482
9–9.9	1,723	1,788	1,976	2,227	2,571	2,987	3,112	642	690	933	1,219	1,584	2,171	2,524
10–10.9	1,740	1,784	2,019	2,296	2,583	2,873	3,093	616	702	842	1,141	1,608	2,500	3,005
11–11.9	1,784	1,987	2,316	2,612	3,071	3,739	3,953	707	802	1,015	1,301	1,942	2,730	3,690
12–12.9	2,092	2,182	2,579	2,904	3,225	3,655	3,847	782	854	1,090	1,511	2,056	2,666	3,369
13–13.9	2,269	2,426	2,657	3,130	3,529	4,081	4,568	726	838	1,219	1,625	2,374	3,272	4,150
14–14.9	2,418	2,562	2,874	3,220	3,704	4,294	4,850	981	1,043	1,423	1,818	2,403	3,250	3,765
15–15.9	2,426	2,518	2,847	3,248	3,689	4,123	4,756	839	1,126	1,396	1,886	2,544	3,093	4,195
16–16.9	2,308	2,567	2,865	3,248	3,718	4,353	4,946	1,126	1,351	1,663	2,006	2,598	3,374	4,236
17–17.9	2,442	2,674	2,996	3,336	3,883	4,552	5,251	1,042	1,267	1,463	2,104	2,977	3,864	5,159
18–18.9	2,398	2,538	2,917	3,243	3,694	4,461	4,767	1,003	1,230	1,616	2,104	2,617	3,508	3,733
19–24.9	2,538	2,728	3,026	3,406	3,877	4,439	4,940	1,046	1,198	1,596	2,166	2,959	4,050	4,896
25–34.9	2,661	2,826	3,148	3,573	4,138	4,806	5,541	1,173	1,399	1,841	2,548	3,512	4,690	5,560
35–44.9	2,750	2,948	3,359	3,783	4,428	5,240	5,877	1,336	1,619	2,158	2,898	3,932	5,093	5,847
45–54.9	2,784	2,956	3,378	3,858	4,520	5,375	5,964	1,459	1,803	2,447	3,244	4,229	5,416	6,140
55–64.9	2,784	3,063	3,477	4,045	4,750	5,632	6,247	1,345	1,879	2,520	3,369	4,360	5,276	6,152
65–74.9	2,737	3,018	3,444	4,019	4,739	5,566	6,214	1,363	1,681	2,266	3,063	3,943	4,914	5,530

Adapted from Frisancho AR. New norms of upper limb fat and muscle areas for assessment of nutritional status. Am J Clin Nutr 1981;34:2540–45. With permission from the American Society for Nutrition.

Table I-5 Selected Percentiles for 2-month Increments in Weight (Birth to 12 months)

				Percentiles (g/d)						
Age (mo)	Infants (n)	Mean (g/d)	SD (g/d)	5th	10th	25th	50th	75th	90th	95th
Males										
Birth to 2	580	33	7.0	21	24	28	32	38	42	44
1–3	580	31	6.9	20	22	27	31	35	39	43
2–4	65	23	4.7	–	17	19	23	26	29	–
3–5	298	19	3.2	14	15	17	18	20	22	24
4–6	298	16	2.9	12	13	14	16	18	20	21
5–7	233	15	2.4	11	12	13	15	16	18	18
6–8	233	13	2.4	10	11	12	13	15	16	17
7–9	233	12	2.4	9	10	11	12	14	15	16
8–10	233	12	2.4	9	9	10	11	13	15	15
9–11	233	11	2.3	8	8	9	11	12	14	14
10–12	233	10	2.3	7	8	9	10	12	13	14
Females										
Birth to 2	562	28	6.5	17	20	23	28	32	36	38
1–3	562	26	6.3	16	19	22	26	30	34	37
2–4	72	22	5.4	–	16	19	21	24	27	–
3–5	298	18	4.7	13	14	16	17	19	21	22
4–6	298	15	4.6	11	12	14	15	17	18	19
5–7	224	14	4.7	11	11	13	14	15	17	17
6–8	224	13	4.6	10	10	12	13	14	16	16
7–9	224	12	4.5	9	10	11	12	13	15	15
8–10	224	12	4.5	8	9	10	11	13	14	14
9–11	224	11	4.4	8	8	9	10	12	13	14
10–12	224	10	4.3	7	8	9	10	11	13	13

Adapted from Guo S, Roche AF, Fomon SJ, et al. Reference data on gains in weight and length during the first two years of life. J Pediatr 1991;119:355-62. With permission from Elsevier.

Table I-6 Selected Percentiles for 3-month Increments in Length (Birth to 14 months)

				Percentile						
Age (mo)	Infants (n)	Mean (mm/d)	SD (mm/d)	5th	10th	25th	50th	75th	90th	95th
Males										
Birth to 3	580	1.07	0.11	0.89	0.92	0.99	1.06	1.14	1.21	1.26
1–4	65	1.00	0.08	–	0.94	1.01	1.06	1.09	–	
2–5	65	0.84	0.09	–	0.74	0.79	0.84	0.91	0.95	–
3–6	255	0.69	0.08	0.56	0.60	0.64	0.68	0.73	0.79	0.82
4–7	190	0.62	0.06	0.54	0.55	0.58	0.61	0.65	0.73	0.72
5–8	190	0.56	0.05	0.49	0.50	0.53	0.56	0.59	0.69	0.65
6–9	190	0.52	0.05	0.46	0.46	0.49	0.52	0.54	0.58	0.60
7–10	190	0.48	0.05	0.42	0.43	0.45	0.48	0.51	0.54	0.57
8–11	190	0.45	0.04	0.39	0.40	0.43	0.45	0.48	0.51	0.53
9–12	190	0.43	0.04	0.36	0.38	0.40	0.43	0.45	0.48	0.51
10–13	190	0.41	0.04	0.34	0.36	0.38	0.41	0.43	0.46	0.49
11–14	190	0.39	0.04	0.33	0.34	0.36	0.39	0.41	0.44	0.47
Females										
Birth to 3	562	0.99	0.10	0.82	0.86	0.93	0.99	1.06	1.11	1.15
1–4	74	0.95	0.10	–	0.84	0.87	0.95	1.02	1.07	–
2–5	74	0.80	0.10	–	0.67	0.73	0.81	0.87	0.92	–
3–6	241	0.67	0.08	0.55	0.58	0.63	0.67	0.72	0.77	0.79
4–7	167	0.60	0.06	0.53	0.54	0.57	0.61	0.64	0.67	0.69
5–8	167	0.56	0.05	0.49	0.50	0.52	0.56	0.59	0.62	0.63
6–9	167	0.52	0.05	0.45	0.46	0.48	0.52	0.55	0.57	0.58
7–10	167	0.48	0.04	0.42	0.43	0.45	0.49	0.52	0.54	0.55
8–11	167	0.46	0.04	0.39	0.41	0.43	0.46	0.49	0.51	0.52
9–12	167	0.44	0.04	0.37	0.38	0.41	0.44	0.46	0.48	0.49
10–13	167	0.42	0.04	0.35	0.37	0.39	0.42	0.45	0.46	0.48
11–14	167	0.40	0.04	0.34	0.35	0.37	0.40	0.43	0.44	0.46

Adapted from Guo S, Roche AF, Fomon SJ, et al. Reference data on gains in weight and length during the first two years of life. J Pediatr 1991;119:355-62. With permission from Elsevier.

Table I-7 Most Common Classifications of Protein-Energy Malnutrition

	Normal	Mild	Moderate	Severe
Weight for height*	>90	80–90	70 to 80	<70
Weight for height†			$-3 \leq$ SD-score$^{\ddagger} < -2$	SD-score$^{\ddagger} < -3$
Height for age*	>95	87–98	80 to 87	<80
Height for age†			$-3 \leq$ SD-score$^{\ddagger} < -2$	SD-score$^{\ddagger} < -3$

*Adapted from Waterlow JC. Classification and definition of protein-calorie malnutrition. BMJ 1972;3:566–69. With permission from the BMJ Publishing Group.

†Adapted from World Health Organization. Management of Severe Malnutrition: A Manual for Physicians and Other Senior Health Care Workers. Geneva: WHO;1999. p. 4.

$$^{\ddagger}\text{SD-score} = \frac{\text{(Observed valued)} - \text{(Median reference value from NCHS/WHO reference)}}{\text{Standard deviation of reference population}}$$

Table I-8 Growth Charts for Specific Syndromes

Condition	Reference(s)
Achondroplasia	Hagenäs L, Hertel T. Skeletal dysplasia, growth hormone treatment and body proportion: Comparison with other syndromic and non-syndromic short children. Horm Res 2003;60:65–70. Height for boys and girls, 0–20 yr; sitting height to total height ratio in girls, 0–20 yr Horton WA, Rotter JI, Rimoin DL, et al. Standard growth curves for achondroplasia. J Pediatr 1978;93:435–8. Stature, growth velocity, head circumference, upper and lower segments
Brachmann (Cornelia)-de Lange syndrome	Kline AD, Barr M, Jackson LG. Growth manifestations in the Brachmann-de Lange syndrome. Am J Med Genet 1993;47:1042–49. Length- and weight-for-age, birth to 36 mo; height- and weight-for age, 2–18 yr; head circumference-for-age, birth to18 yr
Cerebral palsy quadriplegia	Krick J, Murphy-Miller P, Zeger S, et al. Pattern of growth in children with cerebral palsy. J Am Diet Assoc 1996;96(7):680–5* Stature- and weight-for-age and weight-for-stature, birth to 10 yr Stevenson RD, Conaway M, Chumlea WC, et al. Growth and health in children with moderate-to-severe cerebral palsy. Pediatrics 2006;118:1010–8* Knee height-for-age, weight-for-age, and other measures, 2–18 yr
Down syndrome	Cronk CE. Growth of children with Down's syndrome: Birth to age 3 yr. Pediatrics 1978;61:564–68 and Pediatrics 1988;81:102–10.* Length-for-age and weight-for-age, birth to 36 mo; stature-for-age and weight-for-age, 2–18 yr Palmer CGS, Cronk C, Pueschel SM, et al. Head circumference of children with Down syndrome (0–36 months). Am J Med Genet 1992;42:61–7* Head circumference-for-age, 0–36 mo Styles ME, Cole TJ, Dennis J, et al. New cross sectional stature, weight, and head circumference references for Down's syndrome in the UK and Republic of Ireland. Arch Dis Child 2002;87:104–8. Weight and height, 0–18 yr; head cirumference, 0–5 yr (UK and Ireland)
Marfan's syndrome	Pyeritz RE. Marfan syndrome and other disorders of fibrillin. In: Rimoin DL, Connor JM, Pyeritz RE, editors. Principles and Practice of Medical Genetics. New York: Churchill Livingstone; 1997. Pyeritz RE, Murphy EA, Lin SJ, et al. Growth and anthropometrics in the Marfan syndrome. In: Papadatos CJ, Bartsocas CS, editors. Endocrine Genetics and Genetics of Growth (Prog Clin Biol Res v200). New York: Alan R. Liss, Inc.; 1985. Stature- and weight-for-age, 2–18 yr, 20–24 yr, and >24 yr; upper and lower segment ratios, 2–20 yr and adult
Myelomeningocele	Appendix II, Growth grids for special conditions. In: Ekvall SW, Ekvall VK, editors. Pediatric Nutrition in Chronic Diseases and Developmental Disorders: Prevention, Assessment, and Treatment. New York: Oxford University Press; 2005. Preliminary charts, height- and weight-for-age, 2–18 yr Duval-Beaupere G, Kaci M, Lougovoy J, et al. Growth of trunk and legs of children with myelomeningocele. Dev Med Child Neur 1987;29:225–31. Height, upper segment, lower segment measurements, 1–16 yr Trollmann R, Dorr HG, Strehl E, et al. Growth and pubertal development in patients with meningomyelocele: A retrospective analysis. Acta Paediatr 1996;85:76–80. Arm span
Noonan's syndrome	Witt DR, Biedermann B, Hall JG. Clin Genet 1986;30:150–3. Stature-for-age, birth to 18 yr Ranke MB, Heidemann P, Knupfer C, et al. Noonan syndrome: Growth and clinical manifestations in 144 cases. Eur J Pediatr 1988;148:220–7. Height-for-age
Prader–Willi syndrome	Holm VA. Appendix I. Greenswag LR, Alexander RC, editors. In: Management of Prader-Willi Syndrome. New York: Springer Verlag; 1998. p. 317. Height-for-age, 3–25 yr Butler MG, Meaney FJ. Standards for selected anthropometric measurements in Prader–Willi syndrome. Pediatrics 1991;88:853–60* Weight, height, sitting height, head circumference, triceps and subscapular skinfold, plus other measures, 2–22 yr
Sickle cell disease	Phebus CK, Gloninger MG, Maciak BJ. Growth patterns by age and sex in children with sickle cell disease. J Pediatr 1984;105:28–33. Height- and weight-for-age, birth to 18 yr Tanner JM, Davies PS. Clinical longitudinal standards for height and height velocity for North American children. J Pediatr 1985;107:317–29. Height velocity (cm/yr), 2.5–19 yr Stevens MCG, Maude GH, Cupidore L, et al. Prepubertal growth and skeletal maturation in children with sickle cell disease. Pediatrics 1986;78:124–32. Weight, height, height velocity, bone age, 0–9 yr
Silver–Russell syndrome	Tanner JM, Lejarraga H, Cameron N. The natural history of the Silver-Russell syndrome: A longitudinal study of thirty-nine cases. Pediatr Res 1975;9:611–23. Height- and height velocity-for-age, 2–19 yr (includes periods of treatment with human growth hormone)
Turner syndrome	Lyon AJ, Preece MA, Grant DB. Growth curve for girls with Turner syndrome. Arch Dis Child 1985:60:932–5* Height-for-age, 2–19 yr (girls) Ranke MB, Pfluger H, Rosendahl W, et al. Turner syndrome: Spontaneous growth in 150 cases and review of the literature. Eur J Pediatr 1983;141:81–8* Height- and height velocity-for-age, bone age
Williams–Beuren syndrome	Morris CA, Demsey SA, Leonard CO, et al. Natural history of Williams syndrome: Physical characteristics. J Pediatr 1988;113:318–26. Stature-for-age, birth to 24 mo and birth to 18 yr; weight-for-age, birth to 18 yr; head circumference-for-age, birth to 36 mo and 2–18 yr Pankau R, Partsch CJ, Gosch A, et al. Statural growth in Williams–Beuren syndrome. Eur J Pediatr 1992;151;751–5* Height-for-age, head-circumference-for-age Pankau R, Partsch CJ, Neblung A, et al. Natural history of body mass index in Williams-Beuren syndrome. Am J Med Genet 1994;52:51–4. BMI-for-age, both genders, 0–18 yr

*A copy of the growth chart is included in this appendix.

Table I-9 Clinical Examination in Nutritional Deficiencies and Excesses

	Major Physiologic Functions	Deficiency Signs	Excess Signs	Important Food Sources	Potential Causes of Deficiency	Status Assessment
Nutrient						
Carbohydrate	Supplies energy at an average of 4 kcal/g (sparing protein) and is the major energy source for CNS function; unrefined, complex carbohydrates supply fiber which aids in normal bowel function	Ketosis	May cause diarrhea, obesity	Bread, cereals, crackers, potatoes, corn, simple sugar (sugar, honey), fruits and vegetables, milk, breast milk, infant formula	Malabsorption	Blood sugar, OGTT
Fat	Concentrated calorie source at an average of 9 kcal/g; constitutes part of the membrane structure of every cell; supplies essential fatty acids; provides and carries fat-soluble vitamins (A, D, E, K)	Essential fatty acid deficiency (dry, scaly skin, poor weight gain, hair loss); requirements are increased by cell turnover	Atherosclerosis may be affected by excessive intakes of certain dietary fats; altered blood lipid levels	Shortening, oil, butter, margarine, protein-rich foods (meat, dairy, nuts), breast milk, infant formula	Cystic fibrosis, biliary disease, short bowel syndrome, hereditary lipoprotein disorders	Total cholesterol, LDL, HDL
Protein	Supplies energy at an average of 4 kcal/g; regulates body processes as part of enzymes, hormones, body fluids, and antibodies that increase resistance to infection; provides nitrogen; constitutes part of the membrane structure of every cell	Dry, depigmented, easily pluckable hair; bilateral, dependent edema, cirrhosis, fatty liver, decreased visceral proteins; skin is dry with pellagroid dermatosis in severe cases	Azotemia, acidosis, hyperammonemia	Meat, poultry, fish, legumes, eggs, cheese, milk and other dairy products, nuts, breast milk, infant formula	Protein losing enteropathy, liver disease, gastrointestinal disease, renal disease	Albumin, retinol binding protein, prealbumin
Fat soluble vitamins						
Vitamin A	Formation and maintenance of skin and mucous membranes; necessary for the formation of rhodopsin of the rods governing vision in dim light; regulation of membrane structure and function; necessary for growth and normal immune function	Night blindness, degeneration of the retina, xeropthalmia, follicular hyperkeratosis, poor growth, keratomalacia, Bitot's spots	Fatigue, malaise, lethargy, abdominal pain, hepatomegaly, alopecia, headache with increased intracranial pressure	Carrots, liver, green vegetables, sweet potatoes, butter, margarine, apricots, melons, peaches, broccoli, cod liver oil, breast milk, infant formula	Liver disease, cystic fibrosis, short bowel syndrome, protein deficiency (alters transport)	Plasma retinol (HPLC), plasma retinol-binding protein, relative dose response, dark adaptation test, liver biopsy concentration
Vitamin D	Promotes intestinal absorption of calcium and phosphate, and renal conservation of calcium and phosphorus	Rickets, osteomalacia, costochondral beading, epiphyseal enlargement, cranial bossing, bowed legs, persistently open anterior fontanelle	Hypercalcemia, vomiting, anorexia, diarrhea, convulsions	Cod liver oil, fish, eggs, liver, butter, fortified milk, sunlight (activation of 7-dehydrocholesterol in the skin), infant formula	Liver disease, cystic fibrosis, short bowel syndrome, renal disease	Plasma 25-hydrooxyvitamin D (HPLC), serum alkaline phosphatase, calcium and phosphate, radiography, bone densiometry
Vitamin E	Acts as an antioxidant and free radical scavenger to prevent peroxidation of polyunsaturated fatty acids in the body; neuromuscular function	Hemolytic anemia in the premature and newborn, enhanced fragility of red blood cells, increased peroxidative hemolysis	In anemia, suppresses the normal hematologic response to iron	Oils high in polyunsaturated fatty acids, milk, eggs, breast milk, infant formula	Cystic fibrosis, short bowel syndrome, liver disease	Plasma tocopherol (HPLC) (corrected for total or LDL- cholesterol), hydrogen peroxide hemolysis
Vitamin K	Necessary for prothrombin and the three blood-clotting factors VII, IX, and X; half of the vitamin K in humans is of intestinal origin, synthesized by gut flora; necessary for bone mineralization	Hemorrhagic manifestations (especially in newborns), prolonged clotting	Hemolytic anemia, nerve palsy	Green leafy vegetables, fruits, cereals, dairy products, soybeans, breast milk, infant formula	Liver disease, antibiotic therapy	Prothrombin time (prolonged), plasma phylloquinone, clotting factor levels, proteins induced by vit. K absence or antagonists-II (PIVKA-II)

(*Continued*)

Table I-9 Clinical Examination in Nutritional Deficiencies and Excesses (*Continued*)

	Major Physiologic Functions	Deficiency Signs	Excess Signs	Important Food Sources	Potential Causes of Deficiency	Status Assessment
Water soluble vitamins						
Ascorbic acid (vitamin C)	Forms collagen cross-linkage of proline hydroxylase, thus strengthening tissue and improving wound healing and resistance to infection; aids absorption of iron	Joint tenderness, scurvy (capillary hemorrhaging), impaired wound healing, acute periodontal gingivitis, petechiae, purpura, anemia	Documentation of a chronic high intake may result in "rebound" deficiency symptoms	Heat-labile; broccoli, papaya, orange, mango, grapefruit, strawberries, tomatoes, potatoes, leafy vegetables, breast milk, infant formula	Stress	Plasma level (enzyme assay/HPLC), leukocyte concentration (longer-term), whole blood concentration, urine concentration
Biotin	Component of several carboxylating enzymes; plays an important role in the metabolism of fat and carbohydrate	Anorexia, nausea, vomiting; glossitis; depression; dry, scaly dermatitis; thin hair; loss of eyebrows	None known	Liver, kidney, egg yolk, breast milk, infant formula	Certain inborn errors of metabolism	Plasma (microbiologic plasma lactate, assay), urine organic acids, lymphocyte carboxylase
Cobalamin (B_{12} intrinsic factor required)	Cobalamin-containing coenzymes function in the degradation of certain odd-chain fatty acids and in the recycling of tetrahydrofolate	Megaloblastic anemia, neurologic deterioration	None known	Animal products, breast milk, infant formula	Ileal disease, strict vegetarian, lack of Intrinsic Factor	Plasma level (RIA or microbiologic), Schilling test, plasma homocysteine, deoxyuridine suppression test
Folacin	Utilized in carbon transfer and nucleotide synthesis	Megaloblastic anemia, stomatitis, glossitis, neural tube defects in pregnancy	None known	Liver, leafy vegetables, fruit, yeast, breast milk, infant formula	Liver disease, alcoholism, celiac disease, inflammatory bowel disease	Plasma level (RIA or microbiologic), red cell level
Niacin	Aids in energy utilization as part of a coenzyme (NAD+ and NADP+) in fat synthesis, tissue respiration, and carbohydrate utilization; aids digestion and fosters normal appetite; synthesized from the amino acid tryptophan	Pellagra (dermatitis, diarrhea, dementia, death), cheilosis, angular stomatic inflammation of mucous membranes, weakness	Dilation of the capillaries, vasomotor instability, "flushing" (utilization of muscle glycogen, serum lipids, mobilization of fatty acids during exercise)	Liver, meat, fish, poultry, peanuts, fortified cereal products, yeast, breast milk, infant formula	B_6 deficiency (impairs conversion of tryptophan to niacin)	Urine ratio of metabolites (*N*-methylnicotinamide/2-pyridone), tryptophan load, red cell NAD or NAD/NADP ratio
Pantothenic acid	Component of coenzyme A; plays a role in release of energy from carbohydrates and in synthesis and degradation of fatty acids	Infertility, abortion, slow growth, depression, vomiting, malaise, abdominal stress	Diarrhea, water retention	Meat, fish, poultry, whole grains, legumes, breast milk, infant formula	Severe malnutrition	Urine excretion, whole blood level (RIA/microbiologic)
Pyridoxine (B_6)	Coenzyme component for many of the enzymes of amino acid metabolism; all compounds implicated as neurotransmitters are synthesized and/or metabolized in B_6-dependent reactions	Convulsions, weight loss, abdominal distress, vomiting, hyperirritability, depression, confusion, hypochromic and macrocytic anemia	Neuropathy	Fish, poultry, meat, wheat, breast milk, infant formula	Elderly, high protein intake	Red cell aminotransferase activity, pyridoxal phosphate (HPLC), tryptophan load test, urine 4-pyridoxic acid
Riboflavin (B_2)	Functions primarily as the reactive portion of flavoproteins concerned with biologic oxidations (cellular metabolism)	Cheilosis, glossitis, photophobia, angular stomatitis, corneal, vasculation, scrotal skin changes, seborrhea, magenta tongue	None known	Dairy products, liver, almonds, lamb, pork, breast milk, infant formula	Alcoholism, starvation, chronic diarrhea, malabsorption	Red cell glutathione reductase activity (EGR), red cell flavine adenine dinucleotide, urine riboflavin/creatinine ratio
Thiamine (B_1)	Aids in energy utilization as part of coenzyme component to promote the utilization of carbohydrate; promotes normal functioning of the nervous system; coenzyme for oxidative carboxylation of 2-keto acids	Beriberi, neuritis, cardiac failure, anorexia, restlessness, confusion, loss of vibration sense and deep tendon reflexes, calf tenderness, edema	None known	Lean pork, nuts, whole grain and fortified cereal products, breast milk, infant formula	Alcoholism, refeeding syndrome, prolonged dialysis	Red cell transketolase activity, whole blood level (HPLC), urine thiamine/creatinine ratio

(*Continued*)

Table I-9 Clinical Examination in Nutritional Deficiencies and Excesses (*Continued*)

	Major Physiologic Functions	Deficiency Signs	Excess Signs	Important Food Sources	Potential Causes of Deficiency	Status Assessment
Minerals						
Calcium	Essential for calcification of bone (matrix formation); assists in blood clotting; functions in normal muscle contraction and relaxation and in normal nerve transmission	Osteomalacia, osteoporosis	Hypercalcemia, vomiting, anorexia, lethargy	Dairy products (milk, cheese), sardines, oysters, salmon, herring, greens, breast milk, infant formula	Renal disease, liver disease	Plasma total calcium, plasma free calcium in altered protein binding (e.g. hypoalbuminemia), acidosis, radiographs, CT, photon densitometry
Magnesium	Essential part of many enzyme systems; important for maintaining electrical potential in nerves and muscle membranes and for energy turnover	Tremor, convulsions, hyperexcitability (hypocalcemia tetany)	Diarrhea, transient hypocalcemia	Widely distributed, especially in food of vegetable origin; breast milk, infant formula	Protein calorie malnutrition, refeeding syndrome	Plama total or free magnesium, magnesium loading test
Phosphorus	Important intracellular anion; involved in many chemical reactions within the body; necessary for energy turnover (ATP)	Weakness, anorexia, malaise, bone pain, growth arrest	Hypocalcemia (when parathyroid gland not fully functioning)	Dairy products, fish, legumes, pork, breast milk, infant formula	Renal disease, liver disease, refeeding syndrome	Plasma concentration, alkaline phosphatase activity, radiography, densitometry, renal tubular excretion threshold
Trace elements						
Chromium	Maintenance of normal glucose metabolism, cofactor for insulin	Disturbed glucose metabolism (lower glucose tolerance caused by insulin resistance)		Brewer's yeast, meat products, cheeses	Protein calorie malnutrition, elderly	Plasma chromium, glucose tolerance
Copper	Constituent of proteins and enzymes, some of which are essential for the proper utilization of iron; immunity; skeletal development	Anemia (hemolytic), neutropenia, bone disease	Excess accumulation in the liver, brain, kidney, cornea; anemia, diarrhea	Oysters, nuts, liver, kidney, corn oil margarine, dried legumes	Menke's kinky hair syndrome. Excess: Wilson's disease	Plasma copper, plasma ceruloplamin (ferrochelatase), liver biopsy concentration, superoxide dismutase activity
Fluoride	The main target organs of flouride in man are the enamel of teeth and bones, where flouride is incorporated into the crystalline structure of hydroxyapatite and produces increased carie resistance	Poor dentition, caries, osteoporosis	Mottling, brown staining of teeth (in excess of 4 ppm);fluorosis occurs after prolonged (10–20 yr) ingestion of 20–80 mg/d	Fluoridated water; depends on the geochemical environment and therefore amount in food varies widely	Unfluoridated water, bottled water	
Iodine	Component of thyroid hormones triiodothyronine and thyroxine; important in regulation of cellular oxidation and growth	Goiter, depressed thyroid function, cretinism	Thyroid suppression (thyrotoxicosis)	Iodized table salt, salt water, fish, shellfish (content of most other foods geographically dependent), breast milk, infant formula	Endemic goiter in low iodine areas	Thyroid hormones, TSH, urinary iodide/creatinine ratio
Iron	Part of hemoglobin molecule; prevents nutritional anemia and fatigue; increases resistance to infection; functions as part of enzymes involved in tissue respiration	Anemia, malabsorption, irritability, anorexia, pallor, lethargy	Hemosiderosis. hemochromatosis	Red meats, liver, dried beans and peas, enriched farina, breast milk, infant formula, infant cereal	Protein losing enteropathy, malabsorption, acute or chronic blood loss. Excess: hemochromatosis	Plasma iron and ferritin, total iron-binding capacity, hemoglobin/hematocrit, red cell indices, RBC zinc protoporphyrin: heme ratio, bone marrow aspirate stain

(*Continued*)

Table I-9 Clinical Examination in Nutritional Deficiencies and Excesses (*Continued*)

	Major Physiologic Functions	Deficiency Signs	Excess Signs	Important Food Sources	Potential Causes of Deficiency	Status Assessment
Manganese	Essential part of several enzyme systems involved in protein and energy metabolism and in the formation of mucopolysaccharide	Impaired growth, skeletal abnormalities, lowered reproductive function, neonatal ataxia	In extremely high exposure of contamination: severe psychiatric and neurologic disorders	Nuts, whole grains, dried fruits, fruits, leafy vegetables		Plasma level, whole blood level, mitochondrial superoxide dismutase
Molybdenum	Essential for the function of flavin-dependent enzymes involved in the production of uric acid and in the oxidation of aldehydes and sulfites	Not described in man	Acts as an antagonist to the essential element copper; goutlike syndrome associated with elevated blood levels of molybdenum, uric acid and xanthin oxidase	Varies considerably, depending on growing environment; main contributions come from meat, grains, and legumes		
Selenium	Functions as a part of the enzyme glutathione peroxidase, which protects cellular component from oxidative damage	Cardiomyopathy, probably secondary to oxidative damage	In animals: blindness, abdominal pain	Seafoods, kidney, liver meat, grains (depending on growing enironment)	Cystic fibrosis	Plasma concentration, glutathione peroxidase activity, nail/hair selenium
Zinc	Constituent of enzymes involved in most major metabolic pathways (specifically nucleic acid synthesis for growth and repair)	Growth failure, skin changes, delayed wound healing, hypogeusia, sexual immaturity, hair loss, diarrhea	Acute gastrointestinal upset, vomiting, sweating, dizziness, copper deficiency	Whole grains, legumes, beef, lamb, pork, poultry, nuts, seeds, shellfish, eggs, some cheeses, breast milk, infant formula	Malabsorption, chronic diarrhea, liver disease, sickle cell disease	Plasma concentration, alkaline phosphatase activity, urinary excretion, leukocyte concentration

Appendix II

Nutritional Requirements

Melanie V. Connolly, MSc, RD, LDN, CNSD

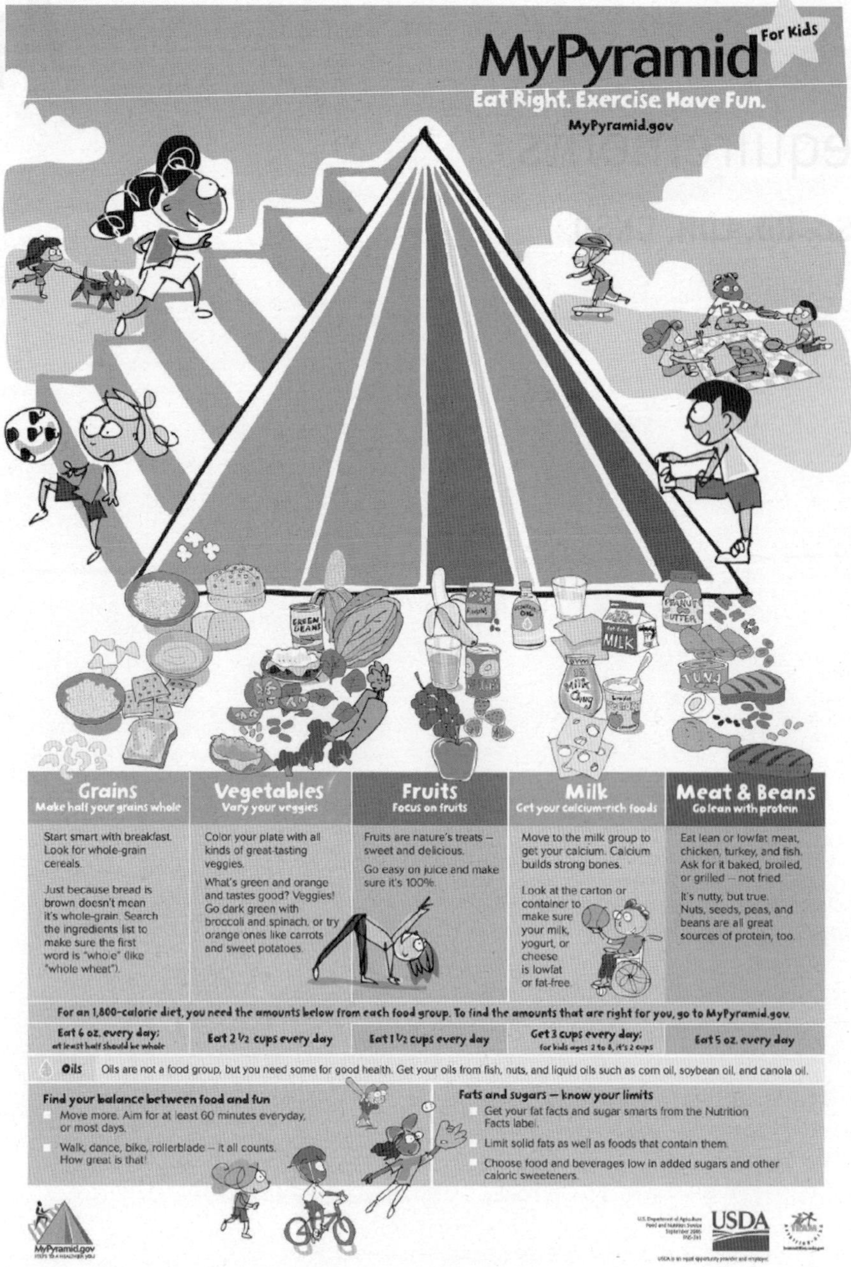

Figure II-1 My Pyramid for Kids. (From the US Department of Agriculture. Available at www.mypyramid.gov/kids.)

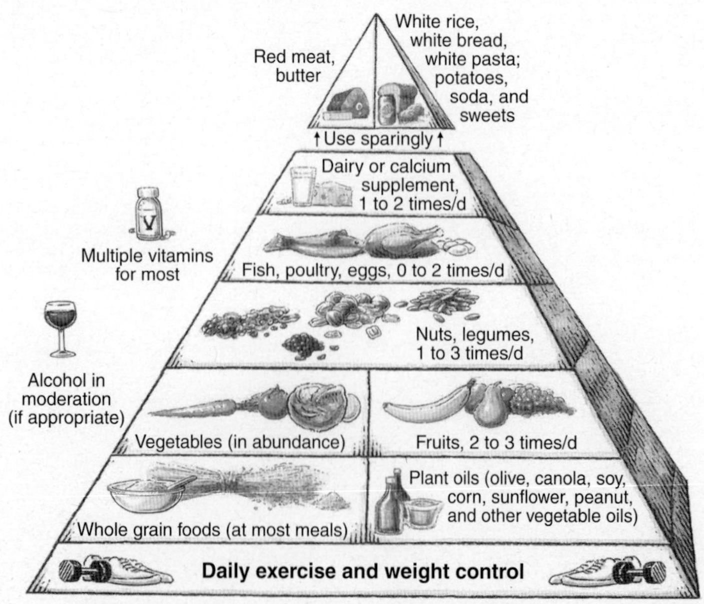

Figure II-2 Healthy eating pyramid. (Reproduced with permission from Willett WC. Eat, Drink, and Be Healthy. New York: Simon & Schuster; 2001. p. 13.)

Table II-1 Dietary Reference Intakes (DRIs): Recommended Intakes for Individuals and Tolerable Upper Intake Levels, Vitamins. Food and Nutrition Board, Institute of Medicine, National Academy of Sciences

		Infants		Children		Males						Females						Pregnancy		Lactation	
		0 to 6 mo	7 to 12 mo	1 to 3 yr	4 to 8 yr	9 to 13 yr	14 to 18 yr	19 to 30 yr	31 to 50 yr	51 to 70 yr	>70 yr	9 to 13 yr	14 to 18 yr	19 to 30 yr	31 to 50 yr	51 to 70 yr	>70 yr	≤18 yr	19 to 50 yr	≤18 yr	19 to 50 yr
Biotin	RDA/AI*	5*	6*	8*	12*	20*	25*	30*	30*	30*	30*	20*	25*	30*	30*	30*	30*	30*	30*	35*	35*
(µg/d)	UL	ND†	ND	ND	ND	ND	ND	ND	ND	ND	ND	ND	ND	ND	ND	ND	ND	ND	ND	ND	ND
Choline	RDA/AI*	125*	150*	200*	250*	375*	550*	550*	550*	550*	550*	375*	400*	425*	425*	425*	425*	450*	450*	550*	550*
(mg/d)	UL	ND	ND	1,000	1,000	2,000	3,000	3,500	3,500	3,500	3,500	2,000	3,000	3,500	3,500	3,500	3,500	3,000	3,500	3,000	3,500
Folate	RDA/AI*	65*	80*	**150**	**200**	**300**	**400**	**400**	**400**	**400**	**400**	**300**	**400**	**400**	**400**	**400**	**400**	**600**	**600**	**500**	**500**
(µg/d)	UL	ND	ND	300	400	600	800	1,000	1,000	1,000	1,000	600	800	1,000	1,000	1,000	1,000	800	1,000	800	1,000
Niacin	RDA/AI*	2*	4*	**6**	**8**	**12**	**16**	**16**	**16**	**16**	**16**	**12**	**14**	**14**	**14**	**14**	**14**	**18**	**18**	**17**	**17**
(mg/d)	UL	ND	ND	10	15	20	30	35	35	35	35	20	30	35	35	35	35	30	35	30	35
Pantothenic Acid	RDA/AI*	1.7*	1.8*	2*	3*	4*	5*	5*	5*	5*	5*	4*	5*	5*	5*	5*	5*	6*	6*	7*	
7* (mg/d)	UL	ND	ND	ND	ND	ND	ND	ND	ND	ND	ND	ND	ND	ND	ND	ND	ND	ND	ND	ND	ND
Riboflavin	RDA/AI*	0.3*	0.4*	**0.5**	**0.6**	**0.9**	**1.3**	**1.3**	**1.3**	**1.3**	**1.3**	**0.9**	**1.0**	**1.1**	**1.1**	**1.1**	**1.1**	**1.4**	**1.4**	**1.6**	**1.6**
(mg/d)	UL	ND	ND	ND	ND	ND	ND	ND	ND	ND	ND	ND	ND	ND	ND	ND	ND	ND	ND	ND	ND
Thiamin	RDA/AI*	0.2*	0.3*	**0.5**	**0.6**	**0.9**	**1.2**	**1.2**	**1.2**	**1.2**	**1.2**	**0.9**	**1.0**	**1.1**	**1.1**	**1.1**	**1.1**	**1.4**	**1.4**	**1.4**	**1.4**
(mg/d)	UL	ND	ND	ND	ND	ND	ND	ND	ND	ND	ND	ND	ND	ND	ND	ND	ND	ND	ND	ND	ND
Vitamin A	RDA/AI*	400*	500*	**300**	**400**	**600**	**900**	**900**	**900**	**900**	**900**	**600**	**700**	**700**	**700**	**700**	**700**	**750**	**770**	**1,200**	**1,300**
(µg/d)	UL	600	600	600	900	1,700	2,800	3,000	3,000	3,000	3,000	1,700	2,800	3,000	3,000	3,000	3,000	2,800	3,000	2,800	3,000
Vitamin B_6	RDA/AI*	0.1*	0.3*	**0.5**	**0.6**	**1.0**	**1.3**	**1.3**	**1.3**	**1.7**	**1.7**	**1.0**	**1.2**	**1.3**	**1.3**	**1.5**	**1.5**	**1.9**	**1.9**	**2.0**	**2.0**
(mg/d)	UL	ND	ND	30	40	60	80	100	100	100	100	60	80	100	100	100	100	80	100	80	100
Vitamin B_{12}	RDA/AI*	0.4*	0.5*	**0.9**	**1.2**	**1.8**	**2.4**	**2.4**	**2.4**	**2.4**	**2.4**	**1.8**	**2.4**	**2.4**	**2.4**	**2.4**	**2.4**	**2.6**	**2.6**	**2.8**	**2.8**
(µg/d)	UL	ND	ND	ND	ND	ND	ND	ND	ND	ND	ND	ND	ND	ND	ND	ND	ND	ND	ND	ND	ND
Vitamin C	RDA/AI*	40*	50*	**15**	**25**	**45**	**75**	**90**	**90**	**90**	**90**	**45**	**65**	**75**	**75**	**75**	**75**	**80**	**85**	**115**	**120**
(mg/d)	UL	ND	ND	400	650	1,200	1,800	2,000	2,000	2,000	2,000	1,200	1,800	2,000	2,000	2,000	2,000	1,800	2,000	1,800	2,000
Vitamin D	RDA/AI*	5*	5*	5*	5*	5*	5*	5*	5*	10*	15*	5*	5*	5*	5*	10*	15*	5*	5*	5*	5*
(µg/d)	UL	25	25	50	50	50	50	50	50	50	50	50	50	50	50	50	50	50	50	50	50
Vitamin E	RDA/AI*	4*	5*	**6**	**7**	**11**	**15**	**15**	**15**	**15**	**15**	**11**	**15**	**15**	**15**	**15**	**15**	**15**	**15**	**19**	**19**
(mg/d)	UL	ND	ND	200	300	600	800	1,000	1,000	1,000	1,000	600	800	1,000	1,000	1,000	1,000	800	1,000	800	1,000
Vitamin K	RDA/AI*	2.0*	2.5*	30*	55*	60*	75*	120*	120*	120*	120*	60*	75*	90*	90*	90*	90*	75*	90*	75*	90*
(µg/d)	UL	ND	ND	ND	ND	ND	ND	ND	ND	ND	ND	ND	ND	ND	ND	ND	ND	ND	ND	ND	ND

Table adapted from the DRI reports: Dietary Reference Intakes for Calcium, Phosphorous, Magnesium, Vitamin D, and Fluoride (1997); Dietary Reference Intakes for Thiamin, Riboflavin, Niacin, Vitamin B_6, Folate, Vitamin B_{12}, Pantothenic Acid, Biotin, and Choline (1998); Dietary Reference Intakes for Vitamin C, Vitamin E, Selenium, and Carotenoids (2000); and Dietary Reference Intakes for Vitamin A, Vitamin K, Arsenic, Boron, Chromium, Copper, Iodine, Iron, Manganese, Molybdenum, Nickel, Silicon, Vanadium, and Zinc (2001). Copyright by The National Academy of Sciences. Complete reports can be accessed at www.nap.edu.

Recommended dietary allowances (RDAs) are represented in bold type.

Adequate intakes (AIs) are represented in regular type and are followed by an asterisk (*).

†ND = Not determinable due to lack of data of adverse effects in this age group and concern with regard to lack of ability to handle excess amounts.

Table II-2 Dietary Reference Intakes (DRIs): Recommended Intakes for Individuals and Tolerable Upper Intake Levels, Elements. Food and Nutrition Board, Institute of Medicine, National Academy of Sciences

		Infants		Children		Males						Females						Pregnancy			Lactation		
		0 to 6 mo	7 to 12 mo	1 to 3 yr	4 to 8 yr	9 to 13 yr	14 to 18 yr	19 to 30 yr	31 to 50 yr	51 to 70 yr	>70 yr	9 to 13 yr	14 to 18 yr	19 to 30 yr	31 to 50 yr	51 to 70 yr	>70 yr	≤ 18 yr	19 to 30 yr	31 to 50 yr	≤ 18 yr	19 to 50 yr	31 to 50 yr
Arsenic	RDA/AI*	ND†	ND	ND	ND	ND	ND	ND	ND	ND	ND	ND	ND	ND	ND	ND	ND	ND	ND	ND	ND	ND	ND
(mg/d)	UL	ND	ND	ND	ND	ND	ND	ND	ND	ND	ND	ND	ND	ND	ND	ND	ND	ND	ND	ND	ND	ND	ND
Boron	RDA/AI*	ND	ND	ND	ND	ND	ND	ND	ND	ND	ND	ND	ND	ND	ND	ND	ND	ND	ND	ND	ND	ND	ND
(mg/d)	UL	ND	ND	3	6	11	17	20	20	20	20	11	17	20	20	20	20	17	20	20	17	20	20
Calcium	RDA/AI*	210*	270*	500*	800*	1,300*	1,300*	1,000*	1,000*	1,200*	1,200*	1,300*	1,300*	1,000*	1,000*	1,200*	1,200*	1,300*	1,000*	1,000*	1,300*	1,000*	1,000*
(mg/d)	UL	ND	ND	2,500	2,500	2,500	2,500	2,500	2,500	2,500	2,500	2,500	2,500	2,500	2,500	2,500	2,500	2,500	2,500	2,500	2,500	2,500	2,500
Chromium	RDA/AI*	0.2*	5.5*	11*	15*	25*	35*	35*	35*	30*	30*	21*	24*	25*	25*	20*	20*	29*	30*	30*	44*	45*	45*
(mg/d)	UL	ND	ND	ND	ND	ND	ND	ND	ND	ND	ND	ND	ND	ND	ND	ND	ND	ND	ND	ND	ND	ND	ND
Copper	RDA/AI*	200*	220*	**340**	**440**	**700**	**890**	**900**	**900**	**900**	**900**	**700**	**890**	**900**	**900**	**900**	**900**	**1,000**	**1,000**	**1,000**	**1,300**	**1,300**	**1,300**
(μg/d)	UL	ND	ND	1,000	3,000	5,000	8,000	10,000	10,000	10,000	10,000	5,000	8,000	10,000	10,000	10,000	10,000	8,000	10,000	10,000	8,000	10,000	10,000
Fluoride	RDA/AI*	0.01*	0.5*	0.7*	1*	2*	3*	4*	4*	4*	4*	2*	3*	3*	3*	3*	3*	3*	3*	3*	3*	3*	3*
(mg/d)	UL	0.7	0.9	1.3	2.2	10	10	10	10	10	10	10	10	10	10	10	10	10	10	10	10	10	10
Iodine	RDA/AI*	110*	130*	**90**	**90**	**120**	**150**	**150**	**150**	**150**	**150**	**120**	**150**	**150**	**150**	**150**	**150**	**220**	**220**	**220**	**290**	**290**	**290**
(μg/d)	UL	ND	ND	200	300	600	900	1,100	1,100	1,100	1,100	600	900	1,100	1,100	1,100	1,100	900	1,100	1,100	900	1,100	1,100
Iron	RDA/AI*	0.27*	**11**	**7**	**10**	**8**	**11**	**8**	**8**	**8**	**8**	**8**	**15**	**18**	**18**	**8**	**8**	**27**	**27**	**27**	**10**	**9**	**9**
(mg/d)	UL	40	40	40	40	40	45	45	45	45	45	40	45	45	45	45	45	45	45	45	45	45	45
Magnesium	RDA/AI*	30*	75*	**80**	**130**	**240**	**410**	**400**	**420**	**420**	**420**	**240**	**360**	**310**	**320**	**320**	**320**	**400**	**350**	**360**	**360**	**310**	**320**
(mg/d)	UL	ND	ND	65	110	350	350	350	350	350	350	350	350	350	350	350	350	350	350	350	350	350	350
Manganese	RDA/AI*	0.003*	0.6*	1.2*	1.5*	1.9*	2.2*	2.3*	2.3*	2.3*	2.3*	1.6*	1.6*	1.8*	1.8*	1.8*	1.8*	2.0*	2.0*	2.0*	2.6*	2.6*	2.6*
(mg/d)	UL	ND	ND	2	3	6	9	11	11	11	11	6	9	11	11	11	11	9	11	11	9	11	11
Molybdenum	RDA/AI*	2*	3*	**17**	**22**	**34**	**43**	**45**	**45**	**45**	**45**	**34**	**43**	**45**	**45**	**45**	**45**	**50**	**50**	**50**	**50**	**50**	**50**
(μg/d)	UL	ND	ND	300	600	1,100	1,700	2,000	2,000	2,000	2,000	1,100	1,700	2,000	2,000	2,000	2,000	1,700	2,000	2,000	1,700	2,000	2,000
Nickel	RDA/AI*	ND	ND	ND	ND	ND	ND	ND	ND	ND	ND	ND	ND	ND	ND	ND	ND	ND	ND	ND	ND	ND	ND
(mg/d)	UL	ND	ND	0.2	0.3	0.6	1.0	1.0	1.0	1.0	1.0	0.6	1.0	1.0	1.0	1.0	1.0	1.0	1.0	1.0	1.0	1.0	1.0
Phosphorus	RDA/AI*	100*	275*	**460**	**500**	**1,250**	**1,250**	**700**	**700**	**700**	**700**	**1,250**	**1,250**	**700**	**700**	**700**	**700**	**1,250**	**700**	**700**	**1,250**	**700**	**700**
(mg/d)	UL	ND	ND	3,000	3,000	4,000	4,000	4,000	4,000	4,000	3,000	4,000	4,000	4,000	4,000	4,000	3,000	3,500	3,500	3,500	4,000	4,000	4,000
Selenium	RDA/AI*	15*	20*	**20**	**30**	**40**	**55**	**55**	**55**	**55**	**55**	**40**	**55**	**55**	**55**	**55**	**55**	**60**	**60**	**60**	**70**	**70**	**70**
(μg/d)	UL	45	60	90	150	280	400	400	400	400	400	280	400	400	400	400	400	400	400	400	400	400	400
Silicon	RDA/AI*	ND	ND	ND	ND	ND	ND	ND	ND	ND	ND	ND	ND	ND	ND	ND	ND	ND	ND	ND	ND	ND	ND
	UL	ND	ND	ND	ND	ND	ND	ND	ND	ND	ND	ND	ND	ND	ND	ND	ND	ND	ND	ND	ND	ND	ND
Vanadium	RDA/AI*	ND	ND	ND	ND	ND	ND	ND	ND	ND	ND	ND	ND	ND	ND	ND	ND	ND	ND	ND	ND	ND	ND
(mg/d)	UL	ND	ND	ND	ND	ND	ND	1.8	1.8	1.8	1.8	ND	ND	1.8	1.8	1.8	1.8	ND	ND	ND	ND	ND	ND
Zinc	RDA/AI*	2*	**3**	**3**	**5**	**8**	**11**	**11**	**11**	**11**	**11**	**8**	**9**	**8**	**8**	**8**	**8**	**12**	**11**	**11**	**13**	**12**	**12**
(mg/d)	UL	4	5	7	12	23	34	40	40	40	40	23	34	40	40	40	40	34	40	40	34	40	40

Table adapted from the DRI reports: Dietary Reference Intakes for Calcium, Phosphorous, Magnesium, Vitamin D, and Fluoride (1997); Dietary Reference Intakes for Thiamin, Riboflavin, Niacin, Vitamin B_6, Folate, Vitamin B_{12}, Pantothenic Acid, Biotin, and Choline (1998); Dietary Reference Intakes for Vitamin C, Vitamin E, Selenium, and Carotenoids (2000); and Dietary Reference Intakes for Vitamin A, Vitamin K, Arsenic, Boron, Chromium, Copper, Iodine, Iron, Manganese, Molybdenum, Nickel, Silicon, Vanadium, and Zinc (2001). Copyright by The National Academy of Sciences. Complete reports can be accessed at www.nap.edu.

Recommended Dietary Allowances (RDAs) are represented in bold type.

Adequate Intakes (AIs) are represented in regular type and are followed by an asterisk (*).

†ND = Not determinable due to lack of data of adverse effects in this age group and concern with regard to lack of ability to handle excess amounts.

Table II-3 Dietary Reference Intakes (DRIs): Recommended Intakes for Individuals and Acceptable Macronutrient Distribution Ranges, Macronutrients. Food and Nutrition Board, Institute of Medicine, National Academy of Sciences

		Infants		Children		Males					Females					Pregnancy	Lactation
		0 to 6 mo	7 to 12 mo	1 to 3 yr	4 to 8 yr	9 to 13 yr	14 to 18 yr	19 to 30 yr	31 to 50 yr	> 50 yr	9 to 13 yr	14 to 18 yr	19 to 30 yr	31 to 50 yr	> 50 yr	≤ 18 to 50 yr	≤ 18 to 50 yr
Carbohydrate (g/d)	RDA/AI*	60*	95*	**130**	**130**	**130**	**130**	**130**	**130**	**130**	**130**	**130**	**130**	**130**	**130**	**175**	**210**
	AMDR	ND†	ND	45 to 65	45 to 65	45 to 65	45 to 65	45 to 65	45 to 65	45 to 65	45 to 65	45 to 65	45 to 65	45 to 65	45 to 65	45 to 65	45 to 65
Total Fiber (g/d)	RDA/AI*	ND	ND	19*	25*	31*	38*	38*	38*	30*	26*	26*	25*	25*	21*	28*	29*
Fat (g/d)	RDA/AI*	31*	30*	ND	ND	ND	ND	ND	ND	ND	ND	ND	ND	ND	ND	ND	ND
	AMDR	ND	ND	30 to 40	25 to 35	25 to 35	25 to 35	20 to 35	20 to 35	20 to 35	25 to 35	25 to 35	20 to 35	20 to 35	20 to 35	20 to 35	20 to 35
Linoleic Acid (g/d)	RDA/AI*	4.4*	4.6*	7*	10*	12*	16*	17*	17*	14*	10*	11*	12*	12*	11*	13*	13*
	AMDR	ND	ND	5 to 10	5 to 10	5 to 10	5 to 10	5 to 10	5 to 10	5 to 10	5 to 10	5 to 10	5 to 10	5 to 10	5 to 10	5 to 10	5 to 10
α to Linolenic Acid	RDA/AI*	0.5*	0.5*	0.7*	0.9*	1.2*	1.6*	1.6*	1.6*	1.6*	1.0*	1.1*	1.1*	1.1*	1.1*	1.4*	1.3*
(g/d)	AMDR	ND	ND	0.6 to 1.2	0.6 to 1.2	0.6 to 1.2	0.6 to 1.2	0.6 to 1.2	0.6 to 1.2	0.6 to 1.2	0.6 to 1.2	0.6 to 1.2	0.6 to 1.2	0.6 to 1.2	0.6 to 1.2	0.6 to 1.2	0.6 to 1.2
Protein (g/d)‡	RDA/AI*	9.1*	**13.5**	**13**	**19**	**34**	**52**	**56**	**56**	**56**	**34**	**46**	**46**	**46**	**46**	**71**	**71**
	AMDR	ND	ND	5 to 20	10 to 30	10 to 30	10 to 30	10 to 35	10 to 35	10 to 35	10 to 30	10 to 30	10 to 35	10 to 35	10 to 35	10 to 35	10 to 35

Table adapted from the DRI reports: Dietary Reference Intakes for Energy, Carbohydrate, Fiber, Fat, Fatty Acids, Cholesterol, Protein, and Amino Acids; 2002. Copyright by The National Academy of Sciences. Complete report can be accessed at www.nap.edu.

Recommended Dietary Allowances (RDAs) are represented in bold type.

Adequate Intakes (AIs) are represented in regular type and are followed by an asterisk (*).

†ND = Not determinable due to lack of data of adverse effects in this age group and concern with regard to lack of ability to handle excess amounts.

‡Based on 1.5 g/kg/d for infants, 1.1 g/kg/d for 1 to 3 yr, 0.95 g/kg/d for 4 to 13 yr, 0.85 g/kg/d for 14 to 18 yr, 0.8 g/kg/d for adults, and 1.1 g/kg/d for pregnant (using prepregnancy weight) and lactating women.

Table II-4 Dietary Reference Intakes (DRIs): Recommended Intakes for Individuals and Tolerable Upper Intake Levels, Macronutrients. Fluids, and Electrolytes. Food and Nutrition Board, Institute of Medicine, National Academy of Sciences

		Infants		Children		Males						Females						Pregnancy		Lactation	
		0 to 6 mo	7 to 12 mo	1 to 3 yr	4 to 8 yr	9 to 13 yr	14 to 18 yr	19 to 30 yr	31 to 50 yr	51 to 70 yr	> 70 yr	9 to 13 yr	14 to 18 yr	19 to 30 yr	31 to 50 yr	51 to 70 yr	> 70 yr	≤ 18 yr	19 to 50 yr	≤ 18 yr	19 to 50 yr
Sodium	AI	0.12	0.37	1.0	1.2	1.5	1.5	1.5	1.5	1.3	1.2	1.5	1.5	1.5	1.5	1.3	1.2	1.5	1.5	1.5	1.5
(g/d)	UL	ND*	ND	1.5	1.9	2.2	2.3	2.3	2.3	2.3	2.3	2.2	2.3	2.3	2.3	2.3	2.3	2.3	2.3	2.3	2.3
Chloride	AI	0.18	0.57	1.5	1.9	2.3	2.3	2.3	2.3	2.0	1.8	2.3	2.3	2.3	2.3	2.0	1.8	2.3	2.3	2.3	2.3
(g/d)	UL	ND	ND	2.3	2.9	3.4	3.6	3.6	3.6	3.6	3.6	3.4	3.6	3.6	3.6	3.6	3.6	3.6	3.6	3.6	3.6
Potassium	AI	0.4	0.7	3.0	3.8	4.5	4.7	4.7	4.7	4.7	4.7	4.5	4.7	4.7	4.7	4.7	4.7	4.7	4.7	5.1	5.1
(g/d)	UL	ND	ND	ND	ND	ND	ND	ND	ND	ND	ND	ND	ND	ND	ND	ND	ND	ND	ND	ND	ND
Water†	AI	0.7	0.8	1.3	1.7	2.4	3.3	3.7	3.7	3.7	3.7	2.1	2.3	2.7	2.7	2.7	2.7	3.0	3.0	3.8	3.8
(L/d)	UL	No UL	No UL	No UL	No UL	No UL	No UL	No UL	No UL	No UL	No UL	No UL	No UL	No UL	No UL	No UL	No UL	No UL	No UL	No UL	No UL
Carbohydrate (total digestible, g/d)	RDA/ AI	60	95	**130**	**130**	**130**	**130**	**130**	**130**	**130**	**130**	**130**	**130**	**130**	**130**	**130**	**130**	**175**	**175**	**210**	**210**
Fat (g/d)	AI	31	30	ND	ND	ND	ND	ND	ND	ND	ND	ND	ND	ND	ND	ND	ND	ND	ND	ND	ND
Fiber (g/d)	AI	ND	ND	19	25	31	38	38	38	30	30	26	26	25	25	21	21	28	28	29	29
	UL	No UL	No UL	No UL	Nc UL	No UL	No UL	No UL	No UL	No UL	No UL	No UL	No UL	No UL	No UL	No UL	No UL	No UL	No UL	No UL	No UL
Protein (g/d)‡	AI	9.1	11.0	13	19	34	52	56	56	56	56	34	46	46	46	46	46	71	71	71	71
	UL	No UL	No UL	No UL	No UL	No UL	No UL	No UL	No UL	No UL	No UL	No UL	No UL	No UL	No UL	No UL	No UL	No UL	No UL	No UL	No UL

Table adapted from the DRI report: Dietary Reference Intakes for Water, Potassium, Sodium, Chloride, and Sulfate; 2004. Copyright by The National Academy of Sciences. Complete report can be accessed at www.nap.edu.

*ND = Not determinable due to lack of data of adverse effects in this age group and concern with regard to lack of ability to handle excess amounts.

†Total water includes all water in food and beverages.

‡Based on 0.8g/kg for the reference body weight.

Table II-5 Dietary Reference Intakes (DRIs): Estimated Energy Requirements. Food and Nutrition Board, Institute of Medicine, National Academy of Sciences

Category	Estimated Energy Requirements (kcal)
Infants and children (0 to 2 yr)	
0 to 3 mo	(89 × wt [kg] − 100) + 175
4 to 6 mo	(89 × wt [kg] − 100) + 56
7 to 12 mo	(89 × wt [kg] − 100) + 22
13 to 35 mo	(89 × wt [kg] − 100) + 20
Males	
3 to 8 yr	88.5 − 61.9 × age [yr] + PA* × (26.7 × wt [kg] + 903 × ht [m]) + 20
9 to 18 yr	88.5 − 61.9 × age [yr] + PA × (26.7 × wt [kg] + 903 × ht [m]) + 25
≥19 yr	662 − 9.53 × age [yr] + PA × (15.91 × wt [kg] + 539.6 × ht [m])
Females	
3 to 8 yr	135.3 − 30.8 × age [yr] + PA × (10.0 × wt [kg] + 934 × ht [m]) + 20
9 to 18 yr	135.3 − 30.8 × age [yr] + PA × (10.0 × wt [kg] + 934 × ht [m]) + 25
≥19 yr	354 − 6.91 × age [yr] + PA × (9.36 × wt [kg] + 726 × ht [m])
Pregnancy	
14 to 18 yr	
First trimester	Adolescent EER
Second trimester	Adolescent EER + 340
Third trimester	Adolescent EER + 452
19 to 50 yr	
First trimester	Adult EER
Second trimester	Adult EER + 340
Third trimester	Adult EER + 452
Lactation	
14 to 18 yr	
First 6 mo	Adolescent EER + 330
Second 6 mo	Adolescent EER + 400
19 to 50 years	
First 6 mo	Adult EER + 330
Second 6 mo	Adult EER + 400

Table adapted from the DRI reports: Dietary Reference Intakes for Energy, Carbohydrate. Fiber, Fat, Fatty Acids, Cholesterol, Protein, and Amino Acids. Washington, DC: National Academy of Sciences; 2002. Copyright by The National Academy of Sciences. Complete report can be accessed at www.nap.edu.

PA = 1.00 if PAL is estimated to be ≥ 1.0 < 1.4 (sedentary).

PA = 1.12 if PAL is estimated to be ≥ 1.4 < 1.6 (low active).

PA = 1.24 if PAL is estimated to be ≥ 1.6 < 1.9 (active).

PA = 1.45 if PAL is estimated to be ≥ 1.9 < 2.5 (very active).

*PA = physical activity coefficient based on physical activity level (PAL).

Table II-6 Criteria and Dietary Reference Intake Values for Energy by Active Individuals by Life Stage Group*

Life Stage Group	Criterion	Active PAL† EER (kcal/d) Male	Active PAL† EER (kcal/d) Female
0 to 6 mo	Energy expenditure plus energy deposition	570	520 (3 mo)
7 to 12 mo	Energy expenditure plus energy deposition	743	676 (9 mo)
1 to 2 yr	Energy expenditure plus energy deposition	1,046	992 (24 mo)
3 to 8 yr	Energy expenditure plus energy deposition	1,742	1,642 (6 yr)
9 to 13 yr	Energy expenditure plus energy deposition	2,279	2,071 (11 yr)
14 to 18 yr	Energy expenditure plus energy deposition	3,152	2,368 (16 yr)
>18 yr	Energy expenditure	3,067‡	2,403‡ (19 yr)
Pregnancy			
14 to 18 yr	Adolescent female EER plus change in TEE plus pregnancy energy deposition		
First trimester	2,368 (16 yr)		
Second trimester	2,708 (16 yr)		
Third trimester	2,820 (16 yr)		
19 to 50 yr	Adult female EER plus change in TEE plus pregnancy energy deposition		
First trimester	2,403‡ (19 yr)		
Second trimester	2,743‡ (19 yr)		
Third trimester	2,855‡ (19 yr)		
Lactation			
14 to 18 yr	Adolescent female EER plus milk energy output minus weight loss		
First 6 mo	2,698 (16 yr)		
Second 6 mo	2,768 (16 yr)		

Adapted from the Institute of Medicine. Dietary Reference Intakes for Energy, Carbohydrate, Fiber, Fat, Fatty Acids, Cholesterol, Protein, and Amino Acids. Washington, DC: National Academy of Sciences; 2002.
*For healthy, active Americans and Canadians.
†EER = estimated energy requirement; PAL = physical activity level; TEE = total energy expenditure. The intake which meets the average energy expenditure of individuals at the reference height, weight, and age.
‡Subtract 10 kcal/d for males and 7 kcal/d for females for each year above 19 yr.

Table II-7 Criteria and Dietary Reference Intake Values for Carbohydrate by Life Stage Group

		EAR (grams per day)*		RDA (grams per day)†		
Life Stage Group	Criterion	Male	Female	Male	Female	AI (g/kg/d)‡
0 to 6 mo	Average content of human milk					60
7 to 12 mo	Average intake from human milk plus complementary foods					95
1 to 3 yr	Extrapolation from adult data	100	100	130	130	
4 to 8 yr	Extrapolation from adult data	100	100	130	130	
9 to 13 yr	Extrapolation from adult data	100	100	130	130	
14 to 18 yr	Extrapolation from adult data	100	100	130	130	
>18 yr	Brain glucose use	100	100	130	130	
Pregnancy						
14 to 18 yr	Adolescent female EAR plus fetal brain glucose use	135	175			
19 to 50 yr	Adult female EAR plus fetal brain glucose use	135	175			
Lactation						
14 to 18 yr	Adolescent female EAR plus average human milk content of carbohydrate	160	210			
19 to 50 yr	Adult female EAR plus average human milk content of carbohydrate	160	210			

*EAR: Estimated average requirement. The intake that meets the estimated nutrient needs of half of the individuals in a group.
†RDA: Recommended dietary allowance. The intake that meets the nutrient need of almost all (97 to 98%) of individuals in a group.
‡AI: Adequate intakes. The observed average or experimentally determined intake by a defined population or subgroup that appears to sustain a defined nutritional status, such as growth rate, normal circulatory nutrient values, or other functional indicators of health. The AI is used if sufficient scientific evidence is not available to derive an EAR. For healthy infants receiving human milk, the AI is the mean intake. The AI is not equivalent to an RDA.

Table II-8 Criteria and Dietary Reference Intake Values for Protein by Life Stage Group

		AI or RDA for Reference Individual (g/d)		EAR (g/kg/d)*		RDA (g/kg/d)†		
Life Stage Group	Criterion	Males	Females	Males	Females	Males	Females	AI (g/kg/d)‡
0 to 6 mo	Average consumption of protein from human milk	9.1 (AI)	9.1 (AI)					1.52
7 to 12 mo	Nitrogen equilibrium + protein deposition	13.5	13.5	1.1	1.1	1.5	1.5	
1 to 3 yr	Nitrogen equilibrium + protein deposition	13	13	0.88	0.88	1.10	1.10	
4 to 8 yr	Nitrogen equilibrium + protein deposition	19	19	0.76	0.76	0.95	0.95	
9 to 13 yr	Nitrogen equilibrium + protein deposition	34	34	0.76	0.76	0.95	0.95	
14 to 18 yr	Nitrogen equilibrium + protein deposition	52	46	0.73	0.71	0.85	0.85	
>18 yr	Nitrogen equilibrium	56	46	0.66	0.66	0.80	0.80	

The EAR and RDA for pregnancy are only for the second half of pregnancy. For the first half of pregnancy, the protein requirements are the same as those of the nonpregnant woman in addition to the EAR and RDA of the nonlactating adolescent or women.

*EAR = Estimated average requirement. The intake that meets the estimated nutrient needs of half of the individuals in a group.

†RDA = Recommended dietary allowance. The intake that meets the nutrient need of almost all (97 to 98%) of individuals in a group.

‡AI = Adequate intakes. The observed average or experimentally determined intake by a defined population or subgroup that appears to sustain a defined nutritional status, such as growth rate, normal circulatory nutrient values, or other functional indicators of health. The AI is used if sufficient scientific evidence is not available to derive an EAR. For healthy infants receiving human milk, the AI is the mean intake. The AI is not equivalent to an RDA.

Table II-9 Estimated Safe and Adequate Daily Dietary Intakes of Selected Minerals

		Trace Elements*				
Category	Age (yr)	Copper (mg)	Manganese (mg)	Fluoride (mg)	Chromium (μg)	Molybdenum (μg)
Infants	0 to 0.5	0.4 to 0.6	0.3 to 0.6	0.1 to 0.5	10 to 40	15 to 30
	0.5 to 1	0.6 to 0.7	0.6 to 1.0	0.2 to 1.0	20 to 60	20 to 40
Children and adolescents	1 to 3	0.7 to 1.0	1.0 to 1.5	0.5 to 1.5	20 to 80	25 to 50
	4 to 6	1.0 to 1.5	1.5 to 2.0	1.0 to 2.5	30 to 120	30 to 75
	7 to 10	1.0 to 2.0	2.0 to 3.0	1.5 to 2.5	50 to 200	50 to 150
	11+	1.5 to 2.5	2.0 to 5.0	1.5 to 2.5	50 to 200	75 to 250
Adults		1.5 to 3.0	2.0 to 5.0	1.5 to 4.0	50 to 200	75 to 250

Adapted from the National Academy of Sciences, Washington, DC.

*Because the toxic levels for many trace elements may be only several times usual intakes, the upper levels for the trace elements given in this table should not be habitually exceeded.

Table II-10 Normal Electrolyte Requirements

Electrolyte	Daily Requirement
Sodium	2 to 4 mEq/kg
Potassium	2 to 3 mEq/kg
Chloride	2 to 3 mEq/kg
Magnesium	0.25 to 0.5 mEq/kg
Calcium	0.5 to 2.5 mEq/kg
Phosphorus	1 to 2 mmol/kg

Adapted from Collier S, Gura KM, Richardson DS, Duggan C. Parenteral nutrition. In: Hendricks KM, Duggan CD, editors. Manual of Pediatric Nutrition, 4th edition. Hamilton (ON): BC Decker; 2005.

Table II-11 Fluid Requirements

Holliday–Segar Method	
1st 10 kg body weight	100 mL/kg
2nd 10 kg body weight	1,000 mL + 50 mL/kg > 10 kg
Each additional kg	1,500 mL + 20 mL/kg > 20 kg
Body Surface Area Method	
	1,500 mL/m^2 24 hr

Adapted from Stone B. Fluid and electrolytes. In: Robertson J, Shilkofski N, editors. The Harriet Lane Handbook, 17th edition. Philadelphia; 2005. p. 284

Table II-12 Milliequivalent–Milligram Conversion Table

Mineral Element	Chemical Symbol	Atomic Weight	Valence
Calcium	Ca	40	2
Chlorine	Cl	35.4	1
Magnesium	Mg	24.3	2
Phosphorus	P	31	2
Potassium	K	39	1
Sodium	Na	23	1
Sulfur	S	32	2
Zinc	Zn	65.4	2
Sulfate	SO_4	96	2

Adapted from Gura KM. Conversion tables. In: Hendricks KM, Duggan CD, editors. Manual of Pediatric Nutrition, 4th edition. Hamilton (ON): BC Decker; 2005.

$$\text{Milliequivalents} = \frac{\text{Milligrams}}{\text{Atomic weight}} \times \text{Valence}$$

Example: Convert 2,000 mg sodium to mEq of sodium

$$\frac{2000}{23} \times 1 = 87 \text{ mEq sodium}$$

To change milliequivalents back to milligrams, multiply the milliequivalents by the atomic weight and divide by the valence.

Example: Convert 20 mEq sodium to mg sodium

$$\frac{20 \times 23}{1} = 460 \text{ mg sodium}$$

Table II-13 Recommended Daily Allowances (RDA) for Energy and Protein

Age	kcal/kg		g Protein/kg	
0 to 6 mo	108		2.2	
6 to 12 mo	98		1.6	
1 to 3 yr	102		1.2	
4 to 6 yr	90		1.1	
7 to 10 yr	70		1.0	
	Males	Females	Males	Females
11 to 14 yr	55	47	1.0	1.0
15 to 18 yr	45	40	0.9	0.8
19 to 24 yr	40	38	0.8	0.8
25 to 50 yr	37	36	0.8	0.8

Adapted from National Academy of Sciences. Recommended Daily Allowances, 10th edition. Washington, DC: National Academy Press; 1989.

Table II-14 Schofield Equations for Calculating Basal Metabolic Rate in Children

Males	
0 to 3 yr	REE = 0.167W + 15.174H − 617.6
3 to 10 yr	REE = 19.59W + 1.303H + 414.9
10 to 18 yr	REE = 16.25W + 1.372H + 515.5
>18 yr	REE = 15.057W + 1.004H + 705.8
Females	
0 to 3 yr	REE = 16.252W + 10.232H − 413.5
3 to 10 yr	REE = 16.969W + 1.618H + 371.2
10 to 18 yr	REE = 8.365W + 4.65H + 200
>18 yr	REE = 13.623W + 23.8H + 98.2

Adapted from Schofield W. Predicting basal metabolic rate, new standards and review of previous work. Hum Nutr Clin Nutr 1985;39C:5–41.

Resting energy expenditure (REE) = kcal/d; W = weight (kg); H = height (cm).

Table II-15 Equations for Predicting Basal Metabolic Rate from Body Weight in Kilograms

Age Range (yr)	kcal/kg/d
Males	
0 to 3	60.9 W − 54
3 to 10	22.7 W + 495
10 to 18	17.5 W + 651
18 to 30	15.3 W + 679
30 to 60	11.6 W + 879
> 60	13.5 W + 487
Females	
0 to 3	61.0 W − 51
3 to 10	22.5 W + 499
10 to 18	22.2 W + 746
18 to 30	14.7 W + 496
30 to 60	8.7 W + 829
> 60	10.5 W + 596

Adapted from World Health Organization. Energy and protein requirements. Report of a Joint FAO/WHO/UNU Expert Consultation, Technical Report Series 724. Geneva: WHO; 1985.

Table II-16 Assessment of Energy Requirements in Hospitalized Pediatric Patients: Step 1. Estimating Basal Metabolic Requirements

Body	kcal/d		Body	kcal/d	
Wt (kg)	Male	Female	Wt (kg)	Male	Female
3.0	120	144	36.0	1,270	1,173
4.0	191	191	38.0	1,305	1,207
5.0	270	274	40.0	1,340	1,241
6.0	330	336	42.0	1,370	1,274
7.0	390	395	44.0	1,400	1,306
8.0	445	448	46.0	1,430	1,338
9.0	495	496	48.0	1,460	1,369
10.0	545	541	50.0	1,485	1,399
11.0	590	582	52.0	1,505	1,429
12.0	625	620	54.0	1,555	1,458
13.0	665	655	56.0	1,580	1,487
14.0	700	687	58.0	1,600	1,516
15.0	725	718	60.0	1,630	1,544
16.0	750	747	62.0	1,660	1,572
17.0	780	775	64.0	1,690	1,599
18.0	810	802	66.0	1,725	1,626
19.0	840	827	68.0	1,765	1,653
20.0	870	852	70.0	1,785	1,679
22.0	910	898	72.0	1,815	1,705
24.0	980	942	74.0	1,845	1,731
26.0	1,070	984	76.0	1,870	1,756
28.0	1,100	1,025	78.0	1,900	1,781
30.0	1,140	1,063	80.0	1,935	1,805
32.0	1,190	1,101	82.0	1,970	1,830
34.0	1,230	1,137	84.0	2,000	1,855

Adapted from Schofield W. Predicting basal metabolic rate, new standards and review of previous work. Hum Nutr Clin Nutr 1985;39C:5–41.

Table II-17 Assessment of Energy Requirements in Hospitalized Pediatric Patients: Step 2. Factors Used in the Calculation of Total Energy Expenditure

Factor	
Activity	
Bedridden	1.20
Ambulatory	1.30
Fever	
Per degree Fahrenheit over normal	1.07
Injury	
Starvation	0.70
Minor surgery	1.00 to 1.20
Peritonitis	1.20 to 1.50
Soft tissue trauma	1.14 to 1.37
Skeletal trauma	1.35
Major sepsis	1.40 to 1.60
Severe thermal injury	2.00

Adapted from Long C, Schaffel N, Geiger J, et al. Response to injury and illness: Estimation of energy and protein needs from indirect calorimetric and nitrogen balance. J Parenter Enteral Nutr 1979;3:452.

Appendix III

Enteral Products

Melanie V. Connolly, MSc, RD, LDN, CNSD

Table III-1 Infant Formulas (per 100 mL)

Product (Manufacturer)	kcal/ mL	Protein g	Protein % kcal	Protein Source	Fat g	Fat % kcal	Fat Source	Carbohydrate g	Carbohydrate % kcal	Carbohydrate Source	Na mEq	K mEq	Ca mg	Fe mg	P mg	Water mOsm/kg	General Comments
Human milk, term, mature	0.67	1.0	5	Whey and casein	3.90	55	Long chain fatty acids high in palmitic, oleic, linoleic, and linolenic oils	7.2	38	Lactose	0.78	1.35	28	0.04	14	255	Preferred nutrition in human infants
Alimentum (Ross)	0.67	1.86	11	Casein hydrolysate, L-cystine, L-tryptophan, L-methionine, L-tyrosine	3.74	48	Safflower oil, MCT oil, soy oil	6.9	41	Sucrose, modified tapioca starch	1.28	2.04	71	1.22	51	370	33% fat as MCT
EleCare (Ross)	0.67	2.0	15	Free amino acids	3.2	42	High-oleic safflower oil, MCT oil, soy oil	7.2	43	Corn syrup solids	1.3	2.6	72	1.2	54	350	100% free amino acid; 33% fat as MCT oil; unflavored or vanilla flavored
Enfacare Lipil 22 kcal/oz (Mead Johnson)	0.74	2.1	11	Whey, nonfat milk	3.9	46	High-oleic vegetable oil, soy oil, MCT oil, coconut oil, DHA, ARA	7.7	43	Liquid: maltodextrin, lactose Powder: lactose, corn syrup solids	1.13	2	89	1.3	49	260	Designed for former premature infants now >2 kg or 40 wks corrected age; additional Ca, P, vitamin A, vitamin D, folate, Zn
Enfamil AR Lipil (Mead Johnson)	0.67	1.67	10	Nonfat milk	3.4	46	Palm olein oil, soy oil, coconut oil, high-oleic sunflower oil	7.4	44	Lactose, rice starch, maltodextrin	1.17	1.84	52	1.2	36	240	Thickened with rice starch
Enfamil Human Milk Fortifier (4 pkts added to 100 mL human milk) (Mead Johnson)	0.82	2.1	10	Milk protein isolate, whey protein isolate hydrolysate	4.9	54	MCT oil, soy oil	7.6	37	Corn syrup solids	1.47	2.10	118	1.48	64		70% MCT oil; 60:40 whey/casein ratio; 1.8:1 Ca/P ratio
Enfamil LactoFree Lipil (Mead Johnson)	0.67	1.4	9	Milk protein isolate	3.5	48	Palm olein oil, soy oil, coconut oil, high-oleic sunflower oil	7.3	43	Corn syrup solids	0.87	43	55	1.2	31	200	Lactose free
Enfamil Lipil With Iron (Mead Johnson)	0.67	1.4	8.5	Whey, nonfat milk	3.6	48	Palm olein oil, soy oil, coconut oil, high-oleic sunflower oil, single cell oil blend rich in DHA and ARA	7.3	44	Lactose	0.78	1.8	52	1.2	29	300	
Enfamil Lipil 24 (Mead Johnson)	0.81	1.7	8.5	Reduced minerals whey, nonfat milk	4.3	48	Palm olein oil, soy oil, coconut oil, high-oleic sunflower oil, single cell oil blend rich in DHA and ARA	8.8	43.5	Lactose	0.95	2.25	63	1.46	43	360	
Enfamil Nutramigen Lipil (Mead Johnson)	0.67	1.88	11	Casein hydrolysate, amino acids	3.6	48	Palm olein oil, soy oil, coconut oil, high-oleic sunflower oil, DHA, ARA	6.9	41	Corn syrup solids, modified cornstarch	1.39	1.89	63	1.2	35	320	Lactose free; sucrose free
Enfamil Pregestimil 20 (Mead Johnson)	0.67	1.8	11	Casein hydrolysate, L-cystine, L-tyrosine, L-tryptophan	3.8	48	Liquid: MCT, soy oil, high-oleic safflower oils Powder: MCT, soy oil, corn oil, high-oleic oils	6.8	41	Liquid: corn syrup solids, modified corn starch powder: corn syrup solids, dextrose, modified corn starch	1.35	1.9	77	1.2	50	330	Lactose free; 55% fat as MCT
Enfamil Pregestimil 24 (Mead Johnson)	0.80	2.2	12	Casein hydrolysate, L-cystine, L-tyrosine, L-trytophan	4.5	48	Liquid: MCT, soy oil, high-oleic safflower oil	8.1	41	Liquid: corn syrup solids, modified corn starch	1.6	2.23	92	1.5	60	330	Lactose free; 84% water

(continued)

Table III-1 Infant Formulas (per 100 mL) *(continued)*

Product (Manufacturer)	kcal/ mL	Protein g	Protein % kcal	Protein Source	Fat g	Fat % kcal	Fat Source	Carbohydrate g	Carbohydrate % kcal	Carbohydrate Source	Na mEq	K mEq	Ca mg	Fe mg	P mg	Water mOsm/kg	General Comments
Enfamil Premature Lipil (Mead Johnson)	0.67	2.0	12	Whey Protein concentrate, nonfat milk	3.4	44	MCT, soy oil, and high-oleic vegetable oil, single cell oil blend rich in DHA and ARA	7.4	44	Corn syrup solids, lactose	1.69	1.69	112	1.22	56	240	Designed for premature and LBW infants; additional Ca, P, vitamin A, vitamin D, folate, Zn; Ca/P ratio of 2:1; high in protein; 40% fat as MCT
Enfamil Premature Lipil 24 (Mead Johnson)	0.8	2.4	12	Whey Protein concentrate, nonfat milk	4.1	44	MCT, soy oil, high-oleic vegetable oil, single cell oil blend rich in DHA and ARA	8.8	44	Corn syrup solids, lactose	2.04	2.05	132	1.4	66	300	Designed for premature and LBW infants; additional Ca, P, vitamin A, vitamin D, folate, Zn; Ca/P ratio of 2:1; high in protein; 40% fat as MCT
Enfamil Prosobee Lipil (Mead Johnson)	0.67	1.68	10	Soy protein isolate, L-methionine	3.6	48	Palm olein oil, soy oil, coconut oil, high-oleic sunflower oil, single cell oil blend rich in DHA and ARA	7.1	42	Corn syrup solids	1.04	2.07	70	1.22	46	200	Lactose free, milk-free
Good Start Essentials (Nestle)	0.67	1.5	9	Whey and casein	3.4	46	Palm olein oil, soy oil, coconut oil, high-oleic safflower oil	7.5	45	Lactose, corn syrup	0.7	1.87	50	1.02	28	295	60:40 whey/casein ratio
Good Start 2 Essentials (Nestle)	0.67	1.75	10	Whey and casein	2.7	36	Palm olein oil, soy oil, coconut oil, high-oleic safflower oil	8.8	53	Corn syrup, corn maltodextrin	1.1	2.3	80	1.25	54	325	For infants >4 mo of age
Good Start Supreme (Nestle)	0.67	1.5	9	Hydrolyzed whey protein	3.4	46	Palm olein oil, soy oil, coconut oil, high-oleic safflower oil	7.5	45	Lactose, corn maltodextrin	0.7	1.7	43	1.0	24	250	100% whey protein
Good Start Supreme DHA and ARA (Nestle)	0.67	1.5	9	Hydrolyzed whey protein	3.4	46	Palm olein, soy, coconut and safflower oils, alpina oil, *c. cohnii* oil	7.6	45	Lactose, corn maltodextrin	0.7	1.7	43	1.02	24	250	100% whey protein
Good Start 2 Supreme, DHA and ARA (Nestle)	0.67	1.5	9	Hydrolyzed whey protein	3.4	46	Palm olein, soy, coconut and safflower oils, alpina oil, *c. cohnii* oil	7.6	45	Lactose, corn maltodextrin	0.79	1.87	127	1.01	71	180	100% whey protein
Good Start Supreme Soy DHA and ARA (Nestle)	0.67	1.6	11	Soy protein isolate	3.4	46	Palm olein oil, soy oil, coconut oil, high-oleic safflower oil, DHA, ARA	7.4	44	Corn maltodextrin, sucrose	1.1	2.0	127	1.01	71	180	Lactose free; milk free
Good Start 2 Supreme Soy (Nestle)	0.67	1.9	11	Soy protein isolate	3.4	46	Palm olein oil, soy oil, coconut oil, high-oleic safflower oil	7.3	44	Corn maltodextrin, sucrose	1.2	2.0	127	1.3	71	175	Lactose free; for 9 to 24 mo of age
Neocate Infant (Nutricia)	0.67	2.08 pro eq.	12	Free amino acids	3.01	41	High-oleic safflower oil, refined vegetable oil (coconut oil, soy oil)	7.8	47	Corn syrup solids	1.07	2.67	83	1.24	62	375	Severe protein allergy; 5% MCT; also available with DHA and ARA
Portagen (Mead Johnson)	1.01	3.54	14	Sodium caseinate	4.79	40	MCT oil, corn oil	11.5	46	Corn syrup solids, sucrose	2.4	3.2	94	1.9	71	350	87% fat from MCT; long-term use not recommended due to low essential fat content; 82% free water; lactose free
RCF (Ross)	0.81	4	20	Soy protein isolate, L-methionine	7.2	80	High-oleic safflower, soy oil, coconut oil	N/A	N/A	To be selected by practitioner	2.57	3.73	140	2.43	100	Depends on type of CHO selected	Carbohydrate free; contains L-carnitine, taurine; 87% water

(continued)

Table III-1 Infant Formulas (per 100 mL) *(continued)*

Product (Manufacturer)	kcal/ mL	Protein g	Protein % kcal	Protein Source	Fat g	Fat % kcal	Fat Source	Carbohydrate g	Carbohydrate % kcal	Carbohydrate Source	Na mEq	K mEq	Ca mg	Fe mg	P mg	Water mOsm/kg	General Comments
Similac Advance (Ross)	0.67	1.39	8	Nonfat milk, whey protein concentrate	3.62	49	High-oleic safflower oil, coconut oil, soy oil, MCT	7.24	43	Lactose, corn syrup solids	0.67	1.8	52	1.22	28	300	With DHA, ARA
Similac 2 Advance (Ross)	0.67	1.39	8	Nonfat milk, whey protein concentrate	3.68	49	High-oleic safflower oil, coconut oil, soy oil, MCT	7.24	43	Lactose, corn syrup solids	0.67	1.8	79	1.22	43	300	With DHA, ARA; for 9–24 months of age
Similac Human Milk Fortifier (4 pkts added to 100 mL human milk) (Ross)	0.81	2	10	Nonfat milk, whey protein concentrate	4.26	47	MCT, soy lecithin	9	44	Corn syrup solids	1.48	2.95	145	0.44	81		To add to preterm human milk for LBW infants
Similac Isomil Advance (Ross)	0.67	1.64	10	Soy protein isolate, L-methionine	3.66	49	High-oleic safflower oil, coconut oil, soy oil	6.90	41	Corn syrup, sucrose	1.27	1.87	70	1.22	50	200	With DHA, ARA; lactose free
Similac Isomil 2 Advance (Ross)	0.67	1.64	10	Soy protein isolate, L-methionine	3.66	49	High-oleic safflower oil, coconut oil, soy oil	6.90	41	Corn syrup, sucrose	1.27	1.88	90	1.22	60	200	With DHA, ARA; lactose free; for 9–24 mo of age
Similac Isomil DF (Ross)	0.67	1.78	11	Soy protein isolate, L-methionine	3.66	49	Soy oil, coconut oil	6.78	40	Corn syrup, sucrose, soy fiber	1.27	1.88	71	1.22	51	240	0.6 gm fiber/100 mL
Similac Lactose Free Advance (Ross)	0.67	1.43	9	Milk protein isolate	3.62	49	High-oleic safflower, soy oil, coconut oil	7.17	43	Maltodextrin, sucrose	0.87	1.85	56	1.22	38	200	With DHA, ARA
Similac Natural Care (Ross)	0.81	2.19	11	Nonfat milk, whey protein concentrate	4.48	47	MCT oil, soy oil, coconut oil	8.6	42	Corn syrup solids, lactose	1.51	2.7	70	1.22	94	280	With DHA, ARA
Similac NeoSure Advance (Ross)	0.74	2.07	11	Nonfat milk, whey protein concentrate	4.07	49	Soy oil, MCT oil, coconut oil	7.47	41	Lactose, maltodextrin	1.04	2.66	78	1.34	46	250	Designed for former premature infants >2 kg or >40 wk corrected age; additional Ca, P, vitamin A, vitamin D, folate, Zn; 25% fat as MCT
Similac PM 60/40 (Ross)	0.67	1.49	9	Whey protein concentrate, sodium caseinate	3.75	50	Corn oil, coconut oil, soy oil	6.83	41	Lactose	0.71	1.47	38	0.5	19	280	For infants with hypocalcemia due to hyperphosphatemia or those with impaired renal function; low iron; lower in Ca, P, maintaining 2:1 ratio; lower in K; 60:40 whey/casein ratio
Similac Special Care Advance with Iron 20 (Ross)	0.67	1.82	11	Nonfat milk, whey protein concentrate	3.64	49	MCT oil, soy oil, coconut oil	6.9	41	Corn syrup solids, lactose	1.27	2.2	121	1.21	67	235	Designed for growing low-birth-weight and premature infants; additional Ca, Phos, vitamin A, vitamin D, folate, Zn; Ca/P ratio of 2:1; with DHA, ARA
Similac Special Care Advance with Iron 24 (Ross)	0.81	2.43	11	Nonfat milk, whey protein concentrate	4.40	47	MCT oil, soy oil, coconut oil	8.43	41	Corn syrup solids, lactose	1.54	2.67	146	1.46	81	280	Designed for growing low-birth-weight and premature infants after they have reached 3,600 g; additional Ca, Phos, vitamin A, vitamin D, folate, Zn; Ca/P ratio of 2:1; with DHA, ARA

Table III-2 Noninfant Formulas (per 1,000 mL)

Product (Manufacturer)	kcal/ mL	Protein g	Protein % kcal	Protein Source	Fat g	Fat % kcal	Fat Source	Carbohydrate g	Carbohydrate % kcal	Carbohydrate Source	Na mEq	K mEq	Ca mg	P mg	Water mOsm/kg	General Comments
Boost Drink (Novartis)	1.01	42	17	Milk protein concentrate	18	16	Canola oil, high-oleic sunflower oil, corn oil	173	67	Corn syrup solids, sucrose	24	43	1,390	1,310	610–670	85% free water; gluten, and lactose free; low residue; kosher
Boost High Protein (Novartis)	1.01	61	24	Milk protein concentrate, sodium, and calcium caseinates	23	21	Canola oil, high-oleic sunflower oil, corn oil	139	55	Corn syrup solids, sucrose	31	41	1,390	1,310	650–690	85% free water; gluten, and lactose free; kosher; low residue
Boost Plus (Novartis)	1.52	59	16	Milk protein concentrate, sodium, and calcium caseinates	58	34	Canola oil, high-oleic sunflower oil, corn oil	190	50	Corn syrup solids, sugar	31	41	1,390	1,310	630–670	78% free water; gluten, and lactose free; kosher; low residue
Carnation Instant Breakfast Junior (Nestle)	1.0	32	13	Nonfat milk	48	44	Soybean oil, canola oil	108	43	Sucrose, maltodextrin, oligofructose, inulin	36	52	1,120	1,120	580	Ready-to-drink; kosher; low sodium; contains fiber; vanilla and chocolate flavors
Carnation Instant Breakfast Lactose Free (Nestle)	1.0	35	14	Calcium caseinate	37	33	Corn oil, canola oil	132	53	Corn syrup solids, sucrose	38	32	500	500	550	Kosher; lactose free, gluten free; low sodium; vanilla, chocolate, strawberry flavors; 85% free water
Carnation Instant Breakfast Ready-to-Drink (Nestle)	0.76	41	22	Nonfat milk	16	19	Soybean oil, canola oil	108	57	Sucrose, maltodextrin	25	26	1,585	1,585	580	Kosher; low sodium; french vanilla, chocolate, strawberry creme flavors; 84% free water
Compleat (Novartis)	1.07	43	16	Chicken, sodium caseinate	37	31	Canola oil, chicken	140	53	Corn syrup, maltodextrin, fruits, vegetables	43	44	760	760	340	85% free water; 6 g/L fiber; unflavored; gluten free, lactose free
Compleat Pediatric (Novartis)	1.0	38	15	Sodium caseinate, chicken, pea puree	39	35	Canola oil, MCT oil, chicken	130	50	Corn syrup solids, cranberry juice, vegetables, fruits	33	41	1,440	1,000	380	82% free water; blenderized formula for children aged 1–10 yr, contains real food; 6.7 g/L fiber; unflavored; lactose and gluten free
Crucial (Nestle)	1.5	94	25	Enzymatically hydrolyzed casein	68	39	MCT, fish oil, soybean oil, soy lecithin	134	36	Maltodextrin, cornstarch	51	48	1,000	1,000	490	50% fat as MCT; lactose and gluten free; high protein for wound healing; 15 g/L arginine
Diabetisource AC (Novartis)	1.2	60	20	Soy protein, L-arginine	59	44	Canola oil	100	36	Corn syrup, fructose, vegetables, fruits	46	44	800	800	450	82% free water; 15 g fiber/L; 7.2 g/L arginine; unflavored
EleCare (Ross)	1.0	30	12	Free amino acids	48	43	High-oleic safflower oil, soy oil, MCT oil	107	43	Corn syrup solids	20	39	1,080	808	560	100% free amino acids for protein sensitivities and allergy for children aged 1–10 yr; 33% fat as MCT; unflavored or vanilla flavor
Ensure (Ross)	1.06	37	14	Sodium and calcium caseinates, soy protein isolate, whey protein concentrate	26	22	Canola oil, corn oil	169	64	Corn syrup, sucrose, maltodextrin	37	40	1,266	1,055	600	80% free water; multiple flavors available; high protein and high calcium versions available; gluten and lactose free; kosher; low residue
Ensure Fiber (Ross)	1.06	37	14	Soy protein isolate, sodium and calcium caseinates	25	22	Corn oil, canola oil, soy oil	175	64	Maltodextrin, sucrose, oat fiber, soy fiber	36	39	1,460	1,250	500	81% free water; gluten and lactose free; kosher; 11.8 g/L fiber; multiple flavors available

(continued)

Table III-2 Noninfant Formulas (per 1,000 mL) *(continued)*

Product (Manufacturer)	kcal/mL	Protein g	Protein % kcal	Protein Source	Fat g	Fat % kcal	Fat Source	Carbohydrate g	Carbohydrate % kcal	Carbohydrate Source	Na mEq	K mEq	Ca mg	P mg	Water mOsm/kg	General Comments
Ensure Plus (Ross)	1.5	54	15	Sodium and calcium caseinates, soy protein isolate	48	32	Corn oil, canola oil, high-oleic safflower oil	208	53	Corn syrup, maltodextrin, sucrose	42	47	833	833	690	75% free water; gluten, and lactose free; kosher; low residue; multiple flavors available
EO28 Splash (Nutricia)	1.0	30	10	L-Amino acids	35	32	MCT oil, canola oil, high-oleic safflower oil	146	58	Maltodextrin, sucrose, corn syrup solids	8.6	24	620	620	820	35% fat as MCT; orange-pineapple flavored; ready-to-drink in 8-oz box
Fibersource HN (Novartis)	1.2	53	18	Soy protein isolate, soy protein concentrate	39	29	Canola oil, MCT oil	160	53	Corn syrup, maltodextrin	52	51	1,000	1,000	490	81% free water; 50% fat as MCT; 10 g/L fiber; gluten and lactose free
Glucerna (Ross)	1.0	42	17	Sodium and calcium caseinates	54	49	High-oleic safflower oil, canola oil, soy lecithin	96	34	Maltodextrin, fructose	40	40	705	705	355	85% free water; low carbohydrate content; 14 g/L fiber
Hepatic-Aid II (Hormel Healthlabs)	1.2	44	15	Branch chain amino acids	36.2	27.7	Hydrogenated soybean oil, lecithin, mono- and diglycerides	168	57.3	Maltodextrin, sucrose	<5	n/a	n/a	n/a	560	High in branched chain amino acids; low in aromatic amino acids and methionine
Hi-Cal (Ross)	2.0	83	17	Sodium and calcium caseinates	88	40	Corn oil, soy lecithin	214	43	Corn syrup solids, corn, maltodextrin, sucrose	63	62	844	844	705	70% free water; gluten and lactose free; low residue; kosher; vanilla flavor
Impact (Novartis)	1.0	56	22	Sodium and calcium caseinates, L-arginine	28	25	Structured lipid from palm kernel and sunflower oil, menhaden fish oil	130	53	Hydrolyzed cornstarch	48	36	800	800	375	85% free water; contains dietary nucleotides and fish oil; 14 g/L arginine; fiber containing, glutamine containing, and high calorie versions available; low residue; gluten and lactose free
Isocal (Novartis)	1.06	34	13	Calcium and sodium caseinates, soy protein isolate	44	37	Soybean oil, MCT oil	135	50	Maltodextrin	23	34	630	530	270	84% free water; gluten, and lactose free; kosher; low residue; unflavored
IsoSource (Novartis)	1.2	43	14	Soy protein isolate	39	29	Canola oil, MCT oil	170	57	Corn syrup, maltodextrin	48	49	1,200	1,100	490	82% free water; 50% fat as MCT; higher protein version available; gluten and lactose free; low residue
Jevity 1 Cal (Ross)	1.06	44	17	Sodium and calcium caseinates	35	29	High-oleic safflower oil, canola oil, MCT oil, soy lecithin	155	54	Maltodextrin, corn syrup, soy fiber	40	40	910	760	300	84% free water; 14.4 g/L fiber; higher calorie versions available; gluten and lactose free; kosher
Kindercal (Mead Johnson)	1.06	30	11	Milk protein concentrate	44	37	Canola oil, high-oleic sunflower oil, MCToil, corn oil	135	52	Sucrose, maltodextrin	16	34	1,010	850	440–520	85% free water; gluten and lactose free; kosher; low residue; fiber formulation with 6.3 g/L; 12% fat as MCT; vanilla and chocolate flavors
Neocate One+ (Nutricia)	1.0	30	10	L-Amino acids	35	32	MCT oil, canola oil, high-oleic safflower oil	146	58	Corn syrup solids	9	24	620	620	610	Free amino acids; for severe protein allergy; contains 4.4 g/L arginine, 3.45 g/L glutamine; 35% fat as MCT; flavor packets available
Neocate Junior (Nutricia)	1.0	30	12	L-Amino acids	50	46	MCT oil, canola oil, high-oleic safflower oil	104	42	Corn syrup solids	17	35	1,130	940	607–690	Free amino acids; for severe protein allergy; 35% fat as MCT; also available in Tropical Fruit flavor
Nepro (Ross)	2.0	70	14	Calcium, magnesium, and sodium caseinates, milk protein isolate	96	43	High-oleic safflower oil, canola oil, soy lecithin	223	43	Corn syrup, sucrose, FOS	37	32	1,370	685	665	70% free water; low vitamin A, vitamin D, K, P; 15.6 g/L fiber; multiple flavors available; gluten and lactose free; kosher

(continued)

Table III-2 Noninfant Formulas (per 1,000 mL) *(continued)*

Product (Manufacturer)	kcal/ mL	Protein g	Protein % kcal	Protein Source	Fat g	Fat % kcal	Fat Source	Carbohydrate g	Carbohydrate % kcal	Carbohydrate Source	Na mEq	K mEq	Ca mg	P mg	Water mOsm/kg	General Comments
Novasource 2.0 (Novartis)	2.0	90	18	Calcium and sodium caseinates	88	39	MCT oil and canola oil	220	43	Corn syrup, sugar, maltodextrin	35	39	1,050	1,050	790	70% free water; 3.4% protein as arginine; lactose free, gluten free; low residue
Nutren Glytrol (Nestle)	1.0	45	18	Calcium-potassium caseinates	47.6	42	High-oleic safflower oil, MCT oil, canola oil	100	40	Maltodextrin, cornstarch, oligofructose, gum arabic, pea fiber, inulin	32	36	720	720	380	84% free water; 20% fat as MCT; 15 g/L fiber; kosher, lactose, gluten, and sucrose free; vanilla flavor
Nutren Junior (Nestle)	1.0	30	12	Isolated casein and whey protein	42	37	Soybean oil, canola oil, MCT oil, soy lecithin	128	51	Maltodextrin, sucrose	20	34	1,000	800	350	85% free water; fiber containing version available (5.6 g/L); vanilla flavor; 20 % MCT oil; kosher; lactose, and gluten free; low residue
Nutren ProBalance (Nestle)	1.2	54	18	Calcium potassium caseinate	40.8	30	Canola oil, MCT oil, corn oil, soy lecithin	156	52	Maltodextrin, corn syrup solids, gum arabic	33	40	1,250	1,000	350–450	81% free water; unflavored or vanilla; 20% fat as MCT; kosher; lactose, and gluten free
Nutren Pulmonary (Nestle)	1.5	68	18	Calcium potassium caseinate	95	55	MCT and canola oil, soy lecithin, corn oil	100	27	Maltodextrin	51	48	1,200	1,200	330–450	40% fat as MCT; unflavored and vanilla; kosher; lactose and gluten free; low residue
Nutren 1.0 (Nestle)	1.0	40	16	Milk protein concentrate, whey protein concentrate	38	33	Canola oil, MCT oil, soybean oil, soy lecithin	127	51	Maltodextrin, corn syrup solids, sucrose	37	32	670	670	300–360	Fiber containing version available (14 g/L); unflavored and vanilla; 25% MCT oil; kosher; lactose, and gluten free; low residue
Nutren 1.5 (Nestle)	1.5	60	16	Calcium-potassium caseinate	68	39	MCT, canola, corn oil, soy lecithin	170	45	Maltodextrin, sucrose	50	49	1,000	1,000	430–520	78% free water; 50% fat as MCT; vanilla flavored
Nutren 2.0 (Nestle)	2.0	80	16	Calcium-potassium caseinate	110	44	MCT and canola oil, soy lecithin, corn oil	200	40	Corn syrup solids, maltodextrin, sucrose	57	49	1,340	1,340	720	70% free water; 75% fat as MCT; kosher; lactose, and gluten free; low residue; vanilla flavored
Nutrihep (Nestle)	1.5	40	11	L- amino acids, whey protein	21	12	MCT oil, canola oil, soy lecithin, corn oil	290	77	Maltodextrin, modified corn starch	7	34	956	1,000	690	76% free water; 70% fat as MCT; high in BCAA; unflavored, flavor packets available; kosher; lactose, and gluten free; low residue
Optimental (Ross)	1.0	51	20.5	Soy protein hydrolysate, partially hydrolyzed sodium caseinate, arginine	28	25	Interesterified sardine oil, MCT oil, canola oil, soybean oil	139	54.5	Maltodextrin, sucrose, FOS	46	45	1,060	1,060	540	83% free water; contains EPA, DHA; 5.5 g/L arginine; 5 g/L fiber
Osmolite (Ross)	1.06	37	14	Sodium and calcium caseinates, soy protein isolate	35	29	High-oleic safflower oil, canola oil, MCT oil, soy lecithin	151	57	Maltodextrin	28	26	535	535	300	84% free water; 20% fat as MCT; unflavored; lactose and gluten free; low residue; kosher; high calorie versions available
Oxepa (Ross)	1.5	63	17	Sodium and calcium caseinates	94	55	Canola oil, MCT oil, sardine oil, borage oil	106	28	Sucrose, maltodextrin	57	50	1,060	1,060	493	79% free water; fortified with Vitamin E, C, and beta carotene; 25% fat as MCT; unflavored
PediaSure Enteral (Ross)	1.0	30	12	Milk protein concentrate	40	35	High-oleic safflower oil, soy oil, MCT oil	133	53	Maltodextrin, sucrose	17	34	970	844	335	84% free water; designed for children aged 1–10 yr; multiple flavors available; lactose and gluten free; low residue

(continued)

Table III-2 Noninfant Formulas (per 1,000 mL) *(continued)*

Product (Manufacturer)	kcal/ mL	Protein g	Protein % kcal	Protein Source	Fat g	Fat % kcal	Fat Source	Carbohydrate g	Carbohydrate % kcal	Carbohydrate Source	Na mEq	K mEq	Ca mg	P mg	Water mOsm/kg	General Comments
PediaSure with Fiber Enteral (Ross)	1.0	30	12	Milk protein concentrate	40	35	High-oleic safflower oil, soy oil, MCT oil, soy lecithin	138	53	Maltodextrin, sucrose, dextrose	16	34	970	844	345	85% free water; fiber containing formula for children aged 1–10 yr (8 g/L); 19.5% fat as MCT
Pediatric Peptinex DT (Novartis)	1.0	30	12	Casein hydrolysate, free amino acid	39	33	MCT oil, soybean oil	138	55	Maltodextrin, modified cornstarch	30	26	1,140	1,000	290	85% free water; 50% fat as MCT; fiber containing version available (6 g/L); lactose and gluten free; low residue
Pepdite One + (Nutricia)	1.0	31	12	L-Amino acids, hydrolyzed protein (pork, soy)	50	46	MCT oil, canola oil, high-oleic safflower oil	106	42	Corn syrup solids	18	35	1,130	940	430–440	44% free amino acids; 35% fat as MCT; banana flavored version available
Peptamen (Nestle)	1.0	40	16	Enzymatically hydrolyzed whey protein	39	33	MCT oil, soybean oil, soy lecithin	127	51	Maltodextrin, corn starch	24	39	800	700	270–380	85% free water; unflavored and vanilla available; fiber containing version available
Peptamen Junior (Nestle)	1.0	30	12	Enzymatically hydrolyzed whey protein	38	33	MCT oil, canola oil, soybean oil	138	55	Maltodextrin, corn starch	20	34	1,000	800	260–360	85% free water; unflavored, vanilla, and flavor packets available; 60% fat as MCT; gluten and lactose free; fiber containing version available
Peptamen 1.5 (Nestle)	1.5	68	18	Enzymatically hydrolyzed whey protein	56	33	MCT oil, soybean oil, soy lecithin	188	49	Maltodextrin, corn starch	44	48	1,000	1,000	550	77% free water; unflavored and vanilla; lactose and gluten free
Peptinex (Novartis)	1.0	50	20	Whey protein hydrolysate	17	15	MCT oil, soybean oil, soy lecithin	160	65	Maltodextrin	44	38	70	670	320	83% free water; 100% peptide; lactose and gluten free; low residue
Peptinex DT (Novartis)	1.0	50	20	Casein hydrolysate, free amino acids	17	15	MCT oil, soybean oil	164	65	Maltodextrin, modified cornstarch	48	31	670	670	460	83% free water; 100% peptides and free amino acids; 50% fat as MCT; lactose and gluten free; 10 g/L fiber
Perative (Ross)	1.3	67	20	Hydrolyzed sodium caseinate, hydrolyzed lactalbumin	37	25	Canola oil, MCT oil, corn oil	180	55	Maltodextrin, FOS	45	44	870	870	460	79% free water; 6.5 g/L fiber; 8 g/L arginine; lactose and gluten free; kosher; unflavored
Pivot 1.5 Cal (Ross)	1.5	94	25	Partially hydrolyzed sodium caseinate, whey protein isolate	51	30	Sardine oil, MCT oil, soy oil, canola oil, soy lecithin	172	45	Corn syrup solids, FOS	61	51	1,000	1,000	595	76% free water; arginine 13 g/L; glutamine 6.5 g/L; fiber 7.5 g/L; low residue; lactose and gluten free
Promote (Ross)	1.0	62.5	25	Sodium and calcium caseinates, soy protein isolate	26	23	High-oleic safflower oil, canola oil, MCT oil, soy lecithin	130	52	Corn maltodextrin, sucrose	44	51	1,200	1,200	340	84% free water; 19% fat as MCT; fiber containing version available; kosher; lactose and gluten free; unflavored or vanilla
ProSure Shake (Ross)	1.27	71	23	Sodium caseinate, whey protein concentrate	29	21	Soy oil, sardine oil, MCT oil, canola oil, lecithin	183	57	Corn syrup solids, sucrose, maltodextrin	65	42	1,460	1,043	635	79% free water; 12.5 g/L fiber; lactose and gluten free; vanilla and banana flavors; not for sole-source nutrition
Pulmocare (Ross)	1.5	63	17	Sodium and calcium caseinates	93	55	Canola oil, MCT oil, corn oil, high-oleic safflower oil, soy lecithin	106	28	Sucrose, maltodextrin	57	50	1,060	1,060	475	79% free water; 20% fat as MCT; low carbohydrate formula; available in vanilla and strawberry flavors; lactose and gluten free; kosher; low residue

(*continued*)

Table III-2 Noninfant Formulas (per 1,000 mL) *(continued)*

Product (Manufacturer)	kcal/ mL	Protein g	Protein % kcal	Protein Source	Fat g	Fat % kcal	Fat Source	Carbohydrate g	Carbohydrate % kcal	Carbohydrate Source	Na mEq	K mEq	Ca mg	P mg	Water mOsm/kg	General Comments
Resource Breeze (Novartis)	1.06	38	14	Whey protein isolate	0			230	86	Corn syrup, sucrose	15	2.2	42	680	750	83% free water; clear liquid, fat-free, protein-containing supplement
Resource Diabetic TF (Novartis)	1.06	58	22	Sodium and calcium caseinates, soy protein isolates, L-arginine	50	42	Canola oil	85	36	Tapioca dextrin, fructose, corn syrup solids	51	43	1,160	1,050	400	85% free water; 14.9 g/L fiber; gluten and lactose free
Resource Just for Kids (Novartis)	1.0	30	12	Sodium and calcium caseinates, whey protein concentrate	50	44	High-oleic sunflower oil, soybean oil, MCT oil	110	44	Maltodextrin, sucrose (fructose in chocolate flavor only)	26	29	1,140	800	440	85% free water; 20% fat as MCT oil; multiple flavors available; fiber-containing version available; lactose and gluten free; low residue
Resource Support Drink (Novartis)	1.5	89	47	Calcium and sodium caseinate, free amino acids	51	30	Canola oil, MCT oil, sunflower oil, marine oil	177	47	Corn syrup, sucrose, maltodextrin	46	39	844	844	800	12.7 g/L fiber; lactose and gluten free; not intended as sole-source nutrition
Subdue (Novartis)	1.0	50	20	Hydrolyzed whey protein concentrate	34	30	MCT oil, canola oil, High-oleic sunflower oil, milk fat, corn oil	130	50	Maltodextrin, modified corn starch, sucrose	48	41	1,100	1,050	525	84% free water; low residue; flavored version only; peptide based
Subdue Plus (Novartis)	1.5	76	20	Hydrolyzed whey protein concentrate	51	30	MCT oil, high-oleic sunflower oil, milk fat, corn oil	130	50	Maltodextrin, modified corn starch	51	51	1,390	1,310	400	76% free water; low residue; lactose and gluten free; kosher
Suplena (Ross)	2.0	30	6	Sodium and calcium caseinates	96	43	High-oleic safflower oil, soy oil, soy lecithin	255	51	Maltodextrin, sucrose	34	29	1,390	730	600	Low protein formula; kosher; lactose and gluten free; low residue; vanilla flavored
Tolerex (Novartis)	1.0	21	8	Free amino acids	1.5	1.0	Safflower oil	230	91	Maltodextrin, modified cornstarch	20	30	560	560	550	86% free water; free amino acid, high carbohydrate, low fat; flavor packets available; lactose and gluten free; low residue
Traumacal (Novartis)	1.5	82	22	Calcium and sodium caseinates	68	40	MCT oil, soy oil	144	38	Corn syrup, sucrose	51	36	750	750	560	78% free water; vanilla flavored version available;higher amounts of vitamins C, B complex, E, copper, and zinc; lactose and gluten free; low residue
TwoCal HN (Ross)	2.0	84	17	Sodium and calcium caseinates	91	41	High-oleic safflower oil, MCT oil, canola oil, soy lecithin	219	43	Corn syrup solids, maltodextrin, sucrose, FOS	63	63	1,050	1,050	725	70% free water; 19% fat as MCT oil; 5 g/L fiber; vanilla, butter pecan, or unflavored; kosher; lactose and gluten free; low residue
Ultracal (Novartis)	1.06	45	17	Milk protein concentrate, casein	39	33	Canola, MCT oil, high-oleic sunflower, corn oil	142	50	Maltodextrin, microcrystalline cellulose, soy fiber, acacia	59	47	1,000	1,000	300	83% free water; 14.2 g/L fiber; lactose and gluten free
Vital HN (Ross)	1.0	42	17	Partially hydrolyzed whey, meat, soy	11	9	Safflower oil, MCT oil, soy lecithin	185	74	Maltodextrin, sucrose	25	36	667	667	500	Hydrolyzed protein; high carbohydrate, low fat formula; 45% fat as MCT; gluten free; low residue; vanilla flavored
Vivonex T.E.N. (Novartis)	1.0	38	15	Free amino acids	2.8	3	Safflower oil	210	82	Maltodextrin, modified corn starch	26	24	500	500	630	85% free water; free amino acids; high carbohydrate, low fat; high protein version available; flavor packets available; lactose and gluten free; low residue

(continued)

Table III-2 Noninfant Formulas (per 1,000 mL) *(continued)*

Product	kcal/	Protein			Fat			Carbohydrate			Na	K	Ca	P	Water	
(Manufacturer)	mL	g	% kcal	Source	g	% kcal	Source	g	% kcal	Source	mEq	mEq	mg	mg	mOsm/kg	General Comments
Vivonex Pediatric (Novartis)	0.8	24	12	Free amino acids	24	25	MCT oil, soybean oil	130	63	Maltodextrin, modified cornstarch	17	31	970	800	360	89% free water; 68% fat as MCT; flavor packets available; lactose and gluten free; low residue

At the time of publication, every effort was made to ensure that all product information was accurate. The most current information can always be obtained by referring to the package label.

Web sites and phone numbers:

Mead Johnson: http://www.meadjohnson.com or 1-800-457-3550

Nestle Clinical Nutrition: http://www.verybestbaby.com or 1-800-628-2229

Novartis Nutrition: http://www.novartisnutrition.com or 1-800-622-2689

Nutricia (formerly SHS): http://www.shsna.com or 1-800-636-2283

Ross: http://www.ross.com or 1-800-227-5767

Table III-3 Selected Modular Additives Used in Pediatrics

Product (Manufacturer)	kcal/g or mL	g/tbsp or mL/tbsp	Energy Source	Comments
Canola oil	8.0	15	Canola	
Corn oil	8.4	15	Corn	Nonemulsified
Cornstarch	3.75			30 kcal/tbsp
Corn Syrup (Karo)	3.8	15		60 kcal/tbsp
Duocal (Nutricia)	4.92	8.5	Hydrolyzed cornstarch, blend of refined vegetable oils (corn, coconut), MCT, mono- and diglycerides	59% carbohydrate; 41% fat (35% MCT, 65% LCT); 310 mOsm/kg water; carbohydrate and fat source used to increase caloric density of formula/foods; 42 kcal/tbsp
MCT oil	7.7	15	Lipid fraction of coconut oil	Bile salts and lipase not necessary for digestion and absorption; does not contain essential fatty acids; nonemulsified; 115 kcal/tbsp
Microlipid (Novartis)	4.5	15	Safflower oil	High in linoleic acid; 50% fat emulsion that mixes easily and stays mixed with enteral formulas, beverages, and table food; 68 kcal/tbsp
Polycose liquid (Ross)	2	15	Glucose polymers from cornstarch	70% free water; 900 mOsm/kg water; carbohydrate liquid used to increase caloric density of formulas/foods
Polycose powder (Ross)	4.0	1 tbsp = 5.6 g carbohydrate	Glucose polymers from cornstarch	Carbohydrate powder used to increase caloric density of formulas/foods; 23 kcal/tbsp
Resource Benecalorie (Novartis)	7.3	330 kcal/1.5 oz serving	Calcium caseinate, high-oleic sunflower oil, mono- and diglycerides	9% protein (7 g/1.5 oz serving); 91% fat (33 g/1.5 oz serving)
Resource Beneprotein (Novartis)	3.5	1 scoop = 1.5 tbsp = 7 g, 6 g pro/scoop	Whey protein isolate, soy lecithin	Protein powder used to increase protein in formulas/foods; 25 kcal/scoop
Resource Benefiber powder (Novartis)	4	4 g/tbsp or packet, 3 g fiber/tbsp or packet	Partially hydrolyzed guar gum	100% carbohydrate; 16 kcal/tbsp
Safflower oil	8.4	15	Safflower	Nonemulsified
Scandical (Axcan Pharma)	5.4	6.5	Nonfat milk, corn syrup solids, maltodextrin, vegetable oil, MCT, coconut oil, soy oil	Tasteless powder used to increase calories in hot or cold foods; 35 kcal/tbsp

At the time of publication, every effort was made to ensure that all product information was accurate. The most current information can always be obtained by referring to the package label.

Table III-4 Enhancing the Caloric Density of Pumped Breastmilk

	Quantity of Additive Needed Total Volume of Breastmilk*		
Kcal/oz Desired by Additive	25 mL	50 mL	100 mL
2 HMF	1/4 tsp†	1 pkg	2 pkgs
4 HMF	1 pkg	2 pkgs	4 pkgs
2 Infant formula powder	1/8 tsp	1/4 tsp	1/2 tsp
4 Infant formula powder	1/4 tsp	1/2 tsp	1 tsp
6 Infant formula powder	1/2 tsp	3/4 tsp	1 tsp
2 Polycose powder	1/4 tsp	1/2 tsp	1 tsp
4 Polycose powder	1/2 tsp	3/4 tsp	1 ¾ tsp
6 Polycose powder	3/4 tsp	1 ¼ tsp	2 ⅔ tsp
2 MCT oil	0.2 mL	0.4 ml	0.9 ml
4 MCT oil	0.4 mL	0.9 ml	1.7 ml
2 Corn oil	0.2 mL	0.4 ml	0.8 ml
4 Corn oil	0.4 mL	0.8 ml	1.6 ml
1 Beneprotein powder	1/8 tsp	1/4 tsp	1/2 tsp
2 Beneprotein powder	1/4 tsp	1/2 tsp	1 tsp

*For calories other than HMF, ingredients should be placed in container and breast milk added to make final volume (to account for displacement).

†Level measurements, not heaping, for all teaspoon measurements.

Table III-5 Selected Metabolic Disorders for Which Nutritional Therapy is Used

Disorder	Nutritional Therapy	Enteral Products Used
β-Ketothiolase deficiency	Low protein High carbohydrate	Ketonex-1*
Biotinidase deficiency	Biotin supplementation	
Galactosemia	Galactose restriction ± calcium supplementation	Soy based (Prosobee,† Isomil*)
Glutaricaciduria type 1	Lysine and tryptophan restriction Riboflavin supplementation Carnitine supplementation	XLys XTrp Analog‡ XLys XTrp Maxamaid‡ Glutarex-1,* Glutarex-2,* GA†
Glycogen storage disease types I and III	High carbohydrate (50–60% of kcal) Low fat (15–30%) Protein (5–10% of kcal) Regular feeding regimen Low cholesterol	Cornstarch
Hereditary fructose intolerance	Fructose, sorbitol restriction Vitamin C supplementation	Fructose, sorbitol, sucrose free
Homocystinuria (cystathionine β-synthase deficiency)	Methionine restriction Cystine supplementation ± Vitamin B_6 supplementation ± Betaine supplementation ± Folate supplementation	HOM 2,# XMet Analog‡ XMet Maxamaid,‡ HCY 1,† HCY 2† Hominex-1,* Hominex-2*
Isovaleric acidemia	Leucine restriction Glycine supplementation ± Carnitine supplementation	XLeu Analog,‡ XLeu Maxamaid‡ I-Valex-1,* I-Valex-2*
Long-chain acyl-CoA dehydrogenase (LCAD) deficiency	Low fat MCT acceptable Avoid prolonged fasting ± carnitine supplementation	Portagen† ProViMin* (add fat and carbohydrate) Tolerex, Vivonex§ as overnight glucose source
Long-chain hydroxy acyl-CoA dehydrogenase (LCHAD) deficiency	Low fat MCT acceptable Avoid prolonged fasting ± Carnitine supplementation	ProViMin* (add fat and carbohydrate) Tolerex, Vivonex§ as overnight glucose source
Maple syrup urine disease	Valine, isoleucine, and leucine restriction Thiamin supplementation	MSUD Analog,‡ MSUD Maxamaid‡ MSUD 1,# MSUD 2# BCAD 1,† BCAD 2†
Medium-chain acyl-CoA dehydrogenase (MCAD) deficiency	Low fat Avoid MCT ± Carnitine supplementation Avoid prolonged fasting	
Methylmalonicacidemia	Methionine, valine, threonine, and isoleucine restriction ± Vitamin B_{12} supplementation	XMTVI Analog,‡ XMTVI Maxamaid‡ OA 1,† OA 2,† OS 2# Propimex-1,* Propimex-2*
Multiple acyl-CoA dehydrogenase deficiency (glutaricaciduria type II)	Fat restriction ± Protein restriction Riboflavin supplementation Carnitine supplementation	
Phenylketonuria	Phenylalanine restriction Tyrosine supplementation PKU 3,# Phenex-1,* Phenex-2* ± Tyrosine supplementation	XPhe Analog,‡ XPhe Maxamaid‡ Phenyl-Free,† PKU-1,# PKU 2,#
Propionic acidemia	Valine, isoleucine, methionine, and threonine restriction Carnitine supplementation ± Biotin supplementation	XMTVI Analog,‡ XMTVI Maxamaid‡ OA 1,† OA 2,† OS 2# Propimex-1,* Propimex-2*
Pyruvate dehydrogenase deficiency	High fat (50 + % of kcal) Low carbohydrate (20–30% of kcal) Thiamin supplementation	Product 3232A† Ross Carbohydrate Free (RCF)*
Tyrosinemia	Phenylalanine and tyrosine restriction Regular feeding regimen	XPhe XTyr Analog,‡ XPTM Analog‡ XPhe XTyr Analog‡ XPhe XTyr Maxamaid,‡ TYR 2# Tyros 1,† Tyros 2† Tyrex-1,* Tyrex-2*
Urea cycle disorders	Protein restriction Essential amino acid supplementation Arginine or citrulline supplementation Sodium benzoate and sodium phenylacetate (or sodium phenylbutyrate)	Cyclinex-1,* Cyclinex-2,* UCD 2#

Adapted from Yannicelli S, Camp K. Appendix III: Metabolic medical foods for nutrition therapy of inherited metabolic diseases. In: Baker SS, Baker RD, Davis AM, editors. Pediatric Nutrition Support. Sudbury, MA: Jones and Bartlett; 2007. p. 570–9.

MCT = medium-chain triglyceride.

*Ross Laboratories, Columbus, OH.

†Mead Johnson Nutritional Division, Evansville, IN.

‡Nutricia, Gaithersburg, MD.

§Sandoz Nutrition Corporation, Minneapolis, MN.

#Milupa, Clarksburg, MD.

INDEX